NINTH EDITION

MEDICAL-SURGICAL NURSING

Assessment and Management of Clinical Problems

Sharon L. Lewis, RN, PhD, FAAN
Professor Emerita
University of New Mexico
Albuquerque, New Mexico;
Former Castella Distinguished Professor
School of Nursing
University of Texas Health Science Center at San Antonio
San Antonio, Texas;
Developer and Consultant
Stress-Busting Program for Family Caregivers

Shannon Ruff Dirksen, RN, PhD, FAAN
Associate Professor
College of Nursing and Health Innovation
Arizona State University
Phoenix, Arizona

Margaret McLean Heitkemper, RN, PhD, FAAN
Professor and Chairperson, Biobehavioral Nursing and Health Systems
Elizabeth Sterling Soule Endowed Chair in Nursing
School of Nursing;
Adjunct Professor, Division of Gastroenterology
School of Medicine
University of Washington
Seattle, Washington

Linda Bucher, RN, PhD, CEN, CNE
Emerita Professor
School of Nursing
University of Delaware
Newark, Delaware;
Consultant/Mentor
W. Cary Edwards School of Nursing
Thomas Edison State College
Trenton, New Jersey;
Per Diem Staff Nurse
Emergency Department
Virtua Memorial Hospital
Mt. Holly, New Jersey

Special Editor
Mariann M. Harding, RN, PhD, CNE
Associate Professor of Nursing
Kent State University at Tuscarawas
New Philadelphia, Ohio

ELSEVIER

ELSEVIER
MOSBY

3251 Riverport Lane
St. Louis, Missouri 63043

MEDICAL-SURGICAL NURSING: ASSESSMENT AND MANAGEMENT OF CLINICAL PROBLEMS

ISBN: 978-0-323-08678-3

Notices

Library of Congress Cataloging-in-Publication Data

Lewis, Sharon Mantik, author.
Medical-surgical nursing : assessment and management of clinical problems / Sharon L. Lewis, Shannon Ruff Dirksen, Margaret McLean Heitkemper, Linda Bucher ; special editor, Mariann M. Harding. – Ninth edition.
p. ; cm.
Preceded by: Medical-surgical nursing : assessment and management of clinical problems / Sharon L. Lewis … [et al.]. 8th ed. c2011.
Includes bibliographical references and index.
ISBN 978-0-323-08678-3 (single volume, hardcover : alk. paper)
I. Dirksen, Shannon Ruff, author.   II. Heitkemper, Margaret M. (Margaret McLean), author.   III. Bucher, Linda, author.   IV. Harding, Mariann, editor.   V. Title.
[DNLM: 1. Nursing Care. 2. Nursing Assessment. 3. Perioperative Nursing.   WY 100]
RT41
617'.0231–dc23

2013036087

Executive Content Strategist: Kristin Geen
Content Manager: Jamie Randall
Associate Content Development Specialist: Melissa Rawe
Content Coordinator: Hannah Corrier
Publishing Services Manager: Jeff Patterson
Senior Project Manager: Mary G. Stueck
Designer: Maggie Reid

Printed in Canada

Last digit is the print number: 9 8 7 6 5 4 3 2 1

ABOUT THE AUTHORS

SHARON L. LEWIS, RN, PhD, FAAN

Sharon Lewis received her Bachelor of Science in nursing from the University of Wisconsin–Madison, Master of Science in nursing with a minor in biological sciences from the University of Colorado–Denver, and PhD in immunology from the Department of Pathology at the University of New Mexico School of Medicine. She had a 2-year postdoctoral fellowship from the National Kidney Foundation. Her more than 40 years of teaching experience include inservice education and teaching in associate degree, baccalaureate, master's degree, and doctoral programs in Maryland, Illinois, Wisconsin, New Mexico, and Texas. Favorite teaching areas are pathophysiology, immunology, and family caregiving. She has been actively involved in clinical research for the past 30 years, investigating altered immune responses in various disorders and developing a stress management program for family caregivers. Her primary professional responsibility is disseminating the Stress-Busting for Family Caregivers Program that she developed. Her free time is spent biking, landscaping, gardening, and being a grandmother.

SHANNON RUFF DIRKSEN, RN, PhD, FAAN

Shannon Dirksen is Associate Professor at the College of Nursing and Health Innovation, Arizona State University. She received her Bachelor of Science in nursing from Arizona State University, Master of Science in nursing from the University of Arizona, and doctorate in clinical nursing research with a minor in psychology from the University of Arizona. She has over 25 years of undergraduate and graduate teaching experience at the University of Arizona, Edith Cowan University (Western Australia), Intercollegiate College of Nursing–Washington State University, and University of New Mexico. She has been on the faculty at Arizona State University since 1996. She currently teaches nursing theory and research, including evidence-based practice. Her research for the past 25 years has focused on quality of life among individuals diagnosed with cancer. Her free time is spent traveling, gardening, bicycling, and reading.

MARGARET McLEAN HEITKEMPER, RN, PhD, FAAN

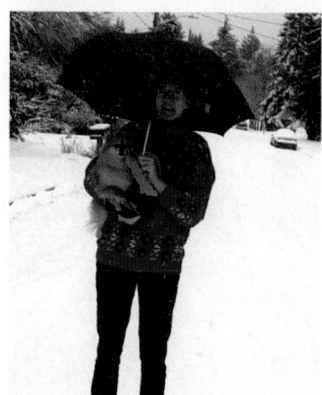

Margaret Heitkemper is Professor and Chairperson, Department of Biobehavioral Nursing and Health Systems at the School of Nursing, and Adjunct Professor, Division of Gastroenterology at the School of Medicine at the University of Washington. She is also Director of the National Institutes of Health-National Institute for Nursing Research–funded Center for Research on Management of Sleep Disturbances at the University of Washington. In the fall of 2006, Dr. Heitkemper was appointed the Elizabeth Sterling Soule Endowed Chair in Nursing. Dr. Heitkemper received her Bachelor of Science in nursing from Seattle University, a Master of Nursing in gerontologic nursing from the University of Washington, and a doctorate in Physiology and Biophysics from the University of Illinois–Chicago. She has been on faculty at the University of Washington since 1981 and has been the recipient of three School of Nursing Excellence in Teaching awards and the University of Washington Distinguished Teaching Award. In addition, in 2002 she received the Distinguished Nutrition Support Nurse Award from the American Society for Parenteral and Enteral Nutrition (ASPEN), in 2003 the American Gastroenterological Association and Janssen Award for Clinical Research in Gastroenterology, and in 2005 she was the first recipient of the Pfizer and Friends of the National Institutes for Nursing Research Award for Research in Women's Health.

LINDA BUCHER, RN, PhD, CEN, CNE

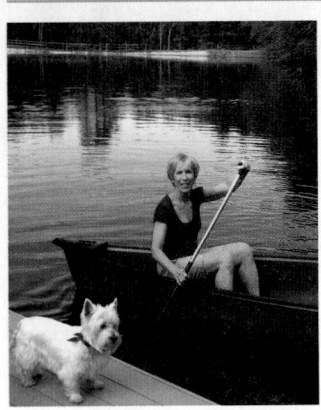

Linda Bucher is an Emerita Professor in the School of Nursing at the University of Delaware in Newark, Delaware. She also is a consultant/mentor in the W. Cary Edwards School of Nursing at Thomas Edison State College. She received her Bachelor of Science in nursing from Thomas Jefferson University in Philadelphia, her Master of Science in adult health and illness from the University of Pennsylvania in Philadelphia, and her doctorate in nursing from Widener University in Chester, Pennsylvania. Her 37 years of nursing experience has spanned staff and patient education, acute and critical care nursing, and teaching in associate, baccalaureate, and graduate nursing programs in New Jersey, Pennsylvania, and Delaware. Her preferred teaching areas include emergency and cardiac nursing and evidence-based practice. She maintains her clinical practice by working as an emergency nurse, is an active member of the American Association of Critical Care Nurses, and enjoys working as a volunteer nurse for Operation Smile. In her free time she enjoys traveling and skiing with her family.

CONTRIBUTORS

Richard Arbour, RN, MSN, CCRN, CNRN, CCNS, FAAN
Critical Care Clinical Nurse Specialist
Albert Einstein Healthcare Network
Philadelphia, Pennsylvania

Margaret Baker, RN, PhD, CNL
Associate Professor
University of Washington School of Nursing
Seattle, Washington

Elisabeth G. Bradley, RN, MS, ACNS-BC
Clinical Leader Cardiovascular Prevention
    Program
Christiana Care Health System
Newark, Delaware

Lucy Bradley-Springer, RN, PhD, ACRN, FAAN
Associate Professor
University of Colorado–Denver, Anschutz
    Medical Campus
Denver, Colorado

Jormain Cady, DNP, ARNP, AOCN
Nurse Practitioner
Virginia Mason Medical Center
Department of Radiation Oncology
Seattle, Washington

Paula Cox-North, RN, PhD, NP-C
Harborview Medical Center
Seattle, Washington

Anne Croghan, MN, ARNP
Nurse Practitioner
Seattle Gastroenterology Associates
Seattle, Washington

Betty Jean Reid Czarapata, MSN, ANP-BC, CUNP
Nurse Practitioner
Urology Wellness Center
Gaithersburg, Maryland

Judi Daniels, PhD, FNP, PNP
Advanced Practice Registered Nurse
Kentucky Polk-Dalton Clinic
Lexington, Kentucky;
Course Coordinator
Frontier Nursing University
Richmond, Kentucky

Rose DiMaria-Ghalili, RN, PhD, CNSC
Associate Professor of Nursing
College of Nursing and Health Professions
Drexel University
Philadelphia, Pennsylvania

Angela DiSabatino, RN, MS
Manager, Cardiovascular Clinical Trials
Christiana Care Health System
Newark, Delaware

Laura Dulski, MSN, RNC-HROB, CNE
Assistant Professor
Resurrection University
Chicago, Illinois

Susan J. Eisel, RN, MSEd
Associate Professor of Nursing
Mercy College of Ohio
Toledo, Ohio

Deborah Hamolsky, RN, MS, AOCNS
Clinical Nurse IV
Carol Franc Buck Breast Care Center
UCSF Helen Diller Family Comprehensive
    Cancer Center
San Francisco, California

Mariann M. Harding, RN, PhD, CNE
Associate Professor of Nursing
Kent State University at Tuscarawas
New Philadelphia, Ohio

Jerry Harvey, RN, MS, BC
Assistant Professor of Nursing
Liberty University
Lynchburg, Virginia

Carol Headley, RN, DNSc, ACNP-BC, CNN
Nephrology Nurse Practitioner
Veterans Affairs Medical Center
Memphis, Tennessee

Teresa E. Hills, RN, MSN, ACNP-BC, CNRN
Neurosurgery Critical Care Nurse
    Practitioner
Christiana Care Health System
Newark, Delaware

Christine Hoch, RN, MSN
Nursing Instructor
Delaware Technical Community College
Newark, Delaware

David M. Horner, CRNA, MS, APN
Nurse Anesthetist
Virtua Hospital
Marlton, New Jersey

Joyce Jackowski, MS, FNP-BC, AOCNP
Nurse Practitioner
Virginia Cancer Specialists
Arlington, Virginia

Kay Jarrell, RN, MS, CNE
Clinical Associate Professor
College of Nursing and Health Innovation
Arizona State University
Phoenix, Arizona

Sharmila Johnson, MSN, ACNS-BC, CCRN
Cardiovascular Clinical Nurse Specialist
Christiana Care Health System
Newark, Delaware

Jane Steinman Kaufman, RN, MS, ANP-BC, CRNP
Advanced Senior Lecturer
University of Pennsylvania School of
    Nursing
Philadelphia, Pennsylvania

Katherine A. Kelly, RN, DNP, FNP-C, CEN
Assistant Professor
School of Nursing
California State University
Sacramento, California

Lindsay L. Kindler, RN, PhD, CNS
Research Associate
Kaiser Permanente Center for Health
    Research
Portland, Oregon

Judy Knighton, RN, MScN
Clinical Nurse Specialist–Burns
Ross Tilley Burn Centre
Sunnybrook Health Sciences Centre
Toronto, Ontario, Canada

Mary Ann Kolis, RN, MSN, ANP-BC, APNP
Instructor
Gateway Technical College
Kenosha, Wisconsin

Catherine N. Kotecki, RN, PhD, APN
Associate Dean
W. Cary Edwards School of Nursing
Thomas Edison State College
Trenton, New Jersey

Nancy Kupper, RN, MSN
Associate Professor
Tarrant County College
Fort Worth, Texas

Jeffrey Kwong, DNP, MPH, ANP-BC
Assistant Professor of Nursing at CUMC
Program Director, Adult-Gerontology Nurse
    Practitioner Program
Columbia University
New York, New York

Carol A. Landis, RN, DNSc
Professor
Biobehavioral Nursing and Health Systems
University of Washington
School of Nursing
Seattle, Washington

Susan C. Landis, RN, MSN
Lecturer
Biobehavioral Nursing and Health Systems
University of Washington School of Nursing
Seattle, Washington

Janice Lazear, DNP, CRNP, CDE
Assistant Professor
School of Nursing
University of Maryland
Baltimore, Maryland

Catherine (Kate) Lein, MS, FNP-BC
Assistant Professor
Michigan State University College of
    Nursing
East Lansing, Michigan

Janet Lenart, RN, MN, MPH
Senior Lecturer
University of Washington School of Nursing
Seattle, Washington

Nancy MacMullen, PhD, APN/CNS, RNC, HR-OB, CNE
Associate Professor
Governors State University
Oak Forest, Illinois

Dorothy (Dottie) M. Mathers, RN, DNP, CNE
Professor
School of Health Sciences
Pennsylvania College of Technology
Williamsport, Pennsylvania

De Ann F. Mitchell, RN, PhD
Professor of Nursing
Tarrant County College
Trinity River East Campus
Fort Worth, Texas

Carolyn Moffa, MSN, FNP-C, CHFN
Clinical Leader
Heart Failure Program
Christiana Care Health System
Newark, Delaware

Janice Neil, RN, PhD
Associate Professor and Chair, Undergraduate
    Nursing Science Junior Division
College of Nursing
East Carolina University
Greenville, North Carolina

DaiWai Olson, RN, PhD, CCRN
Associate Professor of Neurology and
    Neurotherapeutics
University of Texas Southwestern
Dallas, Texas

Rosemary C. Polomano, RN, PhD, FAAN
Associate Professor of Pain Practice
Department of Biobehavioral Health
    Sciences
University of Pennsylvania School of
    Nursing;
Associate Professor of Anesthesiology and
    Critical Care
University of Pennsylvania Perelman School
    of Medicine
Philadelphia, Pennsylvania

Kathleen A. Rich, RN, PhD, CCNS, CCRN-CSC, CNN
Cardiovascular Clinical Specialist
Indiana University Health La Porte Hospital
La Porte, Indiana

Dottie Roberts, RN, MSN, MACI, CMSRN, OCNS-C, CNE
Instructor
University of South Carolina College of
    Nursing
Columbia, South Carolina

Sandra Irene Rome, RN, MN, AOCN, CNS
Clinical Nurse Specialist
Hematology/Oncology/BMT
Cedars-Sinai Medical Center
Los Angeles, California

Jennifer Saylor, RN, PhD, ACNS-BC
Clinical Instructor
University of Delaware
Wilmington, Delaware

Marilee Schmelzer, RN, PhD
Associate Professor
University of Texas at Arlington College of
    Nursing
Arlington, Texas

Maureen A. Seckel, RN, APN, MSN, ACNS-BC, CCNS, CCRN
Clinical Nurse Specialist Medical Pulmonary
    Critical Care
Christiana Care Health System
Newark, Delaware

Virginia (Jennie) Shaw, RN, MSN
Associate Professor
University of Texas Health Science Center
    School of Nursing
San Antonio, Texas

Anita Jo Shoup, RN, MSN, CNOR
Perioperative Clinical Nurse Specialist
Swedish Edmonds
Edmonds, Washington

Dierdre D. Wipke-Tevis, RN, PhD
Associate Professor
PhD Program Director, Coordinator of
    Clinical Nurse Specialist Area of Study
Sinclair School of Nursing
University of Missouri
Columbia, Missouri

Mary Wollan, RN, BAN, ONC
Orthopaedic Nurse Educator
Twin Cities Orthopaedic Education
    Association
Spring Park, Minnesota

Meg Zomorodi, RN, PhD, CNL
Clinical Associate Professor
University of North Carolina at Chapel Hill
    School of Nursing
Chapel Hill, North Carolina

Damien Zsiros, RN, MSN, CNE, CRNP
Nursing Instructor
The Pennsylvania State University School of
    Nursing
Fayette/The Eberly Campus
Uniontown, Pennsylvania

REVIEWERS

Lakshi M. Aldredge, RN, MSN, ANP-BC
Portland, Oregon

Katrina Allen, RN, MSN, CCRN
Fairhope and Bay Minette, Alabama

Carol C. Annesser, RN, MSN, BC, CNE
Toledo, Ohio

Debra Backus, RN, PhD, CNE, NEA-BC
Canton, New York

Jo Ann Baker, RN, MSN, FNP-C
Dover, Delaware

Kathleen M. Barta, RN, EdD
Fayetteville, Arkansas

Cecilia M. Bidigare, RN, MSN
Beavercreek, Ohio

Beth Perry Black, RN, PhD
Chapel Hill, North Carolina

Kathleen Blais, RN, EdD
Wilton Manors, Florida

Mary Blessing, RN, MSN
Albuquerque, New Mexico

Danese M. Boob, MSN/ED, RN-BC
Hershey, Pennsylvania

Barbara S. Broome, RN, PhD, FAAN
Mobile, Alabama

Anna M. Bruch, RN, MSN
Oglesby, Illinois

Carmen Bruni, RN, MSN
Laredo, Texas

Jean Burt, RN, MSN
Chicago, Illinois

Michelle M. Byrne, RN, PhD, CNE, CNOR
Dahlonega, Georgia

Carol Capitano, RN, PhD
Albuquerque, New Mexico

Ronald R. Castaldo, CRNA, MBA, MS, CCRN
New Castle, Delaware

Phyllis Christianson, MN, APRN-BC, GNP
Seattle, Washington

Katie Clark, RD, MPH, CDE
San Diego, California

Bernice Coleman, PhD, ACNP-BC, FAHA
Los Angeles, California

Deborah Marks Conley, RN, MSN, APRN-CNS, GCNS-BC, FNGNA
Omaha, Nebraska

Mary A. Cox, RN, MS
Dayton, Ohio

Paula Cox-North, RN, PhD, NP-C
Seattle, Washington

Betty Jean Reid Czarapata, MSN, ANP-BC, CUNP
Washington, D. C.

Julie Darby, RN, MSN
Memphis, Tennessee

Evelyn Dean, RN, MSN, ACNS-BC, CCRN
Kansas City, Missouri

Fernande E. Deno, RN, MSN, CNE
Coon Rapids, Minnesota

David J. Derrico, RN, MSN
Gainesville, Florida

Julie Dittmer, RN, MSN
Bettendorf, Iowa

Marci Ebberts, RN, BSN, CCRN
Kansas City, Missouri

Susan J. Eisel, RN, MSEd
Toledo, Ohio

Dana R. Epstein, RN, PhD
Phoenix, Arizona

Marianne Ferrin, MSN, ACNP-BC
Philadelphia, Pennsylvania

Shelley Fess, RN, MS, AOCN, CRNI
Rochester, New York

Eleanor Fitzpatrick, RN, MSN, CCRN
Philadelphia, Pennsylvania

Amanda J. Flagg, PhD, ACNS-BC, CNE
San Antonio, Texas

Jan Foecke, RN, MS, ONC
Kansas City, Missouri

Margie Francisco, RN, MSN, EdD
Oglesby, Illinois

Lori Godaire, RN-BC, MS, CCRN, CNL
Norwich, Connecticut

Debra B. Gordon, RN-BC, DNP, ACNS-BC, FAAN
Seattle, Washington

Claudia C. Grobbel, RN, DNP
Rochester, Michigan

Dianne Travers Gustafson, RN, PhD
Omaha, Nebraska

Elizabeth E. Hand, RN, MS
Tulsa, Oklahoma

Carla V. Hannon, MS, APRN, CCRN
New Haven, Connecticut

Mariann M. Harding, RN, PhD, CNE
New Philadelphia, Ohio

Shannon T. Harrington, RN, PhD
Norfolk, Virginia

Jerry Harvey, RN, MS, BC
Lynchburg, Virginia

Mimi Haskins, RN, MS, CMSRN
Buffalo, New York

Kay Helzer, RN, MSN
Phoenix, Arizona

Saundra J. Hendricks, RN, MS, FNP, BC-ADM
Houston, Texas

Margie Hesson, RN, MSN
Rapid City, South Dakota

Kathleen M. Hill, RN, MSN, CCNS
Cleveland, Ohio

Misty Hobart, RN, MSN, ARNP
Spokane, Washington

Patricia Hong, RN, MA
Seattle, Washington

Teressa Sanders Hunter, RN, PhD
Langston, Oklahoma

Janet E. Jackson, RN, MS
Peoria, Illinois

Suzanne L. Jed, MSN, FNP-BC
Los Angeles, California

**Jane Faith Kapustin, PhD, CRNP,
BC-ADM, FAANP**
Baltimore, Maryland

Nancy Karnes, RN, MSN, CCRN, CDE
Bellevue, Washington

Christina D. Keller, RN, MSN
Radford, Virginia

Katherine A. Kelly, RN, DNP, FNP-C, CEN
Sacramento, California

Lisa Kiper, RN, MSN
Morehead, Kentucky

Teri Lynn Kiss, RN, MS, MSSW, CCRN
Fairbanks, Alaska

Tracy H. Knoll, RN, MSN
St. Louis, Missouri

**Mary Ann Kolis, RN, MSN, ANP-BC,
APNP**
Kenosha, Wisconsin

Krista Krause, MSN, FNP-C
Syracuse, New York

Regina Kukulski, RN, MSN, ACNS, BC
Trenton, New Jersey

Vera Kunte, RN-BC, MSN
Trenton, New Jersey

Marci Lagenkamp, RN, MS
Piqua, Ohio

Catherine (Kate) Lein, MS, FNP-BC
East Lansing, Michigan

**Linda R. Littlejohns, RN, MSN, CNRN,
FAAN**
San Juan Capistrano, California

Sarah Livesay, RN, DNP, ACNP, CNS-A
Houston, Texas

Erin M. Loughery, MSN, APRN
Norwich, Connecticut

Beth Lucasey, RN, MA
Kansas City, Missouri

Barbara Lukert, MD
Kansas City, Kansas

Jane A. Madden, RN, MSN
Colorado Springs, Colorado

Laura Mallett, RN, MSN
Laramie, Wyoming

Angela M. Martinelli, RN, PhD, CNOR
Fort Detrick, Maryland

Carole Martz, RN, MS, AOCN, CBCN
Highland Park, Illinois

**Dorothy (Dottie) M. Mathers, RN, DNP,
CNE**
Williamsport, Pennsylvania

**Phyllis A. Matthews, RN, MS, ANCP-BC,
CUNP**
Denver, Colorado

Molly L. McClelland, RN, PhD
Detroit, Michigan

**Tara McMillan-Queen, RN, MSN, ANP,
GNP**
Charlotte, North Carolina

Molly M. McNett, RN, PhD
Cleveland, Ohio

Doreen Mingo, RN, MSN
Waterloo, Illinois

Heidi E. Monroe, RN, MSN, CPAN, CAPA
Green Bay, Wisconsin

Anna Moore, RN, MS
Richmond, Virginia

Amanda Jones Moose, RN, BSN
Taylorsville, North Carolina

Arlene H. Morris, RN, EdD, CNE
Montgomery, Alabama

Brenda C. Morris, RN, EdD, CNE
Phoenix, Arizona

Jason Mott, RN, MSN
Green Bay, Wisconsin

C. Denise Neill, RN, PhD, CNE
Victoria, Texas

Geri B. Neuberger, EdD, APRN-CNS
Kansas City, Kansas

**Lorraine Nowakowski-Grier, MSN, APRN,
BC, CDE**
Newark, Delaware

**Patricia O'Brien, RN, ACNS-BC, MA,
MSN**
Albuquerque, New Mexico

**Margaret Ochab-Ohryn, RN, MS, MBA,
CRNA**
Farmington Hills, Michigan

Devorah Overbay, RN, MSN, CNS
Newberg, Oregon

Judith A. Paice, RN, PhD
Chicago, Illinois

Steven J. Palazzo, RN, PhD
Seattle, Washington

Trevah A. Panek, RN, MSN, CCRN
Loretto, Pennsylvania

Brenda Pavill, RN, PhD, FNP
Dallas, Pennsylvania

Rosalynde D. Peterson, RN, DNP
Tuscaloosa, Alabama

Barbara Pope, RN, MSN, PPCN, CCRN
Philadelphia, Pennsylvania

Tammy Ann Ramon, RN, MSN
University Center, Michigan

Patricia S. Regojo, RN, MSN
Philadelphia, Pennsylvania

Lynn F. Reinke, PhD, ARNP
Seattle, Washington

Tammy C. Roman, RN, EdD, CNE
Rochester, New York

Susan A. Sandstrom, RN, MSN, BC, CNE
Omaha, Nebraska

Marian Sawyier, RN, MSN
Albuquerque, New Mexico

Jennifer Saylor, RN, PhD, ACNS-BC
Wilmington, Delaware

Sally P. Scavone, RN, MS
Buffalo, New York

Mary Scheid, RN, MSN, OCN, CBCN
Greeley, Colorado

Cynthia Schoonover, RN, MS, CCRN
Kettering, Ohio

Teresa J. Seright, RN, PhD, CCRN
Bozeman, Montana

Shellie Simons, RN, PhD
Lowell, Massachusetts

Sarah Smith, RN, MA, CRNO, COT
Oxford, Iowa

Clemma K. Snider, RN, MSN
Richmond, Kentucky

Helen Stegall, RN, BSN, CORLN
Iowa City, Iowa

Elaine K. Strouss, RN, MSN
Monaca, Pennsylvania

Mindy B. Tinkle, RN, PhD, WHNP-BC
Albuquerque, New Mexico

Susan Turner, RN, MSN, FNP
Gilroy, California

Mark R. Van Horn, BS
High Point, North Carolina

Cheryl A. Waklatsi, RN, MSN
Cincinnati, Ohio

Danette Y. Wall, ACRN, MSN, MBA/HCM
Tampa, Florida

Daryle Wane, PhD, ARNP, FNP-BC
New Port Richey, Florida

Lisa A. Webb, RN, MSN, CEN
Charleston, South Carolina

Judith A. Widdoss, RN, MSN, CNE
Bethlehem, Pennsylvania

Sharon A. Willadsen, RN, PhD
Cleveland, Wisconsin

Julie Willenbrink, RN, MSN
Piqua, Ohio

Linda Wilson, RN, PhD, CPAN, CAPA, BC, CNE
Philadelphia, Pennsylvania

Mary Wollan, RN, BAN, ONC
Spring Park, Minnesota

Karen M. Wood, RN, DNSc, CCRN, CNL
Evergreen Park, Illinois

Patricia Worthington, RN, MSN, CNSC
Philadelphia, Pennsylvania

Susan Yeager, RN, MS, CCRN, ACNP
Columbus, Ohio

Amber Young, RN, MSN
Green Bay, Wisconsin

Damien Zsiros, RN, MSN, CNE, CRNP
Uniontown, Pennsylvania

To the Profession of Nursing and to the Important People in Our Lives

Sharon

My husband Peter and our grandchildren Malia, Halle, Aidan, Cian, and Layla

Shannon

My husband John, our children Marshall and Meaghan, my mother Marilyn, and my siblings Michael, Barbara, and Brian

Margaret

My husband David, our daughters Elizabeth and Ellen, and our grandson Jaxon James

Linda

My brother, Rich, who was always so proud of my accomplishments but not near as much as I was of him in his courageous fight against cancer

The ninth edition of *Medical-Surgical Nursing: Assessment and Management of Clinical Problems* has been thoroughly revised to incorporate the most current medical-surgical nursing information in an easy-to-use format. More than just a textbook, this is a comprehensive resource containing essential information that students need to prepare for lectures, classroom activities, examinations, clinical assignments, and the safe, comprehensive care of patients. In addition to the readable writing style and full-color illustrations, the text and accompanying resources include many special features to help students learn key medical-surgical nursing content, including patient and caregiver teaching, gerontology, collaborative care, cultural and ethnic considerations, patient safety, genetics, nutrition and drug therapy, evidence-based practice, and much more.

The comprehensive and timely content, special features, attractive layout, and student-friendly writing style combine to make this the number one medical-surgical nursing textbook used in more nursing schools than any other medical-surgical nursing textbook.

The strengths of the first eight editions have been retained, including the use of the nursing process as an organizational theme for nursing management. Numerous new features have been added to address some of the rapid changes in practice. Contributors have been selected for their expertise in specific content areas; one or more specialists in the subject area have thoroughly reviewed each chapter to increase accuracy. The editors have undertaken final rewriting and editing to achieve internal consistency. All efforts have been directed toward building on the strengths of the previous edition while preparing an even more effective new edition.

ORGANIZATION

Content is organized into two major divisions. The first division, Section 1 (Chapters 1 through 11), discusses general concepts related to adult patients. The second division, Sections 2 through 12 (Chapters 12 through 69), presents nursing assessment and nursing management of medical-surgical problems.

The various body systems are grouped to reflect their interrelated functions. Each section is organized around two central themes: assessment and management. Chapters dealing with assessment of a body system include a discussion of the following:

1. A brief review of anatomy and physiology, focusing on information that will promote understanding of nursing care
2. Health history and noninvasive physical assessment skills to expand the knowledge base on which treatment decisions are made
3. Common diagnostic studies, expected results, and related nursing responsibilities to provide easily accessible information

Management chapters focus on the pathophysiology, clinical manifestations, diagnostic studies, collaborative care, and nursing management of various diseases and disorders. The nursing management sections are organized into assessment, nursing diagnoses, planning, implementation, and evaluation. To emphasize the importance of patient care in various clinical settings, nursing implementation of all major health problems is organized by the following levels of care:

1. Health Promotion
2. Acute Intervention
3. Ambulatory and Home Care

CLASSIC FEATURES

- **Nursing management** is presented in a consistent and comprehensive format, with headings for Health Promotion, Acute Intervention, and Ambulatory and Home Care. Over 60 nursing care plans on the Evolve website and in the text incorporate Nursing Interventions Classification (NIC) and Nursing Outcomes Classification (NOC) in a way that clearly shows the linkages among NIC, NOC, and nursing diagnoses, and applies them to nursing practice.
- **Cultural and ethnic health disparities** content and boxes in the text highlight risk factors and important issues related to the nursing care of various ethnic groups. A special Culturally Competent Care heading denotes cultural and ethnic content related to diseases and disorders. Chapter 2: *Health Disparities and Culturally Competent Care* discusses health status differences among groups of people related to access to care, economic aspects of health care, gender and cultural issues, and disease risk.
- **Collaborative care** is highlighted in special Collaborative Care sections in all management chapters and Collaborative Care tables throughout the text.
- **Coverage on delegation and prioritization** includes the following:
  - Delegation Decisions boxes throughout the text highlight specific topics and skills related to delegation
  - Delegation and priority questions in case studies and Bridge to NCLEX® Examination Questions
  - Nursing interventions throughout the text are listed in order of priority
  - Nursing diagnoses in the nursing care plans are listed in order of priority
- **Focused Assessment boxes** in all assessment chapters provide brief checklists that help students do a more practical "assessment on the run" or bedside approach to assessment. They can be used to evaluate the status of previously identified health problems and monitor for signs of new problems.
- **Safety Alert boxes** highlight important patient safety issues and focus on the National Patient Safety Goals.
- **Pathophysiology Maps** outline complex concepts related to diseases in flowchart format, making them easier to understand.
- **Chapter 8:** *Sleep and Sleep Disorders* expands on this key topic that impacts multiple disorders and body systems as well as nearly every aspect of daily functioning.
- **Patient and caregiver teaching** is an ongoing theme throughout the text. Chapter 4: *Patient and Caregiver Teaching* emphasizes the increasing importance and prevalence of

patient management of chronic illnesses and conditions and the role of the caregiver in patient care.

- **Gerontology and chronic illness** are discussed in Chapter 5: *Chronic Illness and Older Adults,* and included throughout the text under Gerontologic Considerations headings and in Gerontologic Assessment Differences tables.
- **Nutrition** is highlighted throughout the book. Nutritional Therapy tables summarize nutritional interventions and promote healthy lifestyles in patients with various health problems.
- *Healthy People* boxes present health care goals as they relate to specific disorders such as diabetes and cancer.
- **Extensive drug therapy content** includes Drug Therapy tables and concise Drug Alerts highlighting important safety considerations for key drugs.
- **Genetics in Clinical Practice boxes** summarize the genetic basis, genetic testing, and clinical implications for genetic disorders that affect adults.
- **Gender Differences boxes** discuss how women and men are affected differently by conditions such as pain and hypertension.
- A separate chapter on **complementary and alternative therapies** (CAT) addresses current issues in today's health care settings related to these therapies. Complementary & Alternative Therapies boxes expand on this information and summarize what nurses need to know about therapies such as herbal remedies, acupuncture, and biofeedback.
- **Ethical/Legal Dilemmas boxes** promote critical thinking for timely and sensitive issues that nursing students may deal with in clinical practice—topics such as informed consent, advance directives, and confidentiality.
- **Home care/community-based care** is found in special Ambulatory and Home Care sections in the nursing management chapters.
- **Emergency Management tables** outline the emergency treatment of health problems most likely to require emergency intervention.
- **Assessment Abnormalities tables** in assessment chapters alert the nurse to frequently encountered abnormalities and their possible etiologies.
- **Nursing Assessment tables** summarize the key subjective and objective data related to common diseases. Subjective data are organized by functional health patterns.
- **Health History tables** in assessment chapters present key questions to ask patients related to a specific disease or disorder.
- Student-friendly pedagogy includes the following:
  - **Learning Outcomes** and **Key Terms** at the beginning of each chapter help students identify the key content for that chapter.
  - **Evolve website boxes** in chapter openers alert students to supplemental online content and exercises, making it easy for students to facilitate online learning.
  - **Bridge to NCLEX® Examination Questions** at the end of each chapter are matched to the learning outcomes and help students learn the important points in the chapter. Answers are provided just below the questions for immediate feedback, and rationales are provided on the Evolve website.
  - **Case Studies with photos** at the end of chapters bring patients to life. Multiple disorders are incorporated so

students learn how to prioritize care and manage patients in the clinical setting. Discussion questions with a focus on prioritization, delegation, and evidence-based practice are included. Answer guidelines are provided on the Evolve website.

- **Resources** at the end of most chapters include websites for nursing and health care organizations that provide patient teaching and disease and disorder information.
- A **glossary** of key terms and definitions is provided at the back of the text. An expanded version of the glossary with audio pronunciations is included on the Evolve website.

NEW FEATURES

- Once again, each chapter has been carefully revised to ensure a **lower reading level** and more reader-friendly and understandable content than ever. Essential content has been streamlined to help students more effectively learn critical content.
- **Unfolding case studies** in every assessment chapter are an engaging tool that help students apply nursing concepts to real-life patient care.
- **Managing Multiple Patients Case Studies** at the end of each section help students learn to prioritize, delegate, and manage patient care.
- **Informatics boxes** discuss how technology is used by nurses and patients in health care settings.
- **Expanded evidence-based practice content** includes new Applying the Evidence boxes, updated Translating Research Into Practice boxes, and evidence-based practice-focused questions in the case studies.
- **Safety Alerts** have been expanded throughout the book to cover surveillance for high-risk situations.
- New content in Chapter 1 covers **teamwork and interdisciplinary teams,** as this is a key component of QSEN.
- An **increased focus on genetics** includes:
  - A new **genetics chapter** that focuses on practical application of nursing care as it relates to this important topic
  - **Genetic Risk Alerts** in the assessment chapters call attention to important genetic risks
  - **Genetic Link headings** in the management chapters highlight the specific genetic bases of many disorders
- **Expanded coverage of delegation** includes additional Delegation Decision boxes covering issues such as hypertension and postoperative patient care.
- Coverage of **legal considerations has been expanded** in the revised Ethical/Legal Dilemmas boxes.
- **New art** enhances the book's visual appeal and lends a more contemporary look throughout.

LEARNING SUPPLEMENTS FOR STUDENTS

- The handy *Clinical Companion* presents approximately 200 common medical-surgical conditions and procedures in a concise, alphabetical format for quick clinical reference. Designed for portability, this popular reference includes the essential, need-to-know information for treatments and procedures in which nurses play a major role. An attractive and functional two-color design highlights key information for quick, easy reference.

- An exceptionally thorough *Study Guide* contains over 500 pages of review material that reflect the content found in the book. It features a wide variety of clinically relevant exercises and activities, including NCLEX-format multiple choice and alternate format questions, case studies, anatomy review, critical thinking activities, and much more. It features an attractive two-color design and many alternate-item format questions to better prepare students for the NCLEX examination. An answer key is included to provide students with immediate feedback as they study.
- The **Evolve Student Resources** are available online at *http://evolve.elsevier.com/Lewis/medsurg* and include the following valuable learning aids organized by chapter:
  - Printable Key Points summaries for each chapter
  - 1000 NCLEX Examination Review Questions
  - Pre-Tests for every chapter
  - Answer Guidelines to the case studies in the textbook
  - Rationales for the Bridge to NCLEX® Examination Questions in the textbook
  - 55 Interactive Case Studies with state-of-the-art animations and a variety of learning activities, which provide students with immediate feedback. Ten of the case studies are enhanced with photos and narration of the clinical scenarios.
  - Customizable Nursing Care Plans
  - Concept Map Creator and concept maps for selected case studies in the textbook
  - Audio glossary of key terms, available as comprehensive alphabetical glossary and organized by chapter
  - Stress-Busting Kit
  - Animations, video clips, and audio clips
  - Fluids and Electrolytes Tutorial
  - Content Updates
  - Additional resources, including tables, figures, and clinical references
- **Virtual Clinical Excursions** (VCE) is an exciting learning tool that brings learning to life in a "virtual" hospital setting. VCE simulates a realistic, yet safe, nursing environment where the routine and rigors of the average clinical rotation abound. Students can conduct a complete assessment of a patient and set priorities for care, collect data, analyze and interpret data, prepare and administer medications, and reach conclusions about complex problems. Each lesson has a textbook reading assignment and online activities based on "visiting" patients in the hospital. Instructors receive an implementation manual with directions for using VCE as a teaching tool.
- More than just words on a screen, **Pageburst eBooks** come with a wealth of built-in study tools and interactive functionality to help students better connect with the course material and their instructors. Plus, with the ability to fit an entire library of books on one portable device, Pageburst gives students the ability to study when, where, and how they want.

TEACHING SUPPLEMENTS FOR INSTRUCTORS

- The **Evolve Instructor Resources** (available online at *http://evolve.elsevier.com/Lewis/medsurg*) remain the most comprehensive set of instructor's materials available, containing the following:

- **TEACH for Nurses Lesson Plans** with electronic resources organized by chapter to help instructors develop and manage the course curriculum. This exciting resource includes:
  - Objectives
  - Teaching focus
  - Key terms
  - Nursing curriculum standards
  - Student and instructor chapter resource listings
  - Detailed chapter outlines
  - Teaching strategies with learning activities and links to resources in the image collection, PowerPoint presentations, animations, etc.
  - Case studies with answer guidelines
- The **Test Bank** features over 2000 NCLEX Examination test questions with text page references and answers coded for NCLEX Client Needs category, nursing process, and cognitive level. The ninth edition test bank has been completely updated and reviewed, and it now includes hundreds of prioritization, delegation, and multiple patient questions. All alternate item format questions are included. The ExamView software allows instructors to create new tests; edit, add, and delete test questions; sort questions by NCLEX category, cognitive level, nursing process step, and question type; and administer and grade online tests.
- The **Image Collection** contains more than 800 full-color images from the text for use in lectures.
- An extensive collection of **PowerPoint Presentations** includes over 125 different presentations focused on the most common diseases and disorders. The presentations have been thoroughly revised to include helpful instructor notes/teaching tips, unfolding case studies, new illustrations and photos not found in the book, new animations, and updated audience response questions for use with iClicker and other audience response systems.
- Course management system.
- Access to all student resources listed above.
- The **Simulation Learning System (SLS)** is an online toolkit that helps instructors and facilitators effectively incorporate medium- to high-fidelity simulation into their nursing curriculum. Detailed patient scenarios promote and enhance the clinical decision-making skills of students at all levels. The SLS provides detailed instructions for preparation and implementation of the simulation experience, debriefing questions that encourage critical thinking, and learning resources to reinforce student comprehension. Each scenario in the SLS complements the textbook content and helps bridge the gap between lecture and clinical. The SLS provides the perfect environment for students to practice what they are learning in the text for a true-to-life, hands-on learning experience.

ACKNOWLEDGMENTS

The editors are especially grateful to many people at Elsevier who assisted with this major revision effort. In particular, we wish to thank the team of Kristin Geen, Jamie Randall, Mary Stueck, Jeff Patterson, and Maggie Reid. In addition, we want to thank the marketing team of Pat Crowe, Katie Schlesinger, and Becky McBride.

Special thanks and appreciation go to Peter Bonner who assisted with many details of manuscript preparation and review and photography for the book and interactive case studies.

We are particularly indebted to the faculty, nurses, and student nurses who have put their faith in our book to assist them on their path to excellence. The increasing use of this book throughout the United States, Canada, Australia, and other parts of the world has been gratifying. We appreciate the many users who have shared their comments and suggestions on the previous editions. All feedback is welcome.

We also wish to thank our contributors and reviewers for their assistance with the revision process. We sincerely hope that this book will assist both students and clinicians in practicing truly professional nursing.

Sharon L. Lewis
Shannon Ruff Dirksen
Margaret McLean Heitkemper
Linda Bucher

AUTHORS OF TEACHING AND LEARNING RESOURCES

TEST BANK

Barbara Bartz, MN, ARNP, CCRN
Nursing Instructor
Yakima Valley Community College
Yakima, Washington

Linda Bucher, RN, PhD, CEN, CNE
Emerita Professor
School of Nursing, University of Delaware
Newark, Delaware;
Consultant/Mentor
W. Cary Edwards School of Nursing
Thomas Edison State College
Trenton, New Jersey;
Per Diem Staff Nurse
Emergency Department,
Virtua Memorial Hospital
Mt. Holly, New Jersey

Debra Hagler, RN, PhD, ACNS-BC, CNE, CHSE, ANEF, FAAN
Clinical Professor
College of Nursing and Healthcare Innovation
Arizona State University
Phoenix, Arizona

Christina D. Keller, RN, MSN
Instructor
Radford University School of Nursing
Clinical Simulation Center
Radford, Virginia

Jo A. Voss, RN, PhD, CNS
Associate Professor
South Dakota State University
Rapid City, South Dakota

PRE-TESTS

Debra Hagler, RN, PhD, ACNS-BC, CNE, CHSE, ANEF, FAAN
Clinical Professor
College of Nursing and Healthcare Innovation
Arizona State University
Phoenix, Arizona

CASE STUDIES

Interactive, Managing Multiple Patients, and Assessment Case Studies
Dorothy (Dottie) M. Mathers, RN, DNP, CNE
Professor
School of Health Sciences
Pennsylvania College of Technology
Williamsport, Pennsylvania

TEACH for Nurses Case Studies
Elizabeth Day, RN, MSN, CHPN
Nursing Faculty
Fresno City College and Madera Center
Fresno, California

Heidi E. Monroe, RN-BC, MSN, CPAN, CAPA
Assistant Professor of Nursing
Bellin College
Green Bay, Wisconsin

POWERPOINT PRESENTATIONS

Dorothy (Dottie) M. Mathers, RN, DNP, CNE
Professor
School of Health Sciences
Pennsylvania College of Technology
Williamsport, Pennsylvania

Jane E. Oehme, RN, MS
Associate Professor of Nursing
Pennsylvania College of Technology
Williamsport, Pennsylvania

Michelle A. Latshaw, RN, MSN
Associate Professor of Nursing
Williamsport, Pennsylvania

PowerPoint Presentations and Glossaries
Cory Shaw Retherford, MOM, LAc.
Former Research Assistant
University of Texas Health Science Center at San Antonio
San Antonio, Texas

TEACH FOR NURSES

Mariann M. Harding, RN, PhD, CNE
Associate Professor of Nursing
Kent State University at Tuscarawas
New Philadelphia, Ohio

AUDIENCE RESPONSE QUESTIONS

Jo A. Voss, RN, PhD, CNS
Associate Professor
South Dakota State University
Rapid City, South Dakota

NCLEX® EXAMINATION REVIEW QUESTIONS

Susan A. Sandstrom, RN, MSN, BC, CNE
Associate Professor in Nursing, Retired
College of Saint Mary
Omaha, Nebraska

STUDY GUIDE

Susan A. Sandstrom, RN, MSN, BC, CNE
Associate Professor in Nursing, Retired
College of Saint Mary
Omaha, Nebraska

CLINICAL COMPANION

Shannon Ruff Dirksen, RN, PhD, FAAN
Associate Professor
College of Nursing and Health Innovation
Arizona State University
Phoenix, Arizona

Sharon L. Lewis, RN, PhD, FAAN
Professor Emerita
University of New Mexico
Albuquerque, New Mexico;
Former Castella Distinguished Professor
School of Nursing
University of Texas Health Science Center at San Antonio
San Antonio, Texas;
Developer and Consultant
Stress-Busting Program for Family Caregivers

ETHICAL/LEGAL DILEMMAS BOXES

Kathy Lucke, RN, PhD
Clinical Professor
University at Buffalo
School of Nursing
Buffalo, New York

Rosemary J. Mann, RN, CNM, MS, JD, PhD
Clinical Professor
School of Nursing
University at Buffalo
Buffalo, New York

DELEGATION DECISIONS BOXES

Barbara Bartz, MN, ARNP, CCRN
Nursing Instructor
Yakima Valley Community College
Yakima, Washington

EVIDENCE-BASED PRACTICE BOXES

Applying the Evidence Boxes

Linda Bucher, RN, PhD, CEN, CNE
Emerita Professor
School of Nursing
University of Delaware
Newark, Delaware;
Consultant/Mentor
W. Cary Edwards School of Nursing
Thomas Edison State College
Trenton, New Jersey;
Per Diem Staff Nurse
Emergency Department
Virtua Memorial Hospital
Mt. Holly, New Jersey

Translating Research Into Practice Boxes

Shannon Ruff Dirksen, RN, PhD, FAAN
Associate Professor
College of Nursing and Health Innovation
Arizona State University
Phoenix, Arizona

INFORMATICS BOXES

Mariann M. Harding, RN, PhD, CNE
Associate Professor of Nursing
Kent State University at Tuscarawas
New Philadelphia, Ohio

NURSING CARE PLANS

Patricia O'Brien, RN, ACNS-BC, MA, MSN
Albuquerque, New Mexico

SPECIAL PROJECTS

Peter Bonner, MS
DSI
Placitas, New Mexico

CONTENTS

SECTION 7
Problems of Oxygenation:
Perfusion

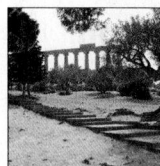

SECTION 8
Problems of Ingestion,
Digestion, Absorption, and
Elimination

SECTION 9
Problems of Urinary Function

SECTION 10
Problems Related to
Regulatory and Reproductive
Mechanisms

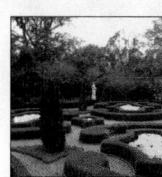

SECTION 11
Problems Related to Movement and Coordination

SECTION 12
Nursing Care in Critical Care Settings

APPENDIXES

SPECIAL FEATURES

COMPLEMENTARY & ALTERNATIVE THERAPIES BOXES

CULTURAL & ETHNIC HEALTH DISPARITIES BOXES

DELEGATION DECISIONS BOXES

DIAGNOSTIC STUDIES TABLES

DRUG THERAPY TABLES

EMERGENCY MANAGEMENT TABLES

ETHICAL/LEGAL DILEMMAS BOXES

EVIDENCE-BASED PRACTICE

Applying the Evidence Boxes

EVIDENCE-BASED PRACTICE

Translating Research Into Practice Boxes

FOCUSED ASSESSMENT BOXES

GENDER DIFFERENCES BOXES

GENETICS IN CLINICAL PRACTICE BOXES

GERONTOLOGIC ASSESSMENT DIFFERENCES TABLES

NURSING CARE PLANS

NUTRITIONAL THERAPY TABLES

PATIENT & CAREGIVER TEACHING GUIDE TABLES

*evolve On Evolve website.

Concepts in Nursing Practice

Peter Bonner

The journey is the reward.
Tao saying

1

The road to knowledge begins
with the turn of the page.
Anonymous

Professional Nursing Practice

Mariann M. Harding

⊖volve WEBSITE

http://evolve.elsevier.com/Lewis/medsurg

- NCLEX Review Questions
- Key Points
- Pre-Test
- Rationales for Bridge to NCLEX Examination Questions
- Concept Map Creator

- Glossary
- Content Updates

eFigures

- eFig. 1-1: Screen from a patient's electronic health record
- eFig. 1-2: Decision tree for delegation to unlicensed assistive personnel (UAP)

eTables

- eTable 1-1: Practice Settings for Transitional Care
- eTable 1-2: Practice Settings for Long-Term Care
- eTable 1-3: Overview of Delegation, Assignment, and Supervision

LEARNING OUTCOMES

1. Describe professional nursing practice in terms of domain, definitions, and recipients of care.
2. Compare the different scopes of practice available to professional nurses.
3. Analyze the effect of expanding technology and knowledge, changing populations, consumerism, and evolving health care systems on professional nursing practice.
4. Describe the role of critical thinking skills and use of the nursing process to provide patient-centered care.

5. Explain how standardized nursing terminologies for nursing diagnoses, patient outcomes, and nursing interventions can be used and linked.
6. Evaluate the role of informatics and technology in nursing practice.
7. Apply concepts of evidence-based practice to nursing practice.
8. Discuss the role of integrating safety and quality improvement processes into nursing practice.
9. Explore the role of the professional nurse in delegating care to licensed practical/vocational nurses and unlicensed assistive personnel.

KEY TERMS

advanced practice nurse (APN), p. 3
case management, p. 14
clinical (critical) pathway, p. 15
clinical reasoning, p. 6
collaborative problems, p. 8
concept map, p. 8

critical thinking, p. 6
delegation, p. 15
electronic health record (EHR), p. 10
evidence-based practice (EBP), p. 11
Healthy People, p. 5
nursing, p. 3

nursing informatics, p. 10
nursing process, p. 6
telehealth, p. 11
unlicensed assistive personnel (UAP), p. 15

This chapter presents an overview of professional nursing practice, discussing the wide variety of roles and responsibilities nurses fulfill to meet the health care needs of society.

PROFESSIONAL NURSING PRACTICE

Domain of Nursing Practice

Nursing practice today consists of a wide variety of roles and responsibilities necessary to meet society's health care needs. As a nurse, you are the frontline professional of health care (Fig. 1-1). You practice in virtually all health care settings and communities across the country. You have never been more important to health care than you are today. As a nurse, you

(1) offer skilled care to those recuperating from illness or injury, (2) advocate for patients' rights, (3) teach patients so that they can make informed decisions, (4) support patients and their caregivers at critical times, and (5) help them navigate the increasingly complex health care system. Although the majority of nurses are employed in acute care facilities, many nurses practice in long-term care, home care, primary and preventive care, ambulatory clinics, and community health. Wherever you practice, recipients of your care include individuals, groups, families, or communities.

The American Nurses Association (ANA) declares that the authority for the practice of nursing is based on a contract with society that acknowledges professional rights and respon-

Reviewed by Claudia C Grobbel, RN, DNP, Assistant Professor, Oakland University, Rochester, Michigan; Elizabeth E. Hand, RN, MS, Adjunct Faculty, Tulsa Community College, School of Nursing, Tulsa, Oklahoma; and Patricia O'Brien, RN, ACNS-BC, MA, MSN, Retired Instructor, University of New Mexico, College of Nursing and Central New Mexico Community College, Albuquerque, New Mexico.

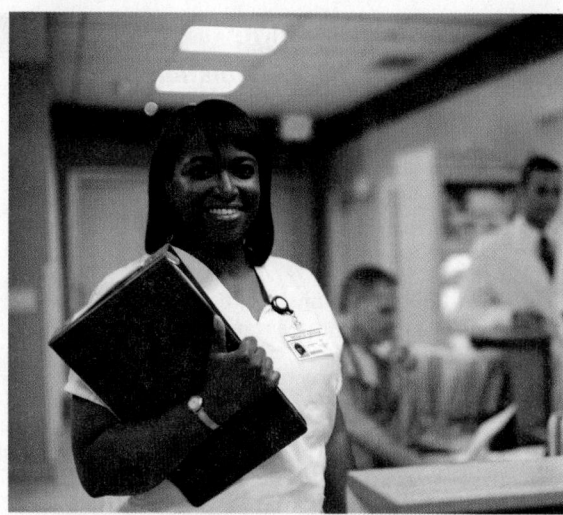

FIG. 1-1 Nurses are frontline professionals of health care. (Thomas Northcut/Digital Vision/Thinkstock)

sibilities, as well as mechanisms for public accountability.[1] The knowledge and skills that comprise nursing practice are derived from society's expectations and needs. Nursing practice continues to evolve according to society's health needs and as knowledge and technology expand. This chapter introduces concepts and factors that affect professional nursing practice.

Definitions of Nursing

Several well-known definitions of nursing indicate that the basic themes of health, illness, and caring have existed since Florence Nightingale described nursing. Following are two such examples:

- Nursing is putting the patient in the best condition for nature to act (Nightingale).[2]
- The nurse's unique function is to assist patients, sick or well, in the performance of those activities contributing to health or its recovery (or to peaceful death) that they would perform unaided if they had the necessary strength, will, or knowledge—and to do this in such a way as to help them gain independence as rapidly as possible (Henderson).[3]

In 1980 the ANA defined **nursing** as "the diagnosis and treatment of human responses to actual and potential health problems."[1] In this context, a nurse caring for a person with a fractured hip would focus on the patient's possible responses to immobility, pain, and loss of independence.

The widely accepted ANA definition of nursing was reaffirmed in the 2010 edition of the ANA's *Nursing: A Social Policy Statement* to reflect the continuing evolution of nursing practice:

> ***Nursing*** *is the protection, promotion, and optimization of health and abilities, prevention of illness and injury, alleviation of suffering through the diagnosis and treatment of human response, and advocacy in the care of individuals, families, communities, and populations.*[1]

This definition reflects nurses' increasing role in promoting health and wellness and advocating for the recipients of care.

Nursing's View of Humanity

Nursing theorists are in widespread agreement that an individual has physiologic (or biophysical), psychologic (or emotional),

sociocultural (or interpersonal), spiritual, and environmental components or dimensions. In this text the human individual is considered "a biopsychosocial spiritual being in constant interaction with a changing environment."[4] The individual is composed of dimensions that are interrelated and not separate entities. Thus a problem in one dimension may affect one or more of the other dimensions. An individual's behavior is meaningful and oriented toward fulfilling needs, coping with stress, and developing one's self. However, at times an individual needs help to meet these needs, cope successfully, or develop his or her unique potential.

Scope of Nursing Practice

Like all health care professions, nursing's scope of practice has a flexible boundary that reflects the changing needs of society and advancement of knowledge. The essential core of nursing practice is to deliver holistic, patient-centered care. It includes assessment and evaluation, administration of a variety of interventions, patient and family teaching, and being a member of the interdisciplinary (also referred to as the interprofessional) health care team.

The extent that individual nurses engage in the scope of practice depends on their educational preparation, experience, and role, and is guided by individual state laws. To enter into practice, a nurse must complete an accredited program and pass an examination verifying the nurse has the skills necessary to provide competent care. Entry-level nurses with associate or baccalaureate degrees are prepared to function as generalists. At this level, nurses provide direct health care and focus on ensuring coordinated and comprehensive care to patients in a variety of settings. They work collaboratively with other health care providers to manage the needs of individuals and groups.[5,6]

With experience and continued study, nurses may specialize in an area of practice. Certification is a formal way for nurses to obtain professional recognition for their expertise in a specialty area. A variety of nursing organizations offer certification in a number of nursing specialties.[7] Certification usually requires a certain amount of clinical experience and successful completion of an examination. Recertification usually requires ongoing clinical experience and continuing education. Common nursing specialties include ambulatory care; cardiovascular care; critical care; women's health; diabetes education; nursing informatics; and geriatric, medical-surgical, perinatal, emergency, psychiatric/mental health, and community health nursing.

Additional formal education and experience can prepare nurses for advanced practice. An **advanced practice nurse (APN)** or *advanced practice registered nurse (APRN)* is a nurse with at least a master's degree in nursing; advanced education in pathophysiology, pharmacology, and health assessment; and expertise in a specialized area of practice. Examples of APNs/APRNs are clinical nurse specialists, clinical nurse leaders, nurse practitioners, nurse midwives, and nurse anesthetists. In addition to managing and delivering direct patient care, APNs/APRNs have roles in health promotion, case management, administration, research, and interdisciplinary health systems.[7] Nurses with a PhD typically serve as faculty in schools of nursing, policy analysts, and researchers. However, they are being increasingly employed in clinical settings as clinical experts and health care system executives.

In response to patient care needs and in anticipation of the needs of the current and future health care system, the doctorate of nursing practice (DNP) degree was endorsed in 2004 by the American Association of Colleges of Nursing (AACN). The DNP moves the educational preparation for advanced nursing practice from the master's degree to the doctoral level. It is designed for nurses seeking a practice-focused terminal degree in nursing. The DNP degree moves nursing in the direction of other health professions that offer practice doctorates (e.g., pharmacy [PharmD], psychology [PsyD], and physical therapy [DPT]).[8]

INFLUENCES ON PROFESSIONAL NURSING PRACTICE

Complex Health Care Environments

Expanding Knowledge and Technology. Rapidly changing technology and dramatically expanding knowledge are adding to the complexity of health care environments. Advanced communication technologies have created a more global environment that affects the delivery of health care worldwide. The number and complexity of patient care technologies are transforming how care is delivered. The human genome project and advances in genetics affect the prevention, diagnosis, and treatment of health problems. With advances in knowledge, ethical dilemmas and controversy arise regarding the use of new scientific knowledge and the disparities that exist in patients' access to more technologically advanced health care. Throughout this book, expanding knowledge and technology's impact on nursing practice are highlighted in genetics, informatics, and ethical/legal boxes.

Diverse Populations. Patient populations are more diverse than ever. Americans are living longer, in part due to advances in medical science, technology, and health care delivery. As the population ages, the number of patients with chronic conditions increases. Unlike those who receive acute, episodic care, patients with chronic conditions have a multitude of needs. They see a variety of health care providers in various settings over an extended period. Nurses are also caring for a more culturally and ethnically diverse population. Immigrants, particularly undocumented immigrants and refugees, often lack the resources necessary to access health care. Inability to pay for health care is associated with a tendency to delay seeking care, resulting in illnesses that are more serious. Boxes throughout this book emphasize the influence of such factors as gender, culture, and ethnicity on nursing practice.

Consumerism. Health care is a consumer-focused business. Patients today are active participants in their health care and expect high-quality, coordinated, and financially reasonable care. Health information is readily available. Many patients eagerly seek information about their health problems and health care from media and Internet sources. They gather information so that they can have a voice in making decisions about their health care. As a nurse, you must be able to help patients access and use appropriate health care information (Fig. 1-2).

Influences on Health Care Systems

Health Care Financing. Many changes in health care systems that influence nursing care delivery were initiated by the government, employers, insurance companies, and regulating agencies in an effort to provide more cost-effective health care. Historically, the most notable event related to changing reimbursement patterns was the institution of prospective payment systems in the Medicare program. With these changes, hospitals

FIG. 1-2 The patient, family, and nurse collaborate as part of coordinating high-quality care. (Hemera/Thinkstock)

were no longer reimbursed for all costs. Instead, payment for hospital services for Medicare patients was based on flat fees determined by the diseases and problems treated during the admission. Private and other public health care systems followed suit by introducing managed care systems that use prospective payment as a means of offering cost-effective health care delivery. In health maintenance organizations (HMOs) and preferred provider organizations (PPOs), charges are negotiated in advance of the delivery of care using predetermined reimbursement rates or capitation fees for medical care, hospitalization, and other health care services.

These same third-party payers demand outcome-based quality care that is provided at a price affordable for both individuals and society. Payment for health care services or pay-for-performance programs reimburse hospitals for their performance on quality-of-care measures. These measures include clinical outcomes, patient safety, patient satisfaction, adherence to evidence-based practice, and adoption of information technology. Payment for care can be withheld if a patient develops certain health care conditions during a hospital stay (e.g., pressure ulcer) or if something happens to the patient that is considered preventable (e.g., acquiring a catheter-related urinary tract infection).[9]

***Healthy People* Initiative.** For the past 30 years the U.S. government has been active in establishing goals and objectives for promoting health and health care delivery for the nation through an initiative known as *Healthy People*.[10] The vision of *Healthy People* is a society in which all people live long, healthy lives. *Healthy People* is a broad-based program that involves government, private, public, and nonprofit organizations. Individuals, groups, and organizations are encouraged to integrate *Healthy People* goals and focus areas into current programs, special events, publications, and meetings. These activities can further the health of all members of a community. The overarching goals of the *Healthy People 2020* initiative are presented in Table 1-1. *Healthy People* boxes related to these goals are integrated throughout this book.

The *Healthy People* initiative is a significant challenge for nursing. Both nursing education programs and clinical nursing practice must respond to major trends in health care. Educational programs for entry-level nurses now place a greater emphasis on health promotion; maintenance; and cost-effective care that responds to the needs of older adults, culturally diverse groups, and underserved populations. Today's nurses must address the identified health problems, developments in health care delivery, research outcomes, and new technologies in order to meet *Healthy People* goals. As a reflection of nursing's contract with society, you are responsible for improving the health status of the public and reducing health disparities. (Health disparities are discussed in Chapter 2.)

Supporting Professional Practice

Professional Nursing Organizations. The American Nurses Association is the primary professional nursing organization. There are numerous professional specialty organizations, such as the American Association of Critical-Care Nurses (AACN),

Association of periOperative Registered Nurses (AORN), and Oncology Nursing Society (ONS). Professional organizations have numerous roles in promoting quality patient care and professional nursing practice. These include developing standards of practice and codes of ethics, supporting research, and lobbying for legislation and regulations. Major nursing organizations also promote research into the causes of errors, develop strategies to prevent future errors, and address nursing issues that affect the nurse's ability to deliver patient care safely. Many nurses join a professional organization to keep current in their practice and network with others who are interested in a particular practice area.

QSEN. In 2003 the Institute of Medicine (IOM) commissioned an interdisciplinary task force to study the educational preparation of health care professionals to see whether new graduates were prepared for today's reality of practice.[11] What they found was that all health professions, including nursing, needed to review and revise their curricula and focus on developing specific competencies that serve as a basis for practice. In nursing this is done through a project known as *Quality and Safety Education for Nurses (QSEN) (www.qsen.org)*. QSEN consists of six core competencies: (1) patient-centered care, (2) informatics and technology, (3) evidence-based practice, (4) quality improvement, (5) safety, and (6) teamwork and collaboration. The remainder of this chapter discusses how professional nursing practice is focusing on acquiring the knowledge, skills, and attitudes within each competency.

PATIENT-CENTERED CARE

Nurses have long demonstrated that they truly deliver patient-centered care based on each patient's unique needs and understanding of the patient's preferences, values, and beliefs. Patient-centered care is interrelated with both quality and safety. In the patient-centered care model, patients and caregivers seek care from competent and knowledgeable health care professionals. Patients and caregivers are involved in making care decisions and managing the patient's care.

Delivery of Nursing Care

Nurses deliver patient-centered care in collaboration with the interdisciplinary health care team and within the framework of a care delivery model. Today a variety of care delivery models are being used in view of nursing shortages, state-mandated nurse-patient ratios, economic issues, and increased acuity of patient conditions.

A *team nursing* model uses a professional nurse as a team leader. As a team leader, you organize and manage the care for a group of patients with other ancillary workers such as licensed practical/vocational nurses (LPN/LVNs) and unlicensed assistive personnel (UAP). In this model, you have the authority and accountability for the quality of care delivered by team members during a work period.

In a *total patient care* model, you assume accountability for the complete care of a patient or group of patients during the assigned shift. In this model, you are responsible for planning and providing all care.

In a *primary nursing* model, you are responsible for a patient or caseload of patients over a period of time.[12] You provide care during assigned shifts, and coordinate and communicate all aspects of patient care with other disciplines and those who provide care when you are absent. Care delivered within a

TABLE 1-1 *HEALTHY PEOPLE 2020*
Overarching Goals
• Attain high quality, longer lives free of preventable disease, disability, injury, and premature death.
• Achieve health equity, eliminate disparities, and improve the health of all groups.
• Create social and physical environments that promote good health for all.
• Promote quality of life, healthy development, and healthy behaviors across all life stages.

Source: US Department of Health and Human Services: *Healthy People* 2020. Retrieved from *www.healthypeople.gov*.

primary care model strengthens the nurse-patient relationship through a focus on continuity of care and interdisciplinary collaboration.

Continuum of Patient Care

Depending on their health status, patients often move among a multitude of different health care settings. Decisions regarding the most appropriate setting for obtaining health care frequently depend on the cost of care and constraints of a patient's health care insurance plan. Although the hospital remains the mainstay for acute care interventions within this continuum, community-based settings offer patients the opportunity to live or recover in settings that maximize their independence and preserve human dignity. For example, a person may be hospitalized in a trauma unit of an acute care hospital following a motor vehicle crash. After the person is stabilized, he or she may be transferred to a general medical-surgical unit and then to an acute rehabilitation facility. After a period of rehabilitation the person may be discharged to his or her home to continue with outpatient rehabilitation, with follow-up by home health care nurses and care in an outpatient clinic.

The continuum of care does not always include hospitalization. Some patients receive community-based care without experiencing an acute problem requiring hospitalization. Community-based settings where health care is provided include ambulatory care, transitional care, and long-term care. Transitional care settings provide care in between the acute care and the home or long-term care setting (see eTable 1-1 on the website for this chapter). Patients may receive transitional care at an acute rehabilitation facility after head trauma or a spinal cord injury. Long-term care refers to the care of patients for a period greater than 30 days (see eTable 1-2 on the website for this chapter). It may be required for individuals who are severely developmentally disabled, are mentally impaired, or have physical deficits requiring continuous medical or nursing management (e.g., patients who are ventilator dependent or have Alzheimer's disease). Long-term care facilities include skilled nursing facilities, intermediate care facilities, retirement communities, and residential care facilities.

Critical Thinking

Complex health care environments require that you use critical thinking and clinical reasoning skills to make decisions that lead to the best patient outcomes. Although no standard definitions of critical thinking or methods of teaching and evaluating critical thinking have been accepted, critical thinking is recognized as a broad term for a learned skill. Critical thinking has been described as knowing how to learn, reason, think creatively, generate ideas, make decisions, and solve problems.[13] Critical thinking is not memorizing a list of facts or the steps of a procedure; instead it is the ability to solve problems by making sense of information. Learning and using critical thinking is a continual process that occurs inside and outside of the clinical setting.

Clinical reasoning is a problem-solving activity in which critical thinking is used to examine patient care issues. It is a process that involves using knowledge from many fields to understand the medical and nursing implications of a patient situation when making decisions regarding patient care.[14] You use clinical reasoning when you identify a change in a patient's status, take into account the context and concerns of the patient and caregiver, and decide what to do about it.

Given the complexity of patient care today, nurses are required to learn and implement critical thinking and clinical reasoning skills long before they gain those skills through the experience of professional practice. Clinical experiences during nursing education provide opportunities for you to learn and make decisions about patient care. To promote practice in critical thinking and clinical reasoning, various education models and techniques have been developed, including exercises in simulation laboratories and interactive scenarios. Throughout this book, select boxes, case studies, and review questions promote your use of critical thinking and clinical reasoning skills.

Nursing Process

Nurses provide patient-centered care using an organizing framework called the nursing process. The nursing process is a problem-solving approach to the identification and treatment of patient problems that is the foundation of nursing practice. The nursing process framework provides a structure for the delivery of nursing care and the knowledge, judgments, and actions that nurses use to achieve best patient outcomes. Once started, the nursing process is not only continuous but also cyclic in nature.

The nursing process consists of five phases: assessment, diagnosis, planning, implementation, and evaluation (Fig. 1-3).

FIG. 1-3 Nursing process.

There is a basic order to the nursing process, beginning with assessment. *Assessment* is the collection of subjective and objective patient information on which to base the plan of care. *Nursing diagnosis* is the act of analyzing the assessment data and making a judgment about the nature of the data. It includes identifying and labeling human responses to actual or potential health problems or life processes. During *planning* the nursing diagnosis directs the development of patient outcomes or goals and identification of nursing interventions to accomplish the outcomes. *Implementation* is the activation of the plan with the use of nursing interventions. *Evaluation* is a continual activity in the nursing process. Evaluation determines whether the patient outcomes have been met as a result of nursing interventions. If the outcomes were not met, a review of the steps of the process is necessary to determine why not. Revision may be needed in assessment (data collection), the nursing diagnosis, planning (determining patient outcomes), or implementation (nursing interventions).

Standardized Nursing Terminologies

The demands of the current health care system challenge the nursing profession to define its practice and its impact on the health and health care of individuals, families, and communities. The nursing profession is asking questions such as the following: What do nurses do? How do they do it? Does it make a measurable difference in the health of those for whom they care? How can nurses best document their care? What happens as a result of their care?

In response to these questions, nursing has moved toward using standardizing nursing terminology (also called *nomenclatures, classification systems,* and *taxonomies*) to clearly define and evaluate nursing care. This can promote continuity of patient care and provide data to support the value of the profession. Instead of using a wide variety of words and methods to describe the same patient problems and nursing interventions, nurses use a readily understood common language to improve communication among themselves. In addition, standardized languages help identify the most effective nursing interventions.[15] For example, do the patient problems of pressure ulcer, decubitus ulcer, and skin breakdown all mean the same thing? What interventions can prevent these problems? Does turning the patient every 2 hours mean the same thing as repositioning the patient every 2 hours? If the patient is turned or repositioned every 2 hours, what happens as a result? How are the results described? Are the results different if a patient is placed on a pressure-relieving mattress or placed on a standard mattress and only turned? How are the results documented, and how do you know what works best?

Standardized terminologies offer ways to organize and describe nursing phenomena. A variety of languages have been developed that address different areas of nursing. Table 1-2 lists the classification systems recognized and approved by the ANA. The Omaha System and the Home Health Care Classification have been developed for community-based and home health care nursing, respectively. The Perioperative Nursing Dataset (discussed in Chapter 19) is used by perioperative nurses. The Nursing Management Minimum Data Set is available for use by nurse managers and administrators.

Three of the nursing terminologies recognized by the ANA are used to describe patient responses, patient outcomes, and nursing interventions: (1) NANDA International: Nursing Diagnoses, Definitions, and Classification; (2) the Nursing Out-

TABLE 1-2	ANA-RECOGNIZED NURSING TERMINOLOGIES

- NANDA International Nursing Diagnoses
- Nursing Interventions Classification (NIC)
- Nursing Outcomes Classification (NOC)
- Clinical Care Classification (CCC)
- Omaha System
- Nursing Management Minimum Data Set (NMMDS)
- PeriOperative Nursing Data Set (PNDS)
- SNOMED CT
- Nursing Minimum Data Set (NMDS)
- International Classification for Nursing Practice (ICNP)
- Logical Observation Identifiers Names and Codes (LOINC)

Source: American Nurses Association: *Recognized languages for nursing,* Washington, DC, 2010, The Association. Retrieved from *www.nursingworld.org/Terminologies.*

comes Classification (NOC); and (3) the Nursing Interventions Classification (NIC). Each of these classification systems focuses on one component of the nursing process. Patients' responses or problems can be labeled using the nursing diagnoses classified and defined by NANDA-I.[16] Nursing interventions, or treatments, can be selected and implemented from NIC,[17] and nursing-sensitive patient outcomes can be identified and evaluated by selecting appropriate NOC outcomes.[18]

NANDA-I Nursing Diagnoses. NANDA International (NANDA-I) is a nursing organization that develops a standardized nursing terminology for identifying, defining, and classifying patients' actual or potential responses to health problems.[16] The two main purposes of NANDA-I are to develop a diagnostic classification system or taxonomy and to identify and accept nursing diagnoses. The use of the standardized terminology of nursing diagnoses documents the analysis and synthesis required in making a nursing diagnosis. It verifies nursing's contribution to cost-effective, efficient, quality health care.

The current NANDA-I nursing diagnoses are listed in Appendix B (NANDA-I nursing diagnoses are updated every 2 years). The nursing diagnoses used in this textbook are NANDA-I approved. The NANDA-I list is continually evolving as research results are interpreted and as nurses identify new human responses.

Nursing Outcomes Classification (NOC). Nursing Outcomes Classification (NOC) is a list of concepts, definitions, and measures that describe patient outcomes influenced by nursing interventions. A nursing-sensitive patient outcome is defined as an individual, family, or community state, behavior, or perception that is measured along a continuum in response to a nursing intervention(s).[18] The impact of your nursing practice on patient outcomes can be identified and measured when you choose a NOC outcome. Currently more than 385 coded outcomes have been organized into 7 domains and 34 classes. Each outcome has a label, a definition, a set of specific indicators to be used in rating the outcomes, and a five-point scale for rating the overall outcome and the specific indicators.

Nursing Interventions Classification (NIC). Nursing Interventions Classification (NIC) includes independent and collaborative interventions that you carry out, or direct others to carry out, on behalf of patients. It includes treatments that you perform in all settings and in all specialties. Because each intervention has a coded number, the use of NIC interventions facilitates electronic collection of standardized nursing data to evaluate the effectiveness of the interventions.

TABLE 1-3	**EXAMPLE OF NANDA-NOC-NIC LINKAGE**

NANDA-I Nursing Diagnosis: *Impaired skin integrity:* A state in which the individual has altered epidermis and/or dermis

NANDA-I–Related Factors	NOC Outcomes	NIC Interventions
Pressure	Tissue integrity: skin and mucous membranes	Pressure management Skin surveillance
Nutritional deficit	Nutritional status: food and fluid intake	Nutrition monitoring Nutrition therapy
Knowledge deficit	Knowledge: illness care	Teaching: disease process

Source: Nursing Diagnoses—Definitions and Classification 2012-2014. © 2012, 1994-2012 by NANDA International. Used by arrangement with Blackwell Publishing Limited, a company of John Wiley & Sons, Inc.
NANDA-I, NANDA International; *NIC,* Nursing Interventions Classification; *NOC,* Nursing Outcomes Classification.

FIG. 1-4 Integration of NANDA, NIC, and NOC into the nursing process.

NIC includes more than 500 interventions with a label name, a definition, and a set of activities for you to choose from to carry out the intervention. The interventions are grouped into 7 domains and 30 classes. Although more than 500 interventions may seem overwhelming, you will soon discover those interventions that are used most often in your particular specialty or with your patient population.[17] When planning care for a patient, choose specific interventions from the domain or class that is appropriate for the patient based on the nursing diagnosis and patient outcomes. Each intervention has a list of activities, and you select the appropriate activities from the list to implement the intervention. NIC does not prescribe interventions for specific situations. You are responsible for making the important decision of when and which interventions to use for a specific patient and situation based on your knowledge of the patient and the patient's condition.

NANDA-NOC-NIC Linkages. NANDA, NOC, and NIC (NNN) linkages show how the three distinct nursing terminologies can be connected and used together when planning care for patients. Linkages may assist in determination of a nursing diagnosis, projection of a desired outcome, and selection of interventions to achieve the desired outcome. Because each outcome or intervention has a coded number, the use of NNN facilitates electronic collection of standardized nursing data to evaluate the effectiveness of nursing care. An example of an NNN linkage is found in Table 1-3. The integration of NNN into the nursing process is illustrated in Fig. 1-4.

Nursing Care Plans

The nursing process is usually recorded and documented differently in nursing education when compared to clinical nursing practice. In nursing education the nursing process is frequently recorded in nursing care plans similar to those presented in this textbook. You practice and learn the nursing process by collecting assessment data, identifying nursing diagnoses, and selecting patient outcomes and nursing interventions—all of which are recorded on specific forms. Rationales for the selected interventions are also identified. These nursing care plans are used as teaching and learning tools.

In clinical practice, nursing care plans are often adapted for a specific setting. Electronic and written standardized care plans are used as guides for routine nursing care and are individualized to each patient's unique needs and problems.

The nursing care plans presented throughout this book use the NANDA-I–approved nursing diagnoses, listed in order of priority, with NOC outcomes and NIC interventions (NCP 1-1). When any of these care plans are used, they should be individualized for a specific patient. You must use critical thinking to continually evaluate the situation and revise the diagnoses, outcomes, and interventions to fit each patient's unique care needs. All of the nursing care plans for this textbook are available in electronic format on the website at *http://evolve.elsevier.com/Lewis/medsurg.*

Collaborative problems are potential or actual complications of disease or treatment that nurses treat with other health care providers (e.g., physicians, APNs, speech therapists).[19] During the diagnosis phase of the nursing process, you identify these risks for physiologic complications in addition to nursing diagnoses. Identification of collaborative problems requires knowledge of pathophysiology and possible complications of medical treatment. Collaborative problem statements are usually written as "potential complication: _____" or "PC: _____" without a *"related to"* statement. An example is PC: pulmonary embolism. When potential complications are used in this textbook, *"related to"* statements have been added to increase understanding and relate the potential complication to possible causes.

A **concept map** is another method of recording a nursing care plan. In a concept map care plan the nursing process is recorded in a visual diagram of patient problems and interventions that illustrates the relationships among clinical data. Concept mapping is most useful in nursing education to teach nursing process and care planning.

Various formats are used for concept maps, and a variety of shapes, colors, and connecting arrows are used to identify concepts and relationships. In one example, assessment data are used to identify the patient's primary reason for seeking health care. That health state (often a medical diagnosis) is positioned centrally on the map. Positioned around the reason for seeking health care are nursing diagnoses that represent the patient's responses to the health state. Listed with each nursing diagnosis

◎ NURSING CARE PLAN 1-1

*Patient with Heart Failure**

NURSING DIAGNOSIS **Activity intolerance** *related to* imbalance between oxygen supply and demand secondary to cardiac insufficiency and pulmonary congestion *as evidenced by* dyspnea, shortness of breath, weakness, increase in heart rate on exertion, and/or patient's statement, "I am too tired to get out of bed. I have no energy."

PATIENT GOAL Achieves a realistic program of activity that balances physical activity with energy-conserving activities

Outcomes (NOC)	Interventions (NIC) and *Rationales*
Activity Tolerance	**_Energy Management_**
• Pulse rate with activity _____	• Encourage alternate rest and activity periods *to reduce cardiac workload and conserve energy.*
• O₂ saturation with activity _____	• Provide calming diversionary activities to promote relaxation *to reduce O₂ consumption and to relieve dyspnea and fatigue.*
• Respiratory rate with activity _____	• Monitor patient's O₂ response (e.g., pulse rate, cardiac rhythm, and respiratory rate) to self-care or nursing activities *to determine level of activity that can be performed.*
• Systolic BP with activity _____	• Teach patient and caregiver techniques of self-care *that will minimize O₂ consumption* (e.g., self monitoring and pacing techniques for performance of ADLs).
• Diastolic BP with activity _____	
• Ease of breathing with activity _____	
• Ease of performing ADLs _____	
• Skin color _____	**_Activity Therapy_**
	• Collaborate with occupational and/or physical therapists *to plan and monitor activity and exercise program.*
Measurement Scale	• Determine patient's commitment to increasing frequency and/or range of activities and exercise *to provide patient with obtainable goals.*
1 = Severely compromised	
2 = Substantially compromised	
3 = Moderately compromised	
4 = Mildly compromised	
5 = Not compromised	

ADLs, Activities of daily living; *NIC,* Nursing Interventions Classification; *NOC,* Nursing Outcomes Classification.
*This example presents one nursing diagnosis for heart failure. The complete nursing care plan for heart failure is NCP 35-1 on pp. 780-781.

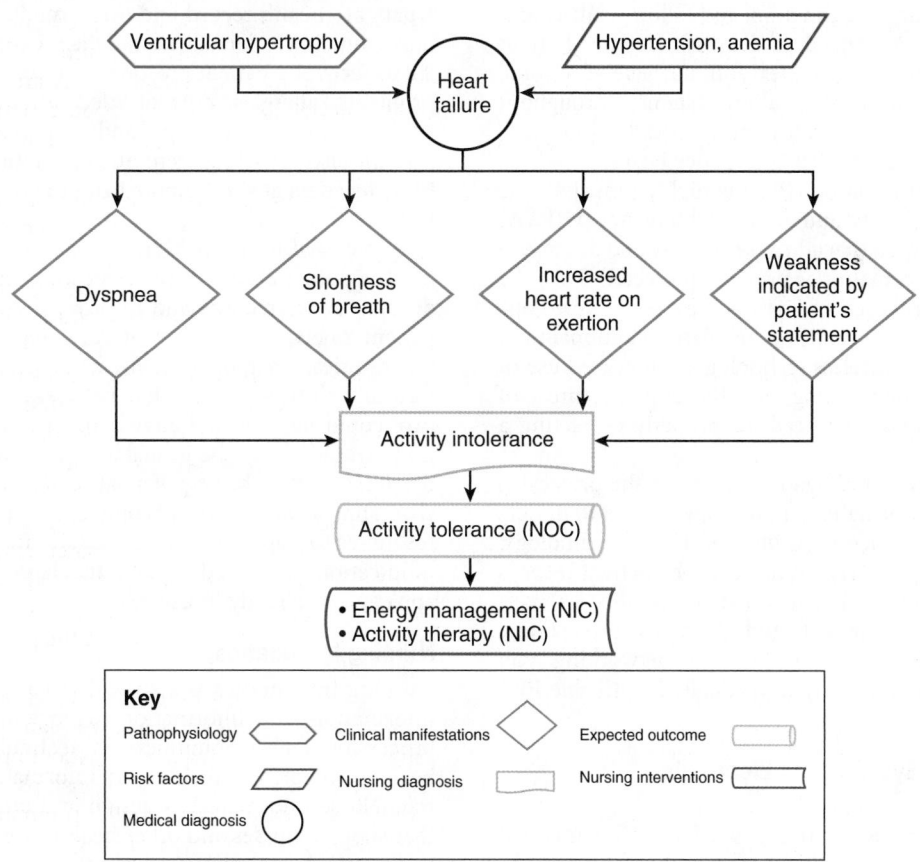

FIG. 1-5 Concept map.

are the assessment data that support the nursing diagnosis. Diagnostic testing data, treatments, medications, and nursing interventions may be listed with the nursing diagnoses or may be identified in separate areas and connected to the nursing diagnoses with arrows.[20] Fig. 1-5 illustrates a simplified version of a concept map for the patient with heart failure. For selected case studies at the end of the management chapters, related concept maps are available on the website at *http://evolve. elsevier.com/Lewis/medsurg.* In addition, a concept map builder is available online on the website.

INFORMATICS AND TECHNOLOGY

Information and Technology in Practice

Nursing is an information-intense profession. Advances in health information technology have changed the way nurses plan, deliver, document, and evaluate care. All nurses, regardless of their setting or role, use informatics and technology every day in practice. The incorporation of technologies into practice has changed how you obtain and review diagnostic information, make clinical decisions, communicate with patients and caregivers, and provide clinical interventions.[21]

Using information technology is becoming increasingly important in providing safe, quality patient care. For example, medication administration applications have been shown to improve patient safety by flagging potential errors, such as look-alike and sound-alike medications and adverse drug interactions, before they can occur. Computerized provider order entry (CPOE) systems can eliminate errors caused by misreading or misinterpreting handwritten instructions. Sensor technology is used to decrease the incidence of falls in high-risk patients.

Being able to use technology skills to communicate and access information is now an essential component of your professional nursing practice. You must be able to use word processing software, communicate by e-mail and text messaging, access the Internet to find information, and follow security and confidentiality rules.[22] You need to demonstrate the skills to safely use patient care technologies and navigate electronic health records and clinical information systems. Throughout this book suggestions on how to use informatics in your practice are highlighted in Informatics in Practice boxes.

Protected health information (PHI) is highly sensitive. The Health Insurance Portability and Accountability Act (HIPAA) is part of federal legislation that addresses the use and disclosure of PHI so that such information is properly protected. With the increased use of informatics and technology come new concerns for how to comply with HIPAA regulations and maintain a patient's privacy. New wireless technologies, increased use of e-mail and computer networking, and the ongoing threat of computer viruses increase the need for properly protecting a patient's privacy.

As a nurse, you have an obligation to ensure the privacy of your patient's health information. To do so, you need to understand your agency's policies regarding the use of technology. You need to know the rules regarding accessing patient records and releasing PHI, know what to do if information is accidently or intentionally released, and diligently protect any passwords you use. If you are using social networking, you must be careful not to place any individually identifiable PHI online.

Clinical Information Systems and Electronic Health Records

A clinical information system (CIS) is a large computerized system that integrates various information technology applications into a centralized repository of information related to patient care.[23] These systems support many types of activities related to patient care, including care documentation, order entry, and the retrieval of results, across various locations. Some examples of CISs including laboratory, nursing, pharmacy, long-term care, and emergency department systems and electronic health records.

An **electronic health record (EHR)** is a computerized record of PHI generated by one or more encounters in any care delivery setting.[24] Information that should be in an EHR includes patient demographics, progress notes, problems, medications, vital signs, past medical history, immunizations, laboratory data, and radiology reports (eFig. 1-1 available on the website for this chapter).

An *electronic medical record (EMR)* is a set of computerized data collected by a health care agency, such as an individual hospital or physician's office, which contributes to a record that is owned and used by that agency. In turn, an EHR is created when information from records created by a variety of agencies under different ownership is made available to other health care providers regardless of the location or affiliation of the health care provider. In practice, the terms *EHR* and *EMR* are often used interchangeably.[25]

The federal government was instrumental in the early adoption of EHRs because of its role in the delivery and payment of health care for millions of Americans through Medicare, the armed services, and the Department of Veterans Affairs (VA). The VA EHR system was one of the first implemented nationwide and today is a prototype for other providers. Patient records in the VA's electronic health system are fully electronic, portable, and readily accessible. The VA's EHR system provides a single place for health care providers to review and update a patient's health record and order medications, special procedures, nursing orders, diets, and diagnostic and laboratory tests. All aspects of a patient's record are integrated, including active problems, allergies, current medications, laboratory results, vital signs, hospitalizations, and outpatient clinic history. The system also provides reminders, cautions, and the ability to review data at sites remote from the original site of data collection.[26]

A national uniform EHR similar to the VA's health record has the potential to reduce medical errors associated with traditional paper records and improve clinical decision making, patient safety, and quality of care. As EHRs, entry systems, laboratories, imaging systems, and pharmacies are all linked into one clinical information network, many types of patient care could be provided anywhere, at anytime, since the "care grid" would always be available.[11] Unfortunately, a number of barriers stand in the way of a national system. EHRs are expensive and technologically complex, requiring a number of resources to implement and maintain. In addition, better communication is needed among the large number of software applications already in use.

Nursing Informatics

Nursing informatics is a specialty that integrates nursing, its information, and information management with information processing and communication technology to support the health of people worldwide.[27] An informatics nurse has a diverse role. Nurse informatacists design and build computer systems that support nurses and other health care providers in all roles and settings to improve decision making and enhance the quality of patient care. Other responsibilities of a nurse informatacist may include training health care providers and implementing, evaluating, and maintaining computer systems.

Computer Languages

When using applications such as an EHR, it is important to use a comprehensive, standardized medical vocabulary. One such standardized vocabulary is the Systematized Nomenclature of Medicine—Clinical Terms (SNOMED CT). In 2004 the federal government's licensure of SNOMED CT made the vocabulary available, free of charge, to all health care providers through the National Library of Medicine.[28] Uses for SNOMED CT include EHRs, intensive care monitoring, clinical decision support, medical research studies, clinical trials, CPOE, disease surveillance, and consumer health information services.

The use of SNOMED CT is of significant value to nursing in that the vocabulary includes the NANDA-I, NIC, and NOC (NNN) terminologies of nursing. With the use of SNOMED CT, nursing diagnoses, interventions, and outcomes can be recorded using the NNN terminologies. Following the links among diagnosis, interventions, and outcomes will greatly advance evidence-based practice (EBP). For example, when you choose the NANDA-I diagnosis of *fatigue* on a computer, the code 00093 is added to a database. Then you might select the NOC outcome of *endurance,* and the code 0001 would also be added to the database. You could select the NIC interventions of *energy management (0180)* and *exercise promotion (0200),* and these codes would also be incorporated. The coded data can be separated from the patient's name, thus providing for patient anonymity. Links that result from these data can be analyzed and serve not only to improve practice, but also to demonstrate the effectiveness of nursing interventions and formulate nursing research questions. This provides a continuing evaluation of nursing's efficacy.

Today many informatics nurses are concerned that, unless nursing care data are stored electronically, CISs or EHRs will contain no data about the decisions that nurses make. As a result, nursing data will not be used in health care planning and policies. Information about identified nursing problems, independent nursing interventions, and improved patient outcomes will not be apparent, and nursing's role in and contribution to health care will be invisible.[29]

Documenting the nursing process is a critical part of the patient's record. This is important because it provides evidence that nursing practice standards related to the nursing process have been maintained during the care of the patient.

All nurses must work to ensure that nursing data are stored electronically and become part of the EHR. Many different electronic documentation methods and formats are used. However, few agencies have implemented the use of standardized nursing terminologies for documenting nursing care. Using nursing terminologies for documenting nursing practice provides an efficient, consistent way to communicate nursing knowledge. It allows nurses to track, improve, and report on the outcomes of nursing care.[15] If nursing data are to be part of the data analyzed from EHRs, nurses need to decide what data should be included in the EHR and what terminology should be used to record the data so that the meaning is clear, consistent, and valuable.

Telehealth

Increasingly, technology is allowing nurses and other health care providers to deliver patient care services in a wider range of settings. Telehealth is the use of videoconferencing or other communication technologies to provide care when patients and health care providers are geographically separated. Telehealth care has many applications, not only in the assessment, diagnosis, and treatment of illness, but also in health promotion, follow-up, and coordination of care. Nurses engaged in telehealth nursing practice continue to assess, plan, intervene, and

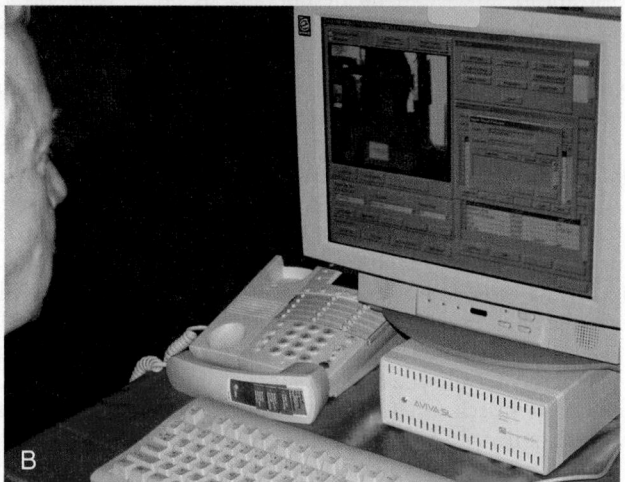

FIG. 1-6 Telemonitoring. **A,** Remote blood pressure monitoring. **B,** Videoconference with health care provider.

evaluate the outcomes of nursing care. However, they do so using technologies such as the Internet, computers, telephones, digital assessment tools, and telemonitoring equipment[30] (Fig. 1-6).

Home care is seeing significant changes as the result of rapidly expanding remote patient monitoring. A growing number of biomedical devices can collect, monitor, and report patient data in real time. These devices include blood glucose monitors, peak flow meters, scales, stethoscopes, and automated blood pressure cuffs. Video cameras with magnifying capabilities are used to assess wounds and monitor the status of healing. Nurses practicing telehealth can provide patient and caregiver teaching and emotional support through videoconferencing.

EVIDENCE-BASED PRACTICE

Evidence-based practice (EBP) is a problem-solving approach to clinical decision making. It involves the use of the best available evidence (e.g., research findings, data from quality improvement projects, professional organization standards) in combination with clinician expertise and patient preferences and values to achieve desired patient outcomes.[31] The most important reason to use EBP is the delivery of the highest quality of care for the best patient outcomes. Expectations for high-quality, cost-effective care and the increased accessibility of health information have contributed to a need for all health disciplines to provide care based on the best evidence. Regulatory and accrediting agencies, including The Joint Commission (TJC), require documentation of the effective use of evidence in clinical care decisions.

EBP does not mean that you need to conduct a research study. Instead, EBP is a process that involves finding, appraising, and applying research conducted by others in an effort to answer a specific clinical question. The use of technology supports EBP by providing you with access to data. You can easily search a number of online resources and collect large amounts of clinical information or evidence to identify the best patient care practices.

Steps of EBP Process

The EBP process has seven critical steps (Table 1-4).

Step 0 of EBP. Creating a spirit of inquiry, or an ongoing curiosity about what are the best nursing practices, is important to support the other stages of EBP. Positive patient outcomes depend on you taking an active role in using the best available evidence when delivering care. When you possess a spirit of inquiry, you routinely ask questions about your patient's care and recognize when more information is needed. When your practice is based on valid evidence, you are solving problems and supporting best patient outcomes.[32]

Step 1 of EBP. Step 1 of the EBP process is asking a clinical question in the PICOT format. Formulating the clinical question is the most important step in the EBP process.[33] A well-formulated clinical question that is searchable and answerable creates the context for integrating best available evidence, clinical judgment, and patient preferences. In addition, the question guides the search for the most current literature and the evidence required.

An example of a clinical question in PICOT format is, "In adult cardiac surgery patients (**P** = patients/population) is morphine (**I** = intervention) or fentanyl (**C** = comparison) more effective in reducing pain (**O** = outcome) on the first postoperative day (**T** = time period)?" A properly stated clinical question may not have all components of PICOT in the statement. Some may only include the first four components, PICO without the T, because the (T) timing for the (I) intervention to support the (O) outcome is not always pertinent. The (C) component of PICOT might include a comparison with a specific intervention, the usual standard of care, or no intervention at all.

Step 2 of EBP. Step 2 of the EBP process is a thorough search for and collection of evidence based on the clinical question.

The content and type of question direct the clinician to the most appropriate databases. The search begins with the strongest external evidence to answer the question. Preappraised evidence such as systematic reviews and evidence-based clinical practice guidelines are time- and effort-saving resources in the EBP process (see Table 1-4).

Systematic reviews of randomized controlled trials (RCTs) are considered the strongest level of evidence to answer questions about interventions (i.e., cause and effect). Systematic reviews, which include the critical analysis and synthesis of methods and findings from multiple studies, are available for only a limited number of clinical topics and may not suit all types of clinical questions. If the clinical question involves how a patient experiences or copes with a health change, searching for a meta-synthesis of qualitative evidence may be the appropriate approach.

Clinical practice guidelines are helpful for translating research findings into specific interventions. However, these published guidelines vary in comprehensiveness and credibility. Guidelines are produced by a variety of authoring groups such as professional health care societies, patient advocacy organizations, and government agencies.

When insufficient research exists to guide practice, recommendations from expert committees, authority figures, and opinion authorities may be the best evidence available. When care decisions must depend on this type of evidence, ongoing and rigorous outcome data should be collected to provide stronger evidence.

Step 3 of EBP. Step 3 of the EBP process is critically appraising and synthesizing evidence found in the search. The purpose of critical appraisal is to determine the value of the research in actual practice. A successful critical appraisal process focuses on three essential questions: (1) What are the results? (2) Are the results reliable and valid? and (3) Will the results help me in caring for my patients? You must determine the strength of the evidence and synthesize the findings related to the clinical question to conclude what is the best practice.

Step 4 of EBP. Step 4 of the EBP process may differ depending on the strength and breadth of the evidence to answer the question. Recommendations from sufficient, strong evidence such as the meta-analysis of well-designed RCTs can be implemented into practice interventions in combination with clinicians' expertise and patient preferences. For example, although evidence supports the use of morphine as an effective analgesic, it may not be appropriate to use in a patient with renal failure. In another example, although their concerns are not supported by evidence, patients may be worried about perceived addictive effects of morphine and prefer an alternative to opioids for their pain management. These types of decisions must be made by combining knowledge of the best available evidence, clinician judgment, and application if the recommendations to the individual patient's circumstances and preferences.

Many areas in practice do not have an established evidence base or have inconsistent evidence. When evidence is insufficient to guide practice, the fourth step would be to generate data to answer the question. One way for data to be gathered is through the conduct of rigorous research. Health care providers can collaborate with researchers to conduct research and generate knowledge that identifies the best patient care practices.

Step 5 of EBP. Step 5 of the EBP process is evaluation of identified outcomes in the clinical setting. Outcomes to be measured must match the clinical project objective that has been

---

TABLE 1-4	STEPS OF EVIDENCE-BASED PRACTICE (EBP) PROCESS

0. Cultivate a spirit of inquiry.
1. Ask the burning clinical question using the **PICO** or **PICOT** format:
   Patients/population
   Intervention
   Comparison or comparison group
   Outcome(s)
   Time period (as applicable)
2. Collect the most relevant best evidence.
3. Critically appraise and synthesize the evidence.
4. Integrate all evidence with clinical expertise and patient preferences and values in making a practice decision or change.
5. Evaluate the practice decision or change.
6. Share the outcomes of the decision or change.

implemented. For example, evaluating only the cost of each medication for pain control does not provide data about clinical effectiveness. Outcomes must reflect all aspects of the implementation and capture the interdisciplinary contributions obtained by the EBP process. For example, an EBP initiative related to pain control might involve patients and caregivers, nurses, physicians, pharmacists, physical and respiratory therapists, and other team members. Some outcomes expectations may be shared, whereas other goals may be different for each team member.

Step 6 of EBP. The last step in EBP is to share the outcomes of the EBP change. If you do not share the outcomes of EBP, then other health care providers and patients cannot benefit from what you learned from your experience. Information is shared locally using unit- or hospital-based newsletters and posters and regionally and nationally through journal publications and presentations at conferences.

Implementing EBP

To implement EBP, you must develop the skills to continually seek and then incorporate into practice the scientific evidence that supports best patient outcomes. The incorporation of evidence, balanced with clinical expertise, should take into account the patient's unique circumstances and preferences. EBP closes the gap between research and practice, providing more reliable and predictable care than that based on tradition, opinion, and trial and error. It provides you with an effective process to manage the wealth of information and newly introduced technologies, while balancing concerns about health care costs and an increasing emphasis on quality and patient outcomes.

Throughout this book, two different types of EBP boxes are used to show how EBP is used in nursing practice. The Translating Research into Practice boxes provide initial answers to specific clinical questions. These boxes contain the clinical question, critical appraisal of the supportive evidence, implications for nursing practice, and the source of the evidence. Applying the Evidence boxes provide an opportunity for you to practice your critical thinking skills in applying EBP to patient scenarios.

To assist you in identifying the use of evidence incorporated throughout this book, an asterisk (*) is used in the reference list at the end of each chapter to indicate evidence-based information for clinical practice.

SAFETY AND QUALITY IMPROVEMENT

As the complexity of the environments in which health care is delivered increases, patient safety and communication among health care professionals are affected. In 1999 the IOM issued a report that indicated that at least 44,000 people, and perhaps as many as 98,000 people, die in hospitals each year as a result of preventable medical errors. The report described medical errors as an epidemic and concluded that it was not acceptable for patients to be harmed by a health care system that is supposed to offer healing and comfort.[34]

Since the IOM report, a series of organizations and commissions have provided safety goals for health care organizations and identified a number of safety competencies for health professionals. By implementing various procedures and systems to improve communication and health care delivery to meet safety goals, health care systems are creating a culture of safety that minimizes the risk of harm to the patient. Because you

FIG. 1-7 Quality improvement system.

have the greatest amount of interaction with patients, you are a vital part of promoting this culture of safety by providing care in a manner that reduces errors and actively promotes patient safety.

Patient-centered care is interrelated with both quality and safety—the higher the culture of safety, the better the quality of care. Health care systems focused on quality outcomes use practice standards and protocols based on best evidence while considering the patient's unique preferences and needs at the moment. Your role is to coordinate and integrate the complex aspects of patient care, including the care delivered by others, and identify issues that are associated with poor quality and unsafe care.

As part of professional nursing practice, you are responsible for collecting data, using data to monitor patient outcomes, and implementing interventions to improve quality of care. An example of a quality improvement system is shown in Fig. 1-7. You need to be able to assess current practices and compare them with relevant better practices elsewhere as a means of identifying areas for improving care and formulating clinical questions for EBP.

National Patient Safety Goals

The Joint Commission (TJC), the accrediting agency for health care organizations, issues National Patient Safety Goals (NPSGs) for each of its accreditation programs.[35] The NPSGs promote specific improvements in patient safety by providing health care organizations with evidence-based solutions to persistent safety problems. The 2013 goals are listed in Table 1-5. Safety alerts that highlight safety information related to patient care and the NPSGs are integrated throughout the textbook.

TEAMWORK AND COLLABORATION

Interdisciplinary Team Members

To deliver high-quality care, you need to establish effective working relationships with members of the health care team. A

TABLE 1-5	NATIONAL PATIENT SAFETY GOALS*
Safety Goal	**Examples**
1. Improve the accuracy of patient identification.	• Use at least two ways to identify patients (e.g., have them state full name and date of birth).
2. Improve the effectiveness of communication among caregivers.	• Use SBAR (see Table 1-7) for communication among health care professionals. • Verify telephone or verbal orders by "write down and read back" procedure. • Quickly get important test results to the right staff person.
3. Improve the safety of using medications.	• Label all medicines that are not already labeled. Discard any found unlabeled. • Take extra care with patients who take anticoagulant drugs.
4. Reduce the risk of health care–associated infections.	• Use soap, water, and hand sanitizer before and after every patient contact. • Use evidence-based practices to prevent infections caused by multidrug-resistant organisms.
5. Accurately and completely reconcile medications across the continuum of care.	• Find out what medications each patient is taking. Make certain that it is safe for the patient to take any new medicines with his or her current medicines. • Give a list of the patient's medicines to his or her next caregiver. Give the list to the patient's regular physician before the patient goes home. • Give a list of the patient's medicines to the patient and caregiver before they go home. Explain the list.
6. Reduce the risk of patient harm resulting from falls.	• Evaluate patients for fall risk. • Take action to reduce risk of injury.
7. Prevent health care–related pressure ulcers (decubitus ulcers).	• Assess patients at risk for pressure ulcers on admission and on a regular basis throughout their care.
8. The organization identifies safety risks inherent in its patient population.	• Assess patients at risk for suicide. • Assess any risks for patients who are getting home oxygen therapy, such as fires.

Universal Protocol (UP)

• Preprocedure verification	• Conduct a time-out before the start of any invasive or surgical procedure,
• Mark procedure site	• Confirm correct patient, procedure, and site.
• Performance of time-out	

health care team may consist of physicians, nurses, pharmacists, occupational and physical therapists, social workers, and others (Table 1-6). As part of your interdisciplinary nursing practice, you will collaborate in many ways by exchanging knowledge, sharing responsibility for problem solving, and making patient care decisions. You may be responsible for coordinating care among the team members and initiating appropriate referrals when you anticipate that expertise in specialized areas is needed to help the patient. To do so, you need to be aware of the knowledge and skills of other team members and be able to communicate effectively among them.

TABLE 1-6	INTERDISCIPLINARY TEAM MEMBERS
Team Member	**Description of Services Provided**
Dietitian	Provides general nutrition services, including dietary consultation regarding health promotion or specialized diets
Home health aide	Assists patients with their personal care needs, such as bathing, dressing, and hair washing, or with some homemaking activities (e.g., meal preparation or light housekeeping)
Occupational therapist (OT)	May assist patient with fine motor coordination, performance of activities of daily living, cognitive-perceptual skills, sensory testing, and the construction or use of assistive or adaptive equipment
Pastoral care	Offers spiritual support and guidance to patients and caregivers
Pharmacist	Prepares medications and infusion products
Physical therapist (PT)	Works with patients on improving strength and endurance, gait training, transfer training, and developing a patient education program
Physician (medical doctor [MD])	Practices medicine and treats illness and injury by prescribing medication, performing diagnostic tests and evaluations, performing surgery, and providing other medical services and advice
Respiratory therapist	May assist with oxygen therapy in the home, provide specialized respiratory treatments, and instruct patient or caregiver regarding the proper use of respiratory equipment
Social worker	Assists patients with developing coping skills, meeting caregiver concerns, securing adequate financial resources or housing assistance, or making referrals to social service or volunteer agencies
Speech therapist	Focuses on treatment of speech defects and disorders, especially through the use of physical exercises to strengthen muscles used in speech, speech drills, and audiovisual aids that develop new speech habits

Coordinating Care Among Health Care Team Members

Communication. Communication is a key component of facilitating teamwork and care across the care continuum, which is essential for fostering a culture of safety. There is evidence that the majority of patient safety issues result from breakdown in communication.[35] Enhancing communication among the health care team requires a systematic approach. One model used for reporting and hand-off communications is the **SBAR (Situation-Background-Assessment-Recommendation)** technique (Table 1-7). This technique provides a mechanism for framing critical communication about a patient's condition between members of the health care team.[36] Other ways to enhance communication include "time-outs" before surgical procedures or during a busy day on a nursing unit to identify risks and develop a plan for delivering care.

Case Management. Case management is a collaborative process that involves assessing, planning, facilitating, and advocating for health services to meet an individual's and/or caregiver's needs through communication and use of available resources to promote cost-effective quality outcomes. Although health care agencies define case management in various ways, the concept of case management involves managing the patient's

TABLE 1-7	GUIDELINES FOR COMMUNICATING USING SBAR

Purpose: SBAR is a model for effective transfer of information by providing a standardized structure for concise factual communications from nurse-to-nurse, nurse-to-physician, or nurse-to–other health professionals.

Steps to Use: Before speaking with a physician or other health care professional about a patient problem, assess the patient yourself, read the most recent physician progress and nursing notes, and have the patient chart available.

S Situation	What is the situation you want to discuss? What is happening at the present time? • Identify self, unit. **State:** I am calling about: *patient, room number.* • Briefly state the problem: what it is, when it happened or started, and how severe it is. **State:** I have just assessed the patient and I am concerned about: *identify why you are concerned.*
B Background	What is the background or circumstances leading up to the situation? **State** pertinent background information related to the situation that may include • Admitting diagnosis and date of admission • List of current medications, allergies, IV fluids • Most recent vital signs • Date and time of any laboratory testing and results of previous tests for comparison • Synopsis of treatment to date • Code status
A Assessment	What do you think the problem is? What is your assessment of the situation? **State** what you think the problem is: • Changes from prior assessments • Patient condition unstable or worsening
R Recommendation/ Request	What should we do to correct the problem? What is your recommendation or request? **State** your request. • Specific treatments • Tests needed • Patient needs to be seen now

Source: Kaiser Permanente of Colorado: SBAR technique for communication: a situational briefing model, Institute for Health Care Improvement. Retrieved from *www.ihi.org/knowledge/Pages/Tools/SBARTechniqueforCommunicationASituational BriefingModel.aspx.*

care across multiple care settings and levels of care.[37] The goals of case management are to provide quality care along a continuum, decrease fragmentation of care across many settings, enhance the patient's quality of life, and contain costs.

A professional nurse often serves as the case manager. The nurse assesses the needs of an individual or caregiver, coordinates services for them, makes referrals as appropriate, and evaluates progress to ensure that short- and long-term goals are met. For example, a patient with severe coronary artery disease may be assigned a nurse as a case manager in an outpatient clinic. When the patient is hospitalized for coronary artery bypass graft surgery, the same case manager coordinates care so that all health care providers understand the patient's unique needs. When the patient is discharged, the case manager determines whether home health care or other services are necessary for the patient.

Clinical Pathways. Care related to common health problems experienced by many patients is delineated and documented using clinical (critical) pathways. A **clinical (critical) pathway** directs the entire health care team in the daily care goals for select health care problems. It includes an interdisciplinary care plan, and goals and interventions specific for each day of hospitalization. The case types selected for clinical pathways are usually those that occur in high volume and are highly predictable, such as myocardial infarction and surgical procedures, including joint replacements, cholecystectomies, and appendectomies.

The clinical pathway describes the patient care required at specific times. An interdisciplinary approach moves the patient toward desired outcomes within an estimated length of stay. The exact content and format of clinical pathways vary among institutions. If clinical pathways are used by an institution, they are usually evidence based and specifically developed by that institution. Nurse- and physician-initiated interventions designed to achieve the patient outcomes are identified throughout the pathway. The interdisciplinary approach can be seen in the referral to and consultation with other health professionals. If a nursing-specific care plan is included in the clinical pathway, it is usually documented with the use of nursing diagnoses and evaluation of patient outcomes. Many pathways are computerized, making them a permanent part of the patient's record.

Delegation and Assignment. As a registered nurse (RN), you will delegate nursing care and supervise others who are qualified to deliver care. **Delegation** is transferring the authority or responsibility to perform a selected nursing task in a selected situation to a competent individual.[38] The delegation and assignment of nursing activities from the professional nurse (the RN) to nonprofessional and/or unlicensed health care personnel is a process that, when used appropriately, can result in safe, effective, and efficient nursing care. Delegating can allow you more time to focus on complex patient care needs.

Delegation typically involves tasks and procedures that **unlicensed assistive personnel (UAP)** and licensed practical/vocational nurses (LPN/LVNs) perform. Nursing interventions that require independent nursing knowledge, skill, or judgment such as assessment, patient teaching, and evaluation of care are your responsibility and cannot be delegated. UAP are unlicensed individuals who assist the RN, the professional nurse. UAP may include nursing aides, orderlies, nursing assistants, attendants, or technicians. Professional nurses are responsible for supervising the education, training, and use of UAP in providing direct patient care. As a nurse, you use professional judgment to determine appropriate activities to delegate based on the patient's needs, the UAP's education and training, and extent of supervision required.[38] In addition, some state boards of nursing identify specific activities that may be delegated to UAP such as obtaining routine vital signs on stable patients, feeding and assisting patients at mealtimes, ambulating stable patients, and helping patients with bathing and hygiene. eFig. 1-2 (available on the website for this chapter) shows a decision tree for delegation to UAP.

Delegation may also involve the LPN/LVN, whose scope and standards of practice are defined by the state nursing practice act and regulated by state agencies. However, you may also delegate specific tasks to the LPN/LVN. You must know the legal scope of practical/vocational nursing practice and delegate and assign nursing functions appropriately. In most states, LPN/LVNs may administer medications, perform sterile

TABLE 1-8	**FIVE RIGHTS OF NURSING DELEGATION**

1. The *right* task
2. Under the *right* circumstances
3. To the *right* person
4. With the *right* direction and communication
5. Under the *right* supervision and evaluation

Source: Joint Statement on Delegation: American Nurses Association (ANA) and the National Council of State Boards of Nursing (NCSBN), 2007. Retrieved from *https://www.ncsbn.org/Joint_statement.pdf*.

procedures, and provide a wide variety of interventions planned by the RN.

Assignment is different from delegation in that assignment is the distribution of work that each staff member is responsible for during a given work period. Therefore the term *assign* is used when you direct a person to do something that he or she is authorized to do. Assignments occur when an RN directs other RNs, LPN/LVNs, or UAP to perform care that is within their scope of practice. Whether you delegate or are working with staff to which you assign tasks, you are responsible for the patient's total care during your work period. You are responsible for the supervision of the UAP or LPN/LVN and remain accountable for ensuring that the delegated tasks are completed in a competent manner. This supervision includes guidance and direction, oversight, evaluation, and follow-up by the RN.[38]

Delegation is a skill that is learned and must be practiced for you to be proficient in managing patient care. You need to use critical thinking and professional judgment to ensure that the Five Rights of Nursing Delegation are implemented (Table 1-8). This book presents delegation decisions in boxes in appropriate chapters and provides delegation questions in case studies at the end of the management chapters.

DELEGATION DECISIONS
Delegation Decisions Boxes Throughout Book

Title	Chapter	Page
Assessment and Data Collection	3	38
Blood Transfusions	31	676
Cardiac Catheterization and Percutaneous Coronary Intervention (PCI)	34	758
Caring for the Incontinent Patient	46	1091
Caring for the Patient Receiving Bladder Irrigation	55	1320
Caring for the Patient Requiring Mechanical Ventilation	66	1625
Caring for the Patient With an Acute Stroke	58	1405
Caring for the Patient With Alzheimer's Disease	60	1455
Caring for the Patient With a Cast or Traction	63	1514
Caring for the Patient With Chronic Venous Insufficiency	38	858
Caring for the Patient With Diabetes Mellitus	49	1185
Caring for the Patient With Hypertension	33	724
Caring for the Patient With Neutropenia	31	661
Caring for the Patient With a Seizure Disorder	59	1426
Caring for the Patient With Venous Thromboembolism (VTE)	38	855
Corrective Lenses and Hearing Aids	22	411
Intravenous Therapy	17	309
Nasogastric and Gastric Tubes and Enteral Feedings	40	900
Ostomy Care	43	994
Oxygen Administration	29	592
Pain	9	134
Postoperative Patient	20	354
Skin Care	24	446
Suctioning and Tracheostomy Care	27	518
Urinary Catheters	46	1093
Wound Care	12	183

BRIDGE TO NCLEX EXAMINATION

The number of the question corresponds to the same-numbered outcome at the beginning of the chapter.

1. An example of a nursing activity that reflects the American Nurses Association's definition of nursing is
   a. diagnosing a patient with a feeding tube as being at risk for aspiration.
   b. establishing protocols for treating patients in the emergency department.
   c. providing antianxiety drugs for a patient who has disturbed sleep patterns.
   d. identifying and treating dysrhythmias that occur in a patient in the coronary care unit.

2. A nurse working on the medical-surgical unit at an urban hospital would like to become certified in a medical-surgical specialty. The nurse knows that this process would most likely require
   a. a bachelor's degree in nursing.
   b. formal education in advanced nursing practice.
   c. experience for a specific period in medical-surgical nursing.
   d. membership in a medical-surgical nursing specialty organization.

3. A nurse is providing care to a patient after right hip surgery. Within a pay-for-performance system, a critical role of the nurse is to
   a. ensure that care is provided using a minimal amount of supplies.
   b. discharge the patient at completion of the number of approved days of care.
   c. implement measures to decrease the risk of the patient acquiring an infection.
   d. assess the patient's ability to pay for health care services at the time of admission.

4. The nurse is assigned to care for a newly admitted patient. Number in order the steps for using the nursing process to prioritize care. (Number 1 is the first step, and number 5 is the last step.)
   ___ Evaluate whether the plan was effective.
   ___ Identify any health problems.
   ___ Collect patient information.
   ___ Carry out the plan.
   ___ Determine a plan of action.

5. The linkages among NANDA-I nursing diagnoses, NOC patient outcomes, and NIC nursing interventions can be used to
   a. evaluate patient outcomes.
   b. provide guides for planning care.
   c. predict the results of nursing care.
   d. shorten written care plans for individual patients.
6. Advantages of the use of informatics in health care delivery are (*select all that apply*)
   a. reduced need for home care nurses in rural areas.
   b. increased patient anonymity and confidentiality.
   c. the ability to achieve and maintain high standards of care.
   d. improved communication of the patient's health status to the health care team.
   e. access to standardized plans of care that are available for most types of health problems.
7. When using evidence-based practice, the nurse
   a. must use clinical practice guidelines developed by national health agencies.
   b. should use findings from randomized controlled trials to plan care for all patient problems.
   c. uses clinical decision making and judgment to determine what evidence is appropriate for a specific clinical situation.
   d. statistically analyzes the relationship of nursing interventions to patient outcomes to establish evidence for the most appropriate patient interventions.

8. The nurse's role in addressing the National Patient Safety Goals established by The Joint Commission includes (*select all that apply*)
   a. using side rails and alarm systems as necessary to prevent patient falls.
   b. memorizing and implementing all the rules published by The Joint Commission.
   c. verifying telephone and verbal orders using the "write down and read back" procedure.
   d. encouraging patients to be actively involved in and question their own health care.
   e. obtaining a complete list of the patient's medications and monitoring their use throughout the continuum of care.
9. The nurse is caring for a diabetic patient in the ambulatory surgical unit who has just undergone debridement of an infected toe. Which task is most appropriate for the nurse to delegate to unlicensed assistive personnel (UAP)?
   a. Check the patient's vital signs.
   b. Evaluate the patient's awareness.
   c. Monitor the site of the patient's IV catheter.
   d. Evaluate the patient's tibial and pedal pulses.

1. a, 2, c, 3, c, 4, 5, 2, 1, 4, 3, 5, b, 6, c, d, e, 7, c, 8, a, c, e, 9, a.

🅔volve

For rationales to these answers and even more NCLEX review questions, visit *http://evolve.elsevier.com/Lewis/medsurg.*

REFERENCES

1. American Nurses Association: *Nursing: a social policy statement,* ed 3, Washington, DC, 2010, The Association. (Classic)
2. Nightingale F: *Notes on nursing: what it is and what it is not (facsimile edition),* Philadelphia, 1946, Lippincott. (Classic)
3. Henderson V: *The nature of nursing,* New York, 1966, Macmillan. (Classic)
4. Roy S, Andrews H: *The Roy adaptation model,* ed 2, Stamford, Conn, 1999, Appleton & Lange. (Classic)
5. American Association of Colleges of Nursing: Essentials of baccalaureate education for professional nursing practice. Retrieved from *www.aacn.nche.edu.*
6. Sportsman S: Competency education and validation in the United States: what should nurses know? *Nurs Forum* 45:140, 2010.
7. American Nurses Credentialing Center: Certification. Retrieved from *www.nursecredentialing.org/certification.aspx.*
8. American Association of Colleges of Nursing: The essentials of doctoral education for advanced nursing practice. Retrieved from *www.aacn.nche.edu/DNP/index.htm.*
9. Cromwell J, Trisolini MG, Pope GC, et al: *Pay for performance in health care: methods and approaches,* Research Triangle Park, NC, 2011, RTI Press Publications.
10. US Department of Health and Human Services: Healthy People 2020. Retrieved from *www.healthypeople.gov.*
11. Committee on the Robert Wood Johnson Foundation Initiative on the Future of Nursing at the Institute of Medicine: *The future of nursing: leading change, advancing health,* Washington, DC, 2011, National Academies Press.
12. Jost SG, Bonnell M, Chacko SJ, et al: Integrated primary nursing: a care delivery model for the 21st-century knowledge worker, *NAQ* 34:208, 2010.
13. Alfaro-LeFevre R: *Critical thinking and clinical judgment,* ed 5, St Louis, 2012, Saunders.
14. Benner P, Sutphen M, Leonard D, et al: *Educating nurses: a call for radical transformation,* San Francisco, 2009, Jossey-Bass.
15. Jones D, Lunney M, Keenan G, et al: Standardized nursing languages: essential for the nursing workforce, *Annu Rev Nurs Res* 28:253, 2010.
16. NANDA International: *Nursing diagnoses: definitions and classification 2012-2014,* Kaukauna, Wisc, 2011, The Association.
17. Bulechek GM, Butcher HK, Dochterman JM: *Nursing interventions classification (NIC),* ed 5, St Louis, 2008, Mosby.
18. Moorhead S, Johnson M, Maas M, et al: *Nursing outcomes classification (NOC),* ed 4, St Louis, 2008, Mosby.
19. Carpenito-Moyet L: *Nursing diagnosis: application to clinical practice,* ed 13, Philadelphia, 2009, Lippincott Williams & Wilkins.
20. Kostovich CT, Poradzisz M, Wood K, et al: Learning style preference and student aptitude for concept maps, *J Nurs Educ* 46:225, 2007.
21. McGonigle D, Mastrian K: *Nursing informatics and the foundation of knowledge,* ed 2, Burlington, Mass, 2012, Jones & Bartlett Learning.
22. QSEN: Informatics. Retrieved from *www.qsen.org/ksas_prelicensure.php#informatics.*
23. Zerwekh J, Garneau A: *Nursing today: transitions and trends,* ed 7, St Louis, 2011, Saunders.
24. Thomes J: Avoiding the trap in the HITECH Act's incentive timeframe for implementing the EHR, *J Health Care Finance* 37:91, 2010.
25. Staggers N, Weir C, Phanaslkar S: Patient safety and health information technology: role of the electronic health record. In *Patient safety and quality: an evidence-based handbook for*

nurses, Rockville, Md, 2008, Agency for Healthcare Research and Quality. Retrieved from *www.ahrq.gov/qual/nurseshdbk*.

26. World VistA: About VistA. Retrieved from *http://worldvista.org*.

27. American Nurses Association: *Scope and standards for nursing informatics practice*, Washington, DC, 2008, The Association.

28. International Health Terminology Standards Development Organization: *Introducing SNOMED CT*, Copenhagen, 2010, The Organization.

29. Thede L: Informatics: the electronic health record: will nursing be on board when the ship leaves? *OJIN* 13:3, 2008. Retrieved from *www.nursingworld.org/MainMenuCategories/ ANAMarketplace/ANAPeriodicals/OJIN/Columns/Informatics/ ElectronicHealthRecord.aspx*.

30. Schlachta-Fairchild L, Elfrink V, Deickman A: Patient safety, telenursing, and telehealth. In *Patient safety and quality: an evidence-based handbook for nurses*, Rockville, Md, 2008, Agency for Healthcare Research and Quality. Retrieved from *www.ahrq.gov/qual/nurseshdbk*.

31. Melnyk B, Fineout-Overholt E: *Evidence-based practice in nursing and healthcare: a guide to best practice*, ed 2, Philadelphia, 2010, Lippincott Williams & Wilkins.

32. Malloch K, Porter-O'Grady T: *Introduction to evidence-based practice in nursing and health care*, Sudbury, Mass, 2010, Jones & Bartlett.

33. Stillwell S, Fineout-Overholt E, Melnyk B, et al: Asking the clinical question: a key step in evidence-based practice, *Am J Nurs* 110:58, 2010.

34. Institute of Medicine: *To err is human: building a safer health system*, Washington, DC, 2000, National Academy Press. (Classic)

35. The Joint Commission: National patient safety goals. Retrieved from *www.jointcommission.org/standards_information/npsgs.aspx*.

36. Kaiser Permanente of Colorado: SBAR technique for communication: a situational briefing model. Retrieved from *www.ihi.org/knowledge/Pages/Tools/SBARTechniquefor CommunicationASituationalBriefingModel.aspx*.

37. Case Management Society of America: Definition of case management. Retrieved from *www.cmsa.org*.

38. American Nurses Association: Joint statement on delegation: American Nurses Association (ANA) and the National Council of State Boards of Nursing (NCSBN). Retrieved from *www.ncsbn.org/Joint_statement.pdf*.

RESOURCES

American Nurses Association
www.nursingworld.org
American Nursing Informatics Association
www.ania.org
Canadian Nurses Association
www.cna-nurses.ca
Center for Nursing Classification and Clinical Effectiveness
www.nursing.uiowa.edu/center-for-nursing-classification-and-clinical-effectiveness
Healthy People
www.healthypeople.gov
NANDA International
www.nanda.org
National Association of Hispanic Nurses
www.thehispanicnurses.org
National Black Nurses Association, Inc.
www.nbna.org
National Student Nurses' Association
www.nsna.org
QSEN (Quality and Safety Education for Nurses)
www.qsen.org

*Injustice anywhere is a threat
to justice everywhere.*
Dr. Martin Luther King, Jr.

Health Disparities and Culturally Competent Care

Janet Lenart

evolve WEBSITE

http://evolve.elsevier.com/Lewis/medsurg

- NCLEX Review Questions
- Key Points
- Pre-Test
- Answer Guidelines for Case Study on p. 33

- Rationales for Bridge to NCLEX Examination Questions
- Concept Map Creator
- Glossary
- Content Updates

eTables
- eTable 2-1: Ethnic Differences in Response to Drugs
- eTable 2-2: Cultural Assessment Guide

LEARNING OUTCOMES

1. Identify the key determinants of health and equity.
2. Describe the primary factors that contribute to health disparities and health equity.
3. Define the terms *culture, values, acculturation, ethnicity, race, stereotyping, ethnocentrism, cultural imposition, transcultural nursing, cultural competency, folk healer,* and *culture-bound syndrome.*
4. Explain how culture and ethnicity may affect a person's physical and psychologic health.
5. Describe strategies for successfully communicating with a person who speaks a language that you do not understand.
6. Apply strategies for incorporating cultural information in the nursing process when providing care for patients from different cultural and ethnic groups.
7. Describe the role of nursing in reducing health disparities.
8. Examine ways that your own cultural background may influence nursing care when working with patients from different cultural and ethnic groups.

KEY TERMS

acculturation, p. 24
cultural competence, p. 24
culture, p. 23
culture-bound syndromes, p. 30
determinants of health, p. 19
ethnicity, p. 21

ethnocentrism, p. 24
folk healers, p. 26
health disparities, p. 20
health equity, p. 20
health status, p. 19
place, p. 21

race, p. 21
sexuality, p. 22
stereotyping, p. 24
transcultural nursing, p. 24

This chapter addresses health disparities and cultural issues. Nursing has a key role in recognizing and reducing health disparities and providing culturally competent care.

DETERMINANTS OF HEALTH

Why are there differences in the health status of people in America? How do these differences occur? The determinants of health are factors that (1) influence the health of individuals and groups (Fig. 2-1) and (2) help explain why some people experience poorer health than others.[1] Where people are born,

grow up, live, work, and age helps determine their health status, behaviors, and care.

Health status describes the health of a person or a community. Many measures make up the concept of health status. For individuals, this means the sum of their current health problems plus their coping resources (e.g., family, financial resources). For a community, health status is the combination of health measures for all individuals living in the community. Community health measures include birth and death rates, life expectancy, access to care, and morbidity and mortality rates related to disease and injury.

Reviewed by Michelle M. Byrne, RN, PhD, CNE, CNOR, Professor of Nursing, North Georgia College & State University, Dahlonega, Georgia; Doreen Mingo, RN, MSN, Assistant Professor, Coordinator, Office of Diversity Services, Nursing Workforce Diversity Grant Project Director, Allen College, Waterloo, Illinois; and Kathleen M. Barta, RN, EdD, Associate Professor, University of Arkansas, Eleanor Mann School of Nursing, Fayetteville, Arkansas.

Factors in a person's social and physical environment, including personal relationships, workplace, housing, transportation, and neighborhood violence, all contribute to health status.[1] For example, the risk of youth homicide is much higher in neighborhoods with gang activity and high crime rates. The physical environment in which one lives, works, and plays may expose a person to such risks as environmental hazards (workplace injuries), toxic agents (chemical spills, industrial pollution), unsafe traffic patterns (lack of sidewalks), or absence of fresh and healthy food choices.

An individual's behavior is influenced by his or her environment, education, and economic status. Behaviors such as tobacco and illicit drug use are strongly linked to a number of health conditions (e.g., lung cancer, liver disease). An individual's biologic makeup such as genetics and family history of disease (e.g., heart disease) can increase the risk for specific diseases.

The amount and quality of health care available also contribute to an individual's health. For example, in some states, health care organizations have reduced the number of Medicaid patients they will cover. Although the use of emergency departments (EDs) for health care is increasing, they are not usually set up to provide primary or long-term follow-up care. In addition, the number of EDs, particularly in rural areas, is decreasing.[2] These determinants of health can either improve a person's health status or put an individual at risk for disease, injury, and mental illness.

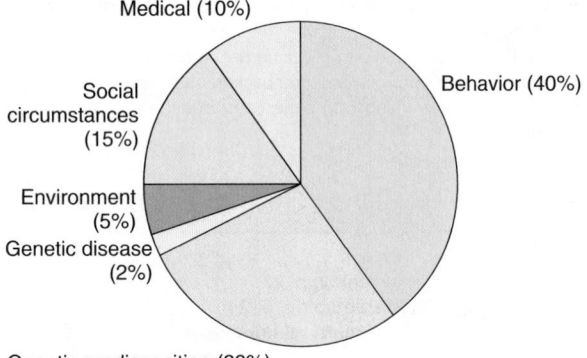

FIG. 2-1 Determinants of health.

Medical (10%)
Social circumstances (15%)
Environment (5%)
Genetic disease (2%)
Behavior (40%)
Genetic predisposition (28%)

HEALTHY PEOPLE

Access to Health Services

- Increase the proportion of people
  - With health insurance.
  - With a usual primary care provider.
  - Who receive appropriate evidence-based clinical preventive services.
- Increase the proportion of insured people with coverage for clinical preventive services.
- Ensure that all people have access to rapidly responding, prehospital emergency medical services.
- Reduce the proportion of individuals who are unable to obtain or delay in obtaining necessary medical care, dental care, or prescription medicines.
- Decrease the time people
  - Spend waiting in physicians' offices and emergency departments.
  - Wait between identifying a need for specific tests and treatments and actually receiving those services.

The vision of the government's *Healthy People 2020* is to create a society in which all people live long, healthy lives (see Table 1-1). This report (discussed in Chapter 1 on p. 5) includes measures that can be used to reflect the health status of the U.S. population.[3]

HEALTH DISPARITIES AND HEALTH EQUITY

Health disparities are differences in the incidence, prevalence, mortality rate, and burden of diseases that exist among specific population groups in the United States because of social, economic, or environmental disadvantages. Health disparities can affect population groups based on gender, age, ethnicity, socioeconomic status, geography, sexual orientation, disability, or special health care needs.[4,5] **Health equity** is achieved when every person has the opportunity to attain his or her health potential and no one is disadvantaged.

Factors and Conditions Leading to Health Disparities

Many factors and conditions can lead to the development of health disparities (Table 2-1). Awareness of these factors will assist you in providing optimal care for your patients.

ETHICAL/LEGAL DILEMMAS
Health Disparities

Situation

E.M., a 47-year-old Mexican American woman with type 2 diabetes mellitus, comes to the clinic to have her blood glucose measured. It has been 12 months since her last visit. At that time the nurse requested that she bring along her glucometer and strips to demonstrate how she checks her blood glucose because her glucose values were high at her previous visits.

When you check E.M.'s equipment and glucose strips, it is clear that the strips are for a different machine and they expired more than 2 years ago. When you inquire about the situation, E.M. explains that she cannot afford to come to the clinic or to buy new equipment and supplies to check her blood glucose level. During the day E.M. cares for her three grandchildren so her daughter can work. E.M. spends most of her income on food for her family, so little money is left over for her own health care.

Ethical/Legal Points for Consideration

- Ethnic minorities and other vulnerable or disadvantaged groups experience certain chronic illnesses at higher rates. Limited access to high-quality, accessible, and affordable health care services is clearly associated with an increased incidence of illness and complications, as well as a reduced life span.
- People with certain health problems such as diabetes may have difficulty obtaining health care insurance. These issues must be considered in the broader context of social justice.
- In many states the legal definition of the role of the professional nurse includes patient advocacy. Advocacy includes the obligation to provide adequate follow-up care for all patients, especially those who are experiencing health care disparities.
- When disparities are observed in an individual patient and family, as a nurse you must consider the possibilities of discrimination and abuse. Professional nurses are legally and ethically responsible for patient advocacy. When failure to fulfill this obligation results in harm to the patient, the nurse may incur legal liability.

Discussion Questions

1. How would you work with E.M. to help her obtain the necessary resources and knowledge to care for her diabetes?
2. What can you do to begin working on the problems of health disparities in your community?

TABLE 2-1	FACTORS AND CONDITIONS LEADING TO HEALTH DISPARITIES

- Ethnicity and race
- Place
- Income status
- Education
- Occupation or unemployment
- Health literacy
- Gender
- Age
- Sexual orientation
- Disability status
- Health care provider attitudes
- Lack of health care services access
- Language barrier

CULTURAL & ETHNIC HEALTH DISPARITIES

Cultural & Ethnic Health Disparities Boxes Throughout Book

Title	Chapter	Page
Arthritis and Connective Tissue Disorders	65	1569
Brain Tumors	57	1375
Breast Cancer	52	1253
Cancer	16	282
Cancers of the Female Reproductive System	54	1292
Cancers of the Male Reproductive System	55	1315
Chronic Kidney Disease	47	1108
Colorectal Cancer	43	986
Coronary Artery Disease	34	732
Diabetes Mellitus	49	1170
Heart Failure	35	767
Hematologic Problems	31	633
Hypertension	33	710
Immunizations in Hispanics	27	504
Inflammatory Bowel Disease	43	976
Integumentary Problems	24	429
Liver, Pancreas, and Gallbladder Disorders	44	1017
Lung Cancer	28	536
Obesity	41	908
Obstructive Pulmonary Diseases	29	561
Oral, Pharyngeal, and Esophageal Problems	42	929
Osteoporosis	64	1554
Sexually Transmitted Infections	53	1262
Stroke	58	1390
Tuberculosis	28	528
Urologic Disorders	46	1065
Visual and Auditory Problems	22	388

Ethnicity and Race. The terms ethnicity and race are subjective and based on self-report. These terms are used interchangeably in conversation and cannot be defined by genetic markers. Social context and lived experiences influence people's decision about the ethnic and race category to which they belong. For example, ethnic and race categories may differ on a person's birth and death certificates.

People are asked to identify their own ethnicity and race for the purpose of health data collection (e.g., for birth and death certificates). Collection of health data based on self-reported ethnic and race categories is important for research, to inform policy, and to understand and eliminate disparities. For example, federal agencies are required to list a minimum of two ethnicities for people who self-identify as either *Hispanic or Latino* and *Not Hispanic or Latino*. A Hispanic or Latino is typically a person of Cuban, Mexican, Puerto Rican, South or Central American, or other Spanish descent, regardless of race.

In addition, federal agencies are required to list a minimum of five race categories: white, black or African American, American Indian or Alaska Native, Asian, and Native Hawaiian or other Pacific Islander.[6] People are asked to identify their race using one or more categories. In this book the terms *ethnicity* and *race* are used interchangeably or together.

Despite dramatic improvements in treatments to prolong life and improve quality of life for most individuals, racial and ethnic minorities have benefited far less from these advances. Disparities are generally determined by comparing population groups. Currently in the United States, based on the latest census, racial and ethnic minority groups include Hispanics/Latinos 16.3%, African Americans 12.6%, Asian Americans 4.8%, Native Hawaiians and other Pacific Islanders 0.2%, Native Americans and Native Alaskans 0.9%, and two or more races 2.9% of the U.S. population.[7] The percentages for most of these groups are expected to increase in the coming decades.

Obesity and chronic illness rates for diabetes, hypertension, chronic obstructive pulmonary diseases, cancer, and stroke are higher among minority people. Racial, ethnic, and cultural differences exist in health services, treatments provided, and access to health care providers. For example, African American men are less likely to be offered intervention procedures for cardiovascular disease and stroke.[8,9] African American and Hispanic women are less likely to have mammography for breast cancer screening.[6] Differences in access to screening and treatment exist even when minority groups are insured at the same level as whites. When patient groups are given the same care, the treatment outcomes are similar across racial and ethnic groups.[8,9]

Disease risk and outcomes are also influenced by race and ethnicity. For example, compared with U.S. white and African American populations, Native Americans have a higher incidence of stroke and are more likely to die as a consequence.[9]

Breast and cervical cancer mortality rates are higher in Hispanic and African American women than in other American women.[10-12] African Americans are three times more likely to die from heart disease compared with whites. Fortunately, numerous strategies are underway to promote health equity and reduce disparities.

Place and Health. Place refers to the geographic and environmental location where a person is born, grows, lives, works, and ages. Place affects the use of health services, health status, and health behaviors.

Approximately 25% of Americans live in nonurban or rural areas.[7] Three percent of Americans live in designated frontier counties. Differences in access to health care services among frontier, rural, and urban settings can create geographic health disparities. For example, rural populations and Native Americans living on reservations may need to travel long distances to receive health care. This can result in inadequate or less frequent access to health care services. Some parts of the rural United States are considered "medically underserved" because of decreased numbers of health care providers per population.

People living in rural areas have higher rates of cancer, heart disease, diabetes, depression, and injury-related deaths than people living in urban areas. For example, in rural Appalachia the rates of lung, colon, cervical, and rectal cancer are higher than the national average.[13] Rural populations tend to be older than urban populations. Many rural areas have higher rates of obesity and chronic disease. Rural Americans are less likely to work for employers who provide health insurance.[12,13] As a group, rural populations have lower literacy rates and poorer health behaviors (e.g., increased smoking rates, increased substance abuse, higher rates of obesity, lower rates of physical activity). Generally, smaller and more isolated rural communities with low economic resources experience greater difficulties accessing high-quality health care.

Living in urban centers may also predispose a person to health disparities. Concerns about personal safety (e.g., clinics located in high-crime neighborhoods) can make patients reluctant to visit health care providers. At the same time, health care providers such as home health nurses working in high-risk areas may experience distress when they witness crime, drug use, or other illegal activities.[14] Among the most obvious health behaviors affected by place are physical activity and nutrition. Safe, walkable neighborhoods with playgrounds and sources of healthy foods promote physical activity and healthy eating. Social support and networks are related to health and coping with illness. Social networks are more likely to be found in communities where neighbors interact and rely on one another. Place may have more influence on the incidence of hypertension, diabetes, and obesity for women than race or ethnicity.[15]

Income, Education, and Occupation. People of lower income, education, or occupational status experience worse health. In addition, they die at a younger age than those who are more affluent. In fact, adults without a high school diploma or equivalent are three times more likely to die before age 65 than those with a college degree.[16] Health care costs are one of the important factors that contribute to health disparities. Individuals who have no insurance, are underinsured, or lack financial resources to pay for treatment of diseases may forgo health care visits and treatments (Fig. 2-2). Patients who lack the knowledge to apply for government assistance programs (e.g., Medicaid) are also at risk. The number of uninsured Americans has increased over the past decade.[17] Hazardous work environments and high-risk occupations of laborers also increase health risk and contribute to higher rates of illness, injury, and death.

Health literacy is defined as the degree to which individuals have the capacity to obtain, process, and understand basic health information and services needed to make appropriate health decisions. This includes the ability to read, comprehend, and analyze information; understand instructions; weigh risks and benefits; and ultimately make decisions and take action. Approximately 80 million Americans have limited healthy literacy.[16,18] Low health literacy is associated with more hospitalizations, greater use of emergency department care, decreased use of cancer screening and influenza vaccine, decreased ability

to use medications correctly, and higher mortality rates among older adults. On a daily basis, patients need to self-manage conditions such as diabetes and asthma. For example, patients with diabetes may not be able to maintain adequate blood glucose levels if they cannot read or understand the numbers on the home glucose monitoring system. The inability to read and understand medication labels can result in taking medications at the wrong time or in the wrong dose. Health literacy is discussed further in Chapter 4.

Gender. Health disparities exist between men and women. Adult women use health care services more than men. At the same time, women are less likely than men to have medical insurance. Women may not receive the same quality of care (Fig. 2-3). For example, women are less likely than men to receive procedures (e.g., coronary angiography) for cardiovascular disease.[19] When gender is combined with racial and ethnic differences, the disparities are even greater. (Gender Differences boxes are presented throughout this book that highlight gender differences in disease risk, manifestations, and treatment.)

Age. Older adults are at risk for experiencing health disparities in the number of diagnostic tests performed and aggressiveness of treatments used. Biases toward older adults that affect their care, or *ageism*, are discussed in Chapter 5. Older women are less likely to be offered mammograms. Older people of low socioeconomic status experience greater disability, more limitations in activities of daily living, and more frequent and rapid cognitive decline.[20] Older adults who belong to minority groups are less likely than their white counterparts to receive screening for prostate and colorectal cancer.[21]

Sexual Orientation. Sexuality is defined as a person's romantic, emotional, or sexual attraction to another person. Gay, lesbian, and bisexual orientation places an individual at risk for health disparities due to their social, economic, or environmental disadvantages. With the repeal of the military's "don't ask, don't tell" legislation in 2010, the focus on the rights and specific health care needs of lesbian, gay, bisexual, and transgender (LGBT) individuals has increased.

Lesbian women are more likely to be obese when compared with their heterosexual counterparts. Lesbian and bisexual

FIG. 2-2 Percentage of adults ages 18 to 64 years old who skipped or delayed medical care because of cost. The data are displayed by disability and insurance coverage status.

FIG. 2-3 Older Asian women are especially at risk for health disparities. (iStockphoto/Thinkstock)

women have increased risk factors for cardiovascular disease.[22] Gay men have higher rates of human immunodeficiency virus and hepatitis infections than other groups. Gay men and lesbian women have higher smoking rates than heterosexuals.

Understanding the cause of these disparities among LGBT individuals is essential to providing safe and high-quality care. One of the barriers to accessing high-quality health care by LGBT adults is the current lack of providers who are knowledgeable about their health needs. LGBT patients may also experience fear of discrimination in health care settings.[23] Within many, but not all, health care settings, LGBT health care issues are now more visible. The Joint Commission requires that patients be allowed the presence of the support individual of their choice. In addition, hospitals need to adopt policies that bar discrimination based on factors such as sexual orientation and gender identification and expression. *Healthy People 2020* has added an objective on LGBT health *(www.healthypeople.gov/2020/topicsobjectives2020/overview.aspx?topicid=25)*.

Health Care Provider Attitudes. Certain behaviors and biases of the health care provider can contribute to health disparities. Factors such as bias and prejudice can affect health care–seeking behavior in minority populations.[24] The health care system itself may also contribute to the problem of health disparities. For example, a clinic located in an area with a large Vietnamese immigrant population that does not provide translators or educational materials and financial forms in Vietnamese may limit these families' ability to understand how to access health care.

Discrimination and *bias* based on a patient's race, ethnicity, gender, age, sexual orientation, or ability to pay are likely to result in less aggressive or negative treatment practices. Sometimes discrimination is difficult to identify, especially when it occurs at the institutional level. Because a health care provider's overt discriminatory behavior may not be immediately evident to the patient or yourself, it may be difficult to confront. Even well-intentioned providers who try to eliminate bias in their care can demonstrate their prior beliefs or prejudices through nonverbal communication. Many policies are in place to eliminate discrimination, but it still exists.[25]

CULTURE

Culture is a way of life for a group of people. It includes the behaviors, beliefs, values, traditions, and symbols that the group accepts, generally without thinking about them. This way of life is passed along by communication and imitation from one generation to the next. You can also think of culture as cultivated behavior that is acquired through social learning. It is the totality of a person's learned, accumulated experience that is socially transmitted. The four classic characteristics of culture are described in Table 2-2.

Values are the sets of rules by which individuals, families, groups, and communities live. They are the principles and standards that serve as the basis for beliefs, attitudes, and behaviors. Although all cultures have values, the types and expressions of those values differ from one culture to another. These cultural values develop over time, guide decision making and actions, and may affect a person's self-esteem. Cultural values are often unconsciously developed early in life as a child learns about acceptable and unacceptable behaviors. The extent to which a person's cultural values are internalized influences that person's tendency toward judging other cultures, while usually using his

TABLE 2-2	BASIC CHARACTERISTICS OF CULTURE

- *Dynamic* and ever-changing
- *Not always shared* by all members of a cultural group
- *Adapted* to specific conditions such as environmental factors
- *Learned* through oral and written histories, as well as socialization

TABLE 2-3	DISTINCT CULTURAL CHARACTERISTICS OF DIFFERENT ETHNIC GROUPS IN THE UNITED STATES

Native American
- Folk healing
- Living in harmony with people and nature
- Respect for all things living
- Returning what is taken from nature
- Doing the honorable thing
- Respect for tribal elders and children
- Spiritual guidance

Hispanic/Latino
- Cultural foods
- Folk healing
- Extended family valued
- Involvement of family in social activities
- Religion and spirituality highly valued
- Respect for elders and authority
- Interdependence and collectivism

African American
- Cultural foods
- Family networks
- Folk healing
- Importance of religion
- Interdependence within ethnic group
- Music and physical activities valued

European American
- Individualistic and competitive
- Equal rights of genders
- Independence and freedom
- Materialistic
- Self-reliance valued
- Technology dependent
- Youth and beauty valued

Asian American
- Cultural foods
- Folk healing
- Respect for one's parents and ancestors
- Family loyalty
- Respect for elders
- Harmonious relationships
- Harmony and balance within body vital for preservation of life energy

Pacific Islander American
- Kinship alliance among nuclear and extended family
- Natural order and balanced relationships
- Collective concern and involvement
- Knowledge is collective; belongs to group, not individual

Adapted from Andrews MM, Boyle JS: *Transcultural concepts in nursing care*, ed 5, Philadelphia, 2008, Wolters Kluwer-Lippincott Williams & Wilkins; and Giger JN, Davidhizar RE: *Transcultural nursing: assessment and intervention*, ed 6, St Louis, 2012, Mosby.

or her own culture as the accepted standard. Table 2-3 provides some examples of cultural characteristics of different ethnic groups in the United States.

Although individuals within a cultural group have many similarities through their shared values, beliefs, and practices, there is also diversity within groups (Fig. 2-4). Each person is culturally unique. Such diversity may result from different perspectives and interpretations of situations. These differences may be based on age, gender, marital status, family structure, income, education level, religious views, and life experiences. Within any cultural group, there are smaller groups that may not hold all of the values of the dominant culture. These smaller cultural groups have experiences that differ from those of the dominant group. These differences may be related to ethnic background, residence, religion, occupation, health, age, gender,

FIG. 2-4 Members of this family share a common heritage. (Jupiterimages/Photos.com/Thinkstock)

education, or other factors that unite the group. Members of a subculture share certain aspects of culture that are different from those of the overall cultural group. For example, among Hispanics, some seek professional health care immediately when symptoms appear, other Hispanics rely first on folk healers, and yet other Hispanics first seek the opinion of family and friends before seeking formal health care.

Cultural beliefs about symptom tolerance and health care–seeking behavior can contribute to health disparities. Some cultures consider pain something to be endured or ignored, and as a result, the patient does not seek help. Some cultures may view diseases or problems fatalistically; that is, people see no reason to seek treatment because they believe it is unlikely to have any benefit. Some cultures view the signs and symptoms of an illness as "God's will" or as a punishment for some prior behavior.[26]

Fatalism is higher in individuals with lower socioeconomic status. Fatalistic beliefs are associated with reduced cancer prevention activities such as exercising, not smoking, and following a healthy diet.[27] In some cultures it may not be acceptable to see a health care provider who is not of the same gender or ethnic group. Such beliefs can result in delays in seeking health care or inadequate treatment.

Acculturation is the life-long process of incorporating cultural aspects of the contexts in which a person grows, lives, works, and ages.[28,29] Acculturation is often bidirectional. In other words, the context also changes as it is influenced by a person's culture. Change may be in attitudes, behaviors, and values. For example, a sedentary person who loves to cook may change his or her attitude toward exercise when living with athletic roommates, who in turn also change as they begin to appreciate cooking. Behaviors change when an immigrant child learns the local language while also influencing the conduct of classmates. Lastly, a deeply held value such as self-sufficiency may change for a person exposed to a culture where reliance on others dominates.

Newcomers may adopt both the strengths and the limitations of the dominant culture. This is relevant when considering health behaviors of individuals and the quality of health care delivered by professionals. For example, an immigrant may be negatively influenced by a dominant cultural context in which unhealthy eating habits prevail. As a new nurse, you may be negatively or positively influenced by the culture of care that is most prevalent in the workplace.[30]

The result of acculturation for the individual may be new cultural variations in attitudes, behaviors, and values. All people participate in this process over their lives. People who move to a new cultural context are more aware of the acculturation experience than people who are not exposed to new experiences. Exposure to new cultural contexts increases the cultural competency of nurses.

Stereotyping refers to an over-generalized viewpoint that members of a specific culture, race, or ethnic group are alike and share the same values and beliefs. This oversimplified approach does not take into account the individual differences that exist within a culture. Being a member of a particular cultural, ethnic, or racial group does not make the person an expert on other members of that same group. Such stereotyping can lead to false assumptions and affect a patient's care. For example, it would be inappropriate for you to assume that just because a nurse is Mexican American, he would know how a Mexican American patient's beliefs might affect that patient's health care practices. A young nurse born and raised in a large city has experienced a different culture than the older patient who was born and raised in a rural area of Mexico.

Ethnocentrism refers to the belief that one's own culture and worldview are superior to those of others from different cultural, ethnic, or racial backgrounds.[31] Comparing others' ways to your own can lead to seeing others as different or inferior. Health care providers' ethnocentrism can result in poor communication, patient alienation, and potentially inadequate treatment. To avoid ethnocentrism, you need to remain open to a variety of perspectives and maintain a nonjudgmental view of the values, beliefs, and practices of others. Failure to do this can result in ethnic stereotyping or cultural imposition.

Cultural imposition occurs when one's own cultural beliefs and practices are imposed on another person or group of people. In health care it can result in disregarding or trivializing a patient's health care beliefs or practices. Cultural imposition may happen when a health care provider is unaware of the patient's cultural beliefs and plans and implements care without taking them into account.

Cultural safety describes care and advocacy that prevent cultural imposition. Culturally safe practice requires cultural competency and action to ensure that cultural histories, experiences, and traditions of patients, their families, and communities are valued and shape health care approaches and policies.[29,31]

The term **transcultural nursing** was coined by Madeleine Leininger in the 1950s. Transcultural nursing is a specialty that focuses on the comparative study and analysis of cultures and subcultures. The goal of transcultural nursing is the discovery of culturally relevant facts that can guide the nurse in providing culturally appropriate care.[31]

CULTURAL COMPETENCE

Cultural competence is the ability to understand, appreciate, and work with individuals from cultures other than your own. It involves an awareness and acceptance of cultural differences, self-awareness, knowledge of the patient's culture, and adaptation of skills to meet the patient's needs. The four components of cultural competence are (1) cultural awareness, (2) cultural knowledge, (3) cultural skill, and (4) cultural encounter[31] (Table 2-4).

Specific information is presented throughout this book to assist you in developing an awareness of cultural differences and learning assessment skills for different cultural groups. Table 2-7 (later in this chapter) presents a cultural assessment guide. Review cultural characteristics associated with a group when preparing to interview a patient. However, it is essential to seek information from patients about their culture because they may not exhibit the typical cultural characteristics.

Providing culturally competent care increases patient satisfaction, reduces health disparities, increases patient safety, and prevents misunderstandings between you and your patients. It also involves integrating cultural practices into Western medicine. For example, before some diagnostic procedures and interventions, it is typical to have patients remove personal objects that are worn on the body. Ask patients whether they wear personal objects and the significance of their removal, since they may have cultural or spiritual significance. You also need to know whether wearing these objects will compromise patient safety, test results, or outcomes of the intervention.

CULTURAL DIVERSITY IN THE HEALTH CARE WORKPLACE

Poorer health outcomes for minorities are linked to the shortage of culturally and ethnically diverse health care providers, who have historically been underrepresented in the health professions.[32] A diversity gap exists between the ethnic composition of the health care workforce and the overall population in the United States (Fig. 2-5). The diversity of nurses in the United States is increasing but still lags behind that of the population. African Americans, Hispanic/Latino Americans, and Native Americans make up more than 27% of the population but only 17% of the nation's nurses.

Cultural differences exist in how well patients believe they can communicate with their health care provider. Communication issues include not understanding the health care provider, feeling that they are not listened to, and having questions but not asking them. In the United States approximately 25% to 33% of minority patients have difficulty communicating with their health care provider, compared with 16% of white patients. Similarly, minority patients are less likely than whites to have a regular health care provider. African Americans are more likely to receive outpatient care in the emergency department (ED) and have fewer physician visits.[33]

When health care providers from different cultures work together as members of the health care team, opportunities for miscommunication and conflict can occur. This is termed *cultural conflict*. The cultural origins of miscommunication and

TABLE 2-4   HOW TO DEVELOP CULTURAL COMPETENCE

Description	Role of Nurse
Cultural Awareness	
• Ability to understand patients' unique cultural needs	• Identify your own cultural background, values, and beliefs, especially as related to health and health care. • Examine your own cultural biases toward people whose cultures differ from your own culture.
Cultural Knowledge	
• Process of learning key aspects of a group's culture, especially as it relates to health and health care practices • Patients as the best source of information about their culture	• Learn basic general information about predominant cultural groups in your geographic area. Cultural pocket guides can be a good resource. • Assess patients for presence or absence of cultural traits based on an understanding of generalizations about a cultural group. • Do not make assumptions based on cultural background because the degree of acculturation varies among individuals. • Read research studies that describe cultural differences. • Read ethnic newspaper articles and books. • View documentaries about cultural groups.
Cultural Skill	
• Ability to collect relevant cultural data • Performance of a cultural assessment	• Be alert for unexpected responses with patients, especially as related to cultural issues. • Become aware of cultural differences in predominant ethnic groups. • Develop assessment skills to do a competent cultural assessment for any patient.* • Learn assessment skills for different cultural groups, including cultural beliefs and practices.
Cultural Encounter	
• Direct cross-cultural interactions between people from culturally diverse backgrounds • Extended contact with a cultural group to enhance understanding of its values and beliefs	• Create opportunities to interact with predominant cultural groups. • Attend cultural events, such as religious ceremonies, significant life passage rituals, social events, and demonstrations of cultural practices. • Visit markets and restaurants in ethnic neighborhoods. • Explore ethnic neighborhoods, listen to different types of ethnic music, and learn games of various ethnic groups. • Visit or volunteer at health fairs in local ethnic neighborhoods. • Learn about prominent cultural beliefs and practices, and incorporate this knowledge into planning nursing care.

*See Table 2-7 later in the chapter.

FIG. 2-5 Nurses working together in a multicultural health care environment. (Fuse/Thinkstock)

conflict in the workplace are often interconnected with cultural beliefs, values, and etiquette. Seeking clarification about misperceptions and misunderstandings is a communication strategy to foster effective teamwork among a multicultural health care team. To ensure the recruitment and retention of nurses from minority populations, all members of the health care team and leadership must create an environment that promotes effective cross-cultural communication and reduces bias and discrimination.

CULTURAL FACTORS AFFECTING HEALTH AND HEALTH CARE

Many cultural factors affect the patient's health and health care. Several potential factors are presented in Table 2-5.

Folk Healers

Many cultures have **folk healers,** who are also known as *traditional healers*. Most folk healers speak the person's native language and cost less than conventional health care providers. Among the many folk healers found worldwide, Hispanics may turn to a *curandero* (or *curandera*), African Americans may visit a *hougan*, Native Americans may seek help from a medicine man or *shaman*, and Asian Americans may use the services of a Chinese herbal therapist. In addition to folk healers, some cultures involve lay midwives (e.g., *parteras* for Hispanic women) in the care of pregnant women.

Folk medicine is a form of prevention and treatment that is culturally based and traditionally relies on oral transmission of healing techniques from one generation to the next. The patient may not use the term *folk medicine* but thinks of these as cultural home remedies or treatment practices. Folk medicine may be practiced in the home without the guidance of a folk healer. It is important to assess whether the patient is practicing traditional or folk healing.

Spirituality and Religion

Spirituality and religion are aspects of culture that may affect a person's beliefs about health, illness, and end-of-life care. They may also play a role in nutrition and decisions related to health, wellness, and how to respond to or treat an illness.

Spirituality refers to a person's effort to find purpose and meaning in life. It is influenced by a person's unique life experiences and reflects one's personal understanding of life's mysteries. Spirituality relates to the soul or spirit more than to the body, and it may provide hope and strength for an individual during an illness.

Religion is a more formal and organized system of beliefs, including belief in or worship of God or gods. Religious beliefs include the cause, nature, and purpose of the universe and involve prayer and rituals. Religion is based on beliefs about life, death, good, and evil. You can use several interventions to meet a patient's religious and spiritual needs, including prayer, scripture reading, listening, and referral to a chaplain, rabbi, or priest.[34]

Many patients find that rituals help them during times of illness. Rituals help a person make sense of life experiences and may take the form of prayer, meditation, or other rituals that the patient may create. With appropriate training, you may

---

TABLE 2-5 CULTURAL FACTORS AFFECTING HEALTH AND HEALTH CARE

Time Orientation
- For some cultures it is more important to attend to a social role than to arrive on time for an appointment with a health care provider.
- Some cultures are future oriented; others are past or present oriented.

Language and Communication
- Patients may not speak English and may not be able to communicate with the health care provider.
- Even with interpreters, communication may be difficult.

Economic Factors
- Patients may not get health care because they cannot pay for it or because of the costs associated with travel for health care.
- Refugee or undocumented immigrant status may deter some patients from using the health care system.
- Immigrant women who are heads of households or single mothers may not seek health care for themselves because of child care costs.
- Patients may lack health insurance.

Health Care System
- Patients may not make or keep appointments because of the time lag between the onset of an illness and an available appointment.
- Hours of operation of health care facilities may not accommodate patients' need to work or use public transportation.
- Requirements to access some types of care may discourage some patients from taking the steps to qualify for health care or health care payment assistance.
- Some patients have a general distrust of health care professionals and health care systems.
- Lack of ethnic-specific health care programs may deter some individuals from seeking health care.

- Transportation may be a problem for patients who have to travel long distances for health care.
- Adequate interpreter services may be unavailable.
- Patients may not have a primary health care provider and may use emergency departments or urgent care centers for health care.
- Shortages of health care providers from specific ethnic groups may deter some people from seeking health care.
- Patients may lack knowledge about the availability of existing health care resources.
- Facility policies may not be culturally competent (e.g., hospital policy may limit the number of visitors, which is problematic for cultures that value having many family members present).

Beliefs and Practices
- Care provided in established health care programs may not be perceived as culturally relevant.
- Religious reasons, beliefs, or practices may affect a person's decision to seek (or not seek) health care.
- Patients may delay seeking health care because of fear or dependence on folk medicine and herbal remedies.
- Patients may stop treatment or discontinue visits for health care because the symptoms are no longer present, and they believe that further care is not required.
- Some patients associate hospitals and extended care facilities with death.
- The patient may have had a previous negative experience with culturally incompetent health care providers or discriminatory practices.
- Some people mistrust the majority population and institutions dominated by them.
- Some patients may feel apprehensive about unfamiliar diagnostic procedures and treatment options.

include spiritual questions in the complete assessment of the patient and plan care based accordingly. (Table 10-5 has a spiritual assessment guide that may be used with patients.) Table 2-6 summarizes health-related beliefs and practices of selected religious groups.

Cross-Cultural Communication

Communication refers to an organized, patterned system of behavior that may be verbal or nonverbal (Fig. 2-6). *Verbal communication* includes not only one's language or dialect, but also voice tone, volume, timing, and ability to share thoughts and feelings. More than 45 million people in the United States speak a language other than English in their home, with Spanish being the most common. Hispanics who do not speak English at home are less likely to receive a variety of health care services regardless of whether they are comfortable speaking English.[35]

Nonverbal communication may take the form of writing, gestures, body movements, posture, and facial expressions. Nonverbal communication also includes eye contact, use of touch, body language, style of greeting, and spatial distancing. Eye

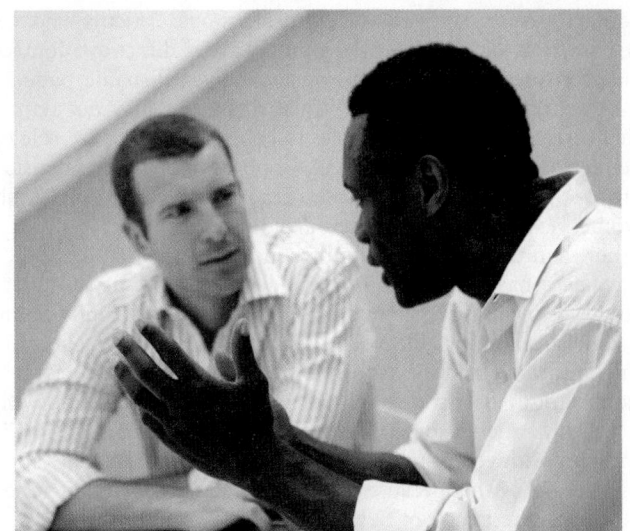

FIG. 2-6 Co-workers from different cultures communicate with verbal and nonverbal cues. (BananaStock/Thinkstock)

TABLE 2-6 HEALTH-RELATED BELIEFS AND PRACTICES OF SELECTED RELIGIOUS GROUPS

Amish
- Alcoholic beverages and drugs are prohibited unless prescribed by health care professional.
- Abortion, artificial insemination, and stem cell use are prohibited.
- Amish seldom purchase commercial health insurance.

Catholicism
- Many fast and abstain from meat and meat products on Ash Wednesday and the Fridays of Lent.
- Artificial contraception and direct abortion are prohibited. Indirect abortion (e.g., treatment of uterine cancer in a pregnant woman) may be morally justified.
- Sacrament of the Sick includes anointing of sick with oil, blessing by a priest, and communion (unleavened wafer made of flour and water).

Church of Jesus Christ of Latter-Day Saints (Mormons)
- Strict dietary code called Word of Wisdom prohibits all alcoholic beverages, hot drinks (nonherbal teas and coffee), tobacco, and illegal or recreational drugs.
- Fasting for 24-hour period occurs monthly on "Fast Sunday."
- During hospitalization or serious illness, an elder anoints the ill person with oil while a second elder seals the anointing with a prayer and blessing (laying on of hands).
- Abortion is prohibited except when the mother's life is in danger.

Hinduism
- Eating meat is prohibited because it involves harming a living creature.
- Cremation is most common form of body disposal, but fetuses or newborns are sometimes buried.

Islam
- Fasting during daytime hours occurs during a month-long period called Ramadan.
- Ritual cleansing with water before eating and before prayer is practiced.
- Eating pork or taking medicines with pork derivatives is prohibited.
- Drinking alcoholic beverages is prohibited.
- Artificial insemination is permissible only if from the husband to his own wife.

Jehovah's Witness
- Transfusions of blood in any form or agents in which blood is an ingredient are not acceptable. Blood volume expanders are acceptable if they are not derivatives of blood.
- Transplants that involve bodily mutilation are prohibited.
- Therapeutic and on-demand abortions are prohibited.
- Artificial insemination is prohibited for both donors and recipients.

Judaism
- Strictly observant Jews never eat pork, shellfish, or predatory fowl and never mix milk dishes and meat dishes in preparing foods. Fish with fins and scales are permissible.
- Certain foods and drink are designated as kosher, which means "proper." All animals must be ritually slaughtered.
- On the eighth day after birth, boys are circumcised in a ritual called Brit Milah, and girls are given a dedication ceremony involving prayers and blessings.
- Abortion is morally unacceptable except when the mother's life is in danger.
- Organized support system for the sick includes a visit from the rabbi. The rabbi may pray with the sick person alone or in a minyan, a group of 10 adults over age 13.
- If an autopsy is performed, all body parts must be returned for burial.

Seventh-Day Adventism
- Vegetarian diet encouraged.
- Nonvegetarian members refrain from eating foods derived from any animal having a cloven hoof that chews its cud (e.g., pigs, goats). Eating fish with fins and scales is acceptable, but consuming shellfish is prohibited.
- Consumption of alcoholic beverages is prohibited.
- Fasting is practiced and involves abstaining from food or liquids by healthy members of the church.

Buddhism*
- Consumption of alcoholic beverages and illicit drugs is prohibited.
- Moderation in diet and avoidance of extremes are practiced.
- Central tenets are maintaining right views, intentions, speech, actions, livelihood, effort, mindfulness, and concentration.

*Data from Andrews MM: Religion, culture, and nursing. In MM Andrews, JS Boyle, editors: *Transcultural concepts in nursing care*, ed 6, Philadelphia, 2012, Lippincott Williams & Wilkins.

contact varies greatly among cultural groups. Patients who are Asian, Arab, or Native American may avoid direct eye contact and consider it disrespectful or aggressive. Hispanic patients may expect you to look directly at them, but may not return that direct gaze. Other variables to consider include the role of gender, age, acculturation, status, or position on what is considered appropriate eye contact. For example, Muslim-Arab women exhibit modesty when avoiding eye contact with men other than their husbands and when in public situations.

Silence has many meanings, and it is important to understand the meaning of silence for different cultural groups. Some people are comfortable with silence, whereas others become uncomfortable and may speak to decrease the silent times. It is important to clarify what silence means in an interaction with a patient. Patients sometimes nod their head or say "yes" as if agreeing with you or to indicate they understand. Actually, they may be doing this because it is a culturally acceptable manner of showing respect, not because they understand or agree.

Many Native Americans are comfortable with silence and interpret silence as essential for thinking and carefully considering a response. In these interactions, silence shows respect for the other person and demonstrates the importance of the remarks. In traditional Japanese and Chinese cultures, the speaker may stop talking and leave a period of silence for the listener to think about what has been said before continuing. Silence may be intended to show respect for the speaker's privacy, whereas in some cultures (e.g., French, Spanish, Russian) the person may interpret silence as meaning agreement. Asian Americans may use silence to demonstrate respect for elders, whereas African Americans may use silence as a response to what is perceived to be an inappropriate question.

Family Roles and Relationships

Family roles differ from one culture to another (Fig. 2-7). It is important for you to determine who should be involved in communication and decision making related to health care. Some cultural groups emphasize interdependence rather than independence. In the United States many in the mainstream culture have strong beliefs related to autonomy. An individual is expected to sign consent forms when receiving health care. In other cultural groups a family member may be expected to make health care decisions. When you encounter a family that

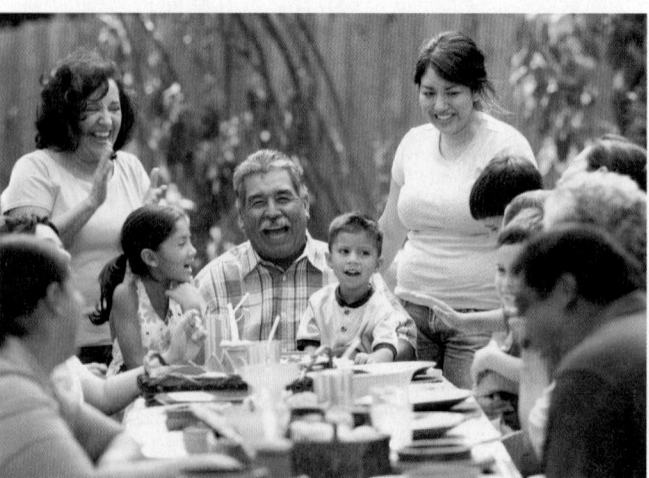

FIG. 2-7 Family roles and relationships differ from one culture to another. (Jack Hollingsworth/Photodisc/Thinkstock)

values interdependence over independence, the health care system may have difficulty adapting to how decisions are made. Treatment may need to be delayed while the patient waits for significant family members to arrive before giving consent for a procedure or treatment. In other instances the patient may make a decision that is best for the family despite adverse outcomes for the patient. Being aware of such values will better prepare you to advocate for the patient.

Some cultural differences relate to expectations of family members in providing care. In some cultures, family members expect to provide care for the patient even in the hospital. The patient may expect that the family, along with the health care providers, will provide all care. This view is the opposite of the predominant Western expectation that the patient will assume self-care as quickly as possible.

Ask about culturally relevant gender relationships. For example, in some cultures, such as many Arab groups, it is not appropriate for a man to be alone with a woman other than his wife. Nor is it appropriate for a woman other than a man's wife to provide physical care for him. The clinical implication of this cultural belief is that for many patients from Arab cultures, nurses cannot provide direct physical care for patients of the opposite gender. In some instances, procedures or treatments may be carried out for patients from the opposite gender but only if a third party is present.

Personal Space

Personal space zones refer to the preferred distances between two individuals. Personal space distances vary from culture to culture, as well as within a culture. For European Americans in the United States, the *intimate distance* ranges from 0 to 18 inches, and the *personal distance* ranges from 18 inches to 4 feet. The personal distance is the one experienced with friends. Social distance ranges from 4 to 12 feet, and public distance is 12 feet or more.[36] As a nurse, you often interact with patients in the intimate or personal zones, which might be uncomfortable for the patient.

Cultural groups have wide variations in their perception of appropriate distances. Whereas an American nurse of European descent may be comfortable with a certain distance, a person from a Hispanic or Middle Eastern background may believe that the distance is too far and will move closer, perhaps causing you to feel uncomfortable. If you then move away to a more comfortable distance, this may cause the other person to think that you are unfriendly, or the person may be offended. Personal space distance also varies within cultures.

Touch

Physical contact with patients conveys various meanings depending on the culture. To do a comprehensive assessment, touching a patient is necessary. Many people of Asian and Hispanic heritage believe that touching a person's head is a sign of disrespect, especially because the head is believed to be the source of one's strength and/or soul. Numerous people in the world believe in the evil eye, or *mal ojo*. In one culture-bound syndrome the illness, usually in a child or a woman, is believed to result from excessive admiration by another person. In some cultures the proper way to ward off the evil eye is to touch the area of admiration. For example, if the person admires the hair, the top of the head may be touched. It is important for you to ask permission before touching anyone, particularly if it is necessary to touch the person's head.

Nutrition

An important part of cultural practices is food, including both the foods that are eaten and rituals and practices associated with food. Muslims fast during the daytime during the Islamic month of Ramadan. Such practices may affect when and how medications are taken. Patients may be asked to make major changes in their diets because of health problems, or alternatively food may be used to cope with life changes such as homesickness. Specific foods may be considered essential to good health during pregnancy or other life stages. It is important that the health care provider take into account food-related cultural beliefs, practices, and habits when discussing nutrition with patients and planning their diets.

When individuals and families immigrate to an area that is very different from their country of origin, they may experience unfamiliar foods, food-storage systems, and food-buying habits. They also may come from countries that have limited food supplies because of poverty, wars, and poor sanitation. They may arrive with conditions such as general poor nutrition, hypertension, diarrhea, and dental caries. Other problems may develop after the person arrives in the new country. For example, second-generation Hispanic immigrants have a greater chance of becoming overweight than their first-generation counterparts. The increase in weight is related to the degree of acculturation experienced by the immigrant.[37]

Immigrants and Immigration

Migration is driven by a number of conditions, such as overcrowding, natural disasters, geopolitical conflict, persecution, and economic forces. Because of these migrations, a rich diversity of cultures exists in many communities and countries today (Fig. 2-8).

Recent immigrants may be at risk for physical and mental health problems for many reasons. Conditions in their countries of origin (e.g., malnutrition, poor sanitation, civil war) may have resulted in chronic health problems. In addition, recent immigrants are at increased risk for health problems after arriving in a new area. Relocation is associated with many losses and can cause economic hardship, physical stress, and mental distress.

As new immigrants go through the acculturation process, many experience cultural stress as they adjust to their new environment, especially if they have left relatives behind or are unable to return to their home country. Older immigrants are especially affected by changes in role and social position. This may result in depression. Posttraumatic stress disorder is seen in immigrants who have survived wars and violence. Immigrants may face barriers to social acceptance, such as prejudice or discrimination, and experience a lack of ethnic and cultural resources. For some, it may mean loss of the social status that they experienced in their countries of origin.

Another potential problem is tuberculosis (TB). More than half of the TB cases in the United States occur in individuals born outside the country. Individuals who have recently immigrated from areas that have a high endemic rate of TB are more likely to have TB.[38] Foreign-born Hispanics and Asians combined account for 48% of the nation's TB cases. The top five countries of origin of foreign-born people with TB were Mexico, Philippines, Vietnam, India, and China. The *Refugee Health Guidelines* from the Centers for Disease Control and Prevention supports early identification and treatment.[39]

During the past 40 years, the migration pattern of North America has shifted. Whereas once most immigrants came from Europe, now most immigrants originate from Asia, Latin America, and Africa. Additionally, an increased number of first- and second-generation immigrants enter the United States after visiting friends and relatives. These individuals have a higher risk for malaria, typhoid fever, cholera, and hepatitis A than native-born Americans. Many immigrants lack health insurance and may primarily obtain their health care in emergency departments and urgent care clinics. Therefore nurses in all settings need to be aware of refugee health screening, treatment recommendations, and resources for access to health care.

Medications

Genetic differences among people from diverse ethnic or racial groups may explain differences in medication selection, dosage, or administration. For example, some medicines are more effective in certain ethnic groups than others. Side effects may vary among individuals from diverse backgrounds. eTable 2-1 on the website for this chapter highlights some ethnic differences in reaction to medications.

Genetic variations can affect how the body processes a drug and the overall effect of selected drugs on the body. Although race and ethnicity are imprecise indicators of genetic differences, they can be helpful in anticipating variations in the response to medications. (Genetics and drug metabolism are discussed in Chapter 13.)

Regardless of their cultural origins, many people use both cultural remedies and prescription drugs to treat their illnesses. Problems can result from interactions of these substances. For example, Chinese Americans who take ginseng as a stimulant and an antihypertensive drug may suffer adverse effects. Some Mexican Americans may treat gastrointestinal problems with preparations that contain lead. Individuals may self-treat their depression with St. John's wort, which can result in adverse effects if prescription antidepressants are also taken.

Patients may avoid standard Western medicine until herbal and other remedies become ineffective or the illness becomes acute. The challenge for you is to try to accommodate the patient's desire for traditional aspects of care while also using evidence-based approaches as appropriate and as acceptable to the patient. Evaluate the safety and appropriateness of the patient's traditional cultural healing therapies.

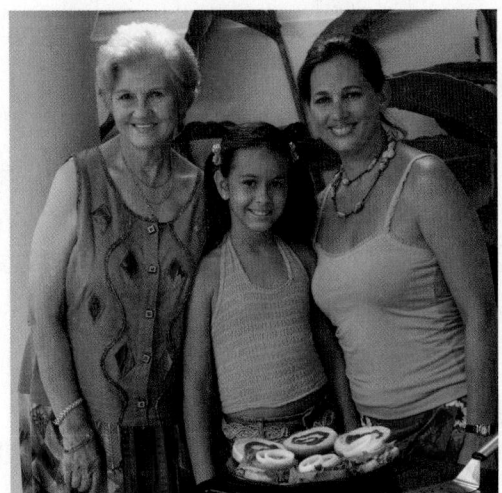

FIG. 2-8 Recently arrived immigrants join a neighbor for a barbecue, a common American tradition. (Jack Hollingsworth/Photodisc/Thinkstock)

Develop a collaborative, trusting relationship with patients and encourage them to discuss their traditional approaches to healing. Seek out information on potential drug and herbal product interaction from the pharmacist. Honor the patient's choices, if safe and effective, since this will enhance collaboration and may have a positive impact on health outcomes.

Psychologic Factors

Symptoms are interpreted through a person's cultural norms and may vary from the recognized interpretations of Western medicine. All symptoms have meaning, and the meanings may vary from one culture to another. It is important to ask patients what their illness means to them, what they believe is the cause, and what they think is the best treatment (Table 2-7).

Culture-bound syndromes are illnesses or afflictions that are recognized only within a cultural group (Table 2-8). The symptoms, course of the illness, and people's reactions to the illness are limited to specific cultures. Culture-bound syndromes are expressed through psychologic or physical symptoms.

TABLE 2-7   CULTURAL ASSESSMENT*

A cultural assessment should include the following:
- Brief history of the cultural group with which person identifies
- Values orientation
- Cultural sanctions and restrictions
- Communication
- Health-related beliefs and practices
- Nutrition
- Socioeconomic considerations
- Organizations providing cultural support
- Educational background
- Religious affiliation
- Spiritual considerations

Adapted from Jarvis C: *Physical examination and health assessment*, ed 6, Philadelphia, 2012, Saunders.
*A comprehensive cultural assessment guide is available (eTable 2-2) on the website for this chapter.

NURSING MANAGEMENT
REDUCING HEALTH DISPARITIES AND INCREASING CULTURAL COMPETENCY

NURSE'S SELF-ASSESSMENT

The first step in reducing health disparities and providing culturally competent care is for you to assess your own cultural background, values, and beliefs, especially those that are related to health and health care. Many tools are available to assist you with this process (*http://nccc.georgetown.edu*).

Table 2-4 suggests ways for you to improve your cultural competence. This information can help you better understand patients and provide culturally competent care. It is important to understand that cultures evolve and change over time. Culturally competent care requires continual learning and self-reflection.[40] Many other important aspects of culture related to

TABLE 2-8   CULTURE-BOUND SYNDROMES

Syndrome	Description
Hispanics/Latinos	
Bilis or *colera*	Caused by strong anger or rage. Many Hispanic/Latino groups believe that anger affects the body balance of hot and cold. Symptoms include acute nervous tension, headache, trembling, screaming, stomach disturbances, and, in severe cases, loss of consciousness.
Ataque de nervios	Brought on by a stressful family event (e.g., death, divorce). Symptoms may include uncontrollable shouting, crying and trembling, and verbal or physical aggression.
Empacho	Condition described as food forming into a ball that clings to the stomach or intestines, causing pain and cramping.
Susto	Sometimes referred to as "fright sickness" or "soul loss." A traumatic anxiety-depressive state that may result from a frightening experience, such as a loud sound or some threat. Can cause anxiety, insomnia, listlessness, loss of appetite, and social withdrawal. One treatment is to have the affected person lie on the floor. The healer then sweeps indigenous herbs over the person's body while praying to release the evil wind.
Native Americans	
Ghost sickness	Condition sometimes associated with witchcraft and a preoccupation with death. Symptoms include general weakness, loss of appetite, a feeling of suffocation, recurring nightmares, and a pervasive feeling of terror.
Chinese	
Shenjing shuairuo	Characterized by physical and mental fatigue, headaches and other pains, dizziness, sleep disturbances, and concentration difficulties.

Syndrome	Description
European Americans (Appalachians)	
States of blood	Blood can exist in four states that are arranged into two sets of extremes: high and low blood, and thick and thin blood. The healthy person has blood that is balanced among these four states. A person with an imbalance lacks vitality; symptoms are fatigue, dizziness, pale complexion, and listlessness.
African Americans	
Brain fag	Term describing brain "fatigue" caused by the challenges of school. Symptoms include difficulties concentrating, remembering, and thinking.
Thin blood	Affects older adults, women, and children. Generally weakens an individual and increases susceptibility to illness.
Caribbean and Southern United States	
Falling out	Characterized by a sudden collapse, which may sometimes be preceded by dizziness or "swimming" in the head. The person can hear but is unable to move.
Cambodians	
Koucharang or *Kit chroeun*	Translates as "thinking too much," brought about by having witnessed or experienced a horrific trauma. Characterized by physical and emotional exhaustion, immobilization, and constant preoccupation with past suffering and loss.
Koreans	
Hwa-byung	Ailment characterized by resentment that is brought about by bitterness and discontent.

health care are included in the Culturally Competent Care sections throughout this book.

In today's increasingly multicultural environment, you will meet patients, families, significant others, and members of the health care team from many different cultures. You will find yourself in patient care situations that require an understanding of the patient's cultural beliefs and practices. Even when you provide care for patients from your own cultural background, you may be from a different subculture than the patient. For example, there are more than 550 federally recognized Native American tribes in the United States, so it would be inappropriate for you to assume that a Native American nurse can give culturally appropriate care to a Native American patient when both may be from different tribes. A white nurse from an urban upbringing may find cultural differences with a white patient from a rural community.

PATIENT ASSESSMENT

Health care providers play an important role in reducing health disparities. However, the causes of health disparities are not always easy to identify. Assess patients for their risk for reduced health care services because of limited access, inadequate resources, age, or low health literacy.

A cultural assessment should be included in the nursing process. Table 2-7 lists important components of the assessment. A comprehensive cultural assessment guide is available in eTable 2-2, which is available on the website for this chapter. Determine (1) the patient's health beliefs and health care practices; and (2) the patient's perspective of the meaning, cause, and preferred treatment of illness.[41] Ask questions that you are comfortable with based on your own culture.

How can you be aware of the differences among ethnic groups? Using guides to cultural assessment will facilitate the nursing process when working with patients, families, or other groups who are from different cultures. Although guides can assist in this process, you need to be careful not to stereotype or assume that common cultural characteristics pertain to each individual patient. Use guides to explore the degree to which patients share commonalities with the traits generally attributed to their cultural group. You need to be informed about traditional characteristics of cultural groups while recognizing that culture is constantly evolving and unique for each individual.

NURSING IMPLEMENTATION

Although the issues associated with health disparities can seem overwhelming, a number of strategies are available to reduce and ultimately eliminate health disparities. Table 2-9 presents nursing interventions to reduce health disparities.

ADVOCACY. The solutions to reduce health disparities often rest with the policy makers. Economic issues often determine health care delivery. Access and public policy decisions determine who is eligible for federal and state health insurance coverage. You, along with the social worker, can help by identifying key resources in the community, including transportation services, reduced-fee screening programs, and appropriate federal and state offices for Medicaid and Medicare.

You can be an advocate by finding and evaluating information on appropriate and individualized treatment and in navigating the health care system. One powerful strategy for reducing health disparities is to increase the number of underrepresented populations in the health care professions (Fig. 2-9).

TABLE 2-9	NURSING INTERVENTIONS TO REDUCE HEALTH DISPARITIES

- Treat all patients equally.
- Be aware of your own biases or prejudices and work toward eliminating them.
- Learn about services and programs that focus on specific cultural/ethnic groups.
- Inform patients about health care services available for their specific cultural/ethnic group.
- Make sure the same standards of care are followed for all patients regardless of culture or ethnicity.
- Identify health care practices and cultural practices that are important to cultural and ethnic identity.
- Participate in research focused on understanding and improving care to culturally and ethnically diverse populations.
- Identify stereotypic attitudes toward a culture/ethnic group that may interfere with getting appropriate health care.
- Support patients of specific cultural/ethnic groups who are fearful about traveling outside the accepted neighborhood for health care services.
- Advocate for patients of specific cultural/ethnic groups to receive health care services that pay special attention to English-language limitations and cultural health practices.
- Learn advocacy and interpersonal strategies from leaders of specific cultural/ethnic groups. For example, African Americans may respond to themes such as "do it for your loved ones." Asian Americans may respond to fear of dependency themes.
- Ensure availability of culturally appropriate patient educational resources.

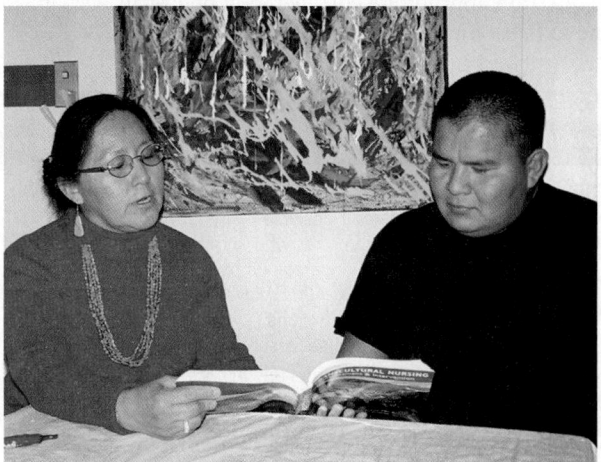

FIG. 2-9 A Navajo nurse instructs a Navajo patient.

STANDARDIZED GUIDELINES. The use of standardized evidence-based care guidelines can reduce disparities in diagnosis and treatments. For example, guidelines for the management of hypertension are based on the patient's blood pressure, symptoms, history, and laboratory values rather than other characteristics such as gender, age, or culture. Racial or cultural differences in outcomes are reduced when the guidelines are followed. In addition, recommendations related to cultural competency will guide you in your learning and practice.[41]

The National Standards for Culturally and Linguistically Appropriate Services in Health Care (CLAS standards) are guidelines that improve the quality of health care. The CLAS standards provide practical guidance for care of people with limited English proficiency and of diverse cultural backgrounds. These recommendations and resources for health care providers and organizations are available at the Think Cultural Health website listed in the Resources at the end of this chapter.

COMMUNICATION. Improving interpersonal skills is an important first step in reducing health disparities and providing culturally competent care. Effective communication between you and your patient is most likely to occur when both parties understand the meaning of that communication, whether it is through gestures, spoken words, or voice tones. To show respect for the patient, you should take into account the patient's usual communication style. For instance, a health history should start out in an unhurried manner and in a way that is appropriate for the culture. In some cultures it is best to start with general rather than direct questions. For some cultures it is most effective to engage in "small talk," with the discussion including answers that may seem to be unrelated to the questions. If you appear to be "too busy," communication may be impaired.

When meeting a patient or family member, introduce yourself and indicate how you would like them to address you—whether they should use first names; Mr., Ms., or Mrs.; or a title, such as nurse. Also ask the patient how he or she prefers to be addressed. This shows respect and will help you begin the relationship in a culturally appropriate manner.

If you need to gather personal information, it is important to understand the most effective approach to use. For instance, when talking with people from some cultural groups, it is imperative that you take time to establish trust and listen to the patient's responses to questions. There may be long silences as the person thinks about the question, showing respect by giving the question appropriate consideration before answering. Take time to listen and help establish trust.

Some cultures, such as the Hmong, rely on oral communication. When working with patients who are from an oral culture, it is important to include oral instructions during the teaching-learning process.

Do not try to serve as an interpreter if your patient does not understand English because this could lead to misunderstandings. Get the assistance of a person who is qualified to do medical interpretation when you cannot speak the patient's primary language (Table 2-10). Interpreters are available by phone anywhere in the United States through a fee-based service and should be used rather than a family member. Table 2-11 provides guidelines for communicating when no interpreter is available. With the large number of immigrants and the many

---

TABLE 2-10   USING A MEDICAL INTERPRETER

Choosing an Interpreter
- Use an agency interpreter if possible.
- Use a trained medical interpreter who knows how to interpret, has a health care background, understands patients' rights, and can help with advice about the cultural relevance or appropriateness of the health care plan and instructions.
- Use a family member only if necessary. Be aware of limitations if the family member does not understand medical terms, is younger or a different gender than the patient, or is not aware of the health care procedures or medical ethics.
- Interpreter should be able to do the following:
  - Translate the patient's nonverbal as well as verbal communication.
  - Translate the message into understandable terms.
  - Act as a patient advocate to represent the patient's needs to the health care team.
  - Be culturally competent and understand how to provide teaching instructions.

Strategies for Working With an Interpreter
- If possible, have the interpreter meet with the patient ahead of time to establish rapport before the interpreting begins.
- Speak slowly.
- Maintain eye contact with the patient.
- Talk to the patient, not the interpreter.
- Use simple language with as few medical terms as possible.
- Speak one or two sentences at a time to allow for easier translation.
- Avoid raising your voice during the interaction.
- Obtain feedback to be certain the patient understands.
- Plan on taking twice as long to complete the interaction.

TABLE 2-11   GUIDELINES FOR COMMUNICATING WHEN NO INTERPRETER IS AVAILABLE

1. Be polite and formal.
2. Pronounce name correctly. If unsure, ask about the correct pronunciation of the name. Use proper titles of respect, such as "Mr.," "Mrs.," "Ms.," "Dr." Greet the person using the last or complete name.
   Gesture to yourself and say your name.
   Offer a handshake or nod. Smile.
3. Proceed in an unhurried manner. Pay attention to any effort by the patient or family to communicate.
4. Speak in a low, moderate voice and avoid excessive hand gestures. Remember that there is a tendency to raise the volume and pitch of your voice when the listener appears not to understand. The listener may perceive that you are shouting or angry.
5. Use any words that you might know in the person's language. This indicates that you are aware of and respect his or her culture.
6. Use simple words, such as "pain" instead of "discomfort." Avoid medical jargon, idioms, and slang. Avoid using contractions (e.g., don't, can't, won't). Use nouns repeatedly instead of pronouns.
   Example:
   Do not say: "He has been taking his medicine, hasn't he?"
   Do say: "Does Juan take medicine?"
7. Pantomime words and simple actions while you verbalize them.
8. Give instructions in the proper sequence.
   Example:
   Do not say: "Before you rinse the bottle, sterilize it."
   Do say: "First, wash the bottle. Second, rinse the bottle."
9. Discuss one topic at a time. Avoid using conjunctions.
   Example:
   Do not say: "Are you cold and in pain?"
   Do say: "Are you cold [while pantomiming]? Are you in pain?"
10. Validate whether the person understands by having him or her repeat instructions, demonstrate the procedure, or act out the meaning.
11. Write out several short sentences in English and determine the person's ability to read them.
12. Try a third language. Many Indochinese people speak French. Europeans often know two or more languages. Try Latin words or phrases. Use English words that have Latin roots (e.g., use precipitation instead of rain).
13. Ask the person's family and friends who could serve as an interpreter.
14. Use websites that translate words from one language to another. Some of them also have audio to help you know how to say the word correctly.
15. Obtain phrase books from a library or bookstore, make or purchase flash cards, contact hospitals for a list of interpreters, and use both a formal and an informal network to locate a suitable interpreter.

Source: Jarvis C: *Physical examination and health assessment*, ed 6, Philadelphia, 2012, Saunders.

different cultural groups, it is highly likely that you will encounter patients who do not speak English.

A dictionary that translates from both your language and the patient's language (e.g., Spanish-English and English-Spanish dictionary) is helpful. You can look up questions and potential answers in several languages using these types of dictionaries. Many websites translate words and documents from one language into another (see Informatics in Practice box).

It is helpful to have resources for those cultural groups who frequently use the health care facility. This is especially beneficial when a qualified medical interpreter is not readily available and you need to learn important phrases in another language.

INFORMATICS IN PRACTICE

Use of Translation Applications

- Communication barriers can negatively affect the type of care received by non–English-speaking patients.
- Use a language translation app to help you translate one language into another language.
- Some apps allow you to speak critical phrases and have the translation immediately spoken back to you or the patient in a natural human voice with the proper accent.
- Check the policy of the health care institution on the use of medical interpreters or translators, including the use of apps for translation.

CASE STUDY

Health Disparities

iStockphoto/
Thinkstock

Patient Profile
A.Z. is a 75-year-old woman who came to the United States from Russia 10 years ago with her daughter, her son-in-law, and their five children. She has a number of health problems, including coronary artery disease, osteoarthritis in her left hip, and diabetes. Her daughter is the primary caregiver and frequently brings her to the urban community health clinic for a variety of health-related complaints. Recently A.Z. has been experiencing memory problems.

The visits to the clinic tend to be chaotic and time consuming for the clinic staff. The entire family comes to the health clinic with A.Z. Because English is a second language for all of the adult family members, the staff relies on the oldest granddaughter to translate.

At this clinic visit A.Z. is complaining of shortness of breath. Through her granddaughter's translation, she tells the nurse that she is having trouble walking up the stairs in the apartment building and can no longer attend her Russian Orthodox church. The nurse does the history and assessment; checks her blood glucose, which is within normal limits; and advises that she get more exercise. Given A.Z.'s memory problems and limited English, the nurse does not complete a 24-hour dietary recall or counsel her or the family about diabetes management. A.Z. is scheduled for an appointment with the cardiologist for an evaluation of her

cardiac disease. Two weeks later, when she is seen by the cardiologist, her shortness of breath is much worse and she is having chest pain. She is hospitalized immediately.

Meanwhile, the clinic supervisor is completing a chart audit for the clinic's quality review program. She is reviewing A.Z.'s chart and notices that, although she has been a patient in the clinic for 3 years, she has never received instructions on blood glucose monitoring or general diabetes management. The clinic has a nurse diabetes educator who teaches individual patients and groups of patients with diabetes. The clinic manager reviews these findings with the nurse and asks why she has not recommended that A.Z. see the diabetes educator. The nurse states that with all of the chaos in the family, A.Z.'s memory problems, and the language barrier, she just assumed that A.Z. would not benefit from the consultation.

Discussion Questions
1. What type of health disparity has A.Z. experienced?
2. What factors led to her not receiving the standard of care?
3. What additional assessment should have been done at the initial visit?
4. What strategies might have worked to enhance patient education?
5. How would you assess A.Z.'s religious and spiritual needs?
6. If you were the clinic manager, how would you recommend that the nurse improve her practice?

evolve Answers available at *http://evolve.elsevier.com/Lewis/medsurg.*

BRIDGE TO NCLEX EXAMINATION

The number of the question corresponds to the same-numbered outcome at the beginning of the chapter.

1. What is the leading determinant of a patient's health?
   a. Behavior
   b. Family history of disease
   c. Home and work environment
   d. Type and quality of medical care received
2. In identifying patients at the greatest risk for health disparities, the nurse would note that
   a. patients who live in urban areas have readily available access to health care services.
   b. cultural differences exist in patients' ability to communicate with their health care provider.
   c. a patient receiving care from a health care provider of a different culture would have decreased quality of care.
   d. men are more likely than women to have their cardiovascular disease symptoms ignored by their health care provider.

3. Forcing one's own cultural beliefs and practices on another person is an example of
   a. stereotyping.
   b. ethnocentrism.
   c. cultural relativity.
   d. cultural imposition.
4. Which statement most accurately describes cultural factors that may affect health?
   a. Diabetes and cancer rates differ by cultural/ethnic groups.
   b. Most patients find that religious rituals help them during times of illness.
   c. There are limited ethnic variations in physiologic responses to medications.
   d. Silence during a nurse-patient interaction usually means that the patient understands the instructions.

5. When communicating with a patient who speaks a language that the nurse does not understand, it is important to first attempt to
   a. have a family member translate.
   b. use a trained medical interpreter.
   c. use specific medical terminology so there will be no mistakes.
   d. focus on the translation rather than nonverbal communication.
6. As part of the nursing process, cultural assessment is best accomplished by
   a. judging the patient's cultural values based on observations.
   b. using a cultural assessment guide as part of the nursing process.
   c. seeking guidance from a nurse from the patient's cultural background.
   d. relying on the nurse's previous experience with patients from that cultural group.
7. Nurses play an important role in reducing health disparities. One important mechanism to do this is to
   a. discourage use of evidence-based practice guidelines.
   b. insist that patients adhere to the *Healthy People 2020* guidelines.
   c. teach patients to use the Internet to find resources related to their health.
   d. engage in active listening and establish relationships with patients and families.

8. What is the first step in developing cultural competence?
   a. Create opportunities to interact with a variety of cultural groups.
   b. Examine the nurse's own cultural background, values, and beliefs about health and health care.
   c. Learn about a multitude of folk medicines and herbal substances that different cultures use for self-care.
   d. Learn assessment skills for different cultural groups, including cultural beliefs and practices and physical assessments.

1. a, 2. b, 3. d, 4. a, 5. b, 6. b, 7. d, 8. b.

⊜volve

For rationales to these answers and even more NCLEX review questions, visit *http://evolve.elsevier.com/Lewis/medsurg*.

REFERENCES

1. World Health Organization: Health impact assessment. Retrieved from *www.who.int/hia/en*.
2. Hsia RY, Kellerman AL, Shen YC: Factors associated with closures of emergency departments in the United States, *JAMA* 305:1978, 2011.
3. US Department of Health and Human Services: Healthy People 2020. Retrieved from *www.healthypeople.gov*.
4. National Partnership for Action to End Health Disparities. Retrieved from *http://minorityhealth.hhs.gov/npa*.
5. Centers for Disease Control and Prevention: Chronic disease prevention and health promotion. Retrieved from *www.cdc.gov/chronicdisease/healthequity*.
6. Heurtin-Roberts S: Race and ethnicity in health and vital statistics, presented to National Committee on Health and Vital Statistics, Washington, DC. Retrieved from *www.ncvh.hhs.gov/040902p1*.
7. US Census Bureau: Population estimates. Retrieved from *www.census.gov/popest/estimates.php*.
8. Bhalla R, Yongue BG, Currie BP, et al: Improving primary percutaneous coronary intervention performance in an urban minority population using a quality improvement approach, *Am J Med Qual* 25:370, 2010.
*9. Cruz-Flores S, Rabinstein A, Biller J, et al: Racial-ethnic disparities in stroke care: the American experience: a statement for healthcare professionals from the American Heart Association/American Stroke Association, *Stroke* 42:2091, 2011.
*10. Byrne SK, Mary ES, DeShields T: Factors associated with why African-American women from one urban county use mammography services less, *J Natl Black Nurses Assoc* 22:8, 2011.
11. Health policy brief: achieving equity in health, *Health Affairs*. Retrieved from *www.healthaffairs.org/healthpolicybriefs/brief.php?brief_id=53*.
*12. National Cancer Institute, Center to Reduce Cancer Health Disparities: Examples of health disparities. Retrieved from *http://crchd.cancer.gov/disparities/examples.html#C4*.
13. Pfeifer G: Finding solutions to advance rural health, *Am J Nurs* 111:15, 2011.
14. Galinsky T, Feng HA, Streit J, et al: Risk factors associated with patient assaults of home healthcare workers, *Rehabil Nurs* 35:206, 2010.
*15. LaVeist T, Pollack K, Thorpe R, et al: Place, not race: disparities dissipate in southwest Baltimore when blacks and whites live under similar conditions, *Health Affairs* 30:1880, 2011.
16. Robert Woods Johnson Foundation: Health policy brief: achieving equity in health, *Health Affairs*. Retrieved from *http://rwjf.org/files/research/72893.disparities.pdf*.
17. Henry Kaiser Family Foundation: The uninsured: key facts about Americans without health insurance. Retrieved from *www.kff.org/uninsured/upload/7451-07.pdf*.
18. Centers for Disease Control and Prevention: Health disparities in cancer. Retrieved from *www.cdc.gov/cancer/healthdisparities/index.htm*.
19. Kones R: Recent advances in the management of chronic stable angina I: approach to the patient, diagnosis, pathophysiology, risk stratification, and gender disparities, *Vasc Health Risk Manag* 9:635, 2010.
*20. Choi NG, Ha JH: Relationship between spouse/partner support and depressive symptoms in older adults: gender differences, *Aging Ment Health* 15:307, 2011.
21. He J, Efron JE: Screening for colorectal cancer, *Adv Surg* 45:31, 2011.
22. Institute of Medicine of The National Academies: *The health of lesbian, gay, bisexual, and transgender people: building a foundation for better understanding*, Washington, DC, 2011, National Academies Press. Retrieved from *www.nap.edu*.
23. Narayan MC: Culture's effects on pain assessment and management, *Am J Nurs* 110:38, 2010.
24. Bralock AR, Farr NB, Kay J, et al: Issues in community-based care among homeless minorities, *J Natl Black Nurses Assoc* 22:57, 2011.

*Evidence-based information for clinical practice.

25. Centers for Disease Control and Prevention, Office of Minority Health & Health Disparities: American Indian and Alaska Native (AI/AN) populations. Retrieved from *www.cdc.gov/omhd/Populations/AIAN/AIAN.htm.*

26. Royse D, Dignan M: Fatalism and cancer screening in Appalachian Kentucky, *Fam Community Health* 34:126, 2011.

27. Li C, Balluz LS, Okoro CA, et al: Surveillance of certain health behaviors and conditions among states and selected local areas—Behavioral Risk Factor Surveillance System, United States, 2009, *MMWR Surveill Summ* 19:1, 2011.

28. Lopez-Class M, Castro FG, Ramirez AG: Conceptions of acculturation: a review and statement of critical issues, *Soc Sci Med* 72:1555, 2011.

29. Giger JN, Davidhizar RE: *Transcultural nursing: assessment and intervention*, ed 6, St Louis, 2012, Mosby.

30. Douglas MK, Pierce JU, Rosenkoetter M, et al: Standards of practice for culturally competent nursing care: 2011 update, *J Transcult Nurs* 22:317, 2011.

31. Andrews MM, Boyle JS: *Transcultural concepts in nursing care*, ed 5, Philadelphia, 2008, Lippincott Williams & Wilkins.

32. Gilliss CL, Powell DL, Carter B: Recruiting and retaining a diverse workforce in nursing: from evidence to best practice to policy, *Policy Polit Nurs Pract* 11:294, 2010.

*33. Karve SJ, Balkishnan R, Mohammad YM: Racial/ethnic disparities in emergency department waiting time for stroke patients in the United States, *J Stroke Cerebrovasc Dis* 20:30, 2011.

34. Sartori P: Exploring how to address patients' spiritual needs in practice, *Nurs Times* 106:23, 2010.

35. Maxwell J, Cortes DE, Schneider KL, et al: Massachusetts' health care reform increases access to care for Hispanics, but disparities remain, *Health Affairs* (Millwood) 30:1451, 2011.

36. Hall E: Proxemics: the study of man's spatial relationships. In Gladstone I, editor: *Man's image in medicine and anthropology*, New York, 1963, New York International University Press. (Classic)

*37. Singh GK, Siahpush M, Hiatt RA, et al: Dramatic increases in obesity and overweight prevalence and body mass index increase among ethnic-immigrant and social class groups in the United States, 1976-2008, *J Community Health* 36:94, 2011.

*38. Guh A, Sosa L, Hadler L, et al: Missed opportunities to prevent tuberculosis in foreign-born people, Connecticut, 2005-2008, *Int J Tuberc Lung Dis* 15:1044, 2011.

39. Centers for Disease Control and Prevention: Refugee health guidelines. Retrieved from *www.cdc.gov/immigrantrefugeehealth/guidelines/refugee-guidelines.html.*

40. Clark L, Calvillo E, dela Cruz F, et al: Cultural competencies for graduate nursing education, *J Profess Nurs* 127:133, 2011.

41. Higginbottom GM, Richter MS, Mogale RS, et al: Identification of nursing assessment models/tools validated in clinical practice for use with diverse ethno-cultural groups: an integrative review of the literature, *BMC Nurs* 10:16, 2011.

RESOURCES

American Association of Colleges of Nursing, Cultural Competency in Nursing Education
www.aacn.nche.edu/education-resources/cultural-competency
Center for Cross-Cultural Research
www.wwu.edu/culture
Cross Cultural Health Care Program
www.xculture.org
Health Literacy Universal Precautions Toolkit
www.nchealthliteracy.org/toolkit
National Center for Cultural Competence
http://nccc.georgetown.edu
National Partnership for Action to End Health Disparities
https://minorityhealth.hhs.gov/npa
Office of Minority Health
https://minorityhealth.hhs.gov
Think Cultural Health: Advancing Health Equity at Every Point of Contact
https://www.thinkculturalhealth.hhs.gov
Transcultural C.A.R.E. Associates
www.transculturalcare.net
Transcultural Nursing Society
www.tcns.org

Strength does not come from physical capacity.
It comes from an indomitable will.
Mahatma Gandhi

Health History and Physical Examination

Jennifer Saylor and Linda Bucher

evolve WEBSITE

LEARNING OUTCOMES

1. Explain the purpose, components, and techniques related to a patient's health history and physical examination.
2. Obtain a nursing history using a functional health pattern format.
3. Select appropriate techniques of inspection, palpation, percussion, and auscultation for physical examination of a patient.
4. Differentiate among comprehensive, focused, and emergency types of assessment in terms of indications, purposes, and components.

KEY TERMS

auscultation, p. 42
database, p. 36
functional health patterns, p. 38

inspection, p. 41
nursing history, p. 37
objective data, p. 37

palpation, p. 41
percussion, p. 41
subjective data, p. 37

You will obtain a patient's health history and perform a physical examination during the assessment phase of the nursing process. The findings of your assessment (1) contribute to a database that identifies the patient's current and past health status and (2) provide a baseline against which future changes can be evaluated. The purpose of the nursing assessment is to enable you to make clinical judgments or diagnoses about your patient's health status.[1] Assessment is identified as the first step of the nursing process, but it is performed continually throughout the nursing process to validate nursing diagnoses, evaluate nursing interventions, and determine whether patient outcomes and goals have been met.

The language of assessment is complex, with many overlapping and confusing terms. In this text, *assessment* describes a hands-on data collection process, whereas a *database* identifies a specific list of information (data) to be collected. For example, a *comprehensive database* would be completed for a patient who is being admitted to a hospital by doing a physical examination, a health history, and a psychosocial assessment.

DATA COLLECTION

In the broadest sense, the database is all the health information about a patient. This includes the nursing history and physical examination, the medical history and physical examination, results of laboratory and diagnostic tests, and information contributed by other health professionals. The nurse and physician both perform a patient history and a physical examination, but they use different formats and analyze the data based on their discipline's focus.

Medical Focus

A *medical history* is designed to collect data to be used primarily by the physician to determine risk for disease and diagnose medical conditions. The medical history is usually collected by a member of the health care team (e.g., physician, advanced practice nurse [APN], resident, physician's assistant, medical student). The health care provider's physical examination and laboratory and diagnostic tests assist in establishing medical

Reviewed by Misty Hobart, RN, MSN, ARNP, Department Chair, Nursing, Spokane Community College, Spokane, Washington; and Vera Kunte, RN-BC, MSN, Nurse Educator, Thomas Edison State College, Cary Edwards School of Nursing, Trenton, New Jersey.

diagnoses and evaluating treatments. The information collected and reported by the health care provider is also used by nurses and other members of the health care team (e.g., pharmacist, physical therapist, dietitian, social worker) within the focus of their care. For example, the abnormal results of a neurologic examination by an APN may assist in the diagnosis of a stroke. You may use the same results of the neurologic examination to identify a nursing diagnosis of risk for falls. A physical therapist may also use this information to plan therapy involving exercise and ambulatory aids.

Nursing Focus

The focus of nursing care is the diagnosis and treatment of human responses to actual or potential health problems or life processes. The information obtained from the nursing history and physical examination is used to determine the patient's strengths and responses to a health problem. For example, for the patient with a medical diagnosis of diabetes mellitus, the patient's responses may include anxiety or a lack of knowledge about self-management of the condition. This patient may also experience the physical response of fluid volume deficit because of the abnormal fluid loss caused by hyperglycemia. These human responses to the condition of diabetes are diagnosed and treated by nurses. During the nursing history interview and physical examination, you will obtain and record the necessary data to support the identification of nursing diagnoses (Fig. 3-1).

Types of Data

The database includes both subjective and objective data. Subjective data, also known as *symptoms,* are collected by interviewing the patient and/or caregiver during the nursing history. This type of data includes information that can be described or verified only by the patient or caregiver. It is what the person tells you either spontaneously or in response to direct questioning.

Objective data, also known as *signs,* are data that can be observed or measured. You obtain this type of data using inspection, palpation, percussion, and auscultation during the physical examination. Objective data are also acquired by diagnostic testing. Usually subjective data are obtained by interview, and objective data are obtained by physical examination.

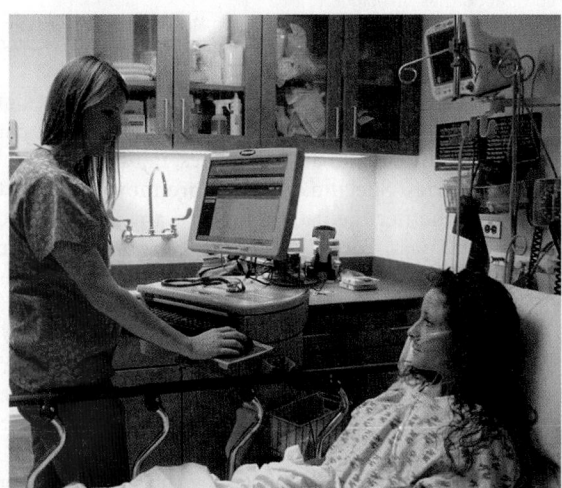

FIG. 3-1 Obtaining and recording data from a nursing history and physical examination using a computer.

However, patients often provide subjective data while you are performing the physical examination. You will also observe objective signs while interviewing the patient. All of the findings related to a specific problem, whether subjective or objective, are known as *clinical manifestations* of that problem.

Interview Considerations

The purpose of the patient interview is to obtain a health history (i.e., subjective data) about the patient's past and present health state. Effective communication is a key factor in the interview process. Creating a climate of trust and respect is critical to establishing a therapeutic relationship.[2] You need to communicate acceptance of the patient as an individual by using an open, responsive, nonjudgmental approach. You communicate not only through language but also in your manner of dress, gestures, and body language. Modes of communication are learned through one's culture, influencing not only the words, gestures, and postures one uses, but also the nature of information that is shared with others (see Chapter 2). In addition to understanding the principles of effective communication, you need to develop a personal style of relating to patients. Although no single style fits all people, your wording of questions can increase the probability of eliciting the needed information. The ease of asking questions, particularly those related to sensitive areas such as sexual functioning, comes with experience.

The amount of time you need to complete a nursing history varies with the format used and your experience. The nursing history may be completed in one or several sessions, depending on the setting and the patient. For example, you may need to plan several short sessions for an older adult patient with a low energy level to allow time for the patient to provide the needed information. You must also make a judgment about the amount of information collected on initial contact with the patient. In interviews with patients with chronic disease, patients in pain, and patients in emergency situations, ask only those questions that are pertinent to a specific problem. You can complete the health history interview at a more appropriate time.

Judge the reliability of the patient as a historian. An older adult may give a false impression about his or her mental status because of a prolonged response time or visual and hearing impairments. The complexity and long duration of health problems may make it difficult for an older adult or a chronically ill younger patient to be an accurate historian.

It is important for you to determine the patient's priority concerns and expectations, since your priorities may be different from the patient's. For example, your priority may be to complete the health history, whereas the patient is interested only in relief from symptoms. Until the patient's priority need is met, you will probably be unsuccessful in obtaining complete and accurate data.

Symptom Investigation

At any time during the assessment the patient may report a symptom such as pain, fatigue, or weakness. Symptoms experienced by the patient are not necessarily observed, so the symptom must be investigated. Table 3-1 shows a mnemonic (PQRST) to help you remember the areas to investigate if a symptom is reported. The information you receive may help determine the cause of the symptom. A common symptom that you will assess is pain (see Chapter 9). For example, if a patient states that he has "pain in his leg," you would assess and record the data using PQRST.

TABLE 3-1　INVESTIGATION OF PATIENT-REPORTED SYMPTOM

	Factor	Questions for Patient and Caregiver	Record
P	Precipitating and Palliative	Were there any events that came before the symptom? What makes it better? Worse? What have you done for the symptom? Did this help?	Influence of physical and emotional activities. Patient's attempts to alleviate (or treat) the symptom.
Q	Quality	Tell me what the symptom feels like (e.g., aching, dull, pressure, burning, stabbing).	Patient's own words (e.g., "Like a pinch or stabbing feeling").
R	Radiation	Where do you feel the symptom? Does it move to other areas?	Region of the body. Local or radiating, superficial or deep.
S	Severity	On a scale of 0-10, with 0 meaning no pain and 10 being the worst pain you could imagine, what number would you give your symptom?	Pain rating number (e.g., 5/0-10 scale).
T	Timing	When did the symptom start? Any particular time of day, week, month, or year? Has the symptom changed over time? Where are you and what are you doing when the symptom occurs?	Time of onset, duration, periodicity, and frequency. Course of symptoms. Where patient is and what patient is doing when the symptom occurs.

Has right midcalf pain that usually occurs at work when climbing stairs after lunch (**P**). Pain is alleviated by stopping and resting for 2 to 3 minutes. Patient states he has been "eating a banana every day for extra potassium" but "it hasn't helped" (**P**). Pain is described as "stabbing" and is non-radiating (**Q, R**). Pain is so severe (rating 9 on 0-10 scale) that patient cannot continue activity (**S**). Onset is abrupt, occurring once or twice daily. It last occurred yesterday while cutting the lawn (**T**).

Data Organization

Assessment data must be systematically obtained and organized so you can readily analyze and make judgments about the patient's health status and any health problems. Some assessment forms are organized using body systems. Although helpful, these types of forms may be incomplete because they omit areas such as health promotion behaviors, sleep, coping, and values.

Functional health patterns, developed by Gordon,[3] provide the framework used throughout this textbook for obtaining a nursing history. This format includes an initial collection of important health information followed by assessment of 11 areas of health status or function (see Table 3-2). Data organized in this format promote the identification of areas of wellness (or positive function), as well as health problems.[2]

CULTURALLY COMPETENT CARE

ASSESSMENT

The process of obtaining a health history and performing a physical examination is an intimate experience for both you and the patient. As noted earlier in the chapter, one's culture influences patterns of communication and what information is shared with others. During the interview and physical examination, be sensitive to issues of eye contact, space, modesty, and touching, as discussed in Chapter 2. Adhering to cultural practices related to male-female relationships and gender identification is especially important during the physical examination. To avoid violating any culturally based practices, ask the patient about cultural values and whether the patient would like to have someone present during the history or physical examination.[1]

NURSING HISTORY: SUBJECTIVE DATA

Important Health Information

Important health information provides an overview of past and present medical conditions and treatments. Past health history, medications, allergies, and surgery or other treatments are included in this part of the history.

DELEGATION DECISIONS

Assessment and Data Collection

Ongoing data collection is expected of all members of the health care team. In acute care the initial (admission) nursing assessment must be completed by the registered nurse (RN).

Role of Registered Nurse (RN)
- On admission, do a comprehensive assessment (see Table 3-6).
- Obtain patient's health history by interviewing patient and/or caregiver.
- Perform physical examination using inspection, palpation, percussion, and auscultation as appropriate.
- Document findings from the health history and physical examination in the patient's record.
- Organize patient data into functional health patterns.
- Develop and prioritize nursing diagnoses and collaborative problems for the patient.
- Throughout hospitalization, perform focused assessments based on patient's history or clinical manifestations (see Table 3-6).

Role of Licensed Practical/Vocational Nurse (LPN/LVN)
- Collect and document specific patient data as delegated by the RN (after the RN has developed the plan of care based on the admission assessment).
- Perform focused assessment based on patient's history, clinical manifestations, or as instructed by the RN (see Table 3-6).

Role of Unlicensed Assistive Personnel (UAP)
- Take and document vital signs.
- Measure and document patient's height and weight.
- Report abnormal vital signs to RN.
- Report patient's subjective complaints to RN.

Past Health History. The past health history provides information about the patient's prior state of health. Ask the patient about major childhood and adult illnesses, injuries, hospitalizations, and surgeries. Specific questions are more effective than simply asking whether the patient has had any illness or health problems in the past. For example, "Do you have a history of diabetes?" will elicit better information than "Do you have any chronic illnesses?"

Medications. Ask the patient for specific details related to past and current medications, including prescription drugs, over-the-counter drugs, vitamins, herbal products, and dietary supplements. Patients frequently do not consider herbal products and dietary supplements as drugs. It is important to specifically ask about their use because they can interact adversely with existing or newly prescribed medications (Complementary & Alternative Therapies box).

COMPLEMENTARY & ALTERNATIVE THERAPIES

Assessment of Use of Herbs and Dietary Supplements

Why Assessment Is Important
- Herbal products and dietary supplements may have side effects or may interact adversely with prescription or OTC medications.
- Patients at high risk for drug-herb interactions include those taking anticoagulant, antihypertensive, antidepressant-psychotic, or immune-regulating therapy and patients undergoing anesthesia.
- Many patients do not tell health care providers that they are using herbal products and dietary supplements. They may fear health care professionals will disapprove of their use.
- Many herbal preparations contain a variety of ingredients. Ask the patient or caregiver to bring labeled containers to the health care site to determine the composition of the products.

Nurse's Role
- Patients typically share this information with you if they are specifically asked.
- Create an accepting and nonjudgmental attitude when assessing use of or interest in herbal products or dietary supplements.
- Use open-ended questions such as, "What types of herbs, vitamins, or supplements do you take?" and "What effects have you noticed from using them?"
- Respond to patients with comments that invite an open-minded discussion.
- Document the use of any herbal product(s) or dietary supplements in the patient record.

Question older adult and chronically ill patients about medication routines. Polypharmacy; changes in absorption, metabolism, reaction to drugs, and elimination of drugs; and surgery and concurrent disease can pose serious potential problems for these patients.[4]

Allergies. Fully explore the patient's history of allergies to medications, contrast media, food, and the environment (e.g., latex, pollen). Include a detailed description of any allergic reaction(s) reported by the patient.

Surgery or Other Treatments. Record all surgeries along with the date of the event, the reason for the surgery, and the outcome. The outcome includes whether the problem was completely resolved or has residual effects. Be sure to ask about and record any blood products the patient received.

Functional Health Patterns

Assess the patient's functional health patterns to identify positive, dysfunctional, and potential dysfunctional health patterns. Dysfunctional health patterns result in nursing diagnoses, and potential dysfunctional patterns identify risk conditions for problems. In addition, you may identify patients with effective health function who express a desire for a higher level of wellness. Examples of specific questions to ask the patient related to the functional health patterns are presented in Table 3-2.

Health Perception–Health Management Pattern. Assessment of the health perception–health management functional health pattern focuses on the patient's perceived level of health and well-being and on personal practices for maintaining health. Ask the patient to describe his or her personal health and any concerns about it. Explore the patient's feelings of effectiveness at staying healthy by asking what helps and what hinders his or her well-being. Ask the patient to rate his or her health as excellent, good, fair, or poor. Be sure to record this information in the patient's own words.

Next, while being culturally sensitive, ask about the type of health care provider the patient uses. For example, if the patient is Native American, a medicine man may be considered the primary health care provider. If the patient is of Hispanic origin, a *curandero* (Hispanic healer who uses folk medicine, herbal products, or magic to treat patients) may be the primary health care provider (see Chapter 2).

The questions for this pattern also seek to identify risk factors by obtaining a thorough family history (e.g., cardiac disease, cancer, genetic disorders), history of personal health habits (e.g., tobacco, alcohol, drug use), and history of exposure to environmental hazards (e.g., asbestos). If the patient is hospitalized, ask about the expectations for this experience. Have the patient describe his or her understanding of the current health problem, including its onset, course, and treatment. These questions obtain information about a patient's knowledge of the health problem and ability to use appropriate resources to manage the problem.

Nutritional-Metabolic Pattern. The processes of ingestion, digestion, absorption, and metabolism are assessed in this pattern. Obtain a 24-hour diet recall from the patient to evaluate the quantity and quality of foods and fluids consumed. If a problem is identified, ask the patient to keep a 3-day food diary for a more careful analysis of dietary intake. Assess the impact of psychologic factors such as depression, anxiety, stress, and self-concept on nutrition. Additionally, determine socioeconomic and cultural factors such as food budget, who prepares the meals, and food preferences. Determine whether the patient's present condition has interfered with eating and appetite by exploring any symptoms of nausea, intestinal gas, or pain. Food allergies should be differentiated from food intolerances, such as lactose or gluten intolerance.

Elimination Pattern. Assess bowel, bladder, and skin function in this pattern. Ask the patient about the frequency of bowel and bladder activity, including laxative and diuretic use. The skin is assessed in the elimination pattern in terms of its excretory function.

Activity-Exercise Pattern. Assess the patient's usual pattern of exercise, work activity, leisure, and recreation. Question the patient about his or her ability to perform activities of daily living and note any specific problems. Table 3-2 includes a scale for rating the functional levels of common activities.

Sleep-Rest Pattern. This pattern describes the patient's perception of his or her pattern of sleep, rest, and relaxation in a 24-hour period. This information can be elicited by asking, "Do you feel rested when you wake up?"

Cognitive-Perceptual Pattern. Assessment of this pattern involves a description of all of the senses and cognitive functions. In addition, assess pain as a sensory perception in this pattern. (See Chapter 9 for details on pain assessment.) Ask the patient about any sensory deficits that affect the ability to perform activities of daily living. Discuss and record ways in which the patient compensates for any sensory-perceptual problems. To plan for patient teaching, ask the patient how he or she communicates best and what he or she understands about the illness and treatment plan. (See Chapter 4 for details on patient teaching.)

Self-Perception–Self-Concept Pattern. This pattern describes the patient's self-concept, which is critical in determining the way the person interacts with others. Included are attitudes about self, perception of personal abilities, body image, and general sense of worth. Ask the patient for a self-description

TABLE 3-2   HEALTH HISTORY

Functional Health Pattern Format

Demographic Data
Name, address, age, occupation, gender
Race, ethnicity, culture

Important Health Information
Past health history
Medications, supplements
Allergies
Surgery or other treatments

Health Perception–Health Management Pattern
1. Reason for visit?
2. General state of health?
3. Number of colds in past year?
4. Most important things done to keep healthy? Testicular self-examination? Colorectal cancer, hypertension, and cardiac disease risk screening? Papanicolaou (Pap) test? Immunizations such as tetanus, pneumonia, hepatitis, and flu vaccines?
5. Who is your primary care physician or health care provider?
6. Health compliance problems?
7. Cause of illness? Action taken? Results?
8. Things important to you while here?
9. Family health history (e.g., cardiovascular disease, hypertension, cancer, diabetes mellitus, psychiatric illness, genetic disorders)?
10. Illness and injury risk factors (e.g., sexual abuse, intimate partner abuse, violence, use of cigarettes or alcohol, substance abuse)?

Nutritional-Metabolic Pattern
1. Typical daily food intake (describe)? Supplements?
2. Typical daily fluid intake (describe)?
3. Weight loss or gain (amount, time span)?
4. Desired weight?
5. Appetite?
6. Food or eating: Discomfort? Diet restrictions?
7. Change in appetite with anxiety?
8. Heal well or poorly?
9. Skin problems: Lesions? Dryness?
10. Dentition: Dental problems? Well-fitting dentures?
11. Food preferences?
12. Food allergies?

Elimination Pattern
1. Bowel elimination pattern (describe): Frequency? Character? Discomfort? Laxatives? Enemas?
2. Urinary elimination pattern (describe): Frequency? Problem in control? Diuretics?
3. Any external devices?
4. Excess perspiration? Odor problems? Itching?

Activity-Exercise Pattern
1. Sufficient energy for desired or required activities?
2. Exercise pattern? Type? Regularity?
3. Spare time (leisure) activities?
4. Dyspnea? Chest pain? Palpitations? Stiffness? Aching? Weakness?
5. Perceived ability for (rate Functional Level 0-III for each):
   Feeding __ Cooking __ Grooming __
   Bed mobility __ Bathing __ Dressing __
   Toileting __ Shopping __ General mobility __

   Functional Levels
   Level 0: Full self-care
   Level I: Requires use of equipment or device
   Level II: Requires assistance or supervision from another person
   Level III: Is dependent and does not participate

Sleep-Rest Pattern
1. Generally rested and ready for daily activities after sleep?
2. Sleep onset problems? Aids? Dreams (nightmares)? Early awakening?
3. Usual sleep rituals?
4. Usual sleep pattern?

Cognitive-Perceptual Pattern
1. Hearing difficulty? Hearing aids?
2. Vision? Wear glasses? Last checked?
3. Any change in taste? Any change in smell?
4. Any recent change in memory?
5. Easiest way to learn things?
6. Any discomfort? Pain (rating on scale of 0-10)? How managed?
7. Ability to communicate?
8. Understanding of illness?
9. Understanding of treatments?

Self-Perception–Self-Concept Pattern
1. Self-description? Self-perception?
2. Effect of illness on self-image?
3. Relieving factors?

Role-Relationship Pattern
1. Live alone? Family/caregiver? Family structure diagram?
2. Difficult family problems?
3. Family problem solving?
4. Family dependence on you for things? How managing?
5. Family's and others' feelings about illness or hospitalization?*
6. Problems with children? Difficulty handling?*
7. Belong to social groups? Have close friends? Feel lonely (frequency)?
8. Work (school) satisfaction? Income sufficient for needs?*
9. Feel part of or isolated from neighborhood where living?

Sexuality-Reproductive Pattern
1. Any changes or problems in sexual relations?*
2. Effect of illness?
3. Use of contraceptives? Problems?
4. When menstruation started? Last menstrual period? Menstrual problems? Gravida? Para?†
5. Effect of present condition or treatment on sexuality?
6. Sexually transmitted infections?

Coping–Stress Tolerance Pattern
1. Tense a lot of the time? What helps? Use any medications, drugs, alcohol?
2. Have someone to confide in? Available to you now?
3. Recent life changes?
4. Problem-solving techniques? Effective?

Value-Belief Pattern
1. Satisfied with life?
2. Religion important in your life?
3. Conflict between treatment and beliefs?

Other
1. Other important issues?
2. Questions?

Modified from Gordon M: *Manual of nursing diagnosis*, ed 12, Boston, 2010, Jones & Bartlett.
*If appropriate.
†For women.

and about how his or her health condition affects self-concept. Patients' expressions of hopelessness or loss of control frequently reflect an inability to care for oneself.

Role-Relationship Pattern. This pattern reveals the patient's roles and relationships, including major responsibilities. Ask the patient to describe family, social, and work roles and relationships and to rate his or her performance of the expected behaviors related to these. Determine whether patterns in these roles and relationships are satisfactory or whether strain is evident. Note the patient's feelings about how the present condition affects his or her roles and relationships.

Sexuality-Reproductive Pattern. This pattern describes satisfaction or dissatisfaction with personal sexuality and describes reproductive issues. Assessing this pattern is important because many illnesses, surgical procedures, and medications affect sexual function. A patient's sexual and reproductive concerns may be expressed, teaching needs and treatable problems may be identified, and normal growth and development may be monitored through information obtained in this pattern.

Obtaining information related to sexuality may be difficult for you. However, it is important to take a health history and screen for sexual function and dysfunction in order to provide information or refer the patient to a more experienced professional.

Coping–Stress Tolerance Pattern. This pattern describes the patient's general coping pattern and the effectiveness of the coping mechanisms. Assessment of this pattern involves analyzing the specific stressors or problems that confront the patient, the patient's perception of the stressors, and the patient's response to the stressors. Document any major losses or stressors experienced by the patient in the previous year. Note strategies used by the patient to deal with stressors and relieve tension, as well as individuals and groups that make up the patient's social support networks.

Value-Belief Pattern. This pattern describes the values, goals, and beliefs (including spiritual) that guide health-related choices. Document the patient's ethnic background and the effects of culture and beliefs on health practices. Note and honor the patient's wishes about continuation of religious or spiritual practices and the use of religious articles.

PHYSICAL EXAMINATION: OBJECTIVE DATA

General Survey

After the nursing history, make a *general survey statement*. This is your general impression of a patient, including behavioral observations. This initial survey is considered a scanning procedure that begins with your first encounter with the patient and continues during the health history interview.

Although you may include other data that seem pertinent, the major areas included in the general survey statement are (1) body features, (2) mental state, (3) speech, (4) body movements, (5) obvious physical signs, (6) nutritional status, and (7) behavior. Vital signs and body mass index (BMI) (calculated from height and weight [kg/m^2]) may be included. The following is a sample of a general survey statement:

A.H. is a 34-year-old Hispanic woman, BP 130/84, P 88, R 18. No distinguishing body features. Alert but anxious. Speech rapid with trailing thoughts. Wringing hands and shuffling feet during interview. Skin flushed, hands clammy. Overweight rela-

tive to height (BMI = 28.3 kg/m^2). Sits with eyes downcast and shoulders slumped and avoids eye contact.

Physical Examination

The *physical examination* is the systematic assessment of a patient's physical status. Throughout the physical examination, explore any positive findings using the same criteria used during the investigation of a symptom in the nursing history (see Table 3-1). A *positive finding* indicates that the patient has or has had the particular problem or sign under discussion (e.g., if the patient with jaundice has an enlarged liver, it is a positive finding). Relevant information about this problem should then be gathered.

Negative findings may also be significant. A *pertinent negative* is the absence of a sign or symptom usually associated with a problem. For example, peripheral edema is common with advanced liver disease. If edema is not present in a patient with advanced liver disease, this should be specifically noted as "no peripheral edema."

Techniques. Four major techniques are used in performing the physical examination: inspection, palpation, percussion, and auscultation. The techniques are usually performed in this sequence, except for the abdominal examination (inspection, auscultation, percussion, and palpation). Performing percussion and palpation of the abdomen before auscultation can alter bowel sounds and produce false findings. Not every assessment area requires the use of all four assessment techniques (e.g., musculoskeletal system requires only inspection and palpation).

Inspection. Inspection is the visual examination of a part or region of the body to assess normal conditions or deviations. Inspection is more than just looking. This technique is deliberate, systematic, and focused. Compare what is seen with the known, generally visible characteristics of the body part that you are inspecting. For example, most 30-year-old men have hair on their legs. Absence of hair may indicate a vascular problem and the need for further investigation, or it may be normal for a patient of a particular ethnicity (e.g., Filipino men have little body hair). Always compare one side of the patient's body to the other to assess bilaterally for any abnormal findings.

Palpation. Palpation is the examination of the body using touch. Using light and deep palpation can yield information related to masses, pulsations, organ enlargement, tenderness or pain, swelling, muscular spasm or rigidity, elasticity, vibration of voice sounds, crepitus, moisture, and texture. Different parts of the hand are more sensitive for specific assessments. For example, use the palmar surface (base of fingers) to feel vibrations, the dorsa (backs) of your hands and fingers to assess temperature, and tips of your fingers to palpate the abdomen[1] (Fig. 3-2).

Percussion. Percussion is a technique that produces a sound and vibration to obtain information about the underlying area (Fig. 3-3). Evaluate the sounds and vibrations relative to the underlying structures. Deviation from an expected sound may indicate a problem. For example, the usual percussion sound in the right lower quadrant of the abdomen is tympany. Dullness in this area may indicate a problem that should be investigated. (Specific percussion sounds of various body parts and regions are discussed in the appropriate assessment chapters.)

Auscultation. Auscultation is listening to sounds produced by the body with a stethoscope to assess normal conditions and deviations from normal. This technique is particularly useful in evaluating sounds from the heart, lungs, abdomen, and vascular

FIG. 3-2 Palpation is the examination of the body using touch. (From Jarvis C: *Physical examination and health assessment*, ed 6, St Louis, 2012, Saunders.)

FIG. 3-3 Percussion technique. Tapping the interphalangeal joint. Only the middle finger of the nondominant hand should be in contact with the skin surface.

FIG. 3-4 Auscultation is listening to sounds produced by the body to assess normal conditions and deviations from normal.

TABLE 3-3	EQUIPMENT FOR PHYSICAL EXAMINATION*
• Stethoscope (with bell and diaphragm or a dual-purpose diaphragm; tubing 15-18 inches [38-46 cm]) • Watch (with second hand or digital) • Blood pressure cuff • Eye chart (wall chart or Snellen pocket eye card)	• Pocket flashlight • Tongue blades • Cotton balls • Percussion hammer • Alcohol swabs • Patient gown • Paper cup with water • Examining table or bed

*These are examples of commonly used equipment; other equipment may be used depending on the situation.

system. The bell of the stethoscope is more sensitive to low-pitched sounds (e.g., heart murmurs). The diaphragm of the stethoscope is more sensitive to high-pitched sounds (e.g., bowel sounds). Some stethoscopes have only a diaphragm, designed to transmit low- and high-pitched sounds. To listen for low-pitched sounds, hold the diaphragm lightly on the skin. For high-pitched sounds, press the diaphragm firmly on the skin[1] (Fig. 3-4). (Specific auscultatory sounds and techniques are discussed in the appropriate assessment chapters.)

Equipment. The equipment needed for the physical examination should be easily accessible (Table 3-3). Organizing equipment before the examination saves time and energy for you and the patient. (The uses of specific equipment are discussed in the appropriate assessment chapters.)

Organization of Examination. Perform the physical examination systematically and efficiently. Provide explanations to the patient as the examination proceeds, and consider the patient's comfort, safety, and privacy. You are less likely to forget a procedure, a step in the sequence, or a portion of the body if you follow the same sequence every time. Table 3-4 presents an outline for a physical examination that is organized and complete.

Adaptations of the physical examination are often useful for the older adult patient, who may have age-related problems such as decreased mobility, limited energy, and perceptual changes.[5] An outline listing some of the useful adaptations is found in Table 3-5.

Recording Physical Examination. Only record abnormal findings during the actual examination. At the conclusion of the examination, combine the normal and abnormal findings in a carefully compiled record. An example of how to record findings of a physical examination of a healthy adult can be found in eTable 3-1 on the website for this chapter. See Table 5-6 to locate age-related assessment findings in the book.

TYPES OF ASSESSMENT

Various types of assessment are used to obtain information about a patient. These approaches can be divided into three types: comprehensive, focused, and emergency (Table 3-6 on p. 45). You need to decide what type of assessment to perform based on the clinical situation (e.g., admission history and physical examination, start of shift, throughout shift). Sometimes the health care agency provides guidelines, and other times it is a nursing judgment.

Comprehensive Assessment

A *comprehensive assessment* includes a detailed health history and physical examination of one body system or many body systems (see Table 3-6). This is typically done on admission to the hospital or onset of care in a primary care setting.

TABLE 3-4 OUTLINE FOR PHYSICAL EXAMINATION

1. General Survey
Observe general state of health (patient is seated).
- Body features
- Level of consciousness and orientation
- Speech
- Body movements and carriage
- Physical appearance
- Nutritional status
- Stature

2. Vital Signs
Record vital signs.
- Blood pressure—both arms for comparison
- Apical/radial pulse
- Respiration
- Temperature
- Record height and weight; calculate body mass index (BMI)

3. Integument
Inspect and palpate skin for the following:
- Color
- Breakdown, lacerations, lesions
- Scars, tattoos, piercings
- Bruises, rash
- Edema
- Moisture
- Texture
- Temperature
- Turgor
- Vascularity

Inspect and palpate nails for the following:
- Color
- Lesions
- Size
- Flexibility
- Shape
- Angle
- Capillary refill time

4. Head and Neck
Inspect and palpate head for the following:
- Shape and symmetry of skull
- Masses
- Tenderness
- Hair
- Scalp
- Skin
- Temporal arteries
- Temporomandibular joint
- Sensory (CN V, light touch, pain)
- Motor (CN VII, shows teeth, purses lips, raises eyebrows)
- Looks up, wrinkles forehead (CN VII)
- Raises shoulders against resistance (CN XI)

Inspect and palpate (occasionally auscultate) neck for the following:
- Skin (vascularity and visible pulsations)
- Symmetry
- Range of motion
- Pulses and bruits (carotid)
- Midline structure (trachea, thyroid gland, cartilage)
- Lymph nodes (preauricular, postauricular, occipital, mandibular, tonsillar, submental, anterior and posterior cervical, infraclavicular, supraclavicular)

Inspect and lightly palpate eyes for the following:
- Visual acuity
- Eyebrows
- Position and movement of eyelids (CN VII)
- Visual fields
- Extraocular movements (CN III, IV, VI)
- Cornea, sclera, conjunctiva
- Pupillary response (CN III)
- Red reflex

Inspect and palpate nose and sinuses for the following:
- External nose: shape, blockage
- Internal nose: patency of nasal passages, shape, turbinates or polyps, discharge
- Frontal and maxillary sinuses

Inspect and palpate ears for the following:
- Placement
- Pinna
- Auditory acuity (whispered voice, ticking watch) (CN VIII)
- Mastoid process
- Auditory canal
- Tympanic membrane

Inspect and palpate mouth for the following:
- Lips (symmetry, lesions, color)
- Buccal mucosa (Stensen's and Wharton's ducts)
- Teeth (absence, state of repair, color)
- Gums (color, receding from teeth)
- Tongue for strength (asymmetry, ability to stick out tongue, side to side, fasciculations) (CN XII)
- Palates
- Tonsils and pillars
- Uvular elevation (CN IX)
- Posterior pharynx
- Gag reflex (CN IX and X)
- Jaw strength (CN V)
- Moisture
- Color
- Floor of mouth

5. Extremities
Observe size and shape, symmetry and deformity, involuntary movements. Inspect and palpate arms, fingers, wrists, elbows, shoulders for the following:
- Strength
- Range of motion
- Joint pain
- Swelling
- Pulses (radial, brachial)
- Sensation (light touch, pain, temperature)
- Test reflexes: triceps, biceps, brachioradialis

Inspect and palpate legs for the following:
- Strength
- Range of motion
- Joint pain
- Swelling, edema
- Hair distribution
- Sensation (light touch, pain, temperature)
- Pulses (dorsalis pedis, posterior tibialis)
- Test reflexes: patellar, achilles, plantar

6. Posterior Thorax
Inspect for muscular development, scoliosis, respiratory movement, approximation of AP diameter.
- Palpate for symmetry of respiratory movement, tenderness of CVA, spinous processes, tumors or swelling, tactile fremitus
- Percuss for pulmonary resonance
- Auscultate for breath sounds
- Auscultate for egophony, bronchophony, and whispered pectoriloquy

7. Anterior Thorax
- Assess breasts for configuration, symmetry, dimpling of skin
- Assess nipples for rash, direction, inversion, retraction
- Inspect for apical impulse, other precordial pulsations
- Palpate the apical impulse and the precordium for thrills, lifts, heaves, tenderness
- Inspect neck for venous distention, pulsations, waves
- Palpate lymph nodes in the subclavian, axillary, and brachial areas
- Palpate breasts
- Auscultate for rate and rhythm; character of S_1 and S_2 in the aortic, pulmonic, Erb's point, tricuspid, mitral areas; bruits at carotid, epigastrium

AP, Anteroposterior; *CN,* cranial nerve; *CVA,* costovertebral angle.

Continued

TABLE 3-4   OUTLINE FOR PHYSICAL EXAMINATION—cont'd

8. Abdomen
- Inspect for scars, shape, symmetry, bulging, muscular position and condition of umbilicus, movements (respiratory, pulsations, presence of peristaltic waves)
- Auscultate for peristalsis (i.e., bowel sounds), bruits
- Percuss then palpate to confirm positive findings; check liver (size, tenderness), spleen, kidney (size, tenderness), urinary bladder (distention)
- Palpate femoral pulses, inguinofemoral nodes, and abdominal aorta

9. Neurologic

Observe motor status.
- Gait
- Toe walk
- Heel walk
- Drift

Observe coordination:
- Finger to nose
- Romberg sign
- Heel to opposite shin

Observe the following:
- Proprioception (position sense of great toe)

10. Genitalia*

Male External Genitalia
- Inspect penis, noting hair distribution, prepuce, glans, urethral meatus, scars, ulcers, eruptions, structural alterations, discharge
- Inspect epidermis of perineum, rectum
- Inspect skin of scrotum; palpate for descended testes, masses, pain

Female External Genitalia
- Inspect hair distribution; mons pubis, labia (minora and majora); urethral meatus; Bartholin's, urethral, Skene's glands (may also be palpated, if indicated); introitus; any discharge
- Assess for presence of cystocele, prolapse
- Inspect perineum, rectum

*If the nurse has the appropriate education, the speculum and bimanual examination of women and the prostate gland examination of men would be performed after this inspection.

TABLE 3-5   GERONTOLOGIC ASSESSMENT DIFFERENCES

Adaptations in Physical Assessment Techniques

General Approach
Keep patient warm and comfortable because loss of subcutaneous fat decreases ability to stay warm. Adapt positioning to physical limitations. Avoid unnecessary changes in position. Perform as many activities as possible in the position of comfort for the patient.

Skin
Handle with care because of fragility and loss of subcutaneous fat.

Head and Neck
Provide a quiet environment free from distraction because of possible sensory impairments (e.g., decreased vision, hearing).

Extremities
Use gentle movements and reinforcement techniques. Avoid having patient hop on one foot or perform deep knee bends because of patient's limited range of motion of the extremities, decreased reflexes, and diminished sense of balance.

Thorax
Adapt examination for changes related to decreased force of expiration, weakened cough reflex, and shortness of breath.

Abdomen
Use caution in palpating patient's liver because it is readily accessible because of a thinner, softer abdominal wall. The older adult patient may have diminished pain perception in the abdominal wall.

Focused Assessment

A *focused assessment* is a more abbreviated history and examination. It is used to evaluate the status of previously identified problems and monitor for signs of new problems. It can be done when a specific problem (e.g., pneumonia) is identified. The patient's clinical manifestations should alert you to the appropriate focused assessment. For example, abdominal pain indicates the need for a focused assessment of the abdomen. Some problems necessitate a focused assessment of more than one body system. A complaint of headache may indicate the need to do musculoskeletal, neurologic, and head and neck examinations. Examples of focused assessments for various body systems can be found in eTable 3-3 on the website for this chapter.

Emergency Assessment

In an emergency or critical situation an *emergency assessment* may be done. This involves the rapid examination and specific questioning of a patient while maintaining vital functions.

Using Assessment Approaches

Assessment in a hospital inpatient setting, particularly in acute care, is markedly different from assessment in other settings. Focused assessment of the hospitalized patient is frequent and performed by many different people. Such a team approach demands a high degree of consistency among different health care professionals.

As you provide ongoing care for a patient, you will be constantly refining your mental image of the patient. As you gain experience, you will form a mental image of a patient's status from a few basic details, such as "85-year-old woman admitted for COPD [chronic obstructive pulmonary disease] exacerbation." Your picture of her becomes clearer as you receive a more complete verbal report, such as length of stay, recent laboratory results, physical findings, and vital signs. Next, perform your own assessment using a focused approach. During your assessment, you will confirm or revise the findings that you read in the medical record and what you heard from other health care professionals.

Keep in mind that the process does not end once you have done your first assessment on a patient during your rounds. You will continue to gather information about all your patients throughout your shift. Everything that you learned previously about each patient is considered in the light of new information. For example, when you are doing a respiratory assessment on your patient with COPD, you hear crackles in her lungs. This finding should lead you to do a cardiovascular assessment because cardiac problems (e.g., heart failure) can also cause crackles. As you gain experience, the importance of new findings will be more obvious to you. Assessment case

TABLE 3-6   TYPES OF ASSESSMENT

The following describes types of assessment that you may use in various situations.

Description	When and Where Performed	Where to Find in Book
Comprehensive • Detailed assessment of one body system or many body systems, including those not directly involved in presenting problem or admission diagnosis • Used for head-to-toe assessment	• Onset of care in primary or ambulatory care setting • On admission to hospital or long-term care setting • On initial home care visit	• Assessment chapters for each body system • Outline for physical examination (see Table 3-4) • Head-to-toe (total body) assessment checklist (see eTable 3-2, available on the website for this chapter)
Focused • Abbreviated assessment that focuses on one or more body systems that are the focus of care • Includes an assessment related to a specific problem (e.g., pneumonia, specific abnormal laboratory findings) • Monitors for signs of new problems	• Throughout hospital admission—at beginning of a shift and as needed throughout shift • Revisited in ambulatory care setting or home care setting	• Focused assessment boxes in each assessment chapter (all boxes available in eTable 3-3 on website) • Tables on nursing assessment of specific diseases throughout book
Emergency • Limited to assessing life-threatening conditions (e.g., inhalation injuries, anaphylaxis, myocardial infarction, shock, stroke) • Conducted to ensure survival; focuses on airway, breathing, circulation, and disability • After lifesaving interventions are initiated, perform brief systematic assessment to identify any and all other injuries or problems	• Performed in any setting when signs or symptoms of a life-threatening condition appear (e.g., emergency department, critical care unit, surgical setting)	• Chapter 69, Table 69-3 and Table 69-5 • Emergency management tables throughout the book and listed in Table 69-1

studies are integrated into all of the assessment chapters for this book to help you develop your assessment skills and knowledge.

Table 3-7 shows how you can perform different types of assessments based on a patient's progress through a given hospitalization. When a patient arrives at the emergency department in acute distress, you will perform an emergency assessment based on the principles of airway, breathing, circulation, disability, and exposure/environmental control (see Chapter 69, Table 69-3). Once the patient is stabilized, you can begin a focused assessment of the respiratory and related body systems. Once the patient is admitted, a comprehensive assessment of all body systems, whether or not they are involved in the current clinical problem, is obtained.

PROBLEM IDENTIFICATION AND NURSING DIAGNOSES

After completing the history and physical examination, analyze the data to develop a list of nursing diagnoses and collaborative problems. See Chapter 1 for a description of the nursing process, including the identification of nursing diagnoses and collaborative problems.

TABLE 3-7   CLINICAL APPLICATION OF VARIOUS TYPES OF ASSESSMENT

The following is an example of how various types of assessment would be used for a patient progressing from the emergency department to a clinical unit of a hospital.

Timeline	Type of Assessment
Emergency Department (ED)	
Patient arrives in acute respiratory distress.	Perform emergency assessment (see Table 69-3).
Problem is identified and critical interventions are performed; patient stabilizes.	Conduct a focused assessment of the respiratory and related body systems (e.g., cardiovascular). May begin comprehensive assessment of all body systems.
Clinical Unit	
Patient is admitted to a monitored clinical unit.	Complete comprehensive assessment of all body systems within proper timeframe.
Reassess throughout shift. New nurse arrives at change of shift.	Perform focused assessment of respiratory system and other related body systems (to determine if new problems have arisen).

BRIDGE TO NCLEX EXAMINATION

The number of the question corresponds to the same-numbered outcome at the beginning of the chapter.

1. The patient health history and physical examination provide the nurse with information to primarily
   a. diagnose a medical problem.
   b. investigate a patient's signs and symptoms.
   c. classify subjective and objective patient data.
   d. identify nursing diagnoses and collaborative problems.

2. The nurse would place information about the patient's concern that his illness is threatening his job security in which functional health pattern?
   a. Role-relationship
   b. Cognitive-perceptual
   c. Coping–stress tolerance
   d. Health perception–health management

3. The nurse is preparing to examine a patient's abdomen. Identify the proper order of the steps in the assessment of the abdomen, using the numbers 1-4 with 1 = the first technique and 4 = the last technique:
   ___Inspection
   ___Palpation
   ___Percussion
   ___Auscultation

4. Which situation would require the nurse to obtain a focused assessment *(select all that apply)*?
   a. A patient denies a current health problem.
   b. A patient reports a new symptom during rounds.
   c. A previously identified problem needs reassessment.
   d. A baseline health maintenance examination is required.
   e. An emergency problem is identified during physical examination.

1. d, 2. a, 3. 1, 4, 3, 2, 4. b, c.

⊖volve

For rationales to these answers and even more NCLEX review questions, visit *http://evolve.elsevier.com/Lewis/medsurg*.

REFERENCES

1. Jarvis C: *Physical examination and health assessment*, ed 6, St Louis, 2012, Saunders.
2. Wilson S, Giddens J: *Health assessment for nursing practice*, ed 4, St Louis, 2009, Mosby.
3. Gordon M: *Manual of nursing diagnosis*, ed 12, Boston, 2010, Jones & Bartlett.
4. Lehne R: *Pharmacology for nursing care*, ed 7, St Louis, 2010, Mosby.
5. Eliopoulos C: *Gerontological nursing*, ed 7, Philadelphia, 2009, Lippincott Williams & Wilkins.

*Tell me and I'll forget;
show me and I may remember;
involve me and I'll understand.*
Chinese proverb

Patient and Caregiver Teaching

Linda Bucher and Catherine N. Kotecki

evolve WEBSITE

http://evolve.elsevier.com/Lewis/medsurg

- NCLEX Review Questions
- Key Points
- Pre-Test
- Rationales for Bridge to NCLEX Examination Questions

- Concept Map Creator
- Glossary
- Content Updates

eFigures
- eFig. 4-1: Plan of care and education record

- eFig. 4-2: Supplemental plan of care—deficient knowledge

eTable
- eTable 4-1: Writing Learning Objectives/Goals

LEARNING OUTCOMES

1. Prioritize patient teaching goals for diverse patients and caregivers.
2. Analyze teaching implications related to the diverse needs of adult learners.
3. Apply strategies to manage challenges to nurse-teacher effectiveness.
4. Evaluate the role of the caregiver in patient teaching.
5. Apply the teaching-learning process to diverse patient populations.
6. Relate the physical, psychologic, and sociocultural characteristics of the patient and caregiver to the teaching-learning process.
7. Select appropriate teaching strategies for diverse patient populations.
8. Select appropriate methods to evaluate patient and caregiver teaching.

KEY TERMS

caregivers, p. 50
health literacy, p. 53
learning, p. 48
learning needs, p. 54

motivational interviewing, p. 48
positive reinforcement, p. 54
self-efficacy, p. 49

teaching, p. 48
teaching plan, p. 48
teaching process, p. 52

This chapter describes the process of patient and caregiver teaching. In addition, it discusses the strategies and methods that contribute to successful teaching and learning experiences.

ROLE OF PATIENT AND CAREGIVER TEACHING

Patient and caregiver (family member or significant other) teaching is an interactive and dynamic process that involves a change in a patient's knowledge, behavior, and/or attitude to maintain or improve health. You will find that teaching is one of your most challenging and rewarding roles. Teaching patients is a key nursing intervention that makes a difference in their lives.

General goals of patient teaching include health promotion, prevention of disease, management of illness, and appro-priate selection and use of treatment options. In patients with acute and chronic health problems, teaching can prevent complications and promote recovery, self-care, and independence. Seventy percent of the deaths in the United States are due to chronic illnesses, illnesses with which patients often live for many years.[1] Whether patients adequately manage their health problems and maintain quality of life depends on what they learn about their conditions and what they choose to do with this knowledge. Patients who understand their discharge teaching, including how to take their medicines and when to follow-up with their health care providers, are 30% less likely to be readmitted or visit the emergency department than patients who did not receive this information.[2]

Teaching may occur wherever you work. Although institutions may employ advanced practice nurses and patient educators to establish and oversee patient teaching programs, you

Reviewed by Kathleen M. Barta, RN, EdD, Associate Professor, University of Arkansas, Eleanor Mann School of Nursing, Fayetteville, Arkansas; Regina Kukulski, RN, MSN, ACNS, BC, Nurse Educator Consultant, Thomas Edison State College, Capital Health Medical Center, Trenton, New Jersey; and C. Denise Neill, RN, PhD, CNE, Assistant Professor and RN-BSN and MSN Program Coordinator, University of Houston–Victoria, Victoria, Texas.

are always responsible for patient and caregiver teaching.[3-5] It is a responsibility that cannot be delegated to unlicensed assistive personnel.

Every interaction with a patient and a caregiver is a potential *teachable moment*. On any given day, more informal opportunities to teach will occur than formal opportunities. Take advantage of all of these moments. For example, when you teach a patient with asthma how to use a peak flow meter, you do not require a formal teaching plan. However, when your patient has a specific learning need about health promotion or management of a health problem, you should develop a teaching plan. A teaching plan includes (1) assessment of the patient's ability, need, and readiness to learn; and (2) identification of problems that can be resolved with teaching. Then develop goals with the patient, provide teaching interventions, and evaluate the effectiveness of the teaching.

TEACHING-LEARNING PROCESS

Teaching is not just imparting information. Teaching is a process of deliberately arranging conditions to promote learning that results in a change in behavior.[6] Teaching can be a planned or informal experience. It uses a combination of methods such as instruction, counseling, and behavior modification.

Learning is acquiring knowledge and/or skills. It can result in a permanent change in a person.[6] Observation of this change is an indication that learning has occurred. Learning may also result in a potential or capability to change behavior. This is seen in a patient who understands the instruction and is fully informed, but chooses not to change behavior. In this case, teaching gives the patient the capability to make a decision to change behavior, but the decision is the patient's.

Although learning may occur without teaching, teaching helps to organize information and skills to make learning more efficient. In patient teaching the teaching-learning process involves the patient, the patient's caregiver(s), and you.

Adult Learner

Adult Learning Principles. Understanding how and why adults learn is important for you to effectively teach patients and their caregivers. Many of the theories of adult learning have risen from the work of Malcolm Knowles, who identified six principles of *andragogy* (adult learning) that are important for you to consider when teaching adults[7] (Table 4-1).

Models to Promote Health. When a change in health behaviors is recommended, patients and their caregivers may progress through a series of steps before they are willing or able to accept the change. Prochaska and Velicer proposed six stages of change in their *Transtheoretical Model of Health Behavior Change*[8] (Table 4-2). This model is frequently used to help patients stop smoking, manage diabetes, and lose weight.

Motivational interviewing (see *www.motivationalinterview.org*) uses nonconfrontational interpersonal communication techniques to motivate patients to change behavior.[9] This strategy includes the use of any intervention that enhances the

TABLE 4-1	ADULT LEARNING PRINCIPLES APPLIED TO PATIENT AND CAREGIVER TEACHING	
Principles	**Teaching Implications for the Nurse**	**Examples**
The learner's need to know	• Patients need to know why they should learn something, what they need to learn, and how it will benefit them. • Ask the patient questions such as, "What do you think you need to learn about this topic?"	Your patient and his caregiver have requested specific information on exercise guidelines after a heart attack.
The learner's readiness to learn	• Readiness and motivation to learn are high when facing new tasks. • Health crises provide opportunities for patients to learn and change behavior. • Stress and anxiety may interfere with learning, thus requiring frequent reinforcement of content.	While recovering from a transient ischemic attack, your patient tells you that she is ready to learn about the changes she needs to take to reduce her risk for stroke.
The learner's prior experiences	• Motivation is increased when patients already know something about the subject from past experiences. • Identification of past knowledge and experiences can help find familiar ground to increase patients' confidence.	Your patient needs to begin injections of enoxaparin (Lovenox). She tells you that she gives her father insulin injections and is ready to learn how to administer this medication.
The learner's motivation to learn	• Patients prefer to apply learning immediately. • Long-term goals may have less appeal than short-term goals. • Focus teaching on information that the patient views as being needed right now.	Your patient is scheduled to be discharged in the morning. Both she and her caregiver have received instruction on wound care and have watched the procedure. The caregiver tells you that he wants to perform the wound care this evening.
The learner's orientation to learning	• Patients seek out various resources for specific learning and prefer to have choices. • When the patient does not recognize the relevancy of the teaching, offer explanations of the value of the learning. • Teaching should target the specific problem or circumstance.	Your patient, who is newly diagnosed with diabetes mellitus, tells you that he is worried about the diet changes he will need to make. Share several options with him to learn about diet changes (e.g., cooking classes, Internet-based tutorials, individual sessions with the dietitian, brochures).
The learner's self-concept	• Patients need control and self-direction (sense of autonomy) to maintain their sense of self-worth. • Patients do not learn when they are treated like children and told what they must do.	Your patient has a temporary colostomy. She says she is not ready to look at the stoma. Work out a schedule with her for learning colostomy care that meets her need for control and prepares her for self-care.

TABLE 4-2   STAGES OF CHANGE IN TRANSTHEORETICAL MODEL

Stage	Patient Behavior	Nursing Implications
1. Precontemplation	Is not considering a change. Is not ready to learn.	Provide support, increase awareness of condition. Describe benefits of change and risks of not changing.
2. Contemplation	Thinks about a change. May verbalize recognition of need to change; says "I know I should," but identifies barriers.	Introduce what is involved in changing the behavior. Reinforce the stated need to change.
3. Preparation	Starts planning the change, gathers information, sets a date to initiate change, shares decision to change with others.	Reinforce the positive outcomes of change, provide information and encouragement, develop a plan, help set priorities, and identify sources of support.
4. Action	Begins to change behavior through practice. Tentative and may experience relapses.	Reinforce behavior with reward, encourage self-reward, discuss choices to help minimize relapses and regain focus. Help patient plan to deal with potential relapses.
5. Maintenance	Practices the behavior regularly. Able to sustain the change.	Continue to reinforce behavior. Provide additional teaching on the need to maintain change.
6. Termination	Change has become part of lifestyle. Behavior no longer considered a change.	Evaluate effectiveness of the new behavior. No further intervention needed.

Adapted from Prochaska J, Velicer W: The transtheoretical model of health behavior change, *Am J Health Promot* 12:38, 1997. (Classic)

patient's motivation for change (Table 4-3). The techniques used in motivational interviewing are linked to the stages of change as identified by Prochaska and Velicer.

During the process of change, relapse and recycling through the stages are expected. Sometimes patients do not change behaviors or return to previous behaviors after a period of change. This may indicate that the interventions used did not consider the patient's stage of change.[10] Identify the patient's current stage of readiness for change and the stage to which the patient is moving. Patients who are in the early stages of change need and use different kinds of motivational support than patients at later stages of change.

For example, a patient who smokes cigarettes who is hospitalized is often in the *precontemplation* or *contemplation* stage of change. In the precontemplation stage, patients are not concerned about their substance use and are not considering changing their behavior. During this stage, help the patient increase awareness of risks and problems related to smoking and create doubt about the use of cigarettes. Ask the patient what he or she thinks could happen if the behavior is continued, provide evidence of the problem (e.g., x-ray changes), and offer factual information about the risks of smoking. Although patients may not be ready to change behavior while experienc-

TABLE 4-3   KEY ASPECTS OF MOTIVATIONAL INTERVIEWING

- Listen rather than tell.
- Adjust to, rather than oppose, patient resistance.
- Express empathy through reflective listening.
- Focus on the positive. Do not criticize the patient.
- Gently persuade with the understanding that change is up to the patient.
- Focus on the patient's strengths to support the hope and optimism needed to make changes.
- Avoid argument and direct confrontation, which can cause defensiveness and a power struggle.
- Help the patient recognize the "gap" between where he or she is and where he or she hopes to be.

ing an acute health problem, the seeds of doubt are sown. In other cases, such as when a patient experiences a life-threatening condition (e.g., heart attack), there may be an immediate awareness of the problem and motivation to change.

A patient in the *contemplation* stage of change often experiences ambivalence. The patient understands that the behavior is a problem and that change is necessary. However, he or she believes that change is too difficult or that the pleasures of the behavior are worth the risks. This is seen in the patient who says, "I know that I have to stop smoking. This heart attack really scared me. I know I need to lose weight and start exercising, but I can't change everything all at once. Smoking helps me control my eating—I can't stop until I lose some weight." During this stage of change, help the patient consider the positive and negative aspects of his or her behavior (e.g., substance use), gently trying to tip the balance in favor of positive behavior. Helping the patient discover internal motivators in addition to those external motivators (e.g., second heart attack, lung disease) that push the patient toward change can move the patient from contemplating change to preparation and action. Throughout this process, emphasize the patient's personal choices and responsibilities for change.

As the patient moves from contemplation to *preparation*, a commitment to change is strengthened by helping the patient develop self-efficacy, which is the belief that one can succeed in a given situation. In this case it is the patient's belief that substance-use behaviors can be changed. Support even the smallest effort to change. Movement through action and maintenance stages of change requires continued support to increase the patient's involvement and participation in treatment. A comprehensive discussion of motivational interviewing is presented in the Treatment Improvement Protocols available at *www.ncbi.nlm.nih.gov/books/NBK14856*.

The resolution of acute health problems or discharge from the hospital often occurs before the patient moves to the preparation and action stages of change. As the patient develops readiness to change in the contemplative stage of change, continue to support him or her with referral to appropriate community and outpatient resources.

Nurse as Teacher

Required Competencies

Knowledge of Subject Matter. Although it is impossible to be an expert in all subject areas, develop confidence as a teacher by becoming knowledgeable about the subject to be taught. Information can be obtained through reliable sources such as journals and books. For example, if you are teaching patients about the management of hypertension, you must be able to explain what hypertension is and why it is important to treat it. Also teach patients what they need to know about exercise, diet, and side effects of medications. Teach the patient and the caregiver how to use blood pressure (BP) equipment to monitor BP and to identify situations that need to be reported to health care providers. Finally, provide the patient with additional resources, such as written brochures, appropriate websites, and information about support organizations (e.g., American Heart Association).

Sometimes you will not be able to answer patients' or caregivers' questions. Clarifying their questions may help if you are unsure of what they are asking. When it is apparent that you do not have the knowledge to answer the question, admit this to the patient and caregiver and seek help from co-workers, patient educators, and other reliable sources.

Communication Skills. Patient teaching depends on effective communication between you and the patient or caregiver. *Medical jargon* is intimidating and frightening to most patients and their caregivers. Introduce medical words with definitions of their meaning. Consider carefully before using acronyms (e.g., CABG for coronary artery bypass graft) and abbreviations (e.g., IV) when talking with patients. Have the patient and caregiver clarify their understanding of the disease process. Have them explain what they know in their own words. For example, if a patient is told that he has leukopenia, explain this diagnosis in words that mean something to him. Use word roots, explaining that *leuko* refers to a leukocyte, a white blood cell that fights infections, and that *penia* means deficiency or shortage. To enhance learning, use a brief explanation such as, "You have a shortage of white blood cells, the cells that fight infection."

Nonverbal communication is critical when teaching. Nonverbal communication is often guided by cultural practices. For example, in Western culture, sitting in an open, relaxed position facing the patient with eyes at the same level delivers a positive, nonverbal message (Fig. 4-1). In a hospital setting this may require raising the patient's bed or sitting in a chair at the bedside. Open body gestures communicate interest and a willingness to share. With patients from Eastern cultures, you may need to avoid direct eye contact and provide health information to a family spokesperson rather than directly to the patient.

Also develop the art of *active listening* by paying attention to what is said, observing the patient's nonverbal cues, and not interrupting. Nod in response to the patient's statements and rephrase and reflect what the patient is saying to help clarify communication.

Empathy is the courage to enter into the world of another in a manner that does not judge or correct but where understanding is the goal. Empathy means putting aside your own self and stepping into the patient's shoes. When combined with the skill of empathy, active listening is a powerful way to communicate caring and prepare the patient to learn.

Challenges to Nurse-Teacher Effectiveness. Teaching patients and caregivers has many challenges, including (1) lack of time, (2) your own feelings as a teacher, (3) nurse-patient dif-

FIG. 4-1 Open, relaxed positioning of patient, spouse, and nurse at eye level promotes communication in teaching and learning. (Jupiterimages/Photos.com/Thinkstock.)

ferences in learning goals, and (4) early discharge from the health care system.

Lack of time can be a barrier to effective teaching. For example, the patient's physical needs may compete for time that could be used for teaching. To make the most of limited time, it is critical to set learning priorities with the patient. Tell the patient at the beginning of the interaction how much time you can devote to the session. Teaching can be delivered or reinforced during every contact with the patient or caregiver. For example, when giving medications, explain the purpose and side effects of each drug. Reinforcing small pieces of information over time is an effective teaching strategy, especially if information is new or complex.

Additional barriers are your *own feelings as a teacher* and insecurity about your own knowledge and competence. Teaching is a skill that takes time to master. Become familiar with the various resources for patient teaching that are available at your agency. Consult with nurse educators for further help with developing your teaching skills.

Also, disagreements can arise among the patient, the caregiver, and you regarding the expectations or outcomes of teaching. Having realistic discussions about discharge plans, identifying timelines, and exploring home care options can bring urgency to the teaching situation. For example, after a diagnosis of chronic heart failure as a result of aortic valve insufficiency and subsequent emergent valve surgery, the patient and the caregiver may reject teaching efforts until they accept and realize the seriousness of the patient's health problem.

Finally, another important challenge to patient teaching relates to patients having early and quick discharges from the health care system. Shortened lengths of hospital stays and hurried outpatient clinic visits have resulted in patients only having basic teaching plans implemented.

Caregiver Support in the Teaching-Learning Process

The teaching and learning process is applicable to the caregiver as well as the patient. Caregivers are people who care for those who cannot care for themselves. Most common, caregivers are family members or significant others who (1) give or assist with direct patient care; (2) provide emotional, social, spiritual, and possibly financial support for the patient; and (3) manage and coordinate health care services.

Approximately one in four American adults provides care to someone on a daily basis. Caregivers are often categorized by their relationship to the patient. The most common types of caregivers are spouses, adult children, parents, grandparents, and life partners. Although older adult women are the most common family caregivers, other examples include husbands who care for wives with Alzheimer's disease, adult children who care for a parent with a stroke, grandparents who care for a grandchild with a developmental disorder, parents who care for an adult child with a spinal cord injury, and life partners who care for loved ones with a variety of health problems.[11]

Identify the key caregiver(s) for the patient. Assess the caregiver's roles and relationships to the patient. The patient's health problem affects family roles and functions. Identify the needs of caregivers, whether it is in the acute care setting, during the transition to home, or in a home setting[12] (Table 4-4).

Consider cultural differences when assessing the caregiver. In some cultures a male family member may be the designated spokesperson. This person would receive and communicate information among family members and the patient. In planning for discharge to home, it is important to include caregivers who will actually provide the care for the patient, along with the family spokesperson.[12]

As much as possible, teach the caregiver along with the patient. Explain the goals of the teaching plan clearly to both of them. Caregivers may need assistance to learn the physical and technical requirements of care, find resources for home care, locate equipment and supplies, and rearrange the home environment to accommodate the patient. Sources of support for the transition from hospital to home include community-based agencies, Medicare and Medicaid offices, and case managers at the hospital and insurance companies.[13] Patients and caregivers may have different teaching needs. For example, the first priority of an older diabetic patient with a large leg ulcer may be to learn how to transfer from a bed to a chair in the least painful manner. On the other hand, the caregiver may be most concerned about learning the technique for dressing changes. Both the patient's and the caregiver's learning needs are important. The patient and the caregiver may also have differing or conflicting views of the illness and treatment options. Developing a successful teaching plan requires you to view the patient's needs within the context of the caregiver's needs. For instance,

you may teach a patient with right-sided *paresis* (weakness) self-feeding techniques with special implements, but at a home visit you find the patient being fed by the caregiver. On questioning, the caregiver reveals that it is too difficult to watch the patient struggle with feeding, it takes too long, and it is messy. As a result, the caregiver decides that it is easier to just feed the patient. This is an example of a situation in which both the patient and caregiver need additional teaching about the goals of self-care.

Finally, discuss the potential that support groups, networks of family and friends, and community resources have for providing ongoing support and continuing education. Support groups help by sharing experiences and information, offering understanding and acceptance, and suggesting solutions to common problems and concerns. Encourage the caregiver to seek help from the formal social support system on matters such as housing, health coverage, finances, and respite care. Respite care, which is planned temporary care for the patient, includes adult day care, in-home care, and assisted living services.

Caregiver Stress. Caregiver responsibilities are usually taken on gradually with the progression of the patient's illness. As the caregiving responsibilities become more demanding, caregivers often realize that their lives have changed because of this experience. Overwhelmingly, caregivers want to continue their usual activities (e.g., work) despite the hardships they face in caring for acute and chronically ill patients.[14,15]

Prolonged periods of caregiving coupled with a patient's life-limiting illness can contribute to stress and burnout. Some common caregiver stressors are listed in Table 4-5. As caregiving progresses, stressors may change. For example, a caregiver may initially need only to adjust work schedules to accommodate a patient's health care appointments. Later, as the patient's condition worsens, the caregiver may have to reduce work hours, incurring financial hardships.

Caregiving is an experience for which most people are not prepared. It is common for caregivers to become physically, emotionally, and economically overwhelmed by the responsibilities and demands of caring for a family member. The stress of caregiving may result in emotional problems such as depression, anger, and resentment. Signs of caregiver stress include irritability, inability to concentrate, fatigue, and sleeplessness. The caregiver often experiences decreased social interactions and may be at risk for social isolation. Multiple commitments, fatigue, and, at times, the patient's socially inappropriate behaviors contribute to the caregiver's social isolation. Stress can progress to burnout and result in negligence and abuse of the

---

TABLE 4-4	ASSESSMENT OF CAREGIVER NEEDS

Assess caregivers using the following questions:
1. How are you coping with your caregiver role?
2. Do you have any difficulties performing your caregiver responsibilities?
3. How much support do you get from outside sources (e.g., other family members, friends)?
4. Are you aware of and do you use community resources (e.g., disease-specific professional organizations [such as Alzheimer's Association, American Heart Association], adult day care centers, church, synagogue)?
5. Do you know about resources that are available for respite (someone caring for your loved one while you have time to yourself)?
6. What kind of help or services do you need now and in the near future?
7. How can I or other health care professionals help you in your caregiving role?

TABLE 4-5	CAREGIVER STRESSORS

- Change in roles and relationships within family unit
- Lack of respite or relief from caregiving responsibilities
- Need to juggle day-to-day activities, decisions, and caregiving
- Change in living conditions to accommodate family member
- Conflict in the family unit related to decisions about caregiving
- Other people's lack of understanding of the time and energy needed for caregiving
- Inability to meet personal self-care needs, such as socialization, sleep, eating, exercise, and rest
- Financial depletion of resources as a result of a caregiver's inability to work and the increased cost of health care
- Inadequate information or skills related to specific caregiving tasks, such as bathing, drug administration, wound care

patient by the caregiver. See Chapter 5 for information on elder mistreatment and abuse.

In the family system an illness experienced by one family member affects the entire family and alters family interactions. Often family members do not communicate with each other about the patient's needs, and this results in tension. Family conflicts regarding how patient care should be given can lead to disagreements and conflict within the family.

At the same time, many family members involved in direct caregiver activities also identify rewards associated with this role. Positive aspects of caregiving include (1) knowing that their loved one is receiving good care (often in a home environment), (2) learning and mastering new skills, and (3) finding opportunities for intimacy. The tasks involved in caregiving often provide opportunities for family members to gain greater insights into each other and strengthen their relationships.

Encourage caregivers to take care of themselves.[16] Suggest journaling or joining a support group (also available online) to help them share feelings that may be difficult to express. Remind caregivers that getting regular exercise and eating balanced meals at regular times will enhance their well-being. Encourage contact with others to provide emotional support. Finally, humor is important, and sometimes its use by caregivers can provide distraction and relieve stress-filled situations.

Regulatory Mandates for Patient Teaching

Several important agencies have provided specific mandates related to teaching hospitalized patients. The Joint Commission's (TJC's) accreditation standards, National Patient Safety Goals,[3] and the American Hospital Association's Patient Care Partnership[17] clearly state that patients have a fundamental right to receive written information about their care. This information includes their diagnosis, treatment, and prognosis in terms that they can reasonably be expected to understand. For example, this means that written materials must be appropriate for the patient's reading level. One program initiated by TJC, called Speak Up, was developed to encourage patients to become more involved and informed about their plan of care[18] (Table 4-6). Another program proposed by the National Patient Safety Foundation is called **Ask Me 3**.[19] A variety of resources that prompt patients to ask specific questions about their care are available as a part of these initiatives *(www.*

jointcommission.org/speakup.aspx, www.npsf.org/for-healthcare-professionals/programs/ask-me-3).

PROCESS OF PATIENT TEACHING

Many different models and approaches are used in the process of patient teaching. However, the approach used most frequently by nurses parallels the nursing process. The teaching process and the nursing process both involve the development of a plan that includes assessment, setting of patient goals or outcomes, intervention, and evaluation. The teaching process, like the nursing process, may not always flow in sequential order, but the steps serve as checkpoints.

Assessment

During the general nursing assessment, gather data to determine if the patient has learning needs. For example, what does the patient know about the health problem? How does he or she perceive the problem? If a learning need is identified, a more detailed assessment is needed, and that problem is addressed with the teaching plan. Assessment also includes the caregivers to determine their role and ability to care for the patient at home.[12] Key questions to use in the assessment are included in Table 4-7.

Physical Factors. The patient's age is an important factor to consider in the teaching plan. Age affects the patient's experiences, rate of learning, and ability to retain information.[20] The effects of increased age may be obvious, but the inexperience of younger individuals can also affect learning. For example, a man in his twenties who has never thought about his own mortality may be unable to accept the long-term health implications of diabetes mellitus.

Sensory impairments (e.g., hearing or vision loss) decrease sensory input and can alter learning. Magnifying glasses, bright lighting, and materials printed in a large font may help the patient with impaired vision read teaching materials. Hearing loss can be helped with hearing aids and teaching techniques that use more visual stimuli. Cognitive function may be affected by disorders of the nervous system, such as stroke and head trauma, and also by other diseases, such as liver impairment and heart failure. Patients with alterations in cognitive function may have difficulty learning and may require greater caregiver involvement in the teaching process. Manual dexterity is needed to perform procedures such as self-administration of injections or BP monitoring. Problems performing manual procedures might be resolved by using adaptive equipment.

Pain, fatigue, and certain medications also influence the patient's ability to learn. No one can learn effectively when in pain. When the patient is experiencing pain, provide only brief explanations and follow up with more detailed instruction when the pain has been managed. A fatigued and weakened patient cannot learn effectively because of the inability to concentrate. Sleep disruption is common during hospitalization, and patients are frequently exhausted at the time of discharge. Drugs that cause central nervous system depression, such as opioids and sedatives, cause a general decrease in mental alertness and can affect the patient's ability to learn new information. Adjust the teaching plan to accommodate these factors by setting high-priority goals based on need-to-know information and realistic expectations. The patient may need a referral for follow-up teaching so that learning is continued and reinforced after discharge.

TABLE 4-6   THE JOINT COMMISSION'S SPEAK UP™ INITIATIVE

Speak up if you have questions or concerns. If you still do not understand, ask again. It is your body and you have a right to know.

Pay attention to the care you get. Always make sure you are getting the right treatments and medicines by the right health care professionals. Do not assume anything.

Educate yourself about your illness. Learn about the medical tests you get and your treatment plan.

Ask a trusted family member or friend to be your advocate (advisor or supporter).

Know what medicines you take and why you take them. Medicine errors are the most common health care mistakes.

Use a hospital, clinic, surgery center, or other type of health care organization that has been carefully checked out.

Participate in all decisions about your treatment. You are the center of the health care team.

Source: The Joint Commission: To prevent health care errors, patients are urged to Speak Up (poster). Retrieved from *http://www.jointcommission.org/assets/1/18/SpeakUp_Poster.pdf.*

TABLE 4-7 ASSESSMENT OF FACTORS AFFECTING PATIENT TEACHING

Factors and Key Questions

Physical
- What is the patient's age and gender?
- Is the patient acutely ill?
- Is the patient fatigued or in pain?
- What is the primary diagnosis?
- Are there additional medical problems?
- What is the patient's current mental status?
- What is the patient's hearing ability? Visual ability? Motor ability?
- What drugs does the patient take that may affect learning?

Psychologic
- Does the patient appear anxious, afraid, depressed, defensive?
- Is the patient in a state of denial?
- What is the patient's level of motivation? Self-efficacy?

Sociocultural
- What are the patient's beliefs regarding his or her illness or treatment?
- Is proposed teaching consistent with the patient's cultural values?
- What is the patient's educational experience, reading ability, primary language?
- What is the patient's present or past occupation?
- How does the patient describe his or her financial status?
- What is the patient's living arrangement?
- Does the patient have family or close friends?

Learner
- What does the patient already know?
- What does the patient think is most important to learn first?
- What prior learning experiences establish a frame of reference for current learning needs?
- What has the patient's health care provider told the patient about the health problem?
- Is the patient ready to change behavior or learn?
- Can the patient identify behaviors and habits that would make the problem better or worse?
- How does the patient learn best? Through reading, listening, doing things?
- In what kind of environment does the patient learn best? Formal classroom? Informal setting, such as home or office? Alone or among peers?
- In what way should the caregiver(s) be involved in patient teaching?

Psychologic Factors. Psychologic factors have a major influence in the patient's ability to learn. Anxiety and depression are common reactions to illness. Although mild anxiety increases the learner's perceptual and learning abilities, moderate or severe anxiety limits learning. Both anxiety and depression can negatively affect the patient's motivation and readiness to learn. For instance, the patient newly diagnosed with diabetes mellitus who is depressed about the diagnosis may not listen or respond to instructions about blood glucose testing. Discussions with the patient about these concerns or referrals to an appropriate support group may enable the patient to learn that management of diabetes is possible.

Patients also respond to the stress of illness with a variety of defense mechanisms such as denial, rationalization, or even humor. A patient who denies having cancer will not be receptive to information related to treatment options. Similarly, a caregiver may have difficulty accepting a terminal diagnosis. A patient using rationalization will imagine any number of reasons for avoiding change or for rejecting instruction. For example, a patient with heart disease who does not want to change dietary habits will relate stories of people who have eaten bacon and eggs every morning and lived to be 100. Some patients also use humor to filter reality or decrease anxiety. They may use laughter to escape from the experience of facing threatening situations. Humor in the teaching process is important and useful, but determine when humor is used excessively or inappropriately to avoid reality.

One important determinant of successful adoption of new behaviors is the patient's sense of self-efficacy. There is a strong relationship between self-efficacy and outcomes of illness management.[21,22] Self-efficacy increases when a person gains new skills in managing a threatening situation, but decreases when the individual experiences repeated failure, especially early in the course of events. Plan easily attainable goals early in the teaching sessions. Proceed from simple to more complex content to establish a feeling of success.

Sociocultural Factors

Health Literacy. *Literacy* is the ability to use printed and written information to function in society. The recent focus on the literacy rates of the U.S. population and their effects on health and health care have major implications for patient and caregiver teaching. The most recent national literacy survey reported that 43% of the general population and 66% of people older than 60 have basic to below basic literacy skills, and another 5% are nonliterate in English.[4] Assessment of literacy is challenging, since patients rarely admit they have difficulty reading because of feelings of inadequacy and low self-esteem.[23]

Health literacy is the degree to which individuals have the capacity to obtain and understand basic health information needed to make appropriate health decisions.[3] Patients with limited literacy have trouble understanding and acting on health information, leading to health illiteracy. Even patients with higher general literacy can have low health literacy when trying to understand complex health information. Health illiteracy results in poor patient outcomes, nonadherence with treatment plans, limited self-management skills, and increased health disparities.[24]

Easy-to-use assessment tools are available to determine a patient's health literacy. The Single-Item Literacy Screener (SILS) uses one question to identify adults who need help with reading.[25] The question is, "How often do you need to have someone help you when you read instructions, pamphlets, or other written material from your doctor or pharmacy?"

Patient teaching materials should be written at the fifth-grade or lower reading level.[23-25] TJC has established that patient teaching should be tailored to the patient's literacy needs. For example, patients should be taught in their primary language. This is accomplished using medical interpreters (translators)[26] (Fig. 4-2). (Medical interpreters are discussed in Chapter 2 on pp. 32 to 33.) Many patient teaching materials are currently available in languages other than English.

Cultural Considerations. Learning is influenced by the wider culture to which a patient belongs. Health practices, beliefs, and behavior are influenced by one's cultural traditions. These traditions, which can affect patient teaching, can be identified in a cultural assessment (see Table 2-7). TJC requires that patient teaching be tailored to the patient's cultural needs.[26] To prevent stereotyping patients, it is important to simply ask if there is a cultural group with which the patient identifies. Ask patients to describe their beliefs regarding health and illness.

FIG. 4-2 Nurse communicating with a non-English-speaking patient using a translation phone service.

One cultural element that specifically affects the teaching-learning process is a conflict between the patient's cultural beliefs and values and the behaviors promoted by the health care team. For example, a patient who values a trim figure can be taught to use diet and exercise to retain that figure while at the same time improving BP control. However, in another patient's culture, being heavier may be valued as a sign of financial success and sexuality. This patient may have more difficulty accepting the need for diet and exercise unless the importance of BP control is understood.

Also assess the patient's use of cultural remedies and folk healers. For teaching to be effective, incorporate cultural health practices into the teaching plan. Also consider the cultural remedies that may interfere with or are contraindicated by the treatment plan.

In addition, it is important to know who has authority in the patient's culture. The patient may defer to the authority, such as an elder or a spiritual leader, for decisions. In this case, identify and work with the decision makers in the patient's cultural group. (See Chapter 2 for more information on cultural competence.)

Socioeconomic Considerations. A variety of socioeconomic factors are considered when preparing to teach patients. Knowing the patient's present or past occupation may assist you in determining the vocabulary to use during teaching. For example, an auto mechanic might understand the volume overload associated with heart failure as flooding an engine. An engineer may understand the principles of physics associated with gravity and pressures when discussing vascular problems.

Ask the patient about living arrangements. Whether the patient lives alone, with friends, or with family will influence who is included in the teaching process. You may need to modify the teaching plan if the patient does not have access to electricity or phones. If the patient has unmet learning needs by the time of discharge, arrange for continued teaching after discharge.

Learner Factors. Finally, assess learner factors, including the patient's learning needs, readiness to learn, and learning style.

Learning Needs. Learning needs are the new knowledge and skills that an individual must have to meet a goal. The assessment of learning needs should first determine what the patient already knows, whether the patient has misinformation, and any past experiences with health problems. Patients with long-standing health problems may have different learning needs from those patients with newly diagnosed health problems.

What a patient should learn about managing an illness or what behaviors need to be changed to promote health may seem obvious to you. However, what you think is important may be different from what patients want to know. Remember that adults learn best when the teaching provides information that they view as being needed immediately (see Table 4-1). Ask patients to prioritize what they see as the most critical information. For example, give the patient a list of the recommended topics to choose from. Also ask the patient to identify other topics not on the list. Having patients prioritize their own learning needs allows you to begin with the patient's most important needs. When information regarding life-threatening complications is needed, promote the priority of learning this content by explaining why the information is "need to know." Tailor your teaching to meet your patient's individual learning needs, especially when time is limited.

Readiness to Learn. Readiness to learn and motivation depend on multiple factors, such as perceived need, attitudes, and beliefs. When teaching adults, identify what information the person values. Readiness to learn is increased if the patient perceives a need for information, has a belief that a behavior change has value, or perceives the learning activities as new and stimulating.[27]

Before implementing the teaching plan, determine where the patient is in the stages of change process (see Table 4-2). If the patient is only in the precontemplation stage, just provide support and increase the patient's awareness of the problem until the patient is ready to consider a change in behavior. Nurses in outpatient settings and home health care can continue to evaluate the patient's readiness to learn and implement the teaching plan as the patient moves through the stages of change. Reinforcement is a strong motivational factor for achieving a desired behavior and needs to be incorporated throughout the change process. Positive reinforcement involves rewarding the target behavior with positive feedback or other rewards to maintain the behavior.[8]

Learning Style. Each person has a distinct style of learning that is as individual as his or her personality. The three general learning styles are (1) *visual* (reading, pictures), (2) *auditory* (listening), and (3) *physical* (doing things). People often use more than one learning style to acquire new information or skills. To assess a patient's learning style, ask how the patient prefers to learn and how the patient has learned in the past.[28] During assessment of the patient's learning style, identify the patient who does not read or who has limited health literacy. For example, the patient may tell you that he or she does not read much, but likes to learn from television programs. If possible, always use auditory and visual methods (e.g., CDs/DVDs) when patients specifically identify them as preferred methods of learning.

Planning

Prioritize the patient's learning needs and agree on learning goals. If the patient's physical or psychologic condition interferes with his or her participation, the patient's caregiver(s) can assist you in the planning phase.

Setting Goals. It is important to write clear, attainable, and measurable learning objectives or goals. Learning goals relate to the intended outcome of the learning process, guide the selection of teaching strategies, and help evaluate the patient's progress. Learning goals are parallel to patient outcomes in the nursing care plan (NCP). Many settings provide standardized NCPs that contain preset goals and interventions for specific learning needs. Modify these NCPs based on the patient's unique sociocultural and learner characteristics.

Standardized teaching plans are often included in care management guides and clinical practice guidelines. Standardized teaching plans frequently contain evidence-based information and skills that a patient and caregiver need to know concerning a specific health problem or procedure. However, as with NCPs, individualize these plans to meet the patient's specific needs. (See eFig. 4-1, eFig. 4-2, and eTable 4-1 on the website for this chapter for information on writing objectives or goals and examples of standardized teaching plans.)

EVIDENCE-BASED PRACTICE

Translating Research Into Practice

Are Decision Aids Helpful in Making Decisions About Health Care?

Clinical Question
For patients (P) with treatment and screening decisions, what is the effect of decision aids (I) versus usual teaching interventions (C) on outcomes associated with decisions about health care (O)?

Best Available Evidence
Systematic review of randomized controlled trials (RCTs).

Critical Appraisal and Synthesis of Evidence
- 86 RCTs (n = 20,209) of adults comparing use of decision aids versus usual care interventions on decision making attributes and behavioral outcomes.
- Decision aids provide information about treatment or screening options that may be valued differently by patients. Aids may be pamphlets, videos, or Internet-based tools.
- Knowledge, decisional conflict, patient-provider communication, and effect on behavior and health care system were measured.
- Decision aids significantly improved knowledge; reduced patient passivity and feelings of being uninformed; positively affected patient-provider communication; and reduced patient elective choices for invasive surgery, prostate specific antigen (PSA) screening, and menopausal hormone usage.

Conclusion
- Decision aids are valuable in helping patients decide among various treatments and screening options.

Implications for Nursing Practice
- Provide decision-making aids and collaboratively engage in communication with patients who face choices in treatment and screening.
- Involve patients in the decision-making process by sharing realistic perceptions of benefits and harms of options.
- Clarify with patients their personal values when exploring health care choices.

Reference for Evidence
Stacy D, Bennett C, Barry M, et al: Decision aids for people facing health treatment or screening decisions, *Cochrane Database Syst Rev* 10: CD00143, 2011.

P, Patient population of interest; I, intervention or area of interest; C, comparison of interest or comparison group; O, outcomes of interest; T, timing (see p. 12).

Selecting Teaching Strategies. Three factors that determine teaching strategies are (1) patient characteristics (e.g., age, educational background, culture, language skills), (2) subject matter, and (3) available resources. Table 4-8 provides a summary of the various learner characteristics and recommended teaching strategies based on the generation of the patient or caregiver.[29,30]

Various teaching strategies are used to enhance learning (Table 4-9). Frequently, several teaching strategies are used together (Fig. 4-3). Discussion is the most common type of interaction used in teaching patients and caregivers. Another type of group teaching involves *peer teaching*, as found in support groups. Patients dealing with common problems such as cancer, alcoholism, and eating disorders can benefit from peer teaching.

Learning Materials. Use learning materials that are provided in multiple formats (see Table 4-9). To use this strategy, know what materials are available within the facility, from support agencies, and from professional groups. The use of CDs/DVDs is extremely beneficial, particularly when teaching content that is largely visual, such as the steps of a procedure (e.g., suctioning a tracheostomy). The health care facility's television system may also deliver patient teaching programs (see Fig. 4-3). A

TABLE 4-8 LEARNER CHARACTERISTICS AND TEACHING STRATEGIES BY GENERATION

Birth Year	Learner Characteristics	Recommended Teaching Strategies
Millennials 1981-2000	• Autonomous • Multitaskers • Prefer interactive and virtual environments • Technologically focused • Integrative thinking • Short attention span	• Provide access to Internet in patient's room. • Discuss reliable websites. • Download health information to cell phones, iPods, or similar devices. • Use video games and game systems to teach health behaviors (e.g., Wii Fit).
Generation X 1965-1980	• Interaction with groups • Self-directed learning • Self-reliant	• Use group teaching sessions. • Recommend support groups. • Suggest role playing. • Provide Internet-based education materials.
Baby Boomers 1946-1964	• Emphasis on self-knowledge • Acquisition of knowledge from authoritative sources	• Consider lecture or lecture-discussion (e.g., PowerPoint presentation). • Use patient education TV channels. • Provide printed materials.
Veterans Born before 1946	• Emphasis on rote learning • Memorization of knowledge	• Consider lecture or lecture-discussion. • Use pictures and printed materials such as books.

Compiled from Rose J: Designing training for Gen Y: learning style and values of Generation Y, 2007. Retrieved from *http://trainingpd.suite101.com/article.cfm/designing_training_for_gen_y;* and Educational strategies in generational designs, *Prog Transplant* 16(1):8, 2006.

TABLE 4-9   COMPARISON OF TEACHING STRATEGIES

Description	Advantages	Limitations
Discussion ("Teach Back") • Purpose is to exchange points of view about a topic or to arrive at a decision or conclusion. • Can be done with patient, with patient and caregiver, or with group. *Example:* Weight loss	• Allows for an active exchange of information and previous experiences among participants. • Good choice when patients have previous experience with subject and have information to share. • Nonthreatening format. • Can use peers (patients with common problems) to teach.	• May require additional time depending on topic and number of participants.
Lecture-Discussion • Commonly used when group of patients and caregivers can benefit from basic information. • Lecture portion is short (i.e., 15-20 minutes). • Discussion ("teach back") follows lecture. *Example:* Basic principles of cardiac rehabilitation (e.g., exercise, nutrition)	• Combines short lecture to present basic information with time for discussion. • Provision of printed material related to lecture content is useful and recommended.	• Need to limit number of lecture topics to 5-7. • May require additional time depending on topic and number of participants.
Demonstration/Return Demonstration ("Show Back") • Purpose is to teach patient and caregiver to perform a skill. • Through return demonstration ("show back") can evaluate patient's ability to perform skill (see Fig. 4-4). *Examples:* Dressing change, injection	• Provides for learning and practice of physical skills. • Dividing skill into series of smaller steps facilitates mastery and provides reinforcement.	• May require additional time for practice needed to master skill. • Patients with limited manual dexterity may have difficulty.

Role Play
• Used when patients need to
  • Examine attitudes and behaviors
  • Understand viewpoints of others
  • Practice carrying out ideas or decisions
Example: Wife who rehearses how to talk with husband about need to quit smoking
	• Allows participants to rehearse variety of situations involving difficult decisions, attitudes, behaviors, etc.
	• Practicing ahead of time may increase self-efficacy.
		• May not be appropriate for all learners, since a certain level of maturity, confidence, and flexibility is required.
		• Requires adequate time for feedback and evaluation.

Learning Materials
• Use of audiovisual materials to supplement teaching including
  • Printed materials (e.g., brochures)
  • CDs/DVDs
• Hospital-based TV
• Internet-based programs
	• Enhance the presentation through visual and/or auditory stimulation.
	• Best used in combination with other teaching strategies.
	• Use of the Internet for health information is the preferred choice for many.
	• Internet access in hospitals (including patient rooms) is increasing.
		• Materials must be previewed and evaluated (e.g., accuracy, completeness, reading level) before using.
		• Sites must be previewed and evaluated for validity of information.
		• Problems include limited access and inaccurate information.
		• May not be appropriate for all learners (e.g., lack of interest, decreased mental capacity).

FIG. 4-3 Effective teaching using a variety of strategies (written materials, video-based patient education programs).

dedicated channel may be available and contain high-quality, professionally produced programs provided on demand or on a rotating schedule. Alternatively, education programs produced by the health care facility may be available on a hospital-based channel and provide content tailored to the patient experience.

Printed educational materials are widely used for teaching patients and caregivers. These materials are most often used in combination with previously discussed teaching strategies. For instance, after a discussion on the effects of smoking on heart disease, you might use a pamphlet from the American Cancer Society to reinforce the pathophysiologic effects of smoking. For a patient who has had surgery for breast cancer, you might provide a book or magazine article written by a woman who has had a mastectomy. Suggest that the patient read this material to prepare for other teaching sessions. Recommend written materials for patients whose preferred learning style is reading.

Before using written materials with patients, evaluate the readability level if it is not indicated on the materials. Several word processing programs (e.g., Microsoft Word) can assess the readability level of written materials. The use of Internet-based programs (e.g., *www.wordscount.info*) also can help you determine the readability and grade level of printed materials.

When writing teaching materials, use several techniques to keep the reading level at a fifth-grade level, including the following: (1) give key information first using bold or italics; (2) use short, common words of one or two syllables; (3) define medical words in simple language if they must be used; (4) keep sentences under 10 words if possible, and 15 at the most; (5) use pictures or drawings; and (6) use an active voice in the manner you would normally say something.[31] Pictographs (simple line drawings) combined with simplified text are an effective tool to improve discharge education for older adults with low literacy.[32]

Major resources for acquiring relevant printed material include the hospital or care facility library, pharmacies, public libraries, federal and state agencies, universities, voluntary organizations, research centers, and websites. Review written materials, including computer-based programs, before using them. In addition to reading level, review the material to determine whether it (1) is accurate, (2) is complete, (3) meets specific learning goals, (4) uses pictures and diagrams to stimulate interest, (5) uses one main idea or concept per pamphlet or program, (6) contains information the patient would like to know, and (7) is culture and gender sensitive and appropriate.[4]

Patients' use of the Internet to obtain health information continues to increase. Patients can quickly do an Internet search and have access to information about their disease, medications, treatments, and surgeries. Your job is to help the patient sift through the wide variety of information to find information that is valid, reliable, and usable. Understanding the principles of web searching for medical information and instructing the patient in finding valid information are critical. An estimated 80% of the people who use the Internet use it to gather health information. Factors that predict use of the Internet for this purpose include access to high-speed connections, younger age, some college education, and confidence in using technology.[33,34] Patients who are chronically ill are more likely to base health decisions on information that they find on the Internet.[33] Encourage patients to use Internet sites established by the government, universities, or reputable health-related associations (e.g., American Diabetes Association, American Heart Association, National Institutes of Health, U.S. Food and Drug Administration). Resources at the end of the chapter identify selected reliable websites for you to review and use for patient teaching.

Although older adults are using the Internet in greater numbers, many may not have the mental capacity, patience, or technical skills to successfully find information. Organizations dedicated to improving the quality of life for older adults are promoting the development of user-friendly websites (available at *www.nlm.nih.gov/pubs/checklist.pdf*) and publishing guides to help older adults evaluate web-based health information.

Obstacles to successful use of the Internet by many patients include limited access, lack of interest, and inaccurate information.[35] The presence of Internet connections in many hospital rooms provide an opportunity for you to teach patients about their illness and how to use the Internet to find health-related information.

The quantity and complexity of health care technology that patients and you have access to for patient teaching are increas-

ing. Telehealth, interactive video, wireless technology, and podcasting are just some of the current technologies that patients may use to manage their health care. *Telehealth* is the delivery of health-related services and information via telecommunications technologies. Telehealth is used to monitor patients' cardiac rhythms, weights, and vital signs and to provide education (see Fig. 35-6). Wireless technology also may be used to monitor patients' blood glucose levels. Always educate yourself about these technologies before teaching patients.

Implementation

During the implementation phase, use the planned teaching strategies to present information and teach new skills (see Table 4-9). Incorporate verbal and nonverbal communication skills, active listening, and empathy into the process. Based on the assessment of the patient's physical, psychologic, sociocultural, and learner characteristics, determine how much the patient can participate. Whenever possible and appropriate, involve the patient's caregiver(s) in the teaching-learning process.

In implementing the teaching plan, remember the principles and characteristics of the adult learner. Reinforcement and reward are important, but be aware that phrases such as "Aren't you doing well?" in a tone one would use with a child can be condescending to adult learners.

Evaluation

Evaluation, the final step in the learning process, is a measure of the degree to which the patient has achieved the learning goals. Various evaluation techniques can be used (Table 4-10). Use techniques such as "teach back" and "show back" to determine the knowledge and skill levels of the patient and/or caregiver throughout the teaching and learning process[27,36] (Fig. 4-4). If certain goals are not reached, reassess the patient and revise the teaching plan accordingly.

For example, an older man with diabetes mellitus entered the hospital with a blood glucose level of 550 mg/dL (30.53 mmol/L). When the student nurse began to prepare his insulin injection, the nurse asked, "Are you going to have him give his own insulin and observe his technique?" "Oh, no," replied the student nurse, "He has been diabetic for 20 years!" The assumption was that a patient with diabetes would know how to perform this task

FIG. 4-4 Teaching using demonstration and return demonstration ("show back") increases successful learning by the patient.

TABLE 4-10	**TECHNIQUES TO EVALUATE PATIENT AND CAREGIVER LEARNING**		
Technique	**Strategy and Examples**	**Technique**	**Strategy and Examples**

Observe patient or caregiver directly.	• Ask person to show you how to change the dressing.
	• Return demonstration ("show back") determines whether
	  • Skill has been mastered.
	  • Further instruction is needed.
	  • Patient and caregiver are ready for new or additional content.
		Ask open-ended questions ("teach back").	• Open-ended questions provide more information about understanding than close-ended questions that require only a "yes" or "no."
			• Ask questions such as
			  • "How often do you need to change the dressing?"
			  • "What will you do if you develop chest pain after returning home?"

Observe verbal and nonverbal cues.	• Teaching may need to be delayed, further teaching is needed, or different strategy should be used if patient or caregiver
	  • Asks you to repeat instructions
	  • Loses eye contact
	  • Begins to doze in chair or bed
	  • Becomes restless or fidgety
	  • Does not speak English
		Talk with caregiver ("teach back").	• Involve caregiver in the evaluation process.
			• Ask questions such as
			  • "What medications is she taking?"
			  • "How often does he use his oxygen?"

		Seek the patient's self-evaluation of progress.	• Ask patient's opinion about his or her progress. • What evidence does the patient have that the goals are being met? • Is the patient ready to go forward with learning new material?

correctly. The nurse and the student nurse returned to the patient's room and asked him to prepare an insulin injection ("show back"). The patient filled the syringe with 30 units of insulin and 10 units of air, instead of 40 units of insulin. After correcting the dose and questioning the patient more fully ("teach back"), the nurses concluded that the patient knew his correct dosage of insulin but could not accurately see the markings on the syringe. The patient most likely had been administering insufficient insulin to himself for some time. The patient's vision was not as good as it had been 20 years ago, and special equipment was now necessary for him to safely and accurately administer the insulin. The lesson here is that assumptions regarding a patient's knowledge and skills are dangerous. Evaluate all past and new learning as well as present abilities.

Long-term evaluation of learning goals often requires follow-up after discharge. Provide a written schedule of visits and other appropriate referrals for the patient before he or she leaves the hospital or clinic. The patient's caregiver(s) also must be familiar with the follow-up plan, so that everyone involved in the patient's long-term progress is on the same page.[18,37]

Documentation is an essential and required component throughout the entire teaching-learning process. Record everything from the assessment through plans for evaluation and follow-up. Because various members of the health care team use these records in different settings and for different reasons, the teaching goals, strategies, and evaluation results need to be clear, complete, and available to all members of the health care team.

CASE STUDY

Patient and Caregiver Teaching

Thomas M Perkins/
Shutterstock.com

Patient Profile

M.L., a 60-year-old Asian woman, is admitted to the hospital with a diagnosis of exacerbation of chronic obstructive pulmonary disease (COPD).

Subjective Data

• History of COPD for 10 years; reports a chronic cough, and denies any recent change in color of sputum; states "I stopped smoking last year but my son-in-law smokes"
• Past medical history: gastroesophageal reflux disease; macular degeneration in right eye
• Social history: widowed 5 years ago and since then has lived with daughter and son-in-law who work full time; cares for two young grandchildren after school; English is M.L.'s second language

Objective Data

Physical Examination

• Alert, cognitively intact, anxious, thin woman with dyspnea on minimal exertion; speaking in short phases or sentences; states "I have no energy"
• Using oxygen via nasal cannula at 2 L/min
• Weight 100 lb, height 5 ft 2 in
• Wears glasses

Diagnostic Studies

• Chest x-ray negative for acute infection
• Arterial blood gases on room air: pH 7.35, $PaCO_2$ 47 mm Hg, PaO_2 75 mm Hg, HCO_3^- 30 mEq/L
• O_2 saturation (via pulse oximetry) during 6-minute walk test on room air = 83%
• Forced expiratory volume in 1 second of expiration (FEV_1) = 60% of predicted

Collaborative Care

• Medications: bronchodilator therapy (inpatient nebulizer therapy, inhalers on discharge), oral corticosteroids
• Long-term home O_2 therapy: O_2 at 2 L/min via nasal cannula
• Pulmonary rehabilitation: inpatient and outpatient

Discussion Questions

1. *Priority Decision:* Given M.L.'s history, what are the priority learning needs?
2. What factors (e.g., sociocultural, physical, psychologic) may influence M.L.'s response to teaching?
3. What potential challenges might you expect when planning to teach M.L.? How would you manage them?
4. *Priority Decision:* Identify two priority nursing diagnoses. Develop a teaching plan for M.L. based on these nursing diagnoses.

BRIDGE TO NCLEX EXAMINATION

The number of the question corresponds to the same-numbered outcome at the beginning of the chapter.

1. What would be the priority teaching goal for a middle-aged Hispanic woman regarding methods to relieve symptoms of menopause?
   a. Prevent the development of future disease.
   b. Maintain the patient's current state of health.
   c. Change the patient's cultural belief regarding the use of herbs.
   d. Provide information for selection and use of treatment options.

2. When planning teaching with consideration of the diverse learning needs of adults, the nurse's best approach would include
   a. presenting material in an efficient lecture format.
   b. recognizing that adults enjoy learning regardless of the relevance to their personal lives.
   c. providing opportunities for the patient to learn from other adults with similar experiences.
   d. postponing practice of new skills until the patient can independently practice the skill at home.

3. Which is the priority patient teaching strategy when limited time is available?
   a. Setting realistic goals that have high priority for the patient
   b. Referring the patient to a nurse educator in private practice for teaching
   c. Observing more experienced nurse-teachers to learn how to teach faster and more efficiently
   d. Providing reading materials for the patient instead of discussing information the patient needs to learn

4. The nurse needs to include caregivers in patient teaching primarily because (select all that apply)
   a. they provide most of the care for patients after discharge.
   b. they might feel rejected if they are not included in the teaching.
   c. patients have better outcomes when their caregivers are involved.
   d. the patient may be too ill or too stressed to fully understand the teaching.
   e. caregivers are responsible for the overall management of the patient's care.

5. Which technique is most appropriate when using motivational interviewing with a patient who tells you that he is ready to start a weight loss program?
   a. Confirm that the patient is serious about losing weight.
   b. Insist that the patient consider an organized group weight loss program.
   c. Focus on the patient's strengths to support his optimism that he can successfully lose weight.
   d. Ask a prescribed set of questions to increase the patient's awareness of his dietary behaviors.

6. Which patient characteristic enhances the teaching-learning process?
   a. Moderate anxiety
   b. High self-efficacy
   c. Being in the precontemplative stage of change
   d. Being able to laugh about the current health problem

7. A patient tells the nurse that she enjoys talking with others and sharing experiences, but easily falls asleep when reading. Which teaching strategy would be most effective with this patient?
   a. Role play
   b. Group teaching
   c. Lecture-discussion
   d. Discussion supplemented with computer programs

8. The nurse has taught a patient's caregiver how to administer insulin to her husband. Evaluation of the nurse's teaching effectiveness before discharge would include
   a. arranging for follow-up with a home care nurse.
   b. monitoring the patient's glucose readings before discharge.
   c. asking the caregiver to "show back" her ability to administer insulin.
   d. asking the caregiver what she found helpful about the teaching experience.

1. d, 2. c, 3. a, 4. c, d, 5. c, 6. b, 7. b, 8. c.

⊖volve

For rationales to these answers and even more NCLEX review questions, visit *http://evolve.elsevier.com/Lewis/medsurg*.

REFERENCES

1. National Center for Chronic Disease Prevention and Health Promotion: *Chronic disease overview*, Washington, DC, 2010, Centers for Disease Control and Prevention. Retrieved from *www.cdc.gov/nccdphp/overview.htm*.

2. Jack BW, Chetty VK, Anthony D, et al: A reengineered hospital discharge program to decrease rehospitalization: a randomized trial, *Ann Intern Med* 150:178, 2009.

3. The Joint Commission: 2011 Hospital national patient safety goals. Retrieved from *www.jointcommission.org/assets/1/6/HAP_NPSG_6-10-11.pdf*.

4. The Joint Commission: What did the doctor say? Improving health literacy to protect patient safety, 2007. Retrieved from *www.jointcommission.org/assets/1/18/improving_health_literacy.pdf*.

5. American Nurses Credentialing Center, Magnet Recognition Program Model: Exemplary professional practice: nurses as teachers, 2011. Retrieved from *http://nursecredentialing.org/Magnet/ProgramOverview/New-Magnet-Model.aspx#ExemplaryProfessionalPractice*.

6. Redman BK: *The practice of patient education*, ed 10, St Louis, 2007, Mosby.

7. Knowles MS, Holton EF, Swanson RA: *The adult learner: the definitive classic in adult education and human resource development*, ed 7, St Louis, 2011, Mosby.

8. Cancer Prevention Research Center: Detailed overview of the transtheoretical model. Retrieved from *www.uri.edu/research/cprc/TTM/detailedoverview.htm.*

9. Rollnick S, Miller WR, Yahne CE: *Motivational interviewing in health care: helping patients change behavior*, New York, 2008, Builford Press.

10. Miller WR: *Enhancing motivation for change in substance abuse treatment: Treatment Improvement Protocol (TIP) series 35, DHHS pub no (SMA) 99-3354*, Rockville, Md, 1999, US Department of Health and Human Services. Retrieved from *www.ncbi.nlm.nih.gov/books/NBK14856.* (Classic)

11. Feinberg L, Reinhard SC, Houser A, et al: Valuing the invaluable: 2011 update—the growing contributions and costs of family caregiving, AARP Public Policy Institute. Retrieved from *http://assets.aarp.org/rgcenter/ppi/ltc/i51-caregiving.pdf.*

12. Levine C: Supporting family caregivers: the hospital nurse's assessment of family caregiver needs, *Am J Nurs* 111:47, 2011.

13. Naylor MD, Aiken LH, Kurtzman ET, et al: The care span: the importance of transitional care in achieving health reform, *Health Affairs* 30:746, 2011.

*14. White K, D'Andrew N, Auret K, et al: Learn now: live well: an educational programme for caregivers, *Int J Palliative Nurs* 14(10):497, 2008.

15. Caregiver stress, 2011. Retrieved from *www.caregiversupport.org/caregiver_stress.cfm.*

16. Pagan CN: A caregiver's guide to staying well, *Arthritis Today* 25(6):80, 2011.

17. American Hospital Association: The patient care partnership: understanding expectations, rights and responsibilities, 2003. Retrieved from *www.aha.org/advocacy-issues/communicatingpts/pt-care-partnership.shtml.*

18. The Joint Commission: Speak up initiatives, 2011. Retrieved from *www.jointcommission.org/speakup.aspx.*

19. National Patient Safety Foundation: Ask me 3. Retrieved from *www.npsf.org/for-healthcare-professionals/programs/ask-me-3.*

*20. Kelley K, Abraham C: Health promotion for people aged over 65 years in hospitals: nurses' perceptions about their role, *J Clin Nurs* 16(3):569, 2007.

*21. Farrell K, Wicks MN, Martin JC: Chronic disease self-management improved with enhanced self-efficacy, *Clin Nurs Res* 13(4):289, 2004. (Classic)

*22. Resnick B: A longitudinal analysis of efficacy expectations and exercise in older adults, *Res Theory Nurs Pract* 18(4):331, 2004. (Classic)

23. Barclay L: Screening questions may help predict limited health literacy, *Ann Fam Med* 7:24, 2009.

*24. Villaire M, Mayer G: Low health literacy: the impact on chronic illness management, *Prof Case Manage* 12(4):213, 2007.

25. Morris NS, MacLean CD, Chew LD, et al: The single item literacy screener: evaluation of a brief instrument to identify limited reading ability, *BMC Fam Pract* 7:21, 2006. (Classic)

26. Wilson-Stronks A, Lee KK, Cordero CL, et al: One size does not fit all: meeting the health care needs of diverse populations, Oakland Terrace, Ill, 2008, The Joint Commission. Retrieved from *www.jointcommission.org/assets/1/6/HLCOneSizeFinal.pdf.*

27. Nigolian CJ, Miller KL: Teaching essential skills to family caregivers, *Am J Nurs* 111:52, 2011.

28. Inott T, Kennedy BB: Assessing learning styles: practical tips for patient education, *Nurs Clin North Am* 46:313, 2011.

29. Rose J: Designing training for Gen Y: learning style and values of Generation Y, 2007. Retrieved from *http://trainingpd.suite101.com/article.cfm/designing_training_for_gen_y.*

30. Educational strategies in generational designs, *Prog Transplant* 16(1):8, 2006.

31. Medline Plus: How to write easy-to-read health materials, 2011. Retrieved from *www.nlm.nih.gov/medlineplus/etr.html.*

32. Choi J: Literature review: using pictographs in discharge instructions for older adults with low-literacy skills, *J Clin Nurs* 20:2984, 2011.

33. Fox S: Pew Internet and American Life Project: the engaged e-patient population, 2008. Retrieved from *www.pewinternet.org/Reports/2008/The-Engaged-Epatient-Population.aspx.*

34. Watson A, Bell A, Kvedar J, et al:. Reevaluating the digital divide: current lack of Internet use is not a barrier to adoption of novel health information technology, *Diabetes Care* 31(3):433, 2008.

35. Anderson A, Klemm P: The Internet: friend or foe when providing patient education? *Clin J Oncol Nurs* 12(1):55, 2008.

36. National Center for Ethics in Health Care: "Teach back": a tool for improving provider-patient communication, *In Focus: Topics in Health Care Ethics*, 2006. Retrieved from *www.ethics.va.gov/docs/infocus/InFocus_20060401_teach_Back.pdf.*

37. Agency for Healthcare Research and Quality: Implementing re-engineered hospital discharges (Project RED): frequently asked questions, 2009. Retrieved from *www.ahrq.gov/news/kt/red/redfaq.htm.*

RESOURCES

Family Caregiver Alliance
www.caregiver.org
GetWellNetwork
www.getwellnetwork.com/index.asp
Implementing Re-engineered Hospital Discharges (Project Red)
www.ahrq.gov/news/kt/red/redfaq.htm
The Joint Commission—Speak Up Initiatives
www.jointcommission.org/speakup.aspx
Mayo Clinic Health Information
www.mayoclinic.com/health-information
National Family Caregivers Association
www.nfcacares.org
U.S. Department of Health and Human Resources—Healthfinder
www.healthfinder.gov
U.S. National Library of Medicine and National Institutes of Health—MedlinePlus
www.nlm.nih.gov/medlineplus
WebMD
www.webmd.com

*Evidence-based information for clinical practice.

Aging is not "lost youth" but a new stage of opportunity and strength.
Betty Friedan

Chronic Illness and Older Adults

Margaret Baker and Margaret McLean Heitkemper

evolve WEBSITE

http://evolve.elsevier.com/Lewis/medsurg

- NCLEX Review Questions
- Key Points
- Pre-Test
- Answer Guidelines for Case Study on p. 76
- Rationales for Bridge to NCLEX Examination Questions

- Concept Map Creator
- Glossary
- Content Updates

eTable
- eTable 5-1: Geriatric Depression Scale (Short Form)

LEARNING OUTCOMES

1. Describe the prevention and major causes of chronic illness.
2. Explain the characteristics of a chronic illness.
3. Define *ageism*.
4. Explain the needs of special populations of older adults.
5. Describe nursing interventions to assist older adults with chronic conditions.

6. Describe common problems of older adults related to hospitalization and acute illness and the nurse's role in assisting them.
7. Differentiate among care alternatives to meet needs of older adults.
8. Describe the nurse's role in health promotion, disease prevention, and managing the special needs of older adults.

KEY TERMS

ageism, p. 65
chronic illness, Table 5-1, p. 61
elder mistreatment, p. 68
ethnogeriatric, p. 67

frail older adult, p. 64
gerontologic nursing, p. 71
Medicaid, p. 69

Medicare, p. 68
old-old adult, p. 64
young-old adult, p. 64

This chapter discusses issues related to chronic illness and aging. The population of older adults is growing quickly and they often have increased health care needs and problems that you need to consider.

CHRONIC ILLNESS

Illness can be categorized as either acute or chronic (Table 5-1). Today the U.S. health care system faces a growing burden of chronic illness as the population ages. Chronic diseases account for 70% of all deaths in the United States.[1] Chronic illness results in limitations in physical functioning, work productivity, and quality of life for nearly 1 out of 10 Americans, or about 31 million people. Older adults often live with more than one chronic illness. A significant portion of U.S. health care dollars go toward the treatment of chronic illnesses.[1] The management of a chronic illness can profoundly affect the lives and identities of the patient, family, and caregiver. Table 5-2 presents the impact of some chronic illnesses.

TABLE 5-1	CHARACTERISTICS OF ACUTE AND CHRONIC ILLNESS	
Description	**Characteristics**
Acute Illness	
Diseases that have a rapid onset and short duration *Examples:* colds, influenza, acute gastroenteritis	• Usually self-limiting • Responds readily to treatment • Complications infrequent • After illness, return to previous level of functioning
Chronic Illness	
Diseases that are prolonged, do not resolve spontaneously, and are rarely cured completely *Examples:* see Table 5-2	• Permanent impairments or deviations from normal • Irreversible pathologic changes • Residual disability • Special rehabilitation required • Need for long-term medical and/or nursing management

Reviewed by Kathleen Blais, RN, EdD, Professor Emerita, Florida International University, College of Nursing and Health Sciences, Wilton Manors, Florida; Deborah Marks Conley, RN, MSN, APRN-CNS, GCNS-BC, FNGNA, Gerontological Clinical Nurse Specialist, Nebraska Methodist Hospital and Assistant Professor of Nursing, Nebraska Methodist College, Omaha, Nebraska; and Mary A. Cox, RN, MS, Professor, Nursing, Sinclair Community College, Dayton, Ohio.

TABLE 5-2   IMPACT OF CHRONIC ILLNESSES

Chronic Illness	Impact	Content in Book	
		Chapter	Page
Alzheimer's disease	• Affects 5.4 million people • 6th leading cause of death	60	1445
Arthritis	• Affects 1 in 5 people • One of most common chronic illnesses	65	1562
Cancer	• 2nd leading cause of death	16	247
Chronic obstructive pulmonary disease	• Affects many older adults • 3rd leading cause of death	29	579
Coronary artery disease	• Affects about 17 million adults • Leading cause of death	34	731
Diabetes	• Affects >25.8 million Americans • 7.0 million do not know they have the disease • 7th leading cause of death	49	1153
Heart failure	• Most common reason older adults are hospitalized	35	766
Obesity	• Affects >35% of adults • Major contributor to other health problems	41	906
Stroke	• Affects about 7 million adults, 15%-30% disabled • 4th leading cause of death	58	1388

Data from Centers for Disease Control and Prevention: Quick facts: economic and health burden of chronic disease. Retrieved from *www.cdc.gov/nccdphp/press/ index.htm#3*; and Heart Disease and Stroke Statistics—2011 update.

TABLE 5-3   CHRONIC ILLNESS TRAJECTORY

Phases	Description
Onset	• Signs and symptoms are present. • Disease diagnosed.
Stable	• Illness course and symptoms controlled by treatment regimen. • Person maintains everyday activities.
Acute	• Active illness with severe and unrelieved symptoms or complications. • Hospitalization may be required for management.
Comeback	• Gradual return to an acceptable way of life.
Crisis	• Life-threatening situation occurs. • Emergency services are necessary.
Unstable	• Unable to keep symptoms or disease course under control. • Life becomes disrupted while patient works to regain stability. • Hospitalization not required.
Downward	• Gradual and progressive deterioration in physical or mental status. • Accompanied by increasing disability and symptoms. • Continuous alterations in everyday life activities.
Dying	• Patient has to relinquish everyday life interests and activities, let go, and die peacefully. • Immediate weeks, days, hours preceding death.

Source: Woog P: *The chronic illness trajectory framework: the Corbin and Strauss nursing model*, New York, 1992, Springer.

In addition to people living longer, other societal changes have contributed to the increase in chronic illnesses, including insufficient physical activity, lack of access to fresh fruits and vegetables, tobacco use, and alcohol consumption.[1]

Trajectory of Chronic Illness

Chronic illnesses may have acute exacerbations in which an individual moves from a level of optimum functioning, with the illness well controlled, to a period of instability during which the individual may need assistance. Corbin and Strauss proposed a view of chronic illness as a trajectory (Fig. 5-1) with overlapping phases[2] (Table 5-3). This trajectory characterizes the common course of most chronic illnesses. In addition,

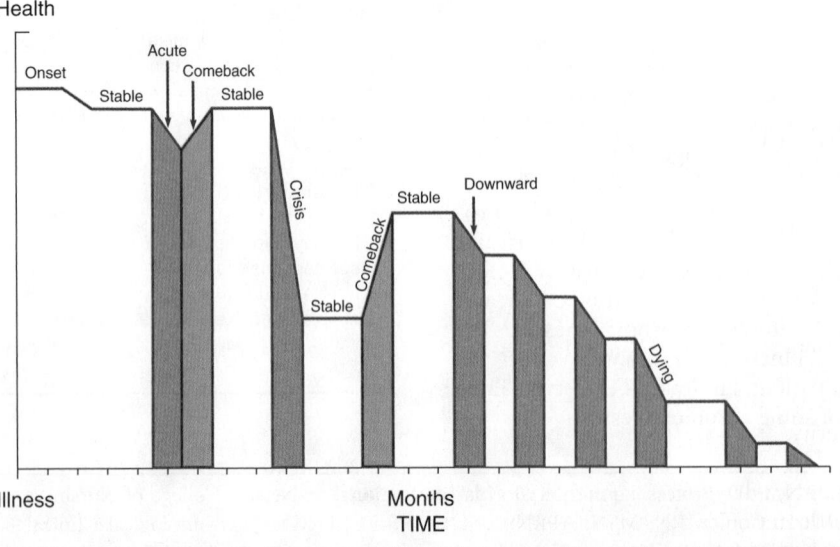

FIG. 5-1 The Chronic Illness Trajectory is a theoretical model of chronic illness. The trajectory model of chronic illness recognizes that chronic illness will have many phases (see Table 5-3).

TABLE 5-4   SEVEN TASKS OF PEOPLE WITH CHRONIC ILLNESS

1. Prevent and manage a crisis.
2. Carry out prescribed treatment regimen.
3. Control symptoms.
4. Reorder time.
5. Adjust to changes in course of disease.
6. Prevent social isolation.
7. Attempt to normalize interactions with others.

Source: Corbin JM, Strauss A: A nursing model for chronic illness management based upon the trajectory framework, *Sch Inq Nurs Pract* 5:155, 1991.

TABLE 5-5   CHARACTERISTICS OF TREATMENT REGIMENS

Characteristic	Example
Difficult	Managing a home hemodialysis unit
Time consuming	Dressing changes done four times daily
Painful or uncomfortable	Injecting heparin daily in the abdomen
Unsightly appearance	Tracheostomy
Slow rate of effectiveness	Lowering blood cholesterol level with medication or diet

---

Corbin and Strauss identified the seven tasks of those who are chronically ill[2] (Table 5-4). These tasks are discussed in the following sections.

Preventing and Managing a Crisis. Most chronic illnesses have the potential for an acute exacerbation of symptoms, which may result in further disability or death. Examples include the patient with heart disease who has another myocardial infarction or the patient with asthma who has a severe attack. A major task for both the patient and the caregiver is to learn to prevent or manage the crisis. First, the patient and caregiver need to understand the potential for the crisis to occur. Second, they need to know ways to prevent or modify the threat. This often involves adherence to a prescribed medical regimen. Patients also need to know the signs and symptoms of the onset of a crisis. Depending on the chronic illness, signs and symptoms may occur suddenly (e.g., seizure in a patient with seizure disorder) or slowly (e.g., heart failure in a patient with untreated hypertension). It is important for the patient and caregiver to develop a plan to manage a crisis that is likely to occur.

Carrying Out Prescribed Treatment Regimens. Treatment regimens vary in degree of difficulty and the impact that they have on the person's lifestyle. Characteristics of treatment regimens are included in Table 5-5.

Controlling Symptoms. An important task for those with chronic illnesses is to learn to control symptoms so that desired activities may be continued. Some individuals redesign their lifestyle by learning to plan ahead, such as the person with irritable bowel syndrome choosing to go only to events where there are restrooms near the seating area. Others may redesign their living space. Patients and their families or caregivers need to learn about the pattern of symptoms, such as typical onset, duration, and severity, so that lifestyle can be changed accordingly.

Reordering Time. Patients with chronic illness often report having too much or too little time. Treatment plans that require large amounts of time for the patient, as well as caregivers, may necessitate changing schedules or eliminating other activities.

Adjusting to Changes in Course of Disease. Some diseases, such as multiple sclerosis, have unpredictable courses that make planning activities difficult. Part of the patient's task is to develop a personal identity that includes the chronic illness and adjust to the lifestyle changes it necessitates.

Preventing Social Isolation. Social isolation may occur with chronic illness because the individual chooses to withdraw from previous activities or because others withdraw from the chronically ill person. An example is a man who has aphasia secondary to a stroke who may be unwilling to go out in public because he is embarrassed because of communication problems.

Attempting to Normalize Interactions With Others. Most individuals with chronic illness attempt to manage symptoms so that they can hide their disabilities or disfigurement. This may involve wearing a prosthesis or demonstrating that they can function the same as a person without a disability or chronic illness. An example of this is the man with chronic lung problems who stops walking to catch his breath, but appears to be inspecting a plant or looking in a store window.

Prevention of Chronic Illness

Chronic illnesses are often preventable. *Primary prevention* refers to measures such as proper diet, proper exercise, and immunizations that prevent the occurrence of a specific disease. *Secondary prevention* refers to actions aimed at early detection of disease that can lead to interventions to prevent disease progression. *Tertiary prevention* refers to activities that limit disease progression, such as rehabilitation.[3]

NURSING MANAGEMENT
CHRONIC ILLNESS

Diagnosis and treatment of the acute phase or acute exacerbations of a chronic illness are sometimes done in a hospital. Other phases of a chronic illness are managed in an ambulatory care setting, at home, in an assisted living facility, or in a skilled nursing facility. The course of chronic illness is often unpredictable. The management of a chronic illness can profoundly affect the lives of the patient, caregiver, and family.

An assessment of health status includes an individual's level of daily functioning and his or her perception of relative health or illness. This health assessment includes activities of daily living (ADLs), such as bathing, dressing, eating, toileting, and transfer. It also includes instrumental ADLs (IADLs), such as using a phone, shopping, preparing food, housekeeping, doing laundry, arranging transportation, taking medications, and handling finances.

Because the majority of chronic illnesses are treated in an ambulatory care setting, it is increasingly important for patients and caregivers to understand and manage their own health. The term *self-management* refers to the individual's ability to manage his or her symptoms, treatment, physical and psychosocial consequences, and lifestyle changes in response to living with a long-term disorder.[4]

You play an important role in the management of individuals with chronic illness. This begins with planning care, teaching the patient and caregiver regarding the treatment plan, implementing strategies for symptom management, and assessing patient outcomes.

Family caregivers (e.g., spouses, adult children, partners) often have important roles in the life of the chronically ill person. The ideal situation is one in which family caregivers work together with the patient to manage the illness. This collaboration begins under the direction of the health care team at the time of diagnosis. When the caregiver is a spouse who is also older, he or she may have a chronic illness as well, which complicates the situation.[5] The stresses and needs of family caregivers are discussed in Chapter 4 and Table 4-5.

OLDER ADULTS

DEMOGRAPHICS OF AGING

In the past three decades the older adult population (those 65 years of age and older) has grown twice as fast as the rest of the population. Almost 40 million people, or 13% of the population, are age 65 or older.[6] Nearly one in five U.S. residents is expected to be 65 or older by 2030. The number of Americans age 85 or older is expected to more than triple, from 5.8 million to 19 million, between 2010 and 2050.[6] This dramatic increase is in part due to aging of the *Baby Boomers* (those born between 1946 and 1964) who began to turn 65 in 2011.

Upcoming cohorts of older adults will be better educated than previous cohorts and have greater access to technology and resources. In the United States 13% of people over age 65 are people of color, including 8% African Americans; 3% Asian/Pacific Islanders; and less than 1% American Indians, Eskimos, and Aleuts. People of Hispanic/Latino ethnicity (who may be of any race) represent 7% of the older population.[1] By 2030 the proportion of older adults who are people of color will increase 160% (Latinos 202%; African Americans 114%; American Indians, Eskimos, and Aleuts 145%; and Asian/Pacific Islanders 145%), while growth in the European-American population will increase by only 59%.[6]

Other factors add to the overall increase in the older population. Common diseases of the early to mid-twentieth century that killed many people before they reached older age, such as influenza and diarrhea, are now less common. Declining infant mortality, new drug therapies, mechanical devices, improved surgical interventions, health promotion, and earlier detection and treatment of diseases have contributed to the increase in life span.

The U.S. Census Bureau predicts life expectancy to continue to increase for both men and women. Men and women born in 1950 who reach age 65 can expect, on average, another 12.8 and 15.8 years of life, respectively.[1,7] Whether this gender difference is due to differences in health behaviors (e.g., smoking, alcohol use) or occupation is not known.[8]

The fastest-growing segment of older Americans is people ages 85 or older. Since the 1960s, this group has increased 250%. The terms young-old adult (65 to 74 years of age) and old-old adult (85 years of age and older) describe two groups of older adults with different characteristics and needs. The old-old adult is often a woman who is widowed, divorced, or single and dependent on family for support. Many have outlived children, spouses or partners, and siblings. Old-old adults are often characterized as hardy, elite survivors. Because old-old adults have lived so long, they may have become the family icon, the symbol of family tradition and legacy.

Nearly 6% of individuals age 65 to 74 and 25% of those 85 and older live in nursing homes.[8] The frail older adult is usually over age 75 and has physical, cognitive, or mental dysfunctions that may interfere with independently performing ADLs.[9] (Older frail adults are discussed later in this chapter.)

ATTITUDES TOWARD AGING

Who is old? The answer to this question often depends on the respondent's age and attitude. It is important to understand that aging is normal and is not related to pathology or disease. Age is established by a date in time and is influenced by many factors, including emotional and physical health, developmental stage, socioeconomic status, culture, and ethnicity.[10]

As people age, they are exposed to new and different life experiences. The accumulation of these differences makes older adults more diverse than any other age-group. As you assess older adults, consider and value their diversity and life history. Also assess their own perceptions of what it means to be an older adult. Older adults with poor health report a higher perceived age and lower sense of well-being when compared with healthy older adults. The majority of older adults report having good-to-excellent health despite having a chronic illness. Age is important, but it may not be the most relevant factor in determining appropriate care of an individual older adult patient.

Myths and stereotypes about aging are often supported by media reports of older adults who are "problematic." These commonly held misconceptions may lead to errors in assessment and unnecessary limitations or interventions. For example, if you think that all older people are rigid in their thinking, you

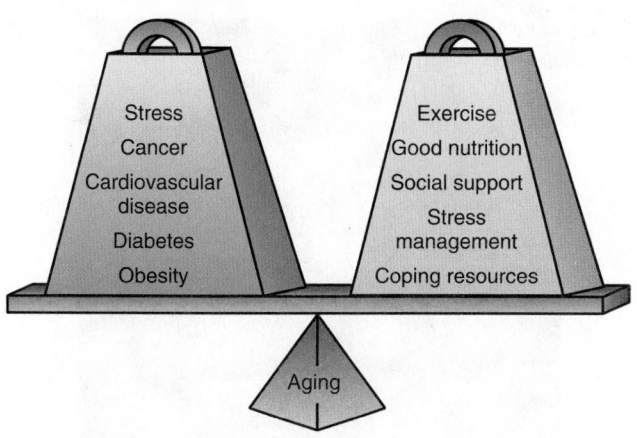

FIG. 5-2 The aging process can be viewed as a balance between negative and positive factors.

TABLE 5-6 GERONTOLOGIC ASSESSMENT DIFFERENCES

Summary of Tables

Body System	Table Number	Page
Visual	21-1	371
Auditory	21-7	380
Integumentary	23-1	417
Respiratory	26-4	481
Hematologic	30-3	619
Cardiovascular	32-1	691
Gastrointestinal	39-5	871
Urinary	45-2	1051
Endocrine	48-3	1141
Reproductive	51-3	1225
Nervous	56-4	1344
Musculoskeletal	62-1	1494

may not present new ideas to a patient.[11] **Ageism** is a negative attitude based on age. Ageism leads to discrimination and disparities in the care given to older adults. If you demonstrate negative attitudes, it may be because you fear your own aging process or you are not knowledgeable about aging and the health care needs of the older adult. Therefore it is important to gain knowledge about normal aging and have increased contact with older adults who are healthy and live independently. Also, it is your role as a nurse to dispel myths of aging.

BIOLOGIC AGING

From a biologic view, *aging* is defined as the progressive loss of function. The exact cause of biologic aging is unknown. Biologic aging is a multifactorial process involving genetics, diet, and environment.[12] In part, biologic aging can be viewed as a balance of positive and negative factors (Fig. 5-2).

Research is directed at increasing both the average life span and the quality of life of older adults. The hope is that new antiaging therapies will be developed to slow down or reverse age-related changes that result in chronic illness and disability. Based on numerous laboratory studies in rodents, caloric restriction (reducing dietary intake by 25% to 50%) has been consistently shown to significantly extend the life span.[13] It may be that caloric restriction results in changes in body composition, metabolism, and hormones that are conducive to long life. Caloric restriction in humans is associated with decreases in the incidence of obesity, diabetes, hypertension, and cancer, all of which are associated with aging.[13,14]

A number of nutrients have been tested for their potential benefits in reducing the impact of aging. Examples include β-carotene, selenium, vitamin C, and vitamin E. To date, research has failed to show that large doses of these supplements prevent chronic illness, such as heart disease or diabetes.[15] However, much more research is needed before it is determined whether any of these substances will delay aging or enhance the functional ability of older adults.

AGE-RELATED PHYSIOLOGIC CHANGES

Age-related changes affect every body system. These changes are normal and occur as people age. However, the age at which specific changes occur differs from person to person and within the same person. For instance, a person may have gray hair at

age 45 but relatively unwrinkled skin at age 80. In your role as a nurse, assess for age-related changes. Table 5-6 presents a list of tables where specific age-related assessment findings can be found throughout the book.

SPECIAL OLDER ADULT POPULATIONS

Chronically Ill Older Adults

Daily living with chronic illness is a reality for many older adults. The incidence of chronic illness triples after age 45. Most people 65 years of age and older have at least one chronic condition, and many have multiple conditions.[1] The most common chronic conditions in older adults are hypertension, osteoarthritis, heart disease, cancer, and diabetes. Other common chronic conditions include Alzheimer's disease, vision and hearing deficits, osteoporosis, hip fractures, stroke, Parkinson's disease, and depression.

Older Adult Women

For the aging woman, the impact of an aging body and being a woman is considered double jeopardy. Many factors have a significant negative impact on the health of older women (see Gender Differences box). Many of these factors are directly

GENDER DIFFERENCES

Older Adults

Men
- More likely to be living with spouse
- More likely to have health insurance
- Higher income after retirement
- Less likely to be involved in caregiving activities
- Generally have fewer chronic health problems than women

Women
- More likely to live alone
- Loss of spouse more common
- Less likely to have health insurance
- More likely to live in poverty
- Poverty rates highest among minority women
- Lack of formal work experience leading to lower income
- More likely to rely on Social Security as major source of income
- More likely to be caregiver of ill spouse
- Have a higher incidence of chronic health problems such as arthritis, hypertension, stroke, and diabetes

TABLE 5-7	GERONTOLOGIC ASSESSMENT DIFFERENCES

Cognitive Function

Cognitive Function	Effect of Aging
Fluid intelligence	Declines during middle age
Crystallized intelligence	Improves
Vocabulary and verbal reasoning	Improves
Spatial perception	Constant visuospatial perception Declines in spatial navigation tasks
Synthesis of new information	Declines during middle age
Mental performance speed	Declines during middle age
Short-term recall memory	Declines during old age
Long-term recall memory	Constant

FIG. 5-3 Older adults living in rural areas often enjoy outside activities, such as gardening. (iStockphoto/Thinkstock)

related to reduced financial resources and the greater longevity of women compared with men. Thus older women often experience disparities, including unequal access to quality health care. (Health disparities are discussed in Chapter 2.) As a nurse, you are in an excellent position to be an advocate for equity for older women in the health care system. Advocacy organizations, such as the Older Women's League (OWL) and the Society for Women's Health Research, can be helpful in this process.

Cognitively Impaired Older Adults

Most healthy older adults have no noticeable decline in cognitive abilities (Table 5-7). Older adults may experience memory lapses or benign forgetfulness, which is significantly different from cognitive impairment. This is also referred to as *age-associated memory impairment.* Encourage older adults with memory loss to be evaluated by their primary care provider, and to use memory aids, attempt recall in a calm and quiet environment, and actively engage in memory improvement techniques. Memory aids include clocks, calendars, notes, marked pillboxes, safety alarms on stoves, and identity necklaces or bracelets. Memory techniques include word association, mental imaging, and mnemonics.

Declining physical health is an important factor that influences cognitive impairment. Older adults who experience sensory loss, heart failure, or cerebrovascular disease may show a decline in cognitive functioning.[16] Cognitive impairment, delirium, and dementia are discussed in Chapter 60.

Rural Older Adults

People over age 65 are less likely to live in metropolitan areas than younger people. Five barriers to health care access for older adults are transportation, limited supply of health care workers and facilities, lack of quality health care, social isolation, and financial limitations.[17,18] Rural older adults are often stressed by declining self-care abilities. Particularly vulnerable are older adults of color living in rural areas, who have even less access to health care providers. In addition, older adults who live in rural areas may be less likely to engage in health-promoting activities.

When you work with older adults in rural areas, recognize lifestyle values and practices of rural life (Fig. 5-3). In planning care, be aware that transportation is the number one barrier to health care for rural older adults. Alternative service approaches such as computer-based Internet sources and chat rooms, DVDs, radio, community centers, and church social events can be used to promote healthful practices or to conduct health screening (Fig. 5-4). The development of telehealth devices for

FIG. 5-4 Older adults are using computers more frequently and accessing health care information on the Internet. (Comstock Images/Thinkstock)

INFORMATICS IN PRACTICE

Older Adults and Internet Use

- Forty percent of older adults use the Internet to look for health information.
- Older adults are more likely to accept as true what they read on a Web page. This is related to a lack of Internet experience and confusion from the large amounts of available information.
- Teach patients who use the Internet as a source of information how to assess the credibility of a website.
- Suggest the use of websites that include senior-friendly design elements.

monitoring patients in their home environments has enhanced the ability to provide care to isolated individuals.[19] Innovative models of nursing practice must continue to be developed to assist the rural older adult.[20]

Homeless Older Adults

The number of older adults who are homeless is increasing. Key factors associated with homelessness include (1) having a low income, (2) having reduced cognitive capacity, (3) living alone, and (4) living in a community that lacks affordable housing. Homeless older adults may be chronically homeless or recently homeless because of a crisis in either health or economic status.[21]

Mortality rates for homeless older adults are three times higher than for older adults who have housing. Older adults who are homeless have more health problems and appear older. They are also at additional risk because many aging network services are not designed to reach out to people who are homeless. Older people who are homeless are less likely to use shelters or meal site services than younger homeless people.[22] Long-term care placement is often an alternative to homelessness, especially when the person is cognitively impaired and alone. Fear of institutionalization may explain why homeless older adults do not use shelter and meal site services. Care for homeless older adults requires an interdisciplinary approach (including nurses, physicians, social workers, clerical workers, and transporters) that links shelters with outreach, primary care clinics, Medicare and Medicaid offices, and pharmacies.

Frail Older Adults

Frailty is a geriatric syndrome in which three or more of the following are present: advanced age, unplanned weight loss (10 lb or more in the past year), weakness, poor endurance and energy, slowness, and low activity levels. Risk factors include disability, multiple chronic illnesses, and dementia. People are more likely to become frail if they smoke, have a history of depression or long-term medical health problems, or are underweight. The old-old population (85 years of age or older) is most at risk for frailty, although many in this age-group remain healthy and robust.

Older frail adults have difficulty coping with declining functional abilities and decreasing daily energy. When stressful life events (e.g., death of a pet) and daily strain (e.g., caring for an ill spouse) occur, frail older adults often cannot cope with the effects of stress and, as a result, may become ill. Common health problems of frail older adults include mobility limitations, sensory impairment, cognitive decline, falls, and increasing frailty.[23]

Frail older adults tire easily; have little physical reserve; and are at risk for disability, elder mistreatment, and institutionalization. Frail older adults are especially at risk for malnutrition and dehydration, which are related to factors such as living alone, depression, and low income. Other factors, such as declining cognitive status, inadequate dental care, sensory decreases, physical fatigue, and limited mobility, increase the risks of malnutrition and dehydration. Monitor frail older adults for adequate calorie, protein, iron, calcium, vitamin D, and fluid intake. Because medications may interfere with nutrition, perform a thorough medication review, including prescription drugs, over-the-counter drugs, vitamins, minerals, supplements, herbal remedies, and cultural remedies.

TABLE 5-8	**SCALES: NUTRITIONAL ASSESSMENT OF OLDER ADULTS**
The acronym SCALES can remind you to assess important nutritional indicators:
Sadness, or mood change
Cholesterol, high
Albumin, low
Loss or gain of weight
Eating problems (e.g., mechanical problems such as impaired swallowing, poor dentition)
Shopping and food preparation problems

A tool to assess the risk factors for poor nutritional status in older adults is presented in Table 5-8. Once an older adult's nutritional needs are identified, common interventions include home-delivered meals, dietary supplements, food stamps, dental referrals, and vitamin supplements.

CULTURALLY COMPETENT CARE

OLDER ADULTS

The term **ethnogeriatric** describes the specialty area of providing culturally competent care to older adults.[24] As American society changes, ethnic institutions and neighborhoods may also change. For the older adult with strong ethnic and cultural roots, there may be a loss of friends who speak the "mother tongue," a loss of the religious institution that supports social ethnic activities, and a loss of stores that carry desired ethnic foods. This sense of loss is increased when children and others deny or ignore ethnic and cultural practices. Support for older adults of color is most frequently found in the family, religious practices, and isolated geographic or community ethnic clusters. In the old-old population, members of an ethnically diverse group often live with extended family and continue to speak their native language.

Ethnic populations of older adults face unique problems. Because older adults often live in older neighborhoods, physical security and personal safety related to crime may be a concern. Individuals with ethnic identities often have disproportionately lower incomes and may not be able to afford Medicare deductibles or drugs needed to treat chronic illnesses.[25] Perceptions of health may also differ by ethnic group. Among older adults, fewer African Americans and Hispanic/Latinos rate their health as excellent or good as compared with white older adults.[26]

Assess each older adult's ethnic and cultural orientation. Do not assume that ethnicity and culture are or are not of value to the patient and the patient's family until you do an assessment. For you to be effective with the ethnic older adult, a sense of respect and clear communication are critical. Nursing interventions to assist in meeting the needs of ethnic populations are described in Table 2-9. (Culturally competent care is discussed in Chapter 2.)

SOCIAL SUPPORT FOR OLDER ADULTS

Social support for older adults occurs at three levels. First, family members are the primary and preferred providers of social support. Second, a semiformal level of support is found in clubs, religious (or faith-based) organizations, neighborhoods, and senior citizen centers. Third, older adults may be linked to formal systems of social welfare agencies, health facilities, and government support. Generally, you, as a nurse, are part of the formal support system.

Family Caregivers

Many older adults require caregiving by family members. Other older adults may take on the role of caregiver for someone in their family, usually their spouse or partner. Many family caregivers caring for older adults are themselves age 65 or over.[27] The challenges of caregiving are discussed in Chapter 4 on pp. 51 to 52.

Elder Mistreatment or Abuse

Elder mistreatment (EM) describes intentional acts of omission or commission by a caregiver or "trusted other" that cause harm or serious risk of harm to a vulnerable older adult. EM may occur in community (home or assisted living facility) or long-term care (institutional) settings.

Approximately 2% to 10% of community-dwelling older adults in the United States are abused, neglected, or exploited by trusted others.[28] The prevalence of EM in institutional settings is unknown, but it is thought to be widespread. Although EM rates are similar in women and men, the majority of victims are women because of the predominance of women in older age cohorts. Victims of EM have a mortality risk that is three times higher than that of nonmistreated peers. The higher mortality risk is not due to the abuse or neglect itself, but rather may be due to stress-related illnesses associated with prolonged mistreatment.[29]

EM is a hidden problem. For every reported case in the community setting, more than five cases go unreported. Underreporting may be higher based on immigration status, ethnic background, or sexual orientation. Victims are unlikely to report mistreatment by "trusted others" because of isolation; impaired cognitive or physical function; feelings of shame, guilt, or self-blame; fear of reprisal; pressure from family members; fear of nursing home placement; or cultural norms. Health care providers also underreport, possibly because of failure to suspect or recognize EM, perceived inability to successfully intervene, desire to avoid responsibility for further action, or ageism.

Much of domestic EM is family violence that involves power and control dynamics. Family members are responsible for up to 90% of domestic EM. Adult children who abuse, neglect, or exploit their parents are usually dependent on their parent(s) for housing and financial support, have a history of violence, are unemployed, and/or are disabled from substance abuse or mental illness. Abusive spouses or partners may either initiate intimate partner violence in older age or continue a lifelong pattern of abuse.[30]

Many factors put community-dwelling older adults at risk for domestic EM. These include (1) physical or cognitive dysfunction that leads to an inability to perform ADLs (and therefore produces dependence on others for care), (2) any psychiatric diagnoses (especially dementia and depression), (3) alcohol abuse, and (4) decreased social support.[31] In long-term care settings the same factors that lead to institutionalization are risk factors for mistreatment by staff, visitors, and others. These include dependence on others for care because of physical or cognitive dysfunction (especially conditions that produce aggressive behaviors). Residents of long-term care facilities are also at risk for harmful aggression by other residents.[32]

Types of EM, characteristics, and manifestations are shown in Table 5-9. EM types frequently co-occur, and up to 70% of cases involve neglect. In institutional settings EM includes the types described in Table 5-9, but also includes failure to follow the plan of care, unauthorized use of physical or chemical restraints, overuse or underuse of medication, or isolation as punishment.

Assess for and consider EM if you observe any of these characteristics or manifestations. Perform a thorough history and physical examination that includes screening for mistreatment. Follow your organization's protocols for EM screening and interventions. Tools that are helpful in assessment include the Elder Mistreatment Assessment and the American Medical Association's Diagnostic and Treatment Guidelines on Elder Abuse and Neglect (see Resources at the end of this chapter).

It is important that you interview patients alone because, if mistreatment is occurring, they may not disclose in the presence of the person who accompanied them, especially if that person is the abuser. Be especially attentive to explanations about injuries that are not consistent with what you observe, contradictory explanations between the patient and the caregiver, or behavioral clues that suggest the patient is being threatened or intimidated. Additional nursing interventions are listed in Table 5-10. In most states, health care workers and others are mandated to report suspected or actual EM to Adult Protective Services and/or law enforcement. Know your legal responsibilities by checking the laws in your state.

Self-Neglect

Despite the prevalence of mistreatment of older adults by trusted others, the majority of referrals made to Adult Protective Services are for self-neglect. Older adults who self-neglect are likely to live alone; refuse or are unable to meet their basic needs; have multiple, untreated medical or psychiatric conditions; and live in squalor. Like EM, older community-dwelling adults who self-neglect face a higher risk of mortality than peers who do not self-neglect. Nursing interventions include assessment for possible self-neglect, referrals for long-term multidisciplinary case management, and referral to Adult Protective Services.[33]

SOCIAL SERVICES FOR OLDER ADULTS

A network of services supports older adults both in the community and in health care facilities. In the United States most older adults are the beneficiaries of at least one social or governmental service. To understand the older adult's situation, learn about government structures that fund and regulate programs for older adults. The Administration on Aging (AoA), which is part of the Department of Health and Human Services, is the federal agency responsible for many older adult programs. Funding from the AoA is funneled to state and local Area Agencies on Aging.[34]

MEDICARE AND MEDICAID

Medicare is a federally funded health insurance program for people ages 65 years or older, as well as for people under age 65 with certain disabilities and people of any age with end-stage kidney disease requiring dialysis or a kidney transplant. Nursing documentation is critically important for adequate reimbursement of services.

TABLE 5-9   TYPES OF ELDER MISTREATMENT

Characteristics	Manifestations
Physical Abuse	
Slapping, striking; restraining; incorrect positioning; oversedation with medications	Bruises, bilateral injuries (ankles, wrists), repeated injuries in various stages of healing; oversedation; use of several emergency departments
Neglect	
Failure or refusal to provide basic life needs, including food, water, medications, clothing, hygiene; failure to provide physical aids such as dentures, eyeglasses, hearing aid; failure to ensure safety	Older adult's reports of being neglected; untreated or infected pressure ulcers on sacral area, heels; loss of body weight; laboratory values showing dehydration (e.g., ↑ Hct, ↑ serum sodium), malnutrition (↓ serum protein); poor personal hygiene; lack of adherence with medical treatment
Failure to provide social stimulation; leaving alone for long periods; failure to provide companionship	Depression, withdrawn behavior; agitation; ambivalent attitude toward caregiver or family member
Psychologic Abuse	
Berating verbally; harassment; intimidation; threats of punishment or deprivation; childlike treatment; isolation	Depression, withdrawn behavior; agitation; ambivalent attitude toward caregiver or family member
Sexual Abuse	
Nonconsensual sexual contact, including touching inappropriately; forced sexual contact	Older adult's report of sexual abuse; unexplained vaginal or anal bleeding; bruised breasts; unexplained STIs or genital infections
Financial Abuse	
Denying access to personal resources, stealing money or possessions; coercing to sign contracts or durable power of attorney; making changes in will or trust	Living situation below level of personal resources; sudden change in personal finances; sudden transfer of assets
Violation of Personal Rights	
Denying right to privacy or right to make decisions regarding health care or living environment; forcible eviction	Sudden inexplicable changes in living situation; confusion
Abandonment	
Desertion of an older person by an individual who has assumed responsibility for providing care or by a person with physical custody	Older adult's reports of being abandoned; desertion of an older adult at a hospital or nursing facility, shopping center, or other public place

Hct, Hematocrit; *STIs,* sexually transmitted infections.

TABLE 5-10   NURSING ASSESSMENT

Mistreatment

- Screen for possible elder mistreatment, including domestic violence.
- Conduct a thorough history and head-to-toe assessment. Document your findings, including any statements made by the older adult or accompanying adult.
- If the older adult appears to be in immediate danger, develop and implement a safety plan in collaboration with the interdisciplinary team involved in the person's care.
- Identify, collect, and preserve physical evidence (e.g., dirty or bloody clothing, dressings, or sheets).
- After obtaining consent, take photographs to document physical findings of suspected abuse or neglect. If possible and appropriate, do this before treating or bathing the alleged victim.
- If you suspect that mistreatment is occurring, report your findings to the appropriate state agency and/or law enforcement as mandated by the laws in your state.
- Initiate social work, forensic nursing, and other consultations as appropriate.

Medicare has four options for coverage: A, B, C, and D. Part A covers inpatient hospital care and partially covers skilled nursing facility care, hospice, and home health care. Part A coverage is "free" because workers support Medicare through payroll taxes.[35] Medicare Part B partially covers outpatient care, physicians' services, and home health care. It also covers some preventive services, such as mammograms. Medicare Part B is voluntary and has a monthly premium and an annual deduct-

ible before payment begins. Medicare Advantage Plans, sometimes called "Part C" or "MA Plans," are offered by private companies approved by Medicare to provide Part A and Part B benefits. Part D is available to Medicare enrollees and provides a prescription drug benefit. Members pay a yearly deductible, a monthly premium, and a copayment. People with lower incomes and limited assets may qualify for extra help to pay for prescriptions.

Medicare does not cover long-term care, custodial ADLs or IADLs care, dental care or dentures, hearing aids, or eyeglasses. (More information is available at *www.Medicare.gov.*) These costs, plus the Medicare deductible, account for the fact that some older adults pay for 50% of their health care costs yearly.

Medicaid is a state-administered, needs-based program to assist eligible low-income people, including Medicare beneficiaries, with certain medical expenses. Individuals who qualify for both Medicare and Medicaid are frequently referred to as "dual-eligibles." Eligibility and coverage vary by state. For Qualified Medicare Beneficiaries, Medicaid pays Medicare premiums, deductibles, and co-insurance, as well as long-term care and home health expenses. In the United States the majority of long-term care is paid for by Medicaid or private pay. (More information is available at *www.medicaid.gov.*)

CARE ALTERNATIVES FOR OLDER ADULTS

Older adults with special care needs include people who are homeless, in need of assistance with ADLs, cognitively impaired, homebound, or no longer able to live at home. Older adults may be served by adult day care, adult day health care, home health care, and long-term care.

Adult Day Care and Adult Day Health Care

Adult day care centers provide social, recreational, and health-related services to individuals in a safe, community-based environment (Fig. 5-5). This includes daily supervision, social activities, opportunities for social interaction, and ADLs assistance for two major groups of adults: those who are cognitively impaired, and those who have problems independently performing ADLs. Services offered in adult day care programs are individualized based on need. Programs designed for adults who are cognitively impaired offer therapeutic recreation, support for family, family counseling, and social involvement.

Adult day health care centers are similar to adult day care but are designed to meet the needs of older adults and people with disabilities who need a higher level of care. This might include health monitoring, therapeutic activities, one-on-one ADLs training, and personal services.

Adult day care centers and adult day health care centers may provide respite to allow continued employment for the caregiver and delay institutionalization of older adults. Centers are regulated, and standards are set by the state. Medicare does not cover costs. Adult day health care is tax deductible as dependent care. Appropriate placement in adult care programs that match participants' needs is important. Caregivers and adults with self-care deficits are often uninformed about adult day centers and their services as an alternative care option. You can assist by knowing the available centers in your area and assessing the needs of older adults and their families. You will then be in a position to assist older adults and their families in making good decisions about their care.

Home Health Care. Home health care (HHC) can be a cost-effective care alternative for older adults who are homebound, have health needs that are intermittent or acute, and have supportive caregiver involvement. HHC is not an alternative for adults in need of 24-hour ADLs assistance or continuous safety supervision. (Private duty care may be an alternative in these situations.) HHC services require physician orders and skilled nursing care for Medicare reimbursement. Unless these requirements are met, assistance by home health aides for ADLs management or assistance by a homemaker for IADLs management will not be paid by Medicare.

In addition to HHC, respite, personal care, and homemaker services are often sought by caregivers through organizations that provide nonmedical assistance. These services help older adults stay at home.

Long-Term Care Facilities

Practice settings for long-term care are presented in eTable 1-2. Three factors appear to precipitate placement in a long-term care facility: (1) rapid patient deterioration, (2) caregiver inability to continue care because of stress and burnout, and (3) an alteration in or loss of the family support system. Deteriorating cognition, incontinence, or a major health event (e.g., stroke) can accelerate placement.

The conflicts and fears faced by older adults and their families make placement a difficult transition. Common caregiver concerns include: (1) Will the older adult resist the admission process?; (2) Will the level of care given by staff be insufficient?; (3) Will the resident be lonely?; and (4) Will nursing care be affordable?

This time of disruption is exacerbated by the physical relocation of the older adult and may result in adverse health effects for them. *Relocation stress syndrome* is a nursing diagnosis that is associated with the disruption, confusion, and challenges that older adults face when moving from one environment to a new environment. Older adults may experience anxiety, depression, and disorientation. Appropriate interventions can reduce the effects of relocation. Whenever possible, involve older adults in the decision to move and fully inform them about the location. Caregivers can share information, pictures, or a video recording of the new location. Personnel at the institution can send a welcome message. On arrival, new residents can be greeted by staff members to provide orientation. To bridge the relocation, new residents can be "buddied" with seasoned residents (Fig. 5-6).

LEGAL AND ETHICAL ISSUES

Legal assistance is a concern for many older adults. Legal concerns include advance directives, estate planning, taxation issues, appeals for denied services (e.g., disability), financial decisions, or exploitation by strangers or "trusted others." Legal aid is available to older adults with low income by contacting a local senior center.

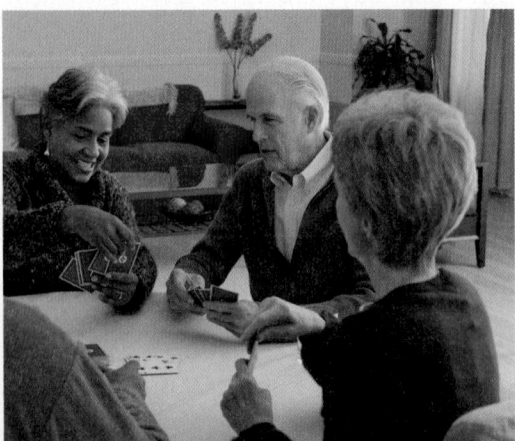

FIG. 5-5 Senior centers offer places for older adults who live independently to meet and gather with friends. (Jupiterimages/Comstock/Thinkstock)

FIG. 5-6 Social interaction and acceptance are important for older adults. (Hemera/Thinkstock)

Advance directives are written statements of a person's wishes regarding medical care. These documents allow patients to more specifically direct their own care at end of life. Advance directives are discussed in detail in Chapter 10 and Table 10-6.

When working with older adults, you may find several ethical issues that influence practice, such as use of physical or chemical restraints or the assessment of older adults' ability to make decisions. Other ethical issues related to end-of-life care include decisions about resuscitation, treatment of infections, nutrition and hydration, and transfer to more intensive treatment units. These situations are often complex and emotionally charged. You can assist the patient, family, and other health care workers by (1) acknowledging when an ethical dilemma is present, (2) keeping current on the ethical issues, and (3) advocating for an institutional ethics committee to help in the decision-making process.

NURSING MANAGEMENT
OLDER ADULTS

Gerontologic nursing is the care of older adults based on the specialty body of knowledge of gerontology and nursing. These specialty nurses approach older adults with a whole-person (physical, psychologic, developmental, socioeconomic, cultural) perspective. Care of older adults is complex and presents challenges that require skilled assessment and creative nursing interventions tailored to this population.

Diseases and conditions in older adults may be difficult to accurately assess and diagnose. Older adults may underreport symptoms and "treat" these symptoms by altering their functional status. For example, a man having loss of feeling in his feet because of neuropathy may start using a walker to get around. At the same time, he does not report the symptom to his health care provider. The older adult may attribute a new symptom to "aging" and ignore it. The older adult may eat less, sleep more, or "wait it out."

In older adults, disease symptoms are often atypical. Complaints of an "aching joint" may actually be a broken hip. Asymptomatic cardiac disease may be diagnosed when the patient is being treated for a urinary tract infection. Pathologic conditions with similar symptoms are often confused. For example, depression may be misdiagnosed and treated as dementia.

In older adults a *cascade disease pattern* may occur. For example, a patient who experiences insomnia treats the condition with a hypnotic medication, becomes lethargic and confused, falls, breaks a hip, and subsequently develops pneumonia. You play a vital role in preventing this downward trajectory.

Older adults may face health problems with fear and anxiety. They may view health care workers as helpful, but perceive institutions as negative and potentially harmful places. Communicate a sense of concern and care by use of direct and simple statements, appropriate eye contact, direct touch, and gentle humor. These actions help the older adult relax in this stressful situation.

NURSING ASSESSMENT

Before beginning the assessment process, first attend to primary needs. For example, make certain that the patient is comfortable and does not need to urinate. Place all assistive devices, such as glasses and hearing aids, within reach. Evaluate your patient's level of fatigue and stop the interview if necessary. Allow adequate time to offer information to the patient and time for the patient to respond to questions. Interview both the older adult and his or her family or caregivers. This can be done separately unless the patient is cognitively impaired or specifically requests the caregiver's presence. The medical history may be lengthy. Review medical records and determine what information is relevant.

The focus of a comprehensive geriatric assessment is to determine appropriate interventions to maintain and enhance the functional abilities of older adults. Comprehensive geriatric assessment is interdisciplinary and, at a minimum, includes the medical history, physical examination, functional assessment, medication review, cognitive and mood evaluation, and social resources. Comprehensive geriatric assessment is often conducted by an interdisciplinary geriatric assessment team. The interdisciplinary team may include many disciplines, but at least a nurse, a physician, and a social worker. After the assessment is complete, the interdisciplinary team meets with the patient and family to present the team's findings and recommendations.[32]

Elements in a comprehensive nursing assessment include a history using a functional health pattern format (see Chapter 3), physical assessment, mood assessment, assessment of ADLs and IADLs, mental status evaluation, and a social-environmental assessment. Evaluation of mental status is particularly important for older adults because these results often determine the potential for independent living. SPICES, an effective tool for obtaining assessment data in older adults, should be the basis of nursing assessment when working in any setting (Fig. 5-7).

Evaluation of the results of a comprehensive nursing assessment helps determine the service and placement needs of older adults. Collect data regarding community resources that are needed to assist older adults and their caregivers in maintaining maximal functioning. The goal is to plan and implement actions that help older adults remain as functionally independent as possible.

PLANNING

When setting goals with older adults, it is helpful to identify their strengths and abilities. Include caregivers in planning. Priority goals for older adults might include gaining a sense of control, feeling safe, and reducing stress.

NURSING IMPLEMENTATION

When carrying out a plan of action for older adults, modify your approach and actions based on their physical and mental status. Small body size, common in older adults who are frail,

Patient name:		Date:	
		EVIDENCE	
SPICES		Yes	No
Sleep disorders			
Problems with eating or feeding			
Incontinence			
Confusion			
Evidence of falls			
Skin breakdown			

FIG. 5-7 SPICES.

may necessitate the use of pediatric equipment (e.g., blood pressure cuff). As with all patient groups, safety is a primary concern when caring for an older adult. Bone and joint changes often require transfer assistance, altered positioning, and use of gait belts and lift devices. Older adults with declining energy reserves may require additional time to complete tasks. A slower approach and the use of other adaptive equipment may be necessary.

Cognitive impairment, if present, requires that you offer careful explanations and a calm approach to avoid producing anxiety and resistance in the older adult. Depression can result in apathy and poor cooperation with the treatment plan.

HEALTH PROMOTION. Health promotion and prevention of health problems for older adults focus on three areas: (1) reduction in diseases and problems, (2) increased participation in health promotion activities (Fig. 5-8), and (3) increased targeted services that reduce health hazards. Programs have been successfully developed for screening for chronic health conditions, tobacco cessation, geriatric foot care, vision and hearing screening, stress reduction, exercise programs, drug usage, crime prevention, elder mistreatment, and home hazards assessment. You can carry out and teach older adults about the need for specific preventive services.

Health promotion and prevention can be included in nursing interventions at any location or level where nurses and older adults interact. You can use health promotion activities to increase self-care, personal responsibility for health, and independent functioning that will enhance the well-being of older adults. Resources available to you are listed at the end of the chapter. Teaching is an important tool for you to use to enhance self-care practices by older adults. (Patient teaching is discussed in Chapter 4.)

ACUTE CARE. Frequently the hospital is the first point of contact for older adults and the formal health care system. Conditions that most commonly result in hospitalization include falls, dysrhythmias, heart failure, stroke, fluid and electrolyte imbalances (e.g., hyponatremia, dehydration), pneumonia, urosepsis, and hip fractures. Older adults are often hospitalized with multiple system problems.

When older adults are being cared for in the acute care setting, both patients and caregivers need assistance with a variety of functions (Table 5-11). The outcome of hospitalization for older adults varies. Of particular concern are problems of high surgical risk, acute confusional state, health care–

associated infection, and premature discharge in an unstable condition. Geriatric nursing considerations sections throughout this book emphasize special needs and interventions for older adult patients.

Care Transitions. At the time of a care transition to another setting (e.g., acute care hospital to rehabilitation), many older adults are in an unstable condition. (Transitional care settings are presented in eTable 1-1.) Frail older adults and patients over 85 years of age are particularly vulnerable during care transitions. Most of these patients are transitioned under Medicare regulations that require a registered nurse or qualified person to develop a plan for discharge. Care transition plans are periodically reassessed, and caregivers and patients must be counseled to prepare the patient for posthospital care. Safe, effective, and efficient care transitions are most likely to occur when interdisciplinary team members work together to coordinate care.

Rehabilitation. The goal of rehabilitation is to help older adults adapt to or recover from disability. Rehabilitation may occur in acute inpatient rehabilitation or long-term care settings. With proper training, assistive equipment, and attendant personal care, people with disabilities often live independently. Older adults, primarily through Medicare reimbursement, can receive rehabilitative assistance through acute inpatient rehabilitation (limited days) and home health care programs (Fig. 5-9).

TABLE 5-11	CARE OF THE HOSPITALIZED OLDER ADULT

- Identify adults over age 85 with or without frailty and patients at risk for iatrogenic (due to medical/surgical treatment) problems.
- Consider discharge needs early in the hospital stay, especially assistance with ADLs, IADLs, and medications.
- Encourage the development and use of interdisciplinary teams, special care units, and individuals who focus on the special needs of older patients.
- Implement standard protocols to screen for at-risk conditions commonly present in the hospitalized older adult, such as urinary tract infection and delirium.
- Implement mobility programs to prevent functional decline. ("The bed is not your friend.")
- Advocate for referral of the patient to appropriate community-based services.

ADLs, Activities of daily living; *IADLs,* instrumental activities of daily living.

FIG. 5-8 Water aerobics is an example of a health promotion activity for older adults. (Jupiterimages/Photos.com/Thinkstock)

FIG. 5-9 The nurse assists a patient in a geriatric rehabilitation facility. (Keith Brofsky/Photodisc/Thinkstock)

Older adults with chronic conditions, such as stroke, arthritis, and heart disease, have increased risk of becoming functionally limited. These disabilities lead to increased self-care deficits, higher mortality rates, increased rates of institutionalization, and decreased life span. Reducing disability through geriatric rehabilitation is important to the quality of life of older adults.

Often older adults have specific fears and anxieties related to falling. Older adults are limited in the rehabilitation process by sensory-perceptual deficits, other health problems, impaired cognition, poor nutrition, and financial problems. Encouragement, support, and acceptance from all members of the health care team and their caregivers can assist older adults in remaining motivated for the hard work of rehabilitation.

Rehabilitation of older adults is influenced by several factors. First, preexisting problems associated with reaction time, visual acuity, fine motor ability, physical strength, cognitive function, and motivation affect the rehabilitation potential of older adults.

Second, older adults often lose function because of inactivity and immobility. This *deconditioning* can occur as a result of unstable acute medical conditions, environmental barriers that limit mobility, and a lack of motivation to stay in condition. The effect of inactivity clearly leads to "use it or lose it" consequences. Older adults can improve flexibility, strength, and aerobic capacity even into very old age. Passive and active range-of-motion exercises are used with all older adults to prevent deconditioning and subsequent functional decline.

Last, the goal of rehabilitation is to strive for maximal function and physical capabilities considering the individual's current health status. When an older adult demonstrates suboptimal health, screen and evaluate for risk behaviors. For example, on admission to any acute or long-term care facility and home health services, assess for fall risk, initiate appropriate fall prevention interventions, and evaluate for ongoing risk. Conduct accurate and comprehensive foot assessments for older adults with diabetes and arrange appropriate follow-up care.

Assistive Devices. Consider the use of assistive devices as interventions for older adults. Using appropriate assistive devices such as dentures, glasses, hearing aids, walkers, wheelchairs, adult briefs or protectors, adaptive utensils, elevated toilet seats, and skin protective devices can decrease disability. Include these tools and devices in the older adult's care plan when appropriate, and provide instruction in the proper use of the devices. For example, using a cane inappropriately may increase the risk for a fall.

Technology can assist with rehabilitation and living with functional impairments.[36] For example, electronic monitoring equipment can be used to monitor heart rhythms and blood pressure. Monitoring can also locate a person with dementia who has wandered away from home or a long-term care facility. Computerized assistive devices can be used to help patients with speech difficulties following stroke, and small electronic devices can serve as memory aids.

Safety. Safety is crucial in the health maintenance of older adults. When compared to younger adults, older adults are at higher risk for accidents because of normal sensory changes, slowed reaction time, decreased thermal and pain sensitivity, changes in gait and balance, and medication effects. Most accidents occur in or around the home. Falls, motor vehicle accidents, and fires are common causes of accidental death in older adults. Another environmental problem arises from the older person's impaired thermoregulation system that cannot adapt to extremes in environmental temperatures. The bodies of older adults can neither conserve nor dissipate heat as efficiently as younger adults. Therefore both hypothermia and hyperthermia occur more readily. This age-group accounts for the majority of deaths during severe cold spells and heat waves.

You can provide valuable counsel regarding environmental changes, which may improve safety for older adults. Measures such as colored step strips, tub and toilet grab bars, and stairway handrails can be effective in "safety-proofing" the living spaces of older adults. You can also advocate for home fire and security alarms. Uncluttered floor space, railings, and increased lighting and night-lights are some of the easiest and most practical adaptations.

Older adults who are new to inpatient or long-term care settings need a thorough orientation to the environment. Reassure the older adult that he or she is safe, and attempt to answer all questions. Foster orientation by displaying large-print clocks, avoiding complex or visually confusing wall designs, clearly designating doors and exits, and using simple bed and nurse-call controls. Provide diffuse lighting while avoiding glare. Environments that provide consistent caregivers and an established daily routine increase an older adult's sense of comfort and safety.

Medication Use. Medication use in older adults requires thorough and regular assessment, care planning, and evaluation. Nonadherence to medication regimens by older adults is common. Four of ten older adults are unable to read prescription drug labels, and two thirds are unable to understand the health information that is provided to them.[37]

Age-related changes alter the pharmacodynamics and pharmacokinetics of drugs. Drug-drug, drug-food, and drug-disease interactions all influence the absorption, distribution, metabolism, and excretion of drugs. The most dramatic changes with aging are related to drug metabolism (Fig. 5-10). Overall, by age 75 to 80, there is a 50% decline in the renal clearance of drugs. Hepatic blood flow decreases markedly with aging, and the enzymes largely responsible for drug metabolism are decreased as well. As a result, drug half-life is increased in older adults as compared with younger adults. This leads to drug toxicity and adverse drug events.

In addition to changes in the metabolism of drugs, older adults may have difficulty due to cognitive impairment, altered sensory perceptions, limited hand mobility, and the high cost of many prescriptions. Common reasons for drug errors made by older adults are listed in Table 5-12. *Polypharmacy* (the use of multiple medications by a person who has more than one health problem), overdose, and addiction to prescription drugs are recognized as major causes of illness in older adults.[37]

The effects of medications in older adults with multiple health problems are particularly challenging to assess and manage. As one disease is treated, another may be affected. For

TABLE 5-12 DRUG THERAPY
Common Causes of Medication Errors by Older Adults
• Decreased vision • Forgetting to take drugs • Use of nonprescription over-the-counter drugs • Use of medications prescribed for someone else • Lack of financial resources to obtain prescribed medication • Failure to understand instructions or importance of drug treatment • Refusal to take medication because of undesirable side effects

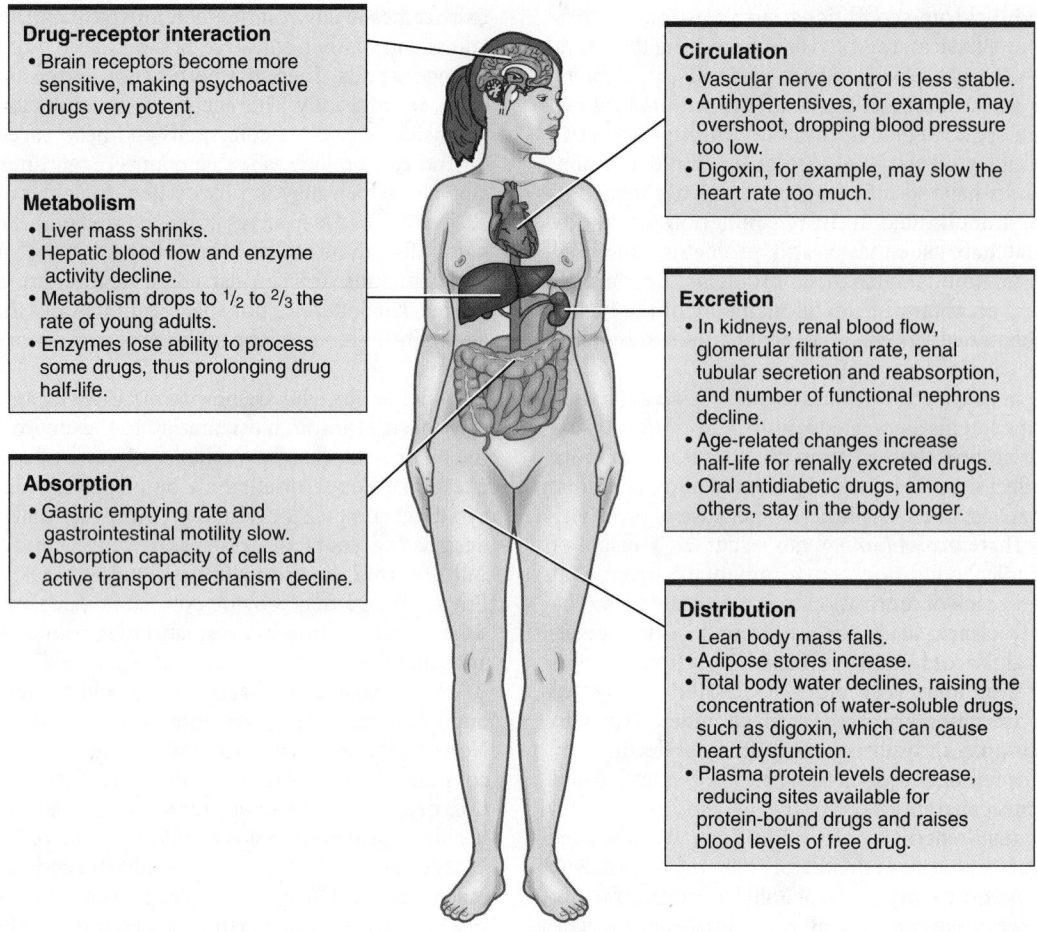

Drug-receptor interaction
- Brain receptors become more sensitive, making psychoactive drugs very potent.

Metabolism
- Liver mass shrinks.
- Hepatic blood flow and enzyme activity decline.
- Metabolism drops to $\frac{1}{2}$ to $\frac{2}{3}$ the rate of young adults.
- Enzymes lose ability to process some drugs, thus prolonging drug half-life.

Absorption
- Gastric emptying rate and gastrointestinal motility slow.
- Absorption capacity of cells and active transport mechanism decline.

Circulation
- Vascular nerve control is less stable.
- Antihypertensives, for example, may overshoot, dropping blood pressure too low.
- Digoxin, for example, may slow the heart rate too much.

Excretion
- In kidneys, renal blood flow, glomerular filtration rate, renal tubular secretion and reabsorption, and number of functional nephrons decline.
- Age-related changes increase half-life for renally excreted drugs.
- Oral antidiabetic drugs, among others, stay in the body longer.

Distribution
- Lean body mass falls.
- Adipose stores increase.
- Total body water declines, raising the concentration of water-soluble drugs, such as digoxin, which can cause heart dysfunction.
- Plasma protein levels decrease, reducing sites available for protein-bound drugs and raises blood levels of free drug.

FIG. 5-10 The effects of aging on drug metabolism.

example, the use of a drug such as oxybutynin (Ditropan), which is prescribed for overactive bladder, may cause confusion. To accurately assess medication use and knowledge, ask older adults to bring all medications (over-the-counter drugs, prescription drugs, vitamins and supplements, and herbal remedies) that they take regularly or occasionally to their health care appointment. You will then be able to accurately assess all medications the patient is taking, including drugs that the person may have omitted or thought unimportant. Additional nursing interventions to assist older adults in following a safe medication routine are listed in Table 5-13.

Depression. Depression is not a normal part of aging. However, it is often an underrecognized problem in older adults. Approximately 15% of older adults living in their homes have symptoms of depression. Rates of depressive symptoms in older adults in institutional settings are higher. Older adults commit 20% of the suicides in the United States, and older men who are white have the highest rate of suicide.[38]

Depression is associated with female gender, divorced or separated marital status, low socioeconomic status, poor social support, and a recent adverse and unexpected event. Depression in older adults tends to arise from a loss of self-esteem and may be related to life situations, such as retirement or loss of a spouse or partner. Problems such as physical complaints, insomnia,

TABLE 5-13   **DRUG THERAPY**
Medication Use by Older Adults

- Evaluate cognitive function and ensure ability to self-administer medication.
- Attempt to reduce medication use that is not essential by consulting the health care provider and pharmacist.
- Assess medication use, including prescription drugs; over-the-counter drugs; antihistamines; cough syrups; vitamins, minerals, and supplements; and herbal remedies.
- Assess alcohol and illicit drug use.
- Encourage the use of written or electronic medication-reminder systems.
- Encourage the use of one pharmacy.
- Work with health care providers and pharmacists to establish routine drug profiles on all older adult patients.
- Advocate (with drug companies) for low-income prescription support services.

lethargy, agitation, weight loss, decreased memory, and inability to concentrate are common.

Late-life depression often co-occurs with medical conditions, such as heart disease, stroke, diabetes, and cancer. Depression can exacerbate medical conditions by affecting adherence with diet, exercise, or drug regimens. It is important that your assessment include physical examination and interpretation of laboratory results for physical disorders that may have symptoms similar to those of depression (e.g., thyroid disorders, vitamin deficiencies). The Geriatric Depression Scale is easy to administer and is the gold standard assessment tool (see eTable 5-1 on the website for this chapter).

Encourage older adults who exhibit depressive symptoms to seek treatment. Because older adults with depression may feel unworthy, withdrawn, and isolated, the support of the family or others in encouraging older adults to seek treatment is important. Assist older adult caregivers who exhibit depressive symptoms to seek medical attention, and assist them in securing respite services and support for their caregiving role. (Family caregiving is discussed in Chapter 4 on pp. 50 to 52.)

Use of Restraints. *Physical restraints* are devices, materials, and equipment that physically prevent individuals from moving freely, such as walking, standing, lying, transferring, or sitting. *Chemical restraints* are medications that prevent a patient's voluntary movement.

Restraints may be used only to ensure the person's safety or the safety of others. Physical and chemical restraints are a last resort in the care of older adults. If physical or chemical restraints are used in the hospital or long-term care setting, use of the least restrictive restraint is required. Restraints require an order from a physician or an independently licensed advance practice nurse. In addition, frequent scheduled reviews of the ongoing necessity of the restraint are needed. There are additional regulatory requirements for restraint use, including time limit, observation and care, and alternatives to the use of restraints. Long-term care regulations and The Joint Commission set standards for restraint usage.

Carefully document restraint use and the behaviors that require this intervention. It is not appropriate to use restraints based on fall risk or irritating behaviors, such as calling out. The current standard is to provide safe care without using restraints of any form, whether physical or chemical.[39]

To achieve this standard, evaluate the patient's behavior. Behavioral symptoms, such as crying and shouting, may arise from co-morbidities, pain, medication toxicity, unmet needs, or environmental factors. When behavioral symptoms are evident, ask the following questions to better understand the patient's behavior: Is the person able to verbalize what she or he needs and wants? People with dementia may respond by speaking, gesturing, nodding, or making eye contact.[38] Questions that use "yes" or "no" answers are better than open-ended questions for gathering assessment information. Ask family, friends, or staff members from previous care settings about the patient's history; usual communication style and cues to indicate pain, fatigue,

hunger, or a need to urinate or defecate; abilities in ADLs; and daily routines (e.g., "Is he often awake at night or an early riser?" "Does she prefer breakfast before dressing? Take an afternoon nap? Have a routine for dressing?").

Evaluate whether disruptive behaviors signal unmet physiologic or psychosocial needs. For example, a patient who tries to get out of bed without help may be trying to reach the toilet. A toileting schedule will help to curtail such attempts and prevent incontinence. In critical care settings, patients emerging from sedation may be alarmed by an inability to speak or the presence of inserted tubes. Consider how treatments feel to the patient and pay attention to gestures, actions, and words to ascertain their meaning.

Restraint alternatives require vigilant, creative, and sensitive nursing care. Restraint alternatives include low beds, body props, and electronic devices (such as bed alarm signaling). Such approaches support the development of a "restraint-free" environment.

Sleep. Adequacy of sleep is often a concern for older adults because of altered sleep patterns. Older people experience a marked decrease in deep sleep and are easily aroused. Many older adults report difficulty initiating sleep and maintaining prolonged sleep; they may state they feel "unrefreshed" after sleep. (Sleep problems of older adults are discussed in Chapter 8.)

EVALUATION

The evaluation phase of the nursing process is similar for all patients. The results of evaluation direct you to continue the plan of care or revise as indicated. When evaluating nursing care with older adults, focus on functional improvement. Useful questions to consider when evaluating the plan of care for older adults are included in Table 5-14.

TABLE 5-14	EVALUATING NURSING CARE FOR OLDER ADULTS

Use the following questions to evaluate the effectiveness of care for older adults.
- Is there an identifiable change in ADLs, IADLs, mental status, or disease signs and symptoms?
- Does the patient consider his or her health state to be improved?
- Does the patient think the treatment is helpful?
- Do the patient and caregiver think the care is worth the time and cost?
- Can you document positive changes that support the interventions?
- Does change adequately meet the required mandates for reimbursement?

ADLs, Activities of daily living; *IADLs,* instrumental activities of daily living.

CASE STUDY

Older Adults

iStockphoto/Thinkstock

Patient Profile

L.X., a 79-year-old Chinese woman, was admitted through the emergency department with shortness of breath. She was diagnosed with community-acquired pneumonia. Her history also indicates she has chronic obstructive pulmonary disease (COPD), hypertension, diabetes, mild cognitive impairment, depression, macular degeneration, and significant hearing loss.

Subjective Data

- Had a stroke 5 years ago and has right-sided weakness
- Has a 100 pack-year history of tobacco use but quit smoking after her stroke
- Has not seen primary care physician in 1 year
- In past year has had an unplanned weight loss of 20 pounds
- Spends her days either in bed or in a recliner watching television

Psychosocial Data

- Came to the United States 15 years ago from China.
- Speaks Mandarin with limited English proficiency.
- Lives with her unemployed adult son who provides assistance with ADLs and IADLs.
- Has three daughters who live within a 2-hour drive.
- Has limited financial resources but has Medicare and Medicaid benefits.
- Her son has not visited her in the hospital, but her daughters raise concerns about their mother's care and safety at home, given their brother's history of anger issues and a gambling addiction.
- When daughters ask their brother about how he is caring for his mother, he says, "I'm doing the best I can. She refuses help. She refuses to go to the doctor. What do you want me to do? She's old. She's crazy. She's going to die anyway!"

Objective Data

- Matted hair, poor oral hygiene, overgrown toenails
- Two stage III sacral ulcers
- Unstageable right heel ulcer
- Multiple small bruises on her forearms and shins
- 5 × 10-cm bruise in the middle of her back

Discussion Questions

1. Compare L.X.'s experience as an older woman to known gender differences for older adults.
2. Identify the stage(s) of Corbin and Strauss chronic illness trajectory that describe L.X.'s current status. Which stage(s) is the goal of your nursing care?
3. Given the tasks of people with chronic illness as described by Corbin and Strauss, what is your assessment of L.X.'s ability to successfully complete these tasks? What will you include in your care planning to optimize her ability to complete these tasks?
4. Define *ageism,* and explain how it may be manifested in this case.
5. What risk factors does L.X. have for development of frailty? Which of these factors are modifiable?
6. **Priority Decision:** Based on your assessment of L.X., what are the priority nursing diagnoses?
7. **Priority Decision:** What are the priority nursing interventions for L.X.?
8. Explain ethnogeriatrics considerations that affect L.X. and how they will influence your nursing care.
9. Based on your knowledge of care alternatives for older adults, what setting(s) might be appropriate for L.X. on hospital discharge?
10. What risk factors does L.X. have for becoming a victim of elder mistreatment?

ⓔvolve   Answers available at *http://evolve.elsevier.com/Lewis/medsurg.*

BRIDGE TO NCLEX EXAMINATION

The number of the question corresponds to the same-numbered outcome at the beginning of the chapter.

1. Examples of primary prevention strategies include
   a. colonoscopy at age 50.
   b. avoidance of tobacco products.
   c. intake of a diet low in saturated fat in a patient with high cholesterol.
   d. teaching the importance of exercise to a patient with hypertension.
2. A characteristic of a chronic illness is that it *(select all that apply)*
   a. has reversible pathologic changes.
   b. has a consistent, predictable clinical course.
   c. results in permanent deviation from normal.
   d. is associated with many stable and unstable phases.
   e. always starts with an acute illness and then progresses slowly.
3. Ageism is characterized by
   a. denial of negative stereotypes regarding aging.
   b. positive attitudes toward the elderly based on age.
   c. negative attitudes toward the elderly based on age.
   d. negative attitudes toward the elderly based on physical disability.

4. An ethnic older adult may feel a loss of self-worth when the nurse
   a. informs the patient about ethnic support services.
   b. allows a patient to rely on ethnic health beliefs and practices.
   c. has to use an interpreter to provide explanations and teaching.
   d. emphasizes that a therapeutic diet does not allow ethnic foods.
5. An important nursing action to help a chronically ill older adult is to
   a. avoid discussing future lifestyle changes.
   b. assure the patient that the condition is stable.
   c. treat the patient as a competent manager of the disease.
   d. encourage the patient to "fight" the disease as long as possible.
6. Older adults who become ill are more likely than younger adults to
   a. complain about the symptoms of their problems.
   b. refuse to carry out lifestyle changes to promote recovery.
   c. seek medical attention because of limitations on their lifestyle.
   d. alter their daily living activities to accommodate new symptoms.

7. An appropriate care choice for an older adult who lives with an employed daughter but requires help with activities of daily living is
   a. adult day care.
   b. long-term care.
   c. a retirement center.
   d. an assisted living facility.

8. Nursing interventions directed at health promotion in the older adult are primarily focused on
   a. disease management.
   b. controlling symptoms of illness.
   c. teaching positive health behaviors.
   d. teaching regarding nutrition to enhance longevity.

1. b, 2. c, d, 3. c, 4. d, 5. c, 6. d, 7. a, 8. c.

evolve

For rationales to these answers and even more NCLEX review questions, visit *http://evolve.elsevier.com/Lewis/medsurg.*

REFERENCES

1. Centers for Disease Control and Prevention: Chronic diseases and health promotion, Retrieved from *www.cdc.gov/chronicdisease/overview/index.htm.*

2. Corbin JM, Strauss A: A nursing model for chronic illness management based upon the Trajectory Framework, *Sch Inq Nurs Pract* 5:155, 1991. (Classic)

3. Centers for Disease Control and Prevention: Skin cancer module: practice exercises. Retrieved from *www.cdc.gov/excite/skincancer/mod13.htm.*

*4. Inouye J, Braqinsky N, Kataoka-Yahiro M: Randomized clinical trials of self-management with Asian/Pacific Islanders, *Clin Nurs Res* 20:366, 2011.

5. Stajduhar KI, Funk L, Wolse F, et al: Core aspects of "empowering" caregivers as articulated by leaders in home health care: palliative and chronic illness contexts, *Can J Nurse Res* 43:78, 2011.

6. Administration on Aging: A profile of older Americans. Retrieved from *www.aoa.gov/aoaroot/aging_statistics/Profile/2010/3.aspx.*

7. US Census Bureau: Facts for features and special editions. Retrieved from *www.census.gov/newsroom/releases/archives/facts_for_features_special_editions.*

8. Administration on Aging: Projected future growth of the older population. Retrieved from *www.aoa.gov/AoARoot/AgingStatistics.*

*9. Vermeulen J, Neyens JC, van Rossum E, et al: Predicting ADL disability in community-dwelling elderly people using physical frailty indicators: a systematic review, *BMC Geriatr* 11:33, 2011.

10. Luo Y, Waite LJ: Mistreatment and psychological well-being among older adults: exploring the role of psychosocial resources and deficits, *J Gerontol B Psychol Sci Soc Sci* 66:217, 2011.

11. Scott G: Ageism is rife in health care, *Nurs Stan* 25:1, 2011.

12. Kourtis N, Tavernarakis N: Cellular stress response pathways and ageing: intricate molecular relationships, *EMBO J* 30:2520, 2011.

13. Barnes SK, Ozanne SE: Pathways linking the early environment to long-term health and lifespan, *Prog Biophys Mol Biol* 106:323, 2011.

14. Weiss EP, Fontana L: Caloric restriction: powerful protection for the aging heart and vasculature, *Am J Physiol Heart Circ Physiol* 301:H1205, 2011.

*15. Dunn-Lewis C, Karemer WJ, Kupchak BR, et al: A multi-nutrient supplement reduced markers of inflammation and improved physical performance in active individuals of middle to older age: a randomized, double-blind, placebo-controlled study, *Nutr J* 10:90, 2011.

16. Nowrangi MA, Rao V, Lyketsos CG: Epidemiology, assessment, and treatment of dementia, *Psychiatr Clin North Am* 34:277, 2011.

*17. Thorpe JM, Thorpe CT, Kennelty KA, et al: Patterns of perceived barriers to medical care in older adults: a latent class analysis, *BMC Health Serv Res* 3:11, 2011.

18. Griffin SF, Williams JE, Hickman P, et al: A university, community coalition, and town partnership to promote walking, *J Public Health Manag Pract* 17:358, 2011.

19. McIlhenny CV, Guzic BL, Knee DR, et al: Using technology to deliver healthcare education to rural patients, *Rural Remote Health* 11:1798, 2011.

*20. Nkosi ZZ, Asah F, Pillay P: Post-basic nursing students' access to and attitudes toward the use of information technology in practice: a descriptive analysis, *J Nurs Manag* 19:876, 2011.

21. Fargo J, Metraux S, Byrne T, et al: Prevalence and risk of homelessness among US veterans: a multisite investigation: the selected works of Dennis P. Culhane. Retrieved from *www.works.bepress.com/dennis_culhane/107.*

22. Brown RT, Kiely DK, Bharel M, et al: Geriatric syndromes in older homeless adults, *J Gen Internal Med* 27:16, 2012.

23. Xue QL: The frailty syndrome: definition and natural history, *Clin Geriatr Med* 27:1, 2011.

24. McBride M: Ethnogeriatrics and cultural competence for nursing practice. Retrieved from *consultgerirn.org/topics/ethnogeriatrics_and_cultural_competence_for_nursing_practice/want_to_know_more.*

*25. Kim G, Worley CB, Allen RS, et al: Vulnerability of older Latino and Asian immigrants with limited English proficiency, *J Am Geriatr Soc* 59:1246, 2011.

26. August KJ, Sorkin DH: Racial and ethnic disparities in indicators of physical health status: do they still exist throughout late life? *J Am Geriatr Soc* 58:2009, 2010.

27. National Family Caregivers Association: Who are America's family caregivers? Retrieved from *www.nfcacares.org/who_are_family_caregiver.*

*28. Acierno R, Hernandez MA, Amstadter AB, et al: Prevalence and correlates of emotional, physical, sexual, and financial abuse and potential neglect in the United States: the National Elder Mistreatment Study, *Am J Public Health* 100:292, 2010.

*29. Lachs M, Bachman R, Williams CS, et al: Resident-to-resident elder mistreatment and police contact in nursing homes:

*Evidence-based information for clinical practice.

findings from a population-based cohort, *J Am Geriatr Soc* 55:840, 2007. (Classic)

30. US Department of Health and Human Services: The national elder abuse incidence study. Retrieved from *http://purl.access.gpo.gov/GPO/LPS104188.*

*31. Cisler JM, Amstadter AB, Begle AM, et al: Elder mistreatment and physical health among older adults: the South Carolina Elder Mistreatment Study, *J Trauma Stress* 23:461, 2010.

*32. Ellis G, Whitehead MA, O'Neill D, et al: Comprehensive geriatric assessment for older adults admitted to hospital, *Cochrane Database Syst Rev* 7:CD006211, 2011.

33. Mosqueda L, Dong X: Elder abuse and self-neglect: "I don't care anything about going to the doctor, to be honest…," *JAMA* 306:532, 2011.

34. HealthCare.gov: Improving care transitions. Retrieved from *www.healthcare.gov/compare/partnership-for-patients/safety/transitions.html#BackgroundonCareTransitions.*

35. Medicare.gov: Medicare basics. Retrieved from *www.medicare.gov/navigation/medicare-basics/medicare-basics-overview.aspx.*

36. Thompson HJ, Demiris G, Rue T, et al: A holistic approach to assess older adults' wellness using e-health technologies, *Telemed J E Health* 17(10):794, 2011.

37. Medication Use Safety Training for Seniors: Facts: older adults and medicine use. Retrieved from *www.mustforseniors.org/facts.jsp.*

38. National Institute of Mental Health: Older adults: depression and suicide facts. Retrieved from *www.nimh.nih.gov/health/publications/older-adults-depression-and-suicide-facts-fact-sheet/index.shtml.*

*39. Enmarker I, Olsen R, Hellzen O: Management of person with dementia with aggressive and violent behavior: a systematic literature review, *Int J Older People Nurs* 6:153, 2011.

RESOURCES

AARP
www.aarp.org

Administration on Aging
www.aoa.gov

American Geriatrics Society
www.americangeriatrics.org

American Society on Aging
www.asaging.org

Best Practices in Nursing Care to Older Adults
www.consultgerirn.org

Centers for Disease Control and Prevention—Healthy Aging
www.cdc.gov/aging

Centers for Medicare and Medicaid Services
www.cms.gov

Hartford Institute for Geriatric Nursing
www.hartfordign.org

National Caucus and Center on Black Aged
www.ncba-aged.org

National Center on Elder Abuse
www.ncea.aoa.gov/ncearoot/Main_Site/index.aspx

National Gerontological Nursing Association
www.NGNA.org

National Hispanic Council on Aging
www.nhcoa.org

National Indian Council on Aging
www.nicoa.org

National Institute on Aging
www.nia.nih.gov

It's supposed to be a secret, but I'll tell you anyway.
We doctors do nothing. We only help and
encourage the doctor within.
Albert Schweitzer, MD

Complementary and Alternative Therapies

Virginia (Jennie) Shaw

evolve WEBSITE

http://evolve.elsevier.com/Lewis/medsurg

- NCLEX Review Questions
- Key Points
- Pre-Test
- Rationales for Bridge to NCLEX Examination Questions

- Concept Map Creator
- Glossary
- Stress-Busting Kit for Nursing Students
- Content Updates

LEARNING OUTCOMES

1. Compare and contrast the conventional model and the integrative model for health care.
2. Describe four categories of complementary and alternative therapies.
3. Choose the key concepts to include when teaching patients about herbal supplements.
4. Name three commonly used herbal products and their indications for use.

5. Describe the nurse's role related to complementary and alternative therapies.
6. Explain how the nurse can assess a patient's use of complementary and alternative therapies.
7. Describe ways that the nurse can use complementary and alternative therapies to provide self-care.

KEY TERMS

acupuncture, p. 83
complementary and alternative therapies, p. 80
herbal therapy, p. 81

holistic nursing, p. 80
massage, p. 83

Historically wellness has been viewed as incorporating the physical, emotional, mental, and spiritual realms. Hippocrates, the father of medicine, advised a daily aromatic bath and fragrant massage for the maintenance of health. Florence Nightingale believed that nursing puts patients in the best condition for nature to act on them. The concepts of holism and balance guided the belief that the body heals itself and works to maintain homeostasis. The concepts of spirituality and harmony with nature were inseparable from the concepts of health and wellness.

This view of "wholeness" began to change with the works of René Descartes (1596–1650) and Sir Isaac Newton (1642–1727). They postulated that the body is a series of parts that can be broken down and studied. This mechanistic approach views the body as a machine; whatever part is broken is analyzed and then repaired, without regard for other aspects of the person involved. The *conventional model* of health care is based on this approach. Health care focuses on the physical body, often to the exclusion of the mind and the spirit.

Emphasis is placed on what can be seen, measured, and quantified.

This conventional model has guided American health care for more than 100 years. About 40 years ago Americans began to explore health care therapies that were outside this model. This consumer-led movement fostered development of a new model of health care, a more "integrative" model. In this model, consumers combine the use of complementary and alternative therapies with conventional therapies. The conventional and integrative health care models are compared in Table 6-1.

The *integrative model* focuses on (1) personal responsibility for health; (2) joining of mind-body-spirit; and (3) use of natural, less invasive modalities. This model promotes health and wellness, not just treatment of diseases. Consumers desire more involvement in their health care decisions. They desire modalities that are more natural, less costly, and safer. The rise of chronic diseases and stress-related disorders has also led to consumers' interest in complementary and alternative therapies.

Reviewed by Jane A. Madden, RN, MSN, Professor of Nursing, Pikes Peak Community College, Colorado Springs, Colorado.

TABLE 6-1	COMPARISON OF CONVENTIONAL AND INTEGRATIVE HEALTH CARE MODELS	
Conventional Health Care Model	**Integrative Health Care Model**	
• Focus on physical body	• Focus on mind-body-spirit	
• Focus on treatment of symptoms using medications and surgery	• Focus on self-healing of the body using herbs, exercise, nutrition, stress management	
• Health care provider directs care	• Individual directs care; personal responsibility for health encouraged	
• Focus on disease states	• Focus on health and wellness	
• Technologic, invasive	• Noninvasive	
• Increasing cost	• Lower cost	
• Little focus on prevention	• Focus on prevention	

COMPLEMENTARY AND ALTERNATIVE THERAPIES

Complementary and alternative therapies (CAT) are a group of diverse medical and health care systems, practices, and products that are not generally considered part of conventional medicine.[1] This definition highlights what might be considered "complementary and alternative" in one country or at one period of history might be considered "conventional" in another place or time. What is classified as complementary and alternative therapies is constantly changing. When these therapies are proven safe and effective, they are often adopted into conventional medicine.

Terms frequently used to describe health-related approaches that are outside the dominant system of health care include *alternative, complementary,* and *integrative. Alternative therapies* are therapies used in place of conventional medicine, whereas *complementary therapies* are used in conjunction with conventional medicine. *Integrative therapies* combine treatments from conventional medicine with complementary and alternative therapies that have evidence of safety and effectiveness.

Many complementary and alternative therapies are harmonious with the values of nursing. Nurses emphasize healing, recognize the provider-patient relationship as a partnership, and focus on health promotion and illness prevention. The American Holistic Nurses Association (AHNA) was established to focus nursing care on the whole person—recognizing the interconnectedness of body, mind, spirit, and environment. The AHNA highlights the practice of holistic nursing.

Holistic nursing is based on a body of knowledge; evidence-based research; sophisticated skill sets; defined standards of practice; and a philosophy of living and being that is grounded in caring, relationship, and interconnectedness.[2] AHNA *(www.ahna.org)* advances the profession of holistic nursing by providing continuing education in holistic nursing, helping to improve the health care workplace through the incorporation of the concepts of holistic nursing, educating professionals and the public about holistic nursing and integrative health care, and promoting research and scholarship in the field of holistic nursing.[3]

Health care professionals have raised important questions about the effectiveness and safety of complementary and alternative approaches in the face of their increased use. In response to this need, the National Center for Complementary and Alternative Medicine (NCCAM) was established *(http://nccam.nih.gov).* A branch of the National Institutes of Health (NIH),

NCCAM serves as the federal government's lead agency for scientific research on complementary and alternative therapies. The mission of NCCAM is to define, through rigorous scientific investigation, the usefulness and safety of complementary and alternative medicine interventions and their roles in improving health and health care.[4]

NCCAM has four areas of focus: (1) advancing scientific research, (2) training CAM researchers, (3) sharing news and information, and (4) supporting integration of proven CAM therapies. The website provides a wealth of information for consumers and professionals, including clinical practice guidelines and literature reviews for the health care professional.

A large study conducted by NCCAM and the National Center for Health Statistics (as a part of the National Health Interview Survey [NHIS]) showed that approximately 38% of adults used CAT within the past 12 months.[5] In another survey Americans were asked why they use CAT, and 55% responded they believed their health would be improved if conventional medical treatments were combined with CAT.[6] Because of this growing use of CAT, you need to have a basic understanding of this topic and know where to find reliable in-depth information. A list of helpful websites is provided at the end of the chapter.

NCCAM CATEGORIES

Because the field of CAT is broad and ever changing, it is helpful to place therapies into broad categories. NCCAM groups these therapies into four broad categories, recognizing that one therapy may fit into more than one category (Table 6-2).

TABLE 6-2	NCCAM CATEGORIES OF COMPLEMENTARY AND ALTERNATIVE THERAPIES	
Category	**Description**	**Examples**
Natural products	Practices that use substances found in nature for their impact on health and wellness.	Herbal therapy, dietary supplements, vitamins, minerals, probiotics, aromatherapy
Mind-body medicine	Techniques that enhance mind's ability to affect the physical body. Science of psychoneuroimmunology demonstrates strength of mind-body connection.	Meditation, yoga, acupuncture, relaxation breathing, guided imagery, hypnotherapy, prayer, journaling, art therapy
Manipulative and body-based practices	Practices that are based on the manipulation and/or movement of one or more parts of the body.	Massage, chiropractic therapy, yoga
Other CAT practices	Wide variety of practices.	Movement therapies (e.g., Pilates), traditional healers, manipulation of energy fields (e.g., Healing Touch), whole medical systems (Table 6-3)

Source: *http://nccam.nih.gov.*
CAT, Complementary and alternative therapies; *NCCAM,* National Center for Complementary and Alternative Medicine.

Natural Products

The category of natural products includes herbal therapy, dietary supplements, vitamins, minerals, and other "natural products." The NHIS found that 17.7% of American adults had used a natural product in the previous year. These products were the most commonly used CAT.[5]

Herbal therapy is the use of individual herbs or combinations of herbs for therapeutic benefit. An *herb* is a plant or plant part (bark, roots, leaves, seeds, flowers, or fruit) that produces and contains chemical substances that act on the body. It is estimated that approximately 25,000 plant species are used medicinally throughout the world, and approximately 30% of modern prescription drugs are derived from plants. Botanical medicine is the oldest form of medicine; archaeologic evidence suggests that Neanderthals used plant-based remedies 60,000 years ago. Today about 80% of the world's population relies extensively on plant-derived remedies.

Medicinal plants work in much the same way as drugs; both are absorbed and trigger biologic effects that can be therapeutic. Many have more than one physiologic effect and thus have more than one condition for which they can be used. The range of action of herbs is extensive.

Overall the use of herbal therapy continues to increase. Although most herbal products can safely be used without professional assistance, side effects and interactions with prescription drugs have been described. There is concern that side effects from the use of herbal products are underreported, thus promoting the impression that herbal products are completely safe to use.

Because consumers tend not to share their use of herbal products with their primary health care provider, herb-drug interactions may also be underreported. Patients who are scheduled for surgery should be advised to stop taking herbal products 2 to 3 weeks before surgery. Patients who are being treated with conventional drug therapy should be advised to discontinue herbal products with similar pharmacologic effects because the combination may lead to an excessive reaction or to unknown interaction effects. Patient teaching guidelines related to herbal therapy are presented in Table 6-4.

TABLE 6-3 WHOLE MEDICAL SYSTEMS

Examples	Description
Traditional Chinese Medicine (TCM)	Based on restoring and maintaining balance of vital energy (*Qi*). One of the world's oldest, most complete medical systems.
Ayurveda	Based on balance of mind, body, and spirit. Developed in India. Views disease as an imbalance between a person's life force (*prana*) and basic metabolic condition (*dosha*).
Homeopathy	Based on "like cures like." Remedies are specially prepared from the same substance that causes the symptom or problem. Extremely small amounts of the substance are used for the remedy. Remedies are believed to work through an energy transfer.
Naturopathy	Based on promotion of health rather than symptom management. Focuses on enhancing the body's natural healing response using a variety of individualized interventions such as nutrition, herbology, homeopathy, physical therapies, and counseling. Naturopathic physicians are graduates of accredited naturopathic medical schools, and licensing varies by state.

TABLE 6-4 PATIENT & CAREGIVER TEACHING GUIDE

Herbal Therapies

- Ask the patient about use of herbal therapies. Take a complete history of herbal use, including amounts, brand names, and frequency of use. Ask the patient about allergies.
- Investigate whether herbs are used instead of or in addition to traditional medical treatments. Find out whether herbal therapies are used to prevent disease or to treat an existing problem.
- Instruct the patient to inform health care provider before taking any herbal treatments.
- Make the patient aware of the risks and benefits associated with herbal use, including drug reactions when taken in combination with other drugs.
- Advise the patient using herbal therapies to be aware of any side effects while taking herbal treatments and to immediately report them to health care provider.
- Make the patient aware that moisture, sunlight, and heat may alter the components of herbal treatments.
- Advise the patient to determine the reputation of the manufacturers of herbal products and the safety of the product before buying herbal treatments.
- Encourage the patient to read labels of herbal therapies carefully. Advise the patient not to take more of an herb than is recommended.
- Inform the patient that most herbal therapies should be discontinued at least 2 to 3 weeks before surgery.
- Inform the patient that the employees of health food stores are not trained health care professionals.

COMPLEMENTARY & ALTERNATIVE THERAPIES

Complementary & Alternative Therapies Boxes Throughout Book

Information related to various complementary and alternative therapies can be found in the following boxes throughout the book.

Title	Chapter	Page
Acupuncture	65	1565
Assessment of Use of Herbs and Dietary Supplements	3	39
Biofeedback	46	1087
Echinacea	27	502
Fish Oil and Omega-3 Fatty Acids	33	716
Ginger	42	927
Glucosamine and Chondroitin	65	1565
Hawthorn	35	777
Herbal and Dietary Supplements That May Affect Clotting	38	851
Herbal Products and Surgery	18	320
Herbs and Supplements for Menopause	54	1285
Herbs and Supplements That May Affect Blood Glucose	49	1174
Imagery	52	1255
Kava	7	97
Lipid-Lowering Agents	34	738
Melatonin	8	104
Milk Thistle (Silymarin)	44	1012
Music Therapy	19	337
St. John's Wort	7	96
Yoga	6	83
Zinc	27	505

TABLE 6-5   COMMONLY USED HERBS*

Name	Uses Based on Scientific Evidence	Comments
Aloe	Constipation	• Short-term use only. • May cause electrolyte imbalances. • May lower blood glucose.
Cranberry	Prevention of urinary tract infection	• Drinking cranberry juice appears to be safe. • Excessive amounts can lead to gastrointestinal upset or diarrhea.
Echinacea	May reduce incidence and duration of upper respiratory tract infections	• Short-term use is recommended. • Use with caution in patients with conditions affecting immune system. • Use cautiously in patients with asthma because of increased risk of allergic reaction.
Evening primrose	Eczema, skin irritation	• Contraindicated in individuals with seizure disorders.
Feverfew	Migraine headache prevention	• May increase risk of bleeding. • Long-term users may experience withdrawal symptoms.
Garlic	May decrease cholesterol and low-density lipoproteins (studies have been inconsistent)	• May increase risk of bleeding. • May lower blood glucose.
Ginger	Nausea and vomiting of pregnancy	• May increase risk of bleeding. • May lower blood glucose. • Use in pregnancy should not exceed 1 g/day. • Supervision by health care provider is recommended for pregnant women considering use of ginger.
Ginkgo biloba	Symptoms of claudication	• Generally well tolerated in recommended dosages for up to 6 months. • May increase risk of stroke. • May increase risk of bleeding. • May affect blood glucose levels.
Ginseng (*Panax* species)	May improve mental performance May enhance immune system May lower blood glucose	• May increase or decrease blood pressure. • May increase risk of bleeding. • Avoid use in patients with hormone-sensitive conditions such as breast cancer.
Hawthorn	Mild to moderate heart failure	• May add to the effects of cardiac glycosides, antihypertensives, and cholesterol-lowering agents.
Kava	Anxiety	• FDA has issued warning of severe liver damage linked to use. • Avoid use in patients with liver problems and patients taking medications that affect liver. • May increase drowsiness. • Use cautiously with herbs or supplements that are metabolized by kidneys.
St. John's wort	Short-term treatment of depression (studies on benefits of use are contradictory)	• Well tolerated in recommended dosages for 1–3 months. • May lead to serious interactions with herbs, supplements, OTC drugs, or prescription drugs. • Interferes with metabolism of drugs that use cytochrome P450 enzyme system. • May lead to increased side effects when taken with other antidepressants. • Advise patients to consult health care professional before self-medicating with St. John's wort.
Zinc	Upper respiratory tract infections	• Relatively safe. • Should not be taken with dairy products or caffeine, which will reduce its absorption.

Source: Data from *www.naturalstandard.com.*
*Advise patients who are pregnant or lactating to consult a health care practitioner before using any herbs. There is limited scientific evidence for the use of most herbs during pregnancy or lactation.
FDA, Food and Drug Administration; *OTC,* over-the-counter.

Commonly used herbs are presented in Table 6-5. Although herbs are derived from plants, most individuals administer them in the form of a pill or capsule (Fig. 6-2). Commonly used dietary supplements are found in Table 6-6 on p. 84. Complementary and alternative therapy boxes related to specific herbs and dietary supplements are found throughout the book (see summary box on previous page).

Mind-Body Medicine

Mind-body medicine therapies focus on the interaction between the mind, the body, and behavior, with the intent to promote health. Examples of these therapies include meditation, yoga, relaxation breathing, guided imagery, and acupuncture. Because some of these therapies are used in stress management, they are discussed in Chapter 7.

FIG. 6-1 Yoga is an example of both mind-body medicine and manipulative and body-based practices. (Jupiterimages/Comstock/Thinkstock)

FIG. 6-2 Herbs are most commonly administered as a pill or capsule, but the source is a plant, such as echinacea. (iStockphoto/Thinkstock)

🌿 **COMPLEMENTARY & ALTERNATIVE THERAPIES**

Yoga

Yoga is an ancient system of relaxation, exercise, and healing with its origins in Indian philosophy. The goal of yoga is physical and mental well-being achieved through the use of stretching, postures, breathing practices, and meditation.

Scientific Evidence

There is evidence to support use of yoga to treat hypertension and to reduce stress and anxiety.*

Nursing Implications
- Regardless of the type of yoga, deep abdominal relaxation breathing is a main component and helps one to focus on the inner self and to promote the relaxation response (Fig. 6-1).
- Yoga is often used to promote relaxation, decrease stress, improve flexibility, and enhance overall health.
- Yoga is generally considered safe. Some postures should not be used by patients with certain medical conditions or illnesses.

*Based on a systematic review of scientific literature, available at www.naturalstandard.com.

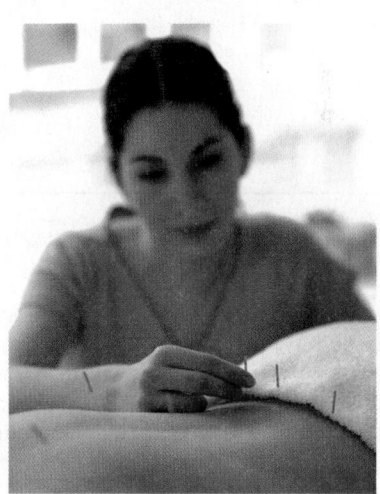

FIG. 6-3 Acupuncture showing the placement of acupuncture needles. (Creatas/Thinkstock)

Acupuncture. Acupuncture involves the insertion of fine needles into the circulation of Qi underneath the skin's surface (Fig. 6-3). Specific points are selected based on the diagnosis and nature of the complaint. With proper point selection and manipulation, acupuncture corrects disruptions in the flow of Qi.

Acupuncture has benefits for osteoarthritis, chronic pain, postoperative pain, headaches, fibromyalgia, postoperative nausea, and nausea and vomiting after chemotherapy.[7]

Acupuncture is considered a safe therapy when the practitioner has been appropriately trained and uses disposable needles. Patients should review their practitioner's credentials. The practitioner should have at least a master's degree in Oriental Medicine and be registered to practice acupuncture in that state. The practitioner should have passed the National Certification Commission for Acupuncture and Oriental Medicine examinations.

Manipulative and Body-Based Practices

Manipulative and body-based practices include interventions and approaches that are based on manipulation or movement of the body. Massage is one of the body-based methods commonly used by nurses.

Massage. Massage includes a range of techniques that manipulate the soft tissues and joints of the body. Involving touch and movement, massage is typically delivered with the hands, although elbows, forearms, feet, or various devices may be used. Massage techniques are used in bodywork, sports training, physical therapy, nursing, chiropractic therapy, osteopathy, and naturopathy.

Benefits of massage relate to its effects on the musculoskeletal, circulatory, lymphatic, and nervous systems. Massage also positively affects mental and emotional states. Massage therapy continues to grow in popularity, with most people using it as a means to reduce stress.

Until the 1970s, nurses were taught to perform "PM care," which consisted of a back rub and other measures to promote

TABLE 6-6   **COMMONLY USED DIETARY SUPPLEMENTS***

Name	Uses Based on Scientific Evidence	Comments
Chondroitin sulfate	Osteoarthritis	• Well tolerated for up to 3 years. • Avoid in patients with prostate cancer or those at increased risk for prostate cancer. • Use with caution in patients with bleeding disorders or those taking anticoagulants.
Coenzyme Q₁₀	Hypertension	• May decrease blood glucose levels.
Fish oil/omega-3 fatty acids	Hypertriglyceridemia Hypertension	• May increase risk of bleeding. • May increase blood glucose levels.
Glucosamine	Osteoarthritis	• Use with caution in patients taking insulin or diabetes medications. • May increase risk of bleeding.
Melatonin	Jet lag Decrease sleep latency (time to fall asleep)	• May increase risk of bleeding. Use with caution in patients with bleeding disorders or those taking anticoagulant drugs. • May decrease blood pressure. • Use with caution in patients with diabetes. • Avoid in patients taking antiseizure medications or central nervous system depressants.
Probiotics (live bacteria or yeast)	Acute diarrhea related to antibiotic therapy Upper respiratory tract infections	• Use with caution in patients with compromised immune systems or gastrointestinal disorders.
Red yeast rice	High cholesterol and high triglycerides	• Some products contain monacolin K, which is the active ingredient in the cholesterol-lowering drug lovastatin.
Soy	High cholesterol	• Use with caution in patients with hormone-sensitive cancers. • May interact with medications taken for diabetes, diarrhea, hypertension, high cholesterol, obesity, or cardiovascular disorders. • Advise patients to consult a health care professional.

Data from *www.naturalstandard.com.*
*Advise patients who are pregnant or lactating to consult a health care professional before using any supplements. There is limited scientific evidence for use during pregnancy or lactation.

relaxation and sleep. After that time, PM care and back rubs became the exception rather than the rule. Yet today, with the increased focus on providing holistic care, nurses are again recognizing the benefits of massage. Massage is an important form of touch. It is also a form of caring, communication, and comfort. Your role related to massage differs from that of the registered massage therapist. Whereas massage therapists can provide more comprehensive therapies, nurses can use specific massage techniques as part of nursing care. For example, you can give a back massage to help promote sleep. For a bedridden patient, gentle massage can stimulate circulation and help prevent skin breakdown.

When you have determined that massage may be useful in meeting a patient goal, first assess the patient's preference regarding touch and massage. Consider cultural and social beliefs, and discuss potential benefits with the patient. Then you can implement the indicated plan of care (e.g., hand massage, back massage) with reassessment after the massage.

Massage Techniques. Nursing use of massage typically begins with *effleurage,* or gliding strokes, to promote relaxation. Stroking is done from distal to proximal, along the long axis of the muscle. After relaxing the muscles with effleurage, you may use *petrissage,* or a "kneading" stroke, to gently lift and knead the muscle. Gently scented lotions or diluted essential oils may be included in the massage.

A simple hand massage (Fig. 6-4) can have a calming and relaxing effect, especially for patients who are anxious or agitated. When a patient is frustrated or agitated, a hand massage can provide a distraction and calm the patient.

Family members can be taught to perform massage on their loved one, providing an excellent way for them to participate in

FIG. 6-4 Hand massage can be a helpful tool to calm down an agitated or nervous patient. (Jupiterimages/Photos.com/Thinkstock)

patient care. This can be therapeutic for both the patient and the family, even when the loved one is cognitively impaired or unresponsive. Massage is beneficial throughout the life continuum. During end-of-life care, hospice nurses may incorporate massage into their nursing care, since the massaging touch can lessen pain and restlessness.

Massage is contraindicated in patients who have recent injuries or trauma, recent surgery, open wounds, deep vein thrombosis, inflammation or infections, bleeding, edema, or decreased sensation. Massage is also contraindicated when someone has used alcohol or recreational drugs.

Other CAT Practices

This broad category incorporates many practices, including movement therapies, practices of traditional healers, energy therapies, and whole body systems (see Table 6-3).

Energy Therapies. Energy therapies involve the manipulation of energy fields. They focus on energy fields originating within the body (biofields) or those from other sources (electromagnetic fields). Biofield therapies are based on the theory that energy systems in and around the body need to be balanced to enhance healing. Examples of energy therapies include Healing Touch, Therapeutic Touch, and Reiki.

Healing Touch (HT) is a nurse-based program founded in the 1980s by a nurse, Janet Mentgen. In HT, the nurse gently places his or her hands on or near the patient's clothed body. Based on established guidelines, the nurse assesses the patient's energy field, realigns energy flow, eliminates energy blockages, reactivates the mind-body-spirit connection, and then evaluates the process. It is an organized system designed to assist the patient to self-heal. The patient, not the nurse, determines effectiveness.

Information on classes, resources, and research findings is available at the Healing Touch International website (www.healingtouchinternational.org).

GERONTOLOGIC CONSIDERATIONS

COMPLEMENTARY AND ALTERNATIVE THERAPIES

Older adults with non–life-threatening, chronic conditions are likely to use complementary and alternative therapies. For the older adult, safety concerns involve herb-drug interactions or toxicity related to polypharmacy and age-related changes in pharmacokinetics. Decreased renal or liver function may slow metabolism and excretion of herbs and dietary supplements. Since older adults are a more vulnerable population, it is critical that you discuss the risks and benefits of using herbal products, while encouraging patients to inform their health care provider of any herbal product or dietary supplement they are taking.

NURSING MANAGEMENT
COMPLEMENTARY AND ALTERNATIVE THERAPIES

The professional nurse can use complementary and alternative therapies in professional practice and also in self-care practice.

PROFESSIONAL PRACTICE

In professional practice, be knowledgeable of these therapies, assess their use in patients, and promote their safety. You can incorporate many of these therapies into your professional nursing practice.

KNOWLEDGE OF THERAPIES. The use of complementary and alternative therapies continues to grow, and your patients expect you to know about them. Nursing schools are incorporating content relating to complementary and alternative therapies into their curriculum. Questions related to this topic are on the National Council Licensure Examination (NCLEX).

It is important for you to understand the commonly used CAT. This includes their clinical uses and scientific-based evidence for their uses. In addition, you need to know about the personal, cultural, and spiritual dimensions related to these therapies. As a nurse, you have been educated as a critical thinker and problem solver. You need to seek ongoing education regarding complementary and alternative therapies and to continually evaluate the evidence for use of these therapies.

You need to provide information on both conventional therapies and complementary and alternative therapies. Advise patients that complementary and alternative therapies do not replace conventional therapies, but can often be used in combination with them. By providing this information, you help patients make informed decisions. You are well positioned to become the "link" between conventional therapy and complementary and alternative therapies.

ASSESSMENT OF COMPLEMENTARY AND ALTERNATIVE THERAPY USE. Because many patients use these therapies, you need to collect data on the use of complementary and alternative therapies as part of your nursing assessment. This is important because most patients do not voluntarily tell their health care provider about their use of these therapies. However, they usually share this information when asked. Ask general, open-ended questions, while remaining nonjudgmental and respectful of the patient's response.

Examples of assessment questions include the following:
- Do you have any conditions that have not responded to conventional medicine? If so, have you tried any other approaches?
- Are you using any vitamin, mineral, dietary, or herbal supplements?
- Are you interested in obtaining information about complementary and alternative therapies?

Additional specific questions for assessing the use of herbs and dietary supplements are presented in the Complementary & Alternative Therapies box in Chapter 3 on p. 44.

PROMOTING SAFE USE OF THERAPIES. The American Nurses Association Code of Ethics states: "The nurse promotes, advocates for, and strives to protect the health, safety, and rights of the patient." A wide variety of therapies are considered complementary and alternative, and some of these therapies may be ineffective or even harmful. However, patients self-select use of these therapies, generally without consulting a health care professional. Safety concerns encompass the reliability of information, the safety and effectiveness of therapies, and the regulation of practitioners. Patients usually get their information from health food stores, friends, books, magazines, and the Internet. Encourage patients to seek professional assistance with these decisions.

There is a lack of regulation of providers of complementary and alternative therapies. For example, in most states massage therapists and acupuncturists are licensed by the state. However, this practice varies by state. Practitioners of some other therapies are more loosely regulated. Along with the challenge of obtaining accurate information, patients may be unable to assess the competency of practitioners. You can serve as a resource to guide patients in the safe use of therapies and in the safe choice of health care practitioners.

INCORPORATING THERAPIES IN PRACTICE. Nursing has a long history of providing therapies that have been considered complementary and alternative. These include massage, relaxation therapy, music therapy, humor, and other strategies to promote comfort, reduce stress, improve coping, and promote symptom relief (Table 6-7). Although these therapies are generally included within the scope of nursing practice, they are not specifically addressed in some state board of nursing practice acts.

TABLE 6-7	NURSES CAN USE COMPLEMENTARY AND ALTERNATIVE THERAPIES

If you have the training and experience, you can use the following:

- Acupressure
- Animal-assisted therapy
- Aromatherapy
- Healing Touch
- Humor
- Imagery
- Journaling
- Massage
- Meditation
- Music
- Prayer
- Reiki
- Relaxation breathing
- Therapeutic Touch

Some of these therapies require additional education, training, or supervision. Check with the board of nursing in your state to determine what therapies fall within the nursing domain. You are expected to obtain the necessary additional education and experience to be competent to use a selected therapy. In addition, institutional or workplace policies must be in place supporting the use of these therapies.

You are responsible for ensuring that the patient has given consent for a given therapy. The patient must be aware of the proposed benefit and any potential risks involved. Document the effectiveness of the intervention and evaluate the outcome.

SELF-CARE PRACTICE

Learning about complementary and alternative therapies can be one road to self-care. Initially, you may be eager to learn about complementary and alternative therapies so you can provide better patient care and be a holistic practitioner. At the same time, you may find that these therapies can enhance your own level of health and wellness. With the many different complementary and alternative therapies available, you should be able to find some that will promote your personal well-being. Examples of therapies that nurses commonly use for personal well-being include deep-breathing exercises, meditation, prayer, yoga, aromatherapy, massage, and music. It is essential that you, as the caregiver, first care for yourself before you can help the patients who need your care.

BRIDGE TO NCLEX EXAMINATION

The number of the question corresponds to the same-numbered outcome at the beginning of the chapter.

1. One characteristic of the integrative model of health care is
   a. increased cost.
   b. a focus on physical disease states.
   c. an integration of mind-body-spirit.
   d. the plan of care is directed by the health care provider.

2. The nurse is preparing to teach a patient about stress management. Which category of complementary and alternative therapies can guide the nurse in preparing this intervention?
   a. Natural products
   b. Energy therapies
   c. Mind-body medicine
   d. Manipulative and body-based practices

3. The nurse is teaching a patient about safe use of herbal therapies. Which statement indicates that the teaching has been effective?
   a. "I can increase the dose if I need to, since these pills are natural."
   b. "I don't have to tell my physician about this herb that I am taking."
   c. "I must remember to stop taking these herbs 2 to 3 weeks before I have surgery."
   d. "I can stop taking my blood pressure medication now that I am taking these herbs."

4. Which herbs can increase a patient's risk of bleeding (*select all that apply*)?
   a. Aloe
   b. Kava
   c. Garlic
   d. Ginger
   e. Feverfew

5. The nurse decides to incorporate complementary and alternative therapies into her practice. Which is the best source of information?
   a. Internet websites
   b. Board of nursing for her state
   c. Salesperson at the health food store
   d. Another nurse who claims his practice is holistic

6. The nurse is preparing to collect data on an older patient's use of complementary and alternative therapies. Which guidelines should the nurse follow?
   a. The patient's culture will probably dictate which therapies are used.
   b. Begin by asking general questions, and then move to more specific questions.
   c. Obtain this information from the medical record. It is not necessary to ask the patient.
   d. Older patients do not use complementary and alternative therapies because of age-related changes in pharmacokinetics.

7. The nurse is experiencing work-related stress and desires to develop a holistic plan of self-care. What is the best source of reliable information?
   a. A self-help book
   b. Internet websites
   c. Another nurse who does not seem stressed
   d. Professional nursing organizations such as AHNA

1, c, 2, c, 3, c, 4, c, d, e, 5, b, 6, b, 7, d.

@volve

For rationales to these answers and even more NCLEX review questions, visit *http://evolve.elsevier.com/Lewis/medsurg*.

REFERENCES

1. National Center for Complementary and Alternative Medicine: What is CAM? Retrieved from *http://nccam.nih.gov/health/ whatiscam*.
2. American Holistic Nurses Association: What is holistic nursing? Retrieved from *www.ahna.org/home/FAQs*.
3. American Holistic Nurses Association: Mission statement. Retrieved from *www.ahna.org/AboutUs/MissionStatement*.
4. National Center for Complementary and Alternative Medicine: Facts at a glance. Retrieved from *www.nccam.nih.gov/about/ ataglance*.
5. National Center for Complementary and Alternative Medicine: Statistics on Complementary and Alternative Medicine National Health Interview Survey. Retrieved from *http://nccam.nih.gov/ news/camstats/NHIS.htm*.
6. American Holistic Nurses Association: Integrative healthcare. Retrieved from *www.ahna.org/Resources/IntegratedHealthcare*.
7. Natural Standard: Acupuncture. Retrieved from *www. naturalstandard.com*.

RESOURCES

American Holistic Nurses Association
  www.ahna.org
Cochrane CAM Field
  www.compmed.umm.edu/cochrane.asp
Dietary Supplements Labels Database
  http://dietarysupplements.nlm.nih.gov/dietary
Evidence-Based Complementary and Alternative Medicine
  www.hindawi.com/journals/ecam
HerbMed
  www.herbmed.org
National Center for Complementary and Alternative Medicine
  http://nccam.nih.gov

I am an old man and have known a great many troubles,
but most of them never happened.
Mark Twain

Stress and Stress Management

Sharon L. Lewis

evolve WEBSITE

http://evolve.elsevier.com/Lewis/medsurg
- NCLEX Review Questions
- Key Points
- Pre-Test
- Answer Guidelines for Case Study on p. 97

- Rationales for Bridge to NCLEX Examination Questions
- Concept Map Creator
- Glossary
- Stress-Busting Kit for Nursing Students
- Content Updates

eTable
- eTable 7-1: Stages of the General Adaptation Syndrome

LEARNING OUTCOMES

1. Differentiate between the terms *stressor* and *stress*.
2. Explain the role of coping in managing stress.
3. Describe the role of the nervous and endocrine systems in the stress process.
4. Describe the effects of stress on the immune system.

5. Discuss the effects of stress on health.
6. Describe the coping and relaxation strategies that can be used by you or a patient experiencing stress.
7. Describe the nursing assessment and management of a patient experiencing stress.

KEY TERMS

coping, p. 92
emotion-focused coping, p. 92
imagery, p. 94

meditation, p. 94
problem-focused coping, p. 92
psychoneuroimmunology (PNI), p. 91

relaxation breathing, p. 93
stress, p. 88
stressors, p. 88

High levels of stress and anxiety are common among patients and their caregivers. How they deal with their stress is critical to their well-being. As a nurse, you have an important role in helping them manage stressful events.

Stress has a powerful effect on the mind, and therefore a significant effect on one's health and well-being. This chapter focuses on how stress can affect the mind and the body and how a person can effectively deal with stress.

DEFINITION OF STRESS

Stress is the inability to cope with perceived (real or imagined) demands or threats to one's mental, emotional, or spiritual well-being.[1] Because demands are perceived differently based on the person and situation, what is emotionally or psychologically stressful to one person may not be stressful to another. Individual responses to the same stressor vary greatly. *Perception* of the potential stressor influences the way an individual responds to that stressor (Fig. 7-1). This is demonstrated in the following examples.

- B.J., a 43-year-old woman, becomes depressed after a laparoscopic hysterectomy for fibroids. She is unwilling to participate in normal self-care activities. You are sur-

prised by her response and think that this is fairly simple surgery and she should get on with her life. After further assessment, you discover that the removal of her uterus is a great psychologic stressor because she perceives it as a loss of her womanhood and femininity.

- K.R., a 52-year-old woman, has just been told by her physician of her new diagnosis of type 2 diabetes. After the physician's visit to her, you are prepared to provide emotional support. However, you are puzzled when she is smiling and breathing a sigh of relief. You think that this diagnosis should be stressful. However, K.R. tells you that she is so relieved because for weeks she has worried that her symptoms were related to terminal cancer.

Many different events or factors can be stressors. They can be physiologic or emotional/psychologic (see Fig. 7-1). The emotional/psychologic stressors can be positive or negative. For example, the birth of a baby is a positive stressor. Marital discord is a negative stressor.

The key aspect of stressors is that they require an individual to adapt. In addition, differences in the behavioral and physiologic adaptive responses to a stressor can be based on the duration of a stressor (acute or chronic) and intensity of a stressor (mild, moderate, or severe). For example, an

Reviewed by Margie Hesson, RN, MSN, Certified Holistic Stress Management Instructor, Instructor of Nursing, South Dakota State University, Rapid City, South Dakota.

Stressors

Physiologic
- Pain
- Excessive noise
- Starvation
- Infection

Emotional/Psychologic
- Diagnosis of cancer
- Death of spouse
- Caring for disabled child
- Marital problems

→ Perception → **Stress**

FIG. 7-1 Stressors can be physiologic or emotional/psychologic. Your perception of these stressors will determine whether they cause stress. Events or circumstances become stressful when you perceive them to be.

TABLE 7-1	FACTORS AFFECTING PERSON'S RESPONSE TO STRESS
Internal	**External**
• Age	• Cultural and ethnic influences
• Health status	• Socioeconomic status
• Personality characteristics	• Social support
• Previous experience with stressors	• Religious or spiritual influences
• Genetic background	• Timing of stressors
• Resilience	• Number of stressors already experiencing
• Hardiness	
• Attitude	
• Optimistic outlook	
• Nutritional status	
• Sleep status	

FIG. 7-2 During stressful situations, the demands seem to exceed the resources. (iStockphoto/Thinkstock)

individual dealing with the chronic stress of caring for a loved one may also be exposed to many acute episodic stressors (e.g., car accident, influenza). Therefore the type, duration, and intensity of a stressor are important variables that can influence an individual's adaptive response (Fig. 7-2).

FACTORS AFFECTING RESPONSE TO STRESS

Why do people respond so differently to stress? Why do some people cope better with stress than others? Interestingly, some individuals experience significant adverse life events but do not succumb to the effects of stress. Factors that affect an individual's response to stress include internal and external influences (Table 7-1). These factors indicate the importance of using a holistic approach when assessing the impact of stress on a person.

Four key personal characteristics that buffer the effects of stress are resilience, hardiness, attitude, and optimism. *Resilience* is being resourceful and flexible and having good problem-solving skills. Individuals who possess a high degree of resilience are not as likely to perceive an event as stressful or taxing.

Hardiness is a combination of three characteristics: commitment, control, and openness to change. Together they provide the courage and motivation needed to turn stressful circumstances from potential calamities into opportunities for personal growth.[2]

Attitude can also influence the effect of stress on a person. People with positive attitudes view situations differently from those with negative attitudes. A person's attitude also influences how he or she manages stress. To some extent, positive emotional attitudes can prevent disease and prolong life.[3]

PATHOPHYSIOLOGY MAP

Stressors
↓
Central nervous system

Neuropeptides
Endocrine hormones
Neuropeptides
Cytokines

Endocrine system ← Endocrine hormones → Immune system
← Cytokines →

FIG. 7-3 Neurochemical links among the nervous, endocrine, and immune systems. The communication among these three systems is bidirectional.

Optimists are able to cope more effectively with stress. Optimism also reduces a person's chances of developing stress-related illnesses. When optimistic people do become ill, they tend to recover more quickly. Pessimists are likely to deny the problem, distance themselves from the stressful event, focus on stressful feelings, or allow the stressor to interfere with achieving a goal. People with a more pessimistic attitude tend to report poorer health than people with optimistic attitudes.[3]

In addition to personal characteristics, external factors play an important role in one's ability to cope with stress. Being surrounded by a strong social support system and receiving positive support from friends and family have a large impact on an individual's ability to cope with stressors.

PHYSIOLOGIC RESPONSE TO STRESS

The following section discusses the roles of the nervous, endocrine, and immune systems. These systems are interrelated, and that interrelationship is reflected in a person's physiologic response to stress (Fig. 7-3). Further, stress activation of these systems affects other body systems, such as the cardiovascular, respiratory, gastrointestinal, renal, and reproductive systems.

The complex process by which an event is perceived as a stressor and the body responds is not fully understood. A person's response to a stressor (real or imagined, and physiologic or emotional/psychologic) determines the impact that stress will have on the body.[4]

Hans Selye, a pioneer in stress research more than 70 years ago, showed that stressors from different sources produced a similar physical response. He termed this physical response to stress the *general adaptation syndrome* (GAS), which has three stages: alarm reaction, stage of resistance, and stage of exhaustion.[5] The GAS is presented in eTable 7-1 on the website for this chapter.

Nervous System

Cerebral Cortex. The cerebral cortex evaluates the emotional/psychologic event (stressor) in light of past experiences and future consequences, and thus plans a course of action. These functions are involved in the perception of a stressor.

Limbic System. The *limbic system* lies in the inner midportion of the brain near the base of the brain. The limbic system is an important mediator of emotions and behavior. When the limbic system is stimulated, emotions, feelings, and behaviors can occur that ensure survival and self-preservation.

Reticular Formation. The *reticular formation* is located between the lower end of the brainstem and the thalamus. It contains the *reticular activating system* (RAS), which sends impulses contributing to alertness to the limbic system and to the cerebral cortex. When the RAS is stimulated, it increases its output of impulses, leading to wakefulness. Stress usually increases the degree of wakefulness and can lead to sleep disturbances.

Hypothalamus. The hypothalamus, which lies at the base of the brain just above the pituitary gland, has many functions that assist in adaptation to stress. Stress activates the limbic system, which in turn stimulates the hypothalamus. Because the hypothalamus secretes neuropeptides that regulate the release of hormones by the anterior pituitary, it is central to the connection between the nervous and endocrine systems in responding to stress (Fig. 7-4).

The hypothalamus plays a primary role in the stress response by regulating the function of both the sympathetic and parasympathetic branches of the autonomic nervous system. When an individual perceives a stressor, the hypothalamus sends signals that initiate both the nervous and endocrine responses to the stressor. It does this primarily by sending signals via nerve fibers to stimulate the sympathetic nervous system (SNS) and by releasing corticotropin-releasing hormone (CRH), which stimulates the pituitary to release adrenocorticotropic hormone (ACTH) (see Chapter 48).

Endocrine System

Once the hypothalamus is activated in response to stress, the endocrine system becomes involved. The SNS stimulates the adrenal medulla to release epinephrine and norepinephrine (catecholamines). The effect of catecholamines and the SNS, including the response of the adrenal medulla, is referred to as the *sympathoadrenal response*. Epinephrine and norepinephrine prepare the body for the *fight-or-flight response* (Fig. 7-5).

Stress activates the hypothalamic-pituitary-adrenal (HPA) axis. In response to stress, the hypothalamus releases CRH, which stimulates the anterior pituitary to release proopiomelanocortin (POMC). Both ACTH (a hormone) and β-endorphin (a neuropeptide) are derived from POMC. Endorphins have analgesic-like effects and blunt pain perception during stress situations involving pain stimuli. ACTH, in turn, stimulates the

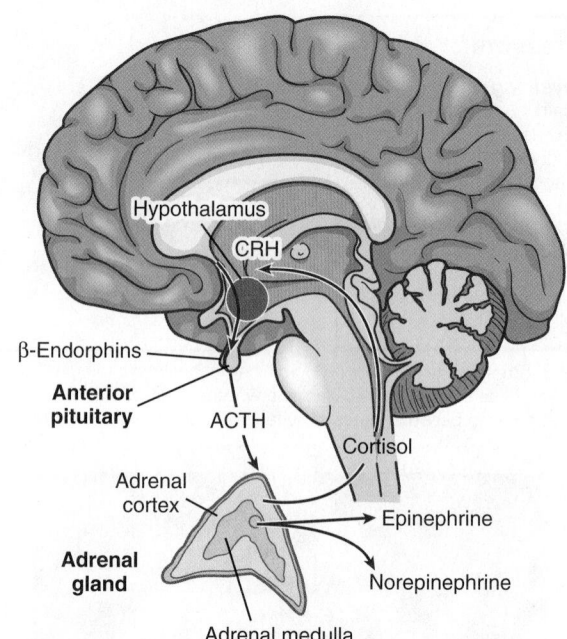

FIG. 7-4 Hypothalamic-pituitary-adrenal axis. *ACTH,* Adrenocorticotropic hormone; *CRH,* corticotropin-releasing hormone.

adrenal cortex to synthesize and secrete corticosteroids (e.g., cortisol) and, to a lesser degree, aldosterone.

Corticosteroids are essential for the stress response. Cortisol produces a number of physiologic effects, such as increasing blood glucose levels, potentiating the action of catecholamines on blood vessels, and inhibiting the inflammatory response. Corticosteroids play an important role in "turning off" or blunting aspects of the stress response, which if uncontrolled can become self-destructive. This is exemplified by corticosteroids' ability to suppress the release of proinflammatory mediators, such as the cytokines tumor necrosis factor (TNF) and interleukin-1 (IL-1). The persistent release of such mediators is believed to initiate organ dysfunction in conditions such as sepsis. Thus corticosteroids act not only to support the body's adaptive response to a stressor, but also to suppress an overzealous and potentially self-destructive response.

The stress response involves increases in (1) cardiac output (resulting from the increased heart rate and increased stroke volume), (2) blood glucose levels, (3) oxygen consumption, and (4) metabolic rate (see Fig. 7-5). In addition, dilation of skeletal muscle blood vessels increases blood supply to the large muscles and provides for quick movement. Increased cerebral blood flow increases mental alertness. The increased blood volume (from increased extracellular fluid and the shunting of blood away from the gastrointestinal system) helps maintain adequate circulation to vital organs in case of traumatic blood loss.

Summary of Stress Response

In summary, the fight-or-flight response is an important adaptive mechanism of the body to acute stress. This response to stressors is activated regardless of whether they are physiologic (e.g., acute pain) or emotional/psychologic (e.g., death of a child, loss of a home through fire, fear).

The acute stress response is a state of physiologic and psychologic arousal characterized by increased SNS activity that leads to increased heart and respiratory rate, increased blood

PATHOPHYSIOLOGY MAP

FIG. 7-5 "Fight-or-flight" reaction. Alarm reaction responses resulting from increased sympathetic nervous system (SNS) activity.

pressure, increased muscle tension, increased brain activity, and decreased skin temperature.

Immune System

Stress also has an impact on the immune system. **Psychoneuroimmunology (PNI)** is an interdisciplinary science that studies the interactions among psychologic, neurologic, and immune responses.[6] Because the brain is connected to the immune system by neuroanatomic and neuroendocrine pathways, stressors have the potential to lead to alterations in immune function (Fig. 7-6).

Nerve fibers extend from the nervous system and synapse on cells and tissues of the immune system (i.e., spleen, lymph nodes). In turn, the cells of the immune system have receptors for many neuropeptides and hormones, which permit them to respond to nervous and neuroendocrine signals. As a result, the mediation of stress by the central nervous system leads to corresponding changes in immune cell activity.

Both acute and chronic stress can cause immunosuppression. Stress affects immune function by (1) decreasing the number and function of natural killer cells; (2) decreasing lymphocyte proliferation; (3) altering production of *cytokines* (soluble factors secreted by white blood cells and other cells), such as interferon and interleukins; and (4) decreasing phagocytosis by neutrophils and monocytes.[7] (Natural killer cells, lymphocytes, and cytokines are discussed in Chapter 14.)

Importantly, the network that links the brain and immune system is bidirectional (see Fig. 7-3). Signals from these systems travel back and forth, allowing for communication among these systems. Consequently, not only do emotions modify the immune response, but products of immune cells send signals back to the brain and alter its activity. Many of the communication signals sent from the immune system to the brain are mediated by cytokines, which are central to the coordination of the immune response. For example, IL-1 (a cytokine made by monocytes) acts on the temperature regulatory center of the hypothalamus and initiates the febrile response to infectious pathogens (see Fig. 12-3).

PATHOPHYSIOLOGY MAP

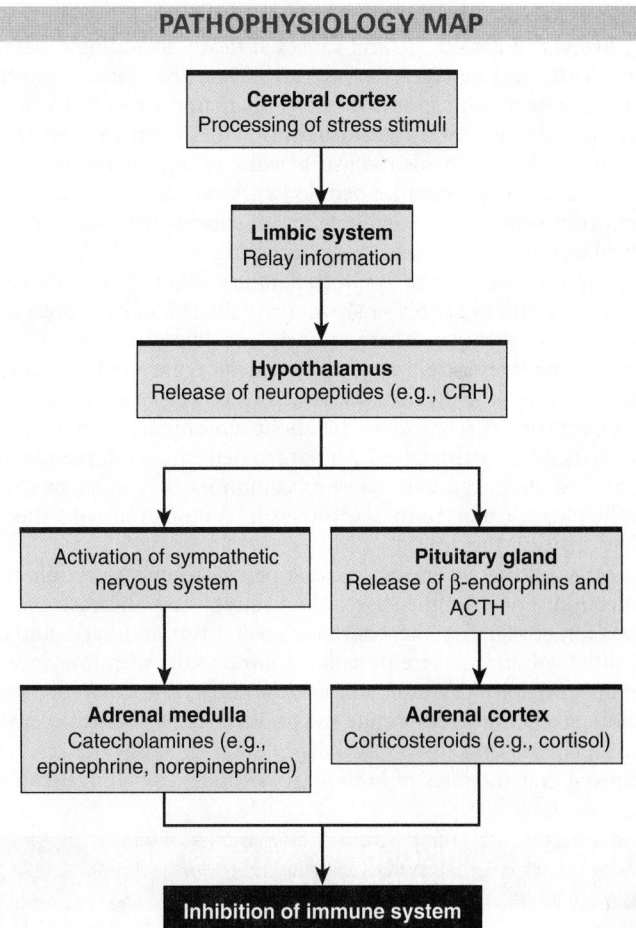

FIG. 7-6 The cerebral cortex processes stressful stimuli and relays the information via the limbic system to the hypothalamus. Corticotropin-releasing hormone *(CRH)* stimulates the release of adrenocorticotropic hormone *(ACTH)* from the pituitary gland. ACTH stimulates the adrenal cortex to release corticosteroids. The sympathetic nervous system is also stimulated, resulting in the release of epinephrine and norepinephrine from the adrenal medulla. The end result is the inhibition of the immune system.

The central nervous system is capable of influencing the function of the immune system. Stress-induced immunosuppression may exacerbate or increase the risk of progression of immune-based diseases such as multiple sclerosis, asthma, rheumatoid arthritis, and cancer.[7-9]

Many questions about stress and the immune response remain unanswered. For example, it is not known how much stress is needed to cause changes or how much of an alteration in the immune system is necessary before disease susceptibility occurs. A current challenge for researchers in the field of PNI is to study stress-induced immune changes and their relationship to health and to illness outcomes.

EFFECTS OF STRESS ON HEALTH

Acute stress leads to physiologic changes that are important to a person's adaptive survival. This is your "alarm system." It puts you on high alert. However, if stress is excessive or prolonged, these same physiologic responses can be maladaptive and lead to harm and disease. Your body was not meant to be on high alert all of the time. When a person sustains chronic, unrelieved stress, the body's defenses can no longer keep up with the demands. Therefore stress plays a role in the development or progression in the diseases of adaptation, or stress-related illnesses (Table 7-2).

Stress is linked to leading causes of death, including cancer, accidents, and suicides. Stress can have effects on cognitive function, including poor concentration, memory problems, distressing dreams, sleep disturbances, and impaired decision making. Stress can also cause a wide variety of changes in behavior. These include people withdrawing from others, becoming quiet or unusually talkative, changing eating habits, drinking alcohol excessively, or becoming irritable.[4,8-10]

Long-term exposure to catecholamines resulting from excessive activation of the SNS may increase the risk of cardiovascular diseases such as atherosclerosis and hypertension. Other conditions that are either precipitated or aggravated by stress include migraine headaches, irritable bowel syndrome, and peptic ulcers.[9,10] Control of metabolic conditions, such as diabetes mellitus, is also affected by stress. Behavioral interventions aimed at stress reduction and relaxation have been successful in helping to manage these diseases in conjunction with standard medical therapy.

Stressful life events can make a person more susceptible to infection. For example, psychologic stress may increase one's risk for developing the common cold. In a landmark study, healthy volunteers were inoculated intranasally with low doses of upper respiratory tract viruses. The subjects underwent psychologic testing to determine the occurrence of stressful events in their lives and their reactions to such stresses. The results showed that the rates of both viral infection and clinical colds increased with the degree of psychologic stress. In this study, social support buffered the harmful effects of stress.[11]

Obesity and depression are often exacerbated by stress. Those who suffer from these conditions report that they are unable to take the necessary steps to relieve their stress or improve their health and therefore engage in maladaptive coping behaviors.[12]

At the cellular level, stress may promote earlier onset of age-related diseases. There is a link between stress and telomere length. Telomeres are the protective end caps on chromosomes, and their diminishing size is an indication of age. Telomeres are highly susceptible to stress and depression. Telomeres are shorter in people who are stressed and depressed than in healthy people. Thus chronic stress can have a long-term effect on our overall health by changing our DNA and accelerating the rate at which our cells age.[13,14]

Adverse experiences early in life have an impact on brain functions. Early life stress can program the development of the hypothalamic-pituitary-adrenal axis and eventually result in neurobehavioral changes.[15] People exposed to major psychologic stressors in early life have elevated rates of morbidity and mortality from chronic diseases of aging. Children raised in poverty or mistreated by their parents have increased risk for vascular disease, autoimmune disorders, and premature death.[16]

Chronic stress is a major driver of chronic illness, which in turn is a major driver of escalating health care costs. It is critical that the entire health care community recognize the role of stress and unhealthy behaviors in causing and exacerbating chronic health conditions.[12]

COPING

Coping is a person's cognitive and behavioral efforts to manage stressors that seem to exceed available resources.[17] Coping can be either positive or negative. Positive coping includes activities such as exercise and spending time with friends and family. Negative coping may include substance abuse and denial.

The availability of coping resources affects an individual's ability to cope with stressful situations. *Coping resources* are characteristics or behaviors drawn on to manage stress. They include factors within the person or the environment, such as health status, belief systems, problem-solving skills, social skills, social support, and financial resources. Knowledge of a patient's coping resources can assist you in supporting existing resources and developing strategies to expand the patient's coping resources.

Coping strategies can be divided into two broad categories: emotion-focused coping and problem-focused coping. **Emotion-focused coping** involves managing the emotions that an individual feels when a stressful event occurs. Examples of emotion-focused coping include discussing feelings with a friend or taking a hot bath. **Problem-focused coping** involves attempts to resolve the problems causing the stress. Setting priorities or collecting information and seeking advice are examples of problem-focused coping.

Both strategies can be used to cope with stressors, and a combination of these strategies can be used to cope with the same stressor. Table 7-3 provides examples of emotion- and problem-focused coping when applied to the same stressful situation. Table 7-4 contains examples of coping strategies.

TABLE 7-2	DISORDERS WITH A STRESS COMPONENT*	
• Depression	• Hypertension	
• Dyspepsia	• Insomnia	
• Eating disorders	• Irritable bowel syndrome	
• Erectile dysfunction	• Low back pain	
• Fatigue	• Menstrual irregularities	
• Fibromyalgia	• Peptic ulcer disease	
• Headaches	• Sexual dysfunction	

*List is not all inclusive.

> *You cannot always choose your destiny in life, but you can choose how you cope with it.*
> *Norman Vincent Peale*

TABLE 7-3	PROBLEM- AND EMOTION- FOCUSED COPING	
Stressor	**Problem-Focused Coping**	**Emotion-Focused Coping**
Failing an examination	Obtaining a tutor	Going for a run
Being diagnosed with diabetes	Attending diabetic education classes	Getting a massage
Receiving questionable mammogram results	Scheduling follow-up testing for ultrasound	Expressing feelings of anxiety to friends and nurse

TABLE 7-4	COPING STRATEGIES
Strategy	**Description**
Social support	• Self-help groups and professional help • Relationships with family and friends
Exercise	• Any form of movement, especially aerobic movement • Can be viewed as meditation in motion • Results in improved circulation, increased release of endorphins, and an enhanced sense of well-being
Journaling	• Allows an individual to express self in writing • Can write about personal events, thoughts, feelings, memories, and perceptions • Allows an individual to reduce stress, enhance coping, and increase self-awareness
Art therapy	• Allows an individual to nonverbally express and communicate feelings, emotions, and thoughts • Can reduce stress, promote relaxation, and help process experiences • Based on the belief that creative process is healing and life enhancing
Humor	• Can take the form of laughter, cartoons, funny movies, videos, riddles, comic books, and joke books • Humor carts set up in many clinical settings to be used by patients and families

When a situation is unchangeable or uncontrollable, emotion-focused coping may predominate. The primary purpose of emotion-focused coping is to help decrease negative emotions and create a feeling of well-being. Although it may not seem to be working toward a solution, emotion-focused coping is a valid and appropriate way to deal with different stressful situations.

If a problem can be changed or controlled, problem-focused coping is the most helpful coping strategy. Problem-focused coping strategies allow an individual to look at a challenge objectively, take action to address the problem, and thereby reduce the stress.

A key aspect of successful coping is *coping flexibility*, which involves the ability to change and adapt coping strategies over time and across different stressful conditions. Stressful circumstances are handled best when an individual uses coping flexibility because certain strategies work more effectively than others depending on the circumstances.

RELAXATION STRATEGIES

The *relaxation response* is a state of physiologic and psychologic rest. It is the opposite of the stress response. The relaxation response is characterized by decreased SNS activity, which leads to decreased heart and respiratory rate, decreased blood pressure, decreased muscle tension, decreased brain activity, and increased skin temperature.[18]

TABLE 7-5	RELAXATION BREATHING TECHNIQUES*

Breathing Assessment
• Begin by placing one hand gently on your abdomen below your waistline.
• Place the other hand on the center of your chest on the sternum.
• Without changing the normal breathing pattern, take several breaths. During inhalation notice which hand rises the most.
• When relaxation breathing is performed properly, the hand on the abdomen should rise more than the hand on the chest.

4 × 4 Technique
• Sit up straight with your back flush to the support of the chair and your feet flat on the floor.
• Rest your arms on your lap, thighs, or arms of the chair.
• Take in a deep breath through your nose to a count of four (1 ... 2 ... 3 ... 4).
• Hold your breath to a count of four (1 ... 2 ... 3 ... 4).
• Release your breath through your mouth to a count of four (1 ... 2 ... 3 ... 4).
• Rest for a count of four (1 ... 2 ... 3 ... 4).
• Repeat the cycle four times.

*evolve Video demonstrations of these techniques are available in the Stress-Busting Kit for Nursing Students on the website for this book.

The relaxation response can be elicited through a variety of relaxation strategies, including relaxation breathing, meditation, imagery, muscle relaxation, prayer, and physical exercise. The most common relaxation strategies are described here. Regular elicitation of the relaxation response has been proven to be an effective treatment for a wide range of stress-related disorders, including chronic pain, insomnia, and hypertension. Individuals who regularly engage in relaxation strategies are able to deal better with their stressors, increase their sense of control over stressors, and reduce their tension.[19]

Relaxation Breathing

The way one breathes affects every aspect of one's life. When a person is stressed, muscles tense and breathing becomes shallow and rapid. Therefore one of the simplest and most effective ways to stop the stress response is to breathe deeply and slowly. It is difficult to maintain tension when breathing in a slow, deep, and relaxed pattern.

Relaxation (abdominal) breathing can be performed while sitting, standing, or lying down. It is especially useful during a stressful or anxious situation to reduce stress. Relaxation breathing forms the basis for most relaxation strategies.

Before practicing relaxation breathing, it is important to assess one's normal breathing pattern (Table 7-5). Chest breathing, which involves the upper chest and shoulders, is inefficient. This type of breathing is often used during times of anxiety and distress. Relaxation breathing, which involves the diaphragm, is natural for newborns and sleeping adults. It is a more efficient type of breathing.

Relaxation breathing involves the primary use of the diaphragm and less use of the upper chest and shoulders to assist in each breath. In this type of breathing, the abdomen gently moves in and out during exhalation and inhalation. The breaths should be slow, steady, and deep.

One basic technique for relaxation breathing is as follows: (1) Inhale slowly and deeply, pushing the abdomen out, thinking about breathing in peace. (2) Exhale slowly, letting the abdomen come in and all the muscles relax. (3) Repeat these deep breaths 10 times without interruption. As with any breathing exercise, if a light-headed feeling arises, stop for 30 seconds and then start again.

A common method used to teach relaxation breathing is the 4×4 technique (see Table 7-5). Other breathing techniques are discussed in the Stress-Busting Kit for Nursing Students available on the website for this book.

Initially, relaxation breathing may feel unusual. With practice it becomes easier, and its relaxing benefits are soon obvious. You should personally learn to use relaxation breathing before teaching it to patients. Once learned, relaxation breathing can be easily taught to patients in a variety of settings, particularly when they are undergoing stressful and painful procedures.

Meditation

Meditation is a state of being with increased concentration and awareness. Meditation can be used to create a sustained period during which one focuses attention and increases self-awareness. Many seek out meditation in response to a deep human need for something transcendental or beyond everyday experiences. However, meditation can also be used to reduce stress.

Three basic ways to practice meditation are (1) concentration methods, (2) guided meditation, and (3) mindfulness practices. The *concentration technique* (e.g., Zen meditation) directs the mind to a single focus, such as the breath, an object, or a *mantra.* A *guided meditation* is similar to guided imagery (described below), where the mind and imagination are focused on a conscious goal. *Mindfulness practices* (e.g., transcendental meditation) are not restricted to any one object but rather attend to any and all sensations, perceptions, thoughts, and emotions as they arise moment to moment in the field of awareness.

Although meditation can be performed anywhere, it is best to practice meditation in a quiet place, free of distractions. Table 7-6 provides some basic guidelines on how to meditate. Meditation is often practiced while seated, and it is important to maintain a comfortable posture. Meditation can also be performed while walking and focusing on a single action such as the movement of the feet. In the beginning, individuals typically start with just 5 to 10 minutes of meditation at a time and often increase the time as the practice becomes more comfortable.

In people who meditate regularly, the brain is reoriented from a stressful fight-or-flight mode to one of acceptance, a shift that increases contentment.[20] Similarly, long-term meditation practices create structural differences in the lower brainstem, which could account for some of the cardiovascular and respiratory parasympathetic effects, as well as cognitive, emotional, and immunoreactive changes. Meditation has many positive health benefits, including reversal of coronary artery disease, decreased levels of cortisol, decreased cholesterol levels, increased airflow to the lungs, and increased immune functions.[21]

Imagery

Imagery is the use of one's mind to generate images that have a calming effect on the body. It involves focusing the mind and incorporates all the senses to create physiologic and emotional changes. It is a simple relaxation technique that requires no equipment other than an active imagination. *Guided imagery* is a variation of imagery in which images are suggested by another person (either live or on a CD or MP3 file).

Imagery can be used in many clinical settings for stress reduction and pain relief. Benefits of imagery include anxiety reduction, decreased muscle tension, improved comfort during medical procedures, enhanced immune function, decreased recovery time after surgery, and reduction in sleeping problems. You can use imagery in your own life or use guided imagery with your patients. One of the uses of imagery is to create a safe and special place for mental retreat to elicit the relaxation response. Table 7-7 describes the steps involved in creating a special place.

When imagery is performed, it is best to find a comfortable position. Take slow, deep breaths. Focus should involve all senses (sight, hearing, touch, smell). For example, one can use an image such as Fig. 7-7, engaging all the senses as one focuses on the image.

Imagery can also be used to specifically target a disease, problem, or stressor. Table 7-8 describes some suggestions for using imagery in specific diseases or disorders.

TABLE 7-6   GUIDE TO MEDITATION*

You can teach yourself the basics of meditation by following a few simple steps:
- Find a quiet place.
- Make sure there are no distractions.
- Sit in a comfortable position.
- Close your eyes.
- Shut out the world so your brain can stop processing information coming from your senses.
- Pick a word or phrase. Find a word or phrase that means something to you, whose sound or rhythm is soothing when repeated (e.g., one, peace, shalom, the Lord is my shepherd, Hail Mary full of grace).
- Breathe slowly and practice relaxation breathing.
- Say the word or phrase again and again.
- Try saying the word or phrase silently to yourself with every exhalation. The monotony will help you focus.
- Do not be concerned when other thoughts come to mind. Just acknowledge them and return calmly to your word or phrase.
- Continue for 10 to 20 minutes, but even 5 minutes can leave you feeling calm and refreshed.
- Rise slowly.

Practice once or twice daily.

*evolve Meditation exercises are available in the Stress-Busting Kit for Nursing Students on the website for this book.

TABLE 7-7   IMAGERY: CREATING YOUR SPECIAL PLACE*

- Begin by closing your eyes and taking several slow, deep breaths.
- Imagine a place where you feel completely comfortable and peaceful. It may be a real place or one you imagine; one from your past or some place you have always wanted to go.
- Allow this special place to take form, slowly. As it takes form, look around, to your left, to your right. Enjoy the scenery: the colors, the texture, the shapes.
- Listen carefully to the sounds of your place. What do you hear?
- Is there a gentle breeze or sunshine warming your face? Pick up or touch some favorite objects from your special place.
- Take in a deep breath through your nose, and notice the rich smells around you. Perhaps your favorite flower is in bloom, or you smell the scents of the ocean.
- Take another deep breath and relax. Enjoy the peace, comfort, and safety of your special place.
- This is your special place. You relax and feel thankful that you are here, in your special place.
- You can return to this place any time that you wish.

*evolve Imagery exercises are available in the Stress-Busting Kit for Nursing Students on the website for this book.

Imagery can also be used to enhance performance or process stressful or difficult tasks. For example, an athlete or musician can use imagery to achieve greater success. Imagery allows one to mentally rehearse the difficult or challenging situation. Imagery can help a fearful nurse start an IV line or perform a difficult procedure. It can also be used with a patient who is afraid to have a stressful procedure performed (e.g., radiation therapy).

Music for Relaxation

Music can help achieve relaxation and bring about healthy changes in emotional or physical states. Listening to relaxing music may divert one's focus from a stressful situation. In addition, healing vibrations from music can return the mind and body to a deeper level of balance.

FIG. 7-7 In imagery, special places are created involving all the senses, such as a place where one can hear rustling water, smell flowers, feel the wind, and see a colorful landscape. (iStockphoto/Thinkstock)

TABLE 7-8 EXAMPLES OF IMAGERY

Imagery can be used to relieve stress and promote health and healing in conjunction with regular medical care. Special images can be created to alleviate symptoms or treat diseases or disorders. The image should be strong and vivid for the person, using many senses to create the image. Below are some examples that some people have found useful.

Disease or Disorder	Images
Infection	• White blood cells with flashing red sirens arrest and imprison harmful germs.
Cancer	• Shark gobbles up cancer cells. • Radiation or chemotherapy treatments enter the body like healing rays of light; they destroy cancer cells.
Coronary artery disease	• Water flows freely through a wide, open river.
Weakened immune system	• White blood cells rapidly multiply like millions of seeds bursting from ripe seed pod.
Asthma	• Tiny elastic rubber bands that constrict the airways pop open.
Depression	• Troubles and feelings of sadness are attached to big colorful helium balloons and are floating off into a clear blue sky.
Pain	• Pain is washed away by a cool calm river flowing through the entire body.

Adapted from Sobel DS, Ornstein R: *Healthy mind, healthy body*, New York, 1996, Patient Education Materials, Time Life.

Music has been used in many clinical settings. Music decreases anxiety and evokes the relaxation response. This relaxation helps people with insomnia go to sleep. In oncology patients it has succeeded in decreasing muscular tension, pain sensation, and emotional stress associated with cancer. In general, music affects the heart rate, blood pressure, gastrointestinal secretions and motility, muscle tone, sweat glands, and skin temperature.[22]

Music that contains approximately 60 to 80 beats/min is considered soothing. Low-pitched tones and music without words is recommended for relaxation. Mozart's music is a popular form of music used for relaxation. On the other hand, fast-tempo music can stimulate and uplift a person. Each person considers different types of music to be relaxing, so it is important to find the music that best matches the person's needs and circumstance. To achieve optimal relaxation, minimize all interruptions and assume a comfortable posture while listening to music.

Music can be incorporated into clinical practice. It is noninvasive, safe, inexpensive, and easy to use. First, it is important to establish the purpose and benefit of using music with patients in a given clinical setting. Then assess each individual patient's interest and preference in music. Create a listening environment, encouraging the patient to find a comfortable position. Headphones or earphones and an MP3 or CD player can be used. Music can be played for 20 to 30 minutes per day at least twice a day. Evaluate patients' response to the music, asking them how it sounds and how it makes them feel.

Massage

Massage is another important relaxation strategy. It involves the systematic manipulation of the soft tissue of the body to reduce tension and enhance health and healing. It also meets an essential human need: touch. Massage can be implemented as back rubs for patients. Massage is discussed in more detail in Chapter 6.

> *You may not be able to change the stressors in your life, but you can change your reaction or response to them.*
> *Florence Nightingale*

NURSING MANAGEMENT
STRESS

NURSING ASSESSMENT

As a nurse, you are in a key position to assess stress in patients and their caregivers, to assist them in identifying high-risk periods for stress, and to implement stress management strategies that can prevent the negative consequences of stress on their health (Fig. 7-8). Assess the number of stressors, the duration of these stressors, and previous experience with similar demands. Also assess the personal meaning attached to the stressful situation to provide useful insight for planning stress management strategies with the patient. Also consider family responses to the demands on the patient.

The patient faces many potential stressors that can have health consequences. Be aware of situations that are likely to result in stress, and determine the patient's perception of these situations. In addition to the stressor itself, specific coping strategies have health consequences and therefore must be included in the assessment.

Although the manifestations of stress may vary from person to person, assess the patient for the signs and symptoms of the stress response, including an increased heart rate and blood pressure, hyperventilation, sweating, headache, musculoskeletal pain, gastrointestinal upset, loss of appetite, skin disorders, insomnia, and fatigue. In addition, the patient may exhibit some of the stress-related illnesses or diseases of adaptation (see Table 7-2).

Behavioral manifestations may include an inability to concentrate, accident proneness, impaired speech, anxiety, crying, frustration, and irritability. Work-related responses to stress may include absenteeism or tardiness at work, decreased productivity, and job dissatisfaction. Cognitive responses include self-reports of an inability to make decisions and forgetfulness. Some of these responses may also be apparent to significant others.

Another major source of stress relates to the patient's illness, which often also causes stress for the caregiver and other family members. Assess what aspects of the illness are the most stressful for the patient. These may include the patient's physical health, job responsibilities, finances, and children. This information is valuable because it gives you the patient's perspective of the stressors. Knowledge of stressors, the feelings these stressors invoke, and the psychologic sequelae they can produce will assist you in identifying potential and actual sources of stress and their effect on the patient.

NURSING IMPLEMENTATION

The first step in managing stress is to become aware of its presence. This includes identifying and expressing stressful feelings. Your role is to facilitate and enhance the patient's coping and adaptation. Nursing interventions depend on the severity of the stress experience. For example, a patient with multiple traumas expends energy in an attempt to physically survive. As a nurse, your efforts are directed to life-supporting interventions and to approaches aimed at reducing additional stressors for the patient. The patient with multiple traumas is much less likely to adapt or recover if faced with additional stressors such as sleep deprivation or an infection.

Coping resources and strategies that are used should be adaptive and not a source of additional stress for the patient. Coping resources and strategies were previously discussed in this chapter.

You can assume a primary role in implementing stress management strategies. Some personal tips for handling stress are presented in Table 7-9. These tips will benefit you personally and can be shared with patients. Ideas for how to incorporate stress management strategies into nursing practice are presented in Table 7-10. Although some may require additional training, many stress management strategies are within the scope of nursing practice. These include relaxation breathing, imagery, music for relaxation, exercise, massage, meditation, art therapy, and journaling. (Additional resources are listed at the

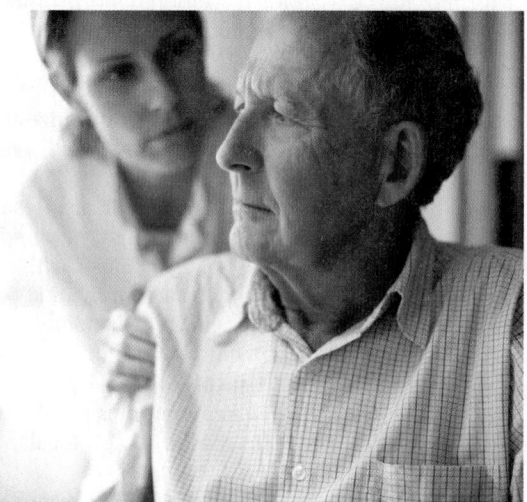

FIG. 7-8 As a nurse, you have an important role in helping patients deal with stress. (Hemera/Thinkstock)

🌿 COMPLEMENTARY & ALTERNATIVE THERAPIES

St. John's Wort

Scientific Evidence
- Although some studies of St. John's wort have reported benefits for depression, others have not.
- For treating major depression of moderate severity, a large study found that the herb was no more effective than a placebo.*
- For symptoms of minor depression, a study found that neither St. John's wort nor citalopram (Celexa), a prescription antidepressant, relieved symptoms better than a placebo.†

Nursing Implications
- Depression is a serious illness. Advise patients to consult with a health care provider before self-medicating with St. John's wort.
- St. John's wort is not a proven therapy for depression. If depression is not adequately treated, it can become severe. Anyone who may have depression should see a health care provider. Effective proven therapies are available.
- Serious interactions can occur with numerous herbs, supplements, over-the-counter drugs, or prescription drugs.
- St. John's wort interferes with the metabolism of drugs that use the cytochrome P450 enzyme system, including birth control pills, cyclosporine, carbamazepine, warfarin, midazolam, nifedipine, tricyclic antidepressants, simvastatin, and HIV drugs.
- Use of St. John's wort may lead to increased side effects when taken with other antidepressants.

*Hypericum Depression Trial Study Group: Effect of *Hypericum perforatum* (St. John's wort) in major depressive disorder: a randomized controlled trial, *JAMA* 287(14):1807, 2002.
†Rapaport MH, Nierenberg AA, Howland R, et al: The treatment of minor depression with St. John's wort or citalopram: failure to show benefit over placebo, *J Psych Res* 45:931, 2011.

TABLE 7-9	PERSONAL TIPS FOR HANDLING STRESS

- Do not try to be superhuman.
- Learn to "let go" of things that are outside of your control.
- Learn acceptance of yourself.
- Exercise regularly.
- Share your feelings.
- Keep a sense of humor; laugh often.
- Learn relaxation breathing.
- Use imagery.
- Meditate or pray.
- Get adequate sleep.
- Live a healthy lifestyle.
- Try to look at change as a positive challenge, not as a threat.
- Solve the little problems, since this can help you gain a feeling of control.
- Work to resolve conflicts with other people.
- If needed, get professional counseling.

end of the chapter and in the Stress-Busting Kit for Nursing Students on the website for this book.)

Before teaching stress management strategies to patients, you need to personally become familiar with them. Most relaxation strategies can be taught to patients in 10 to 15 minutes. To prepare for a relaxation training session, have the patient wear loose-fitting clothing, and ensure that the setting is private, comfortable, and free from distractions or noises. Choose a relaxation strategy to best suit the patient and the situation. Give directions calmly and slowly in short, simple sentences. End the session gradually so as to not disrupt the relaxation that was just elicited. Say a phrase such as, "I am going to count backward from five to one. With each number, you will feel more alert, but still feel at peace." After counting backward, instruct the patient to slowly open his or her eyes.

Effective stress management provides an individual a sense of control of the stressful situation. As stress management practices are incorporated into daily activities, the individual is able to increase his or her confidence and self-reliance and limit the emotional response to the stressful circumstances. Possessing a sense of control can deter the harmful effects from the stress response.

As a nurse, you are in an ideal situation to integrate stress management in clinical practice. You are also well equipped to develop and test the effectiveness of new approaches to manage stress and promote positive health outcomes. However, it is important to recognize when the patient or caregiver needs to be referred to a professional with advanced training in counseling.

TABLE 7-10   HOW TO IMPLEMENT STRESS MANAGEMENT IN PRACTICE

- Learn relaxation breathing. It is the easiest method of relaxation to use.
- Practice teaching relaxation breathing with peers, then patients.
- Pick coping strategies (see Table 7-4) and relaxation strategies that are appropriate for your clinical area.
- Practice using the strategy yourself. It becomes easier with time.
- Take advantage of opportunities to teach coping and relaxation strategies to patients.
- Anticipate setbacks. They provide feedback about what you are doing wrong. Do NOT quit!
- Attend seminars and workshops on stress management to learn more.

✿ COMPLEMENTARY & ALTERNATIVE THERAPIES
Kava

Scientific Evidence
Although scientific studies provide some evidence that kava may be beneficial for the management of anxiety, the U.S. Food and Drug Administration (FDA) has issued a warning that use of kava supplements has been linked to a risk of severe liver damage.

Nursing Implications
- Kava has been reported to cause liver damage, including hepatitis and liver failure (which can cause death).
- It should be avoided by patients with liver problems and patients taking medications that affect the liver.
- Kava has been associated with several cases of abnormal muscle spasm or involuntary muscle movements. Kava may interact with several drugs, including drugs used for Parkinson's disease.
- Long-term or heavy use of kava may result in scaly, yellowed skin.
- Avoid driving and operating heavy machinery while taking kava because the herb has been reported to cause drowsiness.

Source: National Center for Complementary and Alternative Medicine: Kava. Retrieved from *http://nccam.nih.gov/health/kava.*

CASE STUDY

Stress-Induced Complaints

iStockphoto/Thinkstock

Patient Profile
K.F., a 43-year-old woman, recently moved to the United States from Turkey with her two teenage children. She has no family in the country and was recently divorced. She has taken a job as a waitress in a hectic restaurant and works as a seamstress out of her home in the evenings.

She has developed some unusual symptoms and comes to see the nurse practitioner at a community clinic. Although she states that she was in good health when she left Turkey, she now complains of fatigue, inability to sleep, and aches all over her body.

Even when she is able to get some extra sleep, she still feels exhausted. Her co-worker told her she has fibromyalgia.

Discussion Questions
1. Consider K.F.'s situation and describe the stressors with which she is dealing. Describe the possible effects of these stressors on her health.
2. *Priority Decision:* What are the priority coping strategies that you should include in K.F.'s plan of care?
3. What limitations should be considered when discussing specific coping strategies?
4. What cultural considerations should be included in the plan of care?

Ⓔvolve Answers available at *http://evolve.elsevier.com/Lewis/medsurg.*

▌ BRIDGE TO NCLEX EXAMINATION

The number of the question corresponds to the same-numbered outcome at the beginning of the chapter.

1. Determination of whether an event is a stressor is based on a person's
   a. tolerance.
   b. perception.
   c. adaptation.
   d. stubbornness.

2. The nurse recognizes that a patient with newly diagnosed breast cancer is using an emotion-focused coping process when she
   a. joins a support group for women with breast cancer.
   b. considers the pros and cons of the various treatment options.
   c. delays treatment until her family can take a weekend trip together.
   d. tells the nurse that she has a good prognosis because the tumor is small.

3. The nurse would expect which findings in a patient as a result of the physiologic effect of stress on the reticular formation?
   a. An episode of diarrhea while awaiting painful dressing changes
   b. Refusal to communicate with nurses while awaiting a cardiac catheterization
   c. Inability to sleep the night before beginning to self-administer insulin injections
   d. Increased blood pressure, decreased urine output, and hyperglycemia after a car accident

4. The nurse uses knowledge of the effects of stress on the immune system by encouraging patients to
   a. sleep for 10 to 12 hours per day.
   b. avoid exposure to upper respiratory tract infections.
   c. receive regular immunizations when they are stressed.
   d. use emotion-focused rather than problem-focused coping strategies.

5. The nurse recognizes that a person who is subjected to chronic stress could be at higher risk for
   a. osteoporosis.
   b. colds and flu.
   c. low blood pressure.
   d. high serum cholesterol.

6. During a stressful circumstance that is uncontrollable, which type of coping strategy is the most effective?
   a. Avoidance
   b. Coping flexibility
   c. Emotion-focused coping
   d. Problem-focused coping

7. An appropriate nursing intervention for a hospitalized patient who states she cannot cope with her illness is
   a. controlling the environment to prevent sensory overload and promote sleep.
   b. encouraging the patient's family to offer emotional support by frequent visiting.
   c. arranging for the patient to phone family and friends to maintain emotional bonds.
   d. asking the patient to describe previous stressful situations and how she managed to resolve them.

1. b, 2. a, 3. c, 4. b, 5. b, 6. c, 7. d.

ⓔvolve

For rationales to these answers and even more NCLEX review questions, visit *http://evolve.elsevier.com/Lewis/medsurg*.

REFERENCES

1. Seward BL: *Managing stress: principles and strategies for health and well-being*, ed 7, Burlington, Mass, 2012, Jones & Bartlett.
2. Maddi SR: Hardiness: the courage to grow from stresses, *J Pos Psych* 1(3):160, 2006. (Classic)
3. Williams G: Attitude and stress: effects on the body. Retrieved from *http://ezinearticles.com/?Attitude-And-Stress,-Effects-On-The-Body&id=702403*.
4. National Institute of Mental Health: Fact sheet on stress. Retrieved from *www.nimh.nih.gov/health/publications/stress/fact-sheet-on-stress.shtml*.
5. Selye H: The stress concept: past, present, and future. In Cooper CL, editor: *Stress research: issues for the eighties*, New York, 1983, Wiley. (Classic)
6. Segerstrom SC: Resources, stress, and immunity: an ecological perspective on human psychoneuroimmunology, *Ann Behav Med* 40(1):114, 2010.
7. Heffner KL: Neuroendocrine effects of stress on immunity in the elderly: implications for inflammatory disease, *Immunol Allergy Clin North Am* 31(1):95, 2011.
8. Conti CM, Angelucci D, Ferri M, et al: Relationship between cancer and psychology: an updated history, *J Biol Regul Homeost Agents* 25(3):331, 2011.
9. Janusek LW, Cooper DT, Matthews HL: Stress, immunity, and health outcomes. In Rice VH, editor: *Handbook of stress, coping, and health*, Thousand Oaks, Calif, 2012, Sage.
10. Koenig JI, Walker CD, Romeo RD, et al: Effects of stress across the lifespan, *Stress* 14(5):475, 2011.
11. Cohen S, Tyrrell DA, Smith AP: Psychological stress and susceptibility to the common cold. *N Engl J Med* 325:606, 1991. (Classic)
12. American Psychological Association: Stress in America: our health at risk. Retrieved from *www.apa.org/news/press/releases/stress/2011/final-2011.pdf*.
13. Peres J: Telomere research offers insight on stress-disease connection, *J Natl Cancer Inst* 103(11):848, 2011.
14. Effros RB: Telomere/telomerase dynamics within the human immune system: effect of chronic infection and stress, *Exp Gerontol* 46(2-3):135, 2011.
15. Lai MC, Huang LT: Effects of early life stress on neuroendocrine and neurobehavior: mechanisms and implications, *Pediatr Neonatol* 52(3):122, 2011.
16. Miller GE, Chen E, Parker KJ: Psychological stress in childhood and susceptibility to the chronic diseases of aging: moving toward a model of behavioral and biological mechanisms, *Psychol Bull* 137(6):959, 2011.
17. Lazarus R, Folkman S: *Stress, appraisal, and coping*, New York, 1984, Springer. (Classic)
18. Benson H: *The relaxation response*, New York, 1975, Avon. (Classic)
19. Fjorback LO, Arendt M, Ornbøl E, et al: Mindfulness-based stress reduction and mindfulness-based cognitive therapy: a systematic review of randomized controlled trials, *Acta Psychiatr Scand* 124(2):102, 2011.
20. Fortney L, Taylor M: Meditation in medical practice: a review of the evidence and practice, *Prim Care* 37(1):81, 2010.
21. Young LA: Mindfulness meditation: a primer for rheumatologists, *Rheum Dis Clin North Am* 37(1):63, 2011.
22. Chan MF, Wong ZY, Thayala NV: The effectiveness of music listening in reducing depressive symptoms in adults: a systematic review, *Comp Therap Med* 19(6):332, 2011.

RESOURCES

Academy for Guided Imagery
www.academyforguidedimagery.com
American Institute of Stress
www.stress.org
American Music Therapy Association
www.musictherapy.org
Centre for Stress Management
www.managingstress.com/index.html
International Stress Management Association
www.isma.org.uk
Medline Plus: Stress Resources
www.nlm.nih.gov/medlineplus/stress.html
Stress Management Resources
www.mentalhealth.about.com/cs/stressmanagement

*The best bridge between despair and hope is
a good night's sleep.*
E. Joseph Cossman

Sleep and Sleep Disorders

Carol A. Landis and Margaret McLean Heitkemper

evolve WEBSITE

LEARNING OUTCOMES

1. Define *sleep.*
2. Describe stages of sleep.
3. Explain the relationship of various diseases/disorders and sleep
   disorders.
4. Describe the etiology, clinical manifestations, and collaborative and
   nursing management of insomnia.
5. Describe the etiology, clinical manifestations, and collaborative and
   nursing management of narcolepsy.

6. Describe the etiology, clinical manifestations, collaborative care, and
   nursing management of obstructive sleep apnea.
7. Describe parasomnias, including sleepwalking, sleep terrors, and
   nightmares.
8. Select appropriate strategies for managing sleep problems
   associated with shift work sleep disorder.

KEY TERMS

cataplexy, p. 106
circadian rhythms, p. 101
insomnia, p. 101
narcolepsy, p. 106

obstructive sleep apnea (OSA), p. 107
parasomnias, p. 110
sleep-disordered breathing (SDB), p. 107
sleep disorders, p. 99

sleep disturbance, p. 99
sleep hygiene, p. 103
wake behavior, p. 100

SLEEP

Sleep is a state in which an individual lacks conscious awareness of environmental surroundings, but can be easily aroused. Sleep is distinct from unconscious states such as coma in which the individual cannot be aroused. Sleep is a basic, dynamic, highly organized, and complex behavior that is essential for healthy functioning and survival. Over a life span of 80 years, an individual who sleeps 7 hours each night will spend approximately 24 years sleeping. Sleep influences both behavioral and physiologic functions, including memory, mood, hormone secretion, glucose metabolism, immune function, and body temperature.

Most adults require 7 to 8 hours of sleep within a 24-hour period. Adequate sleep is defined as the amount of sleep one needs to be fully awake and alert the next day. *Insufficient sleep* refers to obtaining less than recommended amounts of sleep.

Fragmented sleep refers to frequent arousals or actual awakenings that interrupt sleep continuity.

Sleep disturbance is a term used to indicate conditions of poor sleep quality. Sleep disorders are abnormalities unique to sleep. They can be classified as dyssomnias or parasomnias (Table 8-1). *Dyssomnia* is a term used to describe problems associated with initiating or maintaining sleep. Parasomnias are discussed later in this chapter on p. 110.

More than 70 million people in the United States have a sleep disorder, and many are unaware that they have a problem[1,2] (Fig. 8-1). On average most Americans report sleeping $6\frac{1}{2}$ hours on workdays and $7\frac{1}{2}$ hours on non-workdays. Seventy percent of adults report habitually sleeping less than 7 hours a night.

Insufficient sleep is a serious problem with health consequences. In the 2011 National Sleep Foundation survey, 87% of Americans reported at least one sleep problem such as

Reviewed by Dana R. Epstein, RN, PhD, Adjunct Faculty, College of Nursing and Health Innovation, Arizona State University, Phoenix, Arizona;
and Jo Ann Baker, RN, MSN, FNP-C, Department Chair, Nursing, Delaware Technical and Community College, Terry Campus, Dover, Delaware.

FIG. 8-1 Sleep disorders are common in our society. (Jupiterimages/Creatas/Thinkstock)

FIG. 8-2 Excessive daytime sleepiness can occur in people with sleep disorders. (iStockphoto/Thinkstock)

TABLE 8-1   SELECTED SLEEP DISORDERS

Dyssomnias	Parasomnias

• Insomnia
  • Acute
  • Chronic
    • Primary
    • Secondary (co-morbid)
• Hospital-acquired sleep disorders
• Narcolepsy
• Circadian rhythm disorders
• Sleep-disordered breathing
  • Obstructive sleep apnea
• Periodic limb movement disorder
• Restless legs syndrome
	• Sleepwalking
	• Sleep terrors
	• Nightmares

Source: Based on American Academy of Sleep Medicine: International classification of sleep disorders, 2nd ed: Diagnostic and coding manual, Westchester, Ill., The Academy, 2005. Retrieved from *www.esst.org/adds/ICSD.pdf*.

difficulty falling asleep, fragmented sleep, or snoring a few nights per week.[3] Daytime sleepiness can be so severe that it interferes with work and social functioning (Fig. 8-2). People with chronic illnesses are at the greatest risk for sleep disturbances.

Many sleep disorders go untreated because health care providers do not ask and patients do not talk about sleep problems. Untreated sleep disorders pose considerable health and economic consequences. Driving while drowsy is related to 100,000 accidents and 1500 traffic fatalities per year.[4] Each year, sleep disorders, sleep loss, and excessive daytime sleepiness cost the United States billions of dollars from the cost of health care, work-related accidents, and lost productivity.[1]

PHYSIOLOGIC SLEEP MECHANISMS

Sleep-Wake Cycle

The brain controls the cyclic changes between sleep and waking, but no single structure regulates these states. Rather, complex networks in the brainstem, hypothalamus, and thalamus interact to regulate the sleep and wake cycle.

Wake Behavior. Wake behavior is maintained by an integrated network of arousal systems from the brainstem and basal forebrain. A cluster of neuronal structures in the middle of the brainstem, called the reticular activating system (RAS), is associated with generalized cortical activation and behavioral arousal. Various neurotransmitters (glutamate, acetylcholine, norepinephrine, dopamine, histamine, serotonin) promote wake behavior.[5]

People with Alzheimer's disease have a loss of cholinergic neurons in the basal forebrain, which results in sleep disturbances. People with Parkinson's disease have degeneration of dopamine neurons in the substantia nigra, leading to excessive daytime sleepiness. Histamine neurons in the hypothalamus stimulate cortical activation and wake behavior. The sedating properties of many over-the-counter (OTC) medications result from inhibiting one of these arousal systems.

Orexin (also called hypocretin), a neuropeptide, is found in the lateral hypothalamus. Orexin activates arousal systems and simultaneously inhibits sleep active neurons. Decreased levels of orexin or its receptors lead to difficulties staying awake and the syndrome called *narcolepsy*. (Narcolepsy is discussed later in this chapter on pp. 106-107.)

Sleep Behavior. An area in the hypothalamus just above the optic chiasm contains many sleep-promoting neurons. These neurons act to inhibit the RAS and promote sleep.[5] Sleep is stimulated by a variety of sleep-promoting neurotransmitters and peptides, including γ-aminobutyric acid (GABA), galanin, melatonin, adenosine, somatostatin, growth hormone–releasing hormone, delta-sleep–inducing peptide, prostaglandins, and proinflammatory cytokines (interleukin-1, tumor necrosis factor, interleukin-6). Proinflammatory cytokines are important in mediating sleepiness and lethargy associated with infection. Peptides, such as cholecystokinin, released by the gastrointestinal tract after food ingestion may mediate the sleepiness (*postprandial sleepiness*).

Melatonin is an endogenous hormone produced by the pineal gland in the brain from the amino acid tryptophan. Melatonin secretion is tightly linked to the environmental light-dark cycle. Under normal day-night conditions, melatonin is released in the evening as it gets dark. Light exposure at night can suppress melatonin secretion.[6]

Circadian Rhythms. Many biologic rhythms of behavior and physiology fluctuate within a 24-hour period. Because the **circadian** (*circa dian*, about a day) **rhythms** are controlled by internal clock mechanisms, they persist when people are placed in environments free of external time cues. The suprachiasmatic nucleus (SCN) in the hypothalamus is the master clock of the body. The 24-hour cycle of sleep and wake is synchronized to the environmental light and dark periods through specific light detectors in the retina. Pathways from the retina reach the SCN, and pathways from the SCN innervate brain regions controlling wake and sleep behavior.[5]

Light is the strongest time cue for the sleep-wake rhythm. Thus light can be used as a therapy to shift the timing of the sleep-wake rhythm. For example, bright light used early in the morning will cause the sleep-wake rhythm to move to an earlier time; bright light used in the evening will cause the sleep-wake rhythm to move to a later time.

Sleep Architecture

Sleep architecture refers to the pattern of nighttime sleep recorded from physiologic measures of brain waves, eye movements, and muscle tone called *polysomnography* (PSG). Sleep consists of two basic states: rapid eye movement (REM) sleep and non–rapid eye movement (NREM) sleep (see eFig. 8-1 on the website for this chapter). During sleep, the body cycles between NREM and REM sleep. Once asleep, a person goes through four to six NREM and REM sleep cycles.[7]

NREM Sleep. In healthy adults the largest percentage of total sleep time, approximately 75% to 80%, is spent in NREM sleep. NREM sleep is subdivided into three stages:[8]

Stage 1 occurs in the beginning of sleep, with slow eye movements, and is a transition phase from wakefulness to sleep. During this period the person can be easily awakened.

Stage 2 encompasses most of the night's sleep. The heart rate slows down, and the body temperature drops. This stage is associated with specific electroencephalographic (EEG) wave forms that help to maintain sleep.

Stage 3 is deep sleep or slow-wave sleep (SWS). This stage is associated with large EEG wave forms, called delta waves, which are used as a measure of sleep intensity. SWS sleep declines as people age such that most adults over 60 years of age have little NREM stage 3 sleep.

REM Sleep. REM sleep accounts for 20% to 25% of sleep. REM sleep follows NREM sleep in a sleep cycle (see eFig. 8-1). In this stage brain waves resemble wakefulness and postural muscles are inhibited, leading to greatly reduced skeletal muscle tone. During REM sleep an individual cannot stand up and move around. REM sleep is the period when the most vivid dreaming occurs.

INSUFFICIENT SLEEP AND SLEEP DISORDERS

Insufficient sleep and sleep disorders are associated with changes in body function (Fig. 8-3) and health problems (Table 8-2). Impaired cognitive function and impaired performance on simple behavioral tasks occur within 24 hours of sleep loss. The effects of sleep loss are cumulative. Individuals who report less than 6 hours of sleep a night have a higher body mass index (BMI) and are more likely to be obese. The risk for developing glucose intolerance and diabetes is increased in individuals with a history of insufficient sleep.[9,10] Chronic loss of sleep

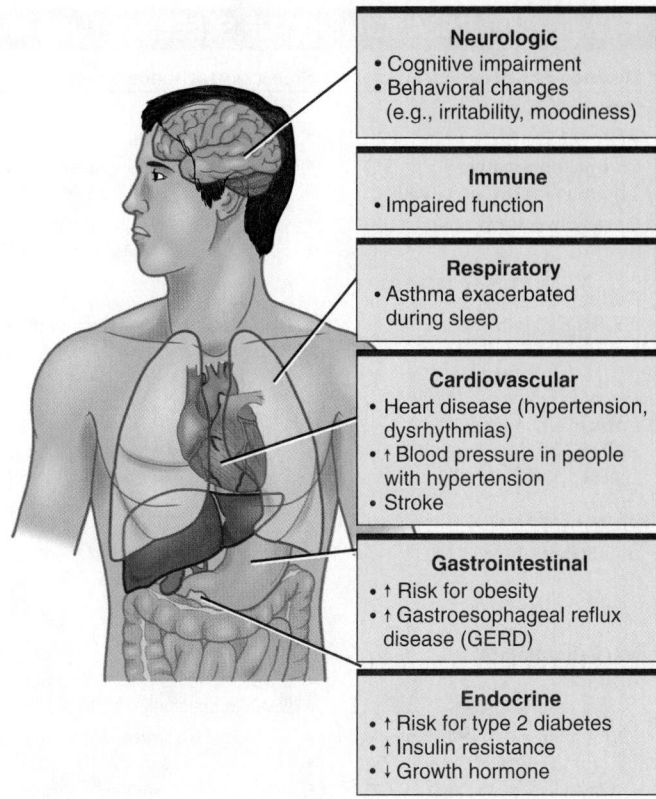

FIG. 8-3 Effects of sleep deprivation and sleep disorders on the body.

- **Neurologic**
  - Cognitive impairment
  - Behavioral changes (e.g., irritability, moodiness)
- **Immune**
  - Impaired function
- **Respiratory**
  - Asthma exacerbated during sleep
- **Cardiovascular**
  - Heart disease (hypertension, dysrhythmias)
  - ↑ Blood pressure in people with hypertension
  - Stroke
- **Gastrointestinal**
  - ↑ Risk for obesity
  - ↑ Gastroesophageal reflux disease (GERD)
- **Endocrine**
  - ↑ Risk for type 2 diabetes
  - ↑ Insulin resistance
  - ↓ Growth hormone

places older adults at risk for depression, impaired daytime functioning, social isolation, and overall reduction in quality of life. In patients with chronic illnesses, especially cardiovascular disease and stroke, insomnia and sleep-disordered breathing are associated with increased morbidity and mortality.[11,12]

INSOMNIA

The most common sleep disorder is insomnia. **Insomnia** is characterized by difficulty falling asleep, difficulty staying asleep, waking up too early, or complaints of waking up feeling unrefreshed. Insomnia is a common problem; one in three adults experiences insomnia.

Acute insomnia refers to difficulties falling or remaining asleep at least 3 nights per week for less than a month. *Chronic insomnia* is defined by the same symptoms and a daytime complaint (e.g., fatigue, poor concentration, interference with social or family activities) that persist for 1 month or longer. Chronic insomnia occurs in 10% to 15% of Americans and is more common in women than men.[13] Chronic insomnia increases with age up to about age 65. Insomnia rates are higher in divorced, widowed, and separated individuals than in those who are married. Insomnia is more prevalent in individuals with low socioeconomic status and less education.[12,13]

Etiology and Pathophysiology

Behaviors, lifestyle, diet, physical and mental conditions, and medications contribute to insomnia. *Inadequate sleep hygiene* refers to those practices or behaviors that are inconsistent with good quality sleep. Intake of stimulants (e.g., caffeine, nicotine, methamphetamine), especially in the evening hours, predisposes a person to insomnia. Insomnia is a common side effect

TABLE 8-2   RELATIONSHIP OF SLEEP DISTURBANCES TO DISEASES AND DISORDERS

Disease or Disorder	Sleep Disturbance
Respiratory	
Asthma	• Exacerbated during sleep.
Chronic obstructive pulmonary disease (COPD)	• Associated with poor sleep quality, nocturnal oxygen desaturation, and coexisting sleep apnea.
Obstructive sleep apnea	• Linked with heart disease (hypertension, stroke, coronary artery disease, dysrhythmias).
	• Results in impaired glucose control similar to that which occurs in type 2 diabetes.
Renal	
End-stage kidney disease	• Disrupted nocturnal sleep with excessive daytime sleepiness.
	• Patients on dialysis have a high incidence of SDB and RLS, which are both significant predictors of mortality in these patients.
Immune Disorders	
Human immunodeficiency virus (HIV)	• Sleep disturbances and fatigue highly prevalent and associated with survival.
Endocrine	
Diabetes	• Insufficient sleep linked to increased risk for type 2 diabetes.
	• Sleep deprivation in healthy people increases insulin resistance.
	• Sleep duration and quality are predictors of Hb A1C levels, an important marker of blood glucose control.
Musculoskeletal	
Arthritis	• Increased rates of RLS and SDB.
	• Disease activity linked to sleep complaints.
Fibromyalgia	• Co-morbid insomnia, especially complaint of nonrestorative sleep.
	• Increased rates of PLMD and RLS.
	• Lower concentrations of sleep-dependent hormones (growth hormone, prolactin).
Chronic fatigue syndrome	• Co-morbid insomnia.
	• Increased rates of SDB.
Cardiovascular (CV)	
	• People with sleep apnea or sleep disorders are at increased risk for CV disorders, including hypertension, dysrhythmias, and coronary artery disease.
Heart failure (HF)	• Sleep disturbances (insomnia, PLMD, SDB) are common.
	• Cheyne-Stokes breathing and central apnea are signs of HF exacerbation related to fluid overload.
Hypertension	• Inadequate sleep in people with hypertension can lead to further elevations in BP.
Gastrointestinal	
Obesity	• Association between short sleep duration and excess body weight. Short sleep duration may result in metabolic changes that are linked to obesity.
	• Higher BMI in people who sleep <6 hours, compared with people who sleep >8 hours.
	• Risk factor for SDB.
Gastroesophageal reflux disease (GERD)	• Reflux of gastric contents into the esophagus occurs during sleep because of incompetent lower esophageal sphincter.
	• Swallowing is depressed during sleep.
Chronic liver disease	• Associated with excessive sleepiness, nocturnal arousal, and RLS.
Neurologic	
Parkinson's disease	• Associated with difficulty initiating or maintaining sleep, parasomnias, and excessive daytime sleepiness.
Alzheimer's disease	• Many have SDB (frequently sleep apnea).
	• Circadian rhythm alterations with nocturnal wandering, daytime sleepiness, and sleep disruption and awakening.
Pain (acute and chronic)	• Decreased quantity and quality of sleep. Poor sleep can intensify pain.
Cancer	• Higher rates of insomnia.
	• Chemotherapy for cancer treatment associated with fragmented sleep and fatigue.

Source: National Center on Sleep Disorders and National Heart, Lung, and Blood Institute: National Sleep Disorders Research Plan: section 4, sleep and health. Retrieved from *www.cdc.gov/sleep/about_sleep/chronic_disease.htm.*
BMI, Body mass index; *PLMD,* periodic limb movement disorder; *RLS,* restless legs syndrome; *SDB,* sleep-disordered breathing.

of many medications (e.g., antidepressants, antihypertensives, corticosteroids, psychostimulants, analgesics). Insomnia is exacerbated or perpetuated by drinking alcohol to help induce sleep, smoking close to bedtime, taking long naps in the afternoon, sleeping late in the morning, having nightmares, exercising near bedtime, and having jet lag.

Chronic insomnia is classified as primary or co-morbid. *Primary insomnia* is difficulty in initiating and maintaining sleep, resulting in poor daytime functioning that is not explained by other causes. The diagnosis of primary insomnia occurs after medical, neurologic, and psychiatric causes have been excluded.[14] The cause of primary insomnia is not known.

Certain individuals may be genetically predisposed or have psychologic traits that make them vulnerable to insomnia. Often individuals report that the onset occurred after a stressful life event (e.g., loss of loved one).

Co-morbid insomnia is common. It is associated with psychiatric illnesses, medical conditions (see Table 8-2), medications, or substance abuse. Patients with psychiatric or medical conditions are 2 times more likely to have insomnia than individuals without these conditions.[15]

Once chronic insomnia manifests, symptoms are likely to persist over time. Individuals may perpetuate disturbed sleep by keeping irregular sleep-wake schedules, using OTC medications or alcohol as sleep aids, and spending more time in bed trying to sleep. Increased attention to one's environment, worry or fear about not obtaining sufficient sleep, and poor sleep habits can lead to arousal that becomes associated with the bed and bedroom. This is called *conditioned arousal*.

Clinical Manifestations

Manifestations of insomnia include one or more of the following symptoms: (1) difficulty falling asleep *(long sleep latency)*, (2) frequent awakenings *(fragmented sleep)*, (3) prolonged nighttime awakenings or awakening too early and not being able to fall back to sleep, and (4) awakening feeling unrefreshed, called *nonrestorative sleep*. Daytime consequences of insomnia include feeling tired, having trouble concentrating at work or school, and having an altered mood. Falling asleep during the day or complaints of sleepiness are common. Behavioral manifestations of poor sleep include irritability, forgetfulness, confusion, and anxiety.

Diagnostic Studies

Self-Report. The diagnosis of insomnia is made based on subjective complaints and on an evaluation of a 1- or 2-week sleep diary completed by the patient. In ambulatory care settings the evaluation of insomnia requires a comprehensive sleep history to establish the type of insomnia and to screen for possible psychiatric, medical, or other sleep disorders that would require specific treatment. Questionnaires such as the Pittsburgh Sleep Quality Index (see eTable 8-1 on the website for this chapter), Insomnia Severity Index (see eTable 8-2), and Epworth Sleepiness Scale (see eTable 8-3) are commonly used to assess sleep quality.[16-18]

Actigraphy. Actigraphy is a relatively noninvasive method of monitoring rest and activity cycles. A small actigraph watch can be worn on the wrist to measure gross motor activity. The unit continuously records the patient's movements, producing data that are downloaded to a computer and analyzed.

Polysomnography. A clinical PSG study is not required to establish a diagnosis of insomnia. A PSG study is done only if there are symptoms or signs of another sleep disorder, such as sleep-disordered breathing (discussed later in the chapter). In a PSG study, electrodes simultaneously record physiologic measures that define the main stages of sleep and wakefulness.[7,8] These measures include (1) muscle tone recorded using an electromyogram (EMG), (2) eye movements recorded with an electro-oculogram (EOG), and (3) brain activity recorded through EEG. To determine additional characteristics of specific sleep disorders, other measures made during PSG include airflow at the nose and mouth, respiratory effort around the chest and abdomen, heart rate, noninvasive oxygen saturation, and EMG of the anterior tibialis muscles (used to detect peri-odic leg movements). Finally, a patient's gross body movements are monitored continuously by audiovisual means.

Collaborative Care

Insomnia treatments are oriented toward symptom management (Table 8-3). A key to management is to change behaviors that perpetuate insomnia. An important first step is to provide teaching about sleep along with behavioral strategies. **Sleep hygiene** is a variety of different practices that are important to have normal, quality nighttime sleep and daytime alertness (Table 8-4).

Cognitive-Behavioral Therapy for Insomnia. Although teaching about sleep hygiene practices is useful, individuals with chronic insomnia require more in-depth cognitive-behavioral therapy for insomnia (CBT-I).[14] CBT-I is based on structured treatment plans that could include relaxation training, guided imagery, cognitive strategies to address misconceptions about sleep, and behavioral strategies. Behavioral strategies for insomnia include instructions to (1) limit the amount of time an individual can stay in bed, (2) maintain a scheduled

TABLE 8-3 COLLABORATIVE CARE

Insomnia

Diagnostic	Collaborative Therapy
History	Nondrug
• Self-report sleep log or diary	• Sleep hygiene (see Table 8-4)
• Sleep assessment (see Table 8-6)	• Cognitive behavioral therapies for insomnia (CBT-I)
• Pittsburgh Sleep Quality Index (see eTable 8-1*)	Drugs (see Table 8-5)
• Insomnia Severity Index (see eTable 8-2*)	• Benzodiazepines
• Epworth Sleepiness Scale (see eTable 8-3*)	• Benzodiazepine-receptor–like agents
Physical assessment	• Melatonin-receptor agonist
• Polysomnography	• Antidepressants
	• Antihistamines
	Complementary and alternative therapies
	• Melatonin

*○evolve Available on website for this chapter.

TABLE 8-4 PATIENT TEACHING GUIDE

Sleep Hygiene

Include the following instructions when teaching a patient who has a sleep disturbance or disorder.
• Don't go to bed unless you are sleepy.
• If you are not asleep after 20 minutes, get out of the bed.
• Adopt a regular pattern in terms of bedtime and awakening.
• Begin rituals (e.g., warm bath, light snack, reading) that help you relax each night before bed.
• Get a full night's sleep on a regular basis.
• Make your bedroom quiet, dark, and a little bit cool.
• Don't read, write, eat, watch TV, talk on the phone, or play cards in bed.
• Avoid caffeine, nicotine, and alcohol at least 4 to 6 hours before bedtime.
• Don't go to bed hungry, but don't eat a big meal near bedtime either.
• Avoid strenuous exercise within 6 hours of your bedtime.
• Avoid sleeping pills, or use them cautiously.
• Practice relaxation techniques (e.g., relaxation breathing) to help you cope with stress in your life (see Chapter 7).

Adapted from American Academy of Sleep Medicine: Sleep hygiene: the healthy habits of good sleep, 2010. Retrieved from *http://yoursleep.aasmnet.org/hygiene.aspx.*

TABLE 8-5   DRUG THERAPY

Insomnia

Benzodiazepines	Melatonin-Receptor Agonist
• diazepam (Valium)	• ramelteon (Rozerem)
• flurazepam (Dalmane)	
• lorazepam (Ativan)	**Antidepressants**
• quazepam (Doral)	• amitriptyline (Elavil)
• triazolam (Halcion)	• bupropion (Wellbutrin)
	• doxepin (Sinequan)
Benzodiazepine-Receptor–	• fluoxetine (Prozac)
like Agents	• trazodone (Desyrel)
• zolpidem (Ambien, Ambien CR,	
Intermezzo, Edluar, ZolpiMist)	**Antihistamines**
• zaleplon (Sonata)	• diphenhydramine (Benadryl,
• eszopiclone (Lunesta)	Nytol, Sominex)

time to get up in the morning, (3) go to bed only when an individual feels sleepy, and (4) get out of bed when unable to sleep. CBT-I also includes teaching about sleep hygiene practices (see Table 8-4). CBT-I requires individuals to change behavior, which sometimes is difficult.

Encourage individuals with insomnia not to watch television or read in bed. Time in bed is limited to the actual time that the individual can sleep. Teach the person with insomnia to avoid naps and consumption of large meals, alcohol, and stimulants, especially a few hours before bedtime. Naps are less likely to affect nighttime sleep if they are limited to 15 to 20 minutes, once per day, and scheduled 7 to 9 hours after morning awakening. Regular exercise (performed several hours before bedtime) may enhance sleep quality.

Drug Therapy. Hypnotic and anxiolytic medications are effective for improving sleep, but the benefits for improving daytime functioning are less certain. Few studies have evaluated the use of hypnotics for chronic insomnia, and their use in older adults is controversial.[19] Many individuals with insomnia become used to taking OTC or prescription medications to treat insomnia and risk becoming dependent on them, both psychologically and physically.[20] *Rebound insomnia* is common with abrupt withdrawal of some hypnotic medications. The resulting daytime fatigue can negatively influence the patient's efforts to use nondrug approaches. Classes of medications used to treat insomnia include benzodiazepines, benzodiazepine-receptor–like agents, melatonin-receptor agonists, and antidepressant and antihistamine medications (Table 8-5).

Benzodiazepines. Benzodiazepines such as diazepam (Valium) activate the γ-aminobutyric acid (GABA) receptors to promote sleep. The prolonged half-life of some of these agents (e.g., flurazepam [Dalmane]) can result in daytime sleepiness, amnesia, dizziness, and rebound insomnia. Tolerance to these agents develops, and there is risk for dependence. It is recommended that the use of benzodiazepines be limited to 2 to 3 weeks. All benzodiazepines have the potential for abuse. In addition, benzodiazepines interact with alcohol and other central nervous system (CNS) depressants. These agents are no longer recommended as first-line therapy for insomnia.

Benzodiazepine-Receptor–like Agents. Zolpidem (Ambien), zaleplon (Sonata), and eszopiclone (Lunesta) are the drugs of first choice for insomnia. Because they are benzodiazepine-receptor agonists, they work similarly to benzodiazepines.[20] These drugs are effective and safe for use from 6 months to a year. Food has the potential to delay onset of action and should

not be taken with these agents. These agents have short half-lives, making their duration of action short. The extended-release formulation of zolpidem (Ambien CR) is used for problems of sleep onset and sleep maintenance. A dissolvable tablet form of zolpidem (Edluar) and an oral spray formulation (ZolpiMist) may be useful for individuals who have difficulty swallowing pills or are on restricted oral fluid intake.[20] Zolpidem tartrate (Intermezzo), a sublingual tablet, is used for patients with insomnia characterized by middle-of-the-night waking followed by difficulty returning to sleep.

Melatonin-Receptor Agonist. Ramelteon (Rozerem) is a melatonin-receptor agonist. It has a rapid onset that is effective for sleep onset but a short duration of action. Unlike benzodiazepines, ramelteon does not cause tolerance, but the drug is not always effective in improving sleep quality.[19]

Antidepressants. Trazodone (Desyrel) is an atypical antidepressant that has sedative properties. It is one of the most common agents prescribed in the United States to treat insomnia, especially in older adults. The insomnia dose of antidepressants like trazodone is much lower than the antidepressant dose. The administration of this drug to older adults is controversial. Daytime sleepiness is a common side effect. Tolerance can develop within a few weeks.

Doxepin (Sinequan) is another antidepressant used to treat insomnia. In very low doses doxepin inhibits histamine receptors in the brain. Doxepin improves sleep without next-day drowsiness in older and middle-aged adults with chronic primary insomnia.[21]

Antihistamines. Many individuals with insomnia self-medicate with OTC sleep aids. Most OTC agents include diphenhydramine (Benadryl, Nytol, Sominex). These agents are less effective than benzodiazepines, and tolerance develops quickly. In addition, antihistamines have anticholinergic side effects, including daytime sleepiness, impaired cognitive function, blurred vision, urinary retention, constipation, and risk of increased intraocular pressure. Agents with diphenhydramine are not intended for long-term use and should not be used by older adults.[11,19]

Complementary and Alternative Therapies. Many types of complementary therapies and herbal products are used as sleep aids. As noted earlier in the chapter, melatonin is a hormone produced by the pineal gland[22] (see Complementary & Alternative Therapies box). Melatonin is effective for improving sleep disturbance associated with jet lag. It also helps night shift

🌿 COMPLEMENTARY & ALTERNATIVE THERAPIES

Melatonin

Scientific Evidence

Overall, the scientific evidence suggests the benefits of melatonin in people who take it for jet lag. The majority of scientific evidence suggests that it may decrease the time it takes to fall asleep (sleep latency).

Nursing Implications

- Regarded as safe in recommended doses for short-term use.
- Avoid in patients using warfarin (Coumadin).
- Avoid in patients using central nervous system depressants.
- May cause a drop in blood pressure. Caution is advised in patients taking drugs that may also lower blood pressure.

Source: Based on a systematic review of scientific literature. Retrieved from *www.naturalstandard.com*.

workers sleep during the daytime. However, melatonin is not considered effective for improving nighttime sleep. Valerian is an herb that has been used for many years as a sleep aid and to relieve anxiety. Although valerian is safe, it is not effective in treating insomnia.[23]

NURSING MANAGEMENT
INSOMNIA

NURSING ASSESSMENT

As a nurse, you are in a key position to assess sleep problems in patients and their caregivers. Sleep assessment is important in helping patients identify personal habits and environmental factors that contribute to poor sleep. Family caregivers may experience sleep disruptions due to the necessity of providing care to patients in the home. These sleep disruptions can increase the burden of caregiving.

Both self-report and objective data are used to assess sleep duration and quality. Many patients do not tell their health care provider about their sleep problems. Therefore all patients should be asked about their sleep on a regular basis. A sleep history includes characteristics of sleep such as the duration, the pattern of sleep, and daytime alertness. Before using any questionnaire, assess the patient's cognitive function, reading level (if a paper form is used), and language ability (Table 8-6). Also assess the diet. Question the patient about the intake of caffeine and other food stimulants (chocolate). Ask about alcohol consumption and whether it is used as a sleep aid.

Ask the patient about sleep aids. This includes both OTC and prescription medications. Note the drug dose, frequency of use, and any side effects (e.g., daytime drowsiness, dry mouth). Many individuals also consume herbal or dietary supplements that they believe improve sleep, including valerian, melatonin, hops, lavender, passion flower, kava, and skullcap. Inform the patient that many of these products are sold as dietary supplements and do not have U.S. Food and Drug Administration (FDA) approval or regulatory oversight. The exact components

TABLE 8-6 NURSING ASSESSMENT

Sleep

Use the following questions to do an initial assessment regarding sleep.
1. What time do you normally go to bed at night? What time do you normally wake up in the morning?
2. Do you often have trouble falling asleep at night?
3. About how many times do you wake up at night?
4. If you do wake up during the night, do you usually have trouble falling back asleep?
5. Does your bed partner say or are you aware that you frequently snore, gasp for air, or stop breathing?
6. Does your bed partner say or are you aware that you kick or thrash about while asleep?
7. Are you aware that you ever walk, eat, punch, kick, or scream during sleep?
8. Are you sleepy or tired during much of the day?
9. Do you usually take one or more naps during the day?
10. Do you usually doze off without planning to during the day?
11. How much sleep do you need to feel alert and function well?
12. Are you currently taking any type of medication or other preparation to help you sleep?

Source: Bloom HG, Ahmed I, Alessi CA, et al: Evidence-based recommendations for the assessment and management of sleep disorders in older people, *J Am Geriatr Soc* 57:761, 2009.

and concentrations of herbs and supplements often are unknown, and patients may experience adverse effects. Certain agents such as kava are associated with liver toxicity. Additional sleep aids include white noise devices or relaxation strategies.

Encourage individuals to keep a sleep diary for 2 weeks. In the diary they record when they go to sleep, when they wake up, and how long they were awake during the night (see eTable 8-4 on the website for this chapter). The number and duration of naps are also recorded. Standardized questionnaires such as the Epworth Sleepiness Scale (see eTable 8-3) may be used to assess daytime sleepiness.[18]

The patient's medical history can also provide important information about factors that contribute to poor sleep. For example, men with benign prostatic hyperplasia often report frequent awakenings during the night for voiding. Psychiatric problems (e.g., depression, anxiety, posttraumatic stress disorder [PTSD], drug abuse) are associated with sleep disturbances. Sleep disturbances often develop as a consequence or complication of a chronic or terminal condition (e.g., heart disease, dementia, cancer).[14]

Ask about work schedules and cross-country and international travel. Shift work contributes to reduced or poor-quality sleep. Work-related behaviors resulting from poor sleep may include poor performance, decreased productivity, and job absenteeism.

NURSING DIAGNOSES

Specific nursing diagnoses related to sleep include insomnia, sleep deprivation, disturbed sleep pattern, and readiness for enhanced sleep.

NURSING IMPLEMENTATION

Nursing interventions depend on the severity and duration of the sleep problem, as well as individual characteristics. Optimally, healthy adults should have 7 to 8 hours of sleep a night. Individuals with longer (more than 9 hours) and shorter (less than 6 hours) sleep durations have increased morbidity and mortality risks. Those with short sleep duration have increased risk for weight gain, impaired glucose tolerance and diabetes, hypertension, cardiovascular disease, and stroke. Occasional difficulty getting to sleep or awakening during the night is not unusual. However, sleep disturbances longer than 1 month are problematic.

Although teaching about sleep hygiene practices (see Table 8-4) is beneficial, individuals with chronic insomnia require more in-depth intervention using CBT-I strategies. An important component of sleep hygiene is reducing dietary intake of substances containing caffeine (Table 8-7). Caffeine has a half-life of about 6 hours, perhaps as long as 9 hours, in older adults. Consuming caffeinated beverages after 12 o'clock should be avoided.

Suggest and implement changes in home and institutional environments to enhance sleep. Reducing light and noise levels enhances sleep. Awareness of time passing and watching the clock adds to anxieties about not falling asleep or returning to sleep. Keeping the bedroom dark and cool is conducive to good sleep.

Teach patients about sleeping medications. With the benzodiazepines, benzodiazepine receptor–like agents, and melatonin-receptor agonists, teach the patient to take the drug right before bedtime, be prepared to get a full night's sleep of at least 6 to 8 hours, and not plan activities the next morning that require

TABLE 8-7   CAFFEINE CONTENT OF SELECTED FOODS AND BEVERAGES

Food or Beverage	Caffeine (mg)
Coffee, brewed (8 oz)	95-200
Coffee, instant (8 oz)	27-173
Coffee, decaffeinated	5
Tea, leaf or bag (8 oz)	50
Celestial Seasoning herbal tea, all varieties	0
Diet Coke (12 oz)	47
Coca-Cola (12 oz)	35
Dr. Pepper (12 oz)	54
Pepsi-Cola (12 oz)	37
7-Up, Sprite, or Diet 7-Up (12 oz)	0
A&W Root Beer (12 oz)	0
Red Bull (12 oz)	80
Mountain Dew (12 oz)	55
Ben & Jerry's no-fat coffee fudge frozen yogurt (1 cup)	85
Dannon coffee yogurt (8 oz)	45
Hershey's special dark chocolate bar (1.5 oz)	31
Hershey bar (milk chocolate) (1.5 oz)	12
Hot chocolate (8 oz)	5

highly skilled psychomotor coordination. Advise patients not to take these medications with high-fat food (delays absorption), alcohol, or other CNS depressants.

Patient follow-up regarding medications is important. Ask about daytime sleepiness, nightmares, and any difficulties in activities of daily living.

SLEEP DISTURBANCES IN THE HOSPITAL

Hospitalization, especially in the intensive care unit (ICU), is associated with decreased total sleep time and decreased SWS and REM sleep.[24] Because of the nature of a critical illness and its treatment, sleep loss may be inevitable for patients in ICUs. Preexisting sleep disorders may be aggravated or triggered in the hospital. Patients with sleep apnea should use continuous positive airway pressure (CPAP) in the hospital. Sleep-disordered breathing is a major concern in the ICU.

Environmental sleep-disruptive factors, psychoactive medications, and acute and critical illness all contribute to poor sleep. Patient symptoms, including pain, dyspnea, and nausea, can also contribute to sleep loss in the acutely ill patient. Medications commonly used in acutely and critically ill patients can further contribute to sleep loss. Hospitalized patients are also at risk for poor sleep because of circadian rhythm disruptions and reduced melatonin levels. The hospital is a new environment and thus normal cues linked to sleep are absent.

Hospital and ICU noise (e.g., staff paging system, respirator alarms, bedside monitors, infusion alarms) and especially staff conversations near patients (e.g., in hallways) during both the day and night disturb sleep. Bright lights during the night also disrupt sleep and reduce melatonin levels. Patient care activities (e.g., dressing changes, blood draws, vital sign monitoring) disrupt sleep. Inactivity, boredom, and certain medications lead to napping during the day and evening that can affect nighttime sleep.

Decreased sleep duration and sleep loss influence pain perception.[25] Psychologic factors, such as anxiety and depression, also modify the sleep-pain relationship. Adequate pain management may improve total sleep time, but medications commonly used to relieve pain, especially opioids, also alter sleep and place an individual at risk for sleep-disordered breathing. Withdrawal of opioids is associated with rebound effects on sleep architecture.

You have an important role in creating an environment conducive to sleep. This includes the scheduling of medications and procedures. Reducing light and noise levels can promote opportunities for sleep. Hypnotic medications are often available on an as-needed basis. Ask patients if they would like medication to help them sleep.

NARCOLEPSY

Narcolepsy is a chronic neurologic disorder caused by the brain's inability to regulate sleep-wake cycles normally. At various times throughout the day, people with narcolepsy experience uncontrollable urges to sleep. As the urge becomes overwhelming, individuals fall asleep for periods lasting from a few seconds to several minutes. Patients with narcolepsy often go directly into REM sleep from wakefulness. This is a unique feature of narcolepsy. Patients with narcolepsy also experience fragmented and disturbed nighttime sleep.[26]

In both genders the onset of narcolepsy typically occurs in adolescence or early in the third decade. However, approximately 25% of the patients are not diagnosed until after 40 years of age. Head trauma, a sudden change in sleep-wake habits, and infection may trigger the onset of narcolepsy symptoms. Patients with narcolepsy are included in the Americans with Disabilities Act, which requires employers to provide reasonable accommodations for all employees with disabilities.

Narcolepsy has two categories: with and without cataplexy. Cataplexy is a brief and sudden loss of skeletal muscle tone or muscle weakness. It can manifest as a brief episode of muscle weakness or complete postural collapse and falling. Laughter, anger, or surprise often triggers episodes. Approximately 30% to 50% of patients with narcolepsy experience cataplexy.[27]

Etiology and Pathophysiology

The cause of narcolepsy remains unknown. It is associated with a deficiency of orexin (hypocretin), a neuropeptide linked to waking, from the destruction of orexin neurons. The reason for the loss of neurons is not well understood, but an autoimmune process is suspected.

Clinical Manifestations and Diagnostic Studies

Manifestations in some patients include brief episodes of sleep paralysis, hallucinations, cataplexy, and fragmented nighttime sleep. *Sleep paralysis* is a temporary (few seconds to minutes) paralysis of skeletal muscles (except respiratory and extraocular muscles) that occurs in the transition from REM sleep to waking. The loss of muscle tone, often triggered by strong emotions, usually lasts less than 2 minutes. During the period of muscle tone loss, the individual remains conscious.

With narcolepsy, unwanted episodes of REM sleep occur throughout the day. These sleep episodes are usually of short duration, but can last for more than 1 hour, and patients feel refreshed afterward. Patients may complain of feeling drowsy and being unable to remain awake while watching a movie, sitting in a classroom, reading, or performing other sedentary activities. As a result, they often show poor performance at work, have reduced quality of life, and experience poor interpersonal relationships.

TABLE 8-8 DRUG THERAPY
Narcolepsy

Wakefulness Promoting
- dextroamphetamine (Dexedrine)
- methamphetamine (Desoxyn)
- methylphenidate (Concerta)
- modafinil (Provigil)

Gabaminergic
- sodium oxybate or γ-hydroxybutyrate (Xyrem)

Antidepressants
Tricyclic
- atomoxetine (Strattera)
- protriptyline (Vivactil)
- desipramine (Norpramin)

Selective Serotonin Reuptake Inhibitors (SSRIs)
- fluoxetine (Prozac)
- venlafaxine (Effexor)

Narcolepsy is diagnosed based on a history of sleepiness, PSG, and daytime *multiple sleep latency tests* (MSLTs). For the MSLT, patients undergo an overnight PSG evaluation followed by four or five naps scheduled every 2 hours during the next day. Short sleep latencies and onset of REM sleep in more than two MSLTs are diagnostic signs of narcolepsy.

Nursing and Collaborative Management
Management of narcolepsy is focused on symptom management (see Table 8-3). Provide teaching about sleep and sleep hygiene. Advise the patient with narcolepsy to take three or more short (15 minute) naps throughout the day and to avoid large or heavy meals and alcohol. You can play a key role in ensuring patient safety by teaching safety behaviors and encouraging adherence to the prescribed medication regimen.

Drug Therapy. Narcolepsy cannot be cured. However, excessive daytime sleepiness and cataplexy (the most disabling manifestation of the disorder) can be controlled in most patients with drug treatment. A nonamphetamine wake-promotion drug, modafinil (Provigil), is considered a first-line drug therapy for narcolepsy. Other agents, including amphetamine drugs such as dextroamphetamine (Dexedrine), methamphetamine (Desoxyn), and methylphenidate (Concerta), are used to manage daytime sleepiness[28] (Table 8-8). Tricyclic antidepressant drugs such as atomoxetine (Strattera), protriptyline (Vivactil), and desipramine (Norpramin) are effective in the management of cataplexy. High doses of selective serotonin reuptake inhibitors (SSRIs) such as fluoxetine (Prozac) and venlafaxine (Effexor) may be prescribed for management of cataplexy. Sodium oxybate, or γ-hydroxybutyrate (Xyrem), a metabolite of GABA, is also used in the treatment of narcolepsy.[28]

Behavioral Therapy. None of the current drug therapies cures narcolepsy or allows patients to consistently maintain a full, normal state of alertness. As a result, drug therapy needs to be combined with various behavioral strategies. The behavioral therapies for insomnia (discussed earlier in this chapter) are also used for patients with narcolepsy.

Safety precautions, especially when driving, are critically important for patients with narcolepsy. Excessive daytime sleepiness and cataplexy can result in serious injury or death if not treated. Individuals with untreated narcolepsy symptoms are involved in automobile accidents roughly 10 times more frequently than the general population. Among those receiving appropriate treatment, the accident rate is normal.[27,28]

Patient support groups are also useful for patients with narcolepsy and their family members. Social isolation can occur because of symptoms. Patients with narcolepsy can be stigma-tized as being lazy and unproductive because of lack of understanding about this disorder.

CIRCADIAN RHYTHM DISORDERS

Circadian rhythm disorders can occur when the circadian time-keeping system loses synchrony with the environment. Lack of synchrony between the circadian time-keeping system and the environment disrupts the sleep-wake cycle and affects the patient's ability to have quality sleep. The two common symptoms are insomnia and excessive sleepiness. *Jet lag disorder* and *shift work sleep disorder* (see Special Sleep Needs of Nurses section on p. 110) are the most common types of circadian rhythm disorders.[29]

Jet lag disorder occurs when a person travels across multiple time zones. One's body time is not synchronized with environmental time. Most individuals crossing at least three time zones experience jet lag. The number of time zones crossed affects the severity of symptoms and the time it takes to recover. Resynchronization of the body's clock occurs at a rate of about 1 hr/day when traveling eastward and 1.5 hr/day when traveling westward. Melatonin is effective as a sleep aid to help synchronize the body's rhythm. Exposure to daylight assists synchronization of the body clock to environmental time.

Several strategies may help to reduce the risk of developing jet lag. Before travel the individual can start to get in harmony with the time schedule of the destination. When time at destination is brief (i.e., 2 days or less), keeping home-based sleep hours rather than adopting destination sleep hours may reduce sleepiness and jet lag symptoms.

SLEEP-DISORDERED BREATHING

The term **sleep-disordered breathing (SDB)** indicates abnormal respiratory patterns associated with sleep.[30] These include snoring, apnea, and hypopnea with increased respiratory effort leading to frequent arousals. SDB results in frequent sleep disruptions and alterations in sleep architecture. Obstructive sleep apnea is the most commonly diagnosed SDB problem.[31]

Obstructive Sleep Apnea
Obstructive sleep apnea (OSA), also called *obstructive sleep apnea–hypopnea syndrome* (OSAHS), is characterized by partial or complete upper airway obstruction during sleep. *Apnea* is the cessation of spontaneous respirations lasting longer than 10 seconds. *Hypopnea* is a condition characterized by shallow respirations (30% to 50% reduction in airflow). Airflow obstruction occurs because (1) narrowing of the air passages with relaxation of muscle tone during sleep leads to apnea and hypopnea or (2) the tongue and the soft palate fall backward and partially or completely obstruct the pharynx (Fig. 8-4).

Each obstruction may last from 10 to 90 seconds. During the apneic period the patient can experience *hypoxemia* (decreased PaO_2 or SpO_2) and *hypercapnia* (increased $PaCO_2$). These changes are ventilatory stimulants and cause brief arousals, but the patient may not fully awaken. The patient has a generalized startle response, snorts, and gasps, which cause the tongue and soft palate to move forward and the airway to open. Apnea and arousal cycles occur repeatedly, as many as 200 to 400 times during 6 to 8 hours of sleep.

Sleep apnea occurs in 2% to 10% of Americans but is considered to be underreported. The risk increases with obesity

FIG. 8-4 How sleep apnea occurs. **A,** The patient predisposed to obstructive sleep apnea (OSA) has a small pharyngeal airway. **B,** During sleep, the pharyngeal muscles relax, allowing the airway to close. Lack of airflow results in repeated apneic episodes. **C,** Continuous positive airway pressure *(CPAP)* splits the airway open, preventing airflow obstruction.

INFORMATICS IN PRACTICE

Sleep Apnea Diagnosis and Monitoring

- Home respiratory monitoring is a cost-effective alternative for diagnosing sleep-related breathing disorders that allows patients the convenience of sleeping in their own home.
- Home respiratory monitoring is used as part of a comprehensive sleep evaluation and in patients likely to have moderate to severe obstructive sleep apnea but without heart failure, obstructive lung disease, or neuromuscular disease.
- Home respiratory monitoring is used to monitor the effectiveness of non-CPAP therapies for patients with sleep-related breathing disorders.
- Wireless monitors can detect changes in vital signs and pulse oximetry, raising an alarm if values fall outside of set parameters.
- Your patient may benefit from telehealth to diagnose and monitor for sleep apnea in the home.

CPAP, Continuous positive airway pressure.

(BMI greater than 28 kg/m²), age greater than 65 years, neck circumference greater than 17 inches, craniofacial abnormalities that affect the upper airway, and acromegaly.[12,31] Smokers are more likely to have OSA. OSA is more common in men than in women until after menopause, when the prevalence of the disorder is equal.[13] Women with OSA have higher mortality rates than men with OSA. OSA patients with excessive daytime sleepiness have increased mortality.[31] Hypoxemia associated with OSA is greater in those patients with chronic obstructive pulmonary disease (COPD).[32]

Clinical Manifestations and Diagnostic Studies. Clinical manifestations of sleep apnea include frequent arousals during sleep, insomnia, excessive daytime sleepiness, and witnessed apneic episodes. The patient's bed partner may complain about the patient's loud snoring. Other symptoms include morning headaches (from hypercapnia or increased blood pressure that causes vasodilation of cerebral blood vessels), personality changes, and irritability.

Complications that can result from untreated sleep apnea include hypertension, right-sided heart failure from pulmonary hypertension caused by chronic nocturnal hypoxemia, and cardiac dysrhythmias. Chronic sleep loss predisposes the person to diminished ability to concentrate, impaired memory, failure to accomplish daily tasks, and interpersonal difficulties. The male patient may experience impotence. Driving accidents are more common in habitually sleepy people. Family life and the patient's ability to maintain employment are often compromised. As a result, the patient may experience severe depres-

sion. Cessation of breathing reported by the bed partner is usually a source of great anxiety because of the fear that breathing may not resume.

Assessment of the patient with OSA includes a thorough sleep and medical history. Symptoms of OSA, including daytime sleepiness, snoring, and witnessed apnea, are obvious characteristics of the disorder. Less obvious symptoms may include cardiovascular manifestations, muscle pain, and mood changes. Patients with OSA frequently have co-morbidities, including a history of stroke and cardiovascular disease.

PSG is used to make the diagnosis of sleep apnea. The patient's chest and abdominal movement, oral and nasal airflow, SpO₂, ocular movement, and heart rate and rhythm are monitored. A diagnosis of sleep apnea requires documentation of apneic events (no airflow with respiratory effort) or hypopnea (airflow diminished 30% to 50% with respiratory effort) of at least 10 seconds' duration. OSA is defined as more than five apnea/hypopnea events per hour accompanied by a 3% to 4% decrease in oxygen saturation. Severe apnea can be associated with apneic events of more than 30 to 50 per hour of sleep.[8]

Typically, PSG is done in a clinical sleep laboratory with technicians monitoring the patient. In some instances, portable sleep studies are conducted in the home setting. Overnight pulse oximetry assessment may be done to determine whether nocturnal oxygen supplementation is indicated.

NURSING AND COLLABORATIVE MANAGEMENT SLEEP APNEA

CONSERVATIVE TREATMENT

Mild sleep apnea (5 to 10 apnea/hypopnea events per hour) may respond to simple measures. Conservative treatment at home begins with sleeping on one's side rather than on the back. Elevating the head of the bed may eliminate OSA in some patients. Instruct the patient to avoid taking sedatives or consuming alcoholic beverages for 3 to 4 hours before sleep. Sleep medications often make OSA worse. OSA is a potentially life-threatening disorder. Because excessive weight worsens sleep apnea, referral to a weight loss program may be indicated. Weight loss and bariatric surgery reduce OSA.[33] Instruct the patient on the dangers of driving or using heavy equipment.

Symptoms may resolve in up to half of patients with OSA who use a special mouth guard, also called an oral appliance, during sleep to prevent airflow obstruction. Oral appliances bring the mandible and tongue forward to enlarge the airway

FIG. 8-5 Examples of positive airwave pressure devices for sleep apnea. **A,** Patient wearing a nasal mask and headgear (positive pressure only through nose). **B,** Patient wearing nasal pillows (positive pressure only through nose). **C,** Patient wearing a full face mask (positive pressure to both nose and mouth).

space, thereby preventing airway occlusion.[34] Some individuals find a support group beneficial, where they can express concerns and feelings and discuss strategies for resolving problems.

In patients with more severe symptoms (more than 15 apnea/hypopnea events per hour), continuous positive airway pressure (CPAP) by mask is the treatment of choice. With CPAP, the patient applies a nasal mask that is attached to a high-flow blower (Fig. 8-5). The blower is adjusted to maintain sufficient positive pressure (5 to 25 cm H_2O) in the airway during inspiration and expiration to prevent airway collapse. Some patients cannot adjust to wearing a mask over the nose or mouth or to exhaling against the high pressure. A technologically more sophisticated therapy, bilevel positive airway pressure (BiPAP), can deliver a higher inspiration pressure and a lower pressure during expiration. With BiPAP, the apnea can be relieved with a lower mean pressure and may be better tolerated.

CPAP reduces apnea episodes, daytime sleepiness, and fatigue. It improves quality of life ratings and returns cognitive functioning to normal.[35] Although CPAP is a highly effective treatment, compliance and adherence are poor. Approximately two thirds of patients using CPAP report side effects such as nasal stuffiness. First assess the patient's knowledge about OSA and CPAP, and involve the bed partner in teaching. Evaluate the patient for nasal resistance. Patient-centered selection of mask and device and exposure to CPAP before initiation of therapy are associated with successful adherence to CPAP treatment.[33] If necessary, facilitate referral for evaluation of equipment. For anxiety related to CPAP, the patient may be referred to a psychologist for desensitization therapy.

When patients with a history of OSA are hospitalized, be aware that the administration of opioid analgesics and sedating medications (benzodiazepines, barbiturates, hypnotics) may worsen OSA symptoms by depressing respiration. This will necessitate that the patient wear the CPAP or BiPAP when resting or sleeping. Many patients are able to use their own CPAP equipment, but hospital policy should be checked to be certain it can be used.

SURGICAL TREATMENT

If other measures fail, sleep apnea can be managed surgically. The two most common procedures are uvulopalatopharyngoplasty (UPPP or UP3) and genioglossal advancement and hyoid myotomy (GAHM). UPPP involves excision of the tonsillar pillars, uvula, and posterior soft palate to remove the obstructing tissue.[34] GAHM involves advancing the attachment of the muscular part of the tongue on the mandible. When GAHM is performed, UPPP is generally performed as well. Depending on the site of the obstruction, symptoms are relieved in up to 80% of patients. Radiofrequency ablation (RFA) alone or in combination with other surgical techniques is also used. RFA is the least invasive surgical intervention.[34]

Complications of airway obstruction or hemorrhage occur most often in the immediate postoperative period. Patients can usually be discharged home within 1 day after the procedure. Before going home the patient is taught what to expect during the postoperative recovery period. Tell patients that their throat will be sore. They may have a foul breath odor that may be reduced by rinsing with diluted mouthwash and then salt water after several days. Snoring may persist until the inflammation has subsided. Follow-up of patients after surgery is important. A repeat PSG is performed 3 to 4 months after surgery.

PERIODIC LIMB MOVEMENT DISORDER

Periodic limb movement disorder (PLMD) is characterized by involuntary, continual movement of the legs and/or arms that affects people only during sleep. PLMD rarely involves the arms. Sometimes abdominal, oral, and nasal movement accompanies PLMD. Movements typically occur for 0.5 to 10 seconds, in intervals separated by 5 to 90 seconds. PLMD causes poor-quality sleep, which may lead to excessive daytime sleepiness. PLMD occurs in 80% to 90% of individuals with restless legs syndrome (RLS).[36] (RLS is a disorder that is discussed in Chapter 59.)

PLMD is diagnosed using a detailed history from the patient and/or bed partner and doing a PSG. PLMD is treated by medications aimed at reducing or eliminating the limb movements or the arousals. Dopamine agonists (pramipexole [Mirapex] and ropinirole [Requip]) are preferred.

GERONTOLOGIC CONSIDERATIONS

SLEEP

With aging, the most notable changes are a decrease in the amount of deep sleep and an increase in arousals and awakenings. Older adults report greater problems getting to and main-

FIG. 8-6 Many older people have sleep problems. (Photodisc/Thinkstock)

taining sleep as compared with younger adults (Fig. 8-6). Older age is associated with overall shorter total sleep time, decreased sleep efficiency, and more awakenings.[37]

A common misconception is that older people need less sleep than younger people. In fact, the amount of sleep needed as a person ages remains relatively constant.[38]

Healthy older adults who do not complain of sleep disturbance often have fragmented sleep, nocturnal wakefulness, and reduced sleep efficiency when studied with PSG. Because older adults may attribute their disturbed sleep to normal aging, they may fail to report symptoms of sleep disorders to their health care providers.[37] Use a sleeping assessment (see Table 8-6) to detect sleep disturbances in older adults.

Multiple factors impair older adults' ability to obtain quality sleep. Insomnia symptoms in older adults frequently occur with depression, heart disease, body pain, and cognitive problems. Insomnia may have detrimental effects on cognitive function in healthy older adults. Older women report more trouble falling asleep and, especially, staying asleep. Other sleep disorders (e.g., sleep-disordered breathing) also increase with age and may manifest with insomnia symptoms.[37,38]

Awakening and getting out of bed during the night (e.g., to use the bathroom) increase the risk for falls. Older adults may use OTC medications or alcohol as a sleep aid. This practice can further increase the risk of falls at night. Chronic disturbed sleep in older adults can result in disorientation, delirium, impaired intellect, disturbed cognition, and increased risk of accidents and injury.[38]

Chronic conditions that are more common in older adults (COPD, diabetes, dementia, chronic pain, cancer) can affect sleep quality.[38] Medications used to treat these conditions can contribute to sleep problems. OTC medications also can lead to sleep disturbance. Cough and cold medications, especially those containing pseudoephedrine; caffeine-containing drugs; and drugs containing nicotine (e.g., nicotine gum, transdermal patches), are stimulants. Diphenhydramine, alone or in combination with other drugs, is sedating with anticholinergic effects. Any OTC medication labeled "PM" probably has diphenhydramine and should be used cautiously by older adults.[39]

Metabolism of most hypnotic drugs decreases with aging. Older adults have increased sensitivity to hypnotic and sedative medications. Thus drug therapies for sleep disturbances are started at lower doses and monitored carefully. Whenever possible, long-acting benzodiazepines should be avoided. Older adults receiving benzodiazepines are at increased risk of daytime sedation, falls, and cognitive and psychomotor impairment.

PARASOMNIAS

Parasomnias are unusual and often undesirable behaviors that occur while falling asleep, transitioning between sleep stages, or arousing from sleep. They are due to CNS activation and often involve complex behaviors. The parasomnia is generally goal directed, although the person is not aware or conscious of the act. Parasomnias may result in fragmented sleep and fatigue.

Sleepwalking and sleep terrors are arousal parasomnias that occur during NREM sleep. *Sleepwalking* behaviors can range from sitting up in bed, moving objects, and walking around the room to driving a car. During a sleepwalking event the individual may not speak and may have limited or no awareness of the event. On awakening, the individual does not remember the event. In the ICU a parasomnia may be misinterpreted as ICU psychosis. Sedated ICU patients can exhibit manifestations of a parasomnia.

Sleep terrors (night terrors) are characterized by a sudden awakening from sleep along with a loud cry and signs of panic. The person has marked increases in heart rate and respiration and diaphoresis. Factors in the ICU such as sleep disruption and deprivation, fever, stress, and exposure to noise and light can contribute to sleep terrors.

Nightmares are a parasomnia characterized by recurrent awakening with recall of a frightful or disturbing dream. These normally occur during the final third of sleep and in association with REM sleep. In critically ill patients nightmares are common and are most likely due to medications. Drug classes most likely to cause nightmares are sedative-hypnotics, β-adrenergic antagonists, dopamine agonists, and amphetamines.

SPECIAL SLEEP NEEDS OF NURSES

Nursing is one of several professions that necessitates night shift and rotating shift schedules. In many settings, nurses are asked to or volunteer to work a variety of day and night shifts, often alternating and rotating them. Unfortunately, nurses who do shift work often report less job satisfaction and more job-related stress. A large number of nurses who work the night shift report episodes of nodding off while driving home after work.[40]

Nurses on permanent night or rapidly rotating shifts are at increased risk of experiencing *shift work sleep disorder,* characterized by insomnia, sleepiness, and fatigue. Nurses on rotating shifts get the least amount of sleep. With repeated periods of inadequate sleep, the sleep debt grows. Poor sleep is the strongest predictor of chronic fatigue in nurses doing shift work. As a result, rotating and night shift schedules pose challenges for the individual nurse's health and patient safety.[40]

Shift work alters the synchrony between circadian rhythms and the environment, leading to sleep disruption. Nurses working the night shift are often too sleepy to be fully alert at work and too alert to sleep soundly the next day. Sustained alterations in circadian rhythms such as those imposed by rotating shift work have been linked to increased morbidity and mortality risks associated with cardiovascular problems. In addition, mood disorders such as anxiety are higher in nurses who work rotating shifts.

From a safety perspective, disturbed sleep and subsequent fatigue can result in errors and accidents for nurses as well as for their patients.[41] Fatigue diminishes or distorts perceptual skills, judgment, and decision-making capabilities. Lack of sleep reduces the ability to cope and handle stress and may result in physical, mental, and emotional exhaustion.

The problem of sleep disruption is critically important to nursing. Several strategies may help reduce the distress associ-ated with rotating shift work. These include brief periods of on-site napping. Maintaining a consistent sleep-wake schedule even on days off is optimum but perhaps unrealistic. For night shift work, scheduling the sleep period just before going to work increases alertness and vigilance, improves reaction times, and decreases accidents during night shift work. Nurses who have control over their work schedules appear to experience less sleep disruption than those whose schedule is imposed. As a nurse, you need to manage the impact of sleep disruption through the use of sleep hygiene practices.

CASE STUDY

Insomnia

iStockphoto/Thinkstock

Patient Profile
G.P., a 49-year-old African American woman, is seen in the primary care clinic for complaints of chronic fatigue. She is postmenopausal based on self-report. In the past year, since the end of her periods, she has experienced daily hot flashes and sleep problems. She denies any other health problems. On a usual workday she drinks two cups of hot tea in the morning and one can of diet cola in the late afternoon. Cur-rently she is taking OTC diphenhydramine for sleep. Her partner, who has accompanied her to the clinic, states that her snoring has gotten worse and it is interfering with his sleep.

Subjective Data
• Complains of hot flashes and nighttime sweating
• Complains of daytime tiredness and fatigue
• States she has trouble getting to sleep and staying asleep

Objective Data
Physical Examination
• Laboratory evaluations within normal limits
• Overweight (20% over ideal body weight for height)
• BP 155/92 mm Hg

Diagnostic Studies
• Nighttime polysomnography study reveals episodes of obstructive sleep apnea

Collaborative Care
• CPAP nightly
• Referred for weight reduction counseling
• Follow-up to rule out other potential sleep disturbances

Discussion Questions
1. What are G.P.'s risk factors for sleep apnea?
2. What specific sleep hygiene practices could G.P. use to improve the quality of her sleep?
3. How does CPAP work?
4. Based on the data above, what are the major health risks for G.P. from sleep apnea?
5. *Priority Decision:* What are the priority nursing interventions for G.P.? What collaborative care treatment ought to be added to the treatment plan?
6. *Delegation Decision:* For the interventions that you identified in the above question, which of the following personnel could be responsible for implementing them: RN, LPN, UAP?
7. *Priority Decision:* Based on the assessment data provided, what are the priority nursing diagnoses? Are there any collaborative problems?

⊜volve Answers available at *http://evolve.elsevier.com/Lewis/medsurg.*

BRIDGE TO NCLEX EXAMINATION

The number of the question corresponds to the same-numbered outcome at the beginning of the chapter.

1. Sleep is best described as a
   a. loosely organized state similar to coma.
   b. state in which pain sensitivity decreases.
   c. quiet state in which there is little brain activity.
   d. state in which an individual lacks conscious awareness of the environment.

2. Which statement is true regarding rapid eye movement (REM) sleep?
   a. The EEG pattern is quiescent.
   b. It occurs only once in the night.
   c. It is separated by distinct physiologic stages.
   d. The most vivid dreaming occurs during this phase.

3. Insufficient sleep is associated with *(select all that apply)*
   a. increased body mass index.
   b. increased insulin resistance.
   c. impaired cognitive functioning.
   d. increased immune responsiveness.
   e. increased daytime body temperature.

4. When teaching the patient with primary insomnia about sleep hygiene, the nurse should emphasize
   a. the importance of daytime naps.
   b. the need to exercise before bedtime.
   c. the need for long-term use of hypnotics.
   d. avoiding caffeine-containing beverages 6 to 9 hours before bedtime.

5. While caring for a patient with a history of narcolepsy with cata-plexy, the nurse can delegate which activity to the unlicensed assis-tive personnel (UAP)?
   a. Teaching about the timing of medications
   b. Walking the patient to and from the bathroom
   c. Developing a plan of care with a family member
   d. Planning an appropriate diet that avoids caffeine-containing foods

6. A patient with sleep apnea would like to avoid using a nasal CPAP device if possible. To help him reach this goal, the nurse suggests that the patient
  a. lose excess weight.
  b. take a nap during the day.
  c. eat a high-protein snack at bedtime.
  d. use mild sedatives or alcohol at bedtime.

7. A patient on the surgical unit has a history of parasomnia (sleep-walking). What statement describes parasomnia?
  a. Hypnotic medications reduce the risk of sleepwalking.
  b. The patient is often unaware of the activity on awakening.
  c. The patient should be restrained at night to prevent personal harm.
  d. The potential for sleepwalking is reduced by exercise before sleep.

8. Strategies to reduce sleepiness during nighttime working include
  a. exercising before work.
  b. taking melatonin before working the night shift.
  c. sleeping for at least 2 hours immediately before work time.
  d. walking for 10 minutes every 4 hours during the night shift.

1. d, 2. d, 3. a, b, c, 4. d, 5. b, 6. a, 7. b, 8. c.

Ⓔvolve

For rationales to these answers and even more NCLEX review questions, visit *http://evolve.elsevier.com/Lewis/medsurg*.

REFERENCES

1. Redeker NS, McEnany GP: The nature of sleep disorders and their impact. In Redeker NS, McEnany GP, editors: *Sleep disorders and sleep promotion in nursing practice*, New York, 2011, Springer.
2. National Sleep Foundation: Can't sleep? Learn about insomnia. Retrieved from *www.sleepfoundation.org/site*.
3. National Sleep Foundation: 2011 sleep in America poll: communications technology and sleep. Retrieved from *www.sleepfoundation.org/2011poll*.
4. National Sleep Foundation: DrowsyDriving.org. Retrieved from *www.drowsydriving.org/tag/national-sleep-foundation*.
5. España RA, Scammell TE: Sleep neurobiology from a clinical perspective, *Sleep* 34:845, 2011.
*6. Rea MS, Brons JA, Figueiro MG: Measurements of light at night (LAN) for a sample of female school teachers, *Chronobiol Intern* 28:673, 2011.
7. Landis CA: Physiological and behavioral aspects of sleep. In Redeker NS, McEnany GP, editors: *Sleep disorders and sleep promotion in nursing practice*, New York, 2011, Springer.
8. Iber C, Ancoli-Israel S, Chesson A, et al: *The American Academy of Sleep Medicine: The AASM manual for the scoring of sleep and associated events: rules, terminology and technical specifications*, Westchester, Ill, 2007, The Academy. (Reference Manual)
9. Van Cauter E: Sleep disturbances and insulin resistance, *Diabetic Med* 28:1455, 2011.
*10. Anic GM, Titus-Ernstoff L, Newcomb PA, et al: Sleep duration and obesity in a population study, *Sleep Med* 11:47, 2010.
*11. Bloom HG, Ahmed I, Alessi CA, et al: Evidence-based recommendations for the assessment and management of sleep disorders in older people, *J Am Geriatr Soc* 57:761, 2009. (Classic)
12. Partinen M: Epidemiology of sleep disorders, *Handb Clin Neurol* 98:275, 2011.
13. Walsleben JA: Women and sleep, *Handb Clin Neurol* 98:639, 2011.
14. Jungquist C: Insomnia. In Redeker NS, McEnany GP, editors: *Sleep disorders and sleep promotion in nursing practice*, New York, 2011, Springer.
15. Budhiraja R, Roth T, Hudgel DW, et al: Prevalence and polysomnographic correlates of insomnia comorbid with medical disorders, *Sleep* 34:859, 2011.

16. Buysse DJ, Reynolds CF, Monk TH, et al: The Pittsburgh Sleep Quality Index: a new instrument for psychiatric practice and research, *Psychiatry Res* 28:193, 1989. (Classic)
17. Morin CM, Belleville G, Belanger L, et al: The Insomnia Severity Index: psychometric indicators to detect insomnia cases and evaluate treatment response, *Sleep* 34:601, 2011.
18. Johns MW: A new method for measuring daytime sleepiness: the Epworth Sleepiness Scale, *Sleep* 14:540, 1991. (Classic)
19. Sullivan SS: Insomnia pharmacology, *Med Clin North Am* 94:563, 2010.
*20. Roehrs TA, Randall S, Harris E, et al: Twelve months of nightly zolpidem does not lead to dose escalation: a prospective placebo-controlled study, *Sleep* 34:207, 2011.
*21. Krystal AD, Lankford A, Durrence HH, et al: Efficacy and safety of doxepin 3 and 6 mg in a 35-day sleep laboratory trial in adults with chronic primary insomnia, *Sleep* 34:1433, 2011.
22. Ferguson SA, Rajaratnam SM, Dawson D: Melatonin agonists and insomnia, *Expert Rev Neurother* 10:305, 2010.
*23. Taibi DM, Vitiello MV, Barsness S, et al: A randomized clinical trial of valerian fails to improve self-reported, polysomnographic, and actigraphic sleep in older women with insomnia, *Sleep Med* 10:319, 2008. (Classic)
24. Redeker NS, Hedges C, Booker KJ: Sleep in adult acute and critical care settings. In Redeker NS, McEnany GP, editors: *Sleep disorders and sleep promotion in nursing practice*, New York, 2011, Springer.
25. Landis CA: Sleep, pain, fibromyalgia, and chronic fatigue syndrome, *Handb Clin Neurol* 98:613, 2011.
26. Rodgers A: Narcolepsy. In Redeker NS, McEnany GP, editors: *Sleep disorders and sleep promotion in nursing practice*, New York, 2011, Springer.
27. National Institutes of Health: Narcolepsy fact sheet. Retrieved from *www.nhlbi.nih.gov/health/health-topics/topics/nar*.
28. Hiria N, Nishino S: Recent advances in the treatment of narcolepsy, *Curr Treatment Options Neurol* 13:437, 2011.
29. Dowling G, Mastick J: Circadian rhythm disorders. In Redeker NS, McEnany GP, editors: *Sleep disorders and sleep promotion in nursing practice*, New York, 2011, Springer.
30. Sawyer AM, Weaver TE: Sleep related-breathing disorders. In Redeker NS, McEnany GP, editors: *Sleep disorders and sleep promotion in nursing practice*, New York, 2011, Springer.
*31. Gooneratne NS, Richards KC, Joffe M, et al: Sleep disordered breathing with excessive daytime sleepiness is a risk factor for mortality in older adults, *Sleep* 34:435, 2011.
32. Tamisier R, Pepin JL, Levy P: Sleep and pulmonary disorders, *Handb Clin Neurol* 98:471, 2011.

*Evidence-based information for clinical practice.

33. Tomfohr LM, Ancoli-Israel S, Loredo JS, et al: Effects of continuous positive airway pressure on fatigue and sleepiness in patients with obstructive sleep apnea: data from a randomized controlled trial, *Sleep* 34:121, 2011.

34. Fleetham JA: Medical and surgical treatment of obstructive sleep apnea syndrome, including dental appliances, *Handb Clin Neurol* 98:441, 2011.

*35. Antic NA, Catcheside P, Buchan C, et al: The effect of CPAP in normalizing daytime sleepiness, quality of life, and neurocognitive function in patients with moderate to severe OSA, *Sleep* 34:111, 2011.

36. eMedicinehealth: Periodic limb movement disorder. Retrieved from *www.emedicinehealth.com/periodic_limb_movement _disorder/article_em.htm*.

37. Cole CS: Sleep and primary care in adults and older adults. In Redeker NS, McEnany GP, editors: *Sleep disorders and sleep promotion in nursing practice*, New York, 2011, Springer.

38. Klerman EB, Dijk DJ: Age-related reduction in the maximal capacity for sleep—implications for insomnia, *Curr Biol* 18:1118, 2008.

39. Cooke JR, Ancoli-Israel S: Normal and abnormal sleep in the elderly, *Handb Clin Neurol* 98:653, 2011.

*40. Scott LD, Hwang WT, Rogers AE, et al: The relationship between nurse work schedules, sleep duration, and drowsy driving, *Sleep* 30:1801, 2007.

*41. Scott LD, Hofmeister N, Rogness N, et al: An interventional approach for patient and nurse safety, *Nurs Res* 59:250, 2010.

RESOURCES

American Academy of Sleep Medicine
www.aasmnet.org
American Sleep Apnea Association
www.sleepapnea.org
Better Sleep Council
www.bettersleep.org
Narcolepsy Network
www.narcolepsynetwork.org
National Institutes of Health
http://health.nih.gov/topic/SleepDisorders
www.nhlbi.nih.gov/health/public/sleep/healthy_sleep.htm
National Sleep Foundation
www.sleepfoundation.org

9

Pain

Lindsay L. Kindler and Rosemary C. Polomano

Pain is inevitable. Suffering is optional.
Anonymous

evolve WEBSITE

LEARNING OUTCOMES

1. Define pain.
2. Describe the neural mechanisms of pain and pain modulation.
3. Differentiate between nociceptive and neuropathic types of pain.
4. Explain the physical and psychologic effects of unrelieved pain.
5. Interpret the subjective and objective data that are obtained from a comprehensive pain assessment.
6. Describe effective interdisciplinary pain management techniques.
7. Describe drug and nondrug methods of pain relief.
8. Explain your role and responsibility in pain management.
9. Discuss ethical and legal issues related to pain and pain management.
10. Evaluate the influence of one's own knowledge, beliefs, and attitudes about pain assessment and management.

KEY TERMS

analgesic ceiling, p. 123
breakthrough pain, p. 121
complex regional pain
   syndrome (CRPS), p. 119

equianalgesic dose, p. 129
modulation, p. 118
neuropathic pain, p. 119
nociception, p. 116

nociceptive pain, p. 119
pain, p. 115
patient-controlled analgesia
   (PCA), p. 131

transduction, p. 116
transmission, p. 117
trigger point, p. 132

Pain is a complex, multidimensional experience that can cause suffering and decreased quality of life. Pain is one of the major reasons that people seek health care. To effectively assess and manage patients with pain, you need to understand the physiologic and psychosocial dimensions of pain. This chapter presents evidence-based information to help you assess and manage pain successfully in collaboration with other health care providers.

MAGNITUDE OF PAIN PROBLEM

Every year, millions of people suffer from pain. Annually in the United States, at least 25 million people experience acute pain as a result of injury or surgery.[1] Common chronic pain conditions such as arthritis, migraine headache, and back pain affect approximately 116 million American adults.[2] Seventy percent of all cancer patients experience significant pain during their illness.[3] The financial impact of pain is staggering. In the United States, unrelieved pain and inadequate management of pain costs an estimated $560 billion to $635 billion each year in direct medical treatment costs and lost work productivity.[2]

Despite the high prevalence and costs of acute and chronic pain, inadequate pain management occurs. For example, approximately a third of patients enrolled in hospice reported pain at their last hospice visit.[4] Cancer pain is often undertreated.[5]

Consequences of untreated pain include unnecessary suffering, physical and psychosocial dysfunction, immunosup-

Reviewed by Judith A. Paice, RN, PhD, Director, Cancer Pain Program, Division Hematology-Oncology, Northwestern University, Feinberg School of Medicine, Chicago, Illinois; Debra B. Gordon, RN-BC, DNP, ACNS-BC, FAAN, Teaching Associate, Department of Anesthesiology and Pain Medicine, University of Washington, Seattle, Washington; Jo Ann Baker, RN, MSN, FNP-C, Department Chair, Nursing, Delaware Technical and Community College, Terry Campus, Dover, Delaware; Susan Turner, RN, MSN, FNP, Professor of Nursing, Gavilan College, Gilroy, California; and Linda Wilson, RN, PhD, CPAN, CAPA, BC, CNE, Assistant Dean for Special Projects, Simulation and CNE Accreditation, Drexel University, College of Nursing and Health Professions, Philadelphia, Pennsylvania.

TABLE 9-1 HARMFUL EFFECTS OF UNRELIEVED ACUTE PAIN

Response	Possible Consequences
Endocrine and Metabolic	
↑ Adrenocorticotropic hormone (ACTH)	Weight loss (from ↑ catabolism)
↑ Cortisol	↑ Respiratory rate
↑ Antidiuretic hormone (ADH)	↑ Heart rate
↑ Epinephrine and norepinephrine	Shock
↑ Renin, ↑ aldosterone	Glucose intolerance
↓ Insulin	Hyperglycemia
Gluconeogenesis	Fluid overload
Glycogenolysis	Hypertension
Muscle protein catabolism	Urinary retention, ↓ urine output
Cardiovascular	
↑ Heart rate	Hypertension
↑ Cardiac output	Unstable angina
↑ Peripheral vascular resistance	Myocardial infarction
↑ Myocardial oxygen consumption	Deep vein thrombosis
↑ Coagulation	
Respiratory	
↓ Tidal volume	Atelectasis
Hypoxemia	Pneumonia
↓ Cough, sputum retention	
Renal and Urologic	
↓ Urine output	Fluid imbalance
Urinary retention	Electrolyte disturbance
Gastrointestinal	
↓ Gastric and intestinal motility	Constipation
	Anorexia
	Paralytic ileus
Musculoskeletal	
Muscle spasm	Immobility
Impaired muscle function	Weakness and fatigue
Neurologic	
Impaired cognitive function	Confusion
	Impaired ability to think, reason, and make decisions
Immunologic	
↓ Immune response	Infection

TABLE 9-2 DIMENSIONS OF PAIN

Dimension	Description
Physiologic	• Genetic, anatomic, and physical determinants of pain influence how painful stimuli are processed, recognized, and described.
Affective	• Emotional responses to pain include anger, fear, depression, and anxiety. • Negative emotions impair patient's quality of life.
Cognitive	• Beliefs, attitudes, memories, and meaning attributed to pain influence the ways in which a person responds to pain.
Behavioral	• Observable actions (e.g., grimacing, irritability) are used to express or control pain. • People unable to communicate may have behavioral changes (e.g., agitation, combativeness).
Sociocultural	• Age and gender influence nociceptive processes and responses to opioids. • Families and caregivers influence patient's response to pain through their beliefs, behaviors, and support. • Culture affects pain expression, medication use, and pain-related beliefs and coping methods.

GENDER DIFFERENCES

Pain

Men
• Men are less likely to report pain than women.
• Men report more control over pain.
• Men are less likely than women to use alternative treatments for pain.

Women
• Women experience more chronic pain than men.
• Even when they have the same condition as men, women have higher levels of pain. Women more frequently experience migraine headache, back pain, arthritis, fibromyalgia, irritable bowel syndrome, neuropathic pain, abdominal pain, and foot ache.
• Women are more likely to be diagnosed with a nonspecific, somatic diagnosis and less likely to receive analgesics for symptoms of chest and abdominal pain.

pression, and sleep disturbances[2] (Table 9-1). The varied reasons for the undertreatment of pain are discussed in this chapter.

DEFINITIONS AND DIMENSIONS OF PAIN

In 1968 Margo McCaffery, a nurse and pioneer in pain management, defined pain as "whatever the person experiencing the pain says it is, existing whenever the person says it does."[6] The International Association for the Study of Pain (IASP) defines pain as "an unpleasant sensory and emotional experience associated with actual or potential tissue damage, or described in terms of such damage."[2]

Note that these definitions emphasize the subjective nature of pain, in which the patient's self-report is the most valid means of assessment. Although understanding the patient's experience and relying on his or her self-report is essential, this view is problematic for many patients. For example, patients who are comatose or who suffer from dementia, patients who are men-

tally disabled, and patients with expressive aphasia possess varying abilities to report pain. In these instances, you must incorporate nonverbal information such as behaviors into your pain assessment.

With pain defined as a human experience, successful pain assessment and treatment must incorporate multiple dimensions.[7] The biopsychosocial model of pain includes the physiologic, affective, cognitive, behavioral, and sociocultural dimensions of pain (Table 9-2).

The emotional distress of pain can cause *suffering*, which is the state of distress associated with loss. Suffering can result in a profound sense of insecurity and lack of control. When suffering occurs, people can experience spiritual distress. Achieving pain relief is an essential step in relieving suffering. In addition, the assessment of ways in which a person's spirituality influences and is influenced by pain is important.[8]

The meaning of the pain can be critical. For example, a woman in labor may experience severe pain but can manage it without analgesics because for her it is associated with a joyful event. Moreover, she may feel control over her pain because of the training she received in prenatal classes and the knowledge that the pain is time-limited. In contrast, a woman with chronic, undefined musculoskeletal pain may be plagued by thoughts that her pain is "not real," is uncontrollable, or is caused by her own actions. These perceptions will influence the ways in which a person responds to pain and must be incorporated into a comprehensive treatment plan.

Some people cope with pain by distracting themselves, whereas others convince themselves that the pain is permanent, untreatable, and overwhelming. People who believe that their pain is uncontrollable and overwhelming are more likely to have poor outcomes.[9]

Families and caregivers influence the patient's response to pain through their beliefs and behaviors. For example, families may discourage the patient from taking opioids because they fear the patient will become addicted.

Pain Mechanisms

Nociception is the physiologic process by which information about tissue damage is communicated to the central nervous system (CNS). It involves four processes: (1) transduction, (2) transmission, (3) perception, and (4) modulation (Fig. 9-1).

Transduction. Transduction involves the conversion of a noxious mechanical, thermal, or chemical stimulus into an electrical signal called an action potential. Noxious (tissue-damaging) stimuli, including thermal (e.g., sunburn), mechanical (e.g., surgical incision), or chemical (e.g., toxic substances) stimuli, cause the release of numerous chemicals such as hydrogen ions, substance P, and adenosine triphosphate (ATP) into the damaged tissues. Other chemicals are released from mast cells (e.g., serotonin, histamine, bradykinin, prostaglandins) and macrophages (e.g., interleukins, tumor necrosis factor [TNF]). These chemicals activate nociceptors, which are specialized receptors, or free nerve endings, that respond to painful stimuli. Activation of nociceptors results in an action potential that is carried from the nociceptors to the spinal cord primarily via small, rapidly conducting, myelinated A-delta fibers and slowly conducting unmyelinated C fibers.

In addition to stimulating nociceptors to fire, inflammation and the subsequent release of chemical mediators lower nociceptor thresholds. As a result, nociceptors may fire in response to stimuli that previously were insufficient to elicit a response. They may also fire in response to non-noxious stimuli, such as light touch. This increased susceptibility to nociceptor activation is called *peripheral sensitization*. Leukotrienes, prostaglandins, cytokines, and substance P are involved in peripheral sensitization. Cyclooxygenase (COX), an enzyme produced in the inflammatory response, also plays an important role in peripheral sensitization. A clinical example of this process is sunburn. This thermal injury causes inflammation that results in a sensation of pain when the affected skin is lightly touched. Peripheral sensitization also amplifies signal transmission, which in turn contributes to central sensitization (discussed under Dorsal Horn Processing). The pain produced from activation of peripheral nociceptors is called *nociceptive pain* (described later in the chapter on p. 119).

Therapies that alter either the local environment or sensitivity of the peripheral nociceptors can prevent transduction and initiation of an action potential. Decreasing the effects of chemicals released at the periphery is the basis of several drug approaches to pain relief. For example, nonsteroidal antiinflammatory drugs (NSAIDs), such as ibuprofen (Advil, Motrin) and naproxen (Naprosyn, Aleve), and corticosteroids, such as dexamethasone (Decadron), exert their analgesic effects by blocking pain-sensitizing chemicals. NSAIDs block the action of COX, thereby interfering with the production of prostaglandins. Corticosteroids reduce the production of both prostaglandins and leukotrienes (see Fig. 12-2).

Drugs that stabilize the neuronal membrane and inactivate peripheral sodium channels inhibit production of the nerve impulse. These medications include local anesthetics (e.g., injectable or topical lidocaine, bupivacaine [Sensorcaine], and

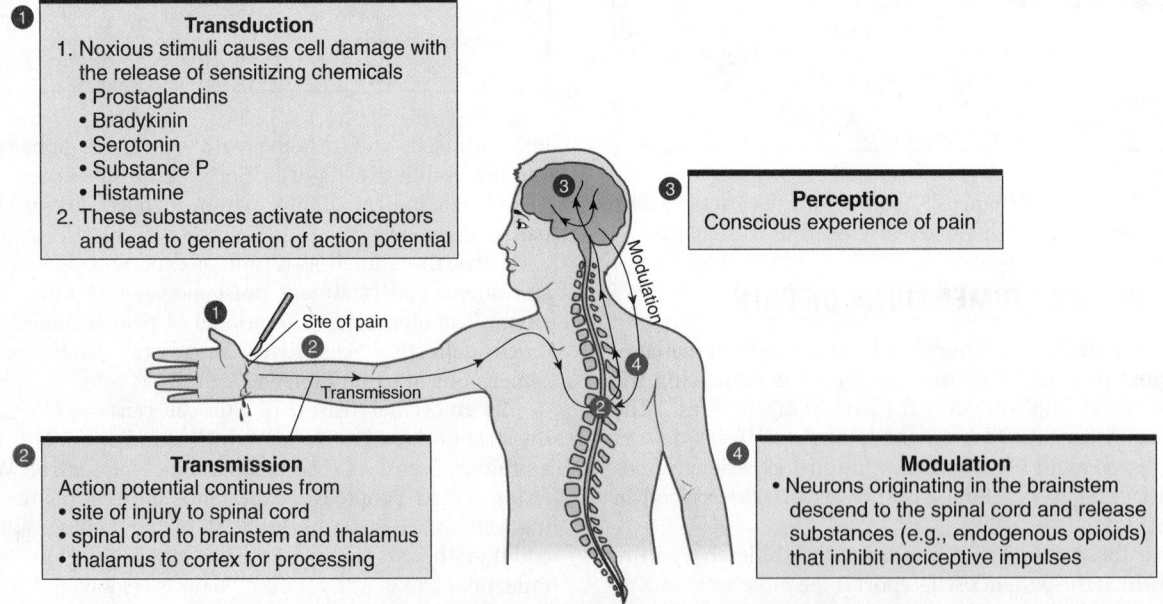

FIG. 9-1 Nociceptive pain originates when the tissue is injured. *1,* Transduction occurs when there is release of chemical mediators. *2,* Transmission involves the conduct of the action potential from the periphery (injury site) to the spinal cord and then to the brainstem, thalamus, and cerebral cortex. *3,* Perception is the conscious awareness of pain. *4,* Modulation involves signals from the brain going back down the spinal cord to modify incoming impulses.

ropivacaine [Naropin]) and antiseizure drugs (e.g., carbamaze-pine [Tegretol] and lamotrigine [Lamictal]).

Transmission. Transmission is the process by which pain signals are relayed from the periphery to the spinal cord and then to the brain. The nerves that carry pain impulses from the periphery to the spinal cord are called primary afferent fibers. These include A-delta and C fibers, each of which is responsible for a different pain sensation. As previously mentioned, A-delta fibers are small, myelinated fibers that conduct pain rapidly and are responsible for the initial, sharp pain that accompanies tissue injury. C fibers are small, unmyelinated fibers that transmit painful stimuli more slowly and produce pain that is typically aching or throbbing in quality. Primary afferent fibers terminate in the dorsal horn of the spinal cord. Activity in the dorsal horn integrates and modulates pain inputs from the periphery.

The propagation of pain impulses from the site of transduction to the brain is shown in Fig. 9-1. Three segments are involved in nociceptive signal transmission: (1) transmission along the peripheral nerve fibers to the spinal cord, (2) dorsal horn processing, and (3) transmission to the thalamus and the cerebral cortex.

Transmission to Spinal Cord. The first-order neuron extends the entire distance from the periphery to the dorsal horn of the spinal cord with no synapses. For example, an afferent fiber from the great toe travels from the toe through the fifth lumbar nerve root into the spinal cord; it is one cell. Once generated, an action potential travels all the way to the spinal cord unless it is blocked by a sodium channel inhibitor (e.g., local anesthetic) or disrupted by a lesion such as a dorsal root entry zone lesion.

The manner in which nerve fibers enter the spinal cord is central to the notion of spinal dermatomes. Dermatomes are areas on the skin that are innervated primarily by a single spinal cord segment. The distinctive pattern of the rash caused by herpes zoster (shingles) across the back and trunk is determined by dermatomes (see Fig. 24-7). Different dermatomes and their innervations are illustrated in eFig. 9-1 (available on the website for this chapter) and Fig. 56-6.

Dorsal Horn Processing. Once a nociceptive signal arrives in the spinal cord, it is processed within the dorsal horn. Neurotransmitters released from the afferent fiber bind to receptors on nearby cell bodies and dendrites of cells. Some of these neurotransmitters (e.g., glutamate, aspartate, substance P) produce activation, whereas others (e.g., γ-aminobutyric acid [GABA], serotonin, norepinephrine) inhibit activation of nearby cells. In this area, exogenous and endogenous opioids also play an important role by binding to opioid receptors and blocking the release of neurotransmitters, particularly substance P. Endogenous opioids include enkephalin and β-endorphin. They are capable of producing analgesic effects similar to those of exogenous opioids such as morphine.

Increased sensitivity and hyperexcitability of neurons in the CNS is called central sensitization. Peripheral tissue damage or nerve injury can cause central sensitization, and continued nociceptive input from the periphery is necessary to maintain it. As a result of the increased excitability of neurons within the CNS, normal sensory inputs cause abnormal sensing and responses to painful and other stimuli. This explains why some people experience significant pain from touch or tactile stimulation in and around the areas of tissue or nerve injury. This is called allodynia. With central sensitization, the central process-

ing circuits are altered. In some cases, central sensitization can be long-lasting due to changes in the synapse.[10]

With ongoing stimulation of slowly conducting unmyelinated C-fiber nociceptors, firing of specialized dorsal horn neurons gradually increases. These inputs create many problems, including the sprouting of wide dynamic range (WDR) neurons and induction of glutamate-dependent N-methyl-D-aspartate (NMDA) receptors. WDR neurons respond to both nociceptive and non-nociceptive inputs that are of varying levels of stimulus intensity. When these neuron dendrites sprout, they grow into areas where pain-receiving nerve cell bodies are located. This results in the capacity to transmit a broader range of stimuli-producing signals, which are then passed up the spinal cord and brain. This process is known as windup and depends on the activation of NMDA receptors. NMDA receptor antagonists, such as ketamine (Ketalar), potentially interrupt or block mechanisms that lead to or sustain central sensitization. Windup, like central sensitization and hyperalgesia (increased pain responses to noxious stimuli), is induced by C-fiber inputs. Windup is different, however, in that it can be short lasting, whereas central sensitization and hyperalgesia persist over time.[11]

It is important for you to understand that acute, unrelieved pain leads to chronic pain through the process of central sensitization. Acute tissue injury produces a cascade of events that involve the release of certain excitatory neurotransmitters (e.g., glutamate) and neuropsychologic responses. Even brief intervals of acute pain are capable of inducing long-term neuronal remodeling and sensitization (plasticity), chronic pain, and lasting psychologic distress.

Neuroplasticity refers to processes that allow neurons in the brain to compensate for injury and adjust their responses to new situations or changes in their environment.[12] Neuroplasticity contributes to adaptive mechanisms for reducing pain but also can result in maladaptive mechanisms that enhance pain. Genetic variability among individuals may have an important effect on the plasticity of the CNS.[12] Understanding this phenomenon helps explain individual differences in response to pain and why some patients develop chronic pain conditions whereas others do not. Clinically, central sensitization of the dorsal horn results in (1) hyperalgesia, (2) painful responses to normally innocuous stimuli (allodynia), (3) prolonged pain after the original noxious stimulus ends (called persistent pain), and (4) the extension of tenderness or increased pain sensitivity outside of an area of injury to include uninjured tissue (i.e., expansion of nociceptive receptive fields, or secondary hyperalgesia).[13]

Referred pain must be considered when interpreting the location of pain reported by the person with an injury or a disease involving visceral organs. The location of a stimulus may be distant from the pain location reported by the patient (Fig. 9-2). For example, pain from liver disease is frequently located in the right upper abdominal quadrant, but can also be referred to the anterior and posterior neck region and to a posterior flank area. If referred pain is not considered when evaluating a pain location report, diagnostic tests and therapy could be misdirected.

Transmission to Thalamus and Cortex. From the dorsal horn, nociceptive stimuli are communicated to the third-order neuron, primarily in the thalamus, and several other areas of the brain. Fibers of dorsal horn projection cells enter the brain through several pathways, including the spinothalamic tract and spinoreticular tract. Distinct thalamic nuclei receive nociceptive input from the spinal cord and have projections to several regions in the cerebral cortex, where the perception of pain is presumed to occur.

Therapeutic approaches that target pain transmission include opioid analgesics that bind to opioid receptors on primary afferent and dorsal horn neurons. These agents mimic the inhibitory effects of endogenous opioids. Another medication, baclofen (Lioresal), inhibits transmission by binding to GABA receptors, thus mimicking the inhibitory effects of GABA.

Perception. *Perception* occurs when pain is recognized, defined, and assigned meaning by the individual experiencing the pain. In the brain, nociceptive input is perceived as pain. There is no single, precise location where pain perception occurs. Instead, pain perception involves several brain struc-

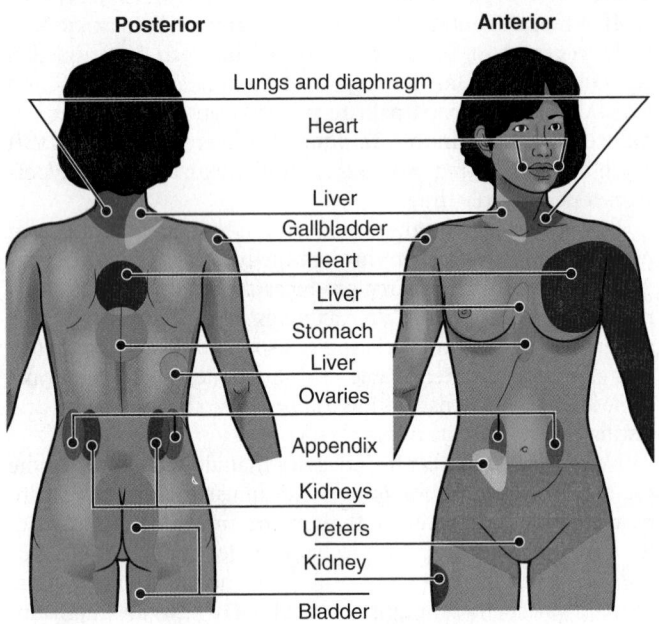

FIG. 9-2 Typical areas of referred pain.

Posterior   Anterior

Lungs and diaphragm
Heart
Liver
Gallbladder
Heart
Liver
Stomach
Liver
Ovaries
Appendix
Kidneys
Ureters
Kidney
Bladder

tures. For example, it is believed that the reticular activating system (RAS) is responsible for warning the individual to attend to the pain stimulus; the somatosensory system is responsible for localization and characterization of pain; and the limbic system is responsible for the emotional and behavioral responses to pain. Cortical structures also are crucial to constructing the meaning of the pain.

Therefore behavioral strategies such as distraction and relaxation are effective pain-reducing therapies for many people. By directing attention away from the pain sensation, patients can reduce the sensory and affective components of pain. Opioids and other classes of analgesics such as some types of antiseizure drugs and antidepressants modify pain perception.

Modulation. Modulation involves the activation of descending pathways that exert inhibitory or facilitatory effects on the transmission of pain (see Fig. 9-1). Depending on the type and degree of modulation, nociceptive stimuli may or may not be perceived as pain. Modulation of pain signals can occur at the level of the periphery, spinal cord, brainstem, and cerebral cortex. Descending modulatory fibers release chemicals such as serotonin, norepinephrine, GABA, and endogenous opioids that can inhibit pain transmission.

Several antidepressants exert their effects through the modulatory systems. For example, tricyclic antidepressants (e.g., amitriptyline [Elavil]) and serotonin norepinephrine reuptake inhibitors (SNRIs) (e.g., venlafaxine [Effexor] and duloxetine [Cymbalta]) are used in the management of chronic nonmalignant and cancer pain. These agents interfere with the reuptake of serotonin and norepinephrine, thereby increasing their availability to inhibit noxious stimuli.

CLASSIFICATION OF PAIN

Pain can be categorized in several ways. Most commonly, pain is categorized as nociceptive or neuropathic based on underlying pathology (Table 9-3). Another useful scheme is to classify pain as acute or chronic (Table 9-4).

TABLE 9-3	**COMPARISON OF NOCICEPTIVE AND NEUROPATHIC PAIN**	
	Nociceptive Pain	**Neuropathic Pain***
Definition	Normal processing of stimulus that damages normal tissue or has the potential to do so if prolonged.	Abnormal processing of sensory input by the peripheral or central nervous system.
Treatment	Usually responsive to nonopioid and/or opioid drugs.	Treatment usually includes adjuvant analgesics.
Types	**Superficial Somatic Pain** Pain arising from skin, mucous membranes, subcutaneous tissue. Tends to be well localized. *Examples:* sunburn, skin contusions **Deep Somatic Pain** Pain arising from muscles, fasciae, bones, tendons. Localized or diffuse and radiating. *Examples:* arthritis, tendonitis, myofascial pain **Visceral Pain** Pain arising from visceral organs, such as the GI tract and bladder. Well or poorly localized. Often referred to cutaneous sites. *Examples:* appendicitis, pancreatitis, cancer affecting internal organs, irritable bowel and bladder syndromes	**Central Pain** Caused by primary lesion or dysfunction in the CNS. *Examples:* poststroke pain, pain associated with multiple sclerosis **Peripheral Neuropathies** Pain felt along the distribution of one or many peripheral nerves caused by damage to the nerve. *Examples:* diabetic neuropathy, alcohol-nutritional neuropathy, trigeminal neuralgia, postherpetic neuralgia **Deafferentation Pain** Pain resulting from a loss of afferent input. *Examples:* phantom limb pain, postmastectomy pain, spinal cord injury pain **Sympathetically Maintained Pain** Pain that persists secondary to sympathetic nervous system activity. *Examples:* phantom limb pain, complex regional pain syndrome

Adapted from National Institute of Neurological Disorders and Stroke: Complex regional pain syndrome fact sheet. Retrieved from *www.ninds.nih.gov/disorders/reflex_sympathetic _dystrophy/detail_reflex_sympathetic_dystrophy.htm.*
*Note: Some types of neuropathic pain (e.g., postherpetic neuralgia) are caused by more than one neuropathologic mechanism.
CNS, Central nervous system; *GI,* gastrointestinal.

Nociceptive Pain

Nociceptive pain is caused by damage to somatic or visceral tissue. *Somatic pain* often is further categorized as superficial or deep. *Superficial pain* arises from skin, mucous membranes, and subcutaneous tissues. It is often described as sharp, burning, or prickly. *Deep pain* is often characterized as deep, aching, or throbbing and originates in bone, joint, muscle, skin, or connective tissue.

Visceral pain comes from the activation of nociceptors in the internal organs and lining of the body cavities such as the thoracic and abdominal cavities. Visceral nociceptors respond to inflammation, stretching, and ischemia. Stretching of hollow viscera in the intestines and bladder that occurs from tumor involvement or obstruction can produce distention and intense cramping pain. Examples of visceral nociceptive pain include pain from a surgical incision, pancreatitis, and inflammatory bowel disease.

Neuropathic Pain

Neuropathic pain is caused by damage to peripheral nerves or structures in the CNS.[14] Typically described as numbing, hot, burning, shooting, stabbing, sharp, or electric shock–like, neuropathic pain can be sudden, intense, short lived, or lingering. Paroxysmal firing of injured nerves is responsible for shooting and electric shock–like sensations. Common causes of neuropathic pain include trauma, inflammation (e.g., secondary to a

herniated disc inflaming the adjacent nerve and dorsal root ganglion), metabolic diseases (e.g., diabetes mellitus), alcoholism, infections of the nervous system (e.g., herpes zoster, human immunodeficiency virus), tumors, toxins, and neurologic diseases (e.g., multiple sclerosis).

Deafferentation pain results from loss of afferent input secondary to either peripheral nerve injury (e.g., amputation) or CNS damage, including a spinal cord injury. *Sympathetically maintained pain* is associated with dysregulation of the autonomic nervous system, and *central pain* is caused by CNS lesions or dysfunction. Painful peripheral polyneuropathies (pain felt along the distribution of multiple peripheral nerves) and painful mononeuropathies (pain felt along the distribution of a damaged nerve) arise from damage to peripheral nerves and generate pain that may be described as burning, paroxysmal, or shock-like. The patient may have associated positive or negative motor and sensory signs, including numbness, allodynia, or change in reflexes and motor strength. No single quality descriptor or sign or symptom is diagnostic for neuropathic pain. Examples of neuropathic pain include postherpetic neuralgia, phantom limb pain, diabetic neuropathies, and trigeminal neuralgia.

One particularly debilitating type of neuropathic pain is complex regional pain syndrome (CRPS). Typical features include dramatic changes in the color and temperature of the skin over the affected limb or body part, accompanied by intense burning pain, skin sensitivity, sweating, and swelling. CRPS type I is frequently triggered by tissue injury, surgery, or a vascular event such as stroke.[14] CRPS type II includes all these features in addition to a peripheral nerve lesion.

Neuropathic pain often is not well controlled by opioid analgesics alone. Treatment frequently necessitates a multimodal approach combining various adjuvant analgesics, including tricyclic antidepressants (e.g., nortriptyline [Pamelor], desipramine [Norpramin]), SNRIs (e.g., venlafaxine, duloxetine, bupropion [Wellbutrin, Zyban]), antiseizure drugs (e.g., gabapentin [Neurontin], pregabalin [Lyrica]), transdermal lidocaine, and α_2-adrenergic agonists (e.g., clonidine [Catapres]). NMDA receptor antagonists such as ketamine have shown promise in alleviating neuropathic pain refractory to other drugs.[14]

Acute and Chronic Pain

Acute pain and chronic pain differ in their cause, course, manifestations, and treatment (see Table 9-4). Examples of *acute pain* include postoperative pain, labor pain, pain from trauma (e.g., lacerations, fractures, sprains), pain from infection (e.g., dysuria from cystitis), and pain from acute ischemia. For acute pain, treatment includes analgesics for symptom control and treatment of the underlying cause (e.g., splinting for a fracture, antibiotic therapy for an infection). Normally, acute pain diminishes over time as healing occurs. However, acute pain that persists can ultimately lead to disabling chronic pain states. For example, pain associated with herpes zoster (shingles) subsides as the acute infection resolves, usually within a month. However, sometimes the pain persists and develops into a chronic pain state called *postherpetic neuralgia*.

Chronic pain, or *persistent pain*, lasts for longer periods, often defined as longer than 3 months or past the time when an expected acute pain or acute injury should subside. The severity and functional impact of chronic pain often are disproportionate to objective findings because of changes in the nervous

TABLE 9-4	DIFFERENCES BETWEEN ACUTE AND CHRONIC PAIN	
	Acute Pain	**Chronic Pain**
Onset	Sudden.	Gradual or sudden.
Duration	<3 mo or as long as it takes for normal healing to occur.	>3 mo. May start as acute injury or event but continues past the normal time for recovery.
Severity	Mild to severe.	Mild to severe.
Cause of pain	Generally can identify a precipitating event (e.g., illness, surgery).	May not be known. Original cause of pain may differ from mechanisms that maintain the pain.
Course of pain	Decreases over time and goes away as recovery occurs.	Typically pain does not go away. Characterized by periods of increasing and decreasing pain.
Typical physical and behavioral manifestations	Manifestations vary but can reflect sympathetic nervous system activation: • ↑ Heart rate, respiratory rate, blood pressure • Diaphoresis, pallor • Anxiety, agitation, confusion • Urine retention	Predominantly behavioral manifestations: • Flat affect • ↓ Physical activity • Fatigue • Withdrawal from social interaction
Usual goals of treatment	Pain control with eventual elimination.	Pain control to the extent possible. Focus on enhancing function and quality of life.

TABLE 9-5 CORE PRINCIPLES OF PAIN ASSESSMENT

Principles	Nursing Implications
1. Patients have the right to appropriate assessment and management of pain.	• Assess pain in *all* patients.
2. Pain is always subjective.	• Patient's self-report of pain is the single most reliable indicator of pain. • Accept and respect this self-report unless there are clear reasons for doubt.
3. Physiologic and behavioral signs of pain (e.g., tachycardia, grimacing) are not reliable or specific for pain.	• Do not rely primarily on observations and objective signs of pain unless the patient is unable to self-report pain.
4. Pain is an unpleasant sensory and emotional experience.	• Address both physical and psychologic aspects of pain when assessing pain.
5. Assessment approaches, including tools, must be appropriate for the patient population.	• Special considerations are needed for assessing pain in patients with difficulty communicating. • Include family members in the assessment process (when appropriate).
6. Pain can exist even when no physical cause can be found.	• Do not attribute pain that does not have an identifiable cause to psychologic causes.
7. Different patients experience different levels of pain in response to comparable stimuli.	• A uniform pain threshold does not exist.
8. Patients with chronic pain may be more sensitive to pain and other stimuli.	• Pain tolerance varies among and within individuals depending on various factors (e.g., heredity, energy level, coping skills, prior experience with pain).
9. Unrelieved pain has adverse consequences. Acute pain that is not adequately controlled can result in physiologic changes that increase the likelihood of developing persistent pain.	• Encourage patients to report pain, especially patients who are reluctant to discuss pain, deny pain when it is probably present, or fail to follow through on prescribed treatments.

system not detectable with standard tests. Whereas acute pain functions as a signal, warning the person of potential or actual tissue damage, chronic pain does not appear to have an adaptive role. Chronic pain can be disabling and often is accompanied by anxiety and depression. As previously discussed, untreated acute pain leads to chronic pain through central sensitization and neuroplasticity. Consequently, it is imperative to treat acute pain aggressively and effectively to help prevent chronic pain.

PAIN ASSESSMENT

Assessment is an essential, though often overlooked, step in pain management. Regularly screen all patients for pain and, when present, perform a more thorough pain assessment. The key to accurate and effective pain assessment is to consider the core principles of pain assessment (Table 9-5).

The goals of a nursing pain assessment are to (1) describe the patient's pain experience in order to identify and implement appropriate pain management techniques and (2) identify the patient's goal for therapy and resources for self-management.

Elements of a Pain Assessment

Most components of a pain assessment involve direct interview or observation of the patient. Diagnostic studies and physical examination findings complete the initial assessment. Although the assessment differs according to the clinical setting, patient population, and point of care (i.e., whether the assessment is part of an initial workup or a reassessment of pain following therapy), the evaluation of pain should always be multidimensional (Table 9-6).

Before beginning any assessment, recognize that patients may use words other than "pain." For example, older adults may deny that they have pain but respond positively when asked if they have soreness or aching. Document the specific words that the patient uses to describe pain. Then consistently ask the patient about pain using those words.

Pain Pattern. Assessing pain *onset* involves determining when the pain started. Patients with acute pain resulting from

TABLE 9-6 NURSING ASSESSMENT

Pain

Subjective Data
Important Health Information
Health history: Pain history includes onset, location, intensity, quality, patterns, aggravating and alleviating factors, and expression of pain; coping strategies; past treatments and their effectiveness; review of health care utilization related to the pain problem (e.g., emergency department visits, treatment at pain clinics, visits to primary health care providers and specialists)
Medications: Use of any prescription or over-the-counter, illicit, or herbal products for pain relief; alcohol use

Functional Health Patterns
Health perception–health management: Social and work history; mental health history; smoking history; effects of pain on emotions, relationships, sleep, and activities; interviews with family members; records from psychiatric treatment related to the pain
Elimination: Constipation related to opioid drug use
Activity-exercise: Fatigue, limitations in activities, pain related to muscle use
Sexuality-reproductive: Decreased libido
Coping–stress tolerance: Psychologic evaluation using standardized measures to examine coping style, depression, anxiety

Objective Data
Physical examination, including evaluation of functional limitations
Psychosocial evaluation, including mood

injury, acute illness, or treatment (e.g., surgery) typically know exactly when their pain began. Those with chronic pain may be less able to identify when the pain started. Establish the *duration* of the pain (how long it has lasted). This information helps to determine whether the pain is acute or chronic and assists in identifying the cause of the pain. For example, a patient with advanced cancer who also has chronic low back pain from spinal stenosis reports a sudden, severe pain in the back that began 2 days ago. Knowing the onset and duration can lead to a diagnostic workup that may reveal new metastatic disease in the spine.

Pain pattern also provides clues about the cause of the pain and directs its treatment. Many types of chronic pain (e.g., arthritis pain) increase and decrease over time. A patient may have pain all the time (constant, around-the-clock pain), as well as discrete periods of intermittent pain.

Breakthrough pain (BTP) is transient, moderate to severe pain that occurs in patients whose baseline persistent pain is otherwise mild to moderate and fairly well controlled. The average peak of BTP can be 3 to 5 minutes, and can last up to 30 minutes or even longer. BTP can either be predictable or unpredictable, and patients can have one to many episodes per day. Several transmucosal fentanyl products are specifically used to treat BTP.

End-of-dose failure is pain that occurs before the expected duration of a specific analgesic. It should not be confused with BTP. Pain that occurs at the end of the duration of an analgesic often leads to a prolonged increase in the baseline persistent pain. For example, in a patient on transdermal fentanyl (Duragesic patches) the typical duration of action is 72 hours. An increase in pain after 48 hours on the drug would be characterized as end-of-dose failure. End-of-dose failure signals the need for changes in the dose or scheduling of the analgesic. Episodic, procedural, or *incident pain* is a transient increase in pain that is caused by a specific activity or event that precipitates pain. Examples include dressing changes, movement, position changes, and procedures such as catheterization.

Location. Determining the *location* of pain assists in identifying possible causes and treatment. Some patients may be able to specify the precise location(s) of their pain, whereas others may describe general areas or comment that they "hurt all over." The location of the pain may also be referred from its origin to another site (see Fig. 9-2). For example, myocardial infarction can result in pain in the left shoulder. Pain may also radiate from its origin to another site. For example, angina pectoris can radiate from the chest to the jaw or down the left arm. This is referred to as radiating pain. *Sciatica* is pain that follows the course of the sciatic nerve. It may originate from joints or muscles around the back or from compression or damage to the sciatic nerve. The pain is projected along the course of the peripheral nerve, causing painful shooting sensations down the back of the thigh and inside of the leg to the foot.

Obtain information about the location of pain by asking the patient to (1) describe the site(s) of pain, (2) point to painful areas on the body, or (3) mark painful areas on a pain map (see eFig. 9-2, available on the website for this chapter). Because many patients have more than one site of pain, make certain that the patient describes every location.

Intensity. Assessing the severity, or *intensity*, of pain provides a reliable measure to determine the type of treatment and its effectiveness. Pain scales help the patient communicate pain intensity. Choice of a scale to use should be based on the patient's developmental needs and cognitive status. Most adults can rate the intensity of their pain using numeric scales (e.g., 0 = no pain, 10 = the worst pain) or verbal descriptor scales (e.g., none, a little, moderate, severe). These tools are sometimes easier for patients to use if they are oriented vertically or include a visual component. The Pain Thermometer Scale is an example of this type of scale[15] (Fig. 9-3). Other visual pain measures or scales include the Wong-Baker FACES Pain Rating Scale (see eFig. 9-3 on the website for this chapter) and the FACES Pain Scale–Revised (see eFig. 9-4 on the website for this chapter). These and other pain scales may be useful for patients with cognitive

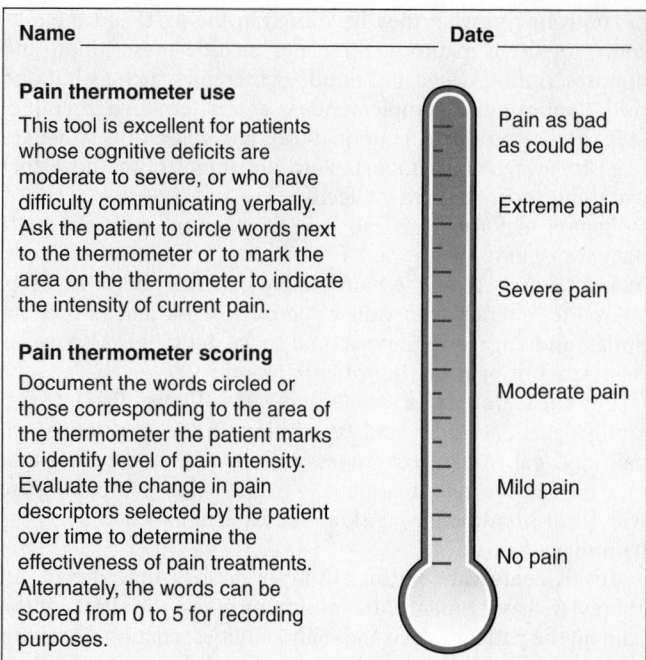

Name _____   **Date** _____

Pain thermometer use
This tool is excellent for patients whose cognitive deficits are moderate to severe, or who have difficulty communicating verbally. Ask the patient to circle words next to the thermometer or to mark the area on the thermometer to indicate the intensity of current pain.

Pain thermometer scoring
Document the words circled or those corresponding to the area of the thermometer the patient marks to identify level of pain intensity. Evaluate the change in pain descriptors selected by the patient over time to determine the effectiveness of pain treatments. Alternately, the words can be scored from 0 to 5 for recording purposes.

Pain as bad as could be
Extreme pain
Severe pain
Moderate pain
Mild pain
No pain

FIG. 9-3 Pain thermometer scale. Ask the patient to circle words next to the thermometer or to mark the area on the thermometer to indicate the intensity of pain. (Used with permission of Keela Herr, RN, PhD, AGSF, FAAN, The University of Iowa.)

or language barriers to describe their pain.[16] Pain assessment measures for cognitively impaired adults and nonverbal adults are addressed later in this chapter.

Although intensity is an important factor in determining analgesic approaches, do not dose patients with opioids solely based on reported pain scores.[17] Opioid "dosing by numbers" without taking into account a patient's sedation level and respiratory status can lead to unsafe practices and serious adverse events. Safer analgesic administration can be achieved by balancing an amount of pain relief with analgesic side effects. Adjustments in therapy can be made to promote better pain control and minimize adverse outcomes.

Quality. The pain *quality* refers to the nature or characteristics of the pain. For example, patients often describe neuropathic pain as burning, numbing, shooting, stabbing, electric shock–like, or itchy. Nociceptive pain may be described as sharp, aching, throbbing, dull, and cramping. Since the quality of pain relates to some degree to the classification of pain (e.g., neuropathic, nociceptive, or visceral), these descriptors can help to guide treatment options that best address the specific mechanism of pain.

Associated Symptoms. *Associated symptoms* such as anxiety, fatigue, and depression may exacerbate or be exacerbated by pain. Ask about activities and situations that increase or alleviate pain. For example, musculoskeletal pain may be increased or decreased with movement and ambulation. Resting or immobilizing a painful body part can decrease pain. Knowing what makes pain better or worse can help characterize the type of pain and be helpful in selecting treatments.

Management Strategies. As people experience and live with pain, they may cope differently and be more or less willing to try different strategies to manage it. Some strategies are successful, whereas others are not. To maximize the effectiveness of the pain treatment plan, ask patients what they are using now to control pain, what they have used in the past, and the outcomes of these methods. Strategies include prescription and nonprescription drugs and nondrug therapies such as hot and cold applications, complementary and alternative therapies (e.g., herbal products, acupuncture), and relaxation strategies (e.g., imagery). It is important to document both those that work and those that are ineffective.

Impact of Pain. Pain can have a profound influence on a patient's quality of life and functioning. In your assessment, include the effect of the pain on the patient's ability to sleep, enjoy life, interact with others, perform work and household duties, and engage in physical and social activities. Also assess the impact of pain on the patient's mood.

Patient's Beliefs, Expectations, and Goals. Patient and family beliefs, attitudes, and expectations influence responses to pain and pain treatment. Assess for attitudes and beliefs that may hinder effective treatment (e.g., the belief that opioid use will result in addiction). Ask about expectations and goals for pain management.

In an acute care setting, time limitations may dictate an abbreviated assessment. At a minimum, assess the effects of the pain on the patient's sleep and daily activities, relationships with others, physical activity, and emotional well-being. In addition, include the ways in which the patient describes the pain and the strategies used to cope with and control the pain.

Documentation

Document the pain assessment, since this is critical to ensure effective communication among team members. Many health care facilities and agencies have adopted specific tools to record an initial pain assessment, treatment, and reassessment. (An example of an initial pain assessment tool appears in eFig. 9-2 on the website for this chapter.) There also are many multidimensional pain assessment tools, such as the Brief Pain Inventory, the McGill Pain Questionnaire, the Memorial Pain Assessment Card, and the Neuropathic Pain Scale.

Reassessment

It is critical for you to reassess pain at appropriate intervals. The frequency and scope of reassessment are guided by factors such as pain severity, physical and psychosocial condition, type of intervention and risks of adverse effects, and institutional policy. For example, reassessment for a postoperative patient is done within 30 minutes of an IV dose of an analgesic. In a long-term care facility, residents with chronic pain are reassessed at least quarterly or with a change in condition or functional status.

PAIN TREATMENT

Basic Principles

All pain treatment plans are based on the following 10 principles and practice standards:

1. *Follow the principles of pain assessment* (see Table 9-5). Remember that pain is a subjective experience. The patient is not only the best judge of his or her own pain, but also the expert on the effectiveness of each pain treatment.
2. *Use a holistic approach to pain management.* The experience of pain affects all aspects of a person's life. Thus a holistic approach to assessment, treatment, and evaluation is required.[18]
3. *Every patient deserves adequate pain management.* Many patient populations, including ethnic minorities, older adults, and people with past or current substance abuse, are at risk for inadequate pain management. Be aware of your own biases and ensure that all patients are treated respectfully.
4. *Base the treatment plan on the patient's goals.* Discuss with the patient realistic goals for pain relief during the initial pain assessment. Although goals can be described in terms of pain intensity (e.g., the desire for average pain to decrease from "8/10" to "3/10"), with chronic pain conditions functional goal setting should be encouraged (e.g., a goal of performing certain daily activities, such as socializing and hobbies). Over the course of prolonged therapy, reassess these goals and progress made toward meeting them. The patient, in collaboration with the health care team, determines new goals. If the patient has unrealistic goals for therapy, such as wanting to be completely rid of all chronic arthritis pain, work with the patient to establish a more realistic goal.
5. *Use both drug and nondrug therapies.* Although drugs are often considered the mainstay of therapy, incorporate self-care activities and nondrug therapies to increase the overall effectiveness of therapy and to allow for the reduction of drug dosages to minimize adverse drug effects.[19]
6. *When appropriate, use a multimodal approach to analgesic therapy. Multimodal analgesia* is the use of two or more classes of analgesic medications to take advantage of the various mechanisms of action. This approach achieves superior pain relief, enhances patient satisfaction, and decreases adverse effects of individual drugs.[20]
7. *Address pain using an interdisciplinary approach.* The expertise and perspectives of an interdisciplinary team are often necessary to provide effective evaluation and therapies for patients with pain, especially chronic pain. Interdisciplinary teams frequently include psychology, physical and occupational therapy, pharmacy, spiritual care, and multiple medical specialties (e.g., neurology, palliative care, oncology, surgery, anesthesiology). Some pain teams also include massage therapists, music therapists, acupuncturists, and art therapists.
8. *Evaluate the effectiveness of all therapies to ensure that they are meeting the patient's goals.* Achievement of an effective treatment plan often requires trial and error. Adjustments in drug, dosage, or route are common to achieve maximal benefit while minimizing adverse effects. This trial-and-error process can become frustrating for the patient and caregivers. Reassure them that pain relief, if not pain cessation, is possible and that the health care team will continue to work with them to achieve adequate pain relief.
9. *Prevent and/or manage medication side effects.* Side effects are a major reason for treatment failure and nonadherence. Side effects are managed in one of several ways, as described in Table 9-7. You play a key role in monitoring for and treating side effects, and in teaching patients and caregivers how to minimize these effects.
10. *Incorporate patient and caregiver teaching throughout assessment and treatment.* Content should include information about the causes of the pain, pain assessment methods, treatment goals and options, expectations of pain management, proper use of drugs, side effect management, and nondrug and self-help pain relief measures. Document the teaching, and include evaluation of patient and caregiver comprehension.

TABLE 9-7 DRUG THERAPY
Managing Side Effects of Pain Medications

Side effects can be managed in one or more of the following methods.
- Decreasing the dose of analgesic by 10%-15%
- Changing to a different medication in the same class
- Adding a drug to counteract the adverse effect of the analgesic (e.g., using a stool softener for patients experiencing opioid-induced constipation)
- Using an administration route that minimizes drug concentrations (e.g., intraspinal administration of opioids used to minimize high drug levels that produce sedation, nausea, and vomiting)

Drug Therapy for Pain

Pain medications generally are divided into three categories: nonopioids, opioids, and adjuvant drugs. Treatment regimens may include medications from one or more of these groups. Mild pain often can be relieved using nonopioids alone. Moderate to severe pain usually requires an opioid. Certain types of pain, such as neuropathic pain, typically require adjuvant drug therapy alone or in combination with an opioid or another class of analgesics. Pain caused by specific medical conditions, such as cancer, may be treated with chemotherapy or radiation therapy as well as pain medications.

Nonopioids. Nonopioid analgesics include acetaminophen, aspirin and other salicylates, and NSAIDs (Table 9-8). These agents are characterized by the following: (1) their analgesic properties have an analgesic ceiling; that is, increasing the dose beyond an upper limit provides no greater analgesia; (2) they do not produce tolerance or physical dependence; and (3) many are available without a prescription. Monitor over-the-counter (OTC) analgesic use to avoid serious problems related to drug interactions, side effects, and overdose.

Nonopioids are effective for mild to moderate pain. They are often used in conjunction with opioids because they allow for effective pain relief using lower opioid doses (thereby causing fewer opioid side effects). This phenomenon is called the *opioid-sparing effect.*[21]

Aspirin is effective for mild pain, but its use is limited by its common side effects, including increased risk for bleeding, especially gastrointestinal (GI) bleeding. Other salicylates such as choline magnesium trisalicylate (Trilisate) cause fewer GI disturbances and bleeding abnormalities. Similar to aspirin, acetaminophen (Tylenol) has analgesic and antipyretic effects, but unlike aspirin, it has no antiplatelet or antiinflammatory effects. Although acetaminophen is well tolerated, it is metabolized by the liver. Hepatotoxicity may result from chronic dosing of more than 4 g/day, acute overdose, or use by patients with severe preexisting liver disease. The addition of acetaminophen to opioid therapy produces an opioid-sparing effect, lower pain scores, and fewer side effects, which is the reason for opioid-acetaminophen combinations such as Percocet and Lortab.[22] IV acetaminophen (OFIRMEV) is used for the treatment of acute mild to moderate pain and moderate to severe pain as an adjunct to opioid analgesics or part of a multimodal analgesic regimen, and reduction of fever. IV acetaminophen is administered over 15 minutes, and the daily dose should also not exceed 4 g/day.

NSAIDs represent a broad class of drugs with varying efficacy and side effects. All NSAIDs inhibit cyclooxygenase

TABLE 9-8 DRUG THERAPY
Selected Nonopioid Analgesics

Drug	Nursing Considerations
Nonsalicylate	
acetaminophen (Tylenol)	• Rectal suppository and injectable form (OFIRMEV) available; sustained-release preparations available; maximum daily dose of 3-4 g. • Doses >4 g/day may cause hepatotoxicity. • Acute overdose: acute liver failure. • Chronic overdose: liver toxicity.
Salicylates	
aspirin	• Rectal suppository and sustained-release preparations available. • Possibility of upper GI bleeding. • Used more commonly in low doses as a cardioprotective measure than for its analgesic properties.
choline magnesium trisalicylate (Trilisate)	• Unlike aspirin and NSAIDs, does not increase bleeding time.
Nonsteroidal Antiinflammatory Drugs (NSAIDs)	
ibuprofen (Motrin, Nuprin, Advil)	• Use lowest effective dose for shortest possible duration. • Increased risk of serious GI adverse events (bleeding, ulceration, perforation), especially in older adults. • May increase risk of serious cardiovascular thrombotic events, myocardial infarction, and stroke. • May increase risk of hypertension and renal insufficiency.
naproxen (Naprosyn, Aleve)	• Use lowest effective dose for shortest possible duration. • Increased risk of serious GI adverse events (bleeding, ulceration, perforation), especially in older adults. • Contraindicated for the treatment of perioperative pain in setting of coronary artery bypass graft (CABG) surgery.
ketorolac (Toradol)	• Limit treatment to 5 days. • May precipitate renal failure in dehydrated patients.
diclofenac K (Cataflam)	• Use lowest effective dose for shortest possible duration. • Available in oral, ophthalmic, topical preparations.
celecoxib (Celebrex)	• Causes fewer GI side effects (e.g., bleeding) than other NSAIDs but risk still present. Is more costly than other NSAIDs. • May increase risk of serious cardiovascular thrombotic events, myocardial infarction, and stroke. • Risks may increase with duration of use, preexisting cardiovascular disease, or risk factors for cardiovascular disease.

(COX), the enzyme that converts arachidonic acid into prostaglandins and related compounds. The enzyme has two forms: COX-1 and COX-2. COX-1 is found in almost all tissues and is responsible for several protective physiologic functions. In contrast, COX-2 is produced mainly at the sites of tissue injury, where it mediates inflammation (Fig. 9-4). Inhibition of COX-1 causes many of the untoward effects of NSAIDs, such as

FIG. 9-4 Arachidonic acid is oxidized by two different pathways: lipoxygen-ase and cyclooxygenase. The cyclooxygenase pathway leads to two forms of the enzyme cyclooxygenase: COX-1 and COX-2. COX-1 is known as *constitutive* (always present), and COX-2 is known as *inducible* (its expression varies markedly depending on the stimulus). Nonsteroidal antiinflammatory drugs (NSAIDs) differ in their actions, with some having more effects on COX-1 and others more on COX-2. Indomethacin acts primarily on COX-1, whereas ibuprofen is equipotent on COX-1 and COX-2. Celecoxib primarily inhibits COX-2.

impairment of renal function, bleeding tendencies, GI irritation, and ulceration. Inhibition of COX-2 is associated with the therapeutic, antiinflammatory effects of NSAIDs. (Celecoxib [Celebrex] is a COX-2 inhibitor.) Older NSAIDs, such as ibuprofen, inhibit both forms of COX and are referred to as nonselective NSAIDs.

Patients vary greatly in their responses to a specific NSAID, so when one NSAID does not provide relief, another should be tried. NSAIDs are associated with many side effects, including GI problems ranging from dyspepsia to life-threatening ulceration and hemorrhage. NSAIDs can also cause cognitive impairment and hypersensitivity reactions with asthma-like symptoms.

Individuals at risk for NSAID-associated GI toxicity include those who have a recent history of peptic ulcer disease, patients who are older than 65, and those concurrently using corticosteroids or anticoagulants. If NSAIDs are used in patients at risk for GI bleeding, they should have concomitant therapy with a misoprostol (Cytotec) or a proton pump inhibitor (PPI) such as omeprazole (Prilosec). NSAIDs should not be administered concurrently with aspirin, since this increases the risk for GI bleeding.[23]

DRUG ALERT
Nonsteroidal Antiinflammatory Drugs (NSAIDs)
- NSAIDs (except aspirin) have been linked to a higher risk for cardiovascular events such as myocardial infarction, stroke, and heart failure.
- Patients who have just had heart surgery should not take NSAIDs.

Opioids. Opioids (Table 9-9) produce their effects by binding to receptors in the CNS. This results in (1) inhibition of the transmission of nociceptive input from the periphery to the spinal cord, (2) altered limbic system activity, and (3) activation of the descending inhibitory pathways that modulate transmis-

sion in the spinal cord. Thus opioids act on several nociceptive processes.

Types of Opioids. Opioids are categorized according to their physiologic action (i.e., agonist and antagonist) and binding at specific opioid receptors (e.g., mu, kappa, and delta). The most commonly administered subclass of opioids is the opioid pure agonists, or morphine-like opioids, which bind to mu receptors.

Opioid agonists are used for both acute and chronic pain. Although nociceptive pain appears to be more responsive to opioids than neuropathic pain, opioids are used to treat both types of pain. Pure opioid agonists include morphine, oxycodone (OxyContin), hydrocodone, codeine, methadone, hydromorphone (Dilaudid), oxymorphone (Opana, Opana ER), and levorphanol (Levo-Dromoran) (see Table 9-9). These drugs are effective for moderate to severe pain because they are potent, have no analgesic ceiling, and can be administered through several routes. When opioids are prescribed for moderate pain, they are usually combined with a nonopioid analgesic such as acetaminophen (e.g., codeine plus acetaminophen [Tylenol #3], or hydrocodone plus acetaminophen [Vicodin] or ibuprofen [Vicoprofen]). Addition of acetaminophen or NSAIDs limits the total daily dose that can be given.

Methadone is a unique mu opioid receptor agonist. When methadone is first administered, it has a relatively short analgesic action (4 to 6 hours) and can be titrated every few days, similar to other short-acting oral opioids. However, after 3 or 4 days of regular dosing, the drug's half-life can become prolonged (90 to 120 hours). Doses should not be increased more than once every 1 to 2 weeks to avoid accumulation. Overdose can result in respiratory depression, leading to death.

DRUG ALERT
Morphine
- Morphine may cause respiratory depression.
- If respirations are 12 or less breaths per minute, withhold medication and contact the health care provider.

DRUG ALERT
Methadone (Dolophine)
- Methadone may cause respiratory depression.

Mixed *agonist-antagonists* (e.g., nalbuphine [Nubain], pentazocine [Talwin], butorphanol [Stadol]) bind as agonists on kappa receptors and as weak antagonists or partial agonists on mu receptors. Because of this difference in binding, mixed agonist-antagonists produce less respiratory depression than drugs that act only at mu receptors. These drugs cause more dysphoria and agitation. In addition, opioid agonist-antagonists have an analgesic ceiling and can precipitate withdrawal if used by a patient who is physically dependent on mu agonist drugs. Partial opioid agonists (e.g., buprenorphine [Buprenex]) bind weakly to mu and kappa receptors, which decreases their analgesic efficacy. Agonist-antagonists and partial agonists currently have limited clinical application in pain management.

Mixed Mu Agonist Opioid and Dual Mechanism Agents. Some analgesics have two distinct actions, or dual mechanisms. Tramadol (Ultram) is a weak mu agonist and also inhibits the reuptake of norepinephrine and serotonin. It is effective in low back pain, osteoarthritis, fibromyalgia, diabetic peripheral neuropathic pain, polyneuropathy, and postherpetic neuralgia. The most common side effects are similar to those of other opioids, including nausea, constipation, dizziness, and sedation. As with other medications that increase serotonin and norepinephrine,

TABLE 9-9 DRUG THERAPY

Opioid Analgesics

Drug	Routes of Administration	Nursing Considerations
Mu Agonists		
morphine (Roxanol, MSIR, MS Contin, Avinza, Kadian, Epimorph, Oramorph SR)	PO (short-acting and sustained-release forms), rectal, IV, subcutaneous, epidural, intrathecal, sublingual	• Standard of comparison for opioid analgesics (Table 9-10). • Indicated for moderate to severe pain. • Can stimulate histamine release, leading to pruritus, with systemic administration. • Tablets for sustained-release preparations are to be swallowed whole, and must not be broken, chewed, dissolved, or crushed. • Preparations for neuraxial* administration must be preservative free.
hydromorphone (Dilaudid)	PO (short-acting and sustained-release forms), rectal, IV, subcutaneous, epidural, intrathecal	• Slightly shorter duration than morphine. • Indicated for moderate to severe pain. • Preparations for neuraxial* administration must be preservative free.
methadone (Dolophine)	PO, IV, IM	• High oral and rectal bioavailability. • Accumulates with repeated dosing. • Use with caution in older adults. • Risk of QT interval prolongation with high doses.
levorphanol (Levo-Dromoran)	PO, IV, IM, subcutaneous	• Accumulates with repeated dosing.
fentanyl (Sublimaze [IV], Duragesic [transdermal], Actiq [transmucosal]), buccal tablet (Fentora), sublingual (Abstral), buccal soluble film (Onsolis), nasal spray (Lazanda)	IV, epidural, intrathecal, transmucosal, transdermal	• Immediate onset after IV route; 7-8 min after IM route; 5-15 min after transmucosal route; up to 6 hr after transdermal route. • For procedures, IV fentanyl often combined with benzodiazepines for analgesia and sedation. • Very potent—dosage is in micrograms (mcg). • Transdermal fentanyl only indicated for chronic pain and should not be administered to opioid-naive patients.
oxymorphone (Opana, Opana ER)	IV, PO (short-acting and extended-release forms)	• Tablets for extended-release forms are to be swallowed whole, and must not be broken, chewed, dissolved, or crushed. • Use with caution in older and debilitated patients and patients with hepatic and renal impairment.
oxycodone (Roxicodone, OxyContin) oxycodone plus acetaminophen (Percocet, Endocet, Tylox) oxycodone plus aspirin (Percodan) oxycodone plus ibuprofen (Combunox)	PO (short-acting and sustained-release forms)	• Available as single entity and in combination with a nonopioid. • Can be used similarly to oral morphine for moderate to severe pain. • Often combined with a nonopioid for acute, moderate pain.
hydrocodone (with acetaminophen [Lortab, Vicodin, Zydone])	PO (short acting) Only available in combination with co-analgesics (acetaminophen, aspirin, or ibuprofen)	• Used for moderate or moderately severe pain. • Generally indicated for short-term management of acute pain (e.g., trauma, musculoskeletal).
codeine oral (with acetaminophen [Tylenol #3]), codeine injectable	PO, subcutaneous	• Associated with higher incidence of nausea and constipation than other mu agonists. • Many codeine preparations are combined with acetaminophen. • 5%-10% of European Americans lack the enzyme to metabolize codeine to morphine.
tramadol (Ultram)	PO, short acting and extended release	• Dual mechanism of action: mu opioid agonist and blocks reuptake of norepinephrine and serotonin. • Used for moderate pain.
tapentadol (Nucynta)	PO, short acting and extended release	• Dual mechanism of action: mu opioid agonist and blocks reuptake of norepinephrine and serotonin.
Mixed Agonist-Antagonists		
pentazocine (Talwin) pentazocine plus naloxone (Talwin NX)	Formulated in combination with acetaminophen, aspirin, ibuprofen Abuse-deterrent preparation includes naloxone to discourage parenteral abuse	• May cause psychotomimetic effects (e.g., hallucinations) and may precipitate withdrawal in opioid-dependent patients. • Not recommended for treatment of chronic pain and rarely for acute pain.
butorphanol (Stadol)	Available in a nasal spray and injectable form Not available orally	• Psychotomimetic effects lower than with pentazocine. • May precipitate withdrawal in opioid-dependent patients. • Injectable used for acute pain. • Nasal spray indicated for migraine headaches.
Partial Agonists		
buprenorphine injectable (Buprenex) buprenorphine plus naloxone sublingual (Suboxone)	Sublingual and injectable forms	• Should not be chewed or swallowed. • Lower abuse potential than morphine. Does not produce psychotomimetic effects. • Buprenorphine plus naloxone used as a sublingual preparation to treat opioid dependence for easier withdrawal when necessary to taper from opioids. • May precipitate withdrawal in opioid-dependent patients. Not readily reversed by naloxone.

*Neuraxial anesthesia pertains to local anesthetics placed around the nerves of the central nervous system such as spinal and epidural anesthesia.

TABLE 9-10   OPIOID EQUIANALGESIC DOSES*

Drug	Dose Equal to Parenteral Morphine 10 mg	
	Oral (mg)	Parenteral (IM, IV, Subcutaneous) (mg)
Morphine	30	10
Codeine	200	120-130
Fentanyl	NA	0.1 (100 mcg)
Hydrocodone	30	NA
Hydromorphone	7.5	1.5
Levorphanol	4	2
Meperidine	300	75
Methadone	20	10
Oxycodone	15-30	NA
Oxymorphone	NA	1

*All equivalencies should be considered approximations. These amounts can be affected by many factors, including interpatient variability, type of pain, and tolerance. Monitor patients for effectiveness and adverse reactions and adjust the dose accordingly
NA, Not available.

this drug should be avoided in patients with a history of seizures because it lowers seizure threshold.

Tapentadol (Nucynta) is a centrally acting analgesic that works at mu receptors and inhibits norepinephrine reuptake.[24] It is approved for management of moderate to severe acute pain. For chronic moderate to severe pain, an extended-release formula is available. The side effects are similar to those of conventional opioids, except that this drug is associated with less nausea and constipation.

Opioids to Avoid. Some opioids should be avoided for pain relief because of limited efficacy and/or toxicities. Meperidine (Demerol) or pethidine is associated with neurotoxicity (e.g., seizures) caused by accumulation of its metabolite, normeperidine. Its use is limited for very short-term (i.e., less than 48 hours) treatment of acute pain when other opioid agonists are contraindicated.[25]

DRUG ALERT
Meperidine (Demerol)
The American Pain Society does not recommend the use of meperidine as an analgesic.

Side Effects of Opioids. Common side effects of opioids include constipation, nausea and vomiting, sedation, respiratory depression, and pruritus. With continued use, many side effects diminish; the exception is constipation. Less common side effects include urinary retention, myoclonus, dizziness, confusion, and hallucinations. *Constipation* is the most common side effect of opioids. Left untreated, constipation may increase the individual's pain and can lead to fecal impaction and paralytic ileus.

Because tolerance to opioid-induced constipation does not develop, a bowel regimen should be instituted at the beginning of opioid therapy and continued for as long as the person takes opioids. Although dietary roughage, fluids, and exercise should be encouraged, these measures alone may not be sufficient. Most patients should use a gentle stimulant laxative (e.g., senna) plus a stool softener (e.g., docusate sodium [Colace]). Other agents (e.g., milk of magnesia, bisacodyl [Dulcolax], polyethylene glycol [MiraLAX], or lactulose [Constulose]) can be added if necessary.

Methylnaltrexone (Relistor) is a peripheral opioid receptor antagonist used for opioid-induced constipation in patients with advanced disease (e.g., incurable cancer, heart failure, chronic obstructive pulmonary disease) when the response to traditional laxative therapy is insufficient. It is generally administered subcutaneously once a day every other day or less frequently, but not more frequently that once daily.

Nausea is often a problem in opioid-naive patients. The use of an antiemetic such as ondansetron (Zofran), metoclopramide (Reglan), transdermal scopolamine (Transderm Scōp), hydroxyzine (Vistaril), or a phenothiazine (e.g., prochlorperazine [Compazine]) can prevent or minimize nausea and vomiting until tolerance develops, usually within 1 week. Opioids delay gastric emptying (patient complains of gastric fullness), and this effect can be reduced by metoclopramide. If nausea and vomiting are severe and persistent, changing to a different opioid may be necessary.

Sedation is usually seen in opioid-naive patients being treated for acute pain. Hospitalized patients receiving opioid analgesics for acute pain should be monitored regularly, especially in the first few days after surgery. Be aware that the risk for unintended advancing sedation in postoperative patients is greatest within 4 hours after leaving the postanesthesia care unit. Opioid-induced sedation resolves with the development of tolerance. Persistent sedation with chronic opioid use can be effectively treated with psychostimulants such as caffeine, dextroamphetamine (Dexedrine), methylphenidate (Ritalin), or the anticataleptic drug modafinil (Provigil).

The risk of *respiratory depression* is also higher in opioid-naive, hospitalized patients who are treated for acute pain. Clinically significant respiratory depression is rare in opioid-tolerant patients and when opioids are titrated to analgesic effect. Patients most at risk for respiratory depression include those who are age 65 or older, have a history of snoring or witnessed apneic episodes, report excessive daytime sleepiness, have underlying cardiac or lung disease, are obese (body mass index greater than 30 kg/m^2), have a history of smoking (more than 20 pack-years), or are receiving other CNS depressants (e.g., sedatives, benzodiazepines, antihistamines). For postoperative patients the greatest risk for opioid-related respiratory adverse events is within the first 24 hours after surgery. Clinically significant respiratory depression cannot occur in patients who are fully awake. Frequently monitor both the sedation level and respiratory rate in patients receiving opioid analgesics. An extensive evidence-based, expert consensus report outlines the risks for unintended advancing sedation and respiratory depression with opioids and recommendations for monitoring to deliver quality and safe patient care.[20]

A sedation scale can be used for monitoring and providing appropriate interventions based on the level of sedation (Table 9-11).

SAFETY ALERT
- If the patient's respirations fall below 8 or 10 breaths/minute and the sedation level is 5 or greater, you should vigorously stimulate the patient and try to keep the patient awake.[20]
- If the patient becomes oversedated, administer oxygen.
- In this situation, the opioid dose should be reduced.

For patients who are excessively sedated or unresponsive, naloxone (Narcan), an opioid antagonist that rapidly reverses the effects of opioids, can be administered. Naloxone can be given IV or subcutaneously every 2 minutes. If the patient has been taking opioids regularly for more than a few days, use naloxone judiciously and titrate carefully because it can precipitate severe, agonizing pain; profound withdrawal symptoms;

TABLE 9-11 PASERO OPIOID-INDUCED SEDATION SCALE (POSS) WITH INTERVENTIONS

Level of Sedation	Nursing Intervention
S = Sleep, easy to arouse	• Acceptable • No action necessary • May increase opioid dose if needed
1 Awake and alert	• Acceptable • No action necessary • May increase opioid dose if needed
2 Slightly drowsy, easily aroused	• Acceptable • No action necessary • May increase opioid dose if needed
3 Frequently drowsy, arousable, drifts off to sleep during conversation	• Unacceptable • Monitor respiratory status and sedation level closely until sedation level is stable at less than 3 and respiratory status is satisfactory • Decrease opioid dose 25% to 50% or notify health care provider or anesthesiologist for orders • Consider administering a non-sedating, opioid-sparing nonopioid, such as acetaminophen or an NSAID, if not contraindicated
4 Somnolent, minimal or no response to verbal or physical stimulation	• Unacceptable • Stop opioid • Consider administering naloxone • Notify health care provider or anesthesiologist • Monitor respiratory status and sedation level closely until sedation level is stable at less than 3 and respiratory status is satisfactory

Adapted from Pasero C: Assessment of sedation during opioid administration for pain management, *Journal of PeriAnesthesia Nursing* 24:186, 2009.

hypertension; and pulmonary edema. Because naloxone's half-life is shorter than that of most opiates, monitor the patient's respiratory rate because it can drop again as soon as 20 minutes after naloxone administration.

Pruritus (itching) is another common side effect of opioids and occurs most frequently when opioids are administered via neuraxial (i.e., epidural, intrathecal) routes. Management of opioid-induced pruritus may include low-dose infusions of naloxone.

A rare but concerning problem with long-term and even short-term use of high-dose opioids is *opioid-induced hyperalgesia* (OIH). OIH is a state of nociceptive sensitization caused by exposure to opioids. It is characterized by a paradoxic response in which patients actually become more sensitive to certain painful stimuli and report increased pain with opioid use. The exact mechanism for this phenomenon is not clearly understood, but it may be due to neuroplasticity changes. This may explain why opioids tend to lose their effectiveness in certain patients over time.

Adjuvant Analgesic Therapy. These medications comprise classes of drugs that can be used alone or in conjunction with opioid and nonopioid analgesics. Generally, these agents were developed for other purposes (e.g., antiseizure drugs, antidepressants) and found later to be effective for pain. Commonly used analgesic adjuvants are listed in Table 9-12.

Corticosteroids. These drugs, which include dexamethasone, prednisone, and methylprednisolone (Medrol), are used for management of acute and chronic cancer pain, pain sec-

ondary to spinal cord compression, and inflammatory joint pain syndromes. Mechanisms of action are unknown but may be related to the ability of corticosteroids to decrease edema and inflammation. They also may decrease activation of an inflamed neuron. Because of this effect, corticosteroids are useful when injected epidurally for acute or subacute disc herniations.

Corticosteroids have many side effects, especially when given chronically in high doses. Adverse effects include hyperglycemia, fluid retention, dyspepsia and GI bleeding, impaired healing, muscle wasting, osteoporosis, adrenal suppression, and susceptibility to infection. Because they act through the same final pathway as NSAIDs, corticosteroids should not be given at the same time as NSAIDs.

Antidepressants. Tricyclic antidepressants (TCAs) enhance the descending inhibitory system by preventing the cellular reuptake of serotonin and norepinephrine. Higher levels of serotonin and norepinephrine in the synaptic cleft inhibit the transmission of nociceptive signals in the CNS. Other potential beneficial actions of TCAs include sodium channel modulation, α_1-adrenergic antagonist effects, and a weak NMDA receptor modulation. They appear to be effective for a variety of pain syndromes, especially neuropathic pain syndromes. However, side effects such as sedation, dry mouth, blurred vision, and weight gain limit their usefulness. Antidepressants that selectively inhibit reuptake of serotonin and norepinephrine (in particular the SNRIs) are effective for many neuropathic pain syndromes and have fewer side effects than the TCAs. These agents include venlafaxine, desvenlafaxine (Pristiq), duloxetine, milnacipran (Savella), and bupropion. A disadvantage to their use is higher cost compared with TCAs.

Antiseizure Drugs. Antiseizure drugs affect both peripheral nerves and the CNS in several ways, including sodium channel modulation, central calcium channel modulation, and changes in excitatory amino acids and other receptors. Agents such as gabapentin, lamotrigine, and pregabalin are valuable adjuvant agents in chronic pain therapy and are being increasingly used in the treatment of acute pain.

GABA Receptor Agonist. Baclofen, an analog of the inhibitory neurotransmitter GABA, can interfere with the transmission of nociceptive impulses and is mainly used for muscle spasms. It crosses the blood-brain barrier poorly and is much more effective for spasticity when delivered intrathecally.

α_2-Adrenergic Agonists. Clonidine and tizanidine (Zanaflex) are the most widely used α_2-adrenergic agonists. They are thought to work on the central inhibitory α-adrenergic receptors. These agents may also decrease norepinephrine release peripherally. They are used for chronic headache and neuropathic pain.

Local Anesthetics. For acute pain from surgery or trauma, local anesthetics such as bupivacaine and ropivacaine can be administered epidurally by continuous infusion, but also by intermittent or continuous infusion with regional nerve blocks. Topical applications of local anesthetics are used to interrupt transmission of pain signals to the brain. For example, 5% lidocaine patch (Lidoderm) is recommended as a first-line agent for the treatment of several types of neuropathic pain. In the treatment of chronic severe neuropathic pain that is refractory to other analgesics, oral therapy with mexiletine (Mexitil) may be tried. Systemic lidocaine administered in the form of an IV infusion is also sometimes used for neuropathic and postoperative visceral pain.

TABLE 9-12 **DRUG THERAPY**

Adjuvant Drugs Used for Pain

Drug	Specific Indication	Nursing Considerations
Corticosteroids	Inflammation	• Avoid high doses for long-term use.
Antidepressants ***Tricyclic Antidepressants*** amitriptyline (Elavil) doxepin (Sinequan) imipramine (Tofranil) nortriptyline (Pamelor) desipramine (Norpramin)	Neuropathic pain	• Side-effect profile differs for each agent and is often dose dependent. • Common side effects include anticholinergic effects (e.g., dry mouth) and sedation. • Monitor for anticholinergic side effects. • Titrate slowly over days to weeks to reach optimal therapeutic doses.
Serotonin Norepinephrine Reuptake Inhibitor (SNRI) Antidepressants venlafaxine (Effexor) duloxetine (Cymbalta) bupropion (Wellbutrin) milnacipran (Savella)	Neuropathic pain Multimodal therapy for acute pain (venlafaxine) Fibromyalgia (duloxetine)	• Side effects vary with each agent.
Antiseizure Drugs *First generation:* carbamazepine (Tegretol) phenytoin (Dilantin) *Second generation:* gabapentin (Neurontin) pregabalin (Lyrica) lamotrigine (Lamictal)	Neuropathic pain Multimodal therapy for acute pain (gabapentin, pregabalin) Fibromyalgia (pregabalin)	• Start with low doses, increase slowly. • Side effects vary with each agent.
GABA Receptor Agonist baclofen (Lioresal)	Neuropathic pain Muscle spasms	• Monitor for weakness, urinary dysfunction. • Avoid abrupt discontinuation because of CNS irritability.
α₂-Adrenergic Agonist clonidine (Duraclon) tizanidine (Zanaflex)	Particularly useful for neuropathic pain when administered intrathecally	• Side effects include sedation, orthostatic hypotension, dry mouth. • Often combined with anesthetics (e.g., bupivacaine [Sensorcaine]).
Anesthetics: Oral or Systemic mexiletine (Mexitil)	Diabetic neuropathy Neuropathic pain	• Monitor for side effects: high incidence of nausea, dizziness, perioral numbness, paresthesias, tremor, seizures (at high doses), dysrhythmias, and myocardial depression. • Avoid in patients with preexisting cardiac disease.
5% lidocaine–impregnated transdermal patch (Lidoderm patch)	Postherpetic neuralgia	• Local skin reactions (e.g., change in color, colored spots, irritation, itching, rash, burning) occur at the site of application; typically mild.
Anesthetics: Local lidocaine (L-M-X)	Topical local anesthetic cream applied to intact skin before venipuncture or lumbar puncture. Possible effective for postherpetic neuralgia	• Apply bubble layer to intact skin, wait at least 20-30 minutes before wiping and performing painful procedure. • Duration is approximately 60 minutes after removed from skin. • Available without prescription.
lidocaine 2.5% + prilocaine 2.5% (topical EMLA [eutectic mixture of local anesthetics])	Longer time to take effect than L-M-X	• Apply under an occlusive dressing (e.g., Tegaderm, DuoDerm) or on an anesthetic disk. • Side effects include mild erythema, edema, skin blanching.
capsaicin (Zostrix)	Pain associated with arthritis, postherpetic neuralgia, diabetic neuropathy	• Apply very sparingly onto affected area. Use gloves or wash hands with soap and water after application. • Monitor for side effects: skin irritation (burning, stinging) at application site and cough when inhaled.

CNS, Central nervous system.

Cannabinoids. Cannabinoid-derived medications show promise in the treatment of certain pain syndromes and symptoms. However, these preparations have sparked considerable controversy and confusion, mostly because cannabinoids are related to the cannabis plant, also known as marijuana. Synthetic cannabinoids (e.g., dronabinol [Marinol]) have been approved for medical use in Canada, the United Kingdom, and the United States. Smoking marijuana or cannabis rapidly increases plasma levels of tetrahydrocannabinol (THC), but the amount is highly dependent on composition of the marijuana cigarette and inhalation technique, so this form of use is associated with highly variable results in relief of pain and symptoms.[26] With commercially available oral preparations, the absorption and bioavailability are more reliable and predictable.

Cannabinoids exert their analgesic effects primarily through the cannabinoid-l (CB1) and CB2 receptors. Activation of cannabinoid receptors modulates neurotransmission in the serotoninergic, dopaminergic, and glutamatergic systems, as well as other systems. Cannabinoids also enhance the endogenous opioid system. Other beneficial effects include alleviation of nausea and increased appetite. They may also have opioid-sparing effects, possibly reduce opioid tolerance, and even ameliorate symptoms of opioid withdrawal.[26] In Canada an oromucosal spray, nabiximols (Sativex), is available for adjunctive treatment of neuropathic pain and moderate to severe pain in cancer.[27]

Administration

Scheduling. Appropriate analgesic scheduling focuses on preventing or controlling pain, rather than providing analgesics only after the patient's pain has become severe. A patient should be premedicated before procedures and activities that are expected to produce pain. Similarly, a patient with constant pain should receive analgesics around the clock rather than on an "as needed" (PRN) basis. These strategies control pain before it starts and usually result in lower analgesic requirements. Fast-acting drugs should be used for incident or breakthrough pain, whereas long-acting analgesics are more effective for constant pain. Examples of fast-acting and sustained-release analgesics are described later in this section.

Titration. Analgesic titration is dose adjustment based on assessment of the adequacy of analgesic effect versus the side effects produced. The amount of analgesic needed to manage pain varies widely, and titration is an important strategy in addressing this variability. An analgesic can be titrated upward or downward, depending on the situation. For example, in a postoperative patient the dose of analgesic generally decreases over time as the acute pain resolves. On the other hand, opioids for chronic, severe cancer pain may be titrated upward many times over the course of therapy to maintain adequate pain control. The goal of titration is to use the smallest dose of analgesic that provides effective pain control with the fewest side effects.

Equianalgesic Dosing. The term **equianalgesic dose** refers to a dose of one analgesic that is approximately equivalent in pain-relieving effects to a given dose of another analgesic (see Table 9-10). This equivalence helps guide opioid dosing when changing routes or opioids when a particular drug is ineffective or causes intolerable side effects. Equianalgesic charts and conversion programs are widely available in clinical guidelines, in health care facility pain protocols, and on the Internet. They are useful tools, but you need to understand their limitations, since equianalgesic doses are estimates.[28] All changes in opioid therapy must be carefully monitored and adjusted for an individual patient.

Administration Routes. Opioids and other analgesic agents can be delivered via many routes. This flexibility allows the health care provider to (1) target a particular anatomic source of the pain, (2) achieve therapeutic blood levels rapidly when necessary, (3) avoid certain side effects through localized administration, and (4) provide analgesia when patients are unable to swallow. The following discussion highlights the uses and nursing considerations for analgesic agents delivered through a variety of routes.

Oral. Generally, oral administration is the route of choice for the person with a functioning GI system. Most pain medications are available in oral preparations, such as liquid and tablet.

For opioids, larger oral doses are needed to achieve the equivalent analgesia of doses administered intramuscularly (IM) or IV (see Table 9-10). For example, 10 mg of parenteral morphine is equivalent to approximately 30 mg of oral morphine. The reason larger doses are required is related to the *first-pass effect* of hepatic metabolism. This means that oral opioids are absorbed from the GI tract into the portal circulation and shunted to the liver. Partial metabolism in the liver occurs before the drug enters the systemic circulation and becomes available to peripheral receptors or can cross the blood-brain barrier and access CNS opioid receptors, which is necessary to produce analgesia. Oral opioids are as effective as parenteral opioids if the dose administered is large enough to compensate for the first-pass metabolism.

Many opioids are available in short-acting (immediate-release) and long-acting (sustained-release or extended-release) oral preparations. Immediate-release products are effective in providing rapid, short-term pain relief. Sustained-release preparations generally are administered every 8 to 12 hours, although some preparations (e.g., Kadian, Avinza, Exalgo) may be dosed every 24 hours. Sustained- or extended-release preparations should not be crushed, broken, or chewed.

Transmucosal and Buccal Routes. Although morphine has historically been administered sublingually to people with cancer pain who have difficulty swallowing, little of the drug is actually absorbed from the sublingual tissue. Instead, most of the drug is dissolved in saliva and swallowed, making its metabolism the same as that of oral morphine.

Several transmucosal fentanyl products are used for the treatment of breakthrough pain including oral transmucosal fentanyl citrate (OTFC) (Actiq) with the fentanyl embedded in a flavored lozenge on a stick, absorbed by the buccal mucosa after being rubbed actively over it when administered as the lozenge (not sucked as a lollipop), fentanyl buccal tablet (FBT) (Fentora) in the form of a buccal tablet that disintegrates, fentanyl sublingual (Abstral), and fentanyl buccal soluble film (Onsolis) for application to the buccal membrane. Transmucosal absorption allows the drug to enter the bloodstream and travel directly to the CNS. Pain relief typically occurs 5 to 7 minutes after administration. These formulations of fentanyl should be used only for patients who are already receiving and are tolerant to opioid therapy.

An oromucosal spray delivery of cannabinoid extract (Sativex) is an adjunctive treatment for neuropathic pain and spasticity in patients with multiple sclerosis. It is not currently available in the United States.

Intranasal Route. Intranasal administration allows delivery of medication to highly vascular mucosa and avoids the first-pass effect. Butorphanol is indicated for acute headache and other intense, recurrent types of pain. A transmucosal fentanyl nasal spray (Lazanda) is available for the treatment of breakthrough pain.

Rectal. The rectal route is often overlooked but is particularly useful when the patient cannot take an analgesic by mouth, such as those patients with severe nausea and vomiting. Analgesics that are available as rectal suppositories include hydromorphone, oxymorphone, morphine, and acetaminophen. If rectal preparations are not available, many oral formulations can be given rectally if the patient is unable to take medications by mouth.

Transdermal Route. Fentanyl (Duragesic) is available as a transdermal patch system for application to nonhairy skin. This delivery system is useful for the patient who cannot tolerate oral analgesic drugs. Absorption from the patch is slow, and it takes 12 to 17 hours to reach full effect with the first application. Therefore transdermal fentanyl is not suitable for rapid dose titration but can be effective if the patient's pain is stable and the dose required to control it is known. Patches may need to be changed every 48 hours rather than the recommended 72 hours based on individual patient responses. Rashes caused by the adhesive of the patch may be reduced by preparing the skin 1 hour before placement with a weak corticosteroid cream. Bio-occlusive dressings are available if the patch keeps falling off because of sweating. A transdermal patient-controlled analgesia (PCA) system (iontophoretic transdermal system [ITS]) is available.

DRUG ALERT
Fentanyl Patches
- Fentanyl patches (Duragesic) may cause death from overdose.
- Signs of overdose include trouble breathing or shallow respirations; tiredness, extreme sleepiness, or sedation; inability to think, talk, or walk normally; and faintness, dizziness, or confusion.

An important distinction should be made between transdermal patches designed for systemic drug delivery (e.g., Duragesic) and those for topical or local delivery (e.g., Lidoderm).

A 5% lidocaine-impregnated transdermal patch (Lidoderm patch) is used for postherpetic neuralgia. The patch is placed directly on the intact skin in the area of postherpetic pain and left in place for up to 12 hours. Topical local anesthetics are generally well tolerated and cause few systemic side effects, even with chronic use.

Creams and lotions containing 10% trolamine salicylate (Aspercreme, Myoflex Creme) are available for joint and muscle pain. This aspirin-like substance is absorbed locally. This route of administration avoids GI irritation but not the other side effects of high-dose salicylates. Topical diclofenac solution and a diclofenac patch (Flector) have been shown to be effective for osteoarthritic pain of the knee.

Other topical analgesic agents, such as capsaicin (e.g., Zostrix) and lidocaine (L-M-X cream), also provide analgesia. Derived from red chili pepper, capsaicin acts on C fiber heat receptors. If used three or four times a day for 4 to 6 weeks, it will cause the C nociceptor fibers to become inactive. The result is neuronal resistance to painful stimuli. Capsaicin can control pain associated with diabetic neuropathy, arthritis, and possibly postherpetic neuralgia. L-M-X cream is useful for control of pain associated with venipunctures. Cover the targeted area of intact skin with a layer of L-M-X for at least 20 to 30 minutes before it is wiped off prior to beginning a painful procedure. An occlusive dressing is recommended but not required during this time.

Parenteral Routes. The parenteral routes include subcutaneous, IM, and IV administration. Single, repeated, or continuous dosing (subcutaneous or IV) is possible via parenteral routes. Although it is frequently used, the IM route is not recommended because injections cause significant pain and result in unreliable absorption. With chronic use, IM injections can result in abscesses and fibrosis. Onset of analgesia after subcutaneous administration is slow, and thus the subcutaneous route is rarely used for acute pain management. However, continuous subcutaneous infusions are effective for pain management at the end of life. This route is especially helpful for people with abnormal GI function and limited venous access. IV administration is the best route when immediate analgesia and rapid titration

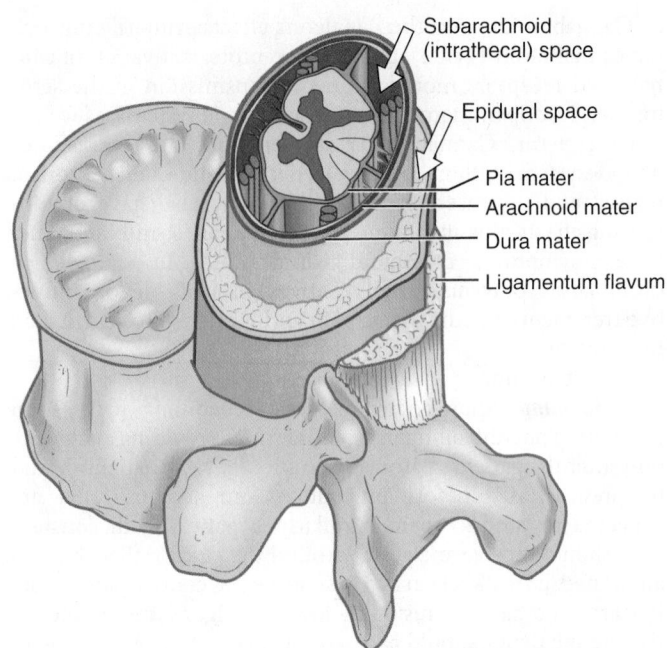

FIG. 9-5 Spinal anatomy. The spinal cord extends from the foramen magnum to the first or second lumbar vertebral space. The subarachnoid space (intrathecal space) is filled with cerebrospinal fluid that continuously circulates and bathes the spinal cord. The epidural space is a potential space filled with blood vessels, fat, and a network of nerve extensions.

are necessary. Continuous IV infusions provide excellent steady-state analgesia through stable blood levels.

Intraspinal Delivery. Intraspinal opioid therapy involves inserting a catheter into the subarachnoid space (*intrathecal delivery*) or the epidural space (*epidural delivery*) (Fig. 9-5). Analgesics are injected either by intermittent bolus doses or continuous infusion.

Percutaneously placed temporary catheters are used for short-term therapy (2 to 4 days), and surgically implanted catheters are used for long-term therapy. Although the lumbar region is the most common site of placement, epidural catheters may be placed at any point along the spinal column (cervical, thoracic, lumbar, or caudal). The tip of the epidural catheter is placed as close to the nerve supplying the painful dermatome as possible. For example, a thoracic catheter is placed for upper abdominal surgery, and a high lumbar catheter is used for lower abdominal surgery. Fluoroscopy is used to ensure correct placement of the catheter.

Intraspinally administered analgesics are highly potent because they are delivered close to the receptors in the spinal cord dorsal horn. Smaller doses of analgesics are needed than with other routes, including IV. For example, 1 mg of intrathecal morphine is approximately equivalent to 10 mg of epidural morphine, 100 mg of IV morphine, and 300 mg of oral morphine. Drugs that are delivered intraspinally include morphine, fentanyl, sufentanil (Sufenta), alfentanil (Alfenta), hydromorphone, ziconotide (Prialt) (a calcium channel receptor modulator for use in neuropathic pain syndromes), and clonidine. Nausea, itching, and urinary retention are common side effects of intraspinal opioids.

Complications of intraspinal analgesia include catheter displacement and migration, accidental infusions of neurotoxic agents, epidural hematomas, and infection. Clinical manifestations of catheter displacement or migration depend on catheter location and the drug being infused. A catheter that migrates out of the intrathecal or epidural space will cause a decrease in pain relief with no improvement with additional boluses or increases in the infusion rate. If an epidural catheter migrates into the subarachnoid space, increased side effects become quickly apparent. Somnolence, confusion, and increased anesthesia (if the infusate contains an anesthetic) occur. Check with institutional policy before aspirating cerebrospinal fluid to determine intrathecal catheter placement. Migration of a catheter into a blood vessel may cause an increase in side effects because of systemic drug distribution.

Many drugs and chemicals are highly neurotoxic when administered intraspinally. These include many preservatives such as alcohol and phenol, antibiotics, chemotherapy agents, potassium, and parenteral nutrition. To avoid inadvertent injection of IV drugs into an intraspinal catheter, the catheter should be clearly marked as an intraspinal access device, and only preservative-free drugs should be injected.

Infection is a rare but serious complication of intraspinal analgesia. Assess the skin around the exit site for inflammation, drainage, or pain. Manifestations of an intraspinal infection include diffuse back pain, pain or paresthesia during bolus injection, and unexplained sensory or motor deficits in the lower limbs. Fever may or may not be present. Acute bacterial infection (meningitis) is manifested by photophobia, neck stiffness, fever, headache, and altered mental status. Infection is avoided by providing regular, meticulous wound care and using sterile technique when caring for the catheter and injecting drugs.

Long-term epidural catheters may be placed for terminal cancer patients or patients with certain pain syndromes that are unresponsive to other treatments. If a long-term indwelling epidural catheter is used, bacterial filters are recommended.

Implantable Pumps. Intraspinal catheters can be surgically implanted for long-term pain relief. The surgical placement of an intrathecal catheter to a subcutaneously placed pump and reservoir allows for the delivery of drugs directly into the intrathecal space. The pump, which is normally placed in a pocket made in the subcutaneous tissue of the abdomen, may be programmable or fixed. Changes are made by either reprogramming the pump or changing the mixture or concentration of drug in the reservoir. The pump is refilled every 30 to 90 days depending on flow rate, mixture, and reservoir size.

Patient-Controlled Analgesia. A specific type of IV delivery system is patient-controlled analgesia (PCA), or demand analgesia. It can also be connected to an epidural catheter (patient-controlled epidural analgesia). With PCA, a dose of opioid is delivered when the patient decides a dose is needed. PCA uses an infusion system in which the patient pushes a button to receive a bolus infusion of an analgesic. PCA is used widely for the management of acute pain, including postoperative pain and cancer pain.

Opioids such as morphine and hydromorphone are commonly administered via IV PCA therapy for both acute and chronic pain management. Fentanyl is less often used for acute pain. Sometimes IV PCA is administered with a continuous or background infusion called a *basal rate*, depending on the patient's opioid requirement. For acute pain (e.g., postoperative pain), basal rates are not recommended when initiating therapy in opioid-naive patients. The addition of a basal rate in opioid-naive patients and those at risk for adverse respiratory outcomes (e.g., older age, obstructive sleep apnea, pulmonary disease) may lead to serious respiratory events.[20]

Use of PCA begins with patient teaching. Help the patient understand the mechanics of getting a drug dose and how to titrate the drug to achieve good pain relief. Teach the patient to self-administer the analgesic before pain is severe. Assure the patient that he or she cannot "overdose" because the pump is programmed to deliver a maximum number of doses per hour. Pressing the button after the maximum dose is administered will not result in additional analgesic. If the maximum doses are inadequate to relieve pain, the pump can be reprogrammed to increase the amount or frequency of dosing. In addition, you can give bolus doses if they are included in the physician's orders. To make a smooth transition from infusion PCA to oral drugs, the patient should receive increasing doses of oral drug as the PCA analgesic is tapered.

Interventional Therapy

Therapeutic Nerve Blocks. Nerve blocks generally involve one-time or continuous infusion of local anesthetics into a particular area to produce pain relief. These techniques are also called *regional anesthesia.* Nerve blocks interrupt all afferent and efferent transmission to the area and thus are not specific to nociceptive pathways. They include local infiltration of anesthetics into a surgical area (e.g., chest incisions, inguinal hernia, joint) and injection of anesthetic into a specific nerve (e.g., occipital or pudendal nerve) or nerve plexus (e.g., brachial or celiac plexus). Nerve blocks often are used during and after surgery to manage pain. For longer-term relief of chronic pain syndromes, local anesthetics can be administered via a continuous infusion.

Adverse effects of nerve blocks are similar to those for local anesthetics delivered via other systemic routes and include systemic toxicity resulting in dysrhythmias, confusion, nausea and vomiting, blurred vision, tinnitus, and metallic taste. Temporary nerve blocks affect both motor function and sensation and typically last 2 to 24 hours, depending on the agent and the site of injection. Motor ability generally returns before sensation.

Neuroablative Techniques. *Neuroablative interventions* are performed for severe pain that is unresponsive to all other therapies. Neuroablative techniques destroy nerves, thereby interrupting pain transmission. Destruction is accomplished by surgical resection or thermocoagulation, including radiofrequency coagulation. Neuroablative interventions that destroy the sensory division of a peripheral or spinal nerve are classified as *neurectomies, rhizotomies,* and *sympathectomies.* Neurosurgical procedures that ablate the lateral spinothalamic tract are classified as *cordotomies* if the tract is interrupted in the spinal cord, or *tractotomies* if the interruption is in the medulla or the midbrain of the brainstem (Fig. 9-6). Both cordotomy and tractotomy can be performed with the aid of local anesthesia by a percutaneous technique under fluoroscopy.

Neuroaugmentation. *Neuroaugmentation* involves electrical stimulation of the brain and the spinal cord. Spinal cord stimulation (SCS) is performed much more often than brain stimulation. The most common use of SCS is for chronic back pain secondary to nerve damage that is unresponsive to other therapies. Other uses include complex regional pain syndrome (CRPS), spinal cord injury pain, and interstitial cystitis. Potential complications include those related to the surgery (bleeding and infection), migration of the generator (which usually is implanted in the subcutaneous tissues of the upper gluteal or pectoralis area), and nerve damage.[29]

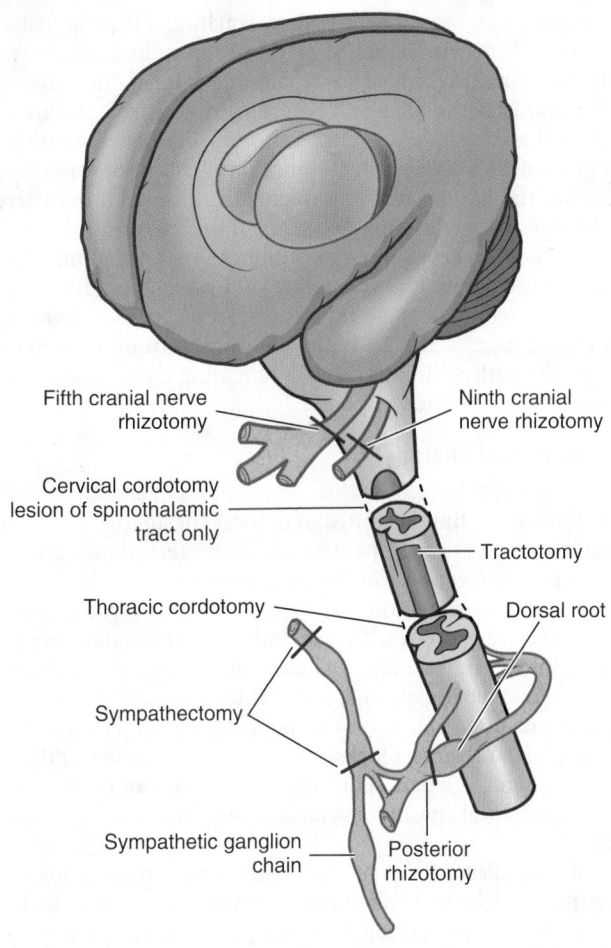

FIG. 9-6 Sites of neurosurgical procedures for pain relief.

TABLE 9-13	**NONDRUG THERAPIES FOR PAIN**
Physical Therapies	**Cognitive Therapies**
• Acupuncture	• Distraction
• Application of heat and cold (see Table 9-14)	• Hypnosis
	• Imagery
• Exercise	• Relaxation strategies (see Chapter 7)
• Massage	• Relaxation breathing
• Transcutaneous electrical nerve stimulation (TENS)	• Imagery
	• Meditation
	• Art therapy
	• Music therapy

Nondrug Therapies for Pain

Nondrug strategies play an important role in pain management (Table 9-13). They can reduce the dose of an analgesic required to relieve pain and thereby minimize side effects of drug therapy. Moreover, they increase the patient's sense of personal control about managing pain and bolster coping skills. Some strategies are believed to alter ascending nociceptive input or stimulate descending pain modulation mechanisms (see discussion on perception on p. 118). These nondrug therapies are especially important in the treatment of chronic pain.[30]

Physical Pain Relief Strategies

Massage. Massage is useful for both acute and chronic pain.[31] Many different massage techniques exist, including moving the hands or fingers over the skin slowly or briskly with long strokes or in circles (superficial massage) or applying firm pressure to the skin to maintain contact while massaging the underlying tissues (deep massage). Another type is trigger point massage. A **trigger point** is a circumscribed hypersensitive area within a tight band of muscle. It is caused by acute or chronic muscle strain and can often be felt as a tight knot under the skin. Trigger point massage is performed by applying either strong, sustained digital pressure; deep massage; or gentler massage with ice followed by muscle heating. (Massage is discussed in Chapter 6.)

Exercise. Exercise is an essential part of the treatment plan for patients with chronic pain, particularly those with musculoskeletal pain.[32] Many patients become physically decondi-

tioned as a result of their pain, which in turn leads to more pain. Exercise acts via many mechanisms to relieve pain. It enhances circulation and cardiovascular fitness, reduces edema, increases muscle strength and flexibility, and enhances physical and psychosocial functioning. An exercise program should be tailored to the patient's physical needs and lifestyle. It may include aerobic exercise, stretching, and strengthening exercises. The program should be supervised by trained personnel (e.g., exercise physiologist, physical therapist).

Transcutaneous Electrical Nerve Stimulation. *Transcutaneous electrical nerve stimulation* (TENS) involves the delivery of an electric current through electrodes applied to the skin surface over the painful region, at trigger points, or over a peripheral nerve. A TENS system consists of two or more electrodes connected by lead wires to a small, battery-operated stimulator (Fig. 9-7). Usually a physical therapist is responsible for administering TENS therapy, although nurses can be trained in the technique.

TENS may be used for acute pain, including postoperative pain and pain associated with physical trauma. The effects of TENS on chronic pain are less clear, but it may be effective in these cases.[33]

Acupuncture. Acupuncture is a technique of Traditional Chinese Medicine in which very thin needles are inserted into the body at designated points. Acupuncture is used for many different kinds of pain. (Acupuncture is discussed in Chapter 6.)

Heat Therapy. Heat therapy is the application of either moist or dry heat to the skin. Heat therapy can be either superficial or deep. Superficial heat can be applied using an electric heating

FIG. 9-7 Transcutaneous electrical nerve stimulation (TENS) treatment being given for treatment of pain after shoulder surgery.

TABLE 9-14   PATIENT & CAREGIVER TEACHING GUIDE

Heat and Cold Therapy

Include the following instructions when teaching the patient and caregiver about superficial heat or cold techniques.

Heat Therapy

- Do not use heat on an area that is being treated with radiation therapy, is bleeding, has decreased sensation, or has been injured in the past 24 hours.
- Do not use any menthol-containing products (e.g., Ben-Gay, Vicks, Icy Hot) with heat applications because this may cause burns.
- Cover the heat source with a towel or cloth before applying to the skin to prevent burns.

Cold Therapy

- Cover the cold source with a cloth or towel before applying to the skin to prevent tissue damage.
- Do not apply cold to areas that are being treated with radiation therapy, have open wounds, or have poor circulation.
- If it is not possible to apply the cold directly to the painful site, try applying it right above or below the painful site or on the opposite side of the body on the corresponding site (e.g., left elbow if the right elbow hurts).

pad (dry or moist), a hot pack, hot moist compresses, warm wax (paraffin), or a hot water bottle. To expose large areas of the body, patients can immerse themselves in a hot bath, shower, or whirlpool. Physical therapy departments provide deep-heat therapy through such techniques as short-wave diathermy, microwave diathermy, and ultrasound therapy. Patient teaching regarding heat therapy is described in Table 9-14.

Cold Therapy. Cold therapy involves the application of either moist or dry cold to the skin. Dry cold can be applied by means of an ice bag, moist cold by means of towels soaked in ice water, cold hydrocollator packs, or immersion in a bath or under running cold water. Icing with ice cubes or blocks of ice made to resemble Popsicles is another technique used for pain relief. Cold therapy is believed to be more effective than heat for a variety of painful conditions, including acute pain from trauma or surgery, acute flare-ups of arthritis, muscle spasms, and headache. Patient teaching regarding cold therapy is described in Table 9-14.

Cognitive Therapies. Techniques to alter the affective, cognitive, and behavioral components of pain include a variety of cognitive strategies and behavioral approaches. For example, patients can identify and challenge negative pain-related thoughts and replace them with more positive coping thoughts. Some of these techniques require little training and often are adopted independently by the patient. For others, a trained therapist is necessary.

Distraction. Distraction involves redirection of attention away from the pain and onto something else. It is a simple but powerful strategy to relieve pain. Distraction can be achieved by engaging the patient in any activity that can hold his or her attention (e.g., watching TV or a movie, conversing, listening to music, playing a game). It is important to match the activity with the patient's energy level and ability to concentrate.

Hypnosis. Hypnotherapy is a structured technique that enables a patient to achieve a state of heightened awareness and focused concentration that can be used to alter the patient's pain perception. Hypnosis should be administered and monitored only by specially trained clinicians.[34]

Relaxation Strategies. Relaxation strategies are varied, but their goal is to reach a state that is free from anxiety and muscle tension. Relaxation reduces stress, decreases acute anxiety, distracts from pain, alleviates muscle tension, combats fatigue, facilitates sleep, and enhances the effectiveness of other pain relief measures.[35] Relaxation strategies include relaxation breathing, music, imagery, meditation, and muscle relaxation. These strategies are described in Chapter 7.

NURSING AND COLLABORATIVE MANAGEMENT PAIN

You are an important member of the interdisciplinary pain management team. You provide input into the assessment and reassessment of pain. You help in planning and implementing treatments, including education, advocacy, and support of the patient and family. Because patients in any care setting can experience pain, you must be knowledgeable about current therapies and flexible in trying new approaches to pain management.

Together with the patient, develop a written agreement or treatment plan that describes the pain management. The plan should ensure that pain will be treated based on the patient's perception and report of pain. In addition, the plan should clearly outline the gradual tapering of the analgesic dose, with eventual substitution of parenteral analgesics with long-acting oral preparations, and possibly cessation of opioids.

Many nursing roles are described earlier in this chapter, including assessing pain, administering treatment, monitoring for side effects, and teaching patients and caregivers. However, the success of these actions depends on your ability to establish a trusting relationship with the patient and caregiver and to address their concerns regarding pain and its treatment.

EFFECTIVE COMMUNICATION

Because pain is a subjective experience, patients need to feel confident that their reporting of pain will be believed and will not be perceived as "complaining." The patient and the caregiver also need to know that you consider the pain significant and understand that pain may profoundly disrupt a person's life. Communicate concern and commit to helping the patient obtain pain relief and cope with any unrelieved pain. Support the patient and the caregiver through the period of trial and error that may be necessary to implement an effective therapeutic plan. It also is important to clarify responsibilities in pain relief. Help the patient understand the role of the health care team members, as well as the patient's roles and expectations.

In addition to addressing specific aspects of pain assessment and treatment, evaluate the impact that the pain has on the lives of the patient and the caregiver. Table 9-15 addresses teaching needs of patients and caregivers related to pain management.

CHALLENGES TO EFFECTIVE PAIN MANAGEMENT

Common challenges to effective pain management include misunderstandings about tolerance, physical dependence, and addiction. It is important for you to understand and be able to explain these concepts.

TOLERANCE. *Tolerance* occurs with chronic exposure to a variety of drugs. In the case of opioids, tolerance to analgesia is characterized by the need for an increased opioid dose to maintain the same degree of analgesia. Although the development of

TABLE 9-15 PATIENT & CAREGIVER TEACHING GUIDE

Pain Management

Include the following information in the teaching plan for the patient with pain and caregiver.

- Self-management techniques.
- Realistic goals for pain control.
- Negative consequences of unrelieved pain.
- Need to maintain a record of pain level and effectiveness of treatment.
- Pain should be treated with drugs and/or nondrug therapies before it becomes severe.
- Medication may stop working after it is taken for a period of time, and dosages may need to be adjusted.
- Potential side effects and complications associated with pain therapies can include nausea and vomiting, constipation, sedation and drowsiness, itching, urinary retention, and sweating.
- Need to report when pain is not relieved to tolerable levels.

TABLE 9-16 MANIFESTATIONS OF OPIOID WITHDRAWAL SYNDROME

	Early Response (6-12 Hr)	Late Response (48-72 Hr)
Psychosocial	• Anxiety	• Excitation
Secretions	• Lacrimation	• Diarrhea
	• Rhinorrhea	
	• Diaphoresis	
Other	• Yawning	• Restlessness
	• Piloerection	• Fever
	• Shaking, chills	• Nausea and vomiting
	• Dilated pupils	• Abdominal cramping pain
	• Anorexia	• Hypertension
	• Tremor	• Tachycardia
		• Insomnia

DELEGATION DECISIONS

Pain

Effective pain management should be a focus for all members of the nursing team.

Role of Registered Nurse (RN)
- Assess pain characteristics (pattern and onset, area or location, intensity, quality, associated symptoms, and management strategies).
- Develop treatment plan for patient's pain (including drug and nondrug therapies).
- Evaluate whether current treatment plan is effective.
- Teach patient and caregiver about treatment plan.
- Implement discharge teaching about pain management.

Role of Licensed Practical/Vocational Nurse (LPN/LVN)
- Administer ordered pain medications (consider the state nurse practice act and agency policy, since LPNs may not be able to give medications by all routes).
- Assess patient's pain.

Role of Unlicensed Assistive Personnel (UAP)
- Assist with screening for pain and notify RN if patient expresses pain.
- Take and report vital signs before and after pain medications are given.
- Note and report if patient is refusing to participate in ordered activities such as ambulation (since this may indicate inadequate pain management).

tolerance to side effects (except constipation) is more predictable, the incidence of clinically significant analgesic opioid tolerance in chronic pain patients is unknown, since dosage needs may increase as the disease (e.g., cancer) progresses. It is essential to assess for increased analgesic needs in patients on long-term therapy. The health care team needs to evaluate and rule out other causes of increased analgesic needs, such as disease progression or infection.

If significant tolerance to opioids develops and it is believed that an opioid is losing its effectiveness, or intolerable side effects are associated with escalation of doses, the practice of *opioid rotation* may be considered. This involves switching from one opioid to another, assuming that the new opioid will be more effective at lower equianalgesic doses. However, very high opioid doses can result in opioid-induced hyperalgesia rather than pain relief. This means that increases in the dose can lead to higher pain levels.

PHYSICAL DEPENDENCE. Like tolerance, physical dependence is a normal physiologic response to ongoing exposure to drugs. It is manifested by a withdrawal syndrome when the drug is abruptly decreased. Manifestations of opioid withdrawal are listed in Table 9-16. When opioids are no longer needed to provide pain relief, a tapering schedule should be used in conjunction with careful monitoring. A typical tapering schedule is determined by calculating the 24-hour dose used by the patient and dividing by 2. Of this decreased amount, 25% is given every 6 hours. After 2 days the daily dose is reduced by an additional 25%; this reduction continues every 2 days until the 24-hour oral dose is 30 mg (morphine equivalent) per day. After 2 days on this minimum dose, the opioid is then discontinued.

PSEUDOADDICTION. Inadequate treatment of pain can lead to a phenomenon called *pseudoaddiction*.[36] This occurs when patients exhibit behaviors commonly associated with addiction (e.g., frequent requests for analgesic refills or higher dosages), but the behaviors resolve with adequate treatment of the patient's pain. These patients are often labeled as drug-seeking, which can result in a crisis of mistrust between the patient and the provider. This phenomenon can be avoided by effective communication strategies and optimal pain management.

ADDICTION. *Addiction* is a complex neurobiologic condition characterized by aberrant behaviors arising from a drive to obtain and take substances for reasons other than the prescribed therapeutic value (see Chapter 11). Tolerance and physical dependence are not indicators of addiction. Rather they are normal physiologic responses to chronic exposure to certain drugs, including opioids. Addiction rarely occurs in patients who receive opioids for pain control. If addiction is suspected, it needs to be investigated and diagnosed, if appropriate, but it should not be implied without evidence because this interferes with pain management. The hallmarks of addiction include (1) compulsive use, (2) loss of control of use, and (3) continued use despite risk of harm.

The risk of developing addiction is associated with certain factors, including younger age, personal or family history of substance abuse, and mood disorders. However, the risk of addiction should not prevent health care providers from using opioids to effectively treat moderate to severe acute and chronic pain. Professional organizations and government agencies have issued joint statements about the roles and responsibilities of health care professionals in the appropriate use of opioids for pain management.[37]

TABLE 9-17 PATIENT & CAREGIVER TEACHING GUIDE

Reducing Barriers to Pain Management

When teaching the patient and caregiver about pain management, discuss the following barriers.

Barrier	Nursing Considerations
Fear of addiction	• Explain that addiction is uncommon in patients taking opioids for pain.
Fear of tolerance	• Teach that tolerance is a normal physiologic response to chronic opioid therapy. If tolerance does develop, the drug may need to be changed (e.g., morphine in place of oxycodone). • Teach that there is no absolute upper limit to pure opioid agonists (e.g., morphine). Dosages can be increased, and patient should not save drugs for when the pain is worse. • Teach that tolerance develops more slowly to analgesic effects of opioids than to side effects (e.g., sedation, respiratory depression). Tolerance does not develop to constipation; thus, a regular bowel program should be started early.
Concern about side effects	• Teach methods to prevent and to treat common side effects. • Emphasize that side effects such as sedation and nausea decrease with time. • Explain that different drugs have unique side effects, and other pain drugs can be tried to reduce the specific side effect.
Fear of injections	• Explain that oral medicines are preferred. • Emphasize that even if oral route becomes unusable, transdermal or indwelling parenteral routes can be used rather than injections.
Desire to be "good" patient	• Explain that patients are partners in their care and that the partnership requires open communication of both the patient and the nurse. • Emphasize to patients that they have a responsibility to keep you informed about their pain.
Desire to be stoic	• Explain that although stoicism is a valued behavior in many cultures, failure to report pain can result in undertreatment and severe, unrelieved pain.
Forgetting to take analgesic	• Provide and teach use of pill containers. • Provide methods of record keeping for drug use. • Recruit caregivers to assist with the analgesic regimen.
Concern that pain indicates disease progression	• Explain that increased pain or the need for analgesics may reflect tolerance. • Emphasize that new pain may come from a non–life-threatening source (e.g., muscle spasm, urinary tract infection). • Institute drug and nondrug strategies to reduce anxiety. • Ensure that patient and caregivers have current, accurate, comprehensive information about the disease and prognosis. • Provide psychologic support.
Sense of fatalism	• Explain that pain can be managed in most patients. • Explain that most therapies require a period of trial and error. • Emphasize that side effects can be managed.
Ineffective medication	• Teach that there are multiple options within each category of medication (e.g., opioids, NSAIDs), and another medication from the same category may provide better relief. • Emphasize that finding the best treatment regimen often requires trial and error. • Incorporate nondrug approaches in treatment plan.

Adapted from Ersek M: Enhancing effective pain management by addressing patient barriers to analgesic use, *J Hospice Palliat Nurs* 1:87, 1999.
NSAIDs, Nonsteroidal antiinflammatory drugs.

In addition to the fears about addiction, physical dependence, and tolerance, other barriers hinder effective pain management. Table 9-17 lists some barriers and strategies to address them.

INSTITUTIONALIZING PAIN EDUCATION AND MANAGEMENT

Besides patient and caregiver barriers, other barriers to effective pain management include inadequate health care provider education and lack of organizational support. Traditionally, medical and nursing school curricula have spent little time teaching future physicians and nurses about pain and symptom management. The lack of emphasis on pain in medical and nursing schools has contributed to inadequate training of health care providers.

Progress has been made in overcoming these barriers. Medical and nursing schools now devote more time to addressing pain. Numerous professional organizations have published evidence-based guidelines for assessing and managing pain in many patient populations and clinical settings.

Researchers and health care providers have documented the central role that institutional commitment and practices have in changing clinical practice. Without institutional support, pain outcomes are unlikely to change. One major step in institutionalizing pain management is the development and adoption of The Joint Commission (TJC) guideline on pain.[37] TJC is the accrediting body for most health care facilities (hospitals, nursing homes, and health care clinics). Under these standards, health care facilities are required to (1) recognize the patient's right to appropriate assessment and management of pain; (2) identify pain in patients during their initial assessment and as needed, during ongoing, periodic reassessments; (3) educate health care providers about pain assessment and management and ensure competency; and, (4) educate patients and their families about pain management.

ETHICAL ISSUES IN PAIN MANAGEMENT

Fear of Hastening Death by Administering Analgesics

A common concern of health care professionals and caregivers is that providing sufficient drug to relieve pain will hasten or precipitate death of a terminally ill person. However, there is no scientific evidence that opioids can hasten death, even among patients at the very end of life. Moreover, as a nurse, you have a moral obligation to provide comfort and pain relief at the end of life. Even if there is a concern about the possibility of hastening death, the rule of double effect provides ethical justification. This rule states that if an unwanted consequence (i.e., hastened death) occurs as a result of an action taken to achieve a moral good (i.e., pain relief), the action is justified if the nurse's intent is to relieve pain and not to hasten death.[38]

Requests for Assisted Suicide

Unrelieved pain is one of the reasons that patients make requests for assisted suicide. Aggressive and adequate pain management may decrease the number of such requests. Assisted suicide is a complex issue that extends beyond pain and pain management. Currently Oregon, Washington, and Montana are the only states where assisted suicide is legal. To address the legal and ethical issues confronting nurses in this unique situation, the Oregon Nurses Association prepared a position paper on this topic.[39]

Use of Placebos in Pain Assessment and Treatment

Placebos are still sometimes used to assess and to treat pain. Using a placebo involves deceiving patients by making them believe that they are receiving an analgesic when in fact they are typically receiving an inert substance such as saline. The use of placebos to assess or treat pain is condemned by several professional organizations.[40]

GERONTOLOGIC CONSIDERATIONS

PAIN

Persistent pain is a common problem in older adults and is often associated with physical disability and psychosocial problems. The prevalence of chronic pain among community-dwelling older adults exceeds 50%, and among older nursing home patients it is approximately 80%. The most common painful conditions among older adults are musculoskeletal conditions such as osteoarthritis and low back pain. Chronic pain often results in depression, sleep disturbance, decreased mobility, increased health care utilization, and physical and social role dysfunction. Despite its high prevalence, pain in older adults is often inadequately assessed and treated.[41]

Several barriers to pain assessment in the older patient exist. Older adults and their health care providers often believe that pain is a normal, inevitable part of aging and that nothing can be done to relieve the pain. Older adults may not report pain for fear of being a "burden" or a "complainer." They may have greater fears of taking opioids than other age-groups. In addition, older patients are more likely to use words such as "aching," "soreness," or "discomfort" rather than "pain." For all these reasons, be persistent in asking older adults about pain. Carry out the assessment in an unhurried, supportive manner.

Another barrier to pain assessment in older adults is the increased prevalence of cognitive, sensory-perceptual, and motor problems that interfere with a person's ability to process information and to communicate. Examples include dementia and delirium, poststroke aphasia, and other communication barriers. Hearing and vision deficits may complicate assessment. Therefore pain assessment tools may need to be adapted for older adults. For example, it may be necessary to use a large-print pain intensity scale. Most older adults, even those with mild to moderate cognitive impairment, can use quantitative scales accurately and reliably.

In older patients with chronic pain, perform a thorough physical examination and history to identify causes of pain, possible therapies, and potential problems. Because depression and functional impairments are common among older adults with pain, they also must be assessed.

Treatment of pain in older adults is complicated by several factors. First, older adults metabolize drugs more slowly than younger people and thus are at greater risk for higher blood levels and adverse effects. The adage "start low and go slow" needs to be applied to analgesic therapy in this age-group. Second, the use of NSAIDs in older adults is associated with a high frequency of GI bleeding. Third, older adults often are taking many drugs for one or more chronic conditions. The addition of analgesics can result in dangerous drug interactions and increased side effects. Fourth, cognitive impairment and ataxia can be exacerbated by analgesics such as opioids, antidepressants, and antiseizure drugs. This requires that health care providers titrate drugs slowly and monitor carefully for side effects.

Treatment regimens for older adults must incorporate nondrug modalities. Exercise and patient teaching are important nondrug interventions for older adults with chronic pain. Also include family and caregivers in the treatment plan (see Table 9-17).

MANAGING PAIN IN SPECIAL POPULATIONS

Patients Unable to Self-Report Pain

Although patient self-report is the gold standard of pain assessment, many illnesses and conditions affect a patient's ability to report pain. These diagnoses and conditions include advanced dementia and other progressive neurologic diseases such as Parkinson's disease and multiple sclerosis, cerebrovascular disease, psychosis, and delirium. For these people, behavioral and physiologic changes may be the only indicators of pain. You must be astute at recognizing behavioral symptoms of pain.

A guide for assessing pain in nonverbal patients is presented in Table 9-18. Several scales have been developed to assess pain-related behaviors in nonverbal patients, particularly those with advanced dementia.[42,43] Several pain assessment tools for people with dementia are available at the City of Hope Pain and Palliative Care Resource Center website (http://prc.coh.org).

TABLE 9-18 ASSESSING PAIN IN NONVERBAL PATIENTS

The following assessment techniques are recommended.
- Obtain a self-report when possible (never assume a person is unable to give verbal report).
- Investigate potential causes of pain.
- Observe patient behaviors that indicate pain (e.g., grimacing, frowning, rubbing a painful area, groaning, restlessness).
- Obtain surrogate reports of pain from professional and family caregivers.
- Try to use analgesics and reassess the patient to observe for a decrease in pain-related behaviors.

Source: Position statement from the American Society for Pain Management Nursing (ASPMN). Modified from Herr K, Coyne PJ, Key T, et al: Pain assessment in the nonverbal patient: position statement with clinical practice recommendations, *Pain Manag Nurs* 7:44, 2006.

Patients With Substance Abuse Problems

Health care providers are often reluctant to administer opioids to substance-abusing patients for fear of promoting or enhancing addictions. However, there is no evidence that providing opioid analgesia to these patients in any way worsens their addictive disease. In fact, the stress of unrelieved pain may contribute to relapse in the recovering patient or increased drug use in the patient who is actively abusing drugs.[44]

Guidelines for pain management in patients with addictive disease have been established by the American Society for Pain Management Nursing.[45] These guidelines reflect your role in a team approach in which patients with addictive disease and pain have the right to be treated with dignity, respect, and the same quality of pain assessment and management as all other patients.

If the patient acknowledges opioid use, it is important to determine the types and amounts of drugs used. It is best to avoid exposing the patient to the drug of abuse, and effective equianalgesic doses of other opioids may be determined if daily drug doses are known. If a history of drug abuse is unknown or if the patient does not acknowledge substance abuse, you should suspect abuse when normal doses of analgesics do not relieve the patient's pain.

Aggressive behavior patterns and signs of withdrawal may also occur. Withdrawal symptoms can exacerbate pain and lead to drug-seeking behavior or illicit drug use. Toxicology screens may be helpful in determining recently used drugs. Discussing these findings with the patient may help gain the patient's cooperation in pain control.

Severe pain should be treated with opioids, and at much higher doses than those used with drug-naive patients. The use of a single opioid is preferred. Avoid using a mixed opioid agonist-antagonist such as butorphanol or a partial agonist such as buprenorphine because these drugs may precipitate withdrawal symptoms. Nonopioid and adjuvant analgesics and nondrug pain relief measures may also be used as appropriate. To maintain opioid blood levels and prevent withdrawal symptoms, provide analgesics around the clock. Use supplemental doses to treat breakthrough pain. IV or PCA infusions may be considered for acute pain management.[38]

Pain management for people with addiction is challenging and requires an interdisciplinary team approach. When possible, the team includes pain management and addiction specialists. Team members need to be aware of their own attitudes about people with substance abuse problems, which may result in undertreatment of pain.

CASE STUDY

Pain

Ryan McVay/Photodisc/
Thinkstock

Patient Profile

K.C. is a 280-lb (127-kg) 68-year-old African American woman with diabetes who was admitted for an incision and drainage of a right abdominal abscess. She is being discharged on her second postoperative day. Her married daughter will assist with dressing changes at home.

Subjective Data

• Lives alone
• Desires 0 pain but will accept 1 or 2 on a scale of 0 to 10
• Reports incision area pain as a 2 or 3 between dressing changes and as a 6 during dressing changes
• States sharp pain persists 1 to 2 hours after dressing change
• Reports pain between dressing changes controlled by two Percocet tablets
• Has history of fibromyalgia and is complaining of pain "everywhere"

Objective Data

• Requires qid dressing changes after discharge
• For discharge, Percocet (two tablets q4hr for pain PRN) is prescribed

Discussion Questions

1. Describe the assessment data that are important for determining whether K.C. has adequate pain management.
2. How long should the daughter wait after the Percocet is given to begin the dressing change?
3. What additional pain therapies might you plan to help K.C. through the dressing change?
4. *Priority Decision:* What are the priority nursing interventions for K.C.?
5. What side effects might she experience because of her pain medication? How can these be managed?
6. *Delegation Decision:* To whom can you delegate teaching K.C. and her daughter the plan of care at home?
7. *Priority Decision:* Based on the data presented, what are the priority nursing diagnoses? Are there any collaborative problems?
8. *Evidence-Based Practice:* K.C.'s daughter asks you if any other strategies could be used to help decrease her mother's incisional pain and her overall fibromyalgia pain.

evolve Answers available at *http://evolve.elsevier.com/Lewis/medsurg.*

BRIDGE TO NCLEX EXAMINATION

The number of the question corresponds to the same-numbered outcome at the beginning of the chapter.

1. Pain is best described as
   a. a creation of a person's imagination.
   b. an unpleasant, subjective experience.
   c. a maladaptive response to a stimulus.
   d. a neurologic event resulting from activation of nociceptors.

2. A patient is receiving a PCA infusion after surgery to repair a hip fracture. She is sleeping soundly but awakens when the nurse speaks to her in a normal tone of voice. Her respirations are 8 breaths/minute. The most appropriate nursing action in this situation is to
   a. stop the PCA infusion.
   b. obtain an oxygen saturation level.
   c. continue to closely monitor the patient.
   d. administer naloxone and contact the physician.

3. Which words are most likely to be used to describe neuropathic pain *(select all that apply)?*
   a. Dull
   b. Mild
   c. Burning
   d. Shooting
   e. Shock-like

4. Unrelieved pain is
   a. expected after major surgery.
   b. expected in a person with cancer.
   c. dangerous and can lead to many physical and psychologic complications.
   d. an annoying sensation, but it is not as important as other physical care needs.

5. A cancer patient who reports ongoing, constant moderate pain with short periods of severe pain during dressing changes is
   a. probably exaggerating his pain.
   b. best treated by referral for surgical treatment of his pain.
   c. best treated by receiving both a long-acting and a short-acting opioid.
   d. best treated by regularly scheduled short-acting opioids plus acetaminophen.

6. An example of distraction to provide pain relief is
   a. TENS.
   b. music.
   c. exercise.
   d. biofeedback.

7. Appropriate nonopioid analgesics for mild pain include *(select all that apply)*
   a. oxycodone.
   b. ibuprofen (Advil).
   c. lorazepam (Ativan).
   d. acetaminophen (Tylenol).
   e. codeine with acetaminophen (Tylenol #3).

8. An important nursing responsibility related to pain is to
   a. leave the patient alone to rest.
   b. help the patient appear to not be in pain.
   c. believe what the patient says about the pain.
   d. assume responsibility for eliminating the patient's pain.

9. Providing opioids to a dying patient who is experiencing moderate to severe pain
   a. may cause addiction.
   b. will probably be ineffective.
   c. is an appropriate nursing action.
   d. will likely hasten the person's death.

10. A nurse believes that patients with the same type of tissue injury should have the same amount of pain. This statement reflects
    a. a belief that will contribute to appropriate pain management.
    b. an accurate statement about pain mechanisms and an expected goal of pain therapy.
    c. a belief that will have no effect on the type of care provided to people in pain.
    d. a lack of knowledge about pain mechanisms, which is likely to contribute to poor pain management.

1. b, 2. c, 3. c, d, e, 4. c, 5. c, 6. b, 7. b, d, 8. c, 9. c, 10. d.

ⓔvolve

For rationales to these answers and even more NCLEX review questions, visit *http://evolve.elsevier.com/Lewis/medsurg*.

REFERENCES

1. National Center of Health Statistics: *Health, United States, 2007, with chartbook on trends in the health of Americans*, Hyattsville, Md, 2007, US Government Printing Office.

2. Institute of Medicine Report from the Committee on Advancing Pain Research, Care, and Education: *Relieving pain in America: a blueprint for transforming prevention, care, education, and research*, Washington, DC, 2011, National Academies Press.

3. American Pain Foundation: Pain facts and figures. Retrieved from *www.painfoundation.org*.

4. Centers for Disease Control and Prevention, National Center for Health Statistics: *Health, United States, 2010, with chartbook on special feature on death and dying*, Hyattsville, Md, 2010, US Government Printing Office.

5. Christo PJ, Mazloomdoost D: Cancer pain and analgesia, *Ann NY Acad Sci* 1138:278, 2008.

6. McCaffery M: *Nursing practice theories related to cognition, bodily pain and man-environmental interactions*, Los Angeles, 1968, UCLA Students Store. (Classic)

7. Keefe FJ: Behavioral medicine: a voyage to the future, *Ann Behav Med* 41:141, 2011.

*8. Lucchetti G, Lucchetti AG, Badan-Neto AM, et al: Religiousness affects mental health, pain and quality of life in older people in an outpatient rehabilitation setting, *J Rehabil Med* 43:316, 2011.

*9. Riddle DL, Keefe FJ, Nay WT, et al: Pain coping skills training for patients with elevated pain catastrophizing who are scheduled for knee arthroplasty: a quasi-experimental study, *Arch Phys Med Rehabil* 92:859, 2011.

10. Tan AM, Waxman SG: Spinal cord injury, dendritic spine remodeling, and spinal memory mechanisms, *Exp Neurol* 235:142, 2012.

11. Cohen SP, Liao W, Gupta A, et al: Ketamine in pain management, *Adv Psychosom Med* 30:139, 2011.

12. Davis KD: Neuroimaging of pain: what does it tell us? *Curr Opin Support Palliat Care* 5:116, 2011.

13. Neziri AY, Haesler S, Petersen-Felix S, et al: Generalized expansion of nociceptive reflex receptive fields in chronic pain patients, *Pain* 151:798, 2010.

14. O'Connor AB, Dworkin RH: Treatment of neuropathic pain: an overview of recent guidelines, *Am J Med* 122:S22, 2009.

15. Herr K, Bjoro K, Decker S: Tools for assessment of pain in nonverbal older adults with dementia: a state-of-the-science review, *J Pain Symptom Manage* 31:170, 2006.

*16. McGuire DB, Reifsnyder J, Soeken K, et al: Assessing pain in nonresponsive hospice patients: development and preliminary testing of the multidimensional objective pain assessment tool (MOPAT), *J Palliat Med* 14:287, 2011.

*Evidence-based information for clinical practice.

*17. Gordon DB, Dahl J, Phillips P, et al: The use of "as-needed" range orders for opioid analgesic in the management of acute pain: a consensus statement of the American Society of Pain Management Nurses and the American Pain Society, *Pain Manag Nurs* 5:53, 2004. (Classic)

18. Kolcaba K: Evolution of the mid range theory of comfort for outcomes research, *Nurs Outlook* 49:86, 2001. (Classic)

19. Fouladbakhsh JM, Szczesny S, Jenuwine ES, et al: Nondrug therapies for pain management among rural older adults, *Pain Manag Nurs* 12:70, 2011.

20. Jarzyna D, Jungquist CR, Pasero C, et al: American Society for Pain Management Nursing guidelines on monitoring for opioid-induced sedation and respiratory depression, *Pain Manag Nurs* 12:118, 2011.

21. Sinatra RS, Jahr JS, Reynolds L, et al: Intravenous acetaminophen for pain after major orthopedic surgery: an expanded analysis, *Pain Pract* 12:357, 2011.

22. Lanza FL, Chan FK, Quigley EM: Guidelines for prevention of NSAID-related ulcer complications, *Am J Gastroenterol* 104:728, 2009.

23. Roth SH, Anderson S: The NSAID dilemma: managing osteoarthritis in high-risk patients, *Phys Sportsmed* 39:62, 2011.

24. Vadivelu N, Timchenko A, Huang Y, et al: Tapentadol extended-release for treatment of chronic pain: a review, *J Pain Res* 4:211, 2011.

25. Micromedex® Healthcare Series [Internet database]. Greenwood Village, Colo: Thomson Reuters (Healthcare) Inc. Updated periodically.

26. Abrams DI, Couey P, Shade SB, et al: Cannabinoid-opioid interaction in chronic pain, *Clin Pharmacol Ther* 90:844, 2011.

27. GW Pharmaceuticals: Sativex. Retrieved from *www.gwpharm.com/Sativex.aspx*.

28. Shaheen PE, Walsh D, Lasheen W, et al: Opioid equianalgesic tables: are they all equally dangerous? *J Pain Symptom Manage* 38:409, 2009.

29. Falowski S, Celii A, Sharan A: Spinal cord stimulation: an update, *Neurotherapeutics* 5:86, 2008.

*30. Reid MC, Papaleontiou M, Ong A, et al: Self-management strategies to reduce pain and improve function among older adults in community settings: a review of the evidence, *Pain Med* 9:409, 2008.

*31. Cherkin DC, Sherman KJ, Kahn J, et al: A comparison of the effects of two types of massage and usual care on chronic low back pain: a randomized, controlled trial, *Ann Intern Med* 155:1, 2011.

*32. Marinko LN, Chacko JM, Dalton D, et al: The effectiveness of therapeutic exercise for painful shoulder conditions: a meta analysis, *J Shoulder Elbow Surg* 20:1351, 2011.

*33. Wanich T, Gelber J, Rodeo S, et al: Percutaneous neuromodulation pain therapy following knee replacement, *J Knee Surg* 24:197, 2011.

*34. Bernardy K, Fuber N, Klose P, et al: Efficacy of hypnosis/guided imagery in fibromyalgia syndrome—a systematic review and meta-analysis of controlled trials, *BMC Musculoskelet Disord* 12:133, 2011.

35. Tracy MF, Chlan L: Nonpharmacological interventions to manage common symptoms in patients receiving mechanical ventilation, *Crit Care Nurse* 31:19, 2011.

36. Bell K, Salmon A: Pain, physical dependence and pseudoaddiction: redefining addiction for 'nice' people? *Int J Drug Policy* 20:170, 2009.

37. The Joint Commission: Standard on pain assessment and management. Retrieved from *www.jointcommission.org*.

38. Beauchamp T, Childress J: *Principles of biomedical ethics*, New York, 2009, Oxford University Press.

39. Oregon Nurses Association: ONA provides guidance on nurses' dilemma. Retrieved from *www.oregonrn.org/associations/3019/files/AssistedSuicide.pdf*.

40. American Society for Pain Management Nursing: Position statement on the use of placebos in pain management. Retrieved from *www.aspmn.org/pdfs/Use%20of%20Placebos.pdf*.

*41. Ersek M, Polissar N, Neradilek MB: Development of a composite pain measure for people with advanced dementia: exploratory analyses in self-reporting nursing home residents, *J Pain Symptom Manage* 41:566, 2011.

*42. Jordon A, Regnard C, O'Brien JT, et al: Pain and distress in advanced dementia: choosing the right tools for the job, *Palliat Med* 26:873, 2012.

*43. Paulson-Conger M, Leske J, Maidl C, et al: Comparison of two pain assessment tools in nonverbal critical care patients, *Pain Manag Nurs* 12:218, 2011.

44. Ling W, Mooney L, Hillhouse M: Prescription opioid abuse, pain, and addiction: clinical issues and implications, *Drug Alcohol Rev* 30:300, 2011.

45. American Society for Pain Management Nursing: Pain management in patients with addictive disease. Retrieved from *www.aspmn.org/Organization/documents/addictions_9pt.pdf*.

RESOURCES

American Academy of Pain Management
www.aapainmanage.org
American Academy of Pain Medicine (AAPM)
www.painmed.org
American Chronic Pain Association
www.theacpa.org
American Pain Society
www.ampainsoc.org
American Society for Pain Management Nursing
www.aspmn.org
City of Hope Pain and Palliative Care Resource Center
http://prc.coh.org
International Association for the Study of Pain (IASP)
www.iasp-pain.org
Pain Link
www2.edc.org/painlink

10

Palliative Care at End of Life

Margaret McLean Heitkemper

> *You matter because you are you. You matter to the last moment of your life, and we will do all we can, not only to help you die peacefully, but also to live until you die.*
>
> *Dame Cicely Saunders*

ⓔvolve WEBSITE

http://evolve.elsevier.com/Lewis/medsurg

- NCLEX Review Questions
- Key Points
- Pre-Test

- Rationales for Bridge to NCLEX Examination Questions
- Case Study
  - Patient With Chronic Myelogenous Leukemia Including End-of-life Care

- Concept Map Creator
- Glossary
- Content Updates

LEARNING OUTCOMES

1. Discuss the purpose of palliative care.
2. Describe the purpose of and services provided by hospice.
3. Describe the physical and psychologic manifestations at the end of life.
4. Explain the process of grief and bereavement at the end of life.
5. Describe the nursing management for the dying patient.
6. Examine the cultural and spiritual issues related to end-of-life care.
7. Discuss ethical and legal issues in end-of-life care.
8. Explore the special needs of family caregivers in end-of-life care.
9. Discuss the special needs of the nurse who cares for dying patients and their families.

KEY TERMS

advance directives, p. 146
bereavement, p. 143
brain death, p. 142
Cheyne-Stokes respiration, p. 142

death, p. 142
death rattle, p. 142
end of life, p. 142
grief, p. 143

hospice, p. 141
palliative care, p. 140
spirituality, p. 144

PALLIATIVE CARE

Palliative care is any form of care or treatment that focuses on reducing the severity of disease symptoms, rather than trying to delay or reverse the progression of the disease itself or provide a cure. The overall goals of palliative care are to (1) prevent and relieve suffering and (2) improve quality of life for patients with serious, life-limiting illnesses (Fig. 10-1). Specific goals of palliative care are listed in Table 10-1.

Palliative care originated as end-of-life (EOL) care in the 1960s. Initially this care focused on providing the relief of symptoms and emotional support to the patient, family, and significant others during the terminal phase of a serious life-limiting disease. Now that phase of palliative care is called palliative care at end-of-life, which is the focus of this chapter. Since its beginning, the scope of palliative care has greatly expanded. Now palliative care focuses on maintaining and improving the quality of life for all patients and their families during any stage of a life-limiting illness, whether acute, chronic, or terminal.

According to the World Health Organization (WHO), palliative care is an approach that improves the quality of life of patients and their families who face problems associated with life-threatening illness. Palliative care aims to prevent and relieve suffering by early identification, assessment, and treatment of pain and other types of physical, psychologic, emotional, and spiritual distress.[1] Ideally, all patients receiving curative or restorative health care should receive palliative care concurrently. Palliative care extends into the period of EOL care; bereavement care follows the patient's death[2] (Fig. 10-2).

To optimize the benefits of palliative care, it should be initiated after a person receives a diagnosis of a life-limiting

TABLE 10-1 GOALS OF PALLIATIVE CARE

- Provide relief from symptoms, including pain.
- Regard dying as a normal process.
- Affirm life and neither hasten nor postpone death.
- Support holistic patient care and enhance quality of life.
- Offer support to patients to live as actively as possible until death.
- Offer support to the family during the patient's illness and in their own bereavement.

Adapted from World Health Organization: WHO definition of palliative care. Retrieved from *www.who.int/cancer/palliative/definition/en.*

Reviewed by Lynn F. Reinke, PhD, ARNP, Research Investigator/Pulmonary Nurse Practitioner, VA Puget Sound Health Care System, Health Services R&D, Seattle, Washington; and Arlene H. Morris, RN, EdD, CNE, Distinguished Teaching Associate Professor of Nursing, Auburn University Montgomery, Montgomery, Alabama.

FIG. 10-1 One goal of palliative care is to improve the quality of the patient's remaining life.

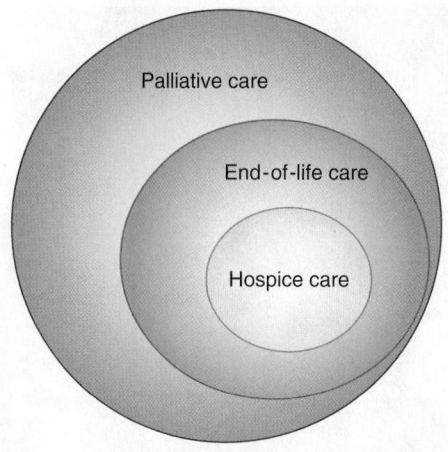

FIG. 10-3 Relationship of palliative care, end-of-life care, and hospice care.

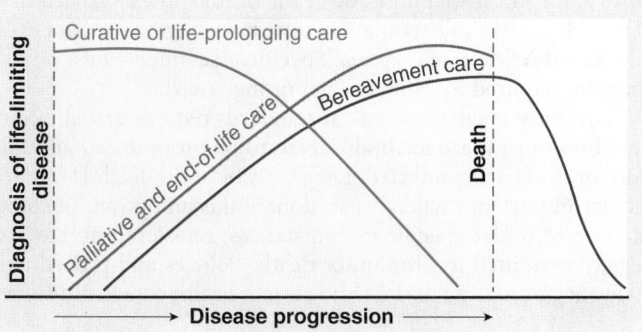

FIG. 10-2 Integrated model of curative care, palliative and end-of-life care, and bereavement care.

FIG. 10-4 Hospice care is designed to provide compassion, concern, and support for the dying.

illness, such as cancer, heart failure, chronic obstructive pulmonary disease, dementia, or end-stage kidney disease. Ideally, the palliative care team is an interdisciplinary collaboration involving physicians, social workers, pharmacists, nurses, chaplains, and other health care professionals. Communication among the patient, family, and palliative health care team is important to provide optimal care. Patients receive palliative care services in the home and in long-term and acute care facilities. More recently, emergency departments and intensive care units (ICUs) have integrated palliative care into the delivery of care. Many institutions have established interdisciplinary palliative and hospice care teams.[3]

HOSPICE CARE

Palliative care often includes hospice care before or at the end of life (Fig. 10-3). **Hospice** is not a place but a concept of care that provides compassion, concern, and support for the dying (Fig. 10-4). Hospice exists to provide support and care for persons in the last phases of a terminal disease so that they might live as fully and as comfortable as possible. Hospice programs provide care with an emphasis on symptom management, advance care planning, spiritual care, and family support.[4]

The major difference between palliative care and hospice care is that palliative care allows a person to simultaneously receive curative and palliative treatments. Hospice care is provided once a person decides to forgo curative treatments.

Approximately 1.5 million patients every year receive services through hospice programs. About 42% of the patients who die in the United States are under the care of a hospice program.[5] More than a third of all hospice patients are 85 years of age or older, and 83% are over 65. Of these patients, the most common diagnosis is cancer. Eighty percent of patients using hospice services are white.[5] Currently the median length of stay in a hospice program is 21 days.

Hospice programs are organized under a variety of models. Some are hospital-based programs, others are part of existing home health care agencies, and others are freestanding or community-based programs. However, regardless of their organization, all hospices emphasize palliative rather than curative care, and quality rather than quantity of life.

Hospice care is provided in a variety of locations, including the home, inpatient settings, and long-term care facilities. Hospice care can be on a part-time, intermittent, on-call, regularly scheduled, or continuous basis. Hospice services are available 24 hours a day, 7 days a week to provide help to patients and families in their homes. The inpatient hospice settings have been deinstitutionalized to make the atmosphere as relaxed and homelike as possible (Fig. 10-5). Staff and volunteers are available for the patient and the family.

A medically supervised interdisciplinary team of professionals and volunteers provides holistic hospice services. The hospice nurse plays a pivotal role in coordination of the hospice team.[6] Hospice nurses work collaboratively with hospice physicians, pharmacists, dietitians, physical therapists, social workers, cer-

FIG. 10-5 Inpatient hospice settings have been deinstitutionalized to make the atmosphere as relaxed and homelike as possible. (Photodisc/Thinkstock)

tified nursing assistants, chaplains and other clergy, and volunteers to provide care and support to the patient and the family. Hospice nurses are educated in pain control and symptom management, spiritual assessment, and assessment and management of family needs. To meet patient and family needs, hospice nurses need excellent teaching skills, compassion, flexibility, cultural competence, and adaptability.

The decision to begin hospice care is difficult for several reasons. Frequently patients, families, physicians, and other health care providers lack information about hospice care. Some cultural/ethnic groups may underutilize hospice because of lack of awareness of hospice services, desire to continue with potentially curative therapies, and concerns about lack of minority hospice workers.[7] Physicians may be reluctant to give referrals because they sometimes view a patient's decline as their personal failure. Some patients or family members see it as giving up.

Admission to a hospice program has two criteria. The first criterion is that the patient must desire the services and agree in writing that only hospice care (and not curative care) can be used to treat the terminal illness. Patients in hospice programs can withdraw from the program at any time (e.g., if their condition unexpectedly improves). Patients can receive care for other health problems that begin after starting hospice.

The second criterion is that the patient must be considered eligible for hospice. Medicare, Medicaid, and other insurers require that two physicians certify that the patient's prognosis is terminal, with less than 6 months to live. It is important to realize that the physician who certified that a hospice patient is terminal does not "guarantee" death within 6 months. Indeed, if a patient in hospice survives beyond 6 months, Medicare and other reimbursement organizations will continue to reimburse for more extended periods of treatment if the patient still meets enrollment criteria. After this initial certification, only one physician (e.g., the hospice medical director) is needed to recertify the patient.

DEATH

Death occurs when all vital organs and body systems cease to function. It is the irreversible cessation of cardiovascular, respiratory, and brain function.

Brain death is an irreversible loss of all brain functions, including those of the brainstem. Brain death is a clinical diagnosis, and it can be made in patients whose hearts continue to beat and who are maintained on mechanical ventilation in the ICU.[8] Brain death occurs when the cerebral cortex stops functioning or is irreversibly destroyed.

Since the development of technology that assists in supporting life, controversies have arisen over the exact definition of death. Questions and discussions have focused on whether brain death occurs when the whole brain (cortex and brainstem) ceases activity or when function of the cortex alone stops. In 1995 the Quality Standards Subcommittee of the American Academy of Neurology recommended diagnostic criteria guidelines for clinical diagnosis of brain death.[9] These criteria for brain death include coma or unresponsiveness, absence of brainstem reflexes, and apnea. Specific assessments by a physician are required to validate each of the criteria.[8,9]

Currently, legal and medical standards require that all brain function must cease for brain death to be pronounced and life support to be disconnected. Diagnosis of brain death is of particular importance when organ donation is an option. In some states and under specific circumstances, registered nurses are legally permitted to pronounce death. Policies and procedures may vary from state to state and among health care institutions.

END-OF-LIFE CARE

End of life generally refers to the final phase of a patient's illness when death is imminent. The time from diagnosis of a terminal illness to death varies considerably, depending on the patient's diagnosis and extent of disease.

The Institute of Medicine defines *end of life* as the period during which an individual copes with declining health from a terminal illness or from the frailties associated with advanced age, even if death is not clearly imminent.[10] In some cases it is obvious to health care providers that the patient is at the end of life, but in other cases they may be uncertain if the end is close at hand. This uncertainty adds to the challenge of answering common questions the patient and family may ask, such as "How much time is left?"

End-of-life care (EOL care) is the term used for issues and services related to death and dying. EOL care focuses on physical and psychosocial needs for the patient and the patient's family. The goals for EOL care are to (1) provide comfort and supportive care during the dying process, (2) improve the quality of the patient's remaining life, (3) help ensure a dignified death, and (4) provide emotional support to the family.

Physical Manifestations at End of Life

As death approaches, metabolism is reduced and the body gradually slows down until all functions end. Respiratory changes are common at the end of life. Respirations may be rapid or slow, shallow, and irregular. Breath sounds may become wet and noisy, both audibly and on auscultation. Noisy, wet-sounding respirations, termed the **death rattle,** are caused by mouth breathing and accumulation of mucus in the airways. **Cheyne-Stokes respiration** is a pattern of breathing characterized by

TABLE 10-2	PHYSICAL MANIFESTATIONS AT END OF LIFE

System	Manifestations
Sensory system	
Hearing	• Usually last sense to disappear
Touch	• Decreased sensation
	• Decreased perception of pain and touch
Taste and smell	• Decreased with disease progression
Sight	• Blurring of vision
	• Sinking and glazing of eyes
	• Blink reflex absent
	• Eyelids remain half-open
Cardiovascular system	• Increased heart rate; later slowing and weakening of pulse
	• Irregular rhythm
	• Decreased blood pressure
	• Delayed absorption of drugs administered intramuscularly or subcutaneously
Respiratory system	• Increased respiratory rate
	• Cheyne-Stokes respiration (pattern of respiration characterized by alternating periods of apnea and deep, rapid breathing)
	• Inability to cough or clear secretions resulting in grunting, gurgling, or noisy congested breathing (death rattle)
	• Irregular breathing, gradually slowing down to terminal gasps (may be described as guppy breathing)
Urinary system	• Gradual decrease in urine output
	• Incontinence of urine
	• Inability to urinate
Gastrointestinal system	• Slowing or cessation of GI function (may be enhanced by pain-relieving drugs)
	• Accumulation of gas
	• Distention and nausea
	• Loss of sphincter control, producing incontinence
	• Bowel movement before imminent death or at time of death
Musculoskeletal system	• Gradual loss of ability to move
	• Sagging of jaw resulting from loss of facial muscle tone
	• Difficulty speaking
	• Swallowing becoming more difficult
	• Difficulty maintaining body posture and alignment
	• Loss of gag reflex
	• Jerking seen in patients on large amounts of opioids
Integumentary system	• Mottling on hands, feet, arms, and legs
	• Cold, clammy skin
	• Cyanosis of nose, nail beds, knees
	• "Waxlike" skin when very near death

TABLE 10-3	PSYCHOSOCIAL MANIFESTATIONS AT END OF LIFE

- Altered decision making
- Anxiety about unfinished business
- Decreased socialization
- Fear of loneliness
- Fear of meaninglessness of one's life
- Fear of pain
- Helplessness
- Life review
- Peacefulness
- Restlessness
- Saying goodbyes
- Unusual communication
- Vision-like experiences
- Withdrawal

TABLE 10-4	KÜBLER-ROSS MODEL OF GRIEF	

Stage	What Person May Say	Characteristics
Denial	No, not me. It cannot be true.	Denies the loss has taken place and may withdraw. This response may last minutes to months.
Anger	Why me?	May be angry at the person who inflicted the hurt (even after death) or at the world for letting it happen. May be angry with self for letting an event (e.g., car accident) take place, even if nothing could have stopped it.
Bargaining	Yes me, but...	May make bargains with God, asking "If I do this, will you take away the loss?"
Depression	Yes me, and I am sad	Feels numb, although anger and sadness may remain underneath.
Acceptance	Yes me, but it is okay	Anger, sadness, and mourning have tapered off. Accepts the reality of the loss.

Adapted from Kübler-Ross E: *On death and dying,* New York, 1969, Macmillan. (Classic)

alternating periods of apnea and deep, rapid breathing. When respirations cease, the heart stops beating within a few minutes. The physical manifestations of approaching death are listed in Table 10-2.

Psychosocial Manifestations at End of Life

A variety of feelings and emotions can affect the dying patient and family at the end of life (Table 10-3). Most patients and families struggle with a terminal diagnosis and the realization that there is no cure. The patient and the family may feel overwhelmed, fearful, powerless, and fatigued. The family's response depends in part on the type and length of the illness and their relationship with the person.

The patient's needs and wishes must be respected. Patients need time to think and express their feelings. Response time to questions may be sluggish because of fatigue, weakness, and confusion.

Bereavement and Grief

Although the terms are often used interchangeably, *bereavement* refers to the state of loss, and *grief* refers to the reaction to loss. Bereavement is the period following the death of a loved one during which grief is experienced and mourning occurs. The time spent in bereavement depends on a number of factors, including how attached one was to the person who died and how much time was spent anticipating the loss.

Grief is a normal reaction to loss. Grief occurs in response to the real loss of a loved one and the loss of what might have been. Grief is dynamic and includes both psychologic and physiologic responses following a loss. Psychologic responses include anger, guilt, anxiety, sadness, depression, and despair. Physiologic reactions include sleeping problems, changes in appetite, physical problems, and illness.

Grief is a powerful emotional state that affects all aspects of a person's life. It is a complex and intense emotional experience. In the Kübler-Ross model of grief, there are five stages[11,12] (Table 10-4). Not every person experiences all the stages of grieving, and they are not always progressive in order. It is common to reach a stage and then go backward. For example, a person may have reached the stage of bargaining, and then revert back to the denial or anger stage.

Another model of grief is the grief wheel (Fig. 10-6). After a person experiences the loss, he or she feels *shock* (numbness, denial, inability to think straight). Then comes the *protest* stage where a person experiences anger, guilt, sadness, fear, and searching. Then comes the *disorganization* stage where a person feels despair, apathy, anxiety, and confusion. The next stage is *reorganization* where a person gradually returns to normal functioning, but he or she feels different. The final stage is the *new normal*. Eventually the destabilization experienced in grief resolves and a normal state can began. However, because of the loss, the normal state is not the same as before. The challenge is to accept the new normal. Trying to go back to the "old" normal (which is not there anymore) is what causes a great deal of anxiety and stress.

The manner in which a person grieves depends on factors such as the relationship with the person who has died (e.g., spouse, parent), physical and emotional coping resources, concurrent life stresses, cultural beliefs, and personality. Additional factors that affect the grief response include mental and physical health, economic resources, religious influences or spiritual beliefs, family relationships, social support, and time spent preparing for the death. Issues that occurred before the death (e.g., marital problems) may affect the grief response.[13]

The grief experience for the caregiver of the patient with a chronic illness often begins long before the actual death event. This is called *anticipatory grief*. Patients at the end of life can also experience anticipatory grief.

Working in a positive way through the grief process helps to adapt to the loss.[14] Grief that assists the person in accepting the reality of death is called *adaptive grief*, which is a healthy response. It may be associated with grieving before a death

actually occurs or when the inevitability of the death is known. Indicators of adaptive grief include the ability to see some good resulting from the death and positive memories of the deceased person.

Dysfunctional reactions to loss can occur, and the physical and psychologic impact of the loved one's death may persist for years. *Prolonged grief disorder,* formerly called *complicated grief,* is a term used to describe prolonged and intense mourning. Prolonged grief disorder can include symptoms such as recurrent and severe distressing emotions and intrusive thoughts related to the loss of a loved one, self-neglect, and denial of the loss for longer than 6 months. Bereaved individuals with prolonged grief disorder may feel "stuck" and unable to move forward after the death of a loved one. It is estimated that one in five bereaved individuals experiences prolonged grief disorder. Those who experience prolonged grief disorder are at great risk for illness and have work and social impairments. Some studies suggest that prolonged grief disorder is less likely to occur after deaths in hospice compared with those in acute care settings.[15]

Bereavement and grief counseling is an important aspect of palliative care. The goal of a bereavement program is to provide support and to assist survivors in the transition to a life without the deceased person. Incorporate grief support into the plan of care for the family and significant others during the patient's illness and after the death.

Priority interventions for grief must focus on providing an environment that allows the patient and the family to express their feelings such as anger, fear, and guilt. Discussion of feelings helps both the patient and the family work toward resolution of the grief process. Respect for the patient's privacy and need or desire to talk (or not to talk) is important. Honesty in answering questions and giving information is essential.

Spiritual Needs
Assessment of spiritual needs in EOL care is a key consideration (Table 10-5). Spiritual needs do not necessarily equate to religion. Spirituality is defined as those beliefs, values, and practices that relate to the search for existential meaning and purpose and that may or may not include a belief in a higher power.[16] A person may not be part of a particular religion but have a deep spirituality. Many times at the end of life, patients question their beliefs about a higher power, their journey through life, religion, and an afterlife (Fig. 10-7). Some patients may choose to pursue

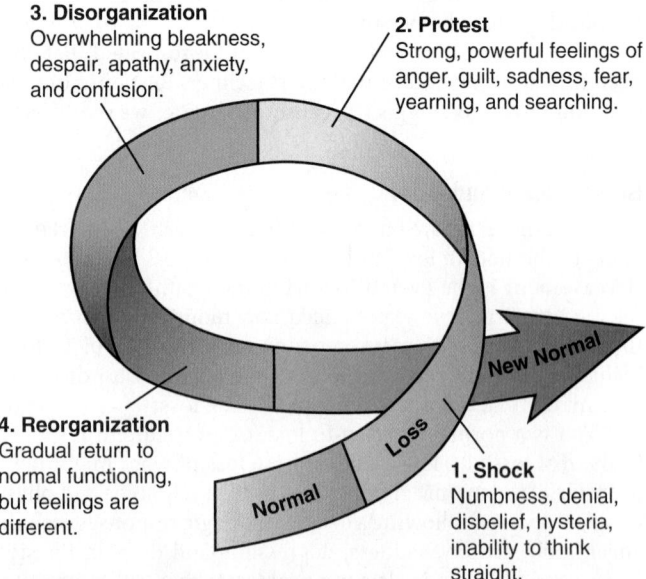

3. Disorganization Overwhelming bleakness, despair, apathy, anxiety, and confusion.

2. Protest Strong, powerful feelings of anger, guilt, sadness, fear, yearning, and searching.

4. Reorganization Gradual return to normal functioning, but feelings are different.

New Normal

Loss

Normal

1. Shock Numbness, denial, disbelief, hysteria, inability to think straight.

FIG. 10-6 The grief wheel model begins with the normal state at the bottom. After a person goes through the grief process, eventually the grief will resolve. However, because of the loss, the normal state is not the same as before. The challenge is to accept the "new normal." (Adapted from Powell TJ: *Stress-free living,* Dorling Kindersley Ltd 2000. © Dorling Kindersley Ltd.)

TABLE 10-5 SPIRITUAL ASSESSMENT
1. Who or what provides you strength and hope?
2. Do you use prayer in your life?
3. How do you express spirituality?
4. How would you describe your philosophy of life?
5. What type of spiritual or religious support do you desire?
6. What is the name of your clergy, minister, chaplain, pastor, rabbi?
7. What does suffering mean to you?
8. What does dying mean to you?
9. What are your spiritual goals?
10. Is there a role of church/synagogue in your life?
11. Has belief in God been important in your life?
12. How does your faith help you cope with illness?
13. How do you keep going day after day?
14. What helps you get through this health care experience?
15. How has illness affected you and your family?

© The Joint Commission. Adapted with permission.

FIG. 10-7 Spiritual needs are an important consideration in end-of-life care. (Photodisc/Thinkstock)

a spiritual path. Some may not. Respect an individual's choice. Assess the patient's and the family's preferences related to spiritual guidance or pastoral care services and make appropriate referrals.[16]

Deep-seated spiritual beliefs may surface for some patients when they deal with their terminal diagnosis and related issues. Spiritual distress may occur.[17] Characteristics of spiritual distress include anger toward God or a higher being, change in behavior and mood, desire for spiritual assistance, or displaced anger toward clergy.[16]

Spirituality has been associated with decreased despair in patients at the end of life. Some dying patients are secure in their faith about the future. It is common to observe patients relinquishing material possessions of life and focusing on values that they believe will lead them on to another place. Many turn to religion because it may provide order to the world even in the presence of physical decline, social losses, suffering, and impending death. Religion may offer an existential meaning that offers a sense of peace and recognition of one's place in the broader cosmic context.[17]

> The loss of a loved person is one of the most intensely painful experiences any human being can suffer.
> John Bowlby

CULTURALLY COMPETENT CARE

END OF LIFE

Culture and ethnicity should be considered throughout the EOL process. Cultural beliefs affect a person's understanding of and reaction to death or loss. In some cultural/ethnic groups, death and dying are private matters shared only with significant others. Often feelings are repressed or internalized. People who believe in "toughing it out" or "being strong" may not express themselves when they are experiencing a loss. Some cultural groups, such as African Americans and Hispanic/Latinos, may easily express their feelings and emotions. Kinship tends to be strong in the Hispanic culture, and both immediate and extended family provide support for one another. Expressing feelings of loss is encouraged and accepted easily.[18,19]

If palliative or hospice care is recommended, some cultural/ethnic groups are less likely to use these resources. For example,

African Americans use hospice care less often because they value "toughness" in times of hardship and rely on God.[18] For Hispanics, often spouses and daughters need to be involved in decisions regarding palliative care and hospice.[20] Consider patient attitudes toward death and suffering and preferences for information. The decision to use palliative care or hospice services may be perceived as "giving up" or receiving second-rate care. Such attitudes are best approached through clear, open discussions with the patient and the family about the philosophy and services of palliative and hospice organizations.[18-21] Culture and ethnicity affect decision making with regard to life support and withholding and withdrawing of treatments.[22] In some cultures, such as the Filipino American culture, it may be appropriate to first discuss a terminal diagnosis with the family before informing the patient.

Rituals associated with dying are part of all cultures.[18] In certain cultures the family may want to keep constant vigil in the room of a dying patient or in the waiting area. For example, some Jewish Americans believe that the spirit should not be alone when it leaves the body at the time of death. Therefore someone who is terminally ill should never be left alone. The Jewish culture believes all body tissues must be buried with the individual. Once a death has occurred, some cultures, such as the Puerto Rican American culture, may want to kiss and touch the body to say goodbye.

Families with non–English-speaking members are at risk for receiving less information about their family member's critical illness and prognosis.[23] Cultural variations also exist in symptom expression (e.g., pain expression) and use of health care services. Providing culturally competent care requires assessment of nonverbal cues such as grimaces, body position, and decreased or guarded movements. Issues related to pain assessment and management are discussed in Chapter 9.

Differences among cultural beliefs and values in relation to death and dying are innumerable. Nursing assessment of beliefs and preferences should be made on an individual basis to avoid stereotyping individuals with different cultural belief systems. This includes assessing and documenting the patient's cultural background, concerns, health practices, and attitudes about suffering. Early in the assessment, ask the patient and family to describe their desires for care before death and care of the body after death. Use open-ended questions related to the patient's perspectives on his or her illness and the patient's expectations of care. Use this assessment to guide the patient's plan of care and evaluation. You can also suggest or plan grief and bereavement counseling for the family. At the same time, accommodations need to be made related to the patient's language, diet, and cultural beliefs and practices. When appropriate, access medical interpreter services so that the patient's wishes are known. (Culturally competent care is discussed in Chapter 2.)

LEGAL AND ETHICAL ISSUES AFFECTING END-OF-LIFE CARE

Patients and families struggle with many decisions during the terminal illness and dying experience. Many people decide that the outcomes related to their care should be based on their own wishes and values. It is important to provide information to assist patients with these decisions. The decisions may involve the choice for (1) organ and tissue donations, (2) advance directives (e.g., medical power of attorney, living wills), (3) resuscitation, (4) mechanical ventilation, and (5) feeding tube placement.

Organ and Tissue Donation

Persons who are legally competent may choose organ donation. Any body part or the entire body may be donated. The decision to donate organs or to provide anatomic gifts may be made by a person before death or by immediate family after death. Family permission must be obtained at the time of donation.[24]

Some people carry donor cards. Some states allow organ donation to be marked on drivers' licenses. The names of agencies that handle organ donation vary by state and community. Common names for such an agency might be the organ bank, organ-sharing network, and organ-sharing alliance. Both organ and tissue donations follow specific legal guidelines. Legal requirements and facility policies for organ or tissue donation must be followed. The physician must be notified immediately when organ donation is intended because some tissues must be used within hours after death.

Advance Care Planning and Advance Directives

Advance care planning is a process that involves having patients (1) think through their values and goals for treatment, (2) talk about their values and goals with others, and (3) document them. Advance directives are the written documents that provide information about the patient's wishes and his or her designated spokesperson (Table 10-6).

The first advance directive was known by laypersons as a *living will.* Most states have replaced the idea of living wills with *natural death acts,* which may include *directives to physicians* (DTPs), *durable power of attorney for health care* (DPAHC), and *medical power of attorney* (MPOA). Under the natural death acts, an individual can tell the physician exactly what treatment is or is not desired. Each state has its own unique requirements. Keep in mind that patients often change their minds about desired treatments as their disease state progresses. Therefore it is important to reassess a patient's advance directives. For cog-

nitively impaired older adults, consider the person's values and manner of life to make health care decisions consistent with decisions they made when they were cognitively intact.

Copies of state-specific forms can be obtained from local medical associations and on the Internet. However, a person may write his or her wishes without special forms. Verbal directives may be given to physicians with specific instructions in the presence of two witnesses. Attorneys and notaries may not be required. If the person is not capable of communicating his or her wishes, the surrogate decision maker (most often family or significant other) determines the measures that will or will not be taken. The physician and the nurse can discuss the options that are available with the family. Then it is important to document the family's decision.

Resuscitation

Cardiopulmonary resuscitation (CPR) has become common practice in health care. Patients who have respiratory or cardiac arrest are given CPR unless a *do-not-resuscitate (DNR) order* is given by the physician. A DNR order is a written medical order that documents a patient's wishes regarding resuscitation and, more important, the patient's desire to avoid CPR.[25]

The patient or the patient's family has the right to decide whether CPR will be used. It is no longer the sole decision of the physician. The American Nurses Association (ANA) supports the patient's right to self-determination and believes that nurses have a primary role in supporting the patient and family's decisions.[26]

A physician's order should be written concerning the patient's or family's wishes for the use of CPR. Several different types of CPR decisions can be made. Complete and total heroic measures, which may include CPR, drugs, and mechanical ventilation, can be referred to as a *full code.* Some people choose variations of the full code. A *chemical code* involves the

TABLE 10-6	COMMON DOCUMENTS USED IN END-OF-LIFE CARE	
Document	**Description**	**Special Considerations**
Advance directive	General term used to describe documents that give instructions about future medical care and treatments and who should make the decisions in the event the person is unable to communicate.	• Should comply with guidelines established by state of residence.
Directive to physicians	Written document specifying the patient's wish to be allowed to die without heroic or extraordinary measures.	• Indicates specific measures to be used or withheld.
Do not resuscitate (DNR)	Written physician's order instructing health care providers not to attempt CPR. DNR order often requested by family. Must be signed by a physician to be valid.	• Must indicate any specific measures to be used or withheld.
Durable power of attorney for health care	Term used by some states to describe a document used for listing the person(s) to make health care decisions should a patient become unable to make informed decisions for self.	• May be the same as medical power of attorney. • Indicates specific measures to be used or withheld.
Living will	Lay term used to describe any documents that give instructions about future medical care and treatments or the wish to be allowed to die without heroic or extraordinary measures should the patient be unable to communicate for self.	• Must identify specific treatments that a person wants or does not want at end of life.
Medical power of attorney	Term used by some states to describe a document used for listing the person(s) to make health care decisions should a patient become unable to make informed decisions for self.	• May be the same as durable power of attorney for health care, health care proxy, or appointment of a health care agent or surrogate. Specifies measures to be used or withheld. • Person appointed may be called a health care agent, surrogate, attorney-in-fact, or proxy.

CPR, Cardiopulmonary resuscitation.

use of drugs for resuscitation without the use of CPR. A "no code," or a DNR order, allows the person to die with comfort measures only and without the interference of technology. Some states have implemented a form called *out-of-hospital DNR* for use by terminally ill patients who wish to have no heroic measures used to prolong life after they leave an acute care facility.[27,28]

Allow natural death (AND) is a term being used to replace "no code" or DNR.[28] This term more accurately conveys what actually happens. It is also sometimes referred to as *"comfort measures only"* status, meaning that all comfort measures associated with pain control and symptom management are carried out, but the natural physiologic progression to death is not delayed or interrupted.

Withholding or withdrawing treatments must be included in an advance directive. The directive must clearly state what is to be done and what is not to be done. The ANA position statement on foregoing nutrition and hydration states that the decision to withhold artificial nutrition and hydration should be made by the patient or surrogate with the health care team.[26] For patients who are no longer receiving artificial nutrition and hydration, it is important to continue to provide expert nursing care.

Euthanasia is the deliberate act of hastening death. The ANA statement on active euthanasia states that the nurse should not participate in active euthanasia because such an act is in direct violation of the Code for Nurses, the ethical traditions and goals of the profession, and its covenant with society. As a nurse, you have an obligation to provide timely, humane, comprehensive, and compassionate EOL care.

You need to be aware of legal issues and the patient's wishes. Advance directives and organ donor information should be located in the medical record and identified on the patient's record and/or the nursing care plan. All caregivers responsible for the patient need to know the patient's wishes. Additionally, you are responsible for becoming familiar with state, local, and agency procedures in EOL care documentation.

NURSING MANAGEMENT
END OF LIFE

Nurses spend more time with patients near the end of life than any other health care professionals. Nursing care of terminally ill and dying patients is holistic and encompasses all psychosocial and physical needs. Respect, dignity, and comfort are important for the patient and the family. In addition, you need to recognize your own needs when dealing with grief and dying.

NURSING ASSESSMENT

Assessment of the terminally ill or dying patient varies with the patient's condition. Be sensitive and do not impose repeated, unnecessary assessments on the dying patient. When possible, use health history data that are available in the medical record rather than tiring the patient with an interview.

Document the specific event or change that brought the patient into the health care setting. Record the patient's medical diagnoses, medication profile, and allergies.

If the patient is alert, do a brief review of the body systems to detect important signs and symptoms. Assess for discomfort, pain, nausea, and dyspnea so that prompt interventions can be implemented. In addition, evaluate and manage co-morbidities

ETHICAL/LEGAL DILEMMAS
End-of-Life Care

Situation
A.P., a terminally ill 50-year-old woman with metastatic breast cancer, has developed severe bone pain that is not adequately controlled by her present dose of IV morphine. She moans at rest and verbalizes severe pain from any movement to reposition her. At the team conference the nurses discuss the need for more effective pain control, but are concerned that additional pain medicine could hasten her death.

Ethical/Legal Points for Consideration
- Adequate pain relief is an important outcome for all patients, especially patients who are terminally ill. The *principle of beneficence* means that care is provided to benefit patients. The goal of adequate pain control in the terminally ill to alleviate suffering is based on the *principle of nonmaleficence:* preventing or reducing harm to the patient. The secondary effect of hastening the patient's death is ethically justified; this is known as the concept of *double effect*.
- Legally, the *standard of care* is used to define the nursing acts that are required for safe and competent nursing practice. When the actual nursing care falls below the standard of care, it is considered negligent and unsafe, and the nurse is at risk for being found incompetent.
- In a court of law the standard of care in nursing is determined by nursing experts and evidence-based practices. The increasing use of technology to access the latest scientific findings is changing the standard of nursing care to a national, if not global, standard defined by research findings and nationally recognized expert testimony.
- In this situation the standard of care is that the patient will experience pain relief. Failure of the nurse to act assertively to achieve pain relief for the patient and failure to effectively use resources to obtain that pain relief will be considered below the standard of care and unsafe and incompetent practice.

Discussion Questions
1. What types of discussions need to occur among the health care team, patient, and family as the terminally ill patient approaches this phase of care?
2. Distinguish between promotion of comfort and relief of pain in dying patients, and between assisted suicide and euthanasia. (Use the American Nurses Association position statements at *www.ana.org*.)

or acute episodes of problems such as diabetes mellitus or headache. Elicit information about the patient's abilities, food and fluid intake, patterns of sleep and rest, and response to the stress of terminal illness. Assess the patient's ability to cope with the diagnosis and prognosis of the illness. Also determine the family's capacity to manage the needed care and to cope with the illness and its consequences.

The physical assessment is abbreviated and focuses on changes that accompany terminal illness and the specific disease process.[29] The frequency of assessment depends on the patient's stability, but assessment is done at least every 8 hours in the institutional setting. For patients cared for in their homes by hospice programs, assessment may occur weekly. As changes occur, assessment and documentation may need to be done more frequently. If the patient is in the final hours of life, the physical assessment may be limited to essential data.

Key elements of a social assessment include determining the relationships and patterns of communication among the family. If multiple family members are present, listen to varying concerns from different members. Differences in expectations and interpersonal conflict can result in family disruptions after the death of the loved one. Social assessment also includes evaluating the goals of the patient and the family.

As death approaches, monitor the patient for multiple systems that often are failing during the EOL period. This requires vigilance and attention to physical changes that are often subtle. Neurologic assessment is especially important and includes level of consciousness, presence of reflexes, and pupil responses. Evaluation of vital signs, skin color, and temperature indicates changes in circulation. Monitor and describe respiratory status, character and pattern of respirations, and characteristics of breath sounds. Monitor nutritional and fluid intake, urine output, and bowel function, since this provides assessment data for renal and gastrointestinal functioning. Assess skin condition on an ongoing basis because skin becomes fragile and may easily break down.

PLANNING

Planning and coordinating care at EOL must focus on the needs of the patient, family, and significant others. In some cases a family conference may be helpful to develop a coordinated plan of care.

Develop a comprehensive plan to support, teach, and evaluate patients and families. Nursing care goals during the last stages of life involve comfort measures and care of the patient's emotional and physical needs. These goals may also include determining where the patient would like to die and whether this is possible. For example, the patient may want to die at home, but the family may object.

The last hours or days of the patient experiencing brain death are frequently spent in the ICU. Planning for EOL care may be particularly challenging in the ICU environment. At this time, some families are approached about organ donation. Consultation from palliative care specialists may help the family plan and cope with EOL issues.

NURSING IMPLEMENTATION

Psychosocial care and physical care are interrelated for both the dying patient and family. Teaching them is an important part of EOL care. Families need ongoing information on the disease, the dying process, and any care that will be provided. They need information on how to cope with the many issues during this period of their lives. Denial and grieving may be barriers to learning and understanding at the end of life for both the patient and family.

PSYCHOSOCIAL CARE. As death approaches, respond appropriately to the patient's psychosocial manifestations at the end of life (Table 10-7).

Anxiety and Depression. Patients often exhibit signs of anxiety and depression during the EOL period. Anxiety is an uneasy feeling whose cause is not easily identified. Anxiety is frequently related to fear.

Causes of anxiety and depression may include uncontrolled pain and dyspnea, psychosocial factors related to the disease process or impending death, altered physiologic states, and drugs used in high dosages. Encouragement, support, and teaching decrease some of the anxiety and depression. Management of anxiety and depression may include both medications and nonpharmacologic interventions. Relaxation strategies such as relaxation breathing, muscle relaxation, music, and imagery may be useful (see Chapter 7).

Anger. Anger is a common and normal response to grief. A grieving person cannot be forced to accept the loss. The surviving family members may be angry with the dying loved one who is leaving them. Encourage the expression of feelings, but

TABLE 10-7   NURSING ASSESSMENT
Psychosocial Care at End of Life

Characteristic	Nursing Management
Withdrawal Patient near death may seem withdrawn from the physical environment, maintaining the ability to hear but unable to respond.	Converse as though the patient were alert, using a soft voice and gentle touch.
Unusual Communication This may indicate that an unresolved issue is preventing the dying person from letting go. Patient may become restless and agitated or perform repetitive tasks (may also indicate terminal delirium).	Encourage the family to talk with and reassure the dying person.
Vision-like Experiences Patient may talk to persons who are not there or see places and objects not visible. Vision-like experiences assist the dying person in coming to terms with meaning in life and transition from it.	Affirm the dying person's experience as a part of transition from this life.
Saying Goodbyes It is important for the patient and family to acknowledge their sadness, mutually forgive one another, and say goodbye.	Encourage the dying person and family to verbalize their feelings of sadness, loss, forgiveness; to touch, hug, cry. Allow the patient and family privacy to express their feelings and comfort one another.
Spiritual Needs Patient or family may request spiritual support such as the presence of a chaplain.	Encourage visit by appropriate spiritual care service provider, chaplain, or family member. Allow patient to express his or her spiritual needs.

at the same time realize how difficult it is to come to terms with loss. As a nurse, you may be the target of the anger. You need to understand what is happening and not react on a personal level.

Hopelessness and Powerlessness. Feelings of hopelessness and powerlessness are common at the EOL. Encourage realistic hope within the limits of the situation. Allow the patient and the family to deal with what is within their control, and help them to recognize what is beyond their control. When possible, support the patient's involvement in decision making about care to foster a sense of control and autonomy.

Fear. Fear is a typical feeling associated with dying. Four specific fears associated with dying are fear of pain, fear of shortness of breath, fear of loneliness and abandonment, and fear of meaninglessness.

Fear of Pain. Many people assume that pain always accompanies death. Physiologically, there is no absolute indication that death is always painful. Psychologically, pain may occur based on the anxieties and separations related to dying. Terminally ill patients who do experience physical pain should have pain-relieving drugs available. Assure the patient and the family that

FIG. 10-8 Dying patients typically want someone whom they know and trust to stay with them. (iStockphoto/Thinkstock)

drugs will be given promptly when needed and that side effects of drugs can and will be managed. Patients can participate in their own pain relief by discussing pain relief measures and their effects. Most patients want their pain relieved without the side effects of grogginess or sleepiness. Pain relief measures do not need to deprive the patient of the ability to interact with others.[30]

Fear of Shortness of Breath. Respiratory distress and dyspnea are common near the end of life. The sensation of air hunger results in anxiety for the patient and family. Current therapies include opioids, bronchodilators, and oxygen, depending on the cause of the dyspnea. Anxiety-reducing agents (e.g., anxiolytics) may help produce relaxation.

Fear of Loneliness and Abandonment. Most terminally ill and dying people fear loneliness and do not want to be alone. Many dying patients are afraid that loved ones who are unable to cope with the patient's imminent death will abandon them. The simple presence of someone provides support and comfort (Fig. 10-8). Holding hands, touching, and listening are important nursing interventions. Providing companionship allows the dying person a sense of security.

Fear of Meaninglessness. Fear of meaninglessness leads people to review their lives. They review their intentions during life, examining actions and expressing regrets about what might have been. *Life review* helps patients recognize the value of their lives. Assist patients and their families in identifying the positive qualities of the patient's life. Practical ways of helping may include looking at photo albums or collections of important mementos. Sharing thoughts and feelings may enhance spirituality and provide comfort for the patient at this time. Respect and accept the practices and rituals associated with the patient's life review while remaining nonjudgmental.[30]

> *What we leave behind is not what is engraved in stone monuments, but what is woven into the lives of others.*
> *Pericles (fifth-century Greek statesman)*

Communication. Communication among health care providers, patient, and family is essential at the end of life. Empathy and active listening are essential components of communication in EOL care. *Empathy* is the identification with and understanding of another's situation, feelings, or motives. *Active listening* is paying attention to what is said, observing the patient's nonverbal cues, and not interrupting.

There may be silence. Frequently silence is related to the overwhelming feelings experienced at the end of life. Silence can also allow time to gather thoughts. Listening to the silence sends a message of acceptance and comfort. Communication also needs to consider the patient's ethnic, cultural, and religious backgrounds.

Patients and family members may have difficulties expressing themselves emotionally. Allow time for them to express their feelings and thoughts. Make time to listen and interact in a sensitive way to enhance the relationship among you, the patient, and the family. A family conference is one way to create a more conducive environment for communication.

Unusual communication by the patient may take place at the end of life. The patient's speech may become confused, disoriented, or garbled. Patients may speak to or about family members or others who have predeceased them, give instructions to those who will survive them, or speak of projects yet to be completed. Active, careful listening allows for the identification of specific patterns in the dying person's communication and decreases the risk for inappropriate labeling of behaviors.

PHYSICAL CARE. Nursing management related to physical care at the end of life focuses on symptom management and comfort rather than treatment for curing a disease or disorder (Table 10-8). The priority is meeting the patient's physiologic and safety needs. Physical care focuses on the needs for oxygen, nutrition, pain relief, mobility, elimination, and skin care. People who are dying deserve and require the same physical care as people who are expected to recover.

Postmortem Care. After the patient is pronounced dead, prepare or delegate preparation of the body for immediate viewing by the family with consideration for cultural customs and in accord with state law and agency policies and procedures. In some cultures and in some types of death, it may be important to allow the family to prepare or assist in preparing the body. In general, close the patient's eyes, replace dentures, wash the body as needed (placing pads under the perineum to absorb urine and feces), and remove tubes and dressings (if appropriate). The body is straightened, leaving the pillow to support the head and prevent pooling of blood and discoloration of the face. Allow the family privacy and as much time as they need with the deceased person. In the case of an unexpected or unanticipated death, preparation of the body for viewing or release to a funeral home depends on state law and agency policies and procedures.

SPECIAL NEEDS OF CAREGIVERS AND NURSES IN END-OF-LIFE CARE

Special Needs of Family Caregivers

Family caregivers are important in meeting the patient's physical and psychosocial needs. The role of caregivers includes working and communicating with the patient and other family members, supporting the patient's concerns, and helping the patient resolve any unfinished business. Families often face emotional, physical, and economic consequences as a result of caring for a family member who is dying. The caregiver's responsibilities do not end when the person is admitted to an acute care, inpatient hospice, or long-term care facility.

TABLE 10-8   NURSING MANAGEMENT

Physical Care at End of Life

Characteristic	Nursing Management
Pain • Pain may be a major symptom associated with terminal illness and the one most feared. • Pain can be acute or chronic. • Physical and emotional irritations can aggravate pain.	• Assess pain thoroughly and regularly to determine the quality, intensity, location, and contributing factors. • Minimize possible irritants such as skin irritations from wetness, heat or cold, and pressure. • Administer medications around the clock in a timely manner and on a regular basis to provide constant relief rather than waiting until the pain is unbearable and then trying to relieve it. • Provide complementary and alternative therapies such as guided imagery, massage, and relaxation techniques as needed (see Chapters 6 and 7). • Evaluate effectiveness of pain relief measures frequently to ensure that the patient is on a correct, adequate drug regimen. • Do not delay or deny pain relief measures to a terminally ill patient.
Delirium • A state characterized by confusion, disorientation, restlessness, clouding of consciousness, incoherence, fear, anxiety, excitement, and often hallucinations. • May be misidentified as depression, psychosis, anger, or anxiety. • Use of opioids or corticosteroids may cause delirium. • Underlying disease process may contribute to delirium. • Generally considered a reversible process.	• Perform a thorough assessment for reversible causes of delirium, including pain, constipation, and urinary retention. • Provide a room that is quiet, well lit, and familiar to reduce the effects of delirium. • Reorient the dying person to person, place, and time with each encounter. • Administer ordered benzodiazepines and sedatives as needed. • Stay physically close to frightened patient. Reassure in a calm, soft voice with touch and slow strokes of the skin. • Provide family with emotional support and encouragement in their efforts to cope with the behaviors associated with delirium. • Encourage the family to participate in care of the patient.
Restlessness • May occur as death approaches and cerebral metabolism slows.	• Assess for spiritual distress as a cause of restlessness and agitation. • Do not restrain. • Use soothing music; slow, soft touch and voice. • Limit the number of persons at the bedside.
Dysphagia • May occur because of extreme weakness and changes in level of consciousness.	• Identify the least invasive alternative routes of administration for drugs needed for symptom management. • Suction orally as needed.
Weakness and Fatigue • Expected at the end of life. • Metabolic demands related to disease process contribute to weakness and fatigue.	• Assess the patient's tolerance for activities. • Time nursing interventions to conserve energy. • Help the patient identify and complete valued or desired activities. • Provide support as needed to maintain positions in bed or chair. • Provide frequent rest periods.
Dehydration • May occur during the last days of life. • Hunger and thirst are rare in the last days of life. • As the end of life approaches, patients tend to take in less food and fluid.	• Assess mucous membranes frequently to prevent excessive dryness, which can lead to discomfort. • Maintain complete, regular oral care to provide for comfort and hydration of mucous membranes. • Do not force the patient to eat or drink. • Encourage consumption of ice chips and sips of fluids or use moist cloths to provide moisture to the mouth. • Use moist cloths and swabs for unconscious patients to avoid aspiration. • Apply lubricant to the lips and oral mucous membranes as needed. • Reassure family that cessation of food and fluid intake is a natural part of the process of dying.
Dyspnea • Subjective symptom. • Accompanied by fear of suffocation and anxiety. • Underlying disease process can exacerbate dyspnea. • Coughing and expectorating secretions become difficult.	• Assess respiratory status regularly. • Elevate the head and/or position patient on side to improve chest expansion. • Use a fan or air conditioner to facilitate movement of cool air. • Administer supplemental oxygen as ordered. • Suction PRN to remove accumulation of mucus from the airways. Suction cautiously in the terminal phase.

TABLE 10-8   NURSING MANAGEMENT—cont'd

Physical Care at End of Life

Characteristic	Nursing Management
Myoclonus • Mild to severe jerking or twitching sometimes associated with use of high dose of opioids. • Patient may complain of involuntary twitching of extremities.	• Assess for initial onset, duration, and any discomfort or distress experienced by patient. • If myoclonus is distressing or becoming more severe, discuss possible drug therapy modifications with the health care provider. • Changes in opioid medication may alleviate or decrease myoclonus.
Skin Breakdown • Skin integrity is difficult to maintain at the end of life. • Immobility, urinary and bowel incontinence, dry skin, nutritional deficits, anemia, friction, and shearing forces lead to a high risk for skin breakdown. • Disease and other processes may impair skin integrity. • As death approaches, circulation to the extremities decreases and they become cool, mottled, and cyanotic.	• Assess the skin for signs of breakdown. • Implement protocols to prevent skin breakdown by controlling drainage and odor and keeping the skin and any wound areas clean. • Perform wound assessments as needed. • Follow appropriate nursing management protocol for dressing wounds. • Follow appropriate nursing management protocol for a patient who is immobile, but consider realistic outcomes of skin integrity vs. maintenance of comfort. • Follow appropriate nursing management to prevent skin irritations and breakdown from urinary and bowel incontinence. • Use blankets to cover for warmth; never apply heat. • Prevent the effects of shearing forces.
Bowel Patterns • Constipation can be caused by immobility, use of opioid medications, lack of fiber in the diet, and dehydration. • Diarrhea may occur as muscles relax or from a fecal impaction related to the use of opioids and immobility.	• Assess bowel function. • Assess for and remove fecal impactions. • Encourage movement and physical activities as tolerated. • Encourage fiber in the diet if appropriate. • Encourage fluids if appropriate. • Use suppositories, stool softeners, laxatives, or enemas if ordered.
Urinary Incontinence • May result from disease progression or changes in the level of consciousness. • As death becomes imminent, the perineal muscles relax.	• Assess urinary function. • Use absorbent pads for urinary incontinence. • Follow appropriate nursing protocol for the consideration and use of indwelling or external catheters. • Follow appropriate nursing management to prevent skin irritations and breakdown from urinary incontinence.
Anorexia, Nausea, and Vomiting • May be caused by complications of disease process. • Drugs contribute to nausea. • Constipation, impaction, and bowel obstruction can cause anorexia, nausea, and vomiting.	• Assess the patient for complaints of nausea or vomiting. • Assess possible contributing causes of nausea or vomiting. • Have family provide the patient's favorite foods. • Discuss modifications to the drug regimen with the health care provider. • Provide antiemetics before meals if ordered. • Offer and provide frequent meals with small portions of favorite foods. • Offer culturally appropriate foods. • Provide frequent mouth care, especially after vomiting.

An understanding of the grieving process as it affects both the patient and family is important. Being present during a family member's dying process can be highly stressful. Recognize signs and behaviors among family members who may be at risk for abnormal grief reactions, and be prepared to intervene if necessary. Warning signs may include dependency and negative feelings about the dying person, inability to express feelings, sleep disturbances, a history of depression, difficult reactions to previous losses, perceived lack of social or family support, low self-esteem, multiple previous bereavements, alcoholism, or substance abuse. Caregivers with concurrent life crises (e.g., divorce) will be especially at risk.

Family caregivers and other family members need encouragement to continue their usual activities as much as possible. They need to discuss their activities and maintain some control over their lives.

Inform caregivers about appropriate resources for support, including respite care. Resources such as community counseling and local support may assist some people in working through their grief. Encourage caregivers to build a support system of extended family, friends, faith community, and clergy. The caregivers should have people to call on at any time to express any feelings they are experiencing. (The stressors and special needs of family caregivers are discussed in Chapter 4 on pp. 51-52.)

Special Needs of Nurses

Many nurses who care for dying patients do so because they are passionate about providing high-quality EOL care. Caring for patients and their families at the end of life is challenging and rewarding, but also intense and emotionally charged. A bond or connection may develop between you and the patient or family. Be aware of how grief personally affects you. When you provide care for terminally ill or dying patients, you are not immune to feelings of loss. It is common to feel helpless and powerless when dealing with death. Express feelings of sorrow, guilt, and frustration.

Interventions are available that may help ease your physical and emotional stress. Be aware of what you can and cannot control. Recognizing personal feelings allows openness in exchanging feelings with the patient and the family. Realizing that it is okay to cry with the patient or family during the end of life may be important for your well-being.

To meet your personal needs, focus on interventions that will help decrease your stress. Get involved in hobbies or other interests, schedule time for yourself, maintain a peer support system, and develop a support system beyond the workplace.[31] Hospice agencies can help you cope through professionally assisted groups, informal discussion sessions, and flexible time schedules.

BRIDGE TO NCLEX EXAMINATION

The number of the question corresponds to the same-numbered outcome at the beginning of the chapter.

1. An 80-year-old female patient is receiving palliative care for heart failure. Primary purpose(s) of her receiving palliative care is (are) to (select all that apply)
   a. improve her quality of life.
   b. assess her coping ability with disease.
   c. have time to teach patient and family about disease.
   d. focus on reducing the severity of disease symptoms.
   e. provide care that the family is unwilling or unable to give.

2. The primary purpose of hospice is to
   a. allow patients to die at home.
   b. provide better quality of care than the family can.
   c. coordinate care for dying patients and their families.
   d. provide comfort and support for dying patients and their families.

3. A 67-year-old woman was recently diagnosed with inoperable pancreatic cancer. Before the diagnosis she was very active in her neighborhood association. Her husband is concerned because his wife is staying at home and missing her usual community activities. Which common EOL psychologic manifestation is she most likely demonstrating?
   a. Peacefulness
   b. Decreased socialization
   c. Decreased decision making
   d. Anxiety about unfinished business

4. For the past 5 years Tom has repeatedly asked his mother to donate his deceased father's belongings to charity, but his mother has refused. She sits in the bedroom closet, crying and talking to her long-dead husband. What type of grief is Tom's mother experiencing?
   a. Adaptive grief
   b. Disruptive grief
   c. Anticipatory grief
   d. Prolonged grief disorder

5. The home health nurse visits a 40-year-old patient with metastatic breast cancer who is receiving palliative care. The patient is experiencing pain at a level of 7 (on a 10-point scale). In prioritizing activities for the visit, the nurse would do which first?
   a. Auscultate for breath sounds.
   b. Administer PRN pain medication.
   c. Check pressure points for skin breakdown.
   d. Ask family about patient's food and fluid intake.

6. While caring for his dying wife, the husband states that his wife is a devout Roman Catholic but he is a Baptist. Who is considered the most reliable source for spiritual preferences concerning EOL care for the dying wife?
   a. A priest
   b. Dying wife
   c. Hospice staff
   d. Husband of dying wife

7. The family attorney informed a patient's adult children and wife that the patient did not have an advance directive after he suffered a serious stroke. Who is responsible for making the decision about EOL measures when the patient cannot communicate his or her specific wishes?
   a. Notary and attorney
   b. Physician and family
   c. Wife and adult children
   d. Physician and nursing staff

8. The children caregivers of an elderly patient whose death is imminent have not left the bedside for the past 36 hours. In the nurse's assessment of the family, what findings indicate the potential for an abnormal grief reaction to occur (select all that apply)?
   a. Family cannot express their feelings to one another.
   b. Dying patient is becoming more restless and agitated.
   c. A family member is going through a difficult divorce.
   d. Family talks with and reassures the patient at frequent intervals.
   e. Siblings who were estranged from each other have now reunited.

9. A nurse has been working full time with terminally ill patients for 3 years. He has been experiencing irritability and mixed emotions when expressing sadness since four of his patients died on the same day. To optimize the quality of his nursing care, he should examine his own
   a. full-time work schedule.
   b. past feelings toward death.
   c. patterns for dealing with grief.
   d. demands for involvement in patient care.

1. a, d. 2. d. 3. b. 4. d. 5. b. 6. b. 7. c. 8. a, c. 9. c.

ⓔvolve

For rationales to these answers and even more NCLEX review questions, visit *http://evolve.elsevier.com/Lewis/medsurg.*

CHAPTER 10 Palliative Care at End of Life 153

End of Life

REFERENCES

1. World Health Organization: Palliative care. Retrieved from *www.who.int/cancer/palliative/en*.

2. Hospice Foundation of America: What is hospice? Retrieved from *www.hospicefoundation.org/hospiceinfo*.

3. National Consensus Project for Quality Palliative Care: Clinical practice guidelines for palliative care, ed 2. Retrieved from *www.nationalconsensusproject.org/guideline.pdf*.

4. American Cancer Society: Hospice care. Retrieved from *www.cancer.org/Treatment/FindingandPayingforTreatment/ChoosingYourTreatmentTeam/HospiceCare/hospice-care-what-is-hospice-care*.

5. National Hospice and Palliative Care Organization: Hospice care in America. Retrieved from *www.nhpco.org/files/public/statistics_research/hospice_facts_figures_oct-2010.pdf*.

6. Hospice and Palliative Nurses Association Care. HPNA Position statement: Value of the professional nurse in palliative care. Copyright by the Hospice and Palliative Nurses Association, Pittsburgh, 2011. Retrieved from *www.hpna.org*.

*7. Johnson KS, Kuchibhatia M, Tulsky JA: Racial differences in self-reported exposure to information about hospice care. *J Palliat Med* 12(10):921, 2009.

8. Teitelbaum J, Shemi SD: Neurologic determination of death, *Neurol Clin* 29:787, 2011.

*9. American Academy of Neurology: Practice parameters: determining brain death in adults. Retrieved from *www.aan.com/professionals/practice/guidelines/pda/Brain_death_adults.pdf*.

10. Field M, Cassel C: *Approaching death: improving care at the end of life*, Washington, DC. 1997, National Academy Press. (Classic)

11. Kübler-Ross E: *On death and dying*, New York, 1969, Macmillan. (Classic)

12. Kübler-Ross E, Kessler D: The five stages of grief. Retrieved from *www.grief.com/the-five-stages-of-grief*

13. A guide to grief: bereavement, mourning, and grief. Retrieved from *www.hospicenet.org/html/grief_guide.html*.

14. Anderson WG, Arnold RM, Angus DC, et al: Posttraumatic stress and complicated grief in family of patients in the intensive care unit, *J Gen Intern Med* 23:1871, 2008.

15. Kacel E, Gao X, Prigerson HG: Understanding bereavement: what every oncology practitioner should know, *J Support Oncol* 9:172, 2011.

16. Selman L, Harding R, Gysels M, et al: The measurement of spirituality in palliative care and the content of tools validated cross-culturally: a systematic review, *J Pain Symptom Manage* 41:728, 2011.

17. Bruce A, Schreiber R, Petrovskaya O, et al: Longing for ground in a ground(less) world: a qualitative inquiry of existential suffering, *BMS Nurs* 27:2, 2011.

18. Zhang AY, Zyzanski SJ, Siminoff LA: Differential patient-caregiver opinions of treatment and care for advanced lung cancer patient, *Soc Sci Med* 70:115, 2010.

19. Liaschenko J, Peden-McAlpine C, Andrews GJ: Institutional geographies in dying: nurses' actions and observations on dying spaces inside and outside intensive care units, *Health Place* 17:814, 2011.

20. Kelley AS, Wenger NS, Sarkisian CA: Opinions: End of life care preferences and planning among older Latinos, *J Am Geriatr Soc* 58:1109, 2010.

21. Sharma RK, Hughes MT, Nolan MT, et al: Family understanding of seriously-ill patient preferences for family involvement in healthcare decision making, *J Gen Intern Med* 26:881, 2011.

22. Carr D: Racial differences in end-of-life planning: why don't Blacks and Latinos prepare for the inevitable? *Omega (Westport)* 63:1, 2011.

23. Thornton JD, Pham K, Engelberg RA, et al: Families with limited English proficiency receive less information and support in interpreted intensive care unit family conferences, *Crit Care Med* 37:89, 2009.

24. DeWispelaere J, Stirton L: Advance commitment: an alternative approach to the family veto problem in organ procurement, *J Med Ethics* 36:180, 2010.

25. Billings JA, Krakauer EL: On patient autonomy and physician responsibility in end of life care, *Arch Intern Med* 171:849, 2011.

26. American Nurses Association: ANA position statements. Retrieved from *http://nursingworld.org/MainMenuCategories/HealthcareandPolicyIssues/ANAPositionStatements/EthicsandHumanRights.aspx*.

27. Iowa Department of Public Health: Out of hospital DNR. Retrieved from *www.idph.state.ia.us/ems/dnr.asp*.

28. Walker KA, Peltier H, Mayo RL, et al: Impact of writing "comfort measures only" orders in a community teaching hospital, *J Palliat Med* 13:241, 2010.

29. Adams JA, Bailey DE, Anderson RA, et al: Nursing roles and strategies in end-of-life decision making in acute care: a systematic review of the literature, *Nurs Res Pract* 2011:527834, 2011. Published online doi:10.1155/2011/527834.

30. Prince-Paul M, Exline JJ: Personal relationships and communication messages at the end of life, *Nurs Clin North Am* 45:449, 2010.

31. Sinclair S: Impact of death and dying on the personal lives and practices of palliative and hospice care professionals, *CMAJ* 183:180, 2011.

RESOURCES

End-of-Life Nursing Education Consortium (ELNEC), American Association of Colleges of Nursing
www.aacn.nche.edu/ELNEC
Hospice and Palliative Nurses Association
www.hpna.org
National Hospice and Palliative Care Organization
www.nhpco.org

*Evidence-based information for clinical practice.

11

Substance Abuse

Mariann M. Harding

If you are on the wrong road, progress means doing an about-turn and walking back to the right road.
C. S. Lewis

evolve WEBSITE

http://evolve.elsevier.com/Lewis/medsurg

- NCLEX Review Questions
- Key Points
- Pre-Test
- Answer Guidelines for Case Study on p. 167
- Rationales for Bridge to NCLEX Examination Questions

- Nursing Care Plan (Customizable)
  - NCP 11-1: Patient in Alcohol Withdrawal
- Concept Map Creator
- Glossary
- Content Updates

eTable
- eTable 11-1: Clinical Institute Withdrawal Assessment of Alcohol Scale, Revised (CIWA-Ar)

LEARNING OUTCOMES

1. Apply the terms *addiction, addictive behavior, substance misuse, substance abuse, dependence, tolerance, withdrawal, craving,* and *abstinence* to clinical situations.
2. Relate the effects of substance abuse to its resulting major health complications.
3. Differentiate among the effects of the use of stimulants, depressants, and cannabis.

4. Explain your role in promoting the cessation of smoking and tobacco use.
5. Summarize the nursing management and collaborative care of patients who experience intoxication, overdose, or withdrawal from stimulants and depressants.
6. Describe the incidence and effects of substance abuse and dependence in the older adult.

KEY TERMS

addiction, Table 11-1, p. 155
addictive behavior, Table 11-1, p. 155
craving, Table 11-1, p. 155
dependence, Table 11-1, p. 154

Korsakoff's psychosis, p. 159
physical dependence, Table 11-1, p. 155
psychologic dependence, Table 11-1, p. 155

substance abuse, Table 11-1, p. 155
tolerance, Table 11-1, p. 155
Wernicke's encephalopathy, p. 159

Substance abuse and addiction are serious problems affecting the health care system and society today. Addiction to chemical substances usually includes dependence on psychoactive agents that result in pleasure or modify thinking and perception. These include substances that are legal for adult use such as alcohol and tobacco, and illicit drugs including marijuana/hashish, cocaine, heroin, hallucinogens, inhalants, and prescription medications used nonmedically. In 2010 an estimated 22.6 million Americans ages 12 or older, or 8.9% of the population, were using illicit drugs monthly.[1] Americans' abuse and misuse of prescription medications such as analgesics, sedative-hypnotics, tranquilizers, and amphetamines have increased and can create harmful effects that are more deadly than the abuse of illicit drugs.[2]

The *Diagnostic and Statistical Manual of Mental Disorders IV* states that substance abuse and dependence (defined in Table 11-1) are specific psychiatric diagnoses.[3] Abused substances are discussed in detail in psychiatric and pharmacologic books and resources. Long-term management of patients who abuse substances is most often provided in specialized treatment facilities that provide both drug and behavior therapies.

Individuals who abuse substances use the health care system more than those who do not.[4] Almost every drug of abuse harms some tissue or organ in addition to the brain. Some health problems are caused by the effects of specific drugs, such as liver damage related to alcohol use or chronic obstructive pulmonary disease (COPD) related to smoking. Other health problems result from behaviors associated with substance abuse, such as injecting drugs or neglecting nutrition and hygiene. Common health complications related to substance abuse are identified in Table 11-2.

This chapter focuses on the role of the medical-surgical nurse in identifying and managing the substance-abusing patient in acute care settings. All nurses care for patients dependent on substances, whether they are identified as dependent or not, simply because of the prevalence of substance abuse and its association with health problems.

Reviewed by Carol Capitano, RN, PhD(C), College of Nursing, University of New Mexico, Albuquerque, New Mexico.

TABLE 11-1   TERMINOLOGY OF SUBSTANCE ABUSE

Term	Definition
Abstinence	Avoidance of substance use.
Addiction	Compulsive, uncontrollable dependence on a substance, behavior, or practice to such a degree that cessation causes severe emotional, mental, or physiologic reactions.
Addictive behavior	Behavior associated with maintaining an addiction.
Craving	Subjective need for a substance, usually experienced after decreased use or abstinence. Cue-induced craving occurs in the presence of experiences previously associated with drug taking.
Dependence	Reliance on a substance to the degree that its absence will cause impairment in function.
• Physical	Altered physiologic state from prolonged substance use; regular use is necessary to prevent withdrawal.
• Psychologic	Compulsive need to experience pleasurable response from the substance.
Overdose	Ingestion of excessive dose of one drug or a combination of similarly acting drugs. Leads to toxic reactions, including respiratory and circulatory arrest.
Relapse	Return to substance use after a period of abstinence.
Substance	Drug, chemical, or biologic entity that is self-administered. The words "drug," "substance," and "chemical" are often used interchangeably.
Substance abuse	Overindulgence in a substance that has a negative impact on an individual's psychologic, physiologic, and/or social functioning.
Substance misuse	Use of a drug for purposes other than those for which it is intended.
Tolerance	Decreased effect of a substance that results from repeated exposure. It is possible to develop cross-tolerance to other substances in the same category.
Withdrawal	Combination of physiologic and psychologic responses that occur when there is abrupt cessation or reduced intake of a substance on which an individual is dependent.

TABLE 11-2   COMMON HEALTH PROBLEMS RELATED TO SUBSTANCE ABUSE

Substance	Health Problems*
Nicotine and smoking	• Chronic obstructive pulmonary disease (COPD) • Cancers of lung, mouth, larynx, esophagus, stomach, pancreas, bladder, prostate, cervix • Coronary artery disease, peripheral artery disease • Peptic ulcer disease, GERD
Cocaine	• Nasal sores, septal necrosis or perforation • Chronic sinusitis • Cardiac dysrhythmias, myocardial ischemia and infarction • Stroke • Psychosis
Amphetamines	• Cardiac dysrhythmias, myocardial ischemia and infarction • Death of brain cells • Mood disturbances, violent behavior, psychoses
Caffeine	• Gastrointestinal irritation, peptic ulcer disease, GERD • Anxiety, insomnia
Alcohol	• See Table 11-7 on p. 160
Sedative-hypnotics	• Possible memory impairment • Respiratory depression • Risk for falls and fractures
Opioids	• Sexual dysfunction • Gastric ulcers • Glomerulonephritis
Cannabis	• Bronchitis, chronic sinusitis • Cardiac dysrhythmias, myocardial ischemia and palpitations • Memory impairment • Impaired immune function
Behaviors	**Health Problems**
Injecting drugs	• Blood clots, phlebitis, skin infections • Hepatitis B and C • HIV/AIDS • Other infections: endocarditis, tuberculosis, pneumonia, meningitis, tetanus, bone and joint infections, lung abscesses
Snorting drugs	• Nasal sores, septal necrosis or perforation • Chronic sinusitis
Risky sexual behavior	• HIV/AIDS • Hepatitis B and C • Other sexually transmitted infections
Personal neglect	• Malnutrition, impaired immunity • Accidental injuries

Source: National Institute on Drug Abuse: Addiction and health. In NIDA: *Drugs, brains, and behavior—the science of addiction*, NIH pub no 07-5605, Rockwell, Md, 2008, National Institutes of Health, US Department of Health and Human Services. Retrieved from *www.nida.nih.gov/scienceofaddiction/health.html*.
*The health problems related to substance abuse are discussed in the appropriate chapters throughout the text where they are identified as risk factors for these problems.
GERD, Gastroesophageal reflux disease.

COMMON DRUGS OF ABUSE

NICOTINE

The addictive behavior that you are most likely to encounter is tobacco use. Nicotine is a stimulant substance in tobacco and is the most rapidly addictive of commonly abused drugs. Cigarette smoking is the predominant form of tobacco abuse in the United States. Tobacco use is the leading cause of preventable illness and death in the United States, claiming 443,000 lives a year.[5]

Effects of Use and Complications

The effects of nicotine are identical to those of other highly addictive stimulant drugs, including cocaine. Although users report that nicotine causes a depressant effect with relaxation

and relief of anxiety, these effects are thought to occur when withdrawal is relieved with more nicotine.

Smoking is the most harmful method of nicotine use and can injure nearly every organ in the body. Smoking causes chronic lung disease, cardiovascular disease, and many cancers, and it is associated with cataracts, pneumonia, periodontitis, and abdominal aortic aneurysm[6] (see Table 11-2). The chronic respiratory irritation caused by exposure to cigarette smoke is a key risk factor in the development of COPD and lung cancer (carcinogens in tobacco are also involved). The toxic gases inhaled in cigarette smoke constrict the bronchi, paralyze the cilia, thicken the mucus-secreting membranes, dilate the distal airways, and destroy the alveolar walls.

Carbon monoxide is a component of cigarette smoke. Its effects, combined with those of nicotine, increase the risk for coronary artery disease. Carbon monoxide has a high affinity for hemoglobin and combines with it more readily than oxygen, reducing the oxygen-carrying capacity of the blood. Smokers inhale less oxygen when smoking, further decreasing the available oxygen. Together with the increased myocardial oxygen consumption that nicotine causes, carbon monoxide significantly decreases the oxygen available to the myocardium. The result is a cycle of increases in heart rate and myocardial oxygen consumption that can lead to myocardial ischemia.

Children whose parents smoke have a higher rate of respiratory illnesses and sudden infant death syndrome. In adults, secondhand smoking is associated with decreased pulmonary function, increased risk for lung cancer, and increased mortality rates from coronary artery disease.

Women appear to be at greater risk than men for smoking-related diseases. Smoking in women is associated with increased menstrual bleeding and dysmenorrhea, early menopause, and infertility. Lung cancer related to smoking has surpassed breast cancer as the leading cause of cancer deaths among women.[7]

Although those who use smokeless tobacco (snuff, plug, and leaf) have less risk of lung disease than smokers, the use of smokeless tobacco is not without complications. Holding tobacco in the mouth increases the risk of cancer of the mouth, the cheek, the tongue, and gingiva nearly 50-fold. Smokeless tobacco users also experience the systemic effects of nicotine on the cardiovascular system, thus increasing the risk for cardiovascular disease.[6]

All users of nicotine in any form may develop complications directly related to the effects of nicotine itself, including an increased risk for peripheral artery disease, delayed wound healing, peptic ulcer disease, and gastroesophageal reflux disease (GERD).[6]

NURSING AND COLLABORATIVE CARE TOBACCO USE

TOBACCO CESSATION

As a nurse, you have a professional responsibility to help individuals stop smoking or using tobacco. The Joint Commission mandates that every health professional is responsible for identifying tobacco users and providing them with information on ways to stop the use of tobacco. Hospitalization offers an ideal opportunity to provide cessation assistance because hospitals are tobacco-free environments, and patients may be more motivated to quit because of their illness. Patients who receive even brief advice and intervention from you are more likely to quit than those who receive no intervention.

Because many health care facilities are tobacco-free environments, an admitted patient who is addicted to nicotine may experience withdrawal symptoms since they are unable to smoke. These symptoms are the same as for the person who stops using tobacco "cold turkey." Ask each patient about his or her tobacco status. Unless contraindicated, offer nicotine replacement therapy to those who desire it to control with-

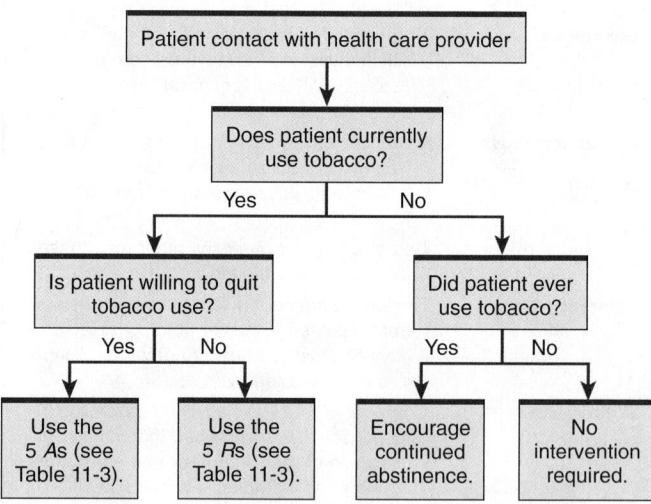

FIG. 11-1 Clinical practice guidelines: treating tobacco use and dependence.

TABLE 11-3	CLINICAL PRACTICE GUIDELINE

Treating Tobacco Use and Dependence

The Five As for Individuals Who Desire to Quit	The Five Rs for Individuals Unwilling to Quit
1. **Ask:** Identify all tobacco users at every contact.	1. **Relevance:** Ask the patient to indicate why quitting is personally relevant (e.g., family, health).
2. **Advise:** Strongly urge all tobacco users to quit.	2. **Risks:** Ask the patient to identify negative consequences of tobacco use (e.g., cough, shortness of breath).
3. **Assess:** Determine willingness to make a quit attempt.	3. **Rewards:** Ask the patient to identify potential benefits of stopping tobacco use (e.g., saving money, feeling better).
4. **Assist:** Aid the patient in developing a plan to quit.	4. **Roadblocks:** Ask patient to identify barriers or impediments to quitting (e.g., weight gain, partner smokes).
5. **Arrange:** Schedule follow-up contact.	5. **Repetition:** Repeat process every clinic visit.

Source: Agency for Healthcare Research and Quality: *AHCPR supported clinical practice guideline: treating tobacco use and dependence: 2008 update,* Washington, DC, 2008, US Public Health Service.

TABLE 11-4	INPATIENT TOBACCO CESSATION INTERVENTIONS

Take the following steps for every hospitalized patient.
- Ask each patient on admission if he or she uses tobacco and document tobacco use status.
- For current tobacco users, list tobacco use status on the admission problem list and as a discharge diagnosis.
- Use counseling and medication to help all tobacco users maintain abstinence and to treat withdrawal symptoms.
- Provide advice and assistance on how to quit during hospitalization and remain abstinent after discharge.
- Arrange for follow-up regarding smoking status. Supportive contact should be provided for at least a month after discharge.

Source: Agency for Healthcare Research and Quality: *AHCPR supported clinical practice guideline: treating tobacco use and dependence: 2008 update,* Washington, DC, 2008, US Public Health Service.

drawal symptoms during their hospitalization. These symptoms include craving, restlessness, depression, headache, hyperirritability, drowsiness or insomnia, decreased BP and heart rate, and increased appetite.

With each patient encounter, encourage the patient to quit and offer specific smoking cessation interventions. The Agency for Healthcare Research and Quality has issued clinical practice guidelines for clinicians, including nurses, to use to motivate users to quit[8] (Tables 11-3 and 11-4 and Fig. 11-1). Use these brief clinical interventions, called the "five As," with each patient encounter. These interventions are designed to identify tobacco users, encourage them to quit, determine their willingness to

quit, assist them in quitting, and arrange for follow-up to prevent relapse.

If a tobacco user is unwilling to quit, *motivational interventions* based on the principles of motivational interviewing have been shown to increase future quit attempts. The content areas that should be addressed in a motivational counseling intervention can be captured by the "five Rs": relevance, risks, rewards, roadblocks, and repetition. A patient teaching guide (Table 11-5) expands on the fourth "A" strategy, "Assist: aid the patient in quitting."

The patient is most likely to achieve long-term tobacco cessation with a combination of nicotine replacement products,

---

TABLE 11-5 PATIENT TEACHING GUIDE

Smoking and Tobacco Use Cessation

The following interventions are methods that work for quitting tobacco use. Tobacco users have the best chance of quitting if they use more than one method.

Develop a Quit Plan
- Set a quit date, ideally within 2 weeks.
- Talk to your health care provider about getting help to quit.
- Tell family, friends, and co-workers about quitting and request understanding and support.
- Anticipate withdrawal symptoms and challenges when quitting.
- Before quitting, avoid smoking in places where you spend a lot of time (work, car, home).
- Throw away all tobacco products from your home, car, and work.
- Do not take even a single puff or dip after the quit date. Total abstinence is essential.

Use Approved Nicotine Replacement Systems
- Use a nicotine replacement agent unless you are a pregnant or nursing woman (see Table 11-6).
- Do not use other forms of tobacco when using nicotine replacement systems.

Dealing With Urges to Use Tobacco
- Identify situations that may cause you to want to smoke or use other tobacco, such as being around other smokers, being under time pressure, getting into an argument, feeling sad or frustrated, and drinking alcohol.
- Avoid difficult situations while you are trying to quit. Try to lower your stress level.
- Exercise can help, such as walking, jogging, or bicycling.
- Distract yourself from thoughts of smoking and the urge to use tobacco by talking to someone, getting busy with a task, or reading a book.
- Drink a lot of water.
- Take a shower or soak in the tub.

Support and Encouragement
- If you have tried to stop using tobacco before, identify what helped and what hurt in previous quit attempts.
- Joining a quit-tobacco support group will increase your chances of stopping permanently.
- If you get the urge for tobacco, call someone to help talk you out of it—preferably an ex-user.
- Do not be afraid to talk about how you feel while quitting, especially fears of not being able to quit for good. Ask your spouse or partner, friends, and co-workers to support you. Self-help materials and hot lines are also available:
  - American Lung Association: 800-586-4872; *www.lungusa.org*
  - American Cancer Society: 800-227-2345; *www.cancer.org*

- National Cancer Institute: 877-448-7848 or 800-784-8669; *www.smokefree.gov*
- Make Smoking History, Massachusetts Department of Public Health: 800-784-8669; *http://makesmokinghistory.org*

Avoiding Relapse
Most relapses occur within the first 3 months after quitting. Do not be discouraged if you start using tobacco again. Remember, most people try several times before they finally quit. Explore different ways to break habits. You may have to deal with some of the following triggers that cause relapse.
- *Change your environment.* Get rid of cigarettes, tobacco (in any form), and ashtrays in your home, car, and place of work. Get rid of the smell of cigarettes in your car and home.
- *Alcohol.* Consider limiting or stopping alcohol use while you are quitting tobacco.
- *Other smokers at home.* Encourage housemates to quit with you. Work out a plan to cope with others who smoke, and avoid being around them.
- *Weight gain.* Tackle one problem at a time. Work on quitting tobacco first. You will not necessarily gain weight, and increased appetite is often temporary.
- *Negative mood or depression.* If these symptoms persist, talk to your health care provider. You may need treatment for depression.
- *Withdrawal symptoms.* Your body will go through many changes when you quit tobacco. You may have a dry mouth, cough, or scratchy throat, and you may feel irritable. The nicotine patch or gum may help with cravings (see Table 11-6).
- *Thoughts.* Get your mind off tobacco. Exercise and do things you enjoy.
- *Keep a list.* Keep a list of "slips" and near-slips, what caused them, and what you can learn from them.
- *Focus on the benefits of quitting:*
  1. At 20 minutes after you quit, blood pressure decreases, pulse rate drops, and the body temperature of your hands and feet increases.
  2. At 12 hours, the carbon monoxide level in your blood drops to normal, and the oxygen level in your blood increases to normal.
  3. At 24 hours, your chance of a heart attack decreases.
  4. At 48 hours, nerve endings start regrowing, and the ability to smell and taste is enhanced.
  5. At 2 weeks to 3 months, your circulation improves; walking becomes easier; lung function increases; and coughing, sinus congestion, fatigue, and shortness of breath decrease.
  6. At 1 year, your risk of heart disease decreases to half that of a smoker.
  7. By 10 to 15 years, your risk of stroke, lung and other cancers, and early death returns to nearly the level of people who have never smoked.

Sources: Agency for Healthcare Research and Quality: *Help for smokers and other tobacco users: consumer guide,* Washington, DC, May 2008, US Public Health Service. Retrieved from *www.ahrq.gov/consumer/tobacco/helpsmokers.htm*; and American Lung Association: Freedom from smoking online. Retrieved from *www.lungusa.org.*

TABLE 11-6   DRUG THERAPY
Smoking Cessation*

Agents	Common Side Effects	Considerations
Nicotine Replacement Agents		
Nicotine Gum (OTC) Nicorette 2 mg, 4 mg • Use 12 wk or more • Use 9-12 pieces/day • Maximum dose: 30 pieces of 2 mg, 20 pieces of 4 mg	Hiccups, mouth ulcers, indigestion, jaw pain	Specific 30-min chewing regimen with periods of holding the gum between cheek and teeth. Avoid food and drink 15 min before and during use.
Nicotine Lozenge (OTC) Commit 2 mg, 4 mg • Use 8-12 wk or more • Use 1 lozenge q1-2hr tapering to 1 lozenge q4-8hr in 12 wk	Nausea and indigestion, hiccups, headache, cough, mouth soreness, flatulence	Dissolves in the mouth in 20-30 min. Chewing and swallowing the lozenge increases GI side effects. Avoid food and drink during use.
Nicotine Patch (OTC) NicoDerm CQ, Habitrol, Nicotine transdermal system • 18- or 24-hr doses • Use ≥8 wk	Transient itching, burning, and redness at patch site. Sleep disturbances with 24-hr patch	Provides steady level of nicotine and is easy to use. Cannot be used by those with adhesive allergies.
Nicotine Nasal Spray Nicotrol NS • Use up to 6 mo	Nose and throat irritation, sneezing, rhinitis, watery eyes, cough	Requires a prescription. Provides fastest nicotine delivery and highest nicotine levels. Most irritating product.
Nicotine Inhaler Nicotrol nicotine inhalation system • Delivers 4 mg • Use up to 6 mo	Cough. Nose, mouth, and throat irritation. Heartburn and nausea	Requires a prescription. Simulates smoking with mouthpiece and nicotine cartridge. May not be advisable for those with asthma or pulmonary disease.
Non-Nicotine Agents		
Bupropion (Zyban) • 150 mg/day for 3 days, then 150 mg bid • Use 12 wk; can use up to 6 mo or longer	Insomnia, dry mouth, irritability, anorexia	Contraindicated with history of seizures or eating disorders. Promotes weight loss. First choice for smokers with depression.
Varenicline (Chantix)† • 0.5 mg/day for 3 days, 0.5 mg bid for 4 days, then 1 mg bid • Use 12 wk; additional 12 wk recommended for those who stop smoking to increase chance of long-term abstinence	Nausea, sleep disturbances, constipation, flatulence, vomiting, headache	If taken concurrently with nicotine replacement therapy, incidence of nausea, headache, vomiting, dizziness, dyspepsia, and fatigue is increased, but nicotine pharmacokinetics not affected.
Nortriptyline (Aventyl)‡ • 25-75 mg/day • Use 12 wk, longer if depressed	Dry mouth, drowsiness, dizziness	Must have stable ECG. Do not use immediately after MI.
Clonidine (Catapres)‡ • 0.1 mg q6hr PRN for craving	Dry mouth, drowsiness, constipation, hypotension	Used to control craving. Change position slowly to prevent postural hypotension.

*OTC nicotine replacement agents are also available in generic forms. Additional information and patient instructions are available from the American Lung Association at *www.lungusa.org.*
†See the Drug Alert for varenicline on p. 157.
‡Nortriptyline and clonidine are not approved by the U.S. Food and Drug Administration for treatment of smoking cessation but have been used successfully for this purpose.

medications, behavioral approaches, and support.[9] Support the patient by providing the resources needed to continue or start a quit attempt.

A variety of nicotine replacement products can be used to reduce the craving and withdrawal symptoms associated with tobacco cessation (Table 11-6). These agents enable a smoker to reduce nicotine previously obtained from cigarettes with a system that delivers the drug more slowly and eliminates the carcinogens and gases associated with tobacco smoke. Nicotine replacement therapy is generally not recommended for pregnant women and people who have experienced an acute myocardial infarction within 2 weeks, have unstable angina, or have life-threatening dysrhythmias.

Varenicline (Chantix) is a drug used to aid smoking cessation. Varenicline is unique in that it has both agonist and antagonist actions at nicotinic receptors. Its agonist activity at one subtype of nicotinic receptors provides some nicotine effects to ease the withdrawal symptoms. It also prevents stimulation of the dopamine system by blocking another subtype of nicotinic receptors. Thus it eases withdrawal symptoms while blocking the effects of nicotine if a person resumes smoking.

Non-nicotine drugs may also be used in smoking cessation. Bupropion (Zyban) is an antidepressant approved as an aid to quit smoking. It reduces the urge to smoke, reduces some symptoms of withdrawal, and helps prevent weight gain associated with smoking cessation. Nortriptyline (Aventyl) and clonidine (Catapres) are not approved by the U.S. Food and Drug Administration (FDA) for use in smoking cessation, but are used in some cases to reduce withdrawal symptoms and promote cessation.[10]

DRUG ALERT: Varenicline (Chantix) and Bupropion (Zyban)
- Serious neuropsychiatric symptoms such as changes in behavior, hostility, agitation, depressed mood, suicidal thoughts and behavior, and attempted suicide can occur.
- Advise patients to stop taking these drugs and contact a health care provider immediately if they experience any of these symptoms.

Participation in tobacco cessation programs is recommended in conjunction with nicotine replacement therapy. You should be aware of community resources that assist individuals who are motivated to quit. Local chapters of the American Lung Association and the American Cancer Society have information on available programs. Cessation programs may involve hypnosis, acupuncture, behavioral interventions, aversion therapy, group support programs, individual therapy, and self-help options. Behavioral approaches teach patients to avoid high-risk situations for smoking relapse, such as those that promote *cue-induced craving.* Cessation programs also promote development of other coping skills, such as cigarette refusal skills, assertiveness, alternative activities to cope with stress, and use of peer support systems.

Women are less successful than men in quitting smoking. Some of the reasons include concern about weight gain, less responsiveness to nicotine replacement therapy, influences of the menstrual cycle, and inadequate emotional support from others. Smoking-associated environmental cues may be more influential in smoking behavior in women than in men. The identification of gender differences in smoking cessation suggests that women who use nicotine replacement do better with nicotine inhalers than the nicotine patch and that women can increase their chances for quitting by timing their attempt to coincide with the first half of their menstrual cycles.[7]

ALCOHOL

Almost half of Americans ages 12 and older consume alcohol (Fig. 11-2). Although most people use alcohol in moderation, it is estimated that alcoholism, or alcohol dependence, affects 7% of the population.[1] Alcoholism is currently viewed as a chronic, progressive, potentially fatal disease if untreated. Alcohol dependence generally occurs over a period of years and may be preceded by heavy social drinking.

Effects of Use and Complications

Alcohol affects almost all cells of the body and has complex effects on the neurons in the central nervous system (CNS). Alcohol, like other addictive substances, causes increased levels of dopamine in the brain, but it also depresses all areas and

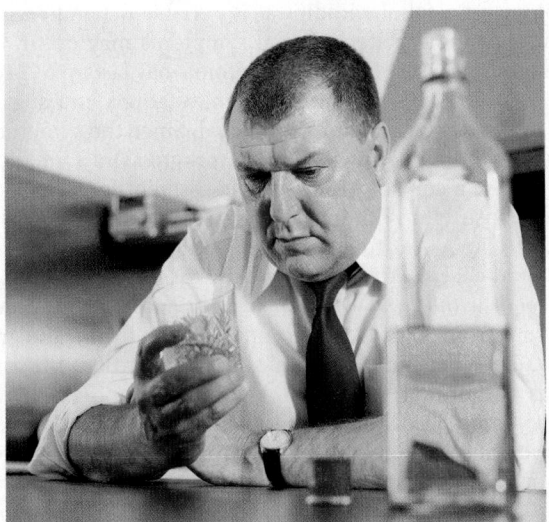

FIG. 11-2 Alcohol is often used to cope with the stresses of life. (Digital Vision/Thinkstock)

functions of the CNS.[11] Alcohol is absorbed directly from the stomach and small intestine. In a moderate drinker the metabolism of alcohol by the liver and the stomach occurs at a relatively constant rate of approximately one drink (7 g of alcohol) per hour. One drink is equal to 12 oz of beer, 5 oz of wine, or 1 oz of distilled spirits. Because women have significantly lower rates of stomach metabolism, they have higher blood alcohol levels than men do after the same amount of alcohol intake.[12]

The effects of alcohol are related to the concentration of alcohol and individual susceptibility to the drug. The concentration of alcohol in the body can be determined by assessing the blood alcohol concentration (BAC). For the person who is not dependent on alcohol, the BAC is generally predictable of alcohol's effects. The relationship between BAC and behavior is different in a person who has developed tolerance to alcohol and its effects. This tolerant individual is usually able to drink large amounts without obvious impairment and perform complex tasks without problems at BAC levels several times higher than levels that would produce obvious impairment in the nontolerant drinker.[12] In the United States the legal limit for intoxication is 0.08 mg% BAC as measured by a breath device, urinalysis, or blood test.

Individuals who abuse alcohol have many health problems (Table 11-7), which frequently are the reasons they seek health care. One serious complication of chronic alcohol abuse is **Wernicke's encephalopathy,** an inflammatory, hemorrhagic, degenerative condition of the brain. Wernicke's encephalopathy is caused by a thiamine deficiency resulting from poor diet and alcohol-induced suppression of thiamine absorption. This syndrome is readily reversible with administration of thiamine. Untreated or progressive Wernicke's encephalopathy may lead to **Korsakoff's psychosis,** an irreversible form of amnesia characterized by loss of short-term memory and an inability to learn.

Complications may also arise from the interaction of alcohol with commonly prescribed or over-the-counter (OTC) drugs. Drugs that interact with alcohol in an additive manner include antihypertensives, antihistamines, and antianginals. Alcohol taken with aspirin may cause or exacerbate GI bleeding. Alcohol taken with acetaminophen may increase the risk of liver damage. Potentiation and cross-tolerance with other CNS depressants also may occur. *Potentiation* occurs when an additional CNS depressant is taken with alcohol, increasing the effect. *Cross-tolerance,* requiring an increased dose for effect, occurs when an alcohol-dependent individual is alcohol free and receives other CNS depressants.

NURSING AND COLLABORATIVE CARE
ALCOHOL DEPENDENCE

ALCOHOL INTOXICATION

Acute alcohol toxicity may occur with binge drinking or the use of alcohol with other CNS depressants. It manifests as an emergency primarily because of the narrow range between the intoxicating, the anesthetic, and the lethal doses of alcohol. Alcohol-induced CNS depression leads to respiratory and circulatory failure.

Obtain as accurate a history as possible and assess for injuries, trauma, diseases, and hypoglycemia. No antidote for alcohol is available. Implement supportive care measures to maintain airway, breathing, and circulation (the ABCs) until detoxification is complete and the alcohol is metabolized. Fre-

TABLE 11-7	EFFECTS OF CHRONIC ALCOHOL ABUSE
Body System	**Effects**
Central nervous system	Alcoholic dementia. Wernicke's syndrome (confusion, nystagmus, paralysis of ocular muscles, ataxia). Korsakoff's psychosis (confabulation, amnesic disorder). Impairment of cognitive function, psychomotor skills, abstract thinking, and memory. Depression, attention deficit, labile moods, seizures, sleep disturbances.
Peripheral nervous system	Peripheral neuropathy, including pain, paresthesias, weakness.
Immune system	Increased risk for tuberculosis and viral infections. Increased risk for cancer of oral cavity, pharynx, esophagus, liver, colon, rectum, and possibly breast.
Hematologic system	Bone marrow depression, anemia, leukopenia, thrombocytopenia, blood clotting abnormalities.
Musculoskeletal system	Painful, tender swelling of large muscle groups. Painless progressive muscle weakness and wasting; osteoporosis.
Cardiovascular system	Elevated pulse and blood pressure. Decreased exercise tolerance. Cardiomyopathy (irreversible). Increased risk for hemorrhagic stroke, coronary artery disease, hypertension, sudden cardiac death.
Hepatic system	Steatosis* (nausea, vomiting, hepatomegaly). Alcoholic hepatitis* (anorexia, nausea, vomiting, fever, chills, abdominal pain). Cirrhosis, hepatocellular cancer.
Gastrointestinal system	Gastritis, gastroesophageal reflux disease (GERD), peptic ulcer, esophagitis, esophageal varices, enteritis, colitis, Mallory-Weiss tear, chronic pancreatitis.
Nutrition	Decreased appetite, indigestion, malabsorption, vitamin deficiencies (especially thiamine).
Urinary system	Diuretic effect from inhibition of antidiuretic hormone.
Endocrine and reproductive systems	Altered gonadal function, testicular atrophy, decreased beard growth, decreased libido, diminished sperm count, gynecomastia, glucose intolerance.
Integumentary system	Palmar erythema, spider angiomas, rosacea, rhinophyma.

*In the early stages of the disease this is reversible if the person quits drinking.

TABLE 11-8	CLINICAL MANIFESTATIONS AND TREATMENT OF ALCOHOL WITHDRAWAL
Clinical Manifestations	**Drug Treatment**
Minor Withdrawal Syndrome	
Tremulousness, anxiety ↑ Heart rate ↑ Blood pressure Sweating Nausea Hyperreflexia Insomnia ↑ Hyperactivity without seizures	Benzodiazepines (such as chlordiazepoxide [Librium], lorazepam [Ativan], or diazepam [Valium]) to stabilize vital signs, reduce anxiety, and prevent seizures and delirium Thiamine (prevents Wernicke's encephalopathy) Multivitamins (folic acid, B vitamins) Magnesium sulfate (if serum magnesium is low) IV glucose solution
Major Withdrawal Syndrome	
Visual or auditory hallucinations Gross tremors Seizures Alcohol withdrawal delirium	Continued use of benzodiazepines Carbamazepine (Tegretol) or phenytoin (Dilantin) to treat seizures Antipsychotic agents (e.g., chlorpromazine [Thorazine], haloperidol [Haldol]) if psychosis persists after benzodiazepine administration

quently monitor vital signs and level of consciousness. Treat alcohol-induced hypotension with IV fluids. Do not give stimulants to an intoxicated patient. In addition, do not give other depressants because of their additive effects.

Patients experiencing hypoglycemia are given glucose-containing IV solutions. Glucose administration may precipitate Wernicke's encephalopathy in a previously unaffected patient. To identify Wernicke's encephalopathy in the patient with chronic alcoholism, assess the patient for eye abnormalities (e.g., nystagmus, paralysis of the lateral rectus muscles), ataxia, and confusion.

Because the intoxicated patient may have symptoms similar to those of encephalopathy and because untreated encephalopathy may progress to Korsakoff's psychosis, administer IV thiamine before or with IV glucose solutions to all intoxicated patients. Many patients also have decreased serum magnesium

levels and other signs of malnutrition, so health care providers frequently add multivitamins and magnesium to the IV fluids.

Agitation and anxiety are common. Stay with the patient as much as possible, orienting to reality as necessary. Assess the patient for increasing belligerence and a potential for violence. Because the patient is also at risk for injury because of lack of coordination and impaired judgment, use protective measures. It is critical to continue assessment and interventions until the BAC has fallen to at least 100 mg/dL (0.10 mg%) and until any associated disorders or injuries have been ruled out.

ALCOHOL WITHDRAWAL SYNDROME

A patient with alcohol dependence who is hospitalized for any condition can develop *alcohol withdrawal syndrome* when the ingestion of alcohol is abruptly stopped. The onset of signs and symptoms of alcohol withdrawal is variable depending on the patient's drinking pattern. Initial symptoms may occur 4 to 6 hours after the last drink, and symptoms may last up to 14 days. Table 11-8 presents the clinical manifestations and suggested drug treatment for alcohol withdrawal. Since the symptoms of alcohol withdrawal do not always progress in a predictable manner, use a clinical withdrawal assessment tool, such as the Clinical Institute Withdrawal Assessment of Alcohol Scale, Revised (CIWA-Ar), to determine treatment (see Table 11-9 on p. 162 and eTable 11-1 on the website for this chapter).

Alcohol withdrawal delirium is a serious complication that can occur from 30 to 120 hours after the last drink. The greater the patient's dependence on alcohol, the greater the risk of serious withdrawal symptoms. Delirium components include disorientation, visual or auditory hallucinations, and increased hyperactivity without seizures. Death may result from hyperthermia, peripheral vascular collapse, or cardiac failure.[13]

Anticipating withdrawal syndrome in patients is important because alcohol withdrawal delirium can usually be prevented or controlled by administration of benzodiazepines such as

◎ NURSING CARE PLAN 11-1

Patient in Alcohol Withdrawal

| NURSING DIAGNOSIS | **Acute confusion** *related to* alcohol abuse and delirium *as evidenced by* increased agitation, hallucinations, fluctuations in level of consciousness and psychomotor activity, disorientation, or misperceptions. |

PATIENT GOALS
1. Demonstrates decrease in alcohol withdrawal severity.
2. Experiences no injury or complications of acute alcohol withdrawal.
3. Experiences no hallucinations.
4. Experiences no seizures.

Outcomes (NOC)

Interventions (NIC) and *Rationales*

Substance Withdrawal Severity
- Substance cravings ___
- Agitation ___
- Hyperreflexia ___
- Tremors ___
- Change in vital signs ___
- Disorientation ___
- Altered level of consciousness ___
- Difficulty interpreting environmental stimuli ___
- Misinterpretation of cues ___
- Sleeplessness ___
- Hallucinations ___
- Seizures ___

Measurement Scale
1 = Severe
2 = Substantial
3 = Moderate
4 = Mild
5 = None

Distorted Thought Self-Control
- Asks for validation of reality ___
- Reports decrease in hallucinations or delusions ___
- Perceives environment accurately ___
- Exhibits logical thought flow patterns ___
- Exhibits reality-based thinking ___
- Exhibits appropriate thought content ___

Measurement Scale
1 = Never demonstrated
2 = Rarely demonstrated
3 = Sometimes demonstrated
4 = Often demonstrated
5 = Consistently demonstrated

Substance Use Treatment: Alcohol Withdrawal
- Monitor vital signs during withdrawal *to identify extreme autonomic nervous system response.*
- Administer antiseizure drugs or sedatives *to prevent alcohol withdrawal delirium and relieve other symptoms during withdrawal.*
- Administer vitamin therapy *to prevent Wernicke's syndrome.*
- Address hallucinations in a therapeutic manner *to provide reality orientation.*
- Determine CIWA-Ar score every 4 hours until it is less than 8 for 24 hours *to assess need for medications.*
- Provide emotional support to patient/family *to decrease anxiety.*

Seizure Precautions
- Keep suction, Ambu-bag, and oral or nasopharyngeal airway at bedside *to establish respiratory function after seizure activity.*
- Use padded side rails and keep side rails up *to prevent injury during seizure activity.*

Delirium Management
- Monitor neurologic status on an ongoing basis *to determine appropriate interventions.*
- Verbally acknowledge the patient's fears and feelings to *decrease anxiety.*
- Provide patient with information about what is happening and what can be expected to occur in the future *to assist in reality orientation.*
- Maintain a well-lit environment that reduces sharp contrasts and shadows *to reduce external stimuli.*
- Remove stimuli, when possible, that create misperception in a particular patient (e.g., pictures on the wall or television) *to reduce misinterpretation of environment.*
- Inform patient of person, place, and time *to promote orientation.*
- Use environmental cues (e.g., signs, pictures, clocks, calendars, and color coding of environment) *to stimulate memory, reorient, and promote appropriate behavior.*

| NURSING DIAGNOSIS | **Ineffective self-health management** *related to* inadequate coping mechanisms and resources *as evidenced by* abuse of alcohol |

PATIENT GOALS
1. Acknowledges a substance abuse problem
2. Commits to alcohol cessation
3. Identifies positive coping mechanisms and resources to use during alcohol abstinence

Outcomes (NOC)

Interventions (NIC) and *Rationales*

Alcohol Abuse Cessation Behavior
- Expresses willingness to stop alcohol use ___
- Develops effective strategies to eliminate alcohol use ___
- Commits to alcohol elimination strategies ___
- Uses strategies to cope with withdrawal symptoms ___
- Uses effective coping mechanisms ___
- Adjusts lifestyle to promote alcohol elimination ___
- Obtains assistance from health professional ___
- Uses available support groups ___
- Eliminates alcohol use ___

Measurement Scale
1 = Never demonstrated
2 = Rarely demonstrated
3 = Sometimes demonstrated
4 = Often demonstrated
5 = Consistently demonstrated

Substance Use Treatment
- Encourage patient to take control over own behavior *to change undesired behaviors.*
- Discuss with patient the impact of substance use on medical condition or general health *to promote acknowledgment of consequences of use.*
- Identify constructive goals with patient *to provide alternatives to the use of substances to reduce stress.*
- Assist patient to learn alternative methods of coping with stress or emotional distress *to reduce substance use.*
- Identify support groups in the community for long-term substance abuse treatment *to promote continued abstinence.*

TABLE 11-9	CLINICAL INSTITUTE WITHDRAWAL ASSESSMENT OF ALCOHOL SCALE, REVISED (CIWA-Ar)*

The CIWA-Ar is a widely used tool for assessing alcohol withdrawal. The categories assessed are:

- Agitation
- Anxiety
- Auditory disturbances
- Headache, fullness in head
- Nausea and vomiting

- Orientation and clouding of sensorium
- Paroxysmal sweats
- Tactile disturbances
- Tremor
- Visual disturbances

Source: University of Maryland School of Medicine. Available at *http://umem.org/files/uploads/1104212257_CIWA-Ar.pdf*.
*⊖volve The complete CIWA-Ar and instructions for how to use it are presented in eTable 11-1 (available on the website for this chapter).

chlordiazepoxide (Librium) or lorazepam (Ativan).[13] A quiet, calm environment is important to prevent exacerbation of symptoms. Avoid the use of restraints and IV lines whenever possible. Supportive care is needed to ensure adequate rest and nutrition. The nursing care for a patient in alcohol withdrawal is presented in NCP 11-1 on p. 161.

OTHER DRUGS OF ABUSE

STIMULANTS

Frequently abused stimulants include cocaine and amphetamines. The use of cocaine is illegal, but amphetamines may be prescribed for the treatment of narcolepsy, attention deficit disorders, and weight control. All stimulants work in part by increasing the amount of dopamine in the brain, producing euphoria, alertness, and rapid dependence (see Table 11-10). Cocaine and amphetamines also stimulate the peripheral nervous and cardiovascular systems, thus creating adrenalin-like effects.[11]

Caffeine is the most widely used psychoactive substance in the world, but it is very weak when compared with the other stimulants. It is not regulated, and its use is safe in most people. Recently, more problems with caffeine have occurred because of high doses in popular "power" drinks. Caffeine dependence in a hospitalized patient can result in withdrawal headaches after general anesthesia or during restrictions on usual coffee or tea intake.

NURSING AND COLLABORATIVE CARE STIMULANT ABUSE

OVERDOSE

Almost 500,000 people are treated each year for cocaine and amphetamine use.[1] At high levels of overdose, the patient experiences restlessness, paranoia, agitated delirium, confusion, and repetitive stereotyped behaviors. Death is often related to stroke, dysrhythmias, or myocardial infarction.[14]

Emergency management of cocaine and amphetamine toxicity depends on the clinical manifestations at the time of treatment (Table 11-11). Therapy may be complicated by the possibility that the patient has combined the use of stimulants with heroin, alcohol, or phencyclidine hydrochloride (PCP). A specific antidote for cocaine and amphetamine toxicity is not available.

WITHDRAWAL

It is unusual for an individual dependent on stimulants to be hospitalized for management of withdrawal symptoms. However, you may identify withdrawal symptoms in a patient dependent on cocaine or amphetamines who is hospitalized for other health problems. Withdrawal from cocaine and amphetamines usually causes few physical symptoms, but fatigue, prolonged sleep, and depression occur in some individuals (see Table 11-10). Craving for the drug is intense during the first hours to days of drug cessation and may continue for weeks. Treatment is supportive.

DEPRESSANTS

Commonly abused depressants include sedative-hypnotics and opioids. With the exception of alcohol and some federally regulated drugs, most CNS depressants are medically useful. These drugs are widely recognized for their rapid development of tolerance and dependence and for medical emergencies involving overdose and withdrawal.

Sedative-Hypnotics

Commonly abused sedative-hypnotic agents include barbiturates, benzodiazepines, and barbiturate-like drugs. Barbiturates are preferred as recreational drugs because they more frequently produce euphoric effects. Sedative-hypnotic drugs depress the CNS, causing sedation at low doses and sleep at high doses. Excessive amounts produce an initial euphoria and an intoxication that resembles that of alcohol. The effects of sedative-hypnotics are presented in Table 11-10.

Tolerance develops rapidly to the effects of the drug, requiring higher doses to achieve euphoria. Tolerance may not develop to the brainstem-depressant effects. As a result, an increased dose may trigger hypotension and respiratory depression, resulting in death.[15]

Health problems resulting from the use of sedative-hypnotics are identified in Table 11-2. Complications associated with IV use of the drugs (e.g., blood-borne infections) also occur. An overdose of sedative-hypnotics can cause death from respiratory depression and arrest.

Opioids

Commonly abused opioids are identified in Table 11-10. Individuals dependent on opioids include those who use illegal drugs sold on the street and those who misuse prescription opioids. Heroin is a commonly used street drug. Misusing medications such as oxycodone (OxyContin) and acetaminophen plus hydrocodone (Vicodin) can result in the same harmful consequences as abusing heroin (Fig. 11-3). By acting on opiate receptors and neurotransmitter systems in the CNS, opioids cause CNS depression and have a major effect on the brain reward system. Cross-tolerance among the opioids is common. Cross-tolerance to other CNS depressants does not occur. However, additive effects of other CNS depressants may cause increased CNS depression.

Opioids are usually injected IV, increasing the user's risk for human immunodeficiency virus (HIV) infection, hepatitis B virus (HBV) infection, and hepatitis C virus (HCV) infection. In addition, drug abuse by any route increases the risk of contracting HIV because of risky sexual behaviors in exchange for drugs or money or because of lack of inhibition. Like all depressants, opioids can cause death from CNS and respiratory

TABLE 11-10 COMMONLY ABUSED ADDICTIVE SUBSTANCES

Substance	Physiologic and Psychologic Effects	Manifestations of Withdrawal	Treatment of Withdrawal
Stimulants *Cocaine and Amphetamines* Cocaine (street names: crack, snow, nose candy, coke, flake) dextroamphetamine (Dexedrine) methamphetamine (Desoxyn) methylphenidate (Ritalin) phentermine (Adipex-P)	*Early:* euphoria, grandiosity, excitation, restlessness, insomnia; tachycardia, hypertension, angina, dysrhythmias; dyspnea, tachypnea; sexual arousal, delayed orgasm; anorexia *Long-term:* depression, hallucinations, tremors, myocardial infarction, heart failure, cardiomyopathy; lung congestion; rhinorrhea; loss of interest in sexual activity	Severe craving, severely depressed mood, exhaustion, prolonged sleep, vivid dreams, apathy, irritability, disorientation	No specific drug therapy is effective in treating withdrawal. Supportive care includes taking measures to decrease agitation and restlessness in the early phase and allowing the patient to sleep and eat as needed in later phases. Refer to psychotherapy or behavioral therapy once stable.
Depressants *Sedative-Hypnotics* *Barbiturates:* secobarbital (Seconal), pentobarbital (Nembutal), amobarbital (Amytal) *Benzodiazepines:* diazepam (Valium), chlordiazepoxide (Librium), alprazolam (Xanax) *Nonbarbiturates-nonbenzodiazepines:* methaqualone (Quaalude), chloral hydrate (Somnote)	Initial relaxation, emotional lability, decreased inhibitions, drowsiness, lack of coordination, impaired judgment, slurred speech, hypotension, bradycardia, bradypnea, constricted pupils	*Early:* Weakness, restlessness, insomnia, hyperthermia, orthostatic hypotension, confusion, disorientation *Days 3-5:* Major convulsive episodes, psychotic delirium, exhaustion, cardiovascular collapse, death	Stabilize on phenobarbital or a long-acting benzodiazepine. Gradually taper dose after stabilization. Supportive care includes measures to ensure patient safety and comfort, frequent assessment of neurologic status and vital signs, and provision of reassurance and orientation. Motivate the patient to engage in long-term treatment and refer to psychotherapy or behavioral therapy once stable.
Opioids Heroin (street names: brown sugar, dope, horse, junk, mud, smack), morphine, opium, codeine, fentanyl (Sublimaze), meperidine (Demerol), hydromorphone (Dilaudid), pentazocine (Talwin), oxycodone (OxyContin), methadone (Dolophine)	Analgesia, euphoria, drowsiness, detachment from environment, relaxation, constricted pupils, constipation, nausea, decreased respiratory rate, slurred speech, impaired judgment, decreased sexual and aggressive drives	Watery eyes, dilated pupils, runny nose, yawning, tremors, muscle and joint pain, chills, fever, diaphoresis, insomnia, tachycardia, hypertension, nausea, vomiting, diarrhea, abdominal cramps, food cravings	Methadone in decreasing doses is used during detoxification to decrease symptoms. Symptom management includes bismuth subsalicylate (Kaopectate) for diarrhea, acetaminophen (Tylenol) for muscle aches, and clonidine (Catapres) for generalized symptoms. Once stable, continued use of opioid agonists (methadone), opioid antagonists (naltrexone [ReVia]), or mixed opioid agonists-antagonists (buprenorphine [Subutex, Suboxone]) is recommended under outpatient supervision.
Cannabis Marijuana (street names: pot, reefer, weed, herb), hashish (street names: hash, hemp)	Euphoria, sedation, hallucinations	Flulike illness, disturbed sleep, irritability, anxiety, insomnia, tremor, anorexia	No specific drug therapy is effective in treating withdrawal. Supportive care includes measures to ensure patient comfort, including analgesics and hydration. Benzodiazepines are used for symptomatic relief. Refer to psychotherapy or behavioral therapy once stable.

depression. Other complications associated with opioid use are presented in Table 11-2.

NURSING AND COLLABORATIVE CARE DEPRESSANT ABUSE

OVERDOSE

Unintentional overdose frequently occurs with recreational use of depressants because of the unpredictability in potency and purity. If the patient has ingested multiple substances, a complex and potentially confusing clinical picture can result. Serum and urine drug screens may be helpful in identifying the type and amounts of drugs present in the body. The first priority of care in overdose is always the patient's ABCs. Continuous monitoring of neurologic status, including level of consciousness, and respiratory and cardiovascular function is critical until the patient is stable.[15] Emergency management of depressant drug overdose is presented in Table 11-12.

SEDATIVE-HYPNOTICS. Overdoses of benzodiazepines are treated with flumazenil (Romazicon), a specific benzodiazepine antagonist. Flumazenil is used with caution because it can cause seizures in patients with physical dependence on benzodiaze-

FIG. 11-3 Use of oxycodone injections has increased rapidly. (Doug Menuez/Photodisc/Thinkstock)

pines. Because flumazenil may have a shorter duration of action than some benzodiazepines, doses may need to be repeated until the benzodiazepine is metabolized.

There are no known antagonists to counteract the effects of barbiturates or other sedative-hypnotic drugs. The patient who has overdosed on sedative-hypnotics other than benzodiazepines must be treated aggressively. Dialysis may be required to decrease the drug level and to prevent irreversible CNS depressant effects and death. Gastric lavage and administration of activated charcoal may be instituted if the drug was taken orally within the previous hour. CNS stimulants are avoided, since their use is associated with higher mortality rates.

OPIOIDS. A patient with an opioid overdose can be seen at the emergency department in a coma and respiratory arrest. A toxicologic blood or urine screen may be helpful to identify the

✚ TABLE 11-11 EMERGENCY MANAGEMENT
Cocaine and Amphetamine Toxicity

Assessment Findings	Interventions
Cardiovascular • Palpitations • Tachycardia • Hypertension • Dysrhythmias • Myocardial ischemia or infarction	• Ensure patent airway. • Anticipate need for intubation if respiratory distress evident. • Establish IV access and initiate fluid replacement as appropriate. • Obtain a 12-lead ECG and initiate ECG monitoring.
Central Nervous System • Feeling of impending doom • Euphoria • Agitation • Combativeness • Seizures • Hallucinations • Confusion • Paranoia • Fever	• Treat ventricular dysrhythmias as appropriate with lidocaine, bretylium (Bretylol), or procainamide (Pronestyl). • Hypertension and chest pain may require administration of nitroprusside (Nipride) or phentolamine (Regitine). • Aspirin may be administered to lower the risk of myocardial infarction. • Administer IV diazepam (Valium) or lorazepam (Ativan) for seizures. • Administer IV antipsychotic drugs for psychosis and hallucinations. • Naloxone (Narcan) IV should be given if CNS depression is present and concurrent opioid use is suspected.
Other • Track marks • Consumption of bags of cocaine	• Monitor vital signs and level of consciousness. • Initiate cooling measures for hyperthermia.

✚ TABLE 11-12 EMERGENCY MANAGEMENT
Depressant Drug Overdose

Assessment Findings	Interventions
• Aggressive behavior • Agitation • Confusion • Lethargy • Stupor • Hallucinations • Depression • Slurred speech • Pinpoint pupils • Nystagmus • Seizures • Needle tracks • Cold, clammy skin • Rapid, weak pulse • Slow or rapid shallow respirations • Decreased oxygen saturation • Hypotension • Dysrhythmias • ECG changes • Cardiac or respiratory arrest	• Ensure patent airway. • Anticipate intubation if respiratory distress evident. • Establish IV access. • Obtain temperature. • Obtain 12-lead ECG and initiate continuous ECG monitoring. • Obtain information about substance (name, route, when taken, amount). • Obtain specific drug levels or comprehensive toxicology screen. • Obtain a health history, including drug use and allergies. • Administer antidotes as appropriate. • Perform gastric lavage if necessary. • Administer activated charcoal and cathartics as appropriate. • Monitor vital signs, level of consciousness, and oxygen saturation.

specific drug, but treatment is not delayed for toxicology results. Death can occur if the overdose is not treated. An opioid antagonist such as naloxone (Narcan) should be given as soon as life support is instituted. Monitor the patient closely because naloxone has a shorter duration of action than most opioids. The patient may have a mixed drug ingestion that does not respond to opioid antagonists.

┃ WITHDRAWAL

SEDATIVE-HYPNOTICS. Withdrawal from sedative-hypnotics can be life threatening. The manifestations are nearly identical to those of alcohol withdrawal (see Table 11-8). Because the patient may experience delirium, seizures, and respiratory and cardiac arrest within 24 hours after the last dose, close monitoring in an inpatient setting is often required[16] (see Table 11-10). Mild to moderate symptoms can persist for 2 to 3 weeks after a 3- to 5-day period of acute symptoms.

OPIOIDS. Withdrawal from opioids occurs with decreased amounts or cessation of the drug after prolonged moderate to heavy use. The administration of an opioid antagonist, such as naloxone, will also cause withdrawal symptoms in dependent individuals. Symptoms of withdrawal are not usually life threatening but can be severe, depending on the potency of the abused opioid, route of administration, and duration of use (see Table 11-10). Treatment is based on symptoms and may require the use of medications. Methadone (Dolophine) in decreasing doses is the drug used most often during detoxification to decrease symptoms.

CANNABIS

Cannabis, called marijuana or hashish, is the most widely used illicit drug in North America.[1] Patterns of use are similar to those of alcohol in that there is occasional use, misuse resulting in temporary problems, and abuse or dependence associated with a high potential for future problems.

The key active ingredient in cannabis responsible for most of the psychoactive effects is tetrahydrocannabinol (THC). Two THC preparations, dronabinol (Marinol) and nabilone (Cesamet), are available by prescription to control nausea and vomiting resulting from cancer chemotherapy. Dronabinol may also be used to stimulate the appetite in patients with acquired immunodeficiency syndrome (AIDS). Some states have legalized marijuana use for specified health problems. At low to moderate doses, THC produces fewer physiologic and psychologic alterations than do other classes of psychoactive drugs, including alcohol. Health problems caused by heavy use are identified in Table 11-2.

In the patient with acute marijuana intoxication, perform a physical examination and a thorough history. An individual with marijuana intoxication is seldom hospitalized. Panic, flashbacks, and toxic reactions related to the use of marijuana are managed by providing a quiet environment and supporting and reassuring the patient by explaining what is happening. The patient needs to understand that the level of intoxication may fluctuate over several days as metabolites are released.

You may identify withdrawal symptoms in a patient dependent on cannabis who is hospitalized for other health problems. Withdrawal usually causes few physical symptoms, but some patients have flu-like illness, disturbed sleep, and tremors[17] (see Table 11-10). Treatment is supportive.

NURSING MANAGEMENT
SUBSTANCE ABUSE

NURSING ASSESSMENT

Any patient with substance dependence who is hospitalized for any condition can develop withdrawal syndrome when the ingestion of the substance is abruptly stopped. Early recognition and identification of withdrawal syndrome are crucial to successful treatment outcomes for any health problem. Hospitalization also provides a chance to address substance use, and for many patients, controlling their health problems requires addressing their substance use.

Question every patient about the use of all substances, including prescribed medications, OTC drugs, caffeine, tobacco, and recreational drugs. Screen for alcohol use using a validated screening questionnaire. Although a variety of screening tools are available, one culturally sensitive tool that is easily used by nurses to identify alcohol dependence is the Alcohol Use Disorders Identification Test (AUDIT) (Table 11-13). A score of 8 points or less is considered nonalcoholic, whereas 9 points or above indicates alcoholism. Another frequently used instrument is the Drug Abuse Screening Test (DAST-10) questionnaire (Table 11-14).

Take a history in a setting that ensures privacy and avoids interruption. To obtain accurate information, use open and nonjudgmental communication with the patient. Ask questions in a way that lets the patient know that you find a behavior normal or at least understandable. You might say, "Given your situation, I wonder if you have been using anything to help relieve your stress." You may also collect a history from any available collateral sources (e.g., spouse) because patients often underreport or minimize their alcohol and drug use.

Reassure the patient that all information will remain confidential and will be used only to provide safe care. The substance-abusing patient may be afraid of losing control of drug

TABLE 11-13 ALCOHOL USE DISORDERS IDENTIFICATION TEST (AUDIT)

Please answer each question by checking one of the circles in the second column.

Question	Response	Score
1. How often do you have a drink containing alcohol?	Never	(0)
	Monthly or less	(1)
	2-4 times per month	(2)
	2-4 times per week	(3)
	4+ times per week	(4)
2. How many drinks containing alcohol do you have on a typical day when you are drinking?	1 or 2	(0)
	3 or 4	(1)
	5 or 6	(2)
	7 to 9	(3)
	10 or more	(4)
3. How often do you have six or more drinks on one occasion?	Never	(0)
	Less than monthly	(1)
	Monthly	(2)
	Weekly	(3)
	Daily or almost daily	(4)
4. How often during the last year have you found that you were not able to stop drinking once you had started?	Never	(0)
	Less than monthly	(1)
	Monthly	(2)
	Weekly	(3)
	Daily or almost daily	(4)
5. How often in the last year have you failed to do what was normally expected of you because you were drinking?	Never	(0)
	Less than monthly	(1)
	Monthly	(2)
	Weekly	(3)
	Daily or almost daily	(4)
6. How often during the last year have you needed a first drink in the morning to get yourself going after a heavy drinking session?	Never	(0)
	Less than monthly	(1)
	Monthly	(2)
	Weekly	(3)
	Daily or almost daily	(4)
7. How often during the last year have you had a feeling of guilt or remorse about drinking?	Never	(0)
	Less than monthly	(1)
	Monthly	(2)
	Weekly	(3)
	Daily or almost daily	(4)
8. How often during the last year have you been unable to remember what happened the night before because you had been drinking?	Never	(0)
	Less than monthly	(1)
	Monthly	(2)
	Weekly	(3)
	Daily or almost daily	(4)
9. Have you or someone else been injured as a result of your drinking?	No	(0)
	Yes, but not in the last year	(2)
	Yes, during the last year	(4)
10. Has a relative, friend, or other health worker been concerned about your drinking or suggested that you cut down?	No	(0)
	Yes, but not in the last year	(2)
	Yes, during the last year	(4)

Scoring for AUDIT: Questions 1 through 8 are scored 0, 1, 2, 3, or 4. Questions 9 and 10 are scored 0, 2, or 4 only. The minimum score (nondrinkers) is 0 and the maximum possible score is 40. A score of 9 or more indicates hazardous or harmful alcohol consumption.
Source: Saunders JB, Aasland OG, Babor TF, et al: Development of the Alcohol Use Disorders Identification Test (AUDIT), WHO collaborative project on early detection of people with harmful alcohol consumption, II, *Addiction* 88:791, 1993. Retrieved from *http://pubs.niaaa.nih.gov/publications/Practitioner/CliniciansGuide2005/clinicians_guide11.htm.*

administration and may be concerned that substance use will be reported to legal authorities. Inform the patient that federal privacy laws prohibit nurses and other health care providers from disclosing any treatment of substance abuse without the patient's specific written consent.

TABLE 11-14	**DRUG ABUSE SCREENING TEST (DAST-10)**		
In the last 12 months:			
1. Have you used drugs other than those required for medical reasons?		No	Yes
2. Do you abuse more than one drug at a time?		No	Yes
3. Are you always able to stop using drugs when you want to?		No	Yes
4. Have you had "blackouts" or "flashbacks" as a result of drug use?		No	Yes
5. Do you ever feel bad or guilty about your drug use?		No	Yes
6. Does your spouse (or parents) ever complain about your involvement with drugs?		No	Yes
7. Have you neglected your family because of your use of drugs?		No	Yes
8. Have you engaged in illegal activities in order to obtain drugs?		No	Yes
9. Have you ever experienced withdrawal symptoms or felt sick when you stopped taking drugs?		No	Yes
10. Have you had medical problems as a result of your drug use?		No	Yes

Copyright 1982 by Harvey A. Skinner, PhD, and the Centre for Addiction and Mental Health, Toronto, Canada. You may reproduce this instrument for non-commercial use (clinical, research, training purposes) as long as you credit the author, Dr. Harvey A. Skinner, Dean, Faculty of Health, York University, Toronto, Canada. Email: harvey.skinner@yorku.ca.

TABLE 11-15	**SIGNS SUGGESTING SUBSTANCE ABUSE**

- Fatigue
- Insomnia
- Headaches
- Seizure disorder
- Changes in mood
- Anorexia, weight loss
- Vague physical complaints
- Overabundant use of mouthwash or toiletries
- Appearing older than stated age, unkempt appearance
- Leisure activities that involve alcohol and/or other drugs
- Sexual dysfunction, decreased libido, erectile dysfunction
- Trauma secondary to falls, auto accidents, fights, or burns
- Driving while intoxicated (more than one citation suggests dependence)
- Failure of standard doses of sedatives to have a therapeutic effect
- Financial problems, including those related to spending for substances
- Defensive or evasive answers to questions about substance use and its importance in the person's life
- Problems in areas of life function (e.g., frequent job changes; marital conflict, separation, or divorce; work-related accidents, tardiness, absenteeism; legal problems; social isolation, estrangement from friends or family)

During your assessment, observe for patient behaviors that influence history taking such as denial, avoidance, underreporting or minimizing of substance use, or provision of inaccurate information. Possible behaviors and physical complaints suggesting substance dependence are listed in Table 11-15, but these behaviors are not all-inclusive. Even if a patient denies addiction or dependence, if there is any indication of alcohol or other CNS depressant use when a patient is hospitalized, always ask when the patient last used the substance. This information will help you anticipate drug interactions or the time of possible onset of withdrawal symptoms if the patient is indeed dependent on a substance.

Problems associated with substance abuse are often revealed through physical assessment, including assessment of the patient's general appearance and nutritional status and examination of the abdomen; the skin; and the cardiovascular, respiratory, and neurologic systems. Urine and blood drug screenings may be performed in some situations to determine drug use. A complete blood count, serum electrolytes, blood urea nitrogen, creatinine, and hepatic function tests may be done to evaluate for electrolyte imbalances or kidney or liver dysfunction.

NURSING DIAGNOSES

Nursing diagnoses for an individual with substance abuse may include, but are not limited to, those presented in NCP 11-1.

PLANNING

The overall goals are that the patient with a substance abuse problem will (1) have normal physiologic functioning, (2) acknowledge a substance abuse problem, (3) explain the psychologic and physiologic effects of substance use, (4) abstain from the use of addicting substances, and (5) cooperate with a proposed treatment plan.

NURSING IMPLEMENTATION

HEALTH PROMOTION. Your role in health promotion includes prevention and early detection of substance abuse. Teaching about the effects and negative outcomes of substance abuse is essential in preventing this problem. When individuals have substance abuse problems, it is critical to motivate them to enter treatment programs.

ACUTE INTERVENTION. Acute intoxication, overdose, and withdrawal may be seen in acute care situations. Intoxication and overdose may require physiologic support until detoxification can occur. During detoxification the patient is treated to diminish or remove drugs or their effects from the body. Treatments may involve administration of antagonistic drugs, promotion of metabolism and elimination of the drug, or intensive supportive care until the drug is naturally eliminated. Be aware that intoxication and overdose could occur in a hospitalized patient dependent on substances if visitors provide the substances.

You are in a unique position to motivate and facilitate behavior change in people who are abusing substances. When patients seek care for health problems related to substance abuse or when hospitalization interferes with the patient's usual pattern of substance use, the patient's awareness of a substance abuse problem is increased. Intervention by nurses at this time can be a crucial factor in promoting behavior change. Take an active role in performing motivational interviewing and providing counseling aimed at promoting cessation. Document all the interventions in the patient's chart.

AMBULATORY AND HOME CARE. Before treatment and rehabilitation for substance abuse are considered, acute health problems must be resolved. Many of the patients with substance abuse problems that you encounter in hospitals and primary care centers seek care for health problems associated with substance abuse, not for their addiction itself. When you are working in a medical-surgical setting, you usually will not be involved in long-term treatment of patients with substance abuse problems. However, it is your responsibility to identify the problem, motivate the patient to change behavior, and be prepared to refer the patient to inpatient and outpatient programs in the community that provide treatment and rehabilitation. Failure to confront the patient's substance abuse problem, thus enabling the behavior, is a breach of your professional responsibility.

GERONTOLOGIC CONSIDERATIONS

SUBSTANCE ABUSE

Health care providers are much less likely to recognize substance misuse, abuse, and dependence in older adults than in younger adults. Older adults do not fit the image of abusers. In addition, their patterns of misuse of prescription psychoactive agents and alcohol are less commonly seen than those of younger populations. Because the effects of alcohol and drug use can be mistaken for medical conditions common among older adults, such as insomnia, depression, poor nutrition, heart failure, and frequent falls, the substance abuse problem is often not diagnosed and not treated.[18]

Older adults' misuse and abuse of psychoactive agents, either alone or in combination, may cause confusion, disorientation, delirium, memory loss, and neuromuscular impairment. Physiologic changes that accompany aging, such as decreased circulation, metabolism, and excretion, may lead to intoxication at levels that may not have been a problem at a younger age. Withdrawal symptoms that occur in the older adult when alcohol, opioids, or sedative-hypnotics are abruptly stopped may be more severe than in younger individuals. Always consider that behavior changes in older adults may be caused by substance use or withdrawal.

Identification of substance misuse, abuse, and dependence in older adults presents a challenge. Family members are important sources of information. As with all patients, it is important for you to discuss all drug and alcohol use with older adult patients, including OTC, herbal, and homeopathic drug use.

Assess the patient's knowledge of medications that are currently being taken.

The older adult may not exhibit the social, legal, and occupational consequences of substance abuse identified by common screening questionnaires. However, the Short Michigan Alcoholism Screening Test–Geriatric Version (SMAST-G) has been developed as a short-form alcoholism-screening instrument for older adults.[19] This tool, available at *http://consultgerirn.org,* can identify those at risk for negative outcomes of alcohol use. The AUDIT and DAST-10 questionnaires (discussed previously) can also be used with or instead of the SMAST-G to identify alcohol and drug abuse or dependence in older adults.

Smoking and other tobacco use is also an issue in older adults. Older adults who have been chronic smokers for decades may feel unable to stop, or they may believe there is no benefit to stopping at an advanced age. However, smoking contributes to and exacerbates many chronic illnesses found in the older adult population. Smoking cessation at any age is beneficial. The clinical practice guideline for treating tobacco use and dependence discussed earlier is appropriate for helping older adults with smoking cessation (see Tables 11-3 to 11-6).

Patient teaching for the older adult includes teaching about the desired effects, possible side effects, and appropriate use of prescribed and OTC drugs. Advise patients not to drink alcohol when using prescribed and OTC drugs. If no medical condition or possible drug interactions preclude the use of alcohol, advise older patients to limit their alcohol intake to one drink per day. When you suspect alcohol or substance dependence in the older patient, refer the patient for treatment. It is a mistaken belief that older people have little to gain from alcohol and drug dependence treatment. The rewards of treatment can lead to greater quality and quantity of life for older adults.

CASE STUDY

Substance Misuse and Abuse

iStockphoto/Thinkstock

Patient Profile
C.M., a 78-year-old white woman, is admitted to the emergency department after falling and injuring her right hip. She has been widowed for 4 years and lives alone. Recently her best friend died. Her only family is a daughter who lives out of town. When contacted by phone, the daughter tells the nurse that her mother has appeared more disoriented and confused over the past few months when she has talked to her on the phone.

Subjective Data
- Is complaining of severe pain in her right hip
- Admits she had some wine in the late afternoon to stimulate her appetite
- Has experienced several falls in the past 2 months
- Reports that she fell after taking her sleeping pill prescribed by her physician because she does not sleep well
- Speech is hesitant and slurred
- Says she smokes about one-half pack of cigarettes a day

Objective Data
Physical Examination
- Oriented to person and place, but not time
- BP 162/94, pulse 92, respirations 24
- Severe pain and tenderness in the right hip region
- Tremors of hands

Diagnostic Tests
- X-ray reveals a subtrochanteric fracture of the right femur requiring surgical repair
- Blood alcohol concentration (BAC) 120 mg/dL (0.12 mg%)
- Complete blood count: hemoglobin 10.6 g/dL, hematocrit 33%

Discussion Questions
1. What other information is needed to assess C.M.'s condition?
2. How should questions regarding substance use be addressed?
3. What factors may contribute to C.M.'s use of psychoactive substances?
4. *Priority Decision:* What are the priority nursing interventions during C.M.'s preoperative period?
5. What possible complications and other health problems may become apparent during C.M.'s postoperative recovery?
6. *Priority Decision:* What are the priority nursing interventions after C.M.'s surgery?
7. *Delegation Decision:* How would you use the following nursing personnel on the postoperative unit to carry out the priority interventions that you identified in question 6: registered nurse (RN), licensed practical nurse (LPN), unlicensed assistive personnel (UAP)?
8. *Priority Decision:* Based on the assessment data presented, what are the priority nursing diagnoses? Are there any collaborative problems?

BRIDGE TO NCLEX EXAMINATION

The number of the question corresponds to the same-numbered outcome at the beginning of the chapter.

1. A person who injects heroin to experience the euphoria that it causes is demonstrating
   a. abuse.
   b. addiction.
   c. tolerance.
   d. addictive behavior.

2. When admitting a patient, the nurse must assess the patient for substance use based on the knowledge that long-term use of addictive substances leads to
   a. the development of coexisting psychiatric illnesses.
   b. a higher risk for complications from underlying health problems.
   c. increased availability of dopamine, resulting in decreased sleep requirements.
   d. potentiation of effects of similar drugs taken when the individual is drug free.

3. The nurse would suspect cocaine overdose in the patient who is experiencing
   a. craving, restlessness, and irritability.
   b. agitation, cardiac dysrhythmias, and seizures.
   c. diarrhea, nausea and vomiting, and confusion.
   d. slow, shallow respirations; hyporeflexia; and blurred vision.

4. The most appropriate nursing intervention for a patient who is being treated for an acute exacerbation of chronic obstructive pulmonary disease who is not interested in quitting smoking is to
   a. accept the patient's decision and not intervene until the patient expresses a desire to quit.
   b. realize that some smokers will never quit, and trying to assist them increases the patient's' frustration.
   c. motivate the patient to quit by describing how continued smoking will worsen the breathing problems.
   d. ask the patient to identify the relevance, risks, and benefits of quitting and what barriers to quitting are present.

5. While caring for a patient who is experiencing alcohol withdrawal, the nurse should (select all that apply)
   a. monitor neurologic status on a routine basis.
   b. provide a quiet, nonstimulating, dimly lit environment.
   c. pad the side rails and place suction equipment at the bedside.
   d. orient the patient to environment and person with each contact.
   e. administer antiseizure drugs and sedatives to relieve symptoms during withdrawal.

6. Substance abuse problems in older adults are usually related to
   a. use of drugs and alcohol as a social activity.
   b. misuse of prescribed and over-the-counter drugs and alcohol.
   c. continuing the use of illegal drugs initiated during middle age.
   d. a pattern of binge drinking for weeks or months with periods of sobriety.

1. d, 2. b, 3. b, 4. d, 5. a, c, d, e, 6. b

⊖volve

For rationales to these answers and even more NCLEX review questions, visit *http://evolve.elsevier.com/Lewis/medsurg.*

REFERENCES

1. Substance Abuse and Mental Health Services Administration: Results from the 2010 national survey on drug use and health. Retrieved from *http://oas.samhsa.gov.*
2. National Institute on Drug Abuse: Prescription drugs: abuse and addiction. Retrieved from *www.nida.nih.gov/PDF/RRPrescription.pdf.*
3. American Psychiatric Association: *The diagnostic and statistical manual of mental disorders (DSM-IV-TR),* ed 4, Arlington, Va, 2000, The Association. (Classic)
4. Robin C, O'Connell E, Samnaliev M: Overview of substance abuse and healthcare costs. Retrieved from *http://saprp.org/knowledgeassets/knowledge_detail.cfm?KAID=21.*
5. Centers for Disease Control and Prevention: Adult smoking in the U.S. Retrieved from *www.cdc.gov/VitalSigns/pdf/2011-09-vitalsigns.pdf.*
6. US Department of Health and Human Services: How tobacco smoke causes disease: the biology and behavioral basis for smoking-attributable disease: a report of the Surgeon General. Retrieved from *www.surgeongeneral.gov/library/tobaccosmoke/index.html.*
7. American Cancer Society: Women and smoking. Retrieved from *www.cancer.org/Cancer/CancerCauses/TobaccoCancer/WomenandSmoking/index.*
8. Agency for Healthcare Research and Quality: Treating tobacco use and dependence: 2008 update. Retrieved from *www.ncbi.nlm.nih.gov/books/bv.fcgi?rid=hstat2.chapter.28163.*
*9. Reynolds S: Combination therapy most effective for helping smokers quit, *NIDA Notes* 23:7, 2011.
*10. Raupach T, van Schayck C: Pharmacotherapy for smoking cessation: current advances and research topics, *CNS Drugs* 25:371, 2011.
11. National Institute on Drug Abuse: Drugs, brains, and behavior: the science of addiction. Retrieved from *www.nida.nih.gov/scienceofaddiction/brain.html.*
12. Keltner NL, Bostrom CE, McGuinness T: *Psychiatric nursing,* ed 7, St Louis, 2010, Mosby.

*Evidence-based information for clinical practice.

*13. Tovar R: Diagnosis and treatment of alcohol withdrawal, *JCOM* 18:361, 2011.

14. Wood DM, Dargan PI: Putting cocaine use and cocaine-associated cardiac arrhythmias into epidemiological and clinical perspective, *Br J Clin Pharmacol* 69:443, 2010.

15. Lehne RA: *Pharmacology for nursing care*, ed 7, St Louis, 2010, Saunders.

16. Tetrault JM, O'Connor PG: Substance abuse and withdrawal in the critical care setting, *Crit Care Clin* 24:767, 2008.

17. Maldonado JR: An approach to the patient with substance use and abuse, *Med Clin North Am* 94:1169, 2010.

18. Frances RJ: Geriatric addictions, *Am J Geriatr Psychiatry* 19: 681, 2011.

19. Naegle M: Alcohol use screening and assessment for older adults. Retrieved from *http://consultgerirn.org/uploads/File/trythis/try_this_17.pdf.*

RESOURCES

American Lung Association
www.lungusa.org
American Psychiatric Nurses Association
www.apna.org
American Society of Addiction Medicine
www.asam.org
National Council on Alcoholism and Drug Dependence, Inc.
www.ncadd.org
National Institute on Drug Abuse
www.nida.nih.gov
Substance Abuse and Mental Health Services Administration
http://www.samhsa.gov/
Tobacco Information and Prevention Source (TIPS)
www.cdc.gov/tobacco

MANAGING MULTIPLE PATIENTS

Introduction

You are assigned to care for the following five patients on a medical-surgical unit. Your team consists of yourself, a new LPN still on orientation, and an unlicensed assistive personnel (UAP).

Patients

A.Z. is a 75-year-old woman who came to the United States from Russia 10 years ago with her daughter, her son-in-law, and their five children. She speaks minimal English, relying on her oldest granddaughter to translate. A.Z., who has a history of diabetes mellitus, was admitted to the hospital yesterday with a diagnosis of heart failure.

iStockphoto/Thinkstock

M.L. is a 60-year-old Asian woman who was admitted to the hospital with a diagnosis of exacerbation of chronic obstructive pulmonary disease (COPD). She is receiving oxygen at 2 L/min via nasal cannula and her condition is currently stable.

Thomas M. Perkins/
Shutterstock.com

L.X. is a 79-year-old Chinese woman who was admitted through the emergency department with a chief complaint of shortness of breath. She was diagnosed with community-acquired pneumonia, which is being treated with IV antibiotics.

iStockphoto/Thinkstock

K.C. is a 280-lb (127-kg) 68-year-old African American woman with diabetes who was admitted for an incision and drainage of a right abdominal abscess. She is being discharged on her second postoperative day. Her married daughter will assist with dressing changes at home.

Ryan McVay/Photodisc/
Thinkstock

C.M. is a 78-year-old white woman who was admitted from the emergency department after falling and fracturing her right hip. She is in Buck's traction and is scheduled to undergo surgical repair later this morning. She has a history of substance abuse and her blood alcohol content (BAC) was 120 mg/dL (0.12 mg%) on admission. The night nurse reports that she has been somewhat confused and restless overnight.

iStockphoto/Thinkstock

Management Discussion Questions

1. *Priority Decision:* After receiving report, which patient should you see first? Provide rationale.
2. *Delegation Decision:* Which morning task(s) could you delegate to the LPN (select all that apply)?
   a. Obtain a capillary blood glucose reading on K.C.
   b. Assess L.X.'s IV site for signs of phlebitis or infiltration.
   c. Access the hospital's available translation services for A.Z.
   d. Titrate M.L.'s oxygen to obtain a pulse oximetry reading of 95%, as ordered by the health care provider.

3. *Priority and Delegation Decision:* When you and the LPN enter A.Z.'s room, you find the patient sitting up in bed with labored respirations. Although you cannot understand what she is saying, you note that she is unable to say more than two words without stopping for a breath. Which initial action would be the most appropriate?
   a. Ask the LPN to get A.Z.'s vital signs while you auscultate her lung sounds.
   b. Administer A.Z.'s cardiac and respiratory medications and reassess her in 30 minutes.
   c. Have the LPN find A.Z.'s granddaughter so that she can translate what A.Z. is trying to tell you.
   d. Ask the LPN to stay with A.Z. while you go to the nurse's station to call A.Z.'s health care provider.

Case Study Progression

A.Z.'s assessment reveals bibasilar crackles, 2+ dependent pitting edema, BP 175/84, pulse 96, RR 32, temp 36.8°C, and pulse oximetry 88% on room air. You administer oxygen at 2 L/min via nasal cannula and obtain an order from A.Z.'s health care provider for furosemide 40 mg IV stat. After administering the diuretic, A.Z.'s granddaughter arrives and you discuss her grandmother's condition. She tells you that her grandmother asked her to bring in potato chips and soda yesterday. She did not think her grandmother should be eating salt, but A.Z. insisted that the dietitian said that she could eat them.

4. On further investigation, the dietitian tells you that a translator was not available when she saw A.Z. yesterday. Because the dietitian did not understand what the patient was saying, she could not respond to any of her questions. She planned to visit A.Z. today when the granddaughter is present. Being a culturally competent nurse, you realize that A.Z. most likely interpreted the dietitian's silence as
   a. agreement with what A.Z. was asking.
   b. demonstrating a lack of respect for A.Z.'s wishes.
   c. a lack of understanding by the dietitian as to what she was asking.
   d. a need for the dietitian to get more information before answering her questions.
5. Which assessment findings might suggest elder mistreatment by L.X.'s son, with whom she lives (select all that apply)?
   a. Two sacral ulcers
   b. Asking when her son is coming to visit
   c. Multiple small bruises on her forearms and shins
   d. Matted hair, poor oral hygiene, overgrown toenails
6. Knowing that C.M.'s reported restlessness overnight may indicate acute alcohol withdrawal, you perform a more thorough assessment. Your assessment reveals a score of 11 on the Clinical Institute Withdrawal Assessment for Alcohol Scale. To prevent alcohol delirium, you plan to administer
   a. IV thiamine.
   b. morphine sulfate.
   c. naloxone (Narcan).
   d. lorazepam (Ativan).
7. *Management Decision:* The UAP informs you that the LPN is not following hospital protocol when caring for patients at risk for falling. What is your most appropriate action?
   a. Notify the unit manager as soon as possible.
   b. Ask the UAP to explain hospital protocol to the LPN.
   c. Write up the LPN's actions so they are included in her evaluation.
   d. Talk to the LPN about the importance of following hospital protocol to prevent injury in patients at risk for falling.

Pathophysiologic Mechanisms of Disease

iStockphoto/Thinkstock

When you arrive at a fork in the road, take it.
Yogi Berra

CHAPTER

12

Unless someone like you cares a whole awful lot, nothing is going to get better. It's not.
Dr. Seuss

Inflammation and Wound Healing

Sharon L. Lewis

⊖volve WEBSITE

http://evolve.elsevier.com/Lewis/medsurg

- NCLEX Review Questions
- Key Points
- Pre-Test
- Answer Guidelines for Case Study on p. 188
- Rationales for Bridge to NCLEX Examination Questions
- Case Study
  - Patient With Pressure Ulcers
- Nursing Care Plans (Customizable)
  - eNCP 12-1: Patient With a Fever
  - eNCP 12-2: Patient With a Pressure Ulcer

- Concept Map Creator
- Glossary
- Content Updates

eFigures
- eFig. 12-1: Margination, diapedesis, and chemotaxis of white blood cells
- eFig. 12-2: Sequential activation and biologic effects of the complement system
- eFig. 12-3: Granulating wound

eTables
- eTable 12-1: Wound Classification by Etiology
- eTable 12-2: Wound Classification Systems
- eTable 12-3: Braden Scale for Predicting Pressure Sore Risk
- eTable 12-4: Pressure Ulcer Scale for Healing (PUSH)

LEARNING OUTCOMES

1. Describe the inflammatory response, including vascular and cellular responses and exudate formation.
2. Explain local and systemic manifestations of inflammation and their physiologic bases.
3. Describe the drug therapy, nutrition therapy, and nursing management of inflammation.
4. Differentiate among healing by primary, secondary, and tertiary intention.
5. Describe the factors that delay wound healing and common complications of wound healing.
6. Describe the nursing and collaborative management of wound healing.
7. Explain the etiology and clinical manifestations of pressure ulcers.
8. Apply a patient risk assessment for pressure ulcers to measures used to prevent the development of pressure ulcers.
9. Discuss nursing and collaborative management of a patient with pressure ulcers.

KEY TERMS

adhesions, Table 12-8, p. 180
dehiscence, Table 12-8, p. 180
evisceration, Table 12-8, p. 180
fibroblasts, p. 178

hypertrophic scars, Table 12-8, p. 180
inflammatory response, p. 172
pressure ulcer, p. 184

regeneration, p. 177
repair, p. 177
shearing force, p. 184

This chapter focuses on inflammation and wound healing. Pressure ulcer prevention and treatment are also described.

INFLAMMATORY RESPONSE

The **inflammatory response** is a sequential reaction to cell injury. It neutralizes and dilutes the inflammatory agent, removes necrotic materials, and establishes an environment suitable for healing and repair. The term *inflammation* is often but incorrectly used as a synonym for the term *infection*. Inflammation is always present with infection, but infection is not always present with inflammation. However, a person who

is neutropenic may not be able to mount an inflammatory response. An infection involves invasion of tissues or cells by microorganisms such as bacteria, fungi, and viruses. In contrast, inflammation can also be caused by heat, radiation, trauma, chemicals, allergens, and an autoimmune reaction.

The mechanism of inflammation is basically the same regardless of the injuring agent. The intensity of the response depends on the extent and severity of injury and on the injured person's reactive capacity. The inflammatory response can be divided into a vascular response, a cellular response, formation of exudate, and healing. Fig. 12-1 illustrates the vascular and cellular response to injury.

Reviewed by Trevah A. Panek, RN, MSN, CCRN, Assistant Professor of Nursing, Saint Francis University, Loretto, Pennsylvania; and Clemma K. Snider, RN, MSN, Assistant Professor, Associate Degree Nursing, Eastern Kentucky University, Richmond, Kentucky.

PATHOPHYSIOLOGY MAP

FIG. 12-1 Vascular and cellular responses to tissue injury.

Vascular Response

After cell injury, local arterioles briefly undergo transient vaso-constriction. After release of histamine and other chemicals by the injured cells, the vessels dilate. Chemical mediators cause increased capillary permeability and facilitate fluid movement from capillaries into tissue spaces. Initially composed of serous fluid, this inflammatory exudate later contains plasma proteins, primarily albumin. These proteins exert oncotic pressure that further draws fluid from blood vessels. Both vasodilation and increased capillary permeability are responsible for redness, heat, and swelling at the site of injury.

As the plasma protein fibrinogen leaves the blood, it is activated to fibrin by the products of the injured cells. Fibrin strengthens a blood clot formed by platelets. In tissue the clot functions to trap bacteria, prevent their spread, and serve as a framework for the healing process. Platelets release growth factors that start the healing process.

Cellular Response

Neutrophils and monocytes move from circulation to the site of injury (see Fig. 12-1). *Chemotaxis* is the directional migration of white blood cells (WBCs) to the site of injury, resulting in an accumulation of neutrophils and monocytes at the site. (eFig. 12-1 showing chemotaxis is available on the website for this chapter.)

Neutrophils. Neutrophils are the first leukocytes to arrive at the injury site (usually within 6 to 12 hours). They phagocytize (engulf) bacteria, other foreign material, and damaged cells. With their short life span (24 to 48 hours), dead neutrophils soon accumulate. In time a mixture of dead neutrophils, digested bacteria, and other cell debris accumulates as a creamy substance termed *pus*.

To keep up with the demand for neutrophils, the bone marrow releases more neutrophils into circulation. This results in an elevated WBC count, especially the neutrophil count. Sometimes the demand for neutrophils increases to the extent that the bone marrow releases immature forms of neutrophils *(bands)* into circulation. (Mature neutrophils are called segmented neutrophils.) The finding of increased numbers of band neutrophils in circulation is called a *shift to the left*, which is commonly found in patients with acute bacterial infections. (See Chapter 30 for a discussion of neutrophils.)

Monocytes. Monocytes are the second type of phagocytic cells that migrate from circulating blood. They usually arrive at the site within 3 to 7 days after the onset of inflammation. On entering the tissue spaces, monocytes transform into macrophages. Together with the tissue macrophages, these newly arrived macrophages assist in phagocytosis of the inflammatory debris. The macrophage role is important in cleaning the area before healing can occur. Macrophages have a long life span;

TABLE 12-1	MEDIATORS OF INFLAMMATION	
Mediator	**Source**	**Mechanisms of Action**
Histamine	Stored in granules of basophils, mast cells, platelets	Causes vasodilation and increased capillary permeability.
Serotonin	Stored in platelets, mast cells, enterochromaffin cells of GI tract	Same as above. Stimulates smooth muscle contraction.
Kinins (e.g., bradykinin)	Produced from precursor factor kininogen as a result of activation of Hageman factor (XII) of clotting system	Cause contraction of smooth muscle and vasodilation. Result in stimulation of pain.
Complement components (C3a, C4a, C5a)	Anaphylatoxic agents generated from complement pathway activation	Stimulate histamine release and chemotaxis.
Prostaglandins (PGs) and leukotrienes (LTs)	Produced from arachidonic acid (see Fig. 12-2)	PGs cause vasodilation. LTs stimulate chemotaxis.
Cytokines	For information on cytokines, see Table 14-3	

FIG. 12-2 Pathway of generation of prostaglandins, thromboxane, and leukotrienes. Corticosteroids, nonsteroidal antiinflammatory drugs (NSAIDs), and acetylsalicylic acid (ASA) act to inhibit various steps in this pathway.

they can multiply and may stay in the damaged tissues for weeks. These long-lived cells are important in orchestrating the healing process.

In cases where particles are too large for a single macrophage, the macrophages accumulate and fuse to form a *multinucleated giant cell*. The giant cell is then encapsulated by collagen, leading to the formation of a granuloma. A classic example of this process occurs in tuberculosis of the lung. While the *Mycobacterium* bacillus is walled off, a chronic state of inflammation exists. The granuloma formed is a cavity of necrotic tissue.

Lymphocytes. Lymphocytes arrive later at the site of injury. Their primary role is related to humoral and cell-mediated immunity (see Chapter 14).

Chemical Mediators

Mediators of the inflammatory response are presented in Table 12-1.

Complement System. The complement system is an enzyme cascade (C1 to C9) consisting of pathways to mediate inflammation and destroy invading pathogens. (eFig. 12-2 showing the complement cascade is available on the website for this chapter.) Major functions of the complement system are enhanced phagocytosis, increased vascular permeability, chemotaxis, and cellular lysis. All of these activities are important mediators of the inflammatory response and healing.

Cell lysis occurs when the final components create holes in the cell membranes and cause targeted cell death by membrane rupture. In autoimmune disorders, healthy tissue can be damaged by complement activation and the resulting inflammatory response. Examples of this include rheumatoid arthritis and systemic lupus erythematosus.

Prostaglandins and Leukotrienes. When cells are activated by injury, the arachidonic acid in the cell membrane is rapidly converted to produce prostaglandins (PGs), thromboxane, and leukotrienes (Fig. 12-2). PGs are generally considered proin-

flammatory and are potent vasodilators contributing to increased blood flow and edema formation.

Some subtypes of PGs are formed when platelets are activated and can inhibit platelet and neutrophil aggregation. PGs also perform a significant role in sensitizing pain receptors to arousal by stimuli that would normally be painless. PGs have a pivotal role as pyrogens when stimulating the temperature-regulating area of the hypothalamus and producing a febrile response.

Thromboxane is a powerful vasoconstrictor and platelet-aggregating agent. It causes brief vasoconstriction and skin pallor at the injury site and promotes clot formation. It has a short half-life, and the pallor soon gives way to vasodilation and redness, which is caused by PGs and histamine.

Leukotrienes form the slow-reacting substance of anaphylaxis (SRS-A), which constricts smooth muscles of bronchi, causing narrowing of the airway, and increases capillary permeability, leading to airway edema.

Exudate Formation

Exudate consists of fluid and leukocytes that move from the circulation to the site of injury. The nature and quantity of exudate depend on the type and severity of the injury and the tissues involved (Table 12-2).

Clinical Manifestations

The *local response* to inflammation includes the manifestations of redness, heat, pain, swelling, and loss of function (Table 12-3). *Systemic* manifestations of inflammation include an increased WBC count with a shift to the left, malaise, nausea and anorexia, increased pulse and respiratory rate, and fever.

Leukocytosis results from the increased release of WBCs from the bone marrow. Although the causes of other systemic manifestations are poorly understood, they may be related to complement activation and the release of *cytokines* (soluble factors secreted by WBCs and other types of cells that act as intercellular and intracellular messengers). Some of these cytokines (e.g., interleukins [ILs], tumor necrosis factor [TNF]) are important in causing the systemic manifestations of inflammation, as well as inducing fever. An increase in pulse and respiration follows the rise in metabolism as a result of an increase in body temperature. (Cytokines are discussed in Chapter 14.)

Fever. The onset of fever is triggered by the release of cytokines, which cause fever by initiating metabolic changes in the

TABLE 12-2 TYPES OF INFLAMMATORY EXUDATE

Type	Description	Examples
Serous	Results from outpouring of fluid. Seen in early stages of inflammation or when injury is mild.	Skin blisters, pleural effusion
Serosanguineous	Found during the midpoint in healing after surgery or tissue injury. Composed of RBCs and serous fluid, which is semiclear pink and may have red streaks.	Surgical drain fluid
Fibrinous	Occurs with increasing vascular permeability and fibrinogen leakage into interstitial spaces. Excessive amounts of fibrin that coats tissue surfaces may cause them to adhere.	Adhesions, gelatinous ribbons seen in surgical drain tubing Frequently covers fluid-exuding wounds such as venous ulcers
Hemorrhagic	Results from rupture or necrosis of blood vessel walls.	Hematoma, bleeding after surgery or tissue trauma
Purulent (pus)	Consists of WBCs, microorganisms (dead and alive), liquefied dead cells, and other debris.	Furuncle (boil), abscess, cellulitis (diffuse inflammation in connective tissue)
Catarrhal	Found in tissues where cells produce mucus. Mucus production is accelerated by inflammatory response.	Runny nose associated with upper respiratory tract infection

TABLE 12-3 LOCAL MANIFESTATIONS OF INFLAMMATION

Manifestations	Cause
Redness (rubor)	Hyperemia from vasodilation.
Heat (calor)	Increased metabolism at inflammatory site.
Pain (dolor)	Change in pH. Nerve stimulation by chemicals (e.g., histamine, prostaglandins). Pressure from fluid exudate.
Swelling (tumor)	Fluid shift to interstitial spaces. Fluid exudate accumulation.
Loss of function (functio laesa)	Swelling and pain.

PATHOPHYSIOLOGY MAP

FIG. 12-3 Production of fever. When monocytes/macrophages are activated, they secrete cytokines such as interleukin-1 *(IL-1)*, interleukin-6 *(IL-6)*, and tumor necrosis factor *(TNF)*, which reach the hypothalamic temperature-regulating center. These cytokines promote the synthesis and secretion of prostaglandin E_2 *(PGE$_2$)* in the anterior hypothalamus. PGE_2 increases the thermostatic set point, and the autonomic nervous system is stimulated, resulting in shivering, muscle contraction, and peripheral vasoconstriction.

production and conservation to raise the body temperature to the new level. At this point the individual feels chilled and shivers. The shivering response is the body's method of raising the body's temperature until the new set point is attained. This seeming paradox is dramatic: the body is hot, yet an individual piles on blankets and may go to bed to get warm. When the body temperature reaches the set point, the chills and warmth-seeking behavior cease.

The released cytokines and the fever they trigger activate the body's defense mechanisms. Beneficial aspects of fever include increased killing of microorganisms, increased phagocytosis by neutrophils, and increased proliferation of T cells. Higher body temperatures may also enhance the activity of interferon, the body's natural virus-fighting substance[1] (see Chapter 14).

Types of Inflammation

The basic types of inflammation are acute, subacute, and chronic. In *acute inflammation* the healing occurs in 2 to 3 weeks and usually leaves no residual damage. Neutrophils are the predominant cell type at the site of inflammation. A *subacute inflammation* has the features of the acute process but lasts longer. For example, infective endocarditis is a smoldering infection with acute inflammation, but it persists for weeks or months (see Chapter 37).

Chronic inflammation lasts for weeks, months, or even years. The injurious agent persists or repeatedly injures tissue. The predominant cell types present at the site of inflammation are lymphocytes and macrophages. Examples of chronic inflammation include rheumatoid arthritis and osteomyelitis. The prolongation and chronicity of any inflammation may be the result of an alteration in the immune response (e.g., autoimmune disease) and can lead to physical deterioration.

temperature-regulating center in the hypothalamus (Fig. 12-3). The synthesis of PGs is the most critical metabolic change. PGs act directly to increase the thermostatic set point. The hypothalamus then activates the autonomic nervous system to stimulate increased muscle tone and shivering and decreased perspiration and blood flow to the periphery. Epinephrine released from the adrenal medulla increases the metabolic rate. The net result is fever.

With the physiologic thermostat fixed at a higher-than-normal temperature, the rate of heat production is increased until the body temperature reaches the new set point. As the set point is raised, the hypothalamus signals an increase in heat

NURSING AND COLLABORATIVE MANAGEMENT INFLAMMATION

NURSING IMPLEMENTATION

HEALTH PROMOTION. The best management of inflammation is the prevention of infection, trauma, surgery, and contact with potentially harmful agents. This is not always possible. A simple mosquito bite causes an inflammatory response. Because occasional injury is inevitable, concerted efforts to minimize inflammation and infection are needed.

Adequate nutrition is essential so that the body has the necessary factors to promote healing when injury occurs. A high fluid intake is needed to replace fluid loss from perspiration. There is a 7% increase in metabolism for every 1°F increase in temperature above 100°F (37.8°C), or a 13% increase for every 1°C increase. The increased metabolic rate increases a patient's need for calories.

Early recognition of the manifestations of inflammation is necessary so that appropriate treatment can begin. This may be rest, drug therapy, or specific treatment of the injured site. Immediate treatment may prevent the extension and complications of inflammation.

ACUTE INTERVENTION

Observation and Vital Signs. The ability to recognize the clinical manifestations of inflammation is important. In the individual who is immunosuppressed (e.g., taking corticosteroids or receiving chemotherapy), the classic manifestations of inflammation may be masked. In this individual, early symptoms of inflammation may be malaise or "just not feeling well."

Vital signs are important to note with any inflammation, especially when an infectious process is present. With infection, the temperature may rise, and pulse and respiration rates may increase.

Fever. An important aspect of fever management is determining its cause. Although fever is usually regarded as harmful, an increase in body temperature is an important host defense mechanism. In the seventeenth century, Thomas Sydenham[1] noted that "fever is a mighty engine which nature brings into the world for the conquest of her enemies."

Steps are frequently taken to lower body temperature to relieve the anxiety of the patient and health care professionals. Because mild to moderate fever usually does little harm, imposes no great discomfort, and may benefit host defense mechanisms, antipyretic drugs are rarely essential to patient welfare. Moderate fevers (up to 103°F [39.4°C]) usually produce few problems in most patients. However, if the patient is very young or very old, is extremely uncomfortable, or has a significant medical problem (e.g., severe cardiopulmonary disease, brain injury), the use of antipyretics should be considered. Fever in the immunosuppressed patient should be treated immediately with antibiotic therapy because infections can rapidly progress to septicemia. (Neutropenia is discussed in Chapter 31 on p. 660.)

Fever (especially if greater than 104°F [40°C]) can damage body cells, and delirium and seizures can occur. At temperatures greater than 105.8°F (41°C), regulation by the hypothalamic temperature control center becomes impaired. Damage can occur to many cells, including those in the brain.

Older adults have a blunted febrile response to infection. The body temperature may not rise to the level expected for a younger adult, or the rise may be delayed in its onset. The blunted response can delay diagnosis and treatment. By the time fever (as defined for younger adults) is present, the illness may be more severe. Patients who are taking nonsteroidal antiinflammatory drugs (NSAIDs) on a regular basis (e.g., for treatment of rheumatoid arthritis) may also have a blunted febrile response.

Although sponge baths increase evaporative heat loss, they may not decrease the body temperature unless antipyretic drugs have been given to lower the set point. Otherwise, the body will initiate compensatory mechanisms (e.g., shivering) to restore body heat. The same principle applies to the use of cooling blanket, which are most effective in lowering body temperature when the set point has also been lowered.

A nursing care plan for the patient with a fever (eNursing Care Plan 12-1) is available on the website for this chapter.

Drug Therapy. Drugs are used to decrease the inflammatory response and lower the body temperature (Table 12-4). Aspirin blocks PG synthesis in the hypothalamus and elsewhere in the body. Acetaminophen acts on the heat-regulating center in the hypothalamus. Some NSAIDs (e.g., ibuprofen [Motrin, Advil]) have antipyretic effects. Corticosteroids are antipyretic through the dual mechanisms of preventing both cytokine production and PG synthesis. The action of these drugs results in dilation of superficial blood vessels, increased skin temperature, and sweating.

Antipyretics should be given around the clock to prevent acute swings in temperature. Chills may be evoked or perpetuated by the intermittent administration of antipyretics. These agents cause a sharp decrease in temperature. When the antipyretic wears off, the body may initiate a compensatory involuntary muscular contraction (i.e., chill) to raise the body

TABLE 12-4 DRUG THERAPY

Inflammation and Healing

Drug	Mechanism of Action
Antipyretic Drugs	
Salicylates (aspirin)	Inhibit synthesis of PGs (see Fig. 12-2). Lower temperature by action on heat-regulating center in hypothalamus, resulting in peripheral vasodilation and heat loss
acetaminophen (Tylenol)	Inhibits synthesis of PGs. Lowers temperature by action on heat-regulating center in hypothalamus
NSAIDs (e.g., ibuprofen [Motrin, Advil])	Inhibit synthesis of PGs
Antiinflammatory Drugs	
Salicylates (aspirin)	Inhibit synthesis of PGs, reduce capillary permeability
Corticosteroids (e.g., prednisone)	Interfere with tissue granulation, induce immunosuppressive effects (decreased synthesis of lymphocytes), prevent liberation of lysosomes
NSAIDs (e.g., ibuprofen, piroxicam [Feldene])	Inhibit synthesis of PGs
Vitamins	
Vitamin A	Accelerates epithelialization
Vitamin B complex	Acts as coenzymes
Vitamin C	Assists in synthesis of collagen and new capillaries
Vitamin D	Facilitates calcium absorption

PGs, Prostaglandins.

temperature back up to its previous level. This unpleasant side effect of antipyretic drugs can be prevented by administering these agents regularly at 2- to 4-hour intervals.

Antihistamine drugs may also be used to inhibit the action of histamine. (Antihistamines are discussed in Chapters 14 and 27.)

RICE. **R**est, **i**ce, **c**ompression, and **e**levation (RICE) is a key concept in treating soft tissue injuries and related inflammation.

Rest. Rest helps the body use its nutrients and O$_2$ for the healing process. The repair process is facilitated by allowing fibrin and collagen to form across the wound edges with little disruption.

Cold and Heat. Cold application is usually appropriate at the time of the initial trauma to promote vasoconstriction and decrease swelling, pain, and congestion from increased metabolism in the area of inflammation. Heat may be used later (e.g., after 24 to 48 hours) to promote healing by increasing the circulation to the inflamed site and subsequent removal of debris. Heat is also used to localize the inflammatory agents. Warm, moist heat may help debride the wound site if necrotic material is present.

Compression and Immobilization. Compression counters the vasodilation effects and development of edema. Compression by direct pressure over a laceration occludes blood vessels and stops bleeding. Compression bandages provide support to injured joints that have tendons and muscles unable to provide support on their own. Assess distal pulses and capillary refill before and after application of compression to evaluate whether compression has compromised circulation (e.g., pale color of skin, loss of feeling).

Immobilization of the inflamed or injured area promotes healing by decreasing the tissues' metabolic needs. Immobilization with a cast or splint supports fractured bones and prevents further tissue injury by sharp bone fragments that could sever nerves or blood vessels (causing hemorrhage). As with compression, evaluate the patient's circulation after application and at regular intervals. Swelling can occur within the closed space of a cast and compromise circulation.

Elevation. Elevating the injured extremity above the level of the heart reduces the edema at the inflammatory site by increasing venous and lymphatic return. Elevation also helps reduce pain associated with blood engorgement at the injury site. Elevation may be contraindicated in patients with significantly reduced arterial circulation.

HEALING PROCESS

The final phase of the inflammatory response is healing. Healing includes two major components: regeneration and repair.

Regeneration

Regeneration is the replacement of lost cells and tissues with cells of the same type. The ability of cells to regenerate depends on the cell type (Table 12-5).

Repair

Repair is healing as a result of lost cells being replaced by connective tissue. Repair is the more common type of healing and usually results in scar formation. Repair is a more complex process than regeneration. Most injuries heal by connective tissue repair. Repair healing occurs by primary, secondary, or tertiary intention (Fig. 12-4).

TABLE 12-5	REGENERATIVE ABILITY OF DIFFERENT TYPES OF TISSUES	
Tissues	**Cell Type**	**Description**
Skin, lymphoid organs, bone marrow, and mucous membranes	Labile cells	Cells divide constantly. Injury to these organs is followed by rapid regeneration.
Liver, pancreas, kidney, and bone cells	Stable cells	Retain their ability to regenerate but do so only if the organ is injured. Regeneration is slow.
Neurons of the central nervous system (CNS) and skeletal and cardiac muscle cells	Permanent cells	Do not divide. Damage to CNS neurons or skeletal or heart muscle can lead to permanent loss. Healing of skeletal and cardiac muscle will occur by repair with scar tissue. If neurons in the CNS are destroyed, the tissue is generally replaced by glial cells. However, neurogenesis may occur from stem cells (see Chapter 56).

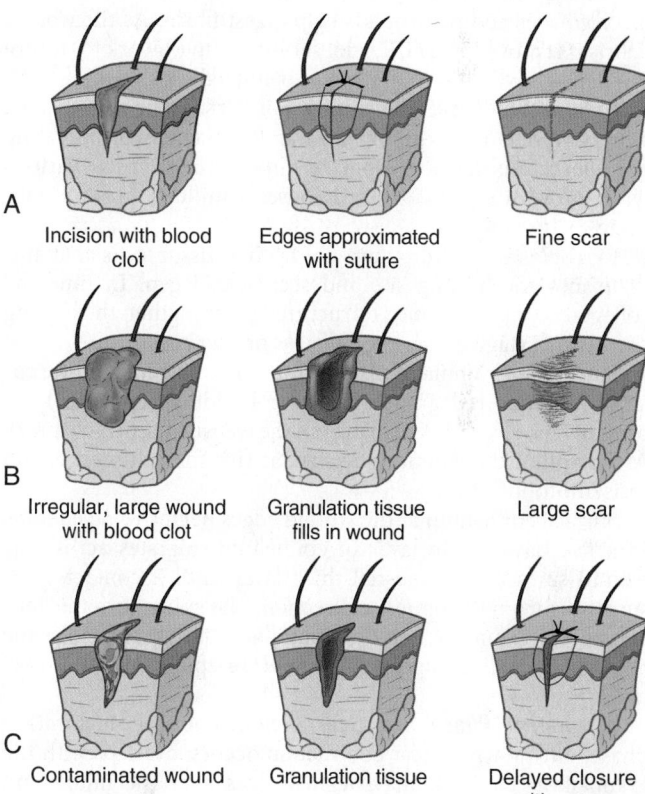

FIG. 12-4 Types of wound healing. **A,** Primary intention. **B,** Secondary intention. **C,** Tertiary intention.

Primary Intention. *Primary intention* healing takes place when wound margins are neatly approximated, as in a surgical incision or a paper cut. A continuum of processes is associated with primary healing (Table 12-6). These processes include three phases.

Initial Phase. In the *initial* (inflammatory) phase, the edges of the incision are first aligned and sutured (or stapled) in place. The incision area fills with blood from the cut blood vessels, blood clots form, and platelets release growth factors to begin

[Figure labels: A — Incision with blood clot; Edges approximated with suture; Fine scar. B — Irregular, large wound with blood clot; Granulation tissue fills in wound; Large scar. C — Contaminated wound; Granulation tissue; Delayed closure with suture]

TABLE 12-6	PHASES IN PRIMARY INTENTION HEALING	
Phase	**Duration**	**Description**
Initial	3-5 days	Approximation of incision edges. Migration of epithelial cells. Clot serving as meshwork for starting capillary growth.
Granulation	5 days to 4 wk	Migration of fibroblasts. Secretion of collagen. Abundance of capillary buds. Wound fragile.
Maturation and scar contraction	7 days to several months	Remodeling of collagen. Strengthening of scar.

the healing process. This forms a matrix for WBC migration. An acute inflammatory reaction occurs.

The area of injury is composed of fibrin clots, erythrocytes, neutrophils (both dead and dying), and other debris. Macrophages ingest and digest cellular debris, fibrin fragments, and red blood cells (RBCs). Extracellular enzymes derived from macrophages and neutrophils help digest fibrin. As the wound debris is removed, the fibrin clot serves as a meshwork for future capillary growth and migration of epithelial cells.

Granulation Phase. The *granulation* phase is the second step. The components of granulation tissue include proliferating fibroblasts; proliferating capillary sprouts *(angioblasts);* various types of WBCs; exudate; and loose, semifluid, ground substance.

Fibroblasts are immature connective tissue cells that migrate into the healing site and secrete collagen. In time the collagen is organized and restructured to strengthen the healing site. At this stage it is termed *fibrous* or *scar tissue.*

During the granulation phase, the wound is pink and vascular. Numerous red granules (young budding capillaries) are present (see eFig. 12-3 available on the website for this chapter). At this point the wound is friable, at risk for dehiscence, and resistant to infection.

Surface epithelium at the wound edges begins to regenerate. In a few days a thin layer of epithelium migrates across the wound surface in a one-cell-thick layer until it contacts cells spreading from the opposite direction. The epithelium thickens and begins to mature, and the wound now closely resembles the adjacent skin. In a superficial wound, re-epithelialization may take 3 to 5 days.

Maturation Phase and Scar Contraction. The maturation phase, during which scar contraction occurs, overlaps with the granulation phase. It may begin 7 days after the injury and continue for several months or years. This is the reason abdominal surgery discharge instructions limit lifting for up to 6 weeks.

Collagen fibers are further organized, and the remodeling process occurs. Fibroblasts disappear as the wound becomes stronger. The active movement of the myofibroblasts causes contraction of the healing area, helping to close the defect and bring the skin edges closer together. A mature scar is then formed. In contrast to granulation tissue, a mature scar is virtually avascular and pale. The scar may be more painful at this phase than in the granulation phase.

Secondary Intention. Wounds that occur from trauma, ulceration, and infection have large amounts of exudate and wide, irregular wound margins with extensive tissue loss. These wounds may have edges that cannot be *approximated* (brought together). The inflammatory reaction may be greater than in primary healing. This results in more debris, cells, and exudate. The debris may have to be cleaned away *(debrided)* before healing can take place.

The process of healing by secondary intention is essentially the same as healing by primary intention. The major differences are the greater defect and the gaping wound edges. Healing and granulation take place from the edges inward and from the bottom of the wound upward until the defect is filled. There is more granulation tissue, and the result is a much larger scar.

Tertiary Intention. *Tertiary intention* (delayed primary intention) healing occurs with delayed suturing of a wound in which two layers of granulation tissue are sutured together. This occurs when a contaminated wound is left open and sutured closed after the infection is controlled. It also occurs when a primary wound becomes infected, is opened, is allowed to granulate, and is then sutured. Tertiary intention usually results in a larger and deeper scar than primary or secondary intention.

Wound Classification

Identifying the etiology of a wound is essential to classifying the wound properly. Wounds can be classified by their cause (surgical or nonsurgical; acute or chronic) or depth of tissue affected (superficial, partial thickness, or full thickness). A *superficial wound* involves only the epidermis. *Partial-thickness* wounds extend into the dermis. *Full-thickness* wounds have the deepest layer of tissue destruction because they involve the subcutaneous tissue and sometimes even extend into the fascia and underlying structures such as the muscle, tendon, or bone (see Fig. 25-3). (Wound classification systems are described in eTables 12-1 and 12-2, available on the website for this chapter.)

Another system used to classify open wounds is based on the color of the wound (red, yellow, black) rather than on the depth of tissue destruction (Table 12-7). The red-yellow-black classification can be applied to any wound allowed to heal by secondary intention, including surgically induced wounds left to heal without skin closure because of a risk for infection. A wound may have two or three colors at the same time. In this situation the wound is classified according to the least-desirable color present.

Complications of Healing

The shape and location of the wound determine how well the wound will heal. Certain factors can interfere with wound healing and lead to complications (Table 12-8 on p. 180).

NURSING AND COLLABORATIVE MANAGEMENT WOUND HEALING

NURSING ASSESSMENT

Observe and record the characteristics of the wound. Thoroughly assess the wound on admission (or first clinic visit) and on a regular basis thereafter. Deterioration in the wound will require you to assess and document changes more frequently. Various methods exist for measuring wounds. One method is presented in Fig. 12-9 on p. 181.

Record the consistency, color, and odor of any drainage and report if abnormal for the situation. *Staphylococcus* and *Pseudomonas* are common organisms that cause purulent, draining wounds.

TABLE 12-7   RED-YELLOW-BLACK CONCEPT OF WOUND CARE

Red Wound	Yellow Wound	Black Wound
Description and Characteristics		
Can be a superficial or deep wound if it is clean and pink in appearance, possible presence of serosanguineous drainage, pink to bright or dark red healing, or chronic wound with granulating tissue.	Presence of slough or soft necrotic tissue. Liquid to semiliquid slough with exudate ranging from creamy ivory to yellow-green.	Black, gray, or brown adherent necrotic tissue called eschar. Possible presence of purulent drainage. Risk of wound infection increases in proportion to amount of necrotic tissue present.
Examples		
Skin tears, pressure ulcers (stage II), partial-thickness or second-degree burns, and wounds created by trauma or surgery that are allowed to heal by secondary intention.	Wounds with nonviable necrotic tissue, which creates an ideal situation for bacterial growth and therefore must be removed.	Full-thickness or third-degree burns, pressure ulcers (stages III and IV), and gangrenous ulcers.
Purpose of Treatment		
Protection and gentle atraumatic cleansing.	Wound cleansing to remove nonviable tissue and absorb excess drainage.	Debridement of eschar and nonviable tissue.
Dressings and Therapy		
Transparent film dressing (e.g., Tegaderm, OpSite), hydrocolloid dressing (e.g., DuoDerm), hydrogels (e.g., Tegagel), gauze dressing with antimicrobial ointment or solution, Telfa dressing with antibiotic ointment.	Absorptive dressing, hydrocolloidal dressing, hydrogel covered with gauze, wound irrigations, hydrotherapy, moist gauze dressing with or without antibiotic or antimicrobial agent.	Topical debridement (enzyme, surgical, chemical) (see Table 12-11), hydrotherapy, moist gauze dressing, hydrogel covered with gauze, absorptive dressing covered with gauze.

In healthy people, wounds heal at a normal, predictable rate. Identify factors that may delay wound healing and contribute to chronic nonhealing wounds (Table 12-9, p. 181).

Chronic wounds are those that do not heal within the normal time (approximately 3 months). If a wound fails to heal in a timely manner, assess and identify factors that may delay healing. Refer the patient to a health care provider specializing in wound management. Time does not heal all wounds. While caring for patients during the healing process, you need to continually assess for complications (e.g., infection) associated with healing[2] (see Table 12-8).

NURSING IMPLEMENTATION

The type of wound management and dressings required depend on the type, extent, and characteristics of the wound and the phase of healing. The purposes of wound management include (1) cleaning a wound to remove any dirt and debris from the wound bed, (2) treating infection to prepare the wound for healing, and (3) protecting a clean wound from trauma so it can heal normally.

Superficial skin injuries may only need cleansing. Adhesive strips (e.g., Steri-Strips, butterflies), sutures (stitches), or tissue adhesives (fibrin sealants) are used to close wounds. Adhesive strips may be used instead of *sutures* in some injuries because

they decrease *scarring* and are easier to care for. Sutures are used to close wounds because suture material provides the mechanical support necessary to sustain closure. A wide variety of suturing materials are available. In contrast, tissue adhesives are a biologic adhesive that can be used by themselves or in conjunction with sutures or tape.

If the wound is contaminated, it must be converted into a clean wound before healing can occur normally. Debridement of a wound that has multiple fragments or devitalized tissue may be necessary. If the source of inflammation is an internal organ (e.g., appendix, ruptured spleen), surgical removal of the organ is the treatment of choice.

For wounds that heal by primary intention, it is common to cover the incision with a dry, sterile dressing that is removed as soon as the drainage stops or in 2 to 3 days. Medicated sprays that form a transparent film on the skin may be used for dressings on a clean incision or injury. Transparent film dressings are also commonly used. Sometimes a surgeon will leave a surgical wound uncovered.

Sometimes drains are inserted into the wound to facilitate removal of fluid. The Jackson-Pratt drain is a suction drainage device consisting of a flexible plastic bulb connected to an internal plastic drainage tube (Fig. 12-10).

Topical antimicrobials and antibactericidals (e.g., povidone-iodine [Betadine], Dakin's solution [sodium hypochlorite],

TABLE 12-8   COMPLICATIONS OF WOUND HEALING

Adhesions
- Bands of scar tissue that form between or around organs.
- Adhesions may occur in the abdominal cavity or between the lungs and the pleura.
- Adhesions in abdomen may cause an intestinal obstruction.

Contractions
- Wound contraction is a normal part of healing.
- Complications occur when excessive contraction results in deformity.
- Shortening of muscle or scar tissue, especially over joints, results from excessive fibrous tissue formation (see Fig. 25-14).

Dehiscence
- Separation and disruption of previously joined wound edges (Fig. 12-5).
- Usually occurs when a primary healing site bursts open.
- May be caused by the following:
  - Infection causing an inflammatory process
  - Granulation tissue not strong enough to withstand forces imposed on wound
  - Obesity placing individuals at high risk for dehiscence because adipose tissue has less blood supply and may slow healing
  - Pocket of fluid (seroma, hematoma) developing between tissue layers and preventing the edges of the wound from coming together

Evisceration
- Occurs when wound edges separate to the extent that intestines protrude through wound.

Excess Granulation Tissue ("Proud Flesh")
- Excess granulation tissue may protrude above surface of healing wound.
- If the granulation tissue is cauterized or cut off, healing continues in normal manner.

Fistula Formation
- An abnormal passage between organs or a hollow organ and skin (abdominal or perianal fistula).

Infection (Fig. 12-6)
- ↑ Risk of infection when wound contains necrotic tissue or blood supply is ↓, patient's immune function is ↓ (e.g., from immunosuppressive drugs such as corticosteroids), undernutrition, multiple stressors, and hyperglycemia in diabetes.

Hemorrhage
- Bleeding is normal immediately after tissue injury and ceases with clot formation.
- Hemorrhage occurs as abnormal internal or external blood loss caused by suture failure, clotting abnormalities, dislodged clot, infection, or erosion of a blood vessel by a foreign object (tubing, drains) or infection process.

Hypertrophic Scars
- Inappropriately large, raised red and hard scars (Fig. 12-7).
- Occur when an overabundance of collagen is produced during healing.

Keloid Formation
- Great protrusion of scar tissue that extends beyond wound edges and may form tumor-like masses of scar tissue (Fig. 12-8).
- Permanent without any tendency to subside.
- Patients often complain of tenderness, pain, and hyperparesthesia, especially in early stages.
- Thought to be a hereditary condition occurring most often in dark-skinned people, particularly African Americans.

FIG. 12-5 Dehiscence following a cholecystectomy.

FIG. 12-6 Postoperative deep wound infection following wrist surgery.

FIG. 12-7 Hypertrophic scarring.

FIG. 12-8 Keloid scarring.

hydrogen peroxide [H₂O₂], and chlorhexidine [Hibiclens]) should be used with caution in wound care because they can damage the new epithelium of healing tissue and delay healing. Therefore they should never be used in a clean granulating wound.

RED, YELLOW, AND BLACK WOUNDS. The management of wounds that heal by secondary intention depends on the cause of the injury and type of tissue in the wound. The red-yellow-black concept of wound care presented in Table 12-7 provides a method of dressing selection based on the wound tissue color. Examples of types of wound dressings are presented in Table 12-10, p. 182.

Red Wounds. In red wounds the purpose of treatment is protection of the wound and gentle cleansing (if indicated). Clean wounds that are granulating and re-epithelializing should be kept slightly moist and protected from further trauma until they

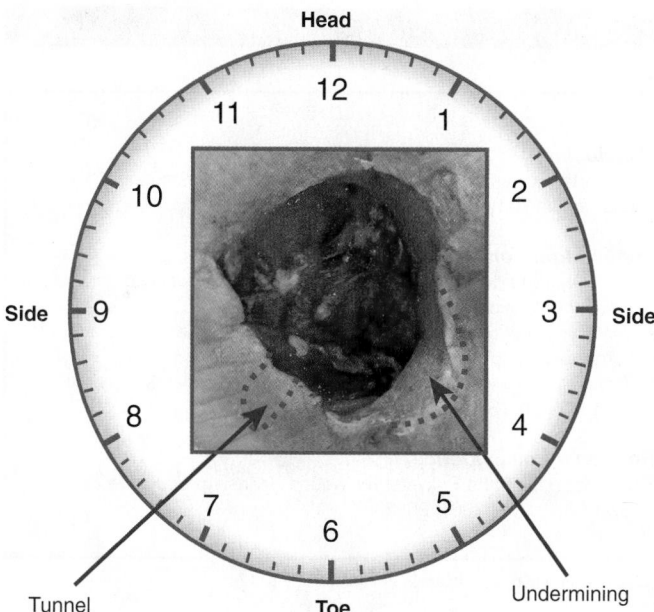

FIG. 12-9 Wound measurements are made in centimeters. The first measurement is oriented from head to toe, the second is from side to side, and the third is the depth (if any). If there is any tunneling (when cotton-tipped applicator is placed in wound, there is movement) or undermining (when cotton-tipped applicator is placed in wound, there is a "lip" around the wound), this is charted in respect to a clock, with 12 o'clock being toward the patient's head. This wound would be charted as a full-thickness, red wound, $7 \times 5 \times 3$ cm, with a 3-cm tunnel at 7 o'clock and 2 cm undermining from 3 o'clock to 5 o'clock.

FIG. 12-10 Jackson-Pratt drainage device.

TABLE 12-9	FACTORS DELAYING WOUND HEALING
Factor	**Effect on Wound Healing**
Nutritional deficiencies	
• Vitamin C	Delays formation of collagen fibers and capillary development
• Protein	Decreases supply of amino acids for tissue repair
• Zinc	Impairs epithelialization
Inadequate blood supply	Decreases supply of nutrients to injured area, decreases removal of exudative debris, inhibits inflammatory response
Corticosteroid drugs	Impair phagocytosis by WBCs, inhibit fibroblast proliferation and function, depress formation of granulation tissue, inhibit wound contraction
Infection	Increases inflammatory response and tissue destruction
Smoking	Nicotine, a potent vasoconstrictor, impedes blood flow to healing areas
Mechanical friction on wound	Destroys granulation tissue, prevents apposition of wound edges
Advanced age	Slows collagen synthesis by fibroblasts, impairs circulation, requires longer time for epithelialization of skin, alters phagocytic and immune responses
Obesity	Decreases blood supply in fatty tissue
Diabetes mellitus	Decreases collagen synthesis, retards early capillary growth, impairs phagocytosis (result of hyperglycemia), reduces supply of O_2 and nutrients secondary to vascular disease
Poor general health	Causes generalized absence of factors necessary to promote wound healing
Anemia	Supplies less O_2 at tissue level

heal naturally. Do not let a wound dry out. Dryness is an enemy of wound healing. "Airing out" a wound is a great mistake. Wounds need a moist environment to heal.

A dressing material that keeps the wound surface clean and slightly moist is optimal to promote epithelialization. Transparent film or adhesive semipermeable dressings (e.g., OpSite, Tegaderm) are occlusive dressings that are permeable to oxygen. The wound is then usually covered with a sterile dressing. Unnecessary manipulation during dressing changes may destroy new granulation tissue and break down fibrin formation.

Yellow Wounds. A type of dressing used in yellow wounds is an absorption dressing that absorbs exudate and cleanses the wound surface. Absorption dressings work by drawing excess drainage from the wound surface. The amount of wound secretions determines the number of dressing changes.

Hydrocolloid dressings such as DuoDerm are also used to treat yellow wounds. The inner part of these dressings interacts with the exudate, forming a hydrated gel over the wound. When the dressing is removed, the gel separates and stays over the wound. The wound must be cleansed gently to prevent damage to newly formed tissue. These types of dressings are designed to be left in place for up to 7 days or until leakage occurs around the dressing.

Black Wounds. The immediate treatment is debridement of the nonviable, eschar tissue. The debridement method used depends on the amount of debris and the condition of the wound tissue (Table 12-11, p. 183).

NEGATIVE-PRESSURE WOUND THERAPY. Negative-pressure wound therapy *(vacuum-assisted wound closure)* is a type of therapy that uses suction to remove drainage and speed wound healing.[3] In this therapy the wound is cleaned, and a gauze or foam dressing is cut to the dimensions of the wound. A large occlusive dressing is applied, and a small hole is made over the gauze or foam dressing where the tubing is attached (Fig. 12-11, p. 183). The tubing is connected to a pump, which creates a negative pressure in the wound bed.

EVIDENCE-BASED PRACTICE
Translating Research Into Practice

What Is the Effect of Tap Water on Wound Cleansing?

Clinical Question
In patients with an infected wound (P), what is the effect of tap water (I) versus normal saline or no cleansing (C) on infection and healing rates (O)?

Best Available Evidence
Randomized controlled trials (RCTs) and quasi-randomized controlled trials

Critical Appraisal and Synthesis of Evidence
• Ten trials (n = 35 to 705/trial) with people who had acute infected wounds. Seven trials compared infection and healing rates with water versus normal saline. Three trials compared wound cleansing with various solutions versus no cleansing at all.
• No significant differences were found in infection rate and healing in wounds cleansed with tap water versus not cleansed at all.
• Tap water was more effective than saline in reducing wound infection rate.

Conclusion
• Using tap water to cleanse acute wounds does not increase infection rate and, in some cases, it may reduce infection.

Implications for Nursing Practice
• Carefully consider the option of using tap water when other wound cleansing solutions are not accessible.
• Evaluate water quality, type of wound, and the patient's overall health before using tap water.
• If potable tap water is not available, boiled water that is cooled or distilled water may be used in wound cleansing.

Reference for Evidence
Fernandez R, Griffiths R: Water for wound cleansing, *Cochrane Database Syst Rev* 2:CD003861, 2012.

P, Patient population of interest; *I*, intervention or area of interest; *C*, comparison of interest or comparison group; *O*, outcomes of interest (see p. 12).

TABLE 12-10 TYPES OF WOUND DRESSINGS

Type	Description	Uses	Examples
Gauzes and nonwovens	Provide absorption of exudates. Support debridement if applied and kept moist.	Maintaining moist wound surface. Cleansing, packing, and covering a variety of wounds.	Numerous products available (e.g., Curity, Kling, Kerlix)
Nonadherent dressings	Woven or nonwoven dressings. May be impregnated with saline, petrolatum, or antimicrobials. Are minimally absorbent.	Minor wounds or as a second dressing.	Adaptic, Vaseline gauze, Xeroform
Semipermeable transparent films	Semipermeable membrane of polyurethane with acrylic adhesive. Transparency allows visualization of the wound. Minimally absorbent.	Dry, uninfected wounds or wounds with minimal drainage.	Bioclusive, Blisterfilm, OpSite, Polyskin, Suresite, Tegaderm, Transeal
Hydrocolloids	Gelatin, pectin, or carboxymethylcellulose bonded to a film or sheet. Produce a flat occlusive dressing that forms a gel on wound surface. Occlusion does not interfere with wound healing. Support debridement and prevent secondary infections.	Wounds with moderate to heavy drainage.	Aquacel, Combiderm, Comfeel, DuoDerm, Tegasorb
Foams	Sheets and other shapes of foamed polyurethane or silicone. Able to hold large amounts of exudate. Some come with adhesive backings; others require gauze wrapping.	Wounds with moderate to heavy drainage. Often used on new wounds.	Allevyn, Curafoam, Hydrasorb, Lyofoam, PolyMem
Hydrogels	Available in gels, gel-covered gauze, or sheets. Donate moisture to a dry wound and maintain a moist environment. Can rehydrate wound tissue. Debridement because of moisturizing effects. Require a secondary dressing.	Wounds with minimal drainage. Necrotic wounds.	Aquaform, Curasol, GranuGel, IntraSite, Nu-Gel, Purilon, Tegagel
Alginates	Derived from seaweed. Form a nonsticky gel on contact with draining wound. Easy to use over irregular-shaped wounds. Generally require a secondary dressing.	Wounds with moderate to heavy exudates (e.g., pressure ulcers, infected wounds).	AlgiSite, Algosteril, Kaltostat, Melgisorb, SeaSorb, Sorbsan
Antimicrobials	Wound covers that deliver agents such as silver and iodine, and polyhexamethylene biguanide (PHMB), which have antibacterial properties. Bacteria are not able to develop resistance to metals. Available as sponges, impregnated woven gauzes, film dressings, absorptive products, nylon fabric, nonadherent barriers, or a combination of materials.	Partial- and full-thickness wounds, over surgical incisions, or around tracheostomies.	Acticoat, Curity AMD, Iodoflex, Iodosorb, SilverDerm, Silverlon

For more information, see *http://search.woundsource.com.*

Although the exact mechanism for promoting healing is not known, it is thought that this therapy pulls excess fluid from the wound, reduces bacterial load, and encourages blood flow into the wound base. Monitor the patient's serum protein levels and fluid and electrolyte balance because of losses from the wound. Additionally, monitor the patient's coagulation studies (platelet count, prothrombin time [PT], partial thromboplastin time [PTT]).

HYPERBARIC OXYGEN THERAPY. Hyperbaric O_2 therapy (HBOT) is the delivery of O_2 at increased atmospheric pressures. It can be given systemically with the patient placed in an enclosed chamber where 100% O_2 is administered at 1.5 to 3 times the normal atmospheric pressure. HBOT allows O_2 to diffuse into the serum, rather than RBCs, and be transported to the tissues. By increasing the O_2 content in the serum, HBOT moves the O_2 past narrowed arteries and capillaries where RBCs cannot go.[4]

In addition, elevated O_2 levels stimulate *angiogenesis* (the production of new blood vessels), kill anaerobic bacteria, and increase the killing power of WBCs and certain antibiotics (e.g.,

FIG. 12-11 Negative-pressure wound therapy. **A,** Femoral wound that is not healing. **B,** Negative-pressure wound therapy in place. **C,** Granulation tissue formation after therapy.

DELEGATION DECISIONS

Wound Care

In general, wound care for complex or nonhealing wounds should be managed by the registered nurse (RN). State nurse practice acts vary in the wound care actions allowed by licensed practical/vocational nurses (LPN/LVNs) and unlicensed assistive personnel (UAP).

Role of Registered Nurse (RN)
- Assess patients for pressure ulcer risk and develop a plan of care to prevent the development of pressure ulcers.
- Assess patients for factors that might delay wound healing and develop a plan of care to address these factors.
- Assess and document initial wound appearance, including wound size, depth, color, and drainage.
- Plan nursing actions to assist with wound healing, including wound care, positioning, and nutritional interventions.
- Choose dressings and therapies for wound treatment (in conjunction with the health care provider and/or wound care specialist).
- Implement wound care for complex or new wounds, including negative-pressure wound therapy and hyperbaric O_2 therapy.
- Evaluate whether wound care is effective in promoting wound healing.
- Provide teaching to patient and caregivers about home wound care and pressure ulcer prevention.

Role of Licensed Practical/Vocational Nurse (LPN/LVN)
- Perform sterile dressing changes on acute and chronic wounds.
- Apply ordered topical antimicrobials and antibactericidals to wounds.
- Apply prescribed dressings or medications for wound debridement.
- Collect and record data about wound appearance.
- Reinforce teaching that was provided by the RN.

Role of Unlicensed Assistive Personnel (UAP)
- Perform dressing changes for chronic wounds using clean technique (need to consider state nurse practice act and agency policy).
- Empty wound drainage containers and document drainage on intake and output record.
- Report changes in wound appearance or drainage to RN.

TABLE 12-11	**TYPES OF DEBRIDEMENT**
Type	**Description**
Surgical debridement	• Quick method of debridement to prevent, control, or remove infection. • Used when large amounts of nonviable tissue are present. • Prepares wound bed for healing, skin grafting, or flaps.

Mechanical debridement	• Three methods:
	  • *Wet-to-dry dressings* in which open-mesh gauze is moistened with normal saline, packed on or into wound surface, and allowed to dry. Wound debris adheres to dressing and then dressing is removed.
	  • *Wound irrigation.* Make certain bacteria are not accidentally driven into wound with high irrigation pressure.
	  • *Whirlpool.* Should not be used in a clean granulating wound. Used when minimal debris is present. Nonselective and will also debride some healthy tissue.

Autolytic debridement	• Semiocclusive or occlusive dressings (see Table 12-10) used to soften dry eschar by autolysis. • Assess area around wound for maceration when using these dressings. • Malodorous.
Enzymatic debridement	• Drugs applied topically to dissolve necrotic tissue and then covered with moist dressing (e.g., saline-moistened gauze). • Examples of these drugs include collagenase and papain and urea (e.g., Panafil, Gladase). • Process can be slow, and thick eschar may need to be scored with scalpel.

DRUG THERAPY. Platelet-derived growth factor is released from the platelets and stimulates cell proliferation and migration. Becaplermin (Regranex), a recombinant human platelet–derived growth factor gel, actively stimulates wound healing. This product should be used only when the wound is free of devitalized tissue and infection. It should not be used if cancer is suspected in the wound.

NUTRITIONAL THERAPY. Special nutritional measures facilitate wound healing. A high fluid intake is needed to replace fluid loss from perspiration and exudate formation. An increased metabolic rate intensifies water loss. Individuals at risk for wound healing problems are those with malabsorption problems (e.g., Crohn's disease, gastrointestinal [GI] surgery, liver disease), deficient intake or high energy demands (e.g., malignancy, major trauma or surgery, sepsis, fever), and diabetes.

Undernutrition puts a person at risk for poor healing. A diet high in protein, carbohydrate, and vitamins with moderate fat intake is necessary to promote healing. Protein is needed to correct the negative nitrogen balance resulting from the increased metabolic rate. Protein is also necessary for synthesis of immune factors, leukocytes, fibroblasts, and collagen, which are the building blocks for healing. Carbohydrate is needed for the increased metabolic energy required in inflammation and healing. If there is a carbohydrate deficit, the body will break down protein for the needed energy. Fats are also a necessary component in the diet to help in the synthesis of fatty acids and triglycerides, which are part of the cellular membrane.

Vitamin C is needed for capillary synthesis and collagen production by fibroblasts. The B-complex vitamins are necessary as coenzymes for many metabolic reactions. If a vitamin B

fluoroquinolones, aminoglycosides). HBOT accelerates granulation tissue formation and wound healing.

An alternative approach is to topically administer hyperbaric O_2 by creating a chamber around the injured limb. Most systemic treatments last from 90 to 120 minutes, and the number of treatments may vary from 10 to 60 depending on the condition being treated. The topical treatments can last 20 minutes twice daily or 4 to 6 hours daily. The number of treatments is highly variable.

deficiency develops, a disruption of protein, fat, and carbohydrate metabolism will occur. Vitamin A is also needed in healing because it aids in the process of epithelialization. It increases collagen synthesis and tensile strength of the healing wound.

If the patient is unable to eat, enteral feedings and supplements should be the first choice if the GI tract is functional. Parenteral nutrition is indicated when enteral feedings are contraindicated or not tolerated. (Enteral and parenteral nutrition is discussed in Chapter 40.)

INFECTION PREVENTION AND CONTROL. You and the patient must scrupulously follow aseptic procedures for keeping the wound free from infection. Do not allow the patient to touch a recently injured area. The patient's environment should be as free as possible from contamination from items introduced by roommates and visitors. Antibiotics may be administered prophylactically to some patients.

If an infection develops, a culture and sensitivity test should be done to determine the organism and the most effective antibiotic for that specific organism. The culture should be taken before the first dose of antibiotic is given. Cultures can be obtained by needle aspiration, tissue culture, or swab technique. Physicians will obtain needle and tissue punch biopsy samples. As a nurse, you can obtain cultures using the swab technique.

Concurrent swab specimens are obtained from wounds using (1) wound exudates, (2) Z-technique, and (3) Levine's technique. The first technique samples visible wound exudates from the wound bed before cleansing. The Z-technique involves rotating a culture swab over the cleansed wound bed surface in a 10-point Z-track fashion. Levine's technique involves rotating a culture swab over a cleansed 1-cm² area near the center of the wound using sufficient pressure to extract wound fluid from deep tissue layers. Finally, a specimen of viable wound tissue is removed from the center of the wound using sterile technique. When collecting samples, do not take the specimen from exudate or eschar and do not use cotton-tipped swabs.

PSYCHOLOGIC IMPLICATIONS. The patient may be distressed at the thought or sight of an incision or wound because of fear of scarring or disfigurement. Drainage and odor from a wound often cause increased alarm. The patient needs to understand the healing process and the normal changes that occur as the wound heals. When changing a dressing, avoid inappropriate facial expressions that might alert the patient to problems with the wound or raise doubts about your ability to care for it. Wrinkling your nose may convey disgust to the patient. Be careful not to focus on the wound to the extent that the patient is not treated as a total person.

PATIENT TEACHING. Because patients are being discharged earlier after surgery and many have surgery as outpatients, it is important that the patient, the family, or both know how to care for the wound and perform dressing changes. Wound healing may not be complete for 4 to 6 weeks or longer. Adequate rest and good nutrition should be continued throughout this time. Physical and emotional stress should be minimal. Observing the wound for complications such as contractures, adhesions, and secondary infection is important. The patient should understand the signs and symptoms of infection. The patient should note changes in wound color and the amount of drainage. Teach the patient to notify the health care provider of any signs of abnormal wound healing.

Drugs are often taken for a time after recovery from the acute infection. Review drug-specific side effects and adverse effects with the patient, as well as methods to prevent side effects (e.g.,

taking with food or not). Teach the patient to contact the health care provider if any of these effects occur. Inform the patient of the need to continue the drugs for the specified time. For example, a patient who is instructed to take an antibiotic for 10 days may stop taking the drug after 5 days because of decreased or absent symptoms. However, the organism may not be entirely eliminated, and it may also become resistant to the antibiotic if the drug is not continued.

PRESSURE ULCERS

Etiology and Pathophysiology

A **pressure ulcer** is localized injury to the skin and/or underlying tissue (usually over a bony prominence) as a result of pressure or pressure in combination with shear and/or friction.

Pressure ulcers generally fall under the category of healing by secondary intention. The most common site for pressure ulcers is the sacrum, with heels being second. Factors that influence the development of pressure ulcers include the amount of pressure (intensity), the length of time the pressure is exerted on the skin (duration), and the ability of the patient's tissue to tolerate the externally applied pressure. Besides pressure, other factors that contribute to pressure ulcer formation include **shearing force** (pressure exerted on the skin when it adheres to the bed and the skin layers slide in the direction of body movement [e.g., when pulling patient up in bed]), *friction* (two surfaces rubbing against each other), and *excessive moisture.*

Factors that put a patient at risk for the development of pressure ulcers are presented in Table 12-12. Individuals at risk include those who are older, incontinent, bed- or wheelchair-bound, or recovering from spinal cord injuries.

Clinical Manifestations

The clinical manifestations of pressure ulcers depend on the extent of the tissue involved. Pressure ulcers are graded or staged according to their deepest level of tissue damage. Table 12-13 illustrates the pressure ulcer stages based on the National Pressure Ulcer Advisory Panel (NPUAP) guidelines. A pressure ulcer may be unstageable (see Table 12-13).

If the pressure ulcer becomes infected, the patient may display signs of infection (e.g., leukocytosis, fever). In addition, the pressure ulcer may increase in size, odor, and drainage; have necrotic tissue; and be indurated, warm, and painful. Untreated ulcers may lead to cellulitis, chronic infection, sepsis, and possibly death. The most common complication of a pressure ulcer is recurrence. Therefore it is important to note the location of previously healed pressure ulcers on a patient's initial admission assessment.

TABLE 12-12	RISK FACTORS FOR PRESSURE ULCERS
• Advanced age	• Low diastolic blood pressure (<60 mm Hg)
• Anemia	
• Contractures	• Mental deterioration
• Diabetes mellitus	• Neurologic disorders
• Elevated body temperature	• Obesity
• Immobility	• Pain
• Impaired circulation	• Prolonged surgery
• Incontinence	• Vascular disease

NURSING AND COLLABORATIVE MANAGEMENT PRESSURE ULCERS

In 1859 Florence Nightingale wrote, "If he has a bedsore, it's generally not the fault of the disease, but of the nursing."[5] Her comment emphasizes the critical role that nurses have in prevention and treatment of pressure ulcers.

Nursing and collaborative management are discussed together because the activities are interrelated. In addition to the nurse, other members of the health team, such as the wound care specialist, plastic surgeon, dietitian, physical therapist, and occupational therapist, can provide valuable input into the complex treatment necessary to prevent and treat pressure ulcers.

TABLE 12-13   STAGING OF PRESSURE ULCERS

Suspected Deep Tissue Injury
Purple or maroon localized area of discolored intact skin or blood-filled blister caused by damage of underlying soft tissue from pressure and/or shear. The area may be painful, firm, mushy, boggy, warmer, or cooler compared with adjacent tissue.

Stage I
Intact skin with nonblanchable redness of a localized area, usually over a bony prominence. Darkly pigmented skin may not have visible blanching. Its color may differ from the surrounding area.

Stage II
Partial-thickness loss of dermis manifesting as a shallow open ulcer with a red-pink wound bed, without slough. May also manifest as an intact or open/ruptured serum-filled blister.

Stage III
Full-thickness tissue loss. Subcutaneous fat may be visible, but bone, tendon, and muscle are not exposed. Slough may be present but does not obscure the depth of tissue loss. May include undermining and tunneling.

Stage IV
Full-thickness tissue loss with exposed bone, tendon, or muscle. Slough or eschar may be present on some parts of the wound bed. Often includes undermining and tunneling.

Unstageable Ulcer
Full-thickness tissue loss in which the base of the ulcer is covered by slough (yellow, tan, gray, green, or brown) and/or eschar (tan, brown, or black) in the wound bed.

The true depth and stage of the ulcer cannot be determined until enough slough and eschar are removed. Stable (dry, adherent, intact without erythema or fluctuance) eschar on the heels provides a natural biologic cover and should not be removed.

Photos used with permission of the National Pressure Ulcer Advisory Panel.

NURSING ASSESSMENT

Assess patients for pressure ulcer risk initially on admission and at periodic intervals based on the patient's condition.

SAFETY ALERT
- In acute care, reassess patients for pressure ulcers every 24 hours.
- In long-term care, reassess residents weekly for the first 4 weeks after admission and then at least monthly or quarterly.
- In home care, reassess patients at every nurse visit.

Risk assessment should be done using a validated assessment tool such as the Braden Scale (available at *www.bradenscale.com* or in eTable 12-3 on the website for this chapter). Knowing the level of risk can help determine how aggressive preventive measures should be.

Conduct a thorough head-to-toe assessment on admission to identify and document a pressure ulcer. Thereafter conduct periodic reassessment of the skin and wounds. Identification of skin changes may be difficult in patients with dark skin. Table 12-14 presents techniques to help assess darker skin.

Subjective and objective data that should be obtained from a person with or at risk for a pressure ulcer are presented in Table 12-15.

NURSING DIAGNOSES

Nursing diagnoses for the patient with a pressure ulcer may include, but are not limited to, the following:

- Impaired skin integrity *related to* mechanical factors and physical immobilization
- Impaired tissue integrity *related to* impaired circulation and imbalanced nutritional state

PLANNING

The overall goals are that the patient with a pressure ulcer will (1) have no deterioration of the ulcer, (2) reduce or eliminate the factors that lead to pressure ulcers, (3) not develop an infection in the pressure ulcer, (4) have healing of pressure ulcers, and (5) have no recurrence.

NURSING IMPLEMENTATION

HEALTH PROMOTION. A primary nursing responsibility is the identification of patients at risk for developing pressure ulcers (see Tables 12-12 and 12-15) and implementation of pressure ulcer prevention strategies for those who are at risk. Prevention remains the best treatment for pressure ulcers.[6,7]

SAFETY ALERT
- Reposition patients frequently to prevent pressure ulcers (usually every 2 hours).
- Use devices to reduce pressure and shearing force (e.g., low-air-loss mattresses, foam mattresses, wheelchair cushions, padded commode seats, boots [foam, air], lift sheets) as appropriate.
- These devices do not replace the need for frequent repositioning.

ACUTE INTERVENTION. Care of a patient with a pressure ulcer requires local care of the wound and support measures of the whole person, such as adequate nutrition, pain management, control of other medical conditions, and pressure relief. Both conservative and surgical strategies are used in the treatment of pressure ulcers, depending on the stage and condition of the ulcer.

Once a pressure ulcer has developed, initiate interventions based on the ulcer characteristics (e.g., stage, size, location, amount of exudate, type of wound, presence of infection or pain) and the patient's general status (e.g., nutritional state, age, cardiovascular status, level of mobility). Carefully document the

---

TABLE 12-14 ASSESSING PATIENTS WITH DARK SKIN

- Look for changes in skin color, such as skin that is darker (purplish, brownish, bluish) than surrounding skin.
- Use natural or halogen light source to accurately assess the skin color. Fluorescent light casts blue color, which can make skin assessment difficult.
- Assess the area for the skin temperature using your hand. The area may feel initially warm, then cooler.
- Touch the skin to feel its consistency. Boggy or edematous feel may indicate a stage I pressure ulcer.
- Ask the patient if he or she has any pain or itchy sensation.

TABLE 12-15 NURSING ASSESSMENT

Pressure Ulcers

Subjective Data
Important Health Information
Past health history: Stroke, spinal cord injury; prolonged bed rest or immobility; circulatory impairment; poor nutrition; altered level of consciousness; prior history of pressure ulcer; immunologic abnormalities; advanced age; diabetes; anemia; trauma
Medications: Use of opioids, hypnotics, systemic corticosteroids
Surgery or other treatments: Recent surgery

Functional Health Patterns
Nutritional-metabolic: Obesity, emaciation; decreased fluid, calorie, or protein intake; vitamin or mineral deficiencies; clinically significant malnutrition as indicated by low serum albumin, decreased total lymphocyte count, and decreased body weight (15% less than ideal body weight)
Elimination: Incontinence of urine, feces, or both
Activity-exercise: Weakness, debilitation, inability to turn and position body; contractures
Cognitive-perceptual: Pain or altered cutaneous sensation in pressure ulcer area; decreased awareness of pressure on body areas; capacity to follow treatment plan

Objective Data
General
Fever

Integumentary
Diaphoresis, edema, and discoloration, especially over bony areas such as sacrum, hips, elbows, heels, knees, ankles, shoulders, and ear rims, progressing to increased tissue damage characteristic of ulcer stages*

Possible Diagnostic Findings
Leukocytosis, positive cultures for microorganisms from pressure ulcer

*See Table 12-13.

---

size of the pressure ulcer. A wound-measuring card or tape can be used to note the ulcer's maximum length and width in centimeters. To find the depth of the ulcer, take a sterile cotton-tipped applicator and soak it with saline. Gently place it into the deepest part of the ulcer, and then measure the length of the portion of the applicator that probed the ulcer. Documentation of the healing wound can be done using several available pressure ulcer healing tools such as the NPUAP Pressure Ulcer Scale for Healing (PUSH) tool[8] (eTable 12-4; available at *www.npuap.org/PDF/push3.pdf*).

Some agencies require that pictures of the pressure ulcer be taken initially and at regular intervals during the course of treatment. The informatics box on p. 187 has suggestions for digital imaging.

EVIDENCE-BASED PRACTICE

Applying the Evidence

You are caring for S.W., an obese 86-year-old woman with a history of diabetes, hypertension, and chronic kidney disease. S.W. spends most of her time in bed or a wheelchair and now has a stage I pressure ulcer on her sacral area. You are doing discharge teaching with her daughter, who is her primary caregiver. You explain the importance of preventing further skin breakdown and that she needs to reposition her mother every 2 to 3 hours during the night. S.W.'s daughter tells you that she will reposition her mother during the night if her mother wakes up to use the commode. Otherwise, she needs her sleep because she watches her two young grandchildren during the day.

Best Available Evidence	Clinician Expertise	Patient Preferences and Values
Repositioning remains the primary method of reducing risk for pressure ulcers. Pressure-reducing devices (e.g., foam mattress, padded commode seats) can also be used but should not be a substitute for repositioning.	You know that patients with pressure ulcers should be repositioned at least every 2 hours while in bed and every hour when in a chair. You also know that stage I pressure ulcers can rapidly deteriorate to stage II if proper care is not taken.	S.W.'s caregiver expresses the need to have a certain amount of uninterrupted sleep to maintain multiple family responsibilities. States she will reposition her mother at least every 2 hours while she is in bed during the day and every hour when she is in a wheelchair. S.W.'s caregiver states she will purchase a foam mattress, wheelchair cushion, and padded commode seat to help prevent further skin issues.

Your Decision and Action

You discuss the importance of repositioning as the primary method to prevent pressure ulcers and decrease the progression of existing pressure ulcers to more serious ones. S.W.'s daughter reiterates that she will not reposition her mother every 2 hours during the night. You can understand her decision and document this discussion in the patient's discharge teaching record.

Reference for Evidence

European Pressure Ulcer Advisory Panel and National Pressure Ulcer Advisory Panel: *Pressure ulcer treatment: quick reference guide*, Washington, DC, 2009, National Pressure Ulcer Advisory Panel. Retrieved from *www.npuap.org/wp-content/uploads/2012/03/Final_Quick_Treatment_for_web_2010.pdf*.

INFORMATICS IN PRACTICE

Digital Images

To monitor wound progress, use digital photography. For the best images:

- Include a ruler with date, length, width, and depth of the wound in each photo.
- Position the patient the same way for each photo.
- Take the photo from the same angle each time. Pointing perpendicularly at the wound is best.
- Use natural light, without flash, whenever possible.
- Show the wound on a solid background, avoiding shiny underpads.

TABLE 12-16   PATIENT & CAREGIVER TEACHING GUIDE

Pressure Ulcer

When teaching the patient and caregiver to prevent and care for pressure ulcers do the following.

1. Identify and explain risk factors and etiology of pressure ulcers to patient and caregiver.
2. Assess all at-risk patients at time of first hospital and/or home visit or whenever the patient's condition changes. Thereafter assess at regular intervals based on care setting (every 24 hours for acute care or every visit in home care).
3. Teach the caregiver techniques for incontinence. If incontinence occurs, cleanse skin at time of soiling and use absorbent pads or briefs.
4. Demonstrate correct positioning to decrease risk of skin breakdown. Instruct caregiver to reposition a bed-bound patient at least every 2 hours, a chair-bound patient every hour. NEVER position the patient directly on the pressure ulcer.
5. Assess resources (i.e., caregiver's availability and skill, finances, equipment) of patients requiring pressure ulcer care at home. When selecting ulcer care dressing, consider cost and amount of caregiver time required.
6. Teach patient and/or caregiver to place clean dressings over sterile dressings using "no touch" technique when changing dressings. Instruct caregiver on disposal of contaminated dressings.
7. Teach patient and caregiver to inspect skin daily. Tell them to report any significant changes to the health care provider.
8. Teach patient and caregiver the importance of good nutrition to enhance ulcer healing.
9. Evaluate program effectiveness.

Local care of the pressure ulcer may involve debridement, wound cleaning, application of a dressing, and relief of pressure. It is important to select the appropriate pressure-relieving technique (e.g., pad, overlay, mattress, specialty bed) to relieve pressure and keep the patient off of the pressure ulcer. Whenever possible, do not turn the patient onto a body surface that is still reddened. Massage is contraindicated in the presence of acute inflammation and where there is the possibility of damaged blood vessels or fragile skin.[7]

Sliding down in bed causes friction and sheer. Encourage patients to reposition themselves by lifting rather than sliding and to use a trapeze if indicated. Lift sheets may be used to move patients up in bed or to transfer them.[9]

A pressure ulcer that has necrotic tissue or eschar (except for dry, stable necrotic feet or heels) must have the tissue removed by surgical, mechanical, enzymatic, or autolytic debridement methods. Once the pressure ulcer has been successfully debrided and has a clean granulating base, the goal is to provide an appropriate wound environment that supports moist wound healing and prevents disruption of the newly formed granulation tissue. Reconstruction of the pressure ulcer site by operative repair, including skin grafting, skin flaps, musculocutaneous flaps, or free flaps, may be necessary.

Clean pressure ulcers with noncytotoxic solutions that do not kill or damage cells, especially fibroblasts. Solutions such as Dakin's solution (sodium hypochlorite solution), acetic acid, povidone-iodine, and hydrogen peroxide are cytotoxic and therefore should not be used to clean pressure ulcers. It is also important to use enough irrigation pressure to adequately clean the pressure ulcer (4 to 15 psi) without causing trauma or damage to the wound. To obtain this pressure, use a 30-mL syringe and a 19-gauge needle.

After the pressure ulcer has been cleansed, cover it with an appropriate dressing. The current trend is to keep a pressure ulcer slightly moist, rather than dry, to enhance re-epithelialization. Some factors to consider when selecting a dressing are maintenance of a moist environment, prevention of the wound from drying out, ability to absorb the wound drainage, location of the wound, amount of caregiver time required to change the dressing, cost of the dressing, presence of infection, clean versus sterile dressings, and care delivery setting. A wet-to-dry dressing should never be used on a clean granulating pressure ulcer. This type of dressing should be used only for mechanical debridement of the wound. (Dressings are discussed in Table 12-10.)

Stages II through IV pressure ulcers are considered contaminated or colonized with bacteria. Remember that in people who have chronic wounds or are immunocompromised, the clinical signs of infection (purulent exudate, odor, erythema, warmth, tenderness, edema, pain, fever, and elevated WBC count) may not be present even though the pressure ulcer is infected.[10]

The maintenance of adequate nutrition is an important nursing responsibility for the patient with a pressure ulcer. Often, the patient is debilitated and has a poor appetite secondary to inactivity. Oral feedings must be adequate in calories, protein, fluids, vitamins, and minerals to meet the patient's nutritional requirements. The caloric intake needed to correct and maintain nutritional balance may be 30 to 35 calories/kg/day and 1.25 to 1.50 g of protein/kg/day.

Enteral feedings can be used to supplement the oral feedings. When oral and enteral feedings are inadequate, parenteral nutrition consisting of amino acid and glucose solutions is used. (Parenteral and enteral nutrition is discussed in Chapter 40.)

AMBULATORY AND HOME CARE. Pressure ulcers affect the quality of life of patients and their caregivers. Because pressure ulcers commonly recur, teaching prevention techniques to both the patient and the caregiver is extremely important (Table 12-16, p. 187). A sixth-grade-level version of the patient guide to pressure ulcer prevention is available for use in patient teaching *(www.npuap.org/PU_Prev_Points.pdf)*. The caregiver needs to know the etiology of pressure ulcers, prevention techniques, early signs, nutritional support, and care techniques for actual pressure ulcers. Because the patient with a pressure ulcer often requires extensive care for other health problems, it is important that the nurse support the caregiver with the added responsibility for pressure ulcer treatment. eNursing Care Plan 12-2 (available on the website for this chapter) outlines the care for the patient with a pressure ulcer.

EVALUATION

The expected outcomes are that the patient with a pressure ulcer will have
- Healing of pressure ulcer(s)
- Intact skin with no further breakdown

CASE STUDY

Inflammation and Infection

iStockphoto/Thinkstock

Patient Profile

G.N., a 58-year-old African American man, was admitted to the hospital emergency department with partial-thickness burns that involved his face, neck, and upper trunk. He also had a lacerated right leg. His injuries occurred about 36 hours earlier when he fell out of a tree onto his gas grill (which was lit) while trying to get his cat.

Subjective Data
- Complains of slightly hoarse voice and irritated throat
- States that he tried to treat himself because he does not have health insurance
- Has been coughing up sooty sputum
- Complains of severe pain in left hip

Objective Data
Physical Examination
- Leg wound is gaping and has drainage: temperature 101.1°F (38.4°C).
- X-rays reveal a fractured right tibia and fractured left hip.

Laboratory Studies
- WBC count 26,400/μL (26.4 × 10⁹/L) with 80% neutrophils (10% bands)

Collaborative Care
- Surgery is performed to repair the left hip.

Discussion Questions
1. What clinical manifestations of inflammation did G.N. exhibit, and what are their pathophysiologic mechanisms?
2. What type of exudate formation did he develop?
3. What is the basis for the development of the temperature?
4. What is the significance of his WBC count and differential?
5. Because his wound was deep, primary tissue healing was not possible. How would you expect healing to take place? What complications could he develop?
6. What risk factors does G.N. have to develop a pressure ulcer?
7. ***Priority Decision:*** Based on the assessment data provided, what are the priority nursing diagnoses? Are there any collaborative problems?
8. ***Delegation Decision:*** What nursing activities related to wound care can be delegated to unlicensed assistive personnel (UAP)?

Evolve Answers available at *http://evolve.elsevier.com/Lewis/medsurg.*

BRIDGE TO NCLEX EXAMINATION

The number of the question corresponds to the same-numbered outcome at the beginning of the chapter.

1. A patient 1 day postoperative after abdominal surgery has incisional pain, 99.5°F temperature, slight erythema at the incision margins, and 30 mL serosanguineous drainage in the Jackson-Pratt drain. Based on this assessment, what conclusion would the nurse make?
   a. The abdominal incision shows signs of an infection.
   b. The patient is having a normal inflammatory response.
   c. The abdominal incision shows signs of impending dehiscence.
   d. The patient's physician needs to be notified about her condition.

2. The nurse assessing a patient with a chronic leg wound finds local signs of erythema and pain at the wound site. What would the nurse anticipate being ordered to assess the patient's systemic response?
   a. Serum protein analysis
   b. WBC count and differential
   c. Punch biopsy of center of wound
   d. Culture and sensitivity of the wound

3. A patient in the unit has a 103.7° F temperature. Which intervention would be most effective in restoring normal body temperature?
   a. Use a cooling blanket while the patient is febrile.
   b. Administer antipyretics on an around-the-clock schedule.
   c. Provide increased fluids and have the UAP give sponge baths.
   d. Give prescribed antibiotics and provide warm blankets for comfort.

4. A nurse is caring for a patient who has a pressure ulcer that is treated with debridement, irrigations, and moist gauze dressings. How should the nurse anticipate healing to occur?
   a. Tertiary intention
   b. Secondary intention
   c. Regeneration of cells
   d. Remodeling of tissues

5. A nurse is caring for a patient with diabetes who is scheduled for amputation of his necrotic left great toe. The patient's WBC count is $15.0 \times 10^6/\mu L$, and he has coolness of the lower extremities, weighs 75 lb more than his ideal body weight, and smokes two packs of cigarettes per day. Which priority nursing diagnosis addresses the primary factor affecting the patient's ability to heal?
   a. Imbalanced nutrition: more than body requirements *related to* high-fat foods
   b. Impaired tissue integrity *related to* decreased blood flow secondary to diabetes and smoking
   c. Ineffective peripheral tissue perfusion *related to* narrowed blood vessels secondary to diabetes and smoking
   d. Ineffective individual coping *related to* indifference and denial of the long-term effects of diabetes and smoking

6. Which one of the orders should a nurse question in the plan of care for a patient with a stage III pressure ulcer?
   a. Pack the ulcer with foam dressing.
   b. Turn and position the patient every 2 hours.
   c. Clean the ulcer every shift with Dakin's solution.
   d. Assess for pain and medicate before dressing change.

7. An 85-year-old patient is assessed to have a score of 16 on the Braden Scale. Based on this information, how should the nurse plan for this patient's care?
   a. Implement a q2hr turning schedule with skin assessment.
   b. Place DuoDerm on the patient's sacrum to prevent breakdown.
   c. Elevate the head of bed to 90 degrees when the patient is supine.
   d. Continue with weekly skin assessments with no special precautions.

8. A 65-year-old stroke patient with limited mobility has a purple area of suspected deep tissue injury on the left greater trochanter. Which nursing diagnoses is/are most appropriate *(select all that apply)?*
   a. Acute pain *related to* tissue damage and inflammation
   b. Impaired skin integrity *related to* immobility and decreased sensation
   c. Impaired tissue integrity *related to* inadequate circulation secondary to pressure
   d. Risk for infection *related to* loss of tissue integrity and undernutrition secondary to stroke

9. An 82-year-old man is being cared for at home by his family. A pressure ulcer on his right buttock measures $1 \times 2 \times 0.8$ cm in depth, and pink subcutaneous tissue is completely visible on the wound bed. Which stage would the nurse document on the wound assessment form?
   a. Stage I
   b. Stage II
   c. Stage III
   d. Stage IV

1. b, 2. b, 3. b, 4. b, 5. b, 6. c, 7. a, 8. b, c, 9. c

ⓔvolve

For rationales to these answers and even more NCLEX review questions, visit *http://evolve.elsevier.com/Lewis/medsurg.*

REFERENCES

1. Atkins E: Fever: its history, cause, and function, *Yale J Biol Med* 55:283, 1982. (Classic)
2. Reddy M, Gill SS, Wu W, et al: Does this patient have an infection of a chronic wound? *JAMA* 307(6):605, 2012.
3. Martindell D: The safe use of negative-pressure wound therapy, *Am J Nurs* 112:59, 2012.
4. Kranke P, Bennett MH, Martyn-St James M, et al: Hyperbaric oxygen therapy for chronic wounds, *Cochrane Database Syst Rev* 4:CD004123, 2012.
5. Nightingale F: *Notes on nursing*, Philadelphia, 1859, Lippincott. (Classic)
6. Lynch S, Vickery P: Steps to reduce hospital-acquired pressure ulcers, *Nursing* 40:61, 2010.
7. European Pressure Ulcer Advisory Panel and National Pressure Ulcer Advisory Panel: *Pressure ulcer prevention: quick reference guide*, Washington, DC, 2009, National Pressure Ulcer Advisory Panel. Retrieved from *www.npuap.org/wp-content/uploads/2012/03/Final_Quick_Prevention_for_web_2010.pdf.*
8. National Pressure Ulcer Advisory Panel: PUSH tool. Retrieved from *www.npuap.org/resources/educational-and-clinical-resources/push-tool/push-tool.*
9. Blaney WD: Taking steps to prevent pressure ulcers, *Nursing* 40:45, 2010.
10. Pham B, Stern A, Chen W: Preventing pressure ulcers in long-term care: a cost-effective analysis, *Arch Intern Med* 171:1839, 2011.

RESOURCES

Braden Scale for Predicting Pressure Sore Risk
www.bradenscale.com/images/bradenscale.pdf
National Pressure Ulcer Advisory Panel
www.npuap.org
Wound Ostomy and Continence Nurses Society
www.wocn.org

13

Genetics and Genomics

Sharon L. Lewis

*The laws of genetics apply even if you refuse
to learn them.*
Allison Plowden

evolve WEBSITE

http://evolve.elsevier.com/Lewis/medsurg

- NCLEX Review Questions
- Key Points
- Pre-Test
- Rationales for Bridge to NCLEX
  Examination Questions

- Concept Map Creator
- Glossary
- Content Updates

eFigure
- eFig. 13-1: Transcription and translation

LEARNING OUTCOMES

1. Differentiate the common terms related to genetics and genetic disorders: *autosomal, carrier, heterozygous, homozygous, mutation, recessive,* and *X-linked gene.*
2. Differentiate between the two common causes of genetic mutations.
3. Compare and contrast the three most common inheritance patterns of genetic disorders.
4. Describe the most common classifications of genetic disorders.
5. Explore the complex ethical and social implications of genetic testing.
6. Analyze the role of pharmacogenetics in developing personalized drug therapy.
7. Discuss your role in assisting the patient and family in dealing with genetic issues.

KEY TERMS

genetics, p. 190
genomics, p. 190
hereditary, Table 13-1, p. 191

heterozygous, Table 13-1, p. 191
homozygous, Table 13-1, p. 191
mutation, Table 13-1, p. 191

pharmacogenetics, p. 198
pharmacogenomics, p. 198

GENETICS AND GENOMICS

In the 1860s an Austrian monk named Gregor Mendel, while experimenting with pea plants, discovered how traits are transmitted from parents to offspring. This discovery laid the foundation for modern **genetics**, the study of genes and their role in inheritance. Genetics determines the way that certain traits or conditions are passed down from one generation to another. **Genomics** is the study of all of a person's genes (the *genome*), including interactions of these genes with each other and with the person's environment. (Common terms used in genetics and genomics are defined in Table 13-1.) Genomics includes the study of complex diseases such as heart disease, asthma, diabetes mellitus, and cancer because these diseases are typically caused by a combination of genetic and environmental factors rather than by a single gene.

A person's genes can have a profound impact on health and disease. More than 4000 diseases are thought to be related to altered genes. Genomic factors play a role in 9 of the 10 leading causes of death in the United States, including heart disease, cancer, diabetes, stroke, and Alzheimer's disease.[1]

Genomics may help us understand why some people who eat healthy diets and exercise regularly still die at a young age of cancer, whereas some people eat unhealthy diets and never exercise, and yet live to an old age.

The identification of a genetic basis for many human diseases has the potential to strongly influence the care of patients at risk for or diagnosed with a disease that has a genetic link. You need to know the basic principles of genetics, be familiar with the impact that genetics and genomics have on health and disease, and be prepared to assist the patient and family with genetic issues.

Basic Principles of Genetics

Genes. *Genes* are the basic units of heredity. There are approximately 20,000 to 25,000 genes in each person's genetic makeup, or *genome*. Genes encode (carry the instructions) for proteins that direct the activities of cells and functions of the

Reviewed by Mindy B. Tinkle, RN, PhD, WHNP-BC, Associate Professor and Chair, Research and PhD Studies, University of New Mexico, College of Nursing, Albuquerque, New Mexico; Laura Mallett, RN, MSN, Assistant Lecturer, University of Wyoming, Fay W. Whitney School of Nursing, Laramie, Wyoming; and Bernice Coleman, PhD, ACNP-BC, FAHA, Nurse Practitioner, Heart Transplantation and Ventricular Assist Device Programs, Cedars Sinai Medical Center, Los Angeles, California.

TABLE 13-1   GLOSSARY OF GENETIC AND GENOMIC TERMS

Term	Definition
Allele	An alternative form of a gene. Each person receives two alleles of a gene, one from each biologic parent. Different alleles produce variations in inherited traits such as eye color and blood type.
Autosome	Any chromosome that is not a sex chromosome. Humans have 22 pairs of autosomes.
Carrier	Individual who carries a copy of a mutated gene for a recessive disorder.
Chromosome	A compact structure containing DNA and proteins present in nearly all cells of the body. Normally each cell has 46 chromosomes in 23 pairs. Each biologic parent contributes one of each pair of chromosomes.
Codominance	Two dominant versions of a trait that are both expressed in the same individual.
Congenital disorder	Condition present at birth.
Dominant allele	Gene that is expressed in the phenotype of a heterozygous individual.
Familial disorder	Condition that affects more than one person in a family.
Gene	The basic unit of heredity information located on a specific part of a chromosome. Genes direct cells to make proteins and guide almost every aspect of operation and repair of cells.
Genetic risk factor	A change in a gene that increases a person's risk of developing a disease.
Genetics	Study of genes and their role in inheritance.
Genome	All the DNA contained in an individual.
Genome-wide association study (GWAS)	A study approach that involves scanning complete sets of DNA (genomes) of many individuals to find genetic variations associated with a particular disease.
Genomics	Study of how genes interact and influence people's biologic and physical characteristics.

Term	Definition
Genotype	Genetic identity of an individual. This identity does not show as outward characteristics.
Hereditary	Transmission of a disease, condition, or trait from parent to children.
Heterozygous	Having two different alleles for one given gene, one inherited from each parent.
Homozygous	Having two identical alleles for one given gene, one inherited from each parent.
Locus	Position of a gene on a chromosome.
Mutation	A change in DNA or a gene. Sometimes these changes are passed from parent to children.
Oncogene	Gene that is able to initiate and contribute to the conversion of normal cells to cancer cells.
Pedigree	Family tree that contains the genetic characteristics and disorders of that particular family.
Pharmacogenetics	Study of variability of responses to drugs related to variations in single genes.
Pharmacogenomics	Study of variability of responses to drugs related to variations in and interactions of multiple genes.
Phenotype	Observable traits or characteristics of an individual (e.g., hair color).
Protooncogene	Normal cellular genes that are important regulators of normal cellular processes. Mutations can activate them to become oncogenes.
Recessive allele	Allele that has no noticeable effect on the phenotype in a heterozygous individual.
Trait	Physical characteristic that one inherits, such as hair or eye color.
X-linked gene	Gene located on the X chromosome. In general, sex-linked disorders are only seen in males.

body. Genes control how a cell functions, including how quickly it grows, how often it divides, and how long it lives. To control these functions, genes produce proteins that perform specific tasks and act as messengers for the cell. Therefore it is essential that each gene have the correct instructions or "code" for making its protein so that the protein can perform the proper function for the cell.[2]

Genes are arranged in a specific linear formation along a chromosome (Fig. 13-1). Each gene has a specific location on a chromosome, termed a *locus*. An *allele* is one of two or more alternative forms of a gene that occupy corresponding loci on *homologous chromosomes* (a pair of chromosomes having corresponding deoxyribonucleic acid [DNA] sequences, with one coming from the mother and the other from the father). Each allele codes for a specific inherited characteristic.

When there are two different alleles, the allele that is fully expressed is the *dominant allele*. The other allele that lacks the ability to express itself in the presence of a dominant allele is the *recessive allele*. Physical traits expressed by an individual are termed the *phenotype*, and the actual genetic makeup of the individual is termed the *genotype*.

Chromosomes. *Chromosomes* are contained in the nucleus of a cell and occur in pairs. Humans have 23 pairs of chromosomes; 22 of the 23 pairs of chromosomes are *homologous* and are termed *autosomes*. Autosomes are the same in both males and females. The sex chromosomes make up the twenty-third pair of chromosomes. A female has two X chromosomes, and a male has one X and one Y chromosome. One chromosome of each pair is inherited from the mother and one from the father. One half of each child's chromosomes (and therefore the genetic makeup) comes from his or her father and one half from his or her mother.

DNA. Genes are made up of a nucleic acid called *deoxyribonucleic acid* (DNA). DNA stores genetic information and encodes the instructions for synthesizing specific proteins needed to maintain life. DNA also dictates the rate at which proteins are made. Every somatic cell in a person's body has the same DNA.

The information in DNA is stored as a code made up of four nitrogenous bases: adenine (A), guanine (G), cytosine (C), and thymine (T). Human DNA consists of about 3 billion bases, and more than 99% of those bases are the same in all people. The

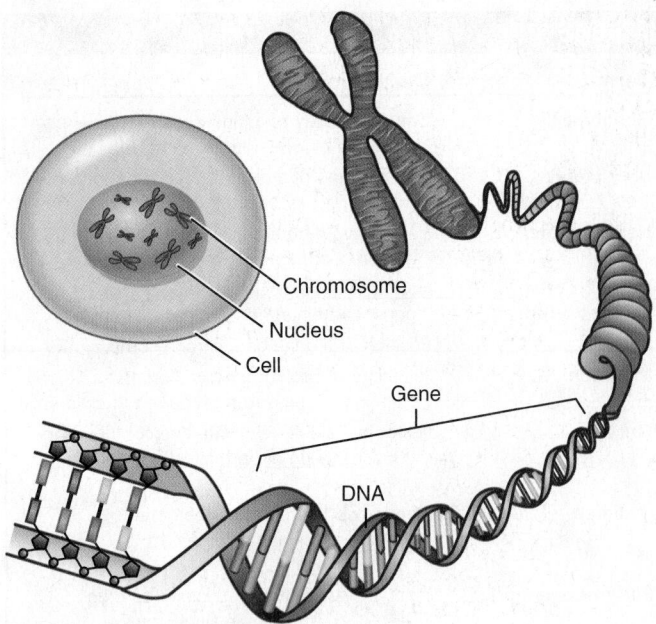

FIG. 13-1 The long, stringy DNA that makes up genes is spooled within chromosomes inside the nucleus of a cell. (Note that a gene would actually be a much longer stretch of DNA than what is shown here.)

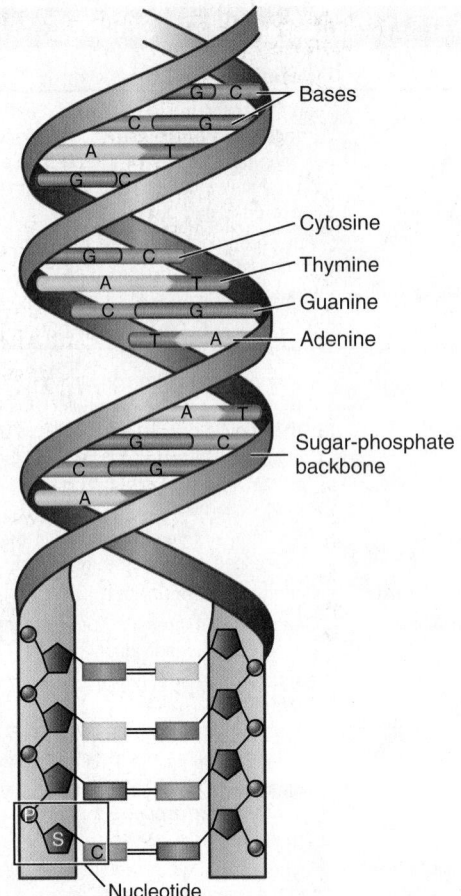

FIG. 13-2 DNA consists of two long, twisted chains made up of nucleotides. Each nucleotide contains one base, one phosphate molecule *(P)*, and the sugar molecule deoxyribose *(S)*. The bases in DNA nucleotides are adenine *(A)*, thymine *(T)*, cytosine *(C)*, and guanine *(G)*.

order (or sequence) of these bases determines the information for building and maintaining an organism. This is similar to the way letters of the alphabet are used to create words and sentences.

DNA bases pair up with each other, A with T and C with G, to form units called *base pairs*. Each base is also attached to a sugar molecule and a phosphate molecule (Fig. 13-2). Together, a base, sugar, and phosphate are called a *nucleotide*. Nucleotides are arranged in two long strands that form a spiral called a *double helix*. The structure of the double helix is somewhat like a ladder, with the base pairs forming the ladder's rungs and the sugar and phosphate molecules forming the ladder's vertical sidepieces.

DNA can *replicate* (make copies of itself). Each strand of DNA in the double helix can serve as a pattern for duplicating the sequence of bases. When cells divide, each new cell needs to have an exact copy of the DNA that was in the parent (original) cell.

If the chromosomes in one of your cells were uncoiled and placed end-to-end, the DNA would be about 6 feet long. If all of the DNA in your body were connected, it would stretch about 67 billion miles.[3]

RNA. Ribonucleic acid (RNA) is similar to DNA, but with some significant differences. Like DNA, RNA contains the nitrogenous bases adenine, guanine, and cytosine. However, RNA lacks the nitrogenous base thymine and instead contains uracil. RNA is single stranded and contains ribose instead of deoxyribose sugar. RNA transfers the genetic information obtained from DNA to the proper location for protein synthesis.

Protein Synthesis. Protein synthesis, or the making of proteins, occurs in two steps: *transcription* and *translation*. (Transcription and translation are shown in eFig. 13-1 on the website for this chapter.) Transcription is the process by which messenger RNA (mRNA) is synthesized from single-stranded DNA. The mRNA becomes attached to a ribosome, where translation occurs. At this point another specialized type of RNA, transfer RNA (tRNA), arranges the amino acids in the correct sequence

to assemble the protein. Once the protein is completed, it is released from the ribosome and is able to perform its specific function in the cell.

Mitosis. *Mitosis* is a type of cell division that results in the formation of genetically identical daughter cells. Before cell division the chromosomes duplicate, and each new cell (called daughter cells) receives an exact replica of the chromosomes from the original cell (called the parent cell).

Meiosis. *Meiosis* occurs only in sexual reproductive cells. In meiosis the number of chromosomes is reduced, resulting in half of the usual number of chromosomes. Therefore oocytes and sperm contain only a single copy of each chromosome, whereas all other body cells contain duplicates of each chromosome.

Genetic Mutations

A *mutation* is any change in the usual DNA sequence. Subtle variations in DNA are called *polymorphisms* (meaning *many forms*). Many of these *gene* polymorphisms account for slight variations among people such as hair and eye color. However, some gene variations may result in disease or an increased risk for disease. These gene variations or changes are referred to as *mutations*.

A genetic mutation is like a spelling error in a gene's sequence. For example, in people with sickle cell disease, a substitution of a single base (adenine is replaced by thymine) in a single gene

FIG. 13-3 In sickle cell disease a single gene mutation leads to mutant (incorrect) protein. The substitution of valine *(VAL)* for glutamic acid on the β-globin chain of hemoglobin produces abnormal hemoglobin, hemoglobin S (Hb S). In response to low O_2 levels, the erythrocytes with Hb S stiffen and elongate, taking on a sickle shape (see Fig. 31-3).

(β-globin gene) causes the disease (Fig. 13-3). Mutations range in size from a single DNA base (building block) to a large segment of a chromosome.

The change in gene structure may alter the type and/or amount of protein produced. The protein may not work at all, or it may work incorrectly. In some cases, genetic mutations do not have an obvious effect on the people who have them.

Types of Mutations. Genetic mutations occur in two ways. They can be inherited from a parent (germline mutation) or acquired (somatic mutation) during a person's lifetime.

Germline mutations are passed from parent to child. These mutations are present in the oocyte and sperm cells. This type of mutation is present throughout a person's life in virtually every cell in the body.

Acquired (somatic) mutations occur in the DNA of a cell at some time during a person's life. An acquired mutation is passed on to all cells that develop from that single cell. These mutations in somatic cells cannot be passed on to the next generation. Acquired mutations can occur if (1) a mistake is made as DNA replicates during cell division or (2) environmental factors alter the DNA.

Mutations can occur when a cell is dividing. Considering that 3 billion base pairs are replicated in each cell division, DNA replication is very accurate. However, during replication occasionally mistakes such as deletions, insertions, or duplication of DNA material can occur. Although DNA repair enzymes can correct replication errors, mistakes can go uncorrected.[4]

In addition to cell division, DNA damage can also occur from environmental factors. For example, ultraviolet (UV) radiation can cause DNA damage, leading to skin cancer. Toxins in cigarettes can lead to lung cancer. Many chemotherapy drugs used to treat cancer target the DNA of both cancer cells and healthy cells. In the process these drugs increase a person's risk of developing secondary cancers (see Chapter 16).

Cells have built-in mechanisms that catch and repair most of the changes that occur during DNA replication or from environmental damage. However, as we age, our DNA repair does not work as effectively and we accumulate changes in our DNA.

Inheritance Patterns

Genetic disorders can be categorized into autosomal dominant, autosomal recessive, or X-linked (sex-linked) recessive disorders (Table 13-2). If the mutant gene is located on an autosome, the genetic disorder is called *autosomal*. If the mutant gene is on the X chromosome, the genetic disorder is called *X-linked*.

TABLE 13-2	**COMPARISON OF GENETIC DISORDERS**	
Characteristics	**Examples**
Autosomal Dominant	
Males and females are affected* equally. More common than recessive disorders and usually less severe. Affected individuals show variable expression. Affected individuals may have an affected parent. Children of a heterozygous (affected) parent have a 50% chance of being affected. Individuals are affected in successive generations.	Breast and ovarian cancer related to *BRCA* genes Familial hypercholesterolemia Hereditary nonpolyposis colorectal cancer Huntington's disease Neurofibromatosis Marfan's syndrome
Autosomal Recessive	
Males and females are affected equally. Heterozygotes are carriers and usually asymptomatic. Affected individuals may have unaffected† parents who are heterozygous for trait. Children of two heterozygous parents have 25% chance of being affected and 50% chance of being carriers (see Fig. 13-9). Frequently there is a no family history of disease.	Cystic fibrosis Phenylketonuria Sickle cell disease Tay-Sachs disease Thalassemia
X-Linked Recessive	
Most affected individuals have unaffected parents. Affected individuals are usually males. Daughters of affected male are carriers. Sons of affected male are unaffected (unless mother is a carrier).	Duchenne muscular dystrophy Hemophilia Wiskott-Aldrich syndrome

*Have the disease.
†Do not have the disease.

Family pedigrees for autosomal recessive and dominant disorders and X-linked recessive disorders are shown in Figs. 13-4 and 13-5.

Autosomal dominant disorders are caused by a mutation of a single gene pair (heterozygous) on a chromosome. A dominant allele prevails over a normal allele. Autosomal dominant disorders show variable expression. *Variable expression* means that the symptoms expressed by the individuals with the mutated gene vary from person to person even though they have the same mutated gene. Although autosomal dominant disorders have a high probability of occurring in families, sometimes these disorders cause a new mutation or skip a generation. This is termed *incomplete penetrance.*

Autosomal recessive disorders are caused by mutations of two gene pairs (homozygous) on a chromosome. A person who inherits one copy of the recessive allele does not develop the disease because the normal allele predominates. However, this person is a *carrier.*

X-linked recessive disorders are caused by a mutation on the X chromosome. Usually only men are affected by this disorder because women who carry the mutated gene on one X chromosome have another X chromosome to compensate for the mutation. However, women who carry the mutated gene can transmit it to their offspring. It is possible for women to have X-linked recessive disorders, and this can occur when an affected male mates with an unaffected female carrier. This points to the

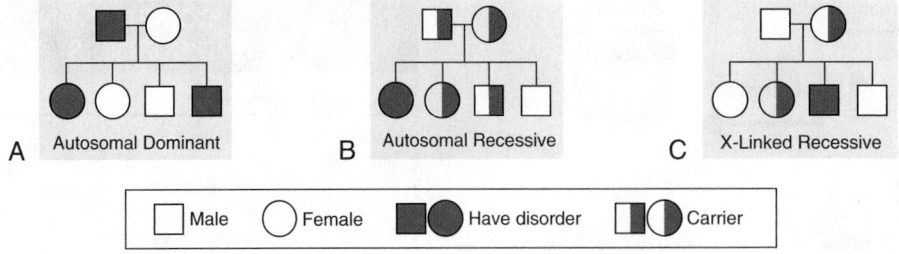

FIG. 13-4 Examples of family pedigrees showing inheritance of **(A)** autosomal dominant, **(B)** autosomal recessive, and **(C)** X-linked recessive disorders.

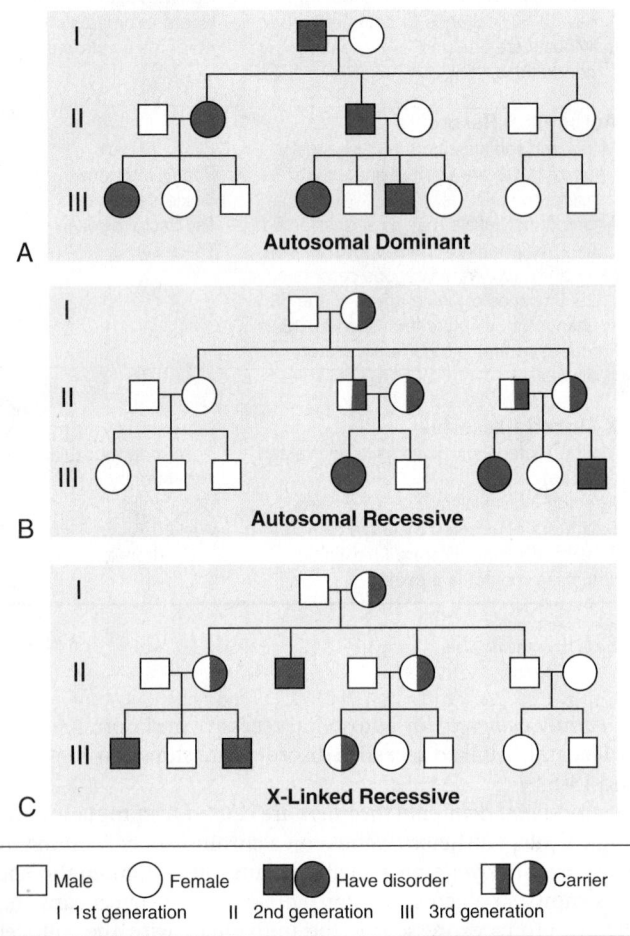

FIG. 13-5 Family pedigrees showing three generations. **A,** Family pedigree suggestive of an autosomal dominant disorder. **B,** Family pedigree suggestive of an autosomal recessive disorder. **C,** Family pedigree suggestive of an X-linked recessive disorder.

importance of testing the carrier status of the female partner of affected males. *X-linked dominant disorders* do exist but are rare.

Multifactorial inherited conditions are caused by a combination of genetic and environmental factors. These disorders run in families but do not show the same inherited characteristics as the single gene mutation conditions. Multifactorial conditions include diabetes mellitus, obesity, hypertension, cancer, and coronary artery disease.

Human Genome Project

The Human Genome Project (HGP), which was completed in 2003, mapped the entire human genome.[5] Analysis of the data

will continue for many years. The knowledge gained through the HGP will (1) help improve the diagnosis of diseases, (2) allow for earlier detection of genetic predisposition to diseases, and (3) play a critical role in determining risk assessment for genetic-related diseases. In addition, the results of the HGP assist in matching organ donors with transplant recipients.

GENETIC DISORDERS

A *genetic disorder* is caused in whole or in part by an alteration in the DNA sequence. As discussed in the section on genetic mutations (pp. 192-193), genetic disorders can be inherited (person born with altered genetic code) or they can be acquired (e.g., replication errors, damage to DNA from toxins). Genetic disorders can be caused by (1) a mutation in one gene (single gene disorder); (2) mutations in multiple genes (multifactorial inheritance disorder), which are often related to environmental factors; or (3) damage to chromosomes (changes in the number or structure of entire chromosomes).

Classification of Genetic Disorders

Single Gene Disorders. Some genetic disorders result from a single gene mutation (Fig. 13-6, *A*). Examples of these diseases include cystic fibrosis, sickle cell disease, and polycystic kidney disease. The pattern of inheritance for single gene disorders can be autosomal dominant, autosomal recessive, or X-linked. Single gene disorders are relatively rare compared with more commonly occurring multifactorial genetic disorders such as diabetes mellitus and heart disease.

Multifactorial Genetic Disorders. Multifactorial genetic disorders are complex diseases that result from small inherited variations in genes, often acting together with environmental factors (Fig. 13-6, *B*). Heart disease, diabetes, and most cancers are examples of such disorders.

Although many common diseases are usually caused by inheritance of mutations in multiple genes, such diseases can also be caused by rare hereditary mutations in a single gene. In these cases, genetic mutations that cause or strongly predispose a person to these diseases run in a family. These mutations can significantly increase each family member's risk of developing the disease. One example is breast cancer, where inheritance of a mutated *BRCA1* or *BRCA2* gene confers significant risk of developing the disease.

Epigenetics. Environmental factors can alter the way our genes are expressed (i.e., which genes are "switched" on or off). Identical twins, who have the same genetic makeup, do not always develop the same diseases or at the same rate.[6]

Genetic and environmental factors interact to influence a person's predisposition to different diseases. *Epigenetics* is the study of changes in gene function that do not involve a change

A   **Mutation in a single gene**

B   **Mutations in multiple genes**

FIG. 13-6 A, Genetic disorders can be caused by a mutation in a single gene (e.g., sickle cell disease, cystic fibrosis, hemophilia). **B,** Most genetic disorders are multifactorial genetic disorders caused by a combination of mutations in multiple genes, often interacting with environmental factors. Examples include cancer, diabetes mellitus, obesity, and hypertension.

GENETICS IN CLINICAL PRACTICE

Genetics in Clinical Practice Boxes Throughout Book

GENETIC DISORDER	CHAPTER	PAGE
α₁-Antitrypsin (AAT) Deficiency	29	582
Alzheimer's Disease (AD)	60	1446
Ankylosing Spondylitis	65	1580
Breast Cancer	52	1244
Cystic Fibrosis (CF)	29	602
Duchenne and Becker Muscular Dystrophy (MD)	64	1545
Familial Adenomatous Polyposis (FAP)	43	985
Familial Hypercholesterolemia	34	733
Genetic Information Nondiscrimination Act (GINA)	13	196
Hemochromatosis	31	648
Hemophilia A and B	31	655
Hereditary Nonpolyposis Colorectal Cancer (HNPCC) or Lynch Syndrome	43	986
Huntington's Disease	59	1440
Ovarian Cancer	54	1295
Polycystic Kidney Disease (PKD)	46	1083
Sickle Cell Disease	31	645
Types 1 and 2 Diabetes Mellitus	49	1155

in DNA sequence. Epigenetics focuses on how and when particular genes are expressed. The expression of genes can be affected both positively and negatively by environmental factors, such as exercise, diet, chemicals, toxins, or smoking. Epigenetic changes can be inherited.

Chromosome Disorders. *Chromosome disorders* are caused by structural changes within chromosomes or by an excess or deficiency of the genes that are located on chromosomes. For example, Down syndrome is caused by an extra copy of chromosome 21 (called trisomy 21), so there are three copies of this chromosome instead of two. In Down syndrome there is no individual abnormal gene on the chromosome.

Chronic myelocytic leukemia can be caused by a chromosomal translocation, in which portions of two chromosomes (chromosomes 9 and 22) are exchanged. This translocation is called the Philadelphia chromosome.

Throughout the book, genetic disorders are highlighted in Genetics in Clinical Practice boxes, Genetic Risk Alert boxes (in the assessment chapters), and Genetic Links content (in the management chapters).

GENETIC TESTING

Genetic testing includes any procedure done to analyze chromosomes, genes, or any gene product that can determine whether a mutation or predisposition to a condition exists. Genetic tests have been developed for more than 2000 diseases. Samples from a person's blood, skin, hair, or saliva can be used to obtain samples for genetic testing. Tissues and cells can also be obtained prenatally.

Genetic testing has been very useful in health care (Table 13-3). Most tests assess single genes and are used to diagnose genetic disorders such as cystic fibrosis or Duchenne muscular dystrophy.[7] Some genetic tests look at rare inherited mutations of otherwise protective genes, such as *BRCA1* and *BRCA2*, which are responsible for some types of hereditary breast and ovarian cancers.

The results of these tests are used in diagnosing an illness or risk for a disorder, and provide the basis for appropriate treatments. Other genetic tests identify people at high risk for conditions that may be preventable. For example, monitoring for and removing polyps or the entire colon in those inheriting a gene for familial adenomatous polyposis (FAP) has saved many lives. (FAP is discussed in Chapter 43 on p. 985.)

Genetic testing of individuals may raise both ethical and social issues. People considering genetic testing should be aware that test results in their medical records might not be kept private. However, the Genetic Information Nondiscrimination Act (GINA) protects people from discrimination by employers and health insurance companies.

If an individual has genetic testing, it may uncover information that may also affect a family member who was not tested. These individuals are frequently not a part of the decision-making process to undergo testing. Similarly, if a whole family is tested, the results may indicate that the biologic relationship is not what the family believed it to be. Some tests are used to help guide health care providers' recommendations for treatment in consultation with the patient (e.g., *BRCA* testing). Other tests allow families to make the decision about not having children with devastating diseases (e.g., cystic fibrosis) or identify people at high risk for conditions that may be prevented by monitoring or having prophylactic surgery (e.g., familial adenomatous polyposis [FAP]).

Currently, many genetic tests are available from testing laboratories. In most cases insurance companies will not cover the cost of genetic testing. For more information about genetic testing, see *www.cdc.gov/dls/moleculartesting*.

TABLE 13-3   USE OF GENETIC TESTS*

Type of Test	Description	Examples
Diagnostic testing	• Used to diagnose, rule out, or confirm a specific genetic or chromosomal condition. • Used to confirm findings when patient's signs and symptoms suggest a genetic disorder. • Can be performed at any time during a person's life, but is not available for all genes or all genetic conditions.	Cystic fibrosis Sickle cell disease Polycystic kidney disease Hemophilia Familial hypercholesterolemia
Carrier screening	• Can be used to identify unaffected individuals who carry one copy of a gene. • Offered to individuals who have a family history of a genetic disorder and to people in ethnic groups with an increased risk of specific genetic conditions. • If both parents are tested, the test can provide information about a couple's risk of having a child with a genetic condition.	Cystic fibrosis Sickle cell disease Hemophilia
Preimplantation genetic diagnosis (PGD)	• Fertilized embryos tested before implantation and pregnancy. • Allows embryos free of particular disorders to be placed into the uterus. • Embryos that test positive for genetic disorders can be destroyed.	For individuals known to have or be a carrier for a genetic mutation (e.g., Huntington's disease)
Prenatal diagnostic testing	• Fluid obtained from amniocentesis or tissue from chorionic villus used to obtain fetal cells. • Used to detect changes in genes or chromosomes of fetus before birth. • Type of testing offered to couples with an increased risk of having a baby with a genetic or chromosomal disorder. • Can decrease a couple's uncertainty or help them decide whether to terminate the pregnancy.	Down syndrome or other genetic alterations in fetuses
Newborn screening	• Most widespread use of genetic testing. • Early intervention to treat these disorders can eliminate or reduce symptoms that might otherwise cause a lifetime of disability.	Phenylketonuria Congenital hypothyroidism Cystic fibrosis
Presymptomatic testing	• Used to detect genetic mutations associated with disorders that appear later in life. • Can be helpful to people who have a family member with a genetic disorder, but who have no features of the disorder themselves at the time of testing. • Results can provide information about a person's risk of developing a specific disorder and help with making decisions about treatment.	Huntington's disease Adult polycystic kidney disease Hemochromatosis Familial adenomatous polyposis Hereditary nonpolyposis colorectal cancer syndrome
Predictive testing	• Can identify mutations that increase a person's risk of developing disorders. • If results are positive, person can have prophylactic measures (e.g., mastectomy, oophorectomy) to prevent development of cancer.	Breast cancer Ovarian cancer
Forensic testing	• Done to identify an individual for legal purposes.	Identify crime or victims in catastrophic situations Rule out or implicate a crime suspect
Parental testing	• Establish biologic relationships between people.	Paternity testing
Pharmacogenetic testing	• Identifies genetic variations that influence a person's response to drugs. • Results provide information to help select drug therapy that is best for the person.	warfarin (Coumadin) dose

*The laboratory performing the tests must, by law, keep your personal information and test results confidential.

GENETICS IN CLINICAL PRACTICE

Genetic Information Nondiscrimination Act (GINA)

What Is GINA?
The Genetic Information Nondiscrimination Act (GINA) prohibits discrimination in health care coverage and employment based on genetic information.

Why Was GINA Needed?
• Decreases concerns about discrimination that might prevent people from getting genetic tests.
• Enables people to take part in research studies without fear that their DNA information might be used against them in the workplace or prevent them from getting health insurance.

What Is a Genetic Test?
• An analysis of human genes (DNA, RNA), chromosomes, proteins, or metabolites that detects genotypes, mutations, or chromosomal changes.

What Is Genetic Information?
• Any information about a person's genetic tests, family members' genetic tests, and family history of a genetic disease or disorder.

• Referral of a person or family for, or use of, genetic services and participation in clinical research that involves genetic services.

What Does GINA Do?
• Prevents health insurers from denying health insurance coverage, adjusting premiums, and discriminating against a person based solely on his or her genetic or family history information.
• Prevents health insurers from requesting that a person have a genetic test.
• Prohibits most employers from using genetic information for hiring, firing, or promotion decisions, and for any decisions regarding terms of employment.
• GINA's health coverage nondiscrimination protection does not extend to life insurance, disability insurance, and long-term care insurance.

For more information see
• www.genome.gov/Pages/PolicyEthics/GeneticDiscrimination/GINA InfoDoc.pdf
• Frequently Asked Questions about GINA at www.dnapolicy.org/gina/faqs.html

Interpreting Genetic Test Results

The results of genetic tests are not always straightforward, which often makes them challenging to interpret and explain. When interpreting test results, health care professionals need to consider a person's medical history, family history, and the type of genetic test that was done.

A *positive test* result means that the laboratory found a change in a particular gene, chromosome, or protein that was being tested. Depending on the purpose of the test, this result may confirm a diagnosis (e.g., Huntington's disease), indicate that a person is a carrier of a particular genetic mutation (e.g., cystic fibrosis), identify an increased risk of developing a disease (e.g., breast cancer), or suggest a need for further testing. A positive result of a predictive or presymptomatic genetic test usually cannot establish the absolute risk of developing a disorder. In addition, a positive test cannot predict the course or severity of a condition.

In some situations it is difficult to interpret a positive result because some people who have the genetic mutation being tested never develop the disease. For example, having the apolipoprotein E-4 *(Apo E-4)* allele increases the risk of developing Alzheimer's disease. However, many people who test positive for *Apo E-4* never develop Alzheimer's disease (see Chapter 60).

A *negative test* result means that the laboratory did not find an altered form of the gene, chromosome, or protein under consideration. This result can indicate that a person is not affected by a particular disorder, is not a carrier of a specific genetic mutation, or does not have an increased risk of developing a certain disease. However, it is possible that the test missed a disease-causing genetic alteration, since many tests cannot detect all the genetic changes that cause a particular disorder. Further testing may be required to confirm a negative result.

ETHICAL/LEGAL DILEMMAS

Genetic Testing

Situation
A 30-year-old woman informs you that she is 3 months' pregnant. She has two children with her current husband. This pregnancy was unplanned, and her youngest child has cystic fibrosis (CF). She expresses concern regarding the possibility of having another child with CF. She mentions that she would like to have genetic testing on her fetus. Her husband asks you what the likelihood is of having another child with CF.

Ethical/Legal Points for Consideration
- With genetic testing, the patient and her family can find out whether their child will have CF. The woman and her husband can then make an informed decision.
- Genetic counseling is recommended before and after obtaining genetic testing because of the complexity of the information and the emotional issues involved with implications and options.
- Knowing that CF is an autosomal recessive condition, you can use Punnett squares (see Fig. 13-9) or a family pedigree (see Figs. 13-4 and 13-5) to show the woman and her husband the probability of having another child with CF.

Discussion Questions
1. What information would you give the patient and her husband regarding genetic testing in order for them to make an informed decision?
2. What options are available for this couple?
3. How would you assist this couple as they are considering terminating the pregnancy if the results of the genetic testing reveal that the fetus will have CF?

Direct-to-Consumer Genetic Tests

Direct-to-consumer genetic tests (at-home testing) are marketed directly to people (consumers) via television, print advertisements, or the Internet. The test kit is mailed to the person instead of being ordered through a health care provider's office. The test typically involves collecting a DNA sample at home, often by swabbing the inside of the cheek, and mailing the sample back to the laboratory. In some cases the person must visit a health clinic to have blood drawn.

Consumers are notified of their results by mail or over the telephone, or the results are posted online. In some cases a genetic counselor or other health care provider is available to explain the results and answer questions. The price for at-home genetic testing ranges from several hundred dollars to more than $1000.

Direct-to-consumer genetic tests have significant risks and limitations. Consumers are vulnerable to being misled by the results of unproven or invalid tests. Without guidance from a health care provider, they may make important decisions about disease treatment or prevention based on inaccurate, incomplete, or misunderstood information about their health. Consumers may also experience an invasion of genetic privacy if testing companies use their genetic information in an unauthorized way.

If your patients are considering using these kinds of genetic tests, let them know that they first need to discuss the issue with their health care provider or a genetic counselor. Patient teaching related to genetic testing is presented in Table 13-4.

Genetic Technology

DNA Finger Printing. DNA (genetic) finger printing begins by extracting DNA from the cells in a sample of blood, saliva, semen, or other appropriate fluid or tissue. *Polymerase chain reaction* (PCR) is a quick, easy method to provide unlimited copies of a DNA or RNA sequence using only a small amount of sample. PCR involves the artificial replication of a DNA or RNA sequence. The DNA or RNA strands can be separated to form new templates that are used for replication.[8]

PCR is a key element in *genetic finger printing*. It is an essential technique to finding mutations in genes. It is also used extensively in forensic medicine to identify DNA of criminal suspects by using samples from blood, hair, saliva, and semen. PCR has also been used in finding evidence to free innocent prisoners and in paternity testing.

PCR can also be used as a confirmatory test in HIV testing. This is especially important when an infant of a mother who is HIV-antibody positive also tests HIV positive. In this situation it is not known whether the antibodies from the infant's blood are from the baby or the mother. PCR techniques can be used on the baby's lymphocytes to determine whether the baby is infected with HIV.

DNA Microarray (DNA Chip). Although all of a person's somatic cells contain identical genetic material, the same genes are not active in every cell. Studying which genes are active and which are inactive in different cell types helps to understand (1) how these cells function normally and (2) how they are affected when various genes do not perform properly.

Gene expression profiling uses a technology called *DNA microarrays* (DNA chips). This technology is used to measure the expression levels of large numbers of genes simultaneously or to genotype multiple regions of a genome. The chips are laid

TABLE 13-4	**PATIENT & FAMILY TEACHING GUIDE**

Genetic Testing

Genetic Counselors
- Individuals who are considering genetic testing should meet with a genetic counselor who is specially trained in medical genetics and counseling.
- Counseling is advised to help you understand the purpose of genetic testing, considerations before testing, and the emotional and medical impact of the test results.
- Genetic counseling can help you understand the pros and cons of genetic testing before making a decision to undergo a genetic test.

General Information
The following includes some important general information about genetic testing.
- Genetic testing can be expensive and may not be included in your medical insurance policy.
- Genetic testing may determine whether you are predisposed to developing an inherited disease.
- A particular genetic test will only tell you whether there is a specific genetic variant or mutation. Positive tests do not mean you will develop that disease or disorder. Neither can the results tell you when you will develop the disease.
- If a genetic test demonstrates a genetic predisposition to an inherited disorder, the news can be depressing.
- Knowledge of a genetic predisposition to a disease may give you the motivation to take preventive measures (e.g., taking drugs for familial hypercholesterolemia) or make lifestyle changes to lower the risk of a disease (e.g., exercising to decrease the risk of type 2 diabetes).
- If a genetic test reveals a strongly negative result, you probably will not develop that disease.
- If a genetic test reveals you are at risk for a specific genetic disorder, there is the possibility that other family members may also be at risk.
- If a genetic test reveals you are at risk for developing an inherited disease, whether or not you decide to share that information with family members is both a personal and an ethical decision that you will have to make.
- Genetic testing may provide important information that you can use when making decisions about having children.

out by robots that can position DNA fragments so precisely that more than 20,000 of them can fit on one microscope slide.

Then fluorescent-tagged molecules are washed over the DNA fragments. Some molecules (with green fluorescent tags) bind to their complementary sequence. These molecules can be identified because they glow under fluorescent light when scanned using automated equipment. Complete patterns of gene activity can be captured with this technology.

Genome-Wide Association Study (GWAS)

Genome-wide association study (GWAS) is an approach that involves rapidly scanning complete sets of DNA, or genomes, of many individuals to find genetic variations associated with the development or progression of a particular disease.

Until recently, researchers looked at single genes and the proteins that they encode. With GWAS, researchers study large numbers of genes and proteins, including how they act and interact. This provides a more complete picture of what goes on in a person. After the genetic associations are identified, researchers may be able to learn how to stop or jump-start genes on demand, change the course of a disease, or prevent it from

ever happening.[4,8] GWAS is particularly useful in finding genetic variations that contribute to multifactorial inherited disorders such as asthma, cancer, diabetes, and heart disease.

To carry out a GWAS, researchers use two groups of participants: people with the disease being studied and similar people without the disease. Each person's complete set of DNA, or genome, is then purified from the blood or cells, placed on tiny chips, and scanned on automated laboratory machines. The machines quickly survey each participant's genome for strategically selected markers of genetic variation.

If certain genetic variations are found to be significantly more common in people with the disease compared to people without the disease, the variations are said to be "associated" with the disease. The associated genetic variations can serve as powerful pointers to the region of the human genome where the disease-causing problem resides.

The potential impact of GWAS is substantial, since it lays the groundwork for personalized medicine, in which the current one-size-fits-all approach to health care gives way to more customized strategies. Tools such as GWAS can provide patients with individualized information about their risks of developing certain diseases. The information will help health care professionals tailor prevention programs to each person's unique genetic makeup.

PHARMACOGENETICS AND PHARMACOGENOMICS

Patients vary widely in their response to drugs. Although the reasons for this are complex, genetic factors may account for a large percentage of patient variability in response to individual drugs. **Pharmacogenetics** is the study of genetic variability of drug responses related to variations in single genes. **Pharmacogenomics** is similar to pharmacogenetics except that it involves multiple genes associated with variability in drug response. These two terms are frequently used interchangeably in describing the relationship between pharmacology and genetic variability in determining an individual's response to drugs.

Pharmacogenetic and pharmacogenomic studies can potentially lead to drugs that can be tailor-made or adapted to each person's particular genetic makeup.[9] Table 13-5 has examples of pharmacogenetics.

One important area of study has been focused on the cytochrome P450 (CYP450) family of major enzymes, which are important in *drug metabolism*. Alterations in the *CYP450* gene can affect how the liver breaks down certain drugs, such as warfarin (Coumadin). People with a less active form of the enzyme (who metabolize the drug slowly) might get too much of the drug, whereas people with a more active form of the enzyme (who metabolize the drug quickly) might get too little of the drug. Too much warfarin can lead to internal bleeding, whereas too little warfarin may still allow blood clots to form. Pharmacogenetic testing can assist health care providers in prescribing the right amount of a medicine based on a patient's particular genetic makeup (Fig. 13-7).

Currently a genetic test for identifying *CYP450* polymorphisms is available that has been approved by the U.S. Food and Drug Administration (FDA). In addition to maximizing the safety and effectiveness of drugs, this type of genetic testing can lead to individualized drug therapy.

Health care providers are starting to use pharmacogenomic information to prescribe drugs, but at this time such tests are

TABLE 13-5 EXAMPLES OF PHARMACOGENETICS

Drug	Role of Pharmacogenetics
trastuzumab (Herceptin)	• In breast cancer, drug only works for women whose tumors have genes that lead to the overproduction of a protein called HER-2. • Drug is a monoclonal antibody to HER-2. After the antibody attaches to the antigen, it kills the cells. • Genetic testing provides information on which patients are good candidates for treatment with drug. • Drug does not work for patients whose tumor genes do not express HER-2.
crizotinib (Xalkori)	• Drug used to treat patients with late-stage (locally advanced or metastatic), non–small cell lung cancers (NSCLC) who express the abnormal anaplastic lymphoma kinase *(ALK)* gene. • *ALK* gene abnormality causes cancer development and growth. • Crizotinib works by blocking certain proteins called kinases, including the protein produced by the abnormal *ALK* gene. • Drug was approved for use with a companion genetic diagnostic test that determines whether a patient with NSCLC has the abnormal *ALK* gene.
vemurafenib (Zelboraf)	• Approved for patients with late-stage (metastatic) or unresectable melanoma. • Indicated for the treatment of patients with melanoma whose tumors express a gene mutation called *BRAF V600E*. • To be considered for treatment, patients must first have genetic testing to determine whether melanoma cells have the *BRAF V600E* mutation.

Drug	Role of Pharmacogenetics
warfarin (Coumadin)	• Genetic variants in the genes *VKORC1* and cytochrome P450 2C9 *(CYP2C9)* have a significant impact on people's sensitivity to warfarin. • Individuals with particular variations in these genes require a lower warfarin dose to maintain therapeutic levels of anticoagulation. • Individuals with other variations require higher doses. • Together these genetic variations explain about 50% of the required dose difference between individuals. • Testing for patient's *CYP2C9* and *VKORC1* genotype information can assist in selecting the starting dose.
abacavir (Ziagen)	• Some people are at greater risk for serious allergic reactions when first starting treatment with this drug. • Genetic testing for *HLA-B*5701* before taking the drug can identify people who carry a genetic marker that is associated with life-threatening hypersensitivity reactions.
clopidogrel (Plavix)	• For clopidogrel to work, cytochrome P450 enzymes in the liver (particularly CYP2C19) must convert the drug to its active form. • About 2% to 14% of the population are poor metabolizers, and these patients may not receive the full benefits of the drug. • Genetic tests are available to identify genetic differences in CYP2C19 function.

Metabolism of Drug	Genetic Variants of Cytochrome P450	Drug Dose Based on Genetic Testing of Cytochrome P450
Normal metabolism		Normal dose
Some people metabolize the drug quickly (fast metabolizers) and need higher doses		Higher dose
Some people metabolize the drug slowly (slow metabolizers) and need lower doses		Lower dose

FIG. 13-7 Individuals respond differently to the drug warfarin (Coumadin). The diversity of responses is partially due to genetic variants in one of the cytochrome *P450* genes.

routine for only a few diseases or disorders (examples are presented in Table 13-5). However, given the field's rapid growth, pharmacogenomics may soon lead to personalized medicine and individualized drug therapy to manage heart disease, cancer, asthma, depression, and many other common diseases.

GENE THERAPY

Gene therapy is an experimental technique that uses genes to treat or prevent disease. Gene therapy is an approach to treating potentially lethal and disabling diseases that are caused by single gene deficiencies. With specialized techniques, gene expression can be manipulated to correct the problem in the particular patient, although the correction will not be passed along to offspring of that person. Approaches to gene therapy include:[10]

- Replacing a mutated gene with a healthy copy of the gene
- Inactivating, or "knocking out," a mutated gene that is functioning improperly
- Introducing a new gene into the body to help fight a disease

A gene that is inserted directly into a cell usually does not function. A carrier molecule called a *vector* must be used to deliver the therapeutic gene to the patient's target cells. Currently, the most common vector is a virus that has been genetically altered to carry normal human DNA. The vector can be injected or given IV directly into specific tissue. The vector unloads its genetic material containing the therapeutic human gene into the target cell. If the treatment is successful, the new gene will make a functional protein and restore the target cell to a normal state. A diagram of gene therapy is depicted in Fig. 13-8.

Although gene therapy is a promising treatment option for a number of diseases (including inherited disorders, some types of cancer, and certain viral infections), the technique remains risky and is still under study to make sure that it will be safe

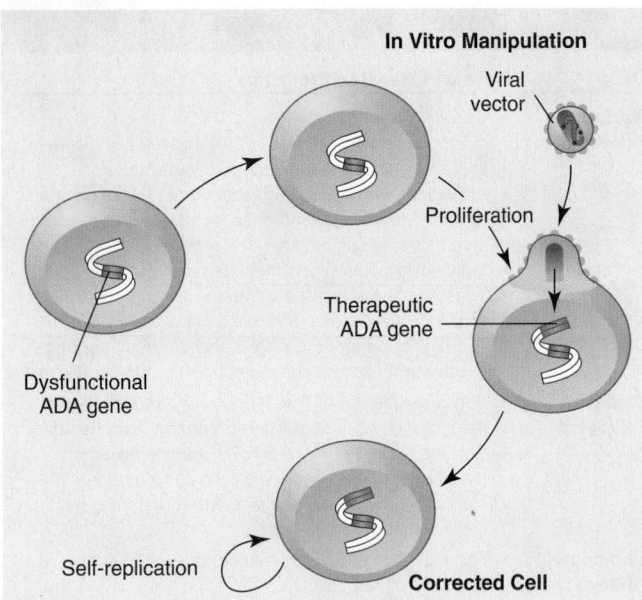

In Vitro Manipulation

Viral vector

Proliferation

Therapeutic ADA gene

Dysfunctional ADA gene

Self-replication

Corrected Cell

FIG. 13-8 Gene therapy for adenosine deaminase *(ADA)* deficiency attempts to correct this immunodeficiency state. The viral vector containing the therapeutic ADA gene is inserted into the patient's lymphocytes. These cells can then make the ADA enzyme.

and effective. Gene therapy is currently only being tested for the treatment of diseases that have no other cures.[10]

STEM CELL THERAPY

Stem cells are the subject of much discussion because they may offer treatment for many diseases. The use of stem cells may allow for the regeneration of lost tissue and restoration of function in various diseases.

Stem cells are unspecialized cells in the body that have the ability to (1) remain in their unspecialized state and divide or (2) differentiate and develop into specialized cells such as a brain cell or a muscle cell. In some body organs such as the gastrointestinal (GI) tract and bone marrow, stem cells divide to repair and replace damaged or old tissues. In other organs such as the pancreas and the heart, stem cells divide only under special conditions.

Stem cells can be divided into two types: embryonic and adult, or somatic. *Embryonic stem cells* come from the embryo at a very early stage in development (4 to 5 days old) and have the ability to become any one of the hundreds of types of cells in the human body. These stem cells can be stimulated to differentiate into any type of tissue (skin, liver, kidney, blood, etc.) found in an adult human.

Adult stem cells are undifferentiated cells that are found in small numbers in many adult organs and tissues, including brain, bone marrow, peripheral blood, blood vessels, skeletal muscle, skin, teeth, heart, GI tract, liver, ovarian epithelium, and testes. They are thought to reside in a specific area of each tissue called a *stem cell niche*. Adult stem cells are more limited than embryonic stem cells in their potential (e.g., stem cells from liver may only develop into more liver cells).

The primary roles of adult stem cells in the body are to maintain and repair tissues in which they are found. They are usually thought of as multipotent cells, giving rise to a closely

related family of cells within the tissue. For example, skin stem cells produce new skin cells. Hematopoietic stem cells found within the bone marrow are capable of forming all of the various blood cells. These cells are prolific by design and are already being used for bone marrow transplants (see Chapter 16).

Medical researchers are investigating the use of stem cells to repair or replace damaged body tissues, similar to whole organ transplants. Currently not enough donated organs are available to meet the demand for transplants. In organ transplants, when tissues from a donor are placed into a patient's body, the patient's immune system may react and reject the donated tissue as "foreign." However, using stem cells presents less risk of this immune rejection, and the therapy may be more successful.

In addition, stem cells could be directed to differentiate into specific cell types. They would then become a renewable source of replacement cells and tissues to treat conditions such as Alzheimer's disease, spinal cord injury, stroke, burns, heart disease, diabetes, osteoarthritis, and rheumatoid arthritis. It may become possible to generate healthy heart muscle cells in the laboratory and then transplant those cells into patients with chronic heart disease. Whether these cells can generate heart muscle cells or stimulate the growth of new blood vessels is under investigation.[11]

NURSING MANAGEMENT GENETICS AND GENOMICS

You need to be knowledgeable about the fundamentals of genetics and genomics.[12,13] By understanding the profound influence that genetics has on health and illness, you can assist the patient and family in making critical decisions related to genetic issues, such as genetic testing. You also need to collaborate with the health care team to involve a genetic nurse or a genetic counselor.

A genetic nurse is a licensed professional nurse with special education and training in genetics. Nurses with GCN after their names are baccalaureate-prepared licensed registered nurses who have received specialty credentialing as a Genetic Clinical Nurse (GCN). Nurses with APNG after their names are licensed registered nurses with a master's degree who have received specialty credentialing as an Advanced Practice Nurse in Genetics (APNG).

As a basic professional nurse, you should be an advocate for patients and families by facilitating access to genetics resources. In addition, you need to provide or reinforce accurate information pertaining to genetics or a genetic disease or concern. This information should be tailored to the patient based on culture, religion, knowledge level, literacy, and preferred language.[14]

You can identify and assess inheritance patterns and explain them to the patient and the family through the use of family pedigrees (see Figs. 13-4 and 13-5) and Punnett squares (Fig. 13-9). Maintain the patient's confidentiality and respect the patient's values and beliefs because genetic information may have major health and social implications.

Genetic testing may raise many psychologic and emotional issues. Knowledge of carrier status of a genetic disorder may influence a person's decisions for a career, marriage, and childbearing. It may also affect significant others in grappling with serious life and health care issues. For example, how should a wife deal with a husband who has tested positive for Hunting-

Autosomal Recessive (e.g., cystic fibrosis)

X-Linked Recessive (e.g., hemophilia)

Autosomal Dominant (e.g., Huntington's disease)

FIG. 13-9 Punnett squares illustrate inheritance possibilities. **A,** If the mother and father are both carriers for cystic fibrosis, there is a 25% chance that offspring will have cystic fibrosis. **B,** If the mother is a carrier for the hemophilia gene and the father has a normal genotype, there is a 50% chance that any male offspring will have hemophilia. There is a 50% chance that any female offspring will be a carrier. **C,** If the mother has a normal genotype and the father has Huntington's disease, there is a 50% chance that offspring will have the disease.

ton's disease and shows early signs of cognitive impairment but does not yet show any other neurologic manifestations of the disease? Should their children be tested for the disease? A 43-year-old woman who has a family history of breast cancer and is now diagnosed with breast cancer wants to know if she and her two teenage daughters should have *BRCA* testing. What do you tell her?

Furthermore, there are ethical concerns. Who should know the results of a genetic test? Who should protect the privacy of individuals' test results and prevent individuals from possible discrimination? Genetic information should not be misused to label individuals or particular ethnic groups. Close attention must be paid to better understand the psychosocial needs of individuals and societal responses and health care policy related to genetic testing.

People may be reluctant to share or disclose information about family history or genetic test results. They fear they are vulnerable to discrimination based on their DNA. Inform your patients about the Genetic Information Nondiscrimination Act (GINA), which protects them from discrimination by employers and health care insurance companies (see Genetics in Clinical Practice Box on p. 196).

Resources on genetics for nurses and nurse educators are available in the list of resources at the end of this chapter.

NURSING ASSESSMENT
FAMILY HISTORY

Family history is one of the strongest influences on a person's risk of developing genetic-related disorders such as heart disease, stroke, diabetes, or cancer. Even though a person cannot change his or her genetic makeup, knowing the family history can help in the prevention or early diagnosis and treatment of a disorder. For example, it is important to monitor cholesterol levels in a person with a family history of familial hypercholesterolemia.

The key features of a family history that may increase a person's risk for genetic-related diseases are
- Disease in more than one close relative
- Disease that does not usually affect a certain gender (e.g., breast cancer in a male)
- Diseases that occur at an earlier age than expected (e.g., myocardial infarction before age 35)
- Certain combinations of diseases within a family (e.g., breast and ovarian cancer, heart disease and diabetes)

If a family has one or more of these features, the family history may hold important clues about a person's risk for a genetic disease. People with a family history of disease may have the most to gain from lifestyle changes and screening tests. People cannot change their genes, but they can change unhealthy behaviors (e.g., smoking, poor eating habits). They can also get screening tests to detect diseases and disease risk factors (e.g., elevated cholesterol, hypertension) that can be treated.

Genetic Risk Alert boxes in the assessment chapters in this book highlight a patient's risks related to genetic diseases and disorders. Use the information in these boxes when obtaining a nursing history.

Family health history is a written or graphic record of the diseases and health conditions present in one's family (see Chapter 3). A useful family health history shows three generations of a person's biologic relatives, the age of diagnosis of a disease, and the age and cause of death of deceased family members. A family health history is a useful tool for understanding health risks and preventing disease in individuals and their close relatives.

Talk with your own family members about your family's health history. Record this information and update it periodically so you and your family members will have organized and accurate information ready to share with your health care provider. Family health history information may help health care providers determine which tests and screenings are recommended to help you and your family know their health risk.

To help individuals collect and organize their family history information, the Centers for Disease Control and Prevention (CDC) has collaborated with the U.S. Surgeon General and other federal agencies to develop a Web-based tool called *My Family Health Portrait (https://familyhistory.hhs.gov/fhh-web/home.action)*.

BRIDGE TO NCLEX EXAMINATION

The number of the question corresponds to the same-numbered outcome at the beginning of the chapter.

1. If a person is heterozygous for a given gene, it means that the person
   a. is a carrier for a genetic disorder.
   b. is affected by the genetic disorder.
   c. has two identical alleles for the gene.
   d. has two different alleles for the gene.

2. Common causes of genetic mutations include *(select all that apply)*
   a. DNA damage from toxins.
   b. DNA damage from UV radiation.
   c. inheritance of altered genes from father.
   d. inheritance of altered genes from mother.
   e. inheritance of somatic mutations from either parent.

3. A father who has an X-linked recessive disorder and a wife with a normal genotype will
   a. pass the carrier state to his male children.
   b. pass the carrier state to all of his children.
   c. pass the carrier state to his female children.
   d. not pass on the genetic mutation to any of his children.

4. What characterizes multifactorial genetic disorders?
   a. Genetic testing available for most disorders
   b. Commonly caused by single gene alterations
   c. Many family members report having the disorder
   d. Caused by complex interactions of genetic and environmental factors

5. If a person tests positive for a genetic mutation, it means *(select all that apply)*
   a. that the laboratory found an alteration in a gene.
   b. that the person is predisposed to develop a genetic disease.
   c. that the person will develop the disease at some point in time.
   d. there is the possibility that other family members may also be at risk.
   e. that the person should not have any children or any additional children.

6. What role does pharmacogenetics have in health care?
   a. It can assess individual variability to many drugs.
   b. It can be used to determine the effectiveness of a drug.
   c. It provides important assessment data for gene therapy.
   d. It can assess the variability of drug responses due to single genes.

7. A couple who recently had a son with hemophilia A is consulting with a nurse. They want to know if their next child will have hemophilia A. The nurse can tell the parents that if their child is a
   a. boy, he will have hemophilia A.
   b. boy, he will be a carrier of hemophilia A.
   c. girl, she will be a carrier of hemophilia A.
   d. girl, there is a 50% chance she will be a carrier of hemophilia A.

1. d, 2. a, b, c, d, 3. c, 4. d, 5. a, d, 6. d, 7. d

ⓔvolve

For rationales to these answers and even more NCLEX review questions, visit *http://evolve.elsevier.com/Lewis/medsurg.*

REFERENCES

1. US Department of Health and Human Services: Genomics. Retrieved from *www.healthypeople.gov/2020/topicsobjectives2020/overview.aspx?topicid=15.*
2. Patton K, Thibodeau GA: *Anatomy and physiology,* ed 8, St Louis, 2013, Mosby.
3. The New Genetics, National Institute of General Medical Sciences, National Institutes of Health, US Department of Health and Human Services. Retrieved from *http://publications.nigms.nih.gov/thenewgenetics/thenewgenetics.pdf.*
4. Jorde LB, Carey JC, Bamshad MJ: *Medical genetics,* ed 4, St Louis, 2010, Mosby.
5. US Department of Energy: Human Genome Project information. Retrieved from *www.ornl.gov/sci/techresources/Human_Genome/home.shtml.*
6. Bell JT, Spector TD: A twin approach to unraveling epigenetics, *Trends Genet* 27(3):116, 2011.
7. National Center for Biotechnology Information: GeneTests. Retrieved from *www.ncbi.nlm.nih.gov/sites/GeneTests.*
8. Ellard S, Turnpenny P: *Emery's elements of medical genetics,* St Louis, 2012, Mosby.
9. Mayo Clinic staff: Personalized medicine and pharmacogenetics. Retrieved from *www.mayoclinic.com/health/personalized-medicine/CA00078.*
10. Lister Hill National Center for Biomedical Communications: Gene therapy. Retrieved from *http://ghr.nlm.nih.gov/handbook/therapy.pdf.*
11. National Institutes of Health: Stem cell basics. Retrieved from *stemcells.nih.gov.*
12. Genetic Science Learning Center, University of Utah: Learning genetics. Retrieved from *http://learn.genetics.utah.edu/content/health/history/genetic.*
13. Beery TA, Workman ML: *Genetics and genomics in nursing and health care,* Philadelphia, 2012, FA Davis.
14. International Society of Nurses in Genetics: *Position statements: Genetic counseling for vulnerable populations: The role of nursing.* Retrieved from *www.isong.org.*

RESOURCES

American Society of Human Genetics (ASHG)
www.ashg.org

Essential Nursing Competencies and Curricula Guidelines for Genetics and Genomics
www.genome.gov/17517146

GeneTests
www.ncbi.nlm.nih.gov/sites/GeneTests

Genetics Home Reference, National Library of Medicine
http://ghr.nlm.nih.gov

International Society of Nurses in Genetics (ISONG)
www.isong.org

National Coalition for Health Professional Education in Genetics (NCHPEG)
www.nchpeg.org

National Human Genome Research Institute
www.genome.gov

Nursing Competencies Relating to Genetics
www.genome.gov/27527634

Understanding Gene Testing
www.accessexcellence.org/AE/AEPC/NIH

A cloudy day is no match for a sunny disposition.
William Arthur Ward

Altered Immune Responses and Transplantation

Sharon L. Lewis

evolve WEBSITE

http://evolve.elsevier.com/Lewis/medsurg

- NCLEX Review Questions
- Key Points
- Pre-Test
- Rationales for Bridge to NCLEX Examination Questions

- Concept Map Creator
- Glossary
- Animations
  - Function of B Cells
  - Function of T Cytotoxic Cells
- Content Updates

eFigures
- eFig. 14-1: Production of interferon
- eFig. 14-2: Monoclonal antibodies

eTables
- eTable 14-1: Mediators of Inflammation
- eTable 14-2: Technologies in Immunology

LEARNING OUTCOMES

1. Describe the functions and components of the immune system.
2. Compare and contrast humoral and cell-mediated immunity, including lymphocytes involved, types of reactions, and effects on antigens.
3. Characterize the five types of immunoglobulins.
4. Differentiate among the four types of hypersensitivity reactions in terms of immunologic mechanisms and resulting alterations.
5. Identify the clinical manifestations and emergency management of a systemic anaphylactic reaction.
6. Describe the assessment and collaborative care of a patient with chronic allergies.
7. Explain the relationship between the human leukocyte antigen system and certain diseases.
8. Describe the etiologic factors, clinical manifestations, and treatment modalities of autoimmune diseases.
9. Describe the etiologic factors and categories of immunodeficiency disorders.
10. Differentiate among the types of rejections following transplantation.
11. Identify the types and side effects of immunosuppressive therapy.

KEY TERMS

anergy, p. 209
antigen, p. 203
autoimmunity, p. 217
cell-mediated immunity, p. 208

cytokines, p. 206
human leukocyte antigen (HLA), p. 219
humoral immunity, p. 207
hypersensitivity reactions, p. 209

immunocompetence, p. 209
immunodeficiency, p. 218
immunosuppressive therapy, p. 221

This chapter discusses the normal immune response and the altered immune responses of hypersensitivity (including allergies), autoimmunity, and immunodeficiency. Histocompatibility, organ transplantation, and immunosuppressive therapy are also presented.

NORMAL IMMUNE RESPONSE

Immunity is the body's ability to resist disease. Immune responses serve the following three functions:

1. *Defense:* The body protects against invasions by microorganisms and prevents the development of infection by attacking foreign antigens and pathogens.

2. *Homeostasis:* Damaged cellular substances are digested and removed. Through this mechanism, the body's different cell types remain uniform and unchanged.

3. *Surveillance:* Mutations continually arise in the body but are normally recognized as foreign cells and destroyed.

Antigens

An **antigen** is a substance that elicits an immune response. Most antigens are composed of protein. However, other substances such as large polysaccharides, lipoproteins, and nucleic acids can act as antigens. All of the body's cells have antigens on their surface that are unique to that person and enable the body to recognize itself. The immune system normally

Reviewed by Bernice Coleman, PhD, ACNP-BC, FAHA, Nurse Practitioner, Heart Transplantation and Ventricular Assist Device Programs, Cedars Sinai Medical Center, Los Angeles, California; Devorah Overbay, RN, MSN, CNS, Assistant Nursing Professor and NCLEX Education Specialist ATI Testing, George Fox University, Department of Nursing, Newberg, Oregon; and Laura Mallett, RN, MSN, Assistant Lecturer, University of Wyoming, Fay W. Whitney School of Nursing, Laramie, Wyoming.

becomes "tolerant" to the body's own molecules. Therefore it is nonresponsive to "self" antigens.

Types of Immunity

Immunity is classified as innate or acquired.

Innate Immunity. *Innate immunity* is present at birth, and its primary role is first-line defense against pathogens. This type of immunity involves a nonspecific response, and neutrophils and monocytes are the primary white blood cells (WBCs) involved. Innate immunity is not antigen specific so it can respond within minutes to an invading microorganism without prior exposure to that organism.

Acquired Immunity. *Acquired immunity* is the development of immunity, either actively or passively (Table 14-1).

Active Acquired Immunity. *Active acquired immunity* results from the invasion of the body by foreign substances such as microorganisms and subsequent development of antibodies and sensitized lymphocytes. With each reinvasion of the microorganisms, the body responds more rapidly and vigorously to fight off the invader. Active acquired immunity may result naturally from a disease or artificially through immunization with a less virulent antigen. Because antibodies are synthesized, immunity takes time to develop but is long lasting.

Passive Acquired Immunity. *Passive acquired immunity* implies that the host receives antibodies to an antigen rather than synthesizing them. This may take place naturally through the transfer of immunoglobulins across the placental membrane from mother to fetus. Artificial passive acquired immunity occurs through injection with gamma globulin (serum antibodies). The benefit of this immunity is its immediate effect. Unfortunately, passive immunity is short lived because the person does not synthesize the antibodies and consequently does not retain memory cells for the antigen.

Lymphoid Organs

The lymphoid system is composed of central (or primary) and peripheral lymphoid organs. The *central lymphoid organs* are

the thymus gland and bone marrow. The *peripheral lymphoid organs* are the lymph nodes; tonsils; spleen; and gut-, genital-, bronchial-, and skin-associated lymphoid tissues (Fig. 14-1).

Lymphocytes are produced in the bone marrow and eventually migrate to the peripheral organs. The thymus is involved in the differentiation and maturation of T lymphocytes and is therefore essential for a cell-mediated immune response. During childhood the thymus is large. It shrinks with age, and in the older person the thymus is a collection of reticular fibers, lymphocytes, and connective tissue.

When antigens are introduced into the body, they may be carried by the bloodstream or lymph channels to regional lymph nodes. The antigens interact with B and T lymphocytes and macrophages in the lymph nodes. The two important functions of lymph nodes are (1) filtration of foreign material brought to the site and (2) circulation of lymphocytes.

The tonsils are an example of lymphoid tissue. The spleen, a peripheral lymph organ, is important as the primary site for filtering foreign antigens from the blood. It consists of two kinds of tissue: white pulp containing B and T lymphocytes and red pulp containing erythrocytes. Macrophages line the pulp and sinuses of the spleen.

Lymphoid tissue is found in the submucosa of the gastrointestinal (GI) (gut-associated), genitourinary (genital-associated), and respiratory (bronchial-associated) tracts. This tissue protects the body surface from external microorganisms.

The skin-associated lymph tissue primarily consists of lymphocytes and Langerhans' cells (a type of dendritic cell) found in the epidermis of skin. When Langerhans' cells are depleted, the skin can neither initiate an immune response nor support a skin-localized delayed hypersensitivity reaction.

Cells Involved in Immune Response

Mononuclear Phagocytes. The *mononuclear phagocyte system* includes monocytes in the blood and macrophages found

TABLE 14-1 TYPES OF ACQUIRED SPECIFIC IMMUNITY

Type	Natural	Artificial
Active	Natural contact with antigen through clinical infection (e.g., recovery from chickenpox, measles, mumps)	Immunization with antigen (e.g., immunization with live or killed vaccines)
Passive	Transplacental and colostrum transfer from mother to child (e.g., maternal immunoglobulins in neonate)	Injection of serum from immune human (e.g., injection of human gamma globulin)

HEALTHY PEOPLE

Health Impact of Immunization

- Can help control the spread of infections within communities.
- Can prevent disability and death from infectious disease for individuals.
- Reduces and can possibly eliminate polio, measles, and other diseases with widespread use.
- Decreased incidence of infectious diseases (e.g., influenza, pneumonia) when more people are vaccinated against these diseases.

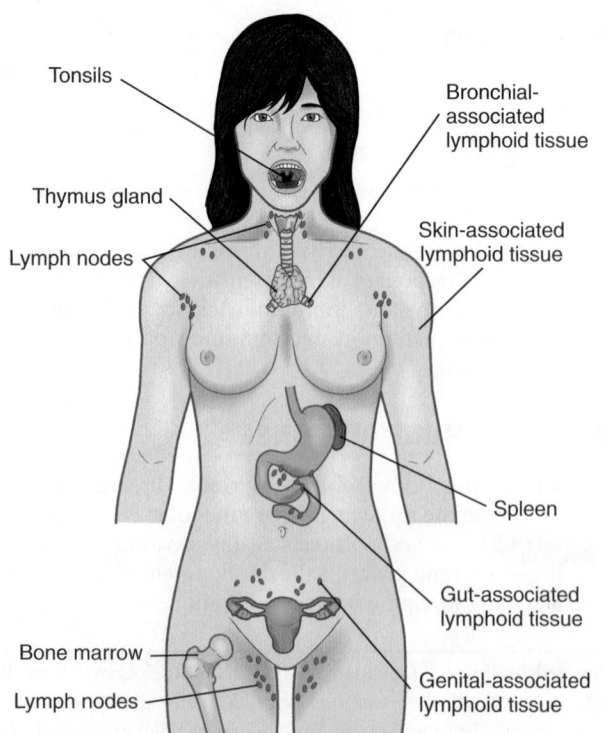

FIG. 14-1 Organs of the immune system.

throughout the body. Mononuclear phagocytes have a critical role in the immune system. They are responsible for capturing, processing, and presenting the antigen to the lymphocytes. This stimulates a humoral or cell-mediated immune response. Capturing is accomplished through phagocytosis. The macrophage-bound antigen, which is highly immunogenic, is presented to circulating T or B lymphocytes and thus triggers an immune response (Fig. 14-2).

Lymphocytes. Lymphocytes are produced in the bone marrow (Fig. 14-3). They then differentiate into B and T lymphocytes.[1]

B Lymphocytes. In the early research on *B lymphocytes* (bursa-equivalent lymphocytes) in birds, it was discovered that they mature under the influence of the bursa of Fabricius, hence the name *B cells.* However, this lymphoid organ does not exist in humans. The bursa-equivalent tissue in humans is the bone marrow. B cells differentiate into *plasma cells* when activated. Plasma cells produce antibodies (immunoglobulins) (Table 14-2).

T Lymphocytes. Cells that migrate from the bone marrow to the thymus differentiate into *T lymphocytes* (thymus-dependent cells). The thymus secretes hormones, including thymosin, that stimulate the maturation and differentiation of T lymphocytes. T cells make up 70% to 80% of the circulating lymphocytes and are primarily responsible for immunity to intracellular viruses, tumor cells, and fungi. T cells live from a few months to the life span of an individual and account for long-term immunity.

T lymphocytes can be categorized into T cytotoxic and T helper cells. Antigenic characteristics of WBCs have now been classified using monoclonal antibodies. These antigens are classified as *clusters of differentiation,* or *CD antigens.* Many types of WBCs, especially lymphocytes, are referred to by their CD designations. All mature T cells have the CD3 antigen.

T Cytotoxic Cells. T cytotoxic (CD8) cells are involved in attacking antigens on the cell membrane of foreign pathogens and releasing cytolytic substances that destroy the pathogen. These cells have antigen specificity and are sensitized by exposure to the antigen. Much like B lymphocytes, some sensitized T cells do not attack the antigen but remain as memory T cells. As in the humoral immune response, a second exposure to the antigen results in a more intense and rapid cell-mediated immune response.

T Helper Cells. T helper (CD4) cells are involved in the regulation of cell-mediated immunity and the humoral antibody response. T helper cells differentiate into subsets of cells that produce distinct types of cytokines (discussed in a later section). These subsets are called T_H1 cells and T_H2 cells. T_H1 cells stimulate phagocyte-mediated ingestion and killing of microbes, the key component of cell-mediated immunity. T_H2 cells stimulate eosinophil-mediated immunity, which is effective against parasites and is involved in allergic responses.

Natural Killer Cells. Natural killer (NK) cells are also involved in cell-mediated immunity. These cells are not T or B cells but are large lymphocytes with numerous granules in the cyto-

FIG. 14-2 The immune response to a virus. **A,** A virus invades the body through a break in the skin or another portal of entry. The virus must make its way inside a cell to replicate itself. **B,** A macrophage recognizes the antigens on the surface of the virus. The macrophage digests the virus and displays pieces of the virus (antigens) on its surface. **C,** A T helper cell recognizes the antigen displayed and binds to the macrophage. This binding stimulates the production of cytokines (interleukin-1 *[IL-1]* and tumor necrosis factor *[TNF]*) by the macrophage and interleukin-2 *(IL-2)* and γ-interferon *(γ-IFN)* by the T cell. These cytokines are intracellular messengers that provide communication among the cells. **D,** IL-2 instructs other T helper cells and T cytotoxic cells to proliferate (multiply). T helper cells release cytokines, causing B cells to multiply and produce antibodies. **E,** T cytotoxic cells and natural killer cells destroy infected body cells. **F,** The antibodies bind to the virus and mark it for macrophage destruction. **G,** Memory B and T cells remain behind to respond quickly if the same virus attacks again.

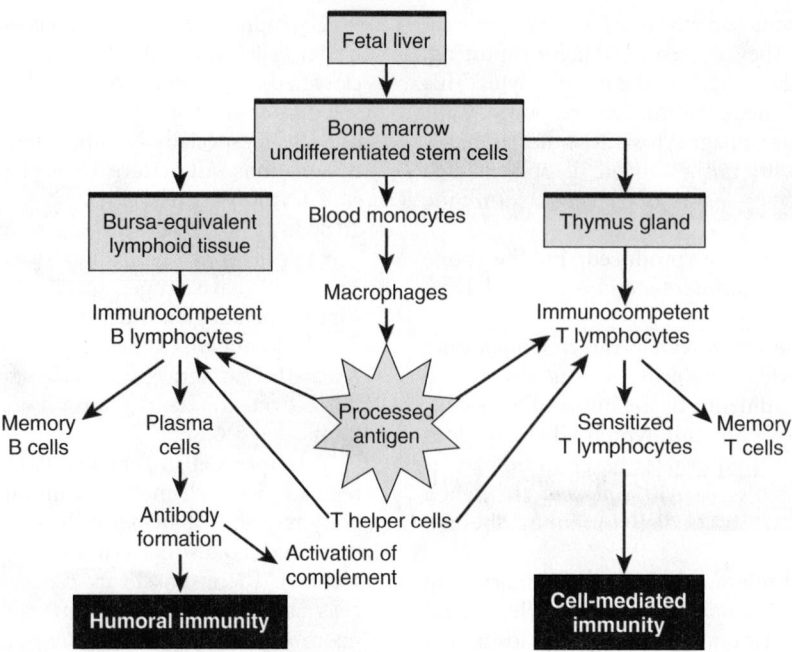

FIG. 14-3 Relationships and functions of macrophages, B lymphocytes, and T lymphocytes in an immune response.

TABLE 14-2	CHARACTERISTICS OF IMMUNOGLOBULINS		
Class	**Serum Concentration**	**Location**	**Characteristics**
IgG	76%	Plasma, interstitial fluid	Is only immunoglobulin that crosses placenta. Is responsible for secondary immune response
IgA	15%	Body secretions, including tears, saliva, breast milk, colostrum	Lines mucous membranes and protects body surfaces
IgM	8%	Plasma	Is responsible for primary immune response. Forms antibodies to ABO blood antigens
IgD	1%	Plasma	Is present on lymphocyte surface. Assists in the differentiation of B lymphocytes
IgE	0.002%	Plasma, interstitial fluids	Causes symptoms of allergic reactions. Fixes to mast cells and basophils. Assists in defense against parasitic infections

plasm. NK cells do not require prior sensitization for their generation. These cells are involved in recognition and killing of virus-infected cells, tumor cells, and transplanted grafts. The mechanism of recognition is not fully understood. NK cells have a significant role in immune surveillance for malignant cell changes.

Dendritic Cells. *Dendritic cells* make up a system of cells that are important to the immune system, especially the cell-mediated immune response. They have an atypical shape with extensive dendritic processes that form and retract. They are found in many places in the body, including the skin (where they are called Langerhans cells) and the lining of the nose, the lungs, the stomach, and the intestine. Especially in the immature state, they are found in the blood.[2]

They primarily function to capture antigens at sites of contact with the external environment (e.g., skin, mucous membranes) and then transport an antigen until it encounters a T cell with specificity for the antigen. In this role, dendritic cells can have an important function in activating the immune response.

Cytokines

The immune response involves complex interactions of T cells, B cells, monocytes, and neutrophils. These interactions depend on **cytokines** (soluble factors secreted by WBCs and a variety of other cells in the body) that act as messengers between the cell types. Cytokines instruct cells to alter their proliferation, differentiation, secretion, or activity.

Currently more than 100 different cytokines are known, and they can be classified into distinct categories. Some of these cytokines are listed in Table 14-3. In general, the interleukins act as immunomodulatory factors, colony-stimulating factors act as growth-regulating factors for hematopoietic cells, and interferons are antiviral and immunomodulatory.

The net effect of an inflammatory response is determined by a balance between proinflammatory and antiinflammatory mediators. Sometimes cytokines are classified as proinflammatory or antiinflammatory (see Table 14-3). However, it is not that clear-cut, since many other factors (e.g., target cells, environment) influence the inflammatory response to a given injury or insult.

Cytokines have a beneficial role in hematopoiesis and immune function. They can also have detrimental effects such as those seen in chronic inflammation, autoimmune diseases,

TABLE 14-3   TYPES AND FUNCTIONS OF CYTOKINES*

Type	Primary Functions	Type	Primary Functions
Interleukins (ILs)		**Interferons (IFNs)**	
IL-1	Proinflammatory mediator. Promotes maturation and clonal expansion of B cells, enhances activity of NK cells, activates T cells, activates macrophages.	α-IFN β-IFN	Inhibit viral replication, activate NK cells and macrophages, antiproliferative effects on tumor cells.
IL-2	Induces proliferation and differentiation of T cells; activation of T cells, NK cells, and macrophages. Stimulates release of other cytokines (α-IFN, TNF, IL-1, IL-6).	γ-IFN	Proinflammatory mediator: activates macrophages, neutrophils, and NK cells; promotes B cell differentiation. Inhibits viral replication.
IL-3 (multicolony colony-stimulating factor)	Hematopoietic growth factor for hematopoietic precursor cells.	**Tumor Necrosis Factor (TNF)**	Proinflammatory mediator; activates macrophages and granulocytes; promotes the immune and inflammatory responses; kills tumor cells; responsible for weight loss associated with chronic inflammation and cancer.
IL-4	Antiinflammatory mediator. B-cell growth factor, stimulates proliferation and differentiation of B cells. Induces differentiation into T_H2 cells. Stimulates growth of mast cells.		
IL-5	B cell growth and differentiation. Promotes growth and differentiation of eosinophils.	**Colony-Stimulating Factors (CSFs)**	
IL-6	Proinflammatory mediator: T- and B-cell growth factor, promotes differentiation of B cells into plasma cells, stimulates antibody secretion, induces fever, synergistic effects with IL-1 and TNF.	Granulocyte colony-stimulating factor (G-CSF)	Stimulates proliferation and differentiation of neutrophils, enhances functional activity of mature PMNs.
IL-7	Promotes growth of T and B cells.	Granulocyte-macrophage colony-stimulating factor (GM-CSF)	Stimulates proliferation and differentiation of PMNs and monocytes.
IL-8	Chemotaxis of neutrophils and T cells, stimulates superoxide and granule release.		
IL-9	Enhances T cell survival, mast cell activation.	Macrophage colony-stimulating factor (M-CSF)	Promotes proliferation, differentiation, and activation of monocytes and macrophages.
IL-10	Antiinflammatory mediator, inhibits cytokine production by T cells and NK cells, promotes B cell proliferation and antibody responses, potent suppressor of macrophage function.	**Erythropoietin**	Stimulates erythroid progenitor cells in bone marrow to produce red blood cells.

*A more comprehensive presentation of cytokines is available at *www.rndsystems.com/molecule_group.aspx?g=704&;r=4.*
NK, Natural killer; *PMNs,* polymorphonuclear neutrophils.

and sepsis. Cytokines such as erythropoietin (see Chapter 47), colony-stimulating factors (see Table 16-14), interferons (see Table 16-13), and interleukin-2 (see Table 16-13) are used clinically to (1) stimulate hematopoiesis, (2) stimulate the bone marrow to make WBCs, and (3) treat various malignancies. In addition, inhibitors of cytokines such as soluble tumor necrosis factor receptor antagonist and interleukin-1 are used as antiinflammatory agents. (Clinical uses of cytokines are listed in Table 14-4.)

Interferon helps the body's natural defenses attack tumors and viruses. Three types of interferon have now been identified (see Table 14-3). In addition to their direct antiviral properties, interferons have immunoregulatory functions. These include enhancement of NK cell production and activation, and inhibition of tumor cell growth.

Interferon is not directly antiviral but produces an antiviral effect in cells by reacting with them and inducing the formation of a second protein termed *antiviral protein* (Fig. 14-4). This protein mediates the antiviral action of interferon by altering the cell's protein synthesis and preventing new viruses from becoming assembled.

Comparison of Humoral and Cell-Mediated Immunity

Humans need both humoral and cell-mediated immunity to remain healthy. Each type of immunity has unique properties, different methods of action, and reactions against particular antigens. Table 14-5 compares humoral and cell-mediated immunity.

FIG. 14-4 Mechanism of action of interferon *(IFN).* When a virus attacks a cell, the cell begins to synthesize viral DNA and interferon. Interferon serves as an intercellular messenger and induces the production of antiviral proteins. Then the virus is not able to replicate in the cell.

Humoral Immunity. Humoral immunity consists of antibody-mediated immunity. The term *humoral* comes from the Greek word *humor,* which means body fluid. Since antibodies are produced by plasma cells (differentiated B cells) and found in plasma, the term *humoral immunity* is used. Production of antibodies is an essential component in a humoral immune response. Each of the five classes of immunoglobulins (Igs)— that is, IgG, IgA, IgM, IgD, and IgE—has specific characteristics (see Table 14-2).

TABLE 14-4   CLINICAL USES OF CYTOKINES

Cytokine	Clinical Uses
α-Interferon (Roferon-A, Intron A)*	Hairy cell leukemia, chronic myelogenous leukemia, malignant melanoma, renal cell carcinoma, ovarian cancer, multiple myeloma, Kaposi sarcoma, hepatitis B and C
β-Interferon (Betaseron, Avonex, Rebif)	Multiple sclerosis
Colony-Stimulating Factors *G-CSF*	
• filgrastim (Neupogen) • pegfilgrastim (Neulasta)	Chemotherapy-induced neutropenia
GM-CSF	
• sargramostim (Leukine)	Neutropenia, myeloid recovery after bone marrow transplantation
Soluble TNF Receptor etanercept (Enbrel)	Rheumatoid arthritis
Interleukin-2 aldesleukin (Proleukin)	Metastatic renal cell carcinoma, metastatic melanoma
Interleukin 11 (platelet growth factor) oprelvekin (Neumega)	Prevention of thrombocytopenia after chemotherapy
Erythropoietin epoetin alfa (Epogen, Procrit) darbepoetin alfa (Aranesp)	Anemia of chronic cancer, anemia related to chemotherapy, anemia of chronic kidney disease
IL-1 Receptor Antagonist anakinra (Kineret)	Rheumatoid arthritis

*eFig. 14-1 on the website for this chapter shows how interferon is commercially made.
G-CSF, Granulocyte colony-stimulating factor; *GM-CSF,* granulocyte-macrophage colony-stimulating factor; *IL,* interleukin; *TNF,* tumor necrosis factor.

TABLE 14-5   COMPARISON OF HUMORAL AND CELL-MEDIATED IMMUNITY

Characteristics	Humoral Immunity	Cell-Mediated Immunity
Cells involved	B lymphocytes	T lymphocytes, macrophages
Products	Antibodies	Sensitized T cells, cytokines
Memory cells	Present	Present
Protection	Bacteria Viruses (extracellular) Respiratory and GI pathogens	Fungus Viruses (intracellular) Chronic infectious agents Tumor cells
Examples	Anaphylactic shock Atopic diseases Transfusion reaction Bacterial infections	Tuberculosis Fungal infections Contact dermatitis Graft rejection Destruction of cancer cells

FIG. 14-5 Primary and secondary immune responses. The introduction of antigen induces a response dominated by two classes of immunoglobulins, IgM and IgG. IgM predominates in the primary response, with some IgG appearing later. After the host's immune system is primed, another challenge with the same antigen induces the secondary response, in which some IgM and large amounts of IgG are produced.

that antigen. When the antigen comes in contact with the cell surface receptor, the B cell becomes activated, and most B cells differentiate into plasma cells (see Fig. 14-3). The mature plasma cell secretes immunoglobulins. Some stimulated B lymphocytes remain as memory cells.

The primary immune response becomes evident 4 to 8 days after the initial exposure to the antigen (Fig. 14-5). IgM is the first type of antibody formed. Because of the large size of the IgM molecule, this immunoglobulin is confined to the intravascular space. As the immune response progresses, IgG is produced, and it can move from intravascular to extravascular spaces.

When the individual is exposed to the antigen the second time, a secondary antibody response occurs. This response occurs faster (1 to 3 days), is stronger, and lasts for a longer time than a primary response. Memory cells account for the memory of the first exposure to the antigen and the more rapid production of antibodies. IgG is the primary antibody found in a secondary immune response.

IgG crosses the placental membrane and provides the newborn with passive acquired immunity for at least 3 months. Infants may also get some passive immunity from IgA in breast milk and colostrum.

Cell-Mediated Immunity. Immune responses that are initiated through specific antigen recognition by T cells are termed cell-mediated immunity. Several cell types and factors are involved in cell-mediated immunity. The cell types involved include T lymphocytes, macrophages, and NK cells. Cell-mediated immunity is of primary importance in (1) immunity against pathogens that survive inside of cells, including viruses and some bacteria (e.g., mycobacteria); (2) fungal infections; (3) rejection of transplanted tissues; (4) contact hypersensitivity reactions; and (5) tumor immunity.

GERONTOLOGIC CONSIDERATIONS

EFFECTS OF AGING ON THE IMMUNE SYSTEM

With advancing age, there is a decline in the function of the immune response (Table 14-6). The primary clinical evidence of *immunosenescence* is the high incidence of malignancies in

When a pathogen (especially bacteria) enters the body, it may encounter a B lymphocyte that is specific for antigens located on that bacterial cell wall. In addition, a monocyte or macrophage may phagocytize the bacteria and present its antigens to a B lymphocyte. The B lymphocyte recognizes the antigen because it has receptors on its cell surface specific for

TABLE 14-6 GERONTOLOGIC ASSESSMENT DIFFERENCES

Effects of Aging on the Immune System

- Thymic involution
- ↓ Cell-mediated immunity
- ↓ Delayed hypersensitivity reaction
- ↓ IL-1 and IL-2 synthesis
- ↓ Expression of IL-2 receptors
- ↓ Proliferative response of T and B cells
- ↓ Primary and secondary antibody responses
- ↑ Autoantibodies

IL, Interleukin.

older adults. Older people are also more susceptible to infections (e.g., influenza, pneumonia) from pathogens that they were relatively immunocompetent against earlier in life. Bacterial pneumonia is the leading cause of death from infections in older adults. The antibody response to immunizations (e.g., flu vaccine) in older adults is considerably lower than in younger adults.

The bone marrow remains relatively unaffected by increasing age. Immunoglobulin levels decrease with age and therefore lead to a suppressed humoral immune response in older adults. Thymic involution (shrinking) occurs with aging, along with decreased numbers of T cells. These changes in the thymus gland are a primary cause of immunosenescence. Both T and B cells show deficiencies in activation, transit time through the cell cycle, and subsequent differentiation. However, the most significant alterations involve T cells. As thymic output of T cells diminishes, the differentiation of T cells increases. Consequently, there is an accumulation of memory cells rather than new precursor cells responsive to previously unencountered antigens.

The delayed hypersensitivity reaction, as determined by skin testing with injected antigens, is frequently decreased or absent in older adults. This altered response reflects **anergy** (an immunodeficient condition characterized by lack of or diminished reaction to an antigen or a group of antigens).

ALTERED IMMUNE RESPONSE

Immunocompetence exists when the body's immune system can identify and inactivate or destroy foreign substances. When the immune system is incompetent or underresponsive, severe infections, immunodeficiency diseases, and malignancies may occur. When the immune system overreacts, hypersensitivity disorders such as allergies and autoimmune diseases may develop.

Hypersensitivity Reactions

Sometimes the immune response is overreactive against foreign antigens or reacts against its own tissue, resulting in tissue damage. These responses are termed **hypersensitivity reactions.** *Autoimmune diseases,* a type of hypersensitivity response, occur when the body fails to recognize self-proteins and reacts against self-antigens.

Hypersensitivity reactions can be classified according to the source of the antigen, the time sequence (immediate or delayed), or the basic immunologic mechanisms causing the injury. Four types of hypersensitivity reactions exist (Table 14-7). Types I, II, and III are immediate and are examples of humoral immunity. Type IV is a delayed hypersensitivity reaction and is related to cell-mediated immunity.

Type I: IgE-Mediated Reactions. *Anaphylactic reactions* are type I reactions that occur only in susceptible people who are highly sensitized to specific allergens. IgE antibodies, produced in response to the allergen, have a characteristic property of attaching to mast cells and basophils (Fig. 14-6; see Fig. 29-2). Within these cells are granules containing potent chemical mediators (histamine, serotonin, leukotrienes, eosinophil chemotactic factor of anaphylaxis [ECF-A], kinins, and bradyki-

TABLE 14-7 TYPES OF HYPERSENSITIVITY REACTIONS

	Type I: IgE-Mediated	Type II: Cytotoxic	Type III: Immune-Complex	Type IV: Delayed Hypersensitivity
Antigen	Exogenous pollen, food, drugs, dust	Cell surface of RBCs Cell basement membrane	Extracellular fungal, viral, bacterial	Intracellular or extracellular
Antibody Involved	IgE	IgG, IgM	IgG, IgM	None
Complement Involved	No	Yes	Yes	No
Mediators of Injury	Histamine Mast cells Leukotrienes Prostaglandins	Complement lysis Macrophages in tissues	Neutrophils Complement lysis Monocytes, macrophages Lysosomal enzymes	Cytokines T cytotoxic cells
Examples	Allergic rhinitis Asthma	Transfusion reaction Goodpasture syndrome Immune thrombocytopenic purpura Graves' disease	Systemic lupus erythematosus Rheumatoid arthritis	Contact dermatitis to poison ivy
Skin Test	Wheal and flare	None	Erythema and edema in 3-8 hr	Erythema and edema in 24-48 hr (e.g., TB test)

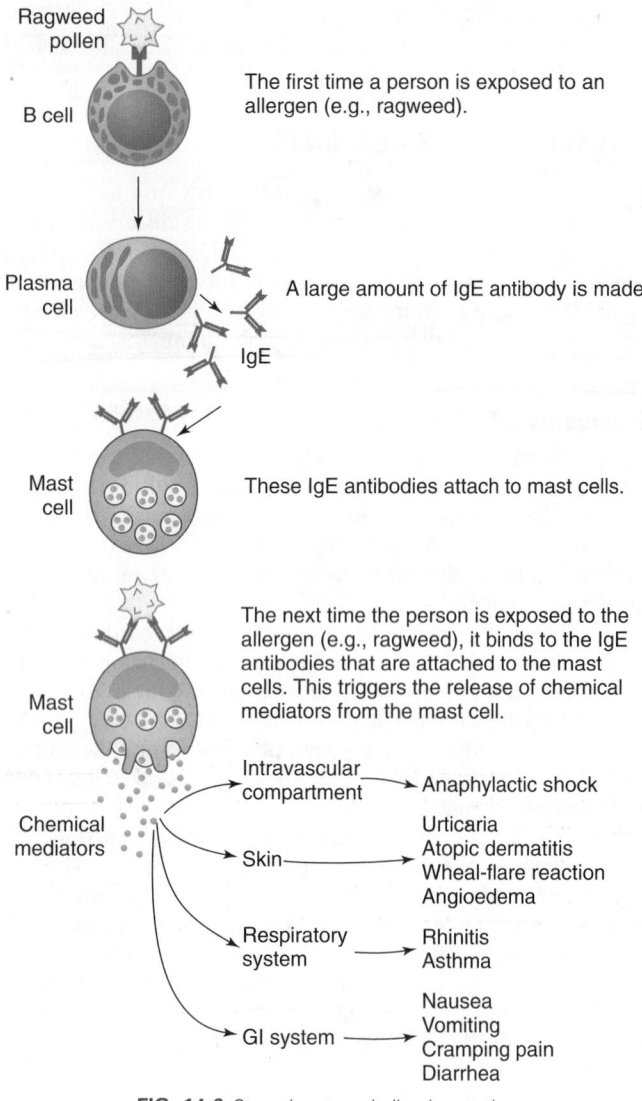

The first time a person is exposed to an allergen (e.g., ragweed).

A large amount of IgE antibody is made.

These IgE antibodies attach to mast cells.

The next time the person is exposed to the allergen (e.g., ragweed), it binds to the IgE antibodies that are attached to the mast cells. This triggers the release of chemical mediators from the mast cell.

Ragweed pollen

B cell

Plasma cell

IgE

Mast cell

Mast cell

Chemical mediators

Intravascular compartment → Anaphylactic shock

Skin → Urticaria / Atopic dermatitis / Wheal-flare reaction / Angioedema

Respiratory system → Rhinitis / Asthma

GI system → Nausea / Vomiting / Cramping pain / Diarrhea

FIG. 14-6 Steps in a type I allergic reaction.

TABLE 14-8   **MEDIATORS OF ALLERGIC RESPONSE** *
• Histamine
• Leukotrienes†
• Prostaglandins
• Platelet-activating factor
• Kinins
• Serotonin
• Anaphylatoxins (C3a, C4a, C5a from complement activation)

*eTable 14-1 is an enhanced version of this table explaining biologic activity and clinical outcomes of these mediators.
†See Chapter 12, Fig. 12-2.

nin). (Chemical mediators of inflammation are discussed in Chapter 12 and Table 12-1.)

On the first exposure to the allergen, IgE antibodies are produced and bind to mast cells and basophils. On any subsequent exposures, the allergen links with the IgE bound to mast cells or basophils and triggers degranulation of the cells and the release of chemical mediators from the granules. In this process the mediators that are released attack target tissues, causing clinical allergy symptoms. These effects include smooth muscle contraction, increased vascular permeability, vasodilation, hypotension, increased secretion of mucus, and itching. Fortunately, the mediators are short acting and their effects are reversible. (The mediators and their effects are summarized in Table 14-8.)

A genetic predisposition to the development of allergic diseases exists. The capacity to become sensitized to an allergen, rather than the specific allergic disorder, appears to be the inherited trait. For example, a father with asthma may have a son who has allergic rhinitis.

The clinical manifestations of an anaphylactic reaction depend on whether the mediators remain local or become systemic, or whether they affect particular organs. When the

mediators remain localized, a cutaneous response termed the *wheal-and-flare reaction* occurs. This reaction is characterized by a pale wheal containing edematous fluid surrounded by a red flare from the hyperemia. The reaction occurs in minutes or hours and is usually not dangerous. A classic example of a wheal-and-flare reaction is the mosquito bite. The wheal-and-flare reaction serves a diagnostic purpose as a means of demonstrating allergic reactions to specific allergens during skin tests.

Common allergic reactions include anaphylaxis and atopic reactions.

Anaphylaxis. Anaphylaxis can occur when mediators are released systemically (e.g., after injection of a drug, after an insect sting). The reaction occurs within minutes and can be life threatening because of bronchial constriction and subsequent airway obstruction and vascular collapse. The target organs affected are seen in Fig. 14-7. Initial symptoms include edema and itching at the site of exposure to the allergen. Shock can occur rapidly and is manifested by rapid, weak pulse; hypotension; dilated pupils; dyspnea; and possibly cyanosis. This is compounded by bronchial edema and angioedema. Death will occur if emergency treatment is not initiated. Some of the important allergens that can cause anaphylactic shock in hypersensitive people are listed in Table 14-9.

Atopic Reactions. An estimated 20% of the population is *atopic,* having an inherited tendency to become sensitive to environmental allergens. The atopic diseases that can result are allergic rhinitis, asthma, atopic dermatitis, urticaria, and angioedema.

Allergic rhinitis, or hay fever, is the most common type I hypersensitivity reaction. It may occur year-round (perennial allergic rhinitis), or it may be seasonal (seasonal allergic rhinitis). Airborne substances such as pollens, dust, and molds are the primary causes of allergic rhinitis. Perennial allergic rhinitis may be caused by dust, molds, and animal dander. Seasonal allergic rhinitis is commonly caused by pollens from trees, weeds, or grasses. The target areas affected are the conjunctiva of the eyes and the mucosa of the upper respiratory tract. Symptoms include nasal discharge; sneezing; lacrimation; mucosal swelling with airway obstruction; and pruritus around the eyes, nose, throat, and mouth. (Treatment of allergic rhinitis is discussed in Chapter 27 on p. 500.)

Many patients with *asthma* have an allergic component to their disease. These patients frequently have a history of atopic disorders (e.g., infantile eczema, allergic rhinitis, food intolerances). Inflammatory mediators produce bronchial smooth muscle constriction, excessive secretion of viscoid mucus, edema of the mucous membranes of the bronchi, and decreased

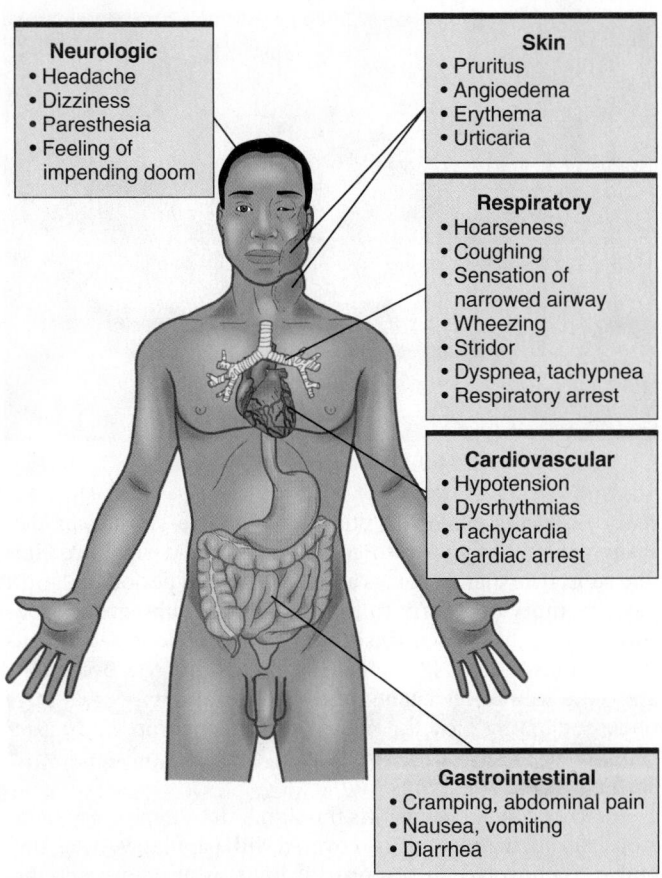

Neurologic
• Headache
• Dizziness
• Paresthesia
• Feeling of impending doom

Skin
• Pruritus
• Angioedema
• Erythema
• Urticaria

Respiratory
• Hoarseness
• Coughing
• Sensation of narrowed airway
• Wheezing
• Stridor
• Dyspnea, tachypnea
• Respiratory arrest

Cardiovascular
• Hypotension
• Dysrhythmias
• Tachycardia
• Cardiac arrest

Gastrointestinal
• Cramping, abdominal pain
• Nausea, vomiting
• Diarrhea

FIG. 14-7 Clinical manifestations of a systemic anaphylactic reaction.

TABLE 14-9 ALLERGENS CAUSING ANAPHYLACTIC SHOCK

Drugs
• Penicillins
• Sulfonamides
• Insulins
• Aspirin
• Tetracycline
• Local anesthetics
• Chemotherapeutic agents
• Cephalosporins
• Nonsteroidal antiinflammatory drugs

Foods
• Eggs, milk, nuts, peanuts, shellfish, fish, chocolate, strawberries

Treatment Measures
• Blood products (whole blood and components)
• Iodine-contrast media for IVP or angiogram test
• Allergenic extracts in hyposensitization therapy

Insect Venoms
• Wasps, hornets, yellow jackets, bumblebees, ants

Animal Sera
• Tetanus antitoxin
• Rabies antitoxin
• Diphtheria antitoxin
• Snake venom antitoxin

IVP, Intravenous pyelogram.

lung compliance. Because of these physiologic alterations, patients manifest dyspnea, wheezing, coughing, tightness in the chest, and thick sputum. (Pathophysiology and management of asthma are discussed in Chapter 29.)

Atopic dermatitis is a chronic, inherited skin disorder characterized by exacerbations and remissions. It is caused by several environmental allergens that are difficult to identify. Although patients with atopic dermatitis have elevated IgE levels and positive skin tests, the histopathologic features do not represent the typical, localized wheal-and-flare type I reactions.

FIG. 14-8 Atopic dermatitis of the lower leg.

The skin lesions are more generalized and involve vasodilation of blood vessels, resulting in interstitial edema with vesicle formation (Fig. 14-8). (Dermatitis is discussed in Chapter 24.)

Urticaria (hives) is a cutaneous reaction against systemic allergens occurring in atopic people. It is characterized by transient wheals (pink, raised, edematous, pruritic areas) that vary in size and shape and may occur all over the body. Urticaria develops rapidly after exposure to an allergen and may last minutes or hours. Histamine causes localized vasodilation (erythema), transudation of fluid (wheal), and flaring. Flaring is due to dilated blood vessels on the edge of the wheal. Histamine is responsible for the pruritus associated with the lesions. (Urticaria is discussed in Chapter 24.)

Angioedema is a localized cutaneous lesion similar to urticaria but involving deeper layers of the skin and the submucosa. The principal areas of involvement include the eyelids, lips, tongue, larynx, hands, feet, GI tract, and genitalia. Swelling usually begins in the face and then progresses to the airways and other parts of the body. Dilation and engorgement of the capillaries secondary to the release of histamine cause the diffuse swelling. Welts are not apparent as in urticaria. The outer skin appears normal or has a reddish hue. The lesions may burn, sting, or itch, and can cause acute abdominal pain if in the GI tract. The swelling may occur suddenly or over several hours and usually lasts for 24 hours.

Type II: Cytotoxic and Cytolytic Reactions. Cytotoxic and cytolytic reactions are type II hypersensitivity reactions involving the direct binding of IgG or IgM antibodies to an antigen on the cell surface. Antigen-antibody complexes activate the complement system, which mediates the reaction. Cellular tissue is destroyed in one of two ways: (1) activation of the complement system resulting in cytolysis or (2) enhanced phagocytosis.

Target cells frequently destroyed in type II reactions are erythrocytes, platelets, and leukocytes. Some of the antigens involved are the ABO blood group, Rh factor, and drugs. Pathophysiologic disorders characteristic of type II reactions include ABO incompatibility transfusion reaction, Rh incompatibility transfusion reaction, autoimmune and drug-related hemolytic anemias, leukopenias, thrombocytopenias, erythroblastosis fetalis (hemolytic disease of the newborn), and Goodpasture syndrome. The tissue damage usually occurs rapidly.

Hemolytic Transfusion Reactions. A classic type II reaction occurs when a recipient receives ABO-incompatible blood from a donor. Naturally acquired antibodies to antigens of the ABO blood group are in the recipient's serum but are not present on the erythrocyte membranes (see Table 30-8). For example, a person with type A blood has anti-B antibodies, a person with type B blood has anti-A antibodies, a person with type AB blood has no antibodies, and a person with type O blood has both anti-A and anti-B antibodies.

If the recipient is transfused with incompatible blood, antibodies immediately coat the foreign erythrocytes, causing *agglutination* (clumping). The clumping of cells blocks small blood vessels in the body, uses existing clotting factors, and depletes them, leading to bleeding. Within hours, neutrophils and macrophages phagocytize the agglutinated cells. The complement system is activated (see eFig. 12-2), and cell lysis occurs, which causes the release of hemoglobin into the urine and plasma. In addition, a cytotoxic reaction causes vascular spasms in the kidney that further block the renal tubules. Acute kidney injury can result from the hemoglobinuria. (Blood transfusions are discussed in Chapter 31.)

Goodpasture Syndrome. *Goodpasture syndrome* is a disorder involving the lungs and kidneys. An antibody-mediated autoimmune reaction occurs involving the glomerular and alveolar basement membranes. The circulating antibodies combine with tissue antigen to activate the complement system, which causes deposits of IgG to form along the basement membranes of the lungs or kidneys. This reaction may result in pulmonary hemorrhage and glomerulonephritis. (Goodpasture syndrome is discussed in Chapter 46.)

Type III: Immune-Complex Reactions. Tissue damage in immune-complex reactions, which are type III reactions, occurs secondary to antigen-antibody complexes. Soluble antigens combine with immunoglobulins of the IgG and IgM classes to form complexes that are too small to be effectively removed by the mononuclear phagocyte system. Therefore the complexes deposit in tissue or small blood vessels. They cause activation of the complement system and release of chemotactic factors that lead to inflammation and destruction of the involved tissue.

Type III reactions may be local or systemic and immediate or delayed. The clinical manifestations depend on the number of complexes and the location in the body. Common sites for deposit are the kidneys, skin, joints, blood vessels, and lungs. Severe type III reactions are associated with autoimmune disorders such as systemic lupus erythematosus, acute glomerulonephritis, and rheumatoid arthritis. (Systemic lupus erythematosus and rheumatoid arthritis are discussed in Chapter 65, and acute glomerulonephritis is discussed in Chapter 46.)

Type IV: Delayed Hypersensitivity Reactions. A *delayed hypersensitivity reaction*—a type IV reaction—is also called a *cell-mediated immune response*. Although cell-mediated responses are usually protective mechanisms, tissue damage occurs in delayed hypersensitivity reactions.

The tissue damage in a type IV reaction does not occur in the presence of antibodies or complement. Rather, sensitized T lymphocytes attack antigens or release cytokines. Some of these cytokines attract macrophages into the area. The macrophages and enzymes released by them are responsible for most of the tissue destruction. In the delayed hypersensitivity reaction, it takes 24 to 48 hours for a response to occur.

Clinical examples of a delayed hypersensitivity reaction include contact dermatitis (Fig. 14-9); hypersensitivity reactions to bacterial, fungal, and viral infections; and transplant rejections. Some drug sensitivity reactions also fit this category.

Contact Dermatitis. *Allergic contact dermatitis* is an example of a delayed hypersensitivity reaction involving the skin. The

FIG. 14-9 Contact dermatitis to rubber.

reaction occurs when the skin is exposed to substances that easily penetrate the skin to combine with epidermal proteins. The substance then becomes antigenic. Over a period of 7 to 14 days, memory cells form to the antigen. On subsequent exposure to the substance, a sensitized person develops eczematous skin lesions within 48 hours. The most common potentially antigenic substances encountered are metal compounds (e.g., those containing nickel or mercury); rubber compounds; catechols present in poison ivy, poison oak, and poison sumac; cosmetics; and some dyes.

In acute contact dermatitis the skin lesions appear erythematous and edematous and are covered with papules, vesicles, and bullae. The involved area is pruritic but may also burn or sting. When contact dermatitis becomes chronic, the lesions resemble atopic dermatitis because they are thickened, scaly, and lichenified. The main difference between contact dermatitis and atopic dermatitis is that contact dermatitis is localized and restricted to the area exposed to the allergens, whereas atopic dermatitis is usually widespread.

Microbial Hypersensitivity Reactions. The classic example of a microbial cell-mediated immune reaction is the body's defense against the tubercle bacillus. Tuberculosis results from invasion of lung tissue by the highly resistant tubercle bacillus. The organism itself does not directly damage the lung tissue. However, antigenic material released from the tubercle bacilli reacts with T lymphocytes, initiating a cell-mediated immune response. The resulting response causes extensive caseous necrosis of the lung.

After the initial cell-mediated reaction, memory cells persist, so subsequent contact with the tubercle bacillus or an extract of purified protein from the organism causes a delayed hypersensitivity reaction. This is the basis for the purified protein derivative (PPD) tuberculosis skin test, which is read 48 to 72 hours after the PPD is injected intradermally. (Tuberculosis is discussed in Chapter 28.)

ALLERGIC DISORDERS

Although an alteration of the immune system may be manifested in many ways, allergies, or type I hypersensitivity reactions, are seen most frequently.

Assessment

For a thorough assessment of a patient with allergies, a comprehensive patient history, physical examination, diagnostic workup, and skin testing for allergens should be done. Obtain information from the patient about family allergies, past and present allergies, and social and environmental factors.

Family history, including information about atopic reactions in relatives, is especially important in identifying at-risk patients. Assess the specific disorder, clinical manifestations, and treatments prescribed.

Note past and present allergies. Identifying the allergens that may have triggered a reaction is essential to control allergic reactions. The time of year when an allergic reaction occurs can be a clue to a seasonal allergen. Also obtain information about any over-the-counter or prescription medications used to treat the allergies.

In addition to identifying the allergen, also obtain information about the clinical manifestations and course of allergic reaction. For women patients, assessment of symptoms during pregnancy, menstruation, or menopause may be important.

Social and environmental factors, especially the physical environment, are important. Questions about pets, trees and plants on the property, pollutants in the air, floor coverings, houseplants, and cooling and heating systems in the home and workplace can provide valuable information about allergens. In addition, a daily or weekly food diary with a description of any untoward reactions is important. Of particular interest is a screening for any reaction to medication. Finally, ask about the patient's lifestyle and stress level in connection with the appearance of allergic symptoms.

Do a comprehensive head-to-toe physical examination, with particular attention focused on the site of the allergic manifestations. Obtain a comprehensive assessment that includes subjective and objective data (Table 14-10).

Diagnostic Studies

Many specialized immunologic techniques can be performed to detect abnormalities of lymphocytes, eosinophils, and immunoglobulins. A complete blood count (CBC) with WBC differential is done, with an absolute lymphocyte count and eosinophil count. Immunodeficiency is diagnosed if the lymphocyte count is below 1200/μL (1.2×10^9/L). T cell and B cell quantification is used to diagnose specific immunodeficiency syndromes. The eosinophil count is elevated in type I hypersensitivity reactions involving IgE. The serum IgE level is also generally elevated in type I hypersensitivity reactions and serves as a diagnostic indicator of atopic diseases.

Sputum and nasal and bronchial secretions may also be tested for the presence of eosinophils. If asthma is suspected, pulmonary function tests for vital capacity, forced expiratory volume, and maximum midexpiratory flow rates are helpful.

Allergy skin testing is the preferred method, but in some cases blood testing may be ordered. Allergy blood tests for IgE antibodies to specific allergens can be done using an enzyme-linked immunosorbent assay (ELISA). Allergy blood testing is recommended if a person (1) is using a drug that interferes with skin test results (e.g., antihistamines, corticosteroids) and cannot stop taking it for a few days, (2) cannot tolerate the many needle scratches required for skin testing, or (3) has a skin disorder (e.g., severe eczema, dermatitis, psoriasis).

Skin Tests. Skin testing is used to identify the specific allergens that are causing the allergy symptoms. With the use of empiric allergy medications as the treatment of choice for most allergic rhinitis, it has become common practice to omit skin testing for specific allergens in these patients. However, diag-

TABLE 14-10	NURSING ASSESSMENT

Allergies

Subjective Data
Important Health Information

Past health history: Recurrent respiratory problems, seasonal exacerbations; unusual reactions to insect bites or stings; past and present allergies

Medications: Unusual reactions to any medications; use of over-the-counter drugs, use of medications for allergies

Functional Health Patterns

Health perception–health management: Family history of allergies; malaise

Nutritional-metabolic: Food intolerances; vomiting

Elimination: Abdominal cramps, diarrhea

Activity-exercise: Fatigue; hoarseness, cough, dyspnea

Cognitive-perceptual: Itching, burning, stinging of eyes, nose, throat, or skin; chest tightness

Role-relationship: Altered home and work environment, presence of pets

Objective Data
Integumentary

Rashes, including urticaria, wheal and flare, papules, vesicles, bullae; dryness, scaliness, scratches, irritation

Eyes, Ears, Nose, and Throat

Eyes: Conjunctivitis; lacrimation; rubbing or excessive blinking; dark circles under the eyes ("allergic shiner")

Ears: Diminished hearing; immobile or scarred tympanic membranes; recurrent ear infections

Nose: Nasal polyps; nasal voice; nose twitching; itchy nose; rhinitis; pale, boggy mucous membranes; sniffling; repeated sneezing; swollen nasal passages; recurrent, unexplained nosebleeds; crease across the bridge of nose ("allergic salute")

Throat: Continual throat clearing; swollen lips or tongue; red throat; palpable neck lymph nodes

Respiratory

Wheezing, stridor; thick sputum

Possible Diagnostic Findings

Eosinophilia of serum, sputum, or nasal and bronchial secretions; ↑ serum IgE levels; positive skin tests; abnormal chest and sinus x-rays

nosing an allergy to a specific antigen enables the patient to avoid an allergen and makes him or her a candidate for immunotherapy. Unfortunately, skin testing cannot be done on patients who cannot be removed from medications that suppress the histamine response or patients with food allergies.

Procedure. Skin testing may be done by three different methods: (1) a scratch or prick test, (2) an intradermal test, or (3) a patch test. The areas of the body usually used in skin testing are the arms and the back. Allergen extracts are applied to the skin in rows with a corresponding control site opposite the test site. Saline or another diluent is applied to the control site. In the *scratch test* a drop of allergen is placed on the skin, and then a pricking device is used so the allergen can enter the skin. In the *intradermal test* the allergen extract is injected under the skin, similar to a PPD test for TB. In the *patch test* an allergen is applied to a patch that is placed on the skin (see Fig. 23-10).

Results. In the scratch and intradermal tests the reaction occurs in 5 to 10 minutes. In the patch test the patches need to be worn for 48 to 72 hours. If the person is hypersensitive to the allergen, a positive reaction will occur within minutes after insertion in the skin and may last for 8 to 12 hours. A positive reaction is manifested by a local wheal-and-flare response.

The size of the positive reaction does not always correlate with the severity of allergy symptoms. False-positive and false-negative results may occur. Negative results from skin testing do not necessarily mean the person does not have an allergic disorder, and positive results do not necessarily mean that the allergen was causing the clinical manifestations. Positive results imply that the person is sensitized to that allergen. Therefore correlating skin test results with the patient's history is important.

Precautions. A highly sensitive person is always at risk for developing an anaphylactic reaction to skin tests. Therefore a patient should never be left alone during the testing period. Sometimes skin testing is completely contraindicated and blood allergy testing is used. If a severe reaction does occur with a skin test, the extract is immediately removed and antiinflammatory topical cream is applied to the site. For intradermal testing, the arm is used so that a tourniquet can be applied during a severe reaction. A subcutaneous injection of epinephrine may also be necessary.

Collaborative Care

After an allergic disorder is diagnosed, treatment is aimed at reducing exposure to the offending allergen, treating the symptoms, and, if necessary, desensitizing the person through immunotherapy.

Anaphylaxis. Anaphylactic reactions occur suddenly in hypersensitive patients after exposure to the offending allergen. They may occur after parenteral injection of drugs (especially antibiotics) or blood products, and after insect stings. The cardinal principle in management is speed in (1) recognition of signs and symptoms of an anaphylactic reaction, (2) maintenance of a patent airway, (3) prevention of spread of the allergen by using a tourniquet, (4) administration of drugs, and (5) treatment for shock. Table 14-11 summarizes the emergency treatment of anaphylactic shock.

Severe cases of anaphylaxis may result in hypovolemic shock because of the loss of intravascular fluid into interstitial spaces that occurs secondary to increased capillary permeability. Peripheral vasoconstriction and stimulation of the sympathetic nervous system occur to compensate for the fluid shift. However, unless shock is treated early, the body will no longer be able to compensate, and irreversible tissue damage will occur, leading to death. (Hypovolemic shock is discussed in Chapter 67.)

All health care workers must be prepared for the rare but life-threatening anaphylactic reaction, which requires immediate medical and nursing interventions. It is extremely important to list all of a patient's allergies on the chart, the nursing care plan, and the medication record.

Chronic Allergies. Most allergic reactions are chronic and are characterized by remissions and exacerbations of symptoms. Treatment focuses on identification and control of allergens, relief of symptoms through drug therapy, and hyposensitization of a patient to an offending allergen.

Allergen Recognition and Control. You play an important role in helping the patient make lifestyle adjustments so that there is minimal exposure to offending allergens. Reinforce that, even with drug therapy and immunotherapy, the patient will never be totally desensitized or completely symptom free. Help the

---

TABLE 14-11   EMERGENCY MANAGEMENT

Anaphylactic Shock

Etiology
- Injection of, inhalation of, ingestion of, or topical exposure to substance that produces profound allergic response (See Table 14-9 for more complete listing.)

Assessment Findings
See Fig. 14-7.

Interventions
Initial
- Ensure patent airway.
- Administer high-flow O_2 via non-rebreather mask.
- Remove insect stinger if present.
- Establish IV access.
- epinephrine 1:1000, 0.01 mL/kg (0.3-0.5 mL) IM into midanterior lateral thigh; repeat every 5-15 min.*
- Nebulized albuterol (Proventil).
- Diphenhydramine (Benadryl) IM or IV.
- Corticosteroids: methylprednisolone (Solu-Medrol) IV.

Hypotension
- Place recumbent and elevate legs.
- epinephrine 1:10,000, 0.1 mL/kg IV every 2-5 min.
- Maintain blood pressure with fluids, volume expanders, vasopressors (e.g., dopamine [Intropin]).

Ongoing Monitoring
- Monitor vital signs, respiratory effort, O_2 saturation, level of consciousness, and cardiac rhythm.
- Anticipate intubation with severe respiratory distress.
- Anticipate cricothyrotomy or tracheostomy with severe laryngeal edema.

*Patients receiving β-blockers may be resistant to treatment with epinephrine and can develop refractory hypotension and bradycardia. Glucagon should be administered in this setting because it has inotropic and chronotropic effects that are not mediated through β-receptors.

---

patient initiate various preventive measures to control the allergic symptoms.

Of primary importance is the need to identify the offending allergen. Sometimes this is done through skin testing. In the case of food allergies an elimination diet is sometimes valuable. If an allergic reaction occurs, all foods eaten shortly before the reaction should be eliminated and gradually reintroduced one at a time until the offending food is detected.

Many allergic reactions, especially asthma and urticaria, may be aggravated by fatigue and emotional stress. Assist the patient in planning a stress management program. Relaxation techniques can be practiced when the patient comes for frequent immunotherapy treatments.

Sometimes control of allergic symptoms requires environmental control, including changing an occupation, moving to a different climate, or giving up a favorite pet. In the case of airborne allergens, sleeping in an air-conditioned room, damp dusting daily, covering mattresses and pillows with hypoallergenic covers, and wearing a mask outdoors may be helpful.

If the allergen is a drug, instruct the patient to avoid the drug. The patient also has the responsibility to make his or her allergies well known to all health care providers. The patient should wear a Medic Alert bracelet listing the particular drug allergy and have the offending drug listed on all medical and dental records.

For a patient allergic to insect stings, commercial bee-sting kits containing preinjectable epinephrine and a tourniquet are available. Instruct the patient and the family about the technique of applying the tourniquet and self-injecting the subcutaneous epinephrine. This patient also should wear a Medic Alert bracelet and carry a bee-sting kit whenever going outdoors.

Drug Therapy. The major categories of drugs used for symptomatic relief of chronic allergic disorders include antihistamines, sympathomimetic/decongestant drugs, corticosteroids, antipruritic drugs, and mast cell–stabilizing drugs. Many of these drugs can be obtained over the counter and are often misused by patients.

Antihistamines. Antihistamines are the best drugs for treatment of allergic rhinitis and urticaria (see Chapter 27, Table 27-2). They are less effective for severe allergic reactions. They act by competing with histamine for H_1-receptor sites and thus blocking the effect of histamine. Best results are achieved if they are taken as soon as allergy symptoms appear. Antihistamines can be used effectively to treat edema and pruritus but are relatively ineffective in preventing bronchoconstriction. With seasonal rhinitis, antihistamines should be taken during peak pollen seasons. (Antihistamines are discussed in Chapter 27.)

Sympathomimetic/Decongestant Drugs. The major sympathomimetic drug is epinephrine (Adrenalin), which is the drug of choice to treat an anaphylactic reaction. Epinephrine is produced by the adrenal medulla and stimulates α- and β-adrenergic receptors. Stimulation of the α-adrenergic receptors causes vasoconstriction of peripheral blood vessels. β-Receptor stimulation relaxes bronchial smooth muscles. Epinephrine also acts directly on mast cells to stabilize them against further degranulation. The action of epinephrine lasts only a few minutes. For the treatment of anaphylaxis, the drug must be given parenterally (intramuscular [IM], IV).

Several specific, minor sympathomimetic drugs differ from epinephrine because they can be taken orally or nasally and last for several hours. Included in this category are phenylephrine (Neo-Synephrine) and pseudoephedrine (Sudafed). The minor sympathomimetic drugs are used primarily to treat allergic rhinitis.

Corticosteroids. Nasal corticosteroid sprays are effective in relieving the symptoms of allergic rhinitis (see Chapter 27 and Table 27-2). Occasionally patients have such severe manifestations of allergies that they are truly incapacitated. In these situations a brief course of oral corticosteroids can be used.

Antipruritic Drugs. Topically applied antipruritic drugs are most effective when the skin is not broken. These drugs protect the skin and provide relief from itching. Common over-the-counter drugs include calamine lotion, coal tar solutions, and camphor. Menthol and phenol may be added to other lotions to produce an antipruritic effect. Some more potent drugs that require a prescription include methdilazine (Tacaryl) and trimeprazine (Temaril). These drugs should be used with great caution because of the associated risk of agranulocytosis.

Mast Cell–Stabilizing Drug. Cromolyn (Intal, NasalCrom) is a mast cell–stabilizing agent that inhibits the release of histamines, leukotrienes, and other agents from the mast cell after antigen-IgE interaction. It is available as an inhalant nebulizer solution or a nasal spray. Cromolyn is used in the management of allergic rhinitis (see Chapter 27).

Leukotriene Receptor Antagonists. Leukotriene receptor antagonists (LTRAs) block leukotriene, one of the major mediators of the allergic inflammatory process (see Table 27-2). These medications can be taken orally. They may be used in the treatment of allergic rhinitis and asthma.

Immunotherapy. Immunotherapy is the recommended treatment for control of allergic symptoms when the allergen cannot be avoided and drug therapy is not effective.[3] Relatively few patients with allergies have symptoms so intolerable that they require allergy immunotherapy. (In individuals with anaphylactic reactions to insect venom, immunotherapy is definitely indicated.)

Immunotherapy involves administration of small titers of an allergen extract in increasing strengths until hyposensitivity to the specific allergen is achieved. For best results, teach the patient to avoid the offending allergen whenever possible because complete desensitization is impossible. Unfortunately, not all allergy-related conditions respond to immunotherapy. Food allergies cannot be safely treated with this therapy, and eczema may worsen with immunotherapy.

Mechanism of Action. The IgE level is elevated in atopic individuals. When IgE combines with an allergen in a hypersensitive person, a reaction occurs, releasing histamine in various body tissues. Allergens more readily combine with IgG than with other immunoglobulins. Therefore immunotherapy involves injecting allergen extracts that will stimulate increased IgG levels. The binding of IgG to allergen-reactive sites interferes with allergen binding to mast cell–bound IgE, preventing mast cell degranulation, and thus reduces the number of reactions that cause tissue damage. The goal of long-term immunotherapy is to keep "blocking" IgG levels high. In addition, allergen-specific T suppressor cells develop in individuals receiving immunotherapy.

Method of Administration. The allergens included in immunotherapy are chosen based on the results of skin testing with a panel of allergens.

Subcutaneous Immunotherapy. *Subcutaneous immunotherapy* involves the subcutaneous injection of titrated amounts of allergen extracts biweekly or weekly. The dose is small at first and is increased slowly until a maintenance dosage is reached. Generally it takes 1 to 2 years of immunotherapy to reach the maximal therapeutic effect. Therapy may be continued for about 5 years. After that, discontinuing therapy is considered. In many patients a decrease in symptoms is sustained after the treatment is discontinued. For patients with severe allergies or sensitivity to insect stings, maintenance therapy is continued indefinitely. Best results are achieved when immunotherapy is administered throughout the year.

Sublingual Immunotherapy. *Sublingual immunotherapy* involves allergen extracts taken under the tongue. This method of immunotherapy has a lower risk of severe adverse reaction than the traditional subcutaneous administration. Today in Europe, sublingual immunotherapy accounts for 40% of allergy treatment. In the United States, although some allergists are using sublingual immunotherapy, it is considered an investigational therapy. Most insurance plans do not cover sublingual immunotherapy. It is considered a U.S. Food and Drug Administration (FDA) "off-label" use. An advantage of this form of immunotherapy is that patients can do it at home.[3]

NURSING MANAGEMENT
IMMUNOTHERAPY

You will often be the person responsible for administering subcutaneous immunotherapy. Always anticipate adverse reactions, especially when using a new-strength dose, after a previous reaction, or after a missed dose. Early manifestations of a systemic reaction include pruritus, urticaria, sneezing, laryngeal edema, and hypotension. Emergency measures for anaphylactic shock should be initiated immediately. Describe a local reaction according to the degree of redness and swelling at the injection site. If the area is greater than the size of a quarter in an adult, report the reaction to the health care provider so that the allergen dosage may be decreased.

Immunotherapy always carries the risk of a severe anaphylactic reaction. Therefore a health care provider, emergency equipment, and essential drugs should be available whenever injections are given.

Record keeping must be accurate and can be invaluable in preventing an adverse reaction to the allergen extract. Before giving an injection, check the patient's name against the name on the vial. Next, determine the vial strength, amount of last dose, date of last dose, and any reaction information.

Always administer the allergen extract in an extremity away from a joint so that a tourniquet can be applied for a severe reaction. Rotate the site for each injection. Aspirate for blood before giving an injection to ensure that the allergen extract is not injected into a blood vessel. An injection directly into the bloodstream can potentiate an anaphylactic reaction. After giving the injection, carefully observe the patient for 20 minutes, since systemic reactions are most likely to occur immediately. However, warn the patient that a delayed reaction can occur as long as 24 hours later.

Latex Allergies

Allergies to latex products have become an increasing problem, affecting both patients and health care professionals. The increase in allergic reactions has coincided with the sharp increase in glove use. It is estimated that 5% to 18% of health care workers regularly exposed to latex are sensitized. The more frequent and prolonged the exposure to latex, the greater the likelihood of developing a latex allergy.[4]

In addition to gloves, many latex-containing products are used in health care, such as blood pressure cuffs, stethoscopes, tourniquets, IV tubing, syringes, electrode pads, O_2 masks, tracheal tubes, colostomy and ileostomy pouches, urinary catheters, anesthetic masks, and adhesive tape. Latex proteins can become aerosolized through powder on gloves and can result in serious reactions when inhaled by sensitized individuals. It is recommended that all health care facilities use powder-free gloves to avoid respiratory exposure to latex proteins.

Types of Latex Allergies. Two types of latex allergies can occur: type IV allergic contact dermatitis and type I allergic reactions. *Type IV contact dermatitis* is caused by the chemicals used in the manufacturing process of latex gloves. It is a delayed reaction that occurs within 6 to 48 hours. Typically the person first has dryness, pruritus, fissuring, and cracking of the skin, followed by redness, swelling, and crusting at 24 to 48 hours. Chronic exposure can lead to lichenification, scaling, and hyperpigmentation. The dermatitis may extend beyond the area of physical contact with the allergen.

A *type I allergic reaction* is a response to the natural rubber latex proteins and occurs within minutes of contact with the proteins. The manifestations of these allergic reactions can vary from skin redness, urticaria, rhinitis, conjunctivitis, or asthma to full-blown anaphylactic shock. Systemic reactions to latex may result from exposure to latex protein via various routes, including the skin, mucous membranes, inhalation, and blood.[5]

Latex-Food Syndrome. Because some proteins in rubber are similar to food proteins, some foods may cause an allergic reaction in people who are allergic to latex. This is called *latex-food syndrome*. The most common of these foods are banana, avocado, chestnut, kiwi, tomato, water chestnut, guava, hazelnut, potato, peach, grape, and apricot. In people with latex allergy, most have a positive allergy test to at least one related food.

NURSING AND COLLABORATIVE MANAGEMENT LATEX ALLERGIES

Identifying patients and health care workers sensitive to latex is crucial to prevent adverse reactions. Obtain a thorough health history and history of any allergies, especially for patients with any complaints of latex contact symptoms. Not all latex-sensitive individuals can be identified, even with a careful and thorough history. The greatest risk factor is long-term multiple exposures to latex products (e.g., health care personnel, individuals who have had multiple surgeries, rubber industry workers). Additional risk factors include a patient history of hay fever, asthma, and allergies to certain foods (listed earlier).

Use latex precaution protocols for those patients identified as having a positive latex allergy test or a history of signs and symptoms related to latex exposure.[6] Many health care facilities have created latex-free product carts that can be used for patients with latex allergies. The National Institute for Occupational Safety and Health (NIOSH) has published recommendations for preventing allergic reactions to latex in the workplace (Table 14-12).

Because of the potential for severe symptoms of food allergy, teach patients to avoid those foods. Other recommendations for people with latex and food allergies include wearing a Medic Alert bracelet or necklace and carrying an injectable epinephrine pen.

Multiple Chemical Sensitivity

Multiple chemical sensitivity (MCS) is a chronic condition characterized by symptoms that the affected person attributes to low-level chemical exposure. Commonly accused substances

---

TABLE 14-12   GUIDELINES FOR PREVENTING ALLERGIC LATEX REACTIONS
• Use nonlatex gloves for activities that are not likely to involve contact with infectious materials (e.g., food preparation, housekeeping).
• Use powder-free gloves with reduced protein content.
• Do not use oil-based hand creams or lotions when wearing gloves.
• After removing gloves, wash hands with mild soap and dry thoroughly.
• Frequently clean work areas that are contaminated with latex-containing dust.
• Know the symptoms of latex allergy, including skin rash; hives; flushing; itching; nasal, eye, or sinus symptoms; asthma; and shock.
• If symptoms of latex allergy develop, avoid direct contact with latex gloves and products.
• Wear a Medic Alert bracelet and carry an epinephrine pen (e.g., EpiPen).

Source: National Institute for Occupational Safety and Health (NIOSH) (www.cdc.gov/niosh).

include smoke, pesticides, plastics, synthetic fabrics, scented products, petroleum products, and paint fumes. Women between the ages of 30 and 50 are more likely to develop the symptoms. Symptoms have also been reported among military personnel, particularly Gulf War veterans. MCS is a controversial diagnosis and is not recognized as a chemical-caused illness by the American Medical Association or other authorities.[7,8]

The symptoms that people report are wide ranging and not specific. They include headache, fatigue, dizziness, nausea, congestion, itching, sneezing, sore throat, chest pain, breathing problems, muscle pain or stiffness, skin rash, diarrhea, bloating, gas, confusion, difficulty concentrating, memory problems, and mood changes. These symptoms are usually subjective, and there is no evidence of a pathologic condition or physiologic dysfunction.

Diagnosis is usually made based on a patient's health history. There is no established test to diagnose MCS. The most effective treatment for MCS is to avoid the chemicals that may trigger the symptoms and create a chemical-free and odor-free home and workplace. Antidepressants, including selective serotonin reuptake inhibitors (SSRIs) (e.g., citalopram [Celexa]), have been used for treatment. Drugs for anxiety and sleep have also been used.

AUTOIMMUNITY

Autoimmunity is an immune response against self in which the immune system no longer differentiates self from nonself. For some unknown reason, immune cells that are normally unresponsive (tolerant to self-antigens) are activated. In autoimmunity, autoantibodies and autosensitized T cells cause pathophysiologic tissue damage.

The cause of autoimmune diseases is still unknown. Age is thought to play some role because the number of circulating autoantibodies increases in people over age 50. However, the principal factors in the development of autoimmunity are (1) the inheritance of susceptibility genes, which may contribute to the failure of self-tolerance; and (2) initiation of autoreactivity by triggers, such as infections, which may activate self-reactive lymphocytes.

Autoimmune diseases tend to cluster, so that a given person may have more than one autoimmune disease (e.g., rheumatoid arthritis, Addison's disease), or the same or related autoimmune diseases may be found in other members of the same family. This observation has led to the concept of genetic predisposition to autoimmune disease. Most of the genetic research in this area correlates certain human leukocyte antigen (HLA) types with an autoimmune condition. (HLAs and disease association are discussed later in this chapter on p. 219.)

Even in a genetically predisposed person, some trigger is required for the initiation of autoreactivity. This may include infectious agents such as a virus. Viral infections can cause an alteration of cells or tissues that are not normally antigenic. The virally induced changes can make the cells or tissues antigenic. Viruses may be involved in the development of diseases such as type 1 diabetes mellitus.[9] Rheumatic fever and rheumatic heart disease are autoimmune responses triggered by streptococcal infection and mediated by antibodies against group A β-hemolytic streptococci that cross-react with heart muscles and valves and synovial membranes.

Drugs can also be precipitating factors in autoimmune disease. Hemolytic anemia can result from methyldopa

TABLE 14-13	EXAMPLES OF AUTOIMMUNE DISEASES*
Systemic Diseases • Mixed connective tissue disease • Progressive systemic sclerosis (scleroderma) • Rheumatoid arthritis • Systemic lupus erythematosus **Organ-Specific Diseases** *Blood* • Autoimmune hemolytic anemia • Immune thrombocytopenic purpura • Hemochromatosis *Central Nervous System* • Guillain-Barré syndrome • Multiple sclerosis *Muscle* • Myasthenia gravis *Heart* • Rheumatic fever	***Endocrine System*** • Addison's disease • Graves' disease • Hypothyroidism • Thyroiditis • Type 1 diabetes mellitus ***Gastrointestinal System*** • Celiac disease • Pernicious anemia • Ulcerative colitis *Kidney* • Glomerulonephritis • Goodpasture syndrome *Liver* • Autoimmune hepatitis • Primary biliary cirrhosis *Eye* • Uveitis

*These diseases are discussed in various chapters throughout the book.

(Aldomet) administration. Procainamide (Pronestyl) can induce the formation of antinuclear antibodies and cause a lupus-like syndrome.

Gender and hormones also have a role in autoimmune disease. More women than men have autoimmune disease. During pregnancy, many autoimmune diseases get better. After delivery, the woman with an autoimmune disease frequently has an exacerbation.

Autoimmune Diseases

Generally, autoimmune diseases are grouped according to organ-specific and systemic diseases (Table 14-13). Systemic lupus erythematosus (SLE) is a classic example of a systemic autoimmune disease characterized by damage to multiple organs. It occurs most frequently in women ages 20 to 40 years. The cause is unknown, but there appears to be a loss of self-tolerance for the body's own DNA antigens.

In SLE, tissue injury appears to be the result of the formation of antinuclear antibodies. For some reason (possibly a viral infection), the cell membrane is damaged and deoxyribonucleic acid (DNA) is released into the systemic circulation, where it is viewed as nonself. This DNA is normally sequestered inside the nucleus of cells. On release into the circulation, the DNA antigen reacts with an antibody. Some antibodies are involved in immune complex formation, and others may cause damage directly. Once the complexes are deposited, the complement system is activated and further damages the tissue, especially the renal glomerulus. (SLE is discussed in Chapter 65.)

Apheresis

Apheresis has been effectively used to treat autoimmune diseases and other diseases and disorders. *Apheresis* is a procedure to separate components of the blood followed by the removal of one or more of these components. Compound words are often used to describe any particular apheresis procedure, depending on the blood components being collected. *Platelet-pheresis* is the removal of platelets, usually for collection from normal individuals to infuse into patients with low platelet counts (e.g., patients taking chemotherapy who develop thrombocytopenia). *Leukocytapheresis* is a general term indicating the removal of WBCs and is used in chronic myelogenous leukemia to remove high numbers of leukemic cells.

Apheresis is also used in peripheral stem cell transplantation to collect stem cells from peripheral blood. These stem cells can then be used to repopulate a person's bone marrow after high-dose chemotherapy (see section on hematopoietic stem cell transplants in Chapter 16).

Plasmapheresis. *Plasmapheresis* is the removal of plasma containing components causing or thought to cause disease. It can also be used to obtain plasma from healthy donors to administer to patients as replacement therapy.

When plasma is removed, it is replaced by substitute fluids such as saline, fresh-frozen plasma, or albumin. Thus the term *plasma exchange* more accurately describes this procedure.

Plasmapheresis has been used to treat autoimmune diseases such as SLE, glomerulonephritis, Goodpasture syndrome, myasthenia gravis, thrombocytopenic purpura, rheumatoid arthritis, and Guillain-Barré syndrome. Many disorders for which plasmapheresis is used are characterized by circulating autoantibodies (usually of the IgG class) and antigen-antibody complexes. The rationale for performing therapeutic plasmapheresis in autoimmune disorders is to remove pathologic substances present in plasma. Immunosuppressive therapy has been used to prevent recovery of IgG production, and plasmapheresis has been used to prevent antibody rebound.

In addition to removing antibodies and antigen-antibody complexes, plasmapheresis may also remove inflammatory mediators (e.g., complement) that are responsible for tissue damage. In the treatment of SLE, plasmapheresis is usually reserved for the patient having an acute attack who is unresponsive to conventional therapy.

Plasmapheresis involves the removal of whole blood through an IV device, and then the blood circulates through the apheresis machine. Inside the machine the blood is divided into plasma and its cellular components by centrifugation or membrane filtration. The plasma is generally replaced with normal saline, lactated Ringer's solution, fresh-frozen plasma, plasma protein fractions, or albumin. When blood is manually removed, only 500 mL can be taken at one time. However, with the use of apheresis procedures, more than 4 L of plasma can be pheresed in 2 to 3 hours.

As with administration of other blood products, be aware of side effects associated with plasmapheresis. The most common complications are hypotension and citrate toxicity. Hypotension is usually the result of a vasovagal reaction or transient volume changes. Citrate is used as an anticoagulant and may cause hypocalcemia, which may manifest as headache, paresthesias, and dizziness.

IMMUNODEFICIENCY DISORDERS

When the immune system does not adequately protect the body, immunodeficiency exists. Immunodeficiency disorders involve an impairment of one or more immune mechanisms, which include (1) phagocytosis, (2) humoral response, (3) cell-mediated response, (4) complement, and (5) a combined humoral and cell-mediated deficiency. Immunodeficiency disorders are *primary* if the immune cells are improperly developed or absent and *secondary* if the deficiency is caused by illnesses or treatment. Primary immunodeficiency disorders are

rare and often serious, whereas secondary disorders are more common and less severe.

Primary Immunodeficiency Disorders

The basic categories of primary immunodeficiency disorders are (1) phagocytic defects, (2) B cell deficiency, (3) T cell deficiency, and (4) a combined B cell and T cell deficiency (Table 14-14).

Secondary Immunodeficiency Disorders

Some of the important factors that may cause secondary immunodeficiency disorders are listed in Table 14-15. Drug-induced immunosuppression is the most common. Immunosuppressive therapy is prescribed for patients to treat autoimmune disorders and to prevent transplant rejection. In addition, immunosuppression is a serious side effect of drugs used in cancer chemotherapy. Generalized leukopenia often results, leading to a decreased humoral and cell-mediated response. Therefore secondary infections are common in immunosuppressed patients.

TABLE 14-14	PRIMARY IMMUNODEFICIENCY DISORDERS	
Disorder	**Affected Cells**	**Genetic Basis**
Chronic granulomatous disease	PMNs, monocytes	X-linked
Job syndrome	PMNs, monocytes	—
Bruton's X-linked agammaglobulinemia	B	X-linked
Common variable hypogammaglobulinemia	B	—
Selective IgA, IgM, or IgG deficiency	B	Some X-linked
DiGeorge syndrome (thymic hypoplasia)	T	—
Severe combined immunodeficiency disease	Stem, B, T	X-linked or autosomal recessive
Ataxia-telangiectasia	B, T	Autosomal recessive
Wiskott-Aldrich syndrome	B, T	X-linked
Graft-versus-host disease	B, T	—

PMNs, Polymorphonuclear neutrophils.

TABLE 14-15	CAUSES OF SECONDARY IMMUNODEFICIENCY
Drug-Induced Immunodeficiency	**Diseases or Disorders**
• Chemotherapy drugs	• Acquired immunodeficiency syndrome (AIDS)
• Corticosteroids	• Cirrhosis
Age	• Chronic kidney disease
• Infants	• Diabetes mellitus
• Older adults	• Hodgkin's lymphoma
	• Malignancies
Malnutrition	• Systemic lupus erythematosus
• Dietary deficiency	• Burns
• Cachexia	• Trauma
	• Severe infection
Therapies	**Stress**
• Radiation	• Chronic stress
• Surgery	• Trauma (physical or emotional)
• Anesthesia	

Malnutrition alters cell-mediated immune responses. When protein is deficient over a prolonged period, the thymus gland atrophies and lymphoid tissue decreases. In addition, an increased susceptibility to infections always exists.

Hodgkin's lymphoma greatly impairs the cell-mediated immune response, and patients may die from severe viral or fungal infections. (Hodgkin's lymphoma is discussed in Chapter 31.) Viruses, especially rubella, may cause immunodeficiency by direct cytotoxic damage to lymphoid cells. Systemic infections can place such a demand on the immune system that resistance to a secondary or subsequent infection is impaired.

Radiation can destroy lymphocytes either directly or through depletion of stem cells. As the radiation dose is increased, more bone marrow atrophies, leading to severe pancytopenia and suppression of immune function. Splenectomy in children is especially dangerous and may lead to septicemia simply from respiratory tract infections.

Stress may alter the immune response. This response involves interrelationships among the nervous, endocrine, and immune systems (see Chapter 7).

HUMAN LEUKOCYTE ANTIGEN SYSTEM

The antigens responsible for rejection of genetically unlike tissues are called the *major histocompatibility antigens*. These antigens are products of histocompatibility genes. In humans they are called the **human leukocyte antigen (HLA)** system. The genes for the HLA antigens are linked and occur together on the sixth chromosome. HLAs are present on all nucleated cells and platelets. The HLA system is primarily used in matching organs and tissues for transplantation.

An important characteristic of HLA genes is that they are highly polymorphic (variable). Each HLA locus can have many different possible alleles, and thus many combinations exist. Each person has two alleles for each locus, one inherited from each parent. Both alleles of a locus are expressed independently (i.e., they are codominant). The proteins encoded by certain genes are known as *antigens*. The entire set of A, B, C, D, and DR genes (the HLA genes) located on one chromosome is termed a *haplotype*. A complete set is inherited as a unit (haplotype). One haplotype is inherited from each parent (Fig. 14-10). This means that a person has HLA genes that are one-half identical to those of each parent. The HLA genes have a 25% chance of being identical to the HLA genes of a sibling.

In organ transplantation A, B, and DR are primarily used for compatibility matching. The specific allele at each locus is identified by a number. For example, a person could have an HLA of A2, A6, B7, B27, DR4, and DR7. Currently more than 8000 HLA alleles have been identified for the various HLA genes.[10]

Human Leukocyte Antigen and Disease Associations

The early interest in HLAs was stimulated by the role of HLAs in matching donors and recipients of organ transplants. Since that time the interest in the association between HLAs and disease has grown.

A number of diseases show significant associations with specific HLA alleles. People who have these alleles are much more likely to develop the associated disease than those who do not have the allele. However, the possession of a particular HLA allele does not mean that the person will necessarily develop the associated disease—only that the relative risk is greater than in the general population.

FIG. 14-10 Patterns of human leukocyte antigen *(HLA)* inheritance. **A,** HLA genes are located on chromosome 6. **B,** The two haplotypes of the father are labeled P^1 and P^2, and the haplotypes of the mother are labeled M^1 and M^2. Each child inherits two haplotypes, one from each parent. **C,** Therefore only four combinations—P^1M^1, P^1M^2, P^2M^1, and P^2M^2—are possible, and 25% of the offspring will have identical HLA haplotypes.

Most of the HLA-associated diseases are classified as autoimmune disorders. Examples of HLA types and disease associations include (1) HLA-B27 and ankylosing spondylitis, (2) HLA-DR2 and HLA-DR3 and SLE, (3) HLA-DR3 and HLA-DR4 and diabetes mellitus, and (5) HLA-DR2 and narcolepsy.

The discovery of HLA associations with certain diseases is a major breakthrough in understanding the genetic bases of these diseases. It is now known that at least part of the genetic bases of HLA-associated diseases lies in the HLA region, but the actual mechanisms involved in these associations are still unknown. However, most individuals who inherit a specific HLA type (e.g., HLA-DR3) that is associated with a disease will never develop that disease.

Currently the association between HLAs and certain diseases is of minimal practical clinical importance. Nevertheless, there is promise for the development of clinical applications in the future. For example, with certain autoimmune diseases, it may be possible to identify members of a family at greatest risk for developing the same or a related autoimmune disease. These people would need close medical supervision, implementation of preventive measures (if possible), and early diagnosis and treatment to prevent chronic complications.

ORGAN TRANSPLANTATION

Transplantation success has improved with advances in surgical technique, advances in histocompatibility testing, and more effective immunosuppressants. Common tissue transplants include corneas, skin, bone marrow, heart valves, bone, and connective tissues (Fig. 14-11). Cornea transplants can prevent or correct blindness. Skin grafts are used in managing burn patients. Bone marrow is donated to help patients with leukemias and other malignancies.

Transplanted organs currently come from many different body systems. These organs include the heart, lung, liver, kid-

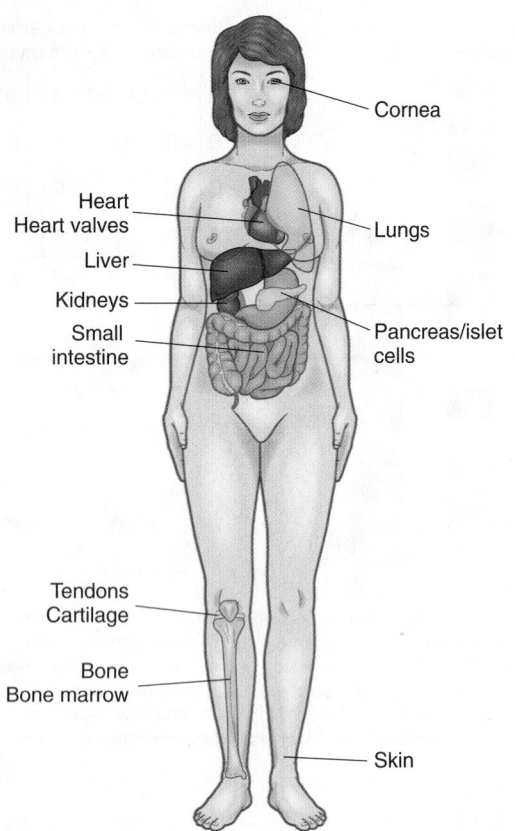

FIG. 14-11 Tissues and organs that can be transplanted.

Cornea

Heart
Heart valves

Lungs

Liver

Kidneys

Small
intestine

Pancreas/islet
cells

Tendons
Cartilage

Bone
Bone marrow

Skin

ney, pancreas, and intestine. Certain organs can be transplanted together, such as kidney and pancreas, kidney and liver, and kidney and heart. For example, many diabetic patients who receive a pancreas transplant also receive a kidney transplant because the diabetes has not only impaired the pancreas, but also led to renal failure.

Some organs can be transplanted in parts or segments instead of transplanting an entire organ. Liver and lung lobes (rather than the whole organ) may be transplanted, or an intestine may be used in segments, thus allowing for one person's organ donation to benefit many recipients. This technique also enables living donors to donate part of an organ (or one of their organs in the case of kidneys).

Organ donations are taken from two sources: deceased (cadaver) and living donors. Most organs and tissues currently come from deceased donors. However, because of the shortage of organs from deceased donors, the use of both related and living unrelated donor organs is increasing.[11]

Individuals can make a decision to become a donor when they sign a donor card, the back of their driver's license, or a donor registry (depending on the state) and indicate their wish to donate organs. However, on their death or imminent death, ultimately the person's legal next of kin must consent to the donation regardless of whether the donor card is signed. That is why it is extremely important for people to notify their next of kin about their willingness to donate organs or tissues at the time of death.

Currently more than 115,000 people are on the organ procurement and transplantation network's national waiting list, which is maintained by the United Network for Organ Sharing (UNOS). However, fewer than 30,000 people receive transplants

annually. The organs in highest demand are kidneys, hearts, and livers. These are also the most commonly transplanted organs.[12]

Organ and tissue donations are regulated by the Uniform Anatomical Gift Act to allow for fair and consistent transplantation laws among all states.[13] Patients are matched to available donors based on a number of factors: ABO blood and HLA typing, medical urgency, time on the waiting list, and geographic location.

Tissue Typing

The recipient usually receives a transplant from an ABO blood group–compatible donor (see Table 30-8). The donor and recipient do not need to share the same Rh factor.

HLA Typing. HLA typing is done on potential donors and recipients. Currently only the A, B, and DR antigens are thought to be clinically significant for transplantation. Because each locus has two alleles that encode for antigens, a total of six antigens are identified. In transplantation an attempt is made to match as many antigens as possible between the HLA-A, HLA-B, and HLA-DR loci. Antigen matches of five and six antigens and certain four-antigen matches have been found to have better clinical outcomes (i.e., the patient is less likely to reject the transplanted organ), especially in kidney and bone marrow transplants.

The degree of HLA matching required or deemed suitable for successful solid organ transplantation depends on the type of organ. Certain organ and tissue transplants require a closer histocompatibility match than other organs. For example, a cornea transplant can be accepted by nearly any individual because corneas are avascular and therefore no antibodies reach the cornea to cause rejection. In kidney and bone marrow transplantation, HLA matching is very important, since these transplants are at high risk for graft rejection. On the other hand, for liver transplants, HLA mismatches have little impact on graft survival. For heart and lung transplants, they fall somewhere in between, but minimizing HLA mismatches significantly improves survival. In addition, for liver, lung, and heart transplants, few donors are available and it is difficult to get good HLA matches.

Transporting and storing donated organs can take time. The "best" match may live many miles from the "ideal" recipient. The need to have the "best" matches has to be balanced against the time it takes to harvest and transport a donated organ and then transplant it.

Panel of Reactive Antibodies. A *panel of reactive antibodies (PRA)* indicates the recipient's sensitivity to various HLAs before receiving a transplant. To detect preformed antibodies to HLA, the recipient's serum is mixed with a randomly selected panel of donor lymphocytes to determine reactivity. The potential recipient may have been exposed to HLA antigens by means of previous blood transfusions, pregnancy, or a previous organ transplant.

For the PRA, the results are calculated in percentages. A high PRA indicates that the person has a large number of cytotoxic antibodies and is highly sensitized, which means there is a poor chance of finding a crossmatch-negative donor. In patients awaiting transplantation, a PRA panel is usually done on a regular basis. Plasmapheresis and IV immune globulin have been used to lower the number of preformed HLA antibodies in highly sensitized patients.

Crossmatch. A *crossmatch* uses serum from the recipient mixed with donor lymphocytes to test for any preformed anti-

HLA antibodies to the potential donor organ. The crossmatch can be used as a screening test when multiple possible living donors are being considered or once a cadaver donor is selected. A final crossmatch is done just before transplant.

A positive crossmatch indicates that the recipient has cytotoxic antibodies to the donor and is an absolute contraindication to transplantation. If transplanted, the organ would undergo hyperacute rejection. A negative crossmatch indicates that no preformed antibodies are present and it is safe to proceed with transplantation. Crossmatching, which is especially important for kidney transplants, may not be done for lung, liver, and heart transplants.

Transplant Rejection

Rejection is one of the major problems following organ transplantation. Rejection of organs occurs as a normal immune response to foreign tissue. The rejection can be prevented by using immunosuppression therapy, performing ABO and HLA matching, and ensuring that the crossmatch is negative. Unfortunately, many different HLAs exist, and a perfect match is nearly impossible unless the tissue is from oneself, an identical twin, or in some cases a sibling. Rejection can be hyperacute, acute, or chronic. Prevention, early diagnosis, and treatment of rejection are essential for long-term graft function.

Hyperacute Rejection. *Hyperacute rejection* occurs minutes to hours after transplantation because the blood vessels are rapidly destroyed. It occurs because the person had preexisting antibodies against the transplanted tissue or organ. There is no treatment for hyperacute rejection, and the transplanted organ is removed.

Fortunately hyperacute rejection is a rare event because the final crossmatch just before transplant usually determines whether the recipient is sensitized to any of the donor HLAs. On occasion, for unclear reasons, the final crossmatch does not detect these preformed antibodies, and hyperacute rejection occurs.

Acute Rejection. *Acute rejection* most commonly manifests in the first 6 months after transplantation. This type of rejection is usually mediated by the recipient's lymphocytes, which have been activated against the donated (foreign) tissue or organ (Fig. 14-12). In addition to cell-mediated rejection, another type of acute rejection occurs when the recipient develops antibodies to the transplanted organ.

It is not uncommon to have at least one rejection episode, especially with organs from deceased donors. These episodes are usually reversible with additional immunosuppressive therapy, which may include increased corticosteroid doses or polyclonal or monoclonal antibodies. Unfortunately, immunosuppressants increase the risk for infection. To combat acute rejection, all patients with transplants require long-term use of immunosuppressants, putting them at a high risk for infection, especially in the first few months after transplant when the immunosuppressive doses are highest.

Chronic Rejection. *Chronic rejection* is a process that occurs over months or years and is irreversible. Chronic rejection can occur for unknown reasons or from repeated episodes of acute rejection. The transplanted organ is infiltrated with large numbers of T and B cells characteristic of an ongoing, low-grade, immune-mediated injury. Chronic rejection results in fibrosis and scarring. In heart transplants it manifests as accelerated coronary artery disease. In lung transplants it manifests as bronchiolitis obliterans. In liver transplants it is characterized

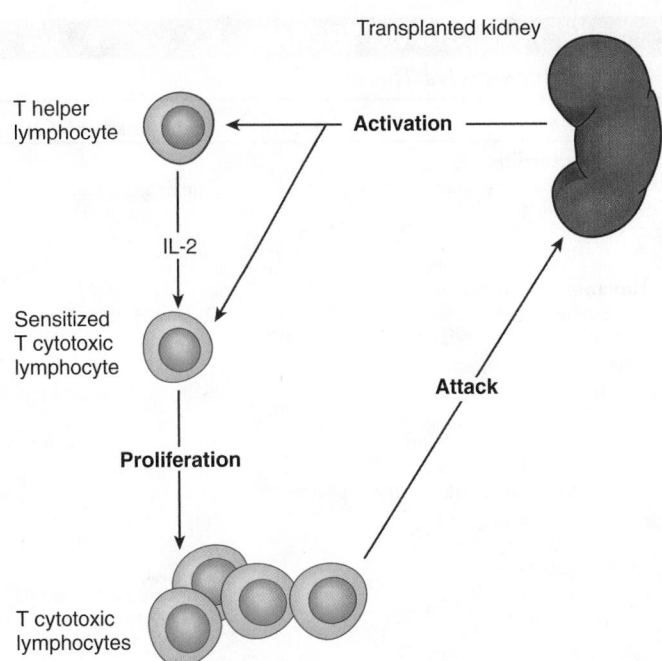

FIG. 14-12 Mechanism of action of T cytotoxic lymphocyte activation and attack of transplanted tissue. The transplanted organ (e.g., kidney) is recognized as foreign and activates the immune system. T helper cells are activated to produce interleukin-2 *(IL-2)*, and T cytotoxic lymphocytes are sensitized. After the T cytotoxic cells proliferate, they attack the transplanted organ.

by loss of bile ducts. In kidney transplants it manifests as fibrosis and glomerulopathy.

There is no definitive therapy for this type of rejection. Treatment is primarily supportive. This type of rejection is difficult to manage and is not associated with the optimistic prognosis of acute rejection.

Immunosuppressive Therapy

Immunosuppressive therapy requires a balance. On one hand, the immune response needs to be suppressed to prevent rejection of the transplanted organ. On the other hand, an adequate immune response needs to be maintained to prevent overwhelming infection and the development of malignancies.[14]

Many of the drugs used to achieve immunosuppression have significant side effects. Because transplant recipients must take immunosuppressants for life, the risk of toxicity continues for the rest of their lives.[15]

Immunosuppressant drugs are listed in Table 14-16. With use of a combination of agents that work during different phases of the immune response (Fig. 14-13), lower doses of each drug can be given to produce effective immunosuppression while minimizing side effects.

The major immunosuppressive agents are (1) calcineurin inhibitors, including cyclosporine (Sandimmune, Neoral, Gengraf) and tacrolimus (Prograf, FK506); (2) corticosteroids (prednisone, methylprednisolone [Solu-Medrol] IV); (3) mycophenolate mofetil (CellCept); and (4) sirolimus (Rapamune). Azathioprine (Imuran) and cyclophosphamide (Cytoxan) can also be used. Antilymphocyte globulin (ALG) and muromonab-CD3 (Orthoclone OKT3) are IV medications used for short periods to prevent early rejection or reverse acute rejection.

Immunosuppression protocols are highly variable among transplant centers, with different combinations of medications

TABLE 14-16 DRUG THERAPY

Immunosuppressive Therapy

Agent	Route	Mechanism of Action	Side Effects
Corticosteroids			
prednisone, methylprednisolone (Solu-Medrol)	PO, IV	Suppress inflammatory response. Inhibit cytokine production (IL-1, IL-6, TNF) and T cell activation and proliferation.	Peptic ulcers, hypertension, osteoporosis, Na$^+$ and H$_2$O retention, muscle weakness, easy bruising, delayed healing, hyperglycemia, ↑ risk for infection.
Calcineurin Inhibitors			
cyclosporine (Sandimmune,* Neoral,* Gengraf*) (Neoral and Gengraf are microemulsions with better absorption than Sandimmune.)	PO, IV	Acts on T helper cells to prevent production and release of IL-2 and γ-interferon. Inhibits production of T cytotoxic lymphocytes and B cells.	Nephrotoxicity, ↑ risk for infection, neurotoxicity (tremors, seizures), hepatotoxicity, lymphoma, hypertension, tremors, hirsutism, leukopenia, gingival hyperplasia.
tacrolimus (Prograf, FK506)	PO, IV	Same as cyclosporine but more effective.	Same as cyclosporine.
Cytotoxic (Antiproliferative) Drugs			
mycophenolate mofetil (CellCept) mycophenolate acid (Myfortic)	PO, IV	Inhibits purine synthesis. Suppresses proliferation of T and B cells.	Diarrhea, nausea and vomiting, severe neutropenia, thrombocytopenia, ↑ risk for infection, ↑ incidence of malignancies.
cyclophosphamide (Cytoxan, Neosar)	PO, IV	Cross-links DNA, leading to cell injury and death. Results in decrease in number and activity of T and B cells.	Neutropenia, hemorrhagic cystitis.
azathioprine (Imuran)	PO, IV	Blocks purine synthesis. Suppresses cell-mediated and humoral immune responses by inhibiting proliferation of T and B cells.	Bone marrow suppression: neutropenia, anemia, thrombocytopenia.
sirolimus (Rapamune)	PO	Binds to mammalian target of rapamycin (mTOR), thereby suppressing T cell activation and proliferation.	↑ Risk for infection, leukopenia, anemia, thrombocytopenia, hyperlipidemia, hypercholesterolemia, arthralgias, diarrhea. ↑ incidence of malignancies. Not used in liver and lung transplants.
everolimus (Zortress)	PO	Same as above	Peripheral edema, constipation, hypertension, nausea, anemia, urinary tract infection, hyperlipidemia.
Monoclonal Antibodies			
muromonab-CD3 (Orthoclone OKT3)	IV push	Monoclonal antibody that binds to CD3 receptors on T cells, causing cell lysis. Inhibits function of cytotoxic T cells.	Fever, chills, dyspnea, chest pain, nausea and vomiting. Anaphylactic reactions include pulmonary edema, cardiac or respiratory arrest.
daclizumab (Zenapax)	IV	Monoclonal antibody that acts as IL-2 receptor antagonist by inhibiting the binding of IL-2. Inhibits T cell activation and proliferation.	Can cause acute hypersensitivity reaction, including anaphylaxis.
basiliximab (Simulect)	IV	Same as daclizumab.	Same as daclizumab.
Polyclonal Antibody			
Lymphocyte immune globulin (Atgam)	IV	Prepared by immunizing horse with human T cells. Polyclonal antibodies directed against T cells, thus depleting them.	Serum sickness (fever, chills, muscle and joint pain), tachycardia, back pain, shortness of breath, hypotension, anaphylaxis, leukopenia, thrombocytopenia, rash, ↑ risk for infection.
Other			
belatacept (Nulojix)	IV	Prevents the activation of T cells.	Anemia, constipation, urinary tract infection, peripheral edema.

*Not bioequivalent and cannot be interchanged.
IL, Interleukin; *TNF,* tumor necrosis factor.

being used. Most patients are initially on triple therapy. The standard triple therapy usually includes a calcineurin inhibitor, a corticosteroid, and mycophenolate mofetil.

The doses of immunosuppressant drugs are reduced over time after the transplant. Patients taking corticosteroids may be weaned off after a few years. The trend in many transplant centers is to use immunosuppression protocols that do not contain corticosteroids because of their many side effects.

Calcineurin Inhibitors. This group of drugs, including tacrolimus and cyclosporine, is the foundation of most immunosuppression regimens. As the most effective immunosuppressants, these drugs prevent a cell-mediated attack against the transplanted organ (see Fig. 14-13). These drugs do not cause bone marrow suppression or alterations of the normal inflammatory response. They are generally used in combination with corticosteroids, mycophenolate mofetil, and sirolimus. Tacrolimus is the most widely used calcineurin inhibitor.[15]

FIG. 14-13 Sites of action for immunosuppressive agents.

Many of the side effects of calcineurin inhibitors are dose related. These drugs are potentially nephrotoxic. Drug levels are monitored closely to prevent toxicity.

DRUG ALERT: Tacrolimus and Cyclosporine
- A substance in grapefruit and grapefruit juice prevents metabolism of these drugs.
- Consuming grapefruit or grapefruit juice while using these drugs could increase their toxicity.

Sirolimus. Sirolimus is an immunosuppressive agent approved for use in renal transplant recipients. It is used in combination with corticosteroids and cyclosporine. It is also used in combination with tacrolimus.

Mycophenolate Mofetil. Mycophenolate mofetil is a lymphocyte-specific inhibitor of purine synthesis with suppressive effects on both T and B lymphocytes. This drug appears to be most effective when used in combination with tacrolimus or cyclosporine. Its effects are additive because it acts later in the lymphocyte activation pathway by a different mechanism. It has also been shown to decrease the incidence of late graft loss. The major limitation of this drug is its GI toxicities, including nausea, vomiting, and diarrhea. In many cases the side effects can be diminished by lowering the dose or giving smaller doses more frequently.

DRUG ALERT: Mycophenolate Mofetil
- When given IV, it must be reconstituted in D_5W and no other solution.
- Do not give as IV bolus. Give over 2 or more hours.

Monoclonal Antibodies. Monoclonal antibodies are used for preventing and treating acute rejection episodes. (eFig. 14-2, showing how monoclonal antibodies are made, is available on the website for this chapter.) Muromonab-CD3 was the first of these monoclonal antibodies to be used in clinical transplantation. It is a mouse monoclonal antibody that binds with the CD3 antigen found on the surface of human thymocytes and mature T cells. It is an anti-antigen receptor antibody that interferes with the function of the T lymphocyte, the pivotal cell in the response to graft rejection. It is administered via IV bolus. All T cells are affected, rather than just the subset active in graft rejection. Within minutes after the initial infusion of muromonab-CD3, the number of circulating T cells decreases significantly.

A flulike syndrome occurs during the first few days of treatment because of cytokine release. Side effects include fever,

rigors, headache, myalgias, and various GI disturbances. To reduce the expected side effects of muromonab-CD3, give patients acetaminophen (Tylenol), diphenhydramine (Benadryl), and IV methylprednisolone before administering the dose.

Newer generation monoclonal antibodies include daclizumab (Zenapax) and basiliximab (Simulect). These monoclonal antibodies are a hybrid of mouse and human antibodies and have fewer side effects than muromonab-CD3 because they have been "humanized."

Polyclonal Antibody. Lymphocyte immune globulin (Atgam) is used as induction therapy or to treat acute rejection. The purpose of induction therapy is to severely immunosuppress an individual immediately after transplantation to prevent early rejection. The drug is made by immunizing horses with human lymphocytes. The antibody made against the human lymphocytes is then purified and administered IV.

Allergic reactions to the foreign proteins from the host animal, manifested by fever, arthralgias, and tachycardia, are common but usually not severe enough to preclude use. These side effects can be attenuated by administering the preparation slowly, over 4 to 6 hours, and premedicating patients with acetaminophen, diphenhydramine, and methylprednisolone. The main toxicities of polyclonal antibodies are lymphopenia and thrombocytopenia caused by antibody contaminants that are not completely removed during preparation of the antibodies.

GRAFT-VERSUS-HOST DISEASE

Graft-versus-host disease (GVHD) occurs when an immuno-incompetent (immunodeficient) patient receives immunocompetent cells.[16] A GVHD response may result from the infusion of any blood product containing viable lymphocytes, as in therapeutic blood transfusions, and from the transplantation of fetal thymus, fetal liver, or bone marrow. In most transplantation situations the biggest concern is the patient's (host's) rejection of the organ or transplant. However, in GVHD disease, the graft (donated tissue) rejects the host (recipient) tissue.

The GVHD response may begin 7 to 30 days after transplantation. Once the reaction is started, little can be done to modify its course. The exact mechanism involved in this reaction is not completely understood. However, it involves donor T cells attacking and destroying vulnerable host cells.

The target organs for the GVHD phenomenon are the skin, liver, and GI tract. The skin disease may be a maculopapular rash, which may be pruritic or painful. It initially involves the palms and soles of the feet but can progress to a generalized erythema with bullous formation and desquamation (shedding of the outer layer of skin). The liver disease may range from mild jaundice with elevated liver enzymes to hepatic coma. The intestinal disease may be manifested by mild to severe diarrhea, severe abdominal pain, GI bleeding, and malabsorption.

The biggest problem with GVHD is infection, with different types of infections seen in different periods. Bacterial and fungal infections predominate immediately after transplantation when granulocytopenia exists. The development of interstitial pneumonitis is the primary concern later in the course of the disease.

There is no adequate treatment of GVHD once it is established. Although corticosteroids are often used, they enhance the susceptibility to infection. The use of immunosuppressive agents (e.g., methotrexate, cyclosporine) has been most effective as a preventive rather than a treatment measure. Radiation of blood products before they are administered is another measure to prevent T cell replication.

BRIDGE TO NCLEX EXAMINATION

The number of the question corresponds to the same-numbered outcome at the beginning of the chapter.

1. The function of monocytes in immunity is related to their ability to
   a. stimulate the production of T and B lymphocytes.
   b. produce antibodies on exposure to foreign substances.
   c. bind antigens and stimulate natural killer cell activation.
   d. capture antigens by phagocytosis and present them to lymphocytes.

2. One function of cell-mediated immunity is
   a. formation of antibodies.
   b. activation of the complement system.
   c. surveillance for malignant cell changes.
   d. opsonization of antigens to allow phagocytosis by neutrophils.

3. The reason newborns are protected for the first 6 months of life from bacterial infections is because of the maternal transmission of
   a. IgG.
   b. IgA.
   c. IgM.
   d. IgE.

4. In a type I hypersensitivity reaction the primary immunologic disorder appears to be
   a. binding of IgG to an antigen on a cell surface.
   b. deposit of antigen-antibody complexes in small vessels.
   c. release of cytokines used to interact with specific antigens.
   d. release of chemical mediators from IgE-bound mast cells and basophils.

5. The nurse is alerted to possible anaphylactic shock immediately after a patient has received intramuscular penicillin by the development of
   a. edema and itching at the injection site.
   b. sneezing and itching of the nose and eyes.
   c. a wheal-and-flare reaction at the injection site.
   d. chest tightness and production of thick sputum.

6. The nurse advises a friend who asks him to administer his allergy shots that
   a. it is illegal for nurses to administer injections outside of a medical setting.
   b. he is qualified to do it if the friend has epinephrine in an injectable syringe provided with his extract.
   c. avoiding the allergens is a more effective way of controlling allergies, and allergy shots are not usually effective.
   d. immunotherapy should only be administered in a setting where emergency equipment and drugs are available.

7. Association between HLA antigens and diseases is most commonly found in what disease conditions?
   a. Malignancies
   b. Infectious diseases
   c. Neurologic diseases
   d. Autoimmune disorders

8. A patient is undergoing plasmapheresis for treatment of systemic lupus erythematosus. The nurse explains that plasmapheresis is used in her treatment to
   a. remove T lymphocytes in her blood that are producing antinuclear antibodies.
   b. remove normal particles in her blood that are being damaged by autoantibodies.
   c. exchange her plasma that contains antinuclear antibodies with a substitute fluid.
   d. replace viral-damaged cellular components of her blood with replacement whole blood.

9. The most common cause of secondary immunodeficiencies is
   a. drugs.
   b. stress.
   c. malnutrition.
   d. human immunodeficiency virus.

10. What accurately describes rejection following transplantation?
    a. Hyperacute rejection can be treated with OKT3.
    b. Acute rejection can be treated with sirolimus or tacrolimus.
    c. Chronic rejection can be treated with tacrolimus or cyclosporine.
    d. Hyperacute reaction can usually be avoided if crossmatching is done before the transplantation.

11. In a person having an acute rejection of a transplanted kidney, what would help the nurse understand the course of events (select all that apply)?
    a. A new transplant should be considered.
    b. Acute rejection can be treated with OKT3.
    c. Acute rejection usually leads to chronic rejection.
    d. Corticosteroids are the most successful drugs used to treat acute rejection.
    e. Acute rejection is common after a transplant and can be treated with drug therapy.

1. d, 2. c, 3. a, 4. d, 5. a, 6. d, 7. d, 8. c, 9. a, 10. d, 11. b, e

ⓔvolve

For rationales to these answers and even more NCLEX review questions, visit *http://evolve.elsevier.com/Lewis/medsurg.*

REFERENCES

1. Kaufman C: The secret lives of lymphocytes, *Nursing* 41:50, 2011.
2. Abbas A, Lichtman A, Pillai S: *Cellular and molecular immunology*, ed 7, Philadelphia, 2012, Saunders.
3. Frati F, Incorvaia C, Lombardi C, et al: Allergen immunotherapy: 100 years, but it does not look like, *Eur Ann Allergy Clin Immunol* 44(3):99, 2012.
4. Mota AN, Turrini RN: Perioperative latex hypersensitivity reactions: an integrative literature review, *Rev Lat Am Enfermagem* 20(2):411, 2012.
5. Wade J: Care of the type 1 latex allergy patient, *Aust Nurs J* 19(9):30, 2012.
6. American Academy of Allergy, Asthma, and Immunology: Latex allergies: tips to remember. Retrieved from *www.aaaai.org/conditions-and-treatments/Library/At-a-Glance/Latex-Allergy.aspx*.
7. Multiple chemical sensitivity. Retrieved from *www.webmd.com/allergies/multiple-chemical-sensitivity*.
8. National Institute of Environmental Health Sciences: Allergies/multiple chemical sensitivity. Retrieved from *www.niehs.nih.gov/research/resources/library/consumer/conditions*.
9. National Institute of Diabetes and Digestive and Kidney Diseases: Autoimmunity and viral etiology of type 1 diabetes. Retrieved from *www2.niddk.nih.gov/Research/ScientificAreas/Diabetes/Type1Diabetes*.
10. HLA nomenclature. Retrieved from *www.hla.alleles.org/alleles/index.html*.
11. Lennerling A, Forsberg A: Donors self-reported experiences of live kidney donation: a prospective study, *J Ren Care* 38(4):207, 2012.
12. United Network of Organ Sharing (UNOS). Retrieved from *www.unos.org*.
13. Uniform Anatomical Gift Act. Retrieved from *http://uniformlaws.org/ActSummary.aspx?title=Anatomical%20Gift%20Act%20 (2006)*.
14. Engels EA, Pfeiffer RM, Fraumeni JF, et al: Spectrum of cancer risk among US solid organ transplant recipients, *JAMA* 306:1891, 2011.
15. Schroeder KS: Pharmacology of immunosuppressive medications in solid organ transplantation. In Lovasik D: Transplant, *Crit Care Nurs Clin North Am* 23:405, 2011.
16. Blazar BR, Murphy WJ, Abedi M: Advances in graft-versus-host disease biology and therapy, *Nat Rev Immunol* 12(6):443, 2012.

RESOURCE

National Institute of Allergy and Infectious Diseases (NIAID)
www.niaid.nih.gov

15

Infection and Human Immunodeficiency Virus Infection

Jeffrey Kwong and Lucy Bradley-Springer

evolve WEBSITE

http://evolve.elsevier.com/Lewis/medsurg
- NCLEX Review Questions
- Key Points
- Pre-Test
- Answer Guidelines for Case Study on p. 244
- Rationales for Bridge to NCLEX Examination Questions
- Case Study
  - Patient With Human Immunodeficiency Virus (HIV) Infection and Acquired Immunodeficiency Syndrome (AIDS)
- Concept Map Creator

- Glossary
- Content Updates

eTables
- eTable 15-1: Centers for Disease Control and Prevention (CDC) Guidelines for Isolation Precautions
- eTable 15-2: Treatment of Common Opportunistic Diseases Associated With HIV Infection
- eTable 15-3: Drug Therapy: Side Effects of Antiretroviral Agents Used in Human Immunodeficiency Virus (HIV) Infection

- eTable 15-4: Patient Teaching Guide: Proper Use and Placement of Male Condom
- eTable 15-5: Patient Teaching Guide: Proper Use and Placement of Female Condom
- eTable 15-6: Patient Teaching Guide: Proper Use of Drug-Using Equipment
- eTable 15-7: Nursing Interventions in HIV Infection

LEARNING OUTCOMES

1. Evaluate the impact of emerging and reemerging infections on health care.
2. Identify ways to decrease the development of resistance to antibiotics.
3. Explain the ways human immunodeficiency virus (HIV) is transmitted and the factors that affect transmission.
4. Describe the pathophysiology of HIV infection.
5. Chart the spectrum of untreated HIV infection.
6. Identify the diagnostic criteria for acquired immunodeficiency syndrome (AIDS).
7. Describe methods used to test for HIV infection.
8. Discuss the collaborative management of HIV infection.
9. Summarize the characteristics of opportunistic diseases associated with AIDS.
10. Describe the potential complications associated with long-term treatment of HIV infection.
11. Compare and contrast HIV prevention methods.
12. Describe the nursing management of HIV-infected patients and HIV-at-risk patients.

KEY TERMS

acquired immunodeficiency syndrome (AIDS), p. 234
antiretroviral therapy (ART), p. 237
emerging infection, p. 228

human immunodeficiency virus (HIV), p. 231
integrase, p. 232
opportunistic diseases, p. 233

postexposure prophylaxis (PEP), p. 241
protease, p. 232
retroviruses, p. 232
reverse transcriptase, p. 232

seroconversion, p. 234
viral load, p. 234
viremia, p. 232
window period, p. 235

This chapter presents a brief overview of infections (both emerging and health care–associated infections). In addition, this chapter provides a comprehensive discussion of human immunodeficiency (HIV) infection focusing on transmission, pathophysiology, collaborative care, and nursing management.

INFECTIONS

Infections, such as lower respiratory tract infections, malaria, HIV, and tuberculosis (TB), are responsible for a significant number of deaths worldwide.[1] Infection occurs when a *pathogen* (a microorganism that causes disease) invades the body, begins to multiply, and produces disease, usually causing harm to the host. The signs and symptoms of infection are a result of specific pathogen activity, which triggers inflammation and other immune responses.[2]

Infections can be divided into localized, disseminated, and systemic disease. A *localized* infection is limited to a small area. A *disseminated* infection has spread to areas of the body beyond the initial site of infection. *Systemic* infections have spread extensively throughout the body, often via the blood.

Reviewed by Danette Y. Wall, ACRN, MSN, MBA/HCM, ISO9001 Lead Auditor, Regional Nurse, Department of Veterans Affairs–Veterans Health Administration, Tampa, Florida.

TYPES OF PATHOGENS

The many different kinds of pathogens can be classified into several groups, including bacteria, viruses, fungi, protozoa, and prions.[3] *Bacteria* are one-celled organisms that are common throughout nature. Many bacteria are normal flora. They live harmoniously in or on the human body without causing disease under normal circumstances. Normal flora protect the human body by preventing the overgrowth of other microorganisms. For example, *Escherichia coli* is a bacteria that is part of the normal flora in the large intestine.

Bacteria cause disease in two ways: by entering the body and growing inside human cells (e.g., TB) or by secreting toxins that damage cells (e.g., *Staphylococcus aureus*). Bacteria are divided into categories based on the shape of their cells. *Cocci*, such as streptococci and staphylococci, are round. *Bacilli* are rod shaped

and include tetanus and TB. *Curved rods* include *Vibrio* bacteria, one of which causes cholera. *Spirochetes* are spiral shaped and include the organisms that cause leprosy and syphilis. Table 15-1 lists common pathogenic bacteria and the diseases that they cause.

Viruses, unlike bacteria, do not have a cellular structure. They are simple infectious particles that consist of a small amount of genetic material (either ribonucleic acid [RNA] or deoxyribonucleic acid [DNA]) and a protein envelope. Viruses can reproduce only after releasing their genetic material into the cell of another living organism. Examples of diseases caused by viruses are shown in Table 15-2.

Fungi are organisms similar to plants, but they lack chlorophyll. *Mycosis* is any disease caused by a fungus. Pathogenic fungi cause infections that are usually localized but can become disseminated in an immunocompromised person. Tinea pedis

TABLE 15-1 DISEASE-CAUSING BACTERIA

Bacteria	Diseases Caused
Clostridia	
• *Clostridium botulinum*	Food poisoning with progressive muscle paralysis
• *Clostridium tetani*	Tetanus (lockjaw)
Corynebacterium diphtheriae	Diphtheria
Escherichia coli	Urinary tract infections, peritonitis, hemolytic-uremic syndrome
Haemophilus	
• *Haemophilus influenzae*	Nasopharyngitis, meningitis, pneumonia
• *Haemophilus pertussis*	Pertussis (whooping cough)
Helicobacter pylori	Peptic ulcers, gastritis
Klebsiella-Enterobacter organisms	Urinary tract infections, peritonitis, pneumonia
Legionella pneumophila	Pneumonia (Legionnaires' disease)
Mycobacteria	
• *Mycobacterium leprae*	Hansen's disease (leprosy)
• *Mycobacterium tuberculosis*	Tuberculosis
Neisseriae	
• *Neisseria gonorrhoeae*	Gonorrhea, pelvic inflammatory disease
• *Neisseria meningitidis*	Meningococcemia, meningitis
Proteus species	Urinary tract infections, peritonitis
Pseudomonas aeruginosa	Urinary tract infections, meningitis
Salmonella	
• *Salmonella typhi*	Typhoid fever
• Other *Salmonella* organisms	Food poisoning, gastroenteritis
Shigella	Shigellosis; diarrhea, abdominal pain, and fever (dysentery)
Staphylococcus aureus	Skin infections, pneumonia, urinary tract infections, acute osteomyelitis, toxic shock syndrome
Streptococci	
• *Streptococcus faecalis*	Genitourinary infection, infection of surgical wounds
• *Streptococcus pneumoniae*	Pneumococcal pneumonia
• *Streptococcus pyogenes* (group A β-hemolytic streptococci)	Pharyngitis, scarlet fever, rheumatic fever, acute glomerulonephritis, erysipelas, pneumonia
• *S. pyogenes* (group B β-hemolytic streptococci)	Urinary tract infections
• *Streptococcus viridans*	Bacterial endocarditis
Treponema pallidum	Syphilis

TABLE 15-2 DISEASE-CAUSING VIRUSES

Virus	Diseases Caused
Adenoviruses	Upper respiratory tract infection, pneumonia
Arbovirus	Syndrome of fever, malaise, headache, myalgia; aseptic meningitis; encephalitis
Coronavirus	Upper respiratory tract infection
Coxsackieviruses A and B	Upper respiratory tract infection, gastroenteritis, acute myocarditis, aseptic meningitis
Echoviruses	Upper respiratory tract infection, gastroenteritis, aseptic meningitis
Hepatitis A, B, C	Viral hepatitis
Herpesviruses	
• Cytomegalovirus (CMV)	Gastroenteritis; pneumonia and retinal damage in immunosuppressed individuals, infectious mononucleosis–like syndrome
• Epstein-Barr	Mononucleosis, Burkitt's lymphoma (possibly)
• Herpes simplex type 1	Herpes labialis ("fever blisters"), genital herpes infection
• Herpes simplex type 2	Genital herpes infection
• Varicella-zoster	Chickenpox, shingles
Human immunodeficiency virus (HIV)	HIV infection, AIDS
Influenza A and B	Upper respiratory tract infection, H1N1 (swine) flu, avian (bird) flu
Mumps	Parotitis, orchitis in postpubertal males
Papillomavirus	Warts
Parainfluenza 1-4	Upper respiratory tract infection
Parvovirus	Gastroenteritis
Poliovirus	Poliomyelitis
Pox viruses	Smallpox
Reoviruses 1, 2, 3	Upper respiratory tract infection
Respiratory syncytial virus	Gastroenteritis, respiratory tract infection
Rhabdovirus	Rabies
Rhinovirus	Upper respiratory tract infection, pneumonia
Rotaviruses	Gastroenteritis
Rubella	German measles
Rubeola	Measles
West Nile virus	Flulike symptoms, meningitis, encephalitis

TABLE 15-3   DISEASE-CAUSING FUNGI

Fungi	Diseases Caused	Organs Affected
Aspergillus fumigatus	Aspergillosis	Lungs*
	Otomycosis	Ears
Blastomyces dermatitidis	Blastomycosis	Lungs, various organs
Candida albicans	Candidiasis	Intestines
	Vaginitis	Vagina
	Thrush	Skin,† mouth
Coccidioides immitis	Coccidioidomycosis	Lungs*
Pneumocystis jiroveci	Pneumocystis pneumonia (PCP)	Lungs*
Sporothrix schenckii	Sporotrichosis	Skin, lymph vessels
Trichophyton	Tinea pedis	Skin†
Microsporum	Tinea capitis	Skin†
Epidermophyton	Tinea corporis	Skin†

*See Table 28-14: Fungal Infections of the Lung.
†See Table 24-6: Common Fungal Infections of the Skin.

TABLE 15-4   EMERGING INFECTIONS

Microorganism	Related Disease
Bacteria	
Borrelia burgdorferi	Lyme disease
Campylobacter jejuni	Diarrhea
Escherichia coli O157:H7	Hemorrhagic colitis, hemolytic-uremic syndrome
Helicobacter pylori	Peptic ulcer disease
Legionella pneumophila	Pneumonia (Legionnaires' disease)
Vibrio cholerae O139	New strain associated with epidemic cholera
Virus	
Ebola virus	Ebola hemorrhagic fever
H1N1	H1N1 (swine) flu
Hantavirus	Hemorrhagic fever associated with severe pulmonary syndrome
Hepatitis C virus	Parenterally transmitted hepatitis
Hepatitis E virus	Enterically transmitted hepatitis
Human immunodeficiency virus (HIV)	HIV infection and AIDS
Human herpesvirus 6 (HHV-6)	Roseola subitum
Human herpesvirus 8 (HHV-8)	Associated with Kaposi sarcoma in immunosuppressed patients, including people with HIV infection
West Nile virus	West Nile fever
Parasite	
Cryptosporidium parvum	Acute and chronic diarrhea

(athlete's foot) and tinea corporis (ringworm) are two common mycotic infections. Some fungi are normal flora in the body, but when overgrowth occurs, disease can result. Overgrowth of *Candida albicans,* for example, can cause candidiasis in the mouth (thrush), esophagus, intestines, and vagina. Other fungi and their respective mycotic infections are listed in Table 15-3.

Protozoa are single-cell, animal-like microorganisms. Protozoa normally live in soil and bodies of water. When introduced into the human body, they can cause infection. Amebic dysentery and giardiasis are caused by protozoal parasites. Malaria is caused by a sporozoa called *Plasmodium malariae.*

Prions are infectious particles that contain abnormally shaped proteins. Not all prions cause disease, but those that do typically affect the nervous system. They can cause a group of illnesses called transmissible spongiform encephalopathies (TSEs). Some of the more common TSEs are Creutzfeldt-Jakob disease and bovine spongiform encephalopathy in cattle (also known as mad cow disease).[4]

EMERGING INFECTIONS

An **emerging infection** is an infectious disease that has recently increased in incidence or that threatens to increase in the immediate future. Examples of emerging infections are described in Table 15-4. Emerging infectious diseases can originate from unknown sources or from contact with animals, changes in known diseases, or biologic warfare. For example, severe acute respiratory syndrome (SARS) and the West Nile virus come from animal sources. Others emerged when a previously treatable organism (e.g., *S. aureus*) developed resistance to antibiotics.

The battle against infection is not new, but modern technologies have changed the rules of the game. Global travel, population density, encroachment into new environments, misuse of antibiotics, and bioterrorism have increased the risk for widespread distribution of emerging infections.[5]

Not too long ago many believed that science had conquered infectious disease. However, newly recognized infectious diseases have emerged in recent decades. These include HIV, Lyme disease, hepatitis C, SARS, Ebola virus, and influenza A (H1N1)

virus. Some diseases once thought to be under control, such as TB, measles, and pertussis, have reemerged.[6]

Studies in *zoonosis* (the science of transmission of diseases from animals to humans) have shown that many known infectious diseases come from animal and insect vectors. The SARS outbreak in China in 2003, for instance, was linked to the civet cat, a small carnivorous mammal found throughout much of Asia and Africa. (SARS is discussed in Chapter 68.)

West Nile virus is carried and transmitted by mosquitoes. Mosquitoes acquire the virus as they draw blood from infected animals and people. The virus does not cause illness in the mosquito, but can be transferred to uninfected animals and humans as the mosquito continues to feed. Bird deaths are an early warning sign of a West Nile virus outbreak, which can spread quickly if action is not taken in a timely manner. (West Nile virus is discussed in Chapter 57.)

Influenza viruses are examples of how disease can spread between animals and humans. Variants of influenza A viruses were responsible for influenza epidemics. These include the 2009 influenza A (H1N1) outbreak that was traced back to pigs, hence the name *swine flu.* In 1997 and 2003 outbreaks of the influenza A (H5N1) strain of avian flu resulted from transmission of influenza virus from chickens to humans.[7]

Ebola virus has presented an ongoing challenge to public health since it was first seen in 1976. Ebola virus causes severe hemorrhagic fever and is usually lethal. Therapeutic and preventive measures are extremely limited. The natural reservoir and path of transmission are unknown, which makes it impossible to effectively combat Ebola virus and the disease it causes.[8]

Reemerging Infections

Vaccines and proper medications have led to the near eradication of some infections (e.g., smallpox and polio), but infective

TABLE 15-5   REEMERGING INFECTIONS

Microorganism	Infection	Description
Bacteria		
Corynebacterium diphtheriae	Diphtheria	Localized infection of mucous membranes or skin.
Bordetella pertussis	Pertussis	Acute, highly contagious respiratory disease characterized by loud whooping inspiration. Also known as whooping cough.
Yersinia pestis	Plague	*Bubonic:* swollen glands, fever, chills, headache, and extreme exhaustion. *Pneumonic:* overwhelming pneumonia with high fever, cough, bloody sputum, and chills.
Mycobacterium tuberculosis	Tuberculosis	Chronic infection transmitted by inhalation of infected droplets (see Chapter 28).
Virus		
Dengue viruses (flaviviruses)	Dengue fever	Acute infection transmitted by mosquitoes and occurring mainly in tropical and subtropical regions.
Parasite		
Giardia	Giardiasis	Diarrheal illness that usually originates in water contaminated with fecal matter. Also known as traveler's diarrhea.

TABLE 15-6   ANTIBIOTIC-RESISTANT ORGANISMS AND TREATMENT

Bacteria	Resistant To	Preferred Treatment
Staphylococcus aureus	methicillin*	vancomycin (Vancocin)
Staphylococcus epidermidis	methicillin*	vancomycin
Enterococcus faecalis	vancomycin streptomycin gentamicin (Garamycin)	penicillin G or ampicillin
Enterococcus faecium	vancomycin streptomycin gentamicin	penicillin G or ampicillin
Streptococcus pneumoniae	penicillin G	ceftriaxone (Rocephin) cefotaxime (Claforan)
Klebsiella pneumoniae	Third-generation cephalosporins (e.g., ceftazidime [Ceptaz, Fortaz])	imipenem and cilastatin (Primaxin) meropenem (Merrem IV)

*This drug is no longer available in the United States.

inactivate the drugs. Drug target sites are then altered so that the antibiotic cannot bind to or enter the bacteria. If the drug cannot enter the cell, it cannot kill the bacteria. Table 15-6 describes the most common antibiotic-resistant bacteria.

Methicillin-resistant *S. aureus* (MRSA), vancomycin-resistant enterococci (VRE), and penicillin-resistant *Streptococcus pneumoniae* are examples of emerging strains of antibiotic-resistant organisms. These drug-resistant bacteria were initially seen primarily in health care settings, but are becoming more prevalent in the community. For example, MRSA, a form of *S. aureus* that does not respond to methicillin- or penicillin-based therapies, was initially considered a health care–associated infection (HA-MRSA). However, over the past decade a variant strain of MRSA that is primarily acquired in the community (community-acquired MRSA [CA-MRSA]) has emerged.[11] This strain of MRSA is more *virulent* (able to cause disease or infection) compared with HA-MRSA. CA-MRSA has been known to cause rapidly forming skin infections and systemic diseases, including pneumonia and sepsis. Rates of CA-MRSA infections appear to be on the rise. Conversely, there has been a reduction in HA-MRSA with the implementation of strict hygiene measures in health care settings.

VRE is another antibiotic-resistant bacteria that has become a concern for patients and health care workers. VRE is more virulent than MRSA and can remain viable on environmental surfaces for weeks.[12] Although antibiotic-resistant bacteria can infect anyone, patients who are hospitalized and those with immunosuppression are more likely to be exposed to these bacteria and to develop infection.

Health care providers have contributed to the development of drug-resistant organisms by (1) administering antibiotics for viral infections, (2) succumbing to pressures from patients to prescribe unnecessary antibiotic therapy, (3) using inadequate drug regimens to treat infections, or (4) using broad-spectrum or combination agents for infections that should be treated with first-line medications. Patients can also contribute to resistance development by (1) skipping doses, (2) not taking antibiotics for the full duration of prescribed therapy, or (3) saving unused antibiotics "in case I need them later." In addition, limited

agents can reemerge if conditions are right. Table 15-5 presents some diseases that have shown resurgence in recent decades.

For example, the incidence of TB began to steadily decrease in the mid-1950s, but in 1984 TB cases began to rise. The growing HIV epidemic in the 1970s and 1980s contributed to the increase in TB as people with depressed immune systems developed new cases of TB or reactivated dormant TB infections. The emergence of multidrug-resistant forms of TB (MDR-TB) also contributed to the increase. Local and federal governments took measures to address the problem, and the rates of TB are now slowly declining again.[9] (TB is discussed in Chapter 28.)

International travel has created a new obstacle for the local eradication of diseases. For example, measles is no longer considered endemic in the United States, but it remains a leading cause of morbidity in developing countries, and outbreaks have occurred in the United States, typically in areas with low vaccination rates. Some measles cases in the United States have been found in people who have recently traveled to measles-endemic areas.[10]

Antibiotic-Resistant Organisms

Resistance occurs when pathogenic organisms change in ways that decrease the ability of a drug (or a family of drugs) to treat disease.[3] Microorganisms can become resistant to classic treatments (e.g., penicillin), as well as to newer antibiotics and antiviral agents. Microorganisms are highly adaptable. They have evolved genetic and biochemical mechanisms to defend against antimicrobial actions. Genetic mechanisms include mutation and acquisition of new DNA or RNA. Biochemically, bacteria can resist antibiotics by producing enzymes that destroy or

TABLE 15-7 PATIENT & CAREGIVER TEACHING GUIDE

Decrease Risk for Antibiotic-Resistant Infection

Include the following instructions when teaching patients or their caregivers how to decrease the risk for antibiotic-resistant infection.

1. Do Not Take Antibiotics to Prevent Illness (unless prescribed)
Doing this increases your risk for developing resistant infection. Exceptions include taking antibiotics as prescribed before certain surgeries and dental work or in the presence of immune dysfunction.

2. Wash Your Hands Frequently
Hand washing is the single most important thing you can do to prevent infection.

3. Follow Directions When Taking Antibiotics
Not taking your antibiotic as prescribed or skipping doses can allow antibiotic-resistant bacteria to develop.

4. Do Not Request an Antibiotic for Flu or Colds
If your health care provider says that you do not need an antibiotic, chances are you do not. Antibiotics are effective against bacterial infections but not viruses, which cause colds and flu.

5. Finish Your Antibiotic
Do not stop taking your antibiotic when you feel better. If you stop taking your antibiotic early, the hardiest bacteria survive and multiply. Eventually you could develop an infection resistant to many antibiotics. You should never have leftover antibiotics.

6. Do Not Take Leftover Antibiotics
Do not save unfinished antibiotics for later use or borrow leftover drugs from family or friends. This is dangerous because (1) the leftover antibiotic may not be appropriate for you, (2) your illness may not be a bacterial infection, (3) old antibiotics can lose their effectiveness and in some cases can even be fatal, and (4) there will not be enough doses in a leftover bottle to provide full treatment.

TABLE 15-8 OSHA REQUIREMENTS FOR PERSONAL PROTECTIVE EQUIPMENT

The following equipment is used to minimize exposure to blood-borne pathogens.

Equipment	Indications for Use
Gloves	• Must be used when the employee can reasonably anticipate having contact with blood or other potentially infectious materials, when performing vascular access procedures, and when handling or touching contaminated items or surfaces. • Gloves must be replaced if torn, punctured, or contaminated or their ability to function as a barrier is compromised.
Clothing (gowns, aprons, caps, boots)	• Must be used when occupational exposure is anticipated. • The type and characteristics depend on the task and degree of exposure anticipated.
Face protection (mask and glasses with solid side shields or a chin-length face shield)	• Must be used when splashes, sprays, spatters, or droplets of blood or other potentially infectious materials pose a hazard to the eyes, nose, or mouth.

Source: Occupational Safety and Health Administration: Bloodborne pathogens and needlestick prevention. Retrieved from *www.osha.gov/SLTC/bloodbornepathogens*. NOTE: Employers must provide, make accessible, and require the use of personal protective equipment (PPE) at no cost to the employee. PPE also must be provided in appropriate sizes. Hypoallergenic gloves or similar alternatives must be made available to employees who have an allergic sensitivity to gloves.
OSHA, Occupational Safety and Health Administration.

resources and access to medications make it difficult for some patients to get adequate treatment for infections. Teaching patients and their families the proper use of antibiotics (Table 15-7) is crucial to treatment success and prevention of drug-resistant pathogens. The Centers for Disease Control and Prevention (CDC), the Infectious Diseases Society of America, and many health care organizations have been campaigning for greater vigilance in minimizing the misuse of antibiotics in reaction to this growing concern.

HEALTH CARE–ASSOCIATED INFECTIONS

Health care–associated infections (HAIs), formerly referred to as *nosocomial infections,* are infections that are acquired as a result of exposure to a microorganism in a health care setting. Approximately 2 million HAIs and 99,000 HAI-associated deaths occur in the United States each year. Antibiotic-resistant organisms cause half of these infections.[13] Up to 10% of hospitalized patients will acquire an HAI. Surgical and immunocompromised patients are at highest risk. Any organism can cause HAIs, but certain bacteria, including *E. coli, S. aureus, Enterobacter aerogenes,* and various types of streptococci, are the more common culprits. Some bacteria that do not normally cause disease can cause infections in high-risk patients as a result of illness or treatment of illness.[14]

Approximately one third of HAIs are preventable. Health care providers often transmit HAIs from patient to patient through direct contact. Hand washing (or using an alcohol-based hand sanitizer) between patients and procedures and the appropriate use of protective equipment such as gloves remain the first lines of defense to prevent the spread of HAIs. Isolated infections can also be caused when bacteria that normally stay in one area of the body are introduced into another area. Therefore care must be taken to change gloves and wash hands when moving from one task to another, even when working with the same patient.[15] The Occupational Safety and Health Administration (OSHA) and the CDC recommend that precautions be followed to control the spread of disease, especially of antibiotic-resistant organisms (Table 15-8).

GERONTOLOGIC CONSIDERATIONS

INFECTIONS IN OLDER ADULTS
For older adults the rate of HAIs is two or three times higher than for younger patients.[13,16] Individuals in long-term care facilities are at special risk for HAI. Age-related changes (e.g., impaired immune function, co-morbidities such as diabetes, physical disabilities) can contribute to higher infection rates.[17]

Infections common in older adults include pneumonia, urinary tract infections, skin infections, and TB. Urinary tract infections are more common in older adults who reside in long-term care facilities. Patients with indwelling catheters are at particular risk. Infections in older adults often have atypical manifestations, such as cognitive and behavioral changes, before the emergence of fever, pain, or alterations in laboratory values.

Suspicion of disease should typically begin if a patient demonstrates changes in the ability to perform daily activities or in cognitive function. In addition, underlying diseases, increased frequency of drug reactions, and institutionalization can all complicate the management of the older adult with infection.

> **SAFETY ALERT**
> • Do not rely on the presence of fever to indicate infection in older adults because many have lower core body temperatures and decreased immune responses.

INFECTION PREVENTION AND CONTROL

Occupational Safety and Health Administration (OSHA) Guidelines

OSHA is a federal agency that protects workers from injury and illness in places of employment and supports activities that minimize or eliminate exposure to infectious materials in the workplace. OSHA mandates that any employer whose employees could be exposed to potentially infectious materials implement standard policies and procedures for protection of those employees. Employees must be provided with appropriate personal protective equipment (PPE) and safety equipment. These include gloves, gowns, facial protection, and disposal systems for sharps (see Table 15-8). Appropriate PPE varies depending on the situation, and as a nurse, you need to use sound judgment when deciding when and how to use protective equipment.

Infection Precautions

If a patient is admitted with or develops an infection that is considered a risk to others, infection precautions may be needed. The CDC has established guidelines with two levels of precautions: (1) *standard precautions*, designed for the care of all patients in hospitals and health care facilities; and (2) *transmission-based precautions,* designed for specific diseases.[15] The purpose of these precautions is to prevent the transmission of organisms from patients to health care providers, from health care providers to patients, from patients to other patients, and from providers and patients to people outside of the hospital. (CDC guidelines for isolation precautions are summarized in eTable 15-1 on the website for this chapter.)

The *standard precautions* system applies to (1) blood; (2) all body fluids, secretions, and excretions; (3) nonintact skin; and (4) mucous membranes. Standard precautions are designed to reduce the risk of transmission of microorganisms in hospitals. Standard precautions should be applied to all patients regardless of diagnosis or presumed infection status. The CDC's standard precautions incorporate all of the OSHA blood-borne pathogens standard requirements.

Transmission-based precautions are used for patients known to be or suspected of being infected with highly transmissible or epidemiologically important pathogens that require additional precautions to interrupt transmission and prevent infection. Transmission-based precautions include airborne precautions, droplet precautions, and contact precautions. *Airborne precautions* are used if the organism can cause infection over long distances when suspended in the air (e.g., TB, rubeola). *Droplet precautions* are used to minimize contact with pathogens that are spread through the air at close contact and that affect the respiratory system or mucous membranes (e.g., influenza, pertussis). *Contact precautions* are used to minimize the spread of pathogens that are acquired from direct or indirect contact, especially multidrug-resistant organisms (e.g., MRSA, VRE). Transmission-based precautions may be combined for diseases that have multiple routes of transmission. Whether used alone or in combination, transmission-based precautions should always be used in conjunction with standard precautions.

HUMAN IMMUNODEFICIENCY VIRUS INFECTION

Human immunodeficiency virus (HIV) infection is caused by HIV, which is a retrovirus that causes immunosuppression. The viral infection causes the person to be susceptible to infections that would normally be controlled through immune responses. The term *HIV disease* is used interchangeably with HIV infection. With advances in treatment, HIV is managed as a chronic disease, since people are living longer.

Significance of Problem

HIV has caused a global pandemic and affected millions. In the past 30 years, important advances have been made in HIV prevention, testing, and treatment. In developed countries the result has been decreases in the number of HIV-related deaths, improved quality of life, and a significant decrease in the number of children born with HIV.[18]

More than 1 million people are currently living with HIV in the United States, with an estimated 50,000 new infections occurring annually. With the availability of effective treatment, people with HIV infection can live for a longer time, resulting in a dramatic drop in the number of deaths attributable to HIV.[19-21]

In North America HIV has been most prevalent among men who have sex with men. However, increasing numbers of new HIV infections are occurring in women, people of color, people who live in poverty, and adolescents. For the most part, HIV remains a disease of marginalized individuals: those who are disenfranchised by virtue of gender, race, sexual orientation, poverty, drug use, or lack of access to health care.[21,22]

Transmission of HIV

HIV can be transmitted as a result of contact with infected blood, semen, vaginal secretions, or breast milk. Transmission of HIV occurs through sexual intercourse with an infected partner; exposure to HIV-infected blood or blood products; and perinatal transmission during pregnancy, at delivery, or through breastfeeding.[19]

HIV-infected individuals can transmit HIV to others within a few days after becoming infected. The ability to transmit HIV continues for life. Transmission of HIV is subject to the same requirements as other microorganisms (i.e., a large enough amount of the virus must enter the body of a susceptible host).

Variables that influence whether infection will be established after an exposure include (1) duration and frequency of contact with the organism; (2) volume, virulence, and concentration of the organism; and (3) host immune status. The concentration of virus is an important variable. Large amounts of HIV can be found in the blood, and to a lesser extent in the semen, during the first 6 months of infection and again during the late stages of the disease (Fig. 15-1). Although unprotected sexual intercourse or blood exposure to an infected individual during these

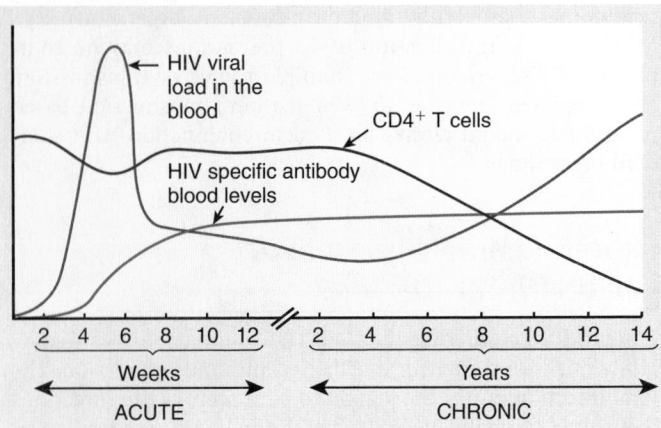

FIG. 15-1 Viral load in the blood in relationship to number of CD4+ T cells over the spectrum of untreated HIV infection.

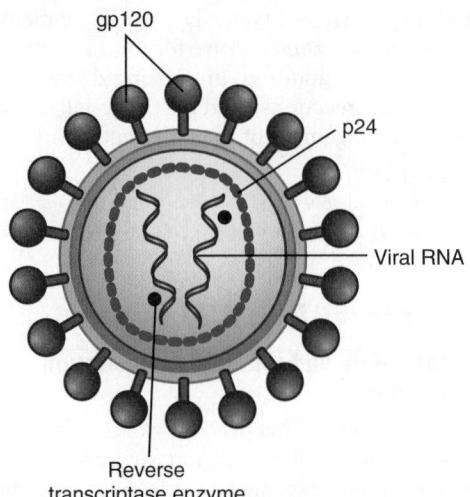

FIG. 15-2 HIV is surrounded by an envelope made up of proteins (including gp120) and contains a core of viral RNA and proteins.

periods is more risky, HIV can be transmitted during all phases of the disease.

HIV is not spread casually. The virus cannot be transmitted through hugging, dry kissing, shaking hands, sharing eating utensils, using toilet seats, or casual encounters in any setting.[19] It is not spread by tears, saliva, urine, emesis, sputum, feces, sweat, respiratory droplets, or enteric routes. Health care workers have a low risk of acquiring HIV at work, even after a needle-stick injury.[23]

Sexual Transmission. The most common mode of HIV transmission is unprotected sexual contact with an HIV-infected partner. Sexual activity involves contact with semen, vaginal secretions, and/or blood, all of which have lymphocytes that may contain HIV. During any form of sexual intercourse (anal, vaginal, or oral), the risk of infection is greater for the partner who receives the semen, although infection can also be transmitted to the inserting partner. This occurs because the receiver has prolonged contact with infected fluids, and it helps explain why it is easier to infect women than men during heterosexual intercourse. Sexual activities that cause trauma to local tissues can increase the risk of transmission. In addition, genital lesions from other sexually transmitted infections (e.g., herpes, syphilis) significantly increase the likelihood of transmission.

Contact With Blood and Blood Products. HIV can be transmitted during exposure to blood through drug-using equipment. Used equipment may be contaminated with HIV and other blood-borne organisms, and sharing that equipment can result in disease transmission.

In North America, transfusion of infected blood and blood products has caused only 1% of adult AIDS cases.[22] Routine screening of blood donors to identify at-risk individuals and testing donated blood for the presence of HIV have improved the safety of the blood supply. In countries that routinely test donated blood, HIV infection as a result of blood transfusions or hemophilia clotting factors is now unlikely.

Puncture wounds are the most common means of work-related HIV transmission. The risk of infection after a needle-stick exposure to HIV-infected blood is 0.3% to 0.4% (or 3 to 4 out of 1000).[23] The risk is higher if the exposure involves blood from a patient with a high level of circulating HIV, a deep puncture wound, a needle with a hollow bore and visible blood, a device used for venous or arterial access, or a patient who dies within 60 days. Splash exposures of blood on skin with an open

lesion present some risk, but it is much lower than from a puncture wound.

Perinatal Transmission. Perinatal transmission from an HIV-infected mother to her infant can occur during pregnancy, delivery, or breastfeeding. On average, 25% of infants born to women with untreated HIV infection are born with HIV. Fortunately, the risk of transmission can be reduced to less than 2% in settings where pregnant women are routinely tested for HIV infection and, if found to be infected, treated with antiretroviral therapy (ART).[24]

Pathophysiology

HIV is an RNA virus. RNA viruses are called **retroviruses** because they replicate in a "backward" manner (going from RNA to DNA). Like all viruses, HIV cannot replicate unless it is inside a living cell. HIV enters a cell when the gp120 "knobs" (Fig. 15-2) on the viral envelope bind to specific CD4 and chemokine receptor sites on the cell's surface (*fusion*) (Fig. 15-3). Chemokine receptors are proteins normally found in cell membranes that respond to chemokines outside the cell and trigger a response inside the cell. HIV uses the chemokine receptors CXCR4 and CCR5 as co-receptors (CD4 is the main receptor) to support binding and entry into the CD4+ T cell.[25]

Once bound, viral RNA enters the CD4+ T cell, where it is transcribed into a single strand of viral DNA with the assistance of **reverse transcriptase**, an enzyme made by retroviruses. This strand copies itself, becoming double-stranded viral DNA, which then enters the cell's nucleus and, using another enzyme called **integrase,** splices itself into the human genome, becoming a permanent part of the cell's genetic structure. This action has two consequences: (1) because all genetic material is replicated during cell division, all daughter cells are also infected and (2) viral DNA in the genome directs the cell to make new HIV. HIV production in the cell starts with long strands of HIV RNA. These are cut into appropriate lengths in the presence of the enzyme **protease** during the budding sequence.[25]

Initial infection with HIV results in **viremia** (large amounts of virus in the blood). This is followed within a few weeks by a prolonged period in which HIV levels in the blood remain low even without treatment (see Fig. 15-1). During this time, which may last for more than 10 years, clinical symptoms can be

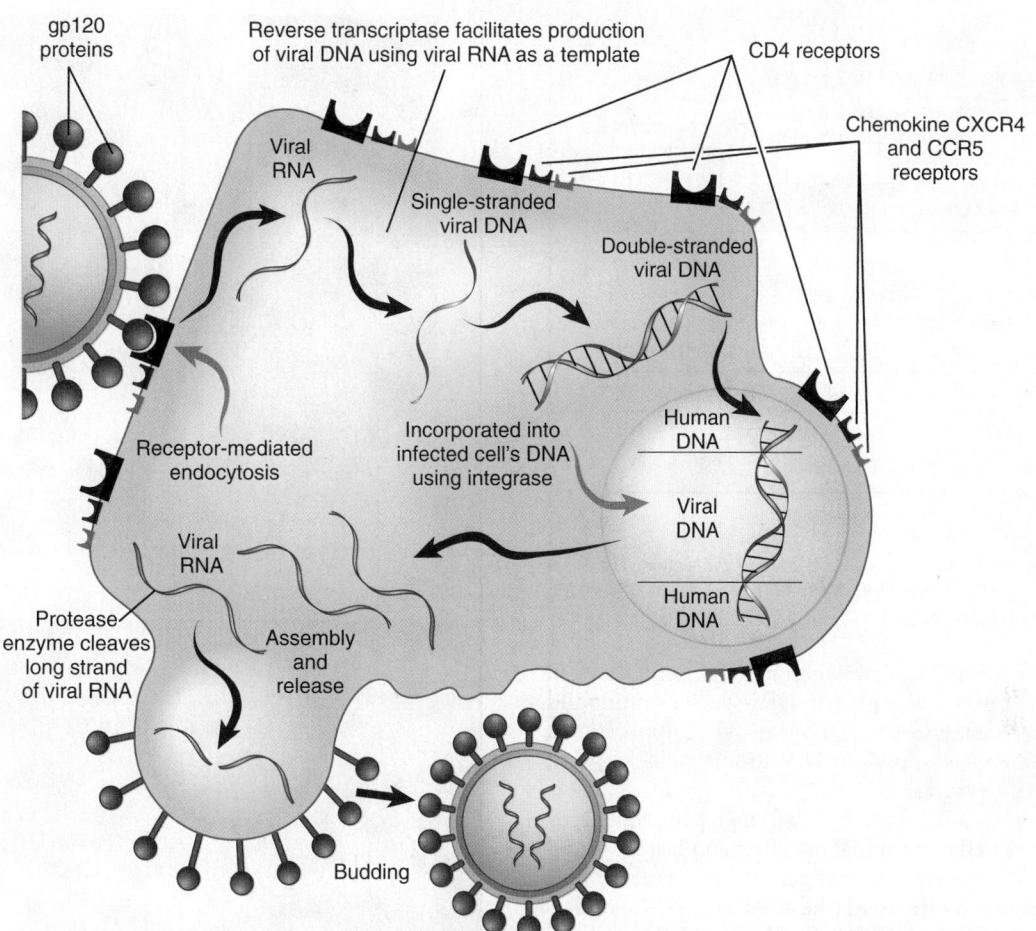

FIG. 15-3 HIV has gp120 glycoproteins that attach to CD4 and chemokine CXCR4 and CCR5 receptors on the surface of CD4⁺ T cells. Viral RNA then enters the cell, produces viral DNA in the presence of reverse transcriptase, and incorporates itself into the cellular genome in the presence of integrase, causing permanent cellular infection and the production of new virions. New viral RNA develops initially in long strands that are cut in the presence of protease and leave the cell through a budding process that ultimately contributes to cellular destruction.

limited. Even without symptoms, HIV replication occurs at a rapid and constant rate in the blood and lymph tissues. A major consequence of rapid replication is that errors can occur in the copying process, causing mutations that can contribute to resistance to ART and limit treatment options.

In the initial stages of HIV infection, B cells and T cells respond and function normally. B cells make HIV-specific antibodies that are effective in reducing viral loads in the blood. Activated T cells mount a cellular immune response to viruses trapped in the lymph nodes.[25]

HIV infects human cells with CD4 receptors on their surfaces, including lymphocytes, monocytes/macrophages, astrocytes, and oligodendrocytes. However, immune dysfunction in HIV infection is predominantly the result of damage to and destruction of CD4⁺ T cells (also known as T helper cells or CD4⁺ T lymphocytes). These cells are targeted because they have more CD4 receptors on their surfaces than the other CD4 receptor–bearing cells. CD4⁺ T cells play a key role in the immune system's ability to recognize and defend against pathogens.

Adults without immune dysfunction normally have 800 to 1200 CD4⁺ T cells per microliter (μL) of blood. The normal life span of a CD4⁺ T cell is about 100 days, but HIV-infected CD4⁺ T cells die after an average of only 2 days.

HIV destroys about 1 billion CD4⁺ T cells every day. The body can produce new CD4⁺ T cells to replace the destroyed cells for many years. However, eventually the ability of HIV to destroy CD4⁺ T cells exceeds the body's ability to replace the cells. The decline in the CD4⁺ T cell count impairs immune function. Generally, the immune system remains healthy with more than 500 CD4⁺ T cells/μL. Immune problems start to occur when the count drops below 500 CD4⁺ T cells/μL. Severe problems develop with fewer than 200 CD4⁺ T cells/μL. With HIV, a point is eventually reached where so many CD4⁺ T cells have been destroyed that not enough are left to regulate immune responses (see Fig. 15-1). This allows **opportunistic diseases** (infections and cancers that occur in immunosuppressed patients) to develop. Opportunistic diseases are the main cause of disease, disability, and death in patients with HIV infection.

Clinical Manifestations and Complications

The typical course of untreated HIV infection follows the pattern shown in Fig. 15-4. It is important to remember that (1) disease progression is highly individualized, (2) treatment can significantly alter this pattern, and (3) an individual's prognosis is unpredictable.

Acute Infection. A mononucleosis-like syndrome of fever, swollen lymph glands, sore throat, headache, malaise, nausea,

FIG. 15-4 Timeline for the spectrum of untreated HIV infection. The time-line represents the course of untreated illness from the time of infection to clinical manifestations of disease.

FIG. 15-5 Oral thrush involving hard and soft palate.

FIG. 15-6 Kaposi sarcoma (KS). The malignant vascular lesions of KS can appear anywhere on the skin surface or on internal organs. Lesions vary in size from pinpoint to large and may appear in a variety of shades.

muscle and joint pain, diarrhea, and/or a diffuse rash often accompanies **seroconversion** (when HIV-specific antibodies develop). Some people also develop neurologic complications, such as aseptic meningitis, peripheral neuropathy, facial palsy, or Guillain-Barré syndrome.

These symptoms, called *acute HIV infection,* generally occur within 2 to 4 weeks after the initial infection and last for 1 to 3 weeks, although some symptoms may persist for several months. During this time a high **viral load** (the amount of HIV circulating in the blood) is noted, and CD4$^+$ T cell counts fall temporarily but quickly return to baseline or near-baseline levels (see Fig. 15-1). Many people, including health care providers, mistake acute HIV symptoms for a bad case of the flu.[26]

Chronic HIV Infection

Asymptomatic Infection. The interval between untreated HIV infection and a diagnosis of AIDS is about 10 years. During this time, CD4$^+$ T cell counts remain above 500 cells/μL (normal or only slightly decreased), and the viral load in the blood is low. This phase has been referred to as *asymptomatic infection,* although fatigue, headache, low-grade fever, night sweats, *persistent generalized lymphadenopathy* (PGL), and other symptoms may be present.[27]

Because most of the symptoms during early infection are vague and nonspecific for HIV, people may not be aware that they are infected. During this time, infected people continue their usual activities, which may include high-risk sexual and drug-using behaviors. This is a public health problem because infected individuals can transmit HIV to others even though they have no symptoms. Personal health is also affected because people who do not know that they are infected have little reason to seek treatment and are less likely to make behavior changes that could improve the quality and length of their lives.

Symptomatic Infection. As the CD4$^+$ T cell count drops to 200 to 500 cells/μL and the viral load increases, HIV advances to a more active stage. Symptoms seen in earlier phases become worse, leading to persistent fever, frequent drenching night sweats, chronic diarrhea, recurrent headaches, and fatigue severe enough to interrupt normal routines. Other problems may include localized infections, lymphadenopathy, and nervous system manifestations.[27]

The most common infection associated with this phase of HIV infection is oropharyngeal candidiasis, or thrush (Fig. 15-5). *Candida* organisms rarely cause problems in healthy adults, but are more common in HIV-infected people. Other infections that can occur at this time include shingles (caused by the varicella-zoster virus); persistent vaginal candidal infections; outbreaks of oral or genital herpes; bacterial infections; and Kaposi sarcoma (KS), which is caused by human herpesvirus 8 (Fig. 15-6). *Oral hairy leukoplakia,* an Epstein-Barr virus infection that causes painless, white, raised lesions on the lateral aspect of the tongue (Fig. 15-7), is another indicator of disease progression.[28]

AIDS. A diagnosis of **acquired immunodeficiency syndrome (AIDS)** is made when an HIV-infected patient meets criteria established by the CDC.[29] These criteria occur when the immune system becomes severely compromised (Table 15-9). As the viral load increases, the absolute number and percentage of T cells decrease and the risk of developing opportunistic diseases increases.

Opportunistic diseases generally do not occur in the presence of a functioning immune system. Many infections, a variety of malignancies, wasting, and HIV-related dementia can occur in patients with immune impairment (Table 15-10).

FIG. 15-7 Oral hairy leukoplakia on the lateral aspect of the tongue.

TABLE 15-9   DIAGNOSTIC CRITERIA FOR AIDS

AIDS is diagnosed when an individual with HIV develops at least one of the following conditions:

1. CD4+ T cell count drops below 200 cells/μL.
2. One of the following opportunistic infections (OIs):
   - *Fungal*: candidiasis of bronchi, trachea, lungs, or esophagus; *Pneumocystis jiroveci* pneumonia (PCP); disseminated or extrapulmonary coccidioidomycosis; disseminated or extrapulmonary histoplasmosis
   - *Viral*: cytomegalovirus (CMV) disease other than liver, spleen, or nodes; CMV retinitis (with loss of vision); herpes simplex with chronic ulcer(s) or bronchitis, pneumonitis, or esophagitis; progressive multifocal leukoencephalopathy (PML); extrapulmonary cryptococcosis
   - *Protozoal*: toxoplasmosis of the brain, chronic intestinal isosporiasis, chronic intestinal cryptosporidiosis
   - *Bacterial: Mycobacterium tuberculosis* (any site); any disseminated or extrapulmonary mycobacteria, including *Mycobacterium avium* complex (MAC) or *Mycobacterium kansasii;* recurrent pneumonia; recurrent *Salmonella* septicemia
3. One of the following opportunistic cancers:
   - Invasive cervical cancer
   - Kaposi sarcoma (KS)
   - Burkitt's lymphoma
   - Immunoblastic lymphoma
   - Primary lymphoma of the brain
4. Wasting syndrome. *Wasting* is defined as a loss of 10% or more of ideal body mass.
5. AIDS dementia complex (ADC).

Modified from Centers for Disease Control and Prevention: 1993 Revised classification system for HIV infection and expanded surveillance case definition for AIDS among adolescents and adults, 1993. Retrieved from *www.cdc.gov/mmwr/ preview/mmwrhtml/rr5710a1.htm?s_cid=rr5710a1_e.*

Organisms that do not cause severe disease in people with functioning immune systems can cause debilitating, disseminated, and life-threatening infections during this stage. Several opportunistic diseases may occur at the same time, compounding the difficulties of diagnosis and treatment. Advances in HIV treatment have decreased the occurrence of opportunistic diseases.

Diagnostic Studies

Diagnosis of HIV Infection. Diagnosis of HIV infection is made by testing for HIV antibodies and/or antigen in the blood. HIV-antibody tests detect HIV-specific antibodies, but typically it takes several weeks after the infection before antibodies can

be detected on a screening test (see Fig. 15-1). This delay is known as the window period.

Standard antibody tests can be completed on blood or oral fluid specimens. They are sent to a laboratory, and results are reported back to the provider anywhere from a day to a week later. *Rapid* HIV-antibody tests are done in the office, and results can be shared with patients before they leave the office. They can also be done at home using a self-administered HIV test kit. A positive antibody test should be followed by a confirming test (usually the Western blot) (Table 15-11).

Laboratory Studies in HIV Infection. The progression of HIV infection is monitored by two important laboratory assessments: CD4+ T cell counts and viral load. CD4+ T cell counts provide a marker of immune function. As the disease progresses, the number of CD4+ T cells usually decreases (see Fig. 15-1). The normal range for CD4+ T cells is 800 to 1200 cells/μL. Laboratory tests that measure viral levels provide an assessment of disease progression. The lower the viral load, the less active the disease. In HIV, viral loads are reported as real numbers (e.g., 1260 copies/μL) or as undetectable. "Undetectable" indicates that the viral load is lower than the test is able to report. "Undetectable" does *not* mean that the virus has been eliminated from the body or that the individual can no longer transmit HIV to others.

Abnormal blood test results are common in HIV infection and may be caused by HIV, opportunistic diseases, or complications of therapy. Decreased white blood cell (WBC) counts, especially below-normal numbers of lymphocytes (lymphopenia) and neutrophils (neutropenia), are often seen. Low platelet counts (thrombocytopenia) may be caused by HIV, antiplatelet antibodies, or drug therapy. Anemia is associated with the chronic disease process and with adverse effects of ART. Altered liver function, caused by HIV infection, drug therapy, or co-infection with a hepatitis virus, is common. Early identification of co-infection with hepatitis B virus (HBV) or hepatitis C virus (HCV) is extremely important because these infections have a more serious course in patients with HIV, may ultimately limit options for ART, and can cause liver-related morbidity and mortality.[27]

Two types of resistance tests can determine if a patient's HIV is resistant to drugs used for ART. The *genotype assay* detects drug-resistant viral mutations that are present in reverse transcriptase and protease genes. The *phenotype assay* measures the growth of HIV in various concentrations of antiretroviral drugs (much like bacteria-antibiotic sensitivity tests). These assays help determine new drug combinations for patients who are not responding to therapy.

Collaborative Care

Collaborative care of the HIV-infected patient focuses on (1) monitoring HIV disease progression and immune function, (2) initiating and monitoring ART, (3) preventing the development of opportunistic diseases, (4) detecting and treating opportunistic diseases, (5) managing symptoms, (6) preventing or decreasing complications of treatment, and (7) preventing further transmission of HIV. To accomplish these objectives, ongoing assessment, clinician-patient interactions, and patient teaching and support are required.

The initial patient visit provides an opportunity to gather baseline data and to start establishing rapport. A complete history and physical examination, including an immunization history and psychosocial and dietary evaluations, should be

TABLE 15-10 OPPORTUNISTIC DISEASES ASSOCIATED WITH HIV INFECTION*

Organism or Disease	Clinical Manifestations
Candida albicans	Thrush (see Fig. 15-5), esophagitis, vaginitis; whitish yellow patches in mouth, esophagus, GI tract, vagina
Coccidioides immitis	Pneumonia and fever, weight loss, cough
CNS lymphoma	Cognitive dysfunction, motor impairment, aphasia, seizures, personality changes, headache
Cryptococcus neoformans	Meningitis, cognitive impairment, motor dysfunction, fever, seizures, headache
Cryptosporidium muris	Gastroenteritis, watery diarrhea, abdominal pain, weight loss
Cytomegalovirus (CMV)	*Retinitis:* retinal lesions, blurred vision, loss of vision *Esophagitis, stomatitis:* difficulty swallowing; colitis or gastritis: bloody diarrhea, pain, weight loss *Pneumonitis:* respiratory symptoms *Neurologic disease:* CNS manifestations
Hepatitis B virus (HBV)	Jaundice, fatigue, abdominal pain, loss of appetite, nausea, vomiting, joint pain; 30% may have no signs or symptoms
Hepatitis C virus (HCV)	Jaundice, fatigue, abdominal pain, loss of appetite, nausea, vomiting, dark urine; 80% may have no signs or symptoms
Herpes simplex	*HSV-1 (type 1):* orolabial and mucocutaneous vesicular and ulcerative lesions; keratitis; visual disturbances; encephalitis; CNS manifestations *HSV-2 (type 2):* genital and perianal vesicular and ulcerative lesions
Histoplasma capsulatum	*Pneumonia:* fever, cough, weight loss *Meningitis:* CNS manifestations, disseminated disease

Organism or Disease	Clinical Manifestations
Influenza virus	Fever (usually high), headache, extreme tiredness, dry cough, sore throat, runny or stuffy nose, muscle aches; nausea, vomiting, and diarrhea can occur
JC papovavirus	Progressive multifocal leukoencephalopathy (PML), CNS manifestations, mental and motor declines
Kaposi sarcoma (KS) caused by human herpesvirus 8 (HHV-8)	Vascular lesions on the skin (see Fig. 15-6), mucous membranes, and viscera with wide range of presentation: firm, flat, raised, or nodular; pinpoint to several cm in size; hyperpigmented, multicentric; can cause lymphedema and disfigurement, particularly when confluent; usually not serious unless occurring in the respiratory or gastrointestinal system
Mycobacterium avium complex (MAC)	Gastroenteritis, watery diarrhea, weight loss
Mycobacterium tuberculosis (MTB, TB)	Respiratory and disseminated disease; productive cough, fever, night sweats, weight loss
Pneumocystis jiroveci pneumonia (PCP)	Pneumonia, nonproductive cough, hypoxemia, progressive shortness of breath, fever, night sweats, fatigue
Toxoplasma gondii	Encephalitis, cognitive dysfunction, motor impairment, fever, altered mental status, headache, seizures, sensory abnormalities
Varicella zoster virus (VZV)	*Shingles:* erythematous maculopapular rash along dermatomal planes, pain, pruritus *Ocular:* progressive outer retinal necrosis (PORN)

*Treatment of opportunistic diseases is presented in eTable 15-2 on the website for this chapter.

TABLE 15-11 HIV-ANTIBODY TESTS

1. A highly sensitive enzyme immunoassay (EIA) is done to detect serum antibodies that bind to HIV antigens on test plates. Blood samples that are negative on this test are reported as negative.
   - If the patient reports recent risky behaviors, encourage retesting at 3 wk, 6 wk, and 3 mo.
2. If the blood is EIA-antibody positive, repeat the test.
3. If the blood is repeatedly EIA-antibody positive, a more specific confirming test, such as the Western blot (WB) or immuno-fluorescence assay (IFA), is done.
4. Blood that is reactive in all of the first three steps is reported as HIV-antibody positive.
5. If the results are indeterminate, the following steps are taken:
   - If in-depth risk assessment reveals that the individual does not have a history of high-risk activities, reassure the patient that HIV infection is extremely unlikely and suggest retesting in 3 mo.
   - If in-depth risk assessment reveals that the individual does have a history of high-risk activities, consider tests that detect HIV antigen.

Rapid HIV-Antibody Testing

1. Rapid testing is strongly recommended by the Centers for Disease Control and Prevention. Results are highly accurate, and it can be done in a variety of settings (mobile health units, physicians' offices, or even in the privacy of an individual's home). Results are typically available within 20 min.
2. In-home use HIV test kits are available. Testing is done on an oral fluid sample.
3. Rapid tests are screening tests for antibodies, not for antigen.
4. Negative rapid tests should be followed by a risk assessment to determine the need for repeat tests.
5. Positive rapid tests can be disclosed to the patient, but need to be confirmed with the more specific WB or IFA (as above). This step necessitates a blood draw and a return appointment to get results.

Combined Antibody/Antigen Testing

1. The combined antibody/antigen test allows for diagnosis of HIV infection, especially during the window period when antibody may be undetectable but viral loads are generally high.

conducted. Findings from the history, assessment, and laboratory tests help to determine patient needs. This is also a good time to complete the case reports required by the state health department. Patient teaching about the spectrum of HIV disease, treatment, prevention of transmission to others, improvements in health, and family planning can be initiated at this meeting. Use patient input to develop a plan of care and determine the need for referrals. Remember that a newly diagnosed patient may not be able to retain or understand information. Be prepared to repeat and clarify information over the course of several months.

Drug Therapy for HIV Infection. The goals of drug therapy in HIV infection are to (1) decrease the viral load, (2) maintain or increase CD4$^+$ T cell counts, (3) prevent HIV-related symptoms and opportunistic diseases, (4) delay disease progression, and (5) prevent HIV transmission. HIV cannot be cured, but antiretroviral therapy (ART) can delay disease progression by decreasing viral replication. When taken consistently and correctly, ART can reduce viral loads by 90% to 99%, which makes adherence to treatment regimens extremely important.

Drugs used to treat HIV work at various points in the HIV replication cycle (Table 15-12). The major advantage of using drugs from different classes is that combination therapy can inhibit viral replication in several different ways, making it more difficult for the virus to recover and decreasing the likelihood of drug resistance. A major problem with most drugs used in ART is that resistance develops rapidly when they are used alone *(monotherapy)* or taken in inadequate doses.[27,28] For that reason, combinations of three or more drugs should be used.

Many antiretroviral drugs have dangerous and potentially lethal interactions with other commonly used drugs, including over-the-counter drugs and herbal therapies. For example, St. John's wort, an herb used to alleviate depression, can interfere with ART. Encourage patients to discuss the use of all over-the-counter and herbal products with their health care providers.

TABLE 15-12 DRUG THERAPY

HIV Infection

Drug Classification	Mechanism of Action	Examples*
Entry Inhibitors	Prevent binding of HIV to cells, thus preventing entry of HIV into cells where replication would occur	enfuvirtide (Fuzeon) maraviroc (Selzentry)
Reverse Transcriptase Inhibitors		
Nucleoside Reverse Transcriptase Inhibitors (NRTIs)	Insert a piece of DNA into the developing HIV DNA chain, blocking further development of the chain and leaving the production of the new strand of HIV DNA incomplete	zidovudine (AZT, ZDV, Retrovir) didanosine (ddI, Videx, Videx-EC [time-released]) stavudine (d4T, Zerit) lamivudine (3TC, Epivir) abacavir (Ziagen) emtricitabine (FTC, Emtriva)
Nonnucleoside Reverse Transcriptase Inhibitors (NNRTIs)	Inhibit the action of reverse transcriptase	nevirapine (Viramune) delavirdine (Rescriptor) efavirenz (Sustiva) etravirine (Intelence) rilpivirine (Edurant)
Nucleotide Reverse Transcriptase Inhibitor (NtRTI)	Combines with reverse transcriptase enzyme to block the process needed to convert HIV RNA into HIV DNA	tenofovir (Viread)
Integrase Inhibitors	Bind with integrase enzyme and prevent HIV from incorporating its genetic material into the host cell	raltegravir (Isentress) elvitegravir† dolutegravir (Tivicay)
Protease Inhibitors (PIs)	Prevent the protease enzyme from cutting HIV proteins into the proper lengths needed to allow viable virions to assemble and bud out from the cell membrane	saquinavir (Fortovase, Invirase) indinavir (Crixivan) ritonavir (Norvir)‡ nelfinavir (Viracept) atazanavir (Reyataz) fosamprenavir (Lexiva) tipranavir (Aptivus) darunavir (Prezista) lopinavir + ritonavir (Kaletra)
Fixed-Dose Combination Products	More than one drug combined into a single tablet. Drugs may be from the same or different classes.	Atripla (tenofovir DF + emtricitabine + efavirenz) Combivir (lamivudine + zidovudine) Complera (tenofovir DF + emtricitabine + rilpivirine) Epzicom (abacavir + lamivudine) Trizivir (abacavir + lamivudine + zidovudine) Truvada (tenofovir DF + emtricitabine) Stribild (tenofovir DF + emtricitabine + elvitegravir + cobicistat§)

*Side effects of these drugs are listed in eTable 15-3 available on the website for this chapter.
†Part of the combination pill Stribild (see below)
‡Most often used in low doses with other PIs to boost effect.
§Cobicistat is a pharmacologic booster that enhances the potency of some HIV antiretrovirals. It has no direct effects against HIV.
DF, Disoproxil fumarate.

DRUG ALERT: Efavirenz (Sustiva)
- Do not use in pregnancy, because large doses could cause fetal anomalies.
- Once-a-day doses should be taken at bed time (at least initially) to help patients cope with side effects, including dizziness and confusion.
- Inform patients that many people who use the drug have reported vivid and sometimes bizarre dreams.

Drug Therapy for Opportunistic Diseases. Management of HIV is complicated by the many opportunistic diseases that can develop as the immune system deteriorates (see Table 15-10). Prevention is the preferred approach to opportunistic diseases. A number of opportunistic diseases associated with HIV can be delayed or prevented with adequate ART, vaccines (including hepatitis B, influenza, and pneumococcal), and disease-specific prevention measures. Although it is usually not possible to eradicate opportunistic diseases once they occur, prophylactic medications can significantly decrease morbidity and mortality rates.[30] Advances in the prevention, diagnosis, and treatment of opportunistic diseases have contributed significantly to increased life expectancy. (Drug therapy for opportunistic infections is presented in eTable 15-2 on the website for this chapter.)

Preventing Transmission of HIV. Preexposure prophylaxis (PrEP) is a comprehensive HIV prevention strategy to reduce the risk of sexually acquired HIV infection in adults at high risk.[31] PrEP includes safe sex practices, risk reduction counseling, and regular HIV testing. In addition, emtricitabine and tenofovir (Truvada) can be used for PrEP.

Truvada is the first drug approved to reduce the risk of HIV infection in uninfected individuals who are at high risk of HIV infection and who may engage in sexual activity with HIV-infected partners. Truvada is also currently used in combination with other antiretroviral agents for the treatment of HIV-infected people. Guidelines for PrEP for HIV prevention are available at *www.cdc.gov/hiv/prep/pdf/PrEPfactsheet.pdf*.

NURSING MANAGEMENT
HIV INFECTION

NURSING ASSESSMENT
Nursing assessment for individuals not known to be infected with HIV should focus on behaviors that put the person at risk for HIV and other sexually transmitted and blood-borne infections. Assess patients for risky behaviors on a regular basis. Do not assume that someone is without risk because he or she is too old or too young, is married, or sings in the church choir.

Help individuals assess risk by asking some basic questions: (1) Have you ever had a blood transfusion or used clotting factors? If so, was it before 1985? (2) Have you ever shared drug-using equipment with another person? (3) Have you ever had a sexual experience in which your penis, vagina, rectum, or mouth came into contact with another person's penis, vagina, rectum, or mouth? and (4) Have you ever had a sexually transmitted infection? These questions provide the minimum information needed to initiate a risk assessment. A positive response to any of these questions should be followed by an in-depth exploration of issues related to the identified risk.

Specific assessments are needed for an individual who has been diagnosed with HIV infection. Subjective and objective data that should be obtained are presented in Table 15-13. Repeated nursing assessments over time are essential because people's circumstances change. Early recognition and treatment

can slow the progression of HIV infection and prevent new infections. A complete history and thorough systems review can help identify and address problems in a timely manner.

PLANNING
Nursing interventions can help the patient (1) adhere to drug regimens; (2) adopt a healthy lifestyle that includes avoiding exposure to other sexually transmitted infections and blood-borne diseases; (3) protect others from HIV; (4) maintain or develop healthy and supportive relationships; (5) maintain activities and productivity; (6) explore spiritual issues; (7) come to terms with issues related to disease, disability, and death; and (8) cope with symptoms caused by HIV and its treatments.

NURSING IMPLEMENTATION
The complexity of HIV disease is related to its chronic nature. As with most chronic and infectious diseases, primary preven-

ETHICAL/LEGAL DILEMMAS
Individual Versus Public Health Protection

Situation
A nurse in a community clinic is having a follow-up visit with V.T., a 38-year-old woman, who was found to have HIV during her annual examination 2 wk ago. During the visit, V.T. discloses that she has been verbally and physically abused by her partner. V.T. also indicates that she had not yet told her partner about the HIV diagnosis because she is afraid that he will hurt her. She has not used any protection during sex with him since she learned of her test results because she suspects he infected her.

Ethical/Legal Points for Consideration
- You face a conflict between preventing further harm to V.T. (possible increase in intimate partner violence), providing care to her partner (his need for an HIV test, diagnosis, and treatment), and protecting the public health (potential spread of HIV infection to her partner or from her partner to others in the community). Patient teaching and support are paramount because your primary obligation is to the patient.
- Because relevant law varies from state to state, your first step is to be familiar with your state law concerning mandated reporting for domestic partner abuse and infectious diseases.
- Laws regarding protection of privacy in HIV testing are federal and apply everywhere.
- In many states, reporting domestic abuse is mandatory only when the abuse is actually witnessed by the reporter or when the immediate effects of the abuse (e.g., wounds, contusions, broken bones) are witnessed.
- You should be familiar with crisis counseling services for V.T. and offer her the following advice: collect and stash a set of car keys or taxi money in a safe place, keep a bag packed and hidden or even stored in a locker somewhere accessible, develop a code phrase to use with a friend or family member to call for help, keep a cell phone charged and hidden with the money.

Discussion Questions
1. Within the parameters of your state's requirements for reportable conditions, how can you protect the patient's confidentiality to prevent further intimate partner violence?
2. What services are offered by your state to notify a partner without disclosing the source patient's name? How would V.T. access those services in your state?
3. How can you protect the partner from possible infection while also protecting V.T. from further violence?
4. How can you best address the issue of intimate partner violence? What resources would V.T. have in your community?
5. Discuss the benefits of universal, voluntary testing in light of V.T.'s case.

tion and health promotion are the most effective health care strategies. When prevention fails, disease results. Table 15-14 presents a synopsis of nursing goals, assessments, and interventions at each stage of HIV infection.

HEALTH PROMOTION. Even with recent successes in HIV treatment, prevention is the only way to eventually control the epidemic. In addition, health promotion encourages early detection of the disease so that, if primary prevention has failed, early intervention can be initiated.

Prevention of HIV Infection. HIV infection is preventable. Avoiding or modifying risky behaviors is the most effective prevention tool.[32] Nursing interventions to prevent disease transmission are based on an assessment of the individual's risky behaviors. Although changing behaviors is difficult, encourage the patient to adopt safer, healthier, and less risky behaviors. Provide culturally sensitive, language appropriate, and age-specific teaching and behavior change counseling. Nurses who are comfortable with and know how to talk about

---

HEALTHY PEOPLE

Prevention and Early Detection of HIV

- Increase safe sexual practices, including condom use.
- Decrease equipment sharing among IV drug users.
- Increase clinician skills to assess for risk factors for HIV infection, recommend HIV testing, and provide counseling for behavior change.
- Make voluntary HIV testing a routine part of health care.
- Increase access to new HIV testing technologies, especially rapid testing.
- Increase access to HIV testing facilities in traditional health care settings, as well as in alternative sites such as drug and alcohol treatment facilities and community-based organizations.
- Increase risk assessment and individualized behavior change messages to people with HIV to prevent new infections.
- Decrease perinatal HIV infection by offering voluntary HIV testing as a part of routine prenatal care.
- Provide counseling and appropriate HIV therapy to those who are infected.

TABLE 15-13 NURSING ASSESSMENT

HIV-Infected Patient

Subjective Data
Important Health Information
Past health history: Route of infection; hepatitis; other sexually transmitted infections; tuberculosis; frequent viral, fungal, and/or bacterial infections
Medications: Use of immunosuppressive drugs

Functional Health Patterns
Health perception–health management: Perception of illness; alcohol and drug use; malaise
Nutritional-metabolic: Weight loss, anorexia, nausea, vomiting; lesions, bleeding, or ulcerations of lips, mouth, gums, tongue, or throat; sensitivity to acidic, salty, or spicy foods; difficulty swallowing; abdominal cramping; skin rashes, lesions, or color changes; wounds that don't heal
Elimination: Persistent diarrhea, change in character of stools; painful urination, low back pain
Activity-exercise: Chronic fatigue, muscle weakness, difficulty walking; cough, shortness of breath
Sleep-rest: Insomnia, night sweats, fatigue
Cognitive-perceptual: Headaches, stiff neck, chest pain, rectal pain, retrosternal pain; blurred vision, photophobia, diplopia, loss of vision; hearing impairment; confusion, forgetfulness, attention deficit, changes in mental status, memory loss, personality changes; paresthesias, hypersensitivity in feet, pruritus
Role-relationship: Support system(s), career or job, financial resources
Sexuality-reproductive: Lesions on genitalia (internal or external), pruritus or burning in vagina, penis, or anus; painful sexual intercourse, rectal pain or bleeding, changes in menstruation, vaginal or penile discharge; use of birth control measures, pregnancies, desire for future children
Coping–stress tolerance: Stress levels, previous losses, coping patterns, self-concept; social withdrawal

Objective Data
General
Lethargy, persistent fever, lymphadenopathy, peripheral wasting, fat deposits in truncal areas and upper back

Integumentary
Decreased skin turgor, dry skin, diaphoresis; pallor, cyanosis; lesions, eruptions, discolorations, bruises of skin or mucous membranes; vaginal or perianal excoriation; alopecia; delayed wound healing

Eyes
Presence of exudates, retinal lesions or hemorrhage, papilledema

Respiratory
Tachypnea, dyspnea, intercostal retractions; crackles, wheezing, productive or nonproductive cough

Cardiovascular
Pericardial friction rub, murmur, bradycardia, tachycardia

Gastrointestinal
Mouth lesions, including blisters (HSV), white-gray patches (*Candida* infection), painless white lesions on lateral aspect of the tongue (hairy leukoplakia), discolorations (KS); gingivitis, tooth decay or loosening; redness or white patchy lesions of throat; vomiting, diarrhea, incontinence; rectal lesions; hyperactive bowel sounds, abdominal masses, hepatosplenomegaly

Musculoskeletal
Muscle wasting, weakness

Neurologic
Ataxia, tremors, lack of coordination; sensory loss; slurred speech, aphasia; memory loss, peripheral neuropathy, apathy, agitation, depression, inappropriate behavior; decreasing levels of consciousness, seizures, paralysis, coma

Reproductive
Genital lesions or discharge, abdominal tenderness secondary to pelvic inflammatory disease (PID)

Possible Diagnostic Findings
Positive HIV antibody assay (EIA, confirmed by WB or IFA); detectable viral load; ↓ CD4⁺ T cell count, ↓ WBC count, lymphopenia, anemia, thrombocytopenia; electrolyte imbalances; abnormal liver function tests; ↑ cholesterol, triglycerides, and blood glucose

---

EIA, Enzyme immunoassay; *HSV,* herpes simplex virus; *IFA,* immunofluorescence assay; *KS,* Kaposi sarcoma; *WB,* Western blot; *WBC,* white blood cell.

TABLE 15-14   PATIENT & CAREGIVER TEACHING GUIDE

Antiretroviral Drugs

Resistance to antiretroviral drugs is a major problem in treating HIV infection. Include the following instructions when teaching the patient and/or caregiver to decrease the risk of developing resistance.

1. Discuss options with your health care provider to find the best regimen for you. Your provider should order at least three different antiretroviral drugs from at least two different drug groups.
2. Know the drugs you are taking and how to take them (some have to be taken with food, some must be taken on an empty stomach, some cannot be taken together). If you do not understand, ask. Have your nurse write the instructions clearly for you.
3. Take the full dose prescribed, and take it on schedule. If you cannot take the drug because of side effects or other problems, report it to your health care provider immediately.
4. Take all of your medications as prescribed. Do not quit taking one drug while continuing the others. If you cannot tolerate even one of your drugs, talk to your health care provider, who will recommend a way to deal with the side effects or a new set of drugs.
5. Many antiretroviral drugs interact with other drugs, including a number of common drugs you can buy without a prescription. Be sure your health care provider and pharmacist know all of the drugs that you are taking, and do not take any new drugs without checking for possible interactions.
6. The goals of antiretroviral therapy are to decrease the amount of virus in your blood (your viral load) and to keep your $CD4^+$ T cell count high. The best results reduce your viral load below detectable levels and keep your $CD4^+$ T cell count high. Most health care providers do routine laboratory work every 3 to 6 mo whether you are taking antiretroviral agents or not.
7. Two to 4 wk after you start on drug therapy (or change your therapy), your health care provider will test your viral load to find out how the drugs are working.
   - Your viral load is reported in absolute numbers or in logarithms (a mathematical concept). All you need to know is that you want to see the viral load drop. If reports are in logarithms, you want to see a drop of at least 1 unit, which means that 90% of your viral load has been eliminated. If your viral load drops by 2 units, your viral load will have decreased by 95%. If your viral load drops by 3 units, your viral load will have decreased by 99%.
   - Your $CD4^+$ T cell count is reported in absolute numbers or percentages. It is best for your $CD4^+$ T cell count to be above 500 to 600 cells/μL. If reported in percentages, you would like your $CD4^+$ T cell value to be above 14%.
8. An undetectable viral load means that the amount of virus is extremely low and HIV cannot be found in the blood using current testing technology. It does not mean that the virus is gone because the virus can be in lymph nodes and organs that blood tests cannot detect. It also does not mean that you are no longer able to transmit HIV to others. You will need to continue protecting all of your sexual and drug-using partners from HIV.

EVIDENCE-BASED PRACTICE

Applying the Evidence

As a nurse in an HIV clinic, you are counseling P.S., a 25-year-old gay man, and his partner. P.S. is on antiretroviral therapy. His viral load is very low, and his $CD4^+$ T cell count is normal. He tells you that since the medications are working, he and his partner (who is not infected with HIV) have decided to forgo the use of condoms. They tell you that they are in a committed relationship and have no other partners. You spend time explaining to both of them the risks of unprotected sex: his partner may get infected with HIV even with a low viral load (although the risk is decreased).

Best Available Evidence	Clinician Expertise	Patient Preferences and Values
One of the best ways to prevent HIV transmission from an infected person to an uninfected person is by using condoms.	You know that risk-reducing sexual activities in this situation include the continued use of condoms. However, you also know that a very low viral load decreases the risk of HIV transmission.	After listening, the patient tells you that he and his partner do not like using condoms. They both understand the risks and believe that while the medications are working, the risk is low and worth it.

Your Decision and Action

As his nurse, you respect his decision. You remind him of the importance of maintaining his medication regimen and attending his appointments at the clinic. You explain that this will be even more important now to keep P.S.'s infection under control.

Reference for Evidence

Cohen MS, McCauley M, Gamble RT: HIV treatment as prevention and HPTN 052, *Curr Opin HIV AIDS* 7(2):99, 2012.

---

sensitive topics such as sexuality and drug use are best prepared to provide prevention teaching.

A wide variety of activities can reduce the risk of HIV infection. Individuals will choose the methods that best fit their needs and circumstances. Prevention techniques can be divided into *safe sexual activities* (those that eliminate risk) and *risk-reducing sexual activities* (those that decrease, but do not eliminate, risk).

The goal is to develop safer, healthier, and less risky behaviors. The more consistently and correctly prevention methods are used, the more effective they are in preventing HIV infection. It is also a good idea to use a combination of prevention methods (e.g., using condoms and decreasing the number of sex partners) to increase the prevention effect.

Decreasing Risks Related to Sexual Intercourse. *Safe sexual activities* eliminate the risk of exposure to HIV in semen and vaginal secretions.[33] Abstaining from all sexual activity is an effective way to accomplish this goal, but there are safe options for those who cannot or do not wish to abstain. Limiting sexual behavior to activities in which the mouth, penis, vagina, or rectum does not come into contact with a partner's mouth, penis, vagina, or rectum eliminates contact with blood, semen, or vaginal secretions. Safe activities include masturbation, mutual masturbation ("hand job"), and other activities that meet the "no contact" requirements. *Insertive sex* between partners who are not infected with HIV and not at risk of becoming infected with HIV is also considered safe.

Risk-reducing sexual activities decrease the risk of contact with HIV through the use of barriers. Barriers should be used when engaging in insertive sexual activity (oral, vaginal, or anal) with a partner who has HIV or whose HIV status is not known. The most commonly used barrier is the male condom. The *efficacy* (protection provided under ideal circumstances) of male condoms is essentially 100%. Their *effectiveness* (protection provided in actual or "real life" circumstances) is better than 90%. Male condoms can be used for protection during anal, vaginal, and oral intercourse. (The proper use and placement of the male condom are presented in eTable 15-4 on the website for this chapter.)

Female condoms provide an alternative to male condoms. Female condom efficacy is also close to 100%, and effectiveness

INFORMATICS IN PRACTICE

Use of Internet and Mobile Devices to Manage HIV

- The Internet offers resources and support for patients that can assist them in coping with their illness and educate them about signs and symptoms of serious illness.
- By monitoring their health and quickly spotting warning signs of serious illnesses, patients are able to alert their physicians and receive earlier treatment.
- These systems can help the patient manage antiretroviral therapy by sending medication reminders by text or e-mail.

is 94% to 97% against HIV and other sexually transmitted infections. (The proper use and placement of the female condom are presented in eTable 15-5 on the website for this chapter.) In addition, squares of latex (known as dental dams) can be used to cover the external female genitalia during oral sexual activity.

Decreasing Risks Related to Drug Use. Drug use, including alcohol and tobacco, is harmful. It can cause immunosuppression, poor nutrition, and a host of psychosocial problems, but drug use does not cause HIV infection. The major risk for HIV related to using drugs involves sharing equipment or having unsafe sexual experiences while under the influence of drugs. Basic risk reduction rules are (1) do not use drugs; (2) if you use drugs, do not share equipment; and (3) do not have sexual intercourse when under the influence of any drug (including alcohol) that impairs decision making.[34]

The safest method is to abstain from drugs, but this may not be a viable option for users who are not prepared to quit or have no access to drug treatment services. The risk of HIV for these individuals can be eliminated if they do not share equipment. Injecting equipment ("works") includes needles, syringes, cookers (spoons or bottle caps used to mix the drug), cotton, and rinse water. Equipment used to snort (straws) or smoke (pipes) drugs can also be contaminated with blood and should not be shared.

Access to sterile equipment is an important risk elimination tactic. Some communities have needle and syringe exchange programs (NSEPs) that provide sterile equipment in exchange for used equipment. Opposition to these programs is related to the fear that access to injecting supplies will increase drug use. However, studies have shown that, in communities with NSEPs, drug use does not increase, rates of HIV and other blood-borne infections are controlled, and an overall cost benefit results.[35] Cleaning equipment before use can also reduce risk by decreasing the chance of blood contact. (The proper use of drug equipment is presented in eTable 15-6 on the website for this chapter.)

Decreasing Risks of Perinatal Transmission. The best way to prevent HIV infection in infants is to prevent HIV infection in women. Women who are already infected with HIV should be asked about their reproductive desires. Those who choose not to have children need to have family planning methods discussed in detail. Should they become pregnant, abortion may be desired and should be discussed in conjunction with other options, including the possibility of maintaining the pregnancy and using ART to decrease the risk of transmission. If HIV-infected pregnant women are appropriately treated during pregnancy, the rate of perinatal transmission can be decreased from 25% to less than 2%.[24] ART has significantly decreased the risk for infants born to HIV-infected women, and more of these women are now becoming mothers. The current standard of care is for all women who are pregnant or contemplating preg-

nancy to be counseled about HIV, routinely offered access to voluntary HIV-antibody testing, and, if infected, offered optimal ART.[24]

Decreasing Risks at Work. The risk of infection from occupational exposure to HIV is small but real. OSHA requires employers to protect workers from exposure to blood and other potentially infectious materials (see Table 15-8). Precautions and safety devices decrease the risk of direct contact with blood and body fluids. Should exposure to HIV-infected fluids occur, **postexposure prophylaxis (PEP)** with combination ART can significantly decrease the risk of infection.[23] The need for timely treatment and counseling makes it even more critical for nurses to report all blood exposures.

HIV Testing. An estimated 21% of people living with HIV in the United States are not aware that they are infected. People who do not know they are infected are more likely to transmit the infection to others.[36,37] The CDC recommends universal, voluntary testing for all people ages 13 to 64 regardless of the patient's risk or perceived risk. The CDC recommends an "opt out" process in which the patient is given the opportunity to decline a test, but it is offered as "routine." The goal is to normalize the test, decrease the stigma related to HIV testing, find hidden cases, get infected individuals into care, and prevent new cases of infection.[38]

ACUTE INTERVENTION

Early Intervention. Early intervention after detection of HIV infection can promote health and limit disability. The nursing assessment in HIV disease should focus on early detection of symptoms, opportunistic diseases, and psychosocial problems[39] (see Tables 15-13 and eTable 15-7).

Initial Response to Diagnosis of HIV. Reactions to an HIV diagnosis are similar to the reactions of people who are diagnosed with any life-threatening, debilitating, or chronic illness. They include anxiety, panic, fear, depression, denial, hopelessness, anger, and guilt.[40] Unfortunately, all these emotions are overlaid with the stigma and discrimination that continue to pervade societal reactions to HIV. Many of these reactions are also seen in the patient's family members, friends, and caregivers. As time passes, patients and their loved ones will be confronted with complex treatment decisions; feelings of loss, anger, powerlessness, depression, and grief; social isolation; the possibility of death; and/or thoughts of suicide.

Antiretroviral Therapy. ART can significantly slow the clinical progression of HIV.[28] However, treatment regimens can be complex, the drugs have side effects, ART does not work for everyone, and it is expensive. These factors can contribute to problems with adherence to treatment, a dangerous situation because of the high risk of developing drug resistance.

As a nurse, you are often the person who works most closely with patients who are trying to cope with these issues. Interventions include teaching about (1) advantages and disadvantages of new treatments, (2) dangers of poor adherence to therapeutic regimens, (3) how and when to take each drug, (4) drug interactions to avoid, and (5) side effects that must be reported to the health care provider. Table 15-14 provides guidance for patient teaching in these areas.

Guidelines on when and how to initiate ART are based on the degree of immune suppression.[28] Issues to consider when selecting an initial drug regimen include the ability of the patient's HIV to resist specific drugs (assessed by the resistance tests discussed on p. 235), potential medication side effects, existing co-morbidities, and dosing schedules. This is a critical

TABLE 15-15   PATIENT & CAREGIVER TEACHING GUIDE

Improving Adherence to Antiretroviral Therapy

The following are strategies that you can use to improve a patient's adherence to using antiretroviral therapy:

- Determine whether the patient understands the importance of adherence and is ready to start therapy.
- Provide teaching on medication dosing.
- Review potential side effects of drugs.
- Assure the patient that side effects can be treated. If not, medication regimens can be changed.
- Use teaching and memory aids, including pictures, pillboxes, and calendars.
- Engage family and friends in the teaching process. Solicit their support to help the patient take treatment.
- Simplify regimens, dosing, and food requirements as much as possible.
- Use a team of nurses, physicians, pharmacists, case managers, and mental health and peer counselors to support the patient.
- Help the patient integrate the medication regimen into his or her typical life activities and work schedules.

Modified from Centers for Disease Control and Prevention: Guidelines for the use of antiretroviral agents in HIV-1-infected adults and adolescents, 2012. Retrieved from *http://aidsinfo.nih.gov.*

decision because the first treatment regimen is generally the patient's best chance for success. However, the most important consideration for initiating therapy is patient readiness.[39]

Adherence to ART is a critical component of successful drug therapy for people with HIV infection. Nurses are uniquely prepared to provide assistance with adherence to the drug regimen[39,41] (Table 15-15). Taking drugs as prescribed (right dose and time) is important for all drug therapy, but with HIV infection, missing even a few doses can lead to drug resistance. Patients can be helped to adhere to difficult treatment regimens with electronic reminders, beepers, timers on pillboxes, and calendars. Group support and individual counseling can also help, but the best approach is to learn about the patient's life and assist with problem solving related to taking medications within the confines of that life.

Delaying Disease Progression. HIV disease progression may be delayed by promoting a healthy immune system, whether the patient chooses to use ART or not. Useful interventions for HIV-infected patients include (1) getting nutritional support to maintain lean body mass and ensure appropriate levels of vitamins and micronutrients; (2) moderating or eliminating alcohol, tobacco, and drug use; (3) keeping up to date with recommended vaccines; (4) getting adequate rest and exercise; (5) reducing stress; (6) avoiding exposure to new infectious agents; (7) accessing mental health counseling; (8) getting involved in support groups and community activities; and (9) developing a consistent relationship with health care providers, including attendance at regular appointments.

Teach patients to recognize symptoms that may indicate disease progression and/or drug side effects so that prompt medical care can be initiated. Table 15-16 provides an overview of symptoms that patients should report.

Acute Exacerbations. Chronic diseases are characterized by acute exacerbations of recurring problems. This is especially true in HIV disease where infections, cancers, debility, and psychosocial or economic issues may interact to overwhelm the patient's ability to cope. Nursing care becomes more complex as the patient's immune system deteriorates and new problems

TABLE 15-16   PATIENT & CAREGIVER TEACHING GUIDE

Signs and Symptoms HIV Patients Need to Report

Teach the patient with HIV infection and the caregiver to report the following signs and symptoms.

Report Immediately
- Any change in level of consciousness: lethargic, hard to arouse, unable to be aroused, unresponsive, unconscious
- Headache accompanied by nausea and vomiting, changes in vision, changes in ability to perform coordinated activities, or after any head trauma
- Vision changes: blurry or black areas in vision field, new floaters, double vision
- Persistent shortness of breath related to activity and not relieved by a short rest period
- Nausea and vomiting accompanied by abdominal pain
- Vomiting blood
- Dehydration: unable to eat or drink because of nausea, diarrhea, or mouth lesions; severe diarrhea or vomiting; dizziness when standing
- Yellow discoloration of the skin
- Any bleeding from the rectum that is not related to hemorrhoids or trauma (e.g., from anal sexual intercourse)
- Pain in the flank with fever and inability to urinate for more than 6 hr
- Blood in the urine
- New onset of weakness in any part of the body, new onset of numbness that is not obviously related to pressure, new onset of difficulty speaking
- Chest pain not obviously related to cough
- Seizures
- New rash accompanied by fever
- New oral lesions accompanied by fever
- Severe depression, anxiety, hallucinations, delusions, or thoughts of causing danger to self or others

Report the Following Signs and Symptoms Within 24 Hr
- New or different headache; constant headache not relieved by over-the-counter medication
- Headache accompanied by fever, nasal congestion, or cough
- Burning, itching, or discharge from the eyes
- New or productive cough
- Vomiting 2-3 times a day
- Vomiting accompanied by fever
- New, significant, or watery diarrhea (more than 6 times a day)
- Painful urination, bloody urine, urethral discharge
- Significant new rash (widespread; painful; or following a path down the leg or arm, around the chest, or on the face)
- Difficulty eating or drinking because of mouth lesions
- Vaginal discharge, pain, or itching

arise to compound existing difficulties.[39] When opportunistic diseases or difficult treatment side effects develop, symptom management, teaching, and emotional support are needed.

Nursing care can help prevent the many opportunistic diseases associated with HIV infection. The best way to prevent opportunistic disease is to ensure that the patient is adhering to an effective ART regimen and, if appropriate, taking prophylactic medications for opportunistic infections. Should an opportunistic disease occur, nursing care can be an essential part of helping the patient adhere to medications and providing supportive care specific to the opportunistic disease. For example, if the patient has *Pneumocystis jiroveci* pneumonia (PCP) (Fig. 15-8), nursing interventions can ensure adequate oxygenation. If the patient has cryptococcal meningitis, an important nursing concern is maintaining a safe environment for a confused patient.

FIG. 15-8 Chest x-ray showing interstitial infiltrates as the result of *Pneumocystis jiroveci* pneumonia.

FIG. 15-9 Lipodystrophy manifestations.

AMBULATORY AND HOME CARE. HIV infection has no cure, continues for life, causes physical disability, and contributes to impaired health. In many cases it can lead to death. HIV infection affects the entire range of a person's life from physical health to social, emotional, economic, and spiritual well-being.

Stigma of HIV. HIV-infected patients share problems experienced by all individuals with chronic diseases, but these problems are exacerbated by negative social constructs surrounding HIV.[42] HIV-infected people may be thought to lack control over urges to have sex or use drugs. Some people then conclude that people with HIV brought the disease on themselves and deserve to be sick. Behaviors associated with HIV infection are viewed by some as immoral (e.g., homosexuality, having many sexual partners) and are sometimes illegal (e.g., using drugs, sex work). The fact that infected individuals can transmit HIV to others creates fear, which leads to stigma and discrimination in all facets of life.

In the United States, HIV-infected people have lost jobs, homes, and insurance, although these forms of discrimination are prohibited by the Americans with Disabilities Act (ADA).[43] HIV-related stigma is a global problem that is often more severe for women. Discrimination can lead to social isolation, dependence, frustration, low self-image, loss of control, and economic pressures.

Disease and Drug Side Effects. Physical problems related to HIV or its treatment can interfere with the patient's ability to maintain a desired lifestyle. HIV-infected patients frequently experience anxiety, fear, depression, diarrhea, peripheral neuropathy, pain, nausea, vomiting, and fatigue. Nursing interventions for these symptoms are similar to what they would be for the patient who does not have HIV infection. For example, nursing management of diarrhea includes helping patients collect specimens, recommending dietary changes, encouraging fluid and electrolyte replacement, instructing the patient about skin care, and managing skin breakdown around the perianal area. Nursing approaches for fatigue in HIV include teaching patients to assess fatigue patterns; determine contributing factors; set

activity priorities; conserve energy; schedule rest periods; exercise regularly; and avoid substances such as caffeine, nicotine, alcohol, and other drugs that may disturb sleep.

Some HIV-infected patients, especially those who have been infected and on ART for a long time, develop a set of metabolic disorders that include changes in body shape (fat deposits in the abdomen, upper back, and breasts along with fat loss in the arms, legs, and face) because of lipodystrophy (Fig. 15-9), hyperlipidemia (elevated triglycerides, elevated low-density lipoproteins, and decreased high-density lipoproteins), insulin resistance and hyperglycemia, bone disease (osteoporosis, osteopenia, avascular necrosis), lactic acidosis, renal disease, and cardiovascular disease.[31]

It is still not clear why these disorders develop, but it is probably a combination of factors such as long-term infection with HIV, side effects of ART, genetic predisposition, and chronic stress. Management of metabolic disorders focuses on detecting problems early, dealing with symptoms, and helping the patient cope with emerging problems and changes to treatment regimens. It is important to recognize and treat these problems early, especially because cardiovascular disease and lactic acidosis are potentially fatal complications.

A frequent first intervention is to change ART medications because some drugs are more often associated with these disorders. Lipid abnormalities are generally treated with lipid-lowering drugs (see Table 34-5), dietary changes, and exercise. Insulin resistance is treated with hypoglycemic drugs and weight loss. Bone disease may be improved with exercise, dietary changes, and calcium and vitamin D supplements.

End-of-Life Care. Despite new developments in the treatment of HIV infection, many patients eventually experience disease progression, disability, and death. Sometimes these occur because treatments do not work for the patient. Sometimes the patient's HIV becomes resistant to all available drug therapies. In addition, ART is now allowing people living with HIV to live longer and to develop diseases of aging, such as cardiovascular and endocrine problems that lead to death.

Nursing care during the terminal phase of any disease should focus on keeping the patient comfortable, facilitating emotional and spiritual acceptance of the finite nature of life, helping the patient's significant others deal with grief and loss, and maintaining a safe environment. As a nurse, you are the pivotal care provider during this phase of illness, whether at home, through hospice, or in a health care facility.[39] (End-of-life care is discussed in Chapter 10.)

EVALUATION

The expected outcomes are that the patient at risk for HIV infection will
- Analyze personal risk factors
- Develop and implement a personal plan to decrease risks
- Get tested for HIV

The expected outcomes are that the patient with HIV infection will
- Describe basic aspects of the effects of HIV on the immune system
- Compare and contrast various treatment options for HIV disease
- Work with a team of health care providers to achieve optimal health
- Prevent transmission of HIV to others

GERONTOLOGIC CONSIDERATIONS

HIV INFECTION

The number of older adults who have HIV disease is increasing because (1) HIV treatment has been effective in reducing the number of deaths from HIV-related opportunistic infections and (2) people 60 and older are being infected at increasing rates. The number of people over the age of 60 living with HIV is expected to grow.

Remember that older people living with HIV are susceptible to the same diseases as non-HIV-infected older people. These include heart disease, cancer, diabetes, bone disease, arthritis, hypertension, kidney disease, and cognitive impairment. However, people with HIV infection may experience these diseases at an earlier age (compared with non-HIV-infected people) and may be at higher risk of co-morbidities related to the medications used to treat HIV. For example, some of the HIV medications are associated with increased lipids and altered insulin metabolism. Focusing nursing care on early identification of these complications, and assisting patients in reducing their risk for heart disease, diabetes, or other chronic disease, are critical aspects of caring for the older HIV patient.

Another consideration with the aging HIV population is the impact of polypharmacy. In general, older adults are often prescribed multiple medications to manage various chronic diseases. Some of these medications may interact with or be potentiated by HIV medications. Therefore careful monitoring and assessment of possible drug interactions is important when providing care to this population.

Older adults may be ashamed and hesitate to tell anyone that they have an HIV infection. This may make it difficult for them to get the appropriate health care and support. As a nurse, you need to recognize that HIV is a chronic disease that will affect more and more older adults and be prepared to help the older person who is living with HIV infection.

CASE STUDY

HIV Infection

iStockphoto/Thinkstock

Patient Profile
J.N., a 35-year-old African American woman, was admitted to the hospital in respiratory distress. AIDS and *Pneumocystis jiroveci* pneumonia (PCP) were both diagnosed 2 days ago.

Subjective Data
- Seen by a physician 6 years ago for pain behind the sternum and difficulty swallowing, diagnosed as esophageal candidiasis; positive HIV-antibody test at that time
- Has consistently refused ART because, "We can't afford it"
- Married to Jim, a former IV drug user, for 15 years until his recent death from AIDS-related complications
- Has two children, ages 8 and 10; neither has been tested for HIV infection
- Experiences fatigue and frequent oral and vaginal candidiasis outbreaks
- Expresses concern about the welfare of her children, who are at home with her sister, and says, "Maybe I should take better care of myself for them"

Objective Data
Physical Examination
- 5 ft 6 in tall, 100 lb, temperature 100.4° F (38° C), O₂ saturation 92% on 3 L of O₂ via nasal cannula

Laboratory Studies
- CD4+ T cell count 185 cells/μL
- Viral load 55,328 copies/μL
- Hematocrit 30%

Collaborative Care
- Trimethoprim/sulfamethoxazole
- Combination antiretroviral therapy: tenofovir and emtricitabine (Truvada), darunavir (Prezista), ritonavir (Norvir)

Discussion Questions
1. Why did J.N.'s initial medical problem (esophageal candidiasis) lead to an HIV test?
2. Why was trimethoprim/sulfamethoxazole ordered, and what are its common side effects?
3. What diagnostic criteria for AIDS are present in J.N.?
4. Is there a potential advantage to J.N.'s refusal to take antiretroviral drugs in the past? If so, why or why not?
5. Women often put their children's welfare first. What barriers could this cause for J.N.'s treatment? How can these problems be resolved?
6. *Priority Decision:* What priority teaching needs should be covered before J.N. is discharged from the hospital to return home? What referrals need to be made?
7. How can J.N. be helped to adhere to her medication schedule?
8. *Priority Decision:* What are the priority nursing interventions? What plans need to be made for continued nursing care after discharge?
9. *Evidence-Based Practice:* J.N. asks you if her kids should be tested. She is afraid of what the results may be. How should you respond?

BRIDGE TO NCLEX EXAMINATION

The number of the question corresponds to the same-numbered outcome at the beginning of the chapter.

1. Emerging infections can affect health care by *(select all that apply)*
   a. revealing antibiotic resistance.
   b. generating scientific discoveries.
   c. creating a strain on limited resources.
   d. challenging established medical traditions.
   e. limiting travel options for nursing personnel.
2. Which antibiotic-resistant organisms cannot be killed by normal hand soap?
   a. Vancomycin-resistant enterococci
   b. Methicillin-resistant *Staphylococcus aureus*
   c. Penicillin-resistant *Streptococcus pneumoniae*
   d. β-Lactamase–producing *Klebsiella pneumoniae*
3. Transmission of HIV from an infected individual to another most commonly occurs as a result of
   a. unprotected anal or vaginal sexual intercourse.
   b. low levels of virus in the blood and high levels of CD4⁺ T cells.
   c. transmission from mother to infant during labor and delivery and breastfeeding.
   d. sharing of drug-using equipment, including needles, syringes, pipes, and straws.
4. During HIV infection
   a. the virus replicates mainly in B-cells before spreading to CD4⁺ T cells.
   b. infection of monocytes may occur, but antibodies quickly destroy these cells.
   c. the immune system is impaired predominantly by the eventual widespread destruction of CD4⁺ T cells.
   d. a long period of dormancy develops during which HIV cannot be found in the blood and there is little viral replication.
5. Which statements accurately describe HIV infection *(select all that apply)*?
   a. Untreated HIV infection has a predictable pattern of progression.
   b. Late chronic HIV infection is called acquired immunodeficiency syndrome (AIDS).
   c. Untreated HIV infection can remain in the early chronic stage for a decade or more.
   d. Untreated HIV infection usually remains in the early chronic stage for 1 year or less.
   e. Opportunistic diseases occur more often when the CD4⁺ T cell count is high and the viral load is low.
6. A diagnosis of AIDS is made when an HIV-infected patient has
   a. a CD4⁺ T cell count below 200/μL.
   b. a high level of HIV in the blood and saliva.
   c. lipodystrophy with metabolic abnormalities.
   d. oral hairy leukoplakia, an infection caused by Epstein-Barr virus.

7. Screening for HIV infection generally involves
   a. laboratory analysis of blood to detect HIV antigen.
   b. electrophoretic analysis for HIV antigen in plasma.
   c. laboratory analysis of blood to detect HIV antibodies.
   d. analysis of lymph tissues for the presence of HIV RNA.
8. Antiretroviral drugs are used to
   a. cure acute HIV infection.
   b. decrease viral RNA levels.
   c. treat opportunistic diseases.
   d. decrease pain and symptoms in terminal disease.
9. Opportunistic diseases in HIV infection
   a. are usually benign.
   b. are generally slow to develop and progress.
   c. occur in the presence of immunosuppression.
   d. are curable with appropriate drug interventions.
10. Which statement about metabolic side effects of ART is true *(select all that apply)*?
    a. These are annoying symptoms that are ultimately harmless.
    b. ART-related body changes include central fat accumulation and peripheral wasting.
    c. Lipid abnormalities include increases in triglycerides and decreases in high-density cholesterol.
    d. Insulin resistance and hyperlipidemia can be treated with drugs to control glucose and cholesterol.
    e. Compared to uninfected people, insulin resistance and hyperlipidemia are more difficult to treat in HIV-infected patients.
11. Which strategy can the nurse teach the patient to eliminate the risk of HIV transmission?
    a. Using sterile equipment to inject drugs
    b. Cleaning equipment used to inject drugs
    c. Taking zidovudine (AZT, ZDV, Retrovir) during pregnancy
    d. Using latex or polyurethane barriers to cover genitalia during sexual contact
12. What is the most appropriate nursing intervention to help an HIV-infected patient adhere to a treatment regimen?
    a. "Set up" a drug pillbox for the patient every week.
    b. Give the patient a video and a brochure to view and read at home.
    c. Tell the patient that the side effects of the drugs are bad but that they go away after a while.
    d. Assess the patient's routines and find adherence cues that fit into the patient's life circumstances.

11, a, 12, d

1, a, b, c, d, 2, a, 3, a, 4, c, 5, a, b, c, 6, a, 7, c, 8, b, 9, c, 10, b, c, d,

ⓔvolve

For rationales to these answers and even more NCLEX review questions, visit *http://evolve.elsevier.com/Lewis/medsurg.*

REFERENCES

1. World Health Organization: The top 10 causes of death. Retrieved from *www.who.int/mediacentre/factsheets.*
2. Huether SE, McCance K: *Understanding pathophysiology,* ed 5, St Louis, 2012, Mosby.
3. Pommerville JC: *Alcamo's fundamentals of microbiology,* ed 9, Sudsbury, Mass, 2011, Jones & Bartlett.
4. Centers for Disease Control and Prevention: Prion diseases. Retrieved from *www.cdc.gov/ncidod/dvrd/prions.*
5. United Nations Environmental Program: Environmental change and new infectious diseases. Retrieved from *www.grida.no.*
6. Hall-Baker PA, Groseclose SL, Jajosky RA, et al: Summary of notifiable diseases—United States 2009, *MMWR* 58:53, 2011.
7. World Health Organization: Disease outbreak news. Retrieved from *www.who.int.*
8. Centers for Disease Control and Prevention: Questions and answers about Ebola hemorrhagic fever, 2009. Retrieved from *www.cdc.gov/ncidod.*

9. Centers for Disease Control and Prevention: Reported cases of tuberculosis: United States, 2010. Retrieved from *www.cdc.gov/tb*.

10. Centers for Disease Control and Prevention: Measles update travel notice. Retrieved from *wwwnc.cdc.gov/travel*.

11. Mostofsky E, Lipsitch M, Regev-Yochay G: Is methicillin-resistant *Staphylococcus aureus* replacing methicillin-sensitive *S. aureus*? *J Antimicrob Chemother* 66(10):2199, 2011.

12. Calfee DP: Methicillin-resistant *Staphylococcus aureus* and vancomycin-resistant enterococci, and other gram-positives in healthcare, *Curr Opin Infect Dis*;25(4):385, 2012.

13. Centers for Disease Control and Prevention: Healthcare-associated infections: the burden. Retrieved from *www.cdc.gov/HAI*.

14. US Department of Health and Human Services Agency for Healthcare Research & Quality: Healthcare-associated infections. Retrieved from *www.ahrq.gov*.

*15. Centers for Disease Control and Prevention: Guidelines for isolation precautions: preventing transmission of infectious agents in healthcare settings, 2007. Retrieved from *www.cdc.gov/hicpac*.

*16. Centers for Disease Control and Prevention: Top CDC recommendations to prevent healthcare-associated infections. Retrieved from *www.cdc.gov/HAI*.

17. Mattison M, Marcantonio ER: Hospital care of the older adult. Retrieved from *www.uptodate.com*.

18. DeCock DM, Jaffe HW, Curran JW: Reflections on 30 years of AIDS, *Emerg Infect Dis* 17(6):1044, 2011.

19. Centers for Disease Control and Prevention: Basic information about HIV and AIDS. Retrieved from *www.cdc.gov/hiv*.

20. Prejean J, Song R, Hernandez A, et al: Estimated HIV incidence in the United States, 2006-2009, *PLOS ONE* 6(8):e17502, 2011.

21. Centers for Disease Control and Prevention: HIV surveillance report 2010, 22. Retrieved from *www.cdc.gov/hiv/surveillance/resources/reports*.

22. World Health Organization: HIV/AIDS data and statistics. *www.who.int/hiv/data/en*.

*23. Centers for Disease Control and Prevention: Updated US Public Health Service guidelines for the management of occupational exposures to HIV and recommendations for postexposure prophylaxis, 2005. Retrieved from *www.aidsinfo.nih.gov*.

*24. Centers for Disease Control and Prevention: US Public Health Service Task Force recommendations for use of antiretroviral drugs in pregnant HIV-1-infected women for maternal health and interventions to reduce perinatal HIV transmission in the United States—July 31, 2012. Retrieved from *www.aidsinfo.nih.gov*.

25. The HIV life cycle: fact sheet 106, New Mexico AIDS InfoNet, 2012. Retrieved from *www.aidsinfo.nih.gov*.

26. Cohen MS, Shaw GM, McMichael AJ, et al: Acute HIV-1 infection, *N Engl J Med* 364:1943, 2011.

27. Longo DL, Fauci AS, Kasper DL, et al: *Harrison's principles of internal medicine*, ed 18, New York, 2012, McGraw Hill.

*28. Centers for Disease Control and Prevention: Guidelines for the prevention and treatment of opportunistic infections in HIV-infected adults and adolescents, *MMWR* 58(RR-4), 2009. Retrieved from *www.aidsinfo.nih.gov*.

29. Centers for Disease Control and Prevention: Revised surveillance case definitions for HIV infection among adults, adolescents and children <18 months and for HIV infection and AIDS among children aged 18 months to <13 years—United States, 2008. Retrieved from *www.cdc.gov/mmwr*.

30. Luetkemeyer AF, Havlir DV, Currier JS: Complications of HIV disease and antiretroviral therapy, *Top Antivir Med* 20(2):48, 2012.

31. Buchbinder SP, Liu A: Pre-exposure prophylaxis and the promise of combination prevention approaches, *AIDS Behav* 25:S72, 2011.

*32. Centers for Disease Control and Prevention: Sexually transmitted diseases treatment guidelines, 2010. Retrieved from *www.cdc.gov/std/treatment/2010/default.htm*.

33. Fisher JD, Smith LR, Lenz EM: Secondary prevention of HIV in the United States: past, current, and future perspectives, *JAIDS* 55:106, 2010.

34. Drug use and HIV: fact sheet 154, New Mexico AIDS InfoNet, 2011. Retrieved from *www.aidsinfonet.org*.

35. Arkin E: Studies confirm effectiveness of harm reduction for people who inject drugs, *HIV AIDS Policy Law Rev* 15:29, 2011.

36. Gardner EM, McLees MP, Steiner JF, et al: The spectrum of engagement in HIV care and its relevance to test-and-treat strategies for prevention of HIV infection, *CID* 52:793, 2011.

37. Hunter E, Perry M, Leen C, et al: HIV testing: getting the message across—a survey of knowledge, attitudes, practice of non-HIV specialist physicians, *Postmed Grad J* 88(1036):59, 2012.

*38. Centers for Disease Control and Prevention: Revised guidelines for HIV testing of adults, adolescents, and pregnant women in health-care settings—September 22, 2006. Retrieved from *www.aidsinfo.nih.gov*.

39. Smith B: *ANAC's core curriculum HIV/AIDS nursing*, ed 3, Sudbury, Mass, 2010, Jones & Bartlett.

40. Nachega JB, Morroni C, Zuniga JM, et al: HIV-related stigma, isolation, and serostatus disclosure: a global survey of 2035 HIV-infected adults, *J Int Assoc Physicians AIDS Care* 3:172, 2012.

41. Enriquez M, McKinsey DS: Strategies to improve HIV treatment adherence in developed countries: clinical management at the individual level, *HIV/AIDS* 3:45, 2011.

42. Holzemer WL, Human S, Arudo J, et al: Exploring HIV stigma and quality of life for persons living with HIV infection, *J Assoc Nurses AIDS Care* 20:161, 2009. (Classic)

43. Americans with Disabilities Act, 42 U.S.C. §1201 et seq (1992 and 1994).

RESOURCES

AIDS Education and Training Centers National Resource Center
www.aidsetc.org
AIDS Info
http://aidsinfo.nih.gov
AIDS InfoNet
www.aidsinfonet.org
Association of Nurses in AIDS Care (ANAC)
www.nursesinaidscare.org
Centers for Disease Control and Prevention HIV/AIDS Information
www.cdc.gov/hiv
Journal of the Association of Nurses in AIDS Care
www.janacnet.org
National Association of People with AIDS (NAPWA)
www.napwa.org
National Minority AIDS Council (NMAC)
www.nmac.org
National Native American AIDS Prevention Center (NNAAPC)
www.nnaapc.org
Office of National AIDS Policy
www.whitehouse.gov/administration/eop/onap

*Evidence-based information for clinical practice.

Never, never, never give up.
Winston Churchill

Cancer

Jormain Cady and Joyce A. Jackowski

⊖volve WEBSITE

LEARNING OUTCOMES

1. Describe the prevalence, incidence, survival, and mortality rates of cancer in the United States.
2. Describe the processes involved in the biology of cancer.
3. Differentiate the three phases of cancer development.
4. Describe the role of the immune system related to cancer.
5. Differentiate among the various classifications of drugs used to treat cancer.
6. Discuss the role of the nurse in the prevention, detection, and diagnosis of cancer.
7. Explain the use of surgery, chemotherapy, radiation therapy, and biologic and targeted therapies in the treatment of cancer.
8. Identify the classifications of chemotherapy agents and methods of administration.
9. Differentiate between teletherapy (external beam radiation) and brachytherapy (internal radiation).
10. Describe the effects of radiation therapy and chemotherapy on normal tissues.
11. Identify the types and effects of biologic and targeted therapy agents.
12. Describe the nursing management of patients receiving chemotherapy, radiation therapy, and biologic and targeted therapy.
13. Describe nutritional therapy for patients with cancer.
14. Identify the various complications associated with advanced cancer.
15. Describe the psychologic support interventions for cancer patients, cancer survivors, and their caregivers.

KEY TERMS

Cancer is a group of more than 200 diseases characterized by uncontrolled and unregulated growth of cells. Although cancer is often considered a disease of aging, with the majority of cases (77%) diagnosed in those over age 55 years, it occurs in people of all ages. An estimated 1,660,290 people in the United States are diagnosed annually with invasive carcinoma (excluding basal and squamous cell skin cancers).[1]

Overall the incidence of cancer has been declining since the 1990s. The mortality rate for the most common cancers (prostate, breast, lung, and colorectal) is also declining.[2] The incidences of many cancers, such as colorectal, lung, breast, and oropharyngeal cancers, have declined largely as a result of preventive efforts. However, the incidence of other types of cancers, such as leukemia, liver cancer, and skin cancers, has

Reviewed by Shelley Fess, RN, MS, AOCN, CRNI, Assistant Professor in Nursing, Monroe Community College, Rochester, New York.

TABLE 16-1   CANCER INCIDENCE BY SITE AND GENDER*

Male		Female	
Type	%	Type	%
Prostate	28	Breast	29
Lung	14	Lung	14
Colon/rectum	9	Colon/rectum	9
Urinary bladder	6	Uterus	6
Melanoma	5	Thyroid	6
Kidney and renal pelvis	5	Non-Hodgkin's lymphoma	4
Non-Hodgkin's lymphoma	4	Melanoma	4
Oropharynx	3	Ovary	3

Source: American Cancer Society: *Cancer facts and figures*, Atlanta, 2012,
The Society. Retrieved from *www.cancer.org/acs/groups/content/
@epidemiologysurveilance/documents/document/acspc-036845.pdf.*
*Numbers are estimates excluding basal and squamous cell skin cancers and
carcinoma in situ.

TABLE 16-2   CANCER DEATHS BY SITE AND GENDER*

Male		Female	
Type	%	Type	%
Lung and bronchus	28	Lung and bronchus	26
Prostate	10	Breast	14
Colon/rectum	9	Colon/rectum	9
Pancreas	6	Pancreas	7
Liver and intrahepatic bile ducts	5	Ovary	5
		Leukemia	4
Leukemia	4	Non-Hodgkin's lymphoma	3
Esophagus	4	Uterus	3
Urinary bladder	3	Liver and intrahepatic bile ducts	2
Non-Hodgkin's lymphoma	3	Brain and other nervous system	2
Kidney and renal pelvis	3		

Source: American Cancer Society: *Cancer facts and figures*, Atlanta, 2012,
The Society. Retrieved from *www.cancer.org/acs/groups/content/
@epidemiologysurveilance/documents/document/acspc-031941.pdf.*
*Numbers are estimates based on 2008 statistics.

GENDER DIFFERENCES

Cancer

Men
- More men than women die from cancer-related deaths each year.
- Mortality rate from lung cancer is higher in men than in women.
- Esophageal cancer is more prevalent in men than in women.
- Cancer with the highest incidence among men is prostate cancer.
- Men are more likely to develop liver cancer than women.
- Head and neck cancer occurs more frequently in men than in women.
- Bladder cancer is at least three times more common in men than in women.

Women
- Cancer with the highest death rate among women is lung cancer.
- Nonsmoking women are at a greater risk than nonsmoking men of developing lung cancer.
- Cancer with the highest incidence among women is breast cancer.
- Thyroid cancer is more prevalent in women than in men.
- Women are less likely to have colon cancer screenings than men.

INFORMATICS IN PRACTICE

Managing Cancer Patients' Symptoms

- When patients arrive at some clinics, they are handed a tablet computer. While in the waiting room or chemotherapy infusion unit, with the touch of a finger they select the symptoms they have been experiencing.
- Health care providers can review the information and provide care aimed at managing the patient's specific symptoms.
- After the visit, the notes are stored in the patient's electronic health record. This system can assist with quality of care by determining if standards of care were followed.

been on the rise. Notably, the incidence of melanoma rose faster than that for any other malignancy in the United States.[1]

Cancer incidence overall is higher in men than women. Gender differences in incidence and in death rates for specific cancers are presented in Tables 16-1 and 16-2 and the Gender Differences box. Although mortality rates from all cancers combined are on the decline, cancer is still the second most common cause of death in the United States (heart disease is the most common). However, in people less than 85 years of age, cancer is the leading cause of death. Annually about 580,350 Americans are expected to die as a result of cancer, which is more than 1500 people per day.[1]

Considerable progress has been made in controlling cancer for long periods. More than 13.7 million Americans are alive today who have a history of cancer. The overall 5-year survival rate is now 68% (19% increase over the past 30 years).[1] This statistic represents Americans living with cancer, including those who are disease free, in remission, or undergoing treatment. (Cancer survivors are discussed in this chapter on p. 281.)

Statistics are helpful in describing the scope of cancer as a public health problem, but they cannot describe the combined physiologic, psychologic, and social impact of cancer on individual patients and their caregivers pand families. Considerable apprehension is associated with a cancer diagnosis, proportion-

ately more than with other chronic diseases such as heart disease. Despite advances in treatment and care, a great deal of anxiety and fear continue to be associated with a diagnosis of cancer. Education of health care professionals and the public is essential to promote realistic attitudes about cancer and cancer treatment.

You are in a strategic position to lead efforts at changing attitudes about cancer. Furthermore, you can also (1) assist individuals in decreasing their risk of cancer development, (2) help patients comply with cancer management regimens, and (3) support patients and their families as they cope with the effects of cancer and related treatment. You need to be knowledgeable about specific types of cancer, treatment options, management of side effects of therapy, and supportive therapies for cancer.

BIOLOGY OF CANCER

Two major dysfunctions in the process of cancer development are defective cell proliferation (growth) and defective cell differentiation.

Defect in Cell Proliferation

Normally, most tissues contain a population of undifferentiated cells known as stem cells. These stem cells ultimately differentiate and become mature, functioning cells of that tissue and only that tissue.

Cell proliferation originates in the stem cell and begins when the stem cell enters the cell cycle (Fig. 16-1). The time from

FIG. 16-1 Cell life cycle and metabolic activity. Generation time is the period from *M* phase to *M* phase. Cells not in the cycle but capable of division are in the resting phase *(G₀).*

when a cell enters the cell cycle to when the cell divides into two identical cells is called the *generation time of the cell.* A mature cell continues to function until it degenerates and dies.

All of the body's cells are controlled by an intracellular mechanism that determines when cell proliferation is necessary. Under normal conditions, a state of dynamic equilibrium is constantly maintained (i.e., cell proliferation equals cell degeneration or death). Normally the process of cell division and proliferation is activated only in the presence of cell degeneration or death. Cell proliferation also occurs if the body has a physiologic need for more cells. For example, a normal increase in white blood cell (WBC) count occurs in the presence of infection.

Another mechanism for proliferation control in normal cells is *contact inhibition.* Normal cells respect the boundaries and territory of the cells surrounding them. They will not invade a territory that is not their own. The neighboring cells are thought to inhibit cell growth through the physical contact of the surrounding cell membranes. Cancer cells grown in tissue culture are characterized by loss of contact inhibition. These cells have no regard for cell boundaries and grow on top of one another and also on top of or between normal cells.

The rate of normal cell proliferation (from the time of cell birth to the time of cell death) differs in each body tissue. In some tissues, such as bone marrow, hair follicles, and epithelial lining of the gastrointestinal (GI) tract, the rate of cell proliferation is rapid. In other tissues, such as myocardium and cartilage, cell proliferation does not occur or is slow.

A common misconception regarding the characteristics of cancer cells is that the rate of proliferation is more rapid than that of normal body cells. Cancer cells usually proliferate at the same rate as the normal cells of the tissue from which they arise. However, cancer cells respond differently than normal cells to the intracellular signals that regulate the state of dynamic equilibrium. The difference is that proliferation of the cancer cells is indiscriminate and continuous. Sometimes they produce more than two cells at the time of mitosis. In this way, there is con-

tinuous growth of a tumor mass: $1 \times 2 \times 4 \times 8 \times 16$ and so on. This is termed the *pyramid effect.* The time required for a tumor mass to double in size is known as its *doubling time.*

Defect in Cell Differentiation

Cell differentiation is normally an orderly process that progresses from a state of immaturity to a state of maturity. Because all body cells are derived from the fertilized ova, all cells have the potential to perform all body functions. As cells differentiate, this potential is repressed, and the mature cell is capable of performing only specific functions (see eFig. 16-1 on the website for this chapter). With cell differentiation, there is a stable and orderly phasing out of cell potential. Under normal conditions the differentiated cell is stable and will not *dedifferentiate* (i.e., revert to a previous undifferentiated state).

Genetic Link

Cancer involves the malfunction of genes that control differentiation and proliferation. Two types of normal genes that can be affected by mutation are *protooncogenes* and *tumor suppressor genes.* **Protooncogenes** are normal cell genes that are important regulators of normal cell processes. Protooncogenes promote growth, whereas tumor suppressor genes suppress growth. Mutations that alter the expression of protooncogenes can activate them to function as **oncogenes** (tumor-inducing genes).

The protooncogene has been described as the genetic lock that keeps the cell in its mature functioning state. When this lock is "unlocked," as may occur through exposure to *carcinogens* (agents that cause cancer) or oncogenic viruses, genetic alterations and mutations occur. The abilities and properties that the cell had in fetal development are again expressed. Oncogenes can change a normal cell to a malignant one. This cell regains a fetal appearance and function. For example, some cancer cells produce new proteins, such as those characteristic of the embryonic and fetal periods of life. These proteins, located on the cell membrane, include carcinoembryonic antigen (CEA) and α-fetoprotein (AFP). They can be detected in human blood by laboratory studies (see Role of the Immune System later in this chapter). Other cancer cells, such as small cell carcinoma of the lung, produce hormones (see Complications Resulting from Cancer later in this chapter) that are ordinarily produced by cells arising from the same embryonic cells as the tumor cells.

Tumor suppressor genes function to regulate cell growth. They prevent cells from going through the cell cycle. Mutations that alter tumor suppressor genes make them inactive, resulting in a loss of their tumor-suppressing action. Examples of tumor suppressor genes are *BRCA1* and *BRCA2*. Alterations in these genes increase a person's risk for breast and ovarian cancer. Another tumor suppressor gene is the *APC* gene. Alterations in this gene increase a person's risk for familial adenomatous polyposis, which is a precursor for colorectal cancer (see Chapter 43). Mutations in the *p53* tumor suppressor gene have been found in many cancers, including bladder, breast, colorectal, esophageal, liver, lung, and ovarian cancers.

Development of Cancer

The following is a theoretical model of the development of cancer. The cause and development of each type of cancer are likely to be multifactorial. A common misbelief is that the development of cancer is a rapid, haphazard event. However, cancer is usually an orderly process that occurs over time and has several stages: initiation, promotion, and progression[2] (Fig. 16-2).

Initiation. Cancer cells arise from normal cells as a result of changes in genes. The first stage, *initiation*, involves a mutation in the cell's genetic structure. A *mutation* is any change in the usual DNA sequence.

Genetic Link

Gene mutations can occur in two different ways: *inherited* from a parent (passed from one generation to the next) or *acquired* during a person's lifetime. (Mutations are discussed in Chapter 13.)

About 5% of all cancers or the predisposition to the cancer is inherited from one's parents. These genetic alterations lead to a high risk of developing a specific type of cancer. However, most cancers do not result from inherited genes but are acquired from damage to genes occurring during one's lifetime.[1] An acquired mutation is passed on to all cells that develop from that single cell. The damaged cell may die or repair itself. However, if cell death or repair does not occur before cell division, the cell will replicate into daughter cells, each with the same genetic alteration.

Carcinogens. Many **carcinogens** (cancer-causing agents capable of producing cell alterations) are detoxified by protective enzymes and are harmlessly excreted. If this protective mechanism fails, carcinogens can enter the cell's nucleus and alter deoxyribonucleic acid (DNA). Carcinogens may be chemical, radiation, or viral.

Chemical Carcinogens. Chemicals were identified as cancer-causing agents in the latter part of the eighteenth century when Percival Pott noted that chimney sweeps had a higher incidence of cancer of the scrotum associated with exposure to soot residue in chimneys. As the years passed, many chemical agents have been identified as carcinogens. People exposed to certain chemicals over time have a greater incidence of certain cancers than others. The long latency period from the time of exposure

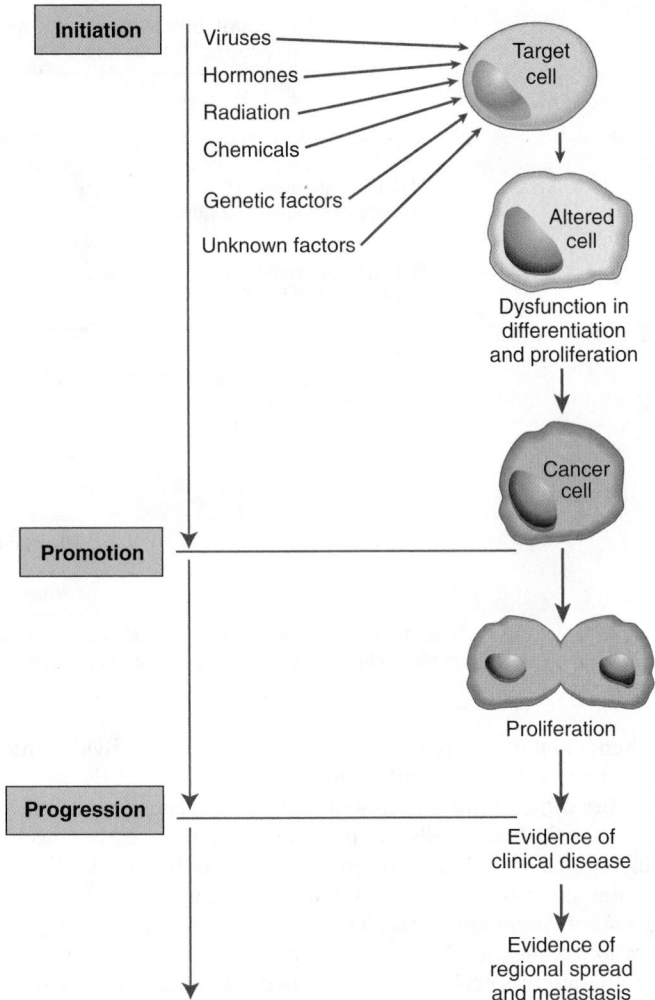

FIG. 16-2 Process of cancer development.

to the development of cancer makes it difficult to identify cancer-causing chemicals.

Certain drugs have also been identified as carcinogens. Drugs that are capable of interacting with DNA (e.g., alkylating agents) and immunosuppressive agents have the potential to cause cancer. The use of alkylating agents (e.g., cyclophosphamide [Cytoxan]), either alone or in combination with radiation therapy, has been associated with an increased incidence of acute myelogenous leukemia in people treated for Hodgkin's lymphoma, non-Hodgkin's lymphoma, and multiple myeloma. These *secondary leukemias* are resistant to chemotherapy. Secondary leukemia has also been observed in people who have undergone transplant surgery and taken immunosuppressive drugs.

Radiation. Radiation can cause cancer in almost any body tissue. When cells are exposed to a source of radiation, damage occurs to DNA. Certain malignancies have been correlated with radiation as a carcinogenic agent:

- Leukemia, lymphoma, thyroid cancer, and other cancers increased in incidence in the general population of Hiroshima and Nagasaki after the atomic bomb explosions.
- A higher incidence of bone cancer occurs in people exposed to radiation in certain occupations, such as radiologists, radiation chemists, and uranium miners.

Ultraviolet (UV) radiation has long been associated with melanoma and squamous and basal cell carcinoma of the skin. Skin cancer is the most common type of cancer among whites in the United States. Of great concern is the increase in the incidence of melanoma. Although the cause of melanoma is probably multifactorial, UV radiation secondary to sunlight exposure is linked to the development of melanoma.

Viral Carcinogens. Certain DNA and ribonucleic acid (RNA) viruses, termed *oncogenic,* can transform the cells they infect and induce malignant transformation. Viruses have been identified as causative agents of cancer in animals and humans. Burkitt's lymphoma has consistently shown evidence of Epstein-Barr virus (EBV) in vitro. People with acquired immunodeficiency syndrome (AIDS), which is caused by human immunodeficiency virus (HIV), have a high incidence of Kaposi sarcoma (see Chapter 15). Other viruses that have been linked to the development of cancer include hepatitis B virus, which is associated with hepatocellular carcinoma; and human papillomavirus, which is believed to induce lesions that progress to squamous cell carcinomas, such as cervical, anal, and head and neck cancers.[3]

Promotion. A single alteration of the genetic structure of the cell is not sufficient to result in cancer. However, the odds of cancer development are increased with the presence of promoting agents. *Promotion,* the second stage in the development of cancer, is characterized by the reversible proliferation of the altered cells. An increase in the altered cell population further increases the likelihood of additional mutations.

An important distinction between initiation and promotion is that the activity of promoters is reversible. This is a key concept in cancer prevention. Promoting factors include such agents as dietary fat, obesity, cigarette smoking, and alcohol consumption. Changing a person's lifestyle to modify these risk factors can reduce the chance of cancer development. Approximately half of cancer-related deaths in the United States are related to tobacco use, unhealthy diet, physical inactivity, and obesity.[1]

Several promoting agents have activity against specific types of body tissues. Therefore these agents tend to promote specific kinds of cancer. For example, cigarette smoke is a promoting agent in bronchogenic carcinoma and, in conjunction with alcohol intake, promotes esophageal and bladder cancers.

Some carcinogens, termed *complete carcinogens,* are capable of both initiating and promoting the development of cancer. Cigarette smoke is an example of a complete carcinogen capable of initiating and promoting cancer.

A period of time, ranging from 1 to 40 years, elapses between the initial genetic alteration and the actual clinical evidence of cancer. This period, called the *latent* period, includes both the initiation and the promotion stages in the natural history of cancer. The variation in the length of time that elapses before the cancer becomes clinically evident is associated with the mitotic rate of the tissue of origin and environmental factors. In most cancers the process of developing cancer is years or even decades in length.

For the disease process to become clinically evident, the cells must reach a critical mass. A tumor that is 1.0 cm (0.4 inch) (the size usually detectable by palpation) contains 1 billion cancer cells. A 0.5-cm tumor is the smallest that can be detected by current diagnostic measures, such as magnetic resonance imaging (MRI).

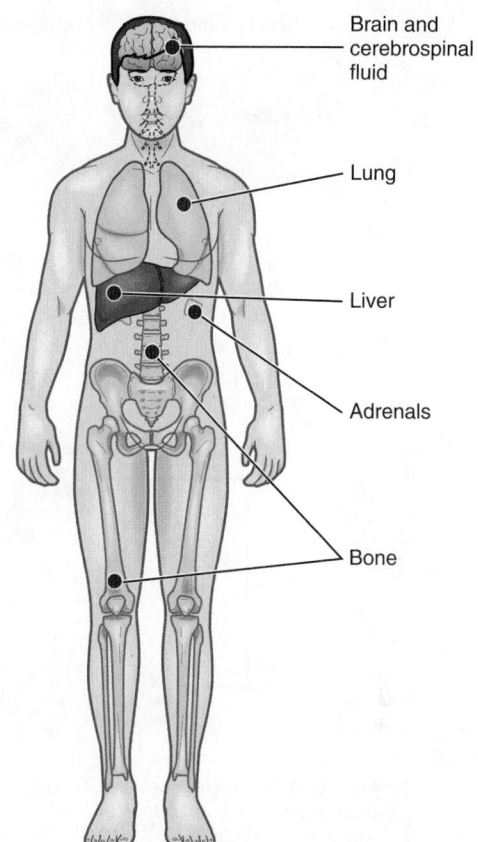

Brain and cerebrospinal fluid

Lung

Liver

Adrenals

Bone

FIG. 16-3 Main sites of metastasis.

Progression. *Progression* is the final stage in the natural history of a cancer. This stage is characterized by increased growth rate of the tumor, increased invasiveness, and **metastasis**—spread of the cancer to a distant site. Certain cancers seem to have an affinity for a particular tissue or organ as a site of metastasis (e.g., colon cancer often spreads to the liver). Other cancers (e.g., melanoma) are unpredictable in their pattern of metastasis. The most frequent sites of metastasis are lungs, liver, bone, brain, and adrenal glands (Fig. 16-3).

Metastasis is a multistep process beginning with the rapid growth of the primary tumor (Fig. 16-4). As the tumor increases in size, development of its own blood supply is critical to its survival and growth. The process of the formation of blood vessels within the tumor itself is termed **tumor angiogenesis** and is facilitated by tumor angiogenesis factors produced by the cancer cells.

Tumor cells are able to detach from the primary tumor, invade the tissue surrounding the tumor, and penetrate the walls of lymph or vascular vessels for metastasis to a distant site. Once free from the primary tumor, metastatic tumor cells frequently travel to distant organ sites via lymphatic and hematogenous routes.

Hematogenous metastasis involves several steps beginning with primary tumor cells penetrating blood vessels. These tumor cells then enter the circulation, travel through the body, and adhere to and penetrate small blood vessels of distant organs. Most tumor cells do not survive this process and are destroyed by mechanical mechanisms (e.g., turbulence of blood flow) and cells of the immune system. However, the formation of a combination of tumor cells, platelets, and fibrin deposits may protect some tumor cells from destruction in blood vessels.

FIG. 16-4 The pathogenesis of cancer metastasis. To produce metastases, tumor cells must detach from the primary tumor and enter the circulation, survive in the circulation to arrest in the capillary bed, adhere to capillary basement membrane, gain entrance into the organ parenchyma, respond to growth factors, proliferate and induce angiogenesis, and evade host defenses.

In the lymphatic system, tumor cells may be "trapped" in the first lymph node confronted or they may bypass regional lymph nodes and travel to more distant lymph nodes, a phenomenon termed *skip metastasis*. This phenomenon is exhibited in malignancies such as esophageal cancers. It also raises questions about the effectiveness of dissection of regional lymph nodes for the prevention of distant metastases.[4]

Tumor cells that do survive the process of metastasis must create an environment in the distant organ site that is conducive to their growth and development. Growth and development are facilitated by the tumor cells' ability to evade cells of the immune system and to produce a vascular supply within the metastatic site similar to that developed in the primary tumor site. Vascularization is critical to the supply of nutrients to the metastatic tumor and to the removal of waste products. Vascularization of the metastatic site is also facilitated by tumor angiogenesis factors produced by the cancer cells.

Role of the Immune System

This section is limited to a discussion of the role of the immune system in the recognition and destruction of tumor cells. (For a detailed discussion of immune system function, see Chapter 14.)

The immune system has the potential to distinguish cells that are normal (self) from abnormal (nonself) cells. For example, cells of transplanted organs can be recognized by the immune system as *nonself* and thus elicit an immune response. This response can ultimately result in the rejection of the organ. Similarly, cancer cells can be perceived as nonself and elicit an immune response resulting in their rejection and destruction. However, unlike transplanted cells, cancer cells arise from

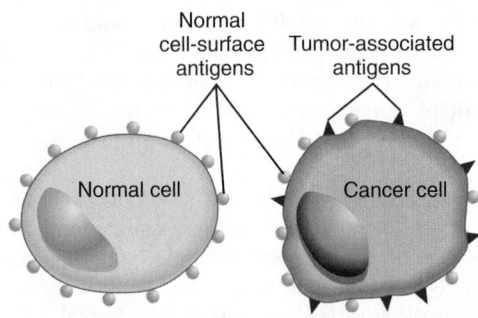

FIG. 16-5 Tumor-associated antigens appear on the cell surface of malignant cells.

normal human cells and, although they are mutated and thus different, the immune response that is mounted against cancer cells may be inadequate to effectively kill them.

Cancer cells may display altered cell-surface antigens as a result of malignant transformation. These antigens are termed **tumor-associated antigens (TAAs)** (Fig. 16-5). It is believed that one of the functions of the immune system is to respond to TAAs. The immune system's response to antigens of the malignant cells is termed **immunologic surveillance**. In this process lymphocytes continuously check cell-surface antigens and detect and destroy cells with abnormal or altered antigenic determinants. Under most circumstances, immune surveillance prevents these transformed cells from developing into clinically detectable tumors.

Immune response to malignant cells involves cytotoxic T cells, natural killer (NK) cells, macrophages, and B cells. *Cytotoxic T cells* play a dominant role in resisting tumor growth.

These cells are capable of killing tumor cells. T cells are also important in the production of cytokines (e.g., interleukin-2 [IL-2] and γ-interferon), which stimulate T cells, NK cells, B cells, and macrophages.

Natural killer (NK) cells are able to directly lyse tumor cells spontaneously without any prior sensitization. These cells are stimulated by γ-interferon and IL-2 (released from T cells), resulting in increased cytotoxic activity.

Monocytes and *macrophages* have several important roles in tumor immunity. Macrophages can be activated by γ-interferon (produced by T cells) to become nonspecifically lytic for tumor cells. Macrophages also secrete cytokines, including interleukin-1 (IL-1), tumor necrosis factor (TNF), and colony-stimulating factors (CSFs). The release of IL-1, coupled with the presentation of the processed antigen, stimulates T lymphocyte activation and production. α-Interferon augments the killing ability of NK cells. TNF causes hemorrhagic necrosis of tumors and exerts cytocidal or cytostatic actions against tumor cells. CSFs regulate the production of various blood cells in the bone marrow and stimulate the function of various WBCs.

B cells can produce specific antibodies that bind to tumor cells. These antibodies are often detectable in the patient's serum and saliva.

Escape Mechanisms From Immunologic Surveillance. The process by which cancer cells evade the immune system is termed *immunologic escape*. Theorized mechanisms by which cancer cells can escape immunologic surveillance include (1) suppression of factors that stimulate T cells to react to cancer cells; (2) weak surface antigens allowing cancer cells to "sneak through" immunologic surveillance; (3) the development of tolerance of the immune system to some tumor antigens; (4) suppression of the immune response by products secreted by cancer cells; (5) the induction of suppressor T cells by the tumor; and (6) blocking antibodies that bind TAAs, thus preventing their recognition by T cells (Fig. 16-6).

Oncofetal Antigens and Tumor Markers. *Oncofetal antigens* are a type of tumor antigen. They are found on both the surfaces and the inside of cancer cells and fetal cells. These antigens are an expression of the shift of cancerous cells to a more immature metabolic pathway, an expression usually associated with embryonic or fetal periods of life. The reappearance of fetal antigens in malignant disease is not well understood, but it is believed to occur as a result of the cell regaining its embryonic capability to differentiate into many different cell types.

Examples of oncofetal antigens are carcinoembryonic antigen (CEA) and α-fetoprotein (AFP). CEA is found on the surfaces of cancer cells derived from the GI tract and from normal cells from the fetal gut, liver, and pancreas. Normally, it disappears during the last 3 months of fetal life. CEA was originally isolated from colorectal cancer cells. However, elevated CEA levels have also been found in nonmalignant conditions (e.g., cirrhosis of the liver, ulcerative colitis, heavy smoking).

These oncofetal antigens can be used as *tumor markers* that may be clinically useful to monitor the effect of therapy and indicate tumor recurrence. However, oncofetal antigens are not 100% specific for tumor recurrence. Tumor markers are affected by various factors that need to be accounted for when reviewing these results. For example, the persistence of elevated preoperative CEA titers after surgery indicates that the tumor is not completely removed. A rise in CEA levels after chemotherapy or radiation therapy may indicate recurrence or spread of the cancer and may be affected by chronic lung or liver disease and smoking.

AFP is produced by malignant liver cells and fetal liver cells. AFP levels have also been found to be elevated in some cases of testicular carcinoma, viral hepatitis, and nonmalignant liver disorders. AFP has diagnostic value in primary cancer of the liver (hepatocellular cancer), but it is also produced when metastatic liver growth occurs. The detection of AFP is of value in tumor detection and determination of tumor progression.

Other examples of oncofetal antigens are CA-125 (found in ovarian carcinoma), CA-19-9 (found in pancreatic and gallbladder cancer), prostate-specific antigen (PSA) (found in prostate cancer), and CA-15-3 and CA-27-29 (found in breast cancer). Molecular markers for specific tumors include kRAS (expression of oncogene in colon cancer), epidermal growth factor receptor (EGFR) often overexpressed in lung cancer, and human epidermal growth factor receptor 2 (HER-2) expression in breast cancer.

BENIGN VERSUS MALIGNANT NEOPLASMS

Tumors can be classified as benign or malignant. In general, *benign neoplasms* are well differentiated, and malignant neoplasms range from well differentiated to undifferentiated. The ability of malignant tumor cells to invade and metastasize is the major difference between benign and malignant neoplasms. Other differences are presented in Table 16-3.

CLASSIFICATION OF CANCER

Tumors can be classified according to anatomic site, histology (grading), and extent of disease (staging). Tumor classification

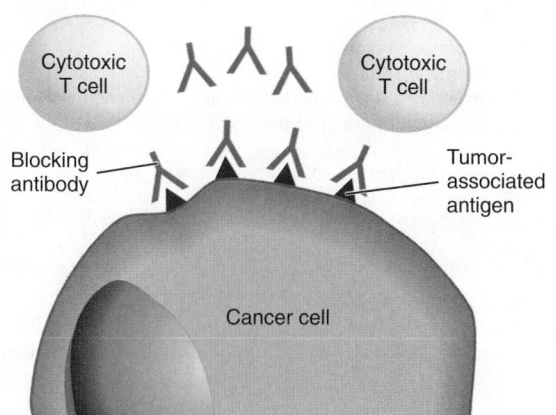

FIG. 16-6 Blocking antibodies prevent T cells from interacting with tumor-associated antigens and from destroying the malignant cell.

TABLE 16-3	COMPARISON OF BENIGN AND MALIGNANT NEOPLASMS	
Characteristic	**Benign**	**Malignant**
Encapsulated	Usually	Rarely
Differentiated	Normally	Poorly
Metastasis	Absent	Capable
Recurrence	Rare	Possible
Vascularity	Slight	Moderate to marked
Mode of growth	Expansive	Infiltrative and expansive
Cell characteristics	Fairly normal, similar to parent cells	Cells abnormal, become more unlike parent cells

systems are intended to stratify risk. Classification systems provide a standardized way to (1) communicate the status of the cancer to all members of the health care team, (2) assist in determining the most effective treatment plan, (3) evaluate the treatment plan, (4) predict prognosis, and (5) compare like groups for statistical purposes.

Anatomic Site Classification

In the *anatomic classification* of tumors, the tumor is identified by the tissue of origin, the anatomic site, and the behavior of the tumor (i.e., benign or malignant) (Table 16-4). *Carcinomas* originate from embryonal *ectoderm* (skin and glands) and *endoderm* (mucous membrane linings of the respiratory tract, GI tract, and genitourinary [GU] tract) (see eFig. 16-1 on the website for this chapter). *Sarcomas* originate from embryonal *mesoderm* (connective tissue, muscle, bone, and fat). Lymphomas and leukemias originate from the hematopoietic system.

Histologic Classification

In **histologic grading** of tumors, the appearance of cells and the degree of differentiation are evaluated pathologically. For many tumor types, four grades are used to evaluate abnormal cells based on the degree to which the cells resemble the tissue of origin. Tumors that are poorly differentiated (undifferentiated) have a worse prognosis than those that are closer in appearance to the normal tissue of origin (well differentiated):

Grade I: Cells differ slightly from normal cells (mild dysplasia) and are well differentiated (low grade).

Grade II: Cells are more abnormal (moderate dysplasia) and moderately differentiated (intermediate grade).

Grade III: Cells are very abnormal (severe dysplasia) and poorly differentiated (high grade).

Grade IV: Cells are immature and primitive *(anaplasia)* and undifferentiated; cell of origin is difficult to determine (high grade).

Grade X: Grade cannot be assessed.

Extent of Disease Classification

Classifying the extent and spread of disease is termed **staging**. This classification system is based on the anatomic extent of disease rather than on cell appearance. Although there are similarities in the staging of various cancers, there are many differences for specific types of cancer.

Clinical Staging. The clinical staging classification system determines the anatomic extent of the malignant disease process by stages:

Stage 0: cancer in situ

Stage I: tumor limited to the tissue of origin; localized tumor growth

Stage II: limited local spread

Stage III: extensive local and regional spread

Stage IV: metastasis

Clinical staging has been used as a basis for staging a variety of tumor types, including cancer of the cervix (see Table 54-11) and Hodgkin's lymphoma (see Fig. 31-14). Other malignant diseases (e.g., leukemia) do not use this staging approach.

TNM Classification System. The *TNM classification system* (Table 16-5) is used to determine the anatomic extent of the disease involvement according to three parameters: tumor size and invasiveness (T), presence or absence of regional spread to the lymph nodes (N), and metastasis to distant organ sites (M). (Examples of the TNM classification system can be found in Tables 28-17 and 52-6.) TNM staging cannot be applied to all malignancies. For example, the leukemias are not solid tumors and therefore cannot be staged using these guidelines. **Carcinoma in situ (CIS)** refers to a neoplasm whose cells are localized and show no tendency to invade or metastasize to other tissues. CIS has its own designation in the system (T_{is}), since it has all the histologic characteristics of cancer except invasion—a primary feature of the TNM staging system.

Staging of the disease can be performed initially and at several evaluation points. Clinical staging is done at the completion of the diagnostic workup to guide effective treatment selection. Examples of diagnostic studies that may be performed to assess for extent of disease include radiologic studies, such as bone and liver scans; ultrasonography; and computed tomography (CT), MRI, and positron emission tomography (PET) scans.

Surgical staging refers to the extent of the disease as determined by surgical excision, exploration, and/or lymph node

TABLE 16-4 ANATOMIC CLASSIFICATION OF TUMORS

Site	Benign	Malignant
Epithelial Tissue Tumors*	-oma	-carcinoma
Surface epithelium	Papilloma	Carcinoma
Glandular epithelium	Adenoma	Adenocarcinoma
Connective Tissue Tumors†	-oma	-sarcoma
Fibrous tissue	Fibroma	Fibrosarcoma
Cartilage	Chondroma	Chondrosarcoma
Striated muscle	Rhabdomyoma	Rhabdomyosarcoma
Bone	Osteoma	Osteosarcoma
Nervous Tissue Tumors	-oma	-oma
Meninges	Meningioma	Meningeal sarcoma
Nerve cells	Ganglioneuroma	Neuroblastoma
Hematopoietic Tissue Tumors		
Lymphoid tissue	—	Hodgkin's lymphoma, non-Hodgkin's lymphoma
Plasma cells	—	Multiple myeloma
Bone marrow	—	Lymphocytic and myelogenous leukemia

*Body surfaces, lining of body cavities, and glandular structures.
†Supporting tissue, fibrotic tissue, and blood vessels.

TABLE 16-5 TNM CLASSIFICATION SYSTEM

Primary Tumor (T)

T_0	No evidence of primary tumor
T_{is}	Carcinoma in situ
T_{1-4}	Ascending degrees of increase in tumor size and involvement
T_x	Tumor cannot be measured or found

Regional Lymph Nodes (N)

N_0	No evidence of disease in lymph nodes
N_{1-4}	Ascending degrees of nodal involvement
N_x	Regional lymph nodes unable to be assessed clinically

Distant Metastases (M)

M_0	No evidence of distant metastases
M_{1-4}	Ascending degrees of metastatic involvement, including distant nodes
M_x	Cannot be determined

NOTE: For examples of TNM classification system applied to diseases, see Fig. 31-14 and Table 28-17.

sampling. For example, a laparotomy and a splenectomy may be performed in staging of Hodgkin's lymphoma. During a staging laparotomy, lymph node biopsies may be done, and margins of any masses may be marked with metal clips for use during radiation therapy. However, exploratory surgical staging is being used less frequently as noninvasive diagnostic technology becomes increasingly sophisticated.

After the extent of the disease is determined, the stage classification is not changed. The original description of the extent of the tumor remains part of the record. If additional treatment is needed, or if treatment fails, retreatment staging is done to determine the extent of the disease process before retreatment. "Restaging" classification (rTNM) is differentiated from the stage at diagnosis, since the clinical significance may be quite different.

In addition to tumor classification systems, other rating scales can be used to describe and document the status of patients with cancer at the time of diagnosis, treatment, and retreatment and at each follow-up examination. For example, the Karnofsky Functional Performance Scale and the Katz Index of Independence in Activities of Daily Living describe patient performance in terms of function. (These scales are presented in eTables 16-1 and 16-2 available on the website for this chapter.)

PREVENTION AND EARLY DETECTION OF CANCER

As a nurse, you have an essential role in the prevention and early detection of cancer. Eliminating risk factors reduces the incidence of cancer. For example, rates of smoking-related cancers (e.g., lung and head and neck cancers) have declined following reduction in smoking rates.[1] Early detection and prompt treatment are responsible for increased survival rates in patients with cancer. Colonoscopy is important in reducing colon cancer mortality both by early detection of colon cancers and by prevention (e.g., excision of adenomatous polyps).[5]

Teach patients and the public about cancer prevention and early detection, including the following:

- Reduce or avoid exposure to known or suspected carcinogens and cancer-promoting agents, including cigarette smoke and sun exposure.
- Eat a balanced diet that includes vegetables and fresh fruits (see Fig. 40-1 and Table 40-1), whole grains, and adequate amounts of fiber. Reduce dietary fat and preservatives, including smoked and salt-cured meats containing high nitrite concentrations.
- Limit alcohol intake.
- Participate in regular exercise (i.e., 30 minutes or more of moderate physical activity five times weekly).
- Maintain a healthy weight.
- Obtain adequate, consistent periods of rest (at least 6 to 8 hours per night).
- Eliminate, reduce, or change the perception of stressors and enhance the ability to effectively cope with stressors (see Chapter 7).
- Have a regular physical examination that includes a health history. Be familiar with your own family history and your risk factors for cancer.
- Learn and follow the American Cancer Society's recommended cancer screening guidelines for breast, colon, cervical, and prostate cancer. (See eTable 16-3 on the website for this chapter.)

TABLE 16-6   SEVEN WARNING SIGNS OF CANCER

C hange in bowel or bladder habits
A sore that does not heal
U nusual bleeding or discharge from any body orifice
T hickening or a lump in the breast or elsewhere
I ndigestion or difficulty in swallowing
O bvious change in a wart or mole
N agging cough or hoarseness

HEALTHY PEOPLE

Prevention and Early Detection of Cancer

- Limit alcohol use.
- Get regular physical activity.
- Maintain a normal body weight.
- Obtain regular colorectal screenings.
- Avoid cigarette smoking and other tobacco use.
- Get regular mammography screening and Pap tests.
- Use sunscreen with a sun protection factor of 15 or higher.
- Practice healthy dietary habits, such as reduced fat consumption and increased fruit and vegetable consumption.

- Learn and practice self-examination (e.g., breast or testicular self-examination).
- Know the seven warning signs of cancer, and inform the health care provider if they are present (Table 16-6). (These actually detect fairly advanced disease.)
- Seek immediate medical care if you notice a change in what is normal for you and if cancer is suspected.

The goals of public education are to (1) motivate people to recognize and modify behaviors that may negatively affect health and (2) encourage awareness of and participation in health-promoting behaviors. When you teach about cancer, try to minimize the fear that surrounds the diagnosis.

Diagnosis of Cancer

When a patient has a possible diagnosis of cancer, it is a stressful time for the patient and the family. Patients may undergo several days to weeks of diagnostic studies. During this time, fear of the unknown may be more stressful than the actual diagnosis of cancer. Patients may also be overwhelmed or confused by the need for multiple diagnostic studies and consultations. Help to coordinate care between multiple specialists and explain the purpose of required tests and any special preparation needed for them.

While patients are waiting for the results of diagnostic studies, be available to actively listen to their concerns. Their anxiety may arise from myths and misconceptions about cancer (e.g., cancer is a "death sentence," cancer treatment is worse than the illness). Correcting those misconceptions can help to minimize their anxiety.

Learn to recognize your own discomfort during difficult conversations. Avoid communication patterns that may hinder exploration of feelings and meaning, such as providing false reassurances (e.g., "It's probably nothing"), redirecting the discussion (e.g., "Let's discuss that later"), generalizing (e.g., "Everyone feels this way"), and using overly technical language as a means of distancing yourself from the patient. These self-protective strategies deny patients the opportunity to share the meaning of their experience. In addition, they can jeopardize your ability to build a trusting relationship with your patients.

During this time of high anxiety, the patient may need repeated explanations of the diagnostic workup. Include as much information as needed by the patient and the family. Give clear, understandable explanations and reinforce them as needed. Written information is helpful for reinforcement of verbal information.

A diagnostic plan for the person suspected of having cancer includes the health history (including a history of present illness), identification of risk factors, the physical examination, and specific diagnostic studies. For many people, cancer is initially diagnosed after the findings of an abnormal screening test (e.g., mass on mammogram). For others, they are alerted to the presence of cancer by a presenting symptom or cluster of symptoms (e.g., cough and hemoptysis, anorexia and weight loss).

Concentrate on risk factors for malignancy such as family or personal history of cancer, exposure to or use of known carcinogens (e.g., cigarette smoking, occupational pollutants or chemicals, radiation exposure), diseases characterized by chronic inflammation or immunosuppression (e.g., ulcerative colitis), and drug ingestion (e.g., hormone therapy, previous anticancer therapies). Also assess factors that may warrant additional supportive care during therapy, including alcohol or recreational drug use, living situation, social support, and coping strategies for perceived stressors.

Diagnostic studies depend on the suspected primary or metastatic site(s) of the cancer. (Specific procedures as they relate to each body system are discussed in the respective assessment chapters.) Examples of diagnostic studies include the following:

- Cytology studies (e.g., Papanicolaou [Pap] test, bronchial washings)
- Tissue biopsy
- Chest x-ray
- Complete blood count, chemistry profile
- Liver function studies (e.g., aspartate aminotransferase [AST])
- Endoscopic examination: upper GI, sigmoidoscopy, or colonoscopy (including guaiac test for occult blood)
- Radiographic studies (e.g., mammography, ultrasound, CT scan, MRI)
- Radioisotope scans (e.g., bone, lung, liver, brain)
- PET scan (Fig. 16-7)
- Tumor markers (e.g., CEA, AFP, PSA, CA-125)
- Genetic markers (e.g., *BRCA1, BRCA2*)
- Molecular receptor status (e.g., estrogen and progesterone receptors)
- Bone marrow examination (if a hematolymphoid malignancy is suspected or to document metastatic disease)

Biopsy. A *biopsy* is the removal of a tissue sample for pathologic analysis. Various methods are used to obtain a biopsy depending on the location and size of the suspected tumor. *Percutaneous biopsy* is commonly performed for tissue that can be safely reached through the skin. *Endoscopic biopsy* may be used for lung or other intraluminal lesions (esophageal, colon, bladder). When a tumor is not easily accessible, a *surgical procedure* (laparotomy, thoracotomy, craniotomy) is often necessary to obtain a piece of the tumor tissue. Many radiographic techniques may be used in conjunction with the biopsy procedure (e.g., CT, MRI, ultrasound-guided biopsy, stereotactic biopsy, fluoroscopic-assisted biopsy) to improve tissue localization.

FIG. 16-7 Positron emission tomography (PET) scan before treatment **(A)** indicating metastasis throughout the body. PET scan after treatment **(B)** indicates the effects of therapy. More radioactive material accumulates in areas that have higher levels of activity. This often corresponds to areas of disease and shows up as brighter spots on the PET scan.

Various types and sizes of biopsy needles are available and are selected according to the type of tissue to be sampled. *Fine-needle aspiration* (FNA) may be accomplished with a small-gauge aspiration needle that provides cells from the mass for cytologic examination. *Large-core biopsy* cutting needles deliver an actual piece of tissue (core) that can be analyzed with the advantage of preserving the histologic architecture of the tissue specimen. *Excisional biopsy* involves the surgical removal of the entire lesion, lymph node, nodule, or mass. Therefore it is therapeutic as well as diagnostic. If an excisional biopsy is not feasible, an *incisional biopsy* (partial excision) may be performed with a scalpel or dermal punch.

Pathologic evaluation of a tissue sample is the only definitive means to diagnose a malignancy. The pathologist examines the tissue to determine whether it is benign or malignant, the anatomic tissue from which the tumor arises *(histology),* and the degree of cell differentiation *(histologic grade).* Other information that can be obtained includes the extent of malignant involvement (size of tumor and depth), evidence of invasiveness (extracapsular, lymphatic), adequacy of surgical excision (positive or negative surgical margin status), nuclear grade (mitotic rate), and special staining techniques that may provide insight into responsiveness of the tumor to treatment or disease behavior (receptor status, tumor markers).

COLLABORATIVE CARE

Treatment Goals

The goals of cancer treatment are cure, control, and palliation (Fig. 16-8). Primary factors that determine what therapy is used are the tumor histology and staging outcomes. Other important factors are the patient's physiologic status (e.g., presence of

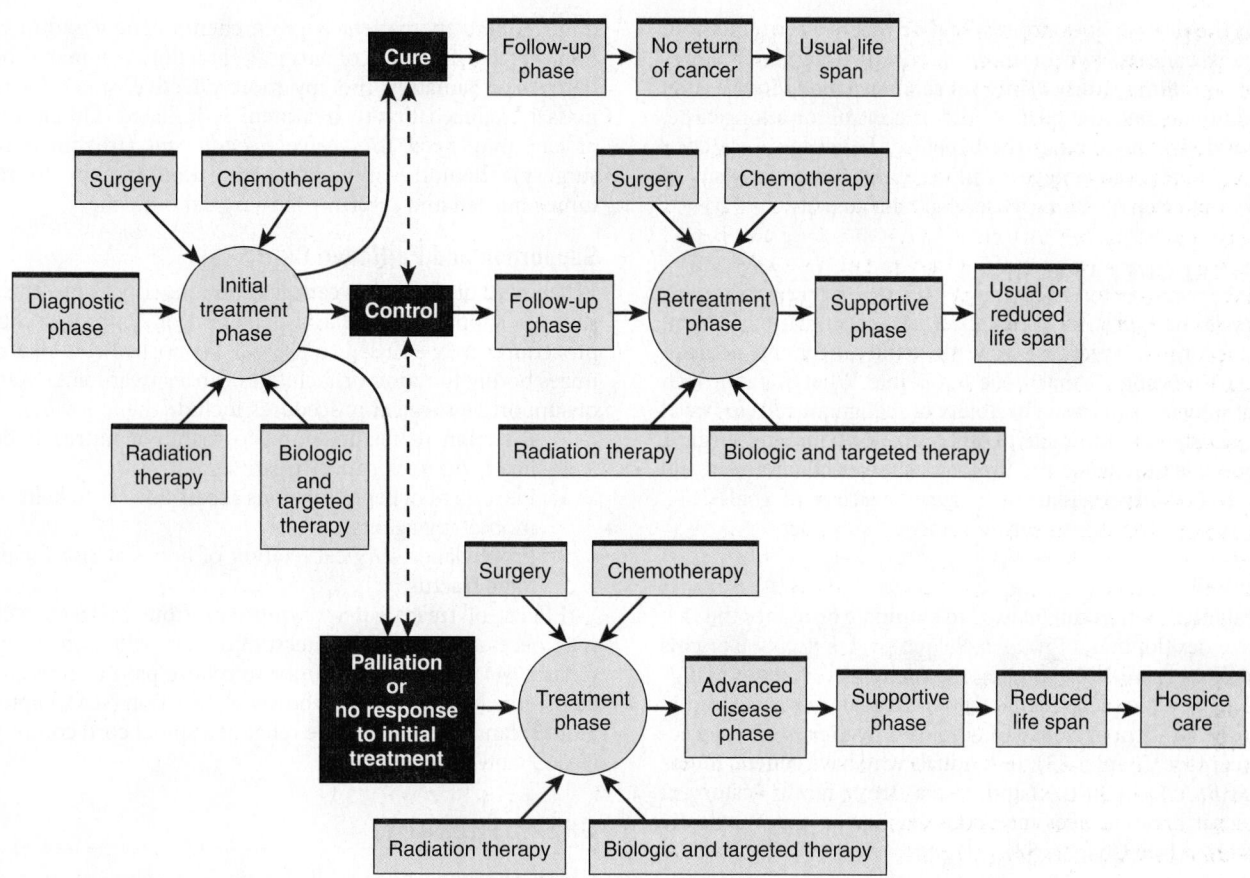

FIG. 16-8 Goals of cancer treatment.

co-morbid illnesses), psychologic status, and personal desires (e.g., active treatment versus palliation of symptoms). These factors influence the modalities chosen for treatment (i.e., surgery, radiation therapy, chemotherapy, biologic and targeted therapy), how therapies are sequenced, and the length of time the treatment is prescribed.

A variety of evidence-based cancer treatment guidelines have been developed to guide the appropriate treatment recommendations for individual patients. Some examples include guidelines of the American Society of Clinical Oncology (ASCO) *(www.asco.org)* and the National Comprehensive Cancer Network (NCCN) *(www.nccn.org).*

Cure. When caring for the patient and family with cancer, know the treatment goals to appropriately communicate with, teach, and support the patient. When *cure* is the goal, treatment is expected to have the greatest chance of disease eradication. Curative cancer therapy differs according to the particular cancer being treated and may involve local therapies (i.e., surgery or radiation) alone or in combination, with or without periods of adjunctive systemic therapy (i.e., chemotherapy). For example, basal cell carcinoma of the skin is usually cured by surgical removal of the lesion and/or several weeks of radiation therapy. In the treatment plan for acute promyelocytic leukemia (which has curative potential), several chemotherapy drugs are given on a scheduled basis over many months to several years. Testicular cancer can be cured with a combination of surgery, chemotherapy, and radiation.

Although there is no benchmark that ensures "cure" for most malignancies, in general the risk for recurrent disease is highest after treatment completion, and gradually decreases the longer the patient remains disease free following treatment. Cancers with a higher mitotic rate (e.g., testicular cancer) are less likely to recur than cancers with slower mitotic rates (e.g., postmenopausal breast cancer). Therefore the timeframe to consider a person "cured" may differ according to the tumor and its characteristics.

Control. *Control* is the goal of the treatment plan for many cancers that cannot be completely eradicated, but are responsive to anticancer therapies. As with other chronic illnesses (e.g., diabetes mellitus, heart failure), cancer can be maintained for long periods with therapy. Examples include multiple myeloma and chronic lymphocytic leukemia (see Chapter 31). Patients may undergo an initial course of treatment followed by maintenance therapy for as long as the disease is responding. Patients are monitored closely for early signs and symptoms of disease recurrence or progression and the cumulative effects of therapy. Evidence of tumor resistance (such as disease progression) may warrant changing to an alternative therapy.

Palliation. *Palliation* is the treatment goal when relief or control of symptoms and the maintenance of a satisfactory quality of life are the primary objectives. An example of treatment in which palliation is the primary goal includes using radiation therapy or chemotherapy to reduce tumor size and relieve subsequent symptoms such as the pain of bone metastasis.

The goals of cure, control, and palliation are achieved through the use of four treatment modalities for cancer: surgery, radiation therapy, chemotherapy, and biologic and targeted therapy. Each can be used alone or in any combination during initial treatment or as maintenance therapy, as well as in retreatment if the disease does not respond or recurs after remission. For many cancers, two or more of the treatment modalities (known as *multimodality therapy* or *combined modality therapy*) are used to achieve the goal of cure or control for a long time. Multimodality therapy has the benefit of being more effective (because it takes advantage of more than one mechanism of action), but often at the expense of greater toxicity.

SURGICAL THERAPY

Surgery is the oldest form of cancer treatment. The treatment of choice for many years was to remove the cancer and as much of the surrounding normal tissue as possible. What this approach did not fully consider was the ability of malignant cells to travel from the original tumor site to other locations, making surgical cure possible only when the tumor was localized and relatively small. Today surgery is used to meet a variety of goals (Fig. 16-9), and the trend is toward less radical surgeries.

Prevention

Surgical intervention can be used to eliminate or reduce the risk of cancer development. Prophylactic removal of nonvital organs has been successful in reducing the incidence of some malignancies. For example, patients who have adenomatous familial polyposis may benefit from a total colostomy to prevent colorectal cancer (see Chapter 43). Individuals who have genetic mutations of *BRCA1* or *BRCA2* and have a strong family history of early-onset breast cancer may consider having a prophylactic mastectomy (see Chapter 52).

Cure or Control

When the goal is cure or control, the objective is to remove all or as much resectable tumor as possible while sparing normal tissue. Examples of surgical procedures used for cure or control of cancer include radical neck dissection, mastectomy, orchiectomy, thyroidectomy, nephrectomy, hysterectomy, and oophorectomy.

A *debulking* or *cytoreductive procedure* may be used if the tumor cannot be completely removed (e.g., a tumor attached to a vital organ). When this occurs, as much tumor as possible is removed and the patient is given chemotherapy and/or radiation therapy. This type of surgical procedure can make chemotherapy or radiation therapy more effective, since the tumor mass is reduced before treatment is initiated. Other times, a patient may need to receive *neoadjuvant* (treatment before surgery) chemotherapy and/or radiation therapy to reduce tumor burden and improve the surgical outcome.

Supportive and Palliative Care

When cure or control of cancer is no longer possible, the focus shifts to supportive care and palliation of symptoms. Surgical procedures may be used to provide supportive care that maximizes bodily function or facilitates cancer treatment. Examples of supportive surgical procedures include the following:

- Insertion of feeding tube to maintain nutrition during head and neck cancer treatment
- Placement of central venous access devices to deliver chemotherapy agents
- Prophylactic surgical fixation of bones at risk for pathologic fracture

Effects of treatment or symptoms from metastatic cancer may necessitate surgical intervention for palliation. Examples include (1) debulking of tumor to relieve pain or pressure, (2) colostomy for the relief of a bowel obstruction (see Chapter 43), and (3) laminectomy for the relief of a spinal cord compression (see Chapter 61).

CHEMOTHERAPY

Chemotherapy is the use of chemicals as a systemic therapy for cancer. In the 1940s nitrogen mustard, a chemical warfare agent used in World Wars I and II, was used in the treatment of lymphoma and acute leukemia. In the 1970s chemotherapy was established as an effective treatment modality for cancer. Chemotherapy is now a mainstay of cancer treatment for most solid tumors and hematologic malignancies (e.g., leukemias, lymphomas). Chemotherapy can offer cure for some cancers, control other cancers for long periods, and in some instances offer palliative relief of symptoms when cure or control is no longer possible (Fig. 16-10).

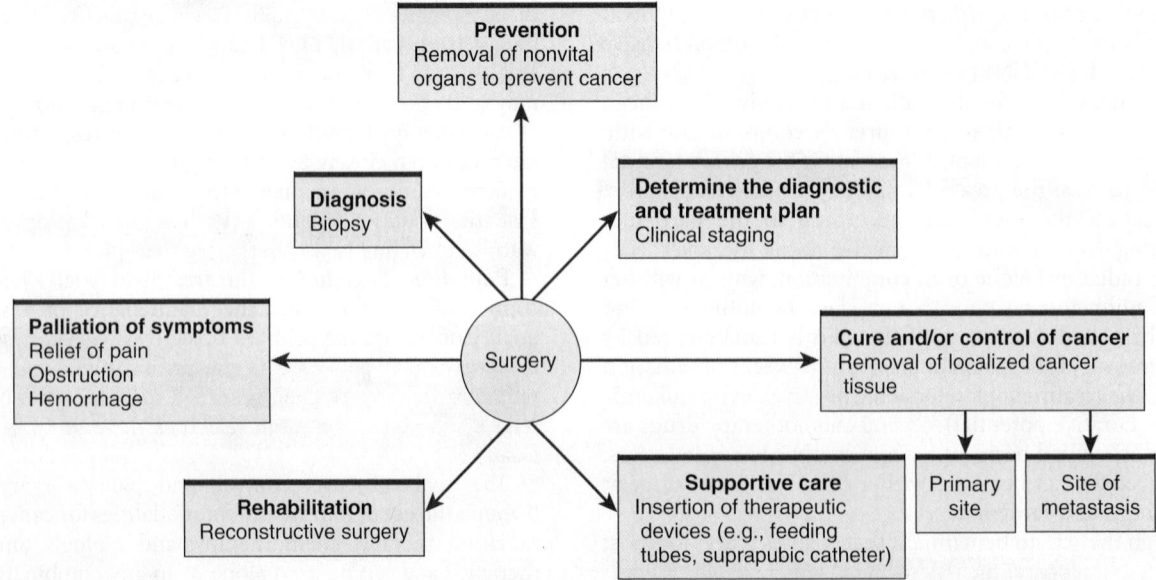

FIG. 16-9 Role of surgery in the treatment of cancer.

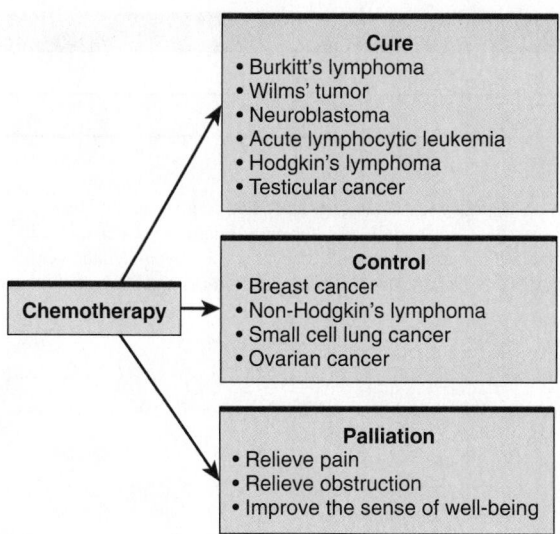

FIG. 16-10 Goals of chemotherapy.

The two major categories of chemotherapy drugs are cell cycle phase–nonspecific and cell cycle phase–specific drugs. *Cell cycle phase–nonspecific chemotherapy drugs* have their effect on the cells during all phases of the cell cycle, including the process of cell replication and proliferation and the resting phase (G_0). *Cell cycle phase–specific chemotherapy drugs* exert their most significant effects during specific phases of the cell cycle (i.e., when cells are in the process of cell replication or proliferation during G_1, S, G_2, or M). Cell cycle phase–specific and cell cycle phase–nonspecific agents are often administered in combination to maximize effectiveness by using agents that function by differing mechanisms and throughout the cell cycle.

When cancer first begins to develop, most of the cells are actively dividing. As the tumor increases in size, more cells become inactive and convert to a resting state (G_0). Because most chemotherapy agents are most effective against dividing cells, cells can escape death by staying in the G_0 phase. A major challenge is to overcome the effect of resistant resting and non-cycling cells.

Effect on Cells

The goal of chemotherapy is to eliminate or reduce the number of malignant cells in the primary tumor and metastatic tumor site(s). All cells (cancer cells and normal cells) enter the cell cycle for replication and proliferation (see Fig. 16-1). The effects of the chemotherapy drugs are described in relation to the cell cycle.

Classification of Chemotherapy Drugs

Chemotherapy drugs are classified in general groups according to their molecular structure and mechanisms of action (Table 16-7). Each drug in a particular classification has many similarities. However, there are major differences in how the drugs work and the unique side effects associated with drugs in each class.

TABLE 16-7   DRUG THERAPY

Chemotherapy Drugs

Mechanisms of Action	Examples
Alkylating Agents *Cell Cycle Phase–Nonspecific Agents* Damage DNA by causing breaks in the double-stranded helix. If repair does not occur, cells will die immediately (cytocidal) or when they attempt to divide (cytostatic).	bendamustine (Treanda), busulfan (Myleran), chlorambucil (Leukeran), cyclophosphamide (Cytoxan, Neosar), dacarbazine (DTIC-Dome), ifosfamide (Ifex), mechlorethamine (Mustargen), melphalan (Alkeran), temozolomide (Temodar), thiotepa (Thioplex)
Nitrosoureas *Cell Cycle Phase–Nonspecific Agents* Like alkylating agents, break DNA helix, interfering with DNA replication. Cross blood-brain barrier.	carmustine (BiCNU, Gliadel), lomustine (CeeNU), streptozocin (Zanosar)
Platinum Drugs *Cell Cycle Phase–Nonspecific Agents* Bind to DNA and RNA, miscoding information and/or inhibiting DNA replication, and cells die.	carboplatin (Paraplatin), cisplatin (Platinol-AQ), oxaliplatin (Eloxatin)
Antimetabolites *Cell Cycle Phase–Specific Agents* Mimic naturally occurring substances, thus interfering with enzyme function or DNA synthesis. Primarily act during S phase. Purine and pyrimidine are building blocks of nucleic acids needed for DNA and RNA synthesis. • Interfere with purine metabolism. • Interfere with pyrimidine metabolism. • Interfere with folic acid metabolism. • Interfere with DNA synthesis.	 cladribine (Leustatin), clofarabine (Clolar), fludarabine (Fludara), mercaptopurine (Purinethol), nelarabine (Arranon), pentostatin (Nipent), thioguanine capecitabine (Xeloda); cytarabine (ara-C [Cytosar-U, DepoCyt]), floxuridine (FUDR), 5-fluorouracil (5-FU [Adrucil]), gemcitabine (Gemzar) methotrexate (Rheumatrex, Trexall), pemetrexed (Alimta) hydroxyurea (Hydrea, Droxia)

NOTE: Many of these drugs are irritants or vesicants that require special attention during administration to avoid extravasation. It is important to know this information about a drug before administering it.

Continued

TABLE 16-7 DRUG THERAPY—cont'd

Chemotherapy Drugs

Mechanisms of Action	Examples
Antitumor Antibiotics *Cell Cycle Phase–Nonspecific Agents* Bind directly to DNA, thus inhibiting the synthesis of DNA and interfering with transcription of RNA.	bleomycin (Blenoxane), dactinomycin (Cosmegen), daunorubicin (Cerubidine, DaunoXome), doxorubicin (Adriamycin, Rubex, Doxil), epirubicin (Ellence), idarubicin (Idamycin), mitomycin (Mutamycin), mitoxantrone (Novantrone), plicamycin (Mithracin), valrubicin (Valstar)
Mitotic Inhibitors *Cell Cycle Phase–Specific Agents* *Taxanes* Antimicrotubule agents that interfere with mitosis. Act during the late G_2 phase and mitosis to stabilize microtubules, thus inhibiting cell division.	albumin-bound paclitaxel (Abraxane), docetaxel (Taxotere), paclitaxel (Taxol)
Vinca Alkaloids Act in M phase to inhibit mitosis.	vinblastine (Velban), vincristine (Oncovin), vinorelbine (Navelbine)
Others Microtubular inhibitors.	estramustine (Emcyt), ixabepilone (Ixempra), eribulin (Halaven)
Topoisomerase Inhibitors *Cell Cycle Phase–Specific Agents* Inhibit topoisomerases (normal enzymes) that function to make reversible breaks and repairs in DNA that allow for flexibility of DNA in replication.	etoposide (VePesid), irinotecan (Camptosar), teniposide (Vumon), topotecan (Hycamtin)
Corticosteroids *Cell Cycle Phase–Nonspecific Agents* Disrupt the cell membrane and inhibit synthesis of protein. Decrease circulating lymphocytes, inhibit mitosis, depress immune system, increase sense of well-being.	cortisone (Cortone), dexamethasone (Decadron), hydrocortisone (Cortef), methylprednisolone (Medrol), prednisone
Hormone Therapy *Cell Cycle Phase–Nonspecific Agents* *Antiestrogens* Selectively attach to estrogen receptors, causing down-regulation of them and inhibiting tumor growth. Also known as selective estrogen receptor modulators (SERMs).	fulvestrant (Faslodex), raloxifene (Evista), tamoxifen (Nolvadex), toremifene (Fareston)
Estrogens Interfere with hormone receptors and proteins.	estradiol (Estrace), estramustine (Emcyt), estrogen (Menest)
Aromatase Inhibitors Inhibit aromatase, an enzyme that converts adrenal androgen to estrogen.	anastrozole (Arimidex), exemestane (Aromasin), letrozole (Femara)
Miscellaneous Enzyme derived from the yeast Erwinia used to deplete the supply of asparagine (amino acid) for leukemic cells that are dependent on an exogenous source of this amino acid. Inhibits protein synthesis.	Erwinia asparaginase, L-asparaginase (Elspar)
Causes changes in DNA in leukemia cells and leads to cell death. Suppresses mitosis. Appears to alter DNA, RNA, and protein.	arsenic trioxide (Trisenox) procarbazine (Matulane, Natulan)

Preparation of Chemotherapy

It is important to know the specific guidelines for administration of chemotherapy drugs. In addition, it is important to understand that drugs may pose an occupational hazard to health care professionals who do not follow safe handling guidelines. A person preparing, transporting, or administering chemotherapy may absorb the drug through inhalation of particles when reconstituting a powder and through skin contact from exposure to droplets or powder from oral agents. There may also be some risk in handling the body fluids and excretions of people receiving chemotherapy immediately after administration for 48 hours. Only those personnel specifically trained in

chemotherapy handling techniques should be involved with the preparation and administration of antineoplastic agents.

Guidelines for the safe handling of chemotherapy agents have been developed by the National Institute for Occupational Safety and Health (available at *www.cdc.gov/niosh/docs/2004-165*) and the Occupational Safety and Health Administration (OSHA) and the Oncology Nursing Society (ONS).[6]

Methods of Administration

Chemotherapy can be administered by multiple routes (Table 16-8). With advances in drug formulation techniques, more oral chemotherapy agents are available.

TABLE 16-8 DRUG THERAPY

Methods of Chemotherapy Administration

Method	Examples
Oral	cyclophosphamide (Cytoxan), capecitabine (Xeloda), temozolomide (Temodar)
Intramuscular	bleomycin (Blenoxane)
Intravenous	doxorubicin (Adriamycin), vincristine (Oncovin), cisplatin (Platinol), 5-fluorouracil (5-FU), paclitaxel (Taxol)
Intracavitary (pleural, peritoneal)	Radioisotopes, alkylating agents, methotrexate
Intrathecal	methotrexate (preservative free), cytarabine
Intraarterial	dacarbazine, 5-FU, methotrexate
Perfusion	Alkylating agents
Continuous infusion	5-FU, methotrexate, cytarabine
Subcutaneous	cytarabine
Topical	5-FU cream

FIG. 16-11 Extravasation injury from infiltration of chemotherapy drug.

The IV route is most common. Major concerns associated with the IV administration of antineoplastic drugs include venous access difficulties, device- or catheter-related infection, and *extravasation* (infiltration of drugs into tissues surrounding the infusion site) causing local tissue damage (Fig. 16-11).

Many chemotherapy drugs are either irritants or vesicants. *Irritants* will damage the intima of the vein, causing phlebitis and sclerosis and limiting future peripheral venous access, but will not cause tissue damage if infiltrated. However, vesicants, if inadvertently infiltrated into the skin, may cause severe local tissue breakdown and necrosis. It is extremely important to monitor for and promptly recognize symptoms associated with extravasation of a vesicant and to take immediate action if it occurs. Immediately turn off the infusion and follow protocols for drug-specific extravasation procedures to minimize further tissue damage.

Although pain is the cardinal symptom of extravasation, it can occur without causing pain. Other signs of extravasation are swelling, redness, and vesicles on the skin. After a few days the tissue may begin to ulcerate and necrose. Complications of extravasation include sepsis, scarring, contractures, joint pain, and nerve loss.[6] Vesicants may cause partial- or full-thickness loss of skin. Patients may need surgical intervention varying from debridement to skin grafting.

To minimize the associated physical discomforts, emotional distress, and risks of infection and infiltration, IV chemotherapy can be administered by a *central venous access device* (CVAD).

CVADs are placed in large blood vessels and permit frequent, continuous, or intermittent administration of chemotherapy, biologic and targeted therapy, and other products, thus avoiding multiple venipunctures for vascular access. (CVADs are discussed in Chapter 17 on p. 309.)

Regional Chemotherapy Administration

Regional treatment with chemotherapy involves delivery of the drug directly to the tumor site. The advantage of this method is that higher concentrations of the drug can be delivered to the tumor with reduced systemic toxicity. Several regional delivery methods have been developed, including intraarterial, intraperitoneal, intrathecal or intraventricular, and intravesical bladder chemotherapy.

Intraarterial Chemotherapy. Intraarterial chemotherapy delivers the drug to the tumor via the arteries supplying the tumor. This method has been used for the treatment of osteogenic sarcoma; cancers of the head and neck, bladder, brain, and cervix; melanoma; primary liver cancer; and metastatic liver disease. One method of intraarterial drug delivery involves the surgical placement of a catheter that is subsequently connected to an external infusion pump or an implanted infusion pump for infusion of the chemotherapy agent.

Intraperitoneal Chemotherapy. Intraperitoneal chemotherapy involves the delivery of chemotherapy to the peritoneal cavity for treatment of peritoneal metastases from primary colorectal and ovarian cancers and malignant ascites. Temporary Silastic catheters (Tenckhoff, Hickman, and Groshong) are percutaneously or surgically placed into the peritoneal cavity for short-term administration of chemotherapy. Alternatively, an implanted port can be used to administer chemotherapy intraperitoneally. Chemotherapy is generally infused into the peritoneum in 1 to 2 L of fluid and allowed to *dwell* in the peritoneum for 1 to 4 hours. After the *dwell time*, the fluid is drained from the peritoneum.

Intrathecal or Intraventricular Chemotherapy. Cancers that metastasize to the central nervous system (CNS) are difficult to treat because the blood-brain barrier often prevents distribution of chemotherapy to this area. One method used to treat metastasis to the CNS is intrathecal chemotherapy. This method involves a lumbar puncture and injection of chemotherapy into the subarachnoid space. However, this method has resulted in incomplete distribution of the drug in the CNS.

To ensure more uniform distribution of chemotherapy, an Ommaya reservoir is often inserted. An Ommaya reservoir is a Silastic, dome-shaped disk with an extension catheter that is surgically implanted through the cranium into a lateral ventricle. In addition to more consistent drug distribution, the Ommaya reservoir precludes the need for repeated, painful lumbar punctures.

Intravesical Bladder Chemotherapy. *Intravesical bladder chemotherapy* involves instillation of chemotherapy into the bladder. The chemotherapy agent is instilled into the bladder via a urinary catheter and retained for 1 to 3 hours.

Effects of Chemotherapy on Normal Tissues

Chemotherapy agents cannot selectively distinguish between normal cells and cancer cells. Chemotherapy-induced side effects are the result of the destruction of normal cells, especially those that are rapidly proliferating such as those in the bone marrow, the lining of the GI system, and the integumentary system (skin, hair, and nails)[7] (Table 16-9). The general and

TABLE 16-9 CELLS WITH RAPID RATE OF PROLIFERATION

Cells and Generation Time	Effect of Cell Destruction
Bone marrow stem cell, 6-24 hr	Myelosuppression (infection, bleeding, anemia)
Neutrophils, 12 hr	Leukopenia, infection
Epithelial cells lining the gastrointestinal tract, 12-24 hr	Anorexia, mucositis (including stomatitis, esophagitis), nausea and vomiting, diarrhea
Cells of the hair follicle, 24 hr	Alopecia
Ova or testes, 24-36 hr	Reproductive dysfunction

drug-specific adverse effects of these drugs are classified as acute, delayed, or chronic.

Acute toxicity occurs during and immediately after drug administration and includes anaphylactic and hypersensitivity reactions, extravasation or a flare reaction, anticipatory nausea and vomiting, and cardiac dysrhythmias.

Delayed effects are numerous and include delayed nausea and vomiting, mucositis, alopecia, skin rashes, bone marrow suppression, altered bowel function (diarrhea or constipation), and a variety of cumulative neurotoxicities.

Chronic toxicities involve damage to organs such as the heart, liver, kidneys, and lungs. Chronic toxicities can be either long-term effects that develop during or immediately after treatment and persist, or late effects that are absent during treatment and manifest later.

Some side effects fall into more than one category. For example, nausea and vomiting can be both acute and delayed.

Treatment Plan

Although single-drug chemotherapy is sometimes prescribed, combining agents in multidrug regimens has proven to be more effective in managing most cancers. The regimens with multiple agents involve drugs with different mechanisms of action and varying toxicity profiles. However, when chemotherapy agents are used in combination, patients can experience an increase in toxicities.

Drug regimens are selected based on evidence supporting their use in specific cancers. Sometimes they are customized to meet the needs of an individual patient. Chemotherapy is most effective when the tumor burden is low, therapy is not interrupted, and the patient receives the intended dose. The dose of each drug is based on the individual's body weight and height using the body surface area calculation.

Mutation of cancer cells within the tumor can result in cells that are resistant to chemotherapy. With the use of multiple drugs that work at different places in the cell cycle, cancer cells can be more effectively killed. Thus mutation and resistance of cancer cells can be prevented.

RADIATION THERAPY

Along with surgery, radiation therapy is one of the oldest methods of cancer treatment. It was first used by Emil Grubbe (a medical student) to treat an ulcerating breast cancer in 1896 (although the patient responded locally, she died later of metastatic disease). The observation that radiation exposure caused tissue damage led scientists to explore the use of radiation to treat tumors. The hypothesized association was that if radiation

exposure resulted in the destruction of highly mitotic skin cells, it could be used in a controlled way to prevent the continued growth of cancer cells.

It was not until the 1960s that sophisticated equipment and treatment planning facilitated the delivery of adequate radiation doses to tumors and tolerable doses to normal tissues. Currently, about half of all cancer patients receive radiation therapy at some point in their treatment.[8]

Effects of Radiation

Radiation is energy that is emitted from a source and travels through space or some material. Delivery of high-energy beams, when absorbed into tissue, produces ionization of atomic particles. The energy in ionizing radiation acts to break the chemical bonds in DNA. The DNA is damaged, resulting in cell death.

Different types of ionizing radiation are used to treat cancer, including *electromagnetic radiation* (i.e., x-rays, gamma rays) and *particulate radiation* (alpha particles, electrons, neutrons, protons). High-energy x-rays (photons) are generated by an electric machine, such as a linear accelerator (sometimes referred to as a *linac*).

Technologic advances have expanded and refined the sources and methods of delivering radiation therapy, thus offering more accurate and less invasive radiation treatment options. Most radiation centers in the United States currently use megavoltage linear accelerator technology. Larger radiation facilities may offer a combination of machines that permit expanded options for patients at one treatment site.

Principles of Radiobiology

As the radiation beam passes through the treatment field, energy is deposited. *Low-energy beams* (such as electrons) expend energy quickly on impact with matter. Therefore they penetrate only a short distance. (They are clinically useful in treating superficial skin lesions.) *High-energy beams* (such as photons) have greater depth of penetration, not attaining full intensity until they reach a certain depth. Therefore they are suitable for delivering optimal doses to internal targets while sparing the skin. The principles of radiation therapy are guided by cell response to radiation, known as the four *R*s of radiobiology (see eTable 16-4 on the website for this chapter).

Technically, all cancer cells could be killed with radiation given in high enough doses. However, to avoid serious toxicity and long-term complications of treatment, radiation to surrounding healthy tissue must be limited to the *maximal tolerated dose* for that specific tissue. Advances in planning and in delivery technology (such as *intensity-modulated radiation therapy [IMRT]* and *image-guided radiation therapy [IGRT]*) have greatly improved the ability to deliver maximal doses to the target volume while sparing critical structures (e.g., spinal cord, carotid arteries, optic chiasm) as much as possible.

Historically, the radiation dose was expressed in units called *rads* (radiation absorbed doses). Current nomenclature is *gray* (Gy) or centigray (cGy). A *centigray* is equivalent to 1 rad, and 100 centigray equals 1 gray.

Once the total dose to be delivered is determined, that dose is divided into daily *fractions*. Doses between 180 and 200 cGy/day are considered *standard fractionation*, typically delivered once a day Monday through Friday for a period of 2 to 8 weeks (depending on the desired total dose). Other treatment schedules may be prescribed based on principles of radiobiologic effect. High daily doses of radiation may be given with fewer

TABLE 16-10 TUMOR RADIOSENSITIVITY*

High Radiosensitivity
- Ovarian dysgerminoma
- Testicular seminoma
- Hodgkin's lymphoma
- Non-Hodgkin's lymphoma
- Wilms' tumor
- Neuroblastoma

Moderate Radiosensitivity
- Oropharyngeal carcinoma
- Esophageal carcinoma
- Breast adenocarcinoma
- Uterine and cervical carcinoma
- Prostate carcinoma
- Bladder carcinoma

Mild Radiosensitivity
- Soft tissue sarcomas (e.g., chondrosarcoma)
- Gastric adenocarcinoma
- Renal adenocarcinoma
- Colon adenocarcinoma

Poor Radiosensitivity
- Osteosarcoma
- Malignant melanoma
- Malignant glioma
- Testicular nonseminoma

*Radiosensitivity is the relative susceptibility of cells and tissues to the effects of radiation.

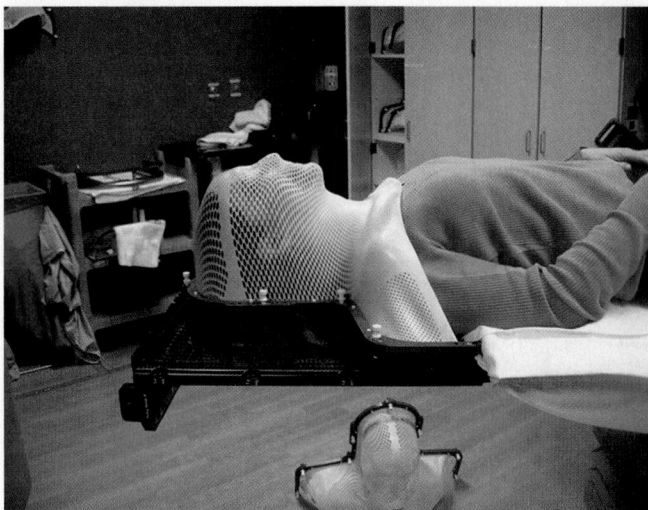

FIG. 16-12 Immobilization device. A head holder and an immobilization mask may be used to ensure accurate positioning for daily treatment of head and neck cancer.

fractions *(hypofractionated),* lower doses may be given more than once daily *(hyperfractionated),* or standard doses may be delivered twice daily over a shortened treatment time *(accelerated fractionation).*

The amount of time required for the manifestations of radiation damage is determined by the mitotic rate of the tissue, with rapidly proliferating tissues being more sensitive. Rapidly dividing cells in the GI tract, oral mucosa, and bone marrow die quickly and exhibit early acute responses to radiation. Tissues with slowly proliferating cells, such as cartilage, bone, and kidneys, manifest later responses to radiation. This differential rate of cell death explains the timing of clinical manifestations related to radiation therapy.

Certain cancers are more susceptible to the effects of radiation than others (Table 16-10). In responsive tumors (such as lymphomas), even a large tumor burden is affected by radiation therapy. In less responsive tumors, a large tumor burden may result in a slower and perhaps incomplete response. Localized prostate cancer responds very slowly to radiation (several months after treatment is completed).

Simulation and Treatment Planning

Simulation is a process by which the radiation treatment fields are defined, filmed, and marked out on the skin. The radiation oncologist specifies the dose and volume of area to be treated. Treatment volumes include the (1) *gross target v*olume (GTV), which is the gross extent of the tumor identified by examination or imaging; (2) the *clinical target* volume (CTV), which is the GTV plus additional margin to encompass any potential microscopic or subclinical disease; and (3) the *planning target volume* (PTV), which is the GTV/CTV plus additional margin to allow for organ motion or variance in daily set-up position.[9]

During the simulation, goals of the radiation plan are met by determining the orientation and size of radiation beams, defining the location of field-shaping blocks, and outlining the field on the patient's skin. The patient is positioned on a simulator, which is a diagnostic x-ray machine that re-creates the actions of the linear accelerator. Immobilization devices (e.g., casts, bite blocks, thermoplastic face masks) are typically used to help the patient maintain a stable position (Fig. 16-12).

The target is defined using a variety of possible imaging techniques (e.g., x-rays; CT, MRI, PET scans), physical examination, and surgical reports. Under fluoroscopy or with CT-based treatment planning, the critical normal structures that will be included in the treatment field (or portal) are identified so they can be protected. A film is taken to verify the field, and marks are placed on the skin to delineate the "treatment port." Small tattoos may be placed to ensure the patient position is precisely reproduced on a daily basis.

Treatment

Radiation is used to treat a carefully defined area of the body. Since radiation only has an effect on tissues within the treatment field, it is not appropriate as the primary treatment for systemic disease. However, radiation may be used by itself, in combination with chemotherapy or surgery to treat primary tumors, or for palliation of metastatic lesions (see eTable 16-5 on the website for this chapter).

External Radiation. Radiation can be delivered externally (known as *teletherapy* or *external beam radiation therapy*) or internally *(brachytherapy).* Teletherapy *(external beam radiation)* is the most common form of radiation treatment delivery. With this technique, the patient is exposed to radiation from a megavoltage treatment machine. A linear accelerator, which generates ionizing radiation from electricity and can have multiple energies, is the most commonly used machine for delivering external beam radiation (Fig. 16-13). *Gamma knife technology* (used to deliver highly accurate stereotactic treatment to a localized treatment volume) uses a cobalt source. A cyclotron produces particulate energy, such as neutrons or protons. Proton therapy requires significant energy to generate, and only a small number of facilities in the United States are equipped to provide this treatment.

A linear accelerator may be used to deliver different types of treatment techniques (or plans). A *two-dimensional* plan is the simplest type of therapy, designed using x-rays, bony landmarks, and a simple beam arrangement. *Three-dimensional-conformal therapy* plans treatment based on three-dimensional anatomy using CT and/or other imaging, with the goal of improved dose distribution around the target volume. *Intensity-modulated radiation therapy* (IMRT) involves an inverse planning process, in which multiple beams of varying intensity deliver tailored treatment doses to a precise treatment field. It

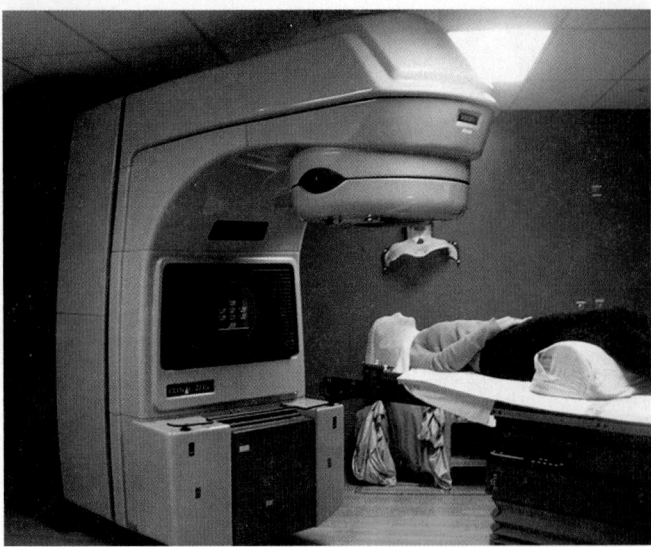

FIG. 16-13 Linear accelerator. Varian Clinac EX linear accelerator with multiple photon and electron energies available for use according to the treatment plan. Patient is positioned on radiation treatment table for treatment of head and neck cancer.

is more labor intensive to plan but has the advantage of tailoring beam intensity to optimize dose delivery to the target volume while minimizing dose to critical structures. It is particularly well suited to treating irregularly shaped fields and fields adjacent to sensitive structures (e.g., head and neck cancers).

Volumetric-modulated arc therapy (VMAT) and *tomotherapy* build on IMRT to further improve accuracy of dose delivery. With VMAT, the dose is delivered in one to three continuous arcs around the patient. An advantage of VMAT over standard IMRT is dramatically reduced treatment time, often delivering treatments in 3 to 5 minutes that previously would have taken 20 to 30 minutes.

Tomotherapy is a similar concept, but is done with a specialized linear accelerator built into a round gantry (similar to a CT scanner). The gantry rotates spirally around the patient advancing through the "doughnut," and treatment is thus delivered in "slice by slice" fashion. Dosimetry with tomotherapy appears to be comparable or superior to standard IMRT or VMAT, but is not as time efficient as VMAT.

Image-guided radiation therapy (IGRT) (sometimes referred to as *four-dimensional-conformal* therapy) further optimizes the delivery of conformal or IMRT treatment plans by addressing the element of physiologic movement over time. IGRT incorporates methods to control for physiologic movement during therapy, or anatomic changes (such as tumor shrinkage or weight loss), on a daily basis or over time during the treatment course. Imaging (usually CT, fluoroscopy, or ultrasound) may be performed in conjunction with the radiation treatment to detect any variations in tumor position or organ movement. Images are taken daily before treatment and compared with the original treatment plan so that "shifts" can be made if necessary to accommodate for any variations in target localization. Such tracking and visualization of tumor position during treatment may further improve the accuracy of dose delivery to the intended target volume. Although it is unclear how much these technologies will affect survival, IMRT treatment planning can reduce treatment toxicity, especially for prostate and head and neck cancers.

Internal Radiation. Radiation can also be delivered as brachytherapy, which means "close" or internal radiation treatment. It consists of the implantation or insertion of radioactive materials directly into the tumor (interstitial) or in close proximity to the tumor (intracavitary or intraluminal). This allows for direct delivery of radiation to the target with minimal exposure to surrounding healthy tissues. (In external radiation, the beam has to pass through external tissues to reach the internal target.) Brachytherapy is commonly used in combination with external radiation as a supplemental "boost" treatment, but may also be used as primary or adjuvant therapy.

Sources of radiation for brachytherapy include temporary sealed sources such as iridium-192 and cesium-137 and permanent sealed sources such as iodine-125, gold-198, and palladium-103. These are supplied in the form of seeds or ribbons. With a temporary implant, the source may be placed into a special catheter or metal tube that has been inserted into the tumor area. It is left in place until the prescribed dose of radiation has been reached in the calculated number of hours.

Brachytherapy may be delivered as high-dose-rate (HDR) treatment (i.e., several doses administered at varying intervals over a few minutes each time) or low-dose-rate (LDR) treatment (i.e., continuous treatment over several hours or days). A remote "afterloading" technique (i.e., the source is inserted after the applicator is in place) is designed to enhance physician and patient safety and is used for HDR brachytherapy with iridium-192. These methods are commonly used for head and neck, lung, breast, and gynecologic malignancies.

Permanent implants, such as for prostate brachytherapy, involve the insertion of radioactive seeds directly into the tumor tissue, where they remain permanently. As interstitial seeds used for treatment emit low energies with limited tissue penetration, patients are not considered radioactive. However, some initial radiation precautions may be recommended because of a small risk of seed dislodgement. Over time, the isotopes that are used decay and are no longer radioactive. The timeframe for side effects induced by treatment can be predicted based on the rate of decay for the specific isotope used.

Radiopharmaceutical therapy employs unsealed liquid radioactive sources that are administered orally as a drink, such as iodine-131 for thyroid cancer, or IV as with yttrium-90 given for refractory lymphomas or samarium-153 used to treat bone metastases.

Caring for the person undergoing brachytherapy or receiving radiopharmaceuticals requires that you be aware that the patient is emitting radioactivity. Patients with temporary implants are radioactive only while the source is in place. In patients with permanent implants, because the sources have fairly short half-lives and are weak emitters, the radioactive exposure to the outside and to others is low. These patients may be discharged with minimal precautions.

The principles of *ALARA (as low as reasonably achievable)* and *time, distance,* and *shielding* are vital to health care professional safety when caring for the person with a source of internal radiation. Organize care to limit the time spent in direct contact with the patient. To minimize anxiety and confusion, tell the patient the reason for time and distance limitations before the procedure.

The radiation safety officer will indicate how much time at a specific distance can be spent with the patient. This is determined by the dose delivered by the implant. Because the source is nonpenetrating, small differences in distance are critical.

Only care that must be delivered near the source, such as checking placement of the implant, is performed in close proximity. Use shielding, if available, and do not deliver care without wearing a film badge indicating cumulative radiation exposure. Do not share the film badge, do not wear it anywhere but at work, and return it according to the agency's protocol.

NURSING MANAGEMENT
CHEMOTHERAPY AND RADIATION THERAPY

You have an important role in helping patients deal with the side effects of chemotherapy and radiation therapy. Before initiating teaching, assess the patient's ability to process information. Customize teaching to meet the patient's and the family's learning needs.

Common side effects of chemotherapy and radiation are presented in Table 16-11. Bone marrow suppression, fatigue, GI disturbances, integumentary and mucosal reactions, and pulmonary and reproductive effects are discussed in this section.

NURSING IMPLEMENTATION
BONE MARROW SUPPRESSION. Myelosuppression is one of the most common effects of chemotherapy and, to a lesser extent, it can also occur with radiation. Treatment-induced reductions in blood cell production can result in life-threatening and distressing effects, including infection, hemorrhage, and overwhelming fatigue. The major difference in manifestations between radiation therapy and chemotherapy is that with radiation (a local therapy), only bone marrow within the treatment field is affected, whereas chemotherapy (a systemic therapy) affects bone marrow function throughout the body. Therefore effects are more profound with chemotherapy and when the two therapies are combined.

In general, the onset of bone marrow suppression is related to the life span of the type of blood cell. WBCs (especially neutrophils) are affected most acutely (within 1 to 2 weeks), platelets in 2 to 3 weeks, and red blood cells (RBCs), with a longer life span of 120 days, at a later time. The severity of myelosuppression depends on the chemotherapy drugs used, dosages of drugs, and the specific radiation treatment field. Radiation to large marrow-containing regions of the body produces the most clinically significant myelosuppression. In the adult, most of the active marrow is in the pelvis or thoracic and lumbar vertebrae.

Monitor the complete blood count, particularly the neutrophil, platelet, and RBC counts, in patients receiving chemotherapy or radiation. Typically patients experience the lowest blood cell counts (called the **nadir**) between 7 and 10 days after initiation of therapy. However, the exact onset depends on the particular drug regimen.

Neutropenia is more common in patients receiving chemotherapy than radiation therapy. Neutropenia is a serious risk factor for life-threatening infection and sepsis. Significant neutropenia will prompt treatment delay or modification (i.e., lower dosages). Take every possible measure to prevent infections in these patients. Hand hygiene is the mainstay of patient protection. Patients and their contacts (including hospital staff) should follow hand-washing guidelines. Other precautions to minimize risks from neutropenia are presented in eTable 16-6, available on the website for this chapter.

Monitor temperature routinely. Any sign of infection should be treated promptly, since fever in the setting of neutropenia is a medical emergency. WBC growth factors (i.e., filgrastim [Neupogen], pegfilgrastim [Neulasta]) are routinely used to reduce the duration of chemotherapy-induced neutropenia. They are also used as a prophylactic measure to prevent neutropenia when highly myelosuppressive chemotherapy drugs are used.[10] (Neutropenia is discussed in Chapter 31; see also the patient teaching guide in Table 31-24 and eNursing Care Plan 31-2 on the website for that chapter.)

Thrombocytopenia can result in spontaneous bleeding or major hemorrhage. Avoid invasive procedures and advise patients to avoid activities that place them at risk for injury or bleeding (including excessive straining). Risk of serious bleeding is generally not apparent until the platelet count falls below 50,000/μL. Platelet transfusions may be necessary and are usually administered when platelet counts fall below 20,000/μL. (Thrombocytopenia is discussed in Chapter 31; see also the patient teaching guide in Table 31-16 and eNursing Care Plan 31-1 on the website for that chapter.)

Anemia is common in patients undergoing either radiation therapy or chemotherapy. It generally has a later onset (about 3 to 4 months after treatment initiation). For patients with low hemoglobin levels, RBC growth factors (i.e., darbepoetin [Aranesp], epoetin [Procrit]) may be given according to clinical guidelines for use. In extreme circumstances (i.e., symptomatic anemia), RBC transfusions may also be indicated. However, in general, RBC transfusions should be avoided. (Hematopoietic growth factors are discussed later in this chapter and presented in Table 16-14 on p. 274.)

FATIGUE. *Fatigue* is the persistent subjective sense of tiredness associated with cancer and its treatment that interferes with usual day-to-day functioning. Fatigue is a nearly universal symptom affecting most patients with cancer. It is commonly reported by patients as the most distressful of treatment-related side effects. Furthermore, it may persist long after treatment has ended.

Anemia is one cause of fatigue. Other causes may be related to (1) the accumulation of toxic substances that are left in the body after cells are killed by cancer treatment, (2) the need for extra energy to repair and heal body tissue damaged by treatment, and (3) lack of sleep caused by some chemotherapy drugs. Assess for reversible causes of fatigue, such as anemia, hypothyroidism, depression, anxiety, insomnia, dehydration, or infection.[11]

Help patients recognize that fatigue is a common side effect of therapy, and encourage energy conservation strategies. Help individuals identify days or times during the day when they typically feel better, and encourage them to remain more active during that time period. Resting before activity and having others assist with work or home management may be necessary. Ignoring the fatigue or overstressing the body when fatigue is tolerable may lead to an increase in symptoms. However, maintaining exercise and activity within tolerable limits is often helpful in managing fatigue. Walking programs are a way for most patients to keep active without overtaxing themselves. Remaining active helps to improve mood and avoid the debilitating cycle of fatigue-depression-fatigue that can occur in patients with cancer.

Published guidelines for the evaluation and management of cancer-related fatigue have been developed by the NCCN[11] and are available at *www.nccn.org*.

GASTROINTESTINAL EFFECTS. The cells of the mucosal lining of the GI tract are highly proliferative, with epithelial cells being replaced every 2 to 6 days. The intestinal mucosa is one of the

TABLE 16-11   NURSING MANAGEMENT OF PROBLEMS CAUSED BY CHEMOTHERAPY AND RADIATION THERAPY

Etiology	Nursing Management	Etiology	Nursing Management
Gastrointestinal System ***Stomatitis, Mucositis, Esophagitis*** • Epithelial cells are destroyed by chemotherapy or radiation treatment when located in field (e.g., head and neck, stomach, esophagus). • Inflammation and ulceration occur due to rapid cell destruction.	• Assess oral mucosa daily and teach patient to do this. • Encourage nutritional supplements (e.g., Ensure, Carnation Instant Breakfast) if intake decreasing. • Be aware that eating, swallowing, and talking may be difficult (may require analgesics). • Instruct in diet modification as necessary (avoidance of irritating spicy or acidic foods; selection of moist, bland, and softer foods). • Encourage patient to keep oral cavity clean and moist by performing frequent oral rinses with saline or salt and soda solution. • Encourage patient to use artificial saliva to manage dryness (radiation). • Discourage use of irritants such as tobacco and alcohol. • Apply topical anesthetics (e.g., viscous lidocaine, oxethazaine).	***Constipation*** • Decreased intestinal motility is related to autonomic nervous system dysfunction. • Caused by neurotoxic effects of plant alkaloids (vincristine, vinblastine). ***Hepatotoxicity*** • Toxic effects from chemotherapy drugs (usually transient and resolve when drug is stopped).	• Instruct patient to take stool softeners as needed, eat high-fiber foods, and increase fluid intake. • Instruct patient to increase activity (e.g., walking) if tolerated. • Monitor liver function tests.
Nausea and Vomiting • Release of intracell breakdown products stimulates vomiting center in brain. • Drugs also stimulate vomiting center in brain (see Fig. 42-1). • GI lining destroyed with radiation and chemotherapy.	• Encourage patient to eat and drink when not nauseated. • Administer antiemetics prophylactically before chemotherapy and also on as-needed basis. • Instruct patient to take antiemetics on a scheduled basis for 2-3 days after highly emetogenic chemotherapy. • Use diversional activities (if appropriate).	**Hematologic System** ***Anemia*** • Bone marrow depressed secondary to therapy. • Malignant infiltration of bone marrow by cancer. ***Leukopenia*** • Depression of bone marrow secondary to chemotherapy or radiation therapy. • Infection most frequent cause of morbidity and death in cancer patients. • Respiratory and genitourinary system usual sites of infection.	• Monitor hemoglobin and hematocrit levels. • Administer iron supplements and erythropoietin. • Encourage intake of foods that promote RBC production (see Table 31-5). • Monitor WBC count, especially neutrophils. • Tell patient to report temperature elevation and any other manifestations of infection. • Teach patient to avoid large crowds and people with infections. • Administer WBC growth factors (see Table 16-14). • For patient teaching, see Table 31-24.
Anorexia • Release of TNF and IL-1 from macrophages has appetite-suppressant effect. • Therapy-induced GI effects (mucositis, nausea and vomiting, bowel disturbances) and anxiety reduce appetite.	• Monitor weight. • Encourage patient to eat small, frequent meals of high-protein, high-calorie foods. • Gently encourage patient to eat, but avoid nagging. • Recommend keeping a food diary to track daily calories and fluids. • Serve food in pleasant environment.	***Thrombocytopenia*** • Bone marrow depressed secondary to chemotherapy. • Malignant infiltration of bone marrow crowds out normal marrow. • Spontaneous bleeding can occur with platelet counts ≤20,000/μL.	• Observe for signs of bleeding (e.g., petechiae, ecchymosis). • Monitor platelet counts. • For patient teaching, see Table 31-16.
Diarrhea • From denuding of epithelial lining of intestines. • Side effect of chemotherapy. • Follows radiation to abdomen, pelvis, lumbosacral areas.	• Give antidiarrheal drugs as needed. • Encourage low-fiber, low-residue diet. • Encourage fluid intake of at least 3 L/day.	**Integumentary System** ***Alopecia*** • Destruction of hair follicles by chemotherapy or radiation to scalp. • Hair loss usually is temporary with chemotherapy, but usually permanent in response to radiation.	• Suggest ways to cope with hair loss (e.g., hair pieces, scarves, wigs). • Cut long hair before therapy. • Avoid excessive shampooing, brushing, and combing of hair. • Avoid use of electric hair dryers, curlers, and curling rods. • Discuss impact of hair loss on self-image.

TABLE 16-11   NURSING MANAGEMENT OF PROBLEMS CAUSED BY CHEMOTHERAPY AND RADIATION THERAPY—cont'd

Etiology	Nursing Management	Etiology	Nursing Management

Radiation Skin Changes (dry to moist desquamation)
• Radiation damages skin.
	• See Table 16-12 for patient management details.	**Cognitive Changes ("chemo brain")**
		• Occur during and after treatment (especially with chemotherapy).
		• Difficulties in concentration, memory lapses, trouble remembering details, taking longer to finish tasks.
		• May happen quickly and last a short time. Sometimes people have mild long-term effects.
			• Teach patients to do the following:
			  • Use detailed daily planner.
			  • Get enough sleep and rest.
			  • Exercise brain (learn something new, do word puzzles).
			  • Focus on one thing (no multitasking).

Chemotherapy-Induced Skin Changes • Hyperpigmentation • Telangiectasia • Photosensitivity • Acneiform eruptions • Acral erythema	• Alert patient to potential skin changes. • Encourage patient to avoid sun exposure. • Implement symptomatic management as needed depending on specific skin effect (e.g., application of lotions, benzoyl peroxide for acne, corticosteroid creams).	**Respiratory System** **Pneumonitis** • Radiation pneumonitis develops 2-3 mo after start of treatment. • After 6-12 mo, fibrosis occurs and is evident on x-ray. • Side effect of some chemotherapy drugs.	• Monitor for dry, hacking cough; fever; and exertional dyspnea.
Genitourinary Tract **Hemorrhagic Cystitis** • Cells lining bladder are destroyed by chemotherapy (e.g., cyclophosphamide, ifosfamide). • Side effect of radiation when located in treatment field.	• Encourage increased fluid intake 24-72 hr after treatment as tolerated. • Monitor manifestations such as urgency, frequency, and hematuria. • Administer cytoprotectant agent (mesna [Mesnex]) and hydration. • Administer supportive care agents to manage symptoms (e.g., flavoxate [Urispas]).	**Cardiovascular System** **Pericarditis and Myocarditis** • Inflammation secondary to radiation injury. • Complication when chest wall is irradiated. May occur up to 1 yr after treatment. • Side effect of some chemotherapy drugs.	• Monitor for clinical manifestations of these disorders (e.g., dyspnea).
Reproductive Dysfunction • Cells of testes or ova are damaged by therapy.	• Discuss possibility with patients before treatment initiation. • Offer opportunity for sperm and ova banking before treatment for patients of childbearing age.	**Cardiotoxicity** • Some chemotherapy drugs (e.g., anthracyclines, taxanes) can cause ECG changes and rapidly progressive heart failure.	• Monitor heart with ECG and cardiac ejection fractions. • Drug therapy may need to be modified for symptoms or deteriorating cardiac function studies.
Nephrotoxicity • Direct renal cell damage from exposure to nephrotoxic agents (cisplatin and high-dose methotrexate). • Precipitation of metabolites of cell breakdown (tumor lysis syndrome [TLS]).	• Monitor BUN and serum creatinine levels. • Avoid potentiating drugs. • Alkalinize the urine with sodium bicarbonate and administer allopurinol (Zyloprim) or rasburicase for TLS prevention.	**Biochemical** **Hyperuricemia** • Increased uric acid levels due to chemotherapy-induced cell destruction. • Can cause secondary gout and obstructive uropathy.	• Monitor uric acid levels. • Allopurinol may be given as a prophylactic measure. • Encourage increased fluid intake.
Nervous System **Increased Intracranial Pressure** • May result from radiation edema in central nervous system.	• Monitor neurologic status. • May be controlled with corticosteroids.	**Psychoemotional** **Fatigue** • Anabolic processes result in accumulation of metabolites from cell breakdown.	• Assess for reversible causes of fatigue, and address them as indicated. • Reassure patient that fatigue is a common side effect of therapy. • Encourage patient to rest when fatigued, to maintain usual lifestyle patterns as much as possible, and to pace activities in accordance with energy level. • Encourage moderate exercise as tolerated.
Peripheral Neuropathy • Paresthesias, areflexia, skeletal muscle weakness, and smooth muscle dysfunction can occur as a side effect of plant alkaloids, taxanes, and cisplatin.	• Monitor for these manifestations in patients on these drugs. • Consider temporary chemotherapy dose interruption or reduction until symptoms improve. • Antiseizure drugs (e.g., gabapentin [Neurontin]) may be considered.		

BUN, Blood urea nitrogen; *IL-1,* interleukin-1; *TNF,* tumor necrosis factor.

most sensitive tissues to radiation and chemotherapy. The etiology of GI reactions is related to a variety of mechanisms, including (1) the release of serotonin from the GI tract, which then stimulates the chemoreceptor trigger zone (CTZ) and the vomiting center in the brain; and (2) cell death and resulting damage to GI mucosa. Additionally, radiation to treatment fields that contain GI structures (i.e., abdominopelvic, lumbosacral, and lower thoracic areas) and selected chemotherapy agents produce direct injury to GI epithelial cells. These injuries result in a variety of GI effects, including nausea and vomiting, diarrhea, mucositis, and anorexia. These problems can significantly affect the patient's hydration and nutritional status and sense of well-being.

Nausea and Vomiting. Nausea and vomiting are common sequelae of chemotherapy and, in some instances, radiation therapy. Vomiting may occur within 1 hour of chemotherapy administration or a few hours after radiation therapy to the chest or abdomen and may persist for 24 hours or more. Several antiemetic drugs are available (see Table 42-1). Metoclopramide (Reglan), prochlorperazine (Compazine), serotonin (5-HT_3) receptor antagonists (ondansetron [Zofran], granisetron [Kytril], dolasetron [Anzemet], and palonosetron [Aloxi]), and dexamethasone (Decadron) have been used to decrease nausea and vomiting caused by chemotherapy. Aprepitant (Emend), a neurokinin-1 receptor antagonist, is effective in preventing nausea and vomiting on the day of chemotherapy, as well as for delayed symptoms.[12,13]

Patients may also develop *anticipatory nausea and vomiting* if they experience poorly controlled nausea and vomiting after chemotherapy administration. In this phenomenon, encountering the cues even without receiving treatment may precipitate nausea and vomiting. Aggressive emesis control, including the prophylactic administration of antiemetic and antianxiety medication 1 hour before treatment, is recommended. The patient may find that eating a light meal of nonirritating food before treatment is also helpful.

Delayed nausea and vomiting can develop 24 hours to a week after treatment. Assess patients experiencing nausea and vomiting for signs and symptoms of dehydration and metabolic alkalosis. Nausea and vomiting can be successfully managed with antiemetic regimens, dietary modification, and other nondrug interventions (e.g., relaxation breathing).

Diarrhea. Diarrhea is a reaction of the bowel mucosa to radiation and to certain chemotherapy drugs. It is characterized by an increase in frequency and liquidity of stool. The small bowel is extremely sensitive and does not tolerate significant radiation doses. With pelvic radiation, patients may be treated with a full bladder to move the small bowel out of the treatment field. Both radiation- and chemotherapy-induced diarrhea are best managed with diet modification, antidiarrheals, antimotility agents, and antispasmodics (see Table 43-2).

Recommend a diet low in fiber and residue before treatment with chemotherapy known to cause diarrhea. This includes limiting foods that are high in roughage (e.g., fresh fruits, vegetables, seeds, nuts) (see Table 43-6). To prevent diarrhea, other foods to avoid include fried, fatty, or highly seasoned foods and other foods that are gas producing. Bowel mucosal injury from radiation may also result in temporary lactose intolerance. Therefore avoiding milk products is helpful for some patients during and immediately after treatment.

Depending on the severity of the diarrhea, hydration and electrolyte supplementation are also recommended. Lukewarm

sitz baths may alleviate discomfort and cleanse the rectal area if significant rectal irritation has developed. The rectal area must be kept clean and dry to maintain skin integrity. You should visually inspect the perianal area for evidence of skin breakdown. Systemic analgesia may be warranted for the painful skin irritations that may develop. Note the number, volume, consistency, and character of stools per day. Teach patients to maintain a diary or log to record episodes and aggravating and alleviating factors.[14]

Mucositis. Mucositis (irritation, inflammation, and/or ulceration of the mucosa) is a common complication in almost all patients receiving radiation to the head and neck and in many patients receiving certain antineoplastic agents, especially 5-fluorouracil (5-FU). Similar to the bowel mucosa, the mucosal linings of the oral cavity, oropharynx, and esophagus are extremely sensitive to the effects of radiation and chemotherapy.

Certain factors can compound the problem. For example, patients undergoing head and neck radiation may face the additional challenge of radiation-induced parotid gland dysfunction. This may result in decreased salivary flow, causing acute or chronic *xerostomia* (dry mouth). Dryness or thick saliva compromises the protective salivary functions of assisting with cleansing teeth, moistening food, and swallowing. Meticulous oral care during and for a long time after treatment reduces the risk of cavities related to the radiation, which may develop as a result of diminished saliva. Advise patients to continue regular dental follow-up every 6 months and to use fluoride supplements as recommended by their dentist. Saliva substitutes may be offered to patients with xerostomia, although many patients find that drinking small amounts of water frequently has a similar effect.

Amifostine (a cytoprotectant) may be used during radiation treatment if a significant radiation dose to the parotid glands is expected. It may help to reduce radiation-related mucositis.

Dysgeusia (taste loss) may develop during therapy, and by the end of treatment patients often report that all food has lost its flavor. Ultimately, nutritional status may be compromised. *Dysphagia* (difficulty swallowing), which characterizes pharyngeal and/or esophageal involvement, further impedes eating. Patients may report feeling that they have a "lump" as they swallow and that "foods get stuck." *Odynophagia* (painful swallowing) caused by oropharyngeal or esophageal irritation and ulceration may require the use of analgesics before meals.

Oral assessment and meticulous intervention to keep the oral cavity moist, clean, and free of debris are essential to prevent infection and to facilitate nutritional intake. Implementing standard oral care protocols that address prevention and management of mucositis facilitates routine assessment, patient and family education, and intervention.

Routinely assess the oral cavity, mucous membranes, characteristics of saliva, and ability to swallow. Having a dentist perform all necessary dental work before the initiation of treatment is also recommended. Teach patients to self-examine the oral cavity and also how to perform oral care (proper tooth brushing with a soft-bristle toothbrush, flossing, and use of fluoride trays to prevent caries). Oral care should be performed at least before and after each meal, at bedtime, and as needed through the day. A saline solution of 1 tsp of salt in 1 L of water is an effective cleansing agent. One tsp of sodium bicarbonate may be added to the oral care solution to decrease odor, alleviate pain, and dissolve mucin.

Mucositis or pain in the throat can be alleviated by systemic and/or topical analgesics and antibiotics if infection is present. Monitor and get prompt treatment for oral candidiasis (which often occurs with mucositis). Frequent cleansing with saline and water and topical application of anesthetic gels directly to the lesions are standard care.

Palifermin (Kepivance), a synthetic version of keratinocyte growth factor, is available to prevent or shorten the duration of mucositis. It is given IV and stimulates growth of cells on the surface layer of the mouth. This leads to faster replacement of these cells when killed by cancer treatment. It may also speed up the healing process of mouth ulcers. Palifermin is currently recommended for mucositis prevention in patients with hematologic malignancies undergoing treatment. The safety and efficacy of palifermin have not been established in patients with nonhematologic malignancies.

Anorexia. Anorexia (loss of appetite) is a common occurrence in patients with cancer. It is a side effect of the cancer itself as well as of cancer treatment. Anorexia may be related to an inflamed mouth or esophagus, which creates difficulty chewing or swallowing, or to emotions such as anxiety or depression.

Patients experiencing nausea and vomiting, bowel disturbances, mucositis, and taste alterations typically have little desire to eat. Although it is highly individual, anorexia seems to peak at about 4 weeks of treatment and to resolve more quickly than fatigue when treatment ends.

Monitor the patient with anorexia during and after treatment to ensure that weight loss does not become excessive. Also observe for dehydration. Small, frequent meals of high-protein, high-calorie foods are better tolerated than large meals. Nutritional supplements can be helpful as well. Enteral or parenteral nutrition may be indicated if the patient is severely malnourished, if symptoms are expected to interfere with nutrition for a time, or if the bowel is being rested. Monitor for and manage other symptoms that may interfere with appetite (e.g., nausea, vomiting, pain, depression).[15]

SKIN REACTIONS

Radiation Skin Changes. With radiation, skin effects are local, occurring only in the treatment field. Radiation-induced skin changes can be acute or chronic depending on the area irradiated, dosage, and technique. The skin-sparing ability of modern radiation equipment limits the severity of these reactions. Erythema may develop 1 to 24 hours after a single treatment, but generally occurs progressively as the treatment dose accumulates. Erythema is an acute response followed by dry desquamation (Fig. 16-14). If the rate of cell sloughing is faster than the

ability of the new epidermal cells to replace dead cells, a wet desquamation occurs with exposure of the dermis and weeping of serous fluid (Fig. 16-15). Skin reactions are particularly evident in areas of skinfolds or where skin is subjected to pressure, such as behind the ear; in gluteal folds; or on the perineum, breast, collar line, and bony prominences.

Although skin care protocols vary among institutions, basic skin care principles apply. The goal is to prevent infection and facilitate wound healing. Protect radiated skin from temperature extremes. Do not use heating pads, ice packs, and hot water bottles in the treatment field. Avoid constricting garments, rubbing, harsh chemicals, and deodorants, since they may traumatize the skin. Dry reactions are uncomfortable and result in pruritus. Lubricate dry skin with a nonirritating lotion emollient that contains no metal, alcohol, perfume, or additives, since these can be irritating. Calendula ointment and topical hyaluronic acid cream are effective for the management of radiation dermatitis. Aloe vera gel is also used, especially for prevention of skin problems.[16]

Wet desquamation of tissues generally produces pain, drainage, and increased risk of infection. Skin care to manage most desquamation includes keeping tissues clean with normal saline compresses or modified Burow's solution soaks and protected from further damage with moisture vapor–permeable dressings or Vaseline petrolatum gauze. Because protocols vary widely, the guidelines presented in Table 16-12 should be verified with your institution's radiation oncology department before using.

Chemotherapy Skin Changes. Chemotherapy produces a wide range of skin toxicities. These can range from mild erythema and hyperpigmentation to more distressing effects such as acral erythema and *erythrodysesthesia syndrome* (also called palmar-plantar erythrodysesthesia or hand-foot syndrome). Erythrodysesthesia syndrome can cause mild symptoms of redness and tingling of the palms of the hands and soles of the feet. It may also cause severe symptoms of painful moist desquamation, ulceration, blistering, and pain.

Alopecia is an easily recognizable effect of cancer therapy. It is frequently associated with varying degrees of emotional distress. Hair loss associated with radiation is local, whereas chemotherapy affects hair throughout the body. The degree and duration of hair loss experienced by patients depend on the type and dose of the chemotherapy agent.

Alopecia caused by the administration of chemotherapy agents is usually reversible. Sometimes the hair grows back while the patient is still receiving chemotherapy agents, but generally the hair does not grow back until 3 to 4 weeks after

FIG. 16-14 Dry desquamation.

FIG. 16-15 Wet desquamation.

TABLE 16-12 PATIENT & CAREGIVER TEACHING GUIDE

Radiation Skin Reactions

Include the following instructions when teaching the patient and the caregiver to clean and protect the skin in a radiation treatment area.

1. Gently cleanse the skin in the treatment field using a mild soap (Ivory, Dove), tepid water, a soft cloth, and a gentle patting motion. Rinse thoroughly and pat dry.
2. Apply nonmedicated, nonperfumed, moisturizing lotion or cream, such as calendula ointment, aloe gel, Aquaphor, or Biafine cream, to alleviate dry skin. Some substances must be gently cleansed from the treatment field before each treatment and reapplied. Over-the-counter hydrocortisone cream 1% may reduce itching.
3. Rinse the area with saline solution. Expose the area to air as often as possible. If copious drainage is present, use astringent compresses (such as Domeboro solution) and nonadhesive absorbent dressings (they must be changed as soon as they become wet). Observe the area daily for signs of infection.
4. Avoid wearing tight-fitting clothing such as brassieres and belts over the treatment field.
5. Avoid wearing harsh fabrics, such as wool and corduroy. A lightweight cotton garment is best. If possible, expose the treatment field to air.
6. Use gentle detergents such as Dreft and Ivory Snow to wash clothing that will come in contact with the treatment field.
7. Avoid direct exposure to the sun. If the treatment field is in an area that is exposed to the sun, wear protective clothing such as a wide-brimmed hat when out in the sun and apply sunscreen lotion.
8. Avoid all sources of excessive heat (hot water bottles, heating pads, sunlamps) on the treatment field.
9. Avoid exposing the treatment field to cold temperatures (ice bags or cold weather).
10. Avoid swimming in saltwater or in chlorinated pools during the time of treatment.
11. Avoid the use of potential irritants (e.g., perfumes, powders, or cosmetics) on the skin in the treatment field; review use of other topical medications or lotions with your health care provider during treatment. Also avoid tape, dressings, and adhesive bandages unless permitted by the radiation therapist. Avoid shaving the hair in the treatment field.
12. Continue to protect sensitive skin after the treatment is completed. Do the following:
    - Avoid direct exposure to the sun. A sunscreen agent and protective clothing must be worn if the potential of exposure to the sun is present.
    - Use an electric razor if shaving is necessary in the treatment field.

the drugs are discontinued. Often the new hair has a different color and texture than the hair that was lost.

Patients experience a range of emotions at the prospect of losing their hair and when hair loss actually occurs. These may include anger, grief, embarrassment, or fear. Hair loss is a visible reminder of their cancer and the challenges of treatment. For some people, the loss of hair is one of the most stressful events experienced during the course of treatment. The American Cancer Society's "Look Good, Feel Better" program is an excellent support and resource for people experiencing not just hair loss but body image changes in general.

PULMONARY EFFECTS. Both chemotherapy and radiation have the potential to produce pulmonary tissue damage that is irreversible and progressive. Distinguishing between the complications of treatment and those related to disease is challenging. The effects of radiation on the lung include both acute and late

reactions. Immediate pulmonary effects of radiation can be alarming to patients because they may mimic symptoms (e.g., cough, dyspnea) that precipitated the cancer diagnosis.

Pneumonitis is a delayed acute inflammatory reaction that may occur within 1 to 3 months after completion of thoracic radiation. This reaction is often asymptomatic, although an increase in cough, fever, and night sweats may occur. Some patients may develop pulmonary fibrosis (with or without prior pneumonitis), which is a late effect of therapy.

The most common pulmonary toxicities associated with chemotherapy include pulmonary edema (noncardiogenic) related to capillary leak syndrome or fluid retention, hypersensitivity pneumonitis, interstitial fibrosis, and pneumonitis produced by an inflammatory reaction or destruction of alveolar-capillary endothelium.

CARDIOVASCULAR EFFECTS. Radiation to the thorax can damage the pericardium, myocardium, valves, and coronary blood vessels. The pericardium is most commonly involved, with pericardial effusion or pericarditis the key problems. Patients with preexisting coronary artery disease are especially vulnerable.

Anthracyclines (e.g., doxorubicin [Adriamycin], daunorubicin) cause cardiotoxicity. Acute cardiotoxicities may cause electrocardiographic (ECG) abnormalities. Late effects of anthracyclines are left ventricular dysfunction and heart failure.

5-FU can cause cardiac ischemic syndrome. Trastuzumab (Herceptin), which is used in the treatment of breast cancer, is cardiotoxic and may result in ventricular dysfunction and heart failure. Baseline and periodic echocardiograms to monitor left ventricular function during treatment are usually done.

REPRODUCTIVE EFFECTS. Reproductive dysfunction secondary to radiation and chemotherapy varies according to the radiation treatment field and dosage, the particular chemotherapy agent and dose, and host factors (e.g., age). Treatment can cause temporary or permanent gonadal failure. Reproductive effects occur most often when reproductive organs are included in the radiation treatment field and when alkylating agents are used.

The testes are highly sensitive to radiation, and they should be protected with a testicular shield whenever possible. Pretreatment status may be a significant factor because a low sperm count and loss of motility are seen in individuals with testicular cancer and Hodgkin's lymphoma before any therapy is begun. Combined modality treatment or prior chemotherapy with alkylating agents enhances and prolongs the effects of radiation on the testes. When radiation is used alone with conventional doses and appropriate shielding, testicular recovery often occurs. Compromise of reproductive function in men may also result from erectile dysfunction after pelvic radiation.

The radiation dose that induces ovarian failure changes with age. Unlike the testes, there is no way to repair ovarian function. When radiation therapy is given, the ovaries are shielded whenever possible. Other factors that influence reproductive or sexual functioning in women include reactions in the cervix and endometrium. These tissues withstand a high radiation dose with minimal sequelae, accounting for the ability to treat endometrial and cervical cancer with high external and brachytherapy doses. Acute reactions such as tenderness, irritation, and loss of lubrication compromise sexual activity. Late effects of combined internal and external radiation therapy include vaginal shortening related to fibrosis and loss of elasticity and lubrication.

The patient and her or his partner require information about the expected effects of treatment relative to reproductive and sexual issues. Potential infertility can be a significant consequence for the individual, and counseling may be indicated. However, in no case should the patient think that conception is not possible during treatment. Pretreatment harvesting of sperm, ova, or ovarian tissue may be considered. Specific suggestions to manage side effects that have an impact on sexual functioning include using a water-soluble vaginal lubricant and routinely using a vaginal dilator after pelvic irradiation. Encourage discussion of issues related to sexuality, offer specific suggestions, and make referrals for ongoing counseling when indicated.

COPING WITH THERAPY. You have a key role in assisting patients in coping with the psychoemotional issues associated with cancer treatment. Anxiety is common—anxieties about various aspects of treatment administration (e.g., repeated venipuncture), dependency on others, ability to pay, potential side effects, and poor outcomes. Repetitive office visits or hospitalizations, continuing medications, and frequent laboratory testing force the individual to confront the cancer on a daily basis. Treatment-related uncertainties and fears are often most evident at the beginning of therapy, but anxiety may surface again when therapy is completed (e.g., fear of recurrence, less available support).

Telling patients that they will be followed and that support is ongoing can be reassuring. Providing information and support can help minimize the negative impact of cancer therapy on a person's quality of life. Patient teaching, symptom management, and interventions to help patients self-manage their illness (e.g., adjusting treatment schedules to permit patients to work when possible, making referrals to support groups) facilitate coping. Arranging for patients to meet with individuals who have successfully completed therapy can increase their hopefulness and confidence. In addition, make regular supportive telephone contacts between office visits and assist with planning for transportation, nutrition, and emotional support with available resources such as the American Cancer Society, Cancer Lifeline, churches, and other community resources.

LATE EFFECTS OF RADIATION AND CHEMOTHERAPY

Cancer survivors are achieving long-term remission and survival with advancements in treatment modalities. However, these forms of therapy (especially radiation therapy and chemotherapy) may produce long-term sequelae termed *late effects* that occur months to years after cessation of therapy. Every body system can be affected to some extent by chemotherapy or radiation therapy.

Acute radiation effects generally manifest as transient inflammatory changes in highly proliferative cells (e.g., epithelial tissues). In contrast, late radiation effects occur most commonly in post-mitotic cells (e.g., liver, kidney, lung, heart, muscle, bone, and connective tissues). Once they occur, the late effects may be progressive and generally are permanent. Examples range from skin telangiectasias to strictures, fistulas, or radiation necrosis. Alteration of the lymphatic channels (e.g., axillary lymph node dissection) may contribute to lymphedema. Secondary malignancies (particularly skin cancers) are other late radiation effects.

Long-term effects of chemotherapy include cataracts, arthralgias, endocrine alterations, renal insufficiency, hepatitis, osteoporosis, neurocognitive dysfunction, or other effects depending on the agents. The additive effects of multiagent chemotherapy before, during, or after a course of radiation therapy can significantly increase the resulting late effects.

The cancer survivor may also be at risk for secondary malignancies, including leukemia, angiosarcoma, and skin cancer. Approximately 8% of cancer survivors (most commonly breast and colon cancer survivors) face a secondary malignancy. Alkylating agents and high-dose radiation are the most frequent causes of secondary malignancies.

In general, the overall risk of developing neoplastic complications is low, and the latency period may be long. The potential risk for developing a secondary malignancy does not contraindicate the use of cancer treatment. Smoking may significantly increase the risk of secondary malignancies following some cancer treatment. Therefore counsel all patients about smoking cessation.

BIOLOGIC AND TARGETED THERAPY

Biologic and targeted therapy is the fourth cancer treatment modality. Biologic and targeted therapy can be effective alone or in combination with surgery, radiation therapy, and chemotherapy. **Biologic therapy,** or *biologic response modifier* therapy, consists of agents that modify the relationship between the host and the tumor by altering the biologic response of the host to the tumor cells. Biologic agents may affect host-tumor response in three ways: (1) they have direct antitumor effects; (2) they restore, augment, or modulate host immune system mechanisms; and (3) they have other biologic effects, such as interfering with the cancer cells' ability to metastasize or differentiate.

Targeted therapy interferes with cancer growth by targeting specific cell receptors and pathways that are important in tumor growth. Targeted therapies work at sites that are on the cell surface, at the intracellular level, or in the extracellular domain (Fig. 16-16 and Table 16-13). The targeted therapies are more selective for specific molecular targets than cytotoxic anticancer drugs. Thus they are able to kill cancer cells with less damage to normal cells compared with chemotherapy.

Targeted therapies include epidermal growth factor receptor (EGFR)–tyrosine kinase inhibitors, BCR-ABL tyrosine kinase inhibitors, CD20 monoclonal antibodies (MoAb), angiogenesis inhibitors, and proteasome inhibitors. As more oncogene targets are identified, such as BRAF (B-type Raf kinase) or ALK

FIG. 16-16 Sites of action of targeted therapy. *EGFR,* Epidermal growth factor receptor; *HER-2,* human epidermal growth factor receptor 2; *VEGF,* vascular endothelial growth factor.

TABLE 16-13   DRUG THERAPY

Biologic and Targeted Therapy*

Drug	Mechanism of Action	Indications
α-interferon (Roferon-A, Intron A)	Inhibits DNA and protein synthesis Suppresses cell proliferation Increases cytotoxic effects of natural killer (NK) cells	Hairy cell leukemia, chronic myelogenous leukemia, malignant melanoma, renal cell carcinoma, ovarian cancer, multiple myeloma, Kaposi sarcoma
interleukin-2 (aldesleukin [Proleukin])	Stimulates proliferation of T and B cells Activates NK cells	Metastatic renal cell cancer, metastatic melanoma
BCG vaccine (TheraCys)	Induces an immune response that prevents angiogenesis of tumor	In situ bladder cancer
Epidermal Growth Factor Receptor (EGFR)–Tyrosine Kinase (TK) Inhibitors		
cetuximab (Erbitux)	Inhibits EGFR	Colorectal cancer, head and neck cancer
erlotinib (Tarceva)	Inhibits EGFR-TK	Non–small cell lung cancer, advanced pancreatic cancer
lapatinib (Tykerb)	Inhibits EGFR-TK and binds HER-2	Advanced breast cancer that is HER-2 positive
panitumumab (Vectibix)	Inhibits EGFR	Colorectal cancer
BCR-ABL Tyrosine Kinase Inhibitors		
dasatinib (Sprycel)	Inhibits BCR-ABL TK	Chronic myeloid leukemia
imatinib (Gleevec)	Inhibits BCR-ABL TK	Chronic myeloid leukemia, GI stromal tumors (GIST)
nilotinib (Tasigna)	Inhibits BCR-ABL TK	Chronic myeloid leukemia
CD20 Monoclonal Antibodies		
ibritumomab tiuxetan/yttrium-90 (Zevalin)	Binds CD20 antigen, causing cytotoxicity and radiation injury	Non-Hodgkin's lymphoma (B cell)
ofatumumab (Arzerra)	Binds CD20 antigen, causing cytotoxicity	Chronic lymphocytic leukemia
rituximab (Rituxan)	Binds CD20 antigen, causing cytotoxicity	Non-Hodgkin's lymphoma (B cell)
tositumomab/^{131}I tositumomab (Bexxar)	Binds CD20 antigen, causing immune attack and radiation injury	Non-Hodgkin's lymphoma (B cell)
Angiogenesis Inhibitors		
bevacizumab (Avastin)	Binds vascular endothelial growth factor (VEGF), thereby inhibiting angiogenesis	Colorectal cancer, non–small cell lung cancer, renal cell carcinoma
pazopanib (Votrient)	Binds VEGF, thereby inhibiting angiogenesis	Advanced renal cell carcinoma
Proteasome Inhibitors		
bortezomib (Velcade)	Inhibits proteasome activity, which functions to regulate cell growth	Multiple myeloma
carfilzomib (Kyprolis)	Inhibits proteasome activity, which functions to regulate cell growth	Multiple myeloma
Other Targeted Therapies		
alemtuzumab (Campath)	Binds CD52 antigen (found on T and B cells, monocytes, NK cells, neutrophils)	Chronic lymphocytic leukemia (B cell), GIST
axitinib (Inlyta)	Inhibits multiple TKs	Advanced renal cell carcinoma
crizotinib (Xalkori)	Inhibits anaplastic lymphoma kinase (ALK)	Locally advanced or metastatic non–small cell lung cancer that is ALK positive
everolimus (Afinitor)	Inhibits a specific protein known as the mammalian target of rapamycin (mTOR)	Advanced renal cell carcinoma, advanced breast cancer
ipilimumab (Yervoy)	Binds with CTLA-4 causing an antitumor-mediated immune response	Metastatic melanoma or unresectable melanoma
pertuzumab (Perjeta)	Binds HER-2	Breast cancer (HER-2 positive)
sorafenib (Nexavar)	Inhibits multiple TKs	Advanced renal cell carcinoma
sunitinib (Sutent)	Inhibits multiple TKs	Advanced renal cell carcinoma, GIST
temsirolimus (Torisel)	Inhibits a specific protein known as the mammalian target of rapamycin (mTOR)	Advanced renal cell carcinoma
trastuzumab (Herceptin)	Binds HER-2	Breast cancer (HER-2 positive)
vandetanib (Caprelsa)	Inhibits multiple TKs	Medullary thyroid cancer
vemurafenib (Zelboraf)	Inhibits BRAF serine threonine kinase	BRAF V600E mutated metastatic melanoma

*An enhanced version of this table listing side effects (eTable 16-7) is available on the website for this chapter.
BRAF, B-type Raf; *CTLA-4,* cytotoxic T lymphocyte antigen 4; *HER-2,* human epidermal growth factor receptor 2.

(anaplastic lymphoma kinase), agents are being developed that target specific oncogenes. Targeted therapies provide for use of personalized therapy based on the biology of an individual's tumor.[17]

EGFR is a transmembrane molecule that works through activation of intracellular tyrosine kinase (TK). Overexpression of EGFR is associated with unregulated cell growth and poor prognosis. Drugs that inhibit EGFR suppress cell proliferation and promote *apoptosis* (programmed cell death).

EGFRs belong to the same receptor family as human epidermal growth factor receptor 2 (HER-2), the target for trastuzumab (Herceptin). HER-2 is overexpressed in certain cancers (especially breast cancers) and is associated with more aggressive disease and decreased survival. Trastuzumab is a MoAb that binds to HER-2 and is given IV to inhibit the growth of breast cancer cells that overexpress the HER-2 protein. Lapatinib (Tykerb) is an oral agent used for breast cancer that overexpresses HER-2.

Chronic myeloid leukemia (CML) cells make an abnormal active enzyme called *BCR-ABL tyrosine kinase*. Drugs (e.g., imatinib [Gleevec]) that inhibit this enzyme suppress proliferation of CML cells and promote apoptosis.

Angiogenesis inhibitors work by preventing the mechanisms and pathways necessary for vascularization of tumors. Bevacizumab (Avastin), a recombinant human MoAb, binds with vascular endothelial growth factor (VEGF), a compound that stimulates blood vessel growth. When bevacizumab binds with VEGF, it prevents VEGF from binding with its receptors on vascular endothelial cells and promoting new vessel formation. As a result, further tumor growth is inhibited.

Proteasomes are intracellular multienzyme complexes that degrade proteins. In cancer cells, proteasome inhibitors (e.g., bortezomib [Velcade]) promote accumulation of proteins that lead to cell death.

Side Effects of Biologic and Targeted Therapy

The administration of one biologic agent usually induces the endogenous release of other biologic agents. The release and action of these biologic agents result in systemic immune and inflammatory responses. The toxicities and side effects of biologic agents are related to dose and schedule. (eTable 16-7 summarizes the potential side effects associated with specific biologic and targeted therapies.)

Common side effects include constitutional flu-like symptoms, including headache, fever, chills, myalgias, fatigue, malaise, weakness, photosensitivity, anorexia, and nausea. With interferon therapy, these flu-like symptoms almost invariably appear, but their severity generally decreases over time. Acetaminophen administered every 4 hours, as prescribed, often reduces the severity of the flu-like syndrome. The patient is commonly premedicated with acetaminophen in an attempt to prevent or decrease the intensity of these symptoms. In addition, large amounts of fluids help decrease the symptoms.

Tachycardia and orthostatic hypotension are also commonly reported. IL-2 and MoAbs can cause *capillary leak syndrome,* which can result in pulmonary edema. Other toxic and side effects may involve the CNS, renal and hepatic systems, and cardiovascular system. These effects are found particularly with interferons and IL-2.

A wide range of neurologic deficits has been observed with interferon and IL-2 therapy. The nature and extent of these problems are not yet completely understood. However, these problems are understandably frightening to the patient and the family, who must be taught to observe for neurologic problems (e.g., confusion, memory loss, difficulty making decisions, insomnia), report their occurrence, and institute appropriate safety and support measures.

MoAbs are administered by infusion. Patients may experience infusion-related symptoms, which can include fever, chills, urticaria, mucosal congestion, nausea, diarrhea, and myalgias. There is also a risk, although rare, of anaphylaxis associated with the administration of MoAbs. This potential exists because most MoAbs are produced by mouse lymphocytes and thus represent a foreign protein to the human body. The risk is significantly decreased with human MoAbs. Onset of anaphylaxis can occur within 5 minutes of administration and can be a life-threatening event. If this occurs, stop administration of the MoAb immediately, obtain emergency assistance, and implement resuscitation measures. (See Chapter 14 for a discussion of nursing management of anaphylaxis.)

Skin rashes are common in patients receiving EGFR inhibitors and manifest generally as erythema and acneiform-like rash that can cover up to 50% of the upper body. Angiogenesis inhibitors can cause problems of arterial thrombi, hemorrhage, hypertension, impaired wound healing, and proteinuria. Other toxicities of MoAbs include hepatotoxicity, bone marrow depression, and CNS effects. Individuals who receive rituximab may have a reactivation of hepatitis. Patients who receive trastuzumab may also experience cardiac dysfunction, especially when it is administered in higher doses or in combination with anthracycline antibiotics such as doxorubicin.

NURSING MANAGEMENT
BIOLOGIC AND TARGETED THERAPY

Some problems experienced by the patient receiving biologic and targeted therapy are different from those observed with more traditional forms of cancer therapy. These effects occur more acutely and are dose limited (i.e., effects resolve when the agent is discontinued). Capillary leak syndrome and pulmonary edema are problems that require critical care nursing. Bone marrow depression occurring with biologic therapy administration is generally more transient and less severe than that observed with chemotherapy. Fatigue associated with biologic therapy can be so severe that it constitutes a dose-limiting toxicity. As these agents are increasingly combined with cytotoxic therapies, the spectrum of therapy-related effects expands.

Nursing interventions for flu-like syndrome include the administration of acetaminophen before treatment and every 4 hours after treatment. IV meperidine (Demerol) has been used to control the severe chills or rigors associated with some biologic agents. Other nursing measures include monitoring vital signs and temperature, planning for periods of rest for the patient, assisting with activities of daily living (ADLs), and monitoring for adequate oral intake.

Many new targeted therapies are being developed and used more frequently. You need to become familiar with side effects associated with each agent.

HEMATOPOIETIC GROWTH FACTORS

Hematopoietic growth factors are used to support cancer patients through the treatment of the disease (Table 16-14). Colony-stimulating factors (CSFs) are a family of glycoproteins

TABLE 16-14 DRUG THERAPY

Hematopoietic Growth Factors Used in Cancer Treatment

Growth Factor	Drug Name	Indications	Side Effects
Granulocyte-macrophage colony-stimulating factor (GM-CSF)	sargramostim (Leukine)	Myeloid cell recovery after bone marrow transplantation	Nausea, vomiting, diarrhea, fever, chills, myalgia, headache, fatigue
Granulocyte colony-stimulating factor (G-CSF)	filgrastim (Neupogen), pegfilgrastim (Neulasta), tbo-filgrastim	Chemotherapy-induced neutropenia	Bone pain, nausea, vomiting
Erythropoietin	epoetin α (Epogen, Procrit)	Anemia of chronic cancer	Hypertension, thrombosis, headache
	darbepoetin α (Aranesp)	Anemia related to chemotherapy	Hypertension, thrombosis, headache
Interleukin-11 (platelet growth factor)	oprelvekin (Neumega)	Thrombocytopenia related to chemotherapy	Fluid retention, peripheral edema, dyspnea, tachycardia, nausea, mouth sores

TABLE 16-15 INDICATIONS FOR HEMATOPOIETIC STEM CELL TRANSPLANTATION

Malignant Diseases	Nonmalignant Diseases
• Acute and chronic myelogenous leukemia • Acute lymphocytic leukemia • Hodgkin's lymphoma • Multiple myeloma • Myelodysplastic syndrome • Neuroblastoma • Non-Hodgkin's lymphoma • Ovarian cancer • Sarcoma • Testicular cancer	• Hematologic diseases • Aplastic anemia • Chronic granulomatous disease • Fanconi's anemia • Sickle cell disease (severe) • Thalassemia • Immunodeficiency diseases • Severe combined immunodeficiency disease (SCID) • Wiskott-Aldrich syndrome

produced by various cells. CSFs stimulate production, maturation, regulation, and activation of cells of the hematologic system. The name of the CSF is based on the specific cell line it affects (see Table 16-14).

Erythropoiesis-stimulating agents (ESAs) should be used only when treating anemia specifically caused by chemotherapy. ESA use is avoided in patients receiving chemotherapy with the intent to cure the disease. Use of these agents has raised safety concerns because they can cause thromboembolic events and increase the risk for death and for serious cardiovascular events when administered to achieve a target hemoglobin of greater than 12 g/dL. Therefore the lowest dose should be used that will gradually increase hemoglobin to the lowest level sufficient to avoid the need for blood transfusion. Monitor the hemoglobin level regularly.

HEMATOPOIETIC STEM CELL TRANSPLANTATION

Bone marrow transplantation (BMT) and peripheral stem cell transplantation (PSCT) are effective, lifesaving procedures for the treatment of a number of malignant and nonmalignant diseases (Table 16-15). BMT and PSCT allow for the safe use of very high doses of chemotherapy agents and/or radiation therapy in patients whose tumors have developed resistance or failed to respond to standard doses of chemotherapy and radiation. Although these procedures are lifesaving, patients may have long-term or delayed complications that can affect their quality of life.[18,19]

This therapeutic approach was typically referred to as BMT because the bone marrow was the original source of stem cells when the procedure was first developed. However, advances in

harvesting and cryopreservation technologies have opened new pathways to the collection of stem cells from the peripheral blood. Consequently, the terminology has changed, and the procedure is now referred to as hematopoietic stem cell transplantation (HSCT). Whether the diagnosis is a malignant or nonmalignant disease, the goal of HSCT is cure. Overall cure rates are still low but are steadily increasing. Even when cure is not achieved, transplantation can result in a period of remission.

The approach in HSCT is to eradicate diseased tumor cells and/or clear the marrow of its components to make way for engraftment of the transplanted, healthy stem cells. This is accomplished by administering higher than usual dosages of chemotherapy with or without radiation therapy, which can produce life-threatening consequences associated with pancytopenia and other adverse effects. After chemotherapy and radiation therapy are completed, healthy stem cells are infused. These healthy stem cells "rescue" the damaged bone marrow through subsequent proliferation and differentiation of the donated stem cells in the recipient.

HSCT is an intensive procedure with many risks. Some patients die from treatment-related complications or from recurrence of the original disease. Because it is a highly toxic therapy, the patient must weigh the significant risks of treatment-related death or treatment failure (relapse) against the hope of cure.

Types of Hematopoietic Stem Cell Transplants

HSCTs are categorized as allogeneic, syngeneic, or autologous. The sources of stem cells include the bone marrow, peripheral circulating blood, and umbilical cord blood. In *allogeneic transplantation,* stem cells are acquired from a donor who, through human leukocyte antigen (HLA) tissue typing, has been determined to be HLA matched to the recipient. HLA typing involves testing WBCs to identify genetically inherited antigens common to both donor and recipient that are important in compatibility of transplanted tissue. (HLA tissue typing is discussed in Chapter 14.) The donor is often a family member but may be an unrelated donor found through a national or international bone marrow registry (e.g., National Marrow Donor Program). Although more risks and toxicities may be associated with an unrelated allogeneic transplant, a benefit of this type of transplant is that it not only eradicates tumor cells with high-dose therapy, but also may stimulate the graft-versus-tumor effect in which donor WBCs identify and attack malignant cells in the

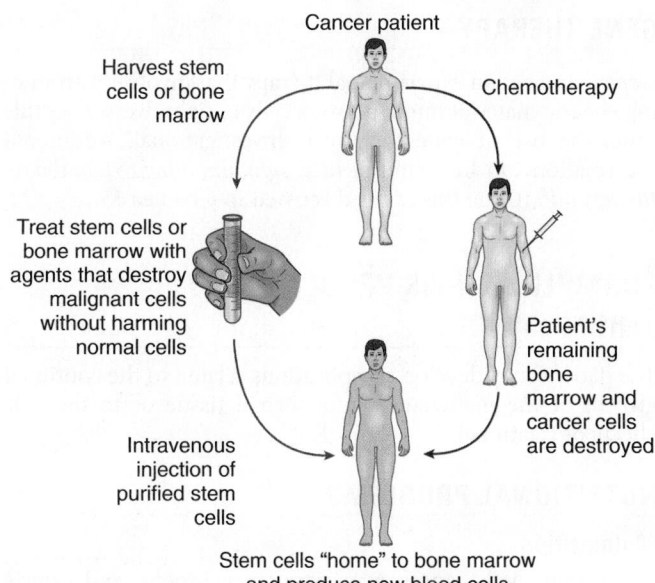

Cancer patient

Harvest stem cells or bone marrow

Chemotherapy

Treat stem cells or bone marrow with agents that destroy malignant cells without harming normal cells

Patient's remaining bone marrow and cancer cells are destroyed

Intravenous injection of purified stem cells

Stem cells "home" to bone marrow and produce new blood cells

FIG. 16-17 Autologous stem cell transplant.

recipient. Common indications for allogeneic transplant are certain leukemias, multiple myeloma, and lymphoma.

Syngeneic transplantation is a type of allogeneic transplant that involves obtaining stem cells from one identical twin and infusing them into the other. Identical twins have identical HLA types and are a perfect match. Therefore neither the graft-versus-host nor the graft-versus-tumor effect occurs.

In *autologous transplantation*, patients receive their own stem cells back after *myeloablative* (destroying bone marrow) chemotherapy (Fig. 16-17). The aim of this approach is purely "rescue." It enables patients to receive intensive chemotherapy and/or radiation by supporting them with their previously harvested stem cells until their marrow generates blood cells again on its own. Restoration usually takes about 4 to 6 weeks. Autologous transplants are typically used to treat hematologic malignancies if there is no suitable donor or the patient cannot undergo allogeneic transplantation.

The newer, nonmyeloablative or reduced intensity transplant uses lower doses of radiation or chemotherapy that result in less toxicity and myelosuppression. HSCT continues to be investigated in the management of some solid tumors refractory to treatment.

Procedures

Harvest Procedures. Hematopoietic stem cells are *harvested* from a donor (for allogeneic transplantation) or from the recipient (for autologous transplantation) via two different methods. In one type of procedure, used for harvesting stem cells residing in bone marrow (as the process was originally developed), the procedure is performed in the operating room using general or spinal anesthesia. Multiple bone marrow aspirations (usually from the iliac crest, but sometimes from the sternum) are carried out to obtain stem cells. The entire bone marrow harvest procedure takes about 1 to 2 hours, and the patient can be discharged after recovery. Postharvest, the donor may experience pain at the collection site that lasts up to 7 days and can be treated with mild analgesics. The donor's body will replenish the removed bone marrow in a few weeks.

In the other type of procedure, peripheral stem cell transplants are obtained from the peripheral blood in an outpatient procedure. It is done using cell separator equipment that automatically separates the stem cells from the blood circulating through the machine and returns the remaining blood components to the donor. The process averages about 2 to 4 hours but can sometimes take longer depending on donor factors and the quality of the venous access. Often it takes more than one procedure to obtain enough stem cells. Because the blood has fewer stem cells than the bone marrow, "mobilization" of stem cells from the bone marrow into the peripheral blood can be accomplished using chemotherapy and/or hematopoietic growth factors.

Common growth factors that are used are granulocyte-macrophage colony-stimulating factor (GM-CSF) and granulocyte colony-stimulating factor (G-CSF) (see Table 16-14), but chemotherapy agents, typically cyclophosphamide, can also be used if there is a need to reduce tumor burden. When patients are given growth factors for mobilization, stem cells are harvested after 4 or 5 days of growth factor injections.

Plerixafor (Mozobil) is a drug given subcutaneously that, when used in combination with G-CSF, boosts the number of stem cells released from the bone marrow into the bloodstream. Plerixafor is intended to be used in combination with G-CSF for treatment of multiple myeloma or non-Hodgkin's lymphomas; it is not to be used for leukemia.

Harvested marrow is processed to strain out bone fragments (this is not necessary with peripheral collections). The marrow or peripherally collected stem cells are then bagged with preservative for cryopreservation and storage until they are needed, or they are used immediately. Since it is coming from the patient, autologous stem cells are sometimes treated (purged) to remove undetected cancer cells. Many different pharmacologic, immunologic, physical, and chemical agents have been used for this purpose.

Umbilical cord blood is also rich in hematopoietic stem cells, and successful allogeneic transplants have been performed using this source. Cord blood can be HLA-typed and cryopreserved. A disadvantage of cord blood is the possibility of insufficient numbers of stem cells to permit transplant to adults. Considerable research is currently ongoing to define the optimal application of this technology.

Preparative Regimens and Stem Cell Infusions. In malignant diseases, patients receive myeloablative dosages of chemotherapy with or without adjunctive radiation to treat underlying disease. Total-body irradiation (TBI) can be used for immunosuppression or to treat the disease. These preparative therapies are known as the *conditioning regimen*.

The timing of stem cell harvest and reinfusion is critical, particularly with autologous transplantation. To ensure the collection of optimally functioning stem cells in adequate numbers, conditioning is begun only after stem cells have already been harvested. They are thawed and reinfused only after chemotherapy has been eliminated from the body (i.e., usually about 24 to 48 hours) to avoid damage to newly infused cells.

Stem cell infusions are administered IV, and can be injected via the slow bolus method or infused much like a blood transfusion. The infused stem cells reconstitute the bone marrow elements, "rescuing" the recipient's hematopoietic system. Usually 2 to 4 weeks are required for the transplanted marrow to start producing hematopoietic blood cells. During this period, when the patient has pancytopenia, it is critical to protect the patient from exposure to infectious agents and support the patient with electrolyte supplements, nutrition, and blood component transfusions (as needed) to maintain adequate levels of circulating RBCs and platelets.

Complications. Bacterial, viral, and fungal infections are common after HSCT. Prophylactic antibiotic therapy may reduce their incidence. A potentially serious complication of allogeneic transplant is graft-versus-host disease. This occurs when the T lymphocytes from the donated marrow (graft) recognize the recipient (host) as foreign and begin to attack certain organs such as the skin, liver, and GI tract. (Graft-versus-host disease is discussed in Chapter 14.) The occurrence and severity of posttransplant complications also depend on the drugs used in the patient's particular conditioning regimen (some are more toxic than others) and the stem cell source. Because stem cells in the peripheral blood are more mature than those harvested from the marrow, the hematologic recovery period in PSCT is shorter, and fewer, less severe complications are seen.

TABLE 16-16   NUTRITIONAL THERAPY

Protein Foods With High Biologic Value

Milk

Whole milk (1 cup) = 9 g protein

Double-strength milk: 1 quart of whole milk plus 1 cup of dried skim milk blended and chilled: 1 cup = 14 g protein

Milk shake: 1 cup of ice cream plus 1 cup of milk = 15 g protein, 416 calories

Use evaporated milk, double-strength milk, or half-and-half to make casseroles, hot cereals, sauces, gravies, puddings, milk shakes, and soups.

Yogurt (regular and frozen): check labels and purchase brand with highest protein content: 1 cup = 10 g protein

Eggs

Egg = 6 g protein

Eggnog (1 cup) = 15.5 g protein

Add eggs to salads, casseroles, and sauces. Deviled eggs are especially well tolerated.

Desserts that contain eggs include angel food cake, sponge cake, custard, and cheesecake.

Cheese

Cottage	½ cup	15 g protein
American	1 slice	3 g protein
Cheddar	1 slice	6 g protein
Cream	1 tbs	1 g protein

Use cheese in a sandwich or as a snack.

Add cheese to salads, casseroles, sauces, and baked potatoes.

Cheese spread with crackers is a wholesome snack that can be made and stored in the refrigerator for easy accessibility.

Advise patient that cheese can be constipating.

Meat, Poultry, Fish

Pork	3 oz	approx. 19 g protein
Chicken	½ breast	approx. 26 g protein
Fish	3 oz	approx. 30 g protein
Tuna fish	6½ oz	approx. 44.5 g protein

Add meat, poultry, and fish to salads, casseroles, and sandwiches.

Add strained and junior baby meats to soups and casseroles.

Cocktail wieners and deviled ham on crackers are wholesome snacks. These snacks can be made and stored in the refrigerator for easy accessibility.

GENE THERAPY

Gene therapy is an experimental therapy that involves introducing genetic material into a person's cells to fight disease. At this time, the use of gene therapy is investigational. Additional information can be found at *http://ghr.nlm.nih.gov/handbook/therapy.pdf*. (Gene therapy is discussed in Chapter 13.)

COMPLICATIONS RESULTING FROM CANCER

The patient may develop complications related to the continual growth of the malignancy into normal tissue or to the side effects of treatment.

NUTRITIONAL PROBLEMS

Malnutrition

The patient with cancer may experience protein and calorie malnutrition characterized by fat and muscle depletion. (Assessment of malnutrition is discussed in Chapter 40.)

Soft, nonirritating high-protein and high-calorie foods should be eaten throughout the day. Foods suggested for increasing the protein intake are presented in Table 16-16. High-calorie foods that provide energy and minimize weight loss are presented in Table 16-17. (A sample high-calorie, high-protein diet is presented in Table 40-10.)

Teach the patient to avoid extremes of temperature, tobacco, alcohol, spicy or rough foods, and other irritants. Encourage nutritional supplements (e.g., Ensure) as an adjunct to meals and fluid intake. Weigh the patient at least twice each week to monitor for weight loss.

Suggest a referral for individualized nutritional counseling to the patient or the health care provider as soon as a 5% weight loss is noted or if the patient has the potential for protein and calorie malnutrition. Monitor albumin and prealbumin levels. Once a 10-lb (4.5-kg) weight loss occurs, it is difficult to maintain the nutritional status.

Teach the patient to use nutritional supplements in place of milk when cooking or baking. Foods to which nutritional supplements can be easily added include scrambled eggs, pudding, custard, mashed potatoes, cereal, and cream sauces. Packages of Instant Breakfast can be used as indicated or sprinkled on cereals, desserts, and casseroles.

Families are an integral part of the health care team. As symptom severity increases, the family's role in helping the patient eat becomes increasingly critical.

TABLE 16-17   NUTRITIONAL THERAPY

High-Calorie Foods

Mayonnaise	1 tbs	=	101 cal
Butter or margarine	1 tsp	=	35 cal
Sour cream	1 tbs	=	72 cal
Peanut butter	1 tbs	=	94 cal
Whipped cream	1 tbs	=	53 cal
Corn oil	1 tbs	=	119 cal
Jelly	1 tbs	=	49 cal
Ice cream	1 cup	=	256 cal
Honey	1 tbs	=	64 cal

If the malnutrition cannot be treated with dietary intake, it may be necessary to use enteral or parenteral nutrition. (Enteral and parenteral nutrition are discussed in Chapter 40.)

Altered Taste Sensation (Dysgeusia)

Cancer cells may release substances that stimulate the bitter taste buds. The patient may also experience an alteration in the sweet, sour, and salty taste sensations. Meat may taste bitter or bland. At this time, the physiologic basis of these varied taste alterations is unknown.

Teach the patient with an altered taste problem to avoid foods that are disliked. Frequently the patient may feel compelled to eat certain foods that are believed to be beneficial. Tell the patient to experiment with spices and other seasoning agents in an attempt to mask the taste alterations. Lemon juice, onion, mint, basil, and fruit juice marinades may improve the taste of certain meats and fish. Bacon bits, onion, and ham may enhance the taste of vegetables. Increasing the amount of spice or seasoning agent is usually not an effective way to enhance the taste.

INFECTION

Infection is a primary cause of death in the patient with cancer. The usual sites of infection include the lungs, GU system, mouth, rectum, peritoneal cavity, and blood (septicemia). Infection occurs as a result of the ulceration and necrosis caused by the tumor, compression of vital organs by the tumor, and neutropenia caused by the disease process or the treatment of cancer.

Instruct patients with a risk for neutropenia to call their health care provider if they have a temperature of 100.4° F (38° C) or greater. Assessment most often includes signs and symptoms of fever, determination of possible etiology (e.g., sinuses, mucous membranes, respiratory, GI, urinary, sites of any tubes or lines), and complete blood count.

Many patients are neutropenic when an infection develops. In these individuals, infection may cause significant morbidity and may be rapidly fatal if not treated promptly. The classic manifestations of infection are often subtle or absent in a patient with neutropenia and a depressed immune system. (Neutropenia is discussed in Chapter 31.)

ONCOLOGIC EMERGENCIES

Oncologic emergencies are life-threatening emergencies that can occur as a result of cancer or cancer treatment. These emergencies can be obstructive, metabolic, or infiltrative.

Obstructive Emergencies

Obstructive emergencies are primarily caused by tumor obstruction of an organ or blood vessel. Obstructive emergencies include superior vena cava syndrome, spinal cord compression syndrome, third space syndrome, and intestinal obstruction. (Chapter 43 presents a discussion of intestinal obstruction.)

Superior Vena Cava Syndrome. *Superior vena cava syndrome* (SVCS) results from obstruction of the superior vena cava by a tumor or thrombosis. The clinical manifestations include facial edema; periorbital edema; distention of veins of the head, neck, and chest (Fig. 16-18); headache; and seizures. A mediastinal mass is often visible on chest x-ray. The most common causes are lung cancer, non-Hodgkin's lymphoma, and

FIG. 16-18 Superior vena caval obstruction in bronchial carcinoma. Note the swelling of the face and neck and the development of collateral circulation in the veins.

metastatic breast cancer. The presence of a central venous catheter and previous radiation therapy to the mediastinum increase the risk for development of SVCS.

SVCS is considered a serious medical problem. Management usually involves radiation therapy to the site of obstruction. However, chemotherapy may be administered for tumors more sensitive to this form of therapy.

Spinal Cord Compression. *Spinal cord compression* (SCC) is a neurologic emergency caused by a malignant tumor in the epidural space of the spinal cord. The most common cancers that cause this problem are breast, lung, prostate, GI, and renal tumors and melanomas. Lymphomas also pose a risk if diseased lymph tissue invades the epidural space.

Symptoms of SCC are back pain that is intense, localized, and persistent, accompanied by vertebral tenderness and aggravated by the Valsalva maneuver; motor weakness and dysfunction; sensory paresthesia and loss; and autonomic dysfunction. One of the clinical symptoms that reflects autonomic dysfunction is a reported change in bowel or bladder function.

The use of radiation therapy in conjunction with corticosteroids is generally associated with some initial improvement. Surgical decompressive laminectomy is used for those with tumors that are not responsive to radiation or when the tumor is in a previously irradiated area. Activity limitations and pain management are important nursing interventions.

Third Space Syndrome. *Third space syndrome* involves a shifting of fluid from the vascular space to the interstitial space that generally occurs secondary to extensive surgical procedures, biologic therapy, or septic shock. Initially patients exhibit signs of hypovolemia, including hypotension, tachycardia, low central venous pressure, and decreased urine output. Treatment includes fluid, electrolyte, and plasma protein replacement. During recovery hypervolemia can occur, resulting in hypertension, elevated central venous pressure, weight gain, and shortness of breath. Treatment generally involves reduction in fluid administration and fluid balance monitoring.

Metabolic Emergencies

Metabolic emergencies are caused by the production of ectopic hormones directly from the tumor or are secondary to metabolic alterations caused by the tumor or by cancer treatment.

Ectopic hormones arise from tissues that do not normally produce these hormones. Cancer cells return to a more embryonic form, thus allowing the cells' stored potential to become evident.

Metabolic emergencies include syndrome of inappropriate antidiuretic hormone secretion, hypercalcemia, tumor lysis syndrome, septic shock, and disseminated intravascular coagulation. (Septic shock is discussed in Chapter 67, and disseminated intravascular coagulation is discussed in Chapter 31.)

Syndrome of Inappropriate Antidiuretic Hormone Secretion. Syndrome of inappropriate antidiuretic hormone (SIADH) results from abnormal or sustained production of antidiuretic hormone (ADH) by tumor cells with resultant water retention and hyponatremia (hypotonic hyponatremia) (see Chapter 50).

SIADH occurs most frequently in carcinoma of the lung (especially small cell lung cancer), but can also occur in cancer of the pancreas, duodenum, brain, esophagus, colon, ovary, prostate, bronchus, and nasopharynx; leukemia; and Hodgkin's lymphoma. Cancer cells in these tumors are actually able to manufacture, store, and release ADH. Many chemotherapy agents may also contribute to ectopic ADH production, or potentiate ADH effects, including vincristine, cyclophosphamide, vinblastine, and cisplatin.[20]

Symptoms of SIADH include weight gain without edema, weakness, anorexia, nausea, vomiting, personality changes, seizures, oliguria, decrease in reflexes, and coma. Treatment of SIADH includes treating the underlying malignancy and measures to correct the sodium-water imbalance, including fluid restriction, oral salt tablets or isotonic (0.9%) saline administration, and, in severe cases, IV administration of 3% sodium chloride solution. Furosemide (Lasix) may also be a helpful treatment in the initial phases of SIADH. Demeclocycline (Declomycin) may be needed on an ongoing basis for moderate SIADH. Monitor the sodium level because correcting SIADH rapidly may result in seizures or death.

Hypercalcemia. Hypercalcemia can occur in metastatic disease of the bone or multiple myeloma, or when a parathyroid hormone–like substance is secreted by cancer cells. It occurs in approximately 10% to 20% of patients with advanced cancer.[21] Hypercalcemia resulting from malignancies that have metastasized occurs most frequently in patients with lung, breast, kidney, colon, ovarian, or thyroid cancer. Hypercalcemia resulting from secretion of parathyroid hormone–like substance occurs most frequently in squamous cell carcinoma of the lung; head and neck, cervical, and esophageal cancer; lymphomas; and leukemia. Immobility and dehydration can contribute to or exacerbate hypercalcemia.

The primary manifestations of hypercalcemia include apathy, depression, fatigue, muscle weakness, ECG changes, polyuria and nocturia, anorexia, nausea, and vomiting. Serum levels of calcium in excess of 12 mg/dL (3 mmol/L) often produce symptoms, and significant calcium elevations can be life threatening.

Serum calcium levels are affected by a low albumin level. A low albumin level will give a false-normal calcium level. Therefore the calcium level must be corrected for serum albumin values, or an ionized calcium level should be obtained.

Chronic hypercalcemia can result in nephrocalcinosis and irreversible renal failure. The long-term treatment of hypercalcemia is aimed at the primary disease. Acute hypercalcemia is treated by hydration (3 L/day) and bisphosphonate therapy. When hydration therapy is used in the frail or older adult, diuretics (particularly loop diuretics) may be used to avoid heart failure or edema. Bisphosphonates (the mainstay of treatment) are drugs that inhibit the action of osteoclasts and therefore reduce serum calcium levels. Infusion of the bisphosphonate zoledronate (Zometa) or pamidronate (Aredia) is the treatment of choice. Bisphosphonates are also used to prevent bone complications in patients with bone metastasis.

Tumor Lysis Syndrome. Acute *tumor lysis syndrome* (TLS) is a metabolic complication characterized by rapid release of intracellular components in response to chemotherapy. It occurs less commonly with radiation therapy. TLS is often associated with large tumors that have high growth rates and are sensitive to the effects of chemotherapy.[22] Massive cell destruction, associated with aggressive chemotherapy for rapidly growing tumors, releases a host of intracellular components into the bloodstream, including potassium, phosphate, and DNA and RNA components (which are metabolized to uric acid by the liver).

A rise in serum phosphate drives serum calcium levels down, with resultant hypocalcemia. Metabolic abnormalities and concentrated uric acid (which crystallizes in the distal tubules of the kidneys) lead quickly to acute renal failure if not identified and treated early.

The four hallmark signs of TLS are hyperuricemia, hyperphosphatemia, hyperkalemia, and hypocalcemia. Early symptoms include weakness, muscle cramps, diarrhea, nausea, and vomiting. TLS usually occurs within the first 24 to 48 hours after the initiation of chemotherapy and may persist for approximately 5 to 7 days.

The primary goal of TLS management is preventing renal failure and severe electrolyte imbalances. Patients at risk for TLS should be identified early, and preventive measures implemented concurrently with chemotherapy. The primary treatment includes increasing urine production using hydration therapy and decreasing uric acid concentrations using allopurinol.

Infiltrative Emergencies

Infiltrative emergencies occur when malignant tumors infiltrate major organs or secondary to cancer therapy. The most common infiltrative emergencies are cardiac tamponade and carotid artery rupture.

Cardiac Tamponade. *Cardiac tamponade* results from fluid accumulation in the pericardial sac, constriction of the pericardium by tumor, or pericarditis secondary to radiation therapy to the chest. Manifestations include a heavy feeling over the chest, shortness of breath, tachycardia, cough, dysphagia, hiccups, hoarseness, nausea, vomiting, excessive perspiration, decreased level of consciousness, distant or muted heart sounds, and extreme anxiety. Emergency management is aimed at reduction of fluid around the heart and includes surgical establishment of a pericardial window or an indwelling pericardial catheter. Supportive therapy includes administration of oxygen therapy, IV hydration, and vasopressor therapy.

Carotid Artery Rupture. Rupture of the carotid artery occurs most frequently in patients with cancer of the head and neck secondary to invasion of the arterial wall by tumor or to erosion following surgery or radiation therapy. Bleeding can manifest as minor oozing to spurting of blood in the case of a "blowout" of the artery. In the presence of a blowout, apply pressure to the site with a finger. IV fluids and blood products are administered in an attempt to stabilize the patient for surgery. Surgical management involves ligation of the carotid artery above and below the rupture site and reduction of local tumor.

CANCER PAIN

Moderate to severe pain occurs in approximately 50% of patients who are receiving active treatment for their cancer and in 80% to 90% of patients with advanced cancer. What is concerning is that these statistics have not changed in the past 30 years. Undertreatment of cancer pain is common and causes needless suffering, decreases quality of life, and increases the burden on family caregivers.[23]

Pain Assessment

Inadequate pain assessment is the single greatest barrier to effective pain management. Data such as vital signs and patient behaviors are not reliable indicators of pain, especially long-standing, chronic pain. It is important to distinguish between persistent and episodic, positional, or breakthrough pain. Therefore it is essential that a comprehensive pain assessment include a detailed history to elicit the following characteristics of pain: quality, location, intensity, duration, and precipitating and alleviating factors. Differentiating between types of pain (e.g., visceral, bone, neuropathic) is important in developing an effective pain management plan.

Assess pain on an ongoing basis to determine the effectiveness of the treatment plan. Obtain data and document at regular intervals the location and intensity of the pain, what it feels like, and how it is relieved. Assess change in pain (e.g., a significant change in the intensity, character, or location of pain) to determine the cause (e.g., progression of disease).

Always believe the patient report and accept it as the primary source of assessment data. Table 16-18 presents assessment questions that may facilitate data collection.

Pain Management

Pain management for the cancer patient needs to address both persistent and breakthrough components of pain if they are present. Adjuvant therapies need to be developed specific to the type or nature of the pain. In addition, teach patients how to keep a pain management diary.

Drug therapy, including nonsteroidal antiinflammatory drugs, opioids, and adjuvant pain medications, should be used and selected based on the character and/or cause of the pain. Opioids normally are prescribed for the treatment of moderate to severe cancer pain. Analgesic medications (e.g., morphine, fentanyl) should be given on a regular schedule (around the clock) with additional doses available as needed for breakthrough pain. In general, oral administration of the medication is preferred, but other routes (e.g., transdermal, transmucosal) are also available.

It is critical for you to pay attention to common side effects of pain medications (e.g., constipation) to ensure the patient's well-being and adherence with the pain management program. Nonsteroidal antiinflammatories (acetaminophen, ibuprofen) often serve as helpful adjuncts to opioid therapy, particularly for bone pain. Other adjuvant therapies, such as antidepressant and antiseizure drugs, may beneficial in neuropathic pain, which is often resistant to opioids.

Radiopharmaceuticals (e.g., samarium-153) may benefit patients with diffuse bone pain (particularly if no further chemotherapy is planned). Patients may experience an initial pain *flare* after administration. Nerve blocks or epidural or intrathecal analgesia may also be used to treat patients with unrelieved pain or to minimize the requirements for opioids.

Remember that with opioid drugs (e.g., morphine) the appropriate dosage is whatever is necessary to control the pain with the fewest side effects. Fear of addiction is not warranted. However, it must be addressed as part of patient teaching, since it is a significant barrier for both patients and nurses in appropriate pain management. Discuss the goals of analgesic therapy with patients, especially those requiring large or chronic doses of opioids. Treatment plans should be developed that balance analgesia and side effects to maintain optimal functional status.

Patient teaching should clarify myths and misconceptions and reassure patients and family caregivers that cancer pain can be effectively relieved. Furthermore, addiction and tolerance are not problems associated with effective cancer pain management. Nondrug interventions, including relaxation therapy and imagery, can be effectively used to manage pain (see Chapter 7). Additional strategies to relieve pain are discussed in Chapter 9.

PSYCHOLOGIC SUPPORT

Psychologic support of a patient with cancer is an important aspect of cancer care. The patient may experience a variety of psychosocial concerns, including fears of dependency, loss of control, family and relationship stress, financial burden, and fear of death. Distress may be experienced at many points throughout the cancer continuum, including at diagnosis, during or after treatment, and in association with long-term follow-up visits.

Adaptation and coping with a cancer diagnosis may be influenced by a variety of patient factors, including demographics, prior coping skills and strategies, social support, and religious and spiritual beliefs (Table 16-19). You are in a key position to assess the patient's and family's responses and support positive coping strategies.

To facilitate the development of effective coping and to support the patient and the family during the various stages of cancer, you should do the following.

TABLE 16-18	PAIN ASSESSMENT IN CANCER PATIENTS
Characteristic	**Questions to Ask**
Location	• Where is the pain? • Is the pain in more than one place? Is the pain in a new location? • Does location of pain correlate with known diagnosis?
Intensity	• How bad is the pain? • Rate the pain on a scale of 0-10. (See Chapter 9 for rating scales.)
Quality	• What does the pain feel like—sharp, dull, burning, shooting, aching, or other? (See Chapter 9 for descriptors.)
Pattern	• Has the pain changed? • Is the pain getting better, worse, or unchanged? • What makes the pain better or worse?
Relief measures	• What do you do to control your pain? • Do you use medications? • Do the relief measures help much? How much?

TABLE 16-19	FACTORS AFFECTING HOW PATIENTS COPE WITH CANCER
Factor	**Description**
Ability to cope with stressful events in the past	How patients coped with previous stressful events (e.g., loss of job, major disappointment, significant traumatic event) affects how they cope with diagnosis of cancer.
Availability of significant others	Patients who have effective support systems cope more effectively than those who do not.
Ability to express feelings and concerns	Patients who express feelings and needs and ask for help cope more effectively than those who internalize feelings and needs.
Age at the time of diagnosis	Age determines coping strategies to a great degree. For example, a young mother with cancer may have concerns that differ from those of a 70-year-old woman with cancer.
Extent of disease	Cure or control of the disease process is usually easier to cope with than the reality of terminal illness.
Disruption of body image	Disruption of the body image (e.g., radical neck dissection, alopecia, mastectomy) may intensify the psychologic impact of cancer.
Presence of symptoms	Symptoms such as fatigue, nausea, diarrhea, and pain may intensify the psychologic impact of cancer.
Past experience with cancer	Negative experiences with cancer (personal or in others) influence perceptions about the current situation.
Attitude associated with the cancer	Patients who feel in control and have a positive attitude about cancer and cancer treatment cope better with the diagnosis and treatment of cancer than those who feel hopeless, helpless, and out of control.

- Be available and continue to be available, especially during difficult times.
- Exhibit a caring attitude.
- Listen actively to fears and concerns.
- Help provide relief from distressing symptoms.
- Provide essential information regarding cancer and cancer care that is accurate and establishes realistic expectations about what the patient will experience.
- Maintain a relationship based on trust and confidence. Be open, honest, and caring in the approach.
- Use touch to exhibit caring. A squeeze of the hand or a hug may at times be more effective than words.
- Assist the patient in setting realistic, reachable short-term and long-term goals.
- Assist the patient in maintaining usual lifestyle patterns.
- Maintain hope, which is the key to effective cancer care. Hope varies, depending on the patient's status—hope that the symptoms are not serious, hope that the treatment is curative, hope for independence, hope for relief of pain, hope for a longer life, hope to achieve meaningful goals, or hope for a peaceful death. Hope provides control over what is occurring and is the basis of a positive attitude toward cancer and cancer care.

Many patients with cancer benefit from a variety of psychosocial interventions, such as supportive listening, stress management techniques, individual or group counseling, and cognitive-behavioral therapy. Assess the psychosocial concerns and emotional responses of patients and their families so you

ETHICAL/LEGAL DILEMMAS
Medical Futility

Situation

D.M., a 65-year-old Jewish woman, has breast cancer with metastasis to the liver and bone. The family asks you why their mother is not receiving chemotherapy. In addition, they want to make sure that she will be resuscitated should her heart stop. They are aware of her diagnosis and that she may have only a few months to live. In morning rounds you were told that D.M. does not want any treatment that would prolong her life.

Ethical/Legal Points for Consideration

- Although court decisions have varied, legally there is substantial consensus concerning right to privacy (a constitutional right), right to informed consent and refusal of treatment, and rights pertaining to end-of-life decision making.
- A patient who is an adult and is competent (defined as capable of understanding and interpreting information and making choices) solely retains the right to make personal health care decisions.
- The Patient Self-Determination Act requires that the patient be asked on admission whether he or she has an advance directive. It is placed in the medical record if available. If the patient does not have an advance directive, it must be documented.
- Often families have difficulty accepting the finality of a terminal diagnosis.
- Sometimes family members have conflicting interests (e.g., finances, property, inheritance rights) that influence their decision-making abilities.

Discussion Questions

1. How can you help D.M. communicate her wishes to her family?
2. How can you and the health care team assist the family in planning end-of-life care that incorporates the wishes of their mother?
3. What are the cultural issues in D.M.'s case?

can connect patients with appropriate supportive care resources. Organizations are listed in the Resources section at the end of this chapter. In many cities, local units of the American Cancer Society provide a wide variety of services.

GERONTOLOGIC CONSIDERATIONS

CANCER

Cancer is usually a disease of aging, with most cancers occurring in people over age 65. The cancer mortality rate is exceedingly high in older adults, with 70% of all deaths due to malignancies occurring in those over age 65. This is especially important since the normal life span is lengthening and the proportion of the population who are older than 65 years is increasing.[24,25]

Clinical manifestations of cancer in older adults may be mistakenly attributed to age-related changes and ignored by the person.[25] Older adults are particularly vulnerable to the complications of both cancer and cancer therapy. This is due to their decline in physiologic functioning, social and emotional resources, and cognitive function.

The older adult's functional status should be taken into consideration when developing a treatment plan. Age alone is not a good predictor of tolerance or response to treatment. Advances in the treatment of cancer are making cancer therapies beneficial to an increasing number of older adults, including patients with suboptimal health.

Conduct a Comprehensive Geriatric Assessment (CGA) at the time of diagnosis to identify important issues that might affect decisions about treatment options. Issues to assess include projected life expectancy, estimate of morbidity from cancer, co-morbidities that would affect treatment, and patient decision-making capacity and wishes.[24] The CGA also includes assessment of functional status, socioeconomic issues, psychosocial distress, cognitive function, nutrition, and medication-polypharmacy review.

Some important questions to consider when an older person is diagnosed with cancer include the following: Will the treatment provide more benefits than harm? Will he or she be able to tolerate the treatment safely? Is there need to optimize other co-morbidities or nutritional or functional status before starting treatment? What are the patient's preferences and wishes?

CANCER SURVIVORSHIP

It is estimated that there are currently more than 13.7 million cancer survivors in the United States, with breast cancer patients making up the largest portion of this group. Some of these individuals are cancer free, whereas others still have evidence of cancer and may be undergoing treatment.[1]

Over the past 20 years, the number of cancer survivors has increased threefold. With progressive advances in early detection and treatment, further increases in the number of cancer survivors are expected.[26]

The rapid increase in cancer survivors has been accompanied by a greater awareness of the long-term health and quality-of-life issues that a cancer diagnosis imposes. Cancer survivors experience a variety of long-term and late sequelae following treatment (discussed earlier in this chapter on pp. 265-271). The impact of cancer and its treatment confers greater risk of non-cancer-related death and co-morbidities (e.g., heart disease, diabetes, metabolic syndrome, endocrine dysfunction, osteoporosis) among cancer survivors. Furthermore, cancer survivors may continue to experience symptoms or functional impairment related to treatment for years after treatment.

The impact of a cancer diagnosis can affect many aspects of a patient's life, with cancer survivors commonly reporting financial, vocational, marital, and emotional concerns even long after treatment is over. These psychosocial effects can play a profound role in a patient's life after cancer, with issues related to living in uncertainty being frequently encountered.

To better assist cancer survivors, try to understand the meaning of the cancer experience from the individual's perspective.[27] Some patients may wish to return to their normal lives as soon as possible, and they might fail to attend scheduled follow-up appointments. Other survivors may become cancer advocates or active members of a cancer support group. Still others may allow their lives to revolve around the cancer and may even resist giving up the illness role. Some resources for survivors are listed in Table 16-20. Connecting diverse cancer survivors to culturally appropriate, evidence-based online support and resources is a strategy to enhance health outcomes.[28]

An important question that cancer survivors may ask is whether they should have children or whether their children will have genetic abnormalities. Recent and ongoing research suggests that children of cancer survivors are not at increased risk for genetic or congenital abnormalities. It is unknown whether humans have the ability to repair damage to germ cell DNA or whether processes such as infertility or miscarriages filter out any problems.[29]

TABLE 16-20	RESOURCES FOR CANCER SURVIVORS
Resource	**Website**
National Coalition for Cancer Survivorship (NCCS)	www.canceradvocacy.org
Office of Cancer Survivorship (OCS)	http://cancercontrol.cancer.gov/ocs/office-survivorship.html
Livestrong Survivor Care	www.livestrong.org
Cancer Survivors Network of the American Cancer Society	http://csn.cancer.org
Resources for Cancer Survivors	www.cancerinformation.com/survivorship/resources.aspx

You can help cancer survivors by doing the following:
- Provide all cancer patients with a treatment summary and care plan outlining treatment exposures, risk of late effects, preventive care recommendations, and follow-up surveillance plan after completion of treatment. Care plans should clearly identify all members of the care team and their responsibilities for follow-up care. Also include referrals to appropriate supportive care and community resources that would benefit the patient in recovery or ongoing care.
- Coordinate care among the oncology team, primary health care provider, and other specialists. Teach health care providers about the needs of cancer survivors, including long-term effects of cancer and cancer treatments.
- Teach cancer survivors to look for and report any ongoing symptoms resulting from treatment, including late effects of radiation therapy and chemotherapy.
- Promote healthy behaviors:
  - *Prevention:* good nutrition, exercise, smoking avoidance, maintenance of proper weight, cardiac risk reduction, bone health
  - *Early detection:* routine health screenings (e.g., breast, colon), cholesterol, diabetes, osteoporosis screening as recommended
- Encourage cancer survivors to have regular follow-up examinations with an identified primary health care provider.
- Assess for psychoemotional, financial, health insurance, or vocational problems related to cancer. Assist patients in getting appropriate help if necessary.

CULTURALLY COMPETENT CARE

CANCER
Both cancer incidence and death rates are disproportionately higher in African Americans than in whites and other minority groups (see Cultural and Ethnic Health Disparities box). Although overall racial disparities in cancer death rates have been declining, death rates continue to be 33% higher among African American men and 16% higher among African American women than whites. In addition, African Americans are more likely to have later stage disease at the time of diagnosis than whites.[30,31]

Differences in survival rates from cancer are attributed primarily to a combination of factors, including poverty, difficult access to and poorer quality of health care, more co-morbid conditions, and differences in tumor biology. Disparities in cancer care exist throughout the continuum from cancer pre-

⊕ CULTURAL & ETHNIC HEALTH DISPARITIES

Cancer

- Cancer incidence and death rates for men are highest among African Americans, followed by whites, Hispanics, and Asians/Pacific Islanders.
- Cancer incidence rates for women are highest among whites, followed by African Americans, Hispanics, and Asians/Pacific Islanders.
- However, cancer death rates for women are highest among African Americans, followed by whites, Hispanics, and Asians/Pacific Islanders.

vention and screening to end-of-life care and survivorship. The disparity in prevention and screening results in cancer being in advanced stages at the time of diagnosis.[32]

Culturally competent care in oncology is needed to meet the needs of diverse groups. Culturally competent care involves awareness of personal background, how culture affects care delivery, and how to adapt to meet cultural needs. Nurses need to actively seek to understand cultural differences to meet the individualized needs. (Culturally competent care related to specific cancers is presented in the chapters where the cancer is discussed.)

▌ BRIDGE TO NCLEX EXAMINATION

The number of the question corresponds to the same-numbered outcome at the beginning of the chapter.

1. Trends in the incidence and death rates of cancer include the fact that
   a. lung cancer is the most common type of cancer in men.
   b. a higher percentage of women than men have lung cancer.
   c. breast cancer is the leading cause of cancer deaths in women.
   d. African Americans have a higher death rate from cancer than whites.

2. What features of cancer cells distinguish them from normal cells *(select all that apply)*?
   a. Cells lack contact inhibition.
   b. Cells return to a previous undifferentiated state.
   c. Oncogenes maintain normal cell expression.
   d. Proliferation occurs when there is a need for more cells.
   e. New proteins characteristic of embryonic stage emerge on cell membrane.

3. A characteristic of the stage of progression in the development of cancer is
   a. oncogenic viral transformation of target cells.
   b. a reversible steady growth facilitated by carcinogens.
   c. a period of latency before clinical detection of cancer.
   d. proliferation of cancer cells in spite of host control mechanisms.

4. The primary protective role of the immune system related to malignant cells is
   a. surveillance for cells with tumor-associated antigens.
   b. binding with free antigen released by malignant cells.
   c. production of blocking factors that immobilize cancer cells.
   d. responding to a new set of antigenic determinants on cancer cells.

5. The primary difference between benign and malignant neoplasms is the
   a. rate of cell proliferation.
   b. site of malignant tumor.
   c. requirements for cell nutrients.
   d. characteristic of tissue invasiveness.

6. The nurse is caring for a 59-year-old woman who had surgery 1 day ago for removal of a suspected malignant abdominal mass. The patient is awaiting the pathology report. She is tearful and says that she is scared to die. The most effective nursing intervention at this point is to use this opportunity to
   a. motivate change in an unhealthy lifestyle.
   b. teach her about the seven warning signs of cancer.
   c. instruct her about healthy stress relief and coping practices.
   d. allow her to communicate about the meaning of this experience.

7. The goals of cancer treatment are based on the principle that
   a. surgery is the single most effective treatment for cancer.
   b. initial treatment is always directed toward cure of the cancer.
   c. a combination of treatment modalities is effective for controlling many cancers.
   d. although cancer cure is rare, quality of life can be increased with treatment modalities.

8. The most effective method of administering a chemotherapy agent that is a vesicant is to
   a. give it orally.
   b. give it intraarterially.
   c. use an Ommaya reservoir.
   d. use a central venous access device.

9. The nurse explains to a patient undergoing brachytherapy of the cervix that she
   a. must undergo simulation to locate the treatment area.
   b. requires the use of radioactive precautions during nursing care.
   c. may experience desquamation of the skin on the abdomen and upper legs.
   d. requires shielding of the ovaries during treatment to prevent ovarian damage.

10. A patient on chemotherapy and radiation for head and neck cancer has a WBC count of $1.9 \times 10^3/\mu L$, hemoglobin of 10.8 g/dL, and a platelet count of $99 \times 10^3/\mu L$. Based on the CBC results, what is the most serious clinical finding?
    a. Cough, rhinitis, and sore throat
    b. Fatigue, nausea, and skin redness at site of radiation
    c. Temperature of 101.9° F, fatigue, and shortness of breath
    d. Skin redness at site of radiation, headache, and constipation

11. To prevent fever and shivering during an infusion of rituximab (Rituxan), the nurse should premedicate the patient with
    a. aspirin.
    b. acetaminophen.
    c. sodium bicarbonate.
    d. meperidine (Demerol).

12. The nurse counsels the patient receiving radiation therapy or chemotherapy that
    a. effective birth control methods should be used for the rest of the patient's life.
    b. if nausea and vomiting occur during treatment, the treatment plan will be modified.
    c. after successful treatment, a return to the person's previous functional level can be expected.
    d. the cycle of fatigue-depression-fatigue that may occur during treatment can be reduced by restricting activity.

13. A patient on chemotherapy for 10 weeks started at a weight of 121 lb. She now weighs 118 lb and has no sense of taste. Which nursing intervention would be a priority?
   a. Advise the patient to eat foods that are fatty, fried, or high in calories.
   b. Discuss with the physician the need for parenteral or enteral feedings.
   c. Advise the patient to drink a nutritional supplement beverage at least three times a day.
   d. Advise the patient to experiment with spices and seasonings to enhance the flavor of food.

14. A 70-year-old male patient has multiple myeloma. His wife calls to report that he sleeps most of the day, is confused when awake, and complains of nausea and constipation. Which complication of cancer is this most likely caused by?
   a. Hypercalcemia
   b. Tumor lysis syndrome
   c. Spinal cord compression
   d. Superior vena cava syndrome

15. A patient has recently been diagnosed with early stages of breast cancer. What is most appropriate for the nurse to focus on?
   a. Maintaining the patient's hope
   b. Preparing a will and advance directives
   c. Discussing replacement child care for the patient's children
   d. Discussing the patient's past experiences with her grandmother's cancer

1. d, 2. a, b, e, 3. d, 4. a, 5. d, 6. d, 7. c, 8. d, 9. b, 10. c, 11. b, 12. c, 13. d, 14. a, 15. a

⊖volve

For rationales to these answers and even more NCLEX review questions, visit *http://evolve.elsevier.com/Lewis/medsurg*.

REFERENCES

1. American Cancer Society: *Cancer facts and figures* 2012. Retrieved from *www.cancer.org/research/cancerfactsfigures/cancerfactsfigures/cancer-facts-figures-2013*.
2. Casey G: The biology of cancer, *Nurs N Z* 18(1):20, 2012.
3. Wu X, Watson M, Wilson R, et al: Human papillomavirus–associated cancers—United States, 2004-2008, *MMWR* 61(15):258, 2012.
4. Prenzel KL, Bollschweiler E, Schröder W, et al: Prognostic relevance of skip metastases in esophageal cancer, *Ann Thorac Surg* 90:1662, 2010.
*5. Zauber AG, Winawer SJ, O'Brien MJ, et al: Colonoscopic polypectomy and long-term prevention of colorectal-cancer deaths, *N Engl J Med* 366:687, 2012.
*6. Polovitch M, Whitford J, Olsen M: *Chemotherapy and biotherapy guidelines and recommendations for practice*, ed 3, Pittsburgh, 2009, Oncology Nursing Society. Retrieved from *www.ons.org*.
7. Held-Warmkessel J: Taming the three high-risk chemotherapy complications, *Nursing* 41:30, 2011.
8. National Cancer Institute: Radiation therapy for cancer Q&A. Retrieved from *www.cancer.gov/cancertopics/coping/radiation-therapy-and-you/page2*.
*9. Ma CM: The practice of radiation oncology. In Iwamoto RR, Haas ML, Gosselin TK, editors: *Manual for radiation oncology nursing practice and education*, ed 4, Pittsburgh, 2011, Oncology Nursing Society.
*10. National Comprehensive Cancer Network: NCCN clinical practice guidelines—myeloid growth factors. Retrieved from *www.nccn.org/professionals/physician_gls/pdf/myeloid_growth.pdf*.
*11. National Comprehensive Cancer Network: NCCN clinical practice guidelines—cancer related fatigue v1. 2012. Retrieved from *www.nccn.org*.
*12. Ettinger DS, Armstrong DK, Barbour S, et al: NCCN clinical practice guidelines in oncology: antiemesis, *J Natl Compr Cancer Network* 7:572, 2009.
*13. Feyer P, Maranzano E, Molassiotis A, et al: Radiotherapy-induced nausea and vomiting (RINV): MASCC/ESMO guideline for antiemetics in radiotherapy: update 2009, *Support Care Cancer* 19(Suppl 1):S5, 2011.
*14. Muehlbauer PM, Thrope D, Davis A: Putting evidence into practice: evidence-based interventions to prevent, manage, and treat chemotherapy- and radiotherapy-induced diarrhea, *Clin J Oncol Nurs* 13:336, 2009.
15. Cady J: Gastrointestinal/abdomen. In Iwamoto RR, Haas ML, Gosselin TK, editors: *Manual for radiation oncology nursing practice and education*, ed 4, Pittsburgh, 2012, Oncology Nursing Society.
16. Feight D, Baney T, Bruce S, et al: Putting evidence into practice: evidence-based interventions for radiation dermatitis, *Clin J Oncol Nurs* 15(5):481, 2011.
17. Camidge D, Doebele R: Treating Alk-positive lung cancer: early successes and future challenges, *Nature Rev Clin Oncol* 9:268, 2012.
18. National Cancer Institute: Bone marrow transplantation and peripheral blood stem cell transplantation, 2010. Retrieved from *http://cancer.gov.cancertopics/factsheet/Therapy/bone-marrow-transplant*.
19. Antin JH, Yolin DS: *Manual of cell and bone marrow transplantation*, Cambridge, Mass, 2009, Cambridge University Press.
20. Esposito P, Piotti G, Bianzina S, et al: The syndrome of inappropriate antidiuresis: pathophysiology, clinical management and new therapeutic options, *Nephron Clin Pract* 119:c62, 2011.
21. LeGrand S: Modern management of malignant hypercalcemia, *Am J Hospice Palliative Care* 28:515, 2011.
22. Held-Warmkessel J: How to prevent and manage tumor lysis syndrome, *Nursing* 40:27, 2010.
23. National Cancer Institute: Pain (PDQ). Retrieved from *www.cancer.gov/cancertopics/pdq/supportivecare/pain/HealthProfessional*.
24. National Comprehensive Cancer Network: NCCN clinical practice guidelines—senior adult oncology v2. 2012. Retrieved from *www.nccn.org*.
25. Hurria A, Cohen HJ: *Practical geriatric oncology*, Cambridge, Mass, 2009, Cambridge University Press.

*Evidence-based information for clinical practice.

26. Vachani C, Hampshire MK, Hill-Kayser CE, et al: Preparing patients for life after cancer treatment, *Am J Nurs* 111:51, 2011.

27. Stanton AL: What happens now? Psychosocial care for cancer survivors after medical treatment completion, *J Clin Oncol* 30:1215, 2012.

*28. Hong Y, Peña-Purcell NC, Ory MG: Outcomes of online support and resources for cancer survivors: a systematic literature review, *Patient Educ Couns* 86(3):288, 2012.

29. Signorella LB: Congenital anomalies in the children of cancer survivors: a report from the childhood cancer survivor study, *J Clin Oncol* 30:239, 2012.

30. National Cancer Institute: *Cancer trends progress report update, 2009/2010*, Bethesda, Md, 2010, National Institutes of Health. Retrieved from *http://progressreport.cancer.gov*.

31. American Cancer Society: *Cancer facts and figures for African Americans, 2011-2012*, Atlanta, 2012, The Society. Retrieved from *www.cancer.org/acs/groupscontent/@epidemiology surveilance/documents/document/acspc-027765.pdf*.

32. Pluth Yeo T, Phillips J, Delengowski A, et al: Oncology nursing: educating advanced practice nurses to provide culturally competent care, *J Professional Nurs* 27(4):245, 2011.

RESOURCES

American Association for Cancer Education (AACE)
  www.aaceonline.com
American Cancer Society
  www.cancer.org

American Society of Clinical Oncology (ASCO)
  www.asco.org
Association of Community Cancer Centers (ACCC)
  www.accc-cancer.org
Cancer Care, Inc.
  www.cancercare.org
Cancer Guide
  http://cancerguide.org
Cancer Hotlines
  800-525-3777
  800-638-6070 (Alaska)
  800-636-5700 (District of Columbia)
  800-524-1234 (Hawaii; call collect)
Cancer Information Service (CIS), a Program of the National Cancer Institute (NCI)
  www.cancer.gov/aboutnci/cis
International Society of Nurses in Cancer Care (ISNCC)
  www.isncc.org
National Cancer Institute (NCI)
  www.cancer.gov
National Coalition for Cancer Survivorship (NCCS)
  www.canceradvocacy.org
OncoLink (cancer information site)
  www.oncolink.org
Oncology Nursing Society (ONS)
  www.ons.org

We never know the worth of water
till the well is dry.
Thomas Fuller

Fluid, Electrolyte, and Acid-Base Imbalances

Mariann M. Harding

evolve WEBSITE

http://evolve.elsevier.com/Lewis/medsurg

- NCLEX Review Questions
- Key Points
- Pre-Test
- Answer Guidelines for Case Study on p. 313

- Rationales for Bridge to NCLEX Examination Questions
- Case Studies
  - Patient With Hyponatremia/Fluid Volume Imbalance

- Concept Map Creator
- Glossary
- Fluids and Electrolytes Tutorial
- Content Updates

LEARNING OUTCOMES

1. Describe the composition of the major body fluid compartments.
2. Define processes involved in the regulation of movement of water and electrolytes between the body fluid compartments.
3. Describe the etiology, laboratory diagnostic findings, clinical manifestations, and nursing and collaborative management of the following disorders:
   a. Extracellular fluid volume imbalances: fluid volume deficit and fluid volume excess
   b. Sodium imbalances: hypernatremia and hyponatremia
   c. Potassium imbalances: hyperkalemia and hypokalemia
   d. Magnesium imbalances: hypermagnesemia and hypomagnesemia
   e. Calcium imbalances: hypercalcemia and hypocalcemia
   f. Phosphate imbalances: hyperphosphatemia and hypophosphatemia
4. Identify the processes to maintain acid-base balance.
5. Discuss the etiology, laboratory diagnostic findings, clinical manifestations, and nursing and collaborative management of the following acid-base imbalances: metabolic acidosis, metabolic alkalosis, respiratory acidosis, and respiratory alkalosis.
6. Describe the composition and indications of common IV fluid solutions.
7. Discuss the types and nursing management of commonly used central venous access devices.

KEY TERMS

acidosis, p. 302
active transport, p. 287
alkalosis, p. 302
anions, p. 286
buffers, p. 303
cations, p. 286

central venous access devices (CVADs), p. 309
electrolytes, p. 286
fluid spacing, p. 289
hydrostatic pressure, p. 288
hypertonic, p. 288

hypotonic, p. 288
isotonic, p. 288
oncotic pressure, p. 288
osmolality, p. 288
osmosis, p. 287
osmotic pressure, p. 287

HOMEOSTASIS

Body fluids and electrolytes play an important role in maintaining *homeostasis*, the stable internal environment of the body.[1] Body fluids are in constant motion transporting nutrients, electrolytes, and oxygen to cells and carrying waste products away from cells. The body uses a number of adaptive responses associated with these activities to keep the composition and volume of body fluids and electrolytes within the narrow limits of normal to maintain homeostasis and promote health.

Many diseases and their treatments can affect fluid and electrolyte balance. For example, a patient with metastatic breast or lung cancer may develop hypercalcemia because of bone destruction from tumor invasion. Chemotherapy prescribed to treat the cancer may result in nausea and vomiting and, subsequently, dehydration and acid-base imbalances. When correcting dehydration with IV fluids, the patient requires close monitoring to prevent fluid overload.

It is important for you to anticipate the potential for alterations in fluid and electrolyte balance associated with certain disorders and medical therapies, recognize the signs and symptoms of imbalances, and intervene with the appropriate action. This chapter describes the (1) normal control of fluids, electrolytes, and acid-base balance; (2) conditions that disrupt homeostasis and resultant manifestations; and (3) actions that

Reviewed by Dorothy (Dottie) M. Mathers, RN, DNP, CNE, Professor, School of Health Sciences, Pennsylvania College of Technology, Williamsport, Pennsylvania; and Jason Mott, RN, MSN, Instructor of Nursing, Bellin College: School of Nursing, Green Bay, Wisconsin.

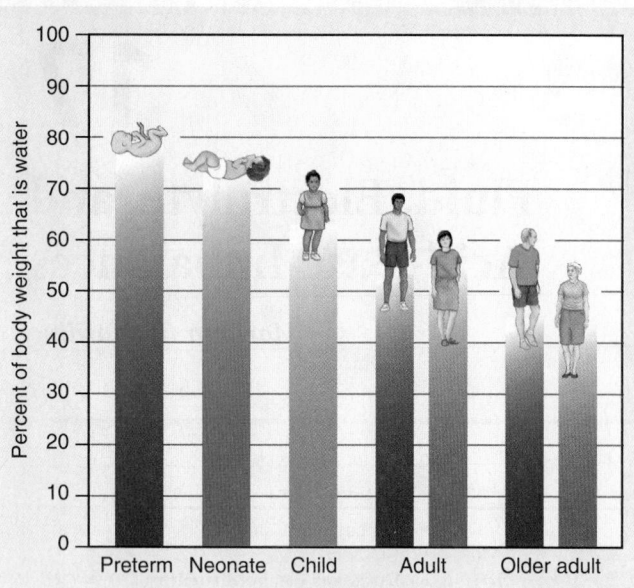

FIG. 17-1 Body water over the life span.

FIG. 17-2 Relative volumes of three body fluids. Values represent fluid distribution in a young male adult.

the health care provider and you can take to prevent fluid, electrolyte, and acid-base imbalances and restore homeostasis.

WATER CONTENT OF THE BODY

Water is the primary component of the body, accounting for approximately 50% to 60% of body weight in the adult. The water content varies with gender, body mass, and age (Fig. 17-1). The percentage of body weight that is composed of water is generally greater in men than in women because men tend to have more lean body mass. The more fat present in the body, the less the total water content. Therefore obese individuals have a lower percentage of body water than slender people do. Older adults, with less muscle mass and more fat content, have less body water for this same reason. In the older adult, body water content averages 45% to 55% of body weight, leaving them at a higher risk for fluid-related problems than young adults.

Body Fluid Compartments

The two fluid compartments in the body are the *intracellular space* (inside the cells) and the *extracellular space* (outside the cells) (Fig. 17-2). Approximately two thirds of the body water is located within cells and is termed *intracellular fluid* (ICF); ICF constitutes approximately 40% of body weight of an adult. The body of a 70-kg young man would contain approximately 42 L of water, of which 28 L would be located within cells.

The extracellular fluid (ECF) consists of *interstitial fluid* (the fluid in the spaces between cells), *plasma* (the liquid part of blood), and *transcellular fluid* (a very small amount of fluid contained within specialized cavities of the body). Transcellular fluids include cerebrospinal fluid; fluid in the gastrointestinal (GI) tract; and pleural, synovial, peritoneal, intraocular, and pericardial fluid. ECF consists of one third of the body water; this would amount to about 14 L in a 70-kg man. About 20% of ECF is in the intravascular space as plasma (3 L in a 70-kg man), and 70% is in the interstitial space (10 L in a 70-kg man). The fluid in the transcellular spaces totals about 1 L at any given time. However, because 3 to 6 L of fluid is secreted into and reabsorbed from the GI tract every day, loss of this fluid from

vomiting or diarrhea can produce serious fluid and electrolyte imbalances.

Calculation of Fluid Gain or Loss

One liter of water weighs 2.2 lb (1 kg). Body weight change, especially sudden change, is an excellent indicator of overall fluid volume loss or gain. For example, if a patient drinks 240 mL (8 oz) of fluid, weight gain will be 0.5 lb (0.23 kg). A patient receiving diuretic therapy who loses 4.4 lb (2 kg) in 24 hours has experienced a fluid loss of approximately 2 L. An adult patient who is fasting might lose approximately 1 to 2 lb/day. A weight loss exceeding this is likely due to loss of body fluid.

ELECTROLYTES

Electrolytes are substances whose molecules dissociate, or split into ions, when placed in water. *Ions* are electrically charged particles. **Cations** are positively charged ions. Examples include sodium (Na^+), potassium (K^+), calcium (Ca^{2+}), and magnesium (Mg^{2+}) ions. **Anions** are negatively charged ions. Examples include bicarbonate (HCO_3^-), chloride (Cl^-), and phosphate (PO_4^{3-}) ions. Most proteins bear a negative charge and are thus anions.

Measurement of Electrolytes

The milliequivalent (mEq) is the commonly used unit of measure for electrolytes. Electrolytes in body fluids are active chemicals that unite in varying combinations, so it is more practical to express their concentration as a measure of chemical activity (or milliequivalents) rather than as a measure of weight. Ions combine milliequivalent for milliequivalent. For example, 1 mEq (1 mmol) of sodium combines with 1 mEq (1 mmol) of chloride.

Electrolyte Composition of Fluid Compartments

Electrolyte composition varies between ECF and ICF. The overall concentration of electrolytes is approximately the same in the two compartments. However, concentrations of specific ions differ greatly (Fig. 17-3). In ECF the main cation is sodium, with small amounts of potassium, calcium, and magnesium. The primary ECF anion is chloride, with small amounts of bicarbonate, sulfate, and phosphate anions. In ICF the most

FIG. 17-3 The relative concentrations of the major cations and anions in the intracellular space and the plasma.

TABLE 17-1	NORMAL SERUM ELECTROLYTE VALUES
Electrolyte	**Reference Interval**
Anions	
Bicarbonate (HCO_3^-)	22-26 mEq/L (22-26 mmol/L)
Chloride (Cl^-)	96-106 mEq/L (96-106 mmol/L)
Phosphate (PO_4^{3-})*	2.4-4.4 mg/dL (0.78-1.42 mmol/L)
Cations	
Potassium (K^+)	3.5-5.0 mEq/L (3.5-5.0 mmol/L)
Magnesium (Mg^{2+})	1.5-2.5 mEq/L (0.75-1.25 mmol/L)
Sodium (Na^+)	135-145 mEq/L (135-145 mmol/L)
Calcium (Ca^{2+}) (total)	8.6-10.2 mg/dL (2.15-2.55 mmol/L)
Calcium (ionized)	4.6-5.3 mg/dL (1.16-1.32 mmol/L)

*The majority of the phosphorus (P) in the body is found as phosphate (PO_4^{3-}). The terms are used interchangeably in this text.

prevalent cation is potassium, with small amounts of magnesium and sodium. The prevalent ICF anion is phosphate, with some protein and a small amount of bicarbonate. (Normal serum electrolyte values are presented in Table 17-1.)

MECHANISMS CONTROLLING FLUID AND ELECTROLYTE MOVEMENT

The movement of electrolytes and water between ICF and ECF involves many different processes, including simple diffusion, facilitated diffusion, and active transport. Water moves as driven by two forces: hydrostatic pressure and osmotic pressure.

Diffusion

Diffusion is the movement of molecules from an area of high concentration to one of low concentration (Fig. 17-4). It occurs in liquids, gases, and solids. Net movement of molecules across a membrane stops when the concentrations are equal in both areas. The membrane separating the two areas must be perme-

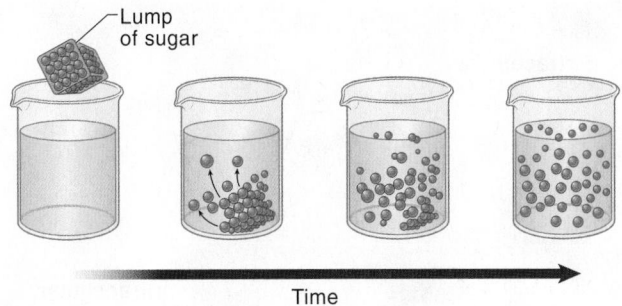

FIG. 17-4 Diffusion is the movement of molecules from an area of high concentration to an area of low concentration. Eventually the sugar molecules are evenly distributed.

able to the diffusing substance for the process to occur. Simple diffusion requires no external energy.

Facilitated Diffusion

Facilitated diffusion involves the use of a protein carrier in the cell membrane. The protein carrier combines with a molecule, especially one too large to pass easily through the cell membrane, and assists in moving the molecule across the membrane from an area of high concentration to one of low concentration. Like simple diffusion, facilitated diffusion is passive and requires no energy. Glucose transport into the cell is an example of facilitated diffusion. The large glucose molecule must combine with a carrier molecule to be able to cross the cell membrane and enter most cells.

Active Transport

Active transport is a process in which molecules move against the concentration gradient. External energy is required for this process. An example is the sodium-potassium pump. The concentrations of sodium and potassium differ greatly intracellularly and extracellularly (see Fig. 17-3). To maintain this concentration difference, the cell uses active transport to move sodium out of the cell and potassium into the cell (Fig. 17-5). The energy source for this mechanism is adenosine triphosphate (ATP), produced in the cell's mitochondria.

Osmosis

Osmosis is the movement of water "down" a concentration gradient, that is, from a region of low solute concentration to one of high solute concentration, across a semipermeable membrane.[2] Imagine a chamber with two compartments separated by a semipermeable membrane, one that allows only the movement of water (Fig. 17-6). Water will move from the less concentrated side (has more water) to the more concentrated side of the chamber water (has less water). Osmosis requires no outside energy sources and stops when the concentration differences disappear or when hydrostatic pressure builds and is sufficient to oppose any further movement of water.

Whenever dissolved substances are contained in a space with a semipermeable membrane, they can pull water into the space by osmosis. The concentration of the solution determines the strength of the osmotic pull. The higher the concentration, the greater the solution's pulling, or osmotic pressure. Osmotic pressure is measured in milliosmoles (mOsm) and may be expressed as either fluid osmolarity or fluid osmolality. Although the terms *osmolarity* and *osmolality* are often used interchangeably, they are different measurements. *Osmolarity* measures the

FIG. 17-5 Sodium-potassium pump. As sodium *(Na⁺)* diffuses into the cell and potassium *(K⁺)* diffuses out of the cell, an active transport system supplied with energy delivers Na⁺ back to the extracellular compartment and K⁺ to the intracellular compartment. *ATP,* Adenosine triphosphate.

FIG. 17-6 Osmosis is the process of water movement through a semipermeable membrane from an area of low solute concentration to an area of high solute concentration.

total milliosmoles per liter of solution, or the concentration of molecules per volume of solution (mOsm/L). **Osmolality** measures the number of milliosmoles per kilogram of water, or the concentration of molecules per weight of water. Osmolality is the test typically performed to evaluate the concentration of plasma and urine.[2]

Measurement of Osmolality. Osmolality is approximately the same in the various body fluid spaces. Determining osmolality is important because it indicates the body's water balance. To assess the state of the body's water balance, one can measure or estimate plasma osmolality. Normal plasma osmolality is between 275 and 295 mOsm/kg. A value greater than 295 mOsm/kg indicates that the concentration of particles is too great or that the water content is too little. This condition is termed *water deficit*. A value less than 275 mOsm/kg indicates too little solute for the amount of water or too much water for the amount of solute. This condition is termed *water excess*. Both conditions are clinically significant. Because the major determinants of plasma osmolality are sodium and glucose, one can calculate the effective plasma osmolality based on the concentrations of those substances.

Osmolality of urine can range from 100 to 1300 mOsm/kg, depending on fluid intake and the amount of antidiuretic hormone (ADH) in circulation and the renal response to it.

Osmotic Movement of Fluids. The osmolality or tonicity of the fluid surrounding the cells affects them. Fluids with the

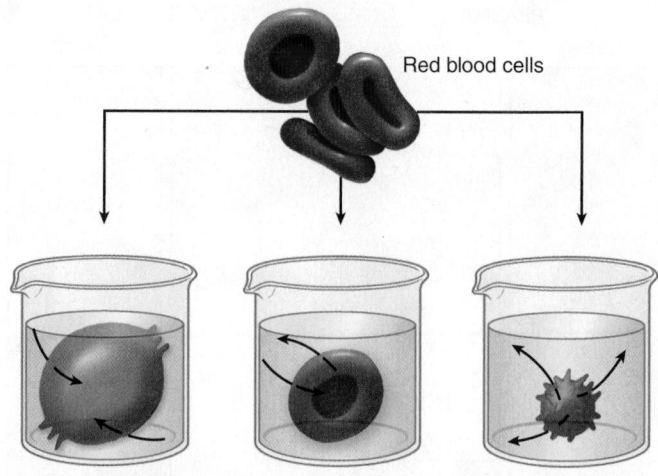

A Hypotonic solution **B** Isotonic solution **C** Hypertonic solution

FIG. 17-7 Effects of water status on red blood cells. **A,** Hypotonic solution (H₂O excess) results in cellular swelling. **B,** Isotonic solution (normal H₂O balance) results in no change. **C,** Hypertonic solution (H₂O deficit) results in cellular shrinking.

same osmolality as the cell interior are termed **isotonic**. Normally, ECF and ICF are isotonic to one another, so no net movement of water occurs.

Changes in the osmolality of ECF alter the volume of cells. Solutions in which the solutes are less concentrated than in the cells are termed **hypotonic** (hypoosmolar). If a cell is surrounded by hypotonic fluid, water moves into the cell, causing it to swell and possibly to burst. Fluids with solutes more concentrated than in cells, or an increased osmolality, are termed **hypertonic** (hyperosmolar). If hypertonic fluid surrounds a cell, water leaves the cell to dilute ECF; the cell shrinks and may eventually die (Fig. 17-7).

Hydrostatic Pressure

Hydrostatic pressure is the force within a fluid compartment. In the blood vessels, hydrostatic pressure is the blood pressure generated by the contraction of the heart. Hydrostatic pressure in the vascular system gradually decreases as the blood moves through the arteries until it is about 30 mm Hg in the capillary bed. At the capillary level, hydrostatic pressure is the major force that pushes water out of the vascular system and into the interstitial space.

Oncotic Pressure

Oncotic pressure (colloidal osmotic pressure) is the osmotic pressure caused by plasma colloids in solution. The major colloid in the vascular system contributing to the total osmotic pressure is protein. Plasma has substantial amounts of protein, whereas the interstitial space has very little. The plasma protein molecules attract water, pulling fluid from the tissue space to the vascular space. Under normal conditions, plasma oncotic pressure is approximately 25 mm Hg. The small amount of protein found in the interstitial space exerts an oncotic pressure of approximately 1 mm Hg.

FLUID MOVEMENT IN CAPILLARIES

As plasma flows through the capillary bed, four factors determine if fluid moves out of the capillary and into the interstitial

FIG. 17-8 Dynamics of fluid exchange between a capillary and tissue. An equilibrium exists between forces filtering fluid out of the capillary and forces absorbing fluid back into the capillary. Note that the hydrostatic pressure is greater at the arterial end of the capillary than at the venous end. The net effect of pressures at the arterial end of the capillary causes a movement of fluid into the tissue. At the venous end of the capillary, there is net movement of fluid back into the capillary.

space or if fluid moves back into the capillary from the interstitial space. The amount and direction of movement are determined by the interaction of (1) capillary hydrostatic pressure, (2) plasma oncotic pressure, (3) interstitial hydrostatic pressure, and (4) interstitial oncotic pressure.

Capillary hydrostatic pressure and interstitial oncotic pressure move water out of the capillaries. Plasma oncotic pressure and interstitial hydrostatic pressure move fluid into the capillaries. At the arterial end of the capillary, capillary hydrostatic pressure exceeds plasma oncotic pressure, and fluid moves into the interstitial space. At the venous end of the capillary, the capillary hydrostatic pressure is lower than plasma oncotic pressure, drawing fluid back into the capillary by the oncotic pressure created by plasma proteins (Fig. 17-8).

Fluid Shifts

If capillary or interstitial pressures change, fluid may abnormally shift from one compartment to another, resulting in edema or dehydration.

Shifts of Plasma to Interstitial Fluid. *Edema,* an accumulation of fluid in the interstitial space, occurs if venous hydrostatic pressure rises, plasma oncotic pressure decreases, or interstitial oncotic pressure rises. Edema may also develop if an obstruction of lymphatic outflow causes decreased removal of interstitial fluid.

Elevation of Venous Hydrostatic Pressure. Increasing the pressure at the venous end of the capillary inhibits fluid movement back into the capillary, which results in edema. Causes of increased venous pressure include fluid overload, heart failure, liver failure, obstruction of venous return to the heart (e.g., tourniquets, restrictive clothing, venous thrombosis), and venous insufficiency (e.g., varicose veins).

Decrease in Plasma Oncotic Pressure. Fluid remains in the interstitial space if the plasma oncotic pressure is too low to draw fluid back into the capillary. Low plasma protein content decreases oncotic pressure. This can result from excessive protein loss (renal disorders), deficient protein synthesis (liver disease), and deficient protein intake (malnutrition).

Elevation of Interstitial Oncotic Pressure. Trauma, burns, and inflammation can damage capillary walls and allow plasma proteins to accumulate in the interstitial space. This increases inter-

stitial oncotic pressure, draws fluid into the interstitial space, and holds it there.

Shifts of Interstitial Fluid to Plasma. An increase in the plasma osmotic or oncotic pressure draws fluid into the plasma from the interstitial space. This could happen with administration of colloids, dextran, mannitol, or hypertonic solutions. Increasing the tissue hydrostatic pressure is another way of causing a shift of fluid into plasma. Wearing elastic compression gradient stockings or hose to decrease peripheral edema is a therapeutic application of this effect.

FLUID SPACING

Fluid spacing is a term used to describe the distribution of body water. *First spacing* describes the normal distribution of fluid in ICF and ECF compartments. *Second spacing* refers to an abnormal accumulation of interstitial fluid (i.e., edema). *Third spacing* occurs when fluid accumulates in a portion of the body from which it is not easily exchanged with the rest of the ECF. Third-spaced fluid is trapped and unavailable for functional use. Examples of third spacing are ascites; sequestration of fluid in the abdominal cavity with peritonitis; and edema associated with burns, trauma, or sepsis.[3]

REGULATION OF WATER BALANCE

Hypothalamic-Pituitary Regulation

Water balance is maintained via the finely tuned balance of water intake and excretion. Water ingestion will equal water loss in the individual who has free access to water, a normal thirst and ADH mechanism, and normally functioning kidneys.

An intact thirst mechanism is critical because it is the primary protection against the development of hyperosmolality. Osmoreceptors in the hypothalamus sense a body fluid deficit or increase in plasma osmolality, which in turn stimulates thirst and ADH release. Thirst causes the patient to drink water. The distal tubules and collecting ducts in the kidneys respond to ADH by becoming more permeable to water. The result is increased water reabsorption from the tubular filtrate into the blood and decreased excretion in the urine. Together these factors result in increased free water in the body and decreased plasma osmolality.

The patient who cannot recognize or act on the sensation of thirst is at risk for fluid deficit and hyperosmolality. Other factors that stimulate ADH release include stress, nausea, nicotine, and morphine. A decreased plasma osmolality or water excess suppresses secretion of ADH, resulting in urinary excretion of water. It is common for the postoperative patient to have a lower plasma osmolality, possibly because of the stress of surgery and opioid analgesia. Social and psychologic factors not related to fluid balance also affect the desire to consume fluids. A dry mouth will cause the patient to drink, even when there is no measurable body water deficit.

Renal Regulation

The kidneys are the primary organs for regulating fluid and electrolyte balance (see Chapter 45). The kidneys regulate water balance by adjusting urine volume and the urinary excretion of most electrolytes to maintain a balance between overall intake and output. The kidneys filter the total plasma volume many times each day. In the average adult the kidneys reabsorb 99% of this filtrate, producing approximately 1.5 L of urine per day.

As the filtrate moves through the renal tubules, selective reabsorption of water and electrolytes and secretion of electrolytes result in the production of urine that is greatly different in composition and concentration from plasma. This process helps maintain normal plasma osmolality, electrolyte balance, blood volume, and acid-base balance. The renal tubules are the site for the actions of ADH and aldosterone.

With severely impaired renal function, the kidneys cannot maintain fluid and electrolyte balance. This condition results in edema, potassium and phosphorus retention, acidosis, and other electrolyte imbalances (see Chapter 47).

Adrenal Cortical Regulation

Glucocorticoids and mineralocorticoids secreted by the adrenal cortex help regulate both water and electrolytes. The glucocorticoids (e.g., cortisol) primarily have an antiinflammatory effect and increase serum glucose levels, whereas the mineralocorticoids (e.g., aldosterone) enhance sodium retention and potassium excretion (Fig. 17-9). When sodium is reabsorbed, water follows because of osmotic changes.

Cortisol is the most abundant glucocorticoid. In large doses, cortisol has both glucocorticoid (glucose elevating and antiinflammatory) and mineralocorticoid (sodium-retention) effects. Normally cortisol secretion is in a diurnal or circadian pattern. Increased cortisol secretion occurs in response to physical and psychologic stress, affecting many body functions, including fluid and electrolyte balance (Fig. 17-10).

Aldosterone is a mineralocorticoid with potent sodium-retaining and potassium-excreting capabilities. Decreased renal perfusion or decreased sodium delivery to the distal portion of the renal tubule activates the renin-angiotensin-aldosterone system (RAAS), which results in aldosterone secretion (see Fig. 45-4). In addition to the RAAS, increased plasma potassium, decreased plasma sodium, and adrenocorticotropic hormone (ACTH) from the anterior pituitary act directly on the adrenal cortex to stimulate the secretion of aldosterone (see Fig. 17-9).

Cardiac Regulation

Natriuretic peptides, including atrial natriuretic peptide (ANP) and b-type natriuretic peptide (BNP), are hormones produced by cardiomyocytes. They are natural antagonists to the RAAS. They are produced in response to increased atrial pressure (increased volume, such as occurs in heart failure) and high serum sodium levels. They suppress secretion of aldosterone, renin, and ADH, and the action of angiotensin II. In the renal tubules these peptides promote excretion of sodium and water, resulting in a decrease in blood volume and blood pressure.

Gastrointestinal Regulation

Daily water intake and output are normally between 2000 and 3000 mL (Table 17-2). Oral intake of fluids accounts for most

TABLE 17-2	NORMAL FLUID BALANCE IN THE ADULT	
Intake		
Fluids		1200 mL
Solid food		1000 mL
Water from oxidation		300 mL
Total		2500 mL
Output		
Insensible loss (skin and lungs)		900 mL
In feces		100 mL
Urine		1500 mL
Total		2500 mL

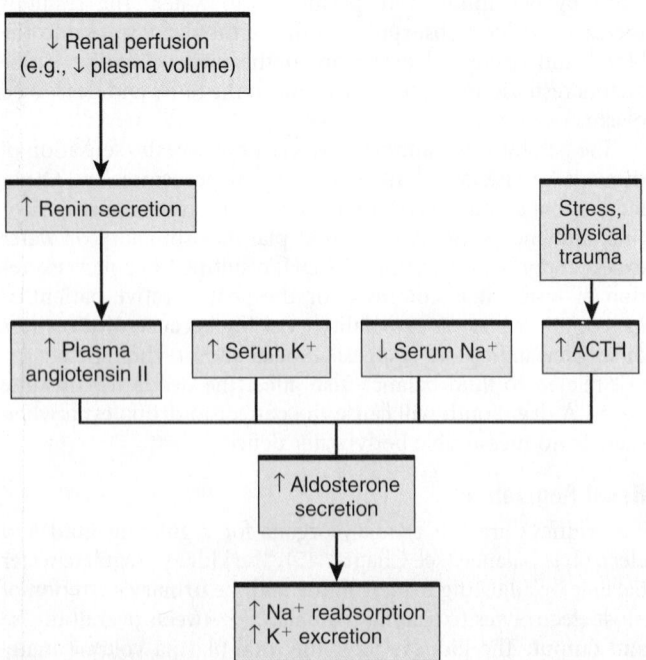

FIG. 17-9 Factors affecting aldosterone secretion. *ACTH,* Adrenocorticotropic hormone.

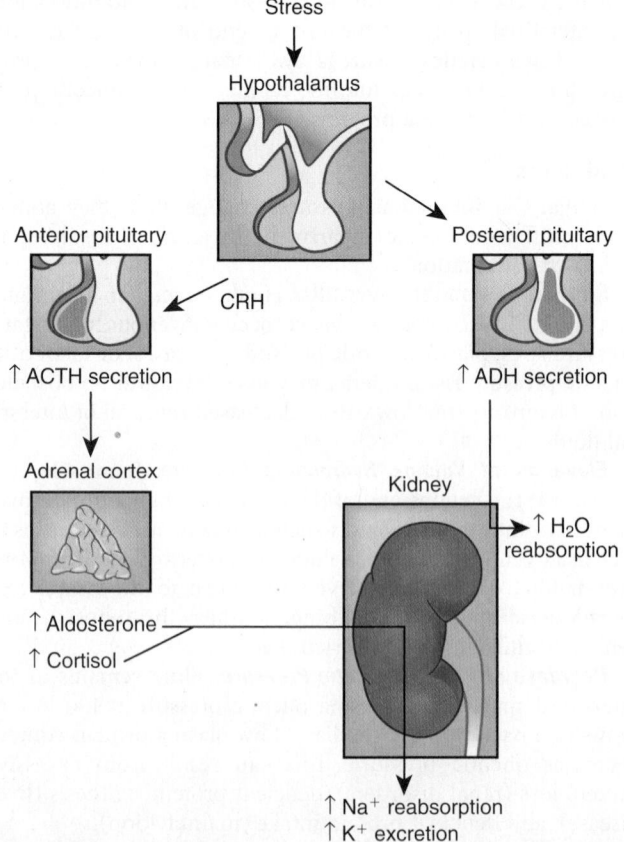

FIG. 17-10 Effects of stress on fluid and electrolyte balance. *ACTH,* Adrenocorticotropic hormone; *ADH,* antidiuretic hormone; *CRH,* corticotropin-releasing hormone.

of the water intake. Water intake also includes water from food metabolism and water present in solid foods. Lean meat is approximately 70% water, whereas the water content of many fruits and vegetables approaches 100%.

In addition to oral intake, the GI tract normally secretes approximately 8000 mL of digestive fluids each day. Most of this fluid is reabsorbed in the GI tract; only a small amount is normally eliminated in feces. Diarrhea and vomiting, which prevent GI reabsorption of this secreted fluid, can lead to significant fluid and electrolyte loss.

Insensible Water Loss

Insensible water loss, which is invisible vaporization from the lungs and skin, assists in regulating body temperature. Normally, about 600 to 900 mL/day is lost. Accelerated body metabolism, which occurs with increased body temperature and exercise, increases the amount of water loss.

Do not confuse water loss through the skin with the vaporization of water excreted by sweat glands. Insensible perspiration causes only water loss. Excessive sweating (*sensible perspiration*) caused by exercise, fever, or high environmental temperatures may lead to large losses of water and electrolytes.

GERONTOLOGIC CONSIDERATIONS

FLUID AND ELECTROLYTES

The older adult experiences normal physiologic changes with aging that increase susceptibility to fluid and electrolyte imbalances. Structural changes to the kidneys and a decrease in the renal blood flow lead to decreased glomerular filtration rate, decreased creatinine clearance, and loss of the ability to concentrate urine and conserve water. Hormonal changes include a decrease in renin and aldosterone and an increase in ADH and ANP.[4] Loss of subcutaneous tissue and thinning of the dermis lead to increased loss of moisture through the skin and an inability to respond to heat or cold quickly.

Older adults experience a decrease in the thirst mechanism, resulting in decreased fluid intake despite increases in osmolality and serum sodium level. Older adults, especially if they are ill, are at increased risk of free-water loss and subsequent development of hypernatremia secondary to impairment of the thirst mechanism and barriers to obtaining fluids to drink.[5]

Healthy older adults usually consume adequate fluids to remain well hydrated. However, functional changes may occur that affect the ability to independently obtain fluids. For example, musculoskeletal changes, such as stiffness of the hands and fingers, can lead to a decreased ability to hold a glass or cup. Mental status changes, such as confusion or disorientation, or changes in ambulation status may lead to a decreased ability to obtain fluids. To reduce incontinent episodes, the older adult may intentionally restrict fluid intake.

You should not automatically attribute older patients' fluid and electrolyte problems to the natural processes of aging. Adapt your assessment and nursing interventions to account for these physiologic and functional changes. Suggestions for alterations in nursing care for the older adult are presented throughout this chapter.

FLUID AND ELECTROLYTE IMBALANCES

Fluid and electrolyte imbalances occur to some degree in most patients with a major illness or injury because illness dis-

rupts the normal homeostatic mechanism. Some fluid and electrolyte imbalances are directly caused by illness or disease (e.g., burns, heart failure). At other times, therapeutic measures (e.g., IV fluid replacement, diuretics) cause or contribute to fluid and electrolyte imbalances. Perioperative patients are at risk for the development of fluid and electrolyte imbalances because of fluid restrictions, blood or fluid loss, and the stress of surgery.[6]

Imbalances are commonly classified as *deficits* or *excesses.* Although each imbalance is discussed separately in this chapter, it is common for more than one imbalance to occur in the same patient. For example, a patient with prolonged nasogastric suction will lose sodium, potassium, hydrogen, and chloride ions. These imbalances may result in a deficiency of both sodium and potassium, a fluid volume deficit, and metabolic alkalosis caused by loss of hydrochloric acid.

EXTRACELLULAR FLUID VOLUME IMBALANCES

ECF volume deficit (*hypovolemia*) and ECF volume excess (*hypervolemia*) are common clinical conditions. ECF volume imbalances are typically accompanied by one or more electrolyte imbalances, particularly changes in the serum sodium level.

Fluid Volume Deficit

Fluid volume deficit can occur with abnormal loss of body fluids (e.g., diarrhea, fistula drainage, hemorrhage, polyuria), inadequate intake, or a shift of fluid from plasma into interstitial fluid. The term *fluid volume deficit* is not interchangeable with the term *dehydration. Dehydration* refers to loss of pure water alone without a corresponding loss of sodium. Causes and clinical manifestations of fluid volume deficit are listed in Table 17-3.

Collaborative Care

The goal of treatment for fluid volume deficit is to correct the underlying cause and to replace both water and any needed electrolytes. Balanced IV solutions, such as lactated Ringer's solution, are usually given. Isotonic (0.9%) sodium chloride is used when rapid volume replacement is indicated. Blood is administered when volume loss is due to blood loss.

Fluid Volume Excess

Fluid volume excess may result from excessive intake of fluids, abnormal retention of fluids (e.g., heart failure, renal failure), or a shift of fluid from interstitial fluid into plasma fluid. Although fluid shifts between the interstitial space and plasma do not alter the overall volume of ECF, these shifts result in changes in the intravascular volume. Causes and clinical manifestations of fluid volume excess are listed in Table 17-3.

Collaborative Care

The goal of treatment for fluid volume excess is removing fluid without producing abnormal changes in the electrolyte composition or osmolality of ECF. The primary cause must be identified and treated. Diuretics and fluid restriction are the primary forms of therapy. Restriction of sodium intake may also be indicated. If the fluid excess leads to ascites or pleural

TABLE 17-3	EXTRACELLULAR FLUID IMBALANCES: CAUSES AND CLINICAL MANIFESTATIONS	

ECF Volume Deficit	ECF Volume Excess
Causes	
• ↑ Insensible water loss or perspiration (high fever, heatstroke) • Diabetes insipidus • Osmotic diuresis • Hemorrhage • GI losses: vomiting, NG suction, diarrhea, fistula drainage • Overuse of diuretics • Inadequate fluid intake • Third-space fluid shifts: burns, intestinal obstruction	• Excessive isotonic or hypotonic IV fluids • Heart failure • Renal failure • Primary polydipsia • SIADH • Cushing syndrome • Long-term use of corticosteroids
Clinical Manifestations	
• Restlessness, drowsiness, lethargy, confusion • Thirst, dry mucous membranes • Decreased skin turgor, ↓ capillary refill • Postural hypotension, ↑ pulse, ↓ CVP • ↓ Urine output, concentrated urine • ↑ Respiratory rate • Weakness, dizziness • Weight loss • Seizures, coma	• Headache, confusion, lethargy • Peripheral edema • Jugular venous distention • Bounding pulse, ↑ BP, ↑ CVP • Polyuria (with normal renal function) • Dyspnea, crackles, pulmonary edema • Muscle spasms • Weight gain • Seizures, coma

CVP, Central venous pressure; *ECF,* extracellular fluid; *SIADH,* syndrome of inappropriate antidiuretic hormone.

effusion, an abdominal paracentesis or thoracentesis may be necessary.

NURSING MANAGEMENT
EXTRACELLULAR FLUID VOLUME IMBALANCES

NURSING DIAGNOSES

Nursing diagnoses and collaborative problems for the patient with fluid imbalances include, but are not limited to, the following:

ECF volume deficit:

- Deficient fluid volume *related to* excessive ECF losses or decreased fluid intake
- Decreased cardiac output *related to* excessive ECF losses or decreased fluid intake
- Risk for deficient fluid volume *related to* excessive ECF losses or decreased fluid intake
- Potential complication: hypovolemic shock

ECF volume excess:

- Excess fluid volume *related to* increased water and/or sodium retention
- Impaired gas exchange *related to* water retention leading to pulmonary edema
- Risk for impaired skin integrity *related to* edema
- Activity intolerance *related to* increased water retention, fatigue, and weakness
- Disturbed body image *related to* altered body appearance secondary to edema
- Potential complications: pulmonary edema, ascites

NURSING IMPLEMENTATION

INTAKE AND OUTPUT. The use of 24-hour intake and output records gives valuable information regarding fluid and electrolyte problems. An accurately recorded intake-and-output flow sheet can identify sources of excessive intake or fluid losses. Intake should include oral, IV, and tube feedings and retained irrigants. Output includes urine, excess perspiration, wound or tube drainage, vomitus, and diarrhea. Estimate fluid loss from wounds and perspiration. Measure the urine specific gravity according to agency policy. Readings of greater than 1.025 indicate concentrated urine, whereas those of less than 1.010 indicate dilute urine.

CARDIOVASCULAR CHANGES. Monitoring the patient for cardiovascular changes is necessary to prevent or detect complications from fluid and electrolyte imbalances. Signs and symptoms of ECF volume excess and deficit are reflected in changes in blood pressure, pulse force, and jugular venous distention. In fluid volume excess the pulse is full, bounding, and not easily obliterated. Increased volume causes distended neck veins (jugular venous distention) and increased blood pressure.

In mild to moderate fluid volume deficit, compensatory mechanisms include sympathetic nervous system stimulation of the heart and peripheral vasoconstriction. Stimulation of the heart increases the heart rate and, combined with vasoconstriction, maintains the blood pressure within normal limits. A change in position from lying to sitting or standing may elicit a further increase in the heart rate or a decrease in the blood pressure (orthostatic hypotension). If vasoconstriction and tachycardia provide inadequate compensation, hypotension occurs when the patient is recumbent. Severe fluid volume deficit can cause flattened neck veins and a weak, thready pulse that is easily obliterated. Severe, untreated fluid deficit will result in shock.

RESPIRATORY CHANGES. Both fluid excess and fluid deficit affect respiratory status. ECF excess can result in pulmonary congestion and pulmonary edema as increased hydrostatic pressure in the pulmonary vessels forces fluid into the alveoli. The patient will experience shortness of breath and moist crackles on auscultation. The patient with ECF deficit will demonstrate an increased respiratory rate because of decreased tissue perfusion and resultant hypoxia.

NEUROLOGIC CHANGES. Changes in neurologic function may occur with fluid volume excesses or deficits. ECF excess may result in cerebral edema from increased hydrostatic pressure in cerebral vessels. Alternatively, profound volume depletion may cause an alteration in sensorium secondary to reduced cerebral tissue perfusion.

Assessment of neurologic function includes evaluation of (1) the level of consciousness, which includes responses to verbal and painful stimuli and determination of a person's orientation to time, place, and person; (2) pupillary response to light and equality of pupil size; and (3) voluntary movement of the extremities, degree of muscle strength, and reflexes. Nursing care focuses on maintaining patient safety.

DAILY WEIGHTS. Accurate daily weights provide the easiest measurement of volume status. An increase of 1 kg (2.2 lb) is equal to 1000 mL (1 L) of fluid retention (provided the person has maintained usual dietary intake or has not been on nothing-by-mouth [NPO] status). Obtain the weight under standardized conditions, that is, weigh the patient at the same time every day, wearing the same garments, and on the same carefully calibrated scale. Remove excess bedding and empty all drainage

FIG. 17-11 Assessment of skin turgor. **A** and **B,** When normal skin is pinched, it resumes shape in seconds. **C,** If the skin remains wrinkled for 20 to 30 seconds, the patient has poor skin turgor.

bags before the weighing. If the patient has items present that are not there every day, such as bulky dressings or tubes, note this along with the weight.

SKIN ASSESSMENT AND CARE. Detect clues to ECF volume deficit and excess by inspecting the skin. Examine the skin for turgor and mobility. Normally a fold of skin, when pinched, will readily move and, on release, rapidly return to its former position. Skin areas over the sternum, abdomen, and anterior forearm are the usual sites for evaluation of tissue turgor (Fig. 17-11). In older people, decreased skin turgor is less predictive of fluid deficit because of the loss of tissue elasticity.[4] In ECF volume deficit, skin turgor is diminished, and there is a lag in the pinched skinfold's return to its original state (referred to as *tenting*).

The skin may be cool and moist if there is vasoconstriction to compensate for the decreased fluid volume. Mild hypovolemia usually does not stimulate this compensatory response. Consequently, the skin will be warm and dry. Volume deficit may also cause the skin to appear dry and wrinkled. These signs may be difficult to evaluate in the older adult because the patient's skin may be normally dry, wrinkled, and nonelastic. Oral mucous membranes will be dry, the tongue may be furrowed, and the individual often complains of thirst. Routine oral care is critical for the comfort of a patient who is dehydrated or fluid restricted for management of fluid volume excess.

Edematous skin may feel cool because of fluid accumulation and a decrease in blood flow secondary to the pressure of the fluid. The fluid can also stretch the skin, causing it to feel taut and hard. Assess edema by pressing with a thumb or forefinger over the edematous area. A grading scale is used to standardize the description if an indentation (ranging from 1+ [slight edema; 2-mm indentation] to 4+ [pitting edema; 8-mm indentation]) remains when pressure is released. Evaluate for edema in areas where soft tissues overlie a bone, with preferred sites being the tibia, fibula, and sacrum.

Good skin care for the person with ECF volume excess or deficit is important. Protect edematous tissues from extremes of heat and cold, prolonged pressure, and trauma. Frequent skin care and changes in position will prevent skin breakdown. Elevate edematous extremities to promote venous return and fluid reabsorption. Dehydrated skin needs frequent care without the use of soap. Applying moisturizing creams or oils increases moisture retention and stimulates circulation.

OTHER NURSING MEASURES. Carefully monitor the rates of infusion of IV fluid solutions. Be cautious about any attempts to "catch up," particularly when large volumes of fluid or certain electrolytes are involved. This is especially true in patients with cardiac, renal, or neurologic problems. Patients receiving tube feedings need supplementary water added to their enteral formula. The amount of additional water depends on the osmolarity of the feeding and the patient's condition.

Do not allow the patient with nasogastric suction to drink water because it will increase the loss of electrolytes. Occasionally the patient may be given small amounts of ice chips to suck. Irrigate nasogastric tubes with isotonic saline solution, not with water. Water causes diffusion of electrolytes into the gastric lumen from mucosal cells. The suction then removes the electrolytes, increasing the risk of electrolyte imbalances.

Nurses in hospitals and long-term care facilities should encourage and help the older or debilitated patient to maintain adequate oral intake. Assess the patient's ability to obtain adequate fluids independently, express thirst, and swallow effectively.[4] Fluids should be easily accessible. Assist older adults with physical limitations, such as arthritis, to open and hold containers. A variety of types of fluids should be available, and assess for individual preferences. Serve fluids at the temperature preferred by the patient. Seventy percent to 80% of the daily intake of fluids should be with meals, with fluid supplements between meals. Older adults may choose to decrease or eliminate fluids 2 hours before bedtime to decrease nocturia or incontinence. The unconscious or cognitively impaired patient is at increased risk because of an inability to express thirst and act on it. In these patients, accurately document fluid intake and losses and carefully evaluate the adequacy of intake and output.[4]

SODIUM IMBALANCES

Sodium, the main cation of ECF, plays a major role in maintaining the concentration and volume of ECF and influencing water distribution between ECF and ICF. Sodium plays an important role in the generation and transmission of nerve impulses, muscle contractility, and the regulation of acid-base balance.

Because sodium is the primary determinant of ECF osmolality, sodium imbalances are typically associated with parallel changes in osmolality. Serum sodium is measured in milliequivalents per liter (mEq/L) or millimoles per liter (mmol/L). The serum sodium level reflects the ratio of sodium to water, not necessarily the loss or gain of sodium. Changes in the serum sodium level may reflect a primary water imbalance, a primary sodium imbalance, or a combination of the two. Sodium imbalances are typically associated with imbalances in ECF volume (Figs. 17-12 and 17-13).

The GI tract absorbs sodium from foods. Typically, daily intake of sodium far exceeds the body's daily requirements. Sodium leaves the body through urine, sweat, and feces. The kidneys are the primary regulator of sodium balance. The kidneys regulate the ECF concentration of sodium by excreting or retaining water under the influence of ADH. Aldosterone

FIG. 17-12 Differential assessment of extracellular fluid *(ECF)* volume.

also plays a role in sodium regulation by promoting sodium reabsorption from the renal tubules.

Hypernatremia

Hypernatremia, an elevated serum sodium, may occur with water loss or sodium gain. Because sodium is the major determinant of the ECF osmolality, hypernatremia causes hyperosmolality. In turn, ECF hyperosmolality causes a shift of water out of the cells, which leads to cellular dehydration. As discussed earlier, the primary protection against the development of hyperosmolality is thirst. Hypernatremia is not a problem in an alert person who has access to water, can sense thirst, and is able to swallow. Hypernatremia secondary to water deficiency is often the result of an impaired level of consciousness or an inability to obtain fluids.

Several clinical states can produce hypernatremia from water loss (Table 17-4). A deficiency in the synthesis or release of ADH from the posterior pituitary gland (central diabetes insipidus) or a decrease in kidney responsiveness to ADH (neph-

rogenic diabetes insipidus) can result in profound diuresis, thus producing a water deficit and hypernatremia. Hyperosmolality with osmotic diuresis can result from administration of concentrated hyperosmolar tube feedings and hyperglycemia associated with uncontrolled diabetes mellitus. Other causes of hypernatremia include excessive sweating and increased sensible losses from high fever.

Excessive sodium intake with inadequate water intake can also lead to hypernatremia. Examples of sodium gain include IV administration of hypertonic saline or sodium bicarbonate, use of sodium-containing drugs, excessive oral intake of sodium (e.g., ingestion of seawater), and *primary aldosteronism* (hypersecretion of aldosterone) caused by a tumor of the adrenal glands.

Clinical Manifestations. The manifestations of hypernatremia are primarily the result of water shifting out of cells into ECF with resultant dehydration and shrinkage of cells (see Table 17-4). Dehydration of brain cells results in neurologic manifestations such as intense thirst, agitation, and decreased alertness, ranging from sleepiness to coma.[7] If there is any accompanying

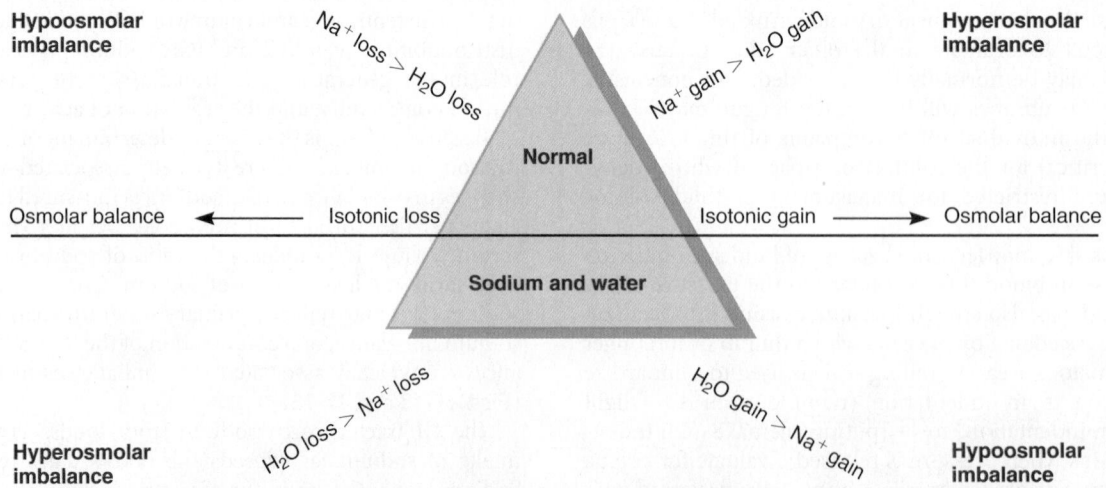

FIG. 17-13 Isotonic gains and losses affect mainly the extracellular fluid (ECF) compartment with little or no water movement into the cells. Hypertonic imbalances cause water to move from inside the cell into ECF to dilute the concentrated sodium, causing cell shrinkage. Hypotonic imbalances cause water to move into the cell, causing cell swelling.

TABLE 17-4 SODIUM IMBALANCES: CAUSES AND CLINICAL MANIFESTATIONS

Hypernatremia (Na⁺ >145 mEq/L [mmol/L])	Hyponatremia (Na⁺ <135 mEq/L [mmol/L])
Causes	
Excessive Sodium Intake	***Excessive Sodium Loss***
• IV fluids: hypertonic NaCl, excessive isotonic NaCl, IV sodium bicarbonate • Hypertonic tube feedings without water supplements • Near-drowning in salt water	• *GI losses:* diarrhea, vomiting, fistulas, NG suction • *Renal losses:* diuretics, adrenal insufficiency, Na⁺ wasting renal disease • *Skin losses:* burns, wound drainage
Inadequate Water Intake	***Inadequate Sodium Intake***
• Unconscious or cognitively impaired individuals	• Fasting diets
Excessive Water Loss (↑ sodium concentration)	***Excessive Water Gain (↓ sodium concentration)***
• ↑ Insensible water loss (high fever, heatstroke, prolonged hyperventilation) • Osmotic diuretic therapy • Diarrhea	• Excessive hypotonic IV fluids • Primary polydipsia
Disease States	***Disease States***
• Diabetes insipidus • Primary hyperaldosteronism • Cushing syndrome • Uncontrolled diabetes mellitus	• SIADH • Heart failure • Primary hypoaldosteronism
Clinical Manifestations	
Hypernatremia With Decreased ECF Volume	***Hyponatremia With Decreased ECF Volume***
• Restlessness, agitation, twitching, seizures, coma • Intense thirst. Dry, swollen tongue. Sticky mucous membranes • Postural hypotension, ↓ CVP, weight loss, ↑ pulse • Weakness, lethargy	• Irritability, apprehension, confusion, dizziness, personality changes, tremors, seizures, coma • Dry mucous membranes • Postural hypotension, ↓ CVP, ↓ jugular venous filling, ↑ pulse, thready pulse • Cold and clammy skin
Hypernatremia With Normal or Increased ECF Volume	***Hyponatremia With Normal or Increased ECF Volume***
• Restlessness, agitation, twitching, seizures, coma • Intense thirst, flushed skin • Weight gain, peripheral and pulmonary edema, ↑ BP, ↑ CVP	• Headache, apathy, confusion, muscle spasms, seizures, coma • Nausea, vomiting, diarrhea, abdominal cramps • Weight gain, ↑ BP, ↑ CVP

CVP, Central venous pressure; *ECF,* extracellular fluid; *SIADH,* syndrome of inappropriate antidiuretic hormone.

ECF volume deficit, manifestations such as postural hypotension, weakness, and decreased skin turgor occur.

NURSING AND COLLABORATIVE MANAGEMENT HYPERNATREMIA

NURSING DIAGNOSES

Nursing diagnoses and collaborative problems for the patient with hypernatremia include, but are not limited to, the following:

• Risk for injury *related to* altered sensorium and seizures
• Risk for fluid volume deficit *related to* excessive intake of sodium and/or loss of water
• Risk for electrolyte imbalance *related to* excessive intake of sodium and/or loss of water
• Potential complication: seizures and coma leading to irreversible brain damage

NURSING IMPLEMENTATION

The primary goal of treatment of hypernatremia is to treat the underlying cause. In primary water deficit, fluid replacement is provided either orally or IV with isotonic or hypotonic fluids such as 5% dextrose in water or 0.45% sodium chloride saline solution.[8] The goal of treatment for sodium excess is to dilute the sodium concentration with sodium-free IV fluids, such as 5% dextrose in water, and to promote excretion of the excess sodium by administering diuretics. (See Chapter 50 for specific treatment of diabetes insipidus.)

Monitor serum sodium levels and the patient's response to therapy. Quickly reducing serum sodium levels can cause a rapid shift of water back into the cells, resulting in cerebral edema and neurologic complications. This risk is greatest in the patient who has developed hypernatremia over several days or longer. Dietary sodium intake is often restricted.

Hyponatremia

Hyponatremia (low serum sodium) may result from a loss of sodium-containing fluids, water excess in relation to the amount of sodium (dilutional hyponatremia), or a combination of both (see Table 17-4). Common causes of hyponatremia from loss of sodium-rich body fluids include profuse diaphoresis, draining wounds, excessive diarrhea or vomiting, and trauma with significant blood loss. Hyponatremia causes hypoosmolality with a shift of water into the cells.

A common cause of hyponatremia from water excess is inappropriate use of sodium-free or hypotonic IV fluids. This may occur in patients after surgery or major trauma or during administration of fluids in patients with renal failure. Patients with psychiatric disorders may have an excessive water intake. Syndrome of inappropriate antidiuretic hormone secretion (SIADH) will result in dilutional hyponatremia caused by abnormal retention of water. (See Chapter 50 for a discussion of the causes of SIADH.)

Clinical Manifestations. Manifestations of hyponatremia are due to cellular swelling and first manifested in the central nervous system (CNS) (see Table 17-4). The excess water lowers plasma osmolality, shifting fluid into brain cells, causing irritability, headache, confusion, seizures, and even coma. Severe acute hyponatremia, if untreated, can cause irreversible neurologic damage or death.[7]

NURSING AND COLLABORATIVE MANAGEMENT HYPONATREMIA

NURSING DIAGNOSES

Nursing diagnoses and collaborative problems for the patient with hyponatremia include, but are not limited to, the following:

• Risk for acute confusion *related to* electrolyte imbalance
• Risk for injury *related to* altered sensorium and decreased level of consciousness

- Risk for electrolyte imbalance *related to* excessive loss of sodium and/or excessive intake or retention of water
- Potential complication: severe neurologic changes

NURSING IMPLEMENTATION

In hyponatremia caused by water excess, fluid restriction is often the only treatment. If severe symptoms (seizures) develop, small amounts of IV hypertonic saline solution (3% sodium chloride) can restore the serum sodium level while the body is returning to a normal water balance. Treatment of hyponatremia associated with abnormal fluid loss includes fluid replacement with sodium-containing solutions.

The drugs conivaptan (Vaprisol) and tolvaptan (Samsca) are given to block the activity of ADH. Conivaptan results in increased urine output without loss of electrolytes such as sodium and potassium. It should not be used in patients with hyponatremia from excess water loss. Tolvaptan is used to treat hyponatremia associated with heart failure, liver cirrhosis, and SIADH.[9] Treatment with these drugs is started in a hospital setting so the patient's clinical status and serum sodium levels can be carefully monitored.

POTASSIUM IMBALANCES

Potassium is the major ICF cation, with 98% of the body potassium being intracellular. For example, potassium concentration within muscle cells is approximately 140 mEq/L; potassium concentration in ECF is 3.5 to 5.0 mEq/L. The sodium-potassium pump in cell membranes maintains this concentration difference by pumping potassium into the cell and sodium out. Because the ratio of ECF potassium to ICF potassium is the major factor in the resting membrane potential of nerve and muscle cells, neuromuscular and cardiac function are commonly affected by potassium imbalances.

Disruptions in the dynamic equilibrium between ICF and ECF potassium often cause clinical problems. Potassium regulates intracellular osmolality and promotes cellular growth. Potassium is required for glycogen to be deposited in muscle and liver cells. Potassium also plays a role in acid-base balance (discussed in the section on acid-base regulation later in this chapter).

Diet is the source of potassium. The typical Western diet contains approximately 50 to 100 mEq of potassium daily, mainly from fruits, dried fruits, and vegetables. Many salt substitutes used in low-sodium diets contain substantial potassium. Patients may receive potassium from parenteral sources, including IV fluids; transfusions of stored, hemolyzed blood; and medications (e.g., potassium penicillin).

The kidneys are the primary route for potassium loss, eliminating about 90% of the daily potassium intake. The remainder is lost in the stool and sweat. There is an inverse relationship between sodium and potassium reabsorption in the kidneys. Factors that cause sodium retention (e.g., low blood volume, increased aldosterone level) cause potassium loss in the urine. Large urine volumes can be associated with excess loss of potassium in the urine. If kidney function is significantly impaired, retained potassium can lead to toxic levels.

Hyperkalemia

Hyperkalemia (high serum potassium) may result from impaired renal excretion, a shift of potassium from ICF to ECF, a massive intake of potassium, or a combination of these factors (Table

TABLE 17-5	POTASSIUM IMBALANCES: CAUSES AND CLINICAL MANIFESTATIONS
Hyperkalemia (K⁺ >5.0 mEq/L [mmol/L])	**Hypokalemia** (K⁺ <3.5 mEq/L [mmol/L])
Causes	
Excess Potassium Intake	***Potassium Loss***
• Excessive or rapid parenteral administration	• *GI losses:* diarrhea, vomiting, fistulas, NG suction
• Potassium-containing drugs (e.g., potassium penicillin)	• *Renal losses:* diuretics, hyperaldosteronism, magnesium depletion
• Potassium-containing salt substitute	• *Skin losses:* diaphoresis
	• Dialysis
Shift of Potassium Out of Cells	***Shift of Potassium Into Cells***
• Acidosis	• Increased insulin (e.g., IV dextrose load)
• Tissue catabolism (e.g., fever, sepsis, burns)	• Alkalosis
• Crush injury	• Tissue repair
• Tumor lysis syndrome	• ↑ Epinephrine (e.g., stress)
Failure to Eliminate Potassium	***Lack of Potassium Intake***
• Renal disease	• Starvation
• Potassium-sparing diuretics (e.g., amiloride [Midamor])	• Diet low in potassium
• Adrenal insufficiency	• Failure to include potassium in parenteral fluids if NPO
• ACE inhibitors	
• NSAIDs	
Clinical Manifestations	
• Irritability	• Fatigue
• Anxiety	• Muscle weakness, leg cramps
• Abdominal cramping, diarrhea	• Nausea, vomiting, paralytic ileus
• Weakness of lower extremities	• Soft, flabby muscles
• Paresthesias	• Paresthesias, decreased reflexes
• Irregular pulse	• Weak, irregular pulse
• Cardiac arrest if hyperkalemia sudden or severe	• Polyuria
	• Hyperglycemia
Electrocardiogram Changes	***Electrocardiogram Changes***
• Tall, peaked T wave	• ST segment depression
• Prolonged PR interval	• Flattened T wave
• ST segment depression	• Presence of U wave
• Loss of P wave	• Prolonged QRS
• Widening QRS	• Ventricular dysrhythmias (e.g., PVCs)
• Ventricular fibrillation	• Bradycardia
• Ventricular standstill	

ACE, Angiotensin-converting enzyme; *PVCs,* premature ventricular contractions.

17-5). The most common cause of hyperkalemia is renal failure. Adrenal insufficiency with a subsequent aldosterone deficiency leads to retention of potassium ions. Factors that cause potassium to move from ICF to ECF include acidosis, massive cell destruction (as in burn or crush injury, tumor lysis, severe infections), and exercise. In metabolic acidosis, potassium ions shift from ICF to ECF in exchange for hydrogen ions moving into the cell.

Both digoxin-like drugs and β-adrenergic blockers (beta blockers) (e.g., propranolol [Inderal]) can impair entry of potassium into cells, resulting in a higher ECF potassium concentration.[10] Certain drugs, such as potassium-sparing diuretics (e.g., amiloride [Midamor]), aldosterone receptor blockers (e.g., spi-

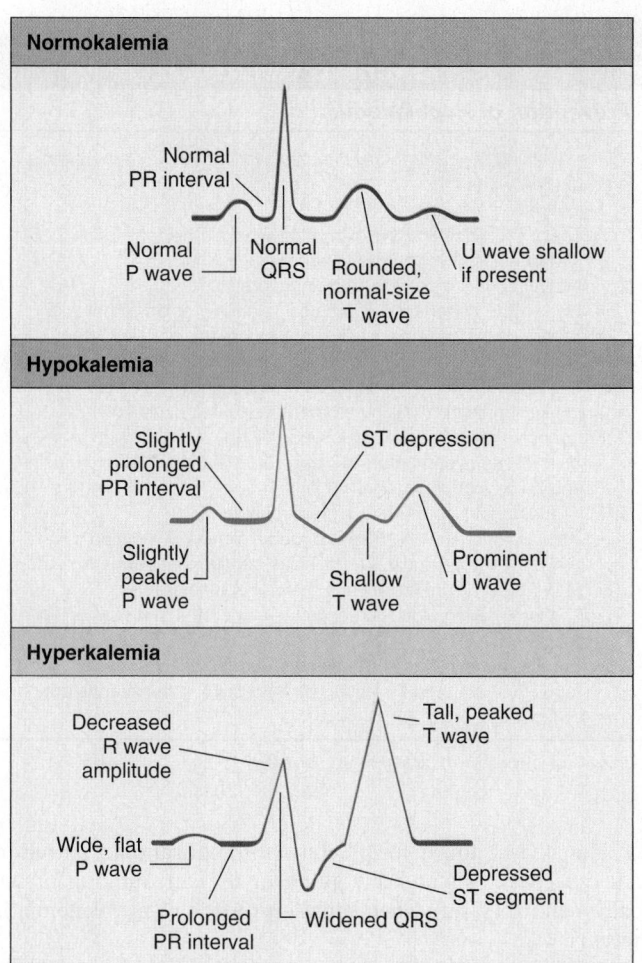

FIG. 17-14 Electrocardiographic changes associated with alterations in potassium status.

ronolactone [Aldactone]), and angiotensin-converting enzyme (ACE) inhibitors (e.g., enalapril [Vasotec], lisinopril [Prinivil]), may contribute to the development of hyperkalemia by reducing the kidney's ability to excrete potassium.

Clinical Manifestations. Hyperkalemia increases the concentration of potassium outside of the cell, altering the normal ECF and ICF ratio and resulting in increased cellular excitability (see Table 17-5). Initially, as the levels of potassium increase, the patient may experience cramping leg pain and weakness, followed by weakness or paralysis of other skeletal muscles, including the respiratory muscles. Abdominal cramping and diarrhea occur from hyperactivity of smooth muscles.

The most clinically significant manifestations of hyperkalemia are the disturbances in cardiac conduction[8] (Fig. 17-14). Cardiac depolarization is decreased, leading to flattening of the P wave and widening of the QRS complex. Repolarization occurs more rapidly, resulting in shortening of the QT interval and a T wave that is narrower and more peaked. Ventricular fibrillation or cardiac standstill may occur.

NURSING AND COLLABORATIVE MANAGEMENT
HYPERKALEMIA

NURSING DIAGNOSES

Nursing diagnoses and collaborative problems for the patient with hyperkalemia include, but are not limited to, the following:

- Risk for activity intolerance *related to* lower extremity muscle weakness
- Risk for electrolyte imbalance *related to* excessive retention or cellular release of potassium
- Risk for injury *related to* lower extremity muscle weakness and seizures
- Potential complication: dysrhythmias

NURSING IMPLEMENTATION

Treatment of hyperkalemia consists of the following:

1. Eliminate oral and parenteral potassium intake (see Table 47-11).
2. Increase elimination of potassium. This is accomplished with diuretics, dialysis, and ion-exchange resins such as sodium polystyrene sulfonate (Kayexalate). Kayexalate, administered orally or rectally, binds potassium in exchange for sodium, and the resin is excreted in feces (see Chapter 47).
3. Force potassium from ECF to ICF. This is accomplished by IV administration of regular insulin (along with glucose so the patient does not become hypoglycemic) or IV sodium bicarbonate for the correction of acidosis. Occasionally, a β-adrenergic agonist (e.g., nebulized albuterol) is administered. This therapy is not indicated for patients with tachycardia or coronary artery disease.
4. Reverse the membrane potential effects of the elevated ECF potassium by administering IV calcium gluconate. Calcium ions can immediately reverse the membrane excitability.

In cases in which the elevation of potassium is mild and the kidneys are functioning, it may be sufficient to (1) withhold potassium from the diet and IV sources and (2) increase renal potassium elimination by administering fluids and loop or thiazide diuretics. Patients with moderate hyperkalemia should additionally receive one of the treatments to force potassium into cells, usually IV insulin and glucose. Monitor the electrocardiograms (ECGs) of all patients with clinically significant hyperkalemia to detect dysrhythmias and to monitor the effects of therapy. The patient experiencing dangerous cardiac dysrhythmias should receive IV calcium gluconate immediately. Monitor blood pressure because rapid administration of calcium can cause hypotension. Hemodialysis is an effective means of removing potassium from the body in the patient with renal failure.

Hypokalemia

Hypokalemia (low serum potassium) can result from increased loss of potassium, from an increased shift of potassium from ECF to ICF, or rarely from deficient dietary potassium intake. The most common causes of hypokalemia are abnormal losses from either the kidneys or the GI tract. GI tract losses of potassium are associated with diarrhea, laxative abuse, vomiting, and ileostomy drainage. Renal losses occur when the patient has a low magnesium level or is diuresing, particularly in the patient with an elevated aldosterone level. Aldosterone is released when the circulating blood volume is low, thus causing sodium retention in the kidneys with a loss of potassium in the urine. Low plasma magnesium stimulates renin release and subsequent increased aldosterone levels, which results in potassium excretion.

Among the factors causing potassium to move from ECF to ICF are insulin therapy (especially in conjunction with diabetic ketoacidosis) and β-adrenergic stimulation (catecholamine release in stress, coronary ischemia, delirium tremens, administration of β-adrenergic agonist drugs). Alkalosis can cause a shift of potassium into cells in exchange for hydrogen, thus lowering the potassium in ECF and causing symptomatic hypokalemia.

Clinical Manifestations. Hypokalemia alters the resting membrane potential, resulting in hyperpolarization (an increased negative charge within the cell) and impaired muscle contraction. Therefore the manifestations of hypokalemia involve changes in cardiac and muscle function (see Table 17-5).

The most serious clinical problems are cardiac changes, including impaired repolarization, resulting in a flattening of the T wave and eventually in emergence of a U wave. The P waves peak, and the QRS complex is prolonged (see Fig. 17-14). There is an increased incidence of potentially lethal ventricular dysrhythmias.

Skeletal muscle weakness and paralysis may occur with hypokalemia. As with hyperkalemia, hypokalemia initially affects leg muscles. Severe hypokalemia can cause weakness or paralysis of respiratory muscles, leading to shallow respirations and respiratory arrest. Alterations in smooth muscle function may lead to decreased GI motility (e.g., paralytic ileus), decreased airway responsiveness, and impaired regulation of arteriolar blood flow, possibly contributing to smooth muscle cell breakdown. Finally, hypokalemia can impair function in nonmuscle tissue by impairing insulin secretion, leading to hyperglycemia.

NURSING AND COLLABORATIVE MANAGEMENT HYPOKALEMIA

NURSING DIAGNOSES

Nursing diagnoses and collaborative problems for the patient with hypokalemia include, but are not limited to, the following:
- Risk for activity intolerance *related to* lower extremity muscle weakness
- Risk for electrolyte imbalance *related to* excessive loss of potassium
- Risk for injury *related to* muscle weakness and hyporeflexia
- Potential complication: dysrhythmias

NURSING IMPLEMENTATION

Treatment of hypokalemia consists of oral or IV potassium chloride (KCl) supplements and increased dietary intake of potassium. Except in severe deficiencies, KCl is not given unless there is urine output of at least 0.5 mL/kg of body weight per hour.

SAFETY ALERT
- IV KCl must always be diluted and never given in concentrated amounts.
- Never give KCl via IV push or as a bolus.
- Invert IV bags containing KCl several times to ensure even distribution in the bag.
- Never add KCl to a hanging IV bag to prevent giving a bolus dose.

The preferred maximum concentration is 40 mEq/L. However, stronger concentrations (up to 80 mEq/L) may be given for severe hypokalemia, with continuous cardiac monitoring.[11] The rate of IV administration of KCl should not exceed 10 mEq/hr and must be given by infusion pump to ensure correct administration rate. Because KCl is irritating to the vein, assess

---

Prevention of Hypokalemia

When teaching the patient and the caregiver to prevent hypokalemia, do the following.
1. For all patients at risk:
   - Teach the signs and symptoms of hypokalemia (see Table 17-5) and to report them to the health care provider.
2. For patients taking potassium-losing diuretics:*
   - Explain the importance of increasing dietary potassium intake.
   - Teach which foods are high in potassium (see Table 47-11).
   - Explain that salt substitutes contain approximately 50 to 60 mEq of potassium per teaspoon, and help patients raise their potassium levels if taking a potassium-losing diuretic.
3. For patients taking potassium-sparing diuretics:*
   - Instruct the patient and the caregiver to avoid salt substitutes and foods high in potassium.
4. For patients taking oral potassium supplements:
   - Instruct the patient to take the medication as prescribed to prevent overdosage and to take the supplement with a full glass of water to help it dissolve in the GI tract.
5. For patients taking digitalis preparations and others at risk for hypokalemia:
   - Explain the importance of having serum potassium levels regularly monitored because low potassium enhances the action of digitalis.

*For specific information on diuretics, see Table 33-7.

IV sites at least hourly for phlebitis and infiltration. Infiltration can cause necrosis and sloughing of the surrounding tissue. Use a central IV line when rapid correction of hypokalemia is necessary.

Patients at risk for hypokalemia and those who are critically ill should have cardiac monitoring to detect cardiac changes related to potassium imbalances. Monitor serum potassium levels and urine output as appropriate. Because patients on digoxin therapy have an increased risk of toxicity if their serum potassium level is low, monitor the patient for digitalis toxicity.

Teach patients methods to prevent hypokalemia (Table 17-6). Foods high in potassium are identified in Table 47-11. Patients at risk for hypokalemia should have regular serum potassium levels monitored.

CALCIUM IMBALANCES

Calcium is necessary for many metabolic processes. It is the major cation in the structure of bones and teeth. Other functions of calcium include blood clotting, transmission of nerve impulses, myocardial contractions, and muscle contractions. The source of calcium is dietary intake. Calcium absorption requires the active form of vitamin D. Vitamin D is either ingested in the diet or formed in the skin in the presence of sunlight.

The total body content of calcium is about 1200 g. More than 99% of the body's calcium is found in bones; the remainder is in plasma and body cells. Of the calcium in plasma, 50% is bound to plasma proteins (primarily albumin); 40% is in the free or ionized form; and the remainder is bound with phosphate, citrate, or carbonate. Ionized calcium is the biologically active form.

Calcium is measured in milligrams per deciliter (mg/dL) and milliequivalents per liter (mEq/L). Serum calcium levels usually

TABLE 17-7	CALCIUM IMBALANCES: CAUSES AND CLINICAL MANIFESTATIONS
Hypercalcemia (Ca²⁺ >10.2 mg/dL [2.55 mmol/L])	**Hypocalcemia (Ca²⁺ <8.6 mg/dL [2.15 mmol/L])**

Hypercalcemia (Ca^{2+} >10.2 mg/dL [2.55 mmol/L])	Hypocalcemia (Ca^{2+} <8.6 mg/dL [2.15 mmol/L])
Causes	
Increased Total Calcium	*Decreased Total Calcium*
• Multiple myeloma	• Chronic kidney disease
• Malignancies with bone metastasis	• Elevated phosphorus
• Prolonged immobilization	• Primary hypoparathyroidism
• Hyperparathyroidism	• Vitamin D deficiency
• Vitamin D overdose	• Magnesium deficiency
• Thiazide diuretics	• Acute pancreatitis
• Milk-alkali syndrome	• Loop diuretics (e.g., furosemide [Lasix])
	• Chronic alcoholism
	• Diarrhea
	• ↓ Serum albumin (patient is usually asymptomatic due to normal ionized calcium level)
Increased Ionized Calcium	*Decreased Ionized Calcium*
• Acidosis	• Alkalosis
	• Excess administration of citrated blood
Clinical Manifestations	
• Lethargy, weakness	• Easy fatigability
• Depressed reflexes	• Depression, anxiety, confusion
• Decreased memory	• Numbness and tingling in extremities and region around mouth
• Confusion, personality changes, psychosis	• Hyperreflexia, muscle cramps
• Anorexia, nausea, vomiting	• Chvostek's sign
• Bone pain, fractures	• Trousseau's sign
• Polyuria, dehydration	• Laryngeal spasm
• Nephrolithiasis	• Tetany, seizures
• Stupor, coma	
Electrocardiogram Changes	*Electrocardiogram Changes*
• Shortened ST segment	• Elongation of ST segment
• Shortened QT interval	• Prolonged QT interval
• Ventricular dysrhythmias	• Ventricular tachycardia
• Increased digitalis effect	

reflect the total calcium level (all three forms). Ionized calcium levels are analyzed and reported separately. The levels listed in Table 17-7 reflect total calcium levels. Changes in serum pH alter the level of ionized calcium without altering the total calcium level. A decreased plasma pH (acidosis) decreases calcium binding to albumin, leading to more ionized calcium. An increased plasma pH (alkalosis) increases calcium binding, leading to decreased ionized calcium. Alterations in serum albumin levels affect the interpretation of total calcium levels. Low albumin levels result in a drop in the total calcium level, although the level of ionized calcium is not affected.

Calcium balance is controlled by parathyroid hormone (PTH) and calcitonin. Since the bones serve as a readily available store of calcium, the body is usually able to maintain normal serum calcium levels by regulating the movement of calcium into or out of the bone. PTH is produced by the parathyroid gland. Its production and release are stimulated by low serum calcium levels. PTH increases bone resorption (movement of calcium out of bones), increases GI absorption of calcium, and increases renal tubule reabsorption of calcium.

Calcitonin is produced by the thyroid gland and is stimulated by high serum calcium levels. It opposes the action of PTH and lowers the serum calcium level by decreasing GI absorption, increasing calcium deposition into bone, and promoting renal excretion.

Hypercalcemia

Hypercalcemia (high serum calcium) is caused by hyperparathyroidism in about two thirds of the cases. Malignancy, especially from myeloma and breast, lung, and kidney cancers, causes the remaining third.[12] Malignancies lead to hypercalcemia through bone destruction from tumor invasion or through tumor secretion of a parathyroid-related protein, which stimulates calcium release from bones. Hypercalcemia is also associated with prolonged immobilization, which results in bone mineral loss and increased plasma calcium concentration. Rare causes include vitamin D overdose or increased calcium intake (e.g., ingestion of antacids containing calcium, excessive administration during cardiac arrest).

Excess calcium leads to reduced excitability of both muscles and nerves. Table 17-7 outlines the causes and clinical manifestations of hypercalcemia.

NURSING AND COLLABORATIVE MANAGEMENT HYPERCALCEMIA

NURSING DIAGNOSES

Nursing diagnoses and collaborative problems for the patient with hypercalcemia include, but are not limited to, the following:

- Risk for activity intolerance *related to* generalized muscle weakness
- Risk for electrolyte imbalance *related to* excessive bone destruction
- Risk for injury *related to* neuromuscular and sensorium changes
- Potential complication: dysrhythmias

NURSING IMPLEMENTATION

The basic treatment for hypercalcemia is promoting urinary excretion of calcium by administering a loop diuretic (e.g., furosemide [Lasix]) and hydrating the patient with isotonic saline infusions. The patient must drink 3000 to 4000 mL of fluid daily to promote the renal excretion of calcium and decrease the possibility of kidney stone formation. Other supportive measures include a diet low in calcium and an increase in weight-bearing activity to enhance bone mineralization.

Bisphosphonates (e.g., pamidronate [Aredia], zoledronic acid [Zometa]) are the most effective agents in treating hypercalcemia caused by a malignancy.[12] They inhibit the activity of osteoclasts (cells that break down bone and result in calcium release). Synthetic calcitonin given intramuscularly (IM) or subcutaneously lowers serum calcium levels; the intranasal form is not effective.

Hypocalcemia

Hypocalcemia (low serum calcium) can be caused by any condition that decreases the production of PTH. This may occur with surgical removal of a portion of or injury to the parathyroid glands during thyroid or neck surgery. Acute pancreatitis is

FIG. 17-15 Tests for hypocalcemia. **A,** Chvostek's sign is contraction of facial muscles in response to a light tap over the facial nerve in front of the ear. **B,** Trousseau's sign is a carpal spasm induced by, **C,** inflating a blood pressure cuff above the systolic pressure for a few minutes.

another potential cause of hypocalcemia. Lipolysis, a consequence of pancreatitis, produces fatty acids that combine with calcium ions, decreasing serum calcium levels. The patient who receives multiple blood transfusions can become hypocalcemic because the citrate used to anticoagulate the blood binds with the calcium. Sudden alkalosis may result in symptomatic hypocalcemia despite a normal total serum calcium level. The high pH increases calcium binding to protein, decreasing the amount of ionized calcium. Hypocalcemia can occur if there is increased loss of calcium due to laxative abuse and malabsorption syndromes. (See Table 17-7 for the causes of hypocalcemia.)

Low calcium levels allow sodium to move into excitable cells, decreasing the threshold of action potentials with subsequent depolarization of the cells. This results in increased nerve excitability and sustained muscle contraction, or *tetany*. Clinical signs of tetany include Chvostek's sign and Trousseau's sign. *Chvostek's sign* is contraction of facial muscles in response to a tap over the facial nerve in front of the ear (Fig. 17-15, *A*). *Trousseau's sign* refers to carpal spasms induced by inflating a blood pressure cuff on the arm (Fig. 17-15, *B* and *C*). After the cuff is inflated above the systolic pressure, carpal spasms occur within 3 minutes if hypocalcemia is present. Other manifestations of tetany are laryngeal stridor, dysphagia, and numbness and tingling around the mouth or in the extremities.

Cardiac effects of hypocalcemia include decreased cardiac contractility and ECG changes. A prolonged QT interval may develop into ventricular tachycardia. Table 17-7 outlines the clinical manifestations of hypocalcemia.

NURSING AND COLLABORATIVE MANAGEMENT HYPOCALCEMIA

NURSING DIAGNOSES

Nursing diagnoses and collaborative problems for the patient with hypocalcemia include, but are not limited to, the following:

- Acute pain *related to* sustained muscle contractions
- Ineffective breathing pattern *related to* laryngospasm
- Risk for electrolyte imbalance *related to* decreased production of PTH
- Risk for injury *related to* tetany and seizures
- Potential complications: fracture, respiratory arrest

NURSING IMPLEMENTATION

The primary goal of treatment of hypocalcemia is to treat the underlying cause. When severe manifestations of hypocalcemia occur, IV preparations of calcium (e.g., calcium gluconate, calcium chloride) are given. Treatment of mild hypocalcemia involves a diet high in calcium-rich foods along with vitamin D supplementation. Oral calcium supplements, such as calcium carbonate, can be used when patients are unable to consume enough dietary calcium, such as those who cannot tolerate dairy products. Measures to promote CO_2 retention, such as breathing into a paper bag or sedating the patient, can control muscle spasm and other symptoms of tetany until the calcium level is corrected. Adequately treat pain and anxiety because hyperventilation-induced respiratory alkalosis can precipitate hypocalcemic symptoms. Closely observe any patient who has had thyroid or neck surgery in the immediate postoperative period for manifestations of hypocalcemia because of the proximity of the surgery to the parathyroid glands.

PHOSPHATE IMBALANCES

Phosphorus is the primary anion in ICF and the second most abundant element in the body, second to calcium. Most phosphorus is in the bones and teeth as calcium phosphate. The remaining phosphorus is metabolically active and essential to the function of muscle, red blood cells (RBCs), and the nervous system. It is also involved in the acid-base buffering system; the mitochondrial formation of ATP; cellular uptake and use of glucose; and the metabolism of carbohydrates, proteins, and fats.

PTH maintains serum phosphorus levels and balance. Regulation of phosphate balance requires adequate renal functioning because the kidneys are the major route of phosphate excretion. When the phosphate level in the glomerular filtrate falls below the normal level or PTH levels are low, the kidneys reabsorb additional phosphorus. A reciprocal relationship exists between phosphorus and calcium in that a high serum phosphate level tends to cause a low calcium concentration in the serum. Low serum calcium levels stimulate the release of PTH, which decreases reabsorption of phosphorus.

Hyperphosphatemia

Hyperphosphatemia (high serum phosphate) is commonly caused by acute kidney injury or chronic kidney disease, which results in an altered ability of the kidneys to excrete phosphate. Other causes include chemotherapy for leukemia or lymphoma, excessive ingestion of milk or phosphate-containing laxatives, and large intakes of vitamin D that increase GI absorption of phosphorus. Table 17-8 summarizes causes and clinical manifestations of hyperphosphatemia.

Mild hyperphosphatemia is often asymptomatic. The clinical manifestations of more severe hyperphosphatemia primarily relate to the low serum calcium levels often associated with high serum phosphate levels. These include tetany, muscle cramps, paresthesias, and seizures. Increased levels of phosphate readily

TABLE 17-8	PHOSPHATE IMBALANCES: CAUSES AND CLINICAL MANIFESTATIONS

Hyperphosphatemia (PO_4^{3-} >4.4 mg/dL [1.42 mmol/L])	Hypophosphatemia (PO_4^{3-} <2.4 mg/dL [0.78 mmol/L])
Causes	
• Renal failure • Chemotherapy drugs • Enemas containing phosphorus (e.g., Fleet Enema) • Excessive ingestion (e.g., milk, phosphate-containing laxatives) • Hypoparathyroidism • Sickle cell anemia	• Malabsorption syndromes • Recovery from malnutrition or refeeding • Glucose or insulin therapy • Total parenteral nutrition • Alcohol withdrawal • Phosphate-binding antacids • Recovery from diabetic ketoacidosis • Respiratory alkalosis
Clinical Manifestations	
• Hypocalcemia • Numbness and tingling in extremities and region around mouth • Hyperreflexia, muscle cramps • Tetany, seizures • Deposition of calcium-phosphate precipitates in skin, soft tissue, cornea, viscera, blood vessels	• CNS depression (confusion, coma) • Muscle weakness, including respiratory muscle weakness and difficulty weaning from ventilator • Polyneuropathy, seizures • Cardiac problems (dysrhythmias, decreased stroke volume) • Osteomalacia • Rhabdomyolysis

precipitate with calcium, and calcified deposits occur outside of the bones. These metastatic calcium precipitates can be found in soft tissues such as joints, arteries, skin, kidneys, and corneas and produce organ dysfunction, notably renal failure (see Chapter 47).

The primary management of hyperphosphatemia is identifying and treating the underlying cause. Ingestion of foods and fluids high in phosphorus (e.g., dairy products) should be restricted. Phosphate-binding agents or gels (e.g., calcium carbonate) limit intestinal phosphate absorption and increase phosphate secretion into the intestine. With severe hyperphosphatemia, hemodialysis or an insulin and glucose infusion can rapidly decrease levels. If hypocalcemia is present, providing adequate hydration and instituting measures to correct calcium levels assist with returning phosphorus levels to normal.

Hypophosphatemia

Hypophosphatemia (low serum phosphate) is rare, but may occur in the patient who is malnourished or has a malabsorption syndrome. Other causes include alcohol withdrawal and use of phosphate-binding antacids. Hypophosphatemia may also occur during parenteral nutrition with inadequate phosphorus replacement. Table 17-8 summarizes causes and clinical manifestations of hypophosphatemia.

Most clinical manifestations of hypophosphatemia result from impaired cellular energy and O_2 delivery due to low levels of cellular ATP and 2,3-diphosphoglycerate (2,3-DPG), an enzyme in RBCs that facilitates O_2 delivery to the tissues. Mild to moderate hypophosphatemia is often asymptomatic. Severe hypophosphatemia may be fatal because of decreased cellular function. Acute manifestations include CNS depression, confu-

sion, and other mental changes. Other manifestations include muscle weakness and pain, dysrhythmias, and cardiomyopathy.

Management of a mild phosphorus deficiency may involve oral supplementation (e.g., Neutra-Phos) and ingestion of foods high in phosphorus (e.g., dairy products). Symptomatic hypophosphatemia can be fatal and often requires IV administration of sodium phosphate or potassium phosphate.[13] Frequent monitoring of serum phosphate and calcium levels is necessary to guide IV therapy. Sudden symptomatic hypocalcemia, secondary to increased calcium phosphorus binding, is a potential complication of IV phosphorus administration.

MAGNESIUM IMBALANCES

Magnesium is the second most abundant intracellular cation. Magnesium plays an important role in many essential cellular processes. The most notable is the activation of a wide variety of enzyme systems. Magnesium is a coenzyme in the metabolism of carbohydrates and protein and is required for the synthesis of nucleic acids and proteins. Magnesium plays a role in maintaining normal calcium and potassium balance. Adequate intracellular magnesium is necessary for normal function of the sodium-potassium pump. Because magnesium acts directly on the myoneural junction, alterations in serum magnesium levels profoundly affect neuromuscular excitability and contractility.

Approximately 50% to 60% of the body's magnesium is contained in bone. Only a small amount (2%) is in ECF, with the remainder inside the cell. Magnesium is regulated by GI absorption and renal excretion. The kidneys are able to conserve magnesium in times of need and excrete excesses. Factors that regulate calcium balance (e.g., PTH) similarly influence magnesium balance. Manifestations of magnesium imbalance are often mistaken for calcium imbalances. Because magnesium, calcium, and potassium balance are closely related, assess all three cations together.[14]

Hypermagnesemia

Hypermagnesemia (high serum magnesium level) usually occurs only with an increase in magnesium intake accompanied by renal insufficiency or failure. (Table 17-9 lists the causes of hypermagnesemia.) A patient with chronic kidney disease who ingests products containing magnesium (e.g., Maalox, milk of magnesia) will have a problem with excess magnesium. Magnesium excess could develop in the pregnant woman who receives magnesium sulfate for the management of eclampsia.

Hypermagnesemia depresses neuromuscular and CNS functions. Initial clinical manifestations of a mildly elevated serum magnesium concentration include lethargy, nausea, and vomiting. As the levels of serum magnesium increase, deep tendon reflexes are lost, followed by somnolence, and then respiratory and, ultimately, cardiac arrest can occur (see Table 17-9).

Management of hypermagnesemia should focus on prevention. People with chronic kidney disease should not take magnesium-containing drugs and should limit ingestion of magnesium containing foods (e.g., green vegetables, nuts, bananas, oranges, peanut butter, chocolate).

The emergency treatment of hypermagnesemia is IV administration of calcium chloride or calcium gluconate to oppose the effects of the magnesium on cardiac muscle. If renal function is adequate, promoting urinary excretion with oral and parenteral fluids and IV furosemide decreases magnesium levels. The

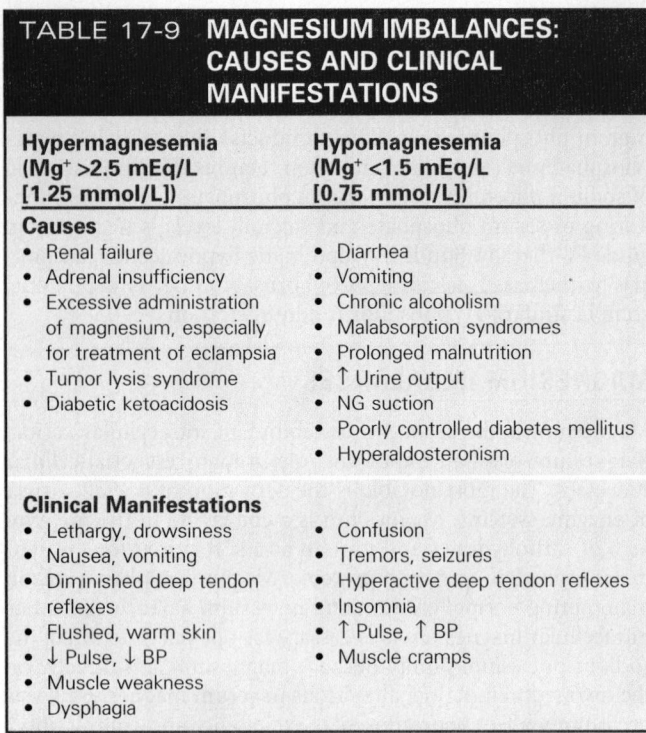

TABLE 17-9	MAGNESIUM IMBALANCES: CAUSES AND CLINICAL MANIFESTATIONS	
	Hypermagnesemia (Mg+ >2.5 mEq/L [1.25 mmol/L])	**Hypomagnesemia (Mg+ <1.5 mEq/L [0.75 mmol/L])**
Causes	• Renal failure • Adrenal insufficiency • Excessive administration of magnesium, especially for treatment of eclampsia • Tumor lysis syndrome • Diabetic ketoacidosis	• Diarrhea • Vomiting • Chronic alcoholism • Malabsorption syndromes • Prolonged malnutrition • ↑ Urine output • NG suction • Poorly controlled diabetes mellitus • Hyperaldosteronism
Clinical Manifestations	• Lethargy, drowsiness • Nausea, vomiting • Diminished deep tendon reflexes • Flushed, warm skin • ↓ Pulse, ↓ BP • Muscle weakness • Dysphagia	• Confusion • Tremors, seizures • Hyperactive deep tendon reflexes • Insomnia • ↑ Pulse, ↑ BP • Muscle cramps

FIG. 17-16 The normal range of plasma pH is 7.35 to 7.45. A normal pH is maintained by a ratio of 1 part carbonic acid to 20 parts bicarbonate.

patient with impaired renal function requires dialysis because the kidneys are the major route of excretion for magnesium.

Hypomagnesemia

Hypomagnesemia (low serum magnesium level) occurs in patients with limited magnesium intake or increased renal losses. Major causes of hypomagnesemia from insufficient food intake include prolonged fasting or starvation and chronic alcoholism. Fluid loss from the GI tract interferes with magnesium absorption. Another potential cause of hypomagnesemia is prolonged parenteral nutrition without magnesium supplementation. Many diuretics increase the risk of magnesium loss through renal excretion.[14] In addition, osmotic diuresis caused by high glucose levels in uncontrolled diabetes mellitus increases renal excretion of magnesium.

Hypomagnesemia produces neuromuscular and CNS hyperirritability. Clinical manifestations include confusion, hyperactive deep tendon reflexes, muscle cramps, tremors, and seizures. Magnesium deficiency predisposes to cardiac dysrhythmias, such as premature ventricular contractions and ventricular fibrillation. Clinically, hypomagnesemia resembles hypocalcemia and may contribute to the development of hypocalcemia resulting from the decreased action of PTH. Hypomagnesemia may also be associated with hypokalemia that does not respond well to potassium replacement. This occurs because intracellular magnesium is critical to normal function of the sodium-potassium pump.

The primary goal of treatment of hypomagnesemia is to treat the underlying cause. Management of mild magnesium deficiencies involves oral supplements and increased dietary intake of foods high in magnesium. If hypomagnesemia is severe or if hypocalcemia is present, IV magnesium (e.g., magnesium sulfate) is given. Monitor vital signs and use an infusion pump, since too rapid administration of magnesium can lead to cardiac or respiratory arrest.

ACID-BASE IMBALANCES

The body normally maintains a steady balance between the acids produced during normal metabolism and the bases that neutralize and promote the excretion of the acids. Because these acids alter the body's internal environment, their regulation is necessary to maintain homeostasis and acid-base balance. Many health problems may lead to acid-base imbalances. Patients with diabetes mellitus, chronic obstructive pulmonary disease, and kidney disease frequently develop acid-base imbalances. Remember that an acid-base imbalance is not a disease but a symptom of an underlying health problem. Always consider the possibility of acid-base imbalance in patients with serious illnesses.

pH and Hydrogen Ion Concentration

The acidity or alkalinity of a solution depends on its hydrogen ion (H^+) concentration. An increase in H^+ concentration leads to acidity; a decrease leads to alkalinity. Despite the fact that acids are produced by the body daily, the H^+ concentration of body fluids is small (0.0004 mEq/L) and maintained within a narrow range to ensure optimal cellular function.

H^+ concentration is usually expressed as a negative logarithm (symbolized as *pH*) rather than in milliequivalents. The use of the negative logarithm means that the lower the pH, the higher the H^+ concentration. In contrast to a pH of 7, a pH of 8 represents a 10-fold decrease in H^+ concentration.

The pH of a chemical solution may range from 1 to 14. A solution with a pH of 7 is considered neutral. An acid solution has a pH less than 7, and an alkaline solution has a pH greater than 7. Blood is slightly alkaline (pH 7.35 to 7.45). Yet if it drops below 7.35, the person has acidosis, even though the blood may never become truly acidic. If the blood pH is greater than 7.45, the person has alkalosis (Fig. 17-16).

Acid-Base Regulation

Normally the body has three mechanisms by which it regulates the acid-base balance to maintain the arterial pH between 7.35 and 7.45. These mechanisms are the buffer systems, the respiratory system, and the renal system. The regulatory mechanisms react at different speeds. Buffers react immediately. The respiratory system responds in minutes and reaches maximum effectiveness in hours. The renal response takes 2 or 3 days to respond maximally, but the kidneys can maintain balance indefinitely in patients with chronic imbalances.

Buffer System. The buffer system is the fastest-acting system and the primary regulator of acid-base balance. Buffers act chemically to change strong acids into weaker acids or to bind acids to neutralize their effect. This minimizes the effect of acids on blood pH until their excretion from the body. The body buffers an acid load better than it neutralizes base excess. Buffers cannot maintain pH without the adequate functioning of the respiratory and renal systems.

A buffer consists of a weakly ionized acid or a base and its salt. The buffers in the body include carbonic acid–bicarbonate, monohydrogen–dihydrogen phosphate, intracellular and plasma protein, and hemoglobin buffers. The cell can also act as a buffer by shifting hydrogen in and out of the cell. With an accumulation of H^+ in ECF, the cells can accept H^+ in exchange for another cation (e.g., potassium ion).

The carbonic acid–bicarbonate (H_2CO_3/HCO_3^-) buffer system neutralizes hydrochloric acid (HCl) in the following manner:

$$HCl \; + \; NaH_2CO_3 \; \rightarrow \; NaCl \; + \; H_2CO_3$$

Strong acid   Strong base   Salt   Weak acid

In this way, combining a strong acid with a strong base prevents the acid from making a large change in the blood's pH. The carbonic acid is broken down to H_2O and CO_2. The lungs excrete CO_2, either combined with insensible H_2O as carbonic acid, or alone as CO_2. In this process, the buffer system maintains a 20:1 ratio between bicarbonate and carbonic acid and the normal pH.

The phosphate buffer system is composed of sodium and other cations in combination with monohydrogen phosphate (HPO_4^{2-}) or dihydrogen phosphate ($H_2PO_4^-$). This intracellular buffer system acts in the same manner as the bicarbonate system. Bases neutralize strong acids, forming sodium chloride (NaCl) and sodium biphosphate (NaH_2PO_4), a weaker acid. Conversely, if a strong base, such as sodium hydroxide (NaOH), is present, sodium dihydrogen phosphate (NaH_2PO_4) neutralizes it to a weaker base (Na_2HPO_4) and H_2O.

The intracellular and extracellular protein buffering system acts like the bicarbonate system. Some of the amino acids of proteins contain free acid radicals (–COOH), which can dissociate into CO_2 and H^+. Other amino acids have basic radicals (NH_3OH [ammonium hydroxide]), which can dissociate into NH_3^+ (ammonia) and OH^- (hydroxide). The OH^- can combine with an H^+ to form H_2O. Hemoglobin is a protein and assists in regulation of pH by shifting chloride in and out of RBCs in exchange for bicarbonate.

Respiratory System. The lungs help maintain a normal pH by excreting CO_2 and water, which are by-products of cellular metabolism. When released into the circulation, CO_2 enters RBCs and combines with H_2O to form H_2CO_3. This carbonic acid dissociates into H^+ and HCO_3^-. Hemoglobin buffers the free H^+, and the HCO_3^- diffuses into the plasma. This process is reversed in the pulmonary capillaries, forming CO_2 that is then excreted by the lungs. The overall reversible reaction is expressed in the following manner:

$$CO_2 + H_2O \rightarrow H_2CO_3 \rightarrow H^+ + HCO_3^-$$

The amount of CO_2 in the blood directly relates to carbonic acid concentration and subsequently to H^+ concentration. With increased respirations, more CO_2 is expelled and less remains in the blood. This leads to less carbonic acid and less H^+. With decreased respirations, more CO_2 remains in the blood. This leads to increased carbonic acid and more H^+.

The respiratory center in the medulla in the brainstem controls the rate of excretion of CO_2. If increased amounts of CO_2 or H^+ are present, the respiratory center stimulates an increased rate and depth of breathing. If the center senses low H^+ or CO_2 levels, respirations are inhibited.

As a compensatory mechanism, the respiratory system acts on the $CO_2 + H_2O$ side of the reaction by altering the rate and depth of breathing to "blow off" (through hyperventilation) or "retain" (through hypoventilation) CO_2. If a respiratory problem (e.g., respiratory failure) is the cause of an acid-base imbalance, the respiratory system loses its ability to correct a pH alteration. The older adult has impaired compensatory ability because of decreased respiratory function.

Renal System. Under normal conditions, the body depends on the kidneys to reabsorb and conserve all of the HCO_3^- they filter and excrete a portion of the acid produced by cellular metabolism. The three mechanisms of acid elimination are (1) secretion of small amounts of free hydrogen into the renal tubule, (2) combination of H^+ with ammonia (NH_3) to form ammonium (NH_4^+), and (3) excretion of weak acids.

The kidneys normally excrete acidic urine (average pH is 6). As a compensatory mechanism, the pH of the urine can decrease to 4 or increase to 8. To compensate for acidosis, the kidneys can reabsorb additional HCO_3^- and eliminate excess H^+. Thus the pH of the blood increases and the pH of the urine decreases. If the renal system is the cause of an acid-base imbalance (e.g., renal failure), it loses its ability to correct a pH alteration. In the older adult the kidneys are less able to compensate for an acid load.

Alterations in Acid-Base Balance

An acid-base imbalance results when there is an alteration in the ratio of 20:1 between base and acid content. This occurs when a primary disease or process alters one side of the ratio (e.g., CO_2 retention in pulmonary disease) and the compensatory processes that maintain the other side of the ratio (e.g., increased renal HCO_3^- reabsorption) either fail or are inadequate. The compensatory process may be inadequate because either the pathophysiologic process is overwhelming or there is insufficient time for the compensatory process to function.

Acid-base imbalances are classified as respiratory or metabolic. *Respiratory imbalances* result from the retention or an excess of CO_2 altering carbonic acid concentrations; *metabolic imbalances* affect the base HCO_3^-. Therefore acidosis is caused by an increase in carbonic acid (respiratory acidosis) or a decrease in HCO_3^- (metabolic acidosis). Alkalosis is caused by a decrease in carbonic acid (respiratory alkalosis) or an increase in HCO_3^- (metabolic alkalosis). Imbalances may be further classified as acute or chronic. Chronic imbalances allow greater time for compensatory changes.

Respiratory Acidosis. *Respiratory acidosis* (carbonic acid excess) occurs whenever the person hypoventilates (Table 17-10). Hypoventilation leads to a buildup of CO_2, resulting in an accumulation of carbonic acid in the blood. Carbonic acid dissociates, liberating H^+, and there is a decrease in pH. If CO_2

TABLE 17-10 ACID-BASE IMBALANCES

Common Causes	Pathophysiology	Laboratory Findings
Respiratory Acidosis		
Chronic obstructive pulmonary disease	CO_2 retention from hypoventilation	↓ Plasma pH
		↑ $PaCO_2$
Barbiturate or sedative overdose	Compensatory response is HCO_3^- retention by kidney	HCO_3^- normal (uncompensated)
Chest wall abnormality		↑ HCO_3^- (compensated)
Severe pneumonia		
Atelectasis		*Sample ABG*
Respiratory muscle weakness (e.g., Guillain-Barré syndrome)		Uncompensated:
		pH 7.31
		$PaCO_2$ 54 mm Hg
Mechanical hypoventilation		HCO_3^- 25 mEq/L
Respiratory Alkalosis		
Hyperventilation (e.g., hypoxia, pulmonary emboli, anxiety, fear, pain, exercise, fever)	Increased CO_2 excretion from hyperventilation	↑ Plasma pH
		↓ $PaCO_2$
	Compensatory response is HCO_3^- excretion by kidney	HCO_3^- normal (uncompensated)
Stimulated respiratory center (e.g., septicemia, encephalitis, brain injury, salicylate poisoning)		↓ HCO_3^- (compensated)
		Sample ABG
		Uncompensated:
		pH 7.52
		$PaCO_2$ 27 mm Hg
Mechanical hyperventilation		HCO_3^- 24 mEq/L
Metabolic Acidosis		
Diabetic ketoacidosis	Gain of fixed acid, inability to excrete acid or loss of base	↓ Plasma pH
Lactic acidosis		$PaCO_2$ normal (uncompensated)
Starvation		
Severe diarrhea		↓ $PaCO_2$ (compensated)
Renal tubular acidosis	Compensatory response is CO_2 excretion by lungs	↓ HCO_3^-
Renal failure		*Sample ABG*
Gastrointestinal fistulas		Uncompensated:
Shock		pH 7.29
		$PaCO_2$ 38 mm Hg
		HCO_3^- 18 mEq/L
Metabolic Alkalosis		
Severe vomiting	Loss of strong acid or gain of base	↑ Plasma pH
Excess gastric suctioning		$PaCO_2$ normal (uncompensated)
Diuretic therapy	Compensatory response is CO_2 retention by lungs	↑ $PaCO_2$ (compensated)
Potassium deficit		↑ HCO_3^-
Excess NaHCO$_3$ intake		*Sample ABG*
		Uncompensated:
Excessive mineralocorticoids		pH 7.50
		$PaCO_2$ 40 mm Hg
		HCO_3^- 34 mEq/L

ABG, Arterial blood gas.

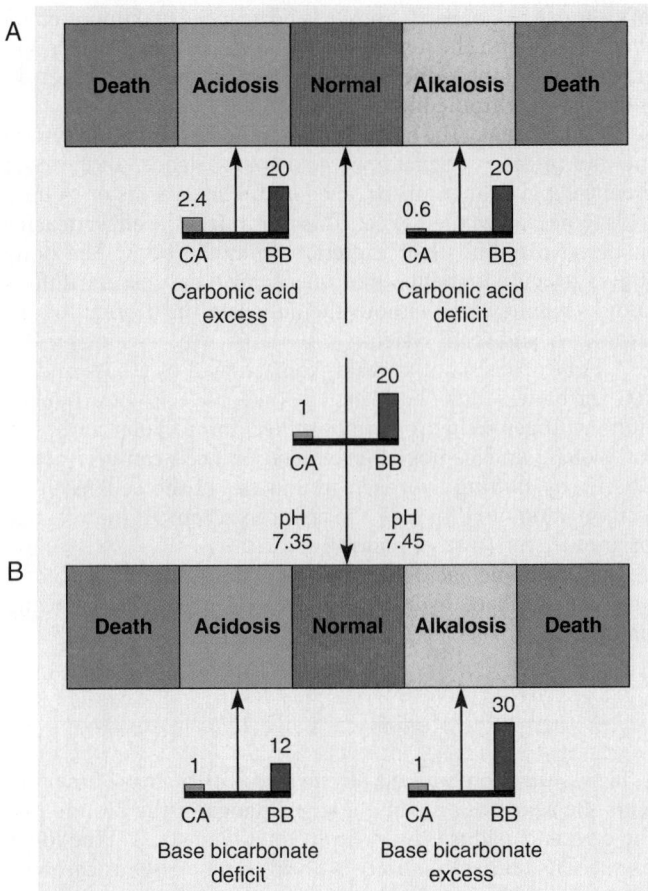

FIG. 17-17 Kinds of acid-base imbalances. **A,** Respiratory imbalances caused by carbonic acid *(CA)* excess and carbonic acid deficit. **B,** Metabolic imbalances caused by base bicarbonate *(BB)* deficit and base bicarbonate excess.

Respiratory Alkalosis. *Respiratory alkalosis* (carbonic acid deficit) occurs with hyperventilation (see Table 17-10). The primary cause of respiratory alkalosis is hypoxemia from acute pulmonary disorders. Anxiety, CNS disorders, and mechanical overventilation also increase the ventilation rate. The decrease in the partial pressure of arterial CO_2 ($PaCO_2$) level leads to decreased carbonic acid concentration and alkalosis (see Fig. 17-17, *A*).

Compensated respiratory alkalosis is rare. In acute respiratory alkalosis, aggressive treatment of the causes of hypoxemia is essential and usually does not allow time for compensation to occur. However, buffering of acute respiratory alkalosis may occur with shifting of HCO_3^- into cells in exchange for chloride ions (Cl^-). In chronic respiratory alkalosis that occurs with pulmonary fibrosis or CNS disorders, compensation may include renal excretion of HCO_3^-.

Metabolic Acidosis. *Metabolic acidosis* (base bicarbonate deficit) occurs when an acid other than carbonic acid accumulates in the body or when bicarbonate is lost from body fluids (see Table 17-10 and Fig. 17-17, *B*). Ketoacid accumulation in diabetic ketoacidosis and lactic acid accumulation with shock are examples of accumulation of acids. Severe diarrhea results in loss of HCO_3^-. In renal disease the kidneys lose their ability to reabsorb HCO_3^- and secrete H^+.

The compensatory response to metabolic acidosis is to increase CO_2 excretion by the lungs. The patient often develops

is not eliminated from the blood, acidosis results from the accumulation of carbonic acid (Fig. 17-17, *A*).

To compensate, the kidneys conserve HCO_3^- and secrete increased concentrations of H^+ into the urine. During acute respiratory acidosis, the renal compensatory mechanisms begin to operate within 24 hours. Until the renal mechanisms have an effect, the serum HCO_3^- level will usually be normal.

Kussmaul respiration (deep, rapid breathing). In addition, the kidneys attempt to excrete additional acid.

If metabolic acidosis is present, calculating the anion gap can help determine the source of the acidosis. The *anion gap* is the difference between the cations and the anions in ECF that are routinely measured. You calculate an anion gap by summing the chloride and bicarbonate levels and subtracting this number from the plasma sodium concentration. Ordinarily, the sum of the measured cations is greater than the sum of the measured anions. The anion gap is normally 10 to 14 mmol/L. The anion gap is increased in metabolic acidosis associated with acid gain (e.g., lactic acidosis, diabetic ketoacidosis) but remains normal in metabolic acidosis caused by bicarbonate loss (e.g., diarrhea).

Metabolic Alkalosis. *Metabolic alkalosis* (base bicarbonate excess) occurs when a loss of acid (e.g., from prolonged vomiting or gastric suction) or a gain in bicarbonate (e.g., from ingestion of baking soda) occurs (see Table 17-10 and Fig. 17-17, *B*). Renal excretion of bicarbonate occurs in response to metabolic alkalosis. The compensatory response to metabolic alkalosis is limited. There is a decreased respiratory rate to increase plasma CO_2. However, once plasma CO_2 reaches a certain level, stimulation of chemoreceptors results in ventilation.

Mixed Acid-Base Disorders. A mixed acid-base disorder occurs when two or more disorders are present at the same time. The pH depends on the type, severity, and acuity of each of the disorders involved and any compensatory mechanisms at work. Respiratory acidosis combined with metabolic alkalosis (e.g., a patient with chronic obstructive pulmonary disease also treated with a thiazide diuretic) may result in a near-normal pH, whereas respiratory acidosis combined with metabolic acidosis will cause a greater decrease in pH than either disorder alone. An example of a mixed acidosis is a patient in cardiopulmonary arrest. An example of a mixed alkalosis is a patient who is hyperventilating because of postoperative pain and losing acid secondary to nasogastric suctioning.

Clinical Manifestations

Clinical manifestations of acidosis and alkalosis are summarized in Tables 17-11 and 17-12. In both respiratory and metabolic acidosis, the CNS is depressed. Headache, lethargy, weakness, and confusion develop, leading eventually to coma and death. In both types of alkalosis, irritability of the CNS causes tingling and numbness of the fingers, restlessness, and tetany. If the severity of alkalosis increases, convulsions and coma may occur.[7]

The compensatory mechanisms also produce specific clinical manifestations. For example, the deep, rapid respirations of a patient with metabolic acidosis are an example of respiratory compensation. In alkalosis, hypocalcemia occurs due to increased calcium binding with albumin, lowering the amount of ionized, biologically active calcium. The hypocalcemia accounts for many of the clinical manifestations of alkalosis.

Blood Gas Values. Arterial blood gas (ABG) values provide objective information about a patient's acid-base status, the underlying cause of an imbalance, the body's ability to regulate pH, and the patient's overall O_2 status. Knowledge of the patient's clinical situation and the physiologic extent of renal and respiratory compensation enables you to identify acid-base disorders, as well as the patient's ability to compensate. Blood gas analysis also shows the partial pressure of arterial O_2 (PaO_2) and O_2 saturation. These values are used to identify hypoxemia.

TABLE 17-11	CLINICAL MANIFESTATIONS OF ACIDOSIS	
Respiratory (↑ $PaCO_2$)		**Metabolic (↓ HCO_3^-)**
Neurologic		
Drowsiness		Drowsiness
Confusion		Confusion
Dizziness		Dizziness
Headache		Headache
Coma		Coma
Cardiovascular		
↓ BP		↓ BP
Ventricular fibrillation (related to hyperkalemia from compensation)		Dysrhythmias (related to hyperkalemia from compensation)
Warm, flushed skin (related to peripheral vasodilation)		Warm, flushed skin (related to peripheral vasodilation)
Gastrointestinal		
No significant findings		Nausea, vomiting, diarrhea, abdominal pain
Neuromuscular		
Seizures		No significant findings
Respiratory		
Hypoventilation with hypoxia (lungs are unable to compensate when there is a respiratory problem)		Deep, rapid respirations (compensatory action by the lungs)

TABLE 17-12	CLINICAL MANIFESTATIONS OF ALKALOSIS	
Respiratory (↓ $PaCO_2$)		**Metabolic (↑ HCO_3^-)**
Neurologic		
Dizziness		Dizziness
Light-headedness		Light-headedness
Confusion		Confusion
Headache		Headache
Cardiovascular		
Tachycardia		Tachycardia
Dysrhythmias (related to hypokalemia from compensation)		Dysrhythmias (related to hypokalemia from compensation)
Gastrointestinal		
Nausea		Nausea
Vomiting		Vomiting
Epigastric pain		Anorexia
Neuromuscular		
Tetany		Tetany
Numbness		Tremors
Tingling of extremities		Tingling of fingers and toes
Hyperreflexia		Muscle cramps, hypertonic muscles
Seizures		Seizures
Respiratory		
Hyperventilation (lungs are unable to compensate when there is a respiratory problem)		Hypoventilation (compensatory action by the lungs)

To interpret the results of an ABG, perform the following six steps:

1. Determine whether the pH is acidotic or alkalotic. Label values less than 7.35 as acidotic and values greater than 7.45 as alkalotic.
2. Analyze the $PaCO_2$ to determine if the patient has respiratory acidosis or alkalosis. Since the lungs control $PaCO_2$, it is the respiratory component of the ABG. Because CO_2 forms carbonic acid when dissolved in blood, high $PaCO_2$ levels indicate acidosis, and low $PaCO_2$ levels indicate alkalosis.
3. Analyze the HCO_3^- level to determine if the patient has metabolic acidosis or alkalosis. Since the kidneys primarily control HCO_3^-, it is the metabolic component of the ABG. Because HCO_3^- is a base, high levels of HCO_3^- result in alkalosis and low levels result in acidosis.
4. At this point, if the pH is between 7.35 and 7.45, and the CO_2 and the HCO_3^- are within normal limits, the ABGs are normal.
5. Determine if the CO_2 or the HCO_3^- matches the acid or base alteration of the pH. For example, if the pH is acidotic (less than 7.35) and the CO_2 is high (respiratory acidosis) but the HCO_3^- is high (metabolic alkalosis), the CO_2 is the parameter that matches the pH alteration of acidosis. The patient's acid-base imbalance is diagnosed as respiratory acidosis.
6. Determine if the body is attempting to compensate for the pH change. If the parameter that does not match the pH is moving in the opposite direction, the body is attempting to compensate. In the example in step 5, the HCO_3^- level is alkalotic; this is in the opposite direction of respiratory acidosis and considered compensation. If compensatory mechanisms are functioning, the pH will return toward 7.40. When the pH is within normal limits, the patient has *full compensation*.

Table 17-13 lists normal blood gas values, and Table 17-14 explains how to analyze ABG results. The laboratory findings section of Table 17-10 provides ABG findings of the four major acid-base disturbances. Table 17-15 shows ROME, a quick memory device (mnemonic) for understanding acid-base imbalances. See Chapter 26 for further discussion of blood gases.

ASSESSMENT OF FLUID, ELECTROLYTE, AND ACID-BASE IMBALANCES

Assessing patients for fluid, electrolyte, and acid-base imbalances is an important part of your nursing practice. Clinical manifestations for specific imbalances are presented earlier in this chapter. In addition to assessing for those clinical manifestations, obtain subjective and objective data from any patient with suspected fluid, electrolyte, or acid-base imbalances as outlined below.

Subjective Data
Important Health Information
Past Health History. Question the patient about any past history of problems involving the kidneys, heart, GI system, or lungs that could affect the present fluid, electrolyte, and acid-base balance. Obtain information about specific diseases such as diabetes mellitus, diabetes insipidus, chronic obstructive pulmonary disease, renal failure, ulcerative colitis, and Crohn's disease. Ask the patient about any prior fluid, electrolyte, or acid-base disorders.

Medications. Assess the patient's current and past use of medications. The ingredients in many drugs, especially over-the-counter drugs, are often missed as sources of sodium, potassium, calcium, magnesium, and other electrolytes. Many prescription drugs, including diuretics, corticosteroids, and electrolyte supplements, can cause fluid and electrolyte imbalances.

Surgery or Other Treatments. Ask the patient about past or present renal dialysis, kidney surgery, or bowel surgery resulting

TABLE 17-14	ARTERIAL BLOOD GAS (ABG) ANALYSIS
ABG Values	**Analysis**
pH 7.30 $PaCO_2$ 25 mm Hg HCO_3^- 16 mEq/L	1. pH <7.35 indicates acidosis. 2. $PaCO_2$ is low, indicating respiratory alkalosis. 3. HCO_3^- is low, indicating metabolic acidosis. 4. Metabolic acidosis matches the pH. 5. The CO_2 does not match, but is moving in the opposite direction, which indicates the lungs are attempting to compensate for the metabolic acidosis.

Interpretation
This ABG is interpreted as metabolic acidosis with partial compensation. If the pH returns to the normal range, the patient is said to have full compensation.

TABLE 17-13	NORMAL ARTERIAL BLOOD GAS VALUES*	
Parameter		**Reference Interval**
pH		7.35-7.45
$PaCO_2$		35-45 mm Hg
Bicarbonate (HCO_3^-)		22-26 mEq/L (mmol/L)
PaO_2†		80-100 mm Hg
SaO_2		>95%
Base excess		±2.0 mEq/L

*Venous blood gas reference intervals are listed in Table 26-1.
†Decreases above sea level and with increasing age.
$PaCO_2$, Partial pressure of CO_2 in arterial blood; *PaO_2,* partial pressure of O_2 in arterial blood; *SaO_2,* arterial O_2 saturation.

TABLE 17-15	ROME: MEMORY DEVICE FOR ACID-BASE IMBALANCES

For acid-base imbalances a quick memory device (mnemonic) can be used.
In **Respiratory** conditions, the pH and the $PaCO_2$ go in **Opposite** directions.
- In respiratory alkalosis, the pH is ↑ and the $PaCO_2$ is ↓.
- In respiratory acidosis the pH is ↓ and the $PaCO_2$ is ↑.
In **Metabolic** conditions, the pH and the HCO_3^- go in the same direction (equal or **Equivalent**). The $PaCO_2$ may also go in the same direction.
- In metabolic alkalosis, pH and HCO_3^- are ↑ and the $PaCO_2$ is ↑ or normal.
- In metabolic acidosis, pH and HCO_3^- are ↓ and the $PaCO_2$ is ↓ or normal.

Respiratory		pH	$PaCO_2$
Opposite	Acidosis	↓	↑
	Alkalosis	↑	↓
Metabolic		pH	HCO_3^-
Equivalent	Acidosis	↓	↓
	Alkalosis	↑	↑

in a temporary or permanent external collecting system such as a colostomy.

Functional Health Patterns

Health Perception–Health Management Pattern. If the patient is currently experiencing a problem related to fluid, electrolyte, and acid-base balance, obtain a careful description of the illness, including onset, course, and treatment. Question the patient about any recent changes in body weight.

Nutritional-Metabolic Pattern. Ask the patient about diet and any special dietary practices. Weight reduction diets, fad diets, or any eating disorders, such as anorexia or bulimia, can lead to fluid and electrolyte problems. If the patient is on a special diet, such as low sodium or high potassium, assess the ability to adhere to the dietary prescription.

Elimination Pattern. Make note of the patient's usual bowel and bladder habits. Carefully document any deviations from the expected elimination pattern, such as diarrhea, oliguria, nocturia, polyuria, or incontinence.

Activity-Exercise Pattern. Inquire about the patient's exercise pattern and any complaints of excessive perspiration. Determine if the patient is exposed to extremely high temperatures as a result of leisure or work activity. Ask the patient what he or she does to replace fluid and electrolytes lost through excessive perspiration. Assess the patient's activity level to determine any functional problems that could lead to lack of ability to obtain food or fluids.

Cognitive-Perceptual Pattern. Ask about any changes in sensations, such as numbness, tingling, *fasciculations* (uncoordinated twitching of a single muscle group), or muscle weakness, that could indicate a fluid and electrolyte problem. Additionally, ask both the patient and the caregiver if there have been any changes in mentation or alertness, such as confusion, memory impairment, or lethargy.

Objective Data

Physical Examination. A complete physical examination is needed because fluid, electrolyte, and acid-base balance affects all body systems. As you assess each system, check for manifestations that you would expect with an imbalance. Common abnormal assessment findings of major body systems offer clues to possible imbalances (Table 17-16).

Laboratory Values. Assessment of serum electrolyte values is a good starting point for identifying fluid and electrolyte imbalance (see Table 17-1). However, serum electrolyte values often provide only limited information. They reflect the concentration of that electrolyte in ECF but not necessarily in ICF. For example, most of the potassium in the body is found intracellularly. Changes in serum potassium values may be the result of a true deficit or excess of potassium or may reflect the movement of potassium into or out of the cell during acid-base imbalances. An abnormal serum sodium level may reflect a sodium problem or, more likely, a water problem.

In addition to arterial and venous blood gases, serum electrolytes can provide important information about a patient's acid-base balance. Changes in the serum HCO_3^- (often reported as total CO_2 or CO_2 content on an electrolyte panel) indicate metabolic acidosis (low HCO_3^- level) or alkalosis (high HCO_3^- level).

Other laboratory tests helpful in evaluating the presence of or risk for fluid, electrolyte, and acid-base imbalances include serum and urine osmolality, serum glucose, blood urea nitrogen, serum creatinine, venous blood gas sampling, urine specific gravity, and urine electrolytes.

TABLE 17-16 **ASSESSMENT ABNORMALITIES**
Fluid and Electrolyte Imbalances

Finding	Possible Etiology
Skin	
Poor skin turgor	Fluid volume deficit
Cold, clammy skin	Na^+ deficit, shift of plasma to interstitial fluid
Pitting edema	Fluid volume excess
Flushed, dry skin	Na^+ excess
Pulse	
Bounding pulse	Fluid volume excess, shift of interstitial fluid to plasma
Rapid, weak, thready pulse	Shift of plasma to interstitial fluid, Na^+ deficit, fluid volume deficit
Weak, irregular, rapid pulse	Severe K^+ deficit
Weak, irregular, slow pulse	Severe K^+ excess
Blood Pressure	
Hypotension	Fluid volume deficit, shift of plasma to interstitial fluid, Na^+ deficit
Hypertension	Fluid volume excess, shift of interstitial fluid to plasma
Respirations	
Deep, rapid breathing	Compensation for metabolic acidosis
Shallow, slow, irregular breathing	Compensation for metabolic alkalosis
Shortness of breath	Fluid volume excess
Moist crackles	Fluid volume excess, shift of interstitial fluid to plasma
Restricted airway	Ca^{2+} deficit
Skeletal Muscles	
Cramping of exercised muscle	Ca^{2+} deficit, Mg^{2+} deficit, alkalosis
Carpal spasm (Trousseau's sign)	Ca^{2+} deficit, Mg^{2+} deficit, alkalosis
Flabby muscles	K^+ deficit
Positive Chvostek's sign	Ca^{2+} deficit, Mg^{2+} deficit, alkalosis
Behavior or Mental State	
Picking at bedclothes	K^+ deficit, Mg^{2+} deficit
Indifference	Fluid volume deficit, Na^+ deficit
Apprehension	Shift of plasma to interstitial fluid
Extreme restlessness	K^+ excess, Na^+ excess, fluid volume deficit
Confusion and irritability	K^+ deficit, fluid volume excess, Ca^{2+} excess, Mg^{2+} excess, H_2O excess, Na^+ deficit
Decreased level of consciousness	Na^+ deficit, H_2O excess

ORAL FLUID AND ELECTROLYTE REPLACEMENT

In all cases of fluid, electrolyte, and acid-base imbalances, the primary treatment involves correction of the underlying cause. Oral rehydration solutions containing water, potassium, sodium, and glucose may be used to correct mild fluid and electrolyte deficits. Glucose not only provides calories but also promotes sodium and water absorption in the small intestine. Commercial oral rehydration solutions are now available for home use.

Cola drinks are avoided because they do not contain adequate electrolyte replacement and the sugar content may lead to osmotic diuresis.

INTRAVENOUS FLUID AND ELECTROLYTE REPLACEMENT

IV fluid and electrolyte therapy is necessary to treat many different fluid and electrolyte imbalances. Many patients need maintenance IV fluid therapy while they cannot take oral fluids (e.g., during and after surgery). Other patients need corrective or replacement therapy for losses that have already occurred. The amount and type of solution are determined by the normal daily maintenance requirements and by imbalances identified by laboratory results. IV replacement solutions are classified by their concentration or tonicity (Table 17-17). Tonicity is an important factor in determining the appropriate solution to correct water and solute imbalances.

Solutions

Hypotonic. A hypotonic solution provides more water than electrolytes, diluting the ECF. Osmosis then produces a movement of water from ECF to ICF. After achieving osmotic equilibrium, ICF and ECF have the same osmolality and both compartments are expanded. Table 17-17 gives examples of commonly used hypotonic fluids. Maintenance fluids are usually hypotonic solutions (e.g., 0.45% NaCl) because normal daily losses are hypotonic. Additional electrolytes (e.g., KCl) may be added to maintain normal levels. Because hypotonic solutions have the potential to cause cellular swelling, monitor patients for changes in mentation that may indicate cerebral edema.[15]

Although 5% dextrose in water is considered an isotonic solution, the dextrose is quickly metabolized, and the net result is the administration of free water (hypotonic) with proportionately equal expansion of ECF and ICF. One liter of a 5% dextrose solution provides 50 g of dextrose, or 170 calories. Although this amount of dextrose is not enough to meet caloric requirements, it helps prevent ketosis associated with starvation.

Isotonic. Administration of an isotonic solution expands only ECF. There is no net loss or gain from ICF. An isotonic solution is the ideal fluid replacement for a patient with an ECF volume deficit. Examples of isotonic solutions include lactated Ringer's solution and 0.9% NaCl. Lactated Ringer's solution

TABLE 17-17 COMMONLY USED CRYSTALLOID SOLUTIONS

Solution	Tonicity	mOsm/kg	Glucose (g/L)	Indications and Considerations
Dextrose in Water				
5%	Isotonic, but physiologically hypotonic	278	50	• Provides free water necessary for renal excretion of solutes • Used to replace water losses and treat hypernatremia • Provides 170 cal/L • Does not provide any electrolytes
10%	Hypertonic	556	100	• Provides free water only, no electrolytes • Provides 340 cal/L
Saline				
0.45%	Hypotonic	154	0	• Provides free water in addition to Na+ and Cl- • Used to replace hypotonic fluid losses • Used as maintenance solution, although it does not replace daily losses of other electrolytes • Provides no calories
0.9%	Isotonic	308	0	• Used to expand intravascular volume and replace extracellular fluid losses • Only solution that may be administered with blood products • Contains Na+ and Cl- in excess of plasma levels • Does not provide free water, calories, other electrolytes • May cause intravascular overload or hyperchloremic acidosis
3.0%	Hypertonic	1026	0	• Used to treat symptomatic hyponatremia • Must be administered slowly and with extreme caution because it may cause dangerous intravascular volume overload and pulmonary edema
Dextrose in Saline				
5% in 0.225%	Isotonic	355	50	• Provides Na+, Cl-, and free water • Used to replace hypotonic losses and treat hypernatremia • Provides 170 cal/L
5% in 0.45%	Hypertonic	432	50	• Same as 0.45% NaCl except provides 170 cal/L
5% in 0.9%	Hypertonic	586	50	• Same as 0.9% NaCl except provides 170 cal/L
Multiple Electrolyte Solutions				
Ringer's solution	Isotonic	309	0	• Similar in composition to plasma except that it has excess Cl-, no Mg2+, and no HCO3- • Does not provide free water or calories • Used to expand the intravascular volume and replace extracellular fluid losses
Lactated Ringer's (Hartmann's) solution	Isotonic	274	0	• Similar in composition to normal plasma except does not contain Mg2+ • Used to treat losses from burns and lower GI • May be used to treat mild metabolic acidosis but should not be used to treat lactic acidosis • Does not provide free water or calories

contains sodium, potassium, chloride, calcium, and lactate (the precursor of bicarbonate) in about the same concentrations as those of ECF. It is contraindicated in patients with hyperkalemia and lactic acidosis because they have a decreased ability to convert lactate to bicarbonate.

Isotonic saline (0.9% NaCl) has a sodium concentration (154 mEq/L) somewhat higher than that of plasma (135 to 145 mEq/L) and a chloride concentration (154 mEq/L) significantly higher than the plasma chloride level (96 to 106 mEq/L). Thus excessive administration of isotonic saline can result in elevated sodium and chloride levels. Isotonic saline may be used when a patient has experienced both fluid and sodium losses or as vascular fluid replacement in hypovolemic shock.

Hypertonic. A hypertonic solution initially raises the osmolality of ECF and expands it. In addition, the higher osmotic pressure draws water out of the cells into ECF. It is useful in the treatment of hypovolemia and hyponatremia. Table 17-17 lists commonly used hypertonic solutions. Hypertonic solutions require frequent monitoring of blood pressure, lung sounds, and serum sodium levels because of the risk for intravascular fluid volume excess.[15]

Although concentrated dextrose and water solutions (10% dextrose or greater) are hypertonic solutions, once the dextrose is metabolized, the net result is the administration of water. The free water provided by these solutions ultimately expands both ECF and ICF. The primary use of these solutions is the provision of calories as part of parenteral nutrition. Parenteral nutrition is composed of concentrated dextrose solutions with amino acids, electrolytes, vitamins, and trace elements (see Chapter 40). You may administer solutions containing 10% dextrose or less through a peripheral line. However, you must use a central line to administer solutions with concentrations greater than 10% dextrose. (Central lines are discussed at right.)

Intravenous Additives. In addition to the basic solutions that provide water, electrolytes, and a minimum amount of calories, there are additives to replace specific losses. KCl, CaCl, $MgSO_4$, and HCO_3^- are common additives to the basic IV solutions. The use of these additives is mentioned previously in the discussion of the specific electrolyte deficiencies.

Plasma Expanders. Plasma expanders stay in the vascular space and increase the osmotic pressure. Plasma expanders include colloids, dextran, and hetastarch (Hespan). Colloids are protein solutions such as plasma, albumin, and commercial plasmas (e.g., Plasmanate). Albumin is available in 5% and 25% solutions. The 5% solution has an albumin concentration similar to that of plasma and results in plasma volume expansion equal to the volume infused. This makes the 5% concentration useful in treating hypovolemic patients. In contrast, 25% albumin solution is hypertonic and draws additional fluid from the interstitial space. The main use of the 25% concentration is as a volume expander following a paracentesis for ascites.[16] Dextran is a complex synthetic sugar. Because dextran metabolizes slowly, it remains in the vascular system for a prolonged period (but not as long as the colloids). It pulls additional fluid into the intravascular space. Hetastarch is a synthetic colloid that works similarly to dextran to expand plasma volume. (See Chapter 67 for a discussion of plasma volume expanders.)

If the patient has lost blood, whole blood or packed RBCs are necessary. Packed RBCs have the advantage of giving the patient primarily RBCs. Thus the blood bank can use the plasma for blood components. Although packed RBCs have a decreased plasma volume, they increase the oncotic pressure and pull fluid

DELEGATION DECISIONS
Intravenous Therapy

Although many states permit licensed practical nurses (LPNs) to administer IV fluids and medications, administration of IV fluids or medications to unstable or critically ill patients should be done by the registered nurse (RN).

Role of Registered Nurse (RN)
- Assess patient for clinical manifestations of fluid and electrolyte disturbances.
- Determine whether ordered IV therapies are still appropriate based on monitoring of patient hydration and electrolyte levels.
- Choose and insert appropriate IV catheters and infusion devices.
- Administer IV fluids and medications to unstable and critically ill patients.
- Evaluate patient for clinical manifestations of fluid overload or hypovolemia and initiate appropriate changes in IV fluids.
- Evaluate whether patient fluid and electrolyte needs are being addressed with IV therapies.

Role of Licensed Practical/Vocational Nurse (LPN/LVN)
- Administer IV fluids and medications to stable patients (consider state nurse practice act and agency policy).
- Adjust IV flow rate for stable patients according to health care provider orders (consider state nurse practice act and agency policy).
- Insert IV catheters (consider state nurse practice act and agency policy).
- Monitor for clinical manifestations of adverse reactions to IV fluids or medications.

Role of Unlicensed Assistive Personnel (UAP)
- Measure and record oral intake and output.
- Report swelling or redness at IV site or patient complaints of discomfort at IV site to RN.

into the intravascular space. The use of whole blood, with its additional fluid volume, may cause circulatory overload, particularly in patients who are susceptible to complications from excess circulating volume (e.g., heart failure). To prevent manifestations of fluid volume excess, loop diuretics may be administered with blood. (See Chapter 31 for more information on the administration of blood and blood products.)

CENTRAL VENOUS ACCESS DEVICES

Central venous access devices (CVADs) are catheters placed in large blood vessels (e.g., subclavian vein, jugular vein) of people who require frequent or special access to the vascular system. There are three main types of CVADs: centrally inserted catheters, peripherally inserted central catheters (PICCs), and implanted ports. A physician may place any of these devices; a nurse with specialized training can insert PICCs.

Advantages of CVADs include immediate access to the central venous system, a reduced need for multiple venipunctures, and decreased risk of extravasation injury. CVADs permit frequent, continuous, rapid, or intermittent administration of fluids and medications. They allow for the administration of drugs that are potential vesicants, blood and blood products, and parenteral nutrition. CVADs can provide a means to perform hemodynamic monitoring and obtain venous blood samples. They are useful with patients who have limited peripheral vascular access or who have a projected need for long-term vascular access. Table 17-18 provides examples of conditions where CVADs are used.

TABLE 17-18	INDICATIONS FOR CENTRAL VENOUS ACCESS DEVICE (CVAD)*	
Medical Condition	**Indications for Use**	
Medication administration		
• Cancer	• Chemotherapy, infusion of irritating or vesicant medications	
• Infection	• Long-term administration of antibiotics	
• Pain	• Long-term administration of pain medication	
• Drugs at risk for causing phlebitis	• epoprostenol (Flolan) • calcium chloride • potassium chloride • amiodarone (Cordarone)	
Nutritional replacement	• Infusion of parenteral nutrition • Able to infuse higher dextrose solutions through CVAD than peripheral line	
Blood samples	• Multiple blood draws for diagnostic tests over time	
Blood transfusions	• Infusion of blood or blood products	
Renal failure	• Perform hemodialysis (especially on an acute basis) or continuous renal replacement therapy	
Shock, burns	• Infusion of high volumes of fluid and electrolyte replacement	
Hemodynamic monitoring	• Used to measure central venous pressure to assess fluid balance	
Heart failure	• Perform ultrafiltration	
Autoimmune disorders	• Perform plasmapheresis	

*This list is not all-inclusive, and these are examples only.

Specifically indicated CVADs are safe for injections of radiopaque contrast media at high pressures and controlled rates. For patients who already have poor peripheral venous access, using the port to inject contrast media decreases discomfort from venipuncture and helps lower the risk for extravasation of vesicant contrast media.[17]

The major disadvantages of CVADs are an increased risk of systemic infection and the invasiveness of the procedure. Extravasation can still occur if there is displacement of or damage to the device.

Centrally Inserted Catheters

Centrally inserted catheters (also called central venous catheters [CVCs]) are inserted into a vein in the neck or chest (subclavian or jugular) or groin (femoral) with the tip resting in the distal end of the superior vena cava (Fig. 17-18). The other end of the catheter is either nontunneled or tunneled through subcutaneous tissue and exits through a separate incision on the chest or abdominal wall. A Dacron cuff serves to stabilize the catheter and may decrease the incidence of infection by impeding bacteria migration along the catheter beyond the cuff. Do not use a newly place CVAD until the tip position is verified with a chest x-ray.

These catheters are single-, double-, triple-, or quad-lumen catheters. Multi-lumen catheters are useful in the critically ill patient because all of the lumens can provide a different therapy simultaneously. For example, incompatible drugs infuse in separate lumens without mixing while a third lumen provides access for blood sampling. Specific types of long-term central

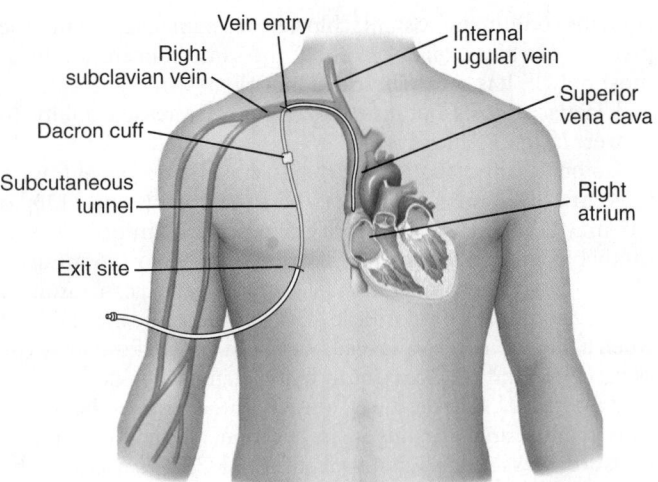

FIG. 17-18 Tunneled central venous catheter. Note tip of the catheter in the superior vena cava.

catheters are Hickman catheters, which require clamps to make sure the valve is closed, and Groshong catheters, which have a valve that opens as fluid is withdrawn or infused and remains closed when not in use.

Peripherally Inserted Central Catheters

PICCs are central venous catheters inserted into a vein in the arm rather than a vein in the neck or chest. They are inserted at or just above the antecubital fossa (usually cephalic or basilic vein) and advanced to a position with the tip ending in the distal one third of the superior vena cava. PICCs are single- or multiple-lumen, are nontunneled, and are up to 60 cm in length with gauges ranging from 24 to 16 (Fig. 17-19). They are used with patients who need vascular access for 1 week to 6 months but can be in place for longer periods.

Advantages of the PICC over a central venous catheter are lower infection rate, fewer insertion-related complications, decreased cost, and insertion at the bedside or outpatient area. Complications of PICCs include catheter occlusion and phlebitis (Table 17-19). If phlebitis occurs, it usually appears within 7 to 10 days after insertion. Do not use the arm with the PICC to obtain a blood pressure reading or draw blood.

FIG. 17-19 Peripherally inserted central catheter (*PICC*) can be inserted using the basilic or cephalic vein.

TABLE 17-19 COMPLICATIONS OF CENTRAL VENOUS ACCESS DEVICES (CVADs)

Possible Cause	Clinical Manifestations	Management
Catheter Occlusion • Clamped or kinked catheter • Tip against wall of vessel • Thrombosis • Precipitate buildup in lumen	• Sluggish infusion or aspiration • Inability to infuse and/or aspirate	• Instruct patient to change position, raise arm, and cough. • Assess for and alleviate clamping or kinking. • Flush with normal saline using a 10-mL syringe. Do not force flush. • Perform fluoroscopy to determine cause and site. • Administer anticoagulant or thrombolytic agents.
Embolism • Catheter breaking • Dislodgment of thrombus • Entry of air into circulation	• Chest pain • Respiratory distress (dyspnea, tachypnea, hypoxia, cyanosis) • Hypotension • Tachycardia	• Administer O₂. • Clamp catheter. • Place patient on left side with head down (air emboli). • Notify physician.
Catheter-Related Infection (local or systemic) • Contamination during insertion or use • Migration of organisms along catheter • Immunosuppressed patient	• *Local:* redness, tenderness, purulent drainage, warmth, edema • *Systemic:* fever, chills, malaise	**Local** • Culture drainage from site. • Apply warm, moist compresses. • Remove catheter if indicated. **Systemic** • Take blood cultures. • Give antibiotic therapy. • Give antipyretic therapy. • Remove catheter if indicated.
Pneumothorax • Perforation of visceral pleura during insertion	• Decreased or absent breath sounds • Respiratory distress (cyanosis, dyspnea, tachypnea) • Chest pain • Distended unilateral chest	• Administer O₂. • Position in semi-Fowler's position. • Prepare for chest tube insertion.
Catheter Migration • Improper suturing • Insertion site trauma • Changes in intrathoracic pressure • Forceful catheter flushing • Spontaneous	• Sluggish infusion or aspiration • Edema of chest or neck during infusion • Patient complaint of gurgling sound in ear • Dysrhythmias • Increased external catheter length	• Perform fluoroscopy to verify position. • Assist with removal and new CVAD placement.

Implanted Infusion Ports

Implanted infusion ports consist of a central venous catheter connected to an implanted, single or double subcutaneous injection port (Fig. 17-20, *A*). The catheter tip lies in the desired vein, and the other end is connected to a port that is surgically implanted in a subcutaneous pocket on the chest wall. The port consists of a metal sheath with a self-sealing silicone septum. To access these devices, a special Huber-point needle with a deflected tip is used to prevent damage to the rubber septum that could make the port useless (Fig. 17-20, *B*). Huber-point needles are also available with the tip at a 90-degree angle for longer infusions.

Drugs are placed in the port's reservoir either by a direct injection or through injection into an established IV line. After being filled, the reservoir slowly releases the medicine into the bloodstream. Implanted ports are good for long-term therapy and have a low risk of infection. The hidden port offers the patient cosmetic advantages and overall has less maintenance than other types of CVADs. Regular flushing is required to avoid the formation of "sludge" (clotted blood and drug precipitate) within the port septum.

Complications

CVADs always have a potential for complications. Astute monitoring and assessment may assist in early identification of potential complications. Table 17-19 lists common possible complications, potential causes, clinical manifestations, and interventions.

NURSING MANAGEMENT
CENTRAL VENOUS ACCESS DEVICES

Nursing management of CVADs includes assessment, dressing changes and cleansing, injection cap changes, and maintenance of catheter patency. The exact frequency and procedures for these requirements vary by type of CVAD and institution, so it is important to follow your specific institution's policies and procedures. The following section discusses some general guidelines.

Catheter and insertion site assessment includes inspection of the site for redness, edema, warmth, drainage, and tenderness or pain. Observation of the catheter for misplacement or slippage is important. Perform a comprehensive pain assessment,

FIG. 17-20 A, Cross section of implantable port displaying access of the port with the Huber-point needle. Note the deflected point of the Huber-point needle, which prevents coring of the port's septum. **B,** Two Huber-point needles used to enter the implanted port. The 90-degree needle is used for top-entry ports for continuous infusion.

particularly noting any complaints of chest or neck discomfort, arm pain, or pain at the insertion site.[17] Before manipulating a catheter for any reason, perform hand hygiene.

Perform dressing changes and cleanse the catheter insertion site using strict sterile technique. Typical dressings include transparent semipermeable dressings or gauze and tape. If the site is bleeding, a gauze dressing may be preferable. Otherwise, transparent dressings are preferred. They allow observation of the site without having to remove the dressing. Transparent dressings may be left in place for up to 1 week if clean, dry, and intact. Change any dressing immediately if it becomes damp, loose, or visibly soiled.

Cleanse the skin around the catheter insertion site according to institution policy. A chlorhexidine-based preparation is the cleansing agent of choice. Its effects last longer than either povidone-iodine or isopropyl alcohol, offering improved killing of bacteria. When using chlorhexidine, cleansing the skin with friction is critical to infection prevention. When applying a new dressing, allow the area to air dry completely before application for chlorhexidine to be effective.[18] Secure the lumen ports to the skin above the dressing site. Document the date and time of the dressing change and initial the dressing.

Change injection caps at regular intervals according to institution policy or if they are damaged from excessive punctures. Use strict sterile technique. Teach the patient to turn the head to the opposite side of the CVAD insertion site during cap change. If the catheter cannot be clamped, instruct the patient to lie flat in bed and perform the Valsalva maneuver whenever the catheter is open to air to prevent an air embolism.

Flushing is one of the most effective ways to maintain lumen patency and to prevent occlusion of the CVAD.[19] It also keeps incompatible drugs or fluids from mixing. Use a normal saline solution in a syringe that has a barrel capacity of 10 mL or more to avoid excess pressure on the catheter. If you feel resistance, do not apply force. This could result in a ruptured catheter or create an embolism if a thrombus is present. Because of the risk of contamination and infection, prefilled syringes or single-dose vials are preferred over multiple-dose vials. If you are not using a positive-pressure valve cap, clamp any unused lines after flushing.

Use the push-pause technique when flushing all catheters. Push-pause creates turbulence within the catheter lumen, promoting the removal of debris that adheres to the catheter lumen and decreasing the chance of occlusion. This technique involves injecting saline with a rapid alternating push-pause motion, instilling 1 to 2 mL with each push on the syringe plunger. If you are using a negative-pressure cap or neutral pressure cap, clamp the catheter while maintaining positive pressure while instilling the last 1mL of saline in order to prevent reflux of blood back into the catheter. If a positive-pressure valve cap is present, it works to prevent the reflux of blood and resultant catheter lumen occlusion. Remove the syringe before clamping the catheter to allow the positive pressure valve to work correctly. Clamping the catheter during flushing with this cap may actually promote blood reflux.[19]

REMOVAL OF CVADs

Removal of CVADs is done according to institution policy and the nurse's scope of practice. In many agencies, nurses with demonstrated competency can remove PICCs and nontunneled central venous catheters. The procedure involves removing any sutures and then gently withdrawing the catheter. Instruct the patient to perform the Valsalva maneuver as the last 5 to 10 cm of the catheter is withdrawn. Immediately apply pressure to the site with sterile gauze to prevent air from entering and to control bleeding. Inspect the catheter tip to determine that it is intact. After bleeding has stopped, apply an antiseptic ointment and sterile dressing to the site.

CASE STUDY

Fluid and Electrolyte Imbalance

iStockphoto/Thinkstock

Patient Profile

S.S., a 63-year-old white woman with lung cancer, has been receiving chemotherapy on an outpatient basis. She completed her third treatment 5 days ago and has been experiencing nausea and vomiting for 2 days even though she has been using ondansetron (Zofran). S.S.'s daughter brings her to the hospital, where she is admitted to the medical unit. As the admitting nurse, you perform a thorough assessment.

Subjective Data

- Complains of lethargy, weakness, dizziness, and dry mouth
- States she has been too nauseated to eat or drink anything for 2 days

Objective Data

- Heart rate 110 beats/min, pulse thready
- BP 100/65
- Weight loss of 5 lb since she received her chemotherapy treatment 5 days ago
- Dry oral mucous membranes

Discussion Questions

1. Based on her clinical manifestations, what fluid imbalance does S.S. have?
2. What additional assessment data should you obtain?
3. What are her risk factors for fluid and electrolyte imbalances?
4. You draw blood for a serum chemistry evaluation. What electrolyte imbalances are likely and why?
5. S.S. is at risk for which acid-base imbalance? Describe the changes that would occur in S.S.'s ABGs with this acid-base imbalance. How would the body compensate?
6. The physician orders dextrose 5% in 0.45% saline to infuse at 100 mL/hr. What type of solution is this, and how will it help S.S.'s fluid imbalance?
7. *Priority Decision:* What are the priority nursing interventions for S.S.?
8. *Evidence-Based Practice:* S.S. has a double-lumen PICC in her left arm. One lumen is connected to the IV infusion; the other is unused. What is the recommended practice for maintaining the patency of the unused lumen?

⊜volve Answers available at *http://evolve.elsevier.com/Lewis/medsurg.*

■ BRIDGE TO NCLEX EXAMINATION

The number of the question corresponds to the same-numbered outcome at the beginning of the chapter.

1. During the postoperative care of a 76-year-old patient, the nurse monitors the patient's intake and output carefully, knowing that the patient is at risk for fluid and electrolyte imbalances primarily because
   a. older adults have an impaired thirst mechanism and need reminding to drink fluids.
   b. water accounts for a greater percentage of body weight in the older adult than in younger adults.
   c. older adults are more likely than younger adults to lose extracellular fluid during surgical procedures.
   d. small losses of fluid are more significant because body fluids account for only about 50% of body weight in older adults.

2. During administration of a hypertonic IV solution, the mechanism involved in equalizing the fluid concentration between ECF and the cells is
   a. osmosis.
   b. diffusion.
   c. active transport.
   d. facilitated diffusion.

3a. An older woman was admitted to the medical unit with dehydration. Clinical indications of this problem are *(select all that apply)*
   a. weight loss.
   b. dry oral mucosa.
   c. full bounding pulse.
   d. engorged neck veins.
   e. decreased central venous pressure.

3b. The nursing care for a patient with hyponatremia includes
   a. fluid restriction.
   b. administration of hypotonic IV fluids.
   c. administration of a cation-exchange resin.
   d. increased water intake for patients on nasogastric suction.

3c. The nurse should be alert for which manifestations in a patient receiving a loop diuretic?
   a. Restlessness and agitation
   b. Paresthesias and irritability
   c. Weak, irregular pulse and poor muscle tone
   d. Increased blood pressure and muscle spasms

3d. Which patient would be at greatest risk for the potential development of hypermagnesemia?
   a. 83-year-old man with lung cancer and hypertension
   b. 65-year-old woman with hypertension taking β-adrenergic blockers
   c. 42-year-old woman with systemic lupus erythematosus and renal failure
   d. 50-year-old man with benign prostatic hyperplasia and a urinary tract infection

3e. It is especially important for the nurse to assess for which clinical manifestation(s) in a patient who has just undergone a total thyroidectomy *(select all that apply)*?
   a. Confusion
   b. Weight gain
   c. Depressed reflexes
   d. Circumoral numbness
   e. Positive Chvostek's sign

3f. The nurse anticipates that treatment of the patient with hyperphosphatemia secondary to renal failure will include
   a. fluid restriction.
   b. calcium supplements.
   c. loop diuretic therapy.
   d. magnesium supplements.

4. The lungs act as an acid-base buffer by
   a. increasing respiratory rate and depth when CO_2 levels in the blood are high, reducing acid load.
   b. increasing respiratory rate and depth when CO_2 levels in the blood are low, reducing base load.
   c. decreasing respiratory rate and depth when CO_2 levels in the blood are high, reducing acid load.
   d. decreasing respiratory rate and depth when CO_2 levels in the blood are low, increasing acid load.

5. A patient has the following arterial blood gas results: pH 7.52; $PaCO_2$ 30 mm Hg; HCO_3^- 24 mEq/L. The nurse determines that these results indicate
   a. metabolic acidosis.
   b. metabolic alkalosis.
   c. respiratory acidosis.
   d. respiratory alkalosis.

6. The typical fluid replacement for the patient with a fluid volume deficit is
   a. dextran.
   b. 0.45% saline.
   c. lactated Ringer's.
   d. 5% dextrose in 0.45% saline.

7. The nurse is unable to flush a central venous access device and suspects occlusion. The best nursing intervention would be to
   a. apply warm moist compresses to the insertion site.
   b. attempt to force 10 mL of normal saline into the device.
   c. place the patient on the left side with head-down position.
   d. instruct the patient to change positions, raise arm, and cough.

1. d, 2. a, 3a. a, b, e, 3b. a, 3c. c, 3d. c, 3e. a, d, e, 3f. b, 4. a, 5. d, 6. c, 7. d

⊜volve

For rationales to these answers and even more NCLEX review questions, visit *http://evolve.elsevier.com/Lewis/medsurg.*

REFERENCES

1. Huether SE, McCance KL: *Understanding pathophysiology*, ed 5, St Louis, 2012, Mosby.
2. McCance K, Huether SE: *Pathophysiology: the biologic basis for disease in adults and children*, ed 6, St Louis, 2010, Mosby.
3. Herlihy B: *The human body in health and illness*, ed 5, St Louis, 2011, Saunders.
4. Touhy TA, Jett KF: *Gerontologic nursing and healthy aging*, ed 3, St Louis, 2010, Mosby.
5. Fillit H, Rockwood K, Woodhouse K, et al: *Brocklehurst's textbook of geriatric medicine and gerontology*, ed 7, St Louis, 2010, Mosby.
6. Rothrock J: *Alexander's care of the patient in surgery*, ed 14, St Louis, 2011, Mosby.
*7. Yee AH, Rabinstein AA: Neurologic presentations of acid-base imbalance, electrolyte abnormalities and endocrine emergencies, *Neurol Clin* 28:1, 2010.
8. Crawford A, Harris H: Balancing act: sodium and potassium, *Nursing* 41:44, 2011.
*9. Cyr PL, Slawsky KA, Olchanski N, et al: Effect of serum sodium concentration and tolvatapan treatment on length of hospitalization in patients with heart failure, *Am J Health System Pharm* 68:328, 2011.
10. Lehnhardt A, Kemper MJ: Pathogenesis, diagnosis and management of hyperkalemia, *Pediatr Nephrol* 26:377, 2011.
11. Gahart BL, Nazareno AR: *Intravenous medications*, ed 27, St Louis, 2011, Mosby.
12. Lewis MA, Hendrickson AW, Moynihan TJ: Oncologic emergencies, *CA-Cancer J Clin* 61:287, 2011.
*13. Geerse DA, Bindels AJ, Kuiper MA, et al: Treatment of hypophosphatemia in the intensive care unit: a review, *Crit Care* 14:147, 2010.
14. Crawford A, Harris H: Balancing act: hypermagnesemia and hypomagnesemia, *Nursing* 41:52, 2011.
15. Bope ET, Kellerman RD: *Conn's current therapy 2012*, St Louis, 2012, Saunders.
*16. Nieme TT, Miyashita R, Yamakage M: Colloid solutions: a clinical update, *J Anesth* 24:913, 2010.
*17. Earhart A, McMahon P: Vascular access and media, *J Infusion Nurs* 34:97, 2011.
18. Eisenberg S: Accessing implanted ports, *Clin J Oncol Nurs* 15:324, 2011.
19. Mathers D: Evidence-based practice: improving outcomes for patients with a central venous access device, *JAVA* 16:64, 2011.

*Evidence-based information for clinical practice.

RESOURCE

Infusion Nurses Society
www.ins1.org

CASE STUDY

Managing Multiple Patients

You are assigned to care for the following three patients in the intensive care unit (ICU). There are two other RNs and two unlicensed assistive personnel (UAP) on duty to care for a total of 12 patients currently in the unit.

Patients

iStockphoto/Thinkstock

G.N., a 58-year-old African American man, was admitted to the ICU after falling out of a tree onto a lit gas grill. He has partial-thickness burns on his face, neck, and upper trunk. He has undergone surgical repair of right tibia and left hip fractures as well as debridement of a severely lacerated right leg. His voice is slightly hoarse and he is coughing up sooty sputum. He is receiving O_2 at 4 L/min via nasal cannula and his O_2 saturation is 93%. His WBC count is 26,400/μL (26.4 × 10^9/L) with 80% neutrophils (10% bands).

iStockphoto/Thinkstock

J.N., a 35-year-old African American woman, was transferred to the ICU from the clinical unit last evening with acute respiratory failure. She was diagnosed 2 days ago with AIDS and *Pneumocystis jiroveci* pneumonia (PCP). Prior to this hospital admission she had consistently refused antiretroviral therapy (ART) because she could not afford it. She was started on oral trimethoprim/sulfamethoxazole (Bactrim) and combination antiretroviral therapy. However, her respiratory distress worsened and she was transferred to the ICU for intubation and mechanical ventilation. She is started on IV Bactrim and corticosteroid therapy.

iStockphoto/Thinkstock

S.S., a 63-year-old white woman with lung cancer, has been receiving chemotherapy on an outpatient basis. She completed her third treatment 5 days ago and has been experiencing nausea and vomiting for 2 days even though she has been using ondansetron (Zofran). She was initially admitted to the medical unit but was transferred to the ICU for closer monitoring after becoming severely hypotensive overnight. Her most recent blood pressure was 98/50.

Management Discussion Questions

1. **Priority Decision:** After receiving report, which patient should you see first? Provide rationale.
2. **Delegation Decision:** Which of the following morning tasks should you delegate to the UAP (*select all that apply*)?
   a. Take blood pressure readings on S.S.
   b. Perform neurovascular checks on G.N.
   c. Document strict intake and output on S.S.
   d. Provide oral care around the endotracheal tube for J.N.
   e. Titrate S.S.'s IV infusion rate based on her blood pressure reading.

3. **Priority and Delegation Decision:** When you enter J.N.'s room, the ventilator alarms are going off. The UAP had just finished providing oral care and she tells you that J.N. has become increasingly agitated within the last 5 minutes. Which initial action would be most appropriate?
   a. Suction J.N.'s endotracheal tube.
   b. Have the UAP stay with J.N. while you obtain IV sedation for her.
   c. Ask the UAP to describe exactly what she did when she was performing oral care.
   d. Assess the ventilator to identify what alarm is going off and to make sure all connections are secure.

Case Study Progression

J.N.'s ventilator tubing had become disconnected. You quickly reconnect her tubing and she settles down as her oxygenation improves. You ask the UAP to obtain vital signs on all your patients while you begin a more thorough assessment of J.N.

4. During your assessment of J.N., you note grey-white patches on the inside of her mouth. You recognize these as most likely caused by
   a. *Candida albicans*.
   b. poor oral hygiene.
   c. *Coccidioides immitis*.
   d. irritation from recent mouth care.
5. G.N.'s family asks you why surgery was performed on his leg wound. Your response is based on the knowledge that debridement (*select all that apply*)
   a. is used to remove infected tissue.
   b. is used to remove nonviable tissue.
   c. prepares the wound bed for healing.
   d. can only be accomplished with surgery.
6. S.S.'s morning laboratory results reveal a serum potassium level of 2.8 mEq/L. You notify the health care provider and obtain an order for IV potassium. During infusion of the potassium aliquots, you prioritize assessment of S.S.'s
   a. bowel function.
   b. cardiac rhythm.
   c. muscle strength.
   d. level of consciousness.
7. **Management Decision:** While sitting at the computer charting your patients' morning assessments, you overhear the UAP telling a nursing student that J.N. deserves what she got because HIV is God's way of punishing those who sin. Your most appropriate response would be to
   a. report the UAP's actions to your supervisor.
   b. ask the UAP to keep her opinions to herself.
   c. ignore the conversation as it does not impact patient care.
   d. talk to the UAP and student about keeping personal feelings separate from patient care.

SECTION 3

Perioperative Care

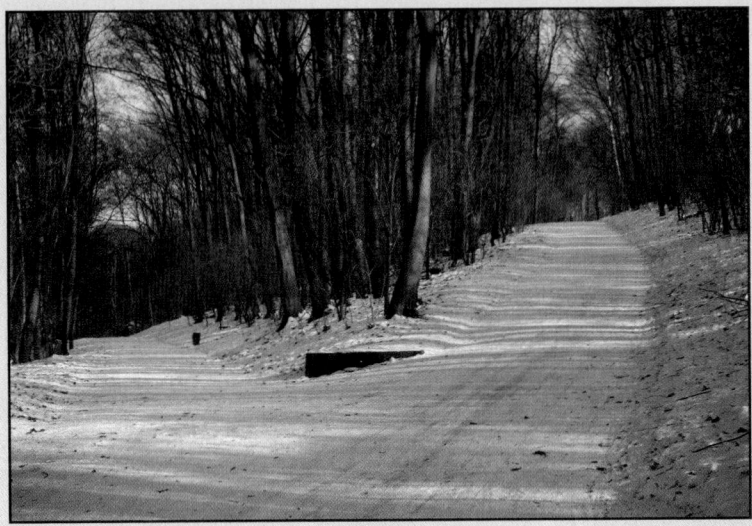

iStockphoto/Thinkstock

Two roads diverged in a wood, and I—I took the one less traveled by,
and that has made all the difference.
Robert Frost

Nursing Management
Preoperative Care

Janice Neil

e‍volve WEBSITE

http://evolve.elsevier.com/Lewis/medsurg

- NCLEX Review Questions
- Key Points
- Pre-Test

- Answer Guidelines for Case Study on p. 330
- Rationales for Bridge to NCLEX Examination Questions

- Concept Map Creator
- Glossary
- Content Updates

The very first requirement in a hospital is that it should do the sick no harm.
Florence Nightingale

LEARNING OUTCOMES

1. Differentiate the common purposes and settings of surgery.
2. Apply knowledge of the purpose and components of a preoperative nursing assessment.
3. Interpret the significance of data related to the preoperative patient's health status and operative risk.
4. Analyze the components and purpose of informed consent for surgery.
5. Examine the nursing role in the physical, psychologic, and educational preparation of the surgical patient.
6. Prioritize the nursing responsibilities related to day-of-surgery preparation for the surgical patient.
7. Differentiate the purposes and types of common preoperative medications.
8. Apply knowledge of the special considerations of preoperative preparation for the older adult surgical patient.

KEY TERMS

ambulatory surgery, p. 318
elective surgery, p. 318

emergency surgery, p. 318
informed consent, p. 325

same-day admission, p. 318
surgery, p. 317

Preparation of patients for surgery is an important nursing role. This chapter includes a discussion of preoperative care that is applicable to all surgical patients regardless of where the surgery is performed. Preparation measures for specific surgical procedures (e.g., abdominal, thoracic, or orthopedic surgery) are discussed in appropriate chapters of this text.

Surgery is the art and science of treating diseases, injuries, and deformities by operation and instrumentation. The surgical experience involves a multidisciplinary interaction among the patient, surgeon, anesthesia care provider (ACP), nurse, and other health care team members as needed. Surgery may be performed for any of the following purposes:

- *Diagnosis:* Determination of the presence and extent of a pathologic condition (e.g., lymph node biopsy, bronchoscopy).

- *Cure:* Elimination or repair of a pathologic condition (e.g., removal of ruptured appendix or benign ovarian cyst).
- *Palliation:* Alleviation of symptoms without cure (e.g., cutting a nerve root [rhizotomy] to remove symptoms of pain, creating a colostomy to bypass an inoperable bowel obstruction).
- *Prevention* (e.g., removal of a mole before it becomes malignant, removal of the colon in a patient with familial polyposis to prevent cancer).
- *Cosmetic improvement* (e.g., repairing a burn scar, breast reconstruction after a mastectomy).
- *Exploration:* Surgical examination to determine the nature or extent of a disease (e.g., laparotomy). With the advent of advanced diagnostic tests, exploration is less common because problems can be identified earlier and easier.

Reviewed by Lisa Kiper, RN, MSN, Assistant Professor of Nursing, Morehead State University, Morehead, Kentucky; Margaret Ochab-Ohryn, RN, MS, MBA, CRNA, Associate Professor, Oakland Community College, Farmington Hills, Michigan; and Cynthia Schoonover, RN, MS, CCRN, Associate Nursing Professor, Sinclair Community College, Dayton, Ohio and PACU Staff Nurse, Kettering Medical Center, Kettering, Ohio.

TABLE 18-1	SUFFIXES DESCRIBING SURGICAL PROCEDURES	
Suffix	**Meaning**	**Example**
-ectomy	Excision or removal of	Appendectomy
-lysis	Destruction of	Electrolysis
-orrhaphy	Repair or suture of	Herniorrhaphy
-oscopy	Looking into	Endoscopy
-ostomy	Creation of opening into	Colostomy
-otomy	Cutting into or incision of	Tracheotomy
-plasty	Repair or reconstruction of	Mammoplasty

Specific suffixes are commonly used in combination with a body part or organ in naming surgical procedures (Table 18-1).

SURGICAL SETTINGS

Surgery may be a carefully planned event (elective surgery) or may arise with unexpected urgency (emergency surgery). Both elective and emergency surgery may be performed in a variety of settings. The setting in which a surgical procedure may be safely and effectively performed is influenced by the type of surgery, potential complications, and the patient's general health status.

For inpatient surgery, patients who are going to be admitted to the hospital are usually admitted on the day of surgery (same-day admission). Patients who are in the hospital before surgery are usually there because of acute or chronic medical conditions.

The majority of surgical procedures are performed as ambulatory surgery (also called same-day or outpatient surgery). Many of these surgeries use minimally invasive techniques (e.g., laparoscopic techniques). (The surgeries are described in chapters throughout the text in discussions of interventions for specific problems.) Ambulatory surgery may be conducted in endoscopy clinics, physicians' offices, freestanding surgical clinics, and outpatient surgery units in hospitals. These procedures can be performed using general, regional, or local anesthetic; have an operating time of less than 2 hours; and require less than a 24-hour stay postoperatively. Many patients go home with a caregiver within hours of surgery.

Ambulatory surgery is often preferred by patients and physicians. Generally, it involves minimal laboratory tests, requires fewer preoperative and postoperative medications, and reduces the patient's risk for health care–associated infections. Patients like the convenience of recovering at home, physicians prefer the flexibility in scheduling, and the cost is usually less for both the patient and the insurer.

Regardless of where the surgery is performed, you play an essential role in preparing the patient for surgery, caring for the patient during surgery, and facilitating the patient's recovery after surgery. To perform these functions effectively, first know the nature of the disorder requiring surgery and any coexisting medical problems. Second, identify the individual patient's response to the stress of surgery. Third, know the results of appropriate preoperative diagnostic tests. Finally, identify potential risks and complications associated with the surgical procedure and any coexisting medical problems that should be included in the plan of care. The nurse caring for the patient preoperatively is likely to be different from the nurse in the operating room (OR), postanesthesia care unit (PACU), surgical intensive care unit (SICU), or surgical unit. Thus communication and documentation of important preoperative assessment findings are essential for the continuity of care.

PATIENT INTERVIEW

One of the most important nursing actions is the preoperative interview. The nurse who works in the physician's office, the ambulatory surgery center, or the hospital preoperative area may do the interview. The site of the interview and the time before surgery dictate the depth and completeness of the interview. Important findings must be documented and communicated to others to maintain continuity of care.

The preoperative interview can occur in advance or on the day of surgery. The primary purposes of the patient interview are to (1) obtain the patient's health information; (2) provide and clarify information about the planned surgery, including anesthesia; and (3) assess the patient's emotional state and readiness for surgery, including his or her expectations about the surgical outcomes. Ensure that the patient's consent form for surgery has been signed and witnessed and that the appropriate laboratory and diagnostic tests have been ordered or completed.

The interview also provides the patient and the caregiver an opportunity to ask questions about surgery, anesthesia, and postoperative care. Often patients ask about taking their routine medications, such as insulin, anticoagulants, or cardiac medications, and if they will experience pain. By being aware of the patient's and caregiver's needs, you can provide the information and support needed during the perioperative period.

NURSING ASSESSMENT OF PREOPERATIVE PATIENT

The overall goal of the preoperative assessment is to identify risk factors and plan care to ensure patient safety throughout the surgical experience. Goals of the assessment are to

- Determine the patient's psychologic status in order to reinforce the use of coping strategies during the surgical experience.
- Determine physiologic factors directly or indirectly related to the surgical procedure that may contribute to operative risk factors.
- Establish baseline data for comparison in the intraoperative and postoperative period.
- Participate in the identification and documentation of the surgical site and/or side (of body) on which the surgical procedure will be performed.
- Identify prescription drugs, over-the-counter medications, and herbal supplements taken by the patient that may result in drug interactions affecting the surgical outcome.
- Document the results of all preoperative laboratory and diagnostic tests in the patient's record, and communicate this information to appropriate health care providers.
- Identify cultural and ethnic factors that may affect the surgical experience.
- Determine if the patient has received adequate information from the surgeon to make an informed decision to have surgery and that the consent form is signed and witnessed.

Subjective Data

Psychosocial Assessment. Surgery is a stressful event, even when the procedure is considered minor. The psychologic and physiologic reactions to surgery and anesthesia may elicit the stress response (e.g., elevated blood pressure [BP] and heart rate). The stress response enables the body to prepare to meet the demands in the perioperative period. If stressors or the responses to the stressors are excessive, the stress response can be magnified and may affect recovery. Many factors influence the patient's susceptibility to stress, including age, past experiences with illness and pain, current health, and socioeconomic status. Identifying a patient's perceived or actual stressors allows you to provide support during the preoperative period so that stress does not become distress.

The use of common language and avoidance of medical jargon are essential. Use words and language that are familiar to the patient to increase the patient's understanding of surgical consent and the surgery. Familiar language also helps reduce preoperative anxiety.

Your role in psychologically preparing the patient for surgery is to assess the patient for potential stressors that could negatively affect surgery (Table 18-2). Communicate all concerns to the appropriate surgical team member, especially if the concern requires intervention later in the surgical experience. Because many patients are admitted directly into the preoperative area

from their homes, you must be skilled in assessing important psychologic factors in a short time. The most common psychologic factors are anxiety, fear, and hope.

Anxiety. Most people are anxious when facing surgery because of the unknown. This is normal and is an inborn survival mechanism. However, if the anxiety level is high, cognition, decision making, and coping abilities are reduced.

Anxiety can arise from lack of knowledge, which may range from not knowing what to expect during surgery to uncertainty about the outcome. This may be a result of past experiences or stories heard through friends or the media. You can decrease some anxiety for the patient by providing information about what to expect. This is often done through classes, or web-based or audiovisual educational materials before surgery. Inform the surgeon if the patient requires any additional information or if anxiety is excessive.

The patient may experience anxiety when surgery is in conflict with his or her religious and cultural beliefs. In particular, identify, document, and communicate the patient's religious and cultural beliefs about the possibility of blood transfusions. For example, Jehovah's Witnesses may choose to refuse blood or blood products.[1]

Common Fears. Patients fear surgery for a number of reasons. The most common fear is the risk of death or permanent disability resulting from surgery. Sometimes the fear arises after hearing or reading about the risks during the informed consent process. Other fears are related to pain, change in body image, or results of diagnostic procedures.

Fear of death can be extremely harmful. Notify the physician if the patient has a strong fear of death. A patient's strong fear of impending death may prompt the physician to delay the surgery until the situation improves because the emotional state influences the stress response, and thus the surgical outcome.

Fear of pain and discomfort during and after surgery is common. If the fear is extreme, notify the ACP or the surgeon. Reassure the patient that drugs are available for both anesthesia and analgesia during surgery. For pain after surgery, tell patients to ask for pain medication before pain becomes severe. Instruct the patient on the use of a pain intensity scale (e.g., 0 to 10, FACES [see eFig. 9-3, available on the website for Chapter 9]). (Pain scales are explained in Chapter 9.)

Drugs may also be given that provide an amnesic effect so the patient will not remember what occurs during surgery. Tell the patient that this effect assists in decreasing anxiety after surgery.

Fear of mutilation or alteration in body image can occur whether the surgery is radical, such as amputation, or minor, such as a bunion repair. Even a small scar on the body can be upsetting to some, and others fear keloid development (overgrowth of a scar). Listen to and assess the patient's concern about this fear with an accepting attitude.

Fear of anesthesia may arise from the unknown, personal experience, or tales of others' bad experiences. These concerns can also result from information about the risks (e.g., brain damage, paralysis) of anesthesia. Many patients fear losing control while under anesthesia. If these fears are identified, inform the ACP immediately so that he or she can talk further with the patient. Reassure the patient that a nurse and the ACP will be present at all times during surgery.

Fear of disruption of life functioning may be present in varying degrees. It can range from fear of permanent disability to concern about not being able to engage in activities of daily

TABLE 18-2 PSYCHOSOCIAL ASSESSMENT OF PREOPERATIVE PATIENT

Situational Changes
- Identify support systems, including family, other caregivers, group and institutional structures, and religious and spiritual groups.
- Define current degree of personal control, decision making, and independence.
- Consider the impact of surgery and hospitalization and the possible effects on lifestyle.
- Determine the presence of hope and anticipation of positive results.

Concerns With the Unknown
- Identify specific areas and degree of anxiety and fears related to the surgery (e.g., pain).
- Identify expectations of surgery, changes in current health status, effects on daily living, and sexual activity (if appropriate).

Concerns With Body Image
- Identify current roles or relationships and view of self.
- Determine perceived or potential changes in roles or relationships and their impact on body image.

Past Experiences
- Review previous surgical experiences, hospitalizations, and treatments.
- Determine responses to those experiences (positive and negative).
- Identify current perceptions of surgical procedure in relation to the above and information from others (e.g., a friend's view of a personal surgical experience).

Knowledge Deficit
- Identify the amount and type of preoperative information the patient wants.
- Assess understanding of the surgical procedure, including preparation, care, interventions, preoperative activities, restrictions, and expected outcomes.
- Identify the accuracy of information the patient has received from others, including health care team, family, friends, and the media.

living for a few weeks. Concerns about loss of role function, separation from family, and how the family will manage may be revealed. Financial concerns may be related to an anticipated loss of income or the costs of surgery.

If you identify any of these fears, a consult with the patient's caregiver, a social worker, a spiritual or cultural advisor, or a psychologist may be appropriate. Financial advisors at the hospital may be able to provide information about financial support.

Hope. Although many psychologic factors related to surgery seem to be negative, hope is a positive attribute.[2] Hope may be the patient's strongest method of coping. To deny or minimize hope may negate the positive mental attitude necessary for a quick and full recovery. Some surgeries are hopefully anticipated. These can be the surgeries that repair (e.g., plastic surgery for burn scars), rebuild (e.g., total joint replacement to reduce pain and improve function), or save and extend life (e.g., repair of aneurysm, organ transplant). Assess and support the presence of hope and the patient's anticipation of positive results.

Past Health History. Ask the patient about any previous medical problems and surgeries. Determine if the patient understands the need for surgery. For example, the patient scheduled for a total knee replacement may indicate that increasing pain and immobility are the reasons for the surgery.

Document the reason for any past hospitalizations, including previous surgeries and the dates. Also identify any problems with previous surgeries. For example, the patient may have experienced a wound infection or a reaction to a medication.

Ask women about their menstrual and obstetric history. This includes the date of their last menstrual period, the number of pregnancies, and any history of cesarean section.

When obtaining a family health history, ask both patient and caregiver about any inherited traits, since they may contribute to the surgical outcome. Record any family history of cardiac and endocrine diseases. For example, if a patient reports a parent with hypertension, sudden cardiac death, or myocardial infarction, this should alert you to the possibility that the patient may have a similar predisposition or condition. Also obtain information about the patient's family history of adverse reactions to or problems with anesthesia. For example, malignant hyperthermia has a genetic predisposition. Measures to decrease complications associated with this condition can be taken. (For further information on malignant hyperthermia, see Chapter 19.)

Medications. Document all current routine and intermittent medication use, including over-the-counter drugs and herbal supplements. In many ambulatory surgery centers, patients are asked to bring their medications with them when reporting for surgery. This helps to accurately assess and document both the name and the dosage of medications.

The interaction of the patient's current medications and anesthetics can increase or decrease the desired physiologic effect of anesthetics. Consider the effects of opioids and prescribed medications for chronic health conditions (e.g., heart disease, hypertension, depression, epilepsy, diabetes mellitus). For example, certain antidepressants can potentiate the effect of opioids, agents that can be used for anesthesia. Antihypertensive drugs may predispose the patient to shock from the combined effect of the drug and the vasodilator effect of some anesthetic agents. Insulin or oral hypoglycemic agents may require dose or agent adjustments during the perioperative period because of increased body metabolism, decreased oral intake, stress, and anesthesia. Antiplatelet drugs (e.g., aspirin,

clopidogrel [Plavix]) and nonsteroidal antiinflammatory drugs (NSAIDs) inhibit platelet aggregation and may contribute to postoperative bleeding. Surgeons may instruct patients to withhold these medications before surgery. Specific timeframes for withholding drugs depend on the drug and the patient. Patients on long-term anticoagulation therapy (e.g., warfarin [Coumadin]) present a unique challenge. The options for these patients include (1) continuing therapy, (2) withholding therapy for a time before and after surgery, or (3) withholding the therapy and starting subcutaneous or IV heparin therapy during the perioperative period. The management strategy selected is determined by patient characteristics and the nature of the surgery.[3]

Ask about the use of herbs and dietary supplements because their use is so common. Many patients do not think to include supplements in their list of medications. They believe that herbal and dietary supplements are "natural" and do not pose a surgical risk.[4] (See the Complementary & Alternative Therapies box in Chapter 3 on p. 39 on how to assess for the use of herbal supplements.) Excessive use of vitamins and herbs can cause harmful effects in patients undergoing surgery. In patients taking anticoagulants or antiplatelets, herbal supplements can produce excessive postoperative bleeding that may require a return to the OR.[5] The effects of specific herbs that are of concern during the perioperative period are listed below in the Complementary & Alternative Therapies box.

Also ask the patient about possible recreational drug use, abuse, and addiction. The substances most likely to be abused include tobacco, alcohol, opioids, marijuana, cocaine, and amphetamines. Ask questions about the use of these substances in a frank manner. Stress that recreational drug use may affect the type and amount of anesthesia that will be needed. When patients become aware of the potential interactions of these substances with anesthetics, most patients respond honestly about using them. Chronic alcohol use can place the patient at risk because of lung, gastrointestinal, or liver damage. When liver function is decreased, metabolism of anesthetic agents is prolonged, nutritional status is altered, and the potential for postoperative complications is increased. Alcohol withdrawal can also occur during lengthy surgery or in the postoperative period. Although this can be a life-threatening event, it can be

---

🌸 COMPLEMENTARY & ALTERNATIVE THERAPIES

Herbal Products and Surgery

The following can be used as a guide for patient teaching:
- Notify your health care provider of all vitamins, herbal products, and dietary supplements that you are or have been taking.
- Avoid astragalus and ginseng, since they can increase blood pressure before and during surgery.
- Avoid garlic, vitamin E, ginkgo, and fish oils because they can increase bleeding.
- Avoid kava and valerian because they can cause excess sedation.
- In general, discontinue all herbal supplements 2 to 3 weeks before any surgical procedure. Consult your health care provider for specific instructions.

Helpful Herbs and Vitamins
- Ginger can be useful for preventing nausea associated with anesthesia. Consider ginger ale, crystallized ginger, or ginger tea.
- Arnica is a homeopathic remedy useful in soft tissue healing.
- Multivitamins can be taken until the day before surgery. Taking them on the day of surgery, on an empty stomach, may contribute to nausea and vomiting after surgery.

avoided with appropriate planning and management (see Chapter 11).

Document and communicate all findings of the medication history to the perioperative health care team. The ACP will determine the appropriate schedule and dose of the patient's routine medications before and after surgery. Ensure that all of the patient's medications are identified, implement any changes in the medication plan, and monitor the patient for potential interactions and complications.

Allergies. Question the patient about drug intolerances and drug allergies. Drug intolerance usually results in side effects that are uncomfortable or unpleasant for the patient but are not life threatening. These effects can include nausea, constipation, diarrhea, or *idiosyncratic* (opposite than expected) reactions. A true drug allergy produces hives and/or an anaphylactic reaction, causing cardiopulmonary compromise (e.g., hypotension, tachycardia, bronchospasm). Being aware of drug intolerances and drug allergies aids the health care team to maintain patient comfort and safety. For example, some anesthetic agents contain sulfur, so notify the ACP if a history of allergy to sulfur is reported. Document all drug intolerances and drug allergies and, if appropriate, place an allergy identification band on the patient on the day of surgery.

Also inquire about nondrug allergies, specifically food and environmental (e.g., latex, pollen, animals) allergies. The patient with a history of any allergic reactions has a greater potential for hypersensitivity reactions to drugs given during anesthesia. Patients need to be screened specifically for latex allergies by gathering data in the following areas:

- Risk factors
- Contact dermatitis
- Contact urticaria (e.g., hives)
- Aerosol reactions
- History of reactions that suggest an allergy to latex

Risk factors for latex allergy include long-term, multiple exposures to latex products, such as those experienced by health care and rubber industry workers. Additional risk factors include a history of hay fever, asthma, and allergies to certain foods (e.g., eggs, avocados, bananas, chestnuts, potatoes, peaches).[6] (Latex allergies are discussed in Chapter 14.)

Review of Systems. The last component of the patient history is the body systems review. Ask specific questions to confirm the presence or absence of any diseases. Current medical problems can alert you to areas that should be more closely examined in the preoperative physical examination. The combined review of systems and the patient history provide essential data to determine the specific preoperative tests that need to be ordered.

Cardiovascular System. Evaluate cardiovascular (CV) function to determine preexisting disease or problems (e.g., coronary artery disease, prosthetic heart valve). In reviewing the CV system, you may find a history of hypertension, angina, dysrhythmias, heart failure, or myocardial infarction. Inquire about the patient's current treatment for any CV condition (e.g., medications) and the level of functioning. A cardiology consult is often required before surgery if the patient has a significant CV history (e.g., recent myocardial infarction, valvular heart disease, implantable cardioverter-defibrillator).

If indicated, a 12-lead electrocardiogram (ECG) and coagulation studies should be ordered, and the results should be on the chart before surgery. The CV assessment provides data on what other measures need to be done. For example, the patient who is on diuretic therapy will need to have a serum potassium level drawn preoperatively. If the patient has a history of hypertension, the ACP may administer vasoactive drugs to maintain adequate BP during surgery. If the patient has a history of valvular heart disease, antibiotic prophylaxis often is given before surgery to decrease the risk of bacterial endocarditis (see Chapter 37).

Postoperative venous thromboembolism (VTE), a condition that includes deep vein thrombosis and pulmonary embolism, is a concern for any surgical patient. Patients at high risk for VTE include those with a history of previous thrombosis, blood-clotting disorders, cancer, varicosities, obesity, smoking, heart failure, or chronic obstructive pulmonary disease (COPD).[7] People are also at risk for developing a VTE because of immobility and positioning during the operative procedure. Antiembolism stockings or sequential compression devices may be applied to the legs in the preoperative holding area.

Respiratory System. Ask the patient about any recent or chronic respiratory disease or infections. Elective surgery may need to be postponed if the person has an upper respiratory tract infection. Upper airway infections increase the risk of bronchospasm, laryngospasm, decreased O_2 saturation, and problems with respiratory secretions. Also report a patient's history of dyspnea at rest or with exertion, coughing (dry or productive), or hemoptysis (coughing blood) to the ACP and the surgeon.

If a patient has a history of asthma, inquire about the use of inhaled or oral corticosteroids and bronchodilators, as well as the frequency and triggers of asthma attacks. The patient with a history of COPD is at high risk for postoperative pulmonary complications, including hypoxemia and atelectasis.

Encourage the patient who smokes to stop at least 6 weeks preoperatively to decrease the risk of intraoperative and postoperative respiratory complications. The greater the patient's pack-years of smoking (packs smoked per day times years), the greater the risk for pulmonary complications during or after surgery. Report conditions likely to affect respiratory function such as sleep apnea; obesity; and spinal, chest, and airway deformities. For example, patients may be asked to bring their sleep apnea devices with them to the hospital or surgical center. Depending on the patient's history and physical examination, baseline pulmonary function tests and arterial blood gases may be ordered preoperatively.

Neurologic System. Preoperative evaluation of neurologic functioning includes assessing the patient's ability to respond to questions, follow commands, and maintain orderly thought patterns. Alterations in the patient's hearing and vision may affect responses and the ability to follow directions throughout the perioperative assessment and evaluation. Document the patient's ability to pay attention, concentrate, and respond appropriately to establish a preoperative baseline for postoperative comparison.

If you note deficits in cognitive function, determine the extent of the problems and whether they can be corrected before surgery. If the problems cannot be corrected, it is important to involve a legal guardian or person with durable power of attorney for health care to assist the patient and provide informed consent for surgery.

Preoperative assessment of the older person's baseline cognitive function is especially crucial for intraoperative and postoperative evaluation.[8] The older adult may have intact mental abilities preoperatively, but is more prone to adverse outcomes during and after surgery than the younger adult. This is due to the additional stressors of the surgical procedure, dehydration, hypothermia, and anesthesia and adjunctive medications. These factors may contribute to the development of emergence delirium ("waking up wild"), a condition that may be falsely labeled as senility or dementia. Thus preoperative findings are critical for postoperative comparison.

In the review of the neurologic system, inquire about any history of strokes, transient ischemic attacks, or spinal cord injury. Also ask about neurologic diseases, such as myasthenia gravis, Parkinson's disease, and multiple sclerosis, and any treatments used.

Genitourinary System. Assess the preoperative patient for a history of renal or urinary tract diseases, such as glomerulonephritis, chronic kidney disease, or repeated urinary tract infections. Document the present disease state and treatment used to control the disease. Renal dysfunction is associated with a number of alterations, including fluid and electrolyte imbalances, coagulopathies, increased risk for infection, and impaired wound healing. Because many drugs are metabolized and excreted by the kidneys, a decrease in renal function can lead to an altered response to drugs and unpredictable drug elimination. Renal function tests, such as serum creatinine and blood urea nitrogen (BUN), are commonly ordered preoperatively.

Document and report to the perioperative team if the patient has problems voiding (e.g., incontinence, hesitancy). Male patients may have physical conditions, such as an enlarged prostate, that can interfere with the insertion of a urinary catheter during surgery or impair voiding in the postoperative period.

For women of childbearing age, determine if they are pregnant or think they could be pregnant. Most institutions require a pregnancy test for all women of childbearing age before surgery.[9] Immediately inform the surgeon if the patient states that she might be pregnant, since maternal and subsequent fetal exposure to anesthetics during the first trimester should be avoided.

Hepatic System. The liver is involved in glucose homeostasis, fat metabolism, protein synthesis, drug and hormone metabolism, and bilirubin formation and excretion. The liver detoxifies many anesthetics and adjunctive drugs. The patient with hepatic dysfunction may have an increased perioperative risk for clotting abnormalities and adverse responses to medications. Consider the presence of liver disease if there is a history of jaundice, hepatitis, alcohol abuse, or obesity.

Integumentary System. Inquire about a history of skin problems. Assess the current condition of the skin, especially at the incision site, for rashes, breakdown, or other dermatologic conditions. A patient with a history of pressure ulcers may require extra padding during surgery. Skin problems can affect postoperative healing.

Body art such as tattoos and piercings are increasingly common. When possible, select pigment-free areas for injections, IV sites, and laboratory draws.

Musculoskeletal System. Note any musculoskeletal and mobility problems, especially in the older adult. If the patient has arthritis, identify all affected joints. Mobility restrictions may influence intraoperative and postoperative positioning and ambulation. Spinal anesthesia may be difficult if the patient cannot flex his or her lumbar spine adequately to allow easy needle insertion. If the neck is affected, intubation and airway management may be difficult. Any mobility aids (e.g., cane, walker) should be brought with the patient on the day of surgery.

Endocrine System. The patient with diabetes is especially at risk for adverse effects of anesthesia and surgery. Hypoglycemia, hyperglycemia, delayed wound healing, and infection are common complications of diabetes during the perioperative period. Clarify with the patient's surgeon or ACP whether the patient should take the usual dose of insulin or oral hypoglycemic agents on the day of surgery. ACPs may vary the usual insulin dose based on the patient's current status and history of glucose control. Regardless of the preoperative insulin orders, determine serum or capillary glucose levels the morning of surgery to establish baseline levels. Assess the patient's glucose levels periodically and manage, if necessary, with short-acting or rapid-acting insulin.

Determine if the patient has a history of thyroid dysfunction. Hyperthyroidism or hypothyroidism can place the patient at surgical risk because of alterations in metabolic rate. If the patient takes a thyroid replacement drug, check with the ACP about administration of the drug on the day of surgery. If the patient has a history of thyroid dysfunction, laboratory tests may be ordered to determine current levels of thyroid function.

The patient with Addison's disease also requires special consideration during surgery. Addisonian crisis or shock can occur if a patient abruptly stops taking replacement corticosteroids, and the stress of surgery may require additional IV corticosteroid therapy[10] (see Chapter 50).

Immune System. If the patient has a history of a compromised immune system or takes immunosuppressive drugs, document it. Corticosteroids used in immunosuppressive doses may be tapered before surgery. Impairment of the immune system can lead to delayed wound healing and increased risk for postoperative infections.[11] If the patient has an acute infection (e.g., upper respiratory tract infection, sinusitis, influenza), elective surgery is often canceled. Patients with active chronic infections such as hepatitis B or C, acquired immunodeficiency syndrome, or tuberculosis may have surgery if indicated. However, when preparing the patient for surgery, remember to take infection control precautions for the protection of the patient and staff.[12] (Infection control guidelines are discussed in Chapter 15 and eTable 15-1, available on the website for Chapter 15.)

Fluid and Electrolyte Status. Ask the patient about any recent conditions that increase the risk for fluid and electrolyte imbalances, such as vomiting, diarrhea, or preoperative bowel preps. For example, surgery may be planned for a patient with cholecystitis who has been vomiting for several days. Also identify drugs that alter fluid and electrolyte status, such as diuretics. Serum electrolyte levels are often assessed before surgery. Many patients may have restricted fluids for some time before surgery. If the surgery is delayed, they could develop dehydration. A patient with or at risk for dehydration may require additional fluids and electrolytes before or during surgery.

Although a preoperative fluid balance history should be completed for all patients, it is especially critical for older adults. Their reduced adaptive capacity leaves a narrow margin of safety between overhydration and underhydration.

Nutritional Status. Nutritional deficits include overnutrition and undernutrition, both of which require considerable time to correct. However, knowing that a patient has a nutritional deficit can help the perioperative team provide more individualized care. For example, if the patient is thin, provide more padding than usual (pressure points on all patients are protected routinely) on the OR table. Notify the team if a patient is morbidly obese (body mass index [BMI] greater than 40 kg/m^2) to allow time to obtain special equipment needed for the patient's care (e.g., longer instruments for abdominal surgery).

Obesity stresses both the cardiac and pulmonary systems and makes access to the surgical site and anesthesia administration more difficult.[13] It predisposes the patient to wound dehiscence, wound infection, and incisional herniation postoperatively. Adipose tissue is less vascular than other types of tissue. In addition, the patient may be slower to recover from anesthesia because inhalation agents are absorbed and stored by adipose tissue, thus leaving the body more slowly. (See Chapter 41 for special needs of obese patients undergoing surgery.)

Nutritional deficiencies impair the ability to recover from surgery. Remember that the obese patient and the very thin patient can also be protein and vitamin deficient. If the nutritional problem is severe, surgery may be postponed. Protein and vitamins A, C, and B complex deficiencies are particularly significant because these substances are essential for wound healing.[14] Supplemental nutrition may be administered during the perioperative period to patients who are malnourished. The older adult is often at risk for malnutrition and fluid volume deficits.[8]

Identify patients who consume large quantities of coffee or soft drinks containing caffeine. In many cases, withholding caffeinated beverages preoperatively or for some time postoperatively can lead to severe withdrawal headaches.[15] Caffeine withdrawal headaches can be confused with spinal headaches if the preoperative data are not documented. Giving caffeinated beverages postoperatively, when possible, may prevent these headaches.

Objective Data

Physical Examination. The Joint Commission requires that all patients admitted to the OR have a documented history and physical examination (H&P) in their chart.[16] This may be done in advance of surgery or on the day of surgery. It may be performed by any qualified person, including advanced practice nurses, physicians, physician assistants, or ACPs. Findings from the patient's H&P will enable the ACP to assign the patient a physical status rating for anesthesia administration (Table 18-3). This rating is an indicator of the patient's perioperative risk and may influence perioperative decisions.

TABLE 18-3	**AMERICAN SOCIETY OF ANESTHESIOLOGISTS' PHYSICAL CLASSIFICATION SYSTEM**
Rating	**Definition**
P1	Normal healthy person
P2	Patient with mild systemic disease
P3	Patient with severe systemic disease
P4	Patient with severe systemic disease that is a constant threat to life
P5	Moribund patient who is not expected to survive without surgery
P6	Declared brain-dead patient whose organs are being removed for donor purposes

Source: American Society of Anesthesiologists: ASA physical status classification system, 2012. Retrieved from *www.asahq.org/clinical/physicalstatus.htm*.
NOTE: Patients selected for surgery in ambulatory or outpatient settings generally have ratings of P1, P2, or P3.

In addition to the health assessment, also complete a physical examination of the patient before surgery (Table 18-4). Review the documentation already present in the patient's chart, including the H&P, to better proceed with your examination. Document all findings and communicate any relevant findings immediately to the surgeon or the ACP.

Laboratory and Diagnostic Testing. Obtain and assess the results of laboratory and diagnostic tests ordered preoperatively (Table 18-5). For example, if the patient is taking an antiplatelet medication (e.g., aspirin), a coagulation profile will be ordered; if the patient is on diuretic therapy, a potassium level is assessed; if the patient is of childbearing age, a pregnancy test should be ordered; or if the patient is taking medications for dysrhythmias, a preoperative ECG is obtained. Blood glucose monitoring is done for patients with diabetes. In some settings, tests for methicillin-resistant *Staphylococcus aureus* are done preoperatively. Patients with positive results are prescribed antibiotics for several days before surgery.[17]

Ideally, preoperative tests are ordered based on the patient's H&P. However, many facilities and insurers have a written protocol for preoperative tests, which may not include all the identified areas. In addition, the preoperative tests may be done days before surgery. Ensure that all laboratory and diagnostic reports are in the patient's chart. Missing reports may result in a delay or cancellation of the surgery.

NURSING MANAGEMENT PREOPERATIVE PATIENT

Preoperative nursing interventions are derived from the nursing assessment and must reflect each patient's specific needs. Physical preparations are determined by the pending surgery and the routines of the surgery setting. Preoperative teaching may be minimal or extensive. The Association of periOperative Registered Nurses (AORN) provides standards and recommended practices to guide nursing interventions in all perioperative settings.[7]

PREOPERATIVE TEACHING

The patient has a right to know what to expect and how to participate effectively during the surgical experience. Preoperative teaching increases patient satisfaction and may reduce postoperative fear, anxiety, and stress.[18] Teaching may also decrease the development of complications, the length of hospitalization, and the recovery time after discharge.

In most surgical settings, patients often arrive only a short time before surgery is scheduled. Preoperative teaching for these patients is generally done in the surgeon's office or a preadmission surgical clinic and reinforced on the day of surgery. After ambulatory surgery the patient usually goes home several hours after recovery, depending on the patient's progress and procedure-specific needs. Teaching must include information that focuses on the patient's safety. Provide written materials for patients and caregivers to use for review and reinforcement at home. Discharge teaching is required for all patients[19,20] and is discussed in Chapter 20.

When doing preoperative teaching for a patient, provide a balance between explaining so much that the patient is overwhelmed and telling so little that the patient is unprepared. If you observe carefully and listen sensitively to the patient, you can usually determine how much information is enough. Remember that anxiety and fear may decrease learning ability.

TABLE 18-4 HEALTH ASSESSMENT AND PHYSICAL EXAMINATION OF PREOPERATIVE PATIENT*

Cardiovascular System
- Identify acute or chronic problems. Note presence of angina, hypertension, heart failure, recent myocardial infarction, renal disease, diabetes.
- Identify any drugs (e.g., aspirin) or herbal supplements (e.g., ginkgo) that may affect coagulation.
- Identify patients with prosthetic heart valves, pacemakers, or implantable cardioverter-defibrillators.
- Assess for edema (including dependent areas), noting location and severity.
- Inspect neck veins for distention.
- Obtain bilateral baseline blood pressures.
- Assess pulses (bilaterally when appropriate) for rate, rhythm, and quality: apical, radial, and pedal.

Respiratory System
- Identify acute or chronic problems. Note the presence of infection, chronic obstructive pulmonary disease, or asthma. Note use of CPAP machine.
- Assess history of smoking, including the time since the last cigarette and the number of pack-years.
- Determine baseline respiratory rate and rhythm and regularity of pattern.
- Observe for cough, dyspnea, and use of accessory muscles of respiration.
- Auscultate lungs for normal and adventitious breath sounds.

Neurologic System
- Determine orientation to person, place, and time.
- Assess baseline mental status. Note presence of confusion, disorderly thinking, or inability to follow commands.
- Identify past history of strokes, transient ischemic attacks, or neurologic diseases (e.g., Parkinson's disease, multiple sclerosis).

Genitourinary System
- Identify any infection or preexisting disease.
- Determine ability to void.
- Note color, amount, and characteristics of urine (if appropriate).
- Determine pregnancy status (if appropriate).

Hepatic System
- Review past history of substance abuse, especially alcohol and IV drug use.
- Inspect skin color and sclera of eyes for any signs of jaundice.

Integumentary System
- Identify any current or previous skin disorders (e.g., pressure ulcers, eczema).
- Determine skin status. Note drying, bruising, or breaks in surface.
- Inspect skin for rashes, boils, or infection, especially around the planned surgical site.
- Inspect the mucous membranes and skin turgor for signs of dehydration.
- Assess skin moisture and temperature.

Musculoskeletal System
- Examine skin around bone pressure points.
- Assess for limitations in joint range of motion and muscle strength.
- Assess for joint or muscle pain.
- Assess mobility, gait, and balance.

Gastrointestinal System
- Determine patterns of food and fluid intake and any recent changes in weight.
- Determine usual pattern of bowel movements, including date of last bowel movement.
- Assess for the presence of dentures and bridges (loose dentures or teeth may be dislodged during intubation).
- Weigh patient.
- Auscultate abdomen for presence of bowel sounds.

Immune System
- Identify any immunodeficiency or autoimmune disorders.
- Assess for use of corticosteroids or other immunosuppressant drugs.

Laboratory and Diagnostic Tests
- Review results of all laboratory and diagnostic tests completed preoperatively (see Table 18-5).

*See specific body system chapters for more detailed assessments and related laboratory studies.
CPAP, Continuous positive airway pressure.

Also assess what the patient wants to know and give priority to those concerns.

Generally, preoperative teaching includes three types of information: sensory, process, and procedural. Different patients, with varying cultures, backgrounds, and experience, may want different types of information.

With *sensory information*, patients find out what they will see, hear, smell, and feel during the surgery. For example, you may tell them that the OR will be cold, but they can ask for a warm blanket; the lights in the OR are bright; or many unfamiliar sounds and specific smells will be present.

Patients wanting *process information* may not want specific details but just the general flow of what is going to happen. This information would include the patient's transfer to the holding area, visits by the nurse and the ACP before transfer to the OR, and waking up in the PACU.

With *procedural information*, patients desire details that are more specific. For example, this information would include that an IV line will be started while the patient is in the holding area and the surgeon will mark the operative area with an indelible marker to verify site and side.[7]

Share the preoperative teaching provided to the patient with the nurses providing postoperative care to evaluate learning and avoid duplication of teaching. Because the time for teaching is limited, the team approach is often used. For example, teaching may be started in the outpatient setting. Your responsibility is to assess the patient's understanding of this teaching and fill in the gaps. The discharge nurse provides written instructions and additional information for reinforcement. Home care nurses may be involved if patients have complex learning needs that must be addressed after discharge.

Document all teaching in the patient's chart. A Patient & Caregiver Teaching Guide for preoperative preparation is presented in Table 18-6. Additional information related to patient and caregiver teaching is found in Chapter 4.

GENERAL SURGERY INFORMATION. Unless contraindicated (e.g., after craniotomy, tonsillectomy), all patients should receive instruction about deep breathing, coughing, and early ambulation (moving) postoperatively. This is essential because patients may not want to do these activities postoperatively unless they are taught the reason for them and practice them preoperatively. Tell patients and caregivers if tubes, drains, monitoring devices, or special equipment will be used after surgery. Explain that these devices help you to safely care for the patient. Examples of individualized teaching may include how to use incentive spirometers or postoperative patient-controlled analgesia

TABLE 18-5	COMMON PREOPERATIVE LABORATORY AND DIAGNOSTIC TESTS

Test	Assessment
ABGs, pulse oximetry	Respiratory and metabolic function, oxygenation status
Blood glucose	Metabolic status, diabetes mellitus
Blood urea nitrogen, creatinine	Renal function
Chest x-ray	Pulmonary disorders, cardiac enlargement, heart failure
Complete blood count: RBCs, Hgb, Hct, WBCs, WBC differential	Anemia, immune status, infection
Electrocardiogram	Cardiac disease, dysrhythmias
Electrolytes	Metabolic status, renal function, diuretic side effects
hCG	Pregnancy status
Liver function tests	Liver status
PT, PTT, INR, platelet count	Coagulation status
Pulmonary function studies	Pulmonary status
Serum albumin	Nutritional status
Type and crossmatch	Blood available for replacement (elective surgery patients may have own blood available)
Urinalysis	Renal status, hydration, urinary tract infection

hCG, Human chorionic gonadotropin; *Hct,* hematocrit; *Hgb,* hemoglobin; *INR,* international normalized ratio; *PT,* prothrombin time; *PTT,* partial thromboplastin time.

pumps. Patients should have a clear understanding of how to rate their pain intensity and how their pain will be managed.[21] (See Chapter 9 for additional information on pain.)

The patient should also receive accurate surgery-specific information. For example, a patient having a total joint replacement may have an immobilizer after surgery, or a patient with extensive neurosurgery should be told about waking up in the intensive care unit.

AMBULATORY SURGERY INFORMATION. The ambulatory surgery patient or the patient admitted to the hospital the day of surgery needs to receive information before admission. Some ambulatory surgical centers telephone the patients the evening before surgery to answer last-minute questions and to reinforce teaching. Each center has policies and procedures that direct this communication in a timely manner.

In addition to specifics on the procedure, patients need information on day-of-surgery events such as arrival time, registration, parking, what to wear, what to bring, and the need to have a responsible adult present for transportation home after surgery.

Traditionally, patients having elective surgery are instructed to have nothing by mouth (NPO) starting at midnight on the night before surgery. Current guidelines published by the American Society of Anesthesiologists are less strict[22] (Table 18-7). Restriction of fluids and food is designed to reduce the risk of pulmonary aspiration and postoperative nausea and vomiting. Protocols may vary for patients having local anesthesia or surgery scheduled late in the day. Follow the NPO protocol of each surgical facility. The patient who has not followed the NPO instructions may have surgery delayed or canceled. It is critical that the patient understands the reason for and follows all restrictions.

TABLE 18-6	PATIENT & CAREGIVER TEACHING GUIDE

Preoperative Preparation

Include the following information in the preoperative teaching plan for patient and caregiver.

Sensory Information
- Preoperative holding area may be noisy.
- Drugs and cleaning solutions may be cold and odorous.
- Operating room (OR) can be cold. Warm blankets are available and can be requested.
- Talking may be heard in the OR but may be distorted because of masks. Ask questions if something is not understood.
- OR bed will be narrow. A safety strap will be applied over the thighs.
- Lights in the OR may be bright.
- Monitoring machines may be heard (e.g., ticking and beeping noises) when awake.

Procedural Information
- What to bring and what type of clothing to wear to the surgery center.
- Any changes in time of surgery.
- Fluid and food restrictions.
- Physical preparation required (e.g., bowel or skin preparation).
- Purpose of frequent vital signs assessment.
- Pain control and other comfort measures.
- Why turning, coughing, and deep breathing postoperatively are important. Practice sessions need to be done preoperatively.
- Insertion of IV lines.
- Procedure for anesthesia administration.
- Expect surgical site and/or side to be marked with indelible ink or marker.

Process Information
Information About General Flow of Surgery
- Admission area.
- Preoperative holding area, OR, and recovery area.
- Caregivers can usually stay in preoperative holding area until surgery.
- Caregivers will be able to see the patient after discharge from the recovery area or possibly in the recovery area once the patient is awake.
- Identification of any technology that may be present on awakening, such as monitors and central lines.

Where Caregivers Can Wait During Surgery
- Encourage caregivers to ask questions and express any concerns.
- OR staff will update caregivers during surgery and when surgery is completed.
- Surgeon will usually talk with caregivers after surgery.

LEGAL PREPARATION FOR SURGERY

Legal preparation for surgery consists of checking that all required forms have been correctly signed and are present in the patient's chart, and that the patient and the caregiver clearly understand what is going to happen. Standard consent forms include those for the surgical procedure and blood transfusions. Other forms may include advance directives and durable power of attorney for health care (see Chapter 10).

CONSENT FOR SURGERY. Before nonemergency surgery can be legally performed, the patient must voluntarily sign an informed consent form in the presence of a witness. **Informed consent** is an active, shared decision-making process between the health care provider and the recipient of care.[23] Three conditions must be met for consent to be valid. First, there must be *adequate*

TABLE 18-7 PREOPERATIVE FASTING RECOMMENDATIONS*

Liquid and Food Intake	Minimum Fasting Period (Hr)
Clear liquids (e.g., water, clear tea, black coffee, carbonated beverages, fruit juice without pulp)	2
Breast milk	4
Nonhuman milk, including infant formula	6
Light meal (e.g., toast and clear liquids)	6
Regular meal (may include fried or fatty food, meat)	8 or more

Source: Practice guidelines for preoperative fasting and the use of pharmacologic agents to reduce the risk of pulmonary aspiration: application to healthy patients undergoing elective procedures: an updated report by the American Society of Anesthesiologists Task Force on Preoperative Fasting. Retrieved from *http://journals.lww.com/anesthesiology/Fulltext/2011/03000/Practice_Guidelines_for_Preoperative_Fasting_and.13.aspx?WT.mc_id=HPxADx20100319xMP.*
*For healthy patients of all ages undergoing elective surgery (excluding women in labor).

EVIDENCE-BASED PRACTICE
Applying the Evidence

G.L. is a 57-year-old woman scheduled for a knee replacement. She has been NPO since midnight and was scheduled to be the third surgical case of the day. Unfortunately, several emergency surgeries have resulted in delays, and she is not expected to leave for surgery for another 4 hours. She tells you that she has a "headache" from missing her "morning coffee." She says she is hungry and thirsty and, since surgery has been delayed, she would like a cup of coffee.

Best Available Evidence	Clinician Expertise	Patient Preferences and Values
For healthy adults, the minimum fasting period for clear liquids before surgery is 2 hr.	Nothing by mouth (NPO) restrictions are meant to prevent aspiration and vomiting during surgery. Patients who are NPO from midnight frequently complain of hunger and thirst while waiting for surgery. Patients who regularly drink caffeine in the morning often experience a "caffeine withdrawal" headache when fasting. You know that clear liquids consist of water, fruit juices without pulp, carbonated beverages, clear tea, and black coffee.	Patient is requesting something to drink given the extended period of fast due to the delay in surgery.

Your Decision and Action
You know that the current protocol of keeping all patients NPO after midnight for surgery does not reflect the best available evidence. You also know that there is a multidisciplinary task force working to review and revise the protocol. You decide to call the anesthesia care provider to discuss G.L.'s situation and request that clear liquids be ordered for her.

References for Evidence
American Society of Anesthesiologists Committee on Standards and Practice Parameters: Practice guidelines for preoperative fasting and the use of pharmacologic agents to reduce the risk of pulmonary aspiration: application to healthy patients undergoing elective procedures: an updated report by the ASA Committee on Standards and Practice Parameters, *Anesthesiology* 114(3):495, 2011.
Crenshaw JT: Preoperative fasting: will the evidence ever be put into practice? *Am J Nurs* 111:38, 2011.

disclosure of the diagnosis; the nature and purpose of the proposed treatment; the risks and consequences of the proposed treatment; the probability of a successful outcome; the availability, benefits, and risks of alternative treatments; and the prognosis if treatment is not instituted. Second, the patient must demonstrate clear *understanding* of the information being provided before receiving sedating preoperative medications. Third, the recipient of care must *give consent voluntarily.* The patient must not be persuaded or coerced in any way by anyone to undergo the procedure.[24]

The physician is ultimately responsible for obtaining the patient's consent for surgical treatment. You may be responsible for witnessing the patient's signature on the consent form. At this time, you can be a patient advocate, verifying that the patient (or caregiver) understands the information presented in the consent form and the implications of consent, and that consent for surgery is truly voluntary. If the patient is unclear about the surgical plans, contact the surgeon about the patient's need for additional information. The patient should also be aware that consent, even when signed, can be withdrawn at any time.

If the patient is a minor, unconscious, or mentally incompetent to sign the permit, a legally appointed representative or responsible family member may give written permission. An *emancipated minor* is one who is younger than the legal age of consent but is recognized as having the legal capacity to provide consent.[25] Procedures for obtaining consent vary among states and agencies. Follow specifics required by your state's nurse practice act and agency policies that apply to an individual situation.

ETHICAL/LEGAL DILEMMAS
Informed Consent

Situation
J.S., a 72-year-old woman, is waiting in the preoperative holding area. You are discussing her impending surgery when you realize that this competent adult does not fully understand her surgery and was not informed of the alternatives to this surgery. Although she has previously signed a consent form, your assessment is that she was not fully informed about her treatment options or does not recall them.

Ethical/Legal Points for Consideration
- Informed consent requires that patients have complete information about the proposed treatment, as well as alternative treatments, risks and benefits of each treatment option, and possible consequences of the surgical procedure. The person (usually the surgeon) performing the procedure usually has this responsibility.
- An opportunity to have questions answered about the various treatment options and their possible outcomes is also an important element of informed consent.
- A patient can revoke the consent at any time, even at the very last minute. It is essential that you report any circumstance that suggests that the patient does not understand the information or is revoking the informed consent to the person who obtained the consent.
- In most states, the registered nurse's legal role is to witness the signing of the document. This means that as a nurse, you attest to the fact that the patient's signature was valid.

Discussion Questions
1. What do you think you should do next?
2. What is your role as a patient advocate in the informed consent process?
3. What should you do if the patient states that she does not want to know about the surgical procedure or alternatives to surgery?

A true medical emergency may override the need to obtain consent. When immediate medical treatment is needed to preserve life or to prevent serious impairment to life or limb and the patient is incapable of giving consent, the next of kin may give consent. If reaching the next of kin is not possible, the physician may begin treatment without written consent. A note is written in the chart documenting the medical necessity of the procedure. In the case of an emergency where consent cannot be obtained, the perioperative nurse usually needs to complete an event report because it is an occurrence that is inconsistent with routine facility practices.[26]

DAY-OF-SURGERY PREPARATION

NURSING ROLE. Day-of-surgery preparation varies a great deal depending on whether the patient is an inpatient or an ambulatory surgical patient. Your responsibilities immediately before surgery include final preoperative teaching, assessment, and communication of pertinent findings. In addition, ensure that all preoperative orders are done and that the chart is complete and accompanies the patient to the OR. It is especially important to verify the presence of a signed informed consent, laboratory and diagnostic data, an H&P, a record of any consultations, baseline vital signs, and completed nursing notes. In addition, the site and side of the anticipated surgery are identified and marked with an indelible marker by the surgeon and documented to indicate the patient agrees.[9]

Hospitals often require that a patient wear a hospital gown with no underclothes. Surgical centers may allow the patient to wear underwear, depending on the procedure to be performed. The patient should remove any cosmetics, since observation of skin color is important. Nail polish and artificial nails should be removed so that capillary refill and pulse oximetry can be assessed. Place an identification band on the patient and, if applicable, an allergy band (Fig. 18-1). Return all patient valuables to a caregiver or secure according to institutional protocol. All prostheses, including dentures, contact lenses, and glasses, are generally removed to prevent loss or damage. If electrocautery devices will be used during surgery, jewelry in piercings needs to be removed as a safety measure. Hearing aids should

FIG. 18-1 The nurse performs a safety check by verifying that the patient has an identification band (wristband) as part of the preoperative preparations before she goes to surgery.

be left in place to allow the patient to better follow instructions. Return glasses to the patient as soon as possible after surgery. Encourage the patient to void before preoperative medications are given and before transfer to the OR. Many preoperative medications interfere with balance and increase the risk for a fall during ambulation. An empty bladder prevents involuntary elimination under anesthesia and reduces the possibility of urinary retention during the early postoperative recovery.

> **SAFETY ALERT**
> Use a preoperative checklist (Table 18-8) to ensure that all preoperative preparations have been completed before the patient is given any sedating medications.

PREOPERATIVE MEDICATIONS. Preoperative medications are used for a variety of reasons (Table 18-9). A patient may receive a single drug or a combination of drugs. Benzodiazepines are used for their sedative and amnesic properties. Anticholinergics are sometimes given to reduce secretions. Opioids may be given to decrease pain and intraoperative anesthetic requirements. Antiemetics may be given to decrease nausea and vomiting.

Other medications that may be administered preoperatively include antibiotics, eyedrops, and routine prescription drugs. Antibiotics may be administered throughout the perioperative period for patients with a history of congenital or valvular heart disease to prevent infective endocarditis and for patients with previous joint replacement. Antibiotics may also be ordered for the patient undergoing surgery where wound contamination is a potential risk (e.g., gastrointestinal surgery) or where wound infection could have serious postoperative consequences (e.g., cardiac and joint replacement surgery). Antibiotics are most commonly administered IV and are usually started preoperatively (e.g., 30 to 60 minutes before the surgical incision).

β-Adrenergic blockers (β-blockers) are sometimes used in people with known hypertension or coronary artery disease to control BP or reduce the chances of myocardial infarction and cardiac arrest.[27] People with diabetes are also carefully monitored and may receive insulin in the preoperative period.[28] Eyedrops are often ordered and given preoperatively for the patient undergoing cataract and other eye surgery. Many times the patient will require multiple sets of eyedrops given at 5-minute intervals. It is important to give these drugs as ordered and on time to adequately prepare the eye for surgery.

Medications that patients routinely take may or may not be used on the day of surgery. To facilitate patient teaching and eliminate confusion about which medications should be taken, carefully check written preoperative orders and clarify the orders with the surgeon and/or ACP if there is any question.

Preoperative medications may be ordered by mouth (PO), IV, or subcutaneously. Provide PO medications with a small sip

INFORMATICS IN PRACTICE

Computer-Based Timing for Antibiotic Administration

- A patient who receives the appropriate preoperative antibiotic has a decreased risk of a health care–associated infection.
- Using a computer to time the administration of preoperative antibiotics can decrease the incidence of wound infections.
- Computer-based timing systems assist with quality of care by tracking patient outcomes.
- You can look at the time patients received antibiotics and compare the rate of wound infections for those who did and did not receive timely treatment.

TABLE 18-8   PREOPERATIVE CHECKLIST

Preoperative Requirements	Initials	Day of Surgery	Initials
Height _____ Weight _____		Surgical site marked Y or NA	
Isolation Y or N Type _____		ID band on patient Y or N	
Allergies noted on chart Y or N		Allergy band on patient Y or NA	
Vital signs (baseline) T _____ P _____ R _____ BP _____ Pulse Ox _____		Vital signs Time _____ T _____ P _____ R _____ BP _____ Pulse Ox _____	
Chart Review		**Procedures**	
H&P on chart		NPO since _____	
H&P within 30 days? Y or N		Capillary blood glucose Result: _____ NA	
Signed and witnessed informed consent form on chart Y or N		Voided/catheter Time _____	
Signed consent for blood administration Y or NA		Preoperative medications given Time _____ NA	
Blood type and crossmatch Y or NA		Preoperative antibiotics given Time _____ NA	
Name plate on chart Y or N		Preoperative skin prep Y or NA Shower_____ Scrub_____ Clip_____	
Diagnostic Results		Makeup, nail polish, false fingernails, and false eyelashes removed Y or NA	
Hgb/Hct _____ / _____ NA		Hospital gown applied Y or NA	
PT/INR/PTT _____ / _____ / _____ NA		**Valuables**	
CXR _____ NA		Dentures Y or N	
ECG _____ NA hCG _____ Negative _____ Positive _____NA		Wig or hairpiece Y or N	
Other labs		Eyeglasses Y or N	
Final Chart Review		Contact lenses Y or N	
Additional forms attached		Hearing aid Y or N	
		Prosthesis Y or N	
		Jewelry Y or N Piercings with jewelry Y or N	
		Clothing Y or N	
		Disposition of valuables: Hearing aid in place Y or NA	

Time to OR _____ Date _____
Transported to OR by _____
Final check by _____ RN _____

of water 60 to 90 minutes before the patient goes to the OR unless otherwise ordered. Subcutaneous injections (e.g., insulin) and IV medications are usually given to the patient after arrival in the preoperative holding area or OR. Inform the patient about the expected effects of the medications (e.g., drowsiness).

TRANSPORTATION TO THE OPERATING ROOM

For inpatients, transport staff move the patient by stretcher to the OR. Assist the patient in moving from the hospital bed to the stretcher, raise the side rails, and ensure that the completed chart and any ordered preoperative equipment (e.g., sequential compression devices) goes with the patient. In many institutions the caregiver may accompany the patient to the holding area.

In an ambulatory surgical center the patient may be transported to the OR by stretcher or wheelchair. If no sedatives have been given, the patient may even walk accompanied to the OR. In all cases it is important to ensure patient safety during transport. Document the method of transportation and the person who transports the patient to the OR. You are also responsible

for the hand-off communication to the nurse receiving the patient. This provides an opportunity for each of you to ensure that all pertinent information regarding the patient has been shared.[29] To avoid adverse events related to miscommunication, AORN recommends the use of the Situation-Background-Assessment-Recommendation (SBAR) model for the hand-off process in this setting[30,31] (see Table 1-7).

Show the caregiver where to wait for the patient during surgery. Many hospitals have a surgical waiting room where OR personnel communicate the patient's status to the caregiver(s) and notify them when the surgery is complete. The surgeon also can locate the caregiver in this room after surgery to discuss the outcome. Some hospitals provide pagers to caregivers so that they may eat or do errands during the surgery.

CULTURALLY COMPETENT CARE

PREOPERATIVE PATIENT

Include cultural considerations when assessing and implementing care for the patient's preoperative needs. For example,

TABLE 18-9 DRUG THERAPY

Commonly Used Preoperative Medications

Class	Drug	Purpose
Antibiotics	cefazolin (Ancef)	Prevent postoperative infection
Anticholinergics	atropine (Isopto Atropine) glycopyrrolate (Robinul)	↓ Oral and respiratory secretions
	scopolamine (Transderm-Scōp)	Prevent nausea and vomiting Provide sedation
Antidiabetics	insulin (Humulin R)	Stabilize blood glucose
Antiemetics	metoclopramide (Reglan)	↑ Gastric emptying
	ondansetron (Zofran)	Prevent nausea and vomiting
Benzodiazepines	midazolam (Versed) diazepam (Valium) lorazepam (Ativan)	↓ Anxiety, induce sedation, amnesic effects
β-Blockers	labetalol (Normodyne)	Manage hypertension
Histamine (H₂)-receptor antagonists	famotidine (Pepcid) ranitidine (Zantac)	↓ HCl acid secretion, ↑ pH, ↓ gastric volume
Opioids	morphine (Duramorph) fentanyl (Sublimaze)	Relieve pain during preoperative procedures

culture often determines one's expression of pain, family expectations, and ability to verbally express needs. One's culture may require that the family be included in any decision making. For example, many older Hispanic women may defer to their family for the decision to have or not to have surgery. Respect these decisions. If the patient or caregiver does not speak English, it is mandated that a qualified translator or translator communication system be used.[32] (Culturally competent care is discussed in Chapter 2.)

▌GERONTOLOGIC CONSIDERATIONS

PREOPERATIVE PATIENT

Many surgical procedures are performed on patients older than 65 years of age. Surgery on older adults requires careful evaluation.[33] Frequently performed procedures in older adults include cataract extraction, coronary and vascular procedures, prostate surgery, herniorrhaphy, cholecystectomy, and joint repair or replacement.

Be particularly alert when assessing and caring for the older adult surgical patient. An event that has little effect on a younger adult may be overwhelming to the older patient. Emotional reactions to impending surgery and hospitalization often intensify in the older adult. Hospitalization may represent a physical decline and loss of health, mobility, and independence. The older adult may view the hospital as a place to die or as a stepping-stone to nursing home placement. Help to decrease anxieties and fears, as well as maintaining and restoring the self-esteem of the older adult during the surgical experience.

The risks associated with anesthesia and surgery increase in the older patient.[33] In general, the older the patient, the greater the risk of complications after surgery. In planning care, consider the patient's physiologic status, not simply the chronologic age. The surgical risk in the older adult relates to normal physiologic aging and changes that compromise organ function, reduce reserve capacity, and limit the body's ability to adapt to stress. This decreased ability to cope with stress, often compounded by the burden of one or more chronic illnesses, and the surgery itself increase the risk of complications.

When preparing the older adult for surgery, obtain a detailed H&P. Preoperative laboratory tests, an ECG, and a chest x-ray are important in planning the choice and type of anesthesia. The patient's primary physician is usually not the surgeon, and frequently several physicians are involved in the patient's care. Help to coordinate the care for the older adult patient.

Many older adults have sensory deficits. Vision and hearing may be reduced, and bright lights may bother those with eye problems. Thought processes and cognitive abilities may be slowed or impaired. Assess and document baseline sensory and cognitive function. Physical reactions are often slowed as a result of mobility and balance problems. All these changes may require more time for the older adult to complete preoperative testing and understand preoperative instructions. These changes also require attention to promote patient safety and prevent injury. (See Chapter 5 for more discussion about older adults.)

When older adults live in some type of long-term care facility, you may need to coordinate transportation from these agencies so that timely arrival allows for surgery preparation. A legal representative of the patient must be present to provide consent for surgery if the patient cannot sign for himself or herself.

Finally, determine the presence of or need for caregiver support for the older adult undergoing surgery. With the increase in outpatient surgical procedures and shorter postoperative length of stays, caregiver support is often critical in the continuity of care for this population.

CASE STUDY

Preoperative Patient

Ryan McVay/Photodisc/ Thinkstock

Patient Profile

F.D., a 72-year-old Hispanic retired librarian, is admitted to the hospital with compromised circulation of the right lower leg and a necrotic right foot. She has diabetes and takes insulin to maintain appropriate blood glucose levels. In addition, she has hypertension and kidney and peripheral vascular disease. She has been NPO since midnight. It is now 10 AM on the morning of the surgery.

Subjective Data

- History of type 2 diabetes mellitus for 30 years; states "my blood sugar is hard to control" and "I just started taking insulin"
- History of hypertension
- History of stage 2 chronic kidney disease
- History of peripheral vascular disease
- History of macular degeneration in right eye; reports poor vision
- Surgical history: cesarean section at age 30, cholecystectomy at age 65; reports poor wound healing after last surgery
- Social Security checks barely cover the cost of living
- States she often runs out of medications and cannot always afford to refill them right away
- Reports chronic burning pain in both legs and has trouble sleeping at night
- Lives alone but has family who want her to move in with them after surgery
- Uses herbs to control blood glucose levels and frequently skips her insulin

Objective Data
Physical Examination
- Alert, cognitively intact, anxious, older woman with complaints of numbness and lack of feeling in right leg

- Weight 190 lb, height 5 ft 3 in
- BP 180/94, pulse 84 and slightly irregular
- Wears glasses for close work and reading
- Has macular degeneration in right eye

Diagnostic Studies
- Admission serum blood glucose level 272 mg/dL (15.2 mmol/L); glycosylated hemoglobin (Hb A1C) 14%
- Morning capillary blood glucose level 198 mg/dL (11 mmol/L)
- Doppler pulses for right lower leg weak, absent in right foot
- Doppler pulses in left lower leg present, weak in left foot
- Serum creatinine 2.0 mg/dL (176 mmol/L)

Collaborative Care
- Scheduled for a below-the-knee amputation of the right leg at 1 PM today

Discussion Questions
1. What factors may influence F.D.'s response to hospitalization and surgery?
2. *Priority Decision:* Given F.D.'s history, what priority preoperative nursing assessments would you want to complete and why?
3. What potential perioperative complications might you expect for F.D.?
4. *Priority Decision:* What priority topics would you include in F.D.'s preoperative teaching plan?
5. *Priority Decision:* Based on the assessment data presented, identify the priority nursing diagnoses and related interventions. Are there any collaborative problems?
6. *Delegation Decision:* Identify appropriate preoperative interventions that need to be completed and could be delegated to unlicensed assistive personnel (UAP).
7. *Evidence-Based Practice:* F.D. asks you why she received insulin this morning when she has not eaten anything since midnight. How would you respond to her?

ⓔvolve Answers available at *http://evolve.elsevier.com/Lewis/medsurg.*

▐ BRIDGE TO NCLEX EXAMINATION

The number of the question corresponds to the same-numbered outcome at the beginning of the chapter.

1. An overweight patient (BMI 28.1 kg/m²) is scheduled for a laparoscopic cholecystectomy at an outpatient surgery setting. The nurse knows that
   a. surgery will involve multiple small incisions.
   b. this setting is not appropriate for this procedure.
   c. surgery will involve removing a portion of the liver.
   d. the patient will need special preparation because of obesity.

2. The patient tells the nurse in the preoperative setting that she has noticed she has a reaction when wearing rubber gloves. What is the most appropriate intervention?
   a. Notify the surgeon so the case can be cancelled.
   b. Ask additional questions to assess for a possible latex allergy.
   c. Notify the OR staff immediately so that latex-free supplies can be used.
   d. No intervention is needed because the patient's rubber sensitivity has no bearing on surgery.

3. A 59-year-old man is scheduled for a herniorrhaphy in 2 days. During the preoperative evaluation he reports that he takes ginkgo daily. What is the priority intervention?
   a. Inform the surgeon, since the procedure may need to be rescheduled.
   b. Notify the anesthesia care provider, since this herb interferes with anesthetics.
   c. Ask the patient if he has noticed any side effects from taking this herbal supplement.
   d. Tell the patient to continue to take the herbal supplement up to the day before surgery.

4. A 17-year-old patient with a leg fracture is scheduled for surgery. She reports that she is living with a friend and is an emancipated minor. She has a statement from the court for verification. Which intervention is most appropriate?
   a. Witness the permit after consent is obtained by the surgeon.
   b. Call a parent or legal guardian to sign the permit, since the patient is under 18.
   c. Obtain verbal consent, since written consent is not necessary for emancipated minors.
   d. Investigate your state's nurse practice act related to emancipated minors and informed consent.

5. A priority nursing intervention to assist a preoperative patient in coping with fear of postoperative pain would be to
   a. inform the patient that pain medication will be available.
   b. teach the patient to use guided imagery to help manage pain.
   c. describe the type of pain expected with the patient's particular surgery.
   d. explain the pain management plan, including the use of a pain rating scale.

6. A patient is scheduled for surgery requiring general anesthesia at an ambulatory surgical center. The nurse asks him when he ate last. He replies that he had a light breakfast a couple of hours before coming to the surgery center. What should the nurse do first?
   a. Tell the patient to come back tomorrow, since he ate a meal.
   b. Proceed with the preoperative checklist, including site identification.
   c. Notify the anesthesia care provider of when and what the patient last ate.
   d. Have the patient void before administering any preoperative medications.

7. A patient who normally takes 40 units of glargine insulin (long acting) at bedtime asks the nurse what to do about her dose the night before surgery. The best response would be to have her
   a. skip her insulin altogether the night before surgery.
   b. take her usual dose at bedtime and eat a light breakfast in the morning.
   c. eat a moderate meal before bedtime and then take half her usual insulin dose.
   d. get instructions from her surgeon or health care provider on any insulin adjustments.

8. Preoperative considerations for older adults include (select all that apply)
   a. only using large-print educational materials.
   b. speaking louder for patients with hearing aids.
   c. recognizing that sensory deficits may be present.
   d. providing warm blankets to prevent hypothermia.
   e. teaching important information early in the morning.

1.a, 2.b, 3.a, 4.a, 5.d, 6.c, 7.d, 8.c, d

evolve

For rationales to these answers and even more NCLEX review questions, visit *http://evolve.elsevier.com/Lewis/medsurg.*

REFERENCES

1. Jehovah's Witness Official Website: You have the right to choose. Retrieved from *www.watchtower.org/e/hb/article_04.htm.*
*2. Sanatani M, Schreier G, Stitt L: Level and direction of hope in cancer patients: an exploratory longitudinal study, *Support Care Cancer* 16:493, 2008.
3. Levy J, Key N, Azran M: Novel oral anticoagulants: implications in the perioperative setting. Retrieved from *http://journals.lww.com/anesthesiology/Fulltext/2010/09000/Novel_Oral_Anticoagulants__Implications_in_the.38.aspx.*
4. American Society of Anesthesiologists: Common questions by patients preparing for anesthesia. Retrieved from *www.asahq.org/sitecore/content/Lifeline/Anesthesia-Topics/Michigan/Common-Questions-for-Patients-Preparing-for-Anesthesia.aspx.*
5. American Society of Anesthesiologists: What you should know about your patients' use of herbal medicines and other dietary supplements. Retrieved from *https://ecommerce.asahq.org/p-131-considerations-for-anesthesiologists-what-you-should-know-about-your-patients-use-of-herbal-medicines.aspx.*
6. American Academy of Allergy, Asthma, and Immunology: Tips to remember: latex allergy, 2007. Retrieved from *www.aaaai.org/patients/publicedmat/tips/latexallergy.stm.*
7. Association of periOperative Registered Nurses: *Perioperative standards and recommended practices*, Denver, 2010, The Association.

*8. Slor C, de Jonghe J, Vreeswijk R, et al: Anesthesia and postoperative delirium in older adults undergoing hip surgery, *J Am Geriatr Society* 59:7, 2011.
*9. Hepner DL: The role of testing in the preoperative evaluation, *Cleve Clin J Med.* Retrieved from *www.ccjm.org/content/76/Suppl_4/S22.full.*
10. Yalamarthi S: Perioperative steroids in surgical patients. Retrieved from *www.hmjanaesthesia.4t.com/periopsteroid.htm.*
11. Neil JA: Perioperative care of the immunocompromised patient, *AORN J* 85:544, 2007.
12. Neil JA: Perioperative care of the patient with tuberculosis, *AORN J* 88:942, 2008.
13. Ide P, Farber E, Lautz D: Perioperative nursing care of the bariatric surgical patient, *AORN J* 88:30, 2008.
14. Posthauer M, Dorner B, Collins, N, et al: A critical component of wound healing, *Adv Skin Wound Care* 23:12, 2010.
15. Health News Feed, John Hopkins Medical Information: Caffeine withdrawal. Retrieved from *www.hopkinsmedicine.org/hnf/hnf_915.htm.*
16. Code of Federal Regulations for Hospitals: *Surgical services,* §482.45 42 CFR Ch. IV (10-1-04 Edition). Retrieved from *http://edocket.access.gpo.gov/cfr_2004/octqtr/pdf/42cfr482.51.pdf.*
17. Durai R, Ng P, Hogue H: Methicillin-resistant *Staphylococcus aureus*: an update, *AORN J* 91:5, 2010.
*18. Kruzik N: Benefits of preoperative education for adult elective surgery patients, *AORN J* 90:3, 2009.
19. Appendix L—Guidance for surveyors: ambulatory surgical. In *State operations manual*, Survey procedures §416.52(c)(1), US Department of Health and Human Services, Centers for

*Evidence-based information for clinical practice.

Medicare and Medicaid Services. Retrieved from *www.cms.gov/manuals/Downloads/som107ap_l_ambulatory.pdf*.

20. American Hospital Association: The patient care partnership: understanding expectations, rights and responsibilities. Retrieved from *www.aha.org/aha/content/2003/pdf/pcp_english_030730.pdf*.

*21. Odom-Forren J: Postoperative patient care and pain management. In JC Rothrock, editor: *Alexander's care of the patient in surgery*, ed 14, St Louis, 2011, Mosby.

*22. Practice guidelines for preoperative fasting and the use of pharmacologic agents to reduce the risk of pulmonary aspiration: application to healthy patients undergoing elective procedures: an updated report by the American Society of Anesthesiologists Committee on Standards and Practice Parameters, *Anesthesiology* 114:3, 2011.

23. American College of Surgeons: Public information from the American College of Surgeons: principle of informed consent. Retrieved from *www.facs.org/public_info/operation/consent.html*.

24. Phillips NF, Berry EC, Kohn ML: *Berry and Kohn's operating room technique*, ed 12, St Louis, 2013, Mosby.

25. DiFusco LA: Pediatric surgery. In Rothrock JC, editor: *Alexander's care of the patient in surgery*, ed 14, St Louis, 2011, Mosby.

26. Rothrock JC: *Alexander's care of the patient in surgery*, ed 14, St Louis, 2011, Mosby.

*27. Wolf A, McGoldrick K: Cardiovascular pharmacotherapeutic considerations in patients undergoing anesthesia, *Cardiol Rev* 19:1, 2011.

28. DeLamar LM: Anesthesia. In Rothrock JC, editor: *Alexander's care of the patient in surgery*, ed 14, St Louis, 2011, Mosby.

*29. American Society of PeriAnesthesia Nurses: *2010-2012 Perianesthesia nursing and practice recommendations*, Cherry Hill, NJ, 2010, The Society.

30. Association of periOperative Registered Nurses: Perioperative patient hand-off tool kit: AORN practice resources. Retrieved from *www.aorn.org/PracticeResources/ToolKits/PatientHandOff ToolKit*.

31. Murphy EK: Patient safety and risk management. In Rothrock JC, editor: *Alexander's care of the patient in surgery*, ed 14, St Louis, 2011, Mosby.

32. Wilson-Stronks A, Lee KK, Cordero CL, et al: *One size does not fit all: meeting the health care needs of diverse populations*, Washington, DC, 2008, The Joint Commission. Retrieved from *www.jointcommission.org/assets/1/6/HLCOneSizeFinal.pdf*.

33. Chow WB, Ko CY, Rosenthal RA, et al: American College of Surgeons NSQIP®/AGS best practice guidelines: optimal preoperative assessment of the geriatric surgical patient. Retrieved from *www.jhartfound.org/blog/wp-content/upLoads/2012/10/ACS-NSQIP-AGS-Geriatric-2012-Guidelines6.pdf*.

RESOURCES

Resources for this chapter are listed in Chapter 20 on p. 366.

*The ultimate measure of a man is not
where he stands in moments of comfort and
convenience, but where he stands at times
of challenge and controversy.*
Martin Luther King, Jr.

Nursing Management
Intraoperative Care

*Anita Jo Shoup and David M. Horner**

LEARNING OUTCOMES

1. Differentiate the purposes of the various areas of the perioperative/surgery department and the proper attire for each area.
2. Differentiate the roles and responsibilities of the interdisciplinary surgical team members.
3. Prioritize needs of patients undergoing surgery.
4. Analyze the role of the perioperative nurse in the management of the patient undergoing surgery.
5. Apply basic principles of aseptic technique used in the operating room.
6. Evaluate the importance of safety in the operating room relative to patients, equipment, and anesthesia.
7. Differentiate the common types of and delivery systems for anesthesia.

KEY TERMS

anesthesia care provider (ACP), p. 336
anesthesiology, p. 336
epidural block, p. 345

general anesthesia, p. 341
local anesthesia, p. 342
malignant hyperthermia (MH), p. 346

nurse anesthetist, p. 336
regional anesthesia, p. 342
spinal anesthesia, p. 345

Historically, surgery took place in the traditional environment of the hospital operating room (OR). However, now the majority of surgical procedures are performed as ambulatory surgery (outpatient surgery). This chapter includes a discussion of the intraoperative care that is applicable to all surgical patients regardless of where the surgery if performed.

PHYSICAL ENVIRONMENT OF OPERATING ROOM

Department Layout

The *surgical suite* is a controlled environment designed to minimize the spread of pathogens and allow a smooth flow of patients, staff, and equipment needed to provide safe patient care. The suite is divided into three distinct areas: unrestricted, semirestricted, and restricted areas. The *unrestricted area* is where people in street clothes can interact with those in surgical attire. These areas typically include the points of entry for patients (e.g., holding area), staff (e.g., locker rooms), and information (e.g., nursing station or control desk). The *semirestricted area* includes the surrounding support areas and corridors. Only authorized staff are allowed access to the semirestricted areas. All staff in the semirestricted area must wear surgical attire and cover all head and facial hair. In the *restricted area* masks are required to supplement surgical attire.[1] The restricted area can include the OR, scrub sink area, and clean core.

In addition, the physical layout is designed to reduce cross-contamination. The flow of clean and sterile supplies and equipment should be separated from contaminated supplies,

*Contributed section on anesthesia content.
Reviewed by Ronald R. Castaldo, CRNA, MBA, MS, CCRN, Staff Nurse Anesthetist, Anesthesia Services, New Castle, Delaware; Lisa Kiper, RN, MSN, Assistant Professor of Nursing, Morehead State University, Morehead, Kentucky; Angela M. Martinelli, RN, PhD, CNOR, Science Officer, Congressionally Directed Medical Research Programs, Fort Detrick, Maryland; and Cynthia Schoonover, RN, MS, CCRN, Associate Nursing Professor, Sinclair Community College, Dayton, Ohio and PACU Staff Nurse, Kettering Medical Center, Kettering, Ohio.

equipment, and waste by space, time, and traffic patterns. Staff move supplies from clean areas, such as the clean core, through the OR for surgery, and on to the surrounding areas, such as the instrument decontamination area.[2]

Holding Area

The *holding area*, frequently called the *preoperative holding area*, is a special waiting area inside of or adjacent to the surgical suite. The size can range from a centralized area to accommodate numerous patients to a small designated area immediately outside the actual room scheduled for the surgical procedure. The holding area is where you identify and assess the patient before transferring him or her to the OR.

The *Surgical Care Improvement Project* (SCIP) is a national quality partnership of organizations focused on improving surgical care by significantly reducing the number of complications from surgery[3] (refer to *www.jointcommission.org/assets/1/6/Surgical%20Care%20Improvement%20Project.pdf*). Several SCIP measures may be implemented in the holding area, such as drug administration, patient warming, and application of sequential compression devices (SCDs). Many minor procedures (e.g., inserting IV catheters and arterial lines) can also be performed here.

The National Patient Safety Goals (NPSGs) require a preprocedure process, including the verification of relevant documentation (e.g., history and physical examination, signed consent form, nursing and preanesthesia assessment). In addition, any required blood products, implants, devices, and special equipment need to be available. Further, any diagnostic and radiology test results (e.g., x-rays, biopsy reports) need to be properly labeled and displayed.[4]

In addition, the NPSGs require that the surgeon mark the procedure site. If possible, the marking should be done with the patient's involvement.[4]

In some settings, another area for holding is identified as the *admission, observation, and discharge* (AOD) area. This area is designed to allow early-morning admission for outpatient surgery, same-day admission, and inpatient holding before surgery. In this area you can assess preoperative information, observe the patient both before and after surgery, and allow sufficient recovery time before the patient is discharged to either the home or an inpatient room. The AOD area is important in the patient's stay throughout outpatient surgery and prevents unnecessary overnight stays in the inpatient setting.

Separation from caregivers just before surgery can produce anxiety for the patient. This anxiety can be reduced when the caregiver is permitted to wait with the patient in the holding area until the patient is transferred to the OR.

Operating Room

The traditional surgical environment, or OR, is a unique setting removed from other hospital clinical units. It is controlled geographically, environmentally, and bacteriologically, and it is restricted in terms of the inflow and outflow of staff (Fig. 19-1). It is preferable to have the OR located next to the postanesthesia care unit (PACU) and the surgical intensive care unit. This allows for quick transport of the postoperative patient and close proximity to anesthesia staff if complications arise.

Several methods are used to prevent the transmission of infection. Filters and controlled airflow in the ventilating systems provide dust control. Positive air pressure in the rooms prevents air from entering the OR from the halls and corridors.

FIG. 19-1 Typical operating room.

Ultraviolet (UV) lighting may be used because UV radiation reduces the number of microorganisms in the air. Dust-collecting surfaces such as open shelves and tables are omitted. Materials that are resistant to the corroding effects of strong disinfectants are used.

Overall safety and comfort are aided by the use of OR furniture that is adjustable, easy to clean, and easy to move. All equipment is checked frequently to ensure proper functioning and electrical safety. The lighting is designed to provide a low- to high-intensity range for a precise view of the surgical site (see Fig. 19-2). A communication system provides a means for the delivery of routine and emergency messages.[5,6]

SURGICAL TEAM

Registered Nurse

The *perioperative nurse* is a registered nurse (RN) who implements patient care during the perioperative period. Through close collaboration with the other members of the surgical team, you prepare the OR for patients before they arrive. You are usually the first member of the surgical team who meets the patient. You are the patient's advocate throughout the intraoperative experience. This includes maintaining the patient's safety, privacy, dignity, and confidentiality; communicating with the patient; and providing physical care. Assess the patient to determine any additional needs or tasks to complete before surgery. Provide physical and emotional comfort and patient and caregiver teaching regarding the upcoming surgery. In addition, work with the patient's caregivers, keeping them informed and answering questions. This is particularly important in day-surgery areas where caregivers must assume greater responsibility for preoperative and postoperative care.

In the perioperative role, you assume functions that involve either sterile or unsterile activities (Table 19-1). When you serve in the role of *scrub nurse,* you follow the designated scrub procedure, are gowned and gloved in sterile attire, and remain in the sterile field (Fig. 19-2). When you serve in the role of *circu-*

TABLE 19-1 INTRAOPERATIVE ACTIVITIES OF PERIOPERATIVE NURSE

Circulating, Nonsterile Activities

- Reviews anatomy, physiology, and surgical procedure
- Assists in preparing room, ensuring that supplies and equipment are available, in working order, and sterile (if required)
- Maintains aseptic technique in all required activities
- Monitors practices of aseptic technique in self and others
- Checks mechanical and electrical equipment and environmental factors
- Conducts a preprocedure verification process
- Assesses patient's physical and emotional status
- Verifies and implements ordered SCIP measures
- Plans and coordinates intraoperative nursing care
- Checks chart and relates pertinent data to team members
- Participates in the application of monitoring devices and insertion of invasive lines and other devices
- Assists with and ensures patient safety in transferring and positioning patient
- Assists with induction of anesthesia
- Monitors draping procedure
- Participates in surgical time-out
- Documents intraoperative care
- Prepares, records, labels, and sends blood, pathology, and any anatomic specimens to proper locations
- Measures blood, urine output, and other fluid loss
- Verifies, dispenses, and records medications used, including local anesthetics

- Coordinates all intraoperative activities with team members and other health-related staff and departments
- Maintains accurate count of sponges, needles, instruments, and medical devices that could be retained in the patient
- Accompanies patient to PACU
- Provides hand-off report to PACU nurse with information relevant to care of patient

Scrubbed, Sterile Activities

- Reviews anatomy, physiology, and surgical procedure
- Assists in preparing the operating room
- Completes surgical hand and arm scrub, and gowns and gloves self and other members of surgical team
- Prepares instrument table and organizes sterile equipment for functional use
- Assists with draping procedure
- Participates in surgical time-out procedure
- Passes instruments to surgeon and assistants by anticipating their needs
- Maintains accurate count of sponges, needles, instruments, and medical devices that could be retained in the patient
- Monitors practices of aseptic technique in self and others
- Keeps track of irrigation solutions used for calculation of blood loss
- Accepts, verifies, and reports medications used by surgeon and/or ACP, including local anesthetics

ACP, Anesthesia care provider; *PACU,* postanesthesia care unit; *SCIP,* Surgical Care Improvement Project.

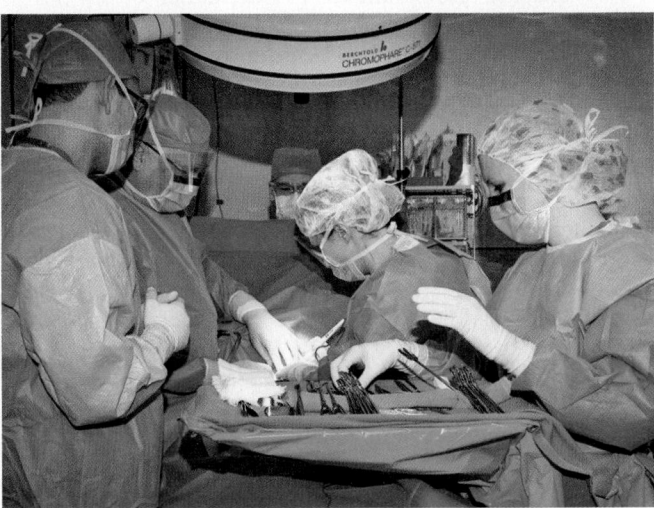

FIG. 19-2 The complexity of surgery requires maintaining asepsis.

lating nurse, you remain in the unsterile field and so you are not gowned and gloved in sterile attire.

Ongoing assessment of the patient is essential because the patient's condition may change quickly. You respond to these changes and revise the plan of care as needed. Examples of nursing activities that characterize each phase surrounding the surgical experience are presented in Table 19-2.

As patients move through the surgical experience, they are cared for by many team members. Opportunities for error are created whenever clinical information is shared among these members.[7] The Joint Commission requires that all health care providers implement a standardized approach to hand-off communication. The perioperative RN ensures that a complete and accurate hand-off using a consistent format, such as SBAR (see Table 1-7), occurs every time the responsibility for patient care

is transferred to another professional. Examples of such transfers include change of shift, surgeon to nurse, and OR nurse to postanesthesia nurse.

You also have the opportunity to become a certified operating room nurse (CNOR). Certification reflects expertise in surgical nursing. The credential is a personal commitment to higher standards that inspires credibility and confidence with patients and peers in the workplace.[8]

Licensed Practical/Vocational Nurse and Surgical Technologist

Depending on your state nurse practice act, the role of the circulating or scrub nurse may be filled by a licensed practical/vocational nurse or a surgical technologist. Surgical technologists may attend an associate degree program, a vocational training program, or a hospital or military training program. The Association of Surgical Technologists is an organization that sets standards for education, provides continuing education opportunities, and offers certification for surgical technologists.[9]

If the circulating nurse is not an RN, the licensed practical/vocational nurse or surgical technologist must have access to an RN at all times. You are responsible for supervising the licensed practical/vocational nurse or surgical technologist in the performance of all delegated nursing tasks.[10]

Surgeon and Assistant

The *surgeon* is the physician who performs the surgical procedure. The surgeon is primarily responsible for the following:

- Preoperative medical history and physical assessment, including need for surgical intervention, choice of surgical procedure, management of preoperative testing, and discussion of the risks of and alternatives to surgical intervention

TABLE 19-2	**NURSING ACTIVITIES DURING SURGICAL EXPERIENCE***	
Before	**During**	**After**
Assessment and Planning	**Implementation**	**Evaluation**
Home, Clinic, Holding Area Initiates preoperative assessment Plans teaching appropriate to patient's needs Involves caregiver **Surgical Unit** Completes preoperative assessment Coordinates patient teaching with staff Develops a plan of care that reflects patient's level of function and ability **Surgical Suite** Conducts preprocedure verification Assesses patient's level of consciousness, skin integrity, mobility, emotional status, and functional limitations Reviews chart Ensures all supplies and equipment needed are available, functioning, and sterile, if appropriate	**Safety Maintenance** Ensures integrity of sterile field Ensures that sponge, needle, instrument, and medical device counts are correct Positions patient to ensure correct alignment, exposure of surgical site, and prevention of injury Prevents chemical injury from prepping solutions, pharmaceuticals, etc. Ensures safe use of electrical equipment Safely administers medications **Monitoring Physical Status** Monitors and reports changes in patient's vital signs Monitors blood loss and urine output **Monitoring Psychologic Status** Provides emotional support to patient Stands near or touches patient during procedures Ensures patient's right to privacy is maintained Communicates patient's emotional status to health care team	**Postanesthesia, Discharge Area** Determines patient's response to surgical intervention Monitors ABCs, vital signs, level of consciousness Safely administers medications **Clinical Unit** Evaluates effectiveness of nursing care in OR using patient outcome criteria Determines patient's level of satisfaction with care given during perioperative period Determines patient's psychologic status Assists with discharge planning **Home, Clinic** Seeks patient's perception of surgery in terms of effects of anesthetic agents, impact on body image, immobilization Determines caregiver's perceptions of surgery

*List of activities is not all-inclusive.
ABCs, Airway, breathing, circulation.

- Patient safety and management in the OR
- Postoperative management of the patient

The surgeon's assistant can be a physician who functions in an assisting role during the surgical procedure. The assistant usually holds retractors to expose surgical areas and assists with hemostasis and suturing. In some instances, especially in educational settings, the assistant may perform some portions of the surgery under the surgeon's direct supervision. In many institutions the surgeon's assistant is a registered nurse first assistant or a physician's assistant (PA) who functions under the physician's direct supervision.

Registered Nurse First Assistant

The *registered nurse first assistant* (RNFA) works in collaboration with the surgeon to produce an optimal surgical outcome for the patient. The Association of periOperative Registered Nurses (AORN) position statement on RNFAs states that the perioperative nurse must have formal education for this role and works collaboratively with the surgeon, patient, and surgical team by handling tissue, using instruments, providing exposure to the surgical site, assisting with hemostasis, and suturing.[6,11] RNFA education programs are designed to provide RNs with the education necessary to assume this expanded role.[12] The RNFA can also obtain certification.

Anesthesia Care Provider

The **anesthesia care provider (ACP)** is a person who administers anesthesia and can be an anesthesiologist, nurse anesthetist, or anesthesiologist assistant (AA). **Anesthesiology** is a discipline within the practice of medicine that specializes in the following.

- Medically managing patients who are unconscious or insensible to pain and emotional stress during surgical and other medical procedures
- Protecting functions and vital organs under the stress of anesthetic, surgical, or other medical procedures

- Managing pain
- Managing cardiopulmonary resuscitation
- Managing problems in pulmonary care
- Managing critically ill patients in special care units

ACPs who are anesthesiologists are responsible for administering anesthetic agents to relieve pain and manage vital life functions (e.g., breathing, blood pressure [BP]) during surgery. After surgery they provide care during recovery.[13]

A **nurse anesthetist** is an RN who has graduated from an accredited nurse anesthesia program (minimally a master's degree program) and successfully completed a national certification examination to become a certified registered nurse anesthetist (CRNA). The CRNA scope of practice includes the following:[14]

- Performing and documenting a preanesthetic assessment and evaluation
- Developing and implementing a plan for delivering anesthesia
- Selecting and initiating the planned anesthetic technique
- Selecting, obtaining, and administering the anesthesia, adjuvant drugs, and fluids
- Selecting, applying, and inserting appropriate noninvasive and invasive monitoring devices
- Managing a patient's airway and pulmonary status
- Managing emergence and recovery from anesthesia
- Releasing or discharging patients from a PACU
- Ordering, initiating, or modifying pain relief therapy
- Responding to emergency situations by providing airway management, and administering emergency fluids and drugs
- Assuming additional responsibilities within the expertise of the individual

An *anesthesiologist assistant* (AA) is a specialty PA who functions under the direction of an anesthesiologist in many states. The AA has graduated from an accredited program (minimally a master's degree program) and successfully completed a national certification examination. AAs participate in the provision of all types of anesthesia, including administering drugs, obtaining vascular access, applying and interpreting monitors, establishing and maintaining airways, and assisting with preoperative assessments.

NURSING MANAGEMENT
PATIENT BEFORE SURGERY

The preoperative assessment of the surgical patient establishes baseline data for intraoperative and postoperative care. Preoperative care of the patient is discussed in Chapter 18. Some additional information is discussed in this chapter.

PSYCHOSOCIAL ASSESSMENT

Knowing about the activities that occur when a patient is moved into the surgical suite allows you to provide explanations and reassurances, especially to the anxious patient. You can usually answer general questions regarding surgery or anesthesia, such as "When will I go to sleep?" "Who will be in the room?" "When will my surgeon arrive?" "How much of my body will be exposed?" "Will I be cold?" "When will I wake up?" Specific questions relating to details of the surgical procedure and anesthesia may be referred to the surgeon or the ACP.

Performing a cultural and spiritual assessment can help you understand the patient's response to the surgical experience (see Tables 2-7 and Table 10-5 for additional information). For example, members of the Jehovah's Witness community may refuse blood transfusions.[15] For Muslims, the left hand is considered unclean, so you should use the right hand to give forms, drugs, and treatments.[16] Some Native American patients may request that surgically removed body tissue be preserved so that it may be buried. Some tattoos and body piercings may also have cultural meaning.[17] Some patients may have a prayer cloth or other traditional or sacred item with them. Consider spiritual needs and beliefs in the individualized plan of care. For patients who do not speak English, a qualified interpreter must be used (see Table 2-10).

PHYSICAL ASSESSMENT

Perform a thorough physical assessment during the preoperative preparation of the patient (see Chapter 18).

CHART REVIEW

Required chart data vary with agency policy, patient condition, and specific surgical procedures. Because ambulatory surgery facilities tend to have a healthier population, fewer tests may be required. Examples of data that are obtained during the preoperative assessment can be found in Tables 18-2 and 18-4. This information contributes to an understanding of past and present history, cardiopulmonary status, and potential for infection and other complications.

ADMITTING THE PATIENT

Hospital policy designates the protocol to be followed when admitting the patient to the holding area and OR. A general routine includes initial greeting, extension of human contact and warmth, and proper identification. A preprocedure verification process is conducted before the start of surgery. In some institutions this takes place in the holding area; in others it takes place in the OR itself.

COMPLEMENTARY & ALTERNATIVE THERAPIES
Music Therapy

Music is an ancient healing tool recognized in the writings of Plato.

Scientific Evidence
Strong scientific evidence for use in reducing stress and anxiety and enhancing mood.*

Nursing Implications
- To be effective, the music selected needs to be appropriate for the situation. Music can have many different physiologic effects.
  - Listening to calming music can result in slower, deeper breathing and a decrease in heart rate and blood pressure. Both of these indicate relaxation.
  - Music with a faster pace can energize a person and promote mental alertness.
- Music therapy is safe in combination with other treatment approaches.

*Based on a systematic review of scientific literature. Retrieved from www.naturalstandard.com.

Complementary and alternative therapies such as therapeutic touch, aromatherapy, music therapy, guided imagery, and even movies may be used for surgical patients. (See the Complementary & Alternative Therapies box above on music and Chapter 6.) These therapies may decrease anxiety, promote relaxation, reduce pain, and accelerate the healing process.[6,18] In some facilities these therapies are initiated before the patient's admission to the OR. In others, such as ambulatory settings, they may be started after the patient's arrival in the holding area.

The admitting procedure is continued with reassessment of the patient and with time allowed for last-minute questions. Complete the chart review for the previously mentioned data and note any abnormalities or changes. Question the patient concerning valuables, prostheses, and last intake of food and fluid. Validate that the correct preoperative medications were given (if ordered). Provide a pillow or position adjustment if the patient is uncomfortable. Most hospitals require the patient's hair to be covered just before transfer to the OR suite to reduce potential shedding. Specific SCIP measures may include a prophylactic antibiotic started within 30 to 60 minutes before the surgical incision, and application of a warming blanket and SCDs.

NURSING MANAGEMENT
PATIENT DURING SURGERY

ROOM PREPARATION

Before transferring the patient into the OR, prepare the room to ensure privacy, prevention of infection, and safety. Individualization of this preparation is essential to achieve the expected patient outcomes. For example, when an obese patient is admitted to the OR, there are several special considerations (see Chapter 41). Ask such questions as, What equipment is needed to safely transfer the patient to and from the OR table? Will extra staff be required for safe transfer and positioning? Is special equipment needed (e.g., extra-long instrumentation)? What special precautions, if any, must be taken to ensure maintenance of the patient's airway? The unique needs of each patient must be addressed for a safe surgical experience.

Surgical attire (pants and shirts, masks, protective eyewear, and caps or hoods) is worn by all people entering the OR (Fig. 19-3). All electrical and mechanical equipment is checked

FIG. 19-3 Surgical attire is worn by all people entering the operating room.

FIG. 19-4 A sterile field is created before surgery.

for proper functioning. Aseptic technique is practiced as each surgical item is opened and placed on the instrument table.[19] Sponges, needles, instruments, and small medical devices (e.g., surgical clip cartridges, universal adapters) are counted according to strict processes to ensure accurate retrieval at the end of the procedure. Any retained surgical supplies, devices, or instruments are sentinel events that can result in negative outcomes for the patient.[20,21]

During room preparation and the surgical procedure, the scrub person performs surgical hand antisepsis, dons sterile gown and gloves, and touches only those items in the sterile field. The circulating nurse remains in the unsterile field and performs those activities that permit touching all unsterile items and the patient. This coordinated effort allows for smooth functioning throughout the procedure.

TRANSFERRING PATIENT

Once the patient's identity has been verified and the OR has been prepared, the patient is transported into the room for the surgery. Each time a patient is transferred from one bed to another, the wheels of the stretcher must be locked, and a sufficient number of personnel should be available to lift, guide, and prevent accidental falling or injury to self, other staff, or the patient. Once the patient is on the OR bed, place safety straps snugly across the patient's thighs. At this time the monitor leads (e.g., electrocardiogram [ECG] leads), BP cuff, and pulse oximeter are usually applied and an IV catheter is inserted if it was not done in the holding area.

SCRUBBING, GOWNING, AND GLOVING

Surgical hand antisepsis is required of all sterile members of the surgical team (scrub nurse, surgeon, and assistant). When the procedure of scrubbing is the chosen method for surgical hand antisepsis (often for the first case of the day), your fingers and hands should be scrubbed first with progression to the forearms and elbows. The hands should be held away from surgical attire and higher than the elbows at all times to prevent contamination from clothing or detergent suds and water from draining from the unclean area above the elbows to the clean and previously scrubbed areas of the hands and fingers.[6,22]

Waterless, alcohol-based agents are replacing traditional soap and water in many facilities. When using an alcohol-based surgical hand-scrub product, prewash hands and forearms with soap and dry completely before applying the alcohol-based product. After application of the alcohol-based product, allow hands and forearms to dry thoroughly before donning sterile gloves.[22,23]

Once surgical hand antisepsis is completed, the team members enter the OR to put on surgical gowns and two pairs of gloves to protect patients and themselves from the transmission of microorganisms.[24,25] Because the gowns and gloves are sterile, those who have scrubbed can manipulate and organize all sterile items for use during the procedure.

BASIC ASEPTIC TECHNIQUE

Aseptic technique is practiced in the OR to prevent infection. This is implemented through the creation and maintenance of a sterile field (Fig. 19-4). The center of the sterile field is the site of the surgical incision. Inanimate items used in the sterile field, including surgical items and equipment, have been sterilized by appropriate sterilization methods.

Team members must understand specific principles to practice aseptic technique (Table 19-3). Unless these principles are followed, the patient's safety is compromised and the potential for postoperative infection is increased.[5,6,19]

In addition to following the principles of aseptic technique, the surgical team is responsible for following the guidelines established by the U.S. Occupational Safety and Health Administration (OSHA) and AORN to protect the patient and the team from exposure to blood-borne pathogens.[26] These guidelines emphasize standard and transmission-based precautions (see eTable 15-1, available on the website for Chapter 15); engineering and work practice controls; and the use of personal protective equipment such as gloves, gowns, caps, face shields, masks, and protective eyewear. This is especially important in the OR because of the high potential for exposure to blood-borne pathogens.

ASSISTING ANESTHESIA CARE PROVIDER

While you check the OR to complete the final preparations, the ACP prepares the patient for the administration of the anesthetic. You need to understand the effects of the anesthetic agents and know the location of all emergency drugs and equipment.

If you are the circulating nurse, you may be involved in placing monitoring devices to be used during the surgical pro-

TABLE 19-3	PRINCIPLES OF ASEPTIC TECHNIQUE IN OPERATING ROOM

- All materials that enter the sterile field must be sterile.
- If a sterile item comes in contact with an unsterile item, it is contaminated.
- Contaminated items are removed immediately from the sterile field. If the unsterile item is small (e.g., unopened suture), once it is removed, the area is marked off (i.e., covered with a sterile drape). If the entire field is contaminated, it should be set up again with all new materials.
- The surgical team working in the operative field must wear sterile gowns and gloves. Once dressed for procedure, they must recognize that the only parts of the gown considered sterile are front from chest to table level and sleeves to 2 inches above elbow.
- A wide margin of safety must be maintained between sterile and unsterile fields.
- Tables are considered sterile only at tabletop level. Items extending beneath this level are considered contaminated.
- The edges of a sterile package are considered contaminated once the package has been opened. If a sterile package (e.g., package of sutures) is placed on the sterile field, that entire package remains sterile even when opened.
- Microorganisms travel on airborne particles and will enter the sterile field with excessive air movements and currents.
- Microorganisms travel by capillary action through moist fabrics, resulting in contamination.
- Microorganisms harbor on the patient's and team members' hair, skin, and respiratory tracts and must be confined by appropriate attire.

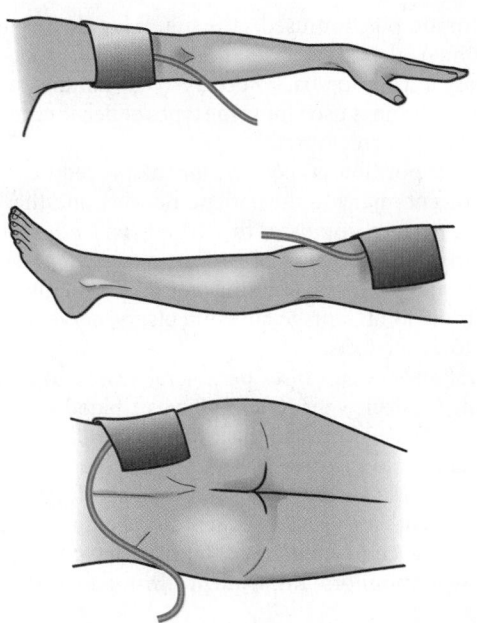

FIG. 19-5 When an electrosurgical unit is used, the patient must be properly grounded to prevent unintended injury. A well-vascularized muscle mass is an optimal site. Safety can be compromised by excessive hair, adipose tissue, bony prominences, fluid (edema), adhesive failure, and scar tissue.

cedure (e.g., ECG leads). If the patient is to have a general anesthetic, remain at the patient's side to ensure safety and to assist the ACP. These responsibilities may include measuring BP and assisting in the maintenance of the patient's airway. During the surgical procedure, you also provide a vital communication link for the ACP to other departments such as the laboratory or the blood bank.

SAFETY CONSIDERATIONS

All surgical procedures, regardless of where they take place, can put the patient at risk for injury. These injuries can be infections, physical trauma from positioning or equipment used, or physiologic effects of surgery itself. Be alert to all safety issues, since the patient in the OR is often compromised from the effects of anesthesia.

Fire in the OR can have devastating consequences for the patient. Fortunately, surgical fires can be prevented with awareness of the hazards and emphasis on safe practices.[27] Care must be taken to correctly place the grounding pad and all electrosurgical equipment to prevent injury from burns or fire[28] (Fig. 19-5).

Smoke particles produced during laser procedures may contain trace hydrocarbons (e.g., acetone, isopropanol, formaldehyde, cyanide). These airborne contaminants can cause respiratory irritation and have mutagenic and carcinogenic potential. Smoke evacuators may be used to minimize this exposure.[29]

The *Universal Protocol*, one of the NPSGs, is followed to prevent wrong site, wrong procedure, and wrong surgery.[30] A patient safety checklist for ORs is the cornerstone of a major focus to make surgery safer around the world (see eFig. 19-1 available on the website for this chapter). The use of the World Health Organization (WHO) Surgical Safety Checklist has

improved compliance with standards and decreased complications from surgery.[31]

Similarly, AORN has developed a position statement regarding correct site surgery and guidelines for implementing the Universal Protocol.[32] All members of the surgical team stop what they are doing during a *surgical time-out* just before the procedure starts to verify patient identification, surgical procedure, and surgical site. In addition, it is becoming more common for OR personnel to complete a fire risk assessment protocol (see eTable 19-1 available on the website for this chapter) to identify and reduce the potential for an OR fire.

SAFETY ALERT: Take a Surgical Time-Out
- Before the induction of anesthesia, ask the patient to confirm name, birth date, operative procedure and site, and consent.
- Compare the hospital ID number with the patient's own ID band and chart.

POSITIONING PATIENT

Positioning the patient is a critical part of every procedure and usually follows administration of the anesthetic. The ACP indicates when to begin the positioning. The patient's position should allow for accessibility to the operative site, administration and monitoring of anesthetic agents, and maintenance of the patient's airway. When positioning for the surgical procedure, take care to (1) provide correct musculoskeletal alignment; (2) prevent undue pressure on nerves, skin over bony prominences, earlobes, and eyes; (3) provide for adequate thoracic excursion; (4) prevent occlusion of arteries and veins; (5) provide modesty in exposure; and (6) recognize and respect individual needs such as previously assessed aches, pains, or deformities. It is your responsibility to secure the extremities, provide adequate padding and support, and obtain sufficient physical or mechanical help to avoid unnecessary straining of self or patient.[33]

The patient may be placed in various positions, including supine, prone, lateral, lithotomy, or sitting. The supine is the most common position used. It is suited for surgery involving the abdomen, the heart, and the breast. The prone position allows easy access for back surgery (e.g., laminectomy). The lithotomy position is used for some types of pelvic organ surgery (e.g., vaginal hysterectomy).

Whatever position is required for the procedure, take great care to prevent injury to the patient. Because anesthesia blocks the sensory nerve impulses, the patient will not feel pain or discomfort or stress being placed on nerves, muscles, bones, and skin. Improper positioning could potentially result in muscle strain, joint damage, pressure ulcers, nerve damage, and other untoward effects.

General anesthesia causes peripheral vessels to dilate. Position changes affect where the pooling of blood occurs. If the head of the OR bed is raised, the lower torso will have increased blood volume and the upper torso may become compromised. Hypovolemia and cardiovascular disease can further compromise the patient's status. Consequently, the entire surgical team carefully plans and implements the patient's positioning, and then closely monitors the patient throughout the surgical procedure.

PREVENTING HYPOTHERMIA

Research has shown a correlation between unintended hypothermia and impaired wound healing, adverse cardiac events, altered drug metabolism, and coagulopathies. One study showed that the rate of culture-positive surgical site infections among those with mild perioperative hypothermia was three times higher than among normothermic patients.[34]

To prevent hypothermia, members of the surgical team need to closely monitor the patient's temperature and may apply a thermal warming blanket to the patient to maintain body temperature.[35,36]

PREPARING SURGICAL SITE

The purpose of skin preparation, or "prepping," is to reduce the number of microorganisms available to migrate to the surgical wound. The task of prepping is completed intraoperatively by the circulating nurse, surgeon, or surgical assistant.

The skin is prepared by mechanically scrubbing or cleansing around the surgical site with an antimicrobial agent identified as one that reduces microorganisms on intact skin, contains a nonirritating antimicrobial agent, has broad-spectrum activity, is fast acting and persistent, and is nonallergenic to the patient. A liberal area is scrubbed in a circular motion. The principle of scrubbing from the clean area (site of the incision) to the dirty area (distal to the incision) is observed at all times.[37,38]

Antiseptic agents used for skin preparation may contain alcohol and be flammable. Skin injury can occur if these agents are allowed to pool under the patient. Care must be taken to ensure that these agents are properly confined and allowed to fully dry. After the skin is prepped and the fumes are allowed to dispel, the sterile members of the surgical team drape the area. Only the site to be incised is left exposed.

PATIENT AFTER SURGERY

Through constant observation of the surgical process, the ACP anticipates the end of the surgical procedure. Appropriate types and doses of anesthetic agents are used so that their effects will be minimal at the end of the surgical procedure. This also allows greater physiologic control of the patient during the transfer to the PACU.

The patient's response to your care is evaluated based on outcome criteria established during the development of the patient's plan of care. These outcome criteria are published as the *Perioperative Nursing Data Set (PNDS)* by AORN. The PNDS reflects standards and recommended practices related to the delivery of nursing care in any perioperative setting.[6,39]

The ACP and you or another member of the surgical team accompany the patient to the PACU. A hand-off of the patient that includes his or her status and the procedure performed is communicated to the nurse receiving the patient in the PACU to promote safe, ongoing care.

ANESTHESIA

The art and science of anesthesia have dramatically changed over time. For example, the Bispectral Index monitor allows ACPs to track the level of patient awareness (i.e., *awareness monitoring*) during surgery and adjust sedation as needed. The use of regional anesthetics facilitates the smooth and rapid transition from patient recovery to early discharge.

The anesthetic technique and agents are selected by the ACP in collaboration with the surgeon and the patient. The ACP has ultimate responsibility for the choice of anesthetic. Factors contributing to the decision include the patient's current physical and mental status, allergy and pain history, expertise of the ACP, and factors relating to the operative procedure (e.g., length, site, discharge plans). An absolute contraindication to any anesthetic technique or agent is patient refusal.

The ACP obtains anesthesia consent, writes orders for preoperative and postoperative medications, and assigns the patient an anesthesia classification. The American Society of Anesthesiologists (ASA) physical status classification system is based on the patient's physiologic status with no regard to the surgical procedure to be performed. A scale of P1 to P6 is used, with a rating of P6 reserved for a brain-dead patient undergoing organ harvest (see Table 18-3). An intraoperative complication is more likely to develop with a higher classification number. Other designations can be added to the ASA status (e.g., "E" to designate an "emergent" procedure). ASA physical status is dynamic and represents the patient's status immediately before surgery. For example, a healthy 26-year-old adult who is severely injured in an automobile collision may be classified as ASA P5E because life-threatening injuries require emergent surgery.

CLASSIFICATION OF ANESTHESIA

The ASA classifies anesthesia according to the effect that it has on the patient's sensorium and pain perception. These classifications include general anesthesia, regional anesthesia, local anesthesia, monitored anesthesia care (MAC), and moderate sedation[40,41] (Table 19-4).

Monitored anesthesia care (MAC) is used for diagnostic or therapeutic procedures performed in or outside of the OR (e.g., eye clinic). It includes varying levels of sedation, analgesia, and anxiolysis. A critical component of MAC is the assessment and management of any physiologic problems that may develop. The provider of MAC must be an ACP, since it may be necessary to convert to general anesthesia during the procedure.

Moderate sedation is used for procedures performed outside of the OR (e.g., reduction of dislocated joints in the emergency department) and does not require the presence of an ACP. RNs

TABLE 19-4 CLASSIFICATION OF ANESTHESIA AND PATIENT EFFECTS

Classification	Anticipated Patient Effects
General anesthesia	• Loss of sensation with loss of consciousness • Combination of hypnosis, analgesia, and amnesia • Usually involves use of inhalation agents • Skeletal muscle relaxation • Elimination of coughing, gagging, vomiting, and sympathetic nervous system responsiveness • Requires advanced airway management
Regional anesthesia	• Loss of sensation to a region of body without loss of consciousness • Involves blocking a specific nerve or group of nerves with administration of a local anesthetic • Includes spinal, caudal, and epidural anesthesia and IV and peripheral nerve blocks (e.g., interscalene, axillary, infraclavicular or supraclavicular, popliteal, femoral, sciatic)
Local anesthesia	• Loss of sensation without loss of consciousness • Induced topically or via infiltration, intracutaneously, or subcutaneously • Topical applications may be aerosolized or nebulized
Monitored anesthesia care (MAC)	• Similar to general anesthesia • Sedative, anxiolytic, and/or analgesic medications used • Does not usually involve inhalation agents • Patients less responsive and may require airway management • Provides maximum flexibility to match sedation level to patient needs and procedural requirements • Often used in conjunction with regional or local anesthesia • Often used for minor therapeutic and diagnostic procedures (e.g., eye surgery, colonoscopy)
Moderate sedation (formerly called conscious sedation)	• Sedative, anxiolytic, and/or analgesic medications used • Does not include use of inhalation agents • Patients responsive and breathe without assistance • Not expected to induce levels of sedation that would impair patients' ability to protect their airway • Most often used for minor therapeutic procedures (e.g., realignment of a fracture in the emergency department)

Sources: American Society of Anesthesiologists: Frequently asked questions. Retrieved from *www.lifelinetomodernmedicine.com/FAQs.aspx*; and American Society of Anesthesiologists: Distinguishing monitored anesthesia care ("MAC") from moderate sedation/analgesia (conscious sedation). Retrieved from *www.asahq.org/~/media/For%20Members/Standards%20and%20Guidelines/DISTINGUISHING%20MONITORED%20ANESTHESIA%20CARE.ashx*.

who receive education in moderate sedation and are permitted by institutional protocols and state nurse practice acts can provide this type of anesthesia.[42] It is administered by the nurse under the direct supervision of a physician.

General Anesthesia

The present goals of anesthesiology include the (1) control of excessive biologic responses induced by a variety of stressors and (2) protection of patients from stress-induced complications. To this end, *total intravenous anesthesia (TIVA)* and newer inhalation agents have a fast onset, fast elimination, and

fewer undesirable side effects than previous agents. These factors facilitate early discharge from the PACU and ambulatory surgery centers.

General anesthesia is the technique of choice for patients who are having surgical procedures that are of significant duration, require skeletal muscle relaxation, require uncomfortable operative positions because of the location of the incision site, or require control of ventilation. Additional reasons for general anesthesia include refusal of local or regional techniques, contraindications to other techniques, and uncooperative patients. Patients may be uncooperative due to intoxication, emotional lability, head injury, impaired cognition, or inability to remain immobile for any length of time. Phases of general anesthesia are presented in Table 19-5.

General anesthesia may be induced IV or by inhalation, and maintained by either one or a combination of the two (Table 19-6, p. 343). A *balanced technique*, using adjunctive drugs to complement the induction, is the most common approach used for general anesthesia.

Intravenous Agents. Virtually all routine general anesthetics begin with an IV induction agent, whether it is a hypnotic, an anxiolytic, or a dissociative agent. When used during the initial period of anesthesia, these agents induce a pleasant sleep with a rapid onset of action that patients find desirable. A single dose lasts only a few minutes, which is long enough for a laryngeal mask airway (LMA) or an endotracheal (ET) tube to be placed. Once this is done, the ACP uses the selected inhalation and IV agent(s).

Recent advances in IV hypnotics and opioids have led to the more frequent use of TIVA. However, the patient may still require advanced airway management (e.g., LMA, ET tube) and will receive oxygen/air mixtures via this route.

Inhalation Agents. Inhalation agents are the cornerstone of general anesthesia. These agents may be volatile liquids or gases. Volatile liquids are administered through a specially designed vaporizer after being mixed with oxygen as a carrier gas. This gas mixture is then delivered to the patient via the anesthesia circuit. Waste gases are removed using negative evacuation pressure venting to the outside of the institution.

Inhalation agents enter the body through the alveoli in the lungs. Ease of administration and rapid excretion by ventilation make them desirable agents. One undesirable trait is the irritating effect some inhalation agents (e.g., desflurane [Suprane]) have on the respiratory tract. Possible complications include coughing, laryngospasm (muscular constriction of the larynx), and increased secretions.[43]

Once the patient has been induced with an IV agent, the choice for delivering inhalation agents is usually through an ET tube or LMA. The ET tube permits control of ventilation and protects the airway from aspiration. LMAs are currently an important option for patients with difficult airways, but they do not provide access to the trachea with the same certainty as ETs. Complications of ET tube or LMA include those primarily associated with insertion and removal. These include failure to intubate, damage to teeth and lips, laryngospasm, laryngeal edema, postoperative sore throat, and hoarseness caused by injury or irritation of the vocal cords or surrounding tissues.

Adjuncts to General Anesthesia. The administration of general anesthesia is rarely limited to one agent. Drugs added to an inhalation anesthetic (other than an IV induction agent) are termed *adjuncts*. These agents are added to the anesthetic

TABLE 19-5	PHASES OF GENERAL ANESTHESIA			
Preinduction	**Induction**	**Maintenance**	**Emergence**	
Description				
• Period starting with preoperative medication, initiation of IV or arterial access, application of monitors (e.g., ECG).	• Initiation of medications that make patient unconscious. • Airway secured with airway assist devices.	• Period during which surgical procedure is performed. • Patient remains in an unconscious state with measures to ensure airway safety.	• Period when surgical procedure is completed. • Patient is prepared for return to consciousness and removal of airway assist devices.	
Role of Anesthesia Care Provider				
• Determine final anesthetic care plan. • Insert and monitor IV or arterial access. • Confirm antibiotic prophylaxis. • Administer drugs for anxiety, aspiration prophylaxis.	• Administer appropriate drugs. • Secure airway. • Position patient appropriately for surgical procedure.	• Monitor patient's physiologic status. • Administer medications and titrate fluids as appropriate.	• Reverse residual neuromuscular blocking agents. • Assess for return of all protective reflexes. • Remove airway assist devices. • Assess pain.	
Role of Perioperative Nurse				
• Complete preoperative assessment. • Check and confirm signed informed consent. • Complete surgical time-out.	• Assist with application of monitors (noninvasive and invasive). • Assist with airway management.	• Adjust patient position as necessary. • Monitor patient safety.	• Assist in placement of dressing. • Protect patient during return of reflexes. • Prepare patient to move to postanesthesia care unit.	
Classes of Drugs Used (see Tables 18-9, 19-6, and 19-7)				

• Benzodiazepines
• Opioids
• Antibiotics
• Aspiration prophylaxis:
  • H$_2$-receptor blockers (e.g., ranitidine [Zantac])
  • Gastric motility agents (e.g., metoclopramide [Reglan])
  • Anticholinergics (e.g., scopolamine [Transderm-Scōp])
	• Benzodiazepines
	• Opioids
	• Barbiturates
	• Hypnotics
	• Volatile gases
		• Benzodiazepines
		• Opioids
		• Barbiturates
		• Hypnotics
		• Volatile gases
		• Neuromuscular blocking agents
			• Reversal agents:
			  • Anticholinesterases (e.g., neostigmine [Prostigmin])
			  • Opioid antagonists (PRN) (e.g., naloxone [Narcan])
			  • Benzodiazepine antagonists (PRN) (e.g., flumazenil [Romazicon])
			• Supplemental opioids (PRN)
			• Antiemetics (PRN)	

regimen specifically to achieve unconsciousness, analgesia, amnesia, muscle relaxation, or autonomic nervous system control. Adjuncts include opioids, benzodiazepines, neuromuscular blocking agents (muscle relaxants), and antiemetics (Table 19-7, p. 344). It is important to know that these drugs are often given in combination and may have synergistic or antagonistic effects. You may observe deeper levels of sedation or more drug-related side effects beyond those seen with inhalation anesthetics alone. If needed, drugs are available to reverse the effects of some of these adjuncts.

Dissociative Anesthesia. Dissociative anesthesia interrupts associative brain pathways while blocking sensory pathways. The patient may appear catatonic, is amnesic, and experiences profound analgesia that lasts into the postoperative period. Ketamine (Ketalar) is a commonly administered dissociative anesthetic. Ketamine (administered IV or intramuscularly) is a potent analgesic and amnesic. It is used in asthmatic patients undergoing surgery because it promotes bronchodilation and in trauma patients requiring surgery because it increases heart rate and helps maintain cardiac output. Because ketamine is a phenylcyclohexylpiperidine (PCP) derivative, the drug may cause hallucinations and nightmares, greatly limiting its usefulness. Concurrent use of midazolam (Versed) can reduce or eliminate hallucinations associated with ketamine. Provide a quiet, unhurried environment in the PACU for all patients receiving dissociative anesthesia.[44]

Local and Regional Anesthesia

Local anesthesia interrupts the generation of nerve impulses by altering the flow of sodium into nerve cells through cell membranes. Volume and concentration of the local anesthetic agent will, in accelerating fashion, first block autonomic, then somatic sensory, and, last, somatic motor impulses. The result is autonomic nervous system blockade, anesthesia, and skeletal muscle flaccidity or paralysis. Local anesthetics are topical, ophthalmic, nebulized, or injectable.

A local anesthetic, such as lidocaine (Xylocaine), is applied to a specific area of the body by the surgeon or ACP and does not require sedation or loss of consciousness. Regional anesthesia (or block) using a local anesthetic is always injected and involves a central nerve (e.g., spinal) or group of nerves (e.g., plexus) that innervate a site remote to the point of injection.

Administration of a local or regional anesthetic may involve concurrent use of MAC or moderate sedation (see Table 19-4), either preinjection or intraoperatively. Regional blocks are used as preoperative analgesia, intraoperatively to manage surgical pain, and postoperatively to control pain. Indwelling catheters that deliver local anesthetic via a pump to the surgical site may be implanted before the patient emerges from anesthesia to provide continuous pain relief up to 72 hours postoperatively.

Certain advantages of local and regional anesthesia include rapid recovery and discharge with continued postoperative analgesia and without any accompanying cognitive dysfunc-

TABLE 19-6   DRUG THERAPY

General Anesthesia

Drugs	Advantages	Disadvantages	Nursing Interventions
Intravenous Agents			
Barbiturates			
thiopental (Pentothal) methohexital (Brevital)	Rapid induction, duration of action <5 min.	Adverse cardiac effects (e.g., myocardial depression), hypotension, respiratory depression. *thiopental:* histamine release. *methohexital:* excitation, involuntary movement.	Usually have minimal postoperative effects because of short duration of action. Increased incidence of postoperative nausea in patients with barbiturate sensitivity, histamine-triggered nausea, vomiting.
Nonbarbiturate Hypnotics			
etomidate (Amidate)	Produces little change in cardiovascular dynamics. Useful for hemodynamically unstable patients. Only minor respiratory depression. No histamine release.	Associated with adverse effects of myoclonia, nausea and vomiting, hiccups, and adrenocortical inhibition.	Observe for transient skeletal muscle movements (myoclonia), nausea and vomiting, hiccups, hypotension, hypoglycemia.
propofol (Diprivan)	Ideal for short outpatient procedures because of rapid onset of action, metabolic clearance. May be used for induction and maintenance of anesthesia.	May cause bradycardia and other dysrhythmias, hypotension, apnea, transient phlebitis, nausea and vomiting, hiccups. May cause hypertriglyceridemia.	Monitor for postoperative hypotension, bradycardia. Monitor serum triglycerides q24hr for sedation >24 hr.
Inhalation Agents			
Volatile Liquids			
isoflurane (Forane) desflurane (Suprane) sevoflurane (Ultane) halothane (Fluothane)	All cause skeletal muscle relaxation. *isoflurane:* No increase in ventricular irritability. Does not cause liver or renal toxicity. Resistant to metabolic breakdown. *desflurane:* Fastest onset and emergence, widely used in ambulatory settings. Least postoperative cognitive dysfunction. Potential airway irritant. *sevoflurane:* Predictable effects on cardiovascular and respiratory systems, rapid acting. Preferred for inhalation induction as nonirritating to respiratory tract. *halothane:* Bronchodilation, nonirritating to respiratory tract.	All cause respiratory depression, hypotension, myocardial depression. *isoflurane and desflurane:* May be unsuitable for patients with coronary artery disease. *sevoflurane:* May be associated with emergence delirium (see Chapter 20). Atypical seizure-like activity has been reported. *halothane:* Ventricular excitability, hepatotoxicity.	Assess and treat pain during early anesthesia recovery. Assess for adverse reactions such as cardiopulmonary depression with hypotension and prolonged respiratory depression. Monitor for nausea and vomiting.
Gaseous Agents			
nitrous oxide	Potentiates volatile agents, thus speeding induction and reducing total dosage and side effects. Good analgesic potency. Produces little or no toxicity at therapeutic concentrations.	Weak anesthetic, rarely used alone. Must be administered with O_2 to prevent hypoxemia. Avoid in patients with strong history of nausea and vomiting.	Avoid in patients with bone marrow depression.
Dissociative Anesthetic			
ketamine (Ketalar)	Can be administered IV or IM. Potent analgesic and amnesic.	May cause hallucinations and nightmares, increased intracranial and intraocular pressure, ↑ heart rate, ↑ blood pressure.	Anticipate administration of a benzodiazepine if agitation and hallucinations occur. Calm, quiet environment is essential in postoperative care.

tion.[45] Patients with co-morbidities that would preclude general anesthesia are now offered surgical solutions with increased safety. Some disadvantages to local and regional anesthesia include the potential for technical difficulties; discomfort at the injection site; and the risk of inadvertent vascular injection leading to refractory hypotension, dysrhythmias, and possible seizures. Finally, the inability to precisely match the agent's duration of action to the duration of the surgical procedure is a limiting factor.

In ambulatory or outpatient procedures, you may assist a physician in the administration of a peripheral or regional block. Consequently, you must be familiar with the drugs, the methods of administration, and adverse and toxic effects of the drugs. Initial assessment of the patient should include detailed questioning of the patient's history with local anesthetics and any adverse events associated with their use by the patient or blood relatives.

Many patients report "allergies" to local anesthetics. Although true allergies to local anesthetics occur, they are rare. Allergies are likely to be a result of additives or preservatives in the preparation. Moreover, many local anesthetics are combined with epinephrine solutions. They may be absorbed in the tissues or inadvertently injected IV. Once the agent enters the general circulation, the patient may experience tachycardia, hyperten-

TABLE 19-7 DRUG THERAPY

Adjuncts to General Anesthesia

Agents	Uses During Anesthesia	Adverse Effects	Nursing Interventions
Opioids fentanyl (Sublimaze) sufentanil (Sufenta) morphine sulfate hydromorphone (Dilaudid) alfentanil (Alfenta) remifentanil (Ultiva) methadone (Dolophine)	Induce and maintain anesthesia, reduce stimuli from sensory nerve endings, provide analgesia during surgery and recovery in PACU.	Respiratory depression, stimulation of vomiting center, possible bradycardia and peripheral vasodilation (when combined with anesthetics). High incidence of pruritus in both regional and IV administration.	Assess respiratory rate and rhythm, monitor pulse oximetry, protect airway in anticipation of vomiting. Use standing orders for antipruritics and antiemetics. Reverse opioid-induced respiratory depression with naloxone (Narcan). If used, reversal of analgesic effects also occurs.
Benzodiazepines midazolam (Versed) diazepam (Valium) lorazepam (Ativan)	Reduce anxiety preoperatively and postoperatively, induce and maintain anesthesia, induce amnesia, treat emergence delirium. Supplement sedation in local and regional anesthesia and MAC.	Synergistic effect with opioids, increasing potential for respiratory depression. Hypotension and tachycardia. Prolonged sedation or confusion.	Monitor level of consciousness. Assess for respiratory depression, hypotension, and tachycardia. Reverse severe benzodiazepine-induced respiratory depression with flumazenil (Romazicon).
Neuromuscular Blocking Agents *Depolarizing agent:* succinylcholine (Anectine) *Nondepolarizing agents:* vecuronium (Norcuron) pancuronium (Pavulon) pipecuronium (Arduan) doxacurium (Nuromax) rocuronium (Zemuron)	Facilitate endotracheal intubation, promote skeletal muscle relaxation (paralysis) to enhance access to surgical sites. Effects of nondepolarizing agents are usually reversed toward end of surgery by administration of anticholinesterase agents (e.g., neostigmine, pyridostigmine).	Apnea related to paralysis of respiratory muscles. Duration of action of nondepolarizing agents may be longer than surgery. Reversal agents may not completely eliminate effects. Confusion and nausea. Recurrence of muscle weakness with correction of hypothermia.	If intubated, monitor return of muscle strength, level of consciousness, and ventilation. Maintain patent airway. Monitor respiratory rate and rhythm until patient able to cough and return to previous levels of muscle strength. Ensure availability of nondepolarizing reversal agents (e.g., neostigmine [Prostigmin]) and emergency respiratory support equipment. Monitor temperature and levels of muscle strength with temperature changes.
Antiemetics ondansetron (Zofran) dolasetron (Anzemet) granisetron (Kytril) metoclopramide (Reglan) prochlorperazine (Compazine) promethazine (Phenergan) scopolamine (Transderm-Scōp) diphenhydramine (Benadryl)	Counteract emetic effects of inhalation agents and opioids. Prophylactic prevention of nausea and vomiting related to histamine release, vagal stimulation, vestibular disturbance, surgical procedure (e.g., abdominal and laparoscopic procedures).	Headache, dizziness, IV irritation, dysrhythmias, dysphoria, dystonia, dry mouth, central nervous system sedation.	Monitor heart rhythm, cardiopulmonary status, level of central nervous system excitation or sedation, ability to move limbs, presence of nausea or vomiting.
Miscellaneous dexamethasone (Decadron)	Counteract emetic effects of inhalation agents and opioids (off-label use).*	Insomnia, nervousness, abdominal distention.	Monitor for possible side effects.

*For an explanation of off-label drug use, see *www.cancer.org/docroot/ETO/content/ETO_1_2x_Off-Label_Drug_Use.asp.*
MAC, Monitored anesthesia care; *PACU,* postanesthesia care unit.

sion, and a general perception of panic. There are two classes of local anesthetics: esters and amides. It is highly unlikely that an individual is allergic to both. Therefore it is important to carefully question the patient concerning the agent and the symptoms experienced so that an agent in the proper class can be selected for the procedure.

Methods of Administration. Local anesthetics are injected at the surgical site, nebulized, or applied topically. Topical applications, with or without compression, of creams, ointments, aerosols, and liquids are all standard methods of administration. The agent is applied directly to the skin, mucous membranes, or open surface. Eutectic mixture of local anesthetics (EMLA cream, a combination of prilocaine and lidocaine) is an example of a cream applied to the site 30 to 60 minutes before the pro-

cedure for analgesia. The success of injected local anesthetics may be limited by prolonged duration of procedure or infection at the injection site, thus interfering with drug absorption.

Whenever a patient is prepared for regional anesthesia, airway equipment, emergency drugs, and a cardiac monitor/defibrillator should be immediately available to provide advanced airway and cardiopulmonary support if necessary. Inadvertent IV injection of the agent or excessive absorption of bupivacaine (Sensorcaine), in particular, may lead to cardiac depression, severe dysrhythmias, or cardiac arrest.[46]

Examples of common regional nerve blocks include brachial plexus block; IV regional anesthesia (IVRA) or Bier block anesthesia; and femoral, axillary, cervical, sciatic, ankle, and retrobulbar blocks. For IVRA or Bier block, the patient has a

Spinal cord
Subarachnoid space
Dura

L2

L3

A

L4

Epidural space with anesthesia

B

C

L5

Sagittal section

FIG. 19-6 Location of needle point and injected anesthetic relative to dura and spinal cord. **A,** Spinal anesthesia. **B,** Single-injection epidural. **C,** Epidural catheter. (Interspaces most commonly used are L2-3, L4-5, L3-4.)

double-cuff tourniquet applied as a safety measure. You can facilitate the success of regional anesthesia by assisting in patient positioning, monitoring vital signs during block delivery, administering oxygen therapy, and using supporting devices (at the direction of the ACP) that contribute to the anesthesia (e.g., ultrasound imaging, nerve stimulator, tourniquets).

Spinal and Epidural Anesthesia. Spinal anesthesia and epidural anesthesia are also types of regional anesthesia. Spinal anesthesia involves the injection of a local anesthetic into the cerebrospinal fluid found in the subarachnoid space, usually below the level of L2 (Fig. 19-6, *A*). The local anesthetic mixes with cerebrospinal fluid. Depending on the extent of its spread, various levels of anesthesia are achieved. Because the local anesthetic is administered directly into the cerebrospinal fluid, a spinal anesthetic produces an autonomic, sensory, and motor blockade. Patients experience vasodilation and may become hypotensive as a result of the autonomic block. They feel no pain as a result of the sensory block. They cannot move as a result of the motor block. The duration of action of the spinal anesthetic depends on the agent selected and the dose administered. A spinal anesthetic may be used for procedures involving the extremities (e.g., joint replacements) and lower gastrointestinal, prostate, and gynecologic surgeries.[47]

An **epidural block** involves injection of a local anesthetic into the epidural space via a thoracic or lumbar approach (see Fig. 19-6, *B*). The anesthetic agent does not enter the cerebrospinal fluid but binds to nerve roots as they enter and exit the spinal cord. With use of a low concentration of local anesthetic, sensory pathways are blocked but motor fibers remain intact. In higher doses, both sensory and motor fibers are blocked. Epidural anesthesia may be used as the sole anesthetic for a surgical procedure. In addition, a catheter may be placed to allow for intraoperative use and continued analgesia in the postoperative period (see Fig. 19-6, *C*). For postoperative analgesia, lower doses of epidurally administered local anesthetic, usually in combination with an opioid, are used.[47] Epidural anesthesia is commonly used for analgesia, or in combination with MAC or general anesthesia, in obstetrics, vascular procedures involving the lower extremities, lung resections, and renal and midab-

dominal surgeries. The desirable effects of vasodilation and analgesia contribute to better surgical outcomes.[48]

When spinal or epidural anesthesia is used, the patient can remain fully conscious, receive MAC, or choose general anesthesia. The onset of spinal anesthesia is more rapid than that of epidural anesthesia. Both spinal and epidural anesthesia may be extended in duration using indwelling catheters, thus allowing administration of additional doses of anesthetic. Closely observe the patient for signs of autonomic nervous system blockade. These include hypotension, bradycardia, nausea, and vomiting. There is less autonomic nervous system blockade with epidural anesthesia than with spinal anesthesia. Should "too high" a block be achieved, the patient may experience tingling in the arms and hands or inadequate breathing and apnea.[47] Other complications of spinal or epidural anesthesia include postdural puncture headache, back pain, isolated nerve injury, and meningitis.

GERONTOLOGIC CONSIDERATIONS

PATIENT DURING SURGERY

Although anesthetic agents have become safer and more predictable, the aging process affects the pharmacokinetics of drugs, specifically the absorption, distribution, and metabolism of medications. This results in alterations in the onset, peak, and duration of medications independent of the route of administration. Because of this, anesthetic drugs should be carefully titrated when given to older adults. Physiologic changes in aging may alter the patient's response not only to the anesthetic but also to blood and fluid loss and replacement, hypothermia, pain, and tolerance of the surgical procedure and positioning. Carefully monitor the older adult's response to all anesthetic agents. Assess the postoperative recovery from these agents before the patient is transferred out of the PACU.

Some older adults may have difficulty communicating and following directions as a result of alterations in hearing or vision. These factors increase the need for clear and concise communication in the OR, especially when preoperative sedation is combined with already existing sensory deficits. Because of decreased ability to perceive discomfort or pressure on vulnerable areas and a loss of skin elasticity, the older adult's skin is at risk for injury from tape, electrodes, warming and cooling blankets, and certain types of dressings. In addition, pooling of solutions used to prepare the skin in dependent areas can quickly create skin burns or abrasions.

The care and vigilance of the entire surgical team are needed in preparing and positioning the older patient. The older adult often has osteoporosis and osteoarthritis. Misalignment, pressure, or other insults to arthritic joints that may be desensitized from administration of an anesthetic may create long-term injury and disability. Older adults are also at a greater risk of perioperative hypothermia. Consider the use of a variety of warming devices and carefully monitor them if used.

CATASTROPHIC EVENTS IN OPERATING ROOM

Unanticipated intraoperative events occasionally occur. Although some might be anticipated (e.g., cardiac arrest in an unstable patient, massive blood loss during trauma surgery), others may occur without warning, demanding immediate intervention by all members of the OR team. Two such events are anaphylactic reactions and malignant hyperthermia.

Anaphylactic Reactions

Anaphylaxis is the most severe form of an allergic reaction, manifesting with life-threatening pulmonary and circulatory complications. The initial clinical manifestations of anaphylaxis may be masked by anesthesia. ACPs administer an array of drugs to patients, such as anesthetics, antibiotics, blood products, and plasma expanders. Because any parenterally administered material can stimulate an allergic response, vigilance and rapid intervention are essential. An anaphylactic reaction causes hypotension, tachycardia, bronchospasm, and possibly pulmonary edema. Antibiotics and latex are responsible for many perioperative allergic reactions. (Anaphylaxis is discussed in Chapter 14.)

Latex allergy has become a particular concern in the perioperative setting, given the use of gloves, catheters, and many other devices containing natural rubber latex. Reactions to natural rubber latex range from urticaria to anaphylaxis with symptoms appearing immediately or at some time during the surgical procedure. Latex allergy protocols should be set up in each institution to provide a latex-safe environment for susceptible individuals.[49] (Latex allergies are discussed in Chapter 14.)

Malignant Hyperthermia

Malignant hyperthermia (MH) is a rare disorder characterized by hyperthermia with rigidity of skeletal muscles that can result in death. It occurs in susceptible people when they are exposed to certain anesthetic agents. Succinylcholine (Anectine), especially when given with volatile inhalation agents, appears to be the primary trigger of the disorder. Other factors, such as stress, trauma, and heat, also have been implicated. When MH does occur, it is usually during general anesthesia, but it may manifest in the recovery period as well.

MH is an autosomal dominant trait but is variable in its genetic manifestation, so predictions based on family history are important but not reliable. (Autosomal dominant disorders are discussed in Chapter 13.) The fundamental defect is hypermetabolism of skeletal muscle resulting from altered control of intracellular calcium. This leads to muscle contracture, hyperthermia, hypoxemia, lactic acidosis, and hemodynamic and cardiac alterations.

Tachycardia, tachypnea, hypercarbia, and ventricular dysrhythmias are generally seen but are nonspecific to MH. MH is generally diagnosed after all other causes of the hypermetabolism are ruled out. The rise in body temperature is not an early sign of MH. Unless promptly detected and treated, MH can result in cardiac arrest and death. The definitive treatment of MH is prompt administration of dantrolene (Dantrium). Dantrolene slows metabolism, reduces muscle contraction, and mediates the catabolic processes associated with MH.[44] A treatment protocol, available from the Malignant Hyperthermia Association of the United States, is often displayed in the OR[50] (see eFig. 19-2 available on the website for this chapter).

To prevent MH, obtain a careful family history and be alert to the development of MH perioperatively. The patient known or suspected to be at risk for this disorder can be anesthetized with minimal risks if appropriate precautions are taken. Patients with MH should be informed of the condition so that family members may be genetically tested.

FUTURE CONSIDERATIONS

Changes in technology and surgical techniques provide new and better treatment modalities for the patient undergoing surgery. For example, the use of *hypothermia,* or the deliberate lowering of body temperature, decreases metabolism and blood loss. This, in turn, reduces both the demand for oxygen and anesthetic requirements. Neurosurgery and selected trauma surgery benefit from this approach.

Transesophageal echocardiography (TEE) is used intraoperatively to assess ventricular function and competency of heart valves and to recognize venous air embolism. TEE is less invasive, inexpensive, and associated with few complications. It is quickly replacing the use of the pulmonary artery catheter during surgery to assess hemodynamics.

Ultrasonic-guided regional anesthesia is the technique of visualizing a nerve or plexus of nerves using ultrasound to place a regional block with more accuracy. This approach results in fewer side effects and increased patient satisfaction.

Minimally invasive surgery (MIS) is rapidly increasing as more procedures are performed using endoscopes. Incisions are smaller, blood loss is reduced, postoperative pain is decreased, and recovery time is shortened with MIS. Similarly, "bloodless surgery" is becoming more of a reality. Techniques to minimize blood loss during and after surgery include drug therapy and techniques for managing low hematocrit, hemostatic agents to enhance clotting and control bleeding, surgical devices and techniques to locate and stop internal bleeding, and surgical and anesthetic techniques to limit blood loss. The goal is to manage blood loss without the need for a blood transfusion.

Hydroxyethyl starch (Voluven, Hespan) is an IV synthetic starch solution approved for use as a blood volume expander during and after surgery. Blood volume expanders are administered to quickly restore some of the volume lost during surgery so that remaining red blood cells can continue to deliver oxygen to the body's tissues. There are also new alternatives to blood transfusions such as the perioperative use of erythropoietin (epoetin α [Epogen, Procrit]) to increase red blood cell count. Research on the development of a synthetic blood substitute (e.g., PolyHeme) is ongoing.

The number of procedures that can be performed using *robotic-assisted surgery* is rapidly growing. For example, laparoscopic procedures using robotics include prostatectomy, cholecystectomy, common bile duct injury repair, small bowel surgery, tubal reanastomosis, internal mammary artery harvesting, and video-assisted thoracoscopic surgery.

More recent technologic advancements have made *telesurgery,* or remote surgery, a reality. In telesurgery, a surgeon at a site separate from the patient performs the surgery using a robotic system located at the patient's site. Telesurgery allows surgeons to perform procedures in areas where their expertise is not readily available. In addition, they can perform procedures on patients in remote or hazardous locations (e.g., war zones).

BRIDGE TO NCLEX EXAMINATION

The number of the question corresponds to the same-numbered outcome at the beginning of the chapter.

1. Proper attire for the semirestricted area of the surgery department is
   a. street clothing.
   b. surgical attire and head cover.
   c. surgical attire, head cover, and mask.
   d. street clothing with the addition of shoe covers.

2. Activities that the nurse might perform in the role of a scrub nurse during surgery include (select all that apply)
   a. checking electrical equipment.
   b. preparing the instrument table.
   c. passing instruments to the surgeon and assistants.
   d. coordinating activities occurring in the operating room.
   e. maintaining accurate counts of sponges, needles, and instruments.

3. The nurse is caring for a patient undergoing surgery for a knee replacement. What is critical to the patient's safety during the procedure (select all that apply)?
   a. Universal protocol is followed.
   b. The ACP is an anesthesiologist.
   c. The patient has adequate health insurance.
   d. The circulating nurse is a registered nurse.
   e. The patient's allergies are conveyed to the surgical team.

4. The nurse's primary responsibility for the care of the patient undergoing surgery is
   a. developing an individualized plan of nursing care for the patient.
   b. carrying out specific tasks related to surgical policies and procedures.
   c. ensuring that the patient has been assessed for safe administration of anesthesia.
   d. performing a preoperative history and physical assessment to identify patient needs.

5. When scrubbing at the scrub sink, the nurse should
   a. scrub from elbows to hands.
   b. scrub without mechanical friction.
   c. scrub for a minimum of 10 minutes.
   d. hold the hands higher than the elbows.

6. When positioning a patient in preparation for surgery, the nurse understands that injury to the patient is most likely to occur as a result of
   a. incorrect musculoskeletal alignment.
   b. loss of perception of pain or pressure.
   c. pooling of blood in peripheral vessels.
   d. disregarding the patient's need for modesty.

7. Intravenous induction for general anesthesia is the method of choice for most patients because
   a. the patient is not intubated.
   b. the agents are nonexplosive.
   c. induction is rapid and pleasant.
   d. emergence is longer but with fewer complications.

1. b, 2. b, c, e, 3. a, e, 4. a, 5. d, 6. a, 7. c

⊖volve

For rationales to these answers and even more NCLEX review questions, visit http://evolve.elsevier.com/Lewis/medsurg.

REFERENCES

*1. Association of periOperative Registered Nurses: Recommended practices for surgical attire. In Perioperative standards and recommended practices, Denver, 2012, The Association.

*2. Association of periOperative Registered Nurses: Recommended practice for traffic patterns in the perioperative practice setting. In Perioperative standards and recommended practices, Denver, 2012, The Association.

3. The Joint Commission: Surgical care improvement project, 2011. Retrieved from www.jointcommission.org/surgical_care_improvement_project.

4. The Joint Commission: National patient safety goals. Retrieved from www.jointcommission.org/assets/1/6/NPSG_Chapter_Jan2012_HAP.pdf.

5. Phillips N: Berry and Kohn's operating room technique, ed 12, St Louis, 2013, Mosby.

6. Rothrock JC: Alexander's care of the patient in surgery, ed 14, St Louis, 2011, Mosby.

7. Agency for Healthcare Research and Quality: Patient safety network. Retrieved from http://psnet.ahrq.gov/primer.aspx?primerID=9.

8. Competency and Credentialing Institute: CNOR certification, 2012. Retrieved from www.cc-institute.org/cnor.

9. Association of Surgical Technologists: About the profession, 2011. Retrieved from www.ast.org/professionals/about_prof.aspx.

10. Association of periOperative Registered Nurses: AORN position statement on allied health care providers and support personnel in the perioperative practice setting, 2012. Retrieved from www.aorn.org/Clinical_Practice/Position_Statements/Position_Statements.aspx.

11. Association of periOperative Registered Nurses: AORN position statement on RN first assistants, 2011. Retrieved from www.aorn.org/Clinical_Practice/Position_Statements/Position_Statements.aspx.

*12. Association of periOperative Registered Nurses: AORN standards for RN first assistant education programs. In Perioperative standards and recommended practices, Denver, 2012, The Association.

13. American Society of Anesthesiologists: About ASA, 2011. Retrieved from www.asahq.org/aboutASA.htm.

14. American Association of Nurse Anesthetists: Nurse anesthetists at a glance. Retrieved from www.aana.com/ceandeducation/becomeacrna/Pages/Nurse-Anesthetists-at-a-Glance.aspx.

15. Jehovah's Witnesses: Teachings on blood transfusions and related procedures, 2008. Retrieved from www.religioustolerance.org/witness5.htm.

*Evidence-based information for clinical practice.

16. 30-Days Prayer Network: Customs and behavior: tips on how to behave in Muslim countries, 2011. Retrieved from *www.30-days.net/reveal/customs.*

17. About.com: The meanings behind common tattoo symbols and designs, 2009. Retrieved from *http://tattoo.about.com/cs/tatfaq/a/symbols_ancient.htm.*

*18. Shabanloei R, Golchin M, Esfahani A, et al: Effects of music therapy on pain and anxiety in patients undergoing bone marrow biopsy and aspiration, *AORN J* 91:746, 2010.

*19. Association of periOperative Registered Nurses: Recommended practice for sterile field-maintaining. In *Perioperative standards and recommended practices*, Denver, 2012, The Association.

*20. Association of periOperative Registered Nurses: Recommended practice for counts—sponge, sharp and instrument. In *Perioperative standards and recommended practices*, Denver, 2012, The Association.

*21. Steelman VM: Designing a safer process to prevent retained surgical sponges: a healthcare failure mode and effect analysis, *AORN J* 94:132, 2011.

*22. Association of periOperative Registered Nurses: Recommended practice for hand antisepsis—surgical. In *Perioperative standards and recommended practices*, Denver, 2012, The Association.

23. World Health Organization: WHO guidelines on hand hygiene in health care, 2009. Retrieved from *http://whqlibdoc.who.int/publications/2009/9789241597906_eng.pdf.*

*24. Centers for Disease Control and Prevention: Guideline for hand hygiene in health-care settings, 2002. Retrieved from *www.cdc.gov/mmwr/PDF/rr/rr5116.pdf.* (Classic)

*25. Association of periOperative Registered Nurses: Recommended practice for prevention of transmissible infections in the perioperative practice setting. In *Perioperative standards and recommended practices*, Denver, 2012, The Association.

*26. Cicconi L, Claypool M, Stevens W: Prevention of transmissible infections in the perioperative setting, *AORN J* 92:519, 2010.

27. ECRI Institute: Surgical fire safety update: best practices for prevention. Retrieved from *www.ecri.org/Conferences/Pages/Surgical_Fires.aspx.*

*28. Association of periOperative Registered Nurses: Recommended practice for electrosurgery. In *Perioperative standards and recommended practices*, Denver, 2012, The Association.

*29. Association of periOperative Registered Nurses: AORN position statement on surgical smoke and bio-aerosols, 2012. Retrieved from *www.aorn.org/Clinical_Practice/Position_Statements/Position_Statements.aspx.*

30. The Joint Commission: Universal protocol, 2012. Retrieved from *www.jointcommission.org/assets/1/6/NPSG_Chapter_Jan2012_HAP.pdf.*

*31. World Health Organization: Safe surgery saves lives. Retrieved from *www.who.int/patientsafety/safesurgery/en.*

32. Association of periOperative Registered Nurses: Preventing wrong-patient, wrong-site, wrong-procedure events. Retrieved from *www.aorn.org/Clinical_Practice/Position_Statements/Position_Statements.aspx.*

*33. Association of periOperative Registered Nurses: Recommended practice for positioning the patient in the perioperative practice setting. In *Perioperative standards and recommended practices*, Denver, 2012, The Association.

*34. American Society of PeriAnesthesia Nurses: ASPAN's evidence-based clinical practice guideline for the promotion of perioperative normothermia. Retrieved from *www.aspan.org/ClinicalPractice/ClinicalGuidelines/Normothermia/tabid/5599/Default.aspx.*

*35. Lynch S, Dixon J, Leary D: Reducing the risk of unplanned perioperative hypothermia, *AORN J* 92:553, 2010.

*36. Jardeleza A, Fleig D, Davis N, et al: The effectiveness and cost of passive warming in adult ambulatory surgery patients, *AORN J* 94:363, 2011.

*37. Association of periOperative Registered Nurses: Recommended practice for skin preparation of patients. In *Perioperative standards and recommended practices*, Denver, 2012, The Association.

*38. Centers for Disease Control and Prevention: Guideline for prevention of surgical site infection, 1999. Retrieved from *www.cdc.gov/hicpac/pdf/guidelines/SSI_1999.pdf.* (Classic)

*39. Association of periOperative Registered Nurses: *Perioperative nursing data set: the perioperative nursing vocabulary*, ed 3, Denver, 2011, The Association.

40. American Society of Anesthesiologists: Frequently asked questions. Retrieved from *www.lifelinetomodernmedicine.com/FAQs.aspx.*

41. American Society of Anesthesiologists: Distinguishing monitored anesthesia care ("MAC") from moderate sedation/analgesia (conscious sedation). Retrieved from *www.asahq.org/.../Distinguishing%20Monitored%20Anesthesia%20Care%20From.ashx.*

42. American Association of Nurse Anesthetists: Considerations for policy development number 4.2 registered nurses engaged in the administration of sedation and analgesia, 2010. Retrieved from *www.aana.com/resources2/professionalpractice/Documents/PPM%20Consid%204.2%20RNs%20Engaged%20in%20Sedation%20Analgesia.pdf.*

43. Kossick MA: Inhalation anesthetics. In Naglehout JJ, Plaus KL, editors: *Nurse anesthesia*, ed 4, St Louis, 2010, Saunders.

44. Hodgson BB, Kizior RJ: *Saunders nursing drug handbook 2012.* St Louis, 2012, Saunders.

45. Silverstein JH, Steinmetz J, Reichenberg A, et al: Postoperative cognitive dysfunction in patients with preoperative cognitive impairment: which domains are most vulnerable? *Anesthesiology* 106:431, 2007.

46. Morrell RC: Intralipid might save lives as a rescue from bupivacaine toxicity, 2007. Retrieved from *www.apsf.org/newsletters/html/2007/summer/03_intralipid.htm.*

47. Olson RL, Pellegrini JE, Movinsky BA: Regional anesthesia. In Naglehout JJ, Plaus KL, editors: *Nurse anesthesia*, ed 4, St Louis, 2010, Saunders.

48. Ballantyne JC: Does epidural analgesia improve surgical outcome? *Br J Anesthesia* 92:4, 2004. (Classic)

49. Shoup AJ: Latex allergy. In Watson DS, editor: *Perioperative safety*, St Louis, 2011, Mosby.

*50. Malignant Hyperthermia Association of the United States: Emergency therapy for malignant hyperthermia, 2008. Retrieved from *http://medical.mhaus.org/PubData/PDFs/treatmentposter.pdf.*

RESOURCES

Resources for this chapter are listed in Chapter 20 on p. 366.

Life moves pretty fast. If you don't stop and look around once in a while, you could miss it.

Ferris Bueller

Nursing Management
Postoperative Care

Christine Hoch

evolve WEBSITE

http://evolve.elsevier.com/Lewis/medsurg

- NCLEX Review Questions
- Key Points
- Pre-Test
- Answer Guidelines for Case Study on p. 364

- Rationales for Bridge to NCLEX Examination Questions
- Case Study
  - Patient Undergoing Surgery
- Nursing Care Plan (Customizable)
  - eNCP 20-1: Postoperative Patient
- Concept Map Creator

- Glossary
- Content Updates

eTable
- eTable 20-1: Modified Aldrete Scoring System

LEARNING OUTCOMES

1. Prioritize nursing responsibilities in admitting patients to the postanesthesia care unit (PACU).
2. Prioritize nursing responsibilities in the prevention of postoperative complications of patients in the PACU.
3. Apply data from the initial nursing assessment to the management of the patient after transfer from the PACU to the general care unit.
4. Select appropriate nursing interventions to manage potential problems during the postoperative period.
5. Differentiate discharge criteria from Phase I and Phase II postanesthesia care.

KEY TERMS

airway obstruction, p. 351
atelectasis, p. 351
delayed emergence, p. 357

emergence delirium, p. 357
fast-tracking, p. 349
patient-controlled analgesia (PCA), p. 358

postoperative ileus, p. 359
rapid postanesthesia care unit progression (RPP), p. 349

The postoperative period begins immediately after surgery and continues until the patient is discharged from medical care. This chapter focuses on the common features of postoperative nursing care of the surgical patient. Specific surgical procedures are discussed in the appropriate chapters of this text.

POSTOPERATIVE CARE OF THE SURGICAL PATIENT

The patient's immediate recovery period is managed in a *postanesthesia care unit (PACU),* which is located adjacent to the operating room (OR). This location minimizes transportation of the patient immediately after surgery and provides ready access to anesthesia and OR personnel. During the three phases of postanesthesia care, different levels of care are provided depending on the patient's needs[1] (Table 20-1).

Postanesthesia Care Unit Admission

The patient's initial admission to the PACU is a joint effort among the anesthesia care provider (ACP), the OR nurse, and the PACU nurse. This collaborative effort fosters a smooth transfer of care to the PACU and helps determine the phase to which the patient is assigned.

PACU Progression. How patients move through the phases of care in the PACU is determined by their condition. If a patient assigned to Phase I care on admission to the PACU is stable and recovering well, the patient may rapidly progress through Phase I to discharge to either Phase II care or an inpatient unit. This accelerated progress is called **rapid postanesthesia care unit progression (RPP).** Another accelerated system of care is **fast-tracking,** which involves admitting ambulatory surgery patients directly to Phase II care.[1] Although both RPP and fast-tracking can potentially result in time and cost savings, the patient's safety is the primary

Reviewed by Lisa Kiper, RN, MSN, Assistant Professor of Nursing, Morehead State University, Morehead, Kentucky; Heidi E. Monroe, RN, MSN, CPAN, CAPA, Assistant Professor of Nursing, Bellin College, Green Bay, Wisconsin; and Cynthia Schoonover, RN, MS, CCRN, Associate Nursing Professor, Sinclair Community College, Dayton, Ohio and PACU Staff Nurse, Kettering Medical Center, Kettering, Ohio.

TABLE 20-1	PHASES OF POSTANESTHESIA CARE

Phase I
- Care during the immediate postanesthesia period
- ECG and more intense monitoring (e.g., arterial BP monitoring, mechanical ventilation)
- *Goal:* Prepare patient for transfer to Phase II or inpatient unit

Phase II
- Ambulatory surgery patients
- *Goal:* Prepare patient for transfer to extended observation, home, or extended care facility

Extended Observation
- Extended care or observation unit
- *Goal:* Prepare patient for self-care

Source: American Society of PeriAnesthesia Nurses: *Perianesthesia nursing standards and practice recommendations 2010-2012,* Cherry Hill, NJ, 2010, The Society.

determining factor of where and at what level postoperative care is provided.[2,3]

Phase I Initial Assessment. On admission of the patient to the PACU, the ACP gives you a complete postanesthesia admission report (Table 20-2). The goal of PACU care is to identify actual and potential patient problems that may occur as a result of anesthesia and surgery and to intervene appropriately. Potential problems in the postoperative period are identified in Fig. 20-1. Table 20-3 identifies key components of a PACU assessment.

Begin the assessment with an evaluation of the patient's airway, breathing, and circulation (ABC) status. During the initial assessment, identify signs of inadequate oxygenation and

TABLE 20-2	PACU ADMISSION REPORT

General Information
- Patient name
- Age
- Anesthesia care provider
- Surgeon
- Surgical procedure
- Type of anesthesia (e.g., general, regional, monitored anesthesia care [MAC])

Patient History
- Indication for surgery
- Medical history, medications, allergies
- Preoperative or baseline vital signs, level of consciousness, orientation

Intraoperative Management
- Anesthetic medications
- Other medications received preoperatively or intraoperatively
- Last dose of opioid administration
- Total fluid replacements, including blood transfusions
- Total fluid losses (e.g., blood, nasogastric drainage)
- Urine output

Intraoperative Course
- Unexpected anesthetic events or reactions
- Unexpected surgical events
- Most recent vital signs and monitoring trends
- Results of intraoperative laboratory tests

PACU, Postanesthesia care unit.

TABLE 20-3	INITIAL PACU ASSESSMENT

Airway
- Patency
- Oral or nasal airway
- Laryngeal mask airway
- Endotracheal tube

Breathing
- Respiratory rate and quality
- Auscultated breath sounds
- Pulse oximetry
- Supplemental O_2

Circulation
- ECG monitoring—rate and rhythm
- Blood pressure
- Temperature
- Capillary refill
- Color and temperature of skin
- Peripheral pulses

Neurologic
- Level of consciousness
- Orientation
- Sensory and motor status
- Pupil size and reaction

Gastrointestinal
- Nausea, vomiting
- Intake (fluids, irrigations)

Genitourinary
- Output (urine, drains)

Surgical Site
- Dressings and drainage

Pain
- Incision
- Other

ventilation (Table 20-4). Any evidence of respiratory compromise requires prompt intervention.

Pulse oximetry monitoring provides a noninvasive means of assessing oxygenation and can provide an early warning of hypoxemia.[4] *Transcutaneous carbon dioxide (PTCCO2) and end-tidal CO2 (PETCO2) (capnography) monitoring* are used to detect respiratory depression.[5-6] (Pulse oximetry, PTCCO2, and PETCO2 are discussed in Chapter 26.)

Note and evaluate deviations in electrocardiographic (ECG) results from preoperative findings. Measure the blood pressure (BP) and compare it with baseline readings. Invasive monitoring (e.g., arterial BP) is initiated if needed. Also assess body temperature, capillary refill, and skin condition (e.g., color, moisture). Any evidence of inadequate circulatory status requires prompt intervention.

The initial neurologic assessment focuses on level of consciousness; orientation; sensory and motor status; and size, equality, and reactivity of the pupils. The patient may be awake, drowsy but arousable, or asleep. Because hearing is the first sense to return in the unconscious patient, explain all activities to the patient from the moment of admission to the PACU. If the patient received a regional anesthetic (e.g., spinal, epidural), sensory and motor blockade may still be present and a

TABLE 20-4	MANIFESTATIONS OF INADEQUATE OXYGENATION

Central Nervous System
- Restlessness
- Agitation
- Confusion
- Muscle twitching
- Seizures
- Coma

Cardiovascular System
- Hypertension
- Hypotension
- Tachycardia
- Bradycardia
- Dysrhythmias
- Delayed capillary refill
- Decreased O_2 saturation

Integumentary System
- Flushed and moist skin
- Cyanosis

Respiratory System
- Increased to absent respiratory effort
- Use of accessory muscles
- Abnormal breath sounds
- Abnormal arterial blood gases

Renal System
- Urine output <0.5 mL/kg/hr

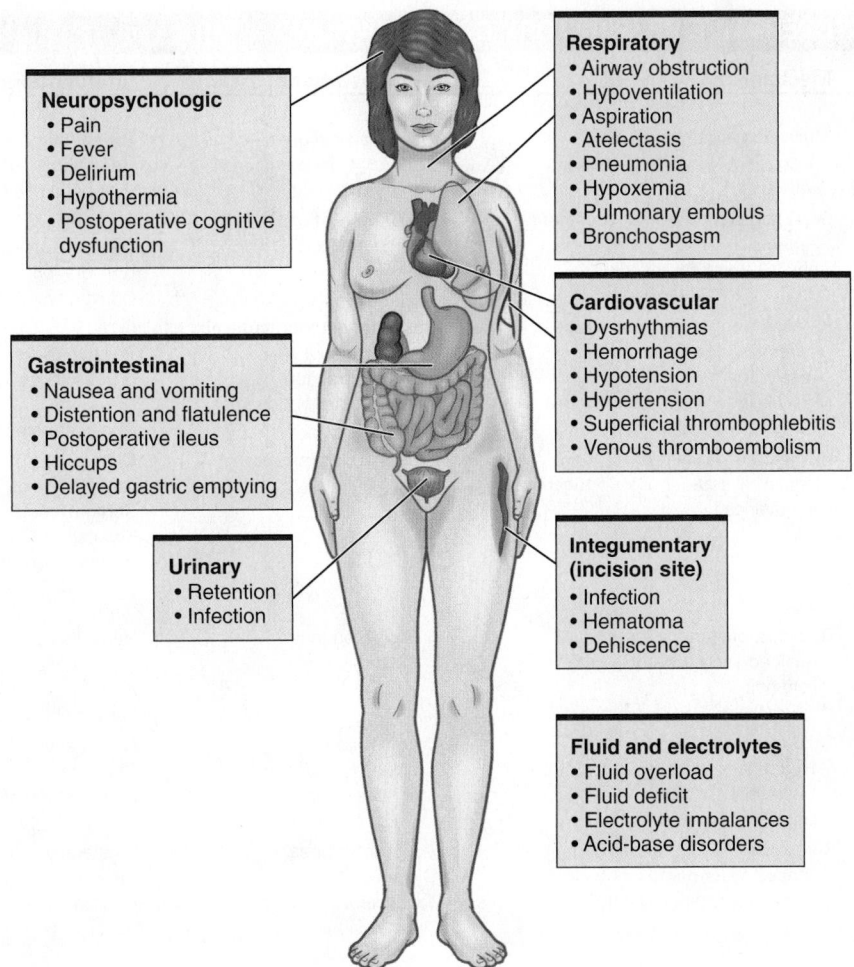

Neuropsychologic
• Pain
• Fever
• Delirium
• Hypothermia
• Postoperative cognitive dysfunction

Respiratory
• Airway obstruction
• Hypoventilation
• Aspiration
• Atelectasis
• Pneumonia
• Hypoxemia
• Pulmonary embolus
• Bronchospasm

Cardiovascular
• Dysrhythmias
• Hemorrhage
• Hypotension
• Hypertension
• Superficial thrombophlebitis
• Venous thromboembolism

Gastrointestinal
• Nausea and vomiting
• Distention and flatulence
• Postoperative ileus
• Hiccups
• Delayed gastric emptying

Urinary
• Retention
• Infection

Integumentary (incision site)
• Infection
• Hematoma
• Dehiscence

Fluid and electrolytes
• Fluid overload
• Fluid deficit
• Electrolyte imbalances
• Acid-base disorders

FIG. 20-1 Potential problems in the postoperative period.

dermatome level should be checked (see eFig. 9-1). (A dermatome is an area of the skin that is supplied by a single spinal nerve.) During recovery from regional anesthesia, sensory and motor function returns from the extremities to the site where the anesthetic was administered. Therefore the areas near the site of injections are the last to recover.

Assessment of the urinary system focuses on intake, output, and fluid balance. Intraoperative fluid totals are part of the anesthesia report. Note the presence of all IV lines; all irrigation solutions and infusions; and all output devices, including catheters and wound drains. Assess the surgical site, noting the condition of any dressings and the type and amount of any drainage. Implement postoperative orders related to incision care.

Nursing management of these problems is discussed in the following pages and can be applied to patients in both the PACU and the clinical unit.

RESPIRATORY PROBLEMS

Etiology

PACU. In the immediate postanesthesia period the most common causes of airway compromise include obstruction, hypoxemia, and hypoventilation (Table 20-5). Patients at high risk include those who have had general anesthesia; are older; have a smoking history; have obstructive sleep apnea or lung disease; are obese; or have undergone airway, thoracic, or abdominal surgery. However, respiratory problems may occur with any patient who has been anesthetized.

Airway obstruction is commonly caused by blockage of the airway by the patient's tongue (Fig. 20-2). The base of the tongue falls backward against the soft palate and occludes the pharynx. It is most pronounced in the supine position and in the patient who is extremely sleepy after surgery.

Hypoxemia, a partial pressure of arterial oxygen (PaO_2) less than 60 mm Hg, is characterized by a variety of nonspecific clinical signs and symptoms, ranging from agitation to somnolence, hypertension to hypotension, and tachycardia to bradycardia. Pulse oximetry will indicate low O_2 saturation (less than 90% to 92%).

The most common cause of postoperative hypoxemia is atelectasis. **Atelectasis** (alveolar collapse) may be the result of bronchial obstruction caused by retained secretions or decreased respiratory excursion. Atelectasis may also result from general anesthesia. Atelectasis occurs when mucus blocks bronchioles or when the amount of alveolar surfactant (the substance that holds the alveoli open) is reduced (Fig. 20-3). As air becomes trapped beyond the plug and is eventually absorbed, the alveoli collapse. Atelectasis may affect a portion of or an entire lobe of the lungs.

Other causes of hypoxemia include pulmonary edema, pulmonary embolism (PE), aspiration, and bronchospasm.

TABLE 20-5	POSTOPERATIVE RESPIRATORY COMPLICATIONS		
Complications	**Mechanisms**	**Manifestations**	**Interventions**
Airway Obstruction			
Tongue falling back	Muscular flaccidity associated with ↓ consciousness and muscle relaxants	Use of accessory muscles Snoring respirations ↓ Air movement	Patient stimulation Head tilt, jaw thrust (see Fig. 20-2) Artificial airway
Retained thick secretions	Secretion stimulation by anesthetic agents Dehydration of secretions	Noisy respirations Coarse crackles	Suctioning Deep breathing and coughing IV hydration Chest physical therapy
Laryngospasm	Irritation from endotracheal tube, anesthetic gases, or gastric aspiration Most likely to occur after removal of endotracheal tube	Inspiratory stridor (crowing respirations) Sternal retraction Acute respiratory distress	O_2 therapy Positive pressure ventilation IV muscle relaxant Lidocaine Corticosteroids
Laryngeal edema	Allergic drug reaction Mechanical irritation from intubation Fluid overload	Similar to laryngospasm	O_2 therapy Antihistamines Corticosteroids Sedatives Possible intubation
Hypoxemia			
Atelectasis	Bronchial obstruction caused by retained secretions or ↓ lung volumes	↓ Breath sounds ↓ O_2 saturation	Humidified O_2 therapy Deep breathing Incentive spirometry Early mobilization
Pulmonary edema	Fluid overload ↑ Hydrostatic pressure ↓ Interstitial pressure ↑ Capillary permeability	↓ O_2 saturation Crackles Infiltrates on chest x-ray	O_2 therapy Diuretics Fluid restriction
Pulmonary embolism	Thrombus dislodged from peripheral venous system and lodged in pulmonary arterial system	Acute tachypnea Dyspnea Tachycardia Hypotension ↓ O_2 saturation Bronchospasm	O_2 therapy Cardiopulmonary support Anticoagulant therapy
Aspiration	Inhalation of gastric contents into lungs	Unexplained tachypnea Bronchospasm ↓ O_2 saturation Atelectasis Interstitial edema Alveolar hemorrhage Respiratory failure	O_2 therapy Cardiac support Antibiotics
Bronchospasm	↑ Smooth muscle tone with closure of small airways	Wheezing Dyspnea Tachypnea ↓ O_2 saturation	O_2 therapy Bronchodilators
Hypoventilation			
Depression of central respiratory drive	Medullary depression from anesthetics, opioids, sedatives	Shallow respirations ↓ Respiratory rate, apnea ↓ PaO_2 ↑ $PaCO_2$	Stimulation Reversal of opioids or benzodiazepines Mechanical ventilation
Poor respiratory muscle tone	Neuromuscular blockade Neuromuscular disease	As above	Reversal of paralysis Mechanical ventilation
Mechanical restriction	Tight casts, dressings, abdominal binders. Positioning and obesity preventing lung expansion	As above	Elevate head of bed Repositioning Loosen dressings
Pain	Shallow breathing to prevent incisional pain	↑ Respiratory rate Hypotension Hypertension ↓ $PaCO_2$ ↓ PaO_2 Complaints of pain Guarding behavior	Opioid analgesic drug therapy Nonsteroidal antiinflammatory drug therapy Adjunctive complementary and alternative therapies (e.g., music therapy, guided imagery)

PaCO₂, Partial pressure of arterial carbon dioxide; *PaO₂,* partial pressure of arterial oxygen.

Tongue

Tongue occluding airway

Manually elevate the jaw
while tilting the head back

Tongue

Airway cleared

FIG. 20-2 Etiology and relief of airway obstruction.

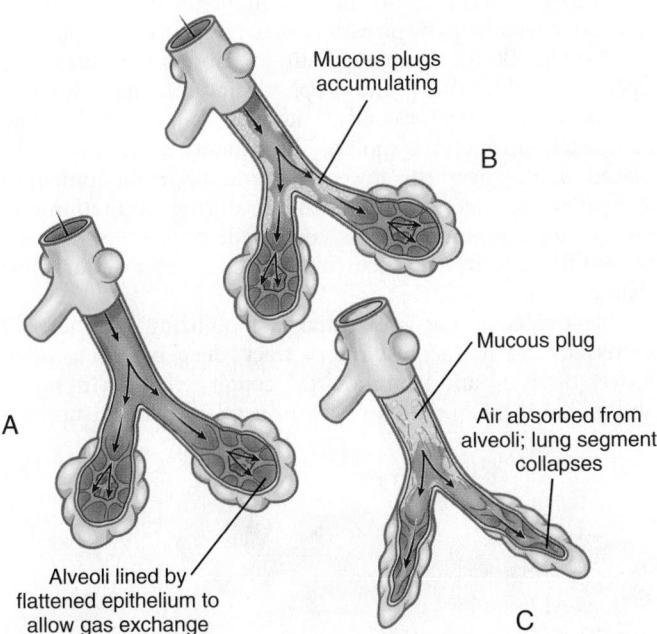

Mucous plugs
accumulating

B

Mucous plug

Air absorbed from
alveoli; lung segment
collapses

A

Alveoli lined by
flattened epithelium to
allow gas exchange

C

FIG. 20-3 Postoperative atelectasis. **A,** Normal bronchiole and alveoli. **B,** Mucous plug in bronchiole. **C,** Collapse of alveoli resulting from atelectasis after absorption of air.

Pulmonary edema is caused by an accumulation of fluid in the alveoli. It may be the result of fluid overload, left ventricular failure, prolonged airway obstruction, sepsis, or aspiration.

Aspiration of gastric contents into the lungs is a potentially serious emergency. Gastric aspiration may also cause laryngospasm, infection, and pulmonary edema. Because of the serious consequences of aspiration of gastric fluids, prevention is the goal.

Bronchospasm is the result of an increase in bronchial smooth muscle tone with resultant closure of small airways. Airway edema develops, causing secretions to build up in the airway. The patient will have wheezing, dyspnea, use of accessory muscles, hypoxemia, and tachypnea. Bronchospasm may be due to aspiration, endotracheal intubation, suctioning, or an allergic response. (Allergic responses are discussed in Chapter 14.) Bronchospasm may occur in any patient but is seen more frequently in patients with asthma and chronic obstructive pulmonary disease (COPD).

Hypoventilation, a common complication in the PACU, is characterized by a decreased respiratory rate or effort, hypoxemia, and an increasing partial pressure of arterial carbon dioxide ($PaCO_2$) *(hypercapnia).* Hypoventilation may result from depression of the central respiratory drive (secondary to anesthesia or pain medication), poor respiratory muscle tone (secondary to neuromuscular blockade or disease), or a combination of both.

Clinical Unit. Common causes of respiratory problems for postoperative patients in the clinical unit are atelectasis and pneumonia, especially after abdominal and thoracic surgery. The postoperative development of mucous plugs and decreased surfactant production is directly related to hypoventilation, immobility and bed rest, ineffective coughing, and history of smoking. Increased bronchial secretions occur when the respiratory passages have been irritated by heavy smoking; acute or chronic pulmonary infection or disease; and the drying of mucous membranes that occurs with intubation, inhalation anesthesia, and dehydration. Without intervention, atelectasis can progress to pneumonia.

NURSING MANAGEMENT
RESPIRATORY PROBLEMS

NURSING ASSESSMENT

For an adequate respiratory assessment, evaluate airway patency; chest symmetry; and the depth, rate, and character of respirations. Observe the chest wall for symmetry of movement. Impaired ventilation may initially be seen as slowed breathing or reduced chest and abdominal movement during breathing. Also assess for the use of abdominal or accessory muscles, which may indicate respiratory distress. Auscultate breath sounds, since decreased or absent breath sounds are found when airflow is diminished or obstructed.

Regular monitoring of vital signs, including pulse oximetry, and a thorough respiratory assessment permit you to recognize early signs of respiratory problems. Manifestations of hypoxemia include tachypnea, gasping, anxiety, restlessness, confusion, and a rapid or thready pulse.

Note and record the characteristics of sputum or mucus. Mucus from the trachea and throat is normally colorless and thin in consistency. Sputum from the lungs and bronchi is normally thick with a pale yellow tinge. Changes in sputum (e.g., color) may indicate a respiratory infection.

DELEGATION DECISIONS
Postoperative Patient

In the PACU, patients require frequent assessment and intervention by RNs. On the clinical units, the RN is responsible for assessment, development of an individualized plan of care, evaluation of the patient, and discharge teaching. Much of the care can be delegated to LPN/LVNs and UAP.

PACU	Clinical Unit
Registered Nurse (RN)	
• Assess patient's initial airway, breathing, and circulation status.	• Assess patient on initial admission to the clinical unit.
• Evaluate for the return to consciousness, ability to maintain airway and breathing.	• Assess for postoperative complications (e.g., atelectasis, hemodynamic instability, cognitive dysfunction, pain, fluid and electrolyte disturbance, fever or hypothermia, nausea and vomiting, urinary retention, wound infection).
• Provide ongoing assessments for postoperative problems (e.g., airway obstruction, hypoventilation, hypotension or hypertension, dysrhythmias, emergence delirium).	
• Evaluate patient's readiness to transfer to the clinical unit or be discharged from ambulatory surgery.	• Develop an individualized plan of care based on identification of patient risk factors and potential complications.
• Provide oral and written report about patient status when transferring patient to RN on the clinical unit.	• Develop and implement individualized patient and caregiver education, including discharge teaching.
• Provide discharge teaching for patient and caregiver after ambulatory surgery.	
Licensed Practical/Vocational Nurse (LPN/LVN)	
• Administer and titrate O₂ based on agency protocols.	• Titrate O₂ administration according to prescribed parameters.
• Administer analgesics and IV fluids (consider state nurse practice act and agency policy).	• Monitor pain level and administer prescribed analgesics.
	• Administer medications (consider state nurse practice act and agency policy for medications).
	• Provide wound care, including dressing changes.
	• Use bladder ultrasound to check for urinary retention.
	• Insert catheter as prescribed for urinary retention.
Unlicensed Assistive Personnel (UAP)	
• Assist with positioning of patients in the "recovery" position.	• Monitor vital signs, pulse oximetry, and intake and output. Report abnormal levels to RN.
• Obtain vital signs and pulse oximetry; report abnormal levels to RN.	• Assist patient with deep breathing and coughing exercises.
• Assist patient with elimination needs.	• Report complaints of pain to RN or LPN/LVN.
• Assist in transfer of patient to clinical unit.	• Reposition and ambulate patients.
	• Provide hygiene, including oral care.
	• Assist with nutrition and elimination needs.

NURSING DIAGNOSES

Nursing diagnoses and collaborative problems related to respiratory problems include, but are not limited to, the following:

- Ineffective airway clearance *related to* ineffective cough, obstruction, pain
- Ineffective breathing pattern *related to* anesthetic agents, pain
- Impaired gas exchange *related to* hypoventilation
- Risk for aspiration
- Potential complication: pneumonia
- Potential complication: atelectasis

NURSING IMPLEMENTATION

In the PACU, nursing interventions are designed to prevent and treat respiratory problems. Proper positioning of the patient facilitates respirations and protects the airway.

> **SAFETY ALERT**
> - Position the unconscious patient in a lateral "recovery" position (Fig. 20-4) to keep the airway open and reduce the risk of aspiration if vomiting occurs.

Once conscious, the patient is usually returned to a supine position with the head of the bed elevated. This position maximizes expansion of the thorax by decreasing the pressure of the abdominal contents on the diaphragm.

Oxygen therapy is used if the patient has had general anesthesia or if ordered. Oxygen is given via nasal cannula or face mask. The oxygen aids in the elimination of anesthetic gases and helps meet the increased demand for oxygen resulting from decreased blood volume or increased cellular metabolism.

Deep breathing is encouraged to aid gas exchange and to promote the return to consciousness. Once the patient is more awake, deep-breathing and coughing techniques help prevent alveolar collapse and move respiratory secretions to larger airway passages for expectoration. One technique, known as *sustained maximal inspiration,* requires the patient to inhale as deeply as possible and, at the peak of inspiration, hold the breath for a few seconds, and then exhale. This should be followed by a second deep breath and cough. The use of an incentive spirometer helps by providing visual feedback of respiratory effort (Fig. 20-5). Diaphragmatic or abdominal breathing involves inhaling slowly and deeply through the nose, holding the breath for a few seconds, and then exhaling slowly and completely through the mouth. The patient's hands should be placed lightly over the lower ribs and upper abdomen so the patient can feel the abdomen rise during inspiration and fall during expiration. Unless contraindicated, encourage the patient to perform these maneuvers 10 times every hour while awake.

Effective coughing is essential in mobilizing secretions. If secretions are in the respiratory tract, deep breathing often moves them up and stimulates the cough reflex. Splinting an abdominal incision with a pillow or a rolled blanket supports

FIG. 20-4 Position of patient during recovery from general anesthesia.

FIG. 20-5 Proper use of an incentive spirometer.

FIG. 20-6 Techniques for splinting incision when coughing.

the incision and aids in coughing and expectorating secretions (Fig. 20-6).

Change the patient's position every 1 to 2 hours to allow full chest expansion and to increase perfusion of both lungs. Sitting in a chair and ambulating should be carried out as soon as physician approval is given. Provide adequate and regular analgesic medication because incisional pain often is the greatest barrier to patient participation in effective breathing exercises and ambulation. Also reassure the patient that these activities will not cause the incision to open. Adequate hydration, either parenteral or oral, is essential to maintain the integrity of mucous membranes and to keep secretions thin and loose for easy expectoration.

Other nursing interventions appropriate for specific respiratory problems are detailed in Table 20-5. A nursing care plan for the postoperative patient (eNursing Care Plan 20-1) is available on the website for this chapter.

CARDIOVASCULAR PROBLEMS

Etiology

PACU. In the immediate postanesthesia period the most common cardiovascular problems include hypotension, hypertension, and dysrhythmias. Patients at greatest risk for alterations in cardiovascular function include those with alterations in respiratory function, those with a history of cardiovascular disease, older adults, the debilitated, and the critically ill.

Hypotension is evidenced by signs of hypoperfusion to the vital organs, especially the brain, heart, and kidneys. Clinical signs of disorientation, loss of consciousness, chest pain, and oliguria reflect hypoperfusion, hypoxemia, and the loss of physiologic compensation. Intervention must be timely to prevent the devastating complications of cardiac ischemia or infarction, cerebral ischemia, renal ischemia, and bowel infarction.

The most common cause of hypotension in the PACU is unreplaced fluid and blood loss, which may lead to hypovolemic shock. Hemorrhage is always a risk of surgery. Marked blood loss is possible when cauterization or sutures fail. Hemorrhage most often occurs internally, requiring assessment for changes in level of consciousness and vital signs. If changes are detected, treatment is directed toward restoring circulating volume. If there is no response to fluid administration, cardiac dysfunction should be considered the cause of hypotension.

Primary cardiac dysfunction, as may occur in myocardial infarction, cardiac tamponade, or PE, results in an acute fall in cardiac output. Secondary myocardial dysfunction occurs as a result of the negative *chronotropic* (rate of cardiac contraction) and negative *inotropic* (force of cardiac contraction) effects of drugs, such as β-adrenergic blockers, digoxin, or opioids. Other causes of hypotension include decreased systemic vascular resistance, dysrhythmias, and measurement errors (e.g., taking BP with an incorrectly sized cuff).

Hypertension, a common finding in the PACU, is most frequently the result of sympathetic nervous system stimulation that may be the result of pain, anxiety, bladder distention, or respiratory compromise. Hypertension may also be the result of hypothermia and preexisting hypertension.

In the PACU, *dysrhythmias* are caused by hypoxemia, hypercapnia, alterations in electrolyte and acid-base status, circulatory instability, and preexisting heart disease. Hypothermia, pain, surgical stress, and many anesthetic agents can also cause dysrhythmias.

Clinical Unit. In the clinical unit, postoperative fluid and electrolyte imbalances are contributing factors to cardiovascular problems. Such imbalances may result from a combination of the body's normal response to the stress of surgery, excessive fluid losses, and improper IV fluid replacement. The body's fluid status directly affects cardiac output.

Fluid retention during postoperative days 1 to 3 can result from the stress response, which serves to maintain both blood volume and BP. Fluid retention is caused by the secretion and release of two hormones by the pituitary—antidiuretic hormone (ADH) and adrenocorticotropic hormone (ACTH)—and activation of the renin-angiotensin-aldosterone system (RAAS). ADH release leads to increased water reabsorption and decreased urine output, increasing blood volume. ACTH stimulates the adrenal cortex to secrete cortisol and, to a lesser degree, aldosterone. Fluid losses resulting from surgery decrease kidney perfusion, stimulating the RAAS and causing marked release of aldosterone (see Chapter 17). Both mechanisms that increase aldosterone lead to significant sodium and fluid retention, thus increasing blood volume.

Fluid overload may occur during this period of fluid retention when IV fluids are administered too rapidly, when chronic (e.g., cardiac, renal) disease exists, or when the patient is an older adult. Fluid deficits from untreated preoperative dehydration, intraoperative blood losses, or slow or inadequate fluid replacement can lead to decreases in cardiac output and tissue perfusion. Postoperative losses from vomiting, bleeding, wound drainage, or suctioning can also contribute to fluid deficits.

Hypokalemia can be a consequence of urinary and gastrointestinal (GI) tract losses. Low serum potassium levels directly affect the contractility of the heart and may contribute to decreases in cardiac output and tissue perfusion. Potassium replacement, usually 40 mEq/day, should not be given until renal function is assessed. A urine output of at least 0.5 mL/kg/hr is generally considered indicative of adequate renal function.

Cardiovascular status is also affected by the state of tissue perfusion or blood flow. The stress response contributes to an increase in clotting tendencies by increasing platelet production. In addition, general anesthesia causes peripheral vasodilation, which may contribute to damage of the vascular lining.

A *venous thromboembolism* (VTE) may form in leg veins as a result of inactivity, body position, and pressure, all of which lead to venous stasis and decreased perfusion. VTE is especially common in older adults, obese individuals, immobilized patients, and patients with a history of PE. It is a potentially life-threatening complication because it may lead to PE and infarction. Suspect PE in any patient with tachypnea, dyspnea, and tachycardia, particularly when the patient is already receiving O_2 therapy. Other manifestations may include agitation, chest pain, hypotension, hemoptysis, dysrhythmias, and heart failure. Superficial thrombophlebitis is an uncomfortable but less serious complication that may develop in a leg vein as a result of venous stasis or in the arm veins as a result of irritation from IV catheters or solutions. (PE and VTE are discussed in Chapters 28 and 38, respectively.)

Syncope (fainting) may indicate decreased cardiac output, fluid deficits, or defects in cerebral perfusion. Syncope frequently occurs as a result of postural hypotension when the patient ambulates. It is more common in the older adult or in the patient who has been immobile for long periods. Normally when the patient stands up quickly, the arterial baroreceptors respond to the accompanying fall in BP with sympathetic nervous system stimulation. This produces vasoconstriction and thereby maintains BP. These sympathetic and vasomotor functions may be diminished in the older adult and the immobile or postanesthesia patient.

NURSING MANAGEMENT CARDIOVASCULAR PROBLEMS

NURSING ASSESSMENT

The most important aspect of the cardiovascular assessment is frequent monitoring of vital signs. They are usually monitored every 15 minutes in Phase I, or more often until stabilized, and then at less frequent intervals in Phase II. Compare postoperative vital signs with preoperative and intraoperative readings to determine when the signs are returning to baseline. Notify the ACP or the surgeon if any of the following occurs:

- Systolic BP less than 90 mm Hg or greater than 160 mm Hg
- Pulse rate less than 60 beats/minute or greater than 120 beats/minute
- Pulse pressure (difference between systolic and diastolic pressures) narrows
- BP trends gradually decrease over several consecutive readings
- Change in cardiac rhythm

ECG monitoring is recommended for patients who have a history of cardiac disease and for all older adult patients who have undergone major surgery, regardless of whether they have cardiac problems. Assess the apical-radial pulse carefully, and report any deficits or irregularities.

Assessment of skin color, temperature, and moisture provides valuable information in detecting cardiovascular problems. Hypotension accompanied by a normal pulse and warm, dry, pink skin usually represents the residual vasodilating effects of anesthesia and suggests only a need for continued observation. Hypotension accompanied by a rapid or weak pulse and cold, clammy, pale skin may indicate impending hypovolemic shock and requires immediate treatment.

NURSING DIAGNOSES

Nursing diagnoses and collaborative problems related to cardiovascular problems include, but are not limited to, the following:

- Decreased cardiac output *related to* hypovolemia, dysrhythmias
- Ineffective peripheral tissue perfusion *related to* prolonged immobility, venous stasis
- Risk for imbalanced fluid volume
- Potential complication: hypovolemic shock
- Potential complication: venous thromboembolism

NURSING IMPLEMENTATION

PACU. Treatment of hypotension should always begin with O_2 therapy to promote oxygenation of hypoperfused organs. Inspect the surgical incision to determine if excessive bleeding is the cause of volume loss. Because the most common cause of hypotension is fluid loss, IV fluid boluses are given to normalize BP. Primary cardiac dysfunction may require drug intervention. Peripheral vasodilation and hypotension may require vasoconstrictive agents to increase systemic vascular resistance.

Treatment of hypertension centers on eliminating the cause of sympathetic nervous system stimulation. Treatment may include the use of analgesics, assistance in voiding, and correction of respiratory problems. Rewarming corrects hypothermia-induced hypertension. If the patient has preexisting hypertension or has undergone cardiac or vascular surgery, drug therapy to reduce BP is usually required.

Because the majority of dysrhythmias seen in the PACU have identifiable causes, treatment is directed toward removing the cause. Correction of these physiologic alterations usually corrects the dysrhythmias. In the event of life-threatening dysrhythmias (e.g., ventricular tachycardia), protocols for advanced cardiac life support are followed.

CLINICAL UNIT. Maintaining an accurate intake and output record, monitoring laboratory findings (e.g., electrolytes, hematocrit), and managing IV therapy are key nursing responsibilities during the postoperative period. Ongoing assessment of the potential complications associated with IV potassium, such as cardiac dysrhythmias and pain at the infusion site, is essential.

Early ambulation is the most significant general nursing measure to prevent postoperative complications. The exercise associated with walking (1) increases muscle tone; (2) stimulates circulation, which prevents venous stasis and VTE, and speeds wound healing; and (3) increases vital capacity and maintains normal respiratory function.

Recommendations for the prevention of VTE for patients who undergo a major surgical procedure or who have multiple risk factors for VTE (e.g., nonambulatory, older, history of VTE) include prophylaxis with low-molecular-weight heparin (LMWH) (e.g., dalteparin [Fragmin], enoxaparin [Lovenox]) or low-dose unfractionated heparin. In addition, sequential compression devices (SCDs) are often used in combination with drug prophylaxis.[7] (SCDs are discussed in Chapter 38.)

You can prevent syncope by slowly making changes in the patient's position. Progression to ambulation can be achieved by first raising the head of the patient's bed for 1 to 2 minutes and then assisting the patient to sit, with legs dangling, while monitoring the pulse rate. If no changes or complaints are noted, start ambulation with ongoing monitoring of the pulse. If changes in the pulse are noted or dizziness occurs, sit the patient in a nearby chair. The patient should remain in this location until the BP and pulse are stable. Then help the patient back to the bed. If dizziness occurs, it is often frightening for the patient and you. Injury can result from a fall, so take measures to ensure patient safety.

NEUROLOGIC AND PSYCHOLOGIC PROBLEMS

Etiology

PACU. Postoperatively, emergence delirium, or *waking up wild,* is the neurologic alteration that causes the most concern. It is manifested by behaviors such as restlessness, agitation, disorientation, thrashing, and shouting. This condition may be caused by hypoxia, anesthetic agents, bladder distention, pain, residual neuromuscular blockade, or the presence of an endotracheal tube.[8] If delirium occurs, first suspect hypoxia.

Delayed emergence may also be a problem postoperatively. Fortunately, the most common cause of delayed emergence is prolonged drug action, particularly of opioids, sedatives, and inhalation anesthetics, as opposed to neurologic injury. Normal awakening can be predicted by the ACP based on the drugs used in surgery.

Clinical Unit. Two types of postoperative cognitive impairments seen in surgical patients are *postoperative cognitive dysfunction* (POCD) and *delirium.* POCD is a decline in the patient's cognitive function (e.g., memory, ability to concentrate) for weeks or months after surgery. POCD is primarily seen in the older surgical patient. Preexisting cognitive impairment, age, duration of anesthesia, intraoperative complications, and postoperative infections are related to the development of POCD.[9]

Postoperative delirium is more common in the older patient, but it can occur in patients of any age. Delirium may be the result of severe postoperative pain, fluid and electrolyte imbalances, hypoxemia, drug effects, sleep deprivation, and sensory deprivation or overload. It is characterized by cognitive dysfunction, varying levels of consciousness, altered psychomotor activity, and a disturbed sleep/wake cycle. (Delirium is discussed in Chapter 60.)

Anxiety and depression may also occur in postoperative patients. Any patient may experience these responses as part of grieving for lost body parts or functions or for decreased independence during the recovery and rehabilitation process.

Alcohol withdrawal delirium occurs as a result of alcohol withdrawal in a postoperative patient. It is characterized by restlessness, insomnia and nightmares, irritability, and auditory or visual hallucinations. Identification and management of alcohol withdrawal delirium are discussed in Chapter 11.

NURSING MANAGEMENT
NEUROLOGIC AND PSYCHOLOGIC PROBLEMS

NURSING ASSESSMENT

Assess the patient's level of consciousness, orientation, memory, and ability to follow commands. Determine the size, reactivity, and equality of the pupils. Also assess the patient's sleep/wake cycle and sensory and motor status. If the neurologic status is altered, try to determine possible causes. If the patient was mentally alert before surgery and becomes cognitively impaired postoperatively, you should suspect delirium or POCD.

NURSING DIAGNOSES

Nursing diagnoses related to neurologic or psychologic problems include, but are not limited to, the following:

- Acute confusion *related to* hypoxia, postoperative cognitive dysfunction, delirium
- Anxiety *related to* change in health status, hospital environment
- Disturbed body image *related to* loss of body part(s), function
- Disturbed sleep pattern *related to* pain, hospital environment

NURSING IMPLEMENTATION

PACU. The most common cause of postoperative agitation in the PACU is hypoxemia. As a result, focus your attention on evaluating respiratory function. Once you have ruled out hypoxemia or other known causes of postoperative delirium, sedation may be beneficial in controlling the agitation. Because the most common cause of delayed emergence is prolonged drug action, delays in awakening usually spontaneously resolve with time. If necessary, benzodiazepines and opioids may be reversed with drug antagonists.

Until the patient is awake and able to communicate effectively, be a patient advocate and maintain patient safety at all times. This includes having the side rails up, securing equipment (e.g., IV lines, artificial airways), monitoring physiologic status, and verifying the presence of identification and allergy bands.

Clinical Unit. To prevent or manage postoperative delirium or POCD, address factors that are known to contribute to the condition. Maintenance of normal physiologic function is important and includes fluid and electrolyte balance, adequate nutrition and sleep, pain management, proper bowel and bladder function, and early mobilization. To help orient the patient, use specific aids, such as clocks, calendars, and photos.

To prevent or limit psychologic problems, provide adequate support for the patient. This includes listening to and talking with the patient, offering explanations and reassurance, and encouraging the presence and assistance of the patient's caregiver(s). Evaluate the patient's behavior to distinguish a normal reaction to a stressful situation from one that is becoming abnormal or excessive. The recognition of alcohol withdrawal delirium presents a particular challenge. Document and report any unusual or disturbed behavior so that a diagnosis and treatment may be made.

PAIN AND DISCOMFORT

Etiology

Despite the availability of pain-relieving drugs and techniques, pain remains a common problem and a significant fear for patients. Postoperative pain is caused by the interaction of a number of physiologic and psychologic factors. The skin and underlying tissues have been traumatized by the incision and retraction during surgery. In addition, there may be reflex muscle spasms around the incision. Anxiety and fear, sometimes related to the anticipation of pain, create tension and further increase muscle tone and spasm. Positioning during surgery or the use of internal devices such as an endotracheal tube or catheters may also result in pain. The effort and movement associated with deep breathing, coughing, and ambulating may aggravate pain by creating tension on the incision area.

When the internal viscera are cut, no pain is felt. However, pressure in the internal viscera elicits pain. Therefore deep visceral pain may signal a complication such as intestinal distention, bleeding, or abscess formation. Pain also increases the risk of atelectasis and impaired respiratory function.[10]

NURSING MANAGEMENT
PAIN

NURSING ASSESSMENT

The patient's self-report is the single most reliable indicator of pain. Since this is not always possible in the PACU, observe the patient for other indications of pain (e.g., restlessness, changes in vital signs, diaphoresis). Identifying the location of the pain is important. Incisional pain is to be expected, but other causes of pain, such as a full bladder, may also be present.

The American Society for Pain Management Nursing and American Society of PeriAnesthesia Nurses have developed evidence-based guidelines for the nursing management of pain throughout the perioperative experience.[11,12] In addition, The Joint Commission requires that effective pain management strategies be implemented for all patients experiencing pain.[13] (Pain is discussed in Chapter 9.)

NURSING DIAGNOSES

A nursing diagnoses for the patient experiencing pain includes, but is not limited to, the following:

- Acute pain *related to* inflammation or injury in surgical area

NURSING IMPLEMENTATION

The most effective interventions for postoperative pain management include using a variety of analgesics. IV opioids provide the most rapid relief.[14] More sustained relief may be obtained using epidural catheters, patient-controlled analgesia (PCA), or regional anesthetic blockade.

Orders for analgesic medication and other comfort measures are often written on an as-needed (PRN) basis. During the first 48 hours or longer, opioid analgesics (e.g., morphine) are required to relieve moderate to severe pain. A combination of two analgesics (e.g., an opioid and a nonsteroidal antiinflammatory drug [NSAID]) may be used to provide the lowest dose of medication and decrease side effects.[15] Nonopioid analgesics, such as NSAIDs, may be sufficient as pain decreases.

Time the administration of analgesics to ensure that they are in effect during activities that may be painful, such as walking. Although opioid analgesics are often essential for the postoperative patient's comfort, there are undesirable side effects. The most common include constipation, nausea and vomiting, respiratory and cough depression, and hypotension. Before administering any analgesic, first assess the patient's pain,

including location, quality, and intensity; respiratory rate; and level of consciousness. If it is incisional pain, analgesic administration is appropriate. If it is chest or leg pain, medication may simply mask a complication (e.g., VTE). If it is gas pain, opioids can aggravate it. If the analgesic either fails to relieve the pain or makes the patient excessively lethargic or somnolent, notify the physician and request a change in the order.

Patient-controlled analgesia (PCA) and epidural analgesia are two alternative approaches for pain control. The goals of PCA are to provide immediate analgesia and to maintain a constant, steady blood level of the analgesic agent. PCA involves self-administration of predetermined doses of analgesia by the patient. The route of delivery may be IV, oral, epidural, or transdermal. The transdermal route is designed for short-term pain management and may offer advantages over the IV route (e.g., needleless, low infection risk, decreased medication errors associated with inaccurate pump function or programming).[14] Some advantages of PCA are early ambulation, better pain management than with PRN analgesia, and greater patient satisfaction. (PCA is discussed in Chapter 9.)

Epidural analgesia is the infusion of opioid analgesics through a catheter placed into the epidural space surrounding the spinal cord (see Fig. 19-6). The goal of epidural analgesia is delivery of medication directly to opiate receptors in the spinal cord. Administration methods include intermittent bolus dosing, continuous infusion, and patient-controlled epidural analgesia. This technique results in a constant circulating level and a reduced total dose of medication. The use of epidural analgesia for postoperative pain is increasing. Superior pain relief and improved functional outcomes after major surgery have been found in patients who receive epidural analgesia compared with those who receive IV opioids.[16,17]

Postoperative pain can also be managed by the infiltration of a nonopioid medication into the surgical site. A single dose of bupivacaine liposome injectable suspension (Exparel) provides pain relief with reduced opioid requirements for up to 72 hours.

The acute pain of surgery almost always requires the use of analgesics. However, nondrug approaches such as repositioning, massage, distraction, and deep breathing can enhance pain management. Complementary and alternative therapies such as music therapy, guided imagery, relaxation exercises, and aromatherapy have also been shown to be effective adjuncts in pain management.[18,19]

ALTERATIONS IN TEMPERATURE

Etiology

The patient's temperature in the postoperative period provides valuable information (Table 20-6).

Hypothermia. *Hypothermia*, a core temperature less than 96.8° F (36° C), occurs when heat loss exceeds heat production. Heat loss may occur due to skin exposure by the surgical procedure and the use of cold irrigants and unwarmed inhaled gases.[20] Although all patients are at risk for hypothermia, patients with a systolic BP less than 140 mm Hg, older patients, and female patients are at a higher risk of developing hypothermia postoperatively.[21] Long surgical procedures and prolonged anesthetic administration lead to redistribution of body heat from the core to the periphery. This places the patient at an increased risk for hypothermia.

Hypothermia can affect the patient's perception of the perioperative experience. The complications associated with hypo-

TABLE 20-6 POSTOPERATIVE TEMPERATURE CHANGES

Time After Surgery	Temperature	Possible Causes
Up to 12 hr	Hypothermia: ≤96.8° F (36° C)	Effects of anesthesia, body heat loss during surgical procedure
First 48 hr (postop days 1 and 2)	Mild elevation: ≤100.4° F (38° C)	Inflammatory response to surgical stress
	Moderate elevation: >100.4° F (38° C)	Lung congestion, dehydration
After first 48 hr (postop day 3 and later)	Elevation >100° F (37.8° C)	Infection (e.g., wound, urinary, respiratory)

thermia can include compromised immune function, bleeding, untoward cardiac events, impaired wound healing, altered drug metabolism, and postoperative pain and shivering.[22] Shivering can increase oxygen consumption, carbon dioxide production, and cardiac output, as well as significantly affect the patient's comfort level.

Fever. Fever may occur at any time during the postoperative period (see Table 20-6). Wound infection, particularly from aerobic organisms, is often accompanied by a fever that spikes in the afternoon or evening and returns to near-normal levels in the morning. The respiratory tract may be infected secondary to stasis of secretions in areas of atelectasis. The urinary tract may be infected secondary to catheterization. Superficial thrombophlebitis may occur at the IV site. VTE in the leg veins may produce a temperature elevation.

Surgical patients who receive antibiotics for a period of time are at risk for *Clostridium difficile* infections. Manifestations of *C. difficile* may include fever, diarrhea, and abdominal pain.

Intermittent high fever accompanied by shaking chills and diaphoresis suggests septicemia. This may occur at any time during the postoperative period because microorganisms may have been introduced into the bloodstream during surgery, especially in GI or genitourinary (GU) procedures. Septicemia may also occur later from a wound or urinary tract infection.

NURSING MANAGEMENT ALTERED TEMPERATURE

NURSING ASSESSMENT
Frequent assessment of the patient's temperature is important to detect patterns of hypothermia or fever. Temperature may be taken orally, temporally, or via the tympanic membrane. The same route of temperature measurement should be used while the patient is in the PACU.[21] Also assess the color and temperature of the skin. Observe the patient for early signs of inflammation and infection that may precede a fever so that any complications can be treated in a timely manner.

NURSING DIAGNOSES
Nursing diagnoses related to an altered temperature include, but are not limited to, the following:
- Hypothermia *related to* long surgical procedures, prolonged use of anesthetics
- Risk for imbalanced body temperature

NURSING IMPLEMENTATION
Passive warming measures include the use of warmed cotton blankets, socks, and reflective blankets and limiting skin exposure. *Active warming measures* involve the application of external warming devices, including forced air warmers; heated water mattresses; radiant warmers; heated, humidified oxygen; and warmed IV fluids. When using any external warming device, assess body temperature and the patient's comfort level at 15-minute intervals.[21] In addition, take care to prevent skin injuries. Oxygen therapy via nasal prongs or mask is used to treat the increased demand for oxygen caused by shivering. Shivering can be treated with opioids (e.g., meperidine [Demerol]).

Measure the patient's temperature every 4 hours for the first 24 hours postoperatively and then less frequently if no problem develops. Meticulous asepsis is required with wound and IV site care. Airway clearance is encouraged with deep breathing, coughing, and the use of the incentive spirometer. If fever develops, chest x-rays may be taken and antipyretic drugs given. Depending on the suspected cause of the fever, cultures of the wound, sputum, urine, or blood are obtained. If a bacterial infection is the source of the fever, antibiotics are started as soon as cultures have been obtained. If the fever rises above 103° F (39.4° C), body-cooling measures may be used.

GASTROINTESTINAL PROBLEMS

Etiology
Nausea and vomiting remain the most common postoperative complications. Risk factors include gender (female), history of motion sickness or previous postoperative nausea and vomiting, action of anesthetics or opioids, and duration and type of surgery.[1,21] Delayed gastric emptying and slowed peristalsis that result from handling of the bowel during abdominal surgery also contribute to nausea and vomiting, as does the resumption of oral intake too soon after surgery.

Postoperative ileus, or the temporary impairment of gastric and bowel motility after surgery, is another common problem and is an expected result of major abdominal surgery.[23] It results from the handling or reconstruction of the intestine during surgery and limited dietary intake before and after surgery. After abdominal surgery, motility in the large intestine may be reduced for 3 to 5 days, although motility in the small intestine resumes within 24 hours. Use of opioid analgesia prolongs the duration of postoperative ileus.[23] Abdominal distention and gas pains can occur as a result of decreased bowel motility, swallowed air, and the accumulation of GI secretions.

Hiccups (singultus) are intermittent spasms of the diaphragm caused by irritation of the phrenic nerve, which innervates the diaphragm. The phrenic nerve may be irritated postoperatively by gastric distention, intestinal obstruction, intraabdominal bleeding, and a subphrenic abscess. Indirect irritation of the phrenic nerve may be produced by acid-base and electrolyte imbalances. Reflex irritation may come from drinking hot or cold liquids or from the presence of a nasogastric (NG) tube. Hiccups usually last a short time and subside spontaneously.

NURSING MANAGEMENT GASTROINTESTINAL PROBLEMS

NURSING ASSESSMENT
Ask the patient about feelings of nausea. If vomiting occurs, determine the quantity, characteristics, and color of the vomitus.

Assess the abdomen for distention and the presence of bowel sounds. Because bowel sounds are frequently absent or diminished in the immediate postoperative period, auscultate all four quadrants to determine the presence, frequency, and characteristics of the sounds. The return of normal bowel motility is usually accompanied by the passage of gas or stool and the patient's ability to tolerate oral intake without complaints of nausea or vomiting.[24]

NURSING DIAGNOSES

Nursing diagnoses and collaborative problems related to GI problems include, but are not limited to, the following:

- Nausea *related to* anesthetic agents, manipulation of abdominal contents
- Imbalanced nutrition: less than body requirements *related to* vomiting, decreased appetite, decreased peristalsis
- Risk for imbalanced fluid volume
- Risk for electrolyte imbalance
- Potential complication: hiccups

NURSING IMPLEMENTATION

Postoperative nausea and vomiting are treated with antiemetic or prokinetic drugs (see Chapter 42, Table 42-1). In the PACU, oral fluids should be given only as ordered and tolerated. IV fluids will provide hydration until the patient is able to tolerate oral fluids. Be alert to prevent aspiration if the patient vomits while still sleepy from anesthesia. Position the patient in the lateral recovery position and have suction equipment readily available at the bedside. Complementary and alternative therapy interventions for nausea and vomiting include guided imagery, music therapy, aromatherapy, distraction, and acupressure.[25]

Depending on the type of the surgery, the patient may begin oral intake as soon as the gag reflex returns. The patient who has abdominal surgery is usually allowed nothing by mouth (NPO) until the return of peristalsis. Chewing gum has been found to aid in the return of bowel motility.[26,27] When the patient is NPO, IV infusions are given to maintain fluid and electrolyte balance. An NG tube may be used to decompress the stomach to prevent nausea, vomiting, and abdominal distention. Regular oral care is essential for comfort and stimulation of salivary glands when the patient is NPO or has an NG tube. When oral intake is allowed, clear liquids are offered first and the IV infusion is continued, usually at a reduced rate. If oral intake is well tolerated, the IV infusion is discontinued, and the diet is advanced until a regular diet is tolerated.

Despite limited evidence to support early ambulation for abdominal distention, it is a standard postoperative intervention.[28] Assess the patient regularly to detect the return of peristalsis as evidenced by the passage of gas or stool. The NG tube must be clamped or the suction turned off when the abdomen is auscultated. Resumption of a normal diet after bowel sounds have returned also enhances the return of normal peristalsis.

Encourage the patient to expel gas. Gas pains, which tend to become pronounced on the second or third postoperative day, may be relieved by ambulation and frequent repositioning. Positioning the patient on the right side permits gas to rise along the transverse colon and aids its release. Bisacodyl (Dulcolax) suppositories may be ordered to stimulate colonic peristalsis and expulsion of gas and stool.

URINARY PROBLEMS

Etiology

Low urine output (800 to 1500 mL) in the first 24 hours after surgery may be expected, regardless of fluid intake. This low output is caused by increased aldosterone and ADH secretion resulting from the stress of surgery; fluid restriction before surgery; and fluid loss through surgery, drainage, and diaphoresis. By the second or third day, after fluid has been mobilized and the immediate stress reaction subsides, the patient will begin to have increasing urine output.

Acute urinary retention can occur in the postoperative period for a variety of reasons. Anesthesia depresses the nervous system, including the micturition reflex arc and the higher centers that influence it. This allows the bladder to fill more completely than normal before the urge to void is felt. Anesthesia also impedes voluntary micturition. Anticholinergic and opioid drugs may also interfere with the ability to initiate voiding or to empty the bladder completely.

Urinary retention is more likely to occur after lower abdominal or pelvic surgery because spasms or guarding of the abdominal and pelvic muscles interferes with their normal function in micturition. Pain may alter perception and interfere with the patient's awareness of bladder filling. Voiding ability is probably impaired to the greatest extent by immobility and bed rest. The supine position reduces the ability to relax the perineal muscles and external sphincter.

Oliguria (the diminished output of urine) can be a manifestation of renal failure and is a less common, although more serious, problem after surgery. It may result from renal ischemia caused by inadequate renal perfusion.

NURSING MANAGEMENT URINARY PROBLEMS

NURSING ASSESSMENT

Examine the urine for both quantity and quality. Note the color, amount, and odor of the urine. Assess indwelling catheters for patency. Urine output should be at least 0.5 mL/kg/hr. To decrease the risk of catheter-associated urinary tract infection (CAUTI), remove the catheter as soon as possible or within 24 hours, unless there is a reason to continue its use.[29] Most patients urinate within 6 to 8 hours after surgery. If no voiding occurs, scan or percuss the suprapubic area for signs of bladder fullness or distention.

NURSING DIAGNOSES

Nursing diagnoses and collaborative problems related to urinary problems include, but are not limited to, the following:

- Urinary retention *related to* anesthetic agents, pain
- Potential complication: acute kidney injury

NURSING IMPLEMENTATION

You can aid voiding by normal positioning of the patient—sitting for women and standing for men. Reassure the patient regarding the ability to void. Helpful techniques include providing privacy, running water, offering water for the patient to drink, or pouring warm water over the perineum. Walking, preferably to the bathroom, and the use of a bedside commode are additional helpful measures to assist in voiding.

The surgeon often leaves an order to catheterize the patient in 6 to 8 hours if voiding has not occurred. Because of the possibility of CAUTI, first try to validate that the bladder is actually full. Consider fluid intake during and after surgery and determine bladder fullness (e.g., discomfort when the bladder is palpated). Scan the bladder with a portable ultrasound to assess volume of urine in the bladder and avoid unnecessary catheterization. If catheterization is required, a straight catheterization (as compared to an indwelling catheter) is preferred to limit the possibility of CAUTI.

INTEGUMENTARY PROBLEMS

Etiology

Surgery generally involves an incision through the skin and underlying tissues, disrupting the protective skin barrier. Therefore wound healing is one of the major concerns during the postoperative period.

Wound infection may result from contamination of the wound from three major sources: (1) exogenous flora present in the environment and on the skin, (2) oral flora, and (3) intestinal flora. The incidence of wound sepsis is higher in patients who are malnourished, immunosuppressed, or older, or who have had a long hospital stay or a lengthy surgical procedure (more than 3 hours). Patients needing bowel surgery, particularly after a traumatic injury, are at high risk. Infection may involve the entire incision and may extend downward through deeper tissues. An abscess may form locally, or it may spread throughout entire body cavities, as in peritonitis.

Evidence of wound infection usually does not become apparent before the third to fifth postoperative day. Local manifestations include redness, swelling, and increasing pain and tenderness at the site. Systemic manifestations are fever and leukocytosis.

An accumulation of fluid in a wound may create pressure, impair circulation and wound healing, and predispose the patient to infection. To allow for drainage, the surgeon may place a drain in the incision or make a stab wound adjacent to the incision. These drains may be made of soft rubber and drain into a dressing, or they may be firm catheters attached to a Hemovac or other source of gentle suction.

An adequate nutritional state is essential for wound healing. Obesity affects abdominal wound healing. Wound healing is also a concern for the older adult. The patient who was well nourished preoperatively can tolerate the postoperative delay in nutritional intake for several days. However, the patient with preexisting nutritional deficits that occur with chronic diseases (e.g., diabetes, ulcerative colitis, alcoholism) is more prone to problems of wound healing. The patient who is unable to meet nutritional needs postoperatively may be provided with enteral or parenteral nutrition to promote healing.

NURSING MANAGEMENT SURGICAL WOUNDS

NURSING ASSESSMENT

Nursing assessment of the wound and dressing requires knowledge of the type of wound, the drains inserted, and expected drainage related to the specific type of surgery. A small amount of serous drainage is common from any type of wound. If a drain is in place, a moderate to large amount of drainage may be expected. For example, an abdominal incision with an accompanying drain is expected to have a moderate amount of serosanguineous drainage in the first 24 hours. In contrast, an inguinal herniorrhaphy should have only minimal serous drainage during the postoperative period.

In general, drainage is expected to change from sanguineous (red) to serosanguineous (pink) to serous (clear yellow). The drainage should decrease over hours or days, depending on the type of surgery. Wound infection may be accompanied by purulent drainage. *Wound dehiscence* (separation and disruption of previously joined wound edges) may be preceded by a sudden discharge of brown, pink, or clear drainage. (Wound dehiscence is discussed in Chapter 12.)

NURSING DIAGNOSES

Nursing diagnoses related to surgical wounds include, but are not limited to, the following:
- Impaired skin integrity *related to* surgical incision
- Risk for infection

NURSING IMPLEMENTATION

When drainage appears on the dressing, document the type, amount, color, and odor of drainage. Expected drainage from tubes is outlined in Table 20-7. Also assess the effect of position changes on drainage. Notify the surgeon of any excessive or abnormal drainage or significant changes in vital signs.

TABLE 20-7 DRAINAGE FROM TUBES AND CATHETERS

Substance	Daily Amount	Color	Odor	Consistency
Indwelling Catheter				
Urine	800-1500 mL for first 24 hr Minimum expected output: 0.5 mL/kg/hr	Clear, yellow	Ammonia	Watery
Nasogastric Tube or Gastrostomy Tube				
Gastric contents	<1500 mL/day	Pale, yellow-green Bloody after GI surgery	Sour	Watery
Hemovac				
Wound drainage	Varies with procedure May decrease over hours or days	Varies with procedure Initially, may be sanguineous or serosanguineous, changing to serous	Same as wound dressing	Variable
T Tube				
Bile	500 mL	Bright yellow to dark green	Acid	Thick

The incision may be covered with a dressing immediately after surgery. If there is no drainage after 24 to 48 hours, the dressing may be removed and the incision left open to the air. If the initial operative dressing is saturated, agency policy determines whether you may change the dressing or simply reinforce it.

When a dressing is changed, note the number and type of drains present, and avoid dislodging the drains. Inspect the incision site carefully. The area around the sutures may be slightly reddened and swollen, which is an expected inflammatory response. However, the skin around the incision should be of normal color and temperature. If the wound is healing by primary intention, has little or no drainage, or has no drains in place, a single-layer dressing or no dressing is sufficient. A multilayer dressing is used when drains are in place, when moderate to heavy drainage is occurring, or when healing occurs other than by primary intention. (Wound healing and care are discussed in Chapter 12.)

DISCHARGE FROM THE PACU

The choice of discharge site is based on patient acuity, access to follow-up care, and the potential for postoperative complications. The decision to discharge the patient from the PACU is based on written discharge criteria (Table 20-8). A standardized scoring system, such as the *Modified Aldrete Scoring System,* is often used to determine the patient's general condition and readiness for discharge from the PACU. (The Modified Aldrete Scoring System is presented in eTable 20-1 on the website for this chapter.)

Discharge to the Clinical Unit

Before discharging the patient from the PACU to the clinical unit, provide a verbal report about the patient to the receiving nurse. The report summarizes the operative and postanesthesia period. It should also include information as to where the patient's caregivers are waiting. Nurse-to-nurse communication must be accurate and allow for questions. The use of a standardized communication tool, such as SBAR *(Situation-Background-Assessment-Recommendation),* provides a complete report and

enhances a safe transfer of the patient from PACU to the clinical unit (Table 20-9). (Handoff communication is discussed in Chapter 1, and SBAR is presented in Table 1-7.)

If you are the nurse who receives the patient on the clinical unit, assist the PACU transport staff to move the patient from the stretcher to the bed. Take care to protect IV lines, drains, and traction devices. Use a draw sheet, transfer board or sling, and sufficient staff to facilitate the safe transfer of the patient. Obtain vital signs and compare the patient status with the report provided by the PACU nurse. After this, perform a more in-depth assessment and initiate postoperative orders and nursing care as appropriate (Table 20-10).

AMBULATORY SURGERY

Phase II and Extended Observation

Advances in minimally invasive and noninvasive procedures, anesthesia, and analgesia have resulted in an increase in ambulatory surgical procedures.[30] Ambulatory surgery patients include those patients receiving Phase II and extended observation postoperative care (see Table 20-1). Postoperative nausea and vomiting and pain are significant problems after ambulatory surgery. These can lead to delirium, prolonged PACU stay, delayed discharge, readmission, delayed resumption of usual activities, and decreased patient satisfaction.[31,32]

Ambulatory Surgery Discharge

The patient leaving an ambulatory surgery setting must be mobile and alert to provide a degree of self-care when discharged to home (see Table 20-8). Postoperative pain, nausea,

---

TABLE 20-8 SURGERY DISCHARGE CRITERIA

PACU Discharge Criteria (Phase I)
- Patient awake (or baseline)
- Vital signs at baseline or stable
- No excess bleeding or drainage
- No respiratory depression
- O₂ saturation >90%
- Pain controlled or acceptable
- Minimal nausea and vomiting
- Report given

Ambulatory Surgery Discharge Criteria (Phase II or Extended Observation)
- All PACU discharge criteria (Phase I) met
- No IV opioid drugs for last 30 min
- Voided if appropriate to surgical procedure or orders
- Able to ambulate if not contraindicated
- Responsible adult present to accompany and drive patient home
- Written discharge instructions given and patient and caregiver understanding confirmed

---

TABLE 20-9 POSTOPERATIVE SBAR HANDOFF COMMUNICATION

Situation
Patient transferring to Room # _____ Date _____
Surgeon _____ Anesthesia _____
Procedure _____
Surgical site(s) _____

Background
Allergies _____
Medications received in PACU _____
IV site/fluids _____
Dressings and/or drains _____
Operative comments _____

Assessment
PACU vital signs T _____ P _____ RR ___ BP _____ O₂ Sat _____
Oxygen source _____ FIO₂ _____
Pain rating at discharge _____
Method of pain management _____
Last dose of pain medication _____
Nausea/vomiting at discharge _____
Intake _____ Output _____
Recovery comments _____

Recommendations
Equipment needed _____
Physician orders to be completed _____
Other notes _____
Transferring RN _____ Phone # for questions _____
Receiving RN _____

Modified from Sandlin D: Improving patient safety by implementing a standardized and consistent approach to hand-off communication, *J Perianesth Nurs* 22:290, 2007.

TABLE 20-10 NURSING ASSESSMENT

Care of Patient on Admission to Clinical Unit

1. Record time of patient's return to unit and assess airway, breathing, and circulation.
2. Obtain baseline vital signs, including O_2 saturation.
3. Assess neurologic status, including level of consciousness and movement of extremities.
4. Assess level of pain:
   - Last dose and type of pain control
   - Current pain rating
5. Assess wound, dressing, and drainage tubes:
   - Type and amount of drainage
   - Tubing connected to gravity or suction drainage (per orders)
6. Assess color, temperature, and appearance of skin.
7. Assess urinary status:
   - Time of voiding
   - Presence of catheter, patency, and total output
   - Bladder distention or urge to void
8. Position for airway maintenance, comfort, and safety (bed in low position, side rails up).
9. Check IV infusion:
   - Type of solution
   - Amount of fluid remaining
   - Patency and flow rate
   - Condition of insertion site and size of catheter
10. Position call light within reach, and orient patient to use of call light.
11. Assess for any nausea or vomiting.
    - Availability of emesis basin and tissues
12. Determine emotional state and provide support as needed.
13. Check for presence of caregiver.
    - Patient and caregiver oriented to immediate environment
14. Check and carry out postoperative orders.

INFORMATICS IN PRACTICE

Discharge Teaching

- If you are discharging a patient who requires a complex dressing change and think that written instructions are not adequate, consider using a video. This may be available on the hospital's television system or the Internet (e.g., YouTube). You could also take a series of pictures that show how to perform the procedure.
- If using a video from the Internet, check it to ensure that the procedure is properly done.
- The patient and caregiver can view the video or pictures at home as a reference when performing the procedure.

---

and vomiting must be controlled. Overall, the patient must be stable and near the level of preoperative functioning for discharge from the unit. At discharge, provide teaching for the patient and the caregiver specific to the type of anesthesia and surgery, and reinforce with written instructions. The patient may not drive and must be accompanied by a responsible adult at the time of discharge. A follow-up evaluation of the patient's status is made by telephone, and any specific questions and concerns are addressed.

Carefully assess the patient's readiness for discharge and home care needs. Determine availability of caregivers (e.g., family, friends) and access to a (1) pharmacy for prescriptions, (2) phone in the event of an emergency, and (3) follow-up care.

Discuss the patient's expectations regarding activity and assistance needed after discharge. The patient and caregiver must be included in discharge planning and provided with the information and support to make informed decisions about continuing care.

Planning for Discharge and Follow-up Care

Preparation for the patient's discharge is an ongoing process that begins during the preoperative period. The informed patient is prepared as events unfold and gradually assumes more responsibility for self-care during the postoperative period. As discharge approaches, be certain that the patient and any caregivers have the following information:

- Symptoms to be reported (e.g., fever, increased incisional drainage, unrelieved incisional pain, discomfort in other parts of the body)
- When and how to take drugs, and possible side effects
- Care of incision and any dressings, including bathing recommendations
- Activities allowed and prohibited. When various activities can be resumed safely (e.g., driving a car, returning to work, sexual intercourse, leisure activities)
- Dietary restrictions or modifications
- Where and when to return for follow-up care
- Answers to any individual questions or concerns

Common reasons patients seek help after discharge include unrelieved pain, need for advice about medications, and wound issues (e.g., drainage). Attention to complete discharge instructions may prevent needless distress for the patient and the caregiver. Standardized, preprinted discharge instructions that are surgery specific and easy to read ensure that information is complete.[33,34]

Document the discharge instructions in the medical record. For the patient, the postoperative phase of care continues and extends into the recuperative period. Assessment and evaluation of the patient after discharge may be accomplished by a follow-up call or by a visit from a nurse (e.g., home health nurse).

Increasingly, patients are being discharged from the hospital with many care needs. They may be transferred to transitional care facilities, to long-term care facilities, or directly to their homes. When discharged directly to home, the patient is expected to continue self-care, with assistance from family, friends, or home health care personnel. The care may include dressing changes, wound care, catheter or drain care, home antibiotics, or continued physical therapy. Working with the discharge planner or case manager, facilitate the patient's safe transition from hospital-based care to community- or home-based care.

GERONTOLOGIC CONSIDERATIONS

POSTOPERATIVE PATIENT

The older postoperative patient deserves special consideration. The older adult has decreased respiratory function, including decreased ability to cough and decreased thoracic compliance. These alterations lead to an increase in the work of breathing and a decreased ability to eliminate drugs. Carefully monitor reactions to anesthetic drugs. Pneumonia is a common postoperative complication in older adults.

Vascular function in the older adult is altered due to atherosclerosis and decreased elasticity in the blood vessels. Cardiac function is often compromised, and compensatory responses to changes in BP and volume are limited. Circulating blood volume is decreased, and hypertension is common. Cardiovascular parameters must be closely monitored throughout surgery and the postoperative period.

Drug toxicity is a potential problem in the older adult. Renal perfusion in the older adult normally decreases, with a reduction in the ability to eliminate drugs that are excreted by the kidneys. Decreased liver function also leads to decreased drug metabolism and increased drug activity. Carefully assess renal and liver function in the postoperative phase to prevent drug overdose and toxicity.[35]

Observing for changes in mental status is an important part of postoperative care in older adults. Factors such as age, history of alcohol abuse, poor baseline cognition, hypoxia, severe metabolic derangement, hypotension, and polypharmacy can contribute to postoperative delirium. Anesthetics, especially anticholinergic drugs and benzodiazepines, also increase the risk for delirium. Despite knowledge of risk factors, postoperative delirium in older adults is poorly understood.[36]

Research suggests that recovery from postoperative delirium is delayed in older patients with high pain levels. This may affect the length of hospital stay and the patient's condition at the time of discharge.[37]

Pain control in the older patient is challenging because of possible preexisting cognitive deficits, impaired communication, and physiologic changes that affect how drugs are metabolized. Older patients may hesitate to request pain medication because they believe that pain is an inevitable result of surgery that should be tolerated. Some older patients may be nervous about using PCA machines.

Thoroughly assess pain in a surgical patient who does not report any pain. Encourage the use of analgesics, and explain to the patient and caregiver that untreated pain has a negative effect on recovery.[35]

CASE STUDY

Postoperative Patient

Stockbyte/Thinkstock

Patient Profile
E.G., a 74-year-old African American retired college professor, has just undergone surgery for a fractured hip. He fell off a ladder while painting his house. The surgery, performed while the patient was under general anesthesia, lasted 3 hours.

Subjective Data
- Was in good health before his fall
- Played tennis three times each week
- Smokes 1 pack of cigarettes per day × 58 years
- Always had problems sleeping
- Difficulty hearing, wears hearing aid
- Upset with injury and its impact on activity
- Is a widower and has no relatives nearby or friends to assist with care
- Reports pain is 8 on a 0-10 scale on arrival to PACU

Objective Data
- Admitted to PACU with abduction pillow between his legs, one peripheral IV catheter, a self-suction drain from the hip dressing, an indwelling urinary catheter
- O₂ saturation 91% on 40% O₂ face mask

Collaborative Care
Postoperative Orders
- Vital signs per PACU routine
- Dextrose 5% in 0.45 normal saline at 100 mL/hr
- Morphine via patient-controlled analgesia 1 mg q10min (20 mg max in 4 hr) for pain
- Advance diet as tolerated
- Incentive spirometry q1hr × 10 while awake
- O₂ therapy to keep O₂ saturation >90%
- Neurovascular checks q1hr × 4 hr
- Empty and measure self-suction drain every shift
- Strict intake and output

Discussion Questions
1. What are the potential postanesthesia problems that you might expect with E.G.?
2. **Priority Decision:** What priority nursing interventions would be appropriate to prevent these complications from occurring?
3. **Delegation Decision:** Which of these interventions could you delegate to unlicensed assistive personnel (UAP)?
4. What factors may predispose E.G. to the following problems: atelectasis, infection, pulmonary embolism, nausea and vomiting?
5. How can you determine when E.G. is sufficiently recovered from general anesthesia to be discharged to the clinical unit?
6. What potential postoperative problems on the clinical unit might you expect?
7. What are risk factors for this patient developing postoperative delirium? What are the signs and symptoms of delirium?
8. Why is drug toxicity a potential problem for E.G.?
9. **Priority Decision:** Based on the assessment data presented, identify two priority nursing diagnoses. Are there any collaborative problems?
10. **Evidence-Based Practice:** E.G. asks you why he has to use the incentive spirometer. How would you respond to this question?

evolve Answers available at *http://evolve.elsevier.com/Lewis/medsurg.*

BRIDGE TO NCLEX EXAMINATION

The number of the question corresponds to the same-numbered outcome at the beginning of the chapter.

1. When a patient is admitted to the PACU, what are the priority interventions the nurse performs?
   a. Assess the surgical site, noting presence and character of drainage.
   b. Assess the amount of urine output and the presence of bladder distention.
   c. Assess for airway patency and quality of respirations, and obtain vital signs.
   d. Review results of intraoperative laboratory values and medications received.

2. A patient is admitted to the PACU after major abdominal surgery. During the initial assessment the patient tells the nurse he thinks he is going to "throw up." A priority nursing intervention would be to
   a. increase the rate of the IV fluids.
   b. obtain vital signs, including O₂ saturation.
   c. position patient in lateral recovery position.
   d. administer antiemetic medication as ordered.

3. After admission of the postoperative patient to the clinical unit, which assessment data require the most immediate attention?
   a. Oxygen saturation of 85%
   b. Respiratory rate of 13/min
   c. Temperature of 100.4° F (38° C)
   d. Blood pressure of 90/60 mm Hg

4. A 70-kg postoperative patient has an average urine output of 25 mL/hr during the first 8 hours. The priority nursing intervention(s) given this assessment would be to
   a. perform a straight catheterization to measure the amount of urine in the bladder.
   b. notify the physician and anticipate obtaining blood work to evaluate renal function.
   c. continue to monitor the patient because this is a normal finding during this time period.
   d. evaluate the patient's fluid volume status since surgery and obtain a bladder ultrasound.

5. Discharge criteria for the Phase II patient include (*select all that apply*)
   a. no nausea or vomiting.
   b. ability to drive self home.
   c. no respiratory depression.
   d. written discharge instructions understood.
   e. opioid pain medication given 45 minutes ago.

1. c, 2. c, 3. a, 4. d, 5. c, d, e

ⓔ*volve*

For rationales to these answers and even more NCLEX review questions, visit *http://evolve.elsevier.com/Lewis/medsurg.*

REFERENCES

*1. American Society of PeriAnesthesia Nurses: *Perianesthesia nursing standards and practice recommendations 2010-2012,* Cherry Hill, NJ, 2012, The Society.

2. Varadhan KK, Lobo DN, Ljungqvist O: Enhanced recovery after surgery: the future of improving surgical care, *Crit Care Clin* 26(3):527, 2010.

*3. Larsson G, Holgers K: Fast-track care for patients with suspected hip fracture, *Injury* 42:1257, 2011.

*4. Pedersen T, Hovhannisyan K, Moller AM: Pulse oximetry for perioperative monitoring, *Cochrane Database Syst Rev* 4:CD002013, 2009. doi:10.1002/14651858.CD002013.pub2.

*5. Xue Q, Wu X, Jin J, et al: Transcutaneous carbon dioxide monitoring accurately predicts arterial carbon dioxide partial pressure in patients undergoing prolonged laparoscopic surgery, *Anesth Analg* 111:417, 2010.

6. Godden B: Where does capnography fit into the PACU? *J Perianesth Nurs* 26(6):408, 2011.

*7. Geerts WH, Bergqvist D, Pineo GF, et al: Prevention of venous thromboembolism: American College of Chest Physicians evidence-based clinical practice guidelines, ed 8, *Chest* 133(Suppl 6):381S, 2008.

8. Hudek K: Emergence delirium: a nursing perspective, *JAORN* 89:509, 2009.

9. Rudolph JL, Marcantonio ER: Postoperative delirium: acute change with long-term implications, *Anesth Analg* 112:1202, 2011.

10. Shander A, Fleisher LA, Barie PS, et al: Clinical and economic burden of postoperative pulmonary complications: patient safety summit on definition, risk-reducing interventions, and preventive strategies, *Crit Care Med* 39:2163, 2011.

*11. Czarnecki ML, Turner HN, Collins PM, et al: Procedural pain management: a position statement with clinical practice recommendations, *Pain Manag Nurs* 12:95, 2011.

*12. American Society of PeriAnesthesia Nurses: Pain and comfort clinical guidelines, 2003. Retrieved from *www.aspan.org/Portals/6/docs/ClinicalPractice/Guidelines/ASPAN_Clinical Guideline_PainComfort.pdf.*

13. The Joint Commission: Provision of care, treatment, and services: standard PC 01.02.07. In comprehensive accreditation manual for hospitals E-edition, 2009. Retrieved from *www.educode.com/Images/aacn-pharm04-16.pdf.*

14. Comerford D: Techniques of opioid administration, *Anes Intens Care Med* 12:16, 2011.

15. Buvanendran A, Kroin JS: Multimodal analgesia for controlling acute postoperative pain, *Curr Opin Anaesthesiol* 22:588, 2009.

16. Manion SC, Brennan TJ: Thoracic epidural analgesia and acute pain management, *Anesthesiology* 115:181, 2011.

*17. van Lier F, van der Geest PJ, Hoeks SE, et al: Epidural analgesia is associated with improved health outcomes of surgical patients with chronic obstructive pulmonary disease, *Anesthesiology* 115:315, 2011.

*18. Easter B, DeBoer L, Settlemyre G, et al: The impact of music on the PACU patient's perception of discomfort, *J Perianesth Nurs* 25:70, 2010.

*19. Topcu SY, Findik UY: Effect of relaxation exercises on controlling postoperative pain, *Pain Manag Nurs* 13:11, 2012.

20. Burns SM, Piotrowski K, Caraffa G, et al: Incidence of postoperative hypothermia and the relationship to clinical variables, *J Perianesth Nurs* 25:286, 2010.

*21. Hooper VD, Chard R, Clifford T, et al: ASPAN's evidence-based clinical practice guideline for the promotion of perioperative normothermia: ed 2, *J Perianesth Nurs* 25:346, 2010.

*22. Pikus E, Hooper VD: Postoperative rewarming: are there alternatives to warm hospital blankets? *J Perianesth Nurs* 25:11, 2010.

23. Miaskowski C: A review of the incidence, causes, consequences, and management of gastrointestinal effects associated with postoperative opioid administration, *J Perianesth Nurs* 24:222, 2009.

24. Artinyan A, Nunoo-Mensah JW, Balasubramaniam S, et al: Prolonged postoperative ileus: definition, risk factors, and predictors after surgery, *World J Surg* 32:1495, 2008.

25. Makic MB: Management of nausea, vomiting, and diarrhea during critical illness, *AACN Adv Crit Care* 22:265, 2011.

*26. Hocevar BJ, Robinson B, Gray M: Does chewing gum shorten the duration of postoperative ileus in patients undergoing abdominal surgery and creation of a stoma? *J Wound Ostomy Continence Nurs* 37:140, 2010.

*27. Crainic C, Erickson K, Gardner J, et al: Comparison of methods to facilitate postoperative bowel function, *Medsurg Nurs* 18:235, 2009.

*28. McNicol ED, Boyce D, Schumann R, et al: Mu-opioid antagonists for opioid-induced bowel dysfunction, *Cochrane Database Syst Rev* 2:CD006332, 2008. doi:10.1002/14651858.CD006332.pub2.

*29. Gould CV, Umscheid CA, Agarwal RK, et al: *Health care infection control practices advisory committee: guideline for prevention of catheter-associated urinary tract infections,* 2009, Centers for Disease Control and Prevention. Retrieved from *www.cdc.gov/hicpac/pdf/CAUTI/CAUTIguideline2009final.pdf.*

30. Cullen KA, Hall MJ, Golosinskiy A: Ambulatory surgery in the United States, *Natl Health Stat Report* 11:1, 2009.

*Evidence-based information for clinical practice.

31. Le TP, Gan TJ: Update on the management of postoperative nausea and vomiting and postdischarge nausea and vomiting in ambulatory surgery, *Anesthesiol Clin* 28:225, 2010.

32. Elvir-Lazo OL, White PF: Postoperative pain management after ambulatory surgery: role of multimodal analgesia, *Anesthesiol Clin* 28:217, 2010.

33. Ortoleva C: An approach to consistent patient education, *JAORN* 92:437, 2010.

*34. Shuilain L, Stuenkel DI, Rodriguez L: The impact of diagnosis-specific discharge instructions on patient satisfaction, *J Perianesth Nurs* 24:156, 2009.

35. Coldrey JC, Upton RN, Macintyre PE: Advances in analgesia in the older patient, *Best Pract Res Clin Anaesthesiol* 25:367, 2011.

36. Krenk L, Rasmussen LS: Postoperative delirium and postoperative cognitive dysfunction in the elderly—what are the differences? *Minerva Anestesiol* 77:742, 2011.

37. DeCrane SK, Sands L, Ashland M, et al: Factors associated with recovery from early postoperative delirium, *J Perianesth Nurs* 26:231, 2011.

RESOURCES

American Association of Nurse Anesthetists (AANA)
www.aana.com
American Latex Allergy Association
www.latexallergyresources.org
American Society of Anesthesiologists
www.asahq.org
American Society of PeriAnesthesia Nurses (ASPAN)
www.aspan.org
Association of periOperative Registered Nurses (AORN)
www.aorn.org

CASE STUDY

Managing Multiple Patients

You have been called into work at 10 AM to cover patients for a nurse who had a family emergency. You take over care for the following three patients on an orthopedic surgical unit. You have one UAP available who is assigned to help you and two other RNs.

Patients

E.G., a 74-year-old man, underwent surgery for a fractured hip yesterday. He is currently receiving dextrose 5% in 0.45 normal saline at 100 mL/hr, morphine via patient-controlled analgesia at 1 mg q10min (20 mg max in 4 hr) for pain, and O_2 to keep O_2 saturation >93%. He has a self-suction drain in place at the surgical site. He has good respiratory effort when using his incentive spirometer.

Stockbyte/Thinkstock

F.D., a 72-year-old woman, was admitted to the hospital with compromised circulation of the right lower leg and a necrotic right foot as a complication of her diabetes. She is scheduled for a below-the-knee amputation of the right leg at 1 PM today. She has been NPO since midnight. Her morning capillary blood glucose level was 198 mg/dL. She received 4 units of regular insulin at 8 AM. She has an IV of NSS infusing at 125 mL/hr.

Ryan McVay/Photodisc/Thinkstock

A.T., a 56-year-old man, is 2 days post lumbar laminectomy. He has been ambulating in the hallway without difficulty and his pain is controlled with the prescribed analgesic medication, last administered at 4 AM. His discharge orders have been written but teaching has yet to be completed.

Ryan McVay/Digital Vision/Thinkstock

Management Discussion Questions

1. **Priority Decision:** After receiving report, which patient should you see first? Provide a rationale for your decision.
2. **Delegation Decision:** Which tasks should you delegate to the UAP? *(select all that apply)*
   a. Explain discharge instructions to A.T.
   b. Obtain noon vital signs on E.G. and F.D.
   c. Obtain capillary blood glucose level on F.D.
   d. Remind E.G. and A.T. to use their incentive spirometers every hour.
   e. Confirm E.G.'s understanding of how to use the PCA pump.

3. **Priority and Delegation Decision:** When you enter F.D.'s room, you find her somewhat withdrawn and lethargic. Her face is cool and slightly clammy. What initial action would be most appropriate?
   a. Give 1 ampule of D_{50} IV stat
   b. Increase F.D.'s IV rate to 150 mL/hour.
   c. Ask the UAP to give F.D. a glass of orange juice.
   d. Have the UAP obtain a stat capillary blood glucose level.

Case Study Progression

F.D.'s capillary blood glucose reading was 64 mg/dL. You notify her health care provider and administer IV dextrose as ordered. You also change her IV infusion to D5 ½NS and monitor her capillary blood glucose levels on an hourly basis.

4. A preoperative checklist for F.D. is used to ensure completion of *(select all that apply)*
   a. removal of nail polish and jewelry.
   b. signed and witnessed informed consent.
   c. patient understanding of sensory information.
   d. identification of surgical site with indelible marker.
   e. notifying family of where to wait for surgeon postoperatively.
5. F.D. tells you that she is afraid they might amputate the wrong leg. She tells you she has read stories of that happening at other hospitals. Your best response to F.D. would be to
   a. ask her if she would like a sedative to calm her fears.
   b. reassure her that it has never happened in this hospital.
   c. explain the "time-out" procedure for preventing such errors.
   d. offer to go to the operating room with her to ensure the correct leg is amputated.
6. The UAP reports that E.G.'s blood pressure is 92/54 mm Hg, his heart rate is 110 bpm, his respirations are 30 breaths/min, and his O_2 saturation is 90%. On entering E.G.'s room, you find him clutching his chest, complaining of shortness of breath and chest pain. His lungs are clear to auscultation but you note unilateral swelling of his left leg. You suspect that E.G. is likely experiencing
   a. anxiety.
   b. atelectasis.
   c. pulmonary edema.
   d. pulmonary emboli.
7. **Management Decision:** When providing discharge instructions to A.T., he tells you that the UAP told him that he could do whatever activity he was comfortable doing—to let pain guide his progress. Your initial reaction to this statement should be to
   a. ask the UAP to clarify what was said to A.T.
   b. report the UAP's actions to the nurse manager.
   c. teach A.T. about the reason for activity restrictions.
   d. clarify the discharge instructions with the health care provider.

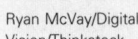

SECTION 4

Problems Related to Altered Sensory Input

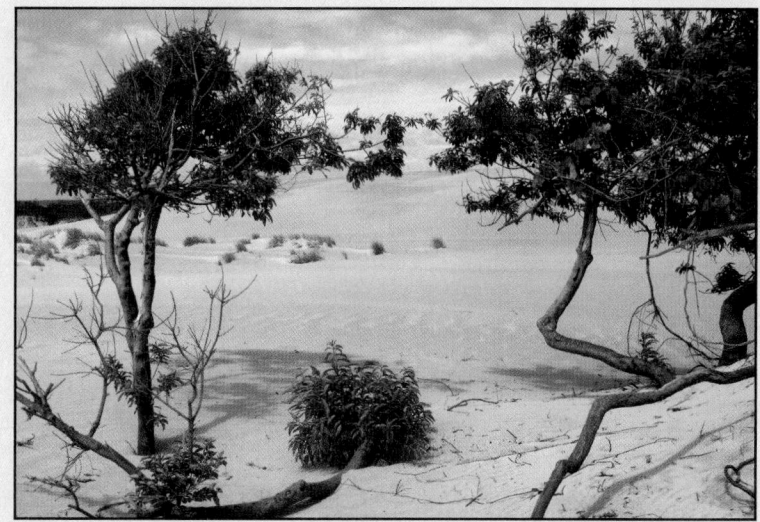

Courtesy Peter Bonner

*It's fun to be a little bit different in the world,
to make a few new trails of your own.*
Dennis Weaver

CHAPTER

21

Nursing Assessment
Visual and Auditory Systems

Mary Ann Kolis

⊖volve WEBSITE

http://evolve.elsevier.com/Lewis/medsurg

- NCLEX Review Questions
- Key Points
- Pre-Test
- Answer Guidelines for Case Study in this chapter
- Rationales for Bridge to NCLEX Examination Questions
- Concept Map Creator
- Glossary
- Animation
  - Weber Test

- Videos
  - Evaluation: Central Vision and Visual Acuity
  - Evaluation: Pupil Responses, Direct and Consensual
  - Inspection and Palpation: External Ear
  - Inspection and Palpation: External Eye
  - Inspection: Ear Canal
  - Physical Examination: Ears
  - Physical Examination: Eyes
- Content Updates

eFigures
- eFig. 21-1: Six cardinal positions of gaze
- eFig. 21-2: Tono-pen tonometry
- eFig. 21-3: Pneumatic otoscopic examination of the adult ear

eTable
- eTable 21-1: Diagnostic Tuning Fork Tests: Auditory System

LEARNING OUTCOMES

1. Describe the structures and functions of the visual and auditory systems.
2. Explain the physiologic processes involved in normal vision and hearing.
3. Evaluate the significant subjective and objective assessment data related to the visual and auditory systems that should be obtained from a patient.
4. Select the appropriate techniques to use in the physical assessment of the visual and auditory systems.
5. Differentiate normal from common abnormal findings of a physical assessment of the visual and auditory systems.
6. Link the age-related changes in the visual and auditory systems to differences in assessment findings.
7. Describe the purpose, significance of results, and nursing responsibilities related to diagnostic studies of the visual and auditory systems.

KEY TERMS

astigmatism, p. 369
conjunctiva, p. 370
hyperopia, p. 369
lens, p. 370

myopia, p. 369
nystagmus, p. 379
presbycusis, p. 379

presbyopia, p. 369
refraction, p. 369
retina, p. 371

sclera, p. 370
tinnitus, p. 379
vertigo, p. 379

VISUAL SYSTEM

STRUCTURES AND FUNCTIONS OF VISUAL SYSTEM

The visual system consists of the external tissues and structures surrounding the eye, the external and internal structures of the eye, the refractive media, and the visual pathway. The external structures are the eyebrows, eyelids, eyelashes, lacrimal system, conjunctiva, cornea, sclera, and extraocular muscles. The internal structures are the iris, lens, ciliary body, choroid, and retina. The entire visual system is important for visual function. Light reflected from an object in the field of vision passes through the transparent structures of the eye and, in doing so, is *refracted* (bent) so that a clear image can fall on the retina. From the retina, the visual stimuli travel through the visual pathway to the occipital cortex, where they are perceived as an image.

Reviewed by Sarah Smith, RN, MA, CRNO, COT, Nurse Manager, Department of Ophthalmology, University of Iowa Health Care, Oxford, Iowa; and Helen Stegall, RN, BSN, CORLN, Nurse Manager of Department of Ophthalmology, University of Iowa Hospitals and Clinics, Iowa City, Iowa.

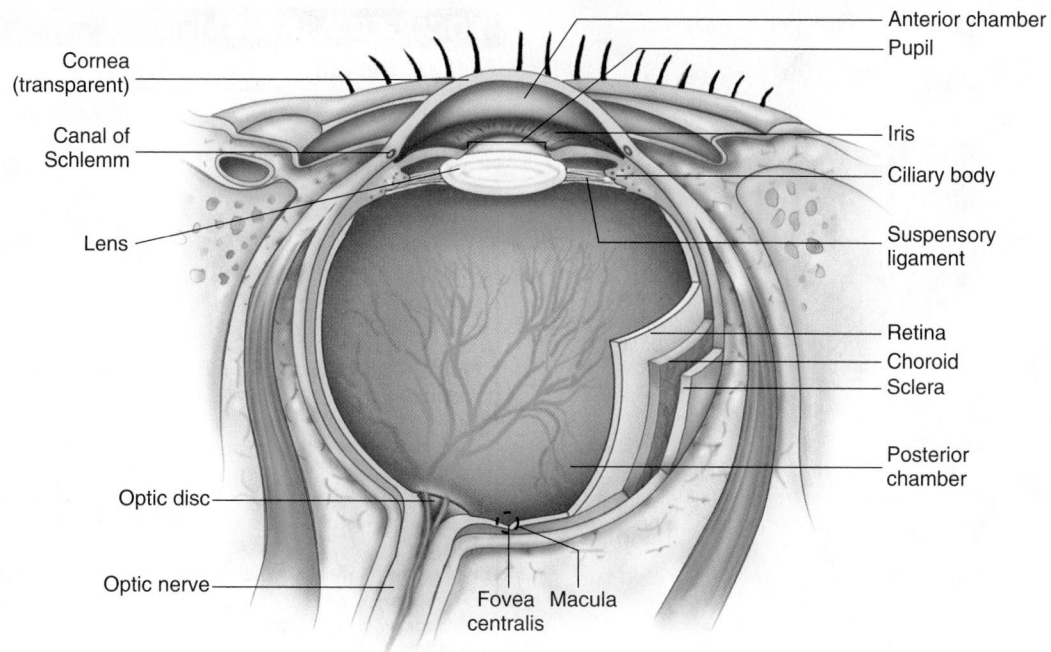

FIG. 21-1 The human eye.

Structures and Functions of Vision

Eyeball. The eyeball, or globe, is composed of three layers (Fig. 21-1). The tough outer layer is composed of the sclera and the transparent cornea. The middle layer consists of the uveal tract (iris, choroid, and ciliary body), and the innermost layer is the retina. The *anterior cavity* is divided into the anterior and posterior chambers. The anterior chamber lies between the iris and the posterior surface of the cornea, and the posterior chamber lies between the anterior surface of the lens and the posterior surface of the iris. The *posterior cavity* lies in the large space behind the lens and in front of the retina.

Refractive Media. For light to reach the retina, it must pass through a number of structures: the cornea, aqueous humor, lens, and vitreous. All these structures must remain clear for light to reach the retina and stimulate the photoreceptor cells. The transparent cornea is the first structure through which light passes. It is responsible for the majority of light refraction necessary for clear vision.

Aqueous humor, a clear watery fluid, fills the anterior and posterior chambers of the anterior cavity of the eye. Aqueous humor is produced from capillary blood in the ciliary body. It is drained away by the scleral veins *(canal of Schlemm),* which enter the circulation of the body. The aqueous humor bathes and nourishes the lens and the endothelium of the cornea. Excess production or decreased outflow can elevate intraocular pressure above the normal 10 to 21 mm Hg, a condition termed *glaucoma.*

The lens is a biconvex structure located behind the iris and supported in place by small fibers collectively called *zonule.* The zonule is a "scaffolding," a series of microscopic wire-like threads that connect the lens to the ciliary body. The primary function of the lens is to bend light rays, allowing the rays to fall onto the retina. The lens shape is modified by action of the ciliary body as part of *accommodation,* a process that allows a person to focus on near objects, such as when reading. Anything altering the clarity of the lens affects light transmission.

Vitreous humor is a transparent gel-like substance that fills the posterior chamber (see Fig. 21-1). Light passing through the vitreous may be blocked by any nontransparent substance within the vitreous. The effect on vision varies, depending on the amount, type, and location of the substance blocking the light.

Refractive Errors. Refraction is the eye's ability to bend light rays so that they fall on the retina. In the normal eye, parallel light rays are focused through the lens into a sharp image on the retina. When the light does not focus properly, it is called a *refractive error.*

The individual with myopia (nearsightedness) can see near objects clearly, but objects in the distance are blurred. The individual with hyperopia (farsightedness) can see distant objects clearly, but close objects are blurred. Astigmatism is caused by unevenness in the cornea, which results in visual distortion. Presbyopia is a loss of accommodation, causing an inability to focus on near objects. It occurs as a normal process of aging, usually around age 40.

Visual Pathways. Once the image travels through the refractive media, it is focused on the retina (Fig. 21-2). From the retina, the impulses travel through the optic nerve to the optic chiasm where the nasal fibers of each eye cross over to the other side. Fibers from the left field of both eyes form the left optic tract and travel to the left occipital cortex. The fibers from the right field of both eyes form the right optic tract and travel to the right occipital cortex. This arrangement of the nerve fibers in the visual pathways allows determination of the anatomic location of abnormalities.

External Structures and Functions

The eyebrows, eyelids, and eyelashes serve an important role in protecting the eye. They provide a physical barrier to dust and foreign particles (Fig. 21-3). The eye is further protected by the surrounding bony orbit and by fat pads located below and behind the *globe,* or eyeball.

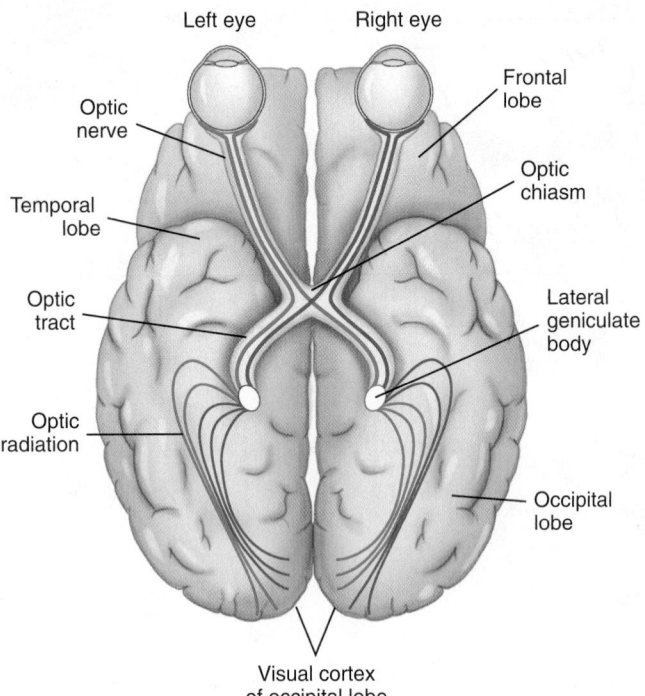

FIG. 21-2 The visual pathway. Fibers from the nasal portion of each retina cross over to the opposite side of the optic chiasma, terminating in the lateral geniculate body of the opposite side. Location of a lesion in the visual pathway determines the resulting visual defect.

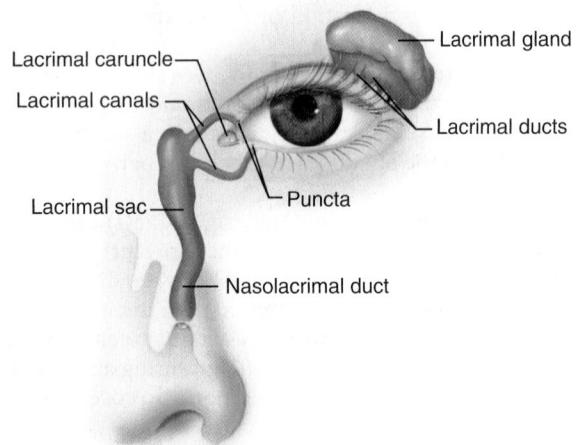

FIG. 21-3 External eye and lacrimal apparatus. Tears produced in the lacrimal gland pass over the surface of the eye and enter the lacrimal canal. From there the tears are carried through the nasolacrimal duct to the nasal cavity.

The upper and lower eyelids join at the medial and lateral canthi. Blinking of the upper eyelid distributes tears over the anterior surface of the eyeball and helps control the amount of light entering the visual pathway. The eyelids open and close through the action of muscles innervated by cranial nerve (CN) VII, the facial nerve.

The conjunctiva is a transparent mucous membrane that covers the inner surfaces of the eyelids and also extends over the sclera, forming a "pocket" under each eyelid. Glands in the conjunctiva secrete mucus and tears. The sclera is composed of collagen fibers meshed together to form an opaque structure

commonly referred to as the "white" of the eye. The sclera forms a tough shell that helps protect the intraocular structures.

The transparent and avascular cornea allows light to enter the eye (see Fig. 21-1). The curved cornea refracts (bends) incoming light rays to help focus them on the retina. The cornea consists of five layers: the epithelium, Bowman's layer, the stroma, Descemet's membrane, and the endothelium. The lacrimal system consists of the lacrimal gland and ducts, lacrimal canals and puncta, lacrimal sac, and nasolacrimal duct (see Fig. 21-3). In addition to the lacrimal gland, other glands provide secretions to make up the mucous, aqueous, and lipid layers of the tear film. The tear film moistens the eye and provides oxygen to the cornea.

Each eye is moved by three pairs of extraocular muscles: (1) superior and inferior rectus muscles, (2) medial and lateral rectus muscles, and (3) superior and inferior oblique muscles. Neuromuscular coordination produces simultaneous movement of the eyes in the same direction.

Internal Structures and Functions

The iris provides the color of the eye. The iris has a small round opening in its center, the *pupil,* which allows light to enter the eye. The pupil constricts via action of the iris sphincter muscle (innervated by CN III [oculomotor nerve]) and dilates via action of the iris dilator muscle (innervated by CN V [trigeminal nerve]) to control the amount of light that enters the eye.

The lens is a biconvex, avascular, transparent structure located behind the iris. The primary function of the lens is to bend light rays so that they fall onto the retina. Accommodation occurs when the eye focuses on a near object and is facilitated by contraction of the ciliary body, which changes the shape of the lens. The ciliary body consists of the ciliary muscles, which surround the lens and lie parallel to the sclera. The ciliary processes lie behind the peripheral part of the iris and secrete aqueous humor. The *choroid* is a highly vascular structure that nourishes the ciliary body, the iris, and the outer portion of the retina. It lies inside and parallel to the sclera (see Fig. 21-1).

TABLE 21-1   GERONTOLOGIC ASSESSMENT DIFFERENCES

Visual System

Changes	Differences in Assessment Findings	Changes	Differences in Assessment Findings
Eyebrows and Eyelashes		**Iris**	
Loss of pigment in hair	Graying of eyebrows, eyelashes	Increased rigidity of iris	Decreased pupil size
		Dilator muscle atrophy or weakness	Slower recovery of pupil size after light stimulation
Eyelids		Loss of pigment	Change of iris color
Loss of orbital fat, decreased muscle tone	Entropion, ectropion, mild ptosis	Ciliary muscle becoming smaller, stiffer	Decrease in near vision and accommodation
Tissue atrophy, prolapse of fat into eyelid tissue	Blepharodermachalasis (excessive upper lid skin)		
		Lens	
Conjunctiva		Biochemical changes in lens proteins, oxidative damage, chronic exposure to ultraviolet light	Cataracts
Tissue damage related to chronic exposure to ultraviolet light or to other chronic environmental exposure	Pinguecula (small yellowish spot usually on medial aspect of conjunctiva)	Increased rigidity of lens	Presbyopia
		Opacities in lens (may also be related to opacities in cornea and vitreous)	Complaints of glare, night vision impaired
Sclera		Accumulation of yellow substances	Yellow color of lens
Lipid deposition	Scleral color yellowish as opposed to bluish		
		Retina	
Cornea		Retinal vascular changes related to atherosclerosis and hypertension	Narrowed, pale, straighter arterioles. Acute branching
Cholesterol deposits in peripheral cornea	Arcus senilis (milky white-gray ring encircling periphery of cornea) (Fig. 21-4)	Decrease in cones	Changes in color perception, especially blue and violet
Tissue damage related to chronic exposure	Pterygium (thickened, triangular bit of pale tissue that extends from inner canthus of eye to nasal border of cornea)	Loss of photoreceptor cells, retinal pigment, epithelial cells, and melanin	Decreased visual acuity
		Age-related macular degeneration as a result of vascular changes	Loss of central vision
Decrease in water content, atrophy of nerve fibers	Decreased corneal sensitivity and corneal reflex		
Epithelial changes	Loss of corneal luster	**Vitreous**	
Accumulation of lipid deposits	Blurring of vision	Liquefaction and detachment of vitreous	Increased complaints of "floaters"
Lacrimal Apparatus			
Decreased tear secretion	Dryness		
Malposition of eyelid resulting in tears overflowing lid margins instead of draining through puncta	Tearing, irritated eyes		

The retina is the innermost layer of the eye that extends and forms the optic nerve. Neurons make up the major portion of the retina. Therefore retinal cells are unable to regenerate if destroyed. The retina lines the inside of the eyeball, extending from the area of the optic nerve to the ciliary body (see Fig. 21-1). It is responsible for converting images into a form that the brain can understand and process as vision. The retina is composed of two types of photoreceptor cells: rods and cones. Rods are stimulated in dim or darkened environments, and cones are receptive to colors in bright environments. The center of the retina is the *fovea centralis*, a pinpoint depression composed only of densely packed cones.[1] This area of the retina provides the sharpest visual acuity. Surrounding the fovea is the *macula*, an area less than 1 mm^2, which has a high concentration of cones and is relatively free of blood vessels.

GERONTOLOGIC CONSIDERATIONS

EFFECTS OF AGING ON VISUAL SYSTEM

Every structure of the visual system is subject to changes as the individual ages. Whereas many of these changes are relatively benign, others may result in severely compromised visual acuity in the older adult. The psychosocial impact of poor vision or blindness can be highly significant. Age-related changes in the visual system and differences in assessment findings are presented in Table 21-1.

ASSESSMENT OF VISUAL SYSTEM

Assessment of the visual system may be as simple as determining a patient's visual acuity or as complex as collecting complete subjective and objective data pertinent to the visual system. To do an appropriate visual evaluation, determine which parts of the data collection are important for each individual patient.

Subjective Data

Important Health Information

Past Health History. Obtain information about the patient's past health history, including both the ocular and nonocular history. Question the patient specifically about systemic diseases, such as diabetes, hypertension, cancer, rheumatoid arthritis, syphilis and other sexually transmitted infections

FIG. 21-4 Arcus senilis, or age-related degeneration of the cornea.

CASE STUDY

Patient Introduction

Jack Hollingsworth/
Photodisc/Thinkstock

F.M. is an 81-year-old Hispanic woman who comes to the emergency department with complaints of visual disturbances. F.M. states that her vision "looks like everything is covered with a spider web." She also reports seeing periodic light flashes and small white spots "floating" in the air.

Critical Thinking

As you read through this assessment chapter, think about F.M. with the following questions in mind:

1. What are the possible causes of F.M.'s visual disturbances?
2. What type of assessment would be most appropriate for F.M.: comprehensive, focused, or emergency?
3. What questions would you ask?
4. What should be included in the physical assessment? What would you be looking for?
5. What diagnostic studies might you expect to be ordered?

evolve Answers available at *http://evolve.elsevier.com/Lewis/medsurg.*

(STIs), acquired immunodeficiency syndrome (AIDS), muscular dystrophy, myasthenia gravis, multiple sclerosis, inflammatory bowel disease, and hypothyroidism or hyperthyroidism; many of these diseases have ocular manifestations. It is particularly important to determine whether the patient has any history of cardiac or pulmonary disease because β-adrenergic blockers are often used to treat glaucoma. These medications can slow heart rate, decrease blood pressure, and exacerbate asthma or chronic obstructive pulmonary disease (COPD).[2]

Obtain a history of tests for visual acuity, including the date of the last examination and change in glasses or contact lenses. Ask the patient about a history of strabismus, amblyopia, cataracts, retinal detachment, refractive surgery, or glaucoma. Note any trauma to the eye, its treatment, and sequelae.

The patient's nonocular history can be significant in assessing or treating the ophthalmic condition. Ask the patient about previous surgeries, treatments, or trauma related to the head.

Medications. If the patient takes medication, obtain a complete list, including dosage and frequency of over-the-counter (OTC) medicines, eyedrops, and herbal therapies or dietary supplements. Many patients do not think of these as "real" drugs and may not mention their use unless specifically questioned. However, many of these drugs have ocular effects. For example, many cold preparations contain a form of epinephrine (e.g., pseudoephedrine) that can dilate the pupil. Note the use of any antihistamine or decongestant, since these drugs can cause ocular dryness. In addition, specifically ask whether the patient uses any prescription drugs such as corticosteroids, thyroid medications, or agents such as oral hypoglycemics and insulin to lower blood glucose levels. Long-term use of corticosteroid preparations can contribute to the development of glaucoma or cataracts. Also note whether the patient is taking any β-adrenergic blockers, since these can be potentiated by the β-adrenergic blockers used to treat glaucoma.

Surgery or Other Treatments. Note any surgical procedures related to the eye or brain. Brain surgery and the subsequent swelling can cause pressure on the optic nerve or tract, resulting in visual alterations. Also document any laser procedures to the eye. The effect of any eye surgery or laser treatment on visual acuity is important information to obtain.

Functional Health Patterns. Ocular problems do not always affect the patient's visual acuity. For example, patients with blepharitis or diabetic retinopathy may not have noticeable visual deficits. The focus of the functional health pattern assessment depends on the presence or absence of vision loss and whether the loss is permanent or temporary. Table 21-2 lists suggested health history questions related to the functional health patterns.

Health Perception–Health Management Pattern. Patient characteristics such as gender, ethnicity, and age are important in assessing ophthalmic conditions. Men are more likely than women to have color blindness. The leading cause of blindness among African Americans is glaucoma.[3] Older individuals are also at greater risk for glaucoma.

The ophthalmic patient in a clinic or office setting is often seeking routine eye care or a change in the prescription of eyewear. However, the patient may have some underlying concerns that he or she does not mention or even recognize. Ask the patient, "Why are you here today?"

The patient's visual health can affect activities at home or at work. It is important to know how the patient perceives the current health problem. As outlined in Table 21-2, guide the patient in describing the current problem. Assess the patient's ability to accomplish necessary self-care, especially any eye care related to the patient's ophthalmic problem.

The patient may not recognize the importance of eye-safety practices such as wearing protective eyewear during potentially hazardous activities or avoiding noxious fumes and other eye irritants. Obtain information about the use of sunglasses in bright light. Prolonged exposure to ultraviolet (UV) light can affect the retina. Ask about night driving habits and any problems encountered. Today, millions of people wear contact lenses, but many do not care for them properly. The type of contact lenses used and the patient's wearing and care habits may provide information for teaching.

Obtain information about allergies. Allergies often cause eye symptoms such as itching, burning, watering, drainage, and blurred vision.

Hereditary systemic diseases (e.g., sickle cell anemia) can significantly affect ocular health. In addition, many refractive errors and other eye problems are hereditary. Specifically, ask whether the patient has a family history of diseases such as atherosclerosis, diabetes, thyroid disease, hypertension, arthritis, or cancer. In addition, determine whether the patient has a family history of ocular problems such as cataracts, tumors,

TABLE 21-2 HEALTH HISTORY
Visual System

Health Perception–Health Management
- Describe the change in your vision. Describe how this affects your daily life.
- Do you wear protective eyewear (sunglasses, safety goggles, hats)?*
- Do you wear contact lenses? If so, how do you take care of them?
- If you use eyedrops, how do you instill them?
- Do you have any allergies that cause eye symptoms?*
- Do you have a family history of cataracts, glaucoma, or macular degeneration?*

Nutritional-Metabolic
- Do you take any nutritional supplements?*
- Does your visual problem affect your ability to obtain and prepare food?*

Elimination
- Do you have to strain to void or defecate?*

Activity-Exercise
- Are your activities limited in any way by your eye problem?*
- Do you participate in any leisure activities that have the potential for eye injury?*

Sleep-Rest
- Is your vision affected by the amount of sleep you get?*
- Does your eye problem affect your sleeping patterns?*

Cognitive-Perceptual
- Does your eye problem affect your ability to read?*
- Do you have any eye pain?* Do you have any eye itching, burning, or foreign body sensation?*

Self-Perception–Self-Concept
- How does your eye problem make you feel about yourself?

Role-Relationship
- Do you have any problems at work or home because of your eyes?*
- Have you made any changes in your social activities because of your eyes?*

Sexuality-Reproductive
- Has your eye problem caused a change in your sex life?*
- For women: Are you pregnant? Do you use birth control pills?*
- For men: Do you use any erectile dysfunction drugs? Any vision problems with their use?*

Coping–Stress Tolerance
- Do you feel able to cope with your eye problem?*
- Are you able to acknowledge the effects of your eye problem on your life?*

Value-Belief
- Do you have any conflicts about the treatment of your eye problem?*

*If yes, describe.

glaucoma, refractive errors (especially myopia and hyperopia), or retinal degenerative conditions (e.g., macular degeneration, retinal detachment).

GENETIC RISK ALERT
Glaucoma
- Certain types of glaucoma have a strong genetic link. Many different glaucoma genes have been discovered.
- People with a family history of glaucoma have a much greater risk of developing it.

Age-Related Macular Degeneration (AMD)
- Some cases of AMD have a genetic link. Multiple genes may be associated with AMD.

Nutritional-Metabolic Pattern. High doses of vitamins containing antioxidants (vitamins C and E and beta-carotene) may be important to ocular health. Some patients with AMD may benefit from supplements of these vitamins.

Elimination Pattern. Straining to defecate (Valsalva maneuver) can raise the intraocular pressure. After eye surgery, many surgeons do not want the patient to strain. Assess the patient's usual pattern of elimination and determine whether there is the potential for constipation in the patient who has had ophthalmic surgical procedures.

Activity-Exercise Pattern. The patient's usual level of activity or exercise may be affected by reduced vision, symptoms accompanying an ocular problem, or activity restrictions after a surgical procedure. Inquire about leisure activities during which the patient may incur an ocular injury. For example, gardening, woodworking, and other craft activities can result in corneal or conjunctival foreign bodies or even penetrating injuries of the globe. Sports activities such as racquetball, baseball, and tennis carry risks for blunt trauma to the eyes. Protection goggles should be worn for these sports.

Sleep-Rest Pattern. In the otherwise healthy person, lack of sleep may cause ocular irritation, especially if the patient

wears contact lenses. Normal sleep patterns may be disrupted in the patient with painful eye problems such as corneal abrasions.

Cognitive-Perceptual Pattern. The entire assessment of the ophthalmic patient focuses on the sense of sight, but do not overlook other cognitive or perceptual problems. For example, the functional ability of a patient with a visual deficit will be further compromised if the patient also has hearing problems. The patient who cannot see to read has increased difficulty following postoperative instructions if he or she also has trouble hearing or remembering verbal instructions. Eye pain is always an important symptom to assess. If eye pain is present, question the patient about treatment and response.

Self-Perception–Self-Concept Pattern. The loss of independence that can follow a partial or complete loss of vision, even if the condition is temporary, can have devastating effects on the patient's self-concept. Carefully evaluate the potential effect of vision loss on the patient's self-image. For instance, disabling glare from a cataract may prevent nighttime driving. In today's highly mobile society, the loss of ability to drive can represent a significant loss of independence and self-esteem.

Role-Relationship Pattern. Ocular problems can negatively affect the patient's ability to maintain the necessary or desired roles and responsibilities in the home, work, and social environments. For example, AMD may decrease visual acuity so that the patient can no longer adequately function at work. Many occupations place workers in conditions in which eye injury may occur. For example, factory workers may be at risk from flying metal debris. Eye-safety practices, such as the use of goggles or safety glasses, are now a legal requirement in the workplace. The patient with diabetes may not be able to see well enough to self-administer insulin. This patient may resent dependence on a family member who takes over this function.

Subjective Data

A focused subjective assessment of F.M. revealed the following information:

- **PMH:** Extraocular extraction of cataract on R eye with implantation of intraocular lens 2 mo ago. Type 2 diabetes mellitus, hypothyroidism, and hypertension.
- **Medications:** Glyburide (DiaBeta) 5 mg/day, levothyroxine (Synthroid) 100 mcg/day, metoprolol (Lopressor) 50 mg PO daily.
- **Health Perception–Health Management:** States she was compliant with postoperative antibiotic and corticosteroid eyedrops and with office follow-up with eye surgeon. Recovery from surgery was uneventful, and eyedrops were discontinued 2 wk ago. Does not have allergies. Had excellent eyesight until today. Is afraid she might be having a stroke.
- **Elimination:** Has had difficulty moving bowels with increased straining. Trying prune juice to help.
- **Activity-Exercise:** Walks in the mall at least ½ mile three times a week. No resistance or isotonic exercises.
- **Cognitive-Perceptual:** Denies eye pain, itching, or tearing. Having difficulty reading.
- **Coping–Stress Tolerance:** Afraid she is having a stroke.

Jack Hollingsworth/ Photodisc/Thinkstock

Sensitively inquire if the ocular problem has affected the patient's preferred roles and responsibilities.

Sexuality-Reproductive Pattern. The patient with severe vision loss may develop such a poor self-image that the ability to be sexually intimate is lost. Assure the patient that low vision or blindness does not affect a person's ability to be sexually expressive. Often touch is more important than vision.

Coping–Stress Tolerance Pattern. The patient with temporary or permanent visual problems may experience emotional stress. Assess the patient's coping level, coping mechanisms, and availability of social and personal support systems.

Value-Belief Pattern. Be sensitive to each patient's individual values and spiritual beliefs, since these may guide the patient's decisions regarding ophthalmic care. It can be difficult to understand why a patient refuses treatment that has potential benefit or wants treatment that may have limited potential benefit.

Objective Data

Physical Examination. Physical examination of the visual system includes inspecting the ocular structures and determining the status of their respective functions. Physiologic functional assessment includes determining the patient's visual acuity, ability to judge closeness and distance, and extraocular muscle (EOM) function; evaluating visual fields; observing pupil function; and measuring the intraocular pressure.[4] Assessment of ocular structures should include examining the ocular adnexa, the external eye, and internal structures. Some structures, such as the retina and blood vessels, must be visualized with the ophthalmoscope.

Assessment of the visual system may include all of the components discussed in the following sections, or it may be as brief as measuring the patient's visual acuity. Assess what is appropriate and necessary for the specific patient. Many of the following assessments are within your scope of practice, but some require special training.

TABLE 21-3   NORMAL PHYSICAL ASSESSMENT OF VISUAL SYSTEM

- Visual acuity 20/20 OU. No diplopia.
- External eye structures symmetric and without lesions or deformities.
- Lacrimal apparatus nontender and without drainage.
- Conjunctiva clear. Sclera white.
- PERRLA.
- Lens clear.
- EOMI.
- Optic nerve margins sharp.
- Retinal vessels normal, with no hemorrhages or spots.

EOMI, Extraocular movements intact; *OU,* both eyes; *PERRLA,* pupils equal, round, reactive to light and accommodation.

Normal physical assessment of the visual system is outlined in Table 21-3. Age-related visual changes and differences in assessment findings are listed in Table 21-1. Assessment techniques related to vision are summarized in Table 21-4, and assessment abnormalities are listed in Table 21-5 on p. 376.

A *focused assessment* is used to evaluate the status of previously identified visual problems and to monitor for signs of new problems (see Table 3-6). A focused assessment of the visual system is presented in the box on p. 370.

Initial Observation. Your initial observation of the patient can provide information that will help focus the assessment. When first encountering the patient, you may observe that the patient is dressed in clothing with unusual color combinations. This may indicate a color-vision deficit. Also note an unusual head position. The patient with diplopia may hold the head in a skewed position in an attempt to see a single image. The patient with a corneal abrasion or photophobia will cover the eyes with the hands to try to block out room light. Make a crude estimate of depth perception by extending a hand for the patient to shake.

During the initial observation, observe the patient's overall facial and ophthalmic appearance. The eyes should be symmetric and normally placed on the face. The globes should not have a bulging or sunken appearance.

Assessing Functional Status

Visual Acuity. Always record the patient's visual acuity for medical and legal reasons. Document the patient's visual acuity before the patient receives any ophthalmic care. Position the person on a mark exactly 20 ft (6 m) from the Snellen eye chart. If the person wears glasses or contacts, leave them on. Cover one eye at a time during the test. Ask the person to read down the lines of the chart to the smallest line of letters possible. Record the result using the numeric fraction at the end of the last successful line read. Indicate whether any letters were missed and if corrective lenses were worn (e.g., "Left eye, 20/30-2, with contacts"). Next ask the patient to cover the other eye, and repeat the process. Normal visual acuity is 20/20. The first number indicates the distance the person is standing or sitting from the chart; the second number gives the distance at which a normal eye can read the particular line. *Legal blindness* is defined as the best-corrected vision in the better eye of 20/200 or less.

If the patient reports near vision difficulty or is 40 years of age or older, you would also use a hand-held vision screener with varying print sizes (e.g., a Jaeger chart). Hold the card at

TABLE 21-4 NURSING ASSESSMENT

Assessment Techniques: Visual System

Description	Purpose
Visual Acuity Testing Patient reads from Snellen chart at 20 ft (distance vision test) or Jaeger chart at 14 in (near vision test). Examiner notes smallest print patient can read on each chart.	Determines distance and near visual acuity
Confrontation Visual Field Test Patient faces examiner, covers one eye, fixates on examiner's face, and counts number of fingers that examiner brings into patient's field of vision.	Determines if patient has a full field of vision, without obvious scotomas
Pupil Function Testing Examiner shines light into patient's pupil and observes pupillary response. Each pupil is examined independently. Examiner also checks for consensual and accommodative response.	Determines if patient has normal pupillary response
Intraocular Pressure Testing: Tono-pen Covered end of probe is gently touched several times to anesthetized corneal surface. Examiner records several readings to obtain a mean intraocular pressure (see eFig. 21-2).	Measures intraocular pressure (normal pressure is 10-21 mm Hg)
Ophthalmoscopy Examiner holds ophthalmoscope close to patient's eye, shining light into back of eye and looking through aperture on ophthalmoscope. Examiner adjusts dial to select one of lenses in ophthalmoscope that produces desired amount of magnification to inspect retina.	Provides magnified view of retina and optic nerve head (see Fig. 21-5)
Color Vision Testing In the Ishihara test, a patient identifies numbers or paths formed by pattern of dots in series of color plates.	Determines ability to distinguish colors
Keratometry Examiner aligns projection and notes readings of corneal curvature.	Measures corneal curvature. Often done before fitting contact lenses, before refractive surgery, or after corneal transplantation

14 in (35 cm) from the eye in good light to assess near vision. Examine each eye separately with glasses on. A normal result is "14/14" in each eye, read without hesitancy and without the patient moving the card.

Hand motion or light perception may be used for distance vision assessment if a specific vision chart for distance assessment is not available. If you must assess near visual acuity without access to a Jaeger eye chart, an accurate assessment is still possible using newsprint or the label on a container. Record the acuity as "reads newspaper headline at X inches."

Extraocular Muscle Functions. Observe the corneal light reflex to evaluate for weakness or imbalance of the extraocular muscles (EOM). In a darkened room, ask the patient to look straight ahead while shining a penlight directly on the cornea. The light reflection should be located in the center of both corneas as the patient faces the light source.

To assess eye movement, hold a finger or an object within 10 to 12 in of the patient's nose. Ask the patient to follow with eyes only the movement of the object or finger in the six cardinal positions of gaze. (This is demonstrated in eFig. 21-1 available on the website for this chapter.) This test can indicate weakness or paralysis in the EOM and cranial nerves (oculomotor nerve [CN III], trochlear nerve [CN IV], and abducens nerve [CN VI]).

Pupil Function and Intraocular Pressure. Pupil function is determined by inspecting the pupils and their reactions to light. The normal finding is commonly abbreviated as PERRL (pupils are equal [in size], round, and reactive to light). To test for accommodation, ask the person to focus on a distant object. This process dilates the eyes. Then have the person shift the focus to a near object (e.g., your finger held about 3 inches from the person's nose). A normal response is constriction of the eyes and convergence (inward movement of both eyes toward each other). When accommodation is assessed in addition to the pupillary light reflex, a normal response is *PERRLA* (pupils are equal, round, and reactive to light and accommodation).

In a small percentage of the population the pupils are unequal in size *(anisocoria)*. The pupils should react to light directly (the pupil constricts when a light shines into the eye) and consensually (the pupil constricts when a light shines into the opposite eye).

Intraocular pressure (see Table 21-4) can be measured by a variety of methods, including the Tono-pen[5] (shown in eFig. 21-2 available on the website for this chapter). Normal intraocular pressure ranges from 10 to 21 mm Hg.

Assessing Structures. The visual system structures are assessed primarily by inspection. The visual system is unique because not only the external structures but also many of the internal structures can be directly inspected. The iris, lens, vitreous, retina, and optic nerve can all be visualized directly through the clear cornea and pupil opening.

This direct inspection requires special observation equipment such as the slit lamp microscope and the ophthalmoscope. This equipment permits examination of the conjunctiva, sclera, cornea, anterior chamber, iris, lens, vitreous, and retina under magnification. The *ophthalmoscope* is a hand-held instrument with a light source and magnifying lenses that is held close to the patient's eye to visualize the posterior part of the eye. Little pain or discomfort is associated with these examinations.

Eyebrows, Eyelashes, and Eyelids. All structures should be present and symmetric, without deformities, redness, or swelling. Eyelashes extend outward from the lid margins. In normal closing the upper and lower eyelid margins just touch. The lacrimal puncta should be open and positioned properly against the globe.

Conjunctiva and Sclera. The conjunctiva and sclera can easily be examined at the same time. Evaluate the color, smoothness, and presence of lesions or foreign bodies. The conjunctiva covering the sclera is normally clear, with fine blood vessels visible. These blood vessels are more common in the periphery.

The sclera is normally white, but it may take on a yellowish hue in the older individual because of lipid deposition. A pale blue cast caused by scleral thinning can also be normal in older adults and in infants (who have naturally thinner sclerae). A

TABLE 21-5   ASSESSMENT ABNORMALITIES

Visual System

Finding	Description	Possible Etiology and Significance
Subjective Data		
Pain	Foreign body sensation	Superficial corneal erosion or abrasion. Can result from contact lens wear or trauma. Conjunctival or corneal foreign body
	Severe, deep, throbbing	Anterior uveitis, acute glaucoma, infection. Acute glaucoma also associated with nausea, vomiting
Photophobia	Persistent abnormal intolerance to light	Inflammation or infection of cornea or anterior uveal tract (iris and ciliary body)
Blurred vision	Gradual or sudden inability to see clearly	Refractive errors, corneal opacities, cataracts, migraine aura, retinal changes (detachment, macular degeneration)
Spots, floaters	Patient describes seeing spots, "spiderwebs," "curtain," or floaters within the field of vision	Most common cause is vitreous liquefaction (benign phenomenon). Other possible causes include hemorrhage into the vitreous humor, retinal holes or tears
Dryness	Discomfort, sandy, gritty, irritation, or burning	Decreased tear formation or changes in tear composition because of aging or various systemic diseases
Diplopia	Double vision	Abnormalities of extraocular muscle action related to muscle or cranial nerve pathologic condition
Objective Data **Eyelids**		
Allergic reactions	Redness, excessive tearing, and itching of lid margins	Many possible allergens. Associated eye trauma can occur from rubbing itchy eyelids
Hordeolum (sty)	Small, superficial white nodule along lid margin	Infection of sebaceous gland of eyelid. Causative organism is usually bacterial (most commonly *Staphylococcus aureus*)
Blepharitis	Redness, swelling, and crusting along lid margins	Bacterial invasion of lid margins. Often chronic
Ptosis	Drooping of upper lid margin, unilateral or bilateral	Mechanical causes as a result of eyelid tumors or excess skin. Myasthenia gravis
Entropion	Inward turning of upper or lower lid margin, unilateral or bilateral	Congenital causes resulting in development abnormalities
Ectropion	Outward turning of lower lid margin	Mechanical causes as a result of eyelid tumors, herniated orbital fat, or extravasation of fluid
Conjunctiva		
Conjunctivitis	Redness, swelling of conjunctiva. May be itchy	Bacterial or viral infection. May be allergic response or inflammatory response to chemical exposure
Subconjunctival hemorrhage	Appearance of blood spot on sclera. May be small or can affect entire sclera	Conjunctival blood vessels rupture, leaking blood into the subconjunctival space
Cornea		
Corneal abrasion	Localized painful disruption of the epithelial layer of cornea. Can be visualized with fluorescein dye	Trauma. Overwear or improper fit of contact lenses
Globe		
Exophthalmos	Protrusion of globe beyond its normal position within bony orbit. Sclera often visible above iris when eyelids are open	Intraocular or periorbital tumors. Hyperthyroidism
Pupil		
Anisocoria	Pupils unequal (constricted)	Central nervous system disorders. Slight difference in pupil size is normal in some people
Abnormal response to light or accommodation	Pupils respond asymmetrically or abnormally to light stimulus or accommodation	Central nervous system disorders, general anesthesia
Extraocular Muscles		
Strabismus	Deviation of eye position in one or more directions	Overaction or underaction of one or more extraocular muscles
Lens		
Cataract	Opacification of lens. Pupil can appear cloudy or white when opacity is visible behind pupil opening	Aging, trauma, diabetes, long-term systemic corticosteroid therapy
Visual Field Defect		
Peripheral	Partial or complete loss of peripheral vision	Glaucoma. Interruption of visual pathway (e.g., tumor). Migraine headache
Central	Loss of central vision	Macular disease

FIG. 21-5 Magnified view of retina through the ophthalmoscope.

Optic disc • Fovea centralis • Retinal blood vessels • Macula

slight yellow cast may also be found in some dark-skinned people, such as African Americans and Native Americans.

Cornea. The cornea should be clear, transparent, and shiny. The iris should appear flat and not bulge toward the cornea. The area between the cornea and the iris should be clear, with no blood or purulent material visible in the anterior chamber.

Iris. Both irides should be of similar color and shape. However, a color difference between the irides occurs normally in a small portion of the population.

Retina and Optic Nerve. An ophthalmoscope is used to magnify the retina and optic nerves and bring them into crisp focus (Fig. 21-5). Examine the optic nerve or disc for size, color, and abnormalities. The optic disc is creamy yellow with distinct margins. A central depression in the disc, called the *physiologic cup,* may be seen. This area is the exit site for the optic nerve. The cup should be less than one half the diameter of the disc. Normally, no hemorrhages or exudates are present in the fundus (retinal background). Careful inspection of the fundus can reveal retinal holes, tears, detachments, or lesions. Small hemorrhages can be associated with diabetes or hypertension and can appear in various shapes, such as dots or flames. Finally, examine the macula for shape and appearance. This area of high reflectivity is devoid of any blood vessels.

Important information about the vascular system and the central nervous system (CNS) can be obtained through direct visualization with an ophthalmoscope. Skilled use of this instrument requires practice.

Special Assessment Techniques

Color Vision. Testing the patient's ability to distinguish colors can be an important part of the overall assessment because some occupations may require accurate color discrimination. The Ishihara color test determines the patient's ability to distinguish a pattern of color in a series of color plates.[6]

Stereopsis. Stereoscopic vision allows a patient to see objects in three dimensions. Any event that causes a patient to have monocular vision (e.g., enucleation, patching) results in the loss of stereoscopic vision. Without stereopsis, the individual's ability to judge distances or the height of a step is impaired. This disability can have serious consequences if the patient trips over a step when walking or follows too closely behind another vehicle when driving.

DIAGNOSTIC STUDIES OF VISUAL SYSTEM

Diagnostic studies provide important information in monitoring the patient's condition and planning appropriate interventions. These studies are considered objective data. Table 21-6 presents the most common diagnostic studies of the visual system.

AUDITORY SYSTEM

STRUCTURES AND FUNCTIONS OF AUDITORY SYSTEM

The auditory system is composed of the peripheral auditory system and the central auditory system. The peripheral system includes the structures of the ear itself: the external, middle, and inner ear (Fig. 21-6). This system is concerned with the reception and perception of sound. The inner ear functions in hearing and balance. The central system integrates and assigns meaning to what is heard. This system includes the vestibulocochlear nerve (CN VIII) and the auditory cortex of the brain. The brain and its pathways transmit and process sound and sensations that maintain a person's equilibrium.

The role of the external and middle portion of the ear is to conduct and amplify sound waves from the environment. This portion of sound conduction is termed *air conduction.* Problems in these two parts of the ear may cause *conductive hearing loss,* resulting in a decrease in sound intensity and/or a distortion in sound.

Disturbances in equilibrium can impair coordination, balance, and orientation. Damage to or an abnormality of the inner ear or along the nerve pathways results in *sensorineural hearing loss.* In addition to causing distortion or faintness of sound, sensorineural hearing loss may affect the ability to understand speech or cause complete hearing loss. Impairment within the auditory pathways of the brain causes *central hearing loss.* This type of hearing loss causes difficulty in understanding the meaning of words that are heard. (Types of hearing loss are discussed in Chapter 22 on pp. 406-407.)

External Ear

The external ear consists of the *auricle* (pinna), external auditory canal, and tympanic membrane (TM). The auricle is composed of cartilage and connective tissue covered with epithelium,

TABLE 21-6   DIAGNOSTIC STUDIES
Visual System

Description and Purpose	Nursing Responsibility*
Refractometry Subjective measure of refractive error. Multiple lenses are mounted on rotating wheels. Patient sits looking through apertures at Snellen acuity chart, and lenses are changed. Patient chooses lenses that make acuity sharpest. Comprehensive examination requires dilation of eyes to visualize retina and optic nerves.	Procedure is painless. Patient may need help to hold head still. Pupil dilation makes it difficult to focus on near objects. Dilation may last 3-4 hr.
Ultrasonography *A-scan* probe is applanated against patient's anesthetized cornea. Used primarily for axial length measurement for calculating power of intraocular lens implanted after cataract extraction. *B-scan* probe is applied to patient's closed lid. Used more often than A-scan for diagnosis of ocular pathologic conditions such as intraocular foreign bodies or tumors, vitreous opacities, retinal detachments.	Procedure is painless (cornea is anesthetized).
Fluorescein Angiography Fluorescein (a nonradioactive, non-iodine dye) injected IV into antecubital or other peripheral vein, followed by serial photographs (over 10-min period) of the retina through dilated pupils. Provides diagnostic information about flow of blood through pigment epithelial and retinal vessels. Often used in diabetic patients to accurately locate areas of diabetic retinopathy before laser destruction of neovascularization.	If extravasation occurs, fluorescein is toxic to tissue. Although systemic allergic reactions are rare, be familiar with emergency equipment and procedures. Tell patient that dye can sometimes cause transient nausea or vomiting. Transient yellow-orange discoloration of urine and skin is normal.
Amsler Grid Test Test is self-administered using a hand-held card printed with a grid of lines (similar to graph paper). Patient fixates on center dot and records any abnormalities of the grid lines, such as wavy, missing, or distorted areas. Used to monitor macular problems.	Regular testing is necessary to identify any changes in macular function.

*Patient teaching regarding the purpose and method of testing is a nursing responsibility for all diagnostic procedures.

which also lines the external auditory canal (see Fig. 21-6). The external auditory canal is a slightly S-shaped tube about 1 in (2.5 cm) in length in the adult. The lining of the canal contains fine hairs (cilia), sebaceous (oil) glands, and ceruminous (wax) glands. The oil and wax lubricate the ear canal, keep it free from debris, and kill bacteria.

The function of the external ear and canal is to collect and transmit sound waves to the *tympanic membrane* (eardrum). This shiny, translucent, pearl-gray membrane is composed of epithelial cells, connective tissue, and mucous membrane. It serves as a partition and an instrument of sound transmission between the external auditory canal and the middle ear.

Middle Ear

The middle ear cavity is an air space located in the temporal bone. Mucous membrane lines the middle ear and is continuous from the nasal pharynx via the eustachian (auditory) tube. The eustachian tube functions to equalize atmospheric air pressure between the middle ear and the throat and allows the tympanic membrane to move freely. It opens during yawning and swallowing. Blockage of this tube can occur with allergies, nasopharyngeal infections, or enlarged adenoids.

The middle ear contains the three smallest bones in the body: *malleus, incus,* and *stapes* (ossicles). Vibrations of the TM cause the ossicles to move and transmit sound waves to the oval window. The superior part of the middle ear is called the *epitympanum,* or the attic. It also communicates with air cells within the mastoid bone. The mastoid is the posterior part of the temporal bone. The facial nerve (CN VII) traverses above the oval window of the middle ear. The thin, bony covering of the facial nerve can become damaged by chronic ear infection, skull fracture, or trauma during ear surgery. Problems may occur related to voluntary facial movements, eyelid closure, and taste discrimination. Permanent damage to the facial nerve can also result.

Inner Ear

The inner ear is composed of a bony labyrinth (maze) surrounding a membrane. Perilymphatic fluid lies between the bone and the membrane. The fluid inside the membrane is called *endolymph.* The inner ear contains the functional organs for hearing and balance. The receptor organ for hearing is the *cochlea,* which is a coiled structure. It contains the *organ of Corti,* whose tiny hair cells respond to stimulation of selected portions of the basilar membrane according to pitch. This stimulus is converted into an electrochemical impulse and then transmitted by the acoustic portion of the vestibulocochlear nerve (CN VIII) to the temporal lobe of the brain to process and interpret the sound.

Three semicircular canals and the vestibule make up the organ of balance. These structures comprise the membranous labyrinth, which is housed within the bony labyrinth. The membranous labyrinth is filled with endolymphatic fluid, and the bony labyrinth is filled with perilymphatic fluid. Nervous stimuli are communicated by the vestibular portion of CN VIII. Debris such as loose crystals of calcium or excessive pressure within the lymphatic fluid can produce disorders such as benign paroxysmal positional vertigo (BPPV).

Transmission of Sound. Sound waves are conducted by air (air conduction) and picked up by the auricles and auditory canal. The TM is struck by the sound waves, causing it to vibrate. The central area of the TM is connected to the malleus, which also starts to vibrate. The malleus transmits the vibration to the incus and then the stapes. As the stapes moves back and forth, it pushes the membrane of the oval window in and out. Movement of the oval window produces waves in the perilymph.

Once sound has been transmitted to the liquid medium of the inner ear, the vibration is picked up by the tiny sensory hair cells of the cochlea, which initiate nerve impulses. These impulses are carried by nerve fibers to the main branch of the acoustic portion of CN VIII and then to the brain.

The bones of the skull can also transmit sound directly to the inner ear (bone conduction). This can be demonstrated by placing the stem of a vibrating tuning fork on the skull.

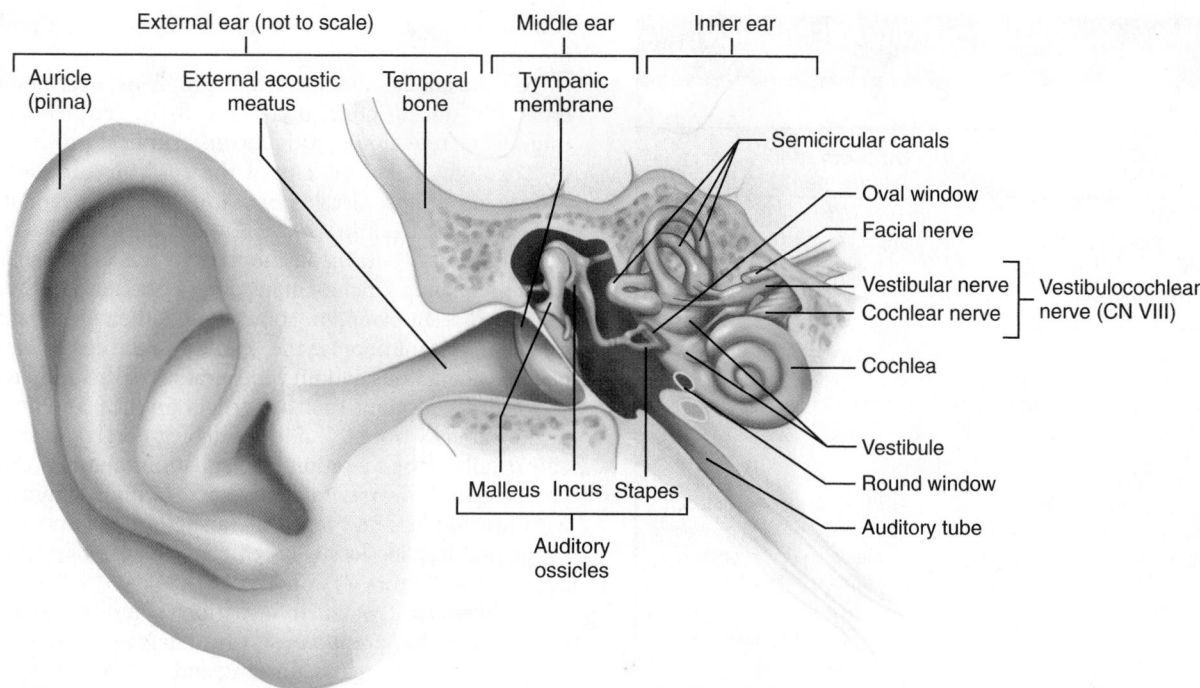

External ear (not to scale) | Middle ear | Inner ear

Auricle (pinna)
External acoustic meatus
Temporal bone
Tympanic membrane
Semicircular canals
Oval window
Facial nerve
Vestibular nerve
Cochlear nerve
Vestibulocochlear nerve (CN VIII)
Cochlea
Vestibule
Round window
Auditory tube
Malleus Incus Stapes
Auditory ossicles

FIG. 21-6 External, middle, and inner ear.

GERONTOLOGIC CONSIDERATIONS

EFFECTS OF AGING ON AUDITORY SYSTEM

Approximately 36 million American adults report some degree of hearing loss, with aging being the primary cause.[7] **Presbycusis,** or hearing loss due to aging, can result from a variety of sources. Noise exposure, systemic diseases, poor nutrition, ototoxic drugs, and pollution exposure over the life span can damage the delicate hair cells of the organ of Corti or atrophy lymph-producing cells. Sound transmission is also diminished by calcification of the ossicles. The loss associated with presbycusis is usually greater for high-pitched sounds. Accumulation of dry cerumen (earwax) in the external canal can also interfere with the transmission of sound.[8] **Tinnitus,** or ringing in the ears, may accompany the hearing loss that results from the aging process. As the average life span increases, the number of people with hearing loss will also increase. Prevention and early identification of problems will ensure a more active and healthy aging population.

Age-related changes in the auditory system and differences in assessment findings are presented in Table 21-7.

ASSESSMENT OF AUDITORY SYSTEM

Assessment of the auditory system should include assessment of hearing and equilibrium because the auditory and *vestibular* (balance) systems are closely related. It is often difficult to separate symptoms related to these two systems. Help the patient describe symptoms and problems to differentiate the source of the problems. Health history questions to ask a patient with an auditory problem are listed in Table 21-8.

Problems with balance may manifest as vertigo or nystagmus. **Vertigo** is a sense that the person or objects around the person are moving or spinning and is usually stimulated by movement of the head. *Dizziness* is a sensation of being off-

FOCUSED ASSESSMENT

Auditory System

Use this checklist to make sure the key assessment steps have been done.

Subjective
Ask the patient about any of the following and note responses.

Changes in hearing	Y	N
Ear pain	Y	N
Ear drainage	Y	N

Objective: Physical Examination
Inspect

Alignment and position of ears on head	✓
Size, shape, symmetry, color, and skin intactness	✓
External auditory meatus for discharge or lesions	✓

Assess

Hearing based on ability to respond to conversation, respond to a whisper, or hear a ticking watch	✓

balance that occurs when standing or walking. **Nystagmus** is an abnormal eye movement that may be observed as a twitching of the eyeball or described by the patient as a blurring of vision with head or eye movement.

Initially try to categorize symptoms related to balance and separate them from symptoms related to hearing loss or tinnitus. The symptoms can be combined later in the assessment to help make the diagnosis and plan for the patient.

Subjective Data

Important Health Information

Past Health History. Many problems related to the ear may result from childhood illnesses or problems of adjacent organs.

TABLE 21-7 GERONTOLOGIC ASSESSMENT DIFFERENCES

Auditory System

Changes	Differences in Assessment Findings
External Ear	
Increased production of and drier cerumen	Impacted cerumen, potential hearing loss
Increased hair growth	Visible hair, especially in men
Loss of elasticity in cartilage	Collapsed ear canal
Middle Ear	
Atrophic changes of tympanic membrane	Conductive hearing loss
Inner Ear	
Hair cell degeneration, neuron degeneration in auditory nerve and central pathways, reduced blood supply to cochlea, calcification of ossicles	Presbycusis, diminished sensitivity to high-pitched sounds, impaired speech reception, tinnitus
Less effective vestibular apparatus in semicircular canals	Alterations in balance and body orientation
Brain	
Decline in ability to filter out unwanted and unnecessary sound	Difficulty hearing in a noisy environment, heightened sensitivity to loud sounds

Consequently, a careful assessment of past health problems is important.

Ask the patient about previous problems regarding the ears, especially during childhood. Record the frequency of acute middle ear infections (otitis media); surgical procedures (e.g., myringotomy); perforations of the eardrum; drainage; and a history of mumps, measles, or scarlet fever. Congenital hearing loss can result from infectious diseases (e.g., rubella, influenza, syphilis), teratogenic medications, or hypoxia in the first trimester of pregnancy. Document head injury because it may result in hearing loss. Information about food and environmental allergies is important because they can cause the eustachian tube to become edematous and prevent aeration of the middle ear.

Record symptoms such as vertigo, tinnitus, and hearing loss in the patient's words. Guide the description by asking for specific details of the sensations and situations that may cause them or make them worse. Information regarding family members with hearing loss and type of hearing loss is important. Some congenital hearing loss is hereditary. The age of onset of presbycusis also follows a familial pattern.

Medications. Obtain information about present or past medications that are *ototoxic* (cause damage to CN VIII) and can produce hearing loss, tinnitus, and vertigo. The amount and frequency of aspirin use are important because tinnitus can result from high aspirin intake. Aminoglycosides, any other antibiotics, salicylates, antimalarial agents, chemotherapeutic drugs, diuretics, and nonsteroidal antiinflammatory drugs

TABLE 21-8 HEALTH HISTORY

Auditory System

Health Perception–Health Management
Hearing
- Have you had a change in your hearing?* If yes, how does this change affect your daily life?
- Do you use any devices to improve your hearing (e.g., hearing aid, special volume control, headphones for television or stereo)?*
- How do you protect your hearing?
- Do you have any allergies that result in ear problems?*

Equilibrium
- When did the dizziness or spinning sensation first occur?
- Does this sensation occur when you first stand up, when you are lying down, or both?
- Have you ever fallen because of the dizziness?*
- Can you drive or walk alone? If no, elaborate.
- Are there any times of the day when your symptoms are worse?*

Tinnitus
- How long have you experienced ringing in your ears? Has it changed?* Describe the ringing (e.g., buzzing, ringing, roaring). Do you also have a feeling of fullness or pressure?*
- When does it bother you the most?
- What things have you tried that help or have not helped?
- What medications are you taking?

Nutritional-Metabolic
- Do you notice any differences in symptoms with changes in diet?*
- Does your ear problem cause nausea that interferes with your food intake?*
- Does chewing or swallowing cause you any ear discomfort?*

Elimination
- Does straining during a bowel movement cause ear pain?*

Activity-Exercise
- Do you need help with certain activities (e.g., lifting, bending, climbing stairs, driving, speaking) because of symptoms?*

Sleep-Rest
- Is your sleep disturbed by noises or ringing in the ears or by a sensation of spinning?*

Cognitive-Perceptual
- Do you experience ear pain?* What relieves the pain? What makes it worse? Does the pain affect your hearing or balance?
- Have you noticed any problem with communicating or understanding what people are saying?*

Self-Perception–Self-Concept
- Have changes in your hearing affected how you feel about yourself or your feeling of independence?*

Role-Relationship
- What effect has your ear problem had on your work, family, or social life?
- Are you able to recognize the effects of your ear problems on your life?*

Sexuality-Reproductive
- Has your ear problem caused a change in your sex life?*

Coping–Stress Tolerance
- Do you consider your ear problem a source of stress?*
- How do you cope when you are experiencing symptoms?

Value-Belief
- Do you have a conflict between what your health care provider would like you to do and what you believe you should do?

*If yes, describe.

(NSAIDs) are groups of drugs that are potentially ototoxic. Monitor for hearing and balance problems in patients receiving these drugs. Many drugs produce hearing loss that may be reversible if treatment is stopped.

Surgery or Other Treatments. Document previous hospitalizations for ear surgery, including *myringotomy* (ventilation holes placed in the TM with or without tubes), *tympanoplasty* (surgical repair of TM), tonsillectomy, and adenoidectomy (removal of tonsils and adenoids). Record the use of and satisfaction with a hearing aid. Also note any problems with impacted cerumen.

Functional Health Patterns. Hearing and balance problems can affect all aspects of a person's life. To assess the impact of hearing loss, ask health history questions based on a functional health patterns approach (see Table 21-8).

Health Perception–Health Management Pattern. Note the onset of hearing loss, whether sudden or gradual, and who noted the onset (e.g., patient, family, significant others). Gradual hearing losses are most often noted by those who communicate with the patient. Sudden losses and those exacerbated by some other condition are most often reported by the patient.

Assess the patient for personal measures used to preserve hearing. The use of protective ear covers or earplugs is good practice for people in high-noise environments. Document if the patient is a swimmer and the frequency and duration of swimming and use of ear protection. Note the type of water (pool, lake, or ocean) in which the swimming takes place to help identify contact with contaminated water. Assess for the placement of any item in the ear, including hearing aids, which can cause trauma to the canal and TM.

Nutritional-Metabolic Pattern. Alcohol, sodium, and dietary supplements affect the amount of endolymph in the inner ear system. Patients with Ménière's disease may notice some improvement in their symptoms with alcohol restriction and a low-sodium diet.[9] Note changes in symptoms with food intake. Question the patient about any ear pain (otalgia) or discomfort associated with chewing or swallowing that might decrease nutritional intake. This situation is often associated with a problem in the middle ear.

Assessment of clenching or grinding of the teeth helps differentiate problems of the ear from referred pain of the temporomandibular joint (TMJ). Ask about dental problems and dentures.

Elimination Pattern. Elimination patterns are mainly of interest in the patient with perilymph fistula and after surgical procedures. Frequent constipation or straining with bowel or bladder elimination may interfere with healing or repair of a perilymph fistula. After middle ear surgery (stapedectomy) the patient needs to prevent increased intracranial (and consequent inner ear) pressure associated with straining during bowel movements. Stool softeners may be ordered postoperatively for the patient who reports chronic problems with constipation.

Activity-Exercise Pattern. A review of the patient's activity-exercise pattern is essential when assessing for equilibrium problems. Question the patient specifically about the onset, duration, and frequency of symptoms. Identify activities that relieve or worsen symptoms and how they relate to the time of the day. For example, patients with Ménière's disease are less able to compensate for environmental input as the day progresses.

Sleep-Rest Pattern. Ask the patient with chronic tinnitus about sleep problems. Find out if the patient has tried any techniques to drown out the tinnitus (e.g., having fan on, using white noise devices). Also assess for snoring because it can be caused by swelling or hypertrophy of tissue in the nasopharynx. This excessive tissue can impair the functioning of the eustachian tube and cause the sensation of ear fullness or pain.

Cognitive-Perceptual Pattern. Pain is associated with some ear problems, particularly those involving the middle ear and auditory canal. If pain is present, ask the patient to describe the pain, presence of drainage (otorrhea), history of teeth grinding, and the treatments used for relief. Note the effect on the pain level when the auricle is moved or the tragus is palpated.

Note the patient's ability to pay attention and follow directions. Problems with these tasks may be an early indicator of hearing loss. The patient may not recognize a gradual hearing loss. Ask significant others if they have noted any change in the patient's hearing.

Self-Perception–Self-Concept Pattern. Ask the patient to describe how the ear problem has affected his or her personal life and feelings about himself or herself. Hearing loss and chronic vertigo are particularly distressing for the patient. Hearing loss can result in embarrassing social situations that affect the patient's self-concept. Sensitively question the patient about such situations.

At times the patient with chronic vertigo may be accused of acting intoxicated. Clarify the symptom history with the patient and consider an evaluation with a hearing specialist.

Role-Relationship Pattern. Question the patient about the effect that the ear problem has had on family life, work responsibilities, and social relationships. Hearing loss can result in strained family relations and misunderstandings.

Also ask about employment or contact with environments that have excessive noise levels, such as work with jet engines and machinery and electronically amplified music. Document the use of preventive devices worn in noisy environments. Many jobs rely on the ability to hear accurately and respond appropriately. If a hearing loss is present, gather detailed information on the effect this has on the patient's job.

The unpredictability of vertigo attacks can have devastating effects on all aspects of a patient's life. Ordinary activities such as driving or cooking and work that requires balance all have an element of danger. Assess the effect of the vertigo on the patient's many roles and responsibilities.

Sexuality-Reproductive Pattern. Determine whether hearing loss or vertigo has interfered with the establishment of a satisfactory sex life. Although intimacy does not depend on the ability to hear, a hearing loss could interfere with establishing or maintaining a relationship.

Coping–Stress Tolerance Pattern. Ask the patient about his or her usual coping style, stress-reducing techniques, and available support. If the patient seems unable to manage the situation, outside intervention may be required. Denial is a common response to a hearing problem and should be assessed.

Value-Belief Pattern. Question the patient about any conflicts produced by the problem or treatment related to values or beliefs. Every effort should be made to resolve the problem so the patient does not experience additional stress. Ask about the use of home remedies such as hot oil in the ear.

Objective Data

Physical Examination. During the health-history interview, collect objective data regarding the patient's ability to hear. Note clues such as posturing of the head and appropriateness of

TABLE 21-9	NORMAL PHYSICAL ASSESSMENT OF AUDITORY SYSTEM

- Ears symmetric in location and shape.
- Auricles and tragus nontender, without lesions.
- Canal clear, tympanic membrane intact, landmarks and light reflex intact.
- Able to hear low whisper at 30 cm. Weber test results, no lateralization. Rinne test results AC > BC.

AC, Air conduction; *BC,* bone conduction.

responses. Does the patient ask to have certain words repeated? Does the patient intently watch the examiner but miss comments when *not* looking at the examiner? Is the patient lip reading? Record these significant observations. This is also important because the patient is often unaware of hearing loss or does not admit to changes in hearing until moderate losses have occurred.

A normal assessment of the auditory system is listed in Table 21-9. Age-related changes of the auditory system and differences in assessment findings are listed in Table 21-7.

A *focused assessment* is used to evaluate the status of previously identified auditory problems and to monitor for signs of new problems (see Table 3-6). A focused assessment of the auditory system is presented in the box on p. 379.

External Ear. Inspect and palpate the external ear before examining the external canal and tympanum.[4] Observe the auricle, preauricular area, and mastoid area for symmetry, color of skin, swelling, redness, and lesions. Then palpate the auricle and mastoid areas for tenderness and nodules. Grasping the auricle or pressing on the tragus may elicit pain, especially if the external ear or canal is inflamed.

External Auditory Canal and Tympanum. Before inserting an otoscope, inspect the canal opening for patency, palpate the tragus, and gently move the auricle to check for discomfort. Select a speculum slightly smaller than the size of the ear canal. Tip the patient's head to the opposite shoulder. Grasp the top of the auricle and gently pull up and backward to straighten the canal. Hold the otoscope while stabilizing it with your fingers on the patient's cheek, and then insert it slowly. A pneumatic otoscope creates negative pressure to pull at the TM and is helpful in confirming TM retraction or fluid behind the membrane (see eFig. 21-3 available on the website for this chapter). A tight seal of the speculum is essential during this step of the examination. Observe the canal for size and shape and the color, amount, and type of cerumen. Be careful when clearing the canal of cerumen. Damage can occur to the middle ear if the TM is perforated.

Inspect the TM for color, fluid behind the membrane, landmarks, contour, and intactness (Fig. 21-7). The TM is normally pearl gray, white, or pink; shiny; and translucent. The handle *(manubrium)* of the malleus and its short process *(umbo)* should be visible through the membrane. The position and dome (concave) shape of the TM causes the light from the otoscope to reflect back in a cone shape with crisp edges. If the TM is bulging or retracted, the edges of the light reflex will be fuzzy (diffuse) and may spread over the TM. The middle and inner ear cannot be examined with the otoscope because of the TM.

Table 21-10 summarizes assessment abnormalities of the auditory system.

FIG. 21-7 The tympanic membrane. **A,** Landmarks of right tympanic membrane. **B,** Normal-appearing tympanic membrane. **C,** Perforated tympanic membrane.

DIAGNOSTIC STUDIES OF AUDITORY SYSTEM

Table 21-11 describes diagnostic studies commonly used to assess the auditory system.

Tests for Hearing Acuity

Tests involving the whispered and spoken voice can provide general screening information about the patient's ability to hear. Audiometric testing provides more detailed information that can be used for diagnosis and treatment.

In the *whisper test,* stand 12 to 24 in (30.5 to 61 cm) to the side of the patient and, after exhaling, speak in a low whisper. Ask the patient to repeat numbers or words or answer questions. Use a louder whisper if the patient does not respond correctly. Test each ear separately. The ear not being tested is covered by the patient.

Tuning Fork Tests. Tuning fork tests aid in differentiating between conductive and sensorineural hearing loss. Tuning forks of 512 Hz are generally used for this examination. Both skill and experience are required to ensure accurate results. If a problem is suspected, further evaluation by pure-tone audiometry is needed. The most common tuning fork tests are the *Weber test* and the *Rinne test*[10] (described in eTable 21-1 available on the website for this chapter). These tests measure hearing by bone conduction or by air conduction. Results of tuning fork tests are subjective. The patient with inconsistent or questionable test results should be referred for more objective audiometric evaluation.

Audiometry. *Audiometry* is beneficial as a screening test for hearing acuity and as a diagnostic test for determining the degree and type of hearing loss. The audiometer produces pure tones at varying intensities to which the patient can respond. Sound is characterized by the number of vibrations or cycles that occur each second. *Hertz* (Hz) is the unit of measurement used to classify the frequency of a tone; the higher the fre-

TABLE 21-10 ASSESSMENT ABNORMALITIES

Auditory System

Finding	Description	Possible Etiology and Significance
External Ear and Canal		
Sebaceous cyst behind ear	Usually within skin, possible presence of black dot (opening to sebaceous gland)	Removal or incision and drainage if painful
Tophi	Hard nodules in the helix or antihelix consisting of uric acid crystals	Associated with gout, metabolic disorder. Further diagnosis needed
Impacted cerumen	Wax that has not normally been excreted from the ear. No visualization of eardrum	Decreased hearing possible, pain, sensation of fullness in auditory canal, removal necessary before otoscopic examination
Discharge in canal	Infection of external ear, usually painful	Swimmer's ear, infection of external ear. Possibly caused by ruptured eardrum and otitis media
Swelling of pinna, pain	Infection of glands of skin, hematoma caused by trauma	Aspiration (for hematoma)
Scaling or lesions	Change in usual appearance of skin	Seborrheic dermatitis, actinic keratosis, basal or squamous cell carcinoma
Exostosis	Bony growth extending into canal causing narrowing of canal	Possible interference with visualization of tympanum. Usually asymptomatic
Tympanum		
Retracted eardrum	Appearance of shorter, more horizontal malleus. Absent or bent cone of light	Vacuum in middle ear, blockage of eustachian tube, negative pressure in middle ear
Hairline fluid level, yellow-amber bubbles above fluid level	Caused by transudate of blood and serum, meniscus of fluid producing hairline appearance	Serous otitis media
Bulging red or blue eardrum, lack of landmarks	Fluid-filled middle ear, pus, blood	Acute otitis media, perforation possible
Perforation of eardrum (see Fig. 21-7)	Previous perforations of the eardrum that have failed to heal. Thin, transparent layer of epithelium surrounding eardrum	Chronic otitis media, mastoiditis, drainage
Recruitment	Disproportionate loudness of sound from malfunction of inner ear	Hearing aid difficult to use

TABLE 21-11 DIAGNOSTIC STUDIES

Auditory System

Study	Description and Purpose	Nursing Responsibility
Auditory		
Pure-tone audiometry	Sounds are presented through earphones in soundproof room. Patient responds nonverbally when sound is heard. Response is recorded on an audiogram. Purpose is to determine patient's hearing range in terms of decibels (dB) and Hertz (Hz) for diagnosing conductive and sensorineural hearing loss. Tinnitus can cause inconsistent results.	Nurse does not usually participate in examination.
One- and two-syllable word lists	Words are presented and recorded at comfortable level of hearing to determine percentage correct and word understanding.	Nurse may perform test.
Auditory evoked potential (AEP)	Procedure is similar to electroencephalogram (see Chapter 56 and Table 56-8). Electrodes are attached to patient in a darkened room. Electrodes are placed typically at vertex, mastoid process, or earlobes and forehead. A computer is used to isolate auditory from other electrical activity of brain.	Explain procedure to patient. Do not leave patient alone in darkened room.
Electrocochleography	Test is useful for uncooperative patient or patient who cannot volunteer useful information. Test records electrical activity in cochlea and auditory nerve.	Nurse does not usually participate in examination.
Auditory brainstem response (ABR)	Study measures electrical peaks along auditory pathway of inner ear to brain and provides diagnostic information related to acoustic neuromas, brainstem problems, and stroke.	Nurse does not usually participate in examination.
Tympanometry (impedance audiometry)	Useful in diagnosis of middle ear effusions. A probe is placed snugly in external ear canal, and positive and negative pressures are then applied. Compliance of middle ear is then noted in response to pressures.	Nurse does not usually participate in examination.

Continued

TABLE 21-11   DIAGNOSTIC STUDIES—cont'd

Auditory System

Study	Description and Purpose	Nursing Responsibility
Vestibular		
Caloric test stimulus	Endolymph of semicircular canals is stimulated by irrigation of cold (68° F [20° C]) or warm (97° F [36° C]) solution into ear. Patient is seated or in supine position. Observation of type of nystagmus, nausea and vomiting, falling, or vertigo is helpful in diagnosing disease of labyrinth. Decreased function is indicated by decreased response and indicates disease of vestibular system. Other ear is tested similarly and results are compared.	Instruct patient to eat light meal before test to avoid nausea. Observe patient for vomiting. Assist if necessary. Ensure patient safety.
Electronystagmography (ENG)	Electrodes are placed near patient's eyes, and movement of eyes (nystagmus) is recorded on graph during specific eye movements and when ear is irrigated. Used to diagnose diseases of vestibular system.	Instruct patient to eat light meal before test to avoid nausea. Observe patient for vomiting. Assist if necessary. Ensure patient safety.
Posturography	Balance test that can isolate one semicircular canal from others to determine site of lesion. Test is done in a boxlike device in which floor moves in response to a correction in balance by patient.	Inform patient that test is time consuming and uncomfortable. Test can be discontinued at any time at patient's request.
Rotary chair testing	Evaluates peripheral vestibular system. Patient is seated in a chair driven by a motor under computer control. Test is usually done in the dark.	Instruct patient to eat light meal before test to avoid nausea. Observe patient for vomiting. Assist if necessary. Ensure patient safety.

quency, the higher the pitch. Hearing loss can affect certain sound frequencies. The specific pattern produced on the audiogram by these losses can assist in the diagnosis of the type of hearing loss. The intensity or strength of a sound wave is expressed in terms of decibels (dB), ranging from 0 to 110 dB. The intensity of a sound required to make any frequency barely audible to the average normal ear is 0 dB. *Threshold* refers to the signal level at which pure tones are detected (pure-tone thresholds) or the signal level at which the patient correctly hears 50% of the signals (speech detection thresholds).

Normal speech is approximately 40 to 65 dB; a soft whisper is 20 dB. Normally, a child and a young adult can hear frequencies from about 16 to 20,000 Hz, but hearing is most sensitive between 500 and 4000 Hz. This is similar to the frequencies of normal speech. A 40- to 45-dB loss in these frequencies causes moderate difficulty in hearing normal speech. A hearing aid may be helpful because it makes sound information louder but not clearer. A hearing aid may not be helpful to the patient who has problems with discrimination of sounds or sound information because the consonants are still not heard enough to make speech understandable.

Screening Audiometry. Screening audiometry is the testing of large numbers of people with a fast, simple test to detect possible hearing problems. A pass-fail criterion is used to screen people who will or will not be given additional diagnostic testing. People who fail the screening should be referred to an audiologist for pure-tone (threshold) audiometry.

Specialized Tests

The more specialized tests of the auditory system are frequently performed in an outpatient setting by an audiologist. An audiologist can perform many additional tests with the use of audiometers and computers that record electrical activity from the middle ear, inner ear, and brain (see Table 21-11). The most common test performed by the audiologist is pure-tone audiometry. A pure-tone audiometer produces pure tones at varied frequencies (pitch) and intensity (volume). Testing determines the patient's hearing range in decibels and Hertz.

More sophisticated tests are available to determine the origin of certain hearing losses. These include evoked potential studies (also called auditory brainstem response) and electrocochleography. Computed tomography (CT) and magnetic resonance imaging (MRI) scans are used to diagnose the site of a lesion, such as a tumor of the auditory nerve.

Test for Vestibular Function

Table 21-11 describes diagnostic studies commonly used to assess vestibular function.

BRIDGE TO NCLEX EXAMINATION

The number of the question corresponds to the same-numbered outcome at the beginning of the chapter.

1. In a patient who has a hemorrhage in the posterior cavity of the eye, the nurse knows that blood is accumulating
   a. in the aqueous humor.
   b. between the lens and the retina.
   c. between the cornea and the lens.
   d. in the space between the iris and the lens.

2. Increased intraocular pressure may occur as a result of
   a. edema of the corneal stroma.
   b. dilation of the retinal arterioles.
   c. blockage of the lacrimal canals and ducts.
   d. increased production of aqueous humor by the ciliary process.

3. Question patients using eyedrops to treat their glaucoma about
   a. use of corrective lenses.
   b. their usual sleep pattern.
   c. a history of heart or lung disease.
   d. sensitivity to opioids or depressants.
4. Always assess the patient with an ophthalmic problem for
   a. visual acuity.
   b. pupillary reactions.
   c. intraocular pressure.
   d. confrontation visual fields.
5. During an assessment of hearing, the nurse would expect to find normal finding of
   a. absent cone of light.
   b. bluish purple tympanic membrane.
   c. midline tone heard equally in both ears.
   d. fluid level at hairline in the tympanum.

6. Age-related changes in the auditory system commonly include (select all that apply)
   a. drier cerumen.
   b. tinnitus in both ears.
   c. auditory nerve degeneration.
   d. atrophy of the tympanic membrane.
   e. greater ability to hear high-pitched sounds.
7. Before injecting fluorescein for angiography, it is important for the nurse to (select all that apply)
   a. obtain an emesis basin.
   b. ask if the patient is fatigued.
   c. administer a topical anesthetic.
   d. inform patient that skin may turn yellow.
   e. assess for allergies to iodine-based contrast media.

1. b, 2. d, 3. c, 4. a, 5. c, 6. a, c, d, 7. a, d

⊖volve

For rationales to these answers and even more NCLEX review questions, visit *http://evolve.elsevier.com/Lewis/medsurg.*

REFERENCES

1. Thibodeau G, Patton K: *Structure and function of the body,* ed 14, St Louis, 2012, Mosby.
2. *Saunders nursing drug handbook 2012,* St Louis, 2012, Saunders.
3. American Foundation for the Blind: AFB senior site. Retrieved from *www.afb.org/seniorsite.asp?SectionID=63&TopicID=286&DocumentID=3198.*
4. Goldman L, Schafer A, editors: *Goldman's Cecil medicine,* ed 24, St Louis, 2011, Saunders.
5. Rakel R, Rakel D, editors: *Textbook of family medicine,* ed 8, St Louis, 2011, Saunders.
*6. Almog Y, Nemet A: The correlation between visual acuity and color vision as an indicator of the cause of visual loss, *Am J Ophthalmol* 149:1000, 2010.

*Evidence-based information for clinical practice.

7. National Institute on Deafness and Other Communication Disorders: Quick statistics. Retrieved from *www.nided.nih.gov/health/statistics.*
8. Ko J: Presbycusis and its management, *Br J Nurs* 19:160, 2010.
9. Bope E, Kellerman R, editors: *Conn's current therapy 2012,* St Louis, 2011, Saunders.
10. Isaacson B: Hearing loss, *Med Clin North Am* 94:973, 2010.

RESOURCES

Resources for this chapter are listed after Chapter 22 on p. 413.

CHAPTER

22

Nursing Management
Visual and Auditory Problems

Mary Ann Kolis

⊖volve WEBSITE

LEARNING OUTCOMES

1. Compare and contrast the types of refractive errors and appropriate corrections.
2. Describe the etiology and collaborative care of extraocular disorders.
3. Explain the pathophysiology, clinical manifestations, and nursing management and collaborative care of the patient with selected intraocular disorders.
4. Discuss the nursing measures that promote the health of the eyes and ears.
5. Elaborate on the general preoperative and postoperative care of patients undergoing surgery of the eye or ear.
6. Summarize the action and uses of drug therapy for treating problems of the eyes and ears.
7. Explain the pathophysiology, clinical manifestations, and nursing and collaborative management of common ear problems.
8. Compare the causes, management, and rehabilitative potential of conductive and sensorineural hearing loss.
9. Explain the use, care, and patient teaching related to assistive devices for eye and ear problems.
10. Describe the common causes and assistive measures for uncorrectable visual impairment and deafness.
11. Describe the measures used to assist the patient in adapting psychologically to decreased vision and hearing.

KEY TERMS

acoustic neuroma, p. 406
age-related macular degeneration (AMD), p. 397
astigmatism, p. 387
benign paroxysmal positional vertigo (BPPV), p. 406
cataract, p. 393
conjunctivitis, p. 390

enucleation, p. 402
external otitis, p. 403
glaucoma, p. 398
hordeolum, p. 389
hyperopia, p. 387
keratitis, p. 391
Ménière's disease, p. 405
myopia, p. 387

otosclerosis, p. 405
presbycusis, p. 410
presbyopia, p. 387
refractive error, p. 387
retinal detachment, p. 396
retinopathy, p. 395
strabismus, p. 392

Reviewed by Sarah Smith, RN, MA, CRNO, COT, Nurse Manager, Department of Ophthalmology, University of Iowa Health Care, Oxford, Iowa; and Helen Stegall, RN, BSN, CORLN, Nurse Manager of Department of Ophthalmology, University of Iowa Hospitals and Clinics, Iowa City, Iowa.

The chapter describes visual and auditory problems, with an emphasis on their pathophysiology, clinical manifestations, collaborative care, and nursing management. Discussion of assistive devices for visual and hearing impairment is also included.

VISUAL PROBLEMS

CORRECTABLE REFRACTIVE ERRORS

The most common visual problem is **refractive error.** This defect prevents light rays from converging into a single focus on the retina. Defects are a result of irregularities of the corneal curvature, the focusing power of the lens, or the length of the eye. The major symptom is blurred vision. In some cases the patient may also complain of ocular discomfort, eyestrain, or headaches. The principal refractive errors of the eye can be corrected by the use of lenses in the form of eyeglasses or contact lenses, refractive surgery, or surgical implantation of an artificial lens. Contrary to popular belief, failure to correct refractive errors does not worsen the error, nor does it cause any further pathologic conditions after age 6.

Myopia (nearsightedness) is an inability to accommodate for objects at a distance. It causes light rays to be focused in front of the retina. Myopia may occur because of excessive light refraction by the cornea or lens or because of an abnormally long eye. (Refractive errors are depicted in eFig. 22-1 available on the website for this chapter.) Myopia is the most common refractive error, with approximately 25% of Americans having this disorder.

Hyperopia (farsightedness) is an inability to accommodate for near objects. It causes the light rays to focus behind the retina and requires the patient to use accommodation to focus the light rays on the retina for near objects. This type of refractive error occurs when the cornea or lens does not have adequate focusing power or when the eyeball is too short.

Presbyopia is the loss of accommodation associated with age. This condition generally appears at about age 40. As the eye ages, the lens becomes larger, firmer, and less elastic. These changes, which progress with aging, result in an inability to focus on near objects.[1]

Astigmatism is caused by an irregular corneal curvature. This irregularity causes the incoming light rays to be bent unequally. Consequently, the light rays do not come to a single point of focus on the retina. Astigmatism can occur in conjunction with any of the other refractive errors.

Aphakia is the absence of the lens. Rarely, the lens may be absent congenitally, or it may be removed during cataract surgery. A lens that is traumatically injured is removed and replaced with an intraocular lens (IOL) implant. The lens accounts for approximately 30% of ocular refractive power. The absence of the lens results in a significant refractive error. Without the focusing ability of the lens, images are projected behind the retina.

Nonsurgical Corrections

Corrective Glasses. Myopia, hyperopia, presbyopia, and astigmatism can be modified by using the appropriate corrective lenses. Glasses for presbyopia are often called "reading glasses" because they are usually worn for close work only. The presbyopic correction may also be combined with a correction for another refractive error, such as myopia or astigmatism. In these combined glasses the presbyopic correction is in the lower portion of the spectacle lens. A traditional bifocal or trifocal has visible lines. However, most lenses today that correct vision at various distances do not have visible lines. The prescription varies throughout the lens, allowing distance focusing in the top two thirds and near focus in the bottom one third of the lens.

Contact Lenses. Contact lenses are another way to correct refractive errors. Contact lenses are made from various plastic and silicone substances that are highly permeable to oxygen and have a high water content. These features allow for increased wearing time with greater comfort. If the oxygen supply to the cornea is decreased, it becomes swollen, visual acuity decreases, and the patient experiences severe discomfort.

Altered or decreased tear formation can make wearing contact lenses difficult. Tear production can be decreased by medications such as antihistamines, decongestants, diuretics, and birth control pills, as well as the hormones produced during pregnancy. Environmental factors such as wind, fans, and dust may also decrease the tear film. Allergic conjunctivitis with itching, tearing, and redness can also affect contact lens wear.

In general, you need to know whether the patient wears contact lenses, the pattern of wear (daily versus extended), and care practices. Shining a light obliquely on the eyeball can help visualize a contact lens. Contact lenses are associated with microbial keratitis, a severe sight-threatening complication. Risk factors for keratitis include poor hand cleaning, poor lens case hygiene, and inadequate lens cleaning.[2] Teach the patient the importance of following recommended cleaning practices and reporting redness, sensitivity, vision problems, and pain to the eye care professional. Instruct the patient to remove contact lenses immediately if any of these problems occur.

Surgical Therapy

Surgical procedures are designed to eliminate or reduce the need for eyeglasses or contact lenses and correct refractive errors by changing the focus of the eye. Surgical management for refractive errors includes laser surgery and IOL implantation.

Laser. *Laser-assisted in situ keratomileusis* (LASIK) may be considered for patients with low to moderately high amounts of myopia or hyperopia, with or without astigmatism. The procedure first involves using a laser or surgical blade to create a flap in the cornea. The flap is folded back on the middle section, or stroma, of the cornea.[3] Pulses from a computer-controlled laser vaporize a part of the stroma. The flap is then repositioned, adhering on its own without sutures in a few minutes.

Photorefractive keratectomy (PRK) is indicated for low to moderate amounts of myopia or hyperopia, with or without astigmatism and is a good option for a patient with insufficient corneal thickness for a LASIK flap. In PRK only the epithelium is removed, and the laser sculpts the cornea to correct the refractive error. *Laser-assisted subepithelial keratomileusis* (LASEK) is similar to PRK except that the epithelium is replaced after surgery.

Implant. *Refractive intraocular lens* (refractive IOL) implantation is an option for patients with a high degree of myopia or hyperopia. Like cataract surgery, it involves removal of the patient's natural lens and implantation of an IOL, which is a small plastic lens to correct a patient's refractive error. Since this requires entering the eye, the risk of complications is higher. New accommodating IOLs correct both myopia and presbyopia.

Phakic intraocular lenses (phakic IOLs) are sometimes referred to as implantable contact lenses. They are implanted into the eye without removing the eye's natural lens. They are used for patients with high degrees of myopia or hyperopia. Unlike refractive IOLs, the phakic IOL is placed in front of the eye's natural lens. Leaving the natural lens in the eye preserves the eye's ability to focus for reading vision. Artisan is one type of phakic IOL used for moderate to severe myopia.

UNCORRECTABLE VISUAL IMPAIRMENT

In the United States, 6.5 million people over age 65 have *severe visual impairment,* which is defined as the inability to read newsprint even with glasses.[4] Of those individuals, 9% have no useful vision, and the remaining 91% are considered partially sighted. The *partially sighted* individual may still have significant visual abilities.

A patient with visual impairment may be categorized by the level of visual loss. *Total blindness* is defined as no light perception and no usable vision. *Functional blindness* is present when the patient has some light perception but no usable vision.

The patient with either total or functional blindness is considered legally blind. *Legal blindness* refers to central visual acuity of 20/200 or less in the better eye with correction, or a peripheral visual field of 20 degrees or less. It is estimated that about 1.3 million people in the United States are legally blind. Almost all blindness in the United States is the result of common eye diseases, including cataracts, glaucoma, age-related macular degeneration, and diabetic retinopathy. Less than 4% of blindness is the result of injuries.[4]

NURSING MANAGEMENT
VISUAL IMPAIRMENT

NURSING ASSESSMENT

It is important to assess how long the patient has had a visual impairment, since recent loss of vision has different implications for nursing care. Determine how the patient's visual impairment affects normal functioning. Question the patient about the level of difficulty involved in doing certain tasks. For example, ask how much difficulty the patient has when reading a newspaper, writing a check, moving from one room to the next, or viewing television. Other questions can help determine the personal meaning that the patient attaches to the visual impairment. Ask how the vision loss has affected specific aspects of the patient's life, whether the patient has lost a job, or what activities the patient does not engage in because of the visual impairment. The patient may attach many negative meanings

to the impairment because of societal views of blindness. For example, the patient may view the impairment as punishment or view himself or herself as useless and burdensome. Determine the patient's primary coping strategies, the patient's emotional reactions, and the availability and strength of the patient's support systems.

PLANNING

The overall goals are that the patient with recently impaired vision or the patient with poor adjustment to long-standing visual impairment will (1) make a successful adjustment to the impairment, (2) verbalize feelings related to the loss, (3) identify personal strengths and external support systems, and (4) use appropriate coping strategies. If the patient has been functioning at an appropriate or acceptable level, the goal is to maintain the current level of function.

NURSING IMPLEMENTATION

HEALTH PROMOTION. Encourage the partially sighted patient with preventable causes of further visual impairment to seek appropriate health care. For example, the patient with vision loss from glaucoma may prevent further visual impairment by complying with prescribed therapies and suggested ophthalmic evaluations.

ACUTE INTERVENTION. Provide emotional support and direct care to the patient with recent visual impairment. Allow the patient to express anger and grief, and help the patient identify fears and successful coping strategies. The family is intimately involved in the experiences that follow vision loss. With the patient's knowledge and permission, include family members in discussions and encourage them to express their concerns.

Many people are uncomfortable around a blind or partially sighted individual because they are not sure what behaviors are appropriate. Being sensitive to the patient's feelings without being overly worried or smothering the patient's independence is vital in creating a therapeutic nursing presence. Always communicate in a normal conversational tone and manner with the patient, and address the patient, not the caregiver. Common courtesy dictates introducing oneself and any other people who approach the blind or partially sighted patient and saying goodbye on leaving. Making eye contact with the partially sighted patient accomplishes several objectives. It ensures that you are speaking while facing the patient so the patient has no difficulty hearing. Your head position validates that you are attentive to the patient. In addition, establishing eye contact ensures that you can observe the patient's facial expressions and reactions.

Assist the patient using a *sighted-guide technique.* Stand slightly in front and to one side of the patient, and offer an elbow for the patient to hold. Serve as the sighted guide, walking slightly ahead of the patient with the patient holding the back of your arm. As you walk, describe the environment to help orient the patient. For example, "We're going through an open doorway and approaching two steps down." Help the patient sit by placing one of his or her hands on the seat of the chair.

AMBULATORY AND HOME CARE. In working with the visually impaired patient, remember that a person classified as legally blind may have some useful vision. Rehabilitation after partial or total loss of vision can foster independence, self-esteem, and productivity. Know what services and devices are available for the partially sighted or blind patient, and make appropriate referrals. For the legally blind patient the primary resource for services is the state agency for rehabilitation of the blind. Legally blind individuals are eligible for federal and state assistance and income tax benefits. A list of agencies that serve the partially sighted or blind patient is available from the American Foundation for the Blind (www.afb.org). Many of these agencies are listed in the resources section at the end of the chapter.

Braille or audio books for reading and a cane or guide dog for ambulation are examples of vision substitution techniques. These are usually most appropriate for the patient with no functional vision. For most patients who have some remaining vision, vision enhancement techniques can provide help in learning to ambulate, read printed material, and accomplish activities of daily living (ADLs).

Optical Devices for Vision Enhancement. A wide range of newer technologies are available to assist people with low vision.[5] These devices include desktop video magnification/closed circuit units, electronic hand-held magnifiers, text-to-speech scanners (material read aloud to you), E-readers, and computer tablets (material read aloud, magnification, image zooming, brighter screen, voice recognition). Many of these devices require some training by an assistive technology professional. Encourage patients to practice with the technologic device to ensure they can use it successfully.

Nonoptical Methods for Vision Enhancement. Approach magnification is a simple way to enhance the patient's residual vision. Recommend that the patient sit closer to the television or hold books closer to the eyes. Contrast enhancement techniques include watching television in black and white, using a black felt-tip marker, and using contrasting colors (e.g., a red stripe at the edge of steps or curbs). Increased lighting can be provided by halogen lamps, direct sunlight, or gooseneck lamps that can be aimed directly at the reading material or other near objects.[6] Large type is often helpful, especially in conjunction with other optical or nonoptical vision enhancements.

EVALUATION

The overall expected outcomes are that the patient with severe visual impairment will
- Have no further loss of vision
- Be able to use adaptive coping strategies
- Not experience a decrease in self-esteem or social interactions
- Function safely within her or his own environment

GERONTOLOGIC CONSIDERATIONS

VISUAL IMPAIRMENT

The older adult is at an increased risk for vision loss caused by eye disease. This older person may have other deficits, such as cognitive impairment or limited mobility, that further affect the ability to function in usual ways. Societal devaluation of the elderly may compound the self-esteem or isolation issues associated with the older patient's visual impairment. Financial resources may meet normal needs but can be inadequate to meet the increased demands of vision services or assistive devices.

The older patient may become confused or disoriented when visually compromised. The combination of decreased vision and confusion increases the risk of falls, which have potentially serious consequences for the older adult. Decreased vision may compromise the older patient's ability to function, resulting in concerns about maintaining independence and a diminished self-image. Decreased manual dexterity may make the instillation of prescribed eyedrops difficult for some older adults.

EYE TRAUMA

Although the eyes are well protected by the bony orbit and fat pads, everyday activities can result in ocular trauma. In the United States an estimated 2.5 million eye injuries occur each year. Of those injured, more than 10% will lose useful vision in the affected eye. Table 22-1 outlines emergency management of the patient with an eye injury. The most common ocular injuries in the United States occur in the home due to gardening, power tool use, and home repair work.[7] Sport and work-related injuries are additional causes of eye trauma.

Trauma is often a preventable cause of visual impairment. Many eye injuries could be prevented by wearing protective eyewear. Your role in individual and community education is extremely important in reducing the incidence of ocular trauma.

EXTRAOCULAR DISORDERS

INFLAMMATION AND INFECTION

One of the most common conditions encountered by the ophthalmologist is inflammation or infection of the external eye. Many external irritants or microorganisms can affect the eye, conjunctiva, and avascular cornea. It is your responsibility to teach the patient appropriate interventions related to the specific disorder.

An external **hordeolum** (commonly called a *sty*) is an infection of the sebaceous glands in the lid margin (Fig. 22-1). The most common bacterial infective agent is *Staphylococcus aureus.* A red, swollen, circumscribed, and acutely tender area develops rapidly. Instruct the patient to apply warm, moist compresses at least four times a day until it improves. This may be the only treatment necessary. If it tends to recur, teach the patient to perform lid scrubs daily. In addition, appropriate antibiotic ointments or drops may be indicated.

A *chalazion* is a chronic inflammatory granuloma of the meibomian (sebaceous) glands in the lid. It may evolve from a hordeolum or occur in response to the material released into the lid when a blocked gland ruptures. The chalazion usually appears on the upper lid as a swollen, tender, reddened area that may be painful. Initial treatment is similar to that for a hordeolum. If warm, moist compresses are ineffective in promoting spontaneous drainage, the ophthalmologist may surgically remove the lesion (this is normally an office procedure) or inject the lesion with corticosteroids.

Blepharitis is a common chronic bilateral inflammation of the lid margins.[8] The lids are red rimmed with many scales or

✚ TABLE 22-1   EMERGENCY MANAGEMENT

Eye Injury

Etiology	Assessment Findings	Interventions
Trauma • Blunt (e.g., fist) • Penetrating (e.g., glass, metal, or wood fragments. Knife, stick, or other object) **Chemical Burn** • Alkaline • Acid **Thermal Burn** • Direct burn from hot surface • Indirect burn from UV light (e.g., welding torch, looking directly at sun) **Foreign Bodies** • Glass • Metal • Wood • Plastic • Ceramics	• Pain • Photophobia • Redness—diffuse or localized • Swelling • Ecchymosis • Tearing • Blood in the anterior chamber • Absent eye movements • Fluid drainage from eye (e.g., blood, CSF, aqueous humor) • Abnormal or decreased vision • Visible foreign body • Prolapsed globe • Abnormal intraocular pressure • Visual field defect	**Initial** • Determine mechanism of injury. • Ensure airway, breathing, circulation. • Assess for other injuries. • Assess for chemical exposure. • Begin ocular irrigation *immediately* in case of chemical exposure. Do not stop until emergency personnel arrive to continue irrigation. Use sterile saline or water if saline is unavailable. • Assess visual acuity. • Do not put pressure on the eye. • Instruct patient not to blow nose. • Do not attempt to treat the injury (except as noted above for chemical exposure). • Stabilize foreign objects. • Cover the eye(s) with dry, sterile patches and a protective shield. • Do not give the patient food or fluids. • Elevate head of bed 45 degrees. • Do not put medication or solutions in the eye unless ordered by physician. • Administer analgesia as appropriate. **Ongoing Monitoring** • Reassure the patient. • Monitor pain. • Anticipate surgical repair for penetrating injury, globe rupture, or globe avulsion.

CSF, Cerebrospinal fluid; *UV*, ultraviolet.

FIG. 22-1 Hordeolum (sty) on the upper eyelid caused by staphylococcal infection.

crusts on the lid margins and lashes. The patient may primarily complain of itching but may also experience burning, irritation, and photophobia. Conjunctivitis may occur simultaneously.

If the blepharitis is caused by a staphylococcal infection, collaborative care includes the use of an appropriate ophthalmic antibiotic ointment. Often blepharitis is caused by both staphylococcal and seborrheal microorganisms, and the treatment must be more vigorous to avoid hordeolum, *keratitis* (inflammation of the cornea), and other eye infections. Emphasize thorough cleaning practices of the skin and scalp. Gentle cleansing of the lid margins with baby shampoo can effectively soften and remove crusting.

Conjunctivitis

Conjunctivitis is an infection or inflammation of the conjunctiva. These infections may be caused by bacteria or viruses. Conjunctival inflammation may result from exposure to allergens or chemical irritants. The tarsal conjunctiva (lining the interior surface of the lids) may become inflamed as a result of a chronic foreign body in the eye, such as a contact lens. Careful hand washing and use of individual or disposable towels help prevent spreading the condition.

Bacterial Infections. Acute bacterial conjunctivitis *(pinkeye)* is a common infection. Although it occurs in every age-group, epidemics are common among children because of their poor hygienic habits. *S. aureus* is the most common cause. The patient with bacterial conjunctivitis may complain of discomfort, pruritus, redness, and a mucopurulent drainage.[9] Although this typically occurs initially in one eye, it generally spreads to the unaffected eye. It is usually self-limiting, but treatment with antibiotic drops (e.g., besifloxacin [Besivance]) shortens the course of the disorder.

Viral Infections. Conjunctival infections may be caused by many different viruses. The patient with viral conjunctivitis may complain of tearing, foreign body sensation, redness, and mild photophobia. This condition is usually mild and self-limiting. However, it can be severe, with increased discomfort and subconjunctival hemorrhaging. Adenovirus conjunctivitis may be contracted in contaminated swimming pools and through direct contact with an infected patient. Treatment is usually palliative. If the patient is severely symptomatic, topical corticosteroids can provide temporary relief but have no effect on the final outcome. Antiviral drops are ineffective and therefore not indicated.

Chlamydial Infections. Trachoma is a chronic conjunctivitis caused by *Chlamydia trachomatis* (serotypes A through C). It is a major cause of blindness worldwide. An estimated 84 million people have active disease in need of treatment if blindness is to be prevented, with 8 million people already living with irreversible vision loss.[10]

This preventable eye disease is transmitted mainly by the hands and by flies. Adult inclusion conjunctivitis (AIC) is caused by *C. trachomatis* (serotypes D through K). AIC is becoming more prevalent in the United States because of the increase in sexually transmitted chlamydial infection.

Manifestations of both trachoma and AIC are mucopurulent ocular discharge, irritation, redness, and lid swelling. For unknown reasons, AIC does not carry the long-term consequences of trachoma. AIC also differs from trachoma in that it is common in economically developed countries, whereas trachoma is most commonly seen in underdeveloped countries. Antibiotic therapy is usually effective for trachoma and AIC.

Although antibiotic treatment may be successful, patients with AIC have a high risk of concurrent chlamydial genital infection, as well as other sexually transmitted infections. In your teaching plan for these patients, include the sexual implications of AIC.

Allergic Conjunctivitis. Conjunctivitis caused by exposure to an allergen can be mild and transitory, or it can be severe enough to cause significant swelling, sometimes ballooning the conjunctiva beyond the eyelids. The defining symptom of allergic conjunctivitis is itching. The patient may also complain of burning, redness, and tearing. In addition to pollens, the patient may develop allergic conjunctivitis in response to animal dander, ocular solutions, and medications. Instruct the patient to avoid the allergen if it is known. Artificial tears can be effective in diluting the allergen and washing it from the eye. Effective topical medications include antihistamines and corticosteroids.

Keratitis

Keratitis is an inflammation or infection of the cornea that can be caused by a variety of microorganisms or by other factors. The condition may involve the conjunctiva and/or the cornea. When it involves both, the disorder is termed *keratoconjunctivitis*.

Bacterial Infections. The cornea can become infected by a variety of bacteria. Topical antibiotics are generally effective, but eradicating the infection may require subconjunctival antibiotic injection or, in severe cases, IV antibiotics. Risk factors include mechanical or chemical corneal epithelial damage, contact lens wear, nutritional deficiencies, immunosuppressed states, and contaminated products (e.g., lens care solutions and cases, topical medications, cosmetics).

Viral Infections. Herpes simplex virus (HSV) keratitis is the most frequently occurring infectious cause of corneal blindness in the Western hemisphere. It is a growing problem, especially with immunosuppressed patients. The corneal ulcer has a characteristic dendritic (tree-branching) appearance. Pain and photophobia are common. Up to 40% of patients with herpetic keratitis heal spontaneously.

Antiviral treatments include trifluridine drops (Viroptic), oral acyclovir (Zovirax), and topical vidarabine (Vira-A) ointment.[11] Therapy may also involve corneal debridement. Topical corticosteroids are usually contraindicated because they contribute to a longer course and possible deeper ulceration of the cornea.

The varicella-zoster virus (VZV) causes both chickenpox and herpes zoster ophthalmicus (HZO). HZO may occur by reactivation of an endogenous infection that has persisted in a latent form after an earlier attack of varicella or by contact with a patient with chickenpox or herpes zoster. It occurs most frequently in the older adult and in the immunosuppressed patient. Collaborative care of the patient with acute HZO may include analgesics for the pain, topical corticosteroids to reduce inflammation, antiviral agents such as acyclovir to reduce viral replication, mydriatic agents to dilate the pupil and relieve pain, and topical antibiotics to combat secondary infection. The patient may apply warm compresses and povidone-iodine gel to the affected skin (gel should not be applied near the eye).

Epidemic keratoconjunctivitis (EKC) is the most serious ocular adenoviral disease. EKC is spread by direct contact, including sexual activity. In the medical setting, contaminated hands and instruments can be the source of spread. The patient may complain of tearing, redness, photophobia, and foreign body sensation. In most patients the disease involves only one eye. Treatment is primarily palliative and includes ice packs and dark glasses. In severe cases therapy can include mild topical corticosteroids to temporarily relieve symptoms and topical antibiotic ointment. Teach the patient and the caregiver the importance of good hygiene practices to avoid spreading the disease.

Other Causes of Keratitis. Keratitis may also be caused by fungi (most commonly *Aspergillus, Candida,* and *Fusarium* species), especially in the case of ocular trauma in an outdoor setting where fungi are prevalent in the soil and moist organic matter.

Acanthamoeba keratitis is caused by a parasite that is associated with contact lens wear, probably as a result of contaminated lens care solutions or cases. Homemade saline solution is particularly susceptible to *Acanthamoeba* contamination. Instruct the patient who wears contact lenses about good lens care practices. Medical treatment of *Acanthamoeba* keratitis is difficult, since the organism is resistant to most drugs. Only one antifungal eyedrop (natamycin [Natacyn]) is approved by the U.S. Food and Drug Administration (FDA). If antimicrobial therapy fails, the patient may require a corneal transplant.

Exposure keratitis occurs when the patient cannot adequately close the eyelids. The patient with *exophthalmos* (protruding eyeball) from thyroid eye disease or masses posterior to the globe is susceptible to exposure keratitis.

Corneal Ulcer. Tissue loss caused by infection of the cornea produces a *corneal ulcer* (infectious keratitis) (Fig. 22-2). The infection can be due to bacteria, viruses, or fungi. Corneal ulcers are often painful, and patients may feel as if there is a foreign body in their eye. Other symptoms can include tearing, purulent or watery discharge, redness, and photophobia. Treatment is generally aggressive to avoid permanent loss of vision.

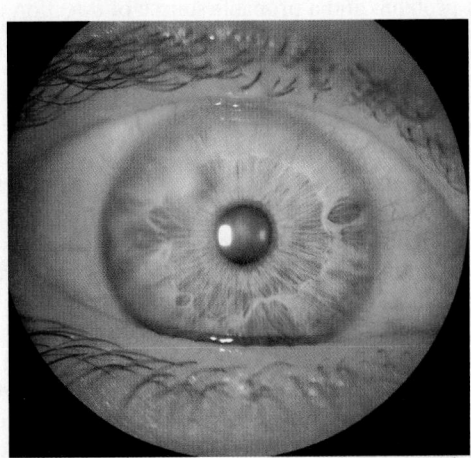

FIG. 22-2 Corneal ulcer. Infection associated with poor contact lens care.

Antibiotic, antiviral, or antifungal eyedrops may be prescribed as frequently as every hour night and day for the first 24 hours. An untreated corneal ulcer can result in corneal scarring and perforation (hole in the cornea). A corneal transplant may be indicated.

NURSING MANAGEMENT INFLAMMATION AND INFECTION

Assess ocular changes, such as edema, redness, decreased visual acuity, feelings that a foreign body is present, or discomfort. Document the findings in the patient's record. Also consider the psychosocial aspects of the patient's condition, especially when vision is impaired.

Careful asepsis and frequent, thorough hand washing are essential to prevent spreading organisms from one eye to the other, to other patients, to family members, and to health care professionals. Teach the patient and the family about avoiding sources of ocular irritation or infection and responding appropriately if an ocular problem occurs. Inform the patient about appropriate use and care of lenses and lens care products. The patient with infective disorders that may have a sexual mode of transmission needs specific information about those disorders.

Apply warm or cool compresses if indicated for the patient's condition. Darkening the room and providing an appropriate analgesic are other comfort measures. If the patient's visual acuity is decreased, modify the patient's environment or activities for safety.

The patient may require eyedrops as frequently as every hour. If the patient receives two or more different drops, stagger the eyedrops to promote maximum absorption. For example, if two different eyedrops are ordered hourly, administer one drop on the hour and one drop on the half hour (unless otherwise prescribed). The patient who needs frequent eyedrop administration may experience sleep deprivation.

The patient's primary need in the home environment is for information about required care and how to accomplish that care. Also instruct the patient and the caregiver about the proper techniques for medication administration. If the patient's vision is compromised, suggest alternative ways to accomplish necessary daily activities and self-care. Inform the patient who wears contact lenses and develops infections to discard all opened or used lens care products and cosmetics to decrease the risk of reinfection from contaminated products (a common problem and a probable source of infection for many patients).

DRY EYE DISORDERS

Keratoconjunctivitis sicca (dry eyes) is a common complaint, particularly of older adults and individuals with certain systemic diseases such as scleroderma and systemic lupus erythematosus. Patients with dry eyes complain of irritation or "sand in my eye" and that the sensation typically worsens through the day. This condition is caused by a decrease in the quality or quantity of the tear film, and treatment is directed at the underlying cause. With decreased tear secretion, the patient may use artificial tears or ointments. In severe cases, closure of the lacrimal puncta may be necessary. Patients with dry eyes associated with dry mouth may have Sjögren's syndrome (see Chapter 65).

STRABISMUS

Strabismus is a condition in which the patient cannot consistently focus two eyes simultaneously on the same object. One eye may deviate in *(esotropia)*, out *(exotropia)*, up *(hypertropia)*, or down *(hypotropia)* (see eFig. 22-2 available on the website for this chapter). Strabismus in the adult may be caused by thyroid disease, neuromuscular problems of the eye muscles, retinal detachment repair, or cerebral lesions. In the adult the primary complaint with strabismus is double vision.

CORNEAL DISORDERS

Corneal Scars and Opacities

The cornea is an optically transparent tissue that allows light rays to enter the eye and focus on the retina, thus producing a visual image. Any wound causes the cornea to become abnormally hydrated and decreases the normal transparency. The treatment for corneal scars or opacities is *penetrating keratoplasty* (corneal transplant). The ophthalmic surgeon removes the full thickness of the patient's cornea and replaces it with a donor cornea that is sutured into place (Fig. 22-3). Vision may not be restored for up to 12 months. Newer procedures in which only the damaged cornea epithelial layer is replaced are Descemet's stripping endothelial keratoplasty (DSEK) and Descemet's membrane endothelial keratoplasty (DMEK).[12] Patients report faster visual recovery with less astigmatism and changes in their glass lens prescription with these surgeries.

Approximately 40,000 corneal transplants are performed in the United States each year. The surgery is one of the fastest and safest of all tissue or organ transplant surgeries. The time between the donor's death and the removal of the tissue should be as short as possible. The eye banks test donors for human immunodeficiency virus (HIV) and hepatitis B and C. The tissue is preserved in a special nutritive solution. Improved methods of tissue procurement and preservation, postoperative topical corticosteroids, and careful follow-up have decreased graft rejection. Matching the blood type of the donor and the recipient may also improve the success rate.

Keratoconus

Keratoconus is a noninflammatory, usually bilateral disease that has a familial tendency. Keratoconus usually appears during adolescence and slowly progresses between ages 20 and 60

FIG. 22-3 Sutures on a donated cornea after penetrating keratoplasty (corneal transplant).

years. The anterior cornea thins and protrudes forward, taking on a cone shape. The only symptom is blurred vision. The astigmatism may be corrected with glasses or rigid contact lenses.

Intacs inserts are two clear plastic lenses surgically inserted on the cornea perimeter to reduce astigmatism and myopia. Intacs are generally used to delay the need for a corneal transplant when contact lenses or glasses no longer help a patient achieve adequate vision.

The cornea can perforate as central corneal thinning progresses. In advanced cases a penetrating keratoplasty is indicated before perforation.

INTRAOCULAR DISORDERS

CATARACT

A cataract is an opacity within the lens. The patient may have a cataract in one or both eyes. If cataracts are present in both eyes, one may affect the patient's vision more than the other. Almost 22 million Americans ages 40 years and older have cataracts, and by age 80 more than 50% have cataracts. Direct medical costs for cataract treatment are estimated at $6.8 billion annually. Cataract removal is the most common surgical procedure in the United States.[13]

Etiology and Pathophysiology

Although most cataracts are age related (senile cataracts), they can be associated with other factors. These include blunt or penetrating trauma, congenital factors such as maternal rubella, radiation or ultraviolet (UV) light exposure, certain drugs such as systemic corticosteroids or long-term topical corticosteroids, and ocular inflammation. The patient with diabetes mellitus tends to develop cataracts at a younger age.

Cataract development is mediated by a number of factors. In senile cataract formation it appears that altered metabolic processes within the lens cause an accumulation of water and alterations in the lens fiber structure. These changes affect lens transparency, causing vision changes.

Clinical Manifestations and Diagnostic Studies

The patient with cataracts may complain of a decrease in vision, abnormal color perception, and glare. Glare is due to light scatter caused by the lens opacities, and it may be significantly worse at night when the pupil dilates. The visual decline is gradual, but the rate of cataract development varies from patient to patient. Diagnosis is based on decreased visual acuity or other complaints of visual dysfunction. The opacity is directly observable by ophthalmoscopic or slit lamp microscopic examination. As noted earlier, a totally opaque lens creates the appearance of a white pupil. Table 22-2 lists other diagnostic studies that may be helpful in evaluation of a cataract.

Collaborative Care

The presence of a cataract does not necessarily indicate a need for surgery. For many patients the diagnosis is made long before they actually decide to have surgery. Nonsurgical therapy may postpone the need for surgery. Collaborative care for cataracts is presented in Table 22-2.

Nonsurgical Therapy. Currently, no treatment is available to "cure" cataracts other than surgical removal. Often changing the patient's eyewear prescription can improve visual acuity, at least temporarily. Other visual aids, such as strong reading glasses or

TABLE 22-2   COLLABORATIVE CARE
Cataract

Diagnostic	Acute Care: Surgical Therapy
• History and physical examination	**Preoperative**
• Visual acuity measurement	• Mydriatic, cycloplegic agents
• Ophthalmoscopy (direct and indirect)	• Nonsteroidal antiinflammatory drugs
• Slit lamp microscopy	• Topical antibiotics
• Glare testing, potential acuity testing in selected patients	• Antianxiety medications
• Keratometry and A-scan ultrasound (if surgery is planned)	**Surgery**
• Other tests (e.g., visual field perimetry) to determine cause of visual loss	• Removal of lens
	• Phacoemulsification
	• Extracapsular extraction
	• Correction of surgical aphakia
Collaborative Therapy	• Intraocular lens implantation (most frequent type of correction)
Nonsurgical	• Contact lens
• Change in glasses prescription	
• Strong reading glasses or magnifiers	**Postoperative**
• Increased lighting	• Topical antibiotic
• Lifestyle adjustment	• Topical corticosteroid or other antiinflammatory agent
	• Mild analgesia if necessary
	• Eye shield and activity as preferred by patient's surgeon

magnifiers of some type, may help the patient with close vision. Increasing the amount of light to read or accomplish other near-vision tasks is another useful measure. The patient may be willing to adjust his or her lifestyle to adjust to visual decline. For example, if glare makes it difficult to drive at night, a patient may elect to drive only during daylight hours or to have a family member drive at night. Sometimes informing and reassuring the patient about the disease process makes the patient comfortable about choosing nonsurgical measures, at least temporarily.

Surgical Therapy. When palliative measures no longer provide an acceptable level of visual function, the patient is an appropriate candidate for surgery. The patient's occupational needs and lifestyle changes are also factors affecting the decision to have surgery. In some instances, factors other than the patient's visual needs may influence the need for surgery. Lens-induced problems such as increased intraocular pressure (IOP) may require lens removal. Opacities may prevent the ophthalmologist from obtaining a clear view of the retina in the patient with diabetic retinopathy or other sight-threatening pathologic conditions. In those cases the cataract may be removed to allow visualization of the retina and adequate management of the problem.

Preoperative Phase. The patient's preoperative preparation should include an appropriate history and physical examination. Because almost all patients have local anesthesia, many physicians and surgical facilities do not require an extensive preoperative physical assessment. However, most patients with cataracts are older adults who may have several medical problems that should be evaluated and controlled before surgery. Almost all patients with cataracts are admitted to a surgical facility on an outpatient basis. The patient is normally admitted several hours before surgery to allow time for preoperative procedures.

The patient receives dilating drops and a nonsteroidal antiinflammatory eyedrop to reduce inflammation. One type of drug used for dilation is a *mydriatic,* an α-adrenergic agonist that produces pupillary dilation by contraction of the iris dilator muscle. Another type of drug is a *cycloplegic,* an anticholinergic agent that produces paralysis of accommodation (cycloplegia) by blocking the effect of acetylcholine on the ciliary body muscles. Cycloplegics (tropicamide [Mydriacyl, Tropicacyl]) produce pupillary dilation (mydriasis) by blocking the effect of acetylcholine on the iris sphincter muscle. The patient often receives preoperative antianxiety medication before the local anesthesia injection.

DRUG ALERT: Cycloplegics and Mydriatics
- Instruct patient to wear dark glasses to minimize photophobia.
- Monitor for signs of systemic toxicity (e.g., tachycardia, central nervous system [CNS] effects).

Intraoperative Phase. Cataract extraction is an intraocular procedure. The anterior capsule is opened and the lens nucleus and cortex are removed, leaving the remaining capsular bag intact. In extracapsular extraction the surgeon removes the lens nucleus by *phacoemulsification,* in which the nucleus is fragmented by ultrasonic vibration and aspirated from inside the capsular bag.[14] The remaining cortex is aspirated with an irrigation and aspiration instrument. Larger incisions require closure with sutures, whereas smaller incisions are self-sealing and may require no closing suture.

Almost all patients now have an IOL implanted at the time of cataract extraction surgery (Fig. 22-4). The lens of choice is a posterior chamber lens that is implanted in the capsular bag behind the iris. At the end of the procedure, additional medications such as antibiotics and corticosteroids may be administered. Depending on the type of anesthesia, the patient's eye may be covered with a patch or protective shield, which is usually worn overnight and removed during the first postoperative visit.

Postoperative Phase. Unless complications occur, the patient is usually ready to go home as soon as the effects of sedative agents have worn off. Postoperative medications usually include antibiotic drops to prevent infection and corticosteroid drops to decrease the postoperative inflammatory response. Although postoperative activity restrictions and nighttime eye shielding are probably unnecessary, many ophthalmologists still prefer that the patient avoid activities that increase the IOP, such as bending or stooping, coughing, or lifting.

During each postoperative examination the surgeon measures the patient's visual acuity, checks anterior chamber depth,

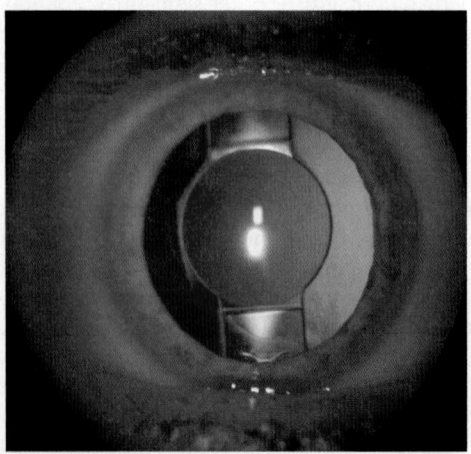

FIG. 22-4 Intraocular lens implant after cataract surgery.

assesses corneal clarity, and measures IOP. Even on the operative day the patient's uncorrected visual acuity in the operative eye may be good. However, it is not unusual or indicative of any problem if the patient's visual acuity is reduced immediately after surgery.

The postoperative eyedrops are gradually reduced in frequency and finally discontinued when the eye has healed. When the eye is fully recovered, the patient receives a final prescription for glasses. The newest innovation is a multifocal IOL that corrects for both near and far vision. Regardless of the type of IOL used, patients may still need glasses to achieve their best visual acuity.

NURSING MANAGEMENT CATARACTS

NURSING ASSESSMENT

Assess the patient's distance and near visual acuity. If the patient is going to have surgery, especially note the visual acuity in the patient's unoperated eye. Use this information to determine how visually compromised the patient may be while the operative eye is healing. In addition, assess the psychosocial impact of the patient's visual disability and the level of knowledge regarding the disease process and therapeutic options. Postoperatively, assess the patient's level of comfort and ability to follow the postoperative regimen.

NURSING DIAGNOSES

Nursing diagnoses for the patient with a cataract include, but are not limited to, the following:
- Self-care deficits *related to* visual deficit
- Anxiety *related to* lack of knowledge about the surgical and postoperative experience

PLANNING

Preoperatively, the overall goals are that the patient with a cataract will (1) make informed decisions regarding therapeutic options and (2) experience minimal anxiety. Postoperatively, the overall goals are that the patient with a cataract will (1) understand and comply with postoperative therapy, (2) maintain an acceptable level of physical and emotional comfort, and (3) remain free of infection and other complications.

NURSING IMPLEMENTATION

HEALTH PROMOTION. There are no proven measures to prevent cataract development. However, it is probably wise (and certainly does no harm) to suggest that the patient wear sunglasses, avoid extraneous or unnecessary radiation, and maintain appropriate intake of antioxidant vitamins (e.g., vitamins C and E) and good nutrition. Also provide information about vision enhancement techniques for the patient who chooses not to have surgery.

ACUTE INTERVENTION. Preoperatively, the patient with cataracts needs accurate information about the disease process and the treatment options, especially because cataract surgery is considered an elective procedure. Be available to give the patient and the family information to help them make an informed decision about appropriate treatment. For the patient who elects to have surgery, provide information, support, and reassurance about the surgical and postoperative experience to reduce or alleviate anxiety.

TABLE 22-3 PATIENT & CAREGIVER TEACHING GUIDE

After Eye Surgery

Include the following information in the teaching plan for the patient and the caregiver after eye surgery.

- Proper hygiene and eye care techniques to ensure that medications, dressings, and/or surgical wound is not contaminated during eye care
- Signs and symptoms of infection and when and how to report these to allow for early recognition and treatment of possible infection
- Importance of complying with postoperative restrictions on head positioning, bending, coughing, and Valsalva maneuver to optimize visual outcomes and prevent increased intraocular pressure
- How to instill eye medications using aseptic techniques and adherence with prescribed eye medication routine to prevent infection
- How to monitor pain, take pain medication, and report pain not relieved by medication
- Importance of continued follow-up as recommended to maximize potential visual outcomes

Source: Lamb P, Simms-Eaton S: *Core curriculum for ophthalmic nursing*, ed 3, Dubuque, 2008, Kendall-Hunt.

Photophobia is common when administering pupil dilation medications. Therefore decreasing the room lighting is helpful. These medications produce transient stinging and burning. Table 22-3 outlines patient and caregiver teaching after eye surgery. Inform patients with a patch that they will not have depth perception until the patch is removed. This necessitates special considerations to avoid falls or other injuries. The patient with significant visual impairment in the unoperated eye requires more assistance while the operative eye is patched. Some patients may require 1 or 2 weeks for the visual acuity in the operated eye to reach an adequate level for most visual needs. These patients also need some special assistance until the vision improves.

After cataract surgery the patient usually experiences little or no pain but may have some scratchiness in the operative eye. Mild analgesics are usually sufficient to relieve any pain. If the pain is intense, the patient should notify the surgeon because this may indicate hemorrhage, infection, or increased IOP. Also instruct the patient to notify the surgeon if there is increased or purulent drainage, increased redness, or any decrease in visual acuity. A nursing care plan for the patient after eye surgery (eNursing Care Plan 22-1) is available on the website for this chapter.

AMBULATORY AND HOME CARE. Patients with cataracts who have surgery remain in the surgical facility for only a few hours. The patient and caregiver are responsible for almost all postoperative care. Give them written and verbal instructions before discharge, including information about postoperative eye care, activity restrictions, medications, follow-up visit schedule, and signs and symptoms of possible complications. Include the patient's caregiver in the instruction because some patients may have difficulty with self-care activities, especially if the vision in the unoperated eye is poor. Provide an opportunity for the patient and the caregiver to perform return demonstrations of any self-care activities.

Most patients experience little visual impairment after surgery.[15] IOL implants provide immediate visual rehabilitation,

and many patients achieve a usable level of visual acuity within a few days after surgery.

A few patients may have significant visual impairment postoperatively. These include patients who do not have an IOL implanted at the time of surgery, those who require several weeks to achieve a usable level of visual acuity following surgery, or those with poor vision in their unoperated eye. For those patients the time between surgery and receiving glasses or contacts can be a period of significant visual disability. Suggest ways the patient and caregiver can modify activities and the environment to maintain an adequate level of safe functioning. Suggestions may include getting assistance with steps, removing area rugs and other potential obstacles, preparing meals for freezing before surgery, or obtaining audio books for diversion until visual acuity improves.

EVALUATION

The overall expected outcomes are that the patient following cataract surgery will

- Have improved vision
- Be better able to take care of self
- Have minimal to no pain
- Be optimistic about expected outcomes

GERONTOLOGIC CONSIDERATIONS

CATARACTS

Most patients with cataracts are older. When the older patient is visually impaired, even temporarily, the patient may experience a loss of independence, lack of control over her or his life, and a significant change in self-perception. Societal devaluation of the older individual complicates these experiences. The older patient often needs emotional support and encouragement, as well as specific suggestions to allow a maximum level of independent function. Assure the older patient that cataract surgery can be accomplished safely and comfortably with minimal sedation.

RETINOPATHY

Retinopathy is a process of microvascular damage to the retina. It can develop slowly or rapidly and lead to blurred vision and progressive vision loss. Retinopathy occurs most often in adults with diabetes mellitus or hypertension.

Diabetic retinopathy is a common complication of diabetes mellitus, especially in patients with long-standing uncontrolled diabetes. It is estimated that 40% of patients with diabetes over the age of 40 years have some evidence of retinopathy. (Diabetes is discussed in Chapter 49.) *Nonproliferative retinopathy* is the most common form of diabetic retinopathy and is characterized by capillary microaneurysms, retinal swelling, and hard exudates. Macular edema represents a worsening of the retinopathy as plasma leaks from macular blood vessels. As capillary walls weaken, they can rupture, leading to intraretinal "dot or blot" hemorrhaging (Fig. 22-5). A severe loss in central vision can result. As the disease advances, *proliferative retinopathy* may occur. New blood vessels grow, but they are abnormal, fragile, and predisposed to leak, thus causing severe vision loss. Fluorescein angiography is used to detect retinopathy, which may be treated with laser photocoagulation.[16]

Hypertensive retinopathy is caused by high blood pressure creating blockages in retinal blood vessels. (Hypertension is

FIG. 22-5 Diabetic retinopathy. Intraretinal dot or blot hemorrhages.

TABLE 22-5	**COLLABORATIVE CARE**

Retinal Detachment

Diagnostic	Surgery
• History and physical examination	• Laser photocoagulation
• Visual acuity measurement	• Cryotherapy (cryopexy)
• Ophthalmoscopy (direct and indirect)	• Scleral buckling procedure
• Slit lamp microscopy	• Vitrectomy
• Ultrasound if cornea, lens, or vitreous is hazy or opaque	• Intravitreal bubble
	Postoperative
Collaborative Therapy Preoperative	• Topical antibiotic
• Mydriatic, cycloplegic agents	• Topical corticosteroid
• Photocoagulation of retinal break that has not progressed to detachment	• Analgesia
	• Mydriatics
	• Positioning and activity as preferred by patient's surgeon

discussed in Chapter 33.) These changes may not initially affect a person's vision. On a routine eye examination, retinal hemorrhages, anoxic cotton-wool spots, and macular swelling can be noted. Sustained, severe hypertension can cause sudden visual loss from swelling of the optic disc and nerve (*papilledema*). Treatment, which may be an emergency, focuses on lowering the blood pressure. Normal vision is restored in most patients with treatment of the underlying cause of the hypertension.

RETINAL DETACHMENT

A **retinal detachment** is a separation of the sensory retina and the underlying pigment epithelium, with fluid accumulation between the two layers. The incidence of retinal detachment is approximately 1 out of every 15,000 individuals each year. In the patient with no other risk factors who has had a retinal detachment in one eye, the risk of detachment in the second eye is 2% to 25%. Almost all patients with an untreated, symptomatic retinal detachment become blind in the involved eye.

Etiology and Pathophysiology

Retinal detachment has many causes, the most common of which is a retinal break. *Retinal breaks* are an interruption in the full thickness of the retinal tissue, and they can be classified as tears or holes. *Retinal holes* are atrophic retinal breaks that occur spontaneously. *Retinal tears* can occur as the vitreous humor shrinks during aging and pulls on the retina. The retina tears when the traction force exceeds the strength of the retina. Once the retina has a break, liquid vitreous can enter the subretinal space between the sensory layer and the retinal pigment epithelium layer, causing a *rhegmatogenous* retinal detachment. Risk factors for retinal detachment are listed in Table 22-4.

Clinical Manifestations and Diagnostic Studies

Patients with a detaching retina describe symptoms that include *photopsia* (light flashes); floaters; and a "cobweb," "hairnet," or ring in the field of vision. Once the retina has detached, the patient describes a painless loss of peripheral or central vision, "like a curtain" coming across the field of vision. The area of visual loss corresponds to the area of detachment. If the detachment is small or develops slowly, the patient may not be aware of a visual problem. Visual acuity measurements should be the first diagnostic procedure with any complaint of vision loss

(Table 22-5). The retinal detachment can be directly visualized using direct and indirect ophthalmoscopy or slit lamp microscopy in conjunction with a special lens to view the far periphery of the retina. Ultrasound may be useful in identifying a retinal detachment if the retina cannot be directly visualized (e.g., when the cornea, lens, or vitreous is hazy or opaque).

Collaborative Care

Some retinal breaks are not likely to progress to detachment. In these situations the ophthalmologist simply monitors the patient, giving precise information about the warning signs and symptoms of impending detachment and instructing the patient to seek immediate evaluation if any of those signs or symptoms is recognized. The ophthalmologist usually refers the patient with a detachment to a retinal specialist. Treatment objectives are to seal any retinal breaks and to relieve inward traction on the retina. Several techniques are used to accomplish these objectives.[17]

Surgical Therapy

Laser Photocoagulation and Cryopexy. These techniques seal retinal breaks by creating an inflammatory reaction that causes a chorioretinal adhesion or scar. *Laser photocoagulation* involves using an intense, precisely focused light beam to create an inflammatory reaction. The light is directed at the area of the retinal break. For retinal breaks accompanied by significant detachment, the retinal specialist may use photocoagulation intraoperatively in conjunction with scleral buckling. Tears or holes without accompanying retinal detachment may be treated prophylactically with laser photocoagulation if there is a high risk of progression to a retinal detachment. When used alone, laser therapy is an outpatient procedure that usually requires only topical anesthesia. The patient may experience minimal adverse symptoms during or after the procedure.

Another method used to seal retinal breaks is cryotherapy (also called *cryopexy*). This procedure involves using extreme cold to create the inflammatory reaction that produces the sealing scar. The ophthalmologist applies the cryoprobe instrument to the external globe in the area over the tear. This is usually done on an outpatient basis and using local anesthesia. As with photocoagulation, cryotherapy may be used alone or during scleral buckling surgery. The patient may experience significant discomfort and eye pain after cryotherapy. Encourage the patient to take the prescribed pain medication.

Scleral Buckling. *Scleral buckling* is an extraocular surgical procedure that involves indenting the globe so that the pigment epithelium, the choroid, and the sclera move toward the detached retina. The retinal surgeon sutures a silicone implant against the sclera, causing the sclera to buckle inward. The surgeon may place an encircling band over the implant if there are multiple retinal breaks, if suspected breaks cannot be located, or if there is widespread inward traction on the retina (Fig. 22-6). If present, subretinal fluid may be drained by inserting a small-gauge needle to facilitate contact between the retina and the buckled sclera. Scleral buckling is usually done with the patient under local anesthesia as an outpatient procedure.

Intraocular Procedures. In addition to the extraocular procedures described, retinal surgeons may also use one or more intraocular procedures in treating some retinal detachments. *Pneumatic retinopexy* is the intravitreal injection of a gas to form a temporary bubble in the vitreous that closes retinal breaks and provides apposition of the separated retinal layers.

Retinal break with detachment — Sclera — Choroid

Silicone implant — Encircling band

Retinal tear — Silicone implant — Encircling band

FIG. 22-6 Retinal break with detachment and surgical repair by scleral buckling technique.

Because the intravitreal bubble is temporary, this technique is combined with laser photocoagulation or cryotherapy (also called cryopexy). The patient with an intravitreal bubble must position the head so that the bubble is in contact with the retinal break. The patient may need to maintain this position as much as possible for up to several weeks.

Vitrectomy (surgical removal of the vitreous) may be used to relieve traction on the retina, especially when the traction results from proliferative diabetic retinopathy. Vitrectomy may be combined with scleral buckling to provide a dual effect in relieving traction.

Postoperative Considerations. Reattachment is successful in 90% of retinal detachments.[17] Visual prognosis varies, depending on the extent, length, and area of detachment. Postoperatively, the patient may be on bed rest and may require special positioning to maintain proper position of an intravitreal bubble. The patient may need multiple topical medications, including antibiotics, antiinflammatory agents, or dilating agents. The level of activity restriction after retinal detachment surgery varies greatly. Verify the prescribed level of activity with each patient's surgeon, and help the patient plan for any necessary assistance related to activity restrictions.

In most cases, retinal detachment is an urgent situation, and the patient is confronted suddenly with the need for surgery. The patient needs emotional support, especially during the immediate preoperative period when preparations for surgery can lead to additional anxiety. When the patient experiences postoperative pain, administer prescribed pain medications and teach the patient to take the medication as necessary after discharge. The patient may go home within a few hours of surgery or may remain in the hospital for several days, depending on the surgeon and the type of repair.

Discharge planning and teaching are important and should begin as early as possible because the patient does not remain hospitalized long. Patient and caregiver teaching after eye surgery is discussed in Table 22-5. The patient is at risk for retinal detachment in the other eye. Therefore teach the patient the signs and symptoms of retinal detachment. Also promote the use of proper protective eyewear to help avoid retinal detachments related to trauma.

AGE-RELATED MACULAR DEGENERATION

Age-related macular degeneration (AMD) is the most common cause of irreversible central vision loss in people over age 60 in the United States. AMD is divided into two forms: dry (nonexudative) and wet (exudative). People with *dry AMD*, which is the more common form (90% of all cases), often notice that close vision tasks are becoming more difficult. In this form the macular cells start to atrophy, leading to a slowly progressive and painless vision loss.

Wet AMD is the more severe form. Wet AMD accounts for 90% of the cases of AMD-related blindness. Wet AMD has a more rapid onset and is characterized by the development of abnormal blood vessels in or near the macula. Patients with wet AMD had dry AMD first.[18]

Etiology and Pathophysiology

AMD is related to retinal aging. Genetic factors also play a major role, and family history is a major risk factor for AMD. A gene responsible for some cases of AMD has been recently identified.

Long-term exposure to UV light, hyperopia, cigarette smoking, and light-colored eyes may be additional risk factors. Nutritional factors may play a role in the progression of AMD. A dietary supplement of vitamin C, vitamin E, beta-carotene, and zinc decreases the progression of advanced AMD but has no effect on people with minimal AMD or those with no evidence of AMD.[19] Eating lots of dark green, leafy vegetables containing lutein (e.g., kale and spinach) may help reduce the risk of AMD (*www.nei.nih.gov/health/maculardegen/armd_facts.asp*).

The dry form of AMD starts with the abnormal accumulation of yellowish extracellular deposits called *drusen* in the retinal pigment epithelium. The atrophy and degeneration of macular cells then result. Wet AMD is characterized by the growth of new blood vessels from their normal location in the choroids to an abnormal location in the retinal epithelium. As the new blood vessels leak, scar tissue gradually forms. Acute vision loss may occur in some cases with bleeding from sub-retinal neovascular membranes.

Clinical Manifestations and Diagnostic Studies

The patient may complain of blurred and darkened vision, *scotomas* (blind spots in the visual field), and *metamorphopsia* (distortion of vision). If patients have only one eye affected, they may not notice early changes in their vision. In addition to visual acuity measurement, the primary diagnostic procedure is ophthalmoscopy. The examiner looks for drusen and other fundus changes associated with AMD. The Amsler grid test may help define the involved area, and it provides a baseline for future comparison. Fundus photography and IV angiography with fluorescein and/or indocyanine green dyes may help to further determine the extent and type of AMD.

Collaborative Care

Vision does not improve for most people with AMD. Limited treatment options for patients with wet AMD include several medications that are injected directly into the vitreous cavity. Ranibizumab (Lucentis), bevacizumab (Avastin), aflibercept (Eylea), and pegaptanib (Macugen) are selective inhibitors of endothelial growth factor, thus helping to slow vision loss in wet AMD. Side effects can include blurred vision, eye irritation, eye pain, and photosensitivity. The injections are given at 4- to 6-week intervals, depending on which drug is used. Retinal stability is determined by ocular coherence tomography (OCT). OCT allows the physician to identify fluid in the central retina that determines the need for continued intravitreal injections.

Photodynamic therapy (PDT) uses verteporfin (Visudyne) IV and a "cold" laser to excite the dye. This procedure is used in wet AMD and destroys the abnormal blood vessels without permanent damage to the retinal pigment epithelium and photoreceptor cells. Verteporfin is a photosensitizing drug that becomes active when exposed to the low-level laser light wave. Until the drug is completely excreted by the body, it can be activated by exposure to sunlight or other high-intensity light such as halogen. Therefore caution patients to avoid direct exposure to sunlight and other intense forms of light for 5 days after treatment. After receiving therapy, patients must be completely covered because any exposure of the skin to sunlight could activate the drug in that area, resulting in a thermal burn.

People at risk for developing advanced AMD should consider supplements of vitamins and minerals (in consultation with their health care provider). The cessation of smoking may also help in halting the progression of dry AMD to a more advanced stage.

Many patients with low-vision assistive devices can continue reading and retain a license to drive during the daytime and at lowered speeds. The permanent loss of central vision has significant psychosocial implications for nursing care. Management of the patient with uncorrectable visual impairment is discussed on p. 388 and is appropriate for the patient with AMD. Avoid giving the impression that "nothing can be done" about the problem when caring for the patient with AMD. Although therapy will not recover lost vision, much can be done to augment the remaining vision.

GLAUCOMA

Glaucoma is a group of disorders characterized by increased IOP and the consequences of elevated pressure, optic nerve atrophy, and peripheral visual field loss. Glaucoma is the second leading cause of permanent blindness in the United States and the leading cause of blindness among African Americans. At least 2 million people have glaucoma, and, of these, more than 50% are unaware of their condition. Another 10 million people have elevated IOP, placing them at increased risk of developing the disease. The incidence of glaucoma increases with age. Blindness from glaucoma is largely preventable with early detection and appropriate treatment. Genetic factors have been identified in some types of glaucoma.[20]

Etiology and Pathophysiology

A proper balance between the rate of aqueous production (referred to as *inflow*) and the rate of aqueous reabsorption (referred to as *outflow*) is essential to maintain the IOP within normal limits. The place where the outflow occurs is called the *angle* because it is the angle where the iris meets the cornea. When the rate of inflow is greater than the rate of outflow, IOP can rise above the normal limits. If IOP remains elevated, permanent vision loss may occur.

Primary open-angle glaucoma (POAG) is the most common type of glaucoma. In POAG the outflow of aqueous humor is decreased in the trabecular meshwork. The drainage channels become clogged, like a clogged kitchen sink. Damage to the optic nerve can then result.

Primary angle-closure glaucoma (PACG) is due to a reduction in the outflow of aqueous humor that results from angle closure. Usually this is caused by the lens bulging forward as a result of the aging process. Angle closure may also occur as a result of pupil dilation in the patient with anatomically narrow angles. An acute attack may be precipitated by situations in which the pupil remains partially dilated long enough to cause an acute and significant rise in the IOP. This may occur because of drug-induced mydriasis, emotional excitement, or darkness. Drug-induced mydriasis may occur not only from topical ophthalmic preparations but also from many systemic medications (both prescription and over-the-counter [OTC] drugs). Check drug records and documentation before administering medications to the patient with angle-closure glaucoma, and instruct the patient not to take any mydriatic medications.

Clinical Manifestations

POAG develops slowly and without symptoms of pain or pressure. The patient usually does not notice the gradual visual field loss until peripheral vision has been severely compromised.

Eventually the patient with untreated glaucoma has "tunnel vision" in which only a small center field can be seen, and all peripheral vision is absent.

Acute angle-closure glaucoma causes definite symptoms, including sudden, excruciating pain in or around the eye. This is often accompanied by nausea and vomiting. Visual symptoms include seeing colored halos around lights, blurred vision, and ocular redness.

Manifestations of subacute or chronic angle-closure glaucoma appear more gradually. The patient who has had a previous, unrecognized episode of subacute angle-closure glaucoma may report a history of blurred vision, seeing colored halos around lights, ocular redness, or eye or brow pain.

Diagnostic Studies

IOP is usually elevated in glaucoma (normal is 10 to 21 mm Hg). In the patient with elevated pressures, the ophthalmologist usually repeats the measurements over time to verify the elevation. In open-angle glaucoma, IOP is usually between 22 and 32 mm Hg. In acute angle-closure glaucoma, IOP may be over 50 mm Hg.

In open-angle glaucoma, slit lamp microscopy reveals a normal angle. In angle-closure glaucoma the examiner may note a markedly narrow or flat anterior chamber angle, an edematous cornea, a fixed and moderately dilated pupil, and ciliary injection (hyperemia of the ciliary blood vessels produces a red color).

Measures of peripheral and central vision provide other diagnostic information. Whereas central acuity may remain 20/20 even in the presence of severe peripheral visual field loss, visual field perimetry may reveal subtle changes in the peripheral retina early in the disease process, long before actual scotomas develop. In acute angle-closure glaucoma, central visual acuity is reduced if the patient has corneal edema, and the visual fields may be markedly decreased. As glaucoma progresses, *optic disc cupping* may be one of the first signs of chronic open-angle glaucoma. The optic disc becomes wider, deeper, and paler (light gray or white), which is visible with direct or indirect ophthalmoscopy (Fig. 22-7).

Collaborative Care

The primary focus of glaucoma therapy is to keep the IOP low enough to prevent the patient from developing optic nerve damage. Therapy varies with the type of glaucoma. The diagnostic and collaborative care of glaucoma is summarized in Table 22-6.

Chronic Open-Angle Glaucoma

Initial treatment in chronic open-angle glaucoma is with drugs (Table 22-7). The patient must understand that continued treatment and supervision are necessary because the drugs control, but do not cure, glaucoma.

Argon laser trabeculoplasty (ALT) is a noninvasive option to lower IOP when medications are not successful or when the patient either cannot or will not use the drug therapy as recommended. ALT is an outpatient procedure that requires only topical anesthetic. The laser stimulates scarring and contraction of the trabecular meshwork, which opens the outflow channels. ALT reduces IOP approximately 75% of the time. The patient uses topical corticosteroids for 3 to 5 days after the procedure. The most common postoperative complication is an acute rise in IOP. The ophthalmologist examines the patient 1 week and again at 4 to 6 weeks after surgery.

FIG. 22-7 A, In the normal eye the optic cup is pink with little cupping. **B,** In glaucoma the optic cup is bleached and optic cupping is present. (Note the appearance of the retinal vessels, which travel over the edge of the optic cup and appear to dip into it.)

TABLE 22-6 COLLABORATIVE CARE

Glaucoma

Diagnostic
- History and physical examination
- Visual acuity measurement
- Tonometry
- Ophthalmoscopy (direct and indirect)
- Slit lamp microscopy
- Gonioscopy
- Visual field perimetry

Collaborative Therapy
Chronic Open-Angle Glaucoma
Drug Therapy (see Table 22-7)
- β-Adrenergic blockers
- α-Adrenergic agonists
- Cholinergic agents (miotics)
- Carbonic anhydrase inhibitors

Surgical Therapy
- Argon laser trabeculoplasty (ALT)
- Trabeculectomy with or without filtering implant

Acute Angle-Closure Glaucoma
- Topical cholinergic agent
- Hyperosmotic agent
- Laser peripheral iridotomy
- Surgical iridectomy

Filtration surgery, also called a *trabeculectomy,* may be indicated if medical management and laser therapy are not successful. The success rate of this surgery is 75% to 85%.

Acute Angle-Closure Glaucoma. Acute angle-closure glaucoma is an ocular emergency that requires immediate intervention. Miotics (see Table 22-7) and oral or IV hyperosmotic agents, including glycerin liquid (Ophthalgan), isosorbide solution (Ismotic), and mannitol solution (Osmitrol), are usually successful in immediately lowering the IOP. A laser peripheral iridotomy or surgical iridectomy is necessary for long-term treatment and prevention of subsequent episodes. These procedures allow the aqueous humor to flow through a newly created opening in the iris and into normal outflow channels. One of these procedures may also be performed on the other eye as a

TABLE 22-7   DRUG THERAPY

Acute and Chronic Glaucoma

Drug	Action	Side Effects	Nursing Considerations
β-Adrenergic Blockers			
betaxolol (Betoptic)	β_1 Cardioselective blocker. ↓ IOP, ↓ aqueous humor production	Transient discomfort. Systemic reactions rarely reported but include bradycardia, heart block, pulmonary distress, headache, depression	Topical drugs. Minimal effect on pulmonary and cardiovascular parameters. Contraindicated in patient with bradycardia, cardiogenic shock, or overt cardiac failure. Systemic absorption can have additive effect with systemic β_1-blocking agents.
carteolol (Ocupress) levobunolol (Betagan) metipranolol (OptiPranolol) timolol maleate (Timoptic, Istalol)	β_1 and β_2 noncardioselective blockers. ↓ IOP, ↓ aqueous humor production	Transient ocular discomfort, blurred vision, photophobia, bradycardia, decreased BP, bronchospasm, headache, depression	Topical drops. Same as betaxolol. These noncardioselective β_2-blockers are also contraindicated in patients with asthma or COPD.
α-Adrenergic Agonists			
dipivefrin (Propine)	α- and β-adrenergic agonist. Converted to epinephrine inside the eye. ↓ aqueous humor production, enhances outflow facility	Ocular discomfort and redness, tachycardia, hypertension	Topical drops. Contraindicated in patient with narrow-angle glaucoma. Teach punctal occlusion if patient at risk of systemic reactions.
epinephrine (Epifrin, Eppy, Glaucon, Epitrate, Epinal, Eppy/N)	Same as dipivefrin	Same as dipivefrin, but can be more pronounced	Topical drops. Same as dipivefrin.
apraclonidine (Iopidine) brimonidine (Alphagan)	α-Adrenergic agonists. ↓ aqueous humor production	Ocular redness. Irregular heart rate	Topical drops. Used to control or prevent acute postlaser IOP rise (used before and immediately after ALT and iridotomy, Nd:YAG laser capsulotomy). Teach patient at risk of systemic reactions to occlude puncta.
latanoprost (Xalatan) travoprost (Travatan) bimatoprost (Lumigan)	Prostaglandin F analogs	Increased brown iris pigmentation, ocular discomfort and redness, dryness, itching, and foreign body sensation	Topical drops. Teach patient to not exceed 1 drop per evening. Have patient remove contact lens 15 min before instilling.
Cholinergic Agents (Miotics)			
carbachol (Isopto Carbachol)	Parasympathomimetic. Stimulates iris sphincter contraction, causing miosis and opening of trabecular meshwork, facilitating aqueous outflow. Also partially inhibits cholinesterase	Transient ocular discomfort, headache, blurred vision, decreased adaptation to the dark, syncope, salivation, dysrhythmias, vomiting, diarrhea, hypotension	Topical drops. Caution patient about ↓ visual acuity caused by miosis, particularly in dim light.
pilocarpine (Akarpine, Isopto Carpine, Pilocar, Pilopine-HS, Piloptic, Pilostat)	Parasympathomimetic. Stimulates iris sphincter contraction, causing miosis and opening of trabecular meshwork, facilitating aqueous humor outflow	Same as carbachol	Topical drops. Same as carbachol.
Carbonic Anhydrase Inhibitors			
Systemic			
acetazolamide (Diamox) dichlorphenamide (Daranide) methazolamide (Neptazane)	↓ Aqueous humor production	Paresthesias, especially "tingling" in extremities. Hearing dysfunction or tinnitus. Loss of appetite, taste alteration, GI disturbances. Drowsiness, confusion	Oral nonbacteriostatic sulfonamides. Anaphylaxis and other sulfa-type allergic reactions may occur in patient allergic to sulfa. Diuretic effect can ↓ electrolyte levels. Should not be given to patient on high-dose aspirin therapy.
Topical			
brinzolamide (Azopt) dorzolamide (Trusopt)	—	Transient stinging, blurred vision, redness	Same as above.

ALT, Argon laser trabeculoplasty; *IOP,* intraocular pressure.

precaution because many patients often experience an acute attack in the other eye.

DRUG ALERT: Miotics
- Warn patients about decreased visual acuity, especially in dim light.

NURSING MANAGEMENT
GLAUCOMA

NURSING ASSESSMENT

Because glaucoma is a chronic condition requiring long-term management, assess the patient's ability to understand and adhere to the rationale and regimen of the prescribed therapy. In addition, assess the patient's psychologic reaction to the diagnosis of a potentially sight-threatening chronic disorder. Include the patient's caregiver in the assessment process because the chronic nature of this disorder affects the family in many ways. Some families may become the primary providers of necessary care, such as eyedrop administration, if the patient is unwilling or unable to accomplish these self-care activities.

NURSING DIAGNOSES

Nursing diagnoses for the patient with glaucoma include, but are not limited to, the following:
- Risk for injury *related to* visual acuity deficits
- Self-care deficits *related to* visual acuity deficits
- Acute pain *related to* pathophysiologic process and surgical correction
- Noncompliance *related to* the inconvenience and side effects of glaucoma medications

PLANNING

The overall goals are that the patient with glaucoma will (1) have no progression of visual impairment, (2) understand the disease process and rationale for therapy, (3) comply with all aspects of therapy (including medication administration and follow-up care), and (4) have no postoperative complications.

NURSING IMPLEMENTATION

HEALTH PROMOTION. Loss of vision as a result of glaucoma is a preventable problem. Teach the patient and the caregiver about the risk of glaucoma and that it increases with age. Stress the importance of early detection and treatment in preventing visual impairment. A comprehensive ophthalmic examination is important in identifying people with glaucoma or those at risk of developing glaucoma. The current recommendation is for an ophthalmologic examination every 2 to 4 years for people between ages 40 and 64 years, and every 1 to 2 years for people age 65 years or older. African Americans in every age category should have examinations more often because of the increased incidence and more aggressive course of glaucoma in these individuals.[21]

ACUTE INTERVENTION. Acute nursing interventions are directed primarily toward the patient with acute angle-closure glaucoma and the surgical patient. The patient with acute angle-closure glaucoma requires immediate medication to lower the IOP. It must be administered in a timely and appropriate manner according to the ophthalmologist's prescription. Most surgical procedures for glaucoma are outpatient procedures. Acutely, the patient needs postoperative instructions and may require nursing measures to relieve discomfort related to the procedure. Patient and caregiver teaching after eye surgery is discussed in Table 22-3.

AMBULATORY AND HOME CARE. Because of the chronic nature of glaucoma, remind the patient to follow the therapeutic regimen and follow-up recommendations prescribed by the ophthalmologist. Provide accurate information about the disease process and treatment options, including the rationale underlying each option. In addition, the patient needs information about the purpose, frequency, and technique for administration of antiglaucoma drugs. Encourage adherence by helping the patient identify the most convenient and appropriate times for medication administration or advocating a change in therapy if the patient reports unacceptable side effects.

EVALUATION

The overall expected outcomes are that the patient with glaucoma will
- Have no further loss of vision
- Adhere to the recommended therapy
- Safely function within own environment
- Obtain relief from pain associated with the disease and surgery

GERONTOLOGIC CONSIDERATIONS

GLAUCOMA

Many older patients with glaucoma have systemic illnesses or take systemic medications that may affect their therapy. In particular, the patient using a β-adrenergic blocking glaucoma agent may experience an additive effect if a systemic β-adrenergic blocking drug is also being taken. All β-adrenergic blocking glaucoma agents are contraindicated in the patient with bradycardia, heart block greater than first-degree heart block, cardiogenic shock, and overt cardiac failure. The noncardioselective β-adrenergic blocking glaucoma agents are also contraindicated in the patient with chronic obstructive pulmonary disease (COPD) or asthma. The hyperosmolar agents may precipitate heart failure or pulmonary edema in the susceptible patient. The older patient on high-dose aspirin therapy for rheumatoid arthritis should not take carbonic anhydrase inhibitors. The α-adrenergic agonists can cause tachycardia or hypertension, which may have serious consequences in the older patient. Teach the older patient to occlude the puncta to limit the systemic absorption of glaucoma medications.

INTRAOCULAR INFLAMMATION AND INFECTION

The term *uveitis* is used to describe inflammation of the uveal tract, retina, vitreous body, or optic nerve. This inflammation may be caused by bacteria, viruses, fungi, or parasites. *Cytomegalovirus retinitis* (CMV retinitis) is an opportunistic infection that occurs in patients with acquired immunodeficiency syndrome (AIDS) and in other immunosuppressed patients. The etiology of sterile intraocular inflammation includes autoimmune disorders, AIDS, malignancies, or those disorders associated with systemic diseases such as inflammatory bowel disease. Pain and photophobia are common symptoms.

Endophthalmitis is an extensive intraocular inflammation of the vitreous cavity. Bacteria, viruses, fungi, or parasites can all induce this serious inflammatory response. The mechanism of infection may be endogenous, in which the infecting agent arrives at the eye through the bloodstream, or exogenous, in which the infecting agent is introduced through a surgical wound or a penetrating injury. Although rare, endophthalmitis is a devastating complication of intraocular surgery or penetrating ocular injury. It can lead to irreversible blindness within hours or days. Manifestations include ocular pain, photophobia, decreased visual acuity, headaches, reddened and swollen conjunctiva, and corneal edema.

Treatment of intraocular inflammation depends on the underlying cause. Intraocular infections require antimicrobial agents, which may be delivered topically, subconjunctivally, intravitreally, systemically, or in some combination. Sterile inflammatory responses require antiinflammatory medications such as corticosteroids. The patient with intraocular inflammation is usually uncomfortable and may be noticeably anxious and frightened. Provide accurate information and emotional support to the patient and family. In severe cases, enucleation may be necessary. When the patient has lost visual function or even the entire eye, the patient will grieve the loss. Your role includes helping the patient through the grieving process.

OCULAR TUMORS

Benign and malignant tumors can occur in many areas of the eye, including the conjunctiva, retina, and orbit. Malignancies of the eyelid include basal cell and squamous cell carcinomas (see Chapter 24).

Uveal melanoma is a cancerous neoplasm of the iris, choroid, or ciliary body. It is the most common primary intraocular malignancy in adults with an incidence of 2610 new cases diagnosed annually in the United States.[22] It is more frequently found in light-skinned people over age 60 with chronic UV exposure. Genetic factors such as a mutated gene may also increase a person's risk. Uveal melanoma can arise from preexisting nevi in the eye. Tumors may be asymptomatic or associated with vision loss depending on their size and location and presence of hemorrhage and retinal detachment. As with other cancers, cancer stage and cell type are important variables in the patient's prognosis. Diagnostic testing may include ultrasonography, magnetic resonance imaging (MRI), and fine-needle aspiration biopsy. Uveal melanoma commonly appears as a dome-shaped, well-circumscribed, solid brown to golden colored pigment in the iris, choroid, or ciliary body (Fig. 22-8). Many patients do not lose their eye, and some may experience good vision after treatment in the affected eye.

FIG. 22-8 Uveal melanoma. A large tumor in the choroid, the most common location in the eye for melanoma.

Depending on the status of the involved eye, treatment options can include enucleation, plaque radiation therapy (brachytherapy), external beam radiation, transpupillary photocoagulation, eye wall resection, and exenteration. Within 15 years, about 50% of all patients with uveal melanoma will develop metastases, with the liver the most common site.

ENUCLEATION

Enucleation is the removal of the eye. The primary indication for enucleation is a blind, painful eye. This may result from glaucoma, infection, or trauma. Enucleation may also be indicated in ocular malignancies. The surgical procedure includes severing the extraocular muscles close to their insertion on the globe, inserting an implant to maintain the intraorbital anatomy, and suturing the ends of the extraocular muscles over the implant. The conjunctiva covers the joined muscles, and a clear conformer is placed over the conjunctiva until the permanent prosthesis is fitted. A pressure dressing helps prevent postoperative bleeding.

Postoperatively, observe the patient for signs of complications, including excessive bleeding or swelling, increased pain, displacement of the implant, or temperature elevation. Patient teaching should include the instillation of topical ointments or drops and wound cleansing. Instruct the patient in the method of inserting the conformer into the socket in case it falls out. The patient is often devastated by the loss of an eye, even when enucleation occurs after a lengthy period of painful blindness. Recognize and validate the patient's emotional response and provide support to the patient and the family.

Approximately 6 weeks after surgery the wound is sufficiently healed for the permanent prosthesis. The prosthesis is fitted by an ocularist and designed to match the remaining eye. Teach the patient how to remove, cleanse, and insert the prosthesis. Special polishing is required periodically to remove dried protein secretions.

OCULAR MANIFESTATIONS OF SYSTEMIC DISEASES

Many systemic diseases have significant ocular manifestations. Ocular signs and symptoms may be the first finding or complaint in the patient with a systemic disease. One example is the patient with undiagnosed diabetes who seeks ophthalmic care for blurred vision. A careful history and examination of the patient can reveal that the underlying cause of the blurred vision is lens swelling caused by hyperglycemia. Another example is the patient who seeks care for a conjunctival lesion. The ophthalmologist may be the first health care professional to make the diagnosis of AIDS based on the presence of a conjunctival Kaposi sarcoma (KS). eTable 22-1 (available on the website for this chapter) lists some systemic diseases and disorders and the associated ophthalmic manifestations.

AUDITORY PROBLEMS
EXTERNAL EAR AND CANAL

TRAUMA

Trauma to the external ear can cause injury to the subcutaneous tissue that may result in a hematoma. If the hematoma is not aspirated, inflammation of the membranes of the ear cartilage (perichondritis) can result. Blows to the ear can also cause conductive hearing loss if the ossicles in the middle ear are damaged or the tympanic membrane (TM) is perforated. Head trauma that injures the temporal lobe of the cerebral cortex can impair the ability to understand the meaning of sounds.

EXTERNAL OTITIS

The skin of the external ear and canal is subject to the same problems as skin anywhere on the body. **External otitis** involves inflammation or infection of the epithelium of the auricle and ear canal. Swimming may alter the flora of the external canal because of chemicals and contaminated water. This can result in an infection often referred to as "swimmer's ear." Trauma from picking the ear or using sharp objects (e.g., hairpins) frequently causes the initial break in the skin. Piercing of cartilage in the upper part of the auricle also places the patient at higher risk for infection.

Infections and skin conditions may cause external otitis. Bacteria or fungi may be the cause. *Pseudomonas aeruginosa* is the most common bacterial cause. Fungi, including *Candida albicans* and *Aspergillus,* especially thrive in warm, moist climates. The warm, dark environment of the ear canal provides a good growth medium for microorganisms.

Malignant external otitis is a serious infection caused by *P. aeruginosa.* It occurs mainly in older patients with diabetes. The infection, which can spread from the external ear to the parotid gland and temporal bone (osteomyelitis), is usually treated with antibiotics.

Ear pain *(otalgia)* is one of the first signs of external otitis. Even in mild cases, the patient may experience significant discomfort with chewing, moving the auricle, or pressing on the tragus. Swelling of the ear canal can muffle hearing. There may be serosanguineous (blood-tinged fluid) or purulent (white to green thick fluid) drainage. Fever occurs when the infection spreads to surrounding tissue.

NURSING AND COLLABORATIVE MANAGEMENT EXTERNAL OTITIS

Diagnosis of external otitis is made by otoscopic examination of the ear canal. Care must be taken to avoid pain when pulling on the pinna to straighten out the canal or when inserting the otoscope speculum. The eardrum may be difficult to see due to swelling in the canal. Culture and sensitivity studies of the drainage may be done. Moist heat, mild analgesics, and topical anesthetic drops usually control the pain. Topical treatments may include antibiotics for infection and corticosteroids for inflammation. If the surrounding tissue is involved, systemic antibiotics are prescribed.[23] Improvement should occur in 48 hours, but the patient needs to adhere to the prescribed therapy for 7 to 14 days for complete resolution.

Hands should be washed before and after administration of otic drops (eardrops). The drops should be administered at room temperature. Cold drops can cause vertigo due to stimulation of the semicircular canals, and heated drops can burn the tympanum. The tip of the dropper should not touch the ear during administration to prevent contamination of the entire bottle of drops. The ear is positioned so that the drops can run into the canal. The patient should maintain this position for 2 minutes to allow the drops to spread. Sometimes the drops are

TABLE 22-8	PATIENT & CAREGIVER TEACHING GUIDE

Prevention of External Otitis

Include the following instructions when teaching the patient and caregiver.
1. Do not put anything in your ear canal unless requested by your health care provider.
2. Report itching if it becomes a problem.
3. Earwax is normal.
   - It lubricates and protects the canal.
   - Report chronic excessive cerumen if it impairs your hearing.
4. Keep your ears as dry as possible.
   - Use earplugs if you are prone to swimmer's ear.
   - Turn your head to each side for 30 seconds at a time to help water run out of the ears.
   - Do not dry with cotton-tipped applicators.
   - A hair dryer set to low and held at least 6 in from the ear can speed water evaporation.

placed onto a wick of cotton that is placed in the canal. Instruct the patient not to push the cotton farther into the ear. Careful handling and disposal of material saturated with drainage are important. Instruct the patient on methods to reduce the risk of external otitis (Table 22-8).

CERUMEN AND FOREIGN BODIES IN EXTERNAL EAR CANAL

Impacted cerumen (earwax) can cause discomfort and decreased hearing. In the older person the cerumen becomes dense and drier. The hair in the ear becomes thicker and coarser, entrapping the hard, dry cerumen in the canal. Symptoms of cerumen impaction include hearing loss, otalgia, tinnitus, and vertigo.

Management involves irrigation of the canal with body-temperature solutions to soften the cerumen. Special syringes can be used and vary from a simple bulb syringe to special irrigating equipment. Place the patient in a sitting position with an emesis basin under the ear. Pull the auricle up and back, and direct the flow of solution above or below the impaction. It is important that the ear canal not be completely occluded with the syringe tip. If irrigation does not remove the wax, mild lubricant drops may be used to soften the earwax. Severe impactions may need to be removed by the health care provider.

Attempts to remove a foreign object from the ear may result in pushing it farther into the canal. Vegetable matter in the ear tends to swell and may create a secondary inflammation, making removal more difficult. Mineral oil or lidocaine drops can be used to kill an insect before removal with microscope guidance. Removal of impacted objects should be performed by the health care provider.

Ears should be cleaned with a washcloth and finger. Cotton-tipped applicators should be avoided. Penetration of the middle ear by a cotton-tipped applicator can cause serious injury to the TM and ossicles. The use of cotton-tipped applicators can also cause cerumen to become impacted against the TM and impair hearing.

MALIGNANCY OF EXTERNAL EAR

Skin cancers are the only common malignancies of the ear. Rough sandpaper-like changes to the upper border of the auricle are premalignant lesions (actinic keratoses) associated with chronic sun exposure. They are often removed with liquid nitrogen. Malignancies in the external ear canal include basal cell carcinoma in the pinna and squamous cell carcinoma in the ear canal. If left untreated, they can invade underlying tissue. Teach the patient about the dangers of sun exposure and the importance of using hats and sunscreen when outdoors.

MIDDLE EAR AND MASTOID

OTITIS MEDIA

Acute Otitis Media

Acute otitis media is an infection of the tympanum, ossicles, and space of the middle ear. Swelling of the auditory tube from colds or allergies can trap bacteria, causing a middle ear infection. Pressure from the inflammation pushes on the TM, causing it to become red, bulging, and painful. Acute otitis media is usually a childhood disease because, in children, the auditory tube that normally drains fluid and mucus from the middle ear is shorter and narrower and its position is flatter than in adults. Infection can be due to viruses or bacteria. Pain, fever, malaise, and reduced hearing are signs and symptoms of infection. Referred pain from the temporomandibular joint, teeth, gums, sinuses, or throat may also cause ear pain.

Collaborative care involves the use of antibiotics if an infection is present.[24] Surgical intervention is generally reserved for the patient who does not respond to medical treatment. A *myringotomy* involves an incision in the tympanum to release the increased pressure and exudate from the middle ear. A tympanostomy tube may be placed for short- or long-term use. Prompt treatment of an episode of acute otitis media generally prevents spontaneous perforation of the TM. If allergies are a causative factor, antihistamines may also be prescribed.

Otitis Media With Effusion

Otitis media with effusion is an inflammation of the middle ear with a collection of fluid in the middle ear space. The fluid may be thin, mucoid, or purulent. If the auditory tube does not open and allow equalization of atmospheric pressure, negative pressure within the middle ear pulls fluid from surrounding tissues. This problem commonly follows upper respiratory tract or chronic sinus infections, barotrauma (caused by pressure change), or otitis media.

Complaints include a feeling of fullness of the ear, a "plugged" feeling or popping, and decreased hearing. The patient does not experience pain, fever, or discharge from the ear. It is common to have otitis media with effusion for weeks to months after an episode of acute otitis media. It usually resolves without treatment but may recur.

Chronic Otitis Media and Mastoiditis

Repeated attacks of otitis media may lead to chronic otitis media, especially in adults who have a history of recurrent otitis in childhood. Because the mucous membrane of the middle ear is continuous with the air cells of the mastoid bone, both can be involved in the chronic infectious process.

Chronic otitis media is characterized by a purulent exudate and inflammation that can involve the ossicles, the auditory tube, and the mastoid bone. It is often painless. Hearing loss, nausea, and episodes of dizziness can occur. Hearing loss is a

complication from inflammatory destruction of the ossicles, a TM perforation, or accumulation of fluid in the middle ear space. A mass of epithelial cells and cholesterol in the middle ear *(cholesteatoma)* may also develop. The cholesteatoma enlarges and can destroy the adjacent bones. Unless removed surgically, it can cause extensive damage to the ossicles and impair hearing.

Otoscopic examination of the TM may reveal changes in color and mobility or a perforation (Fig. 22-9). Culture and sensitivity tests of the drainage are necessary to identify the organisms involved so that appropriate antibiotic therapy can be prescribed. The audiogram may demonstrate a hearing loss as great as 50 to 60 dB if the ossicles have been damaged or separated. Sinus x-rays, MRI, or a computed tomography (CT) scan of the temporal bone is done to assess for bone destruction and the presence of a mass.

NURSING AND COLLABORATIVE MANAGEMENT CHRONIC OTITIS MEDIA

The aims of treatment are to clear the middle ear of infection, repair any perforations, and preserve hearing (Table 22-9). Otic and systemic (oral and IV) antibiotic therapy is started based on the culture and sensitivity results. In many cases of chronic otitis media, antibiotic resistance is present. The patient may need to undergo frequent evacuation of drainage and debris in an outpatient setting.

Often chronic TM perforations do not heal with conservative treatment, and surgery is necessary. *Tympanoplasty (myringoplasty)* involves reconstruction of the TM and/or the ossicles. A *mastoidectomy* is often performed with a tympanoplasty to

TABLE 22-9 COLLABORATIVE CARE
Chronic Otitis Media

Diagnostic	Collaborative Therapy
• History and physical examination	• Ear irrigations
• Otoscopic examination	• Otic, oral, or parenteral antibiotics
• Culture and sensitivity of middle ear drainage	• Analgesics
• Mastoid x-ray	• Antiemetics
	• Surgery
	• Tympanoplasty (see eTable 22-2)
	• Mastoidectomy

FIG. 22-9 Perforation of the tympanic membrane (TM).

remove infected portions of the mastoid bone. Removal of tissue stops at the middle ear structures that appear capable of conducting sound. Sudden pressure changes in the ear and postoperative infections can disrupt the surgical repair during the healing phase or cause facial nerve paralysis.

Impaired hearing is expected during the postoperative period if there is packing in the ear. A cotton ball dressing is used for the incision made through the external auditory canal (endaural). Instruct the patient to change the cotton packing as needed. If a postauricle (behind the ear) incision is used and a drain is in place, place a dressing over the mastoid area. A small gauze pad is cut to fit behind the ear, and soft dressing material is applied over the ear to prevent the outer circular head dressing from placing pressure on the auricle. Monitor the tightness of the dressing to prevent tissue necrosis and assess the amount and type of drainage. Keep the suture line dry. Postoperative teaching is presented in eTable 22-2, available on the website for this chapter.

OTOSCLEROSIS

Otosclerosis is a hereditary autosomal dominant disease. It is the most common cause of hearing loss in young adults.[25] Spongy bone develops from the bony labyrinth, preventing movement of the footplate of the stapes in the oval window. This reduces the transmission of vibrations to the inner ear fluids and results in conductive hearing loss. Although otosclerosis is typically bilateral, one ear may show faster progression of hearing loss. The patient is often unaware of the problem until the loss becomes so severe that communication is difficult.

Otoscopic examination may reveal a reddish blush of the tympanum (Schwartz's sign) caused by the vascular and bony changes within the middle ear. Tuning fork tests and an audiogram demonstrate good hearing by bone conduction but poor hearing by air conduction (air-bone gap). Usually a difference of at least 20 to 25 dB between air and bone conduction levels of hearing is seen in otosclerosis.

The hearing loss associated with otosclerosis may be stabilized by the oral administration of sodium fluoride with vitamin D and calcium carbonate. These medications retard bone resorption and encourage the calcification of bony lesions. Amplification of sound by a hearing aid can be effective because the inner ear function is normal.

Collaborative care of otosclerosis is shown in Table 22-10. Microdrill or laser surgical treatment involves opening the footplate (stapedotomy) or replacing the stapes with a metal or Teflon substitute (prosthesis). These procedures are usually performed with the patient under conscious sedation. The ear with poorer hearing is repaired first, and the other ear may be operated on within a year. Immediately after surgery the patient often reports a significant improvement in hearing in the operative ear. Because of the accumulation of blood and fluid in the middle ear during the postoperative period, the hearing level decreases initially, but it improves gradually with healing.

Nursing management of the patient undergoing surgery to correct otosclerosis is similar to that for the patient having a tympanoplasty. Use Gelfoam on the incision flap to limit bleeding. Place a cotton ball in the ear canal, and cover the ear with a small dressing. The patient may experience dizziness, nausea, and vomiting as a result of stimulation of the labyrinth during surgery. Some patients demonstrate nystagmus because of disturbance of the perilymph fluid. The patient should take care to avoid sudden movements that may bring on or exacerbate vertigo. Actions that increase inner ear pressure, such as coughing, sneezing, lifting, bending, and straining during bowel movements, should be avoided.

INNER EAR PROBLEMS

Three symptoms that indicate disease of the inner ear are vertigo, sensorineural hearing loss, and tinnitus. Symptoms of vertigo arise from the vestibular labyrinth, whereas hearing loss and tinnitus arise from the auditory labyrinth. There is an overlap between manifestations of inner ear problems and CNS disorders.

MÉNIÈRE'S DISEASE

Ménière's disease (endolymphatic hydrops) is characterized by symptoms caused by inner ear disease, including episodic vertigo, tinnitus, fluctuating sensorineural hearing loss, and aural fullness. The patient experiences significant disability because of sudden, severe attacks of vertigo with nausea, vomiting, sweating, and pallor. Symptoms usually begin between 30 and 60 years of age.

The cause of the disease is unknown, but it results in an excessive accumulation of endolymph in the membranous labyrinth. The volume of endolymph increases until the membranous labyrinth ruptures. Attacks may be preceded by a sense of fullness in the ear, increasing tinnitus, and muffled hearing. The patient may experience the feeling of being pulled to the ground ("drop attacks"). Some patients report that they feel like they are whirling in space. Attacks may last hours or days and may occur several times a year. The clinical course of the disease is highly variable.

NURSING AND COLLABORATIVE MANAGEMENT MÉNIÈRE'S DISEASE

Collaborative care of Ménière's disease (Table 22-11) includes diagnostic tests to rule out other causes of the symptoms, including CNS disease. Results that suggest Ménière's disease include a mild, low-frequency sensorineural hearing loss on audiogram and abnormalities with vestibular tests. A glycerol test may aid in diagnosis. An oral dose of glycerol is given, followed by serial audiograms over 3 hours. Improvement in hearing or speech discrimination supports a diagnosis of Ménière's disease. The improvement is attributed to the osmotic effect of glycerol that pulls fluid from the inner ear.

During the acute attack, antihistamines (e.g., diphenhydramine [Benadryl]), anticholinergics (e.g., atropine), and benzodiazepines (e.g., lorazepam [Ativan]) can be used to decrease

TABLE 22-10	**COLLABORATIVE CARE**

Otosclerosis

Diagnostic	Collaborative Therapy
• History and physical examination	• Hearing aid
• Otoscopic examination	• Surgery (stapedectomy or stapes prosthesis)
• Rinne test	• Drug therapy
• Weber test	• Sodium fluoride with vitamin D
• Audiometry	• Calcium carbonate
• Tympanometry	

TABLE 22-11   COLLABORATIVE CARE

Ménière's Disease

Diagnostic	**Surgical Therapy**
• History and physical examination	• Endolymphatic sac decompression
• Audiometric studies (including speech discrimination, tone decay)	• Endolymphatic shunt
• Vestibular tests (including caloric test, positional test)	• Vestibular nerve section
• Electronystagmography	• Labyrinthectomy
• Neurologic examination	
• Glycerol test	**Ambulatory or Home Care**
	• Diuretics
Collaborative Therapy	• Antihistamines
Acute Care	• Calcium channel blockers
Drug Therapy (one or more)	• Sedatives
• Sedatives	• Hydrops diet: restriction of sodium, caffeine, nicotine, alcohol, and foods with monosodium glutamate (MSG)
• Benzodiazepines	
• Anticholinergics	
• Antihistamines	
• Antiemetics	

the abnormal sensation and lessen nausea and vomiting. Acute vertigo is treated symptomatically with bed rest, sedation, and antiemetics (e.g., prochlorperazine [Compazine]) or antivertigo drugs (e.g., meclizine [Antivert]) for motion sickness. The patient requires reassurance and counseling that the condition is not life threatening. Management between attacks may include diuretics, antihistamines, calcium channel blockers, and a low-sodium diet. Diazepam (Valium), meclizine, and fentanyl with droperidol (Innovar) may be used to reduce the vertigo. Over time, most patients respond to the prescribed medications but must learn to live with the unpredictability of the attacks and the loss of hearing.

Frequent and incapacitating attacks are indications for surgical intervention. Decompression of the endolymphatic sac and shunting are performed to reduce the pressure on the cochlear hair cells and to prevent further damage and hearing loss. If relief is not achieved, vestibular nerve section (cutting the nerve) may be performed. When involvement is unilateral, surgical ablation of the labyrinth, resulting in loss of the vestibular and hearing cochlear function, is performed. Some patients with severe attacks of vertigo have shown improvement with the injection of gentamicin through the TM.[26] This results in inner ear damage and a reduction in endolymph production.

Plan nursing interventions to minimize vertigo and provide for patient safety. During an acute attack keep the patient in a quiet, darkened room in a comfortable position. Teach the patient to avoid sudden head movements or position changes. Fluorescent or flickering lights or a television may exacerbate symptoms and should be avoided. Make an emesis basin available because vomiting is common. To minimize the risk of falling, keep the side rails up and the bed in a low position when the patient is in bed. Instruct the patient to call for assistance when getting out of bed. Medications and fluids are administered parenterally, and intake and output are monitored. When the attack subsides, assist the patient with ambulation because unsteadiness may remain.

BENIGN PAROXYSMAL POSITIONAL VERTIGO

Benign paroxysmal positional vertigo (BPPV) is a common cause of vertigo. Approximately 50% of the cases of vertigo may

be due to BPPV. In BBPV, free-floating debris in the semicircular canal causes vertigo with specific head movements, such as getting out of bed, rolling over in bed, and sitting up from lying down. The debris ("ear rocks") is composed of small crystals of calcium carbonate that derive from the utricle in the inner ear. The utricle may be injured by head trauma, infection, or degeneration from the aging process. However, for many patients a cause cannot be found.

Symptoms include nystagmus, vertigo, light-headedness, loss of balance, and nausea. There is no hearing loss, and symptoms tend to be intermittent. The symptoms of BPPV may be confused with those of Ménière's disease. Diagnosis is based on the results of auditory and vestibular tests.

Although BPPV is bothersome, it is rarely serious unless a person falls. The Epley maneuver, or canalith repositioning procedure, is effective in providing symptom relief for many patients.[27] In this maneuver the ear debris is moved from areas in the inner ear that cause symptoms and repositioned into less sensitive areas where they do not cause these problems. The Epley maneuver does not address the actual presence of debris but rather changes their location. A trained health care provider can instruct the patient in how to perform the maneuver.

ACOUSTIC NEUROMA

An **acoustic neuroma** is a unilateral benign tumor that occurs where the vestibulocochlear nerve (cranial nerve [CN] VIII) enters the internal auditory canal. Early diagnosis is important because the tumor can compress the trigeminal and facial nerves and arteries within the internal auditory canal. Symptoms usually begin between 40 and 60 years of age.

Early symptoms are associated with CN VIII compression and destruction. They include unilateral, progressive, sensorineural hearing loss; reduced touch sensation in the posterior ear canal; unilateral tinnitus; and mild, intermittent vertigo. Diagnostic tests include neurologic, audiometric, and vestibular tests; CT scans; and MRI.

Surgery to remove small tumors generally preserves hearing and vestibular function. Large tumors (larger than 3 cm) and the surgery required to remove them can leave the patient with permanent hearing loss and facial paralysis. Stereotactic radiosurgery may slow tumor growth and preserve the facial nerve. Instruct the patient to report any clear, colorless discharge from the nose. This may be cerebrospinal fluid (CSF), which increases the risk of infection. Teach the importance of follow-up care after surgery to monitor hearing and for recurrence of the tumor.

HEARING LOSS AND DEAFNESS

Hearing disorders are a common cause of disability in the United States. Nearly half of the people who need assistance with hearing disorders are 65 years of age or older. With the aging of the population, the incidence of hearing loss is increasing. Causes of hearing loss are shown in Fig. 22-10.

Types of Hearing Loss

Conductive Hearing Loss. *Conductive hearing loss* occurs when conditions in the outer or middle ear impair the transmission of sound through air to the inner ear. A common cause is otitis media with effusion. Other causes are impacted cerumen,

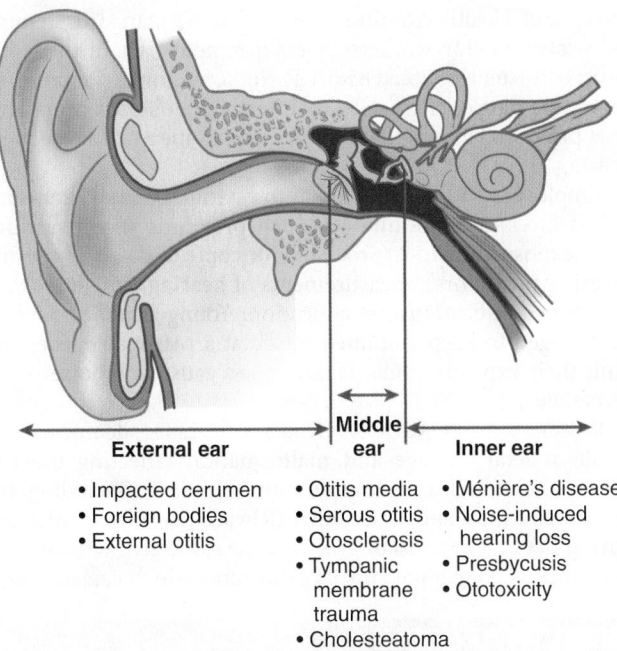

- External ear
  - Impacted cerumen
  - Foreign bodies
  - External otitis
- Middle ear
  - Otitis media
  - Serous otitis
  - Otosclerosis
  - Tympanic membrane trauma
  - Cholesteatoma
  - Acoustic neuroma
- Inner ear
  - Ménière's disease
  - Noise-induced hearing loss
  - Presbycusis
  - Ototoxicity

FIG. 22-10 Causes of hearing loss.

TABLE 22-12	CLASSIFICATION OF HEARING LOSS
Decibel (dB) Loss	Meaning
0-15	Normal hearing
16-25	Slight hearing loss
26-40	Mild impairment
41-55	Moderate impairment
56-70	Moderately severe impairment
71-90	Severe impairment
>90	Profound deafness*

*Most people in this category have been deaf since birth (congenitally deaf).

perforation of the TM, otosclerosis, and narrowing of the external auditory canal.[28]

The audiogram demonstrates better hearing through bone than through air (air-bone gap). The patient often speaks softly because hearing his or her own voice (which is conducted by bone) seems loud. This patient hears better in a noisy environment. The first step is to identify and treat the cause if possible. If correction of the cause is not possible, a hearing aid may help if the loss is greater than 40 to 50 dB.

Sensorineural Hearing Loss. *Sensorineural hearing loss* is caused by impairment of function of the inner ear or the vestibulocochlear nerve (CN VIII). Congenital and hereditary factors, noise trauma over time, aging (presbycusis), Ménière's disease, and ototoxicity can cause sensorineural hearing loss. Ototoxic drugs include aspirin, nonsteroidal antiinflammatory drugs, antibiotics (aminoglycosides, erythromycin, vancomycin), loop diuretics, and chemotherapy drugs (e.g., vincristine [Oncovin], cisplatin [Platinol]).

Systemic infections, such as Paget's disease of the bone, immune diseases, diabetes mellitus, bacterial meningitis, and trauma, are associated with this type of hearing loss. The main problems are the ability to hear sound but not to understand speech, and the lack of understanding of the problem by others. The ability to hear high-pitched sounds, including consonants, diminishes. Sounds become muffled and difficult to understand. An audiogram demonstrates a loss in decibel levels of the 4000-Hz range and eventually the 2000-Hz range. A hearing aid may help some patients, but it only makes sounds and speech louder, not clearer.

Mixed Hearing Loss. Mixed hearing loss occurs due to a combination of conductive and sensorineural causes. Careful evaluation is needed if corrective surgery for conductive loss is planned because the sensorineural component of the hearing loss will still remain.

Central and Functional Hearing Loss. Central hearing loss involves an inability to interpret sound, including speech, because of a problem in the brain (CNS). A careful history is helpful because there are usually cases of deafness in the family. Refer the patient to a qualified hearing and speech service if indicated.

Functional hearing loss may be caused by an emotional or a psychologic factor. The patient does not seem to hear or respond to pure-tone subjective hearing tests, but no physical reason for hearing loss can be identified. Psychologic counseling may help.

Classification of Hearing Loss. Hearing loss can also be classified by the decibel (dB) level or loss as recorded on the audiogram. Normal hearing is in the 0- to 15-dB range. Table 22-12 describes the levels of hearing loss.

Clinical Manifestations

Common early signs of hearing loss are answering questions inappropriately, not responding when not looking at the speaker, asking others to speak up, and showing irritability with others who do not speak up. Other behaviors that suggest hearing loss include straining to hear, cupping the hand around the ear, reading lips, and an increased sensitivity to slight increases in noise level. Often the patient is unaware of minimal hearing loss. Family and friends who get tired of repeating or talking loudly are often the first to notice hearing loss. Pressure exerted by significant others is a significant factor in whether the patient seeks help for hearing impairment.

Deafness is often called the "unseen handicap" because the difficulty in communication with a deaf person is not realized until you initiate a conversation with that person. You need to thoroughly validate the deaf person's understanding of health teaching. Descriptive visual aids can be helpful. If the significantly hearing-impaired individual uses sign language to communicate, the Americans with Disabilities Act[29] requires providing an interpreter when significant information is presented such as for patient consent or discharge teaching.

Interference in communication and interaction with others can be the source of many problems for the patient and caregiver. Often the patient refuses to admit or may be unaware of impaired hearing. Irritability is common because the patient must concentrate so hard to understand speech. The loss of clarity of speech in the patient with sensorineural hearing loss is most frustrating. The patient may hear what is said but not understand it. Withdrawal, suspicion, loss of self-esteem, and insecurity are commonly associated with advancing hearing loss.

Tinnitus and Hearing Loss. *Tinnitus* is the perception of *sound* in the ears where no external source is present. It is "ringing in the ears" or "head noise" (see *www.ata.org*). Tinnitus is sometimes the first symptom of hearing loss, especially in older people. It may be soft or loud, high pitched or low pitched.

Tinnitus and hearing loss are directly related. Both are caused by inner ear nerve damage. The main difference between tinnitus and hearing loss is the extent of the damage (since tinnitus can still be heard).

Although the most common cause of tinnitus is noise, it can also be a side effect of medications (see discussion on drugs causing sensorineural hearing loss on p. 407). More than 200 drugs are known to cause tinnitus.

NURSING AND COLLABORATIVE MANAGEMENT
HEARING LOSS AND DEAFNESS

HEALTH PROMOTION

ENVIRONMENTAL NOISE CONTROL. Noise is the most preventable cause of hearing loss. (Fig. 22-11 lists the levels of environmental noise generated by common indoor and outdoor sounds.) Sudden severe loud noise (acoustic trauma) and chronic exposure to loud noise (noise-induced hearing loss) can damage hearing. Acoustic trauma causes hearing loss by destroying the hair cells of the organ of Corti. Sensorineural hearing loss as a result of increased and prolonged environmental noise, such as amplified sound, is occurring in young adults at an increasing rate. Amplified music (e.g., on iPods or MP3 players) should not exceed 50% of maximum volume. Ear protection should be worn when firing a gun and during other recreational pursuits with high noise levels. Health teaching regarding avoidance of continued exposure to noise levels greater than 70 dB is essential.

In work environments known to have high noise levels (more than 85 dB), ear protection should be worn. Occupational Safety and Health Administration (OSHA) standards require ear protection for workers in environments where the noise levels consistently exceed 85 dB. Periodic audiometric screening should be part of the health maintenance policies of industry. This provides baseline data on hearing to measure subsequent hearing loss.

Employees should participate in hearing conservation programs in work environments. Such programs should include noise exposure analysis, provision for control of noise exposure (hearing protectors), measurements of hearing, and employee-employer notification and education. Young adults should be encouraged to keep amplified music at a reasonable level and limit their exposure time. Hearing loss caused by noise is not reversible.

IMMUNIZATIONS. Various viruses can cause deafness as a result of fetal damage and malformations affecting the ear. Promote childhood and adult immunizations, including the measles, mumps, and rubella (MMR) vaccine. Rubella infection during the first 8 weeks of pregnancy is associated with an 85% incidence of congenital rubella syndrome, which causes senso-

HEALTHY PEOPLE
Health Impact of Wearing Ear Protection

- Ear protection should be worn during all recreational and work activities involving high noise levels.
- Ear protection can greatly reduce the damage to the ear from loud noise.
- Periodic audiometric screening is important to detect loss before it progresses.

Outdoor sounds	NOISE LEVEL (dB)	Indoor sounds
	110	Rock concert
B-747-200 takeoff		
	100	Indoor subway
Gas lawnmower at 3 ft		
	90	Blender at 3 ft
Noisy urban daytime		
	80	Shouting at 3 ft
	70	Vacuum cleaner at 10 ft / Normal speech at 3 ft
Commercial area		
	60	
Quiet urban daytime		Large business office
	50	
		Small theater
	40	
Quiet suburban nighttime		Library
	30	
	20	
Quiet rural nighttime		Broadcast and recording studio
	10	

Hearing threshold

FIG. 22-11 Range of common environmental sounds.

rineural deafness. Women of childbearing age should be tested for antibodies to these viral diseases. Women should avoid pregnancy for at least 3 months after being immunized. Immunization must be delayed if the woman is pregnant. Women who are susceptible to rubella can be vaccinated safely during the postpartum period.

OTOTOXIC SUBSTANCES. Drugs commonly associated with ototoxicity include salicylates, loop diuretics, cancer chemotherapy drugs, and antibiotics.[30] Chemicals used in industry (e.g., toluene, carbon disulfide, mercury) may damage the inner ear. The patient who is receiving ototoxic drugs or is exposed to ototoxic chemicals should be monitored for signs and symptoms associated with ototoxicity, including tinnitus, diminished hearing, and changes in equilibrium. If these symptoms develop, immediate withdrawal of the drug may prevent further damage and may cause the symptoms to disappear.

ASSISTIVE DEVICES AND TECHNIQUES

HEARING AIDS. The patient with a suspected hearing loss should have a hearing assessment by a qualified audiologist. If a hearing aid is indicated, it should be fitted by an audiologist or a speech and hearing specialist. Many types of hearing aids

are available, each with advantages and disadvantages (Table 22-13). The conventional hearing aid serves as a simple amplifier. For the patient with bilateral hearing impairment, binaural hearing aids provide the best sound lateralization and speech discrimination.

The goal of hearing aid therapy is improved hearing with consistent use. Patients who are motivated and optimistic about using a hearing aid are more successful users. Determine the patient's readiness for hearing aid therapy, including acknowledgment of a hearing problem, the patient's feelings about wearing a hearing aid, the degree to which the hearing loss affects life, and any difficulties the patient has manipulating small objects such as putting a battery in a hearing aid.

Initially, use of the hearing aid should be restricted to quiet situations in the home. The patient must first adjust to voices (including the patient's own voice) and household sounds. The patient should also experiment by increasing and decreasing the volume as situations require. As the patient adjusts to the increase in sounds and background noise, he or she can progress to situations where several people will be talking simultaneously. Next, the environment can be expanded to the outdoors and then the shopping mall or grocery store. Adjustment to

TABLE 22-13 TYPES OF HEARING AIDS

Type	Advantages	Disadvantages	Type	Advantages	Disadvantages
Completely in the canal (mild to moderate hearing loss)	Smallest and least visible aid. Protected from sounds such as wind noise.	Costly. No space for add-ons such as directional microphones or volume controls. Small, short-lived batteries.	**In the ear** (mild to severe hearing loss)	Powerful amplification. Inserts and adjusts easily. Longer-lasting batteries.	Visible. May pick up wind noise readily.
In the canal (mild to severe hearing loss)	More powerful than aids completely in the canal. Has adjustable features such as noise reduction.	Small size of aid with its additional features may be difficult to operate for patients with visual loss or arthritis.	**Behind the ear** (all types of hearing loss)	Most powerful aid. Adjusts easily. Longest battery life.	Largest, most visible aid. Newer models may be smaller and less obvious.

TABLE 22-14	COMMUNICATION WITH HEARING-IMPAIRED PATIENT

Nonverbal Aids	Verbal Aids
• Draw attention with hand movements.	• Speak normally and slowly.
• Have speaker's face in good light.	• Do not overexaggerate facial expressions.
• Avoid covering mouth or face with hands.	• Do not overenunciate.
• Avoid chewing, eating, smoking while talking.	• Use simple sentences.
• Maintain eye contact.	• Rephrase sentence. Use different words.
• Avoid distracting environments.	• Write name or difficult words.
• Avoid careless expression that the patient may misinterpret.	• Do not shout.
• Use touch.	• Speak in normal voice directly into better ear.
• Move close to better ear.	
• Avoid light behind speaker.	

FIG. 22-12 Cochlear implant.

different environments occurs gradually, depending on the individual patient.

When the hearing aid is not being worn, it should be placed in a dry, cool area where it will not be inadvertently damaged or lost. The battery should be disconnected or removed when not in use. Battery life averages 1 week, and patients should be advised to purchase only a month's supply at a time. Ear molds should be cleaned weekly or as needed. Toothpicks or pipe cleaners may be used to clear a clogged ear tip.

An implanted hearing system (i.e., Esteem) is available to treat moderate to severe sensorineural hearing loss. The system consists of external testing and programming instruments and three implantable components: a sound processor, sensor, and driver. The device does not have external components that are visible. Criteria for placement of the device include a stable bilateral sensorineural hearing loss, a normally functioning eustachian tube, and normal middle ear anatomy.

SPEECH READING. *Speech reading,* commonly called *lip reading,* can be helpful in increasing communication. It allows for approximately 40% understanding of the spoken word. The patient is able to use visual cues associated with speech, such as gestures and facial expression, to help clarify the spoken message. In speech reading, many words look alike to the patient (e.g., rabbit, woman). Help the patient by using and teaching verbal and nonverbal communication techniques as described in Table 22-14.

SIGN LANGUAGE. *Sign language* is used as a form of communication for people with profound hearing impairment. It involves gestures and facial features such as eyebrow motion and lip-mouth movements. Sign language is not universal. American Sign Language (ASL) is used in the United States and the English-speaking parts of Canada.

COCHLEAR IMPLANT. The *cochlear implant* is used as a hearing device for people with severe to profound sensorineural hearing loss in one or both ears. The ideal candidate is one who has become deaf after acquiring speech and language. The system consists of an external microphone placed behind the ear, a speech processor and a transmitter implanted under the skin that change sounds into electrical impulses, and a group of electrodes placed within the cochlea that stimulate the auditory nerves in the ear (Fig. 22-12). Cochlear implants send information that covers the entire range of sound frequencies.[31] The cochlear implant electrodes are inserted as far as possible into the cochlea to send both high- and low-frequency information.

For patients with conductive and mixed hearing loss, the cochlear Baha system may be surgically implanted. The system works through direct bone conduction and integrates with the skull bone over time.

Extensive training and rehabilitation are essential to receive maximum benefit from these implants. The positive aspects of a cochlear implant include providing sound to the person who heard none, improving lip-reading ability, monitoring the loudness of the person's own speech, improving the sense of security, and decreasing feelings of isolation. With continued research, the cochlear implant may offer the possibility of aural rehabilitation for a wider range of hearing-impaired individuals.

The FDA has an information website on cochlear implants.[32] The website includes an animated movie to help visualize the implants and how they work.

ASSISTED LISTENING DEVICES. Numerous devices are now available to assist the hearing-impaired person. Direct amplification devices, amplified telephone receivers, alerting systems that flash when activated by sound, an infrared system for amplifying the sound of the television, and a combination FM receiver and hearing aid are all devices that you can explore based on patient needs. People with profound deafness may be assisted by text-telephone alerting systems that flash when activated by sound, closed captioning on television, and a specially trained dog. The dogs are trained to alert their owners to specific sounds within the environment, thus increasing the person's safety and independence.

GERONTOLOGIC CONSIDERATIONS

HEARING LOSS

Presbycusis, hearing loss associated with aging, includes the loss of peripheral auditory sensitivity, a decline in word recognition ability, and associated psychologic and communication issues. Because consonants (high-frequency sounds) are the letters by which spoken words are recognized, the older person with presbycusis has a diminished ability to understand the spoken word. Vowels are heard, but some consonants fall into the high-frequency range and cannot be differentiated. This may lead to confusion and embarrassment because of the difference in what was said and what was heard.

The cause of presbycusis is related to degenerative changes in the inner ear. Noise exposure is thought to be a common factor. Table 22-15 describes the classification of specific causes and associated hearing changes of presbycusis. Often a person may have more than one type of presbycusis. The prognosis for hearing depends on the cause of the loss. Sound amplification

with the appropriate device is often helpful in improving the understanding of speech. In other situations an audiologic rehabilitation program can be valuable.

The older adult is often reluctant to use a hearing aid for sound amplification.[30] Reasons cited most often include cost, appearance, insufficient knowledge about hearing aids, amplification of competing noise, and unrealistic expectations. Most hearing aids and batteries are small, and neuromuscular changes such as stiff fingers, enlarged joints, and decreased sensory perception often make the care and handling of a hearing aid difficult and frustrating for an older person. Some older adults may also tend to accept their losses as part of getting older and believe there is no need for improvement.

TABLE 22-15   CLASSIFICATION OF PRESBYCUSIS

Type	Hearing Change and Prognosis
Sensory Atrophy of auditory nerve. Loss of sensory hair cells	Loss of high-pitched sounds. Little effect on speech understanding. Good response to sound amplification.
Neural Degenerative changes in cochlea and spinal ganglion	Loss of speech discrimination. Amplification alone not sufficient.
Metabolic Atrophy of blood vessels in wall of cochlea with interruption of essential nutrient supply	Uniform loss for all frequencies accompanied by recruitment.* Good response to hearing aid.
Cochlear Stiffening of basilar membrane, which interferes with sound transmission in the cochlea	Hearing loss increases from low to high frequencies. Speech discrimination affected with higher-frequency losses. Helped by appropriate forms of amplification.

*Abnormally rapid increase in loudness as sound intensity increases.

DELEGATION DECISIONS
Corrective Lenses and Hearing Aids

Role of Registered Nurse (RN)
- Assess patient vision and hearing with and without corrective devices.
- Teach patient about the use of and care for corrective lenses and hearing aids.
- Evaluate whether corrective lenses or hearing aids are effective in maintaining or improving vision or hearing.
- Evaluate for problems that may occur with contact lenses (e.g., conjunctivitis) or with hearing aids (e.g., external ear irritation).

Role of Licensed Practical/Vocational Nurse (LPN/LVN)
- Perform Snellen and/or Jaeger testing as delegated by the RN (consider state nurse practice act and agency policy).
- Monitor for adverse effects of contact lenses (e.g., redness, complaints of irritation) and report these to the RN.

Role of Unlicensed Assistive Personnel (UAP)
- Clean corrective lenses with ordered solutions.
- Help patients with hearing aid placement.
- Clean and replace batteries in hearing aids.

CASE STUDY
Glaucoma and Diabetic Retinopathy

Kevin Peterson/ Stockbyte/Thinkstock

Patient Profile
J.K. is a 68-year-old African American woman who has been diagnosed with osteoarthritis and type 2 diabetes mellitus for the past 15 years. She now has diabetic retinopathy. She returns to the eye clinic with her daughter for continued care of primary open-angle glaucoma (POAG) and reexamination for changes in diabetic retinopathy. Her current medical regimen for POAG includes topical timolol maleate 0.5% extended (Timoptic-XE) once daily OU and latanoprost (Xalatan) 0.005% OU hs. At her last examination it was noted that she had microaneurysms and hard exudates of the retina.

Subjective Data
- She can no longer read the newspaper and reports that medication labels are difficult to read.
- States she is not always successful in getting the eyedrops instilled because her hands are gnarled and painful from osteoarthritis.

Objective Data
- Distant and near visual acuity are stable at 20/60 (OD) and 20/50 (OS). This is a reduction from 20/40 (OU) at her last visit.

- Intraocular pressures are stable at 20 mm Hg (OU). There is a new scotoma on visual field testing in the OS.
- Fluorescein angiography reveals diabetic macular edema OU.

Collaborative Care
- Brimonidine (Alphagan) 0.15% (OS) 15 min before and immediately after argon laser trabeculoplasty (ALT)
- Argon laser (OU) to seal leaking microaneurysms from macular edema
- Check intraocular pressure (IOP) 1 hr after ALT
- Continue previous glaucoma drop regimen
- Follow-up examination for glaucoma in 2 wk for possible ALT (OD)
- Follow-up examination for diabetic macular edema in 8 wk

Discussion Questions
1. Explain the etiology of the new scotoma.
2. Why might ALT be an appropriate therapy for J.K.?
3. What is the purpose of the eyedrops before and immediately after ALT?
4. **Priority Decision:** What are the priority topics that should be discussed in discharge teaching with J.K.?
5. What is the etiology of the vision loss from diabetic retinopathy?
6. **Priority Decision:** What are the priority nursing interventions for J.K.?
7. **Priority Decision:** Based on the assessment data, what are the priority nursing diagnoses? Are there any collaborative problems?
8. **Evidence-Based Practice:** J.K. wants to know if her glaucoma is related to her diabetes. How would you respond to her question?

BRIDGE TO NCLEX EXAMINATION

The number of the question corresponds to the same-numbered outcome at the beginning of the chapter.

1. Presbyopia occurs in older individuals because
   a. the eyeball elongates.
   b. the lens becomes inflexible.
   c. the corneal curvature becomes irregular.
   d. light rays are focusing in front of the retina.

2. The most important intervention for the patient with epidemic keratoconjunctivitis is
   a. cleansing the affected area with baby shampoo.
   b. monitoring spread of infection to the opposing eye.
   c. regular instillation of artificial tears to the affected eye.
   d. teaching the patient and family members good hygiene techniques.

3. Inflammation and infection of the eye
   a. are caused by irritants and microorganisms.
   b. have a higher incidence in sexually active patients.
   c. are chronic problems that result in a loss of vision.
   d. are frequently treated with cold compresses and antibiotics.

4. Which patient behaviors would the nurse promote for healthy eyes and ears (select all that apply)?
   a. Wearing protective sunglasses when bicycling
   b. Supplemental intake of B vitamins and magnesium
   c. Playing amplified music at 75% of maximum volume
   d. Patient notifying the health care provider of tinnitus while on antibiotics
   e. A woman avoiding pregnancy for 4 weeks after receiving measles, mumps, rubella (MMR) immunization

5. What should be included in the postoperative teaching of the patient who has undergone cataract surgery (select all that apply)?
   a. Eye discomfort is often relieved with mild analgesics.
   b. A decline in visual acuity is common for the first week.
   c. Stay on bed rest and limit activity for the first few days.
   d. Notify surgeon if an increase in redness or drainage occurs.
   e. Nighttime eye shielding and activity restrictions are essential to prevent eyestrain.

6. What should be included in the nursing plan for a patient who needs to administer antibiotic eardrops?
   a. Cool the drops so that they decrease swelling in the canal.
   b. Avoid placing a cotton wick to assist in administering the drops.
   c. Be careful to avoid touching the tip of the dropper bottle to the ear.
   d. Keep the head tilted 5 to 7 minutes after administration of the drops.

7. What is important for the nurse to include in the postoperative care of the patient following tympanoplasty?
   a. Check the gag reflex.
   b. Encourage independence.
   c. Avoid changing the cotton padding.
   d. Instruct patient to refrain from forceful nose blowing.

8. The patient who has a conductive hearing loss
   a. hears better in a noisy environment.
   b. hears sound but does not understand speech.
   c. often speaks loudly because his or her own voice seems low.
   d. experiences clearer sound with a hearing aid if the loss is less than 30 dB.

9. Instruct the patient who is newly fitted with bilateral hearing aids to (select all that apply)
   a. replace the batteries monthly.
   b. clean the ear molds weekly or as needed.
   c. clean ears with cotton-tipped applicators daily.
   d. disconnect or remove the batteries when not in use.
   e. initially restrict usage to quiet listening in the home.

10. Which strategies would best assist the nurse in communicating with a patient who has a hearing loss (select all that apply)?
    a. Overenunciate speech.
    b. Speak normally and slowly.
    c. Exaggerate facial expressions.
    d. Raise the voice to a higher pitch.
    e. Write out names or difficult words.

11. Patients with permanent visual impairment
    a. feel most comfortable with other visually impaired people.
    b. may feel threatened when others make eye contact during a conversation.
    c. usually need others to speak louder so they can communicate appropriately.
    d. may experience the same grieving process that is associated with other losses.

1. b, 2. d, 3. a, 4. a, d, 5. a, d, 6. c, 7. d, 8. a, 9. b, d, e, 10. b, e, 11. d

ⓔvolve

For rationales to these answers and even more NCLEX review questions, visit *http://evolve.elsevier.com/Lewis/medsurg*.

REFERENCES

1. Shagam JY: Diagnosis and treatment of ocular disorders, *Radiol Technol* 81:565, 2010.
*2. Wu Y, Carnt N, Stapleton F: Contact lens user profile, attitudes and level of compliance to lens care, *Contact Lens Anterior Eye* 33:183, 2010.
3. US Food and Drug Administration: LASIK. Retrieved from *www.fda.gov/MedicalDevices/ProductsandMedicalProcedures/SurgeryandLifeSupport/LASIK/default.htm*.

*Evidence-based information for clinical practice.

4. American Foundation for the Blind: Aging and vision fact sheet. Retrieved from *www.afb.org/seniorsite*.
5. Johns Hopkins University: New technologies brighten up low vision, *Johns Hopkins Med Lett Health After 50* 28:3, 2011.
6. American Foundation for the Blind: Maximize your lighting. Retrieved from *www.afb.org/seniorsite.asp?SectionID=66&TopicID=321&SubTopicID=206&DocumentID=4813*.
7. Boyle E: Preparedness critical to minimizing ocular trauma in emergencies, *Ocular Surgery News* 28:1, 2010.
8. Bernardes T, Bonfioli A: Blepharitis, *Semin Ophthalmol* 25:79, 2010.
9. Selby M: The red and painful eye, *Practice Nurse* 41:34, 2011.

10. World Health Organization: Trachoma and world-wide blindness. Retrieved from *www.who.int/blindness/causes/trachoma*.

*11. Wilhelmus K: Antiviral treatment and other therapeutic interventions for herpes simplex virus epithelial keratitis, *Cochrane Database Syst Rev* vol. 1, CD002898, 2010.

12. John T: Descemet's membrane endothelial keratoplasty: a useful technique for selective tissue corneal transplantation, *Ocular Surgery News* 28:4, 2010.

13. Chan E, Mahroo O, Spalton D: Complications of cataract surgery, *Clin Experiment Optometry* 93:379, 2010.

14. Mayo Clinic: Cataract surgery. Retrieved from *www.mayoclinic.com/health/cataract-surgery/MY00164/DSECTION=what-you-can-expect*.

15. National Eye Institute, National Institutes of Health: Facts about cataracts. Retrieved from *www.nei.nih.gov/health/cataract/cataract_facts.asp#5a*.

16. Bressler N, Beck R, Ferris F: Panretinal photocoagulation for proliferative diabetic retinopathy, *N Engl J Med* 365:1520, 2011.

17. Schaal S, Sherman M, Barr C, et al: Primary retinal detachment repair: comparison of 1-year outcomes of four surgical techniques, *Retina* 31:1500, 2011.

18. National Eye Institute, National Institutes of Health: Age-related macular degeneration. Retrieved from *www.nei.nih.gov/health/maculardegen/armd*.

19. Age-Related Eye Disease Study Research Group: A randomized, placebo-controlled, clinical trial of high-dose supplementation with vitamins C and E, beta-carotene, and zinc for age-related macular degeneration and vision loss, *Arch Ophthalmol* 119:1417, 2001. (Classic)

20. Khan A: Genetics of primary glaucoma, *Curr Opin Ophthalmol* 22:347, 2011.

*21. Wise L, Rosenberg L, Radin R, et al: A prospective study of diabetes, lifestyle factors, and glaucoma among African-American women, *Ann Epidemiol* 21:430, 2011.

22. American Cancer Society: Eye cancer (melanoma and lymphoma). Retrieved from *www.cancer.org/acs/groups/cid/documents/webcontent/003100-pdf.pdf*.

23. Centers for Disease Control and Prevention: Estimated burden of acute otitis externa—United States 2003-2007, *MMWR* 60:605, 2011.

*24. Ebell M: Short course of antibiotics for acute otitis media treatment, *Am Fam Physician Cochrane Briefs* 83:37, 2011.

25. Ferri F: *Ferri's clinical advisor 2012*, St Louis, 2011, Mosby.

26. Vibert D, Caversaccio M, Hausler R: Ménière's disease in the elderly, *Otolaryngol Clin North Am* 43:1041, 2010.

27. Balatsouras D: Subjective benign paroxysmal positional vertigo, *Otolaryngol Head Neck Surg* 146:98, 2012.

28. Harkin H, Kelleher C: Caring for older adults with hearing loss, *Nursing Older People* 23:9, 2011.

29. American Disabilities Act. Retrieved from *www.ada.gov/pubs/ada.htm*.

30. Laubach G: Speaking up for older patients with hearing loss, *Nursing* 40:60, 2010.

31. National Institute on Deafness and Other Communication Disorders: Cochlear implants. Retrieved from *www.nidcd.nih.gov/health/hearing/coch.asp*.

32. Cochlear implants. Retrieved from *www.fda.gov/MedicalDevices/ProductsandMedicalProcedures/ImplantsandProsthetics/CochlearImplants/default.htm*.

RESOURCES

Alexander Graham Bell Association for the Deaf and Hard of Hearing
www.agbell.org

American Academy of Audiology
www.audiology.org

American Academy of Ophthalmology
www.aao.org

American Foundation for the Blind
www.afb.org

American Society of Cataract and Refractive Surgery
www.ascrs.org

American Society of Ophthalmic Registered Nurses
www.asorn.org

Association for Education and Rehabilitation of the Blind and Visually Impaired
www.aerbvi.org

Guide Dogs for the Blind
www.guidedogs.com

Hearing Loss Association of America
www.hearingloss.org

International Hearing Dog, Inc.
www.ihdi.org

International Hearing Society
www.ihsinfo.org

Lighthouse International
http://lighthouse.org

National Association of the Deaf
www.nad.org

National Braille Association
www.nationalbraille.org

National Institute on Deafness and Other Communication Disorders, National Institutes of Health
www.nidcd.nih.gov

TDI (telecommunications for the deaf and hard of hearing)
www.tdi-online.org

23

Nursing Assessment
Integumentary System

Shannon Ruff Dirksen

> *Nobody grows old merely by living a number of years. We grow old by deserting our ideals. Years may wrinkle the skin, but to give up enthusiasm wrinkles the soul.*
>
> *Samuel Ullman*

evolve WEBSITE

http://evolve.elsevier.com/Lewis/medsurg

- NCLEX Review Questions
- Key Points
- Pre-Test
- Answer Guidelines for Case Study in this chapter

- Rationales for Bridge to NCLEX Examination Questions
- Concept Map Creator
- Glossary
- Content Updates

- Videos
  - Physical Examination: Back and Posterior Chest
  - Physical Examination: Feet, Legs, and Hips
  - Physical Examination: Head and Face

LEARNING OUTCOMES

1. Describe the structures and functions of the integumentary system.
2. Link the age-related changes in the integumentary system to differences in assessment findings.
3. Select the significant subjective and objective data related to the integumentary system that should be obtained from a patient.
4. Describe specific assessments to be made during the physical examination of the skin and the appendages.
5. Compare and contrast the critical components for describing primary and secondary lesions.

6. Select appropriate techniques to use in the physical assessment of the integumentary system.
7. Specify the structural and assessment differences in light- and dark-skinned individuals.
8. Differentiate normal from common abnormal findings of a physical assessment of the integumentary system.
9. Describe the purpose, significance of results, and nursing responsibilities related to diagnostic studies of the integumentary system.

KEY TERMS

alopecia, Table 23-8, p. 422
dermis, p. 415
epidermis, p. 414
erythema, Table 23-8, p. 422

hirsutism, Table 23-8, p. 422
intertriginous, p. 419
keloid, p. 423
keratinocytes, p. 415

melanocytes, p. 414
mole (nevus), Table 23-8, p. 422
pruritus, p. 419
sebaceous glands, p. 416

The integumentary system is the largest body organ and is composed of the skin, hair, nails, and glands. The skin is further divided into two layers: the epidermis and the dermis. The subcutaneous tissue is immediately under the dermis (Fig. 23-1).

STRUCTURES AND FUNCTIONS OF SKIN AND APPENDAGES

Structures

The epidermis is the outermost layer of the skin. The dermis, the second skin layer, contains collagen bundles and supports the nerve and vascular network. The subcutaneous layer is composed primarily of fat and loose connective tissue.

Epidermis. The **epidermis,** the thin avascular superficial layer of the skin, is made up of an outer dead cornified portion that serves as a protective barrier and a deeper, living portion that folds into the dermis. Together these layers measure 0.05 to 0.1 mm in thickness. The epidermis is nourished by blood vessels in the dermis. The epidermis regenerates with new cells every 28 days. The two major types of epidermal cells are melanocytes (5%) and keratinocytes (90%).

Melanocytes are contained in the deep, basal layer (stratum germinativum) of the epidermis. They contain melanin, a pigment that gives color to the skin and hair and protects the body from damaging ultraviolet (UV) sunlight. Sunlight and hormones stimulate the melanosome (within the melanocyte) to increase the production of melanin.[1] The wide range of skin

---

Reviewed by Brenda C. Morris, RN, EdD, CNE, Senior Director, Baccalaureate Nursing and Clinical Associate Professor, College of Nursing and Health Innovation, Arizona State University, Phoenix, Arizona; and Rosalynde D. Peterson, RN, DNP, Nursing Instructor, Shelton State Community College, Tuscaloosa, Alabama.

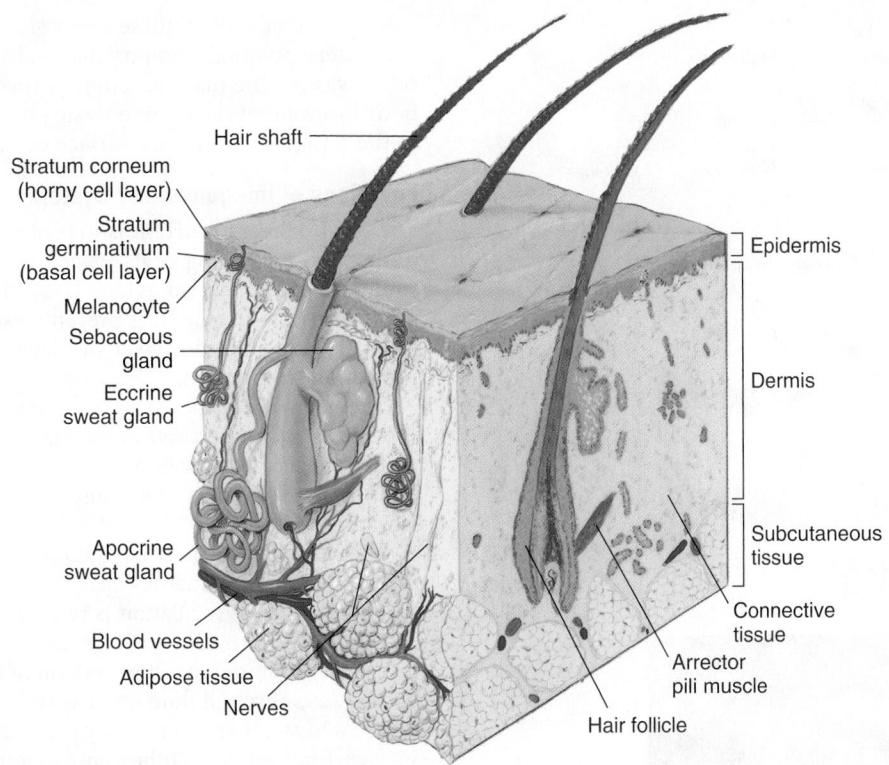

Hair shaft

Stratum corneum
(horny cell layer)

Stratum
germinativum
(basal cell layer)

Melanocyte

Sebaceous
gland

Eccrine
sweat gland

Apocrine
sweat gland

Blood vessels

Adipose tissue

Nerves

Epidermis

Dermis

Subcutaneous
tissue

Connective
tissue

Arrector
pili muscle

Hair follicle

FIG. 23-1 Microscopic view of the skin in longitudinal section. From Jarvis C: *Physical examination and health assessment,* ed 6, St Louis, 2012, Saunders.

color is caused by the amount of melanin produced; more melanin results in darker skin color.[2]

Keratinocytes are synthesized from epidermal cells in the basal layer. Initially these cells are undifferentiated. As they mature (keratinize), they move to the surface, where they flatten and die to form the outer skin layer (stratum corneum). Keratinocytes produce a fibrous protein, keratin, which is vital to the skin's protective barrier function. The upward movement of keratinocytes from the basement membrane to the stratum corneum takes approximately 4 weeks. If dead cells slough off too rapidly, the skin will appear thin and eroded. If new cells form faster than old cells are shed, the skin becomes scaly and thickened. Changes in this cell cycle are reflected in many skin problems, such as psoriasis.

Dermis. The **dermis** is the connective tissue below the epidermis. Dermal thickness varies from 1 to 4 mm. The dermis is very vascular.

The dermis is divided into two layers, an upper thin papillary layer and a deeper, thicker reticular layer. The papillary layer is folded into ridges, or papillae, which extend into the upper epidermal layer. These exposed surface ridges form congenital patterns called fingerprints and footprints. The reticular layer contains collagen and elastic and reticular fibers.

Collagen forms the greatest part of the dermis and is responsible for the skin's mechanical strength. The primary cell type in the dermis is the *fibroblast.* Fibroblasts produce collagen and elastin fibers and are important in wound healing. Nerves, lymphatic vessels, hair follicles, and sebaceous glands are also found in the dermis.

Subcutaneous Tissue. The subcutaneous tissue lies below the dermis and is not part of the skin. The subcutaneous tissue is often discussed with the skin because it attaches the skin to

underlying tissues such as muscle and bone. The subcutaneous tissue contains loose connective tissue and fat cells that provide insulation. The anatomic distribution of subcutaneous tissue varies according to gender, heredity, age, and nutritional status. This layer also stores lipids, regulates temperature, and provides shock absorption.

Skin Appendages. Appendages of the skin include the hair, nails, and glands (sebaceous, apocrine, and eccrine). These structures develop from the epidermal layer and receive nutrients, electrolytes, and fluids from the dermis. Hair and nails form from specialized keratin that becomes hardened.

Hair grows on most of the body except for the lips, the palms of the hands, and the soles of the feet.[3] The color of the hair is a result of heredity and is determined by the type and amount of melanin in the hair shaft. Hair grows approximately 1 cm per month. On average 100 hairs are lost each day. The rate of growth is not affected by cutting.[2] When lost hair is not replaced, baldness results. The absence of hair may be related to disease, treatment, or heredity.

Nails grow from the matrix. The nail matrix is located at the proximal area of the nail plate. The matrix is commonly called the *lunula,* which is the white crescent-shaped area visible through the nail plate (Fig. 23-2). The nail bed that is under the nail matrix and nail plate is normally pink and contains blood vessels. The nail plate adheres to and is supported by the nail bed. The cuticle is part of the skin that extends a small distance on the nail plate before being shed (like the stratum corneum). The nail root is bordered by the cuticle and hidden by a fold of skin. Fingernails grow at a rate of 0.7 to 0.84 mm per week, with toenail growth 30% to 50% slower. Nails can be injured by direct trauma. A lost fingernail usually regenerates in 3 to 6 months, whereas a lost toenail may require 12 months or longer for

FIG. 23-2 Structure of a nail.

FIG. 23-3 Pigmented nail bed normally seen with dark skin color.

regeneration. Nail growth may vary according to the person's age and health. Nail color ranges from pink to yellow or brown depending on skin color. Pigmented longitudinal bands (melanonychia striata) may commonly occur in the nail bed in approximately 90% or more of all people with dark skin (Fig. 23-3).

Two major types of glands are associated with the skin: sebaceous and sweat (apocrine and eccrine) glands. The **sebaceous glands** secrete *sebum,* which is emptied into the hair follicles. Sebum prevents the skin and hair from becoming dry. Sebum is somewhat bacteriostatic and fungistatic and consists mainly of lipids. These glands depend on sex hormones, particularly testosterone, to regulate sebum secretion and production. Sebum secretion varies across the life span according to sex hormone levels. Sebaceous glands are present on all areas of the skin except the palms and the soles. These glands are most abundant on the face, scalp, upper chest, and back.

The *apocrine sweat glands* are located in the axillae, breast areolae, umbilical and anogenital areas, external auditory canals, and eyelids. They secrete a thick milky substance of unknown composition that becomes odoriferous when altered by skin surface bacteria. These glands enlarge and become active at puberty because of reproductive hormones.

The *eccrine sweat glands* are widely distributed over the body, except in a few areas, such as the lips. One square inch of skin contains about 3000 of these sweat glands. Sweat is a transparent watery solution composed of salts, ammonia, urea, and other wastes. The main function of these glands is to cool the body by evaporation, excrete waste products through the pores of the skin, and moisturize surface cells.

Functions of Integumentary System

The skin's primary function is to protect the underlying tissues of the body by serving as a surface barrier to the external environment. The skin also acts as a barrier against invasion by bacteria and viruses, and it prevents excessive water loss. The fat of the subcutaneous layer insulates the body and provides protection from trauma.

The skin with its nerve endings and special receptors provides sensory perception for environmental stimuli. These highly specialized nerve endings supply information to the brain related to pain, heat and cold, touch, pressure, and vibration.

The skin controls heat regulation by responding to changes in internal and external temperature with vasoconstriction or vasodilation. Heat regulation is related to the skin's function of excretion. Between 600 and 900 mL of water is lost daily through insensible perspiration. This function of the skin helps maintain homeostasis through fluid and electrolyte balance. In addition, sebum and sweat are secreted by the skin and lubricate the skin surface. Endogenous synthesis of vitamin D, which is critical to calcium and phosphorus balance, occurs in the epidermis. Vitamin D is synthesized by the action of UV light on vitamin D precursors in epidermal cells.

The esthetic functions of the skin include the expression of various emotions, such as anger or embarrassment, and the person's individual appearance. The skin is also used as a system for the delivery of drugs. An increasing number of systemic drugs are effectively delivered via patches or creams applied directly to the skin.

GERONTOLOGIC CONSIDERATIONS

EFFECTS OF AGING ON INTEGUMENTARY SYSTEM

Many skin changes are associated with aging. Although many changes are not serious except for their cosmetic value, others are more serious and need careful evaluation. Age-related changes of the integumentary system and differences in assessment findings are listed in Table 23-1.

The rate of age-related skin changes is influenced by heredity, a personal history of sun exposure, hygiene practices, nutrition, and general state of health. Skin changes that are related to aging include decreased turgor, thinning, dryness, wrinkling, vascular lesions, increased skin fragility, and benign neoplasms.

The junction between the dermis and the epidermis becomes flattened and the epidermis contains fewer melanocytes, which decreases the production of melanin, resulting in gray or white hair. In addition, the dermis loses volume and has fewer blood vessels. Scalp, pubic, and axillary hair becomes depigmented and thinner. The nail plate thins, and nails become brittle and more prone to splitting and yellowing. Nails, especially the toenails, may also thicken with age.

Chronic UV exposure is the major contributor to the photoaging and wrinkling of skin.[4] Sun damage to the skin is cumulative (Fig. 23-4). The wrinkling of sun-exposed areas such as the face and hands is more marked than that of a sun-shielded area such as the buttocks. Poor nutrition, with decreased intake

TABLE 23-1 GERONTOLOGIC ASSESSMENT DIFFERENCES

Integumentary System

Changes	Differences in Assessment Findings
Skin	
Decreased subcutaneous fat, muscle laxity, degeneration of elastic fibers, collagen stiffening	Increased wrinkling, sagging breasts and abdomen, redundant flesh around eyes, slowness of skin to flatten when pinched (tenting).
Decreased extracellular water, surface lipids, and sebaceous gland activity	Dry, flaking skin with possible signs of excoriation caused by scratching.
Decreased activity of apocrine and sebaceous glands	Dry skin with minimal to no perspiration, skin color uneven.
Increased capillary fragility and permeability	Bruising.
Increased focal melanocytes in basal layer with pigment accumulation	Solar lentigines on face and back of hands.
Diminished blood supply	Decrease in rosy appearance of skin and mucous membranes. Skin cool to touch. Diminished awareness of pain, touch, temperature, peripheral vibration.
Decreased proliferative capacity	Diminished rate of wound healing.
Decreased immunocompetence	Increase in neoplasms.
Hair	
Decreased melanin and melanocytes	Gray or white hair.
Decreased oil	Dry, coarse hair. Scaly scalp.
Decreased density of hair	Thinning and loss of hair. Loss of hair in outer half or outer third of eyebrow and back of legs.
Cumulative androgen effect; decreasing estrogen levels	Facial hirsutism, baldness.
Nails	
Decreased peripheral blood supply	Thick, brittle nails with diminished growth.
Increased keratin	Longitudinal ridging.
Decreased circulation	Prolonged return of blood to nails on blanching.

FIG. 23-4 Photoaging. Irregular pigmentation and keratoses occur on sun-damaged skin on forehead.

TABLE 23-2 NORMAL PHYSICAL ASSESSMENT OF INTEGUMENTARY SYSTEM

Skin	• Evenly pigmented; no petechiae, purpura, lesions, or excoriations. • Warm, good turgor.
Nails	• Pink, oval, adhere to nail bed with 160-degree angle.
Hair	• Shiny and full; amount and distribution appropriate for age and gender. • No flaking of scalp, forehead, or pinna.

In older adults decreased subcutaneous fat leads to an increased risk of traumatic injury, hypothermia, and skin shearing, which may lead to pressure ulcers. With aging, the apocrine and eccrine sweat glands atrophy, causing dry skin and decreased body odor. The growth rate of the hair and nails decreases as a result of atrophy of the involved structures. Hormonal and vitamin deficiencies can cause dry, thin hair and alopecia (partial or complete lack of hair).

The visible effects of aging on the skin and hair may have a profound psychologic effect. A youthful look may be tied to a person's self-image. Although fine wrinkling of the skin, thinning hair, and brittle nails are normal changes with aging, they may result in an altered self-image.[5]

ASSESSMENT OF INTEGUMENTARY SYSTEM

A general assessment of the skin begins at the initial contact with the patient and continues throughout the examination. Specific areas of the skin are assessed during the examination of other body systems unless the chief complaint is a dermatologic problem. Record a general statement about the skin's physical condition (Table 23-2). In addition, ask the health history questions presented in Table 23-3 when a skin problem is noted.

Subjective Data

Individuals with skin problems may have complaints that are not readily observed. A thorough health history yields information about possible causes and the effect of the problem on the individual's life.

Important Health Information

Past Health History. Past health history indicates previous trauma, surgery, or disease that involves the skin. Determine if the patient has noticed any dermatologic manifestations of systemic problems such as jaundice (liver disease), delayed wound

of protein, calories, and vitamins, also contributes to aging of the skin. With aging, collagen fibers stiffen, elastic fibers degenerate, and the amount of subcutaneous tissue decreases. These changes, with the added effects of gravity, lead to wrinkling.

Benign neoplasms related to the aging process can occur on the skin. These growths include seborrheic keratoses, vascular lesions such as cherry angiomas, and skin tags. *Actinic keratoses* appear on areas of chronic sun exposure, especially in the person who has a fair complexion and light eyes (blue, green, or hazel). These premalignant cutaneous lesions place an individual at increased risk for squamous cell and basal cell carcinomas. The photoaged person is more susceptible to skin cancers because UV exposure decreases the capacity to repair cellular damage (especially deoxyribonucleic acid [DNA]). Chronic UV exposure from tanning beds causes the same damage as UV from the sun.

- Inherited genetic factors can also increase the risk for skin cancer. A person has an increased risk for developing melanoma if he or she has a first-degree relative (e.g., parent, full sibling) who had a melanoma.
- The risk for skin cancer is increased for people who have a fair complexion (light-colored skin that easily freckles, red or blond hair, and blue or light-colored eyes).

Obtain information about the family history of any skin diseases, including congenital and familial diseases (e.g., alopecia, psoriasis) and systemic diseases with dermatologic

CASE STUDY

Patient Introduction

iStockphoto/Thinkstock

D.A. is a 74-year-old woman who comes to the medical clinic with concerns related to various "spots" on her face. She says they have been there for a while and she thought they were just "age spots" but got concerned after her friend was diagnosed with a malignant melanoma.

Critical Thinking

As you read through this assessment chapter, think about D.A. with the following questions in mind:

1. What are the possible causes of D.A.'s facial lesions?
2. What questions would you ask D.A. to determine the possible causes?
3. What should be included in the physical assessment? What specific characteristics of the skin lesions would you be looking for?
4. What diagnostic studies might you expect to be ordered?

evolve Answers available at *http://evolve.elsevier.com/Lewis/medsurg*.

healing (diabetes mellitus), cyanosis (respiratory disorder), or pallor (anemia). eTable 24-1 lists diseases with dermatologic manifestations. Obtain specific information related to food sensitivities, pet or drug allergies, and skin reactions to insect bites and stings. Note any history of chronic or unprotected exposure to UV light, including tanning bed use and radiation treatments.

Medications. Ask the patient about skin-related problems that occurred as a result of taking prescription or over-the-counter (OTC) medications. A thorough medication history is important, especially in relation to vitamins, hormones, antibiotics, corticosteroids, and antimetabolites because these may cause side effects that are manifested in the skin.

Document the use of prescription or OTC medications used specifically to treat a primary skin problem such as acne or a secondary skin problem such as itching. If a medication is used, record the name, length of use, method of application, and effectiveness.

Surgery or Other Treatments. Determine if any surgical procedures, including cosmetic surgery, were performed on the skin. If a biopsy was done, record the result. Note any treatments specific for a skin problem (e.g., phototherapy) or for a health problem (e.g., radiation therapy). In addition, document any treatments undergone primarily for cosmetic purposes, such as tanning booth use, laser resurfacing, or cosmetic "peels."

Functional Health Patterns

Health Perception–Health Management Pattern. Question the patient about health practices related to the integumentary system, such as self-care habits related to daily hygiene. Document the frequency of use and sun protection factor (SPF) of sunscreen products. Assess the use of personal care products (e.g., shampoos, moisturizing agents, cosmetics), including brand name, quantity, and frequency. Record a description of any current skin problem, including onset, symptoms, course, and treatment. Note any medications used for treating hair loss.

GENETIC RISK ALERT

- The primary risk factor leading to skin cancer and melanoma is environmental exposure to UV radiation. UV radiation damages DNA, causing an error in the genetic code and resulting in abnormal skin cells.

TABLE 23-3 HEALTH HISTORY

Integumentary System

Health Perception–Health Management
- Describe your daily hygiene practices.
- What skin products are you currently using?
- Describe any current skin condition, including onset, course, and treatment (if any).

Nutritional-Metabolic
- Describe any changes in the condition of your skin, hair, nails, and mucous membranes.
- Have you noticed any recent changes in the way sores or wounds heal?*
- Have you had any weight loss or dietary changes, including supplemental vitamins and minerals?*

Elimination
- Have you noticed recent changes in your skin related to excessive sweating, dryness, or swelling?*

Activity-Exercise
- Do your leisure or work activities involve the use of any chemicals that are irritating to your skin?*
- Do you do anything to protect yourself from the sun?*

Sleep-Rest
- Does your skin condition keep you awake or awaken you after you have fallen asleep?*

Cognitive-Perceptual
- Do you have any unusual sensations of heat, cold, or touch?*
- Do you have any pain associated with your skin condition?*
- Do you have any joint pain?*

Self-Perception–Self-Concept
- How does your skin condition make you feel about yourself?

Role-Relationship
- Has your skin condition changed your relationships with others?*
- Have you changed your lifestyle because of your skin condition?*

Sexuality-Reproductive
- Has your skin condition changed your intimate relationships with others?*
- Has your birth control method (if used) caused a skin problem?*

Coping–Stress Tolerance
- Are you aware of any situation or stressor that changes your skin condition?*
- Do you think that stress plays a role in your skin condition?*
- How do you handle stress?

Value-Belief
- Are there any cultural beliefs that influence your thinking or feelings about your skin condition?*
- Are there any treatment options that you would be opposed to using?

*If yes, describe.

manifestations (e.g., diabetes, thyroid disease, cardiovascular diseases, immune disorders). In addition, note any family and personal history of skin cancer, particularly melanoma.

Nutritional-Metabolic Pattern. Question the patient about any changes in the condition of skin, hair, nails, and mucous membranes and whether they are related to dietary changes. A diet history reveals the adequacy of nutrients essential to healthy skin such as vitamins A, D, E, and C; dietary fat; and protein. Note any food allergies that cause a skin reaction. Ask obese patients if they have areas of chafing or a rash in **intertriginous** areas, where skin surfaces overlap and rub on each other (e.g., below the breasts, axillae, and groin). Note any excessive or absent sweating. Question the patient about poor or delayed wound healing.

Elimination Pattern. Ask the patient about conditions of the skin such as dehydration, edema, and **pruritus** (itching), which can indicate alterations in fluid balance. If urinary or fecal incontinence is a problem, determine the condition of the skin in the anal and perineal areas.

Activity-Exercise Pattern. Obtain information about environmental hazards in relation to hobbies and recreational activities, including exposure to known carcinogens, chemical irritants, and allergens. Ask the patient if any changes occur in the skin during exercise or other activities.

Sleep-Rest Pattern. Question the patient about disturbances in sleep patterns caused by a skin condition. For example, pruritus can be distressing and cause major alterations in normal sleep patterns. Also, poor sleep and resulting tiredness are often reflected in a patient's face by dark circles under the eyes and a decreased firmness in the facial skin.

Cognitive-Perceptual Pattern. Determine the patient's perception of the sensations of heat, cold, pain, and touch. Note any discomfort associated with a skin condition, especially when observed in intact skin. Assess and record any joint pain. Assess the mobility of the joints, since the patient's skin condition may cause alterations in mobility.

Self-Perception–Self-Concept Pattern. Assess any feelings related to the patient's skin condition such as sadness, anxiety, despair, or altered body image. These feelings can occur with visible skin problems such as acne, rosacea, and psoriasis, which alter a person's physical appearance.

Role-Relationship Pattern. Determine how the patient's skin condition affects relationships with family members, peers, and work associates. In addition, question the patient regarding the effect of environmental factors on the skin such as occupational exposure to irritants, sun, and unusually cold or unhygienic conditions. Contact dermatitis caused by allergies and irritants is a common skin problem associated with occupation.

Sexuality-Reproductive Pattern. Tactfully question and assess the effect of the patient's skin condition on sexual activity. In particular, note the reproductive status of the female patient relative to possible therapeutic interventions. For example, isotretinoin (Accutane), used to treat acne, and topical fluorouracil (Efudex, Fluoroplex), used to treat actinic keratoses, are teratogenic drugs that may cause abnormal fetal development. These medications should not be used by pregnant women or women who could become pregnant.

Coping–Stress Tolerance Pattern. Assess and question the patient about the role that stress may play in creating or exacerbating the skin condition. Ask the patient what coping strategies are used to manage the skin condition.

CASE STUDY—cont'd

Subjective Data

iStockphoto/Thinkstock

A focused subjective assessment of D.A. reveals the following:
- **PMH:** Negative except for an appendectomy at age 16.
- **Medications:** None at present. NKA.
- **Health Perception–Health Management:** Currently washes her face with a skin cleanser in the morning and nighttime. After cleansing, she applies a moisturizer with SPF 15. She has used these facial products for the past 3 years since she first started noticing small age spots appearing. Before that she just used soap and water.
- **Nutritional:** D.A. reports that her skin seems to be drier as she ages but otherwise no changes besides the "age spots" or "whatever they are." Denies any changes in the way cuts or sores heal. No weight loss. Does not take any supplemental vitamins or minerals.
- **Elimination:** Although skin is a little dry, D.A. does not perceive it to be excessively dry. Denies excessive sweating or any swelling.
- **Activity-Exercise:** Loves to garden and go for walks outdoors. Reports a history of frequent, sometimes severe, sunburns as a child. No use of sunscreen growing up but does remember her mother making her wear T-shirts over her bathing suits to help prevent sunburn. Has used sunscreen for the past 20 years when outdoors. Reapplies as needed.
- **Cognitive-Perceptual:** Denies any pain or discomfort associated with skin lesions.
- **Coping–Stress Tolerance:** Fearful that she might have skin cancer.

Value-Belief Pattern. Ask about cultural or religious beliefs that could influence the patient's self-image as related to the skin condition. Also, assess values and beliefs that might influence or limit the choice of treatment options.

Objective Data

Physical Examination. Primary skin lesions develop on previously unaltered skin. The common characteristics of primary skin lesions are shown in Table 23-4. Secondary skin lesions are lesions that change with time or occur because of factors such as scratching or infection. Secondary skin lesions are shown in Table 23-5. General principles when assessing the skin are as follows:
- Have a private examination room of moderate temperature with good lighting; a room with exposure to daylight is preferred.
- Ensure that the patient is comfortable and in a dressing gown that allows easy access to all skin areas.
- Be systematic and proceed from head to toe.
- Compare symmetric parts.
- Perform a general inspection and then a lesion-specific examination.
- Use the metric system when taking measurements.
- Use appropriate terminology and nomenclature when reporting or documenting.

Photographs are useful when accurate findings are needed. Follow clinical agency protocol regarding obtaining a patient's consent to photograph skin lesions for inclusion in the medical record.

Inspection. Inspect the skin for general color and pigmentation, vascularity, bruising, and lesions or discolorations. The critical factor in assessment of skin color is change. A skin color

TABLE 23-4	**PRIMARY SKIN LESIONS**

Lesion	Description
Macule 	Circumscribed, flat area with a change in skin color; <0.5 cm in diameter; if lesion >0.5 cm, it is a *patch* *Examples:* freckles, petechiae, measles, flat mole (nevus), café-au-lait spots, vitiligo (complete depigmentation)
Papule 	Elevated, solid lesion; <0.5 cm in diameter; if lesion is >0.5 cm in diameter, it is a *nodule* *Examples:* wart (verruca), elevated moles, lipoma, basal cell carcinoma
Vesicle 	Circumscribed, superficial collection of serous fluid; <0.5 cm in diameter *Examples:* varicella (chickenpox), herpes zoster (shingles), second-degree burn
Plaque 	Circumscribed, elevated, superficial, solid lesion; >0.5 cm in diameter *Examples:* psoriasis, seborrheic and actinic keratoses
Wheal 	Firm, edematous, irregularly shaped area; diameter variable *Examples:* insect bite, urticaria
Pustule 	Elevated, superficial lesion filled with purulent fluid *Examples:* acne, impetigo

TABLE 23-5	**SECONDARY SKIN LESIONS**

Lesion	Description
Fissure 	Linear crack or break from the epidermis to the dermis; dry or moist *Examples:* athlete's foot, cracks at corner of the mouth
Scale 	Excess, dead epidermal cells produced by abnormal keratinization and shedding *Examples:* flaking of skin after a drug reaction or sunburn
Scar 	Abnormal formation of connective tissue that replaces normal skin *Examples:* surgical incision, healed wound
Ulcer 	Loss of the epidermis, extending into the dermis; crater-like, irregular shape *Examples:* pressure ulcer, chancre
Atrophy 	Depression in skin resulting from thinning of the epidermis or dermis *Examples:* aged skin, striae
Excoriation	Area in which epidermis is missing, exposing the dermis *Examples:* abrasion, scratch

that is normal for a particular patient can be a sign of a pathologic condition in another patient. The skin color depends on the amount of melanin (brown), carotene (yellow), oxyhemoglobin (red), and reduced hemoglobin (bluish red) present at a particular time. The most reliable areas to assess erythema, cyanosis, pallor, and jaundice are the areas of least pigmentation, such as the sclerae, conjunctivae, nail beds, lips, and buccal mucosa. The true skin color is best observed in photo-protected areas such as the buttocks. Activity, sun (UV) exposure, emotions, cigarette smoking, and edema, as well as respiratory, renal, cardiovascular, and hepatic disorders, can all directly affect skin color. Table 23-6 describes assessment variations in light- and dark-skinned individuals.

TABLE 23-6   NURSING ASSESSMENT

Assessment Variations in Light- and Dark-Skinned Individuals

Light Skin	Dark Skin
Cyanosis	
Grayish blue tone, especially in nail beds, earlobes, lips, mucous membranes, palms, and soles	Ashen or gray color most easily seen in the conjunctiva of the eye, mucous membranes, and nail beds
Ecchymosis	
Dark red, purple, yellow, or green color, depending on age of bruise	Purple to brownish black. Difficult to see unless occurring in an area of light pigmentation
Erythema	
Reddish tone, possibly accompanied by increased skin temperature secondary to localized inflammation	Deeper brown or purple skin tone with evidence of increased skin temperature secondary to inflammation
Jaundice	
Yellowish color of skin, sclera, fingernails, palms, and oral mucosa	Yellowish green color most obviously seen in sclera of eye (do not confuse with yellow eye pigmentation, which may be evident in dark-skinned patients), palms, and soles
Pallor	
Pale skin color that may appear white or ashen; also evident on lips, nail beds, and mucous membranes	Lack of underlying red tone in brown or black skin. In light-skinned African Americans, yellowish brown skin. In dark-skinned African Americans, ashen or gray skin
Petechiae	
Lesions appearing as small, reddish purple pinpoints, best observed on abdomen and buttocks	Difficult to see. May be evident in the buccal mucosa of the mouth or conjunctiva of the eye
Rash	
May be visualized and felt with light palpation	Not easily visualized, but may be felt with light palpation
Scar	
Generally heals, showing narrow scar line	Higher incidence of keloid development, resulting in a thickened, raised scar (see Table 23-5)

In your general inspection, note the presence of body art such as piercings and tattoos. The nose, ears, eyebrows, lips, navel, and nipples are common sites of piercing. Tattoo pigments deposited in the skin may cause itching, pain, and sensitivity for several weeks after the tattoo is placed.

Examine the skin for possible problems related to vascularity, including bruising and vascular and purpuric lesions such as *angioma* (benign tumor of blood or lymph vessels), *petechiae* (tiny purple spots on skin), or *purpura* (bleeding disorder caused by ecchymosis or petechiae). Note the reaction to direct pressure. If a lesion blanches on direct pressure and then refills, the redness is due to dilated blood vessels. If the discoloration remains, it is the result of subcutaneous or intradermal bleeding or a nonvascular lesion. Note any pattern of bruising such as discoloration in the shape of the hand or fingers or bruises at different stages of resolution. These may indicate other health problems or abuse and should be further investigated.

If lesions are found on the skin, record their color, size, distribution, location, and shape. Skin lesions are usually described in terms related to the lesions' configuration (solitary or pattern in relation to other lesions) and distribution (arrangement of lesions over an area of skin) (Table 23-7).

During systematic inspection, note any unusual odors. Skin sites with lesions, such as rashes, may be colonized with yeast or bacteria, which can be associated with distinctive odors in intertriginous areas (Fig. 23-5). Examine tattoos and needle-track marks and note the location and characteristics of the surrounding skin area.

TABLE 23-7   LESION DISTRIBUTION TERMINOLOGY

Term	Description
Asymmetric	Unilateral distribution
Confluent	Merging together
Diffuse	Wide distribution
Discrete	Separate from other lesions
Generalized	Diffuse distribution
Grouped	Cluster of lesions
Localized	Limited areas of involvement that are clearly defined
Solitary	A single lesion
Symmetric	Bilateral distribution
Zosteriform	Bandlike distribution along a dermatome area

FIG. 23-5 Intertrigo. Rash in body folds with *Candida* infection.

TABLE 23-8   ASSESSMENT ABNORMALITIES

Integumentary System

Finding	Description	Possible Etiology and Significance
Alopecia	Loss of hair (localized or general)	Heredity, friction, rubbing, traction, trauma, stress, infection, inflammation, chemotherapy, pregnancy, emotional shock, tinea capitis, immunologic factors
Angioma	Tumor consisting of blood or lymph vessels	Normal increase in incidence with aging, liver disease, pregnancy, varicose veins
Carotenemia (carotenosis)	Yellow discoloration of skin, no yellowing of sclerae, most noticeable on palms and soles	Vegetables containing carotene (e.g., carrots, squash), hypothyroidism
Comedo (acne lesion)	Enlarged hair follicle plugged with sebum, bacteria, and skin cells; can be open (blackhead) or closed (whitehead)	Heredity, certain drugs, hormonal changes with puberty and pregnancy
Cyanosis	Slightly bluish gray or dark purple discoloration of the skin and mucous membranes caused by excessive amounts of reduced hemoglobin in capillaries	Cardiorespiratory problems, vasoconstriction, asphyxiation, anemia, leukemia, and malignancies
Cyst	Sac containing fluid or semisolid material	Obstruction of a duct or gland, parasitic infection
Ecchymosis	Large, bruise-like lesion caused by collection of extravascular blood in dermis and subcutaneous tissue	Trauma, bleeding disorders
Erythema	Redness occurring in patches of variable size and shape	Heat, certain drugs, alcohol, ultraviolet rays, any problem that causes dilation of blood vessels to the skin
Hematoma	Extravasation of blood of sufficient size to cause visible swelling	Trauma, bleeding disorders
Hirsutism	Male distribution of hair in women	Abnormality of ovaries or adrenal glands, decrease in estrogen level, familial trait
Hypopigmentation	Loss of pigmentation resulting in lighter patches than the normal skin	Chemical agents, nutritional factors, burns, inflammation, infection
Intertrigo	Dermatitis of overlying surfaces of the skin	Moisture, irritation, obesity; may be complicated by *Candida* infection (see Fig. 23-5)
Jaundice	Yellow (in white patients) or yellowish brown (in African Americans) discoloration of the skin, best observed in the sclera, secondary to increased bilirubin in the blood	Liver disease, red blood cell hemolysis, pancreatic cancer, common bile duct obstruction
Keloid	Hypertrophied scar beyond wound margins (see Fig. 23-6)	Predisposition more common in African Americans
Lichenification	Thickening of the skin with accentuated normal skin markings	Repeated scratching, rubbing, and irritation usually as a result of pruritus or neurosis
Mole (nevus)	Benign overgrowth of melanocytes	Defects of development; excessive numbers and large, irregular moles; often familial
Petechiae	Pinpoint, discrete deposits of blood <1-2 mm in the extravascular tissues and visible through the skin or mucous membrane	Inflammation, marked vasodilation, blood vessel trauma, blood dyscrasia that results in bleeding tendencies (e.g., thrombocytopenia)
Telangiectasia	Visibly dilated, superficial, cutaneous small blood vessels, commonly found on face and thighs	Aging, acne, sun exposure, alcohol, liver failure, corticosteroids, radiation, certain systemic diseases, skin tumors
Tenting	Failure of skin to return immediately to normal position after gentle pinching	Aging, dehydration, cachexia
Varicosity	Increased prominence of superficial veins	Interruption of venous return (e.g., from tumor, incompetent valves, inflammation), commonly found on lower legs with aging
Vitiligo	Complete absence of melanin (pigment) resulting in chalky white patch (see Fig. 23-7)	Autoimmune, familial, thyroid disease

Inspection of the hair should include an examination of all body hair. Note the distribution, texture, and quantity of hair. Changes in the normal distribution of body hair and growth may indicate an endocrine or vascular disorder. Carefully inspect the nails, including nail shape, thickness, curvature, and surface. Note any grooves, pitting, ridges, or detachment from nail bed. Changes in nail smoothness or thickness can occur with anemia, psoriasis, thyroid problems, decreased vascular circulation, and some infections.

Palpation. Palpate the skin to obtain information about temperature, turgor, moisture, and texture. Temperature of the patient's skin is best assessed using the back of your hand. The skin should be warm without being hot. The temperature of the skin increases when blood flow to the dermis is increased. A localized temperature increase occurs with burns and local inflammation. A generalized increase in skin temperature occurs when a person has a fever. A decreased body temperature may occur when shock or other circulatory problems, chilling, or infection is present.

Turgor refers to the elasticity of the skin. Assess turgor by gently pinching an area of skin under the clavicle or on the back of the hand. Skin with good turgor should move easily when lifted and should immediately return to its original position when released. In patients with dehydration and aging, a loss of turgor occurs and can cause tenting of the skin (Table 23-8).

Moisture of the skin (the dampness or dryness of the skin) increases in intertriginous areas and with high humidity. Skin moisture varies with environmental temperature, muscular activity, body weight, and body temperature. The skin should be intact with no flaking, scaling, or cracking. Skin generally becomes drier with increasing age.

FOCUSED ASSESSMENT
Integumentary System

Use this checklist to make sure the key assessment steps have been done.

Subjective
Ask the patient about any of the following and note responses.

Hair loss (unusual or rapid)	Y	N
Changes in skin (e.g., lesions, bruising)	Y	N
Nail discoloration	Y	N

Objective: Diagnostic
Check the following for results and critical values.

Biopsy results	✓
Albumin	✓

Objective: Physical Examination
Inspect

Skin for color, integrity, scars, lesions, signs of breakdown	✓
Facial and body hair for distribution, color, quantity, hygiene	✓
Nails for shape, contour, color, thickness, cleanliness	✓
Dressings if present	✓

Palpate

Skin for temperature, texture, moisture, thickness, turgor, mobility	✓

FIG. 23-6 Keloid. Hypertrophic scarring after skin injury, which is more common in dark-skinned individuals.

FIG. 23-7 Vitiligo. Total loss of pigment in the affected area.

Texture refers to the fineness or coarseness of the skin. The skin should feel smooth and firm with the surface evenly thin in most areas. Thickened callus areas are normal on the soles and palms and relate to weight bearing. Increased thickness is often work related and the result of excessive pressure.

A *focused assessment* is used to evaluate the status of previously identified integumentary problems and to monitor for signs of new problems (see Table 3-6). A focused assessment of the integumentary system is presented in the box on this page. Assessment abnormalities of the skin are described in Table 23-8.

Assessment of Dark Skin

A normal range of differences occurs in the physical examination of skin, hair, and nails. Genetic factors determine a person's skin color, which can vary from white to dark brown with overtones of yellow, olive, and red. The darker skin tones result from the reflection of light as it strikes the underlying skin pigment. An increased amount of melanin pigment produced by the melanocytes causes the darker skin color. This increased melanin forms a natural sun shield for dark skin and results in a decreased incidence of skin cancer in these individuals.

The structures of dark skin are no different from those of lighter skin, but they are often more difficult to assess (see Table 23-6). Color is more easily assessed in areas where the epidermis is thin and pigmentation is not influenced by sun exposure such as the lips, mucous membranes, nail beds, and protected areas (e.g., buttocks). Palmar and plantar surfaces are lighter than other skin areas in darker-skinned individuals. Rashes are often more difficult to observe and may need to be palpated.[6] Wrinkling is more apparent in light-skinned individuals than in dark-skinned individuals.

Individuals with dark skin are predisposed to certain skin and hair conditions. **Keloid** is an overgrowth of collagenous tissue at the site of a skin injury (e.g., ear piercing) (Fig. 23-6).

Vitiligo is total loss of pigment in the affected area (Fig. 23-7). In *dermatosis papulosa nigra*, small, pigmented wartlike papules are commonly found on the face. *Nevus of Ota* is a slate-gray or blue-gray birthmark located on the forehead and face around the eye area; it may also involve the sclera (Fig. 23-8). *Traction alopecia* may be noted due to trauma from hair rollers or from tight braiding of the hair (Fig. 23-9). The hair loss may be temporary or permanent. *Pseudofolliculitis* is an inflammatory response to ingrown hairs that occurs after shaving too closely in the beard area. It is characterized by pustules and papules.

Because of the darkness of the skin of some individuals, color often cannot be used as an indicator of systemic conditions (e.g., flushed skin with fever). Cyanosis may be difficult to determine because a normal bluish hue occurs in dark-skinned people.

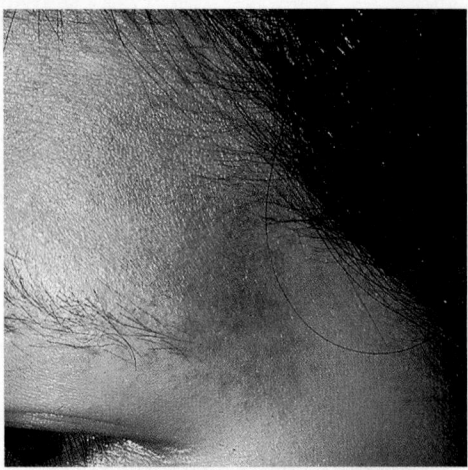

FIG. 23-8 Nevus of Ota. Flat gray to blue pigmentation in the upper trigeminal area, which is more common in dark-skinned individuals.

FIG. 23-9 Traction alopecia. Hair loss in scalp because of prolonged tension from hair rollers, braiding, or straightening combs.

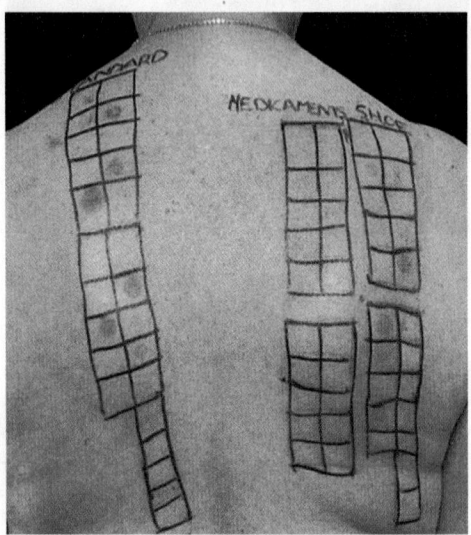

FIG. 23-10 Patch test. Results from an application of possible allergens to the skin shows positive reactions in the sites labeled "standard" and "shoe."

CASE STUDY—cont'd
Objective Data

iStockphoto/Thinkstock

Physical Examination

Physical examination findings of D.A.'s skin are as follows:

- Complexion fair. Wrinkles around eyes, above upper lip, and on sides of cheeks bilaterally. Normal skin temperature and turgor.
- Lesion on upper right forehead measuring 2 × 3 mm; on left forehead near hairline measuring 1 × 2 mm; and on left lower cheek measuring 2 × 2.5 mm.
- All lesions are slightly erythematous but do not blanch when direct pressure is applied. Borders distinct. Minimal elevation noted on palpation.
- No other skin lesions noted on rest of body.

As you continue to read this chapter, consider diagnostic studies you would anticipate being performed for D.A. Also identify patient problems and appropriate nursing interventions for D.A. while she is a patient in the clinic.

Diagnostic Studies

The health care provider examines the lesion via dermatoscopy and also uses a Wood's lamp to rule out a fungal infection. The provider suspects basal cell carcinoma, which is confirmed by a shave biopsy.

DIAGNOSTIC STUDIES OF INTEGUMENTARY SYSTEM

Diagnostic studies provide important information in monitoring the patient's condition and planning interventions. These studies are considered to be objective data. Table 23-9 contains diagnostic studies commonly used for the integumentary system.

The main diagnostic techniques related to skin problems are inspection of an individual lesion and a careful history related to the problem. If a definitive diagnosis cannot be made by these techniques, additional tests may be indicated, such as *dermatoscopy* (examination of the skin through a lighted instrument with optical magnification).[6]

Biopsy is one of the most common diagnostic tests used to evaluate a skin lesion. A biopsy is indicated in all conditions in which a malignancy is suspected or a specific diagnosis is questionable. Techniques include punch, incisional, excisional, and shave biopsies. The method used is related to factors such as the site of the biopsy, the cosmetic result desired, and the type of tissue to be obtained.

Other diagnostic procedures include stains and cultures for fungal, bacterial, and viral infections. Direct immunofluorescence is a special diagnostic technique used on biopsy specimens and may be indicated in certain conditions such as bullous diseases and systemic lupus erythematosus. Indirect immunofluorescence is performed on a sample of blood. Patch testing (Fig. 23-10) and photopatch testing may be used to evaluate allergic dermatitis and photoallergic reactions.[2]

TABLE 23-9 DIAGNOSTIC STUDIES
Integumentary System

Study	Description and Purpose	Nursing Responsibility
Biopsy		
Punch	Special punch biopsy instrument of appropriate size used. Instrument rotated to appropriate level to include dermis and some fat. Suturing may or may not be done. Provides full-thickness skin for diagnostic purposes.	Verify that consent form is signed (if needed). Assist with preparation of site, anesthesia, procedure, and hemostasis. Apply dressing, give postprocedure instructions to patient. Properly identify specimen.
Excisional	Used when good cosmetic results and/or entire lesion removal desired. Skin closed with subcutaneous and skin sutures.	Same as above.
Incisional	Wedge-shaped incision made in lesion too large for excisional biopsy. Useful when larger specimen than shave or punch biopsy is needed.	Same as above.
Shave	Single-edged razor blade used to shave off superficial lesions or small sample of a large lesion. Provides thin specimen for diagnostic purposes.	Same as above.
Microscopic Tests		
Potassium hydroxide (KOH)	Hair, scales, or nails examined for superficial fungal infection. Specimen put on glass slide and 10%-20% concentration of KOH added.	Instruct patient regarding purpose of test. Prepare slide.
Tzanck test (Wright's and Giemsa's stain)	Fluid and cells from vesicles examined. Used to diagnose herpes infections. Specimen put on slide, stained, and examined microscopically.	Inform patient of purpose of test. Use sterile technique for collection of fluid.
Culture	Test identifies fungal, bacterial, and viral organisms. For *fungi*, scraping or swab of skin performed. For *bacteria*, material obtained from intact pustules, bullae, or abscesses. For *viruses*, vesicle or bulla and exudate taken from base of lesion.	Instruct patient regarding purpose and procedure. Properly identify specimen. Follow instructions for storage of specimen if not immediately sent to laboratory.
Mineral oil slides	To check for infestations, scrapings are placed on slide with mineral oil and viewed microscopically.	Instruct patient about purpose of test. Prepare slide.
Immunofluorescent studies	Some skin diseases have specific, abnormal antibody proteins that can be identified by fluorescent studies. Both skin tissue and serum can be examined.	Inform patient about purpose of test. Assist in obtaining specimen. For punch biopsy of tissue, place specimen in special fixative (e.g., Michel's) and not formalin.
Miscellaneous		
Wood's lamp (black light)	Examination of skin with long-wave ultraviolet light causes specific substances to fluoresce (e.g., *Pseudomonas* organisms, fungal infections, vitiligo).	Explain purpose of examination. Inform patient it is not painful. Room is darkened for examination.
Patch test	Used to determine whether patient is allergic to specific testing material. Small amount of potentially allergenic material applied, usually to skin on back.	Explain purpose and procedure to patient. Instruct patient to return in 48-72 hr for removal of allergens and at 96 hr for preliminary evaluation (see Fig. 23-10).

BRIDGE TO NCLEX EXAMINATION

The number of the question corresponds to the same-numbered outcome at the beginning of the chapter.

1. The primary function of the skin is
   a. insulation.
   b. protection.
   c. sensation.
   d. absorption.
2. Age-related changes in the hair and nails include *(select all that apply)*
   a. oily scalp.
   b. scaly scalp.
   c. thinner nails.
   d. thicker, brittle nails.
   e. longitudinal nail ridging.
3. When assessing the nutritional-metabolic pattern in relation to the skin, the nurse questions the patient regarding
   a. joint pain.
   b. the use of moisturizing shampoo.
   c. recent changes in wound healing.
   d. self-care habits related to daily hygiene.

4. During the physical examination of a patient's skin, the nurse would
   a. use a flashlight in a poorly lit room.
   b. note cool, moist skin as a normal finding.
   c. pinch up a fold of skin to assess for turgor.
   d. perform a lesion-specific examination first and then a general inspection.
5. The nurse assessed the patient's skin lesions as firm, edematous, irregularly shaped with a variable diameter. They would be called
   a. wheals.
   b. papules.
   c. pustules.
   d. plaques.
6. To assess the skin for temperature and moisture, the most appropriate technique for the nurse to use is
   a. palpation.
   b. inspection.
   c. percussion.
   d. auscultation.

7. Individuals with dark skin are more likely to develop
   a. keloids.
   b. wrinkles.
   c. skin rashes.
   d. skin cancer.

8. On inspection of a patient's dark skin, the nurse notes a blue-gray birthmark on the forehead and eye area. This assessment finding is called
   a. vitiligo.
   b. intertrigo.
   c. telangiectasia.
   d. Nevus of Ota.

9. Diagnostic testing is recommended for skin lesions when
   a. a health history cannot be obtained.
   b. a more definitive diagnosis is needed.
   c. percussion reveals an abnormal finding.
   d. treatment with prescribed medication has failed.

1. b, 2. b, d, e, 3. c, 4. c, 5. a, 6. a, 7. a, 8. d, 9. b.

⊖volve

For rationales to these answers and even more NCLEX review questions, visit *http://evolve.elsevier.com/Lewis/medsurg*.

REFERENCES

1. Patton KT, Thibodeau GA, Douglas M: *Essentials of anatomy and physiology*, St Louis, 2012, Mosby.
2. Goldsmith L, Katz S, Gilcrest B, et al: *Fitzpatrick's dermatology in general medicine*, ed 8, New York, 2012, McGraw-Hill.
3. Thibodeau GA, Patton KT: *Structure and function of the body*, ed 14, St Louis, 2011, Mosby.
4. Burnett C, Ozog D: Aging gracefully, *Dermatol Nurs* 22:11, 2010.
5. Jarvis C: *Physical examination and health assessment*, ed 6, Philadelphia, 2012, Saunders.
6. Micali MD, Lacarrubba F, Massimino D, et al: Dermatoscopy: alternative daily uses in clinical practice, *J Am Acad Dermatol* 64:1135, 2011.

RESOURCES

Resources for this chapter are listed after Chapter 24 on p. 449.

Though we travel the world over to find the beautiful, we must carry it with us or we will not find it.
Ralph Waldo Emerson

Nursing Management
Integumentary Problems

Shannon Ruff Dirksen

evolve WEBSITE

http://evolve.elsevier.com/Lewis/medsurg

- NCLEX Review Questions
- Key Points
- Pre-Test
- Answer Guidelines for Case Study on p. 447
- Rationales for Bridge to NCLEX Examination Questions
- Nursing Care Plans (Customizable)
  - eNCP 24-1: Patient With Chronic Skin Lesions

- Concept Map Creator
- Glossary
- Content Updates

eFigures
- eFig. 24-1: Squamous cell carcinoma of the finger
- eFig. 24-2: Candidiasis in interdigital cleft

- eFig. 24-3: Scabies infestation on hand
- eFig. 24-4: Seborrheic keratosis
- eFig. 24-5: PUVA unit for phototherapy
- eFig. 24-6: Curettage

eTable
- eTable 24-1: Diseases With Dermatologic Manifestations

LEARNING OUTCOMES

1. Specify health promotion practices related to the integumentary system.
2. Explain the etiology, clinical manifestations, and nursing and collaborative management of common acute dermatologic problems.
3. Summarize the psychologic and physiologic effects of chronic dermatologic conditions.
4. Explain the etiology, clinical manifestations, and nursing and collaborative management of malignant dermatologic disorders.
5. Explain the etiology, clinical manifestations, and nursing and collaborative management of bacterial, viral, and fungal infections of the integument.
6. Describe the etiology, clinical manifestations, and nursing and collaborative management of infestations and insect bites.
7. Explain the etiology, clinical manifestations, and nursing and collaborative management of allergic dermatologic disorders.
8. Explain the etiology, clinical manifestations, and nursing and collaborative management related to benign dermatologic disorders.
9. Distinguish the dermatologic manifestations of common systemic diseases.
10. Explain the indications and nursing management related to common cosmetic procedures and skin grafts.

KEY TERMS

acne vulgaris, Table 24-9, p. 439
actinic keratosis, p. 431
basal cell carcinoma (BCC), p. 431
cellulitis, Table 24-4, p. 434
cryosurgery, p. 442

curettage, p. 442
dysplastic nevi (DN), p. 434
herpes zoster, Table 24-5, p. 436
impetigo, Table 24-4, p. 434
lichenification, p. 444

malignant melanoma, p. 432
psoriasis, p. 437
squamous cell carcinoma (SCC), p. 431
sun protection factor (SPF), p. 428
urticaria, Table 24-8, p. 438

In this chapter health promotion of the skin, common dermatologic conditions, and malignant skin neoplasms are discussed. Nursing management of patients with dermatologic conditions is emphasized.

HEALTH PROMOTION

Health promotion practices related to the skin often parallel practices for general good health. The skin reflects both phys-

ical and psychologic well-being. Specific health promotion activities appropriate to good skin health include avoidance of environmental hazards, adequate hygiene and nutrition, and skin self-examination.

Environmental Hazards

Sun Exposure. Years of exposure to the sun are cumulative and damaging. The ultraviolet (UV) rays of the sun cause degenerative changes in the dermis, resulting in premature

Reviewed by Lakshi M. Aldredge, RN, MSN, ANP-BC, Nurse Practitioner, Dermatology Service, Portland VA Medical Center, Portland, Oregon; and Brenda C. Morris, RN, EdD, CNE, Senior Director, Baccalaureate Nursing and Clinical Associate Professor, College of Nursing and Health Innovation, Arizona State University, Phoenix, Arizona.

aging (e.g., loss of elasticity, thinning, wrinkling, drying of the skin). Prolonged and repeated sun exposure is a major factor in precancerous and cancerous lesions. Actinic keratosis, basal cell carcinoma, squamous cell carcinoma, and malignant melanoma are dermatologic problems that are associated with direct or indirect sun exposure.

Safe sun practices are important for you to emphasize to the patient. Specific wavelengths of the sun (Table 24-1) have different effects on the skin. Sunlight is composed of visible light and UV light. There are two types of UV light: UVA and UVB. UVA light is responsible for tanning and UVB for sunburn. Both types can damage the skin and increase the risk of skin cancer. Both UVA and UVB can cause collagen damage and accelerate the aging of skin. Tanning is the skin's response to injury and is caused by the increased production of melanin. When sun exposure is excessive, the turnover time of the skin becomes shortened, which can result in peeling. Fair-skinned persons should be especially cautious about excessive sun exposure because they have less melanin and thus less natural protection.

Patients should recognize that sun safety guidelines include sun avoidance (especially during the midday hours), protective clothing, and sunscreen. Advise the patient on ways to avoid the damaging effects of the sun, such as wearing a large-brimmed hat, sunglasses, and a long-sleeved shirt of a lightly woven fabric or carrying an umbrella. Patients need to know that the rays of the sun are most dangerous between 10:00 AM and 2:00 PM standard time or 11:00 AM and 3:00 PM daylight saving time, regardless of the latitude. Even on overcast days, serious sunburn can occur because up to 80% of the sun's UV rays can penetrate the clouds.

Other factors that increase the possibility of sunburn include being at high altitude, being in snow (reflects 80% of the sun's rays), or being in or near water. Warn people of the dangers of tanning booths and sun lamps, which are UVA. Tanning booths increase the risk of sunburn and contribute to the development of skin cancer.[1]

Sunscreens can filter both UVA and UVB wavelengths. The two types of topical sunscreens are chemical and physical. Chemical sunscreens are light creams or lotions designed to absorb or filter UV light, resulting in diminished UV light penetration. Physical sunscreens are thick, opaque, heavy creams that reflect UV radiation.

The U.S. Food and Drug Administration (FDA) rates sunscreen products on their **sun protection factor (SPF)**. The SPF

TABLE 24-1 WAVELENGTHS OF SUN AND EFFECTS ON SKIN

Wavelength	Effect
Long (ultraviolet A [UVA])	Can produce elastic tissue damage and actinic skin damage. Contributes to formation of skin cancer.
Middle (ultraviolet B [UVB])	Causes sunburn and cumulative effect of sun damage. Major factor in development of skin cancer.
Short (ultraviolet C [UVC])	Does not reach earth, since it is blocked by atmosphere.

EVIDENCE-BASED PRACTICE
Applying the Evidence

You are a nurse helping in a skin cancer screening clinic. W.S., a 24-year-old woman with a fair skin type (blond hair and blue eyes), is completing her health history before her screening examination. She indicates that she visits an indoor tanning salon every other week. She tells you that being tan makes her feel "more attractive." You spend time explaining the increased risk of skin cancer associated with the use of tanning booths.

Best Available Evidence	Clinician Expertise	Patient Preferences and Values
American Academy of Dermatology reports a strong link between exposure to indoor tanning devices and development of skin cancer and melanoma.	You note that W.S. has the following skin cancer risk factors: fair skin, blond hair, blue eyes, frequent use of tanning booths.	After listening, the patient tells you that she will consider reducing the frequency of her visits—going only when she has an important event to attend.

Your Decision and Action
As her nurse, you accept her decision, tell her that this is a step in the right direction, and encourage her to consider completely stopping her usage of the tanning booth.

Reference for Evidence
American Academy of Dermatology: The dangers of indoor tanning. Retrieved from *www.aad.org/skin-care-and-safety/skin-cancer-prevention/indoor-tanning.*

EVIDENCE-BASED PRACTICE
Translating Research Into Practice

Is Sun-Protective Counseling Effective?
Clinical Question
In adults (P) does sun-protective counseling (I) improve safe sun behaviors (O)?

Best Available Evidence
Systematic review of randomized controlled trials (RCTs)

Critical Appraisal and Synthesis of Evidence
- Five RCTs (n = 6949) of middle-aged white men and women and three RCTS (n = 897) of young adults examined the effect of counseling on sun-protective behaviors. Trials ranged from one to several sessions of in-person counseling, phone counseling, or tailored risk written feedback.
- Counseling with tailored feedback influenced sun-protective behaviors in older adults.
- Appearance-focused counseling reduced indoor tanning use among young adult women.

Conclusion
- Relevant counseling by primary health care providers can increase sun-protective behaviors and decrease indoor tanning.

Implications for Nursing Practice
- Promote safe sun behaviors for patients to decrease ultraviolet exposure, including sunscreen use, sun avoidance hours, and protective clothing.
- Emphasize the dangers of tanning booth use among college students.
- Tailor sun safety interventions to the target population.

Reference for Evidence
Lin J, Eder M, Weinmann S: Behavioral counseling to prevent skin cancer: a systematic review for the U.S. Preventive Services Task Force, *Ann Intern Med* 154:190, 2011.

P, Patient population of interest; I, intervention or area of interest; O, outcomes of interest (see p. 12).

measures the effectiveness of a sunscreen in filtering and absorbing UV radiation. All sunscreen labels in the United States must state which rays they protect against. Products labeled with "broad protection" block both UVA and UVB.[2] Sunscreen broad protection labeling is allowed only if the product has an SPF of at least 15. Sunscreen should no longer be labeled as "waterproof" and "sweat proof." The product should only state if it is "water resistant."

Consumers need to select the sunscreen most appropriate for their needs. Para-aminobenzoic acid (PABA) and PABA esters, cinnamates, salicylates, and methyl anthranilate block UVB rays. PABA has been removed from many sunscreen products because it stains clothing and can cause allergic reactions, including contact dermatitis. Avobenzone (Parsol) blocks UVA rays and has been added to some sunscreens. The benzophenones block both UVA and UVB rays.

The general recommendation is that everyone should use a sunscreen with a minimum SPF of 15 daily. Teach patients to look for the term *broad spectrum* on sunscreen packaging. Sunscreens with an SPF of 15 or more filter 92% of the UVB rays that are responsible for erythema, and make sunburn unlikely when applied appropriately. Patients who have a history of skin cancer or problems with sun sensitivity should use a product with an SPF of at least 30. Sunscreens should be applied 20 to 30 minutes before going outdoors, even in cloudy weather. The SPF value of all sunscreens decreases with time after application, and therefore sunscreen should be reapplied every 2 hours in a sufficient amount. One ounce per total body application is recommended. The ears, toes, and lips also need sunscreen. Sunscreens are not "waterproof" and should be reapplied immediately after swimming. Regular sunscreen use decreases the rate of developing melanoma.[3]

Certain topical and systemic medications potentiate the effect of the sun, even with brief exposure. Categories of drug therapy that may contain common photosensitizing medications are listed in Table 24-2. Be aware that many drugs are included in these categories. Examine the photosensitivity of each individual drug. The chemicals in these medications absorb light when exposed to natural sunlight and release energy that harms cells and tissues. The clinical manifestations of drug-induced photosensitivity (Fig. 24-1) are similar to those of exaggerated sunburn. These include swelling; erythema; vesicles; and papular, plaquelike lesions. Skin that is at risk for photosensitivity reactions can be protected by the use of sunscreen products. Teach patients who are taking these drugs about their photosensitizing effect.

Irritants and Allergens. Patients can seek treatment for irritant or allergic dermatitis, which are two types of contact dermatitis. *Irritant contact dermatitis* is produced by direct chemical injury to the skin. *Allergic contact dermatitis* is an antigen-specific, type IV delayed hypersensitivity response. This response requires sensitization and occurs only in individuals who are predisposed to react to a particular antigen (see Chapter 14).

Counsel patients to avoid known irritants (e.g., ammonia, harsh detergents). Skin patch testing (application of allergens) can sometimes help determine the most likely sensitizing agent. Sometimes the health care provider is the first to detect a contact

TABLE 24-2 DRUG THERAPY

Drugs That May Cause Photosensitivity

Categories	Examples
Anticancer drugs	methotrexate, vinorelbine (Navelbine)
Antidepressants	amitriptyline (Elavil), clomipramine (Anafranil), doxepin (Sinequan)
Antidysrhythmics	quinidine, amiodarone (Cordarone)
Antihistamines	diphenhydramine (Benadryl), chlorpheniramine, clemastine (Tavist)
Antimicrobials	tetracycline, sulfamethoxazole, azithromycin (Zithromax), ciprofloxacin (Cipro)
Antifungals	griseofulvin, ketoconazole (Nizoral)
Antipsychotics	chlorpromazine (Thorazine), haloperidol (Haldol)
Diuretics	furosemide (Lasix), hydrochlorothiazide (HydroDIURIL)
Hypoglycemics	tolbutamide (Orinase), glipizide (Glucotrol), chlorpropamide (Diabinese)
Nonsteroidal antiinflammatory drugs	diclofenac (Voltaren), piroxicam (Feldene), sulindac (Clinoril)

CULTURAL & ETHNIC HEALTH DISPARITIES

Integumentary Problems

- African Americans and Native Americans have a lower incidence of skin cancer than whites.
- Melanoma can occur in dark-skinned individuals, but often goes unrecognized until the advanced stages.
- Skin assessment may be difficult in individuals with darker skin. The oral mucous membranes and conjunctiva are areas where pallor, cyanosis, and jaundice are more readily detected. The palms of the hands and soles of the feet can also be used for assessment of the skin of darker individuals.
- When darker skin heals after injury or inflammation, it tends to be hypopigmented or hyperpigmented.

FIG. 24-1 Intense eruption in areas exposed to sunlight after patient started on hydrochlorothiazide.

allergy to various metals, gloves (latex), and adhesives. Prescribed and over-the-counter (OTC) topical and systemic medications used to treat a variety of conditions may contain fragrances and preservatives that can cause dermatologic reactions.

Radiation. Although most radiology departments are extremely cautious in protecting both themselves and their patients from the effects of excessive radiation, it is important for you to help the patient make decisions about radiologic procedures. X-rays are valuable in both diagnosis and therapy but can cause serious side effects to the skin, including erythema, dry and moist desquamation, edema, and hypopigmentation or hyperpigmentation. In the past (30 years ago), acne and hirsutism were treated with radiation. This information is important for you to obtain because of an increased incidence of carcinoma for these patients.

Rest and Sleep

Sleep is restorative to the skin, as well as to the rest of the body. Pruritic skin diseases often interfere with sleep. Therefore helping patients obtain high-quality sleep is an important health-promotion consideration. Adequate rest increases the patient's ability to tolerate itching, thereby decreasing skin damage from the resultant scratching.

Exercise

Exercise increases circulation and dilates the blood vessels. In addition to the healthy glow produced by exercise, the psychologic effects can also improve one's appearance and mental outlook. However, caution must be used to prevent overexposure to heat, cold, and sun during outdoor exercise.

Hygiene

Hygienic practices are influenced by the patient's skin type, lifestyle, culture, age, and gender. The normal acidity of the skin and perspiration protect against bacterial overgrowth. Most soaps are alkaline and neutralize the skin surface, leading to a loss of protection. The use of mild, moisturizing soaps (e.g., Ivory) and lipid-free cleansers, plus avoidance of hot water and vigorous scrubbing, can noticeably decrease local skin irritation and inflammation. Skin piercings where jewelry has been inserted can be cared for with antibacterial soaps that do not contain sulfites.

In general, the skin and hair should be washed often enough to remove excess oil and excretions and to prevent odor. Older persons should avoid harsh soaps and shampoos and frequent bathing because of the dryness of their skin and scalp. Moisturizers should be used immediately after a bath or shower while the skin is still damp to seal in this moisture.

Nutrition

A well-balanced diet adequate in all food groups can produce healthy skin, hair, and nails. Important elements of skin nutrition include the following:

- *Vitamin A:* Essential for maintenance of normal cell structure, specifically epithelial cells. It is necessary for normal wound healing. The absence of vitamin A causes dryness of the conjunctiva and poor wound healing.
- *Vitamin B complex:* Essential for complex metabolic functions. Deficiencies of niacin and pyridoxine (B_6) manifest as dermatologic symptoms such as erythema, bullae, and seborrhea-like lesions.
- *Vitamin C (ascorbic acid):* Essential for connective tissue formation and normal wound healing. Absence of vitamin C causes symptoms of scurvy, including petechiae, bleeding gums, and purpura.
- *Vitamin D_3 (cholecalciferol):* Essential for bone health. It is produced naturally by cutaneous photosynthesis after UVB exposure. A deficiency manifests as bone and muscle weakness and pain.
- *Vitamin K:* Essential for synthesizing blood clotting factors. A deficiency interferes with normal prothrombin synthesis in the liver and can lead to bruising.
- *Protein:* Necessary in amounts adequate for cell growth and maintenance. It is also necessary for normal wound healing.
- *Unsaturated fatty acids:* Necessary to maintain the function and integrity of cellular and subcellular membranes in tissue metabolism. Linoleic and arachidonic acids are particularly important.

A deficiency of biotin, a water-soluble B-complex vitamin, may result in rashes and alopecia. The effectiveness of biotin supplements has not been proven. Foods high in biotin include liver, cauliflower, salmon, carrots, bananas, soy flour, cereals, and yeast.

Obesity has adverse effects on the skin. The increase in subcutaneous fat can lead to stretching and overheating (see Chapter 41). Overheating secondary to the greater insulation provided by fat causes increased sweating, which inflames and dries the skin. Obesity is also a risk factor for poor wound healing. Obesity can be associated with the development of type 2 diabetes mellitus, which may cause skin symptoms such as velvety dark skin of neck and body folds (*acanthosis nigricans*), rash in intertriginous sites (*intertrigo*), skin tags (*acrochordons*), and impaired arterial and venous flow (see Chapter 49).

Self-Treatment

Determine if the patient is aware of the dangers of self-diagnosis and treatment. The increasing variety of OTC skin preparations can be confusing.

In your general instructions to the patient, stress the duration of the treatment and the need to closely follow package directions. Skin problems may be slow to produce symptoms and slow to resolve. If the package insert of an OTC drug says its use should not exceed 7 days, patients should heed this warning. Tell the patient to always follow package directions for use of OTC drugs. If any systemic signs of inflammation or extensions of the skin problem (e.g., an increased number of lesions or increased erythema or swelling) develop, the patient should stop self-care and seek the help of a health care provider.

MALIGNANT SKIN NEOPLASMS

Skin cancer is the most commonly diagnosed cancer.[4] Skin cancers are either nonmelanoma or melanoma. A persistent skin lesion that does not heal is highly suspicious for malignancy and should be examined by a health care provider. Early detection and treatment can often lead to a highly favorable prognosis. The fact that skin lesions are so visible increases the likelihood of early detection and diagnosis.

Teach patients to self-examine their skin at least on a monthly basis. The cornerstone of skin self-examination is the ABCDE rule,[5] which is easy to teach and remember. Examine skin lesions for *Asymmetry*, *Border* irregularity, *Color* change and

FIG. 24-2 The ABCDEs of melanoma. **A,** Asymmetry: one half unlike the other half. **B,** Border irregularity: edges are ragged, notched, or blurred. **C,** Color: varied pigmentation; shades of tan, brown, and black. **D,** Diameter: greater than 6 mm (diameter of a pencil eraser). **E,** (not pictured) Evolving; changing appearance (change in shape, size, color, or other characteristic is noted over time).

variation, *Diameter* of 6 mm or more, and *Evolving* in appearance (Fig. 24-2). Emphasize that lesions once flat and now raised, or once small and recently growing or changing in appearance, are warning signs and should be examined by a health care provider.

Risk Factors

Risk factors for skin malignancies include having a fair skin type (blond or red hair and blue or green eyes), history of chronic sun exposure, family history of skin cancer, and exposure to tar and systemic arsenicals.[6] Environmental factors that increase the risk of skin malignancies include living near the equator, outdoor occupations, and frequent outdoor recreational activities. Behavioral factors such as using indoor tanning booths and outdoor sunbathing are controllable risk factors for skin malignancies. Patients treated with oral methoxsalen (psoralen) and psoralen plus ultraviolet A radiation (PUVA) may be at greater risk for melanoma.

Dark-skinned persons are less susceptible to skin cancer because of the naturally occurring increased melanin, which is a sunscreen. However, although dark skin lowers the risk of melanoma, people with dark skin can develop melanoma, most often on the palms, soles, and mucous membranes.

The Fitzpatrick classification of skin type can assist you in determining how a patient will respond or react to facial treatments, and how likely they are to get skin cancer. This system classifies skin into six different skin types, skin color, and reaction to sun exposure.

- Type I (very white or freckled): Always burn
- Type II (white): Usually burn
- Type III (white to olive): Sometimes burn
- Type IV (brown): Rarely burn
- Type V (dark brown): Very rarely burn
- Type VI (black): Never burn

NONMELANOMA SKIN CANCERS

Nonmelanoma skin cancers, either basal cell or squamous cell carcinoma, are the most common forms of skin cancer.[7] More than 2.2 million new cases are diagnosed every year. Nonmelanoma skin cancers develop in the epidermis. They do not develop from melanocytes, the skin cells that make melanin, as melanoma skin cancers do. The most common sites for the development of nonmelanoma skin cancer are in sun-exposed areas, such as the face, head, neck, back of the hands, and arms.

Although relatively few deaths are attributable to nonmelanoma skin cancer, the tumors have an inherent potential for severe local destruction, permanent disfigurement, and disability. The most common etiologic factor is sun exposure. Avoidance of exposure to the midday sun and the use of protective clothing and sunscreens beginning early in life can prevent the formation of skin malignancies later in life.

Actinic Keratosis

Actinic keratosis, also known as solar keratosis, consists of hyperkeratotic papules and plaques on sun-exposed areas. Actinic keratoses are premalignant skin lesions that affect nearly all of the older white population. These are the most common of all precancerous skin lesions. The clinical appearance of actinic keratoses can be highly varied. The typical lesion is an irregularly shaped, flat, slightly erythematous papule with indistinct borders and an overlying hard keratotic scale or horn (Table 24-3).

Many forms of treatment are used, including cryosurgery, fluorouracil (5-FU), surgical removal, tretinoin (Retin-A), imiquimod (Aldara), diclofenac (Solaraze), chemical peeling agents, dermabrasion, laser resurfacing, and photodynamic therapy (PDT, with 5-aminolevulinic acid [5-ALA] or methyl aminolevulinate [MAL] followed by light irradiation). (These treatments are discussed later in this chapter.) Any lesion that persists should be evaluated for a possible biopsy.

Basal Cell Carcinoma

Basal cell carcinoma (BCC) is a locally invasive malignancy arising from epidermal basal cells. It is the most common type of skin cancer and also the least deadly. BCC usually occurs in middle-aged to older adults. Clinical manifestations are described in Table 24-3. The cancerous cells of BCC almost never spread beyond the skin (Fig. 24-4). However, if BCC is left untreated, massive tissue destruction may result. Some BCCs are pigmented with curled borders and an opaque appearance and may be misinterpreted as a melanoma. A tissue biopsy is needed to confirm the diagnosis.[8]

Multiple treatment modalities are used depending on the tumor location and histologic type, history of recurrence, and patient characteristics. Treatment modalities include surgical excision, electrodesiccation and curettage, cryosurgery, radiation therapy, topical or systemic chemotherapy, and photodynamic therapy. (These treatments are discussed later in this chapter.) Electrodesiccation and curettage, cryosurgery, and surgical excision all have a cure rate of greater than 90% when used correctly on primary lesions. Location and size are important factors in determining the best treatment.

Squamous Cell Carcinoma

Squamous cell carcinoma (SCC) is a malignant neoplasm of keratinizing epidermal cells (see eFig. 24-1 available on the website for this chapter). It frequently occurs on sun-exposed skin at the base of an actinic keratosis or another lesion. SCC is less common than BCC. SCC can be highly aggressive, has the potential to metastasize, and may lead to death if not treated early and correctly. Pipe, cigar, and cigarette smoking contribute

TABLE 24-3   PREMALIGNANT AND MALIGNANT CONDITIONS OF THE SKIN

Etiology and Pathophysiology	Clinical Manifestations	Treatment and Prognosis
Actinic Keratosis Actinic (sun) damage. Premalignant skin lesions. Common in older whites.	Flat or elevated, dry, hyperkeratotic scaly papule. Possibly flat, rough, or verrucous (wartlike). Adherent scale, which returns when removed. Often multiple. Rough scale on red base. Often on erythematous sun-exposed area. Increase in number with age.	Cryosurgery, chemical peels, laser resurfacing, topical application of 5-FU over entire area for 14-28 days or topical application of imiquimod (Aldara) for 16 wk, photodynamic therapy followed by light irradiation. Recurrence possible even with adequate treatment.
Atypical or Dysplastic Nevi Morphologically between common acquired nevi and melanoma. May be precursor of malignant melanoma.	Often >5 mm. Irregular border, possibly notched. Variegated color of tan, brown, black, red, or pink within single mole. Presence of at least one flat portion, often at edge of mole. Frequently multiple. Most common site on back, but possible in uncommon mole sites such as scalp or buttocks (Fig. 24-3).	Increased risk for melanoma. Careful monitoring of persons suspected of familial tendency to melanoma or dysplastic nevi. Excisional biopsy for suspicious lesions.
Basal Cell Carcinoma Change in basal cells. No maturation or normal keratinization. Continuing division of basal cells and formation of enlarging mass. Related to excessive sun exposure, genetic skin type, x-ray radiation, scars, and some types of nevi.	*Nodular and ulcerative:* Small, slowly enlarging papule. Borders semitranslucent or "pearly," with overlying telangiectasia. Erosion, ulceration, and depression of center. Normal skin markings lost (see Fig. 24-2). *Superficial:* Erythematous, pearly, sharply defined, barely elevated plaques.	Surgical excision, chemosurgery, electrosurgery, chemotherapy, cryosurgery. 90% cure rate. Slow-growing tumor that invades local tissue. Metastasis rare. 5-FU and imiquimod for superficial lesions, photodynamic therapy for small lesions, vismodegib (Erivedge) for metastatic or recurrent locally invasive lesions.
Squamous Cell Carcinoma Frequent occurrence on previously damaged skin (e.g., from sun, radiation, scar). Malignant tumor of squamous cell of epidermis. Invasion of dermis, surrounding skin.	*Superficial:* Thin, scaly erythematous plaque without invasion into the dermis. *Early:* Firm nodules with indistinct borders, scaling and ulceration (see eFig. 24-1). *Late:* Covering of lesion with scale or horn from keratinization, ulceration. Most common on sun-exposed areas such as face and hands.	Surgical excision, cryosurgery, radiation therapy, chemotherapy, electrodesiccation and curettage. Untreated lesion may metastasize to regional lymph nodes and distant organs. High cure rate with early detection and treatment.
Malignant Melanoma Neoplastic growth of melanocytes anywhere on skin, eyes, or mucous membranes. Classification according to major histologic mode of spread. Potential invasion and widespread metastases.	Irregular color, surface, and border. Variegated color, including red, white, blue, black, gray, brown. Flat or elevated. Eroded or ulcerated. Often <1 cm in size. Most common sites in males are back, then chest. In females are legs, then back (see Fig. 24-2).	Surgical excision and possible sentinel lymph node evaluation depending on the depth. Correlation of survival rate with depth of invasion. Poor prognosis unless diagnosed and treated early. Spreading by local extension, regional lymphatic vessels, and bloodstream. Possible use of adjuvant therapy after surgery if lesion >1.5 mm in depth.
Cutaneous T-Cell Lymphoma Origination in skin. Localized chronic, slowly progressing disease. Possibly related to environmental toxins and chemical exposure. Mycosis fungoides (MF) is most common form. Sézary syndrome is an advanced form of MF. Prevalence twice as high in men as in women in United States.	Classic presentation involves three stages— patch (early), plaque, and tumor (advanced). History of persistent macular eruption followed by gradual appearance of indurated erythematous plaques on the trunk that appear similar to psoriasis. Pruritus, lymphadenopathy.	Treatment usually controls symptoms, not curative. UVB, PUVA, corticosteroids, topical nitrogen mustard, radiation therapy in patch and plaque stage disease. Interferon, systemic chemotherapy, extracorporeal photopheresis, romidepsin (Istodax) for progressive disease. Bexarotene (Targretin), denileukin diftitox (Ontak), and vorinostat (Zolinza) for advanced disease. Disease course is unpredictable, 10% will have progressive disease.

5-FU, Fluorouracil; *PUVA,* psoralen ultraviolet A; *UVB,* ultraviolet B.

to the formation of SCC on the mouth and lips. The clinical manifestations of SCC are described in Table 24-3. A biopsy should always be performed when a lesion is suspected to be SCC.

MALIGNANT MELANOMA

Malignant melanoma is a tumor arising in melanocytes, which are the cells producing melanin. Melanoma causes the majority of skin cancer deaths. More than 132,000 new cases are diagnosed every year worldwide. Melanoma has the ability to metastasize to any organ, including the brain and the heart. The death rate of melanoma is 10 times higher in white persons than in African Americans.[4]

Although the exact cause of melanoma is unknown, a combination of environmental and genetic factors is involved. The use of immunosuppressive drugs and a history of dysplastic nevi also increase a person's risk. UV radiation from the sun is

FIG. 24-3 Dysplastic nevus. Irregular border and color.

FIG. 24-4 Basal cell carcinoma. Rolled, well-defined border and central erosion.

FIG. 24-5 Breslow measurement of tumor thickness. **A,** Thin (0.08 mm) superficial spreading melanoma, good prognosis. **B,** Thick nodular melanoma with lymph node involvement, poor prognosis.

the main cause of melanomas and other skin cancer, but artificial sources of UV radiation, such as sunlamps and tanning booths, also play a role. UV radiation damages the deoxyribonucleic acid (DNA) in skin cells, creating "misspellings" in their genetic code. As a result, these cells are altered.

Although anyone can develop melanoma, the risk is greatest for people who have red or blond hair, blue or light-colored eyes, and light-colored skin that freckles easily. These people have less melanin and thus less protection from UV radiation.

A person may have a genetic predisposition toward getting melanoma. Between 5% and 10% of people who develop melanoma have a first-degree relative (e.g., parent, full sibling) who developed melanoma. This risk increases significantly if multiple relatives have a history of melanoma. Mutated genes have been identified in some families who have a high familial incidence of melanoma.

Clinical Manifestations

About one fourth of melanomas occur in existing nevi or moles; about 20% occur in dysplastic nevi (see Table 24-3). Melanoma frequently occurs on the lower legs and backs in women and on the trunk, head, and neck in men. Because most melanoma cells continue to produce melanin, melanoma tumors are often dark brown or black. Individuals should consult their health care provider immediately if their moles or lesions show any of the clinical signs (ABCDEs) of melanoma (see Fig. 24-2). Any sudden or progressive change or increase in the size, color, or shape of a mole should be evaluated.

When melanoma begins in the skin, it is called *cutaneous melanoma.* Melanoma can also occur in the eye (see Fig. 22-8), meninges, lymph nodes, digestive tract, and anywhere else in the body where melanocytes are found.

Collaborative Care

Pigmented lesions suspicious for melanoma should not be shave-biopsied, shave-excised, or electrocauterized. Handheld screening devices (e.g., MelaFind) can assist the health care provider in determining if a lesion without the obvious ABCDE signs should be biopsied. All suspicious lesions should be biopsied using an excisional biopsy technique.

The most important prognostic factor is tumor thickness at the time of diagnosis. Two methods to determine thickness are currently being used. The *Breslow measurement* indicates the depth of the tumor in millimeters (Fig. 24-5), and the *Clark level* indicates the depth of invasion of the tumor; the higher the number, the deeper the melanoma.

Treatment depends on the site of the original tumor, the stage of the cancer, and the patient's age and general health. The staging of melanoma (stages 0 to IV) is based on tumor size (thickness), nodal involvement, and metastasis. In stage 0 the melanoma is confined to one place (in situ) in the epidermis. Melanoma is nearly 100% curable by excision if diagnosed at stage 0. The 5-year survival rate depends on sentinel node biopsy results, which indicate if metastasis has occurred. If metastasis to other organs is found (stage IV), treatment then becomes palliative.

Initial treatment of malignant melanoma is surgical excision, which may require a skin graft to close (discussed later in the chapter). Melanoma that has spread to the lymph nodes or nearby sites usually requires additional (adjuvant) therapy such as chemotherapy, biologic therapy (e.g., α-interferon, interleukin-2), and/or radiation therapy. Examples of chemotherapy agents used are dacarbazine (DTIC), temozolomide (Temodar), procarbazine (Matulane), carmustine (BCNU), and lomustine (CCNU).

Newer treatment options for patients with metastatic melanoma are ipilimumab (Yervoy), vemurafenib (Zelboraf), dabrafenib (Tafinlar), and trametinib (Mekinist). Ipilimumab, a type of immunotherapy, is a monoclonal antibody that locks onto CTLA-4, a protein that normally helps keep T cells in check. By blocking the action of CTLA-4, ipilimumab boosts the immune response against melanoma cells.[9] Vemurafenib, dabrafenib, and trametinib are used for patients whose melanoma tumors express a gene mutation called *BRAF V600*.

Atypical or Dysplastic Nevus

An abnormal nevus pattern called *dysplastic nevus syndrome* identifies an individual at increased risk of melanoma. Approximately 2% to 8% of the white population has moles classified as atypical or dysplastic nevi. **Dysplastic nevi (DN),** or atypical moles, are nevi that are larger than usual (greater than 5 mm across) with irregular borders and various shades of color (see

TABLE 24-4 COMMON BACTERIAL INFECTIONS OF THE SKIN		
Etiology and Pathophysiology	**Clinical Manifestations**	**Treatment and Prognosis**
Impetigo Group A β-hemolytic streptococci, staphylococci, or combination of both. Associated with poor hygiene. Primary or secondary infection. Contagious.	Vesiculopustular lesions that develop thick, honey-colored crust surrounded by erythema. Pruritic. Most common on face as primary infection.	*Systemic antibiotics:* Oral penicillin, benzathine penicillin, erythromycin. *Local treatment:* Warm saline or aluminum acetate soaks followed by soap-and-water removal of crusts. Topical antibiotic cream or ointment (mupirocin [Bactroban], retapamulin [Altabax]). With no treatment, glomerulonephritis possible when streptococcal strain nephritogenic. Meticulous hygiene essential.
Folliculitis Usually staphylococci. Present in areas subjected to friction, moisture, rubbing, or oil. Increased incidence in patients with diabetes mellitus.	Small pustule at hair follicle opening with minimal erythema. Development of crusting. Most common on scalp, beard, extremities in men. Tender to touch.	Antistaphylococcal soap (e.g., Hibiclens, Lever 2000, Dial) and water cleansing. Topical antibiotics (e.g., mupirocin). Warm compresses of water or aluminum acetate solution. Healing usually without scarring. If lesions extensive and deep, possible scarring, loss of involved hair follicles, and treatment with systemic antibiotics.
Furuncle Deep infection with staphylococci around hair follicle, often associated with severe acne or seborrheic dermatitis.	Tender erythematous area around hair follicle. Draining pus and core of necrotic debris on rupture. Most common on face, back of neck, axillae, breasts, buttocks, perineum, thighs. Painful.	Incision and drainage, possibly with packing, antibiotics, meticulous care of involved skin, frequent application of warm, moist compresses.
Furunculosis Increased incidence in patients who are obese, diabetic, chronically ill, or regularly exposed to moisture, pressure.	Lesions as above. Malaise, regional adenopathy, elevated body temperature.	Incision and drainage of painful nodules. Warm, moist compresses to erythematous plaques. Systemic antibiotic after culture and sensitivity study of drainage (usually semisynthetic, penicillinase-resistant, oral penicillin such as cloxacillin and oxacillin). Measures to reduce surface staphylococci include antimicrobial cream to nares, armpits, and groin and antiseptic to entire skin. Often recurrent with scarring. Prevention or correction of predisposing factors. Meticulous personal hygiene.
Carbuncle Multiple, interconnecting furuncles.	Many pustules appearing in erythematous area, most common at nape of neck.	Treatment same as for furuncles. Often recurrent despite production of antibodies. Healing slow with scar formation.
Cellulitis Inflammation of subcutaneous tissues. Possibly secondary complication or primary infection. Often following break in skin. *Staphylococcus aureus* and streptococci usual causative agents. Deep inflammation of subcutaneous tissue from enzymes produced by bacteria.	Hot, tender, erythematous, and edematous area with diffuse borders. Chills, malaise, and fever (Fig. 24-6).	Moist heat, immobilization and elevation, systemic antibiotic therapy, hospitalization if severe. Progression to gangrene possible if untreated.
Erysipelas Superficial cellulitis primarily involving the dermis. Group A β-hemolytic streptococci.	Red, hot, sharply demarcated plaque that is indurated and painful. Bacteremia possible. Most common on face and extremities. Toxic signs, such as fever, ↑ white blood cell count, headache, malaise.	Systemic antibiotics, usually penicillin. Hospitalization often required.

Fig. 24-3). These nevi may have the same ABCDE characteristics as melanoma, but they are less pronounced. The earliest clinically detectable abnormality associated with DN is an increase in the number of morphologically normal-looking nevi that occur in children between 2 and 6 years of age. Another proliferation occurs around adolescence, and new nevi continue to appear throughout the person's life. The average number of normal nevi in adults is about 40. Individuals with DN may have more than 100 normal-appearing nevi. Obtain a detailed family history related to melanoma and DN. The risk of developing melanoma doubles with the presence of one DN, and having multiple DN increases the risk up to 12-fold.

SKIN INFECTIONS AND INFESTATIONS

Bacterial Infections

The skin provides an ideal environment for bacterial growth with an abundant supply of nutrients, water, and warm temperature. Bacterial infection occurs when the balance between the host and the microorganisms is altered. This can occur as a primary infection after a break in the skin. It can also occur as a secondary infection to already damaged skin or as a sign of a systemic disease (Table 24-4). *Staphylococcus aureus* and group A β-hemolytic streptococci are the major types of bacteria responsible for primary and secondary skin infections.

Healthy persons can develop bacterial skin infections. Predisposing factors such as moisture, obesity, atopic dermatitis, systemic corticosteroids and antibiotics, and chronic disease such as diabetes mellitus all increase the likelihood of infection. Good hygiene practices and general good health inhibit bacterial infections. If an infection is present, the resulting drainage is infectious. Good skin hygiene and infection control practices are necessary to prevent the spread of the infection.

Viral Infections

Viral infections of the skin are as difficult to treat as viral infections anywhere in the body. When a virus infects a cell, a skin lesion may develop. Lesions can also result from an inflammatory response to viral infections. Herpes simplex, herpes zoster (Fig. 24-7), and warts (Fig. 24-8) are the most common viral infections affecting the skin (Table 24-5).

FIG. 24-6 Cellulitis with characteristic erythema, tenderness, and edema.

FIG. 24-7 Herpes zoster (shingles) on the anterior chest, classic dermatomal distribution.

FIG. 24-8 Plantar wart. **A,** Keratotic lesion. **B,** After excision.

Fungal Infections

Because of the large number of fungi that are present everywhere, exposure to some pathologic varieties may occur. Skin, hair, and nails may all become infected with fungi, including candidiasis (see eFig. 24-2 available on the website for this chapter) and tinea unguium (Fig. 24-9). Common fungal infections of the skin are presented in Table 24-6. Most infections are relatively harmless in healthy adults, but they can be embarrassing and distressing to the patient.[10]

The microscopic examination of the scraping of suspicious scaly skin lesions in 10% to 20% potassium hydroxide (KOH) is an inexpensive diagnostic measure to determine the presence of a fungus. The appearance of microscopic hyphae (threadlike structures) is indicative of a fungal infection.

FIG. 24-9 Tinea unguium (onychomycosis). Fungal infection of toenails. Crumbly, discolored, and thickened nails.

TABLE 24-5   COMMON VIRAL INFECTIONS OF THE SKIN

Etiology and Pathophysiology	Clinical Manifestations	Treatment and Prognosis
Herpes Simplex Virus (HSV) Types 1 and 2 Oral or genital HSV infections can be serotyped as either HSV-1 or HSV-2. Both are recurrent lifelong viral infections. Exacerbated by sunlight, trauma, menses, stress, and systemic infection. Contagious to those not previously infected. Transmission by respiratory droplets or virus-containing fluid (e.g., saliva, cervical secretions). Infection in one area is readily transmitted to another site by contact.	*First episode:* Symptoms occurring 3-7 days or more after contact, Painful local reaction. Single or grouped vesicles on erythematous base. Systemic symptoms (e.g., fever, malaise) possible or no symptoms possible. *Recurrent:* Small. Recurrence in similar spot. Characteristic grouped vesicles on erythematous base.	Symptomatic medication. Soothing, moist compresses. White petrolatum to lesions. Scarring not usual result. Antiviral agents such as acyclovir (Zovirax), famciclovir (Famvir), and valacyclovir (Valtrex). Vaccine not currently available for HSV-1 or HSV-2.
Herpes Zoster (Shingles) Activation of the varicella-zoster virus. Incidence increases with age. Potentially contagious to anyone who has not had varicella or who is immunosuppressed. >1 million cases annually in the United States.	Linear distribution along a dermatome of grouped vesicles and pustules on erythematous base resembling chickenpox. Usually unilateral on trunk, face, and lumbosacral areas. Burning, pain, and neuralgia preceding outbreak. Mild to severe pain during outbreak (see Fig. 24-7).	Symptomatic. Antiviral agents such as acyclovir, famciclovir, and valacyclovir within 72 hr to prevent postherpetic neuralgia. Wet compresses, silver sulfadiazine (Silvadene) to ruptured vesicles. Analgesia. Mild sedation at bedtime. Gabapentin (Neurontin) to treat postherpetic neuralgia. Usually heals without complications, but scarring and postherpetic neuralgia possible. Vaccine (Zostavax) to prevent shingles is available for adults ≥50 yr.
Verruca Vulgaris Caused by human papillomavirus (HPV). Spontaneous disappearance in 1-2 yr possible. Mildly contagious by autoinoculation. Specific response dependent on body part affected. Prevalence greater in youth and immunosuppressed.	Circumscribed, hypertrophic, flesh-colored papule limited to epidermis. Painful on lateral compression.	Multiple treatments, including surgery using blunt dissection with scissors or curette. Liquid nitrogen therapy. Blistering agent (cantharidin). Keratolytic agent (salicylic acid). CO_2 laser destruction.
Plantar Warts Caused by HPV.	Wart on bottom surface of foot, growing inward because of pressure of walking or standing. Painful when pressure applied. Interrupted skin markings. Cone shaped with black dots (thrombosed vessels) when wart removed (see Fig. 24-8).	Topical immunotherapy (imiquimod), cryosurgery, salicylic acid, duct tape.

TABLE 24-6   COMMON FUNGAL INFECTIONS OF THE SKIN

Etiology and Pathophysiology	Clinical Manifestations	Treatment and Prognosis
Candidiasis Caused by *Candida albicans*. Also known as moniliasis. 50% of adults symptom-free carriers. Appears in warm, moist areas such as groin area, oral mucosa, and submammary folds. HIV infection, chemotherapy, radiation, and organ transplantation related to depression of cell-mediated immunity that allows yeast to become pathogenic.	*Mouth:* White, cheesy plaque, resembles milk curds. *Vagina:* Vaginitis with red, edematous, painful vaginal wall, white patches. Vaginal discharge. Pruritus. Pain on urination and intercourse. *Skin:* Diffuse papular erythematous rash with pinpoint satellite lesions around edges of affected area (see eFig. 24-2).	Microscopic examination and culture. Azole antifungals (e.g., fluconazole, ketoconazole) or other specific medication such as vaginal suppository or oral lozenge. Sexual abstinence or use of condom. Skin hygiene to keep area clean and dry. Powder is effective on nonmucosal surfaces of skin to prevent recurrence.
Tinea Corporis Various dermatophytes, commonly referred to as ringworm.	Typical annular (ringlike) scaly appearance, well-defined margins. Erythematous.	Cool compresses. Topical antifungals for isolated patches. Creams or solutions of miconazole, ketoconazole, clotrimazole, butenafine.
Tinea Cruris Various dermatophytes, commonly referred to as jock itch.	Well-defined scaly plaque in groin area. Does not affect mucous membranes.	Topical antifungal cream or solution.
Tinea Pedis Various dermatophytes, commonly referred to as athlete's foot.	Interdigital scaling and maceration. Scaly plantar surfaces sometimes with erythema and blistering. May be pruritic. Possibly painful.	Topical antifungal cream, gel, solution, spray, or powder.
Tinea Unguium (Onychomycosis) Various dermatophytes. Incidence increases with age.	Only few nails on one hand may be affected. Toenails more commonly affected. Scaliness under distal nail plate. Brittle, thickened, broken, or crumbling nails with yellowish discoloration (see Fig. 24-9).	Oral antifungal (terbinafine [Lamisil], itraconazole [Sporanox]). Topical antifungal cream or solution (minimal effectiveness) if unable to tolerate systemic treatment. Thinning of toenails if needed. Nail avulsion (removal) is an option.

TABLE 24-7 COMMON INFESTATIONS AND INSECT BITES

Etiology and Pathophysiology	Clinical Manifestations	Treatment and Prognosis
Bees and Wasps *Hymenoptera* species.	Intense, burning, local pain. Swelling and itching. Severe hypersensitivity possibly leading to anaphylaxis.	Cool compresses. Local application of antipruritic lotion. Antihistamines if indicated. Usually uneventful recovery.
Bedbugs *Cimicidae* species. Feeding periodic, usually at night. Present in furniture, walls during day.	Wheal surrounded by vivid flare. Firm urticaria transforming into persistent lesion. Severe pruritus. Often grouped in threes appearing on uncovered parts of body.	Bedbug controlled by chlorocyclohexane. Lesions usually requiring no treatment. Severe itching possibly requiring use of antihistamines or topical corticosteroids.
Pediculosis (Head Lice, Body Lice, Pubic Lice) *Pediculus humanus* var. *capitis, Pediculus humanus* var. *corporis, Phthirus pubis.* Obligate parasites that suck blood, leave excrement and eggs on skin and hair, live in seams of clothing (if body lice) and in hair as nits. Transmission of pubic lice often by sexual contact.	Minute, red, noninflammatory. Points flush with skin. Progression to papular wheal-like lesions. Pruritus. Secondary excoriation, especially parallel linear excoriations in intrascapular region. Firmly attached to hair shaft in head and body lice.	γ-Benzene hexachloride or pyrethrins to treat various parts of body. Application as directed. Spinosad (Natroba) topical suspension 0.9% to treat scalp and hair. Close contacts (e.g., bed partners and playmates) should be screened and treated. Do not share head gear.
Scabies *Sarcoptes scabiei.* Mite penetrates stratum corneum, deposits eggs. Allergic reaction to eggs, feces, mite parts. Transmission by direct physical contact, only occasionally by shared personal items. Rarely seen in dark-skinned people.	Severe itching, especially at night, usually not on face. Presence of burrows, especially in interdigital webs, flexor surface of wrists, genitalia, and anterior axillary folds. Erythematous papules (may be crusted), possible vesiculation, interdigital web crusting (see eFig. 24-3).	5% permethrin topical lotion, one overnight application with second application 1 wk later, may yield 95% eradication. Treat all family members, treat environment with plastic covering for 5 days, launder all clothes and linen with bleach. Treat sexual partner. Antibiotics if secondary infections present. Possible residual pruritus up to 4 wk after treatment. Recurrence possible if inadequately treated.
Ticks *Borrelia burgdorferi* (spirochete transmitted by ticks in certain areas) causes Lyme disease. Endemic areas include Northeast, Mid-Atlantic states, parts of Midwest and West (see Chapter 65).	Spreading, ringlike rash 3-4 wk after bite (see Fig. 65-7). Rash commonly in groin, buttocks, axillae, trunk, and upper arms and legs. Warm, itchy, or painful rash. Flu-like symptoms. Cardiac, arthritic, and neurologic manifestations possible. Unreliable laboratory test. No acquired immunity.	Oral antibiotics, such as doxycycline, tetracycline. IV antibiotics for arthritic, neurologic, and cardiac symptoms. Rest and healthy diet. Most patients recover.

Infestations and Insect Bites

The possibilities for exposure to *infestations* (harboring insects or worms) and insect bites are numerous. In many instances an allergy to the venom plays a major role in the reaction. In other cases the clinical manifestations are a reaction to the eggs, feces, or body parts of the invading organism. Some individuals react with a severe hypersensitivity (anaphylaxis), which can be life threatening. (Anaphylaxis is discussed in Chapter 14.)

Prevention of insect bites by avoidance or by the use of repellents is somewhat effective. Meticulous hygiene related to personal articles, clothing, bedding, and examination and care of pets, as well as careful selection of sexual partners, can reduce the incidence of infestations. Routine skin inspection is necessary in geographic areas where there is a risk of tick bites (Table 24-7). (Lyme disease, which is caused by a tick, is discussed in Chapter 65.)

ALLERGIC DERMATOLOGIC PROBLEMS

Dermatologic problems associated with allergies and hypersensitivity reactions may present a challenge to the clinician (Table 24-8). The pathophysiology related to allergic and contact dermatitis is discussed in Chapter 14. A careful family history and discussion of exposure to possible offending agents can provide valuable data. Patch testing involves the application of allergens to the patient's skin (usually on the back) for 48 hours with reevaluation at 96 hours. Test sites are examined for erythema, papules, vesicles, or all of these. Patch testing is used to aid in determining possible causative agents (see Fig. 23-10). The best treatment of allergic dermatitis is avoidance of the causative agent. The extreme pruritus of contact dermatitis and its potential for chronicity make it a frustrating problem for you and the patient, especially if the offending agent cannot be identified.

BENIGN DERMATOLOGIC PROBLEMS

Although the list of benign dermatoses is extensive, some of the most commonly seen and distressing problems include acne vulgaris (Fig. 24-10), psoriasis (Fig. 24-11), and seborrheic keratoses (see eFig. 24-4 available on the website for this chapter). Benign problems are summarized in Table 24-9.

Psoriasis is a common benign disorder that currently affects 125 million people worldwide.[11] The disease usually develops in individuals between 15 and 35 years old. One third of people

TABLE 24-8 COMMON ALLERGIC CONDITIONS OF THE SKIN

Etiology and Pathophysiology	Clinical Manifestations	Treatment and Prognosis
Allergic Contact Dermatitis Manifestation of delayed hypersensitivity, absorbed agent acting as antigen, sensitization after one or more exposures, appearance of lesions 2-7 days after contact with allergen.	Red papules and plaques. Sharply circumscribed with occasional vesicles. Usually pruritic. Area of dermatitis frequently takes shape of causative agent (e.g., metal allergy and bandlike dermatitis on ring finger) (see Fig. 14-9).	Topical or oral corticosteroids, antihistamines. Skin lubrication. Elimination of contact allergen. Avoidance of irritating affected area. Systemic corticosteroids if sensitivity severe.
Urticaria Usually allergic phenomenon. Erythema and edema in upper dermis resulting from a local increase in permeability of capillaries (usually from histamine release).	Spontaneously occurring, raised or irregularly shaped wheals, varying size, usually multiple. A single lesion usually resolves in 24 hr. Can occur anywhere on the body.	Removal of triggering agent, if known. Oral antihistamine therapy. Possibly systemic corticosteroids.
Drug Reaction May be caused by any drug that acts as antigen and causes hypersensitivity reaction. Certain drugs (e.g., penicillin) more likely to cause reactions. Not all reactions are allergic, some are intolerance (e.g., gastric upset).	Rash of any morphology. Often red, macular and papular, semiconfluent, generalized rash with abrupt onset. Appearance as late as 14 days after cessation of drug. Possibly pruritic. Some reactions may be life threatening requiring immediate and intensive care.	Withdrawal of drug if possible. Antihistamines, topical or systemic corticosteroids may be necessary depending on severity of symptoms.
Atopic Dermatitis Genetically influenced, chronic, relapsing disease associated with immunologic irregularity involving inflammatory mediators, exaggerated by a cutaneous response to environmental allergens. Associated with allergic rhinitis and asthma.	Multiple presentations, including acute, subacute, and chronic stages. All are pruritic. *Acute stage* with bright erythema, oozing vesicles, with extreme pruritus. *Subacute stage* with scaly, light red to red-brown plaques. *Chronic stage* with thickened skin with accentuation of skin markings (lichenification), possible hypopigmentation or hyperpigmentation. Dry skin. Common in antecubital and popliteal space.	Lubrication of dry (xerotic) skin, restoration of skin barrier function. Topical immunomodulators (pimecrolimus [Elidel], tacrolimus [Protopic]). Corticosteroids, phototherapy for severe inflammation and pruritus. Reduction of stress reduces flares. Antibiotics for secondary infection as needed.

with psoriasis have at least one relative with the disease. Diagnosis is often based on the appearance of the skin (see Fig. 24-11). Most people have mild disease that affects at least 3% of the body. Severe disease is when psoriasis affects more than 10% of the body. Patients with severe disease often have a weakened immune system and are at risk for cardiovascular disease. Monitor the laboratory values (e.g., cholesterol, triglycerides) of patients with severe psoriasis to assist in early detection and intervention strategies for cardiovascular disease.

The chronicity of psoriasis can be severe and disabling as people withdraw from social contacts because of visible lesions. Quality of life is also negatively affected. Psoriatic arthritis affects 10% to 30% of all persons with psoriasis. (Psoriatic arthritis is discussed in Chapter 65.)

DRUG ALERT: Isotretinoin (Accutane)
- Can cause serious damage to fetus
- Blood donation prohibited for those taking the drug and for 1 month after treatment ends
- Contraindicated in women who are pregnant or who are intending to become pregnant while on the drug
- Linked to liver function test abnormalities

DISEASES WITH DERMATOLOGIC MANIFESTATIONS

Dermatologic manifestations of various diseases are listed in eTable 24-1 (available on the website for this chapter). Always consider the possibility that a particular skin manifestation is a clue to an internal, less obvious disease or disorder.

FIG. 24-10 Acne vulgaris. Papules and pustules.

FIG. 24-11 Psoriasis. Characteristic inflammation and scaling.

TABLE 24-9   COMMON BENIGN CONDITIONS OF THE SKIN

Etiology and Pathophysiology	Clinical Manifestations	Treatment and Prognosis
Acne Vulgaris Inflammatory disorder of sebaceous glands. More common in teenagers but possible development and persistence in adulthood. Flare can occur with use of corticosteroids and androgen-dominant birth control pills and before menses.	Noninflammatory lesions, including open comedones (blackheads) and closed comedones (whiteheads). Inflammatory lesions, including papules and pustules. Most common on face, neck, and upper back (see Fig. 24-10).	Mechanical removal of multiple lesions with comedo extractor. Topical benzoyl peroxide or other antimicrobials. Veltin gel (clindamycin and tretinoin). Topical retinoids, systemic antibiotics. Aim of treatment to suppress new lesions and minimize scarring. Spontaneous remission possible. Often improvement with exposure to sun. May last many years. Use of isotretinoin (Accutane) for severe nodulocystic acne to possibly provide lasting remission (see Drug Alert on p. 438 for contraindications). Pregnancy tests, monitoring of liver function, cholesterol, triglycerides, and for depression essential.
Nevi (Moles) Grouping of normal cells derived from melanocyte-like precursor cells.	Hyperpigmented areas that vary in form and color. Flat, slightly elevated, verrucoid, polypoid, dome-shaped, sessile, or papillomatous. Preservation of normal skin markings. Hair growth possible.	No treatment necessary except for cosmetic reasons. Skin biopsy for suspicious nevi.
Psoriasis Autoimmune chronic dermatitis that involves excessively rapid turnover of epidermal cells. Family predisposition. Usually develops before age 40.	Sharply demarcated silvery scaling plaques on reddish colored skin commonly on the scalp, elbows, knees, palms, soles, and fingernails. Itching, burning, pain. Localized or general, intermittent or continuous. Symptoms vary in intensity from mild to severe (see Fig. 24-11).	Goal to reduce inflammation and suppress rapid turnover of epidermal cells. No cure, but control is possible. *Topical treatments:* corticosteroids, tar, calcipotriene, anthralin. Intralesional injection of corticosteroids for chronic plaques. *Systemic treatments:* natural or artificial UVB. PUVA (UVA with topical or systemic photosensitizer [psoralen]). Antimetabolite (methotrexate), retinoid (acitretin), immunosuppressant (cyclosporine), biologic therapy (adalimumab [Humira], alefacept [Amevive], etanercept [Enbrel], infliximab [Remicade], ustekinumab [Stelara]) for moderate to severe plaque disease.
Seborrheic Keratoses Benign, familial, exact etiology unknown. Usually occur after age 40, increase in number with age.	Irregularly round or oval, often verrucous papules or plaques. Well-defined shape, appearance of being stuck on. Increase in pigmentation with time. Usually multiple and possibly itchy (see eFig. 24-4).	Removal by curettage or cryosurgery for cosmetic reasons or to eliminate source of irritation. Biopsy if unable to distinguish from melanoma.
Acrochordons (Skin Tags) Common after midlife. Appearance on neck, axillae, and upper trunk secondary to mechanical friction or redundant skin (associated with obesity).	Small, skin-colored, soft, pedunculated papules. May become irritated.	No treatment medically necessary. Surgical removal when needed. Usually just snipping without anesthesia.
Lipoma Benign tumor of adipose tissue, often encapsulated, most common in 40- to 60-yr-old age-group.	Rubbery, compressible, round mass of adipose tissue. Single or multiple. Variable in size, possibly extremely large. Most common on trunk, back of neck, and forearms.	Usually no treatment, biopsy to differentiate from liposarcoma, excision usual treatment (when indicated).
Lentigo Increased number of normal melanocytes in basal layer of epidermis related to sun exposure and aging. Also called "liver spots" or "age spots."	Hyperpigmented, brown to black macule or patch (flat lesion) on sun-exposed areas.	Evaluate carefully for progression. Treatment only for cosmetic purposes: liquid nitrogen, laser resurfacing. May recur. Biopsy when suspicious of melanoma.

PUVA, Psoralen ultraviolet A; *UBA,* ultraviolet A; *UVB,* ultraviolet B.

COLLABORATIVE CARE DERMATOLOGIC PROBLEMS

Diagnostic Studies

A careful history is of prime importance in the diagnosis of skin problems. The clinician must be skilled at detecting any evidence that could lead to the cause of many different skin diseases and conditions. After a careful history and physical examination, inspect individual lesions. Based on the history, physical examination, and appropriate diagnostic tests, either medical, surgical, or combination therapy is planned.

Collaborative Therapy

Many different treatment methods are used in dermatology. Advances in this field have brought relief to many previously chronic, untreatable conditions. Many of the specific therapeutic treatments require specialized equipment and are usually reserved for use by the dermatologist. Many clinicians prescribe drug therapy. The effectiveness of topical therapy can often be related to the base (or vehicle) in which the medication is prepared. Table 24-10 summarizes the common agents used as bases for topical preparations and their therapeutic considerations.

Phototherapy. Ultraviolet light (UVL) of different wavelengths may be used to treat many dermatologic conditions, including psoriasis, cutaneous T-cell lymphoma, atopic dermatitis, vitiligo, and pruritus. Light sources available to treat skin problems include broadband UVB, narrowband UVB, and long-wave UV (UVA1). One form of phototherapy involves the use of psoralen plus UVA light (PUVA). The photosensitizing drug psoralen is given to patients for a prescribed amount of time before exposure to UVA (see eFig. 24-5 available on the website for this chapter).

Treatments are generally given two to four times a week. Side effects of oral psoralen include nausea and vomiting, sunburn, and persistent pruritus. Perform frequent skin assessments on all patients receiving phototherapy, since erythema is a side effect of treatment. Topical corticosteroids may be given for painful erythema. Psoralen should be used with extreme caution in patients with liver or renal disease because slower metabolism and excretion can lead to prolonged photosensitivity.

Caution patients about the potential hazards of using photosensitizing chemicals and further exposure to UV rays from sunlight or artificial UVL during the course of phototherapy.

Protective eyewear that blocks 100% of UVL is prescribed for patients receiving PUVA because psoralen is absorbed by the lens of the eye. The eyewear is used to prevent cataract formation. Instruct patients to use the eyewear for 24 hours after taking the medication when outdoors or near a bright window because UVA penetrates glass. Ongoing monitoring of these patients is essential because of the immunosuppressive effects of PUVA, including an increased risk of squamous and basal cell carcinomas and melanoma.

Photodynamic therapy is a special type of phototherapy that may be used in the treatment of actinic keratosis and malignant skin tumors.[12] This therapy uses a photosensitizing agent in a different way than some phototherapy treatments to selectively cause tumor necrosis.

Radiation Therapy. The use of radiation for the treatment of basal and squamous cell carcinomas and malignant melanoma varies greatly according to local practice and availability.[13] Even if radiation therapy is planned, a biopsy must first be performed to obtain a pathologic diagnosis.

Radiation to malignant cutaneous lesions may be given to reduce tumor size or in palliative treatment. One advantage of this therapy is minimal damage to surrounding tissue, which is of prime consideration in locations such as the nose, eyelids, and canthal areas. Careful shielding is necessary to prevent ocular lens damage if the irradiated area is around the eyes. Radiation therapy is particularly effective for the older adult or debilitated patient who cannot tolerate even a minor surgical procedure.

Radiation therapy usually requires multiple visits to a radiology department. It can produce permanent hair loss (*alopecia*) of the irradiated areas. Other adverse effects, depending on anatomic location and dose of radiation delivered, include telangiectasia, atrophy, hyperpigmentation, depigmentation, ulceration, hearing loss, ocular damage, atrophy, and mucositis. (Radiation therapy is discussed in Chapter 16.)

Total-body skin irradiation (body is bombarded with high-energy electrons) is one treatment for cutaneous T-cell lymphoma. Treatment follows a lengthy course and causes premature aging of the skin. Patients experience varying degrees of permanent alopecia and radiation dermatitis with a transient loss of sweat gland function.

Laser Technology. Laser treatment is expanding rapidly as an efficient surgical tool for many types of dermatologic problems (Table 24-11). Lasers are able to produce measurable, repeatable, consistent zones of tissue damage. They can cut, coagulate, and vaporize tissue to some degree. The wavelength determines the type of delivery system used and the intensity of the energy delivered.

The surgical use of laser energy requires a focusing device to produce a small, high-density spot of energy. Written policies and procedures should cover laser safety and be reviewed by all personnel working with laser equipment. Laser light does not

---

TABLE 24-10 DRUG THERAPY

Common Bases for Topical Medications

Agent	Therapeutic Considerations
Powder	Promotion of dryness. Lubricates skinfold areas to prevent irritation. Base for antifungal preparations. Protect patient from inhaling
Lotion	Oil and water emulsions. Cooling and drying. Some leave residual powder film after evaporation of water. Useful in subacute pruritic eruptions
Cream	Emulsions of oil and water. Most common base for topical medications. Lubrication and protection
Ointment	Oil with differing amounts of water added in suspension. Lubrication and prevention of dehydration. Petrolatum most common
Paste	Mixture of powder and ointment, used when drying effect necessary because moisture is absorbed
Gel	Nongreasy combination of propylene glycol and water. May contain alcohol

---

TABLE 24-11 SKIN CONDITIONS TREATED BY LASER

• Acne scars	• Port wine stain
• Skin lesions	• Vascular lesions
• Hemangiomas	• Tattoo removal
• Leg veins	• Resurfacing of skin
• Rosacea	• Psoriasis
• Pigmented nevi	• Wrinkles
• Hair removal	• Pigment discoloration in epidermis

accumulate in body cells and cannot cause cumulative cellular changes or damage.

Several types of lasers are available in most offices and hospitals. The CO_2 laser, the most common, has numerous applications as a vaporizing and cutting tool for most tissues. The argon laser emits light that is primarily absorbed by hemoglobin and helps in the treatment of vascular and other pigmented lesions. Other, less common lasers include the use of copper and gold vapors and neodymium:yttrium-aluminum-garnet (Nd:YAG).

Drug Therapy

Antibiotics. Antibiotics are used both topically and systemically to treat dermatologic problems, and are often used in combination. When using topical antibiotics, apply a thin film lightly to clean skin. Common OTC topical antibiotics include bacitracin-neomycin-polymyxin (Neosporin), bacitracin, and polymyxin B. Many health care providers do not recommend Neosporin because it often causes allergic contact dermatitis. Prescription topical antibiotics include mupirocin (for superficial *Staphylococcus* infections such as impetigo), gentamicin (used for *Staphylococcus* and most gram-negative organisms), and erythromycin (used for gram-positive cocci [staphylococci and streptococci] and gram-negative cocci and bacilli). Topical erythromycin and clindamycin (Cleocin solutions or gels) are used in the treatment of acne vulgaris. Topical metronidazole is used to treat rosacea and bacterial vaginosis. Many of the more popular systemic antibiotics are not used topically because of the danger of allergic contact dermatitis.

If there are manifestations of systemic infection, a systemic antibiotic should be used. Systemic antibiotics are useful in the treatment of bacterial infections and acne vulgaris. The most frequently used are synthetic sulfur, penicillin, minocycline, erythromycin, and tetracycline (or doxycycline). These drugs are particularly useful for erysipelas, cellulitis, carbuncles, and severe infected eczema. Culture and sensitivity of the lesion can guide the choice of antibiotic. Patients require drug-specific instructions on the proper technique of taking or applying antibiotics. For instance, oral tetracycline must be taken on an empty stomach. It should never be taken within 1 hour before consuming a dairy product or 2 hours after, since this would interfere with its absorption.

Corticosteroids. Corticosteroids are particularly effective in treating a wide variety of dermatologic conditions and can be used topically, intralesionally, or systemically. Topical corticosteroids are used for their local antiinflammatory and antipruritic effects. Attempts to diagnose a skin problem should be made *before* a corticosteroid preparation is applied, since corticosteroids may alter the clinical manifestations. Once a sufficient amount of medication is dispensed, limits should be set on the duration and frequency of application.

The potency of a particular preparation is related to the concentration of active drug. With prolonged use, more potent corticosteroid formulations can cause adrenal suppression, especially if a large surface area is covered and occlusive dressings are used. Over time, high-potency corticosteroids may produce side effects, including atrophy of the skin resulting from impaired cell mitosis, capillary fragility, and susceptibility to bruising. In general, dermal and epidermal atrophy does not occur until a corticosteroid has been used for 2 to 3 weeks. If drug use is discontinued at the first sign of atrophy, recovery usually occurs in several weeks. Rosacea eruptions and severe exacerbations of acne vulgaris may also occur. Rebound dermatitis is not uncommon when therapy is stopped. This can be

reduced by tapering the use of high-potency topical corticosteroids when improvement is noted.

Low-potency corticosteroids such as hydrocortisone act more slowly but can be used for a longer time without producing serious side effects. Low-potency corticosteroids are safe to use on the face and intertriginous areas, such as the axillae and groin.

The most potent delivery system for a topical corticosteroid is an ointment form. Creams and ointments should be applied in thin layers and slowly massaged into the site one to three times a day as prescribed. Accurate and adequate topical therapy is often the key to a successful outcome.

Intralesional corticosteroids are injected directly into or just beneath the lesion. This method provides a reservoir of medication with an effect lasting several weeks to months. Intralesional injection is commonly used in the treatment of psoriasis, alopecia areata (patchy hair loss), cystic acne, hypertrophic scars, and keloids. Triamcinolone acetonide (Kenalog) is the most common drug used for intralesional injection.

Systemic corticosteroids can have remarkable results in the treatment of dermatologic conditions. However, they often have undesirable systemic effects (see Chapter 50). Corticosteroids can be administered as short-term therapy for acute conditions such as contact dermatitis caused by poison ivy. Long-term corticosteroid therapy for dermatologic conditions is reserved for severe disease such as bullous (blistering) disorders.

Antihistamines. Oral antihistamines are used to treat conditions that exhibit urticaria, angioedema, and pruritus.[14] Dermatologic problems such as atopic dermatitis, allergic dermatitis, and other allergic cutaneous reactions can be reduced with the use of histamine blockers. Antihistamines compete with histamine for the receptor site, thus preventing its effect. Antihistamines may have anticholinergic and/or sedative effects. Several different antihistamines may have to be tried before the satisfactory therapeutic effect is achieved. Sedating antihistamines, such as hydroxyzine (Atarax) and diphenhydramine (Benadryl), are often preferred for pruritic conditions because the tranquilizing and sedative effects offer symptomatic relief. Warn the patient about sedative effects, a particular problem when driving or operating heavy machinery. Antihistamines such as loratadine (Claritin), fexofenadine (Allegra), and cetirizine (Zyrtec) bind to peripheral histamine receptors, providing antihistamine action without sedation. These nonsedating antihistamines are not effective for controlling pruritus. Antihistamines should be used with particular caution in older adults because of their long half-life and their anticholinergic effects.

Topical Fluorouracil. Fluorouracil (5-FU) is a topical cytotoxic agent with selective toxicity for sun-damaged cells. 5-FU is available in four strengths (0.5%, 1%, 2%, and 5%) and is used for the treatment of premalignant (especially actinic keratosis) and some malignant skin diseases. Because systemic absorption of the drug is minimal, systemic side effects are virtually nonexistent. Patient compliance is a consideration in the use of 5-FU. The medication produces erythema and pruritus within 3 to 5 days and painful, eroded areas over the damaged skin within 1 to 3 weeks, depending on skin thickness at the site. Low-potency topical corticosteroids are often prescribed to be applied 20 minutes after 5-FU to reduce erythema and pruritus and increase patient adherence with therapy. Treatment must continue with applications one (only in the 0.5% strength) or two times a day for 2 to 6 weeks. Healing may take up to 4 weeks after medication is stopped.

Because 5-FU is a photosensitizing drug, instruct the patient to avoid sunlight during treatment. Teach patients about the effect of the medication and that they will look worse before they look better. Adherence depends on thoroughness of your instruction, which should include a written handout. After effective treatment, treated skin is smooth and free of actinic keratosis. Actinic keratosis may recur in treated areas, and multiple courses of chemotherapy may be necessary over the years for individuals with severely sun-damaged skin.

Immunomodulators. Topical immunomodulators, such as pimecrolimus (Elidel) and tacrolimus (Protopic), are used to treat atopic dermatitis. They work by suppressing an overreactive immune system. The side effects are minimal and may include a transient burning or feeling of heat at the application site. An increased risk of skin cancer and precancerous lesions may be associated with these drugs.

Another topical immunomodulator, imiquimod, acts to stimulate the production of α-interferon and other cytokines to enhance cell-mediated immunity. It boosts the immune response only where applied and is safe for transplant patients. This medication is used for external genital warts, actinic keratoses, and superficial BCC. Most patients using this cream experience skin reactions, including redness, swelling, blistering, excoriations, peeling, itching, and burning.

Diagnostic and Surgical Therapy

Skin Scraping. Scraping is done with a scalpel blade to obtain a sample of surface cells (stratum corneum) for microscopic inspection and diagnosis. The most common tests of skin scrapings are potassium hydroxide (KOH) for fungus and mineral oil examination for scabies.

Electrodesiccation and Electrocoagulation. Electrical energy can be converted to heat with the tip of an electrode. This results in tissue being destroyed by burning. The major uses of this type of therapy are coagulation of bleeding vessels to obtain hemostasis and destruction of small *telangiectasias* (dilation of groups of superficial capillaries and venules). *Electrodesiccation* usually involves more superficial destruction, and a monopolar electrode is used. *Electrocoagulation* has a deeper effect, with better hemostasis and an increased possibility of scarring. A dipolar electrode is used for electrocoagulation.

Curettage. Curettage is the removal and scooping away of tissue using an instrument with a circular cutting edge attached to a handle (see eFig. 24-6 available on the website). Although the curette is not usually strong enough to cut normal skin, it is useful for removing many types of small, soft skin tumors and superficial lesions, such as warts, actinic keratoses, and small basal and squamous cell carcinomas. The area to be curetted is anesthetized before the procedure. Hemostasis is obtained by one of several methods: electrodesiccation, ferric subsulfate (Monsel solution), gelatin foam, aluminum chloride (Drysol), or a gauze pressure dressing. A small scar and hypopigmentation can result. The curetted tissue should be sent for biopsy.

Punch Biopsy. Punch biopsy is a common dermatologic procedure used to obtain a tissue sample for histologic study or to remove small lesions (Fig. 24-12). It is generally reserved for lesions smaller than 0.5 cm.[15] Before local anesthesia is used, the biopsy area is outlined so that landmarks will not be obscured by the anesthetizing agent. The punch biopsy instrument is twirled between the fingers, and its sharp edge cores out a small cylinder of skin. The core of skin is snipped from the subcutaneous fat and appropriately preserved for examination

FIG. 24-12 Punch biopsy. **A,** Removal of skin for diagnostic purposes. **B,** Specimen obtained.

in a fixative solution. Hemostasis is achieved by using methods similar to those used with curettage, but sites of 4 mm or larger are usually closed with sutures. Other types of biopsies are discussed in Table 23-9 and Chapter 23.

Cryosurgery. Cryosurgery is the use of subfreezing temperatures to destroy epidermal lesions. Cryosurgery is a useful treatment for common benign, precancerous conditions, including common and genital warts, cutaneous tags, thin seborrheic keratoses, lentigines, actinic keratoses, and nonmelanoma skin cancers. Topical liquid nitrogen (−196° F) is the agent most commonly used for cryosurgery.[15] The mechanism of injury involves direct cellular freezing and vascular stasis (stoppage or slowdown in the flow of blood), which develops after thawing. Intracellular ice formation causes the cell to rupture during thaw, leading to cell death and necrosis of the treated tissue.

Liquid nitrogen can be applied topically (directly onto the lesion) with a direct spray or a cotton-tipped applicator. Patients are informed that they will feel a stinging cold sensation. The lesion first becomes swollen and red, and it may blister. A scab forms and falls off in 1 to 3 weeks. The skin lesion is sloughed along with the scab. Growth of new skin follows.

Because of the temperature of the liquid nitrogen, melanocytes can easily be destroyed, leaving an area of hypopigmentation resembling a scar. The size of an affected area to be treated may limit the use of cryotherapy. The disadvantages of this treatment are (1) the lack of a tissue specimen for histologic confirmation of cell type before destruction and (2) the potential for destruction of adjacent healthy tissue.

Excision. Excision should be considered if the lesion to be removed involves the dermis. Complete closure of the excised area usually results in a good cosmetic result.

A specific type of excision is *Mohs' surgery,* which is a microscopically controlled removal of a cutaneous malignancy. This procedure sections the surgical specimen horizontally, so that

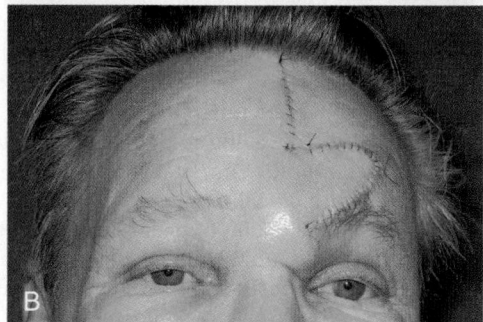

FIG. 24-13 A, Removal of melanoma by Mohs' surgery. **B,** After plastic surgery using a skin flap to repair defect.

100% of the surgical margin can be examined. Tissue is removed in thin layers, and all margins of the specimen are mapped to determine whether any malignant cells remain (Fig. 24-13). Any residual tumor not removed by the first surgical excision can be removed in serial excisions performed the same day. The benefits of this treatment are preserving normal tissue, producing the smallest possible wound, and completely removing the cancer before surgical closure. Although this can become a lengthy procedure, it is performed in an outpatient setting with the patient under local anesthesia.

NURSING MANAGEMENT
DERMATOLOGIC PROBLEMS

AMBULATORY AND HOME CARE

Dermatologic conditions are not usually the primary reason for hospitalization. Nevertheless, many hospitalized patients exhibit concurrent skin problems that warrant nursing intervention and patient education.

If the patient is in an acute care setting, you both administer and teach the appropriate treatments. In an outpatient setting the focus is on patient teaching, with opportunities provided for demonstration and repeated demonstration. Subsequent visits allow you to evaluate patient understanding and treatment effectiveness.

Nursing interventions related to dermatologic conditions fall into broad categories. They are applicable to many skin problems in both inpatient and outpatient settings. (A nursing care plan for the patient with chronic skin lesions [eNursing Care Plan 24-1] is available on the website for this chapter.)

WET DRESSINGS. Wet dressings are commonly used when there is oozing from the skin. Oozing usually indicates an infection and/or inflammation. Salt water or a prescribed solution (e.g., Domeboro powder) is used on the skin by soaking (a foot or hand) or applying compresses to a larger area. Wet dressings

are also used to relieve itching, suppress inflammation, and debride a wound. In addition, wet dressings increase penetration of topical medications; promote sleep by relieving discomfort; and enhance removal of scales, crusts, and exudate. Materials such as thin sheeting, gauze sponges, thermal underwear, or tube socks can be used for dressings. Ingenuity is sometimes required when odd-shaped body parts must be covered.

Place the prescribed dressing material into fresh solution, and squeeze until it is no longer dripping. Then apply it to the affected area, avoiding normal skin tissue. If the desired effect is drying, soaks or compresses are left in place for 20 minutes, three times daily for 2 or 3 days. Take care to avoid overdrying, since new problems such as fissuring may result. Wet dressings for uses other than drying should be left in place 10 to 30 minutes, two to four times a day as ordered. If the skin appears *macerated* (softens and turns white), discontinue the dressings for 2 to 3 hours. Protect the patient from discomfort and chilling by using linens and bedclothes with pads or plastic.

Wet dressings do not need to be sterile. Tap water at room temperature is the most common solution where water quality is adequate. Filtered or sterile water may be indicated in some locations. Wet dressings should be cool when an antiinflammatory effect is desired and tepid when the purpose is to debride an infected, crusted lesion. These treatments are excellent ways to remove the scabs left by the collection of debris at a wound site.

BATHS. Baths are appropriate when large body areas need to be treated. They also have sedative and antipruritic effects. Some agents, such as oilated oatmeal (Aveeno) and sodium bicarbonate, can be added directly to bath water. Fill the tub to cover the affected areas. Both the bath water and the prescribed solution should be at a lukewarm (tepid) temperature. Have the patient soak for 15 to 20 minutes three or four times a day, depending on the severity of the dermatitis and the patient's discomfort. Stress to the patient that the skin must not be rubbed dry with a towel but gently patted to prevent increased irritation and inflammation. The addition of oils makes the bathtub extremely slippery and should be avoided. If oils are used in the tub, use caution in transferring patients to prevent accidents. To sustain the hydrating effect, apply cream or ointment emollients (moisturizers) or other prescribed topical agents after the bath. This helps retain the moisture in the hydrated cells and increases the absorption of a prescribed topical medication.

TOPICAL MEDICATIONS. A thin layer of ointment, cream, lotion or solution, or gel should be applied to clean skin and spread evenly in a downward motion. Thickly applied topical medications waste medication and leave the skin greasy. An alternative method is for you to apply the medication directly onto a dressing. Pastes are designed to protect the affected area. Apply pastes thickly with a tongue blade or a gloved hand. Draining lesions and lesions with oily medication can be covered with a light dressing to avoid soiling clothes. Provide specific directions to patients on the proper application technique of prescribed topical medications.

CONTROL OF PRURITUS. *Pruritus* (itching) can be caused by dry skin, almost any physical or chemical stimulus to the skin (such as drugs or insects), and any scaling skin disorder. The itch sensation is carried by the same nonmyelinated nerve fibers as pain. If the epidermis is damaged or absent, the sensation will be felt as pain rather than an itch.

The itch/scratch cycle must be broken to prevent excoriation and lichenification. Control of pruritus is also important because it is difficult to diagnose a lesion that is excoriated and inflamed. Certain circumstances make itching worse. Anything that causes vasodilation, such as heat or rubbing, should be avoided. Dryness of the skin lowers the itch threshold and increases the itch sensation.

Inform the patient of the various methods that may be helpful in breaking the itch/scratch cycle. A cool environment may cause vasoconstriction and decrease itching. Topically applied menthol, camphor, or phenol can be used to numb the itch receptors.[16] Systemic antihistamines may provide relief while the underlying cause of the patient's pruritus is diagnosed and treated. The principal side effect of most antihistamines is sedation. This may be desirable because pruritus is often worse at night and can interfere with sleep.

Wet dressings may also relieve pruritus. Thin cotton sheets or thermal underwear should be placed in warm water, wrung out, and placed over the pruritic area. After 10 to 15 minutes remove the dressing, pat the skin dry, and then apply a lubricant or medication. This procedure can be repeated as necessary for comfort.

Lichenification is a thickening of skin as a result of the proliferation of keratinocytes with accentuation of the normal markings of the skin. Lichenification is caused by chronic scratching or rubbing of the skin and is often associated with atopic dermatoses and pruritic conditions. Although any area of the body may be affected, the hands, forearms, shins, and nape of the neck are common sites. Excoriations may be evident in the lichenified skin as a result of persistent pruritus and scratching. Treatment of the cause of the itching is the key to prevention of lichenification.

PREVENTION OF SPREAD. Although most skin problems are not contagious, infection control precautions indicate the need for gloves with open or bleeding wounds or any lesion with purulent drainage. Explain procedures to the patient to avoid provoking undue anxiety. Careful hand washing and the safe disposal of soiled dressings are the best means of preventing the spread of skin problems. The most common contagious lesions include impetigo, staphylococcal infections, pyoderma, fungal infections, primary chancre, scabies, and pediculosis.

PREVENTION OF SECONDARY INFECTIONS. Open lesions on the skin are susceptible to invasion by other viral, bacterial, or fungal organisms. Meticulous hygiene, hand washing, and dressing changes are important to minimize the potential for secondary infections. Warn the patient about scratching the lesions, which can cause excoriations and create a portal of entry for pathogens. Trim the patient's nails short to minimize trauma from scratching.

SPECIFIC SKIN CARE. You are often in a position to advise patients regarding care of the skin after simple dermatologic surgical procedures, such as skin biopsy, excision, and cryosurgery. Patient follow-up should be individualized. In general, your instructions should include dressing changes, use of topical antibiotics, and the signs and symptoms of infection. After a dermatologic procedure, any oozing wound should be cleansed with a saline solution twice daily or as ordered by the provider. A wound that is not oozing may be washed with soap and plain water. An antibiotic ointment or plain petrolatum ointment may then be applied with a dressing that is both absorbent and nonadherent.

Wounds that are kept moist and covered heal more rapidly and with less scarring. The initial crust that forms should be left undisturbed as a protective coating for the damaged skin beneath it. Healing crusts that have been moisturized and protected will separate naturally from healed epidermis.

A wound that required sutures can be covered with a variety of different dressings. Sutures are generally removed in 4 to 14 days, depending on the placement site. Sometimes alternating sutures are removed after the third day. Incision lines may require daily cleansing, usually with plain tap water. If necessary, a topical antibiotic is applied and the wound is either covered with a dry sterile dressing or left open to air. The patient may experience some swelling and discomfort in the first 24 hours, during the first phase of wound healing. Ice packs may be applied over the surgical dressing to reduce edema. Mild analgesics such as acetaminophen or a nonsteroidal antiinflammatory medication should control the discomfort. Teach the patient the manifestations of inflammation, such as redness, fever, or increased pain or swelling, and signs of infection, such as purulent drainage. If these manifestations occur, they should be reported to the health care provider.

PSYCHOLOGIC EFFECTS OF CHRONIC DERMATOLOGIC PROBLEMS. Emotional stress can occur for persons who suffer from chronic skin problems such as psoriasis, atopic dermatitis, or acne. The sequelae of chronic skin problems could result in social and employment problems with subsequent financial implications, a poor self-image, problems with sexuality, and increasing and progressive frustration. The usual lack of systemic overt illness coupled with the visibility of the skin lesions often presents a real problem to the patient.

Help the patient comply with the prescribed regimen. The patient must be allowed to verbalize the "Why me?" question, even though there is no ready answer. Dermatology patient support groups are listed on the American Academy of Dermatology website *(www.aad.org)*. These groups are extremely helpful for patient support and accurate education materials.

Many lesions can be camouflaged with the skillful use of cosmetics. Individual sensitivity to product ingredients must always be considered in the selection of a cosmetic product. Oil-free, hypoallergenic cosmetics are available and may be beneficial to the allergic patient. Rehabilitative cosmetics are available to help camouflage and deemphasize such lesions as *vitiligo* (loss of pigmentation), *melasma* (tan to brown patches on the face), or healed postoperative wound sites. These commercially available products are opaque, smudge resistant, and water resistant.

In addition to specific skin conditions that tend to be chronic, other factors affecting the outcome of long-term dermatologic problems include skin type, history of previous exacerbations, family history, complications, intolerance to therapy, environmental factors, lack of adherence to the prescribed regimen, endocrine factors, and psychologic factors.

PHYSIOLOGIC EFFECTS OF CHRONIC DERMATOLOGIC PROBLEMS. Scarring and lichenification are the results of chronic dermatologic problems. Scars occur when ulceration takes place. Scars are pink and vascular at first. With time, they become avascular and white (scars on individuals with darker skin may be hyperpigmented) with increasing strength. Different regions of the body scar differently. For example, the face and neck heal fairly rapidly because they are well vascularized. Regions of the lower body with less vascularization tend to scar more easily and heal more slowly. Scar formation is described in Chapter 12.

The location of the scar is the determining factor with respect to its cosmetic implications. Facial scars are the most damaging

TABLE 24-12 COMMON COSMETIC TOPICAL PROCEDURES

Tretinoin (Retin-A, Renova)	Chemical Peels	Microdermabrasion	α-Hydroxy Acids (e.g., Glycolic Acid, Lactic Acid)
Indications			
Improves appearance of photodamaged skin, especially fine wrinkling. Reduces actinic keratoses.	Improves appearance of photodamaged skin, acne scarring, actinic and seborrheic keratoses.	Smoothes appearance of photodamaged and wrinkled skin, acne scarring.	Similar indications as microdermabrasion. Also called a "light chemical peel."
Description			
Applied initially qod, nightly applications as tolerated, since preparation is inactivated by light. Treatment stopped if severe inflammation occurs. Maximum response in 8-12 mo.	Solution applied (e.g., trichloroacetic acid, phenol) in varying amounts to the skin, causing a controlled burn with a loss of melanin.	Epidermis and top dermal layer removed by applying aluminum oxide or baking soda crystals. Re-epithelialization of abraded surface then occurs.	Low concentrations (<10%) in many skin care products consumers can apply to the skin. Higher concentrations (50%-70%) given only by a health care provider.
Side Effects			
Erythema, swelling, flaking, pigmentation changes. Teratogenic. Increases phototoxicity if also taking other photosensitive drugs (see Table 24-2).	Moderate swelling and crusting for 1 wk. Redness for 6-8 wk. Pink tone possible for several mo. Photosensitivity.	Light pink tone that resolves within 24 hr. Photosensitivity.	Photosensitivity, slight irritation at lower concentrations, severe redness, oozing, and flaking skin possible with higher concentrations.
Patient Teaching			
Apply emollients, use sunscreen (SPF 15 or higher), use sun avoidance measures, avoid use of abrasive or drying facial cleansers for severe sensitivity (e.g., excess irritation).	Use sunscreen, avoid sun for 6 mo to prevent hyperpigmentation.	Generous application of emollients and sunscreen.	Use sunscreen.

qod, Every other day; *SPF,* sun protection factor.

psychologically, because they are so visible. Creative use of cosmetics can do much to mask the scarring of chronic skin conditions. The best treatment is the prevention of scarring by controlling the problem in the acute phase.

COSMETIC PROCEDURES

A vast array of cosmetic procedures is available, including chemical peels, toxin injections, fillers, laser surgery, breast enlargement and reduction (see Chapter 52), face-lift, eyelid-lift, and liposuction. Common cosmetic topical procedures are presented in Table 24-12. Other types of cosmetic procedures include the injection of botulinum toxin (Botox), calcium hydroxylapatite (Radiesse), collagen (Zyplast), and hyaluronic acid fillers (Restylane, Perlane). Transitory side effects may occur such as mild redness, pain, swelling, and bruising. Uncommon side effects from cosmetic procedures include allergic reaction, infection, or lumps at the injection sites; undercorrection or overcorrection of wrinkles; and reactivation of human papillomavirus (HPV). Instruct the patient that he or she will need to repeat the procedure at prescribed intervals to maintain the appearance desired.

The reasons for undergoing these procedures are as varied as the techniques. The most common reason that people suffer the discomfort and financial expense (most are not covered by health insurance) of a cosmetic procedure is to improve their body image. If they feel better about themselves after having cosmetic procedures, they often act more confident and self-assured. Often social position and economic considerations are part of the decision. Increased longevity provides a larger population to whom cosmetic procedures are especially appealing.

Regardless of the patient's reasons for seeking cosmetic procedures, maintain a supportive, nonjudgmental attitude about these procedures. If the patient wishes to change or enhance a body feature perceived as unattractive and has realistic expectations about the outcome, you should support this decision.

Elective Surgery

Laser Surgery. When a laser beam enters the skin, the light can affect skin structures by scattering, absorbing, or passing through different layers. The spectrum of clinical application for each laser depends on the depth of the wavelength emitted and the operator technique. Alterations in technique, such as pulse duration and the number of passes over the skin, vary the result. New handpiece technology with multiple spot size and cooling device additions has also generated new flexibility in laser surgery.

Lasers can reduce scarring and fine wrinkles around the lips or eyes and remove facial lesions[17] (see Table 24-11). Swelling, redness, and bruising are common after treatment. The treated areas usually are kept moist with ointment or occlusive dressings (surgical bandages) for the first few days. The treated skin must be protected from the sun.

Face-Lift. A face-lift *(rhytidectomy)* is the lifting and repositioning of the lower two thirds of the face and neck to improve appearance (Fig. 24-14). Indications for this procedure include the following:
- Redundant soft tissue or scarring resulting from disease (e.g., acne scarring)
- Asymmetric redundancy of soft tissues (e.g., facial palsy)
- Redundant soft tissue resulting from trauma
- Preauricular lesions

FIG. 24-14 Face-lift. **A,** Preoperative. **B,** Postoperative.

- Redundant soft tissues resulting from *solar elastosis* (sagging of the skin as a result of sun damage), changes in body weight, and the effects of gravity
- Restoration of body image

The surgical approach and lines of incisions vary according to the desired correction and the position of the hairline. Eyelid-lifts *(blepharoplasty)* with similar indications are performed to remove redundant tissue and possibly improve the field of vision. Prevention of hematoma formation is the most important postoperative consideration. Ice packs are usually applied for the first 24 to 48 hours to reduce swelling and decrease the possibility of hematoma formation. Complications can occur if the person smokes or is involved in vigorous exercise. Usually the pain is minimal. Antibiotics are used at the surgeon's discretion.

Liposuction. Liposuction is a technique for removing sub-cutaneous fat to improve facial and body contours. Although not a substitute for diet and exercise, it can be successful in removing areas of fat from virtually any body area that is resistant to other techniques.

Liposuction is relatively free of complications, but possible contraindications include use of anticoagulants, uncontrolled hypertension, diabetes mellitus, and poor cardiovascular status. Persons under 40 years of age with good skin elasticity are the best candidates. However, patients ranging in age from 16 to 70 years can be treated successfully.

The procedure is usually performed on an outpatient basis with the aid of local anesthesia. One or more sessions may be necessary, depending on the size of the area to be treated. A blunt-tipped cannula is inserted through a 0.5-in incision and pushed into the fat to break it loose from the fibrous stroma. Multiple repeated thrusts disrupt the fat and create tunnels. The loosened fat is removed with a powerful suction. The incision sites are taped because firm, absorbent bandaging reduces the amount of postoperative bleeding and fluid accumulation.[18] Bandaging also helps to contour the skin. It may take several months for the final results to be evident.

NURSING MANAGEMENT
COSMETIC SURGERY

Many cosmetic surgical procedures are performed in well-equipped day-surgery units or in dermatology surgeons' or plastic surgeons' office surgery suites.

Role of Registered Nurse (RN)
- Assess patient's skin for acute and chronic integumentary problems.
- Assess patient's risk factors for integumentary problems.
- Document skin condition and risk factor assessment, and develop a plan of care.
- Determine whether patient is taking drugs that increase photosensitivity.
- Teach about risks associated with sun exposure and methods for decreasing exposure to the sun.
- Teach about therapies that are used for integumentary disorders, including dressings, baths, and oral or topical medications used on an outpatient basis.
- Evaluate treatment for effectiveness and any adverse effects.

Role of Licensed Practical/Vocational Nurse (LPN/LVN)
- Administer prescribed therapies such as dressings and oral or topical medications.
- Monitor the skin for changes in appearance or texture that may indicate worsening of integumentary problem or adverse reactions to treatment.
- Reinforce teaching done by the RN.

Role of Unlicensed Assistive Personnel (UAP)
- Assist patient with bathing.
- Apply wet dressings to skin or add medications (such as oilated oatmeal) to patient baths (consider state nurse practice act and agency policy).
- Report changes in skin appearance or patient complaints of discomfort to the RN.

PREOPERATIVE MANAGEMENT

A major preoperative management consideration relates to informed consent and realistic expectations of what cosmetic surgery can accomplish. Although the surgeon should provide this information, reinforce it and answer questions and concerns. For instance, a face-lift has little or no effect on deep wrinkling of the forehead and temples, deep nasolabial grooves, or vertical lip wrinkles. Before-and-after treatment photographs of similar cases are often useful in helping the patient to set realistic expectations.

Your teaching plan should include patient understanding of the timeframe for healing. Because wound healing may not be complete for 1 year, immediate, complete results should not be anticipated. Explain the oozing, crusting stage of the abrasive procedure so the patient can plan time off from work if necessary. The final results of the cosmetic procedure are affected by the patient's age, general state of health, and skin type and the extent (severity) of the condition being treated. If a health problem is present, efforts should be made to correct or control the problem before the procedure is performed.

POSTOPERATIVE MANAGEMENT

Most cosmetic procedures are not extremely painful. Usually mild analgesics are sufficient to keep the patient comfortable.

Although infection is not a common problem after cosmetic surgery, assess the surgical sites for signs of infection. Inform the patient of the signs and symptoms of infection with instructions to report them immediately so that appropriate antibiotic intervention can be started.

If the surgery involved an alteration in the circulation to the skin, as in a face-lift, carefully monitor for adequate circulation.

Warm, pink skin that blanches on pressure indicates that adequate circulation is present in the surgical area. Supportive, compressive dressings and ice packs may be necessary early in the postoperative period.

SKIN GRAFTS

Uses

Skin grafts may be necessary to protect underlying structures or to reconstruct areas for cosmetic or functional purposes. Ideally, wounds heal by primary intention. However, large wounds, surgically created wounds, trauma, and chronic wounds can cause extensive tissue destruction, making primary intention healing impossible. In these cases, skin grafting may be necessary to close the defect. Improved surgical techniques make it possible to graft skin, bone, cartilage, fat, fascia, muscles, and nerves. For cosmetically pleasing results, the color, thickness, texture, and hair-growing nature of skin used for grafting must be chosen to match the recipient site. (Skin grafting is also discussed in Chapter 25.)

Types

The two types of skin grafts are free grafts and skin flaps. Free grafts are further classified according to the method of providing a blood supply to the grafted skin. One method is to transfer the graft (epidermis and part or all of the dermis) to the recipient site from the donor site. If the graft is an *autograft* (from the patient's own body) or an *isograft* (from an identical twin), it will revascularize and become fixed to the new site. Chapter 25 discusses full- and split-thickness skin grafts. Another method of free skin grafting is by *reconstructive*

microsurgery. With the use of an operating microscope, circulation is immediately established in the free flap by anastomosis of the blood vessels from the skin flap to the vessels in the recipient site.

Skin flaps involve moving a section of skin and subcutaneous tissue from one part of the body to another without terminating the vascular attachment.[19] The vascular attachment is called a *pedicle.* Skin flaps are used to cover wounds with a poor vascular bed, to provide padding when needed, and to cover wounds over cartilage and bone. The patient may need intermediate flap placement if the recipient site is far removed from the donor site. For instance, a skin flap from the thigh to the head would require an intermediate graft. The flap is advanced to the recipient site when circulation is well established at the intermediate site. The type of flap and the route of transfer are determined according to the patient's needs and the defect being repaired.

Soft tissue expansion is a technique for providing skin for resurfacing of a defect, such as a burn scar; for removal of a disfiguring mark (e.g., a tattoo); or as a preliminary step in breast reconstruction. A subcutaneous tissue expander of an appropriate size and shape is placed under the skin, usually as an outpatient procedure. Weekly expansion with saline solution can be done in a health care setting or by the patient at home. This expansion procedure is repeated until the skin reaches the size needed for the repair. This may take from several weeks to 3 to 4 months. Once sufficient skin is available, the old incision is opened, the expander is removed, and the soft tissue is ready to be used as an advancement flap. The tissue expander next to a defect retains the primary tissue characteristics such as color and texture.

CASE STUDY
Malignant Melanoma and Dysplastic Nevi

Hemera/Thinkstock

Patient Profile
G.L. is a 59-year-old white fair-skinned man who is a long-distance truck driver. In his leisure time, he enjoys swimming. He comes to the clinic for evaluation of a changing lesion on his left arm.

Subjective Data
- History of a basal cell carcinoma (BCC) on his left ear in the last 4 years
- Father treated for metastatic malignant melanoma in the last 2 years
- First noted the lesion 5 months ago when it started changing size
- Anxious the lesion might have spread and require extensive, disfiguring surgery

Objective Data
Physical Examination
- Has a 4-mm lesion, dark brown, scalloped with vaguely defined borders
- Four dysplastic nevi found on back

Diagnostic Studies
- Excisional biopsy confirmed malignant melanoma.
- Sentinel node biopsy results were negative.
- Diagnostic tests indicate melanoma stage I.

Discussion Questions
1. What risk factors for malignant melanoma does he have?
2. What are the usual clinical manifestations associated with malignant melanoma?
3. What is the prognosis for a patient with this stage of malignant melanoma?
4. What treatment options are available for him?
5. How would you help G.L. deal with his anxiety over the treatment outcomes?
6. *Priority Decision:* What is the priority of care for G.L.?
7. What would you include in his patient teaching plan to address future sun exposure?
8. *Delegation Decision:* Which of the following nursing personnel should be responsible for teaching G.L.: RN, LPN/LVN, or UAP?
9. *Priority Decision:* Based on the assessment data presented, what are the priority nursing diagnoses? Are there any collaborative problems?
10. *Evidence-Based Practice:* G.L. wants to know whether regularly applying sunscreen will reduce his risk for developing a second melanoma. How would you reply?

BRIDGE TO NCLEX EXAMINATION

The number of the question corresponds to the same-numbered outcome at the beginning of the chapter.

1. Which safe sun practices would the nurse include in the teaching care plan for a patient who has photosensitivity *(select all that apply)*?
   a. Wear protective clothing.
   b. Apply sunscreen liberally and often.
   c. Emphasize the short-term use of a tanning booth.
   d. Avoid exposure to the sun, especially during midday.
   e. Wear any sunscreen as long as it is purchased at a drugstore.

2. In teaching a patient who is using topical corticosteroids to treat acute dermatitis, the nurse should tell the patient that *(select all that apply)*
   a. the cream form is the most efficient system of delivery.
   b. short-term use of topical corticosteroids usually does not cause systemic side effects.
   c. creams and ointments should be applied with a glove in small amounts to prevent further infection.
   d. abruptly discontinuing the use of topical corticosteroids may cause a reappearance of the dermatitis.
   e. systemic side effects may be experienced from topical corticosteroids if the person is malnourished.

3. A patient with acne vulgaris tells the nurse that she has quit her job as a receptionist because she believes her facial appearance is unattractive to customers. The nursing diagnosis that best describes this patient response is
   a. ineffective coping related to lack of social support.
   b. impaired skin integrity related to presence of lesions.
   c. anxiety related to lack of knowledge of the disease process.
   d. social isolation related to decreased activities secondary to fear of rejection.

4. In teaching a patient with malignant melanoma about this disorder, the nurse recognizes that the patient's prognosis is most dependent on
   a. the thickness of the lesion.
   b. the degree of asymmetry in the lesion.
   c. the amount of ulceration in the lesion.
   d. how much the lesion has spread superficially.

5. The nurse determines that a patient with a diagnosis of which disorder is most at risk for spreading the disease?
   a. Tinea pedis
   b. Impetigo on the face
   c. Candidiasis of the nails
   d. Psoriasis on the palms and soles

6. A mother and her two children have been diagnosed with pediculosis corporis at a health care center. An appropriate measure in treating this condition is
   a. applying pyrethrins to the body.
   b. topical application of griseofulvin.
   c. moist compresses applied frequently.
   d. administration of systemic antibiotics.

7. A common site for the lesions associated with atopic dermatitis is the
   a. buttocks.
   b. temporal area.
   c. antecubital space.
   d. plantar surface of the feet.

8. During the assessment of a patient, you note an area of red, sharply defined plaques covered with silvery scales that are mildly itchy on the patient's knees and elbows. You recognize this finding as
   a. lentigo.
   b. psoriasis.
   c. actinic keratosis.
   d. seborrheic keratosis.

9. Dermatologic manifestation(s) of Addison's disease can include *(select all that apply)*
   a. urticaria.
   b. loss of body hair.
   c. increased sweating.
   d. generalized hyperpigmentation.
   e. hypopigmentation in the legs and trunk.

10. Important patient teaching after a chemical peel includes
    a. avoidance of sun exposure.
    b. application of firm bandages.
    c. limitation of vigorous exercise.
    d. use of moist heat to relieve discomfort.

1. a, b, d. 2. b, d. 3. d. 4. a. 5. b. 6. a. 7. c. 8. b. 9. b, d. 10. a

⊖volve

For rationales to these answers and even more NCLEX review questions, visit *http://evolve.elsevier.com/Lewis/medsurg*.

REFERENCES

1. Lim HW, James WD, Rigel D, et al: Adverse effects of ultraviolet radiation from the use of indoor tanning equipment: time to ban the tan, *J Am Acad Dermatol* 64:e51, 2011.
2. US Food and Drug Administration: FDA announces changes to better inform consumers about sunscreen. Retrieved from *www.fda.gov/NewsEvents/Newsroom/PressAnnouncements/ucm258940.htm*.
*3. Green A, Williams G, Logan V, et al: Reduced melanoma after regular sunscreen use: randomized trial follow-up, *J Clin Oncol* 29:257, 2010.

4. American Cancer Society: *Cancer facts and figures* 2011, Atlanta, American Cancer Society. Retrieved from *www.cancer.org*.
5. Rigel D, Russak J, Friedman R: The evolution of melanoma diagnosis: 25 years beyond the ABCDs, *CA-Cancer J Clin* 60:301, 2010.
6. Madan V, Lear J, Szeimies R: Non-melanoma skin cancer, *Lancet* 375:673, 2010.
7. Miller SJ, Alam M, Andersen J, et al: Basal cell and squamous cell skin cancers, *J Natl Compr Cancer Network* 8:836, 2010.
8. Pfenninger J: Approach to various lesions. In Pfenninger J, Fowler G, editors: *Pfenninger and Fowler's procedures for primary care*, ed 3, St Louis, 2010, Saunders.
9. US Food and Drug Administration: FDA approves new treatment for a type of late-stage skin cancer. Retrieved from

*Evidence-based information for clinical practice.

www.fda.gov/newsevents/newsroom/pressannouncements/ ucm1193237.htm.

10. Gould D: Diagnosis, prevention and treatment of fungal infections, *Nurs Stand* 33:38, 2011.
11. National Psoriasis Foundation: About psoriasis. Retrieved from *www.psoriasis/org/about.*
12. Agostinis O, Berg K, Cengel K, et al: Photodynamic therapy of cancer, *CA-Cancer J Clin* 61:250, 2011.
13. Hulyalkar R, Rakkhit T, Garcia-Zuazaga J: The role of radiation therapy in the management of skin cancers, *Dermatol Clin* 29:287, 2011.
14. Saunders nursing drug handbook 2012, St Louis, 2012, Mosby.
15. Pfenninger J: Skin biopsy. In Pfenninger J, Fowler G, editors: *Pfenninger and Fowler's procedures for primary care*, ed 3, St Louis, 2010, Saunders.
16. Karim K: Diagnosis, treatment and management of pruritus, *Br J Nurs* 20:356, 2011.
17. Goel A, Krupashankar D, Aurangabadkar S, et al: Fractional lasers in dermatology: current status and recommendations, *Indian J Dermatol Venereol Leprol* 77:369, 2011.
18. Pelosi M, Pelosi M: Liposuction, *Obstet Gynecol Clin* 37:507, 2010.
19. Zhang A, Meine J: Flaps and grafts reconstruction, *Dermatol Clin* 29:217, 2011.

RESOURCES

AcneNet
www.skincarephysicians.com/acnenet
American Academy of Cosmetic Surgery
www.cosmeticsurgery.org
American Academy of Dermatology
www.aad.org
American Academy of Facial Plastic and Reconstructive Surgery
www.aafprs.org
American Society of Plastic Surgical Nurses
https://aspsn.org
Dermatology Foundation
www.dermfnd.org
Dermatology Nurses' Association
www.dnanurse.org
National Institute of Arthritis and Musculoskeletal and Skin Diseases, National Institutes of Health
www.niams.nih.gov
National Psoriasis Foundation
www.psoriasis.org
Skin Cancer Foundation
www.skincancer.org

Holding onto anger is like grasping onto a hot coal with the intent of throwing it at someone else. You are the one who gets burned.
Gautama Buddha

Nursing Management

Burns

Judy Knighton

evolve WEBSITE

http://evolve.elsevier.com/Lewis/medsurg

- NCLEX Review Questions
- Key Points
- Pre-Test
- Answer Guidelines for Case Study on p. 470

- Rationales for Bridge to NCLEX Examination Questions
- Case Study
  - Patient With Burns
- Nursing Care Plan (Customizable)
  - eNCP 25-1: Patient With a Thermal Burn Injury

- Concept Map Creator
- Glossary
- Content Updates

eFigure
- eFig. 25-1: Foot contractures

LEARNING OUTCOMES

1. Relate the causes of and prevention strategies for burn injuries.
2. Differentiate between partial-thickness and full-thickness burns.
3. Apply the tools used to determine the severity of burns.
4. Compare the pathophysiology, clinical manifestations, complications, and collaborative management throughout the three burn phases.
5. Compare the fluid and electrolyte shifts during the emergent and acute burn phases.
6. Differentiate the nutritional needs of the burn patient throughout the three burn phases.
7. Compare the various burn wound care techniques and surgical options for partial-thickness versus full-thickness burn wounds.
8. Prioritize nursing interventions in the management of the burn patient's physiologic and psychosocial needs.
9. Examine the various physiologic and psychosocial aspects of burn rehabilitation.
10. Design a plan of care to prepare the burn patient and caregiver for discharge.

KEY TERMS

burn, p. 450
carboxyhemoglobin, p. 452
chemical burns, p. 451
contracture, p. 468
cultured epithelial autograft (CEA), p. 466

debridement, p. 461
electrical burns, p. 452
escharotomy, p. 458
excision and grafting, p. 465

full-thickness burns, p. 453
partial-thickness burns, p. 453
smoke and inhalation injuries, p. 451
thermal burns, p. 451

The focus of this chapter is the care of patients who have experienced a burn. A **burn** is an injury to the tissues of the body caused by heat, chemicals, electric current, or radiation. The resulting effects are influenced by the temperature of the burning agent, duration of contact time, and type of tissue that is injured.

An estimated 450,000 Americans seek medical care each year for burns.[1,2] Approximately 45,000 people are hospitalized, one half of whom require care in specialized burn centers. About 3500 Americans die annually as a direct result of their injuries. The highest fatality rates occur in children ages 4 years and younger and adults over age 65. Around the world, nearly 11 million people need medical attention annually for burn injuries, and about 300,000 die.[3]

Although burn incidence has decreased over the past 20 years, burn injuries still occur too frequently and mainly to people at a lower socioeconomic level. Most burn incidents should be viewed as preventable. Today, the focus of burn prevention programs has shifted from blaming individuals and changing behaviors to making legislative changes and collecting global burn data to address the unique prevention needs of developing countries.[4]

Coordinated national programs in developed countries have focused on child-resistant lighters, nonflammable children's clothing, tap water anti-scald devices, fire-safe cigarettes, stricter building codes, hardwired smoke detectors and alarms, and fire sprinklers. As a nurse, you can advocate for burn risk reduction strategies in the home and at work, and

Reviewed by Cecilia M. Bidigare, RN, MSN, Associate Professor of Nursing, Sinclair Community College, Beavercreek, Ohio; and Patricia S. Regojo, RN, MSN, Nurse Manager, Burn Center, Temple University Hospital, Philadelphia, Pennsylvania.

TABLE 25-1 SOURCES OF BURN INJURY*

Home Hazards

Kitchen and Bathroom
- Microwaved food
- Steam, hot grease or liquids from cooking
- Hot water heaters set at 140° F (60° C) or higher

General Household
- Fireplaces (e.g., gas, wood)
- Open space heaters
- Radiators (e.g., home, automobile)
- Outdoor grills (e.g., propane, charcoal)
- Frayed or defective wiring
- Multiple extension cords per outlet
- Flammables (e.g., starter fluid, gasoline, kerosene)
- Carelessness with cigarettes, matches, candles

Occupational Hazards
- Tar
- Chemicals
- Hot metals
- Steam pipes
- Combustible fuels
- Fertilizers, pesticides
- Electricity from power lines
- Sparks from live electric sources

*List is not all-inclusive.

TABLE 25-2 STRATEGIES TO REDUCE BURN INJURY

Flame or Contact
- Never leave candles unattended or near open windows or curtains.
- Use "child-resistant" lighters.
- Hold regular home fire exit drills.
- Never use gasoline or other flammable liquids to start a fire.
- Never leave hot oil unattended while cooking.
- Never smoke in bed.
- Consider a flame-retardant smoking apron for older or "at-risk" people.
- Exercise caution when microwaving food and beverages.

Scald
- Lower hot water temperature to the "lowest point" or 120° F (40° C).
- Use "anti-scald" devices with showerhead or faucet fixtures.
- Supervise bathing with small children, older adults, or anyone with impaired physical movement, physical sensation, or judgment.
- After running bath water, check temperature with back of hand or bath thermometer.

Inhalation
- Install smoke and carbon monoxide detectors.

Chemical
- Store chemicals safely in approved containers and label clearly.
- Ensure safety of workers and students handling chemicals (education, protective eyewear, gloves, masks, clothing).

Electrical
- Avoid or repair frayed wiring.
- Ensure electrical power source is shut off before beginning repairs.
- Wear protective eyewear and gloves when making electrical repairs.
- Avoid outdoor activities during electrical (i.e., lightning) storms.

you can teach workers to reduce burn injuries in both settings (Tables 25-1 and 25-2).

TYPES OF BURN INJURY

Thermal Burns

Thermal burns, caused by flame, flash, scald, or contact with hot objects, are the most common type of burn injury (Fig. 25-1). The severity of the injury depends on the temperature of

FIG. 25-1 Types of burn injury. **A,** Partial-thickness thermal hand burn. **B,** Full-thickness thermal hand burn. **C,** Full-thickness scald burn to the buttock and lower back secondary to immersion in hot water.

the burning agent and the duration of contact time. Scald injuries can occur in the bathroom or while cooking. Flash, flame, or contact burns can occur while cooking, smoking, burning leaves in the backyard, or using gasoline or hot oil.

Chemical Burns

Chemical burns are the result of contact with acids, alkalis, and organic compounds. In addition to tissue damage, eyes can be injured if they are splashed with the chemical. Acids are found in the home and at work and include hydrochloric, oxalic, and hydrofluoric acid. Alkali burns can be more difficult to manage than acid burns, since alkalis adhere to tissue, causing protein hydrolysis and liquefaction. Alkalis are found in oven and drain cleaners, fertilizers, and heavy industrial cleansers. Organic compounds, including phenols (chemical disinfectants) and petroleum products (creosote and gasoline), produce contact burns and systemic toxicity.

Smoke and Inhalation Injury

Smoke and inhalation injuries from breathing hot air or noxious chemicals can cause damage to the respiratory tract. Three types of smoke and inhalation injuries can occur: metabolic asphyxiation, upper airway injury, and lower airway injury. Because smoke inhalation injuries are a major predictor of mortality in burn patients, rapid assessment is critical.[5]

TABLE 25-3	MANIFESTATIONS OF LUNG INJURY ASSOCIATED WITH BURNS
Upper Airway	**Lower Airway**
• Blisters, edema • Hoarseness • Difficulty swallowing • Copious secretions • Stridor • Substernal and intercostal retractions • Total airway obstruction	• High degree of suspicion if patient was trapped in a fire in an enclosed space or clothing caught fire • Presence of facial burns or singed nasal or facial hair • Dyspnea • Carbonaceous sputum • Wheezing • Hoarseness • Altered mental status

Metabolic Asphyxiation. The majority of deaths at a fire scene are the result of inhaling certain smoke elements, primarily carbon monoxide (CO) or hydrogen cyanide. Oxygen delivery to or consumption by tissues is impaired. The result is hypoxia and, ultimately, death when **carboxyhemoglobin** (i.e., hemoglobin combined with CO) blood levels are greater than 20%. CO and hydrogen cyanide poisoning may occur in the absence of burn injury to the skin.

Upper Airway Injury. Upper airway injury results from an inhalation injury to the mouth, oropharynx, and/or larynx. The injury may be caused by thermal burns or the inhalation of hot air, steam, or smoke. Mucosal burns of the oropharynx and the larynx are manifested by redness, blistering, and edema (Table 25-3). The swelling can be massive and the onset rapid. Flame burns to the neck and the chest may make breathing more difficult because of the burn eschar, which becomes tight and constricting from the underlying edema. Swelling from scald burns to the face and the neck can also be lethal, as can external pressure from edema pressing on the airway. Mechanical obstruction can occur quickly, presenting a true medical emergency.

Carefully assess the patient for facial burns, singed nasal hair, hoarseness, painful swallowing, darkened oral and nasal membranes, carbonaceous sputum, history of being burned in an enclosed space, and clothing burns around the chest and neck.

Lower Airway Injury. An inhalation injury to the trachea, bronchioles, and alveoli is usually caused by breathing in toxic chemicals or smoke. Tissue damage is related to the duration of exposure to toxic fumes or smoke. Clinical manifestations of lower airway lung injury are presented in Table 25-3. Pulmonary edema may not appear until 12 to 24 hours after the burn, and then it may manifest as acute respiratory distress syndrome (ARDS) (see Chapter 68).

Electrical Burns

Electrical burns result from intense heat generated from an electric current. Direct damage to nerves and vessels, causing tissue anoxia and death, can also occur. The severity of the electrical injury depends on the amount of voltage, tissue resistance, current pathways, surface area in contact with the current, and length of time that the current flow was sustained (Fig. 25-2). Tissue densities offer various amounts of resistance to electric current. For example, fat and bone offer the most resistance, whereas nerves and blood vessels offer the least resistance. Current that passes through vital organs (e.g., brain, heart, kidneys) produces more life-threatening sequelae than

FIG. 25-2 Electrical injury produces heat coagulation of blood supply and contact area as electric current passes through the skin. **A,** Back and buttock (arrows). **B,** Leg (arrow).

that which passes through other tissues. In addition, electric sparks may ignite the patient's clothing, causing a flash injury.

As with inhalation injury, perform a rapid assessment of the patient with electrical injury. Transfer to a burn center is indicated. The severity of an electrical injury can be difficult to determine, since most of the damage is below the skin (known as the *iceberg effect*). Determination of electric current contact points and history of the injury may help determine the probable path of the current and potential areas of injury. Contact with electric current can cause muscle contractions strong enough to fracture the long bones and vertebrae. Another reason to suspect long bone or spinal fractures is a fall resulting from the electrical injury. For this reason, all patients with electrical burns should be considered at risk for a potential cervical spine injury. Cervical spine immobilization must be used during transport and subsequent diagnostic testing completed to rule out any injury.

Electrical injury puts the patient at risk for dysrhythmias or cardiac arrest, severe metabolic acidosis, and myoglobinuria. The electric shock event can cause immediate cardiac standstill or ventricular fibrillation. Delayed cardiac dysrhythmias or arrest may also occur without warning during the first 24 hours after injury. Myoglobin from injured muscle tissue and hemoglobin from damaged red blood cells (RBCs) are released into the circulation whenever massive muscle and blood vessel damage occurs. The released myoglobin pigments travel to the kidneys and can block the renal tubules, which can result in acute tubular necrosis (ATN) and acute kidney injury (see Chapter 47).

Cold Thermal Injury

Cold thermal injury, or frostbite, is discussed in Chapter 69.

TABLE 25-4   BURN CENTER REFERRAL CRITERIA

Burn injuries that should be referred to a burn center include the following:

1. Partial-thickness burns >10% of total body surface area (TBSA).
2. Burns that involve the face, hands, feet, genitalia, perineum, or major joints.
3. Third-degree burns in any age-group.
4. Electrical burns, including lightning injury.
5. Chemical burns.
6. Inhalation injury.
7. Burn injury in patients with preexisting medical disorders that could complicate management, prolong recovery, or affect mortality risk (e.g., heart or kidney disease).
8. Any patients with burns and concomitant trauma (e.g., fractures) in which the burn injury poses the greatest risk of morbidity or mortality. In such cases, if the trauma poses the greater immediate risk, the patient may be initially stabilized in a trauma center before being transferred to a burn center. The health care provider will need to use his or her judgment, in consultation with the regional medical control plan and triage protocols.
9. Burn injury in children in hospitals without qualified personnel or equipment needed to care for them.
10. Burn injury in patients who will require special social, emotional, or long-term rehabilitative intervention.

Source: Guidelines for the operation of burn centers. In American College of Surgeons, Committee on Trauma: Resources for optimal care of the injured patient, 2006. Retrieved from *www.ameriburn.org/Chapter14.pdf*.

CLASSIFICATION OF BURN INJURY

The treatment of burns is related to the severity of the injury.[6] Severity is determined by (1) depth of burn, (2) extent of burn calculated in percent of total body surface area (TBSA), (3) location of burn, and (4) patient risk factors (e.g., age, past medical history). The American Burn Association (ABA) has established referral criteria to determine which burn injuries should be treated in burn centers with specialized facilities (Table 25-4). The majority of patients with minor burn injuries can be managed in community hospitals.[7]

Depth of Burn

Burn injury involves the destruction of the integumentary system. The skin is divided into three layers: epidermis, dermis, and subcutaneous tissue (Fig. 25-3). The *epidermis*, or nonvascular protective outer layer of the skin, is approximately as thick as a sheet of paper. (The structure and function of the skin are discussed in Chapter 23.)

The *dermis*, which lies below the epidermis, is approximately 30 to 45 times thicker than the epidermis. The dermis contains connective tissues with blood vessels, hair follicles, nerve endings, sweat glands, and sebaceous glands.

Under the dermis lies the *subcutaneous tissue,* which contains major vascular networks, fat, nerves, and lymphatics. The subcutaneous tissue acts as a heat insulator for underlying structures, including muscles, tendons, bones, and internal organs.

Burns continue to be defined by degrees: first, second, third, and fourth degree. The ABA recommends a more precise definition and classifies burns according to depth of skin destruction: **partial-thickness burns** and **full-thickness burns** (see Fig. 25-3). Skin-reproducing (re-epithelializing) cells are located along the shafts of the hair follicles, sweat glands, and oil glands.

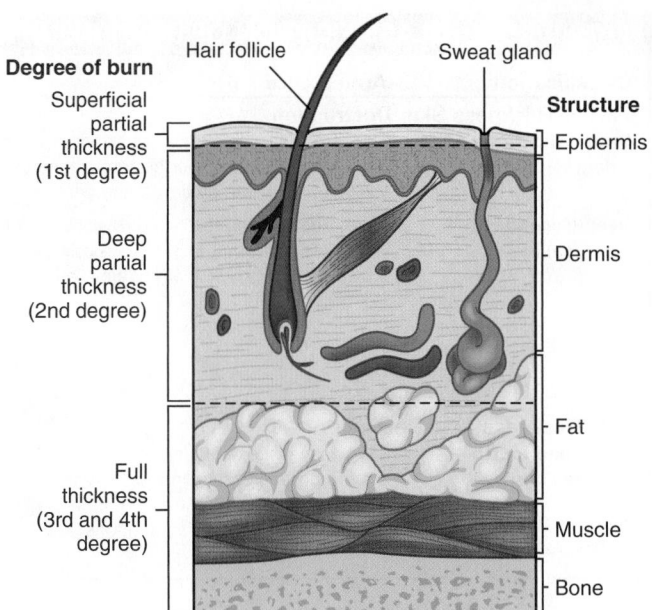

FIG. 25-3 Cross section of skin indicating the depth of burn and structures involved.

If significant damage occurs to the dermis (i.e., a full-thickness burn), not enough skin cells remain to regenerate new skin. A permanent, alternative source of skin needs to be found. Table 25-5 compares the various burn classifications according to the depth of injury.

Extent of Burn

Two commonly used guides for determining the TBSA affected or the extent of a burn wound are the *Lund-Browder chart* (Fig. 25-4, *A*) and the *Rule of Nines* (Fig. 25-4, *B*). (First-degree burns, equivalent to a sunburn, are not included when calculating TBSA.) The Lund-Browder chart is considered more accurate because it considers the patient's age in proportion to relative body-area size. The Rule of Nines is often used for initial assessment of a burn patient because it is easy to remember. For irregular- or odd-shaped burns, the patient's hand (including the fingers) is approximately 1% TBSA. The *Sage Burn Diagram* is a free, Internet-based tool for estimating TBSA burned (*www.sagediagram.com*).

Location of Burn

The severity of the burn injury is also determined by the location of the burn wound. Burns to the face and neck and circumferential burns to the chest or back may interfere with breathing as a result of mechanical obstruction from edema or leathery, devitalized burn tissue *(eschar).* These burns may also indicate possible inhalation injury and respiratory mucosal damage.

Burns to the hands, feet, joints, and eyes are of concern because they make self-care difficult and may jeopardize future function. Burns to the hands and feet are challenging to manage because of superficial vascular and nerve supply systems that need to be protected while the burn wounds are healing.

Burns to the ears and the nose are susceptible to infection because of poor blood supply to the cartilage. Burns to the buttocks or perineum are highly susceptible to infection from urine or feces contamination. Circumferential burns to the extremi-

TABLE 25-5	CLASSIFICATION OF BURN INJURY DEPTH		
Classification	**Appearance**	**Possible Cause**	**Structures Involved**
Partial-Thickness Skin Destruction			
Superficial (first-degree) burn	Erythema, blanching on pressure, pain and mild swelling, no vesicles or blisters (although after 24 hr skin may blister and peel).	Superficial sunburn Quick heat flash	Superficial epidermal damage with hyperemia. Tactile and pain sensation intact.
Deep (second-degree) burn	Fluid-filled vesicles that are red, shiny, wet (if vesicles have ruptured). Severe pain caused by nerve injury. Mild to moderate edema.	Flame Flash Scald Contact burns Chemical Tar Electric current	Epidermis and dermis involved to varying depths. Skin elements, from which epithelial regeneration occurs, remain viable.
Full-Thickness Skin Destruction			
Third- and fourth-degree burns	Dry, waxy white, leathery, or hard skin; visible thrombosed vessels. Insensitivity to pain because of nerve destruction. Possible involvement of muscles, tendons, and bones.	Flame Scald Chemical Tar Electric current	All skin elements and local nerve endings destroyed. Coagulation necrosis present. Surgical intervention required for healing.

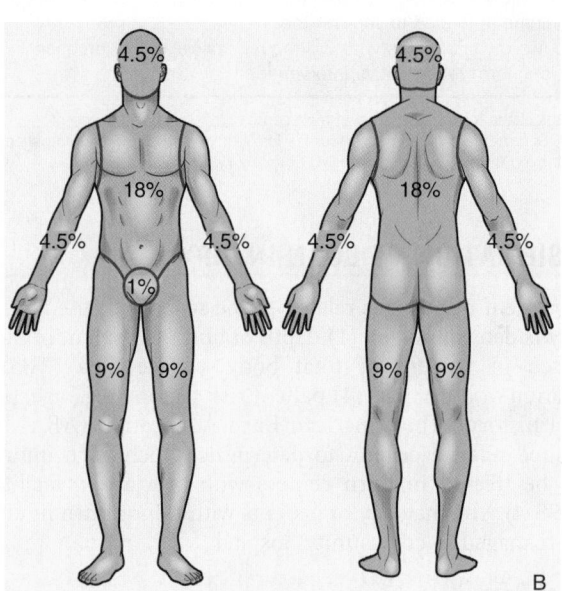

FIG. 25-4 A, Lund-Browder chart. By convention, areas of partial-thickness injury are colored in blue and areas of full-thickness injury in red. Superficial partial-thickness burns are not calculated. **B,** Rule of Nines chart.

ties can cause circulation problems distal to the burn, with possible nerve damage to the affected extremity. Patients may also develop compartment syndrome (see Chapter 63) from direct heat damage to the muscles, swelling, and/or preburn vascular problems.

Patient Risk Factors

Any patient with preexisting cardiovascular, respiratory, or renal disease has a poorer prognosis for recovery because of the tremendous demands placed on the body by a burn injury. The patient with diabetes mellitus or peripheral vascular disease is at high risk for poor healing, especially with foot and leg burns.[8] General physical debilitation from any chronic disease, including alcoholism, drug abuse, or malnutrition, makes it challenging for the patient to fully recover from a burn injury. In addition, the burn patient who has also sustained fractures, head injuries, or other trauma has a more difficult time recovering.

PHASES OF BURN MANAGEMENT

Burn management can be organized chronologically into three phases: emergent (resuscitative), acute (wound healing), and rehabilitative (restorative). Overlap in care does exist. For example, the emergent phase begins at the time of the burn injury, and care often begins in the prehospital phase, depending on the skill level of providers at the scene. Planning for rehabilitation begins on the day of the burn injury or admission to the burn center. Formal rehabilitation begins as soon as functional assessments can be performed. Wound care is the primary focus of the acute phase, but wound care also takes place in both the emergent and rehabilitation phases.

PREHOSPITAL CARE

At the scene of the injury, priority is given to removing the person from the source of the burn and stopping the burning

✚ TABLE 25-6   EMERGENCY MANAGEMENT

Thermal Burns

Etiology	Assessment Findings	Interventions
• Hot liquids or solids • Flash flame • Open flame • Steam • Hot surface • Ultraviolet rays	***Partial-Thickness (superficial; first-degree) Burn*** • Redness • Pain • Moderate to severe tenderness • Minimal edema • Blanching with pressure ***Partial-Thickness (deep; second-degree) Burn*** • Moist blebs, blisters • Mottled white, pink to cherry-red • Hypersensitive to touch or air • Moderate to severe pain • Blanching with pressure ***Full-Thickness (third- and fourth-degree) Burns*** • Dry, leathery eschar • Waxy white, dark brown, or charred appearance • Strong burn odor • Impaired sensation when touched • Absence of pain with severe pain in surrounding tissues • Lack of blanching with pressure	**Initial** • Assess airway, breathing, and circulation. • Stabilize cervical spine. • Assess for inhalation injury. • Provide supplemental O_2 as needed. • Anticipate endotracheal intubation and mechanical ventilation with circumferential full-thickness burns to the neck and chest or large TBSA burn. • Monitor vital signs, level of consciousness, respiratory status, O_2 saturation, and heart rhythm. • Remove nonadherent clothing, shoes, watches, jewelry, glasses or contact lenses (if face was exposed). • Cover burned areas with dry dressings or clean sheet. • Establish IV access with two large-bore catheters if burn >15% TBSA. • Begin fluid replacement. • Insert indwelling urinary catheter if burn >15% TBSA. • Elevate burned limbs above heart to decrease edema. • Administer IV analgesia and assess effectiveness frequently. • Identify and treat other associated injuries (e.g., fractures, head injury). **Ongoing Monitoring** • Monitor airway. • Monitor vital signs, heart rhythm, level of consciousness, respiratory status, and O_2 saturation. • Monitor urine output.

TBSA, Total body surface area.

process. Rescuers must also protect themselves from being injured. In the case of electrical and chemical injuries, initial management involves removal of the patient from contact with the electrical or chemical source.

Small thermal burns (10% or less of TBSA) should be covered with a clean, cool, tap water–dampened towel for the patient's comfort and protection until medical care is available.[9] Cooling of the injured area (if small) within 1 minute helps minimize the depth of the injury. If the burn is large (greater than 10% TBSA) or an electrical or inhalation burn is suspected, first focus your attention on the ABCs:

- *Airway:* Check for patency, soot around nares and on the tongue, singed nasal hair, darkened oral or nasal membranes.
- *Breathing:* Check for adequacy of ventilation.
- *Circulation:* Check for presence and regularity of pulses, and elevate the burned limb(s) above the heart to decrease pain and swelling.

To prevent hypothermia, cool large burns for no more than 10 minutes. Do not immerse the burned body part in cool water because it may cause extensive heat loss. Never cover a burn with ice, since this can cause hypothermia and vasoconstriction of blood vessels, thus further reducing blood flow to the injury. Gently remove as much burned clothing as possible to prevent further tissue damage. Leave adherent clothing in place until the patient is transferred to a hospital. Wrap the patient in a dry, clean sheet or blanket to prevent further contamination of the wound and to provide warmth.

Chemical burns are best treated by quickly removing any chemical particles or powder from the skin. Remove all clothing containing the chemical because the burning process continues while the chemical is in contact with the skin. Flush the affected area with copious amounts of water to irrigate the skin anywhere from 20 minutes to 2 hours postexposure. Tap water is acceptable for flushing eyes exposed to chemicals. Tissue destruction may continue for up to 72 hours after contact with some chemicals.

Observe patients with inhalation injuries closely for signs of respiratory distress. These patients need to be treated quickly and efficiently if they are to survive. If CO poisoning is suspected, treat the patient with 100% humidified O_2. Patients who have both body burns and an inhalation injury must be transferred to the nearest burn center.

Always remember that the burn patient may also have sustained other injuries that could take priority over the burn itself. Individuals involved in the prehospital phase of burn care must adequately communicate the circumstances of the injury to hospital providers. This is especially important when the patient's injury involves being trapped in a closed space, exposure to hazardous chemicals or electricity, or a possible traumatic injury (e.g., fall).

Prehospital care and emergency management are presented in tables that describe thermal burns (Table 25-6), inhalation injury (Table 25-7), electrical burns (Table 25-8), and chemical burns (Table 25-9).

EMERGENT PHASE

The *emergent (resuscitative) phase* is the time required to resolve the immediate, life-threatening problems resulting from the burn injury. This phase usually lasts up to 72 hours from the time the burn occurred. The primary concerns are the onset of hypovolemic shock and edema formation. The emergent phase ends when fluid mobilization and diuresis begin.

➕ TABLE 25-7 **EMERGENCY MANAGEMENT**

Inhalation Injury

Etiology	Assessment Findings	Interventions
• Exposure of respiratory tract to intense heat or flames • Inhalation of noxious chemicals, smoke, or CO	• History of being trapped in an enclosed space, being in an explosion, or having clothing catch fire • Rapid, shallow respirations • Increasing hoarseness • Coughing • Singed nasal or facial hair • Darkened oral or nasal membranes • Smoky breath • Carbonaceous sputum • Productive cough with black, gray, or bloody sputum • Irritation of upper airways or burning pain in throat or chest • Difficulty swallowing • Cherry-red skin color (CO levels >20%) • Restlessness, anxiety • Altered mental status, including confusion, coma • Decreased O_2 saturation • Dysrhythmias	**Initial** • Assess airway, breathing, and circulation. • Stabilize cervical spine. • Assess for thermal burn. • Provide 100% humidified O_2. • Anticipate endotracheal intubation and mechanical ventilation with significant inhalation injury. • Monitor vital signs, level of consciousness, O_2 saturation, and heart rhythm. • Remove nonadherent clothing, jewelry, glasses, or contact lenses (if face was exposed). • Establish IV access with two large-bore catheters if burn >15% TBSA. • Begin fluid replacement. • Insert indwelling urinary catheter if burn >15% TBSA. • Elevate burned limb(s) above heart to decrease edema. • Obtain arterial blood gas, carboxyhemoglobin levels, and chest x-ray. • Administer IV analgesia and assess effectiveness frequently. • Identify and treat other associated injuries (e.g., fractures, pneumothorax, head injury). • Cover burned areas with dry dressings or clean sheet. • Anticipate need for fiberoptic bronchoscopy or intubation. **Ongoing Monitoring** • Monitor airway. • Monitor vital signs, level of consciousness, respiratory status, O_2 saturation, and heart rhythm. • Monitor urine output.

CO, Carbon monoxide; *TBSA,* total body surface area.

➕ TABLE 25-8 **EMERGENCY MANAGEMENT**

Electrical Burns

Etiology	Assessment Findings	Interventions
Alternating Current • Electric wires • Utility wires **Direct Current** • Lightning • Defibrillator	• Leathery, white, or charred skin • Burn odor • Loss of consciousness • Impaired touch sensation • Minimal or absent pain • Dysrhythmias • Cardiac arrest • Location of contact points • Diminished peripheral circulation in injured extremity • Thermal burns if clothing ignites • Fractures or dislocations from force of current • Head or neck injury if fall occurred • Depth and extent of wound difficult to visualize. Assume injury greater than what is seen	**Initial** • Remove patient from electrical source while protecting rescuer. • Assess airway, breathing, and circulation. • Stabilize cervical spine. • Provide supplemental O_2 as needed. • Monitor vital signs, heart rhythm, level of consciousness, respiratory status, and O_2 saturation. • Check pulses distal to burns. • Remove nonadherent clothing, shoes, watches, jewelry, glasses or contact lenses (if face was exposed). • Cover burned areas with dry dressings or clean sheet. • Establish IV access with two large-bore catheters if burn >15% TBSA. • Begin fluid replacement. • Obtain arterial blood gas to assess acid-base balance. • Insert indwelling urinary catheter if burn >15% TBSA. • Elevate burned limb(s) above heart to decrease edema. • Administer IV analgesia and assess effectiveness frequently. • Identify and treat other associated injuries (e.g., fractures, head injury, thermal burns). **Ongoing Monitoring** • Monitor airway. • Monitor vital signs, heart rhythm, level of consciousness, respiratory status, O_2 saturation, and neurovascular status of injured limbs. • Monitor urine output. • Monitor urine for development of myoglobinuria secondary to muscle breakdown and hemoglobinuria secondary to RBC breakdown. • Anticipate possible administration of $NaHCO_3$ to alkalinize the urine and maintain serum pH >6.0.

$NaHCO_3$, Sodium bicarbonate; *TBSA,* total body surface area.

TABLE 25-9 EMERGENCY MANAGEMENT

Chemical Burns

Etiology	Assessment Findings	Interventions
• Acids • Alkalis • Organic compounds	• Burning • Redness, swelling of injured tissue • Degeneration of exposed tissue • Discoloration of injured skin • Localized pain • Edema of surrounding tissue • Tissue destruction continuing for up to 72 hr • Respiratory distress if chemical inhaled • Decreased muscle coordination (if organophosphate) • Paralysis	**Initial** • Assess airway, breathing, and circulation before decontamination procedures. • Stabilize cervical spine. • Provide supplemental O_2 as needed. • Brush dry chemical from skin before irrigation. • Remove nonadherent clothing, shoes, watches, jewelry, glasses or contact lenses (if face was exposed). • Flush chemical from wound and surrounding area with copious amounts of saline solution or water. • For chemical burn of the eye(s), flush from inner to outer corner of eye with water or lactated Ringer's (if available). • Cover burned areas with dry dressings or clean sheet. • Establish IV access with two large-bore catheters if burn >15% TBSA. • Begin fluid replacement. • Insert indwelling urinary catheter if burn >15% TBSA. • Elevate burned limb(s) above heart to decrease edema. • Administer IV analgesia and assess effectiveness frequently. • Contact poison control center for assistance. **Ongoing Monitoring** • Monitor airway if exposed to chemicals. • Monitor urine output. • Consider possibility of systemic impact of identified chemical, and monitor and treat accordingly. • Monitor pH of eye if exposed to chemicals.

TBSA, Total body surface area.

Pathophysiology

Fluid and Electrolyte Shifts. The greatest initial threat to a patient with a major burn is hypovolemic shock (Fig. 25-5). It is caused by a massive shift of fluids out of the blood vessels as a result of increased capillary permeability and can begin as early as 20 minutes postburn. As the capillary walls become more permeable, water, sodium, and plasma proteins (especially albumin) move into the interstitial spaces and other surrounding tissue. The colloidal osmotic pressure decreases with progressive loss of protein from the vascular space. This results in more fluid shifting out of the vascular space into the interstitial spaces (Fig. 25-6). Fluid accumulation in the interstitium is termed *second spacing.*

Fluid also moves to areas that normally have minimal to no fluid, a phenomenon termed *third spacing.* Examples of third spacing in burn injury are exudate and blister formation, as well as edema in nonburned areas.

Other sources of fluid loss are insensible losses by evaporation from large, denuded body surfaces and the respiratory system. The normal insensible loss of 30 to 50 mL/hr is increased in the severely burned patient. The net result of the fluid shifts and losses is termed *intravascular volume depletion.* Clinical signs of hypovolemic shock are decreased blood pressure (BP) and increased heart rate. If hypovolemic shock is not corrected, irreversible shock and death may result. (Shock is discussed in Chapter 67.)

The circulatory system is also affected by the hemolysis of RBCs from circulating factors (e.g., oxygen free radicals) released at the time of the burn, as well as by the direct insult of the burn injury. Thrombosis in the capillaries of burned tissue causes an additional loss of circulating RBCs. An elevated hematocrit is commonly caused by hemoconcentration resulting from fluid loss. After fluid balance has been restored, dilution causes the hematocrit levels to drop.

PATHOPHYSIOLOGY MAP

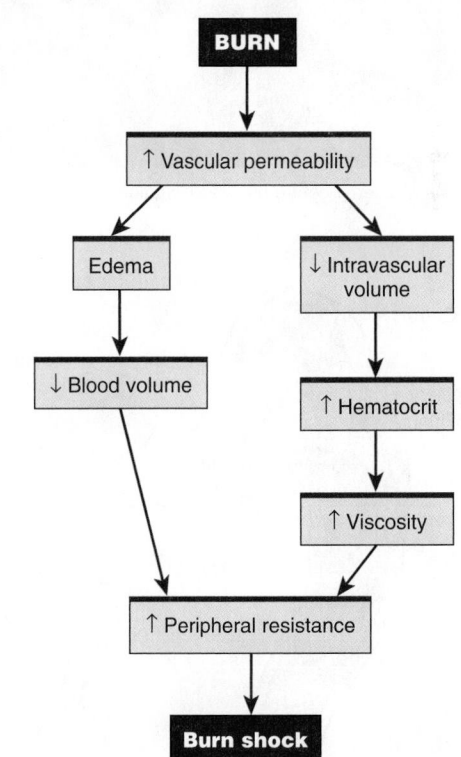

FIG. 25-5 At the time of major burn injury, there is increased capillary permeability. All fluid components of the blood begin to leak into the interstitium, causing edema and a decreased blood volume. Hematocrit increases, and the blood becomes more viscous. The combination of decreased blood volume and increased viscosity produces increased peripheral resistance. Burn shock, a type of hypovolemic shock, rapidly ensues and, if not corrected, can result in death.

Major electrolyte shifts of sodium and potassium also occur during this phase. Sodium rapidly moves to the interstitial spaces and remains there until edema formation ceases (Fig. 25-7). A potassium shift develops initially because injured cells and hemolyzed RBCs release potassium into the circulation.

Toward the end of the emergent phase, capillary membrane permeability is restored if fluid replacement is adequate. Fluid loss and edema formation end. Interstitial fluid gradually returns to the vascular space (see Fig. 25-7). Diuresis occurs, and the urine has a low specific gravity.

Inflammation and Healing. Burn injury to tissues and vessels causes coagulation necrosis. Neutrophils and monocytes accumulate at the site of injury. Fibroblasts and newly formed collagen fibrils appear and begin wound repair within the first 6 to 12 hours after injury. (The inflammatory response is discussed in Chapter 12.)

Immunologic Changes. The body's immune system is challenged when a burn injury occurs. The skin barrier to invading organisms is destroyed, bone marrow depression occurs, and circulating levels of immunoglobulins are decreased. Defects occur in the function of white blood cells (WBCs). The inflammatory cytokine cascade, triggered by tissue damage, impairs the function of lymphocytes, monocytes, and neutrophils. Thus the patient is at a greater risk for infection.

Clinical Manifestations

The patient with severe burns is likely to be in shock from hypovolemia. Frequently the areas of full-thickness and deep partial-thickness burns are initially anesthetic because the nerve endings have been destroyed. Superficial to moderate partial-thickness burns are very painful. Blisters, filled with fluid and protein, are common in partial-thickness burns. The patient with a larger burn area may develop a paralytic ileus, with absent or decreased bowel sounds. Shivering may occur as a result of chilling that is caused by heat loss, anxiety, or pain. The patient may be alert and able to answer questions shortly after admission or until he or she is intubated (if there is an inhalation injury). Patients are often frightened and benefit from your calm reassurances and simple explanations of what to expect as you provide care. Unconsciousness or altered mental status in a burn patient is usually not a result of the burn but of the hypoxia associated with smoke inhalation. Other possibilities include head trauma, substance abuse, or excessive amounts of sedation or pain medication.

Complications

The three major organ systems most susceptible to complications during the emergent phase of burn injury are the cardiovascular, respiratory, and urinary systems.

Cardiovascular System. Cardiovascular system complications include dysrhythmias and hypovolemic shock, which, if untreated, may progress to irreversible shock. Circulation to the extremities can be severely impaired by deep circumferential burns and subsequent edema formation, which act like a tourniquet. If untreated, ischemia, paresthesias, and necrosis can occur. An **escharotomy** (a scalpel or electrocautery incision through the full-thickness eschar) is frequently performed after transfer to a burn center to restore circulation to compromised extremities (Fig. 25-8). Initially, blood viscosity increases because of the fluid loss. Microcirculation is impaired because of the damage to skin structures that contain small capillary systems. These two events result in a phenomenon termed *sludging*. Sludging can be corrected by adequate fluid replacement.

FIG. 25-6 **A,** Facial edema before fluid resuscitation. **B,** Facial edema after 24 hours.

FIG. 25-7 The effects of burn shock are shown above the blue line. As the capillary seal is lost, interstitial edema develops. The cellular integrity is also altered, with sodium *(Na)* moving into the cell in abnormal amounts and potassium *(K)* leaving the cell. The shifts after the resolution of burn shock are shown below the blue line. The water and sodium move back into the circulating volume through the capillary. The albumin remains in the interstitium. Potassium is transported into the cell and sodium is transported out as the cellular integrity returns.

FIG. 25-8 Escharotomies of the chest and arm (indicated by *arrows*).

Respiratory System. The respiratory system is vulnerable to two types of injury: (1) upper airway burns and (2) lower airway injury (see Table 25-3). Upper airway distress may occur with or without smoke inhalation, and airway injury at either level may occur in the absence of burn injury to the skin. (Smoke and inhalation injuries are discussed earlier in this chapter on pp. 451-452.)

The patient may require a fiberoptic bronchoscopy and carboxyhemoglobin blood levels to confirm a suspected inhalation injury. Look in the prehospital notes to see if the patient was exposed to smoke or fumes. Examine any sputum for carbon. Watch for signs of impending respiratory distress, such as increased agitation, anxiety, restlessness, or a change in the rate or character of the patient's breathing, since symptoms may not be present immediately. In general, there is no correlation between the extent of TBSA burn and severity of inhalation injury. In a patient with inhalation injury, a chest x-ray may appear normal on admission, but changes usually occur over the next 24 to 48 hours. Arterial blood gas (ABG) values may also be within the normal range on admission and change over time.

Other Cardiopulmonary Problems. Patients with preexisting heart disease (e.g., myocardial infarction) or lung disease (e.g., chronic obstructive pulmonary disease) are at an increased risk for complications. If fluid replacement is too vigorous, watch for early signs of heart failure or pulmonary edema. Invasive measures (e.g., hemodynamic monitoring) may be necessary to monitor fluid resuscitation.

Patients with preexisting respiratory problems are more likely to develop a respiratory tract infection. Pneumonia, a common complication of major burns, is the leading cause of death in patients with an inhalation injury.

Burn patients are at an increased risk for venous thromboembolism (VTE) if one or more of the following conditions are present: advanced age, morbid obesity, extensive or lower-extremity burns, concomitant lower-extremity trauma, and prolonged immobility.[10] VTE prophylaxis should be started and should include medications such as enoxaparin (Lovenox) unless contraindicated.[11]

Urinary System. The most common complication of the urinary system in the emergent phase is acute tubular necrosis (ATN). If your patient becomes hypovolemic, blood flow to the kidneys is decreased, causing renal ischemia. If this continues, acute kidney injury may develop.

With full-thickness and major electrical burns, myoglobin (from muscle cell breakdown) and hemoglobin (from RBC breakdown) are released into the bloodstream and occlude renal tubules. Carefully monitor the adequacy of fluid replacement because this can counteract obstruction of the tubules.

NURSING AND COLLABORATIVE MANAGEMENT
EMERGENT PHASE

In the emergent phase the patient's survival depends on rapid and thorough assessment and appropriate interventions. Usually the physician and you make an initial assessment of the depth and extent of the burn and coordinate the actions of others on the health care team. In a community hospital, determine whether the patient requires inpatient or outpatient care. In the case of inpatient care, decide whether the patient remains in the hospital or should be transferred to the closest burn center (see Table 25-4).

Nursing and collaborative management predominantly consists of airway management, fluid therapy, and wound care (Table 25-10). Patients often improve and worsen, unpredictably, on an almost daily basis.

Although physical and occupational therapy are important in both the acute and rehabilitation phases, proper positioning and splinting begin on the day of admission. Emotional support and teaching of patients and caregivers begin on admission. A nursing care plan for the patient with burn injury (eNursing Care Plan 25-1) is available on the website for this chapter.

AIRWAY MANAGEMENT

Airway management frequently involves early endotracheal (preferably orotracheal) intubation. Early intubation eliminates the need for emergency tracheostomy after respiratory problems have become apparent. In general, the patient with burns to the face and neck requires intubation within 1 to 2 hours after injury. (Intubation is discussed in Chapter 66.) After intubation the patient is placed on ventilatory support, with the delivered oxygen concentration based on ABG values. Extubation may be indicated when the edema resolves, usually 3 to 6 days after burn injury, unless severe inhalation injury is involved. Escharotomies of the chest wall may be needed to relieve respiratory distress secondary to circumferential, full-thickness burns of the neck and trunk (see Fig. 25-8).

Within 6 to 12 hours after injury in which smoke inhalation is suspected, a fiberoptic bronchoscopy should be performed to assess the lower airway. When intubation is not performed, treatment of inhalation injury includes administration of 100% humidified O_2 as needed. Place the patient in a high Fowler's position, unless contraindicated (e.g., spinal injury), and encourage deep breathing and coughing every hour. Reposition the patient every 1 to 2 hours and provide suctioning and chest physiotherapy (as ordered). If severe respiratory distress (e.g., hoarseness, shortness of breath) develops, intubation and mechanical ventilation are initiated. Positive end-expiratory pressure (PEEP) may be used to prevent collapse of the alveoli and progressive respiratory failure (see Chapters 66 and 68). Bronchodilators may be administered to treat severe bronchospasm. CO poisoning is treated by administering 100% O_2 until carboxyhemoglobin levels return to normal.

FLUID THERAPY

Establishing IV access is critical for fluid resuscitation and drug administration. At least two large-bore IV access sites must be in place for patients with burns that are 15% TBSA or more. It is critical to establish IV access that can handle large volumes of fluid. For patients with burns greater than 30% TBSA, consider a central line for fluid and drug administration and blood sampling (central lines are discussed in Chapter 17). An arterial line is often placed if frequent ABGs or invasive BP monitoring is needed.

Assess the extent of the burn wound using a standardized chart (see Fig. 25-4). Then use a standardized formula to estimate the patient's fluid resuscitation requirements. Fluid replacement is achieved with crystalloid solutions (usually lactated Ringer's), colloids (albumin), or a combination of the two.[12] Paramedics generally give IV saline until the patient's arrival at the hospital.

The Parkland (Baxter) formula for fluid replacement is the most common formula used (Table 25-11, or *www.mdcalc.com/ parkland-formula-for-burns*). Remember that all formulas are

TABLE 25-10   COLLABORATIVE CARE

Burn Injury

Emergent Phase	Acute Phase	Rehabilitation Phase
Fluid Therapy (see Table 25-11) • Assess fluid needs. • Begin IV fluid replacement. • Insert indwelling urinary catheter. • Monitor urine output.	**Fluid Therapy** • Continue to replace fluids, depending on patient's clinical response.	• Continue to counsel and teach patient and caregiver. • Continue to encourage and assist patient in resuming self-care. • Continue to prevent or minimize contractures and assess likelihood for scarring (surgery, physical and occupational therapy, splinting, pressure garments). • Discuss possible reconstructive surgery. • Prepare for discharge home or transfer to rehabilitation hospital.
Wound Care • Start daily shower and wound care. • Debride as necessary. • Assess extent and depth of burns. • Administer tetanus toxoid or tetanus antitoxin.	**Wound Care** • Continue daily shower and wound care. • Continue debridement (if necessary). • Assess wound daily and adjust dressing protocols as necessary. • Observe for complications (e.g., infection).	
Pain and Anxiety • Assess and manage pain and anxiety.	**Early Excision and Grafting** • Provide temporary allografts. • Provide permanent autografts. • Care for donor sites.	
Physical and Occupational Therapy • Place patient in position that prevents contracture formation and reduces edema. • Assess need for splints.	**Pain and Anxiety** • Continue to assess for and treat pain and anxiety.	
Nutritional Therapy • Assess nutritional needs and begin feeding patient by most appropriate route as soon as possible.	**Physical and Occupational Therapy** • Begin daily therapy program for maintenance of range of motion. • Assess need for splints and anticontracture positioning. • Encourage and assist patient with self-care as possible.	
Respiratory Therapy • Assess oxygenation needs. • Provide supplemental O₂ as needed. • Intubate if necessary. • Monitor respiratory status.	**Nutritional Therapy** • Continue to assess diet to support wound healing.	
Psychosocial Care • Provide support to patient and caregiver during initial crisis phase.	**Respiratory Therapy** • Continue to assess oxygenation needs. • Continue to monitor respiratory status. • Monitor for signs of complications (e.g., pneumonia).	
	Psychosocial Care • Provide ongoing support, counseling, and teaching to patient and caregiver about physical and emotional aspects of care and recovery. • Begin to anticipate discharge needs.	
	Drug Therapy (see Table 25-13) • Assess need for medications (e.g., antibiotics). • Continue to monitor effectiveness and adjust dosage as needed.	

TABLE 25-11   FLUID RESUSCITATION

Parkland (Baxter) Formula*
4 mL lactated Ringer's solution per kilogram (kg) of body weight per percent of total body surface area (% TBSA) burned = Total fluid requirements for first 24 hr after burn

Application
½ of total in first 8 hr
¼ of total in second 8 hr
¼ of total in third 8 hr

Example
For a 70 kg patient with a 50% TBSA burn:
  4 mL × 70 kg × 50 TBSA burned = 14,000 mL in 24 hr

½ of total in first 8 hr = 7000 mL (875 mL/hr)
¼ of total in second 8 hr = 3500 mL (437 mL/hr)
¼ of total in third 8 hr = 3500 mL (437 mL/hr)

*Formulas are guidelines. Fluid is administered at a rate to produce 0.5-1.0 mL/kg/hr of urine output. The American Burn Association Consensus Fluid Resuscitation Formula of 2-4 mL lactated Ringer's solution per kg of body weight per %TBSA burned = Total fluid requirements for first 24 hr after burn has been suggested as a strategy to avoid over-resuscitation, or "fluid creep."

estimates, and fluids must be titrated based on the patient's response (e.g., hourly urine output, vital signs). Patients with an electrical injury have greater than normal fluid requirements and generally require an osmotic diuretic (mannitol [Osmitrol]) to increase their urine output and overcome high levels of hemoglobin and myoglobin in the urine. Too much fluid and overestimation of TBSA contribute to the development of "fluid creep."[13] For the first 24 hours, the recommendation is 2 to 4 mL lactated Ringer's/kg/%TBSA burned.

Colloidal solutions (e.g., 5% albumin) may also be given. However, administration is recommended after the first 12 to 24 hours postburn when capillary permeability returns to normal or near normal. After this time, the plasma remains in the vascular space and expands the circulating volume. The replacement volume is calculated based on the patient's body weight and TBSA burned (e.g., 0.3 to 0.5 mL/kg/%TBSA burned).

Hourly assessments of the adequacy of fluid resuscitation are best made using clinical parameters. Urine output, the most commonly used parameter, and cardiac parameters are defined as follows.

- *Urine output:* 0.5 to 1 mL/kg/hr; 75 to 100 mL/hr for electrical burn patient with evidence of hemoglobinuria or myoglobinuria.
- *Cardiac parameters:* Mean arterial pressure (MAP) greater than 65 mm Hg, systolic BP greater than 90 mm Hg, heart rate less than 120 beats/minute. MAP and BP are best measured by an arterial line. Manual BP measurement is often invalid because of edema and vasoconstriction.

WOUND CARE

Once a patent airway, effective circulation, and adequate fluid replacement have been established, priority is given to care of the burn wound. Partial-thickness burn wounds appear pink to cherry-red and are wet and shiny with serous exudate. These wounds may or may not have intact blisters; are painful when touched; and have only minor, localized sensation because nerve endings have been destroyed in the burned dermis.

You and appropriate personnel can perform cleansing and gentle debridement, using scissors and forceps, on a cart shower (Fig. 25-9), regular shower, or patient bed or stretcher.[14] Extensive, surgical debridement is performed in the operating room (OR) (Fig. 25-10). During **debridement,** necrotic skin is removed. Releasing escharotomies and fasciotomies are carried out in the emergent phase, usually in burn centers by burn physicians.

Patients find the initial wound care to be both physically and psychologically demanding. Provide emotional support and begin to build trust during this activity. A once-daily shower and dressing change in the morning, with an evening dressing change in the patient's room, are part of the routine in many burn centers. Others opt to shower the patient on admission and then perform all other dressing changes in the patient's room. Some of the newer antimicrobial dressings can be left in place from 3 to 14 days, thereby decreasing the frequency of dressing changes.

Infection may cause further tissue injury and possible sepsis.[15] The source of infection in burn wounds is likely the patient's own flora, predominantly from the skin, respiratory tract, and gastrointestinal (GI) tract. The prevention of cross-contamination from one patient to another is a priority.

Two approaches to burn wound treatment are (1) the open method and (2) the use of multiple dressing changes (closed method). In the *open method* the patient's burn is covered with a topical antimicrobial and has no dressing over the wound. In the *multiple dressing change,* or *closed method,* sterile gauze dressings are impregnated with or laid over a topical antimicrobial (Fig. 25-11). These dressings are changed anywhere from every 12 to 24 hours to once every 14 days (depending on the product). Most burn centers support the concept of moist wound healing and use dressings to cover the burned areas, with the exception of facial burns.

When the patient's open burn wounds are exposed, always wear personal protective equipment (PPE) (e.g., disposable hats, masks, gowns, gloves). When removing contaminated dressings and washing the dirty wound, use nonsterile, disposable gloves. Use sterile gloves when applying ointments and sterile dressings. In addition, prevent shivering by keeping the room warm (approximately 85° F [29.4° C]). Before leaving one patient, remove your PPE. Don new equipment before you treat another patient. Perform thorough hand washing both before and after patient contact to prevent cross-contamination.

Permanent skin coverage is the primary goal for burn wound care. There is rarely enough unburned skin in the major (greater than 50% TBSA) burn patient for immediate skin grafting. This situation requires the use of temporary wound closure methods. *Allograft (homograft) skin* (from skin donor cadavers) is used, along with newer biosynthetic options. The treatment approaches vary among burn centers (Table 25-12).

FIG. 25-9 Cart shower. Showering presents an opportunity for physical therapy and wound care.

FIG. 25-10 Surgical debridement of full-thickness burns is necessary to prepare the wound for grafting.

FIG. 25-11 Application of silver sulfadiazine cream to saline-moistened gauze.

TABLE 25-12   SOURCES OF GRAFTS

Source	Graft Name	Coverage
Porcine skin	Xenograft (or heterograft) (different species)	Temporary (3 days to 2 wk)
Cadaveric skin	Allograft (or homograft) (same species)	Temporary (3 days to 2 wk)
Patient's own skin	Autograft	Permanent
Patient's own skin and cell cultures	Cultured epithelial autograft (CEA)	Permanent
Porcine collagen bonded to silicone membrane	Biobrane	Temporary (10-21 days)
Bovine collagen and glycosaminoglycan bonded to silicone membrane	Integra	Permanent
Acellular dermal matrix derived from donated human skin	AlloDerm	Permanent

OTHER CARE MEASURES

Certain parts of the body (e.g., face, eyes, hands, arms, ears, perineum) require particularly vigilant nursing care. The face is highly vascular and can become very swollen. It is often covered with ointments and gauze but not wrapped to limit pressure on delicate facial structures. Eye care for corneal burns or edema includes antibiotic ointments. An ophthalmology examination should occur soon after admission for all patients with facial burns. Periorbital edema can prevent eye opening and is often frightening for the patient. Provide assurance that the swelling is not permanent. Instill methylcellulose drops or artificial tears into the eyes for moisture and additional comfort.

Ears should be kept free from pressure because of their poor vascularization and tendency to become infected. Do not use pillows for the patient with ear burns. The pressure on the cartilage may cause chondritis. Further, the ear may stick to the pillowcase, causing pain and bleeding. Elevate your patient's head using a rolled towel placed under the shoulders, being careful to avoid pressure necrosis. Follow the same strategy for the patient with neck burns to hyperextend the neck and prevent neck wound contracture.

Extend your patient's burned hands and arms and elevate them on pillows or plastic-covered foam wedges to minimize edema. Ask the occupational therapist and the physician if splints need to be applied to burned hands and feet to maintain them in positions of function. Remove the splints frequently and inspect the skin and bony prominences to avoid areas of pressure from inappropriate or prolonged application.

Keep your patient's perineum as clean and dry as possible after each voiding or bowel movement. In addition to monitoring hourly urine outputs, an indwelling catheter prevents urine contamination of the perineal area. Regular once- or twice-daily perineal and catheter care, in the presence or absence of a perineal burn wound, is essential. Assess the need for an indwelling urinary catheter on a daily basis and remove when no longer necessary to avoid development of a urinary tract infection. If your patient has frequent, loose stools, consider the temporary insertion of a fecal diversion device.

Perform necessary laboratory tests to monitor fluid and electrolyte balance. Draw ABGs, as necessary, to determine adequacy of ventilation and perfusion in patients with suspected or confirmed inhalation or electrical injury.

Work in collaboration with the physical therapist to perform range-of-motion (ROM) exercises during dressing changes and throughout the day. Movement facilitates mobilization of the leaked fluid back into the vascular bed. Active and passive exercise of body parts also maintains function, prevents contractures, and reassures the patient that movement is still possible.

DRUG THERAPY

ANALGESICS AND SEDATIVES. Promote the use of analgesics for the patient's comfort.[16] Early in the postburn period, IV pain medications should be given because (1) onset of action is fastest with this route; (2) oral medications have a slower onset of action and are not as effective when GI function is slowed or impaired because of shock or paralytic ileus; and (3) intramuscular (IM) injections will not be absorbed adequately in burned or edematous areas, causing pooling of medications in the tissues. Consequently, when fluid mobilization begins, the patient could be inadvertently overdosed from the interstitial accumulation of previous IM medications.

Common opioids used for pain control are listed in Table 25-13. Reevaluate analgesic requirements, since the patient's needs may change and tolerance to medications may develop over time. Initially, opioids are the drug of choice for pain control. When given appropriately, these drugs should provide adequate pain relief. Sedatives/hypnotics and antidepressants can also be given with analgesics to control the anxiety, insomnia, or depression that patients may experience (see Table 25-13). Analgesic requirements can vary widely from one patient to another, so consider a multimodal approach to pain management.[17] Remember that the patient's pain intensity may not directly correlate with the extent and depth of burn.

TETANUS IMMUNIZATION. Tetanus toxoid is given routinely to all burn patients because of the likelihood of anaerobic burn wound contamination. If the patient has not received an active immunization within 10 years before the burn injury, tetanus immunoglobulin should be considered. (Tetanus immunization is discussed in Table 69-6.)

ANTIMICROBIAL AGENTS. After the wound is cleansed, topical antimicrobial agents may be applied (see Fig. 25-11) and covered with a light dressing.[18] Systemic antibiotics are not routinely used to control burn wound flora because the burn eschar has little or no blood supply and consequently little antibiotic is delivered to the wound. In addition, the routine use of systemic antibiotics increases the chance of developing multidrug-resistant organisms. Some topical burn agents penetrate the eschar and inhibit bacterial invasion of the wound. Silver-impregnated dressings (e.g., Acticoat, Silverlon, Aquacel AG) can be left in place from 3 to 14 days, depending on the patient's clinical situation and the particular product. Silver sulfadiazine (Silvadene, Flamazine) and mafenide acetate (Sulfamylon) creams are also used.

SAFETY ALERT
- Check the patient for any allergies to sulfa, since many burn antimicrobial creams contain sulfa.

Sepsis remains a primary cause of death in the patient with major burns and may lead to multiple organ dysfunction syndrome (see Chapter 67). Systemic antibiotic therapy is initiated when the diagnosis of sepsis is made, or when some other source of infection is identified (e.g., pneumonia).[19]

TABLE 25-13   DRUG THERAPY

Burn Care

Drugs	Purpose
Analgesics	
morphine (Avinza)	Relieve pain
sustained-release morphine (MS Contin)	
hydromorphone (Dilaudid)	
sustained-release hydromorphone (Dilaudid CR)	
fentanyl (Sublimaze)	
oxycodone and acetaminophen (Percocet)	
methadone (Dolophine)	
Nonsteroidal antiinflammatory (e.g., ketorolac [Toradol])	
Adjuvant analgesics (e.g., gabapentin [Neurontin])	
Sedatives/Hypnotics	
lorazepam (Ativan)	Reduce anxiety
midazolam (Versed)	Provide short-acting amnesic effects
zolpidem (Ambien)	Promote sleep
Antidepressants	
sertraline (Zoloft)	Reduce depression, improve mood
citalopram (Celexa)	
Anticoagulants	
enoxaparin (Lovenox)	Prevent venous thromboembolism
heparin	
Nutritional Support	
Vitamins A, C, E, and multivitamins	Promote wound healing
Minerals: zinc, iron (ferrous sulfate)	Promote cell integrity and hemoglobin formation
oxandrolone (Oxandrin)	Promote weight gain and preservation of lean body mass
Gastrointestinal Support	
ranitidine (Zantac)	Decrease stomach acid and risk of Curling's ulcer
esomeprazole (Nexium)	
calcium carbonate and magnesium carbonate (Mylanta), aluminum hydroxide and magnesium hydroxide (Maalox)	Neutralize stomach acid
nystatin (Mycostatin)	Prevent overgrowth of *Candida albicans* in oral mucosa

Fungal infections may develop in the patient's mucous membranes (mouth and genitalia) as a result of systemic antibiotic therapy and low resistance. The offending organism is usually *Candida albicans*. Oral infection is treated with nystatin (Mycostatin) mouthwash. When a normal diet is resumed, yogurt or *Lactobacillus* (Lactinex) may be given by mouth to reintroduce the normal intestinal flora that was destroyed by antibiotic therapy.

VENOUS THROMBOEMBOLISM PROPHYLAXIS. Burn patients are at risk for VTE. If there are no contraindications, it is recommended that low-molecular-weight heparin (enoxaparin) or low-dose unfractionated heparin be started as soon as it is considered safe. For burn patients who have a high bleeding risk, VTE prophylaxis with sequential compression devices and/or graduated compression stockings are used until the bleeding

EVIDENCE-BASED PRACTICE

Translating Research Into Practice

Does the Type of Enteral Feeding Affect Outcomes in Burn Patients?

Clinical Question
In patients with burns (P), what is the effect of high-carbohydrate enteral feeding (I) versus high-fat enteral feeding (C) in reducing mortality, days on ventilator, and incidence of pneumonia (O)?

Best Available Evidence
Systematic review of randomized controlled trials (RCTs)

Critical Appraisal and Synthesis of Evidence
• Two RCTs ($n = 93$) of hospitalized patients in the immediate postburn period, with burns covering ≥10% of the total body surface area (TBSA).
• Two types of enteral feeding were compared: high-carbohydrate, high-protein, low-fat feeding (high-carbohydrate formula) and low-carbohydrate, high-protein, high-fat feeding (high-fat formula).
• High-carbohydrate enteral feeding resulted in a reduced incidence of pneumonia compared with high-fat enteral feeding.
• Inconclusive results on type of enteral feeding and patient outcomes of mortality and days on ventilator.

Conclusion
• High-carbohydrate enteral feedings may be of benefit in reducing the risk of pneumonia.

Implications for Nursing Practice
• Further research is needed to determine if enteral feeds are significantly different related to patient outcomes.

Reference for Evidence
Masters B, Aarabi S, Sidhwa F, et al: High-carbohydrate, high-protein, low-fat versus low-carbohydrate, high-protein, high-fat enteral feeds for burns, *Cochrane Database Syst Rev* (1):CD006122, 2012.

P, Patient population of interest; *I*, intervention or area of interest; *C*, comparison of interest or comparison group; *O*, outcomes of interest (see p. 12).

risk decreases and heparin can be started (see Table 25-13). (VTE prophylaxis is discussed in Chapter 38.)

NUTRITIONAL THERAPY

Once fluid replacement needs have been addressed, nutrition takes priority in the initial emergent phase.[20] Early and aggressive nutritional support within several hours of the burn injury can decrease mortality risks and complications, optimize healing of the burn wound, and minimize the negative effects of hypermetabolism and catabolism.[21] Nonintubated patients with a burn of less than 20% TBSA will generally be able to eat enough to meet their nutritional needs.

Intubated patients and those with larger burns require additional support. Enteral feedings (gastric or intestinal) have almost entirely replaced parenteral feeding. Early enteral feeding, usually with smaller-bore tubes, preserves GI function, increases intestinal blood flow, and promotes optimal conditions for wound healing. In general, begin the feedings slowly at a rate of 20 to 40 mL/hr and increase to the goal rate within 24 to 48 hours. If a large nasogastric tube is inserted, gastric residuals should be checked to rule out delayed gastric emptying. Assess bowel sounds every 8 hours.

A *hypermetabolic state* proportional to the size of the wound occurs after a major burn injury.[21] Resting metabolic expenditure may be increased by 50% to 100% above normal in patients with major burns. Core temperature is elevated. Catecholamines, which stimulate catabolism and heat production, are increased. Massive catabolism can occur and is characterized by protein breakdown and increased gluconeogenesis. Failure to supply adequate calories and protein leads to malnutrition and delayed healing. Calorie-containing nutritional supplements and milkshakes are often given to meet the caloric needs. Protein powder can also be added to food and liquids. Supplemental vitamins may be started in the emergent phase, with iron supplements often given in the acute phase (see Table 25-13).

ACUTE PHASE

The *acute phase* of burn care begins with the mobilization of extracellular fluid and subsequent diuresis. It concludes when partial-thickness wounds are healed or full-thickness burns are covered by skin grafts. This may take weeks or months.

Pathophysiology

A healing burn injury causes many pathophysiologic changes in the body. Diuresis from fluid mobilization occurs, and the patient is less edematous. Bowel sounds return. The depth of the burn wounds may be more apparent as they "declare" themselves as partial or full thickness. The patient may now become more aware of the enormity of his or her situation and will benefit from psychosocial support and information.

Some healing begins as WBCs surround the burn wound and phagocytosis occurs. Necrotic tissue begins to slough. Fibroblasts lay down matrices of the collagen precursors that eventually form granulation tissue. A partial-thickness burn will heal, from both the wound edges and the dermal bed below, if kept free from infection and *desiccation* (dryness). However, full-thickness burn wounds, unless extremely small, must have the burn eschar surgically removed (excised) and skin grafts applied in order to heal. In some cases, healing time and length of hospitalization are decreased by early excision and grafting.

Clinical Manifestations

Partial-thickness wounds form eschar, which begins separating fairly soon after injury. Once the eschar is removed, re-epithelialization begins at the wound margins and appears as red or pink scar tissue. Epithelial buds, from the hair follicles and glands in the dermal bed, eventually close the wound. Healing is spontaneous and usually occurs within 10 to 21 days.

Margins of full-thickness eschar take longer to separate. As a result, full-thickness burn wounds require surgical debridement and skin grafting to heal.

Laboratory Values

Because the body is attempting to reestablish fluid and electrolyte balance in the initial acute phase, it is important to follow serum electrolyte levels closely.

Sodium. *Hyponatremia* can develop from excessive GI suction, diarrhea, and water intake. Manifestations of hyponatremia include weakness, dizziness, muscle cramps, fatigue, headache, tachycardia, and confusion. The patient may also develop a dilutional hyponatremia called *water intoxication*. To avoid this condition, encourage the patient to drink fluids other than water, such as juice or nutritional supplements.

Hypernatremia may be seen after successful fluid resuscitation if copious amounts of hypertonic solutions were required. Hypernatremia may also be related to tube feeding therapy or inappropriate fluid administration. Manifestations of hyperna-

tremia include thirst; dried, furry tongue; lethargy; confusion; and possibly seizures. Sodium restrictions may be applied to IV fluids and enteral or oral feedings until levels return to safe limits.

Potassium. *Hyperkalemia* may occur if the patient has renal failure, adrenocortical insufficiency, or massive deep muscle injury (e.g., electrical burn) with large amounts of potassium released from damaged cells. Cardiac dysrhythmias and arrest can occur with elevated potassium levels. Muscle weakness, cramping, and paralysis are found clinically (see Chapters 17 and 36).

Hypokalemia occurs with vomiting, diarrhea, prolonged GI suction, and IV therapy without potassium supplementation. Potassium is also lost through the patient's burn wounds. Signs and symptoms of hypokalemia include fatigue, muscle weakness, leg cramps, cardiac dysrhythmias (e.g., premature ventricular contractions), paresthesias, and decreased reflexes (see Chapter 17).

Complications

Infection. The body's first line of defense, the skin, is destroyed by a burn injury. The burn wound is now colonized with the person's own organisms that were on the skin before the burn. If the levels of bacteria between the eschar and the viable wound bed rise to greater than 10^5/g of tissue, the patient has a burn wound infection. Localized inflammation, induration, and sometimes suppuration can be seen at the burn wound margins. Partial-thickness burns can convert to full-thickness wounds when these organisms invade viable, adjacent, unburned tissue. Invasive wound infections may be treated with systemic antibiotics based on culture and sensitivity wound swab results.

Watch for signs and symptoms, including hypothermia or hyperthermia, increased heart and respiratory rate, decreased BP, and decreased urine output. The patient may have mild confusion, chills, malaise, and loss of appetite. The WBC count usually is between 10,000/μL (10×10^9/L) and 20,000/μL (20×10^9/L). The WBCs have functional defects and the patient remains immunosuppressed for many months after the burn injury.

The causative organisms of sepsis are usually gram-negative bacteria (e.g., *Pseudomonas, Proteus* organisms), putting the patient at further risk for septic shock. When sepsis is suspected, immediately obtain cultures from all possible sources, including the burn wound, blood, urine, sputum, oropharynx and perineal regions, and IV site. Treatment immediately begins with antibiotics appropriate for the usual residual flora of the particular burn center. When the culture and sensitivity results are known, the antibiotic in use may be continued or changed based on the results. At this stage the patient's condition is considered critical, requiring close monitoring of vital signs.

Cardiovascular and Respiratory Systems. The same cardiovascular and respiratory system complications present in the emergent phase may continue into the acute phase of care. In addition, new problems might arise, requiring timely intervention.

Neurologic System. Neurologically, the patient probably has no physical symptoms unless severe hypoxia from respiratory injuries or complications from electrical injuries occur. Probable causes of neurologic complications include electrolyte imbalance, stress, cerebral edema, sepsis, sleep disturbances, and the use of analgesics and antianxiety drugs. However, some patients may demonstrate certain behaviors that are not completely understood. The patient can become extremely disoriented, may withdraw or become combative, and may have hallucinations and frequent nightmare-like episodes. Delirium is more acute at night and occurs more often in the older patient. Use a screening tool to diagnose delirium (see Table 60-16) and initiate appropriate nursing interventions to prevent delirium, whenever possible. Focus on nursing strategies to orient and reassure your patient if he or she is confused or agitated. This state is usually transient, lasting from a day or two to several weeks, but complications and sequelae can last for years and be quite serious.

Musculoskeletal System. The musculoskeletal system is particularly prone to complications during the acute phase, and the involvement of both the physical and occupational therapist is vitally important.[22] As the burns begin to heal and scar tissue forms, the skin is less supple and pliant. ROM may be limited, and contractures can occur. Because of pain, the patient likely prefers a flexed position for comfort. Encourage the patient to stretch and move the burned body parts as much as possible. Consult with the occupational therapist about proper positioning and splinting to prevent or reduce contracture formation.

Gastrointestinal System. The GI system may also experience complications during this phase. Paralytic ileus can be caused by sepsis. Diarrhea may result from the use of enteral feedings or antibiotics. Constipation can occur as a side effect of opioid analgesics, decreased mobility, and a low-fiber diet. *Curling's ulcer* is a type of gastroduodenal ulcer characterized by diffuse superficial lesions (including mucosal erosion). It is caused by a generalized stress response to decreased blood flow to the GI tract. The patient has increased gastric acid secretion. Aim to prevent Curling's ulcer by feeding the patient as soon as possible after the burn injury. Antacids, H_2-histamine blockers (e.g., ranitidine [Zantac]), and proton pump inhibitors (e.g., esomeprazole [Nexium]) are used prophylactically to neutralize stomach acids and inhibit histamine and the secretion of hydrochloric acid (see Table 25-13). Patients with major burns may also have occult blood in their stools during the acute phase and require close monitoring for bleeding.

Endocrine System. Observe for transient increases in the patient's blood glucose levels as a result of stress-mediated cortisol and catecholamine release. There is an increased mobilization of glycogen stores and gluconeogenesis. Subsequently, glucose is produced, along with an increase in insulin production. However, insulin's effectiveness is decreased because of relative insulin insensitivity. This results in an elevated blood glucose level. Hyperglycemia may also be caused by the increased caloric intake necessary to meet some patients' metabolic requirements. When this occurs, the treatment is supplemental IV insulin, not decreased feeding. Check blood glucose levels frequently and give insulin as ordered. Point-of-care testing of glucose can be done, but serum glucose testing is more accurate. As the patient's metabolic demands are met and less stress is placed on the entire system, this stress-induced condition is reversed.

NURSING AND COLLABORATIVE MANAGEMENT ACUTE PHASE

The predominant therapeutic interventions in the acute phase are (1) wound care, (2) excision and grafting, (3) pain management, (4) physical and occupational therapy, and (5) nutritional therapy.

WOUND CARE

The goals of wound care are to (1) prevent infection by cleansing and debriding the area of necrotic tissue that would promote bacterial growth and (2) promote wound re-epithelialization and/or successful skin grafting.

Wound care consists of ongoing observation, assessment, cleansing, debridement, and dressing reapplication. Nonsurgical debridement, dressing changes, topical antimicrobial therapy, graft care, and donor site care are performed as often as necessary, depending on the topical cream or dressing ordered. Enzymatic debriders made of natural ingredients, such as collagen, may be used for *enzymatic debridement* of burn wounds, which speeds up the removal of dead tissue from the healthy wound bed.

Cleanse wounds with soap and water or normal saline-moistened gauze to gently remove the old antimicrobial agent and any loose necrotic tissue, scabs, or dried blood. During the debridement phase, cover the wound with topical antimicrobial creams (e.g., silver sulfadiazine) or silver-impregnated dressings. When the partial-thickness burn wounds have been fully debrided, a protective, coarse or fine-meshed, greasy-based (paraffin or petroleum) gauze dressing is applied to protect the re-epithelializing keratinocytes as they resurface and close the open wound bed.

If grafting is necessary, protect the skin graft (discussed below) with the same greasy gauze dressings next to the graft, followed by saline-moistened middle, and dry gauze outer dressings. With facial grafts the unmeshed sheet graft is left open, so it is possible for *blebs* (serosanguineous exudate) to form between the graft and the recipient bed. Blebs prevent the graft from permanently attaching to the wound bed. The evacuation of blebs is best performed by aspiration with a tuberculin syringe and only by those who have received instruction in this specialized skill. (Dressings are discussed in Table 12-10.)

EXCISION AND GRAFTING

Management of full-thickness burn wounds involves early removal (surgical excision) of the necrotic tissue followed by application of split-thickness autograft skin.[23] This aggressive and definitive approach has improved the management and survival rate of burn patients. In the past, patients with major burns had low rates of survival because healing and wound coverage took so long that the patient usually died of sepsis or malnutrition.

Many patients, especially those with major burns, are taken to the OR for wound excision on day 1 or 2 (emergent phase). The wounds are covered with a biologic dressing or allograft for temporary coverage until permanent grafting can occur (see Table 25-12).

During the procedure of excision and grafting, devitalized tissue (eschar) is excised down to the subcutaneous tissue or fascia, depending on the degree of injury. Surgical excision can result in massive blood loss.[24] To decrease surgical blood loss, topical application of epinephrine or thrombin, injection of saline and epinephrine, application of extremity tourniquets, or application of a new fibrin sealant (Artiss) is used. Once hemostasis has been achieved, a graft is then placed on clean, viable tissue to achieve good adherence. Whenever possible, the freshly excised wound is covered with *autograft* (the person's own) skin (see Table 25-12). Recently, fibrin sealant has been used to attach skin grafts to the wound bed. Grafts can also be stapled or sutured into place (Fig. 25-12, *A*). A temporary

FIG. 25-12 A, Freshly applied split-thickness sheet skin graft to the hand. **B,** Split-thickness skin graft is harvested from a patient's thigh using a dermatome. **C,** Donor site is covered with a hydrophilic foam dressing after harvesting. **D,** Healed donor site.

allograft can be used to test the suitability of the recipient site to accept a graft.[25] The allograft is then removed several days later in the OR and an autograft applied.

With early excision, function is restored and scar tissue formation is minimized. Clots between the graft and the wound keep the graft from adhering to the wound. Outer occlusive dressings apply just enough pressure to promote adherence of the graft to the wound bed and help control bleeding. Protect the grafted area from shearing, friction, and pressure. Facial, neck, and hand burns require skillful nursing care to identify and manage clots quickly for the best functional and esthetic outcomes.

Donor skin is taken from the patient for grafting by means of a *dermatome,* which removes a thin (14/1000 to 16/1000 inch) split-thickness layer of skin from an unburned site (Fig. 25-12, *B*). The donor skin can be meshed (usually ratio of 1.5:1) to allow for greater wound coverage, or it may be applied as an unmeshed sheet for a better cosmetic result when grafting the face, neck, and hands. The donor site now becomes a new open wound.

The goals of donor site care are to promote rapid, moist wound healing; decrease pain at the site; and prevent infection. The choices of dressings for donor sites vary among burn centers and include transparent dressings (e.g., Opsite), xenograft, silver sulfadiazine, silver-impregnated dressings, calcium alginate, and hydrophilic foam dressings (Fig. 25-12, *C*). Nursing care of the donor site is specific to the dressing selected.[26] Several of the newer dressing materials offer decreased healing time, which facilitates earlier reharvesting of skin at the same site. The average healing time for a donor site is 10 to 14 days (Fig. 25-12, *D*).

CULTURED EPITHELIAL AUTOGRAFTS. In the patient with large body burns, only a limited amount of unburned skin may be available as donor sites for grafting, and some of that skin may be unsuitable for harvesting. Cultured epithelial autograft (CEA) is a method of obtaining permanent skin from a person with limited skin available for harvesting. CEA is grown from biopsy specimens obtained from the patient's own unburned skin.[27] This procedure is performed in suitable patients in some burn centers as soon as possible. The specimens are sent to a commercial laboratory, where the biopsied keratinocytes are grown in a culture medium containing epidermal growth factor. After approximately 18 to 25 days, the keratinocytes have expanded up to 10,000 times and form sheets that can be used as skin grafts. The cultured skin is returned to the burn center, where it is placed on the patient's excised burn wounds (Fig. 25-13, *A*). CEA grafts generally form a seamless, smooth replacement skin tissue (Fig. 25-13, *B*). Problems related to CEA include a poor graft take because of thin epidermal skin, graft loss during healing, infection, and contracture development.

ARTIFICIAL SKIN. Artificial skin must replace all functions of the skin and consist of both dermal and epidermal elements.[27] The Integra artificial skin dermal regeneration template is an example of a skin replacement system. As with CEA, it is indicated for use in the treatment of life-threatening, full-thickness or deep partial-thickness burn wounds when conventional autograft is not available or advisable, as in older or high anesthetic-risk patients. It has also been successfully used in reconstructive burn surgery procedures. It needs to be applied within a few days postburn for greatest success.

Integra artificial skin has a bilayer membrane composed of acellular dermis and silicone. The wound is excised, the bilayer membrane is placed dermal layer down, and the wound is wrapped with dressings in the OR. The dermal layer functions as a biodegradable template that induces organized regeneration of new dermis by the body. The silicone layer remains intact for 3 weeks as the dermal layer degrades and epidermal autografts become available. At this point, the silicone is removed during a second surgical procedure and replaced by the patient's own epidermal autografts. Some burn centers use CEA as the source of the epidermis.

Another dermal replacement is AlloDerm, a cryopreserved allogenic dermis. Human allograft dermis, harvested from

FIG. 25-13 Patient with cultured epithelial autograft (CEA). **A,** Intraoperative application of CEA. **B,** Appearance of healed CEA.

cadavers, is decellularized to render it immunogenic and then freeze-dried. Once thawed, AlloDerm is rehydrated with ultrathin epidermal autografts immediately before placement on a freshly excised wound.

PAIN MANAGEMENT

Many aspects of burn care cause pain. However, patients experience moments of relative comfort if they receive adequate analgesia. To provide effective pain management, you must understand both the physiologic and psychologic aspects of pain. (Pain management is discussed in Chapter 9.)

Burn patients experience two kinds of pain: (1) *continuous, background pain* that might be present throughout the day and night; and (2) *treatment-induced pain* associated with dressing changes, ambulation, and rehabilitation activities. The first line of treatment is drugs (see Table 25-13). With background pain, a continuous IV infusion of an opioid (e.g., hydromorphone [Dilaudid]) allows for a steady, therapeutic level of medication. If an IV infusion is not present, slow-release, twice-a-day opioid medications (e.g., morphine [MS Contin]) are indicated. Around-the-clock oral analgesics can also be used. Breakthrough doses of pain medication need to be available regardless of the regimen selected. Anxiolytics, which can potentiate analgesics, are also indicated and include lorazepam (Ativan) and midazolam (Versed). Adjuvant analgesics, such as gabapentin (Neurontin) and pregabalin (Lyrica), also potentiate opioids. The use of these drugs can help reduce the opioid dosage and undesirable side effects.

For treatment-induced pain, premedicate with an analgesic and an anxiolytic via the IV or oral route. For patients with an IV infusion, a potent, short-acting analgesic, such as fentanyl (Sublimaze), is often effective. During treatment and activity, small doses should be given to keep the patient as comfortable as possible. Elimination of all the pain is difficult, and most patients indicate acceptance of "tolerable" levels of discomfort.

Pain management is complex and ever-changing throughout the patient's hospital stay and after discharge.[28] Some pain can be managed using nondrug strategies. Mind-body interventions, such as relaxation breathing, guided imagery, hypnosis, biofeedback, and music therapy, can be effective in helping patients cope with pain (see Chapters 6 and 7).

Remember, the more control the patient has in managing pain, the more successful the chosen strategies will be. Active participation in requesting time-outs and scheduling treat-

ments and rest periods can help the patient manage feelings of anticipatory pain. Patient-controlled analgesia (PCA) is used in selected circumstances in some burn centers, with varying degrees of success. (PCA is discussed in Chapter 9.)

PHYSICAL AND OCCUPATIONAL THERAPY

Continuous physical therapy, throughout burn recovery, is imperative if the patient is to regain and maintain muscle strength and optimal joint function. A good time for exercise is during and after wound cleansing, when the skin is softer and bulky dressings are removed. Passive and active ROM should be performed on all joints. Ensure that the patient with neck burns continues to sleep without pillows or with the head hanging slightly over the top of the mattress to encourage hyperextension. Maintain the occupational therapy schedule for wearing custom-fitted splints, which are designed to keep joints in functional position. Examine the splints frequently to ensure an optimal fit, with no undue pressure that might lead to skin breakdown or nerve damage.

NUTRITIONAL THERAPY

The goal of nutritional therapy during the acute burn phase is to provide adequate calories and protein to promote healing. When the wounds are still open, the burn patient is in a hypermetabolic and highly catabolic state.

The patient may benefit from an antioxidant protocol, which includes selenium, acetylcysteine, ascorbic acid, vitamin E, zinc, and a multivitamin. Meeting daily caloric requirements is crucial and should begin within the first 1 to 2 days postburn. The daily estimated caloric needs must be regularly calculated by a dietitian and readjusted as the patient's condition changes (e.g., wound healing improves, sepsis develops). Monitor laboratory values (e.g., albumin, prealbumin, total protein, transferrin) on a regular basis.

If the patient is on a mechanical ventilator or unable to consume adequate calories by mouth, a small-bore feeding tube is placed and enteral feedings are initiated. When the patient is extubated, contact the speech pathologist to perform a swallowing assessment before an oral diet is started.[29] Encourage the patient to eat high-protein, high-carbohydrate foods to meet caloric needs. Ask caregivers to bring in favorite foods from home. Appetite is usually diminished, and you will need to reinforce whatever steps are necessary to achieve adequate intake. Ideally, weight loss should not be more than 10% of preburn weight. Record the patient's daily caloric intake using calorie count sheets, which are monitored by the dietitian. Weigh your patient weekly to evaluate progress.

REHABILITATION PHASE

The formal *rehabilitation phase* begins when the patient's wounds have healed and he or she is engaging in some level of self-care. This may happen as early as 2 weeks or as long as 7 to 8 months after the burn injury. Goals for the patient now are to (1) work toward resuming a functional role in society and (2) rehabilitate from any functional and cosmetic postburn reconstructive surgery that may be necessary.[30]

Pathophysiologic Changes and Clinical Manifestations

Burn wounds heal either by spontaneous re-epithelialization or by skin grafting. Layers of keratinocytes begin rebuilding the tissue structure destroyed by the burn injury. Collagen fibers, present in the new scar tissue, assist with healing and add strength to weakened areas. The new skin appears flat and pink. In approximately 4 to 6 weeks, the area becomes raised and hyperemic. If adequate ROM is not instituted, the new tissue will shorten, causing a contracture. Mature healing is reached in about 12 months when suppleness has returned, and the pink or red color has faded to a slightly lighter hue than the surrounding unburned tissue.

Counsel patients who have more heavily pigmented skin that it will take longer for it to regain its dark color because many of the melanocytes have been destroyed. Frequently, the skin does not regain its original color. Provide teaching and psychosocial support to assist the patient with grieving about these changes to his or her body image. In particular, teenagers and female patients may need more support, but explore potential body image concerns with everyone.[31] Cosmetic camouflage, the implantation of pigment within the skin, can help even out unequal skin tones and improve the patient's overall appearance and self-image.

Scarring has two characteristics: discoloration and contour. The discoloration of scars fades somewhat with time. However, scar tissue tends to develop altered contours; that is, it is no longer flat or slightly raised but becomes elevated and enlarged above the original burned area. Some burn care providers believe that pressure can eventually help keep a scar flat.[32] Gentle pressure is maintained on the healed burn with custom-fitted pressure garments and clear, thermoplastic face masks. Pressure garments and masks should never be worn over unhealed wounds and, once a wearing schedule has been established, are removed only for short periods while bathing. Pressure garments are worn up to 24 hours a day for as long as 12 to 18 months.

The patient typically experiences discomfort from itching where healing is occurring. Teach your patient about the application of water-based moisturizers and selective, short-term use of oral antihistamines (e.g., hydroxyzine [Atarax]) to help reduce the itching. Massage oil, silicone gel sheeting (e.g., Biodermis), gabapentin, and injectable corticosteroids also may be helpful.[33]

As "old" epithelium is replaced by new cells, flaking occurs. The newly formed skin is extremely sensitive to trauma. Blisters and skin tears are likely to develop from slight pressure or friction. Additionally, these newly healed areas can be hypersensitive or hyposensitive to cold, heat, and touch. Grafted areas are

FIG. 25-14 Neck contractures.

more likely to be hyposensitive until peripheral nerve regeneration occurs. Teach your patients to protect healed burn areas from direct sunlight for about 3 months to prevent hyperpigmentation and sunburn injury. They should always wear sunscreen when they are outside.[34]

Complications

The most common complications during the rehabilitation phase are skin and joint contractures and hypertrophic scarring (Fig. 25-14) and eFig. 25-1 (available on the website for this chapter). A **contracture** (an abnormal condition of a joint characterized by flexion and fixation) develops as a result of the shortening of scar tissue in the flexor tissues of a joint. Areas that are most susceptible to contracture formation include the anterior and lateral neck areas, axillae, antecubital fossae, fingers, groin areas, popliteal fossae, knees, and ankles. Some areas encompass major joints. Not only does the skin over these areas develop contractures, but the underlying tissues, such as the ligaments and tendons, also have a tendency to shorten during the healing process.

Carefully observe the patient for these potential problems. Encourage proper positioning, splinting, and exercise to minimize this complication. Tell the patient to continue with these strategies until the skin matures at around 1 year posthealing. Rehabilitative therapy is aimed at the extension of body parts because the flexors are stronger than the extensors. Burned legs may first be wrapped with elastic (e.g., tensor, Ace) bandages to assist with circulation to leg-graft and donor sites before ambulation. Burned arms can be wrapped with a layer of tubular elastic gauze (e.g., Tubigrip). This interim pressure prevents blister formation, promotes venous return, and decreases pain and itchiness. Once the skin is completely healed and less fragile, custom-fitted pressure garments replace the elastic bandages and tubular gauze.

NURSING AND COLLABORATIVE MANAGEMENT
REHABILITATION PHASE

During the rehabilitation phase, encourage both the patient and the caregiver to participate in care. Since the patient may go home with small, unhealed wounds, teach your patient and caregiver the skills for dressing changes and wound care.[34] Pain management and nutritional needs continue to be based on individual patient status. If needed, arrange home care nursing services to assist with care after discharge. Water-based creams that penetrate into the dermis (e.g., Vaseline Intensive Rescue, Sween, Complex 15) should be used routinely on healed areas to keep the skin supple and well moisturized, which will decrease itching and flaking. Occasionally low-dose antihistamines may be used at bedtime if itching persists.

Postburn reconstructive surgery is frequently required after a major burn. The need for further surgery is reviewed at the outpatient burn clinic appointments after discharge.

Continue to encourage the patient to perform the physical and occupational therapy routines. Constant encouragement and reassurance are necessary to maintain a patient's morale, particularly once the patient realizes that recovery can be slow. Rehabilitation may need to be a primary focus for at least the next 6 to 12 months.

GERONTOLOGIC CONSIDERATIONS

BURNS

The older patient presents many challenges for the burn team. The normal aging process puts the patient at risk for injury because of unsteady gait, limited eyesight, and diminished hearing. As people age, skin becomes drier and more wrinkled. Older adults have thinning of the dermal layer, a loss of elastic fibers, a reduction in subcutaneous adipose tissue, and a decrease in vascularity. As a result, the thinner dermis, with reduced blood flow, sustains deeper burns with poorer rates of healing.[35]

Once injured, the older adult has more complications in the emergent and acute phases of burn resuscitation because of preexisting medical conditions. For example, older patients with diabetes, heart failure, or chronic obstructive pulmonary disease have morbidity and mortality rates exceeding those of healthy, younger patients. In older patients, pneumonia is a frequent complication, burn wounds and donor sites take longer to heal, and surgical procedures are less well tolerated. Weaning from a ventilator can be a challenge. Although usually self-limiting, delirium, if it develops, may be distressing. It usually takes longer for these patients to rehabilitate to the point where they can safely return home.[36] For some, a return home to independent living may not be possible. As the population ages, developing strategies to prevent burn injuries in older adults is a priority.

EMOTIONAL/PSYCHOLOGIC NEEDS OF PATIENTS AND CAREGIVERS

Patients and caregivers have many emotional/psychologic needs during the often lengthy, unpredictable, and complex course of care.[37,38] You have an important supportive and counseling role as patients struggle to get their lives back on track.

To manage the enormous range of emotional responses that the burn patient may exhibit, assess the circumstances of the burn (e.g., cause, people involved), family relationships, and previous coping experiences with stressful stimuli. At any time the patient may experience a variety of emotions such as fear, anxiety, anger, guilt, and depression (Table 25-14).

Burn survivors frequently experience thoughts and feelings that are frightening and disturbing, such as guilt about the burn incident, reliving of the frightening burn experience, fear of dying, concern about future therapy and surgery, frustrations

TABLE 25-14	EMOTIONAL RESPONSES OF BURN PATIENTS*
Emotion	**Possible Verbal Expression**
Fear	Will I die? What will happen next? Will I be disfigured? Will my family and friends still love me?
Anxiety	I feel out of control. What's going to happen to me? When will I look normal again?
Anger	Why did this happen to me? The nurses enjoy hurting me. I hope the person who did this to me dies.
Guilt	If only I'd been more careful. I'm being punished because I did something wrong.
Depression	It's no use going on like this. I don't care what happens to me. I wish people would leave me alone.

*List is not all-inclusive.

with ongoing discomfort and treatment, and hopelessness about the future. During recovery, as more independence is expected from the patient, new fears may occur: "Can I really do this?" "Am I a desirable person?" "How can I go outside looking like this?" These challenges confront patients throughout their recovery and perhaps for years to come.

A person's self-esteem may be adversely affected by a burn injury. Some individuals may fear the loss of relationships because of perceived or actual physical disfigurement. In a society that values physical beauty, alterations in body image can result in psychologic distress.

Open and frequent communication among the patient, caregivers, close friends, and burn team members is essential. Because of the tremendous psychologic impact of a burn injury, be particularly sensitive to the patient's emotions and concerns. Encourage the patient to discuss fears regarding loss of life as he or she once knew it, loss of function, temporary or permanent deformity and disfigurement, return to work and home life, and financial burdens resulting from a long and costly hospitalization and rehabilitation.[39]

Encourage appropriate independence and an eventual return to preburn activities, such as school or work.[40] Peer counseling and informal interactions with other burn survivors may bring comfort and help to restore confidence. Reassure patients that their feelings, during this period of adjustment, are a normal reaction to an extraordinary life event. Their frustration and impatience are to be expected as they work to establish a new life. Assist patients in adapting to a realistic, yet positive appraisal of their particular situation, emphasizing what they *can* do instead of what they *cannot* do.

Caregivers may share some or all of these challenges and feelings. At times, they may feel helpless or too exhausted to assist their loved one. Continued support from trusted and familiar burn team members is essential. Helping caregivers assist with aspects of the patient's care helps them to reconnect with their loved one and eases the transition home. Many burn survivors and their caregivers remark on the powerful learning experience of the burn and a renewed appreciation of life, despite the ongoing challenges of a prolonged recovery. You need to acknowledge that their feelings are real and common. Most burn survivors speak of a real satisfaction with their postburn life and are more empowered as time goes on.

It is important to address individual spiritual and cultural needs because both have a role in treatment decisions and recovery. Pastoral care may be a helpful resource for the patient and the caregiver. The need for support, information, and family involvement may vary among cultures. Identify what is important to your patient and caregiver, and communicate that information in the patient's plan of care. Encourage the burn care team to remain culturally aware of and sensitive to the individual patient's and caregiver's cultural needs.

The difficult issue of sexuality must be met with honesty.[41] Physical appearance is altered in the patient who has sustained a major burn. Acceptance of any changes is difficult at first for the patient and significant other. The nature of skin injury in itself can cause modifications in processing sexual stimuli. Touch is an important part of sexuality, and immature scar tissue may make the sensation of touch unpleasant or may dull it. This may only be transient, but the patient and partner need to know that it is normal and receive anticipatory guidance from the burn team to avoid undue emotional strain.

The stress of the burn injury occasionally precipitates a psychologic crisis. Many patients realize this experience is beyond their ability to cope. Assessment by a psychiatrist who can prescribe appropriate medication, if needed, and begin short-term counseling is frequently helpful. Early psychiatric intervention is essential if the patient has been previously treated for a psychiatric illness or if the injury was a suicide attempt. The diagnosis of posttraumatic stress disorder is made in a number of burn patients. Treatment typically begins in the hospital, but links to community resources must be made before discharge to ensure continuity of psychologic care. A referral to a psychiatrist, psychologist, mental health counselor, social worker, or psychiatric advanced practice nurse (APN) should be discussed if concerns are raised at burn clinic follow-up.

Caregiver and patient support groups may be beneficial in meeting the patient's and caregiver's emotional needs at any phase of the recovery process.[42] Speaking with others who have experienced burn trauma can be beneficial, both in terms of

reaffirming that the patient's feelings are normal and in sharing helpful advice. The Phoenix Society (*www.phoenix-society.org*) is an international, highly respected burn survivors' support group. For many years the society has offered invaluable support and resources (e.g., annual World Burn Congress conference) to burn survivors, caregivers, and burn team personnel.

SPECIAL NEEDS OF NURSES

Warm, trusting, and mutually satisfying relationships frequently develop between burn patients and nursing staff, not only during hospitalization but also during the long-term rehabilitation period.[43] Sometimes the bond can be so strong that the patient has difficulty separating from the hospital and staff. The frequency and intensity of family contact can be rewarding as well as draining to you. You may find it difficult to cope with the deformities caused by the burn injury, the odors, the unpleasant sight of the wound, and the reality of the pain that accompanies the burn and its treatment. Do not hesitate to seek help from co-workers, a manager, or the employee assistance program should you feel the need.

In time, you will come to know that the specialized burn care you provide makes a critical difference in helping patients not only survive, but also cope with and triumph over an intense and multifaceted injury.

Ongoing support services or critical incident stress debriefings led by a psychiatrist, psychologist, psychiatric APN, or social worker may also be helpful. Peer support groups (e.g., ABA, International Society for Burn Injuries) can serve a similar purpose by helping you cope with difficult feelings experienced when caring for burn patients. Because burn nursing is physically, psychologically, and intellectually demanding, it has many challenges and inherent rewards. Attention to your own self-care is important to maintain a positive attitude and healthy work-life balance.[44] Time with family and friends and rest and relaxation at home are essential parts of self-care and a balanced life with purpose and meaning.

CASE STUDY

Burn Injury

Comstock/Thinkstock

Patient Profile
G.M., a 52-year-old married white man, arrives at the emergency department with burns to his face, neck, chest, right arm and hand, and right foot. He was burning brush on his farm when the fire went out of control. He has an 18-gauge IV with NSS running at 100 mL/hr, and he is receiving 100% humidified O₂ by mask.

Subjective Data
• Complains of blurry vision and trouble swallowing
• States his burns are painful and that he is scared
• States he is a "diabetic" and has "high blood pressure"

Objective Data
Physical Examination
• Is awake, alert, and oriented, but in some distress
• Eyes are red, irritated
• Voice is hoarse; nasal hair is singed
• Face is reddened with blisters noted on the nose and forehead

• Right arm, right hand, chest, neck, and right foot have shiny, bright red, wet wounds
• Patient is shivering

Discussion Questions
1. *Priority Decision:* What are the priorities of care in the prehospital environment? How should his airway, breathing, and circulation be managed?
2. *Priority Decision:* What factors place G.M. at high risk for an inhalation injury? What priority interventions can be anticipated?
3. What pain medications might be considered to relieve his pain?
4. Which of the criteria for burn center referral does G.M. meet for admission to the hospital burn unit?
5. What metabolic disturbances would be expected soon after G.M.'s admission? Explain the physiologic basis for these changes.
6. How might G.M.'s co-morbidities affect his burn care and rehabilitation?
7. What measures should be taken to support G.M.'s caregivers?
8. *Priority Decision:* Based on the assessment data presented, develop three priority nursing diagnoses. Identify any collaborative problems.
9. *Evidence-Based Practice:* What are the most effective wound care strategies to manage G.M.'s burn wounds?

BRIDGE TO NCLEX EXAMINATION

The number of the question corresponds to the same-numbered outcome at the beginning of the chapter.

1. Knowing the most common causes of household fires, which prevention strategy would the nurse focus on when teaching about fire safety?
   a. Set hot water temperature at 140° F (60° C).
   b. Use only hardwired smoke detectors.
   c. Encourage regular home fire exit drills.
   d. Never permit older adults to cook unattended.

2. The injury that is least likely to result in a full-thickness burn is
   a. sunburn.
   b. scald injury.
   c. chemical burn.
   d. electrical injury.

3. When assessing a patient with a partial-thickness burn, the nurse would expect to find (select all that apply)
   a. blisters.
   b. exposed fascia.
   c. exposed muscles.
   d. intact nerve endings.
   e. red, shiny, wet appearance.

4. A patient is admitted to the burn center with burns of his head and neck, chest, and back after an explosion in his garage. On assessment, the nurse auscultates wheezes throughout the lung fields. On reassessment, the wheezes are gone and the breath sounds are greatly diminished. Which action is the most appropriate for the nurse to take next?
   a. Obtain vital signs and a STAT arterial blood gas.
   b. Encourage the patient to cough and auscultate the lungs again.
   c. Document the findings and continue to monitor the patient's breathing.
   d. Anticipate the need for endotracheal intubation and notify the physician.

5. Fluid and electrolyte shifts that occur during the early emergent phase of a burn injury include
   a. adherence of albumin to vascular walls.
   b. movement of potassium into the vascular space.
   c. sequestering of sodium and water in interstitial fluid.
   d. hemolysis of red blood cells from large volumes of rapidly administered fluid.

6. To maintain a positive nitrogen balance in a major burn, the patient must
   a. eat a high-protein, low-fat, high-carbohydrate diet.
   b. increase normal caloric intake by about three times.
   c. eat at least 1500 calories/day in small, frequent meals.
   d. eat rice and whole wheat for the chemical effect on nitrogen balance.

7. A patient has 25% TBSA burned from a car fire. His wounds have been debrided and covered with a silver-impregnated dressing. The nurse's priority intervention for wound care would be to
   a. reapply a new dressing without disturbing the wound bed.
   b. observe the wound for signs of infection during dressing changes.
   c. apply cool compresses for pain relief in between dressing changes.
   d. wash the wound aggressively with soap and water three times a day.

8. Pain management for the burn patient is most effective when (select all that apply)
   a. a pain rating tool is used to monitor the patient's level of pain.
   b. painful dressing changes are delayed until the patient's pain is completely relieved.
   c. the patient is informed about and has some control over the management of the pain.
   d. a multimodal approach is used (e.g., sustained-release and short-acting opioids, NSAIDs, adjuvant analgesics).
   e. nonpharmacologic therapies (e.g., music therapy, distraction) replace opioids in the rehabilitation phase of a burn injury.

9. A therapeutic measure used to prevent hypertrophic scarring during the rehabilitation phase of burn recovery is
   a. applying pressure garments.
   b. repositioning the patient every 2 hours.
   c. performing active ROM at least every 4 hours.
   d. massaging the new tissue with water-based moisturizers.

10. A patient is recovering from second- and third-degree burns over 30% of his body and is now ready for discharge. The first action the nurse should take when meeting with the patient would be to
    a. arrange a return-to-clinic appointment and prescription for pain medications.
    b. teach the patient and the caregiver proper wound care to be performed at home.
    c. review the patient's current health care status and readiness for discharge to home.
    d. give the patient written discharge information and websites for additional information for burn survivors.

1. c, 2. a, 3. a, d, e, 4. d, 5. c, 6. a, 7. b, 8. a, c, d, 9. a, 10. c

ⓔvolve

For rationales to these answers and even more NCLEX review questions, visit http://evolve.elsevier.com/Lewis/medsurg.

REFERENCES

1. American Burn Association: Burn incidence and treatment in the US: 2011 fact sheet. Retrieved from www.ameriburn.org/resources_factsheet.php.

2. Centers for Disease Control and Prevention: Fire deaths and injuries: fact sheet, Atlanta, 2011. Retrieved from www.cdc.gov/HomeandRecreationalSafety/Fire-Prevention/fires-factsheet.html.

*3. Peck M: Epidemiology of burns throughout the world—part I: distribution and risk factors, Burns 37:1087, 2011.

*4. Edwards D, Heard J, Latenser B, et al: Burn injuries in Eastern Zambia: impact of multidisciplinary teaching teams, J Burn Care Res 32:31, 2011.

5. Cancio L: Airway management and smoke inhalation injury in the burn patient, Clin Plast Surg 36:555, 2009.

6. Latenser B: Critical care of the burn patient: the first 48 hours, Crit Care Med 37:2819, 2009.

7. Moss L: Treatment of the burn patient in primary care, Skin Wound Care 23:517, 2010.

*8. Schwartz S, Rothrock M, Barron-Vaya Y, et al: Impact of diabetes on burn injury: preliminary results from prospective study, J Burn Care Res 32:435, 2011.

*Evidence-based information for clinical practice.

9. Arnstein P: What's the best way to cool my patient's burn pain, *Nursing* 40:61, 2010.

*10. Pannucci C, Osborne N, Wahl W: Venous thromboembolism in thermally-injured patients: analysis of the National Burn Repository, *J Burn Care Res* 32:6, 2011.

*11. Garcia DA, Baglin TP, Weitz JI, et al: Parenteral anticoagulants: antithrombotic therapy and prevention of thrombosis, ed 9: American College of Chest Physicians evidence-based clinical practice guidelines, *Chest* 141:e24S, 2012.

12. Dries DJ, Mohr WJ: *Yearbook of intensive care and emergency medicine*, Berlin, 2010, Springer-Verlag.

13. Cartotto R: Fluid resuscitation of the thermally-injured patient, *Clin Plast Surg* 36:569, 2009.

*14. Davison P, Loiselle F, Nickerson D: Survey on current hydrotherapy use among North American burn centers, *J Burn Care Res* 31:540, 2010.

*15. Rafla K, Tredget E: Infection control in the burn unit, *Burns* 37:5, 2011.

*16. Trupkovic T, Kinn M, Kleinschmidt S: Analgesia and sedation in the intensive care of burn patients: results of a European survey, *J Intens Care Med* 26:397, 2011.

*17. Wong L, Turner L: Treatment of post-burn neuropathic pain: evaluation of pregabalin, *Burns* 36:769, 2010.

18. Greenhalgh D: Topical antimicrobial agents for burn wounds, *Clin Plast Surg* 36:597, 2009.

*19. Posluszny J, Conrad P, Halerz M, et al: Surgical burn wound infections and their clinical implications, *J Burn Care Res* 32:324, 2011.

*20. Mosier M, Pham T, Klein M, et al: Early enteral nutrition in burns: compliance with guidelines and associated outcomes in a multicenter study, *J Burn Care Res* 32:104, 2011.

*21. Williams I, Herndon D, Jeschke M, et al: The hypermetabolic response to burn injury and interventions to modify this response, *Clin Plast Surg* 36:583, 2009.

*22. Holavanahalli R, Helm P, Parry I, et al: Select practices in management and rehabilitation of a survey report, *J Burn Care Res* 32:210, 2011.

23. Mosier M, Gibran N: Surgical excision of the burn wound, *Clin Plast Surg* 36:617, 2009.

*24. Curinga G, Jain A, Feldman M, et al: RBC transfusion following burns, *Burns* 37:742, 2011.

25. Saffle J: Closure of the excised burn wound: temporary skin substitutes, *Clin Plast Surg* 36:627, 2009.

*26. Demirtas Y, Yagmur C, Soylemez S, et al: Management of split-thickness skin graft donor sites: a prospective clinical trial for comparison of five different dressing materials, *Burns* 36:999, 2010.

27. Sheridan R: Closure of the excised burn wound: autograft, semipermanent skin substitutes and permanent skin substitutes, *Clin Plast Surg* 36:643, 2009.

*28. Tengvall O, Wickman M, Wengstrom Y: Memories of pain after burn injury—the patient's experience, *J Burn Care Res* 31:319, 2010.

*29. Rumbach A, Ward E, Cornwell P, et al: Incidence and predictive factors for dysphagia after thermal burn injury: a prospective cohort study, *J Burn Care Res* 32:608, 2011.

*30. Reeve J, James F, McNeill R, et al: Functional and psychological outcomes following burn injury: reduced income and hidden emotions are predictors of greater distress, *J Burn Care Res* 32:468, 2011.

*31. Sundara D: A review of issues and concerns of family members of adult burn survivors, *J Burn Care Res* 32:349, 2011.

*32. Engrav L, Heimbach D, Rivara F, et al: Twelve-year within-wound study of the effectiveness of custom pressure garment therapy, *Burns* 36:975, 2010.

*33. Gautos I: Burns pruritus—a study of current practices in the UK, *Burns* 36:42, 2010.

*34. Richards R: Burn rehabilitation and research: proceedings of a consensus summit, *J Burn Care Res* 30:543, 2009.

*35. Holavanahalli R, Helm P, Kowalske K, et al: Long-term outcomes in patients surviving large burns: the skin, *J Burn Care Res* 31:631, 2010.

*36. Brown-Guttovz H: Burn injury, *Nursing* 41:68, 2011.

*37. Elsherbiny O, Salem M, El-Sabbagh A, et al: Quality of life of adult burn patients with severe burns, *Burns* 37:776, 2011.

*38. Schneider J, Bassi S, Ryna C: Employment outcomes after burn injury: a comparison of those burned at work and those burned outside of work, *J Burn Care Res* 32:294, 2011.

*39. Klein M, Lezotte D, Heltshe S, et al: Functional and psychosocial outcomes of older adults after burn injury: results from a multicenter database of severe burn injury, *J Burn Care Res* 32:66, 2011.

*40. Solanki N, Greenwood J, Kavanagh S, et al: Social issues prolong elderly burn patient hospitalization, *J Burn Care Res* 32:387, 2011.

*41. Rimmer R, Rutter C, Lessard C, et al: Burn care professionals' attitudes and practices regarding discussions of sexuality and intimacy with adult burn survivors, *J Burn Care Res* 31:579, 2010.

*42. Orcutt T: Developing family support groups in the ICU, *Nurs Crit Care* 5:33, 2010.

43. Greenfield E: The pivotal role of nursing personnel in burn care, *Indian J Plast Surg* 43:594, 2010.

*44. Kornhaber R, Wilson A: Psychosocial needs of burns nurses: a descriptive, phenomenological inquiry, *J Burn Care Res* 32:286, 2011.

RESOURCES

American Burn Association
www.ameriburn.org
Burn Survivor.org
www.burnsurvivor.org
Changing Faces
www.changingfaces.org.uk
International Society for Burn Injuries
www.worldburn.org
Phoenix Society for Burn Survivors
www.phoenix-society.org
World Burn Foundation
www.burnfoundation.com

CASE STUDY

Managing Multiple Patients

Introduction

You are working the day shift on a medical-surgical unit and have been assigned to care for the following five patients. You have 1 UAP who is assigned to work with you. There are 15 other patients on the unit being cared for by an additional 3 RNs and 3 UAPs.

Patients

F.M., an 81-year-old Hispanic woman, had pneumatic retinopexy surgery yesterday to repair a partially detached retina. She has a history of diabetes, hypothyroidism, and hypertension. She is scheduled to be discharged today, but the night nurse is concerned because her blood pressure is elevated at 150/94 mm Hg.

Jack Hollingsworth/
Photodisc/Thinkstock

J.K., a 68-year-old African American woman with osteoarthritis and type 2 diabetes mellitus for the past 15 years, now has diabetic retinopathy. She had argon laser therapy to her right eye yesterday to seal leaking microaneurysms from macular edema. She was admitted with uncontrolled postoperative hyperglycemia.

Kevin Peterson/Stockbyte/
Thinkstock

D.A., a 74-year-old woman, is admitted to the hospital with complaints of chest tightness and shortness of breath. Her past medical history is negative except for a recent diagnosis of basal cell carcinoma (BCC) on her face. She was scheduled to have the BCC surgically removed tomorrow. The health care provider suspects D.A.'s symptoms are caused by anxiety but first needs to rule out any coronary artery disease before surgery.

iStockphoto/Thinkstock

G.L., a 59-year-old white man, just arrived for admission. He is scheduled for surgical removal of malignant melanoma lesions on his face at 1200. He is worried that the surgery will be disfiguring.

Hemera/Thinkstock

G.M., a 52-year-old white man, is transferred from the ICU following burns to his face, neck, chest, right arm and hand, and right foot. He has a tracheostomy and is receiving 35% O_2 via a humidified trach collar. He has a history of diabetes and hypertension. In the ICU he had been on a mechanical ventilator for respiratory failure caused by inhalation injury. His burns are shiny, bright red, and wet. There are a few blisters on his face.

Comstock/Thinkstock

Management Discussion Questions

1. **Priority Decision:** After receiving report, which patient should you see first? Provide rationale.
2. **Delegation Decision:** Which tasks could you delegate to the UAP *(select all that apply)?*
   a. Obtain vital signs on F.M.
   b. Take a blood pressure reading on G.M.
   c. Perform an admission assessment on G.L.
   d. Explain planned diagnostic testing to D.A.
   e. Obtain a capillary blood glucose reading on J.K.
3. **Priority and Delegation Decision:** When you enter G.M.'s room, he tells you he is not feeling well. He says he has a headache and his legs are "cramping up." He is also somewhat confused as he is unaware that he is in the hospital. What initial action would be most appropriate?
   a. Administer acetaminophen for headache relief.
   b. Have the UAP obtain a stat capillary blood glucose reading.
   c. Notify G.M.'s health care provider of his altered level of consciousness.
   d. Have the UAP obtain vital signs on G.M. while you look at his most recent laboratory test results.

Case Study Progression

G.M.'s vital signs are BP 154/88 mm Hg, his heart rate is 112 bpm, his respirations are 18 breaths/min, and his temperature is 98° F (36.8° C). His most recent lab work reveals a serum sodium level of 125 mEq/L (125 mmol/L). You notify his health care provider, who orders a normal saline IV to infuse at 100 mL/hr.

4. G.M. complains of thirst and asks for something to drink. Which fluid would be appropriate to give him *(select all that apply)?*
   a. Gatorade
   b. Tap water
   c. Cola soda
   d. Apple juice
   e. Orange juice
5. In addition to teaching F.M. how to administer postoperative eye drops, you will also explain
   a. position and activity restrictions.
   b. how to change the dressing on her eye.
   c. the necessity for restricting fluid intake.
   d. that protective eyewear will no longer be required.
6. When giving report to your UAP regarding your assigned patients, she asks if there is a significant difference between D.A. and G.L.'s skin cancers. You reply based on knowledge that
   a. basal cell carcinoma is the most deadly form of skin cancer.
   b. malignant melanoma typically appears as red, rough patches on the skin.
   c. basal cell carcinoma typically presents during the second and third decades of life.
   d. melanoma has the ability to metastasize to any organ, including the brain and heart.
7. **Management Decision:** Another RN offers to help you by providing wound care for G.M. Which observed action by the RN would require your immediate intervention?
   a. G.M.'s hands are elevated on pillows.
   b. G.M.'s burns are cleansed with soap and water.
   c. G.M. is promised analgesia as soon as wound care is complete.
   d. G.M.'s burns are covered with a very thin layer of prescribed ointment.

evolve Answers available at *http://evolve.elsevier.com/Lewis/medsurg.*

SECTION 5

Problems of Oxygenation: Ventilation

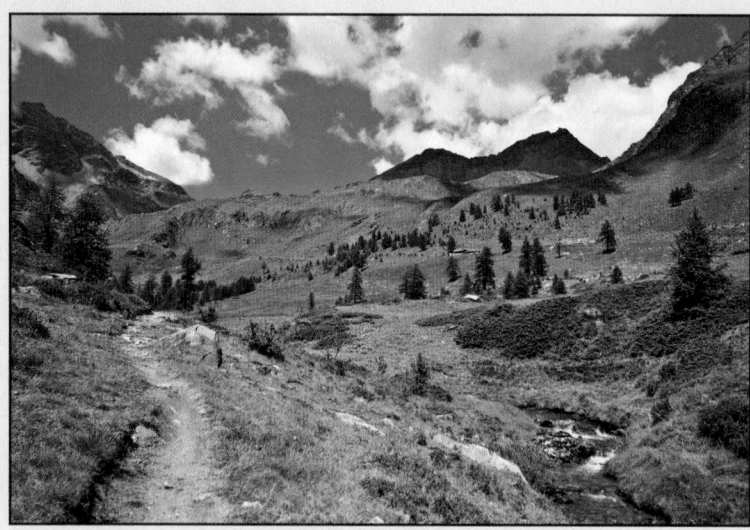

iStockphoto

May your trails be crooked, winding, lonesome, dangerous, leading to the most amazing view. May your mountains rise into and above the clouds.
Edward Abbey

When you own your breath, nobody can steal your peace.
Author Unknown

Nursing Assessment
Respiratory System

Susan J. Eisel

⊘volve WEBSITE

- NCLEX Review Questions
- Key Points
- Pre-Test
- Answer Guidelines for Case Study in this chapter
- Rationales for Bridge to NCLEX Examination Questions
- Concept Map Creator
- Glossary
- Animations
  - Patterns of Respiration
  - Percussion Tones Throughout Chest
  - Pulmonary Circulation
- Videos
  - Inspection and Palpation: Breathing and Respiratory Excursion, Anterior Chest

- Inspection and Palpation: Respirations, Respiratory Excursion, and Tactile Fremitus, Posterior Chest
- Inspection and Percussion: Diaphragmatic Excursion
- Inspection: Nose
- Palpation: Tactile Fremitus, Posterior Chest
- Percussion: Anterior Thorax
- Physical Examination: Anterior Chest, Lungs, Heart
- Physical Examination: Lung
- Content Updates
- Audio
  - Bronchial Breath Sounds
  - Bronchovesicular Breath Sounds
  - High-Pitched Crackles
  - High-Pitched Wheeze

- Low-Pitched Crackles
- Low-Pitched Wheeze
- Pleural Friction Rub
- Stridor
- Vesicular Breath Sounds

eFigures
- eFig 26-1: Oxygen-hemoglobin dissociation curve
- eFig. 26-2: Pulse oximeter
- eFig. 26-3: Finger clubbing
- eFig. 26-4: Relationship of lung volumes and capacities

eTable
- eTable 26-1: Oxygen-Hemoglobin Dissociation Curve

LEARNING OUTCOMES

1. Differentiate among the structures and functions of the upper respiratory tract, the lower respiratory tract, and the chest wall.
2. Describe the process that initiates and controls inspiration and expiration.
3. Describe the process of gas diffusion within the lungs.
4. Identify the respiratory defense mechanisms.
5. Describe the significance of arterial blood gas values in relation to respiratory function.
6. Relate the signs and symptoms of inadequate oxygenation to implications of these findings.

7. Link the age-related changes of the respiratory system to the differences in assessment findings.
8. Select the significant subjective and objective data related to the respiratory system that should be obtained from a patient.
9. Select appropriate techniques to use in the physical assessment of the respiratory system.
10. Differentiate normal from common abnormal findings in a physical assessment of the respiratory system.
11. Describe the purpose, significance of results, and nursing responsibilities related to diagnostic studies of the respiratory system.

KEY TERMS

adventitious sounds, p. 488
chemoreceptor, p. 480
compliance, p. 478
crackles, Table 26-8, p. 489
dyspnea, p. 478

elastic recoil, p. 478
fremitus, p. 486
mechanical receptors, p. 480
pleural friction rub, Table 26-8, p. 490
rhonchi, Table 26-8, p. 489

surfactant, p. 477
tidal volume (V_T), p. 477
ventilation, p. 478
wheezes, Table 26-8, p. 489

STRUCTURES AND FUNCTIONS OF RESPIRATORY SYSTEM

The primary purpose of the respiratory system is gas exchange. This involves the transfer of oxygen (O_2) and carbon dioxide (CO_2) between the atmosphere and the blood. The respiratory system is divided into two parts: the upper respiratory tract and the lower respiratory tract (Fig. 26-1).

Upper Respiratory Tract

The *upper respiratory tract* includes the nose, mouth, pharynx, epiglottis, larynx, and trachea. Air enters into the respiratory tract through the nose. The nose is made of bone and cartilage and is divided into two nares by the nasal septum. The inside of the nose is shaped into three passages by projections called *turbinates*. The turbinates increase the surface area of the nasal

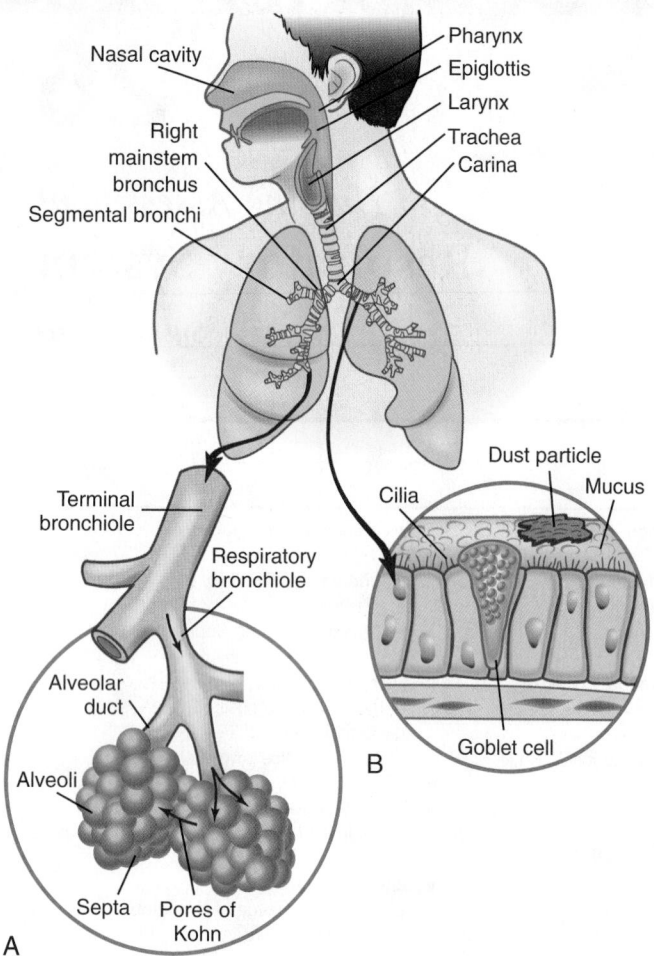

FIG. 26-1 Structures of the respiratory tract. **A,** Pulmonary functional unit. **B,** Ciliated mucous membrane.

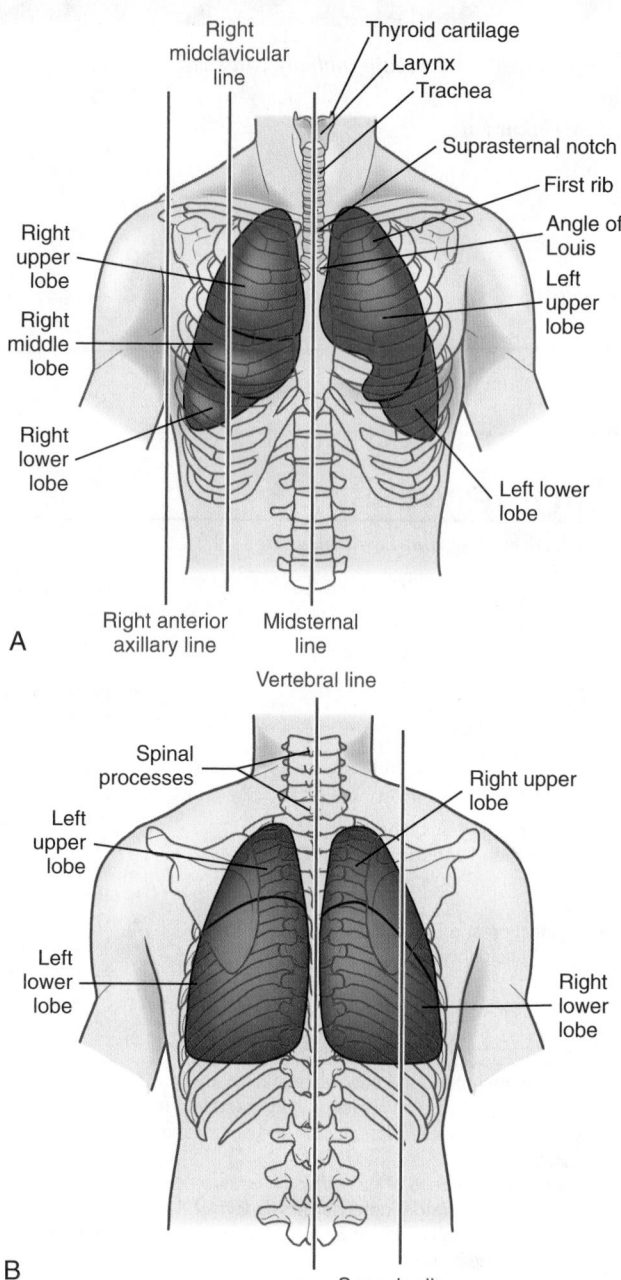

FIG. 26-2 Landmarks and structures of the chest wall. **A,** Anterior view. **B,** Posterior view.

mucosa, which warms and moistens the air as it enters the nose. The internal nose opens directly into the sinuses. The nasal cavity connects with the pharynx, a tubular passageway that is subdivided into three parts: the *nasopharynx, oropharynx,* and *laryngopharynx.*

The nose functions to protect the lower airway by warming and humidifying air and filtering small particles before air enters the lungs. Olfactory nerve endings, located in the roof of the nose, are responsible for the sense of smell.

Air moves through the oropharynx to the laryngopharynx. It then travels through the epiglottis to the larynx before moving into the trachea. The *epiglottis* is a small flap located behind the tongue that closes over the larynx during swallowing. This prevents solids and liquids from entering the lungs. The vocal cords are located in the larynx. Vibrational sounds are made during respiration leading to vocalization. Air passes through the glottis, the opening between the vocal cords, and into the trachea. The trachea is a cylindric tube about 5 in (10 to 12 cm) long and 1 in (1.5 to 2.5 cm) in diameter. U-shaped cartilages keep the trachea open but allow the adjacent esophagus to expand for swallowing. The trachea bifurcates into the right and left mainstem bronchi at a point called the *carina.* The carina is located at the level of the manubriosternal junction, also called the *angle of Louis.* The carina is highly sensitive, and touching it during suctioning causes vigorous coughing.[1]

Lower Respiratory Tract

The *lower respiratory tract* consists of the bronchi, bronchioles, alveolar ducts, and alveoli. With the exception of the right and left mainstem bronchi, all lower airway structures are located inside the lungs. The right lung is divided into three lobes (upper, middle, and lower) and the left lung into two lobes (upper and lower) (Fig. 26-2). The structures of the chest wall (ribs, pleura, muscles of respiration) are also important for respiration.

Once air passes the carina, it is in the lower respiratory tract. The mainstem bronchi, pulmonary vessels, and nerves enter the lungs through a slit called the *hilus.* The right mainstem bronchus is shorter, wider, and straighter than the left mainstem bronchus. For this reason, aspiration is more likely to occur in the right lung than in the left lung.

Conducting airways					Respiratory unit
Trachea	Bronchi, segmental bronchi	Sub-segmental bronchi	Bronchioles		Alveolar ducts, alveoli
			Non-respiratory	Respiratory	
Generations	8	15	21-22	24	28

FIG. 26-3 Structures of lower airways.

The mainstem bronchi subdivide several times to form the lobar, segmental, and subsegmental bronchi. Further divisions form the bronchioles. The most distant bronchioles are called the respiratory bronchioles. Beyond these lie the alveolar ducts and alveolar sacs (Fig. 26-3). The bronchioles are encircled by smooth muscles that constrict and dilate in response to various stimuli. The terms *bronchoconstriction* and *bronchodilation* refer to a decrease or increase in the diameter of the airways caused by contraction or relaxation of these muscles.

Oxygen and carbon dioxide exchange takes place in the alveoli. The trachea and bronchi act as a pathway to conduct gases to the alveoli. The trachea plus the bronchi are called *anatomic dead space* (VD). The air filling this space with every breath is not available for gas exchange. In adults a normal **tidal volume** (VT), or volume of air exchanged with each breath, is about 500 mL (in a 150 lb man). Of each 500 mL inhaled, about 150 mL is VD.

After moving through the VD, air reaches the respiratory bronchioles and alveoli (Fig. 26-4). *Alveoli* are small sacs that are the primary site of gas exchange in the lungs. The alveoli are interconnected by pores of Kohn, which allow movement of air from alveolus to alveolus (see Fig. 26-1). Deep breathing promotes air movement through these pores and assists in moving mucus out of the respiratory bronchioles. Bacteria can also move through these pores, spreading infection to previously uninfected areas. The adult lung has 300 million alveoli. Alveoli have a total volume of about 2500 mL and a surface area for gas exchange that is about the size of a tennis court.

Gases are exchanged at the alveolar-capillary membrane where the alveoli come in contact with pulmonary capillaries (Fig. 26-5). In conditions such as pulmonary edema, excess fluid fills the interstitial space and alveoli, markedly reducing gas exchange.

Surfactant. The lungs are a collection of 300 million alveoli, each 0.3 mm in diameter. Because alveoli are unstable, they have a natural tendency to collapse. Alveolar cells secrete surfactant. **Surfactant** is a lipoprotein that lowers the surface tension in the alveoli. It reduces the amount of pressure needed to inflate the alveoli and makes them less likely to collapse. Normally, each person takes a slightly larger breath, termed a *sigh*, after every five or six breaths. This sigh stretches the alveoli and promotes surfactant secretion.

FIG. 26-4 Scanning electron micrograph of lung parenchyma. **A,** Alveoli *(A)* and alveolar-capillary membrane *(arrow)*. **B,** Effects of atelectasis. Alveoli *(A)* are partially or totally collapsed.

Exhaled
PaO$_2$ 127 mm Hg
PaCO$_2$ 28 mm Hg

Inhaled
PaO$_2$ 159 mm Hg
PaCO$_2$ 0.3 mm Hg

Alveolus
PaO$_2$ 100 mm Hg
PaCO$_2$ 40 mm Hg

Venous blood
PaO$_2$ 40 mm Hg
PaCO$_2$ 46 mm Hg

Arterial blood
PaO$_2$ 100 mm Hg
PaCO$_2$ 40 mm Hg

FIG. 26-5 Partial pressure of respiratory gases in normal respiration. The pressures are shown in inhaled and exhaled air from the lungs and at the level of the alveoli and pulmonary venous and arterial blood vessels.

When not enough surfactant is present, the alveoli collapse. The term *atelectasis* refers to collapsed, airless alveoli (see Fig. 26-4, *B*). The postoperative patient is at risk for atelectasis because of the effects of anesthesia and restricted breathing with pain (see Chapter 20). In acute respiratory distress syndrome (ARDS), lack of surfactant contributes to widespread atelectasis (see Chapter 68).

Blood Supply. The lungs have two different types of circulation: pulmonary and bronchial. The *pulmonary circulation* provides the lungs with blood that participates in gas exchange. The pulmonary artery receives deoxygenated blood from the right ventricle of the heart and delivers it to pulmonary capillaries that are directly connected with alveoli. Oxygen–carbon dioxide exchange occurs at this point. The pulmonary veins return oxygenated blood to the left atrium, which then delivers it to the left ventricle. This oxygenated blood is pumped by the left ventricle into the aorta, which supplies the arteries of the systemic circulation. Venous blood is collected from capillary networks of the body and returned to the right atrium by way of the venae cavae.

The *bronchial circulation* starts with the bronchial arteries, which arise from the thoracic aorta. The bronchial circulation provides oxygen to the bronchi and other pulmonary tissues. Deoxygenated blood returns from the bronchial circulation through the azygos vein into the superior vena cava.

Chest Wall

The chest wall is shaped, supported, and protected by 24 ribs (12 on each side). The ribs and the sternum protect the lungs and the heart from injury and are called the *thoracic cage.*

The chest cavity is lined with a membrane called the *parietal pleura,* and the lungs are lined with a membrane called the *visceral pleura.* The parietal and visceral pleurae join to form a closed, double-walled sac. The visceral pleura does not have any sensory pain fibers or nerve endings, whereas the parietal pleura does have sensory pain fibers. Therefore irritation of the parietal pleura causes pain with each breath.

The space between the pleural layers is called the *intrapleural space.* Normally this space contains 20 to 25 mL of fluid. This fluid serves two purposes: (1) it provides lubrication, allowing the pleural layers to slide over each other during breathing; and (2) it increases cohesion between the pleural layers, thereby facilitating expansion of the pleurae and lungs during inspiration.

Fluid drains from the pleural space by the lymphatic circulation. Several pathologic conditions may cause the accumulation of greater amounts of fluid, termed a *pleural effusion.* Pleural fluid may accumulate because of blockage of lymphatic drainage (e.g., from malignant cells) or because of an imbalance between intravascular and oncotic fluid pressures, as in heart failure. Purulent pleural fluid with bacterial infection is called *empyema.*

The *diaphragm* is the major muscle of respiration. During inspiration the diaphragm contracts, increasing intrathoracic volume and pushing the abdominal contents downward. At the same time the external intercostal muscles and scalene muscles contract, increasing the lateral and anteroposterior (AP) dimension of the chest. This causes the size of the thoracic cavity to increase and intrathoracic pressure to decrease, so air enters the lungs.

The diaphragm is made up of two hemidiaphragms, each innervated by the right and left phrenic nerves. The phrenic nerves arise from the spinal cord between C3 and C5, the third and fifth cervical vertebrae. Injury to the phrenic nerve results in hemidiaphragm paralysis on the side of the injury. Complete spinal cord injuries above the level of C3 result in total diaphragm paralysis and dependence on a mechanical ventilator.

Physiology of Respiration

Ventilation. Ventilation involves *inspiration,* or inhalation (movement of air into the lungs), and *expiration,* or exhalation (movement of air out of the lungs). Air moves in and out of the lungs because intrathoracic pressure changes in relation to pressure at the airway opening. Contraction of the diaphragm and intercostal and scalene muscles increases chest dimensions, thereby decreasing intrathoracic pressure. Gas flows from an area of higher pressure (atmospheric) to one of lower pressure (intrathoracic).[2] When **dyspnea** (shortness of breath) occurs, neck and shoulder muscles can assist the effort. Some conditions (e.g., phrenic nerve paralysis, rib fractures, neuromuscular disease) may limit diaphragm or chest wall movement and cause the patient to breathe with smaller tidal volumes. As a result, the lungs do not fully inflate, and gas exchange is impaired.

In contrast to inspiration, expiration is passive. **Elastic recoil** is the tendency for the lungs to relax after being stretched or expanded. The elasticity of lung tissue is due to the elastin fibers found in the alveolar walls and surrounding the bronchioles and capillaries. The elastic recoil of the chest wall and lungs allows the chest to passively decrease in volume. Intrathoracic pressure rises, causing air to move out of the lungs.

Exacerbations of asthma or chronic obstructive pulmonary disease (COPD) cause expiration to become an active, labored process (see Chapter 29). Abdominal, intercostal, and accessory muscles (e.g., scalene, trapezius) assist in expelling air during labored breathing.

Compliance. Compliance (distensibility) is a measure of the ease of expansion of the lungs. This is a product of the elasticity of the lungs and the elastic recoil of the chest wall. When compliance is decreased, the lungs are more difficult to inflate. Examples include conditions that increase fluid in the lungs (e.g., pulmonary edema, ARDS, pneumonia), conditions that make lung tissue less elastic or distensible (e.g., pulmonary fibrosis, sarcoidosis), and conditions that restrict lung movement (e.g., pleural effusion). Compliance is increased when there is destruction of alveolar walls and loss of tissue elasticity, as in COPD.

Diffusion. Oxygen and carbon dioxide move back and forth across the alveolar-capillary membrane by diffusion. The overall direction of movement is from the area of higher concentration to the area of lower concentration. Thus oxygen moves from alveolar gas (atmospheric air) into the arterial blood and carbon dioxide from the arterial blood into the alveolar gas. Diffusion continues until equilibrium is reached.

The lungs' ability to oxygenate arterial blood adequately is assessed by examination of the partial pressure of oxygen in arterial blood (PaO_2) and arterial oxygen saturation (SaO_2). Oxygen is carried in the blood in two forms: dissolved oxygen and hemoglobin-bound oxygen. The PaO_2 represents the amount of oxygen dissolved in the plasma and is expressed in millimeters of mercury (mm Hg). The SaO_2 is the amount of oxygen bound to hemoglobin in comparison with the amount of oxygen the hemoglobin can carry. The SaO_2 is expressed as a percentage. For example, if the SaO_2 is 90%, this means that 90% of the hemoglobin attachments for oxygen have oxygen bound to them.

Arterial Blood Gases. Two methods are used to assess the efficiency of gas transfer in the lung and tissue oxygenation: analysis of *arterial blood gases* (ABGs) and pulse oximetry. ABGs are measured to determine oxygenation status and acid-base balance. ABG analysis includes measurement of the PaO_2, $PaCO_2$, acidity (pH), and bicarbonate (HCO_3^-) in arterial blood. The SaO_2 is either calculated or measured during this analysis. Normal values for ABGs are given in Table 26-1.

Blood for ABG analysis can be obtained by arterial puncture or from an arterial catheter, usually in the radial or femoral artery. Both techniques allow only intermittent analysis. Con-

TABLE 26-1 NORMAL ARTERIAL AND VENOUS BLOOD GAS VALUES*

Laboratory Value	Arterial Blood Gases Sea Level BP 760 mm Hg	1 Mile Above Sea Level BP 629 mm Hg	Venous Blood Gases Mixed Venous Blood Gases	
pH	7.35-7.45	7.35-7.45	pH	7.32-7.43
PaO₂†	80-100 mm Hg	65-75 mm Hg	PvO₂	38-42 mm Hg
SaO₂†	>95%‡	>95%‡	SvO₂	60%-80%‡
PaCO₂	35-45 mm Hg	35-45 mm Hg	PvCO₂	38-55 mm Hg
HCO₃⁻	22-26 mEq/L (mmol/L)	22-26 mEq/L (mmol/L)	HCO₃⁻	22-26 mEq/L (mmol/L)

*Assumes patient is ≤60 yr of age and breathing room air.
†Values decrease with age.
‡The same normal values apply when SpO_2 and SvO_2 are obtained by oximetry.
BP, Barometric pressure; *HCO₃⁻*, bicarbonate; *PaCO₂*, partial pressure of arterial CO₂; *PvCO₂*, partial pressure of CO₂ in venous blood; *PaO₂*, partial pressure of O₂ in arterial blood; *PvO₂*, partial pressure of O₂ in venous blood; *SaO₂*, arterial O₂ saturation; *SvO₂*, venous O₂ saturation.

TABLE 26-2 MANIFESTATIONS OF INADEQUATE OXYGENATION

Manifestations	Onset Early	Late	Manifestations	Onset Early	Late
Central Nervous System			**Cardiovascular**		
Unexplained apprehension	X		Tachycardia	X	
Unexplained restlessness or irritability	X		Mild hypertension	X	
Unexplained confusion or lethargy	X	X	Dysrhythmias	X	X
Combativeness		X	Hypotension		X
Coma		X	Cyanosis		X
			Cool, clammy skin		X
Respiratory					
Tachypnea	X		**Other**		
Dyspnea on exertion	X		Diaphoresis	X	X
Dyspnea at rest		X	Decreased urine output	X	X
Use of accessory muscles		X	Unexplained fatigue	X	X
Retraction of interspaces on inspiration		X			
Pause for breath between sentences, words		X			

tinuous intraarterial blood gas monitoring is also possible via a fiberoptic sensor or an oxygen electrode inserted into an arterial catheter. An arterial catheter permits ABG sampling without repeated arterial punctures.

The normal PaO_2 decreases with advancing age. It also varies in relation to the distance above sea level. At higher altitudes the barometric pressure is lower, resulting in a lower inspired oxygen pressure and a lower PaO_2 (see Table 26-1).

Mixed Venous Blood Gases. For the patient with a normal or near-normal cardiac status, an assessment of PaO_2 or SaO_2 is usually sufficient to determine the level of oxygenation. The patient with impaired cardiac output or hemodynamic instability may have inadequate tissue oxygen delivery or abnormal oxygen consumption.[3]

The amount of oxygen delivered to the tissues or consumed can be calculated. A catheter positioned in the pulmonary artery, termed a *pulmonary artery (PA) catheter,* is used for mixed venous sampling (see Chapter 66). Blood drawn from a PA catheter is termed a *mixed venous blood gas* sample because it consists of venous blood that has returned to the heart and "mixes" in the right ventricle. Normal mixed venous values are given in Table 26-1. When tissue oxygen delivery is inadequate or when inadequate oxygen is transported to the tissues by the hemoglobin, the PvO_2 and SvO_2 fall.

Oximetry. Arterial oxygen saturation can be monitored noninvasively and continuously using a *pulse oximetry* probe on the finger, toe, ear, or bridge of the nose[4] (see eFig. 26-2 available on the website). The abbreviation SpO_2 is used to indicate the

oxygen saturation of hemoglobin as measured by pulse oximetry. SpO_2 and heart rate are displayed on the monitor as digital readings (see eFig. 26-2).

Pulse oximetry is particularly valuable in intensive care and perioperative situations, in which sedation or decreased consciousness might mask hypoxia (Table 26-2). SpO_2 is assessed with each routine vital sign check in many inpatient areas. Changes in SpO_2 can be detected quickly and treated (Table 26-3). Oximetry is also used during exercise testing and when adjusting flow rates during long-term oxygen therapy.

Values obtained by pulse oximetry are less accurate if the SpO_2 is less than 70%. At this level the oximeter may display a value that is ±4% of the actual value. For example, if the SpO_2 reading is 70%, the actual value can range from 66% to 74%. Pulse oximetry is also inaccurate if hemoglobin variants (e.g., carboxyhemoglobin, methemoglobin) are present. Other factors that can alter the accuracy of pulse oximetry include motion, low perfusion, anemia, cold extremities, bright fluorescent lights, intravascular dyes, thick acrylic nails, and dark skin color. If there is doubt about the accuracy of the SpO_2 reading, obtain an ABG analysis to verify the results.

Oximetry can also be used to monitor SvO_2 via a PA catheter. A decrease in SvO_2 suggests that less oxygen is being delivered to the tissues or that more oxygen is being consumed. Changes in SvO_2 provide an early warning of a change in cardiac output or tissue oxygen delivery. Normal SvO_2 is 60% to 80%.

Carbon Dioxide Monitoring. Carbon dioxide can be monitored using transcutaneous CO₂ ($PTCCO_2$) and end-tidal CO₂

TABLE 26-3		CRITICAL VALUES FOR PaO$_2$ AND SpO$_2$*
PaO$_2$ (%)	SpO$_2$ (%)	**Significance**
≥70	≥94	Adequate unless patient is hemodynamically unstable or hemoglobin (Hgb) has difficulty releasing O$_2$ to the tissues.
60	90	Adequate in almost all patients. Provides adequate oxygenation but with less margin for error than above.
55	88	Adequate for patients with chronic hypoxemia if no cardiac problems occur. These values are also used as criteria for prescription of continuous O$_2$ therapy.
40	75	Inadequate but may be acceptable on a short-term basis if the patient also has CO$_2$ retention. In this situation, respirations may be stimulated by a low PaO$_2$. Thus the PaO$_2$ cannot be raised rapidly.
<40	<75	Inadequate. Tissue hypoxia and cardiac dysrhythmias can be expected.

*The same critical values apply for SpO$_2$ and SaO$_2$. Values pertain to rest or exertion.

(PETCO$_2$) (capnography). Transcutaneous measurement of CO$_2$ is a noninvasive method of estimating arterial pressure of CO$_2$ (PaCO$_2$) using an electrode placed on the skin.

PETCO$_2$ is the noninvasive measurement of alveolar CO$_2$ at the end of exhalation when CO$_2$ concentration is at its peak. It is used to monitor and assess trends in the patient's ventilatory status. Expired gases are sampled from the patient's airway and are analyzed by a CO$_2$ sensor that uses infrared light to measure exhaled CO$_2$. The sensor may be attached to an adaptor on the endotracheal tube or the tracheostomy tube. A nasal cannula with a sidestream capnometer can be used in patients without an artificial airway. Capnography is usually presented as a graph of expiratory CO$_2$ plotted against time.

In the past, capnography was used mainly intraoperatively, postoperatively, and in critical care units. Today's monitors are portable and practical for use on inpatient units and emergency departments.

Measurement of oxygen saturation (oximetry) is primarily used to assess for hypoxia. CO$_2$ monitoring assesses for hypoventilation. The use of both measures together is important in determining patients' oxygenation and ventilatory status.

Control of Respiration

The respiratory center in the medulla (located in the brainstem) responds to chemical and mechanical signals. Impulses are sent from the medulla to the respiratory muscles through the spinal cord and the phrenic nerves.

Chemoreceptors. A chemoreceptor is a receptor that responds to a change in the chemical composition (PaCO$_2$ and pH) of the fluid around it. Central chemoreceptors are located in the medulla and respond to changes in the hydrogen ion (H$^+$) concentration. An increase in the H$^+$ concentration *(acidosis)* causes the medulla to increase the respiratory rate and tidal volume (V$_T$). A decrease in H$^+$ concentration *(alkalosis)* has the opposite effect. Changes in PaCO$_2$ regulate ventilation primarily by their effect on the pH of the cerebrospinal fluid. When the PaCO$_2$ level is increased, more CO$_2$ is available to combine with H$_2$O and form carbonic acid (H$_2$CO$_3$). This lowers the cerebrospinal fluid pH and stimulates an increase in respiratory rate. The opposite process occurs with a decrease in PaCO$_2$ level.

Peripheral chemoreceptors are located in the carotid bodies at the bifurcation of the common carotid arteries and in the aortic bodies above and below the aortic arch. The peripheral chemoreceptors respond to decreases in PaO$_2$ and pH and to increases in PaCO$_2$. These changes also stimulate the respiratory center.

In a healthy person an increase in PaCO$_2$ or a decrease in pH causes an immediate increase in the respiratory rate. The PaCO$_2$ does not vary more than about 3 mm Hg if lung function is normal. Conditions such as COPD alter lung function and may result in chronically elevated PaCO$_2$ levels. In these instances the patient is relatively insensitive to further increases in PaCO$_2$ as a stimulus to breathe and may be maintaining ventilation largely because of a hypoxic drive from the peripheral chemoreceptors (see Chapter 29).

Mechanical Receptors. Mechanical receptors (juxtacapillary and irritant) are located in the lungs, upper airways, chest wall, and diaphragm. They are stimulated by a variety of physiologic factors, such as irritants, muscle stretching, and alveolar wall distortion. Signals from the stretch receptors aid in the control of respiration. As the lungs inflate, pulmonary stretch receptors activate the inspiratory center to inhibit further lung expansion. This is termed the *Hering-Breuer reflex*, and it prevents overdistention of the lungs. Impulses from the mechanical sensors are sent through the vagus nerve to the brain. Juxtacapillary (J) receptors are believed to cause the rapid respiration (tachypnea) seen in pulmonary edema. These receptors are stimulated by fluid entering the pulmonary interstitial space.

Respiratory Defense Mechanisms

Respiratory defense mechanisms are efficient in protecting the lungs from inhaled particles, microorganisms, and toxic gases. The defense mechanisms include filtration of air, the mucociliary clearance system, the cough reflex, reflex bronchoconstriction, and alveolar macrophages.

Filtration of Air. Nasal hairs filter inspired air. In addition, the abrupt changes in direction of airflow that occur as air moves through the nasopharynx and larynx increase air turbulence. This causes particles and bacteria to contact the mucosa lining these structures. Most large particles (greater than 5 μm) are less dangerous because they are removed in the nasopharynx or bronchi and do not reach the alveoli.

The velocity of airflow slows greatly after it passes the larynx, facilitating the deposition of smaller particles (1 to 5 μm). They settle out the way sand does in a river, a process termed *sedimentation*. Particles less than 1 μm in size are too small to settle in this manner and are deposited in the alveoli. An example of small particles that can build up is coal dust, which can lead to pneumoconiosis (see Chapter 28).

Mucociliary Clearance System. Below the larynx, the movement of mucus is accomplished by the mucociliary clearance system, commonly referred to as the *mucociliary escalator*. This term is used to indicate the relationship between the secretion of mucus and the ciliary activity. Mucus is continuously secreted at a rate of about 100 mL/day by goblet cells and submucosal glands. It forms a mucous blanket that contains the impacted particles and debris from distal lung areas (see Fig. 26-1). The small amount of mucus normally secreted is swallowed without being noticed. Secretory immunoglobulin A (IgA) in the mucus helps protect against bacteria and viruses.

Cilia cover the airways from the level of the trachea to the respiratory bronchioles (see Fig. 26-1). Each ciliated cell contains approximately 200 cilia, which beat rhythmically about 1000 times per minute in the large airways, moving mucus toward the mouth. The ciliary beat is slower further down the tracheobronchial tree. As a consequence, particles that penetrate more deeply into the airways are removed less rapidly. Ciliary action is impaired by dehydration; smoking; inhalation of high oxygen concentrations; infection; and ingestion of drugs such as atropine, anesthetics, alcohol, or cocaine. Patients with COPD and cystic fibrosis have repeated lower respiratory tract infections. Cilia are often destroyed during these infections, resulting in impaired secretion clearance; a chronic productive cough; and chronic colonization by bacteria, which leads to frequent respiratory tract infections.

Cough Reflex. The cough is a protective reflex action that clears the airway by a high-pressure, high-velocity flow of air. It is a backup for mucociliary clearance, especially when this clearance mechanism is overwhelmed or ineffective. Coughing is only effective in removing secretions above the subsegmental level (large or main airways). Secretions below this level must be moved upward by the mucociliary mechanism before they can be removed by coughing.

Reflex Bronchoconstriction. *Reflex bronchoconstriction* is another defense mechanism. In response to the inhalation of large amounts of irritating substances (e.g., dusts, aerosols), the bronchi constrict in an effort to prevent entry of the irritants. A person with hyperreactive airways, such as a person with asthma, may experience bronchoconstriction after inhalation of triggers such as cold air, perfume, or other strong odors.

Alveolar Macrophages. Because ciliated cells are not found below the level of the respiratory bronchioles, the primary defense mechanism at the alveolar level is alveolar macrophages. *Alveolar macrophages* rapidly phagocytize inhaled foreign particles such as bacteria. The debris is moved to the level of the bronchioles for removal by the cilia or removed from the lungs by the lymphatic system. Particles (e.g., coal dust, silica) that cannot be adequately phagocytized tend to remain in the lungs for indefinite periods and can stimulate inflammatory responses (see Chapter 28). Because alveolar macrophage activity is impaired by cigarette smoke, the smoker who is employed in an occupation with heavy dust exposure (e.g., mining, foundries) is at an especially high risk for lung disease.

GERONTOLOGIC CONSIDERATIONS

EFFECTS OF AGING ON RESPIRATORY SYSTEM

Age-related changes in the respiratory system can be divided into alterations in structure, defense mechanisms, and respiratory control (Table 26-4). Structural changes include calcification of the costal cartilages, which can interfere with chest expansion. The outward curvature of the spine is marked, especially with osteoporosis, and the lumbar curve flattens. Therefore the chest may appear barrel shaped, and the older person may need to use accessory muscles to breathe. Respiratory muscle strength progressively declines after age 50. Overall, the lungs in the older adult are harder to inflate.[5]

Many older adults lose subcutaneous fat, and bony prominences are pronounced. Within the lung, the number of functional alveoli decreases, and they become less elastic. Small airways in the lung bases close earlier in expiration. As a consequence, more inspired air is distributed to the lung apices and ventilation is less well matched to perfusion, lowering the PaO₂. Therefore older adults have less tolerance for exertion, and

TABLE 26-4 GERONTOLOGIC ASSESSMENT DIFFERENCES

Respiratory System

Changes	Differences in Assessment Findings
Structures	
Chest wall stiffening	Barrel chest appearance, kyphotic
Costal cartilage calcification	posture, ↓ chest wall movement,
↓ Elastic recoil	↓ deep breathing; mucus thickened
↓ Chest wall compliance	↓ Vital capacity, ↑ residual volume,
↑ Anteroposterior diameter	↑ functional residual capacity
↓ Functioning alveoli	Diminished breath sounds, particularly
↓ Respiratory muscle strength	at lung bases; ↓ PaO_2 and SaO_2, normal pH and $PaCO_2$
Defense Mechanisms	
↓ Cell-mediated immunity	↓ Cough effectiveness, ↓ secretion
↓ Specific antibodies	clearance
↓ Cilia function	↑ Risk of upper respiratory aspiration,
↓ Cough force	infection, influenza, pneumonia
↓ Alveolar macrophage function	Respiratory infections may be more severe and last longer
↓ Sensation in pharynx	
Respiratory Control	
↓ Response to hypoxemia	Greater ↓ in PaO_2 and ↑ in $PaCO_2$
↓ Response to hypercapnia	before respiratory rate changes
	↓ Ability to maintain acid-base balance
	Significant hypoxemia or hypercapnia may develop from relatively small incidents
	Retained secretions, excessive sedation, or positioning that impairs chest expansion may substantially alter PaO_2 or SpO_2 values

dyspnea can occur if their activity exceeds their normal exercise.[6]

Respiratory defense mechanisms are less effective because of a decline in both cell-mediated and humoral immunity (ability to produce antibodies). The alveolar macrophages are less effective at phagocytosis. An older patient has a less forceful cough and fewer and less functional cilia. Mucous membranes tend to be drier. Retained mucus predisposes the older adult to respiratory tract infections. Formation of secretory IgA, an important defense mechanism, is diminished. Swallowing is slower because of transit time in the pharyngeal area, and there is reduced sensation in the pharynx. If the older adult patient has a superimposed neurologic condition, aspiration is likely.

Respiratory control is altered, resulting in a more gradual response to changes in blood oxygen or carbon dioxide level. The PaO₂ drops to a lower level and the PaCO₂ rises to a higher level before the respiratory rate changes.

The extent of these changes in people of the same age varies greatly. The older adult who has a significant smoking history, is obese, and is diagnosed with a chronic illness is at greatest risk of adverse outcomes.

ASSESSMENT OF RESPIRATORY SYSTEM

Determining a patient's needs related to the respiratory system requires an accurate health history and a thorough physical examination. A respiratory assessment can be done as part of a comprehensive physical examination or as a focused respiratory

CASE STUDY

Patient Introduction

Kevin Peterson/
Photodisc/Thinkstock

F.T. is a 70-year-old African American man who comes to the emergency department complaining of increased shortness of breath. He states that he started using his albuterol inhaler every 4 hours a few days ago, but it does not seem to be helping. He has been having trouble sleeping or doing any activity because of the shortness of breath.

Critical Thinking

As you read through this assessment chapter, think about F.T. with the following questions in mind:
1. What are the possible causes of F.T.'s shortness of breath?
2. What type of assessment would be most appropriate for F.T.: comprehensive, focused, or emergency?
3. What questions would you ask?
4. What should be included in the physical assessment? What would you be looking for?
5. What diagnostic studies might you expect to be ordered?

ⓔvolve Answers available at *http://evolve.elsevier.com/Lewis/medsurg.*

examination. Use judgment in determining whether all or part of the history and physical examination will be completed based on the patient's problems and degree of respiratory distress. If respiratory distress is severe, only obtain pertinent information and defer a thorough assessment until the patient's condition stabilizes.

Subjective Data

Important Health Information

Past Health History. It is important to determine the frequency of upper respiratory problems (e.g., colds, sore throats, sinus problems, allergies) and whether seasonal changes have an effect on these problems. Question the patient with allergies about possible precipitating factors or triggers such as medications, pollen, smoke, mold, or pet exposure. Document characteristics and severity of the allergic reaction such as runny nose, wheezing, scratchy throat, or chest tightness. Inquire about a past history of lower respiratory problems, such as asthma, COPD, pneumonia, and tuberculosis (TB). Also determine the frequency of asthma exacerbations and triggers, if known. Because respiratory symptoms are often manifestations of problems that involve other body systems, it is important to ask about a history of additional health problems. For example, the patient with cardiac dysfunction may experience dyspnea (shortness of breath) as a consequence of heart failure. The patient with human immunodeficiency virus (HIV) infection may experience frequent respiratory tract infections because immune function is compromised.

Medications. Take a thorough medication history, including both prescription and over-the-counter medications. Ask about the reason for taking the medication, its name, the dose and frequency, length of time taken, its effect, and any side effects. Assess for overuse of short-term bronchodilators as a key indicator of symptom control, since this information will help guide management. Inquire about the use of an angiotensin-converting enzyme (ACE) inhibitor, since cough is a relatively common side effect of this class of drugs. Encourage the patient to bring her or his medication bottles to each visit with a health care provider.

If the patient is using oxygen to ease a breathing problem, document the fraction of inspired oxygen concentration (FIO_2), liter flow, method of administration, number of hours used per day, and effectiveness of the therapy. Assess safety practices, including the patient's mechanical and cognitive ability related to using oxygen.

Surgery or Other Treatments. Determine if the patient has been hospitalized for a respiratory problem. Note the dates, therapy (including surgery), and current status of the problem. Determine if the patient has ever been intubated because of a respiratory problem. Ask about the use and the response to respiratory treatments such as a nebulizer, humidifier, airway clearance modalities (see Chapter 29), high-frequency chest wall oscillation, postural drainage, and percussion.

Functional Health Patterns. Health history questions to ask a patient with a respiratory problem are presented in Table 26-5.

Health Perception–Health Management Pattern. Ask the patient if there has been a perceived change in health status within the last several days, months, or years. In COPD, lung function declines slowly over many years. The patient may not notice this decline because activity is altered to accommodate reduced exercise tolerance. If an upper respiratory tract infection is superimposed on a chronic problem, dyspnea and decreased exercise tolerance may occur very quickly. In asthma, symptoms may occur or worsen during exercise, if animals are present, or following a change in temperature.

Explore and document common signs of respiratory problems (e.g., cough, dyspnea). Also describe the course of the patient's illness, including when it began, the type of symptoms, and factors that alleviate or aggravate these symptoms. Because of the chronic nature of respiratory problems, the patient may relate a change in symptoms rather than the onset of new symptoms when describing the present illness. Carefully document any changes because they often suggest the cause of illness. For example, increased shortness of breath or increased purulence of sputum may suggest an acute exacerbation of COPD.

If a cough is present, evaluate its quality. For example, a loose-sounding cough indicates secretions; a dry, hacking cough indicates airway irritation or obstruction; a harsh, barky cough suggests upper airway obstruction from inhibited vocal cord movement related to subglottic edema. Assess whether the cough is strong enough to clear secretions, and note whether it is productive or nonproductive of secretions. Determine if a cough is acute or chronic (longer than 3 weeks in duration) or if it first began with an upper respiratory tract infection. The pattern and etiology of the cough are determined by asking questions such as the following: What has been the pattern of coughing? Has it been regular or paroxysmal (i.e., sudden, periodic onset), or related to a time of day, the weather, certain activities, talking, or deep breaths? Any change over time? Do you clear your throat a lot? What have you tried to alleviate the coughing? Did you try any prescription or over-the-counter drugs?

If the patient has a productive cough, evaluate the following characteristics of sputum: amount, color, consistency, and odor. Quantify the amount of sputum in teaspoons, tablespoons, or cups per day. Note any recent increases or decreases in the amount. The normal color is clear or slightly whitish. If a patient is a cigarette smoker, the sputum is usually clear to gray with occasional specks of brown. The patient with COPD may exhibit clear, whitish, or slightly yellow sputum, especially in the morning on rising. If the patient reports any change from base-

TABLE 26-5 HEALTH HISTORY

Respiratory System

Health Perception–Health Management
- Describe your daily activities. Have breathing problems changed activities that you could perform in the past several days?* Months?* Years?* Are your breathing problems better, worse, or about the same compared with 6 months ago?
- How do your breathing problems affect your self-care abilities?
- Have you ever smoked? Do you smoke now? If yes, how many cigarettes each day and for how long? Are you interested in stopping smoking? Are there aids we can tell you about that would assist your quitting? Would you be willing to come back for a visit so we can explore your quitting? If you stopped smoking, did you do so because of your health?* How did you stop?
- Have you ever smoked street drugs?*
- Have you had a Pneumovax vaccination? When was your last flu shot?
- What equipment helps you manage your respiratory problems? How often do you use it? Does it help? Cause problems?

Nutritional-Metabolic
- Have you recently lost weight because of difficulty eating secondary to a respiratory problem? How much? Voluntarily?
- Do any particular foods affect your sputum production or breathing?*

Elimination
- Does your respiratory problem make it difficult for you to get to the toilet?*
- Are you inactive because of dyspnea to the point that it causes constipation?*

Activity-Exercise
- Are you ever short of breath during exercise?* At rest?*
- Do you get too short of breath to do the things you want to do?*
- Is your home one story? Two stories? How many steps from the street to your door?
- Can you walk up a flight of steps without stopping?
- Are you able to maintain your typical activity pattern? If not, explain.
- What do you do when you get short of breath?

Sleep-Rest
- Do breathing problems cause you to awaken during the night?*
- Can you lie flat at night? If not, how many pillows do you use?
- Do you need to sleep upright in a chair?*
- Are you or your sleep partner aware of any snoring?
- Do you awaken in the morning feeling rested?
- Do you have a morning headache?*
- Do you fall asleep easily during the day?*

Cognitive-Perceptual
- Do you have any pain associated with breathing?* On a scale from 0 to 10, with 10 being the worst pain you can imagine, where would you rate your pain? Does it hurt more on inspiration?*
- Do you ever feel restless, irritable, or confused without a reason?*
- Do you have difficulty remembering things?*

Self-Perception–Self-Concept
- Describe how your respiratory problems have changed your life.
- If you use oxygen, do you ever go out without bringing it with you? When and why?

Role-Relationship
- Has your respiratory problem caused any difficulties in your work, family, or social relationships?*

Sexuality-Reproductive
- Has your respiratory problem caused a change in your sexual activity?*
- Do you want to discuss ways to decrease dyspnea during sexual activity?

Coping–Stress Tolerance
- How often do you leave your home?
- Would you want to join a support group? Pulmonary rehabilitation program?
- Does stress have an effect on your breathing?*
- What effect does your respiratory problem have on your emotions?

Value-Belief
- What do you believe causes your respiratory problems?
- Do you think the things you have been told to do for your respiratory problems really help? If not, why?

*If yes, describe.

line color, suspect pulmonary complications. Note any changes in consistency of sputum to thick, thin, or frothy and pink tinged. These changes may indicate dehydration, postnasal drip or sinus drainage, or possible pulmonary edema. Normally sputum should be odorless. A foul odor or exceptionally bad breath or taste in the mouth suggests an infectious process. Ask the patient if the sputum was produced along with a change in position (e.g., increased with lying down) or activity.

When assessing mucus, determine if the patient has a history of coughing up blood *(hemoptysis)*. Hemoptysis can range from a slight streaking of blood in the mucus to massive coughing up of blood, in which the patient loses 100 to 600 mL of blood in a 24-hour period. This situation is a medical emergency.

Frequently the patient cannot differentiate between hemoptysis and *hematemesis* (vomiting blood). Carefully question and then test the mucus for an acidic pH (which is present with hematemesis), since this will help differentiate the two. Hemoptysis can be found with a variety of conditions such as pneumonia, TB, lung cancer, and severe bronchiectasis.

Assess for a history of wheezing. *Wheezes* are musical sounds that can be audible. Wheezing indicates some degree of airway obstruction, such as asthma, foreign body aspiration, and emphysema. Assess for any history of family exposure to *Mycobacterium tuberculosis*.

GENETIC RISK ALERT
- Respiratory problems that have a strong genetic link include cystic fibrosis, COPD resulting from α_1-antitrypsin deficiency, and asthma.
- If people have a family history of these respiratory problems, they have a much greater risk of developing them.
- Although cigarette smoking is a major risk factor for COPD, only a minority of cigarette smokers develop symptomatic disease. The risk for COPD related to cigarette smoking is genetically related.
- Determine if there is a family history of any of these respiratory problems that may have genetic or familial tendencies.

Smoking is the most important risk factor for COPD and lung cancer. Discuss current and past smoking habits. Quantify smoking habits in *pack-years*. This is done by multiplying the number of packs smoked per day by the number of years smoked. For example, a person who smoked 1 pack per day for

15 years has a 15 pack-year history. In addition to asking about cigarette use, find out about the use of any tobacco products, including cigars, pipes, chewing tobacco, and smokeless tobacco products. Also find out about exposure to secondhand smoke. Determine if the patient has tried to quit using tobacco products, including using prescription, over-the-counter, and herbal remedies.

Assess if the patient received immunization for influenza (flu) and pneumococcal pneumonia (Pneumovax). Influenza vaccine should be administered yearly in the fall. Pneumovax is administered any time during the year. (The recommendations for use of Pneumovax are presented in Table 28-5.)

Ask where the patient has lived and traveled. Risk factors for TB include prior residence in Asia, Africa, the former Soviet Republic, Latin America, or any third-world country. Other TB risk factors include exposure to people with high rates of TB transmission such as the homeless, injection drug users, and people with HIV infection. Risk factors for fungal infections of the lung include living or traveling in the Southwest (coccidioidomycosis) and the Mississippi River Valley (histoplasmosis).

Ask the patient about the use of equipment to manage respiratory symptoms (e.g., home O_2 therapy equipment, inhalers, devices for sleep apnea). Question the patient about the type of equipment used, cleaning of the device, frequency of use, its effect, and any side effects. Have patients demonstrate the use of their inhalers. Many patients do not know how to use these devices correctly (see Chapter 29).

Nutritional-Metabolic Pattern. Weight loss is a symptom of many respiratory diseases. Determine if weight loss was intentional and, if not, if food intake is altered by anorexia (from medications), fatigue (from hypoxemia, increased work of breathing), or feeling full quickly (from lung hyperinflation). Anorexia, weight loss, and chronic malnutrition are common in patients with COPD, lung cancer, TB, and chronic severe infection (bronchiectasis). Also note fluid intake. Dehydration can cause mucus to thicken and obstruct the airway.

Excessive weight interferes with normal ventilation and may cause sleep apnea (see Chapter 8). Morbidly obese individuals may hypoventilate while awake or asleep, and weight loss can improve ABGs. Rapid weight gain from fluid retention may decrease pulmonary gas exchange.

Elimination Pattern. Healthy elimination habits depend on the ability to reach a toilet when necessary. Activity intolerance secondary to dyspnea could result in incontinence. Dyspnea can also be the cause of limited mobility, which can cause constipation. Question the patient with dyspnea about incontinence and constipation. People with a chronic cough, especially women, may be troubled with urinary incontinence during paroxysms of coughing.

Activity-Exercise Pattern. Determine if the patient's activity is limited by dyspnea at rest or during exercise. Also note whether the patient's residence (e.g., number of steps, levels) poses a problem that increases social isolation. Record and objectively measure the degree of the patient's dyspnea. For example, can the patient walk up one flight of stairs without stopping because of dyspnea? Is dyspnea that is associated with an activity better, worse, or about the same in the last few months? Determine if the patient has difficulty breathing in a certain position, or if relief of dyspnea can be obtained by assuming a different position (e.g., tripod position in COPD).

Discuss whether the patient is able to carry out activities of daily living without dyspnea or other respiratory symptoms. If

unable, document the amount and type of care needed. Immobility and sedentary habits can be risk factors for hypoventilation leading to atelectasis or pneumonia.

Sleep-Rest Pattern. Determine if the patient wakes up because of pulmonary problems. The patient with asthma or COPD may awaken at night with chest tightness, wheezing, or coughing. This suggests a need for adjunct therapy or other medication changes. The patient with cardiovascular disease (e.g., heart failure) may sleep with the head elevated on several pillows to avoid respiratory problems brought on by lying flat (orthopnea). Signs of sleep apnea include snoring, insomnia, abrupt awakenings, daytime drowsiness, and early morning headaches. Night sweats may be a manifestation of TB.

Cognitive-Perceptual Pattern. Because hypoxia can cause neurologic symptoms, ask the patient about apprehension, restlessness, irritability, and memory changes, which can indicate inadequate cerebral oxygenation (see Table 26-2). Hypoxemia interferes with the ability to learn and retain information. For this reason, teaching may be more effective if the caregiver is present during teaching sessions to provide reinforcement at a later date.

Assess the patient's cognitive ability to cooperate with treatment. Failure or inability to participate in needed therapy can result in exacerbation of respiratory problems.

Inquire about any discomfort or pain with breathing. Explore a complaint of chest pain carefully to rule out cardiac involvement. Problems such as pleurisy, fractured ribs, and costochondritis cause chest pain. Pleuritic pain is described as a sharp, localized, stabbing pain associated with movement or deep breathing. Fractured ribs cause localized sharp pain associated with breathing.

Self-Perception–Self-Concept Pattern. Dyspnea limits activity, impairs ability to fulfill normal roles, and often alters self-esteem. A patient may be reluctant to appear in public with a highly visible nasal cannula and O_2 equipment. Discuss with the patient his or her personal body image. A barrel chest, clubbed fingers, pursed-lip breathing, and frequent expectoration of sputum or throat clearing can be embarrassing and can lead to social isolation. Referral to a support group or pulmonary rehabilitation program may be beneficial in developing a support system and coping strategies.

Role-Relationship Pattern. Acute or chronic respiratory problems can seriously affect performance in work or other activities. Discuss the impact of medications, O_2 therapy, and special routines (e.g., pulmonary hygiene for cystic fibrosis) on the patient's family, job, and social life.

Document the nature of the patient's work and the frequency and intensity of exposure to fumes, toxins, asbestos, coal, fibers, or silica. Inquire whether symptoms are worse in specific situations (e.g., home versus work environments). Investigate any patient-specific allergens, such as dust or fumes, that could be present in the work environment. Hobbies such as woodworking (sawdust) or pottery (silica) and exposure to animals (allergies) may also cause respiratory problems. Because of hyperreactive airways, exposure to fumes, smoke, and other chemicals may trigger an attack in the patient with asthma.

Sexuality-Reproductive Pattern. Most patients can continue to have satisfactory sexual relationships despite marked physical limitations. In a tactful manner, determine whether breathing difficulties have caused alterations in sexual activity. If so, provide teaching about positions that decrease dyspnea during sexual activity and alternative strategies for sexual fulfillment.

CASE STUDY—cont'd

Subjective Data

Kevin Peterson/
Photodisc/Thinkstock

A focused subjective assessment of F.T. revealed the following information:

PMH: COPD, hypertension, and benign prostatic hyperplasia. No history of environmental allergies. Denies history of coronary artery disease or heart failure.

Medications: Metoprolol (Lopressor) 50 mg/day PO, finasteride (Proscar) 5 mg/day PO, Advair inhaler (fluticasone and salmeterol) 2 puffs bid, and albuterol inhaler 2 puffs q4hr PRN. Does not use O₂ at home.

Health Perception–Health Management: F.T. states that he usually manages his COPD well with just the Advair inhaler and occasional use of the albuterol inhaler as needed. However, he caught a cold from his granddaughter last week and has had increasing difficulty breathing, even with the use of albuterol.

Has a history of 30 pack-years of smoking, quitting 5 years ago. Had a Pneumovax vaccination 5 years ago and receives the flu vaccine on an annual basis.

Activity-Exercise: States that he can typically walk at least 2 blocks and up and down stairs without getting short of breath. However, at this point, he can't walk 100 feet without feeling short of breath, nor can he walk up one flight of stairs without stopping to catch his breath.

Sleep-Rest: Has been having difficulty sleeping with this most recent episode of shortness of breath. Typically uses just one pillow to sleep with but needed three pillows this week, and last night he slept upright in his recliner.

Cognitive-Perceptual: Denies any pain or confusion associated with shortness of breath. Feels slightly irritable because of lack of sleep.

Coping–Stress Tolerance: Denies any stress or emotional disturbance that could be having an impact on his breathing.

Many patients need to perform good pulmonary hygiene (bronchodilators, coughing and deep breathing) before intimacy. This is similar to what they would do before strenuous physical activity. They may need to use O₂ therapy equipment during intercourse.

Coping–Stress Tolerance Pattern. Dyspnea causes anxiety, and anxiety exacerbates dyspnea. The result is a vicious cycle—the patient avoids activities that cause dyspnea, becoming more deconditioned and more dyspneic. The outcome is often physical and social isolation. Assess how often the patient leaves home and interacts with others. Referral to a support group or pulmonary rehabilitation program may be beneficial.

The chronic nature of many respiratory problems such as COPD and asthma can cause prolonged stress. Inquire about the patient's coping strategies to manage this stress.

Value-Belief Pattern. Determine the patient's adherence to the management regimen. Explore reasons for lack of adherence, including conflict with cultural beliefs, financial constraints (e.g., costs of prescriptions), or failure to understand benefit. Including the patient and the caregiver in the planning of care can improve adherence.

Objective Data

Physical Examination. Vital signs, including temperature, pulse, respirations, blood pressure, and SpO₂ (oxygen saturation obtained by pulse oximetry), are important data to collect before examination of the respiratory system.

Nose. Inspect the nose for patency, inflammation, deformities, symmetry, and discharge. Check each naris for air patency with respiration while the other naris is briefly occluded. Tilt the patient's head backward and push the tip of the nose upward gently. With a nasal speculum and a good light, inspect the interior of the nose. The mucous membrane should be pink and moist, with no evidence of edema (bogginess), exudate, or bleeding.[7] Inspect the nasal septum for deviation, perforations, and bleeding. Some nasal deviation is normal in an adult. Inspect the turbinates for polyps, which are abnormal, fingerlike projections of swollen nasal mucosa. Polyps may result from long-term irritation of the mucosa (e.g., from allergies). Assess any discharge for color and consistency. Purulent and malodorous discharge could indicate the presence of a foreign body. Watery discharge could be secondary to allergies or from cerebrospinal fluid. Bloody discharge could be from trauma or dryness. Thick mucosal discharge could indicate infection.

Mouth and Pharynx. Using a good light source, inspect the interior of the mouth for color, lesions, masses, gum retraction, bleeding, and poor dentition. Inspect the tongue for symmetry and lesions. Observe the pharynx by pressing a tongue blade against the middle of the back of the tongue. If the oropharynx is tight, have the patient yawn, since this usually allows more structures to be visible. The pharynx should be smooth and moist, with no evidence of exudate, ulcerations, swelling, or postnasal drip. Note the color, symmetry, and any enlargement of the tonsils. Stimulate the gag reflex by placing a tongue blade along the side of the pharynx behind the tonsil. A normal response (gagging) indicates that cranial nerves IX (glossopharyngeal) and X (vagus) are intact and that the airway is protected.

Neck. Inspect the neck for symmetry and tender or swollen areas. Palpate the lymph nodes while the patient is sitting erect with the neck slightly flexed. Progression of palpation is from the nodes around the ears, to the nodes at the base of the skull, and then to those located under the angles of the mandible to the midline. The patient may have small, mobile, nontender nodes (shotty nodes), which are not a sign of a pathologic condition. Tender, hard, or fixed nodes indicate disease. Describe the location and characteristics of any palpable nodes.

Thorax and Lungs. Picture imaginary lines on the chest to help identify abnormalities (see Fig. 26-2). Describe abnormalities in terms of their location relative to these lines (e.g., 2 cm from the right midclavicular line).[8]

Chest examination is best performed in a well-lighted, warm room with measures taken to ensure the patient's privacy. Perform all physical assessment maneuvers (inspection, palpation, percussion, auscultation) on either the anterior or the posterior chest rather than moving from anterior to posterior or vice versa with each maneuver. It is best to begin on the posterior chest, particularly with female patients, since more information can be obtained without interference from the breast tissue. In addition, if the patient tires or you are interrupted, baseline data with the most information will have been obtained from examining the posterior of the chest.

Inspection. When inspecting the *anterior chest*, have the patient sit upright or with the head of the bed upright. The patient may need to lean forward for support on the bedside table to facilitate breathing. First, observe the patient's appearance and note any evidence of respiratory distress, such as tachypnea or use of accessory muscles. Next, determine the shape and symmetry of the chest. Chest movement should be equal on both sides, and the AP diameter should be less than the side-to-side or transverse diameter by a ratio of 1:2. An increase in AP diameter (e.g., barrel chest) may be a normal aging change or result from lung hyperinflation. Observe for abnormalities in the sternum (e.g., *pectus carinatum* [a prominent protrusion of the sternum] and *pectus excavatum* [an indentation of the lower sternum above the xiphoid process]).

Next observe the respiratory rate, depth, and rhythm. The normal rate is 12 to 20 breaths/minute; in the older adult, it is 16 to 25 breaths/minute. Inspiration (I) should take half as long as expiration (E) (I:E ratio = 1:2). Observe for abnormal breathing patterns, such as Kussmaul (rapid, deep breathing), Cheyne-Stokes (abnormal respirations characterized by alternating periods of apnea and deep, rapid breathing), or Biot's (irregular breathing with apnea every four to five cycles) respirations.

Skin color provides clues to respiratory status. Cyanosis, a late sign of hypoxemia, is best observed in a dark-skinned patient in the conjunctivae, lips, and palms and under the tongue. Causes of cyanosis include hypoxemia or decreased cardiac output. Inspect the fingers for evidence of long-standing hypoxemia known as *clubbing* (an increase in the angle between the base of the nail and the fingernail to 180 degrees or more, usually accompanied by an increase in the depth, bulk, and sponginess of the end of the finger) (see eFig. 26-3 available on the website for this chapter).

When inspecting the *posterior chest,* ask the patient to lean forward with arms folded. This position moves the scapulae away from the spine, exposing more of the area to be examined. The same sequence of observations that was done on the anterior part of the chest is performed on the posterior part. In addition, any spinal curvature is noted. Spinal curvatures that affect breathing include kyphosis, scoliosis, and kyphoscoliosis.

Palpation. Determine tracheal position by gently placing the index fingers on either side of the trachea just above the suprasternal notch and gently pressing backward. Normal tracheal position is midline; deviation to the left or right is abnormal. Tracheal deviation occurs away from the side of a tension pneumothorax or a neck mass, but toward the side of a pneumonectomy or lobar atelectasis.

Symmetry of chest expansion and extent of movement are determined at the level of the diaphragm. Place your hands over the lower anterior chest wall along the costal margin and move them inward until the thumbs meet at midline. Ask the patient to breathe deeply. Observe the movement of the thumbs away from each other. Normal expansion is 1 in (2.5 cm). Hand placement on the posterior side of the chest is at the level of the tenth rib. Move the thumbs until they meet over the spine (Fig. 26-6). Check expansion anteriorly or posteriorly, but it is not necessary to check both.

Normal chest movement is equal. Unequal expansion occurs when air entry is limited by conditions involving the lung (e.g., atelectasis, pneumothorax) or the chest wall (e.g., incisional pain). Equal but diminished expansion occurs in conditions that produce a hyperinflated or barrel chest or in neuromuscular diseases (e.g., amyotrophic lateral sclerosis, spinal cord lesions). Movement may be absent or unequal over a pleural effusion, an atelectasis, or a pneumothorax.

Fremitus is the vibration of the chest wall produced by vocalization. Tactile fremitus can be felt by placing the palmar surface of the hands with hyperextended fingers against the patient's chest. Ask the patient to repeat a phrase such as "ninety-nine" in a deeper, louder than normal voice. Move your hands from side to side at the same time from top to bottom on

FIG. 26-6 Estimation of thoracic expansion. **A,** Exhalation. **B,** Maximal inhalation.

the patient's chest (Fig. 26-7). When performing percussion, palpate all areas of the chest and compare vibrations from similar areas. Tactile fremitus is most intense adjacent to the sternum and between the scapulae because these areas are closest to the major bronchi. Fremitus is less intense farther away from these areas.

Note an increase, decrease, or absence of fremitus. Increased fremitus occurs when the lung becomes filled with fluid or is denser. As the patient's voice moves through a dense tissue or fluid, you can feel that the vibration is increased. This is found in pneumonia, in lung tumors, with thick bronchial secretions, and above a pleural effusion (the lung is compressed upward). Fremitus is decreased if the hand is farther from the lung (e.g., pleural effusion) or the lung is hyperinflated (e.g., barrel chest). Absent fremitus may be noted with pneumothorax or atelectasis. The anterior of the chest is more difficult to palpate for fremitus because of the large muscles and breast tissue.

Percussion. Percussion is performed to assess the density or aeration of the lungs. Percussion sounds are described in Table 26-6. (The technique for percussion is described in Chapter 3.)

The anterior chest is usually percussed with the patient in a semi-sitting or supine position. Starting above the clavicles, percuss downward, interspace by interspace (see Fig. 26-7). The area over lung tissue should be resonant, with the exception of the area of cardiac dullness (Fig. 26-8). For percussion of the posterior chest, have the patient sit leaning forward with arms

FIG. 26-7 Sequence for examination of the chest. **A,** Anterior sequence. **B,** Lateral sequence. **C,** Posterior sequence. For palpation, place the palms of the hands in the position designated as *"1"* on the right and left sides of the chest. Compare the intensity of vibrations. Continue for all positions in each sequence. For percussion, tap the chest at each designated position, moving downward from side to side. Compare percussion sounds at all positions. For auscultation, place the stethoscope at each position and listen to at least one complete inspiratory and expiratory cycle. Keep in mind that, with a female patient, the breast tissue will modify the completeness of the anterior examination.

TABLE 26-6	PERCUSSION SOUNDS
Sound	**Description**
Resonance	Low-pitched sound heard over normal lungs
Hyperresonance	Loud, lower-pitched sound than normal resonance heard over hyperinflated lungs, such as in chronic obstructive pulmonary disease and acute asthma
Tympany	Sound with drumlike, loud, empty quality heard over gas-filled stomach or intestine, or pneumothorax
Dull	Sound with medium-intensity pitch and duration heard over areas of "mixed" solid and lung tissue, such as over top area of liver, partially consolidated lung tissue (pneumonia), or fluid-filled pleural space
Flat	Soft, high-pitched sound of short duration heard over very dense tissue where air is not present, such as posterior chest below level of diaphragm

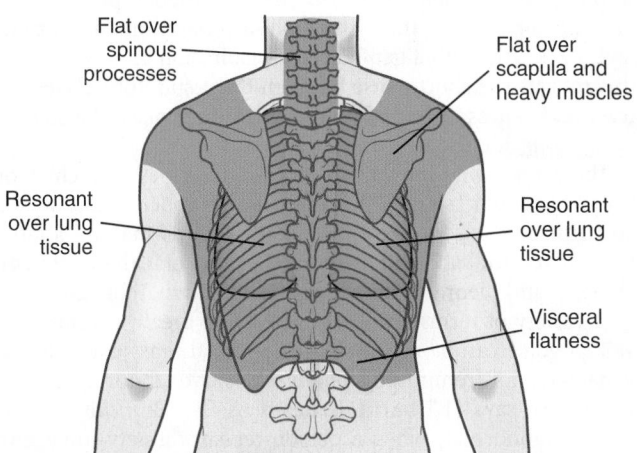

FIG. 26-8 Diagram of percussion areas and sounds in the anterior side of the chest.

folded. The posterior chest should be resonant over lung tissue to the level of the diaphragm (Fig. 26-9).

Auscultation. During chest auscultation, instruct the patient to breathe slowly and a little more deeply than normal through the mouth. Auscultation should proceed from the lung apices to the bases, comparing opposite areas of the chest, unless the patient is in respiratory distress or will tire easily; if so, start at the bases (see Fig. 26-7). Place the stethoscope over lung tissue, not over bony prominences. At each placement of the stethoscope, listen to at least one cycle of inspiration and expiration. Note the pitch (e.g., high, low), duration of sound, and presence of adventitious or abnormal sounds.[9] The location of normal auscultatory sounds is more easily understood by visualization of a lung model (Fig. 26-10).

The lung sounds are heard anteriorly from a line drawn perpendicular to the xiphoid process lateral to the midclavicular line. Palpate inferiorly (down) two ribs in the midaxillary line and around to the posterior chest. This gives you a fairly accurate and easy way to determine the lung fields to be auscultated. When documenting the location of the lung sounds, divide the anterior and posterior lung into thirds (upper, middle,

FIG. 26-9 Diagram of percussion areas and sounds in the posterior side of the chest. Percussion proceeds from the lung apices to the lung bases while comparing sounds in opposite areas of the chest.

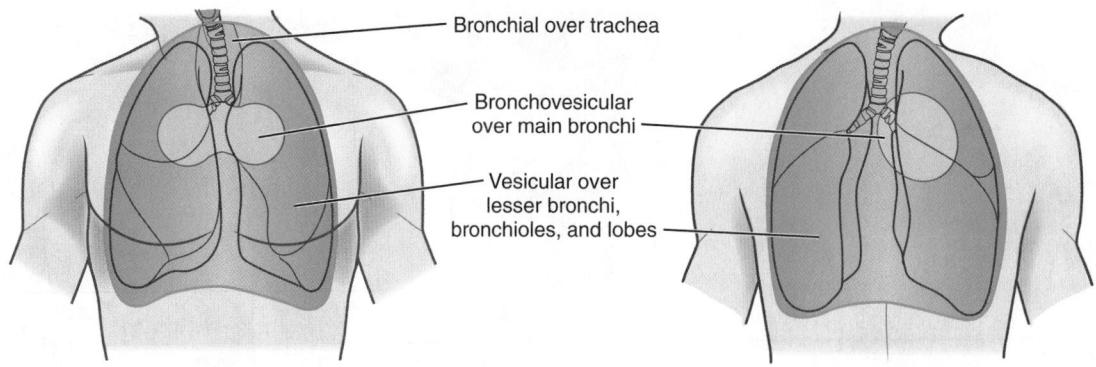

FIG. 26-10 Normal auscultatory sounds.

TABLE 26-7	NORMAL PHYSICAL ASSESSMENT OF THE RESPIRATORY SYSTEM
Nose	• Symmetric with no deformities • Nasal mucosa pink, moist with no edema, exudate, blood, or polyps • Nasal septum straight; nares patent bilaterally
Oral mucosa	• Light pink, moist, with no exudate or ulcerations
Pharynx	• Smooth, moist, and pink
Neck	• Trachea midline
Chest	• Anteroposterior to lateral diameter 1:2 • Respirations nonlabored at 14 breaths/min • Breath sounds vesicular without crackles, rhonchi, or wheezes • Excursion equal bilaterally with no increase in tactile fremitus

and lower) and note, for example, "crackles posterior right lower lung field." You are not expected to define which lobe of the lung has particular lung sounds.

The three normal breath sounds are vesicular, bronchovesicular, and bronchial. *Vesicular sounds* are relatively soft, low-pitched, gentle, rustling sounds. They are heard over all lung areas except the major bronchi. Vesicular sounds have a 3:1 ratio, with inspiration three times longer than expiration. *Bronchovesicular sounds* have a medium pitch and intensity and are heard anteriorly over the mainstem bronchi on either side of the sternum and posteriorly between the scapulae. Bronchovesicular sounds have a 1:1 ratio, with inspiration equal to expiration. *Bronchial sounds* are louder and higher pitched and resemble air blowing through a hollow pipe. Bronchial sounds have a 2:3 ratio with a gap between inspiration and expiration. This reflects the short pause between the respiratory cycles. To hear the likeness of bronchial breath sounds, place the stethoscope alongside the trachea in the neck.

The term *abnormal breath sounds* describes bronchial or bronchovesicular sounds heard in the peripheral lung fields. **Adventitious sounds** are extra breath sounds that are abnormal. Adventitious breath sounds include crackles, rhonchi, wheezes, and pleural friction rub (described in Table 26-7).

A variety of terms are used to describe breath sounds. The spoken voice can be auscultated over the thorax just as it can be palpated for fremitus. *Egophony* is positive (abnormal) when the person says "E" but it is heard as "A." *Bronchophony* is positive (abnormal) when a person repeats "ninety-nine" and the words are easily understood and are clear and loud. *Whispered pectoriloquy* is positive (abnormal) when the patient

FOCUSED ASSESSMENT
Respiratory System

Use this checklist to make sure the key assessment steps have been done.

Subjective
Ask the patient about any of the following and note responses.

Shortness of breath	Y	N
Wheezing	Y	N
Sputum production (color, quantity)	Y	N
Pain with breathing	Y	N
Cough	Y	N

Objective: Diagnostic
Check the following laboratory tests for critical values.

Arterial blood gases	✓
Chest x-ray	✓
Hct, Hgb	✓

Objective: Physical Examination
Observe

Respirations for rate, quality, and pattern	✓

Inspect

Skin and nails for integrity and color	✓
Neck for position of trachea	✓
Shape, symmetry, and movement of chest wall	✓

Palpate

Chest and back for masses	✓

Auscultate

Lung (breath) sounds	✓

Hct, Hematocrit; *Hgb,* hemoglobin.

whispers "one-two-three" and the almost inaudible voice is transmitted clearly and distinctly. Conditions that increase lung density or a consolidated lung (e.g., pneumonia) have positive (abnormal) voice sounds.

A record of the normal physical assessment of the respiratory system is shown in Table 26-7. Assessment abnormalities of the thorax and lungs are presented in Table 26-8. Chest examination findings in common pulmonary problems are presented in Table 26-9. Age-related changes in the respiratory system and assessment findings are presented in Table 26-4.

A *focused assessment* is used to evaluate the status of previously identified respiratory problems and to monitor for signs of new problems (see Chapter 3, Table 3-6). A focused assessment of the respiratory system is presented in the box above.

TABLE 26-8   **ASSESSMENT ABNORMALITIES**

Respiratory System

Finding	Description	Possible Etiology and Significance*
Inspection		
Pursed-lip breathing	Exhalation through mouth with lips pursed together to slow exhalation.	COPD, asthma. Suggests ↑ breathlessness. Strategy taught to slow expiration, ↓ dyspnea.
Tripod position; inability to lie flat	Learning forward with arms and elbows supported on overbed table.	COPD, asthma in exacerbation, pulmonary edema. Indicates moderate to severe respiratory distress.
Accessory muscle use; intercostal retractions	Neck and shoulder muscles used to assist breathing; muscles between ribs pull in during inspiration.	COPD, asthma in exacerbation, secretion retention. Indicates severe respiratory distress, hypoxemia.
Splinting	Voluntary ↓ in tidal volume to ↓ pain on chest expansion.	Thoracic or abdominal incision, chest trauma, pleurisy.
↑ AP diameter	AP chest diameter equal to lateral; slope of ribs more horizontal (90 degrees) to spine.	COPD, asthma, cystic fibrosis, lung hyperinflation, advanced age.
Tachypnea	Rate >20 breaths/min; >25 breaths/min in older adults.	Fever, anxiety, hypoxemia, restrictive lung disease. Magnitude of ↑ above normal rate reflects increased work of breathing.
Kussmaul respirations	Regular, rapid, and deep respirations.	Metabolic acidosis. Increases CO_2 excretion.
Cyanosis	Bluish color of skin best seen in lips and on the palpebral conjunctiva (inside the lower eyelid).	Reflects 5-6 g of hemoglobin not bound with O_2. ↓ O_2 transfer in lungs, ↓ cardiac output. Nonspecific, unreliable indicator.
Finger clubbing	↑ Depth, bulk, sponginess of distal portion of finger (see eFig. 26-3 on the website for this chapter).	Chronic hypoxemia, cystic fibrosis, lung cancer, bronchiectasis.
Abdominal paradox	Inward (rather than normal outward) movement of abdomen during inspiration.	Inefficient and ineffective breathing pattern. Nonspecific indicator of severe respiratory distress.
Palpation		
Tracheal deviation	Leftward or rightward movement of trachea from normal midline position.	Nonspecific indicator of change in position of mediastinal structures. Medical emergency if caused by tension pneumothorax. Trachea deviates to the side opposite the collapsed lung.
Altered tactile fremitus	Increase or decrease in vibrations.	↑ In pneumonia, pulmonary edema. ↓ In pleural effusion, lung hyperinflation. Absent in pneumothorax, atelectasis.
Altered chest movement	Unequal or equal but diminished movement of two sides of chest with inspiration.	Unequal movement caused by atelectasis, pneumothorax, pleural effusion, splinting. Equal but diminished movement caused by barrel chest, restrictive disease, neuromuscular disease.
Percussion		
Hyperresonance	Loud, lower-pitched sound over areas that normally produce a resonant sound.	Lung hyperinflation (COPD), lung collapse (pneumothorax), air trapping (asthma).
Dullness	Medium-pitched sound over areas that normally produce a resonant sound.	↑ Density (pneumonia, large atelectasis), ↑ fluid in pleural space (pleural effusion).
Auscultation		
Fine crackles	Series of short-duration, discontinuous, high-pitched sounds heard just before the end of inspiration. Result of rapid equalization of gas pressure when collapsed alveoli or terminal bronchioles suddenly snap open. Similar sound to that made by rolling hair between fingers just behind ear.	Idiopathic pulmonary fibrosis, interstitial edema (early pulmonary edema), alveolar filling (pneumonia), loss of lung volume (atelectasis), early phase of heart failure.
Coarse crackles	Series of long-duration, discontinuous, low-pitched sounds caused by air passing through airway intermittently occluded by mucus, unstable bronchial wall, or fold of mucosa. Evident on inspiration and, at times, expiration. Similar sound to blowing through straw under water. Increase in bubbling quality with more fluid.	Heart failure, pulmonary edema, pneumonia with severe congestion, COPD.
Rhonchi	Continuous rumbling, snoring, or rattling sounds from obstruction of large airways with secretions. Most prominent on expiration. Change often evident after coughing or suctioning.	COPD, cystic fibrosis, pneumonia, bronchiectasis.
Wheezes	Continuous high-pitched squeaking or musical sound caused by rapid vibration of bronchial walls. First evident on expiration but possibly evident on inspiration as obstruction of airway increases. Possibly audible without stethoscope.	Bronchospasm (caused by asthma), airway obstruction (caused by foreign body, tumor), COPD.
Stridor	Continuous musical or crowing sound of constant pitch. Result of partial obstruction of larynx or trachea.	Croup, epiglottitis, vocal cord edema after extubation, foreign body.
Absent breath sounds	No sound evident over entire lung or area of lung.	Pleural effusion, mainstem bronchi obstruction, large atelectasis, pneumonectomy, lobectomy.

Continued

TABLE 26-8 ASSESSMENT ABNORMALITIES—cont'd

Respiratory System

Finding	Description	Possible Etiology and Significance*
Auscultation—cont'd		
Pleural friction rub	Creaking or grating sound from roughened, inflamed pleural surfaces rubbing together. Evident during inspiration, expiration, or both and no change with coughing. Usually uncomfortable, especially on deep inspiration.	Pleurisy, pneumonia, pulmonary infarct.
Bronchophony, whispered pectoriloquy	Spoken or whispered syllable more distinct than normal on auscultation.	Pneumonia.
Egophony	Spoken "E" similar to "A" on auscultation because of altered transmission of voice sounds.	Pneumonia, pleural effusion.

*Limited to common etiologic factors. (Further discussion of conditions listed may be found in Chapters 27 through 29.)

TABLE 26-9 CHEST EXAMINATION FINDINGS IN PULMONARY PROBLEMS

Problem	Inspection	Palpation	Percussion	Auscultation
Chronic obstructive pulmonary disease	Barrel chest, cyanosis, tripod position, use of accessory muscles	↓ Movement	Hyperresonant or dull if consolidation	Crackles, rhonchi, wheezes, distant breath sounds
Asthma				
In exacerbation	Prolonged expiration, tripod position, pursed lips	↓ Movement	Hyperresonance	Wheezes, ↓ breath sounds ominous sign (severely diminished air movement)
Not in exacerbation	Normal	Normal	Normal	Normal
Pneumonia	Tachypnea, use of accessory muscles, duskiness or cyanosis	↑ Fremitus over affected area	Dull over affected areas	*Early:* Bronchial sounds *Later:* Crackles, rhonchi, egophony, whispered pectoriloquy
Atelectasis	No change unless involves entire segment, lobe	If small, no change If large, ↓ movement, ↓ fremitus	Dull over affected area	Crackles (may disappear with deep breaths) Absent sounds if large
Pulmonary edema	Tachypnea, labored respirations, cyanosis	↓ Movement or normal movement	Dull or normal depending on amount of fluid	Fine or coarse crackles at bases moving upward as condition worsens
Pleural effusion	Tachypnea, use of accessory muscles	↑ Movement ↑ Fremitus above effusion Absent fremitus over effusion	Dull	Diminished or absent over effusion, egophony over effusion
Pulmonary fibrosis	Tachypnea	↓ Movement	Normal	Crackles or sounds like Velcro being pulled apart

DIAGNOSTIC STUDIES OF RESPIRATORY SYSTEM

Numerous diagnostic studies are available to assess the respiratory system. Table 26-10 identifies the most common studies, and select studies are described in more detail below.

Sputum Studies

Sputum samples can be obtained by expectoration, tracheal suction, or bronchoscopy (discussed below). When the patient is unable to expectorate spontaneously, sputum may also be collected by inhalation of an irritating aerosol, usually hypertonic saline. This is called sputum induction. The specimens may be examined for culture and sensitivity to identify an infecting organism (e.g., *Mycobacterium, Pneumocystis jiroveci*) or to confirm a diagnosis (e.g., malignant cells). Regardless of whether specimen tests are ordered, observe the sputum for color, blood, volume, and viscosity.

Skin Tests

Skin tests may be performed to test for allergic reactions (see Chapter 14) or exposure to TB bacilli or fungi. Skin tests involve the intradermal injection of an antigen. A positive result on a TB skin test indicates that the patient has been exposed to the antigen. It does not indicate that TB is currently present. A negative result indicates either no exposure or a depression of cell-mediated immunity such as occurs in HIV infection. Table 26-11 on p. 494 describes reactions that indicate a positive TB skin test.

Nursing responsibilities are similar for all skin tests. First, to prevent a false-negative reaction, be certain that the injection is intradermal and not subcutaneous. After the injection, circle the site(s) and instruct the patient not to remove the marks. When charting administration of the antigen, draw a diagram of the forearm and hand and label the injection sites. The diagram is especially helpful when more than one test is administered.

When reading test results, use a good light. If an induration is present, use a marking pen to indicate the periphery on all four sides of the induration. As the pen touches the raised area, make a mark. Then determine the diameter of the induration in millimeters. Reddened, flat areas are not measured.

Endoscopic Examinations Bronchoscopy. *Bronchoscopy* is a procedure in which the bronchi are visualized through a fiberoptic tube (Fig. 26-11). Bronchoscopy may be used for diagnos-

TABLE 26-10 DIAGNOSTIC STUDIES

Respiratory System

Study	Description and Purpose	Nursing Responsibility
Blood Studies		
Hemoglobin	Test reflects amount of hemoglobin available for combination with O_2. Venous blood is used. *Male:* 13.2-17.3 g/dL (132-173 g/L) *Female:* 11.7-16.0 g/dL (117-160 g/L)	Explain procedure and its purpose.
Hematocrit	Test reflects ratio of red blood cells to plasma. Increased hematocrit (polycythemia) found in chronic hypoxemia. Venous blood is used. *Male:* 39%-50% (0.39-0.50) *Female:* 35%-47% (0.35-0.47)	Explain procedure and its purpose.
Arterial blood gases (ABGs)	Arterial blood is obtained through puncture of radial or femoral artery or through arterial catheter. Performed to assess acid-base balance, ventilation status, need for O_2 therapy, change in O_2 therapy, or change in ventilator settings.* Continuous ABG monitoring is also possible via a sensor or electrode inserted into arterial catheter.	Indicate whether patient is using O_2 (percentage, L/min). Avoid change in O_2 therapy or interventions (e.g., suctioning, position change) for 20 min before obtaining sample. Assist with positioning (e.g., palm up, wrist slightly hyperextended if radial artery is used). Collect blood in heparinized syringe. To ensure accurate results, expel all air bubbles and place sample in ice, unless it will be analyzed in <1 min. Apply pressure to artery for at least 5 min after specimen is obtained to prevent hematoma at the arterial puncture site.
O_2 Monitoring		
Oximetry	Monitors arterial or venous O_2 saturation. Probe attaches to finger, toe, earlobe, bridge of the nose for SpO_2 monitoring (see eFig. 26-2) or is contained in a pulmonary artery catheter for SvO_2 monitoring. Oximetry is used for intermittent or continuous monitoring and exercise testing.	Apply probe. When interpreting SpO_2 and SvO_2 values, first assess patient status and presence of factors that can alter accuracy of pulse oximeter reading. For SpO_2 these include motion, low perfusion, cold extremities, bright lights, acrylic nails, dark skin color, carbon monoxide, and anemia. For SvO_2, these include change in O_2 delivery or O_2 consumption.
CO_2 Monitoring		
End-tidal CO_2 ($PETCO_2$) (capnography)	Assesses the level of CO_2 in exhaled air. Graphically displays partial pressure of CO_2. Expired gases are sampled from the patient's airway and are analyzed by a CO_2 sensor that uses infrared light to measure exhaled CO_2. The sensor may be attached to an adaptor on the endotracheal or tracheostomy tube. A nasal cannula with a sidestream capnometer can be used in patients without an artificial airway. Can be used as a diagnostic measure to detect lung disease and for monitoring patients. Normal difference between $PaCO_2$ and $PETCO_2$ is 2-5 mm Hg ($PaCO_2$: 35-45 mm Hg; $PETCO_2$: 37-50 mm Hg).	Teach patient and caregiver about the purpose of capnography monitoring, emphasizing the benefit of continuous monitoring. Make sure that sensor is properly attached. Record and document data per institution policy.
Sputum Studies		
Culture and sensitivity	Purpose is to diagnose bacterial infection, select antibiotic, and evaluate treatment. Sputum specimen is collected in a sterile container. Takes 48-72 hr for results.	Instruct patient on how to produce a good specimen (see Gram stain). If patient cannot produce specimen, bronchoscopy may be used (see Fig. 26-11).
Gram stain	Staining of sputum permits classification of bacteria into gram-negative and gram-positive types. Results guide therapy until culture and sensitivity results are obtained.	Instruct patient to expectorate sputum into container after coughing deeply. Obtain sputum (mucoidlike), not saliva. Obtain specimen in early morning after mouth care because secretions collect during night. If unsuccessful, try increasing oral fluid intake unless fluids are restricted. Collect sputum in sterile container (sputum trap) during suctioning or by aspirating secretions from the trachea. Send specimen to laboratory promptly.
Acid-fast smear and culture	Assesses sputum for acid-fast bacilli (e.g., *Mycobacterium tuberculosis*). A series of three early-morning specimens is used.	Instruct patient how to produce a good specimen (see Gram stain). Cover specimen and send to laboratory for analysis.
Cytology	Determines presence of abnormal cells that may indicate malignant condition. Single sputum specimen is collected in special container with fixative solution.	Instruct patient on how to produce a good specimen (see Gram stain). If patient cannot produce specimen, bronchoscopy may be used (see Fig. 26-11). Send specimen to laboratory promptly.

*For reference intervals, see Table 26-1.

Continued

TABLE 26-10   DIAGNOSTIC STUDIES—cont'd

Respiratory System

Study	Description and Purpose	Nursing Responsibility
Radiology		
Chest x-ray	Used to screen, diagnose, and evaluate changes in respiratory system. Most common views are anteroposterior (AP) and lateral.	Instruct patient to undress to waist, put on gown, and remove any metal between neck and waist.
Computed tomography (CT)	Performed for diagnosis of lesions difficult to assess (e.g., mediastinum, hilum, pleura) by conventional x-ray studies. Common types are helical or spiral CT (contrast medium is usually used) and high-resolution CT scan (contrast medium is not used). Spiral CT used to diagnose a pulmonary embolism.	Same as for chest x-ray. Contrast medium may be given IV. Evaluation of BUN and serum creatinine is done before contrast to assess renal function. Assess if patient is allergic to shellfish (iodine), since the contrast is iodine based. Be sure the patient is well hydrated before and after procedure (to excrete contrast). Warn patient that contrast injection may cause a feeling of being warm and flushed. Instruct the patient that he or she will need to lie still on a hard table and the scanner will revolve around the body with clicking noises.
Magnetic resonance imaging (MRI)	Used for diagnosis of lesions difficult to assess by CT scan (e.g., lung apex) and for distinguishing vascular from nonvascular structures.	Same as for chest x-ray and CT scan, except contrast medium is not iodine based. If closed MRI is used and patient has claustrophobia, provide with relaxation or other modes to cope. Patient must remove all metal (e.g., jewelry, watch) before test. Patients with pacemakers and implantable cardioverter-defibrillators may not be able to have MRI.
Ventilation-perfusion (V/Q) scan	Used to assess ventilation and perfusion of lungs. IV radioisotope given to assess perfusion. For the ventilation portion, the patient inhales a radioactive gas (xenon or krypton), which outlines the alveoli. Normal scans show homogeneous radioactivity. Diminished or absent radioactivity suggests lack of perfusion or airflow. Ventilation without perfusion suggests a pulmonary embolus.	Same as for chest x-ray. No precautions needed afterward because the gas and isotope transmit radioactivity for only a brief interval.
Pulmonary angiogram	Used to visualize pulmonary vasculature and locate obstruction or pathologic conditions (e.g., pulmonary embolus). Contrast medium is injected through a catheter threaded into pulmonary artery or right side of the heart. Series of x-rays are taken after contrast medium is injected into pulmonary artery. Chest CT is replacing angiography, since it is less invasive.	Same as for chest x-ray. (See CT scan for contrast media precautions.) Check pressure dressing site after procedure. Monitor blood pressure, pulse, and circulation distal to injection site. Report and record significant changes.
Positron emission tomography (PET) scan	Used to distinguish benign and malignant pulmonary nodules. Because malignant lung cells have an increased uptake of glucose, the PET scan, which uses an IV radioactive glucose preparation, can demonstrate increased uptake of glucose in malignant lung cells.	*Preprocedure:* Check the blood glucose levels as high levels may interfere with test. Food and fluids other than water may be restricted for 4-6 hr. *Postprocedure:* Encourage fluids to excrete radioactive substance.
Endoscopy		
Bronchoscopy (see Fig. 26-11)	Flexible fiberoptic scope is used for diagnosis, biopsy, specimen collection, or assessment of changes. It may also be done to suction mucous plugs, lavage the lungs, or remove foreign objects.	Instruct patient to be on NPO status for 6-12 hr before the test. Obtain signed permit. Give sedative if ordered. After procedure, keep patient NPO until gag reflex returns. Monitor for recovery from sedation. Blood-tinged mucus is not abnormal. If biopsy was done, monitor for hemorrhage and pneumothorax.

Fiberoptic bronchoscope

Smaller bronchus

A   B

FIG. 26-11 Fiberoptic bronchoscope. **A,** The transbronchoscopic balloon-tipped catheter and the flexible fiberoptic bronchoscope. **B,** The catheter is introduced into a small airway and the balloon inflated with 1.5 to 2 mL of air to occlude the airway. Bronchoalveolar lavage is performed by injecting and withdrawing 30-mL aliquots of sterile saline solution, gently aspirating after each instillation. Specimens are sent to the laboratory for analysis.

TABLE 26-10   DIAGNOSTIC STUDIES—cont'd

Respiratory System

Study	Description and Purpose	Nursing Responsibility
Mediastinoscopy	Scope is inserted through a small incision in the suprasternal notch and advanced into the mediastinum to inspect and biopsy lymph nodes. Used to diagnose lung cancer, non-Hodgkin's lymphoma, granulomatous infections, and sarcoidosis.	Prepare patient for surgical intervention. Obtain signed informed consent. Performed in the operating room (OR) using a general anesthetic. Afterward, monitor as for bronchoscopy.
Lung Biopsy	Specimens may be obtained by transbronchial or percutaneous biopsy or via transthoracic needle aspiration (TTNA), video-assisted thoracoscopic surgery (VATS), or open lung biopsy. Transbronchial biopsy and VATS can be performed in the bronchoscopy suite. TTNA is done under CT guidance in radiology department. Open lung is performed in the OR. VATS can also be done in the OR. These tests are used to obtain specimens for laboratory analysis.	Same as bronchoscopy if procedure done with bronchoscope, and same as thoracotomy if open lung biopsy done. With TTNA, check breath sounds q4hr for 24 hr and report any respiratory distress. Check incision site for bleeding. A chest x-ray should be done after TTNA or transbronchial biopsy to check for pneumothorax. With VATS a chest tube may be in postprocedure until lung has reexpanded. Monitor breath sounds to follow chest reexpansion. Encourage deep breathing for lung reinflation. Obtain signed informed consent for all procedures.
Thoracentesis	Used to obtain specimen of pleural fluid for diagnosis, to remove pleural fluid, or to instill medication. Chest x-ray is always obtained after procedure to check for pneumothorax.	Explain procedure to patient and obtain signed informed consent before procedure, which is usually performed in the patient's room. Position patient upright with elbows on an overbed table and feet supported. Instruct the patient not to talk or cough, and assist during procedure. Observe for signs of hypoxia and pneumothorax, and verify breath sounds in all fields after procedure. Encourage deep breaths to expand lungs. Send labeled specimens to laboratory.
Pulmonary Function Tests	Used to evaluate lung function. Involves use of spirometer to assess air movement as patient performs prescribed respiratory maneuvers.†	Avoid scheduling immediately after mealtime. Avoid administration of inhaled bronchodilator 6 hr before procedure. Explain procedure to patient. Assess for respiratory distress before procedure and report. Provide rest after the procedure.
Exercise Testing	Used in diagnosis and in determining exercise capacity. A *complete test* involves walking on a treadmill while expired O_2 and CO_2, respiratory rate, heart rate, and heart rhythm are monitored. In a *modified test* (desaturation test) only SpO_2 is monitored.	Instruct patient to wear comfortable shoes. Encourage patient to walk as quickly as possible.
6-Min walk test	Used to measure functional capacity and response to treatment in patients with heart or lung disease. Pulse oximetry is usually monitored during the walk. The distance walked is measured and used to monitor progression of disease or improvement after rehabilitation.	The patient is instructed by a trained practitioner to walk as far as possible during 6 min, stopping when short of breath and continuing when able.

†For reference intervals, see Tables 26-12 and 26-13.

tic purposes to obtain biopsy specimens and assess results of treatment. Small amounts (30 mL) of sterile saline may be injected through the scope and withdrawn and examined for cells, a technique termed *bronchoalveolar lavage* (BAL). Bronchoscopy is also used for treatment, for example, to remove mucous plugs or foreign bodies. Laser therapy, electrocautery, cryotherapy, and stents may be placed through a bronchoscope to achieve patency of an airway that has been completely or partially obstructed by tumors.

Bronchoscopy can be performed in an outpatient procedure room, in a surgical suite, or at the bedside in the intensive care unit or on a medical-surgical unit, with the patient lying down or seated. After the nasopharynx and oropharynx are anesthetized with local anesthetic, the bronchoscope is coated with lidocaine (Xylocaine) and inserted, usually through the nose, and threaded down into the airways. Bronchoscopy can be done on mechanically ventilated patients through the endotracheal tube.

Lung Biopsy

Lung biopsy may be done (1) transbronchially, (2) percutaneously or via transthoracic needle aspiration (TTNA), (3) by video-assisted thoracic surgery (VATS), or (4) as an open lung biopsy. The purpose of a lung biopsy is to obtain tissue, cells, or secretions for evaluation. Transbronchial lung biopsy involves passing a forceps or needle through the bronchoscope for a specimen (Fig. 26-12). Specimens can be cultured or examined for malignant cells. A combination of transbronchial lung biopsy and BAL is used to differentiate infection and rejection in lung transplant recipients.

Percutaneous needle aspiration or TTNA involves inserting a needle through the chest wall, usually under computed tomography (CT) guidance. Because of the risk of a pneumothorax, a chest x-ray is ordered after TTNA.

In VATS a rigid scope with a lens is passed through a trocar placed into the pleura via one or two small incisions in the intercostal muscles. The physician views the lesions on a monitor

TABLE 26-11	INTERPRETING RESPONSES TO TUBERCULIN SKIN TESTING
Types of Responses	**Consider Positive in the Following Groups**
Positive Reactions	
≥5-mm induration	• HIV-infected people • People who had recent contact with a person with TB disease • People with fibrotic lesions on chest x-ray consistent with prior TB • Patients with organ transplants • People who are immunosuppressed (e.g., taking the equivalent of ≥15 mg/day of prednisone for ≥1 mo)
≥10-mm induration	• Recent immigrants (<5 yr) from high-prevalence countries • Injecting drug users • Residents and employees of high-risk congregate settings • Mycobacteriology laboratory personnel • People with clinical conditions (e.g., diabetes mellitus, end-stage kidney disease) that place them at high risk
≥15-mm induration	• All other people who are at low risk
False Reactions	**Possible Causes**
False-negative reactions (do not react even though infected)	• Anergy, immunosuppression • Recent TB infection (within 8-10 wk of exposure) • Overwhelming TB infection • Very old TB infection (many years) • Recent live virus vaccination (e.g., measles, chickenpox)
False-positive reactions (react even though not infected)	• Nontuberculous mycobacteria (e.g., *Mycobacterium avium-intracellulare* [MAI] or *Mycobacterium avium* complex [MAC]) • Previous BCG vaccine

Source: Centers for Disease Control and Prevention: Tuberculosis (TB) fact sheet: tuberculin skin testing. Retrieved from *www.cdc.gov/tb/publications/factsheets/testing/skintesting.htm*.

CASE STUDY—cont'd

Objective Data: Diagnostic Studies

Kevin Peterson/
Photodisc/Thinkstock

The health care provider orders the following diagnostic studies for F.T.:
• CBC, basic metabolic panel (electrolytes, BUN, creatinine)
• ABGs
• Chest x-ray
• Sputum for culture and sensitivity
The ABGs demonstrate a compensated respiratory acidosis with hypoxemia. The WBC is 14,350/µL, and the chest x-ray shows lower lobe pneumonia. F.T. is admitted to the cardiopulmonary medical-surgical nursing unit.

directly via the lens, and biopsy specimens can be taken. A chest tube is kept in place until the lung expands. Lesions in the pleura or peripheral lung are biopsied via VATS. VATS is much less invasive than open lung biopsy and is the procedure of choice when appropriate.

Open lung biopsy is used when pulmonary disease cannot be diagnosed by other procedures. The patient is anesthetized, the chest is opened with a thoracotomy incision, and a biopsy

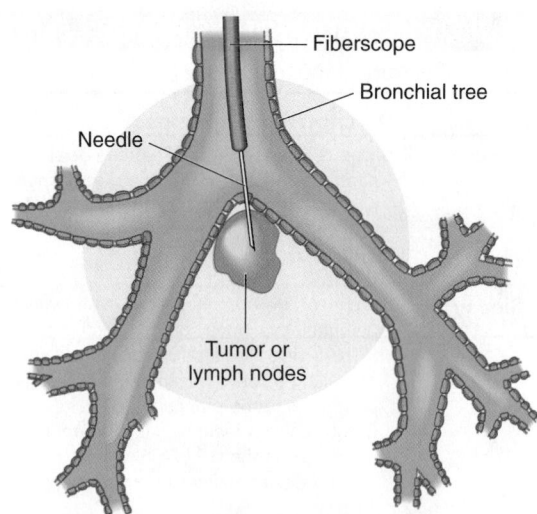

FIG. 26-12 Transbronchial biopsy needle penetrating the bronchial wall and entering a mass of subcarinal lymph nodes or tumor.

FIG. 26-13 Thoracentesis. A catheter is positioned in the pleural space to remove accumulated fluid.

specimen is obtained. Nursing care for the procedure is the same as after thoracotomy (see Chapter 28).

Thoracentesis

Thoracentesis is the insertion of a large-bore needle through the chest wall into the pleural space to obtain specimens for diagnostic evaluation, remove pleural fluid, or instill medication into the pleural space (Fig. 26-13). The patient is positioned sitting upright with elbows on an overbed table and feet supported. The skin is cleansed and a local anesthetic (lidocaine) is instilled subcutaneously. A chest tube may be inserted to permit further drainage of fluid.

Pulmonary Function Tests

Pulmonary function tests (PFTs) measure lung volumes and airflow. The results of PFTs are used to diagnose pulmonary disease, monitor disease progression, evaluate disability, and assess response to bronchodilators. Airflow measurement is administered by trained personnel using a spirometer. The patient inserts a mouthpiece, takes as deep a breath as possible,

TABLE 26-12 LUNG VOLUMES AND CAPACITIES

Parameter	Definitions	Normal Values*
Volumes		
Tidal volume (V_T)	Volume of air inhaled and exhaled with each breath. Only a small proportion of total capacity of lungs.	0.5 L
Expiratory reserve volume (ERV)	Additional air that can be forcefully exhaled after normal exhalation is complete.	1.0 L
Residual volume (RV)	Amount of air remaining in lungs after forced expiration. Air available in lungs for gas exchange between breaths.	1.5 L
Inspiratory reserve volume (IRV)	Maximum volume of air that can be inhaled forcefully after normal inhalation.	3.0 L
Capacities		
Total lung capacity (TLC)	Maximum volume of air that lungs can contain (TLC = IRV + V_T + ERV + RV).	6.0 L
Functional residual capacity (FRC)	Volume of air remaining in lungs at end of normal exhalation (FRC = ERV + RV). Increase or decrease possible with lung disease.	2.5 L
Vital capacity (VC)	Maximum volume of air that can be exhaled after maximum inspiration (VC = IRV + V_T + ERV); higher VC for men (generally).	4.5 L
Inspiratory capacity (IC)	Maximum volume of air that can be inhaled after normal expiration (IC = V_T + IRV).	3.5 L

*Normal values vary with patient's height, weight, age, race, and gender.

TABLE 26-13 COMMON MEASURES OF PULMONARY FUNCTION AIRFLOW

Measure	Description	Normal Value*
Forced vital capacity (FVC)	Amount of air that can be quickly and forcefully exhaled after maximum inspiration.	>80% of predicted
Forced expiratory volume in first second of expiration (FEV$_1$)	Amount of air exhaled in first second of FVC. Grades severity of airway obstruction.	>80% of predicted
FEV$_1$/FVC ratio	Dividing value for FEV$_1$ by value for FVC. Useful in differentiating obstructive and restrictive pulmonary dysfunction.	Age <50: ≥75% of predicted; Age ≥50: ≥70% of predicted
Forced midexpiratory flow rate (FEF$_{25\%-75\%}$)	Measurement of airflow rate in middle half of forced expiration; early indicator of disease of small airways.	Age <50: ≥75% of predicted; Age ≥50: ≥70% of predicted
Maximal voluntary ventilation (MVV)	Deep breathing as rapidly as possible for specified period. Fairly nonspecific test that gives information about exercise capacity. Used in conjunction with exercise stress test.	About 170 L/min
Peak expiratory flow rate (PEFR)	Maximum airflow rate during forced expiration. Aids in monitoring bronchoconstriction in asthma. Can be measured with peak flow meter.	Up to 600 L/min

*Normal values vary with patient's height, age, race, and gender.

and exhales as hard, fast, and long as possible. Verbal coaching is given to ensure that the patient continues blowing out until exhalation is complete.

The computer calculates the patient's percentage of predicted values, that is, how well the performance compares with an average based on age, gender, race, and height. Normal values are approximately 80% to 120% of the predicted value.[10] Normal values for PFTs are shown in Tables 26-12 and 26-13 and in eFig. 26-4, available on the website for this chapter.

Spirometry may be ordered before and after the administration of a bronchodilator to determine the patient's response. This may help document reversibility of airway obstruction (e.g., asthma). A positive response to the bronchodilator is greater than 200 mL increase or greater than 12% increase between preadministration and postadministration values.

Home spirometry may be used to monitor lung function in people with asthma, cystic fibrosis, or COPD, as well as before and after lung transplantation or other thoracic surgeries.[11] A peak flow meter is the instrument used at home. It is a hand-held device through which one blows forcefully and quickly after taking a deep breath. Spirometry changes at home can warn of early lung transplant rejection or infection. Data from a peak flow meter provide important feedback to patients with asthma so they can learn to modify activities and medications in response to changes in peak expiratory flow rates (see Chapter 29).

Pulmonary function parameters can also be used to determine the need for mechanical ventilation or the readiness to be weaned from ventilatory support (see Table 66-13).

BRIDGE TO NCLEX EXAMINATION

The number of the question corresponds to the same-numbered outcome at the beginning of the chapter.

1. To promote the release of surfactant, the nurse encourages the patient to
   a. take deep breaths.
   b. cough five times per hour to prevent alveolar collapse.
   c. decrease fluid intake to reduce fluid accumulation in the alveoli.
   d. sit with head of bed elevated to promote air movement through the pores of Kohn.

2. A patient with a respiratory condition asks "How does air get into my lungs?" The nurse bases her answer on her knowledge that air moves into the lungs because of
   a. contraction of the accessory abdominal muscles.
   b. increased carbon dioxide and decreased oxygen in the blood.
   c. stimulation of the respiratory muscles by the chemoreceptors.
   d. decrease in intrathoracic pressure relative to pressure at the airway.

3. The nurse can best determine adequate arterial oxygenation of the blood by assessing
   a. heart rate.
   b. hemoglobin level.
   c. arterial oxygen tension.
   d. arterial carbon dioxide tension.

4. When teaching a patient about the most important respiratory defense mechanism distal to the respiratory bronchioles, which topic would the nurse discuss?
   a. Alveolar macrophages
   b. Impaction of particles
   c. Reflex bronchoconstriction
   d. Mucociliary clearance mechanism

5. A student nurse asks the RN what can be measured by arterial blood gases (ABGs). The RN tells the student that the ABGs can measure (select all that apply)
   a. acid-base balance.
   b. oxygenation status.
   c. acidity of the blood.
   d. glucose bound to hemoglobin.
   e. bicarbonate (HCO_3^-) in arterial blood.

6. To detect early signs or symptoms of inadequate oxygenation, the nurse would examine the patient for
   a. dyspnea and hypotension.
   b. apprehension and restlessness.
   c. cyanosis and cool, clammy skin.
   d. increased urine output and diaphoresis.

7. During the respiratory assessment of the older adult, the nurse would expect to find (select all that apply)
   a. a vigorous cough.
   b. increased chest expansion.
   c. increased residual volume.
   d. increased breath sounds in the lung apices.
   e. increased anteroposterior (AP) chest diameter.

8. When assessing activity-exercise patterns related to respiratory health, the nurse inquires about
   a. dyspnea during rest or exercise.
   b. recent weight loss or weight gain.
   c. ability to sleep through the entire night.
   d. willingness to wear oxygen equipment in public.

9. When auscultating the chest of an older patient in respiratory distress, it is best to
   a. begin listening at the apices.
   b. begin listening at the lung bases.
   c. begin listening on the anterior chest.
   d. ask the patient to breathe through the nose with the mouth closed.

10. Which assessment finding of the respiratory system does the nurse interpret as abnormal?
   a. Inspiratory chest expansion of 1 in
   b. Percussion resonance over the lung bases
   c. Symmetric chest expansion and contraction
   d. Bronchial breath sounds in the lower lung fields

11. The nurse is preparing the patient for a diagnostic procedure to remove pleural fluid for analysis. The nurse would prepare the patient for which test?
   a. Thoracentesis
   b. Bronchoscopy
   c. Pulmonary angiography
   d. Sputum culture and sensitivity

1. a, 2. d, 3. c, 4. d, 5. a, b, c, e, 6. b, 7. c, e, 8. a, 9. b, 10. d, 11. a

Ⓔvolve

For rationales to these answers and even more NCLEX review questions, visit http://evolve.elsevier.com/Lewis/medsurg.

REFERENCES

1. Thibodeau GA, Patton KT: *Anthony's textbook of anatomy and physiology*, St Louis, 2013, Mosby.
2. Kaneko H, Horie J: Breathing movements of the chest and abdominal wall in healthy subjects, *Respir Care* 57(9):1442, 2012.
3. Kelly AM: Review article: can venous blood gas analysis replace arterial in emergency medical care, *Emerg Med Australas* 22(6):493, 2010.
4. Valdez-Lowe C, Ghareeb SA, Artinian NT: Pulse oximetry in adults, *Am J Nurs* 109(6):52, 2009.
5. Touhy TA: *Ebersole and Hess' toward healthy aging: human needs and nursing response*, ed 8, St Louis, 2012, Mosby.
6. Taylor BJ, Johnson BD: The pulmonary circulation and exercise responses in the elderly, *Semin Respir Crit Care Med* 31(5):528, 2010.
7. Pullen RL: Assessing the paranasal sinuses, *Nursing* 40(5):49, 2010.
8. Jarvis C: *Physical examination and health assessment*, ed 6, St Louis, 2012, Mosby.
9. Page B: Lung sound assessment: the lost art of using a stethoscope, *JEMS* 36(8):26, 2011.
10. Liang BM, Lam DC, Feng YL: Clinical applications of lung function tests: a revisit. *Respirology* 17(4):611, 2012.
11. Lam DC, Hui CK, Ip MS: Issues in pulmonary function testing for the screening and diagnosis of chronic obstructive pulmonary disease, *Curr Opin Pulm Med* 18(2):104, 2012.

RESOURCES

Resources for this chapter are listed after Chapter 29 on p. 610.

For breath is life, and if you breathe well you
will live long on earth.
Sanskrit Proverb

Nursing Management

Upper Respiratory Problems

Dorothy (Dottie) M. Mathers

⊘volve WEBSITE

http://evolve.elsevier.com/Lewis/medsurg

- NCLEX Review Questions
- Key Points
- Pre-Test
- Answer Guidelines for Case Study on p. 519
- Rationales for Bridge to NCLEX Examination Questions

- Case Study
  - Patient With Head and Neck Cancer/ Laryngectomy With Tracheostomy
- Nursing Care Plans (Customizable)
  - eNCP 27-1: Patient With a Tracheostomy
  - eNCP 27-2: Patient Having Total Laryngectomy and/or Radical Neck Surgery

- Concept Map Creator
- Glossary
- Animation
  - Anatomic Location of Sinuses
- Content Updates

eFigure
- eFig. 27-1: Placing posterior nasal pack in epistaxis

LEARNING OUTCOMES

1. Describe the clinical manifestations and nursing and collaborative management of problems of the nose.
2. Discuss the clinical manifestations and nursing and collaborative management of problems of the paranasal sinuses.
3. Describe the clinical manifestations and nursing and collaborative management of problems of the pharynx and larynx.
4. Discuss the nursing management of the patient who requires a tracheostomy.

5. Identify the steps involved in performing tracheostomy care and suctioning an airway.
6. Describe the risk factors and warning symptoms associated with head and neck cancer.
7. Discuss the nursing management of the patient with a laryngectomy.
8. Explain the methods used in voice restoration for the patient with temporary or permanent loss of speech.

KEY TERMS

allergic rhinitis, p. 499
deviated septum, p. 497
epistaxis, p. 498

esophageal speech, p. 516
nasal polyps, p. 506
rhinoplasty, p. 498

sinusitis, p. 504
tracheostomy, p. 507

Disorders of the nose, sinuses, pharynx, and larynx are presented in this chapter. Nursing management of patients with a tracheostomy or total laryngectomy is also discussed.

PROBLEMS OF NOSE AND PARANASAL SINUSES

DEVIATED SEPTUM

Deviated septum is a deflection of the normally straight nasal septum. Although up to 80% of the adult population may have septums that are slightly off center, the diagnosis of deviated septum is generally reserved for those that are severely shifted.[1] Trauma to the nose, either at birth or later in life, is the most common cause of deviated septum.[2] Deviation from midline can interfere with airflow and sinus drainage through the narrowed passageway. Symptoms vary depending on the degree

of deviation. Minor septal deviations may be asymptomatic. Common manifestations of septal deviation include obstruction to nasal breathing, nasal congestion, frequent sinus infections and nosebleeds *(epistaxis),* and facial pain.

Medical management of deviated septum is focused on symptom control of nasal inflammation and congestion (see Table 27-2). For recurrent or severe symptoms, a nasal septoplasty is performed to reconstruct and properly align the deviated septum.

NASAL FRACTURE

Nasal fracture is the most common facial fracture and the third most common fracture of any bone. Fracture of the nose occurs as a result of blunt trauma, such as occurs with fights, automobile accidents, falls, and sports injuries. Many cases of facial trauma can be prevented by using protective sports

Reviewed by Sharon A. Willadsen, RN, PhD, Nursing Instructor, Lakeshore Technical College, Cleveland, Wisconsin.

equipment and protecting against falls. Complications associated with nasal fractures include airway obstruction, epistaxis, meningeal tears causing cerebrospinal fluid (CSF) leakage, septal hematoma, and cosmetic deformity.

Nasal fractures can be classified as simple or complex. *Simple fractures* may be unilateral or bilateral and typically produce little or no displacement.[3] Powerful frontal blows can cause *complex fractures,* which may also involve subsequent damage to adjacent facial structures such as the teeth, eyes, or other facial bones. Orbital fractures may be seen with midfacial trauma.

Diagnosis of a nasal fracture is based on the health history and physical examination. Clinical manifestations suggestive of a nasal fracture include localized pain, crepitus on palpation, swelling, ecchymosis, cosmetic deformity, epistaxis, and difficulty breathing out of the nostrils. Although facial deformity with a nasal fracture is common, often epistaxis may be the only initial sign.

On inspection, assess the patient's ability to breathe through each side of the nose and note the presence of edema, bleeding, or hematoma. Ecchymosis may be under one or both eyes. Ecchymosis involving both eyes is often termed *raccoon eyes* and may suggest an orbital or basilar skull fracture (see Chapter 57). Inspect the nose internally for evidence of septal deviation, hemorrhage, or clear drainage. Clear, pink-tinged, or persistent drainage after control of epistaxis suggests a CSF leak. Perform a quick test at the bedside or send a specimen to the laboratory to determine if glucose is present; the presence of glucose indicates that the fluid is CSF.

Injury of sufficient force to fracture nasal bones results in considerable swelling of soft tissues. With extensive swelling, it may be necessary to wait to repair the fracture until the edema subsides, which may be 5 to 10 days.

Goals of nursing management are to maintain the airway, reduce edema and pain, prevent complications, and provide emotional support. The best way to maintain the airway is to keep the patient in an upright position. Apply ice to the face and nose in 10- to 20-minute intervals to help reduce edema and bleeding. Administer analgesia as ordered to control pain. Acetaminophen is preferred over nonsteroidal antiinflammatory drugs (NSAIDs) or acetylsalicylic acid (ASA; aspirin) for the first 48 hours to avoid prolonging clotting time and increasing the risk for bleeding. Nasal stuffiness may be relieved with nasal decongestants, saline nasal sprays, and a humidifier. Tell the patient to avoid hot showers and alcohol for the first 48 hours to prevent an increase in swelling. Encourage the patient to quit or decrease smoking to maximize tissue healing.

When a fracture is confirmed, the goals are to realign the fracture using closed or open reduction (septoplasty, rhinoplasty) and to ensure that a septal hematoma does not develop, since this increases the patient's risk for infection. In addition to reestablishing cosmetic appearance, these surgical procedures provide an adequate airway and function of the nose.

RHINOPLASTY

Rhinoplasty, the surgical reconstruction of the nose, is performed for cosmetic reasons or to improve airway function when trauma or developmental deformities result in nasal obstruction. When caring for rhinoplasty patients before surgery, assess the patient's expectations of the surgery. Any actual or perceived alteration in body image (e.g., a deformed or enlarged nose) can affect self-esteem and interactions with others. Computerized photographs can be used to show the patient's appearance after the surgery. These images often help patients decide whether to undergo rhinoplasty. Explain expected results of surgery frankly and truthfully to avoid disappointment.

Rhinoplasty is performed as an outpatient procedure using regional or general anesthesia. Sometimes nasal tissue is added or removed, and the nose may be lengthened or shortened. Plastic implants are sometimes used to reshape the nose. Incisions are typically inside the nose and are thus hidden. Sonic rhinoplasty incorporates the use of an ultrasonic device to gently aspirate bone, enabling a refined cosmetic result.[4]

After surgery, nasal packing may be inserted to apply pressure and prevent bleeding or septal hematoma formation. An external plastic splint protects and supports the new shape of the nose during the healing process. Nasal packing is usually removed the day after surgery, and the splint is left in place for approximately 1 week.

NURSING MANAGEMENT NASAL SURGERY

Examples of nasal surgery include rhinoplasty, septoplasty, and nasal fracture reductions. Before surgery, instruct the patient not to take aspirin-containing drugs or NSAIDs for 2 weeks to reduce the risk of bleeding. Encourage preoperative smoking cessation to promote postoperative wound healing. Nursing interventions during the immediate postoperative period include maintenance of the airway; assessment of respiratory status; pain management; and observation of the surgical site for bleeding, infection, and edema. Teaching is important because the patient must be able to detect early and late complications at home. The patient typically experiences temporary edema and ecchymosis. Cold compresses and elevation of the head can help minimize swelling and discomfort. Teach activity restrictions aimed at preventing bleeding and injury (no nose blowing, swimming, heavy lifting, strenuous exercise).[5] Subtle swelling may be slow to resolve, delaying the achievement of a full cosmetic result for up to a year.

EPISTAXIS

Epistaxis (nosebleed) occurs in a bimodal distribution, with children 2 to 10 years of age and adults over age 50 most affected. Epistaxis can be caused by low humidity, allergies, upper respiratory tract infections, sinusitis, trauma, foreign bodies, hypertension, chemical irritants such as street drugs, overuse of decongestant nasal sprays, facial or nasal surgery, anatomic malformation, and tumors.[6] Any condition that prolongs bleeding time or alters platelet counts will predispose the patient to epistaxis. Bleeding time may also be prolonged if the patient takes aspirin, NSAIDs, warfarin, or other anticoagulant drugs.

Approximately 90% of nosebleeds occur in the anterior portion of the nasal cavity and are easily visualized. Posterior bleeding occurs more commonly with older adults secondary to other health problems. Anterior bleeding usually stops spontaneously or can be self-treated. Posterior bleeding may require medical treatment.

NURSING AND COLLABORATIVE MANAGEMENT
EPISTAXIS

Use simple first aid measures to control epistaxis: (1) keep the patient quiet; (2) place the patient in a sitting position, leaning slightly forward with head tilted forward; and (3) apply direct pressure by pinching the entire soft lower portion of the nose against the nasal septum for 10 to 15 minutes. If bleeding does not stop within 15 to 20 minutes, seek medical assistance.

Medical management involves identifying the bleeding site and applying a vasoconstrictive agent, cauterization, or anterior packing. Pledgets (nasal tampon) impregnated with anesthetic solution (lidocaine) and/or vasoconstrictive agents such as cocaine or epinephrine are placed into the nasal cavity and left in place for 10 to 15 minutes. Silver nitrate may be used to chemically cauterize an identified bleeding point after epistaxis is controlled. Thermal cauterization is reserved for more severe bleeding and requires the use of local or general anesthesia.[7]

If bleeding does not stop, packing may be used. Packing with compressed sponges (e.g., Merocel) or epistaxis balloons (e.g., Rapid Rhino) is preferred over the use of traditional Vaseline ribbon gauze because of the ease of placement. Packing is inserted into the nares and advanced along the floor of the nasal cavity. The sponge expands with moisture to fill the nasal cavity and tamponade bleeding. The balloon is inflated with air to achieve the same pressure effect (Fig. 27-1). Alternatively, absorbable materials such as oxidized cellulose (surgical), gelatin foam (Gelfoam), or a gelatin-thrombin combination (Floseal) may be used as packing for anterior bleeds. In addition to providing pressure to stop bleeding, these materials increase clot formation and protect the nasal mucosa from further trauma.[7] A nasal sling (a folded 2 × 2-in gauze pad) may be taped under the nares to absorb drainage.

Nasal packing may impair respiratory status, especially in older adults. Closely monitor respiratory rate, heart rate and rhythm, oxygen saturation using pulse oximetry (SpO_2), and level of consciousness, and observe for signs of aspiration. Because of the risk of complications, all patients with posterior packing should be admitted to a monitored unit to permit closer observation.

Packing is painful because sufficient pressure must be applied to stop the bleeding. Nasal packing predisposes patients to infection from bacteria (e.g., *Staphylococcus aureus*) present in the nasal cavity. The patient should receive a mild opioid analgesic for pain (e.g., acetaminophen with codeine) and an antibiotic effective against staphylococci to protect against infection.

Nasal packing may be left in place for a few days. Before removal, medicate the patient for pain because this procedure is very uncomfortable. After removal, cleanse the nares gently and lubricate them with water-soluble jelly.

Teach the patient about home care before discharge. Instruct the patient to avoid vigorous nose blowing, engaging in strenuous activity, lifting, and straining for 4 to 6 weeks. Teach the patient to use saline nasal spray and/or a humidifier, to sneeze with the mouth open, and to avoid the use of aspirin-containing products or NSAIDs.

ALLERGIC RHINITIS

Allergic rhinitis is the reaction of the nasal mucosa to a specific allergen. Allergic rhinitis can be classified according to the causative allergen (seasonal or perennial) or the frequency of symptoms (episodic, intermittent, or persistent).[8] *Episodic* refers to symptoms related to sporadic exposure to allergens that are not typically encountered in the patient's normal environment, such as exposure to animal dander when visiting another person's home. *Intermittent* means that the symptoms are present less than 4 days a week or less than 4 weeks per year. *Persistent* means that the symptoms are present more than 4 days a week and for more than 4 weeks per year.

Seasonal rhinitis usually occurs in the spring and fall and is caused by allergy to pollens from trees, flowers, or grasses. The typical attack lasts for several weeks during times when pollen counts are high; then it disappears and recurs at the same time the following year. *Perennial rhinitis* occurs from exposure to environmental allergens, such as animal dander, dust mites, indoor molds, or cockroaches. Both seasonal and perennial rhinitis can be classified as episodic, intermittent, or persistent, depending on the duration and frequency of symptoms.

Sensitization to an allergen occurs with initial allergen exposure, which results in the production of antigen-specific immu-

FIG. 27-1 A, Epistaxis balloon. The balloon is inflated after insertion. **B,** Epistaxis balloon in proper position in nares.

noglobulin E (IgE) (see Fig. 14-6). After exposure, mast cells and basophils release histamine, cytokines, prostaglandins, and leukotrienes, which cause the early symptoms of sneezing, itching, rhinorrhea, and congestion. Four to 8 hours after exposure, inflammatory cells infiltrate the nasal tissues, causing and maintaining the inflammatory response. Because symptoms of rhinitis resemble those of the common cold, the patient may believe the condition is a continuous or repeated cold.

Clinical Manifestations

Manifestations of allergic rhinitis are initially sneezing; watery, itchy eyes and nose; altered sense of smell; and thin, watery nasal discharge that can lead to a more sustained mucus production and nasal congestion. The nasal turbinates appear pale, boggy, and swollen. The turbinates may fill the air space and press against the nasal septum. The posterior ends of the turbinates can become so enlarged that they obstruct sinus aeration or drainage and result in sinusitis. With chronic exposure to allergens, the patient's responses include headache, congestion, pressure, nasal polyps, and postnasal drip as the most common cause of cough. The patient may complain of cough, hoarseness, and the recurrent need to clear the throat. Congestion may cause snoring.

NURSING AND COLLABORATIVE MANAGEMENT ALLERGIC RHINITIS

The most important step in managing allergic rhinitis is identifying and avoiding triggers of allergic reactions (Table 27-1). Instruct the patient to keep a diary of times when the allergic reaction occurs and the activities that precipitate the reaction. Patients are often more aware of intermittent exposure to an allergen such as pets than they are of a more persistent exposure to allergens such as dust mites, cockroaches, or mold. Identifying such triggers is the first step toward avoiding them.

The goal of medications is to reduce inflammation associated with allergic rhinitis, reduce nasal symptoms, minimize associated complications, and maximize quality of life. Appropriate oral medication options include H_1-antihistamines, corticosteroids, decongestants, and leukotriene receptor antagonists (LTRAs). Intranasal medications include antihistamines, anticholinergics, corticosteroids, cromolyn, and decongestants[9] (Table 27-2).

Second-generation antihistamines are preferred over first-generation antihistamines because of their nonsedating effects. Remind patients who are taking antihistamines to have adequate fluid intake to reduce adverse symptoms. Nasal corticosteroid sprays are used to decrease inflammation locally with little absorption in the systemic circulation. Therefore systemic side effects are rare. If symptoms are not relieved with monotherapy, a two-drug combination (such as an oral H_1-antihistamine and an intranasal corticosteroid) may be helpful. Immunotherapy (allergy shots) may be used when a specific, unavoidable allergen is identified and drugs are not tolerated or are ineffective in controlling symptoms. Immunotherapy involves controlled exposure to small amounts of the known allergen through frequent (at least weekly) injections with the goal of decreasing sensitivity. Sublingual or intranasal administration of allergen immunotherapy may be appropriate for selected patients. (Immunotherapy is discussed in Chapter 14.)

TABLE 27-1	PATIENT & CAREGIVER TEACHING GUIDE

Avoiding Allergens in Allergic Rhinitis

Include the following instructions when teaching a patient or caregiver about allergic rhinitis.

What to Avoid	Specific Approaches
House dust	• Focus on the bedroom. Remove carpeting. Limit furniture. • Put the pillows, mattress, and springs in airtight vinyl bags or containers. • Limit clothing in the bedroom to items used frequently. Place clothing in airtight, zipper-sealed vinyl clothes bags. • Install an air filter. Close the air conditioning vent into the room. Use blinds rather than draperies.
House dust mites	• Wash bedding in hot water (130° F [54° C]) weekly. • Wear a mask when vacuuming. Install a filter on the outlet port of the vacuum cleaner. • Avoid sleeping or lying on upholstered furniture. • Keep house temperature and conditions cool and dry.
Pet allergens	• Remove pets from interior of home. • Clean the living area thoroughly. • Do not expect instant relief. Symptoms usually do not improve significantly for 2 mo after pet removal.
Mold spores	• The three *D*s that promote growth of mold spores are darkness, dampness, and drafts. • Ventilate closed rooms and open doors. Consider adding windows to dark rooms. Consider keeping a small light on in closets. • Basement light with a timer that provides light several hours a day may decrease mold growth. • Avoid places where humidity is high (e.g., basements, clothes hampers, greenhouses, barns). Dehumidifiers are rarely helpful.
Pollens	• Stay inside with closed doors and windows during high-pollen season. • Install an air conditioner with a good air filter. Wash filters weekly during high-pollen season. • Put the car air conditioner on "recirculate" when driving. • Avoid having plants, especially in the bedroom.
Smoke	• Presence of a smoker will sabotage the best of all possible symptom reduction programs.

DRUG ALERT: Antihistamines
• First-generation antihistamines (e.g., chlorpheniramine [Chlor-Trimeton]) can cause drowsiness and sedation.
• Warn patients that operating machinery and driving may be dangerous because of the sedative effect.

DRUG ALERT: Pseudoephedrine (Sudafed)
• Large doses may produce tachycardia and palpitations, especially in patients with cardiac disease.
• Overdosage in those over 60 years of age may result in central nervous system depression, seizures, and hallucinations.

ACUTE VIRAL RHINITIS

Acute viral rhinitis (common cold or acute coryza) is an infection of the upper respiratory tract that can be caused by more than 200 different viruses. The majority of colds, which are caused by rhinoviruses, are mild and self-limiting. Other

TABLE 27-2 DRUG THERAPY

Rhinitis and Sinusitis

Drug	Mechanism of Action	Side Effects	Nursing Actions
Corticosteroids ***Nasal Spray*** beclomethasone (Beconase) budesonide (Rhinocort) ciclesonide (Omnaris) flunisolide (Nasalide) fluticasone (Flonase) fluticasone furoate (Veramyst) mometasone (Nasonex) triamcinolone (Nasacort)	Inhibits inflammatory response of allergic rhinitis. At recommended dose, systemic side effects are unlikely because of low systemic absorption. Systemic effects may occur with higher than recommended doses.	Mild transient nasal burning and stinging, mucosal drying. In rare instances, localized fungal infection with *Candida albicans*.	• Instruct patient to use on regular basis and not PRN. • Instruct patient to clear nasal passages before use. • Reinforce that spray acts to decrease inflammation and it may take several days or weeks to achieve maximum effects. • Discontinue use if nasal infection develops.
Mast Cell Stabilizer ***Nasal Spray*** cromolyn spray (NasalCrom)	Suppresses release of histamine and other inflammatory mediators from mast cells.	Minimal side effects. Occasional burning or nasal irritation.	• Reinforce that spray prevents symptoms. • Begin 2 wk before pollen season starts and use throughout pollen season. • If isolated allergy, such as cat, use prophylactically (i.e., 10-15 min before exposure to allergen).
Leukotriene Receptor Antagonists (LTRAs) and Inhibitors ***Antagonists*** zafirlukast (Accolate) montelukast (Singulair) ***Inhibitors*** zileuton (Zyflo)	Suppress leukotriene activity, thereby inhibiting airway edema, bronchoconstriction, mucus production, and inflammation (see Fig. 12-2).	Generally well tolerated. May cause headaches, dizziness, rash, altered liver function tests, GI disturbances. *Zafirlukast and zileuton:* Monitor PT levels and theophylline levels if patient is taking warfarin or theophylline.	• Monitor liver function tests periodically while on therapy. Discontinue if elevated. • Administer on empty stomach. • Do not discontinue therapy without consulting health care professional. • Not to be used for acute attacks.
Anticholinergic ***Nasal Spray*** ipratropium bromide (Atrovent)	Blocks nasal cholinergic receptors, reducing nasal secretions in the common cold and nonallergic rhinitis.	Nasal dryness and irritation may occur. Does not cause systemic side effects.	• Need to prime pump with seven actuations before initial use • May reduce the need for other rhinitis medications.

Antihistamines
First-Generation Agents (Oral)
azatadine (Optimine)
brompheniramine
  (Dimetane)
chlorpheniramine
  (Chlor-Trimeton)
clemastine (Tavist)
dexchlorpheniramine
  (Polaramine)
diphenhydramine (Benadryl)
levocetirizine (Xyzal)
	Bind with H_1 receptors on target cells, blocking histamine binding. Relieve acute symptoms of allergic response (itching, sneezing, rhinorrhea).	Cross blood-brain barrier, frequently causing sedation and somnolence.
		Can also cause paradoxical stimulation (restlessness, nervousness, insomnia).
		Anticholinergic side effects (e.g., palpitations, dry mouth, constipation, urinary hesitancy).
			• Warn patient that operating machinery and driving may be dangerous because of sedative effect.
			• Teach patient to report palpitations, change in heart rate, change in bowel or bladder habits.
			• Instruct patient not to use alcohol with antihistamines because of additive depressant effect.
			• Rapid onset of action, no drug tolerance with prolonged use.

Second-Generation Agents (Oral) loratadine (Claritin) cetirizine (Zyrtec) fexofenadine (Allegra) desloratadine (Clarinex) levocetirizine (Xyzal)	Same as above.	Limited affinity for brain H_1 receptors. Cause minimal sedation, few effects on psychomotor activities or bladder function.	• Teach patient to expect few, if any, side effects. • More expensive than classic antihistamines. • Rapid onset of action, no drug tolerance with prolonged use.
Second-Generation Agents (Intranasal) azelastine (Astelin) olopatadine (Patanase)	Same as above.	Headache, bitter taste, somnolence, nasal irritation.	Longer use increases risk of rebound vasodilation, which can increase congestion.

Continued

TABLE 27-2   DRUG THERAPY—cont'd

Rhinitis and Sinusitis

Drug	Mechanism of Action	Side Effects	Nursing Actions
Decongestants **Oral** pseudoephedrine (Sudafed)	Stimulates adrenergic receptors on blood vessels, promotes vasoconstriction, reduces nasal congestion.	CNS stimulation, causing insomnia, excitation, headache, irritability, increased blood and ocular pressure, dysuria, palpitations, tachycardia.	• Advise patient of adverse reactions. • Advise that some preparations are contraindicated for patients with cardiovascular disease, hypertension, diabetes, glaucoma, benign prostatic hyperplasia, hepatic and renal disease.
Topical (Nasal Spray) oxymetazoline (Dristan 12-Hour) phenylephrine (Neo-Synephrine)	Same as above.	Same as above, plus rebound nasal congestion.	• Teach patient that these drugs should not be used for >3 days or >3-4 times/day.
Combination Cold Medications Zutripro oral solution (hydrocodone, chlorpheniramine, and pseudoephedrine) Rezira oral solution (hydrocodone and pseudoephedrine)	Hydrocodone suppresses cough. Mechanism of action of chlorpheniramine and pseudoephedrine discussed above.	See individual drugs above.	• Avoid in patients with head injury or increased intracranial pressure. • Use with caution in patients with acute abdominal conditions.

PT, Prothrombin time.

viruses, such as coxsackieviruses and adenoviruses, can cause a more severe illness. Acute viral rhinitis is the most prevalent infectious disease, with the average adult contracting one to three colds per year.

The virus is spread by airborne droplet sprays emitted by the infected person while breathing, talking, sneezing, or coughing. Because the virus can survive on inanimate objects for up to 3 days, transmission can also occur by direct hand contact. Frequency of the infection increases in the winter months when people stay indoors and overcrowding is more common. Other factors that increase susceptibility include fatigue, physical and emotional stress, allergies that affect the nose and throat, and compromised immune status. Exercise can significantly reduce the number of upper respiratory tract infections.[10]

Symptoms of acute viral rhinitis typically begin 2 or 3 days after infection and may include runny nose, watery eyes, nasal congestion, sneezing, cough, sore throat, fever, headache, and fatigue. Cold symptoms may last 2 to 14 days, with typical recovery in 7 to 10 days.

NURSING AND COLLABORATIVE MANAGEMENT ACUTE VIRAL RHINITIS

Interventions are directed toward relieving symptoms. Rest, fluids, proper diet, antipyretics, and analgesics are recommended. Warm salt water gargles, ice chips, throat lozenges, or throat sprays alleviate a sore throat. Petroleum jelly soothes a raw nose. Saline nasal spray reduces nasal congestion. Antihistamine and decongestant therapy reduces postnasal drip and significantly decreases severity of cough, nasal obstruction, and nasal discharge. Caution patients to use the intranasal decongestant sprays for no more than 3 days to prevent rebound congestion from occurring. Cough suppressants may be used.

 COMPLEMENTARY & ALTERNATIVE THERAPIES

Echinacea

Scientific Evidence
• Echinacea may have some benefit in reducing the incidence and duration of the common cold.
• However, there is conflicting evidence on its use in prevention and treatment of upper respiratory tract infections.

Nursing Implications
• Echinacea is considered safe when used in recommended doses.
• Patients with asthma or allergies to plants in the daisy family (including ragweed, mums, marigolds, and daisies) are more likely to have allergic reactions.
• It may interfere with drugs that suppress the immune system and those that are metabolized by the liver.
• Caution is advised in patients with autoimmune disorders.

Complications of acute viral rhinitis include pharyngitis, sinusitis, otitis media, tonsillitis, and lung infections. Unless symptoms of complications are present, antibiotic therapy is not indicated. Antibiotics have no effect on viruses and, if taken injudiciously, may produce antibiotic-resistant bacteria. If symptoms remain for 10 to 14 days with no improvement, acute bacterial sinusitis may be present, and antibiotics will be prescribed.

Teach the patient to recognize the symptoms of secondary bacterial infection, such as a temperature higher than 100.4° F (38° C); tender, swollen glands; severe sinus or ear pain; or significantly worsening symptoms. Green, purulent nasal drainage during the later stages of a cold is not uncommon and is not considered indicative of bacterial infection. In the patient with pulmonary disease, signs of infection include a change in consistency, color, or volume of the sputum. Because infection

EVIDENCE-BASED PRACTICE

Translating Research Into Practice

Do Probiotics Prevent Upper Respiratory Tract Infections?

Clinical Question

In healthy patients (P) what is the effect of probiotics (I) versus placebo (C) in preventing acute upper respiratory tract infections (O)?

Best Available Evidence

Systematic review of randomized controlled trials (RCTs)

Critical Appraisal and Synthesis of Evidence

- Ten RCTs (n = 3451) including healthy children and adults up to age 40.
- Intervention was ingestion of any probiotic (single or mixture of strains, any dosage regimen or route of administration) for more than 7 days, compared with placebo or no treatment.
- Most common probiotics were lactic acid bacteria and bifidobacteria, often consumed in fermented foods (e.g., yogurt) or as dietary supplements.
- Probiotics were better than placebo in reducing the occurrence of acute URIs.
- The number of URIs requiring antibiotics was lower in patients using probiotics compared with those using placebo.

Conclusion

- Probiotics are effective in reducing the incidence of URIs.

Implications for Nursing Practice

- Encourage continued probiotic use to prevent acute URIs.
- Yogurt is an excellent food source for probiotics.
- Probiotics are also available as a dietary supplement.
- Advise patients with frequent URIs of potential benefit from probiotic ingestion.
- Probiotics are typically well tolerated, but can cause gastrointestinal (GI) side effects
- Counsel patients of minor probiotic side effects, including flatulence and increased GI irritability.

Reference for Evidence

Hao Q, Lu Z, Dong B, et al: Probiotics for preventing acute upper respiratory tract infections, *Cochrane Database Syst Rev* 9:CD006895, 2011.

P, Patient population of interest; *I,* intervention or area of interest; *C,* comparison of interest or comparison group; *O,* outcomes of interest (see p. 12).

can progress rapidly, teach the patient with chronic respiratory disease to immediately report sputum changes, increased shortness of breath, and chest tightness. During the cold season, advise patients with a chronic illness or a compromised immune system to avoid crowded situations and other persons who have obvious cold symptoms. Frequent hand washing and avoiding hand-to-face contact help prevent direct spread.

INFLUENZA

Influenza (flu) is a highly contagious respiratory illness that causes significant morbidity and mortality. Millions of Americans (about 5% to 20% of U.S. population) contract influenza each year. The flu season begins in September and continues through April of each year, peaking anywhere from November to March. More than 200,000 people are hospitalized each year for flu-related complications.[11] Death rates vary from season to season. On average, influenza is responsible for 20,000 deaths annually. Vaccination of high-risk groups can prevent many of these deaths.

Etiology and Pathophysiology

Influenza viruses are classified into three serotypes (A, B, and C), but only A and B cause significant illness in humans. Influenza A is subtyped based on the presence of two surface proteins: hemagglutinin (H) and neuraminidase (N). The H antigens enable the virus to enter the cell, and the N antigens facilitate cell-to-cell transmission. Influenza A viruses are thus named according to their H and N type (e.g., H3N2).

Influenza A can infect a variety of animals as well as humans. More than 100 types of influenza A are found in birds (avian flu), pigs (swine flu), horses, seals, and dogs. The virus mutates to allow it to infect different species. When a new viral strain reaches humans, people do not have immunity, and the virus can spread quickly around the globe, causing a *pandemic.* The type A H1N1 influenza (swine flu) emerged in 2009 having never been seen in humans before. A worldwide pandemic resulted. Pandemics can also be triggered by the reemergence of a viral strain that has not circulated for many years. *Epidemics* are more localized outbreaks, usually occurring yearly, caused by variants of already circulating strains. Influenza A is the most common flu virus and also the most virulent.

Influenza B and C viruses are not divided into subtypes and only infect humans. Outbreaks of influenza B can also cause regional epidemics, but the disease it produces is generally milder than that caused by influenza A. Influenza C causes mild illness and does not cause epidemics or pandemics.

Influenza viruses have a remarkable ability to change over time. This accounts for widespread disease and the need for annual vaccination against new strains. Fewer cases of influenza result when a minor change in the virus occurs because most persons have partial immunity.

Influenza is transmitted from animals to humans by direct contact with infected animals or through exposure to water and surfaces contaminated with animal feces. Influenza is communicable between humans through droplet contact and inhalation of aerosolized particles. The virus has an incubation period of 1 to 4 days, with peak transmission risk starting at approximately 1 day before onset of symptoms and continuing for 5 to 7 days.

Clinical Manifestations

The onset of flu is typically abrupt, with systemic symptoms of chills, fever, anorexia, malaise, and generalized myalgia often accompanied by a headache, cough, rhinorrhea, and sore throat. Physical findings are usually minimal, with normal assessment on chest auscultation. Dyspnea and diffuse crackles are signs of pulmonary complications. In uncomplicated cases, symptoms subside within 7 days. Some patients, particularly older adults, experience weakness or lassitude that persists for weeks. Hyperactive airways and a chronic cough often occur during recovery.

The most common complication of influenza is pneumonia, which can be either primary influenza (viral) pneumonia or secondary bacterial pneumonia. The patient who develops secondary bacterial pneumonia usually experiences gradual improvement of influenza symptoms, then worsening cough and purulent sputum. Treatment with antibiotics is usually effective if started early.

Diagnostic Studies

Important diagnostic factors in influenza include the patient's health history, clinical findings, and other cases of influenza in the community. Although a diagnosis of flu is frequently based on clinical findings, rapid flu tests can help in the diagnosis by detecting the virus in nasal secretions. Depending on the method, the test may be completed in the physician's office in less than 30 minutes or be sent to a laboratory, with results available the same day. The test can help differentiate influenza from other viral and bacterial infections with similar symptoms that may be serious and must be treated differently. Rapid flu tests are best used within the first 48 hours of the onset of symptoms to help diagnose influenza and determine whether antiviral drugs are a treatment option.[12] The main disadvantages of the rapid flu test are that it will miss some cases or occasionally be positive when a person does not actually have the flu.

Viral cultures are considered the "gold standard" for diagnosing influenza, but they can take up to 3 to 10 days for results. A viral culture has the advantage of identifying which virus (A, B, or another respiratory virus) and which strains of virus are present. These data are used in the formulation of the following season's flu vaccine.

NURSING AND COLLABORATIVE MANAGEMENT
INFLUENZA

The most effective strategy for managing influenza is prevention. Two types of flu vaccines are available: inactivated and live attenuated (Table 27-3). The influenza vaccine may be changed on a yearly basis, depending on the virus strains identified by the Centers for Disease Control and Prevention as being most likely to cause illness in the upcoming flu season. The best time to receive the vaccine is in September (before flu exposure) because it takes 2 weeks for full protection to occur. Patients can receive it later if needed.

Vaccination of healthy people decreases the incidence and the risk of transmitting influenza to those who have less ability to cope with the effects of this illness. Despite obvious benefits, many persons are reluctant to be vaccinated. Current vaccines are highly purified, and reactions are extremely uncommon. Soreness at the injection site is usually the only side effect. Contraindications are history of Guillain-Barré syndrome within 6 weeks following a previous influenza vaccine and anaphylactic hypersensitivity to eggs.[13]

The primary nursing goals in influenza are relief of symptoms and prevention of secondary infection. Unless the patient with influenza is at high risk or complications develop, only supportive therapy is necessary. Rest, hydration, analgesics, and antipyretics can provide symptom relief. Older adults and those with a chronic illness may require hospitalization.

Two antiviral medications, zanamivir (Relenza) and oseltamivir (Tamiflu), are available to prevent and treat influenza A and B.[14] These drugs are neuraminidase inhibitors that prevent the virus from budding and spreading to other cells. These drugs shorten the duration of influenza symptoms and reduce the risk of complications. Treatment should be initiated as soon as possible in patients who are hospitalized with influenza, have severe or complicated illness, or are at high risk for complications. For maximum benefit in the treatment of influenza, therapy should begin within 2 days of the onset of symptoms, but it can be started later based on clinical judgment. Zanamivir is administered using an inhaler. Oseltamivir is available as an oral capsule.

SINUSITIS

Sinusitis affects one out of every seven adults in the United States. It develops when inflammation or hypertrophy (swelling) of the mucosa blocks the openings (ostia) in the sinuses through which mucus drains into the nose (Fig. 27-2). *Rhinosinusitis* is concurrent inflammation of the nasal mucosa. Obstruction of mucus drainage can also be caused by nasal polyps, foreign bodies, deviated septa, or tumors. The secretions

TABLE 27-3	TYPES OF INFLUENZA IMMUNIZATION	
Trivalent Inactivated Influenza Vaccine (TIV)	**Live Attenuated Influenza Vaccine (LSIV)**
Given by injection	Given by nasal spray
Approved for use in people ≥6 mo of age	Approved for healthy people ages 2-49 yr
Can be used in people at increased risk:	Should NOT be used in:
• People of any age with chronic medical conditions	• Children <2 yr or adults >50 yr
• Residents of nursing homes and long-term care facilities	• Pregnant women
• People who are immunocompromised	• People with known immunodeficiency
• Pregnant women	• Children or adolescents receiving aspirin or other salicylates
	• People who have medical conditions that place them at increased risk for complications from influenza (chronic cardiovascular, pulmonary, or neurologic diseases; diabetes mellitus; renal or hepatic dysfunction; hemoglobinopathies)
	• Health care providers of high-risk patients because of risk of viral transmission from vaccine (should not care for high-risk patients for 7 days after vaccination)
Most common side effects are injection site reactions, such as pain, redness, and swelling	Most common side effects are runny nose and nasal congestion in all ages, fever in children ages 2-6 yr, and sore throat in adults

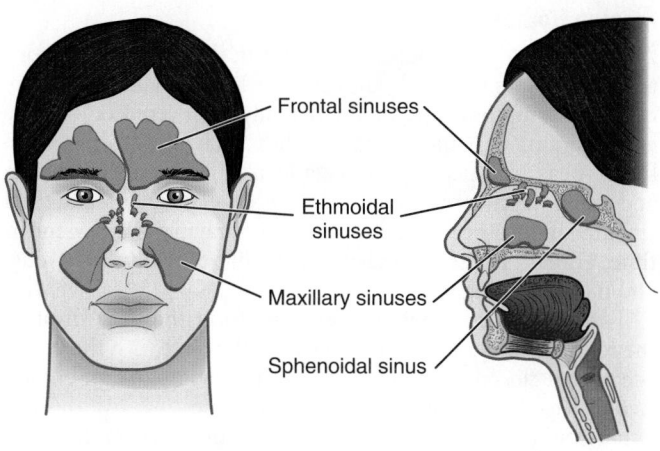

FIG. 27-2 Location of the sinuses.

that accumulate behind the blocked ostia provide a rich medium for growth of bacteria, viruses, and fungi, all of which may cause infection.

Viral sinusitis typically follows an upper respiratory tract infection in which the virus penetrates the mucous membrane and decreases ciliary function. Viral infections usually resolve without treatment in less than 14 days. If symptoms worsen after 3 to 5 days or persist for longer than 10 days, a secondary bacterial infection may be present. Only 5% to 10% of patients with viral sinusitis develop a bacterial infection requiring antibiotic therapy.[15] *Streptococcus pneumoniae, Haemophilus influenzae,* and *Moraxella catarrhalis* are the most common causes of bacterial sinusitis. Fungal sinusitis is uncommon, usually occurring in patients who are debilitated or immunocompromised.

Sinusitis can be classified as acute, subacute, or chronic. *Acute sinusitis* typically begins within 1 week of an upper respiratory tract infection and lasts less than 4 weeks. *Subacute sinusitis* is present when symptoms progress over 4 to 12 weeks. *Chronic sinusitis* (lasting longer than 12 weeks) is a persistent infection usually associated with allergies and nasal polyps. Chronic sinusitis generally results from repeated episodes of acute sinusitis that result in irreversible loss of the normal ciliated epithelium lining the sinus cavity.

🌿 COMPLEMENTARY & ALTERNATIVE THERAPIES
Zinc

Scientific Evidence
- When administered within 24 hr of onset of symptoms, zinc reduces the duration and severity of cold symptoms in healthy people.
- When zinc supplementation is taken for at least 5 mo, the incidence of colds is reduced.

Nursing Implications
- Zinc is regarded as relatively safe when taken at recommended doses.
- Zinc lozenges are more apt to cause adverse effects (bad taste, nausea) than syrup or tablets.
- Oral zinc should not be taken with foods that will reduce its absorption, such as caffeine and dairy products.

Source: Singh M, Das RR: Zinc for the common cold, *Cochrane Database Syst Rev* 16(2):CD001364, 2011.

Clinical Manifestations

Acute sinusitis causes significant pain over the affected sinus, purulent nasal drainage, nasal obstruction, congestion, fever, and malaise. The patient looks and feels sick. Assessment involves inspection of the nasal mucosa and palpation of the sinus points for pain. Findings that indicate acute sinusitis include hyperemic and edematous mucosa, discolored purulent nasal drainage, enlarged turbinates, and tenderness over the involved frontal and/or maxillary sinuses. Some patients have recurrent headaches that change in intensity with position changes or when secretions drain.

Chronic sinusitis is difficult to diagnose because symptoms are often nonspecific. The patient is rarely febrile. The patient may have facial or dental pain, nasal congestion, and increased drainage, but severe pain and purulent drainage are often absent. Some symptoms mimic those seen with allergies. X-rays or computed tomography (CT) scan of the sinuses may be done to confirm the diagnosis. CT scans may show the sinuses to be filled with fluid or a thickened mucous membrane. Nasal endoscopy with a flexible scope may be used to examine the sinuses, obtain drainage for culture, and restore normal drainage.

As many as 50% of patients with moderate to severe asthma have chronic sinusitis. The exact link between these diseases is unclear. Postnasal drip associated with sinusitis may trigger asthma by stimulating bronchoconstriction. Gastroesophageal reflux disease (GERD) and smoking may increase the risk of a person with asthma developing sinusitis. Appropriate treatment of sinusitis often causes a reduction in asthma symptoms.

NURSING AND COLLABORATIVE MANAGEMENT SINUSITIS

If allergies are the precipitating cause of sinusitis, instruct the patient about ways to reduce sinus inflammation and infection, including environmental control of allergens and appropriate drug therapy (see section on allergic rhinitis, earlier in this chapter).

Initial treatment for acute sinusitis focuses on symptom relief. Medications include oral or topical decongestants to promote drainage, nasal corticosteroids to decrease inflammation, analgesics to relieve pain, and saline nasal spray to relieve congestion. Instruct patients using topical decongestants to use the medication for no longer than 3 days to prevent rebound congestion caused by vasodilation. Saline irrigation of the nasal cavity can be used to rinse nasal passages, facilitate drainage, and decrease inflammation. Saline nasal spray is available over the counter as sterile physiologic saline solution in spray bottles. Alternatively, a saline solution can be prepared at home with ¼ tsp of salt dissolved in 8 oz of tap water. Patients may also add a pinch of baking soda to soften the effect of salt. Two to four puffs of nasal saline should be administered at least three times a day. The alternative, more aggressive method is lavage with a squeeze bottle, neti pot, or syringe while leaning over the sink with the mouth open.[16] Repeated full-syringe wash is recommended at least once a day to wash out the secretions if they cannot be effectively removed with saline spray alone. Alternatively, patients can use a Waterpik device on the lowest setting.

If symptoms worsen or persist for longer than 10 days, antibiotic therapy may be prescribed. Antibiotic therapy, consisting of amoxicillin as the first-line drug of choice, is continued for 10 to 14 days to prevent the formation of antibiotic-resistant

TABLE 27-4   PATIENT & CAREGIVER TEACHING GUIDE

Acute or Chronic Sinusitis

Include the following instructions when teaching the patient and caregiver about management of sinusitis.

1. Get plenty of rest to help body fight infection and promote recovery.
2. Keep well hydrated by drinking six to eight glasses of water to loosen secretions.
3. Take hot showers twice daily. Use a steam inhaler (15-min vaporization of boiled water), bedside humidifier, or nasal saline spray to promote secretion drainage.
4. Apply warm, damp towels around nose, cheeks, and eyes to ease facial pain.
5. Sleep with head elevated to help sinuses drain and reduce congestion.
6. Report a temperature of 100.4° F (38° C) or higher, which indicates infection.
7. Follow prescribed medication regimen:
   - Take analgesics to relieve pain.
   - Take decongestants/expectorants to relieve swelling.
   - Take antibiotics (as prescribed) for infection. Be sure to take entire prescription and report continued symptoms or a change in symptoms.
   - Administer nasal sprays correctly.
8. Perform large-volume nasal saline washes once or twice a day to wash sinuses.
9. Do not smoke, and avoid exposure to smoke. Smoke is an irritant and will worsen symptoms.
10. If allergies predispose to sinusitis, follow instructions regarding environmental control, drug therapy, and immunotherapy to reduce the inflammation and prevent sinus infection.

organisms. If symptoms do not resolve, the antibiotic should be changed to a broader spectrum cephalosporin antibiotic. With chronic sinusitis, mixed bacterial flora is often present and infections are difficult to eliminate. Broad-spectrum antibiotics may be used for 4 to 6 weeks. Patient and caregiver teaching for acute and chronic sinusitis is presented in Table 27-4.

Medical therapy may not relieve the symptoms of some patients with persistent or recurrent sinus complaints. They may require nasal endoscopic surgery to relieve blockage caused by hypertrophy or septal deviation. This is an outpatient procedure usually performed using local anesthesia. Propel, a self-expanding dissolvable implant, can be placed directly in the sinus during surgery to maintain postoperative patency and provide localized corticosteroid delivery directly to the sinus lining[17] (see Nursing Management: Nasal Surgery on p. 498).

OBSTRUCTION OF NOSE AND SINUSES

Nasal Polyps

Nasal polyps are soft, painless, benign growths that form slowly in response to repeated inflammation of the sinus or nasal mucosa. Polyps, which appear as gray-blue, semitransparent projections in the naris, can exceed the size of a grape. The patient may be anxious, fearing they are malignant. Small polyps are typically asymptomatic. Clinical manifestations of larger polyps include nasal obstruction, nasal discharge (usually clear mucus), and speech distortion. Topical and systemic corticosteroids are the primary medical therapy used to shrink nasal polyps. Endoscopic or laser surgery can remove nasal polyps, but recurrence is common.

Foreign Bodies

A variety of foreign bodies may lodge in the upper respiratory tract. Inorganic foreign bodies such as buttons and beads may cause no symptoms and be incidentally discovered on routine examination. Organic foreign bodies such as wood, cotton, beans, peas, and paper produce a local inflammatory reaction and nasal discharge, which may become purulent and foul smelling if the object remains in the nasal cavity for an extended time. Foreign bodies can also cause pain, difficulty breathing, and nasal bleeding.

Foreign bodies should be removed from the nose through the route of entry. Sneezing or blowing the nose with the opposite nostril closed is often effective in removing foreign bodies. Avoid irrigating the nose or pushing the object backward, since either could cause aspiration and airway obstruction. If sneezing or blowing the nose does not remove the object, the patient should see a health care provider.

PROBLEMS OF PHARYNX

ACUTE PHARYNGITIS

Acute pharyngitis is an acute inflammation of the pharyngeal walls. It may include the tonsils, palate, and uvula. It can be caused by a viral, bacterial, or fungal infection. Viral pharyngitis accounts for approximately 90% of cases in adults. Bacterial pharyngitis ("strep throat") usually results from β-hemolytic streptococci and accounts for 10% of cases in adults. Fungal pharyngitis, such as candidiasis, can develop with prolonged use of antibiotics or inhaled corticosteroids. It can also occur in immunosuppressed patients, especially those with human immunodeficiency virus (HIV) infection. Other causes of pharyngitis include dry air, smoking, GERD, allergy and postnasal drip, chemicals, neoplasia, and endotracheal intubation.[18]

Clinical Manifestations

Symptoms of acute pharyngitis range in severity from complaints of a "scratchy throat" to pain so severe that swallowing is difficult. Both viral and strep infections appear as a red and edematous pharynx, with or without patchy exudates. Fever, anterior cervical lymph node enlargement, tonsillar exudates, and the absence of cough are highly suggestive of bacterial pharyngitis. However, appearance is not always diagnostic. When two or three of the above criteria are present, a rapid strep antigen test and/or a culture is done to establish the cause and direct appropriate management. White, irregular patches on the oropharynx suggest fungal infection with *Candida albicans*.

NURSING AND COLLABORATIVE MANAGEMENT ACUTE PHARYNGITIS

The goals of nursing management are infection control, symptom relief, and prevention of secondary complications. Penicillin is the drug of choice for bacterial pharyngitis. This antibiotic needs to be taken several times a day for a full 10 days to prevent rheumatic fever, a sequela to the infection. Other antibiotics (amoxicillin, azithromycin [Zithromax], cephalosporins) may also be used. Most people with strep infections are contagious until they have been on antibiotics for 24 to 48 hours.

Candida infections are treated with nystatin (Mycostatin), an antifungal antibiotic. Tell patients to swish the preparation in their mouth as long as possible before swallowing it. Treatment should continue until symptoms are gone. Patients taking inhaled corticosteroids are at risk for infection with *Candida* organisms. Thoroughly rinsing the mouth out with water after using corticosteroids can prevent this infection.

Instruct patients to use ibuprofen or acetaminophen for pain relief. Encourage the patient with pharyngitis to increase fluid intake. To relieve the symptoms, instruct the patient to gargle with warm salt water (½ tsp of salt in 8 oz of water); drink warm or cold liquids; and suck on popsicles, hard candies, or throat lozenges. Cool, bland liquids and gelatin will not irritate the pharynx; citrus juices are often irritating. Encourage the patient to use a cool-mist vaporizer or humidifier.

PERITONSILLAR ABSCESS

Peritonsillar abscess is a complication of acute pharyngitis and is most often caused by β-hemolytic streptococci. The abscess causes pain, swelling, and (when severe) blockage of the throat, threatening airway patency. The patient also experiences a high fever, chills, leukocytosis, difficulty swallowing, and a muffled voice. IV antibiotic therapy is given along with needle aspiration or incision and drainage of the abscess. In some cases an emergency tonsillectomy is performed, or an elective tonsillectomy is scheduled after the infection has subsided.

PROBLEMS OF TRACHEA AND LARYNX

AIRWAY OBSTRUCTION

Acute airway obstruction is a medical emergency. Airway obstruction can be caused by aspiration of food or a foreign body, allergic reactions, edema and inflammation caused by infections or burns, peritonsillar or retropharyngeal abscesses, malignancy, laryngeal or tracheal stenosis, and trauma. Symptoms include choking, stridor, use of accessory muscles, suprasternal and intercostal retractions, flaring nostrils, wheezing, restlessness, tachycardia, cyanosis, and change in level of consciousness. Airway obstruction may be partial or complete. Prompt assessment and treatment are essential because partial obstruction may quickly progress to complete obstruction. Complete airway obstruction can result in permanent brain damage or death if not corrected within 3 to 5 minutes.

Interventions to reestablish a patent airway include the obstructed airway (Heimlich) maneuver (see Appendix A), cricothyroidotomy, endotracheal intubation, and tracheostomy. Unexplained or recurrent symptoms indicate the need for additional tests, such as a chest x-ray, laryngoscopy, and bronchoscopy.

TRACHEOSTOMY

A **tracheostomy** is a surgically created stoma (opening) in the trachea to establish an airway. It is used to (1) bypass an upper airway obstruction, (2) facilitate removal of secretions, or (3) permit long-term mechanical ventilation. Most patients who require mechanical ventilation are initially managed with an endotracheal tube, which can be quickly inserted in an emergency. (Care of the patient with an endotracheal tube is discussed in Chapter 66.)

Most *surgical tracheostomies* are performed in the operating room using general anesthesia. These are typically done elec-

tively on patients already intubated who require prolonged mechanical ventilation. When swelling, trauma, or upper airway obstruction prevents endotracheal intubation, an emergent surgical tracheostomy may be performed at the bedside.

A minimally invasive *percutaneous tracheostomy* can also be performed at the bedside using local anesthesia and sedation. A needle is placed into the trachea, followed by a guide wire. The opening is progressively dilated until it is large enough for insertion of a tracheostomy tube.

A tracheostomy provides a more secure airway, is less likely to be displaced, and allows more freedom of movement than an endotracheal tube. There is less risk of long-term damage to the vocal cords. Airway resistance and work of breathing are decreased, facilitating independent breathing.[19] Patient comfort may be increased because no tube is present in the mouth. The patient can eat with a tracheostomy because the tube enters lower in the airway (Fig. 27-3). Speaking is also permitted once the tracheostomy cuff can be deflated.

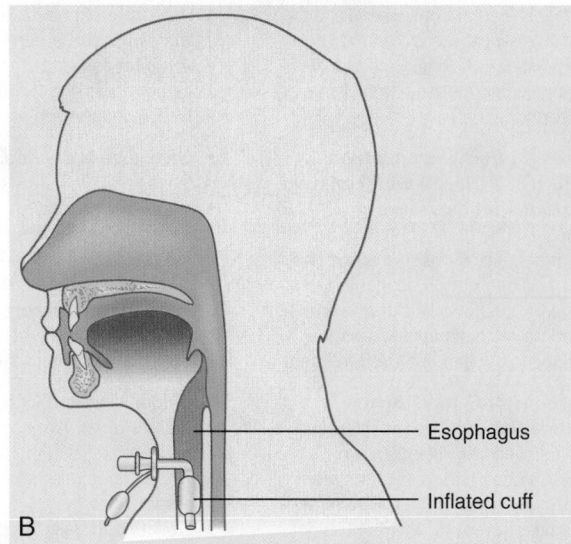

FIG. 27-3 Tracheostomy tube. **A,** Parts of a tracheostomy tube. **B,** Tracheostomy tube inserted in airway with inflated cuff. (See Table 27-5 and eNursing Care Plan 27-1 [on the website for this chapter] for related nursing management.)

NURSING MANAGEMENT
TRACHEOSTOMY

PROVIDING TRACHEOSTOMY CARE

Before the tracheostomy procedure, explain to the patient and the caregiver the purpose of the procedure. Also inform them that the patient will not be able to speak while an inflated cuff is used.

A variety of tubes are available to meet individual patient needs (Table 27-5; see Fig. 27-3). All tracheostomy tubes contain a faceplate, or *flange*, which rests on the neck between the clavicles and outer cannula. In addition, all tubes have an *obturator*, which is used when inserting the tube (see Fig. 27-3, *A*). During insertion of the tube, place the obturator inside the outer cannula with its rounded tip protruding from the end of the tube to ease insertion. After insertion, immediately remove the obturator so air can flow through the tube. Keep the obturator in an easily accessible place at the bedside (e.g., taped to the wall) so that it can be used quickly in case of accidental decannulation.

TABLE 27-5 NURSING MANAGEMENT OF TRACHEOSTOMIES

Tube and Characteristics	Nursing Management
Tracheostomy tube with cuff and pilot balloon (see Fig. 27-3, *A* and *B*) When properly inflated, low-pressure, high-volume cuff distributes cuff pressure over large area, minimizing pressure on tracheal wall.	**Procedure for cuff inflation** • *Mechanically ventilated patient:* Inflate the cuff using *minimal occlusion volume (MOV) technique* by slowly injecting air into the cuff until no leak (sound) is heard at peak inspiratory pressure (end of ventilator inspiration) when a stethoscope is placed over the trachea. An alternative approach, termed *minimal leak technique* (MLT), involves inflating the cuff to minimal occlusion pressure and then withdrawing 0.1 mL of air. • *Spontaneously breathing patient:* Inflate cuff using MOV by slowly injecting air into the cuff until no sound is heard after deep breath or during inhalation with manual resuscitation bag. If using MLT, remove 0.1 mL of air while maintaining seal. MLT should not be used if there is risk of aspiration. • *Immediately after cuff inflation (both groups):* Verify pressure is within accepted range (≤20 mm Hg or ≤25 cm H_2O) with a manometer. Record cuff pressure and volume of air used for cuff inflation in chart. **Care of patients with an inflated cuff** • Monitor and record cuff pressure q8hr. Cuff pressure should be ≤20 mm Hg or ≤25 cm H_2O to allow adequate tracheal capillary perfusion. If needed, remove or add air to the pilot tubing using a syringe and stopcock. Afterward, verify cuff pressure is within accepted range with manometer. • Report inability to keep the cuff inflated or need to use progressively larger volumes of air to keep cuff inflated. Potential causes include tracheal dilation at the cuff site or a crack or slow leak in the housing of the one-way inflation valve. If the leak is due to tracheal dilation, the physician may intubate the patient with a larger tube. Cracks in the inflation valve may be temporarily managed by clamping the small-bore tubing with a hemostat. The tube should be changed within 24 hr.
Fenestrated tracheostomy tube (Shiley, Portex) with cuff, inner cannula, and decannulation plug (see Fig. 27-7, *A*) When nonfenestrated inner cannula is removed, cuff deflated, and decannulation plug inserted, air flows around tube, through fenestration in outer cannula, and up over vocal cords. Patient can then speak. A fenestrated inner cannula can be used to facilitate cleaning.	• Assess risk of aspiration before removing inner cannula. This is best accomplished by consulting with a speech therapist. An alternative but less reliable method is the use of colored liquid (e.g., Kool-Aid). Deflate cuff. Note coughing. Have patient swallow a small amount of colored liquid. Observe secretions for color after patient coughs or is suctioned. Severe coughing or cyanosis after drinking is also indicative of aspiration. If no aspiration is noted, a fenestrated tube may be used. • ***Never*** insert decannulation plug in tracheostomy tube until cuff is deflated and nonfenestrated inner cannula removed. Prior insertion will prevent patient from breathing (no air inflow). This may precipitate a respiratory arrest. • Assess for signs of respiratory distress when a fenestrated cannula is first used. If this occurs, remove the cap, insert a nonfenestrated inner cannula, and reinflate the cuff. • A nonfenestrated inner cannula must be used to suction patient to prevent tracheal damage from suction catheter passing through fenestrated openings. • Cuff management as described above.
Speaking tracheostomy tube (Portex, National) with cuff, two external tubings (see Fig. 27-7, *B*) Has two tubings, one leading to cuff and second to opening above the cuff. When port is connected to air source, air flows out of opening and up over the vocal cords, allowing speech with cuff inflated.	• Once tube is inserted, wait 2 days before use so that the stoma can close around the tube and prevent leaks. • When patient desires to speak, connect port to compressed air (or O_2). Be certain to identify correct tubing. If gas enters the cuff, it will overinflate and rupture, requiring an emergency tube change. Use lowest flow (typically 4-6 L/min) that results in speech. High flows dehydrate mucosa. • Cover port adapter. This will cause the air to flow upward. Instruct patient to speak in short sentences because voice becomes a whisper with long sentences. • Disconnect flow when patient does not want to speak to prevent mucosal dehydration. • Cuff management as described above.
Tracheostomy tube (Bivona Fome-Cuf) with foam-filled cuff Cuff is filled with plastic foam. Before insertion, cuff is deflated. After insertion, cuff is allowed to fill passively with air. Pilot tubing is not capped, and no cuff pressure monitoring is required.	• Before insertion, withdraw all air from the cuff using a 20-mL syringe. Cap pilot balloon tubing to prevent reentry of air. After tracheostomy is inserted, remove cap from pilot tubing, allowing cuff to passively reinflate. • Do not inject air into tubing or cap pilot balloon tubing while it is in patient. Air will flow in and out in response to pressure changes (head turning). Place tag on tubing to alert staff not to cap or inflate cuff. • Deflate cuff daily via pilot balloon to evaluate integrity of cuff. Also assess ability to easily deflate cuff. Difficulty deflating cuff indicates a need for tube change. If aspirate returns with air, cuff is no longer intact. • Tube can be used for up to 1 mo in patients on home mechanical ventilation. • Good choice for patients who require inflated cuff at home, since teaching about cuff pressure is simplified.

Some tracheostomy tubes also have an inner cannula, which can be removed for cleaning (see Fig. 27-3, *A*). The inner cannula can be disposable or nondisposable. If it is disposable, replace per manufacturer and institutional guidelines. If nondisposable, clean the inner cannula at least every 8 hours (Table

TABLE 27-6	SUCTIONING A TRACHEOSTOMY TUBE

1. Assess the need for suctioning q2hr. Indications include coarse crackles or rhonchi over large airways, moist cough, increase in peak inspiratory pressure on mechanical ventilator, and restlessness or agitation if accompanied by decrease in SpO_2 or PaO_2. Do not suction routinely or if patient is able to clear secretions with cough.
2. If suctioning is indicated, explain procedure to patient.
3. Collect necessary sterile equipment: suction catheter (no larger than half the lumen of the tracheostomy tube), gloves, sterile water, cup, and drape. If a closed tracheal suction system is used, the catheter is enclosed in a plastic sleeve and reused (see Fig. 27-4). No additional equipment is needed.
4. Check suction source and regulator. Adjust suction pressure until the dial reads −120 to −150 mm Hg pressure with tubing occluded.
5. Assess SpO_2 and heart rate and rhythm to provide baseline for detecting change during suctioning.
6. Wash hands and put on goggles.
7. Use sterile technique to open package, fill cup with sterile water, put on sterile gloves, and connect catheter to suction tubing. Designate one hand as contaminated for (1) connecting and disconnecting the tubing at the suction catheter, (2) using the resuscitation bag, and (3) operating the suction control. Suction sterile water through the catheter to test the system.
8. Provide preoxygenation for a minimum of 30 seconds by (1) adjusting ventilator to deliver 100% O_2; (2) using a reservoir-equipped manual resuscitation bag (MRB) connected to 100% O_2; or (3) asking the patient to take 5-6 deep breaths while administering O_2. The method chosen depends on the patient's underlying disease and acuity of illness. The patient who has had a tracheostomy for an extended period and is not acutely ill may be able to tolerate suctioning without use of an MRB or the ventilator.
9. Gently insert catheter *without suction* to minimize the amount of O_2 removed from the lungs. Insert the catheter to the point where the patient coughs or resistance is met, or 0.5-1.0 cm beyond the length of the artificial airway. Withdraw the catheter 0.5-1.0 cm before applying suction to prevent trauma to the carina.
10. Apply suction intermittently, while withdrawing catheter in a rotating manner. If secretion volume is large, apply suction continuously. Suction should be applied for as short a time as possible to minimize decreases in arterial oxygenation levels.
11. *Limit suction time to 10 seconds.* Discontinue suctioning if heart rate decreases from baseline by 20 beats/min, increases from baseline by 40 beats/min, a dysrhythmia occurs, or SpO_2 decreases to less than 90%.
12. After each suction pass, oxygenate for at least 30 sec with 5-6 breaths by ventilator or MRB or deep breaths with O_2.
13. Rinse catheter with sterile water between suction passes.
14. Repeat procedure until airway is clear. Limit insertions of suction catheter to as few as needed. If airway is not clear after three suction passes, allow the patient to rest before additional suctioning.
15. Return O_2 concentration to prior setting.
16. Rinse catheter, and suction the oropharynx or use mouth suction.
17. Dispose of catheter by wrapping it around fingers of gloved hand and pulling glove over catheter. Discard equipment in proper waste container.
18. Auscultate to assess changes in lung sounds. Record time, amount, and character of secretions and response to suctioning.

27-6). Cleaning removes mucus from the inside of the tube to prevent airway obstruction. If humidification is adequate, mucus may not accumulate and a tube without an inner cannula can be used. Suction the airway via the tracheostomy tube as needed (Fig. 27-4 and Table 27-6). Also, clean around the stoma at least every 8 hours and change the tracheostomy ties as needed (Fig. 27-5 and Table 27-7). A two-person technique, one to stabilize the tracheostomy and one to change the ties, is best to ensure that the tracheostomy does not become accidentally dislodged during the procedure. Place two fingers underneath the ties to ensure they are not too tight around the neck.[20]

Both cuffed and uncuffed tracheostomy tubes are available. A tracheostomy tube with an inflated cuff is used if the patient is at risk of aspiration or needs mechanical ventilation. Because an inflated cuff exerts pressure on the tracheal mucosa, it is important to inflate the cuff with the minimum volume of air required to obtain an airway seal. Cuff inflation pressure should not exceed 20 mm Hg or 25 cm H_2O because higher pressures may compress tracheal capillaries, limit blood flow, and predispose the patient to tracheal necrosis. The minimal leak technique (MLT) and the minimal occlusion volume (MOV) are two commonly used methods to inflate the tracheostomy cuff (see Table 27-5).

Routine cuff deflation is no longer recommended.[21] When the patient is not at risk for aspiration, the cuff may be deflated to allow the patient to talk and swallow more easily. Before deflation, have the patient cough up secretions, if possible, and suction the tracheostomy tube and then the mouth (see Table 27-6). This step is important to prevent secretions from being aspirated during deflation. The cuff is deflated during exhalation because the exhaled gas helps propel secretions into the mouth. Have the patient cough, and then suction the tube after cuff deflation. Assess the patient's ability to protect the airway from aspiration. Remain with the patient when the cuff is initially deflated. If needed, reinflate the cuff during inspiration.

Retention sutures may be placed in the tracheal cartilage when the tracheostomy is performed. Tape the free ends of the sutures to the skin in a place and manner that leaves them accessible in case the tube is dislodged. Take care not to dislodge the tracheostomy tube during the first 5 to 7 days when the stoma is not mature (healed). Because tube replacement is difficult, several precautions are required: (1) keep a replacement tube of equal or smaller size at the bedside, readily available for emergency reinsertion; (2) do not change tracheostomy tapes for at least 24 hours after the insertion procedure; and (3) a physician

FIG. 27-4 Suctioning tracheostomy with closed system suction catheter.

FIG. 27-5 Changing tracheostomy ties. **A,** A slit is cut about 1 in (2.5 cm) from the end. The slit end is put into the opening of the cannula. **B,** A loop is made with the other end of the tape. **C,** The tapes are tied together with a double knot on the side of the neck. **D,** A Velcro tracheostomy tube holder can be used instead of twill ties to make tracheostomy tube stabilization more secure.

performs the first tube change usually no sooner than 7 days after the tracheostomy.

If the tube is accidentally dislodged, immediately attempt to replace it. Grasp the retention sutures (if present) or use a hemostat to spread the opening to facilitate replacing the tube. Insert the obturator in the replacement tube, lubricated with saline poured over the tip, and insert the tube into the stoma at a 45-degree angle to the neck. Once the tube is inserted, remove the obturator immediately so that air can flow through the tube. Another method is to insert a suction catheter to allow passage of air and to serve as a guide for insertion. Thread the tracheostomy tube over the catheter and remove the suction catheter. If the tube cannot be replaced, assess the level of respiratory distress. Position the patient in the semi-Fowler's position to alleviate minor dyspnea until assistance arrives. Severe dyspnea may progress to respiratory arrest. If this situation occurs, cover the stoma with a sterile dressing, and ventilate the patient with bag-mask ventilation over the nose and mouth until help arrives. If a patient has had a total laryngectomy, there will be complete separation between the upper airway and the trachea. Ventilate this patient through the tracheostomy stoma.

Initially, tracheostomy patients should receive humidified air to compensate for the loss of the upper airway to warm and moisturize secretions. Humidification is essential to prevent retention of tenacious secretions and formation of mucous plugs. Change the tube approximately once a month after the first tube change. When a tracheostomy has been in place for several months, the healed tract will be well formed. Teach the patient to change the tube using a clean technique at home

TABLE 27-7 TRACHEOSTOMY CARE

1. Explain procedure to patient.
2. Use tracheostomy care kit or collect necessary sterile equipment (e.g., suction catheter, gloves, water basin, drape, tracheostomy ties, tube brush or pipe cleaners, 4 × 4 gauze pads, sterile water or normal saline, and tracheostomy dressing [optional]). NOTE: Clean rather than sterile technique is used at home.
3. Position patient in semi-Fowler's position.
4. Assemble needed materials on bedside table next to patient.
5. Wash hands. Put on goggles and clean gloves.
6. Auscultate chest sounds. If rhonchi or coarse crackles are present, suction the patient if unable to cough up secretions (see Table 27-6). Remove soiled dressing and clean gloves.
7. Open sterile equipment, pour sterile H_2O or normal saline into two compartments of sterile container or two basins, and put on sterile gloves. NOTE: Hydrogen peroxide (3%) is no longer recommended unless an infection is present. If it is used, rinse the inner cannula and skin with sterile H_2O or normal saline afterward to prevent trauma to tissue.
8. Unlock and remove inner cannula, if present. Many tracheostomy tubes do not have inner cannulas. Care for these tubes includes all steps except for inner cannula care.
9. If disposable inner cannula is used, replace with new cannula. If a nondisposable cannula is used:
   • Immerse inner cannula in sterile solution and clean inside and outside of cannula using tube brush or pipe cleaners.
   • Rinse cannula in sterile solution. Remove from solution and shake to dry.
   • Insert inner cannula into outer cannula with the curved part downward, and lock in place.
10. Remove dried secretions from stoma using 4 × 4 gauze pad soaked in sterile water or saline. Gently pat area around the stoma dry. Be sure to clean under the tracheostomy faceplate, using cotton swabs to reach this area.
11. Maintain position of tracheal retention sutures (if present) by taping above and below the stoma.
12. Change tracheostomy ties. Use two-person change technique or secure new ties to flanges before removing the old ones. Tie tracheostomy ties securely with room for two fingers between ties and skin (see Fig. 27-5). To prevent accidental tube removal, secure the tracheostomy tube by gently applying pressure to the flange of the tube during the tie changes. *Do not change tracheostomy ties for 24 hr after the tracheostomy procedure.*
13. As an alternative, some patients prefer tracheostomy ties made of Velcro, which are easier to adjust.
14. If drainage is excessive, place dressing around tube (see Fig. 27-5). A tracheostomy dressing or unlined gauze should be used. Do not cut the gauze because threads may be inhaled or wrap around the tracheostomy tube. Change the dressing frequently. Wet dressings promote infection and stoma irritation.
15. Repeat care three times/day and as needed.

(Fig. 27-6). Monitor the patient for potential complications[22] (Table 27-8).

SWALLOWING DYSFUNCTION

The patient with a tracheostomy who cannot protect the airway from aspiration requires an inflated cuff. However, an inflated cuff may result in swallowing dysfunction by interfering with the normal function of muscles used to swallow. It is important to evaluate the patient's swallowing ability and risk for aspiration with the cuff deflated. If the patient is able to swallow without aspiration when the cuff is deflated, the cuff may be left deflated or a cuffless tube substituted. Clinical assessment of the patient's ability to swallow is done by a speech therapist, videofluoroscopy, or fiberoptic endoscopic evaluations.[23]

FIG. 27-6 Changing the tracheostomy tube at home. When a tracheostomy has been in place for several months, the tract will be well formed. The patient can be taught to change the tube using a clean technique at home.

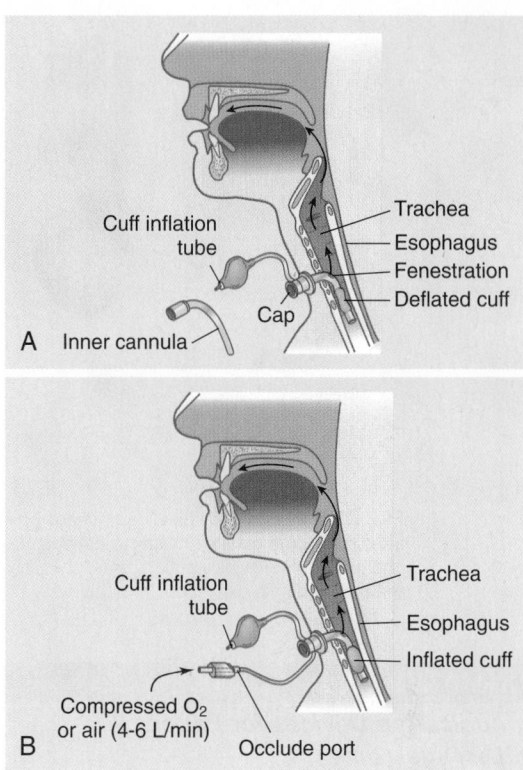

FIG. 27-7 Speaking tracheostomy tubes. **A,** Fenestrated tracheostomy tube with cuff deflated, inner cannula removed, and tracheostomy tube capped to allow air to pass over the vocal cords. **B,** Speaking tracheostomy tube. One tube is used for cuff inflation. The second tube is connected to a source of compressed air or O_2. When the port on the second tube is occluded, air flows up over the vocal cords, allowing speech with an inflated cuff. (See Table 27-5 and eNursing Care Plan 27-1 for related nursing management.)

TABLE 27-8	COMPLICATIONS OF TRACHEOSTOMY

Closely monitor patients with a tracheostomy for the following potential complications:

- Airway obstruction
- Air leak
- Altered body image
- Aspiration
- Bleeding
- Fistula formation
- Impaired cough
- Infection—wound or respiratory tract
- Subcutaneous emphysema
- Tracheal stenosis
- Tracheal necrosis
- Tube displacement

SPEECH WITH A TRACHEOSTOMY TUBE

A number of techniques promote speech in the patient with a tracheostomy. The spontaneously breathing patient may be able to talk by deflating the cuff, which allows exhaled air to flow upward over the vocal cords. This can be enhanced by the patient occluding the tube. However, this method is discouraged because bacteria from the fingers can lead to infection. Specialized tracheostomy tubes and speaking valves are available to facilitate speech. Advocating for the use of these devices will provide psychologic benefits and facilitate self-care for the patient with a tracheostomy.

A *fenestrated tube* has openings on the surface of the outer cannula that permit air from the lungs to flow over the vocal cords (see Fig. 27-7, *A*). A fenestrated tube allows the patient to breathe spontaneously through the larynx, speak, and cough up secretions while the tracheostomy tube remains in place. Air passes from the lungs through the openings in the tracheostomy into the upper airway and out the mouth and nose. Only patients who can swallow without risk of aspiration can use this tube. The inner cannula can be fenestrated or nonfenestrated. Use a nonfenestrated inner cannula when suctioning to decrease the risk of tracheal damage caused by the suction catheter going through the openings. The nonfenestrated inner cannula is also used whenever the patient needs to be mechanically ventilated.

Before using the fenestrated tube, determine the patient's ability to swallow without aspiration (see Table 27-5 and eNursing Care Plan 27-1, available on the website for this chapter). If there is no aspiration, (1) remove the inner cannula (if nonfenestrated), (2) deflate the cuff, and (3) place the decannulation cap in the tube (see Fig. 27-7, *A*). It is important to perform the

steps in order because severe respiratory distress may result if the tube is capped before removing the inner cannula and deflating the cuff. When a fenestrated cannula is first used, frequently assess the patient for signs of respiratory distress. If the patient is not able to tolerate the procedure, remove the cap, insert a nonfenestrated inner cannula, and reinflate the cuff. A disadvantage of fenestrated tubes is the potential for development of tracheal polyps from tracheal tissue granulating into the fenestrated openings.

A speaking tracheostomy tube has two pigtail tubings. One tubing connects to the cuff and is for cuff inflation, and the second connects to an opening just above the cuff (see Fig. 27-7, *B*). When the second tubing is connected to a low-flow (4 to 6 L/minute) air source, sufficient air moves up over the vocal cords to permit speech. This device allows a patient at risk for aspiration to speak with the tracheostomy cuff inflated. However, speech quality is typically poor, with the patient barely speaking above a whisper.

A variety of speaking valves are available that can be attached to the tracheostomy tube (Fig. 27-8). These valves contain a thin plastic diaphragm that opens on inspiration and closes on expiration. During inspiration, air flows in through the valve. During expiration, the valve prevents exhalation and air flows upward over the vocal cords and into the mouth, allowing normal speech patterns. When a speaking tracheostomy valve is used, a cuffless tube must be in place or the cuff needs to be deflated to allow exhalation. Before attaching a speaking valve, evaluate the patient's ability to tolerate cuff deflation without

FIG. 27-8 Passy-Muir speaking tracheostomy valve. The valve is placed over the hub of the tracheostomy tube after the cuff is deflated. Multiple options are available and can be used for ventilated and nonventilated patients. The one-way valve allows air to enter the lungs during inspiration and redirects air upward over the vocal cords into the mouth during expiration.

INFORMATICS IN PRACTICE

Communication Devices for Patient With Laryngectomy

- Assisting with communication will improve a patient's quality of life after a laryngectomy.
- Use an iPad or iPhone and download a text-to-speech application. These applications allow the patient to type in text, and then a computer voice says the text aloud.
- You can also teach the patient how to use a keyboard-based communication program. The patient types on a traditional keyboard and generates speech that is transmitted through hand-held speakers.

aspiration or respiratory distress. Once the speaking valve is in place, carefully assess the patient's ability to breathe. The patient may initially be able to tolerate only short periods of use until he or she becomes acclimated to exhaling through the mouth. Remove the valve immediately if the patient demonstrates any signs of respiratory distress.

If speaking devices are not used, provide the patient with a paper and pencil or Magic Slate. A communication board with pictures of common needs and an alphabet for spelling words is useful for patients who are weak or have difficulty writing.

DECANNULATION

When the patient can adequately exchange air and expectorate secretions, the tracheostomy tube can be removed. Close the stoma with tape strips and cover it with an occlusive dressing. The dressing must be changed if it gets soiled or wet. Instruct the patient to splint the stoma with the fingers when coughing, swallowing, or speaking. Epithelial tissue begins to form in 24 to 48 hours, and the opening closes within 4 or 5 days. Surgical intervention to close the tracheostomy is not required.

LARYNGEAL POLYPS

Laryngeal polyps develop on the vocal cords from vocal abuse (e.g., excessive talking, singing) or irritation (e.g., intubation, cigarette smoking). The most common symptom is hoarseness.

Polyps are treated conservatively with voice rest and adequate hydration. Surgical removal may be indicated for large polyps, which may cause dysphagia, dyspnea, and stridor. Polyps are usually benign but may be removed because they can become malignant.

HEAD AND NECK CANCER

Most head and neck cancers arise from squamous cells that line the mucosal surfaces of the head and neck region. The cancer is identified according to the area of origin (e.g., paranasal sinuses, oral cavity, nasopharynx, oropharynx, larynx). (Cancer of the oral cavity is discussed in Chapter 42.)

An estimated 52,600 new cases of head and neck cancer are diagnosed each year in the United States. Eighty-five percent are caused by tobacco use. Excessive alcohol consumption is also a major risk factor. Head and neck cancer occurs most frequently in patients 50 to 60 years of age. Cancers in patients younger than 50 have been associated with human papillomavirus (HPV) infection. Other risk factors include sun exposure (oral cavity), radiation therapy to the head and neck, exposure to asbestos and other industrial carcinogens, and poor oral hygiene.[24] Men are affected twice as often as women.[25]

Most people have locally advanced disease at the time of diagnosis. Disability from the disease and the treatment is great because of the potential loss of voice, disfigurement, and social consequences.

Clinical Manifestations

Early signs and symptoms of head and neck cancer vary with the tumor location. Cancer of the oral cavity may initially be seen as a white or red patch in the mouth, an ulcer that does not heal, or a change in the fit of dentures. Hoarseness that lasts more than 2 weeks may be a symptom of early laryngeal cancer. Some patients experience what feels like a lump in the throat or a change in voice quality. Other clinical manifestations include a sore throat that does not get better with treatment, unilateral sore throat or otalgia (ear pain), swelling or lumps in the neck, and coughing up blood. Difficulties chewing, swallowing, moving the tongue or jaw, and breathing are typically late symptoms. Unintentional weight loss and pain are also late symptoms of head and neck cancer.

Diagnostic Studies

Early detection is key to patient survival. Thoroughly examine the oral cavity, including the area under the tongue and dentures, with a flashlight. Bimanually palpate the floor of the mouth, tongue, and lymph nodes in the neck. There may be thickening of the normally soft and pliable oral mucosa. *Leukoplakia* (white patch) or *erythroplakia* (red patch) may be seen and should be noted for later biopsy. Both leukoplakia and carcinoma in situ (localized to a defined area) may precede invasive carcinoma by many years.

If lesions are suspected, the upper airways may be examined using indirect laryngoscopy, which involves using a laryngeal mirror or a flexible nasopharyngoscope to visualize the larynx. The larynx and vocal cords are visually inspected for lesions and tissue mobility. A CT scan or magnetic resonance imaging (MRI) may be performed to detect local and regional spread. Neoplastic tissue is identifiable because it has a greater density or because it distorts, displaces, or destroys normal anatomic structures. The use of positron emission tomography (PET) scanning along with CT has been successful in diagnosing recurrent cases of head and neck cancer. Typically, multiple biopsy specimens are obtained to determine the extent of the disease.

Collaborative Care

Head and neck cancer is staged based on tumor size (T), number and location of involved nodes (N), and extent of metastasis (M). TNM staging classifies disease as stage I to stage IV. Choice of treatment is based on exact location of tumor, disease stage, patient age and general health, cosmetic and functional considerations (e.g., ability to talk, swallow, and chew), urgency of treatment, and patient choice. Treatment modalities include surgery, radiation therapy, chemotherapy, and targeted therapy. Stage I and II cancers are potentially curable with single-modality radiation therapy or larynx-sparing surgery. Radiation therapy is often preferred for patients with early laryngeal cancer because it offers the patient good results with voice preservation. Surgery can then be reserved for recurrence or poor response to radiation. Patients with advanced disease (stages III and IV) are treated with various combinations of surgery, radiation, chemotherapy, and targeted therapy. Radiation therapy can be delivered by either external-beam therapy or internal implants (brachytherapy). Brachytherapy is a concentrated and localized method of delivering radiation that involves placing a radioactive source into or near the tumor. The goal is to deliver high doses of radiation to the target area while limiting exposure of surrounding tissues. Thin, hollow, plastic needles are inserted into the tumor area, and radioactive iridium seeds are placed in the needles. The seeds emit continuous radiation. (Radiation therapy and brachytherapy are discussed in Chapter 16.)

Surgical treatment varies depending on tumor location and stage. A *cordectomy* (partial removal of one vocal cord) is used for a superficial tumor involving one cord (Fig. 27-9). If the tumor is deeper but does not involve the entire larynx, one of several partial laryngectomy procedures are available that preserve speech and swallowing functions. A *hemilaryngectomy* involves removal of one side of the larynx. A *supraglottic laryngectomy* involves removing structures above the true cords—the

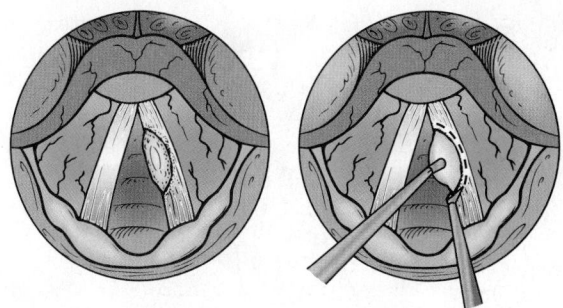

FIG. 27-9 Excision of laryngeal cancer. This cancer of the right vocal cord meets criteria for resection by transoral cordectomy. The cord is fully mobile, and the lesion can be fully exposed. It does not approach or cross the anterior commissure.

false vocal cords and epiglottis. A *supracricoid laryngectomy* involves removal of the entire supraglottis; the false and true vocal cords; and the thyroid cartilage, including the paraglottic and preepiglottic spaces. The patient is at high risk of aspiration after these procedures and requires a temporary tracheostomy. Although speech is preserved, the quality and ease of speech vary. Voice quality is breathy, hoarse, and rough.

Advanced lesions are treated by a total laryngectomy, in which the entire larynx and preepiglottic region are removed and a permanent tracheostomy is performed. Airflow patterns before and after total laryngectomy are shown in Fig. 27-10. *Radical neck dissection* frequently accompanies total laryngectomy to decrease the risk of lymphatic spread. Depending on the extent of involvement, extensive dissection and reconstruction may be performed (Fig. 27-11). This procedure involves wide excision of the lymph nodes and their lymphatic channels. The following structures may also be removed or transected: sternocleidomastoid muscle and other closely associated muscles, internal jugular vein, mandible, submaxillary gland, part of the thyroid and parathyroid glands, and spinal accessory nerve.

A *modified neck dissection* is performed whenever possible as an alternative to a radical neck dissection. The dissection is modified by sparing as many structures as possible to limit disfigurement and functional loss. This usually involves dissection of the major cervical lymphatic vessels and lateral cervical space with preservation of nerves and vessels, including the sympathetic and vagus nerves, spinal accessory nerves, and internal jugular vein. Neck dissection with vocal cord cancer usually involves one side of the neck. However, if the lesion is midline, a bilateral neck dissection may be performed, with a modification on at least one side to minimize structural and functional deficits.

Some patients refuse surgical intervention for advanced lesions because of the extent of the procedure and the potential risk. In this situation, external radiation therapy is used as the sole treatment or in combination with chemotherapy. Your support and counseling are extremely important.

Chemotherapy is used in combination with radiation therapy for patients with stage III or IV cancers. A three-drug chemotherapeutic regimen using cisplatin (Platinol), docetaxel (Taxotere), and fluorouracil (5-FU) is used to treat locally advanced head and neck cancer.[26] Cetuximab (Erbitux), a targeted therapy, is also used in combination with radiation (first-line treatment) or as monotherapy for cancer that has metastasized after stan-

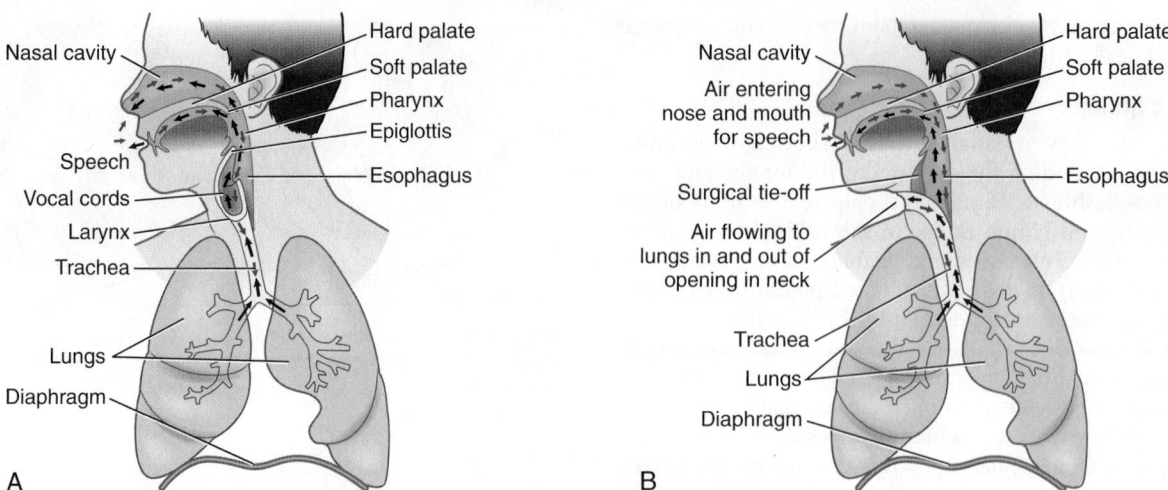

FIG. 27-10 **A,** Normal airflow in and out of the lungs. **B,** Airflow in and out of the lungs after total laryngectomy. Patients using esophageal speech trap air in the esophagus and release it to create sound.

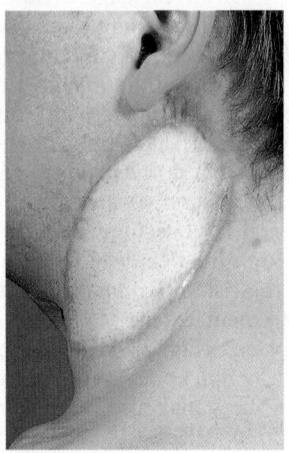

FIG. 27-11 Reconstructive surgery involving skin grafts may be needed after a radical neck dissection.

dard chemotherapy. (Targeted therapy is discussed in Chapter 16 and Table 16-13.)

Isotretinoin (13-*cis*-retinoic acid) is currently under clinical evaluation for use as a chemopreventive agent. This drug is given daily for 1 year to prevent recurrence of head and neck cancer.[27]

Nutritional Therapy. As many as 50% of patients with head and neck cancer are malnourished even before treatment begins.[28] Treatment modalities increase the risk of malnutrition. After radical neck surgery the patient may be unable to take in nutrients orally because of swelling, the location of sutures, or difficulty with swallowing. Side effects from chemotherapy and radiation therapy can impair the patient's ability to maintain adequate nutrition. Painful oral mucositis frequently leads to breaks in treatment if the patient is relying solely on oral intake for nutrition.

A thorough nutritional assessment and prophylactic placement of a gastrostomy tube in high-risk patients are vital to maintaining adequate nutrition. Enteral nutrition may be started before initiation of treatment to obtain and maintain optimal nutritional status needed for tissue repair. (Enteral nutrition is described in Chapter 40.) Observe for tolerance of the feedings and adjust the amount, time, and formula if nausea, vomiting, diarrhea, or distention occurs. Instruct the patient and caregiver about the tube feedings.

Patients who are not candidates for or who refuse enteral feedings need to be monitored closely for weight loss. Antiemetics or analgesics may be given before meals to reduce nausea and mouth pain. Bland foods are easier for patients to tolerate. Patients can increase caloric intake by adding dry milk to foods during preparation, selecting foods high in calories, and using oral supplements. It is helpful to add sauces and gravies to food, which adds calories and moistens food so it is more easily swallowed. Elevate the head of the bed while the patient is eating.

Anticipate swallowing problems when the patient resumes eating after surgery. The type and degree of difficulty vary, depending on the procedure. Videofluoroscopic swallowing studies may be used to evaluate the safety of patient swallowing. When the patient can swallow, give small amounts of thickened liquids or pureed foods with the patient in high Fowler's position. Closely observe for choking. Suctioning may be necessary to prevent aspiration.

Avoid thin, watery fluids because they are difficult to swallow and increase the risk of aspiration. A better choice is nonpourable pureed foods, which are thicker and allow more control during swallowing. Using a commercially available thickening agent (Thick-It) to thicken liquids will enhance swallowing.

When a supraglottic laryngectomy is performed, the upper portion of the larynx is excised, including the epiglottis and false vocal cords. The patient can speak because the true vocal cords remain intact. However, the patient must learn a new technique, the *supraglottic swallow,* to compensate for removal of the epiglottis and minimize the risk of aspiration (Table 27-9). When learning this technique, the patient should start with carbonated beverages because the effervescence helps determine the liquid's position.

NURSING MANAGEMENT
HEAD AND NECK CANCER

NURSING ASSESSMENT
Table 27-10 presents subjective and objective data to obtain from a person with head and neck cancer.

TABLE 27-9   PATIENT TEACHING GUIDE

Supraglottic Swallow

Include the following instructions when teaching a patient to perform a supraglottic swallow.

1. Its purpose is to voluntarily control the closure of the vocal cords before and after swallowing. It protects the trachea from aspiration.
2. To do the technique, take a deep breath and hold it tightly.*
3. Take a bite of food or sip of fluid in your mouth.
4. Swallow while holding your breath. Some food will enter airway and remain on top of closed vocal cords.
4. Cough immediately after swallow to remove food from top of vocal cords.
5. Swallow again.
6. Breathe after cough-swallow sequence to prevent aspiration of food collected on top of vocal cords.

*If patient aspirates with this technique, the super-supraglottic swallow may be useful. This involves having the patient perform the Valsalva maneuver to close the vocal cords while holding breath and during swallow.

TABLE 27-10   NURSING ASSESSMENT

Head and Neck Cancer

Subjective Data
Important Health Information
Past health history: Positive family history; prolonged tobacco use (cigarettes, pipes, cigars, chewing tobacco, smokeless tobacco); prolonged, heavy alcohol use; poor intake of fruits and vegetables
Medications: Prolonged use of over-the-counter medication for sore throat, decongestants

Functional Health Patterns
Health perception–health management: Does not participate in preventive health measures, long history of alcohol and tobacco use
Nutritional-metabolic: Mouth ulcer that does not heal, change in fit of dentures, change in appetite, weight loss, swallowing difficulty (e.g., sensation of lump in throat, pain with swallowing, aspiration when swallowing)
Activity-exercise: Fatigue with minimal exertion
Cognitive-perceptual: Sore throat, pain on swallowing, referred ear pain

Objective Data
Respiratory
Hoarseness, change in voice quality, chronic laryngitis, nasal voice, palpable neck mass and lymph nodes (tender, hard, fixed), tracheal deviation; dyspnea, stridor (late sign)

Gastrointestinal
White (leukoplakia) or red (erythroplakia) patches inside mouth, ulceration of mucosa, asymmetric tongue, exudate in mouth or pharynx, mass or thickening of mucosa

Possible Diagnostic Findings
Mass on direct or indirect laryngoscopy; tumor on soft tissue x-ray, computed tomography (CT) scan, or magnetic resonance imaging (MRI); positive biopsy

NURSING DIAGNOSES

Nursing diagnoses for the patient with head and neck cancer include, but are not limited to, the following:

- Ineffective airway clearance *related to* presence of artificial airway and excessive mucus
- Risk for aspiration *related to* presence of tracheostomy tube and impaired swallowing
- Anxiety *related to* lack of knowledge regarding surgical procedure and pain management
- Acute pain *related to* tissue injury from surgery
- Impaired verbal communication *related to* removal of vocal cords

Additional information on nursing diagnoses for the patient with head and neck cancer is presented in eNursing Care Plan 27-2 on the website for this chapter.

PLANNING

The overall goals are that the patient will have (1) a patent airway, (2) no spread of cancer, (3) no complications related to therapy, (4) adequate nutritional intake, (5) minimal to no pain, (6) the ability to communicate, and (7) an acceptable body image.

NURSING IMPLEMENTATION

HEALTH PROMOTION. Development of head and neck cancer is closely related to personal habits, primarily tobacco use and excessive alcohol ingestion. Although tobacco use (including smokeless tobacco, also called "chewing tobacco" or "snuff") has been linked to most head and neck cancers, people who use both tobacco and alcohol are at greater risk than those who use just one.[24] Poor oral hygiene and HPV infection are also risk factors for head and neck cancer.

Include information about risk factors in health teaching. Encourage good oral hygiene. Teach patients about safe sex practices to prevent HPV infection (e.g., use condoms for every sex act, be in a monogamous relationship, and choose a partner who has had no or few previous partners). If cancer has been diagnosed, tobacco and alcohol cessation is still important. The likelihood of a cure, by any treatment modality, for a patient with head and neck cancer who continues to smoke and ingest alcoholic beverages is diminished. Additionally, risk of a second primary cancer is significantly increased. Give patients information about smoking cessation programs and techniques for success. If necessary, refer to an alcohol treatment program.

ACUTE INTERVENTION. Teach the patient and the caregiver about the type of therapy to be performed and care required. Help prepare them to deal with the psychologic impact of the diagnosis of cancer, alteration of physical appearance, possible need for enteral feedings, and potential for altered methods of communication because of the loss of a voice. The care plan should include assessment of the patient's support system. The patient may not have someone to provide assistance after discharge, may be unemployed, or may have a job that cannot be continued.

Radiation Therapy. Suggest interventions to reduce side effects of radiation therapy. Because the oral mucosa is frequently affected, patients should consult a dentist before starting radiation therapy. Dry mouth (*xerostomia*), the most frequent and annoying problem, typically begins within a few weeks of treatment. The patient's saliva decreases in volume and becomes thick. The change may be temporary or permanent. Pilocarpine hydrochloride (Salagen) is often effective in increasing saliva production and should be started before the initiation of radiation therapy. Amifostine (Ethyol) subcutaneous injection may also be ordered to decrease xerostomia. Patients can get symptom relief by increasing fluid intake, chewing sugarless gum or sugarless candy, using nonalcoholic mouth rinses (baking soda or glycerin solutions), and using artificial saliva. Over-the-counter mucous thinning agents (e.g., guaifenesin) two or three times daily and/or mucous solvents can be used to control thickening secretions. Instruct patients to always carry a water bottle with them. Fluoride gels or treatments can help prevent dental deterioration caused by xerostomia. Acupuncture has also been found to improve discomfort related to xerostomia.[27]

Oral mucositis can cause irritation, ulceration, and pain. Empty fluoride gel trays, along with bite blocks, athletic mouth guards, or gauze pads, can be worn during radiation treatments to prevent radiation scatter to the tongue and cheek from metal work in the mouth that contributes to development of mucositis.[28] Instruct the patient on oral care basics, including the use of a soft toothbrush and regular flossing. Warm bland rinses such as salt and baking soda should be done four to six times daily. Sucking on ice chips can also help with the pain. Encourage patients to eat soft, bland foods. Patients should avoid commercial mouthwashes and hot, spicy, or acidic foods because they are irritating. If the problem is severe, a mixture of equal parts antacid, diphenhydramine (Benadryl), and topical lidocaine can be used. Instruct the patient to rinse the mouth with the mixture without swallowing it.

Fatigue is a common side effect of radiation therapy and usually begins a few weeks into therapy. Encourage patients to walk 15 to 30 minutes each day, since regular exercise can give them more energy. Instruct patients to do activities that are most important to them and to rest during periods of low energy. Identify support systems and encourage patients to ask for help.

Skin over the irradiated area often becomes reddened and sensitive to touch. Instruct patients to use only prescribed lotions and skin products while undergoing radiation therapy, and to not use any lotions within 2 hours before treatment. (Skin care for patients having radiation therapy is discussed in Chapter 16.)

Surgical Therapy. Preoperatively assess the patient's physical and psychosocial needs. Physical preparation is the same as for any major surgery, with an emphasis on oral hygiene. Explanations and emotional support are of special significance and should include postoperative measures relating to communication and feeding. Assess knowledge and understanding of the planned surgical procedure, and clarify information as needed. Include the caregiver in preoperative teaching.

Tailor teaching to the planned surgical procedure. For surgeries that involve a laryngectomy, include information about expected changes in speech. Establish a means of communication for the immediate postoperative period. Magic Slates, alphabet boards, writing materials, pictorial guides, or hand signals are useful methods for communicating. Programmable speech-generating devices allow use of recorded messages that are matched with a graphic representing each message. Integration of this technology into patient care enhances the patient's ability to communicate basic needs postoperatively.[29]

Immediately after surgery, focus your nursing care on airway management, wound care, nutrition, communication, and psychosocial issues related to body-image changes. Maintenance of a patent airway is essential. The inflammation in the surgical area may compress the trachea. A tracheostomy tube will be in place. Keep the patient in semi-Fowler's position to decrease edema and limit tension on the suture lines. The patient with a laryngectomy requires frequent suctioning via the tracheostomy tube. Secretions typically change in amount and consistency over time. The patient may initially have copious blood-tinged secretions that diminish and thicken. Normal saline bolus via the tracheostomy tube is not recommended to assist with removal of thickened secretions, since this causes

hypoxia and damage to the epithelial cells. Maintain adequate fluid intake (IV, enteral, and oral when allowed) and humidification of inspired gases to keep secretions liquid and mucous membranes moist. Encourage deep breathing and coughing. Provide tracheostomy care as needed (see Table 27-7).

Monitor vital signs frequently because of the risk of hemorrhage and respiratory compromise. Pressure dressings, packing, or drainage tubes may be used for wound management, depending on the type of surgical procedure. If skin flaps are employed, dressings are typically not used. This allows better visualization of the incision and avoids excessive pressure on tissue (see Fig. 27-11). When a radical neck dissection is performed, the wound is suctioned with a portable system, such as a Hemovac. The drainage should be serosanguineous and gradually decrease in volume over 24 hours. Monitor patency of drainage tubes every 4 hours to ensure proper functioning. In addition, monitor the amount and character of drainage. If the tubing becomes obstructed, fluid will accumulate under the skin flap and predispose the patient to formation of hematomas or seromas, impair wound healing, and increase the risk for infection. After drainage tubes are removed, closely monitor the area to detect any swelling. If fluid continues to accumulate, aspiration may be necessary. Closely monitor incision sites for signs of infection.

The patient may have a nasogastric tube inserted during surgery to remove gastric contents via intermittent suction for the first 24 to 48 hours until peristalsis returns. Because the nasogastric tube lies close to internal incision lines, do not manipulate or move the tube. When bowel sounds return, enteral feedings may be started slowly and advanced to meet nutritional needs. Monitor daily weights and blood chemistries to evaluate the patient's nutritional status.

After a neck dissection, teach the patient to use the upper extremities to assist with support and movement of the head. After the immediate postoperative period the patient should begin an exercise program to maintain strength and movement in the affected shoulder and neck. This is especially important when the spinal accessory nerve and sternocleidomastoid muscles are removed or damaged. Without exercise, the patient will be left with a "frozen" shoulder and limited range of neck motion. The patient should continue this exercise program after discharge to prevent future functional disabilities.

Voice Rehabilitation. Preoperatively a speech therapist should meet with the patient having a total laryngectomy to discuss voice restoration options. The International Association of Laryngectomees, an association of laryngectomy patients, focuses on helping patients reestablish speech. Local groups, called "Lost Chord" or "New Voice" Clubs, often provide volunteers to visit the patient, preferably preoperatively. Three options are available to restore speech: esophageal speech, electrolarynx, and transesophageal puncture.

Esophageal speech involves swallowing air, trapping it in the esophagus, and releasing it to create sound. The air causes vibration of the pharyngoesophageal segment and sound (which initially is similar to a belch). With practice, many patients develop some speech skills, but few develop fluent speech.

An *electrolarynx* is a hand-held, battery-powered device that creates speech with the use of sound waves. The two most common types of electrolarynx devices are classified as neck and intraoral. The *neck type* is placed against the neck, under the chin (Fig. 27-12, *A*), or on the cheek. The patient moves the lips to articulate sound that is conducted into the oropharynx

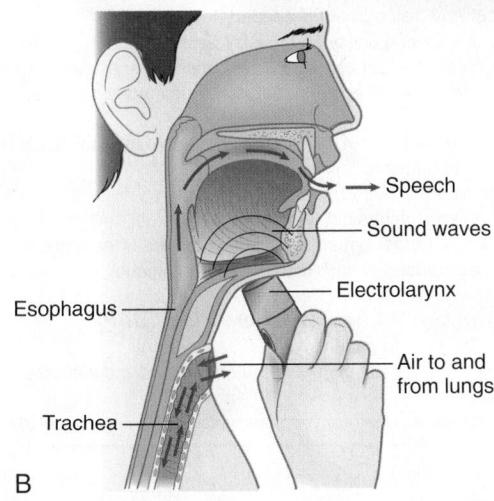

FIG. 27-12 Artificial larynx. **A,** Battery-powered electronic artificial larynx for patient who has had a total laryngectomy. **B,** The sound waves created by the electrolarynx allow the person to speak.

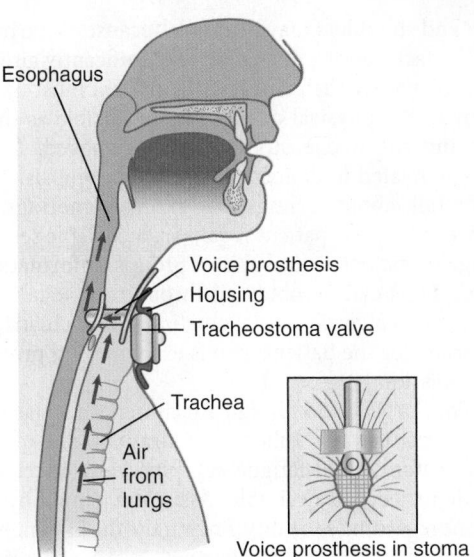

FIG. 27-13 Blom-Singer voice prosthesis and tracheostoma valve. With this prosthesis and valve, patients with a laryngectomy can speak normally. *Inset* shows laryngectomy stoma and voice prosthesis with tracheostoma valve removed.

(Fig. 27-12, *B*). This option allows for speech immediately after surgery, is easy to learn, and requires little maintenance. Intraoral devices are used for patients who cannot achieve adequate sound conduction on the skin. The *intraoral electrolarynx* uses a plastic tube placed in the corner of the roof of the mouth to create vibrations. A hands-free device, using an electromyograph (EMG) transducer in the strap muscles of the neck, is also available.[30] With all devices, voice pitch is low and the sound is mechanical.

Transesophageal puncture, the most common voice rehabilitation method, offers the best speech quality with the highest patient satisfaction.[31] A transesophageal puncture creates a surgical fistula or tract between the esophagus and trachea. The puncture may be created at the same time as the total laryngectomy surgery or afterward if postoperative radiation is planned. A red rubber catheter is placed in the tracheoesophageal puncture as a stent. Several days later, the catheter is removed and a one-way valved prosthesis is placed in the tract. The valve prevents aspiration of food or saliva from the esophagus into the tracheostomy. To speak, the patient manually blocks the stoma with the finger. Air moves from the lungs, through the prosthesis, into the esophagus, and out the mouth. Speech is produced by the air vibrating against the esophagus and is formed into words by moving the tongue and lips. The use of a hands-free external-airflow valve eliminates the need for finger occlusion of the stoma. The prosthesis must be cleaned regularly and replaced when it becomes blocked with mucus. The most commonly used voice prosthesis is the Blom-Singer prosthesis (Fig. 27-13).

Stoma Care. Before discharge, instruct the patient in the care of the laryngectomy stoma. The patient should wash the area around the stoma daily with a moist cloth. A nasal wash spray (e.g., Alkalol) can be used every 1 to 2 hours to keep the stoma moist and prevent crusting. Dried secretions can be removed with tweezers. If a laryngectomy tube is in place, the patient must remove the entire tube at least daily and clean it in the same manner as a tracheostomy tube. The inner cannula may need to be removed and cleaned more frequently. A scarf, a loose shirt, or a crocheted shield can be used to hide the stoma.

The patient should cover the stoma when coughing (because mucus may be expectorated) and during any activity (e.g., shaving, applying makeup) that might lead to inhalation of foreign materials. Because water can easily enter the stoma, the patient should wear a plastic collar when taking a shower. Swimming is contraindicated. Initially, humidification is administered via a tracheostomy mask. After discharge, the patient can use a bedside humidifier. The patient must also maintain a high oral fluid intake, especially in dry weather.

Inform the patient about the importance of wearing a Medic Alert bracelet or other identification that alerts emergency personnel of the neck breathing status. Because the patient no longer breathes through the nose, the ability to smell smoke and food is often lost. Advise the patient to install smoke and carbon monoxide detectors in the home. Encourage preparation of food that is colorful, attractive, and nutritious because taste may also be diminished secondary to the loss of smell and radiation therapy.

Depression. Depression is common in the patient who has had a radical neck dissection. The patient may not be able to speak because of the laryngectomy and cannot control saliva.

The neck and shoulders may be numb because of the transected nerves. The facial appearance may be significantly altered, with swelling, edema, and deformities. The patient must understand that many of the physical changes are reversible as the edema subsides and the tracheostomy tube is removed. Depression may also be related to concern about the prognosis. Allow the patient to talk about feelings and express emotions. Convey acceptance to help the patient regain an acceptable self-concept. Encourage participation in support groups. Information about available groups can be obtained through the local branch of the American Cancer Society. Sometimes a psychiatric referral is appropriate for the patient who is experiencing prolonged or severe depression.

Sexuality. Surgery and foreign attachments such as tracheostomy and gastrostomy tubes may dramatically affect body image. Xerostomia and fatigue can physically affect sexuality. Some patients feel less desirable. Assist the patient by allowing discussions regarding sexuality. Encourage the patient to discuss this problem with his or her partner. It may be difficult for the patient to talk about sexual problems because of the alteration in communication. Assist the patient in planning how to communicate with the sexual partner. Offer support and guidance to the sexual partner. Helping the patient see that sexuality involves much more than appearance may relieve some anxiety.

AMBULATORY AND HOME CARE. The patient is often discharged with a tracheostomy and a nasogastric or gastrostomy feeding tube. Some patients need home health care initially to evaluate the caregiver's or the patient's ability to perform self-care activities. The patient and the caregiver need to learn how to manage tubes and who to call if there are problems. Provide pictorial instructions for tracheostomy care, suctioning, stoma care, and enteral feeding as appropriate. The patient can resume exercise, recreation, and sexual activity when able. Most patients can return to work 1 to 2 months after surgery. However, many never return to full-time employment. The changes that follow a total laryngectomy can be upsetting. Loss of speech, loss of the ability to taste and smell, inability to produce audible sounds (including laughing and weeping), and the presence of a permanent tracheal stoma that produces undesirable mucus are often overwhelming to the patient. Although changes are discussed before surgery, the patient may not be prepared for the extent of these changes. If the patient has a significant other, this person's reaction to the patient's altered appearance is important. Acceptance by another person can promote an improved self-image. Encouraging the patient to participate in self-care is another important part of rehabilitation.

DELEGATION DECISIONS
Suctioning and Tracheostomy Care

Licensed practical nurses (LPNs) may do suctioning and give tracheostomy care to stable patients. In patients who have acute airway problems requiring an endotracheal or tracheostomy tube, these interventions should be done by the registered nurse (RN).

Role of Registered Nurse (RN)
- For unstable patients:
  - Assess for the need for suctioning.
  - Suction the endotracheal or tracheostomy tube.
  - Evaluate for adverse effects of suctioning such as dysrhythmias.
  - Evaluate whether patient status is improved after suctioning.
- Maintain appropriate cuff inflation pressure at 20-25 cm H_2O, or use minimal leak technique to maintain cuff pressure.
- Assess tracheostomy and any retention sutures for evidence of complications (e.g., infection).
- Replace the tracheostomy tube after accidental dislodgment.
- Ventilate the patient with a bag-valve-mask device after accidental tracheostomy dislodgment if needed.
- Assess swallowing ability and risk for aspiration.
- Develop plan to avoid aspiration in a patient with a tracheostomy.
- Teach patient and caregiver about home tracheostomy care.

Role of Licensed Practical/Vocational Nurse (LPN/LVN)
- For stable patients:
  - Determine the need for suctioning.
  - Suction the tracheostomy.
  - Evaluate whether patient status is improved after suctioning.
- Provide tracheostomy care using sterile technique.

Role of Unlicensed Assistive Personnel (UAP)
- Provide oral care to patient with a tracheostomy.
- Suction patient's oropharynx (after being trained and evaluated in this procedure).
- Report increased need for oropharyngeal suctioning to the RN.

EVALUATION

Expected outcomes for the patient with head and neck cancer who is treated surgically are that the patient will
- Demonstrate effective coughing and secretion clearance
- Demonstrate the ability to swallow oral foods without aspiration
- Report satisfaction with pain relief
- Use written and nonverbal techniques to effectively communicate with others

Other outcomes for the patient with head and neck cancer who is treated surgically are addressed in eNursing Care Plans 27-1 and 27-2 on the website for this chapter.

CASE STUDY

Laryngeal Cancer

iStockphoto/Thinkstock

Patient Profile

M.R., a 60-year-old white man, was admitted for evaluation of mild pain on swallowing and a persistent sore throat over the past year. He has a history of type 2 diabetes mellitus.

Subjective Data

- States that his symptoms worsened in the past 2 mo
- Has used various cold remedies to relieve symptoms without relief
- Has lost weight because of decrease in appetite and difficulty swallowing
- Has smoked three packs of cigarettes a day for 40 yr
- Consumes 4-6 cans of beer a day

Objective Data

Laryngoscopy
- Subglottic mass

Physical Examination
- Enlarged cervical nodes

Computed Tomography Scan
- Subglottic lesion with lymph node involvement

Collaborative Care

- Percutaneous gastrostomy tube inserted preoperatively for enteral tube feeding
- Total laryngectomy with tracheostomy with inflated cuff
- Nasogastric tube postoperatively

Discussion Questions

1. What information in the assessment suggests that M.R. is at risk for cancer of the larynx?
2. *Priority Decision:* What are your priority teaching strategies for M.R. before and after laryngectomy?
3. Discuss methods used to restore speech after laryngectomy.
4. Is there anything in his history that may affect wound healing after surgery?
5. *Priority Decision:* While in the recovery room, M.R. develops shortness of breath. What are your priority nursing interventions?
6. What teaching is required to help this patient assume self-care after his surgery? What precautions should the patient take because of his stoma?
7. While on the medical-surgical unit, M.R. is tearful and is staring at the wall. What should you do?
8. *Priority Decision:* Based on the assessment data presented, what are your priority nursing diagnoses? Are there any collaborative problems?
9. *Delegation Decision:* What role can unlicensed assistive personnel (UAP) have in relation to the tracheostomy?
10. *Evidence-Based Practice:* How could you best meet M.R.'s communication needs during the first few postoperative days?

ⓔvolve Answers available at *http://evolve.elsevier.com/Lewis/medsurg.*

▮ BRIDGE TO NCLEX EXAMINATION

The number of the question corresponds to the same-numbered outcome at the beginning of the chapter.

1. A patient was seen in the clinic for an episode of epistaxis, which was controlled by placement of anterior nasal packing. During discharge teaching, the nurse instructs the patient to
   a. use aspirin for pain relief.
   b. remove the packing later that day.
   c. skip the next dose of antihypertensive medication.
   d. avoid vigorous nose blowing and strenuous activity.

2. A patient with allergic rhinitis reports severe nasal congestion; sneezing; and watery, itchy eyes and nose at various times of the year. To teach the patient to control these symptoms, the nurse advises the patient to
   a. avoid all intranasal sprays and oral antihistamines.
   b. limit the usage of nasal decongestant spray to 10 days.
   c. use oral decongestants at bedtime to prevent symptoms during the night.
   d. keep a diary of when the allergic reaction occurs and what precipitates it.

3. A patient is seen at the clinic with fever, muscle aches, sore throat with yellowish exudate, and headache. The nurse anticipates that the collaborative management will include *(select all that apply)*
   a. antiviral agents to treat influenza.
   b. treatment with antibiotics starting ASAP.
   c. a throat culture or rapid strep antigen test.
   d. supportive care, including cool, bland liquids.
   e. comprehensive history to determine possible etiology.

4. The best method for determining the risk of aspiration in a patient with a tracheostomy is to
   a. consult a speech therapist for swallowing assessment.
   b. have the patient drink plain water and assess for coughing.
   c. assess for change of sputum color 48 hours after patient drinks small amount of blue dye.
   d. suction above the cuff after the patient eats or drinks to determine presence of food in trachea.

5. Which nursing action would be of highest priority when suctioning a patient with a tracheostomy?
   a. Auscultating lung sounds after suctioning is complete
   b. Providing a means of communication for the patient during the procedure
   c. Assessing the patient's oxygenation saturation before, during, and after suctioning
   d. Administering pain and/or antianxiety medication 30 minutes before suctioning

6. When planning health care teaching to prevent or detect early head and neck cancer, which people would be the priority to target *(select all that apply)*?
   a. 65-year-old man who has used chewing tobacco most of his life
   b. 45-year-old rancher who uses snuff to stay awake while driving his herds of cattle
   c. 78-year-old woman who has been drinking hard liquor since her husband died 15 years ago
   d. 21-year-old college student who drinks beer on weekends with his fraternity brothers
   e. 22-year-old woman who has been diagnosed with human papilloma virus (HPV) of the cervix

7. While in the recovery room, a patient with a total laryngectomy is suctioned and has bloody mucus with some clots. Which nursing interventions would apply?
   a. Notify the physician immediately.
   b. Place the patient in the prone position to facilitate drainage.
   c. Instill 3 mL of normal saline into the tracheostomy tube to loosen secretions.
   d. Continue your assessment of the patient, including O_2 saturation, respiratory rate, and breath sounds.

8. When using a prosthesis for transesophageal speech, the patient
   a. places a vibrating device in the mouth.
   b. blocks the stoma entrance with a finger.
   c. swallows air using a Valsalva maneuver.
   d. places a speaking valve next to the stoma.

1. d, 2. d, 3. c, 4. d, e, 5. c, 6. a, b, c, 7. d, 8. b

℮volve

For rationales to these answers and even more NCLEX review questions, visit *http://evolve.elsevier.com/Lewis/medsurg.*

REFERENCES

1. American Academy of Otolaryngology–Head and Neck Surgery: Fact sheet: deviated septum. Retrieved from *www.entnet.org/HealthInformation/deviatedSeptum.cfm.*
2. Reitzen SD, Chung W, Shah AR: Nasal septal deviation in the pediatric and adult populations, *Ear Nose Throat J* 90:112, 2011.
*3. Eiff MP, Hatch RL: *Fracture management for primary care*, ed 3, St Louis, 2011, Saunders.
*4. Lewis R: Ultrasound device adds precision to rhinoplasty. Retrieved from *www.medscape.com/viewarticle/750055.*
5. American Academy of Facial, Plastic, and Reconstructive Surgery: Rhinoplasty. Retrieved from *www.aafprs.org/patient/procedures/rhinoplasty.html.*
6. US National Library of Medicine, NIH National Institutes of Health: MedlinePlus: nosebleed. Retrieved from *www.nlm.nih.gov/medlineplus/ency/article/003106.htm.*
7. Bamimore O, Dronen SC: Management of acute epistaxis. Retrieved from *http://emedicine.medscape.com/article/764719-overview.*
*8. Dykewicz MS: Management of rhinitis: guidelines, evidence basis, and systematic clinical approach for what we do, *Immunol Allergy Clin North Am* 31:619, 2011.
*9. Brozek JL, Bousquet J, Baena-Cagnani CE, et al: Allergic rhinitis and its impact on asthma (ARIA) guidelines: 2010 revision, *J Allergy Clin Immunol* 126:466, 2010.
10. National Institute of Allergy and Infectious Diseases: Common cold. Retrieved from *http://niaid.nih.gov/topics/commoncold/Pages/default.aspx.*
11. Centers for Disease Control and Prevention: Seasonal influenza. Retrieved from *www.cdc.gov/flu/about/qa/disease.htm.*
12. American Association for Clinical Chemistry: Influenza tests. Retrieved from *http://labtestsonline.org/understanding/analytes/flu/tab/test.*
13. Centers for Disease Control and Prevention: Key facts about influenza (flu) and flu vaccine. Retrieved from *www.cdc.gov/flu/keyfacts.htm.*
*14. Centers for Disease Control and Prevention: 2011-2012 influenza antiviral medications: a summary for clinicians. Retrieved from *www.cdc.gov/flu/pdf/professionals/antivirals/clinician-antivirals-2011.pdf.*
15. Brook I, Cunha BA, Cohen AJ, et al: Acute sinusitis. Retrieved from *http://emedicine.medscap.com/articl/232670-overview.*
16. WebMD: Nasal irrigation: natural relief for cold and allergy symptoms. Retrieved from *www.webmd.com/allergies/ss/slideshow-nasal-irrigation.*
17. Shantouf R: Intersect ENT's Propel sinus implant receives green light from FDA. Retrieved from *http://medgadget.com/2011/08/intersect-ent%e2%80%99s-propel-sinus-implant-receives-green-light-from-fda.html.*
18. Acerra JR, Dyne PL: Pharyngitis in emergency medicine. Retrieved from *http://emedicine.medscape.com/article/764304-clinical.*
19. Lindman JP, Morgan CE, Schweinfurth J, et al: Tracheostomy. Retrieved from *http://emedicine,medscape.com/article/865968.*
*20. Wiegand DJL, editor: *AACN procedure manual for critical care*, ed 6, St Louis, 2011, Saunders.
21. Frace MA: Tracheostomy care on the medical-surgical unit, *MEDSURG Nurs* 19:58, 2010.
*22. Freman S: Care of adult patients with a temporary tracheostomy, *Nurs Stand* 26:49, 2011.
*23. Regan K, Hunt K: Tracheostomy management: weaning and decannulation. Retrieved from *www.medscape.com/viewarticle/574271.*
24. National Cancer Institute: Head and neck cancer: questions and answers. Retrieved from *www.cancer.gov/cancertopics/factsheet/Sites-Types/head-and-neck.*
25. American Cancer Society: Cancer facts and figures 2011. Retrieved from *www.cancer.org/acs/groups/content/@epidemiologysurveilance/documents/document/acspc-029771.pdf.*
*26. Lowry F: Three-drug combo best for head and neck cancer. Retrieved from *http://medscape.com/viewarticle/735730.*
27. National Cancer Institute: Laryngeal cancer treatment. Retrieved from *www.cancer.gov/cancertopics/pdq/treatment/laryngeal/HealthProfessional/page1.*
28. Lambertz CK, Gruell J, Robenstein V, et al: NO SToPS: reducing treatment breaks during chemoradiation for head and neck cancer, *Clin J Oncol Nurs* 14:585. 2010.
*29. Rodriguez C, Rowe M: Use of a speech-generating device for hospitalized postoperative patients with head and neck cancer experiencing speechlessness, *Oncol Nurs Forum* 37:199, 2010.
30. Lombard LE: Laryngectomy rehabilitation. Retrieved from *http://emedicine.medscape.com/article/883689-overview.*
*31. Xi S, Li Z, Huang X: The effectiveness of voice rehabilitation on vocalization in post-laryngectomy patients: a systematic review, *J Adv Nurs* 66:962, 2010.

RESOURCES

International Association of Laryngectomees
   www.theial.com
National Cancer Institute
   www.cancer.gov

*Evidence-based information for clinical practice.

Breath is the bridge which connects life to
consciousness, which unites your body
to your thoughts.
Thich Nhat Hanh

Nursing Management
Lower Respiratory Problems

Dorothy (Dottie) M. Mathers

evolve WEBSITE

http://evolve.elsevier.com/Lewis/medsurg
- NCLEX Review Questions
- Key Points
- Pre-Test
- Answer Guidelines for Case Study on p. 557
- Rationales for Bridge to NCLEX Examination Questions
- Case Studies
  - Patient With Lung Cancer
  - Patient With Pulmonary Embolism and Respiratory Failure

- Nursing Care Plans (Customizable)
  - eNCP 28-1: Patient With Pneumonia
  - eNCP 28-2: Patient After Thoracotomy
- Concept Map Creator
- Glossary
- Content Updates

eTables
- eTable 28-1: Environmental Lung Diseases
- eTable 28-2: Traumatic Chest Injuries and Mechanisms of Injury
- eTable 28-3: Causes of Restrictive Lung Disease

LEARNING OUTCOMES

1. Compare and contrast the clinical manifestations and collaborative and nursing management of patients with acute bronchitis and pertussis.
2. Differentiate among the types of pneumonia and their etiology, pathophysiology, clinical manifestations, and collaborative care.
3. Prioritize the nursing management of the patient with pneumonia.
4. Describe the pathogenesis, classification, clinical manifestations, complications, diagnostic abnormalities, and nursing and collaborative management of patients with tuberculosis.
5. Describe the causes, clinical manifestations, and collaborative management of patients with pulmonary fungal infections.
6. Explain the pathophysiology, clinical manifestations, and collaborative management of patients with lung abscesses.
7. Identify the causative factors, clinical manifestations, and nursing and collaborative management of patients with environmental lung diseases.
8. Describe the etiology, risk factors, pathophysiology, clinical manifestations, and nursing and collaborative management of lung cancer.

9. Compare and contrast the pathophysiology, clinical manifestations, and nursing and collaborative management of pneumothorax, fractured ribs, and flail chest.
10. Describe the purpose, function, and nursing responsibilities related to chest tubes and various drainage systems.
11. Explain the types of chest surgery and appropriate preoperative and postoperative care.
12. Describe the etiology, clinical manifestations, and nursing and collaborative management of patients with restrictive lung disorders such as pleural effusion, pleurisy, and atelectasis.
13. Describe the pathophysiology, clinical manifestations, and management of pulmonary embolism, pulmonary hypertension, and cor pulmonale.
14. Discuss the use of lung transplantation as a treatment for pulmonary disorders.

KEY TERMS

acute bronchitis, p. 522
community-acquired pneumonia (CAP), p. 523
cor pulmonale, p. 555
empyema, p. 549
flail chest, p. 543
hemothorax, p. 543
lung abscess, p. 534

medical care–associated pneumonia (MCAP), p. 523
pertussis, p. 522
pleural effusion, p. 549
pleurisy (pleuritis), p. 550
pneumoconiosis, p. 535
pneumonia, p. 522
pneumothorax, p. 542

pulmonary edema, p. 551
pulmonary embolism (PE), p. 551
pulmonary hypertension, p. 553
tension pneumothorax, p. 543
thoracentesis, p. 550
thoracotomy, p. 548
tuberculosis (TB), p. 528

Reviewed by Sharon A. Willadsen, RN, PhD, Nursing Instructor, Lakeshore Technical College, Cleveland, Wisconsin.

A wide variety of problems affect the lower respiratory system. Lung diseases that are characterized primarily by an obstructive disorder, such as asthma, chronic obstructive pulmonary disease (COPD), and cystic fibrosis, are discussed in Chapter 29. This chapter discusses other lower respiratory tract diseases, including infectious, oncologic, traumatic, restrictive, and vascular disorders.

LOWER RESPIRATORY TRACT INFECTIONS

Lower respiratory tract infection is both a common and a serious occurrence. It is the third leading cause of death worldwide.[1] Pneumonia and influenza are the eighth leading cause of death in the United States, accounting for more than 56,000 deaths annually.[2]

ACUTE BRONCHITIS

Acute bronchitis is an inflammation of the bronchi in the lower respiratory tract. Up to 90% of acute bronchial infections are viral in origin. Cough, which is the most common symptom, lasts for up to 3 weeks. Clear, mucoid sputum is often present, although some patients produce purulent sputum. The presence of colored (e.g., green) sputum is not a reliable indicator of bacterial infection.[3] Associated symptoms include headache, fever, malaise, hoarseness, myalgias, dyspnea, and chest pain.

Assessment may reveal normal breath sounds or rhonchi, crackles, or wheezes, usually with expiration and exertion. Diagnosis is based on clinical assessment. Evidence of consolidation (e.g., fremitus, rales, egophony), which is suggestive of pneumonia, is absent with bronchitis. (*Consolidation* in the lungs occurs when fluid accumulates, causing the lung tissue to become stiff and unable to exchange gases.) Chest x-rays would be normal and are therefore not indicated unless pneumonia is suspected. (Chronic bronchitis is discussed in Chapter 29.)

Acute bronchitis is usually self-limiting, and treatment is supportive. Cough suppressants, β_2-agonist (bronchodilator) inhalers in patients with wheezing, and high-dose inhaled corticosteroids may be used.[3] Antibiotics generally are not prescribed unless the person has a prolonged infection associated with systemic symptoms. Explain to the patient that antibiotics are not effective in treating a viral infection and that they may cause side effects and antibiotic-resistant germs. Complementary and alternative therapies (e.g., echinacea, honey) may be useful for symptom relief. If the acute bronchitis is due to an influenza virus, treatment with antiviral drugs, either zanamivir (Relenza) or oseltamivir (Tamiflu), can be started. These drugs should be initiated within 48 hours of the onset of symptoms.

PERTUSSIS

Pertussis is a highly contagious infection of the respiratory tract caused by a gram-negative bacillus, *Bordetella pertussis*. Pertussis is characterized by uncontrollable, violent coughing. Despite improved childhood vaccination in the United States, the incidence of pertussis has been steadily increasing since the 1980s, with the largest increase noted in adults.[4] It is thought that immunity resulting from childhood vaccination with DPT (diphtheria, pertussis, tetanus) may wane over time, resulting in a milder infection that is still distressing and contagious. Therefore the Centers for Disease Control and Prevention (CDC) currently recommends that all adults age 18 years and older receive a one-time dose of Tdap (tetanus, diphtheria, and pertussis) vaccination.[4]

Clinical manifestations of pertussis occur in stages. The first (catarrhal) stage manifests as a mild upper respiratory tract infection (URI) with a low-grade or no fever, runny nose, watery eyes, and mild nonproductive cough. The second (paroxysmal) stage is characterized by paroxysms of cough. Inspiration after each cough produces the typical "whooping" sound as the patient tries to breathe in air against an obstructed glottis. Vomiting may also occur with the coughing. Like acute bronchitis, the coughing is more frequent at night. Unlike bronchitis, the cough with pertussis may last from 6 to 10 weeks.

Treatment is antibiotics, usually macrolides (erythromycin, azithromycin [Zithromax]), to minimize symptoms and prevent spread of the disease. Cough suppressants and antihistamines should not be used, since they are ineffective and may induce coughing episodes. Corticosteroids and bronchodilators are not useful in reducing symptoms.

PNEUMONIA

Pneumonia is an acute infection of the lung parenchyma. Until 1936, pneumonia was the leading cause of death in the United States. The discovery of sulfa drugs and penicillin was pivotal in the treatment of pneumonia. Since that time, remarkable progress has been made in the development of antibiotics to treat pneumonia. However, despite new antimicrobial agents, pneumonia is still associated with significant morbidity and mortality rates. Community-acquired pneumonia (CAP) is the sixth leading cause of death for people ages 65 years or older in the United States.[5]

Etiology

Normally, the airway distal to the larynx is protected from infection by various defense mechanisms. Mechanisms that create a mechanical barrier to microorganisms include air filtration, epiglottis closure over the trachea, cough reflex, mucociliary escalator mechanism, and reflex bronchoconstriction (see Chapter 26). Immune defense mechanisms include secretion of immunoglobulins A and G and alveolar macrophages.

Pneumonia is more likely to occur when the defense mechanisms become incompetent or are overwhelmed by the virulence or quantity of infectious agents. Decreased consciousness depresses the cough and epiglottal reflexes, which may allow aspiration of oropharyngeal contents into the lungs. Tracheal intubation interferes with the normal cough reflex and the mucociliary escalator mechanism. Air pollution, cigarette smoking, viral URIs, and normal changes that occur with aging can impair the mucociliary mechanism. Chronic diseases can

TABLE 28-1 RISK FACTORS FOR PNEUMONIA

- Abdominal or thoracic surgery
- Age >65 yr
- Air pollution
- Altered consciousness: alcoholism, head injury, seizures, anesthesia, drug overdose, stroke
- Bed rest and prolonged immobility
- Chronic diseases: chronic lung and liver disease, diabetes mellitus, heart disease, cancer, chronic kidney disease
- Debilitating illness
- Exposure to bats, birds, rabbits, farm animals
- Immunosuppressive disease and/or therapy (corticosteroids, cancer chemotherapy, human immunodeficiency virus [HIV] infection, immunosuppressive therapy after organ transplant)
- Inhalation or aspiration of noxious substances
- Intestinal and gastric feedings via nasogastric or nasointestinal tubes
- IV drug use
- Malnutrition
- Recent antibiotic therapy
- Resident of a long-term care facility
- Smoking
- Tracheal intubation (endotracheal intubation, tracheostomy)
- Upper respiratory tract infection

TABLE 28-2 ORGANISMS CAUSING PNEUMONIA

Community-Acquired Pneumonia	Medical Care–Associated Pneumonia
• *Streptococcus pneumoniae**	• *Pseudomonas aeruginosa*†
• *Mycoplasma pneumoniae*	• *Escherichia coli*†
• *Haemophilus influenzae*	• *Klebsiella pneumoniae*†
• Respiratory viruses	• *Acinetobacter* species†
• *Chlamydophila pneumoniae*	• *Haemophilus influenzae*
• *Chlamydophila psittaci*	• *Staphylococcus aureus*
• *Coxiella burnetti*	• *Streptococcus pneumoniae*
• *Legionella pneumophila*	• *Proteus* species
• Oral anaerobes	• *Enterobacter* species
• *Moraxella catarrhalis*	• Oral anaerobes
• *Staphylococcus aureus*	
• *Pseudomonas aeruginosa*	
• Enteric aerobic gram-negative bacteria (e.g., *Klebsiella* species)	
• Fungi	
• *Mycobacterium tuberculosis*	

*Most common cause of community-acquired pneumonia (CAP).
†Most common causes of medical care–associated pneumonia (MCAP).

TABLE 28-3 ASSESSING PNEUMONIA USING CURB-65

The CURB-65 scale may be used as a supplement to clinical judgment to determine the severity of pneumonia and if patients need to be hospitalized.

Identifying the Level of Risk
Patients receive 1 point for each of the following indicators:
- **C:** Confusion (compared to baseline)
- **U:** BUN >20 mg/dL
- **R:** Respiratory rate ≥30 breaths/min
- **B:** Systolic blood pressure <90 mm Hg or diastolic blood pressure ≤60 mm Hg
- **65:** ≥Age 65 yr

Scoring and Decision Making

Score	Decision
0	Treat at home
1-2	Consider hospital admission
3 or more	Hospital admission
4-5	Consider admission to intensive care unit

Source: Lim WS, van der Eerden MM, Laing R, et al: Defining community acquired pneumonia severity on presentation to hospital: an international derivation and validation study, *Thorax* 58(5):377, 2003.

suppress the immune system's ability to inhibit bacterial growth. The risk factors for pneumonia are listed in Table 28-1.

Organisms that cause pneumonia reach the lung by three methods:

1. *Aspiration* of normal flora from the nasopharynx or oropharynx. Many of the organisms that cause pneumonia are normal inhabitants of the pharynx in healthy adults.
2. *Inhalation* of microbes present in the air. Examples include *Mycoplasma pneumoniae* and fungal pneumonias.
3. *Hematogenous spread* from a primary infection elsewhere in the body. An example is *Staphylococcus aureus*.

Types of Pneumonia

Bacteria, viruses, *Mycoplasma* organisms, fungi, parasites, and chemicals are all potential causes of pneumonia. Although pneumonia can be classified according to the causative organism, a clinically effective way is to classify it as *community-acquired* or *medical care–associated* pneumonia. Classifying pneumonia is important because of the differences in the likely causative organisms (Table 28-2) and the selection of appropriate antimicrobial therapy.

Community-Acquired Pneumonia. Community-acquired pneumonia (CAP) is an acute infection of the lung occurring in patients who have not been hospitalized or resided in a long-term care facility within 14 days of the onset of symptoms.[5] The decision to treat the patient at home or admit him or her to the hospital is based on several factors such as the patient's age, vital signs, mental status, and presence of co-morbid conditions. Clinicians can use tools such as the CURB-65 scale (Table 28-3) or the Pneumonia Patient Outcomes Research Team (PORT) Pneumonia Severity Index (PSI) to supplement clinical judgment. (The PSI calculator is available online at *http://pda.ahrq.gov/clinic/psi/psicalc.asp*). Empiric antibiotic therapy should be started as soon as possible. (*Empiric therapy* is the initiation of treatment before a definitive diagnosis. It is based on experience and knowledge of drugs known to be effective for the likely causative agent.)

Medical Care–Associated Pneumonia. Medical care–associated pneumonia (MCAP) encompasses three forms of pneumonia: hospital-associated pneumonia, ventilator-associated pneumonia, and health care–associated pneumonia.[6]

Hospital-associated pneumonia (HAP) is pneumonia that occurs 48 hours or longer after hospital admission and was not incubating at the time of hospitalization. *Ventilator-associated pneumonia* (VAP) refers to pneumonia that occurs more than 48 hours after endotracheal intubation. (VAP is discussed in Chapter 66.) *Health care–associated pneumonia* (HCAP) is a new-onset pneumonia in a patient who (1) was hospitalized in an acute care hospital for 2 days or longer within 90 days of the infection; (2) resided in a long-term care facility; (3) received IV antibiotic therapy, chemotherapy, or wound care within the past 30 days of the current infection; or (4) attended a hospital or hemodialysis clinic.[6]

These infections cause significant morbidity and increase the risk of death. HAP, VAP, and HCAP also increase health care costs with longer hospital stays and associated costs.

Once the diagnosis is made, empiric treatment of the pneumonia is initiated based on known risk factors, early versus late onset, and probable organism. Antibiotic therapy can be adjusted once the results of sputum cultures identify the exact pathogen.

A major problem in treating MCAP is multidrug-resistant (MDR) organisms. Antibiotic susceptibility tests can identify MDR organisms. The virulence of these organisms can severely limit the available and appropriate antimicrobial therapy. In addition, MDR organisms can increase the morbidity and mortality risks associated with pneumonia. (Chapter 15 discusses MDR organisms.)

Aspiration Pneumonia. *Aspiration pneumonia,* occurring as either CAP or MCAP, results from the abnormal entry of material from the mouth or stomach into the trachea and lungs. Conditions that increase the risk of aspiration include decreased level of consciousness (e.g., seizure, anesthesia, head injury, stroke, alcohol intake), difficulty swallowing, and nasogastric intubation with or without tube feeding. With loss of consciousness, the gag and cough reflexes are depressed, and aspiration is more likely to occur. Other high-risk groups are those who are seriously ill, have poor dentition, or are receiving acid-reducing medications.[7]

The aspirated material (food, water, vomitus, or oropharyngeal secretions) triggers an inflammatory response. The most common form of aspiration pneumonia is a primary bacterial infection. Typically, more than one organism is identified on sputum culture, including both aerobes and anaerobes, since they comprise the flora of the oropharynx. Until the cultures are completed, the choice of antibiotic therapy is based on an assessment of the severity of illness, where the infection was acquired (community versus medical care), and the probable causative organism. In contrast, aspiration of acidic gastric contents causes *chemical (noninfectious) pneumonitis,* which may not require antibiotic therapy. However, secondary bacterial infection can occur 48 to 72 hours later.

Opportunistic Pneumonia. Individuals at risk for opportunistic pneumonia include those with altered immune responses. This can include people with severe protein-calorie malnutrition or immunodeficiencies (e.g., human immunodeficiency virus [HIV] infection), and those receiving radiation therapy, chemotherapy, and any immunosuppressive therapy, including long-term corticosteroid therapy. In addition to the risk of bacterial and viral pneumonia, the immunocompromised person may develop an infection from microorganisms that do not normally cause disease, such as *Pneumocystis jiroveci* (formerly *carinii*) and cytomegalovirus (CMV).

P. jiroveci pneumonia (PCP) rarely occurs in the healthy individual but is the most common form of pneumonia in people with HIV disease. The onset is slow and subtle with symptoms of fever, tachypnea, tachycardia, dyspnea, nonproductive cough, and hypoxemia. The chest x-ray usually shows diffuse bilateral infiltrates. In widespread disease the lungs have massive consolidation. PCP can be life threatening, causing acute respiratory failure and death. Infection can also spread to other organs, including the liver, bone marrow, lymph nodes, spleen, and thyroid. Bacterial and viral pneumonias must first be ruled out because of the vague presentation of PCP. Treatment consists of a course of trimethoprim/sulfamethoxazole

FIG. 28-1 Pathophysiologic course of pneumonia.

(Bactrim, Septra) either IV or orally depending on the severity of disease and the patient's response.

CMV, a herpes virus, can cause viral pneumonia. Most CMV infections are asymptomatic or mild, but severe disease can occur in people with an impaired immune response. CMV is the most common life-threatening infectious complication after hematopoietic stem cell transplantation.[8] Antiviral medications (e.g., ganciclovir [Cytovene], foscarnet [Foscavir], cidofovir [Vistide]) and high-dose immunoglobulin are used for treatment.

Pathophysiology

Specific pathophysiologic changes related to pneumonia vary according to the offending organism. Some viruses cause direct injury and cell death. The majority of organisms, however, trigger an inflammatory response in the lung (Fig. 28-1). A vascular reaction occurs, characterized by an increase in blood flow and vascular permeability. Neutrophils are activated to engulf and kill the offending organisms. The neutrophils, the offending organism, and fluid from surrounding blood vessels fill the alveoli and interrupt normal oxygen transportation, leading to clinical manifestations of hypoxia (e.g., tachypnea, dyspnea, tachycardia). Mucus production is also increased, which can obstruct airflow and further decrease gas exchange. Consolidation, a feature typical of bacterial pneumonia, occurs when the normally air-filled alveoli become filled with fluid and debris. Complete resolution and healing occur if there are no complications. Macrophages lyse and process the debris, normal lung tissue is restored, and gas exchange returns to normal.

Clinical Manifestations

The most common presenting symptoms of pneumonia are cough, fever, shaking chills, dyspnea, tachypnea, and pleuritic chest pain. The cough may or may not be productive. Sputum may appear green, yellow, or even rust colored (bloody). Viral pneumonia may initially be seen as influenza, with respiratory symptoms appearing and/or worsening 12 to 36 hours after onset.[9] The older or debilitated patient may not have classic symptoms of pneumonia. Confusion or stupor (possibly related to hypoxia) may be the only finding. Hypothermia, rather than fever, may also be noted with the older patient. Nonspecific clinical manifestations include diaphoresis, anorexia, fatigue, myalgias, headache, and abdominal pain.

On physical examination, rhonchi and crackles may be auscultated over the affected region. If consolidation is present, bronchial breath sounds, egophony, and increased fremitus (vibration of the chest wall produced by vocalization) may be noted. Patients with pleural effusion may exhibit dullness to percussion over the affected area.

Complications

Complications develop more frequently in older individuals and those with underlying chronic diseases. Potential complications include the following:

- *Pleurisy* (inflammation of the pleura) is relatively common.
- *Pleural effusion* (fluid in the pleural space) can occur. In most cases, the effusion is sterile and is reabsorbed in 1 to 2 weeks. Occasionally, effusions require aspiration by thoracentesis.
- *Atelectasis* (collapsed, airless alveoli) of one or part of one lobe may occur. These areas usually clear with effective coughing and deep breathing.
- *Bacteremia* (bacterial infection in the blood) is more likely to occur in infections with *Streptococcus pneumoniae* and *Haemophilus influenzae*.
- *Lung abscess* is not a common complication of pneumonia. However, it may occur with pneumonia caused by *S. aureus* and gram-negative organisms.
- *Empyema*, the accumulation of purulent exudate in the pleural cavity, occurs in less than 5% of cases and requires antibiotic therapy and drainage of the exudate by a chest tube or open surgical drainage.
- *Pericarditis* results from spread of the infecting organism from infected pleura or via a hematogenous route to the pericardium.
- *Meningitis* can be caused by *S. pneumoniae*. The patient with pneumonia who is disoriented, confused, or drowsy may have a lumbar puncture to evaluate the possibility of meningitis.
- *Sepsis* can occur when bacteria within alveoli enter the bloodstream. Severe sepsis can lead to shock and multisystem organ dysfunction syndrome (MODS) (see Chapter 67).
- *Acute respiratory failure* is one of the leading causes of death in patients with severe pneumonia. Failure occurs when pneumonia damages the lungs' ability to exchange oxygen for carbon dioxide.
- *Pneumothorax* can occur when air collects in the pleura space, causing the lungs to collapse.

Pleurisy, pleural effusion, atelectasis, lung abscess, and pneumothorax are discussed later in this chapter.

Diagnostic Studies

The common diagnostic measures for pneumonia are presented in Table 28-4. History, physical examination, and chest x-ray often provide enough information to make management decisions without costly laboratory tests. Chest x-ray often shows a typical pattern characteristic of the infecting organism and is

TABLE 28-4 **COLLABORATIVE CARE**	
Pneumonia	
Diagnostic	**Collaborative Therapy**
• History and physical examination	• Appropriate antibiotic therapy (see Table 28-6)
• Chest x-ray	• Increased fluid intake (at least 3 L/day)
• Gram stain of sputum	• Limited activity and rest
• Sputum culture and sensitivity test	• Antipyretics
• Pulse oximetry or ABGs (if indicated)	• Analgesics
• Complete blood count, WBC differential, and routine blood chemistries (if indicated)	• O$_2$ therapy (if indicated)
• Blood cultures (if indicated)	

important in the diagnosis of pneumonia. X-ray can also show pleural effusions. A thoracentesis and/or bronchoscopy with washings may be used to obtain fluid samples for patients not responding to initial therapy.

Ideally, a sputum specimen for culture and Gram stain to identify the organism is obtained before beginning antibiotic therapy. However, antibiotic administration should not be delayed if a specimen cannot be readily obtained. Delays in antibiotic therapy can increase morbidity and mortality risks. Blood cultures are done for patients who are seriously ill. Arterial blood gases (ABGs) may be obtained to assess for hypoxemia (partial pressure of oxygen in arterial blood [PaO$_2$] less than 80 mm Hg), hypercapnia (partial pressure of carbon dioxide in arterial blood [PaCO$_2$] greater than 45 mm Hg), and acidosis. Leukocytosis occurs in the majority of patients with bacterial pneumonia; the white blood cell (WBC) count is usually greater than 15,000/μL (15×10^9/L) with the presence of bands (immature neutrophils).

The use of biologic markers of infection to guide clinical decisions for treatment of pneumonia is under investigation. Serum levels of C-reactive protein (CRP) and procalcitonin have shown promise in providing information to guide the duration of antibiotic therapy.[10]

Collaborative Care

Pneumococcal vaccine is used to prevent *S. pneumoniae* (pneumococcus) pneumonia. Vaccination is recommended for individuals 65 years of age or older and younger patients who are at high risk. A one-time repeat vaccination in 5 years is recommended for those who received their initial vaccination when less than 65 years of age (Table 28-5).

Prompt treatment with the appropriate antibiotic almost always cures bacterial and mycoplasmal pneumonia. In uncomplicated cases the patient responds to drug therapy within 48 to 72 hours. Indications of improvement include decreased temperature, improved breathing, and reduced chest pain. Abnormal physical findings can last more than 7 days. A repeat chest x-ray is obtained in 6 to 8 weeks to assess for resolution.

In addition to antibiotic therapy, supportive measures are individualized to the patient's needs. These may include O$_2$ therapy to treat hypoxemia, analgesics to relieve chest pain, and antipyretics such as aspirin or acetaminophen for significantly elevated temperature. Although cough suppressants, mucolytics, bronchodilators, and corticosteroids are often prescribed as adjunctive therapy, there is insufficient evidence to support their use.[11]

Individualize rest and activity to the patient's tolerance. Benefits of mobility include improved diaphragm movement and

TABLE 28-5 PNEUMOVAX VACCINATION

Groups for Which Initial Vaccination Is Recommended

- People age ≥65 yr
- People ages 2-64 yr with long-term health problem (e.g., chronic cardiovascular disease, chronic pulmonary disease, sickle cell disease, diabetes mellitus, alcoholism, cirrhosis, leaks of cerebrospinal fluid, or cochlear implant)
- People ages 19-64 yr who smoke cigarettes or have asthma
- People ages 2-64 yr who have a disease or condition that lowers the body's resistance to infection (e.g., Hodgkin's disease, leukemia, lymphoma, kidney failure, multiple myeloma, HIV infection, nephrotic syndrome; those receiving immunosuppressive chemotherapy, radiation therapy, or long-term corticosteroids; asplenia; and after organ or bone marrow transplantation)
- People living in long-term care facilities

Groups for Which Revaccination Is Recommended

People age ≥65 yr	Patients who received vaccine ≥5 yr previously and were <65 yr at the time of vaccination
People ages 2-64 yr who have a disease or condition that lowers the body's resistance to infection (same as above for initial vaccination)	If ≥5 yr have elapsed since receipt of first dose

Source: Centers for Disease Control and Prevention: Pneumococcal polysaccharide vaccine: what you need to know. Retrieved from *www.cdc.gov/vaccines/pubs/vis/downloads/vis-ppv.pdf.*

TABLE 28-6 DRUG THERAPY
Bacterial Community-Acquired Pneumonia

Patient Variable	Treatment Options
Outpatient	
Previously Healthy	
No recent antibiotic therapy in past 3 mo and no risk for drug-resistant *Staphylococcus pneumoniae* (DRSP)	Macrolide OR doxycycline
Co-morbidities (e.g., COPD; diabetes; chronic heart, liver, lung, or renal disease; malignancy; use of antibiotics in past 3 mo)	Respiratory fluoroquinolone OR β-Lactam plus macrolide (doxycycline may be substituted for macrolide)
Regions with ≥25% Macrolide-Resistant S. pneumoniae	Respiratory fluoroquinolone OR β-Lactam plus macrolide
Inpatient	
Medical Unit	Respiratory fluoroquinolone OR β-Lactam plus macrolide
ICU	β-Lactam plus either azithromycin or respiratory fluoroquinolone
Special Conditions	
• *Pseudomonas* infection	Antipneumococcal, antipseudomonal β-lactam plus either ciprofloxacin or levofloxacin OR Antipneumococcal, antipseudomonal β-lactam plus aminoglycoside and azithromycin OR Antipneumococcal, antipseudomonal β-lactam plus an aminoglycoside and an antipneumococcal fluoroquinolone
• *Pseudomonas* infection but patient has penicillin allergy	Substitute aztreonam for the above β-lactam
• Community-acquired methicillin-resistant *Staphylococcus aureus* (CA-MRSA)	Add vancomycin or linezolid (Zyvox)

Types of Antibiotics	
Macrolides	erythromycin, azithromycin (Zithromax), clarithromycin (Biaxin)
Fluoroquinolones	moxifloxacin (Avelox, Vigamox), levofloxacin (Levaquin), gemifloxacin (Factive)
β-Lactams	High-dose amoxicillin, amoxicillin/clavulanate (Augmentin), cefpodoxime (Vantin), ceftriaxone (Rocephin), cefuroxime (Ceftin)
Antipneumococcal, antipseudomonal β-lactams	imipenem/cilastatin (Primaxin), meropenem (Merrem), cefepime (Maxipime), piperacillin/tazobactam (Zosyn)

Source: Adapted from the Infectious Diseases Society of America Practice Guidelines for CAP. Retrieved from *http://www.idsociety.org/Organ_System/#Community AcquiredPneumoniaCAP.*

chest expansion, mobilization of secretions, and prevention of venous stasis.

Currently, no definitive treatment exists for the majority of viral pneumonias. Care is generally supportive. Antiviral therapy may be used to treat pneumonia caused by influenza (e.g., oseltamivir or zanamivir) and a few other select viruses (e.g., acyclovir [Zovirax] for herpes simplex virus).[12]

Drug Therapy. Once the pneumonia is classified, the health care provider bases empiric therapy on the likely infecting organism (see Table 28-2). Table 28-6 presents the drug therapy for bacterial CAP.

For HAP, VAP, and HCAP, empiric antibiotic therapy is based on whether the patient has risk factors for MDR organisms. The prevalence and resistance patterns of MDR pathogens vary among localities and institutions. Therefore the antibiotic regimen needs to be adapted to the local patterns of antibiotic resistance. Appropriate initial antibiotic therapy for HAP, VAP, and HCAP may also vary markedly. Multiple regimens exist, but all should include antibiotics that are effective against both resistant gram-negative and gram-positive organisms. Clinical improvement usually occurs in 3 to 5 days. Patients who deteriorate or fail to respond to therapy require aggressive evaluation to assess for noninfectious etiologies, complications, coexisting infectious processes, or pneumonia caused by a drug-resistant pathogen.

IV antibiotic therapy should be switched to oral therapy as soon as the patient is hemodynamically stable, is improving clinically, is able to ingest oral medication, and has a normally functioning gastrointestinal (GI) tract. Patients on oral therapy do not need to be observed in the hospital and can be discharged to home. Total treatment time for patients with CAP should be a minimum of 5 days, and the patient should be afebrile for 48 to 72 hours before stopping treatment. Longer treatment time may be needed if initial therapy was not active against the identified pathogen or complications occur.

Nutritional Therapy. Hydration is important in the supportive treatment of pneumonia to prevent dehydration and loosen secretions. Individualize and carefully monitor fluid intake if the patient has heart failure. If the patient cannot maintain adequate oral intake, IV administration of fluids and electrolytes may be necessary.

Weight loss often occurs in patients with pneumonia because of increased metabolic needs and difficulty eating due to shortness of breath and pleuritic pain. Small, frequent meals are easier for dyspneic patients to tolerate. Offer foods high in calories and nutrients.

NURSING MANAGEMENT
PNEUMONIA

NURSING ASSESSMENT

Table 28-7 presents subjective and objective data to obtain from a patient with pneumonia.

NURSING DIAGNOSES

Nursing diagnoses for the patient with pneumonia may include, but are not limited to, the following:

- Impaired gas exchange *related to* fluid and exudate accumulation at the capillary-alveolar membrane
- Ineffective breathing pattern *related to* inflammation and pain
- Acute pain *related to* inflammation and ineffective pain management and/or comfort measures

Additional information on nursing diagnoses for the patient with pneumonia can be found in eNursing Care Plan 28-1 on the website for this chapter.

PLANNING

The overall goals are that the patient with pneumonia will have (1) clear breath sounds, (2) normal breathing patterns, (3) no signs of hypoxia, (4) normal chest x-ray, and (5) no complications related to pneumonia.

NURSING IMPLEMENTATION

HEALTH PROMOTION. To reduce the risk of pneumonia, teach individuals to practice good health habits, such as frequent hand washing, proper nutrition, adequate rest, regular exercise, and coughing or sneezing into the elbow rather than hands. Avoidance of cigarette smoke is one of the most important health-promoting behaviors. If possible, people should avoid exposure to people with URIs. If a URI occurs, it requires prompt attention with supportive measures (e.g., rest, fluids). If symptoms persist for longer than 7 days, the person should seek medical care. Encourage those at risk for pneumonia (e.g., the chronically ill, older adult) to obtain both influenza and pneumococcal vaccines (see Tables 27-3 and Table 28-5).

Identifying patients at risk (see Table 28-1) and taking measures to prevent pneumonia are priority interventions. Place the patient with altered consciousness in positions (e.g., side-lying, upright) that will prevent or minimize the risk of aspiration. Turn and reposition the patient at least every 2 hours to facilitate adequate lung expansion and to discourage pooling of secretions. Encourage and assist with ambulation and positioning in a chair. In the intensive care unit, strict adherence to all aspects of the ventilator bundle (see Table 68-8), a group of interventions aimed at reducing the risk of VAP, has been shown to significantly reduce VAP.[13]

TABLE 28-7 NURSING ASSESSMENT

Pneumonia

Subjective Data
Important Health Information
Past health history: Lung cancer, COPD, diabetes mellitus, chronic debilitating disease, malnutrition, altered consciousness, immunosuppression, exposure to chemical toxins, dust, or allergens
Medications: Antibiotics; corticosteroids, chemotherapy, or any other immunosuppressants
Surgery or other treatments: Recent abdominal or thoracic surgery, splenectomy, endotracheal intubation, or any surgery with general anesthesia; tube feedings

Functional Health Patterns
Health perception–health management: Cigarette smoking, alcoholism; recent upper respiratory tract infection, malaise
Nutritional-metabolic: Anorexia, nausea, vomiting; chills
Activity-exercise: Prolonged bed rest or immobility; fatigue, weakness; dyspnea, cough (productive or nonproductive); nasal congestion
Cognitive-perceptual: Pain with breathing, chest pain, sore throat, headache, abdominal pain, muscle aches

Objective Data
General
Fever, restlessness or lethargy; splinting of affected area

Respiratory
Tachypnea; pharyngitis; asymmetric chest movements or retraction; decreased excursion; nasal flaring; use of accessory muscles (neck, abdomen); grunting; crackles, friction rub on auscultation; dullness on percussion over consolidated areas, increased tactile fremitus on palpation; pink, rusty, purulent, green, yellow, or white sputum (amount may be scant to copious)

Cardiovascular
Tachycardia

Neurologic
Changes in mental status, ranging from confusion to delirium

Possible Diagnostic Findings
Leukocytosis; abnormal ABGs with $\downarrow$ or normal PaO_2, $\downarrow$ $PaCO_2$, and $\uparrow$ pH initially, and later $\downarrow$ PaO_2, $\uparrow$ $PaCO_2$, and $\downarrow$ pH; positive sputum on Gram stain and culture; patchy or diffuse infiltrates, abscesses, pleural effusion, or pneumothorax on chest x-ray*

*In the older dehydrated patient, chest x-ray may not be indicative of pneumonia until patient is rehydrated.

Patients who have orogastric or nasogastric tubes are at risk for aspiration pneumonia (see Chapter 40). Although the feeding tube is small, an interruption in the integrity of the lower esophageal sphincter can allow reflux of gastric contents. To prevent aspiration, elevate the head of the bed 30 to 45 degrees and monitor gastric residual volumes (see Table 40-12).

Elevate the patient's head-of-bed to at least 30 degrees and have patient sit up for all meals. The patient who has difficulty swallowing needs assistance in eating, drinking, and taking medication to prevent aspiration. Assess for a gag reflex before giving food or fluids in patients who have received local anesthesia to the throat. Patients with impaired mobility from any cause need assistance with turning and moving, as well as encouragement to breathe deeply at frequent intervals. Early mobilization, the use of an incentive spirometer, and twice-daily oral hygiene with chlorhexidine swabs have been shown to significantly reduce the incidence of pneumonia in postoperative patients.[14] Treat pain to a comfort level that permits the patient to deep breathe, cough, and achieve optimum mobility.

Practice strict medical asepsis and adherence to infection control guidelines to reduce the incidence of health care–associated infections. Staff and visitors should wash their hands on entering and leaving the patient's room. Staff must wash or use sanitizing hand gel before and after providing care and on removing gloves. Respiratory devices, which can harbor microorganisms, have been associated with outbreaks of pneumonia. Use strict sterile aseptic technique when suctioning the patient's trachea, and use caution when handling ventilator circuits, tracheostomy tubing, and nebulizer circuits that can become contaminated from patient secretions. Avoid inappropriate use of antibiotics to prevent the development of drug-resistant organisms.

ACUTE INTERVENTION. Although many patients with pneumonia are treated on an outpatient basis, the nursing care plan for a patient with pneumonia (see eNursing Care Plan 28-1) applies to both these individuals and in-hospital patients. Essential nursing care for patients with pneumonia includes monitoring physical assessment parameters, providing treatment, and monitoring the patient's response to treatment. Along with physical assessment (including pulse oximetry monitoring), prompt collection of specimens and initiation of antibiotics are critical. Oxygen therapy, hydration, nutritional support, breathing exercises, early ambulation, and therapeutic positioning are part of nursing management. Collaboration with respiratory therapy for postural drainage and chest percussion is important.

AMBULATORY AND HOME CARE. Teach the patient about the importance of taking every dose of the prescribed antibiotic, any drug-drug and food-drug interactions for the prescribed antibiotic, and the need for adequate rest to continue recovery. Instruct the patient to drink plenty of liquids (at least 6 to 10 glasses/day, unless contraindicated) and to avoid alcohol and smoking. A cool mist humidifier or warm bath may help the patient breathe easier. Tell patients that it may be several weeks before their usual vigor and sense of well-being return. Explain that a follow-up chest x-ray will be done in 6 to 8 weeks to evaluate resolution of pneumonia. A prolonged period of convalescence may be necessary for the older adult or chronically ill patient.

Teaching should also include information about available influenza and pneumococcal vaccines. Patients can receive the pneumococcal vaccine and influenza vaccine at the same time in different arms.

EVALUATION

The expected outcomes are that the patient with pneumonia will
- Have effective respiratory rate, rhythm, and depth of respirations
- Lungs clear to auscultation

Additional outcomes for the patient with pneumonia are presented in eNursing Care Plan 28-1.

TUBERCULOSIS

Tuberculosis (TB) is an infectious disease caused by *Mycobacterium tuberculosis*. It usually involves the lungs, but any organ can be infected. TB is a primary cause of death worldwide from a potentially curable infectious disease. It is the leading cause of mortality in patients with HIV infection.[15] The incidence of TB worldwide declined until the mid-1980s when HIV disease

emerged. The major factors contributing to the resurgence of TB were (1) high rates of TB among patients with HIV infection and (2) the emergence of MDR strains of *M. tuberculosis*. Worldwide, more than two billion people (one third of the population) are currently infected with TB. Although the prevalence of TB has increased in Europe, in the United States it has steadily declined since reaching a resurgence peak in 1992.[16,17]

TB occurs disproportionately in the poor, the underserved, and minorities. In the United States, people at risk include the homeless, residents of inner-city neighborhoods, foreign-born people, those living or working in institutions (long-term care facilities, prisons, shelters, hospitals), IV injecting drug users, people at poverty level, and those with poor access to health care. Immunosuppression from any etiology (e.g., HIV infection, malignancy, long-term corticosteroid use) increases the risk of active TB infection. The prevalence of TB in the United States is highest in those of Asian descent (see Cultural & Ethnic Health Disparities box).

Once a strain of *M. tuberculosis* develops resistance to two of the most potent first-line antituberculous drugs (e.g., isoniazid [INH], rifampin [Rifadin]), it is defined as *multidrug-resistant tuberculosis* (MDR-TB). Extensively drug-resistant TB (XDR-TB) occurs when the organism is also resistant to any of the fluoroquinolones plus any injectable antibiotic agent. Resistance results from several problems, including incorrect prescribing, lack of public health case management, and patient nonadherence to the prescribed regimen.[18]

Etiology and Pathophysiology

M. tuberculosis is a gram-positive, acid-fast bacillus (AFB) that is usually spread from person to person via airborne droplets produced by breathing, talking, singing, sneezing, and coughing. A process of evaporation leaves small droplet nuclei, 1 to 5 μm in size, suspended in the air for minutes to hours. These droplet nuclei are then transmitted via inhalation to another person. TB is not highly infectious, and transmission usually requires close, frequent, or prolonged exposure. Brief exposure to a few tubercle bacilli rarely causes an infection. The disease cannot be spread by touching, sharing food utensils, kissing, or any other type of physical contact.

Factors that influence the likelihood of transmission include the (1) number of organisms expelled into the air, (2) concentration of organisms (small spaces with limited ventilation

TABLE 28-8 CLASSIFICATION OF TUBERCULOSIS (TB)

Class	Exposure or Infection	Description
0	No TB exposure	No TB exposure, not infected (no history of exposure, negative tuberculin skin test)
1	TB exposure, no infection	TB exposure, no evidence of infection (history of exposure, negative tuberculin skin test)
2	Latent TB infection, no disease	TB infection without disease (significant reaction to tuberculin skin test, negative bacteriologic studies, no x-ray findings compatible with TB, no clinical evidence of TB)
3	TB, clinically active	TB infection with clinically active disease (positive bacteriologic studies or both a significant reaction to tuberculin skin test and clinical or x-ray evidence of current disease)
4	TB, but not clinically active	No current disease (history of previous episode of TB or abnormal, stable x-ray findings in a person with a significant reaction to tuberculin skin test; negative bacteriologic studies if done; no clinical or x-ray evidence of current disease)
5	TB suspect	TB suspect (diagnosis pending); person should not be in this classification for >3 mo

Source: American Thoracic Society.

TABLE 28-9 LATENT TUBERCULOSIS (TB) INFECTION COMPARED WITH TB DISEASE

Latent TB Infection	TB Disease
Has no symptoms	Has symptoms that may include the following: • Bad cough that lasts ≥3 wk • Pain in the chest • Coughing up blood or sputum • Weakness or fatigue • Weight loss • No appetite • Chills • Fever • Sweating at night
Does not feel sick	Usually feels sick
Cannot spread TB bacteria to others	May spread TB bacteria to others
Usually has a skin test or blood test result indicating TB infection	Usually has a skin test or blood test result indicating TB infection
Has a normal chest x-ray and a negative sputum smear	May have an abnormal chest x-ray or positive sputum smear or culture
Needs treatment for latent TB infection to prevent active TB disease	Needs treatment for active TB disease

Source: Centers for Disease Control and Prevention: Tuberculosis (TB): basic TB facts. Retrieved from *www.cdc.gov/tb/topic/basics/default.htm*.

would mean higher concentration), (3) length of time of exposure, and (4) immune system of the exposed person. Once inhaled, these small particles lodge in the bronchiole and alveolus. A local inflammatory reaction occurs, and the focus of infection is established. This is called the *Ghon focus,* which develops into a *granuloma,* the hallmark of TB. The formation of a granuloma is a defense mechanism aimed at walling off the infection and preventing further spread. Replication of the bacillus is inhibited and the infection is stopped.

Seventy percent of immunocompetent adults infected with TB are able to completely kill the mycobacteria. The rest of them contain the mycobacteria in a nonreplicating dormant state. Of these individuals, 5% to 10% go on to develop active TB infection when the bacteria begin to multiply months or years later. *M. tuberculosis* is aerophilic (oxygen loving) and thus has an affinity for the lungs. However, the infection can spread via the lymphatic system and find favorable environments for growth in other organs, including the kidneys, epiphyses of the bone, cerebral cortex, and adrenal glands.

Classification

Several systems can be used to classify TB. The American Thoracic Society classifies TB based on development of the disease (Table 28-8). TB can also be classified according to its (1) presentation (primary, latent, or reactivated) and (2) whether it is pulmonary or extrapulmonary.

Primary infection occurs when the bacteria are inhaled and initiate an inflammatory reaction. The majority of people mount effective immune responses to encapsulate these organisms for the rest of their lives, preventing primary infection from progressing to disease.

Latent TB infection (LTBI) occurs in a person who does not have active TB disease (Table 28-9). These individuals are asymptomatic and cannot transmit the TB bacteria to others. An estimated 10 million to 15 million Americans have LTBI; of these, 5% to 10% will develop active TB disease at some point. Therefore treatment of LTBI is important (discussed later in this chapter).

If the initial immune response is not adequate, the body cannot contain the organisms, the bacteria replicate, and *active TB disease* results. When active disease develops within the first 2 years of infection, it is termed *primary TB.* Postprimary TB, or *reactivation TB,* is defined as TB disease occurring 2 or more years after the initial infection. Individuals co-infected with HIV are at greatest risk for developing active TB. Immunosuppression, diabetes mellitus, poor nutrition, aging, pregnancy, stress, and chronic disease can also precipitate the reactivation of LTBI.[18] If the site of TB is pulmonary or laryngeal, the individual is considered infectious and can transmit the disease to others.

Clinical Manifestations

People with LTBI have a positive skin test but are asymptomatic (see Table 28-9). Symptoms of pulmonary TB usually do not develop until 2 to 3 weeks after infection or reactivation. The characteristic pulmonary manifestation is an initial dry cough that frequently becomes productive with mucoid or mucopurulent sputum. Active TB disease may initially manifest with constitutional symptoms such as fatigue, malaise, anorexia, unexplained weight loss, low-grade fevers, and night sweats. Dyspnea is a late symptom that may signify considerable pulmonary disease or a pleural effusion. Hemoptysis, which occurs in less than 10% of patients with TB, is also a late symptom.

Sometimes TB has a more acute, sudden presentation. The patient may have a high fever, chills, generalized flu-like symptoms, pleuritic pain, and a productive cough. Auscultation of the lungs may be normal or reveal crackles, rhonchi, and/or bronchial breath sounds.

Immunosuppressed (e.g., HIV-infected) people and older adults are less likely to have fever and other signs of an infection. In patients with HIV, classic manifestations of TB such as fever, cough, and weight loss may be wrongly attributed to PCP or other HIV-associated opportunistic diseases. Clinical manifestations of respiratory problems in patients with HIV must be carefully investigated to determine the cause. A change in cognitive function may be the only initial presenting sign of TB in an older person.

The clinical manifestations of extrapulmonary TB depend on the organs infected. For example, renal TB can cause dysuria and hematuria. Bone and joint TB may cause severe pain. Headaches, vomiting, and lymphadenopathy may be present with TB meningitis.

Complications

Appropriately treated pulmonary TB typically heals without complications except for a scar and residual cavitation within the lung. Significant pulmonary damage, although rare, can occur in patients who are poorly treated or who do not respond to anti-TB treatment.

Miliary TB is the widespread dissemination of the mycobacterium. The bacteria are spread via the bloodstream to distant organs. The infection is characterized by a large amount of TB bacilli and may be fatal if left untreated. It can occur as a result of primary disease or reactivation of latent infection. Clinical manifestations of miliary TB slowly progress over a period of days, weeks, or even months. Symptoms vary depending on which organs are infected. Hepatomegaly, splenomegaly, and generalized lymphadenopathy may be present.

Pleural TB can result from either primary disease or reactivation of a latent infection. A pleural effusion is caused by bacteria in the pleural space, which trigger an inflammatory reaction and a pleural exudate of protein-rich fluid. Empyema is less common than effusion but may occur from large numbers of tubercular organisms in the pleural space.

Acute pneumonia may result when large amounts of tubercle bacilli are discharged from granulomas into the lung or lymph nodes. The clinical manifestations are similar to those of bacterial pneumonia.

Because TB can infect organs throughout the body, various acute and long-term complications can result. TB in the spine (Pott's disease) can lead to destruction of the intervertebral disc and adjacent vertebrae. Central nervous system TB can cause severe bacterial meningitis. Abdominal TB can lead to peritonitis, especially in HIV-positive patients. The kidneys, adrenal glands, lymph nodes, and urogenital tract may also be affected.

Diagnostic Studies

Tuberculin Skin Test. The tuberculin skin test (TST) (Mantoux test) using purified protein derivative (PPD) is the standard method to screen people for *M. tuberculosis*. The test is administered by injecting 0.1 mL of PPD intradermally on the dorsal surface of the forearm. The test is read by inspection and palpation 48 to 72 hours later for the presence or absence of induration. Induration (not redness) at the injection site means the person has been exposed to TB and has developed antibodies. (Antibody formation would occur 2 to 12 weeks after the initial exposure to the organisms.) The indurated area (if present) is measured and recorded in millimeters. Based on the size

of the induration and the risk factors, an interpretation is made according to diagnostic standards for determining a positive test reaction.[15] (The procedure for performing the TST is described in Chapter 26.) Because the immunocompromised patient may have a decreased response to TST, smaller induration reactions (5 mm or larger) are considered positive. (See Table 26-11 for guidelines in interpreting responses to the TST.)

Some people who were previously infected with TB may have a waning immune response to the TST, resulting in a false negative result. However, the repeated TST may stimulate (boost) the body's ability to react to tuberculin in future tests. A positive reaction to a subsequent test could then be misinterpreted as a new infection, rather than the result of the boosted reaction to an old infection. To prevent misinterpretation in future testing, a two-step testing process is recommended for initial testing for health care workers (who get repeated testing) and for individuals who have a decreased response to allergens. A negative two-step TST ensures that any future positive results can be accurately interpreted as being caused by a new infection.[19]

Interferon-γ Release Assays. Interferon-γ (INF-γ) release assays (IGRAs) provide another screening tool for TB. These whole blood assays detect INF-γ released from T lymphocytes in response to mycobacterial antigens. Examples of IGRAs include QuantiFERON-TB test and the T-SPOT.TB test. Test results are available in a few hours.

IGRAs offer several advantages over the TST in that they require only one patient visit, are not subject to reader bias, have no booster phenomenon, and are not affected by prior bacillus Calmette-Guérin (BCG) vaccination.[15] The cost of an IGRA is substantially higher than the TST. Current guidelines suggest that both tests are viable options and that selection should be based on context and reasons for testing. Neither IGRAs nor TST can distinguish between LTBI and active TB infection. LTBI can only be diagnosed by excluding active TB.

Chest X-Ray. Although the findings on chest x-ray examination are important, it is not possible to make a diagnosis of TB solely on chest x-ray findings, since other diseases can mimic the appearance of TB. The chest x-ray may also appear normal in a patient with TB. Findings suggestive of TB include upper lobe infiltrates, cavitary infiltrates, and lymph node involvement.

Bacteriologic Studies. The diagnosis of TB requires the demonstration of tubercle bacilli bacteriologically. The initial testing involves a microscopic examination of stained sputum smears for AFB. Three consecutive sputum specimens collected on different days are obtained and sent for smear and culture. The culture to grow the organisms for confirmatory diagnosis can take up to 8 weeks. Treatment is warranted pending results for patients in whom clinical suspicion of TB is high. Samples for other suspected TB sites can be collected from gastric washings, cerebrospinal fluid (CSF), or fluid from an effusion or abscess.

Collaborative Care

Most patients with TB are treated on an outpatient basis (Table 28-10). Many people can continue to work and maintain their lifestyles with few changes. Patients with sputum smear–positive TB are generally considered infectious for the first 2 weeks after starting treatment. Advise these patients to restrict visitors and avoid travel on public transportation and trips to public places. Hospitalization may be needed for the severely ill or debilitated.

TABLE 28-10 COLLABORATIVE CARE
Pulmonary Tuberculosis

Diagnostic	Collaborative Therapy
• History and physical examination • Tuberculin skin test (TST) • QuantiFERON-TB test • Chest x-ray • Bacteriologic studies • Sputum smear for acid-fast bacilli (AFB) • Sputum culture	• Long-term treatment with antimicrobial drugs (see Tables 28-11 and 28-12) • Follow-up bacteriologic studies and chest x-rays

TABLE 28-11 DRUG THERAPY
Tuberculosis (TB)

Drug	Side Effects*
isoniazid (INH)	Hepatitis, asymptomatic elevation of aminotransferases (ALT, AST) Monitor liver function tests monthly
rifampin (Rifadin)	Hepatitis, thrombocytopenia, orange discoloration of bodily fluids (sputum, urine, sweat, tears)
pyrazinamide (PZA)	Hepatitis, arthralgias, hyperuricemia
ethambutol (Myambutol)	Ocular toxicity (decreased red-green color discrimination) Monitor visual acuity and color discrimination regularly
rifabutin (Mycobutin)	Hepatitis, thrombocytopenia, neutropenia, orange discoloration of bodily fluids (sputum, urine, sweat, tears)
rifapentine (Priftin)	Similar to those of rifampin
streptomycin	Ototoxicity, neurotoxicity, nephrotoxicity
bedaquiline (Sirturo)	Dysrhythmias
aminoglycosides	Ototoxicity, nephrotoxicity

capreomycin (Capastat)
  kanamycin (Kantrex)
  amikacin (Amikin)
	Used in selected cases for treatment of resistant strains

fluoroquinolones
  levofloxacin (Levaquin)
  moxifloxacin (Avelox, Vigamox)
	GI disturbance, neurologic effects (dizziness, headache), rash
	Used in drug-resistant TB

*Only common side effects are listed.
ALT, Alanine transaminase; *AST,* aspartate aminotransferase.

TABLE 28-12 DRUG THERAPY
Tuberculosis Disease Regimens

Initial Phase	Continuation Phase
Option 1 4-drug regimen consisting of INH, rifampin, pyrazinamide, ethambutol Given daily for 56 doses (8 wk) OR 5 days/wk DOT for 40 doses (8 wk)	INH, rifampin daily for 126 doses (18 wk) OR 5 days/wk DOT for 90 doses (18 wk)
Option 2 4-drug regimen consisting of INH, rifampin, pyrazinamide, ethambutol Given daily for 14 doses (2 wk), followed by twice weekly for 12 doses (6 wk) OR 5 days/wk DOT for 10 doses (2 wk), then twice weekly for 12 doses (6 wk)	INH, rifampin twice weekly for 36 doses (18 wk) OR once weekly for 18 doses (18 wk)
Option 3 4-drug regimen consisting of INH, rifampin, pyrazinamide, ethambutol Given 3 times weekly for 24 doses (8 wk)	INH, rifampin 3 times weekly for 54 doses (18 wk)
Option 4 3-drug regimen consisting of INH, rifampin, ethambutol Given daily for 56 doses (8 wk) OR 5 days/wk DOT for 40 doses (8 wk)	INH, rifampin daily for 217 doses (31 wk) OR 5 days/wk DOT for 155 doses (31 wk) OR twice weekly for 62 doses (31 wk)

Source: American Thoracic Society, Centers for Disease Control and Prevention, and Infectious Diseases Society of America: Treatment of tuberculosis. Retrieved from *www.cdc.gov/mmwr/PDF/rr/rr5211.pdf.*
DOT, Directly observed therapy; *INH,* isoniazid.

> **DRUG ALERT: Isoniazid (INH)**
> • Alcohol may increase hepatotoxicity of the drug. Instruct patient to avoid drinking alcohol during treatment.
> • Monitor for signs of liver damage before and while taking drug.

Other drugs can be used if the patient develops a toxic reaction to the primary drugs. The newer rifamycins, rifabutin and rifapentine (Priftin), should be considered first line in special situations: rifabutin for patients receiving medications that have interactions with rifampin or who have an intolerance to rifampin, and rifapentine with INH in once-weekly dosing for selected patients. Treatment for drug-resistant TB is guided by sensitivity testing. MDR-TB therapy typically includes a fluoroquinolone and an injectable antibiotic (see Table 28-11). Bedaquiline (Sirturo), a relatively new drug, is used in combination with other drugs to treat MDR-TB. It works by inhibiting an enzyme needed for *M. tuberculosis* to replicate.

Directly observed therapy (DOT) involves providing the antituberculous drugs directly to patients and watching as they swallow the medications. It is the preferred strategy for all patients with TB to ensure adherence and is recommended for all patients at risk for nonadherence.[15] Nonadherence is a major factor in the emergence of multidrug resistance and treatment failures. Many individuals do not adhere to the treatment program in spite of understanding the disease process and the value of treatment. DOT is an expensive but essential public health measure. The risk for reactivation of TB and MDR-TB is increased in patients who do not complete the full course of therapy. In many areas the public health nurse administers DOT at a clinic site.

The mainstay of TB treatment is drug therapy (Table 28-11). Promoting and monitoring adherence are critical for treatment to be successful.

Drug Therapy

Active TB Disease. Because of the growing prevalence of MDR-TB, it is important to manage the patient with active TB aggressively. Drug therapy is divided into two phases: initial and continuation (Table 28-12). In most circumstances the treatment regimen for patients with previously untreated TB consists of a 2-month initial phase with four-drug therapy (INH, rifampin, pyrazinamide [PZA], and ethambutol). If drug susceptibility test results indicate that the bacteria are susceptible to all drugs, ethambutol may be discontinued. If PZA cannot be included in the initial phase (because of liver disease, pregnancy, etc.), the remaining three drugs are used for the initial phase.

ETHICAL/LEGAL DILEMMAS
Patient Adherence

Situation
The health clinic for the homeless discovers that F.C., a 64-year-old African American man with tuberculosis (TB), has not been taking his prescribed medication. He tells you that it is hard for him to get to the clinic to obtain the medication, much less to keep on a schedule. You are concerned not only about this patient, but also about the risks for the other people at the shelter, in the park, and at the meal sites.

Ethical/Legal Points for Consideration
- Adherence is a complex issue involving a person's culture and values, perceived risk of disease, availability of resources, access to treatment, and perceived consequences of available choices.
- Advocacy for the patient and the community obliges you to involve other members of the health care team, such as social services, to assist in obtaining the necessary resources or support for the patient to complete a course of treatment.
- Legally the constitutionally granted right to control one's own body may be limited by the state and federal obligation to protect public health and safety. Most of these laws have provisions for the protection of constitutional rights such as right to counsel, the right to least restrictive alternative in terms of confinement setting, and the right to prompt judicial review.
- The federal government and many states have provisions for quarantine, detention, and treatment. With the threats of bioterrorism and the globalization of exposure to highly lethal infectious diseases, it seems unlikely that the government's power to detain will be removed.

Discussion Questions
1. What alternatives of care can be offered to F.C.?
2. Under what circumstances are health care providers justified in overriding a patient's autonomy or decision making?

When DOT is not used, fixed-dose combination drugs may enhance adherence. Combinations of INH and rifampin (Rifamate) and of INH, rifampin, and PZA (Rifater) are available to simplify therapy. The therapy for people with HIV follows the same therapy options outlined in Table 28-12. However, alternative regimens that include once-weekly INH plus rifapentine continuation dosing in any HIV-infected patient and twice-weekly INH plus rifampin or rifabutin should not be used if CD4$^+$ counts are less than 100/μL. Health care providers must also be alert for possible drug interactions between antiretrovirals (used to treat HIV) and rifamycins.

Teaching patients about the side effects of these drugs and when to seek prompt medical attention is critical. The major side effect of INH, rifampin, and PZA is nonviral hepatitis. Baseline liver function tests (LFTs) are done at the start of treatment. Monthly monitoring of LFTs is done if baseline tests are abnormal.

Latent Tuberculosis Infection. In people with LTBI, drug therapy helps prevent a TB infection from developing into active TB disease. Because a person with LTBI has fewer bacteria, treatment is much easier. Usually only one drug is needed. Drug therapy regimens for LTBI are presented in Table 28-13.

The standard treatment regimen for LTBI is 9 months of daily INH. It is an effective and inexpensive drug that the patient can take orally. The 9-month regimen is more effective, but adherence issues may make a 6-month regimen preferable. For HIV patients and those with fibrotic lesions on chest x-ray, INH is given for 9 months. An alternative 3-month regimen of INH

TABLE 28-13   DRUG THERAPY
Latent Tuberculosis Infection Regimens

Drugs	Duration	Interval	Minimum Doses
isoniazid	9 mo	Daily	270
		Twice weekly*	76
isoniazid	6 mo	Daily	180
		Twice weekly*	52
isoniazid and rifapentine	3 mo	Once weekly*	12
rifampin	4 mo	Daily	120

Source: Centers for Disease Control and Prevention: Tuberculosis (TB): treatment options for latent tuberculosis infection. Retrieved from *www.cdc.gov/tb/publications/factsheets/treatment/LTBItreatmentoptions.htm.*
* Use directly observed therapy (DOT).

and rifapentine may be used for otherwise healthy patients who are not presumed to be infected with drug-resistant bacilli. Four-month therapy with rifampin may be indicated if the patient is resistant to INH. Because of reports of severe liver injury and deaths, the CDC does not recommend the combination of rifampin and PZA for treatment of LTBI.

Vaccine. BCG vaccine is a live, attenuated strain of *Mycobacterium bovis.* The vaccine is given to infants in parts of the world with a high prevalence of TB. In the United States it is typically not recommended because of the low risk of infection, the vaccine's variable effectiveness against adult pulmonary TB, and potential interference with TB skin test reactivity. The BCG vaccination can result in a false-positive TST. IGRA results are not affected. The BCG vaccine should be considered only for select individuals who meet specific criteria (e.g., health care workers who are continually exposed to patients with MDR-TB and when infection control precautions are not successful).

NURSING MANAGEMENT TUBERCULOSIS

NURSING ASSESSMENT
Ask the patient about a previous history of TB, chronic illness, or any immunosuppressive medications. Obtain a social and occupational history to determine risk factors for transmission of TB. Assess the patient for productive cough, night sweats, afternoon temperature elevation, weight loss, pleuritic chest pain, and abnormal lung sounds. If the patient has a productive cough, early morning is the ideal time to collect sputum specimens for an AFB smear.

NURSING DIAGNOSES
Nursing diagnoses for the patient with TB may include, but are not limited to, the following:
- Ineffective breathing pattern *related to* decreased lung capacity
- Ineffective airway clearance *related to* increased secretions, fatigue, and decreased lung capacity
- Noncompliance *related to* lack of knowledge of disease process, lack of motivation, long-term nature of treatment, and lack of resources
- Ineffective self-health management *related to* lack of knowledge about the disease process and therapeutic regimen

PLANNING

The overall goals are that the patient with TB will (1) comply with the therapeutic regimen, (2) have no recurrence of disease, (3) have normal pulmonary function, and (4) take appropriate measures to prevent the spread of the disease.

NURSING IMPLEMENTATION

HEALTH PROMOTION. The ultimate goal is to eradicate TB worldwide. Screening programs in known risk groups are of value in detecting individuals with TB. Treatment of LTBI reduces the number of TB carriers in the community. The person with a positive TST should have a chest x-ray to assess for active TB disease. Individuals with a diagnosis of TB must be reported to the public health authorities for identification and assessment of contacts and risk to the community.

Programs to address the social determinants of TB are necessary to decrease transmission of TB.[20] Reducing HIV infection, poverty, overcrowded living conditions, malnutrition, smoking, and drug and alcohol abuse can help minimize TB infection rates. Improving access to health care and education is also important.

ACUTE INTERVENTION. Patients admitted to the emergency department or directly to the nursing unit with respiratory symptoms should be triaged for the possibility of TB. Those strongly suspected of having TB should (1) be placed on airborne isolation; (2) receive a medical workup, including chest x-ray, sputum smear, and culture; and (3) receive appropriate drug therapy. Airborne infection isolation is indicated for the patient with pulmonary or laryngeal TB until the patient is noninfectious (defined as effective drug therapy, clinical improvement, and three negative AFB smears). *Airborne infection isolation* refers to isolation of patients infected with organisms spread by the airborne route. It requires a single-occupancy room with negative pressure and airflow of 6 to 12 exchanges per hour.

High-efficiency particulate air (HEPA) masks are worn whenever entering the patient's room. These masks are highly effective at protecting from small particles 5 μm or less in diameter. Health care providers should be "fit tested" to ensure proper mask size. To be effective, the mask must be molded to fit tightly around the nose and mouth.

Teach patients to cover the nose and mouth with paper tissues every time they cough, sneeze, or produce sputum. The tissues should be thrown into a paper bag and disposed of with the trash, burned, or flushed down the toilet. Emphasize careful hand washing after handling sputum and soiled tissues. If patients need to be out of the negative-pressure room, they must wear a standard isolation mask to prevent exposure to others. Minimize prolonged visitation to other parts of the hospital.

Identify and screen close contacts of the person with TB. Anyone testing positive for TB infection will undergo further evaluation and needs to be treated for either LTBI or active TB disease.

AMBULATORY AND HOME CARE. Patients who respond clinically are discharged home (even with positive cultures) if their household contacts have already been exposed and the patient is not posing a risk to susceptible people. Negative cultures are needed to declare the patient not infectious. Monthly sputum collections for AFB are obtained until two consecutive specimens are culture negative.[15]

Teach the patient how to minimize exposure to close contacts and household members. Homes should be well ventilated, especially the areas where the infected person spends a lot of time. While still infectious, the patient should sleep alone, spend as much time as possible outdoors, and minimize time in congregate settings or on public transportation.

Teach the patient and caregiver about adherence with the prescribed regimen. This is important, since most treatment failures occur because the patient neglects to take the drug, discontinues it prematurely, or takes it irregularly. Strategies to improve adherence to drug therapy include teaching and counseling, reminder systems, incentives or rewards, contracts, and DOT.

Notification of the public health department is required. The public health nurse is responsible for follow-up on household contacts and assessment of the patient for adherence. If adherence is an issue, the public health agency may be responsible for DOT. Most individuals can be considered adequately treated when the therapy regimen has been completed and there is evidence of negative cultures, clinical improvement, and improvement on chest x-ray.

Because about 5% of individuals experience relapses, teach the patient to recognize the symptoms that indicate recurrence of TB. If these symptoms occur, the patient should seek immediate medical attention. Instruct the patient about certain factors that could reactivate TB, such as immunosuppressive therapy, malignancy, and prolonged debilitating illness. If the patient experiences any of these events, the health care provider must be told so that reactivation of TB can be closely monitored. In some situations it is necessary to put the patient on anti-TB therapy. Because smoking is associated with poor outcomes in TB, patients should be encouraged to quit. Provide patients with teaching and resources to help them stop smoking.

EVALUATION

The expected outcomes are that the patient with TB will have
- Complete resolution of the disease
- Normal pulmonary function
- Absence of any complications
- No transmission of TB

ATYPICAL MYCOBACTERIA

There are more than 30 varieties of acid-fast mycobacteria that do not cause TB but can cause pulmonary disease, lymphadenitis, skin or soft tissue disease, or disseminated disease. Pulmonary disease is indistinguishable from TB clinically and radiologically but can be differentiated by bacteriologic culture. Atypical mycobacteria are not airborne and thus are not transmitted by droplets.

Mycobacterium avium complex (MAC), found in aerosols generated from baths, hot spas, and swimming pools, is the most common cause of atypical mycobacteria pulmonary infection. Only a small number of people exposed to the organism actually develop MAC lung disease. People who are immunosuppressed (e.g., HIV/AIDS) or have chronic pulmonary disease are most susceptible. Treatment is similar to that for TB.

PULMONARY FUNGAL INFECTIONS

Pulmonary fungal pneumonia is an infectious process in the lungs caused by endemic (native and common) or opportunis-

TABLE 28-14 FUNGAL INFECTIONS OF THE LUNG

Infection	Organism
Endemic Fungal Infections	
Histoplasmosis	*Histoplasma capsulatum*
Coccidioidomycosis	*Coccidioides immitis*
Blastomycosis	*Blastomyces dermatitidis*
Opportunistic Fungal Infections	
Candidiasis	*Candida albicans*
Aspergillosis	*Aspergillus niger* or *Aspergillus fumigatus*
Cryptococcosis	*Cryptococcus neoformans*

tic fungi (Table 28-14). *Endemic* fungal pathogens cause infection in healthy people and in immunocompromised people in certain geographic locations in the United States. For example, *Coccidioides*, which cause coccidioidomycosis, is a fungus found in the soil of dry, low rainfall areas. It is endemic in many areas of the southwestern United States. *Opportunistic* fungal infections occur in immunocompromised patients (e.g., those being treated with corticosteroids, chemotherapy, and immunosuppressive drugs) and in patients with HIV and cystic fibrosis. These infections can be very serious.

Fungal infections are acquired by inhalation of spores. These infections are not transmitted from person to person, and the patient does not have to be placed in isolation. The clinical manifestations are similar to those of bacterial pneumonia. Skin testing, serology, and biopsy methods assist in identifying the infecting organism.

Amphotericin B remains the standard therapy for treating serious systemic fungal infections. It must be given IV to achieve adequate blood and tissue levels because the GI tract does not absorb it well. Less serious infections can be treated with oral antifungals such as ketoconazole (Nizoral), fluconazole (Diflucan), voriconazole (Vfend), and itraconazole (Sporanox). Effectiveness of therapy can be monitored with fungal serology titers.[21]

LUNG ABSCESS

Etiology and Pathophysiology

A lung abscess is caused by necrosis of lung tissue typically resulting from bacteria aspirated from the GI tract or from the oral cavity in patients with periodontal disease. Because oral secretions can contain large amounts of bacteria, even small amounts *(microaspiration)* can cause infection. The abscess usually develops slowly, beginning with an enlarging area of infection that becomes necrotic and eventually forms a cavity filled with purulent material. Lung abscesses can also result from IV drug use, malignancy, pulmonary emboli, TB, and various parasitic and fungal diseases. Abscesses usually contain more than one type of microbe, most commonly reflecting the anaerobic flora of the mouth.

The area of the lung most often affected is the posterior segment of the right upper lobe. The abscess may erode into the bronchial system, causing the production of foul-smelling or sour-tasting sputum. It may grow toward the pleura and cause pleuritic pain. Multiple small abscesses, sometimes referred to as necrotizing pneumonia, can occur within the lung.

Clinical Manifestations and Complications

Clinical manifestations usually occur slowly over a period of weeks to months, especially if anaerobic organisms are the primary cause. Symptoms of abscess caused by aerobic bacteria develop more acutely and resemble bacterial pneumonia. The most common manifestation is cough-producing purulent sputum (often dark brown) that is foul smelling and foul tasting. Hemoptysis is common, especially when an abscess ruptures into a bronchus. Other common manifestations are fever, chills, prostration, night sweats, pleuritic pain, dyspnea, anorexia, and weight loss.

Physical examination of the lungs indicates dullness to percussion and decreased breath sounds on auscultation over the involved segment of lung. Bronchial breath sounds may be transmitted to the periphery if the communicating bronchus becomes patent and the segment begins to drain. Crackles may also be present in the later stages as the abscess drains.

Complications include chronic pulmonary abscess, bronchopleural fistula, bronchiectasis, and empyema from perforation of the abscess into the pleural cavity. The infection can also spread via the bloodstream, resulting in a brain abscess.

Diagnostic Studies

A chest x-ray is often the only test needed. The presence of a solitary cavitary lesion with an air-fluid level and local infiltrate can confirm the diagnosis. Computed tomography (CT) scanning may be helpful if the cavitation is not clear on chest x-ray. As long as there is drainage via the bronchus, sputum will contain the microorganisms that are present in the abscess. However, expectorated sputum samples are contaminated with oral flora, making it difficult to determine the offending organisms. Bronchoscopy may be used (1) to avoid oropharyngeal contamination, (2) to collect a specimen if drainage is delayed, or (3) to investigate if there is a possibility of an underlying malignancy. Pleural fluid and blood cultures may be useful to identify the offending organisms. Although nonspecific, an elevated neutrophil count from a complete blood count (CBC) indicates an infectious process.

NURSING AND COLLABORATIVE MANAGEMENT
LUNG ABSCESS

Monitor the patient's vital signs, level of consciousness, and respiratory status for any signs of hypoxia. Note any cyanosis or clubbing of the fingers. Administer oxygen as needed. Broadspectrum antibiotic coverage is necessary because of mixed bacteria in an abscess. IV antibiotic therapy should be started as soon as possible. Clindamycin is first-line therapy. Parenteral antibiotics are switched to oral antibiotics once the patient shows clinical and x-ray evidence of improvement.

Because of the need for prolonged antibiotic therapy, the patient must be aware of the importance of continuing the medication for the prescribed period. Sometimes the patient is asked to return periodically during the course of antibiotic therapy for repeat cultures and sensitivity tests to ensure that the infecting organism is not becoming resistant to the antibiotic. When antibiotic therapy is completed, the patient is reevaluated.

Teach the patient how to cough effectively (see Table 29-23). Chest physiotherapy and postural drainage are not recommended because they may cause spillage of infection into other bronchi, extending the infection. Rest, good nutrition, and adequate fluid intake are supportive measures to facilitate recovery. If dentition is poor and dental hygiene is not adequate, encourage the patient to obtain dental care. Consider collaboration with the social worker to evaluate available options for dental care if the patient has limited resources.

Percutaneous drainage of the abscess may be necessary if the patient does not adequately respond to antibiotic treatment. A CT- or ultrasound-guided catheter is placed to drain the abscess. Surgery is rarely indicated but occasionally necessary when reinfection of a large cavitary lesion occurs or to establish a diagnosis when there is evidence of an underlying problem such as a neoplasm. The usual procedure in such cases is a lobectomy. A pneumonectomy may be necessary for multiple abscesses.

ENVIRONMENTAL LUNG DISEASES

Environmental or occupational lung diseases result from inhaled dust or chemicals. The extent of lung damage is influenced by the toxicity of the inhaled substance, amount and duration of exposure, and individual susceptibility. Environmentally induced lung disease includes pneumoconiosis, chemical pneumonitis, hypersensitivity pneumonitis, and asthma. (Asthma is discussed in Chapter 29.)

Pneumoconiosis is a general term for a group of lung diseases caused by inhalation and retention of mineral or metal dust particles. The literal meaning of *pneumoconiosis* is "dust in the lungs." These diseases are classified according to the origin of the dust (e.g., silicosis, asbestosis, berylliosis). Black lung is caused by inhalation of large amounts of coal dust, an occupational hazard for underground coal miners. The inhaled substance is ingested by macrophages, which releases substances that cause cell injury and death. Fibrosis occurs as a result of tissue repair. Repeated exposure eventually results in diffuse *pulmonary fibrosis* (excess connective tissue). Fibrosis is the result of tissue repair after inflammation. Pneumoconiosis and other environmental lung diseases are presented in eTable 28-1 available on the website for this chapter.

Chemical pneumonitis results from exposures to toxic chemical fumes. Acutely, there is diffuse lung injury characterized as pulmonary edema. Chronically, the clinical picture is that of *bronchiolitis obliterans* (obstruction of the bronchioles due to inflammation and fibrosis), which is usually associated with a normal chest x-ray or one that shows hyperinflation. An example is silo filler's disease.

Hypersensitivity pneumonitis, or extrinsic allergic alveolitis, is a form of parenchymal lung disease seen when an individual inhales antigens to which he or she is allergic. Examples include bird fancier's lung and farmer's lung.

Lung cancer, either squamous cell carcinoma or adenocarcinoma, is the most frequent cancer associated with asbestos exposure. People with more exposure are at a greater risk of disease. There is a minimum lapse of 15 to 19 years between first exposure and development of lung cancer. Mesotheliomas, both pleural and peritoneal, are also associated with asbestos exposure.

Clinical Manifestations

Symptoms of many environmental lung diseases may not occur until at least 10 to 15 years after the initial exposure to the inhaled irritant. Clinical manifestations common to all pneu-

moconioses include dyspnea, cough, wheezing, and weight loss. Pulmonary function studies often show reduced vital capacity. A chest x-ray often reveals lung involvement specific to the primary problem. CT scans have been useful in detecting early lung involvement.

Cor pulmonale (described later in this chapter) is a late complication, especially in conditions characterized by diffuse pulmonary fibrosis. COPD is the most common complication of environmental lung disease. Other associated disorders include lung cancer, mesothelioma, and TB. Manifestations of these complications are often the reason the patient seeks health care.

Manifestations of acute hypersensitivity pneumonitis occur 4 to 6 hours after exposure and include chills, fever, cough, shortness of breath, and malaise. Symptoms of chronic hypersensitivity pneumonitis include cough, anorexia, and weight loss. Acute pulmonary edema may occur after exposure to chemical fumes.

Collaborative Care

The best approach to management of environmental lung diseases is to try to prevent or decrease environmental and occupational exposure. Teach the public about the risk and the appropriate protective equipment. Using well-designed, effective ventilation systems and wearing masks are appropriate for some occupations and household activities. Inhalation of smoke by nonsmoking workers has led to regulations requiring a smoke-free workplace. Periodic inspections and monitoring of workplaces by agencies such as the Occupational Safety and Health Administration (OSHA) and the National Institute for Occupational Safety and Health (NIOSH) reinforce the employers' obligations to provide a safe work environment. NIOSH is responsible for workplace safety and health regulations in the United States (*www.cdc.gov/niosh/homepage.html*).

Early diagnosis is essential to halting the disease process. Strategies are directed toward preventing disease progression and improving or controlling respiratory symptoms. Discontinuation of exposure to the offending inhalant and smoking cessation may or may not be effective in stopping disease progression. Strategies to improve respiratory status include O_2 therapy, inhaled bronchodilators, percussion therapy, and pulmonary rehabilitation. Patients should also be immunized against pneumococcal pneumonia and influenza.

LUNG CANCER

Lung cancer is the leading cause of cancer-related deaths in the United States. Lung cancer accounts for 28% of all cancer deaths, more than those caused by breast, prostate, and colon cancer combined. An estimated 225,000 new cases of lung cancer are diagnosed and 160,000 deaths occur each year in the United States. Although lung cancer is associated with a high mortality and low cure rate, advances in medical treatment are improving the response to treatment.[22]

Etiology

Smoking is responsible for 80% to 90% of all lung cancers. Tobacco smoke contains 60 carcinogens in addition to substances (carbon monoxide, nicotine) that interfere with normal cell development. Exposure to tobacco smoke causes changes in the bronchial epithelium, which usually returns to normal when smoking is discontinued. The risk of lung cancer gradually

🌐 CULTURAL & ETHNIC HEALTH DISPARITIES

Lung Cancer

African Americans
- Have the highest incidence of lung cancer
- Are more likely to die from lung cancer than any other ethnic group
- Have a higher rate of lung cancer among men than in other ethnic groups

Whites
- Have the second-highest death rate from lung cancer
- Have a higher rate of lung cancer among women than in other ethnic groups

Asian/Pacific Islanders and Hispanics
- Have the lowest rates of lung cancer in both men and women

Other
- Regional variations among ethnic groups may be due to smoking prevalence, exposure to cancer-causing substances, and other factors.
- Cigarette consumption has decreased dramatically in developed countries such as the United States and Canada.
- Cigarette smoking is increasing in developing countries (e.g., nations in Africa, Asia, Latin America).

Source: Centers for Disease Control and Prevention: Racial/ethnic disparities and geographic differences in lung cancer incidence—38 states and the District of Columbia, 1998-2006. Retrieved from *www.cdc.gov/mmwr/PDF/wk/mm5944.pdf.*

GENDER DIFFERENCES

Lung Cancer

Men	Women
• More men than women are diagnosed with lung cancer. • More men than women die from lung cancer. • Male smokers are 10 times more likely to develop lung cancer than nonsmokers. • Men with lung cancer have a worse prognosis than women. • Lung cancer incidence and deaths are decreasing in men.	• Lung cancer incidence and deaths are increasing in women. • Women develop lung cancer after fewer years of smoking than men do. • Women develop lung cancer at a younger age than men. • Women are more likely to develop small cell carcinoma than men. • Nonsmoking women are at greater risk of developing lung cancer than men. • Women with lung cancer live, on the average, 12 months longer than men.

FIG. 28-2 Lung cancer (peripheral adenocarcinoma). The tumor shows prominent black pigmentation, suggestive of having evolved in an anthracotic scar.

decreases with smoking cessation, reaching that of nonsmokers within 10 to 15 years of quitting.

Assessment of the risk of lung cancer is now divided into three categories: (1) smokers, people who are currently smoking; (2) nonsmokers, people who formerly smoked; and (3) never smokers. The Memorial Sloan-Kettering Cancer Center has developed a tool that calculates risk for developing lung cancer for smokers and former smokers who quit 20 years ago or less (*www.mskcc.org/cancer-care/adult/lung/prediction-tools*).

The risk of developing lung cancer is directly related to total exposure to tobacco smoke, measured by total number of cigarettes smoked in a lifetime, age of smoking onset, depth of inhalation, tar and nicotine content, and the use of unfiltered cigarettes. Sidestream smoke (smoke from burning cigarettes, cigars) contains the same carcinogens found in mainstream smoke (smoke inhaled and exhaled by the smoker). This exposure to secondhand smoke creates a health risk to nonsmoking adults and children.

Other common causes of lung cancer include high levels of pollution, radiation (especially radon exposure), and asbestos.[22] Heavy or prolonged exposure to industrial agents such as ionizing radiation, coal dust, nickel, uranium, chromium, formaldehyde, and arsenic can also increase the risk of lung cancer, especially in smokers.

Marked variations exist in a person's propensity to develop lung cancer. Although genetic factors are not yet well understood, mutations in the epidermal growth factor receptor gene (*EGFR*) may be linked to familial lung cancer.[22] It is also theorized that people have different genetic carcinogen-metabolizing pathways. This may explain why some smokers develop lung cancer and others do not.

Differences in lung cancer incidence, risk factors, and survival exist between men and women (see Gender Differences box above). Genetic, hormonal, and molecular influences may contribute to these differences. Female smokers have a higher relative risk of developing lung cancer than male smokers.

Pathophysiology

Most primary lung tumors are believed to arise from mutated epithelial cells. The development of mutations, which are caused by carcinogens, are also influenced by various genetic factors.[23] Once started, continued tumor development is promoted by epidermal growth factor. These cells grow slowly, taking 8 to 10 years for a tumor to reach 1 cm in size, the smallest lesion detectable on an x-ray. Lung cancers occur primarily in the segmental bronchi or beyond and have a preference for the upper lobes of the lungs (Figs. 28-2 and 28-3).

Primary lung cancers are categorized into two broad subtypes (Table 28-15): non–small cell lung cancer (NSCLC) (80%) and small cell lung cancer (SCLC) (20%).[22] Lung cancers metastasize primarily by direct extension and via the blood and lymph system. The common sites for metastasis are the liver, brain, bones, lymph nodes, and adrenal glands.

Paraneoplastic Syndrome. *Paraneoplastic syndrome* is caused by humoral factors (hormones, cytokines) excreted by tumor cells or by an immune response against the tumor.

TABLE 28-15 TYPES OF PRIMARY LUNG CANCER

Type	Growth Rate	Characteristics	Response to Therapy
Non–Small Cell Lung Cancer (NSCLC)			
Squamous cell carcinoma	Slow	Accounts for 20%-30% of lung cancers. More common in men. Centrally located, producing early symptoms of nonproductive cough and hemoptysis. Does not have a strong tendency to metastasize.	Surgical resection may be attempted. Adjuvant chemotherapy and radiation. Depending on the staging, life expectancy is better than for small cell lung cancer.
Adenocarcinoma	Moderate	Accounts for 30%-40% of lung cancers. Most common lung cancer in people who have not smoked; more common in women. Peripherally located. Often has no clinical manifestations until widespread metastasis is present.	Surgical resection may be attempted depending on the staging. Does not respond well to chemotherapy.
Large cell (undifferentiated) carcinoma	Rapid	Accounts for 10% of lung cancers. Composed of large cells that are anaplastic and often arise in the bronchi. Is highly metastatic via lymphatics and blood.	Surgery is not usually attempted because of high rate of metastases. Tumor may be radiosensitive but often recurs.
Small Cell Lung Cancer (SCLC)			
Small cell carcinoma	Very rapid	Accounts for about 20% of lung cancers. Most malignant form of lung cancer. Spreads early via lymphatics and bloodstream; frequent metastasis to brain. Associated with endocrine disturbances.	Chemotherapy mainstay of treatment but overall poor prognosis. Radiation is used as adjuvant therapy and palliative measure.

FIG. 28-3 Lung carcinoma. The gray-white tumor tissue is infiltrating the lung. Histologically this tumor is identified as a squamous cell carcinoma.

Sometimes the symptoms of paraneoplastic syndrome manifest even before the diagnosis of a malignancy.

Examples of paraneoplastic syndrome include hypercalcemia, syndrome of inappropriate antidiuretic hormone (SIADH), adrenal hypersecretion, hematologic disorders, and neurologic syndromes. SCLCs are most often associated with the paraneoplastic syndrome. These conditions may stabilize with treatment of the underlying neoplasm.[24] (These effects are discussed in the section on metabolic emergencies in Chapter 16 on pp. 277-278.)

Clinical Manifestations

The clinical manifestations of lung cancer are usually nonspecific and appear late in the disease process. Symptoms may be masked by a chronic cough attributed to smoking or smoking-related lung disease. Manifestations depend on the type of primary lung cancer, its location, and metastatic spread. Lung

EVIDENCE-BASED PRACTICE

Translating Research Into Practice

Which Interventions Improve Well-Being in Lung Cancer?

Clinical Question
In patients with lung cancer (P), what is the effectiveness of nonpharmacologic interventions (I) on symptoms, psychologic functioning, and quality of life (O)?

Best Available Evidence
Systematic review of randomized controlled trials (RCTs) and quasi-randomized clinical trials

Critical Appraisal and Synthesis of Evidence
- Fifteen trials (n = 1440) of patients diagnosed with lung cancer receiving various nonpharmacologic interventions, including exercise and nutrition, breathlessness and pain management, progressive muscle relaxation, foot reflexology, and counseling.
- Significant benefits resulted from nurse-led breathlessness programs.
- Counseling may assist patients in coping with emotional symptoms.
- Exercise and nutrition interventions did not improve quality of life in the long term.
- Reflexology may provide short-term help for pain and anxiety.

Conclusion
- Nonpharmacologic interventions can improve anxiety, depression, and symptoms such as breathlessness.

Implications for Nursing Practice
- Encourage patients to participate in programs that help reduce breathlessness and other distressful symptoms.
- Follow-up with patients who are self-managing their symptoms.
- Engage in educational programs to increase your ability to deliver high-quality supportive care.

Reference for Evidence
Rueda J, Solà I, Pascual A, et al: Non-invasive interventions for improving well-being and quality of life in patients with lung cancer, *Cochrane Database Syst Rev* 9:CD004282, 2011.

P, Patient population of interest; *I*, intervention or area of interest; *O*, outcomes of interest (see p. 12).

TABLE 28-16   COLLABORATIVE CARE

Lung Cancer

Diagnostic	Collaborative Therapy
• History and physical examination • Chest x-ray • Cytologic study of sputum, bronchial washings, or pleural space fluid • Bronchoscopy • Computed tomography (CT) scan • Magnetic resonance imaging (MRI) • Positron emission tomography (PET) • Mediastinoscopy • Video-assisted thoracoscopic surgery (VATS) • Transbronchial or percutaneous fine-needle aspiration	• Surgery • Radiation therapy • Chemotherapy • Biologic and targeted therapy • Prophylactic cranial radiation • Bronchoscopic laser therapy • Photodynamic therapy • Airway stenting • Cryotherapy

TABLE 28-17   STAGING OF NON–SMALL CELL LUNG CANCER

Stages	Characteristics
I	Tumor is small and localized to lung. No lymph node involvement.
A	Tumor <3 cm.
B	Tumor 3-5 cm and invading surrounding local areas.
II	Increased tumor size, some lymph node involvement.
A	Tumor 3-5 cm with invasion of lymph nodes on same side of chest OR Tumor 5-7 cm without lymph node involvement.
B	Tumor 5-7 cm involving the bronchus and lymph nodes on same side of chest and tissue of other local organs OR Tumor >7 cm without lymph node involvement.
III	Increased spread of tumor
A	Tumor spread to the nearby structures (chest wall, pleura, pericardium) and regional lymph nodes.
B	Extensive tumor involving heart, trachea, esophagus, mediastinum, malignant pleural effusion, contralateral lymph nodes, scalene or supraclavicular lymph nodes.
IV	Distant metastasis.

cancer frequently manifests as a lobar pneumonia that does not respond to treatment.

One of the most common symptoms of lung cancer, and often the one reported first, is a persistent cough. Blood-tinged sputum may be produced because of bleeding caused by the malignancy. The patient may complain of dyspnea or wheezing. Chest pain, if present, may be localized or unilateral, ranging from mild to severe.

Later manifestations include nonspecific systemic symptoms such as anorexia, fatigue, weight loss, and nausea and vomiting. Hoarseness may be present as a result of laryngeal nerve involvement. Unilateral paralysis of the diaphragm, dysphagia, and superior vena cava obstruction may occur because of intrathoracic spread of the malignancy. Sometimes there are palpable lymph nodes in the neck or axillae. Mediastinal involvement may lead to pericardial effusion, cardiac tamponade, and dysrhythmias.

Diagnostic Studies

A chest x-ray is the initial diagnostic test used for patients with suspected lung cancer. Approximately 5% of cases are found incidentally on a chest x-ray performed for unrelated conditions.[22] The x-ray may identify a lung mass or infiltrate. Evidence of metastasis to the ribs or vertebrae and a pleural effusion may also be seen on chest x-ray. CT scanning is used to further evaluate the lung mass. CT scans can identify the location and extent of masses in the chest, any mediastinal involvement, and lymph node enlargement.

Sputum cytologic studies can identify malignant cells, but results are positive in only 20% to 30% of specimens because the malignant cells are not always present in the sputum. Biopsy is necessary for a definitive diagnosis. Cells for biopsy can be obtained by CT-guided needle aspiration, bronchoscopy, mediastinoscopy, or video-assisted thoracoscopic surgery (VATS) (see Chapter 26). If a thoracentesis is performed to relieve a pleural effusion, the fluid is also analyzed for malignant cells.

Accurate assessment of lung cancer is critical for staging and determining appropriate treatment. Bone scans and CT scans of the brain, pelvis, and abdomen are used to determine if metastatic disease is present. A complete history and physical examination, CBC with differential, chemistry panel, LFTs, renal function tests, and pulmonary function tests are necessary. Magnetic resonance imaging (MRI) and/or positron emis-

sion tomography (PET) may also be used to evaluate and stage lung cancer. Table 28-16 summarizes the diagnostic management of lung cancer.

Staging. Staging of NSCLC is performed according to the TNM staging system (see Table 16-5). Under the TNM system, the tumor is grouped into four stages with A or B subtypes. A simplified version of staging of NSCLC is presented in Table 28-17. Patients with stages I, II, and IIIA disease may be surgical candidates. However, stage IIIB or IV disease is usually inoperable and has a poor prognosis.

Staging of SCLC by TNM has not been useful because this cancer is aggressive and is always considered systemic. The stages of SCLC are *limited* and *extensive*. Limited means that the tumor is confined to one side of the chest and regional lymph nodes. Extensive SCLC means that the cancer extends beyond the limited stage. Approximately 65% to 70% of patients with SCLC have extensive disease. On average, patients with extensive SCLC survive only 12 months with treatment and 6 weeks without.[25]

Screening for Lung Cancer. Screening for high-risk patients is supported by the recent National Lung Screening Trial (NLST). This study showed a 20% decrease in deaths from lung cancer in patients who underwent screening with low-dose spiral CT scanning, compared with those who had chest x-rays.[26] Only those patients who meet the following criteria should be considered for screening: 55 to 74 years old, current or former smokers with at least a 30 pack-year smoking history, former smokers who quit within the past 15 years, no history of lung cancer, not on home O_2 therapy.[27-29]

Collaborative Care

Surgical Therapy. Surgical resection is the treatment of choice in NSCLC stages I to IIIA without mediastinal involvement, since resection provides the best chance for a cure. The 5-year survival rate in stage I and II disease ranges from 30% to 50%. Factors that affect survival include the size of the primary tumor and co-morbidities. For other NSCLC stages, patients may require surgery in conjunction with radiation therapy and/or chemotherapy. Fifty percent of NSCLCs are not resectable at the time of diagnosis.

The surgical procedures that may be performed include pneumonectomy (removal of one entire lung), lobectomy (removal of one or more lobes of the lung), or segmental or wedge resection procedures. VATS may be used to treat lung cancers near the outside of the lung. Surgery is generally not indicated for SCLC because of its rapid growth and dissemination at the time of diagnosis.

When the tumor is considered operable, the patient's cardiopulmonary status must be evaluated to determine the ability to withstand surgery. Pulmonary function studies and ABGs are often used to assess the patient's cardiopulmonary status.

Radiation Therapy. Radiation therapy may be used as treatment for both NSCLC and SCLC. Radiation therapy may be given as curative therapy, palliative therapy (to relieve symptoms), or adjuvant therapy in combination with surgery or chemotherapy.

Radiation therapy may be used as primary therapy in the individual who is unable to tolerate surgical resection because of co-morbidities. Radiation therapy also relieves symptoms of dyspnea and hemoptysis resulting from bronchial obstructive tumors and treats superior vena cava syndrome. It can also be used to treat pain that is caused by metastatic bone lesions or cerebral metastasis. Sometimes radiation is used preoperatively to reduce the tumor mass before surgical resection. Complications of radiation therapy include esophagitis, skin irritation, nausea and vomiting, anorexia, and radiation pneumonitis (see Chapter 16).

Stereotactic Body Radiotherapy. Stereotactic body radiotherapy (SBRT), also called stereotactic surgery or radiosurgery, is a new lung cancer treatment. It is a type of radiation therapy that uses high doses of radiation delivered accurately to the tumor. SBRT provides an option for patients with early stage lung cancers who are not surgical candidates for other medical reasons. SBRT is an outpatient procedure that uses special positioning procedures and radiology techniques so that a higher dose of radiation can be delivered to the tumor, and only a small part of the healthy lung is exposed. Therapy is given over 1 to 3 days.

Chemotherapy. Chemotherapy is the primary treatment for SCLC. In NSCLC, chemotherapy may be used in the treatment of nonresectable tumors or as adjuvant therapy to surgery. A variety of chemotherapy drugs and multidrug regimens (i.e., protocols) have been used. Chemotherapy for lung cancer typically consists of combinations of two or more of the following drugs: etoposide (VePesid), carboplatin (Paraplatin), cisplatin (Platinol), paclitaxel (Taxol), vinorelbine (Navelbine), cyclophosphamide (Cytoxan), ifosfamide (Ifex), docetaxel (Taxotere), gemcitabine (Gemzar), and pemetrexed (Alimta).

Targeted Therapy. Targeted therapy uses drugs that block the growth of molecules involved in specific aspects of tumor growth (see Chapter 16). Because it inhibits growth rather than directly kills cancer cells, targeted therapy may be less toxic than chemotherapy. One type of targeted therapy for patients with NSCLC inhibits tyrosine kinase, an enzyme associated with epidermal growth factor receptor. These drugs (e.g., erlotinib [Tarceva]) block signals for growth in the cancer cells.

Another kinase inhibitor, crizotinib (Xalkori), is used to treat patients with NSCLC who have an abnormal anaplastic lymphoma kinase *(ALK)* gene. This drug directly inhibits the kinase protein produced by the *ALK* gene that is responsible for cancer development and growth.

Other drugs, such as bevacizumab (Avastin), inhibit the growth of new blood vessels (angiogenesis) by targeting vascular endothelial growth factor.

Other Therapies

Prophylactic Cranial Radiation. Patients with SCLC have early metastases, especially to the central nervous system. Most chemotherapy does not penetrate the blood-brain barrier. Therefore after successful systemic treatment, the patient is at risk for cerebral metastases. Prophylactic radiation has been shown to decrease the incidence of cerebral metastases and improve the survival rate in patients with limited SCLC.[22]

Bronchoscopic Laser Therapy. Bronchoscopic laser therapy makes it possible to remove obstructing bronchial lesions. The neodymium:yttrium-aluminum-garnet (Nd:YAG) laser is most commonly used for laser resection using either the flexible or the rigid bronchoscope. The laser's thermal energy is transmitted to the target tissue. It is a safe and effective treatment of endobronchial obstructions from tumors. Symptoms of airway obstruction are relieved as a result of thermal necrosis and shrinkage of the tumor. The procedure may be repeated as needed.[27]

Photodynamic Therapy. Photodynamic therapy can be used to treat very early stage lung cancers that are confined to the outer layers of the airways. It can also remove lesions obstructing the airway. Porfimer (Photofrin) is injected IV and selectively concentrates in tumor cells. After a set time (usually 48 hours), the tumor is exposed to laser light via bronchoscopy, activating the drug and causing cell death. Necrotic tissue is removed with bronchoscopy a few days later.[27] This process can also be repeated as needed.

Airway Stenting. Stents are used alone or in combination with other techniques for relief of dyspnea, cough, or respiratory insufficiency. The advantage of an airway stent is that it supports the airway wall against collapse or external compression and can delay extension of tumor into the airway lumen.

Radiofrequency Ablation. Radiofrequency ablation therapy is being used to treat small NSCLC lung tumors that are near the outer edge of the lungs. This therapy is an alternative to surgery in patients who cannot or elect not to have surgery. A thin, needle-like probe is inserted through the skin into the tumor. CT scans are used to guide placement. An electric current is then passed through the probe, which heats and destroys tumor cells. Local anesthesia is used for this outpatient procedure.[27]

NURSING MANAGEMENT LUNG CANCER

NURSING ASSESSMENT

It is important to determine the patient and caregiver's understanding of diagnostic tests (those completed as well as those planned), the diagnosis or potential diagnosis, the treatment options, and the prognosis. At the same time, assess the patient's level of anxiety and support provided by the patient's significant others. Subjective and objective data that should be obtained from a patient with lung cancer are presented in Table 28-18.

NURSING DIAGNOSES

Nursing diagnoses for the patient with lung cancer may include, but are not limited to, the following:

• Ineffective airway clearance *related to* increased tracheobronchial secretions and presence of tumor

TABLE 28-18 NURSING ASSESSMENT

Lung Cancer

Subjective Data

Important Health Information

Past health history: Exposure to secondhand smoke, airborne carcinogens (e.g., asbestos, radon, hydrocarbons), or other pollutants; urban living environment; chronic lung disease (e.g., TB, COPD, bronchiectasis)

Medications: Cough medicines or other respiratory medications

Functional Health Patterns

Health perception–health management: Smoking history, including amount per day and number of years; family history of lung cancer; frequent respiratory tract infections

Nutritional-metabolic: Anorexia, nausea, vomiting, dysphagia (late); weight loss; chills

Activity-exercise: Fatigue; persistent cough (productive or nonproductive); dyspnea at rest or with exertion, hemoptysis (late symptom)

Cognitive-perceptual: Chest pain or tightness, shoulder and arm pain, headache, bone pain (late symptom)

Objective Data

General

Fever, neck and axillary lymphadenopathy, paraneoplastic syndrome (e.g., syndrome of inappropriate ADH secretion)

Integumentary

Jaundice (liver metastasis); edema of neck and face (superior vena cava syndrome), digital clubbing

Respiratory

Wheezing, hoarseness, stridor, unilateral diaphragm paralysis, pleural effusions (late signs)

Cardiovascular

Pericardial effusion, cardiac tamponade, dysrhythmias (late signs)

Neurologic

Unsteady gait (brain metastasis)

Musculoskeletal

Pathologic fractures, muscle wasting (late)

Possible Diagnostic Findings

Observance of lesion on chest x-ray, CT scan, or PET scan; MRI findings of vertebral, spinal cord, or mediastinal invasion; positive sputum or bronchial washings for cytologic studies; positive fiberoptic bronchoscopy and biopsy findings

ADH, Antidiuretic hormone.

- Anxiety *related to* lack of knowledge of diagnosis or unknown prognosis and treatments
- Ineffective self-health management *related to* lack of knowledge about the disease process and therapeutic regimen
- Ineffective breathing pattern *related to* decreased lung capacity
- Impaired gas exchange *related to* tumor obstructing airflow

PLANNING

The overall goals are that the patient with lung cancer will have (1) effective breathing patterns, (2) adequate airway clearance, (3) adequate oxygenation of tissues, (4) minimal to no pain, and (5) a realistic attitude about treatment and prognosis.

NURSING IMPLEMENTATION

HEALTH PROMOTION. The best way to halt the epidemic of lung cancer is to prevent people from starting to smoke and help smokers stop smoking. Because most smokers start in the teenage years, prevention of teen smoking has the most significant role in reducing the incidence of lung cancer. A wealth of material is available to the smoker who is interested in smoking cessation. The CDC provides an index of tools *(www.cdc.gov/tobacco/quit_smoking/cessation/index.htm).* (Smoking cessation is discussed in Chapter 11.)

Modeling healthy behavior by not smoking, promoting smoking cessation programs, and actively supporting education and policy changes related to smoking are important nursing activities. Many changes have occurred as a result of the recognition that passive smoke is a health hazard. Laws prohibit smoking in most public places and limit public smoking to designated areas. Most hospital environments are now completely smoke-free, prohibiting smoking by employees and patients. A new trend is for hospitals to refuse employment to anyone testing positive for nicotine. This includes not only smokers but also nonsmokers who are routinely exposed to secondhand smoke.

ACUTE INTERVENTION. Care of the patient with lung cancer initially involves support and reassurance during the diagnostic evaluation. It is important to recognize the multiple stressors that occur when someone is diagnosed with lung cancer. The stress response is a normal and adaptive response, but can become detrimental when it is overwhelming and intense. Patients suffer the stress of their symptoms, including dyspnea and cough. Diagnostic and therapeutic procedures provide additional stress by placing patients in unfamiliar environments with unusual and perhaps painful results. Emotional stressors include the knowledge of the high mortality rate of lung cancer and the causal effect of cigarette smoking. Worries about role performance and ability to care for their family while undergoing cancer treatment provide further stress. Carefully assess each individual, since he or she will experience unique stressors. The insight gained will help the patient and caregiver cope with the stress of the illness and treatment.[30]

Care of the patient undergoing thoracic surgery is discussed later in this chapter on p. 548. Care of the patient undergoing radiation therapy and chemotherapy is discussed in Chapter 16. Individualized care depends on the plan for treatment. Assessment and intervention in symptom management are pivotal, as is teaching the patient to recognize signs and symptoms that may indicate progression or recurrence of disease. Provide patient comfort, teach methods to reduce pain, monitor for side effects of prescribed medications, foster appropriate coping strategies for the patient and caregiver, assess smoking cessation readiness, and help patients access resources to deal with the illness.

AMBULATORY AND HOME CARE. Teach signs and symptoms to report, such as hemoptysis, dysphagia, chest pain, and hoarseness. Counseling patients on smoking cessation and prevention is essential in decreasing morbidity and mortality risks associated with lung cancer. Encourage the patient and the family to provide a smoke-free environment. This may include smoking cessation for multiple family members. If the treatment plan includes home oxygen, the teaching plan must include the safe use of oxygen.

For many individuals who have lung cancer, little can be done to significantly prolong their lives. Radiation therapy and chemotherapy can provide palliative relief from distressing symptoms. Constant pain may become a major problem. (Measures used to relieve pain are discussed in Chapter 9. Care of the patient with cancer is discussed in Chapter 16.) The palliative care team should be involved as the patient and the family move toward the end of life (see Chapter 10). The team can provide information about disability, financial planning, and community resources for end-of-life care such as hospice.

EVALUATION

The expected outcomes are that the patient with lung cancer will have
- Adequate breathing patterns
- Adequate oxygenation
- Minimal to no pain
- Realistic attitude about prognosis

OTHER TYPES OF LUNG TUMORS

SCLC and NSCLC account for 95% of lung tumors. The other 5% include the following:
- *Hamartomas*, the most common benign tumor, is a slow-growing congenital tumor composed of fibrous tissue, fat, and blood vessels.
- *Mucous gland adenoma* is a benign tumor arising in the bronchi that consists of columnar cystic spaces.
- *Mesotheliomas* are either malignant or benign and originate from the visceral pleura. Malignant mesotheliomas are associated with exposure to asbestos. Benign mesotheliomas are localized lesions.
- Secondary metastases from other malignancies can occur. Malignant cells from another part of the body reach the lungs via the pulmonary capillaries or the lymphatic network. The primary malignancies that spread to the lungs often originate in the GI or genitourinary tract and in the breast. General symptoms of lung metastases are chest pain and nonproductive cough.

CHEST TRAUMA AND THORACIC INJURIES

Traumatic injuries to the chest contribute to 75% of all traumatic deaths.[31] Thoracic injuries range from simple rib fractures to complex life-threatening rupture of organs. The mechanisms of injuries causing chest trauma are separated into two categories: blunt trauma and penetrating trauma.

Blunt trauma occurs when the chest strikes or is struck by an object. The impact can cause deceleration, acceleration, shearing, and compression of thoracic structures. The external injury may appear minor, but internally the organs may have severe injuries. The injuries can occur on the same side as the impact and on the opposite side as the tissue moves back and forth. Rib and sternal fractures can lacerate lung tissue. In a high-velocity impact the shearing force may result in laceration or tearing of the aorta. Compression of the chest may result in contusion, crush injury, and organ rupture.

Penetrating trauma is an open injury in which a foreign body impales or passes through the body tissues, creating an open wound. Examples include knife wounds, gunshot wounds, and injuries with other sharp objects. eTable 28-2 (available on the website for this chapter) describes traumatic injuries as they relate to the categories of trauma and the mechanism of injury. Emergency care of the patient with a chest injury is presented in Table 28-19.

The most common thoracic emergencies and their management are described in Table 28-20.

✚ TABLE 28-19 EMERGENCY MANAGEMENT

Chest Trauma

Etiology	Assessment Findings	Interventions
Blunt • Motor vehicle accident • Pedestrian accident • Fall • Assault with blunt object • Crush injury • Explosion **Penetrating** • Knife • Gunshot • Stick • Arrow • Other missiles	**Respiratory** • Dyspnea, respiratory distress • Cough with or without hemoptysis • Cyanosis of mouth, face, nail beds, mucous membranes • Tracheal deviation • Audible air escaping from chest wound • Decreased breath sounds on side of injury • Decreased O_2 saturation • Frothy secretions **Cardiovascular** • Rapid, thready pulse • Decreased BP • Narrowed pulse pressure • Asymmetric BP values in arms • Distended neck veins • Muffled heart sounds • Chest pain • Crunching sound synchronous with heart sounds • Dysrhythmias **Surface Findings** • Bruising • Abrasions • Open chest wound • Asymmetric chest movement • Subcutaneous emphysema	**Initial** • Ensure patent airway. • Administer O_2 to keep SpO_2 >90%. • Establish IV access with two large-bore catheters. Begin fluid resuscitation as appropriate. • Remove clothing to assess injury. • Cover sucking chest wound with nonporous dressing taped on three sides. • Stabilize impaled objects with bulky dressings. *Do not remove object.* • Assess for other significant injuries and treat appropriately. • Stabilize flail rib segment with hand followed by application of large pieces of tape horizontal across the flail segment. • Place patient in a semi-Fowler's position or position patient on the injured side if breathing is easier *after* cervical spine injury has been ruled out. • Prepare for emergency needle decompression if tension pneumothorax or cardiac tamponade present. **Ongoing Monitoring** • Monitor vital signs, level of consciousness, O_2 saturation, cardiac rhythm, respiratory status, and urine output. • Anticipate intubation for respiratory distress. • Release dressing if tension pneumothorax develops after sucking chest wound is covered.

✚ TABLE 28-20   EMERGENCY MANAGEMENT

Thoracic Injuries

Injury	Definition	Manifestations	Interventionist
Pneumothorax	Air in pleural space (see Fig. 28-4).	Dyspnea, decreased movement of involved chest wall, diminished or absent breath sounds on the affected side, hyperresonance to percussion	Chest tube insertion with flutter valve or chest drainage system.
Hemothorax	Blood in the pleural space, may or may not occur in conjunction with pneumothorax.	Dyspnea, diminished or absent breath sounds, dullness to percussion, decreased Hgb, shock depending on blood volume lost	Chest tube insertion with chest drainage system. Autotransfusion of collected blood, treatment of hypovolemia as necessary.
Tension pneumothorax	Air in pleural space that does not escape. The increased air in the pleural space shifts organs and increases intrathoracic pressure (see Fig. 28-5).	Cyanosis, air hunger, violent agitation, tracheal deviation away from affected side, subcutaneous emphysema, neck vein distention, hyperresonance to percussion	Medical emergency: needle decompression followed by chest tube insertion with chest drainage system.
Flail chest	Fracture of two or more adjacent ribs in two or more places with loss of chest wall stability (see Fig. 28-6).	Paradoxic movement of chest wall, respiratory distress. May be associated hemothorax, pneumothorax, pulmonary contusion	O_2 as needed to maintain O_2 saturation, analgesia. Stabilize flail segment with positive pressure ventilation (CPAP, BiPAP) or intubation and mechanical ventilation. Treat associated injuries. Surgical fixation.
Cardiac tamponade	Blood rapidly collects in pericardial sac, compresses myocardium because the pericardium does not stretch, and prevents ventricles from filling.	Muffled, distant heart sounds, hypotension, neck vein distention, increased central venous pressure	Medical emergency: pericardiocentesis with surgical repair as appropriate.

BiPAP, Bilevel positive airway pressure; *CPAP,* continuous positive airway pressure.

PNEUMOTHORAX

A **pneumothorax** is caused by air entering the pleural cavity. Normally, negative pressure exists between the visceral pleura (surrounding the lung) and the parietal pleura (lining the thoracic cavity), allowing the lung to be filled by chest wall expansion. The pleural space contains only a few milliliters of lubricating fluid to reduce friction when the tissues move. When air enters this space, the change to positive pressure causes a partial or complete lung collapse. As the volume of air in the pleural space increases, the lung volume decreases. This condition should be suspected after any trauma to the chest wall. Pneumothorax can be classified as *open* (air entering through an opening in the chest wall) or *closed* (no external wound).

If a pneumothorax is small, mild tachycardia and dyspnea may be the only manifestations. If the pneumothorax occupies a large area, respiratory distress may be present, including shallow, rapid respirations; dyspnea; air hunger; and oxygen desaturation. Chest pain and a cough with or without hemoptysis may be present. On auscultation, no breath sounds are detected over the affected area. A chest x-ray shows air or fluid in the pleural space and reduction in lung volume.

Types of Pneumothorax

Spontaneous Pneumothorax. A spontaneous pneumothorax typically occurs due to the rupture of small blebs (air-filled blisters) located on the apex of the lung. These blebs can occur in healthy, young individuals (*primary spontaneous pneumothorax*) or as a result of lung disease such as COPD, asthma, cystic fibrosis, and pneumonia (*secondary spontaneous pneumothorax*). Smoking increases the risk for bleb formation. Other risk factors include being tall and thin, male gender, family history, and previous spontaneous pneumothorax.

Iatrogenic Pneumothorax. *Iatrogenic pneumothorax* can occur due to laceration or puncture of the lung during medical procedures. Transthoracic needle aspiration is the leading cause

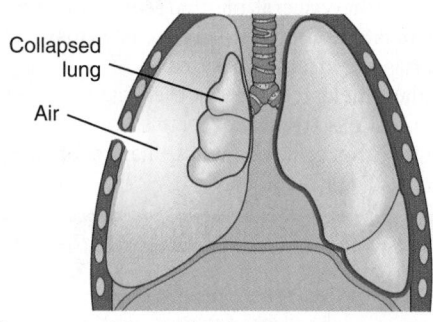

FIG. 28-4 Open pneumothorax resulting from collapse of lung due to disruption of chest wall and outside air entering.

of iatrogenic pneumothorax.[32] Other causes include subclavian catheter insertion, thoracentesis, pleural biopsy, and transbronchial lung biopsy. Barotrauma from excessive ventilatory pressure during manual or mechanical ventilation can rupture alveoli or bronchioles. Esophageal procedures may also be involved in the development of a pneumothorax. Tearing during insertion of a gastric tube can allow air from the esophagus to enter the mediastinum and the pleural space.

Traumatic Pneumothorax. *Traumatic pneumothorax* can occur from either penetrating (open) or nonpenetrating (closed) chest trauma. Penetrating trauma allows air to enter the pleural space through an opening in the chest wall (Fig. 28-4). Examples include stab or gunshot wounds and surgical thoracotomy. A penetrating chest wound may be referred to as a *sucking chest wound*, since air enters the pleural space through the chest wall during inspiration.

Emergency treatment consists of covering the wound with an occlusive dressing that is secured on three sides (vent dressing). During inspiration, as negative pressure is created in the chest, the dressing pulls against the wound, preventing air from entering the pleural space. During expiration, as the pressure rises in the pleural space, the dressing is pushed out and air escapes through the wound and from under the dressing. If the

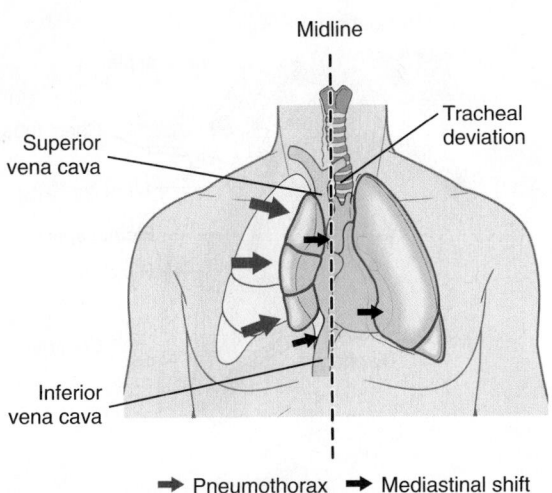

Midline

Superior vena cava

Tracheal deviation

Inferior vena cava

→ Pneumothorax   → Mediastinal shift

FIG. 28-5 Tension pneumothorax. As pleural pressure on the affected side increases, mediastinal displacement ensues with resultant respiratory and cardiovascular compromise. Tracheal deviation is an external manifestation of the mediastinal shift.

object that caused the open chest wound is still in place, do not remove it until a physician is present. Stabilize the impaled object with a bulky dressing.

Nonpenetrating chest trauma, such as rib fractures, can lacerate the lung and cause air to enter the pleural space. Blunt trauma can also cause alveolar rupture secondary to sudden chest compression.

Tension Pneumothorax. Tension pneumothorax occurs when air enters the pleural space but cannot escape. The continued accumulation of air in the pleural space causes increasingly elevated intrapleural pressures. This results in compression of the lung on the affected side and pressure on the heart and great vessels, pushing them away from the affected side (Fig. 28-5). The mediastinum shifts toward the unaffected side, compressing the "good" lung, which further compromises oxygenation. As the pressure increases, venous return is decreased and cardiac output falls. Tension pneumothorax may result from either an open or a closed pneumothorax. In an open chest wound, a flap may act as a one-way valve. Thus air can enter on inspiration but cannot escape. Tension pneumothorax can occur with mechanical ventilation and resuscitative efforts. It can also occur if chest tubes are clamped or become blocked in a patient with a pneumothorax. Unclamping the tube or relieving the obstruction will remedy this situation.

Tension pneumothorax is a medical emergency, with both the respiratory and cardiovascular systems affected. Manifestations include dyspnea, marked tachycardia, tracheal deviation, decreased or absent breath sounds on the affected side, neck vein distention, cyanosis, and profuse diaphoresis.[32] If the tension in the pleural space is not relieved, the patient is likely to die from inadequate cardiac output or severe hypoxemia.

Hemothorax. Hemothorax is an accumulation of blood in the pleural space resulting from injury to the chest wall, diaphragm, lung, blood vessels, or mediastinum.[32] When it occurs with pneumothorax, it is called a *hemopneumothorax*. The patient with a traumatic hemothorax requires immediate insertion of a chest tube for evacuation of the blood, which can be recovered and reinfused for a short time after the injury. (Autotransfusion is discussed in Chapter 31.)

Chylothorax. *Chylothorax* is the presence of lymphatic fluid in the pleural space. The thoracic duct is disrupted either

traumatically or from a malignancy, and the lymphatic fluid fills the pleural space. This milky white fluid is high in lipids. Normal lymphatic flow through the thoracic duct is 1500 to 2500 mL/day. This amount can be increased up to tenfold after ingestion of fats. Fifty percent of cases heal with conservative treatment (chest drainage, bowel rest, and parenteral nutrition). Octreotide has been used with some success to reduce the flow of lymphatic fluid.[29] Surgery and pleurodesis are options if conservative therapy fails. *Pleurodesis* is the artificial production of adhesions between the parietal and visceral pleura, usually done with a chemical sclerosing agent, such as talc or doxycycline.

Collaborative Care

Treatment of a pneumothorax depends on its severity and the underlying disease. If the patient is stable and minimal air and fluid is accumulated in the intrapleural space, no treatment may be necessary, since the condition may resolve spontaneously. The pleural space can also be aspirated with a large-bore needle. This procedure is called a thoracentesis.

The most definitive and common treatment of pneumothorax and hemothorax is to insert a chest tube and connect it to water-seal drainage. Repeated spontaneous pneumothorax may need to be treated surgically by a partial pleurectomy, stapling, or pleurodesis to promote adherence of the pleurae to one another. Tension pneumothorax is a medical emergency, requiring urgent needle decompression followed by chest tube insertion to water-seal drainage.

FRACTURED RIBS

Rib fractures are the most common type of chest injury resulting from blunt trauma. Ribs 5 through 9 are most frequently fractured because they are the least protected by chest muscles. If the fractured rib is splintered or displaced, it may damage the pleura and lungs.

Clinical manifestations of fractured ribs include pain at the site of injury, especially during inspiration and coughing. The patient splints the affected area and takes shallow breaths to try to decrease the pain. Atelectasis and pneumonia may develop because of decreased ventilation and retained secretions.

The main goal in treatment is to decrease pain so that the patient can breathe adequately and clear secretions. Strapping the chest with tape or using a binder is not recommended, since it limits chest expansion and predisposes the individual to atelectasis. Nonsteroidal antiinflammatory drugs (NSAIDs), opioids, and nerve blocks can be used to reduce pain and aid with deep breathing and coughing. Patient teaching should emphasize deep breathing, coughing, incentive spirometry, and appropriate use of pain medications.

FLAIL CHEST

Flail chest results from the fracture of several consecutive ribs, in two or more separate places, causing an unstable segment (Fig. 28-6). It can also be caused by fracture of the sternum and several consecutive ribs. The resultant instability of the chest wall causes paradoxic movement during breathing. The affected (flail) area moves in the opposite direction with respect to the intact portion of the chest. During inspiration, the affected portion is sucked in, and during expiration, it bulges out. This paradoxic chest movement prevents adequate ventilation of the lung in the injured area and increases the work of breathing.

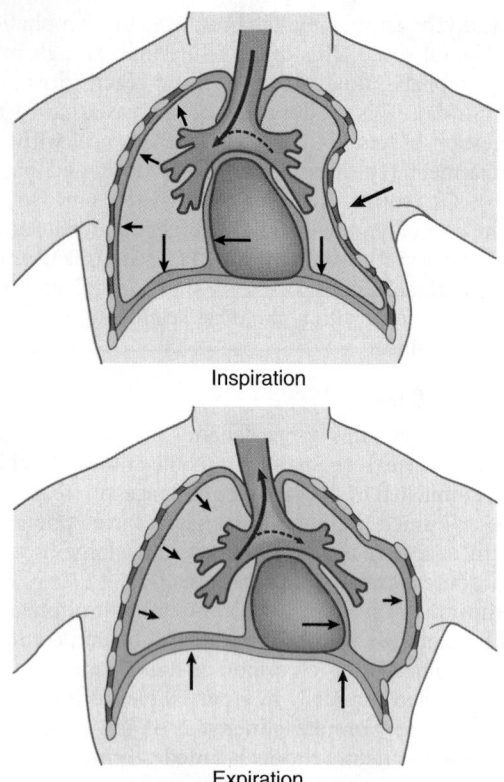

FIG. 28-6 Flail chest produces paradoxic respiration. On inspiration, the flail section sinks in with mediastinal shift to the uninjured side. On expiration, the flail section bulges outward with mediastinal shift to the injured side.

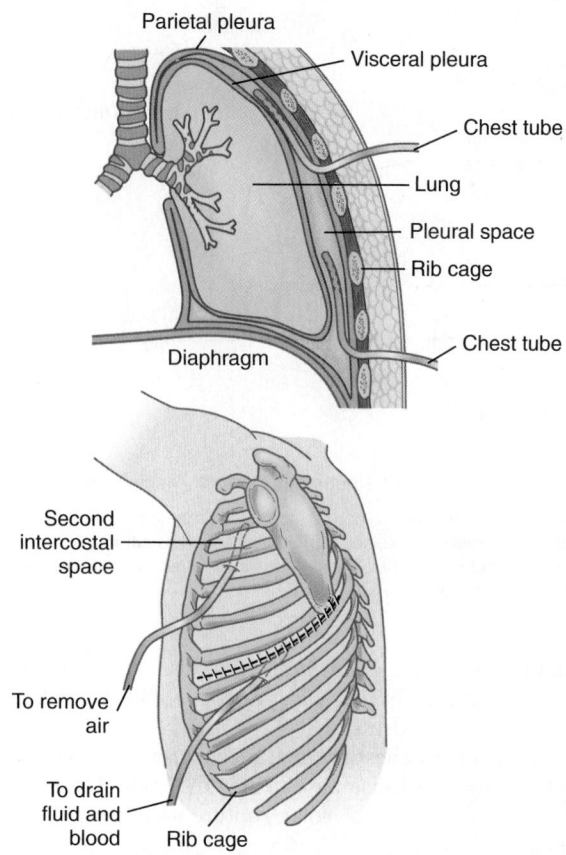

FIG. 28-7 Placement of chest tubes.

The underlying lung may have a pulmonary contusion aggravating hypoxemia.

In an unconscious patient a flail chest is usually apparent on visual examination. The patient manifests rapid, shallow respirations and tachycardia. In a conscious patient a flail chest may not be initially apparent as a result of splinting of the chest wall. The patient moves air poorly, and movement of the thorax is asymmetric and uncoordinated. Palpation of abnormal respiratory movements, evaluation for crepitus near the rib fractures, chest x-ray, and ABGs all assist in the diagnosis.

Initial therapy consists of airway management, adequate ventilation, supplemental oxygen therapy, careful administration of IV solutions, and pain control. The definitive therapy is to reexpand the lung and ensure adequate oxygenation. Although many patients can be managed without mechanical ventilation, intubation and ventilation may be necessary. Surgical fixation of the flail segment may be done.[33] The lung parenchyma and fractured ribs heal with time. Some patients continue to experience intercostal pain after the flail chest has resolved.

CHEST TUBES AND PLEURAL DRAINAGE

Whenever fluid or air accumulates in the pleural space, the pressure becomes positive instead of negative and the lungs collapse. Chest tubes are inserted to drain the pleural space and reestablish negative pressure, allowing for proper lung expansion. Tubes may also be inserted in the mediastinal space to drain air and fluid postoperatively.

Chest tubes are approximately 20 inches (51 cm) long and vary in size from 12F to 40F. The size inserted is determined by the patient's condition. Large (36F to 40F) tubes are used to drain blood, medium (24F to 36F) tubes are used to drain fluid, and small (12F to 24F) tubes are used to drain air.[34] Pigtail tubes are very small (10F to 14F) tubes with a curly end designed to keep them in place. They are a safe and effective alternative to larger-bore chest tubes for treatment of pneumothorax.[35]

Chest Tube Insertion

Insertion of a chest tube can take place in the emergency department, at the patient's bedside, or in the operating room. The patient is positioned with the arm raised above the head on the affected side to expose the midaxillary area, the standard site for insertion. Elevate the patient's head 30 to 60 degrees, when possible, to lower the diaphragm and reduce the risk of injury.

A chest x-ray is used to confirm the affected side. The area is cleansed with an antiseptic solution. The chest wall is prepared with a local anesthetic, and a small incision is made over a rib. The chest tube is advanced up and over the top of the rib to avoid the intercostal nerves and blood vessels that are behind the rib inferiorly (Fig. 28-7). Once inserted, the tube is connected to a pleural drainage system (Fig. 28-8). Two tubes may be connected to the same drainage unit with a Y-connector.

The incision is closed with sutures, and the chest tube is secured. The wound is covered with an occlusive dressing. Some clinicians prefer to seal the wound around the chest tube with petroleum gauze. Proper tube placement is confirmed by chest x-ray.

The insertion of a chest tube and its presence in the pleural space are painful. Monitor the patient's comfort at frequent intervals and use the appropriate pain-relieving interventions.

FIG. 28-8 Chest drainage unit. Both units have three chambers: (1) collection chamber; (2) water-seal chamber; and (3) suction control chamber. Suction control chamber requires a connection to a wall suction source that is dialed up higher than the prescribed suction for the suction to work. **A,** Water suction. This unit uses water in the suction control chamber to control the wall suction pressure. **B,** Dry suction. This unit controls wall suction by using a regulator control dial.

Flutter or Heimlich Valve

A flutter valve (also called the Heimlich valve after its inventor) is used to evacuate air from the pleural space (Fig. 28-9). This device consists of a one-way rubber valve within a rigid plastic tube. It is attached to the external end of the chest tube. The valve opens whenever the pressure in the chest is greater than atmospheric pressure, such as during expiration, and it closes when intrathoracic pressure is less than atmospheric pressure, such as during inspiration.

The flutter valve can be used for emergency transport and for a small- to moderate-sized pneumothorax. It also allows for patient mobility, since the smaller drainage bag can be hidden under the clothes while the patient ambulates. Drainage bags attached to the flutter valve must have a vent to the atmosphere to prevent a potential tension pneumothorax. This can be accomplished by simply cutting a small slit in the top of any drainage bag that does not have a built-in vent. Patients may go home with a flutter valve in place.

FIG. 28-9 A, Heimlich chest drain valve is a specially designed flutter valve that is used in place of a chest drainage unit for small uncomplicated pneumothorax with little or no drainage and no need for suction. The valve allows for escape of air but prevents the reentry of air into the pleural space. **B,** Placement of valve between chest tube and vented drainage bag, which can be worn under a person's clothes.

Pleural Drainage

The second type of chest drainage is larger and less portable, and it contains three basic compartments, each with a separate function (see Fig. 28-8). The *first compartment*, or collection chamber, receives fluid and air from the pleural or mediastinal space. The drained fluid stays in this chamber while the air vents to the second compartment.

The *second compartment*, called the water-seal chamber, contains 2 cm of water, which acts as a one-way valve. The incoming air enters from the collection chamber and bubbles up through the water. The water prevents backflow of air into the patient from the system. Initially, brisk bubbling of air occurs in this chamber when a pneumothorax is evacuated. Intermittent bubbling during exhalation, coughing, or sneezing (when the patient's intrathoracic pressure is increased) will continue as long as there is air in the pleural space. As the source of the air in the pleural space gets smaller, it will take more and more positive intrapleural pressure to force air out. Eventually, the air leak seals and the lung is fully expanded.

Normal fluctuation of the water within the water-seal chamber is called *tidaling*. This up and down movement of water in concert with respiration reflects the intrapleural pressure changes during inspiration and expiration. Investigate any sudden cessation of tidaling, since this may signify an occluded chest tube. Gradual reduction and eventual cessation of tidaling are expected as the lung reexpands. The parietal and visceral pleura will form a tight seal around the chest tube openings, obliterating the response to changes in intrapleural pressures with respiration.

The *third compartment*, the suction control chamber, applies suction to the chest drainage system. There are two types of suction control: water and dry. The water suction control chamber uses a column of water with the top end vented to the atmosphere to control the amount of suction from the wall regulator. The chamber is typically filled with 20 cm of water. When the negative pressure generated by the suction source exceeds the set 20 cm, air from the atmosphere enters the chamber through the vent on top and the air bubbles up through

TABLE 28-21 CHEST TUBES AND WATER-SEAL DRAINAGE

Set-Up and Insertion

1. Make sure patient is aware of the procedure and informed consent is obtained.
2. Gather equipment.
   - Thoracotomy tray
   - Chest drainage unit (CDU)
   - Chest tube
   - Bottle of sterile water
   - 1% lidocaine
   - Suction tubing and collection container
   - Occlusive dressing
3. Prepare CDU.
   - Wet suction: add sterile water to 2-cm mark in water-seal chamber and to 20-cm mark (or as ordered) in suction control chamber.
   - Dry suction: add sterile water to the fill line of the air leak meter. Attach suction tubing and increase suction until the bellows-like float moves across the display window.
4. Position and support the patient to minimize movement during procedure.

Drainage System

1. Keep all tubing loosely coiled below chest level. Tubing should drop straight from bed or chair to drainage unit. Do not let it be compressed.
2. Keep all connections between chest tubes, drainage tubing, and the drainage collector tight, and tape at connections.
3. Observe for air fluctuations (tidaling) and bubbling in the water-seal chamber.
   - If tidaling (rising with inspiration and falling with expiration in the spontaneously breathing patient) is not observed, the drainage system is blocked, the lungs are reexpanded, or the system is attached to suction.
   - If bubbling increases, there may be an air leak in the drainage system or a leak from the patient (bronchopleural leak).
4. If the chest tube is connected to suction, disconnect from wall suction to check for tidaling.
5. Suspect a system leak when bubbling is continuous.
   - Retape tubing connections.
   - Ensure that dressing is air-occlusive.
   - If leak persists, briefly clamp the chest tube at the patient's chest. If the leak stops, then the air is coming from the patient.
   - If the air leak persists, briefly and methodically move the clamps down the tubing away from the patient until the air leak stops. The leak will then be present between the last two clamp points. If the air leak persists all the way to the drainage unit, replace the unit.
6. High fluid levels in the water seal indicate residual negative pressure.
   - The chest system may need to be vented by using the high-negativity release valve available on the drainage system to release residual pressure from the system.
   - Do not lower water-seal column when wall suction is not operating or when patient is on gravity drainage.

Patient's Clinical Status

1. Monitor the patient's clinical status. Assess vital signs, lung sounds, and pain.
2. Assess for manifestations of reaccumulation of air and fluid in the chest ($\downarrow$ or absent breath sounds), significant bleeding (>100 mL/hr), chest drainage site infection (drainage, erythema, fever, $\uparrow$ WBC), or poor wound healing. Notify physician for management plan.
3. Evaluate for subcutaneous emphysema at chest tube site.
4. Encourage the patient to breathe deeply periodically to facilitate lung expansion and encourage range-of-motion exercises to the shoulder on the affected side. Encourage use of incentive spirometry every hour while awake to prevent atelectasis or pneumonia.

Chest Drainage

1. Never elevate the drainage system to the level of the patient's chest because this will cause fluid to drain back into the lungs. Secure the unit to the drainage stand. Change the unit if the collection chamber is full. Do not try to empty it.
2. Mark the time of measurement and the fluid level on the drainage unit according to the unit standards. Report any change in the quantity or characteristics of drainage (e.g., clear yellow to bloody) to the physician and record the change. Notify physician if >100 mL/hr drainage.
3. Check the position of the chest drainage container. If the drainage system is overturned and the water seal is disrupted, return it to an upright position and encourage the patient to take a few deep breaths, followed by forced exhalations and cough maneuvers.
4. If the drainage system breaks, place the distal end of the chest tubing connection in a sterile water container at a 2-cm level as an emergency water seal.
5. Milking or stripping chest tubes is no longer recommended, since these practices can dangerously increase intrapleural pressures and damage lung tissues. Position tubing so that drainage flows freely to negate need for milking or stripping. If ordered by physician to milk or strip tubes, do so GENTLY.
   - *Milking:* Alternately fold or squeeze and then release drainage tubing. Milk only if drainage and evidence of clots or obstruction. Take 15-cm strips of the chest tube and squeeze and release starting close to the chest and repeating down the tube distally.
   - *Stripping:* Squeeze drainage tube with thumb and forefinger and use gentle pulling motion down tube with other hand, then release the tubing.

Monitoring Wet vs. Dry Suction Chest Drainage Systems
Suction Control Chamber in Wet Suction System

1. Keep the suction control chamber at the appropriate water level by adding sterile water as needed to replace water lost to evaporation.
2. Keep the muffler covering the suction control chamber in place to prevent more rapid evaporation of water and to decrease the noise of the bubbling.
3. After filling the suction control chamber to the ordered suction amount (generally 20 cm H_2O suction), connect the suction tubing to the wall suction.
4. Dial the wall suction regulator until continuous gentle bubbling is seen in the suction control chamber (generally 80-120 mm Hg). Vigorous bubbling is not necessary and will increase the rate of evaporation.
5. If no bubbling is seen in the suction control chamber, (1) there is no suction, (2) suction is not high enough, or (3) the pleural air leak is so large that suction is not high enough to evacuate it.

Suction Control Chamber in Dry Suction System (see manufacturer's directions)

1. After connecting patient to system, turn the dial on the chest drainage system to amount ordered (generally −20 cm pressure), connect suction tubing to wall suction source, and increase the suction until the correct amount of negative pressure is indicated.
2. If ordered to decrease suction, turn the dial down, depress the high-negativity vent, and assess for a rise in the water level of the water-seal chamber.

Chest Tube Dressings

1. Change dressing according to unit protocol and physician preference.
2. Remove old dressing carefully to avoid removing unsecured chest tube. Assess the site and culture site as indicated.
3. Cleanse the site according to protocol, maintaining asepsis.
4. Redress with occlusive dressing (e.g., Opsite or gauze with occlusive tape). Some physicians prefer the use of petroleum gauze dressing around the tube to prevent air leak. Date the dressing and document dressing change.

the water, causing a suction-breaker effect. As a result, excess pressure is relieved.

The amount of suction applied is regulated by the amount of water in this chamber and not by the amount of suction applied to the system. An increase in suction does not result in an increase in negative pressure to the system because any excess suction merely draws in air through the vent on the top of the third chamber. The suction pressure is usually ordered to be −20 cm H_2O, although higher pressures (−40 cm H_2O) are sometimes necessary to evacuate the pleural space; lower pressure (−10 cm H_2O) may be used for frail patients at risk for tissue damage with higher pressures.

To initiate suction, turn up the vacuum source until gentle bubbling is present in the chamber. Excessive bubbling does not increase the amount of applied suction, but does increase the rate of evaporation of the column of water and the amount of noise made by the device.

The dry suction control chamber system contains no water. It has a visual alert that indicates if the suction is working. It uses either a restrictive device or a regulator to dial the desired negative pressure; this is internal in the chest drainage system. To increase the suction pressures, turn the dial on the drainage system. Increasing the vacuum source does not increase the pressure. When decreasing suction, depress the manual vent to reduce excess vacuum to the lower prescribed level.

The addition of wall suction (active suction) to the chest drainage unit may actually promote the development of air leaks and thus prolong the number of days the chest tube needs to remain in place.[36] Patients with just water-seal drainage (passive suction) have a shorter duration of air leaks. Although the majority of clinicians continue to use active suction, the use of water-seal drainage alone is gaining popularity.

A variety of commercial disposable plastic chest drainage systems are available. Manufacturers include directions for set-up and use with each unit. Atrium Medical Corporation offers online educational videos of the principles of chest drainage and products at *www.atriummed.com/Products/Chest_Drains/education.asp*.

NURSING MANAGEMENT
CHEST DRAINAGE

General guidelines for nursing care of the patient with chest tubes and water-seal drainage systems are presented in Table 28-21.

Clamping of chest tubes during transport or when the tube is accidentally disconnected is no longer advocated. The danger of rapid accumulation of air in the pleural space, causing tension pneumothorax, is far greater than that of a small amount of atmospheric air entering the pleural space. If a chest tube becomes disconnected, immediately reestablish the water-seal system and attach a new drainage system as soon as possible. In some hospitals, when disconnection occurs, the chest tube is immersed in sterile water (about 2 cm) until the system can be reestablished. It is important to know the unit protocol, individual clinical situation (whether an air leak exists), and physician preference before resorting to prolonged chest tube clamping.

Chest tubes may be momentarily clamped to change the drainage apparatus or to check for air leaks. Appearance of a new air leak warrants assessment of the drainage system to identify whether the air leak is coming from the patient or the system. Although it is controversial, some clinicians clamp the chest tube for a few hours before removal. This is done to assess how the patient will tolerate chest tube removal. Generally this occurs 4 to 6 hours before the tube is removed, and the patient is monitored closely for any signs of respiratory distress.

Closely monitor the patient for complications associated with chest tube placement and drainage. If volumes from 1 to 1.5 L of pleural fluid are removed rapidly, reexpansion pulmonary edema or a vasovagal response with symptomatic hypotension can occur. Subcutaneous emphysema can occur from air leaking into the tissue surrounding the chest tube insertion site. A "crackling" sensation will be felt when palpating the skin. A small amount of subcutaneous air is harmless and will be reabsorbed. However, severe subcutaneous emphysema can cause drastic swelling of the head and the neck with potential airway compromise.[37]

Meticulous sterile technique during dressing changes can reduce the incidence of infected sites. Nursing care and patient teaching can minimize the risk of atelectasis and shoulder stiffness. Encourage coughing, deep breathing, incentive spirometer use, and range-of-motion exercises.

CHEST TUBE REMOVAL

The chest tubes are removed when the lungs are reexpanded and fluid drainage has ceased or is minimal. Generally suction is discontinued and the chest drain is on gravity drainage for 24 hours before the tube is removed. Give the patient pain medication about 30 to 60 minutes before tube removal. Gather dressing supplies and petroleum jelly dressing. Explain the procedure to the patient. The tube is removed by the physician or an advanced practice nurse in most settings. The suture is cut, and a sterile airtight petroleum jelly gauze dressing is prepared. With the patient holding his or her breath or bearing down (Valsalva maneuver), the tube is removed. The site is immediately covered with the airtight dressing to prevent air from entering the pleural space. The pleura will seal off, and the wound usually heals in several days. A chest x-ray is done to evaluate for pneumothorax or reaccumulation of fluid. Observe the wound for drainage, and reinforce the dressing if necessary. Assess the patient for respiratory distress, which may signify a recurrence of the original problem.

CHEST SURGERY

Chest surgery is performed for various reasons, including lung, heart, vascular, and esophageal disorders. The most common types of chest surgery are described in Table 28-22.

Preoperative Care

The patient's cardiopulmonary status is assessed to determine his or her ability to tolerate the surgery and to provide a baseline reference for postoperative care. Diagnostic studies include pulmonary function studies, chest x-ray, electrocardiogram (ECG),

TABLE 28-22   CHEST SURGERIES

Type	Indications	Description
Lobectomy Removal of one lobe of lung	Lung cancer, bronchiectasis, TB, emphysematous bullae, benign lung tumors, fungal infections	Most common lung surgery. Need chest tubes postoperatively. Lung tissue expands to fill up space left by resected lobe.
Pneumonectomy Removal of entire lung	Lung cancer (most common)	Done only when lobectomy or segmental resection will not remove all diseased lung. May have clamped chest tube postoperatively. Fluid will gradually fill space where lung has been removed. Position patient on operative side to facilitate expansion of remaining lung.
Segmental resection Removal of one or more lung segments	Lung cancer, bronchiectasis	Done to remove bronchovascular lung segment. Need chest tubes postoperatively. Remaining lung tissue expands to fill space. Indicated for a patient unable to handle more extensive surgery.
Wedge resection Removal of small, localized lesion that occupies only part of a segment	Lung biopsy, excision of small nodules	Most conservative approach. Need chest tubes postoperatively. Done to remove small peripheral nodules or for patients unable to handle more extensive surgery.
Decortication Removal or stripping of thick, fibrous membrane from visceral pleura	Empyema or other inflammatory process unresponsive to conservative management	Need chest tubes postoperatively.
Exploratory thoracotomy Incision into thorax to look for injured or bleeding tissues	Chest trauma	Need chest tubes postoperatively.
Thoracotomy (not involving lungs) Incision into thorax for surgery on other organs	Hiatal hernia repair, open heart surgery, esophageal surgery, tracheal resection, thoracic aorta repair	Postoperative care related to thoracotomy and to primary reason for surgical procedure; need chest tubes postoperatively.
Video-assisted thoracoscopic surgery (VATS)	VATS done under general anesthesia in operating room Procedures performed using VATS include lung biopsy, lobectomy, resection of nodules, repair of fistulas	Video-assisted technique with a rigid scope with a distal lens inserted into the pleura and image shown on a monitor screen. Allows surgeon to manipulate instruments passed into the pleural space through separate small intercostal incisions. Need one chest tube postoperatively.
Lung volume reduction surgery (LVRS)	Advanced bullous emphysema, α_1-antitrypsin emphysema	Involves reducing lung volume by multiple wedge excisions or VATS.

ABGs, blood urea nitrogen (BUN), serum creatinine, blood glucose, serum electrolytes, prothrombin time/international normalized ratio (PT/INR), activated partial thromboplastin time (aPTT), and CBC. Additional cardiac function studies are often done for the patient who is to undergo a pneumonectomy. An anesthesia consult is also completed.

The patient should be in optimal health and stop smoking, if applicable, before elective surgery. Anxiety associated with anticipated surgery makes smoking cessation more difficult. Provide encouragement, support, and teaching regarding various methods to help stop smoking (see Chapter 11).

Teach the patient what to expect postoperatively, including the use of oxygen, possible intubation, administration of blood and fluids, and the purpose and function of chest tubes. Reassure the patient that adequate medication will be used to reduce pain. Explain how to use patient-controlled analgesia (PCA), if planned. Preoperative teaching also includes exercises for effective deep breathing and use of incentive spirometry. If the patient practices these techniques before surgery, they will be easier to perform postoperatively. Show the patient how to splint the incision with a pillow to facilitate deep breathing. Teach and have the patient provide a return demonstration of range-of-motion exercises on the surgical side (similar to those for the mastectomy patient [see Fig. 52-9]).

The thought of losing part of a vital organ is frequently frightening. Reassure the patient that the lungs have a large degree of functional reserve. Even after the removal of one lung, enough lung tissue is left to maintain adequate oxygenation. Be available to answer the patient and caregiver's questions. Answer questions honestly. Try to facilitate the expression of concerns, feelings, and questions. (General preoperative care and teaching are discussed in Chapter 18.)

Surgical Procedures

Thoracotomy. A **thoracotomy** is a surgical incision into the chest to gain access to the heart, lungs, esophagus, thoracic aorta, or anterior spine. The two most common approaches to a thoracotomy are the medial sternotomy and the lateral thoracotomy. The medial sternotomy involves splitting the sternum and is primarily used for surgery involving the heart. The lateral thoracotomy incision can be done using a posterolateral or anterolateral incision. The *posterolateral incision* is used for most surgeries involving the lung. The incision is made from front to back at the level of the fourth, fifth, or sixth intercostal space. Strong mechanical retractors are used to separate the ribs and gain access to the lung. The *anterolateral incision* is made in the fourth or fifth intercostal space from sternal border to the midaxillary line. This procedure is commonly used for surgery or trauma victims, mediastinal operations, and wedge resections of the upper and middle lobes of the lung.

Video-Assisted Thoracic Surgery. *Video-assisted thoracoscopic surgery* (VATS) is a widely used, minimally invasive surgical approach. It provides a real-time two-dimensional video image of the inside of the chest cavity. It is used for diagnosis and treatment of diseases of the pleura, pulmonary masses and nodules, mediastinal masses, and interstitial lung disease. Through incisions just large enough to insert the instruments, the surgeon can inspect the chest cavity, biopsy suspicious areas, obtain samples of fluids for analysis, and remove tissue. VATS is increasingly being used for patients with thoracic trauma. The surgeon can inspect, diagnose, and manage intrathoracic injuries in both blunt and penetrating trauma, including injuries to the diaphragm. A chest tube is placed in the pleural space through one or more of the incisions at the end of the procedure, secured with sutures, and connected to a drainage unit in the usual manner.

The advantages of minimally invasive surgery include less discomfort, faster return to normal activity level, reduced length of hospital stay, lower postoperative morbidity risk, and fewer complications.[38] Patients who have marginal respiratory reserve or are too debilitated to tolerate an open thoracotomy approach may benefit from the VATS procedure.

Postoperative Care

Postoperative pain after a thoracotomy is typically intense because respiratory muscles are cut during surgery. Adequate pain management is a priority to prevent respiratory compromise. The use of PCA and intercostal nerve blocks enables the patient to breathe deeply, cough, and move the arm and shoulder on the operative side.

For most chest surgeries, chest tubes are placed in the pleural space to allow for lung reexpansion. In a pneumonectomy, chest tubes may or may not be placed in the space from which the lung was removed. If a chest tube is used, it is clamped and only released by the surgeon to adjust the volume of serosanguineous fluid that will fill the space vacated by the lung. If the cavity overfills, it could compress the remaining lung and compromise the cardiovascular and pulmonary function. Daily chest x-rays assess the volume and space.

Nursing care priorities in the postoperative period include assessment of respiratory function, including observation of respiratory rate and effort, sputum volume and color, breath sounds, and chest tube function and drainage. Assessment of pain, monitoring of temperature, and observation of the surgical site are similar to care provided for other postoperative patients (see Chapter 20). Care after thoracotomy is presented in eNursing Care Plan 28-2 (available on the website for this chapter).

RESTRICTIVE RESPIRATORY DISORDERS

Disorders that impair the ability of the chest wall and diaphragm to move with respiration are called *restrictive respiratory disorders*. There are two categories: *extrapulmonary conditions*, in which the lung tissue is normal, and *intrapulmonary conditions*, in which the cause is the lung or the pleura. Examples of extrapulmonary conditions that alter respirations are listed in Table 28-23. These disorders are further described in their respective chapters.

Examples of intrapulmonary causes are listed in Table 28-24. Lung damage can be caused by inflammation and scarring of lung tissue (interstitial lung disease), air spaces (pneumonitis), or pleura (empyema).

Pulmonary function tests are the best means of differentiating between restrictive and obstructive respiratory disorders. Restrictive lung disorders are characterized by reduced vital capacity (VC) and total lung capacity (TLC).[39] Mixed obstruc-

TABLE 28-23	EXTRAPULMONARY CAUSES OF RESTRICTIVE LUNG DISEASE*
Central Nervous System (CNS) • Head injury, CNS lesion (e.g., tumor, stroke) • Opioid and barbiturate use **Neuromuscular System** • Spinal cord injury • Guillain-Barré syndrome • Amyotrophic lateral sclerosis • Myasthenia gravis • Muscular dystrophy	**Chest Wall** • Chest wall trauma (e.g., flail chest, fractured rib) • Obesity-hypoventilation syndrome (Pickwickian syndrome) • Kyphoscoliosis

*See eTable 28-3 for more detailed descriptions on extrapulmonary causes of restrictive lung disease.

TABLE 28-24	INTRAPULMONARY CAUSES OF RESTRICTIVE LUNG DISEASE*
Pleural Disorders • Pleural effusion • Pleurisy (pleuritis) • Pneumothorax	**Parenchymal Disorders** • Atelectasis • Pneumonia • Interstitial lung diseases • Acute respiratory distress syndrome (ARDS)

*See eTable 28-3 for more detailed descriptions on intrapulmonary causes of restrictive lung disease.

tive and restrictive disorders sometimes occur together. For example, a patient may have both chronic bronchitis (an obstructive problem) and pulmonary fibrosis (a restrictive problem).

PLEURAL EFFUSION

Types

The pleural space normally contains 5 to 15 mL of fluid that acts as a lubricant between the chest wall (parietal pleura) and the lung (visceral pleura). **Pleural effusion** is an abnormal collection of fluid in this space. It is not a disease but rather an indication of disease. A balance between hydrostatic pressure, oncotic pressure, and membrane permeability governs movement of fluid in and out of the pleural space. Fluid accumulation can be a result of increased pulmonary capillary pressure, decreased oncotic pressure, increased pleural membrane permeability, or obstruction of lymphatic flow.[40]

Pleural effusion is classified as transudative or exudative according to the protein content. A *transudate* occurs primarily in noninflammatory conditions and is an accumulation of protein-poor, cell-poor fluid. Transudative pleural effusions are clear, pale yellow, and caused by (1) increased hydrostatic pressure found in heart failure or (2) decreased oncotic pressure (from hypoalbuminemia) found in chronic liver or renal disease. An *exudative effusion* results from increased capillary permeability characteristic of the inflammatory reaction. It is most commonly associated with infections and malignancies.

An **empyema** is the collection of purulent fluid in the pleural space. It is caused by conditions such as pneumonia, TB, lung

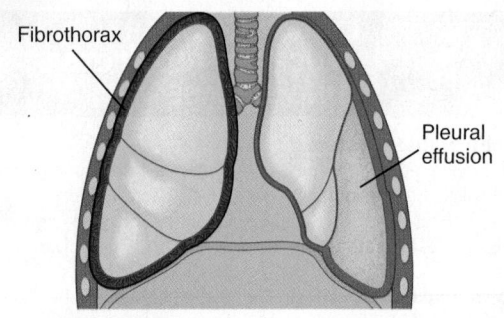

Fibrothorax

Pleural effusion

FIG. 28-10 Fibrothorax resulting from an organization of inflammatory exudate and pleural effusion.

abscess, and infection of surgical wounds of the chest. A complication of empyema is *fibrothorax,* in which there is fibrous fusion of the visceral and parietal pleurae (Fig. 28-10).

Clinical Manifestations

Common clinical manifestations of pleural effusion are dyspnea; cough; and occasional sharp, nonradiating chest pain that is worse on inhalation. Physical examination of the chest may indicate decreased movement of the chest on the affected side, dullness to percussion, and diminished breath sounds over the affected area. A chest x-ray and CT reveal the volume and location of the effusion. Manifestations of empyema include the manifestations of pleural effusion, as well as fever, night sweats, cough, and weight loss.

Thoracentesis

Thoracentesis is aspiration of intrapleural fluid for diagnostic and therapeutic purposes. For a thoracentesis, the patient sits on the edge of a bed and leans forward over a bedside table. Chest x-ray results, ultrasound images, and percussion of chest for maximal dullness are used to determine the optimal puncture site. The skin is cleansed with an antiseptic solution and injected with a local anesthetic. The thoracentesis needle is inserted into the intercostal space. Fluid is aspirated with a syringe, or tubing is connected to the needle to allow fluid to drain into a sterile container. After the fluid is removed, the needle is withdrawn, and a bandage is applied over the insertion site.

Usually only 1000 to 1200 mL of pleural fluid is removed at one time. Rapid removal of a large volume can result in hypotension, hypoxemia, or pulmonary edema. A chest x-ray may be done after the procedure to assess for possible complications such as pneumothorax or pulmonary edema. During and after the procedure, monitor vital signs and pulse oximetry, and observe the patient for any manifestations of respiratory distress.

Collaborative Care

The management of pleural effusions is to treat the underlying cause. For example, adequate treatment of heart failure with diuretics and sodium restriction will result in decreased incidence of pleural effusion. The treatment of pleural effusions secondary to malignant disease represents a more difficult problem. These types of pleural effusions are frequently recurrent and accumulate quickly after thoracentesis.

Chemical pleurodesis is performed to obliterate the pleural space and prevent reaccumulation of effusion fluid in both malignant and nonmalignant pleural effusions. This procedure first requires chest tube drainage of the effusion. Once the fluid is drained, a chemical slurry is instilled into the pleural space. Talc is the most effective agent for pleurodesis.[41] Other agents such as doxycycline and bleomycin can also be used. The chest tube is clamped for 8 hours while the patient is turned in different positions to allow the chemical to contact the entire pleural space. After 8 hours the chest tube is unclamped and attached to a drainage unit. Fever and chest pain are the most common side effects associated with pleurodesis. Chest tubes are left in place until fluid drainage is less than 150 mL/day and no air leaks are noted.

Treatment of empyema is generally with chest tube drainage. Appropriate antibiotic therapy is also necessary to eradicate the causative organism. Intrapleural fibrinolytic therapy (instilled via the chest tube) may be considered for some patients to dissolve fibrous adhesions. If this therapy is unsuccessful, a *decortication* surgical procedure may be needed to remove the pleural peel.

PLEURISY

Pleurisy (pleuritis) is an inflammation of the pleura. Inflammation can be caused by infectious diseases, neoplasms, autoimmune disorders, chest trauma, GI disease, and certain medications. The inflammation usually subsides with adequate treatment of the primary disease. The pain of pleurisy is typically abrupt and sharp in onset and is aggravated by inspiration. The patient's breathing is shallow and rapid to avoid unnecessary movement of the pleura and chest wall. A pleural friction rub may occur, which is the sound over areas where inflamed visceral pleura and parietal pleura rub over one another during inspiration. This sound, like a squeaking door, is usually loudest at peak inspiration but may be heard during exhalation as well.

Treatment of pleurisy is aimed at treating the underlying disease and providing pain relief. Taking NSAIDs or analgesics and lying on or splinting the affected side may provide some relief. Teach the patient to splint the rib cage when coughing. Intercostal nerve blocks may be done if the pain is severe.

ATELECTASIS

Atelectasis is a lung condition characterized by collapsed, airless alveoli. There may be diminished or absent breath sounds and dullness to percussion over the affected area. The most common cause of atelectasis is obstruction of the small airways with secretions. This is common in bedridden patients and in postoperative abdominal and thoracic surgery patients. Normally the pores of Kohn (see Fig. 26-1) provide collateral passage of air from one alveolus to another. Deep inspiration is necessary to open the pores effectively. For this reason, deep-breathing exercises and coughing are important to prevent atelectasis and treat the patient at risk. (The prevention and treatment of atelectasis are discussed in Chapter 20.)

INTERSTITIAL LUNG DISEASES

Interstitial lung disease (ILD), also called *diffuse parenchymal lung disease,* refers to more than 200 lung disorders in which the tissue between the air sacs of the lungs (the interstitium) is affected by inflammation or scarring (fibrosis). ILDs can be caused by inhalation of occupational and environmental toxins, certain medications, radiation therapy, connective tissue disorders, malignancy, and infection. Treatment is aimed at reducing exposure to the causative agent and/or treating the underlying disease process. Although scarring is irreversible, treatment with corticosteroids and immunosuppressant drugs can minimize progression. A lung transplant may be an option for some patients.

Many times the cause of ILD is unknown. The most common ILDs of unknown etiology are idiopathic pulmonary fibrosis and sarcoidosis.

IDIOPATHIC PULMONARY FIBROSIS

Idiopathic pulmonary fibrosis (IPF) is a chronic, progressive disorder characterized by chronic inflammation and formation of scar tissue in the connective tissue. A history of cigarette smoking is a risk factor for IPF. It affects more men than women and typically first appears between the ages of 50 and 70 years.

Clinical manifestations of IPF include exertional dyspnea, nonproductive cough, clubbing of the fingers, and inspiratory crackles. Fatigue, weakness, anorexia, and weight loss may occur as the disease progresses. Chest x-ray shows changes characteristic of IPF. High-resolution CT scan provides detailed images. Pulmonary function tests are abnormal with evidence of restriction (reduced vital capacity) and impaired gas exchange. Open lung biopsy using VATS often helps to confirm the pathology and is considered the "gold standard" for diagnosis.

The clinical course of IPF is variable and the prognosis is poor, with a 5-year survival rate of 30% to 50% after diagnosis. Many people diagnosed with IPF are initially treated with a corticosteroid (prednisone), sometimes in combination with other drugs that suppress the immune system (e.g., methotrexate, cyclosporine). None of these combinations has proved very effective.[42] O$_2$ therapy should be prescribed for all patients. Lung transplantation is an option for those who meet the criteria. (Lung transplantation is discussed later in this chapter on p. 556.)

SARCOIDOSIS

Sarcoidosis is a chronic, multisystem granulomatous disease of unknown cause that primarily affects the lungs. The disease may also involve the skin, eyes, liver, kidney, heart, and lymph nodes. African Americans and those with a family history are at higher risk for developing sarcoidosis. Signs and symptoms vary depending on what organs are affected. Pulmonary symptoms include dyspnea, cough, and chest pain. Many patients do not have symptoms.

The disease is staged and treatment decisions are based on pulmonary function and progression of the disease. Some patients have a spontaneous remission. Treatment is aimed at suppression of the inflammatory response. Patients are followed every 3 to 6 months with pulmonary function tests, chest x-ray, and CT scan to monitor disease progression.

VASCULAR LUNG DISORDERS

PULMONARY EDEMA

Pulmonary edema is an abnormal accumulation of fluid in the alveoli and interstitial spaces of the lungs. It is a complication of various heart and lung diseases (Table 28-25). Pulmonary edema is considered a life-threatening medical emergency.

TABLE 28-25 CAUSES OF PULMONARY EDEMA

- Heart failure
- Overhydration with IV fluids
- Hypoalbuminemia: nephrotic syndrome, hepatic disease, nutritional disorders
- Altered capillary permeability of lungs: inhaled toxins, inflammation (e.g., pneumonia), severe hypoxia, near-drowning
- Malignancies of the lymph system (e.g., non-Hodgkin's lymphoma)
- Respiratory distress syndrome (e.g., O$_2$ toxicity)
- Unknown causes: neurogenic condition, opioid overdose, reexpansion pulmonary edema, high altitude

The most common cause of pulmonary edema is left-sided heart failure. (Pathophysiology, clinical manifestations, and management of pulmonary edema are described in Chapter 35.)

PULMONARY EMBOLISM

Etiology and Pathophysiology

Pulmonary embolism (PE) is the blockage of pulmonary arteries by a thrombus, fat or air embolus, or tumor tissue. The word *embolus* derives from a Greek word meaning "plug" or "stopper." *Emboli* are mobile clots that generally do not stop moving until they lodge at a narrowed part of the circulatory system. A pulmonary embolus consists of material that gains access to the venous system and then to the pulmonary circulation. The embolus travels with the blood flow through ever-smaller blood vessels until it lodges and obstructs perfusion of the alveoli (Fig. 28-11). Because of higher blood flow, the lower lobes of the lung are commonly affected. Approximately 10% of patients with PE die within the first hour. An additional 30% die from recurrent embolism. Treatment with anticoagulants reduces the mortality rate to less than 5%.[43]

More than 90% of pulmonary emboli arise from deep vein thrombosis (DVT) in the deep veins of the legs.[7] *Venous thromboembolism* (VTE) is the preferred term to describe the spectrum of pathologic conditions from DVT to PE (see Table 38-7). Lethal pulmonary emboli most commonly originate in the femoral or iliac veins. Generally, DVTs that are below the knee are not considered a risk factor for PE, since they rarely migrate to the pulmonary circulation without first extending above the knee. The highest rate of DVT is in spinal cord injury patients (60% to 80%).[43]

Other sites of origin of PE include the right side of the heart (especially with atrial fibrillation), the upper extremities (rare),

FIG. 28-11 Large embolus from the femoral vein lying in the main left and right pulmonary arteries.

and the pelvic veins (especially after surgery or childbirth). Upper extremity DVT occasionally occurs in the presence of central venous catheters or cardiac pacing wires. These cases may resolve with the removal of the catheter.

In addition to dislodged thrombi, less common causes of PE include fat emboli (from fractured long bones), air emboli (from improperly administered IV therapy), bacterial vegetations, amniotic fluid, and tumors. Risk factors for PE include immobility or reduced mobility, surgery within the last 3 months (especially pelvic and lower extremity surgery), history of DVT, malignancy, obesity, oral contraceptives and hormone therapy, heavy cigarette smoking, prolonged air travel, heart failure, pregnancy, and clotting disorders.

Clinical Manifestations

The signs and symptoms in PE are varied and nonspecific, making diagnosis difficult. Symptoms may begin slowly or suddenly. Dyspnea is the most common presenting symptom, occurring in 85% of patients with PE.[7] A mild to moderate hypoxemia with a low $PaCO_2$ is a common finding. Other manifestations are tachypnea, cough, chest pain, hemoptysis, crackles, wheezing, fever, accentuation of the pulmonic heart sound, tachycardia, syncope, and sudden change in mental status as a result of hypoxemia.

Clinical manifestations depend on the size and extent of emboli. Massive emboli may produce abrupt hypotension and shock. The mortality rate for massive PE is 30% to 60%, with most deaths occurring within 1 to 2 hours of onset.[43]

Conversely, small emboli may go undetected or produce vague, transient symptoms. The exception to this is the patient with underlying cardiopulmonary disease. In these patients, even small or medium-sized emboli may result in severe cardiopulmonary compromise. Repeated pulmonary emboli gradually cause a reduction in the capillary bed and eventual pulmonary hypertension. Right ventricular hypertrophy can develop secondary to pulmonary hypertension.

Complications

Pulmonary infarction (death of lung tissue) is most likely when the following factors are present: (1) occlusion of a large or medium-sized pulmonary vessel (more than 2 mm in diameter), (2) insufficient collateral blood flow from the bronchial circulation, or (3) preexisting lung disease. Infarction results in alveolar necrosis and hemorrhage. Occasionally the necrotic tissue becomes infected, and an abscess may develop. Concomitant pleural effusion is frequent.

Pulmonary hypertension results from hypoxemia or from involvement of more than 50% of the area of the normal pulmonary bed. As a single event, an embolus does not cause pulmonary hypertension unless it is massive. Recurrent emboli may result in chronic pulmonary hypertension. Pulmonary hypertension eventually results in dilation and hypertrophy of the right ventricle. Depending on the degree of pulmonary hypertension and its rate of development, outcomes can vary, with some patients dying within months of the diagnosis and others living for decades.

Diagnostic Studies

D-dimer is a laboratory test that measures the amount of cross-linked fibrin fragments. These fragments are the result of clot degradation and are rarely found in healthy individuals. The disadvantage of D-dimer is that it is neither specific (other

TABLE 28-26   COLLABORATIVE CARE

Acute Pulmonary Embolism

Diagnostic	Collaborative Therapy
• History and physical examination	• Supplemental O_2, intubation if necessary
• Chest x-ray	• Fibrinolytic agent
• Continuous ECG monitoring	• Unfractionated heparin IV
• ABGs	• Low-molecular-weight heparin (e.g., enoxaparin [Lovenox])
• Venous ultrasound	
• CBC count with WBC differential	• Warfarin (Coumadin) for long-term therapy
• Spiral (helical) CT scan	• Monitoring of aPTT and INR levels
• Ventilation-perfusion (V/Q) lung scan	
• D-dimer level	• Limited activity
• Troponin level, BNP level	• Opioids for pain relief
• Pulmonary angiography	• Inferior vena cava filter
	• Pulmonary embolectomy in life-threatening situation

ABGs, Arterial blood gases; *aPTT,* activated partial thromboplastin time; *BNP,* b-type natriuretic peptide; *INR,* international normalized ratio.

conditions cause elevation) nor sensitive, because up to 50% of patients with small pulmonary emboli have normal results. Patients with suspected PE and an elevated D-dimer level but normal venous ultrasound may need a spiral CT or lung scan.

A *spiral (helical) CT scan* (also known as CT angiography or CTA) is the most frequently used test to diagnose PE (Table 28-26). An IV injection of contrast media is required to view the blood vessels. The scanner continuously rotates while obtaining slices and does not start and stop between each slice. This allows visualization of all anatomic regions of the lungs. The computer reconstructs the data to provide a three-dimensional picture and assist in emboli visualization.

If a patient cannot have contrast media, a ventilation-perfusion (V/Q) scan is done. The V/Q scan has two components and is most accurate when both are performed:

1. *Perfusion scanning* involves IV injection of a radioisotope. A scanning device images the pulmonary circulation.
2. *Ventilation scanning* involves inhalation of a radioactive gas such as xenon. Scanning reflects the distribution of gas through the lung. The ventilation component requires the patient's cooperation and may be impossible to perform in the critically ill patient, particularly if the patient is intubated.

Pulmonary angiography is the most sensitive and specific test for PE. However, it is an expensive and invasive procedure that involves insertion of a catheter through the antecubital or femoral vein, advancement to the pulmonary artery, and injection of contrast medium. The reliability of the spiral CT has greatly diminished the need for pulmonary angiography.

ABG analysis is important, but not diagnostic. The PaO_2 is low because of inadequate oxygenation secondary to an occluded pulmonary vasculature preventing matching of perfusion to ventilation. The pH remains normal unless respiratory alkalosis develops as a result of prolonged hyperventilation or to compensate for lactic acidosis caused by shock. Abnormal findings are usually reported on the chest x-ray (atelectasis, pleural effusion) and the ECG (ST segment and T wave changes), but they are not diagnostic for PE. Serum troponin levels and b-type natriuretic peptide (BNP) levels are frequently elevated. Although not diagnostic, elevated levels of these markers are associated with increased mortality in patients with PE.[44]

Collaborative Care

Prevention of PE begins with prevention of DVT. DVT prophylaxis includes the use of sequential compression devices, early ambulation, and anticoagulant medications.

To reduce mortality risk, treatment is begun as soon as PE is suspected (see Table 28-26). The objectives are to (1) prevent further growth or multiplication of thrombi in the lower extremities, (2) prevent embolization from the upper or lower extremities to the pulmonary vascular system, and (3) provide cardiopulmonary support if indicated.

Supportive therapy for the patient's cardiopulmonary status varies according to the severity of the PE. O_2 can be given via mask or cannula, and the concentration is determined by ABG analysis. In some situations, endotracheal intubation and mechanical ventilation are necessary to maintain adequate oxygenation. Respiratory measures such as turning, coughing, deep breathing, and using incentive spirometry are important to help prevent or treat atelectasis. If manifestations of shock are present, IV fluids are administered followed by vasopressor agents as needed to support perfusion (see Chapter 67). If heart failure is present, diuretics are used (see Chapter 35). Pain resulting from pleural irritation or reduced coronary blood flow is treated with opioids (usually morphine).

Drug Therapy. Immediate anticoagulation is required for patients with PE. Subcutaneous administration of low-molecular-weight heparin (LMWH) (e.g., enoxaparin [Lovenox]) has been found to be safer and more effective than use of unfractionated heparin. It is the recommended choice of treatment for patients with nonmassive PE. Unfractionated IV heparin can be as effective but is more difficult to titrate to therapeutic levels. Monitoring the aPTT is not necessary or useful when using LMWH.

Warfarin (Coumadin) should be initiated within the first 3 days of heparinization and is typically administered for 3 to 6 months. Some health care providers use direct thrombin inhibitors (see Table 38-10) in the treatment of PE. Anticoagulant therapy may be contraindicated if the patient has complicating factors such as blood dyscrasias, hepatic dysfunction causing alteration in the clotting mechanism, injury to the intestine, overt bleeding, a history of hemorrhagic stroke, or neurologic conditions.

Fibrinolytic agents, such as tissue plasminogen activator (tPA) or alteplase (Activase), dissolve the pulmonary embolus and the source of the thrombus in the pelvis or deep leg veins, thereby decreasing the likelihood of recurrent emboli. Indications for thrombolytic therapy in PE include hemodynamic instability and right ventricular dysfunction. (Fibrinolytic therapy is discussed in Chapter 34.)

Surgical Therapy. Hemodynamically unstable patients with massive PE with contraindications for fibrinolytic therapy are candidates for immediate pulmonary embolectomy. This can be achieved via a vascular (catheter) or surgical approach. Pulmonary embolectomy has a high mortality rate and is thus not recommended for patients who can be successfully treated otherwise.

To prevent further emboli, an inferior vena cava (IVC) filter may be the treatment of choice in patients who remain at high risk and patients for whom anticoagulation is contraindicated. This device is percutaneously placed at the level of the diaphragm in the inferior vena cava via the femoral vein. It prevents migration of large clots into the pulmonary system. The complications associated with this device are rare and include misplacement, migration, and perforation.

NURSING MANAGEMENT PULMONARY EMBOLISM

NURSING IMPLEMENTATION

Nursing measures aimed at prevention of PE are similar to those for prophylaxis of DVT (see Chapter 38, pp. 849-850).

The prognosis of a patient with PE is good if therapy is promptly instituted. Keep the patient on bed rest in a semi-Fowler's position to facilitate breathing. Maintain an IV line for medications and fluid therapy. Administer oxygen therapy as ordered. Assess the patient's cardiopulmonary status with careful monitoring of vital signs, cardiac rhythm, pulse oximetry, ABGs, and lung sounds. Monitor laboratory results to ensure therapeutic ranges of INR (for warfarin) and aPTT (for IV heparin). Monitor the patient for complications of anticoagulant and fibrinolytic therapy (e.g., bleeding, hematomas, bruising). Provide appropriate interventions related to immobility and fall precautions.

The patient is usually anxious because of pain, a sense of doom, inability to breathe, and fear of death. Carefully explain the situation and provide emotional support and reassurance to help relieve the patient's anxiety.

Patient teaching regarding long-term anticoagulant therapy is critical. Anticoagulant therapy continues for at least 3 to 6 months. Patients with recurrent emboli are treated indefinitely. INR levels are drawn at intervals and warfarin dosage is adjusted. Some patients are monitored by nurses in an anticoagulation clinic.

Long-term management is similar to that for the patient with DVT (see discussion of DVT in Chapter 38 on pp. 847-856). Discharge planning is aimed at limiting progression of the condition and preventing complications and recurrence. Reinforce the need for the patient to return to the health care provider for regular follow-up examinations.

EVALUATION

The expected outcomes are that the patient who has a PE will have

- Adequate tissue perfusion and respiratory function
- Adequate cardiac output
- Increased level of comfort
- No recurrence of PE

PULMONARY HYPERTENSION

Pulmonary hypertension is characterized by elevated pulmonary artery pressure, resulting from an increase in resistance to blood flow through the pulmonary circulation. Normally the pulmonary circulation is characterized by low resistance and low pressure. In pulmonary hypertension the pulmonary pressures are elevated with the mean pulmonary artery pressure greater than 25 mm Hg at rest (normal is 12 to 16 mm Hg) or greater than 30 mm Hg with exercise.

The disease commonly manifests with shortness of breath and fatigue. Pulmonary hypertension can occur as a primary disease (*idiopathic pulmonary arterial hypertension*) or as a secondary complication of a respiratory, cardiac, autoimmune, hepatic, or connective tissue disorder (*secondary pulmonary arterial hypertension*).

IDIOPATHIC PULMONARY ARTERIAL HYPERTENSION

Idiopathic pulmonary arterial hypertension (IPAH) is pulmonary hypertension that occurs without an apparent cause. (It was previously known as *primary pulmonary hypertension* [PPH].) If untreated, this disorder can be rapidly progressive, causing right-sided heart failure and death within a few years. Although new drug therapy has greatly improved survival, the disease remains incurable.

Etiology and Pathophysiology

The etiology of IPAH is unknown. It affects females more than males. The pathophysiology of IPAH is poorly understood. Some type of insult (e.g., hormonal, mechanical) to the pulmonary endothelium may occur, causing a cascade of events leading to vascular scarring, endothelial dysfunction, and smooth muscle proliferation[44] (Fig. 28-12).

Clinical Manifestations and Diagnostic Studies

Classic symptoms of pulmonary hypertension are dyspnea on exertion and fatigue. Exertional chest pain, dizziness, and exertional syncope are other symptoms. These symptoms are related to the inability of cardiac output to increase in response to increased oxygen demand. Eventually, as the disease progresses, dyspnea occurs at rest. Pulmonary hypertension increases the workload of the right ventricle and causes right ventricular hypertrophy (a condition called *cor pulmonale*) and eventually heart failure.

Right-sided cardiac catheterization is the definitive test to diagnose any type of pulmonary hypertension. In addition to providing an accurate measurement of pulmonary artery pressures, it also determines cardiac output and pulmonary vascular resistance. Confirmation of IPAH requires a thorough workup to exclude conditions that may cause secondary pulmonary hypertension. Diagnostic evaluation includes ECG, chest x-ray, pulmonary function tests, echocardiogram, and CT scans.

The mean time between onset of symptoms and the diagnosis is about 2 years. By the time patients become symptomatic, the disease is already in the advanced stages and the pulmonary artery pressure is two to three times normal.

NURSING AND COLLABORATIVE MANAGEMENT PULMONARY HYPERTENSION

Early recognition of pulmonary hypertension is essential to interrupt the vicious cycle responsible for progression of the disease (see Fig. 28-12). Patients are classified using the New York Heart Association functional classification (see Chapter 35, Table 35-5).

Although IPAH has no cure, treatment can relieve symptoms, improve quality of life, and prolong life. Drug therapy consists of several drug classifications that promote vasodilation of the pulmonary blood vessels, reduce right ventricular overload, and reverse remodeling (Table 28-27). Diuretics are used to manage peripheral edema. The use of anticoagulants is also beneficial in pulmonary complications related to thrombus formation. Because hypoxia is a potent pulmonary vasoconstrictor, low-flow O_2 provides symptomatic relief. The goal is to keep O_2 saturation at 90% or greater.

Surgical interventions for pulmonary hypertension include atrial septostomy (AS) and lung transplantation. AS is a palliative procedure that involves the creation of an intraatrial right-to-left shunt to decompress the right ventricle. It is used for a select group of patients awaiting lung transplantation.

Lung transplantation is indicated for those patients who do not respond to drug therapy and progress to severe right-sided heart failure. Recurrence of the disease has not been reported in individuals who have undergone transplantation. A patient teaching and support website for pulmonary hypertension is located at *www.phassociation.org*.

SECONDARY PULMONARY ARTERIAL HYPERTENSION

Secondary pulmonary arterial hypertension (SPAH) occurs when a primary disease causes a chronic increase in pulmonary artery pressures. SPAH can develop as a result of parenchymal lung disease, left ventricular dysfunction, intracardiac shunts, chronic pulmonary thromboembolism, or systemic connective tissue disease. The specific primary disease pathology can result in anatomic or vascular changes causing the pulmonary hypertension.

The symptoms can reflect the underlying disease, but some are directly attributable to SPAH, including dyspnea, fatigue, lethargy, and chest pain. The initial physical findings can include right ventricular hypertrophy and signs of right ventricular failure (increased pulmonic heart sound, right-sided fourth heart sound, peripheral edema, and hepatomegaly).

Diagnosis of SPAH is similar to that of IPAH. Treatment of SPAH consists mainly of treating the underlying primary disorder. When irreversible pulmonary vascular damage has occurred, therapies used for IPAH are initiated. A pulmonary thromboendarterectomy (PTE) may offer a cure for patients with chronic pulmonary hypertension caused by thromboembolism. It is a technically demanding procedure and is performed only at selected centers.

PATHOPHYSIOLOGY MAP

Insult occurs (hormonal, mechanical, other)

↓

Pulmonary endothelial injury
- Smooth muscle proliferation
- Vascular scarring

↓

Sustained pulmonary hypertension

↓

Right ventricular hypertrophy

↓

Cor pulmonale

↓

Right-sided heart failure

FIG. 28-12 Pathogenesis of pulmonary hypertension and cor pulmonale.

TABLE 28-27 DRUG THERAPY

Pulmonary Hypertension

Drug	Mechanism of Action	Considerations
Calcium Channel Blockers		
nifedipine (Adalat CC, Nifedical XL, Procardia) diltiazem (Cardizem, Cardizem LA, Cartia XT, Tiazac)	• Act on vascular smooth muscle, causing dilation • Lower pulmonary artery pressure	• Can only be used in patients who do not have right-sided heart failure. • Used at high doses in comparison to other uses of calcium channel blockers.
Phosphodiesterase (Type 5) Enzyme Inhibitors		
sildenafil (Revatio) tadalafil (Adcirca)	• Promote selective smooth muscle relaxation in lung vasculature	• Given orally. • Contraindicated in patients taking nitroglycerin, since may cause refractory hypotension.
Vasodilators (Parenteral)		
epoprostenol (Flolan, Veletri) treprostinil (Remodulin) adenosine (Adenocard)	• Prostacyclin analog • Promote pulmonary vasodilation and reduce pulmonary vascular resistance	• Given IV to patients who do not respond to calcium channel blockers or have New York Heart Association (NYHA) class III or IV right-sided heart failure. • Given by continuous IV (central line) or continuous subcutaneous route (see Fig. 28-13). Half life of epoprostenol is short. Potential clinical deterioration from abrupt withdrawal if infusion disrupted.
Vasodilators (Inhaled)		
iloprost (Ventavis) treprostinil (inhaled) (Tyvaso)	• Synthetic analogs of prostacyclin (PGI₂) • Dilate systemic and pulmonary arterial vasculature	• Indicated for patients with NYHA class III or IV heart failure. • Administered 6-9 times a day using a disk inserted into a nebulizer. • Can cause orthostatic hypotension. Do not give to patients with systolic BP <85 mm Hg.
Endothelin Receptor Antagonists		
bosentan (Tracleer) ambrisentan (Letairis)	• Bind to endothelin-1 receptors, causing a reduction in pulmonary artery pressure, pulmonary vascular resistance, and mean atrial pressure • Significantly increase cardiac index	• Given orally. • Indicated for patients with NYHA class II to IV symptoms. • Hepatotoxic. • Monitor liver function tests monthly.

FIG. 28-13 A patient with pulmonary hypertension who is on continuous epoprostenol infusion is being taught how to use the portable infusion pump.

COR PULMONALE

Cor pulmonale is enlargement of the right ventricle caused by a primary disorder of the respiratory system. Pulmonary hypertension is usually a preexisting condition in cor pulmonale. Cor pulmonale may be present with or without overt cardiac failure. The most common cause of cor pulmonale is COPD. Almost any disorder that affects the respiratory system can cause cor pulmonale. Fig. 28-12 outlines the etiology and pathogenesis of pulmonary hypertension and cor pulmonale.

Clinical Manifestations and Diagnostic Studies

Clinical manifestations are subtle and often masked by the symptoms of the pulmonary condition. Common symptoms include exertional dyspnea, tachypnea, cough, and fatigue. Physical signs include evidence of right ventricular hypertrophy on ECG and an increase in intensity of the second heart sound. Chronic hypoxemia leads to polycythemia and increased total blood volume and viscosity of the blood. (Polycythemia is often present in cor pulmonale secondary to COPD.)

If heart failure accompanies cor pulmonale, additional manifestations such as peripheral edema; weight gain; distended neck veins; full, bounding pulse; and enlarged liver will also be found. (Heart failure is discussed in Chapter 35.) Various laboratory tests and imaging studies are used to confirm the diagnosis of cor pulmonale (Table 28-28).

Collaborative Care

The primary management of cor pulmonale is directed at treating the underlying pulmonary problem (see Table 28-28). Long-term O₂ therapy to correct the hypoxemia reduces vasoconstriction and pulmonary hypertension. If fluid, electrolyte, and acid-base imbalances are present, they must be corrected. Diuretics and a low-sodium diet help decrease the plasma volume and reduce the workload on the heart. Bronchodilator therapy is indicated if the underlying respiratory problem is due to an obstructive disorder. Other treatments include those for pulmonary hypertension, such as vasodilator therapy, calcium channel blockers, and anticoagulants. Theophylline may help

TABLE 28-28 COLLABORATIVE CARE

Cor Pulmonale

Diagnostic	Collaborative Therapy
• History and physical examination	• O_2 therapy
• ABGs, SpO_2	• Bronchodilators
• Serum and urine electrolytes	• Diuretics
• b-Type natriuretic peptide (BNP)	• Low-sodium diet
• ECG	• Vasodilators (if indicated)
• Chest x-ray	• Calcium channel blockers
• Echocardiography	(if indicated)
• CT scans	• Inotropic agents
• MRI	
• Cardiac catheterization	

due to its weak inotropic effect on the heart. Digitalis may also be used to increase cardiac contractility. Phlebotomy is indicated in patients with chronic cor pulmonale and chronic hypoxia causing severe polycythemia (hematocrit 65% or greater). Chronic management of cor pulmonale resulting from COPD is similar to that described for COPD (see Chapter 29).

LUNG TRANSPLANTATION

Lung transplantation has become an important mode of therapy for patients with end-stage lung disease. The limiting factor for this therapy is the availability of donors. A variety of pulmonary disorders are potentially treatable with lung transplantation (Table 28-29). Improved patient selection criteria, technical advances, and better methods of immunosuppression have resulted in improved survival rates.

Preoperative Care

Patients being considered for lung transplantation need to undergo extensive evaluation. Absolute contraindications for lung transplant include malignancy within past 2 years (except for skin cancer), chronic active hepatitis B or C, HIV, untreatable advanced dysfunction of another major organ system (e.g., liver or renal failure), current smoker, poor nutritional status, poor rehabilitation potential, and significant psychosocial problems. The patient and the family must be able to cope with a complex postoperative regimen (e.g., strict adherence to immunosuppressive therapy, continuous monitoring for early signs of infection, prompt reporting of manifestations of infection). Many transplant centers require preoperative outpatient pulmonary rehabilitation to maximize physical conditioning.

The United Network for Organ Sharing (UNOS) designates recipients of donor lungs based on a lung allocation score (LAS). The LAS prioritizes waiting list recipients based on the urgency of need and posttransplant survival expectations.

TABLE 28-29 INDICATIONS FOR LUNG TRANSPLANTATION*

- Chronic obstructive pulmonary disease
- Idiopathic pulmonary fibrosis
- Cystic fibrosis
- Idiopathic pulmonary arterial hypertension
- α_1-Antitrypsin deficiency

* These are the most common indications.

Patients who are accepted as good potential transplant candidates must carry a pager with them at all times in case a donor organ becomes available. These patients must be prepared to move to their chosen transplant center at a moment's notice. Such patients may be encouraged to limit their travel within a certain geographic region to facilitate rapid transportation to a transplant center.

Surgical Procedure

Four types of transplant procedures are available: single-lung transplantation, bilateral lung transplantation, heart-lung transplantation, and transplantation of lobes from a living-related donor. *Single-lung transplantation* involves an incision on the side of the chest. The opposite lung is ventilated while the diseased lung is excised. The lung is removed and the donor lung implanted. Three anastomoses are done: the bronchus, the pulmonary artery, and the pulmonary veins. In *bilateral lung transplantation* the incision is made across the sternum, and the donor lungs are implanted separately. A median sternotomy incision is used for a *heart-lung transplant* procedure. *Lobar transplantation* from living donors is reserved for candidates who urgently need transplantation and are unlikely to survive until a donor becomes available. The majority of these transplant recipients are patients with cystic fibrosis, and their parents or relatives are donors. Once anastomosis is complete, the lung is gently reinflated, perfusion is reestablished, two chest tubes are placed, and the surgical incision is closed.

Postoperative Care

Early postoperative care includes ventilatory support, fluid and hemodynamic management, immunosuppression, nutritional support, detection of early rejection, and prevention or treatment of infection. Pulmonary clearance measures, including aerosolized bronchodilators, chest physiotherapy, and deep-breathing and coughing techniques, minimize potential complications. Maintenance of fluid balance is vital in the postoperative phase.

Lung transplant recipients are at high risk for bacterial, viral, fungal, and protozoal infections. Infections are the leading cause of death in the early period after the transplant. Bacterial pneumonia, the most common infection, occurs in more than 35% of patients within the first year posttransplant.[45] Cytomegalovirus (CMV), the second most common cause of pneumonia, is the most common opportunistic infection, usually occurring 1 to 4 months postoperatively. Infection by *Aspergillus* organisms is the most common fungal infection.

Immunosuppressive therapy usually includes a three-drug regimen of tacrolimus, mycophenolate mofetil (CellCept), and prednisone. (The mechanisms of action of these drugs are discussed in Table 14-16 and Fig. 14-13.) Drug levels are monitored on a regular basis. Lung transplant recipients usually receive higher levels of immunosuppressive therapy than other organ recipients.

Acute rejection is fairly common in lung transplantation, typically occurring in the first 5 to 10 days after surgery. Low-grade fever, fatigue, dyspnea, dry cough, and O_2 desaturation are signs of rejection. Accurate diagnosis of rejection is by transtracheal biopsy. Treatment is high doses of IV corticosteroids administered for 3 days, followed by high doses of oral prednisone. In patients with persistent or recurrent acute rejection, antilymphocyte therapy may be useful.

Respiratory System

Bronchiolitis obliterans (BOS) is a manifestation of chronic rejection in lung transplant patients. BOS is characterized by airflow obstruction that progresses over time. The onset is often subacute, with gradual development of exertional dyspnea, nonproductive cough, wheezing, and/or low-grade fever. The airway obstruction is not responsive to bronchodilators and corticosteroid therapy. Although not proven effective, additional immunosuppressive agents are used in the treatment of chronic rejection. Because acute rejection is a major risk factor for BOS, prevention of acute rejection is key to decreasing the incidence of chronic rejection.

Before discharge, the patient needs to be able to perform self-care activities, including medication management and activities of daily living, and to accurately identify when to call the transplant team. Patients are placed in an outpatient rehabilitation program to improve physical endurance. Home spirometry is useful in monitoring trends in lung function. Teach patients to keep medication logs, laboratory results, and spirometry records.

After discharge, the transplant team follows patients for transplant-related issues. Patients return to their primary care team for health maintenance and routine illnesses. As transplant procedures become more frequent, transplant patients will return to hospitals for other routine procedures. Coordination of care between the transplant team, primary care team, and inpatient teams is essential for ongoing successful management of these patients. (Organ transplantation, histocompatibility, rejection, and immunosuppressive therapy are discussed in Chapter 14.)

CASE STUDY

Pneumonia and Lung Cancer

iStockphoto/Thinkstock

Patient Profile
J.H. is a 52-year-old white man who comes to the emergency department complaining of shortness of breath. He has not seen a health care provider for many years.

Subjective Data
- Has a 38 pack-year history of cigarette smoking
- States he has always been slender but has had 25-lb weight loss despite a normal appetite in the past few months
- Admits to a "smoker's cough" for the past 2 to 3 years; recently coughing up blood
- Is married and the father of three adult children

Objective Data
Physical Examination
- Thin, pale man looking older than stated age
- Height 6 ft; weight 135 lb (61.2 kg)
- Intermittently confused and anxious with rapid shallow respirations
- Vital signs: temperature 102.6° F (39.2° C), heart rate 120, respiratory rate 36
- Chest wall has limited excursion on right side; auscultation of left side reveals coarse crackles but clear with cough; right side has diminished breath sounds

Diagnostic Studies
- Arterial blood gases: pH 7.21, PaO_2 58 mm Hg, $PaCO_2$ 82 mm Hg, HCO_3^- 33 mEq/L, O_2 saturation 84%

- Chest x-ray: consolidation of the right lung, especially in the base with possible mass in the area of right bronchus; pleural effusion on the right side
- Bronchoscopy with biopsy of mass: small cell lung carcinoma

Collaborative Care
- Diagnosis: pneumonia with small cell lung cancer
- Follow-up with patient and family to consider treatment options

Discussion Questions
1. How would you classify J.H.'s pneumonia? Why is this important?
2. What is your analysis of J.H.'s arterial blood gas results?
3. **Priority Decision:** Based on the assessment data presented, what are the priority nursing diagnoses? Are there any collaborative problems?
4. **Priority Decision:** What are the priority nursing interventions for J.H.?
5. **Delegation Decision:** Identify activities that can be delegated to unlicensed assistive personnel (UAP).
6. You are planning a meeting with J.H. and his family to discuss their needs. The physician tells you that J.H. is terminally ill. Who will you include in this meeting?
7. **Evidence-Based Practice:** J.H.'s children tell you that they are worried they will get lung cancer, since their father has it and they grew up around his secondhand smoke. They want to know what kind of screening is available for them. How will you respond?
8. What is the goal if radiation therapy is used for J.H.?
9. What issues should be addressed in your teaching of J.H. and his wife as you prepare him for discharge and care at home?

evolve Answers available at *http://evolve.elsevier.com/Lewis/medsurg.*

BRIDGE TO NCLEX EXAMINATION

The number of the question corresponds to the same-numbered outcome at the beginning of the chapter.

1. When caring for a patient with acute bronchitis, the nurse will prioritize
   a. auscultating lung sounds.
   b. encouraging fluid restriction.
   c. administering antibiotic therapy.
   d. teaching the patient to avoid cough suppressants.

2. For which patients with pneumonia would the nurse suspect aspiration as the likely cause of pneumonia (*select all that apply*)?
   a. Patient with seizures
   b. Patient with head injury
   c. Patient who had thoracic surgery
   d. Patient who had a myocardial infarction
   e. Patient who is receiving nasogastric tube feeding

3. An appropriate nursing intervention for a patient with pneumonia with the nursing diagnosis of ineffective airway clearance related to thick secretions and fatigue would be to
   a. perform postural drainage every hour.
   b. provide analgesics as ordered to promote patient comfort.
   c. administer O_2 as prescribed to maintain optimal oxygen levels.
   d. teach the patient how to cough effectively to bring secretions to the mouth.

4. A patient with TB has been admitted to the hospital and is placed in an airborne infection isolation room. What should the patient be taught (select all that apply)?
   a. Expect routine TST to evaluate infection.
   b. Visitors will not be allowed while in airborne isolation.
   c. Take all medications for full length of time to prevent multidrug-resistant TB.
   d. Wear a standard isolation mask if leaving the airborne infection isolation room.
   e. Maintain precautions in airborne infection isolation room by coughing into a paper tissue.

5. A patient has been receiving high-dose corticosteroids and broad-spectrum antibiotics for treatment secondary to a traumatic injury and infection. The nurse plans care for the patient knowing that the patient is most susceptible to
   a. candidiasis.
   b. aspergillosis.
   c. histoplasmosis.
   d. coccidioidomycosis.

6. When caring for a patient with a lung abscess, what is the nurse's priority intervention?
   a. Postural drainage
   b. Antibiotic administration
   c. Obtaining a sputum specimen
   d. Patient teaching regarding home care

7. The emergency department nurse is caring for patients exposed to a chlorine leak from a local factory. The nurse would closely monitor these patients for
   a. pulmonary edema.
   b. anaphylactic shock.
   c. respiratory alkalosis.
   d. acute tubular necrosis.

8. The nurse receives an order for a patient with lung cancer to receive influenza vaccine and pneumococcal vaccines. The nurse will
   a. call the health care provider to question the order.
   b. administer both vaccines at the same time in different arms.
   c. administer the flu shot and tell the patient to come back 1 week later to receive the pneumococcal vaccine.
   d. administer the pneumococcal vaccine and suggest FluMist (nasal vaccine) instead of the influenza injection.

9. The nurse identifies a flail chest in a trauma patient when
   a. multiple rib fractures are determined by x-ray.
   b. a tracheal deviation to the unaffected side is present.
   c. paradoxic chest movement occurs during respiration.
   d. there is decreased movement of the involved chest wall.

10. The nurse notes tidaling of the water level in the tube submerged in the water-seal chamber in a patient with closed chest tube drainage. The nurse should
    a. continue to monitor the patient.
    b. check all connections for a leak in the system.
    c. lower the drainage collector further from the chest.
    d. clamp the tubing at progressively distal points away from the patient until the tidaling stops.

11. An appropriate nursing intervention for a patient postpneumonectomy is
    a. monitoring chest tube drainage and functioning.
    b. positioning the patient on the unaffected side or back.
    c. doing range-of-motion exercises on the affected upper limb.
    d. auscultating frequently for lung sounds on the affected side.

12. A priority nursing intervention for a patient who has just undergone a chemical pleurodesis for recurrent pleural effusion is
    a. administering ordered analgesia.
    b. monitoring chest tube drainage.
    c. sending pleural fluid for laboratory analysis.
    d. monitoring the patient's level of consciousness.

13. When planning care for a patient at risk for pulmonary embolism, the nurse prioritizes
    a. maintaining the patient on bed rest.
    b. using sequential compression devices.
    c. encouraging the patient to cough and deep breathe.
    d. teaching the patient how to use the incentive spirometer.

14. Which statement(s) describe(s) the management of a patient following lung transplantation (select all that apply)?
    a. The lung is biopsied using a transtracheal method.
    b. High doses of oxygen are administered around the clock.
    c. The use of a home spirometer will help to monitor lung function.
    d. Immunosuppressant therapy usually involves a three-drug regimen.
    e. Most patients experience an acute rejection episode in the first 3 days.

1. a, 2. a, b, e, 3. d, 4. c, d, e, 5. a, 6. b, 7. a, 8. b, 9. c, 10. a, 11. c, 12. a, 13. b, 14. a, c, d

⊘volve

For rationales to these answers and even more NCLEX review questions, visit *http://evolve.elsevier.com/Lewis/medsurg.*

REFERENCES

1. World Health Organization: WHO fact sheet, October 2008. Retrieved from *www.who.int/mediacentre/factsheets/fs310/en/index.html.*
2. US Department of Health and Human Services: National vital statistics reports, vol. 59, no. 4, March 16, 2011. Retrieved from *www.cdc.gov/nchs/data/nvsr/nvsr59/nvsr59_04.pdf.*

*3. Albert RH: Diagnosis and treatment of acute bronchitis, *Am Fam Physician* 82:1345, 2010.
*4. Hessen MT, Ferri FF, Pearson RL, et al: Pertussis latest updates: October 6, 2011. Retrieved from *www.mdconsult.com/das/pdxmd/body/308288232-3/0?type=med&eid=9-u1.0-_1_mt_1014575#Contributors.*

*Evidence-based information for clinical practice.

*5. Hessen MT, Thompson A, Murphy P, et al: Community-acquired pneumonia in adults. Retrieved from *www.mdconsult.com/das/pdxmd/body/308841038-3/0?type=med&eid=9-u1.0-_1_mt_5091406*.

*6. Thompson AB, Murphy PJ, Pearson RL, et al: Medical care–associated pneumonia. Retrieved from *www.mdconsult.com/das/pdxmd/body/308841038-4/1247664507?type=med&eid=9-u1.0-_1_mt_5091407*.

7. Ferri FF: *Ferri's clinical advisor*, St Louis, 2012, Mosby.

8. Vigil KJ, Adachi JA, Chemaly RF: Analytic review: viral pneumonias in immunocompromised adult hosts, *J Intens Care Med* 25:307, 2010.

9. US Department of Health and Human Services: How is pneumonia treated? Retrieved from *www.nhlbi.nih.gov/health/health-topics/topics/pnu/treatment.html*.

10. Waterer GW, Rello J, Wunderink RG: Community acquired pneumonia, *Am J Respir Crit Care Med* 183:157, 2010.

*11. Eisenstadt ES: Dysphagia and aspiration pneumonia in older adults, *J Am Acad Nurse Pract* 22:17, 2010.

*12. Vigil KJ, Adachi JA, Chemaly RF: Analytic review: viral pneumonias in immunocompromised adult hosts, *J Intens Care Med* 25:307, 2010.

*13. Pogorzelska M, Stone PW, Furuya EY, et al: Impact of the ventilator bundle on ventilator-associated pneumonia in intensive care unit, *Int J Qual Health Care* 1:7, 2011.

*14. Wren SM, Martin M, Yoon JK, et al: Postoperative pneumonia prevention program for the inpatient surgical ward, *J Am College Surg* 210:492, 2010.

*15. MDConsult: Tuberculosis. Retrieved from *www.mdconsult.com/das/pdxmd/body/310121351-3/0?type=med&eid=9-u1.0-_1_mt_1014609*.

16. Centers for Disease Control and Prevention: Tuberculosis fact sheet. Retrieved from *www.cdc.gov/tb/publications/factsheets/statistics/TBTrends.htm*.

17. Karim K: Tuberculosis and infection control, *Br J Nurs* 20:1128, 2011.

18. Gough A, Kaufman G: Pulmonary tuberculosis: clinical features and patient management, *Nurs Stand* 25:48, 2011.

*19. Centers for Disease Control and Prevention: Tuberculin skin testing. Retrieved from *www.cdc.gov/tb/publications/factsheets/testing/skintesting.htm*.

*20. Hargreaves JR, Boccia D, Evans CA, et al: The social determinants of tuberculosis: from evidence to action, *Am J Pub Health* 101:654, 2011.

21. Hsu LY, Ng ES, Koh LP: Common and emerging fungal pulmonary infections, *Infect Dis Clin North Am* 24:557, 2010.

*22. O'Hanlon KM, Choy E, Sisson SD, et al: Lung cancer. Retrieved from *www.mdconsult.com/das/pdxmd/body/312606682-3/0?type=med&eid=9-u1.0-_1_mt_1014666*.

23. Huethner SE, McCance KL: *Understanding pathophysiology*, ed 5, St Louis, 2012, Mosby.

24. Santacroce L, Harris JE: Paraneoplastic syndromes treatment and management. Retrieved from *http://emedicine.medscape.com/article/280744-treatment*.

25. Winston WD: Small cell lung cancer. Retrieved from *http://emedicine.medscape.com/article/280104-overview*.

*26. Jett JR, Midthun DE: Screening for lung cancer: for patients at increased risk for lung cancer, it works, *Ann Intern Med* 155:541, 2011.

27. American Cancer Society: Lung cancer (non-small cell). Retrieved from *www.cancer.org/acs/groups/cid/documents/webcontent/003115-pdf*.

28. American Cancer Society: Lung cancer (small cell). Retrieved from *www.cancer.org/acs/groups/cid/documents/webcontent/003116-pdf*.

*29. National Comprehensive Cancer Network: NCCN guidelines version 1:2012 lung cancer screening. Retrieved from *www.nccn.org/professionals/physician_gls/pdf/lung_screening.pdf*.

*30. Lehto RH: Identifying primary concerns in patients newly diagnosed with lung cancer, *Oncol Nurs Forum* 38:440, 2011.

31. Manicini MC: Blunt chest trauma. Retrieved from *http://emedicine.medscape.com/article/428723-overview*.

32. Mason RJ, Broaddus VC, Martin TR, et al: *Murray and Nadel's textbook of respiratory medicine*, ed 5, St Louis, 2010, Mosby.

*33. Wendling P: Study supports broader use of rib fixation in flail chest. Retrieved from *www.mdconsult.com/das/news/body/314081249-3/mnfp/1258119330/224596/1.html*.

34. American Association of Critical-Care Nurses: *Procedure manual for critical care*, ed 6, St Louis, 2010, Mosby.

*35. Phillips AM: Pigtail tube drainage as a safe and effective alternative to traditional chest tube thoracostomy in adults with spontaneous pneumothoraces: a systematic review, *School Phys Assist Stud*, paper 266. Retrieved from *http://commons.pacificu.edu/pa/266*.

*36. Cerfolio RJ, Bryant AY: The management of chest tubes after pulmonary resection, *Thorac Surg Clin* 20:399, 2010.

37. Domke MN: Get a positive outcome from negative pressure, *Nursing Made Incredibly Easy* 8:20, 2010.

38. Jarrar D: Video-assisted thoracoscopy. Retrieved from *http://emedicine.medscape.com/article/1970013*.

39. Kanaparthi LK: Restrictive lung disease. Retrieved from *http://emedicine.medscape.com/article/301760*.

*40. McGrath EE, Anderson PB: Diagnosis of pleural effusion: a systematic approach, *Am J Crit Care* 20:119, 2011.

41. Muduly DK, Subi TS, Kallianpur AA, et al: An update in the management of malignant pleural effusion, *Indian J Pall Care* 17:98, 2011.

*42. Lee JS, McLaughlin S, Collard HR: Comprehensive care of the patient with idiopathic pulmonary fibrosis, *Curr Opin Pulm Med* 17:348, 2011.

43. Ouellette DR: Pulmonary embolism. Retrieved from *http://emedicine.medscape.com/article/300901-overview*.

44. Oudiz RJ: Primary pulmonary hypertension. Retrieved from *http://emedicine.medscape.com/article/301450*.

45. Moffatt-Bruce SD: Lung transplantation. Retrieved from *http://emedicine.medscape.com/article/429499*.

RESOURCES

American Lung Association
  www.lungusa.org
Centers for Disease Control and Prevention, Smoking and Tobacco Use
  www.cdc.gov/tobacco
Pulmonary Fibrosis Foundation
  www.pulmonaryfibrosis.org
Pulmonary Hypertension Association (PHA)
  www.phassociation.org

29

Nursing Management

Obstructive Pulmonary Diseases

Jane Steinman Kaufman

Ⓔvolve WEBSITE

http://evolve.elsevier.com/Lewis/medsurg

- NCLEX Review Questions
- Key Points
- Pre-Test
- Answer Guidelines for Case Study on p. 607
- Rationales for Bridge to NCLEX Examination Questions
- Case Studies
  - Patient With Asthma
  - Patient With Chronic Obstructive Pulmonary Disease (COPD)
  - Patient With Cystic Fibrosis

- Nursing Care Plans (Customizable)
  - NCP 29-1: Patient With Asthma
  - NCP 29-2: Patient With Chronic Obstructive Pulmonary Disease
- Concept Map Creator
- Concept Map for Case Study on p. 607
- Glossary
- Content Updates

eFigures
- eFig. 29-1: Postural drainage positions
- eFig. 29-2: Flutter mucus clearance device

eTables
- eTable 29-1: Drug Therapy: Asthma and Chronic Obstructive Pulmonary Disease (enhanced)
- eTable 29-2: Asthma Action Plan (Spanish)
- eTable 29-3: COPD Assessment Test (CAT)
- eTable 29-4: Modified Medical Research Council (mMRC) Dyspnea Scale
- eTable 29-5: Home Oxygen Delivery Systems

LEARNING OUTCOMES

1. Describe the etiology, pathophysiology, clinical manifestations, and collaborative care of asthma.
2. Describe the nursing management of the patient with asthma.
3. Describe the etiology, pathophysiology, clinical manifestations, and collaborative care of the patient with chronic obstructive pulmonary disease (COPD).
4. Describe the effects of cigarette smoking on the lungs.
5. Identify the indications for O_2 therapy, methods of delivery, and complications of O_2 administration.
6. Explain the nursing management of the patient with COPD.
7. Describe the pathophysiology, clinical manifestations, collaborative care, and nursing management of the patient with cystic fibrosis.
8. Describe the pathophysiology, clinical manifestations, collaborative care, and nursing management of the patient with bronchiectasis.

KEY TERMS

α_1-antitrypsin (AAT) deficiency, p. 582
asthma, p. 561
bronchiectasis, p. 606
chest physiotherapy (CPT), p. 594
chronic bronchitis, p. 580

chronic obstructive pulmonary disease (COPD), p. 580
cor pulmonale, p. 584
cystic fibrosis (CF), p. 601
emphysema, p. 580

O_2 toxicity, p. 592
postural drainage, p. 594
pursed-lip breathing (PLB), p. 593

Imagine needing to consciously think about every breath that you take for minutes, hours, or days. Many individuals with obstructive lung disease have this experience. Approximately 31.5 million adult Americans are living with asthma or chronic obstructive pulmonary disease (COPD).[1,2]

Obstructive pulmonary disease, the most common chronic lung disease, is characterized by increased resistance to airflow as a result of airway obstruction or airway narrowing. Types of obstructive lung diseases include asthma, COPD, cystic fibrosis (CF), and bronchiectasis. *Asthma* is a chronic inflammatory lung disease that results in variable episodes of airflow obstruction, but it is usually reversible. *COPD* is an obstructive pulmonary disease with progressive limitation in airflow that is not fully reversible. The patient with asthma has

Reviewed by Danese M. Boob, MSN/ED, RN-BC, Nursing Instructor, Pennsylvania State University, Hershey Campus, Hershey, Pennsylvania; Marianne Ferrin, MSN, ACNP-BC, Coordinator Penn Lung Center, Adult Cystic Fibrosis Program, Philadelphia, Pennsylvania; Mark R. Van Horn, BS, Respiratory Therapist, High Point Regional Hospital, High Point, North Carolina; and Karen M. Wood, RN, DNSc, CCRN, CNL, Associate Professor, Saint Xavier University, Evergreen Park, Illinois.

Obstructive Pulmonary Diseases

Asthma
- Asthma prevalence rates are more than 38% higher among African Americans than whites.
- Puerto Ricans have higher asthma prevalence rates and age-adjusted death rates than all other racial and ethnic subgroups.
- Female African Americans have the highest mortality rates from asthma among all ethnic/gender groups.

Chronic Obstructive Pulmonary Disease (COPD)
- Whites have the highest incidence of COPD in spite of higher rates of smoking among other ethnic groups.
- Hispanics have lower death rates related to COPD than other ethnic groups.

Cystic Fibrosis
- Whites have the highest incidence of cystic fibrosis.
- Cystic fibrosis is uncommon among African Americans, Hispanics, and Asian Americans.

variations in airflow over time, usually with normal lung function between exacerbations, whereas the limitation in expiratory airflow in the patient with COPD is generally more constant. The pathology of asthma and the response to therapy differ from those associated with COPD. However, the patient with a diagnosis of obstructive pulmonary disease may have features of both asthma and COPD. Patients with asthma who have less responsive reversible airflow obstruction are difficult to distinguish from COPD patients.

Cystic fibrosis, another form of obstructive pulmonary disease, is a genetic disorder that produces airway obstruction because of changes in exocrine glandular secretions, resulting in increased mucus production. *Bronchiectasis* is an obstructive disease characterized by dilated bronchioles. It most frequently results from untreated or poorly treated pulmonary infections that cause an increase in sputum production.

ASTHMA

Asthma is a chronic inflammatory disorder of the airways. The chronic inflammation leads to recurrent episodes of wheezing, breathlessness, chest tightness, and cough, particularly at night or in the early morning. These episodes are associated with widespread but variable airflow obstruction that is usually reversible, either spontaneously or with treatment. The clinical course of asthma is unpredictable, ranging from periods of adequate control to exacerbations with poor control of symptoms.[3]

GENDER DIFFERENCES

Asthma

Men	Women
• Before puberty, more boys are affected than girls.	• After puberty and into adulthood, more women are affected than men. • Women who are admitted to the emergency department are more likely to need hospitalization than men. • Death rate from asthma is greater in women than in men.

Asthma affects an estimated 18.8 million adult Americans. Among adults, women are 62% more likely to have asthma than men. Asthma is a public health concern, with more than 14.2 million lost workdays in adults. However, the good news is that after a long period of an increasing incidence of asthma, the mortality and use of health care services are continuing to plateau and/or decrease. Despite the decline in the number of deaths from asthma over the past 10 years, more than 3300 people still die from asthma yearly.[1]

Risk Factors for Asthma and Triggers of Asthma Attacks

Risk factors for asthma and triggers of asthma attacks can be related to the patient (e.g., genetic factors) or the environment (e.g., pollen) (Table 29-1). Male gender is a risk factor for asthma in children (but not adults). Obesity is also a risk factor for asthma.[4] Other factors and triggers are discussed in this section.

Genetics. Asthma has a component that is inherited, but the genetics are complex. Numerous genes may be involved in the development of asthma and a person's response to various asthma medications.[3,4] *Atopy,* the genetic predisposition to develop an allergic (immunoglobulin E [IgE]–mediated) response to common allergens, is a major risk factor for asthma.

TABLE 29-1	TRIGGERS OF ASTHMA ATTACKS

Allergen inhalation
- Animal dander (e.g., cats, mice, guinea pigs)
- House dust mite
- Cockroaches
- Pollens
- Molds

Air pollutants
- Exhaust fumes
- Perfumes
- Oxidants
- Sulfur dioxides
- Cigarette smoke
- Aerosol sprays

Inflammation and infection
- Viral upper respiratory tract infection
- Sinusitis, allergic rhinitis

Drugs
- Aspirin
- Nonsteroidal antiinflammatory drugs
- β-Adrenergic blockers

Occupational exposure
- Agriculture, farming
- Paints, solvents
- Laundry detergents
- Metal salts
- Wood and vegetable dusts
- Industrial chemicals and plastics
- Pharmaceutical agents

Food additives
- Sulfites (bisulfites and metabisulfites)
- Beer, wine, dried fruit, shrimp, processed potatoes
- Monosodium glutamate
- Tartrazine

Other factors
- Exercise and cold, dry air
- Stress
- Hormones, menses
- Gastroesophageal reflux disease (GERD)

Immune Response. The *hygiene hypothesis* suggests that a newborn baby's immune system must be educated so it will function properly during infancy and the rest of life. People who are exposed to certain infections early in life, use few antibiotics, are exposed to other children (e.g., siblings, day care), or live in the country or with pets have a lower incidence of asthma. People for whom these factors are not present in childhood have a higher incidence of asthma.[3]

Allergens. Indoor and outdoor allergens, such as cockroaches, furry animals, fungi, and molds, can trigger asthma attacks. However, their role in the actual development of asthma is not as clear.[3,4]

Exercise. Asthma that is induced or exacerbated during physical exertion is called *exercise-induced asthma* (EIA). Typically, EIA occurs after vigorous exercise, not during it (e.g., jogging, aerobics, walking briskly, climbing stairs). Symptoms of EIA are pronounced during activities where there is exposure to cold, dry air. For example, swimming in an indoor heated pool is less likely to produce symptoms than downhill skiing. Airway obstruction may occur due to changes in the airway mucosa caused by hyperventilation during exercise, with either cooling or rewarming of air and capillary leakage in the airway wall.

Air Pollutants. Various air pollutants, such as cigarette or wood smoke or vehicle exhaust, can trigger asthma attacks. In heavily industrialized or densely populated areas, climatic conditions often lead to concentrated pollution in the atmosphere, especially with thermal inversions and stagnant air masses. Ozone alert days are regularly noted on the news reports, and patients should minimize outdoor activity during these times. Cigarette smoking is associated with an accelerated decline of lung functioning in a person with asthma, increases the severity of the disease, may cause the patient to be less responsive to treatment, and reduces the chance of the asthma being controlled. Despite the relationship of pollutants in triggering asthma attacks, the role of outdoor air pollution as a cause of asthma development remains controversial.[4]

Occupational Factors. *Occupational asthma* is the most common occupational respiratory disorder, with up to 15% of new asthma cases arising from job-related exposures to more than 300 agents.[4,5] Irritants cause a change in the responsiveness of the airways. However, the development of symptoms from this alteration may not occur until the patient has had months to years of exposure. Agricultural worker, baker, hospital worker, plastics manufacturer, and beautician are occupations with a high risk of occupational asthma. Characteristically people with occupational asthma give a history of arriving at work feeling well but gradually develop symptoms by the end of the day.

Respiratory Tract Infections. Respiratory tract infections (i.e., viral and not bacterial) are often the major precipitating factor of an acute asthma attack. Acute infection can increase airway narrowing and airway hyperresponsiveness. Viral-induced alterations of epithelial cells, increased inflammatory cell accumulation, edema of airway walls, and exposure of airway nerve endings contribute to altered airway function. These alterations in airway function may exacerbate asthma.

Nose and Sinus Problems. Most patients with asthma have a history of allergic rhinitis. Treatment of allergic rhinitis usually improves the symptoms of asthma. Additional information on the relationship of rhinitis and asthma can be found at *www.whiar.org*.

Acute and chronic sinusitis may worsen asthma. Some patients with asthma have chronic sinus problems that cause inflammation of the mucous membranes. Sinusitis must be treated and large nasal polyps removed for an asthma patient to have good control. (Sinusitis is discussed in Chapter 27.)

Drugs and Food Additives. Sensitivity to specific drugs may occur in some people, especially those with nasal polyps and sinusitis. Some people with asthma have what is termed the *asthma triad*: nasal polyps, asthma, and sensitivity to aspirin and nonsteroidal antiinflammatory drugs (NSAIDs). Salicylic acid can be found in many over-the-counter (OTC) drugs and some foods, beverages, and flavorings. Some asthmatics who use aspirin or NSAIDs (e.g., ibuprofen [Motrin]) develop wheezing within 2 hours. In addition, there is usually profound rhinorrhea, congestion, tearing, and even angioedema. Avoidance of aspirin and NSAIDs is required. However, patients with aspirin sensitivity under the care of an allergist can be desensitized by daily administration of the drug.

β-Adrenergic blockers in oral form (e.g., metoprolol [Toprol]) or topical eyedrops (e.g., timolol) may trigger asthma because they can cause bronchospasm. Angiotensin-converting enzyme (ACE) inhibitors (e.g., lisinopril [Prinivil]) may produce cough in susceptible individuals, thus making asthma symptoms worse.

Other agents that may precipitate asthma in the susceptible patient are tartrazine (yellow dye no. 5, found in many foods) and sulfiting agents widely used in the food and pharmaceutical industries as preservatives and sanitizing agents. Sulfiting agents are commonly found in fruits, beer, and wine and used extensively in salad bars to protect vegetables from oxidation. Asthma exacerbations have been reported after the use of sulfite-containing preservatives found in topical ophthalmic solutions, IV corticosteroids, and some inhaled bronchodilator solutions.

Food allergies triggering asthma reactions in adults are rare. Avoidance diets are not recommended until an allergy has been demonstrated, usually by oral challenges.

Gastroesophageal Reflux Disease. Gastroesophageal reflux disease (GERD) is more common in people with asthma than in the general population. GERD may worsen asthma symptoms. Reflux may trigger bronchoconstriction and cause aspiration. On the other hand, asthma medications may worsen GERD symptoms. β$_2$-Agonists (especially given orally), which are used to treat asthma, relax the lower esophageal sphincter, thus allowing stomach contents to reflux into the esophagus and possibly be aspirated into the lungs. Medications used to treat GERD usually do not reduce asthma symptoms in most people.[4,6] (GERD is discussed in Chapter 42.)

Psychologic Factors. Asthma is not a psychosomatic disease. However, many people with asthma report that symptoms worsen with stress. Certainly psychologic factors cause bronchoconstriction via stimulation of the cholinergic reflex pathways. Extreme emotional expressions (e.g., crying, laughing, anger, fear) can lead to hyperventilation and hypocapnia, which can cause airway narrowing.[4]

An asthma attack caused by any triggering event can produce panic, stress, and anxiety. However, it varies from patient to patient and in the same patient from episode to episode.

Pathophysiology

The primary pathophysiologic process in asthma is persistent but variable inflammation of the airways. The airflow is limited

PATHOPHYSIOLOGY MAP

FIG. 29-1 Pathophysiology of asthma. *IL,* Interleukin.

because the inflammation results in bronchoconstriction, airway hyperresponsiveness (hyperreactivity), and edema of the airways. Exposure to allergens or irritants initiates the inflammatory cascade (Fig. 29-1). A variety of inflammatory cells are involved, including mast cells, macrophages, eosinophils, neutrophils, T and B lymphocytes, and epithelial cells of the airways.[3]

As the inflammatory process begins, mast cells (found beneath the basement membrane of the bronchial wall) degranulate and release multiple inflammatory mediators (Fig. 29-2). IgE antibodies are linked to mast cells, and the allergen cross-links the IgE. Then inflammatory mediators such as leukotrienes, histamine, cytokines, prostaglandins, and nitric oxide are released. Some inflammatory mediators have effects on the blood vessels, causing vasodilation and increasing capillary permeability. Some mediators result in the airways being infiltrated by eosinophils, lymphocytes, and neutrophils. The resulting inflammatory process causes vascular congestion, edema, production of thick and tenacious mucus, bronchial muscle spasm, thickening of airway walls, and increased bronchial hyperresponsiveness (Fig. 29-3). This whole process is sometimes referred to as the *early-phase response* in asthma. Clinically it can occur within 30 to 60 minutes after exposure to an allergen or irritant.

Symptoms can recur 4 to 6 hours after the early response because of the influx of many inflammatory cells, which are set

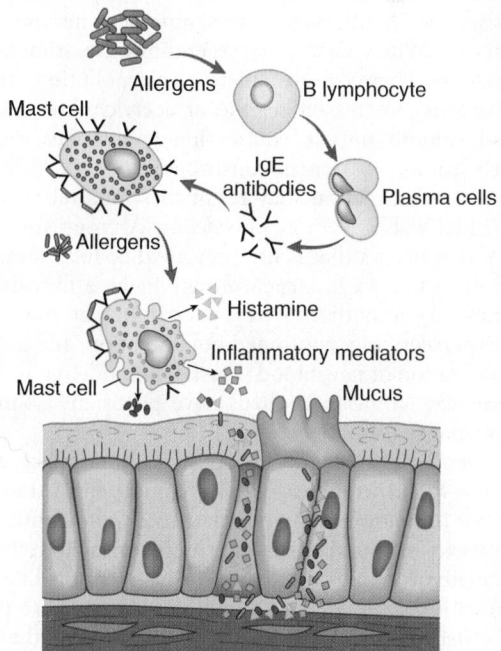

FIG. 29-2 Allergic asthma is triggered when an allergen cross-links IgE receptors on mast cells, which are then activated to release histamine and other inflammatory mediators (early-phase response). A late-phase response may occur due to further inflammation.

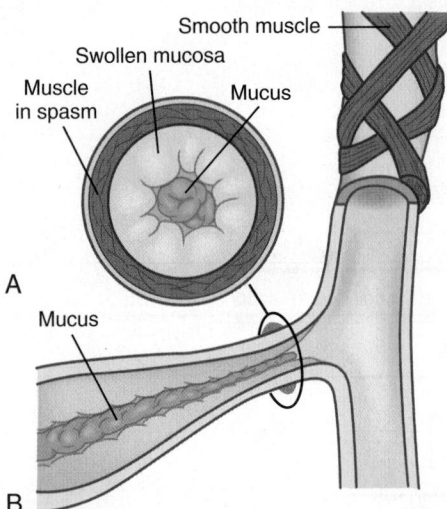

FIG. 29-3 Factors causing obstruction (especially expiratory obstruction) in asthma. **A,** Cross section of a bronchiole occluded by muscle spasm, swollen mucosa, and mucus in the lumen. **B,** Longitudinal section of a bronchiole.

in motion by the initial response. At this later time the patient may develop symptoms again or worsening of symptoms. This is called the *late-phase response,* which occurs in about 50% of individuals with asthma. In this late-phase response, more inflammatory cells are recruited and activated, with continuing inflammation of the airways. Thus bronchoconstriction with symptoms persists for 24 hours or more. Corticosteroids are effective in treating this inflammation.

Alterations in the neural control of the airways also occur in asthma. The autonomic nervous system, consisting of the parasympathetic and sympathetic systems, innervates the bronchi. Airway smooth muscle tone is regulated by the parasympathetic nervous system. In asthma the parasympathetic nervous system is overactive. When airway nerve endings are stimulated by mechanical or chemical stimuli (e.g., air pollution, cold air, dust, allergens), increased release of acetylcholine results in increased smooth muscle contraction and mucus secretion, ultimately leading to bronchoconstriction.

Chronic inflammation may result in structural changes in the bronchial wall known as *remodeling.* A progressive loss of lung function occurs that is not prevented or fully reversed by therapy. The changes in structure may include fibrosis of the subepithelium, smooth muscle hypertrophy of the airways, mucus hypersecretion, continued inflammation, and *angiogenesis* (proliferation of new blood vessels). Remodeling is thought to explain why some individuals have persistent asthma and limited response to therapy.[3,4]

Hyperventilation occurs during an asthma attack as lung receptors respond to increased lung volume from trapped air and airflow limitation. Decreased perfusion and ventilation of the alveoli and increased alveolar gas pressure lead to ventilation-perfusion abnormalities in the lungs. The patient is hypoxemic early on with decreased $PaCO_2$ and increased pH (respiratory alkalosis) because he or she is hyperventilating. As the airflow limitation worsens with air trapping, the patient works much harder to breathe. The $PaCO_2$ normalizes as the patient tires, and then it increases to produce respiratory acidosis, which is an ominous sign of respiratory failure.[6]

Clinical Manifestations

Asthma is characterized by an unpredictable and variable course, with a person's asthma attacks ranging from seemingly minor interferences in breathing to life-threatening episodes. Depending on an individual's response, asthma can rapidly progress from normal breathing to acute severe asthma. Recurrent episodes of wheezing, breathlessness, chest tightness, and cough, particularly at night and in the early morning, are typical in asthma.

An attack of asthma may have an abrupt onset, but usually symptoms occur more gradually. Attacks may last for a few minutes to several hours. Between attacks the patient may be asymptomatic with normal or near-normal pulmonary function, depending on the severity of disease. However, in some people, compromised pulmonary function may result in a state of continuous symptoms and chronic debilitation characterized by irreversible airway disease.

The characteristic clinical manifestations of asthma are wheezing, cough, dyspnea, and chest tightness after exposure to a precipitating factor or trigger. Expiration may be prolonged. Instead of a normal inspiratory-expiratory ratio of 1:2, it may be prolonged to 1:3 or 1:4. Normally the bronchioles constrict during expiration. However, as a result of bronchospasm, edema, and mucus in the bronchioles, the airways become narrower than usual. Thus it takes longer for the air to move out of the bronchioles. This produces the characteristic wheezing, air trapping, and hyperinflation.

Wheezing is an unreliable sign to gauge the severity of an attack. Many patients with minor attacks wheeze loudly, whereas others with severe attacks do not wheeze. The patient with severe asthma attacks may have no audible wheezing because of the marked reduction in airflow. For wheezing to occur, the patient must be able to move enough air to produce the sound. Wheezing usually occurs first on exhalation. As asthma progresses, the patient may wheeze during inspiration and expiration. The term *wheezing* may also be used to describe sounds arising from the nose and upper airways.[7]

In some patients with asthma, cough is the only symptom, and this is termed *cough variant asthma.* The bronchospasm may not be severe enough to cause airflow obstruction, but it can increase bronchial tone and cause irritation with stimulation of the cough receptors. The cough may be nonproductive. Secretions may be thick, tenacious, white, gelatinous mucus, which makes their removal difficult.

The person with asthma has difficulty with air movement in and out of the lungs, which creates a feeling of suffocation. Patients may express, "I can't get a deep breath." Therefore during an acute attack, the person with asthma usually sits upright or slightly bent forward using the accessory muscles of respiration to try to get enough air. The more difficult the breathing becomes, the more anxious the patient feels.

Examination of the patient during an acute attack usually reveals signs of hypoxemia, which may include restlessness, anxiety, inappropriate behavior, and increased pulse and blood pressure (BP). As the patient worsens, it becomes difficult to speak in complete sentences. The respiratory rate is significantly increased (greater than 30 breaths/minute) with the use of accessory muscles. Percussion of the lungs indicates hyperresonance, and auscultation indicates inspiratory or expiratory wheezing. As the episode resolves, coughing produces thick, stringy mucus.

TABLE 29-2 CLASSIFICATION OF ASTHMA SEVERITY

| | | Asthma Severity | | |
| | | | Persistent | |
Components of Severity	Intermittent	Mild	Moderate	Severe
Impairment				
Symptoms	≤2 days/wk	>2 days/wk, not daily	Daily	Continuous
Nighttime awakenings	≤2/mo	3-4/mo	>1/wk, not nightly	Often, 7/wk
SABA use for symptoms	≤2 days/wk	>2 days/wk, not daily	Daily	Several times per day
Interference with normal activity	None	Minor limitation	Some limitation	Extremely limited
Lung function*	Normal FEV_1 between exacerbations FEV_1 >80% FEV_1/FVC normal	FEV_1 >80% predicted FEV_1/FVC normal	FEV_1 60%-80% predicted FEV_1/FVC reduced by 5%	FEV_1 <60% predicted FEV_1/FVC reduced by 5%
Risk				
Exacerbations requiring oral corticosteroids	0-1/yr	≥2/yr even in the absence of impairment ⟶		
	Consider severity and interval since last exacerbation ⟶			
	Frequency and severity may fluctuate over time ⟶			
	Relative annual risk of exacerbation may be related to FEV_1 ⟶			
Recommended Step for Initiating Treatment	Step 1	Step 2	Step 3†	Step 4 or 5†
	Reevaluate asthma control in 2-6 wk and adjust therapy accordingly			

Guidelines for Using Table

- Patients should be assigned to the most severe step in which any feature occurs. Clinical features for individual patients may overlap across steps. Determine level of severity by assessment of both impairment and risk. Assess impairment by patient's recall of previous 2-4 wk and spirometry results.
- An individual's classification should change over time as treatment is initiated. After treatment, the focus switches to level of control, not the classification of severity.
- Patients at any level of severity of chronic asthma can have mild, moderate, or severe exacerbations of asthma. Some patients with intermittent asthma experience severe and life-threatening exacerbations separated by long periods of normal lung function and no symptoms.

Source: Adapted from National Asthma Education and Prevention Program, National Heart, Lung, and Blood Institute: *Expert Panel Report 3: guidelines for the diagnosis and management of asthma*, NIH pub no 08-4051, Bethesda, Md, 2007, National Institutes of Health. Retrieved from *www.nhlbi.nih.gov/guidelines*.
*Percent predicted values for FEV_1 or ratio of FEV_1/FVC. Normal FEV_1/FVC: 8-19 yr, 85%; 20-39 yr, 80%; 40-59 yr, 75%; 60-80 yr, 70%.
†Consider short-term corticosteroid therapy.
FEV_1, Forced expiratory volume in 1 sec; *FVC*, forced vital capacity; *SABA*, short-acting β₂-adrenergic agonist.

Diminished or absent breath sounds may indicate a significant decrease in air movement resulting from exhaustion and an inability to generate enough muscle force to ventilate. Severely diminished breath sounds, often referred to as the "silent chest," are an ominous sign, indicating severe obstruction and impending respiratory failure.

Classification of Asthma

Asthma can be classified as intermittent, mild persistent, moderate persistent, or severe persistent (Table 29-2). The classification system is used to determine the treatment. Patients may move to different asthma classifications over the course of their disease.

Complications

Severe and Life-Threatening Asthma Exacerbations. Severe asthma exacerbations occur when the patient is dyspneic at rest and the patient speaks in words, not sentences, because of the difficulty of breathing. The patient is usually sitting forward to maximize the diaphragmatic movement with prominent wheezing, a respiratory rate higher than 30 breaths/minute, and pulse greater than 120 beats/minute. Accessory muscles in the neck are straining to lift the chest wall, and the patient is often agitated. The peak flow (peak expiratory flow rate [PEFR]) is 40% of the personal best or less than 150 L/minute. Arterial blood gas (ABG) changes are listed in Table 29-3. Neck vein distention

may result. These patients usually are seen in emergency departments (EDs) or hospitalized.[6]

A few patients perceive asthma symptoms poorly and may have a significant decrease in lung function without any change in symptoms. Patients with life-threatening asthma are typically too dyspneic to speak and perspire profusely. They may even be drowsy or confused as the ABGs further deteriorate. The breath sounds may be difficult to hear, and no wheezing is apparent because the airflow is exceptionally limited. Peak flow is less than 25% of the personal best. They become bradycardic and are close to respiratory arrest. These patients require ED or hospital care and are often admitted to an intensive care unit.

SAFETY ALERT
- If the patient has been wheezing and then there is an absence of a wheeze (i.e., silent chest) and the patient is obviously struggling, this is a life-threatening situation that may require mechanical ventilation.

Diagnostic Studies

Underdiagnosis of asthma is common. A detailed history is important to determine if a person has had similar attacks, which are often precipitated by a known trigger. (Triggers are discussed on pp. 561-562.) Because wheezing and cough are seen with a variety of disorders (e.g., COPD, GERD, vocal cord dysfunction, heart failure), it is important to determine if asthma is the cause of these problems.

TABLE 29-3   COMPARISON OF ASTHMA AND COPD*

	Asthma	COPD
Clinical Features		
Age	Usually <40 yr (onset).	Usually 40-50 yr (onset).
Smoking history	Not causal.	Often long history (>10-20 pack-years).
Health and family history	Presence of allergy, rhinitis, eczema. Family history of asthma.	Infrequent allergies. May have exposure to environmental pollutants. With α_1-antitrypsin deficiency, family history of lung or liver disease without smoking history.
Clinical symptoms	Intermittent, vary day to day, at night or early morning.	Slowly progressive and persistent.
Dyspnea	Absent except in exacerbations or poor control.	Dyspnea during exercise.
Sputum	Infrequent.	Often.
Disease course	Stable (with exacerbations).	Progressive worsening (with exacerbations).
Diagnostic Study Results		
ABGs	Normal between exacerbations.	Between exacerbations in advanced COPD • Often low-normal pH and PaO_2 • High-normal $PaCO_2$ with high HCO_3^- (compensated respiratory acidosis)
pH	↑ Early in exacerbation, then ↓ if prolonged or severe exacerbation.	N→↓
PaO_2	↓	N→↓
$PaCO_2$	↓ Early in exacerbation, then ↑ if prolonged or severe exacerbation.	N→↑
Chest x-ray	May reveal hyperinflation.	Hyperinflation. May have cardiac enlargement, flattened diaphragm.
Lung volumes	Often normalizes.	Never normalizes.
• Total lung capacity	Increased.	Increased.
• Residual volume	Increased.	Increased.
• FEV_1	Decreased.	Decreased.
• FEV_1/FVC	Normal to decreased.	Decreased (<70%).

*Individuals may have features of both asthma and COPD.
ABGs, Arterial blood gases; *FEV_1,* forced expiratory volume in 1 sec; *FVC,* forced vital capacity.

TABLE 29-4   COLLABORATIVE CARE

Asthma

Diagnostic
- History and physical examination
- Pulmonary function studies, including response to bronchodilator therapy
- Peak expiratory flow rate (PEFR)
- Chest x-ray
- Measurement of oximetry
- Allergy skin testing (if indicated)
- Blood level of eosinophils and IgE (if indicated)

Collaborative Therapy
Intermittent or Persistent Asthma
- Identification and avoidance or elimination of triggers
- Patient and caregiver teaching
- Drug therapy (see Tables 29-6 and 29-7 and Fig. 29-4)
- Asthma action plan (see Table 29-12)
- Desensitization (immunotherapy) if indicated
- Assess for control (e.g., Asthma Control Test [ACT])*

Severe or Life-Threatening Asthma Exacerbation
- SaO_2 monitoring
- ABGs
- Inhaled β_2-adrenergic agonists
- Inhaled anticholinergic agents (only in the initial treatment)
- O_2 by mask or nasal prongs
- IV or oral corticosteroids
- IV fluids
- IV magnesium and/or heliox
- Intubation and assisted ventilation

*See *www.qualitymetric.com/demos/TP_Launch.aspx?SID=52461.*
ABGs, Arterial blood gases; *IgE,* immunoglobulin E; *SaO_2,* O_2 saturation.

in 1 second [FEV_1]). PEFR should be compared with patients' own previous best measurements using their own meter, since types of peak flow meters vary.

PFTs are usually normal between asthma attacks if the patient has no other underlying pulmonary disease. However, the patient with asthma may show an obstructive pattern with asthma, including a decrease in forced vital capacity (FVC), FEV_1, PEFR, and FEV_1 to FVC ratio (FEV_1/FVC). (The normal values for PFTs are discussed in Chapter 26.)

When PFTs are scheduled, ask the patient to stop taking any bronchodilator medications for 6 to 12 hours before the tests. PFTs can be done before and after the administration of a bronchodilator to determine the degree of the response. This may help determine reversibility of airway obstruction, which is critical information for diagnosing asthma. A positive response to the bronchodilator is an increase of more than 200 mL and an increase of more than 12% between preadministration and postadministration values.

During an exacerbation of asthma, lung function parameters fall from their baseline levels. Some patients with symptoms of asthma have normal lung function. Therefore measures of airway responsiveness to known bronchial irritants (e.g., methacholine, histamine, exercise) may help establish a diagnosis of asthma.

An elevated serum eosinophil count and elevated serum IgE levels are highly suggestive of *atopy* (genetic predisposition to develop an allergic response), which may be a risk factor for asthma. Allergy skin testing may be of some value to determine sensitivity to specific allergens. However, a positive skin test does not necessarily mean that the allergen is causing the

Some controversy exists about how to best diagnose asthma. Common diagnostic measures are presented in Table 29-4. In general, the health care provider should consider the diagnosis of asthma if various indicators (i.e., clinical manifestations, health history, peak flow variability or spirometry) are positive. Pulmonary function tests (PFTs) can be used to determine the reversibility of bronchoconstriction (using bronchodilators) and thus establish the diagnosis of asthma.

The peak expiratory flow rate (PEFR) measured by the peak flow meter is an aid to diagnose and monitor asthma. However, PEFR measurements are not interchangeable with other lung measurements of lung function (e.g., forced expiratory volume

TABLE 29-5   COMPONENTS OF ASTHMA CONTROL

Components of Control	Classification of Asthma Control		
	Well Controlled	Not Well Controlled	Very Poorly Controlled
Impairment			
Symptoms	≤2 days/wk	>2 days/wk	Throughout the day
Nighttime awakenings	≤2/mo	1-3/wk	≥4/wk
Interference with normal activity	None	Some limitation	Extremely limited
SABA use	≤2 days/wk	>2 days/wk	Several times/day
FEV_1 or peak flow	>80% predicted/personal best	60%-80% predicted/personal best	<60% predicted/personal best
Risk			
Exacerbations requiring oral corticosteroids	0-1/yr	≥2/yr	≥2/yr
	Consider severity and interval since last exacerbation. ⟶		
Progressive loss of lung function	Evaluation requires long-term follow-up. ⟶		
Treatment-related adverse effects	Can vary in intensity from none to very troublesome and worrisome. Level of intensity does not correlate to specific levels of control but should be considered in the overall assessment of risk. ⟶		
Recommended Action for Treatment (Based on assessment of control)	• Maintain current step. • Regular follow-up every 1-6 mo to maintain control. • Consider step down if well controlled for at least 3 mo.	• Step up one step. • Reevaluate in 2-6 wk. • For side effects, consider alternative treatment options.	• Consider oral corticosteroids. • Step up one or two steps and reevaluate in 2 wk. • For side effects, consider alternative treatment options.

Source: Adapted from National Asthma Education and Prevention Program, National Heart, Lung, and Blood Institute: *Expert Panel Report 3: guidelines for the diagnosis and management of asthma*, NIH pub no 08-4051, Bethesda, Md, 2007, National Institutes of Health. Retrieved from *www.nhlbi.nih.gov/guidelines*.
FEV_1, Forced expiratory volume in 1 sec; *SABA*, short-acting β_2-adrenergic agonist.

asthma attack. On the other hand, a negative allergy test does not mean that the asthma is not allergy related. (Allergy testing is discussed in Chapter 14.)

A chest x-ray in an asymptomatic patient with asthma is usually normal, but needs to be obtained as a baseline on initial diagnosis. A chest x-ray obtained during an acute attack usually shows hyperinflation and may reveal other complications of asthma such as mucoid impaction, pneumothorax, or atelectasis.

If the patient has wheezing and acute distress, it is not feasible to obtain a detailed health history (although a family member may supply some pertinent information). During an acute attack of asthma, bedside spirometry (specifically FEV_1 or FVC, but usually PEFR) may be used to monitor obstruction. PFT results, serial spirometric parameters, oximetry, and measurement of ABGs provide information about the severity of the attack and the response to therapy. A complete blood cell count (CBC) and serum electrolytes are also obtained to help monitor the course of therapy.

A sputum specimen for culture and sensitivity may be obtained to rule out bacterial infection, especially if the patient has purulent sputum, a history of upper respiratory tract infection, a fever, or an elevated white blood cell (WBC) count. However, the vast majority of asthma exacerbations are viral, and sputum cultures are rarely done on an outpatient basis.

A hand-held, point-of-care device, called Niox Mino, measures airway inflammation related to asthma. It measures fractional exhaled nitric oxide (FENO). Nitric oxide levels are increased in the breath of people with asthma and decreased with oral and inhaled corticosteroid and leukotriene treatment. This allows the health care provider to rely on FENO measures versus a patient's symptoms and lung function. FENO may be used to assess a patient's' adherence to therapy or to determine if he or she needs more antiinflammatory medication. FENO is also a predictor of loss of asthma control and exacerbations.[8]

Collaborative Care

The National Asthma Education and Prevention Program (NAEPP) of the National Heart, Lung, and Blood Institute (NHLBI) convened expert panels to prepare guidelines for the diagnosis and management of asthma.[3] The first NAEPP report served as a basis for the development of reports prepared by asthma experts worldwide, and the Global Initiative for Asthma (GINA) was created. The goals of GINA are to decrease asthma morbidity and mortality rates and improve the management of asthma worldwide.[4] Although the reports of NAEPP and GINA are similar, GINA is updated every year. The NAEPP guidelines are presented in this chapter (e.g., Tables 29-2 and 29-5 and Fig. 29-4).

The goal of asthma treatment is to achieve and maintain control of the disease. Once the patient is diagnosed, the guidelines provide direction on classification of asthma severity (see Table 29-2) and which medications (based on steps 1 through 6) the patient requires (Table 29-5 and Fig. 29-4). The current guidelines focus on (1) assessing the severity of the disease at diagnosis and initial treatment and then (2) monitoring periodically to control the disease.

At the initial diagnosis a patient may have severe asthma and require step 4 or 5 of asthma medication. After treatment the patient's level of control is assessed (i.e., well controlled, not well controlled, or very poorly controlled) (see Table 29-5). The health care provider steps down the medication as the patient achieves control of the symptoms, or steps it up if the symptoms worsen. Achieving rapid control of the symptoms is the goal to return the patient to his or her daily functioning at the best possible level (see Fig. 29-4).

Validated questionnaires (e.g., Asthma Control Test [ACT], *www.qualitymetric.com/demos/TP_Launch.aspx?SID=52461*) can be used to assess quality-of-life issues in asthma patients. The level of control is determined by the patient's current peak

Intermittent Asthma	**Persistent Asthma: Daily Medication** Consult with asthma specialist if step 4 care or higher is required. Consider consultation at step 3.

Step 1
Preferred
SABA
as needed

Step 2
Preferred
Low-dose ICS
Alternative
LTRA or
theophylline

Step 3
Preferred
Low-dose ICS
+ LABA
OR
Medium-dose
ICS
Alternative
Low-dose ICS
+ either LTRA,
theophylline,
or zileuton

Step 4
Preferred
Medium-dose
ICS + LABA
Alternative
Medium-dose
ICS +
either LTRA,
theophylline,
or zileuton

Step 5
Preferred
High-dose
ICS + LABA
AND
Consider
omalizumab
for patients
who have
allergies

Step 6
Preferred
High-dose ICS
+ LABA + oral
corticosteroid
AND
Consider
omalizumab
for patients
who have
allergies

Step up if needed
(first, check adherence, environmental control, and co-morbid conditions)

Assess control

Step down if possible
(and asthma is well controlled at least 3 months)

Each step: Patient education, environmental control, and management of co-morbidities.

Quick-Relief Medication for All Patients
- SABA as needed for symptoms. Intensity of treatment depends on severity of symptoms: up to three treatments at 20-minute intervals as needed. Short course of oral systemic corticosteroids may be needed.
- Use of SABA >2 days a week for symptom relief (not prevention of EIB) generally indicates inadequate control and the need to step up treatment.

Key: *EIB*, Exercise-induced bronchospasm; *ICS*, inhaled corticosteroid; *LABA*, long-acting inhaled β_2-agonist; *LTRA*, leukotriene receptor antagonist; *SABA*, short-acting inhaled β_2-agonist.

FIG. 29-4 Drug therapy: stepwise approach for managing asthma. Modified from *Expert Panel Report 3: Guidelines for the Diagnosis and Management of Asthma*. Bethesda, Md, 2007, National Asthma Education and Prevention Program, National Heart, Lung, and Blood Institute.

TABLE 29-6   DRUG THERAPY

Long-Term Control Versus Quick Relief of Asthma

Long-Term Control Medications
Antiinflammatory Drugs
Corticosteroids
- Inhaled (e.g., fluticasone [Flovent Diskus or HFA])
- Oral (e.g., prednisone)

Leukotriene modifiers (e.g., montelukast [Singulair])
Anti-IgE (omalizumab [Xolair])

Bronchodilators
Long-acting inhaled β_2-adrenergic agonists (e.g., salmeterol [Serevent])
Long-acting oral β_2-adrenergic agonists (e.g., albuterol [VoSpire ER])
Methylxanthines (e.g., theophylline [Theo-24])

Quick-Relief Medications
Bronchodilators
Short-acting inhaled β_2-adrenergic agonists (e.g., albuterol [Proventil HFA])
Anticholinergics (inhaled) (e.g., ipratropium [Atrovent HFA])*

Antiinflammatory Drugs
Corticosteroids (systemic) (e.g., prednisone)†

*Used as alternative if patient has intolerable side effects to albuterol or in emergency department for moderate to severe exacerbations.
†Considered quick-relief drugs when used in a short burst (3-10 days) at the start of therapy or during a period of gradual deterioration. Corticosteroids are not used for immediate relief of an ongoing attack.

---

flow or FEV$_1$. In addition, any exacerbations or adverse effects of treatment will determine the level of control.

Intermittent and Persistent Asthma. The classification of severity of asthma at initial diagnosis helps determine which types of drugs are best suited to control the asthma symptoms (see Tables 29-2 and 29-5). Patients in all classifications of asthma require a short-term (rescue or reliever) medication. The most effective ones are the short-acting β_2-adrenergic agonists (SABAs) (e.g., albuterol [ProAir HFA, Proventil HFA, Ventolin HFA]). Patients with persistent asthma must also be on a long-term or controller medication (Table 29-6). Inhaled corticosteroids (ICSs) (e.g., fluticasone [Flovent Diskus or HFA]) are the most effective class of drugs to treat the inflammation. (See later section on drug therapy in this chapter.)

Acute Asthma Exacerbations. Asthma exacerbations may be mild to life threatening. With *mild exacerbations* the patient has difficulty breathing only with activity and may feel that he or she "can't get enough air." The peak flow is greater than 70% of the patient's personal best, and usually the symptoms are relieved at home promptly with an SABA such as albuterol delivered via a nebulizer or metered-dose inhaler (MDI) with a spacer. For any classification of asthma in a "rescue plan," patients are instructed to take 2 to 4 puffs of albuterol every 20 minutes three times to gain rapid control of symptoms. Occasionally a short course of oral corticosteroids is needed to decrease airway inflammation.

With a *moderate exacerbation*, dyspnea interferes with usual activities and peak flow is 40% to 60% of personal best. In this situation the patient usually comes to the ED or a health care provider's office to get help. Relief is provided with the SABA delivered as in the mild exacerbation, and oral corticosteroids are needed. Oral routes are usually as effective as IV routes, as well as being less invasive and less expensive. The patient's symptoms may persist for several days even after the corticosteroids are started. Oxygen can be used with both mild and moderate exacerbations to maintain SpO_2 at 90% or greater. The patient's symptoms and peak flow are monitored and lung auscultation is done to ensure the patient is moving air. A good response would be measured by the peak flow (or FEV_1) returning to 70% of personal best, normal airflow on physical examination, alleviation of patient's distress, and findings sustained more than 1 hour after the last treatment.[3]

Severe and Life-Threatening Asthma Exacerbations.

Severe and life-threatening asthma exacerbations are discussed on p. 565. Management of the patient with severe and life-threatening asthma focuses on correcting hypoxemia and improving ventilation. The goal is to keep the O_2 saturation at 90% or greater. Continuous monitoring of the patient is critical. Obtaining a peak flow reading during a severe asthma attack is usually not possible. However, if it can be obtained and it is less than 200 L/min, it indicates severe obstruction in all but very small adults.

Many of the therapeutic measures are the same as those for acute asthma. Repetitive or continuous SABA administration is provided in the ED. Initially three treatments of SABA are given, 20 to 30 minutes apart. Then more SABA is given depending on the patient's airflow, improvement, and side effects from the SABA. The person with a severe asthma exacerbation usually has partial relief from the SABA plus ipratropium (Atrovent). However, the patient with life-threatening asthma has minimal if any relief from the same medications.

After the initial treatment, ipratropium is not given during the inpatient stay, since it has not been found to deliver any added benefit. Nebulized SABAs are continued for several days even after clinical improvement is noted.

In severe asthma, oral systemic corticosteroids are given to patients who do not respond to the initial SABA. In life-threatening asthma, IV corticosteroids are administered and are usually tapered rapidly. IV corticosteroids (e.g., methylprednisolone) are administered every 4 to 6 hours, although their peak effect is not apparent for 4 to 12 hours. Then the patient is started on oral corticosteroids. The length of oral prednisone treatment for both severe and life-threatening asthma is usually about 10 days after discharge. ICSs are usually added while the patient is still in the hospital. High-dose ICSs prevent asthma relapse and may be prescribed until the patient can step down to lower doses.

In severe and life-threatening asthma, adjunctive medications such as IV magnesium sulfate may be administered to adults with a very low FEV_1 or peak flow (less than 40% of predicted or personal best) or those who fail to respond to initial treatment. In addition, for hospitalized patients who do not respond to the usual therapy, heliox (a mixture of helium and oxygen) may be used to deliver the nebulized albuterol. Helium has a low density and may improve the bronchodilation effect of albuterol.

Supplemental O_2 is given by mask or nasal prongs to achieve a PaO_2 of at least 60 mm Hg or O_2 saturation greater than 90%. An arterial catheter may be inserted to facilitate frequent ABG monitoring. Because the patient's insensible loss of fluids and metabolic rate are increased, moderate rates of IV fluids are given to provide optimal hydration.

Sodium bicarbonate administration is usually limited to treatment of severe metabolic or respiratory acidosis (pH less than 7.29) in the mechanically ventilated patient because effective bronchodilation by β-adrenergic agonists is not possible if the patient has extreme acidosis. Bronchoscopy, although rarely performed during an acute attack, may be necessary to remove thick mucus plugs.

Occasionally, asthma exacerbations are life threatening and respiratory arrest is pending or actually occurring. The patient requires intubation and mechanical ventilation if there is no response to treatment. The patient is provided with 100% oxygen, hourly or continuously nebulized SABA, IV corticosteroids, and possibly other adjunctive therapies as noted previously.

Theophylline, mucolytics, and sedatives are no longer recommended for asthma exacerbations. Sedatives can result in depression of the respiratory drive and possible death. Antibiotics are not recommended for asthma treatment unless there are signs of pneumonia, fever, and purulent sputum, suggesting bacterial infections. Chest physiotherapy is generally not recommended for asthma because it is too stressful for the breathless patient.[3]

Epinephrine is not routinely indicated for treatment in asthma exacerbations. However, a subcutaneous or intramuscular (IM) injection of epinephrine may be indicated for acute treatment of anaphylaxis. If epinephrine is administered, patients need their BP and electrocardiogram (ECG) monitored closely.

Bronchial thermoplasty is a novel approach that may be used in addition to traditional therapy in those with severe asthma. Via a fiberoptic bronchoscope, a catheter directly applies heat and reduces the muscle mass in the bronchial wall. This benefits the patient by reversing the accumulation of excessive tissue that is part of the remodeling process that causes narrowing of the airway size and adds to bronchoconstriction.[9]

Drug Therapy

A stepwise approach to drug therapy is based initially on the asthma severity and then on the level of control. Persistent asthma requires daily long-term therapy in addition to appropriate medications to manage acute symptoms. Medications are divided into two general classifications: (1) *quick-relief* or *rescue medications* to treat symptoms and exacerbations, such as SABAs; and (2) *long-term control medications* to achieve and maintain control of persistent asthma, such as ICSs (see Table 29-6). Some of the controllers are used in combination to gain better asthma control (e.g., fluticasone and salmeterol [Advair]) (Table 29-7).

Antiinflammatory Drugs

Corticosteroids. Chronic inflammation is a primary component of asthma. Corticosteroids are antiinflammatory medications that reduce bronchial hyperresponsiveness, block the late-phase response, and inhibit migration of inflammatory cells. Corticosteroids are more effective in improving asthma control than any other long-term drug. ICSs are first-line therapy for patients with persistent asthma requiring step 2 through 6 therapies (see Fig. 29-4). Usually, ICSs must be administered for 1 to 2 weeks before maximum therapeutic effects can be seen. Some ICSs (e.g., fluticasone, budesonide [Pulmicort]) begin to have a therapeutic effect

TABLE 29-7 DRUG THERAPY

Asthma and Chronic Obstructive Pulmonary Disease (COPD)*

Drug	Route of Administration	Comments†
Antiinflammatory Agents		
Corticosteroids		
hydrocortisone (Solu-Cortef)	IV	Alternate-day therapy minimizes side effects. Oral dose should be taken in morning with food or milk. When given in high dosages, observe for epigastric distress. Long-term corticosteroid therapy requires supplementation with vitamin D and calcium to prevent osteoporosis. Discontinue gradually over time to prevent adrenal insufficiency. If symptoms recur during tapering, notify health care provider.
methylprednisolone (Medrol, Solu-Medrol)	Oral, IV	
prednisone	Oral	
fluticasone (Flovent HFA, Flovent Diskus)	MDI, DPI	Not recommended for acute asthma attack. Rinse mouth with water or mouthwash after use to prevent oral fungal infections. Use of spacer device with MDI may decrease incidence of oral candidiasis. With ICSs, may not see effects until after at least 2 wk of regular treatment.
beclomethasone (Qvar)	MDI	Same as fluticasone except less oral candidiasis because of very small particle size, which is deposited deeper in the airways.
budesonide (Pulmicort Flexhaler)	DPI	Same as above.
mometasone (Asmanex Twisthaler)	DPI	Same as above.
ciclesonide (Alvesco)	MDI	Oral candidiasis and other localized oropharyngeal effects (e.g., hoarseness). Fewer side effects than other ICSs because of small particle size with minimal activation in oropharynx.
Phosphodiesterase Inhibitor Type 4 (PDE-4)		
roflumilast (Daliresp)	Oral	Only used in severe COPD to reduce exacerbation frequency. Not to be used for acute bronchospasm. GI symptoms occur within 6 mo of initiating medication. Patients to report any psychiatric symptoms (e.g., anxiety, depression, suicidal thoughts). Not to be used with theophylline.
Anticholinergics		
Short Acting		
ipratropium (Atrovent HFA)	Nebulizer, MDI	Approved for COPD. May provide additive benefit to SABA in moderate to severe asthma exacerbations (used in emergency department with no benefit beyond that). Use in asthma as alternative for patients with intolerable side effects with SABA. Temporary blurred vision if sprayed in eyes. Use cautiously in patients with narrow-angle glaucoma or prostatic enlargement.
aclidinium bromide (Tudorza, Pressair)	DPI	Only approved for COPD. Do not administer with other anticholinergics. Not for acute relief of bronchospasm.
Long Acting		
tiotropium (Spiriva HandiHaler)	DPI	Only approved for COPD. Blurred vision if powder comes in contact with eyes. Must discontinue use of ipratropium while on tiotropium. Patients with COPD must use SABA or short-acting anticholinergics for quick-relief medication. Maximum effect 1 wk after initiation of drug.
Anti-IgE		
omalizumab (Xolair)	Subcutaneous injection	Only for moderate to severe persistent allergic asthma with symptoms not adequately controlled by ICSs. Not for acute bronchospasm. Administer only under direct medical supervision and observe patient for a minimum of 2 hr after administration, since anaphylaxis has been reported with use.
Leukotriene Modifiers		
Leukotriene Receptor Blocker		
zafirlukast (Accolate)	Oral tablets	Take at least 1 hr before or 2 hr after meals. Affects metabolism of erythromycin and theophylline. Not used to treat acute asthma episodes.
montelukast (Singulair)	Oral tablets, chewable tablets, oral granules	Not used to treat acute asthma episodes.
Leukotriene Inhibitor		
zileuton (Zyflo, Zyflo CR)	Oral tablets	Monitor liver enzymes. May interfere with metabolism of warfarin (Coumadin) and theophylline. Not used to treat acute asthma episodes.
β_2-Adrenergic Agonists		
Inhaled: Short Acting (SABA)		
albuterol (Proventil HFA, Ventolin HFA, ProAir HFA, AccuNeb, VoSpire ER [oral only])	Nebulizer, MDI, oral tablets, including extended release NOTE: Oral tablets not for acute use, only long acting	Use with caution in patients with cardiac disorders, since β-agonists may cause ↑ BP and heart rate, CNS stimulation/excitation, and ↑ risk of dysrhythmias. Has rapid onset of action (1-3 min). Duration of action is 4-8 hr. Ventolin HFA is the only albuterol MDI with a counter.
levalbuterol (Xopenex, Xopenex HFA)	Nebulizer, MDI	Too frequent use can result in loss of effectiveness. Efficacy no better than other SABA.

*An enhanced version of this table listing side effects of drugs (eTable 29-1) is available on the website.

TABLE 29-7   DRUG THERAPY—cont'd

Asthma and Chronic Obstructive Pulmonary Disease (COPD)*

Drug	Route of Administration	Comments†
Inhaled: Long Acting (LABA)		*In asthma:* Never use as monotherapy. Use in combination with ICSs.
		In COPD: Can be used as monotherapy. Not used for rapid relief of dyspnea.
salmeterol (Serevent Diskus)	DPI	Not to exceed 2 puffs q12hr. Not used for acute exacerbations. Has a counter.
formoterol (Foradil Aerolizer, Perforomist)	DPI, nebulizer (Perforomist)	Can affect blood glucose levels. Use with caution in patients with diabetes.
arformoterol (Brovana)	Nebulizer	See formoterol. For chronic COPD use.
indacaterol (Arcapta Neohaler)	DPI	Only once-daily LABA. For chronic COPD use. Not intended to treat asthma.
Methylxanthines		
IV agent: aminophylline (second-line therapy)	Oral tablets, IV, elixir, sustained-release tablets	Wide variety of response to drug metabolism exists. Half-life is ↓ by smoking and ↑ by heart failure and liver disease. Cimetidine, ciprofloxacin, erythromycin, and other drugs may rapidly ↑ theophylline levels. Taking drug with food or antacids may help GI effects. Use usually limited to situations when other long-term bronchodilation not available or not affordable.
Oral: theophylline		
Combination Agents		Also see each component of medications for SE.
ipratropium/albuterol (Combivent Respimat, DuoNeb)	Nebulizer (DuoNeb), inhalation spray (Combivent Respimat)	Patients must be careful not to overuse. Respimat is an inhaler, but propellant free, unlike an MDI. Respimat is independent of inspiratory flow. Has dose indicator.
fluticasone/salmeterol (Advair Diskus or HFA)	DPI, MDI	See salmeterol and fluticasone. Has a counter. Comes in three different strengths.
budesonide/formoterol (Symbicort)	MDI	See budesonide and formoterol. Has a counter.
mometasone furoate/formoterol fumarate (Dulera)	MDI	
fluticasone/vilanterol (Breo Ellipta)	DPI	Vilanterol is an LABA.

†For patient instructions in English and Spanish for the devices, see *www.chestnet.org/accp/patient-guides/patient-instructions-inhaled-devices-english-and-spanish*.
DPI, Dry powder inhaler; *HFA*, hydrofluoroalkane (propellant); *ICSs*, inhaled corticosteroids; *MDI*, metered-dose inhaler.

in 24 hours. These drugs need to be administered on a fixed schedule.

When ICSs are administered, asthma can usually be controlled without significant systemic side effects, since little systemic drug absorption occurs from these devices. However, ICSs at the highest dosage levels have been associated with side effects (e.g., easy bruising, decreased bone mineral density).[4] Oropharyngeal candidiasis, hoarseness, and dry cough are local side effects caused by inhalation of corticosteroids. These problems can be reduced or prevented by using a spacer (Fig. 29-5) with the MDI and by gargling with water or mouthwash after each use. Using a spacer or holding device for inhalation of corticosteroids can be helpful in getting more medication into the lungs. However, drugs that are activated in the lungs (not the pharynx) (e.g., ciclesonide [Alvesco]) appear to minimize these side effects without the need for a spacer or mouth rinsing.[4]

To gain prompt control, short courses of orally administered corticosteroids are indicated for acute exacerbations of asthma. Maintenance doses of oral corticosteroids may be necessary to control asthma in a minority of patients with severe chronic asthma when long-term therapy is required. A single dose in the morning to coincide with endogenous cortisol production and alternate-day dosing are associated with fewer side effects. (Side effects of long-term corticosteroid therapy are discussed in Chapter 50.)

Women, especially postmenopausal women, who have asthma and who use corticosteroids should take adequate amounts of calcium and vitamin D and participate in regular weight-bearing exercise. (Osteoporosis is discussed in Chapter 64.)

FIG. 29-5 Example of an AeroChamber spacer used with a metered-dose inhaler.

Leukotriene Modifiers. Leukotriene modifiers include leukotriene receptor blockers (antagonists) (zafirlukast [Accolate], montelukast [Singulair]) and leukotriene synthesis inhibitors (zileuton [Zyflo CR]). These drugs interfere with the synthesis or block the action of leukotrienes. Leukotrienes are inflammatory mediators produced from arachidonic acid metabolism (see Fig. 12-2). Leukotrienes are potent bronchoconstrictors, and some also cause airway edema and inflammation, thus contributing to the symptoms of asthma. Because these drugs block the release of some substances from mast cells and eosinophils, they have both bronchodilator and antiinflammatory effects.

These drugs are not indicated for use in the reversal of bronchospasm in acute asthma attacks. They are used for prophylactic and maintenance therapy. One advantage of leukotriene modifiers is that they are administered orally.

Anti-IgE. Omalizumab (Xolair) is a monoclonal antibody to IgE that decreases circulating free IgE levels. Omalizumab prevents IgE from attaching to mast cells, thus preventing the release of chemical mediators. This drug is indicated for patients with moderate to severe persistent, allergic asthma or those requiring step 5 or 6 care with persistent asthma that cannot be controlled with ICSs. Omalizumab is administered subcutaneously every 2 to 4 weeks. The drug has a risk of anaphylaxis, and patients must receive the medication in a health care provider's office where this potential emergency problem can be handled.

Bronchodilators. Three classes of bronchodilator drugs currently used in asthma therapy are β₂-adrenergic agonists (also referred to as β₂-agonists), methylxanthines and derivatives, and anticholinergics (see Table 29-7).

β₂-Adrenergic Agonist Drugs. These drugs may be short-acting β₂-adrenergic agonists (SABAs) or long-acting β₂-adrenergic agonists (LABAs). Because inhaled SABAs are the most effective drugs for relieving acute bronchospasm (as seen in acute exacerbations of asthma), they are known as rescue medications. Examples of these drugs include albuterol and pirbuterol (Maxair Autohaler). These drugs have an onset of action within minutes and are effective for 4 to 8 hours. These drugs act by stimulating β-adrenergic receptors in the bronchioles, thus producing bronchodilation. They also increase mucociliary clearance.

> **DRUG ALERT:** β₂-Adrenergic Agonists
> - Use with caution in patients with cardiac disorders, since both SABAs and LABAs may cause elevated BP and heart rate, central nervous system stimulation or excitation, and increased risk of dysrhythmias.
> - Overuse of SABAs may cause rebound bronchospasms.

β₂-Adrenergic agonists are also useful in preventing bronchospasm precipitated by exercise and other stimuli because they prevent the release of inflammatory mediators from mast cells. They do not inhibit the late-phase response of asthma or have antiinflammatory effects. If used frequently, inhaled β₂-adrenergic agonists may produce tremors, anxiety, tachycardia, palpitations, and nausea. Too frequent use of β₂-adrenergic agonists indicates poor asthma control, may mask asthma severity, and may lead to reduced drug effectiveness. The goal in asthma therapy is that the patient with persistent asthma will never need to use SABAs for rescue, but that effective control is achieved with a long-term controller medication.

SABAs are not used for long-term control, and they should not be used alone for persistent asthma. They are used in any stage of asthma for quick relief and should be with the patient at all times for that purpose. Oral β₂-agonists are rarely used because of the cardiovascular side effects, skeletal muscle tremor, and anxiety. However, they may be used for long-term control, but they should not be used alone or as first-line therapy in treating asthma.

LABAs, including salmeterol (Serevent Diskus) and formoterol (Foradil), are effective for 12 hours. LABAs are added to a daily dose of ICSs for long-term control of moderate to severe persistent asthma (i.e., step 3 or higher for long-term control) and prevention of symptoms, particularly at night. When LABAs are added to a patient's daily regimen of corticosteroids, they decrease the need for SABAs and allow patients to achieve better asthma control with a lower dosage of ICSs.[3,4]

LABAs should never be used as monotherapy for asthma, and should only be used if the patient is on ICS. Tell patients that these drugs should not be used to treat acute symptoms or to obtain quick relief from bronchospasm. Teach the patient that these drugs are used only once every 12 hours.

> **DRUG ALERT:** Long-Acting β₂-Adrenergic Agonists (LABAs)
> - Should not be the first medicine used to treat asthma.
> - Should never be used as the only medication to treat asthma but should be added to the treatment plan only if other controller medicines do not control asthma.
> - Should not be used to treat wheezing that is getting worse.
> - Always use a SABA to treat sudden wheezing.

Combination therapy using an ICS and LABA is available in several inhalers (e.g., Advair and budesonide/formoterol [Symbicort]). The combinations are more convenient, improve adherence, and ensure that patients receive the LABA together with an ICS.

Methylxanthines. Sustained-release methylxanthine (theophylline) preparations are not a first-line controller medication. They are used only as an alternative therapy for step 2 care in mild persistent asthma. Methylxanthine is a bronchodilator with mild antiinflammatory effects, but the exact mechanism of action is unknown.

> **DRUG ALERT:** Theophylline
> - Instruct patient to report signs of toxicity: nausea, vomiting, seizures, insomnia.
> - Avoid caffeine to prevent intensifying adverse effects.

The main problems with theophylline are the relatively high incidence of interaction with other drugs and the side effects, which include nausea, headache, insomnia, gastrointestinal distress, tachycardia, dysrhythmias, and seizures. Because theophylline has a narrow margin of safety, monitor serum blood levels regularly to determine if the drug is within therapeutic range.

Anticholinergic Drugs. Anticholinergic agents (e.g., ipratropium) block the bronchoconstricting effect of the parasympathetic nervous system. These drugs are less effective than β₂-adrenergic agonists. Anticholinergic drugs are used for quick relief in those patients unable to tolerate SABAs. In addition, they are used for the patient in severe asthma exacerbation in emergency situations, often nebulized with an SABA. Other than these indications, they have no role in the treatment of asthma.

The onset of action of ipratropium is slower than that of β₂-adrenergic agonists, peaking at 30 minutes to 1 hour and lasting up to 4 to 6 hours. Systemic side effects of inhaled anticholinergics are uncommon because they are poorly absorbed. The most common side effect is a dry mouth.

Inhalation Devices for Drug Delivery. The multiple devices for asthma drug administration can be confusing. The majority of asthma drugs are administered only or preferably by inhalation because systemic side effects are reduced and the onset of action is faster. Inhalation devices include metered-dose inhalers (MDIs), dry powder inhalers (DPIs), and nebulizers.

Inhalers. MDIs are small, hand-held, pressurized devices that deliver a measured dose of drug with each activation.

Dosing is usually accomplished with one or two puffs. Depending on the specific MDI, a spacer or holding chamber (e.g. AeroChamber or InspirEase [see Fig. 29-5]) is used to reduce the amount of drug delivered to the oropharynx and improve the amount of drug delivered to the lungs. In addition, spacers assist people who have hand-breath coordination problems.[10]

All MDIs are mandated by international law to have an ozone-friendly propellant, which is a hydrofluoroalkane (HFA). This propellant is nontoxic, evaporates almost instantly once it forces medicine out of the MDI canister, and is not harmful to the patient. The number of times an MDI needs to be primed and the frequency of priming vary widely, so read the package insert with the patient.[10]

The MDI should be cleaned by removing the dust cap and rinsing the holder (not the medication chamber) in warm water at least two times per week (Fig. 29-6). The patient who needs to use several MDIs is often unclear about the order in which to take the medications. Historically it had been recommended that SABAs should be used first to open up the airway and improve the delivery of subsequent medications. However, this technique is not evidence based. It is a potential source of confusion to patients because the SABAs are usually used on an as-needed (PRN) basis.

One of the major problems with metered-dose drugs is the potential for overuse (more than two canisters per month) rather than seeking needed medical care (Table 29-8). As a patient develops additional asthmatic symptoms, he or she may use the β_2-adrenergic agonist MDI repeatedly. β_2-Adrenergic agonists help by relieving bronchospasm. They do not treat the inflammatory response. Therefore teach the patient the correct therapeutic use of these drugs. The patient also needs to know the correct way to determine whether the MDI is empty (see

---

Using an inhaler seems simple, but most patients do not use it the right way. When you use your inhaler the wrong way, less medicine gets to your lungs. (Your physician may give you other types of inhalers.)

For the next 2 weeks, read these steps aloud as you do them or ask someone to read them to you. Ask your physician or nurse to check how well you are using your inhaler.

Use your inhaler in one of the three ways pictured below (**A** or **B** is best, but **C** can be used if you have trouble with **A** or **B**).

Steps for Using Your Inhaler

Getting ready
1. Take off the cap and shake the inhaler.
2. Breathe out all the way.
3. Hold your inhaler the way your doctor said (**A, B,** or **C** below).

Breathe in slowly 4. As you start breathing in **slowly** through your mouth, press down on the inhaler **one** time. (If you use a holding chamber, first press down on the inhaler. Within 5 seconds, begin to breathe in slowly.)
5. Keep breathing in **slowly,** as deeply as you can.

Hold your breath 6. Hold your breath as you count to 10 slowly, if you can.
7. For inhaled quick-relief medicine (β_2-agonists), wait about 1 minute between puffs. There is no need to wait between puffs for other medicines.

A. Hold inhaler 1 to 2 inches in front of your mouth (about the width of two fingers).

B. Use a spacer/holding chamber. These come in many shapes and can be useful to any patient.

C. Put the inhaler in your mouth.

Clean Your Inhaler as Needed

Look at the hole where the medicine sprays out from your inhaler. If you see "powder" in or around the hole, clean the inhaler. Remove the metal canister from the L-shaped plastic mouthpiece. Rinse only the mouthpiece and cap in warm water. Let them dry over night. In the morning, put the canister back inside. Put the cap on.

Know When to Replace Your Inhaler

For medicines you take each day (an example): Say your new canister has 200 puffs (number of puffs is listed on canister) and you are told to take 8 puffs per day.

$$8 \text{ puffs per day} \overline{)\,200 \text{ puffs in canister}}^{\,25 \text{ days}}$$

So this canister will last 25 days. If you started using this inhaler on May 1, replace it on or before May 25. You can write the date on your canister.

For **quick-relief medicine take as needed** and count each puff.

Do not put your canister in water to see if it is empty as water may enter MDI and impair inhaler.

FIG. 29-6 How to use your metered-dose inhaler correctly.

TABLE 29-8   PROBLEMS USING A METERED-DOSE INHALER (MDI)

- Failing to coordinate activation with inspiration
- Activating MDI in the mouth while breathing through nose
- Inspiring too rapidly
- Not holding the breath for 10 sec (or as close to 10 sec as possible)
- Holding MDI upside down or sideways
- Inhaling more than 1 puff with each inspiration
- Not shaking MDI before use
- Not waiting a sufficient amount of time between each puff
- Not opening mouth wide enough, causing medication to bounce off teeth, tongue, or palate
- Not having adequate strength to activate MDI
- Being unable to understand and follow directions

FIG. 29-7 Example of a dry powder inhaler (DPI).

TABLE 29-9   PATIENT TEACHING GUIDE

How to Use a Dry Powder Inhaler (DPI)

Include the following instructions when teaching a patient to use a DPI.
1. Remove mouthpiece cap or open the device according to manufacturer's instructions. Check for dust or dirt. If there is an external counter, note the number of doses remaining.
2. Load the medicine into the inhaler or engage the lever to allow the medicine to become available. Some DPIs should be held upright while loading. Others should be held sideways or in a horizontal position.
3. Do not shake your medicine.
4. Tilt your head back slightly and breathe out, getting as much air out of your lungs as you can. Do not breathe into your inhaler because this could affect the dose.
5. Close your lips tightly around the mouthpiece of the inhaler.
6. Breathe in deeply and quickly. This will ensure that the medicine moves down deeply into your lungs. You may not taste or sense the medicine going into your lungs.
7. Hold your breath for 10 seconds or as long as you can to disperse the medicine into your lungs.
8. If there is an external counter, note the number of doses remaining. It should be one less than the number in step 1 above.
9. Do not keep your DPI in a humid place such as a shower room because the medicine may clump.

TABLE 29-10   COMPARISON OF METERED-DOSE AND DRY POWDER INHALERS

	Metered-Dose Inhaler (MDI)	Dry Powder Inhaler (DPI)
Shake before use	Yes, shake well*	No
Inspiration	Slow	Rapid
Spacer	Yes, at least with inhaled corticosteroids*	None permitted
Counting device	Few have external device	Most preloaded forms include counter
Inhalations/dose	Often 2/dose	Often 1/dose
Cleaning	Use water for plastic case	Avoid moisture

Source: National Jewish Health: Inhaled medication instructional videos: asthma and general lung diseases. Retrieved from *www.nationaljewish.org/healthinfo/ medications/lung-diseases/devices/instructional-videos.*
*MDIs use hydrofluoroalkane (HFA) as a propellant, and shaking or a spacer may not be needed.

Fig. 29-6). In the past, floating the MDI in water was an appropriate way to determine if medication remained in the MDI. Now this is not recommended because it is not accurate and water can enter the MDI. Teach patients that shaking the canister is not an accurate way to determine if the MDI is empty because they may be hearing only the propellant.

DPIs are simpler to use than MDIs (Fig. 29-7 and Table 29-9). The DPI contains dry, powdered medication and is breath activated. No propellant is used. Instead an aerosol is created when the patient inhales through a reservoir containing a dose of powder. The convenient-to-carry diskus has several advantages over MDIs: (1) less manual dexterity is needed, (2) there is no need to coordinate device puffs with inhalation, (3) an easily visible color or number system indicates the number of doses left in the diskus, and (4) no spacer is required. Disadvantages are that commonly prescribed drugs are not yet available in DPIs and the medication may clump if exposed to humidity. Since the medicine is delivered only by the patient's inspiratory effort, patients with a low FEV$_1$ (less than 1 L) may not be able to inspire the medication adequately.

Differences between MDIs and DPIs are presented in Table 29-10. Aerosolized medication delivery systems, when used with comparable drug doses, provide equivalent efficacy. Therefore patients should use the device best suited to their needs.

Nebulizers. Nebulizers are small machines used to convert drug solutions into mists. The mist can be inhaled through a face mask or mouthpiece held between the teeth. Nebulizers are usually used for individuals who have severe asthma or difficulty with the MDI inhalation.

Nebulizers are usually powered by a compressed air or O_2 generator. At home the patient may have an air-powered compressor. In the hospital, wall O_2 or compressed air is used to power the nebulizer.

Aerosolized medication orders must include the medication, dose, diluent, and whether it is to be nebulized with O_2 or compressed air. The advantage of nebulization therapy is that it is easy to use. Medications that are routinely nebulized include albuterol and ipratropium.

The patient is placed in an upright position that allows for most efficient breathing to ensure adequate penetration and deposition of the aerosolized medication. The patient must breathe slowly and deeply through the mouth and hold inspirations for 2 or 3 seconds. Deep diaphragmatic breathing helps ensure deposition of the medication. Instruct the patient to breathe normally in between these large forced breaths to prevent alveolar hypoventilation and dizziness. After the treatment instruct the patient to cough effectively.

A disadvantage of nebulizer equipment use is the potential for bacterial growth. Review cleaning procedures for home respiratory equipment with the patient. A frequently used, effective home-cleaning method is to wash the nebulizer daily in soap and water, rinse it with water, and soak it for 20 to 30 minutes in a 1:1 white vinegar–water solution, followed by a water rinse and air drying. Commercial respiratory cleaning agents may also be used if directions are followed carefully. Cleaning the nebulizer in the top shelf of an automatic dishwasher saves time, and the hot water destroys most organisms.

Patient Teaching Related to Drug Therapy. Information about medications should include the name, purpose, dosage, method of administration, and schedule, taking into consideration activities of daily living (ADLs) that require energy expenditure and thus oxygen (e.g., bathing). Teaching should also include side effects, appropriate action if side effects occur, how to properly use and clean devices, how to prime and the frequency, and consequences of not taking medications as prescribed. One of the major factors determining success in asthma management is the correct administration of drugs.

Several factors can affect the correct use of these devices. These include advanced age, alterations in physical dexterity (e.g., arthritis in hands, coordination), psychologic state (e.g., cognition), affordability, convenience, and administration time and preference.[10]

Poor adherence with asthma therapy is a major challenge in the long-term management of chronic asthma. Lack of adherence often occurs in chronic asthma because the patient is symptom free and does not use the long-term therapy (e.g., ICS) regularly because no immediate benefit is felt. The patient does not realize that ICSs are needed to treat the ongoing inflammatory process.

Explain to the patient the importance and purpose of taking the long-term therapy regularly, emphasizing that maximum improvement may take longer than 1 week. Tell the patient that, without regular use, the swelling in the airways may progress and the asthma will likely worsen over time. Become familiar with the vast array of compassionate use programs offered by pharmaceutical companies to help lower-income patients obtain medications (e.g., www.needymeds.com).

In addition to the typical MDI and DPI devices, a variety of other devices are used to deliver inhalant pulmonary medications. Be certain that patients understand exactly how to use the device, and give them printed instructions. (For instructions, see www.nationaljewish.org/healthinfo/medications/lung-diseases/devices.) Most inhalant drugs have clear patient instructions, but you need to either use a placebo device or the actual drug to assess the patient's ability to deliver the medication. At every clinic visit or hospitalization reassess the patient's inhaler technique.

New drug delivery devices are becoming available at a rapid pace, and you must keep informed of the correct operation of these. If package inserts are available, you can review them before teaching the patient. The drug company websites have numerous excellent teaching videos available.

Nonprescription Combination Drugs. Several nonprescription combination drugs are available OTC. They are usually combinations of a bronchodilator (ephedrine) and an expectorant (guaifenesin). Inhalers containing epinephrine are also available.[11] These agents are advertised as medications to relieve bronchospasm. Often patients seek OTC drugs because they are less expensive than prescription medication. Many people consider these drugs safe because they can be obtained without a prescription. In general, they should be avoided.

Drugs containing ephedrine and epinephrine are dangerous because they stimulate the central nervous and cardiovascular systems, causing nervousness, heart palpitations and dysrhythmias, tremors, insomnia, and increases in BP. Many respiratory products containing ephedrine are located behind the counter at pharmacies or require a prescription. This limited access is to prevent the diversion of ephedrine to the production of methamphetamine. Also many of the OTC products have been reformulated with phenylephrine, instead of ephedrine, which works well topically but has modest effects in the oral form.

An important teaching responsibility is to warn patients about the dangers associated with nonprescription combination drugs. These drugs are especially dangerous to a patient with underlying cardiac problems because elevated BP and tachycardia often occur. Caution the patient who persists in taking these medications to read and follow the directions on the label.

NURSING MANAGEMENT
ASTHMA

NURSING ASSESSMENT

If a patient can speak and is not in acute distress, take a detailed health history, including identification of any precipitating factors and what has helped alleviate attacks in the past. The patient may be using herbs and supplements to treat asthma.[12] When doing the health history, ask about specific herbs or supplements that a patient may be using.

Subjective and objective data that should be obtained from a patient with asthma are presented in Table 29-11. You may also assess the patient's asthma control using one of the validated self-administered questionnaires (e.g., ACT at www.qualitymetric.com/demos/TP_Launch.aspx?SID=52461).

NURSING DIAGNOSES

Nursing diagnoses for the patient with asthma may include, but are not limited to, those presented in Nursing Care Plan 29-1.

PLANNING

The overall goals are that the patient with asthma will have asthma control as evidenced by (1) minimal symptoms during the day and night, (2) acceptable activity levels (including

◎ NURSING CARE PLAN 29-1

Patient With Asthma

NURSING DIAGNOSIS* **Ineffective airway clearance** *related to* bronchospasm, excessive mucus production, tenacious secretions, and fatigue *as evidenced by* ineffective cough, inability to raise secretions, and/or adventitious breath sounds

PATIENT GOALS
1. Maintains clear airway with removal of excessive secretions
2. Experiences normal breath sounds and respiratory rate

Outcomes (NOC)	Interventions (NIC) and *Rationales*
Respiratory Status: Airway Patency • Respiratory rate _____ • Respiratory rhythm _____ • Ability to clear secretions _____ **Measurement Scale** 1 = Severe deviation from normal range 2 = Substantial deviation from normal range 3 = Moderate deviation from normal range 4 = Mild deviation from normal range 5 = No deviation from normal range	**Asthma Management** • Determine baseline respiratory status *to use as a comparison point.* • Monitor rate, rhythm, depth, and effort of respiration *to determine need for intervention and evaluate effectiveness of interventions.* • Observe chest movement, including symmetry, use of accessory muscles, and supraclavicular and intercostal muscle retractions, *to evaluate respiratory status.* • Auscultate breath sounds, noting areas of decreased or absent ventilation and adventitious sounds, *to evaluate respiratory status.* • Administer medication as appropriate and/or per policy and procedural guidelines *to improve respiratory function.* • Coach in breathing and relaxation techniques *to improve respiratory rhythm and rate.* • Offer warm fluids to drink *to liquefy secretions and promote bronchodilation.*

NURSING DIAGNOSIS **Anxiety** *related to* difficulty breathing, perceived or actual loss of control, and fear of suffocation *as evidenced by* restlessness and elevated pulse, respiratory rate, and blood pressure

PATIENT GOALS
1. Reports decreased anxiety with increased control of respirations
2. Experiences vital signs within normal limits

Outcomes (NOC)	Interventions (NIC) and *Rationales*
Anxiety Level • Restlessness _____ • Increased blood pressure _____ • Increased pulse rate _____ • Increased respiratory rate _____ • Verbalized anxiety _____ • Facial tension _____ **Measurement Scale** 1 = Severe 2 = Substantial 3 = Moderate 4 = Mild 5 = None	**Anxiety Reduction** • Identify when level of anxiety changes *to determine possible precipitating factors.* • Use calm, reassuring approach *to provide reassurance.* • Stay with patient *to promote safety and reduce fear.* • Encourage verbalization of feelings, perceptions, and fears *to identify problem areas so appropriate planning can take place.* • Provide factual information concerning diagnosis, treatment, and prognosis *to help patient know what to expect.* • Instruct patient in the use of relaxation techniques *to relieve tension and to promote ease of respirations.*

NURSING DIAGNOSIS **Deficient knowledge** *related to* lack of information and education about asthma and its treatment *as evidenced by* frequent questioning regarding all aspects of long-term management

PATIENT GOALS
1. Describes the disease process and treatment regimen
2. Demonstrates correct administration of aerosol medications
3. Expresses confidence in ability for long-term management of asthma

Outcomes (NOC)	Interventions (NIC) and *Rationales*
Asthma Self-Management • Describes causal factors _____ • Initiates action to avoid and manage personal triggers _____ • Seeks early treatment of infections _____ • Monitors peak flow routinely _____ • Monitors peak flow when symptoms occur _____ • Makes appropriate medication choices _____ • Demonstrates appropriate use of inhalers, spacers, and nebulizers _____ • Self-manages exacerbations _____ • Reports uncontrolled symptoms to health care provider _____ **Measurement Scale** 1 = Never demonstrated 2 = Rarely demonstrated 3 = Sometimes demonstrated 4 = Often demonstrated 5 = Consistently demonstrated	**Asthma Management** • Determine patient and family understanding of disease and management *to assess learning needs.* • Teach patient to identify and avoid triggers if possible *to prevent asthma attacks.* • Encourage verbalization of feelings about diagnosis, treatment, and impact on lifestyle *to offer support and increase adherence with treatment.* • Teach patient about the use of the peak expiratory flow rate (PEFR) meter at home *to promote self-management of symptoms.* • Instruct patient and family on antiinflammatory and bronchodilator medications and their appropriate use *to promote understanding of effects.* • Teach proper techniques for using medication and equipment (e.g., inhaler, nebulizer, peak flow meter) *to promote self-care.* • Assist in the recognition of signs and symptoms of impending asthmatic reaction and implementation of appropriate response measures *to prevent escalation of attacks.* • Establish a written plan with the patient for managing exacerbations *to plan adequate treatment of future exacerbations.*

*Nursing diagnoses listed in order of priority.

TABLE 29-11 NURSING ASSESSMENT
Asthma

Subjective Data
Important Health Information
Past health history: Allergic rhinitis, sinusitis, or skin allergies; previous asthma attack and hospitalization or intubation; symptoms worsened by triggers in the environment; gastroesophageal reflux disease (GERD); occupational exposure to chemical irritants (e.g., paints, dust)
Medications: Adherence to medication, inhaler technique; use of antibiotics; pattern and amount of short-acting β₂-adrenergic agonist used per week; medications that may precipitate an attack in susceptible asthmatics such as aspirin, nonsteroidal antiinflammatory drugs, β-adrenergic blockers

Functional Health Patterns
Health perception–health management: Family history of allergies or asthma; recent upper respiratory tract or sinus infection
Activity-exercise: Fatigue, decreased or absent exercise tolerance; dyspnea, cough (especially at night), productive cough with yellow or green sputum or sticky sputum; chest tightness, feelings of suffocation, air hunger, talking in short sentences or words or phrases, sitting upright to breathe
Sleep-rest: Awakened from sleep because of cough or breathing difficulties, insomnia
Coping–stress tolerance: Emotional distress, stress in work environment or home

Objective Data
General
Restlessness or exhaustion, confusion, upright or forward-leaning body position

Integumentary
Diaphoresis, cyanosis (circumoral, nail bed), eczema

Respiratory
Nasal discharge, nasal polyps, mucosal swelling; wheezing, crackles, diminished or absent breath sounds, and rhonchi on auscultation; hyperresonance on percussion; sputum (thick, white, tenacious); ↑ work of breathing with use of accessory muscles; intercostal and supraclavicular retractions; tachypnea with hyperventilation; prolonged expiration

Cardiovascular
Tachycardia, pulsus paradoxus, jugular venous distention, hypertension or hypotension, premature ventricular contractions

Possible Diagnostic Findings
Abnormal ABGs during attacks, ↓ O₂ saturation, serum and sputum eosinophilia, ↑ serum IgE, positive skin tests for allergens, chest x-ray demonstrating hyperinflation with attacks, abnormal pulmonary function tests showing ↓ flow rates; FVC, FEV₁, PEFR, and FEV₁/FVC ratio that improve between attacks and with bronchodilators

ABGs, Arterial blood gases; *FEV₁,* forced expiratory volume in 1 sec; *FVC,* forced vital capacity; *IgE,* immunoglobulin E; *PEFR,* peak expiratory flow rate.

exercise and other physical activity), (3) maintenance of greater than 80% of personal best PEFR or FEV₁, (4) few or no adverse effects of therapy, (5) no recurrent exacerbations of asthma, and (6) adequate knowledge to participate in and carry out management.

NURSING IMPLEMENTATION
HEALTH PROMOTION. Your role in preventing asthma attacks or decreasing their severity focuses primarily on teaching the patient and caregiver. Teach the patient to identify and avoid known personal triggers for asthma (e.g., cigarette smoke, pet dander) and irritants (e.g., cold air, aspirin, foods, cats, indoor air pollution) (see Table 29-1). Although special dust covers on mattresses and pillows may reduce exposure to dust mites and improve symptoms, the evidence does not support making this a definitive recommendation.[13] Washing bedclothes in hot water or cooler water with detergent and bleach has some effect on allergen levels. Avoidance of furred animals is suggested, but the allergen of pets is nearly impossible to avoid. Pet allergen can be found in many public areas for months even after removal of the animal. Many people are allergic to cockroach remains and the dried droppings, so measures to avoid or control cockroaches are partly effective in removing allergens.

If cold air cannot be avoided, dressing properly with scarves or using a mask helps reduce the risk of an asthma attack. Aspirin and NSAIDs should be avoided if they are known to precipitate an attack. Many OTC drugs contain aspirin. Therefore teach the patient to read the labels carefully. Nonselective β-blockers (e.g., propranolol [Inderal]) are contraindicated because they inhibit bronchodilation. Selective β-blockers (e.g., atenolol [Tenormin]) should be used with caution. Desensitization (immunotherapy) may be partially effective in decreasing the patient's sensitivity to known allergens (see Chapter 14).

Prompt diagnosis and treatment of upper respiratory tract infections and sinusitis may prevent an exacerbation of asthma. If occupational irritants are involved as etiologic factors, the patient may need to consider changing jobs. Individuals who are obese often find that weight loss improves control of asthma. Encourage the patient to maintain a fluid intake of 2 to 3 L/day, good nutrition, and adequate rest. If exercise is planned or if the patient has asthma only with exercise, the health care provider can suggest a medication regimen for pretreatment or long-term control of symptoms to prevent bronchospasm.

ACUTE INTERVENTION. A goal in asthma care is to maximize the patient's ability to safely manage acute asthma exacerbations using an asthma action plan developed in conjunction with the health care provider (Table 29-12). Action plans are particularly important for individuals with moderate to severe persistent asthma or severe exacerbations. The action plan dictates what symptoms or peak flow reading necessitates a change in asthma care to gain control.

The patient can take 2 to 4 puffs of an SABA every 20 minutes three times as a rescue plan. Depending on the response with alleviation of symptoms or improved peak flow, continued SABA use and/or oral corticosteroids may be a part of the home management plan at this point. If symptoms persist or if the patient's peak flow is less than 50% of the personal best, the health care provider or emergency medical services (EMS) needs to be immediately contacted.

When the patient is in the health care facility with an acute exacerbation, it is important to monitor the patient's respiratory and cardiovascular systems. This includes auscultating lung sounds; taking the heart and respiratory rates and BP; and monitoring ABGs, pulse oximetry, and peak flow.

Louder wheezing may actually occur in airways that are responding to the therapy as airflow increases. As improvement continues and airflow increases, breath sounds increase and wheezing decreases. Remember that, despite the disappearance of most of the bronchospasms, the edema and cellular infiltration of the airway mucosa and the viscous mucous plugs may take several days to improve. Thus intensive therapy must be continued even after clinical improvement.

An important nursing goal during an acute attack is to decrease the patient's sense of panic. A calm, quiet, reassuring attitude may help the patient relax. Position the patient comfortably (usually sitting) to maximize chest expansion. Stay with the patient and be available to provide additional comfort. A technique called "talking down" can help the patient remain calm. In talking down, you gain eye contact with the patient. In a firm, calm voice coach the patient to use pursed-lip breathing, which keeps the airways open by maintaining positive pressure (Table 29-13), and abdominal breathing, which slows the respiratory rate and encourages deeper breaths (see Table 7-5). You or the caregiver should stay with the patient until the respiratory rate (with the assistance of the medications) has slowed.

When the acute attack subsides, provide rest and a quiet, calm environment for the patient. When the patient has recovered from exhaustion, try to obtain the health history and pattern of asthma along with a physical assessment. If the caregiver and other family members are present, they may be able to provide information about the patient's health history (see Table 29-11). This information, which is important in planning an individualized nursing care plan, helps the patient with the goal of control.

AMBULATORY AND HOME CARE. Control of symptoms can also be achieved by teaching the patient about medications. The drug regimen itself can be confusing and complex. Teach patients the importance of monitoring their response to medication. It is easy to undermedicate or overmedicate unless careful monitoring is ongoing. Some patients may benefit from keeping a diary to record medication use, wheezing or coughing, peak flow, the drug's side effects, and activity level. This information will help the health care provider adjust the medication.

TABLE 29-12   ASTHMA ACTION PLAN*

General Information
- Name _____
- Emergency contact _____
- Physician/health care provider _____
- Physician signature _____

Phone numbers _____
Phone numbers _____
Date _____

Severity Classification	**Triggers**			**Exercise**
○ Intermittent	○ Colds	○ Smoke	○ Weather	1. Premedication (how much and when) _____
○ Mild persistent	○ Exercise	○ Dust	○ Air pollution	_____
○ Moderate persistent	○ Animals	○ Food		2. Exercise modifications _____
○ Severe persistent	○ Other _____			

Green Zone: Doing Well
Symptoms
- Breathing is good
- No cough or wheeze
- Can work and play
- Sleeps all night

Peak Flow Meter
More than 80% of personal best or
_____

Peak Flow Meter Personal Best =
Control Medications:

Medicine	How Much to Take	When to Take It
_____	_____	_____
_____	_____	_____

Yellow Zone: Getting Worse
Symptoms
- Some problems breathing
- Cough, wheeze, or chest tight
- Problems working or playing
- Wake at night

Peak Flow Meter
Between 50% and 80% of personal best or _____ and _____

Contact Physician If Using Quick Relief More Than 2 Times per Week
Continue Control Medicines and Add:

Medicine	How Much to Take	When to Take It
_____	_____	_____
_____	_____	_____

IF your symptoms (and peak flow, if used) return to Green Zone after 1 hour of the quick-relief treatment, THEN
○ Take quick-relief medication every 4 hours for 1 to 2 days
○ Change your long-term control medicines by
_____
○ Contact your physician for follow-up care

IF your symptoms (and peak flow, if used) DO NOT return to the Green Zone after 1 hour of the quick-relief treatment, THEN
○ Take quick-relief treatment again
○ Change your long-term control medicines by

○ Call your physician/health care provider within
_____ hours of modifying your medication routine

Red Zone: Medical Alert
Symptoms
- Lots of problems breathing
- Cannot work or play
- Getting worse instead of better
- Medicine is not helping

Peak Flow Meter
Between 0% and 50% of personal best or _____ and _____

Ambulance/Emergency Phone Number:
Continue Control Medicines and Add:

Medicine	How Much to Take	When to Take It
_____	_____	_____
_____	_____	_____

Go to the hospital or call for an ambulance if
○ Still in the red zone after 15 minutes
○ You have not been able to reach your physician/health care provider for help

Call an ambulance immediately if the following danger signs are present
○ Trouble walking/talking due to shortness of breath
○ Lips or fingernails are blue

Source: American Lung Association. Retrieved from *www.lungusa.org*.
*Available in Spanish (eTable 29-2) on the website for this chapter.

TABLE 29-13 PATIENT TEACHING GUIDE

Pursed-Lip Breathing (PLB)

Teach the patient how to do PLB using the following guidelines.
1. Use PLB before, during, and after any activity causing you to be short of breath.
2. Inhale slowly and deeply through the nose.
3. Exhale slowly through pursed lips, almost as if whistling.
4. Relax your facial muscles without puffing your cheeks—like whistling—while you are exhaling.
5. Make breathing out (exhalation) three times as long as breathing in (inhalation).
6. The following activities can help you get the "feel" of PLB:
   - Blow through a straw in a glass of water with the intent of forming small bubbles.
   - Blow a lit candle enough to bend the flame without blowing it out.
   - Steadily blow a table-tennis ball across a table.
   - Blow a tissue held in the hand until it gently flaps.
7. Practice 8-10 repetitions of PLB three or four times a day.

Good nutrition is important. Physical exercise (e.g., swimming, walking, stationary cycling) within the patient's limit of tolerance is also beneficial and may require pretreatment with an SABA, as noted previously. Sleep that is uninterrupted by asthma symptoms is an important goal. If patients with asthma wake up because of asthma symptoms, their asthma is not under good control and their therapeutic plan should be reevaluated.

Together with the patient and caregiver, develop written asthma action plans (see Table 29-12). Base these plans on the patient's asthma symptoms and PEFR. To follow the management plan, the patient must measure his or her peak flow at least daily. Some patients may want to just monitor symptoms for self-management. Patients with asthma frequently do not perceive changes in their breathing. Therefore peak flow monitoring, when done correctly, can be a reliable, objective measurement of asthma control (Table 29-14).

TABLE 29-14 PATIENT TEACHING GUIDE

How to Use Your Peak Flow Meter

Include the following instructions when teaching the patient to use a peak flow meter.

Why Use a Peak Flow Meter?
- Peak flow meters are used to check your asthma the way that blood pressure cuffs are used to check blood pressure. A peak flow meter is a device that measures how well air moves out of your lungs.
- During an asthma episode, the airways of the lungs usually begin to narrow slowly. The peak flow meter may tell you if there is narrowing in the airways hours, sometimes even days, before you have any asthma symptoms.
- By taking your medicines early (before symptoms), you may be able to stop the episode quickly and avoid a severe asthma episode.
- The peak flow meter also can be used to help you and your health care provider:
  - Learn what makes your asthma worse.
  - Decide if your treatment plan is working well.
  - Decide when to add or stop medicine.
  - Decide when to seek emergency care.

How to Use Your Peak Flow Meter
- Do the following five steps with your peak flow meter:
  1. Move the indicator to the bottom of the numbered scale.
  2. Stand up.
  3. Take a deep breath, filling your lungs completely.
  4. Place the mouthpiece in your mouth and close your lips around it. Do not put your tongue inside the hole.
  5. Blow out as hard and fast as you can in a single blow.
- Write down the number you get. But if you cough or make a mistake, do not write down the number. Do it over again.
- Repeat steps 1 through 5 two more times, and write down the best of the three blows in your asthma diary.

Find Your Personal Best Peak Flow Number
- Your personal best peak flow number is the highest peak flow number you can achieve over a 2-week period when your asthma is under good control. Good control is when you feel good and do not have any asthma symptoms.
- Each patient's asthma is different, and your best peak expiratory flow (PEF) may be higher or lower than the peak flow of someone of your same height, weight, and gender. This means that it is important for you to find your own personal best peak flow number, which is the basis for your treatment plan.

- To find your personal best peak flow number, take peak flow readings:
  - At least twice a day for 2-3 wk, between 12 noon and 2 PM when your peak flow is the highest
  - 15-20 min after taking inhaled short-acting β₂-agonist (SABA) for quick relief
  - As instructed by your health care provider

The Peak Flow Zone System
Once you know your personal best peak flow number, your health care provider will put the peak flow numbers into zones that are set up like a traffic light. This will help you know what to do when your peak flow number changes. For example:

Green Zone (more than __L/min [80% of your personal best number]) signals good control. No asthma symptoms are present. Take your medicines as usual.

Yellow Zone (between __ and __L/min [50% to <80% of your personal best number]) signals caution. If you remain in the yellow zone after several measures of peak flow, take an inhaled SABA. If you continue to register peak flow readings in the yellow zone, your asthma may not be under good control. Ask your physician if you need to change or increase your daily medicines.

Red Zone (<__L/min [<50% of your personal best number]) signals a medical alert. Take an inhaled SABA (quick-relief medicine) right away. Call your health care provider or the emergency department and ask what to do, or go directly to the emergency department.

Use the Diary to Keep Track of Your Peak Flow
- Record your personal best peak flow number and peak flow zones in your asthma diary.
- Measure your peak flow when you wake up, *before* taking medicine. Write down your peak flow number in the diary every day, or as instructed by your health care provider.

Actions to Take When Peak Flow Numbers Change
- PEF goes between __ and __L/min (50% to <80% of personal best, yellow zone).
  ACTION: Take an inhaled SABA (quick-relief medicine) as prescribed by your health care provider.
- PEF increases ≥20% when measured before and after taking an inhaled SABA (quick-relief medicine).
  ACTION: Talk to your physician about adding more medicine to control your asthma better (e.g., an antiinflammatory medication).

Source: Adapted from National Asthma Education and Prevention Program, National Heart, Lung, and Blood Institute: *Expert Panel Report 3: guidelines for the diagnosis and management of asthma,* NIH pub no 08-4051, Bethesda, Md, 2007, National Institutes of Health. Retrieved from *www.nhlbi.nih.gov/guidelines.*

If a patient's PEFR is within the green zone (usually 80% to 100% of the person's personal best), the patient should remain on her or his usual medications. If the PEFR is within the yellow zone (usually 50% to 80% of personal best), it indicates caution. Something is triggering the patient's asthma (e.g., viral infection).

The patient should have a written asthma action plan that prescribes a step increase in medications during the acute phase of the infection. The dose is stepped down once the viral infection symptoms subside. Based on the asthma management plan, the patient can use different strategies, such as using the SABA more frequently.

If the PEFR is in the red zone (50% or less of personal best), it indicates a serious problem. A rescue plan should be a part of the asthma action plan. Teach the patient and caregiver to take definitive action, as noted previously. Emphasize to the patient the need to monitor PEFR daily or several times a day to have an objective measure that can be correlated with symptoms. Although it may happen, it is unusual for a patient's PEFR to drop from the green zone to the red zone quickly. Usually the patient has time to make changes in medications, avoid triggers, and notify the health care provider.

It is important to involve the patient's caregiver or family. They should know where the patient's inhalers, oral medications, and emergency phone numbers are located. Instruct the caregiver or family on how to decrease the patient's anxiety if an asthma attack occurs. When the patient is stabilized or controlled, the caregiver can gently remind the patient about doing daily PEFR by asking questions such as, "What zone are you in? How's your peak flow today?" A patient and caregiver teaching guide for the patient with asthma is presented in Table 29-15.

An increased number of older adults are diagnosed with asthma. This is a special concern because they have more complicated health issues than younger patients with asthma. Issues that face older adults (especially urban and minority people) are costly medications, nonadherence to medical regimen, and difficulty accessing the health system. Keep these factors in mind when implementing a management plan for older adults.

A variety of factors may contribute to African Americans and Hispanics (especially those from Puerto Rico) having higher rates of poorly controlled asthma and deaths compared with whites. Some factors may be disparities in socioeconomic status and access to proper health care, cultural beliefs about the management of asthma, and underutilization of the long-term controller medications because of high costs. Seek to explore and eliminate any barriers to health care. Also seek out culturally appropriate resources and educational material in languages other than English to improve the asthma control of these individuals.

Relaxation therapies (e.g., yoga, meditation, relaxation techniques, breathing techniques) may help a patient relax respiratory muscles and decrease the respiratory rate. (Chapter 7 discusses relaxation breathing and other relaxation strategies.) A healthy emotional outlook can also be important in preventing future asthma attacks.[14] A variety of websites have excellent resources for patient teaching (see Resources at the end of the chapter). Some communities have asthma support groups.

EVALUATION

The expected outcomes for the patient with asthma are presented in Nursing Care Plan 29-1.

CHRONIC OBSTRUCTIVE PULMONARY DISEASE

Chronic obstructive pulmonary disease (COPD) is a preventable and treatable disease characterized by persistent airflow limitation that is slowly progressive. COPD is associated with an enhanced chronic inflammatory response of the airways and lungs to noxious particles or gases, primarily caused by cigarette smoking. COPD exacerbations and other coexisting illnesses contribute to the overall severity of the disease.[15,16]

Previous definitions of COPD encompassed two types of obstructive airway diseases: chronic bronchitis and emphysema. Chronic bronchitis is the presence of chronic productive cough for 3 months in each of 2 consecutive years in a patient in whom other causes of chronic cough have been excluded. Emphysema is an abnormal permanent enlargement of the air spaces distal to the terminal bronchioles, accompanied by destruction of their walls and without obvious fibrosis. Only about 10% of patients with COPD have pure emphysema. Patients may have a predominance of chronic bronchitis or emphysema, but it is often difficult to determine because the conditions usually coexist. COPD is discussed in this section as one disease state from the viewpoint of pathophysiology and management.[16]

Patients with COPD may have asthma. Although the evidence is not conclusive, asthma may be a risk factor for COPD development. An estimated 12.7 million adults in the United States over age 18 have COPD.[2,15] An additional 24 million people have evidence of impaired lung function. The number of people with COPD is greatly underestimated because the disease is usually not diagnosed until it is moderately advanced. COPD is the third leading cause of death in the United States, killing more than 133,000 Americans each year.[17,18]

Etiology

The many factors involved in the etiology of COPD are discussed in this section.

Cigarette Smoking. Worldwide the major risk factor for developing COPD is cigarette smoking.[18,19] COPD affects about 15% of smokers.[20] An intriguing question is why some smokers develop COPD and others do not. In people over age 40 with a smoking history of 10 or more pack-years, COPD should be considered.[21]

GENDER DIFFERENCES

Chronic Obstructive Pulmonary Disease (COPD)

Men	Women
• COPD is more common in men than in women, but the incidence is not increasing in men. • Fewer men die from COPD than women.	• The number of women with COPD is increasing. • Increase is probably due to increased number of women smoking cigarettes and increased susceptibility (e.g., smaller lungs and airways, lower elastic recoil). • Women with COPD have lower quality of life, more exacerbations, increased dyspnea, and better response to O_2 therapy compared with men.

TABLE 29-15 PATIENT & CAREGIVER TEACHING GUIDE

Asthma

Include the following information in a teaching plan for the patient with asthma and the caregiver. It will help to improve the patient's quality of life and promote lifestyle changes that support successful living with asthma.

Teaching Topic	Resources
What Is Asthma? • Basic anatomy and physiology of lung • Pathophysiology of asthma • Relationship of pathophysiology to signs and symptoms • Measurement and correlation of pulmonary function tests and peak expiratory flow rate	*What Is Asthma?* (National Heart, Lung, and Blood Institute) Retrieved from *www.nhlbi.nih.gov/health/dci/Diseases/ Asthma/Asthma_WhatIs.html.* *What Is Asthma?* (Global Initiative for Asthma). Retrieved from *www. ginasthma.org/q-a-general-information -about-asthma.html.* *Asthma: Overview* (National Jewish Health). Retrieved from *www.njhealth. org/healthinfo/conditions/asthma/index. aspx.*
What Is Good Asthma Control?	Resource for patient on personal ideas of good control. *Asthma Control Test.* Retrieved from *www.qualitymetric.com/demos/ TP_Launch.aspx?SID=52461.*
Hindrances to Asthma Treatment and Control • Intermittent nature of symptoms • Role of denial • Poor perception of asthma severity by patient	Discussion with patient and caregiver about possible hindrances.
Environmental and Trigger Control • Identifications of possible triggers and possible preventive measures • Avoidance of allergens and other triggers • Need to maintain good hydration	*Environmental Management* (National Jewish Health). Retrieved from *www. nationaljewish.org/healthinfo/conditions/ asthma/lifestyle-management/ environmental.* *Pollen Count Report* (sign up for daily notification about a particular area) (American Academy of Asthma Allergy and Immunology). Retrieved from *www.aaaai.org/nab.* Trigger diary kept by patient.

Medications
Types (include mechanism of action)
  • β₂-Agonists
  • Corticosteroids
  • Methylxanthines
  • Anti-IgE
  • Leukotriene modifiers
  • Combination drugs
Establishing medication schedule
Use of preventive and maintenance agents (e.g., antiinflammatory agents)
	Asthma: Treatment (National Jewish Health). Available at *www. nationaljewish.org/healthinfo/conditions/ asthma/treatment.*
	Asthma Action Plan (see Table 29-12).
	Write out medication list and schedule.

Teaching Topic	Resources
Correct Use of Inhalers, Spacer, and Nebulizer	Demonstration–return demonstration with placebo devices (see Figs. 29-5 to 29-7 and Tables 29-8 to 29-10). *Inhaled Medication Instructional Videos: Asthma and General Lung Disease* (National Jewish Health). Retrieved from *www.nationaljewish.org/ healthinfo/medications/lung-diseases/ devices/instructional-videos.* Patient instructions for inhaled devices in English and Spanish (American College of Chest Physicians). Retrieved from *www.chestnet.org/accp/patient-guides/ patient-instructions-inhaled-devices- english-and-spanish.*
Breathing Techniques • Pursed-lip breathing	See Table 29-13.
Correct Use of Peak Flow Meter	See Table 29-14. *Measuring Your Peak Flow Rate (text and video)* (American Lung Association). Retrieved from *www.lung.org/ lung-disease/asthma/living-with-asthma/ take-control-of-your-asthma/measuring- your-peak-flow-rate.html.*
Asthma Action Plan • Peak flow zones • Individualize plan • Early recognition of infection • Building a partnership with your health care provider • Questions patients may have about asthma, but patient cannot reach the provider	See Table 29-12. Patient completes asthma action plan and discusses it with health care provider. *Asthma Clinical Research Centers* (American Lung Association). Retrieved from *www.lung.org/finding-cures/ our-research/acrc.* *My Asthma Wallet Card* (National Heart, Lung, and Blood Institute). Retrieved from *www.nhlbi.nih.gov/health/public/ lung/asthma/asthma_walletcard.htm.* *Asthma Profiler* (online decision support tool to assist patients in understanding treatment options and side effects; includes personalized questions to ask the provider and research reports) (American Lung Association). Retrieved from *www.lung.org/lung-disease/ asthma/living-with-asthma/ making-treatment-decisions.* *Lung Line* (ask a specialized nurse questions about early detection, care, and prevention of respiratory diseases) (National Jewish Health). Telephone: 800-222-LUNG or *www.njhealth.org/ about/contact/lung-line.aspx.*

Cigarette smoke has several direct effects on the respiratory tract (Table 29-16). The irritating effect of the smoke causes hyperplasia of cells, including goblet cells, thereby increasing the production of mucus. Hyperplasia reduces airway diameter and increases the difficulty in clearing secretions. Smoking reduces the ciliary activity and may cause actual loss of cilia. Smoking also produces abnormal dilation of the distal air space with destruction of alveolar walls. Many cells develop large, atypical nuclei, which are considered a precancerous condition. Smoking causes chronic, enhanced inflammation of various parts of the lung with structural changes and repair (called remodeling). The reasons for the inflammatory response are not clearly understood, but may be genetically determined, since patients who have never smoked can develop COPD.

Cigarette smoking causes oxidative stress, as well as an imbalance between proteases that break down connective tissue in the lung and antiproteases that protect the lungs.[16] These changes resulting from cigarette smoking increase with more severe disease and even persist with smoking cessation. (See Chapter 11 for more detail about cigarette smoking.)

Passive smoking is the exposure of nonsmokers to cigarette smoke, also known as *environmental tobacco smoke* (ETS) or secondhand smoke. In adults, involuntary smoke exposure is associated with decreased pulmonary function, increased respiratory symptoms, and severe lower respiratory tract infections (e.g., pneumonia). ETS is also associated with increased risk for lung cancer and nasal sinus cancer.

Occupational Chemicals and Dusts. If a person has intense or prolonged exposure to various dusts, vapors, irritants, or fumes in the workplace, symptoms of lung impairment consistent with COPD can develop. If a person has occupational exposure and smokes, the risk of COPD increases.[16]

Air Pollution. High levels of urban air pollution are harmful to people with existing lung disease. However, the effect of outdoor air pollution as a risk factor for the development of COPD is unclear. Another risk factor for COPD development is coal and other biomass fuels that are used for indoor heating and cooking. Many people who have never smoked are at significant risk for developing COPD because of cooking with these fuels in poorly ventilated areas.[16]

Infection. Infections are a risk factor for developing COPD. Severe recurring respiratory tract infections in childhood have been associated with reduced lung function and increased respiratory symptoms in adulthood. It is unclear whether the development of COPD can be related to recurrent infections in adults. People who smoke and also have human immunodeficiency virus (HIV) have an accelerated development of COPD. Tuberculosis is also a risk factor for COPD development.

Genetics. The fact that a relatively small percentage of smokers get COPD strongly suggests that genetic factors influence which smokers get the disease. Because of the genetic-environmental interaction, two people may have the same smoking history, but only one develops COPD. To date, one genetic factor has been clearly identified (see next section).[16]

α_1-Antitrypsin (AAT) Deficiency. α_1-Antitrypsin (AAT) deficiency is an autosomal recessive disorder that may affect the lungs or liver. AAT deficiency is a genetic risk factor for COPD. Approximately 3% of all people diagnosed with COPD may have undetected AAT deficiency. AAT is a serum protein produced by the liver and normally found in the lungs. The main function of AAT, an α_1-protease inhibitor, is to protect normal lung tissue from attack by proteases during inflammation related to cigarette smoking and infections. Severe AAT deficiency leads to premature bullous emphysema in the lungs found on x-ray. Smoking greatly exacerbates the disease process in these patients.[22]

🧬 Genetic Link

AAT deficiency is an autosomal recessive disorder (see Figs. 13-4 and 13-5 and the Genetics in Clinical Practice box). The

TABLE 29-16	EFFECTS OF TOBACCO SMOKE ON RESPIRATORY SYSTEM	
Area of Defect	**Acute Effects**	**Long-Term Effects**
Respiratory mucosa		
• Nasopharyngeal	↓ Sense of smell	Cancer
• Tongue	↓ Sense of taste	Cancer
• Vocal cords	Hoarseness	Chronic cough, cancer
• Bronchus and bronchioles	Bronchospasm, cough	Chronic bronchitis, asthma, cancer
Cilia	Paralysis, sputum accumulation, cough	Chronic bronchitis, cancer
Mucous glands	↑ Secretions, ↑ cough	Hyperplasia and hypertrophy of glands, chronic bronchitis
Alveolar macrophages	↓ Function	↑ Incidence of infection
Elastin and collagen fibers	↑ Destruction by proteases	Emphysema
	↓ Function of antiproteases (α_1-antitrypsin)	
	↓ Synthesis and repair of elastin	

🧬 GENETICS IN CLINICAL PRACTICE

α_1-Antitrypsin (AAT) Deficiency

Genetic Basis
- Autosomal recessive disorder.
- Mutations in *SERPINA1* gene (located on chromosome 14) cause AAT deficiency.
- Gene provides instructions for the liver to make the protein AAT, which protects the lungs and liver from powerful proteolytic enzymes.
- Without enough functional AAT, proteolytic enzymes destroy alveoli and cause lung disease.

Incidence
- Occurs in 1 in 1700 to 3500 live births in the United States.
- People of northern European descent most affected.

Genetic Testing
- DNA testing is available.
- Screening of siblings is useful.
- Serum assay is available to measure the amount of AAT.

Clinical Implications
- AAT deficiency can cause lung and liver disease.
- Onset of disease is between ages 20 and 40 yr.
- Treatment includes AAT replacement (Prolastin).
- Disease predisposes to early-onset emphysema.

severity of AAT deficiency depends on which forms of the gene are inherited. The most common abnormal genes are the S and Z alleles. The normal genotype is MM. The most common genotype associated with AAT disease is ZZ (also referred to as PI-ZZ). Other variations include MZ (slightly increased risk of poor lung function) and SZ (higher risk of lung and liver problems in smokers). Some individuals with MZ and SZ genotypes may never seek health care because they have minimal manifestations of the disorder.[22]

Although 100,000 people in the United States are suspected of having the ZZ phenotype, fewer than 10% have been detected. Clues to AAT deficiencies are the onset of symptoms often occurring by age 40, minimal to no tobacco use, and family history of emphysema and/or liver disease.[23] Chronic liver disease as an infant or adult with increased liver enzyme levels may also be seen. Individuals with this type of emphysema are primarily of northern European origin.

A simple blood test can determine low levels of AAT. Those with borderline or low levels can then be genetically tested.

IV-administered AAT (e.g., Prolastin-C) augmentation therapy is used for people with AAT deficiency. The infusions are usually administered weekly. Its effectiveness in slowing the progression of the disease and the results of this treatment continue to be evaluated.

Aging. Although aging is often considered a risk factor for COPD, the evidence is unclear. Does the aging process lead to COPD, or is COPD a result of the cumulative exposures that occur over a long life?[16] Normal aging results in loss of elastic recoil, stiffening of the chest wall, gas exchange alteration, and decrease in exercise tolerance. As people age, the lungs gradually lose their elastic recoil. Thoracic cage changes result from osteoporosis and calcification of the costal cartilages. The thoracic cage becomes stiff and rigid, and the ribs are less mobile. The shape of the rib cage gradually changes because of the increased residual volume (RV), causing it to expand and become rounded. Decreased chest compliance and elastic recoil of the lungs caused by aging affect the mechanical aspects of ventilation and increase the work of breathing.[24]

As one ages, the number of functional alveoli decreases as peripheral airways lose supporting tissues. The surface area for gas exchange decreases, and the PaO_2 decreases. Changes in the elasticity of the lungs reduce the ventilatory reserve.[24] These changes are similar to those seen in the patient with emphysema.

Pathophysiology

COPD is characterized by chronic inflammation of the airways, lung parenchyma (respiratory bronchioles and alveoli), and pulmonary blood vessels (Fig. 29-8). The pathogenesis of COPD is complex and involves many mechanisms. The defining feature of COPD is not fully reversible airflow limitation during forced exhalation. This is caused by loss of elastic recoil and airflow obstruction caused by mucus hypersecretion, mucosal edema, and bronchospasm.

In COPD various processes occur such as airflow limitation, air trapping, gas exchange abnormalities, and mucus hyperse-

FIG. 29-8 Pathophysiology of chronic obstructive pulmonary disease *(COPD)*.

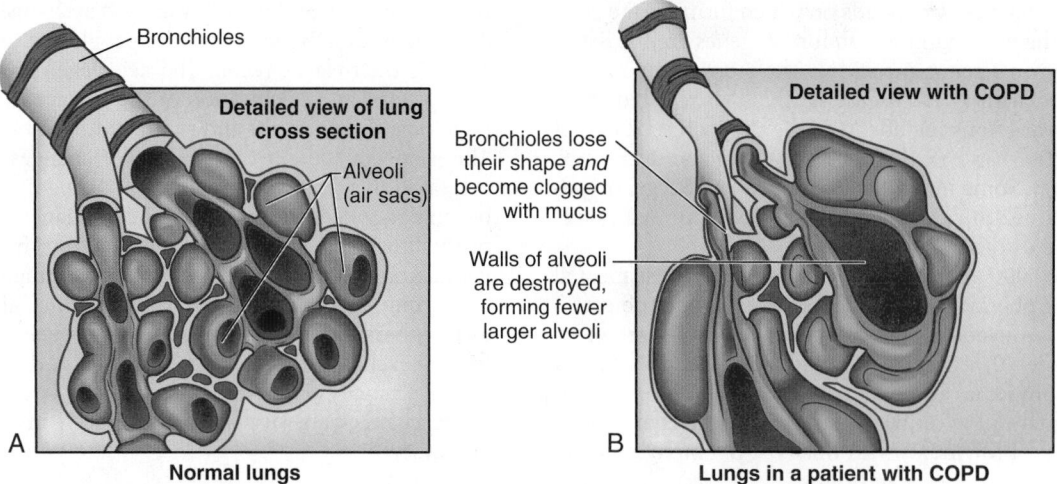

FIG. 29-9 A, Normal lungs showing bronchioles and alveoli. **B,** Changes in the bronchioles and alveoli in the lungs of a patient with chronic obstructive pulmonary disease *(COPD).*

cretion. In severe disease, pulmonary hypertension and systemic manifestations occur (see Fig. 29-8). COPD has an uneven distribution of pathologic changes, with severely destroyed lung areas existing together with areas of relatively normal lung.

The inflammatory process starts with inhalation of noxious particles and gases (e.g., cigarette smoke), but is magnified in the person with COPD. The abnormal inflammatory process causes tissue destruction and disrupts the normal defense mechanisms and repair process of the lung. The mechanisms for the enhanced inflammatory response are not clearly understood, but may be genetically determined.[16]

The predominant inflammatory cells in COPD are neutrophils, macrophages, and lymphocytes. This pattern of inflammatory cells is different from that in asthma. (In asthma the inflammatory cells are eosinophils, mast cells, neutrophils, lymphocytes, and macrophages.) These inflammatory cells attract other inflammatory mediators (e.g., leukotrienes) and proinflammatory cytokines (e.g., tumor necrosis factor). The end result of the inflammatory process is structural changes in the lungs.[16]

The inflammatory process may also be magnified by oxidants, which are produced by cigarette smoke and other inhaled particles and released from the inflammatory cells. The oxidants adversely affect the lungs as they inactivate antiproteases (which prevent the natural destruction of the lungs), stimulate mucus secretion, and increase fluid in the lungs.

After the inhalation of oxidants in tobacco or air pollution, the activity of proteases (which break down the connective tissue of the lungs) increases and the antiproteases (which protect against the breakdown) are inhibited. Therefore the natural balance of protease/antiprotease is tipped in favor of destruction of the alveoli and loss of the lungs' elastic recoil.[16,24]

Inability to expire air is a main characteristic of COPD. The primary site of the airflow limitation is in the smaller airways. As the peripheral airways become obstructed, air is progressively trapped during expiration. The volume of residual air becomes greatly increased in severe disease as alveolar attachments to small airways (similar to rubber bands) are destroyed. The residual air, combined with the loss of elastic recoil, makes passive expiration of air difficult. As air is trapped in the lungs,

the chest hyperexpands and becomes barrel shaped, since the respiratory muscles are not able to function effectively. The functional residual capacity is increased. The patient is now trying to breathe in when the lungs are in an "overinflated" state; thus the patient appears dyspneic and exercise capacity is limited.

Gas exchange abnormalities result in hypoxemia and hypercapnia (increased CO_2) as the disease worsens. As the air trapping increases, walls of alveoli are destroyed (Fig. 29-9), and bullae (large air spaces in the parenchyma) and blebs (air spaces adjacent to pleurae) can form.

Bullae and blebs are not effective in gas exchange, since they do not contain the capillary bed that normally surrounds each alveolus. Therefore a significant ventilation-perfusion (V/Q) mismatch and hypoxemia result. Peripheral airway obstruction also results in V/Q imbalance and, combined with the respiratory muscle impairment, can lead to CO_2 retention, particularly in severe disease.

Excess mucus production, resulting in a chronic productive cough, is a feature of individuals with predominant chronic bronchitis. However, not all COPD patients have sputum production. Excess mucus production is a result of an increased number of mucus-secreting goblet cells and enlarged submucosal glands. In addition, dysfunction of cilia leads to chronic cough and sputum production. Some of the inflammatory mediators also stimulate mucus production.

Pulmonary vascular changes resulting in mild to moderate pulmonary hypertension may occur late in the course of COPD. The small pulmonary arteries vasoconstrict due to hypoxia. As the disease advances, the structure of the pulmonary arteries changes, resulting in thickening of the vascular smooth muscle. Because of the loss of alveolar walls and the capillaries surrounding them, pressure in the pulmonary circulation increases.

Typically, the patient does not have difficulty with hypoxemia at rest until late in the disease. However, hypoxemia may develop during exercise, and the patient may benefit from supplemental O_2. Pulmonary hypertension may progress and lead to hypertrophy of the right ventricle of the heart (**cor pulmonale**). The right ventricle dilates and may eventually lead to right-sided heart failure.[25]

In addition to lung disease, COPD is a systemic disease. Chronic inflammation is an underlying etiology for these systemic effects. Cardiovascular diseases commonly exist in COPD (smoking is a primary risk factor for both of them). Other common systemic diseases include cachexia (skeletal muscle wasting), osteoporosis, diabetes, and metabolic syndrome, which cannot be readily related to smoking.[16,26]

Clinical Manifestations

Clinical manifestations of COPD typically develop slowly, but COPD should be considered in all patients over age 40 with 10 or more pack-years of cigarette smoking.[21] A diagnosis of COPD should be considered in any patient who has symptoms of cough, sputum production, or dyspnea and/or a history of exposure to risk factors for the disease.

A chronic intermittent cough, which is often the first symptom to develop, may later be present every day as the disease progresses. The cough is often dismissed by patients as they expect it with smoking or environmental exposures. The cough may be unproductive of mucus. However, significant airflow limitation may exist without sputum or cough.[16] Typically dyspnea is progressive, usually occurs with exertion, and is present every day.

Patients may complain of not being able to take a deep breath, heaviness in the chest, gasping, increased effort to breathe, and air hunger. Patients usually ignore the symptoms and rationalize that "I'm getting older" and "I'm out of shape." They change behaviors to avoid dyspnea, such as taking the elevator. Gradually the dyspnea interferes with daily activities, such as carrying grocery bags. They cannot walk as fast as their partner or peers. However, as symptoms worsen and interfere with daily activity or they have their first COPD exacerbation, patients usually seek medical care.

In late stages of COPD, dyspnea may be present at rest. As more alveoli become overdistended, increasing amounts of air are trapped. This causes a flattened diaphragm, and the patient must breathe from partially inflated lungs. Effective abdominal breathing is decreased because of the flattened diaphragm from the overinflated lungs. The person becomes more of a chest breather, relying on the intercostal and accessory muscles. However, chest breathing is not efficient.

Wheezing and chest tightness may be present, but may vary by time of the day or from day to day, especially in patients with more severe disease. Wheezes may arise from the laryngeal area, or wheezes may not be present on auscultation. Chest tightness, which often follows activity, may feel similar to muscular contraction.

The person with advanced COPD frequently experiences fatigue, weight loss, and anorexia. Even with adequate caloric intake, the patient still loses weight. Fatigue is a highly prevalent symptom that affects the patient's activities of daily living. Paroxysms of coughing may be so severe the patient faints or fractures a rib.

During physical examination a prolonged expiratory respiratory phase, wheezes, or decreased breath sounds are noted in all lung fields. The patient may need to breathe louder than normal for auscultated breath sounds to be heard. The anteroposterior diameter of the chest is increased ("barrel chest") from the chronic air trapping. The patient may sit upright with arms supported on a fixed surface such as an overbed table (tripod position). The patient may naturally purse lips on expiration (pursed-lip breathing) and use accessory muscles, such as those

in the neck, to aid with inspiration. Edema in the ankles may be the only clue to right-sided heart involvement (cor pulmonale).

Over time, hypoxemia (PaO_2 less than 60 mm Hg or O_2 saturation less than 88%) may develop with hypercapnia ($PaCO_2$ over 45 mm Hg). The bluish red color of the skin results from polycythemia and cyanosis. Polycythemia develops as a result of increased production of red blood cells as the body attempts to compensate for chronic hypoxemia. Hemoglobin concentrations may reach 20 g/dL (200 g/L) or more. However, the person may also have lowered hemoglobin and hematocrit because of chronic anemia.

Clinically it is common for a person to have a combination of emphysema and chronic bronchitis, often with one condition predominating. It is sometimes difficult to distinguish COPD from asthma, especially if the individual has a history of cigarette smoking. However, some clinical features are different (see Table 29-3).

Classification of COPD. COPD should be considered in any person with a chronic cough and dyspnea who has smoked cigarettes or been exposed to environmental or occupational pollutants. The diagnosis is confirmed by spirometry.

COPD can be classified as mild, moderate, severe, and very severe (Table 29-17). An FEV_1/FVC ratio of less than 70% establishes the diagnosis of COPD, and the severity of obstruction (as indicated by FEV_1) determines the stage of COPD. The management of COPD is based on the patient's symptoms, classification, and exacerbation history.

Complications

Cor Pulmonale. Cor pulmonale results from pulmonary hypertension, which is caused by diseases affecting the lungs or pulmonary blood vessels (Fig. 29-10). In North America 50% of the cases of cor pulmonale are due to COPD. Cor pulmonale is a late manifestation of COPD, yet not all patients with COPD develop cor pulmonale. Once the patient develops cor pulmonale, the prognosis worsens.[27]

In COPD, pulmonary hypertension is caused primarily by constriction of the pulmonary vessels in response to alveolar hypoxia, with acidosis further potentiating the vasoconstriction. Chronic alveolar hypoxia causes vascular remodeling. Chronic hypoxia also stimulates erythropoiesis, which causes polycythemia. This results in increased viscosity of the blood. An anatomic reduction of the pulmonary vascular bed, as seen in emphysema with bullae, may occur. These patients have increased pulmonary vascular resistance and thus develop pulmonary hypertension.

TABLE 29-17	CLASSIFICATION OF COPD SEVERITY*	
The following classification is based on postbronchodilator FEV_1.		
Classification	**Level of Severity**	**FEV_1 Results**
GOLD 1	Mild	FEV_1 ≥80% predicted
GOLD 2	Moderate	FEV_1 50%-80% predicted
GOLD 3	Severe	FEV_1 30%-50% predicted
GOLD 4	Very severe	FEV_1 <30% predicted

Adapted from Global Initiative for Chronic Obstructive Lung Disease: Global strategy for the diagnosis, management, and prevention of chronic obstructive pulmonary disease (updated 2013). Retrieved from www.goldcopd.org.
*A diagnosis of COPD is made when a patient has a FEV_1/FVC <0.70.
COPD, Chronic obstructive pulmonary disease; FEV_1, forced expiratory volume in 1 sec; FVC, forced vital capacity.

PATHOPHYSIOLOGY MAP

FIG. 29-10 Mechanisms involved in the pathophysiology of pulmonary hypertension and cor pulmonale secondary to chronic obstructive pulmonary disease.

Normally the right ventricle and pulmonary circulatory system are low-pressure systems compared with the left ventricle and systemic circulation. When pulmonary hypertension develops, the pressures on the right side of the heart must increase to push blood into the lungs. Eventually, right-sided heart failure develops.

Dyspnea is the most common symptom of chronic cor pulmonale. Lung sounds are normal, or crackles may be heard in the bases of the lungs bilaterally. Heart sound changes occur but are usually masked by the underlying lung disease. Other manifestations of right-sided heart failure may develop, including distended neck veins (jugular venous distention), hepatomegaly with right upper quadrant tenderness, peripheral edema, and weight gain.

ECG changes indicating right ventricular hypertrophy may be seen in severe cases. Typically the patient has large pulmonary vessels on chest x-ray and increased pressure on a right-sided heart cardiac catheterization. Echocardiogram may reflect right-sided heart enlargement. B-type natriuretic peptide (BNP) levels, which are used to diagnose heart failure, may be elevated in cor pulmonale secondary to the stretching of the right ventricle. Normally BNP levels are used to distinguish cardiac from respiratory causes of dyspnea, but in cor pulmonale the cause of the heart failure is the lung disease.[27]

Treatment of cor pulmonale is initially targeted at managing the COPD (e.g., bronchodilation). Continuous low-flow, long-term O_2 therapy (for more than 15 hr/day) improves survival.[28] Diuretics are generally used, similar to their use with chronic heart failure. (Cor pulmonale is also discussed in Chapter 28.)

COPD Exacerbations. According to the Global Initiative for Chronic Obstructive Lung Disease (GOLD) guidelines, a *COPD exacerbation* is an acute event in the natural course of the disease. The primary causes of exacerbations are bacterial or viral infections.[16,29] Exacerbations are signaled by an acute change in the patient's usual dyspnea, cough, and/or sputum (i.e., something different from the usual daily patterns). Exacerbations of COPD are typical and increase in frequency (average one or two a year) as the disease progresses. It may take several weeks for a patient to recover from an exacerbation.

Assess patients for the classic signs of exacerbation such as an increase in dyspnea, sputum volume, or sputum purulence. They may also have nonspecific complaints of malaise, insomnia, fatigue, depression, confusion, decreased exercise tolerance, increased wheezing, or fever without other causes.[30]

As the severity of COPD increases, exacerbations of COPD are associated with poorer outcomes. Exacerbations may be treated at home or in the hospital, depending on the severity. The severity is determined by the patient's medical history before the exacerbation, the presence of other diseases, symptoms, ABGs, and other laboratory tests. Typically in the later stages of COPD the patient has a low-normal pH, high-normal or above-normal $PaCO_2$, and high-normal bicarbonate (HCO_3^-). This indicates compensated respiratory acidosis as the patient has chronically retained CO_2 and the kidneys have conserved HCO_3^- to increase the pH to within the normal range (see Table 29-3).

Carefully assess the patient's ABGs for any movement toward respiratory acidosis and further hypoxemia, indicating respiratory failure. Also assess the patient's medical history for the stage of COPD as noted by the level of FEV_1. Assess for new symptoms or worsening of usual symptoms. Determine the number of previous exacerbations per year and if treatment occurred in the home or hospital. The presence of other co-morbid conditions complicates the exacerbation. In addition, the current treatment affects its management. Be alert for signs of severity such as use of accessory muscles, central cyanosis, edema in the lower extremities, unstable BP, right-sided heart failure, and altered alertness. These manifestations affect whether the patient is treated as an inpatient or outpatient.

Short-acting bronchodilators, oral systemic corticosteroids, and antibiotics are the typical therapies for exacerbations. SABAs with or without short-acting anticholinergics are preferred for those who are breathless. Drug administration via MDI or nebulizer works equally well, although sicker patients often prefer the nebulizer. Antibiotic use remains somewhat controversial. However, the presence of green or purulent sputum (as opposed to white sputum) is one of the best ways to determine if antibiotics are needed.[16,29]

Therapies used to treat exacerbations of COPD in the hospital are similar to home management, except supplemental O_2 therapy titrated by ABG measurement may be used. Attempts are made to use noninvasive mechanical methods (e.g., continuous positive airway pressure [CPAP] to support ventilation rather than invasive ventilatory support [e.g., intubation and mechanical ventilation]). Teach the patient and the caregiver early recognition of the three cardinal symptoms of exacerbations (increase in dyspnea, sputum volume, or sputum purulence) to promote early treatment and thus prevent hospitalization and possible respiratory failure.

Acute Respiratory Failure. Patients with severe COPD who have exacerbations are at risk for respiratory failure. Frequently, COPD patients wait too long to contact their health care provider when they first develop symptoms suggestive of exacerbation. Discontinuing bronchodilator or corticosteroid medication may also precipitate respiratory failure.

Cardioselective β-adrenergic blockers (e.g., atenolol, metoprolol) can be safely used. Chronic treatment with β-blockers may improve survival and reduce the risk of exacerbations of COPD.[16,31]

Indiscriminate use of sedatives, benzodiazepines, and opioids, especially in the preoperative or postoperative patient who retains CO_2, may suppress the ventilatory drive and lead to respiratory failure. The person with COPD who retains CO_2 is usually treated with low-flow rates of O_2 with careful monitoring of ABGs to avoid hypercapnia. It is vital to provide adequate O_2 while assessing the ABGs, rather than risk not providing O_2 because of the fear of CO_2 narcosis (discussed on p. 592).

In patients with COPD, surgery or severe, painful illness involving the chest or abdominal organs may lead to splinting and ineffective ventilation and respiratory failure. To prevent postoperative pulmonary complications, careful preoperative screening, which includes PFTs and ABG assessment, is important in the patient with a heavy smoking history and/or COPD. (Respiratory failure is discussed in Chapter 68.)

Depression and Anxiety. Patients with COPD experience many losses as the disease progresses. Because many patients with COPD experience depression and anxiety, assess for both. Ask patients if they "feel down or blue" most of the time. Do they appear anxious about being able to control their breathlessness or know what to do if they have an exacerbation? Are they

exhibiting concern over more difficulty in self-care activities such as bathing? How is the family coping with the patient's disease?

Help the patient with muscle relaxation exercises that can reduce anxiety (see Chapter 7). In addition, teach patients about the treatment and disease, which can give them a sense of control of their disease and complex treatment regimens. It is important to include the patient's caregiver in the teaching so he or she can help the patient cope physically and emotionally.

A consultation with a mental health specialist may be needed for proper screening and diagnosis of depression or other mental health problems. Cognitive and behavioral therapy along with COPD teaching may improve the quality of life. Medications may be used to treat both depression and anxiety. Buspirone (BuSpar), which is used to treat anxiety, has few if any respiratory depression effects. Benzodiazepines should be avoided because they may depress the respiratory drive and may be habit forming. When the patient becomes anxious because of dyspnea, the use of pursed-lip breathing (see Table 29-13) and short-acting bronchodilators may be appropriate.

Diagnostic Studies

Spirometry is required to confirm the diagnosis in individuals suspected of having COPD. Spirometry confirms the presence of airflow obstruction and determines the severity of COPD. The patient is given a short-acting bronchodilator, and post-bronchodilator values are compared with a normal reference value.

A diagnosis of COPD is made when the FEV_1/FVC ratio is less than 70% along with the appropriate symptoms. The value of FEV_1 provides a guideline for the degree of severity of COPD. FEV_1 can be expressed as a percentage compared with a normal reference value (percent predicted). The lower the FEV_1, the sicker the patient.

In addition to spirometry, other diagnostic studies are performed (Table 29-18). Chest x-rays are not diagnostic but may show a flat diaphragm because of the hyperinflated lungs. Computed tomography (CT) scans are not routinely used to diagnose COPD. However, in individuals with predominant emphysema, enlarged air spaces in the apices may be seen on the CT scan.

Other tests may be used to assess the response to therapy, disease severity, and quality of life. Two validated questionnaires are the COPD Assessment Test (CAT) and modified Medical Research Council (mMRC) Dyspnea Scale. The CAT (see eTable 29-3 on the website for this chapter) measures the daily impact of COPD on a person's life and can help the health care team make better management decisions.[32] This test is found online in more than 50 languages with scoring and easy to understand guidelines (www.catestonline.org). The mMRC measures the patient's level of dyspnea (see eTable 29-4).

Patients often have exercise-induced hypoxemia, and thus a 6-minute walk test should be done by a physical or respiratory therapist, with pulse oximetry readings taken when the patient is walking and at rest. If values of O_2 saturation are 88% or lower when at rest and the patient is breathing room air, he or she qualifies for supplemental O_2.[16] Later in the disease the findings presented in Table 29-3 may be present.

A history and physical examination are extremely important in a diagnostic workup.

The BODE index can be used to assess not only the risk of death from COPD, but also the pulmonary and systemic mani-

---

TABLE 29-18   COLLABORATIVE CARE

Chronic Obstructive Pulmonary Disease (COPD)

Diagnostic
- History and physical examination
- Pulmonary function tests
- Chest x-ray
- Serum α_1-antitrypsin levels
- ABGs
- Six-minute walk test
- COPD Assessment Test (CAT)* or modified Medical Research Council (mMRC) Dyspnea Scale†
- BODE Index‡

Collaborative Therapy
- Cessation of cigarette smoking
- Treatment of exacerbations
- Drug therapies (see Tables 29-7 and 29-19)
- Airway clearance techniques
- Breathing exercises and retraining
- Hydration of 3 L/day (if not contraindicated)
- Patient and caregiver teaching
- Influenza immunization yearly
- Pneumovax immunization
- Long-term O_2 (if indicated)
- Progressive plan of exercise, especially walking and upper body strengthening
- Pulmonary rehabilitation program
- Nutritional supplementation if low BMI
- Surgery
  - Lung volume reduction
  - Lung transplantation

*See eTable 29-3 or *www.catestonline.org*.
†See eTable 29-4 or *copd.about.com/od/copdbasics/a/MMRCdyspneascale.htm*.
‡See *www.qxmd.com/calculate-online/respirology/bode-index*. Index is a tool to help predict COPD mortality after diagnosis.
ABGs, Arterial blood gases; *BMI,* body mass index.

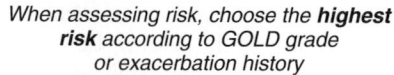

*When assessing risk, choose the **highest risk** according to GOLD grade or exacerbation history*

FIG. 29-11 Rubric for chronic obstructive pulmonary disease *(COPD)* showing the association between symptoms, spirometric classification, and future risk of exacerbations. The following factors are considered in the rubric: (1) current level of patient's symptoms as measured by one of two validated questionnaires (modified Medical Research Council *[mMRC]* Dyspnea Scale [see eTable 29-4] or the COPD Assessment Test *[CAT]* [see eTable 29-3]); (2) severity of the disease as measured by the FEV_1; (3) exacerbation risk as reflected in the spirometric classification or patient's history of exacerbations; and (4) presence of co-morbidities. Source: Global Initiative for Chronic Obstructive Lung Disease: Global strategy for the diagnosis, management, and prevention of chronic obstructive pulmonary disease (updated 2013). Retrieved from *www.goldcopd.org*.

festations (see *www.qxmd.com/calculate-online/respirology/bode-index*).

ABGs are usually assessed in the severe stages (FEV_1 less than 50%) and monitored in patients hospitalized with acute exacerbations. In the later stages of COPD, typical findings are low PaO_2, elevated $PaCO_2$, decreased or low-normal pH, and increased HCO_3^- levels. In early stages, there may be a normal or only slightly decreased PaO_2 and a normal $PaCO_2$. An ECG may be normal or show signs of right ventricular failure. An echocardiogram or multigated acquisition (MUGA) (cardiac blood pool) scan (see Table 32-6) can be used to evaluate right- and left-sided ventricular function. Sputum for culture and sensitivity may be obtained if the patient is hospitalized for an acute exacerbation and has not responded to empiric therapy with antibiotics.

Collaborative Care

Two major evidence-based references related to the care of COPD patients are (1) GOLD (*www.goldcopd.org*) and (2) clinical guidelines from the American College of Physicians.[15,16] Most patients are treated as outpatients. They are hospitalized for exacerbations and potential complications when respiratory failure, pneumonia, and cor pulmonale occur.

The GOLD guidelines present a rubric for assessing and diagnosing COPD (Fig. 29-11). You may be a part of the health care team that administers the mMRC or CAT and inquires about exacerbations. This information is used to detect COPD patients who are at risk for problems.[16]

Evaluate the patient's exposure to environmental or occupational irritants, and determine ways to control or avoid them. For example, teach the patient to avoid aerosol hair sprays and smoke-filled rooms. The patient with COPD is extremely susceptible to pulmonary infections. The patient with COPD and anyone who smokes should receive an influenza virus vaccine yearly. The pneumococcal vaccine (Pneumovax) is recommended for all smokers ages 19 or older and all patients with COPD.[21,33] (The guidelines for Pneumovax are presented in Table 28-5.)

Exacerbations of COPD should be treated as soon as possible, especially if the patient is in the severe stages. Some patients are given a prescription for antibiotics and are instructed to begin taking them when the first symptoms or signs of an exacerbation occur.[34]

Smoking Cessation. Cessation of cigarette smoking in any person with COPD at any level of severity is the most important intervention that can impact the natural history of COPD.[16] After a person discontinues smoking, the accelerated decline in pulmonary function found with smoking slows to almost nonsmoking levels.[21,29] Thus the sooner the smoker stops, the less pulmonary function is lost and the sooner the symptoms decrease, especially cough and sputum production. (Smoking cessation techniques are discussed in Chapter 11 and in Tables 11-4 to 11-6.)

Drug Therapy. Medications for COPD can reduce symptoms, increase exercise capacity, improve overall health, and reduce the number and severity of exacerbations. Bronchodilator drug therapy relaxes smooth muscles in the airway and improves the ventilation of the lungs, thus reducing the degree of breathlessness. Patients with COPD do not respond as dra-

TABLE 29-19 DRUG THERAPY

Medication Guidelines for Stable COPD

The treatment guidelines are based on the FEV_1 results.

FEV₁ Results	Treatment Guidelines*
FEV₁ 60%-80% predicted (with respiratory symptoms)	Treatment with inhaled bronchodilators may be used.
FEV₁ <60% predicted (with respiratory symptoms)	Treat with inhaled bronchodilators: anticholinergics or long-acting β₂–agonist OR Monotherapy with long-acting inhaled anticholinergics or long-acting β₂-agonist OR Combination therapy with long-acting inhaled anticholinergics, long-acting β₂-agonist, or inhaled corticosteroids

*NOTE: Occasional use of short-acting inhaled bronchodilator for acute symptoms are not addressed in these recommendations.
Source: Qaseem A, Wilt T, Weinberger S, et al: Diagnosis and management of stable chronic obstructive pulmonary disease: a clinical practice guideline update from the American College of Physicians, American College of Chest Physicians, American Thoracic Society, and European Respiratory Society, *Ann Intern Med* 155:179, 2011. FEV_1, Forced expiratory volume in 1 sec.

matically to bronchodilator therapy as those with asthma. However, bronchodilator therapy reduces dyspnea and increases FEV_1. The inhaled route of medication is preferred and given on a PRN or regular basis.

Patients commonly do not properly administer inhaled medications. Therefore it is important for you to demonstrate and talk with patients about inhaler use. Give the patient clear, readable instructions.[10]

Medications are given in a stepwise fashion according to the level of airflow obstruction determined from spirometry (FEV_1) and symptoms (see Fig. 29-11). Medications are stepped up but usually not stepped down, as in asthma, because in COPD continual symptoms are probably present (Table 29-19).

Bronchodilator medications commonly used are β₂-adrenergic agonists; anticholinergic agents; and, to a much lesser extent, methylxanthines (see Table 29-7). The choice of a bronchodilator depends on the patient's response. These medications are given on a PRN or scheduled basis. When the patient has mild COPD or fewer symptoms, a short-acting bronchodilator is used.[21] Albuterol or ipratropium may be used as single agents, but combining bronchodilators improves their effect and decreases the risk of adverse effects.[29] Albuterol and ipratropium can be nebulized together (DuoNeb) or delivered by inhalation spray (Combivent Respimat).

In the moderate stage of COPD (FEV_1 less than 60%), a long-acting bronchodilator may be used (see Tables 29-7 and 29-19). A short-acting bronchodilator may still be used PRN as a "rescue" for dyspnea. Salmeterol and formoterol are widely used LABAs, and they can be used in COPD as monotherapy (unlike drug therapy for asthma).[21] Indacaterol (Arcapta Neohaler) is the newest LABA with a duration of action of 24 hours, and thus it can be used just once a day.[16] Tiotropium (Spiriva), a long-acting anticholinergic, is used once a day.

The addition of an ICS to long-acting bronchodilator therapy is often prescribed in COPD patients with FEV_1 of less than 60%. Examples of combinations of ICSs with LABAs are fluticasone/salmeterol (Advair) and budesonide/formoterol

(Symbicort). Inhaled long-acting anticholinergics, LABAs, or ICSs all reduce COPD exacerbations. However, in COPD, unlike asthma, ICSs are not used as monotherapy because of the concerns about side effects. Some patients are on triple therapy with Advair and tiotropium.[21] Oral corticosteroids should not be used for long-term therapy in COPD, but are effective for short-term use to treat exacerbations.

The use of long-acting theophylline in the treatment of COPD is controversial because it interacts with many drugs. A low dose of theophylline with an ICS may benefit a few patients with COPD who do not respond to other inhaled medications.

Roflumilast (Daliresp) is an oral medication used to decrease the frequency of exacerbations in severe COPD. This drug is a phosphodiesterase inhibitor, which is an antiinflammatory drug that suppresses the release of cytokines and other inflammatory mediators, and inhibits the production of reactive oxygen radicals.[21,35]

New drug delivery devices are becoming available at a rapid pace. One example is Respimat, which is an easy-to-use handheld device that provides a high deposition of drug to the lungs and low mouth and throat deposition. Respimat simplifies coordination between activation of the medication and inhalation without propellant, and it is independent of inspiratory flow. It also has a dose indicator. Combivent Respimat (ipratropium and albuterol) inhalation aerosol is now available.[36]

Oxygen Therapy. O_2 therapy is frequently used in the treatment of COPD and other problems associated with hypoxemia. Long-term continuous (more than 15 hr/day) O_2 therapy (LTOT) increases survival and improves exercise capacity and mental status in hypoxemic patients.[15,21]

Oxygen is a colorless, odorless, tasteless gas that constitutes 21% of the atmosphere. Administering supplemental O_2 increases the partial pressure of O_2 (PO_2) in inspired air. Used clinically, it is considered a drug. For reimbursement purposes, Medicare pays for oxygen when certain clinical criteria are met (i.e., the patient's O_2 saturation is 88% or less, and PaO_2 is 55 mm Hg or less).

Indications for Use. Goals for O_2 therapy are to keep the SaO_2 greater than 90% during rest, sleep, and exertion, or the PaO_2 greater than 60 mm Hg. O_2 is usually administered to treat hypoxemia caused by a variety of problems such as (1) respiratory disorders (e.g., COPD, pulmonary hypertension, cor pulmonale, pneumonia, lung cancer, pulmonary emboli); (2) cardiovascular disorders (e.g., myocardial infarction, dysrhythmias, angina pectoris, and cardiogenic shock); and (3) central nervous system disorders (e.g., overdose of opioids, head injury, sleep disorders [sleep apnea]).

Methods of Administration. The goal of O_2 administration is to supply the patient with adequate O_2 to maximize the oxygen-carrying ability of the blood. There are various methods of O_2 administration (Table 29-20 and Fig. 29-12). The method selected depends on factors such as the fraction of inspired O_2 (FIO_2) required by the patient and delivered by the device, the patient's mobility, humidification required, patient cooperation, comfort, cost, and financial resources.

O_2 delivery systems are classified as low- or high-flow systems. Most methods of O_2 administration are low-flow devices that deliver O_2 in concentrations that vary with the person's respiratory pattern. In contrast, the Venturi mask is a high-flow device that delivers fixed concentrations of O_2 (e.g., 24%, 28%) independent of the patient's respiratory pattern.

TABLE 29-20 METHODS OF OXYGEN ADMINISTRATION

Description	**Nursing Interventions**

Low-Flow Delivery Devices
Nasal Cannula

- Most commonly used device.
- O_2 delivered via plastic nasal prongs.
- Safe and simple method that allows some freedom of movement. Patient can eat, talk, or cough while wearing device.
- Useful for a patient requiring low O_2 concentrations.
- O_2 concentrations of 24% (at 1 L/min) to 44% (at 6 L/min) can be obtained.

- Stabilize nasal cannula when caring for a restless patient.
- Amount of O_2 inhaled depends on room air and patient's breathing pattern.
- Most patients with COPD can tolerate 2 L/min via cannula.
- Assess patient's nares and ears for skin breakdown. May need to pad cannula where it sits on ears.
- If flow rates are >5 L/min, nasal membranes may dry and may cause pain in frontal sinuses.

Simple Face Mask

- Covers patient's nose and mouth.
- Used only for short periods, especially when transporting patients.
- Longer use is typically not tolerated because of tight seal and heat generated around nose and mouth from mask.
- O_2 concentrations of 35%-50% can be achieved with flow rates of 6-12 L/min.
- Mask provides adequate humidification of inspired air.

- Wash and dry under mask q2hr.
- Mask must fit snugly.
- Nasal cannula may be provided while patient is eating.
- Watch for pressure necrosis at top of ears from elastic straps if patient wears for a longer time. (Gauze or other padding may alleviate this problem.)

Partial and Non-Rebreather Masks

- Useful for short-term (24 hr) therapy for patients needing higher O_2 concentrations (60%-90% at 10-15 L/min).
- O_2 flows into reservoir bag and mask during inhalation.
- This bag allows patient to rebreathe about first third of exhaled air (rich in O_2) in conjunction with flowing O_2.
- Vents remain open on partial mask only. Some facilities prefer this over non-rebreather as a safety issue.

- O_2 flow rate must be sufficient to keep bag from collapsing during inspiration to avoid CO_2 buildup.
- If deflation occurs, increase liter flow to keep bag inflated.
- Mask should fit snugly.
- With non-rebreather masks, make sure valves are open during expiration and closed during inhalation to prevent drastic decrease in FIO_2.
- Monitor patient closely, since more advanced interventions may be required such as CPAP, BiPAP, or intubation with mechanical ventilation.

Oxygen-Conserving Cannula

- Generally indicated for long-term O_2 therapy at home vs. during hospitalization (e.g., pulmonary fibrosis, pulmonary hypertension).
- May be "moustache" (Oxymizer) or "pendant" type.
- Cannula has a built-in reservoir that ↑ O_2 concentration and allows patient to use lower flow, usually 30%-50%, which increases comfort, lowers cost, and can be increased with activities.
- Can deliver up to 8 L/min O_2.

- May cause necrosis over tops of ears. Can be padded.
- Cannula cannot be cleaned. Manufacturer recommends changing cannula every week.
- It is more expensive than standard cannulas and requires evaluation with ABGs and oximetry to determine correct flow for patient.
- Cannula is highly visible.

Pendant-type O_2-conserving cannula.

TABLE 29-20 METHODS OF OXYGEN ADMINISTRATION—cont'd

Description	Nursing Interventions
High-Flow Delivery Devices ***Tracheostomy Collar*** • Collar attaches to neck with elastic strap and can deliver high humidity and O_2 via tracheostomy. • O_2 concentration is lost into atmosphere because collar does not fit tightly. • Venturi device can be attached to flow meter and thus can deliver exact amounts of O_2 via collar.	• Secretions collect inside collar and around tracheostomy. Remove collar and clean at least q4hr to prevent aspiration of fluid and infection. • Because condensation occurs in tubing, periodically drain distally to tracheostomy.	
Tracheostomy T Bar • Almost identical to tracheostomy collar, but it has a vent and a T connector that allow an inline catheter (e.g., Ballard catheter) to be connected for suctioning. • Tight fit allows better O_2 and humidity delivery than tracheostomy collar.	• Empty as necessary. • Because T bars disconnect easily, monitor closely. • T bar may pull on a patient's tracheostomy tube, causing irritation and potential tissue damage. Monitor this closely. • See tracheostomy collar above.	
Venturi Mask • Mask can deliver precise, high-flow rates of O_2. • Lightweight plastic, cone-shaped device is fitted to face. • Masks are available for delivery of 24%, 28%, 31%, 35%, 40%, and 50% O_2. • Method is especially helpful for administering low, constant O_2 concentrations to patients with COPD. • Adaptors can be applied to increase humidification.	• Entrainment device on mask must be changed to deliver higher concentrations of O_2. • Air entrainment ports must not be occluded. • Mask is uncomfortable. Remove when patient eats. • Patient can talk but voice may be muffled. • See other applicable nursing interventions under simple face mask above.	

ABGs, Arterial blood gases; *BiPAP*, biphasic positive airway pressure; *CPAP*, continuous positive airway pressure; *FIO₂*, fraction of inspired O_2.

FIG. 29-12 Golfer uses Helios liquid portable O_2 system.

Mechanical ventilators are another example of a high-flow O_2 delivery system. Because room air is mixed with O_2, in low-flow systems the percentage of O_2 delivered to the patient is not as precise as with high-flow systems.

Humidification and Nebulization. O_2 obtained from cylinders or wall systems is dry. Dry O_2 has an irritating effect on mucous membranes and dries secretions. Therefore it is important that a high liter flow of O_2, delivering more than 35% to 50% O_2, be humidified, either by humidification or nebulization. A common device used for humidification when the patient has a cannula or a mask is a bubble-through humidifier. It is a small plastic jar filled with sterile distilled water that is attached to the O_2 source by means of a flow meter. O_2 passes into the jar, bubbles through the water, and then goes through tubing to the patient's cannula or mask. The purpose of the bubble-through humidifier is to restore the humidity conditions of room air. However, the need for bubble-through humidifiers at flow rates between 1 and 4 L/minute is based on the patient's comfort.

Another means of administering humidified O_2 is via a nebulizer. It delivers particulate water mist (aerosols) with nearly 100% humidity. The humidity can be increased by heating the water, which increases the gas's ability to hold moisture. Humidified (100%) gas is required when the upper airway is bypassed in acute care. However, patients with established tracheostomies do not always require 100% humidity. When nebulizers are used, large tubing should be employed to connect the device to a face mask or T bar. If small tubing is used, condensation can occlude the flow of O_2. Vapotherm Precision Flow can deliver high flows (up to 40 L/minute) of warm humidified gas (air/O_2) with precise percentages to the patient through a nasal cannula, and it is noninvasive.[37]

Complications

Combustion. O_2 supports combustion and increases the rate of burning, so it is important to prohibit smoking in the area in which O_2 is being used. A "No Smoking" sign should be prominently displayed on the patient's door. Also caution the patient against smoking cigarettes with an O_2 cannula in place.

Carbon Dioxide Narcosis. The chemoreceptors in the respiratory center that control the drive to breathe respond to CO_2 and O_2. Normally, CO_2 accumulation is the major stimulant of the respiratory center. Over time some COPD patients develop a tolerance for high CO_2 levels (the respiratory center loses its sensitivity to the elevated CO_2 levels). Theoretically, for these individuals the "drive" to breathe is hypoxemia. Thus there has been concern regarding the dangers of administering O_2 to COPD patients and reducing their drive to breathe. However, the "hypoxic drive" is complex and involves other factors, including ventilation and perfusion. In addition, not all patients with COPD retain CO_2.

The key concern is not providing adequate oxygen to these patients, since this is much more detrimental because it may lead to hypoxia. It is much easier to reverse high CO_2 than low O_2. Although O_2 administration should be titrated to the lowest effective dose, many patients who have end-stage COPD require high flow rates and higher concentrations for survival. They may exhibit higher than normal levels of CO_2 in their blood, but this is not a major concern. What is important is careful, ongoing assessment when providing O_2 to these patients, monitoring both the physical and cognitive effects of O_2 levels.

It is critical to start O_2 at low flow rates until ABGs can be obtained. ABGs are used as a guide to determine what FIO_2 level is sufficient and can be tolerated. Assess the patient's mental status and vital signs before starting O_2 therapy and frequently thereafter.

Oxygen Toxicity. Pulmonary O_2 toxicity may result from prolonged exposure to a high level of O_2 (PaO_2). High concentrations of oxygen can result in a severe inflammatory response because of oxygen radicals and damage to alveolar-capillary membranes resulting in severe pulmonary edema, shunting of blood, and hypoxia. These individuals develop acute respiratory distress syndrome (ARDS) (see Chapter 68). Fortunately, O_2 toxicity is relatively rare.

Prevention of O_2 toxicity is important for the patient who is receiving O_2. The amount of O_2 administered should be just enough to maintain the PaO_2 within a normal or acceptable range for the patient. Monitor ABGs frequently to evaluate the effectiveness of therapy and to guide the tapering of supplemental O_2. A safe limit of O_2 concentrations has not yet been established. All levels above 50% and O_2 used for longer than 24 hours should be considered potentially toxic. Levels of 40% and below used for short periods may be regarded as relatively nontoxic and probably will not result in significant O_2 toxicity.

Absorption Atelectasis. Normally, nitrogen (which constitutes 79% of the air that is breathed) is not absorbed into the bloodstream. This prevents alveolar collapse. When high concentrations of O_2 are given, nitrogen is washed out of the alveoli and replaced with O_2. If airway obstruction occurs, the O_2 is absorbed into the bloodstream and the alveoli collapse. This process is called *absorption atelectasis*.

Infection. Infection can be a major hazard of O_2 administration. Heated nebulizers present the highest risk. The constant use of humidity supports bacterial growth, with the most common organism being *Pseudomonas aeruginosa*. Disposable equipment that operates as a closed system, such as the Ballard closed suctioning system, should be used. Each hospital has a policy on the required frequency of equipment changes based on the type of equipment used.

Chronic Oxygen Therapy at Home. Improved survival occurs in patients with COPD who receive long-term O_2 therapy (LTOT) (more than 15 hr/day) to treat hypoxemia.[16,21] The improved prognosis results from preventing progression of the disease and subsequent cor pulmonale. The benefits of LTOT include improved mental acuity, sleep, and exercise tolerance; decreased hematocrit; and reduced pulmonary hypertension.

Some patients fear becoming "addicted" to O_2 and are reluctant to use it. Tell them that it is not "addicting" and that it needs to be used because of the positive effects on the heart, lungs, and brain. Evaluate the need for LTOT when the patient's condition has stabilized. The goal of O_2 therapy is to maintain SaO_2 greater than 90% during rest, sleep, and exertion.

Short-term home O_2 therapy (1 to 30 days) may be indicated for the patient in whom hypoxemia persists after discharge from the hospital. For example, a patient with underlying COPD who develops a serious respiratory tract infection may need continued O_2 therapy to treat hypoxemia for 4 to 6 weeks after discharge from the hospital. Measure the patient's oxygenation status by SaO_2 30 to 90 days after an acute episode to determine if the O_2 is still needed.

TABLE 29-21	HOME OXYGEN DELIVERY SYSTEMS*

- Liquid O_2
- Compressed O_2 cylinders
- Concentrator or extractor
- Portable O_2 concentrator
- O_2 conserving or pulsed devices

*Detailed descriptions of these delivery systems are presented in eTable 29-5 (available on the website for this chapter).

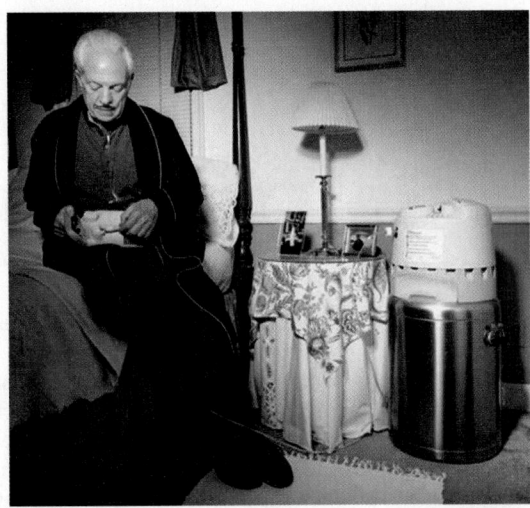

FIG. 29-13 A portable liquid O_2 unit can be refilled from a liquid O_2 reservoir unit.

Patients may receive O_2 only during exercise and/or sleep. Evaluate the need for O_2 during these periods with a 6-minute walk test or overnight oximetry. (Pulse oximetry is discussed in Chapter 26.)

Periodic reevaluations are necessary for the patient who is using chronic supplemental O_2. Generally, the patient should be reevaluated every 30 to 90 days during the first year of therapy and annually after that, as long as the patient remains stable.

Nasal cannulas, either regular or the O_2-conserving type (see Table 29-20), are usually used to deliver O_2 from a central source in the home. The source may be a liquid O_2 storage system, compressed O_2 in tanks, or an O_2 concentrator or extractor, depending on the patient's home environment, insurance coverage, activity level, and proximity to an O_2 supply company (Table 29-21). To increase mobility in the home, the patient can use extension tubing (up to 50 ft) without adversely affecting the O_2 flow delivery. Small, portable systems, such as liquid O_2, may be provided for the patient who remains active outside the home (see Fig. 29-12).

Home O_2 systems are usually rented from a company that sends a respiratory therapist to the patient's home (Fig. 29-13). The therapist teaches the patient and caregiver how to use the O_2 system, how to care for it, and how to recognize when the supply is running low and needs to be reordered. A patient and caregiver teaching guide for the use of O_2 at home is presented in Table 29-22.

Encourage the patient who uses home O_2 to remain active and travel normally. If travel is by automobile, arrangements can be made for O_2 to be available at the destination point. O_2 supply companies can often assist in these arrangements. If a patient wishes to travel by bus, train, or airplane, the patient

TABLE 29-22	PATIENT & CAREGIVER TEACHING GUIDE

Home Oxygen Use

The company that provides the prescribed O_2 therapy equipment will instruct the patient on equipment care. The following are some general instructions that you may include when teaching the patient and caregiver about the use of home O_2.

Decreasing Risk for Infection

- Brush teeth or use mouthwash several times a day.
- Wash nasal cannula (prongs) with a liquid soap and thoroughly rinse once or twice a week.
- Replace cannula every 2-4 wk.
- If you have a cold, replace the cannula after your symptoms pass.
- Always remove secretions that are coughed out.
- If you use an O_2 concentrator, every day unplug the unit and wipe down the cabinet with a damp cloth and dry it.
- Ask the company providing the equipment how often to change the filter.

Safety Issues

- Post "No Smoking" warning signs outside the home.
- O_2 will not "blow up," but it will increase the rate of burning, since it is a fuel for the fire.
- Do not allow smoking in the home, and do not smoke yourself while wearing O_2. Nasal cannulas and masks can catch fire and cause serious burns to face and airways.
- Do not use flammable liquids such as paint thinners, cleaning fluids, gasoline, kerosene, oil-based paints, or aerosol sprays while using O_2.
- Do not use blankets or fabrics that carry a static charge, such as wool or synthetics.
- Inform your electric company if you are using a concentrator. In case of a power failure, it will know the medical urgency of restoring your power.

Adapted from *www.YourLungHealth.org.*

should inform the appropriate people when reservations are made that O_2 will be needed for travel. If there is a potential for the patient to become hypoxic, O_2 needs for flying can be determined via a hypoxia inhalation test or through a mathematical formula. Portable oxygen concentrators are a ready source of renewable O_2 and can be available by recharging at home or with a DC (e.g., auto) power supply. These systems are widely approved by airlines for in-flight use. The patient should contact the airline to determine the particular accommodations and policies for in-flight O_2.

Breathing Retraining. The patient with COPD has dyspnea with an increased respiratory rate. In addition, the accessory muscles of breathing in the neck and upper part of the chest are used excessively to promote chest wall movement. These muscles are not designed for long-term use, and as a result, the patient experiences increased fatigue.

The main types of breathing retraining exercises are (1) pursed-lip breathing and (2) diaphragmatic breathing. The purpose of **pursed-lip breathing (PLB)** is to prolong exhalation and thereby prevent bronchiolar collapse and air trapping. PLB is simple and easy to teach and learn, and it gives the patient more control over breathing, especially during exercise and periods of dyspnea[38] (see Table 29-13). Patients should be taught to use "just enough" positive pressure with the pursed lips because excessive resistance may increase the work of breathing.

Diaphragmatic (abdominal) breathing focuses on using the diaphragm instead of the accessory muscles of the chest to (1) achieve maximum inhalation and (2) slow the respiratory rate.[39] However, the use of diaphragmatic breathing in patients with COPD may increase the work of breathing and dyspnea. Patients with moderate to severe COPD with marked hyperinflation may be poor candidates for diaphragmatic breathing.[40]

PLB slows the respiratory rate and is easier to learn than diaphragmatic breathing. In the setting of extreme acute dyspnea, it is most important to focus on helping the patient slow the respiratory rate by using the principles of PLB. Other techniques that decrease breathing frequency, such as yoga, may also be used to reduce dyspnea.[40]

Airway Clearance Techniques. Many patients with COPD or other conditions (e.g., cystic fibrosis, bronchiectasis) who retain secretions require help to adequately clear their airways. Airway clearance techniques (ACTs) loosen mucus and secretions so they can be cleared by coughing. A variety of safe techniques can be used to achieve airway clearance. When ACTs are compared, it is primarily patient preference that determines which one is used.[41]

ACTs are especially beneficial in patients who have a COPD exacerbation.[42] Respiratory therapists, physical therapists, and nurses are involved in performing these techniques. ACTs are often used with other treatments. Typically the patient receives bronchodilator therapy via an inhaled device (e.g., nebulization) before ACT. Then the ACT is used, followed by effective coughing (e.g., huff coughing). ACTs include effective coughing, chest physiotherapy, airway clearance devices, and high-frequency chest ventilation.

Effective Coughing. Many patients with COPD have developed ineffective coughing patterns that do not adequately clear their airways of sputum. They also fear developing spastic coughing, resulting in increased dyspnea. Although other techniques (e.g., chest physiotherapy) are used to loosen secretions and mucus, the patient must cough effectively to bring the secretions to the central airways to expectorate them.

Huff coughing is an effective forced expiratory technique that you can easily teach the patient. Before starting, ensure that the patient is breathing deeply from the diaphragm. Place the patient's hands on the lower lateral chest wall, and then ask the patient to breathe deeply through the nose. You should feel the patient's hands move outward, which represents a breath from the diaphragm. Guidelines for effective huff coughing are presented in Table 29-23.

Chest Physiotherapy. Chest physiotherapy (CPT) is primarily used for patients with excessive bronchial secretions who have difficulty clearing them (e.g., cystic fibrosis, bronchiectasis). CPT consists of postural drainage, percussion, and vibration. CPT should be performed by an individual who has been properly trained.

Percussion and *vibration* are manual or mechanical techniques used to augment postural drainage. These techniques are used after the patient has assumed a postural drainage position to assist in loosening the mobilized secretions (see eFig. 29-1 on the website for this chapter). Percussion, vibration, and postural drainage assist in bringing secretions into larger, more central airways. Effective coughing (huff coughing) is then necessary to help raise these secretions.

Complications associated with improperly performed CPT include fractured ribs, bruising, hypoxemia, and discomfort.

TABLE 29-23   PATIENT & CAREGIVER TEACHING GUIDE

Effective Huff Coughing

When teaching effective huff coughing:
1. Help the patient assume a sitting position with head slightly flexed, shoulders relaxed, knees flexed, forearms supported by pillow, and, if possible, feet on the floor.

Then you should instruct the patient to:
2. Inhale slowly through the mouth while breathing deeply from the diaphragm.
3. Hold the breath for 2-3 seconds.
4. Forcefully exhale quickly as if one is fogging up a mirror with one's breath (thus creating a "huff"). (This moves the secretions to larger airways.)
5. Repeat the "huff" one or two more times while refraining from a "regular" cough.
6. Cough when mucus is felt in the breathing tubes.
7. Rest for five to ten regular breaths.
8. Repeat the huffs (three to five cycles) until you feel you have cleared mucus or you become tired.

CPT may be stressful for some patients, and some may develop hypoxemia and bronchospasms.

Postural Drainage. Postural drainage is the use of positioning techniques that drain secretions from specific segments of the lungs and bronchi into the trachea. The postural drainage positions used depend on the areas of lung that are involved. This is determined by patient assessment (including the patient's preference), chest x-rays, and chest auscultation. For example, some patients with left lower lobe involvement require postural drainage of only the affected region, whereas a person with cystic fibrosis may require postural drainage of all segments.

The purpose of various positions in postural drainage is to drain each segment toward the larger airways. A side-lying position can be used for the patient who cannot tolerate a head-down position. Aerosolized bronchodilators and hydration therapy are usually administered before postural drainage. The chosen postural drainage position is maintained for about 5 minutes during percussion and vibration. A common order is two to four times a day. In acute situations, postural drainage may be performed as frequently as every 4 hours. Schedule the procedure to be completed at least 1 hour before meals or 3 hours after meals.

Beds are available that can rotate and percuss in various postural drainage positions, and these are quite effective. Some positions for postural drainage (e.g., Trendelenburg) should not be performed on the patient with chest trauma, hemoptysis, heart disease, pulmonary embolus, or head injury, and in other situations where the patient's condition is not stable.

Percussion. *Percussion* is performed in the appropriate postural drainage position with the hands in a cuplike position, with the fingers and thumbs closed (Fig. 29-14). The cupped hand should create an air pocket between the patient's chest and the hand. Both hands are cupped and used in an alternating rhythmic fashion. Percussion is accomplished with flexion and extension of the wrists. If it is performed correctly, a hollow sound should be heard. The air-cushion impact facilitates the movement of thick mucus. Place a thin towel over the area to be percussed, or the patient may choose to wear a T-shirt or hospital gown.

Vibration. *Vibration* is accomplished by tensing the hand and arm muscles repeatedly and pressing mildly with the flat of

FIG. 29-14 Cupped-hand position for percussion. The hand should be cupped as though scooping up water.

FIG. 29-15 Acapella airway clearance device.

the hand on the affected area while the patient slowly exhales a deep breath. The vibrations facilitate movement of secretions to larger airways. Mild vibration is tolerated better than percussion and can be used in situations where percussion may be contraindicated. Commercial vibrators are available for hospital and home use.

Airway Clearance Devices. Various *airway clearance devices* are available to mobilize secretions, are easier to tolerate than CPT, and take less time than conventional CPT sessions. These devices include the Flutter, Acapella, and TheraPEP Therapy System. These devices use the principle of positive expiratory pressure (PEP) and may provide greater benefit to patients with COPD than other ACTs.[42]

The Flutter mucus clearance device is a hand-held device that is shaped like a small, fat pipe (see eFig. 29-2 available on the website for this chapter). It provides PEP treatment for patients with mucus-producing conditions. The Flutter has a mouthpiece, a high-density stainless steel ball, and a cone that holds the ball. When the patient exhales through the Flutter, the steel ball moves, which causes oscillations (vibrations) in the airways and loosens mucus. It helps move mucus up through the airways to the mouth where the mucus can be expectorated. The patient must be upright, and the angle at which the Flutter is held is critical. The Acapella is another small hand-held device (Fig. 29-15) that combines the benefits of both PEP therapy and airway vibrations to mobilize pulmonary secretions. It can be used in virtually any setting, since patients are free to sit, stand, or recline. The patient may also inhale through the Acapella, and nebulizers can be attached to it. This saves time because the treatment does not have to be preceded by the nebulizer.

TheraPEP Therapy System can also provide sustained PEP and can simultaneously deliver aerosols so the patient can inhale and exhale through it. TheraPEP has a mouthpiece attached to tubing connected to a small cylindric resistor and a pressure indicator. The pressure indicator provides visual feedback about the pressure that the patient needs to hold in an exhalation to receive the PEP. The therapist initially determines the pressure, and you can reinforce the treatment. (A description and photo of this system are available at *www*

.smiths-medical.com/catalog/bronchial-hygiene/therapep/ therapep-system.html.)

High-Frequency Chest Wall Oscillation. High-frequency chest wall oscillation uses an inflatable vest (e.g., the Vest Airway system or the SmartVest) with hoses connected to a high-frequency pulse generator. (A description and photo are available at *www.thevest.com/products.*) The pulse generator delivers air to the vest, which vibrates the chest. The high-frequency airwaves dislodge mucus from the airways, mobilize the mucus, and move it toward larger airways. The vest can be used without the aid of another person. The units weigh 23 to 30 lb and are quiet. They come in a suitcase and are portable.

Nutritional Therapy. Many COPD patients in the advanced stages are underweight with loss of muscle mass and cachexia. Weight loss is a predictor of a poor prognosis and increased frequency of COPD exacerbations. Weight gain after nutritional support can decrease the risk of mortality.

The cause of weight loss is not entirely known. To some extent, loss of muscle mass is associated with aging. (Most people with COPD are older.) If the patient is on high doses of corticosteroids, the net effect is protein catabolism and loss of muscle mass. Eating becomes an effort because of the dyspnea related to the energy expended to chew, the reduction of airflow while swallowing, and O_2 desaturation.

Decreased appetite and weight loss also occur because of the systemic inflammatory process in COPD. The inflammation results in increased metabolism, which could explain why some individuals with COPD lose weight despite adequate nutritional intake.[43] Other factors that contribute to malnutrition in COPD include altered taste caused by chronic mouth breathing, excessive sputum, fatigue, anxiety, depression, increased energy needs, numerous infections, and side effects of polypharmacy.[44]

To decrease dyspnea and conserve energy, the patient should rest for at least 30 minutes before eating and use a bronchodilator before meals. Teach the patient to avoid exercise and treatments for at least 1 hour before and after eating. If a patient has O_2 therapy prescribed, use of supplemental O_2 by nasal cannula while eating may be beneficial. Assess the patient's dentition because broken or missing teeth or loose dentures make eating more difficult. Activity such as walking or getting out of bed during the day can stimulate the appetite and promote weight gain. Sensations of bloating and early satiety when eating can be attributed to swallowing air while eating, side effects of medication (especially corticosteroids and theophylline), and the abnormal position of the diaphragm relative to the stomach in association with hyperinflation of the lungs.

Fluid intake should be at least 3 L/day unless contraindicated by other medical conditions. Fluids should be taken between meals (rather than with them) to prevent excess stomach distention and to decrease pressure on the diaphragm. Sodium restriction may be indicated if there is accompanying heart failure.

Getting the patient to eat adequate amounts of nutritionally sound foods may be difficult even though well-balanced meals are available. Give the patient or meal preparer printed information that can make mealtime easier and more nutritious (Table 29-24).

Underweight patients with COPD need extra protein and calories. They may need 25 to 45 kcal/kg body weight and more than 1.5 g of protein/kg body weight to maintain their weight.[45] The patient with excessive malnutrition may need up to 2.5 g of protein/kg of body weight to restore muscle mass.

TABLE 29-24   NUTRITIONAL THERAPY

Maximizing Food Intake in COPD

Sometimes it is difficult for patients with COPD to consume adequate amounts of nutrients. Teach the patients to make mealtimes easier and more nutritious by increasing calories and protein without increasing the amount of food eaten.

- Eat high-calorie foods first.
- Limit liquids at mealtimes.
- Rest before meals.
- Try more frequent meals and snacks.
- Increase calories by adding margarine, butter, mayonnaise, sauces, gravies, and peanut butter to foods.
- Keep favorite foods and snacks on hand.
- Try cold foods, which can make you feel less full than hot foods.
- Keep ready-prepared meals available for times when you have increased shortness of breath.
- Eat larger meals when you are not as tired.
- Avoid foods that you know cause gas (e.g., cabbage, beans, cauliflower).
- Add skim milk powder (2 tbs) to regular milk (8 oz) to add protein and calories.
- Use milk or half-and-half instead of water when making soups, cereals, instant puddings, cocoa, or canned soups.
- Add grated cheese to sauces, vegetables, soups, and casseroles.
- Choose dessert recipes that contain egg (e.g., sponge cake, angel food cake, egg custard, bread pudding, rice pudding).

Source: Grodner M, Roth S, Walkingshaw B: *Nutritional foundations and clinical applications: a nursing approach*, ed 5, St Louis, 2011, Mosby.

A diet high in calories and protein, moderate in carbohydrate, and moderate to high in fat is recommended and can be divided into five or six small meals a day.[46] High-protein, high-calorie nutritional supplements can be offered between meals. Nonprotein calories should be divided evenly between fat and carbohydrate, but avoid overfeeding the patient (see Table 29-24).

The dietitian is the best resource to determine what combination of nutrients and what supplements are best for the patient.[44] (Nutritional supplements are discussed in Chapter 40.)

Surgical Therapy for COPD. Three different surgical procedures have been used in severe COPD. One type of surgery is *lung volume reduction surgery* (LVRS). The goal of this surgery is to reduce the size of the lungs by removing the most diseased lung tissue so the remaining healthy lung tissue can perform better. The rationale for LVRS is that reducing the size of the hyperinflated emphysematous lungs results in decreased airway obstruction and increased room for the remaining normal alveoli to expand and function. The procedure reduces lung volume and improves lung and chest wall mechanics. LVRS is being explored as a therapy that can be performed via a bronchoscope (BLVR).[16]

The second surgical procedure is *bullectomy*. This procedure is used for carefully selected patients with emphysematous COPD who have large bullae (larger than 1 cm). The bullae are usually resected via thoracoscope.

The third surgical procedure is *lung transplantation*, which benefits carefully selected patients with advanced COPD. Although single-lung transplant is the most commonly used technique because of a shortage of donors, bilateral transplantation can be performed. (Lung transplantation is discussed in Chapters 14 and 28.)

A novel approach is being explored for patients with emphysema. Airway bypass is a bronchoscopic procedure currently under evaluation to determine if creating small extra-anatomic openings between the diseased lung and the distal bronchi can reduce hyperinflation. This is a minimally invasive treatment that improves pulmonary function and reduces dyspnea by enabling trapped air to exit the lungs.[47]

NURSING MANAGEMENT
CHRONIC OBSTRUCTIVE PULMONARY DISEASE

NURSING ASSESSMENT

Subjective and objective data that should be obtained from a person with COPD are presented in Table 29-25.

NURSING DIAGNOSES

The nursing diagnoses for the patient with COPD may include, but are not limited to, those presented in Nursing Care Plan 29-2.

PLANNING

The overall goals are that the patient with COPD will have (1) prevention of disease progression, (2) ability to perform ADLs and improved exercise tolerance, (3) relief from symptoms, (4) no complications related to COPD, (5) knowledge and ability to implement a long-term treatment regimen, and (6) overall improved quality of life.

NURSING IMPLEMENTATION

HEALTH PROMOTION. The incidence of COPD would decrease dramatically if people would not begin smoking or would stop smoking. (Techniques to help patients stop smoking are discussed in Chapter 11 and Tables 11-4 to 11-6.) Avoiding or controlling exposure to occupational and environmental pollutants and irritants is another preventive measure to maintain healthy lungs. (These factors are discussed in the section on nursing management of lung cancer in Chapter 28.)

Counseling the patient in smoking cessation is vital, because it is the only way to slow the progression of COPD. As health care professionals, nurses who smoke should reevaluate their own smoking behavior and its relationship to their health. Nurses and other health care providers who smoke should be aware that the odor of smoke is obvious on their clothes, and it can be offensive or tempting to patients.

Early diagnosis and treatment of respiratory tract infections and exacerbations of COPD help prevent progression of the disease. People with COPD should avoid others who are sick, practice good hand-washing techniques, take medications as prescribed, exercise regularly, and maintain a healthy weight. Influenza and pneumococcal pneumonia vaccines are recommended for patients with COPD.

Families with a history of COPD, as well as AAT deficiency, should be aware of the genetic nature of the disease. These individuals should consult a pulmonologist about regular spirometry screening even though they do not have symptoms. Genetic counseling is appropriate for the patient with AAT deficiency who is planning to have children.

ACUTE INTERVENTION. The patient with COPD requires acute intervention for complications such as exacerbations of COPD, pneumonia, cor pulmonale, and acute respiratory failure. (The nursing care for these conditions is discussed in Chapters 28 and 68.) Once the crisis in these situations has been resolved, assess the degree and severity of the underlying respiratory problem. The information obtained will help in planning the nursing care.

TABLE 29-25 NURSING ASSESSMENT

Chronic Obstructive Pulmonary Disease

Subjective Data
Important Health Information
Past health history: Long-term exposure to chemical pollutants, respiratory irritants, occupational fumes, dust; recurrent respiratory tract infections; previous hospitalizations
Medications: Use of O_2 and duration of O_2 use, bronchodilators, corticosteroids, antibiotics, anticholinergics, OTC drugs, herbs, medications purchased outside United States

Functional Health Patterns
Health perception–health management: Smoking (pack-years, including passive smoking, willingness to stop smoking, and previous attempts); family history of respiratory disease (especially α_1-antitrypsin deficiency)
Nutritional-metabolic: Anorexia, weight loss or gain
Activity-exercise: Increasing dyspnea and/or increase in sputum volume or purulence (to detect exacerbation); fatigue, ability to perform ADLs; swelling of feet; progressive dyspnea, especially on exertion; ability to walk up one flight of stairs without stopping; wheezing; recurrent cough; sputum production (especially in the morning); orthopnea
Elimination: Constipation, gas, bloating
Sleep-rest: Insomnia; sitting up position for sleeping, paroxysmal nocturnal dyspnea
Cognitive-perceptual: Headache, chest or abdominal soreness
Coping–stress tolerance: Anxiety, depression

Objective Data
General
Debilitation, restlessness, assumption of upright position

Integumentary
Cyanosis (bronchitis), pallor or ruddy color, poor skin turgor, thin skin, digital clubbing, easy bruising; peripheral edema (cor pulmonale)

Respiratory
Rapid, shallow breathing; inability to speak; prolonged expiratory phase; pursed-lip breathing; wheezing; rhonchi, crackles, diminished or bronchial breath sounds; ↓ chest excursion and diaphragm movement; use of accessory muscles; hyperresonant or dull chest sounds on percussion

Cardiovascular
Tachycardia, dysrhythmias, jugular venous distention, distant heart tones, right-sided S_3 (cor pulmonale), edema (especially in feet)

Gastrointestinal
Ascites, hepatomegaly (cor pulmonale)

Musculoskeletal
Muscle atrophy, ↑ anteroposterior diameter (barrel chest)

Possible Diagnostic Findings
Abnormal ABGs (compensated respiratory acidosis, ↓ PaO_2 or SaO_2, ↑ $PaCO_2$), polycythemia, pulmonary function tests showing expiratory airflow obstruction (e.g., low FEV_1, low FEV_1/FVC, large RV), chest x-ray showing flattened diaphragm and hyperinflation or infiltrates

ABGs, Arterial blood gases; *FEV₁,* forced expiratory volume in 1 sec; *FVC,* forced vital capacity; *RV,* residual volume.

AMBULATORY AND HOME CARE. By far the most important aspect in the long-term care of the patient with COPD is teaching. (A patient and caregiver teaching guide is presented in Table 29-26.)

Pulmonary Rehabilitation. Pulmonary rehabilitation (PR) is an evidence-based intervention that includes many disciplines working together to individualize treatment of the symptomatic COPD patient. PR is designed to reduce symptoms and improve quality of life. PR is an effective intervention to improve exercise capacity and decrease hospitalizations, anxiety, and depression.[48,49] PR should no longer be viewed as a "last ditch" effort for patients with severe COPD.

PR can be done in an inpatient or outpatient setting or in the home. Components of PR vary, but usually include exercise training, smoking cessation, nutrition counseling, and education. A mandatory component of any PR program is exercise that focuses on the muscles used in ambulation, but upper limb exercises may be included also. Smoking cessation is critical to the patient's success. Some rehabilitation programs do not accept patients who are current smokers and not committed to quitting. Physical therapists or nurses who have experience in pulmonary care are often responsible for the management of pulmonary rehabilitation centers. A large part of your role is to teach patients self-management of their disease.

The minimum length of an effective program is 6 weeks with many insurance plans paying for it, but the longer the program, the more effective the results. Other important topics include health promotion, psychologic counseling, and vocational rehabilitation. One benefit of group PR appears to be the develop-

INFORMATICS IN PRACTICE

Texting for Chronic Obstructive Pulmonary Disease (COPD) Patients

- Sometimes patients with COPD or those requiring O_2 therapy experience difficulty speaking because of shortness of breath.
- Encourage your patient to use typed messages displayed on a monitor to communicate.
- Texting and instant messaging family and friends are good alternatives to having phone conversations.

ment of social relationships and support from peers and health care providers that boost patient's self-confidence, coping, and motivation for self-care.[50]

PR groups may be inaccessible to many because of cost, disability, transportation, or geographic location. One alternative program uses the Internet to deliver daily motivational messages that are linked with individualized walking goals and feedback related to pedometer use.[51] Another program uses telehealth for homebound older adults with COPD with daily objective measures of health (e.g., weight, O_2 saturation). This information is received centrally by a nurse who calls back the patient for further evaluation if parameters are abnormal.[52]

Activity Considerations. Exercise training leads to energy conservation, which is an important component in COPD rehabilitation. The patient with severe COPD typically uses upper thoracic and neck muscles to breathe rather than the diaphragm. Thus the patient has difficulty performing upper-extremity

Patient With Chronic Obstructive Pulmonary Disease

NURSING DIAGNOSIS* **Ineffective breathing pattern** *related to* alveolar hypoventilation, anxiety, chest wall alterations, and hyperventilation *as evidenced by* assumption of three-point position, dyspnea, increased anteroposterior diameter of chest, nasal flaring, orthopnea, prolonged expiration, pursed-lip breathing, use of accessory muscles to breathe

PATIENT GOALS 1. Returns to baseline respiratory function
2. Demonstrates an effective rate, rhythm, and depth of respirations

Outcomes (NOC)	Interventions (NIC) and *Rationales*
Respiratory Status: Ventilation	**Ventilation Assistance**
• Respiratory rate ____	• Monitor respiratory and oxygenation status *to assess need for intervention.*
• Respiratory rhythm ____	• Auscultate breath sounds, noting areas of decreased or absent ventilation and presence of adventitious sounds *to obtain ongoing data on patient's response to therapy.*
• Depth of inspiration ____	• Encourage slow, deep breathing; turning; and coughing *to promote effective breathing techniques and secretion mobilization.*
• Pulmonary function tests ____	• Administer medications (e.g., bronchodilators and inhalers) that promote airway patency and gas exchange.
Measurement Scale	• Position to minimize respiratory efforts (e.g., elevate head of the bed and provide overbed table for patient to lean on) *to save energy for breathing.*
1 = Severe deviation from normal range	• Monitor for respiratory muscle fatigue *to determine a need for ventilatory assistance.*
2 = Substantial deviation from normal range	• Initiate a program of respiratory muscle strength and/or endurance training *to establish effective breathing patterns and techniques.*
3 = Moderate deviation from normal range	
4 = Mild deviation from normal range	
5 = No deviation from normal range	
• Accessory muscle use ____	
• Pursed-lip breathing ____	
• Orthopnea ____	
• Impaired expiration ____	
Measurement Scale	
1 = Severe	
2 = Substantial	
3 = Moderate	
4 = Mild	
5 = None	

NURSING DIAGNOSIS **Ineffective airway clearance** *related to* expiratory airflow obstruction, ineffective cough, decreased airway humidity, and tenacious secretions *as evidenced by* ineffective or absent cough, presence of abnormal breath sounds, or absence of breath sounds

PATIENT GOALS 1. Maintains clear airway by effectively coughing
2. Experiences clear breath sounds

Outcomes (NOC)	Interventions (NIC) and *Rationales*
Respiratory Status: Airway Patency	**Cough Enhancement**
• Adventitious breath sounds ____	• Assist patient to sitting position with head slightly flexed, shoulders relaxed, and knees flexed *to allow for adequate chest expansion.*
• Anxiety ____	• Instruct patient to inhale deeply, bend forward slightly, and perform three or four huffs (against an open glottis) *to prevent airway collapse during exhalation.*†
• Gasping ____	• Instruct patient to inhale deeply several times, exhale slowly, and cough at the end of exhalation *to loosen secretions before coughing.*
• Choking ____	• Instruct the patient to follow coughing with several maximal inhalation breaths *to reoxygenate the lungs.*
Measurement Scale	**Airway Management**
1 = Severe	• Encourage slow, deep breathing; turning; and coughing *to mobilize pulmonary secretions.*
2 = Substantial	• Position patient *to maximize ventilation potential.*
3 = Moderate	• Regulate fluid intake to optimize fluid balance *to liquefy secretions for easier expectoration.*
4 = Mild	• Perform endotracheal or nasotracheal suctioning as appropriate *to clear the airway.*
5 = None	• Administer bronchodilators and use airway clearance devices *to facilitate clearance of retained secretions and increase ease of breathing.*

NURSING DIAGNOSIS **Impaired gas exchange** *related to* alveolar hypoventilation *as evidenced by* headache on awakening, $PaCO_2$ ≥45 mm Hg, PaO_2 <60 mm Hg, or SaO_2 <90% at rest

PATIENT GOALS 1. Returns to baseline respiratory function
2. $PaCO_2$ and PaO_2 return to levels normal for patient

Outcomes (NOC)	Interventions (NIC) and *Rationales*
Respiratory Status: Gas Exchange	**Oxygen Therapy**
• PaO_2 ____	• Administer supplemental O_2 as ordered.
• $PaCO_2$ ____	• Set up O_2 equipment and administer through a heated, humidified system to provide moist O_2.
• Arterial pH ____	• Periodically check O_2 delivery device *to ensure that the prescribed concentration is being delivered.*
• Chest x-ray findings ____	• Monitor the effectiveness of O_2 therapy (e.g., pulse oximetry, ABGs) *to evaluate patient response to therapy.*
Measurement Scale	• Observe for signs of O_2-induced hypoventilation *because this occurs with CO_2 narcosis.*
1 = Severe deviation from normal range	• Instruct patient and family about use of O_2 at home *to promote safe long-term O_2 therapy.*
2 = Substantial deviation from normal range	
3 = Moderate deviation from normal range	
4 = Mild deviation from normal range	
5 = No deviation from normal range	

---

*Nursing diagnoses listed in order of priority.
†Guidelines for effective huff coughing are presented in Table 29-23.

TABLE 29-26 PATIENT & CAREGIVER TEACHING GUIDE

Chronic Obstructive Pulmonary Disease

Include the following information in the teaching plan to assist the patient and caregiver to improve quality of life through teaching and promotion of lifestyle practices that support successful living with chronic obstructive pulmonary disease (COPD).

Teaching Topic	Resources	Teaching Topic	Resources
Overall Guide	*Patient Guide: What You Can Do About a Lung Disease Called COPD* (Global Initiative for Lung Disease). Retrieved from *www.goldcopd.org/uploads/users/files/GOLD_Patient_RevJan10.pdf*. (Also available in other languages.)	**Home Oxygen** • Explanation of rationale for use • Guide for home O₂ use and equipment	*Oxygen Therapy* (National Jewish Health). Retrieved from *www.nationaljewish.org/healthinfo/medications/lung-diseases/treatments/oxygen-therapy*. *Traveling With Oxygen* (American College of Chest Physicians). Retrieved from *www.chestnet.org/accp/patient-guides/traveling-oxygen*.
What Is COPD? • Basic anatomy and physiology of lung • Basic pathophysiology of COPD • Signs and symptoms of COPD, exacerbation, cold, flu, pneumonia • Tests to assess breathing	*COPD Statement: Patient Education Section* (American Thoracic Society [ATS]). Retrieved from *www.thoracic.org*. (Also available in Spanish.) *How Lungs Work* (American Lung Association [ALA]). Available under "Your Lungs" at *www.lung.org/your-lungs*.	**Psychosocial/Emotional Issues** Concerns about interpersonal relationships • Dependency • Intimacy Problems with emotions • Depression, anxiety, panic Treatment decisions • Support and rehabilitation groups End-of-life issues	Open discussion (sharing with patient, significant other, and family). *Living With COPD: Get Social Support* (ALA help line, Better Breathers Club, and printed materials). Retrieved from *www.lung.org/lung-disease/copd/living-with-copd/get-social-support.html*. *Questions About Pulmonary Rehabilitation* (ATS). Retrieved from *patients.thoracic.org/materials/index.php*. (Available in English and Spanish.)
Breathing and Airway Clearance Exercises • Pursed-lip breathing • Airway clearance technique—huff cough	See Table 29-13. See Table 29-23.		
Energy Conservation Techniques • Daily activities (e.g., waking up, bathing, grooming, shopping, traveling)	Consult with physical therapist and occupational therapist. *COPD: Lifestyle Management* (National Jewish Health). Retrieved from *www.nationaljewish.org/healthinfo/conditions/copd-chronic-obstructive-pulmonary-disease/lifestyle-management*.	**COPD Management Plan** • Focus on self-management • Need to report changes • Cause of flare-ups or exacerbation • Recognition of signs and symptoms of respiratory infection, heart failure • Reduce risk factors, especially smoking cessation • Exercise program of walking and arm strengthening • Yearly follow-up	Nurse and patient develop and write up COPD management plan that meets individual needs. *COPD Management Tools* (ALA). Retrieved from *www.lung.org/lung-disease/copd/living-with-copd/copd-management-tools.html*.
Medications Types (include mechanism of action and types of devices) • Methylxanthines • β₂-Adrenergic agonists • Corticosteroids • Anticholinergics • Antibiotics • Other medications Establishing medication schedule	*COPD Statement: Patient Education Section: Medications and Other Treatments OR Patient Information Series: Medicines to Treat COPD* (ATS). Retrieved from *www.thoracic.org*. OR *COPD Medicines* (ALA). Retrieved from *www.lungusa.org*. OR *COPD Medications* (National Jewish Health). Search "COPD medications." Also has link to medication chart to take to provider. Retrieved from *www.nationaljewish.org/healthinfo*.	**Healthy Nutrition** • Strategies to lose weight (if overweight) • Strategies to gain weight (if underweight)	Consultation with dietitian. See Table 29-24. *Nutrition* (ALA). Retrieved from *www.lung.org/lung-disease/copd/living-with-copd/nutrition.html*.
Correct Use of Inhalers, Spacer, and Nebulizer	See Figs. 29-5 to 29-7. See Tables 29-8 to 29-10. See Table 29-15 for links to videos on medication devices.		

activities, particularly those that require raising the arm above the head. Exercise training of the upper extremities may improve muscle function and help to reduce dyspnea.

Frequently the patient has already adapted alternative energy-saving practices for ADLs. Alternative methods of hair care, shaving, showering, and reaching may need to be explored. An occupational therapist may help with ideas in these areas. Assuming a tripod posture (elbows supported on a table, chest in fixed position) and placing a mirror on the table while using

an electric razor or hair dryer conserve much more energy than when the patient stands in front of a mirror to shave or blow-dry hair.

If the patient uses home O₂ therapy, O₂ should be used during activities of hygiene because these are energy consuming. Encourage the patient to make a schedule and plan daily and weekly activities to leave plenty of time for rest periods. The patient should also try to sit as much as possible when performing activities. Another energy-saving tip is to exhale when pushing, pulling, or exerting effort during an activity and inhale during rest.

Regular physical exercise is important for patients with COPD. To ensure long-term adherence, the exercise must be individualized and easy to perform. Walking or other endurance exercises (e.g., cycling) combined with strength training are likely the best interventions to strengthen muscles and improve the patient's endurance. Teach the patient coordinated walking with slow, pursed-lip breathing—breathing in through the nose while taking one step, then breathing out through pursed lips while taking two to four steps.

When patients are home, the adherence to exercise may wane. A simple but effective way to sustain optimal exercise intensity with positive outcomes (i.e., no exacerbations) in home settings is to use a metronome. The level of exercise intensity is established on a treadmill by the appropriate health care provider using a metronome. The patient then uses the clip-on metronome to maintain the rate and intensity of walking (instead of trying to walk a certain amount of time).[48]

At times patients may need rest periods and sit or lean against an object such as a tree or post. The patient may need to ambulate using O_2. Walk with the patient, giving verbal reminders when necessary regarding breathing (inhalation and exhalation) and steps. Walking with the patient helps decrease anxiety and helps maintain a slow pace. It also enables you to observe the patient's actions and physiologic responses to the activity. Many patients with moderate or severe COPD are anxious and fearful of walking or performing exercise. These patients and their caregivers require support while they build the confidence they need to walk or to perform daily exercises.

In many situations PR programs are not an option, and patients are advised to exercise on their own. If possible, arrange a one-time consult with the physical therapist to outline an exercise program for the patient that can be followed at home and that you can reinforce in the outpatient setting. Encourage the patient to walk 15 to 20 minutes a day at least three times a week with gradual increases. Severely disabled patients can begin at a slow pace by walking for 2 to 5 minutes three times a day and slowly building up to 20 minutes a day, if possible.

Some patients benefit from using their β_2-adrenergic agonist approximately 10 minutes before exercise. Parameters that may be monitored in the patient with mild COPD are resting pulse and pulse rate after walking. Pulse rate after walking should not exceed 75% to 80% of the maximum heart rate (maximum heart rate is age in years subtracted from 220). In some patients, exercise is limited by dyspnea and the limitation in breathing, rather than increased heart rate. Thus it is better to use the patient's perceived sense of dyspnea as an indication of exercise tolerance.

Tell the patient that shortness of breath will probably increase during exercise (as it does for a healthy individual) but that the activity is not being overdone if this increased shortness of breath returns to baseline within 5 minutes after cessation of exercise. Instruct the patient to wait 5 minutes after completion of exercise before using the β_2-adrenergic agonist to allow a chance to recover. During this time, slow, pursed-lip breathing should be used. If it takes longer than 5 minutes to return to baseline, the patient most likely has overdone it and should proceed at a slower pace during the next exercise period. The patient may benefit from keeping a diary or log of the exercise program. The diary can help provide a realistic evaluation of the patient's progress. In addition, the diary can help motivate the patient and add to the patient's sense of accomplishment. Stationary cycling can also be used either alone or with walking. Cycles and treadmills are particularly good when weather prevents walking outside.

Fatigue, sleep disturbances, and dyspnea are common complaints of patients with COPD. Of these symptoms, dyspnea appears to be the only one that affects the patient's ability to carry out daily activities. Therefore you and other health team members should focus your interventions on improving dyspnea, which would then improve the patient's functional performance. Nutritional counseling (discussed previously) is integral to a PR program. Teaching is an important component of PR and should include information on self-management and prevention and treatment of exacerbations (see Table 29-26).

Sexuality and Sexual Activity. Modifying but not abstaining from sexual activity can also contribute to a healthy psychologic well-being. Most patients with COPD are older. Assess and reflect on your own attitudes and feelings about sexuality, sexual functioning, and aging before exploring sexual issues with the older COPD patient. First assess the patient's concerns related to sexuality and functioning. Ask open-ended questions to determine if the patient wants to discuss any of these concerns. You could ask, "How has your breathing problem affected how you see yourself as a woman or man?" Another question could be, "How does your shortness of breath affect your desire for intimacy with your partner?" These types of questions give the person an opening to discuss concerns. Much of the sexual performance issues experienced by the patient with COPD are changes related to aging, and if you are aware of these changes, you can teach the patient the "normalcy" of the changes.

Dyspnea, the predominant symptom in COPD, should not be a major problem with success in sexual functioning, except for those patients in severe stages. If the patient can walk up two flights of stairs or walk briskly, he or she likely has sufficient energy for sexual activity. Erectile dysfunction can occur with COPD as with many chronic diseases. Using an inhaled bronchodilator before sexual activity can help ventilation. The patient with COPD may also find these suggestions helpful: (1) plan sexual activity during the part of the day when breathing is best, which is usually late morning or early afternoon (plus older men often achieve an erection more easily in the morning); (2) use slow pursed-lip breathing; (3) refrain from sexual activity after eating or drinking alcohol; (4) choose less stressful positions during intercourse (missionary position for men is the worst); (5) use O_2 if prescribed; and (6) understand that cigarettes can increase male impotence. Often the patient has coexisting cardiac disease and should obtain advice from a health care provider related to appropriate levels of activity. These aspects of sexual activity require open communication between partners regarding their needs and expectations and the changes that may be necessary as the result of a chronic disease (e.g., changes in body image, role reversal).[53,54]

Sleep. Adequate sleep is extremely important to maintain quality of life and productivity. Patients with COPD have an increased prevalence of sleep disorders. The hyperinflation of the lungs and the reduction in ventilation can result in severe drops in O_2 saturation (down to 60% or less) during sleep. This leads to a strain on the heart. In addition, hypercapnia may develop with more frequent awakening. The net result is sleeping poorly and awakening unrefreshed and fatigued.

Current tobacco use, depression, and anxiety are all common in COPD and lead to more trouble sleeping. β_2-Agonists may

ETHICAL/LEGAL DILEMMAS
Advance Directives

Situation

L.H., a 79-year-old man with COPD, is in respiratory failure when he is admitted to the hospital. He is placed on a ventilator and responds occasionally by opening his eyes. His advance directives (ADs) were drawn up 5 years ago, and copies were given to his wife and health care provider at that time. The patient's wife brings the documents to the intensive care unit and tells you that the hospital must stop treating her husband and allow him to die as he requested. However, the patient's oldest son is threatening the hospital with a lawsuit if the staff does not provide full care to his father.

Ethical/Legal Points for Consideration

- A Living Will, one form of AD, permits individuals to state their own preferences and refusals should the individual become terminally ill or be in a situation where there is no hope of recovery, and the person is not able to speak for himself or herself.*
- The Durable Power Attorney for Health Care, another form of AD, permits individuals to identify a proxy to make health care decisions in the event the individual is incapacitated.
- AD laws vary from state to state concerning the need for witnesses and who the proxy is.
- Some families are deeply divided about decisions for their loved ones, and conflicts often arise when money and property are involved.
- Health care providers are obligated to follow the patient's ADs when a patient is no longer able to speak for himself or herself.
- In your scope of nursing practice, you need to (1) be informed about the decision-making laws and regulations in your state, (2) make AD documents available to patients, (3) teach patients and their families about ADs, (4) determine if all involved health care providers are aware of the existence of ADs, (5) assist the patient and the family in communicating with the health care providers when a "no code" order is requested, and (6) assist the conflicted family in obtaining appropriate counseling whenever necessary.

Discussion Questions

1. What should you do next with the information provided by L.H.'s wife?
2. How should you address the needs of each member of this family in L.H.'s plan of care?
3. What resources can you use to facilitate decision making in this situation?

*Advance directives are listed in Table 10-6.

cause restlessness and insomnia. Many patients with COPD have postnasal drip or nasal congestion that may cause coughing and wheezing at night. Nasal saline sprays or rinses before sleep and in the morning may help. If the patient is prescribed O_2 therapy, using it at night will decrease insomnia. If the patient is a restless sleeper, snores, stops breathing while asleep, and has a tendency to fall asleep during the day, the patient may need to be tested for sleep apnea[55] (see Chapter 8).

Psychosocial Considerations. Healthy coping is a challenge for the COPD patient and the family. People with COPD frequently have to deal with many lifestyle changes that may involve decreased ability to care for themselves, decreased energy for social activities, and loss or change in a job.

When a patient with COPD is first diagnosed or has complications that require hospitalization, expect a variety of emotional responses. Emotions frequently encountered include guilt, loneliness from social isolation, denial, and frustration from increased dependence. Guilt may result from the knowledge that the disease was caused largely by cigarette smoking. Many patients struggle with depression and anxiety. It is impor-

tant to convey a sense of understanding and caring to the patient. The patient with COPD may benefit from stress management techniques (e.g., massage, muscle relaxation) and referral to a therapist[16] (see Chapter 7). Support groups at local American Lung Association chapters (such as the Better Breathers Club), hospitals, and clinics can also be helpful.

Patients frequently ask whether moving to a warmer or drier climate will help. In general, such a move is not significantly beneficial. Discourage moves to places with an elevation of 4000 ft or more because of the lower partial pressure of O_2 found in the air at higher elevations. A disadvantage of moving may be that a person leaves a job, friends, and familiar environment, which could be psychologically stressful. Any advantage gained from a different climate may be outweighed by the psychologic effects of the move.

Patients need to know that symptoms can be managed, but COPD cannot be cured. End-of-life issues and advance directives are important topics for discussion in the terminal stages of COPD. However, this may be difficult for the patient and family to consider because of the uncertainty of the disease. (Palliative care and end-of-life care are discussed in Chapter 10.)

EVALUATION

The expected outcomes for the patient with COPD are presented in Nursing Care Plan 29-2.

CYSTIC FIBROSIS

Cystic fibrosis (CF) is an autosomal recessive, multisystem disease characterized by altered transport of sodium and chloride ions in and out of epithelial cells. This defect primarily affects the lungs, gastrointestinal tract (pancreas and biliary tract), and reproductive tract.[56]

CF was first described in 1938 when autopsies of young children revealed multiple cysts in the pancreas, so the disease was called "cystic fibrosis of the pancreas."[57] Once advances in care allowed children to live into later childhood, the lung disease became the more significant problem.

Approximately 30,000 children and adults in the United States have CF. About 10 million (about 1 in every 31) Americans are carriers of the CF gene but do not have the disease. Of the CF patients in the Cystic Fibrosis Patient Registry, more than 48% are 18 years of age or older. The first signs and symptoms typically occur in children, but some patients are not diagnosed until they are adults; some live to over 80 years old. The severity and progression of the disease vary. With early diagnosis and improvements in therapy, the prognosis of patients with CF has significantly improved. The median predicted survival was 16 years in 1970, but has increased to more than 37 years.[58] Nurses who work in adult care settings increasingly manage patients with CF.

Etiology and Pathophysiology
Genetic Link

CF is an autosomal recessive disorder (see Figs. 13-4 and 13-5 and the Genetics in Clinical Practice box). The CF gene is located on chromosome 7 and produces a protein called CF transmembrane regulator (CFTR). The CFTR protein localizes to the epithelial surface of the airways, gastrointestinal tract, and ducts of the liver, pancreas, and sweat glands. CFTR regulates sodium and chloride channels. Mutations in the *CFTR*

GENETICS IN CLINICAL PRACTICE

Cystic Fibrosis (CF)

Genetic Basis
- Autosomal recessive disorder.
- Caused by mutations in CF transmembrane regulator (*CFTR*) gene on chromosome 7.
- Many different mutations of *CFTR* gene have been identified.
- *CFTR* gene provides instructions for making protein that controls the channel that transports sodium and chloride.
- Mutations in the *CFTR* gene disrupt the function of the channels, preventing them from regulating the flow of sodium, chloride, and water across cell membranes.

Incidence
- In the United States 1 in 3000 white births.
- Less common in other ethnic populations (1 in 17,000 African Americans and 1 in 31,000 Asian Americans).
- One in 20-25 whites are carriers of the gene.
- If both parents carry the affected gene, there is a 25% chance each offspring will have the disease (see Figs. 13-4 and 13-5).

Genetic Testing
- Blood-based DNA testing is available for disease and carrier states.
- All 50 states have passed legislation requiring that all newborns be screened for CF.
- Testing is usually done in children if CF is suspected or if parents are possible carriers.
- In parents who are known carriers, amniocentesis or chorionic villus sampling in pregnant women may be useful for prenatal testing.

Clinical Implications
- CF is the most common autosomal recessive disease in whites.
- CF has a wide range of clinical expression of disease.
- CF requires long-term medical management.
- Advances in medical care have improved life expectancy.
- Most people who have a child with CF are not aware of a family history of disease.
- CF screening should be offered to all individuals of reproductive age regardless of family history.

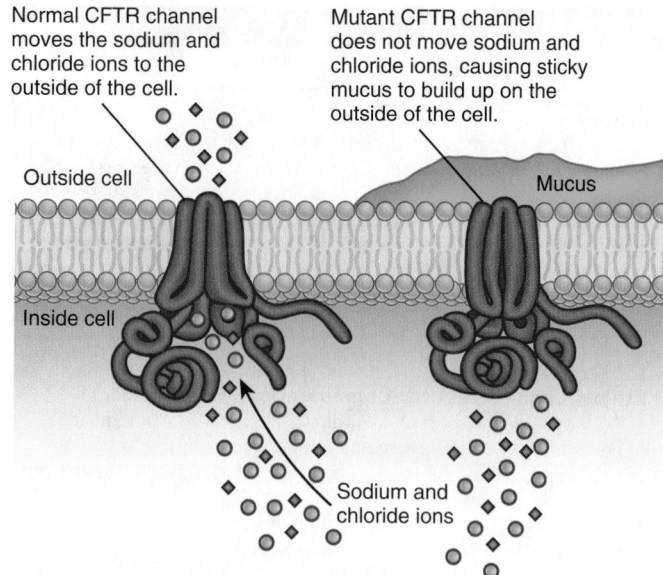

FIG. 29-16 People with cystic fibrosis inherit a defective gene on chromosome 7 called cystic fibrosis transmembrane regulator (*CFTR*). The protein produced by this gene normally helps sodium and chloride move in and out of cells. If the protein does not work correctly, then the movement of sodium and chloride is blocked and an abnormally thick sticky mucus is produced on the outside of the cell.

gene alter this protein in such a way that the channels are blocked. As a result, cells that line the passageways of the lungs, pancreas, intestines, and other organs produce secretions that are low in sodium chloride content (thus low in water content), making mucus abnormally thick and sticky (Fig. 29-16). This mucus fills (plugs up) the glands in these organs and causes the glands to atrophy, ultimately resulting in organ failure. The high concentrations of sodium and chloride in the sweat of the patient with CF result from decreased chloride reabsorption in the sweat duct.[59]

In the respiratory system, both the upper and lower respiratory tracts can be affected. Upper respiratory tract manifestations may include chronic sinusitis and nasal polyposis. The hallmark of respiratory involvement in CF is its effect on the airways. The disease progresses from being a disease of the small airways (*chronic bronchiolitis*) to involvement of the larger airways, and finally causes destruction of lung tissue. The mucus becomes dehydrated and tenacious due to the defect in the chloride secretion and excess sodium absorption. Cilia motility is decreased, thus allowing mucus to adhere to the airways. The bronchioles become obstructed with thick mucus, leading to air trapping and hyperinflation of the lungs.

CF is characterized by chronic airway infection that cannot be eradicated. Organisms commonly cultured from the sputum of a patient with CF are *Staphylococcus aureus, Haemophilus influenzae,* and *Pseudomonas aeruginosa,* and less commonly but more seriously, *Burkholderia cepacia. Pseudomonas* is by far the most common organism. Antibiotic resistance often develops. Pulmonary inflammation may precede the chronic infection and can cause a decrease in respiratory function. Inflammatory mediators (e.g., interleukins, oxidants, proteases released by neutrophils) are increased and contribute to the progression of lung disease.

Lung disorders that initially occur are chronic bronchiolitis and bronchitis. However, after months or years, changes in the bronchial walls lead to bronchiectasis (Fig. 29-17). Over a long period, pulmonary vascular remodeling occurs because of local hypoxia and arteriolar vasoconstriction; pulmonary hypertension and cor pulmonale result in the later phases of the disease. Blebs and large cysts in the lung are also severe manifestations of lung destruction, and pneumothorax may develop. Other pulmonary complications include hemoptysis caused by erosion of enlarged pulmonary arteries. Hemoptysis may range from scant streaking to major bleeding, which can sometimes be fatal.

The sweat glands of CF patients secrete normal volumes of sweat, but sodium chloride cannot be absorbed from sweat as it moves through the sweat duct. Therefore four times the normal amount of sodium and chloride is excreted in sweat. This abnormality usually does not affect the person's general health, but it is the main diagnostic test for CF (explained later in the diagnostic studies section).

Pancreatic insufficiency is caused primarily by mucous plugging of the pancreatic exocrine ducts, which results in atrophy of the gland and progressive fibrotic cyst formation. The pancreas's exocrine function may be completely lost. Because of the exocrine dysfunction, pancreatic enzymes such as lipase, amylase, and the proteases (trypsin, chemotrypsin) are not made in sufficient amounts to allow for absorption of nutrients.

FIG. 29-17 Pathologic changes in bronchiectasis. **A,** Longitudinal section of bronchial wall where chronic infection has caused damage. **B,** Collection of purulent material in dilated bronchioles, leading to persistent infection. **C,** Bronchiectasis in a patient with cystic fibrosis who underwent lung transplantation. Cut surfaces of lung show markedly distended peripheral bronchi filled with mucopurulent secretions.

Malabsorption of fat, protein, and fat-soluble vitamins (A, D, E, and K) occurs. Fat malabsorption results in steatorrhea, and protein malabsorption results in failure to grow and gain weight.

CF-related diabetes mellitus (CFRD) is thought to be related to destruction of islet cells in the pancreas.[58] CFRD is a unique type of diabetes with characteristics of both type 1 and type 2 diabetes. The pancreas in people with CF produces insulin, but too late to fully respond to carbohydrate intake.

Other common disorders that develop in CF include osteopenia and osteoporosis. These disorders are related to malnutrition, malabsorption of vitamin D, insufficient testosterone levels, chronically elevated inflammatory cytokines, and the direct effect of the *CFTR* mutation on the development of bone.

Individuals with CF often have other gastrointestinal problems, including abdominal pain, which may be caused by conditions such as GERD. The liver and gallbladder can be damaged by mucus deposits. The liver enzymes may become chronically elevated, with cirrhosis developing over time. Gallstones, pancreatitis, and portal hypertension can also occur.[56] Distal intes-tinal obstruction syndrome (DIOS) results from intermittent obstruction commonly occurring in the terminal ileum. It is usually caused by thickened, dehydrated stool and mucus. The patient may appear to have a small bowel obstruction. DIOS develops because of chronic malabsorption related to exocrine dysfunction, nonadherence to enzyme supplementation, dehydration, swallowing of mucus, and use of opioids.

Clinical Manifestations

The clinical manifestations of CF vary depending on the severity of the disease. Carriers are not affected by the mutation. The disease severity may vary greatly, both within families and among different families.

The median age of diagnosis of CF is 5 months of age.[58] An initial finding of meconium ileus in the newborn infant prompts the diagnosis in 20% of people with CF. Other signs that suggest a CF diagnosis are acute or persistent respiratory symptoms (wheezing, coughing, frequent pneumonia), failure to thrive or malnutrition, steatorrhea (large, oily, frequent bowel movements), and family history. Without treatment, a large, protuberant abdomen may develop with an emaciated appearance of the extremities. A diagnosis may also be prompted by findings of bronchiectasis.

One of the most common symptoms of CF in the adult is frequent cough. With time, the cough becomes persistent and produces viscous, purulent, often yellow or greenish sputum. Although the most common bacteria in the airways in childhood is *S. aureus*, as the patient ages, the prevalence of *Pseudomonas* organisms increases. Other respiratory problems are recurring lung infections such as bronchiolitis, bronchitis, and pneumonia. As the disease progresses, periods of clinical stability are interrupted by exacerbations characterized by increased cough, weight loss, increased sputum, and decreased pulmonary function. Over time the exacerbations become more frequent, bronchiectasis worsens, and the recovery of lost lung function is less complete, which may ultimately lead to respiratory failure.

If the patient with CF develops DIOS, he or she may have right lower quadrant pain (the area of the ileocecal valve), loss of appetite, nausea, emesis, and often a palpable mass. Insufficient pancreatic enzyme release causes the typical pattern of protein and fat malabsorption with a person being thin with a low body mass index (BMI) and frequent, bulky, foul-smelling stools.

Both males and females have delayed puberty. Nearly all men with CF have reproductive issues because their vas deferens fails to develop in utero, so there is no transport of sperm from storage in the testes to the penile urethra. However, they make sperm normally, and with assisted reproductive technology are capable of fathering a child.

Some women with CF have difficulty conceiving; the cervical mucus is thought to be thickened. During exacerbations, menstrual irregularities and secondary amenorrhea are common. A majority of women with CF are able to become pregnant. Most pregnancies result in viable infants with mothers who are able to breastfeed normally.[60]

Complications

Complications in CF include CFRD, bone disease, sinus disease, and liver disease. Pneumothorax, a relatively uncommon but serious complication, is caused by the formation of bullae and blebs. A small amount of blood in sputum is common in the

CF patient because of chronic lung infection. Massive hemoptysis, which is relatively uncommon, can be life threatening.[58] With advanced lung disease, digital clubbing occurs. Respiratory failure and cor pulmonale caused by pulmonary hypertension are late complications of CF.

Diagnostic Studies

The diagnostic criteria for CF include a combination of clinical presentation, family history, laboratory testing, and genetic testing. The sweat chloride test is considered the gold standard for the diagnosis of CF. However, the diagnosis is not clear-cut in all individuals, especially in adults. The sweat chloride test is performed with the pilocarpine iontophoresis method. Pilocarpine is placed on the skin and carried by a small electric current to stimulate sweat production. This part of the process takes about 5 minutes, and the patient feels a slight tingling or warmth. The sweat is collected on filter paper or gauze and then analyzed for sweat chloride concentrations. The test takes approximately 1 hour. Sweat chloride values above 60 mmol/L are considered positive for the diagnosis of CF. Usually a second sweat chloride test is obtained at the same time (one test in each arm) to confirm the diagnosis.

A genetic test is often used if the results from a sweat chloride test are unclear. A blood sample or cells taken inside the cheek (buccal smear) are sent to a laboratory that specializes in genetic testing. Most laboratories test for only the most common mutations of the CF gene. Because more than 1700 mutations cause CF, screening for all mutations is difficult and is performed in a specialty laboratory.

Collaborative Care

A multidisciplinary team should be involved in the care of a patient with CF. The Cystic Fibrosis Foundation provides funding for and accredits more than 100 CF care centers nationwide. The high quality of specialized care available throughout the care center network has led to the improved length and quality of life for people with CF. These care centers offer the best care, treatments, and support for those with CF (see *www.cff.org/LivingWithCF/CareCenterNetwork/CFFoundation-accreditedCareCenters*). The teams at these care centers include a nurse, physician, respiratory therapist, physical therapist, dietitian, social worker, and often a nurse practitioner.

Management of pulmonary problems in CF aims at relieving airway obstruction and controlling infection. Drainage of thick bronchial mucus is assisted by aerosol and nebulization treatments of medications used to dilate the airways, liquefy mucus, and facilitate clearance. The abnormal viscosity of CF secretions is increased by concentrated deoxyribonucleic acid (DNA) from neutrophils involved in chronic infection. Agents that degrade the DNA in CF sputum (e.g., dornase alfa [Pulmozyme]) increase airflow and reduce the number of acute pulmonary exacerbations. Inhaled hypertonic saline (7%) is effective in clearing mucus and also decreases the frequency of exacerbations. Hypertonic saline is safe, but some patients require concomitant bronchodilators to avoid bronchospasm. Bronchodilators (e.g., β_2-adrenergic agonists) may be used to control bronchospasm, but the long-term benefit is not proven.

Airway clearance techniques are critical, since the normal ciliary motion in CF airways is impaired. CPT (including postural drainage with percussion and vibration) and high-frequency chest wall oscillation loosen mucus. Clearance is achieved by the specialized expiratory techniques aimed at using airflow to remove the loosened secretions. Examples of clearance techniques and devices are PEP devices (e.g., Flutter device [see eFig. 29-2], Acapella [see Fig. 29-15]), breathing exercises (autogenic drainage [see *http://hospitals.unm.edu/cf/autogenic_drainage.shtml*]), pursed-lip breathing (see Table 29-13), and huff coughing (see Table 29-23). Individuals with CF may prefer a certain technique or device that works well for them in a daily routine. No clear evidence exists that any of the airway clearance techniques are superior to the others (see Table 29-18). (Airway clearance techniques are discussed on p. 594.)

More than 95% of patients with CF die of complications from lung infection.[60] Standard treatment of infections includes antibiotics for exacerbations and may include chronic suppressive therapy in conjunction with airway clearance. The use of antibiotics should be carefully guided by sputum culture results. Early intervention with antibiotics is useful, and long courses of antibiotics are the usual treatment. Prolonged high-dose therapy may be necessary because many drugs are abnormally metabolized and rapidly excreted in the patient with CF. There is no evidence to support the chronic use of oral antibiotics in adults with CF.

Most patients have *Pseudomonas* infection, which can be difficult to treat because over time the organism develops resistance to antibiotics. It also has the ability to form a biofilm that must be penetrated to kill the organism. One commonly used antibiotic to treat patients who are chronically infected with *Pseudomonas* organisms is aerosolized tobramycin (TOBI) given every other month, every day, twice a day. This treatment regimen increases lung function and decreases the frequency of exacerbations. Oral agents commonly used for mild exacerbations (i.e., increased cough and sputum) are oral antibiotics such as a semisynthetic penicillin or trimethoprim/sulfamethoxazole (to treat *S. aureus*) or oral quinolones, especially ciprofloxacin (Cipro) (to treat *P. aeruginosa*). The quinolones are used judiciously because of the rapid development of resistant strains. More severe exacerbations require a 2- to 4-week course of IV antimicrobial therapy. Azithromycin, used chronically (longer than 6 months), decreases the frequency of pulmonary exacerbations in CF, especially in those infected with *Pseudomonas*. The effectiveness of this drug is probably related to its antiinflammatory effect.[61]

If home support and resources are adequate, the CF patient and caregiver may choose to continue IV antibiotic therapy at home.[62] The usual treatment is two antibiotics with different mechanisms of action (e.g., cephalosporin and an aminoglycoside). The patient with cor pulmonale or hypoxemia may require home O_2 therapy. (O_2 therapy is discussed on p. 589.) Patients with a large pneumothorax require chest tube drainage, perhaps repeatedly. Sclerosing of the pleural space or partial pleural stripping and pleural abrasion performed surgically may be indicated for recurrent episodes of pneumothorax. With massive hemoptysis, bronchial artery embolization is performed. CF has become a leading indication for lung transplantation.[58] (Lung transplants are discussed in Chapter 28.)

The management of pancreatic insufficiency includes pancreatic enzyme replacement of lipase, protease, and amylase (e.g., pancrelipase [Pancreaze, Creon, Ultresa, Viokase, Zenpep]) administered before each meal and snack. Adequate intake of fat, calories, protein, and vitamins is important. Fat-soluble vitamins (A, D, E, and K) must be supplemented, since they are malabsorbed. Use of caloric supplements improves nutritional status. Added dietary salt is indicated whenever sweating is excessive, such as during hot weather, when fever is present, or from intense physical activity. Hyperglycemia may require insulin treatment.

If the patient develops DIOS with complete bowel obstruction, gastric decompression may be needed. This complication is most often managed medically. If DIOS does not resolve with medical treatment, surgery may be needed to prevent the development of ischemic bowel. Partial and uncomplicated episodes of DIOS are treated with ingestion of a balanced polyethylene glycol (PEG) electrolyte solution (MiraLax, GoLYTELY) used to hydrate bowel contents. In addition, water-soluble contrast enemas may be used.[50] Careful monitoring of bowel habits and patterns is essential for CF patients.

Ivacaftor (Kalydeco) is used to treat patients who have a specific *G551D* mutation in the *CFTR* gene. About 4% of those with CF, or roughly 1200 people, have the *G551D* mutation. Ivacaftor is effective only in patients with CF who have this mutation. It is not effective in patients with CF who have two copies of the *F508* mutation in the *CFTR* gene, which is the most common mutation that results in CF. If a patient's mutation status is not known, a CF mutation test should be done to determine whether the *G551D* mutation is present. Ivacaftor, rather than treating the effects of the basic chloride ion channel defect (e.g., pancreatic insufficiency), targets the function of the gene itself, assisting this mutation to open the chloride channel. This drug proves that it is possible to alter the function of a mutation. Further research is ongoing to develop a drug that targets a more common mutation.[63]

Aerobic exercise is effective in clearing the airways. Important needs to consider when planning an aerobic exercise program for the patient with CF are (1) meeting increased nutritional demands of exercise, (2) observing for dehydration, and (3) drinking large amounts of fluid and replacing salt losses.

There is a higher incidence of depression among individuals with CF than their unaffected peers. CF imposes a significant burden on the individual and family. Issues related to fertility, decreased life expectancy, costs of health care, and career choices may lead to depression.[58]

NURSING MANAGEMENT
CYSTIC FIBROSIS

NURSING ASSESSMENT
Subjective and objective data that should be obtained from the patient with CF are presented in Table 29-27.

NURSING DIAGNOSES
Nursing diagnoses for the patient with CF may include, but are not limited to, the following:
- Ineffective airway clearance *related to* abundant, thick bronchial mucus, weakness, and fatigue
- Ineffective breathing pattern *related to* bronchoconstriction, anxiety, and airway obstruction
- Impaired gas exchange *related to* recurring lung infections
- Imbalanced nutrition: less than body requirements *related to* dietary intolerances, intestinal gas, and altered pancreatic enzyme production
- Ineffective coping *related to* multiple life stressors such as decreased life expectancy, cost of treatment, and limitation on career choices

---

TABLE 29-27 NURSING ASSESSMENT

Cystic Fibrosis

Subjective Data
Important Health Information
Past health history: Recurrent respiratory and sinus infections, persistent cough with excessive sputum production
Medications: Use of and compliance with bronchodilators, antibiotics, herbs

Functional Health Patterns
Health perception–health maintenance: Family history of cystic fibrosis; diagnosis of cystic fibrosis in childhood, genetic testing in offspring
Nutritional-metabolic: Dietary intolerances, voracious appetite, weight loss, heartburn
Elimination: Intestinal gas; large, frequent bowel movements, constipation
Activity-exercise: Fatigue, ↓ exercise tolerance, amount and type of exercise; dyspnea, cough, excessive mucus or sputum production, coughing up blood, airway clearance techniques
Cognitive-perceptual: Abdominal pain
Sexuality-reproductive: Delayed menarche, menstrual irregularities, problems conceiving or fathering a child
Coping–stress tolerance: Anxiety, depression, problems adapting to diagnosis

Objective Data
General
Restlessness; failure to thrive

Integumentary
Cyanosis (circumoral, nail bed), digital clubbing; salty skin

Eyes
Scleral icterus

Respiratory
Sinus difficulties; persistent runny nose; diminished breath sounds, sputum (thick, white or green, tenacious), hemoptysis, ↑ work of breathing, use of accessory muscles of respiration, barrel chest

Cardiovascular
Tachycardia

Gastrointestinal
Protuberant abdomen; abdominal distention; foul, fatty stools

Possible Diagnostic Findings
Abnormal ABGs and pulmonary function tests; abnormal sweat chloride test, chest x-ray, fecal fat analysis

ABGs, Arterial blood gases.

PLANNING
The overall goals are that the patient with CF will have (1) adequate airway clearance, (2) reduced risk factors associated with respiratory infections, (3) adequate nutritional support to maintain appropriate BMI, (4) ability to perform ADLs, (5) recognition and treatment of complications related to CF, and (6) active participation in planning and implementing a therapeutic regimen.

NURSING IMPLEMENTATION
Assist young adults in gaining independence by helping them assume responsibility for their care and for their vocational or school goals. An important issue to discuss is sexuality. Delayed or irregular menstruation is not uncommon. There may be

delayed development of secondary sex characteristics such as breasts in girls. The person with CF may use the illness to avoid certain events or relationships. Other crises and life transitions that must be dealt with in the young adult include building confidence and self-respect on the basis of achievements, persevering with employment goals, developing motivation to achieve, learning to cope with the treatment program, and adjusting to the need for dependence if health fails. Disclosing the CF diagnosis to friends, potential spouses, or employers may pose emotional and financial challenges.

The issue of marrying and having children is difficult. Genetic counseling may be an appropriate suggestion for the couple considering having children. Another concern is the uncertainty surrounding the shortened life span of the parent with CF. In addition, the parent's ability to care for the child must be taken into consideration.

Acute intervention for the patient with CF includes relief of bronchoconstriction, airway obstruction, and airflow limitation. Interventions include aggressive CPT, antibiotics, and O_2 therapy in severe disease. Good nutrition is important. Advances in long-term vascular access (e.g., implanted ports) and inhaled antibiotics have made administration of medication much easier. This has also eased the transition for treatment at home.

The family and the person with CF have a great financial and emotional burden. The cost of drugs, special equipment, and health care is often a financial hardship. Because most CF patients now live to childbearing age, family planning and genetic counseling are important. The burden of living with a chronic disease at a young age can be emotionally overwhelming. Community resources are often available to help the family. In addition, the Cystic Fibrosis Foundation can be of assistance. As the person continues toward and into adulthood, you and other skilled health professionals should be available to help the patient and the family cope with complications resulting from the disease.

BRONCHIECTASIS

Etiology and Pathophysiology

Bronchiectasis is characterized by permanent, abnormal dilation of medium-sized bronchi that is a result of inflammatory changes that destroy elastic and muscular structures supporting the bronchial wall. Infection is the primary reason for the continuing cycle of inflammation, airway damage, and remodeling. Bronchiectasis can follow a single episode of severe pneumonia, with a wide variety of infectious agents initiating the condition. Airways can become colonized with microorganisms (e.g., *Pseudomonas* species), which cause the bronchial walls to weaken, and pockets of infection begin to form (see Fig. 29-17).

When the walls of the bronchial system are injured, the mucociliary mechanism is damaged, allowing bacteria and mucus to accumulate within the pockets. Stasis of thickened mucus occurs due to impaired clearance of mucus by the cilia. This results in a reduced ability to clear mucus from the lungs and decreased expiratory airflow. Thus bronchiectasis is classified as an obstructive lung disease. Large connections (anastomoses) develop between the blood vessels in the lungs, and hemoptysis is often the result.[59]

A variety of pathophysiologic processes can result in bronchiectasis.[64] CF is the main cause of bronchiectasis in children. In adults the main cause is bacterial infections of the lungs

that are either not treated or receive delayed treatment. Other causes of bronchiectasis are obstruction of an airway with mucus plugs or generalized impairment of pulmonary defenses. A number of systemic diseases such as inflammatory bowel disease, rheumatoid arthritis, or immune disorders (e.g., acquired immunodeficiency syndrome [AIDS]) may be associated with bronchiectasis.[25]

Clinical Manifestations

The hallmark of bronchiectasis is persistent cough with consistent production of thick, tenacious, purulent sputum. However, some patients with severe disease and upper lobe involvement may have no sputum production and little cough. Recurrent infections injure blood vessels, and hemoptysis occurs. In severe cases it may be life threatening. The other manifestations of bronchiectasis are pleuritic chest pain, dyspnea, wheezing, clubbing of digits, weight loss, and anemia. On auscultation of the lungs, a variety of adventitious sounds can be heard (e.g., crackles, wheezes, rhonchi).[65,66]

Diagnostic Studies

An individual with a chronic productive cough with copious purulent sputum (which may be blood streaked) should be suspected of having bronchiectasis. Chest x-rays may show some nonspecific abnormalities. A high-resolution CT (HRCT) scan of the chest is the preferred method for diagnosing bronchiectasis.

Sputum may provide additional information regarding the severity of impairment and the presence of active infection. Patients are frequently found to have *H. influenzae, Streptococcus pneumoniae, S. aureus,* or *P. aeruginosa,* with the latter leading to more frequent exacerbations and rapid decline in lung function. PFTs usually show an obstructive pattern, including a decrease in FEV_1 and FEV_1/FVC.[65,66]

Collaborative Care

Bronchiectasis is difficult to treat. Therapy is aimed at treating acute flare-ups and preventing a decline in lung function. Antibiotics are the mainstay of treatment and are often given empirically, but attempts are made to culture the sputum. Long-term suppressive therapy with antibiotics is reserved for those patients who have symptoms that recur a few days after stopping antibiotics. Antibiotics may be given orally, IV, or inhaled. Inhaled tobramycin is effective in treating patients with *P. aeruginosa.*

Concurrent bronchodilator therapy with LABAs, SABAs, or anticholinergics is given to prevent bronchospasm and stimulate mucociliary clearance. Hyperosmolar agents (e.g., hypertonic saline) may be given via a nebulizer to liquefy secretions. In addition, oral and inhaled corticosteroids may be used.

Maintaining good hydration is important to liquefy secretions. CPT and other airway clearance techniques are important to facilitate expectoration of sputum. Teach the patient to reduce exposure to excessive air pollutants and irritants, avoid cigarette smoking, and obtain pneumococcal and influenza vaccinations.

Surgical resection of parts of the lungs, which was common in the past, has largely been replaced by more effective supportive and antibiotic therapy. For selected patients who are disabled in spite of maximal therapy, lung transplantation is an option. Massive hemoptysis may require surgical resection or embolization of the bronchial artery.[66]

NURSING MANAGEMENT
BRONCHIECTASIS

Early detection and treatment of lower respiratory tract infections helps prevent complications such as bronchiectasis. Any obstructing lesion or foreign body should be removed promptly.

An important nursing goal is to promote drainage and removal of mucus. Various airway clearance techniques can be effectively used to facilitate secretion removal. CPT with postural drainage is widely used.

Administration of the prescribed medications is important. The patient needs to understand the importance of taking the prescribed regimen of drugs to obtain maximum effectiveness. Rest is important to prevent overexertion.

If hemoptysis occurs, patients should be given explicit instructions on when they should contact the health care provider. Some patients may periodically expectorate a "spot" of blood that is usual for them. In the acute care setting, if the patient has hemoptysis, contact the health care provider immediately, elevate the head of the bed, and place the patient in a side-lying position with the suspected bleeding side down.

Good nutrition is important and may be difficult to maintain because the patient is often anorexic. Oral hygiene to cleanse the mouth and remove dried sputum crusts may improve the patient's appetite. Offer foods that are appealing, since they may increase the patient's desire to eat.

Adequate hydration to help liquefy secretions and thus make it easier to remove them is extremely important. Unless there are contraindications, instruct the patient to drink at least 3 L of fluid daily. To accomplish this, advise the patient to increase fluid consumption by increasing intake by one glass per day until the goal is reached. Generally, the patient should be counseled to use low-sodium fluids to avoid systemic fluid retention.

Direct hydration of the respiratory system may also prove beneficial in the expectoration of secretions. Often nebulized hypertonic saline may be ordered for a more aggressive effect. At home, a steamy shower can prove effective. Expensive equipment that requires frequent cleaning is usually unnecessary. Teach the patient and caregiver to recognize significant clinical manifestations to report to the health care provider. These manifestations include increased sputum production, bloody sputum, increasing dyspnea, fever, chills, and chest pain.

CASE STUDY

Chronic Obstructive Pulmonary Disease

iStockphoto/Thinkstock

Patient Profile

H.M. is a 68-year-old white, married, female, retired traffic police officer. She has been in the hospital for 3 days with a COPD exacerbation and will be discharged tomorrow.

Subjective Data

- Before admission had 7 days of exceptional shortness of breath and increased volume of sputum, which turned greenish
- Had increased Ventolin HFA use at home to five or six times a day for dyspnea
- Had jitters and racing heart
- Had three or four bouts of bronchitis in the past year that she treated at home
- Thirty pack-year history of smoking; smokes half a pack per day now to "clear out lungs" in the morning
- Eats a regular diet but "gets full fast"
- Cannot climb one flight of stairs without stopping; walks down the flat driveway 10 yards without difficulty
- Awakens two or three times per night coughing and short of breath

Objective Data
Physical Examination
- Weight 129 lb, height 5 ft 8 in, BMI 20 kg/m²
- BP 136/76 mm Hg, pulse 86, respiratory rate 28
- Increased anteroposterior diameter of chest (barrel shaped)
- Slight use of accessory (neck) muscles with breathing
- Distant breath sounds with occasional rhonchi
- No peripheral edema

Diagnostic Studies
- Last PFT: decreased FEV_1 (48%) and FEV_1/FVC (62%)
- ABGs on admission: pH 7.34, $PaCO_2$ 49 mm Hg, HCO_3^- 27 mEq/L, PaO_2 70 mm Hg
- WBC: 14,000/µL on admission
- Chest x-ray: hyperinflation, flat diaphragm, no sign of pneumonia

Collaborative Care
- GOLD 3 (severe) COPD with acute exacerbation
- O_2 2 L via nasal catheter while in hospital
- Prednisone 30 mg daily PO for 3 days, 20 mg for 3 days, 10 mg for 10 days
- Azithromycin 250 mg PO: take two tablets day 1, then take one tablet days 2 through 4
- Ipratropium HFA MDI 2 puffs four times a day
- At discharge: Advair Diskus 250/50 one inhalation q12hr

Discussion Questions
1. What classic manifestations indicate the patient had a COPD exacerbation?
2. What are some likely causes of her COPD?
3. What symptoms indicate the overuse of inhalers, and which drug would cause the symptoms described?
4. What is the only way H.M. can halt the progression of her lung disease?
5. Why would H.M. "feel full fast" when eating? What could you do to minimize this issue?
6. Interpret the ABGs. What pattern do you see?
7. ***Priority Decision:*** What are nursing priorities for discharge planning and teaching?
8. ***Priority Decision:*** Based on the assessment data presented, what are the priority nursing diagnoses? Are there any collaborative problems?
9. ***Evidence-Based Practice:*** H.M.'s son has been trying to convince his mother to quit smoking for many years without success. He asks you to tell his mother the results of her PFTs to convince her it is time to quit. Will this approach work?

BRIDGE TO NCLEX EXAMINATION

The number of the question corresponds to the same-numbered outcome at the beginning of the chapter.

1. A patient is concerned that he may have asthma. Of the symptoms that he relates to the nurse, which ones suggest asthma or risk factors for asthma (select all that apply)?
   a. Allergic rhinitis
   b. Prolonged inhalation
   c. History of skin allergies
   d. Cough, especially at night
   e. Gastric reflux or heartburn

2. In evaluating an asthmatic patient's knowledge of self-care, the nurse recognizes that additional instruction is needed when the patient says,
   a. "I use my corticosteroid inhaler when I feel short of breath."
   b. "I get a flu shot every year and see my health care provider if I have an upper respiratory tract infection."
   c. "I use my inhaler before I visit my aunt who has a cat, but I only visit for a few minutes because of my allergies."
   d. "I walk 30 minutes every day but sometimes I have to use my bronchodilator inhaler before walking to prevent me from getting short of breath."

3. A plan of care for the patient with COPD could include (select all that apply)
   a. exercise such as walking.
   b. high flow rate of O_2 administration.
   c. low-dose chronic oral corticosteroid therapy.
   d. use of peak flow meter to monitor the progression of COPD.
   e. breathing exercises such as pursed-lip breathing that focus on exhalation.

4. The effects of cigarette smoking on the respiratory system include
   a. hypertrophy of capillaries causing hemoptysis.
   b. hyperplasia of goblet cells and increased production of mucus.
   c. increased proliferation of cilia and decreased clearance of mucus.
   d. proliferation of alveolar macrophages to decrease the risk for infection.

5. The major advantage of a Venturi mask is that it can
   a. deliver up to 80% O_2.
   b. provide continuous 100% humidity.
   c. deliver a precise concentration of O_2.
   d. be used while a patient eats and sleeps.

6. Which guideline would be a part of teaching patients how to use a metered-dose inhaler (MDI)?
   a. After activating the MDI, breathe in as quickly as you can.
   b. Estimate the amount of remaining medicine in the MDI by floating the canister in water.
   c. Disassemble the plastic canister from the inhaler and rinse both pieces under running water every week.
   d. To determine how long the canister will last, divide the total number of puffs in the canister by the puffs needed per day.

7. Which treatments in CF would the nurse expect to implement in the management plan of patients with CF (select all that apply)?
   a. Sperm banking
   b. IV corticosteroids on a chronic basis
   c. Airway clearance techniques (e.g., Acapella)
   d. GoLYTELY given PRN for severe constipation
   e. Inhaled tobramycin to combat *Pseudomonas* infection

8. A patient who has bronchiectasis asks the nurse, "What conditions would warrant a call to the clinic?"
   a. Blood clots in the sputum
   b. Sticky sputum on a hot day
   c. Increased shortness of breath after eating a large meal
   d. Production of large amounts of sputum on a daily basis

1. a, c, d; 2. a; 3. a, e; 4. b; 5. c; 6. d; 7. a, c, d, e; 8. a

ⓔvolve

For rationales to these answers and even more NCLEX review questions, visit *http://evolve.elsevier.com/Lewis/medsurg*.

REFERENCES

1. American Lung Association: Trends in asthma morbidity and mortality, Epidemiology and Statistics Unit, Research and Health Education Division, Sept. 2012. Retrieved from *www.lungusa.org*.

2. American Lung Association: Trends in COPD (chronic bronchitis and emphysema): morbidity and mortality, Epidemiology and Statistics Unit, Research and Health Education Division, March 2013. Retrieved from *www.lungusa.org*.

*3. National Heart, Lung, and Blood Institute and National Asthma Education and Prevention Program: *Expert Panel Report 3: guidelines for the diagnosis and management of asthma*, NIH pub no 08-4051, Bethesda, Md, 2007, National Institutes of Health. Retrieved from *www.nhlbi.nih.gov/guidelines*.

*4. Global Initiative for Asthma: Global strategy for asthma management and prevention, 2012. Retrieved from *www.ginasthma.org*.

5. American Academy of Allergy, Asthma, and Immunology: Tips to remember: occupational asthma. Retrieved from *www.aaaai.org/patients/publicedmat/tips/occupationalasthma.stm*.

*6. Barnes P: Asthma. In Longo D, Fauci A, Kasper A, et al, editors: *Harrison's principles of internal medicine*, ed 18, New York, 2012, McGraw-Hill.

*7. Fanta C, Fletcher S: Diagnosis of asthma in adolescents and adults, 2011. Retrieved from *www.uptodate.com*.

*8. Sandrini A, Taylor D, Thomas P, et al: Fractional exhaled nitric oxide in asthma: an update, *Respirology* 13:57, 2010.

*9. Cox G: Bronchial thermoplasty for severe asthma, *Curr Opin Pulm Med* 17:34, 2011.

*10. Lareau SC, Hodder R: Teaching inhaler use in chronic obstructive pulmonary disease patients, *J Am Acad Nurs Pract* 24:113, 2012.

11. US Food and Drug Administration: Epinephrine cfc metered-dose inhalers: questions and answers. Retrieved from *www.fda.gov/Drugs/DrugSafety/InformationbyDrugClass/ucm080427.htm*.

*12. Zayas L, Wisniewski A, Cadzow R, et al: Knowledge and use of ethnomedical treatments for asthma among Puerto Ricans in

*Evidence-based information for clinical practice.

an urban community, *Ann Fam Med* 9: 2011. Retrieved from *www.annfammed.org*.

*13. Gøtzsche PC, Johansen HK: House dust mite control measures for asthma, *Cochrane Database Syst Rev* 3:CD001187, 2008.

*14. Moerman D: Meaningful placebos—controlling the uncontrollable, *N Engl J Med* 365:171, 2012.

*15. Qaseem A, Wilt T, Weinberger S, et al: Diagnosis and management of stable chronic obstructive pulmonary disease: a clinical practice guideline update from the American College of Physicians, American College of Chest Physicians, American Thoracic Society, and European Respiratory Society, *Ann Intern Med* 155:179, 2011.

*16. Global Initiative for Chronic Obstructive Lung Disease: Global strategy for the diagnosis, management, and prevention of chronic obstructive pulmonary disease (updated 2013). Retrieved from *www.goldcopd.org*.

17. Murphy S, Xu J, Kochanek M: Deaths: preliminary data for 2010, *Natl Vital Stat Rep* 60(4), 2012. Retrieved from *www.cdc.gov/nchs/data/nvsr/nvsr60/nvsr60_04.pdf*.

18. National Heart, Lung, and Blood Institute: COPD: are you at risk? Retrieved from *www.nhlbi.nih.gov/health/public/lung/copd/campaign-materials/html/copd-atrisk.htm*.

19. National Institute on Drug Abuse: Info facts: cigarettes and other tobacco products. Retrieved from *www.drugabuse.gov/publications/infofacts/cigarettes-other-tobacco-products*.

20. Health 24: How many smokers develop COPD? Retrieved from: *www.health24.com/medical/Condition_centres/777-792-805-1535,28674.asp*.

*21. Corbridge S, Wilken L, Kapella M, et al: An evidence-based approach to COPD, *Am J Nurs* 112:46, 2012.

22. Alpha-1 Foundation: Healthcare providers: what is alpha-1? Retrieved from *www.alphaone.org*.

*23. Stoller J: Clinical manifestations, diagnosis, and natural history of alpha-1 antitrypsin deficiency, 2011, *UpToDate*. Retrieved from *www.uptodate.com*.

24. Brashers V: Structure and function of the pulmonary system. In Huether S, McCance K, editors: *Understanding pathophysiology*, ed 5, St Louis, 2012, Mosby.

25. Brashers V: Alterations of pulmonary function. In McCance K, Huether S, Brashers V, et al, editors: *Pathophysiology: the biologic basis for disease in adults and children*, ed 6, St Louis, 2010, Mosby.

*26. Nussbaumer-Ochsner Y, Rabe K: Systemic manifestations and comorbidities of COPD, *Chest* 139:165, 2011.

27. Mann DL, Chakinala M: Heart failure and cor pulmonale. In Longo C, Fauci A, Kasper D, et al, editors: *Harrison's principles of internal medicine*, ed 18, New York, 2012, McGraw-Hill.

*28. Stoller J, Panos R, Krachman S, et al: Oxygen therapy for patients with COPD: current evidence and the long-term oxygen treatment trial, *Chest* 138:179, 2010.

*29. Decramer M, Janssens W, Miravitlles M: Chronic obstructive pulmonary disease, *Lancet* 379(9823:7-13):1341-1351, 2012. Retrieved from *www.sciencedirect.com/science/article/pii/S0140673611609689*.

*30. Anthonisen N, Manfreda F, Warren C, et al: Antibiotic therapy in exacerbations of chronic obstructive pulmonary disease, *Ann Intern Med* 106:196, 1987. (Classic)

*31. Rutten F, Zuithoff N, Hak E, et al: β-Blockers may reduce mortality and risk of exacerbations in patients with chronic obstructive pulmonary disease, *Arch Intern Med* 170:880, 2010.

32. GlaxoSmithKline: CAT: COPD assessment test: healthcare professional user guide. Retrieved from *www.catestonline.org/images/UserGuides/CATHCPUser%20guideEn.pdf*.

33. Centers for Disease Control and Prevention: Recommended adult immunization schedule—quickguide 2012, *MMWR* 61(4), 2012. Retrieved from *www.cdc.gov/vaccines/recs/schedules/downloads/adult/mmwr-adult-schedule.pdf*.

*34. Bartlett J, Sethi S: Management of infection in acute exacerbation of COPD, 2012, *UpToDate*. Retrieved from *www.uptodate.com*.

35. US Food and Drug Administration: FDA approves new drug to treat chronic obstructive pulmonary disease (news release), 2011. Retrieved from *www.fda.gov/NewsEvents/newsroom/PressAnnouncements/ucm244989.htm*.

36. Boehringer Ingelheim Pharmaceuticals: FDA approves Combivent Respimat (ipratropium bromide and albuterol) inhalation spray for the treatment of patients with chronic obstructive pulmonary disease. Retrieved from *www.prnewswire.com/news-releases/fda-approves-combivent-respimat-ipratropium-bromide-and-albuterol-inhalation-spray-for-the-treatment-of-patients-with-chronic-obstructive-pulmonary-disease-131368648.html*.

37. Vapotherm: Clinical resources. Retrieved from *www.vtherm.com/forclinicians*.

*38. Facchiano L, Snyder C, Nuñez D: A literature review on breathing retraining as a self-management strategy operationalized through Rosswurm and Larrabee's evidence based practice model, *J Am Acad Nurs Pract* 23:421, 2011.

39. Canadian Lung Association: COPD breathing techniques. Retrieved from *www.lung.ca/diseases-maladies/copd-mpoc/breathing-respiration/index_e.php*.

*40. Celli B, Stoller J: Pulmonary rehabilitation in COPD, 2012, *UpToDate*. Retrieved from *www.uptodate.com*.

*41. Main E, Prasad A, van der Schans C: Conventional chest physiotherapy compared to other airway clearance techniques for cystic fibrosis, *Cochrane Database Syst Rev* 2:CD002011, 2009.

*42. Osadnik CR, McDonald CF, Jones AP, et al: Airway clearance techniques for chronic obstructive pulmonary disease, *Cochrane Database Syst Rev* 2:CD008328, 2012.

*43. Bellini L: Nutritional support in advanced lung disease, 2012, *UpToDate*. Retrieved from *www.uptodate.com*.

44. Grodner M, Roth S, Walkingshaw B: *Nutritional foundations and clinical applications: a nursing approach*, ed 5, St Louis, 2012, Mosby.

*45. Burtin C, Decramer M, Gosselink R, et al: Rehabilitation and acute exacerbations, *Eur Respir J* 38:702, 2011.

*46. Payne C, Wiffen PJ, Martin S: Interventions for fatigue and weight loss in adults with advanced progressive illness, *Cochrane Database Syst Rev* 2:CD008427, 2012.

*47. Shah P, Slebos D, Cardoso P, et al: Design of the exhale airway stents for emphysema (EASE) trial: an endoscopic procedure for reducing hyperinflation, *BMC Pulm Med* 11:1, 2011.

*48. Pomidori L, Contoli M, Mandolesi G, et al: A simple method for home exercise training in patients with chronic obstructive pulmonary disease: 1 year study, *J Cardiopulm Rehabil Prev* 32:53, 2012.

*49. Harrison S, Greening N, Williams J, et al: Have we underestimated the efficacy of pulmonary rehabilitation in improving mood? *Respir Med* 106:838, 2012.

*50. Halding A, Wahl A, Heggdal K: "Belonging": patients' experiences of social relationships during pulmonary rehabilitation, *Disabil Rehabil* 32:1272, 2010.

*51. Moy M, Janney A, Nguyen H, et al: Use of pedometer and internet-mediated walking program in patients with chronic obstructive pulmonary disease, *J Rehabil Res Devel* 47:485, 2010.

*52. Gellis Z, Kenaley B, McGinty J, et al: Outcomes of a telehealth intervention for homebound older adults with heart or chronic respiratory failure: a randomized controlled trial, *Gerontologist* 52:541, 2012.

53. Leader D: Sex and COPD, 2010. Retrieved from *copd.about.com/od/livingwithcopd/a/sexandcopd.htm.*

54. Kam K: COPD and sex: nine tips for better sex and intimacy when you have COPD, 2010. Retrieved from *www.webmd.com/lung/copd/features/copd-sex.*

*55. Budhiraja R, Parthasarathy S, Budhiraja P, et al: Insomnia in patients with COPD, *Sleep* 35:369, 2012.

56. Gott K, Froh D: Alterations of pulmonary function in children. In McCance K, Huether S, Brashers V, et al, editors: *Pathophysiology: the biologic basis for disease in adults and children,* ed 6, St Louis, 2010, Mosby.

*57. Andersen D: Cystic fibrosis of the pancreas and its relation to celiac disease, *Am J Dis Child* 56:344, 1938. (Classic)

58. Cystic Fibrosis Foundation Patient Registry: *2011 annual data report,* Bethesda, Md, 2012, Cystic Fibrosis Foundation. Retrieved from *www.cff.org.*

59. Gott K, Brashers V: Alterations of pulmonary function in children. In Huether S, McCance K, editors: *Understanding pathophysiology.* ed 5, St Louis, 2012, Mosby.

60. Boucher R: Cystic fibrosis. In Longo D, Fauci A, Kasper D, et al, editors: *Harrison's principles of internal medicine,* ed 18, New York, 2012, McGraw-Hill.

*61. Sanders D, Farrell P: Transformative mutation specific pharmacotherapy for cystic fibrosis, *Br Med J* 344:e79, 2012.

*62. Yousef AA, Jaffe A: The role of azithromycin in patients with cystic fibrosis, *Paediatr Respir Rev* 11:108, 2010.

63. Ramsey B, Davies J, McElvaney NG, et al: A CFTR potentiator in patients with cystic fibrosis and the *G551D* mutation, *N Engl J Med* 365:1663, 2011.

64. Barker A: Clinical manifestations and diagnosis of bronchiectasis in adults, 2011, *UpToDate.* Retrieved from *www.uptodate.com.*

*65. Chesnutt M, Prendergast T: Pulmonary disorders. In McPhee S, Papadakis M, Rabow M, editors: *Current medical diagnosis and treatment,* ed 51, New York, 2012, McGraw-Hill.

66. Baron R, Bartlett J: Bronchiectasis and lung abscess. In Longo D, Fauci A, Kasper D, et al, editors: *Harrison's principles of internal medicine,* ed 18, New York, 2012, McGraw-Hill.

RESOURCES

American Lung Association
   www.lung.org
Cystic Fibrosis Foundation
   www.cff.org
Global Initiative for Asthma (GINA)
   www.ginasthma.com
Global Initiative for Chronic Obstructive Lung Disease (GOLD)
   www.goldcopd.com

Managing Multiple Patients

Introduction
You are assigned to care for the following four patients on a medical-surgical unit. You are sharing one unlicensed assistive personnel (UAP) assigned with another RN.

Patients

F.T. is a 70-year-old man admitted yesterday with left-lower lobe pneumonia. He is receiving oxygen at 2 L/min via nasal cannula and IV antibiotics. His last pulse oximetry reading was 92%.

Kevin Peterson/
Photodisc/Thinkstock

M.R. is a 60-year-old man who is 4 days postoperative following a total laryngectomy with tracheostomy for treatment of laryngeal cancer. He is receiving intermittent tube feeding via a percutaneous gastrostomy (PEG) tube and last received pain medication 4 hours ago.

iStockphoto/Thinkstock

J.H. is a 52-year-old man admitted with right lower lobe pneumonia. A bronchoscopy with biopsy done on admission revealed small cell lung carcinoma. He is intermittently confused and anxious with rapid, shallow respirations. He is currently considering his treatment options.

iStockphoto/Thinkstock

H.M. is a 68-year-old white woman admitted 3 days ago with a COPD exacerbation who is anticipating discharge later today. She is on oral prednisone and had been given a new inhaler to use. She will also be started on home oxygen.

iStockphoto/Thinkstock

Management Discussion Questions
1. **Priority Decision:** After receiving report, which patient should you see first? Provide a rationale for your decision.
2. **Delegation Decision:** Which morning tasks can you delegate to the UAP *(select all that apply)*?
   a. Take a pulse oximetry reading on F.T.
   b. Assess M.R.'s pain level and show him how to administer his tube feeding.
   c. Assist H.M. with AM care and gather belongings in anticipation of discharge.
   d. Teach F.T. how to use the incentive spirometer and titrate oxygen to obtain pulse oximetry >95%.
   e. Provide coffee and emotional support for J.H.'s family as they await a family meeting with the physician.

3. **Priority and Delegation Decision:** While you are assessing J.H., the UAP tells you that H.M. is complaining of chest pain and worsening shortness of breath. M.R. is also requesting pain medication. What should you do first?
   a. Ask the UAP to get H.M.'s vital signs while you give M.R. pain medication.
   b. Ask the UAP to increase H.M.'s oxygen to 4L/minute while you assess M.R.'s pain.
   c. Ask the UAP to obtain a stat 12-lead ECG on H.M. while you perform a focused assessment.
   d. Ask the UAP to have another RN give M.R. his pain medication while you go directly to H.M.'s room.

Case Study Progression
After assessing H.M., you notify her health care provider. A stat 12-lead ECG is obtained and a blood sample is drawn to check cardiac enzymes. H.M.'s chest pain is not relieved by sublingual nitroglycerin. You then administer 4 mg IV morphine. H.M. states that her pain is "a little better" but continues to complain of dyspnea. The 12-lead ECG and cardiac enzyme results are all within normal limits.

4. Because of H.M.'s reduced mobility, you recognize that she is at risk for pulmonary emboli and anticipate the health care provider will order which tests to determine the cause of her current symptoms?
   a. BNP and echocardiogram
   b. D-dimer and spiral CT scan
   c. CBC and abdominal flat-plate
   d. Serum electrolytes and renal ultrasound
5. While the charge nurse accompanies H.M. to radiology, you turn your attention back to your remaining three patients. Prior to administering M.R.'s 8 AM tube feeding, you aspirate 300 mL of gastric contents from his PEG tube. Which action should you take next?
   a. Discard the aspirated contents and administer the tube feeding as ordered.
   b. Replace the aspirated contents and administer half of ordered tube feeding volume.
   c. Discard the aspirated contents and withhold the next two scheduled tube feedings.
   d. Replace the aspirated contents and notify the health care provider prior to administering any further tube feedings.
6. When preparing F.T.'s AM medications, you note that he is scheduled to receive the following antibiotics at 8 AM: levofloxacin (Levaquin) 750 mg in 150 mL normal saline over 90 minutes (give once every 24 hours) and cefazolin (Kefzol) 1 g in 100 mL normal saline over 30 minutes (give q8hr). He has only one IV site. Which action is most appropriate?
   a. Obtain a second peripheral IV site.
   b. Call the health care provider to change the administration times.
   c. Check with pharmacy to see if they can be mixed together in the same IV bag.
   d. Administer the cefazolin first because it takes the least amount of time to infuse.
7. **Management Decision:** J.H.'s son calls you on the telephone to inquire about his father's current condition and long-term prognosis. Which initial response would be most appropriate?
   a. Ask the person calling what the code word is to identify themselves as family.
   b. Tell the caller that you are not allowed to discuss any information over the telephone.
   c. Ask J.H. what the physician has explained to him in order to clarify his current understanding of the situation.
   d. Empathize with J.H.'s son's need to know his father's prognosis while acknowledging that no one really knows.

SECTION 6

Problems of Oxygenation: Transport

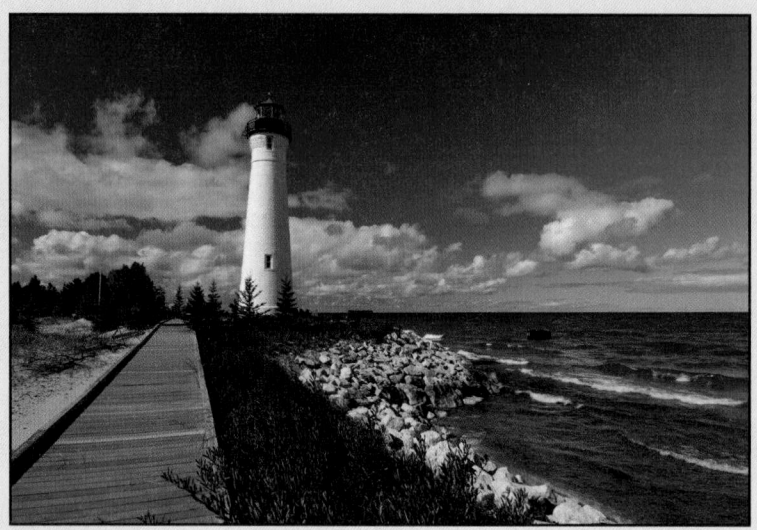

iStockphoto

*There are only two mistakes one can make along the road to truth;
not going all the way, and not starting.*
Buddha

*All the soarings of my mind begin
in my blood.*
Rainer Maria Rilke

Nursing Assessment
Hematologic System

Sandra Irene Rome

℮volve WEBSITE

http://evolve.elsevier.com/Lewis/medsurg

- NCLEX Review Questions
- Key Points
- Pre-Test
- Answer Guidelines for Case Study in this chapter
- Rationales for Bridge to NCLEX Examination Questions
- Concept Map Creator

- Glossary
- Videos
  - Physical Examination: Abdominal Reflexes, Abdominal Muscles, and Inguinal Area
  - Physical Examination: Anterior Chest
  - Physical Examination: Neck
  - Physical Examination: Precordium and Jugular Veins

- Physical Examination: Upper Extremities
- Content Updates

eFigure
- eFig. 30-1: Lymphatic drainage

eTable
- eTable 30-1: Drugs Affecting Hematologic Function

LEARNING OUTCOMES

1. Describe the structures and functions of the hematologic system.
2. Differentiate among the different types of blood cells and their functions.
3. Explain the process of hemostasis.
4. Link the age-related changes in the hematologic system to differences in findings of hematologic studies.
5. Select the significant subjective and objective assessment data related to the hematologic system that should be obtained from a patient.
6. Describe the components of a physical assessment of the hematologic system.
7. Differentiate normal from common abnormal findings of a physical assessment of the hematologic system.
8. Describe the purpose, significance of results, and nursing responsibilities related to diagnostic studies of the hematologic system.

KEY TERMS

ecchymoses, p. 625
erythropoiesis, p. 615
fibrinolysis, p. 618

hematopoiesis, p. 613
hemolysis, p. 615
leukopenia, p. 626

neutropenia, p. 626
pancytopenia, p. 625
petechiae, p. 625

reticulocyte, p. 615
thrombocytopenia, p. 626
thrombocytosis, p. 626

Hematology is the study of blood and blood-forming tissues. This includes bone marrow, blood, spleen, and lymph system. A basic knowledge of hematology is useful in clinical settings to evaluate the patient's ability to transport oxygen and carbon dioxide, maintain intravascular volume, coagulate blood, and combat infections. Assessment of the hematologic system is based on the patient's health history, physical examination, and results of diagnostic studies.

STRUCTURES AND FUNCTIONS OF HEMATOLOGIC SYSTEM

Bone Marrow

Blood cell production (hematopoiesis) occurs within the bone marrow. *Bone marrow* is the soft material that fills the central core of bones. Although there are two types of bone marrow (yellow [adipose] and red [hematopoietic]), it is the red marrow that actively produces blood cells. In the adult the red marrow is found primarily in the flat and irregular bones, such as the ends of long bones, pelvic bones, vertebrae, sacrum, sternum, ribs, flat cranial bones, and scapulae.

All three types of blood cells (red blood cells [RBCs], white blood cells [WBCs], and platelets) develop from a common hematopoietic stem cell within the bone marrow. The hematopoietic *stem cell* is best described as an immature blood cell that is able to self-renew and to differentiate into hematopoietic progenitor cells. As the cells mature and differentiate, several different types of blood cells are formed (Fig. 30-1). The marrow responds to increased demands for various types of blood cells by increasing production via a negative feedback

Reviewed by Katrina Allen, RN, MSN, CCRN, Nursing Instructor, Faulkner State Community College, Division of Nursing, Fairhope and Bay Minette, Alabama; and Mimi Haskins, RN, MS, CMSRN, Nursing Staff Development Instructor, Roswell Park Cancer Institute, Buffalo, New York.

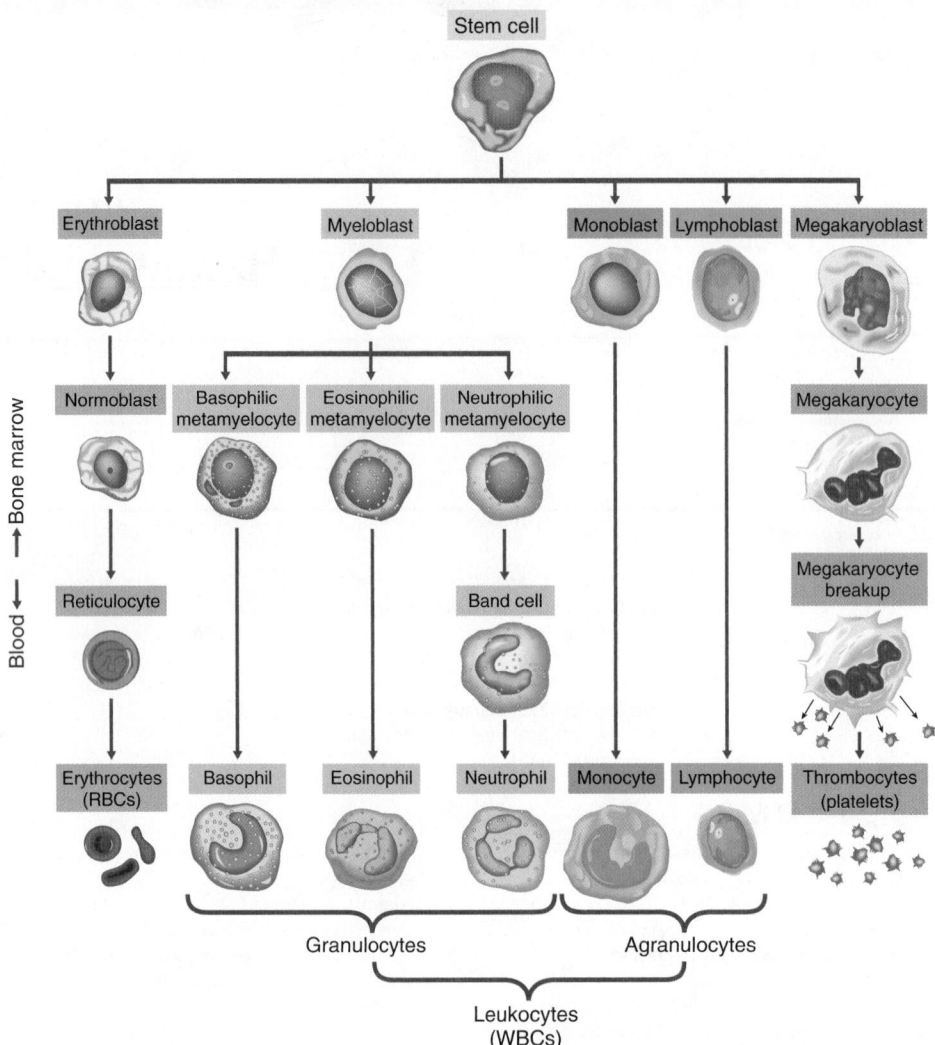

FIG. 30-1 Development of blood cells. *RBCs*, Red blood cells; *WBCs*, white blood cells.

system. The bone marrow is stimulated by various factors or cytokines (e.g., erythropoietin, granulocyte colony-stimulating factor [G-CSF], stem cell factor, thrombopoietin) that cause differentiation of the stem cells into one of the committed hematopoietic cells (e.g., RBC). For example, when tissue hypoxia occurs, erythropoietin is secreted by the kidney and liver. It circulates to the bone marrow and causes differentiation of proerythroblasts in the bone marrow.[1]

Blood

Blood is a type of connective tissue that performs three major functions: transportation, regulation, and protection (Table 30-1). Blood has two major components: plasma and blood cells. In an adult weighing between 150 and 180 lb, the volume of blood is usually between 4.7 and 5.5 L (5 to 6 quarts).

Plasma. Approximately 55% of blood is plasma (Fig. 30-2). Plasma is composed primarily of water, but it also contains proteins, electrolytes, gases, nutrients (e.g., glucose, amino acids, lipids), and waste. The term *serum* refers to plasma minus its clotting factors. Plasma proteins include albumin, globulin, and clotting factors (mostly fibrinogen). Most plasma proteins are produced by the liver, except for antibodies (immunoglobulins), which are produced by plasma cells. Albumin is a protein that helps maintain oncotic pressure in the blood.[1]

TABLE 30-1	**FUNCTIONS OF BLOOD**
Function	**Examples**
Transportation	• O_2 from lungs to cells • Nutrients from gastrointestinal tract to cells • Hormones from endocrine glands to tissues and cells • Metabolic waste products (e.g., CO_2, NH_3, urea) from cells to lungs, liver, and kidneys
Regulation	• Fluid and electrolyte balance • Acid-base balance • Body temperature • Maintaining intravascular oncotic pressure
Protection	• Maintaining homeostasis of blood coagulation • Combating invasion of pathogens and other foreign substances

Blood Cells. About 45% of the blood (see Fig. 30-2) is composed of formed elements, or blood cells. The three types of blood cells are *erythrocytes* (RBCs), *leukocytes* (WBCs), and *thrombocytes* (platelets). The primary function of erythrocytes is oxygen transportation, whereas the leukocytes are involved in protecting the body from infection. Platelets promote blood coagulation.

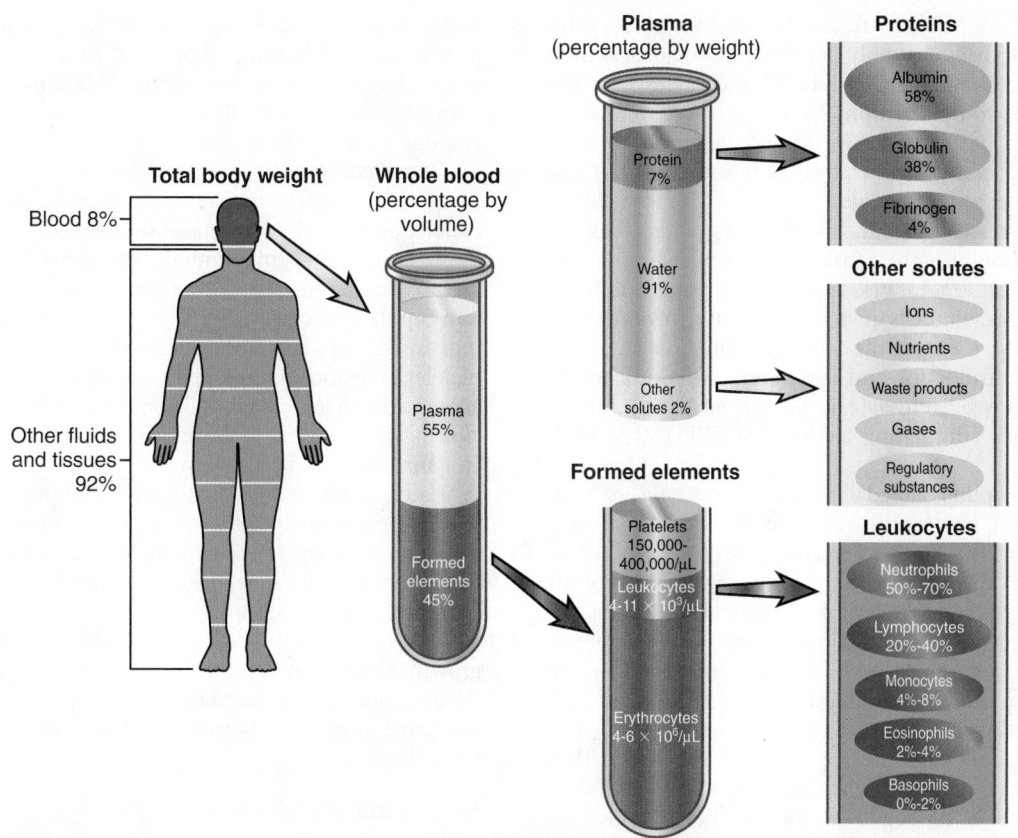

FIG. 30-2 Approximate values for the components of blood in the adult. Normally, 45% of the blood is composed of blood cells and 55% is composed of plasma.

Erythrocytes. The primary functions of RBCs include transport of gases (both oxygen and carbon dioxide) and assistance in maintaining acid-base balance. RBCs are flexible cells with a unique biconcave shape. Flexibility enables the cell to alter its shape so that it can easily pass through tiny capillaries. The cell membrane is thin to facilitate diffusion of gases.

Erythrocytes are primarily composed of a large molecule called hemoglobin. *Hemoglobin,* a complex protein-iron compound composed of heme (an iron compound) and globin (a simple protein), binds with oxygen and carbon dioxide. As RBCs circulate through the capillaries surrounding alveoli within the lung, oxygen attaches to the iron on the hemoglobin. The oxygen-bound hemoglobin is referred to as *oxyhemoglobin* and is responsible for giving arterial blood its bright red appearance. As RBCs flow to body tissues, oxygen detaches from the hemoglobin and diffuses from the capillary into tissue cells. Carbon dioxide diffuses from tissue cells into the capillary, attaches to the globin portion of hemoglobin, and is transported to the lungs for removal. Hemoglobin also acts as a buffer and plays a role in maintaining acid-base balance. This buffering function is described further in Chapter 17.

Erythropoiesis (the process of RBC production) is regulated by cellular oxygen requirements and general metabolic activity. Erythropoiesis is stimulated by hypoxia and controlled by *erythropoietin,* a glycoprotein growth factor synthesized and released primarily by the kidney. Erythropoietin stimulates the bone marrow to increase erythrocyte production. Normally the bone marrow releases 3×10^9 RBC/kg of body weight/day. The normal life span of an erythrocyte is about 120 days. Erythropoiesis is also influenced by the availability of nutrients. Many essential nutrients are necessary for erythropoiesis, including protein, iron, folate (folic acid), cobalamin (vitamin B_{12}), riboflavin (vitamin B_2), pyridoxine (vitamin B_6), pantothenic acid, niacin, ascorbic acid, and vitamin E.[1] Erythrocyte production is also affected by endocrine hormones, such as thyroxine, corticosteroids, and testosterone. For example, hypothyroidism is often associated with anemia.[2]

Several distinct cell types evolve during erythrocyte maturation (see Fig. 30-1). The **reticulocyte** is an immature erythrocyte. The reticulocyte count measures the rate at which new RBCs appear in the circulation. Reticulocytes can develop into mature RBCs within 48 hours of release into the circulation. Therefore assessing the number of reticulocytes is a useful means of evaluating the rate and adequacy of erythrocyte production.

Hemolysis (destruction of RBCs) by monocytes and macrophages removes abnormal, defective, damaged, and old RBCs from circulation. Hemolysis normally occurs in the bone marrow, liver, and spleen. Because one of the components of RBCs is bilirubin, hemolysis of these cells results in increased bilirubin to be processed by the body. When hemolysis occurs via normal mechanisms, the liver is able to conjugate and excrete all bilirubin that is released (see Fig. 31-2).

Leukocytes. *Leukocytes* (WBCs) appear white when separated from blood. Like the RBCs, leukocytes originate from stem cells within the bone marrow (see Fig. 30-1). There are different types of leukocytes, each with a different function. Leukocytes containing granules within the cytoplasm are called *granulocytes* (also known as polymorphonuclear leukocytes). Granulocytes include three types: neutrophils, basophils, and eosinophils. Leukocytes that do not have granules within the cytoplasm are called *agranulocytes* and include lymphocytes and monocytes.

Lymphocytes and monocytes are also referred to as mononuclear cells because they have only one discrete nucleus. Leukocytes have a widely variable life span. Granulocytes may live only for hours, yet some T lymphocytes may live for years.

Granulocytes. The primary function of the granulocytes is *phagocytosis,* a process by which WBCs ingest or engulf any unwanted organism and then digest and kill it. They are able to migrate through vessel walls and to the sites where they are needed. The *neutrophil* is the most common type of granulocyte, accounting for 50% to 70% of all WBCs. Neutrophils are the primary phagocytic cells involved in acute inflammatory responses. Once they engulf the pathogen, they die in 1 to 2 days.[1] Neutrophil production and maturation are stimulated by hematopoietic growth factors (e.g., G-CSF and granulocyte-macrophage colony-stimulating factor [GM-CSF])[1] (see Table 14-3).

A mature neutrophil is called a *segmented neutrophil,* or "seg" or "polysegmented neutrophil," because the nucleus is segmented into two to five lobes connected by strands. An immature neutrophil is called a *band* (for the band appearance of the nucleus). Although band cells are sometimes found in the peripheral circulation of normal people and are capable of phagocytosis, the mature neutrophil is much more effective. An increase in neutrophils in the blood is a common diagnostic indicator of infection and tissue injury.

Eosinophils account for only 2% to 4% of all WBCs. They have a similar but reduced ability for phagocytosis. One of their primary functions is to engulf antigen-antibody complexes formed during an allergic response. An elevated level of eosinophils is also seen in some neoplastic disorders, such as Hodgkin's lymphoma, and in various skin diseases and connective tissue disorders.[3] Eosinophils are also able to defend against parasitic infections.

Basophils make up less than 2% of all leukocytes. These cells have cytoplasmic granules that contain chemical mediators, such as heparin and histamine. If a basophil is stimulated by an antigen or by tissue injury, it responds by releasing substances within the granules. This is part of the response seen in allergic and inflammatory reactions. *Mast cells* are similar to basophils, but they reside in connective tissues and play a central role in inflammation, permeability of blood vessels, and smooth muscle contraction.

Lymphocytes. Lymphocytes, one of the agranular leukocytes, constitute 20% to 40% of the WBCs. Lymphocytes form the basis of the cellular and humoral immune responses (see Chapter 14). Two lymphocyte subtypes are B cells and T cells. Although T cell precursors originate in the bone marrow, these cells migrate to the thymus gland for further differentiation into T cells. *Natural killer (NK) cells* are lymphocytes that do not require prior exposure to antigens to kill virus-infected cells and activate T cells and phagocytes. Most lymphocytes transiently circulate in the blood and also reside in lymphoid tissues. (Details of lymphocyte function are presented in Chapter 14.)

Monocytes. Monocytes, the other type of agranular leukocytes, account for approximately 4% to 8% of the total WBCs. Monocytes are potent phagocytic cells that ingest small or large masses of matter, such as bacteria, dead cells, tissue debris, and old or defective RBCs. These cells are only present in the blood for a short time before they migrate into the tissues and become macrophages (see Chapter 13). In addition to macrophages that have differentiated from monocytes, tissues also contain resident macrophages. These resident macrophages are given special names (e.g., Kupffer cells in the liver, osteoclasts in the bone, alveolar macrophages in the lung). These macrophages protect the body from pathogens at these entry points and are more phagocytic than monocytes. Macrophages also interact with lymphocytes to facilitate the humoral and cellular immune responses (see Chapter 14).

Thrombocytes. The primary function of thrombocytes, or *platelets,* is to initiate the clotting process by producing an initial platelet plug in the early phases of the process. Platelets must be available in sufficient numbers and must be structurally and metabolically sound for blood clotting to occur. Platelets maintain capillary integrity by working as "plugs" to close any openings in the capillary wall. At the site of any capillary damage, platelet activation is initiated. Increasing numbers of platelets accumulate to form an initial platelet plug that is stabilized with clotting factors. Platelets are also important in the process of clot shrinkage and retraction.

Platelets, like other blood cells, originate from stem cells within the bone marrow (see Fig. 30-1). The stem cell undergoes differentiation by transforming into a *megakaryocyte,* which fragments into platelets. About one third of the platelets in the body reside in the spleen.

Platelet production is partly regulated by *thrombopoietin,* a growth factor that acts on bone marrow to stimulate platelet production. It is produced in the liver, kidneys, smooth muscle, and bone marrow. Typically, platelets have a life span of only 8 to 11 days.

Normal Iron Metabolism

Iron is obtained from food and dietary supplements. Approximately 1 mg of every 10 to 20 mg of iron ingested is absorbed in the duodenum and upper jejunum. Therefore only 5% to 10% of ingested iron is absorbed. About two thirds of total body iron is bound to heme in erythrocytes (hemoglobin) and muscle cells (myoglobin).

The other one third of iron is stored as ferritin and hemosiderin (degraded form of ferritin) in the bone marrow, spleen, liver, and macrophages (Fig. 30-3).When the stored iron is not replaced, hemoglobin production is reduced.

Transferrin, which is synthesized in the liver, serves as a carrier plasma protein for iron. The degree to which transferrin is saturated with iron is a reliable indicator of the iron supply for developing RBCs.

As part of normal iron metabolism, iron is recycled after macrophages in the liver and spleen phagocytize, or ingest and destroy, old and damaged RBCs. Iron binds to transferrin in the plasma or is stored as ferritin or hemosiderin (see Fig. 30-3). Only about 3% is lost daily in urine, sweat, bile, and epithelial cells in the gastrointestinal (GI) tract. Therefore there is normally very little iron loss except from blood loss.

Normal Clotting Mechanisms

Hemostasis is a term used to describe the arrest of bleeding. This process is important in minimizing blood loss when various body structures are injured. Four components contribute to normal hemostasis: vascular response, platelet plug formation, the development of the fibrin clot on the platelet plug by plasma clotting factors, and the ultimate lysis of the clot.

Vascular Response. When a blood vessel is injured, an immediate local vasoconstrictive response occurs. Vasoconstriction reduces the leakage of blood from the vessel not only by restricting the vessel size but also by pressing the endothelial surfaces together. The latter reaction enhances vessel wall stickiness and maintains closure of the vessel even after vascon-

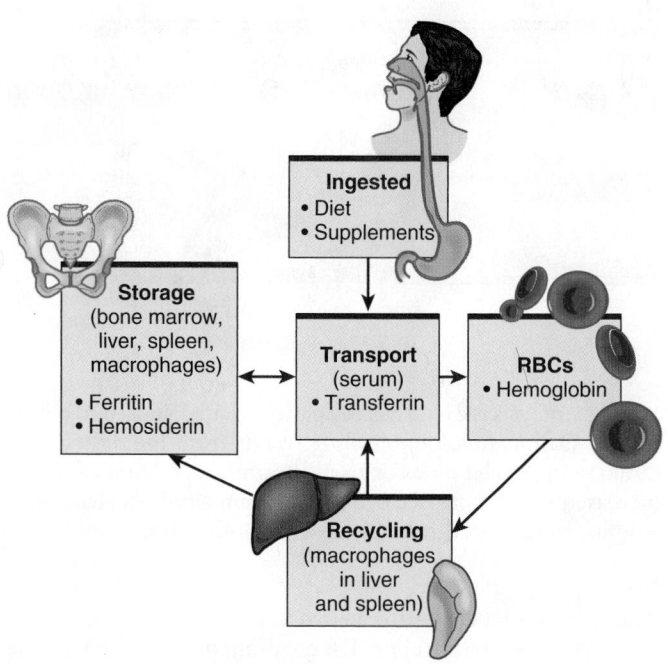

FIG. 30-3 Normal iron metabolism. Iron is ingested in the diet or from supplements. Macrophages break down ingested red blood cells *(RBCs)*. Iron is returned to blood bound to transferrin or stored as ferritin or hemosiderin.

striction subsides. Vascular spasm may last for 20 to 30 minutes, allowing time for the platelet response and plasma clotting factors to be activated. The platelet response and plasma clotting factors are triggered by endothelial injury and the release of substances such as tissue factor (TF).[1]

Platelet Plug Formation. Platelets are activated when they are exposed to interstitial collagen from an injured blood vessel. Platelets stick to one another and form clumps. The stickiness is termed *adhesiveness,* and the formation of clumps is termed *aggregation* or *agglutination.* This interaction causes the platelets to release substances such as platelet factor 3 and serotonin, which facilitate coagulation. At the same time, platelets release adenosine diphosphate, which increases platelet adhesiveness and aggregation, thereby enhancing the formation of a platelet plug. In addition, von Willebrand factor (vWF) is important in forming an adhesive bridge between platelets and vascular subendothelial structures. It is synthesized in endothelial cells and megakaryocytes and acts as a carrier for factor VIII.

In addition to their independent contribution to clotting, platelets also facilitate the reactions of the plasma clotting factors. As Fig. 30-4 shows, platelet lipoproteins stimulate necessary conversions in the clotting process.

Plasma Clotting Factors. The formation of a visible fibrin clot on the platelet plug is the conclusion of a complex series of reactions involving different clotting (coagulation) factors. The plasma clotting factors are labeled with both names and Roman

FIG. 30-4 Coagulation mechanism showing steps in the intrinsic pathway and extrinsic pathway as they would occur in the test tube.

TABLE 30-2 COAGULATION FACTORS

Coagulation Factor		Action
I	Fibrinogen	Source of fibrin to form a clot. Made in liver.
II	Prothrombin	Converted to thrombin, which then activates fibrinogen into fibrin.
III	Tissue factor, tissue thromboplastin	Released from damaged endothelial cells and activates the extrinsic pathway by reacting with factor VII.
IV	Calcium	Required cofactor at several points in the coagulation cascade.
V	Labile factor, proaccelerin	Binds with factor X to activate prothrombin.
VI		Not in use (now obsolete).
VII	Stable factor, proconvertin	Forms a complex with factor III and activates factors IX and X.
VIII	Antihemophilic factor	Works with factor IX and calcium to activate factor X.
IX	Christmas factor, plasma thromboplastin component	Together with factor VIII, activates factor X.
X	Stuart-Prower factor, Stuart factor	Activates conversion of factor II (prothrombin) to thrombin.
XI	Plasma thromboplastin antecedent	Activates factor IX when calcium is present.
XII	Hageman factor	Activates factor XI, which starts the intrinsic pathway.
XIII	Fibrin-stabilizing factor	Cross-links fibrin strands and stabilizes fibrin clot.

FIG. 30-5 Fibrinolytic system.

numerals (Table 30-2). Plasma proteins circulate in inactive forms until stimulated to initiate clotting through one of two pathways, intrinsic or extrinsic (see Fig. 30-4). The *intrinsic pathway* is activated by collagen exposure from endothelial injury when the blood vessel is damaged. The *extrinsic pathway* is initiated when tissue factor or tissue thromboplastin is released extravascularly from injured tissues.

Regardless of whether clotting is initiated by substances internal or external to the blood vessel, coagulation ultimately follows the same final common pathway of the clotting cascade. Thrombin, in the common pathway, is the most powerful enzyme in the coagulation process (see Fig. 30-4). It converts fibrinogen to fibrin, which is an essential component of a blood clot.

Lysis of Clot. Just as some blood elements foster coagulation *(procoagulants),* others interfere with clotting *(anticoagulants).* This counter mechanism to blood clotting serves to keep blood in its fluid state. Anticoagulation may be achieved by antithrombin activity, vessel and platelet activity, and fibrinolysis. As the name implies, antithrombins keep blood in a fluid state by antagonizing thrombin, a powerful coagulant. Endogenous heparin, antithrombin III, protein C, and protein S are examples of anticoagulants.

The second means of maintaining blood in its fluid form is **fibrinolysis**, a process resulting in the dissolution of the fibrin clot. The fibrinolytic system is initiated when plasminogen is activated to plasmin (Fig. 30-5). Thrombin is one of the substances that can activate the conversion of plasminogen to plasmin, thereby promoting fibrinolysis. The plasmin attacks either fibrin or fibrinogen by splitting the molecules into smaller elements known as *fibrin split products* (FSPs) or *fibrin degradation products* (FDPs). (More information about FSPs can be found in Table 30-7 later in this chapter and in the discussion of disseminated intravascular coagulation in Chapter 31.)

If fibrinolysis is excessive, the patient is predisposed to bleeding. In such a situation, bleeding results from the destruction of fibrin in platelet plugs or from the anticoagulation effects of increased FSPs. Increased FSPs lead to impaired platelet aggregation, reduced prothrombin, and an inability to stabilize fibrin.

Spleen

Another component of the hematologic system is the spleen, which is located in the upper left quadrant of the abdomen. The spleen has four major functions: hematopoietic, filtration, immunologic, and storage. *Hematopoietic function* is manifested by the spleen's ability to produce RBCs during fetal development. The *filtration function* is demonstrated by the spleen's ability to remove old and defective RBCs from the circulation by the mononuclear phagocyte system. Filtration also involves the reuse of iron. The spleen is able to catabolize hemoglobin released by hemolysis and return the iron component of the hemoglobin to the bone marrow for reuse. The spleen also plays an important role in filtering circulating bacteria, especially encapsulated organisms such as gram-positive cocci. The *immunologic function* is demonstrated by the spleen's rich supply of lymphocytes, monocytes, and stored immunoglobulins. The *storage function* is reflected in its role as a storage site for RBCs and platelets. More than 300 mL of blood can be stored. About one third of platelets are stored in the spleen. A person who has had a splenectomy has higher circulating levels of platelets than a person who still has his or her spleen.

Lymph System

The lymph system, consisting of lymph fluid, lymphatic capillaries, ducts, and lymph nodes, carries fluid from the interstitial spaces to the blood. It is by means of the lymph that proteins and fat from the gastrointestinal (GI) tract and certain hormones are able to return to the circulatory system. The lymph system also returns excess interstitial fluid to the blood, which is important in preventing edema.

Lymph fluid is pale yellow interstitial fluid that has diffused through lymphatic capillary walls. It circulates through a special vasculature, much as blood moves through blood vessels. The formation of lymph fluid increases when interstitial fluid increases, thereby forcing more fluid into the lymph system. When too much interstitial fluid develops or when something interferes with the reabsorption of lymph, lymphedema develops. Lymphedema that may occur as a complication of mastectomy or lumpectomy with dissection of axillary nodes is often caused by the obstruction of lymph flow from the removal of lymph nodes.

The lymphatic capillaries are thin-walled vessels that have an irregular diameter. They are somewhat larger than blood capillaries and do not contain valves. (eFig. 30-1 shows the lymph drainage throughout the body and is available on the website for this chapter.)

The *lymph nodes,* which are also a part of the lymphatic system, are round, oval, or bean shaped and vary in size according to their location. Structurally, the nodes are small clumps of lymphatic tissue and are found in groups along lymph vessels at various sites. More than 200 lymph nodes are found throughout the body, with the greatest number being in the abdomen surrounding the GI tract. Lymph nodes are situated both superficially and deep. The superficial nodes can be palpated, but evaluation of the deep nodes requires radiologic examination.[4] A primary function of lymph nodes is filtration of pathogens and foreign particles that are carried by lymph to the nodes.

Liver

The liver functions as a filter. It also produces all the procoagulants that are essential to hemostasis and blood coagulation. Additionally, it stores iron that is in excess of tissue needs, which can occur with frequent blood transfusions or diseases that cause iron overload. *Hepcidin,* produced by the liver, is a key regulator of iron balance. The synthesis of hepcidin is stimulated by iron overload or inflammation. Hepcidin reduces the release of stored iron from enterocytes (in the intestines) and macrophages.[5] Thus when iron is deficient, hepatocytes produce less hepcidin. Other functions of the liver are described in Chapters 39 and 44.

GERONTOLOGIC CONSIDERATIONS

HEMATOLOGIC SYSTEM

Physiologic aging is a gradual process that involves cell loss and organ atrophy. Aging leads to a decrease in bone marrow mass and cellularity and an increase in bone marrow fat.[6] However, peripheral blood cell concentrations in healthy older adults are similar to those of younger adults.[7] Although the older adult is still capable of maintaining adequate blood cell levels, the reserve capacity leaves the older adult more vulnerable to possible problems with clotting, transporting oxygen, and fighting infection, especially during periods of increased demand. This results in a diminished ability of an older adult to compensate for an acute or chronic illness.[6,7]

Hemoglobin levels begin to decrease in both men and women after middle age, with the low-normal levels seen in most older people. Total serum iron, total iron-binding capacity, and intestinal iron absorption are all decreased in older adults. Iron deficiency is usually responsible for the low hemoglobin levels. Healthy older patients are not able to produce reticulocytes in response to hemorrhage or hypoxemia as well as younger adults.[1]

The RBC plasma membranes are more fragile in the older person. This may account for a slight increase in mean corpuscular volume (MCV) and a slight decrease in mean corpuscular hemoglobin concentration (MCHC) of RBCs in some older individuals. It is essential to assess for signs of disease processes such as GI bleeding before concluding that decreased hemoglobin levels are caused solely by aging. Thus iron-deficiency anemia is a diagnosis that should be made after other causes have been ruled out.

The total WBC count and differential are generally not affected by aging. However, decreases in humoral antibody response and T cell function may occur.[6,8] During an infection,

TABLE 30-3	GERONTOLOGIC ASSESSMENT DIFFERENCES

Effects of Aging on Hematologic Studies

Study	Changes
CBC Studies	
Hgb	Normal; possibly slight decrease in men
MCV	May be slightly increased
MCHC	May be slightly decreased
WBC count	Diminished response to infection
Platelets	Unchanged but possible increase in adhesiveness
Clotting Studies	
Partial thromboplastin time	Decreased
Fibrinogen	May be elevated
Factors V, VII, IX	May be elevated
ESR	Increased significantly
D-dimers	Increased
Iron Studies	
Serum iron	Decreased
Total iron-binding capacity	Decreased
Ferritin	Increased
Erythropoietin	May be decreased

MCHC, Mean corpuscular hemoglobin concentration; *MCV,* mean corpuscular volume.

the older adult may have only a minimal elevation in the total WBC count. These laboratory findings suggest a diminished bone marrow reserve of granulocytes in older adults and reflect the possible impaired stimulation of hematopoiesis. The number of platelets is unaffected by the aging process, but functionally they may have increased adhesiveness.[9] Changes in vascular integrity related to aging can manifest as easy bruising.

The effects of aging on hematologic studies[9-11] are presented in Table 30-3. Immune changes related to aging are presented in Chapter 14.

ASSESSMENT OF HEMATOLOGIC SYSTEM

Much of the evaluation of the hematologic system is based on a thorough health history. Consequently, you need to be knowledgeable about what to include in the health history so that you can phrase questions to elicit the most information.

Subjective Data

Important Health Information

Past Health History. It is important to learn whether the patient has had prior hematologic problems. Specifically ask about previous problems with anemia, bleeding disorders, and blood diseases such as leukemia. Also document other related medical conditions such as malabsorption or liver (e.g., hepatitis, cirrhosis), kidney, or spleen disorders. Patients may have received a kidney transplant, may have lost a spleen to traumatic injury, or may have a history of IV drug or alcohol use that affects their risk for hematologic disorders. A history of recent or recurrent infections or problems with blood clotting is also important to note.

Medications. A complete medication history of prescription and over-the-counter drugs is an important component of a hematologic assessment. Specifically address the use of vitamins, herbal products, or dietary supplements because many patients may not consider them to be drugs. Many drugs may

CASE STUDY

Patient Introduction

iStockphoto/Thinkstock

A.J. is a 90-year-old white woman who is brought to the emergency department by her son. He came from out of town for a visit and found his mother at home, weak and lying in bed. She says she has been slowly getting more and more "cold and tired" but "that is what happens when you live as long as I do." Her son had not seen her for 6 months and was concerned with how pale and frail she looked. He got scared when he noticed that his mother could not even walk to the bathroom without having to stop to catch her breath.

Critical Thinking

As you read through this assessment chapter, think about A.J. with the following questions in mind:

1. What are the possible causes of A.J.'s weakness, pallor, and shortness of breath?
2. What would be your priority assessment of A.J.?
3. What questions would you ask A.J.?
4. What should be included in the physical assessment? What would you be looking for?
5. What diagnostic studies might you expect to be ordered?

evolve Answers available at *http://evolve.elsevier.com/Lewis/medsurg.*

interfere with normal hematologic function (see eTable 30-1 available on the website for this chapter).[12-14] Herbal therapy can interfere with clotting (see Complementary & Alternative Therapies box in Chapter 38 on p. 851). Antineoplastic agents used to treat malignant disorders (see Chapter 16) and antiretroviral agents used to treat human immunodeficiency virus (HIV) infection (see Chapter 15) may cause bone marrow depression. A patient previously treated with chemotherapy agents, particularly alkylating agents, has a higher risk of developing a secondary malignancy of leukemia or lymphoma. A patient on long-term anticoagulant therapy such as warfarin (Coumadin) could be at risk for bleeding problems.

Surgery or Other Treatments. Ask the patient about specific past surgical procedures, including splenectomy, tumor removal, prosthetic heart valve placement, surgical excision of the duodenum (where iron absorption occurs), partial or total gastrectomy (which removes parietal cells, thus reducing intrinsic factor needed for the absorption of cobalamin [vitamin B_{12}]), gastric bypass (where the duodenum may be bypassed and parietal cell surface area decreased), and ileal resection (where cobalamin absorption takes place). Also assess how wound healing progressed postoperatively and if and when any bleeding problems occurred in relation to the surgery. Discuss wound healing and bleeding as responses to past injuries (including minor trauma) and to dental extractions. Also determine the number of previous blood transfusions and possible complications during administration, since the risk of transfusion reactions and iron overload increases with the number of blood transfusions.

Functional Health Patterns. Key questions to ask a patient with a hematologic problem are presented in Table 30-4.

Health Perception–Health Management Pattern. Ask the patient to describe the usual and present state of health. Gather complete demographic data, including age, gender, race, and ethnic background. Ask if there is any family history of hematologic problems.

- Hematologic problems that have a strong genetic link include sickle cell anemia, hemophilia, thalassemia, and hemochromatosis.
- People with a family history of these hematologic problems have a much greater risk of developing them.
- Other hematologic problems, such as leukemia, pernicious anemia, and clotting disorders, may have a genetic predisposition.

When taking a family health history, explore the following health problems: jaundice, anemia, malignancies, RBC disorders such as sickle cell disease, bleeding disorders such as hemophilia, and clotting disorders.

Assess risk factors such as alcohol and cigarette use that might disrupt the hematologic system. Explore alcohol use tactfully. Alcohol is a caustic agent to the GI mucosa and can cause damage that results in GI bleeding, esophageal varices, and decreased absorption of cobalamin and other nutrients. Chronic alcohol abusers frequently have vitamin deficiencies. Alcohol also exerts a damaging effect on platelet function and the liver, where clotting factors are produced. Consequently, bleeding problems can develop and should be anticipated in cases of known alcohol abuse. Illicit drug use is also important to document, since many of these drugs may affect hematopoiesis.

Cigarette smoking increases low-density lipoprotein (LDL) cholesterol and levels of CO_2, leading to hypoxia and altering the anticoagulant properties of the endothelium. Smoking increases platelet reactivity, plasma fibrinogen, hematocrit, and blood viscosity.

Nutritional-Metabolic Pattern. Obtain the patient's weight and determine if the patient has experienced anorexia, nausea, vomiting, or oral discomfort. A dietary history may provide clues about the cause of anemia. Iron, cobalamin, and folic acid are necessary for the development of RBCs. Iron and folic acid deficiencies are associated with inadequate intake of foods such as liver, meat, eggs, whole-grain and enriched breads and cereals, potatoes, leafy green vegetables, dried fruits, legumes, and citrus fruits. Folic acid deficiencies may be offset by a diet including foods that are also high in iron.[15]

Hematemesis (bright red, brown, or black vomitus) is a symptom of an underlying problem and should always be investigated. Peptic ulcer disease is a common cause of hematemesis.

Explore any changes in the skin's texture or color. Ask about bleeding of gum tissue. Note any *petechiae* or *ecchymotic* areas on the skin and, if present, document the frequency, size, and cause. The location of petechiae can indicate an accumulation of blood in the skin or mucous membranes. Small vessels leak under pressure, and the platelet numbers are insufficient to stop the bleeding. Petechiae are more likely to occur where clothing constricts the circulation.

Also ask about any lumps or swelling in the neck, armpits, or groin. Specifically, ask what the lumps feel like (i.e., hard or soft, tender or nontender) and if they are mobile or fixed. Primary lymph tumors are usually not painful. A nontender, consistently swollen lymph node may be a sign of a malignancy, such as Hodgkin's or non-Hodgkin's lymphoma. Lymph nodes that are enlarged and tender are usually associated with an acute infection.[16] Explore any reports of fever. Determine if the patient currently has a fever, recurring fevers, chills, or night sweats.

Ask patients if they have a history of cardiac or pulmonary diseases. Cardiovascular disorders such as valvular disease or hypertension may predispose patients to hemolysis. Many of the medications used to treat cardiovascular disease can also cause abnormalities in hematopoietic cell production or coagulation.

TABLE 30-4   HEALTH HISTORY

Hematologic System

Health Perception–Health Management
- Do you have any difficulty performing daily activities because of a lack of energy?*
- Do you smoke cigarettes or drink alcohol?*
- Do you take any prescribed or over-the-counter medications?*
- Are you taking any herbal products?* Home remedies?*
- Have you in the past or are you currently consuming illegal drugs? What agents? What route? How frequently? When did you last use?
- Have you ever received a blood transfusion?*
- Is there any family history of anemia, cancer, bleeding, or clotting problems?*
- Have you had any surgeries?*

Nutritional-Metabolic
- Do you have any difficulties with eating, chewing, or swallowing?*
- Have you had any mouth sores, sore tongue, swollen or sore gums, excessive oral bleeding?*
- What kind of diet do you follow? If a vegetarian, do you eat eggs, milk products, fish, chicken?
- How has your appetite been?
- Have you had any changes in your weight in the past year?*
- Do you take any vitamins, nutritional supplements, or iron?*
- Is nausea and vomiting a problem for you?*
- Have you ever experienced any unusual bleeding or bruising?*
- Have there been recent changes in the condition or color of your skin?*
- Have you experienced night sweats or cold intolerance?*
- Have you noticed any swelling in your armpits, neck, or groin?*

Elimination
- Have you had black or tarry stools?* Have you had light, clay-colored stools?*
- Have you noticed any blood or dark "tea color" in your urine?*
- Has your urine had a foul odor or cloudiness?
- Have you had any decrease in urine output?*
- Do you ever have diarrhea or change in bowel patterns?*

Activity-Exercise
- Do you have any shortness of breath at rest? With activity?*
- Do you have any limitations in joint motion?* Have any of your joints been swollen?*
- Do you have a problem with unsteady gait? Have you fallen recently?*
- After activity, do you ever notice bleeding or bruising?*

Sleep-Rest
- Have you experienced excessive fatigue recently?*
- Are you more fatigued than usual?*
- Do you feel rested on awakening? If no, explain.

Cognitive-Perceptual
- Have you experienced any numbness or tingling?*
- Have you had any problems with your vision, hearing, or taste?*
- Have you noticed any changes in your mental function?*
- Do you have any pain, such as bone, joint, or abdominal pain, or abdominal fullness?*
- Do you have pain when moving your joints?*
- Have your muscles been sore or achy recently?*

Self-Perception–Self-Concept
- Does your health problem make you feel differently about yourself?*
- Do you have any physical changes that cause you distress?*

Role-Relationship
- Does your occupation bring you into contact with hazardous substances?*
- Has your present illness caused a change in your roles and relationships?*

Sexuality-Reproductive
- Has your hematologic problem caused any sexual problems that concern you?*
- *Women*: When was your last menses? Do you consider your cycle normal? How long does your bleeding usually last? Have you had any increase in cramping or clotting?* Have there been any changes in the amount of flow?*
- *Men*: Do you experience impotence?*
- Have you had unprotected sex in the past 6 months?* Was your partner someone new or a person with whom you have had a long-term sexual relationship?

Coping–Stress Tolerance
- Do you have a support system to assist you when needed?
- What coping strategies do you use during exacerbation of symptoms?
- Do you experience any specific symptoms when you feel stressed?*

Value-Belief
- Do you have any personal or religious objection to receiving blood or blood products?*
- Do you have any conflicts between your planned therapy and your value-belief system?*

*If yes, describe.

Pulmonary disorders that lead to hypoxemia may cause chronic stimulation of erythropoietin and result in *polycythemia* (excessive RBCs).

Elimination Pattern. Ask if blood has been noted in the urine or stool or if black, tarry stools have occurred. Ask the patient if he or she has had a recent stool Hemoccult (blood) test or colonoscopy. Document any decrease in urine output or diarrhea.

Activity-Exercise Pattern. Because fatigue is a prominent symptom in many hematologic disorders, ask about feelings of tiredness. Also determine any weakness or complaints of heavy extremities. Document symptoms of apathy, malaise, dyspnea, or palpitations. Note any change in the patient's ability to perform activities of daily living (ADLs), especially as they relate to patient safety and a history of falling.

Sleep-Rest Pattern. Determine whether the patient feels rested after a night's sleep. Fatigue secondary to a hematologic problem often does not resolve after sleep.

Cognitive-Perceptual Pattern. *Arthralgia* (joint pain) may be caused by a hematologic problem and should be assessed. Pain in the joint may indicate an autoimmune disorder, such as rheumatoid arthritis, or may be caused by gout secondary to increased uric acid production as a result of a hematologic malignancy or hemolytic anemia. Aching bones may result from pressure of expanding bone marrow with diseases such as leukemia. *Hemarthrosis* (blood in a joint) occurs in the patient with bleeding disorders and can be painful.

Paresthesias, numbness, and tingling may be related to a hematologic disorder and should be noted. Also assess any changes in vision, hearing, taste, or mental status.

Self-Perception–Self-Concept Pattern. Determine the effect of the health problem on the patient's perception of self and personal abilities. Also assess the effect of certain problems, such as bruising, petechiae, and lymph node swelling, on the patient's personal appearance.

Role-Relationship Pattern. Question the patient about any past or present occupational or household exposures to radiation or chemicals. If such exposure has occurred, determine the type, amount, and duration of the exposure.

A person who has been exposed to radiation, as a treatment modality or by accident, has a higher incidence of certain hematologic problems. The same is true of a person who has been exposed to certain chemicals (e.g., benzene, lead, naphthalene, phenylbutazone). These chemicals are commonly used by potters, dry cleaners, and individuals involved with occupations that use adhesives. Ask the patient about a history in the military. Many Vietnam War veterans were exposed to a dioxin-containing defoliant (Agent Orange), which has been linked with leukemia and lymphoma. Also assess the effect of the present illness on the patient's usual roles and responsibilities.

Sexuality-Reproductive Pattern. Obtain a careful menstrual history from women, including the age at which menarche and menopause began, duration and amount of bleeding, incidence of clotting and cramping, and any associated problems. Ask men if they have any problems related to impotence, since this is common in men with hematologic problems. Also question the patient about sexual behavior because HIV infection is potentially a concern, particularly among high-risk groups.

Coping–Stress Tolerance Pattern. The patient with a hematologic problem often needs assistance with ADLs. Ask the patient if adequate support is available to meet daily needs. Determine the patient's usual methods of handling stress. In the patient with platelet disorders or hemophilia, the potential for hemorrhage can be so frightening that usual life patterns may be drastically curtailed, affecting the person's quality of life. Explore the patient's understanding of the problem and provide teaching.

Value-Belief Pattern. Some hematologic problems are treated with blood transfusions or a bone marrow transplant. Determine if these types of treatments conflict with the patient's value-belief system, including the patient's cultural and religious beliefs related to blood and blood transfusions. If conflicts are identified, notify the health care provider.

Objective Data

Physical Examination. A complete physical examination is necessary to accurately examine all systems that affect or are affected by the hematologic system (see Chapter 3). Be aware that disorders of the hematologic system can manifest in various ways. Thus a patient's presenting symptoms may not immediately point to a hematologic problem (Table 30-5). For example, paresthesias of the lower extremities may not immediately appear to reflect a hematologic problem, but when combined with other clinical findings or risk factors, they may indicate cobalamin deficiency and resulting pernicious anemia. Although a full examination should be performed on patients suspected of a hematologic disorder, certain aspects of the physical examination are specifically relevant. These include skin, lymph nodes, spleen, and liver. Examination of the skin is discussed in Chapter 23; spleen and liver examination is found in Chapter 39.

Lymph Node Assessment. Lymph nodes are distributed throughout the body. Superficial lymph nodes can be evaluated by light palpation (Fig. 30-6). Deep lymph nodes cannot be

CASE STUDY

Subjective Data

iStockphoto/Thinkstock

A focused subjective assessment of A.J. revealed the following information:

PMH: History of osteoarthritis. No surgical history. Prefers to take care of self with "natural therapy" and has not seen a health care provider for 10 years.

Medications: Metamucil 1 tbs PO daily; vitamins C, E, and D with calcium.

Health Perception–Health Management: A.J. denies family or personal history of anemia, cancer, or bleeding disorders. She believes she comes from a family with great genes for longevity because they "live off the land." She admits to drinking one glass of red wine with her evening meal "because it's good for your heart." She is a nonsmoker and just can't understand her gradual increase in shortness of breath with exertion. She states she really can't do anything anymore without having to stop and catch her breath. She says "it's tough getting old."

Nutritional-Metabolic: A.J. is living on a fixed income and therefore eats a lot of pasta "because it is cheap." She uses a lot of garlic for flavoring and the "health benefit of it." Although not a vegetarian, she states that she eats little meat.

Elimination: Denies black tarry stool. Occasional constipation. No problems with urination. Urine without odor.

Activity-Exercise: As noted above, A.J. is having difficulty performing ADLs without having to stop and catch her breath. Denies dyspnea at rest. States joints are stiff on arising in morning and after sitting but able to get around OK. States her walking is steady but weak. No history of falling.

Sleep-Rest: Typically sleeps 8-9 hr/night with no difficulty falling asleep. However, she still feels tired and needs to nap on and off during the day.

Cognitive-Perceptual: Denies any numbness or tingling. Admits to being a little hard-of-hearing but can still see "pretty good."

Value-Belief: Prefers natural therapies over traditional medication.

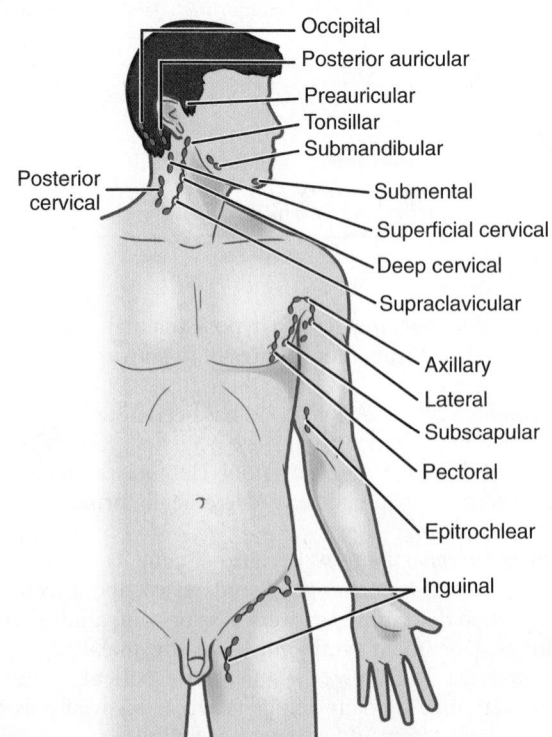

FIG. 30-6 Palpable superficial lymph nodes.

TABLE 30-5 ASSESSMENT ABNORMALITIES

Hematologic System

Finding	Description	Possible Etiology and Significance
Skin		
Pallor of skin or nail beds	Paleness. Decreased or absence of skin coloration.	Low Hgb level (anemia).
Flushing	Transient, episodic redness of skin (usually around face and neck).	Increase in Hgb (polycythemia), congestion of capillaries. Flushing of the palms of the hands or soles of the feet possible indication of anemia.
Jaundice	Yellow appearance of skin and mucous membranes.	Accumulation of bile pigment caused by rapid or excessive hemolysis or liver damage.
Cyanosis	Bluish discoloration of skin and mucous membranes.	Reduced Hgb, excessive concentration of deoxyhemoglobin in blood.
Excoriation	Scratch or abrasion of skin.	Scratching from intense pruritus.
Pruritus	Unpleasant cutaneous sensation that provokes the desire to rub or scratch the skin.	Hodgkin's lymphoma, cutaneous lymphomas, infiltrative leukemias, increased bilirubin.
Leg ulcers	Prominent on the malleoli on the ankles.	Sickle cell disease.
Angioma	Benign tumor consisting of blood or lymph vessels.	Most are congenital. Some may disappear spontaneously.
Telangiectasia	Small angioma with tendency to bleed. Focal red lesions, coarse or fine red lines.	Dilation of small vessels.
Spider nevus	Form of telangiectasia characterized by a round red central portion and branching radiations resembling the profile of a spider. Usually develop on face, neck, or chest.	Elevated estrogen levels as in pregnancy or liver disease.
Purpura	Any of a small group of conditions characterized by ecchymosis or other small hemorrhages in skin and mucous membranes.	Decreased platelets or clotting factors resulting in hemorrhage into the skin. Vascular abnormalities. Break in blood vessel walls resulting from trauma.
Petechiae	Pinpoint, nonraised, perfectly round area >2 mm. Purple, dark red, or brown.	Same as above.
Ecchymosis (bruise)	Small hemorrhagic spot, larger than petechiae; nonelevated. Round or irregular.	Same as above.
Hematoma	A localized collection of blood, usually clotted.	Same as above.
Chloroma	A tumor arising from myeloid tissue and containing a pale green pigment.	Acute myelogenous leukemia that has infiltrated the skin.
Plasmacytoma	A tumor arising from abnormal plasma cells.	Multiple myeloma that has infiltrated tissue.
Eyes		
Jaundiced sclera	Yellow appearance of the sclera.	Accumulation of bile pigment resulting from rapid or excessive hemolysis or liver disease or infiltration.
Conjunctival pallor	Paleness. Decreased or absence of coloration in the conjunctiva.	Low Hgb level (anemia).
Blurred vision, diplopia, visual field cuts	Decreased visual acuity or areas of blindness (field cuts).	Anemia, extreme leukocytosis, polycythemia may cause visual abnormalities. Thrombocytopenia may cause intraocular hemorrhage with visual abnormalities. Excessive clotting may cause thromboses in the circulation to the brain that cause visual field cuts.
Nose		
Epistaxis	Spontaneous bleeding from the nares.	May occur with low platelet counts, especially if the patient bends down for a long time, tries to lift a heavy item, or performs an intense Valsalva maneuver.
Mouth		
Gingival and mucous membrane changes	Pallor. Gingival and mucosal ulceration, swelling, or bleeding.	Low Hgb level (anemia). Neutropenia. Inability of impaired leukocytes to combat oral infections. Thrombocytopenia. Gingival hyperplasia may be present with some types of leukemia.
Smooth tongue	Tongue surface smooth and shiny. Mucosa thin and red from decreased papillae.	Pernicious anemia, iron-deficiency anemia.
Musculoskeletal System		
Bone pain	Pain in pelvis, ribs, spine, sternum.	Multiple myeloma related to enlarged tumors that stretch periosteum; bone invasion by leukemia cells. Bone demineralization resulting from various malignancies. Sickle cell disease.
Joint swelling	Fluid-filled spaces surrounding the joints.	Occurs with hemophilia and sickle cell anemia as bleeding occurs into the joint (hemarthria) causing inflammation.
Arthralgia	Joint pain.	Sickle cell disease from hemarthrosis.

Continued

TABLE 30-5   ASSESSMENT ABNORMALITIES—cont'd

Hematologic System

Finding	Description	Possible Etiology and Significance
Lymph Nodes		
Lymphadenopathy	Lymph nodes enlarged (>1 cm). May be tender to touch.	Infection; foreign infiltrations. Systemic disease such as leukemia, lymphoma, Hodgkin's lymphoma, and metastatic cancer.
Heart and Chest		
Tachycardia	Heart rate >100 beats/min.	Compensatory mechanism in anemia to increase cardiac output.
Palpitations	Feeling the heartbeat, flutter, or pound in the chest.	Anemia, fluid volume overload, hypotension with impending syncope, hypertension, dysrhythmias.
Altered blood pressure	*Orthostasis:* heart rate >20 beats/min increase or blood pressure >20 mm Hg decrease from baseline when moving from a lying position to either sitting or standing.	Orthostasis is a common manifestation in anemia, especially if also accompanied by low blood volume.
	Hypotension: <90 mm Hg systolic or >40 mm Hg drop from baseline.	Hypotension may indicate an infectious process, blood loss, or compromised cardiovascular compensatory mechanisms.
	Hypertension: >140/90 mm Hg.	Hypertension may occur initially as a compensatory mechanism for anemia.
Sternal tenderness	Abnormal sensitivity to touch or pressure on sternum.	Leukemia resulting from increased bone marrow cellularity, causing increase in pressure and bone erosion. Multiple myeloma as a result of stretching of periosteum.
Low O_2 saturation	O_2-carrying capacity as reflected by the O_2 saturation by pulse oximetry.	O_2 saturation may be decreased in cases of severe anemia.
Abdomen		
Hepatomegaly	Palpable liver.	Leukemia, cirrhosis, or fibrosis secondary to iron overload from sickle cell disease or thalassemia.
Splenomegaly	Palpable spleen.	Anemia, thrombocytopenia, leukemia, lymphomas, leukopenia, mononucleosis, malaria, cirrhosis, trauma, portal hypertension.
Distended abdomen	A larger than normal abdominal profile. May be soft or firm, tender or nontender, and accompanied by other symptoms such as nausea, vomiting, or rebound tenderness.	Lymphoma may manifest as abdominal adenopathy, mass(es), or bowel obstruction.
Nervous System		
Paresthesias of feet and hands; ataxia	Numbness sensation and extreme sensitivity experienced in central and peripheral nerves. Impaired muscle movement.	Cobalamin (vitamin B_{12}) deficiency or folate deficiency.
Weakness	Lacking physical strength or energy.	Low Hgb level (anemia).
Headache, nuchal rigidity	Pain in the cranium, potentially involving one area or extending from the frontal area to the back of the neck.	Generalized headache is a common manifestation of mild to moderate anemia. Severe headache with or without visual disturbances may signal intracranial hemorrhage due to thrombocytopenia.

palpated and are best evaluated by radiologic examination. Assess lymph nodes symmetrically and take note of location, size (in centimeters), degree of fixation (e.g., movable, fixed), tenderness, and texture. To assess superficial lymph nodes, lightly palpate the nodes using the pads of the fingers. Then gently roll the skin over the area and concentrate on feeling for possible lymph node enlargement. Ordinarily, lymph nodes are not palpable in adults. If a node is palpable, it should be small (0.5 to 1 cm), mobile, firm, and nontender to be considered a normal finding. A node that is tender, hard, fixed, or enlarged (regardless if it is tender or not) is an abnormal finding and warrants further investigation. Tender nodes are usually a result of inflammation, whereas hard or fixed nodes suggest malignancy.[16]

Develop a sequence when examining the lymph nodes. A convenient sequence is to start at the head and neck. First, palpate the preauricular, posterior auricular, occipital, tonsillar, submandibular, submental, superficial cervical, posterior cervi-cal chain, deep cervical chain, and supraclavicular nodes. Next, palpate the axillary lymph nodes and pectoral, subscapular, and lateral groups of nodes. Then examine the epitrochlear nodes, located in the antecubital fossa between the biceps and triceps muscles. Last, palpate the inguinal lymph nodes, found in the groin.

Palpation of Liver or Spleen. Both the liver and spleen are normally not detectable by palpating the abdomen. When they are enlarged, they may be detectable by percussion or palpation. Measure the degree of enlargement of the liver by the number of fingerbreadths it extends below the rib border. The spleen may be more difficult to detect because of its deep location in the left abdomen. Specific techniques for palpating the liver and spleen are described in Chapter 39.

Skin Assessment. In hematologic disorders, assessment of the skin may be a valuable source of information about the hematologic system. Examine the skin over the entire body in a systematic manner (e.g., starting with the face and oral cavity

FOCUSED ASSESSMENT
Hematologic System

Use this checklist to make sure the key assessment steps have been done.

Subjective
Ask the patient about any of the following and note responses.

Unusual bleeding or bruising	Y	N
Black, tarry stool	Y	N
Blood in vomitus	Y	N
Swelling in neck, armpits, or groin	Y	N
Dark-colored urine	Y	N
Fatigue	Y	N
Heart palpitations	Y	N

Objective: Diagnostic
Check the following laboratory results for critical values.

CBC	✓
White blood cell count with differential	✓
Clotting: PT, INR, aPTT, platelets	✓
Hgb, Hct	✓

Objective: Physical Examination
Inspect

Skin for lesions or color changes	✓

Auscultate

BP for alteration or orthostasis	✓

Palpate

Pulse for tachycardia	✓
Liver and spleen for enlargement	✓
Lymph nodes for lymphadenopathy	✓

aPTT, Activated partial thromboplastin time; *INR*, international normalized ratio; *PT*, prothrombin time.

and moving downward over the body). In patients with RBC disorders the skin may be pale or pasty, or it may have a cyanotic tinge in severe anemia. Erythrocytosis often produces small vessel occlusions causing a purple, mottled appearance of the face, nose, fingers, or toes. Clubbing of the fingers can be seen with chronic anemia such as in patients with sickle cell disease. Leukocyte disorders may cause infectious skin lesions or malignant nodular lesions. These may occur anywhere and have a variable distribution pattern. During the physical assessment of the skin, look carefully for petechiae (small purplish red pinpoint lesions), ecchymoses (bruising), and *spider nevus* (a form of *telangiectasia*) (see Table 30-5) because these can indicate bleeding disorders. In general, skin and mucosal bleeding indicates a platelet disorder, whereas spontaneous bleeding into joints or muscles indicates a coagulation factor problem. Excessive bleeding from trauma can be due to either or both.[17]

A *focused assessment* is used to evaluate the status of previously identified hematologic problems and to monitor for signs of new problems (see Table 3-6). A focused assessment of the hematologic system is presented in the box above.

DIAGNOSTIC STUDIES OF HEMATOLOGIC SYSTEM

The most direct means of evaluating the hematologic system is through laboratory analysis and other diagnostic studies. Diagnostic tests of the hematologic system are presented in Tables 30-6, 30-7, 30-9, and 30-10.

CASE STUDY
Objective Data: Physical Examination

iStockphoto/Thinkstock

Physical examination findings of A.J. are as follows: BP 100/70 (lying), 88/60 (standing); apical pulse 110 (lying), 124 (standing), but regular in rhythm. Respiratory rate 26, temperature 96.8° F (36° C), O₂ saturation 90% on room air. No jugular venous distention. Weight: 106 lb (48 kg). Height: 5 ft 1 in. Skin pale. No jaundice noted. Conjunctiva pale. Tongue smooth and shiny. Lungs clear but diminished breath sounds in the bases bilaterally. No visible bleeding. No enlarged lymph nodes, spleen, or liver noted. General weakness with dyspnea on exertion. No numbness or tingling or peripheral edema.

As you continue to read this chapter, consider diagnostic studies you would anticipate being performed for A.J.

Laboratory Studies

Complete Blood Count. The complete blood count (CBC) involves several laboratory tests (Table 30-6). In addition to the CBC, a *peripheral smear* may be ordered. The smear is used to look at the *morphology* (shape and appearance) of the blood cells and may assist with the diagnosis. For example, a large number of immature *blast* WBCs may indicate acute leukemia.

Although the status of each cell type is important, the entire system may be disrupted by diseases or by treatment of diseases. When the entire CBC is suppressed, a condition termed pancytopenia (marked decrease in the number of RBCs, WBCs, and platelets) exists. The effects of aging on hematologic studies are presented in Table 30-4.

Red Blood Cells. Normal values of some RBC tests are reported separately for men and for women because normal values are based on body mass, and men usually have a larger body mass than women.

The *hemoglobin (Hgb) value* is reduced in cases of anemia, hemorrhage, and hemodilution, such as that occurring when the fluid volume is excessive. Increases in hemoglobin are found in polycythemia or in states of hemoconcentration, which can develop from volume depletion (dehydration).

The *hematocrit (Hct) value* is determined by spinning blood in a centrifuge, which causes RBCs and plasma to separate. The RBCs, being the heavier elements, settle to the bottom. The hematocrit value represents the percentage of RBCs compared with the total blood volume. Reductions and elevations of the hematocrit value are seen in the same conditions that raise and lower the hemoglobin value. The hematocrit value generally is three times the hemoglobin value.

The total RBC count is reported as RBC × 10⁶/µL. However, the total RBC count is not always reliable in determining the adequacy of RBC function. Consequently, other data, such as hemoglobin, hematocrit, and RBC indices, must also be evaluated. The RBC count is altered by the same conditions that raise and lower the hemoglobin and hematocrit values.

RBC indices are special indicators that reflect RBC volume, color, and hemoglobin saturation (see Table 30-6). These parameters may provide insight into the cause of anemia. (The significance of these parameters is discussed further in Chapter 31.)

White Blood Cells. The WBC count provides two different sets of information. The first is a total count of WBCs in 1 µL of peripheral blood. Elevations in WBC count over 11,000/µL are associated with infection, inflammation, tissue injury or death,

TABLE 30-6   DIAGNOSTIC STUDIES

Complete Blood Count Studies

Study	Description and Purpose	Reference Intervals
Hemoglobin (Hgb)	Measurement of gas-carrying capacity of RBC.	*Female:* 11.7-16.0 g/dL (117-160 g/L) *Male:* 13.2-17.3 g/dL (132-173 g/L)
Hematocrit (Hct)	Measure of packed cell volume of RBCs expressed as a percentage of the total blood volume.	*Female:* 35%-47% (0.35-0.47) *Male:* 39%-50% (0.39-0.50)
Total RBC count	Number of circulating RBCs.	*Female:* 3.8-5.1 × 10^6/μL (3.8-5.1 × 10^{12}/L) *Male:* 4.3-5.7 × 10^6/μL (4.3-5.7 × 10^{12}/L)
Red cell indices		
$MCV = \dfrac{Hct \times 10}{RBC \times 10^6}$	Determination of relative size of RBCs. Low MCV reflection of microcytosis, high MCV reflection of macrocytosis.	80-100 fL
$MCH = \dfrac{Hgb \times 10}{RBC \times 10^6}$	Measurement of average weight of Hgb/RBCs. Low MCH indication of microcytosis or hypochromia, high MCH indication of macrocytosis.	27-34 pg
$MCHC = \dfrac{Hgb \times 100}{Hct}$	Evaluation of RBC saturation with Hgb. Low MCHC indication of hypochromia, high MCHC evident in spherocytosis.	32%-37% (0.32-0.37)
RBC morphology	Examination of the shape and size of RBCs.	No variation in RBC morphology
WBC count	Measurement of total number of leukocytes.	4000-11,000/μL (4-11 × 10^9/L)
WBC differential	Determination of whether each kind of WBC is present in proper proportion. Absolute value of each type of WBC can be determined by multiplying the percentage of cell type by total WBC count and dividing by 100.	*Neutrophils:* 50%-70% (0.50-0.70) *Eosinophils:* 0%-4% (0-0.04) *Basophils:* 0%-2% (0-0.02) *Lymphocytes:* 20%-40% (0.20-0.40) *Monocytes:* 4%-8% (0.04-0.08)
Platelet count	Number of platelets available to maintain platelet clotting functions (not measurement of quality of platelet function).	150,000-400,000/μL (150-400 × 10^9/L)

MCH, Mean corpuscular hemoglobin; *MCHC,* mean corpuscular hemoglobin concentration; *MCV,* mean corpuscular volume.

and malignancies (e.g., leukemia, lymphoma). Although the degree of WBC elevation does not necessarily predict the severity of illness, it can provide clues to the etiology. Certain types of leukemias are more likely to produce extremely high WBC counts (e.g., greater than 25,000/μL). A WBC count less than 4000/μL (**leukopenia**) is associated with bone marrow depression, severe or chronic illness, and some types of leukemia.

The second aspect of the WBC count, the *differential count,* measures the percentage of each type of leukocyte. The WBC differential provides valuable clues in determining the cause of illness. When infections are severe, more granulocytes are released from the bone marrow as a compensatory mechanism. To meet the increased demand, many young, immature polymorphonuclear neutrophils (bands) are released into circulation. The usual laboratory procedure is to report the WBCs in order of maturity, with the less mature forms on the left side of the written report. Consequently, the existence of many immature cells is termed a *"shift to the left."*

The WBC differential is of considerable significance because it is possible for the total WBC count to remain essentially normal despite a marked change in one type of leukocyte. For example, a patient may have a normal WBC count of 8800/μL, but the differential count may show that the proportion of lymphocytes is reduced to 10%. This is an abnormal finding that warrants further investigation.

When the lymphocyte count is low, an absolute lymphocyte count (ALC) may be tabulated. If the ALC is low, other diagnostic tests may be performed to look for an underlying reason.

When the bone marrow does not produce enough neutrophils, neutropenia occurs. **Neutropenia** is a condition in which the absolute neutrophil count (ANC) is less than 1000 cells/μL; severe neutropenia is associated with an ANC of less than 500 cells/μL. The ANC is determined by multiplying the total WBC count by the percentage of neutrophils. Neutropenia results from a number of disease processes, such as leukemia, or from bone marrow depression (see Chapter 31), and is associated with a high risk of infection and death from sepsis.

Platelet Count. The platelet count is the number of platelets per microliter of blood. Normal platelet counts are between 150,000 and 400,000/μL. Counts below 100,000/μL signify a condition termed **thrombocytopenia**. Bleeding may occur with thrombocytopenia. Spontaneous hemorrhage is possible once platelet counts fall below 10,000/μL.[18] A more extensive description of clotting studies is presented in Table 30-7.

Thrombocytosis is defined as excessive platelets, a disorder that occurs with inflammation and some malignant disorders (see Chapter 31). The most likely complication related to thrombocytosis is excessive clotting.

Blood Typing and Rh Factor. Blood group antigens (A and B) are found only on RBC membranes and form the basis for the ABO blood typing system. The presence or absence of one or both of the two inherited antigens is the basis for the four blood groups: A, B, AB, and O. Blood group A has A antigens, group B has B antigens, group AB has both antigens, and group O has neither A nor B antigens. Each person has antibodies in the serum termed *anti-A* and *anti-B* that react with A or B antigens. These antibodies are found when the corresponding antigen is absent from the RBC surface. For example, B antibodies are found in the serum of people with blood group A (Table 30-8).

Blood reactions based on ABO incompatibilities result from intravascular hemolysis of the RBCs. RBCs *agglutinate* (or clump) when a serum antibody is present to react with the antigens on the RBC membrane. For example, agglutination would occur in the blood of a person with type A blood when he or she receives blood transfused from a person with B antigens (i.e., type B or AB). The anti-B antibodies in the type A

TABLE 30-7 DIAGNOSTIC STUDIES

Clotting Studies

Study	Description and Purpose	Reference Intervals
Activated clotting time (ACT)	Evaluation of intrinsic coagulation status. More accurate than aPTT. Used during dialysis, coronary artery bypass procedure, arteriograms.	70-120 sec
Activated partial thromboplastin time (aPTT)	Assessment of intrinsic coagulation by measuring factors I, II, V, VIII, IX, X, XI, XII. Longer in patients using heparin.	25-35 sec
Antithrombin	Naturally occurring protein synthesized by liver that inhibits coagulation through inactivation of thrombin and other factors. Depleted in DIC.	21-30 mg/dL (210-300 mg/L) or 80%-120% of standard
Bleeding time	Measurement of timed, small skin incision bleeds. Reflection of ability of small blood vessels to constrict.	2-7 min
Capillary fragility test (tourniquet test, Rumpel-Leede test)	Reflection of capillary integrity when positive or negative pressure is applied to various areas of the body. Positive test indication of thrombocytopenia, toxic vascular reactions.	No petechiae or negative
Clot retraction	Reflection of clot shrinkage or retraction from sides of test tube after 24 hr. Used to confirm a platelet problem.	Begins in 1 hr. Maximum by 24 hr
D-dimer	Assay to measure a fragment of fibrin that is formed as a result of fibrin degradation and clot lysis. Used as an adjunctive measure in diagnosis of hypercoagulable conditions (e.g., DIC, pulmonary embolism).	<250 ng/mL (<250 mcg/L)
Fibrin split products (FSPs), or fibrin degradation products (FDPs)	Reflection of degree of fibrinolysis and predisposition to bleed (if present). Screening test for DIC. Elevated levels associated with DIC, advanced malignancy, severe inflammation.	<10 mcg/mL (<10 mg/L)
Fibrinogen	Reflection of level of fibrinogen. Increase in fibrinogen possible indication of enhancement of fibrin formation, making patient hypercoagulable. Decrease in fibrinogen indicates that patient possibly predisposed to bleeding.	200-400 mg/dL (2-4 g/L)
International normalized ratio (INR)	Standardized system of reporting PT based on a reference calibration model and calculated by comparing the patient's PT with a control value.	2-3*
Platelet count	Number of circulating platelets.	150,000-400,000/μL
Prothrombin time (PT)	Assessment of extrinsic coagulation by measurement of factors I, II, V, VII, X.	11-16 sec
Thrombin time	Reflection of adequacy of thrombin. Prolonged thrombin time indicates that coagulation is inadequate secondary to decreased thrombin activity.	17-23 sec

*Desired therapeutic level with warfarin (Coumadin).
DIC, Disseminated intravascular coagulation.

blood would react with the B antigens, thus initiating the process that results in RBC hemolysis.

The *Rh system* is based on a third antigen, D, which is also on the RBC membrane. Rh-positive people have the D antigen, whereas Rh-negative people do not. Rh-positive blood is indicated with a "+" after the ABO group (e.g., AB+). A Coombs test is used to evaluate the person's Rh status (Table 30-9).

As a result of transfusion therapy or during childbirth, an Rh-negative person may be exposed to Rh-positive blood. After exposure during childbirth the mother forms an antibody, anti-D, which acts against Rh antigens. (Rh-positive people normally have no anti-D.) In subsequent pregnancies the mother's anti-D antibodies can cross the placenta and attack the RBCs of a fetus who is Rh-positive, thus causing hemolysis of the RBCs. A pregnant Rh-negative woman should receive Rho(D) immune

globulin (RhoGAM) injections to prevent anti-D antibodies from forming.

Iron Metabolism. The laboratory tests used to evaluate iron metabolism include serum iron, total iron-binding capacity (TIBC), serum ferritin, and transferrin saturation. Additional tests for nutritional deficiencies leading to defective RBC production may also be done (see Table 30-9).

Serum iron is a measurement of the amount of protein-bound iron circulating in the serum. TIBC provides a measurement of all proteins that act to bind or transport iron between the tissues and bone marrow. Although this indirect measurement is a general reflection of the amount of transferrin present in the circulation, it overestimates transferrin levels by 16% to 20% because it also measures other proteins that can bind iron. These alternative proteins bind iron only when transferrin is

TABLE 30-8 ABO BLOOD GROUPS AND COMPATIBILITIES*

Recipient's Blood Group	A	B	AB (Universal Recipient)	O (Universal Donor)
RBC antigen	A	B	A and B	Neither
Plasma or serum antibody	Anti-B	Anti-A	Neither anti-A nor anti-B	Anti-A and anti-B
Compatible donor for RBC transfusions	A and O	B and O	A, B, AB, and O	O
Compatible donor for plasma transfusions	A and AB	B and AB	AB	A, B, AB, and O
Percent of population	42%	10%	6%	42%

*ABO blood groups are named for the antigen found on the RBCs. Compatibility is based on the antibodies present in the serum.

TABLE 30-9   DIAGNOSTIC STUDIES

Miscellaneous Blood Studies

Study	Description and Purpose	Normal Values
Bilirubin	Measurement of degree of RBC hemolysis or liver's inability to excrete normal quantities of bilirubin. Increase in indirect bilirubin with hemolytic problems.	*Total:* 0.2-1.2 mg/dL (3.0-21.0 μmol/L) *Direct:* 0.1-0.3 mg/dL (1.7-5.1 μmol/L) *Indirect:* 0.1-1.0 mg/dL (1.7-17.0 μmol/L)
Coombs test	Differentiation among types of hemolytic anemias. Detection of immune antibodies and Rh factor.	Negative
• Direct	Detection of antibodies that are attached to RBCs.	Negative
• Indirect	Detection of antibodies in serum.	Negative
Cobalamin (vitamin B$_{12}$)	Level of cobalamin available for production of new RBCs.	200-835 pg/mL (148-616 pmol/L)
Erythropoietin	Measurement of degree of hormonal stimulation to the bone marrow to stimulate the release of RBCs.	5-30 mU/mL (5-30 U/L)
Erythrocyte sedimentation rate (ESR)	Measurement of sedimentation or settling of RBCs in 1 hr. Inflammatory process causes an alteration in plasma proteins, resulting in aggregation of RBCs and making them heavier. The faster the sedimentation rate, the higher the ESR.	<30 mm/hr (some gender variation)
Ferritin	Major iron storage protein. Is normally present in blood in concentrations directly related to iron storage.	10-250 ng/mL (10-250 mcg/L)
Folic acid (folate)	Amount of folic acid (folate) available for RBC production.	3-16 ng/mL (7-36 nmol/L)
Hemoglobin (Hgb) electrophoresis	Proteins involved in development of the Hgb molecule have a definitive pattern of separation on electrophoresis. This pattern is altered with abnormal Hgb synthesis (e.g., thalassemia) or sickle cell anemia (where Hgb S is increased).	*Normal Hb A1:* >95% *Hb A2:* 1.5%-3.7% *Hb F:* <2% *Hb S:* 0% *Hb C:* 0%
Homocysteine	An amino acid formed from methionine. Rapidly metabolized through pathways that require cobalamin (vitamin B$_{12}$) and folic acid. Increased in cobalamin and folic acid deficiency.	*Male:* 5.2-12.9 μmol/L *Female:* 3.7-10.4 μmol/L
Iron		
• Serum iron	Reflection of amount of iron combined with proteins in serum. Accurate indication of status of iron storage and use.	50-175 mcg/dL (9-31.3 μmol/L)
• Total iron-binding capacity (TIBC)	Measurement of all proteins available for binding iron. Transferrin represents the largest quantity of iron-binding proteins. Therefore TIBC is an indirect measure of transferrin, an evaluation of amount of extra iron that can be carried.	250-425 mcg/dL (45-76 μmol/L)
Methylmalonic acid (MMA)	Indirect test for cobalamin. MMA metabolism requires cobalamin. Helps differentiate cobalamin deficiency from folic acid deficiency.	<0.2 μmol/L (<2.4 mcg/dL)
Reticulocyte count	Measurement of immature RBCs, a reflection of bone marrow activity in producing RBCs.	0.5%-1.5% of RBC count (0.005-0.015 of RBC count)
Serum protein electrophoresis (SPEP)	Separates proteins in the blood on basis of electric charge. Helps detect hyperglobulinemic states, such as in multiple myeloma or some lymphomas.	Normal banding pattern of albumin and globulins. Increase in any protein ("protein spike") is abnormal.
Transferrin	The largest of proteins that bind to iron. Increased in most people with iron-deficiency anemia.	190-380 mg/dL (1.9-3.8 g/L)
Transferrin saturation (%)	Decreased in iron-deficiency anemia and increased in hemolytic and megaloblastic anemia.	15%-50%

more than half saturated. Also, TIBC varies inversely with tissue iron stores; it is higher when iron stores are low and lower when iron stores are high.

Transferrin saturation is a better indicator of the availability of iron for erythropoiesis than serum iron because, unlike serum iron, the iron bound to transferrin is readily available for the body to use. Transferrin saturation is calculated by dividing serum iron by TIBC and multiplying by 100. For example, a patient with a serum iron level of 100 mcg/dL and a TIBC of 300 mcg/dL would have a transferrin saturation of about 33%.

Under normal conditions, the serum ferritin concentration correlates closely with body iron stores. In normal patients, 1 ng/mL of ferritin corresponds to 8 to 10 mg of stored iron.

Radiologic Studies

Radiologic studies for the hematology system involve primarily the use of computed tomography (CT) or magnetic resonance imaging (MRI) for evaluating the spleen, liver, and lymph nodes. Nursing responsibilities related to these studies are presented in Table 30-10.

Biopsies

Biopsy procedures specific to hematologic assessment are bone marrow examination and lymph node biopsy. In general, these procedures are done because a peripheral blood smear is nonspecific and usually a diagnosis cannot be established from a peripheral blood smear. Furthermore, a biopsy provides additional information about a hematologic problem that is needed for diagnosis and treatment planning.

Bone Marrow Examination. Bone marrow examination is important in the evaluation of many hematologic disorders. The examination of the marrow may involve aspiration only or aspiration with biopsy. The benefits gained from bone marrow examination are (1) a full evaluation of hematopoiesis and (2)

TABLE 30-10   DIAGNOSTIC STUDIES

Hematologic System

Study	Description and Purpose	Nursing Responsibility
Blood Studies	See Tables 30-6, 30-7, and 30-9.	
Urine Studies		
Bence Jones protein	An electrophoretic measurement is used to detect the Bence Jones protein, which is found in most cases of multiple myeloma. Negative finding is considered normal.	Acquire random urine specimen.
Radioisotope Studies		
Liver and spleen scan	Radioactive isotope is injected IV. Images from the radioactive emissions are used to evaluate the structure of spleen and liver. Patient is not a source of radioactivity.	No specific nursing responsibilities.
Bone scan	Same procedure as for the spleen scan except used for evaluating the structure of the bones.	Patient needs to lie still during the imaging. Patient may be asked to drink 4-6 glasses of water and then void before the imaging (to see pelvic bones).
Radiologic Studies		
Skeletal x-ray	X-rays done as a bone survey to detect lytic lesions associated with multiple myeloma. Bone scans do not identify lesions in this condition because there is no uptake of radioactive isotopes due to lack of blood supply.	No specific nursing responsibilities.
Liver, spleen, or abdominal ultrasound	Noninvasive probe is lubricated and slid across the abdomen to detect the density and borders of the abdominal organs. Can detect irregular borders, masses, vascular structure, and biliary tree.	Patients must be comfortable lying flat and having the probe compress the abdomen.
Positron emission tomography (PET)	A nuclear tracer substance is injected and is taken up by metabolically active cells. The follow-up scan shows different-colored tissues based on the metabolic rate. "Hot spots" reflect increased glucose consumption that is typical of tumors. A valuable diagnostic tool to detect active malignancy because it highlights areas with increased metabolism. PET or CT scanning may also be used.	IV access is required for injection of the tracer substance. Patients should have nothing by mouth, except water and medications, for at least 4 hr before the test. IV solutions containing glucose may be held. Patients who are glucose intolerant or diabetic may need adjustments in their medications. Bowel preparation may also be needed, depending on the area being studied.
Computed tomography (CT)	Noninvasive radiologic examination using computer-assisted x-ray evaluates the lymph nodes. Contrast medium often is used in abdominal studies of liver or spleen. Spiral (helical) CT scans are used to evaluate lymph nodes.	Investigate iodine sensitivity if contrast medium used.
Magnetic resonance imaging (MRI)	Noninvasive procedure produces sensitive images of soft tissue without using contrast media. No ionizing radiation is required. Technique is used to evaluate spleen, liver, and lymph nodes.	Instruct patient to remove all metal objects and ask about any history of surgical insertion of staples, plates, or other metal appliances. Inform patient of need to lie still in small chamber.
Biopsies		
Bone marrow	Technique involves removal of bone marrow through a locally anesthetized site to evaluate the status of the blood-forming tissue. It is used to diagnose multiple myeloma, all types of leukemia, and some lymphomas and to stage some solid tumors (e.g., breast cancer). It is also done to assess efficacy of leukemia therapy (see Chapter 31).	Explain procedure to patient. Obtain signed consent form. Ensure that a *time-out** is done before procedure. Consider preprocedure analgesic administration to enhance patient comfort and cooperation. Apply pressure dressing after procedure. Assess biopsy site for bleeding.
Lymph node biopsy	Purpose is to obtain lymph tissue for histologic examination to determine diagnosis and therapy.	Explain procedure to patient. Obtain signed consent form. Use sterile technique in dressing changes after procedure.
• Open	Performed in the operating room or procedure area using either local or general anesthesia. An incision is made, and the lymph node and surrounding tissue are dissected (excised) whenever possible.	Apply direct pressure to the area after the biopsy procedure to achieve hemostasis. Observe site for bleeding and monitor vital signs, especially if the platelet count is low. The sterile dressing should be changed as ordered, and the wound should be inspected for healing and infection.
• Closed (needle) or fine needle	Performed by a physician at the bedside or in an outpatient area. An extremely small needle is used to reduce the risk of tracking malignant cells through normal subcutaneous tissue.	
Molecular, Cytogenetic, and Gene Analysis Studies		
Fluorescence in situ hybridization (FISH) Comparative genomic hybridization (CGH) Spectral karyotyping (SKY)	Tests are performed on malignant cells, either peripheral blood (e.g., leukemia) or biopsy specimen (bone marrow, lymph node) to assess genetic or chromosomal abnormalities of cancer cells. May be useful in confirming diagnosis and determining treatment modalities and prognosis.	No specific nursing responsibilities. Explain purpose of testing to patient.

*Time-out is done just before the procedure starts to verify patient identification, surgical procedure, and surgical site.

FIG. 30-7 Bone marrow aspiration from the posterior iliac crest.

the ability to obtain specimens for cytopathologic and chromosomal abnormalities. The preferred site for both aspiration and biopsy of bone marrow is the posterior iliac crest.[19] The anterior iliac crest and sternum are alternative sites. However, the sternum is usually used only for aspiration. Bone marrow aspiration and biopsy are performed by a physician or specially credentialed nurse. Local anesthesia and sedation may be used to minimize anxiety and pain that the patient may experience.

For bone marrow aspiration, the skin over the puncture site is cleansed with a bactericidal agent. The skin, subcutaneous tissue, and periosteum are infiltrated with a local anesthetic agent. The patient may be uncomfortable when the periosteum is penetrated. Once the area is anesthetized, a bone marrow needle is inserted through the cortex of the bone. The stylet of the needle is then removed, the hub is attached to a 10-mL syringe, and 0.2 to 0.5 mL of the fluid marrow is aspirated (Fig. 30-7). The patient experiences pain with aspiration. Although it lasts only a few seconds, the pain may be quite uncomfortable. After the marrow aspiration, the needle is removed. Pressure is applied over the aspiration site to ensure hemostasis.

Although complications of bone marrow aspiration are minimal, there is a possibility of damaging underlying structures. This hazard is greatest in aspiration procedures involving the sternum.[20] Other complications include hemorrhage (especially if the patient is thrombocytopenic) and infection (especially if the patient is leukopenic).

The needle aspiration or biopsy site is covered with a sterile pressure dressing. Monitor the patient's vital signs until stable, and assess the site for excess drainage or bleeding. If bleeding is present, advise the patient to lie on the side for 30 to 60 minutes to maintain pressure on the site. If the bed is too soft,

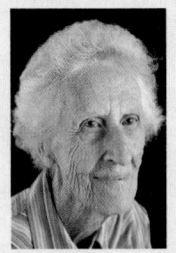
have the patient lie on a rolled towel to provide additional pressure. Analgesics for postprocedure pain may be administered. Soreness over the puncture site for 3 to 4 days after the procedure is normal.[20]

Lymph Node Biopsy. Lymph node biopsy involves obtaining lymph tissue for histologic examination to determine the diagnosis and help plan therapy. This may be accomplished by either an open biopsy or a closed (needle) biopsy.

If the results from a needle biopsy are negative, it may only indicate that the cancer cells were not part of the tissue in the biopsy specimen. However, a positive finding is sufficient evidence for confirming a diagnosis. This technique is rarely used to confirm an initial diagnosis because larger specimens are usually required to perform cytopathologic tests, but it may be used to validate disease recurrence or a new site of disease.

Molecular Cytogenetics and Gene Analysis

Testing for specific genetic or chromosomal variations in hematologic conditions is often helpful in diagnosis and staging. These results also help determine the treatment options and prognosis. If a large number of abnormal cells are circulating in the blood, such as in acute leukemia, these tests may be done by obtaining peripheral blood. However, testing is usually done on samples from bone marrow and lymph node biopsies. For example, fluorescence in situ hybridization (FISH) can identify specific areas by attaching a probe to a targeted region of deoxyribonucleic acid (DNA). It may be used to illuminate an abnormal extra chromosome 8, which is common in certain leukemias. Spectral karyotyping (SKY) allows each set of chromosomes to be painted different colors. It can be used to identify the chromosomal translocation of 22 to 9 in the Philadelphia chromosome of chronic myelogenous leukemia. More information on genetics is in Chapter 13.

▮ BRIDGE TO NCLEX EXAMINATION

The number of the question corresponds to the same-numbered outcome at the beginning of the chapter.

1. An individual who lives at a high altitude may normally have an increased RBC count because
   a. high altitudes cause vascular fluid loss, leading to hemoconcentration.
   b. hypoxia caused by decreased atmospheric oxygen stimulates erythropoiesis.
   c. the function of the spleen in removing old RBCs is impaired at high altitudes.
   d. impaired production of leukocytes and platelets leads to proportionally higher red cell counts.

2. Malignant disorders that arise from granulocytic cells in the bone marrow will have the primary effect of causing
   a. risk for hemorrhage.
   b. altered oxygenation.
   c. decreased production of antibodies.
   d. decreased phagocytosis of bacteria.

3. An anticoagulant such as warfarin (Coumadin) that interferes with prothrombin production will alter the clotting mechanism during
   a. platelet aggregation.
   b. activation of thrombin.
   c. the release of tissue thromboplastin.
   d. stimulation of factor activation complex.

4. When reviewing laboratory results of an 83-year-old patient with an infection, the nurse would expect to find
   a. minimal leukocytosis.
   b. decreased platelet count.
   c. increased hemoglobin and hematocrit levels.
   d. decreased erythrocyte sedimentation rate (ESR).

5. Significant information obtained from the patient's health history that relates to the hematologic system includes
   a. jaundice.
   b. bladder surgery.
   c. early menopause.
   d. multiple pregnancies.

6. While assessing the lymph nodes, the nurse should
   a. apply gentle, firm pressure to deep lymph nodes.
   b. palpate the deep cervical and supraclavicular nodes last.
   c. lightly palpate superficial lymph nodes with the pads of the fingers.
   d. use the tips of the second, third, and fourth fingers to apply deep palpation.

7. If a lymph node is palpated, what is a normal finding?
   a. Hard, fixed nodes
   b. Firm, mobile nodes
   c. Enlarged, tender nodes
   d. Hard, nontender nodes

8. Nursing care for a patient immediately after a bone marrow biopsy and aspiration includes (select all that apply)
   a. administering analgesics as necessary.
   b. preparing to administer a blood transfusion.
   c. instructing on need to lie still with a sterile pressure dressing intact.
   d. monitoring vital signs and assessing the site for excess drainage or bleeding.
   e. instructing on the need for preprocedure and postprocedure antibiotic medications.

9. You are taking care of a male patient who has the following laboratory values from his CBC: WBC $6.5 \times 10^3/\mu L$, Hgb 13.4 g/dL, Hct 40%, platelets $50 \times 10^3/\mu L$. What are you most concerned about?
   a. Your patient is neutropenic.
   b. Your patient has an infection.
   c. Your patient is at risk for bleeding.
   d. Your patient is at fall risk due to his anemia.

1. d, 2. d, 3. b, 4. a, 5. a, 6. c, 7. b, 8. a, c, d, 9. c

Evolve

For rationales to these answers and even more NCLEX review questions, visit *http://evolve.elsevier.com/Lewis/medsurg.*

REFERENCES

1. McCance KL, Huether SE: *Pathophysiology: the biologic basis for disease in adults and children*, ed 6, St Louis, 2010, Mosby.

2. Porter RS, Kaplan JL: *The Merck manual*, Whitehouse Station, NJ, 2011, Merck.

3. Kumar V, Abbas AK: *Pathologic basis of disease*, ed 8, Philadelphia, 2010, Saunders.

4. Monahan FD: *Mosby's expert physician exam handbook*, ed 3, St Louis, 2009, Mosby.

5. Ganz T, Nemeth E: Hepcidin and disorders of iron metabolism, *Ann Rev Med* 62:347, 2011.

6. Beerman I, Maloney WJ, Weissman IL, et al: Stem cells and the aging hematopoietic system, *Curr Opin Immunol* 22:500, 2010.

7. Hurria A, Muss HB, Cohen HG: Cancer and aging. In Hong WK, Bast RC, Hait WN, and Kufe DW, editors: *Holland-Frei cancer medicine*, ed 8, Shelton, Conn, 2010, People's Medical Publishing House.

8. Malaguarnera L, Cristald E, Malaguarnera M: The role of immunity in elderly cancer, *Crit Rev Oncol Hematol* 74:40, 2010.

9. Taffet GE: Normal aging. Retrieved from *www.uptodate.com/contents/normal aging.*

10. Balducci L: Anemia, fatigue, and aging, *Transf Clin Biol* 17:375, 2010.

11. Tita-Nwa F, Bos A, Adjei A, et al: Correlates of D-dimer in older people, *Aging Clin Exper Res* 22(1):20, 2010.

12. Sivilotti MLA: Hematologic principles. In Nelson LS, Lewin NA, Howland MA, et al, editors: *Goldfrank's toxicologic emergencies*, ed 9, New York, 2009, McGraw-Hill.

13. Lopez JA, Lockhart E: Acquired disorders of platelet dysfunction. In Hoffman R, Benz R, Shattil S, et al, editors: *Hematology: basic principles and practice*, ed 5, Philadelphia, 2009, Saunders.

14. Hodgson BB, Kizior RJ: *Saunders nursing drug handbook*, St Louis, 2012, Saunders.

15. American Dietetic Association: Health benefits of folate. Retrieved from *www.eatright.org.*

16. Jarvis C: *Physical examination and health assessment*, ed 6, St Louis, 2012, Saunders.

17. Collar BS, Schneiderman PI: Clinical evaluation of hemorrhagic disorders: the bleeding history and differential diagnosis of purpura. In Hoffman R, Benz R, Shattil S, et al, editors: *Hematology: basic principles and practice*, ed 5, Philadelphia, 2009, Saunders.

18. Babic A, Kaufman RM: Principles of platelet transfusion therapy. In Hoffman R, Benz R, Shattil S, et al, editors: *Hematology: basic principles and practice*, ed 5, Philadelphia, 2009, Saunders.

19. Venes D: *Taber's cyclopedic medical dictionary*, ed 21, Philadelphia, 2009, FA Davis.

20. Fischbach FT, Dunning MB: A manual of laboratory and diagnostic tests, ed 8, Philadelphia, 2009, Lippincott Williams & Wilkins.

RESOURCES

Resources for this chapter are listed in Chapter 31 on p. 683.

I have nothing to offer but blood, toil,
tears, and sweat.
Winston Churchill

Nursing Management
Hematologic Problems

Sandra Irene Rome

LEARNING OUTCOMES

1. Describe the general clinical manifestations and complications of anemia.
2. Differentiate the etiologies, clinical manifestations, diagnostic findings, and nursing and collaborative management of iron-deficiency, megaloblastic, and aplastic anemias and anemia of chronic disease.
3. Explain the nursing management of anemia secondary to blood loss.
4. Describe the pathophysiology, clinical manifestations, and nursing and collaborative management of anemia caused by increased erythrocyte destruction, including sickle cell disease and acquired hemolytic anemias.
5. Describe the pathophysiology and nursing and collaborative management of polycythemia.
6. Explain the pathophysiology, clinical manifestations, and nursing and collaborative management of various types of thrombocytopenia.
7. Describe the types, clinical manifestations, diagnostic findings, and nursing and collaborative management of hemophilia and von Willebrand disease.

8. Explain the pathophysiology, diagnostic findings, and nursing and collaborative management of disseminated intravascular coagulation.
9. Describe the etiology, clinical manifestations, and nursing and collaborative management of neutropenia.
10. Describe the pathophysiology, clinical manifestations, and nursing and collaborative management of myelodysplastic syndrome.
11. Compare and contrast the major types of leukemia regarding distinguishing clinical and laboratory findings.
12. Explain the nursing and collaborative management of acute and chronic leukemias.
13. Compare Hodgkin's lymphoma and non-Hodgkin's lymphomas in terms of clinical manifestations, staging, and nursing and collaborative management.
14. Describe the pathophysiology, clinical manifestations, and nursing and collaborative management of multiple myeloma.
15. Describe the spleen disorders and related collaborative care.
16. Describe the nursing management of the patient receiving transfusions of blood and blood components.

KEY TERMS

anemia, p. 633
aplastic anemia, p. 642
disseminated intravascular coagulation
   (DIC), p. 657
hemochromatosis, p. 647
hemolytic anemia, p. 643
hemophilia, p. 655

Hodgkin's lymphoma, p. 669
iron-deficiency anemia, p. 637
leukemia, p. 664
lymphomas, p. 669
megaloblastic anemias, p. 640
multiple myeloma, p. 673
myelodysplastic syndrome (MDS), p. 663

neutropenia, p. 660
non-Hodgkin's lymphomas (NHLs), p. 671
pernicious anemia, p. 640
polycythemia, p. 648
sickle cell disease (SCD), p. 644
thalassemia, p. 639
thrombocytopenia, p. 650

Reviewed by Mimi Haskins, RN, MS, CMSRN, Nursing Staff Development Instructor, Roswell Park Cancer Institute, Buffalo, New York.

ANEMIA

Definition and Classification

Anemia is a deficiency in the number of erythrocytes (red blood cells [RBCs]), the quantity or quality of hemoglobin, and/or the volume of packed RBCs (hematocrit). It is a prevalent condition with many diverse causes such as blood loss, impaired production of erythrocytes, or increased destruction of erythrocytes (Fig. 31-1). Because RBCs transport oxygen (O_2), erythrocyte disorders can lead to tissue hypoxia. This hypoxia accounts for many of the signs and symptoms of anemia. Anemia is not a specific disease. It is a manifestation of a pathologic process.

Decreased RBC Production

Deficient nutrients
- Iron
- Cobalamin
- Folic acid

Decreased erythropoietin

Decreased iron availability

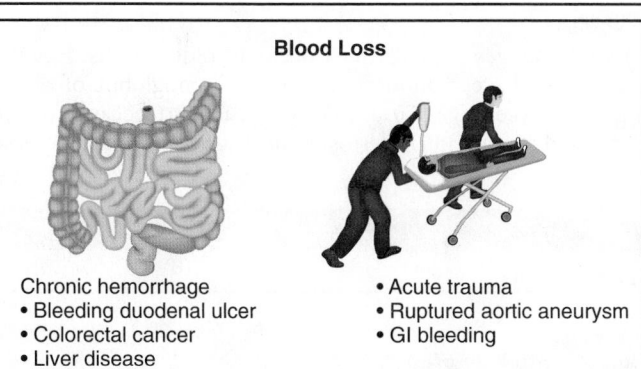

Blood Loss

Chronic hemorrhage
- Bleeding duodenal ulcer
- Colorectal cancer
- Liver disease

- Acute trauma
- Ruptured aortic aneurysm
- GI bleeding

Increased RBC Destruction

Hemolysis
- Sickle cell disease
- Medication (e.g., methyldopa [Aldomet])
- Incompatible blood
- Trauma (e.g., cardiopulmonary bypass)

FIG. 31-1 Causes of anemia.

Anemia is classified by review of the complete blood count (CBC), reticulocyte count, and peripheral blood smear. Once anemia is identified, further investigation is done to determine its specific cause.[1]

Anemia can result from primary hematologic problems or can develop as a secondary consequence of diseases or disorders of other body systems. The various types of anemia can be classified according to either *morphology* (cellular characteristic) or *etiology* (cause). Morphologic classification is based on erythrocyte size and color (Table 31-1). Etiologic classification is related to the clinical conditions causing the anemia[2,3] (Table 31-2). Although the morphologic system is the most accurate means of classifying anemias, it is easier to discuss patient care by focusing on the etiology of the anemia.

Clinical Manifestations

The clinical manifestations of anemia are caused by the body's response to tissue hypoxia. Specific manifestations vary depending on the rate at which the anemia has evolved, its severity, and any coexisting disease. Hemoglobin (Hgb) levels are often used to determine the severity of anemia.

Mild states of anemia (Hgb 10 to 12 g/dL [100 to 120 g/L]) may exist without causing symptoms. If symptoms develop, it is because the patient has an underlying disease or is experiencing a compensatory response to heavy exercise. Symptoms include palpitations, dyspnea, and mild fatigue.[2,3]

In moderate anemia (Hgb 6 to 10 g/dL [60 to 100 g/L]) the cardiopulmonary symptoms are increased. The patient may experience them while resting, as well as with activity.

In severe anemia (Hgb less than 6 g/dL [60 g/L]) the patient has many clinical manifestations involving multiple body systems (Table 31-3).

Integumentary Changes. Integumentary changes include pallor, jaundice, and pruritus. Pallor results from reduced amounts of hemoglobin and reduced blood flow to the skin. Jaundice occurs when hemolysis of RBCs results in an increased concentration of serum bilirubin. Pruritus occurs because of increased serum and skin bile salt concentrations. In addition to the skin, the sclera of the eyes and mucous membranes should be evaluated for jaundice because they reflect the integumentary changes more accurately, especially in a dark-skinned individual.

Cardiopulmonary Manifestations. Cardiopulmonary manifestations of severe anemia result from additional attempts by

TABLE 31-1 MORPHOLOGY AND ETIOLOGY OF ANEMIA

Morphology	Etiology
Normocytic, normochromic (normal size and color) MCV 80-100 fL, MCH 27-34 pg	Acute blood loss, hemolysis, chronic kidney disease, chronic disease, cancers, sideroblastic anemia, endocrine disorders, starvation, aplastic anemia, sickle cell anemia, pregnancy
Microcytic, hypochromic (small size, pale color) MCV <80 fL, MCH <27 pg	Iron-deficiency anemia, vitamin B_6 deficiency, copper deficiency, thalassemia, lead poisoning
Macrocytic (megaloblastic), normochromic (large size, normal color) MCV >100 fL, MCH >34 pg	Cobalamin (vitamin B_{12}) deficiency, folic acid deficiency, liver disease (including effects of alcohol abuse), postsplenectomy

MCH, Mean corpuscular hemoglobin; *MCV,* mean corpuscular volume.

the heart and lungs to provide adequate amounts of oxygen to the tissues. Cardiac output is maintained by increasing the heart rate and stroke volume. The low viscosity of the blood contributes to the development of systolic murmurs and bruits. In extreme cases or when concomitant heart disease is present, angina pectoris and myocardial infarction (MI) may occur if myocardial O_2 needs cannot be met. Heart failure (HF), cardiomegaly, pulmonary and systemic congestion, ascites, and peripheral edema may develop if the heart is overworked for an extended period.

TABLE 31-2 CLASSIFICATION OF ANEMIA

Decreased RBC Production
Decreased Hemoglobin Synthesis
- Iron deficiency
- Thalassemias (decreased globin synthesis)
- Sideroblastic anemia (decreased porphyrin)

Defective DNA Synthesis
- Cobalamin (vitamin B_{12}) deficiency
- Folic acid deficiency

Decreased Number of RBC Precursors
- Aplastic anemia and inherited disorders (e.g., Fanconi syndrome)
- Anemia of myeloproliferative diseases (e.g., leukemia) and myelodysplasia
- Chronic diseases or disorders
- Medications and chemicals (e.g., chemotherapy, lead)
- Radiation

Blood Loss
Acute
- Trauma
- Blood vessel rupture
- Splenic sequestration crisis

Chronic
- Gastritis
- Menstrual flow
- Hemorrhoids

Increased RBC Destruction (Hemolytic Anemias)
Hereditary (Intrinsic)
- Abnormal hemoglobin (sickle cell disease)
- Enzyme deficiency (G6PD)
- Membrane abnormalities (paroxysmal nocturnal hemoglobinuria, hereditary spherocytosis)

Acquired (Extrinsic)
- Macroangiopathic: physical trauma (prosthetic heart valves, extracorporeal circulation)
- Microangiopathic: disseminated intravascular coagulopathy (DIC), thrombotic thrombocytopenic purpura (TTP)
- Antibodies (isoimmune and autoimmune)
- Infectious agents (e.g., malaria) and toxins

G6PD, Glucose-6-phosphate dehydrogenase.

NURSING MANAGEMENT
ANEMIA

This section discusses general nursing management of anemia. Specific care related to various types of anemia is discussed later in this chapter.

NURSING ASSESSMENT
Subjective and objective data that should be obtained from a patient with anemia are presented in Table 31-4.

NURSING DIAGNOSES
Nursing diagnoses for the patient with anemia include, but are not limited to, those presented in Nursing Care Plan 31-1.

PLANNING
The overall goals are that the patient with anemia will (1) assume normal activities of daily living, (2) maintain adequate nutrition, and (3) develop no complications related to anemia.

NURSING IMPLEMENTATION
The numerous causes of anemia necessitate different nursing interventions specific to the patient's needs. Nevertheless, certain general components of care for all patients with anemia are presented in Nursing Care Plan 31-1.

Correcting the cause of the anemia is ultimately the goal of therapy. Acute interventions may include blood or blood product transfusions, drug therapy (e.g., erythropoietin, vitamin supplements), volume replacement, and O_2 therapy to stabilize the patient. Dietary and lifestyle changes (described in sections on specific types of anemia) can reverse some anemias so that the patient can return to the former state of health. Assess the patient's knowledge regarding adequate nutritional intake and adherence to safety precautions to prevent falls and injury.

GERONTOLOGIC CONSIDERATIONS

ANEMIA
Modest changes in RBC mass occur in older adults. Healthy older men have a modest decline in hemoglobin of about 1 g/dL between ages 70 and 88 years, in part because of the decreased production of testosterone. Only a minimal decrease

---

TABLE 31-3 MANIFESTATIONS OF ANEMIA

	Severity of Anemia		
Body System	**Mild** (Hgb 10-12 g/dL [100-120 g/L])	**Moderate** (Hgb 6-10 g/dL [60-100 g/L])	**Severe** (Hgb <6 g/dL [<60 g/L])
Integument	None	None	Pallor, jaundice,* pruritus*
Eyes	None	None	Icteric conjunctiva and sclera,* retinal hemorrhage, blurred vision
Mouth	None	None	Glossitis, smooth tongue
Cardiovascular	Palpitations	Increased palpitations, "bounding pulse"	Tachycardia, increased pulse pressure, systolic murmurs, intermittent claudication, angina, heart failure, myocardial infarction
Pulmonary	Exertional dyspnea	Dyspnea	Tachypnea, orthopnea, dyspnea at rest
Neurologic	None	"Roaring in the ears"	Headache, vertigo, irritability, depression, impaired thought processes
Gastrointestinal	None	None	Anorexia, hepatomegaly, splenomegaly, difficulty swallowing, sore mouth
Musculoskeletal	None	None	Bone pain
General	None or mild fatigue	Fatigue	Sensitivity to cold, weight loss, lethargy

*Caused by hemolysis.

TABLE 31-4 NURSING ASSESSMENT

Anemia

Subjective Data
Important Health Information

Past health history: Recent blood loss or trauma; chronic liver, endocrine, or renal disease (including dialysis); GI disease (malabsorption syndrome, ulcers, gastritis, or hemorrhoids); inflammatory disorders (especially Crohn's disease); smoking, exposure to radiation or chemical toxins (arsenic, lead, benzenes, copper); infectious diseases (HIV) or recent travel with possible exposure to infection; angina, myocardial infarction; history of falling

Medications: Use of vitamin and iron supplements; aspirin, anticoagulants, oral contraceptives, phenobarbital, penicillins, nonsteroidal antiinflammatory drugs, omeprazole, phenacetin, phenytoin (Dilantin), sulfonamides, herbal products

Surgery or other treatments: Recent surgery, small bowel resection, gastrectomy, prosthetic heart valves, chemotherapy, radiation therapy

Dietary history: General dietary patterns, consumption of alcohol

Functional Health Patterns

Health perception–health management: Family history of anemia; malaise

Nutritional-metabolic: Nausea, vomiting, anorexia, weight loss; dysphagia, dyspepsia, heartburn; night sweats, cold intolerance

Elimination: Hematuria, decreased urine output; diarrhea, constipation, flatulence, tarry stools, bloody stools

Activity-exercise: Fatigue, muscle weakness and decreased strength; dyspnea, orthopnea, cough, hemoptysis; palpitations; shortness of breath with activity

Cognitive-perceptual: Headache; abdominal, chest, and bone pain; painful tongue; paresthesias of feet and hands; pruritus; disturbances in vision, taste, or hearing; vertigo; hypersensitivity to cold; dizziness

Sexuality-reproductive: Menorrhagia, metrorrhagia; recent or current pregnancy; male impotence

Objective Data
General
Lethargy, apathy, general lymphadenopathy, fever

Integumentary
Pale skin and mucous membranes; blue, pale white, or icteric sclera; cheilitis (inflammation of the lips); poor skin turgor; brittle, spoon-shaped fingernails; jaundice; petechiae; ecchymoses; nose or gingival bleeding; poor healing; dry, brittle, thinning hair

Respiratory
Tachypnea

Cardiovascular
Tachycardia, systolic murmur, dysrhythmias; postural hypotension, widened pulse pressure, bruits (especially carotid); intermittent claudication, ankle edema

Gastrointestinal
Hepatosplenomegaly; glossitis; beefy, red tongue; stomatitis; abdominal distention; anorexia

Neurologic
Headache, roaring in the ears, confusion, impaired judgment, irritability, ataxia, unsteady gait, paralysis, loss of vibration sense

Possible Diagnostic Findings
↓ RBCs, ↓ Hgb; ↓ Hct; ↑ or ↓ reticulocytes, MCV, serum iron, ferritin, folate, or cobalamin (vitamin B$_{12}$); heme (guaiac)–positive stools; ↓ serum erythropoietin level; ↑ or ↓ LDH, bilirubin, transferrin (see Table 31-6)

LDH, Lactate dehydrogenase; *MCV,* mean corpuscular volume.

⊚ NURSING CARE PLAN 31-1

Patient With Anemia

NURSING DIAGNOSIS* **Fatigue** *related to* inadequate oxygenation of the blood *as evidenced by* increased pulse and blood pressure in response to activity, anorexia, impaired concentration, and/or patient verbalization of an overwhelming lack of energy

PATIENT GOALS
1. Participates in activities of daily living without abnormal increases in blood pressure and pulse
2. Reports increased endurance for activity

Outcomes (NOC)

Fatigue Level
- Exhaustion _____
- Loss of appetite _____
- Decreased motivation _____
- Lassitude _____

Measurement Scale
1 = Severe
2 = Substantial
3 = Moderate
4 = Mild
5 = None

Energy Conservation
- Recognizes energy limitations _____
- Balances activity and rest _____
- Uses energy conservation techniques _____
- Organizes activities to conserve energy _____
- Maintains adequate nutrition _____

Measurement Scale
1 = Never demonstrated
2 = Rarely demonstrated
3 = Sometimes demonstrated
4 = Often demonstrated
5 = Consistently demonstrated

Interventions (NIC) and *Rationales*

Energy Management
- Correct physiologic status deficits (e.g., chemotherapy-induced anemia) as priority items.
- Encourage alternate rest and activity periods *to provide activity without tiring the patient.*
- Monitor cardiorespiratory response to activity (e.g., tachycardia, dysrhythmias, dyspnea, diaphoresis, pallor, respiratory rate) *to evaluate activity intolerance.*
- Limit number of visitors and interruptions by visitors *to provide rest periods.*
- Assist the patient in assigning priority to activities to accommodate energy levels *to promote tolerance for important activities.*
- Arrange physical activities (e.g., avoid activity immediately after meals) *to reduce competition for O$_2$ supply to vital functions.*
- Assist with regular physical activities (e.g., ambulation, transfers, personal care) *to minimize fatigue and risk of injury from falls.*
- Instruct patient and caregiver to recognize signs and symptoms of fatigue that require reduction in activity *to promote self-care.*
- Instruct patient and caregiver to notify health care provider if signs and symptoms of fatigue persist *to review treatment plan.*

*Nursing diagnoses listed in order of priority.

Continued

◎ NURSING CARE PLAN 31-1—cont'd

Patient With Anemia

| NURSING DIAGNOSIS | **Imbalanced nutrition: less than body requirements** *related to* inadequate nutritional intake and anorexia *as evidenced by* weight loss, low serum albumin, decreased iron level, vitamin deficiencies |

| PATIENT GOALS | 1. Maintains dietary intake that provides minimum daily requirements of nutrients
2. Attains normal blood values of nutrients necessary to prevent anemia |

Outcomes (NOC) | **Interventions (NIC) and *Rationales***

Nutritional Status
- Nutrient intake _____
- Weight/height ratio _____

Nutritional Status: Biochemical Measures
- Serum albumin _____
- Serum transferrin _____
- Hemoglobin _____
- Hematocrit _____
- Total iron-binding capacity _____

Measurement Scale
1 = Severe deviation from normal range
2 = Substantial deviation from normal range
3 = Moderate deviation from normal range
4 = Mild deviation from normal range
5 = No deviation from normal range

Nutrition Management
- Determine, in collaboration with dietitian, number of calories and type of nutrients needed to meet nutritional requirements *to plan interventions.*
- Teach patient how to keep a food diary *to help evaluate nutritional intake.*
- Monitor recorded intake for nutritional content and calories *to evaluate nutritional status.*
- Provide appropriate information about nutritional needs and how to meet them *to increase intake of essential nutrients needed.*
- Encourage increased intake of protein, iron, and vitamin C *to provide nutrients needed for maximum iron absorption and hemoglobin production.*
- Encourage increased intake of foods high in iron *to provide nutrient needed for hemoglobin production.*

| NURSING DIAGNOSIS | **Ineffective self-health management** *related to* lack of knowledge about appropriate nutrition and medication regimen *as evidenced by* questioning about lifestyle adjustments, diet, medications |

| PATIENT GOAL | Verbalizes knowledge necessary to maintain adequate nutrition and management of medication regimen |

Outcomes (NOC) | **Interventions (NIC) and *Rationales***

Knowledge: Diet
- Recommended diet _____
- Dietary goals _____
- Healthy nutritional practices _____
- Potential food and medication interactions _____

Knowledge: Medication
- Identification of correct name of medication(s) _____
- Medication therapeutic effects _____
- Medication adverse effects _____
- Correct use of prescribed medication _____
- Required laboratory tests for monitoring medication _____

Measurement Scale
1 = No knowledge
2 = Limited knowledge
3 = Moderate knowledge
4 = Substantial knowledge
5 = Extensive knowledge

Nutritional Counseling
- Facilitate identification of eating behaviors to be changed.
- Use accepted nutritional standards to assist patient in evaluating adequacy of dietary intake *to evaluate adequacy.*
- Discuss nutritional requirements and patient's perceptions of prescribed or recommended diet.
- Provide referral or consultation with other members of the health care team *to help patient maintain gains and adjustments throughout recovery.*
- Review with patient measurements of hemoglobin values *to evaluate response to therapeutic plan.*

Teaching: Prescribed Medication
- Instruct the patient on the purpose and action of each medication.
- Instruct the patient on dosage, route, and duration of each medication *to improve adherence.*
- Instruct the patient on possible adverse effects of each medication *to ensure early detection of untoward responses to medication.*

---

in hemoglobin (about 0.2 g/dL) occurs between these ages in healthy women.

For older adults with anemia, about one third have a nutritional type of anemia (e.g., iron, folate, cobalamin). About another third have renal insufficiency and/or chronic inflammation, and the other third have anemia that is unexplained.

Cobalamin (vitamin B$_{12}$) and folate deficiency may occur in about 14% of older adults because of pernicious anemia, insufficient dietary intake, and malabsorption caused by low stomach acidity.[4] Multiple co-morbid conditions in older adults increase the likelihood of many types of anemia occurring.

Clinical manifestations of anemia in older adults may include pallor, confusion, ataxia, fatigue, worsening angina, and heart failure.[2] Unfortunately, anemia may go unrecognized in older adults because these manifestations may be mistaken for normal aging changes or overlooked because of another health problem. By recognizing signs of anemia, you can play a pivotal role in health assessment and related interventions for older adults.

ANEMIA CAUSED BY DECREASED ERYTHROCYTE PRODUCTION

Normally RBC production (termed *erythropoiesis*) is in equilibrium with RBC destruction and loss. This balance ensures that an adequate number of erythrocytes is available at all times. The normal life span of an RBC is 120 days. Three alterations in erythropoiesis may occur that decrease RBC production: (1) decreased hemoglobin synthesis may lead to iron-deficiency anemia, thalassemia, and sideroblastic anemia; (2) defective deoxyribonucleic acid (DNA) synthesis in RBCs (e.g., cobalamin deficiency, folic acid deficiency) may lead to megaloblastic anemias; and (3) diminished availability of erythrocyte precursors may result in aplastic anemia and anemia of chronic disease (see Table 31-2).

IRON-DEFICIENCY ANEMIA

Iron-deficiency anemia, one of the most common chronic hematologic disorders, is found in 2% to 5% of adult men and postmenopausal women in developed countries. Those most susceptible to iron-deficiency anemia are the very young, those on poor diets, and women in their reproductive years.[5,6] Normally, 1 mg of iron is lost daily through feces, sweat, and urine.[7]

Etiology

Iron-deficiency anemia may develop as a result of inadequate dietary intake, malabsorption, blood loss, or hemolysis. (Normal iron metabolism is discussed in Chapter 30 on p. 616.) Normal dietary iron intake is usually sufficient to meet the needs of men and older women, but it may be inadequate for those individuals who have higher iron needs (e.g., menstruating or pregnant women). Table 31-5 lists nutrients needed for erythropoiesis.[8,9]

Malabsorption of iron may occur after certain types of gastrointestinal (GI) surgery and in malabsorption syndromes. Surgical procedures may involve removal or bypass of the duodenum (see Chapter 42). As iron absorption occurs in the duodenum, malabsorption syndromes may involve disease of the duodenum in which the absorption surface is altered or destroyed.

Blood loss is a major cause of iron deficiency in adults. Two milliliters of whole blood contain 1 mg of iron. The major sources of chronic blood loss are from the GI and genitourinary (GU) systems. GI bleeding is often not apparent and therefore may exist for a considerable time before the problem is identified. Loss of 50 to 75 mL of blood from the upper GI tract is required for stools to appear black (*melena*). The black color results from the iron in the RBCs. Common causes of GI blood loss are peptic ulcer, gastritis, esophagitis, diverticuli, hemorrhoids, and neoplasia. GU blood loss occurs primarily from menstrual bleeding. The average monthly menstrual blood loss is about 45 mL and causes the loss of about 22 mg of iron. Postmenopausal bleeding can contribute to anemia in a susceptible older woman. In addition to anemia of chronic kidney disease, dialysis treatment may induce iron-deficiency anemia because of the blood lost in the dialysis equipment and frequent blood sampling.

Clinical Manifestations

In the early course of iron-deficiency anemia the patient may not have any symptoms. As the disease becomes chronic, any of the general manifestations of anemia may develop (see Table 31-3). In addition, specific clinical manifestations may occur related to iron-deficiency anemia. Pallor is the most common finding, and *glossitis* (inflammation of the tongue) is the second most common. Another finding is *cheilitis* (inflammation of the lips). In addition, the patient may report headache, paresthesias,

TABLE 31-5 NUTRITIONAL THERAPY

Nutrients for Erythropoiesis

Role in Erythropoiesis	Food Sources
Cobalamin (Vitamin B$_{12}$)	
RBC maturation	Red meats, especially liver, eggs, enriched grain products, milk and dairy foods, fish
Copper	
Mobilization of iron from tissues to plasma*	Shellfish, whole grains, beans, nuts, potatoes, organ meats, dark green leafy vegetables, dried prunes
Folic Acid	
RBC maturation	Green leafy vegetables, liver, meat, fish, legumes, whole grains, orange juice, peanuts
Iron	
Hemoglobin synthesis	Liver and muscle meats, eggs, dried fruits, legumes, dark green leafy vegetables, whole-grain and enriched bread and cereals, potatoes
Niacin	
Needed for maturation of RBC	High-protein foods such as peanut butter, beans, meats, avocado; enriched and fortified grains
Pantothenic Acid (Vitamin B$_5$)	
Heme synthesis	Meats, vegetables, cereal grains, legumes, eggs, milk
Pyridoxine (Vitamin B$_6$)	
Hemoglobin synthesis	Meats, fortified cereals, whole grains, legumes, potatoes, cornmeal, bananas, nuts
Riboflavin (Vitamin B$_2$)	
Oxidative reactions	Milk and dairy foods, enriched bread and other grain products, salmon, chicken, eggs, leafy green vegetables
Vitamin E	
Possible role in heme synthesis. Protection against oxidative damage to RBCs	Vegetable oils, salad dressings, margarine, wheat germ, whole-grain products, seeds, nuts, peanut butter
Amino Acids	
Synthesis of nucleoproteins	Eggs, meat, milk and milk products (cheese, ice cream), poultry, fish, legumes, nuts
Ascorbic Acid (Vitamin C)	
Conversion of folic acid to its active forms, aids in iron absorption	Citrus fruits, green leafy vegetables, strawberries, cantaloupe

*Supplementation rarely needed and large amounts of copper are poisonous.

and a burning sensation of the tongue, all of which are caused by lack of iron in the tissues.

Diagnostic Studies

Laboratory abnormalities characteristic of iron-deficiency anemia are presented in Table 31-6. Other diagnostic studies (e.g., stool guaiac test) are done to determine the cause of the

TABLE 31-6 LABORATORY STUDY FINDINGS IN ANEMIAS

Etiology of Anemia	Hgb/Hct	MCV	Reticulocytes	Serum Iron	TIBC	Transferrin	Ferritin	Bilirubin	Serum B$_{12}$	Folate
Iron deficiency	↓	↓	N or slight ↓ or ↑	↓	↑	N or ↓	↓	N or ↓	N	N
Thalassemia major	↓	N or ↓	↑	↑	↓	↓	N or ↑	↑	N	↓
Cobalamin deficiency	↓	↑	N or ↓	N or ↑	N	Slight ↑	↑	N or slight ↑	↓	N
Folic acid deficiency	↓	↑	N or ↓	N or ↑	N	Slight ↑	↑	N or slight ↑	N	↓
Aplastic anemia	↓	N or slight ↑	↓	N or ↑	N or ↑	N	N	N	N	N
Chronic disease	↓	N or ↓	N or ↓	N or ↓	↓	N or ↓	N or ↑	N	N	N
Acute blood loss	↓	N or ↓	N or ↑	N	N	N	N	N	N	N
Chronic blood loss	↓	↓	N or ↑	↓	↓	N	N	N or ↓	N	N
Sickle cell anemia	↓	N	↓	N or ↑	N or ↓	N	N	↑	N	↓
Hemolytic anemia	↓	N or ↑	↑	N or ↑	N or ↓	N	N or ↑	↑	N	N

MCV, Mean corpuscular volume; *N,* normal; *TIBC,* total iron-binding capacity.

TABLE 31-7 COLLABORATIVE CARE

Iron-Deficiency Anemia

Diagnostic
- History and physical examination
- Hct and Hgb levels
- RBC count, including morphology
- Reticulocyte count
- Serum iron
- Serum ferritin
- Serum transferrin
- Total iron-binding capacity (TIBC)
- Stool examination for occult blood

Collaborative Therapy
- Identification and treatment of underlying cause
- Ferrous sulfate or ferrous gluconate
- Iron dextran, sodium ferrous gluconate, iron sucrose IM or IV
- Nutritional and diet therapy (see Table 31-5)
- Transfusion of packed RBCs (symptomatic patient only)

iron deficiency. Endoscopy and colonoscopy may be used to detect GI bleeding. A bone marrow biopsy may be done if other tests are inconclusive.

Collaborative Care

The main goal is to treat the underlying disease that is causing reduced intake (e.g., malnutrition, alcoholism) or absorption of iron. In addition, efforts are directed toward replacing iron (Table 31-7). Teach the patient which foods are good sources of iron (see Table 31-5). If nutrition is already adequate, increasing iron intake by dietary means may not be practical. Consequently, oral or occasionally parenteral iron supplements are used. If the iron deficiency is from acute blood loss, the patient may require a transfusion of packed RBCs.

Drug Therapy. Oral iron should be used whenever possible because it is inexpensive and convenient. Many iron preparations are available. When administering iron, consider the following five factors:

1. Iron is absorbed best from the duodenum and proximal jejunum. Therefore enteric-coated or sustained-release capsules, which release iron farther down in the GI tract, are counterproductive and expensive.
2. The daily dose should provide 150 to 200 mg of elemental iron. This can be ingested in three or four daily doses, with each tablet or capsule of the iron preparation containing between 50 and 100 mg of iron (e.g., a 300-mg tablet of ferrous sulfate contains 60 mg of elemental iron).
3. Iron is best absorbed as ferrous sulfate (Fe^{2+}) in an acidic environment. For this reason and to avoid binding the iron with food, iron should be taken about an hour before meals, when the duodenal mucosa is most acidic. Taking iron with vitamin C (ascorbic acid) or orange juice, which contains ascorbic acid, enhances iron absorption. Gastric side effects, however, may necessitate ingesting iron with meals.
4. Undiluted liquid iron may stain the patient's teeth. Therefore it should be diluted and ingested through a straw.
5. GI side effects of iron administration may occur, including heartburn, constipation, and diarrhea. If side effects develop, the dose and type of iron supplement may be adjusted. For example, many individuals who need supplemental iron cannot tolerate ferrous sulfate because of the effects of the sulfate base. However, ferrous gluconate may be an acceptable substitute. Tell patients that the use of iron preparations will cause their stools to become black because the GI tract excretes excess iron. Constipation is common, and the patient should be started on stool softeners and laxatives, if needed, when started on iron.

DRUG ALERT: Iron
- Some preparations of IV iron have a risk of an allergic reaction, and the patient should be monitored accordingly.
- Oral iron should be taken about 1 hr before meals.
- Vitamin C (ascorbic acid) enhances iron absorption.

In some situations it may be necessary to administer iron parenterally. Parenteral use of iron is indicated for malabsorption, intolerance of oral iron, a need for iron beyond oral limits, or poor patient adherence in taking the oral preparations of iron. Parenteral iron can be given intramuscularly (IM) or IV. An iron-dextran complex (INFeD) contains 50 mg/mL of elemental iron available in 2-mL single-dose vials. Sodium ferrous gluconate and iron sucrose are alternatives and may carry less risk of life-threatening anaphylaxis.[10]

Because IM iron solutions may stain the skin, separate needles should be used for withdrawing the solution and for injecting the medication. Use a Z-track injection technique.

NURSING MANAGEMENT
IRON-DEFICIENCY ANEMIA

Certain groups of individuals are at an increased risk for the development of iron-deficiency anemia. These include premenopausal and pregnant women, persons from low socioeconomic backgrounds, older adults, and individuals experiencing blood loss. Diet teaching, with an emphasis on foods high in iron and ways to maximize absorption, is important for these groups.

Appropriate nursing measures are presented in Nursing Care Plan 31-1. Discuss with the patient the need for diagnostic studies to identify the cause. Reassess the hemoglobin and RBC counts to evaluate the response to therapy. Emphasize adherence with dietary and drug therapy. To replenish the body's iron stores, the patient needs to take iron therapy for 2 to 3 months after the hemoglobin level returns to normal. Patients who require lifelong iron supplementation should be monitored for potential liver problems related to the iron storage.

THALASSEMIA

Etiology

Thalassemia is a group of diseases involving inadequate production of normal hemoglobin, and therefore decreased eryth-rocyte production. Thalassemia is due to an absent or reduced globulin protein. α-Globin chains are absent or reduced in α-thalassemia, and β-globin chains are absent or reduced in β-thalassemia. Hemolysis also occurs in thalassemia, but insufficient production of normal hemoglobin is the predominant problem. Thalassemia is commonly found in members of ethnic groups whose origins are near the Mediterranean Sea and equatorial or near-equatorial regions of Asia, the Middle East, and Africa.

 Genetic Link

Thalassemia has an autosomal recessive genetic basis (see Table 13-2). An individual with thalassemia may have a heterozygous or homozygous form of the disease. A person who is heterozygous has one thalassemic gene and one normal gene and is said to have *thalassemia minor* (or thalassemic trait), which is a mild form of the disease. A homozygous person has two thalassemic genes, causing a severe condition known as *thalassemia major*.[11]

Clinical Manifestations

The patient with thalassemia minor is frequently asymptomatic. The patient has mild to moderate anemia with *microcytosis* (small cells) and *hypochromia* (pale cells).

Thalassemia major is a life-threatening disease in which growth, both physical and mental, is often retarded. The person who has thalassemia major is pale and displays other general symptoms of anemia (see Table 31-3). The symptoms develop in childhood by 2 years of age and can cause growth and developmental deficits. Jaundice from the hemolysis of RBCs is prominent. In addition, the person has pronounced splenomegaly, since the spleen continuously tries to remove the damaged red cells. Hepatomegaly and cardiomyopathy may occur from iron deposition. As the bone marrow responds to the reduced oxygen-carrying capacity of the blood, RBC production is stimulated and the marrow becomes packed with immature erythroid precursors that die. This stimulates further erythropoiesis, leading to chronic bone marrow hyperplasia and expansion of the marrow space. This may cause thickening of the cranium and maxillary cavity. Thrombocytosis after spleen dysfunction and/or removal may occur.

Patients with thalassemia may have hepatitis C because of having received blood transfusions before donated blood was screened for hepatitis C virus (screening started in 1992). Hepatitis C may result in cirrhosis and hepatocellular carcinoma. Cardiac complications from iron overload, pulmonary disease, and hypertension also contribute to early death. Endocrinopathies (hypogonadotrophic hypogonadism) and thrombosis may also be complications of the disease.

Collaborative Care

The laboratory abnormalities of thalassemia major are summarized in Table 31-6. No specific drug or diet therapies are effective in treating thalassemia. Thalassemia minor requires no treatment because the body adapts to the reduction of normal hemoglobin.

Thalassemia major is managed with blood transfusions or exchange transfusions in conjunction with oral deferasirox (Exjade), or deferiprone (Ferriprox) or deferoxamine (Desferal) (chelating agents that bind to iron) is given IV or subcutaneously to reduce the iron overloading (hemochromatosis) that occurs with chronic transfusion therapy.[11] Folic acid is given if there is evidence of hemolysis. Transfusions are administered to keep the hemoglobin level at approximately 10 g/dL (100 g/L) to maintain the patient's own erythropoiesis without causing the spleen to enlarge. Zinc supplementation may be needed, since zinc is reduced with chelation therapy. Ascorbic acid supplementation may be needed during chelation therapy, since it increases urine excretion of iron. Other than during chelation therapy, ascorbic acid should not be taken because it increases the absorption of dietary iron. Iron supplements should not be given.

Because RBCs are sequestered in the enlarged spleen, thalassemia major may be treated by splenectomy. Hepatic, cardiac, and pulmonary organ function should be monitored and treated as appropriate.

Although hematopoietic stem cell transplantation (HSCT) remains the only cure for patients with thalassemia, the risk of this procedure may outweigh its benefits. With proper iron chelation therapy, patients are living longer.

MEGALOBLASTIC ANEMIAS

Megaloblastic anemias are a group of disorders caused by impaired DNA synthesis and characterized by the presence of large RBCs. When DNA synthesis is impaired, defective RBC maturation results. The RBCs are large (macrocytic) and abnormal and are referred to as megaloblasts. Macrocytic RBCs are easily destroyed because they have fragile cell membranes. Although the overwhelming majority of megaloblastic anemias result from cobalamin (vitamin B_{12}) and folic acid deficiencies, this type of RBC deformity can also occur from suppression of DNA synthesis by drugs, inborn errors of cobalamin and folic acid metabolism, and erythroleukemia (malignant blood disorder characterized by a proliferation of erythropoietic cells in bone marrow) (Table 31-8).

Cobalamin (Vitamin B_{12}) Deficiency

Normally, a protein termed intrinsic factor (IF) is secreted by the parietal cells of the gastric mucosa. IF is required for cobalamin (extrinsic factor) absorption. (Cobalamin is normally absorbed in the distal ileum.) Therefore if IF is not secreted, cobalamin will not be absorbed.

Etiology

Pernicious Anemia. The most common cause of cobalamin deficiency is pernicious anemia, which is caused by an absence of IF. In pernicious anemia the gastric mucosa is not secreting IF because of either gastric mucosal atrophy or autoimmune destruction of parietal cells. In the autoimmune process antibodies are directed against the gastric parietal cells and/or IF itself. Because parietal cells also secrete hydrochloric acid (HCl), in pernicious anemia there is a decrease in HCl in the stomach. An acid environment in the stomach is required for the secretion of IF.

Pernicious anemia is a disease of insidious onset that begins in middle age or later (usually after age 40), with 60 years being the most common age at diagnosis. Pernicious anemia occurs frequently in persons of Northern European ancestry (particularly Scandinavians) and African Americans. In African Americans the disease tends to begin early, occurs with higher frequency in women, and is often severe.

TABLE 31-8 CLASSIFICATION OF MEGALOBLASTIC ANEMIA

Cobalamin (Vitamin B_{12}) Deficiency
- Dietary deficiency
- Deficiency of gastric intrinsic factor
  - Pernicious anemia
  - Gastrectomy
- Intestinal malabsorption
- Increased requirement
- Chronic alcoholism

Folic Acid Deficiency
- Dietary deficiency (e.g., leafy green vegetables, citrus fruits)
- Malabsorption syndromes
- Drugs interfering with absorption or use of folic acid
  - Methotrexate
  - Antiseizure drugs (e.g., phenobarbital, phenytoin [Dilantin])
- Increased requirement
- Alcohol abuse
- Anorexia
- Hemodialysis patients (folic acid lost during dialysis)

Drug-Induced Suppression of DNA Synthesis
- Folate antagonists
- Metabolic inhibitors
- Alkylating agents

Inborn Errors
- Defective folate metabolism
- Defective transport of cobalamin

Erythroleukemia

Other Causes of Cobalamin Deficiency. Cobalamin deficiency can also occur in patients who have had GI surgery (e.g., gastrectomy, gastric bypass); patients who have had a small bowel resection involving the ileum; and patients with Crohn's disease, ileitis, celiac disease, diverticuli of the small intestine, or chronic atrophic gastritis (see Table 31-8). In these cases, cobalamin deficiency results from the loss of IF-secreting gastric mucosal cells or impaired absorption of cobalamin in the distal ileum. Cobalamin deficiency is also found in chronic alcoholics, long-term users of H_2-histamine receptor blockers and proton pump inhibitors, and those who are strict vegetarians.[2,3]

Clinical Manifestations

General manifestations of anemia related to cobalamin deficiency develop because of tissue hypoxia (see Table 31-3). GI manifestations include a sore, red, beefy, and shiny tongue; anorexia, nausea, and vomiting; and abdominal pain. Typical neuromuscular manifestations include weakness, paresthesias of the feet and hands, reduced vibratory and position senses, ataxia, muscle weakness, and impaired thought processes ranging from confusion to dementia. Because cobalamin deficiency–related anemia has an insidious onset, it may take several months for these manifestations to develop.

Diagnostic Studies

Laboratory data reflective of cobalamin deficiency anemia are presented in Table 31-6. The RBCs appear large (macrocytic) and have abnormal shapes. This structure contributes to erythrocyte destruction because the cell membrane is fragile. Serum cobalamin levels are reduced.

Serum folate levels are also obtained. If they are normal and cobalamin levels are low, it suggests that megaloblastic anemia is due to a cobalamin deficiency. A serum test for anti-IF antibodies may be done that is specific for pernicious anemia. Because the potential for gastric cancer is increased in patients with pernicious anemia, an upper GI endoscopy and biopsy of the gastric mucosa may also be done.

Testing of serum methylmalonic acid (MMA) (elevated mainly in cobalamin deficiency) and serum homocysteine (elevated in both cobalamin and folic acid deficiencies) helps determine the cause of this type of anemia.

Collaborative Care

Regardless of how much is ingested, the patient is not able to absorb cobalamin if IF is lacking or if absorption in the ileum is impaired. For this reason, increasing dietary cobalamin does not correct this anemia. However, instruct the patient on adequate dietary intake to maintain good nutrition (see Table 31-5).

Parenteral vitamin B_{12} (cyanocobalamin or hydroxocobalamin) or intranasal cyanocobalamin (Nascobal, CaloMist) is the treatment of choice. Without cobalamin administration, these individuals will die in 1 to 3 years. A typical treatment schedule consists of 1000 mcg/day of cobalamin IM for 2 weeks and then weekly until the hemoglobin is normal, and then monthly for life. High-dose oral cobalamin and sublingual cobalamin are also available for those in whom GI absorption is intact. As long as supplemental cobalamin is used, the anemia can be reversed. However, if the person has had long-standing neuromuscular complications, they may not be reversible.

Folic Acid Deficiency

Folic acid (folate) deficiency also causes megaloblastic anemia. Folic acid is required for DNA synthesis leading to RBC formation and maturation. Common causes of folic acid deficiency are listed in Table 31-8.

The clinical manifestations of folic acid deficiency are similar to those of cobalamin deficiency. The disease develops insidiously, and the patient's symptoms may be attributed to other coexisting problems (e.g., cirrhosis, esophageal varices). GI disturbances include dyspepsia and a smooth, beefy red tongue. The absence of neurologic problems is an important diagnostic finding and differentiates folic acid deficiency from cobalamin deficiency.

The diagnostic findings for folic acid deficiency are presented in Table 31-6. In addition, the serum folate level is low (normal is 3 to 25 mg/mL [7 to 57 mol/L]) and the serum cobalamin level is normal.

Folic acid deficiency is treated by replacement therapy. The usual dosage is 1 mg/day by mouth. In malabsorption states or with chronic alcoholism, up to 5 mg/day may be required. The duration of treatment depends on the reason for the deficiency. Encourage the patient to eat foods containing large amounts of folic acid (see Table 31-5).

NURSING MANAGEMENT
MEGALOBLASTIC ANEMIA

Because of the familial predisposition for pernicious anemia, the most common type of cobalamin deficiency, patients who have a positive family history of pernicious anemia should be evaluated for symptoms. Although the disease cannot be prevented, early detection and treatment can lead to reversal of symptoms. Also consider signs and symptoms of other possible megaloblastic anemias and bring them to the attention of the health care provider.

The nursing measures presented in Nursing Care Plan 31-1, for the patient with anemia, are appropriate for the patient with cobalamin or folic acid deficiency anemia. In addition to these measures, ensure that injuries are not sustained because of the diminished sensitivity to heat and pain resulting from the neurologic impairment. Protect the patient from falling, burns, and trauma. If heat therapy is required, evaluate the patient's skin at frequent intervals to detect redness.

Ongoing care focuses on ensuring good patient adherence with treatment. Carefully assess for neurologic difficulties that were not fully corrected by adequate replacement therapy. Because the potential for gastric cancer may be increased in patients with atrophic gastritis-related pernicious anemia, the patient should have frequent and careful appropriate screenings.

ANEMIA OF CHRONIC DISEASE

Anemia of chronic disease (also called anemia of inflammation) can be caused by chronic inflammation, autoimmune and infectious disorders (human immunodeficiency virus [HIV], hepatitis, malaria), HF, or malignant diseases. Bleeding episodes can also contribute to anemia of chronic disease.

Anemia of chronic disease is associated with an underproduction of RBCs and mild shortening of RBC survival. The RBCs are usually normocytic, normochromic, and hypoproliferative. The anemia is usually mild, but it can become more severe if the underlying disorder is not treated.

This type of anemia, which usually develops after 1 to 2 months of disease activity, has an immune basis. The cytokines released in these conditions, particularly interleukin 6 (IL-6), cause an increased uptake and retention of iron within macrophages (see Fig. 30-3). This leads to a diversion of iron from circulation into storage sites with subsequent limited iron available for erythropoiesis. There is also reduced RBC life span, suppressed production of erythropoietin, and an ineffective bone marrow response to erythropoietin.[12]

For any chronic disease, additional factors may contribute to the anemia. For example, with renal disease, the primary factor causing anemia is decreased erythropoietin, a hormone made in the kidneys that stimulates erythropoiesis. With impaired renal function, erythropoietin production is decreased (see Chapter 47).

Anemia of chronic disease must first be recognized and differentiated from anemia of other etiologies. Findings of elevated serum ferritin and increased iron stores distinguish it from iron-deficiency anemia. Normal folate and cobalamin blood levels distinguish it from those types of anemias. The best treatment of anemia of chronic disease is correction of the underlying disorder. If the anemia is severe, blood transfusions may be indicated, but they are not recommended for long-term treatment. Erythropoietin therapy (epoetin alfa [Epogen], darbepoetin) is used for anemia related to renal disease (see Chapter 47) and may be used for anemia related to cancer and its therapies (see Chapter 16 and Table 16-14). However, erythropoietin therapy needs to be used conservatively because of the increased risk of thromboembolism and death in some patients.[12,13] IV iron may be administered, if necessary, to improve the response to therapy with erythropoietin.

APLASTIC ANEMIA

Aplastic anemia is a disease in which the patient has peripheral blood *pancytopenia* (decrease of all blood cell types—RBCs, white blood cells [WBCs], and platelets) and hypocellular bone marrow. The spectrum of the anemia can range from a chronic condition managed with erythropoietin or blood transfusions to a critical condition with hemorrhage and sepsis. The incidence of aplastic anemia is low, affecting approximately 2 of every 1 million persons per year.[14]

Etiology

Aplastic anemia has various etiologic classifications, but is divided into two major groups: *congenital* or *acquired* (Table 31-9). Approximately 75% of the acquired aplastic anemias are idiopathic and thought to have an autoimmune basis.

Clinical Manifestations

Aplastic anemia can manifest abruptly (over days) or insidiously over weeks to months and can vary from mild to severe. Clinically the patient may have symptoms caused by suppression of any or all bone marrow elements. General manifestations of anemia such as fatigue and dyspnea, as well as cardiovascular and cerebral responses, may be seen (see Table 31-3). The patient with neutropenia (low neutrophil count) is susceptible to infection and is at risk for septic shock and death. Even a low-grade fever (above 100.4° F [38° C]) should be considered a medical emergency. Thrombocytopenia is manifested by a predisposition to bleeding (e.g., petechiae, ecchymosis, epistaxis).

Diagnostic Studies

The diagnosis is confirmed by laboratory studies. Because all marrow elements are affected, hemoglobin, WBC, and platelet values are often decreased in aplastic anemia. Other RBC indices are generally normal (see Table 31-6). The condition is therefore classified as a normocytic, normochromic anemia. The reticulocyte count is low. Bleeding time is prolonged.

Aplastic anemia can be further evaluated by assessing various iron studies. The serum iron and total iron-binding capacity (TIBC) may be elevated as initial signs of erythropoiesis suppression. Bone marrow biopsy, aspiration, and pathologic examination may be done for any anemic state. However, the findings are especially important in aplastic anemia because the marrow is hypocellular with increased yellow marrow (fat content).

TABLE 31-9	CAUSES OF APLASTIC ANEMIA
Congenital (Chromosomal Alterations)	**Acquired**
• Fanconi syndrome • Congenital dyskeratosis • Amegakaryocytic thrombocytopenia • Shwachman-Diamond syndrome	• Idiopathic or autoimmune • Chemical agents and toxins (e.g., benzene, insecticides, arsenic, alcohol) • Drugs (e.g., alkylating agents, antiseizure drugs, antimetabolites, antimicrobials, gold) • Radiation • Viral and bacterial infections (e.g., hepatitis, parvovirus)

NURSING AND COLLABORATIVE MANAGEMENT APLASTIC ANEMIA

Management of aplastic anemia is based on identifying and removing the causative agent (when possible) and providing supportive care until the pancytopenia reverses. Nursing interventions appropriate for the patient with pancytopenia from aplastic anemia are presented in Nursing Care Plan 31-1 for anemia and in eNursing Care Plan 31-1 for thrombocytopenia and eNursing Care Plan 31-2 for neutropenia (available on the website for this chapter). Nursing actions are directed at preventing complications from infection and hemorrhage.

The prognosis of severe untreated aplastic anemia is poor. The median survival of untreated severe aplastic anemia is 3 to 6 months (20% survive longer than 1 year).[3] However, advances in medical management, including HSCT and immunosuppressive therapy with antithymocyte globulin (ATG) and cyclosporine or high-dose cyclophosphamide (Cytoxan), have improved outcomes significantly. ATG is a horse serum that contains polyclonal antibodies against human T cells. It can cause anaphylaxis and a serum sickness. The rationale for this therapy is that idiopathic aplastic anemia is considered an autoimmune disorder resulting from activated cytotoxic T cells that target and destroy the patient's own hematopoietic stem cells. (ATG and cyclosporine are discussed in Chapter 14 and Table 14-16.)

The treatment of choice for adults less than 55 years of age who do not respond to the immunosuppressive therapy and who have a human leukocyte antigen (HLA)–matched donor is an HSCT. The best results occur in younger patients who have not had previous blood transfusions. Prior transfusions increase the risk of graft rejection. (HSCT is discussed in Chapter 16.)

For older adults without an HLA-matched donor, the treatment of choice is immunosuppression with ATG or cyclosporine or high-dose cyclophosphamide. High-dose corticosteroids may also be used. However, this therapy may be only partially beneficial. Patients who need ongoing supportive blood transfusion should be on an iron-binding agent to prevent iron overload.

ANEMIA CAUSED BY BLOOD LOSS

Anemia resulting from blood loss may be caused by either acute or chronic problems.

ACUTE BLOOD LOSS

Acute blood loss occurs as a result of sudden hemorrhage. Causes of acute blood loss include trauma, complications of surgery, and conditions or diseases that disrupt vascular integrity. There are two clinical concerns in such situations. First, a sudden reduction in the total blood volume can lead to hypovolemic shock. Second, if the acute loss is more gradual, the body maintains its blood volume by slowly increasing the plasma volume. Although the circulating fluid volume is preserved, the number of RBCs available to carry oxygen is significantly diminished.

Clinical Manifestations

The clinical manifestations of anemia from acute blood loss are caused by the body's attempts to maintain an adequate blood

TABLE 31-10 MANIFESTATIONS OF ACUTE BLOOD LOSS

Volume Lost*		Manifestations
%	**mL**	
10	500	None or rare vasovagal syncope.
20	1000	No detectable signs or symptoms at rest. Tachycardia with exercise and slight postural hypotension.
30	1500	Normal supine blood pressure and pulse at rest. Postural hypotension and tachycardia with exercise.
40	2000	Blood pressure, central venous pressure, and cardiac output below normal at rest; air hunger; rapid, thready pulse and cold, clammy skin.
50	2500	Shock, lactic acidosis, and potential death.

*Based on an adult with a total blood volume of 5 L.

volume and meet oxygen requirements. Table 31-10 summarizes the clinical manifestations of patients with varying degrees of blood volume loss. It is essential to understand that the clinical signs and symptoms the patient is experiencing are more important than the laboratory values. For example, an adult with a bleeding peptic ulcer who had a 750-mL hematemesis (15% of a normal total blood volume) within the past 30 minutes may have postural hypotension, but have normal values for hemoglobin and hematocrit. Over the next 36 to 48 hours, most of the blood volume deficit will be replaced by the movement of fluid from the extravascular into the intravascular space. Only then will the hemoglobin and hematocrit reflect the blood loss.

Assess the patient's expression of pain. Internal hemorrhage may cause pain because of tissue distention, organ displacement, and nerve compression. Pain may be localized or referred. In the case of retroperitoneal bleeding, the patient may not experience abdominal pain. Instead the patient may have numbness and pain in a lower extremity secondary to compression of the lateral cutaneous nerve, which is located in the region of the first to third lumbar vertebrae. The major complication of acute blood loss is shock (see Chapter 67).

Diagnostic Studies

When blood volume loss is sudden, plasma volume has not yet had a chance to increase, the loss of RBCs is not reflected in laboratory data, and values may seem normal or high for 2 to 3 days. However, once the plasma volume is replaced, the RBC mass is less concentrated. At this time, RBC, hemoglobin, and hematocrit levels are low and reflect the actual blood loss.

Collaborative Care

Collaborative care is initially concerned with (1) replacing blood volume to prevent shock and (2) identifying the source of the hemorrhage and stopping the blood loss. IV fluids used in emergencies include dextran, hetastarch, albumin, and crystalloid electrolyte solutions such as lactated Ringer's solution. The amount of infusion varies with the solution used. (Management of shock is discussed in Chapter 67.)

Once volume replacement is established, attention can be directed to correcting the RBC loss. The body needs 2 to 5 days to manufacture more RBCs in response to increased erythropoietin. Consequently, blood transfusions (packed RBCs) may be needed if the blood loss is significant. In addition, if the bleeding is related to a platelet or clotting disorder, replacement of that deficiency is addressed.

The patient may also need supplemental iron because the availability of iron affects the marrow production of erythrocytes. When anemia exists after acute blood loss, dietary sources of iron will probably not be adequate to maintain iron stores. Therefore oral or parenteral iron preparations are administered.

NURSING MANAGEMENT ACUTE BLOOD LOSS

In the case of trauma it may be impossible to prevent the loss of blood. For the postoperative patient, carefully monitor the blood loss from various drainage tubes and dressings and implement appropriate actions. The nursing care for the patient with anemia resulting from acute blood loss most likely includes administration of blood products (described at the end of this chapter).

The anemia should begin to correct itself once the source of hemorrhage is identified, blood loss is controlled, and fluid and blood volumes are replaced. There should be no need for long-term treatment of this type of anemia.

CHRONIC BLOOD LOSS

The sources of chronic blood loss are similar to those of iron-deficiency anemia (e.g., bleeding ulcer, hemorrhoids, menstrual and postmenopausal blood loss). The effects of chronic blood loss are usually related to the depletion of iron stores and considered as iron-deficiency anemia. Management of chronic blood loss anemia involves identifying the source and stopping the bleeding. Supplemental iron may be required.

ANEMIA CAUSED BY INCREASED ERYTHROCYTE DESTRUCTION

The third major cause of anemia is termed hemolytic anemia, a condition caused by the destruction or hemolysis of RBCs at a rate that exceeds production. Hemolysis can occur because of problems intrinsic or extrinsic to the RBCs. *Intrinsic hemolytic anemias,* which are usually hereditary, result from defects in the RBCs themselves (see Table 31-2).

More common are the *acquired hemolytic anemias.* In this type of anemia the RBCs are normal, but damage is caused by external factors (see Table 31-2). The spleen is the primary site of the destruction of RBCs that are old, defective, or moderately damaged. Fig. 31-2 indicates the sequence of events involved in extravascular hemolysis.

The patient with hemolytic anemia has the general manifestations of anemia and specific manifestations related to this type of anemia (see Table 31-3). Jaundice is likely because the increased destruction of RBCs causes an elevation in bilirubin levels. The spleen and liver may enlarge because of their hyperactivity, which is related to macrophage phagocytosis of the defective erythrocytes.

In all causes of hemolysis, a major focus of treatment is to maintain renal function. When RBCs are hemolyzed, the hemoglobin molecule is released and filtered by the kidneys. The accumulation of hemoglobin molecules can obstruct the renal tubules and lead to acute tubular necrosis (see Chapter 47).

FIG. 31-2 Sequence of events in extravascular hemolysis.

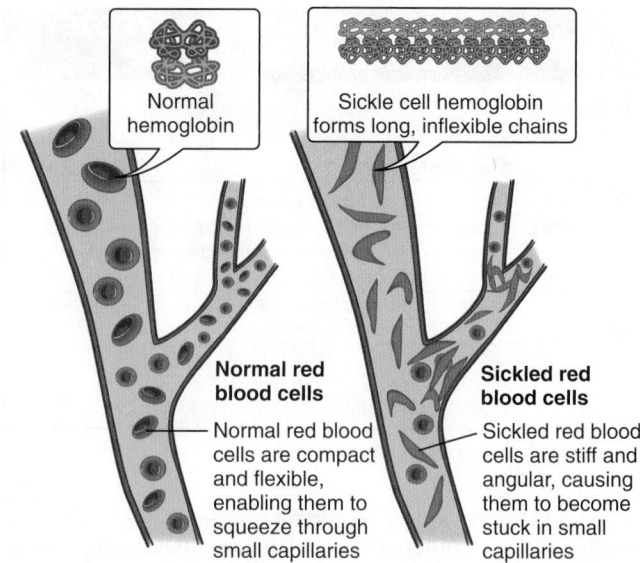

FIG. 31-3 In sickle cell, the hemoglobin forms long inflexible chains and alters the shape of the red blood cells (RBCs). The sickled RBCs can become stuck in the capillaries and occlude the blood flow.

SICKLE CELL DISEASE

Sickle cell disease (SCD) is a group of inherited, autosomal recessive disorders characterized by an abnormal form of hemoglobin in the RBC. (Autosomal recessive genetic disorders are discussed in Chapter 13 and Table 13-2.) Because this is a genetic disorder, SCD is usually identified during infancy or early childhood. It is an incurable disease that is often fatal by middle age because of renal failure, infection, pulmonary failure, and/or stroke.[3]

SCD affects about 100,000 Americans and is predominant in African Americans, occurring in an estimated 1 in about 500 live births. It can also affect people of Mediterranean, Caribbean, South and Central American, Arabian, or East Indian ancestry.[15]

Etiology and Pathophysiology
Genetic Link

In SCD the abnormal hemoglobin, *hemoglobin S* (Hgb S), results from the substitution of valine for glutamic acid on the β-globin chain of hemoglobin (see Fig. 13-3). Hgb S causes the erythrocyte to stiffen and elongate, taking on a sickle shape in response to low oxygen levels (Fig. 31-3).

Types of SCD disorders include sickle cell anemia, sickle cell–thalassemia, sickle cell Hgb C disease, and sickle cell trait. *Sickle cell anemia,* the most severe of the SCD syndromes, occurs when a person is homozygous for hemoglobin S (Hgb SS); the person has inherited Hgb S from both parents. *Sickle cell–thalassemia* and *sickle cell Hgb C* occur when a person inherits Hgb S from one parent and another type of abnormal hemoglobin (such as thalassemia or hemoglobin C) from the other parent. Both of these forms of SCD are less common and less severe than sickle cell anemia. *Sickle cell trait* occurs when a person is heterozygous for hemoglobin S (Hgb AS); the person has inherited hemoglobin S from one parent and normal hemoglobin (Hgb A) from the other parent. Sickle cell trait is typically a mild to asymptomatic condition.

Sickling Episodes. The major pathophysiologic event of SCD is the sickling of RBCs (see Fig. 31-3). Sickling episodes are most commonly triggered by low oxygen tension in the blood. Hypoxia or deoxygenation of the RBCs can be caused by viral or bacterial infection, high altitude, emotional or physical stress, surgery, and blood loss. Infection is the most common precipitating factor. Other events that can trigger or sustain a sickling episode include dehydration, increased hydrogen ion concentration (acidosis), increased plasma osmolality, decreased plasma volume, and low body temperature. A sickling episode can also occur without an obvious cause.

Sickled RBCs become rigid and take on an elongated, crescent shape (see Fig. 31-3). Sickled cells cannot easily pass through capillaries or other small vessels and can cause vascular occlusion, leading to acute or chronic tissue injury. The resulting hemostasis promotes a self-perpetuating cycle of local hypoxia, deoxygenation of more erythrocytes, and more sickling. Circulating sickled cells are hemolyzed by the spleen, leading to anemia. Initially the sickling of cells is reversible with reoxygenation, but it eventually becomes irreversible because of cell membrane damage from recurrent sickling. Thus vaso-occlusive phenomena and hemolysis are the clinical hallmarks of SCD.

Sickle cell crisis is a severe, painful, acute exacerbation of RBC sickling causing a vaso-occlusive crisis. As blood flow is impaired by sickled cells, vasospasm occurs, further restricting blood flow. Severe capillary hypoxia causes changes in membrane permeability, leading to plasma loss, hemoconcentration, thrombi, and further circulatory stagnation. Tissue ischemia, infarction, and necrosis eventually occur from lack of oxygen. Shock is a possible life-threatening consequence of sickle cell crisis because of severe oxygen depletion of the tissues and a reduction of the circulating fluid volume. Sickle cell crisis can begin suddenly and persist for days to weeks.

The frequency, extent, and severity of sickling episodes are highly variable and unpredictable, but largely depend on the percentage of Hgb S present. Individuals with sickle cell anemia have the most severe form because the erythrocytes contain a high percentage of Hgb S.

GENETICS IN CLINICAL PRACTICE

Sickle Cell Disease

Genetic Basis
- Autosomal recessive disorder.
- Mutation in β-globin *(HBB)* gene located on chromosome 11.
- Various versions of β-globin result from different mutations in the *HBB* gene.
- Hgb S variant involves substitution of valine for glutamic acid in the β-globin gene in sickle cell anemia.

Incidence
- Most common inherited blood disorder in the United States.
- Affects 8 of every 100,000 people.
- Affects 1 in 350 to 500 African Americans.
- Affects 1 in 1000 to 1400 Hispanic Americans.
- Also affects people of Mediterranean, Caribbean, Arabian, and East Indian descent.

Genetic Testing
- DNA testing is available.
- Electrophoresis of hemoglobin and sickling screening test are more commonly used.

Clinical Implications
- Requires ongoing continuity of care and extensive patient teaching.
- Sickle cell trait is the carrier state for sickle cell disease and represents a mild type of sickle cell disease; 1 in 10 to 12 African Americans and 1 in 25 Hispanics have sickle cell trait.
- If both parents have the trait, there is a 1 in 4 chance that their baby will have sickle cell disease.
- Management of sickle cell disease should focus on the prevention of sickle cell crisis (e.g., prevention of dehydration and infection).
- Genetic counseling is recommended for individuals with a family history of sickle cell disease. Individuals should understand the risks of transmitting the genetic mutation.

Clinical Manifestations

The effects of SCD vary greatly from person to person, the severity of which may be due to genetic polymorphisms. Many people with sickle cell anemia are in reasonably good health the majority of the time. However, they may have chronic health problems and pain because of organ tissue hypoxia and damage (e.g., involving the kidneys or liver).

The typical patient is anemic but asymptomatic except during sickling episodes. Because most individuals with sickle cell anemia have dark skin, pallor is more readily detected by examining the mucous membranes. The skin may have a grayish cast. Because of the hemolysis, jaundice is common and patients are prone to gallstones (cholelithiasis).

The primary symptom associated with sickling is pain. The pain severity can range from trivial to excruciating. During sickle cell crisis the pain is severe because of ischemia of tissue. The episodes can affect any area of the body or several sites simultaneously, with the back, chest, extremities, and abdomen being most commonly affected. Pain episodes are often accompanied by clinical manifestations such as fever, swelling, tenderness, tachypnea, hypertension, nausea, and vomiting.

Complications

With repeated episodes of sickling, there is gradual involvement of all body systems, especially the spleen, lungs, kidneys, and brain. Organs that have a high need for oxygen are most often affected and form the basis for many of the complications of SCD (Fig. 31-4). Infection is a major cause of morbidity and mortality in patients with SCD. One reason for this is the failure of the spleen to phagocytize foreign substances as it becomes infarcted and dysfunctional (usually by 2 to 4 years of age) from the sickled RBCs. The spleen becomes small because of repeated scarring, a phenomenon termed *autosplenectomy.*

Pneumonia is the most common infection and often is of pneumococcal origin. Infections can be so severe that they cause an aplastic and hemolytic crisis and gallstones. *Aplastic crisis* can be so severe that it causes a temporary shutdown of RBC production in the bone marrow.

Acute chest syndrome is a term used to describe acute pulmonary complications that include pneumonia, tissue infarction, and fat embolism. It is characterized by fever, chest pain, cough, pulmonary infiltrates, and dyspnea. Pulmonary infarctions may cause pulmonary hypertension, MI, HF, and ultimately cor pulmonale. The heart may become ischemic and enlarged, leading to HF. Retinal vessel obstruction may result in hemorrhage, scarring, retinal detachment, and blindness. The kidneys may be injured from the increased blood viscosity and the lack of oxygen, and renal failure may occur. Pulmonary embolism or stroke can result from thrombosis and infarction of cerebral blood vessels. Bone changes may include osteoporosis and osteosclerosis after infarction. Chronic leg ulcers can result from the hypoxia and are especially prevalent around the ankles. *Priapism* (persistent penile erection) may occur if penile veins become occluded.

Diagnostic Studies

A peripheral blood smear may reveal sickled cells and abnormal reticulocytes. The presence of Hgb S can be diagnosed by the sickling test, which uses RBCs (in vitro) and exposes them to a deoxygenation agent.

As a result of the accelerated RBC breakdown, the patient has characteristic clinical findings of hemolysis (jaundice, elevated serum bilirubin levels) and abnormal laboratory test results (see Table 31-6). Hemoglobin electrophoresis may be done to determine the amount of hemoglobin S. Skeletal x-rays demonstrate bone and joint deformities and flattening. Magnetic resonance imaging (MRI) may be used to diagnose a stroke caused by blocked cerebral vessels from sickled cells. Doppler studies may be used to assess for deep vein thromboses. Other tests may be indicated, such as a chest x-ray, to diagnose infection or organ malfunction.

NURSING AND COLLABORATIVE MANAGEMENT SICKLE CELL DISEASE

Collaborative care for a patient with SCD is directed toward (1) alleviating the symptoms from the complications of the disease; (2) minimizing end-organ damage; and (3) promptly treating serious sequelae, such as acute chest syndrome, that can lead to immediate death. Teach patients with SCD to avoid high altitudes, maintain adequate fluid intake, and treat infections promptly. Pneumovax, *Haemophilus influenzae,* influenza, and hepatitis immunizations should be administered. Chronic leg ulcers may be treated with rest, antibiotics, warm saline soaks, mechanical or enzyme debridement, and grafting if necessary.

Priapism is managed with pain medication, fluids, and nifedipine (Procardia). If it does not resolve within a few hours, a urologist can be called to inject the corpus cavernosum with a dilute solution of epinephrine to preserve penile function.

Sickle cell crises may require hospitalization. Oxygen may be administered to treat hypoxia and control sickling. Because

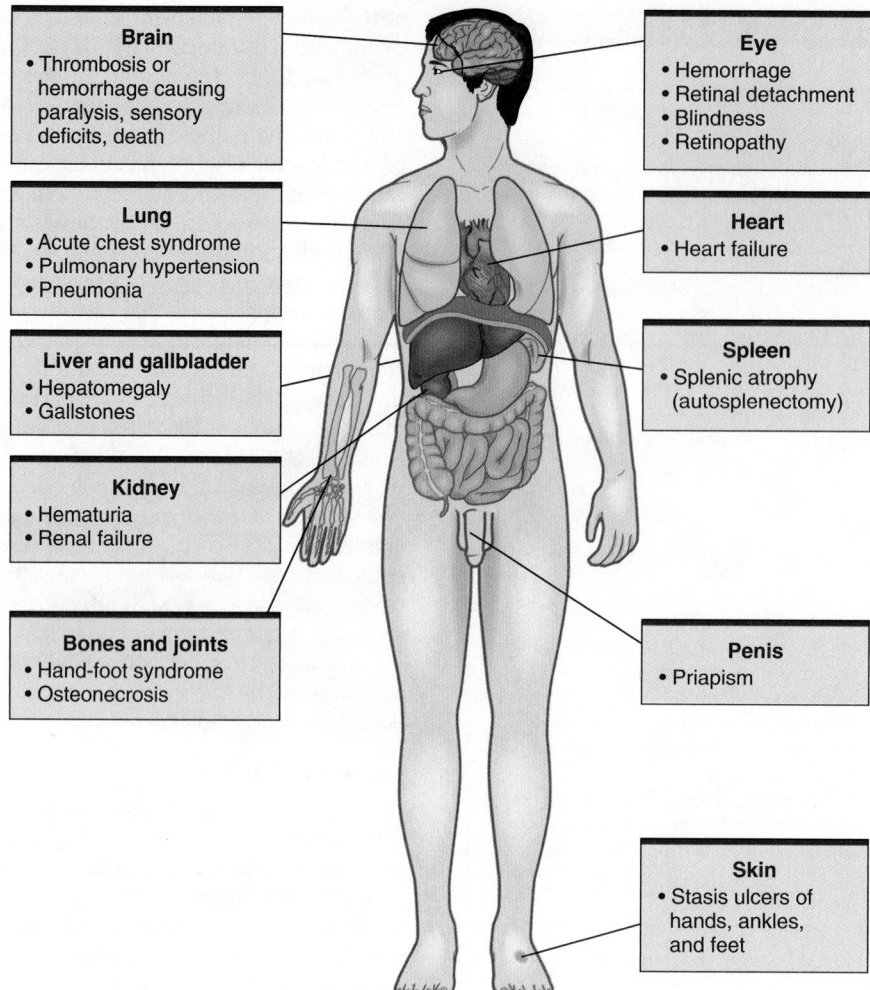

Brain
• Thrombosis or hemorrhage causing paralysis, sensory deficits, death

Lung
• Acute chest syndrome
• Pulmonary hypertension
• Pneumonia

Liver and gallbladder
• Hepatomegaly
• Gallstones

Kidney
• Hematuria
• Renal failure

Bones and joints
• Hand-foot syndrome
• Osteonecrosis

Eye
• Hemorrhage
• Retinal detachment
• Blindness
• Retinopathy

Heart
• Heart failure

Spleen
• Splenic atrophy (autosplenectomy)

Penis
• Priapism

Skin
• Stasis ulcers of hands, ankles, and feet

FIG. 31-4 Clinical manifestations and complications of sickle cell disease.

respiratory failure is the most common cause of death, vigilantly assess for any changes in respiratory status.[16] Rest may be instituted to reduce metabolic requirements, and deep vein thrombosis prophylaxis (using anticoagulants) should be prescribed. Fluids and electrolytes are administered to reduce blood viscosity and maintain renal function. Transfusion therapy is indicated when an aplastic crisis occurs. Aggressive total RBC exchange transfusion programs may be implemented for patients who have frequent crises or serious complications such as acute chest syndrome. These patients, like those with thalassemia major, may require iron chelation therapy to reduce transfusion-produced iron overload.

Undertreatment of sickle cell pain is a major problem. Lack of understanding can lead health care professionals to underestimate how much pain these patients suffer. Patients, because of their prior opioid treatment, may be tolerant, and thus large doses may be needed to reduce the pain to a tolerable level. During an acute crisis, optimal pain control usually includes large doses of continuous (rather than as-needed [PRN]) opioid analgesics along with breakthrough analgesia, often in the form of patient-controlled analgesia (PCA) (PCA is discussed in Chapter 9). Morphine and hydromorphone are the drugs of choice. Meperidine (Demerol) is contraindicated because high doses can lead to the accumulation of a toxic metabolite, normeperidine, which can cause seizures.

Because patients may be experiencing different types and sites of pain, a multimodal and interdisciplinary approach should be used that incorporates emotional aspects of pain (see Chapter 9). Adjunctive measures, such as nonsteroidal antiinflammatory agents, antineuropathic pain medications (e.g., tricyclic antidepressants, antiseizure medications), local anesthetics, or nerve blocks may be used.

Although pain is the most common symptom of patients with SCD seeking medical care, infection is a frequent complication and must be treated. Patients with acute chest syndrome are treated with broad-spectrum antibiotics, O_2 therapy, fluid therapy, and possibly exchange transfusion. Blood transfusions have little if any role in the treatment between crises, since patients develop antibodies to RBCs and iron overload. However, because chronic hemolysis results in increased use of folic acid stores, routine oral folic acid should be taken.

Although many antisickling agents have been tried, hydroxyurea (Hydrea), which is a chemotherapy drug, is the only one that has been shown to be clinically beneficial.[17] This drug increases the production of hemoglobin F (fetal hemoglobin), decreases the reactive neutrophil count, increases RBC volume and hydration, and alters the adhesion of sickle RBCs to the endothelium. The increase in Hgb F is accompanied by a reduction in hemolysis, an increase in hemoglobin concentration, and a decrease in sickled cells and painful crises.[11]

ETHICAL/LEGAL DILEMMAS

Pain Management

Situation

N.C., a 21-year-old African American man, is admitted to the emergency department (ED) in sickle cell crisis with complaints of excruciating pain. He is known to several of the nurses and physicians in the ED. One of the nurses remarks to you that it must be time for his "fix" of pain drugs.

Ethical/Legal Points for Consideration

• The standard of care for pain requires that (1) a pain assessment is done based on the patient's self-report, (2) the best possible relief of pain is provided under the circumstances, and (3) competent and compassionate care is provided to all patients.

• The pain assessment also includes reviewing the patient's medical record to determine if there are health care issues or conditions (e.g., frequent ED visits to request pain medication) that may affect the patient's response to pain and pain management.

• As a nurse, you have a duty to notify the health care professional of those issues or conditions. You also need to document behaviors exhibited by the patient related to pain management. Make sure that the documentation is objective (factual observations) rather than labeling (the patient was in withdrawal).

• When pain relief is inadequate, as a nurse, you are responsible for notifying the health care professional. Efforts to notify must continue and be appropriately documented until the managing health care professional has assessed the patient and made a plan of care based on that assessment.

Discussion Questions

1. How can you educate your colleagues regarding pain assessment and management?
2. What important factors would need to be included in your assessment and management of N.C.?

Hematopoietic stem cell transplantation (HSCT) is the only available treatment that can cure some patients with SCD. The selection of appropriate recipients, scarcity of appropriate donors, risk, and cost-effectiveness limit the use of HSCT for SCD. (HSCT is discussed in Chapter 16.)

Patient teaching and support are important in the long-term care of the patient with SCD. The patient and caregiver must understand the basis of the disease and the reasons for supportive care and ongoing pertinent screening tailored to SCD manifestations, such as eye examinations. Teach the patient ways to avoid crises, including taking steps to avoid dehydration and hypoxia, such as avoiding high altitudes and seeking medical attention quickly to counteract problems such as upper respiratory tract infections. Teaching about pain control is also needed because the pain during a crisis may be severe and often requires considerable analgesia. Minor pain episodes that are not associated with infection or other symptoms warranting medical attention can sometimes be managed at home.

Recurrent episodes of severe acute pain and unrelenting chronic pain can be disabling and depressing. The quality of life of patients with SCD can be profoundly affected. Occupational and physical therapists can help the patient achieve optimum physical functioning and independence. Cognitive behavioral therapy may help patients with SCD cope with anxiety and depression. Support groups may also be helpful.

ACQUIRED HEMOLYTIC ANEMIA

Acquired hemolytic anemia results from hemolysis of RBCs from extrinsic factors. These factors can be separated into four categories: (1) macroangiopathic (physical trauma), (2) micro-angiopathic, (3) antibody reactions, and (4) infectious agents and toxins (see Table 31-2).

Macroangiopathic or physical destruction of RBCs results from the exertion of extreme force on the cells. Traumatic events causing disruption of the RBC membrane include hemodialysis, extracorporeal circulation used in cardiopulmonary bypass, and prosthetic heart valves. In addition, the force needed to push blood through abnormal vessels, such as those that have been burned, irradiated, or affected by vascular disease (e.g., diabetes mellitus), may also physically damage RBCs.

Microangiopathic destruction of RBCs is a result of fragmentation of the cells as they try to pass by abnormal arterial or venous microcirculation. The RBCs are sheared as they try to pass by excessive platelet aggregation and/or fibrin polymer formation, such as is seen in thrombotic thrombocytopenic purpura (TTP) and disseminated intravascular coagulation (DIC) (discussed later in this chapter).

Antibodies may destroy RBCs by the mechanisms involved in antigen-antibody reactions. The reactions may be of an isoimmune or autoimmune type. *Isoimmune reactions* occur when antibodies develop against antigens from another person of the same species. In blood transfusion reactions the recipient's antibodies hemolyze donor cells. *Autoimmune reactions* result when individuals develop antibodies against their own RBCs. Autoimmune hemolytic reactions may be idiopathic, developing with no prior hemolytic history as a result of immunoglobulin G (IgG) covering the RBCs, or secondary to other autoimmune diseases (e.g., systemic lupus erythematosus), leukemia, lymphoma, or medications (penicillin, ibuprofen, metformin, chlorpromazine, procainamide).

Infectious agents and toxins cause the fourth type of acquired hemolytic disorder. Infectious agents cause hemolysis in three ways: (1) by invading the RBC and destroying its contents (e.g., parasites such as in malaria), (2) by releasing hemolytic substances (e.g., *Clostridium perfringens*), and (3) by generating an antigen-antibody reaction (e.g., *Mycoplasma pneumoniae*). Various agents may be toxic to RBCs and cause hemolysis. These hemolytic toxins involve chemicals such as oxidative drugs, arsenic, lead, copper, and bee stings or spider bites.

Laboratory findings in hemolytic anemia are presented in Table 31-6. Treatment and management of acquired hemolytic anemias involve general supportive care until the causative agent can be eliminated or at least made less injurious to the RBCs. Because a hemolytic crisis is a potential consequence, be ready to institute appropriate emergency therapy. This includes aggressive hydration and electrolyte replacement to reduce the risk of kidney injury caused by hemoglobin (from RBC lysis) clogging the kidney tubules and subsequent shock. Additional supportive care may include administering corticosteroids and blood products or removing the spleen.

For chronic hemolytic anemia, folate may need to be replaced. To suppress the RBC destruction, immunosuppressive agents may be used, such as rituximab (Rituxan), a monoclonal antibody to B-cell CD20, and eculizumab (Soliris), a monoclonal antibody to complement protein C5.

OTHER RED BLOOD CELL DISORDERS

HEMOCHROMATOSIS

Hemochromatosis is an iron overload disorder. Although it is primarily caused by a genetic defect, hemochromatosis may

Hemochromatosis

Genetic Basis
- Autosomal recessive disorder.
- Caused by mutations in the *HAMP*, *HFE*, *HFE2*, *SLC40A1*, and *TFR2* genes.
- These genes play an important role in regulating the absorption, transport, and storage of iron.
- Mutations in these genes impair the control of iron absorption during digestion and alter the distribution of iron to other parts of the body. As a result, iron accumulates in tissues and organs.

Incidence
- Most common genetic disease in people of European ancestry.
- One in 8 are carriers of the single HH gene mutation.
- Affects 1 in 200 to 500 in the United States.
- Very low prevalence in other ethnic populations.

Genetic Testing
- DNA testing is available and recommended for all first-degree relatives of people with the disease.
- American Hemochromatosis Society recommends genetic testing regardless of family history.
- Useful diagnostic tests include serum iron concentration, total iron-binding capacity, and transferrin saturation.

Clinical Implications
- Most of the 33 million Americans who have the gene mutation do not know it.
- Clinical expression is variable depending on dietary iron, blood loss, and other modifying factors.
- Early treatment can prevent serious complications.
- If untreated, progressive iron deposits can lead to multiple organ failure.

occur secondary to diseases such as sideroblastic anemia. It may also be caused by liver disease and chronic blood transfusions that are used to treat thalassemia and SCD.[18]

Genetic Link

The genetic disorder *(hereditary hemochromatosis)* is an autosomal recessive disorder characterized by increased intestinal iron absorption and, as a result, increased tissue iron deposition.[18] (Autosomal recessive disorders are discussed in Chapter 13 and Table 13-2.) It is the most common genetic disorder among whites, with an incidence of about 5 per 1000 whites of European ancestry.[19]

The normal range for total body iron is 2 to 6 g. Individuals with hemochromatosis accumulate iron at a rate of 0.5 to 1.0 g/yr and may exceed total iron concentrations of 50 g. Symptoms of hemochromatosis usually develop between 40 and 60 years of age.

Early symptoms are nonspecific and include fatigue, arthralgia, impotence, abdominal pain, and weight loss. Later, the excess iron accumulates in the liver and causes liver enlargement and eventually cirrhosis. Then other organs become affected, resulting in diabetes mellitus, skin pigment changes (bronzing), cardiac changes (e.g., cardiomyopathy), arthritis, and testicular atrophy. Physical examination reveals an enlarged liver and spleen and pigmentation changes in the skin.

Laboratory values demonstrate an elevated serum iron, TIBC, and serum ferritin. Testing for known genetic mutations confirms the diagnosis. Liver biopsy can quantify the amount of iron and establish the degree of organ damage.

The goal of treatment is to remove excess iron from the body and minimize any symptoms the patient may have. Iron removal is achieved by removing 500 mL of blood each week for 2 to 3 years until the iron stores in the body are depleted. Then blood is removed less frequently to maintain iron levels within normal limits.

Iron chelating agents may be used. Deferoxamine, which chelates and removes accumulated iron via the kidneys, can be administered IV or subcutaneously. Deferasirox and deferiprone are oral agents that chelate iron. Chelating agents form a complex with iron and promote its excretion from the body.[20]

Management of organ involvement (e.g., diabetes mellitus, HF) is the same as conventional treatment for these problems. Iron accumulation can also be reduced by dietary modifications such as avoidance of vitamin C and iron supplements, uncooked seafood, and iron-rich foods. The most common causes of death are cirrhosis, liver failure, hepatocellular cancer, and cardiac failure. With early diagnosis and treatment, life expectancy is normal. However, many cases go undetected and untreated.

POLYCYTHEMIA

Polycythemia is the production and presence of increased numbers of RBCs. The increase in RBCs can be so great that blood circulation is impaired as a result of the increased blood viscosity *(hyperviscosity)* and volume *(hypervolemia)*.

Etiology and Pathophysiology

The two types of polycythemia are primary polycythemia, or polycythemia vera, and secondary polycythemia (Fig. 31-5). Their etiologies and pathogenesis differ, although their complications and clinical manifestations are similar.

Primary Polycythemia. *Polycythemia vera* is a chronic myeloproliferative disorder. Therefore not only are RBCs involved, but also WBCs and platelets, leading to increased production of each of these blood cells. The disease develops insidiously and follows a chronic, vacillating course. The median age at diagnosis is 60 years old, with a slight male predominance. In polycythemia vera there is enhanced blood viscosity and blood volume and congestion of organs and tissues with blood. Splenomegaly (which occurs in 90% of patients) and hepatomegaly are common. These patients have hypercoagulopathies that predispose them to clotting.

Genetic Link

Polycythemia vera is associated with mutations in the *Janus kinase-2 (JAK2)* gene. The *JAK2* gene provides instructions for making a protein that promotes proliferation of cells, especially blood cells from hematopoietic stem cells. Polycythemia vera begins with one or more DNA mutations of a single hematopoietic stem cell. Most cases of polycythemia vera are not inherited. This condition is associated with genetic changes that are somatic, which means they are acquired during a person's lifetime and are present only in certain cells.

Secondary Polycythemia. *Secondary polycythemia* can be either hypoxia driven or hypoxia independent. In hypoxia-driven secondary polycythemia, hypoxia stimulates erythropoietin (EPO) production in the kidney, which in turn stimulates RBC production. The need for oxygen may result from high altitude, pulmonary disease, cardiovascular disease, alveolar hypoventilation, defective oxygen transport, or tissue hypoxia. EPO levels may return to normal once the hemoglobin is

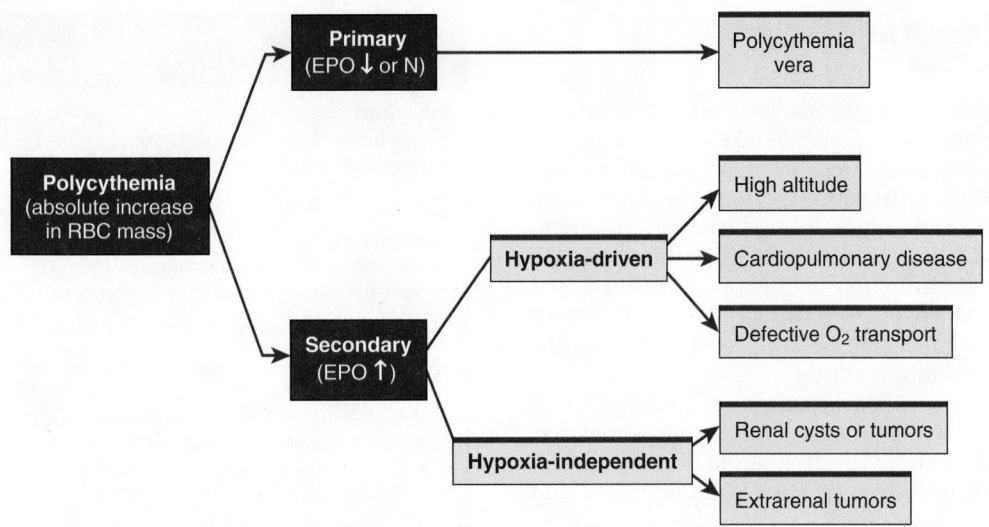

FIG. 31-5 Differentiating between primary and secondary polycythemia. *EPO,* Erythropoietin; *N,* normal.

stabilized at a higher level. In this situation, secondary polycythemia is a physiologic response in which the body tries to compensate for a problem, rather than a pathologic response. (Hypoxia-driven secondary polycythemia is discussed in the section on chronic obstructive pulmonary disease in Chapter 29.)

In hypoxia-independent secondary polycythemia, EPO is produced by a malignant or benign tumor tissue. Serum EPO levels often remain elevated in these situations. Splenomegaly does not accompany secondary polycythemia.

Clinical Manifestations and Complications

Circulatory manifestations of polycythemia vera occur because of the hypertension caused by hypervolemia and hyperviscosity. They are often the first manifestations and include subjective complaints of headache, vertigo, dizziness, tinnitus, and visual disturbances. Generalized pruritus (often exacerbated by a hot bath) may be a striking symptom and is related to histamine release from an increased number of basophils. Paresthesias and *erythromelalgia* (painful burning and redness of the hands and feet) may also be present. In addition, the patient may experience angina, HF, intermittent claudication, and thrombophlebitis, which may be complicated by embolization. These manifestations are caused by blood vessel distention, impaired blood flow, circulatory stasis, thrombosis, and tissue hypoxia caused by the hypervolemia and hyperviscosity. The most common serious acute complication is stroke secondary to thrombosis.

Hemorrhagic phenomena caused by either vessel rupture from overdistention or inadequate platelet function may result in petechiae, ecchymoses, epistaxis, or GI bleeding. Hemorrhage can be acute and catastrophic. Hepatomegaly and splenomegaly from organ engorgement may contribute to patient complaints of satiety and fullness. The patient may also experience pain from peptic ulcer caused either by increased gastric secretions or by liver and spleen engorgement. *Plethora* (ruddy complexion) may also be present. Hyperuricemia is caused by the increase in RBC destruction that accompanies excessive RBC production. Uric acid is one of the products of cell destruction. As RBC destruction increases, uric acid production also increases, thus leading to hyperuricemia and possible gout.

Although the incidence is low, myelofibrosis and leukemia develop in some patients with polycythemia vera. These disorders may be caused by the chemotherapeutic drugs used to treat the disease, or they may be secondary to a disorder in the stem cells that progresses to erythroleukemia. The major cause of morbidity and mortality from polycythemia vera is related to thrombosis (e.g., stroke).

Diagnostic Studies

The following laboratory manifestations are seen in a patient with polycythemia vera: (1) elevated hemoglobin and RBC count with microcytosis; (2) low to normal EPO level (secondary polycythemia has a high level); (3) elevated WBC count with basophilia; (4) elevated platelet count (thrombocytosis) and platelet dysfunction; (5) elevated leukocyte alkaline phosphatase, uric acid, and cobalamin levels; and (6) elevated histamine levels. Bone marrow examination in polycythemia vera shows hypercellularity of RBCs, WBCs, and platelets.

Collaborative Care

Treatment is directed toward reducing blood volume and viscosity and bone marrow activity. Phlebotomy is the mainstay of treatment. The aim of phlebotomy is to reduce the hematocrit and keep it less than 45% to 48%. Generally, at the time of diagnosis 300 to 500 mL of blood may be removed every other day until the hematocrit is reduced to normal levels. An individual managed with repeated phlebotomies eventually becomes deficient in iron, although this effect is rarely symptomatic. Avoid iron supplementation. Hydration therapy is used to reduce the blood's viscosity. Myelosuppressive agents such as hydroxyurea, busulfan (Myleran), and chlorambucil are used.

Ruxolitinib (Jakafi), which is a new drug inhibiting the expression of the *JAK2* mutation, is used for patients who have polycythemia-related myelofibrosis. Low-dose aspirin is used to prevent clotting. α-Interferon (α-IFN) is of particular use in women of childbearing age or those with intractable pruritus. Anagrelide (Agrylin) may be used to reduce the platelet count and inhibit platelet aggregation. Allopurinol (Zyloprim) may reduce the number of acute gouty attacks.[21]

NURSING MANAGEMENT POLYCYTHEMIA VERA

Primary polycythemia (polycythemia vera) is not preventable. When acute exacerbations of polycythemia vera develop, you have several responsibilities. Depending on the institution's policies, you may either assist with or perform the phlebotomy. Evaluate fluid intake and output during hydration therapy to avoid fluid overload (which further complicates the circulatory congestion) and underhydration (which can make the blood even more viscous). If myelosuppressive agents are used, administer the drugs as ordered, observe the patient, and teach the patient about medication side effects.

Assess the patient's nutritional status, since inadequate food intake can result from GI symptoms of fullness, pain, and dyspepsia. Begin activities and/or medications to decrease thrombus formation. Initiate active or passive leg exercises and ambulation when possible.

Because of its chronic nature, polycythemia vera requires ongoing evaluation. Phlebotomy may need to be done every 2 to 3 months, reducing the blood volume by about 500 mL each time. Evaluate the patient for complications.

PROBLEMS OF HEMOSTASIS

Hemostasis involves the vascular endothelium, platelets, and coagulation factors, which normally function together to stop hemorrhage and repair vascular injury. (These mechanisms are described in Chapter 30.) Disruption in any of these components may result in bleeding or thrombotic disorders.

Three major disorders of hemostasis discussed in this section are (1) thrombocytopenia (low platelet count), (2) hemophilia and von Willebrand disease (inherited disorders of specific clotting factors), and (3) disseminated intravascular coagulation (DIC).

THROMBOCYTOPENIA

Etiology and Pathophysiology

Thrombocytopenia is a reduction of platelets below 150,000/μL (150×10^9/L). Acute, severe, or prolonged decreases from this normal range can result in abnormal hemostasis that manifests as prolonged bleeding from minor trauma or spontaneous bleeding without injury.

Platelet disorders can be inherited (e.g., Wiskott-Aldrich syndrome), but the vast majority are acquired (Table 31-11). A common cause of acquired disorders is the ingestion of certain herbs or drugs[22,23] (Table 31-12). Although some agents are directly myelosuppressive (e.g., chemotherapy, ganciclovir [Cytovene]), the usual mechanism of thrombocytopenia caused by herbs or drugs is accelerated platelet destruction caused by drug-dependent antibodies. Antibodies attack the platelets when the offending agent binds to the platelet surface.

A careful review of the patient's history helps to identify the cause of thrombocytopenia. For example, quinine is in tonic water and in many herbal preparations. In addition, some drugs can affect platelet aggregation. Aspirin doses as low as 81 mg (baby aspirin) can alter platelet aggregation. Normal function is restored when new platelets are formed.

Immune Thrombocytopenic Purpura. The most common acquired thrombocytopenia is a syndrome of abnormal destruction of circulating platelets termed *immune thrombocytopenic*

TABLE 31-11 CAUSES OF THROMBOCYTOPENIA

Inherited
- Fanconi syndrome (pancytopenia)
- Hereditary thrombocytopenia

Acquired
Immune
- Immune thrombocytopenic purpura (ITP)
- Neonatal alloimmune thrombocytopenia

Nonimmune
- Shortened circulation (increased consumption)
  - Thrombotic thrombocytopenic purpura (TTP)
  - Disseminated intravascular coagulation (DIC)
  - Heparin-induced thrombocytopenia (HIT)
  - Splenomegaly or splenic sequestration
- Turbulent blood flow (hemangiomas, abnormal cardiac valves, intraaortic balloon pumps)
- Decreased production
  - Drug-induced marrow suppression
  - Chemotherapy
  - Viral infection (hepatitis C virus, HIV, cytomegalovirus)
  - Bacterial infection (sepsis)
  - Alcoholism, bone marrow suppression
  - Myelodysplastic syndrome (MDS)
  - Myelofibrosis
  - Aplastic anemia
  - Hematologic malignancy (leukemias, lymphomas, myeloma)
  - Solid tumor infiltrating bone marrow
  - Radiation to the bone

TABLE 31-12 DRUG AND HERBAL CAUSES OF THROMBOCYTOPENIA*

- Thiazide diuretics
- Alcohol
- Chemotherapeutic drugs
- Digoxin
- Nonsteroidal antiinflammatory drugs: ibuprofen (Advil, Motrin), indomethacin (Indocin), naproxen (Naproxyn, Aleve)
- Antibiotics: penicillins, cephalosporins, sulfonamides
- Other antiinfectives: rifampin (Rifadin), ganciclovir (Cytovene), amphotericin B
- Analgesics: aspirin and aspirin-containing drugs, acetaminophen
- Antipsychotic and antiseizure agents: haloperidol (Haldol), valproate (Depakene), lithium
- Platelet glycoprotein inhibitors: abciximab (ReoPro), tirofiban (Aggrastat), eptifibatide (Integrilin), clopidogrel (Plavix)
- H_2-receptor antagonists: cimetidine (Tagamet), ranitidine (Zantac)
- Gold compounds: auranofin (Ridaura)
- Spices: ginger, cumin, turmeric, cloves
- Vitamins: vitamin C, vitamin E
- Heparin
- Herbs: angelica, bilberry, feverfew, garlic, ginkgo biloba, ginseng
- Quinine compounds: tonic water

*List is not all-inclusive.

---

purpura (ITP). It was originally termed *idiopathic thrombocytopenic purpura* because its cause was unknown. However, it is now known that ITP is primarily an autoimmune disease. In ITP, platelets are coated with antibodies. Although these platelets function normally, when they reach the spleen, the antibody-coated platelets are recognized as foreign and are destroyed by macrophages. Decreased platelet production contributes to ITP.

Sometimes infection, such as *Helicobacter pylori* or viral infection, contributes to this disorder.[23]

Platelets normally survive 8 to 10 days. However, in ITP survival of platelets is shortened. The clinical syndrome manifests as an acute condition in children and a chronic condition in adults. Chronic ITP may occur in women between 15 and 40 years of age or older individuals. Chronic ITP has a gradual onset, and transient remissions may occur.[23]

Thrombotic Thrombocytopenic Purpura. *Thrombotic thrombocytopenic purpura* (TTP) is an uncommon syndrome characterized by hemolytic anemia, thrombocytopenia, neurologic abnormalities, fever (in the absence of infection), and renal abnormalities; not all features are present in all patients. Because it is almost always associated with hemolytic-uremic syndrome (HUS), it is often referred to as TTP-HUS. The disease is associated with enhanced aggregation of platelets, which form microthrombi that deposit in arterioles and capillaries.

In most cases the syndrome is caused by the deficiency of a plasma enzyme (ADAMTS13) that usually breaks down the von Willebrand clotting factor (vWF) into normal size. (vWF is the most important protein mediating platelet adhesion to damaged endothelial cells.) Without the enzyme, unusually large amounts of vWF attach to activated platelets, thereby promoting platelet aggregation.

TTP is seen primarily in adults between 20 and 50 years of age, with a slight female predominance. The syndrome may be idiopathic (thought to be due to an autoimmune disorder against ADAMTS13), but it may be due to certain drug toxicities (e.g., chemotherapy, cyclosporine, quinine, oral contraceptives, valacyclovir [Valtrex], clopidogrel [Plavix]), pregnancy or preeclampsia, infection, or a known autoimmune disorder such as systemic lupus erythematosus or scleroderma. TTP is a medical emergency because bleeding and clotting occur simultaneously.[24]

Heparin-Induced Thrombocytopenia. One of the risks associated with the broad and increasing use of heparin is the development of the life-threatening condition called *heparin-induced thrombocytopenia* (HIT), also called *heparin-induced thrombocytopenia and thrombosis syndrome* (HITTS). Typically, patients develop thrombocytopenia 5 to 10 days after the onset of heparin therapy. HIT should be suspected if the platelet count falls by more than 50% or falls to below 150,000/μL. As many as 5% of patients on heparin therapy develop HIT.[24]

The major clinical problem of HIT is venous thrombosis; arterial thrombosis can also develop. Deep vein thromboses and pulmonary emboli most commonly result as a complication of the thromboses. Additional complications may include arterial vascular infarcts resulting in skin necrosis, stroke, and end-organ damage (e.g., kidneys). Symptoms of bleeding are unusual because the platelet count rarely drops below 60,000/μL.

In HIT, platelet destruction and vascular endothelial injury are the two major responses to an immune-mediated response to heparin. Platelet factor 4 (PF4) binds to heparin (this protein is made and released by platelets). This complex then binds to the platelet surface, leading to further platelet activation and release of more PF4, thus creating a positive feedback loop. Antibodies are created against this complex, and they are removed prematurely from circulation, leading to thrombocytopenia and platelet-fibrin thrombi. Platelet aggregation also induces heparin to be neutralized. Thus more heparin is required to maintain therapeutic activated partial thromboplastin times (aPTT).

FIG. 31-6 Acute idiopathic thrombocytopenic purpura commonly manifests with purpuric lesions of this kind, although they may often be widespread by the time medical attention is sought.

Clinical Manifestations

Many patients with thrombocytopenia are usually asymptomatic. The most common symptom is bleeding, usually mucosal or cutaneous. Mucosal bleeding may manifest as epistaxis and gingival bleeding, and large bullous hemorrhages may appear on the buccal mucosa because of the lack of vessel protection by the submucosal tissue.

Bleeding into the skin is manifested as petechiae, purpura, or superficial ecchymoses (Fig. 31-6). *Petechiae* are small, flat, pinpoint, red or reddish brown microhemorrhages. When the platelet count is low, RBCs may leak out of the blood vessels and into the skin to cause petechiae. When petechiae are numerous, the resulting reddish skin bruise is called *purpura*. Larger purplish lesions caused by hemorrhage are termed *ecchymoses*. Ecchymoses may be flat or raised; pain and tenderness sometimes are present.

Prolonged bleeding after routine procedures such as venipuncture or IM injection may indicate thrombocytopenia. Because the bleeding may be internal, be aware of manifestations that reflect this type of blood loss, including weakness, fainting, dizziness, tachycardia, abdominal pain, and hypotension.

The major complication of thrombocytopenia is hemorrhage. The hemorrhage may be insidious or acute, and internal or external. It may occur in any area of the body, including the joints, retina, and brain. Cerebral hemorrhage may be fatal. Insidious hemorrhage may first be detected by discovering the anemia that accompanies blood loss.

Because thrombocytopenia can be accompanied by vascular thromboses in some of these disorders, signs and symptoms of vascular ischemic problems can manifest (see Chapter 38). For example, subtle confusion, headache, or even serious manifestations such as seizures and coma due to TTP-related thrombosis may be seen. Because signs and symptoms may be subtle, astute and thorough assessment of the patient is essential.

Diagnostic Studies

The platelet count is decreased in thrombocytopenia. Any reduction below 150,000/μL (150 × 10⁹/L) may be termed *thrombocytopenia*. However, prolonged bleeding from trauma or injury does not usually occur until platelet counts are less than 50,000/μL (50 × 10⁹/L). When the count drops below 20,000/μL (20 × 10⁹/L), spontaneous, life-threatening hemorrhages (e.g., intracranial bleeding) can occur. Platelet transfusions are generally not recommended until the count is below 10,000/μL (10 × 10⁹/L) unless the patient is actively bleeding.

TABLE 31-13   LABORATORY RESULTS IN THROMBOCYTOPENIA

Laboratory Test	Immune Thrombocytopenic Purpura	Thrombotic Thrombocytopenic Purpura	Heparin-Induced Thrombocytopenia	Disseminated Intravascular Coagulation
Platelets	↓↓↓	↓↓↓	↓↓	↓↓↓
Hemolysis				
Hgb	N	↓↓	N	N or ↓
LDH	N	↑↑↑	N	↑
Reticulocytes	N	↑	N	N or ↑
Haptoglobin	N	↓	N	↓
Indirect bilirubin	N	↑	N	N or ↑
Schistocytes	N	↑↑↑	N or ↑	N or ↑
Coagulopathy				
PT	N	N	N	↑
aPTT	N	N	N	↑
D-dimer	N	N or ↑	↑	↑↑
Other Tests	ITP platelet antigen-specific assay, ^{14}C-serotonin release assay, *Helicobacter pylori*, bone marrow biopsy	ADAMTS13	^{14}C-serotonin release assay, PF4-heparin complex	

aPTT, Activated partial thromboplastin time; *ITP*, idiopathic thrombocytopenic purpura; *LDH*, lactate dehydrogenase; *N*, normal; *PF4*, platelet factor 4; *PT*, prothrombin time.

Examination of the peripheral blood smear may help distinguish acquired disorders such as ITP and TTP from congenital disorders, which may be indicated by abnormally sized platelets. The patient's medical history and clinical examination, along with comparisons of laboratory parameters, help to determine the etiology of the thrombocytopenia. Table 31-13 compares the types of thrombocytopenia.[23,24]

Laboratory tests that assess secondary hemostasis or coagulation, such as the prothrombin time (PT) and aPTT, can be normal even in severe thrombocytopenia. If they are elevated, this may point toward DIC. Bone marrow examination is done to rule out production problems as the cause of thrombocytopenia (e.g., leukemia, aplastic anemia, other myeloproliferative disorders).

Specific assays, such as ITP antigen-specific assay, ^{14}C-serotonin release assay, or enzyme-linked immunosorbent assay (ELISA) for PF4-heparin complex for HIT, can be done to assist with the diagnosis. In TTP, testing for deficiency of ADAMTS13 is not always diagnostic, so an increase of lactate dehydrogenase (LDH) may help establish the diagnosis.[23,24] When thrombocytopenia occurs with anemia characterized by altered RBC morphology, including *spherocytes* (small, globular, completely hemoglobinated erythrocytes), fragmented cells (schistocytes), and pronounced reticulocytosis, a diagnosis of TTP should be suspected. These findings are partially a result of intravascular fibrin deposition causing a "slicing" of RBCs. In TTP, thrombocytopenia may be severe, but coagulation studies are normal.

Bone marrow analysis is performed if other test results are inconclusive, especially in older patients because of a higher suspicion of an underlying bone marrow disorder. When destruction of circulating platelets is the cause, bone marrow analysis shows *megakaryocytes* (precursors of platelets) to be normal or increased, even though circulating platelets are reduced. The absence or decreased number of megakaryocytes on bone marrow biopsy is consistent with thrombocytopenia caused by decreased bone marrow production (e.g., aplastic anemia). Special blood analyses using flow cytometry and other techniques can detect antiplatelet antibodies as the source of destruction.

Collaborative Care

Collaborative care of thrombocytopenia differs based on the etiology. Removal or treatment of the underlying cause or disorder is sometimes sufficient. The patient with thrombocytopenia should avoid aspirin and other medications that affect platelet function or production. The following sections discuss management strategies for the different causes of thrombocytopenia (Table 31-14).

Immune Thrombocytopenic Purpura. Multiple therapies are used to manage the patient with ITP.[25] If the patient is asymptomatic, therapy may not be used unless the patient's platelet count is below 30,000/μL. Corticosteroids (e.g., prednisone, methylprednisolone) are used initially to treat ITP because of their ability to suppress the phagocytic response of splenic macrophages. This alters the spleen's recognition of platelets and increases the life span of the platelets. In addition, corticosteroids depress antibody formation and reduce capillary leakage.

High doses of IV immunoglobulin (IVIG) and a component of IVIG, anti-Rh$_o$(D) (anti-D, WinRho), may be used in the patient who is unresponsive to corticosteroids or splenectomy, or for whom splenectomy is not an option. It is believed that one way these agents work is by competing with the antiplatelet antibodies for macrophage receptors in the spleen. Rituximab may be used for its ability to lyse activated B cells, therapy reducing the immune recognition of platelets.

Splenectomy may be indicated if the patient does not respond to the above treatments. Splenectomy can usually be done laparoscopically, and 60% to 70% of patients benefit from splenectomy, resulting in a complete or partial remission.[26] The effectiveness of splenectomy is based on four factors. First, the spleen contains an abundance of the macrophages that sequester and destroy platelets. Second, structural features of the spleen enhance the interaction between antibody-coated platelets and macrophages. Third, some antibody synthesis occurs in the spleen; thus antiplatelet antibodies decrease after splenec-

TABLE 31-14 COLLABORATIVE CARE

Thrombocytopenia

Diagnostic
- History and physical examination
- Bone marrow aspiration and biopsy
- CBC, including platelet count
- Specific studies (see Table 31-13)

Collaborative Therapy
Immune Thrombocytopenic Purpura
- Corticosteroids
- IV immunoglobulin (IVIG)
- Anti-Rh$_o$(D)
- Rituximab
- Splenectomy
- Romiplostim (Nplate)
- Eltrombopag (Promacta)
- Danazol
- Immunosuppressives (e.g., cyclosporine, cyclophosphamide [Cytoxan], azathioprine [Imuran], mycophenolate mofetil [CellCept])
- High-dose cyclophosphamide or combination chemotherapy
- Platelet transfusions

Thrombotic Thrombocytopenic Purpura
- Identification and treatment of cause
- Plasmapheresis (plasma exchange)
- High-dose prednisone
- Dextran
- Chemotherapy (vincristine [Oncovin], vinblastine [Velban])
- Immunosuppressives (cyclophosphamide, rituximab [Rituxan])
- Splenectomy

Heparin-Induced Thrombocytopenia
- Direct thrombin inhibitor (lepirudin [Refludan], argatroban [Acova])
- Indirect thrombin inhibitor (fondaparinux [Arixtra])
- Warfarin (Coumadin)
- Plasmapheresis (plasma exchange)
- Protamine sulfate
- Thrombolytic agents

Decreased Platelet Production
- Identification and treatment or removal of cause
- Corticosteroids
- Platelet transfusions

tomy. Fourth, the spleen normally sequesters approximately one third of the platelets, so its removal increases the number of platelets in circulation.

Romiplostim (Nplate) and eltrombopag (Promacta) are used for patients with chronic ITP who have had an insufficient response to the other treatments or who have a contraindication to splenectomy. These drugs are thrombopoietin receptor agonists, thus increasing platelet production.[27] Danazol (Danocrine), an androgen, may be used along with corticosteroids in some patients. Although the mechanism is not totally understood, danazol increases CD4$^+$ T cells, thereby decreasing the immune response. Immunosuppressive therapy may be used in refractory cases[23] (see Table 31-14).

Platelet transfusions may be used to increase platelet counts in cases of life-threatening hemorrhage. Platelets should not be administered prophylactically because of the possibility of antibody formation. The usual indication for administering platelets is for a platelet count less than 10,000/μL or if there is anticipated bleeding before a procedure. Epsilon-aminocaproic

acid (EACA, Amicar), an antifibrinolytic agent, may be used for severe bleeding.

Thrombotic Thrombocytopenic Purpura. TTP may be treated in a variety of ways. The first step is to treat the underlying disorder (e.g., infection) or remove the causative agent, if identified. If untreated, TTP usually results in irreversible renal failure and death. Plasma exchange (plasmapheresis) (see Chapter 14) is used to aggressively reverse platelet consumption by supplying the appropriate vWF and enzyme (ADAMTS13) and removing the large vWF molecules that bind with platelets. Treatment should be continued daily until the patient's platelet counts normalize and hemolysis has ceased. Corticosteroids may be added to this treatment. Recently, rituximab has been used for patients refractory to plasma exchange; it decreases the level of inhibitory ADAMTS13 IgG antibodies. Other immunosuppressants such as cyclosporine or cyclophosphamide may also be used. Splenectomy may be considered in patients refractory to plasma exchange or immunosuppression. The administration of platelets is generally contraindicated because this may lead to new vWF-platelet complexes and increased clotting.

Heparin-Induced Thrombocytopenia. Heparin must be discontinued when HIT is first recognized. Heparin flushes for vascular catheters should also be stopped.

To maintain anticoagulation, the patient should be started on a direct thrombin inhibitor, such as lepirudin (Refludan) or argatroban (Acova). Fondaparinux (Arixtra), a factor Xa inhibitor (indirect thrombin inhibitor), may be used. Warfarin should be started only when the platelet count has reached 150,000/μL. If the clotting is severe, the most commonly used treatment modalities are plasmapheresis to clear the platelet-aggregating IgG from the blood, protamine sulfate to interrupt the circulating heparin, thrombolytic agents to treat the thromboembolic events, and surgery to remove clots. Platelet transfusions are not effective because they may enhance thromboembolic events.

Patients who have had HIT should never be given heparin or low-molecular-weight heparin (LMWH). This should be clearly marked on the patient's medical record.

Acquired Thrombocytopenia From Decreased Platelet Production. The management of acquired thrombocytopenia is based on identifying the cause and treating the disease or removing the causative agent. If the precipitating factor is unknown, the patient may receive corticosteroids. Platelet transfusions are given if life-threatening hemorrhage develops.

Often acquired thrombocytopenia is caused by another underlying condition (e.g., aplastic anemia, leukemia) or therapy used to treat another problem. For example, in acute leukemia all blood cell types may be depressed. Additionally, the patient may receive chemotherapeutic drugs that cause bone marrow suppression. If the patient can be adequately supported throughout the course of chemotherapy-induced thrombocytopenia, the thrombocytopenia will also resolve.

NURSING MANAGEMENT THROMBOCYTOPENIA

NURSING ASSESSMENT

Subjective and objective data that should be obtained from a patient with thrombocytopenia are presented in Table 31-15.

NURSING DIAGNOSES

Nursing diagnoses for the patient with thrombocytopenia may include, but are not limited to, the following.

TABLE 31-15 NURSING ASSESSMENT

Thrombocytopenia

Subjective Data
Important Health Information
Past health history: Recent hemorrhage, excessive bleeding, or viral illness; HIV infection; cancer (especially leukemia or lymphoma); aplastic anemia; systemic lupus erythematosus; cirrhosis; exposure to radiation or toxic chemicals; disseminated intravascular coagulation
Medications: See Table 31-12

Functional Health Patterns
Health perception–health management: Family history of bleeding problems; malaise
Nutritional-metabolic: Bleeding gingiva; coffee-ground or bloody vomitus; easy bruising
Elimination: Hematuria, dark or bloody stools
Activity-exercise: Fatigue, weakness, fainting; epistaxis, hemoptysis; dyspnea
Cognitive-perceptual: Pain and tenderness in bleeding areas (e.g., abdomen, head, extremities); headache
Sexuality-reproductive: Menorrhagia, metrorrhagia

Objective Data
General
Fever, lethargy

Integumentary
Petechiae, ecchymoses, purpura

Gastrointestinal
Splenomegaly, abdominal distention; guaiac-positive stools

Possible Diagnostic Findings
Platelet count <150,000/μL (150 × 10^9/L), prolonged bleeding time, ↓ hemoglobin and hematocrit; normal or ↑ megakaryocytes in bone marrow examination

TABLE 31-16 PATIENT & CAREGIVER TEACHING GUIDE

Thrombocytopenia

Include the following instructions when teaching a patient or caregiver the precautions to take when the platelet count is low.
1. Notify your health care provider of any manifestations of bleeding. These include the following:
   - Black, tarry, or bloody bowel movements
   - Black or bloody vomit, sputum, or urine
   - Bruising or small red or purple spots on the skin
   - Bleeding from the mouth or anywhere in the body
   - Headache or changes in how well you can see
   - Difficulty talking, sudden weakness of an arm or leg, confusion
2. Ask your health care provider regarding restrictions in your normal activities, such as vigorous exercise, lifting weights. Generally, walking can be done safely and should be done with sturdy shoes or slippers. If you are weak and at risk for falling, get help or supervision when getting out of bed or chair.
3. Do not blow your nose forcefully; gently pat it with a tissue if needed. For a nosebleed, keep your head up and apply firm pressure to the nostrils and bridge of your nose. If bleeding continues, place an ice bag over the bridge of your nose and the nape of your neck. If you are unable to stop a nosebleed after 10 min, call your health care provider.
4. Do not bend down with your head lower than your waist.
5. Prevent constipation by drinking plenty of fluids. Do not strain when having a bowel movement. Your health care provider may prescribe a stool softener. Do not use a suppository, an enema, or a rectal thermometer without the permission of your health care provider.
6. Shave only with an electric razor; do not use blades.
7. Do not pluck your eyebrows or other body hair.
8. Do not puncture your skin, such as getting tattoos or body piercing.
9. Avoid using any medication that can prolong bleeding, such as aspirin. Other medications and herbs can have similar effects. If you are unsure about any medication, ask your health care provider or pharmacist about it in relation to your thrombocytopenia.
10. Use a soft-bristle toothbrush to prevent injuring the gums. Flossing is usually safe if it is done gently using the thin tape floss. Do not use alcohol-based mouthwashes, since they can dry your gums and increase bleeding.
11. Women who are menstruating should keep track of the number of pads that are used per day. When you start using more pads per day than usual or bleed more days, notify your health care provider. Do not use tampons; use sanitary pads only.
12. Ask your health care provider before you have any invasive procedures done, such as a dental cleaning, manicure, or pedicure.

- Impaired oral mucous membrane *related to* low platelet counts and/or effects of pathologic conditions and treatment
- Risk for bleeding *related to* decreased platelets
- Deficient knowledge *related to* lack of information regarding the disease process and treatment

PLANNING

The overall goals are that the patient with thrombocytopenia will (1) have no gross or occult bleeding, (2) maintain vascular integrity, and (3) manage home care to prevent any complications related to an increased risk for bleeding.

NURSING IMPLEMENTATION

HEALTH PROMOTION. Discourage excessive use of over-the-counter (OTC) medications known to be possible causes of acquired thrombocytopenia. Many medications contain aspirin as an ingredient. Aspirin reduces platelet adhesiveness, thus contributing to bleeding.

Encourage persons to have a complete medical evaluation if manifestations of bleeding tendencies (e.g., prolonged epistaxis, petechiae) develop. Observe for early signs of thrombocytopenia in the patient receiving cancer chemotherapy drugs.

ACUTE INTERVENTION. The goal during acute episodes of thrombocytopenia is to prevent or control hemorrhage (see eNursing Care Plan 31-1 on the website for this chapter). In the patient with thrombocytopenia, bleeding is usually from super-ficial sites. Deep bleeding (into muscles, joints, and abdomen) usually occurs only when clotting factors are diminished. Emphasize that a seemingly minor nosebleed or new petechiae may indicate potential hemorrhage and the health care provider should be notified.

Bleeding from the posterior nasopharynx may be difficult to detect because the blood may be swallowed. If a subcutaneous injection is unavoidable, the use of a small-gauge needle and application of direct pressure for at least 5 to 10 minutes after injection is indicated, or application of an ice pack may be helpful. Avoid IM injections. Help the patient understand the importance of adherence to self-care measures that reduce the risk of bleeding (Table 31-16).

Note that many of these disorders may be accompanied by vascular clotting, and appropriate assessment and management should be taken (see Chapter 38). As bleeding occurs, red blood cell and coagulation factors are consumed along with platelets, so it is important to monitor all blood cell and coagulation studies.

In a woman with thrombocytopenia, menstrual blood loss may exceed the usual amount and duration. Counting sanitary napkins used during menses is another important intervention to detect excess blood loss. Blood loss of 50 mL will completely soak a sanitary napkin. Suppression of menses with hormonal agents may be indicated during predictable periods of thrombocytopenia (e.g., during chemotherapy and HSCT) to reduce blood loss from menses.

Closely monitor the platelet count, coagulation studies, hemoglobin, and hematocrit. Together these provide important information regarding potential or actual bleeding.

The proper administration of platelet transfusions is an important nursing responsibility. This is discussed under Blood Component Therapy later in this chapter.

AMBULATORY AND HOME CARE. Monitor the patient with ITP who is receiving treatment for the response to therapy. Teach the person with acquired thrombocytopenia to avoid causative agents when possible (see Table 31-12). If the causative agents cannot be avoided (e.g., chemotherapy), teach the patient to avoid injury or trauma during these periods and to be aware of the clinical signs and symptoms of bleeding caused by thrombocytopenia (see Table 31-16).

Patients with either ITP or acquired thrombocytopenia should have planned periodic medical evaluations to assess their status. These regular evaluations can be used to assess and treat situations in which exacerbations and bleeding are likely to occur. The impact of either an acute or a chronic condition on the patient's quality of life should also be addressed appropriately.

EVALUATION

The expected outcomes are that the patient with thrombocytopenia will

- Have no evidence of bleeding or bruising
- Verbalize required knowledge and skills to manage disease process at home

HEMOPHILIA AND VON WILLEBRAND DISEASE

Hemophilia is an X-linked recessive genetic disorder caused by a defective or deficient coagulation factor. The two major types of hemophilia, which can occur in mild to severe forms, are *hemophilia A* (classic hemophilia, factor VIII deficiency) and *hemophilia B* (Christmas disease, factor IX deficiency). *von Willebrand disease* is a related disorder involving a deficiency of the von Willebrand coagulation protein. Factor VIII is synthesized in the liver and circulates as a complex with von Willebrand factor (vWF).

Hemophilia A is the most common form of hemophilia, accounting for about 85% to 90% of all cases. Hemophilia B accounts for about 10% to 15% of all cases. von Willebrand disease is considered the most common congenital bleeding disorder, with estimates as high as 1 or 2 in 100.[28]

Genetic Link

The inheritance patterns of hemophilia and von Willebrand disease are compared in Table 31-17. (X-linked genetic disorders are discussed in Chapter 13 and Table 13-2.)

Clinical Manifestations and Complications

All clinical manifestations relate to bleeding, and any bleeding episode in persons with hemophilia may lead to a life-

TABLE 31-17	**TYPES OF HEMOPHILIA**
Type	**Inheritance Pattern**
Hemophilia A	
Factor VIII	Recessive sex-linked (transmitted by female carriers, displayed almost exclusively in men)
Hemophilia B	
Factor IX	Recessive sex-linked (transmitted by female carriers, displayed almost exclusively in men)
von Willebrand Disease	
vWF, variable factor VIII deficiencies and platelet dysfunction	Autosomal dominant, seen in both genders Recessive (in severe forms of the disease)

vWF, von Willebrand factor.

GENETICS IN CLINICAL PRACTICE

Hemophilia A and B

Genetic Basis
- X-linked recessive disorder.
- *Hemophilia A:* Caused by mutations in the *F8* gene that provides instructions for making coagulation factor VIII.
- *Hemophilia B:* Caused by mutations in the *F9* gene that provides instructions for making coagulation factor IX.
- Mutations in the *F8* or *F9* gene lead to the production of an abnormal version or reduced amounts of these coagulation factors.

Incidence
- *Hemophilia A:* 1 in 5000 to 10,000 male births.
- *Hemophilia B:* 1 in 30,000 to 50,000 male births.

Genetic Testing
- DNA testing is available.

Clinical Implications
- Female carriers transmit the genetic defect to 50% of their sons, and 50% of their daughters are carriers.
- Males with hemophilia do not transmit the genetic defect to their sons, but all of their daughters are carriers.
- Female hemophilia can occur if a male with hemophilia mates with a female carrier. However, this is a rare situation.
- Clinical manifestations of hemophilia A and B are similar.
- Replacement therapy is available for factors VIII and IX (see Table 31-19).

threatening hemorrhage. Clinical manifestations and complications related to hemophilia include (1) slow, persistent, prolonged bleeding from minor trauma and small cuts; (2) delayed bleeding after minor injuries (the delay may be several hours or days); (3) uncontrollable hemorrhage after dental extractions or irritation of the gingiva with a hard-bristle toothbrush; (4) epistaxis, especially after a blow to the face; (5) GI bleeding from ulcers and gastritis; (6) hematuria and potential renal failure from GU trauma and splenic rupture resulting from falls or abdominal trauma; (7) ecchymoses and subcutaneous hematomas (Fig. 31-7); (8) neurologic signs, such as pain, anesthesia, and paralysis, which may develop from nerve compression caused by hematoma formation; and (9) hemarthrosis (bleeding into the joints) (Fig. 31-8), which may lead to joint injury and deformity severe enough to cause crippling (most commonly in knees, elbows, shoulders, hips, and ankles).

FIG. 31-7 Severe ecchymoses in a person with hemophilia after a fall.

FIG. 31-8 Acute hemarthrosis of the knee is a common complication of hemophilia.

TABLE 31-18	**LABORATORY RESULTS IN HEMOPHILIA**
Test	**Results**
Prothrombin time	Normal. No involvement of extrinsic system.
Thrombin time	Normal. No impairment of thrombin-fibrinogen reaction.
Platelet count	Normal. Adequate platelet production.
Partial thromboplastin time	Prolonged because of deficiency in intrinsic clotting system factor.
Bleeding time	Prolonged in von Willebrand disease because of structurally defective platelets. Normal in hemophilia A and B because platelets not affected.
Factor assays	Reductions of factor VIII in hemophilia A, factor IX in hemophilia B, vWF in von Willebrand disease.

vWF, von Willebrand factor.

TABLE 31-19	**DRUG THERAPY**

Replacement Factors for Hemophilia

Factor VIII	Factor IX	For Patients Who Have Inhibitors
Advate	AlphaNine SD	NovoSeven (factor VIIa)
Alphanate	Bebulin VH	Autoplex T
Helixate FS	Benefix	FEIBA (factor VIII inhibitor
Hemofil M	Mononine	bypassing activity)
Humate-P	Profilnine SD	
Koāte-DVI		
Kogenate FS		
Monoclate P		
Recombinate		
Xyntha		

In children these manifestations may lead to the diagnosis. In adults these developments may be the first sign of a newly diagnosed mild form of the disease that escaped detection through a childhood free of major injuries, dental procedures, or surgeries.

Diagnostic Studies

Laboratory studies are used to determine the type of hemophilia present. Any factor deficiency within the intrinsic system (factor VIII, IX, XI, or XII or vWF) will yield the laboratory results presented in Table 31-18.

Collaborative Care

The goals of collaborative care are to prevent and treat bleeding. Collaborative care for persons with hemophilia or von Willebrand disease requires (1) preventive care, (2) the use of replacement therapy during acute bleeding episodes and as prophylaxis, and (3) the treatment of the complications of the disease and its therapy. Today most patients can expect almost normal life spans free of bloodborne illnesses because of improved preparation of replacement products, improved screening of blood donor populations, and use of recombinant replacement factors.[29]

Replacement of deficient clotting factors is the primary means of supporting a patient with hemophilia. In addition to treating acute crises, replacement therapy may be given before surgery and dental care as a prophylactic measure.[30] Examples of replacement therapy are listed in Table 31-19. Fresh frozen plasma, once commonly used for replacement therapy, is rarely used today.

For mild hemophilia A and certain subtypes of von Willebrand disease, desmopressin acetate (also known as DDAVP), a synthetic analog of vasopressin, may be used to stimulate an increase in factor VIII and vWF. This drug acts on platelets and endothelial cells to cause the release of vWF, which subsequently binds with factor VIII, thus increasing their concentration. It can be administered IV, subcutaneously, or by intranasal spray. Beneficial effects (e.g., decreased bleeding time) of DDAVP, when administered IV, are seen within 30 minutes and can last for more than 12 hours. Because the effect of DDAVP is relatively short lived, the patient must be closely monitored and repeated doses may be necessary. It is an appropriate therapy for minor bleeding episodes and dental procedures. The intranasal form may be indicated for home therapy for some patients with mild to moderate forms of the disease.

Antifibrinolytic therapy (tranexamic acid [Cyklokapron] and epsilon-aminocaproic acid) inhibits fibrinolysis by inhibiting plasminogen activation in the fibrin clot, thereby enhancing clot stability. These agents are used to stabilize clots in areas of increased fibrinolysis, such as the oral cavity, and in patients with difficult episodes of epistaxis and menorrhagia.[31]

Complications of the treatment of hemophilia include development of inhibitors to factors VIII or IX, transfusion-transmitted infectious disorders (hepatitis, HIV), allergic reactions, and thrombotic complications with the use of factor IX because it contains activated coagulation factors. Patients with vWF may also develop alloantibodies against vWF concentrates, the infusion of which could cause life-threatening anaphylaxis. Thus replacement factors for these patients should not contain vWF.

The most common difficulties with acute management are starting factor replacement therapy too late and stopping it too soon. Generally, minor bleeding episodes should be treated for at least 72 hours. Surgery and traumatic injuries may need more prolonged therapy. Chronically, development of inhibitors to the factor products has occurred and requires individualized expert patient management. Designated treatment centers in the United States and many other countries provide interdisciplinary care of hemophilia and related disorders. Gene therapy has been used on an experimental basis to treat hemophilia.[32]

NURSING MANAGEMENT
HEMOPHILIA

NURSING IMPLEMENTATION

HEALTH PROMOTION. Because of the hereditary nature of hemophilia, referral of affected persons for genetic counseling before reproduction is an important measure. This is especially important because many persons with hemophilia live into adulthood. Reproductive concerns and long-term effects are issues that you should include in the patient's care plan.

ACUTE INTERVENTION. Interventions are related primarily to controlling bleeding and include the following:

1. Stop the topical bleeding as quickly as possible by applying direct pressure or ice, packing the area with Gelfoam or fibrin foam, and applying topical hemostatic agents such as thrombin.
2. Administer the specific coagulation factor to raise the patient's level of the deficient coagulation factor. Monitor the patient for signs and symptoms, such as hypersensitivity.
3. When joint bleeding occurs, in addition to administering replacement factors, it is important to totally rest the involved joint to prevent crippling deformities from hemarthrosis. Pack the joint in ice. Give analgesics (e.g., acetaminophen, codeine) to reduce severe pain. Aspirin and aspirin-containing compounds should never be used. As soon as bleeding ceases, encourage mobilization of the affected area through range-of-motion exercises and physical therapy. Weight bearing is avoided until all swelling has resolved and muscle strength has returned.
4. Manage any life-threatening complications that may develop as a result of hemorrhage or side effects from coagulation factors. Examples include nursing interventions to prevent or treat airway obstruction from hemorrhage into the neck and pharynx, recognition of compartment syndrome in an extremity, and early assessment and treatment of intracranial bleeding.

AMBULATORY AND HOME CARE. Home management is a primary consideration for the patient with hemophilia because the disease follows a progressive, chronic course. The quality and the length of life may be significantly affected by the patient's knowledge of the illness and how to live with it. The patient and caregiver can be referred to a local chapter of the Hemophilia Federation of America to encourage associations with other individuals who are dealing with the problems of hemophilia. Provide ongoing assessment of the patient's adaptation to the illness. Psychosocial support and assistance should be readily available as needed.

Most of the long-term care measures are related to patient teaching. Teach the patient to recognize disease-related problems and to learn which problems can be resolved at home and which require hospitalization. Immediate medical attention is required for severe pain or swelling of a muscle or joint that restricts movement or inhibits sleep and for a head injury, swelling in the neck or mouth, abdominal pain, hematuria, melena, and skin wounds in need of suturing.

Teach the patient to perform daily oral hygiene without causing trauma. Understanding how to prevent injuries is another consideration. Advise the patient to participate only in noncontact sports (e.g., golf) and to wear gloves when doing household chores to prevent cuts or abrasions from knives, hammers, and other tools. The patient should wear a Medic Alert tag to ensure that health care providers know about the hemophilia in case of an accident. Many patients or their caregivers can be taught to self-administer the factor replacement therapies at home.

EVALUATION

The overall expected outcomes are similar to those for the patient with thrombocytopenia (see p. 655).

DISSEMINATED INTRAVASCULAR COAGULATION

Disseminated intravascular coagulation (DIC) is a serious bleeding and thrombotic disorder that results from abnormally initiated and accelerated clotting. Subsequent decreases in clotting factors and platelets ensue, which may lead to uncontrollable hemorrhage. The term *disseminated intravascular coagulation* can be misleading because it suggests that blood is clotting. However, this condition is characterized by the profuse bleeding that results from the depletion of platelets and clotting factors. DIC is always caused by an underlying disease or condition. The underlying problem must be treated for the DIC to resolve.

Etiology and Pathophysiology

DIC is not a disease. It is an abnormal response of the normal clotting cascade stimulated by a disease process or disorder.[33] The diseases and disorders known to predispose a patient to DIC are listed in Table 31-20. DIC can occur as an acute, catastrophic condition or it may exist at a subacute or chronic level. Each condition may have one or multiple triggering mechanisms to start the clotting cascade. For example, tumors and traumatized or necrotic tissue release tissue factors into circulation. Endotoxin from gram-negative bacteria activates several steps in the coagulation cascade.

Tissue factor is released at the site of tissue injury and by some malignancies, such as leukemia, and enhances normal coagulation mechanisms. Abundant intravascular thrombin, the most powerful coagulant, is produced (Fig. 31-9). It catalyzes the conversion of fibrinogen to fibrin and enhances platelet aggregation. There is widespread fibrin and platelet deposition in capillaries and arterioles, resulting in thrombosis. This process can lead to multiorgan failure.

FIG. 31-9 The sequence of events that occur during disseminated intravascular coagulation (DIC).

In addition, clotting inhibitory mechanisms, such as antithrombin III (AT III) and protein C, are depressed. Excessive clotting activates the fibrinolytic system, which in turn breaks down the newly formed clot, creating fibrin split products (FSPs). These products have anticoagulant properties and inhibit normal blood clotting. Ultimately, as FSPs accumulate and clotting factors are depleted, the blood loses its ability to clot. Therefore a stable clot cannot be formed at injury sites, which predisposes the patient to hemorrhage.

Chronic and subacute DIC is most commonly seen in patients with long-standing illnesses such as malignant disorders or autoimmune diseases. Occasionally these patients have subclinical disease manifested only by laboratory abnormalities. However, the clinical spectrum ranges from easy bruising to hemorrhage, and from hypercoagulability to thrombosis.

Clinical Manifestations

DIC has both bleeding and thrombotic manifestations. Multiple factors cause bleeding manifestations of DIC (see Fig. 31-9) and result from consumption and depletion of platelets and coagulation factors, as well as clot lysis and formation of FSPs that have anticoagulant properties. Bleeding in a person with no previous history or obvious cause should be questioned because it may be one of the first manifestations of acute DIC.

Bleeding manifestations include (1) *integumentary manifestations* such as pallor, petechiae, purpura (Fig. 31-10), oozing

TABLE 31-20	RISK FACTORS FOR DIC
Acute DIC	• Transplant rejections
Shock	• Postoperative damage, especially after extracorporeal membrane oxygenation
• Hemorrhagic	
• Cardiogenic	
• Anaphylactic	• Fat and pulmonary emboli
Septicemia (bacterial, viral, fungal, parasitic)	• Snakebites
	• Glomerulonephritis
Hemolytic processes	• Acute anoxia (e.g., after cardiac arrest)
• Transfusion of mismatched blood	
• Acute hemolysis from infection or immunologic disorders	• Prosthetic devices
	• Fulminant hepatitis
Obstetric conditions	**Subacute DIC**
• Abruptio placentae	Malignancy
• Amniotic fluid embolism	• Myeloproliferative/lymphoproliferative malignancies
• Septic abortion	
• HELLP syndrome	
Malignancies	• Metastatic cancer
• Acute leukemia	Obstetric
• Lymphoma	• Retained dead fetus
• Tumor lysis syndrome	
Tissue damage	**Chronic DIC**
• Extensive burns and trauma	Liver disease
• Heatstroke	Systemic lupus erythematosus
• Severe head injury	Malignancy

DIC, Disseminated intravascular coagulation; *HELLP syndrome,* a life-threatening liver disorder thought to be a type of severe preeclampsia, it is characterized by **H**emolysis (destruction of red blood cells), **E**levated **L**iver enzymes (which indicate liver damage), and **L**ow **P**latelet count.

FIG. 31-10 Disseminated intravascular coagulation (DIC) resulting from staphylococcal septicemia. Note the characteristic skin hemorrhage ranging from small purpuric lesions to larger ecchymoses.

blood, venipuncture site bleeding, hematomas, and occult hemorrhage; (2) respiratory manifestations such as tachypnea, hemoptysis, and orthopnea; (3) cardiovascular manifestations such as tachycardia and hypotension; (4) GI manifestations such as upper and lower GI bleeding, abdominal distention, and bloody stools; (5) urinary manifestations such as hematuria; (6) neurologic manifestations such as vision changes, dizziness, headache, changes in mental status, and irritability; and (7) musculoskeletal complaints such as bone and joint pain.

Thrombotic manifestations are a result of fibrin or platelet deposition in the microvasculature (see Fig. 31-9). They include (1) integumentary manifestations, such as cyanosis, ischemic tissue necrosis (e.g., gangrene), and hemorrhagic necrosis; (2) respiratory manifestations, such as tachypnea, dyspnea, pulmonary emboli, and acute respiratory distress syndrome (ARDS); (3) cardiovascular manifestations, such as electrocardiogram (ECG) changes and venous distention; (4) GI manifestations, such as abdominal pain and paralytic ileus; and (5) kidney damage and oliguria, leading to failure.

Diagnostic Studies

Tests to diagnose acute DIC are listed in Table 31-21. As more clots are made in the body, more breakdown products from fibrinogen and fibrin are also formed. These are termed *fibrin split products* (FSPs), and they interfere with blood coagulation by (1) coating the platelets and interfering with platelet function; (2) interfering with thrombin and thus disrupting coagulation; and (3) attaching to fibrinogen, which interferes with the polymerization process necessary to form a stable clot. D-dimer, a polymer resulting from the breakdown of fibrin (and not fibrinogen), is a specific marker for the degree of fibrinolysis. In general, tests that measure raw materials needed for coagulation (e.g., platelets, fibrinogen) are reduced, and values that measure times to clot are prolonged. Fragmented erythrocytes (schistocytes), indicative of partial occlusion of small vessels by fibrin thrombi, may be found on blood smears.

TABLE 31-21	LABORATORY RESULTS IN ACUTE DIC
Test	**Finding in Acute DIC**
Screening Tests	
Prothrombin time (PT)	Prolonged
Partial thromboplastin time (PTT)	Prolonged
Activated partial thromboplastin time (aPTT)	Prolonged
Thrombin time	Prolonged
Fibrinogen	Reduced
Platelets	Reduced
Special Tests	
Fibrin split products (FSPs)	Elevated
Factor assays (prothrombin and factors V, VIII, X, XIII)	Reduced but may give misleading results, since V and VIII rise with inflammation
D-dimers (cross-linked fibrin fragments)	Elevated
Antithrombin III (AT III)	Reduced
Proteins C and S	Reduced
Plasminogen, tissue plasminogen activator	Reduced
Peripheral blood smear	Schistocytes present
Soluble fibrin monomer	Positive

DIC, Disseminated intravascular coagulation.

Collaborative Care

It is important to diagnose DIC quickly, stabilize the patient if needed (e.g., oxygenation, volume replacement), treat the underlying causative disease or problem, and control the ongoing thrombosis and bleeding. Depending on its severity, a variety of different methods are used to manage DIC (Fig. 31-11). First, if chronic DIC is diagnosed in a patient who is not bleeding, no therapy for DIC is necessary. Treatment of the underlying disease may be sufficient to reverse the DIC (e.g., chemotherapy when DIC is caused by malignancy). Second, when the patient with DIC is bleeding, therapy is directed toward providing support with necessary blood products while treating the primary disorder.

The blood products are administered cautiously based on specific component deficiencies to patients who have serious bleeding, are at high risk for bleeding (e.g., surgery), or require invasive procedures. Blood product support with platelets, cryoprecipitate, and fresh frozen plasma (FFP) is usually reserved for a patient with life-threatening hemorrhage. Therapy stabilizes a patient, prevents exsanguination or massive thrombosis, and permits institution of definitive therapy to treat the underlying cause. In general, platelets are given to correct thrombocytopenia if the platelet count is less than 20,000/μL or less than 50,000/μL with bleeding. Cryoprecipitate replaces factor VIII and fibrinogen and is given if the fibrinogen level is below 100 mg/dL. Fresh frozen plasma replaces all clotting factors except platelets and provides a source of antithrombin.

A patient with manifestations of thrombosis is often treated by anticoagulation with heparin or low-molecular-weight heparin. Heparin is used in the treatment of DIC only when the benefit (reduce clotting) outweighs the risk (further bleeding). Antithrombin III (ATnativ) may be useful in fulminant DIC, although it increases the risk of bleeding. Chronic DIC does not respond to oral anticoagulants, but it can be controlled with long-term use of heparin.

NURSING MANAGEMENT
DISSEMINATED INTRAVASCULAR COAGULATION

NURSING DIAGNOSES

Nursing diagnoses for the patient with DIC may include, but are not limited to, the following:

- Ineffective peripheral tissue perfusion *related to* bleeding and sluggish or diminished blood flow secondary to thrombosis
- Acute pain *related to* bleeding into tissues and diagnostic procedures
- Decreased cardiac output *related to* fluid volume deficit
- Anxiety *related to* fear of the unknown, disease process, diagnostic procedures, and therapy

NURSING IMPLEMENTATION

Be alert to the possible development of DIC and especially to the precipitating factors listed in Table 31-20. Remember that because DIC is secondary to an underlying disease, the causative problem needs to be managed while providing supportive care for the manifestations of DIC.

Appropriate nursing interventions are essential to the survival of a patient with acute DIC. Astute ongoing assessment, active attention to manifestations of DIC, and prompt administration of prescribed therapies are crucial. Table 31-15 and

FIG. 31-11 Intended sites of action for therapies in disseminated intravascular coagulation (DIC). *AT III,* Antithrombin III; *FSPs,* fibrin split products.

eNursing Care Plan 31-1 (available on the website for this chapter) provide assessments and interventions appropriate for the patient with DIC.

Early detection of bleeding, both occult and overt, must be a primary goal. Assess for signs of external bleeding (e.g., petechiae, oozing at IV or injection sites), signs of internal bleeding (e.g., increased heart rate, changes in mental status, increasing abdominal girth, pain), and any indications that microthrombi may be causing clinically significant organ damage (e.g., decreased renal output). Minimize tissue damage and protect the patient from additional foci of bleeding.

An additional nursing responsibility is to administer blood products and medications correctly. (Blood product transfusion is discussed later in this chapter.)

NEUTROPENIA

Leukopenia refers to a decrease in the total WBC count (granulocytes, monocytes, and lymphocytes). *Granulocytopenia* is a deficiency of granulocytes, which include neutrophils, eosinophils, and basophils. The neutrophilic granulocytes, which play a major role in phagocytizing pathogenic microbes, are closely monitored in clinical practice as an indicator of a patient's risk for infection. A reduction in neutrophils is termed **neutropenia.** (Some clinicians use the terms *granulocytopenia* and *neutropenia* interchangeably because the largest constituency of granulocytes is the neutrophils.) The *absolute neutrophil count* (ANC) is determined by multiplying the total WBC count by the percentage of neutrophils. *Neutropenia* is defined as ANC less than 1000 cells/μL (1×10^9/L). (Normally, neutrophils range

from 2200 to 7700 cells/μL.) *Severe neutropenia* is defined as an ANC less than 500 cells/μL.

In considering the clinical significance of neutropenia, it is important to know whether the decrease in the neutrophil count was gradual or rapid, the degree of neutropenia, and the duration. The faster the drop and the longer the duration, the greater the likelihood of life-threatening infection, sepsis, or death. Other factors and co-morbid conditions, such as being older than 60, having an existing infection, being in the hospital, and having diabetes, can increase the risk of a serious infection.

Neutropenia is a clinical consequence that occurs with a variety of conditions or diseases[34,35] (Table 31-22). It can also be an expected effect, a side effect, or an unintentional effect of taking certain drugs. The most common cause of neutropenia is the use of chemotherapy and immunosuppressive therapy in the treatment of malignancies and autoimmune diseases. A term that is often used to describe the lowest point of neutropenia (and other blood cells) in a patient treated with chemotherapy is *nadir*.

Clinical Manifestations

The patient with neutropenia is predisposed to infection with opportunistic pathogens and nonpathogenic organisms from the normal body flora. When the WBC count is depressed or immature WBCs are present, normal phagocytic mechanisms are impaired. Also the classic signs of inflammation—redness, heat, and swelling—may not occur. WBCs are the major component of pus. Therefore in the patient with neutropenia, pus formation (e.g., as a visible skin lesion or as pulmonary infiltrates on a chest x-ray) is also absent.

TABLE 31-22 CAUSES OF NEUTROPENIA

Drugs*
- Antitumor antibiotics (daunorubicin [Cerubidine], doxorubicin [Adriamycin])
- Alkylating agents (nitrogen mustards, busulfan [Myleran])
- Antimetabolites (methotrexate, 6-mercaptopurine [6-MP])
- Antiinflammatory drugs (phenylbutazone)
- Cardiovascular drugs (captopril [Capoten], procainamide [Pronestyl])
- Diuretics (thiazides, furosemide [Lasix])
- Psychotropic and antidepressant agents (clozapine)
- Miscellaneous (gold, penicillamine)
- Antimicrobial agents (ganciclovir, penicillin G, amphotericin B, vancomycin, trimethoprim/sulfamethoxazole [Bactrim])

Hematologic Disorders
- Idiopathic neutropenia
- Congenital (cyclic neutropenia)
- Aplastic anemia
- Fanconi syndrome
- Leukemia
- Myelodysplastic syndrome

Autoimmune Disorders
- Systemic lupus erythematosus
- Felty syndrome
- Rheumatoid arthritis

Infections
- Viral (e.g., hepatitis, influenza, HIV, measles)
- Fulminant bacterial infection (e.g., typhoid fever, miliary tuberculosis)
- Parasitic
- Rickettsial

Others
- Severe sepsis
- Bone marrow infiltration (e.g., carcinoma, tuberculosis, lymphoma)
- Hypersplenism (e.g., portal hypertension, Felty syndrome, storage diseases [e.g., Gaucher disease])
- Nutritional deficiencies (cobalamin, folic acid)
- Transfusion reaction
- Hemodialysis

*Not all inclusive.

SAFETY ALERT
- A low-grade fever in neutropenic patients is of great significance because it may indicate infection and lead to septic shock and death unless treated promptly.
- Neutropenic fever (≥100.4°F [38°C] and a neutrophil count <500/μL) is a medical emergency.
- Blood cultures should be drawn STAT and antibiotics started within 1 hr.

When fever occurs in a neutropenic patient, it is assumed to be caused by infection and requires immediate attention. The immunocompromised, neutropenic patient has little or no ability to fight infection. Thus minor infections can lead rapidly to sepsis. The mucous membranes of the throat and mouth, the skin, the perineal area, and the pulmonary system are common entry points for pathogenic organisms in susceptible hosts.

Clinical manifestations related to infection at these sites include complaints of sore throat and dysphagia, ulcerative lesions of the pharyngeal and buccal mucosa, diarrhea, rectal tenderness, vaginal itching or discharge, shortness of breath, and nonproductive cough. Seriously consider any minor complaint of pain or any other symptom by the patient, and report it to the physician immediately. These seemingly minor com-

DELEGATION DECISIONS

Caring for the Patient With Neutropenia

All members of the health care team have important roles in preventing infection in the patient with neutropenia. Careful hand washing is an important preventive measure and should be done before, during, and after patient care by everyone caring for the patient.

Role of Registered Nurse (RN)
- Determine the type of isolation precautions that need to be initiated, if any.
- Assess patient for subtle signs of infection such as confusion or fatigue.
- Screen visitors for infectious diseases.
- Communicate with nutrition services to eliminate undercooked meats from the patient diet.
- Instruct patient and visitors about hand washing.
- Teach patient and caregivers about how to avoid infection, including the need for skin care and oral hygiene.
- If the patient is managed as an outpatient, teach the patient and the caregivers about signs and symptoms of infection and to report promptly to a health care facility if they occur.

Role of Licensed Practical/Vocational Nurse (LPN/LVN)
- Administer antibiotics and hematopoietic growth factors (consider state nurse practice act and agency policy for IV medications).
- Check the skin, oral mucosa, and perineal area for signs of infection.
- Monitor for signs and symptoms of infection and report them to the RN.

Role of Unlicensed Assistive Personnel (UAP)
- Obtain vital signs and report changes to the RN.
- Assist the patient with oral care and personal hygiene.

plaints can progress to fever, chills, sepsis, and septic shock if not recognized and treated early.

Systemic infections caused by bacterial, fungal, and viral organisms are common in patients with neutropenia. The patient's own flora (normally nonpathogenic) contributes significantly to life-threatening infections such as pneumonia. Organisms known to be common sources of infection include gram-positive coagulase-negative staphylococci and *Staphylococcus aureus* and gram-negative organisms such as *Escherichia coli* and *Pseudomonas aeruginosa*.[36,37] Fungi involved include *Candida* (usually *C. albicans*) and *Aspergillus* organisms. Viral infections caused by reactivation of herpes simplex and zoster are common after prolonged periods of neutropenia, such as in HSCT patients.

Diagnostic Studies

The primary diagnostic tests for assessing neutropenia are the peripheral WBC count and bone marrow aspiration and biopsy (Table 31-23). A total WBC count of less than 4000/μL (4 × 10^9/L) reflects leukopenia. However, only a differential count can confirm the presence of neutropenia (neutrophil count less than 1000/μL [1 × 10^9/L]). If the differential WBC count reflects an absolute neutropenia of 500 to 1000/μL (0.5 to 1.0 × 10^9/L), the patient is at moderate risk for a bacterial infection. An absolute neutropenia of less than 500/μL (0.5 × 10^9/L) places the patient at severe risk.

A peripheral blood smear is used to assess for immature forms of WBCs (e.g., bands). The hematocrit level, reticulocyte count, and platelet count are done to evaluate bone marrow function. Also review the patient's recent past and current drug

TABLE 31-23 COLLABORATIVE CARE

Neutropenia

Diagnostic
- History and physical examination
- WBC count with differential count
- WBC morphology
- Hct and Hgb values
- Reticulocyte and platelet count
- Bone marrow aspiration or biopsy
- Cultures of nose, throat, sputum, urine, stool, obvious lesions, blood (as indicated)
- Chest x-ray

Collaborative Therapy
- Identification and removal of cause of neutropenia (if possible)
- Identification of site of infection (if present) and causative organism
- Antibiotic therapy*
- Blood cultures drawn STAT, immediately before antibiotics
- Hematopoietic growth factors (G-CSF, GM-CSF, pegfilgrastim [Neulasta])
- Strict hand washing and patient hygiene (skin and oral care)
- Single-patient room, positive-pressure or high-efficiency particulate air (HEPA) filtration, depending on risk
- Community isolation and home precautions if outpatient

*Prompt initiation of empiric broad-spectrum antibiotic therapy at any sign of infection, even a low-grade fever (100.4° F [38° C]), is essential.
G-CSF, Granulocyte colony-stimulating factor; *GM-CSF,* granulocyte-macrophage colony-stimulating factor.

history. If the cause of neutropenia is unknown, bone marrow aspirations and biopsies are done to examine cellularity and cell morphology. Additional studies may be done as indicated to assess spleen and liver function.

NURSING AND COLLABORATIVE MANAGEMENT NEUTROPENIA

The factors involved in the nursing and collaborative care of neutropenia include (1) determining the cause of the neutropenia, (2) identifying the offending organisms if an infection has developed, (3) instituting antibiotic therapy, (4) administering hematopoietic growth factors, and (5) implementing protective environmental practices (e.g., strict hand washing)[38] (see Table 31-23).

Occasionally the cause of the neutropenia can be easily treated (e.g., nutritional deficiencies). However, neutropenia can also be a side effect that must be tolerated as a necessary step in therapy (e.g., chemotherapy, radiation therapy). In some situations the neutropenia resolves when the primary disease (e.g., tuberculosis) is treated.

Monitor the neutropenic patient for signs and symptoms of infection (e.g., any fever 100.4° F [38° C] or greater) and early septic shock. Early identification of a potentially infective organism depends on acquiring cultures from various sites. Serial blood cultures (at least two) or one from a peripheral site and one from a venous access device should be done promptly and antibiotics started immediately (within 1 hour). Communicate with the pharmacy regarding the urgency required for dispensing the medication. Cultures of sputum, throat, lesions, wounds, urine, and feces may also be ordered in the surveillance of the patient. Depending on the clinical situation, it may also be necessary to do a tracheal aspiration, bronchoscopy with

bronchial brushings, or lung biopsy to diagnose the cause of pneumonic infiltrates. Invasive diagnostic studies are often contraindicated because of the concern of introducing infection and the fact that these patients are also often thrombocytopenic. Despite these many tests, the causative organism is identified in only approximately one half of neutropenic patients. Thus the priority is to obtain the blood cultures and administer the antibiotic STAT.

When a febrile episode occurs in a neutropenic patient, antibiotic therapy must be initiated immediately (within 1 hour) even before the determination of a specific causative organism by culture. Administration of broad-spectrum antibiotics is usually by the IV route because of the rapidly lethal effects of infection. However, some oral antibiotics are highly effective and routinely used for prophylaxis against infection in some neutropenic patients. The use of a third- or fourth-generation cephalosporin (e.g., cefepime [Maxipime], ceftazidime [Ceptaz]), a carbapenem (e.g., imipenem/cilastatin [Primaxin]), or a combination of an aminoglycoside plus an antipseudomonal offers broad-spectrum coverage for initial management.[37]

Regardless of the combination, you must initiate therapy promptly and observe the patient for side effects of antimicrobial agents. Side effects common to aminoglycosides include nephrotoxicity and ototoxicity. Side effects common to cephalosporins include rashes, fever, and pruritus. Additionally, ongoing febrile episodes or a change in the patient's assessment requires a call to the physician for additional cultures, diagnostic tests, or additional antimicrobial therapies.

The duration of the neutropenia also increases the patient's infection risk. The longer the neutropenia, the greater the risk of a fungal infection. Antifungal therapy is initiated whenever a culture is positive, or in patients who do not become afebrile with broad-spectrum antibiotic coverage.

Granulocyte colony-stimulating factor (G-CSF) (filgrastim [Neupogen], pegfilgrastim [Neulasta]), and granulocyte-macrophage colony-stimulating factor (GM-CSF) (sargramostim [Leukine, Prokine]) (see Table 16-14) can be used to prevent neutropenia or to reduce its severity and duration.[37] Once neutropenia has occurred, these agents are generally not as effective. G-CSF stimulates the production and function of neutrophils. GM-CSF stimulates the production and function of neutrophils and monocytes. These agents can be given IV or subcutaneously. Keratinocyte growth factor (palifermin [Kepivance]) may also be used to reduce the duration and severity of mucositis that may contribute to infection. (G-CSF, GM-CSF, and palifermin are discussed in Chapter 16.)

Determine the best means to protect the patient whose own defenses against infection are compromised. Keep the following principles in mind: (1) the patient's normal flora is the most common source of microbial colonization and infection; (2) transmission of organisms from humans most commonly occurs by direct contact with the hands; (3) air, food, water, and equipment provide additional opportunities for infection transmission; and (4) health care providers with transmissible illnesses and other patients with infections can also be sources of infection transmission under certain conditions.

Hand washing is the single most important preventive measure to minimize the risk of infection in the neutropenic patient. Strict hand washing by staff and visitors using an antiseptic hand wash, before and after contact, is the major method to prevent transmission of harmful pathogens.

TABLE 31-24 PATIENT & CAREGIVER TEACHING GUIDE

Neutropenia

Include the following instructions when teaching a patient or caregiver the precautions to take when the neutrophil count is low.

1. WASH YOUR HANDS frequently and make sure those around you wash their hands frequently, particularly if they help with your care. An antibacterial hand gel may also be used.
2. Notify your nurse or health care provider if you have any of the following:
   - Fever ≥100.4°F (38°C)*
   - Chills or feeling hot
   - Redness, swelling, discharge, or new pain on or in your body
   - Changes in urination or bowel movements
   - Cough, sore throat, mouth sores, or blisters
3. If you are at home, take your temperature as directed and follow instructions on what to do if you have a fever.
4. Avoid crowds and people with colds, flu, or infections. If you are in a public area, wear a mask and use hand sanitizing gel frequently.
5. Avoid uncooked meats, seafood, or eggs and unwashed fruits and vegetables. Ask your health care provider about specific dietary guidelines for you.
6. Bathe or shower daily. A moisturizer may be used to prevent skin from drying and cracking.
7. Brush your teeth with a soft toothbrush four times daily. You may floss once daily if it does not cause excessive pain or bleeding. Avoid alcohol-based mouthwashes.
8. Do not perform gardening or clean up after pets. Feeding and petting your dog or cat are fine as long as you wash your hands well after handling.

*Need to verify cut-off temperature with health care provider.

INFORMATICS IN PRACTICE

Use of Internet to Access Information on Unfamiliar Diseases

- If you are assigned to take care of a patient with a disease or disorder that you are not familiar with, such as thalassemia, access the Internet and perform a quick search.
- Within minutes, you can learn the pathophysiology of thalassemia, treatment options, possible complications that you will need to monitor, and recommended medical and nursing interventions.
- Using this readily available information will help you deliver high-quality, evidence-based care.

Separate immunocompromised patients from those who are infected or have conditions that increase the probability of transmitting infections (e.g., poor hygiene caused by lack of understanding or cognitive dysfunction). Often, patients can be managed on an outpatient basis if the patient and caregiver can astutely monitor for fevers and other signs of infection and then report promptly to a nearby health care facility (Table 31-24). If the patient is hospitalized, a private room should be used. High-efficiency particulate air (HEPA) filtration is an air-handling method with a high-flow filtering system that can reduce or eliminate the number of aerosolized pathogens in the environment. Although it is expensive to install, it is often used for a patient with severe prolonged neutropenia (e.g., bone marrow transplant patients). Care routines in a HEPA environment are essentially the same as care in any other private room. Additional neutropenic precaution guidelines may also be employed, such as prophylactic antibiotics and antifungals or the avoidance of uncooked meat. The nursing measures presented in eNursing Care Plan 31-2 (available on the website for this chapter) are important in the treatment of the patient with neutropenia.

Quality-of-life issues for the patient with neutropenia should not be overlooked. Fatigue, malaise, a decrease in functioning, and social isolation require appropriate interventions.

MYELODYSPLASTIC SYNDROME

Myelodysplastic syndrome (MDS) is a group of related hematologic disorders characterized by peripheral blood cytopenias (from ineffective blood cell production) and changes in the cellularity of the bone marrow with dysplastic changes. In MDS, *hematopoiesis* is disorderly and ineffective. It is estimated that 11,000 new cases of MDS are diagnosed each year in the United States. Although it can occur in all age-groups, the highest prevalence is in men over 80 years of age.[39,40]

Etiology and Pathophysiology

The etiology of MDS is unknown. People who have received radiation therapy, had chemotherapy with alkylating agents (e.g., chlorambucil, cyclophosphamide, melphalan), or been exposed to industrial solvents (e.g., benzene) have a higher risk of developing MDS than people who have not had these exposures. Rarely, genetic disorders are responsible for the disease. Nevertheless, in 60% to 70% of MDS patients, no specific cause can be identified.

MDS is referred to as a *clonal disorder* because some bone marrow stem cells continue to function normally, whereas others (a specific clone) do not. The abnormal clone of the stem cells is usually found in the bone marrow but eventually may be found in the circulation.

Occasionally one type of MDS transforms into another. In about 30% of cases, MDS progresses to acute myelogenous leukemia (AML).[41,42] In contrast to AML, in which the leukemic cells show little normal maturation, the clonal cells in MDS always display some degree of maturity. Disease progression is slower than in AML, and sometimes treatment is not required.

Clinical Manifestations

Manifestations result from neoplastic transformation of the pluripotent hematopoietic stem cells in the bone marrow. MDS commonly manifests as infection and bleeding caused by inadequate numbers of ineffectively functioning circulating granulocytes or platelets. MDS is often discovered in the older adult during testing for the symptoms of anemia, thrombocytopenia, or neutropenia. It may also be diagnosed incidentally from a routine CBC. During the advanced stage of MDS, life-threatening anemia, thrombocytopenia, and neutropenia occur.

Diagnostic Studies

Bone marrow biopsy with aspirate analysis is essential for both the diagnosis and the classification of the specific type of myelodysplasia. In MDS the patient has peripheral cytopenia and changes in the bone marrow (hypocellular or hypercellular). Laboratory data and bone marrow studies help rule out other causes of the dysplasia, such as nonmalignant disorders, cobalamin and folate deficiencies, and infections.[42,43]

NURSING AND COLLABORATIVE MANAGEMENT MYELODYSPLASTIC SYNDROME

Supportive treatment of MDS is based on the premise that the aggressiveness of treatment should match the aggressiveness of the disease. Supportive treatment consists of hematologic monitoring (serial bone marrow and peripheral blood examinations); antibiotic therapy; or transfusions with blood products, along with iron chelators to prevent iron overload.

Low-risk patients can often be treated with erythropoietin and G-CSF. Only about one third of high-risk patients are treated with intensive chemotherapy and/or HSCT. Azacitidine (Vidaza) and decitabine (Dacogen) are drugs that help restore normal growth control and differentiation of hematopoietic cells and reduce the frequency of transformation of MDS to acute leukemia. Side effects include myelosuppression, nausea, vomiting, constipation or diarrhea, renal dysfunction, and injection site erythema.

Lenalidomide (Revlimid) or thalidomide may also be used. Other treatments for MDS include cytarabine (Cytosar, Ara-C) with or without antitumor antibiotics (anthracyclines), antithymocyte globulin, and cyclosporine. High-dose chemotherapy and allogeneic HSCT have been used in an attempt to treat bone marrow dysfunction of MDS and restore it with normal hematopoiesis. However, because of the aggressiveness of this treatment, it is generally recommended for patients less than 55 years old.

Nursing care of a patient with MDS is similar to that of a patient with manifestations of anemia, thrombocytopenia, and neutropenia (see Nursing Care Plan 31-1 for the patient with anemia, and eNursing Care Plan 31-1 for the patient with thrombocytopenia, and eNursing Care Plan 31-2 for the patient with neutropenia. The eNCPs are available on the website for this chapter.)

LEUKEMIA

Leukemia is the general term used to describe a group of malignant disorders affecting the blood and blood-forming tissues of the bone marrow, lymph system, and spleen. Leukemia occurs in all age-groups. It results in an accumulation of dysfunctional cells because of a loss of regulation in cell division. It follows a progressive course that is eventually fatal if untreated. An estimated 43,000 new cases are diagnosed each year. Although often thought of as a disease of children, leukemia affects approximately 10 times more adults than children.[44]

Etiology and Pathophysiology

Regardless of the specific type, leukemia has no single cause. It is now known that all cancers, including leukemia, begin as a mutation in the DNA of certain cells. Most leukemias result from a combination of factors, including genetic and environmental influences. Abnormal genes *(oncogenes)* are capable of causing many types of cancers, including leukemias (see Chapter 16). Chemical agents (e.g., benzene), chemotherapeutic agents (e.g., alkylating agents), viruses, radiation, and immunologic deficiencies have all been associated with the development of leukemia. The incidence of leukemia is increased in radiologists, persons who have lived near nuclear bomb test sites or nuclear reactor accidents (e.g., Chernobyl), and persons previously treated with radiation therapy or chemotherapy.

Although ribonucleic acid (RNA) retroviruses cause a number of leukemias in animals, a viral cause for a human leukemia has been established only for some patients with adult T-cell leukemia. This form of leukemia is endemic in southwestern Japan and parts of the Caribbean and central Africa and is caused by the human T-cell leukemia virus type 1 (HTLV-1).[45]

Classification

Leukemia can be classified based on acute versus chronic disease and on the type of WBC involved. The terms *acute* and *chronic* refer to cell maturity and nature of disease onset. Acute leukemia is characterized by the clonal proliferation of immature hematopoietic cells. The leukemia develops after malignant transformation of a single type of immature hematopoietic cell, followed by cellular replication and expansion of that malignant clone. Chronic leukemias involve more mature forms of the WBC, and the disease onset is more gradual.

Leukemia can also be classified by identifying the type of leukocyte involved, whether it is of myelogenous or lymphocytic origin. By combining the acute and chronic categories with the cell type involved, one can identify four major types of leukemia: acute lymphocytic leukemia (ALL), acute myelogenous leukemia (AML), chronic myelogenous (granulocytic) leukemia (CML), and chronic lymphocytic leukemia (CLL). Other defining features of these leukemic subtypes are presented in Table 31-25.

Acute Myelogenous Leukemia. AML represents only one fourth of all leukemias, but it makes up approximately 80% of the acute leukemias in adults. Its onset is often abrupt and dramatic. A patient may have serious infections and abnormal bleeding from the onset of the disease.[44]

AML is characterized by uncontrolled proliferation of myeloblasts, the precursors of granulocytes. There is hyperplasia of the bone marrow. The clinical manifestations are usually related to replacement of normal hematopoietic cells in the marrow by leukemic myeloblasts and, to a lesser extent, to infiltration of other organs and tissue (see Table 31-25).

Acute Lymphocytic Leukemia. ALL is the most common type of leukemia in children and accounts for about 20% of acute leukemia cases in adults.[44] In ALL, immature small lymphocytes proliferate in the bone marrow; most are of B-cell origin. The majority of patients have fever at the time of diagnosis. Signs and symptoms may appear abruptly with bleeding or fever, or they may be insidious with progressive weakness, fatigue, bone and/or joint pain, and bleeding tendencies.

Central nervous system (CNS) manifestations are especially common in ALL and represent a serious problem. Leukemic meningitis caused by arachnoid infiltration occurs in many patients with ALL.

Chronic Myelogenous Leukemia. CML is caused by excessive development of mature neoplastic granulocytes in the bone marrow. The excess neoplastic granulocytes move into the peripheral blood in massive numbers and ultimately infiltrate the liver and spleen.

The natural history of CML is a chronic stable phase, followed by the development of a more acute, aggressive phase referred to as the *blastic phase*. The chronic phase of CML can last for several years and can usually be well controlled with treatment. Even with treatment, the chronic phase of the disease eventually progresses to the accelerated phase, ending in a blastic phase. Once CML transforms to an acute or blastic

TABLE 31-25 TYPES OF LEUKEMIA

Age of Onset	Clinical Manifestations	Diagnostic Findings
Acute Myelogenous Leukemia (AML)		
Most common cancer in children ages 0-7 yr. Increase in incidence with advancing age after 55 yr.	Fatigue and weakness, headache, mouth sores, anemia, bleeding, fever, infection, sternal tenderness, gingival hyperplasia, mild hepatosplenomegaly (one third of patients).	Low RBC count, Hgb, Hct, platelet count. Low to high WBC count with myeloblasts. High LDH. Hypercellular bone marrow with myeloblasts.
Acute Lymphocytic Leukemia (ALL)		
In children median age at diagnosis is 13 yr. Increases in incidence with advancing age after 60 yr.	Fever, pallor, bleeding, anorexia, fatigue and weakness. Bone, joint, and abdominal pain. Generalized lymphadenopathy, infections, weight loss, hepatosplenomegaly, headache, mouth sores, neurologic manifestations: CNS involvement, increased intracranial pressure (nausea, vomiting, lethargy, cranial nerve dysfunction) secondary to meningeal infiltration.	Low RBC count, Hgb, Hct, platelet count. Low, normal, or high WBC count. High LDH. Transverse lines of rarefaction at ends of metaphysis of long bones on x-ray. Hypercellular bone marrow with lymphoblasts. Lymphoblasts also possible in cerebrospinal fluid. Presence of Philadelphia chromosome (20%-25% of patients).
Chronic Myelogenous Leukemia (CML)		
Increase in incidence with advancing age after 55 yr.	No symptoms early in disease. Fatigue and weakness, fever, sternal tenderness, weight loss, joint pain, bone pain, massive splenomegaly, increase in sweating.	Low RBC count, Hgb, Hct. High platelet count early, lower count later. ↑ Neutrophils, normal number of lymphocytes, and normal or low number of monocytes. Low leukocyte alkaline phosphatase. Presence of Philadelphia chromosome in 90% of patients.
Chronic Lymphocytic Leukemia (CLL)		
Increase in incidence with advancing age after 50 yr, with predominance in men.	Frequently no symptoms. Detection of disease often during examination for unrelated condition, chronic fatigue, anorexia, splenomegaly and lymphadenopathy, hepatomegaly. May progress to fever, night sweats, weight loss, fatigue, and frequent infections.	Mild anemia and thrombocytopenia with disease progression. Total WBC count >100,000/μL. Increase in peripheral lymphocytes and lymphocytes in bone marrow. Hypogammaglobulinemia. May have autoimmune hemolytic anemia, idiopathic thrombocytopenic purpura.

LDH, Lactate dehydrogenase.

phase, it needs to be treated more aggressively, similar to an acute leukemia.

Genetic Link

The *Philadelphia chromosome* originates from the translocation between the *BCR* gene on chromosome 22 and the *ABL* gene on chromosome 9. The protein that is encoded by the newly created *BCR-ABL* gene on the Philadelphia chromosome interferes with normal cell cycle events, such as the regulation of cell proliferation.

The Philadelphia chromosome, which is present in 90% to 95% of patients with CML, is a diagnostic hallmark of CML. In addition, its presence is an important indicator of residual disease or relapse after treatment. However, the presence of the Philadelphia chromosome is not *specific* to diagnose CML, since it is also found in ALL and occasionally in AML.

Chronic Lymphocytic Leukemia. CLL is the most common leukemia in adults. CLL is characterized by the production and accumulation of functionally inactive but long-lived, small, mature-appearing lymphocytes. B cells are usually involved. The lymphocytes infiltrate the bone marrow, spleen, and liver. Lymph node enlargement (lymphadenopathy) is present throughout the body.

Complications are rare in early-stage CLL but may develop as the disease advances. Pressure on nerves from enlarged lymph nodes causes pain and even paralysis. Mediastinal node enlargement leads to pulmonary symptoms. Because CLL is usually a disease of older adults, treatment decisions must be made by considering the progression of the disease and the side effects of treatment. Many individuals in the early stages of CLL require no treatment. Others may be followed closely and receive treatment only when the disease progresses. Approximately one third require immediate intervention at the time of diagnosis.

Other Leukemias. Occasionally the subtype of leukemia cannot be identified. The malignant leukemic cells may have lymphoid, myeloid, or mixed characteristics. Frequently these patients do not respond to treatment and have a poor prognosis. Other rare types include hairy cell and biphenotypic (both abnormal myeloid and lymphoid clones) leukemias.

Overlap Between Leukemia and Lymphoma. Overlap exists between leukemia and non-Hodgkin's lymphoma (NHL) because both involve proliferation of lymphocytes or their precursors. A leukemia-like picture with peripheral lymphocytosis and bone marrow involvement may be present in about 20% of adults with some types of NHL. Although differentiation can be difficult, generally patients with more extensive nodal involvement (especially mediastinal), fewer circulating abnormal cells, and fewer blast forms in the marrow are considered to have lymphoma. A prominent leukemic phase is less common in aggressive lymphomas, except Burkitt's and lymphoblastic lymphomas.[45]

Clinical Manifestations

Although the clinical manifestations of leukemia are varied (see Table 31-25), they relate to problems caused by bone marrow failure and the formation of leukemic infiltrates (Fig. 31-12). Bone marrow failure results from (1) bone marrow overcrowding by abnormal cells and (2) inadequate production of normal marrow elements. The patient is predisposed to anemia, thrombocytopenia, and decreased number and function of WBCs.

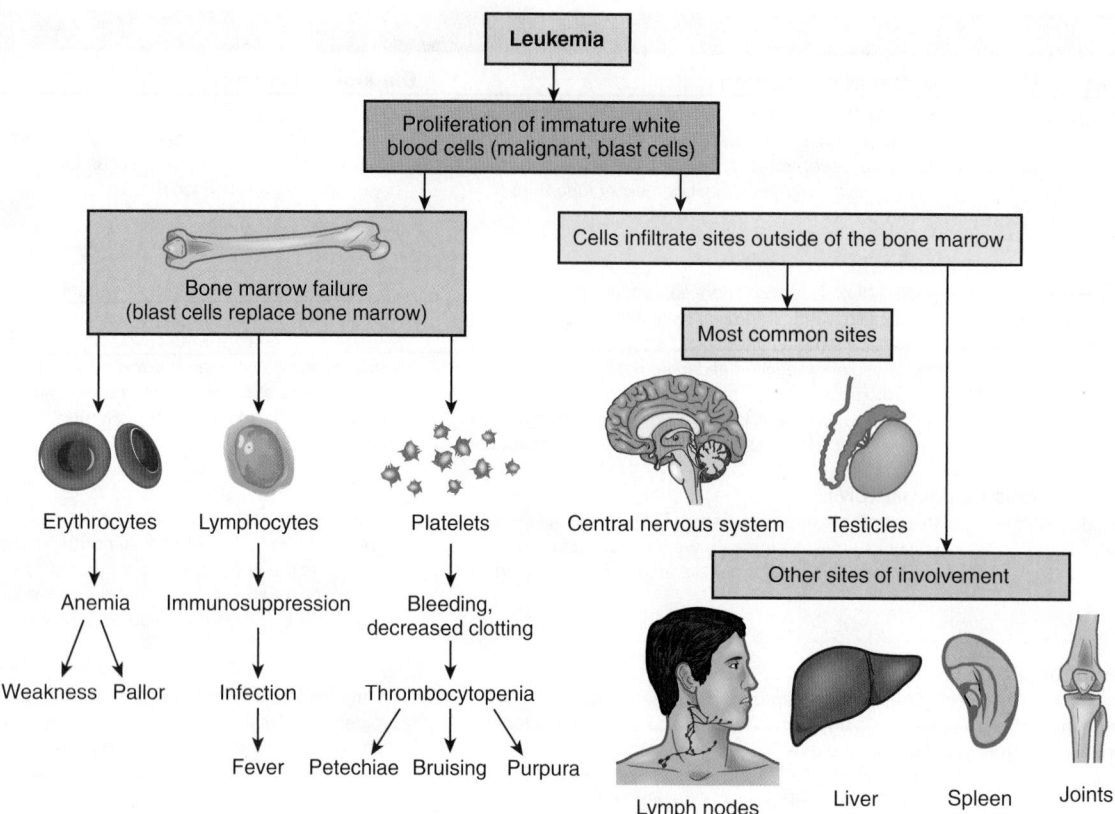

FIG. 31-12 Pathophysiology of leukemia.

As leukemia progresses, fewer normal blood cells are produced. The abnormal WBCs continue to accumulate because they do not go through the normal cell life cycle to death (apoptosis). The leukemic cells may infiltrate the patient's organs, leading to problems such as splenomegaly, hepatomegaly, lymphadenopathy, bone pain, meningeal irritation, and oral lesions. Solid masses resulting from collections of leukemic cells called *chloromas* can also occur. A high leukemic white count in the peripheral blood (more than 100,000 cells/μL) can cause the blood to thicken and potentially block circulatory pathways. This is called *leukostasis* and can be life threatening.

Diagnostic Studies

Peripheral blood evaluation and bone marrow examination are the primary methods of diagnosing and classifying the types of leukemia. Morphologic, histochemical, immunologic, and cytogenetic methods are all used to identify leukemic cell types and stage of development. Identifying the type of leukemia is important because the various types have different prognoses and chemotherapeutic regimens. Other studies such as lumbar puncture and computed tomography (CT) scan can detect leukemic cells outside of the blood and bone marrow.

The malignant cells in most patients with leukemia have specific cytogenetic abnormalities that are associated with distinct subsets of the disease. These cytogenetic abnormalities have diagnostic, prognostic, and therapeutic importance. For example, in CML, the finding of the Philadelphia chromosome has a good prognostic significance, but not so in ALL.

Collaborative Care

Once a diagnosis of leukemia has been made, collaborative care is focused on the initial goal of attaining remission. Age and cytogenetic analysis often help form the basis of important treatment decisions. Because cytotoxic chemotherapy is the mainstay of the treatment, you need to understand the principles of cancer chemotherapy, including cellular kinetics, the use of multiple drugs rather than single agents, and the cell cycle. (See the section on chemotherapy in Chapter 16.)

In some cases, such as nonsymptomatic patients with CLL, watchful waiting with active supportive care may be appropriate. Although a patient may not be cured, attaining remission or disease control is a realistic option for the majority of patients. In some cases, cure is a realistic goal. In *complete remission* there is no evidence of overt disease on physical examination, and the bone marrow and peripheral blood appear normal. A lesser state of control is known as partial remission. *Minimal residual disease* is defined as tumor cells that cannot be detected by morphologic examination, but can be identified by molecular testing. *Partial remission* is characterized by a lack of symptoms and a normal peripheral blood smear, but still evidence of disease in the bone marrow. *Molecular remission* indicates that all molecular studies are negative for residual leukemia. The patient's prognosis is directly related to the ability to maintain a remission. The patient's prognosis becomes more unfavorable with each relapse. After each relapse, the succeeding remission may be more difficult to achieve and shorter in duration.

Sometimes patients have such a high WBC count (e.g., 100,000 cells/μL or more) that initial emergent treatment may include leukapheresis and hydroxyurea. The purpose of these treatments is to reduce the WBC count and risk of leukemia cell–induced thrombosis.

Stages of Chemotherapy. Chemotherapy is often divided into stages: induction, postinduction or postremission, and maintenance.

Induction Therapy. The first stage, *induction therapy,* is the attempt to bring about a remission. Induction is aggressive treatment that seeks to destroy leukemic cells in the tissues, peripheral blood, and bone marrow to eventually restore normal hematopoiesis on bone marrow recovery. During induction therapy, a patient may become critically ill because the bone marrow is severely depressed by the chemotherapeutic agents. Throughout the induction phase, nursing interventions focus on neutropenia, thrombocytopenia, and anemia, as well as providing psychosocial support to the patient and family. Common chemotherapy agents for induction of AML include cytarabine and an antitumor antibiotic (anthracycline) such as daunorubicin (Cerubidine), idarubicin (Idamycin), or mitoxantrone (Novantrone). After one course of induction therapy, approximately 70% of newly diagnosed patients achieve complete remission. It is generally assumed that leukemic cells persist undetected after induction therapy. This could lead to relapse within a few months if no further therapy is administered.[46]

Postinduction or Postremission Therapy. Terms used to describe postinduction or postremission chemotherapy include *intensification* and *consolidation.* *Intensification therapy,* or high-dose therapy, may be given immediately after induction therapy for several months. Other drugs that target the cell in a different way than those administered during induction may also be added.

Consolidation therapy is started after a remission is achieved. It may consist of one or two additional courses of the same drugs given during induction or involve high-dose therapy (intensive consolidation). The purpose of consolidation therapy is to eliminate remaining leukemic cells that may not be clinically or pathologically evident.

Maintenance Therapy. *Maintenance therapy* is treatment with lower doses of the same drugs used in induction or other drugs given every 3 to 4 weeks for a prolonged period. Like consolidation or intensification, the goal is to keep the body free of leukemic cells. Each type of leukemia requires different maintenance therapy. In AML, maintenance therapy is rarely effective and therefore rarely administered.

Drug Therapy Regimens. The therapeutic agents used to treat leukemia vary. Table 31-26 gives examples of treatment regimens used in various types of leukemia.[45-48]

Combination therapy is the mainstay of treatment for leukemia. The three purposes for using multiple drugs are to (1) decrease drug resistance, (2) minimize the drug toxicity to the patient by using multiple drugs with varying toxicities, and (3) interrupt cell growth at multiple points in the cell cycle.

Newer therapeutic drugs are aimed at small molecules that promote the growth and differentiation of leukemic cells. For example, arsenic trioxide (Trisenox), which is used to treat acute promyelocytic leukemia (a type of AML), causes DNA fragmentation and cell death. In addition, it inhibits cell proliferation and angiogenesis (new blood vessel growth). Imatinib targets the *BCR-ABL* protein (discussed above) that is present in nearly all patients with CML. Thus this drug kills only cancer cells, leaving healthy cells alone. (Targeted therapy is discussed in Chapter 16.)

The use of specific targeted therapy in the form of monoclonal antibodies is an important treatment modality in hematopoietic malignancies, but cures with these therapies alone are rare (see Table 16-13 and Fig. 16-16). Rituximab binds to the B-cell antigen (CD20) and has been used with CLL. Alemtu-

TABLE 31-26 DRUG THERAPY	
*Leukemia**	
Drug Therapy	**Other Therapy**
Acute Myelogenous Leukemia	
cytarabine (Cytosar, Ara-C),† daunorubicin (Cerubidine),† idarubicin (Idamycin), 6-thioguanine (6-TG), mitoxantrone (Novantrone), arsenic trioxide (Trisenox),† tretinoin (Vesanoid),† etoposide (VePesid), clofarabine (Clolar), decitabine (Dacogen), fludarabine (Fludara) Combination chemotherapy of cytarabine and antitumor antibiotic (most common)	Autologous or allogeneic hematopoietic stem cell transplant (HSCT) (see Chapter 16)
Acute Lymphocytic Leukemia	
daunorubicin, doxorubicin (Adriamycin), vincristine (Oncovin), prednisone, dexamethasone (Decadron), L-asparaginase (Elspar), ponatinib (Iclusig), pegaspargase (Oncaspar), dasatinib (Sprycel), cyclophosphamide (Cytoxan), methotrexate, 6-mercaptopurine (Purinethol), cytarabine, nelarabine (Arranon), imatinib (Gleevec), clofarabine Combination chemotherapy of several agents is common over a prolonged time	Cranial radiation therapy, intrathecal methotrexate or cytarabine, allogeneic HSCT (see Chapter 16)
Chronic Myelogenous Leukemia	
bosutinib (Bosulif), imatinib, dasatinib, nilotinib (Tasigna), omacetaxine (Synribo), ponatinib, hydroxyurea (Hydrea) Combination chemotherapy including any of the following: cytarabine, thioguanine, daunorubicin, methotrexate, prednisone, vincristine, L-asparaginase, carmustine (BCNU), 6-mercaptopurine	Radiation, HSCT, α-interferon, leukapheresis
Chronic Lymphocytic Leukemia	
chlorambucil (Leukeran), cyclophosphamide, prednisone, vincristine, fludarabine, rituximab (Rituxan), alemtuzumab (Campath), pentostatin (Nipent), bendamustine (Treanda), oxaliplatin (Eloxatin), methotrexate, ofatumumab (Arzerra)	Radiation, splenectomy, colony-stimulating factors, allogeneic HSCT

*The classification and mechanisms of action of these drugs are presented in Table 16-7.
†Used for acute promyelocytic leukemia.

zumab (Campath) binds to CD52, a panlymphocyte antigen present on both T and B cells, and is used to treat CLL.

Other Treatments. In addition to chemotherapy, corticosteroids and radiation therapy can also have a role in the treatment of the patient with leukemia. Total body radiation may be used to prepare a patient for bone marrow transplantation, or radiation may be restricted to certain areas (fields) such as the liver and spleen or other organs affected by infiltrates. In ALL, prophylactic intrathecal methotrexate or cytarabine is given to decrease the chance of CNS involvement, which is common in this type of leukemia. When CNS leukemia does occur, cranial radiation may be given. Biologic and targeted therapy may be indicated for specific leukemias. (Biologic and targeted therapy is discussed in Chapter 16 and Table 16-13.)

Hematopoietic Stem Cell Transplantation. HSCT is another type of therapy used for patients with different forms of leukemia. The goal of HSCT is to totally eliminate leukemic cells from the body using combinations of chemotherapy with or without total body irradiation. This treatment also eradicates the patient's hematopoietic stem cells, which are then replaced with those of an HLA-matched sibling or volunteer donor *(allogeneic)* or an identical twin *(syngeneic)*, or with the patient's own *(autologous)* stem cells that were removed (harvested) before the intensive therapy. (HSCT is discussed in Chapter 16.)

The primary complications for patients with allogeneic HSCT are graft-versus-host disease (GVHD), relapse of leukemia (especially ALL), and infection (especially interstitial pneumonia). GVHD is discussed in Chapter 14. Because HSCT has serious associated risks, the patient must weigh the significant risks of treatment-related death or treatment failure (relapse) with the hope of cure.

NURSING MANAGEMENT LEUKEMIA

NURSING ASSESSMENT

Subjective and objective data that should be obtained from a patient with leukemia are presented in Table 31-27.

NURSING DIAGNOSES

Nursing diagnoses for the patient with leukemia include those for anemia (see Nursing Care Plan 31-1), thrombocytopenia (eNursing Care Plan 31-1), and neutropenia (see eNursing Care Plan 31-2, available on the website for this chapter).

PLANNING

The overall goals are that the patient with leukemia will (1) understand and cooperate with the treatment plan; (2) experience minimal side effects and complications associated with both the disease and its treatment; and (3) feel hopeful and supported during periods of treatment, relapse, or remission.

NURSING IMPLEMENTATION

ACUTE INTERVENTION. The nursing role during acute phases of leukemia is extremely challenging because the patient has many physical and psychosocial needs. As with other forms of cancer, the diagnosis of leukemia can evoke great fear and be equated with death. It may be viewed as a hopeless, horrible disease with many painful and undesirable consequences. The treatment and prognosis of each patient with leukemia are driven by many factors, such as age and type of leukemia. Patients are not the same. Therefore it is important that you understand the patient's type of leukemia, the prognosis, the treatment plan, and the goals. By doing this, you can help the patient realize that, although the future may be uncertain, one can have a meaningful quality of life while in remission or with disease control, and that, in some cases, there is reasonable hope for cure.

The family also needs help adjusting to the stress of this abrupt onset of serious illness and the losses imposed by the sick role (e.g., dependence, withdrawal, changes in role responsibilities, alterations in body image). The diagnosis of leukemia often brings with it the need to make difficult decisions at a time of profound stress for the patient and family.

Patients may have co-morbid conditions that affect treatment decisions. Important nursing interventions include (1) maximizing the patient's physical functioning, (2) teaching patients that acute side effects of treatment are usually temporary, and (3) encouraging patients to discuss their quality-of-life

TABLE 31-27 NURSING ASSESSMENT
Leukemia

Subjective Data
Important Health Information
Past health history: Exposure to chemical toxins (e.g., benzene, arsenic), radiation, or viruses (Epstein-Barr, HTLV-1); chromosome abnormalities (Down syndrome, Klinefelter syndrome, Fanconi syndrome), immunologic deficiencies; organ transplantation; frequent infections; bleeding tendencies
Medications: Use of phenylbutazone (Butazolidin), chloramphenicol, chemotherapy
Surgery or other treatments: Radiation exposure; prior radiation and chemotherapy for cancer

Functional Health Patterns
Health perception–health management: Family history of leukemia; malaise
Nutritional-metabolic: Mouth sores, weight loss; chills, night sweats; nausea, vomiting, anorexia, dysphagia, early satiety; easy bruising
Elimination: Hematuria, decreased urine output; diarrhea, dark or bloody stools
Activity-exercise: Fatigue with progressive weakness; dyspnea, epistaxis, cough
Cognitive-perceptual: Headache; muscle cramps; sore throat; generalized sternal tenderness, bone, joint, abdominal pain; paresthesias, numbness, tingling, visual disturbances
Sexuality-reproductive: Prolonged menses, menorrhagia, impotence

Objective Data
General
Fever, generalized lymphadenopathy, lethargy

Integumentary
Pallor or jaundice; petechiae, ecchymoses, purpura, reddish brown to purple cutaneous infiltrates, macules, and papules

Cardiovascular
Tachycardia, systolic murmurs

Gastrointestinal
Gingival bleeding and hyperplasia; oral ulcerations, herpes and Candida infections; perirectal irritation and infection; hepatomegaly, splenomegaly

Neurologic
Seizures, disorientation, confusion, decreased coordination, cranial nerve palsies, papilledema

Musculoskeletal
Muscle wasting, bone pain, joint pain

Possible Diagnostic Findings
Low, normal, or high WBC count with shift to the left (↑ blast cells); anemia, ↓ hematocrit and hemoglobin, thrombocytopenia, Philadelphia chromosome; hypercellular bone marrow aspirate or biopsy with myeloblasts, lymphoblasts, and markedly ↓ normal cells

HTLV-1, Human T-cell leukemia virus, type 1.

issues. You are an important advocate in helping the patient and family understand the complexities of treatment decisions and manage the side effects and toxicities. A patient may require hospitalization or may need to temporarily relocate to an appropriate treatment center. This situation can lead a patient to feel deserted and isolated at a time when support is most needed. You have contact with a patient many hours a day and can help reverse feelings of abandonment and loneliness by balancing the demanding technical needs with a humanistic, caring approach. The needs of the patient with leukemia are best met by an interdisciplinary team (e.g., psychiatric and oncology clinical nurse specialists, case managers, dietitians, chaplains, and social workers).

From a physical care perspective, you are challenged to make astute assessments and plan care to help the patient manage the severe side effects of chemotherapy. The life-threatening results of bone marrow suppression (neutropenia, thrombocytopenia, and anemia) require aggressive nursing interventions. These patients may be at risk for oncologic emergencies such as tumor lysis syndrome, DIC, and leukostasis. Additional complications of chemotherapy may affect the patient's GI tract, nutritional status, skin and mucosa, cardiopulmonary status, liver, kidneys, and neurologic system. (Nursing interventions related to chemotherapy are discussed in Chapter 16.)

Review all drugs being administered, including the mechanism of action, purpose, routes of administration, usual doses, potential side effects, safe-handling considerations, and toxic effects. Assess laboratory data reflecting the effects of the drugs and sequelae of the disease. Unlike treatments for solid tumors, chemotherapy is administered to patients with leukemia even if they have severe myelosuppression, since the underlying disorder is causing the problem and will not resolve unless treated. Patient survival and comfort during aggressive chemotherapy are significantly affected by the quality of nursing care.

AMBULATORY AND HOME CARE. Ongoing care for the patient with leukemia is necessary to monitor for signs and symptoms of disease control or relapse. For a patient requiring long-term or maintenance chemotherapy, the fatigue of long-term chronic disease management can become arduous and discouraging. Therefore teach the patient and caregiver to understand the importance of continued diligence in disease management and the need for follow-up care. Also teach them about the drugs, self-care measures, and when to seek medical attention.

The goals of rehabilitation for long-term survivors of leukemia are to manage the physical, psychologic, social, and spiritual consequences and delayed effects from the disease and its treatment. (Delayed effects are discussed in Chapter 16.) Assistance may be needed to reestablish the various relationships that are a part of the patient's life. Involving the patient in survivor networks and support groups or services may help the patient adapt to living after a life-threatening illness. Exploring resources in the community (e.g., American Cancer Society, Leukemia & Lymphoma Society) may reduce the financial burden and the feelings of dependence. Also provide the resources for spiritual support.

Vigilant follow-up care helps to ensure that the cancer survivor's unique needs are recognized and treated. Often these needs may require a referral or consultation. For example, physical therapy personnel may be asked to develop an exercise program to prevent posttreatment deficits caused by drug-induced peripheral neuropathy. Most patients should receive the pneumococcal vaccine (Pneumovax) at diagnosis and every 5 years, and an annual influenza vaccine. These needs can also include other concerns such as vocational retraining and reproductive concerns for a patient of childbearing age.

EVALUATION

The expected outcomes are that the patient with leukemia will
- Cope effectively with the diagnosis, treatment regimen, and prognosis

	Hodgkin's Lymphoma	Non-Hodgkin's Lymphoma
Cellular origin	B lymphocytes	B lymphocytes (85%) T or natural killer lymphocytes (15%)
Extent of disease	Localized to regional, but may be more widespread	Disseminated
B symptoms*	Common	40%
Extranodal involvement	Rare	Common

TABLE 31-28 **COMPARISON OF HODGKIN'S AND NON-HODGKIN'S LYMPHOMA**

*B symptoms include fever (>100.4° F [38°C]), drenching night sweats, and weight loss (>10% from baseline within 6 mo).

- Experience no complications related to the disease or its treatment
- Feel comfortable and supported throughout treatment

LYMPHOMAS

Lymphomas are malignant neoplasms originating in the bone marrow and lymphatic structures resulting in the proliferation of lymphocytes. Lymphomas are the fifth most common type of cancer in the United States.[49] Two major types of lymphoma are Hodgkin's lymphoma and non-Hodgkin's lymphoma (NHL). A comparison of these two types of lymphoma is presented in Table 31-28.

HODGKIN'S LYMPHOMA

Hodgkin's lymphoma, also called Hodgkin's disease, makes up about 11% of all lymphomas. It is a malignant condition characterized by proliferation of abnormal giant, multinucleated cells, called *Reed-Sternberg cells,* which are located in lymph nodes. The disease has a bimodal age-specific incidence, occurring most frequently in persons from 15 to 35 years of age and above 50 years of age. In adults, it is twice as prevalent in men as in women. Each year, approximately 9060 new cases of Hodgkin's lymphoma are diagnosed and approximately 1200 deaths occur. However, long-term survival exceeds 85% for all stages.[50]

Etiology and Pathophysiology

Although the cause of Hodgkin's lymphoma remains unknown, several key factors are thought to play a role in its development. The main interacting factors include infection with Epstein-Barr virus (EBV), genetic predisposition, and exposure to occupational toxins. The incidence of Hodgkin's lymphoma is increased among patients who have HIV infection.[50]

Normally, the lymph nodes are composed of connective tissues that surround a fine mesh of reticular fibers and cells. In Hodgkin's lymphoma the normal structure of lymph nodes is destroyed by hyperplasia of monocytes and macrophages. The main diagnostic feature of Hodgkin's lymphoma is the presence of Reed-Sternberg cells in lymph node biopsy specimens. The disease is believed to arise in a single location (it originates in cervical lymph nodes in 70% of patients) and then spreads along adjacent lymphatics. However, in recurrent disease, it may be more diffuse and not necessarily contiguous. It eventually infiltrates other organs, especially lungs, spleen, and liver. When the

FIG. 31-13 Hodgkin's lymphoma (stage IIA). This patient has enlargement of the cervical lymph nodes.

disease begins above the diaphragm, it remains confined to lymph nodes for a variable time. Disease originating below the diaphragm frequently spreads to extralymphoid sites such as the liver.

Clinical Manifestations

The onset of symptoms in Hodgkin's lymphoma is usually insidious. The initial development is most often enlargement of cervical, axillary, or inguinal lymph nodes (Fig. 31-13); a mediastinal node mass is the second most common location. This lymphadenopathy affects discrete nodes that remain movable and nontender. The enlarged nodes are not painful unless they exert pressure on adjacent nerves.

The patient may notice weight loss, fatigue, weakness, fever, chills, tachycardia, or night sweats. A group of initial findings including fever (in excess of 100.4° F [38° C]), drenching night sweats, and weight loss (exceeding 10% in 6 months) are termed *B symptoms* and correlate with a worse prognosis. After the ingestion of even small amounts of alcohol, individuals with Hodgkin's lymphoma may complain of a rapid onset of pain at the site of disease. The cause for the alcohol-induced pain is unknown. Generalized pruritus without skin lesions may develop. Cough, dyspnea, stridor, and dysphagia may all reflect mediastinal node involvement.

In more advanced disease, there may be hepatomegaly and splenomegaly. Anemia results from increased destruction and decreased production of erythrocytes. Other physical signs vary depending on where the disease is located. For example, intrathoracic involvement may lead to superior vena cava syndrome, enlarged retroperitoneal nodes may cause palpable abdominal masses or interfere with renal function, jaundice may occur from liver involvement, spinal cord compression leading to paraplegia may occur with extradural involvement, and bone pain occurs as a result of bone involvement.

Diagnostic and Staging Studies

Peripheral blood analysis, excisional lymph node biopsy, bone marrow examination, and radiologic studies are important means of evaluating Hodgkin's lymphoma. Abnormalities in the CBC, such as a microcytic hypochromic anemia, are variable and not diagnostic. Leukopenia and thrombocytopenia may develop, but they are usually a consequence of treatment, advanced disease, or superimposed hypersplenism. Other blood studies may show hypoferremia caused by excessive iron uptake by the liver and the spleen, elevated leukocyte alkaline phosphatase from liver and bone involvement, hypercalcemia from bone involvement, and hypoalbuminemia from liver involvement.

Radiologic evaluation can help define all sites and determine the clinical stage of the disease. Positron emission tomography (PET) with or without CT scan is used to stage and then assess the response to therapy and to differentiate residual tumor from fibrotic masses after treatment. These scans may show increased uptake (by PET) and masses (by CT) such as mediastinal lymphadenopathy; renal displacement caused by retroperitoneal node enlargement; abdominal lymph node enlargement; and liver, spleen, bone, and brain infiltration.[50]

NURSING AND COLLABORATIVE MANAGEMENT
HODGKIN'S LYMPHOMA

Using all of the information from the various diagnostic studies, one can determine a clinical stage of disease[50,51] (Fig. 31-14). The final staging is based on the clinical stage (extent of the disease) and the presence of B symptoms. Treatment depends on the nature and extent of the disease. The nomenclature used in staging involves an A or B classification, depending on whether symptoms are present when the disease is found, and a Roman numeral (I to IV) that reflects the location and extent of the disease. Additional features that may move an early stage (I or II) to an unfavorable prognosis, warranting more aggressive therapy, include an elevated sedimentation rate; age of 45 years or older; male gender; and the presence of a large mediastinal mass and low serum albumin, hemoglobin, low or high lymphocyte counts.[51]

Once the stage of Hodgkin's lymphoma is established, management focuses on selecting a treatment plan. The standard for chemotherapy is the ABVD regimen: doxorubicin (**A**driamycin), **b**leomycin, **v**inblastine, and **d**acarbazine. Patients with favorable early-stage disease receive two to four cycles of chemotherapy. Patients with early-stage disease but unfavorable prognostic features (e.g., B symptoms) or intermediate-stage disease are treated with four to six cycles of chemotherapy. Advanced-stage Hodgkin's lymphoma is treated more aggressively using six to eight cycles of chemotherapy. A common regimen is BEACOPP (**b**leomycin, **e**toposide, doxorubicin (**A**driamycin), **c**yclophosphamide, vincristine (**O**ncovin), **p**rocarbazine, and **p**rednisone).[51] The role of radiation as a supplement to chemotherapy varies depending on sites of disease and the presence of resistant disease after chemotherapy. Response to therapy is determined by CT and PET scans and other diagnostic tests (e.g., bone marrow biopsy).

A variety of chemotherapy regimens and newer agents, such as brentuximab vedotin (Adcetris), are used to treat patients who have relapsed or refractory disease. Ideally, once remission is obtained, a hope for curative option may be intensive chemotherapy with the use of autologous or allogeneic HSCT.[51] HSCT has allowed patients to receive higher, potentially curative doses of chemotherapy while reducing life-threatening leukopenia (see Chapter 16). Combination chemotherapy works well because, as in leukemia, the drugs used have an additive antitumor effect without increasing side effects. As with leukemia, therapy must be aggressive. Therefore potentially life-threatening problems are encountered in an attempt to achieve a remission.

Maintenance chemotherapy does not contribute to increased survival once a complete remission is achieved. Occasionally, single drugs may be administered palliatively to patients who cannot tolerate intensive combination therapy. A serious consequence of the treatment for Hodgkin's lymphoma is the later

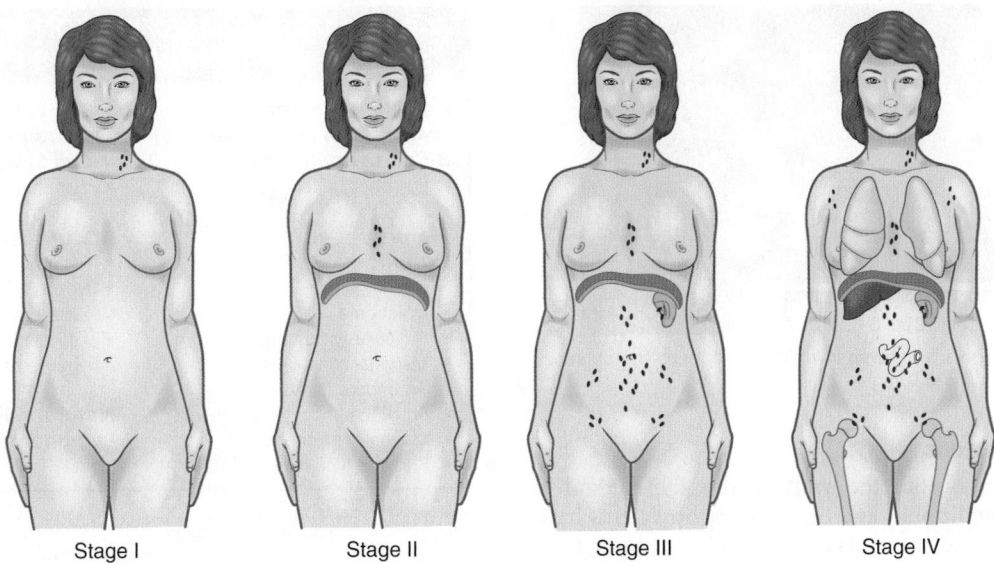

Stage I   Stage II   Stage III   Stage IV

FIG. 31-14 Staging system for Hodgkin's lymphoma and non-Hodgkin's lymphoma. *Stage I,* involvement of single lymph node (e.g., cervical node). *Stage II,* involvement of two or more lymph nodes on one side of diaphragm. *Stage III,* lymph node involvement above and below the diaphragm. *Stage IV,* involvement outside of diaphragm (e.g., liver, bone marrow). The stage is followed by the letter *A* (absence) or *B* (presence) to indicate significant systemic symptoms (e.g., fever, night sweats, weight loss).

development of secondary malignancies (see Chapter 16), as well as potential long-term toxicities from the treatment, such as endocrine, cardiac, and pulmonary dysfunction.[50,51] The estimated risk of a secondary cancer is about 5% and generally occurs within the first 10 years after treatment for Hodgkin's lymphoma.[50] The most common secondary malignancies are AML, NHL, and solid tumors.

The nursing care for Hodgkin's lymphoma is largely based on managing problems related to the disease (e.g., pain caused by a tumor, superior vena cava syndrome), pancytopenia, and other side effects of therapy. Because the survival of patients with Hodgkin's lymphoma depends on their response to treatment, supporting the patient through the consequences of treatment is extremely important.

Psychosocial considerations are as important as they are with leukemia. However, the prognosis for Hodgkin's lymphoma is better than that for many forms of cancer or leukemia. The physical, psychologic, social, and spiritual consequences of the patient's disease must be addressed. Fertility issues may be of particular concern because this disease is frequently seen in adolescents and young adults. Help to ensure that these issues have been addressed soon after diagnosis. Evaluation of patients for long-term effects of therapy is important because delayed consequences of disease and treatment may not be apparent for many years. (Secondary malignancies and delayed effects are discussed in Chapter 16.)

NON-HODGKIN'S LYMPHOMA

Non-Hodgkin's lymphomas (NHLs) are a heterogeneous group of malignant neoplasms of primarily B-, T-, or natural killer (NK) cell origin affecting all ages. B-cell lymphomas constitute about 85% of all NHLs. They are categorized by the level of differentiation, cell of origin, and rate of cellular proliferation.[26] A variety of clinical presentations and courses are recognized, from indolent (slowly developing) to rapidly progressive

disease. NHL is the most commonly occurring hematologic cancer and the fifth leading cause of cancer death. Each year approximately 66,360 new cases of NHL are diagnosed and approximately 19,320 deaths occur.[49]

Etiology and Pathophysiology

As with Hodgkin's lymphoma, the cause of NHL is usually unknown. NHLs may result from chromosomal translocations, infections, environmental factors, and immunodeficiency states. Chromosomal translocations have an important role in the pathogenesis of many NHLs. Some viruses and bacteria are implicated in the pathogenesis of NHL, including HTLV-1, EBV, human herpesvirus 8, hepatitis B and C, *Helicobacter pylori, Chlamydophila psittaci, Campylobacter jejuni,* and *Borrelia burgdorferi.* Environmental factors linked to the development of NHL include chemicals (e.g., pesticides, herbicides, solvents, organic chemicals, wood preservatives). NHL is also more common in individuals who have inherited immunodeficiency syndromes and who have used immunosuppressive medications (e.g., to prevent rejection after an organ transplant or to treat autoimmune disorders) or received chemotherapy or radiation therapy.

NHL does not have a hallmark feature that parallels the Reed-Sternberg cell of Hodgkin's lymphoma. However, all NHLs involve lymphocytes arrested in various stages of development and may mimic a leukemia. For example, small lymphocytic lymphoma (SLL) and chronic lymphocytic leukemia (CLL) result from malignant proliferation of small B lymphocytes, with CLL having the majority of disease within the bone marrow (versus the lymph nodes).[45] (The overlap among leukemia and NHLs is discussed on p. 665.) Diffuse large B-cell lymphoma, the most common aggressive lymphoma, is a neoplasm that originates in the lymph nodes, usually in the neck or abdomen. Burkitt's lymphoma is the most highly aggressive disease and is thought to originate from B-cell blasts in the lymph nodes.

FIG. 31-15 Non-Hodgkin's lymphoma involving the spleen. The presence of an isolated mass is typical.

TABLE 31-29	**CLASSIFICATION OF NON-HODGKIN'S LYMPHOMA***
B-Cell Lymphomas *Precursor or Immature B-Cell Lymphomas* • Lymphoblastic lymphoma	**T-Cell Lymphomas** *Precursor or Immature T-Cell Lymphomas* • Lymphoblastic lymphoma
Mature B-Cell Lymphomas • Diffuse large B-cell lymphoma • Follicular lymphoma • Marginal zone B-cell lymphoma (MALT) • Small lymphocytic lymphoma • Mantle cell lymphoma • Burkitt's lymphoma	*Mature T-Cell Lymphomas* • Peripheral T-cell lymphoma • Mycosis fungoides and Sézary syndrome • Anaplastic large T-cell lymphoma **Natural Killer Cell Lymphomas**

*This is only a partial list.
MALT, Mucosa-associated lymphoid tissue.

Clinical Manifestations

NHLs can originate outside the lymph nodes, the method of spread can be unpredictable, and the majority of patients have widely disseminated disease at the time of diagnosis (Fig. 31-15). The primary clinical manifestation is painless lymph node enlargement. The lymphadenopathy can wax and wane in indolent disease. Because the disease is usually disseminated when it is diagnosed, other symptoms are present depending on where the disease has spread (e.g., hepatomegaly with liver involvement, neurologic symptoms with CNS disease). NHL can also manifest in nonspecific ways, such as an airway obstruction, hyperuricemia and renal failure from tumor lysis syndrome, pericardial tamponade, and GI complaints.

Patients with high-grade lymphomas may have lymphadenopathy and constitutional symptoms (B symptoms) such as fever, night sweats, and weight loss. The peripheral blood is usually normal, but some lymphomas manifest in a "leukemic" phase.

Diagnostic and Staging Studies

Diagnostic studies used for NHL resemble those used for Hodgkin's lymphoma. However, because NHL is more often in extranodal sites, more diagnostic studies may be done, such as an MRI to rule out CNS or bone marrow infiltration, or a barium enema, upper endoscopy, or CT to visualize suspected GI involvement. Clinical staging, as described for Hodgkin's lymphoma, is used to help guide therapy (see Fig. 31-14), but establishment of the precise histologic subtype is extremely important. Lymph node excisional biopsy establishes the cell type and pattern. NHL is classified based on morphologic, genetic, immunophenotypic (cell surface antigens, CD20, CD52), and clinical features.

The World Health Organization has categorized more than 30 unique types of NHL. However, clinical studies have verified that different disease categories can be divided into one of two major categories: *indolent* (low grade) and *aggressive* (high grade), which is useful, along with gene expression patterns, in determining therapy[52] (Table 31-29). Additional factors, known as the International Prognostic Index (IPI), may be considered for each subtype to help select the appropriate treatment for these patients. Factors considered may include the clinical stage, number of extranodal sites, serum LDH, WBC count, hemoglobin, and patient's age and performance status. Immunologic, cytogenetic, and molecular studies are also useful for making therapeutic decisions and assessing prognosis. Other studies might include blood tests for tumor lysis (see Chapter 16); screening for hepatitis, HIV, and *H. pylori*; skin biopsies; bone marrow biopsies; and lumbar punctures. The prognosis for NHL is based on the histopathology.

NURSING AND COLLABORATIVE MANAGEMENT NON-HODGKIN'S LYMPHOMA

Treatment for NHL involves chemotherapy and sometimes radiation therapy (Table 31-30). Ironically, more aggressive lymphomas are more responsive to treatment and more likely to be cured. In contrast, indolent lymphomas have a naturally long course but are difficult to effectively treat.[52]

Patients with low-grade (indolent) lymphoma may live 10 years or more without treatment. However, some initial therapies can be well tolerated and have been shown to reduce the time to progression of the disease. Lymphomas that are infectious driven, such as *H. pylori* gastric lymphomas, may be treated with antibiotic or antiviral therapy. HSCT may have some benefit in certain subtypes of aggressive or refractory lymphomas.[45]

Rituximab, a monoclonal antibody against the CD20 antigen on the surface of normal and malignant B cells, is used to treat NHL. Once bound to the cells, rituximab causes lysis and cell death. Numerous chemotherapy combinations have been used to try to overcome the resistant nature of this disease (see Table 31-30). Complete remissions are uncommon, but the majority of patients respond with improvement in symptoms.

DRUG ALERT: Rituximab (Rituxan)
• Monitor patient for signs of severe hypersensitivity infusion reactions, especially with first infusion.
• Manifestations may include hypotension, bronchospasm, dysrhythmias, angioedema, and cardiogenic shock.
• Screen for history of hepatitis because the drug may reactivate hepatitis.

Other therapies for some types of NHL include the monoclonal antibodies ibritumomab tiuxetan (Zevalin) and tositumomab (Bexxar). These antibodies are linked to a radioactive isotope (yttrium-90 and iodine-131, respectively) (see Table 16-13). The monoclonal antibody targets the CD20 antigen, which is on the surface of mature B cells and B-cell tumors. This targeting allows for the delivery of radiation directly to the malignant cells. Side effects of this type of treatment include pancytopenia. Use radiation precautions in caring for these

TABLE 31-30 TREATMENT OF NON-HODGKIN'S LYMPHOMA*

Recommended Therapies	Common Chemotherapy Combinations
Indolent (Low Grade) (e.g., follicular lymphoma, marginal zone B-cell lymphoma [MALT])	
Observation until disease progression for asymptomatic patients with low-volume tumors and normal blood counts	**R-CHOP: r**ituximab, **c**yclophosphamide, doxorubicin **h**ydrochloride, vincristine (**O**ncovin), **p**rednisone
External beam irradiation for local, limited disease	**FMC: f**ludarabine, **m**itoxantrone, **c**yclophosphamide
Single-agent rituximab (Rituxan)	**R-CVP: r**ituximab, **c**yclophosphamide, **v**incristine, **p**rednisone
Single-agent chemotherapy (chlorambucil, cyclophosphamide, bendamustine, or alemtuzumab)	**FND: f**ludarabine, mitoxantrone [**N**ovantrone], **d**examethasone ± rituximab
Rituximab with another agent (bendamustine, cyclophosphamide, fludarabine, cladribine, pentostatin, chlorambucil, denileukin diftitox)	**FC: f**ludarabine, **c**yclophosphamide
Combination chemotherapy (R-CHOP or other)	
Radioimmunotherapy	
Hematopoietic stem cell transplant (HSCT)	
Aggressive (Intermediate or High Grade) (e.g., mantle cell, diffuse large B-cell, Burkitt's, peripheral T-cell, natural killer cell lymphomas)	
Combination chemotherapy with localized radiation if needed	**R-CHOP** (see above)
Aggressive combination chemotherapy for 3-8 cycles with rituximab with local radiation if needed	**ICE** (or "RICE" with rituximab): **i**fosfamide, **c**yclophosphamide, **e**toposide
Intrathecal chemotherapy if needed	**R-EPOCH: r**ituximab, **e**toposide, **p**rednisone, vincristine (**O**ncovin), **c**yclophosphamide, doxorubicin **h**ydrochloride
HSCT	**ESHAP ± R: e**toposide, methylprednisolone (**S**olu-Medrol), **h**igh-dose cytarabine (**A**ra-C), cisplatin (**P**latinol), with or without rituximab
	Hyper-CVAD ± R: hyperfractionated **c**yclophosphamide, **v**incristine, doxorubicin (**A**driamycin), **d**examethasone alternating with high-dose methotrexate and cytarabine with or without rituximab
	DHAP ± R: dexamethasone, **h**igh-dose cytarabine (**A**ra-C), cisplatin (**P**latinol), with our without rituximab
	CODOX-M: cyclophosphamide, vincristine (**O**ncovin), **dox**orubicin, high-dose **m**ethotrexate, with or without rituximab (includes intrathecal methotrexate)
	FCR: fludarabine, **c**yclophosphamide, **r**ituximab
	SMILE: steroids, **m**ethotrexate, **i**fosfamide, **L**-asparaginase, **e**toposide
	High-dose cytarabine and high-dose methotrexate with leucovorin rescue

*Not all inclusive.
MALT, Mucosa-associated lymphoid tissue.

patients. Teach patients about safety issues and how to minimize the risk of radiation exposure to staff and others.

Peripheral T-cell lymphomas are treated similarly to intermediate-grade or high-grade B-cell lymphomas (without rituximab because they are generally not CD20+). Cutaneous T-cell lymphomas may be treated with topical corticosteroids or topical chemotherapy for limited-stage disease. For more diffuse disease, treatment may include phototherapy, α-interferon, oral bexarotene (Targretin), vorinostat (Zolinza), or denileukin diftitox (Ontak), which is a fusion protein consisting of interleukin-2 and diphtheria toxin.[45,53] (Biologic and targeted therapy is discussed in Chapter 16.)

The nursing care for NHL is similar to that for Hodgkin's lymphoma. It is largely based on managing problems related to the disease (e.g., pain caused by the tumor, spinal cord compression, tumor lysis syndrome), pancytopenia, and other side effects of therapy. However, because NHL can be more extensive and involve specific organs (e.g., CNS, spleen, liver, GI tract, bone marrow), it is important to understand the subtype and extent of the disease. For example, a patient with known involvement of the colon may complain of acute abdominal pain. The patient most likely would have abdominal guarding and an enlarged and tympanic abdomen. This could indicate a bowel perforation and be considered a medical emergency. A patient with a Burkitt's NHL beginning chemotherapy would be at high risk for tumor lysis syndrome and would require frequent laboratory studies and monitoring, as well as strict documentation of intake and output. (Cancer-related therapies and side effects are discussed in Chapter 16.)

The patient undergoing external beam radiation therapy has special nursing needs. The skin in the radiation field requires attention. Concepts related to safety issues regarding radiation therapy are important in the plan of care (see Chapter 16).

Psychosocial considerations are important. Help the patient and family understand the disease, treatment, and expected and potential side effects. Fertility issues may be of concern in young patients. As in Hodgkin's lymphoma, evaluation of patients with NHL for long-term effects of therapy is important because the delayed consequences of disease and treatment may not become apparent for many years. (Secondary malignancies and delayed effects are discussed in Chapter 16.)

MULTIPLE MYELOMA

Multiple myeloma, or *plasma cell myeloma,* is a condition in which neoplastic plasma cells infiltrate the bone marrow and destroy bone. Multiple myeloma accounts for 1% of all malignancies and for about 10% of all hematologic malignancies.[49] The disease is twice as common in men as in women and usually develops after 40 years of age, with an average age of 65 years. Multiple myeloma occurs in African Americans more commonly than in whites. Although it was previously not considered curable, many patients are living 10 or more years because of the variety of treatments that can be provided throughout the course of the disease.[54]

Etiology and Pathophysiology

The cause of multiple myeloma is unknown. It is possible that exposure to radiation, organic chemicals (such as benzene), metals, herbicides, and insecticides may play a role. Genetic factors and viral infection may also influence the risk of developing multiple myeloma.

The disease process involves excessive production of plasma cells. Plasma cells are activated B cells, which produce immunoglobulins (antibodies) that normally serve to protect the body. However, in multiple myeloma instead of a variety of plasma cells producing antibodies to fight different infections, myeloma tumors produce monoclonal antibodies. *Monoclonal* means they are all of one kind, making them ineffective and even harmful. Not only do they not fight infections, but they also infiltrate the bone marrow. These monoclonal proteins (called M proteins) are made up of two light chains and two heavy chains. *Bence-Jones proteins* are the light chain part of these monoclonal antibodies. They show up in the urine in many patients with multiple myeloma.

Furthermore, plasma cell production of excessive and abnormal amounts of cytokines (interleukins [ILs]; IL-4, IL-5, and IL-6) also plays an important role in the pathologic process of bone destruction. As myeloma protein increases, normal plasma cells are reduced, which further compromises the body's normal immune response. Proliferation of malignant plasma cells and the overproduction of immunoglobulin and proteins result in the end-organ effects of myeloma on the bone marrow, bone, and kidneys and possibly the spleen, lymph nodes, liver, and even heart muscle.

Clinical Manifestations

Multiple myeloma develops slowly and insidiously. The patient often does not manifest symptoms until the disease is advanced, at which time skeletal pain is the major manifestation. Pain in the pelvis, spine, and ribs is particularly common and is triggered by movement. Diffuse osteoporosis develops as the myeloma protein destroys bone. Osteolytic lesions are seen in the skull, vertebrae, and ribs. Vertebral destruction can lead to collapse of vertebrae with ensuing compression of the spinal cord. Loss of bone integrity can lead to the development of pathologic fractures.

Bony degeneration also causes calcium to be lost from bones, eventually causing hypercalcemia. Hypercalcemia may cause renal, GI, or neurologic manifestations such as polyuria, anorexia, confusion, and ultimately seizures, coma, and cardiac problems. A serum "hyperviscosity syndrome" leading to cerebral, pulmonary, renal, and other organ dysfunction can occur in some patients. Even without hyperviscosity, high protein levels caused by the myeloma protein can result in renal tubular obstruction, interstitial nephritis, and renal failure. The patient may also display manifestations of anemia, thrombocytopenia, neutropenia, and immune dysfunction, all of which are related to the replacement of normal bone marrow with plasma cells. Neurologic abnormalities may be caused by regional myeloma cell growth compressing the spinal cord or cranial nerves, or by perineuronal or perivascular deposition.

Diagnostic Studies

Evaluating multiple myeloma involves laboratory, radiologic, and bone marrow examination. M protein is found in the blood and urine. Possible findings include pancytopenia, hypercalcemia, Bence Jones protein in the urine, and an elevated serum creatinine.

Skeletal bone surveys, MRI, and/or PET and CT scans show distinct lytic areas of bone erosions; generalized thinning of the bones; or fractures, especially in the vertebrae, ribs, pelvis, and bones of the thigh and upper arms. Bone marrow analysis shows significantly increased numbers of plasma cells in the bone marrow. The simplest measure of staging and prognosis in multiple myeloma is based on blood levels of two markers: β_2-microglobulin and albumin. In general, higher levels of β_2-microglobulin and lower levels of albumin are associated with a poorer prognosis.

Collaborative Care

Collaborative care involves managing both the disease and its symptoms. The current treatment options include watchful waiting (for early multiple myeloma, also called MGUS [monoclonal gammopathy of undetermined significance]), corticosteroids, chemotherapy, targeted therapy, and HSCT. Multiple myeloma is seldom cured, but treatment can relieve symptoms, produce remission, and prolong life. Ambulation and adequate hydration are used to treat hypercalcemia, dehydration, and potential renal damage. Weight bearing helps the bones resorb some calcium, and fluids dilute calcium and prevent protein precipitates from causing renal tubular obstruction. Control of pain and prevention of pathologic fractures are other goals of management. Analgesics, orthopedic supports, and localized radiation help reduce the skeletal pain.

Bisphosphonates, such as pamidronate (Aredia), zoledronic acid (Zometa), and etidronate (Didronel), inhibit bone breakdown and are used for the treatment of skeletal pain and hypercalcemia. They inhibit bone resorption without inhibiting bone formation and mineralization. They are given monthly by IV infusion. Radiation therapy is another important component of treatment, primarily because of its effect on localized lesions. Surgical procedures, such as vertebroplasty, may be done to support degenerative vertebrae.

> **DRUG ALERT: Zoledronic Acid (Zometa)**
> - Patient should be adequately rehydrated before administering drug.
> - Renal toxicity may occur if IV infusion of drug is administered in less than 15 min.

Chemotherapy with corticosteroids is usually the first treatment recommended for multiple myeloma. It is used to reduce the number of plasma cells. Initial treatment depends on whether the patient is a future bone marrow transplant candidate and anticipated tolerance of therapy. The treatment usually includes a corticosteroid (dexamethasone or prednisone) plus one or two therapies, such as cyclophosphamide, lenalidomide, thalidomide, pomalidomide (Pomalyst), doxorubicin, or melphalan. High-dose chemotherapy followed by HSCT has evolved as the standard of care in eligible patients.[55]

Targeted therapy for multiple myeloma may include bortezomib (Velcade) and carfilzomib (Kyprolis). These drugs inhibit proteasomes, which are intracellular multienzyme complexes that degrade proteins. Proteasome inhibitors can cause these proteins to accumulate, thus leading to altered cell function. Normal cells are capable of recovering from proteasome inhibition, but cancer cells undergo death when proteasomes are inhibited.

Drugs may be used to treat complications of multiple myeloma. For example, allopurinol may be given to reduce hyperuricemia, and IV furosemide (Lasix) promotes renal excretion of calcium.

NURSING MANAGEMENT
MULTIPLE MYELOMA

A major focus of care relates to the bone involvement and sequelae from bone breakdown. Maintaining adequate hydration is a primary nursing consideration to minimize problems from hypercalcemia. IV fluids may be administered to attain a urine output of 1.5 to 2 L/day. Although tumor lysis is rare, once chemotherapy is initiated, allopurinol may be given to prevent any renal damage from uric acid accumulation (from cell breakdown). Because of the myeloma proteins, the patient is at additional risk of renal dysfunction and electrolyte and fluid imbalances.

Because of the potential for pathologic fractures, use caution when moving and ambulating the patient. A slight twist or strain in the wrong area (e.g., a weak area in the patient's bones) may be sufficient to cause a fracture. In addition, the development of peripheral neuropathy is common with several therapies for multiple myeloma and can contribute to discomfort, the inability to perform basic activities of daily living, and the risk of injury from falling. Pain medications and therapies can also lead to severe constipation.

Pain management requires innovative and knowledgeable nursing interventions. Analgesics, such as nonsteroidal antiinflammatory drugs, acetaminophen, or an acetaminophen/opioid combination, may be more effective than opioids alone in diminishing bone pain. Braces, especially for the spine, may also help control pain. As in any pain management situation, assess the patient and implement necessary measures to alleviate the pain. (Pain management is discussed in Chapter 9.) Patients may also be at risk for deep vein thrombosis related to chemotherapy and immobility and should have appropriate preventive measures employed.[55]

Assessment and prompt treatment of infection are important in the care of patients with multiple myeloma. These recurrent infections may be due to a decrease in the production of normal immunoglobulins, the ineffectiveness of the overproduced and abnormal immunoglobulins, corticosteroids, and/or neutropenia as a result of the bone marrow infiltration or side effects of treatment.

The patient's psychosocial needs require sensitive, skilled management. Help the patient and significant others adapt to changes fostered by chronic sickness and adjust to the losses related to the disease process, while helping to maximize functioning and quality of life.[56] The patient with multiple myeloma may experience remissions and exacerbations. Patients may be on dialysis because of myeloma-induced renal failure. Consequently acute care is needed at various times during the course of the illness. The final, acute phase is unresponsive to treatment and usually short in duration. The way in which patients and families confront death may be affected by the manner in which they have learned to accept and live with the chronic disease.

DISORDERS OF THE SPLEEN

The spleen can be affected by many illnesses, most of which can cause some degree of *splenomegaly* (enlarged spleen) (Table 31-31). The term *hypersplenism* refers to the occurrence of splenomegaly and peripheral cytopenias (anemia, leukopenia, and thrombocytopenia). The degree of splenic enlargement varies with the disease. For example, massive splenic enlargement occurs with infectious mononucleosis, chronic myelogenous leukemia, and thalassemia major. Mild splenic enlargement occurs with HF and systemic lupus erythematosus. The normal spleen contains 350 mL of blood, and about one third of the platelet mass is sequestered in the spleen.[57]

TABLE 31-31 CAUSES OF SPLENOMEGALY
Hereditary Hemolytic Anemias
• Sickle cell disease
• Thalassemia
Autoimmune Cytopenias
• Acquired hemolytic anemia
• Immune thrombocytopenia
Infections and Inflammations
• Bacterial infections: endocarditis, salmonella
• Mycobacterial infections: tuberculosis
• Spirochetes: syphilis, Lyme disease
• Viral infections: hepatitis, human immunodeficiency virus, cytomegalovirus, mononucleosis
• Parasitic infections: malaria, trypanosomiasis, schistosomiasis, leishmaniasis, toxoplasmosis
• Rickettsial infections: Rocky Mountain spotted fever, typhoid fever
• Fungal infections: histoplasmosis
• Autoimmune diseases: systemic lupus erythematosus, rheumatoid arthritis
Infiltrative Diseases
• Acute and chronic leukemia
• Lymphomas
• Polycythemia vera
• Multiple myeloma, amyloidosis
• Other primary or secondary neoplasms and cysts
• Sarcoidosis
• Gaucher disease
Congestion
• Cirrhosis of the liver
• Heart failure (portal hypertension)
• Portal or splenic vein thrombosis

When the spleen enlarges, its normal filtering and sequestering capacity increases. Consequently, there is often a reduction in the number of circulating blood cells as they engorge the spleen. In addition, there are unusual findings in the peripheral smear, such as pitted or pocked erythrocytes or Howell-Jolly bodies. These findings assist in diagnosing a malfunctioning spleen. A slight to moderate enlargement of the spleen is usually asymptomatic and found during routine examination of the abdomen. Even massive splenomegaly can be well tolerated, but the patient may complain of abdominal discomfort and early satiety. In addition to physical examination, other techniques to assess the size of the spleen include radionuclide colloid liver-spleen scan, CT or PET scan, MRI, and ultrasound scan.

Occasionally laparoscopy or open laparotomy and splenectomy are indicated in the evaluation or treatment of splenomegaly. Another major indication for splenectomy is splenic rupture. The spleen may rupture from trauma; inadvertent tearing during other surgical procedures; and diseases such as mononucleosis, malaria, and lymphoid neoplasms. After a splenectomy, there can be a dramatic increase in peripheral RBC, WBC, and platelet counts.

Nursing responsibilities for the patient with spleen disorders vary depending on the problem. Splenomegaly may be painful and may require analgesic administration; care in moving, turning, and positioning; and evaluation of lung expansion because spleen enlargement may impair diaphragmatic excursion. If anemia, thrombocytopenia, or leukopenia develops from splenic enlargement, institute nursing measures to support the patient and prevent life-threatening complications. If splenectomy is performed, observe the patient for hemorrhage and shock.

After splenectomy, immunologic deficiencies may develop. IgM levels are reduced, while IgG and IgA values remain within normal limits. Postsplenectomy patients have a lifelong risk for infection, especially from encapsulated organisms such as *Pneumococcus* species. This risk is reduced by immunization with pneumococcal vaccine (e.g., Pneumovax).

BLOOD COMPONENT THERAPY

Blood component therapy is frequently used to manage hematologic diseases. Many therapeutic and surgical procedures depend on blood product support. However, blood component therapy only temporarily supports the patient until the underlying problem is resolved. Because transfusions are not free from hazards, they should be used only if necessary.

Avoid developing a complacent attitude about this common but potentially dangerous therapy. Make sure that the physician has discussed the risks, benefits, and alternatives with the patient and that this is documented in the patient's medical record.

Traditionally, the term *blood transfusion* meant the administration of whole blood. Blood transfusion now has a broader meaning because of the ability to administer specific components of blood such as platelets, packed red blood cells (PRBCs), or plasma. Usually a specific component is ordered, although whole blood may be rarely used with massive hemorrhage or for an exchange transfusion[58-60] (Table 31-32).

TABLE 31-32 BLOOD PRODUCTS*

Description	Special Considerations	Indications for Use
Packed RBCs Packed RBCs are prepared from whole blood by sedimentation or centrifugation. One unit contains 250-350 mL. They can be stored up to 35 days depending on processing.	Use of RBCs for treatment allows remaining components of blood (e.g., platelets, albumin, plasma) to be used for other purposes. There is less danger of fluid overload. Packed RBCs are preferred RBC source because they are more component specific. Leukocyte depletion (leukoreduction) by filtration, washing, or freezing frequently used. Decreases hemolytic febrile or mild allergic reactions in patients who receive frequent transfusions.	Severe or symptomatic anemia, acute blood loss. One unit of RBCs can be expected to increase Hgb by 1 g/dL or Hct by 3% in a typical adult. One unit of RBCs can replace a blood loss of 500 mL.
Frozen RBCs Frozen RBCs are prepared from RBCs using glycerol for protection and frozen. They can be stored for 10 yr.	Must be used within 24 hr of thawing. Successive washings with saline solution remove majority of WBCs and plasma proteins.	Autotransfusion. Stockpiling or rare donors for patients with alloantibodies.
Platelets Platelets are prepared from fresh whole blood. One donor unit contains 30-60 mL of platelet concentrate (from whole blood). Platelets also pooled from multiple donors. An apheresed single donation contains 200-400 mL of platelets.	Multiple units of platelets can be obtained from one donor by plateletpheresis. They can be kept at room temperature for 1-5 days depending on type of collection and storage bag used. Bag should be agitated periodically. For patients who receive frequent transfusions and become refractory, may give leukocyte reduced, HLA, or type specific to prevent alloimmunization to HLA antigens.	Bleeding caused by thrombocytopenia; may be contraindicated in thrombotic thrombocytopenic purpura and heparin-induced thrombocytopenia except in life-threatening hemorrhage. Expected increase is 10,000/μL/U. Failure to have an increase may be due to fever, sepsis, splenomegaly, or DIC or development of antibodies *(refractory)*.
Fresh Frozen Plasma Liquid portion of whole blood is separated from cells and frozen. One unit contains 200-250 mL. Plasma is rich in clotting factors but contains no platelets. May be stored for ≥1 yr, depending on storage. Must be used within 24 hr after thawing.	Use of plasma in treating hypovolemic shock is being replaced by pure preparations such as albumin and plasma expanders.	Bleeding caused by deficiency in clotting factors (e.g., DIC, hemorrhage, massive transfusion, liver disease, vitamin K deficiency, excess warfarin).
Albumin Albumin is prepared from plasma. It can be stored for 5 yr. It is available in 5% or 25% solution.	Albumin 25 g/dL is osmotically equal to 500 mL of plasma. Hyperosmolar solution acts by moving water from extravascular to intravascular space. It is heat treated and does not transmit viruses.	Hypovolemic shock, hypoalbuminemia.
Cryoprecipitates and Commercial Concentrates Cryoprecipitate is prepared from fresh frozen plasma, with 10-20 mL/bag. It can be stored for 1 yr. Once thawed, must be used within 5 days.	See Table 31-19.	Replacement of clotting factors, especially factor VIII, von Willebrand factor, and fibrinogen.

*Component therapy has replaced the use of whole blood, which accounts for <10% of all transfusions. Granulocyte transfusions are not included here because they are rarely used.
DIC, Disseminated intravascular coagulation; *HLA*, human leukocyte antigen.

Administration Procedure

Blood components are usually administered with at least a 19-gauge needle, cannula, or catheter. Larger sizes (e.g., 18 or 16 gauge) may be preferred if rapid transfusions are given. Smaller needles can be used for platelets, albumin, and clotting factor replacement. Whatever type of venous access is used, verify its patency before requesting the blood component from the blood bank. Most blood product administration tubing is of a "Y type" with a microaggregate filter (filters out particulate), with one arm of the Y for the isotonic saline solution and the other arm of the Y for the blood product.

> **SAFETY ALERT**
> - Do not use dextrose solutions or lactated Ringer's solution for administering blood because they will cause RBC hemolysis.
> - Do not give any additives (including medications) via the same tubing as the blood unless the tubing is first cleared with saline solution.

After obtaining the blood or blood components from the blood bank, make a positive identification of the donor blood and recipient. Improper product-to-patient identification is the most common cause of hemolytic transfusion reactions, thus placing a great responsibility on nurses to carry out the identification procedure appropriately. Follow the policy and procedures at your place of employment. Many institutions have implemented a dual-checking system with two licensed individuals checking the patient identification with the labeled blood component. The blood bank is responsible for typing and crossmatching the donor's blood with the recipient's blood. The result of the compatibility testing should be noted on the product bag or tag, if pertinent.

ABO compatibility is not a prerequisite for platelet transfusions. However, after multiple platelet transfusions, a patient may develop anti-HLA antibodies to the transfused platelets. With the use of lymphocyte typing to match HLA types of the donor and the recipient, multiple platelet transfusions can be given with fewer complications to those who develop antibodies to platelets. In addition, the patient may be premedicated with an antihistamine (e.g., diphenhydramine [Benadryl]) and hydrocortisone to decrease the possibility of reacting to platelet transfusions.

Take the patient's vital signs before beginning the transfusion so that you have a baseline measure. If the patient has abnormal vital signs (e.g., high fever), call the physician to clarify when the blood component may be administered. Administer the blood as soon as it is brought to the patient. Do not refrigerate it on the nursing unit. If the blood is not used within 30 minutes, return it to the blood bank. During the first 15 minutes or 50 mL of blood infusion, remain with the patient. If there are any untoward reactions, they are most likely to occur at this time. The rate of infusion during this period should be no more than 2 mL/minute. Do not infuse PRBCs quickly except in an emergency. Rapid infusion of cold blood may cause the patient to become chilled. If rapid replacement of large amounts of blood is necessary, a blood-warming device may be used. Other blood components, such as fresh frozen plasma and platelets, may be infused over 15 to 30 minutes. Refer to your institution's policy and procedure.

After the first 15 minutes, vital signs are usually retaken, and the rate of infusion is determined by the patient's clinical condition and the product being infused. Observe the patient periodically throughout the transfusion (e.g., every 30 minutes) and up to 1 hour after the transfusion. Most patients not in danger of fluid overload can tolerate the infusion of 1 unit of PRBCs over 2 hours. The transfusion should not take more than 4 hours to administer because of the increased risk of bacterial growth in the product once it is out of refrigeration. Blood that is unrefrigerated for 4 hours or longer should not be infused and should be returned to the blood bank.

ETHICAL/LEGAL DILEMMAS

Religious Beliefs

Situation

W.D., an 81-year-old woman with dementia, is transferred from a nursing home to a hospital because of gastrointestinal bleeding from an unknown cause. Some of her family members tell you that she is a Jehovah's Witness and must not receive blood products. If she does not have exploratory surgery and transfusions, the surgeon believes that she will die.

Ethical/Legal Points for Consideration

- Competent adults have the right to make health care decisions, including the right to refuse treatment, based on their religious beliefs.
- If the patient is determined to be incompetent and a guardian has been appointed, the guardian has the legal right to make the consent or refusal.
- If the health care professional believes that the treatment is essential to preserve life and health and there is no legal decision maker, a request is made for a legal determination of whether the patient is incapable of consent or refusal. If the judge agrees, the patient is made a ward of the court for this issue. Usually the physician is directed to make a decision based on the patient's best interests.
- Courts tend to defer to any past information coming directly from patients about their own personal desires, even if that information is not in valid advance directives.

Discussion Questions

1. What resources do you have available to consult about religious practices?
2. How could you make a determination if the family were acting in W.D.'s best interest or their own?
3. What nonblood alternatives are available for Jehovah's Witnesses?

DELEGATION DECISIONS

Blood Transfusions

Role of Registered Nurse (RN)

- Ensure that an IV line is being used with a large-bore needle, catheter, or cannula, preferably 19 gauge or larger.
- Double-check patient identification and blood product identification data with another licensed nurse (consider state nurse practice act and agency policy).
- Adjust infusion rate of transfusion according to patient needs.
- Evaluate patient for signs of transfusion reactions.
- Evaluate for therapeutic effect of blood product (improvement in complete blood count, increased blood pressure, improved patient color, decreased bleeding).
- Monitor for signs of circulatory overload (e.g., shortness of breath) if the transfusion must be given rapidly.

Role of Licensed Practical/Vocational Nurse (LPN/LVN)

- Assist with checking patient identification and blood product identification data with the RN (consider state nurse practice act and agency policy).
- Monitor blood transfusion rate (consider state nurse practice act and agency policy).

Role of Unlicensed Assistive Personnel (UAP)

- Obtain blood products from the blood bank as directed by the RN.
- Take vital signs before the transfusion and after the first 15 min.

Blood Transfusion Reactions

A *blood transfusion reaction* is an adverse reaction to blood transfusion therapy that can range in severity from mild symptoms to a life-threatening condition. Because complications of transfusion therapy may be significant, judicious evaluation of the patient is required. Blood transfusion reactions can be classified as acute or delayed (Tables 31-33 and 31-34).

If an acute transfusion reaction occurs, take the following steps: (1) stop the transfusion; (2) maintain a patent IV line with saline solution; (3) notify the blood bank and the health care provider immediately; (4) recheck identifying tags and numbers; (5) monitor vital signs and urine output; (6) treat symptoms per physician order; (7) save the blood bag and tubing and send them to the blood bank for examination;

TABLE 31-33   ACUTE TRANSFUSION REACTIONS

Cause	Manifestations	Management	Prevention
Acute Hemolytic Reaction			
Infusion of ABO-incompatible whole blood, RBCs, or components containing ≥10 mL of RBCs. Antibodies in the recipient's plasma attach to antigens on transfused RBCs, causing RBC destruction.	Reactions usually develop in first 15 min. Chills, fever, low back pain, flushing, tachycardia, dyspnea, tachypnea, hypotension, vascular collapse, hemoglobinuria, acute jaundice, dark urine, bleeding, acute kidney injury, shock, cardiac arrest, DIC, death.	Treat shock and DIC if present. Draw blood samples for serologic testing slowly to avoid hemolysis from the procedure. Send urine specimen to the laboratory. Maintain BP with IV colloid solutions. Give diuretics as prescribed to maintain urine flow. Insert indwelling urinary catheter or measure voided amounts to monitor hourly urine output. Dialysis may be required if renal failure occurs. Do not transfuse additional RBC-containing components until blood bank has provided newly crossmatched units.	Meticulously verify and document patient identification from sample collection to component infusion (e.g., visually compare label on sample collection and blood component with patient identification).
Febrile, Nonhemolytic Reaction (most common)			
Sensitization to donor WBCs (most common), platelets, or plasma proteins.	Sudden chills, rigors, and fever (rise in temperature of >1°C), headache, flushing, anxiety, vomiting, muscle pain.	Give antipyretics as prescribed (acetaminophen). Avoid aspirin in thrombocytopenic patients. Do not restart transfusion unless physician orders.	Consider leukocyte-reduced blood products (filtered, washed, or frozen) for patients with a history of two or more such reactions. Give acetaminophen or diphenhydramine (Benadryl) 30 min before transfusion.
Mild Allergic Reaction			
Sensitivity to foreign plasma proteins. More common in people with history of allergies.	Flushing, itching, pruritus, urticaria (hives).	Give antihistamine, corticosteroid, epinephrine, as ordered. If symptoms are mild and transient, transfusion may be restarted slowly with physician's order. Do not restart transfusion if fever or pulmonary symptoms develop.	Treat prophylactically with antihistamines. Consider washed RBCs and platelets.
Anaphylactic and Severe Allergic Reaction			
Sensitivity to donor plasma proteins. Infusion of IgA proteins to IgA-deficient recipient who has developed IgA antibody.	Anxiety, urticaria, dyspnea, wheezing, progressing to cyanosis, bronchospasm, hypotension, shock, and possible cardiac arrest.	Initiate CPR, if indicated. Have epinephrine ready for injection. Antihistamines, corticosteroids, β₂-agonists may also be prescribed. Do not restart transfusion.	Transfuse extensively washed RBC products from which all plasma has been removed. Use blood from IgA-deficient donor. Use autologous components.
Circulatory Overload Reaction			
Fluid administered faster than the circulation can accommodate. People with cardiac or renal disease at risk.	Cough, dyspnea, pulmonary congestion, adventitious breath sounds, headache, hypertension, tachycardia, distended neck veins.	Place patient upright with feet in dependent position. Obtain chest x-ray STAT if ordered. Administer prescribed diuretics, O₂, morphine. Phlebotomy may be indicated.	Adjust transfusion volume and flow rate based on patient size and clinical status. Have blood bank divide future units into smaller aliquots for better spacing of fluid input.
Sepsis Reaction			
Transfusion of bacterially infected blood components.	Rapid onset of chills, high fever, vomiting, diarrhea, marked hypotension, or shock.	Obtain culture of patient's blood and send bag with remaining blood and tubing to blood bank for further study. Treat septicemia as directed—antibiotics, IV fluids, vasopressors.	Collect, process, store, and transfuse blood products according to blood banking standards and infuse within 4 hr of starting time.

TABLE 31-33 ACUTE TRANSFUSION REACTIONS—cont'd

Cause	Manifestations	Management	Prevention
Transfusion-Related Acute Lung Injury (TRALI) Reaction			
Reaction between transfused antileukocyte antibodies and recipient's leukocytes, causing pulmonary inflammation and capillary leak.	Noncardiogenic pulmonary edema. Fever, hypotension, tachypnea, frothy sputum, dyspnea, hypoxemia, respiratory failure. Leading cause of transfusion-related deaths.	Send bag with remaining blood and tubing to blood bank. Draw blood for arterial blood gases and HLA or antileukocyte antibodies. Obtain chest x-ray STAT. Provide O_2 and administer corticosteroids (diuretics of no value) as ordered. Initiate CPR if needed, and provide ventilatory and BP support if needed.	Provide leukocyte-reduced products. Identify donors who are implicated in TRALI reactions and do not allow them to donate.
Massive Blood Transfusion Reaction			
Can occur when replacement of RBCs or blood exceeds the total blood volume within 24 hr. RBC transfusions do not contain clotting factors, albumin, and platelets.	Hypothermia and cardiac dysrhythmias (from rapid infusion of large quantities of cold blood). Citrate toxicity and hypocalcemia (from the use of citrate as a storage solution). Hypocalcemia (citrate binds calcium) manifested as muscle tremors and ECG changes. Hyperkalemia (from potassium leaking from stored RBCs). Manifested as muscle weakness, diarrhea, paresthesias, paralysis of the cardiac or respiratory muscles, and cardiac arrest.	When patients receive massive transfusions of blood products, monitor clotting status and electrolyte levels.	Use blood-warming equipment. Infusion of 10% calcium gluconate (10 mL with every 1 L of citrated blood).

DIC, Disseminated intravascular coagulation; *HLA,* human leukocyte antigen; *IgA,* immunoglobulin A.

TABLE 31-34 DELAYED TRANSFUSION REACTIONS

Manifestations	Prevention and Management	Manifestations	Prevention and Management
Delayed Hemolytic		**Iron Overload**	
Fever, mild jaundice, decreased hemoglobin. Occurs as early as 3 days or as late as several mo, but usually 5-10 days posttransfusion as the result of destruction of transfused RBCs by alloantibodies not detected during crossmatch.	Generally, no acute treatment is required. But hemolysis may be severe enough to warrant further transfusions.	Excess iron is deposited in heart, liver, pancreas, and joints, causing dysfunction. Heart failure, dysrhythmias, impaired thyroid and gonadal function, diabetes, arthritis, cirrhosis. Commonly occurs in patients receiving >100 units for chronic anemia (e.g., sickle cell anemia, β-thalassemia) over time.	Treat symptomatically. Deferoxamine (Desferal), which chelates and removes accumulated iron via the kidneys, administered IV or subcutaneously. Deferasirox (Exjade) and deferiprone (Ferriprox) are oral agents that chelate iron.
Hepatitis B*			
Elevated liver enzymes (AST and ALT), anorexia, malaise, nausea and vomiting, fever, dark urine, jaundice. Usually resolves spontaneously within 4-6 wk. Chronic carrier state can develop and result in permanent damage to the liver.	Hepatitis B virus can be detected in donated blood by the presence of hepatitis B surface antigen (HBsAg). Treat symptomatically (see Chapter 44).	**Other**	
		Cytomegalovirus (CMV), HIV, human herpesvirus type 6 (HSV-6), Epstein-Barr virus (EBV), human T cell leukemia virus, HTLV-1, and malaria. Most recent threats have been agents that primarily affect animals, but have been transmitted to the blood supply through the food supply, or vectors such as mosquitoes or ticks. These include *Plasmodium* species (malaria), dengue fever virus, West Nile virus, *Trypanosoma cruzi* (Chagas' disease), *Babesia* species (babesiosis), human herpesvirus 8 (KS virus), and variant Creutzfeldt-Jakob disease ("mad cow disease").	Treatment based on the cause. Ways of detecting some of these agents are now available and required, such as the nucleic acid test for West Nile virus and *T. cruzi*. Donor screening has been the only available method to reduce the risk of donor-contaminated blood for others.
Hepatitis C*			
Similar to hepatitis B, but symptoms are usually less severe. Chronic liver disease and cirrhosis may develop.	Before testing of anti-HCV in donated blood, accounted for 90%-95% of all posttransfusion hepatitis. Treat symptomatically (see Chapter 44).		

*New cases of transfusion-related hepatitis B and C are not common.
ALT, Alanine aminotransferase; *AST,* aspartate aminotransferase; *HCV,* hepatitis C virus; *HTLV-1,* human T-cell leukemia virus, type 1; *KS,* Kaposi sarcoma.

(8) collect required blood and urine specimens at intervals based on the hospital policy to evaluate for hemolysis; and (9) document on transfusion reaction form and patient chart. The blood bank and laboratory are responsible for identifying the type of reaction.

Acute Transfusion Reactions. The most common cause of hemolytic reactions is transfusion of ABO-incompatible blood (see Table 31-33). This is an example of a type II cytotoxic hypersensitivity reaction (see Chapter 14). Severe hemolytic reactions are rare. Mislabeling specimens and administering blood to the wrong individual cause most acute hemolytic reactions. This again points to the importance of using proper patient identifiers when drawing blood samples and when administering medications and blood products.

Delayed Transfusion Reactions. Delayed transfusion reactions include delayed hemolytic reactions (discussed previously), infections, and iron overload (see Table 31-34).

Autotransfusion

Autotransfusion, or autologous transfusion, involves removing whole blood from a person and transfusing that blood back into the same person. The problems of incompatibility, allergic reactions, and transmission of disease can be avoided. Methods of autotransfusion include the following:

- *Autologous donation* or *elective phlebotomy* (predeposit transfusion). A person donates blood before a planned surgical procedure. The blood can be frozen and stored for up to 10 years. Usually the blood is stored without being frozen and is given to the person within a few weeks of donation. This technique is especially beneficial to the patient with a rare blood type or for any patient who might be expected to require limited blood product support during a major surgical procedure (e.g., elective orthopedic surgery).
- *Autotransfusion.* A newer method for replacing blood volume involves safely and aseptically collecting, filtering, and returning the patient's own blood lost during a major surgical procedure or from a traumatic injury. This system was originally developed in response to patients' concerns about the safety of blood from blood products. However, today it provides an important way to safely replace volume and stabilize bleeding patients. Collection devices are most often used during surgeries. Some systems allow blood to be automatically and continuously reinfused. Others require collecting the blood for a time (usually no longer than 4 hours) and then reinfusing it.

Drainage after the first 24 hours or drainage that is suspected to contain pathogens should not be reinfused. Anticoagulants may or may not be added before reinfusion. Development of clots after blood is filtered through the collection system can sometimes prevent reinfusion of the blood. Sometimes blood that has been collected has become depleted of its normal coagulation factors. Therefore monitoring coagulation studies in the patient receiving an autotransfusion is important.

CASE STUDY

Leukemia

iStockphoto/Thinkstock

Patient Profile
J.J., a 28-year-old white man, had a bad fall while hiking in the nearby hills. He went to the emergency department because of severe bruising from the fall.

Subjective Data
- Complains of oral pain and white patches covering his tongue
- Has had a 2-month history of extreme fatigue, malaise, and flu symptoms
- Complains of shortness of breath and his heart bounding
- Has taken numerous prescribed antibiotics and increased rest and sleep in the past 2 months without relief of symptoms

Objective Data
Physical Examination
- Has bruises and ecchymoses from fall
- Gingiva has petechiae and patchy white spots
- Temperature 102.2° F (39° C), respiratory rate 26/min, pulse 110/min
- Has splenomegaly

Laboratory Results
- Hct 20%
- Hgb 6.9 g/dL
- WBC count 120,000/µL (120 × 10⁹/L)
- Platelet count 25,000/µL (25 × 10⁹/L)

Bone Marrow Biopsy
- Multiple myeloblasts (>50%)

Collaborative Care
- Consultation with a hematologist-oncologist
- Two units of packed red blood cells

Discussion Questions
1. What components of the laboratory test results suggest acute leukemia?
2. How is acute myelogenous leukemia treated?
3. What is J.J.'s prognosis?
4. What are the life-threatening problems that can occur as a result of this disease and treatment? How can you anticipate and assess for these problems?
5. *Priority Decision:* What are the priority nursing interventions?
6. *Priority Decision:* What are the priorities for patient teaching with a newly diagnosed young adult with leukemia?
7. *Priority Decision:* Based on the assessment data presented, what are the priority nursing diagnoses? Are there any collaborative problems?
8. *Delegation Decision:* What nursing interventions can the registered nurse (RN) delegate to unlicensed assistive personnel (UAP) while J.J. is getting his blood transfusions?
9. *Evidence-Based Practice:* J.J. becomes fatigued after starting chemotherapy. He wants to know if he can still exercise even if he is so fatigued. What is your best advice for him?

Hematologic System

BRIDGE TO NCLEX EXAMINATION

The number of the question corresponds to the same-numbered outcome at the beginning of the chapter.

1. In a severely anemic patient, the nurse would expect to find
   a. dyspnea and tachycardia.
   b. cyanosis and pulmonary edema.
   c. cardiomegaly and pulmonary fibrosis.
   d. ventricular dysrhythmias and wheezing.

2. When obtaining assessment data from a patient with a microcytic, hypochromic anemia, the nurse would question the patient about
   a. folic acid intake.
   b. dietary intake of iron.
   c. a history of gastric surgery.
   d. a history of sickle cell anemia.

3. Nursing interventions for a patient with severe anemia related to peptic ulcer disease include (select all that apply)
   a. monitoring stools for guaiac.
   b. instructions for high-iron diet.
   c. taking vital signs every 8 hours.
   d. teaching self-injection of erythropoietin.
   e. administration of cobalamin (vitamin B$_{12}$) injections.

4. The nursing management of a patient in sickle cell crisis includes (select all that apply)
   a. monitoring CBC.
   b. optimal pain management and O$_2$ therapy.
   c. blood transfusions if required and iron chelation.
   d. rest as needed and deep vein thrombosis prophylaxis.
   e. administration of IV iron and diet high in iron content.

5. A complication of the hyperviscosity of polycythemia is
   a. thrombosis.
   b. cardiomyopathy.
   c. pulmonary edema.
   d. disseminated intravascular coagulation (DIC).

6. When caring for a patient with thrombocytopenia, the nurse instructs the patient to
   a. dab his or her nose instead of blowing.
   b. be careful when shaving with a safety razor.
   c. continue with physical activities to stimulate thrombopoiesis.
   d. avoid aspirin because it may mask the fever that occurs with thrombocytopenia.

7. The nurse would anticipate that a patient with von Willebrand disease undergoing surgery would be treated with administration of vWF and
   a. thrombin.
   b. factor VI.
   c. factor VII.
   d. factor VIII.

8. DIC is a disorder in which
   a. the coagulation pathway is genetically altered, leading to thrombus formation in all major blood vessels.
   b. an underlying disease depletes hemolytic factors in the blood, leading to diffuse thrombotic episodes and infarcts.
   c. a disease process stimulates coagulation processes with resultant thrombosis, as well as depletion of clotting factors, leading to diffuse clotting and hemorrhage.
   d. an inherited predisposition causes a deficiency of clotting factors that leads to overstimulation of coagulation processes in the vasculature.

9. Priority nursing actions when caring for a hospitalized patient with a new-onset temperature of 102.2° F and severe neutropenia include (select all that apply)
   a. administering the prescribed antibiotic STAT.
   b. drawing peripheral and central line blood cultures.
   c. ongoing monitoring of the patient's vital signs for septic shock.
   d. taking a full set of vital signs and notifying the physician immediately.
   e. administering transfusions of WBCs treated to decrease immunogenicity.

10. Because myelodysplastic syndrome arises from the pluripotent hematopoietic stem cell in the bone marrow, laboratory results the nurse would expect to find include a(n)
    a. excess of T cells.
    b. excess of platelets.
    c. deficiency of granulocytes.
    d. deficiency of all cellular blood components.

11. The most common type of leukemia in older adults is
    a. acute myelocytic leukemia.
    b. acute lymphocytic leukemia.
    c. chronic myelocytic leukemia.
    d. chronic lymphocytic leukemia.

12. Multiple drugs are often used in combinations to treat leukemia and lymphoma because
    a. there are fewer toxic and side effects.
    b. the chance that one drug will be effective is increased.
    c. the drugs are more effective without causing side effects.
    d. the drugs work by different mechanisms to maximize killing of malignant cells.

13. The nurse is aware that a major difference between Hodgkin's lymphoma and non-Hodgkin's lymphoma is that
    a. Hodgkin's lymphoma occurs only in young adults.
    b. Hodgkin's lymphoma is considered potentially curable.
    c. non-Hodgkin's lymphoma can manifest in multiple organs.
    d. non-Hodgkin's lymphoma is treated only with radiation therapy.

14. A patient with multiple myeloma becomes confused and lethargic. The nurse would expect that these clinical manifestations may be explained by diagnostic results that indicate
    a. hyperkalemia.
    b. hyperuricemia.
    c. hypercalcemia.
    d. CNS myeloma.

15. When reviewing the patient's hematologic laboratory values after a splenectomy, the nurse would expect to find
    a. leukopenia.
    b. RBC abnormalities.
    c. decreased hemoglobin.
    d. increased platelet count.

16. Complications of transfusions that can be decreased by the use of leukocyte depletion or reduction of RBC transfusion are
    a. chills and hemolysis.
    b. leukostasis and neutrophilia.
    c. fluid overload and pulmonary edema.
    d. transmission of cytomegalovirus and fever.

1. a, 2. b, 3. a, b, 4. a, b, c, d, 5. a, 6. a, 7. d, 8. c, 9. a, b, c, d, 10. d, 11. d, 12. d, 13. c, 14. c, 15. d, 16. d

⊜volve

For rationales to these answers and even more NCLEX review questions, visit *http://evolve.elsevier.com/Lewis/medsurg.*

REFERENCES

1. Marks PW, Glader B: Approach to anemia in the adult and child. In Hoffman R, Silberstein LE, Shattil SJ, et al, editors: *Hematology: basic principles and practice*, ed 5, Philadelphia, 2009, Churchill Livingstone.

2. Rote NS, McCance KL: Alterations of erythrocyte function. In McCance KL, Huether SE, Brashers VL, et al, editors: *Pathophysiology: the biologic basis for disease in adults and children*, ed 6, St Louis, 2010, Mosby.

3. Lichtman MA, Kaushansky K, Kipps TJ, et al: *Williams manual of hematology*, ed 8, New York, 2011, McGraw-Hill.

4. Balducci L: Anemia, fatigue, and aging, *Transf Clin Biol* 17:375, 2010.

5. Goddard AF, James MW, McIntyre AS, et al: Guidelines for the management of iron deficiency anemia, *Gut* 60:1309, 2011.

6. US Department of Health and Human Services, National Heart, Lung, and Blood Institute. Retrieved from *www.nhlbi .nih.gov*.

7. Rote NS, McCance KL: Structure and function of the hematologic system. In McCance KL, Huether SE, Brashers VL, et al, editors: *Pathophysiology: the biologic basis for disease in adults and children*, ed 6, St Louis, 2010, Mosby.

8. American Dietetic Association: B-vitamins and folate: thiamine, riboflavin, and niacin. Retrieved from *www.eatright.org*.

9. US National Library of Medicine, National Institutes of Health, Medline Plus: Copper in diet—pantothenic acid. Retrieved from *www.nlm.nih.gov/medlineplus*.

10. Beutler E: Disorders of iron metabolism. In Lichtman MA, Kipps TJ, Seligsohn U, et al, editors: *Williams hematology*, ed 8, New York, 2010, McGraw-Hill. Retrieved from *www.accessmedicine.com*.

11. Kline NE: Alterations in hematologic function in children. In McCance KL, Huether SE, Brashers VL, et al, editors: *Pathophysiology: the biologic basis for disease in adults and children*, ed 6, St Louis, 2010, Mosby.

12. Ganz T: Anemia of chronic disease. In Lichtman MA, Kipps TJ, Seligsohn U, et al, editors: *Williams hematology*, ed 8, New York, 2010, McGraw-Hill. Retrieved from *www.accessmedicine.com*.

*13. Rogers GM, Becker PS, Bennett CL, et al: Cancer- and chemotherapy-induced anemia, NCCN Clinical Practice Guidelines in Oncology, version 2, 2012. Retrieved from *www.nccn.org*.

14. American Cancer Society: Learn about cancer: aplastic anemia. Retrieved from *www.cancer.org/Cancer/Aplastic Anemia*.

15. Natarajan K, Townes TM, Kutlar A: Disorders of hemoglobin structure: sickle cell anemia and related abnormalities. In Lichtman MA, Kipps TJ, Seligsohn U, et al, editors: *Williams hematology*, ed 8, New York, 2010, McGraw-Hill. Retrieved from *www.accessmedicine.com*.

16. Williams-Johnson J, Williams E: Sickle cell disease and other hereditary hemolytic anemias. In Tintinalli JE, Stapczynski JS, Cline DM, et al, editors: *Tintinalli's emergency medicine: a comprehensive study guide*, ed 7, New York, 2011, McGraw-Hill.

17. Heeney MM, Ware RE: Hydroxyurea for children with sickle cell disease, *Hematol Oncol Clin North Am* 24:199, 2010.

18. Ganz T, Nemeth E: Hepcidin and disorders of iron metabolism, *Ann Rev Med* 62:347, 2011.

19. Doig K: Disorders of iron and heme metabolism. In Rodak BF, Fritsma GA, Keohane EM, editors: *Hematology: clinical principles and application*, ed 4, St Louis, 2012, Mosby.

20. Brittenham GM: Iron-chelating therapy for transfusional iron overload, *N Engl J Med* 364:146, 2011.

21. Prchal JT, Prchal JF: Polycythemia vera. In Lichtman MA, Kipps TJ, Seligsohn U, et al, editors: *Williams hematology*, ed 8, New York, 2010, McGraw-Hill. Retrieved from *www. accessmedicine.com*.

22. Konkle B: Acquired disorders of platelet function, *Hematol Am Soc Hematol Educ Program* 391:391, 2011.

23. Diz-Kucukkaya R, Chen J, Geddis A, et al: Thrombocytopenia. In Lichtman MA, Kipps TJ, Seligsohn U, et al, editors: *Williams hematology*, ed 8, New York, 2010, McGraw-Hill. Retrieved from *www.accessmedicine.com*.

24. Sadler J, Poncz M: Antibody-mediated thrombotic disorders: thrombotic thrombocytopenic purpura and heparin-induced thrombocytopenia. In Lichtman MA, Kipps TJ, Seligsohn U, et al, editors: *Williams hematology*, ed 8, New York, 2010. McGraw-Hill. Retrieved from *www.accessmedicine.com*.

*25. Neunert C, Lim W, Crowther M, et al: The American Society of Hematology 2011 evidence-based practice guidelines for immune thrombocytopenia, *Blood* 117:4190, 2011.

26. Rote NS, McCance KL: Alterations of leukocyte, lymphoid, and hemostatic function. In McCance KL, Huether SE, Brashers VL, et al, editors: *Pathophysiology: the biologic basis for disease in adults and children*, ed 6, St Louis, 2010, Mosby.

27. Imbach P, Crowther M: Thrombopoietin-receptor agonists for primary immune thrombocytopenia, *N Engl J Med* 365:734, 2011.

28. Hemophilia Federation of America: About bleeding disorders. Retrieved from *www.hemophliafed.org*.

29. Roberts HR, Key NS, Escobar MA: Hemophilia A and hemophilia B. In Lichtman MA, Kipps TJ, Seligsohn U, et al, editors: *Williams hematology*, ed 8, New York, 2010, McGraw-Hill. Retrieved from *www.accessmedicine.com*.

30. Fritsma GA: Hemorrhagic coagulation disorders. In Rodak BF, Fritsma GA, Keohane EM: *Hematology: clinical principles and application*, ed 4, St Louis, 2012, Mosby.

31. Chitlur M, Kulkarni R: Hemophilia and related bleeding disorders. In Bope ET, Kellerman RD, editors: *Bope and Kellerman: Conn's current therapy*, Philadelphia, 2012, Saunders.

32. Nathwani AC, Tuddenham EGD, Rangarajan S, et al: Adenovirus-associated virus vector–mediated gene transfer in hemophilia B, *N Engl J Med* 365:2357, 2011.

33. Fritsma GA: Thrombosis risk testing. In Rodak BF, Fritsma GA, Keohane EM, editors: *Hematology: clinical principles and application*, ed 4, St Louis, 2012, Mosby.

34. Baehner RL: Drug-induced neutropenia and agranulocytosis. Retrieved from *www.uptodate.com*.

35. Sivilotti MLA: Hematologic principles. In Nelson LS, Lewin NA, Howland MA, et al, editors: *Goldfrank's toxicologic emergencies*, ed 9, New York, 2011, McGraw-Hill.

36. Klastersky J, Awada A, Paesmans M, et al: Febrile neutropenia: a critical review of the initial management, *Crit Rev Oncol Hematol* 78:185, 2011.

*37. Baden LR, Bensinger W, Angarone M, et al: Prevention and treatment of cancer-related infections, NCCN Clinical Practice Guidelines in Oncology, version 2, 2011. Retrieved from *www.nccn.org*.

*Evidence-based information for clinical practice.

*38. Saria M: Preventing and managing infections in neutropenic stem cell transplantation recipients: evidence-based review, *Clin J Oncol Nurs* 15:133, 2011.

39. Goossen LH: Pediatric and geriatric hematology. In Rodak BF, Fritsma GA, Keohane EM, editors: *Hematology: clinical principles and application*, ed 4, St Louis, 2012, Mosby.

40. Leukemia and Lymphoma Society: Myelodysplastic syndromes. Retrieved from *www.lls.org*.

41. Lindsay M, Beavers J: Myelodysplastic syndromes in older adults, *Clin J Oncol Nurs* 14:545, 2010.

*42. Greenberg PL, Gordeuk V, Issaraqrisil S, et al: Myelodysplastic syndromes, NCCN Clinical Practice Guidelines in Oncology, version 1. 2011, 2012. Retrieved from *www.nccn.org*.

43. Kurtin S: Current approaches to the diagnosis and management of myelodysplastic syndromes, *J Adv Pract Oncol Suppl* 2:7, 2011.

44. Leukemia and Lymphoma Society: Leukemia. Retrieved from *www.lls.org*.

*45. Zelenetz AD, Abramson JS, Advani RH, et al: Non-Hodgkin's lymphomas, NCCN Clinical Practice Guidelines in Oncology, version 4, 2011. Retrieved from *www.nccn.org*.

*46. Estey EH: Acute myeloid leukemia: 2013 update on risk-stratification and management, *Am J Hematol* 88(4):318, 2013.

*47. Jabbour E, Kantarjian H: Chronic myeloid leukemia: 2012 update on diagnosis, monitoring, and management, *Am J Hematol* 87(11):1037, 2012.

48. Pui C: Acute lymphoblastic leukemia. In Lichtman MA, Kipps TJ, Seligsohn U, et al, editors: *Williams hematology*, ed 8, New York, 2010, McGraw-Hill. Retrieved from *www.accessmedicine.com*.

49. Siegel R, Ward E, Brawley O, et al: Cancer statistics, 2011, *CA Cancer J Clin* 61:212, 2011.

50. Horning SJ: Hodgkin lymphoma. In Lichtman MA, Kipps TJ, Seligsohn U, et al: *Williams hematology*, ed 8, New York, 2010, McGraw-Hill. Retrieved from *www.accessmedicine.com*.

*51. Hoppe RT, Advanti RH, Ai WZ, et al: Hodgkin lymphoma, NCCN Clinical Practice Guidelines in Oncology version 3, 2011. Retrieved from *www.nccn.org*.

52. Kipps TJ, Wang H: Acute lymphoblastic leukemia. In Lichtman MA, Kipps TJ, Seligsohn U, et al, editors: *Williams hematology*, ed 8, New York, 2010, McGraw-Hill. Retrieved from *www.accessmedicine.com*.

53. Bragalone DL: *Drug information handbook for oncology*, ed 9, Hudson, Ohio, 2011, Lexicomp.

54. Van Rhee F, Anaissie E, Angtuaco E, et al: Myeloma. In Lichtman MA, Kipps TJ, Seligsohn U, et al, editors: *Williams hematology*, ed 8, New York, 2010, McGraw-Hill. Retrieved from *www.accessmedicine.com*.

*55. Anderson KC, Becker PS, Bennett CL, et al: Multiple myeloma, NCCN Clinical Practice Guidelines in Oncology, version 1, 2012. Retrieved from *www.nccn.org*.

56. Rome SI: Mobility and safety in the multiple myeloma survivor: survivorship care plan of the International Myeloma Foundation Nurse Leadership Board, *Clin J Oncol Nurs* 15(Suppl):41, 2011.

57. Smith L: Hematopoiesis. In Rodak BF, Fritsma GA, Keohane EM, editors: *Hematology: clinical principles and application*, ed 4, St Louis, 2012, Mosby.

58. Nester T, AuBuchon JP: Hemotherapy decisions and their outcomes. In Rodak JD, Grossman BJ, Harris T, et al: *Technical manual: standards for blood banks and transfusion services*, ed 17, Bethesda, Md, 2011, AABB.

59. Lockwood WB, Leonard J, Liles SL: Storage, monitoring, pretransfusion processing, and distribution of blood components. In Rodak JD, Grossman BJ, Harris T, et al: *Technical manual: standards for blood banks and transfusion services*, ed 17, Bethesda, Md, 2011, AABB.

60. Lerner NB, Rafaai MA, Blumberg N: Red cell transfusion. In Lichtman MA, Kipps TJ, Seligsohn U, et al, editors: *Williams hematology*, ed 8, New York, 2010, McGraw-Hill.

RESOURCES

American Hemochromatosis Society
www.americanhs.org
American Sickle Cell Anemia Association
www.ascaa.org
American Society of Hematology
www.hematology.org
Aplastic Anemia & MDS International Foundation, Inc.
www.aamds.org
Hemophilia Federation of America
www.hemophiliafed.org
International Myeloma Foundation
www.myeloma.org
Leukemia and Lymphoma Society
www.lls.org
Managing Myeloma
www.ManagingMyeloma.com
Myelodysplastic Syndromes Foundation
www.mds-foundation.org
National Hemophilia Foundation
www.hemophilia.org
Platelet Disorder Support Association
www.pdsa.org
Sickle Cell Disease Association of America, Inc.
www.sicklecelldisease.org
World Federation of Hemophilia
www.wfh.org

CASE STUDY
Managing Multiple Patients

Introduction
You are working on the oncology unit and have been assigned to care for the following four patients. You have one UAP who is assigned to help you and there are two other RNs on your clinical unit.

Patients

A.J. is a 90-year-old white woman who is admitted with severe anemia (Hgb 5.9 g/dL and Hct 18.2%). She prefers to take care of herself with "natural therapy" and has not seen a health care provider for 10 years. A.J. is having difficulty performing ADLs without having to stop and catch her breath. She received 2 units of RBCs and is undergoing further workup to determine the cause of her anemia.

iStockphoto/Thinkstock

J.J. is a 28-year-old white man newly diagnosed with acute myeloblastic leukemia (AML). His most recent vital signs are BP 100/70, temperature 102.2°F (39°C), respiratory rate 26/min, pulse 110. Lab results reveal hematocrit 20%, Hgb 6.9 g/dL, WBC count 120,000/μL (120 × 10⁹/L), and platelet count 25,000/μL (25 × 10⁹/L). He is admitted for blood transfusions and induction therapy.

iStockphoto/Thinkstock

P.H. is a 45-year-old woman who is currently receiving chemotherapy for treatment of ovarian cancer. She is admitted with fever and chills. Her WBC count is 2200/μL (2.2 × 10⁹/L) with an absolute neutrophil count of 400/μL (0.4 × 10⁹/L). She is admitted for IV antibiotic therapy and is in protective isolation. Her most recent vital signs are BP 118/60, temperature 99.2°F (37.3°C), respiratory rate 20/min, pulse 98.

iStockphoto/Thinkstock

G.L. is a 70-year-old man who came to the emergency department yesterday evening with complaints of abdominal pain. A CT scan of the abdomen revealed several masses in his lymphatic system. The physician suspects non-Hodgkin's lymphoma and admits him for a diagnostic workup. He currently rates his pain as a 3 on a scale of 0-10.

iStockphoto/Thinkstock

Management Discussion Questions
1. *Priority Decision:* After receiving report, which patient should you see first? Provide a rationale for your decision.
2. *Delegation Decision:* Which task could you delegate to the UAP *(select all that apply)?*
   a. Assist A.J. to a chair after completing her AM care.
   b. Obtain the first unit of blood for J.J. from the blood bank.
   c. Explain the importance of protective isolation to P.H. and her family.
   d. Ask A.J. why she has not been willing to get any medical care for 10 years.
   e. Ask G.L. about the presence of additional clinical manifestations of non-Hodgkin's lymphoma.

3. *Priority and Delegation Decision:* When you enter J.J.'s room, you find him somewhat confused and lethargic. His family states he had just had a severe coughing episode. What initial action would be the most appropriate?
   a. Perform a focused neurologic examination.
   b. Call respiratory therapy to give him a breathing treatment.
   c. Ask his family members if they have a copy of his living will.
   d. Have the UAP stay with J.J. while you page the health care provider STAT.

Case Study Progression
J.J.'s health care provider orders a repeat CBC and an emergency CT scan of the head. Your supervisor makes arrangements for another RN to accompany J.J. to the CT scan while you prepare to administer the first unit of RBCs.

4. A.J. is diagnosed with iron-deficiency anemia. The physician orders ferrous sulfate 325 mg TID. You teach A.J. to take her iron *(select all that apply)*
   a. at breakfast time in the morning.
   b. with orange juice to increase absorption.
   c. 1 hour before meals to facilitate absorption.
   d. 2 hours after eating to minimize side effects.
   e. whenever she feels tired or is short of breath with activity.
5. When teaching P.H.'s family about neutropenic precautions, you emphasize that the most important intervention to prevent infection is
   a. hand washing.
   b. wearing a mask.
   c. keeping P.H. in a private room.
   d. limiting the number of visitors in her room.
6. G.L. asks you to explain the diagnostic testing he can expect to undergo related to the suspected lymphoma. Which tests will you explain to him *(select all that apply)?*
   a. PET scan
   b. Bone marrow biopsy
   c. Peripheral blood smear
   d. Excisional lymph node biopsy
   e. Lymphangiography of internal lymph nodes
7. *Management Decision:* An RN from the float pool arrives to accompany J.J. to CT scan at the same time the UAP arrives with his first unit of RBCs. Which intervention would be most appropriate?
   a. Put the unit of RBCs in the refrigerator to start when J.J. returns to the floor.
   b. Ask the RN to verify the correct unit of RBCs with you and start the infusion.
   c. Give the RN a SBAR report on J.J. and ask her to start the blood on route to CT scan.
   d. Ask the RN if she would prefer to give the blood or hold it for J.J.'s return to the unit.

Problems of Oxygenation: Perfusion

David De Lossy/Photodisc/Thinkstock

The trail is the thing, not the end of the trail.
Travel too fast and you miss all you are traveling for.
Louis L'Amour

CHAPTER

32

Let your heart guide you.
It whispers, so listen closely.
Author Unknown

Nursing Assessment
Cardiovascular System

Angela DiSabatino and Linda Bucher

⊖volve WEBSITE

http://evolve.elsevier.com/Lewis/medsurg

- NCLEX Review Questions
- Key Points
- Pre-Test
- Answer Guidelines for Case Study in this chapter
- Rationales for Bridge to NCLEX Examination Questions
- Concept Map Creator
- Glossary
- Animations
  - Auscultation of Heart Valves
  - Blood Flow: Circulatory System
  - Cardiac Cycle During Systole and Diastole
  - Pulse Variations
- Videos
  - Auscultation: Cardiac, With Bell
  - Auscultation: Cardiac, With Diaphragm

- Auscultation: Cardiac, With Diaphragm and Bell
- Auscultation: Carotid Artery
- Inspection and Palpation: Cardiac Auscultatory Landmarks
- Inspection and Palpation: Cardiac, Anterior Chest
- Inspection and Palpation: Pulses, Lower Extremities
- Physical Examination: Anterior Chest, Lungs, and Heart
- Physical Examination: Breasts and Heart
- Physical Examination: Neck
- Physical Examination: Precordium and Jugular Veins
- Physical Examination: Upper Extremities

- Content Updates
- Audio
  - Diastolic Murmur
  - Fourth Heart Sound (S4)
  - Murmurs: Blowing, Harsh or Rough, and Rumble
  - Murmurs: High, Medium, and Low
  - S1 at Various Locations
  - S2 at Various Locations
  - Single S1
  - Single S2
  - Systolic Murmur
- Third Heart Sound (S3)

eFigures
- eFig. 32-1: Types of serum lipids
- eFig. 32-2: Cholesterol delivery

LEARNING OUTCOMES

1. Differentiate the anatomic location and function of the following cardiac structures: pericardial layers, atria, ventricles, semilunar valves, and atrioventricular valves.
2. Relate the coronary circulation to the areas of heart muscle supplied by the major coronary arteries.
3. Differentiate the structure and function of arteries, veins, capillaries, and endothelium.
4. Describe the mechanisms involved in the regulation of blood pressure.
5. Relate the various waveforms on a normal electrocardiogram to the associated cardiac events.

6. Select essential assessment data related to the cardiovascular system that should be obtained from a patient and/or caregiver.
7. Select appropriate techniques to use in the physical assessment of the cardiovascular system.
8. Differentiate normal from abnormal findings of a physical assessment of the cardiovascular system.
9. Link the age-related changes of the cardiovascular system to the differences in assessment findings.
10. Describe the purpose, significance of results, and nursing responsibilities related to diagnostic studies of the cardiovascular system.

KEY TERMS

action potential, p. 687
afterload, p. 689
arterial blood pressure, p. 690
cardiac index (CI), p. 689
cardiac output (CO), p. 689
cardiac reserve, p. 689
coronary angiography, p. 706

diastole, p. 687
diastolic blood pressure (DBP), p. 690
ejection fraction (EF), p. 704
heaves, p. 697
Korotkoff sounds, p. 690
mean arterial pressure (MAP), p. 690

murmur, p. 691
point of maximal impulse (PMI), p. 697
preload, p. 689
pulse pressure, p. 690
systole, p. 689
systolic blood pressure (SBP), p. 690

Reviewed by Jennifer Saylor, RN, PhD, ACNS-BC, Assistant Professor, University of Delaware, Wilmington, Delaware; and Julie Willenbrink, RN, MSN, Assistant Professor of Nursing, Edison State Community College, Piqua, Ohio.

STRUCTURES AND FUNCTIONS OF CARDIOVASCULAR SYSTEM

Heart

Structure. The heart is a four-chambered hollow muscular organ normally about the size of a fist. It lies within the thorax in the mediastinal space that separates the right and left pleural cavities. The heart is composed of three layers: a thin inner lining, the *endocardium;* a layer of muscle, the *myocardium;* and an outer layer, the *epicardium.* The heart is covered by a fibroserous sac called the *pericardium.* This sac consists of two layers: the inside *(visceral)* layer of the pericardium (part of the epicardium) and the outer *(parietal)* layer. A small amount of pericardial fluid (approximately 10 to 15 mL) lubricates the space between the pericardial layers *(pericardial space)* and prevents friction between the surfaces as the heart contracts.[1]

The heart is divided vertically by the septum. The interatrial septum creates a right and left atrium, and the interventricular septum creates a right and left ventricle. The thickness of the wall of each chamber is different. The atrial myocardium is thinner than that of the ventricles, and the left ventricular wall is two or three times thicker than the right ventricular wall.[1] The thickness of the left ventricle is necessary to produce the force needed to pump the blood into the systemic circulation.

Blood Flow Through Heart. The blood flow through the heart is illustrated in Fig. 32-1.

Cardiac Valves. The four valves of the heart serve to keep blood flowing in a forward direction. The cusps of the mitral and tricuspid valves are attached to thin strands of fibrous tissue termed *chordae tendineae* (Fig. 32-2). Chordae are anchored in the papillary muscles of the ventricles. This support system prevents the eversion of the leaflets into the atria during ventricular contraction. The pulmonic and aortic valves (also known as *semilunar valves*) prevent blood from regurgitating into the ventricles at the end of each ventricular contraction.

Blood Supply to Myocardium. The myocardium has its own blood supply, the *coronary circulation* (Fig. 32-3). Blood flow into the two major coronary arteries occurs primarily during **diastole** (relaxation of the myocardium). The left coronary artery arises from the aorta and divides into two main branches: the left anterior descending artery and the left circumflex artery. These arteries supply the left atrium, the left ventricle, the interventricular septum, and a portion of the right ventricle. The right coronary artery also arises from the aorta, and its branches supply the right atrium, the right ventricle, and a portion of the posterior wall of the left ventricle. In 90% of people the atrioventricular (AV) node and the bundle of His receive blood supply from the right coronary artery. For this reason, blockage of this artery often causes serious defects in cardiac conduction.

The divisions of coronary veins parallel the coronary arteries. Most of the blood from the coronary system drains into the coronary sinus (a large channel), which empties into the right atrium near the entrance of the inferior vena cava.

Conduction System. The conduction system is specialized nerve tissue responsible for creating and transporting the electrical impulse, or **action potential.** This impulse starts depolarization and subsequently cardiac contraction (Fig. 32-4, *A*). The electrical impulse is normally started by the sinoatrial (SA) node (the pacemaker of the heart). Each impulse coming from the SA node travels through interatrial pathways to depolarize the atria, resulting in a contraction.

The electrical impulse travels from the atria to the AV node through internodal pathways. The excitation then moves through the bundle of His and the left and right bundle branches. The left bundle branch has two fascicles (divisions): anterior and posterior. The action potential moves through the walls of both ventricles by means of *Purkinje fibers.* The ventricular conduction system delivers the impulse within 0.12 second. This triggers a synchronized right and left ventricular contraction.

The result of the cardiac cycle is the ejection of blood into the pulmonary and systemic circulations. It ends with repolarization when the contractile fiber cells and the conduction pathway cells regain their resting polarized condition. Cardiac

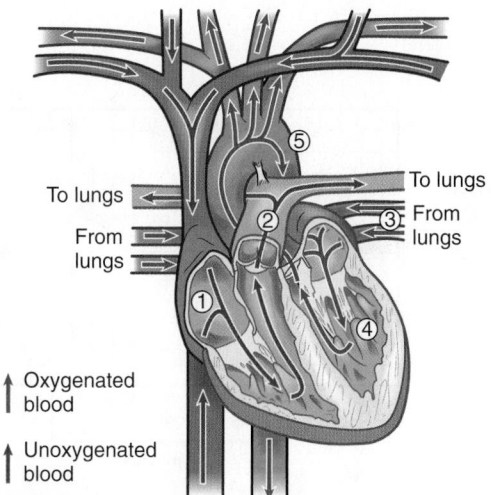

FIG. 32-1 Schematic representation of blood flow through the heart. *Arrows* indicate direction of flow. *1,* The right atrium receives venous blood from the inferior and superior venae cavae and the coronary sinus. The blood then passes through the tricuspid valve into the right ventricle. *2,* With each contraction, the right ventricle pumps blood through the pulmonic valve into the pulmonary artery and to the lungs. *3,* Oxygenated blood flows from the lungs to the left atrium by way of the pulmonary veins. *4,* It then passes through the mitral valve and into the left ventricle. *5,* As the heart contracts, blood is ejected through the aortic valve into the aorta and thus enters the systemic circulation.

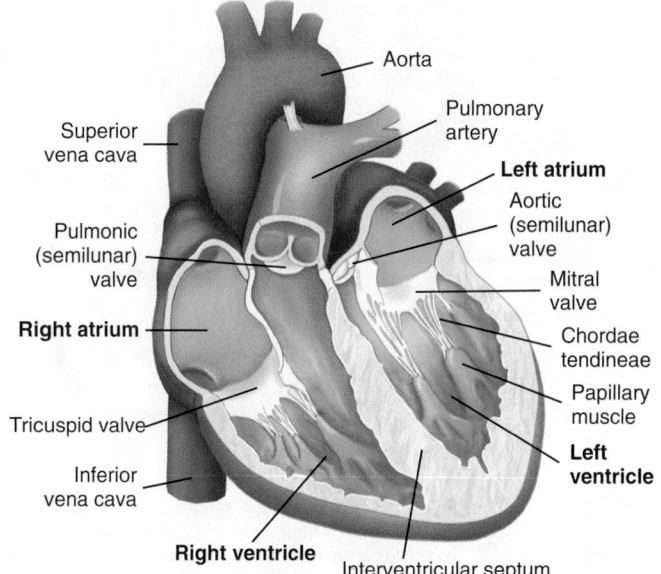

FIG. 32-2 Anatomic structures of the heart and heart valves.

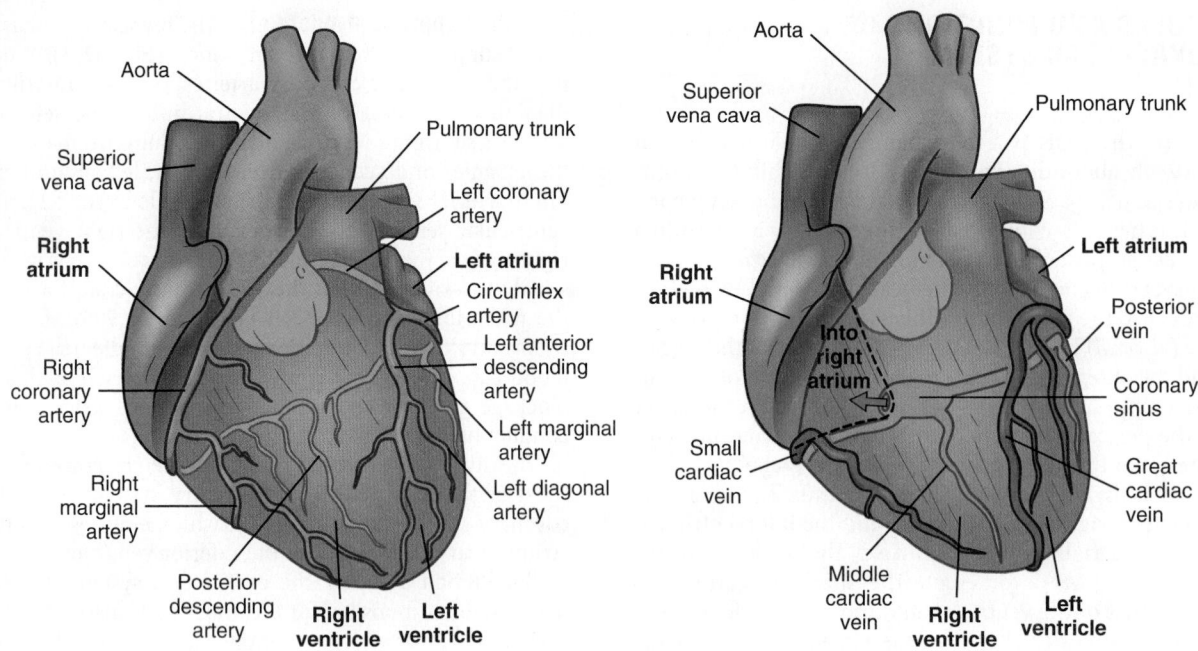

FIG. 32-3 Coronary arteries and veins.

muscle cells have a compensatory mechanism that makes them unresponsive or refractory to restimulation during the action potential. During ventricular contraction, there is an *absolute refractory period* during which cardiac muscle does not respond to any stimuli. After this period, cardiac muscle gradually recovers its excitability, and a *relative refractory period* occurs by early diastole.

Electrocardiogram. The electrical activity of the heart can be detected on the body surface using electrodes and is recorded on an electrocardiogram (ECG). The letters P, QRS, T, and U are used to identify the separate waveforms (Fig. 32-4, *B*). The first wave, P, begins with the firing of the SA node and represents depolarization of the atria. The QRS complex represents depolarization from the AV node throughout the ventricles. There is a delay of impulse transmission through the AV node that accounts for the time between the beginning of the P wave and the beginning of the QRS wave. The T wave represents repolarization of the ventricles. The U wave, if seen, may repre-

FIG. 32-4 A, Conduction system of the heart. *AV,* Atrioventricular; *SA,* sinoatrial. **B,** The normal electrocardiogram (ECG) pattern. The P wave represents depolarization of the atria. The QRS complex indicates depolarization of the ventricles. The T wave represents repolarization of the ventricles. The U wave, if present, may represent repolarization of the Purkinje fibers, or it may be associated with hypokalemia. The PR, QRS, and QT intervals reflect the time it takes for the impulse to travel from one area of the heart to another.

sent repolarization of the Purkinje fibers, or it may be associated with hypokalemia.[2]

Intervals between these waves (PR, QRS, and QT intervals) reflect the time it takes for the impulse to travel from one area of the heart to another. These time intervals can be measured, and changes from these time references often indicate pathologic conditions. (See Chapter 36 for a complete discussion of ECG monitoring.)

Mechanical System. *Depolarization* triggers mechanical activity. Systole, contraction of the myocardium, results in ejection of blood from the ventricles. Relaxation of the myocardium, *diastole*, allows for filling of the ventricles. **Cardiac output (CO)** is the amount of blood pumped by each ventricle in 1 minute. It is calculated by multiplying the amount of blood ejected from the ventricle with each heartbeat—the *stroke volume* (SV)—by the heart rate (HR) per minute:

$$CO = SV \times HR$$

For the normal adult at rest, CO is maintained in the range of 4 to 8 L/min. **Cardiac index (CI)** is the CO divided by the body surface area (BSA). The CI adjusts the CO to the body size. The normal CI is 2.8 to 4.2 L per minute per meter squared $(L/min/m^2)$.

Factors Affecting Cardiac Output. Numerous factors can affect either the HR or the SV, and thus the CO. The HR, which is controlled primarily by the autonomic nervous system, can reach as high as 180 beats/minute for short periods without harmful effects. The factors affecting the SV are preload, contractility, and afterload. Increasing preload, contractility, and afterload increases the workload of the myocardium, resulting in increased oxygen demand.

Frank-Starling law states that, to a point, the more the myocardial fibers are stretched, the greater their force of contraction. The volume of blood in the ventricles at the end of diastole, before the next contraction, is called preload. Preload determines the amount of stretch placed on myocardial fibers. Preload can be increased by a number of conditions such as myocardial infarction, aortic stenosis, and hypervolemia.[3] Contractility can be increased by epinephrine and norepinephrine released by the sympathetic nervous system. Increasing contractility raises the SV by increasing ventricular emptying.

Afterload is the peripheral resistance against which the left ventricle must pump. Afterload is affected by the size of the ventricle, wall tension, and arterial blood pressure (BP). If the arterial BP is elevated, the ventricles meet increased resistance to ejection of blood, increasing the work demand. Eventually this results in *ventricular hypertrophy,* an enlargement of the cardiac muscle tissue without an increase in CO or the size of chambers (see Fig. 35-1, *B*).

Cardiac Reserve. The cardiovascular system must respond to numerous situations in health and illness (e.g., exercise, stress, hypovolemia). The ability to respond to these demands by altering CO is termed **cardiac reserve.**

Vascular System

Blood Vessels. The three major types of blood vessels in the vascular system are the arteries, veins, and capillaries. Arteries, except for the pulmonary artery, carry oxygenated blood away from the heart. Veins, except for the pulmonary veins, carry deoxygenated blood toward the heart. Small branches of arteries and veins are arterioles and venules, respectively. Blood cir-

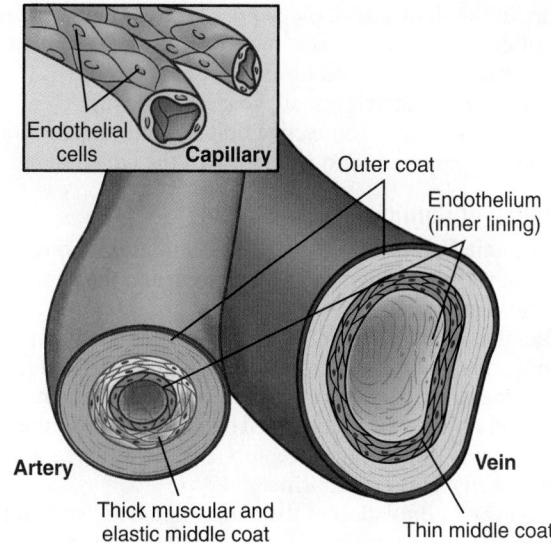

FIG. 32-5 Comparative thickness of layers of the artery, vein, and capillary.

culates from the left side of the heart into arteries, arterioles, capillaries, venules, and veins, and then back to the right side of the heart.

Arteries and Arterioles. The arterial system differs from the venous system by the amount and type of tissue that make up arterial walls (Fig. 32-5). The large arteries have thick walls composed mainly of elastic tissue. This elastic property cushions the impact of the pressure created by ventricular contraction and provides recoil that propels blood forward into the circulation. Large arteries also contain some smooth muscle. Examples of large arteries are the aorta and the pulmonary artery.

Arterioles have relatively little elastic tissue and more smooth muscle. Arterioles serve as the major control of arterial BP and distribution of blood flow. They respond readily to local conditions such as low oxygen (O_2) and increasing levels of carbon dioxide (CO_2) by dilating or constricting.

The innermost lining of the arteries is the endothelium. The endothelium serves to maintain hemostasis, promote blood flow, and, under normal conditions, inhibit blood coagulation. When the endothelial surface is disrupted (e.g., rupture of an atherosclerotic plaque), the coagulation cascade is initiated and results in the formation of a fibrin clot.

Capillaries. The thin capillary wall is made up of endothelial cells, with no elastic or muscle tissue (see Fig. 32-5). The exchange of cellular nutrients and metabolic end products takes place through these thin-walled vessels. Capillaries connect the arterioles and venules.

Veins and Venules. Veins are large-diameter, thin-walled vessels that return blood to the right atrium (see Fig. 32-5). The venous system is a low-pressure, high-volume system. The larger veins contain semilunar valves at intervals to maintain the blood flow toward the heart and to prevent backward flow. The amount of blood in the venous system is affected by a number of factors, including arterial flow, compression of veins by skeletal muscles, alterations in thoracic and abdominal pressures, and right atrial pressure.

The largest veins are the *superior vena cava,* which returns blood to the heart from the head, neck, and arms, and the *inferior vena cava,* which returns blood to the heart from the lower part of the body. These large-diameter vessels are affected by the pressure in the right side of the heart. Elevated right atrial pressure can cause distended neck veins or liver engorgement as a result of resistance to blood flow.

Venules are relatively small vessels made up of a small amount of muscle and connective tissue. Venules collect blood from the capillary beds and channel it to the larger veins.

Regulation of Cardiovascular System

Autonomic Nervous System. The autonomic nervous system consists of the sympathetic nervous system and the parasympathetic nervous system (see Chapter 56).

Effect on Heart. Stimulation of the sympathetic nervous system increases the HR, the speed of impulse conduction through the AV node, and the force of atrial and ventricular contractions. This effect is mediated by specific sites in the heart called beta (β)-adrenergic receptors, which are receptors for norepinephrine and epinephrine.

In contrast, stimulation of the parasympathetic system (mediated by the vagus nerve) slows the HR by decreasing the impulses from the SA node, and thus conduction through the AV node.

Effect on Blood Vessels. The source of neural control of blood vessels is the sympathetic nervous system. The $alpha_1$ (α_1)-adrenergic receptors are located in vascular smooth muscles. Stimulation of α_1-adrenergic receptors results in vasoconstriction. Decreased stimulation to α_1-adrenergic receptors causes vasodilation. (Sympathetic nervous system receptors that influence BP are presented in Table 33-1.)

The parasympathetic nerves have selective distribution in the blood vessels. For example, blood vessels in skeletal muscle do not receive parasympathetic input.

Baroreceptors. *Baroreceptors* in the aortic arch and carotid sinus (at the origin of the internal carotid artery) are sensitive to stretch or pressure within the arterial system. Stimulation of these receptors (e.g., volume overload) sends information to the vasomotor center in the brainstem. This results in temporary inhibition of the sympathetic nervous system and enhancement of the parasympathetic influence, causing a decreased HR and peripheral vasodilation. Decreased arterial pressure causes the opposite effect.

Chemoreceptors. *Chemoreceptors* are located in the aortic and carotid bodies and the medulla. They are capable of causing changes in respiratory rate and BP in response to increased arterial CO_2 pressure (hypercapnia) and, to a lesser degree, decreased plasma pH (acidosis) and arterial O_2 pressure (hypoxia). When the chemoreceptors in the medulla are triggered, they stimulate the vasomotor center to increase BP.[4]

Blood Pressure

The **arterial blood pressure** is a measure of the pressure exerted by blood against the walls of the arterial system. The **systolic blood pressure (SBP)** is the peak pressure exerted against the arteries when the heart contracts. The **diastolic blood pressure (DBP)** is the residual pressure in the arterial system during ventricular relaxation (or filling). BP is usually expressed as the ratio of systolic to diastolic pressure.

The two main factors influencing BP are *cardiac output* (CO) and *systemic vascular resistance* (SVR):

$$BP = CO \times SVR$$

SVR is the force opposing the movement of blood. This force is created primarily in small arteries and arterioles. Normal

blood pressure is SBP less than 120 mm Hg and DBP less than 80 mm Hg[5] (see Chapter 33).

Measurement of Arterial Blood Pressure. BP can be measured by invasive and noninvasive techniques. The invasive technique consists of catheter insertion into an artery. The catheter is attached to a transducer, and the pressure is measured directly (see Chapter 66).

Noninvasive, indirect measurement of BP can be done with a sphygmomanometer and a stethoscope. The sphygmomanometer consists of an inflatable cuff and a pressure gauge. The BP is measured by auscultating for sounds of turbulent blood flow through a compressed artery (termed **Korotkoff sounds**). The brachial artery is the recommended site for taking a BP.

After placing the appropriate size cuff on the upper arm, inflate the cuff to a pressure 20 to 30 mm Hg above the SBP. This causes blood flow in the artery to cease. If the SBP is not known, estimate the pressure by palpating the brachial pulse and inflating the cuff until the pulse ceases. The pressure noted at this time is the estimated SBP. Inflate the BP cuff 20 to 30 mm Hg above this number.

As the pressure in the cuff is lowered, auscultate the artery for Korotkoff sounds. There are five phases of Korotkoff sounds. The first phase is a tapping sound caused by the spurt of blood into the constricted artery as the pressure in the cuff is gradually deflated. This sound is noted as the SBP. The fifth phase occurs when the sound disappears, which is noted as the DBP.[6] BP is recorded as SBP/DBP (e.g., 120/80 mm Hg). Sometimes, an *auscultatory gap* occurs, which is a loss of sound between the SBP and the DBP. Proper BP technique (e.g., using the correct cuff size, positioning arm at heart level) is essential for accurate readings[6] (see Table 33-11).

Another noninvasive way to measure BP indirectly is an automated device that uses oscillometric measurements to assess BP. Though this method does not involve auscultation, the same attention to proper technique is essential for accuracy. Finally, SBP (and pulse) can be assessed using a Doppler ultrasonic flowmeter. The hand-held transducer is positioned over the artery (identified by audible, pulsatile sounds). The cuff is applied above the artery, inflated until the sounds disappear, and then another 20 to 30 mm Hg beyond that point. The cuff is then slowly deflated until sounds return. This point is the SBP.[6]

Pulse Pressure and Mean Arterial Pressure. **Pulse pressure** is the difference between the SBP and DBP. It is normally about one third of the SBP. If the BP is 120/80 mm Hg, the pulse pressure is 40 mm Hg. An increased pulse pressure due to an increased SBP may occur during exercise or in individuals with atherosclerosis of the larger arteries. A decreased pulse pressure may be found in heart failure or hypovolemia.

Another measurement related to BP is **mean arterial pressure (MAP)**. The MAP refers to the average pressure within the arterial system that is felt by organs in the body. It is not the average of the diastolic and systolic pressures because the length of diastole exceeds that of systole at normal HRs. MAP is calculated as follows:

$$MAP = (SBP + 2\,DBP) \div 3$$

A person with a BP of 120/60 mm Hg has an estimated MAP of 80 mm Hg. In patients with invasive BP monitoring, this value is automatically calculated and takes the patient's HR into consideration (see Chapter 66).

An MAP greater than 60 mm Hg is needed to adequately perfuse and sustain the vital organs of an average person under most conditions. When the MAP falls below this number for a period of time, vital organs are underperfused and will become ischemic.

GERONTOLOGIC CONSIDERATIONS

EFFECTS OF AGING ON THE CARDIOVASCULAR SYSTEM

One of the greatest risk factors for cardiovascular disease (CVD) is age. CVD remains the leading cause of death in adults older than age 85. It is the most common cause of hospitalization and the second leading cause of death in adults younger than age 85. The most common cardiovascular problem is coronary artery disease (CAD) secondary to atherosclerosis. It is difficult to separate normal aging changes from the pathophysiologic changes of atherosclerosis. Many of the physiologic changes in the cardiovascular system of older adults are a result of the combined effects of the aging process, disease, environmental factors, and lifetime health behaviors rather than just age alone.[7]

Age-related changes in the cardiovascular system and differences in assessment findings are presented in Table 32-1. With increased age, the amount of collagen in the heart increases and elastin decreases. These changes affect the myocardium's ability to stretch and contract. One of the major changes in the cardiovascular system is the response to physical or emotional stress. In times of increased stress, CO and SV decrease due to reduced

TABLE 32-1	**GERONTOLOGIC ASSESSMENT DIFFERENCES**

Cardiovascular System

Changes	Differences in Assessment Findings
Chest Wall	
Kyphosis	Altered chest landmarks for palpation, percussion, and auscultation. Distant heart sounds.
Heart	
Myocardial hypertrophy, ↑ collagen and scarring, ↓ elastin	↓ Cardiac reserve, heart failure.
Downward displacement	Difficulty in isolating apical pulse
↓ CO, HR, SV in response to exercise or stress	↓ Response to exercise and stress. Slowed recovery from activity.
Cellular aging and fibrosis of conduction system	↓ Amplitude of QRS complex and slight. lengthening of PR, QRS, and QT intervals. Irregular cardiac rhythms, ↓ maximal HR, ↓ HR variability.
Valvular rigidity from calcification, sclerosis, or fibrosis, impeding complete closure of valves	Systolic murmur (aortic or mitral) possible without an indication of cardiovascular disease.
Blood Vessels	
Arterial stiffening caused by loss of elastin in arterial walls, thickening of intima of arteries, and progressive fibrosis of media	↑ In systolic BP and possible ↑ or ↓ in diastolic BP. Possible widened pulse pressure. Pedal pulses diminished. ↑ In intermittent claudication.
Venous tortuosity increased	Inflamed, painful, or cordlike varicosities. Dependent edema.

contractility and HR response. The resting supine HR is not markedly affected by aging. When the patient changes positions (e.g., sits upright), the sympathetic nerve pathway may be affected by fibrous tissue and fatty deposits, resulting in a blunted HR response.[7]

Cardiac valves become thicker and stiffer from lipid accumulation, degeneration of collagen, and fibrosis. The aortic and mitral valves are most frequently affected. These changes result in either regurgitation of blood when the valve should be closed or narrowing of the orifice of the valve (stenosis) when the valve should be open. The turbulent blood flow across the affected valve results in a murmur.

The number of pacemaker cells in the SA node decreases with age. By age 75, a person may have only 10% of the normal number of pacemaker cells. Although this is compatible with adequate SA node function, it may account for the frequency of some sinus dysrhythmias in older adults. Similar decreases also occur in the number of conduction cells in the internodal tracts, bundle of His, and bundle branches. These changes contribute to the development of atrial dysrhythmias and heart blocks. About 50% of older adults have an abnormal resting ECG that shows increases in the PR, QRS, and/or QT intervals.[8]

The autonomic nervous system control of the cardiovascular system changes with aging. The number and function of β-adrenergic receptors in the heart decrease with age. So the older adult not only has a decreased response to physical and emotional stress, but also is less sensitive to β-adrenergic agonist drugs. The lower maximum HR during exercise results in only a twofold increase in CO compared with the three or four times increase seen in younger adults.

Arterial and venous blood vessels thicken and become less elastic with age.[9] Arteries increase their sensitivity to vasopressin (antidiuretic hormone). With aging both of these changes contribute to a progressive increase in SBP and a decrease or no change in DBP. Thus an increase in the pulse pressure is found. Hypertension is not a normal consequence of aging, and should be treated. Valves in the large veins in the lower extremities have a reduced ability to return the blood to the heart, often resulting in dependent edema.

Orthostatic hypotension, which is estimated to be present in more than 30% of patients over age 70 with systolic hypertension, may be related to medications and/or decreased baroreceptor function.[8] *Postprandial hypotension* (decrease in BP of at least 20 mm Hg that occurs within 75 minutes after eating) may also occur in about a third of otherwise healthy older adults. Both orthostatic and postprandial hypotension may be related to falls in older adults. Despite the changes associated with aging, the heart is able to function adequately under most circumstances.

ASSESSMENT OF CARDIOVASCULAR SYSTEM

Subjective Data

A careful health history and physical examination will help you distinguish symptoms that reflect a cardiovascular problem from problems of other body systems. Explore and document all cues that alert you to the possibility of underlying cardiovascular problems.

Important Health Information

History of Present Illness. Ask the patient what problem has brought him or her to the health care facility or provider.

CASE STUDY

Patient Introduction

Jupiterimages/Banana-Stock/Thinkstock

L.P., a 63-year-old Asian American man, is brought to the emergency department by ambulance at 6 AM after calling 911 with complaints of chest pain, shortness of breath (SOB), palpitations, and dizziness. The paramedics have started an IV and oxygen at 2 L/min via nasal cannula. They also administered four chewable baby ASA and a nitroglycerin tablet, and they obtained a 12-lead ECG. L.P. is pain free on arrival but still complains of palpitations and dizziness.

Critical Thinking

As you read through this assessment chapter, think about L.P.'s symptoms with the following questions in mind:
1. What are the possible causes of L.P.'s chest pain, SOB, palpitations, and dizziness?
2. What would be your major focus when assessing L.P.?
3. What questions would you ask L.P.?
4. What should be included in the physical assessment? What would you be looking for?
5. What diagnostic studies would you expect to be ordered?

Ⓔvolve   Answers available at *http://evolve.elsevier.com/Lewis/medsurg.*

Fully explore all symptoms the patient is experiencing (see Table 32-1).

Past Health History. Many illnesses affect the cardiovascular system directly or indirectly. Ask the patient about a history of chest pain, shortness of breath, fatigue, alcohol and tobacco use, anemia, rheumatic fever, streptococcal throat infections, congenital heart disease, stroke, palpitations, dizziness with position changes, syncope, hypertension, thrombophlebitis, intermittent claudication, varicosities, and edema.

Medications. Assess the patient's current and past use of medications. This includes over-the-counter (OTC) drugs, herbal supplements, and prescription drugs. For example, aspirin prolongs the blood clotting time, and is found in many drugs used to treat cold symptoms. List all of the patient's drugs. Include dosage, time of last dose, and the patient's understanding of the drug's purpose and side effects. Many noncardiac drugs can adversely affect the cardiovascular system and should be assessed (Table 32-2).

Surgery or Other Treatments. Ask the patient about specific treatments, past surgeries, or hospital admissions related to cardiovascular problems. Explore any admissions or outpatient procedures for diagnostic workups or cardiovascular symptoms. Note whether an ECG or a chest x-ray has been done for baseline data.

Functional Health Patterns. The strong correlation between components of a patient's lifestyle and cardiovascular health supports the need to review each functional health pattern. Key questions to ask a person with a cardiovascular problem are listed in Table 32-3.

Health Perception–Health Management Pattern. Ask the patient about the presence of major cardiovascular risk factors. These include abnormal serum lipids, hypertension, sedentary lifestyle, diabetes mellitus, obesity, and tobacco use. If a patient uses tobacco, estimate the number of pack-years of tobacco use (number of packs smoked per day multiplied by the number of years the patient has smoked). Document the patient's attitude about tobacco use and attempts and methods used to stop. Record any alcohol use. This information should include type

TABLE 32-2   CARDIOVASCULAR EFFECTS OF NONCARDIAC DRUGS*

Drug Classification	Examples	Cardiovascular Effects
Anticancer agents	daunorubicin (Cerubidine) doxorubicin (Adriamycin)	Dysrhythmias, cardiomyopathy
Antipsychotics	chlorpromazine (Thorazine) haloperidol (Haldol)	Dysrhythmias, orthostatic hypotension
Corticosteroids	cortisone (Cortone) prednisone (Orasone)	Hypotension, edema, potassium depletion
Hormone therapy, oral contraceptives	estrogen + progestin (Ortho-Novum, Prempro, Tri-Norinyl)	Myocardial infarction, thromboembolism, stroke, hypertension
Nonsteroidal antiinflammatory drugs (NSAIDs) †	ibuprofen (Motrin) celecoxib (Celebrex)	Hypertension, myocardial infarction, stroke
Psychostimulants	cocaine amphetamines	Tachycardia, angina, myocardial infarction, hypertension, dysrhythmias
Tricyclic antidepressants	amitriptyline (Elavil) doxepin (Sinequan)	Dysrhythmias, orthostatic hypotension

*List is not all-inclusive.
†Second-generation NSAIDs, known as COX-2 inhibitors, have been linked to an increased risk of serious adverse cardiovascular events.

of alcohol, amount, frequency, and any changes in the reaction to it. Also note any use of habit-forming drugs, including recreational drugs.

Question the patient about any allergies, including food and environmental allergies. Determine whether the patient has ever experienced a drug reaction or an allergic or anaphylactic reaction. Ask specifically about any allergic reaction to contrast media if there is a chance that a cardiac catheterization may be needed.

🧬 GENETIC RISK ALERT
Coronary Artery Disease
- Specific genetic links, especially related to lipoprotein genes, have been identified for some families with CAD.
- The clustering of CAD in families is strong if there is early age of onset affecting several relatives.

Cardiomyopathy
- Hypertrophic cardiomyopathy can be caused by autosomal dominant mutations.
- Dilated cardiomyopathy can be caused by autosomal and X-linked dominant mutations.

Hypertension
- Hypertension results from a complex interplay between genetic and environmental factors.
- Lifestyle choices (e.g., smoking, lack of exercise) may trigger genetic tendencies to hypertension.

Confirmed illnesses of blood relatives can highlight any genetic or familial tendencies toward CAD, peripheral vascular disease, hypertension, bleeding, cardiac disorders, diabetes mellitus, atherosclerosis, and stroke. Note any family members who developed cardiac disease younger than age 55. In addition, disorders affecting the vascular system, such as intermittent claudication and varicosities, may be familial. Finally, assess any family health history of noncardiac problems such as asthma,

TABLE 32-3 HEALTH HISTORY

Cardiovascular System

Health Perception–Health Management
- Do you practice any preventive measures to decrease risk factors for heart disease?*
- Have you noticed an increase in heart symptoms such as chest pain or dyspnea?*
- Does your heart problem cause you to be less able to care for yourself?*
- Do you foresee any potential self-care problems because of your heart problem?*
- Have you ever used tobacco? If yes, in what form, how much, and for how long? Have you tried to quit? If yes, what methods have you tried? Are you interested in more information about quitting?
- How often and how much alcohol do you drink?

Nutritional-Metabolic
- Describe your usual daily diet, including salt, fat, and liquid intake.
- What is your present weight? What was your weight 1 year ago? If different, explain.
- Does eating cause fatigue or shortness of breath?*

Elimination
- Do your feet or ankles ever swell?* If yes, how far up your legs? Does it go away after sleeping all night?
- Have you ever taken medication to help you get rid of excess fluid or to relieve constipation?*
- Are you having any problems related to urination?*
- Do you ever strain to have a bowel movement?

Activity-Exercise
- Are your daily activities or exercise limited because of your heart problem?*
- When were you last able to comfortably perform your usual activities or exercise?
- Do you experience any discomfort or side effects as a result of exercise or any activity?*
- Can you comfortably walk and talk at the same time?
- How often do you attend activities outside your home?
- What was your most strenuous activity in the last few weeks compared with 6 months ago?

Sleep-Rest
- How many pillows do you sleep on at night? Has this changed recently?*
- Do you ever wake up suddenly and feel as if you cannot catch your breath?*
- Do you have a history of sleep apnea?*
- How many times a night do you awaken to urinate?

Cognitive-Perceptual
- Do you ever experience dizziness or fainting?*
- Do you ever find it difficult to verbally express yourself or to remember things?*
- Do you experience any pain (e.g., chest pain, leg pain with activity) as a result of your heart problem?*

Self-Perception–Self-Concept
- Have your perceptions of yourself changed since you were diagnosed with a heart disease?*
- How has your heart disease affected the quality of your life?

Role-Relationship
- Has this illness affected any of the roles that you play in your daily life?*
- How have your significant others been affected by your heart disease?

Sexuality-Reproductive
- Has your heart disease caused a change in your sexual activity?*
- Do you experience any heart-related symptoms during sexual activity?*
- Do any of your medications affect your ability to participate in sexual activities?*
- Females: Are you currently taking oral contraceptives, hormonal therapy, or drug therapy for breast cancer?

Coping–Stress Tolerance
- Describe your normal coping mechanisms during times of stress or anxiety.
- To whom or where would you turn during a time of stress? Are these people or services helping you now?*
- Do you practice any stress reduction techniques?*
- Do you have a history of depression?*
- Do you feel capable of handling your present health situation?
- Do you experience any heart symptoms (e.g., chest pain, palpitations) during times of stress or anger?*

Values-Beliefs
- What influence have your values or beliefs had during your illness?
- Do you feel any conflicts between your values or beliefs and the plan of care?*
- Describe any cultural or religious beliefs that may influence the management of your heart problem.

*If yes, describe.

renal disease, liver disease, and obesity because they can affect the cardiovascular system.

Nutritional-Metabolic Pattern. Being underweight or overweight may indicate potential cardiovascular problems. Thus it is important to assess the patient's weight history (e.g., over the past year) in relation to height. Determine the amount of salt and saturated fats in the patient's typical diet. In addition to actual food habits, which may be influenced by culture, investigate the patient's attitudes and plans relative to diet and weight management.

Elimination Pattern. The patient on diuretics may report increased voiding and/or nocturia. Investigate any history of incontinence or constipation, including any use of medications (prescribed and OTC) for constipation. Teach patients with cardiovascular problems to avoid straining during a bowel movement (Valsalva maneuver). Ask patients if they have any swelling of the lower extremities and if it resolves when their feet are elevated or after an overnight sleep.

Activity-Exercise Pattern. The benefit of exercise for cardiovascular health is clear, with aerobic exercise being most beneficial. Record the types of exercise done and the duration, intensity, and frequency of each. Ask about and note the occurrence of any symptoms during exercise (e.g., chest pain, shortness of breath, claudication) that may indicate a cardiovascular problem.

Sleep-Rest Pattern. Cardiovascular problems often disrupt sleep. *Paroxysmal nocturnal dyspnea* (attacks of shortness of breath, especially ones at night that awaken the patient) and Cheyne-Stokes respiration are associated with heart failure. Many patients with heart failure need to sleep with their head elevated on pillows or in a chair. Note the number of pillows needed to sleep or the need to sleep upright (*orthopnea*) and whether this has changed recently.

Sleep apnea has been associated with an increased risk of life-threatening dysrhythmias, especially in patients with heart failure. Nocturia, a common finding with cardiovascular patients, also interrupts normal sleep patterns. Fully explore both conditions.

Cognitive-Perceptual Pattern. It is important to ask both the patient and the caregiver about cognitive-perceptual problems. Cardiovascular problems such as dysrhythmias, hypertension, and stroke may cause problems with syncope, language, and memory. Report any pain associated with the cardiovascular system (e.g., chest pain, claudication).

Self-Perception–Self-Concept Pattern. If a cardiovascular event is acute, the patient's self-perception may be affected. Invasive diagnostic procedures often lead to body image concerns for the patient. When CVD is chronic, the patient may not be able to identify the cause but can often describe the inability to "keep up" previous levels of activity. This may also affect the patient's quality of life, so inquire about the effects of the illness on the patient.

Role-Relationship Pattern. The patient's gender, race, and age are all related to cardiovascular health. In addition, the patient's marital status, role in the household, employment status, number of children and their ages, living environment, and caregivers help you to identify strengths and support systems in the patient's life. Assess the patient's level of satisfaction or dissatisfaction with life roles, since this may alert you to possible areas of stress or conflict.

Sexuality-Reproductive Pattern. Ask the patient about the effect of the cardiovascular problem on sexual activity. Because older patients often fear sudden death during sexual intercourse, it may lead to changes in their sexual behavior. Fatigue, chest pain, or shortness of breath may also limit sexual activity. Erectile dysfunction (ED) may be a symptom of peripheral vascular disease and/or a side effect of some medications used to treat CVD (e.g., β-adrenergic blockers [beta blockers], diuretics). Ask about the use of drugs for ED (e.g., sildenafil [Viagra]). These drugs are contraindicated if the patient is also taking a nitrate because the combination of ED drugs and nitrates can cause significant hypotension.[10] Determine whether counseling may be helpful.

Ask female patients if they use oral contraceptives, hormone therapy (HT) for symptoms of menopause, or drug therapy for breast cancer. Women who smoke and use oral contraceptives are at increased risk for blood clots (e.g., venous thromboembolism). Similarly, there is an increased risk for CVD with the use of HT and selective estrogen-receptor modulators (e.g., tamoxifen [Novaldex]).[11]

Coping–Stress Tolerance Pattern. Ask the patient to identify areas that cause stress and the usual methods of coping with stress. Potentially stressful areas include health concerns, marital relationships, family and friends, occupation, and finances.

Work-related stress, depression, and inadequate social support are risk factors for CVD and cardiac events.[4] Ask the patient about each of these factors. Information about support systems such as family, extended family and friends, counselors, or religious groups can provide vital insight when planning care.

Values-Belief Pattern. Individual values and beliefs, which are greatly affected by culture, may play a significant role in the

---

CASE STUDY—cont'd

Subjective Data

Jupiterimages/Banana-Stock/Thinkstock

A focused subjective assessment of L.P. revealed the following information:

- ***PMH:*** History of hypertension, mitral valve prolapse with mild regurgitation, heart failure, and type 2 diabetes mellitus.
- ***Medications:*** Lisinopril (Prinivil) 10 mg/day PO, metoprolol (Lopressor) 50 mg PO BID, ASA 325 mg/day PO, furosemide (Lasix) 40 mg/day PO, and glipizide (Glucotrol) 5 mg/day PO.
- ***Health Perception–Health Management:*** L.P. denies any previous history of chest pain or CAD. He was feeling fine until this morning when he awoke and experienced SOB, chest pain, palpitations, and dizziness while walking to the bathroom. He became frightened that he was having a heart attack so called 911. Denies smoking or alcohol intake. SOB and chest pain are now gone, but he continues to feel palpitations and dizziness when he sits up.
- ***Elimination:*** Denies any edema. States takes Lasix in the morning and typically "pees until lunchtime." Denies nocturia.

---

real or potential conflict a patient faces when dealing with a diagnosis of CVD. Some patients may attribute their illness to punishment from God; others may think that a "higher power" may assist them. Information about a patient's values and beliefs will help you intervene during periods of crisis.

Objective Data

Physical Examination

Vital Signs. After you observe the patient's general appearance, obtain vital signs. Measure BP bilaterally. These readings normally vary from 5 to 15 mm Hg. Use the arm with the highest BP for subsequent BP measurements. Take orthostatic (postural) BPs and HRs while the patient is supine, sitting with legs dangling, and standing. SBP should not decrease more than 20 mm Hg from the supine to the standing position. HR should not increase more than 20 beats/minute from the supine to the standing position.

Peripheral Vascular System

Inspection. Inspect the skin for color, hair distribution, and venous pattern. Inspect the extremities for conditions such as edema, dependent rubor, clubbing of the nail beds, varicosities, and lesions such as stasis ulcers. Edema in the extremities can be caused by gravity, interruption of venous return, or right-sided heart failure.

Inspect the large veins in the neck (internal and external jugular) while the patient is gradually elevated from a supine position to an upright (30 to 45 degrees) position. Distention and prominent pulsations of these neck veins, referred to as *jugular venous distention,* can be caused by right-sided heart failure.

Palpation. Palpate the upper and lower extremities for temperature, moisture, pulses, and edema bilaterally to assess for symmetry. Look for edema by depressing the skin over the tibia or medial malleolus for 5 seconds. Normally, there is no depression after releasing pressure. If pitting edema is present, grade it from 1+ (mild pitting, slight brief indentation) to 4+ (very deep pitting, indentation that lasts a long time).[6]

Palpate the pulses in the neck and extremities for information on arterial blood flow. Assess the rhythm (e.g., regular, irregular) and force. It is important to palpate each carotid pulse separately to avoid vagal stimulation and possible dysrhythmias. Compare the characteristics of the arteries on the right and left extremities simultaneously to determine symmetry.

When palpating the arteries identified in Fig. 32-6, rate the force of the pulse using the following scale[6]:

0 = Absent
1+ = Weak
2+ = Normal
3+ = Increased, full, bounding

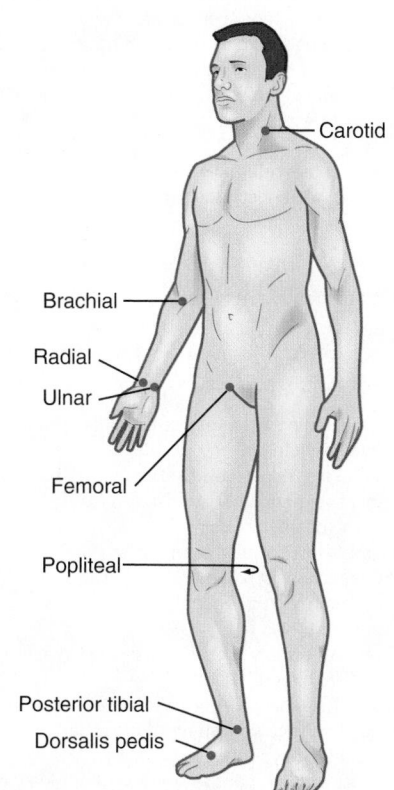

FIG. 32-6 Common sites for palpating arteries.

The rigidity (hardness) of the vessel should also be noted. The normal pulse feels like a tap, whereas a vessel wall that is narrowed or bulging vibrates. The term for a palpable vibration is *thrill*.

Capillary refill is used to assess arterial flow to the extremities. Position the patient's hands near the level of the heart and squeeze a nail bed to produce blanching. Observe for the return of color. This should occur in less than 2 seconds with normal peripheral perfusion and CO.

Auscultation. An artery that is narrowed or has a bulging wall may create turbulent blood flow. This abnormal flow can create a buzzing or humming termed a *bruit*. This is heard with a stethoscope placed over the vessel. Auscultation of major arteries such as the carotid arteries, abdominal aorta, and femoral arteries should be part of the initial cardiovascular assessment. Abnormalities of the cardiovascular system are described in Table 32-4.

Thorax

Inspection and Palpation. An overall inspection and palpation of the bony structures of the thorax are the initial steps in the examination. Next, inspect and palpate the areas where the cardiac valves project their sounds by identifying the intercostal spaces (ICSs). The raised notch, the *angle of Louis*, is where the manubrium and the body of the sternum are joined, and is located at the level of the second rib. It is palpable in the midline of the sternum. It is used to count ICSs and locate specific auscultatory areas (Fig. 32-7).

Locate the following auscultatory areas: the aortic area in the second ICS to the right of the sternum, the pulmonic area in the second ICS to the left of the sternum, the tricuspid area in the fifth left ICS close to the sternum, and the mitral area in the left midclavicular line at the fifth ICS. A fifth auscultatory area is *Erb's point,* located at the third left ICS near the sternum. Normally, no pulsations are felt in these areas unless the patient has a thin chest wall.

A valvular disorder may be suspected if abnormal pulsations or thrills are felt. Next, inspect and palpate the epigastric area, which lies on either side of the midline just below the xiphoid

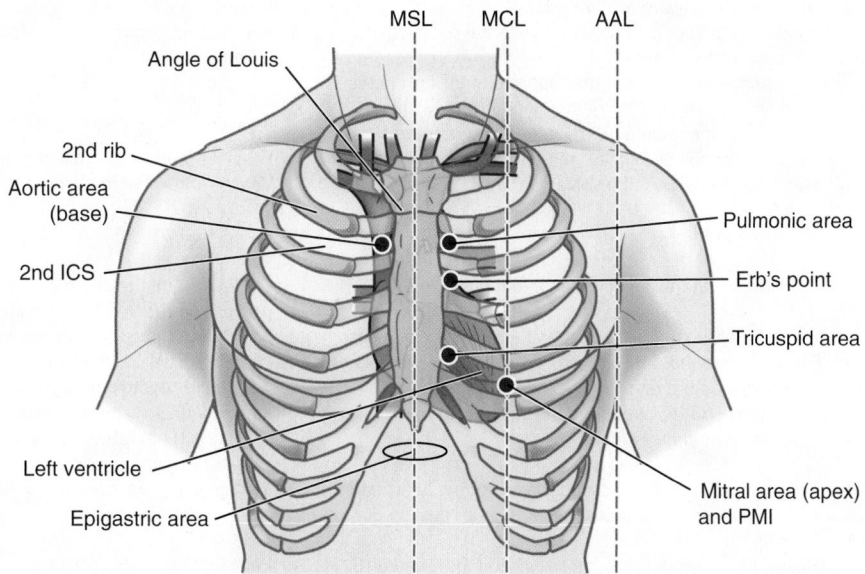

FIG. 32-7 Orientation of the heart within the thorax and cardiac auscultatory areas. *Red lines* indicate the midsternal line *(MSL)*, midclavicular line *(MCL)*, and anterior axillary line *(AAL)*. *ICS*, Intercostal space; *PMI*, point of maximal impulse.

TABLE 32-4　ASSESSMENT ABNORMALITIES

Cardiovascular System

Finding*	Description	Possible Etiology* and Significance
Inspection		
Jugular venous distention	Distended neck (jugular) veins with patient sitting at 30- to 45-degree angle	Elevated right atrial pressure, right-sided heart failure
Central cyanosis	Bluish or purplish tinge in central areas such as tongue, conjunctivae, inner surface of lips	Inadequate O_2 saturation of arterial blood because of pulmonary or cardiac disorders (e.g., congenital defects)
Peripheral cyanosis	Bluish or purplish tinge in extremities or in nose and ears	Reduced blood flow because of heart failure, vasoconstriction, cold environment
Splinter hemorrhages	Small red to black streaks under fingernails	Infective endocarditis (infection of endocardium, usually in area of cardiac valves)
Clubbing of nail beds	Obliteration of normal angle between base of nail and skin	Endocarditis, congenital defects, prolonged O_2 deficiency
Color changes in extremities with postural change	Pallor, cyanosis, mottling of skin after limb elevation. Dependent rubor (reddish blue discoloration). Glossy skin	Chronic decreased arterial perfusion
Ulcers	*Venous:* Necrotic crater-like lesion usually found on lower leg at medial malleolus. Characterized by slow wound healing	Poor venous return, varicose veins, incompetent venous valves. Arteriosclerosis, diabetes
	Arterial: Pale ischemic base, well-defined edges usually found on toes, heels, lateral malleoli	
Varicose veins	Visible dilated, discolored, tortuous vessels in lower extremities	Incompetent valves in vein
Palpation		
Pulse		
Bounding	Sharp, brisk, pounding pulse	Hyperkinetic states (e.g., anxiety, fever), anemia, hyperthyroidism
Thready	Weak, slowly rising pulse easily obliterated by pressure	Blood loss, decreased cardiac output, aortic valve disease, peripheral arterial disease
Irregular	Regularly irregular or irregularly irregular. Skipped beats	Cardiac dysrhythmias
Pulsus alternans	Regular rhythm, but strength of pulse varies with each beat	Heart failure, cardiac tamponade
Absent	Lack of pulse	Atherosclerosis, trauma, embolus
Thrill	Vibration of vessel or chest wall	Aneurysm, aortic regurgitation, arteriovenous fistula
Rigidity	Stiffness or inflexibility of vessel wall	Atherosclerosis
>100 beats/min	Tachycardia	Exercise, anxiety, shock, need for increased cardiac output, hyperthyroidism
<60 beats/min	Bradycardia	Rest or sleeping, SA or AV node damage, athletic conditioning, side effect of drugs (e.g., β-adrenergic blockers), hypothyroidism
Displaced point of maximal impulse (apical pulse)	Point of maximal impulse is palpated (or auscultated) below the fifth ICS and to the left of the MCL	Cardiac enlargement as a result of coronary artery disease, heart failure, cardiomyopathy
Extremities		
Unusually warm extremities	Hands and feet warmer than normal	Possible thyrotoxicosis
Cold extremities	Hands and/or feet cold to touch. External covering necessary for comfort	Intermittent claudication, peripheral arterial disease, low cardiac output, severe anemia
Pitting edema of lower extremities or sacral area	Visible finger indentation after application of firm pressure, weight gain, tightening of clothing, including shoes, marks or indentations from constricting garments	Interruption of venous return to heart, right-sided heart failure
Abnormal capillary refill	Blanching of nail bed for ≥2 sec after release of pressure	Possible reduced arterial capillary perfusion, anemia
Asymmetry in limb circumference	Measurable swelling of involved limb	Venous thromboembolism, varicose veins, lymphedema
Auscultation		
Pulse deficit	Apical heart rate exceeding peripheral pulse rate	Cardiac dysrhythmias, most often atrial fibrillation/flutter or premature ventricular contractions
Arterial bruit	Turbulent flow sound in peripheral artery	Arterial obstruction or aneurysm
Third heart sound (S_3)	Extra heart sound, low pitched, heard in early diastole. Similar to sound of a gallop	Left ventricular failure. Volume overload. Mitral, aortic, or tricuspid regurgitation. Hypertension (possible)
Fourth heart sound (S_4)	Extra heart sound, low pitched, heard in late diastole. Similar to sound of a gallop	Forceful atrial contraction from resistance to ventricular filling (e.g., in left ventricular hypertrophy, aortic stenosis, hypertension, coronary artery disease)
Cardiac murmurs	Turbulent sounds occurring between normal heart sounds. Characterized by loudness, pitch, shape, quality, duration, timing	Cardiac valve disorder, abnormal blood flow patterns
Pericardial friction rub	High-pitched, scratchy sound heard during S_1 and/or S_2 at the apex. Heard best with patient sitting and leaning forward, and at the end of expiration	Pericarditis

*Limited to common assessment findings and etiologic factors. (Further discussion of conditions listed may be found in Chapters 33 to 38, 66, and 67.)

process. In a thin person, you may see the pulsation of the abdominal aorta. Normally, you can palpate it here. Next, inspect the precordium, which is located over the heart, for heaves. **Heaves** are sustained lifts of the chest wall in the precordial area that can be seen or palpated. They may be caused by left ventricular hypertrophy. Normally no pulsations are seen or felt here.

When the patient is supine, palpate the mitral valve area for the **point of maximal impulse (PMI)** (also called the *apical pulse*). This reflects the pulsation of the apex of the heart. The PMI lies medial to the midclavicular line in the fourth or fifth ICS. If the PMI is palpable, record its position in relation to the midclavicular line and ICSs. When the PMI is below the fifth ICS and left of the midclavicular line, the heart may be enlarged.

Auscultation. Normal heart sounds are produced by the movement of blood through the cardiac valves. These sounds can be heard through a stethoscope placed on the chest wall. The first heart sound (S_1) is associated with closure of the tricuspid and mitral valves. It has a soft lubb sound. The second heart sound (S_2) is associated with closure of the aortic and pulmonic valves. It has a sharp dupp sound. S_1 signals the beginning of systole. S_2 signals the beginning of diastole (Fig. 32-8). Listen to the auscultatory areas in sequence (see Fig. 32-7).

S_1 and S_2 are heard best with the diaphragm of the stethoscope because they are high pitched. Extra heart sounds (S_3 or S_4), if present, are heard best with the bell of the stethoscope because they are low pitched. Have the patient lean forward while sitting to enhance the sounds from the second ICSs (aortic and pulmonic areas). Place the patient in a left side-lying position to enhance the sounds at the mitral area.

When auscultating the apical area, simultaneously palpate the radial pulse. Determine whether the rhythm is regular or irregular while listening and feeling. If the apical and radial pulses are not equivalent, count the apical pulse while a second person simultaneously counts the radial pulse for 1 full minute. The difference between the two numbers is called a *pulse deficit* and can indicate cardiac dysrhythmias.

Normally no sound is heard between S_1 and S_2 during the periods of systole and diastole. Sounds that are heard during these periods may represent abnormalities and should be described. An exception to this is a normal splitting of S_2, which is best heard at the pulmonic area during inspiration. Splitting of this heart sound can be abnormal if it is heard during expiration or if it is constant (fixed) during the respiratory cycle.

The S_3 heart sound is a low-intensity vibration of the ventricular walls usually associated with decreased compliance of the ventricles during filling. An S_3 heart sound may be normal (physiologic) in young adults. It is pathologic in patients with left-sided heart failure or mitral valve regurgitation. S_3 is heard

CASE STUDY—cont'd

Objective Data: Physical Examination

Jupiterimages/Banana-Stock/Thinkstock

Physical examination findings of L.P. are as follows:
- BP 98/70, apical pulse 164, pulse irregular, respiratory rate 20, temperature 98.2° F (36.8° C), O_2 saturation 93% on room air
- Awake, alert, and oriented ×3
- Lungs clear on auscultation; systolic murmur present
- Cardiac monitor shows atrial fibrillation with a rapid ventricular response
- +1 pedal pulses bilaterally
- No peripheral edema, jugular venous distention, or heaves noted

As you continue reading this chapter, consider diagnostic studies you would anticipate being ordered for L.P.

closely after S_2 and is known as a *ventricular gallop*. The S_4 heart sound is a low-frequency vibration caused by atrial contraction. It precedes S_1 of the next cycle, and is known as an *atrial gallop*. An S_4 heart sound may be normal in older adults with no evidence of heart disease. It is pathologic in patients with CAD, cardiomyopathy, left ventricular hypertrophy, or aortic stenosis.[6]

Murmurs, produced by turbulent blood flow across diseased heart valves, are graded on a six-point Roman numeral scale of loudness and recorded as a ratio. I/VI indicates a murmur that is barely audible with the stethoscope, heard only in a quiet room and then not easily. VI/VI indicates a murmur that can be heard with the stethoscope lifted just off the chest wall.[6]

Pericardial friction rubs are sounds caused by friction that occurs when inflamed surfaces of the pericardium (pericarditis) move against each other. They are high-pitched, scratchy sounds that may be transient or intermittent and may last several hours to days. Friction rubs are usually heard best at the apex, with the patient upright and leaning forward, and following expiration.[6]

Document any abnormal sounds. This includes the timing (during systole or diastole), location (the anatomic site on the chest where it is heard the loudest), position (heard best when the patient is supine, sitting and leaning forward, or in the left side-lying position), and any other abnormal findings (irregular apical pulse or palpable chest wall heaves) associated with the sound.

Abnormal assessment findings are described in Table 32-4. A method of recording data from the cardiovascular assessment is presented in Table 32-5.

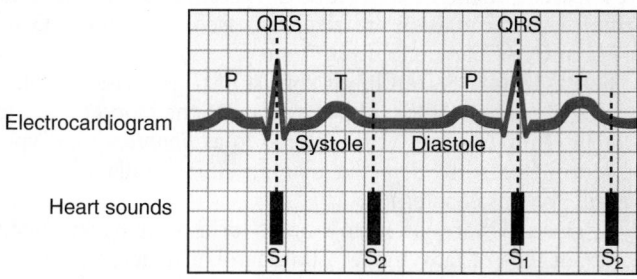

Electrocardiogram

Heart sounds

FIG. 32-8 Relationship of electrocardiogram, cardiac cycle, and heart sounds.

TABLE 32-5	**NORMAL PHYSICAL ASSESSMENT OF CARDIOVASCULAR SYSTEM**
Inspection	Skin warm, normal color. Capillary refill <2 sec. PMI not visible. No JVD with patient at 45-degree angle.
Palpation	PMI palpable in fourth ICS at left MCL. No thrills or heaves. Slight palpable pulsations of abdominal aorta in epigastric area. Carotid and extremity pulses 2+ and equal bilaterally. No pedal edema.
Auscultation	S_1 and S_2 heard. Apical-radial pulse rate equal, 72, and regular. No murmurs or extra heart sounds.

ICS, Intercostal space; *JVD,* jugular venous distention; *MCL,* midclavicular line; *PMI,* point of maximal impulse.

FOCUSED ASSESSMENT

Cardiovascular System

Use this checklist to make certain the key assessment steps have been done.

Subjective
Ask the patient about any of the following and note responses.

Chest pain	Y	N
Palpitations	Y	N
Shortness of breath (especially when lying down or at rest)	Y	N
Edema in legs or any part of body	Y	N
Leg pain during exercise	Y	N
Excess urination at night	Y	N

Objective: Diagnostic
Check the following for critical values or changes.

Cardiac biomarkers (troponin, CK-MB)	✓
Hematocrit and hemoglobin	✓
Electrocardiogram	✓

Objective: Physical Examination
Inspect and Palpate

Anterior chest wall for pulsations and heaves	✓
Pulses for symmetry, quality, and rhythm	✓

Auscultate

Blood pressure	✓
Heart for rate, rhythm, and sounds	✓

CK-MB, Creatine kinase–MB.

A *focused assessment* is used to evaluate the status of previously identified cardiovascular problems and to monitor for signs of new problems (see Table 3-6). A focused assessment of the cardiovascular system is presented in the box above.

DIAGNOSTIC STUDIES OF CARDIOVASCULAR SYSTEM

Numerous diagnostic studies are available to assess the cardiovascular system. Table 32-6 identifies the most common studies. Select studies are described in more detail below.

Blood Studies

Many blood studies provide information about the cardiovascular system. For example, some reflect the O_2-carrying capacity (red blood cell count and hemoglobin) and coagulation properties (clotting times) of the blood. (See Chapter 30 and Tables 30-6 and 30-7 for hematology studies.)

Cardiac Biomarkers. When cells are injured, they release their contents, including enzymes and other proteins, into the circulation. These *biomarkers* are useful in the diagnosis of myocardial injury and infarction.

Cardiac-specific troponin is a myocardial muscle protein released into circulation after injury or infarction. Two subtypes, cardiac-specific troponin T (cTnT) and cardiac-specific troponin I (cTnI), are specific to myocardial tissue. Normally the level in the blood is very low, so a rise in level is diagnostic of myocardial injury. cTnT and cTnI are detectable within hours (on average 4 to 6 hours) of myocardial injury, peak at 10 to 24 hours, and can be detected for up to 10 to 14 days (see Fig.

34-11). Troponin is the biomarker of choice in the diagnosis of myocardial infarction (MI). Recent development of high-sensitivity troponin (hs-cTnT, hs-cTnI) assays may provide even earlier detection of a cardiac event.[12]

Creatine kinase (CK) enzymes are found in a variety of organs and tissues and occur as three isozymes. These isozymes are specific to skeletal muscle (CK-MM), brain and nervous tissue (CK-BB), and the heart (CK-MB). CK-MB elevation is specific for myocardial injury or infarction. CK-MB levels begin to rise 3 to 6 hours after symptom onset, peak in 12 to 24 hours, and return to baseline within 12 to 48 hours after MI.[13] The peak level and return to normal can be delayed in a person who has had a large MI. Levels drop more rapidly in patients who are quickly and successfully treated for an MI. (Fig. 34-11 depicts the changes in cardiac markers related to an MI.)

Myoglobin is a low-molecular-weight heme protein found in cardiac and skeletal muscle. Myoglobin elevation is a sensitive indicator of very early myocardial injury but lacks specificity for MI. Its usefulness in diagnosing MI is limited.[13]

Correct interpretation of diagnostic tests requires consideration of the time from onset of symptoms and the time of the expected presence and elevation of the biomarkers. Additional data (patient symptoms, history, and ECG changes) complete the diagnostic picture for the patient with suspected myocardial injury or MI.

C-Reactive Protein. C-reactive protein (CRP) is a protein produced by the liver during periods of acute inflammation. CRP can be measured using a high-sensitivity test (hs-CRP). An increased level of CRP is an independent risk factor for CAD. The level of CRP may also predict the risk for future cardiac events in patients with unstable angina and MI, but studies have produced conflicting results.[14]

Homocysteine. Homocysteine (Hcy) is an amino acid that is produced during protein catabolism. Elevated Hcy levels can be either hereditary or acquired from dietary deficiencies of vitamin B_6, vitamin B_{12}, or folate. Elevated levels of Hcy have been linked to a higher risk of CAD, peripheral vascular disease, and stroke. It is recommended that Hcy testing be performed in those patients with a familial predisposition for early CVD or a history of CVD in the absence of other common risk factors.[15]

Cardiac Natriuretic Peptide Markers. There are three natriuretic peptides: (1) atrial natriuretic peptide (ANP) from the atrium, (2) b-type natriuretic peptide (BNP) from the ventricles, and (3) c-type natriuretic peptide from endothelial and renal epithelial cells. BNP is the marker of choice for distinguishing a cardiac or respiratory cause of dyspnea. N-terminal pro-brain natriuretic peptide (NT-pro-BNP) is also secreted in the ventricles and is more sensitive but less specific than BNP as a diagnostic marker of heart failure.[13] When diastolic blood pressure increases (e.g., heart failure), BNP and NT-pro-BNP are released and increase natriuresis (excretion of sodium in the urine). (ANP and BNP are also discussed in Chapter 33 on p. 711 and in Chapter 35 on p. 768.)

Serum Lipids. Serum lipids consist of triglycerides, cholesterol, and phospholipids. They circulate in the blood bound to protein. Thus they are often referred to as *lipoproteins*. (Types of serum lipids are depicted in eFig. 32-1, available on the website for this chapter.)

Triglycerides are the main storage form of lipids and make up about 95% of fatty tissue. Cholesterol, a structural component of cell membranes and plasma lipoproteins, is a precursor of corticosteroids, sex hormones, and bile salts. In addition to being absorbed from food in the gastrointestinal tract, cholesterol can also be synthesized in the liver. Phospholipids contain glycerol, fatty acids, phosphates, and a nitrogenous compound. Although formed in most cells, phospholipids usually enter the circulation as lipoproteins synthesized by the liver. Apoproteins are water-soluble proteins that combine with most lipids to form lipoproteins.

Different classes of lipoproteins contain varying amounts of the naturally occurring lipids. These include the following:

1. *Chylomicrons:* primarily exogenous triglycerides from dietary fat
2. *Low-density lipoproteins (LDLs):* mostly cholesterol with moderate amounts of phospholipids
3. *High-density lipoproteins (HDLs):* about 50% protein and 50% phospholipids and cholesterol
4. *Very-low-density lipoproteins (VLDLs):* primarily endogenous triglycerides with moderate amounts of phospholipids and cholesterol

Text continued on p. 704

TABLE 32-6 DIAGNOSTIC STUDIES

Cardiovascular System

Study	Description and Purpose	Nursing Responsibility
Blood Studies*		
Troponin (cardiac)	Contractile proteins that are released after an MI. Both troponin T and troponin I are highly specific to cardiac tissue. *Reference intervals:* **Troponin I (cTnI)** Negative: <0.5 ng/mL (<0.5 mcg/L) Indeterminate or suspicious for injury to myocardium: 0.5-2.3 ng/mL (0.5-2.3 mcg/L) Positive for myocardial injury: >2.3 ng/mL (>2.3 mcg/L) **Troponin T (cTnT)** <0.1 ng/mL (<0.1 mcg/L)	Rapid point-of-care (bedside) assays are available. Explain to patient the purpose of serial sampling (e.g., q6-8hr × 3) in conjunction with CK-MB and serial ECGs.
CK-MB	Cardiospecific isozyme that is released in the presence of myocardial tissue injury. Concentrations >4%-6% of total creatine kinase (CK) are highly indicative of MI. Serum levels increase within 4-6 hr after MI.	Serial sampling often done in conjunction with troponin and ECGs.
Myoglobin	Low-molecular-weight protein that is 99%-100% sensitive for myocardial injury. Serum concentrations rise 30-60 min after MI. *Reference interval:* Male: 15.2-91.2 mcg/L Female: 11.1-57.5 mcg/L	Cleared from the circulation rapidly, limited use in the diagnosis of cardiac injury/infarction.
C-reactive protein (CRP)	Marker of inflammation that can predict risk of cardiac disease and cardiac events, even in patients with normal lipid values. High-sensitivity (hs) CRP assay used. *Lowest risk:* <1 mg/L *Moderate risk:* 1-3 mg/L *High risk:* >3 mg/L	Stable levels that can be measured nonfasting and any time during the day. May be more predictive risk factor of cardiovascular disease than LDLs for women. The average of two assays obtained 2 wk apart provides a more stable measurement than one single measurement.
Homocysteine	Amino acid produced during protein catabolism that has been identified as a risk factor for cardiovascular disease. Homocysteine may cause damage to the endothelium or have a role in formation of thrombi. *Reference interval:* Male: 5.2-12.9 μmol/L Female: 3.7-10.4 μmol/L	Hyperhomocysteinemia resulting from dietary deficiencies is treated with folic acid, vitamin B_6, and vitamin B_{12} supplements.
b-Type natriuretic peptide (BNP)	Peptide that causes natriuresis. Elevation helps to distinguish cardiac vs. respiratory cause of dyspnea. *Reference interval:* BNP (diagnostic for heart failure) >100 pg/mL (28.8 pmol/L)	Infusion of nesiritide (Natrecor) elevates levels temporarily.
NT-Pro-BNP	Aids in assessing the severity of heart failure in symptomatic and asymptomatic patients. *Reference interval:* ≤74 yr: 124 pg/mL >75 yr: 449 pg/mL	In patients with renal insufficiency, NT-pro-BNP concentrations may increase and may not correlate with New York Heart Association functional classification of heart failure.
Serum Lipids		
Cholesterol	A blood lipid. Elevated cholesterol is considered a risk factor for cardiovascular heart disease. *Reference interval:* <200 mg/dL (<5.18 mmol/L) (varies with age and gender)	Cholesterol levels can be obtained in a nonfasting state.

*Reference ranges for the laboratory tests vary by institution because of differences in equipment and reagents used.

Continued

TABLE 32-6   DIAGNOSTIC STUDIES—cont'd

Cardiovascular System

Study	Description and Purpose	Nursing Responsibility
Serum Lipids—cont'd		
Triglycerides	Mixtures of fatty acids. Elevations are associated with cardiovascular disease and diabetes. *Reference interval:* <150 mg/dL (<1.7 mmol/L) (varies with age)	Triglyceride and lipoprotein levels must be obtained in a fasting state (at least 12 hr, except for water). Alcohol should be withheld for 24 hr before testing.
Lipoproteins† (HDL, LDL)	Electrophoresis is done to separate lipoproteins into HDL and LDL. There are marked day-to-day fluctuations in serum lipid levels. More than one determination is needed for accurate diagnosis and treatment. *Reference intervals* (vary with age): **HDL** *Recommended* *Male:* >40 mg/dL (>1.04 mmol/L) *Female:* >50 mg/dL (>1.3 mmol/L) *Low risk for CAD:* ≥60 mg/dL (>1.55 mmol/L) *High risk for CAD:* <40 mg/dL (<1.04 mmol/L) **LDL** *Recommended:* <100 mg/dL (<2.6 mmol/L) *Near optimal:* 100-129 mg/dL (2.6-3.34 mmol/L) *Moderate risk for CAD:* 130-159 mg/dL (3.37-4.12 mmol/L) *High risk for CAD:* >160 mg/dL (>4.14 mmol/L)	Risk for cardiac disease is assessed by dividing the total cholesterol level by the HDL level and obtaining a ratio. *Low risk:* Ratio <3 *Average risk:* Ratio 3-5 *Increased risk:* Ratio >5
Lipoprotein (a) [Lp(a)]	Increased levels are associated with an increased risk of premature CAD and stroke. *Reference interval:* <30 mg/dL (<0.3 g/L)	Lp(a) levels can be obtained in a nonfasting state.
Lipoprotein-associated phospholipase A₂ (Lp-PLA₂)	Elevated levels of Lp-PLA$_2$ are associated with vascular inflammation and increased risk for CAD. Serum levels of Lp-PLA$_2$ are measured by the PLAC test. *Reference interval:* *Male:* 131-376 ng/mL *Female:* 120-342 ng/mL	Lp-PLA$_2$ levels can be obtained in a nonfasting state.
Chest X-Ray	Patient is placed in two upright positions to examine the lung fields and heart size. The two common positions are posteroanterior (PA) and lateral. Normal heart size and contour for the individual's age, sex, and size are noted.	Inquire about frequency of recent x-rays and possibility of pregnancy. Provide lead shielding to areas not being viewed. Remove any jewelry or metal objects that may obstruct the view of the heart and lungs.
12-Lead ECG	Electrodes are placed on the chest and extremities, allowing the ECG machine to record cardiac electrical activity from 12 different views. A resting 12-lead ECG can identify conduction problems, dysrhythmias, position of heart, cardiac hypertrophy, pericarditis, myocardial ischemia or infarction, pacemaker activity, and effectiveness of drug therapy at one point in time.	Prepare skin and apply electrodes and leads. Position patient supine (or with head of bed elevated, if short of breath). Inform patient that no discomfort is involved and to lie still to decrease motion artifact.
Signal-averaged ECG (SAECG)	A high-resolution ECG that can identify electrical activity called late potentials, indicating a patient is at risk for developing ventricular dysrhythmias (e.g., ventricular tachycardia).	Same as for 12-lead ECG.
Ambulatory ECG Monitoring		
Holter monitoring	Recording of ECG rhythm for 24-48 hr and then correlating rhythm changes with symptoms and activities recorded in diary. Normal patient activity is encouraged to simulate conditions that produce symptoms. Electrodes are placed on chest, and a recorder is used to store information until it is recalled, printed, and analyzed for any rhythm disturbance. It can be performed on an inpatient or outpatient basis.	Prepare skin and apply electrodes and leads. Explain importance of keeping an accurate diary of activities and symptoms. Tell patient that no bath or shower can be taken during monitoring. Skin irritation may develop from electrodes.
Event monitor or loop recorder	Records rhythm disturbances that are not frequent enough to be recorded in one 24-hr period. It allows more freedom than a regular Holter monitor. Some units have electrodes that are attached to the chest and have a loop of memory that captures the onset and end of an event. Other types are placed directly on patient's wrist, chest, or fingers and have no loop of memory, but record the patient's ECG in real time. Recordings may be transmitted over the phone to a receiving unit.	Instruct in the use of equipment for recording and transmitting (if appropriate) of transient events. Teach patient about skin preparation for lead placement or steady skin contact for units not requiring electrodes. This will ensure the reception of optimal ECG tracings for analysis. Instruct patient to initiate recording as soon as symptoms begin or as soon thereafter as possible.

†Source: American Heart Association: What your cholesterol levels mean, 2009. Available at *www.americanheart.org/presenter.jhtml?identifier=183#HDL.*

TABLE 32-6   DIAGNOSTIC STUDIES—cont'd

Cardiovascular System

Study	Description and Purpose	Nursing Responsibility
Exercise or Stress Testing	Various protocols are used to evaluate the effect of exercise tolerance on cardiovascular function. A common protocol uses 3-min stages at set speeds and elevation of the treadmill belt. The patient can exercise to either predicted peak HR (calculated by subtracting the person's age from 220) or to peak exercise tolerance, at which time the test is terminated. The test is also terminated for chest discomfort, significant increase or decrease in vital signs from baseline, or significant ECG changes indicating cardiac ischemia. Vital signs and ECG are monitored. The ECG is monitored after exercise for rhythm disturbances or, if ECG changes occurred with exercise, for return to baseline. Continual monitoring of vital signs and ECG rhythms for ischemic changes is important in the diagnosis of CAD. An exercise bike may be used if the patient is unable to walk on the treadmill.	Instruct patient to wear comfortable clothes and shoes that can be used for walking and running. Instruct patient about procedure and importance of reporting any symptoms that occur. Monitor vital signs and obtain 12-lead ECG before exercise, during each stage of exercise, and after exercise until all vital signs and ECG changes have returned to normal. Monitor patient's response throughout procedure. Contraindications include any reasons patient is unable to reach peak exercise tolerance. β-Adrenergic blockers may be held 24 hr before the test because they blunt the HR and limit the patient's ability to achieve maximal HR. Caffeine-containing food and fluids are held for 24 hr. Patients must refrain from smoking and strenuous exercise for 3 hr before test.
6-Minute walk test	Distance patient is able to walk on a flat surface in 6 min. Used to measure response to treatments and determine functional capacity for activities of daily living. Useful in people who are unable to perform treadmill or exercise bike testing. May be a better measure of fitness for older adults than exercise testing.	Instruct patient to wear comfortable shoes. Inform patient to carry or pull oxygen if used routinely. Encourage patient to walk as quickly as possible.
Echocardiogram • Contrast • M-mode • Two-dimensional • Color-flow imaging (duplex) • Real-time three-dimensional	Transducer that emits and receives ultrasound waves is placed in four positions on the chest above the heart. Transducer records sound waves that are bounced off the heart. Also records direction and flow of blood through the heart and transforms it to audio and graphic data that measure valvular abnormalities, congenital cardiac defects, wall motion, EF, and cardiac function. IV contrast agent may be used to enhance images.	Place patient in a left side-lying position facing equipment. Instruct patient about procedure and sensations (pressure and mechanical movement from head of transducer). No contraindications to procedure exist.
Stress echocardiogram	Combination of exercise test and echocardiogram. Resting images of the heart are taken with ultrasound, and then the patient exercises. Postexercise images are taken within 1 min of stopping exercise. Differences in left ventricular wall motion and thickening before and after exercise are evaluated.	Instruct and prepare patient for treadmill or exercise bicycle. Inform patient of importance of timely return to examination table for imaging after exercise. Contraindications include any reasons patient is unable to reach peak exercise tolerance.
Pharmacologic echocardiogram	Used as a substitute for the exercise stress test in individuals unable to exercise. IV dobutamine or dipyridamole is infused, and dosage is increased in 5-min intervals while echocardiogram is performed to detect wall motion abnormalities at each stage.	Start IV infusion. Administer medication per protocol. Monitor vital signs before, during, and after test until baseline achieved. Monitor patient for signs and symptoms of distress during procedure. Observe patient for side effects (e.g., shortness of breath, dizziness, nausea). Aminophylline may be given to prevent or reverse side effects of dipyridamole. Contraindications include any known allergies to medications.
Transesophageal echocardiogram (TEE)	A probe with an ultrasound transducer at the tip is swallowed while the physician controls angle and depth. As it passes down the esophagus, it sends back clear images of heart size, wall motion, valvular abnormalities, endocarditis vegetation, and possible source of thrombi without interference from lungs or chest ribs. A contrast medium may be injected IV for evaluating direction of blood flow if an atrial or ventricular septal defect is suspected. Doppler ultrasound and color-flow imaging can also be used concurrently.	Instruct patient to be NPO for at least 6 hr before test. Remove dentures. IV sedation is administered and throat locally anesthetized. A bite block is placed in the mouth. A designated driver is needed if done in the outpatient department. Monitor vital signs and oxygen saturation levels and perform suctioning as needed during procedure. Assist patient to relax. Patient may not eat or drink until gag reflex returns. Sore throat is temporary.
Nuclear Cardiology	Study involves IV injection of radioactive isotopes (^{99m}technetium-sestamibi [Cardiolite]). Radioactive uptake is counted over the heart by scintillation camera. It supplies information about myocardial contractility, myocardial perfusion, and acute cell injury.	Explain procedure to patient. Women should not wear bras to decrease breast attenuation. Establish IV line for injection of isotopes. Explain that radioactive isotope used is a small, diagnostic amount and will lose most of its radioactivity in a few hours. Inform the patient that he or she will be lying still on back with arms extended overhead for 20 min. Repeat scans are performed within a few minutes to hours after the injection.

Continued

TABLE 32-6 DIAGNOSTIC STUDIES—cont'd

Cardiovascular System

Study	Description and Purpose	Nursing Responsibility
Multigated acquisition (MUGA) (cardiac blood pool) scan	A small amount of the patient's blood is removed, mixed with a radioactive isotope (e.g., ^{99m}technetium-sestamibi), and reinjected IV. With the ECG used for timing, images are acquired during the cardiac cycle. Indicated for patients with MI, heart failure, or valvular heart disease. Can be used to evaluate the effect of various cardiac or cardiotoxic medications on the heart.	Explain procedure to patient. Establish IV line for removal of blood sample and reinjection of isotope. Establish ECG monitoring. Inform patient that procedure involves little risk.
Single-photon emission computed tomography (SPECT)	Used to determine size or risk of infarction and to determine infarction size. Small amounts of a radioactive isotope (e.g., ^{99m}technetium-tetrofosmin [Myoview], thallium-201) are injected IV and recordings are made of the radioactivity emitted over a specific area of the body. Circulation of the isotope can be used to detect coronary artery blood flow, intracardiac shunts, motion of ventricles, EF, and size of the heart chambers.	Explain procedure to patient. Establish IV line for injection of isotope. Establish ECG monitoring. Inform patient that procedure involves little risk.
Exercise (stress) nuclear imaging	Nuclear imaging images are taken at rest and after exercise. The injection is given at maximum HR (usually 85% of age-predicted maximum) on bicycle or treadmill. Patient is then required to continue exercise for 1 min to circulate the radioactive isotope. Scanning is done 15-60 min after exercise. A resting scan is performed 60-90 min after initial infusion or 24 hr later.	Explain procedure to patient. Instruct patient to eat only a light meal between scans. Certain medications may need to be held for 1-2 days before the scan. Patients should not have caffeine 12 hr prior. If targeted maximum HR is not achieved with exercise, test may be changed to pharmacologic imaging.
Pharmacologic nuclear imaging	Dipyridamole or adenosine is used to produce vasodilation when patients are unable to tolerate exercise. Vasodilation increases blood flow to well-perfused coronary arteries. Scanning procedure is same. Aminophylline may be given to prevent or reverse side effects of dipyridamole (e.g., shortness of breath, dizziness, nausea). Dobutamine is used if vasodilators are contraindicated.	Explain procedure to patient. Instruct patient to hold all caffeine products for 12 hr before procedure. Calcium channel blockers and β-adrenergic blockers should be held 24 hr before the test. Observe patient for side effects (e.g., shortness of breath, dizziness, nausea).
Positron emission tomography (PET)	Highly sensitive in distinguishing viable and nonviable myocardial tissue. Uses two radionuclides. Nitrogen-13-ammonia is injected IV first and scanned to evaluate myocardial perfusion. A second radioactive isotope, fluoro-18-deoxyglucose, is then injected and scanned to show myocardial metabolic function. In the normal heart, both scans match, but in an ischemic or damaged heart, they differ. The patient may or may not be stressed. A baseline resting scan is usually obtained for comparison.	Instruct patient on procedure. Explain that patient will be scanned by a machine and will need to stay still for a time. Patient's glucose level must be between 60-140 mg/dL (3.3-7.8 μmol/L) for accurate glucose metabolic activity. If exercise is included as part of testing, patient needs to be NPO and refrain from tobacco and caffeine for 24 hr before test.
Cardiovascular Magnetic Resonance Imaging (CMRI)	Noninvasive imaging technique obtains information about cardiac tissue integrity, aneurysms, EF, cardiac output, and patency of proximal coronary arteries. It does not involve ionizing radiation and is an extremely safe procedure. It provides images in multiple planes with uniformly good resolution.	Explain procedure to patient. Inform patient that the small diameter of the cylinder, along with loud noise of the procedure, may cause panic or anxiety. Antianxiety drugs and distraction strategies (e.g., music) may be recommended. Patient must lie still during test. Contraindicated for persons with implanted metallic devices or other metal fragments unless noted to be MRI safe. Discuss any implants before scan.
Magnetic resonance angiography (MRA)	Used for imaging vascular occlusive disease and abdominal aortic aneurysms. Same as MRI but with use of gadolinium as IV contrast medium.	Contraindications include any known allergies to contrast medium and persons with implanted metallic devices or other metal fragments.
Cardiac Computed Tomography (CT)	Cardiac CT is heart-specific CT imaging technology with or without IV contrast medium used to visualize heart anatomy, coronary circulation, and blood vessels.	
Coronary CT angiography (CTA)	Use of CT with injected IV contrast medium to obtain images of blood vessels and diagnose CAD.	Explain procedure to patient. Metal objects should be removed before examination. Patients should have a regular heart rhythm to allow for accurate testing. A β-adrenergic blocker may need to be administered before the test to control HR. The patient may need to be NPO for several hours before the procedure.

TABLE 32-6 DIAGNOSTIC STUDIES—cont'd

Cardiovascular System

Study	Description and Purpose	Nursing Responsibility
Calcium-scoring CT scan • Electron beam computed tomography (EBCT)	EBCT, also known as ultrafast CT, uses a scanning electron beam to quantify calcification in coronary arteries and heart valves (see Fig. 32-11). Primarily used for risk assessment in asymptomatic patients and to assess for heart disease in patients with atypical symptoms potentially related to cardiac causes.	Explain procedure to patient. Inform patient that procedure is quick and involves little or no risk.
Cardiac Catheterization	Involves insertion of catheter into heart to obtain information about O_2 levels and pressure readings within heart chambers. Contrast medium is injected to assist in seeing structures and motion of heart. Procedure is done by insertion of catheter into a vein (for right side of heart) and/or an artery (for left side of heart).	Check for sensitivity to contrast media. Withhold food and fluids for 6-12 hr before procedure. Give sedative and other drugs, if ordered. Inform patient about use of local anesthesia, insertion of catheter, feeling of warmth when dye is injected, and possible fluttering sensation of heart as catheter is passed. Note that patient may be instructed to cough or take a deep breath when dye is injected and that patient is monitored by ECG throughout procedure. After procedure, frequently assess circulation to extremity used for catheter insertion. Check peripheral pulses, color, and sensation of extremity per agency protocol. Observe puncture site for hematoma and bleeding. Place compression device over arterial site to achieve hemostasis, if indicated. Monitor vital signs and ECG. Assess for hypotension or hypertension, dysrhythmias, and signs of pulmonary emboli (e.g., respiratory difficulty).
Coronary angiography	During a cardiac catheterization, contrast medium is injected directly into coronary arteries. Used to evaluate patency of coronary arteries and collateral circulation.	Same as for cardiac catheterization.
Intracoronary ultrasound (ISUS)	During cardiac catheterization a small ultrasound probe is introduced into coronary arteries. Data are used to assess size and consistency of plaque, arterial walls, and effectiveness of intracoronary artery treatment.	Same as for cardiac catheterization.
Fractional flow reserve (FFR)	During cardiac catheterization a special wire is inserted into coronary arteries to measure pressure and flow. Information is used to determine need for angioplasty or stenting on nonsignificant blockages.	Same as for cardiac catheterization.
Electrophysiology Study (EPS)	Invasive study used to record intracardiac electrical activity using catheters (with multiple electrodes) inserted via the femoral and jugular veins into the right side of the heart. The catheter electrodes record the electrical activity in different cardiac structures. In addition, dysrhythmias can be induced and terminated.	Antidysrhythmic medications may be discontinued several days before study. Keep patient NPO 6-8 hr before test. Give premedication to promote relaxation if ordered. IV sedation often used during procedure. Patient must have frequent vital signs and continuous ECG monitoring after the procedure.
Peripheral Arteriography and Venography	Peripheral vessel blood flow is assessed by injecting contrast media into the appropriate arteries or veins (arteriography and venography). Serial x-ray studies taken to detect and visualize any atherosclerotic plaques, occlusion, aneurysms, venous abnormalities, or traumatic injury.	Check for allergy to contrast media. Give mild sedative, if ordered. Check extremity with puncture site for pulsation, warmth, color, and motion after procedure. Inspect insertion site for bleeding or swelling. Observe patient for allergic reactions to contrast media. See Table 38-9 for additional peripheral vascular diagnostic studies.
Hemodynamic Monitoring	Invasive and minimally invasive bedside hemodynamic monitoring is done using intraarterial, pulmonary artery, and central vein catheters to monitor arterial BP, stroke volume variation, pulmonary artery pressure, pulmonary artery wedge pressure, cardiac output, and central venous pressure. Used to evaluate cardiovascular status and response to treatment.	Patients requiring hemodynamic monitoring are critically ill and are monitored in intensive care units. See Chapter 66 for complete information on hemodynamic monitoring.

A lipid panel usually measures cholesterol, triglyceride, LDL, and HDL. Elevations in triglycerides and LDL are strongly associated with CAD. An increased HDL level is associated with a decreased risk of CAD.[4] High levels of HDLs serve a protective role by mobilizing cholesterol from tissues. (This is shown in eFig. 32-2, available on the website for this chapter.)

Although an association exists between elevated serum cholesterol levels and CAD, a measure of total cholesterol alone is not sufficient for an assessment of CAD. A risk assessment is calculated by comparing the total cholesterol to HDL ratio over time. An increase in the ratio indicates increased risk. This provides more information than either value alone. The patient must fast before blood is drawn for a lipid panel so food intake does not affect the results.

Plasma levels of apolipoprotein A-I (apo A-I) (the major HDL protein) and the ratio of apo A-I to apolipoprotein B (apo B) (the major LDL protein) are stronger predictors of CAD than the HDL cholesterol level alone. Measurements of these lipoproteins can be useful in identifying patients at risk for CAD.[13]

Lipoprotein (a), or Lp(a), has been studied for its role as a risk factor for CAD. Increased levels of Lp(a), especially with increased levels of lactate dehydrogenase (LDH), have been linked with the progression of atherosclerosis, especially in women.[4]

Lipoprotein-Associated Phospholipase A₂. Lipoprotein-associated phospholipase A_2 (Lp-PLA_2) is an inflammatory enzyme expressed in atherosclerotic plaques. Elevated levels of Lp-PLA_2 are related to an increased risk of CAD.[16]

Chest X-Ray

A radiographic picture of the chest can show cardiac contours, heart size, and anatomic changes in individual chambers (Fig. 32-9). The chest x-ray records any displacement or enlargement of the heart, extra fluid around the heart (pericardial effusion), and pulmonary congestion.

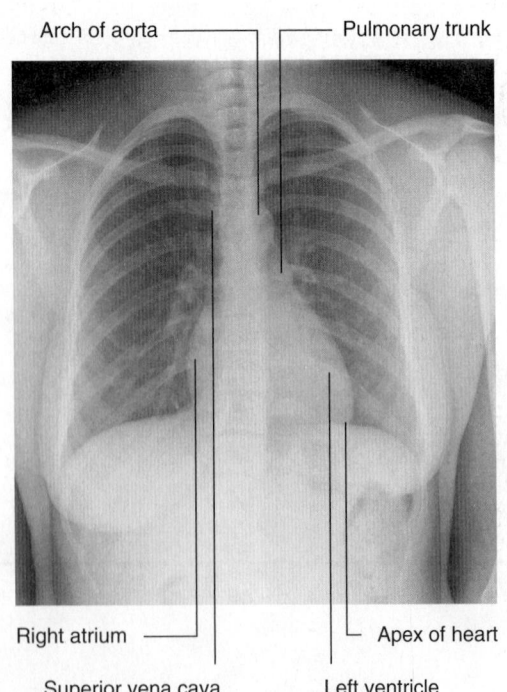

FIG. 32-9 Chest x-ray: standard posterior-anterior view.

Electrocardiogram

The basic P, QRS, and T waveforms (see Fig. 32-4, *B*) are used to assess cardiac activity. Deviations from the normal sinus rhythm can indicate problems in heart function. There are many types of ECG monitoring, including a resting 12-lead ECG, ambulatory ECG monitoring, and exercise or stress testing (see Table 32-6). Continuous ambulatory ECG (Holter monitoring) provides diagnostic information over a period of time. (See Chapter 36 for a complete discussion of ECG monitoring.)

Event Monitor or Loop Recorder. An event monitor or loop recorder is used to document less frequent ECG events. An event monitor is a portable unit that uses electrodes to store ECG data once triggered by the patient. A disadvantage of this type of monitoring is that, if symptoms occur for only a brief time, they may be over before the patient puts on the device and triggers it to record. Likewise, if patients are extremely symptomatic (e.g., syncopal), they may not be physically able to trigger the ECG recording. These devices can be used for routine pacemaker checks over the phone to the health care provider's office.[17]

An implantable loop recorder is used for patients who may have serious yet infrequent dysrhythmias. This small recorder is implanted though a small incision into the chest wall. It is activated to record either by the patient using a remote device or automatically if the HR exceeds or goes below a set rate. External loop recorders are worn for a month, and require electrodes continuously placed on the skin. This device only records when activated by the patient when symptoms occur.

Exercise or Stress Testing

Cardiac symptoms frequently occur only with activity because of the demand on the coronary arteries to provide more oxygen. Exercise testing is used to evaluate the heart's response to physical stress. This helps to assess CVD and set limits for exercise programs. Exercise testing is used for individuals who do not have restrictions related to walking or using a bicycle. It is also helpful for those with normal ECGs that limit diagnostic interpretation (e.g., pacemakers) (see Table 32-6).

Echocardiogram

The echocardiogram uses ultrasound (US) waves to record the movement of the structures of the heart. In the normal heart, ultrasonic sound waves directed at the heart are reflected back in typical configurations. *Contrast echocardiography* involves the addition of an IV contrast agent (e.g., albumin microbubbles, agitated saline) to assist in defining the images, especially in technically difficult patients (e.g., obese).

The echocardiogram provides information about abnormalities of (1) valvular structures and motion, (2) cardiac chamber size and contents, (3) ventricular and septal motion and thickness, (4) pericardial sac, and (5) ascending aorta. The **ejection fraction (EF),** or the percentage of end-diastolic blood volume that is ejected during systole, can also be measured. The EF provides information about the function of the left ventricle during systole.

Two commonly used types of echocardiograms are the *motion-mode (M-mode) echocardiogram* and the *two-dimensional (2-D) echocardiogram.* In the M-mode type, a single ultrasound beam is directed toward the heart, recording the motion of the intracardiac structures and detecting wall thickness and chamber size. The 2-D echocardiogram sweeps

FIG. 32-10 Long-axis images of the aortic and mitral valve with the depth adjusted to optimize evaluation of valve anatomy and motion. The 2-D images *(left)* in diastole *(top)* and systole *(bottom)* show normal aortic and mitral opening and closure. The color flow images *(right)* show normal left ventricular inflow with no aortic regurgitation in diastole *(top)* and normal antegrade flow in the left ventricular outflow tract and no mitral regurgitation in systole *(bottom)*.

the ultrasound beam through an arc, producing a cross-sectional view. This shows correct spatial relationships among the structures.

Doppler technology allows for sound evaluation of the flow or motion of the scanned object (heart valves, ventricular walls, blood flow). *Color-flow imaging (duplex)* is the combination of 2-D echocardiography and Doppler technology (Fig. 32-10). It uses color changes to demonstrate the speed and direction of blood flow. Pathologic conditions, such as valvular leaks and congenital defects, can be diagnosed more effectively.

Real-time three-dimensional (3-D) ultrasound is a technology that uses multiple 2-D echo images with computer technology to provide a reconstruction of the heart. This technique produces information about the structures of the heart and how these structures change during the cardiac cycle.

Stress echocardiography, a combination of treadmill test and ultrasound images, evaluates wall motion abnormalities. By using a digital computer to compare images before and after exercise, wall motion and function are revealed. This test provides the information of an exercise stress test with the information from an echocardiogram. For those individuals unable to exercise, an IV drug (e.g., dobutamine [Dobutrex], dipyridamole [Persantine]) is used to produce pharmacologic stress on the heart while the patient is at rest.

Transesophageal echocardiography (TEE) provides more precise echocardiography of the heart than surface 2-D echocardiography by removing interference from the chest wall and

lungs. The TEE uses a flexible endoscope probe with a ultrasound transducer in the tip for imaging of the heart and great vessels. The probe is passed into the esophagus to the level of the heart, and M-mode, 2-D, Doppler, and color-flow imaging can be obtained.

TEE is used frequently in an outpatient setting for evaluation of mitral valve disease and for identification of endocarditis vegetation, thrombus before cardioversion, or the source of cardiac emboli. In addition, TEE is used in the operating room to assess intraoperative cardiac function and in the emergency department to detect suspected aortic dissection.

The risks of TEE are low. However, complications may include perforation or tearing of the esophagus, hemorrhage, dysrhythmias, vasovagal reactions, and transient hypoxemia. TEE is contraindicated if the patient has a history of esophageal disorders, dysphagia, or radiation therapy to the chest wall. Patients require sedation during a TEE.

Nuclear Cardiology

One of the most common nuclear imaging tests is the multigated acquisition (MUGA) or cardiac blood pool scan. This test provides information on wall motion during systole and diastole, cardiac valves, and EF (see Table 32-6).

Perfusion imaging is also used with exercise testing to determine whether the coronary blood flow changes with increased activity. Stress perfusion imaging may show an abnormality even when a resting image is normal. This procedure is used to diagnose CAD, make a prognosis in existing CAD, differentiate viable myocardium from scar tissue, and determine the potential for success of various interventions (e.g., coronary artery bypass surgery, percutaneous coronary intervention)[18] (see Chapter 34).

Exercise stress perfusion imaging is always preferred but, if a patient cannot exercise, IV dipyridamole or adenosine (Adenocard) can be given to dilate the coronary arteries and simulate the effect of exercise. After the drug takes effect, the isotope is injected and the imaging is done.

Cardiovascular Magnetic Resonance Imaging

Cardiovascular magnetic resonance imaging (CMRI) can detect and find areas of MI in a 3-D view. It is sensitive enough to find even small MIs that are not apparent with single-photon emission computed tomography imaging. CMRI aids in the final diagnosis of MI and the assessment of EF. It also plays a role in prediction of recovery from MI and in the diagnosis of congenital heart and aortic disorders and CAD.[19]

One major advantage of CMRI is that it does not require any radiation to the patient. In general, the use of CMRI in patients with pacemakers and ICDs is discouraged because the magnets can alter the function of the devices. When there is a strong clinical need and the benefits outweigh the risks, CMRI should only be performed in these patients at experienced centers.[19] Some newer models of these devices are approved for use with MRI.

Cardiac Computed Tomography

Cardiac computed tomography (CT) is a heart-imaging test that uses CT technology with or without IV contrast (dye) to see the heart anatomy, coronary circulation, and great blood vessels (e.g., aorta, pulmonary veins, artery). This technology is often called multidetector CT (MDCT) scanning. Types of CT scans used to diagnosis heart disease include coronary CT angiography (CTA) and calcium-scoring CT scan (see Table 32-6).

Coronary CTA is a noninvasive test. It can be done faster than a cardiac catheterization with less risk and discomfort to the patient.[20] Although the use of coronary CTA is increasing, cardiac catheterization (discussed in the next section) remains the gold standard to diagnose coronary artery stenosis. Further, when a cardiac catheterization is done, interventions (e.g., angioplasty, stent placement) can be performed if coronary blockages are found.

The calcium-scoring CT scan is used to find calcium deposits in plaque in the coronary arteries. The most common method used is the electron beam CT (EBCT) (Fig. 32-11). It can detect early coronary calcification before symptoms develop. The amount of coronary calcium is a predictor of future cardiac events.

Cardiac Catheterization

Cardiac catheterization is a common outpatient procedure. It provides information about CAD, coronary spasm, congenital and valvular heart disease, and ventricular function. Cardiac catheterization is also used to measure intracardiac pressures and O₂ levels, as well as CO and EF. With injection of contrast media and fluoroscopy, the coronary arteries can be seen, chambers of the heart can be outlined, and wall motion can be observed.

Cardiac catheterization is done by inserting a radiopaque catheter into the right and/or left side of the heart. For the right

FIG. 32-11 Examples of coronary calcification of the left anterior descending coronary artery *(large arrow)* and left circumflex artery *(small arrow)* as seen on electron beam computed tomography.

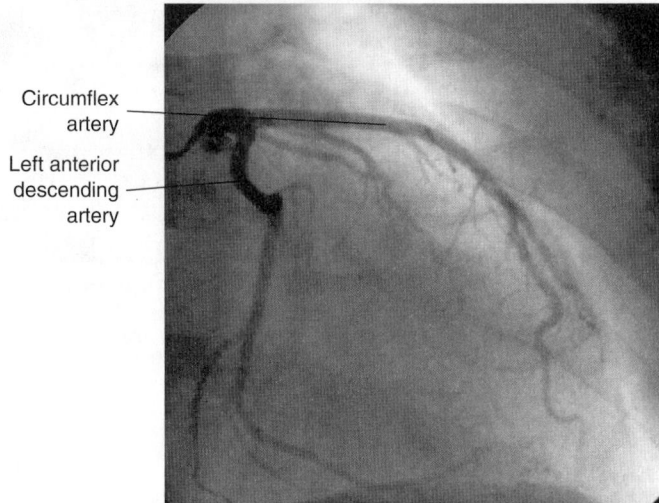

Circumflex artery

Left anterior descending artery

FIG. 32-12 Normal left coronary artery angiogram.

side of the heart, a catheter is inserted through an arm vein (basilic or cephalic) or a leg vein (femoral). Pressures are recorded as the catheter is moved into the vena cava, the right atrium, the right ventricle, and the pulmonary artery. The catheter is then moved until it is wedged or lodged in position. This blocks the blood flow and pressure from the right side of the heart and looks ahead through the pulmonary capillary bed to the pressure in the left side of the heart *(pulmonary artery wedge pressure)*. This pressure is used to assess the function of the left side of the heart.

Left-sided heart catheterization is done by inserting a catheter into a femoral, brachial, or radial artery. The catheter is passed in a retrograde manner up to the aorta, across the aortic valve, and into the left ventricle.

Coronary angiography is done with a left-sided heart catheterization. The catheter is positioned at the origin of the coronary arteries (see Fig. 32-3), and contrast medium is injected into the arteries. Patients often feel a temporary flushed sensation with dye injection. The images identify the location and severity of any coronary blockages (see Figs. 32-12 and 34-7). Complications of cardiac catheterization include bleeding or hematoma at the puncture site; allergic reactions to the contrast media; looping or kinking of the catheter; infection; thrombus formation; aortic dissection; dysrhythmias; MI; stroke; and puncture of the ventricles, cardiac septum, or lung tissue.

Intracoronary Ultrasound. Intracoronary ultrasound (ICUS), also known as intravascular ultrasound (IVUS), is an invasive procedure performed in the catheterization laboratory with coronary angiography. The 2-D or 3-D ultrasound images provide a cross-sectional view of the arterial walls of the coronary arteries. In this procedure a miniature transducer attached to a small catheter is moved to the artery to be studied. Once it is in the artery, ultrasound images are obtained. The health of the arterial layers is assessed, including the composition, location, and thickness of any plaque. ICUS can evaluate vessel response to treatments such as stent placement and atherectomy, as well as any complications that may have occurred during the procedure (see Chapter 34). Patients most often have ICUS in addition to angiography or a coronary intervention. Thus nursing care is similar to that following cardiac catheterization (see Table 32-6).

Fractional Flow Reserve. Fractional flow reserve (FFR) is a procedure that is done during a cardiac catheterization. It involves using a special wire that can measure pressure and flow in the coronary artery. FFR helps to determine the need to perform angioplasty or stenting on nonsignificant blockages.

Electrophysiology Study

The electrophysiology study (EPS) records and manipulates the heart's electrical activity using electrodes placed inside the heart chambers. It provides information on SA node, AV node, and ventricular conduction. It is particularly helpful in determining the source and treatment of dysrhythmias. Patients

---

CASE STUDY—cont'd

Objective Data: Diagnostic Studies

Jupiterimages/Banana-Stock/Thinkstock

The health care provider orders the following initial diagnostic studies for L.P.:
- 12-lead ECG
- CBC, basic metabolic panel (glucose, electrolytes, BUN, creatinine)
- PTT, PT, INR
- Pro-BNP
- Troponin, CK-MB
- TSH, free T₄
- Chest x-ray

L.P.'s initial troponin and CK-MB levels are within normal limits. The ECG demonstrates atrial fibrillation with a rapid ventricular response. Chest x-ray, CBC, basic metabolic panel, pro-BNP, and coagulation studies are all within normal limits. The health care provider orders IV diltiazem (Cardizem) and heparin to be started in the emergency department. L.P. will be admitted to the progressive care unit and will have a consult with a cardiologist.

---

with symptomatic supraventricular or ventricular tachycardias may be at risk for sudden cardiac death. Information from an EPS helps to make an accurate diagnosis and guides treatment decisions.

In EPS, catheters are inserted in a manner similar to that used in a right-sided heart catheterization. These catheters are placed at specific anatomic sites within the heart to record electrical activity. Nursing care for patients after EPS is similar to the care of patients after cardiac catheterization. This includes continuous ECG monitoring and frequent assessment of vital signs and puncture site.

BRIDGE TO NCLEX EXAMINATION

The number of the question corresponds to the same-numbered outcome at the beginning of the chapter.

1. A patient with a tricuspid valve disorder will have impaired blood flow between the
   a. vena cava and right atrium.
   b. left atrium and left ventricle.
   c. right atrium and right ventricle.
   d. right ventricle and pulmonary artery.

2. A patient has a severe blockage in his right coronary artery. Which cardiac structures are most likely to be affected by this blockage *(select all that apply)?*
   a. AV node
   b. Left ventricle
   c. Coronary sinus
   d. Right ventricle
   e. Pulmonic valve

3. The portion of the vascular system responsible for hemostasis is the
   a. thin capillary vessels.
   b. endothelial layer of the arteries.
   c. elastic middle layer of the veins.
   d. smooth muscle of the arterial wall.

4. When a person's blood pressure rises, the homeostatic mechanism to compensate for an elevation involves stimulation of
   a. baroreceptors that inhibit the sympathetic nervous system, causing vasodilation.
   b. chemoreceptors that inhibit the sympathetic nervous system, causing vasodilation.
   c. baroreceptors that inhibit the parasympathetic nervous system, causing vasodilation.
   d. chemoreceptors that stimulate the sympathetic nervous system, causing an increased heart rate.

5. A P wave on an ECG represents an impulse arising at the
   a. SA node and repolarizing the atria.
   b. SA node and depolarizing the atria.
   c. AV node and depolarizing the atria.
   d. AV node and spreading to the bundle of His.

6. When collecting subjective data related to the cardiovascular system, which information should be obtained from the patient *(select all that apply)?*
   a. Annual income
   b. Smoking history
   c. Religious preference
   d. Number of pillows used to sleep
   e. Blood for basic laboratory studies

7. The auscultatory area in the left midclavicular line at the level of the fifth ICS is the best location to hear sounds from which heart valve?
   a. Aortic
   b. Mitral
   c. Tricuspid
   d. Pulmonic

8. When assessing a patient, you note a pulse deficit of 23 beats. This finding may be caused by
   a. dysrhythmias.
   b. heart murmurs.
   c. gallop rhythms.
   d. pericardial friction rubs.

9. When assessing the cardiovascular system of a 79-year-old patient, you might expect to find
   a. a narrowed pulse pressure.
   b. diminished carotid artery pulses.
   c. difficulty in isolating the apical pulse.
   d. an increased heart rate in response to stress.

10. Which nursing responsibilities are priorities when caring for a patient returning from a cardiac catheterization (select all that apply)?
    a. Monitoring vital signs and ECG
    b. Checking the catheter insertion site and distal pulses
    c. Assisting the patient to ambulate to the bathroom to void
    d. Informing the patient that he will be sleepy from the general anesthesia
    e. Instructing the patient about the risks of the radioactive isotope injection

1, c, 2, a, b, d, 3, b, 4, a, 5, b, 6, b, c, d, 7, b, 8, a, 9, c, 10, a, b

ⓔvolve

For rationales to these answers and even more NCLEX review questions, visit http://evolve.elsevier.com/Lewis/medsurg.

REFERENCES

1. Patton KT, Thibodeau GA, Douglas MM: *Essentials of anatomy and physiology*, St Louis, 2012, Mosby.
2. Wesley K: *Huszar's basic dysrhythmias and acute coronary syndromes*, ed 4, St Louis, 2011, Mosby Jems.
3. Watson S, Gorski KA: *Invasive cardiology*, ed 3, Sudbury, Mass, 2011, Jones & Bartlett Learning.
4. Huether S, McCance K: *Understanding pathophysiology*, ed 5, St Louis, 2012, Mosby.
5. American Heart Association: Understand blood pressure readings, 2012. Retrieved from *www.heart.org/HEARTORG/Conditions/HighBloodPressure/AboutHighBloodPressure/Understanding-Blood-Pressure-Readings_UCM_301764_Article.jsp*.
6. Jarvis C: *Physical examination and health assessment*, ed 6, St Louis, 2012, Saunders.
7. Karavidas A, Lazaros G, Tsiachris D, et al: Aging and the cardiovascular system, *Hellenic J Cardiol* 51:421, 2010.
8. Carlson KK: *Advanced critical care nursing*, St Louis, 2009, Saunders.
9. National Institute on Aging: Aging heart and arteries: a scientific quest, 2011. Retrieved from *www.nia.nih.gov/health/publication/aging-hearts-and-arteries-scientific-quest/chapter-2-aging-heart*.
10. Hodgson BB, Kizior RJ: *Saunders nursing drug handbook 2012*, St Louis, 2012, Mosby.
*11. Mosca L, Benjamin EJ, Berry K, et al: Effectiveness-based guidelines for cardiovascular disease prevention in women: 2011 update, *Circulation* 123:1243, 2011.
12. Hughes S: One high-sensitivity troponin test rules out MI, 2011. Retrieved from *www.theheart.org/article/1277167.do*.
13. Malarkey LM, McMorrow ME: *Saunders nursing guide to laboratory and diagnostic tests*, ed 2, St Louis, 2012, Saunders.
14. The Emerging Risk Factors Collaboration: C-reactive protein concentration and risk of coronary heart disease, stroke, and mortality: an individual participant meta-analysis, *Lancet* 375:132, 2010. Original Text
15. American Heart Association: Homocysteine, folic acid and cardiovascular disease, 2012. Retrieved from *www.heart.org/HEARTORG/GettingHealthy/NutritionCenter/Homocysteine-Folic-Acid-and-Cardiovascular-Disease_UCM_305997_Article.jsp*.
*16. The Lp-PLA₂ Studies Collaboration: Lipoprotein-associated phospholipase A₂ and risk of coronary disease, stroke, and mortality: collaborative analysis of 32 prospective studies, *Lancet* 375:1536, 2010.
17. American Heart Association: Common tests for arrhythmia, 2011. Retrieved from *www.heart.org/HEARTORG/Conditions/Arrhythmia/SymptomsDiagnosisMonitoringofArrhythmia/Common-Tests-for-Arrhythmia_UCM_301988_Article.jsp*.
18. Zaret BL, Beller GA: *Clinical nuclear cardiology*, ed 4, St Louis, 2010, Mosby.
*19. Hundley WG, Bluemke DA, Finn JP, et al: ACCF/ACR/AHA/NASCI/SCMR 2010 expert consensus document on cardiovascular magnetic resonance: a report of the American College of Cardiology Foundation Task Force on Expert Consensus Documents, *Circulation* 121:2462, 2010.
*20. Mark DB, Berman DS, Budoff MJ, et al: ACCF/ACR/AHA/NASCI/SAIP/SCAI/SCCT 2010 expert consensus document on coronary computed tomographic angiography: a report of the American College of Cardiology Foundation Task Force on Expert Consensus Documents, *Circulation* 121:2509, 2010.

RESOURCES

Resources for this chapter are listed at the end of Chapter 33 on p. 729 and at the end of Chapter 34 on p. 765.

*Evidence-based information for clinical practice.

One way to get high blood pressure is to go mountain climbing over molehills.
Earl Wilson

Nursing Management
Hypertension

Elisabeth G. Bradley

WEBSITE

http://evolve.elsevier.com/Lewis/medsurg

- NCLEX Review Questions
- Key Points
- Pre-Test
- Answer Guidelines for Case Study on p. 727

- Rationales for Bridge to NCLEX Examination Questions
- Case Study
  - Patient With Hypertension and Stroke
- Concept Map Creator
- Glossary
- Content Updates

eTables
- eTable 33-1: Your Guide to Lowering Your Blood Pressure With DASH
- eTable 33-2: Drug Therapy: Hypertension (expanded)

LEARNING OUTCOMES

1. Relate the pathophysiologic mechanisms associated with primary hypertension to the clinical manifestations and complications.
2. Select appropriate strategies for the prevention of primary hypertension.
3. Describe the collaborative care for primary hypertension, including drug therapy and lifestyle modifications.
4. Explain the collaborative care of the older adult with primary hypertension.
5. Prioritize the nursing management of the patient with primary hypertension.
6. Describe the collaborative care of a patient with hypertensive crisis.

KEY TERMS

blood pressure (BP), p. 710
hypertension, p. 712
hypertensive crisis, p. 726
isolated systolic hypertension (ISH), p. 712

orthostatic hypotension, p. 723
prehypertension, p. 712
primary hypertension, p. 712

secondary hypertension, p. 712
systemic vascular resistance (SVR), p. 710

Hypertension, or high blood pressure (BP), is an important medical and public health problem. There is a direct relationship between hypertension and cardiovascular disease (CVD). As BP increases, so does the risk of myocardial infarction (MI), heart failure, stroke, and renal disease.[1] This chapter discusses the nursing care and collaborative management of patients at risk for or who have hypertension.

One in three adults in the United States has hypertension. Additionally, 30% of adults have prehypertension,[2] and approximately 8% have undiagnosed hypertension.[3] *Healthy People 2020* lists the number of adults with hypertension whose BP is under control as one of the 26 high-priority, leading health indicators for the coming decade.[4] The National Health and Nutrition Examination Survey (NHANES) tracks prevention, treatment, and control of hypertension. Data from

NHANES show that most people 20 years of age and older with hypertension (82%) were aware that they had high BP, and 75% were being treated. However, 53% did not have their BP controlled.[2]

The American College of Cardiology Foundation and the American Heart Association (AHA) provide performance measures for hypertension management that address not only treatment, but also control of BP to target goals. To achieve the measures, patients with hypertension must have a BP of less than 140/90 mm Hg or, if their BP is higher, have at least two antihypertensive medications prescribed.[5]

National guidelines are designed to apply to all racial and ethnic groups. However, certain groups have a higher incidence of risk factors[2,6-8] (see boxes on Cultural & Ethnic Health Disparities and Gender Differences).

Reviewed by Susan J. Eisel, RN, MSEd, Associate Professor of Nursing, Mercy College of Ohio, Toledo, Ohio; Christina D. Keller, RN, MSN, Instructor, Radford University School of Nursing: Clinical Simulation Center, Radford, Virginia; Krista Krause, MSN, FNP-C, Faculty, St. Joseph's College of Nursing, Syracuse, New York; and Erin M. Loughery, MSN, APRN, Acute Care APN, William W. Backus Hospital, Norwich, Connecticut.

🌐 CULTURAL & ETHNIC HEALTH DISPARITIES

Hypertension

African Americans
- Have the highest prevalence of hypertension in the world.
- Develop hypertension at a younger age than whites.
- Have a higher incidence of hypertension among women than among men.
- Hypertension is more aggressive and results in more severe end-organ damage.
- Have a higher death rate resulting from hypertension than whites.
- Produce less renin and do not respond well to renin-inhibiting drugs. They respond better to calcium channel blockers and diuretics.
- Have a higher risk of angioedema with angiotensin-converting enzyme inhibitors than whites.

Mexican Americans
- Are less likely to receive treatment for hypertension than whites and African Americans.
- Have lower rates of BP control than whites and African Americans.
- Have lower levels of awareness of hypertension and its treatment than whites and African Americans.

GENDER DIFFERENCES

Hypertension

Men
- Before age 45, hypertension is more common in men than in women.

Women
- After age 64, hypertension is more common in women than in men.
- Part of the rise in BP in women is attributed to menopause-related factors such as estrogen withdrawal, overproduction of pituitary hormones, and weight gain.
- Older women (ages 70-79) have very poor control of hypertension compared with women ages 50-69, despite having similar rates of treatment.
- Hypertension is two to three times more common in women who take oral contraceptives than in women who do not.
- A history of preeclampsia may be an early sign of risk for cardiovascular disease.

NORMAL REGULATION OF BLOOD PRESSURE

Blood pressure (BP) is the force exerted by the blood against the walls of the blood vessel. It must be adequate to maintain tissue perfusion during activity and rest. The maintenance of normal BP and tissue perfusion requires the integration of both systemic factors and local peripheral vascular effects. BP is primarily a function of cardiac output (CO) and systemic vascular resistance (Fig. 33-1).

CO is the total blood flow through the systemic or pulmonary circulation per minute. It is described as the stroke volume (amount of blood pumped out of the left ventricle per beat [approximately 70 mL]) multiplied by the heart rate (HR) for 1 minute.

Systemic vascular resistance (SVR) is the force opposing the movement of blood within the blood vessels. The radius of the small arteries and arterioles is the principal factor determining vascular resistance. A small change in the radius of the arterioles creates a major change in the SVR. If SVR is increased and CO remains constant or increases, arterial BP will increase.

The mechanisms that regulate BP can affect either CO or SVR, or both. Regulation of BP is a complex process involving both short-term (seconds to hours) and long-term (days to weeks) mechanisms. Short-term mechanisms, including the sympathetic nervous system (SNS) and vascular endothelium, are active within a few seconds. Long-term mechanisms include renal and hormonal processes that regulate arteriolar resistance and blood volume. In a healthy person these regulatory mechanisms function in response to the body's demands.

Sympathetic Nervous System

The nervous system, which reacts within seconds after a drop in BP, increases BP primarily by activating the SNS. Increased SNS activity increases HR and cardiac contractility, produces widespread vasoconstriction in the peripheral arterioles, and promotes the release of renin from the kidneys. The net effect of SNS activation is to increase BP by increasing both CO and SVR.

Specialized nerve cells called *baroreceptors (pressoreceptors)* are located in the carotid arteries and the arch of the aorta. These cells sense changes in BP and transmit this information to the vasomotor centers in the brainstem. The brainstem sends

FIG. 33-1 Factors influencing blood pressure (BP). Hypertension develops when one or more of the BP-regulating mechanisms are defective.

this information through complex networks of neurons that excite or inhibit efferent nerves. SNS efferent nerves innervate cardiac and vascular smooth muscle cells. Under normal conditions, a low level of continuous SNS activity maintains vascular tone. BP may be reduced by withdrawal of SNS activity or by stimulation of the parasympathetic nervous system. This decreases the HR (via the vagus nerve) and thereby decreases CO.

The neurotransmitter norepinephrine (NE) is released from SNS nerve endings. NE activates receptors located in the sinoatrial node, myocardium, and vascular smooth muscle. The response to NE depends on the type of receptors present. SNS receptors are classified as α_1, α_2, β_1, and β_2 (Table 33-1). The smooth muscle of the blood vessels has α-adrenergic and β_2-adrenergic receptors. α-Adrenergic receptors located in the peripheral vasculature cause vasoconstriction when stimulated by NE. β_1-Adrenergic receptors in the heart respond to NE and epinephrine with increased HR *(chronotropic)*, increased force of contraction *(inotropic)*, and increased speed of conduction *(dromotropic)*. β_2-Adrenergic receptors are activated primarily by epinephrine released from the adrenal medulla and cause vasodilation (see Fig. 33-1).

The sympathetic vasomotor center interacts with many areas of the brain to maintain normal BP under various conditions. It is activated during times of pain, stress, and exercise. The SNS response causes an appropriate increase in CO and BP to adjust to the body's increased oxygen demands. During postural change from lying to standing, there is a transient decrease in BP. The vasomotor center is stimulated, and the SNS response causes peripheral vasoconstriction and increased venous return to the heart. If this response did not occur, blood flow to the brain would be inadequate, resulting in dizziness or syncope.

Baroreceptors. Baroreceptors have an important role in the maintenance of BP stability during normal activities. They are sensitive to stretching and, when stimulated by an increase in BP, send inhibitory impulses to the sympathetic vasomotor center. Inhibition of the SNS results in decreased HR, decreased force of contraction, and vasodilation in peripheral arterioles.

When a fall in BP is sensed by the baroreceptors, the SNS is activated. The result is constriction of the peripheral arterioles, increased HR, and increased contractility of the heart. In longstanding hypertension the baroreceptors become adjusted to elevated levels of BP and recognize this level as "normal."

Vascular Endothelium

The vascular endothelium is a single-cell layer that lines the blood vessels. It produces several vasoactive substances and growth factors. Nitric oxide and prostacyclin help maintain low arterial tone, inhibit growth of the smooth muscle layer, and inhibit platelet aggregation. *Endothelin* (ET) is an extremely potent vasoconstrictor. It also causes adhesion and aggregation of neutrophils and stimulates smooth muscle growth (see Fig. 33-1).

Renal System

The kidneys contribute to BP regulation by controlling sodium excretion and extracellular fluid (ECF) volume (see Chapter 45). Sodium retention results in water retention, which causes an increased ECF volume. This increases the venous return to the heart and the stroke volume. Together, these increase CO and BP.

The renin-angiotensin-aldosterone system (RAAS) also plays an important role in BP regulation (see Fig. 33-1). The juxtaglomerular apparatus in the kidney secretes renin in response to SNS stimulation, decreased blood flow through the kidneys, or decreased serum sodium concentration. Renin is an enzyme that converts angiotensinogen to angiotensin I. Angiotensin-converting enzyme (ACE) converts angiotensin I into angiotensin II (A-II). A-II increases BP by two different mechanisms (see Fig. 45-4). First, A-II is a potent vasoconstrictor and increases SVR. This results in an immediate increase in BP. Second, over a period of hours or days, A-II increases BP indirectly by stimulating the adrenal cortex to secrete aldosterone (discussed below).

A-II also acts at a local level within the heart and blood vessels. These effects include vasoconstriction and tissue growth that results in remodeling of the vessel walls. These changes are linked to the development of primary hypertension and also the long-term effects of hypertension (e.g., atherosclerosis, renal disease, cardiac hypertrophy).

Prostaglandins (PGE_2 and PGI_2) secreted by the renal medulla have a vasodilator effect on the systemic circulation. This results in decreased SVR and lowering of BP. (Prostaglandins are discussed in Chapter 12.) The natriuretic peptides (atrial natriuretic peptide [ANP] and b-type natriuretic peptide [BNP]) are secreted by heart cells. They antagonize the effects of antidiuretic hormone (ADH) and aldosterone. This results in *natriuresis* (excretion of sodium in urine) and diuresis, resulting in reduced blood volume and BP.

Endocrine System

Stimulation of the SNS results in release of epinephrine along with a small fraction of NE by the adrenal medulla. Epinephrine increases the CO by increasing the HR and myocardial contractility. Epinephrine activates β_2-adrenergic receptors in peripheral arterioles of skeletal muscle, causing vasodilation. In

TABLE 33-1	SYMPATHETIC NERVOUS SYSTEM RECEPTORS AFFECTING BLOOD PRESSURE	
Receptor	**Location**	**Response When Activated**
α_1	Vascular smooth muscle	Vasoconstriction
	Heart	Increased contractility (positive inotropic effect)
α_2	Presynaptic nerve terminals	Inhibition of norepinephrine release
	Vascular smooth muscle	Vasoconstriction
β_1	Heart	Increased contractility (positive inotropic effect)
		Increased heart rate (positive chronotropic effect)
		Increased conduction (positive dromotropic effect)
	Juxtaglomerular cells of the kidney	Increased renin secretion
β_2	Smooth muscle of blood vessels in heart (e.g., coronary arteries), lungs (e.g., bronchi), and skeletal muscle	Vasodilation
Dopamine receptors	Primarily renal blood vessels	Vasodilation

TABLE 33-2	CLASSIFICATION OF HYPERTENSION		
Category	SBP (mm Hg)		DBP (mm Hg)
Normal	<120	and	<80
Prehypertension	120-139	or	80-89
Hypertension, stage 1	140-159	or	90-99
Hypertension, stage 2	≥160	or	≥100

From the National Heart, Lung, and Blood Institute: Seventh report of the Joint National Committee on Detection, Evaluation, and Treatment of High Blood Pressure (JNC-7), NIH Publication No. 04-5230, Bethesda, Md, 2004, The Institute. Retrieved from *www.nhlbi.nih.gov/guidelines/hypertension/jnc7full.pdf*.
DBP, Diastolic blood pressure; *SBP*, systolic blood pressure.

TABLE 33-3	CAUSES OF SECONDARY HYPERTENSION*

- Cirrhosis
- Coarctation or congenital narrowing of the aorta
- Drug-related: estrogen replacement therapy, oral contraceptives, corticosteroids, nonsteroidal antiinflammatory drugs (e.g., cyclooxygenase-2 inhibitors), sympathetic stimulants (e.g., cocaine, monoamine oxidase)
- Endocrine disorders (e.g., pheochromocytoma, Cushing syndrome, thyroid disease)
- Neurologic disorders (e.g., brain tumors, quadriplegia, traumatic brain injury)
- Pregnancy-induced hypertension
- Renal disease (e.g., renal artery stenosis, glomerulonephritis)
- Sleep apnea

*List is not all inclusive.

peripheral arterioles with only α_1-adrenergic receptors (skin and kidneys), epinephrine causes vasoconstriction.

A-II stimulates the adrenal cortex to release aldosterone. (Release of aldosterone is also regulated by other factors [see Chapters 48 and 50].) Aldosterone stimulates the kidneys to retain sodium and water. This increases blood volume and CO (see Fig. 45-4).

An increased blood sodium and osmolarity level stimulates the release of ADH from the posterior pituitary gland. ADH increases the ECF volume by promoting the reabsorption of water in the distal and collecting tubules of the kidneys. The resulting increase in blood volume causes an increase in CO and BP.

HYPERTENSION

Classification of Hypertension

Hypertension is defined as a persistent systolic BP (SBP) of 140 mm Hg or more, diastolic BP (DBP) of 90 mm Hg or more, or current use of antihypertensive medication.[1] **Prehypertension** is defined as SBP of 120 to 139 mm Hg or DBP of 80 to 89 mm Hg.

Isolated systolic hypertension (ISH) is defined as an average SBP of 140 mm Hg or more, coupled with an average DBP of less than 90 mm Hg.[9] SBP increases with aging. DBP rises until approximately age 55 and then declines. Control of ISH decreases the incidence of stroke, heart failure, and death.

The classification of BP is based on the average of two or more properly measured BP readings on two or more office visits. Table 33-2 presents the BP classification for people 18 years of age and older.

Etiology

Hypertension can be classified as either primary or secondary.

Primary Hypertension. Primary (*essential* or *idiopathic*) hypertension is elevated BP without an identified cause, and it accounts for 90% to 95% of all cases of hypertension. Although the exact cause of primary hypertension is unknown, there are several contributing factors. These include increased SNS activity, overproduction of sodium-retaining hormones and vasoconstricting substances, increased sodium intake, greater-than-ideal body weight, diabetes mellitus, tobacco use, and excessive alcohol consumption. Primary hypertension is the major focus of this chapter because of its prevalence and impact on health.

Secondary Hypertension. Secondary hypertension is elevated BP with a specific cause that often can be identified and corrected (Table 33-3). This type of hypertension accounts for 5% to 10% of hypertension in adults. Secondary hypertension should be suspected in people who suddenly develop high BP, especially if it is severe. Clinical findings that suggest secondary hypertension relate to the underlying cause. For example, an abdominal bruit heard over the renal arteries may indicate renal disease. Treatment of secondary hypertension is aimed at removing or treating the underlying cause. Secondary hypertension is a contributing factor to hypertensive crisis (discussed later in this chapter).

Pathophysiology of Primary Hypertension

BP rises with any increase in CO or SVR. Increased CO is sometimes found in the person with prehypertension. Later in the course of hypertension, the SVR rises and the CO returns to normal. The hemodynamic hallmark of hypertension is persistently increased SVR. This persistent elevation in SVR may occur in various ways. Table 33-4 presents factors that relate to the development of primary hypertension or contribute to its consequences. Abnormalities of any of the mechanisms involved in the maintenance of normal BP can result in hypertension (see Fig. 33-1).

🧬 Genetic Link

Different sets of genes may regulate BP at different times throughout the life span.[2] Genetic abnormalities associated with a rare form of hypertension characterized by excess levels of potassium have been identified. To date, the known contribution of genetic factors to BP in the general population remains very small.[1]

The International Consortium for Blood Pressure Genome-Wide Association Studies is a network of researchers currently working to uncover genetic factors related to hypertension. In practice, you should screen children and siblings of persons with hypertension and strongly advise them to adopt healthy lifestyles to prevent hypertension.

Water and Sodium Retention. Excessive sodium intake is linked to the start of hypertension. Although most people consume a high-sodium diet, only one in three will develop hypertension. When sodium is restricted in many people with hypertension, their BP falls. This suggests that some degree of sodium sensitivity may exist for high sodium intake to trigger the development of hypertension. A high sodium intake may activate a number of pressor mechanisms and cause water retention.

TABLE 33-4	RISK FACTORS FOR PRIMARY HYPERTENSION
Risk Factor	**Description**
Age	• SBP rises progressively with increasing age. • After age 50, SBP >140 mm Hg is a more important cardiovascular risk factor than DBP.
Alcohol	• Excessive alcohol intake is strongly associated with hypertension. • Patients with hypertension should limit their daily intake to 1 oz of alcohol.
Tobacco use	• Smoking tobacco greatly ↑ risk of cardiovascular disease. • People with hypertension who smoke tobacco are at even greater risk for cardiovascular disease.
Diabetes mellitus	• Hypertension is more common in patients with diabetes. • When hypertension and diabetes coexist, complications (e.g., target organ disease) are more severe.
Elevated serum lipids	• ↑ Levels of cholesterol and triglycerides are primary risk factors in atherosclerosis. • Hyperlipidemia is more common in people with hypertension.
Excess dietary sodium	• High sodium intake can 　• Contribute to hypertension in some patients 　• Decrease the effectiveness of certain antihypertensive medications
Gender	• Hypertension is more prevalent in men in young adulthood and early middle age (<55 yr of age). • After age 64, hypertension is more prevalent in women. (See Gender Differences box on p. 710.)
Family history	• History of a close blood relative (e.g., parents, sibling) with hypertension is associated with an ↑ risk for developing hypertension.
Obesity	• Weight gain is associated with increased frequency of hypertension. • The risk is greatest with central abdominal obesity.
Ethnicity	• Incidence of hypertension is 2 times higher in African Americans than in whites. (See Cultural & Ethnic Health Disparities box on p. 710.)
Sedentary lifestyle	• Regular physical activity can help control weight and reduce cardiovascular risk. • Physical activity may ↓ BP.
Socioeconomic status	• Hypertension is more prevalent in lower socioeconomic groups and among the less educated.
Stress	• People exposed to repeated stress may develop hypertension more frequently than others. • People who develop hypertension may respond differently to stress than those who do not develop hypertension.

DBP, Diastolic blood pressure; *SBP*, systolic blood pressure.

In clinical practice, there is not an easy or simple test to identify individuals whose BP will rise with even a small increase in salt intake (*salt sensitive*) versus those who can ingest large amounts of sodium without much change in BP (*salt resistant*). In general, the effect of sodium on BP is greater in African Americans and in middle-aged and older adults.[10]

Altered Renin-Angiotensin-Aldosterone Mechanism. High plasma renin activity (PRA) results in the increased conversion of angiotensinogen to angiotensin I (see Fig. 45-4). This alteration in the RAAS may contribute to the development of hypertension. Any rise in BP inhibits the release of renin from the renal juxtaglomerular cells. Based on this feedback loop, low levels of PRA would be expected in patients with primary hypertension. However, only about 30% have low PRA, 50% have normal levels, and 20% have high PRA. These normal or high PRA levels may be related to excess renin secretion from ischemic nephrons.

Stress and Increased Sympathetic Nervous System Activity. It has long been recognized that BP is influenced by factors such as anger, fear, and pain. Physiologic responses to stress, which are normally protective, may persist to a pathologic degree, resulting in a prolonged increase in SNS activity. Increased SNS stimulation produces increased vasoconstriction, increased HR, and increased renin release. Increased renin activates the RAAS, leading to elevated BP. People exposed to high levels of repeated psychologic stress develop hypertension to a greater extent than those who experience less stress.

Insulin Resistance and Hyperinsulinemia. Abnormalities of glucose, insulin, and lipoprotein metabolism are common in primary hypertension. They are not present in secondary hypertension and do not improve when hypertension is treated. Insulin resistance is a risk factor in the development of hypertension and CVD. High insulin levels stimulate SNS activity and impair nitric oxide–mediated vasodilation. Additional pressor effects of insulin include vascular hypertrophy and increased renal sodium reabsorption.

Endothelium Dysfunction. Endothelium dysfunction may contribute to atherosclerosis and primary hypertension. Some people with hypertension have a reduced vasodilator response to nitric oxide. Others have high levels of ET that produce a pronounced and prolonged vasoconstriction. The role of endothelium dysfunction in the pathogenesis and treatment of hypertension is an area of ongoing investigation.

Clinical Manifestations

Hypertension is often called the "silent killer" because it is frequently asymptomatic until it becomes severe and target organ disease occurs. A patient with severe hypertension may experience a variety of symptoms secondary to the effects on blood vessels in the various organs and tissues or to the increased workload of the heart. These secondary symptoms include fatigue, dizziness, palpitations, angina, and dyspnea. In the past, symptoms of hypertension were thought to include headache and nosebleeds. Unless BP is very high, these symptoms are no more frequent in people with hypertension than in the general population. However, patients with hypertensive crisis (discussed later in the chapter) may experience severe headaches, dyspnea, anxiety, and nosebleeds.[11]

Complications

The most common complications of hypertension are *target organ diseases* occurring in the heart (hypertensive heart disease), brain (cerebrovascular disease), peripheral vessels (peripheral vascular disease), kidneys (nephrosclerosis), and eyes (retinal damage) (Table 33-5).

Hypertensive Heart Disease

Coronary Artery Disease. Hypertension is a major risk factor for coronary artery disease (CAD). The mechanisms by which hypertension contributes to the development of atherosclerosis are not fully known. The "response-to-injury" theory of atherogenesis suggests that hypertension disrupts the coronary artery endothelium (see Fig. 34-1). This results in a stiff arterial wall with a narrowed lumen, and accounts for a high rate of CAD, angina, and MI.

TABLE 33-5 MANIFESTATIONS OF TARGET ORGAN DISEASE

Organ	Manifestations
Cardiac	• Clinical, electrocardiographic, or radiologic evidence of coronary artery disease (e.g., previous myocardial infarction, coronary revascularization) • Left ventricular hypertrophy by ECG or echocardiography • Left ventricular dysfunction or heart failure
Cerebrovascular	• Transient ischemic attack • Stroke
Peripheral vascular	• One or more major pulses in the extremities (except for dorsalis pedis) reduced or absent • Intermittent claudication • Abdominal or carotid bruits or thrills • Aneurysm
Renal	• Serum creatinine ≥1.5 mg/dL (130 μmol/L) • Proteinuria (≥1+) • Microalbuminuria
Retinopathy	• Generalized or focal narrowing of retinal arterioles • Arteriovenous nicking • Hemorrhages or exudates with or without papilledema

Source: National Heart, Lung, and Blood Institute: Seventh report of the Joint National Committee on Detection, Evaluation, and Treatment of High Blood Pressure (JNC-7), NIH Publication No. 04-5230, Bethesda, Md, 2004, The Institute. Retrieved from *www.nhlbi.nih.gov/guidelines/hypertension/jnc7full.pdf.*

FIG. 33-2 A, Massively enlarged heart caused by hypertrophy of the muscle in the left ventricle. **B,** Compare with the thickness of the normal left ventricle. The patient suffered from severe hypertension.

Left Ventricular Hypertrophy. Sustained high BP increases the cardiac workload and produces left ventricular hypertrophy (LVH) (Fig. 33-2). Initially, LVH is a compensatory mechanism that strengthens cardiac contraction and increases CO. However, increased contractility increases myocardial work and oxygen demand. Progressive LVH, especially in the presence of CAD, is associated with the development of heart failure.

Heart Failure. Heart failure occurs when the heart's compensatory mechanisms are overwhelmed and the heart can no longer pump enough blood to meet the body's demands (see Chapter 35). Contractility is depressed, and stroke volume and CO are decreased. The patient may complain of shortness of breath on exertion, paroxysmal nocturnal dyspnea, and fatigue.

Cerebrovascular Disease. Atherosclerosis is the most common cause of cerebrovascular disease. Hypertension is a major risk factor for cerebral atherosclerosis and stroke. Even in mildly hypertensive people, the risk of stroke is four times higher than in normotensive people. Adequate control of BP diminishes the risk of stroke.

Atherosclerotic plaques are commonly found at the bifurcation of the common carotid artery and in the internal and external carotid arteries. Portions of the atherosclerotic plaque or the blood clot that forms with disruption of the plaque may break off and travel to cerebral vessels, producing a thromboembolism. The patient may experience transient ischemic attacks or a stroke. (These conditions are discussed in Chapter 58.)

Hypertensive encephalopathy may occur after a marked rise in BP if the cerebral blood flow is not decreased by autoregulation. Autoregulation is a physiologic process that maintains constant cerebral blood flow despite fluctuations in BP. Normally, as pressure in the cerebral blood vessels rises, the vessels constrict to maintain constant flow. When BP exceeds the body's ability to autoregulate, the cerebral vessels suddenly dilate, capillary permeability increases, and cerebral edema develops. This produces a rise in intracranial pressure. If left untreated, patients die quickly from brain damage. (Chapter 57 discusses cerebral blood flow and autoregulation.)

Peripheral Vascular Disease. Hypertension speeds up the process of atherosclerosis in the peripheral blood vessels. This leads to the development of peripheral vascular disease, aortic aneurysm, and aortic dissection (see Chapter 38). *Intermittent claudication* (ischemic leg pain precipitated by activity and relieved with rest) is a classic symptom of peripheral vascular disease.

Nephrosclerosis. Hypertension is one of the leading causes of chronic kidney disease, especially among African Americans. Some degree of renal disease is usually present in the hypertensive patient, even one with a minimally elevated BP. Renal disease results from ischemia caused by the narrowing of the renal blood vessels. This leads to atrophy of the tubules, destruction of the glomeruli, and eventual death of nephrons. Initially intact nephrons can compensate, but these changes may eventually lead to renal failure. Laboratory indications of renal disease are microalbuminuria, proteinuria, microscopic hematuria, and elevated serum creatinine and blood urea nitrogen (BUN) levels. The earliest manifestation of renal disease is usually nocturia (see Chapter 47).

Retinal Damage. The appearance of the retina provides important information about the severity and duration of hypertension. The blood vessels of the retina can be directly visualized with an ophthalmoscope. Damage to the retinal vessels provides an indication of related vessel damage in the heart, brain, and kidneys. Manifestations of severe retinal damage include blurring of vision, retinal hemorrhage, and loss of vision.

TABLE 33-6 COLLABORATIVE CARE

Hypertension

Diagnostic Studies
History and physical examination, including an ophthalmic examination
Routine urinalysis
Basic metabolic panel (serum glucose, sodium, potassium, chloride, carbon dioxide, BUN, and creatinine)
Complete blood count
Serum lipid profile (total lipids, triglycerides, HDL and LDL cholesterol, total-to-HDL cholesterol ratio)
Serum uric acid
12-lead electrocardiogram (ECG)
Optional:
- 24-hr urinary creatinine clearance
- Echocardiography
- Liver function studies
- Serum thyroid-stimulating hormone (TSH)

Collaborative Therapy
Periodic monitoring of BP
- Home BP monitoring
- Ambulatory BP monitoring (if indicated)
- Every 3-6 mo by health care provider once BP is stabilized
Nutritional therapy (see eTable 33-1)
- Restrict salt and sodium
- Restrict cholesterol and saturated fats
- Maintain adequate intake of potassium
- Maintain adequate intake of calcium and magnesium
Weight management
Regular, moderate physical activity
Tobacco cessation (see Tables 11-4 through 11-6)
Moderation of alcohol consumption
Management of psychosocial risk factors (see Chapter 7)
Antihypertensive drugs (see Tables 33-7 and 33-8)
Patient and caregiver teaching

HDL, High-density lipoprotein; *LDL,* low-density lipoprotein.

Diagnostic Studies

Chapter 32 and the Nursing Management section later in this chapter discuss BP measurement.

Some controversy exists over the diagnostic workup in the initial assessment of a person with hypertension. Because most hypertension is classified as primary hypertension, testing for secondary causes is not routinely done. Basic laboratory studies are performed to (1) identify or rule out causes of secondary hypertension, (2) evaluate target organ disease, (3) determine overall cardiovascular risk, or (4) establish baseline levels before initiating therapy.

Table 33-6 lists basic diagnostic studies performed in a person with hypertension. Routine urinalysis, BUN, and serum creatinine levels are used to screen for renal involvement and to provide baseline information about kidney function. Creatinine clearance reflects the glomerular filtration rate. Decreases in creatinine clearance indicate renal insufficiency. (Chapters 45 and 47 discuss serum creatinine and creatinine clearance.)

Measurement of serum electrolytes, especially potassium, is important to detect hyperaldosteronism, a cause of secondary hypertension. Blood glucose levels assist in the diagnosis of diabetes mellitus. A lipid profile provides information about additional risk factors related to atherosclerosis and CVD. Uric acid levels establish a baseline, since the levels often rise with diuretic therapy. An electrocardiogram (ECG) provides baseline information about cardiac status. It can identify the presence of LVH, cardiac ischemia, or previous MI. If LVH is suspected,

echocardiography is often performed. If the patient's age, history, physical examination, or severity of hypertension points to a secondary cause, further diagnostic testing is indicated.

Ambulatory Blood Pressure Monitoring. Some patients have elevated BP readings in a clinical setting and normal readings when BP is measured elsewhere. This phenomenon is referred to as "white coat" hypertension. Self-monitoring of BP is an easy, cost-effective approach that may be chosen before ambulatory BP monitoring (ABPM). ABPM is a noninvasive, fully automated system that measures BP at preset intervals over a 24-hour period. The equipment includes a BP cuff and a microprocessing unit that fits into a pouch worn on a shoulder strap or belt. Tell patients to hold their arm still by their side when the device is taking a reading. Also ask them to maintain a diary of activities that may affect BP. Other potential applications for ABPM include suspected antihypertensive drug resistance, hypotensive symptoms with antihypertensive drugs, episodic hypertension, or SNS dysfunction.

BP demonstrates diurnal variability expressed as sleep-wakefulness difference. For day-active people, BP is highest in the early morning, decreases during the day, and is lowest at night. BP at night (during sleep) usually drops by 10% or more from daytime (awake) BP.[9] Some patients with hypertension do not show a normal nocturnal dip in BP and are referred to as "nondippers." The absence of diurnal variability has been associated with more target organ disease and an increased risk for CVD. The presence or absence of diurnal variability can be determined by ABPM.

Collaborative Care

Table 33-6 summarizes the collaborative care for a patient with hypertension. Goals include achieving and maintaining goal BP, and reducing cardiovascular risk and target organ disease. Lifestyle modifications are indicated for all patients with prehypertension and hypertension.

Lifestyle Modifications. Lifestyle modifications are directed toward reducing the patient's BP and overall cardiovascular risk. Modifications include (1) weight reduction, (2) Dietary Approaches to Stop Hypertension (DASH) eating plan, (3) dietary sodium reduction, (4) moderation of alcohol consumption, (5) regular physical activity, (6) avoidance of tobacco use (smoking and chewing), and (7) management of psychosocial risk factors.

Weight Reduction. Overweight persons have an increased incidence of hypertension and increased risk for CVD. Weight reduction has a significant effect on lowering BP in many people, and the effect is seen with even moderate weight loss. A weight loss of 22 lb (10 kg) may decrease SBP by approximately 5 to 20 mm Hg.[1] When a person decreases caloric intake, sodium and fat intake are usually also reduced. Although reducing the fat content of the diet has not been shown to produce sustained benefits in BP control, it may slow the progress of atherosclerosis and reduce overall CVD risk (see Chapter 34). Weight reduction through a combination of calorie restriction and moderate physical activity is recommended for overweight patients with hypertension (see Chapter 41).

DASH Eating Plan. The DASH eating plan emphasizes fruits, vegetables, fat-free or low-fat milk and milk products, whole grains, fish, poultry, beans, seeds, and nuts. Compared with the typical American diet, the plan contains less red meat, salt, sweets, added sugars, and sugar-containing beverages[12] (see eTable 33-1 on the website for this chapter). The DASH eating plan significantly lowers BP, and these decreases compare with those achieved with BP-lowering medication.[1] Additional benefits also include lowering of low-density lipoprotein (LDL) cholesterol.[12]

Dietary Sodium Reduction. Healthy adults should restrict sodium intake to less than or equal to 2300 mg/day. African Americans; people middle aged and older; and those with hypertension, diabetes mellitus, or chronic kidney disease should restrict sodium to less than or equal to 1500 mg/day.[10,12] This involves avoiding foods known to be high in sodium (e.g., canned soups, frozen dinners) and not adding salt in the preparation of foods or at meals (see Table 35-8).

Most adults exceed the recommended limits for sodium. Average sodium intake is approximately 4200 mg/day in men and 3300 mg/day in women.[12] The patient and caregiver, especially the person who prepares the meals, need to learn about sodium-restricted diets. Instruction should include reading labels of over-the-counter drugs, packaged foods, and health products (e.g., toothpaste containing baking soda) to identify hidden sources of sodium (see Fig. 35-5). Review the patient's normal diet to identify foods high in sodium.

Sodium restriction may be enough to control BP in some patients. If drug therapy is needed, a lower dosage may be effective if the patient also restricts sodium intake. Further, moderate sodium restriction lessens the risk of hypokalemia associated with diuretic therapy. However, the response differs between patients who are salt sensitive or salt resistant.

The significance of other dietary elements for the control of hypertension is not certain. There is some evidence that greater levels of dietary potassium, calcium, vitamin D, and omega-3 fatty acids are associated with lower BP in the general population and in those with hypertension. People with hypertension should maintain adequate potassium, calcium, and vitamin D intake from food sources. Calcium supplements are not recommended to lower BP. Omega-3 fatty acids found in certain fish oils can contribute to a reduction in BP and triglycerides (see Complementary & Alternative Therapies box).

Moderation of Alcohol Consumption. Excessive alcohol consumption is strongly associated with hypertension. Consumption of three or more alcoholic drinks daily is also a risk factor for CVD and stroke. Men should limit their intake of alcohol to no more than two drinks per day and women and lighter-weight men to no more than one drink per day. One drink is defined as 12 oz of regular beer, 5 oz of wine (12% alcohol), or 1.5 oz of 80-proof distilled spirits. Excessive alcohol consumption that results in cirrhosis is the most frequent cause of secondary hypertension.

Physical Activity. A physically active lifestyle is essential to promote and maintain good health. The AHA and American College of Sports Medicine recommend that adults perform moderate-intensity aerobic physical activity for at least 30 minutes most days (i.e., more than 5 days per week) or vigorous-intensity aerobic activity for at least 20 minutes 3 days a week. The 30-minute goal can be accomplished by performing shorter periods of exercise that last at least 10 minutes. Additionally, combinations of moderate and vigorous activity are acceptable (e.g., walking briskly for 30 minutes on 2 days of the week and jogging for 20 minutes on 2 other days).[13,14]

Separate physical activity guidelines exist for adults age 18 to 65 years, adults over 65 years, and adults age 50 to 64 years with functional limitations. The differences relate to the definition of moderate and vigorous aerobic activity. For adults ages 18 to 65, walking briskly at a pace that noticeably increases the pulse defines moderate-intensity aerobic activity. Jogging at a pace that substantially increases the pulse and causes rapid breathing is an example of vigorous activity for this age-group. For all other adults, individual fitness levels guide aerobic intensity.[13,14]

All adults should perform muscle-strengthening activities using the major muscles of the body at least twice a week. This helps to maintain or increase muscle strength and endurance. Additionally, flexibility and balance exercises are recommended at least twice a week for older adults, especially for those at risk for falls.[14] Moderate-intensity activities can lower BP, promote relaxation, and decrease or control body weight. Regular activity of this type can reduce SBP by approximately 4 to 9 mm Hg.[1]

Generally, physical activity is more likely to be done if it is safe and enjoyable, fits easily into one's daily schedule, and is inexpensive. Many shopping malls open early in the morning and provide a warm, safe, flat area for walking. Some health clubs offer special "off-peak" rates to encourage physical activity among older adults. Cardiac rehabilitation programs offer supervised exercise and education about cardiovascular risk factor reduction.

You can help people with hypertension increase their physical activity by explaining the need for physical activity, describing the different types of physical activities, and assisting in starting an exercise plan. Advise sedentary people to increase activity levels gradually. Individuals with CVD or other serious health problems need a thorough examination and possibly a stress test before beginning an exercise program.

Avoidance of Tobacco Products. Nicotine contained in tobacco causes vasoconstriction and increases BP, especially in people with hypertension. Smoking tobacco is also a major risk factor for CVD. The cardiovascular benefits of stopping tobacco use are seen within 1 year in all age-groups. Strongly encourage everyone, especially patients with hypertension, to avoid tobacco use. Advise those who continue to use tobacco products to monitor their BP during use. (Chapter 11 discusses tobacco use and smoking cessation.)

Management of Psychosocial Risk Factors. Psychosocial risk factors can contribute to the risk of developing CVD, and to a poorer prognosis and clinical course in patients with CVD.

COMPLEMENTARY & ALTERNATIVE THERAPIES

Fish Oil and Omega-3 Fatty Acids

Dietary sources of omega-3 fatty acids include fish oil and certain plant and nut oils. Fish oil contains both docosahexaenoic acid (DHA) and eicosapentaenoic acid (EPA). Some nuts and vegetable oils contain α-linolenic acid (ALA).

Scientific Evidence
- Reduce blood triglyceride levels
- May cause a small reduction in BP
- May reduce the risk of heart attack, stroke, and death among people with cardiovascular disease

Nursing Implications
- For healthy adults with no history of heart disease, the American Heart Association recommends eating fish at least two times per wk. Fatty fish such as anchovies, bluefish, carp, catfish, halibut, lake trout, mackerel, pompano, salmon, striped sea bass, albacore tuna, and whitefish are recommended.
- Fish oil is generally safe in recommended dosages. Higher doses may result in increased risk of bleeding.

Sources: www.naturalstandard.com and http://nccam.nih.gov/health/omega3/introduction.htm.

These risk factors include low socioeconomic status, social isolation and lack of support, stress at work and in family life, and negative emotions such as depression and hostility.[15] Frequently, these risk factors are clustered together. For example, rates of depression tend to be higher in individuals with job stress.

Psychosocial risk factors have direct effects on the cardiovascular system by activating the SNS and stress hormones. This can cause a wide variety of pathophysiologic responses, including hypertension and tachycardia, inflammation, endothelium dysfunction, increased platelet aggregation, insulin resistance, and central obesity.[16]

Psychosocial risk factors can contribute to CVD indirectly as well, simply by their impact on lifestyle behaviors and choices. Screening for psychosocial risk factors is important. Make appropriate referrals (e.g., counseling), when indicated. Suggest behavioral interventions such as relaxation training, stress man-agement courses, support groups, and exercise training for individuals who are not in acute psychologic distress.[16]

Drug Therapy. The goal for treating hypertension is a BP less than 140/90 mm Hg. Persons with high risk for CVD (e.g., diabetes mellitus, kidney disease, tobacco use) have the greatest chance of having a cardiovascular event related to uncontrolled hypertension. For these individuals, a lower goal of 130/80 mm Hg may be appropriate. However, specific guidelines for BP goals for high-risk patients will be published when the Eighth Report of the Joint National Committee on Prevention, Detection, Evaluation, and Treatment of High Blood Pressure (JNC 8) is released.[5]

The drugs currently available for treating hypertension have two main actions: (1) they decrease the volume of circulating blood and (2) they reduce SVR (Table 33-7). The drugs used in the treatment of hypertension include diuretics,

TABLE 33-7 DRUG THERAPY*

Hypertension

Drug	Mechanism of Action	Nursing Considerations
Diuretics		
Thiazide and Related Diuretics		
bendroflumethiazide (Naturetin) chlorothiazide (Diuril) chlorthalidone (Hygroton) hydrochlorothiazide (Microzide, HydroDIURIL) indapamide (Lozol) metolazone (Zaroxolyn)	Inhibit NaCl reabsorption in the distal convoluted tubule. Increase excretion of Na⁺ and Cl⁻. Initial decrease in ECF. Sustained decrease in SVR. Lower BP moderately in 2-4 wk.	Monitor for orthostatic hypotension, hypokalemia, and alkalosis. Thiazides may potentiate cardiotoxicity of digoxin by producing hypokalemia. Dietary sodium restriction reduces the risk of hypokalemia. NSAIDs can decrease diuretic and antihypertensive effect of thiazide diuretics. Advise patient to supplement with potassium-rich foods.
Loop Diuretics		
bumetanide (Bumex) ethacrynic acid (Edecrin) furosemide (Lasix) torsemide (Demadex)	Inhibit NaCl reabsorption in the ascending limb of the loop of Henle. Increase excretion of Na⁺ and Cl⁻. More potent diuretic effect than thiazides, but shorter duration of action. Less effective for hypertension.	Monitor for orthostatic hypotension and electrolyte abnormalities. Loop diuretics remain effective despite renal insufficiency. Diuretic effect of drug increases at higher doses.
Potassium-Sparing Diuretics		
amiloride (Midamor) triamterene (Dyrenium)	Reduce K⁺ and Na⁺ exchange in the distal and collecting tubules. Reduce excretion of K⁺, H⁺, Ca⁺, and Mg⁺.	Monitor for orthostatic hypotension and hyperkalemia. Contraindicated in patients with renal failure. Use with caution in patients on ACE inhibitors or angiotensin II blockers. Avoid potassium supplements.
Aldosterone Receptor Blockers		
spironolactone (Aldactone) eplerenone (Inspra)	Inhibit the Na⁺-retaining and K⁺-excreting effects of aldosterone in the distal and collecting tubules.	Monitor for orthostatic hypotension and hyperkalemia. Do not combine with potassium-sparing diuretics or potassium supplements. Use with caution in patients on ACE inhibitors or angiotensin II blockers. These drugs are also classified as potassium-sparing diuretics.
Adrenergic Inhibitors		
Central-Acting α-Adrenergic Antagonists		
clonidine (Catapres) clonidine patch (Catapres-TTS)	Reduce sympathetic outflow from CNS. Reduce peripheral sympathetic tone, produces vasodilation, decreases SVR and BP.	Sudden discontinuation may cause withdrawal syndrome, including rebound hypertension, tachycardia, headache, tremors, apprehension, sweating. Chewing gum or hard candy may relieve dry mouth. Alcohol and sedatives increase sedation. Transdermal patch may be related to fewer side effects and better adherence.
guanabenz (Wytensin)	Same as clonidine.	Same as clonidine, but not available in transdermal formulation.
guanfacine (Tenex)	Same as clonidine.	Same as clonidine, but not available in transdermal formulation.
methyldopa (Aldomet)	Same as clonidine.	Instruct patient about daytime sedation and avoidance of hazardous activities. Administration of a single daily dose at bedtime minimizes sedative effect.

*An expanded version of this table (eTable 33-2) is available on the website for this chapter.
ACE, Angiotensin-converting enzyme; *AV,* atrioventricular; *CO,* cardiac output; *DBP,* diastolic blood pressure; *ECF,* extracellular fluid; *HDL,* high-density lipoprotein; *LDL,* low-density lipoprotein; *SBP,* systolic blood pressure; *SVR,* systemic vascular resistance.

Continued

TABLE 33-7   **DRUG THERAPY**—cont'd

Hypertension

Drug	Mechanism of Action	Nursing Considerations
Adrenergic Inhibitors—cont'd		
Peripheral-Acting α-Adrenergic Antagonists		
guanethidine (Ismelin)	Prevents peripheral release of norepinephrine, resulting in vasodilation. Lowers CO and reduces SBP more than DBP.	May cause severe orthostatic hypotension. Not recommended for use in patients with cerebrovascular or coronary insufficiency or in older adults. Advise patient to rise slowly and wear support stockings. Hypotensive effect is delayed for 2-3 days and lasts 7-10 days after withdrawal.
guanadrel (Hylorel)	Same as guanethidine	Must be given twice daily. Contraindicated in patients with history of depression. Monitor mood and mental status regularly. Advise patient to avoid barbiturates, alcohol, opioids.
reserpine (Serpasil)	Depletes central and peripheral stores of norepinephrine. Results in peripheral vasodilation (decreases SVR and BP).	
α$_1$-Adrenergic Blockers		
doxazosin (Cardura)	Block α$_1$-adrenergic effects, producing peripheral vasodilation (decreases SVR and BP). Beneficial effects on lipid profile.	Reduced resistance to the outflow of urine in benign prostatic hyperplasia. Taking drug at bedtime reduces risks associated with orthostatic hypotension.
prazosin (Minipress)		
terazosin (Hytrin)		
phentolamine (Regitine)	Blocks α$_1$-adrenergic receptors, resulting in peripheral vasodilation (decreases SVR and BP).	Used in short-term management of pheochromocytoma. Also used locally to prevent necrosis of skin and subcutaneous tissue after extravasation of adrenergic drug. No oral formulation.
β-Adrenergic Blockers		
Cardioselective Blockers	Cardioselective agents block β$_1$-adrenergic receptors (see Table 33-1). Reduce BP by blocking β-adrenergic effects. Decrease CO and reduce sympathetic vasoconstrictor tone. Decrease renin secretion by kidneys.	Monitor pulse and BP regularly. Use with caution in patients with diabetes mellitus because drug may depress the tachycardia associated with hypoglycemia. Esmolol is for IV use only. Cardioselective agents lose cardioselectivity at higher doses.
acebutolol (Sectral)		
atenolol (Tenormin)		
betaxolol (Kerlone)		
bisoprolol (Zebeta)		
esmolol (Brevibloc)		
metoprolol (Lopressor)		
nebivolol (Bystolic)		
Nonselective Blockers	Nonselective agents block β$_1$- and β$_2$-adrenergic receptors (see Table 33-1). Reduce BP by blocking β$_1$- and β$_2$-adrenergic effects.	Same as cardioselective, except nonselective agents may cause bronchospasm, especially in patients with a history of asthma.
carteolol (Cartrol)		
nadolol (Corgard)		
penbutolol (Levatol)		
pindolol (Visken)		
propranolol (Inderal)		
timolol (Blocadren)		
Mixed α- and β-Blockers		
carvedilol (Coreg)	α$_1$-, β$_1$-, and β$_2$-adrenergic blocking properties producing peripheral vasodilation and decreased heart rate (see Table 33-1). Reduce CO, SVR, and BP.	Same as β-adrenergic blockers. IV form available for hypertensive crisis in hospitalized patients. Patients must be kept supine during IV administration. Assess patient tolerance of upright position (severe orthostatic hypotension) before allowing upright activities (e.g., commode).
labetalol (Normodyne, Trandate)		
Direct Vasodilators		
fenoldopam (Corlopam)	Activates dopamine receptors, resulting in systemic and renal vasodilation.	IV use only for hypertensive crisis in hospitalized patients. Use cautiously in patients with glaucoma. Patient should remain supine for 1 hr after administration.
hydralazine (Apresoline)	Reduces SVR and BP by direct arterial vasodilation.	IV use for hypertensive crisis in hospitalized patients. Twice-daily oral dosage. Not used as monotherapy because of side effects. Contraindicated in patients with coronary artery disease.
minoxidil (Loniten)	Reduces SVR and BP by direct arterial vasodilation.	Reserved for treatment of severe hypertension associated with renal failure and resistant to other therapy. Once- or twice-daily dosage.
nitroglycerin (Tridil)	Relaxes arterial and venous smooth muscle, reducing preload and SVR. At low dose, venous dilation predominates; at higher dose, arterial dilation is present.	IV use for hypertensive crisis in hospitalized patients with myocardial ischemia. Administered by continuous IV infusion with pump or control device.

TABLE 33-7   DRUG THERAPY—cont'd

Hypertension

Drug	Mechanism of Action	Nursing Considerations
Direct Vasodilators—cont'd		
sodium nitroprusside (Nipride)	Direct arterial vasodilation reduces SVR and BP.	IV use for hypertensive crisis in hospitalized patients. Administered by continuous IV infusion with pump or control device. Intraarterial monitoring of BP recommended. Wrap IV solutions with an opaque material to protect from light. Stable for 24 hr. Metabolized to cyanide, then thiocyanate. Monitor thiocyanate levels with prolonged use (>3 days) or doses (≥4 mcg/kg/min).
Ganglionic Blockers		
trimethaphan (Arfonad)	Interrupts adrenergic control of arteries, results in vasodilation, and reduces SVR and BP.	IV use for initial control of BP in patient with dissecting aortic aneurysm. Administered by continuous IV infusion with pump or control device.
Angiotensin Inhibitors		
Angiotensin-Converting Enzyme Inhibitors		
benazepril (Lotensin) captopril (Capoten) enalapril (Vasotec) fosinopril (Monopril) lisinopril (Prinivil, Zestril) moexipril (Univasc) perindopril (Aceon) quinapril (Accupril) ramipril (Altace) trandolapril (Mavik)	Inhibit ACE, reduce conversion of angiotensin I to angiotensin II (A-II). Inhibit A-II–mediated vasoconstriction.	Aspirin and NSAIDs may reduce drug effectiveness. Addition of diuretic enhances drug effect. Should not be used with potassium-sparing diuretics. Inhibit breakdown of bradykinin, which may cause a dry, hacking cough. Captopril may be given orally for hypertensive crisis.
enalapril (Vasotec IV)	Inhibits ACE when oral agents not appropriate.	Given IV over 5 min. Monitor BP.
Angiotensin II Receptor Blockers		
candesartan (Atacand) eprosartan (Teveten) irbesartan (Avapro) losartan (Cozaar) olmesartan (Benicar) telmisartan (Micardis) valsartan (Diovan)	Prevent action of A-II and produce vasodilation and increased Na⁺ and water excretion.	Full effect on BP may not be seen for 3-6 wk. Do not affect bradykinin levels, therefore acceptable alternative to ACE inhibitors in people who develop dry cough.
Renin Inhibitors		
aliskiren (Tekturna)	Directly inhibits renin, thus reducing conversion of angiotensinogen to angiotensin I.	May cause angioedema of the face, extremities, lips, tongue, glottis, and/or larynx. Not to be used in pregnancy.
Calcium Channel Blockers		
Non-Dihydropyridines		
diltiazem extended release (Cardizem LA, Dilacor XR) verapamil intermediate release (Isoptin, Calan) verapamil long-acting (Covera-HS, Calan SR) verapamil timed-release (Verelan PM)	Inhibit movement of Ca^{2+} across cell membrane, resulting in vasodilation. Cardioselective resulting in decrease in heart rate and slowing of AV conduction.	Use with caution in patients with heart failure. Serum concentrations and toxicity of certain calcium channel blockers may be increased by grapefruit juice; avoid concurrent use. Used for supraventricular tachydysrhythmias. Avoid in patients with second- or third-degree AV block or left ventricular systolic dysfunction.
Dihydropyridines		
amlodipine (Norvasc) clevidipine (Cleviprex) felodipine (Plendil) isradipine (DynaCirc CR) nicardipine sustained release (Cardene SR) nifedipine long acting (Adalat CC, Procardia XL) nisoldipine (Sular)	Cause vascular smooth muscle relaxation resulting in decreased SVR and arterial BP.	More potent peripheral vasodilators. Clevidipine is for IV use only. Use of sublingual short-acting nifedipine in hypertensive emergencies is unsafe and not effective. Serious adverse events (e.g., stroke, acute MI) have been reported. IV nicardipine available for hypertensive crisis in hospitalized patients. Change peripheral IV infusion sites every 12 hr.

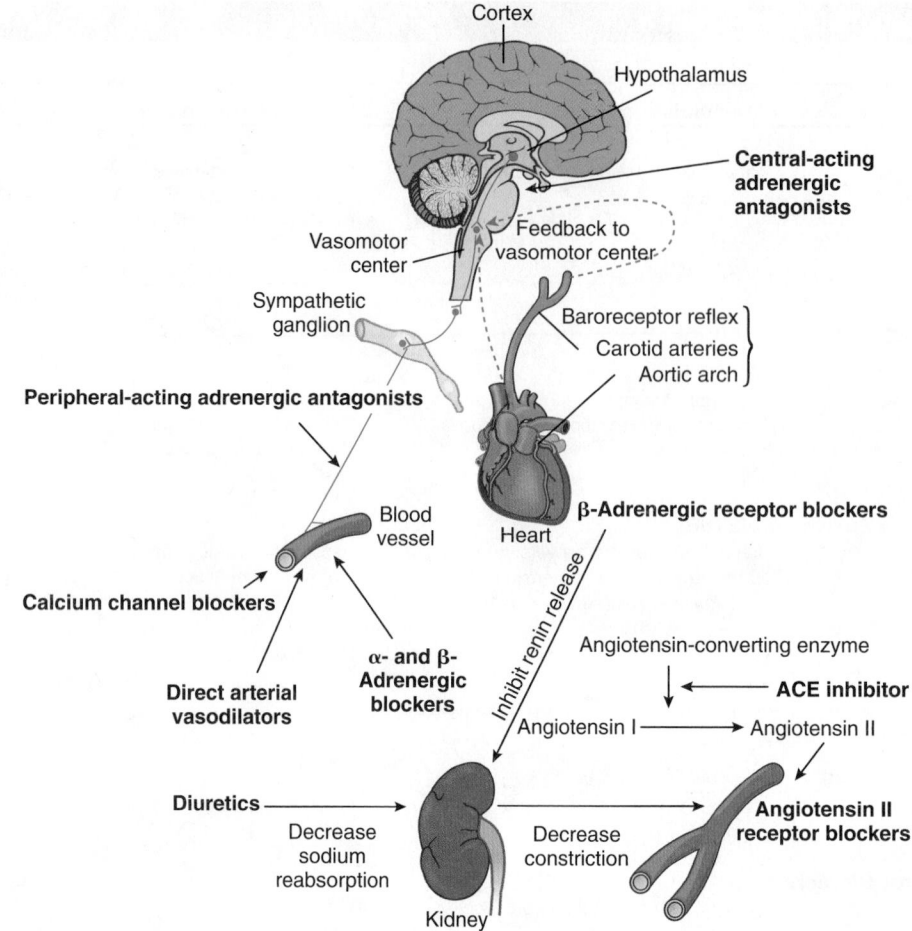

FIG. 33-3 Site and method of action of various antihypertensive drugs *(bold type)*. *ACE*, Angiotensin-converting enzyme.

adrenergic (SNS) inhibitors, direct vasodilators, angiotensin and renin inhibitors, and calcium channel blockers.[17,18] Fig. 33-3 presents the various sites and methods of action of antihypertensive drugs.

Although the precise action of diuretics in the reduction of BP is unclear, it is known that they promote sodium and water excretion, reduce plasma volume, and reduce the vascular response to catecholamines. Adrenergic-inhibiting agents act by decreasing the SNS effects that increase BP. Adrenergic inhibitors include drugs that act centrally on the vasomotor center and peripherally to inhibit NE release or to block the adrenergic receptors on blood vessels. Direct vasodilators decrease the BP by relaxing vascular smooth muscle and reducing SVR. Calcium channel blockers increase sodium excretion and cause vasodilation by preventing the movement of extracellular calcium into cells.

There are two types of angiotensin inhibitors. The first type is angiotensin-converting enzyme (ACE) inhibitors. These prevent the conversion of angiotensin I to A-II and thus reduce A-II-mediated vasoconstriction and sodium and water retention. The second type is A-II receptor blockers (ARBs). These prevent A-II from binding to its receptors in the blood vessel walls.

Most patients who are hypertensive require two or more antihypertensive medications to achieve their goal BP. The addition of a second drug from a different class is started when use of a single drug in adequate doses fails to achieve the goal

BP. These can be separate prescriptions or combination therapy (Table 33-8). If a drug is not tolerated or is contraindicated, then a drug from another class is used.

Once antihypertensive therapy is started, patients should return for follow-up and adjustment of medications at monthly intervals until the goal BP is reached. More frequent visits are necessary for patients with stage 2 hypertension or with co-morbidities. After BP is at goal and stable, follow-up visits can usually be at 3- to 6-month intervals. Co-morbidities (e.g., heart failure), associated diseases (e.g., diabetes mellitus), and the need for ongoing monitoring (e.g., laboratory testing) influence the frequency of visits.

Patient and Caregiver Teaching Related to Drug Therapy. Side effects of antihypertensive drugs are common and may be so severe or undesirable that the patient does not adhere to the therapy[17,18] (see Table 33-7). Patient and caregiver teaching related to drug therapy helps them identify and minimize side effects. This may help the patient adhere to therapy. Side effects may be an initial response to a drug and may decrease over time. Informing the patient about side effects that may decrease with time may enable the person to continue taking the drug. The number or severity of side effects may relate to the dosage. It may be necessary to change the drug or decrease the dosage. Advise the patient to report all side effects to the health care provider who prescribes the medication.

A common side effect of several of these drugs is orthostatic hypotension. This condition results from an alteration of the

TABLE 33-8 DRUG THERAPY

Combination Therapy for Hypertension

Combinations	Trade Names
Angiotensin-Converting Enzyme Inhibitors and Diuretics	
benazepril/hydrochlorothiazide	Lotensin HCT
captopril/hydrochlorothiazide	Capozide
enalapril/hydrochlorothiazide	Vaseretic
fosinopril/hydrochlorothiazide	Monopril-HCT
lisinopril/hydrochlorothiazide	Prinzide, Zestoretic
moexipril/hydrochlorothiazide	Uniretic
quinapril/hydrochlorothiazide	Accuretic
Angiotensin II Receptor Blockers and Diuretics	
azilsartan/chlorthalidone	Edarbyclor
candesartan/hydrochlorothiazide	Atacand HCT
eprosartan/hydrochlorothiazide	Teveten HCT
irbesartan/hydrochlorothiazide	Avalide
losartan/hydrochlorothiazide	Hyzaar
olmesartan medoxomil/hydrochlorothiazide	Benicar HCT
telmisartan/hydrochlorothiazide	Micardis HCT
valsartan/hydrochlorothiazide	Diovan HCT
β-Adrenergic Blockers and Diuretics	
atenolol/chlorthalidone	Tenoretic
bisoprolol/hydrochlorothiazide	Ziac
metoprolol/hydrochlorothiazide	Lopressor HCT
nadolol/bendroflumethiazide	Corzide
propranolol/hydrochlorothiazide	Inderide
timolol/hydrochlorothiazide	Timolide
Centrally Acting Drugs and Diuretics	
methyldopa/hydrochlorothiazide	Aldoril
reserpine/chlorthalidone	Demi-Regroton
reserpine/hydrochlorothiazide	Hydropres
prazosin/polythiazide	Minizide
guanethidine/hydrochlorothiazide	Esimil
clonidine/chlorthalidone	Combipres
Angiotensin-Converting Enzyme Inhibitors and Calcium Channel Blockers	
amlodipine/benazepril	Lotrel
enalapril/felodipine	Lexxel
enalapril/diltiazem	Teczem
trandolapril/verapamil	Tarka
Angiotensin II Receptor Blockers and Calcium Channel Blockers	
telmisartan/amlodipine	Twynsta
valsartan/amlodipine	Exforge
olmesartan/amlodipine	Azor
Diuretics and Diuretics	
amiloride/hydrochlorothiazide	Moduretic
spironolactone/hydrochlorothiazide	Aldactazide
triamterene/hydrochlorothiazide	Dyazide, Maxzide
Angiotensin II Receptor Blocker, Calcium Channel Blocker, and Diuretic	
olmesartan medoxomil/amlodipine/hydrochlorothiazide	Tribenzor

EVIDENCE-BASED PRACTICE

Applying the Evidence

You are caring for P.N., a 46-year-old man with a history of poorly controlled hypertension and chronic kidney disease. You note that he is taking three antihypertensive medications. He tells you that he can no longer live with the side effects of these drugs (e.g., fatigue, dry mouth, erectile dysfunction). He states that he wants to stop taking the medications. He believes that if he changes his lifestyle by reducing salt from his diet, losing weight, and beginning exercise, he can control his hypertension.

Best Available Evidence	Clinician Expertise	Patient Preferences and Values
Uncontrolled BP places persons with concurrent risk for cardiovascular disease (e.g., diabetes, kidney disease) at highest risk for a cardiovascular event (e.g., stroke). Most hypertensive patients will need two or more medications to achieve their goal BP in addition to lifestyle changes.	You know that lifestyle changes can help reduce and control BP in many patients. However, patients with poorly controlled hypertension and target organ disease require medications to control BP and prevent further complications.	P.N. wishes to eliminate antihypertensive medications because of unpleasant and unacceptable side effects that are interfering with his quality of life.

Your Decision and Actions

You discuss the role of lifestyle changes and medications in the treatment of hypertension and prevention of (further) target organ disease with P.N. You support his intention to make lifestyle changes and validate his concerns regarding the side effects of the medications. You discuss the side effects that he is experiencing and explain that it may be possible to change some of his medications to eliminate or reduce the unpleasant side effects. However, given the severity of his hypertension and the chronic kidney disease, he will need to be on medications on a long-term basis. Any of his plans to discontinue medications need to be discussed with his physician.

Reference for Evidence

National Heart, Lung, and Blood Institute: Seventh report of the Joint National Committee on Detection, Evaluation, and Treatment of High Blood Pressure (JNC-7), NIH Publication No. 04-5230, Bethesda, Md, 2004, The Institute. Retrieved from *www.nhlbi.nih.gov/guidelines/hypertension/jnc7full.pdf.*

Sexual problems may occur with many of the antihypertensive drugs and can be a major reason that patients do not adhere to the treatment plan. Problems can range from reduced libido to erectile dysfunction. Rather than discussing a sexual problem with a health care provider, the patient may decide just to stop taking the drug. Approach the patient on this sensitive subject and encourage discussion of any sexual problem that may be experienced. The sexual problems may be easier for the patient to discuss once you explain that the drug may be the source of the problem. Changing to another antihypertensive drug can decrease or remove these side effects. Encourage the patient to discuss sexual issues with the health care provider. If the patient is reluctant to do so, offer to alert the health care provider to the side effects that the patient is experiencing. There are many drug options in treating hypertension. A plan that is acceptable to the patient should be achievable.[19]

Some unpleasant side effects of drugs result from their therapeutic effect, but these can be decreased. For example, diuret-

autonomic nervous system's mechanisms for regulating BP, which are required for position changes. Consequently, the patient may feel dizzy and faint when assuming an upright position after sitting or lying down. Table 33-12 (later in this chapter) presents specific measures to control or decrease orthostatic hypotension.

TABLE 33-9	CAUSES OF RESISTANT HYPERTENSION

Improper BP measurement
Volume overload
- Excess salt intake
- Volume retention from kidney disease
- Inadequate diuretic therapy

Drug-induced or other causes
- Nonadherence
- Illegal drugs (e.g., cocaine, amphetamines)
- Inadequate drug dosages
- Inappropriate combinations of drug therapy
- Nonsteroidal antiinflammatory drugs
- Sympathomimetics (e.g., decongestants, diet pills)
- Oral contraceptives
- Corticosteroids
- Cyclosporine and tacrolimus (Prograf)
- Erythropoietin
- Licorice (including some chewing tobacco)
- Selected over-the-counter dietary or herbal supplements and medicines (e.g., ma huang, bitter orange)

Associated conditions
- Increasing obesity
- Excess alcohol consumption

Identifiable causes of secondary hypertension

Source: National Heart, Lung, and Blood Institute: Seventh report of the Joint National Committee on Detection, Evaluation, and Treatment of High Blood Pressure (JNC-7), NIH Publication No. 04-5230, Bethesda, Md, 2004, The Institute. Retrieved from *www.nhlbi.nih.gov/guidelines/hypertension/jnc7full.pdf.*

ics cause dry mouth and frequent voiding. Sugarless gum or hard candy may help ease the dry mouth. Taking diuretics earlier in the day may limit frequent voiding during the night and preserve sleep. Side effects of vasodilators and adrenergic inhibitors decrease if the drugs are taken in the evening. Remember that BP is lowest during the night and highest shortly after awakening. Therefore drugs with a 24-hour duration of action should be taken as early in the morning as possible (e.g., 4 or 5 AM if the patient awakens to void).

Resistant Hypertension. *Resistant hypertension* is the failure to reach goal BP in patients who are taking full doses of an appropriate three-drug therapy regimen that includes a diuretic. Carefully explore reasons why the patient is not at goal BP (Table 33-9). Studies have shown that the use of *renal denervation* (destruction of overactive renal nerves) reduces BP and muscle sympathetic nerve activity in patients with resistant hypertension. The exact mechanisms underlying sympathetic neural inhibition are not clear.[20]

NURSING MANAGEMENT PRIMARY HYPERTENSION

NURSING ASSESSMENT
Table 33-10 presents subjective and objective data to obtain from a patient with hypertension.

NURSING DIAGNOSES
Nursing diagnoses and collaborative problems for the patient with hypertension include, but are not limited to, the following.
- Ineffective self-health management *related to* lack of knowledge of pathology, complications, and management of hypertension
- Anxiety *related to* complexity of management regimen

TABLE 33-10	NURSING ASSESSMENT

Hypertension

Subjective Data
Important Health Information
Past health history: Known duration and past workup of high BP; cardiovascular, cerebrovascular, renal, or thyroid disease; diabetes mellitus; pituitary disorders; obesity; dyslipidemia; menopause or hormone replacement status
Medications: Use of any prescription or over-the-counter, illicit, or herbal medications or products; previous use of antihypertensive drug therapy

Functional Health Patterns
Health perception–health management: Family history of hypertension or cardiovascular disease; tobacco use, alcohol use; sedentary lifestyle
Nutritional-metabolic: Usual salt and fat intake; weight gain or loss
Elimination: Nocturia
Activity-exercise: Fatigue; dyspnea on exertion, palpitations, exertional chest pain; intermittent claudication, muscle cramps; usual pattern and type of exercise
Cognitive-perceptual: Dizziness; blurred vision; paresthesias
Sexual-reproductive: Erectile dysfunction, decreased libido
Coping–stress tolerance: Stressful life events

Objective Data
Cardiovascular
SBP consistently >140 mm Hg or DBP >90 mm Hg, orthostatic changes in BP and pulse; bilateral BPs significantly different; abnormal heart sounds; laterally displaced, apical pulse; diminished or absent peripheral pulses; carotid, renal, or femoral bruits; peripheral edema

Gastrointestinal
Obesity (BMI ≥30 kg/m^2); abnormal waist-hip ratio

Neurologic
Mental status changes

Possible Diagnostic Findings
Abnormal serum electrolytes (especially potassium); ↑ BUN, creatinine, glucose, cholesterol, and triglyceride levels; proteinuria, microalbuminuria, microscopic hematuria; evidence of ischemic heart disease and left ventricular hypertrophy on ECG; evidence of structural heart disease and left ventricular hypertrophy on echocardiogram; evidence of arteriovenous nicking, retinal hemorrhages, and papilledema on funduscopic examination

BMI, Body mass index; *DBP,* diastolic blood pressure; *SBP,* systolic blood pressure.

- Sexual dysfunction *related to* side effects of antihypertensive medication
- Risk for decreased cardiac tissue perfusion
- Risk for ineffective cerebral tissue perfusion
- Risk for ineffective renal perfusion
- Potential complication: stroke
- Potential complication: MI

PLANNING
The overall goals for the patient with hypertension are that the patient will (1) achieve and maintain the goal BP; (2) understand and follow the therapeutic plan; (3) experience minimal or no unpleasant side effects of therapy; and (4) be confident of the ability to manage and cope with this condition.

NURSING IMPLEMENTATION
HEALTH PROMOTION. Primary prevention of hypertension is a cost-effective approach. Current recommendations for primary

prevention include lifestyle modifications that prevent or delay the rise in BP in at-risk people. Following the DASH diet and reducing sodium can lower BP (see eTable 33-1). This diet is recommended for primary prevention in the general population. Dietary changes by the food industry (e.g., reducing the amount of salt in processed foods) may also be effective.

To raise awareness about the dangers of high BP, the National Heart, Lung, and Blood Institute provides web-based educational materials for health care providers, patients, and the public. (See Your Guide to Lowering High Blood Pressure at *www.nhlbi.nih.gov/hbp*.)

Individual Patient Evaluation. Hypertension is usually identified through routine screening for insurance, preemployment, and military physical examinations. You are in an ideal position to assess for the presence of hypertension, identify the risk factors for hypertension and CAD, and teach the patient about these conditions. In addition to BP measurement, a complete health assessment should include such factors as age, gender, and race; diet history (including sodium and alcohol intake); weight patterns; tobacco use; and family history of heart disease, stroke, renal disease, and diabetes mellitus. Note all medications taken, both prescribed and over-the-counter drugs. Finally, ask the patient about a previous history of high BP and the results of treatment (if any) (see Table 33-10).

Blood Pressure Measurement. BP can be measured using the oscillatory or auscultatory method.[21] Initially, take the BP in both arms to note any differences. Atherosclerosis in the subclavian artery can cause a falsely low reading on the side where the narrowing occurs. Use the arm with the highest BP and take at least two readings, a minimum of 1 minute apart (see Table 33-11). Waiting for at least 1 minute between readings allows the blood to drain from the arm and prevents inaccurate readings. Record the average pressure as the value for that visit.

Proper size and correct placement of the BP cuff are critical for accurate measurement. Place the cuff snugly around the patient's bare upper arm with the midline of the bladder of the cuff (usually marked on the cuff by the manufacturer) placed above the brachial artery. Place the patient's arm at the level of the heart during BP measurement. For BP measurements taken in the sitting position, raise and support the arm at the level of the heart. For measurements taken in a supine position, raise and support (e.g., with a small pillow) the arm at heart level. If the arm is resting on the bed, it will be below heart level.

If neither upper arm can be used to measure the BP (e.g., presence of IV lines, fistula), or if a maximum size BP cuff does not fit the upper arm, use the forearm. In this case, position the proper size cuff midway between the elbow and the wrist. Auscultate Korotkoff sounds over the radial artery or use a Doppler device to note SBP. Use of an oscillometric device on the forearm is acceptable. Forearm and upper arm BPs are not interchangeable.[21]

SAFETY ALERT

- If using the forearm for BP measurement, always document the site.
- BP cuffs that are too small or too large will result in readings that are falsely high or low, respectively.
- If bilateral BP measurements are not equal, document this finding and use the arm with the highest BP for all future measurements.

Assess for orthostatic (or postural) changes in BP and pulse in older adults, in people taking antihypertensive drugs, and in patients who report symptoms consistent with reduced BP on

TABLE 33-11	BLOOD PRESSURE MEASUREMENT

The patient should not have smoked, exercised, or ingested caffeine within 30 min before measurement.

1. Seat patient with legs uncrossed, feet on the floor, and back supported. Bare patient's arm and support it at heart level.
2. Begin measurement after patient has rested quietly for 5 min. Ask patient to relax as much as possible and not to talk during the measurement.
3. Measure and record BP in both arms initially.
4. Select the appropriate cuff size, following instructions for fit and placement according to manufacturer's recommendations.
5. Take the BP with a recently calibrated aneroid or mercury sphygmomanometer, or electronic oscillometric device. Accuracy of oscillometric devices may be limited if patients are hypertensive, are hypotensive, or have heart dysrhythmias (e.g., atrial fibrillation).
6. For auscultatory measurement, estimate SBP by palpating the radial pulse and inflating the cuff until the pulse disappears. Inflate the cuff 20-30 mm Hg above this level.
7. Deflate the cuff at a rate of 2-3 mm Hg/sec.
8. Record the SBP and the DBP. Note the SBP when the first of two or more Korotkoff sounds is heard and the DBP when sound disappears.
9. Average two or more readings (taken at intervals of at least 1 min). Obtain additional readings if the first two readings differ by more than 5 mm Hg.
10. Provide the patient (verbally and in writing) with the BP reading, BP goal, and recommendations for follow-up.

Sources: National Heart, Lung, and Blood Institute: Seventh report of the Joint National Committee on Detection, Evaluation, and Treatment of High Blood Pressure (JNC-7), NIH Publication No. 04-5230, Bethesda, Md, 2004, The Institute. Retrieved from *www.nhlbi.nih.gov/guidelines/hypertension/jnc7full.pdf*; and Seckel MA, Bradley E, Bucher L, et al: AACN practice alert: noninvasive blood pressure monitoring, 2006. Retrieved from *http://classic.aacn.org/AACN/practiceAlert.nsf/Files/NIBP/$file/Noninvasive%20BP%20Monitoring%206-2006.pdf*.
DBP, diastolic blood pressure; *SBP*, systolic blood pressure.

standing (e.g., light-headedness, dizziness, syncope). Measure serial BP and pulse with the patient in the supine, sitting, and standing positions. Initially, measure BP and pulse with the patient in the supine position after at least 2 to 3 minutes of rest. Reposition the patient in the sitting position with legs dangling and measure BP and pulse again within 1 to 2 minutes. Finally reposition the patient to the standing position and measure the BP and pulse within 1 to 2 minutes. Usually the SBP decreases slightly (less than 10 mm Hg) on standing, whereas the DBP and pulse increase slightly. A decrease of 20 mm Hg or more in SBP, a decrease of 10 mm Hg or more in DBP, and/or an increase in the HR of 20 beats/minute or more from supine to standing indicates **orthostatic hypotension**. Common causes of orthostatic hypotension include intravascular volume loss and inadequate vasoconstrictor mechanisms related to disease or medications.

DRUG ALERT: Doxazosin (Cardura)

- Use caution with administration of initial dose.
- Syncope (sudden loss of consciousness) occasionally occurs 30 to 90 min after the initial dose, a too-rapid increase in dose, or addition of another antihypertensive agent to therapy.

In the acute care setting, BP measurement is usually performed to evaluate vital signs, volume status, and effects of medications, rather than to diagnose hypertension. Drugs, acute illness, bed rest, and alterations in usual diet all have an impact on BP values. Inform the health care provider of any patient with a persistent increase in BP. These patients

DELEGATION DECISIONS
Caring for the Patient With Hypertension

Many members of the health care team obtain blood pressure (BP) readings. In patients with stable hypertension, LPN/LVNs and UAP provide most of the routine BP monitoring. For patients in hypertensive crisis, the RN is responsible for titration of medications and ongoing assessment and evaluation of BP.

Role of Registered Nurse (RN)
- Develop and conduct hypertension screening programs.
- Assess patients for hypertension risk factors, and develop risk modification plans.
- Teach patients about lifestyle management and medication use.
- Evaluate the effectiveness of lifestyle management and medications in decreasing BP to acceptable levels.
- Teach about home BP monitoring, including the correct use of automatic BP monitors.
- Make appropriate referrals to other health care professionals, such as dietitians or stress management programs.
- Monitor for complications of hypertension such as coronary artery disease, heart failure, cerebrovascular disease, peripheral vascular disease, and renal disease.
- Assess the patient with hypertensive urgency or crisis for target organ disease (encephalopathy, renal insufficiency, cardiac decompensation).
- Manage the patient with hypertensive crisis, including administration of medications and evaluation for resolution of the emergency.

Role of Licensed Practical Nurse (LPN)
- Administer antihypertensive medications to stable patients.
- Monitor for adverse effects of antihypertensive medications.
- Reinforce teaching about medications and lifestyle management.

Role of Unlicensed Assistive Personnel (UAP)
- Obtain accurate BP readings in outpatient and inpatient settings.
- Report high or low BP readings immediately to RN.
- Check for postural changes in BP as directed.

should be evaluated for hypertension before discharge, if appropriate, or after discharge.[9]

Screening Programs. Screening programs in the community are widely used to check individuals for high BP. At the time of the BP measurement, give each person a written, numeric value of the reading. If necessary, explain why further evaluation is needed. Effort and resources should focus on the following: (1) controlling BP in persons already identified as having hypertension; (2) identifying and controlling BP in at-risk groups such as African Americans, obese people, and blood relatives of people with hypertension; and (3) screening those with limited access to the health care system.

Cardiovascular Risk Factor Modification. Teaching regarding CVD risk factors is appropriate for all individuals and during targeted screening programs. Modifiable cardiovascular risk factors include hypertension, obesity, diabetes mellitus, tobacco use, and physical inactivity. Discuss lifestyle modifications based on identified risk factors. (Table 34-2 discusses health-promoting behaviors for risk factor reduction.)

▌AMBULATORY AND HOME CARE
Your primary responsibilities for long-term management of hypertension are to assist the patient in reducing BP and adhering to the treatment plan. Your nursing actions include evaluating therapeutic effectiveness, detecting and reporting any adverse treatment effects, assessing and enhancing adherence, and patient and caregiver teaching (Table 33-12).

TABLE 33-12   PATIENT & CAREGIVER TEACHING GUIDE
Hypertension

When teaching the patient and/or caregiver about hypertension, include the following information.

General Instructions
1. Provide the patient's BP reading and explain what it means (e.g., high, low, normal, borderline). Encourage patient to monitor BP at home and instruct the patient to call health care provider if BP exceeds high or low limits set by health care provider.
2. Hypertension is usually asymptomatic and symptoms (e.g., nosebleeds) do not reliably indicate BP levels.
3. Hypertension means high BP and does not relate to a "hyper" personality.
4. Long-term therapy and follow-up care are necessary to treat hypertension. Therapy involves lifestyle changes (e.g., weight management, sodium reduction, smoking cessation, regular physical activity) and, in most cases, medications.
5. Therapy will not cure, but should control hypertension.
6. Controlled hypertension usually results in an excellent prognosis and a normal lifestyle.
7. Explain the potential dangers of uncontrolled hypertension (e.g., target organ disease).

Instructions Related to Medications
1. Be specific about the names, actions, dosages, and side effects of prescribed medications.
2. Help the patient plan regular and convenient times for taking medications and measuring BP.
3. Do not stop drugs abruptly because withdrawal may cause a severe hypertensive reaction.
4. Do not double up on doses when a dose is missed.
5. If BP increases, the patient should not increase the medication dosage before consulting with the health care provider.
6. Do not take a medication belonging to someone else.
7. Supplement diet with foods high in potassium (e.g., citrus fruits, green leafy vegetables) if taking potassium-wasting diuretics.
8. Avoid hot baths, excessive amounts of alcohol, and strenuous exercise within 3 hr of taking medications that promote vasodilation.
9. Many medications cause orthostatic hypotension. The effects of orthostatic hypotension can be reduced by rising slowly from bed, sitting on the side of the bed for a few minutes, standing slowly, and beginning to move if no symptoms develop (e.g., dizziness, light-headedness). Do not stand still for prolonged periods, do leg exercises to increase venous return, or sleep with the head of the bed raised. Do lie or sit down when dizziness occurs.
10. Many medications cause sexual problems (e.g., erectile dysfunction, decreased libido). Consult with the health care provider about changing drugs or dosages if sexual problems develop.
11. The side effects of medication(s) may decrease with time.
12. Be careful about taking potentially high-risk over-the-counter medications, such as high-sodium antacids, appetite suppressants, and cold and sinus medications. Read warning labels and consult with a pharmacist.

Home BP Monitoring. Most patients with known or suspected hypertension should monitor their BP at home. Home BP monitoring reduces the white coat effect of measurement by a health care provider. The readings are often lower than those taken in the office setting and are a better predictor of CVD risk.[22]

Patient teaching is critical to ensure accuracy. Tell patients to buy an oscillometric BP monitor that uses a cuff for the upper arm. The patient should bring the BP monitor to the office to verify proper cuff size, accuracy of the device, and the patient's technique.

INFORMATICS IN PRACTICE

Monitoring Blood Pressure

- For patients with hypertension who have a smart phone or computer access, encourage them to use applications aimed at helping them manage their care, including BP self-monitoring and appointment tracking.
- Patients enter their SBP and DBP, heart rate, and other information, including the arm measured. They also indicate whether they were standing, sitting, or lying down and time the BP was taken.
- At appointment time, you can review the reports generated from the application to assist you in determining how well the patient's BP has been controlled.

DBP, Diastolic BP; *SBP*, systolic BP.

Teach the patient to obtain a BP according to the steps in Table 33-11. Tell the patient to measure BP in the nondominant arm, or arm with the higher BP if there is a known difference between arms. Advise the patient to measure BP first thing in the morning (if possible, before taking medications) and at night before going to bed. Tell the patient to keep a log of all BP measurements and to bring the log to office visits.

For clinical decision making (e.g., adjustments in dosage, start of new drug), instruct patients to take BP readings as described for 1 week. Stable, normotensive patients should measure morning and evening BP for at least 1 week every 3 months.[22] Devices that have memory or printouts of the readings are recommended to ensure accurate reporting.[9]

Home BP readings may help achieve patient adherence by reinforcing the need to remain on therapy. However, some patients become overly concerned with the BP readings. Discourage too frequent checking of their BP. Generally, home BP monitoring should reassure the patient that the treatment is effective.

Patient Adherence. A major problem in the long-term management of the patient with hypertension is poor adherence with the prescribed treatment plan. The reasons are many and include inadequate patient teaching, unpleasant side effects of drugs, return of BP to normal range while on medication, lack of motivation, high cost of drugs, lack of insurance, and lack of a trusting relationship between the patient and the health care provider. Also assess the patient's diet, activity level, and lifestyle as additional indicators of adherence.

Individually assess patients to determine the reasons why the patient is not adhering to the treatment and develop a plan with the patient to improve adherence. The plan should be compatible with the patient's personality, habits, and lifestyle. Active patient participation increases the likelihood of adherence to the treatment plan. Measures such as including the patient in the development of a medication schedule, selecting medications that are affordable, and involving caregivers help increase patient adherence.

Substituting combination drugs for multiple drugs once the BP is stable may also facilitate adherence. Combination drugs reduce the number of pills the patient has to take each day and may reduce costs.

It is important to help the patient and caregiver understand that hypertension is a chronic illness that cannot be cured. Emphasize that it can be controlled with drug therapy, diet changes, physical activity, periodic follow-up, and other relevant lifestyle modifications.

EVALUATION

The overall expected outcomes are that the patient with hypertension will
- Achieve and maintain goal BP as defined for the individual
- Understand, accept, and implement the therapeutic plan
- Experience minimal or no unpleasant side effects of therapy

GERONTOLOGIC CONSIDERATIONS

HYPERTENSION

The prevalence of hypertension increases with age. The lifetime risk of developing hypertension is approximately 90% for middle-aged (ages 55 to 65) and older (over 65) normotensive men and women.[17] Isolated systolic hypertension (ISH) is the most common form of hypertension in people over 50 years of age. Additionally, older adults are more likely to have white coat hypertension.[9]

The pathophysiology of hypertension in the older adult involves the following age-related physical changes: (1) loss of elasticity in large arteries from atherosclerosis, (2) increased collagen content and stiffness of the myocardium, (3) increased peripheral vascular resistance, (4) decreased adrenergic receptor sensitivity, (5) blunting of baroreceptor reflexes, (6) decreased renal function, and (7) decreased renin response to sodium and water depletion.

In the older adult who is taking antihypertensive medication, absorption of some drugs may be altered as a result of decreased blood flow to the gut. Metabolism and excretion of drugs may also be prolonged.

Careful technique is important in assessing BP in older adults. Some older people have a wide gap between the first Korotkoff sound and subsequent beats. This is called the *auscultatory gap*. Failure to inflate the cuff high enough may result in underestimating SBP (see Table 33-11).

The recommended BP goals are less than 140/90 mm Hg for people 65 to 79 years of age and an SBP of 140 to 145 mm Hg for those 80 years and older. Lower goals are recommended for older adults with diabetes mellitus, kidney disease, or CAD. Preferred antihypertensive drugs are low-dose thiazides, calcium channel blockers, and RAAS blockers. A diuretic should always be the first or second drug ordered for this age-group.[17]

Because of varying degrees of impaired baroreceptor reflexes, orthostatic hypotension often occurs in older adults, especially in those with ISH. Orthostatic hypotension in this age-group is often associated with volume depletion or chronic disease states, such as decreased renal and hepatic function or electrolyte imbalance. To reduce the likelihood of orthostatic hypotension, antihypertensive drugs should be started at low doses and increased slowly. Measure BP and HR in the supine, sitting, and standing positions at every visit.

Older adults experience postprandial drops in BP. The greatest decrease occurs approximately 1 hour after eating. BP returns to preprandial levels 3 to 4 hours after eating. Avoid giving vasoactive medications with meals.[7]

After CVD, arthritis is the second most prevalent disease in older adults. The most frequently taken drugs by older adults are nonsteroidal antiinflammatory drugs (NSAIDs), both prescription and over-the-counter. Nonselective NSAIDs (e.g., ibuprofen [Advil]) and selective NSAIDs (e.g., celecoxib [Celebrex]) have caused loss of BP control and heart failure. Additionally, there is the potential for adverse renal effects and/or hyperka-

TABLE 33-13	CAUSES OF HYPERTENSIVE CRISIS

- Exacerbation of chronic hypertension
- Renovascular hypertension
- Preeclampsia, eclampsia
- Pheochromocytoma
- Drugs (cocaine, amphetamines)
- Monoamine oxidase inhibitors taken with tyramine-containing foods
- Rebound hypertension (from abrupt withdrawal of some hypertensive drugs such as clonidine [Catapres] or β-adrenergic blockers)
- Head injury
- Acute aortic dissection

FIG. 33-4 Massive retinal exudates (indicated by *arrows*) from hypertensive retinopathy. To see what a normal retina looks like on ophthalmoscopic examination, see Fig. 21-5 on p. 377.

lemia when NSAIDs are used with ACE inhibitors, ARBs, or aldosterone antagonists.[7]

HYPERTENSIVE CRISIS

Hypertensive crisis is a term used to indicate either a hypertensive urgency or emergency. This is determined by the degree of target organ disease and how quickly the BP must be lowered.

A *hypertensive emergency* develops over hours to days. It is a situation in which a patient's BP is severely elevated (often above 220/140 mm Hg) with clinical evidence of target organ disease. Hypertensive emergencies can cause encephalopathy, intracranial or subarachnoid hemorrhage, acute left ventricular failure, MI, renal failure, dissecting aortic aneurysm, and retinopathy.

Hypertensive urgency develops over days to weeks. This is a situation in which a patient's BP is severely elevated (usually above 180/110 mm Hg), but there is no clinical evidence of target organ disease.[23]

The rate of rise of BP is more important than the absolute value in determining the need for emergency treatment. Patients with chronic hypertension can tolerate much higher BPs than normotensive people. Prompt recognition and management of hypertensive crisis are essential to decrease the threat to organ function and life.

Hypertensive crisis occurs more often in patients with a history of hypertension who have not adhered to their medication regimens or who have been undermedicated. In such cases, rising BP is thought to trigger endothelial damage and the release of vasoconstrictor substances. A vicious cycle of BP elevation follows, leading to life-threatening damage to target organs.

Hypertensive crisis related to cocaine or crack use is a frequent problem. Other drugs such as amphetamines, phencyclidine (PCP), and lysergic acid diethylamide (LSD) can also cause hypertensive crisis that may be complicated by drug-induced seizures, stroke, MI, or encephalopathy. Table 33-13 lists causes of hypertensive crisis.

Clinical Manifestations

A hypertensive emergency is often manifested as *hypertensive encephalopathy*, a syndrome in which a sudden rise in BP is associated with severe headache, nausea, vomiting, seizures, confusion, and coma. The manifestations of encephalopathy are the result of increased cerebral capillary permeability. This leads to cerebral edema and a disruption in cerebral function. On

retinal examination, exudates, hemorrhages, and/or papilledema is found[23] (Fig. 33-4).

Renal insufficiency ranging from minor injury to complete renal failure can occur. Rapid cardiac decompensation ranging from unstable angina to MI and pulmonary edema is also possible. Patients can have chest pain and dyspnea. Aortic dissection can develop and will cause sudden, excruciating chest and back pain and possibly reduced or absent pulses in the extremities.

Patient assessment is extremely important. Monitor for signs of neurologic deficits, retinal damage, heart failure, pulmonary edema, and renal failure. The neurologic changes are often similar to those related to a stroke. However, a hypertensive crisis does not show focal or lateralizing signs often seen with a stroke.

NURSING AND COLLABORATIVE MANAGEMENT HYPERTENSIVE CRISIS

BP level alone is a poor indicator of the seriousness of the patient's condition. It is not the major factor in deciding the treatment for a hypertensive crisis. The link between elevated BP and signs of new or progressive target organ disease determines the seriousness of the situation.

Hypertensive emergencies require hospitalization, IV administration of antihypertensive drugs, and intensive care monitoring. In treatment of hypertensive emergencies, the mean arterial pressure (MAP) is often used instead of BP readings to guide and evaluate drug therapy. MAP is calculated as follows:

$$MAP = (SBP + 2\,DBP) \div 3$$

The initial goal is to decrease MAP by no more than 20% to 25%, or to decrease MAP to 110 to 115 mm Hg. If the patient is clinically stable, drugs can be titrated to gradually lower BP over the next 24 hours. Lowering the BP too quickly or too much may decrease cerebral, coronary, or renal perfusion. This could precipitate a stroke, MI, or renal failure.

Special circumstances include patients with aortic dissection. These patients should have their SBP lowered to less than 100 to 120 mm Hg as soon as possible, and if tolerated.[23] Another exception is patients with acute ischemic stroke, in whom BP is lowered to allow the use of thrombolytic agents. Finally, an elevated BP in the immediate poststroke period may be a compensatory response to improve cerebral perfusion to ischemic brain tissue. There is no clear evidence supporting the use of antihypertensive medications in these patients[1] (see Chapter 58).

IV drugs used for hypertensive emergencies include vasodilators (e.g., sodium nitroprusside [Nitropress], fenoldopam [Corlopam], nicardipine [Cardene]), adrenergic inhibitors (e.g., phentolamine [Regitine], labetalol [Normodyne], esmolol [Brevibloc]), the ACE inhibitor enalapril (Vasotec IV), and the calcium channel blocker clevidipine (Cleviprex)[23,24] (see Table 33-7). Sodium nitroprusside is the most effective IV drug to treat hypertensive emergencies. Oral agents may be given along with IV drugs to help make an earlier transition to long-term therapy.

DRUG ALERT: Labetalol (Normodyne)
- Instruct patient not to discontinue drug abruptly, since this may precipitate angina or heart failure.

Antihypertensive drugs administered IV have a rapid (within seconds to minutes) onset of action. Assess the patient's BP and pulse every 2 to 3 minutes during the initial administration of these drugs. Use an intraarterial line (see Chapter 66) or an automated, noninvasive BP machine to monitor the BP. Titrate the drug according to MAP or BP as ordered. Monitor the ECG for heart dysrhythmias and signs of ischemia or MI. Use extreme caution in treating the patient with CAD or cerebrovascular disease. Measure urine output hourly to assess renal perfusion. Patients receiving IV antihypertensive drugs may be restricted to bed. Getting up (e.g., to use the commode) may cause severe cerebral ischemia and fainting.

Ongoing assessment is essential to evaluate the effectiveness of these drugs and the patient's response to therapy. Frequent neurologic checks, including level of consciousness, pupillary size and reaction, and movement of extremities, help detect any changes in the patient's condition. Monitor cardiac, pulmonary, and renal systems for decompensation caused by the severe elevation in BP (e.g., angina, pulmonary edema, renal failure).

Hypertensive urgencies usually do not require IV medications but can be managed with oral agents. The patient with hypertensive urgency may not need hospitalization, but will require follow-up. The oral drugs most frequently used for hypertensive urgencies are captopril (Capoten), labetalol, clonidine (Catapres), and amlodipine (Norvasc)[23] (see Table 33-7). The disadvantage of oral medications is the inability to regulate the dosage moment to moment, as can be done with IV medications. If a patient with hypertensive urgency is not hospitalized, outpatient follow-up care should be arranged within 24 hours.

Once the hypertensive crisis is resolved, it is important to determine the cause. The patient will need appropriate management and teaching to avoid future crises.

DRUG ALERT: Clonidine (Catapres)
Instruct patient to do the following:
- Change positions slowly to limit orthostatic hypotension.
- Avoid hazardous activities, since the drug may cause drowsiness.
- Do not discontinue the medication abruptly to prevent rebound hypertension.

Not every patient with an elevated BP and no target organ disease will require emergent drug therapy or hospitalization. Allowing the patient to sit for 20 or 30 minutes in a quiet environment may significantly reduce BP. Oral drugs may be started or adjusted. Additional nursing interventions include encouraging the patient to verbalize any concerns or fears, answering questions regarding hypertension, and eliminating any adverse stimuli (e.g., excess noise) in the patient's environment.

CASE STUDY

Primary Hypertension

iStockphoto/Thinkstock

Patient Profile
R.L. is a 45-year-old African American man with no previous history of hypertension. At a screening clinic 2 months ago, his BP was found to be 150/95 mm Hg. His primary care provider has followed him for the past month. During this time he has been taking hydrochlorothiazide 12.5 mg/day. He is here today for a follow-up visit.

Subjective Data
- Father died of stroke at age 60
- Mother is alive but has hypertension and a history of MI
- States that he feels fine and is not a "hyper" person
- Smokes one pack of cigarettes daily for the past 28 yr
- Drinks 1-2 six-packs of beer on most Friday and Saturday nights
- Has heard that BP drugs "make you impotent"

Objective Data
Physical Examination
- Mild retinopathy (retinal arteriolar narrowing on ophthalmoscopic examination)
- BP: 166/108 mm Hg (average of two readings, 1 min apart)
- Sustained apical impulse palpable in the fourth intercostal space just lateral to the midclavicular line

Diagnostic Studies
- ECG: mild left ventricular hypertrophy
- Urinalysis: protein 30 mg/dL (0.3 g/L)
- Serum creatinine level: 1.6 mg/dL (141 mmol/L)

Collaborative Care
- Low-sodium, DASH diet
- Hydrochlorothiazide 25 mg/day PO (dosage increase)
- Nicardipine (Cardene) sustained release 30 mg PO bid (second drug added)

Discussion Questions
1. What risk factors for hypertension does R.L. have?
2. What evidence of target organ disease is present?
3. What misconceptions about hypertension should be corrected?
4. *Priority Decision:* Based on the assessment data, what are the priority nursing diagnoses and interventions? What are the collaborative problems?
5. *Evidence-Based Practice:* R.L. wants to know the most effective nonpharmacologic strategies to lower his BP. What would you tell him?

ⓔvolve Answers available at http://evolve.elsevier.com/Lewis/medsurg.

BRIDGE TO NCLEX EXAMINATION

The number of the question corresponds to the same-numbered outcome at the beginning of the chapter.

1. Which BP-regulating mechanism(s) can result in the development of hypertension if defective (select all that apply)?
   a. Release of norepinephrine
   b. Secretion of prostaglandins
   c. Stimulation of the sympathetic nervous system
   d. Stimulation of the parasympathetic nervous system
   e. Activation of the renin-angiotensin-aldosterone system

2. While obtaining subjective assessment data from a patient with hypertension, the nurse recognizes that a modifiable risk factor for the development of hypertension is
   a. a low-calcium diet.
   b. excessive alcohol consumption.
   c. a family history of hypertension.
   d. consumption of a high-protein diet.

3. In teaching a patient with hypertension about controlling the condition, the nurse recognizes that
   a. all patients with elevated BP require medication.
   b. obese persons must achieve a normal weight to lower BP.
   c. it is not necessary to limit salt in the diet if taking a diuretic.
   d. lifestyle modifications are indicated for all persons with elevated BP.

4. A major consideration in the management of the older adult with hypertension is to
   a. prevent primary hypertension from converting to secondary hypertension.
   b. recognize that the older adult is less likely to adhere to the drug therapy regimen than a younger adult.
   c. ensure that the patient receives larger initial doses of antihypertensive drugs because of impaired absorption.
   d. use careful technique in assessing the BP of the patient because of the possible presence of an auscultatory gap.

5. A patient with newly discovered high BP has an average reading of 158/98 mm Hg after 3 months of exercise and diet modifications. Which management strategy will be a priority for this patient?
   a. Medication will be required because the BP is still not at goal.
   b. BP monitoring should continue for another 3 months to confirm a diagnosis of hypertension.
   c. Lifestyle changes are less important, since they were not effective, and medications will be started.
   d. More vigorous changes in the patient's lifestyle are needed for a longer time before starting medications.

6. A patient is admitted to the hospital in hypertensive emergency (BP 244/142 mm Hg). Sodium nitroprusside is started to treat the elevated BP. Which management strategy(ies) would be appropriate for this patient (select all that apply)?
   a. Measuring hourly urine output
   b. Decreasing the MAP by 50% within the first hour
   c. Continuous BP monitoring with an intraarterial line
   d. Maintaining bed rest and providing tranquilizers to lower the BP
   e. Assessing the patient for signs and symptoms of heart failure and changes in mental status

1. a, c, e, 2. b, 3. d, 4. d, 5. a, 6. a, c, e

ⓔvolve

For rationales to these answers and even more NCLEX review questions, visit *http://evolve.elsevier.com/Lewis/medsurg.*

REFERENCES

*1. National Heart, Lung, and Blood Institute: *Seventh report of the Joint National Committee on Detection, Evaluation, and Treatment of High Blood Pressure (JNC-7),* NIH Publication No. 04-5230, Bethesda, Md, 2004, The Institute. Retrieved from *www.nhlbi.nih.gov/guidelines/hypertension/jnc7full.pdf.*

2. Go AS, Mozaffarian D, Roger VL, et al: Heart disease and stroke statistics—2013 update: a report from the American Heart Association, *Circulation* 127:e6, 2013.

3. Fryar CD, Hirsch R, Eberhardt MS, et al: *Hypertension, high serum cholesterol, and diabetes: racial and ethnic prevalence differences in U.S. adults, 1999-2006,* NCHS data brief, no 36, Hyattsville, Md, 2010, National Center for Health Statistics.

4. US Department of Health and Human Services: Healthy people 2020. Retrieved from *www.healthypeople.gov.*

5. Drozda J, Messer JV, Spertus J, et al: ACCF/AHA/AMA-PCPI 2011 performance measures for adults with coronary artery disease and hypertension, *J Am Coll Cardiol* 58:316, 2011.

*6. Mosca L, Benjamin EJ, Berra K, et al: Effectiveness-based guidelines for the prevention of cardiovascular disease in women—2011 update, *Circulation* 123:1243, 2011.

7. Libby P, Bonow R, Zipes D, et al: *Braunwald's heart disease: a textbook of cardiovascular medicine,* ed 8, Philadelphia, 2008, Saunders.

8. Humes KR, Jones NA, Ramirez RR: United States Census Bureau: overview of race and Hispanic origin: 2010 census briefs. Retrieved from *www.census.gov/prod/cen2010/briefs/c2010br-02.pdf.*

*9. Pickering TG, Hall JE, Appel LJ, et al: Recommendations for blood pressure measurement in humans and experimental animals, part 1: blood pressure measurement in humans, *Hypertension* 45:142, 2005. (Classic)

10. Appel LJ: ASH position paper: dietary approaches to lower blood pressure, *J Clin Hypertension* 11:358, 2009.

11. American Heart Association: What are the symptoms of high blood pressure? Retrieved from *www.heart.org/HEARTORG/Conditions/HighBloodPressure/SymptomsDiagnosisMonitoringofHighBloodPressure/What-are-the-Symptoms-of-High-Blood-Pressure_UCM_301871_Article.jsp.*

12. National Heart, Lung, and Blood Institute: *In brief: your guide to lowering your blood pressure with DASH,* NIH Pub No 06-5834, Bethesda, Md, 2006, The Institute. Retrieved from *www.nhlbi.nih.gov/health/public/heart/hbp/dash/dash_brief.pdf.*

*13. Haskell WL, Lee I-M, Pate RR, et al: Physical activity and public health: updated recommendations for adults from the

*Evidence-based information for clinical practice.

American College of Sports Medicine and the American Heart Association, *Circulation* 116:1081, 2007.

*14. Nelson ME, Rejeski WJ, Blair SN, et al: Physical activity and public health in older adults: recommendation from the American College of Sports Medicine and the American Heart Association, *Circulation* 116:1094, 2007.

*15. Graham I, Atar D, Borch-Johnsen K, et al: European guidelines on cardiovascular disease prevention in clinical practice: executive summary; Fourth Joint Task Force of the European Society of Cardiology and other societies on cardiovascular disease prevention in clinical practice, *Eur Heart J* 28:2375, 2007.

16. Rozanski A, Blumenthal JA, Davidson KW, et al: The epidemiology, pathophysiology, and management of psychosocial risk factors in cardiac practice, *J Am Coll Cardiol* 45:637, 2005. (Classic)

*17. Aronow WS, Fleg JL, Pepine CJ, et al: ACCF/AHA 2011 expert consensus document on hypertension in the elderly, *J Am Coll Cardiol* 57:2037, 2011.

18. Olson J: *Clinical pharmacology made ridiculously simple*, ed 4, Miami, 2011, MedMaster.

19. Lehne RA: *Pharmacology for nursing care*, ed 7, St Louis, 2010, Saunders.

20. Hering D, Lambert EA, Marusic P, et al: Substantial reduction in single sympathetic nerve firing after renal denervation in patients with resistant hypertension, *Hypertension* 61:457, 2013.

*21. Seckel MA, Bradley E, Bucher L, et al: AACN practice alert: noninvasive blood pressure monitoring. Retrieved from *http://classic.aacn.org/AACN/practiceAlert.nsf/Files/NIBP/$file/Noninvasive%20BP%20Monitoring%206-2006.pdf*.

*22. Pickering TG, Miller NH, Ogedegbe G, et al: Call to action on use and reimbursement for home blood pressure monitoring: a joint scientific statement from the American Heart Association, American Society of Hypertension, and Preventive Cardiovascular Nurses Association, *Hypertension* 52:10, 2008.

23. Vidt DG: Hypertensive crises, Cleveland Clinic Center for Continuing Education. Retrieved from *www.cleveland clinicmeded.com/medicalpubs/diseasemanagement/nephrology/hypertensive-crises*.

24. Smithburger PL, Kane-Gill SL, Nestor BL, et al: Recent advances in the treatment of hypertensive emergencies, *Crit Care Nurse* 30:24, 2010.

RESOURCES

American Heart Association
www.americanheart.org
American Society of Hypertension
www.ash-us.org
National Heart, Lung, and Blood Institute
www.nhlbi.nih.gov/health/indexpro.htm
WebMD Hypertension and High Blood Pressure Community
www.exchanges.webmd.com/hypertension-and-high-blood-pressure-exchange

34

*I have witnessed the softening of the hardest
of hearts by a simple smile.*
Goldie Hawn

Nursing Management

Coronary Artery Disease and
Acute Coronary Syndrome

Linda Bucher and Sharmila Johnson

evolve WEBSITE

http://evolve.elsevier.com/Lewis/medsurg

- NCLEX Review Questions
- Key Points
- Pre-Test
- Answer Guidelines for Case Study on p. 763
- Rationales for Bridge to NCLEX Examination Questions
- Case Study
  - Patient With Coronary Artery Disease and Acute Coronary Syndrome
- Nursing Care Plan (Customizable)
  - NCP 34-1: Patient With Acute Coronary Syndrome

- Concept Map Creator
- Concept Map for Case Study on p. 763
- Glossary
- Content Updates

eFigures
- eFig. 34-1: Leading causes of death for men and women
- eFig. 34-2: Cardiovascular disease mortality trends for men and women

- eFig. 34-3: Trends in deaths due to cardiovascular disease
- eFig. 34-4: Xanthomas in patients with familial hypercholesterolemia
- eFig. 34-5: What you need to know—antiplatelet therapy

eTable
- eTable 34-1: Genes Known to Contribute to Coronary Artery Disease Risk

LEARNING OUTCOMES

1. Relate the etiology and pathophysiology of coronary artery disease (CAD), angina, and acute coronary syndrome (ACS) to the clinical manifestations of each disorder.
2. Describe the nursing role in the promotion of therapeutic lifestyle changes in patients at risk for CAD.
3. Differentiate the precipitating factors, clinical manifestations, collaborative care, and nursing management of the patient with CAD and chronic stable angina.
4. Explain the clinical manifestations, complications, diagnostic study results, and collaborative care of the patient with ACS.
5. Evaluate commonly used drug therapy in treating patients with CAD and ACS.
6. Prioritize key components to include in the rehabilitation of patients recovering from ACS and coronary revascularization procedures.
7. Differentiate the precipitating factors, clinical presentation, and collaborative care of patients who are at risk for or have experienced sudden cardiac death.

KEY TERMS

acute coronary syndrome (ACS), p. 746
angina, p. 740
atherosclerosis, p. 731
chronic stable angina, p. 741
collateral circulation, p. 732
coronary artery disease (CAD), p. 731

coronary revascularization, p. 745
metabolic equivalent (MET), p. 760
myocardial infarction (MI), p. 747
percutaneous coronary intervention (PCI), p. 745

Prinzmetal's angina, p. 742
silent ischemia, p. 742
stent, p. 746
sudden cardiac death (SCD), p. 762
unstable angina (UA), p. 747

Reviewed by Marci Ebberts, RN, BSN, CCRN, STEMI Program Coordinator, St. Luke's Hospital of Kansas City, Kansas City, Missouri; Kathleen M. Hill, RN, MSN, CCNS, Clinical Nurse Specialist, Surgical Intensive Care Unit, Cleveland Clinic, Cleveland, Ohio; Christina D. Keller, RN, MSN, Instructor, Radford University School of Nursing: Clinical Simulation Center, Radford, Virginia; and Devorah Overbay, RN, MSN, CNS, NCLEX Education Specialist ATI Testing, George Fox University, Department of Nursing, Newberg, Oregon.

Cardiovascular disease is the major cause of death in the United States. (The leading causes of death are shown in eFig. 34-1, available on the website for this chapter.) Coronary artery disease (CAD) is the most common type of cardiovascular disease and accounts for the majority of these deaths.[1] Patients with CAD can be asymptomatic or develop chronic stable angina (or chest pain). Unstable angina (UA) and myocardial infarction (MI) are more serious manifestations of CAD and are termed *acute coronary syndrome* (ACS).

The American Heart Association (AHA) estimates that 1.1 million Americans have an MI each year. About one fourth of these persons die in an emergency department (ED) or before reaching a hospital. Although the mortality rate from MI has decreased because of advances in treatment, it remains the leading cause of death from all cardiovascular diseases and other conditions in general.[1]

CORONARY ARTERY DISEASE

Coronary artery disease (CAD) is a type of blood vessel disorder that is included in the general category of atherosclerosis. The term **atherosclerosis** comes from two Greek words: *athere,* meaning "fatty mush," and *skleros,* meaning "hard." This combination implies that atherosclerosis begins as soft deposits of fat that harden with age. Consequently, atherosclerosis is commonly referred to as "hardening of the arteries." Although this condition can occur in any artery in the body, the *atheromas* (fatty deposits) prefer the coronary arteries. The terms *arteriosclerotic heart disease, cardiovascular heart disease, ischemic heart disease, coronary heart disease,* and *CAD* all describe this disease process.

Etiology and Pathophysiology

Atherosclerosis is the major cause of CAD. It is characterized by deposits of lipids within the intima of the artery. Endothelial injury and inflammation play a central role in the development of atherosclerosis.

The endothelium (the inner lining of the vessel wall) is normally nonreactive to platelets and leukocytes, as well as coagulation, fibrinolytic, and complement factors. However, the endothelial lining can be injured as a result of tobacco use, hyperlipidemia, hypertension, toxins, diabetes, hyperhomocysteinemia, and infection causing a local inflammatory response[2] (Fig. 34-1, *A*).

C-reactive protein (CRP), a protein produced by the liver, is a nonspecific marker of inflammation. It is increased in many patients with CAD[3] (see Table 32-6). The level of CRP rises when there is systemic inflammation. Chronic elevations of CRP are associated with unstable plaques and the oxidation of low-density lipoprotein (LDL) cholesterol.

Developmental Stages. CAD is a progressive disease that develops over many years. When it becomes symptomatic, the disease process is usually well advanced. The stages of development in atherosclerosis are (1) fatty streak, (2) fibrous plaque, and (3) complicated lesion.

Fatty Streak. *Fatty streaks,* the earliest lesions of atherosclerosis, are characterized by lipid-filled smooth muscle cells. As streaks of fat develop within the smooth muscle cells, a yellow tinge appears.[2] Fatty streaks can be seen in the coronary arteries by age 15 and involve an increasing amount of surface area as one ages. Treatment that lowers LDL cholesterol may reverse this process (Fig. 34-1, *B*).

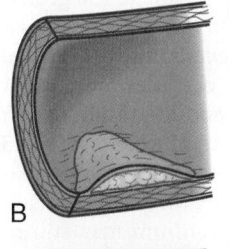

Endothelium   Intima

Chronic endothelial injury
- Hypertension
- Tobacco use
- Hyperlipidemia
- Hyperhomocysteinemia
- Diabetes
- Infections
- Toxins

Damaged endothelium

Fatty streak
- Lipids accumulate and migrate into smooth muscle cells

Fibrous plaque
- Collagen covers the fatty streak
- Vessel lumen is narrowed
- Blood flow is reduced
- Fissures can develop

Complicated lesion
- Plaque rupture
- Thrombus formation
- Further narrowing or total occlusion of vessel

FIG. 34-1 Pathogenesis of atherosclerosis. **A,** Damaged endothelium. **B,** Fatty streak and lipid core formation. **C,** Fibrous plaque. Raised plaques are visible: some are yellow; others are white. **D,** Complicated lesion: thrombus is red; collagen is blue. Plaque is complicated by red thrombus deposition.

Fibrous Plaque. The *fibrous plaque* stage is the beginning of progressive changes in the endothelium of the arterial wall. These changes can appear in the coronary arteries by age 30 and increase with age.

Normally the endothelium repairs itself immediately. This does not happen in the individual with CAD. LDLs and growth factors from platelets stimulate smooth muscle proliferation and thickening of the arterial wall. Once endothelial injury has taken place, lipoproteins (carrier proteins within the bloodstream) transport cholesterol and other lipids into the arterial intima. Collagen covers the fatty streak and forms a fibrous plaque with a grayish or whitish appearance. These plaques can form on one portion of the artery or in a circular fashion involving the entire lumen. The borders can be smooth or irregular with rough, jagged edges. The result is a narrowing of the vessel lumen and a reduction in blood flow to the distal tissues (Fig. 34-1, *C*).

Complicated Lesion. The final stage in the development of the atherosclerotic lesion is the most dangerous. As the fibrous plaque grows, continued inflammation can result in plaque instability, ulceration, and rupture. Once the integrity of the artery's inner wall is compromised, platelets accumulate in large numbers, leading to a thrombus. The thrombus may adhere to the wall of the artery, leading to further narrowing or total occlusion of the artery. Activation of the exposed platelets causes expression of glycoprotein IIb/IIIa receptors that bind fibrinogen. This, in turn, leads to further platelet aggregation and adhesion, further enlarging the thrombus. At this stage the plaque is referred to as a *complicated lesion* (Fig. 34-1, *D*).

Collateral Circulation. Normally some arterial anastomoses or connections, termed collateral circulation, exist within the coronary circulation. Two factors contribute to the growth and extent of collateral circulation: (1) the inherited predisposition to develop new blood vessels *(angiogenesis)* and (2) the presence of chronic ischemia. When a plaque occludes the normal flow of blood through a coronary artery and the resulting *ischemia* is chronic, increased collateral circulation develops (Fig. 34-2). When occlusion of the coronary arteries occurs slowly over a long period, there is a greater chance of adequate collateral circulation developing, and the myocardium may still receive an adequate amount of blood and oxygen.

However, with rapid-onset CAD (e.g., familial hypercholesterolemia) or coronary spasm, time is inadequate for collateral development. Consequently, a diminished blood flow results in a more severe ischemia or infarction.

Risk Factors for Coronary Artery Disease

Risk factors are characteristics or conditions that are associated with a high incidence of a disease. Many risk factors have been associated with CAD. They are categorized as nonmodifiable and modifiable (Table 34-1). *Nonmodifiable risk factors* are age, gender, ethnicity, family history, and genetics. *Modifiable risk factors* include elevated serum lipids, elevated blood pressure, tobacco use, physical inactivity, obesity, diabetes, metabolic syndrome, psychologic states, and elevated homocysteine level.

Data on risk factors for CAD come from several major studies. In the Framingham study (one of the most widely known), men and women were observed for 20 years. Over time, it was noted that elevated serum cholesterol (greater than 240 mg/dL), elevated systolic blood pressure (BP) (greater than 160 mm Hg), and tobacco use (one or more packs a day) were positively correlated with an increased incidence of CAD.[1]

Nonmodifiable Risk Factors

Age, Gender, and Ethnicity. The incidence of CAD and MI is highest among white, middle-aged men. After age 65, the incidence in men and women equalizes, although cardiovascular

FIG. 34-2 Vessel occlusion with collateral circulation. **A,** Open, functioning coronary artery. **B,** Partial coronary artery closure with collateral circulation being established. **C,** Total coronary artery occlusion with collateral circulation bypassing the occlusion to supply blood to the myocardium.

disease causes more deaths in women than men. Additionally, CAD is present in African American women at rates higher than those of their white counterparts.[1] (See Cultural & Ethnic Health Disparities box for additional differences in CAD among ethnic groups.)

Heart disease kills almost 10 times more women than breast cancer and is the leading cause of death in women. Yet most women do not consider CAD their greatest health risk.[4] (Cardiovascular disease mortality trends for both men and women are shown in eFig. 34-2, available on the website for this chapter.) On average, women with CAD are older than men who have

TABLE 34-1	RISK FACTORS FOR CORONARY ARTERY DISEASE
Nonmodifiable Risk Factors	**Modifiable Risk Factors**
Increasing age	**Major**
Gender (more common in men than in women until 65 yr of age)	Serum lipids: • Total cholesterol >200 mg/dL • Triglycerides ≥150 mg/dL* • LDL cholesterol >160 mg/dL
Ethnicity (more common in whites than in African Americans)	• HDL cholesterol <40 mg/dL in men or <50 mg/dL in women*
Genetic predisposition and family history of heart disease	Blood pressure ≥140/90 mm Hg* Diabetes mellitus Tobacco use Physical inactivity Obesity: Waist circumference ≥102 cm (≥40 in) in men and ≥88 cm (≥35 in) in women*
	Contributing Fasting blood glucose ≥100 mg/dL* Psychosocial risk factors (e.g., depression, hostility, anger, stress) Elevated homocysteine levels

*Three or more of these risk factors meet the criteria for metabolic syndrome (as defined by the National Cholesterol Education Program Adult Treatment Panel III). Metabolic syndrome is discussed in Chapter 49.

GENDER DIFFERENCES

Coronary Artery Disease and Acute Coronary Syndrome

Men	Women
Coronary Artery Disease	
• Initial cardiac event for men is more often MI than angina.	• Women experience the onset of heart disease approximately 10 yr later than men.
• Men report more typical signs and symptoms of angina and MI.	• CAD is the leading cause of death for women, regardless of race or ethnicity.
• Men receive more evidence-based therapies (e.g., aspirin, statins, diagnostic catheterization, PCI) when acutely ill from CAD (e.g., MI) than women.	• Initial cardiac event for women is more often angina than MI.
• Mortality rates from CAD have fallen more rapidly for men than women.	• More women than men with MI die of sudden cardiac death before reaching the hospital.
	• Before menopause, women have higher HDL cholesterol levels and lower LDL cholesterol levels than men. After menopause LDL levels increase.
Acute Coronary Syndrome	
• Incidence of MI is highest among white, middle-aged men.	• Women are older than men when seen with first MI and often have more co-morbidities.
• After age 65, the incidence of MI in men and women equalizes.	• Women delay longer in seeking care and are often more ill on presentation than men.
• Men present more frequently than women with an acute MI as the first manifestation of CAD.	• Once a woman reaches menopause, her risk for an MI quadruples.
• Men develop greater collateral circulation than women.	• Fewer women than men manifest the "classic" signs and symptoms of UA or MI.
• Men have larger-diameter coronary arteries than women. Vessel diameter is inversely related to risk of restenosis after interventions.	• Fatigue is often the first symptom of ACS in women.
• Standard screening for risk of sudden cardiac death (e.g., EP studies) is more predictive in men.	• Women experience more "silent" MIs compared with men.
	• Among those who have an MI, women are more likely to suffer a fatal cardiac event within 1 yr than men.
	• Women report more disability after a cardiac event than men.
	• Women who have coronary artery bypass graft surgery have a higher mortality rate and more complications after surgery than men.

ACS, Acute coronary syndrome; *CAD,* coronary artery disease; *EP,* electrophysiology; *HDL,* high-density lipoprotein; *LDL,* low-density lipoprotein; *PCI,* percutaneous coronary intervention, *UA,* unstable angina.

CAD, and women are more likely to have co-morbidities (e.g., hypertension, diabetes). Most women have atypical symptoms of angina rather than MI when they experience their first cardiac event[4] (see Gender Differences box).

Genetic Link

Genetic predisposition is an important factor in the occurrence of CAD. Family history is a risk factor for CAD and MI. Most times, patients with angina or MI can name a parent or sibling who died of CAD.

The genetic basis of CAD/MI is complex and, to date, poorly understood. It is estimated that the genetic contribution to CAD/MI is as high as 40% to 60%. This proportion relates mainly to genes that control known risk factors (e.g., lipid metabolism).[5] (Genes known to contribute to CAD risk are listed in eTable 34-1, available on the website for this chapter.) See the Genetics in Clinical Practice box at right.

Major Modifiable Risk Factors

Elevated Serum Lipids. An elevated serum lipid level is one of the four most firmly established risk factors for CAD.[6] The risk of CAD is associated with a serum cholesterol level greater than 200 mg/dL (5.2 mmol/L) or a fasting triglyceride level greater than 150 mg/dL (3.7 mmol/L). (See Table 32-6 for normal serum lipid values.)

For lipids to be used and transported by the body, they must become soluble in blood by combining with proteins. Lipids combine with proteins to form lipoproteins. Lipoproteins are vehicles for fat mobilization and transport, and vary in composition. They are classified as high-density lipoproteins (HDLs), LDLs, and very-low-density lipoproteins (VLDLs).

HDLs contain more protein by weight and fewer lipids than any other lipoprotein. HDLs carry lipids away from arteries

GENETICS IN CLINICAL PRACTICE

Familial Hypercholesterolemia

Genetic Basis
• Autosomal dominant disorder.
• Mutation in low-density lipoprotein receptor *(LDLR)* gene.
• Gene codes for low-density lipoprotein (LDL) receptor that binds to LDLs.
• LDLs are the primary carriers of cholesterol in the blood. By removing LDLs from the bloodstream, the LDL receptors play a critical role in regulating cholesterol levels.
• Exists in both heterozygous (most common) and homozygous forms.

Incidence
• Heterozygotes: 1 in 500
• Homozygotes: rare

Genetic Testing
• Disorder is characterized by elevated serum LDLs.
• Serum lipid profile can be used to measure total cholesterol, triglycerides, LDLs, and high-density lipoproteins (HDLs).
• DNA testing is available.

Clinical Implications
• Common genetic disease.
• High cholesterol levels are a result of defective function of the LDL receptors.
• Plasma levels of LDLs elevated throughout life.
• Develop severe atherosclerosis in early to middle years.
• Xanthomas (fatty deposits under the surface of the skin) can occur (see eFig. 34-4, available on the website for this chapter).
• Treatment strategies include low-fat diet, exercise, and lipid-lowering medications.
• Homozygous familial hypercholesterolemia is much more severe than the heterozygous form. Cholesterol levels may exceed 600 mg/dL in these patients.

and to the liver for metabolism. This process of HDL transport prevents lipid accumulation within the arterial walls. Therefore high serum HDL levels are desirable and lower the risk of CAD.

There are two types of HDLs: HDL_2 and HDL_3. They differ by their density and apolipoprotein composition. Apolipoproteins are found on lipoproteins and activate enzyme or receptor sites that promote the removal of fat from plasma. Several types of apolipoproteins exist (e.g., apo A-I, apo B-100, apo C-I). Women produce more apo A-I than men, and premenopausal women have HDL_2 levels approximately three times greater than men. This is thought to be related to the protective effects of natural estrogen. After menopause, women's HDL_2 levels decrease and quickly near those of men.

In general, HDL levels are higher in women, decrease with age, and are low in persons with CAD. Physical activity, moderate alcohol consumption, and estrogen administration increase HDL levels.

LDLs contain more cholesterol than any of the lipoproteins and have an attraction for arterial walls. VLDLs contain both cholesterol and triglycerides, and may deposit cholesterol directly on the walls of arteries. Elevated LDL levels correlate closely with an increased incidence of atherosclerosis and CAD. Therefore low serum LDL levels are desirable.[6,7]

Certain diseases (e.g., type 2 diabetes, chronic kidney disease), drugs (e.g., corticosteroids, hormone therapy), and genetic disorders have been associated with elevated triglyceride levels. Lifestyle factors that can contribute to elevated triglycerides include high alcohol consumption, high intake of refined carbohydrates and simple sugars, and physical inactivity. When a high triglyceride level is combined with a high LDL level, a smaller, denser LDL particle is formed, which favors deposition on arterial walls. People with insulin resistance often have this pattern.

Guidelines for treating elevated LDL cholesterol are based on a person's 10-year risk for having a nonfatal MI or dying from a coronary event and his or her LDL levels. The following information generates a risk score: (1) age, (2) gender, (3) use of tobacco, (4) systolic BP, (5) use of BP medications, (6) total cholesterol, and (7) HDL cholesterol level.[7] A 10-year risk calculator is available at *http://hin.nhlbi.nih.gov/atpiii/calculator. asp?usertype=prof.*

In general, individuals with no or only one risk factor are considered at low risk for the development of CAD, and the LDL goal is less than 160 mg/dL (4.14 mmol/L). Those at very high risk have CAD and multiple risk factors. The LDL goal for this group is less than 70 mg/dL (1.8 mmol/L).[7]

Hypertension. The second major risk factor in CAD is hypertension, which is defined as a BP greater than 140/90 mm Hg or greater than 130/80 mm Hg if the patient has diabetes or chronic kidney disease.[8] Hypertension increases the risk of death from CAD 10-fold in all people. In postmenopausal women, hypertension is associated with a higher incidence of CAD than in men and premenopausal women.

Blood pressure is classified as (1) normal (BP less than 120/80 mm Hg), (2) *prehypertension* (BP of 120 to 139/80 to 89 mm Hg), (3) stage 1 hypertension (140 to 159/90 to 99 mm Hg), and (4) stage 2 hypertension (BP greater than 160/100 mm Hg).[8] The cause of hypertension in 90% of those affected is unknown, but it is usually controllable with diet and/or drugs. Therapeutic lifestyle changes should begin in people with prehypertension. Those with stage 1 or 2 hypertension

often require more than one drug to reach therapeutic goals[8] (see Table 33-7). Teach all people with elevated systolic or diastolic BP the importance of achieving and maintaining target BP goals.

The stress of an elevated BP increases the rate of atherosclerotic development. This relates to the shearing stress that causes endothelial injury. Atherosclerosis, in turn, causes narrowed, thickened arterial walls and decreases the distensibility and elasticity of vessels. More force is required to pump blood through diseased arteries, and this increased force is reflected in a higher BP. This increased workload results in left ventricular hypertrophy and decreased stroke volume with each contraction. Salt intake positively correlates with elevated BP, adding volume and increasing systemic vascular resistance (SVR) to the cardiac workload. (See Chapter 33 for a complete discussion of hypertension.)

Tobacco Use. A third major risk factor in CAD is tobacco use. The risk of developing CAD is two to six times higher in those who smoke tobacco or use smokeless tobacco than in those who do not. Further, tobacco smoking decreases estrogen levels, placing premenopausal women at greater risk for CAD. Risk is proportional to the number of cigarettes smoked. Changing to lower nicotine or filtered cigarettes does not affect risk.

Nicotine in tobacco smoke causes catecholamine (i.e., epinephrine, norepinephrine) release. These neurohormones cause an increased heart rate (HR), peripheral vasoconstriction, and increased BP. These changes increase the cardiac workload. Tobacco smoke is also related to an increase in LDL level, a decrease in HDL level, and release of toxic oxygen radicals. All of these add to vessel inflammation and thrombosis.[2]

Carbon monoxide, a byproduct of combustion found in tobacco smoke, affects the oxygen-carrying capacity of hemoglobin by reducing the sites available for oxygen transport. Thus the effects of an increased cardiac workload, combined with the oxygen-depleting effect of carbon monoxide, significantly decrease the oxygen available to the myocardium. There is also some indication that carbon monoxide is a chemical irritant and causes injury to the endothelium.

The benefits of smoking cessation are dramatic and almost immediate. CAD mortality rates drop to those of nonsmokers within 12 months. However, nicotine is highly addictive, and often intensive intervention is required to assist people to quit. Individual and group counseling sessions, nicotine replacement therapy, smoking cessation medications (e.g., bupropion [Zyban], varenicline [Chantix]), and hypnosis are examples of smoking cessation strategies. (See Chapter 11, Tables 11-4 through 11-6 for information on smoking cessation.)

Chronic exposure to environmental tobacco (secondhand) smoke also increases the risk of CAD.[6] People who live in the same household as the patient should be encouraged to stop smoking. This reinforces the individual's effort and decreases the risk of ongoing exposure to environmental smoke. Pipe and cigar smokers, who often do not inhale, have an increased risk of CAD similar to those exposed to environmental tobacco smoke.

Physical Inactivity. Physical inactivity is the fourth major modifiable risk factor. Physical inactivity implies a lack of adequate physical exercise on a regular basis. An example of health-promoting regular physical activity is brisk walking (3 to 4 miles per hour) for at least 30 minutes five or more times a week.[9]

The mechanism by which physical inactivity predisposes a person to CAD is mostly still unknown. Physically active people have increased HDL levels. Exercise improves thrombolytic activity, thus reducing the risk of clot formation. Exercise may also encourage the development of collateral circulation in the heart.

Exercise training for those who are physically inactive decreases the risk of CAD through more efficient lipid metabolism, increased HDL production, and more efficient oxygen extraction by the working muscles, thereby decreasing the cardiac workload. For those individuals with CAD, regular physical activity reduces symptoms, improves functional capacity, and improves other risk factors such as insulin resistance and glucose intolerance.

Obesity. The mortality rate from CAD is statistically higher in obese persons. Obesity is defined as a body mass index (BMI) of greater than 30 kg/m^2 and a waist circumference more than 40 inches for men and more than 35 inches for women. BMI is a measure of body fat based on height and weight. It can be calculated online *(http://nhlbisupport.com/bmi/bmicalc.htm).*

The increased risk for CAD is proportional to the degree of obesity. Obese persons may produce increased levels of LDLs and triglycerides, which are strongly related to atherosclerosis. Obesity is often associated with hypertension. There is also evidence that people who tend to store fat in the abdomen (an "apple" figure) rather than in the hips and buttocks (a "pear" figure) have a higher incidence of CAD (see Table 41-2). As obesity increases, the heart grows and uses more oxygen. In addition, there is an increase in insulin resistance in obese individuals.[2]

Contributing Modifiable Risk Factors

Diabetes Mellitus. The incidence of CAD is two to four times greater among persons who have diabetes, even those with well-controlled blood glucose levels, than the general population. The patient with diabetes manifests CAD not only more frequently but also at an earlier age.[2] There is no age difference between male or female patients with diabetes in the onset of symptoms of CAD. Diabetes virtually eliminates the lower incidence of CAD in premenopausal women.

Undiagnosed diabetes is frequently discovered at the time a person has an MI. The person with diabetes has an increased tendency toward endothelial dysfunction. This may account for the development of fatty streaks in these patients. Diabetic patients also have alterations in lipid metabolism and tend to have high cholesterol and triglyceride levels. Management of diabetes should include lifestyle changes and drug therapy to achieve a glycosylated hemoglobin (A1C or Hb A1C) level of less than 7%.[6]

Metabolic Syndrome. *Metabolic syndrome* refers to a cluster of risk factors for CAD whose underlying pathophysiology may be related to insulin resistance. These risk factors include obesity as defined by increased waist circumference, hypertension, abnormal serum lipids, and an elevated fasting blood glucose[2] (see Table 41-10). These interrelated risk factors of metabolic origin appear to promote the development of CAD. (Chapter 41 discusses metabolic syndrome.)

Psychologic States. The Framingham study provided early evidence that certain behaviors and lifestyles contribute to the development of CAD. Several behavior patterns correlated with CAD. However, the study of these behaviors remains controversial and complex. One type of behavior, referred to as type A, includes perfectionism and a hardworking, driven personality. The type A person often suppresses anger and hostility, has a sense of time urgency, is impatient, and creates stress and tension. This person may be more prone to MIs than a type B person, who is more easygoing, takes upsets in stride, knows personal limitations, takes time to relax, and is not an overachiever. However, findings from studies regarding these relationships are inconsistent.

Studies now are focusing on specific psychologic risk factors thought to increase risk of CAD. These include depression, acute and chronic stress (e.g., poverty, serving as a caregiver), anxiety, hostility and anger, and lack of social support.[10,11] In particular, depression is a risk factor for both the development and worsening of CAD. Depressed patients have elevated levels of circulating catecholamines that may contribute to endothelial injury and inflammation and platelet activation. Higher levels of depression are also associated with an increased number of adverse cardiac events.[10] More research on the treatment of depression and other negative psychologic states (e.g., anger) in patients with or at risk for CAD is needed to improve these patients' emotional and physical health.

Stressful states correlate with the development of CAD.[12] Sympathetic nervous system (SNS) stimulation and its effect on the heart are the physiologic mechanism by which stress predisposes one to the development of CAD. SNS stimulation causes an increased release of catecholamines (i.e., epinephrine, norepinephrine). This stimulation increases HR and intensifies the force of myocardial contraction, resulting in increased myocardial oxygen demand. Also, stress-induced mechanisms can cause elevated lipid and glucose levels and changes in blood coagulation, which can lead to increased atherogenesis.

Homocysteine. High blood levels of homocysteine have been linked to an increased risk for CAD and other cardiovascular diseases.[13] Homocysteine is produced by the breakdown of the essential amino acid methionine, which is found in dietary protein. High homocysteine levels possibly contribute to atherosclerosis by (1) damaging the inner lining of blood vessels, (2) promoting plaque buildup, and (3) altering the clotting mechanism to make clots more likely to occur (see Table 32-6).

Research is ongoing to determine whether a decline in homocysteine can reduce the risk of heart disease. B-complex vitamins (B$_6$, B$_{12}$, folic acid) have been shown to lower blood levels of homocysteine. Generally, a screening test for homocysteine is limited to those suspected of having elevated levels, such as older patients with pernicious anemia or people who develop CAD at an early age.

Substance Abuse. The use of illicit drugs, such as cocaine and methamphetamine, can produce coronary spasm resulting in myocardial ischemia and chest pain. Most people who are seen in the ED with drug-induced chest pain are initially indistinguishable from those with CAD. Although MI can occur, these patients more often have sinus tachycardia, high BP, angina, and anxiety.[14]

The U.S. Food and Drug Administration (FDA) prohibits the sale of dietary supplements containing ephedrine alkaloids. These compounds should be avoided because they can cause high BP, MI, and stroke.

NURSING AND COLLABORATIVE MANAGEMENT
CORONARY ARTERY DISEASE

HEALTH PROMOTION

The appropriate management of risk factors in CAD may prevent, modify, or slow the progression of the disease. In the

United States during the past 30 years, there has been a gradual and persistent decline in cardiovascular-related deaths. (See eFig. 34-3, available on the website for this chapter.) The decline relates to people's efforts to become generally healthier, as well as advances in drugs and technology to treat CAD. Prevention and early treatment of heart disease must involve a multifaceted approach and needs to be ongoing throughout the life span.

IDENTIFICATION OF HIGH-RISK PEOPLE. Clinical manifestations of CAD are not apparent in the early stages of the disease. Therefore regardless of the health care setting, it is extremely important to identify people at risk for CAD. Risk screening involves obtaining a thorough health history. Question the patient about a family history of heart disease in parents and siblings. Note the presence of any cardiovascular symptoms. Assess environmental factors, such as eating habits, type of diet, and level of exercise, to elicit lifestyle patterns. Include a psychosocial history to determine tobacco use, alcohol ingestion, recent stressful events (e.g., loss of a spouse), and any negative psychologic states (e.g., anxiety, depression, anger). The place and type of employment provide important information on the kind of activity performed, exposure to pollutants or noxious chemicals, and the degree of stress associated with work.

Identify the patient's attitudes and beliefs about health and illness. This information can give some indication of how disease and lifestyle changes may affect the patient and can reveal possible misconceptions about heart disease. Knowledge of the patient's educational background can help to decide the level needed for teaching. If the patient is taking medications,

it is important to know the names and dosages and if the patient is compliant with the drug regimen.

MANAGEMENT OF HIGH-RISK PEOPLE. Recommend preventive measures for all persons at risk for CAD. Risk factors such as age, gender, ethnicity, and genetics cannot be modified. However, the person with any of these risk factors can still reduce the risk of CAD by controlling the additive effects of modifiable risk factors. For example, a young man with a family history of heart disease can decrease the risk of CAD by maintaining an ideal body weight, getting adequate physical exercise, reducing intake of saturated fats, and avoiding tobacco use.

Encourage people who have modifiable risk factors to make lifestyle changes to reduce their risk of CAD. You can play a major role in teaching health-promoting behaviors (Table 34-2). For highly motivated persons, knowing how to reduce this risk may be the information they need to get started.

For persons who are less motivated to take charge of their health, the idea of reducing risk factors may be so remote that they are unable to perceive a threat of CAD. Few people desire to make lifestyle changes, especially in the absence of symptoms. First assist these patients in clarifying personal values. Then, by explaining the risk factors and having them identify their vulnerability to various risks, you may help them recognize their susceptibility to CAD. This may help patients set realistic goals and allow them to choose which risk factor(s) to change first. Some persons are reluctant to change until they begin to manifest overt symptoms or actually suffer an MI. Others, having suffered an MI, may find the idea of changing

---

TABLE 34-2 PATIENT & CAREGIVER TEACHING GUIDE

Reducing Risk Factors for Coronary Artery Disease

Include the following instructions when teaching risk reduction for coronary artery disease.

Risk Factor	Health-Promoting Behaviors	Risk Factor	Health-Promoting Behaviors
Hypertension	• Monitor home blood pressure (BP) and attend regular checkups. • Take prescribed medications for BP control. • Reduce salt intake (see eFig. 33-1, Your Guide to Lowering Your Blood Pressure with DASH, available on the website for this chapter). • Stop tobacco use. Avoid exposure to environmental tobacco (secondhand) smoke. • Control or reduce weight. • Perform physical activity daily.	Psychologic state	• Increase awareness of behaviors that are harmful to health. • Alter patterns that are conducive to stress (e.g., get up 30 min earlier so breakfast is not eaten on way to work). • Set realistic goals for self. • Reassess priorities in light of health needs. • Learn effective stress management strategies (see Chapter 7). • Seek professional help if feeling depressed, angry, anxious, etc. • Plan time for adequate rest and sleep (see Chapter 8).
Elevated serum lipids	• Reduce total fat intake. • Reduce animal (saturated) fat intake. • Take prescribed medications for lipid reduction. • Adjust total caloric intake to achieve and maintain ideal body weight. • Engage in daily physical activity. • Increase amount of complex carbohydrates, fiber, and vegetable proteins in diet.	Obesity†	• Change eating patterns and habits. • Reduce caloric intake to achieve body mass index of 18.5-24.9 kg/m². • Increase physical activity to increase caloric expenditure. • Avoid fad and crash diets, which are not effective over time. • Avoid large, heavy meals. Consider smaller, more frequent meals.
Tobacco use*	• Begin a smoking cessation program. • Change daily routines associated with smoking to reduce desire to smoke. • Substitute other activities for smoking. • Ask caregivers to support efforts to stop smoking. • Avoid exposure to environmental tobacco smoke.	Diabetes‡	• Follow the recommended diet. • Control or reduce weight. • Take prescribed antidiabetic medications. • Monitor blood glucose levels regularly.
Physical inactivity	• Develop and maintain at least 30 min of moderate physical activity daily (minimum 5 days a week). • Increase activities to a fitness level.		

*Smoking cessation is discussed in Chapter 11 and Tables 11-4 through 11-6.
†See Chapter 41 for additional health-promoting behaviors.
‡See Chapter 49 for additional health-promoting behaviors.

lifelong habits still unacceptable. Help them identify such choices and respect their final decision.

PHYSICAL ACTIVITY

A physical activity program should be designed to improve physical fitness by following the FITT formula: **F**requency (how often), **I**ntensity (how hard), **T**ype (isotonic), and **T**ime (how long). Everyone should aim for at least 30 minutes of moderate physical activity on most days of the week.[9] In addition, adding weight training to an exercise program two days a week can help treat metabolic syndrome and improve muscle strength. Examples of moderate physical activity include brisk walking, hiking, biking, and swimming. Regular physical activity contributes to weight reduction, reduction in systolic BP, and, in some men more than women, increase in HDL cholesterol. The AHA has developed a program to encourage people, especially women, to increase their daily physical activity (My Heart, My Life at *www.startwalkingnow.org*).

NUTRITIONAL THERAPY

The National Heart, Lung, and Blood Institute recommends therapeutic lifestyle changes for all people to reduce the risk of CAD by lowering LDL cholesterol. These recommendations emphasize a decrease in saturated fat and cholesterol and an increase in complex carbohydrates (e.g., whole grains, fruit, vegetables) and fiber[7] (Tables 34-3 and 34-4). Fat intake should be about 30% of calories, with most coming from mono- and polyunsaturated fats (Fig. 34-3). Red meat, egg yolks, and whole milk products are major sources of saturated fat and cholesterol and should be reduced or eliminated from diets. If the serum triglyceride level is elevated, the guidelines recommend reducing or eliminating alcohol intake and simple sugars.

Omega-3 fatty acids reduce the risks associated with CAD when eaten regularly. For individuals without CAD, the AHA recommends eating fatty fish twice a week because fatty fish such as salmon and tuna contains two types of omega-3 fatty acids: eicosapentaenoic acid (EPA) and docosahexaenoic acid (DHA). Patients with CAD are encouraged to take EPA and DHA supplements with their diet. The AHA also recommends eating tofu and other forms of soybean, canola, walnut, and flaxseed because these products contain alpha-linolenic acid,

which becomes omega-3 fatty acid in the body. For more information on the AHA's nutritional recommendations, see their website listed in the Resources section at the end of this chapter.

Lifestyle changes, including a low-saturated-fat, high-fiber diet; avoidance of tobacco; and increase in physical activity, can promote the reversal of CAD and reduce coronary events.

LIPID-LOWERING DRUG THERAPY

An estimated 31.9 million American adults have cholesterol levels greater than or equal to 240 mg/dL (6.2 mmol/L).[1] A complete lipid profile is recommended every 5 years beginning at age 20. The person with a serum cholesterol level greater than 200 mg/dL is at risk for CAD and should be treated. Treatment usually begins with dietary caloric restriction (if overweight), decreased dietary fat and cholesterol intake, and increased

---

TABLE 34-3   NUTRITIONAL THERAPY

Therapeutic Lifestyle Changes Diet

Nutrient	Recommended Daily Intake
Total fat (includes saturated fat calories)	25%-35% of total daily calories
Saturated fat	<7% of total daily calories
Cholesterol	<200 mg
Plant stanols or sterols (e.g., margarines, nuts, seeds, legumes, vegetable oils)*	2 g
Dietary fiber*	10-25 g of soluble fiber
Total calories	Only enough calories to reach or maintain a healthy weight
Physical activity	At least 30 min of a moderate-intensity physical activity (e.g., brisk walking) on most, and preferably all, days of the week

Source: Your Guide to Lowering Your Cholesterol with TLC. Retrieved from *www.nhlbi.nih.gov/health/public/heart/chol/chol_tlc.pdf*.
*Diet options for additional lowering of low-density lipoprotein (LDL).

TABLE 34-4   NUTRITIONAL THERAPY

Tips to Implement Diet and Lifestyle Recommendations

General Tips

1. Know your caloric needs to achieve and maintain a healthy weight.
2. Know the calorie content of the foods and beverages you consume.
3. Track your weight, physical activity, and calorie intake.
4. Prepare and eat smaller, more frequent meals.
5. Track your activities and, whenever possible, decrease sedentary activities (e.g., watching television, computer time).
6. Incorporate physical movement into daily activities (e.g., take extra steps when possible).
7. Do not smoke or use tobacco products.
8. If you consume alcohol, do so in moderation (i.e., no more than one drink for women or two drinks for men a day).

Tips Related to Food Choices and Preparation

1. Use the Nutrition Facts panel on food labels and ingredients list when choosing foods to buy.
2. Select frozen and canned vegetables and fruits without high-calorie sauces or added salt and sugars.
3. Replace high-calorie foods with fresh fruits and vegetables.
4. Increase fiber intake by eating beans (legumes), whole-grain products, fruits, and vegetables.
5. Use liquid vegetable oils in place of solid fats.
6. Limit beverages and foods high in added sugars (e.g., sucrose, glucose, fructose, maltose, dextrose, corn syrups, concentrated fruit juice, honey).
7. Choose foods made with whole grains (e.g., whole wheat, oats/ oatmeal, rye, barley, corn, popcorn, brown rice, wild rice, buckwheat, cracked wheat, sorghum).
8. Eliminate pastries and high-calorie bakery products (e.g., muffins, doughnuts).
9. Select milk and dairy products that are either fat free or low fat.
10. Reduce salt intake by
    - Comparing the sodium content of similar products (e.g., different brands of tomato sauce) and choosing products with less sodium
    - Choosing versions of processed foods that are reduced in salt, including cereals and baked goods
    - Limiting condiments (e.g., soy sauce, ketchup)
11. Use lean cuts of meat and remove skin from poultry before cooking or eating.
12. Avoid processed meats that are high in saturated fat and sodium (e.g., deli meats).
13. Grill, bake, or broil fish, meat, and poultry.
14. Incorporate vegetable-based meat substitutes into favorite recipes (e.g., soy).
15. Consume whole vegetables and fruits in place of juices.

Adapted from Gidding SS, Lichtenstein AH, Faith MS, et al: Implementing American Heart Association pediatric and adult nutrition guidelines, *Circulation* 119:1161, 2009.

FIG. 34-3 Types of dietary fat.

EVIDENCE-BASED PRACTICE

Translating Research into Practice

Does Dietary Fat Modification Improve Cardiovascular Disease Outcomes?

Clinical Question
For adults (P), what is the effect of dietary fat modification or reduction (I) versus placebo, usual, or control diet (C) on overall mortality and cardiovascular morbidity and mortality (O)?

Best Available Evidence
Systematic review of randomized controlled trials (RCTs)

Critical Appraisal and Synthesis of Evidence
- 48 RCTs with 60 comparisons ($n = 81,327$) of adults with or without existing cardiovascular disease. Intervention was reduced or modified dietary fat intake compared with placebo, usual, or control diet.
- Low-fat diet reduced energy intake to <30% from fat, and partially replaced fats with carbohydrates (simple or complex), protein, or fruit and vegetables.
- Modified fat diet had 30% or more energy intake from total fats with more monounsaturated or polyunsaturated fats than usual diet.

Conclusion
- Reducing saturated fat by reducing and/or modifying dietary fat reduced the risk of cardiovascular events.
- Risk for cardiovascular disease decreased in men (not women) by dietary fat modification.

Implications for Nursing Practice
- Counsel patients on modifying dietary fat intake by substituting monounsaturated or polyunsaturated fats for saturated fats.
- Assist the patient in collaboration with the dietitian to maintain long-term dietary fat changes.

Reference for Evidence
Hooper L, Summerbell C, Thompson R, et al: Reduced or modified dietary fat for preventing cardiovascular disease, *Cochrane Database Syst Rev* 7:CD002137, 2011.

P, Patient population of interest; *I*, intervention or area of interest; *C*, comparison of interest or comparison group; *O*, outcomes of interest; *T*, timing (see p. 12).

COMPLEMENTARY & ALTERNATIVE THERAPIES

Lipid-Lowering Agents*

Agent	Evidence for Use
Garlic	Inconsistent scientific evidence for reductions in total cholesterol and low-density lipoproteins (LDLs) over short periods.
Niacin	Strong scientific evidence for increased high-density lipoproteins. Less dramatic reduction of LDLs.
Omega-3 fatty acids	Strong scientific evidence for reduction of triglyceride levels.
Psyllium	Strong scientific evidence for modest reduction in total cholesterol and LDLs.
Plant sterols	Strong scientific evidence for reduction of total cholesterol.
Red yeast rice	Strong scientific evidence for reduction of total cholesterol, LDLs, and triglycerides.
Soy	Strong scientific evidence for moderate reduction in total cholesterol and LDLs.

Based on a systematic review of scientific literature. Available at *www.naturalstandard.com.*
*Cardiovascular disease is a serious health problem. Herbal or other natural therapy should not be initiated without consultation with a health care provider. This is especially important when conventional drug therapy for cardiovascular disease is also being used.

physical activity. The guidelines for treatment of high cholesterol focus on LDL levels. Serum lipid levels are reassessed after 6 weeks of diet therapy. If they remain elevated, additional dietary options (see the Complementary & Alternative Therapies box above) and drug therapy (Table 34-5) may be considered.

DRUGS THAT RESTRICT LIPOPROTEIN PRODUCTION. The statin drugs are the most widely used lipid-lowering drugs. These drugs inhibit the synthesis of cholesterol in the liver. An unexplained result of the inhibition of cholesterol synthesis is an increase in hepatic LDL receptors. Consequently, the liver is able to remove more LDLs from the blood. In addition, statins

TABLE 34-5 DRUG THERAPY

Hyperlipidemia

Drug	Mechanism of Action	Side Effects	Nursing Considerations
Restrict Lipoprotein Production			
HMG-CoA Reductase Inhibitors (Statins)			
atorvastatin (Lipitor) fluvastatin (Lescol) lovastatin (Mevacor) pitavastatin (Livalo) pravastatin (Pravachol) simvastatin (Zocor) rosuvastatin (Crestor)	Block synthesis of cholesterol and increase LDL receptors in liver ↓ LDL ↓ Triglycerides ↑ HDL	Rash, GI disturbances, elevated liver enzymes, myopathy, rhabdomyolysis	Well tolerated with few side effects. Monitor liver enzymes and creatine kinase (if muscle weakness or pain occurs).
Niacin			
niacin (Nicobid, Niaspan) nicotinic acid (Slo-Niacin, Novo-Niacin)	Inhibits synthesis and secretion of VLDL and LDL ↓ LDL ↓ Triglycerides ↑ HDL	Flushing and pruritus in upper torso and face, GI disturbances (e.g., nausea and vomiting, dyspepsia, diarrhea), orthostatic hypotension, elevated homocysteine levels	Most side effects subside with time. Decreased liver function may occur with high doses. Taking aspirin or NSAID 30 min before drug may prevent flushing. Take drug with food. Treat elevated homocysteine levels with folic acid.
Fibric Acid Derivatives			
fenofibrate (TriCor) gemfibrozil (Lopid)	Decrease hepatic synthesis and secretion of VLDL. Reduce triglycerides by ↓ VLDL ↓ LDL ↓ Triglycerides ↑ HDL	Rashes, mild GI disturbances (e.g., nausea, diarrhea), elevated liver enzymes	May ↑ effects of warfarin (Coumadin) and some antihyperglycemic drugs. When used in combination with statins, may increase adverse effects of statins, especially myopathy.
Omega-3 Fatty Acid			
icosapent ethyl (Vascepa)	Inhibits synthesis and/or secretion of triglycerides	Arthralgia	Used for patients with severe hypertriglyceridemia (levels ≥500 mg/dL).
Increase Lipoprotein Removal			
Bile-Acid Sequestrants			
cholestyramine (Questran) colesevelam (WelChol) colestipol (Colestid)	Bind with bile acids in intestine, forming insoluble complex and excreted in feces Binding results in removal of LDL and cholesterol ↓ LDL	Unpleasant quality to taste, GI disturbances (e.g., indigestion, constipation, bloating)	Effective and safe for long-term use. Side effects diminish with time. Interfere with absorption of many drugs (e.g., digoxin, thiazide diuretics, warfarin, some antibiotics [e.g., penicillins]).
Decrease Cholesterol Absorption			
Cholesterol Absorption Inhibitor			
ezetimibe (Zetia)	Inhibits the intestinal absorption of cholesterol ↓ LDL ↑ HDL	Infrequent, but may include headache and mild GI distress	When used with a statin, LDL is further reduced. Should not be used by patients with liver impairment.

produce a small increase in HDLs and lower CRP levels.[15] Serious adverse effects of these drugs are rare and include liver damage and myopathy that can progress to rhabdomyolysis (breakdown of skeletal muscle). Liver enzymes (e.g., aspartate aminotransferase, alanine aminotransferase) are initially monitored and rechecked with any increase in dosage. Creatine kinase isoenzymes (e.g., CK-MM) are assessed if symptoms of myopathy (e.g., muscle aches, weakness) occur.[15]

DRUG ALERT
Simvastatin (Zocor)
- Increased risk for rhabdomyolysis when also used with gemfibrozil (Lopid) or niacin (Niaspan)
- Signs of rhabdomyolysis: ↑ creatine kinase levels, muscle tenderness

Niacin, a water-soluble B vitamin, is highly effective in lowering LDL and triglyceride levels by interfering with their synthesis. Niacin also increases HDL levels better than many other

lipid-lowering drugs. Unfortunately, side effects of this drug are common and may include severe flushing, pruritus, gastrointestinal (GI) symptoms, and orthostatic hypotension.

DRUG ALERT
Niacin (Niaspan)
- Instruct patient that flushing (especially of face and neck) may occur within 20 minutes after taking drug and may last for 30 to 60 minutes.
- Patient can premedicate with aspirin or nonsteroidal antiinflammatory drug (NSAID) 30 minutes before administration to reduce flushing.
- Use of extended-release niacin may decrease side effects.

The *fibric acid derivatives* (see Table 34-5) work by aiding the removal of VLDLs and increasing the production of apolipoproteins A-I and A-II. They are the most effective drugs for lowering triglycerides and increasing HDL levels. They have no effect on LDLs. Although most patients tolerate the drugs well, complaints may include GI irritability. These drugs should be used with caution when combined with statin medications.

DRUGS THAT INCREASE LIPOPROTEIN REMOVAL. The major route of elimination of cholesterol is by conversion to bile acids in the liver. Bile-acid sequestrants increase conversion of cholesterol to bile acids and decrease hepatic cholesterol. The primary effect is a decrease in total cholesterol and LDLs.

Administration of these drugs can be associated with complaints related to taste and a variety of upper and lower GI symptoms. These include belching, heartburn, nausea, abdominal pain, and constipation. The bile-acid sequestrants interfere with absorption of many other drugs (e.g., warfarin, thiazides, thyroid hormones, β-adrenergic blockers). Separating the time of administration of these drugs from that of other drugs decreases this adverse effect.[15]

DRUGS THAT DECREASE CHOLESTEROL ABSORPTION. Ezetimibe (Zetia) selectively inhibits the absorption of dietary and biliary cholesterol across the intestinal wall. It serves as an adjunct to dietary changes, especially in patients with primary hypercholesterolemia. When it is combined with a statin (e.g., ezetimibe and simvastatin [Vytorin]), even greater reductions in LDLs are found.

Drug therapy for hyperlipidemia often continues for a lifetime. New combination drug therapy (e.g., atorvastatin/ezetimibe [Liptruzet]) is available and may be considered. Concurrent diet modification is essential to minimize the need for drug therapy. The patient must fully understand the rationale and goals of treatment, as well as the safety and side effects of lipid-lowering drug therapy.

ANTIPLATELET THERAPY

Unless contraindicated (e.g., history of GI bleeding), low-dose aspirin (81 mg) is recommended for most people at risk for CAD (see eFig. 34-5, What you need to know—antiplatelet therapy, available on the website for this chapter). Current recommendations include low-dose aspirin for men over 45 years and high-risk women (i.e., those with a calculated 10-year CAD risk of more than 20%) unless contraindicated. For high-risk women who are intolerant of aspirin, clopidogrel (Plavix) can be substituted. In healthy women 65 years or older, aspirin therapy should be considered if BP is controlled and the benefit for MI prevention outweighs the risk of GI bleed or hemorrhagic stroke.[16]

GERONTOLOGIC CONSIDERATIONS

CORONARY ARTERY DISEASE

The incidence of cardiac disease is greatly increased in older adults and is the leading cause of death in older persons.[1] In the older adult, CAD is often a result of the complex interaction of nonmodifiable risk factors (e.g., age) and lifelong modifiable risk behaviors (e.g., inactivity, tobacco use). Strategies to reduce CAD risk and to treat CAD are effective in this age-group.[16]

Aggressive treatment of hypertension and hyperlipidemia stabilizes plaques in the coronary arteries of older adults, and cessation of tobacco use helps decrease the risk for CAD at any age.[16] Similarly, encourage the older patient to consider a planned program of physical activity. Activity performance, endurance, and ability to tolerate stress are improved in the older adult with physical training. Positive psychologic benefits from physical activity can include increased self-esteem and emotional well-being and improved body image. For the older adult who is obese, making modest dietary changes and slowly increasing physical activity (e.g., walking) results in more positive benefits than aiming for a significant weight loss.

When planning a physical activity program for the older adult, recommend the following: (1) longer warm-up periods, (2) longer periods of low-level activity, or (3) longer rest periods between sessions. Heat intolerance in the older adult results from a decreased ability to sweat efficiently. Teach the patient to avoid physical activity in extremes of temperature and to maintain a moderate pace. The older adult should exercise a minimum of 30 minutes on most days of the week as able.[9]

Encouraging the older patient to adopt a healthy lifestyle may increase the quality of life and reduce the risk of CAD and fatal cardiac events. Older adults face many of the same challenges as younger persons when it comes to making lifestyle changes. Older adults are more likely to consider change at two points in time: (1) when hospitalized and (2) when symptoms (e.g., chest pain) are the result of CAD and not normal aging (see Table 32-1). First, assess the older adult for readiness to change, and then help the patient select the lifestyle changes most likely to produce the greatest reduction in risk for CAD.

CHRONIC STABLE ANGINA

CAD is a progressive disease, and patients may be asymptomatic for many years or may develop chronic stable chest pain. When the demand for myocardial oxygen exceeds the ability of the coronary arteries to supply the heart with oxygen, *myocardial ischemia* occurs. Angina, or chest pain, is the clinical manifestation of reversible myocardial ischemia. Either an increased demand for oxygen or a decreased supply of oxygen can lead to myocardial ischemia (Table 34-6). The primary reason for insufficient blood flow is narrowing of coronary arteries by atherosclerosis. For ischemia secondary to atherosclerosis to occur, the artery is usually blocked (stenosed) 75% or more.

On the cellular level, the myocardium becomes hypoxic within the first 10 seconds of coronary occlusion. Myocardial cells are deprived of oxygen and glucose needed for aerobic

TABLE 34-6	FACTORS INFLUENCING MYOCARDIAL OXYGEN NEEDS*
Decreased Oxygen Supply	**Increased Oxygen Demand or Consumption**
Cardiac	
• Coronary artery spasm	• Aortic stenosis
• Coronary artery thrombosis	• Cardiomyopathy
• Dysrhythmias	• Dysrhythmias
• Heart failure	• Tachycardia
• Valve disorders	
Noncardiac	
• Anemia	• Anxiety
• Asthma	• Hypertension
• Chronic obstructive pulmonary disease	• Hyperthermia
• Hypovolemia	• Hyperthyroidism
• Hypoxemia	• Physical exertion
• Pneumonia	• Substance abuse (e.g., cocaine, ephedrine)

*Lists are not all-inclusive.

metabolism and contractility. Anaerobic metabolism begins, and lactic acid accumulates. Lactic acid irritates myocardial nerve fibers and transmits a pain message to the cardiac nerves and upper thoracic posterior nerve roots. This accounts for referred cardiac pain to the shoulders, neck, lower jaw, and arms. In ischemic conditions, cardiac cells are viable for approximately 20 minutes. With restoration of blood flow, aerobic metabolism resumes, contractility is restored, and cellular repair begins.

Chronic stable angina refers to chest pain that occurs intermittently over a long period with the same pattern of onset, duration, and intensity of symptoms. When questioned, some patients may deny feeling pain but describe a pressure or ache in the chest (Table 34-7). It is an unpleasant feeling, often described as a squeezing, heavy, choking, or suffocating sensation. Angina is rarely sharp or stabbing, and it usually does not change with position or breathing. Many people with angina complain of indigestion or a burning sensation in the epigastric region. Although most angina pain appears substernally, the sensation may occur in the neck or radiate to various locations, including the lower jaw, the shoulders, and the arms (Fig. 34-4). Often people complain of pain between the shoulder blades and dismiss it as not being heart related.

The pain usually lasts for only a few minutes (5 to 15 minutes) and commonly subsides when the precipitating factor is resolved (Table 34-8). Pain at rest is unusual. A 12-lead electrocardio-gram (ECG) often shows ST segment depression and/or T wave inversion indicating ischemia (see Chapter 36). The ECG returns to baseline when the pain is relieved.

Chronic stable angina is controlled with medications on an outpatient basis. Because chronic stable angina is often predictable, medications are timed to provide peak effects during the

---

TABLE 34-7   PQRST ASSESSMENT OF ANGINA

Use the following memory aid to obtain information from the patient who has chest pain.

	Factor	Questions to Ask Patient
P	Precipitating events	What events or activities precipitated the pain (e.g., argument, exercise, resting)?
Q	Quality of pain	What does the pain feel like (e.g., pressure, dull, aching, tight, squeezing, heaviness)?
R	Radiation of pain	Where is the pain located? Does the pain radiate to other areas (e.g., back, neck, arms, jaw, shoulder, elbow)?
S	Severity of pain	On a scale of 0 to 10 with 0 indicating no pain and 10 being the most severe pain you could imagine, what number would you give the pain?
T	Timing	When did the pain begin? Has the pain changed since this time? Have you had pain like this before?

TABLE 34-8   PRECIPITATING FACTORS OF ANGINA

Physical Exertion
- Increases HR, reducing the time the heart spends in diastole (the time of greatest coronary blood flow), resulting in an increase in myocardial oxygen demand.
- Isometric exercise of the arms (e.g., raking, lifting heavy objects, snow shoveling) can cause exertional angina.

Temperature Extremes
- Increase the workload of the heart.
- Blood vessels constrict in response to a cold stimulus.
- Blood vessels dilate and blood pools in the skin in response to a hot stimulus.

Strong Emotions
- Stimulate the sympathetic nervous system, activating the stress response.
- Increase the workload of the heart.

Consumption of Heavy Meal
- Can increase the workload of the heart.
- During the digestive process, blood is diverted to the GI system, reducing blood flow in the coronary arteries.

Tobacco Use, Environmental Tobacco Smoke
- Nicotine stimulates catecholamine release, causing vasoconstriction and an increased HR.
- Diminishes available oxygen by increasing the level of carbon monoxide.

Sexual Activity
- Increases the cardiac workload and sympathetic stimulation.
- In a person with CAD, the extra cardiac workload may precipitate angina.

Stimulants (e.g., cocaine, amphetamines)
- Increase HR and subsequent myocardial oxygen demand.

Circadian Rhythm Patterns
- Related to the occurrence of chronic stable angina, Prinzmetal's angina, MI, and sudden cardiac death.
- Manifestations of CAD tend to occur in the early morning after awakening.

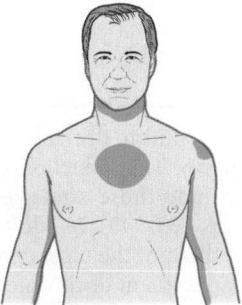

- Mid sternum
- Left shoulder and down both arms
- Neck and arms

- Substernal radiating to neck and jaw
- Substernal radiating down left arm

- Epigastric
- Epigastric radiating to neck, jaw, and arms

- Intrascapular

FIG. 34-4 Common locations and patterns of pain during angina or myocardial infarction.

TABLE 34-9 COMPARISON OF MAJOR TYPES OF ANGINA

Type	Etiology	Characteristics
Chronic stable angina	Myocardial ischemia, usually secondary to CAD	• Episodic pain lasting 5-15 min • Provoked by exertion • Relieved by rest or nitroglycerin
Prinzmetal's angina	Coronary vasospasm	• Occurs primarily at rest • Triggered by smoking and increased levels of some substances (e.g., histamine, epinephrine) • May occur in presence or absence of CAD
Microvascular angina	Myocardial ischemia secondary to microvascular disease affecting the small, distal branches of the coronary arteries	• More common in women • Triggered by activities of daily living (e.g., shopping, work) vs. physical exercise (exertion) • Treatment may include nitroglycerin
Unstable angina	Rupture of thickened plaque, exposing thrombogenic surface	• New-onset angina • Chronic stable angina that increases in frequency, duration, or severity • Occurs at rest or with minimal exertion • Pain refractory to nitroglycerin

TABLE 34-10 TREATMENT OF CHRONIC STABLE ANGINA

Strategies for the patient with chronic stable angina should address all the treatment elements and related patient teaching in the following mnemonic:*

Element	Treatment
A	Antiplatelet/anticoagulant therapy Antianginal therapy ACE inhibitor/angiotensin receptor blocker
B	β-adrenergic blocker Blood pressure control
C	Cigarette smoking cessation Cholesterol (lipid) management Calcium channel blockers Cardiac rehabilitation
D	Diet (weight management) Diabetes management Depression screening
E	Education Exercise
F	Flu vaccination

*Modified from Smith SC, Benjamin EJ, Bonow RO, et al: AHA/ACCF secondary prevention and risk reduction therapy for patients with coronary and other atherosclerotic vascular disease: 2011 update, *J Am Coll Cardiol* 58:2432, 2011.

time of day when angina is likely to occur. For example, if angina occurs when rising, the patient can take medication as soon as awakening and wait 30 minutes to 1 hour before engaging in activity. (See Table 34-9 for a comparison of the major types of angina.)

Silent Ischemia

Silent ischemia refers to ischemia that occurs in the absence of any subjective symptoms. Patients with diabetes have an increased prevalence of silent ischemia. This is most likely due to diabetic neuropathy affecting the nerves that innervate the cardiovascular system. When patients are monitored (e.g., Holter monitor) and silent ischemia occurs, ECG changes are revealed. Ischemia with pain or without pain has the same prognosis.

Nocturnal Angina and Angina Decubitus

Nocturnal angina occurs only at night but not necessarily when the person is in the recumbent position or during sleep. *Angina decubitus* is chest pain that occurs only while the person is lying down and is usually relieved by standing or sitting.

Prinzmetal's Angina

Prinzmetal's angina *(variant angina)* often occurs at rest, usually in response to spasm of a major coronary artery. It is a rare form of angina frequently seen in patients with a history of migraine headaches and Raynaud's phenomenon. The spasm may occur in the absence or presence of CAD. Prinzmetal's angina is not usually precipitated by increased physical demand. Strong contraction (spasm) of smooth muscle in the coronary artery results from increased intracellular calcium.

Factors causing coronary artery spasm include increased myocardial oxygen demand and increased levels of certain substances (e.g., tobacco smoke, alcohol, amphetamines). When spasm occurs, the patient experiences angina and transient ST segment elevation (see Chapter 36). The pain may occur during rapid-eye-movement (REM) sleep when myocardial oxygen consumption increases. The pain may be relieved by moderate exercise, or it may disappear spontaneously. Cyclic, short bursts of pain at a usual time each day may also occur with this type of angina. Calcium channel blockers and/or nitrates are used to control the angina.

Microvascular Angina

In *microvascular angina*, chest pain occurs in the absence of significant coronary atherosclerosis or coronary spasm, especially in women.[2] In these patients, chest pain is related to myocardial ischemia associated with abnormalities of the coronary microcirculation. This is known as coronary microvascular disease (MVD).

Coronary MVD affects the small branches of the distal coronary arteries, whereas CAD affects larger coronary arteries. In coronary MVD, plaque can be diffuse, be evenly distributed, or develop as blockages in the tiny coronary arteries. Prevention and treatment of coronary MVD follow the same recommendations as for CAD.[2]

COLLABORATIVE CARE CHRONIC STABLE ANGINA

The treatment of chronic stable angina aims to decrease oxygen demand and/or increase oxygen supply. The reduction of risk factors is a priority and should include those strategies discussed for patients with CAD (see pp. 735-740). In addition to antiplatelet and lipid-lowering drug therapy, the most common therapeutic interventions for the management of chronic stable angina are the use of nitrates, angiotensin-converting enzyme (ACE) inhibitors, β-adrenergic blockers, and calcium channel blockers to optimize myocardial perfusion[17] (Table 34-10 and Fig. 34-5).

FIG. 34-5 Collaborative care: chronic stable angina and acute coronary syndrome. *ACE,* Angiotensin-converting enzyme; *ARBs,* angiotensin II receptor blockers; *CK,* creatine kinase.

*, see Table 34-11.

†, see Table 34-5.

‡, see Tables 34-2, 34-3, and 34-4.

Drug Therapy

Drug therapy for chronic stable angina aims to prevent MI and death, and reduce symptoms. Aspirin (previously discussed) is given in the absence of contraindications (Table 34-11).

Short-Acting Nitrates. Short-acting nitrates are first-line therapy for the treatment of angina. Nitrates produce their principal effects by the following mechanisms:

Dilating peripheral blood vessels: This results in decreased SVR, venous pooling, and decreased venous blood return to the heart (preload). Therefore myocardial oxygen demand is decreased because of the reduced cardiac workload.

Dilating coronary arteries and collateral vessels: This may increase blood flow to the ischemic areas of the heart. However, when the coronary arteries are severely atherosclerotic, coronary dilation is difficult to achieve.

Sublingual Nitroglycerin. Nitroglycerin (NTG) given sublingually (Nitrostat) or by translingual spray (Nitrolingual) usually relieves pain in about 3 minutes and has a duration of approximately 30 to 40 minutes. The recommended dose for the patient who has been prescribed NTG is one tablet taken sublingually (SL) or one metered spray for symptoms of angina. If symptoms are unchanged or worse after 5 minutes, tell the patient or caregiver to repeat NTG every 5 minutes for a maximum of three doses and contact EMS if symptoms have not resolved completely.[17]

Instruct the patient in the proper use of NTG. It should be easily accessible to the patient at all times. The patient should store the tablets away from light and heat sources, including body heat, to protect them from degradation. Tablets are packaged in light-resistant bottles with metal caps. Once opened, the tablets lose potency and should be replaced every 6 months.

Tell the patient to place a NTG tablet under the tongue and allow it to dissolve. If using the spray, the patient should direct it on the tongue, not inhale it. NTG should cause a tingling sensation when administered; otherwise it may be outdated. Warn the patient that a headache, dizziness, or flushing may occur. Caution the patient to change positions slowly after NTG use because orthostatic hypotension may occur.

Patients can use NTG prophylactically before starting an activity that is known to cause an anginal attack. In these cases the patient can take a tablet or spray 5 to 10 minutes before beginning the activity. Instruct the patient to report any changes in the usual pattern of pain, especially increasing frequency or nocturnal angina, to the health care provider.

Long-Acting Nitrates. Nitrates, such as isosorbide dinitrate (Isordil) and isosorbide mononitrate (Imdur), are longer acting than SL or translingual NTG. They are used to reduce the incidence of anginal attacks. The main side effect of all nitrates is headache from the dilation of cerebral blood vessels. Advise patients to take acetaminophen (Tylenol) with their nitrate to relieve the headache. Over time, the headaches may decrease, but the antianginal effect is still present.

TABLE 34-11   DRUG THERAPY

Chronic Stable Angina and Acute Coronary Syndrome

Drug	Mechanism of Action and Comments	Drug	Mechanism of Action and Comments
Antiplatelet Agents		**Nitrates**	
aspirin	• Inhibits cyclooxygenase, which in turn produces thromboxane A$_2$, a potent platelet activator • Should be administered as soon as ACS is suspected	Sublingual nitroglycerin (Nitrostat) Translingual spray nitroglycerin (Nitrolingual) nitroglycerin ointment (Nitro-Bid) Transdermal nitroglycerin (Transderm-Nitro) isosorbide dinitrate (Isordil) IV nitroglycerin (Tridil)	• Promote peripheral vasodilation, decreasing preload and afterload • Promote coronary artery vasodilation
clopidogrel (Plavix)	• Inhibits platelet aggregation • Alternative for patient who cannot use aspirin or used in combination with aspirin		
prasugrel (Effient)	• Inhibits platelet aggregation • Used as an alternative to clopidogrel or used in combination with aspirin	**Angiotensin-Converting Enzyme (ACE) Inhibitors†**	
ticagrelor (Brilinta)	• Inhibits platelet aggregation • Alternative for patient who cannot use aspirin • If used in combination with aspirin, effectiveness may be decreased by aspirin dosages >100 mg/day (according to a boxed warning)	captopril (Capoten) enalapril (Vasotec) lisinopril (Zestril)	• Prevent conversion of angiotensin I to angiotensin II, resulting in vasodilation • May prevent or limit ventricular remodeling • Decrease endothelial dysfunction • Useful with heart failure, tachycardia, MI, hypertension, diabetes, and chronic kidney disease
Glycoprotein IIb/IIIa Inhibitors		**Angiotensin II Receptor Blockers†**	
abciximab (ReoPro) eptifibatide (Integrilin) tirofiban (Aggrastat)	• Prevent the binding of fibrinogen to platelets, thereby blocking platelet aggregation • Standard antiplatelet therapy in combination with aspirin for patients at high risk for unstable angina	losartan (Cozaar) valsartan (Diovan)	• Inhibit binding of angiotensin II to angiotensin I receptors, resulting in vasodilation • Used for patients intolerant of ACE inhibitors
Anticoagulant Agents **Unfractionated Heparin***		**β-Adrenergic Blockers†**	
heparin (Hep-Lock)	• Prevents conversion of fibrinogen to fibrin and prothrombin to thrombin	atenolol (Tenormin) carvedilol (Coreg) metoprolol (Lopressor) nadolol (Corgard)	• Inhibit sympathetic nervous stimulation of the heart • Reduce heart rate, contractility, and blood pressure • Decrease afterload
Low-Molecular-Weight Heparin*		**Calcium Channel Blockers†**	
dalteparin (Fragmin) enoxaparin (Lovenox)	• Bind to antithrombin III, enhancing its effect • Heparin–antithrombin III complex inactivates activated factor X and thrombin • Prevent conversion of fibrinogen to fibrin	amlodipine (Norvasc) diltiazem (Cardizem) felodipine (Plendil) nicardipine (Cardene) verapamil (Calan)	• Prevent calcium entry into vascular smooth muscle cells and myocytes (cardiac cells) • May prevent or control coronary vasospasm • Promote coronary and peripheral vasodilation • Reduce heart rate, contractility, and blood pressure
Vitamin K Antagonist*		**Opioid Analgesics**	
warfarin (Coumadin)	• Interferes with hepatic synthesis of vitamin K–dependent clotting factors • Alternative for patient who cannot use aspirin or clopidogrel	morphine (morphine sulfate)	• Functions as an analgesic and sedative • Acts as a vasodilator to reduce preload and myocardial O$_2$ consumption
Direct Thrombin Inhibitors		**Thrombolytic Agents**	
bivalirudin (Angiomax) argatroban (Acova)	• Direct inhibition of the clotting factor thrombin	reteplase (Retavase) alteplase (Activase) tenecteplase (TNKase)	• Breaks up fibrin meshwork in clots • Used only in ST-segment-elevation MI

*See Table 38-10.
†See Table 33-7.

Orthostatic hypotension is a complication of all nitrates. Monitor BP after the initial dose, since the venous dilation that occurs may cause a drop in BP, especially in volume-depleted patients. To limit this, patients are often scheduled an 8-hour nitrate-free period every day, usually during the night, unless the patient experiences nocturnal angina.[15] Finally, tolerance to NTG-induced vasodilation can develop.

Nitroglycerin Ointment. Nitropaste is a 2% NTG topical ointment dosed by the inch. It is placed on the upper body or arm, over a flat muscular area that is free of hair and scars. Once absorbed, it produces anginal prophylaxis for 3 to 6 hours. It is especially useful for nocturnal and unstable angina.

Transdermal Controlled-Release Nitrates. Currently two systems are available for transdermal NTG drug administration: reservoir and matrix. The reservoir system delivers the drug using a rate-controlled permeable membrane. The matrix system provides for a slow delivery of the drug through a polymer matrix. Both reservoir and matrix delivery systems offer the advantages of steady plasma levels within the therapeutic range during 24 hours, thus making only one application a day necessary. The reservoir system has the disadvantage of dose dumping if the reservoir seal is punctured or broken. An advantage of the matrix system is that there can be no dose dumping. Both systems achieve steady plasma levels by 2 hours.

DRUG ALERT
Nitroglycerin
- SL tablet must be administered under the tongue. Translingual NTG should be sprayed on the tongue.
- Instruct patient not to combine with drugs used for erectile dysfunction (e.g., sildenafil [Viagra]).
- Monitor for orthostatic hypotension because it may occur after administration.
- Use gloves to apply and remove NTG ointment or transdermal patch to avoid contact with medication.
- Never discharge cardioverter-defibrillator over NTG ointment or transdermal patch.

Angiotensin-Converting Enzyme Inhibitors. Patients with chronic stable angina who are considered high risk for a cardiac event (e.g., ejection fraction [EF] 40% or less, history of diabetes) should take an ACE inhibitor (e.g., captopril [Capoten]) indefinitely.[17] ACE inhibitors are also used for lower risk patients (e.g., patients with mildly reduced EF).

These drugs result in vasodilation and reduced blood volume. Most important, they can prevent or reverse ventricular remodeling (see p. 748). For patients who are intolerant of ACE inhibitors, angiotensin II receptor blockers (e.g., losartan [Cozaar]) are used. (ACE inhibitors and angiotensin II receptor blockers are discussed later in the chapter and in Chapter 33 and Table 33-7.)

β-Adrenergic Blockers. Patients who have left ventricular dysfunction, have elevated BP, or have had an MI should start and continue β-adrenergic blockers indefinitely.[17] These drugs decrease myocardial contractility, HR, SVR, and BP, all of which reduce the myocardial oxygen demand.

β-Adrenergic blockers have many side effects and can be poorly tolerated. Side effects may include bradycardia, hypotension, wheezing, and GI complaints. Many patients also complain of weight gain, depression, and sexual dysfunction. Patients with asthma should avoid β-adrenergic blockers. They are used cautiously in patients with diabetes, since they mask signs of hypoglycemia. β-Adrenergic blockers should not be discontinued abruptly without medical supervision. This may precipitate an increase in the frequency and intensity of angina attacks.

Calcium Channel Blockers. If β-adrenergic blockers are contraindicated, are poorly tolerated, or do not control anginal symptoms, calcium channel blockers are used.[17] These drugs are also used to manage Prinzmetal's angina. The three primary effects of calcium channel blockers are (1) systemic vasodilation with decreased SVR, (2) decreased myocardial contractility, and (3) coronary vasodilation. Most of these agents have sustained-release versions for longer action with the hope of increased patient adherence and stable blood levels of the drug.

Cardiac muscle and vascular smooth muscle cells are more dependent on extracellular calcium than skeletal muscles. Therefore these cells are more sensitive to calcium channel blocking agents. Calcium channel blockers cause smooth muscle relaxation and relative vasodilation of coronary and systemic arteries, thus increasing blood flow.

Calcium channel blockers potentiate the action of digoxin by increasing serum digoxin levels. Therefore serum digoxin levels should be closely monitored after starting calcium channel blockers. Teach the patient the signs and symptoms of digoxin toxicity (see Chapter 35).

Sodium Current Inhibitor. Ranolazine (Ranexa), a sodium current inhibitor, is used to treat chronic angina in those patients who have not achieved adequate response with other antianginals.[17] Because ranolazine prolongs the QT interval, patients with a long QT interval or who are taking QT-prolonging drugs (e.g., fluoxetine [Prozac]) should not use it. Common side effects of ranolazine include dizziness, nausea, constipation, and generalized weakness.[15]

Diagnostic Studies
When a patient has a history of CAD or CAD is suspected, a variety of studies are completed (see Fig. 34-5). After a detailed health history and physical examination, a chest x-ray is done to look for cardiac enlargement, aortic calcifications, and pulmonary congestion. A 12-lead ECG is obtained and compared with a previous tracing when possible. Certain laboratory tests (e.g., lipid profile) and diagnostic studies (e.g., echocardiogram) are done to confirm CAD and identify specific risk factors for CAD.

Measurement of coronary calcification can be useful for predicting adverse cardiac events. The degree of coronary artery calcification correlates with the severity of CAD. The calcium-score screening heart scan locates calcium deposits in atherosclerotic plaque in the coronary arteries (see Fig. 32-11). However, additional testing (e.g., stress testing) is needed to know the impact of the lesion on coronary blood flow.

For patients with known CAD and chronic stable angina, common diagnostic studies include 12-lead ECG, echocardiogram, exercise stress testing, and pharmacologic nuclear imaging. (See Chapter 32 and Table 32-6 for a discussion of these studies, including nursing considerations.)

Cardiac Catheterization. For patients with increasing symptoms or with a significant amount of myocardium that is ischemic under stress, a cardiac catheterization is ordered. Cardiac catheterization and coronary angiography provide images of the coronary circulation and identify the location and severity of any blockage.

If a coronary blockage is amenable to an intervention, coronary revascularization with an elective percutaneous coronary intervention (PCI) is done.[17] During this procedure,

Does Timing of Ambulation Affect Patient Safety After Percutaneous Coronary Intervention?

Clinical Question

Among patients following percutaneous coronary interventions (P), what is the effect of ambulation (I) early versus late (T) on bleeding and hematoma (O)?

Best Available Evidence

Meta-analysis of randomized controlled trials (RCTs)

Critical Appraisal and Synthesis of Evidence

- Five RCTs (*n* = 1854) of patients comparing safety of early versus late ambulation after percutaneous coronary interventions (PCIs) using a femoral artery approach.
- Early ambulation was 2-4 hr after bed rest, with late ambulation 6-20 hr after bed rest.
- Outcomes assessed were hematoma or bleeding.
- Early ambulation was not more harmful than late ambulation.

Conclusion

- Reducing bed rest time from 6-10 hr down to 2-4 hr after PCI is safe.

Implications for Nursing Practice

- Inform nursing personnel that it is safe to ambulate patients 2-4 hr after PCI is done via a femoral artery approach.
- After PCI monitor patients for signs of bleeding at the puncture site.

Reference for Evidence

Tongsai S, Thamlikitkul V: The safety of early versus late ambulation in the management of patients after percutaneous coronary interventions: a meta-analysis, *Int J Nurs Stud* 49(9):1084, 2012.

P, Patient population of interest; *I*, intervention or area of interest; *C*, comparison of interest or comparison group; *O*, outcomes of interest; *T*, timing (see p. 12).

FIG. 34-6 Placement of a coronary artery stent. **A**, The stent is positioned at the site of the lesion. **B**, The balloon is inflated, expanding the stent. The balloon is then deflated and removed. **C**, The implanted stent is left in place.

FIG. 34-7 A, A thrombotic occlusion of the right coronary artery is noted *(arrows)*. **B**, Right coronary artery is opened and blood flow restored following angioplasty and placement of a 4-mm stent.

a catheter with an inflatable balloon tip is inserted into the appropriate coronary artery. When the blockage is located, the catheter is passed through it, the balloon is inflated, and the atherosclerotic plaque is compressed, resulting in vessel dilation. This procedure is called *balloon angioplasty.*

Intracoronary stents are often inserted in conjunction with balloon angioplasty. Stents are used to treat abrupt or threatened abrupt closure and restenosis following balloon angioplasty. A **stent** is an expandable meshlike structure designed to keep the vessel open by compressing the arterial wall (Figs. 34-6 and 34-7). Because stents are thrombogenic, unfractionated heparin (UH) or low-molecular-weight heparin (LMWH) is started to maintain the open vessel. In addition, a direct thrombin inhibitor (e.g., bivalirudin [Angiomax]) and/or a glycoprotein IIb/IIIa inhibitor (e.g., tirofiban [Aggrastat]) is also used during PCI to help prevent the abrupt closure of the stents (see Table 34-11). After PCI, the patient is treated with dual antiplatelet agents (e.g., aspirin [indefinitely] and ticagrelor [Brilinta] for 12 months) until the intimal lining can grow over the stent and provide a smooth vascular surface.

Many stents are drug-eluting stents. This type of stent is coated with a drug (e.g., paclitaxel, sirolimus) that prevents the overgrowth of new intima, the primary cause of stent restenosis. Following drug-eluting stent placement, the patient continues dual antiplatelet therapy to prevent thrombus formation on the stent. Drug therapy may continue for 12 months or longer.[18]

The most serious complications from stent placement are abrupt closure and vascular injury. Other less common com-plications include acute MI, stent embolization, coronary spasm, and emergent coronary artery bypass graft (CABG) surgery. The possibility of dysrhythmias during and after the procedure is always present.

PCI may not be a feasible option for all patients (e.g., patients with three-vessel CAD [three different coronary arteries] and/or significant left main coronary artery disease). Coronary revascularization with CABG surgery may be recommended and is discussed later in the chapter.

ACUTE CORONARY SYNDROME

When ischemia is prolonged and not immediately reversible, **acute coronary syndrome (ACS)** develops and encompasses the spectrum of unstable angina (UA), *non–ST-segment-elevation myocardial infarction* (NSTEMI), and *ST-segment-elevation myocardial infarction* (STEMI) (Fig. 34-8). Although each remains a distinct diagnosis, this nomenclature (ACS) reflects the relationships among the pathophysiology, presentation, diagnosis, prognosis, and interventions for these disorders.

ACS is associated with deterioration of a once stable atherosclerotic plaque. The once stable plaque ruptures, exposing the intima to blood and stimulating platelet aggregation and local vasoconstriction with thrombus formation. This unstable lesion may be partially occluded by a thrombus (manifesting as UA or NSTEMI) or totally occluded by a thrombus (manifesting as

FIG. 34-8 Relationships among coronary artery disease, chronic stable angina, and acute coronary syndrome.

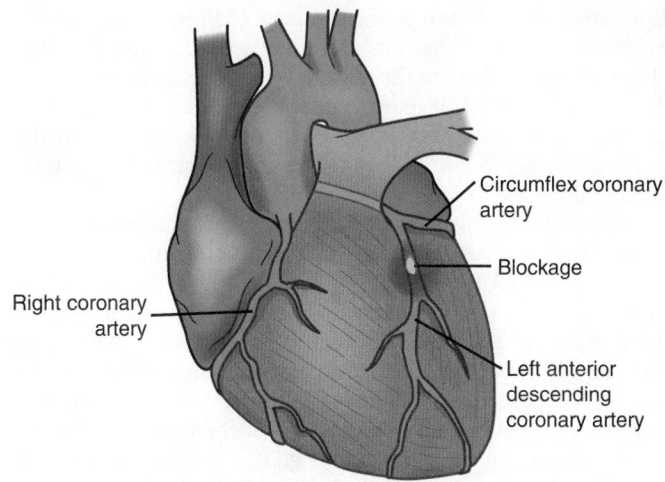

FIG. 34-9 Occlusion of the left anterior descending coronary artery, resulting in a myocardial infarction.

FIG. 34-10 Acute myocardial infarction in the posterolateral wall of the left ventricle. This is demonstrated by the absence of staining in the areas of necrosis *(white arrow)*. Note the scarring from a previous anterior wall myocardial infarction *(black arrow)*.

STEMI).[16] What causes a coronary plaque to suddenly become unstable is not well understood, but systemic inflammation (described earlier) is thought to play a role. Patients with suspected ACS require immediate hospitalization.

UNSTABLE ANGINA

Unstable angina (UA) is chest pain that is new in onset, occurs at rest, or has a worsening pattern. The patient with chronic stable angina may develop UA, or UA may be the first clinical sign of CAD. Unlike chronic stable angina, UA is unpredictable and is an emergency. The patient with previously diagnosed chronic stable angina describes a significant change in the pattern of angina. It occurs with increasing frequency and is easily provoked by minimal or no exertion, during sleep, or even at rest. The patient without previously diagnosed angina describes anginal pain that has progressed rapidly in the past few hours, days, or weeks, often ending in pain at rest.

Women seek medical attention for symptoms of UA more often than men. Despite national efforts to increase awareness, women's symptoms continue to go unrecognized as heart related. These symptoms include fatigue, shortness of breath, indigestion, and anxiety. Fatigue is the most prominent symptom. However, all these symptoms can relate to many different diseases and syndromes. Thus women often present with UA before CAD is diagnosed. (See Gender Differences box on p. 733 earlier in this chapter.)

MYOCARDIAL INFARCTION

A myocardial infarction (MI) occurs because of sustained ischemia, causing irreversible myocardial cell death (necrosis) (Figs. 34-9 and 34-10). Thrombus formation causes 80% to 90% of all acute MIs.[19] When a thrombus develops, there is no blood flow to the myocardium distal to the blockage, resulting in necrosis. Contractile function of the heart stops in the necrotic area(s). The degree of altered function depends on the area of the heart involved and the size of the infarction.

The acute MI process takes time. Cardiac cells can withstand ischemic conditions for approximately 20 minutes before cell death begins. The earliest tissue to become ischemic is the subendocardium (the innermost layer of tissue in the cardiac muscle). If ischemia persists, it takes approximately 4 to 6 hours for the entire thickness of the heart muscle to become necrosed. If the thrombus is not completely blocking the artery, the time to complete necrosis may be as long as 12 hours.

MIs are usually described based on the location of damage (e.g., anterior, inferior, lateral, septal, or posterior wall infarc-

tion). Most involve some portion of the left ventricle. The location of the infarction correlates with the involved coronary circulation. For example, the right coronary artery provides blood supply to the inferior wall. Blockage of the right coronary artery results in an inferior wall MI. Anterior wall infarctions result from blockages in the left anterior descending artery. Blockages in the left circumflex artery usually cause lateral and/or posterior wall MIs. Damage can occur in more than one location, especially if more than one coronary artery is involved (e.g., anterolateral MI, anteroseptal MI).

The degree of preexisting collateral circulation also influences the severity of infarction (see Fig. 34-2). An individual with a long history of CAD develops collateral circulation to provide the area surrounding the infarction site with a blood supply. This is one reason why a younger person may have a more serious first MI than an older person with the same degree of blockage.

Clinical Manifestations of Myocardial Infarction

Pain. Severe, immobilizing chest pain not relieved by rest, position change, or nitrate administration is the hallmark of an MI. Persistent and unlike any other pain, it is usually described as a heaviness, pressure, tightness, burning, constriction, or crushing. Common locations are substernal, retrosternal, or epigastric areas. When epigastric pain is present, the patient may relate it to indigestion and take antacids without relief. The pain may radiate to the neck, lower jaw, and arms or to the back (see Fig. 34-4). It may occur while the patient is active or at rest, asleep or awake. However, it commonly occurs in the early morning hours. It usually lasts for 20 minutes or longer and is more severe than usual anginal pain.

Not everyone has classic symptoms. Some patients may not experience pain but may have "discomfort," weakness, or shortness of breath. Although women and men have more similarities than differences in their acute MI symptoms, some women may experience atypical discomfort, shortness of breath, or fatigue.[20] Patients with diabetes may experience silent (asymptomatic) MIs because of cardiac neuropathy and may manifest atypical symptoms (e.g., dyspnea). An older patient may experience a change in mental status (e.g., confusion), shortness of breath, pulmonary edema, dizziness, or a dysrhythmia.

Sympathetic Nervous System Stimulation. During the initial phase of MI, the ischemic myocardial cells release catecholamines (norepinephrine and epinephrine) that are normally found in these cells. This results in release of glycogen, diaphoresis, and vasoconstriction of peripheral blood vessels. On physical examination, the patient's skin may be ashen, clammy, and cool to touch.

Cardiovascular Manifestations. In response to the release of catecholamines, BP and HR may be elevated initially. Later, the BP may drop because of decreased cardiac output (CO). If severe enough, this may result in decreased renal perfusion and urine output. Crackles, if present, may persist for several hours to several days, suggesting left ventricular dysfunction. Jugular venous distention, hepatic engorgement, and peripheral edema may indicate right ventricular dysfunction.

Cardiac examination may reveal abnormal heart sounds that may seem distant. Other abnormal sounds suggesting ventricular dysfunction are S_3 and S_4. In addition, a loud holosystolic murmur may develop and may indicate a septal defect, papillary muscle rupture, or valve dysfunction.

Nausea and Vomiting. The patient may experience nausea and vomiting. These symptoms can result from reflex stimulation of the vomiting center by the severe pain. They can also result from vasovagal reflexes initiated from the area of the infarcted myocardium.

Fever. The temperature may increase within the first 24 hours up to 100.4° F (38° C). The temperature elevation may last for as long as 1 week. This increase in temperature is due to a systemic inflammatory process caused by myocardial cell death.

Healing Process

The body's response to cell death is the inflammatory process (see Chapter 12). Within 24 hours, leukocytes infiltrate the area. The dead cardiac cells release enzymes that are important diagnostic indicators of MI. (See Serum Cardiac Markers later in this chapter.) The proteolytic enzymes of the neutrophils and macrophages begin to remove necrotic tissue by the fourth day. During this time the necrotic muscle wall is thin. The development of collateral circulation improves areas of poor perfusion and may limit the zones of injury and infarction. Once infarction takes place, catecholamine-mediated lipolysis and glycogenolysis occur. These processes allow the increased plasma glucose and free fatty acids to be used by the oxygen-depleted myocardium for anaerobic metabolism. For this reason, serum glucose levels are frequently elevated after MI.[19]

The necrotic zone is identifiable by ECG changes (e.g., ST segment elevation, pathologic Q wave) and by nuclear scanning after the onset of symptoms. At this point, the neutrophils and monocytes have cleared the necrotic debris from the injured area, and the collagen matrix that will eventually form scar tissue is laid down.

At 10 to 14 days after MI, the new scar tissue is still weak. The myocardium is vulnerable to increased stress during this time because of the unstable state of the healing heart wall. At the same time the patient's activity level may be increasing, so special caution and assessment are necessary. By 6 weeks after MI, scar tissue has replaced necrotic tissue and the injured area is considered healed. The scarred area is often less compliant than the surrounding area. This condition may be manifested by uncoordinated wall motion, ventricular dysfunction, altered conduction patterns, or heart failure (HF).

These changes in the infarcted muscle also cause changes in the unaffected myocardium. In an attempt to compensate for the damaged muscle, the normal myocardium hypertrophies and dilates. This process is called *ventricular remodeling*. Remodeling of normal myocardium can lead to the development of late HF, especially in the individual with atherosclerosis of other coronary arteries and/or an anterior MI.

Complications of Myocardial Infarction

Dysrhythmias. The most common complication after an MI is dysrhythmias, which are present in 80% to 90% of patients. Dysrhythmias are the most common cause of death in patients in the prehospital period. Any condition that affects the myocardial cell's sensitivity to nerve impulses (e.g., ischemia, electrolyte imbalances, SNS stimulation) can cause dysrhythmias. The intrinsic rhythm of the heart is disrupted. This can cause tachycardia, bradycardia, or an irregular HR, all of which adversely affect the ischemic myocardium.

Life-threatening dysrhythmias occur most often with anterior wall infarction, HF, or shock. Complete heart block develops when key portions of the conduction system are destroyed. Ventricular fibrillation, a common cause of sudden cardiac death (SCD), is a lethal dysrhythmia. It most often occurs within the first 4 hours after the onset of pain. Premature ventricular contractions may precede ventricular tachycardia and fibrillation. Life-threatening ventricular dysrhythmias must be treated immediately. (See Chapter 36 for a detailed description of dysrhythmias and their management.)

Heart Failure. *Heart failure* (HF) is a complication that occurs when the heart's pumping action is reduced. Depending on the severity and extent of the injury, HF occurs initially with subtle signs such as mild dyspnea, restlessness, agitation, or slight tachycardia. Other signs indicating the onset of HF include pulmonary congestion on chest x-ray, S_3 or S_4 heart sounds on auscultation, crackles on auscultation of breath sounds, and jugular venous distention. (The treatment of acute decompensated HF is discussed in Chapter 35.)

Cardiogenic Shock. *Cardiogenic shock* occurs when oxygen and nutrients supplied to the tissues are inadequate because of severe left ventricular failure. This occurs less often with the early and rapid treatment of MI with PCI or thrombolytic therapy. When cardiogenic shock does occur, it has a high mortality rate. Cardiogenic shock requires aggressive management. This includes control of dysrhythmias, intraaortic balloon pump (IABP) therapy, and support of contractility with vasoactive drugs. Goals of therapy are to maximize oxygen delivery, reduce oxygen demand, and prevent complications (e.g., acute kidney injury). (Cardiogenic shock is discussed in Chapter 67.)

Papillary Muscle Dysfunction. *Papillary muscle dysfunction* may occur if the infarcted area includes or is near the papillary muscle that attaches to the mitral valve (see Fig. 32-2). You should suspect papillary muscle dysfunction if you auscultate a new murmur at the cardiac apex. An echocardiogram confirms the diagnosis.

Papillary muscle rupture is a rare and life-threatening complication. It causes massive mitral valve regurgitation. Dyspnea, pulmonary edema, and decreased CO result from the back up of blood in the left atrium. This condition aggravates an already damaged left ventricle by reducing CO even further. The patient undergoes rapid clinical deterioration. Treatment includes rapid afterload reduction with nitroprusside (Nipride) and/or IABP therapy, and immediate cardiac surgery with mitral valve repair or replacement.[19] (See Chapter 37 for discussion of valve disorders.)

Ventricular Aneurysm. *Ventricular aneurysm* results when the infarcted myocardial wall is thin and bulges out during contraction. This can develop within a few days, weeks, or months. The patient with a ventricular aneurysm may experience HF, dysrhythmias, and angina. Besides ventricular rupture, which is fatal, ventricular aneurysms harbor thrombi that can lead to an embolic stroke.

Pericarditis. *Acute pericarditis,* an inflammation of the visceral and/or parietal pericardium, may result in cardiac tamponade, decreased ventricular filling and emptying, and HF. It occurs 2 or 3 days after an acute MI as a common complication of the infarction. Pericarditis is characterized by chest pain, which may vary from mild to severe and is aggravated by inspiration, coughing, and movement of the upper body. Sitting in a forward position often relieves the pain. The pain is usually different from pain associated with an MI.

Assess the patient with suspected pericarditis for the presence of a friction rub over the pericardium. The sound may be best heard with the diaphragm of the stethoscope at the mid to lower left sternal border. It may be persistent or intermittent. Fever may also be present. The patient may have hypotension and/or a narrow pulse pressure.

Diagnosis of pericarditis can be made with serial 12-lead ECGs. Typical ECG changes include diffuse ST-segment elevations. This reflects the inflammation of the pericardium. Treatment includes pain relief with NSAIDs, aspirin, or corticosteroids. (Chapter 37 discusses pericarditis.)

Dressler Syndrome. *Dressler syndrome* is pericarditis with effusion and fever that develops 4 to 6 weeks after MI. It may also occur after cardiac surgery. It is thought to be caused by an antigen-antibody reaction to the necrotic myocardium. The patient experiences pericardial pain, fever, a friction rub, pericardial effusion, and arthralgia. Laboratory findings include an elevated white blood cell count and sedimentation rate. Short-term corticosteroids are used to treat this condition.

DIAGNOSTIC STUDIES
ACUTE CORONARY SYNDROME

In addition to the patient's history of pain, risk factors, and health history, the primary diagnostic studies used to determine whether a person has UA or an MI include an ECG and serum cardiac markers (see Fig. 34-5).

Electrocardiogram Findings

The ECG is one of the primary tools to diagnose UA or an MI. Changes in the QRS complex, ST segment, and T wave caused by ischemia and infarction can develop quickly with UA and MI. For diagnostic and treatment purposes, it is important to distinguish between STEMI and UA or NSTEMI. Patients with STEMI tend to have a more extensive MI that is associated with prolonged and complete coronary occlusion; a pathologic Q wave is seen on the ECG. Patients with UA or NSTEMI usually have transient thrombosis or incomplete coronary occlusion and usually do not develop pathologic Q waves. Because MI is a dynamic process that evolves with time, the ECG often reveals the time sequence of ischemia, injury, infarction, and resolution of the infarction.

The ECG must be read carefully, since changes can be subtle at first. It may also be normal or nondiagnostic when the patient comes to the ED with a complaint of chest pain. Within a few hours, the ECG may change to reflect the infarction process. For this reason, when the initial 12-lead ECG is nondiagnostic, serial 12-lead ECGs are done. (See Chapter 36 for discussion of ECG changes associated with ischemia and MI.)

Serum Cardiac Markers

Serum cardiac markers are proteins released into the blood from necrotic heart muscle after an MI (see Table 32-6). These markers are important in the diagnosis of MI. The onset, peak, and duration of levels of these markers are shown in Fig. 34-11.

Cardiac-specific troponin has two subtypes: cardiac-specific troponin T (cTnT) and cardiac-specific troponin I (cTnI). These markers are highly specific indicators of MI and have greater sensitivity and specificity for myocardial injury than creatine kinase (CK) MB (CK-MB). Serum levels of cTnI and cTnT increase 4 to 6 hours after the onset of MI, peak at 10 to 24 hours, and return to baseline over 10 to 14 days.

CK levels begin to rise about 6 hours after an MI, peak at about 18 hours, and return to normal within 24 to 36 hours. The CK enzymes are fractionated into bands. The CK-MB band is specific to myocardial cells and also helps quantify myocardial damage.

Myoglobin is released into the circulation within 2 hours after an MI and peaks in 3 to 15 hours. Although it is one of

FIG. 34-11 Serum cardiac markers found in the blood after myocardial infarction.

TABLE 34-12   EMERGENCY MANAGEMENT
Chest Pain

Etiology	Assessment Findings	Interventions
Cardiovascular • Myocardial ischemia • Myocardial infarction • Dysrhythmia • Pericarditis • Aortic aneurysm • Aortic valve disease **Respiratory** • Costochondritis • Pleurisy • Pneumonia • Pneumothorax, hemothorax • Pulmonary edema • Pulmonary embolus **Chest Trauma** • Rib/sternal fracture • Flail chest • Cardiac tamponade • Hemothorax • Pulmonary contusion • Great vessel injury **Gastrointestinal** • Esophagitis • GERD • Hiatal hernia • Peptic ulcer • Cholecystitis **Others** • Stress • Strenuous exercise • Drugs (e.g., cocaine) • Acute anxiety	• Pain in chest, neck, jaw, arm, or shoulder • Cold, clammy skin • Diaphoresis • Nausea and vomiting • Epigastric pain • Indigestion, heartburn • Dyspnea, tachypnea • Weakness • Anxiety • Feeling of impending doom • Tachycardia, bradycardia • Irregular HR, murmurs • Palpitations • Dysrhythmias • Decreased or increased BP • Narrowed pulse pressure • Unequal BP readings in upper extremities • Syncope, loss of consciousness • Decreased O_2 saturation • Decreased or absent breath sounds • Pericardial friction rub	**Initial** • Assess ABCs. • Position patient upright unless contraindicated and administer O_2 by nasal cannula or non-rebreather mask. • Obtain baseline vital signs, including O_2 saturation. • Auscultate heart and breath sounds. • Obtain 12-lead ECG. • Insert two IV catheters. • Assess pain using PQRST mnemonic (see Table 34-7). • Medicate for pain as ordered (e.g., nitroglycerin, morphine). • Initiate continuous ECG monitoring and identify underlying rhythm. • Obtain baseline blood work (e.g., cardiac markers, serum electrolytes). • Obtain portable chest x-ray. • Assess for contraindications for antiplatelet, anticoagulant, or thrombolytic therapy, or PCI as appropriate. • Administer aspirin for cardiac-related chest pain unless contraindicated. • Administer antidysrhythmic drugs as indicated. **Ongoing Monitoring** • Monitor ABCs, vital signs, level of consciousness, heart and breath sounds, cardiac rhythm, and O_2 saturation. • Assess and record response to medications (e.g., decrease in chest pain) and remedicate or titrate medications (e.g., nitroglycerin) as needed. • Provide reassurance and emotional support to patient and caregiver. • Explain all interventions and procedures to patient and caregiver in simple terms. • Anticipate need for intubation if respiratory distress is evident. • Prepare for CPR and defibrillation if cardiac arrest is evident. • Anticipate need for transcutaneous pacing for symptomatic bradycardia or heart block.

ABCs, Airway, breathing, circulations; *GERD,* gastroesophageal reflux disease; *PCI,* percutaneous coronary intervention.

the first serum cardiac markers to appear after an MI, it lacks cardiac specificity. Its role in diagnosing MI is limited.

Coronary Angiography

The patient with UA or NSTEMI may or may not undergo coronary angiography to evaluate the extent of the disease. Guidelines suggest that it is reasonable to do coronary angiography on stable but high-risk patients with UA or NSTEMI. If appropriate, a PCI is performed at this time. Some patients may be treated with conservative medical management.[21,22] Coronary angiography is the only way to confirm the diagnosis of Prinzmetal's angina.

Other Measures

When the ECG and serum cardiac markers do not confirm MI, other measures for diagnosing UA are considered (see Table 32-6). Exercise or pharmacologic stress testing and echocardiogram are used when a patient has an abnormal but nondiagnostic baseline ECG. A dobutamine (Dobutrex), dipyridamole (Persantine), or adenosine (Adenocard) stress echocardiogram simulates the effects of exercise and is used in patients unable to exercise. (See Chapter 32 for additional information on cardiac assessment.)

COLLABORATIVE CARE
ACUTE CORONARY SYNDROME

It is extremely important to rapidly diagnose and treat a patient with ACS to preserve cardiac muscle. Initial management of the patient with chest pain most often occurs in the ED. Table 34-12 presents the emergency care of the patient with chest pain. Obtain a 12-lead ECG and start continuous ECG monitoring. Position the patient in an upright position unless contraindicated, and initiate oxygen by nasal cannula to keep oxygen saturation above 93%. Establish an IV route to provide an access for emergency drug therapy. Give SL NTG and aspirin (chewable) if not given before arrival at the ED. Morphine sulfate is given for pain unrelieved by NTG. The patient usually receives ongoing care in a critical care unit or telemetry unit, where continuous ECG monitoring is available. Dysrhythmias are treated according to established protocols. Fig. 34-5 on p. 743 presents the collaborative care of ACS.

Monitor vital signs, including pulse oximetry, frequently during the first few hours after admission and closely thereafter. Maintain bed rest and limit activity for 12 to 24 hours, with a gradual increase in activity unless contraindicated.

For patients with ongoing angina and negative cardiac markers, dual antiplatelet therapy (e.g., aspirin and ticagrelor) and heparin (UH or LMWH) is recommended. Coronary angiography with possible PCI is considered once the patient is stabilized and angina is controlled, or if angina returns or increases in severity.[21]

For patients with STEMI or NSTEMI with positive cardiac markers, reperfusion therapy is initiated (see Figs. 34-6 and 34-7). *Reperfusion therapy* can include emergent PCI for STEMI and NSTEMI or thrombolytic (fibrinolytic) therapy for STEMI. Coronary surgical revascularization is considered for select patients (e.g., patients with diabetes and three-vessel disease [involvement of three different coronary arteries]). The goal in the treatment of MI is to salvage as much myocardial muscle as possible.

Emergent PCI

Emergent PCI is the first line of treatment for patients with confirmed MI (i.e., definitive ECG changes and/or positive cardiac markers).[23] The goal is to open the blocked artery within 90 minutes of arrival to a facility that has an interventional cardiac catheterization laboratory. In this situation the patient undergoes a cardiac catheterization to locate the blockage(s), assess the severity of the blockage(s), determine the presence of collateral circulation, and evaluate left ventricular function. During the procedure, treatment modalities (e.g., placement of drug-eluting stents) are selected. Patients with severe ventricular dysfunction may require the addition of intraaortic balloon pump (IABP) therapy, and a small percentage of patients may require emergent CABG surgery.

The advantages of PCI include the following: (1) it provides an alternative to surgical intervention; (2) it is performed with local anesthesia; (3) the patient is ambulatory shortly after the procedure; (4) the length of hospital stay is approximately 1 to 3 days compared with the 4- to 6-day stay with CABG surgery, thus reducing hospital costs; and (5) the patient can return to work several weeks sooner after PCI, compared with a 6- to 8-week convalescence after CABG.

Advances in PCI techniques have significantly reduced the need for emergent CABG. Currently, more PCIs are performed than CABGs.[1] The most serious complication of PCI is dissection of the newly dilated coronary artery.[22] If the damage is extensive, the coronary artery could rupture, causing cardiac tamponade, ischemia and infarction, decreased CO, and possible death. There is also a danger that the infarction could be extended should a portion of the plaque dislodge and block the vessel distal to the catheter. Coronary spasm from the mechanical irritation of the catheter or balloon can occur, as well as chemical irritation from the contrast medium used to see the artery. Abrupt closure is a complication that can occur in the first 24 hours after PCI. Restenosis can also occur. Risk is greatest in the first 30 days after PCI. Nursing care of the patient following PCI is similar to that after cardiac catheterization (see Table 32-6).

Thrombolytic Therapy

Thrombolytic therapy offers the advantages of availability and rapid administration in facilities that do not have an interventional cardiac catheterization laboratory or when one is too far away to transfer the patient safely.[23] Treatment of MI with thrombolytic therapy aims to stop the infarction process by dissolving the thrombus in the coronary artery and reperfusing the myocardium. Thrombolytic therapy is given as soon as possible, ideally within the first hour and preferably within the first 6 hours after the onset of symptoms. Mortality is reduced by 25% if reperfusion occurs within 6 hours.[18,19]

Indications and Contraindications. All thrombolytics are given IV (see Table 34-11). The cost, efficacy, and ease of administration guide the choice of a thrombolytic agent. Although these drugs have different pharmacokinetics, they all open the blocked artery by lysis of the thrombus. The goal is to administer a thrombolytic within 30 minutes of the patient's arrival to a facility without an interventional cardiac catheterization laboratory. (PCI is first-line therapy in a facility with an interventional cardiac catheterization laboratory, as discussed above.)

Because all thrombolytics lyse the pathologic clot, they may also lyse other clots (e.g., a postoperative site). Therefore patient selection is important because minor or major bleeding can be a complication of therapy.[18] Inclusion criteria for thrombolytic therapy include (1) chest pain typical of acute MI 6 hours or less in duration, (2) 12-lead ECG findings consistent with acute MI, and (3) no absolute contraindications (Table 34-13). Although patients with chest pain lasting more than 6 hours and ECG changes supporting MI may be considered for thrombolytic therapy, benefits of this therapy are inconsistent.

Procedure. Each hospital has a protocol for giving thrombolytic therapy, but several factors are common. Draw blood to obtain baseline laboratory values and start two or three lines for IV therapy. All other invasive procedures are done before the thrombolytic agent is given to reduce the possibility of bleeding.

Depending on the drug selected, therapy is administered in one IV bolus or over time (30 to 90 minutes). Note the time at which therapy begins, and monitor the patient during and after administration of the thrombolytic. Evaluate heart rhythm, vital signs, and pulse oximetry and assess the heart and lungs frequently to evaluate the patient's response to therapy. Regularly assess for changes in neurologic status, since this may indicate a cerebral bleed.

TABLE 34-13	**CONTRAINDICATIONS FOR THROMBOLYTIC THERAPY**

Absolute Contraindications
- Active internal bleeding or bleeding diathesis (excluding menstruation)
- Known history of cerebral aneurysm or arteriovenous malformation
- Known intracranial neoplasm (primary or metastatic)
- Previous cerebral hemorrhage
- Recent (within past 3 mo) ischemic stroke
- Significant closed-head or facial trauma within past 3 mo
- Suspected aortic dissection

Relative Contraindications and Cautions
- Active peptic ulcer disease
- Current use of anticoagulants
- Pregnancy
- Prior ischemic stroke (>3 mo ago), dementia, or known intracranial pathologic condition not covered in absolute contraindications
- Recent (within 3 wk) surgery (including eye laser surgery) or puncture of noncompressible vessel
- Recent (within 2-4 wk) internal bleeding
- Serious systemic disease (e.g., advanced or terminal cancer, severe liver or kidney disease)
- Severe uncontrolled hypertension (BP >180/110 mm Hg) on presentation or chronic severe poorly controlled hypertension
- Traumatic or prolonged (>10 min) cardiopulmonary resuscitation

When reperfusion occurs (i.e., the coronary artery that was blocked is opened and blood flow is restored to the myocardium), several clinical markers may be seen. The most reliable marker is the return of the ST segment to baseline on the ECG. Other markers include a resolution of chest pain and an early, rapid rise of the serum cardiac markers within 3 hours of therapy, peaking within 12 hours. These levels increase as the necrotic myocardial cells release proteins into the circulation after perfusion is restored to the area. The presence of *reperfusion dysrhythmias* (e.g., accelerated idioventricular rhythm) is a less reliable marker of reperfusion. These dysrhythmias are generally self-limiting and do not require aggressive treatment. (See Chapter 36 for management of dysrhythmias.)

A major concern with thrombolytic therapy is reocclusion of the artery. The site of the thrombus is unstable, and formation of another clot or spasm of the artery may occur. Because of this possibility, IV heparin therapy is initiated. If another clot develops, the patient will have similar complaints of chest pain, and ECG changes will return. Patients receiving thrombolytic therapy should be transferred to a facility with PCI capabilities as soon as possible. This way, PCI can be performed if thrombolytic therapy fails.[18]

The major complication with thrombolytic therapy is bleeding. Ongoing nursing assessment is essential. Minor bleeding (e.g., surface bleeding from IV sites or gingival bleeding) is expected and controlled by applying a pressure dressing or ice packs.

SAFETY ALERT
- When thrombolytic therapy is used, bleeding may occur.
- If signs and symptoms of major bleeding occur (e.g., drop in BP, an increase in HR, a sudden change in the patient's level of consciousness, blood in the urine or stool), stop the therapy and notify the physician.

Coronary Surgical Revascularization

Coronary revascularization with CABG surgery is recommended for patients who (1) fail medical management, (2) have left main coronary artery or three-vessel disease, (3) are not candidates for PCI (e.g., lesions are long or difficult to access), (4) have failed PCI and continue to have chest pain, (5) have diabetes mellitus, or (6) are expected to have longer term benefits with CABG than with PCI.[24]

Coronary Artery Bypass Graft Surgery. CABG surgery consists of the placement of conduits to transport blood between the aorta, or other major arteries, and the myocardium distal to the blocked coronary artery (or arteries). The procedure may involve one or more grafts using the internal mammary artery, saphenous vein, radial artery, gastroepiploic artery, and/or inferior epigastric artery (Fig. 34-12).

CABG surgery requires a sternotomy (opening of the chest cavity) and *cardiopulmonary bypass* (CPB). During CPB, blood is diverted from the patient's heart to a machine where it is oxygenated and returned (via a pump) to the patient. This allows the surgeon to operate on a quiet, nonbeating, bloodless heart while perfusion to vital organs is maintained.

The internal mammary artery (IMA) is the most common artery used for bypass graft. It is left attached to its origin (the subclavian artery) but then dissected from the chest wall. Next, it is *anastomosed* (connected with sutures) to the coronary artery distal to the blockage. The long-term patency rate for IMA grafts is greater than 90% after 10 years.[24]

Saphenous veins are also used for bypass grafts. The surgeon removes the saphenous vein from one or both legs endoscopically. Sections are attached to the ascending aorta and then to

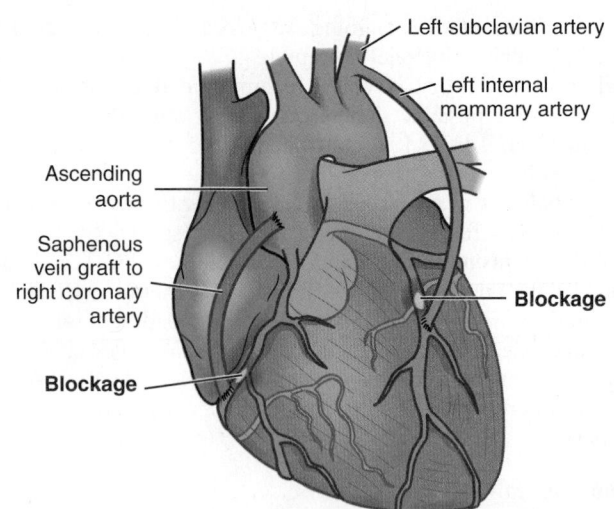

FIG. 34-12 Distal end of the left internal mammary artery is grafted below the area of blockage in the left anterior descending artery. Proximal end of the saphenous vein is grafted to the aorta, and the distal end is grafted below the area of blockage in the right coronary artery.

a coronary artery distal to the blockage. Saphenous vein grafts do develop diffuse intimal hyperplasia. This contributes to future stenosis and graft occlusions. The use of antiplatelet therapy and statins after surgery improves vein graft patency. Patency rates of these grafts are 50% to 60% at 10 years.[24]

The radial artery is another conduit that can be used. It is a thick muscular artery that is prone to spasm. Perioperative calcium channel blockers and long-acting nitrates can control the spasms. Patency rates at 5 years are as high as 84%. There have been no reports of extremity complications (e.g., hand ischemia, wound infection) after removal of this artery.[24]

Other potential conduits include the gastroepiploic or inferior epigastric artery. However, they are rarely used, since the dissection of these arteries is extensive. This increases the length of surgery and the risk for wound complications at the harvest site, especially in an obese or diabetic patient.[24] Like the radial artery, these are also prone to spasms. One-year patency rate for the epigastric artery is 90%, and 10-year patency rate for the gastroepiploic artery is 62%.[24]

CABG surgery remains a palliative treatment for CAD and not a cure. Studies have shown improved patient outcomes, quality of life, and survival after CABG surgery. However, postoperative complications and mortality increase with age.

Women have higher operative mortality rates than men. This has been attributed to the late treatment of CAD in women because women first present with the disease at an older age and are more ill (e.g., decreased left ventricular function) at the time of surgery. Other possible factors include smaller-diameter coronary vessels and the less frequent use of the IMA.

Minimally Invasive Direct Coronary Artery Bypass. *Minimally invasive direct coronary artery bypass* (MIDCAB) offers patients with limited disease an approach to surgical treatment that does not involve a sternotomy and CPB. In many cases these patients are too high risk for traditional bypass surgery.[25] The technique requires several small incisions between the ribs. A thoracoscope is used to dissect the IMA. The heart is slowed using a β-adrenergic blocker (e.g., esmolol [Brevibloc]) or stopped temporarily with adenosine. A mechanical stabilizer immobilizes the operative site. The IMA is then sutured to the left anterior descending or right coronary artery. A radial artery or saphenous vein graft can be used if the IMA is not available.

Off-Pump Coronary Artery Bypass. The *off-pump coronary artery bypass* (OPCAB) procedure uses full or partial sternotomy to access all coronary vessels. OPCAB is performed on a beating heart using mechanical stabilizers and without CPB. It is usually reserved for patients who have limited disease but are at high risk for traditional surgery secondary to multiple co-morbidities. Patients who are typically candidates for OPCAB have a very low EF, severe lung disease, acute or chronic kidney disease, a high risk for stroke, or a calcified aorta.[25]

Robot-Assisted Cardiothoracic Surgery. This technique incorporates the use of a robot in performing CABG or mitral valve replacement. The benefits of robotic surgery include increased precision, smaller incisions, decreased blood loss, less pain, and shorter recovery time.

Transmyocardial Laser Revascularization. *Transmyocardial laser revascularization* (TMR) is an indirect revascularization procedure. It is used for patients with advanced CAD who are not candidates for traditional CABG surgery and who have persistent angina after maximum medical therapy. The procedure involves the use of a high-energy laser to create channels in the heart to allow blood flow to ischemic areas. The procedure is performed during cardiac catheterization as a percutaneous TMR or during surgery using a left anterior thoracotomy incision as an adjunct to CABG.

Drug Therapy

IV NTG, dual antiplatelet therapy (e.g., aspirin and clopidogrel), and systemic anticoagulation with either LMWH given subcutaneously or IV UH are the initial drug treatments of choice for ACS.[18,19] IV direct thrombin inhibitors may also be used if PCI is anticipated. Oral β-adrenergic blockers are given within the first 24 hours of a STEMI if there are no contraindications (e.g., HF, heart block, hypotension). ACE inhibitors are added for select patients following MI (discussed below). Calcium channel blockers or long-acting nitrates are added if the patient is already taking adequate doses of β-adrenergic blockers, cannot tolerate β-adrenergic blockers, or has Prinzmetal's angina.[18,19]

Table 34-11 and Fig. 34-5 present drug therapy for patients with ACS. These drugs are discussed on pp. 743 and 745. ACS-specific discussion of select drugs is presented in this section.

IV Nitroglycerin. IV NTG (Tridil) is used in the initial treatment of the patient with ACS. The goal of therapy is to reduce anginal pain and improve coronary blood flow. IV NTG decreases preload and afterload while increasing the myocardial oxygen supply. The onset of action is immediate. Titrate NTG to control and stop chest pain. Because hypotension is a common side effect, closely monitor BP during this time. Patients who do become hypotensive are often volume depleted and can benefit from an IV fluid bolus. Tolerance is another side effect of IV nitrate therapy. An effective strategy for this phenomenon is to titrate the dose down at night during sleep and titrate the dose up during the day.

Morphine Sulfate. Morphine sulfate is the drug of choice for chest pain that is unrelieved by NTG. As a vasodilator, it decreases cardiac workload by lowering myocardial oxygen consumption, reducing contractility, and decreasing BP and HR. In addition, morphine can help reduce anxiety and fear. In rare situations, morphine can depress respirations. Monitor patients for signs of bradypnea or hypotension, conditions to avoid in myocardial ischemia and infarction.

β-Adrenergic Blockers. β-Adrenergic blockers decrease myocardial oxygen demand by reducing HR, BP, and contractility. The use of these drugs in patients who are not at risk for complications of MI (e.g., cardiogenic shock) reduces the risk of reinfarction and the occurrence of HF. The continuation of β-adrenergic blockers indefinitely is recommended.[23] (See Table 34-11, Chapter 33, and Table 33-7 for a discussion of β-adrenergic blockers.)

Angiotensin-Converting Enzyme Inhibitors. ACE inhibitors should be started within the first 24 hours and continued indefinitely in patients recovering from STEMI of the anterior wall, with heart failure, or an EF of 40% or less.[18] The use of ACE inhibitors can help prevent ventricular remodeling and prevent or slow the progression of HF. For patients who cannot tolerate ACE inhibitors, angiotensin II receptor blockers should be considered (see Table 34-12 and Table 33-7).

Antidysrhythmic Drugs. Dysrhythmias are the most common complications after an MI. In general, they are self-limiting and are not treated aggressively unless they are life threatening (e.g., sustained ventricular tachycardia). (Chapter 36 discusses the drugs used in the treatment of dysrhythmias.)

Lipid-Lowering Drugs. A fasting lipid panel is obtained on all patients admitted with ACS. All patients with elevated triglycerides and LDL cholesterol should receive lipid-lowering drugs (see Table 34-5).

Stool Softeners. After an MI, the patient may be predisposed to constipation because of bed rest and opioid administration. Stool softeners (e.g., docusate sodium [Colace]) are given to facilitate bowel movements. This prevents straining and the resultant vagal stimulation from the Valsalva maneuver. Vagal stimulation produces bradycardia and can provoke dysrhythmias.

Nutritional Therapy

Initially, patients may be NPO (nothing by mouth) except for sips of water until stable (e.g., pain free, nausea resolved). Advance the diet as tolerated to a low-salt, low-saturated-fat, and low-cholesterol diet (see Tables 34-3 and 34-4).

NURSING MANAGEMENT
CHRONIC STABLE ANGINA AND ACUTE CORONARY SYNDROME

NURSING ASSESSMENT

Table 34-14 presents the subjective and objective data to obtain from a patient with ACS.

NURSING DIAGNOSES

Nursing diagnoses for the patient with ACS may include, but are not limited to, those presented in Nursing Care Plan 34-1.

PLANNING

The overall goals for a patient with ACS include (1) relief of pain, (2) preservation of myocardium, (3) immediate and appropriate treatment, (4) effective coping with illness-associated anxiety, (5) participation in a rehabilitation plan, and (6) reduction of risk factors. In addition, the Joint Commission has identified core measures in the management of patients with an acute MI to reflect standards of evidence-based care (available at *www.jointcommission.org/assets/1/6/Acute%20 Myocardial%20Infarction.pdf*).

NURSING IMPLEMENTATION: CHRONIC STABLE ANGINA

HEALTH PROMOTION. Behaviors to reduce the risk for CAD are presented in Table 34-2 and discussed on pp. 735-740.

TABLE 34-14 NURSING ASSESSMENT

Acute Coronary Syndrome

Subjective Data
Important Health Information

Past health history: Previous history of CAD, chest pain/angina, MI, valve disease (e.g., aortic stenosis), heart failure, or cardiomyopathy; hypertension, diabetes, anemia, lung disease; hyperlipidemia

Medications: Use of antiplatelets or anticoagulants, nitrates, angiotensin-converting enzyme inhibitors, β-blockers, calcium channel blockers; antihypertensive drugs; lipid-lowering drugs; over-the-counter drugs (e.g., vitamin and herbal supplements)

History of present illness: Description of events related to current illness, including any self-treatments and response (see Table 34-8)

Functional Health Patterns

Health perception–health management: Family history of heart disease; sedentary lifestyle; tobacco use; exposure to environmental smoke

Nutritional-metabolic: Indigestion, heartburn, nausea, belching, vomiting

Elimination: Urinary urgency or frequency, straining at stool

Activity-exercise: Palpitations, dyspnea, dizziness, weakness

Cognitive-perceptual: Substernal chest pain or pressure (squeezing, constricting, aching, sharp, tingling), possible radiation to jaw, neck, shoulders, back, or arms (see Table 34-7)

Coping–stress tolerance: Stressful lifestyle, depression; anger, anxiety; feeling of impending doom

Objective Data
General

Anxious, fearful, restless, distressed

Integumentary

Cool, clammy, pale skin

Cardiovascular

Tachycardia or bradycardia, pulsus alternans (alternating weak and strong heartbeats), pulse deficit, dysrhythmias (especially ventricular), S_3, S_4, ↑ or ↓ BP, murmur

Possible Diagnostic Findings

Positive serum cardiac markers, ↑ serum lipids; ↑ WBC count; positive exercise or pharmacologic stress test and thallium scans; pathologic Q wave, ST-segment elevation, and/or T wave abnormalities on ECG; cardiac enlargement, calcifications, or pulmonary congestion on chest x-ray; abnormal wall motion with stress echocardiogram; positive coronary angiography

ACUTE INTERVENTION. If your patient experiences angina, institute the following measures: (1) position patient upright unless contraindicated and administer supplemental oxygen, (2) assess vital signs, (3) obtain a 12-lead ECG, (4) provide prompt pain relief first with a nitrate followed by an opioid analgesic if needed, and (5) auscultate heart and breath sounds. The patient will most likely be distressed and may have pale, cool, clammy skin. The BP and HR may be elevated. Auscultation of the heart may reveal an atrial (S_4) or a ventricular (S_3) gallop. A new murmur heard during an anginal attack may indicate ischemia of a papillary muscle of the mitral valve. The murmur is likely to be transient and disappear when symptoms stop.

Ask the patient to describe the pain and to rate it on a scale of 0 to 10 before and after treatment to evaluate the effectiveness of the interventions (see Table 34-7). It is important to use the same words that patients use to describe their pain. Some patients may not report pain. Assess for other manifestations of pain, such as restlessness; ECG changes; elevated HR, respiratory rate, or BP; clutching of the bed linens; or other nonverbal cues. Supportive and realistic assurance and a calm approach help reduce the patient's anxiety during an anginal attack.

AMBULATORY AND HOME CARE. Reassure the patient with a history of angina that a long, active life is possible. Prevention of angina is preferable to its treatment, and this is why teaching is important. Provide the patient with information regarding CAD, angina, precipitating factors for angina, risk factor reduction, and medications.

Patient teaching can be done in a variety of ways. One-on-one contact between you and the patient is often the most effective approach. Time spent providing daily care (e.g., administering medications) offers many teachable moments. Teaching tools such as DVDs or CDs, heart models, and printed information are important components of patient and caregiver teaching (see Chapter 4).

Assist the patient to identify factors that precipitate angina (see Table 34-8). Instruct the patient on how to avoid or control precipitating factors. For example, teach the patient to avoid exposure to extremes of weather and the consumption of large, heavy meals. If a heavy meal is eaten, instruct the patient to rest for 1 to 2 hours after the meal because blood is shunted to the GI tract to aid digestion and absorption.

Assist the patient to identify personal risk factors for CAD. Then discuss the various methods of decreasing any modifiable risk factors (see Table 34-2). Teach the patient and caregiver about diets that are low in salt and saturated fats (see Tables 34-3 and 34-4). Maintaining ideal body weight is important in controlling angina because excess weight increases myocardial workload.

Adhering to a regular, individualized program of physical activity that conditions rather than overstresses the heart is important. For example, advise patients to walk briskly on a flat surface at least 30 minutes a day, most days of the week (minimum 5) if not contraindicated.[6]

It is important to teach the patient and caregiver the proper use of NTG (see pp. 743 and 745). NTG may be used prophylactically before an emotionally stressful situation, sexual intercourse, or physical exertion (e.g., climbing a long flight of stairs).

If needed, arrange for counseling to assess the psychologic adjustment of the patient and caregiver to the diagnosis of CAD and the resulting angina. Many patients feel a threat to their identity and self-esteem and may be unable to fill their usual roles in society. These emotions are normal and real.

NURSING IMPLEMENTATION
ACUTE CORONARY SYNDROME

ACUTE INTERVENTION. Priorities for nursing interventions in the initial phase of ACS include (1) pain assessment and relief, (2) physiologic monitoring, (3) promotion of rest and comfort, (4) alleviation of stress and anxiety, and (5) understanding of the patient's emotional and behavioral reactions. Patients with increased anxiety levels have a greater risk for adverse outcomes such as recurrent ischemic events and dysrhythmias.[2,12] Proper management of these priorities decreases the oxygen needs of a compromised myocardium and reduces the risk of complications. In addition, institute measures to avoid the hazards of immobility while encouraging rest.

Pain. Provide NTG, morphine, and supplemental oxygen as needed to eliminate or reduce chest pain. Ongoing evaluation and documentation of the effectiveness of the interventions are

NURSING CARE PLAN 34-1

Patient With Acute Coronary Syndrome

NURSING DIAGNOSIS* **Decreased cardiac output** *related to* altered contractility and altered heart rate and rhythm *as evidenced by* decrease in BP, elevation in HR, dyspnea, dysrhythmias, diminished pulses, peripheral edema, and/or pulmonary edema

PATIENT GOAL Maintains stable signs of effective cardiac output

Outcomes (NOC)	Interventions (NIC) and *Rationales*
Tissue Perfusion: Cardiac	**Cardiac Care: Acute**
• Angina _____	• Monitor cardiac rhythm and rate and trends in blood pressure and hemodynamic parameters *to monitor for changes in cardiac output, blood pressure, and heart rhythm, which may lead to coronary hypoperfusion.*
• Dysrhythmia _____	• Auscultate lungs for crackles or other adventitious sounds *that can indicate pulmonary edema.*
• Tachycardia _____	
• Bradycardia _____	• Monitor effectiveness of oxygen therapy (e.g., pulse oximetry) *to determine oxygenation of myocardial tissue and prevent further ischemia.*
• Profuse diaphoresis _____	
• Nausea _____	• Monitor serum cardiac markers (troponin, CK-MB levels) *to determine myocardial injury and recovery.*
• Vomiting _____	• Monitor neurologic, renal, and liver function *to evaluate blood perfusion to vital organs.*
Measurement Scale	
1 = Severe	
2 = Substantial	
3 = Moderate	
4 = Mild	
5 = None	

NURSING DIAGNOSIS **Acute pain** *related to* an imbalance between myocardial oxygen supply and demand *as evidenced by* patient's report of severe chest pain and tightness with radiation of pain to the neck and arms, elevated cardiac markers, ECG changes supporting ST elevation MI

PATIENT GOAL Reports relief of pain

Outcomes (NOC)	Interventions (NIC) and *Rationales*
Pain Control	**Cardiac Care**
• Uses preventive measures _____	• Evaluate chest pain (e.g., PQRST [see Table 34-7]) *to accurately evaluate, treat, and prevent further ischemia.*
• Uses analgesics appropriately _____	• Monitor vital signs frequently *to determine baseline and ongoing changes.*
• Reports uncontrolled symptoms to health care professional _____	• Obtain 12-lead ECG during pain episode *to help differentiate angina from extension of MI or pericarditis.*
• Reports pain controlled _____	
Measurement Scale	**Pain Management**
1 = Never demonstrated	• Provide the person optimal pain relief with prescribed analgesics *because pain exacerbates tachycardia and increases blood pressure.*
2 = Rarely demonstrated	• Consider the type and source of pain when selecting pain relief strategy *because angina responds to opioids and measures that increase myocardial perfusion.*
3 = Sometimes demonstrated	
4 = Often demonstrated	
5 = Consistently demonstrated	

NURSING DIAGNOSIS **Anxiety** *related to* perceived or actual threat of death, pain, and/or possible lifestyle changes *as evidenced by* restlessness, agitation, and verbalization of concern over lifestyle changes and prognosis such as patient's statement, "What if I die? Everyone relies on me."

PATIENT GOAL Reports decreased anxiety and increased sense of self-control

Outcomes (NOC)	Interventions (NIC) and *Rationales*
Anxiety Level	**Anxiety Reduction**
• Restlessness _____	• Observe for verbal and nonverbal signs of anxiety *to identify signs of stress and intervene appropriately.*
• Verbalized apprehension _____	• Identify when level of anxiety changes, *since anxiety increases the need for oxygen.*
• Difficulty concentrating _____	• Use a calm, reassuring approach *to avoid increasing patient's anxiety.*
• Distress _____	• Instruct patient in use of relaxation techniques (e.g., relaxation breathing, imagery) *to enhance self-control.*
Measurement Scale	• Encourage caregiver to stay with patient *to provide comfort and support.*
1 = Severe	• Encourage verbalization of feelings, perceptions, and fears *to decrease anxiety and stress.*
2 = Substantial	• Provide factual information concerning diagnosis, treatment, and prognosis *to decrease fear of the unknown.*
3 = Moderate	
4 = Mild	
5 = None	
Acceptance: Health Status	**Coping Enhancement**
• Recognizes reality of health situation _____	• Provide the patient with realistic choices about certain aspects of care *to support decision making.*
• Adjusts to change in health status _____	• Assist the patient in identifying positive strategies *to deal with limitations and manage needed lifestyle or role changes.*
• Makes decisions about health _____	• Help the patient to grieve and work through the losses of chronic illness.
Measurement Scale	
1 = Never demonstrated	
2 = Rarely demonstrated	
3 = Sometimes demonstrated	
4 = Often demonstrated	
5 = Consistently demonstrated	

*Nursing diagnoses listed in order of priority.

Continued

◎ NURSING CARE PLAN 34-1—cont'd

Patient With Acute Coronary Syndrome

NURSING DIAGNOSIS **Activity intolerance** *related to* general weakness secondary to decreased cardiac output and poor lung and tissue perfusion *as evidenced by* patient's report of fatigue with minimal activity, inability to care for self without dyspnea, and increased heart rate

PATIENT GOAL Achieves a realistic program of activity that balances physical activity with energy-conserving activities

Outcomes (NOC)	Interventions (NIC) and *Rationales*
Activity Tolerance • Oxygen saturation with activity _____ • Pulse rate with activity _____ • Ease of breathing with activity _____ • Walking pace _____ • Ease of performing ADLs _____ **Measurement Scale** 1 = Severely compromised 2 = Substantially compromised 3 = Moderately compromised 4 = Mildly compromised 5 = Not compromised	**Cardiac Care** • Monitor patient's response to cardiac medications, *since these medications often affect BP and pulse.* • Arrange exercise and rest periods *to avoid fatigue and to increase activity tolerance without rapidly increasing cardiac workload.* **Energy Management** • Help patient understand energy conservation principles (e.g., the requirement for restricted activity) *to conserve energy and promote healing.* • Teach patient and caregiver techniques of self-care that will minimize oxygen consumption (e.g., self-monitoring and pacing techniques for performance of ADLs) *to promote independence and minimize O_2 consumption.*

NURSING DIAGNOSIS **Ineffective self-health management** *related to* lack of knowledge of disease process, risk factor reduction, rehabilitation, home activities, and medications *as evidenced by* frequent questioning about illness, management, and care after discharge

PATIENT GOAL Describes the disease process, measures to reduce risk factors, and rehabilitation activities necessary to manage the therapeutic regimen

Outcomes (NOC)	Interventions (NIC) and *Rationales*
Knowledge: Cardiac Disease Management • Usual course of disease process _____ • Signs and symptoms of worsening disease _____ • Strategies to reduce risk factors _____ • Importance of completing cardiac rehabilitation program _____ • Rationale for following a low-fat, low-cholesterol diet _____ • Importance of regular exercise _____ **Measurement Scale** 1 = No knowledge 2 = Limited knowledge 3 = Moderate knowledge 4 = Substantial knowledge 5 = Extensive knowledge	**Cardiac Care: Rehabilitative** • Encourage realistic expectations for the patient and caregiver *to promote realistic decision making.* • Instruct the patient and caregiver on appropriate prescribed and over-the-counter medications *to promote compliance with medication regimens.* • Instruct the patient and caregiver on cardiac risk factor modification (e.g., smoking cessation, diet, exercise) *to increase patient's control of the illness.* • Instruct the patient on self-care of chest pain (e.g., take nitroglycerin; if chest pain unrelieved, seek emergency medical care). • Instruct the patient and caregiver on the exercise regimen, including warm-up, endurance, and cool-down, *to reduce cardiac risk factors.* • Instruct the patient and caregiver on wound care and precautions (e.g., sternal incision or catheterization site) *to prevent infection and promote healing after invasive therapies.* • Instruct the patient and caregiver on access to emergency services available in their community *to enable them to obtain immediate care if needed.*

important. Once pain is relieved, you may have to deal with denial in a patient who interprets the absence of pain as an absence of cardiac disease.

Monitoring. Maintain continuous ECG monitoring while the patient is in the ED and intensive care unit and after transfer to a step-down or general unit. Dysrhythmias need to be identified quickly and treated. During the initial period after MI, ventricular fibrillation is the most common lethal dysrhythmia. In many patients, premature ventricular contractions or ventricular tachycardia precedes this dysrhythmia. Monitor the patient for reinfarction or ischemia by monitoring the ST segment for shifts above or below the baseline of the ECG. Silent ischemia can occur without clinical symptoms such as chest pain. Its presence places a patient at higher risk for adverse outcomes and even death. If you note ST segment changes, notify the physician. (See Chapter 36 for a complete discussion of ECG monitoring.)

Perform a physical assessment to detect deviations from the patient's baseline findings. Assess heart and breath sounds and any evidence of early HF (e.g., dyspnea, tachycardia, pulmonary congestion, distended neck veins). In addition to routine vital signs, monitor intake and output at least once a shift.

Assessment of the patient's oxygenation status is important, especially if the patient is receiving oxygen. If a nasal cannula is used to deliver oxygen, check the nares for irritation or dryness, which can cause considerable discomfort.

Rest and Comfort. It is important to promote rest and comfort with any degree of myocardial injury. Bed rest may be ordered for the first few days after an MI that involves a large portion of the ventricle. A patient with an uncomplicated MI (e.g., angina resolved, no signs of complications) may rest in a chair within 8 to 12 hours after the event. The use of a commode or bedpan is based on patient preference.

When sleeping or resting, the body requires less work from the heart than it does when active. It is important to plan nursing and therapeutic interventions to ensure adequate rest periods free from interruption. Comfort measures that can promote rest include a quiet environment, use of relaxation techniques (e.g., relaxation breathing, guided imagery), and assurance that staff are nearby and responsive to the patient's needs.

It is important that the patient understand the reasons why activity is limited but not completely restricted. Gradually increase the patient's cardiac workload through more demand-

TABLE 34-15   PHASES OF REHABILITATION AFTER ACUTE CORONARY SYNDROME

Phase I: Hospital
- Occurs while the patient is still hospitalized.
- Activity level depends on severity of angina or MI.
- Patient may initially sit up in bed or chair, perform range-of-motion exercises and self-care (e.g., washing, shaving), and progress to ambulation in hallway and limited stair climbing.
- Attention focuses on management of chest pain, anxiety, dysrhythmias, and complications.

Phase II: Early Recovery
- Begins after the patient is discharged.
- Usually lasts from 2-12 wk and is conducted in an outpatient facility.
- Activity level is gradually increased under the supervision of the cardiac rehabilitation team and with ECG monitoring.
- Team may suggest that physical activity (e.g., walking) be initiated at home.
- Information regarding risk factor reduction is provided at this time.

Phase III: Late Recovery
- Long-term maintenance program.
- Individual physical activity programs are designed and implemented at home, a local gym, or the rehabilitation center.
- Patient and caregiver possibly restructure lifestyles and roles.
- Therapeutic lifestyle changes should become lifelong habits.
- Medical supervision is still recommended.

TABLE 34-16   PSYCHOSOCIAL RESPONSES TO ACUTE CORONARY SYNDROME

Denial
- May have history of ignoring signs and symptoms related to heart disease
- Minimizes severity of medical condition
- Ignores activity restrictions
- Avoids discussing illness or its significance

Anger and Hostility
- Is commonly expressed as, "Why did this happen to me?"
- May be directed at family, staff, or medical regimen

Anxiety and Fear
- Fears long-term disability and death
- Overtly manifests apprehension, restlessness, insomnia, tachycardia
- Less overtly manifests increased verbalization, projection of feelings to others, hypochondriasis
- Fears activity
- Fears recurrent chest pain, heart attacks, and sudden death

Dependency
- Is totally reliant on staff
- Is unwilling to perform tasks or activities unless approved by health care provider
- Wants to be monitored by ECG at all times
- Is hesitant to leave the intensive care or telemetry unit or hospital

Depression
- Mourns loss of health, altered body function, and changes in lifestyle
- Realizes seriousness of situation
- Begins to worry about future implications of health problem
- Shows manifestations of withdrawal, crying, apathy
- May be more evident after discharge

Realistic Acceptance
- Focuses on optimum rehabilitation
- Plans changes compatible with altered cardiac function
- Actively engages in lifestyle changes to address modifiable risk factors

ing physical tasks so that the patient can achieve a discharge activity level adequate for home care. Table 34-15 outlines the phases of cardiac rehabilitation.

Anxiety. Anxiety is present in all patients with ACS to some degree. Your role is to identify the source of anxiety and assist the patient in reducing it. If the patient is afraid of being alone, allow a caregiver to sit by quietly or check in with the patient frequently. If a source of anxiety is fear of the unknown, explore these concerns with the patient. For anxiety caused by lack of information, provide teaching based on the patient's stated need and level of understanding. Answer the patient's questions with clear, simple explanations.

It is important to start teaching at the patient's level rather than to present a prepackaged program. For example, patients generally are not ready to learn about the pathology of CAD. The earliest questions usually relate to how the disease affects perceived control and independence. Examples include the following.
- When will I leave the intensive care unit?
- When can I be out of bed?
- When will I be discharged?
- When can I return to work?
- How many changes will I have to make in my life?
- Will this happen again?

Tell the patient that a more complete teaching program will begin once the patient is feeling stronger. Frequently the patient may not be able to ask the most serious concern of ACS patients: Am I going to die? Even if a patient denies this concern, it is helpful for you to start a conversation by remarking that fear of dying is a common concern among most patients who have experienced ACS. This gives the patient "permission" to talk about an uncomfortable and fearful topic.

Emotional and Behavioral Reactions. Patients' emotional and behavioral reactions vary but frequently follow a predictable response pattern (Table 34-16). Your role is to understand what the patient is currently experiencing and to support the use of constructive coping styles. Denial may be a positive coping style in the early phase of recovery from ACS.

Assess the support structure of the patient and caregiver. Help to determine how you can help maximize the support system. Often the patient is separated from the most significant support system at the time of hospitalization. Your role can include talking with the caregiver(s), informing them of the patient's progress, allowing the patient and the caregivers to interact as necessary, and supporting the caregivers who will provide the necessary support to the patient. Open visitation is helpful in decreasing anxiety and increasing support for the patient with ACS.[26] Social isolation has been associated with negative outcomes following MI in both men and women. It is important for you to help the patient identify additional support systems (e.g., spiritual care, Mended Hearts) that can assist after discharge.

CORONARY REVASCULARIZATION. Patients with ACS may undergo coronary revascularization with PCI or CABG surgery. The major nursing responsibilities for patient care after PCI involve monitoring for signs of recurrent angina; frequent assessment of vital signs, including HR and rhythm; evaluation of the catheter insertion site for signs of bleeding; neurovascular assessment of the involved extremity; and maintenance of bed rest per institution policy.

For patients having CABG surgery, care is provided in the intensive care unit for the first 24 to 36 hours. Ongoing and intensive monitoring of the patient's hemodynamic status is critical. The patient will have numerous invasive lines for monitoring cardiac status and other vital organs (see Chapter 66). These include (1) a pulmonary artery catheter for measuring CO and other hemodynamic parameters, (2) an intraarterial line for continuous BP monitoring, (3) pleural and mediastinal chest tubes for chest drainage, (4) continuous ECG monitoring to detect dysrhythmias, (5) an endotracheal tube connected to mechanical ventilation, (6) epicardial pacing wires for emergency pacing of the heart, (7) a urinary catheter to monitor urine output, and (8) a nasogastric tube for gastric decompression. Most patients are extubated within 6 hours and transferred to a step-down unit within 24 hours for continued monitoring of cardiac status.

Many of the postoperative complications that develop after CABG surgery relate to the use of CPB. Major consequences of CPB are systemic inflammation, which includes complications of bleeding and anemia from damage to red blood cells and platelets, fluid and electrolyte imbalances, hypothermia as blood is cooled as it passes through the CPB machine, and infections. Focus your nursing care on assessing the patient for bleeding (e.g., chest tube drainage, incision sites), hemodynamic monitoring, checking fluid status, replacing electrolytes as needed, and restoring temperature (e.g., warming blankets).

Postoperative dysrhythmias, specifically atrial dysrhythmias, are common in the first 3 days after CABG surgery. Postoperative atrial fibrillation (AF) occurs in 20% to 50% of patients.[24] β-Adrenergic blockers should be restarted as soon as possible after surgery (unless contraindicated) to reduce the incidence of AF. Discharge is often delayed in these patients in order to begin anticoagulation therapy. (See Chapter 36 for information on treatment of AF.)

Nursing care for the patient with a CABG also involves caring for the surgical sites (e.g., chest, arm, leg). Care of the radial artery harvest site includes monitoring sensory and motor function of the distal hand. The patient with radial artery harvest should take a calcium channel blocker for approximately 3 months to decrease the incidence of arterial spasm at the arm or anastomosis site.

Care of the leg incision is minimal since endoscopy is used to harvest the vein. Management of the chest wound, which involves a sternotomy, is similar to that of other chest surgeries (see Chapter 28). Chest incisions are usually closed with Dermabond and do not require dressings. Other interventions include strategies to manage pain and prevent venous thromboembolism (e.g., early ambulation, sequential compression device) and respiratory complications (e.g., use of incentive spirometer, splinting during coughing and deep-breathing exercises). (See Chapter 20 for care of the postoperative patient.)

Postoperatively, patients may experience some cognitive dysfunction. This includes impairment of memory, concentration, language comprehension, and social integration. Patients may cry or become teary. Postoperative cognitive dysfunction (POCD) can manifest days to weeks after surgery and may remain a permanent disorder. It is seen in 40% of patients several months after cardiac surgery.[27] (POCD is discussed in Chapter 20.)

In the older patient, elective CABG is generally well tolerated. However, the incidence of postoperative complications, including dysrhythmias, stroke, and infection, is high. Although the benefits of treatment may outweigh risks in this population, complications are higher than in younger individuals.

Postoperative nursing care of the patient with a MIDCAB or OPCAB procedure is similar to that for CABG surgery patients. Pain management is important regardless of the procedure. Patients report higher levels of pain with thoracotomy incisions than a sternotomy incision. The recovery time is somewhat shorter with these procedures, and patients often resume routine activities sooner than patients who have CABG surgery.

AMBULATORY AND HOME CARE. *Cardiac rehabilitation* is the restoration of a person to an optimal state of function in six areas: physiologic, psychologic, mental, spiritual, economic, and vocational. Many patients recover from ACS physically, but do not attain psychologic well-being. All patients (e.g., those with ACS, chronic stable angina, cardiac surgery) need to be referred to a cardiac rehabilitation program. In considering rehabilitation, the patient must recognize that CAD is a chronic disease. It is not curable, nor will it disappear by itself. Therefore

EVIDENCE-BASED PRACTICE
Translating Research into Practice

Do Exercise-Based Cardiac Rehabilitation Programs Improve Outcomes?

Clinical Question
In patients with coronary heart disease (P), do exercise-based cardiac rehabilitation programs (I) versus usual care (C) reduce mortality and morbidity and improve quality of life (O)?

Best Available Evidence
Systematic review of randomized controlled trials (RCTs)

Critical Appraisal and Synthesis of Evidence
- 47 RCTs (*n* = 10,794) of patients with myocardial infarction (MI), angina pectoris, coronary artery bypass graft (CABG), or percutaneous transluminal coronary angioplasty (PTCA). Exercise-based cardiac rehabilitation was exercise alone or with psychosocial or educational interventions. Usual care included standard medical care and drug therapy with no structured exercise training.
- Exercise-based rehabilitation reduced overall and cardiovascular mortality, decreased hospital admissions, and improved quality of life.
- Cardiac rehabilitation did not reduce risk of recurrent MI or revascularization (CABG or PTCA).

Conclusion
- Exercise-based cardiac rehabilitation reduces risk of dying from heart disease.

Implications for Nursing Practice
- Provide assistance in accessing cardiac rehabilitation programs.
- Reinforce benefits of adhering to recommended physical activity.
- Reduce program dropout rates by motivating patients to stay engaged.

Reference for Evidence
Heran B, Chen J, Ebrahim S, et al: Exercise-based cardiac rehabilitation for coronary heart disease, *Cochrane Database Syst Rev* 7:CD001800, 2011.

P, Patient population of interest; *I,* intervention or area of interest; *C,* comparison of interest or comparison group; *O,* outcomes of interest; *T,* timing (see p. 12).

EVIDENCE-BASED PRACTICE
Applying the Evidence

J.B. is 56-year-old white man who is being discharged from the hospital after having a myocardial infarction (MI) 4 days ago. You know that he is struggling with the lifestyle changes he must make, including how to kick his cigarette habit. While you are discussing the importance of smoking cessation with him, you share information from both the best available evidence and your clinical expertise. In addition, you describe a variety of smoking cessation interventions available for his consideration.

Best Available Evidence*	Clinician Expertise	Patient Preferences and Values
Combination strategies (e.g., medication plus behavioral support) work best to help patients to stop smoking.	You have heard from several patients who have successfully stopped smoking that they tried more than one intervention at a time to stop smoking (e.g., medication plus support group, hypnotherapy plus support group).	After reviewing all the information, J.B. informs you that he is willing to start with the nicotine patch but does not want to do anything else at this time.

Your Decision and Action
As his nurse, you respect and support his decision. You document your teaching and J.B.'s response. You notify his physician of his choice and request a prescription for the nicotine patch.

References for Evidence
Carpenter MJ, Hughes JR, Gray KM, et al: Nicotine therapy sampling to induce quit attempts among smokers unmotivated to quit: a randomized clinical trial, *Arch Intern Med* 171:1901, 2011.
Joseph AM, Fu SS, Lindgren B, et al: Chronic disease management for tobacco dependence: a randomized, controlled trial, *Arch Intern Med* 171:1894, 2011.

basic changes in lifestyle must be made to promote recovery and future health. These changes often are needed when a person is middle aged or older. The patient must realize that recovery takes time. Resumption of physical activity after ACS or CABG surgery is slow and gradual. However, with appropriate and adequate supportive care, recovery is more likely to occur.

Patient Teaching. Patient teaching needs to occur at every stage of the patient's hospitalization and recovery (e.g., ED, telemetry unit, home care). The purpose of teaching is to give the patient and caregiver the tools they need to make informed decisions about their health. For teaching to be meaningful, the patient must be aware of the need to learn. Careful assessment of the patient's learning needs helps you set goals that are realistic (see Chapter 4).

The timing of the teaching is important. When patients and caregivers are in crisis (either physiologic or psychologic), they may not be interested in learning new information. Answer the patient's questions in simple, brief terms. The answers often require repetition. When the shock and disbelief accompanying a crisis subside, the patient and caregiver are better able to focus on new and more detailed information.

Limit your use of medical terminology. For example, explain that the heart, a four-chambered pump, is a muscle that needs oxygen, like all other muscles, to work properly. When blood vessels supplying the heart muscle with oxygen are blocked by plaque, less oxygen is available to the muscle. As a result, the heart cannot pump normally. It helps to have a model of the heart or to sketch a picture of what you are explaining. Literature written for a nonmedical audience is available through the AHA.

Anticipatory guidance involves preparing the patient and caregiver for what to expect in the course of recovery and rehabilitation. By learning what to expect during treatment and recovery, the patient gains a sense of control over his or her life.

The idea of perceived control is operationalized as the process by which the patient exercises choice and makes decisions by cutting back. Cutting back is one way of minimizing the psychologic and physiologic losses after MI (or any other life-changing event). For example, a middle-aged man who smokes two packs of cigarettes a day, is 20 pounds overweight, and gets no physical exercise has a seemingly overwhelming task. He may decide that he can live with a weight reduction plan and will get more exercise (although perhaps not daily) but that it is not possible for him to quit smoking. He reasons that because he is modifying two of the three risk factors, he will be healthier. Ideally, the tobacco risk factor should be a priority for this patient. If the information regarding risks and effects of tobacco use is not accepted, you must respect the patient's lifestyle choices.

TABLE 34-17   PATIENT & CAREGIVER TEACHING GUIDE

Acute Coronary Syndrome

Include the following information in the teaching plan for the patient with acute coronary syndrome and the caregiver.

- Signs and symptoms of angina and MI and what to do should they occur (e.g., take nitroglycerin)*
- When and how to seek help (e.g., contact EMS)
- Anatomy and physiology of the heart and coronary arteries
- Cause and effect of CAD
- Definition of terms (e.g., CAD, angina, MI, sudden cardiac death, heart failure)
- Identification of and plan to decrease risk factors* (see Tables 34-2, 34-3, and 34-4)
- Rationale for tests and treatments (e.g., ECG monitoring, blood tests, angiography), activity limitations and rest, diet, and medications*
- Appropriate expectations about recovery and rehabilitation (anticipatory guidance)
- Resumption of work, physical activity, sexual activity
- Measures to promote recovery and health
- Importance of the gradual, progressive resumption of activity*

*Identified by patients as most important to learn before discharge.

TABLE 34-18   ENERGY EXPENDITURE IN METABOLIC EQUIVALENTS

Low-Energy Activities (<3 METs or <3 cal/min)
Activities in Hospital
- Resting supine
- Eating
- Washing hands, face

Activities Outside Hospital
- Sweeping floor
- Painting, seated
- Driving a car
- Sewing by machine

Moderate-Energy Activities (3-6 METs or 3-5 cal/min)
Activities in Hospital
- Sitting on bedside commode
- Showering
- Using bedpan
- Walking at 3-4 mph

Activities Outside Hospital
- Ironing, standing
- Cycling at 5.5 mph on level ground
- Golfing
- General gardening
- Painting
- Ascending a flight of stairs

High-Energy Activities (6-8 METs or 6-8 cal/min)
- Walking 5 mph
- Performing carpentry
- Mowing lawn using walking mower

Very-High-Energy Activities (>9 METs or >9 cal/min)
- Cross-country skiing
- Running at >6 mph
- Cycling at >13 mph
- Shoveling heavy snow

In addition to teaching the patient and caregiver what they wish to know, several types of information are essential in achieving optimal health. Table 34-17 presents a teaching guide for the patient with ACS.

Physical Activity. Physical activity, an integral part of rehabilitation, is necessary for optimal physiologic functioning and psychologic well-being. It has a direct, positive effect on maximal oxygen uptake, increasing CO, decreasing blood lipids, decreasing BP, increasing blood flow through the coronary arteries, increasing muscle mass and flexibility, improving the psychologic state, and assisting in weight loss and control. A regular schedule of physical activity, even after many years of sedentary living, is beneficial.[9]

One method of identifying levels of physical activity is through **metabolic equivalent (MET)** units: 1 MET is the amount of oxygen needed by the body at rest—3.5 mL of oxygen per kilogram per minute, or 1.4 cal/kg of body weight per minute. The MET determines the energy costs of various exercises (Table 34-18). Another method to determine levels of physical activity is the *Borg Rating of Perceived Exertion Scale.* This scale focuses on the patient's rating of the effort an activity requires (Table 34-19).

In the hospital the activity level is gradually increased so that by the time of discharge the patient can tolerate moderate-energy activities of 3 to 6 METs or rates activities 12 to 14 on the Borg scale. Many patients with UA that has resolved or an uncomplicated MI are in the hospital for approximately 3 or 4 days. By day 2, the patient can ambulate in the hallway and begin limited stair climbing (e.g., three or four steps). Many physicians order low-level exercise stress tests before discharge to assess readiness for discharge, optimal HR for an exercise program, and potential for ischemia or reinfarction. If tests are positive (i.e., ischemia at a low level of energy expenditure), the patient is evaluated for cardiac catheterization before discharge. If the test is negative, a catheterization may still be done before discharge or several weeks after discharge. Because of the short hospital stay, it is critical to give the patient specific guidelines for physical activity so that overexertion will not occur. It is

TABLE 34-19   BORG RATING OF PERCEIVED EXERTION SCALE®*

Level of Exertion	RPE
No exertion at all	6
Extremely light	7
	8
Very light	9
	10
Light	11
	12
Somewhat hard	13
	14
Hard (heavy)	15
	16
Very hard	17
	18
Extremely hard	19
Maximal exertion	20

9 corresponds to very light exercise. For a healthy person, it is like walking slowly at his or her own pace for some minutes.

13 on the scale is somewhat hard exercise, but it still feels OK to continue.

17 (very hard) is strenuous exercise. A healthy person can still go on, but he or she really has to push himself or herself. It feels very hard, and the person is very tired.

19 on the scale is an extremely strenuous exercise level. For most people this is the most strenuous exercise they have ever experienced.

Source: Borg G: Borg's perceived exertion and pain scales, *Human Kinetics*, 1998, Champaign, Ill. © Gunnar Borg, 1970, 1985, 1994, 1998. For information about scale construction, administration, etc., see Borg's book (Borg G., 1998). Scales and instructions can be obtained for a minor fee from Dr. G. Borg. E-mail: borgperception@telia.com.
*The complete instructions on how to use this scale are available on the website for this chapter.

TABLE 34-20	**PATIENT & CAREGIVER TEACHING GUIDE**

FITT *Activity Guidelines After Acute Coronary Syndrome*

Include the following information in the teaching plan for the patient after an acute coronary syndrome:

Warm-up/Cool-down
Instruct the patient to perform mild stretching for 3-5 min before the physical activity and 5 min after the activity. Activity should not be started or stopped abruptly.

Frequency
Encourage the patient to perform physical activity on most days of the week.

Intensity
Activity intensity is determined by the patient's HR. If an exercise stress test has not been performed, the HR of the patient recovering from an MI should not exceed 20 beats/min over the resting HR.

Type of Physical Activity
Physical activity should be regular, rhythmic, and repetitive, using large muscles to build up endurance (e.g., walking, cycling, swimming, rowing).

Time
Physical activity sessions should be at least 30 min long. Instruct the patient to begin slowly at personal tolerance (perhaps only 5-10 min) and build up to 30 min.

important to tell the patient to "listen to what your body is saying"—the most important aspect of recovery.

Teach patients to check their pulse rate. The patient should know the limits within which to exercise. Tell the patient the maximum HR that should be present at any point. If the HR exceeds this level or does not return to the rate of the resting pulse within a few minutes, instruct the patient to stop and rest. Also instruct the patient to stop exercising and rest if chest pain or shortness of breath occurs.

In a normal, healthy person the minimum threshold for improving cardiopulmonary fitness is 60% of the age-predicted maximum HR (calculate by subtracting the person's age from 220). The ideal training target HR is 80% of maximum HR. The patient who has been physically inactive and is just beginning an exercise program should do so under supervision whenever possible.

The more important factor is the patient's response to physical activity in terms of symptoms rather than absolute HR, especially since many patients are taking β-adrenergic blockers and may not be able to reach a target HR. This point cannot be overstressed. Basic physical activity guidelines for patients after ACS follow the FITT formula (Table 34-20).

The basic categories of physical activity are isometric (static) and isotonic (dynamic). Most daily activities are a mixture of the two. *Isometric activities* involve the development of tension during muscular contraction but produce little or no change in muscle length or joint movement. Lifting, carrying, and pushing heavy objects are isometric activities. Because the HR and BP increase rapidly during isometric work, exercise programs involving isometric exercises should be limited.

Isotonic activities involve changes in muscle length and joint movement with rhythmic contractions at relatively low muscu-

lar tension. Walking, jogging, swimming, bicycling, and jumping rope are examples of activities that are predominantly isotonic. Isotonic exercise can put a safe, steady load on the heart and lungs and improve the circulation in many organs.

Discuss participation in an outpatient cardiac rehabilitation program with all patients (see Table 34-15). These programs are beneficial, but not all patients choose or are able to participate in them (e.g., location and travel limitations). Home-based cardiac rehabilitation programs can provide an alternative. Physical activity guidelines are developed for the patient, and staff maintains ongoing contact with the patient (e.g., telephone, exercise logs, Internet). Maintaining contact with the patient is one key to the success of these programs.

Older women (65 years or older) who experience MI may frequently have poor adherence to a regular physical activity program. Often these women describe continued fatigue post-MI that is poorly understood. Another factor that has been linked to poor adherence to a physical activity program after MI is depression. Depression is common among patients with CAD, especially in women.[28] Routinely screen for depression in all patients with CAD and recommend treatment as appropriate.

Resumption of Sexual Activity. It is important to include sexual counseling for cardiac patients and their partners. This often-neglected area of discussion may be difficult for both the patient and the health care provider to approach. However, the patient's concern about resumption of sexual activity after hospitalization for ACS often produces more stress than the physiologic act itself. Most of these patients change their sexual behavior not because of physical problems, but because they are concerned about sexual inadequacy, death during intercourse, and impotence. A concerned and knowledgeable health care provider could clarify any misconceptions with specific counseling.

Before providing guidelines on resumption of sexual activity, it is important to know the patient's physiologic status, the physiologic effects of sexual activity, and the psychologic effects of having a heart attack. Sexual activity for most middle-aged men and women with their usual partners is considered a moderate-energy activity equivalent to climbing two flights of stairs.[29]

You may be uncertain of how and when to begin counseling about resumption of sex. It is helpful to consider sex as a physical activity and to discuss or explore feelings in this area when other physical activities are discussed. One helpful approach is, "Many people who have had a heart attack wonder when they will be able to resume sexual activity. Has this been of concern to you?" You might also state, "Sexual activity is like other forms of activity and should be gradually resumed after MI. If your ability to perform sexually is concerning you, the energy you use is no more than walking briskly." Facilitate discussion by providing the patient with reading material on resumption of sexual activity. Say something like, "If resuming sexual activity has been of concern to you, this information should be helpful." This type of nonthreatening statement brings up the topic, allows the patient to explore personal feelings, and gives the patient an opportunity to raise questions with you or another health care provider.[28] Common guidelines are presented in Table 34-21.

The patient needs to know that the inability to perform sexually after MI is common and that sexual dysfunction usually disappears after several attempts. Reinforce the idea that

TABLE 34-21   PATIENT TEACHING GUIDE

Sexual Activity After Acute Coronary Syndrome

Include the following information in the teaching plan for the patient and his/her partner after an acute coronary syndrome:

- Sexual activity should be resumed at a level that corresponds to sexual activity before experiencing acute coronary syndrome.
- Physical training may improve the physiologic response to intercourse. Therefore daily physical activity during recovery should be encouraged.
- Consumption of food and alcohol should be reduced before intercourse is anticipated (e.g., waiting 3-4 hr after ingesting a large meal before engaging in sexual activity).
- Familiar surroundings and a familiar partner reduce anxiety.
- Masturbation may be a useful sexual outlet and may reassure the patient that sexual activity is still possible.
- Hot or cold showers should be avoided just before and after intercourse.
- Foreplay is desirable because it allows a gradual increase in heart rate before orgasm.
- Positions during intercourse are a matter of individual choice.
- Orogenital sex places no undue strain on the heart.
- A relaxed atmosphere free of fatigue and stress is optimal.
- Prophylactic use of nitrates to decrease chest pain during sexual activity may be recommended.
- Use of erectile agents (e.g., sildenafil [Viagra]) is contraindicated if taking nitrates in any form.
- Anal intercourse should be avoided because of the possibility of inducing a vasovagal response.

patience and understanding usually solve the problem. However, with the availability of drugs to correct erectile dysfunction, many male patients may be interested in using them. Caution the patient that these drugs are not to be used with nitrates because severe hypotension and even death have been reported.[15] Encourage patients to discuss the use of these drugs with their health care provider.

It is common for a patient who experiences chest pain on physical exertion to have some angina during sexual stimulation or intercourse. The patient may be instructed to take NTG prophylactically.[15] It is also helpful to have the patient avoid sex soon after a heavy meal or after excessive ingestion of alcohol, when extremely tired or stressed, or with unfamiliar partners. Patients should also avoid anal intercourse because of the likelihood of eliciting a vasovagal response.

Tell the patient that resumption of sex depends on the patient and his or her partner's emotional readiness and on the physician's assessment of the extent of recovery. It is generally safe to resume sexual activity 7 to 10 days after an uncomplicated MI.[29] However, some physicians believe that the patient should decide when he or she is ready to resume sex. Others believe that a patient must be asymptomatic when performing moderate-energy activities before resuming sexual activity.[29]

▌EVALUATION

Nursing Care Plan 34-1 presents the expected outcomes for the patient with an ACS.

SUDDEN CARDIAC DEATH

Sudden cardiac death (SCD) is unexpected death resulting from a variety of cardiac causes. An estimated 382,800 people experience SCD yearly.[1]

Etiology and Pathophysiology

In SCD a sudden disruption in cardiac function produces an abrupt loss of CO and cerebral blood flow. The affected person may or may not have a known history of heart disease. SCD is often the first sign of illness for 25% of those who die of heart disease.[30]

Acute ventricular dysrhythmias (e.g., ventricular tachycardia, ventricular fibrillation) cause the majority of cases of SCD. Structural heart disease accounts for 10% of the cases of SCD. Patients in this group include those with left ventricular hypertrophy, myocarditis, and hypertrophic cardiomyopathy. Hypertrophic cardiomyopathy is a risk factor for SCD, especially in young, athletic people.

Approximately 10% to 12% of cases of SCD among people less than age 45 occur in the absence of structural heart disease. These involve disturbances in the conduction system (e.g., prolonged QT syndrome, Wolff-Parkinson-White syndrome).

It is difficult to know who is at high risk for SCD. However, left ventricular dysfunction (EF less than 30%) and ventricular dysrhythmias following MI have been found to be the strongest predictors.[30] Other risk factors include history of syncope, left ventricular outflow tract obstruction (e.g., aortic stenosis), male gender (especially African American men), and family history of ventricular dysrhythmias.

Clinical Manifestations and Complications

Persons who experience SCD because of CAD fall into two groups: (1) those who did not have an acute MI and (2) those who did have an acute MI. The first group accounts for the majority of cases of SCD.[30] These victims usually have no warning signs or symptoms. Patients who survive are at risk for another SCD event because of the continued electrical instability of the heart that caused the initial event to occur.

The second, smaller group of patients includes those who have had an MI and have suffered SCD. Such patients usually have prodromal symptoms, such as chest pain, palpitations, and dyspnea. Death usually occurs within 1 hour of the onset of acute symptoms.

▌NURSING AND COLLABORATIVE MANAGEMENT SUDDEN CARDIAC DEATH

People who survive an episode of SCD require a diagnostic workup to determine whether they have had an MI. Thus serial analysis of cardiac markers and ECGs are done, and the patient is treated accordingly. (See section on collaborative care of ACS.) In addition, because most persons with SCD have CAD, cardiac catheterization is indicated to determine the possible location and extent of coronary artery occlusion. PCI or CABG surgery may be indicated.

Most SCD patients have a lethal ventricular dysrhythmia that is associated with a high incidence of recurrence. Thus it is useful to know when those persons are most likely to have a recurrence and what drug therapy is the most effective treatment. Assessment of dysrhythmias in these patients includes 24-hour Holter monitoring or other type of event recorder, exercise stress testing, signal-averaged ECG, and electrophysiology study (EPS).[30]

EPS is performed under fluoroscopy. Pacing electrodes are placed in selected intracardiac areas, and stimuli are selectively used to attempt to produce dysrhythmias. The patient's response to various antidysrhythmic medications is determined and monitored in a controlled environment. (Chapters 32 and 36 discuss EPS.)

The most common approach to preventing a recurrence is the use of an implantable cardioverter-defibrillator (ICD). It has been shown that an ICD improves survival compared with drug therapy alone.[30,31] (Chapter 36 discusses ICDs.) Drug therapy with amiodarone (Cordarone) may be used in conjunction with an ICD to decrease episodes of ventricular dysrhythmias.

Teaching people about the symptoms of impending cardiac arrest and the actions to take can save lives. Rapid cardiopulmonary resuscitation (CPR) (see Appendix A) and defibrillation with an automatic external defibrillator (AED), combined with early advanced cardiac life support, have greatly improved long-term survival rates for a witnessed arrest.

When caring for these patients, be alert to the patient's psychosocial adaptation to this sudden "brush with death." Many of these patients develop a "time bomb" mentality. They fear the recurrence of cardiac arrest and may become anxious, angry, and depressed. Their caregivers are likely to experience the same feelings. Patients and caregivers also may need to deal with additional issues such as possible driving restrictions, role reversal, and change in occupation. The grief response varies among patients and caregivers. Be attuned to the specific needs of the patient and caregiver and teach them accordingly while providing appropriate emotional support.

CASE STUDY

Myocardial Infarction

iStockphoto/Thinkstock

Patient Profile
D.M., a 51-year-old, white, successful executive, is rushed to the hospital by ambulance after experiencing crushing substernal chest pain that radiates down his left arm. He also complains of dizziness and nausea.

Subjective Data
- Has a history of chronic stable angina and hypertension
- States he is "borderline diabetic"
- Overweight but recently lost 10 pounds
- Rarely exercises
- Has three teenage children who are causing "problems"
- Recently experienced loss of best friend and business partner, who died from cancer

Objective Data
Physical Examination
- Diaphoretic, short of breath, nauseous
- BP 165/100 mm Hg, pulse rate 120/min, respiratory rate 26/min

Diagnostic Studies
- 12-lead ECG shows sinus tachycardia with ST elevation in leads II, III, aVF, V₅, V₆ with occasional premature ventricular contractions
- Cardiac-specific troponin I level elevated
- Cholesterol 350 mg/dL (9.1 mmol/L)
- Hb A1C 9.0%
- Inferolateral wall MI

Collaborative Care
Emergency Department
- Oxygen 2 L/min via nasal cannula, titrate to keep O₂ saturation above 93%
- Continuous ECG monitoring
- Aspirin 325 mg (chewable)
- Eptifibatide (Integrilin) IV
- Weight-based heparin IV
- Nitroglycerin IV, titrate to relieve chest pain; hold for systolic BP below 100 mm Hg
- Morphine 2 to 4 mg IV q5min PRN for chest pain unrelieved by nitroglycerin
- Vital signs, pulse oximetry every 10 minutes
- Preparation of patient for transfer to cardiac catheterization laboratory for possible PCI

Discussion Questions
1. Which coronary artery(ies) is (are) most likely occluded in D.M.'s coronary circulation?
2. Explain the pathogenesis of CAD. What risk factors contribute to its development? What risk factors were present in D.M.'s life?
3. What is angina? How does chronic stable angina differ from angina associated with acute coronary syndrome?
4. Explain the pathophysiologic basis for the clinical manifestations that D.M. exhibited.
5. Explain the significance of the results of the laboratory tests and the 12-lead ECG findings.
6. Provide a rationale for each treatment measure ordered for D.M.
7. *Priority Decision:* Based on the assessment data presented, what are the priority nursing diagnoses? Identify any collaborative problems.
8. *Priority Decision:* What are the priority nursing interventions for D.M. immediately after his MI? Immediately after his PCI?
9. *Delegation Decision:* Identify activities that can be delegated to unlicensed assistive personnel (UAP).
10. *Evidence-Based Practice:* Two days after an uncomplicated PCI and the placement of two stents, D.M. wants to know what the most effective strategies are to prevent another MI. Based on his clinical situation, what would you tell him?

Ⓔvolve Answers and a corresponding concept map available at *http://evolve.elsevier.com/Lewis/medsurg.*

BRIDGE TO NCLEX EXAMINATION

The number of the question corresponds to the same-numbered outcome at the beginning of the chapter.

1. In teaching a patient about coronary artery disease, the nurse explains that the changes that occur in this disorder include *(select all that apply)*
   a. diffuse involvement of plaque formation in coronary veins.
   b. abnormal levels of cholesterol, especially low-density lipoproteins.
   c. accumulation of lipid and fibrous tissue within the coronary arteries.
   d. development of angina due to a decreased blood supply to the heart muscle.
   e. chronic vasoconstriction of coronary arteries leading to permanent vasospasm.

2. After teaching about ways to decrease risk factors for CAD, the nurse recognizes that additional instruction is needed when the patient says
   a. "I would like to add weight lifting to my exercise program."
   b. "I can only keep my blood pressure normal with medication."
   c. "I can change my diet to decrease my intake of saturated fats."
   d. "I will change my lifestyle to reduce activities that increase my stress."

3. A hospitalized patient with a history of chronic stable angina tells the nurse that she is having chest pain. The nurse bases his actions on the knowledge that ischemia
   a. will always progress to myocardial infarction.
   b. will be relieved by rest, nitroglycerin, or both.
   c. indicates that irreversible myocardial damage is occurring.
   d. is frequently associated with vomiting and extreme fatigue.

4. The nurse is caring for a patient who is 2 days post-MI. The patient reports that she is experiencing chest pain. She states, "It hurts when I take a deep breath." Which action would be a priority?
   a. Notify the physician STAT and obtain a 12-lead ECG.
   b. Obtain vital signs and auscultate for a pericardial friction rub.
   c. Apply high-flow oxygen by face mask and auscultate breath sounds.
   d. Medicate the patient with PRN analgesic and reevaluate in 30 minutes.

5. A patient is admitted to the ICU with a diagnosis of unstable angina. Which medication(s) would the nurse expect the patient to receive *(select all that apply)*?
   a. ACE inhibitor
   b. Antiplatelet therapy
   c. Thrombolytic therapy
   d. Prophylactic antibiotics
   e. Intravenous nitroglycerin

6. A patient is recovering from an uncomplicated MI. Which rehabilitation guideline is a priority to include in the teaching plan?
   a. Refrain from sexual activity for a minimum of 3 weeks.
   b. Plan a diet program that aims for a 1- to 2-pound weight loss per week.
   c. Begin an exercise program that aims for at least five 30-minute sessions per week.
   d. Consider the use of erectile agents and prophylactic NTG before engaging in sexual activity.

7. The most common finding in individuals at risk for sudden cardiac death is
   a. aortic valve disease.
   b. mitral valve disease.
   c. left ventricular dysfunction.
   d. atherosclerotic heart disease.

1. b, c, d, 2. a, 3. b, 4. b, 5. a, b, e, 6. c, 7. c

ⓔvolve

For rationales to these answers and even more NCLEX review questions, visit *http://evolve.elsevier.com/Lewis/medsurg*.

REFERENCES

1. Go AS, Mozaffarian D, Roger VL, et al: Heart disease and stroke statistics—2013 update: a report from the American Heart Association, *Circulation* 127:e6, 2013.
2. Huether SE, McCance KL: *Understanding pathophysiology*, ed 5, St Louis, 2012, Mosby.
*3. The Emerging Risk Factors Collaboration: C-reactive protein concentration and risk of coronary heart disease, stroke, and mortality: an individual participant meta-analysis, *Lancet* 375:132, 2010.
4. American Heart Association: Statistical fact sheet 2012 update: women and cardiovascular disease. Retrieved from *www.heart.org/idc/groups/heart-public/@wcm/@sop/@smd/documents/downloadable/ucm_319576.pdf*.
5. Musunuru K, Kathiresan S: Genetics of coronary artery disease, *Annu Rev Genomics Hum Genet* 11:91, 2010.
*6. Smith SC, Benjamin EJ, Bonow RO, et al: AHA/ACCF secondary prevention and risk reduction therapy for patients with coronary and other atherosclerotic vascular disease: 2011 update, *J Am Coll Cardiol* 58:2432, 2011.
*7. Grundy SM, Cleeman JI, Merz MB, et al: Implications of recent clinical trials for the National Cholesterol Education Program Adult Treatment Panel III Guidelines, *Circulation* 110:227, 2004.
*8. National Institutes of Health: *Seventh report of the Joint National Committee on Prevention, Detection, Evaluation, and Treatment of High Blood Pressure (JNC 7)*, pub no 03-5233, Bethesda, Md, 2003, US Department of Health and Human Services.
9. US Department of Health and Human Services (USDHHS): *2008 physical activity guidelines for Americans*, pub no U0036, Bethesda, Md, 2008, The US Department of Health and Human Services.
*10. Thombs BD, de Jonge P, Coyne JC, et al: Depression screening and patient outcomes in cardiovascular care: a systematic review, *JAMA* 300(18):2161, 2008.

*Evidence-based information for clinical practice.

*11. Brydon L, Strike PC, Bhattacharyya MR, et al: Hostility and physiological responses to laboratory stress in acute coronary syndrome patients, *J Psychosom Res* 68:109, 2010.

12. Proietti R, Mapelli D, Volpe B, et al: Mental stress and ischemic heart disease: evolving awareness of a complex association, *Future Cardiol* 7(3):425, 2011.

*13. Humphrey LL, Fu R, Rogers K, et al: Homocysteine level and coronary heart disease incidence: a systematic review and meta-analysis, *Mayo Clin Proc* 83:1203, 2008.

14. National Institute on Drug Abuse: InfoFacts: cocaine. Retrieved from *www.drugabuse.gov/publications/infofacts/cocaine*.

15. Lehne RA: *Pharmacology for nursing care*, ed 7, St Louis, 2010, Saunders.

*16. Mosca L, Benjamin EJ, Berra K, et al: Effectiveness-based guidelines for the prevention of cardiovascular disease in women 2011 update: a guideline from the American Heart Association, *J Am Coll Cardiol* 57:1401, 2011.

*17. Fihn SD, Gardin JM, Abrams J, et al: 2012 ACCF/AHA/ACP/AATS/PCNA/SCAI/STS guideline for the diagnosis and management of patients with stable ischemic heart disease: a report of the American College of Cardiology Foundation/American Heart Association Task Force on Practice Guidelines and the American College of Physicians, American Association for Thoracic Surgery, Preventive Cardiovascular Nurses Association, Society for Cardiovascular Angiography and Interventions, and Society of Thoracic Surgeons, *Circulation* 126:e354, 2012.

*18. O'Gara PT, Kushner FG, Ascheim DD, et al: 2013 ACCF/AHA guideline for the management of ST-elevation myocardial infarction: executive summary, *J Am Coll Cardiol* 61:485, 2013.

19. Bonow RO, Mann DL, Zipes DP, et al: *Braunwald's heart disease: a textbook of cardiovascular medicine*, ed 9, St Louis, 2012, Saunders.

20. Evangelista O, McLaughlin MA: Review of cardiovascular risk factors in women, *Gend Med* 6(Suppl 1):17, 2009.

*21. Jneid H, Anderson JL, Wright RS, Adams CD, et al: 2012 ACCF/AHA focused update of the guidelines for the management of patients with unstable angina/non-ST-elevation myocardial infarction (updating the 2007 guideline and replacing the 2011 focused update), *J Am Coll Cardiol* 126:875, 2012.

*22. Levine GN, Bates ER, Blankenship JC, et al: 2011 ACCF/AHA/SCAI guideline for percutaneous coronary intervention, *J Am Coll Cardiol* 58:1, 2011.

23. Krumholz HM, Anderson JL, Bachelder BL, et al: ACC/AHA 2008 performance measures for adults with ST-elevation and non ST-elevation myocardial infarction, *Circulation* 118:2596, 2008.

*24. Hillis LD, Smith PK, Anderson JL, et al: 2011 ACCF/AHA guideline for coronary artery bypass graft surgery, *J Am Coll Cardiol* 58:1, 2011.

25. Bojar RM: *Manual of perioperative care in adult cardiac surgery*, ed 5, Hoboken, NJ, 2011, Wiley-Blackwell.

26. American Association of Critical-Care Nurses: Family presence: visitation in the adult ICU (2011). Retrieved from *www.aacn.org/WD/practice/content/practicealerts/family-visitation-icu-practice-alert.content*.

27. Caza N, Taha R, Qi Y, et al: The effects of surgery and anesthesia on memory and cognition, *Prog Brain Res* 169:409, 2008.

28. Lichtman JH, Bigger T, Blumenthal JA, et al: Depression and coronary heart disease: recommendations for screening, referral, and treatment, *Circulation* 118:1768, 2008.

*29. Levine GN, Steinke EE, Bakaeen FG, et al: Sexual activity and cardiovascular disease: a scientific statement from the American Heart Association, *Circulation* 125:1058, 2012.

30. Mudawi TO, Albouaini K, Kaye GC: Sudden cardiac death: history, aetiology and management, *Br J Hosp Med* 70:89, 2009.

31. Exner DV: Implantable cardioverter defibrillator therapy for patients with less severe left ventricular dysfunction, *Curr Opin Cardiol* 24:61, 2009.

RESOURCES

American College of Cardiology
www.acc.org
American Heart Association
www.heart.org/HEARTORG/GettingHealthy/GettingHealthy_UCM_001078_SubHomePage.jsp
International Society for Minimally Invasive Cardiothoracic Surgery
www.ismics.org
Mended Hearts
www.mendedhearts.org
National Heart, Lung, and Blood Institute of the National Institutes of Health—Health Topics
www.nhlbi.nih.gov/health/health-topics/by-alpha/#
Preventive Cardiovascular Nurses Association
www.pcna.net

A joyful heart is good medicine, but a crushed spirit dries up the bones.
Proverbs 17:22

Nursing Management
Heart Failure

Carolyn Moffa

evolve WEBSITE

http://evolve.elsevier.com/Lewis/medsurg

- NCLEX Review Questions
- Key Points
- Pre-Test
- Answer Guidelines for Case Study on p. 785
- Rationales for Bridge to NCLEX Examination Questions

- Case Study
  - Patient With Heart Failure
- Nursing Care Plan (Customizable)
  - NCP 35-1: Patient With Heart Failure
- Concept Map Creator
- Concept Map for Case Study on p. 785
- Glossary
- Content Updates

eTable
- eTable 35-1: Who Is the Patient With Heart Failure? Think FACES

LEARNING OUTCOMES

1. Compare the pathophysiology of systolic and diastolic ventricular failure.
2. Relate the compensatory mechanisms involved in heart failure (HF) to the development of acute decompensated heart failure (ADHF) and chronic HF.
3. Select appropriate nursing and collaborative interventions to manage the patient with ADHF.
4. Select appropriate nursing and collaborative interventions to manage the patient with chronic HF.
5. Describe the indications for cardiac transplantation and the nursing management of cardiac transplant recipients.

KEY TERMS

cardiac transplantation, p. 783
diastolic failure, p. 767
heart failure (HF), p. 766

paroxysmal nocturnal dyspnea (PND), p. 771
pulmonary edema, p. 770
systolic failure, p. 767

HEART FAILURE

Heart failure (HF) is an abnormal clinical syndrome that involves inadequate pumping and/or filling of the heart. It is a major health problem in the United States. This chapter discusses the management and nursing care of patients experiencing this syndrome.

HF causes the heart to be unable to provide sufficient blood to meet the oxygen needs of the tissues. In clinical practice, the terms *acute* and *chronic HF* have replaced the term *congestive HF* (CHF) because not all HF involves pulmonary congestion. However, the term *CHF* is still commonly used.[1,2]

HF is associated with numerous cardiovascular diseases, particularly long-standing hypertension, coronary artery disease (CAD), and myocardial infarction (MI). Unlike other cardiovascular diseases, HF is increasing in incidence and prevalence. This is due to improved survival after cardiac events and the growing aging population. Currently, about 5.1 million people in the United States have HF. The American Heart Association (AHA) estimates that over 600,000 new cases are diagnosed each year. HF is primarily a disease of older adults; approximately 10 in every 1000 persons over the age of 65 have HF. The incidence of HF is similar in men and women.[3]

HF is the most common reason for hospital admission in older adults. This places a significant economic burden on the health care system.[1] The complex, progressive nature of HF often results in poor outcomes, the most costly being hospital readmissions.[3]

Reviewed by Evelyn Dean, RN, MSN, ACNS-BC, CCRN, Clinical Nurse Specialist, Heart Failure Department, Mid America Heart Institute, Saint Luke's Hospital of Kansas City, Kansas City, Missouri; Carla V. Hannon, MS, APRN, CCRN, Clinical Nurse Specialist, Intensive Care Unit, Hospital of Saint Raphael, New Haven, Connecticut; Kathleen M. Hill, RN, MSN, CCNS, Clinical Nurse Specialist, Surgical Intensive Care Unit, Cleveland Clinic, Cleveland, Ohio; and Christina D. Keller, RN, MSN, Instructor, Radford University School of Nursing: Clinical Simulation Center, Radford, Virginia.

Etiology and Pathophysiology

Hypertension and CAD are the primary risk factors for HF. Most patients with HF have a history of hypertension. The risk of HF increases with the severity of hypertension. Other factors, such as diabetes, advanced age, tobacco use, obesity, and high serum cholesterol, also contribute to the development of HF.

HF may be caused by any interference with the normal mechanisms regulating cardiac output (CO). CO depends on (1) preload, (2) afterload, (3) myocardial contractility, and (4) heart rate (HR). (Preload and afterload are discussed in Chapter 32.) Any changes in these factors can lead to decreased ventricular function and HF.

The major causes of HF may be divided into two subgroups: (1) primary causes (Table 35-1) and (2) precipitating causes (Table 35-2). Precipitating causes often increase the workload of the ventricles, resulting in an acute condition and decreased heart function.

Genetic Link

Specific genes and gene mutations have been linked to the development of hypertension, CAD, and cardiomyopathy (weakening of the heart muscle) (see Chapters 33, 34, and 37). These cardiovascular diseases are known risk factors for HF. Knowledge of why some people with these diseases are at high risk for developing HF is incomplete. Future research into the effects of these gene mutations will most likely be related to the common causes of HF.[4]

Pathophysiology of Ventricular Failure. HF is classified as systolic or diastolic failure (or dysfunction). Patients can have isolated systolic or diastolic failure or a combination of both.

Systolic Failure. Systolic failure results from an inability of the heart to pump blood effectively. It is caused by impaired contractile function (e.g., MI), increased afterload (e.g., hypertension), cardiomyopathy, and mechanical abnormalities (e.g., valvular heart disease).

The left ventricle (LV) in systolic failure loses its ability to generate enough pressure to eject blood forward through the aorta. Over time, the LV becomes dilated and hypertrophied. The hallmark of systolic failure is a decrease in the left ventricular ejection fraction (EF). The EF is defined as the amount of blood ejected from the LV with each contraction. Normal EF is 55% to 60%. Patients with systolic HF generally have an EF less than 45%. It can be as low as 10%.

Diastolic Failure. Diastolic failure is the inability of the ventricles to relax and fill during diastole. Diastolic failure is often referred to as HF with normal EF. Decreased filling of the ventricles results in decreased stroke volume and CO. Diastolic

TABLE 35-1 PRIMARY CAUSES OF HEART FAILURE

- Coronary artery disease, including myocardial infarction
- Hypertension, including hypertensive crisis
- Rheumatic heart disease
- Congenital heart defects (e.g., ventricular septal defect)
- Pulmonary hypertension
- Cardiomyopathy (e.g., viral, postpartum, substance abuse)
- Hyperthyroidism
- Valvular disorders (e.g., mitral stenosis)
- Myocarditis

TABLE 35-2 PRECIPITATING CAUSES OF HEART FAILURE*

Cause	Mechanism
Anemia	↓ O_2-carrying capacity of the blood stimulating ↑ in CO to meet tissue demands, leading to increase in cardiac workload and increase in size of LV
Infection	↑ O_2 demand of tissues, stimulating ↑ CO
Thyrotoxicosis	Changes the tissue metabolic rate, ↑ HR and workload of the heart
Hypothyroidism	Indirectly predisposes to ↑ atherosclerosis; severe hypothyroidism decreases myocardial contractility
Dysrhythmias	May ↓ CO and ↑ workload and O_2 requirements of myocardial tissue
Bacterial endocarditis	*Infection:* ↑ metabolic demands and O_2 requirements *Valvular dysfunction:* causes stenosis and regurgitation
Pulmonary embolism	↑ Pulmonary pressure resulting from obstruction leads to pulmonary hypertension, ↓ CO
Paget's disease	↑ Workload of the heart by ↑ vascular bed in the skeletal muscle
Nutritional deficiencies	May ↓ cardiac function by ↑ myocardial muscle mass and myocardial contractility
Hypervolemia	↑ Preload causing volume overload on the RV

*List is not all inclusive.
CO, Cardiac output; *LV,* left ventricle; *RV,* right ventricle.

failure is characterized by high filling pressures because of stiff ventricles. This results in venous engorgement in both the pulmonary and systemic vascular systems. Diastolic failure is usually the result of left ventricular hypertrophy from hypertension (most common), myocardial ischemia, valve disease (e.g., aortic, mitral), or cardiomyopathy. However, many patients do not have an identifiable heart disease. The diagnosis of diastolic failure is made based on the presence of HF symptoms with a normal EF.[5] Diastolic failure occurs more frequently in older adults, women, and people who are obese (see Gender Differences box).

Mixed Systolic and Diastolic Failure. Mixed systolic and diastolic failure is seen in disease states such as dilated cardiomyopathy (DCM). DCM is a condition in which poor systolic function is further compromised by dilated left ventricular walls that are unable to relax (see Chapter 37). These patients often have extremely low EFs (less than 35%), high pulmonary pressures, and *biventricular failure* (both ventricles are dilated and have poor filling and emptying capacity).

The patient with ventricular failure of any type may have low blood pressure (BP), low CO, and poor renal perfusion. Poor

Heart Failure

Men	Women
• Men experience systolic failure more frequently than women. • Men with asymptomatic systolic failure experience greater mortality benefit from ACE inhibitor therapy than women.	• Women experience diastolic failure more frequently than men. • Women have a higher risk of ACE inhibitor–related cough than men. • Women experience more digitalis-related death than men. • Women with diabetes are more predisposed to heart failure than men.

ACE, Angiotensin-converting enzyme.

exercise tolerance and heart dysrhythmias are also common. Whether a patient arrives at this point acutely from an MI or chronically from worsening cardiomyopathy or hypertension, the body's response to this low CO is to mobilize its compensatory mechanisms to maintain CO and BP.

Compensatory Mechanisms. HF can have an abrupt onset as with acute MI, or it can be a subtle process resulting from slow, progressive changes. The overloaded heart uses compensatory mechanisms to try to maintain adequate CO. The main compensatory mechanisms include (1) sympathetic nervous system (SNS) activation, (2) neurohormonal responses, (3) ventricular dilation, and (4) ventricular hypertrophy.

Sympathetic Nervous System Activation. SNS activation is often the first mechanism triggered in low-CO states. However, it is the least effective compensatory mechanism. In response to an inadequate stroke volume and CO, SNS activation increases, resulting in the increased release of catecholamines (epinephrine and norepinephrine). This results in increased HR, increased myocardial contractility, and peripheral vasoconstriction. Initially, this increase in HR and contractility improves CO. However, over time these factors are harmful, since they increase the already failing heart's workload and need for oxygen. The vasoconstriction causes an immediate increase in preload, which may initially increase CO. However, an increase in venous return to the heart, which is already volume overloaded, actually worsens ventricular performance.

Neurohormonal Response. As the CO falls, blood flow to the kidneys decreases. This is sensed by the juxtaglomerular apparatus in the kidneys as decreased volume. In response, the kidneys release renin, which converts angiotensinogen to angiotensin I (see Chapter 45 and Fig. 45-4). Angiotensin I is subsequently converted to angiotensin II by a converting enzyme made in the lungs. Angiotensin II causes (1) the adrenal cortex to release aldosterone, which results in sodium and water retention; and (2) increased peripheral vasoconstriction, which increases BP. This response is known as the renin-angiotensin-aldosterone system (RAAS).

Low CO causes a decrease in cerebral perfusion pressure. In response, the posterior pituitary gland secretes antidiuretic hormone (ADH), also called vasopressin. ADH increases water reabsorption in the kidneys, causing water retention. As a result, blood volume is increased in a person who is already volume overloaded.

Other factors also contribute to the development of HF. The production of *endothelin*, a potent vasoconstrictor produced by the vascular endothelial cells, is stimulated by ADH, catecholamines, and angiotensin II. Endothelin results in further arterial

vasoconstriction and an increase in cardiac contractility and hypertrophy.

Locally, proinflammatory cytokines are released by heart cells in response to various forms of cardiac injury (e.g., MI). Two cytokines, tumor necrosis factor (TNF) and interleukin-1 (IL-1), further depress heart function by causing hypertrophy, contractile dysfunction, and cell death. Over time, a systemic inflammatory response also occurs. This accounts for the cardiac and skeletal muscle myopathy and fatigue that accompany advanced HF.

Activation of the SNS and the neurohormonal response lead to elevated levels of norepinephrine, angiotensin II, aldosterone, ADH, endothelin, and proinflammatory cytokines. Together, these factors result in an increase in cardiac workload, myocardial dysfunction, and *ventricular remodeling.* Remodeling involves hypertrophy of the ventricular myocytes, resulting in large, abnormally shaped contractile cells. This altered geometric shape of the ventricles eventually leads to increased ventricular mass, increased wall tension, increased oxygen consumption, and impaired contractility. Although the ventricles become larger, they become less effective pumps. Ventricular remodeling is a risk factor for life-threatening dysrhythmias and sudden cardiac death (SCD).

Dilation. *Dilation* is an enlargement of the chambers of the heart (Fig. 35-1, *A*). It occurs when pressure in the heart chambers (usually the LV) is elevated over time. The heart muscle fibers stretch in response to the volume of blood in the heart at the end of diastole. The degree of stretch is directly related to the force of the contraction (systole) (this is the *Frank-Starling law*). This increased contraction initially leads to increased CO and maintenance of BP and perfusion. Dilation starts as an adaptive mechanism to cope with increasing blood volume. Eventually this mechanism becomes inadequate because the elastic elements of the muscle fibers are overstretched and can no longer contract effectively, thereby decreasing the CO.

Hypertrophy. *Hypertrophy* is an increase in the muscle mass and cardiac wall thickness in response to overwork and strain (Fig. 35-1, *B*). It occurs slowly because it takes time for this increased muscle tissue to develop. Initially, the increased contractile power of the muscle fibers leads to an increase in CO and maintenance of tissue perfusion. Over time, hypertrophic heart muscle has poor contractility, requires more oxygen to perform work, has poor coronary artery circulation (tissue becomes ischemic more easily), and is prone to dysrhythmias.

Counterregulatory Mechanisms. The body's attempts to maintain balance are demonstrated by several counterregulatory processes. Natriuretic peptides (atrial natriuretic peptide [ANP] and brain, or b-type, natriuretic peptide [BNP]) are hormones produced by the heart muscle. ANP is released from the atria and BNP is released from the ventricles in response to increased blood volume in the heart.[6]

The natriuretic peptides have renal, cardiovascular, and hormonal effects. Renal effects include (1) increased glomerular filtration rate and diuresis and (2) excretion of sodium (natriuresis). Cardiovascular effects include vasodilation and decreased BP. Hormonal effects include (1) inhibition of aldosterone and renin secretion and (2) interference with ADH release. The combined effects of ANP and BNP help to counter the adverse effects of the SNS and RAAS in patients with HF.[5]

Nitric oxide (NO) is another counterregulatory substance released from the vascular endothelium in response to the compensatory mechanisms activated in HF. Like the natriuretic

Enlarged atria

Enlarged ventricles

Thickened heart muscle

FIG. 35-1 **A,** Dilated heart chambers. **B,** Hypertrophied heart chambers.

peptides, NO works to relax the arterial smooth muscle, resulting in vasodilation and decreased afterload.

Cardiac compensation occurs when compensatory mechanisms succeed in maintaining an adequate CO that is needed for tissue perfusion. *Cardiac decompensation* occurs when these mechanisms can no longer maintain adequate CO and inadequate tissue perfusion results.

Types of Heart Failure

HF is usually manifested by biventricular failure, although one ventricle may precede the other in dysfunction. Normally the pumping actions of the left and right sides of the heart are synchronized, producing a continuous flow of blood. However, as a result of pathologic conditions, one side may fail while the other side continues to function normally for a time. Because of the prolonged strain, both sides of the heart eventually fail, resulting in biventricular failure (Fig. 35-2).

Left-Sided Heart Failure. The most common form of HF is left-sided HF. Left-sided HF results from left ventricular dysfunction. This prevents normal, forward blood flow and causes blood to back up into the left atrium and pulmonary veins. The increased pulmonary pressure causes fluid leakage from the pulmonary capillary bed into the interstitium and then the alveoli. This manifests as pulmonary congestion and edema.

Right-Sided Heart Failure. Right-sided HF occurs when the right ventricle (RV) fails to contract effectively. Right-sided HF causes a backup of blood into the right atrium and venous circulation. Venous congestion in the systemic circulation results in jugular venous distention, hepatomegaly, splenomegaly, vascular congestion of the gastrointestinal tract, and peripheral edema.

Right-sided HF may result from an acute condition such as right ventricular infarction or pulmonary embolism. *Cor pulmonale* (right ventricular dilation and hypertrophy caused by pulmonary disease) can also cause right-sided HF (see Chapters 28 and 29).

The primary cause of right-sided HF is left-sided HF. In this situation, left-sided HF results in pulmonary congestion and increased pressure in the blood vessels of the lung (pulmonary hypertension). Eventually, chronic pulmonary hypertension (increased right ventricular afterload) results in right-sided hypertrophy and HF.

Clinical Manifestations
Acute Decompensated Heart Failure

In acute decompensated HF (ADHF), an increase in the pulmonary venous pressure is caused by failure of the LV. This results in engorgement of the pulmonary vascular system (Fig. 35-3, *A* and *B*). As a result, the lungs become less compliant, and there is increased resistance in the small airways. In addition, the lymphatic system increases its flow to help maintain a constant volume of the pulmonary extravascular fluid. This early stage is clinically associated with a mild increase in the respiratory rate and a decrease in partial pressure of oxygen in arterial blood (PaO_2).

If pulmonary venous pressure continues to increase, the increase in intravascular pressure causes more fluid to move into the interstitial space than the lymphatics can remove. *Interstitial edema* occurs at this point (Fig. 35-3, *C*). Tachypnea develops, and the patient becomes symptomatic (e.g., short of breath). If the pulmonary venous pressure increases further, the alveoli lining cells are disrupted and a fluid containing red blood cells (RBCs) moves into the alveoli (*alveolar edema*). As the disruption becomes worse from further increases in the pulmonary venous pressure, the alveoli and airways are flooded with fluid. This is accompanied by a worsening of the arterial blood gas values (i.e., lower PaO_2 and possible increased partial pressure of carbon dioxide in arterial blood [$PaCO_2$] and progressive respiratory acidemia).

ADHF can manifest as pulmonary edema. This is an acute, life-threatening situation in which the lung alveoli become filled with serosanguineous fluid (Fig. 35-3, *D*). The most common cause of pulmonary edema is left-sided HF secondary to CAD. (Other etiologic factors for pulmonary edema are listed in Table 28-25.)

Clinical manifestations of pulmonary edema are distinct. The patient is usually anxious, pale, and possibly cyanotic. The skin is clammy and cold from vasoconstriction caused by stimulation of the SNS. The patient has *dyspnea* (shortness of breath) and *orthopnea* (shortness of breath while lying down). Respiratory rate is often greater than 30 breaths/minute, and use of accessory muscles to breathe may be seen. There may be wheezing and coughing with the production of frothy, blood-tinged sputum. Auscultation of the lungs may reveal crackles, wheezes, and rhonchi throughout the lungs. The patient's HR is rapid,

PATHOPHYSIOLOGY MAP

FIG. 35-2 Pathophysiology of heart failure. Elevated systemic vascular resistance results in left-sided heart failure that leads to right-sided heart failure. Systemic vascular resistance and preload are exacerbated by the renin-angiotensin-aldosterone system. *ADH,* Antidiuretic hormone; *LA,* left atrium; *LV,* left ventricle; *LVEDP,* left ventricular end-diastolic pressure; *RV,* right ventricle.

		Congestion (Wet)	
		No	**Yes**
Low Perfusion (Cold)	**No**	**Dry-Warm** • PAWP normal • CO normal • Signs and symptoms: none	**Wet-Warm** • PAWP ↑ • CO normal • Possible signs and symptoms: dyspnea, edema, orthopnea
	Yes	**Dry-Cold** • PAWP ↓ or normal • CO ↓ • Possible signs and symptoms: edema, hypotension, cool extremities	**Wet-Cold** • PAWP ↑ • CO ↓ • Possible signs and symptoms: altered mental status, decreased O₂ saturation, reduced urine output, shock

TABLE 35-3 CLINICAL PROFILE IN ACUTE DECOMPENSATED HEART FAILURE

CO, Cardiac output; *PAWP,* pulmonary artery wedge pressure.

Clinical Manifestations
Chronic Heart Failure

Chronic HF is characterized as a progressive worsening of ventricular function and chronic neurohormonal activation that results in ventricular remodeling. This process involves changes in the size, shape, and mechanical performance of the ventricle. The clinical manifestations of chronic HF depend on the patient's age, the underlying type and extent of heart disease, and which ventricle is failing to pump effectively. Table 35-4 lists the manifestations of right-sided and left-sided chronic HF. The patient with chronic HF usually has manifestations of biventricular failure. The Heart Failure Society of America (HFSA) developed the acronym FACES (*F*atigue, limitation of *A*ctivities, chest *C*ongestion/cough, *E*dema, and *S*hortness of breath) to help teach patients to identify HF symptoms[7] (see eTable 35-1 on the website for this chapter).

Fatigue. Fatigue is one of the earliest symptoms of chronic HF. The patient notes fatigue after usual activities and eventually limits these activities. The fatigue is caused by decreased CO, impaired perfusion to vital organs, decreased oxygenation of the tissues, and anemia. Anemia can result from poor nutrition, renal disease, or drug therapy (e.g., angiotensin-converting enzyme [ACE] inhibitors).

Dyspnea. Dyspnea is a common manifestation of chronic HF. It is caused by increased pulmonary pressures secondary to interstitial and alveolar edema. Dyspnea can occur with mild exertion or at rest. Orthopnea often accompanies dyspnea. Careful questioning of patients often reveals adaptive behaviors such as sleeping with two or more pillows or in a chair to aid breathing.

Paroxysmal nocturnal dyspnea (PND) occurs when the patient is asleep. It is caused by the reabsorption of fluid from dependent body areas when the patient is flat. The patient awakes in a panic, has feelings of suffocation, and has a strong desire to sit or stand up.

A cough is often associated with HF and may be the first clinical symptom. It begins as a dry, nonproductive cough and may be misdiagnosed as asthma or other lung disease. The

and BP may be elevated or decreased depending on the severity of the HF.

Patients with ADHF can be categorized into one of four groups based on hemodynamic and clinical status: dry-warm, dry-cold, wet-warm, and wet-cold[1] (Table 35-3). The most common presentation is the warm and wet patient. This patient has adequate perfusion (warm) but has volume overload (e.g., congestion, dyspnea, edema).

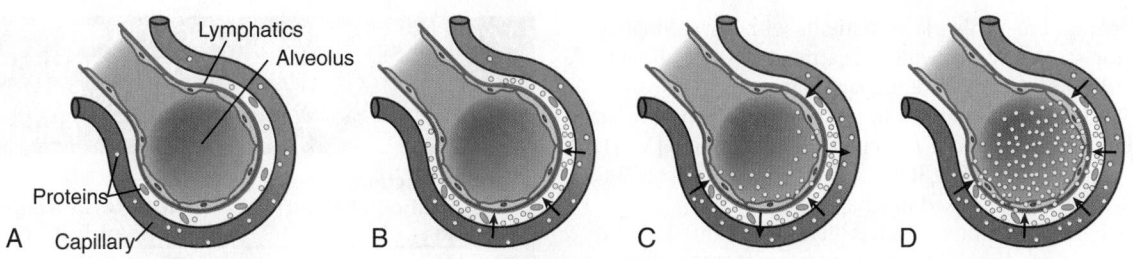

FIG. 35-3 As pulmonary edema progresses, it inhibits oxygen and carbon dioxide exchange at the alveolar-capillary interface. **A,** Normal relationship. **B,** Increased pulmonary capillary hydrostatic pressure causes fluid to move from the vascular space into the pulmonary interstitial space. **C,** Lymphatic flow increases in an attempt to pull fluid back into the vascular or lymphatic space. **D,** Failure of lymphatic flow and worsening of left-sided heart failure result in further movement of fluid into the interstitial space and into the alveoli.

TABLE 35-4	MANIFESTATIONS OF HEART FAILURE	
Right-Sided Heart Failure	**Left-Sided Heart Failure**
Signs	
• RV heaves	• LV heaves
• Murmurs	• Pulsus alternans (alternating pulses: strong, weak)
• Jugular venous distention	
• Edema (e.g., pedal, scrotum, sacrum)	• ↑ HR
	• PMI displaced inferiorly and posteriorly (LV hypertrophy)
• Weight gain	• ↓ PaO₂, slight ↑ PaCO₂ (poor O₂ exchange)
• ↑ HR	
• Ascites	• Crackles (pulmonary edema)
• Anasarca (massive generalized body edema)	• S₃ and S₄ heart sounds
	• Pleural effusion
• Hepatomegaly (liver enlargement)	• Changes in mental status
	• Restlessness, confusion
Symptoms	
• Fatigue	• Weakness, fatigue
• Anxiety, depression	• Anxiety, depression
• Dependent, bilateral edema	• Dyspnea
	• Shallow respirations up to 32-40/min
• Right upper quadrant pain	• Paroxysmal nocturnal dyspnea
• Anorexia and GI bloating	• Orthopnea (shortness of breath in recumbent position)
• Nausea	• Dry, hacking cough
	• Nocturia
	• Frothy, pink-tinged sputum (advanced pulmonary edema)

LV, Left ventricle; *PaCO₂,* partial pressure of CO₂ in arterial blood; *PaO₂,* partial pressure of O₂ in arterial blood; *PMI,* point of maximal impulse; *RV,* right ventricle.

cough is not relieved by position change or over-the-counter cough medicine.

Tachycardia. Tachycardia is an early clinical sign of HF. One of the body's first mechanisms to compensate for a failing ventricle is to increase the HR. Because of reduced CO, the SNS is activated, which increases HR. However, this response may be blocked or reduced in patients taking β-blocker medications.

Edema. Edema is a common sign of HF. It may occur in dependent body areas (peripheral edema), liver (hepatomegaly), abdominal cavity (ascites), and lungs (pulmonary edema and pleural effusion). If the patient is in bed, sacral and scrotal edema may develop. Pressing the edematous skin with the finger may leave a transient depression *(pitting edema).* The development of dependent edema or a sudden weight gain of more than 3 lb (1.4 kg) in 2 days is often a sign of ADHF. It is

important to note that not all lower extremity edema is a result of HF. Hypoproteinemia, immobility, venous insufficiency, and certain medications can cause peripheral edema.

Nocturia. A person with chronic HF who has decreased CO will also have impaired renal perfusion and decreased urine output during the day. However, when the person lies down at night, fluid moves from the interstitial spaces back into the circulatory system. In addition, cardiac workload is decreased at night while resting. These combined effects result in increased renal blood flow and diuresis. The patient may complain of having to void frequently throughout the night.

Skin Changes. Because tissue capillary oxygen extraction is increased in a person with chronic HF, the skin may appear dusky. Often the lower extremities are shiny and swollen, with diminished or absent hair growth. Chronic swelling may result in pigment changes. This causes the skin to appear brown or brawny in areas covering the ankles and lower legs.

Behavioral Changes. Cerebral circulation may be reduced with chronic HF secondary to decreased CO. The patient or caregiver may report unusual behavior, including restlessness, confusion, and decreased attention span or memory. This may also be secondary to poor gas exchange and worsening HF. It is often seen in the late stages of HF.

Chest Pain. HF can precipitate chest pain (angina) because of decreased coronary artery perfusion from decreased CO and increased myocardial work. Chest pain may accompany either ADHF or chronic HF.

Weight Changes. Many factors contribute to weight changes. First, a progressive weight gain may occur because of fluid retention. Renal failure may also contribute to fluid retention. Abdominal fullness from ascites and hepatomegaly frequently causes anorexia and nausea. As HF advances, the patient may have cardiac *cachexia* with muscle wasting and fat loss. This can be masked by the patient's edematous condition and may not be seen until after the edema subsides.

Complications of Heart Failure

Pleural Effusion. *Pleural effusion* results from increasing pressure in the pleural capillaries. A transudation of fluid occurs from these capillaries into the pleural space. (Pleural effusion is discussed in Chapter 28.)

Dysrhythmias. Chronic HF causes enlargement of the chambers of the heart. This enlargement (stretching of the atrial and ventricular walls) can cause changes in the normal electrical pathways. When numerous sites in the atria fire spontaneously and rapidly (atrial fibrillation), the organized atrial depolarization (contraction) no longer occurs. Atrial fibrillation also promotes thrombus formation within the atria. Thrombi may break loose and form emboli. This places patients with atrial fibrillation at risk for stroke. They require treatment with cardioversion, antidysrhythmics, and/or anticoagulants.

Patients with HF are also at risk for ventricular dysrhythmias (e.g., ventricular tachycardia [VT], ventricular fibrillation [VF]). VT and VF can lead to SCD. (SCD is discussed in Chapter 34, and dysrhythmias are discussed in Chapter 36.)

Left Ventricular Thrombus. With ADHF or chronic HF, the enlarged LV and decreased CO combine to increase the chance of thrombus formation in the LV. Once a thrombus has formed, it may also decrease left ventricular contractility, decrease CO, and worsen the patient's perfusion. The development of emboli from the thrombus also places the patient at risk for stroke.

Hepatomegaly. HF can lead to severe hepatomegaly, especially with RV failure. The liver becomes congested with venous blood. The hepatic congestion leads to impaired liver function. Eventually liver cells die, fibrosis occurs, and cirrhosis can develop (see Chapter 44).

Renal Failure. The decreased CO that accompanies chronic HF results in decreased perfusion to the kidneys and can lead to renal insufficiency or failure (see Chapter 47).

Classification of Heart Failure

In 1964 the New York Heart Association (NYHA) developed functional guidelines for classifying people with heart disease based on tolerance to physical activity. Because this system only reflected exercise capacity, the American College of Cardiology Foundation/AHA (ACCF/AHA) developed a staging system that identified disease progression and treatment strategies.[1] This system allows for identification of people at risk for developing HF but who do not currently have heart disease. The ACCF/AHA system encourages clinicians to actively address the patient's risk factors and treat any existing conditions to prevent further disease progression. This may help reduce the growing number of HF patients. The two systems are compared in Table 35-5.

Diagnostic Studies

Diagnosing HF is often difficult, since neither patient signs nor symptoms are highly specific, and both may mimic those associated with many other medical conditions (e.g., anemia, lung disease). Diagnostic tests for ADHF and chronic HF are presented in Table 35-6. A primary goal in diagnosis is to find the underlying cause of HF.

An endomyocardial biopsy (EMB) may be done in patients who develop unexplained, new-onset HF that is unresponsive to usual care.[8] EF is used to differentiate systolic and diastolic HF. This distinction is important to make in the early treatment of HF. EF is measured using echocardiography and/or nuclear imaging studies (see Table 32-6). Other useful diagnostic tests include electrocardiogram (ECG), chest x-ray, and heart catheterization.

Laboratory studies also aid in the diagnosis of HF. In general, BNP levels correlate positively with the degree of left ventricular failure. Many laboratories routinely measure the N-terminal prohormone of BNP (NT-proBNP). This is a more precise assay to aid in the diagnosis of HF (see Table 32-6). Levels are temporarily higher in patients receiving nesiritide (Natrecor) and may be high in patients with chronic, stable HF. Increases in BNP or NT-proBNP levels can be caused by conditions other than HF. These conditions include pulmonary embolism, renal failure, and acute coronary syndrome.

TABLE 35-5	NYHA FUNCTIONAL CLASSIFICATION OF HEART DISEASE AND ACCF/AHA STAGES OF HEART FAILURE	
NYHA Functional Classification of Heart Disease	**ACCF/AHA Stages of Heart Failure**
Class I No limitation of physical activity. Ordinary physical activity does not cause fatigue, dyspnea, palpitations, or anginal pain.	**Stage A** Patients at high risk for HF (e.g., patients with hypertension, diabetes, metabolic syndrome) but without structural heart disease or symptoms of HF.
Class II Slight limitation of physical activity. No symptoms at rest. Ordinary physical activity results in fatigue, dyspnea, palpitations, or anginal pain.	**Stage B** Patients with structural heart disease (e.g., patients with history of MI, valve disease) but who have never shown signs or symptoms of HF.
Class III Marked limitation of physical activity but usually comfortable at rest. Less than ordinary physical activity causes fatigue, dyspnea, palpitations, or anginal pain.	**Stage C** Patients with prior or current symptoms of HF associated with known, underlying structural heart disease.
Class IV Inability to carry on any physical activity without discomfort. Symptoms of cardiac insufficiency or of angina may be present even at rest. If any physical activity is undertaken, discomfort is increased.	**Stage D** Patients with refractory HF (e.g., patients with severe symptoms at rest despite maximal medical therapy) who require specialized interventions.

Sources: The Criteria Committee of the New York Heart Association: *Nomenclature and criteria for diagnosis of diseases of the heart and great vessels*, ed 9, Boston, 1994, Little, Brown & Co. and Yancy CW, Jessup M, Bozkurt B, et al: 2013 ACCF/AHA guideline for the management of heart failure: executive summary, *Circulation* 128:e1, 2013.
ACCF/AHA, American College of Cardiology Foundation/American Heart Association; *HF*, heart failure; *MI*, myocardial infarction; *NYHA*, New York Heart Association.

Collaborative Care
Acute Decompensated Heart Failure

With the addition of new drugs and device therapies, the management of HF has dramatically changed in the past few years. Because of the large number of patients and the high cost of care related to hospital readmissions, strategies to improve outcomes have been developed. One example is the use of guideline-directed medical therapy as defined by the AACF/AHA.[1] Another example is specialized HF inpatient units with transitional programs to the outpatient setting to help manage these patients. These units are staffed with multidisciplinary HF teams, including nurses who are educated in the care of these patients. Table 35-6 lists the collaborative therapy for the patient with ADHF.

Patients with ADHF need continuous monitoring and assessment. This may be done in an intensive care unit (ICU) if the patient is unstable. In the ICU, you will monitor ECG and oxygen saturation continuously. Assess vital signs and urine output at least every hour. The patient may have hemodynamic monitoring, including intraarterial BP and pulmonary artery pressures (PAPs). If a pulmonary artery catheter is placed, eval-

TABLE 35-6   COLLABORATIVE CARE

Heart Failure

Both ADHF and Chronic HF	ADHF	Chronic HF
Diagnostic		
• History and physical examination	• Measurement of LV function	• Exercise stress testing
• Determination of underlying cause	• Endomyocardial biopsy	
• Serum chemistries, cardiac markers, BNP or NT-proBNP level (see Table 32-6), liver function tests, thyroid function tests, CBC, lipid profile, kidney function tests, urinalysis		
• Chest x-ray		
• 12-lead ECG		
• Hemodynamic monitoring		
• 2-dimensional echocardiogram		
• Nuclear imaging studies (see Table 32-6)		
• Cardiac catheterization		
Collaborative Therapy		
• Treatment of underlying cause	• High Fowler's position	• O$_2$ therapy at 2-6 L/min by nasal cannula if indicated
• Circulatory assist devices (e.g., ventricular assist device)	• O$_2$ by mask or nasal cannula	• Rest-activity periods
• Daily weights	• BiPAP	• Cardiac rehabilitation
• Sodium- and, possibly, fluid-restricted diet	• Circulatory assist device: intraaortic balloon pump	• Home health nursing care (e.g., telehealth monitoring)
	• Endotracheal intubation and mechanical ventilation	• Drug therapy (see Table 35-7)
	• Vital signs, urine output at least q1hr	• Cardiac resynchronization therapy with biventricular pacing and internal cardioverter-defibrillator
	• Continuous ECG and pulse oximetry monitoring	• LVAD
	• Hemodynamic monitoring (e.g., intraarterial BP, PAWP, CO)	• Cardiac transplantation
	• Drug therapy (see Table 35-7)	• Palliative and end-of-life care
	• Possible cardioversion (e.g., atrial fibrillation)	
	• Ultrafiltration	

ADHF, Acute decompensated heart failure; *BiPAP*, bilevel positive airway pressure; *BNP*, b-type natriuretic peptide; *CO*, cardiac output; *HF*, heart failure; *LVAD*, left ventricular assist device; *NT-proBNP*, N-terminal prohormone of BNP; *PAWP*, pulmonary artery wedge pressure.

uate CO and pulmonary artery wedge pressure (PAWP). Therapy is titrated to maximize CO and reduce PAWP. A normal PAWP is generally between 8 and 12 mm Hg. Patients with ADHF may have a PAWP as high as 30 mm Hg. (Hemodynamic monitoring is discussed in Chapter 66.)

Supplemental oxygen helps increase the percentage of oxygen in inspired air. (Oxygen therapy is discussed in Chapter 29.) In severe pulmonary edema the patient may need noninvasive ventilatory support (e.g., bilevel positive airway pressure [BiPAP]) or intubation and mechanical ventilation. BiPAP is also effective in decreasing preload. (Ventilatory support is discussed in Chapter 66.)

Some patients with ADHF require hospitalization but are more stable. They are often admitted to a telemetry or stepdown unit for treatment. Assess these patients every 4 hours (e.g., vital signs, pulse oximetry) for adequate oxygenation. Record intake and output and daily weights to evaluate fluid status.

If the patient is dyspneic, place in a high Fowler's position with the feet horizontal in the bed or dangling at the bedside. This position helps decrease venous return because of the pooling of blood in the extremities. This position also increases the thoracic capacity, allowing for improved breathing.

Ultrafiltration (UF), or *aquapheresis,* is an option for the patient with volume overload.[9] It is a process to remove excess salt and water from the patient's blood. UF can rapidly remove intravascular fluid volume while maintaining hemodynamic stability. The ideal patients for UF are those with major pulmonary or systemic volume overload who have shown resistance to diuretics and are hemodynamically stable. UF also may be an appropriate adjunctive therapy for patients with HF and coexisting renal failure. (UF is discussed in Chapter 47.) Once the patient is more stable, determination of the cause of ADHF and pulmonary edema is important. Diagnosis of systolic or diastolic HF will then direct further management protocols.

Circulatory assist devices are used to manage patients with worsening HF. The intraaortic balloon pump (IABP) is a device that increases coronary blood flow to the heart muscle and decreases the heart's workload through a process called counterpulsation. It is useful in hemodynamically unstable patients because it decreases SVR, PAWP, and PAP, leading to improved CO. Ventricular assist devices (VADs) can be used to maintain the pumping action of a heart that cannot effectively contract by itself. A VAD is a battery-operated, mechanical pump that is surgically implanted. (IABPs and VADs are discussed in Chapter 66.)

Coexisting psychologic disorders, especially depression and anxiety, contribute to an increased risk of mortality and higher readmission rates and health care costs in patients with HF.[10] In addition, patients with psychologic disorders have poorer adherence to treatment and self-care.[11] Assess patients with HF for depression and anxiety and, if appropriate, initiate treatment plans.

Drug Therapy. Drug therapy is essential in treating ADHF (Table 35-7).

Diuretics. Diuretics are the mainstay of treatment in patients with volume overload. Diuretics act to decrease sodium reabsorption at various sites within the nephrons, thereby enhancing sodium and water loss. Decreasing intravascular volume with the use of diuretics reduces venous return (preload) and subsequently the volume returning to the LV. This allows the

TABLE 35-7   DRUG THERAPY

Heart Failure

Drug	Mechanism of Action
Diuretics (see Table 33-7) **Loop Diuretics** • furosemide (Lasix) • bumetanide (Bumex)	• Decrease fluid volume • Decrease preload • Decrease pulmonary venous pressure • Relieve symptoms of heart failure (e.g., edema)
Thiazide Diuretics* • hydrochlorothiazide (HCTZ) • metolazone (Zaroxolyn)	
Potassium-Sparing Diuretics • spironolactone (Aldactone) • eplerenone (Inspra)	
Renin-Angiotensin-Aldosterone System Inhibitors (see Table 33-7) **ACE Inhibitors** • captopril (Capoten) • benazepril (Lotensin) • enalapril (Vasotec) **Angiotensin II Receptor Blockers** • losartan (Cozaar) • valsartan (Diovan)	• Dilate venules and arterioles • Improve renal blood flow • Decrease fluid volume • Relieve symptoms of heart failure • Promote reverse remodeling • Decrease morbidity and mortality
Vasodilators • hydralazine (Apresoline)* • isosorbide dinitrate/ hydralazine (BiDil)* • nitrates (e.g., nitroglycerin [Nitro-Bid], isosorbide dinitrate [Isordil]) • nesiritide (Natrecor)† • nitroprusside (Nipride)†	• Reduce cardiac afterload, leading to increased CO • Dilate the arterioles of the kidneys, leading to increased renal perfusion and fluid loss • Decrease BP • Decrease preload • Relieve symptoms of heart failure (e.g., dyspnea)
β-Adrenergic Blockers* (see Table 33-7) • metoprolol (Toprol XL) • bisoprolol (Zebeta) • carvedilol (Coreg)	• Promote reverse remodeling • Decrease afterload • Inhibit SNS • Decrease morbidity and mortality
Positive Inotropes **β-Adrenergic Agonists†** • dopamine (Intropin) • dobutamine (Dobutrex) **Phosphodiesterase Inhibitor†** • milrinone (Primacor) **Digitalis Glycoside*** • digoxin (Lanoxin)	• Increase contractility (positive inotropic effect) • Increase CO • Increase heart rate (positive chronotropic effect) • Produce mild vasodilation • Increase stroke volume and CO • Promote vasodilation
Morphine†	• Decreases anxiety • Decreases preload and afterload
Antidysrhythmic Drugs (see Table 36-9)	• Prevent or treat dysrhythmias
Anticoagulants	• Prevent thromboembolism • Recommended for patients with an ejection fraction <20% and/or atrial fibrillation

*Used for chronic HF only.
†Used for ADHF only.
ACE, Angiotensin-converting enzyme; *ADHF,* acute decompensated heart failure; *CO,* cardiac output; *SNS,* sympathetic nervous system.

LV to contract more efficiently. CO is increased, pulmonary vascular pressures are decreased, and gas exchange is improved. Loop diuretics (e.g., furosemide [Lasix], bumetanide [Bumex]) can be administered by IV push and act rapidly in the kidneys.

Vasodilators. IV nitroglycerin is a vasodilator that reduces circulating blood volume. It also improves coronary artery circulation by dilating the coronary arteries. Therefore nitroglycerin reduces preload, slightly reduces afterload (in high doses), and increases myocardial oxygen supply. When titrating IV nitroglycerin, monitor BP frequently (every 5 to 10 minutes) to avoid symptomatic hypotension.

Sodium nitroprusside (Nipride) is a potent IV vasodilator that reduces both preload and afterload, thus improving myocardial contraction, increasing CO, and reducing pulmonary congestion.[12] Complications of IV sodium nitroprusside include (1) hypotension; and (2) thiocyanate toxicity, which can develop after 48 hours of use. Sodium nitroprusside is administered in an ICU, since symptomatic hypotension is the main adverse effect.

DRUG ALERT: Sodium Nitroprusside (Nipride)
• Assess BP before administration and continuously (every 5-10 min) during administration.
• Too rapid rate of IV administration can reduce BP too quickly.
• Headache, nausea, dizziness, dyspnea, blurred vision, sweating, and restlessness can occur.

Nesiritide, administered IV, is a recombinant form of BNP and causes both arterial and venous dilation. The main hemodynamic effects of nesiritide include (1) a reduction in PAWP and (2) a decrease in systemic BP. Although classified as a vasodilator, nesiritide is also a neurohormonal blocking agent. It can be used for short-term treatment of ADHF.[1,13] Nesiritide does not require titration after the initial IV bolus. It can be given in the emergency department (ED) and non-ICU setting. Because the main adverse effect of nesiritide is symptomatic hypotension, monitor BP closely.

Morphine. Morphine sulfate reduces preload and afterload. It is frequently used in the treatment of acute coronary syndrome and HF. It dilates both the pulmonary and systemic blood vessels. Results include a decrease in pulmonary pressures and myocardial oxygen needs, and an improvement in gas exchange. When morphine is used, the patient often experiences relief from dyspnea and, consequently, the anxiety that often is associated with dyspnea.

Use morphine cautiously in patients with ADHF. Morphine is related to more adverse events, including a greater need for mechanical ventilation, more ICU admissions, prolonged hospitalization, and higher mortality rates.[14]

Positive Inotropes. Inotropic therapy increases myocardial contractility. Drugs include β-adrenergic agonists (e.g., dopamine [Intropin], dobutamine [Dobutrex], epinephrine, norepinephrine [Levophed]), the phosphodiesterase inhibitor milrinone (Primacor), and digitalis. The β-adrenergic agonists are only used as a short-term treatment of ADHF. In addition to increasing myocardial contractility and SVR, dopamine dilates the renal blood vessels and enhances urine output. Unlike dopamine, dobutamine is a selective β-adrenergic agonist and works primarily on the β$_1$-receptors in the heart. Dobutamine does not increase SVR and is preferred for short-term treatment of ADHF.[15]

DRUG ALERT: Dopamine (Intropin)
• Monitor IV site for signs of extravasation.
• Tissue necrosis with sloughing can occur with drug extravasation.
• High dosages may produce ventricular dysrhythmias.

Milrinone is a phosphodiesterase inhibitor that has been called an inodilator. It increases myocardial contractility (inotropic effect) and promotes peripheral vasodilation. Inhibition of phosphodiesterase increases cyclic adenosine monophosphate (cAMP). This enhances calcium entry into the cell and improves myocardial contractility. Milrinone increases CO and reduces BP (decrease afterload). Like dopamine and dobutamine, this drug is available only for IV use. Adverse effects include dysrhythmias, thrombocytopenia, and hepatotoxicity.

Digitalis is a positive inotrope that improves left ventricular function. Digitalis increases contractility but also increases myocardial oxygen consumption. Because digitalis requires a loading dose and time to work, it is not recommended for the initial treatment of ADHF.[15]

Currently, inotropic therapy is only recommended for use in the short-term management of patients with ADHF who have not responded to conventional pharmacotherapy (e.g., diuretics, vasodilators, morphine).[1]

Collaborative Care
Chronic Heart Failure

The main goals in the treatment of chronic HF are to treat the underlying cause and contributing factors, maximize CO, reduce symptoms, improve ventricular function, improve quality of life, preserve target organ function, and improve mortality and morbidity risks (see Table 35-6). The management of hypertension is discussed in Chapter 33, CAD in Chapter 34, dysrhythmias in Chapter 36, and valvular disorders in Chapter 37.

In a person with HF, oxygen saturation of the blood can be reduced because the blood is not adequately oxygenated in the lungs. Administration of oxygen improves saturation and assists in meeting tissue oxygen needs. This helps to relieve dyspnea and fatigue. Optimally pulse oximetry is used to monitor the need for and effectiveness of oxygen therapy.

Physical and emotional rest allows the patient to conserve energy and decreases the need for additional oxygen. The degree of rest recommended depends on the severity of HF. A patient with severe HF may be on bed rest with limited activity. A patient with mild to moderate HF can be ambulatory with restriction of strenuous activity. Instruct the patient to participate in prescribed activities with adequate recovery periods. A structured exercise program, such as cardiac rehabilitation, should be offered to all patients with chronic HF.

Nonpharmacologic therapies are an integral part of the care of HF patients. One therapy is *biventricular pacing* or *cardiac resynchronization therapy* (CRT). Traditional pacemakers pace one or two chambers (e.g., right atrium and/or right ventricle). In HF, neurohormonal effects and cardiac remodeling can result in dyssynchrony of the ventricular contractions. This contributes to poor CO. In CRT an extra pacing lead is placed through the coronary sinus to a coronary vein of the LV. This lead coordinates right and left ventricular contractions through biventricular pacing (Fig. 35-4). The ability to have normal electrical conduction (synchrony) between the RV and the LV increases left ventricular function and CO.

Life-threatening ventricular dysrhythmias (e.g., VT) can cause SCD. The addition of an implantable cardioverter-defibrillator (ICD) with CRT is often warranted. (Pacemakers and defibrillators are discussed in Chapter 36.)

Several mechanical options are available to sustain HF patients with deteriorating conditions, especially those awaiting cardiac transplantation. These include the IABP and VADs.

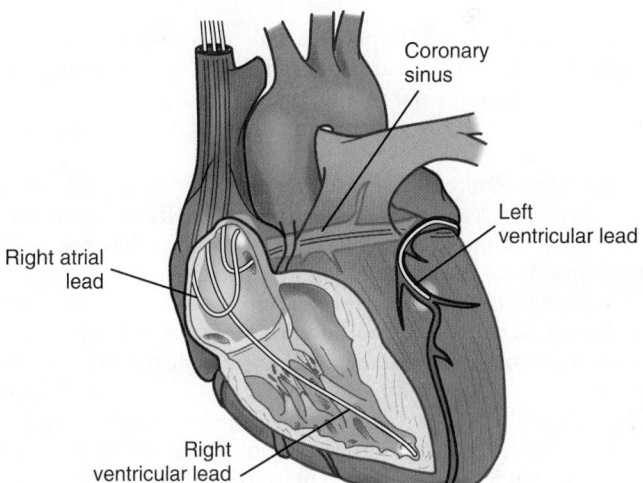

FIG. 35-4 Placement of pacing leads in cardiac resynchronization therapy.

However, the limitations of bed rest and the risk of infection and vascular complications preclude long-term use of IABP. VADs provide highly effective long-term support and have become standard care in many heart transplant centers. VADs are used as a bridge to transplantation. They effectively increase heart function until a donor heart becomes available. The use of a permanent, implantable VAD, known as *destination therapy*,

EVIDENCE-BASED PRACTICE

Applying the Evidence

T.F. is a 62-year-old female patient recovering from an episode of acute decompensated heart failure (ADHF). Her HF is Class III in the New York Heart Association Functional Classification of Heart Disease (see Table 35-5). Her physician has recommended biventricular pacing (cardiac resynchronization therapy) for treatment of her HF symptoms. She tells you that she does not want any artificial implants, and that she has researched the use of hawthorn for treatment of her heart disease.

Best Available Evidence	Clinician Expertise	Patient Preferences and Values
Strong evidence supports the use of biventricular pacing (cardiac resynchronization therapy) to improve symptoms, exercise capacity, quality of life, ejection fraction, and survival and to decrease hospitalizations in patients like T.F.	You know the benefits of and possible complications related to biventricular pacing in patients with T.F.'s situation. You also know that there is strong evidence supporting the use of hawthorn in patients with mild to moderate HF (see Complementary & Alternative Therapies box on p. 777).	Patient does not want any artificial implants. She wants to consider alternative (herbal) therapy.

Your Decision and Action

You review the risks and benefits of biventricular pacing and herbal (hawthorn) therapy for the treatment of HF with T.F. She remains committed to the use of hawthorn—at least for a trial period. You support her decision and inform the physician of her wishes.

Reference for Evidence

Yancy CW, Jessup M, Bozkurt B, et al: 2013 ACCF/AHA guideline for the management of heart failure: executive summary, *Circulation* 128:e1, 2013.

is an option for some HF patients with advanced NYHA Functional Class IV HF who are not candidates for heart transplantation. (IABPs and VADs are discussed in Chapter 66.)

Drug Therapy. Drug therapy for chronic HF is presented in Table 35-7.

Diuretics. Diuretics are used to reduce edema, pulmonary venous pressure, and preload (see Table 33-7). If excess extracellular fluid is removed, blood volume returning to the heart can be reduced and cardiac function improved.

Diuretics act on the kidney by promoting excretion of sodium and water. Many varieties of diuretics are available. Loop diuretics (e.g., furosemide, bumetanide) are potent diuretics. These drugs act on the ascending loop of Henle to promote sodium, chloride, and water excretion. Problems in using loop diuretics include reduction in serum potassium levels, ototoxicity, and possible allergic reaction in patients sensitive to sulfa-type drugs.

Thiazide diuretics inhibit sodium reabsorption in the distal tubule, thus promoting excretion of sodium and water. They can be added to loop diuretics to obtain results if patients become resistant to loop diuretics. Thiazide diuretics also can cause severe reductions in potassium levels.

Diuretics are effective in relieving the congestive symptoms of HF. However, their use does activate the SNS and RAAS, which can exacerbate the HF syndrome. In chronic HF the lowest effective dose of diuretic should be used.

Renin-Angiotensin-Aldosterone System Inhibitors

Angiotensin-Converting Enzyme Inhibitors. ACE inhibitors are the primary drug of choice for blocking the RAAS system in HF patients with systolic failure.[1,16,17] Examples of ACE inhibitors are listed in Table 35-7. Other examples of ACE inhibitors are discussed in Chapter 33 and listed in Table 33-7.

The conversion of angiotensin I to the potent vasoconstrictor angiotensin II requires ACE (see Chapter 45, Fig. 45-4). ACE inhibitors act by blocking this enzyme, resulting in reduced levels of angiotensin II. As a result, plasma aldosterone levels are also reduced. Thus ACE inhibitors serve as neurohormonal blocking agents. Consequently, ACE inhibitors also decrease the development of ventricular remodeling by inhibiting ventricular hypertrophy.

Because CO is dependent on afterload in chronic HF, the reduction in SVR seen with the use of ACE inhibitors causes a significant increase in CO. Although the use of ACE inhibitors may decrease BP, tissue perfusion is maintained or increased as a result of improved CO. In addition, diuresis is enhanced by the suppression of aldosterone.

DRUG ALERT: Captopril (Capoten)
- Excessive hypotension and hyperkalemia may occur.
- Monitor patient for first-dose hypotension (first-dose syncope).
- Skipping doses or discontinuing the drug can result in rebound hypertension.
- Angioedema, a rare adverse effect, can develop suddenly and can be life threatening.

Major side effects of ACE inhibitors include symptomatic hypotension, intractable cough, hyperkalemia, *angioedema* (allergic reaction involving edema of the face and airways), and renal insufficiency (when ACE inhibitors are used in high doses). Aging and baseline renal insufficiency slow the metabolism of ACE inhibitors and may lead to increased serum drug levels. Carefully monitor patients taking ACE inhibitors for potential adverse effects. For example, a cough may be attributed to ACE inhibitors when, in fact, it is also a common symptom of an exacerbation of HF. It is critical that the exact cause of cough and other side effects be confirmed before stopping ACE inhibitor therapy.

Angiotensin II Receptor Blockers. For patients who are unable to tolerate ACE inhibitors, angiotensin II receptor blockers (ARBs) (see Table 33-7) are recommended.[18,19] These agents prevent the vasoconstrictor and aldosterone-secreting effects of angiotensin II by binding to the angiotensin II receptor sites.

Aldosterone Antagonists. Spironolactone (Aldactone) and eplerenone (Inspra) are aldosterone antagonists. They block the harmful neurohormonal effects of aldosterone on the heart blood vessels. They are also potassium-sparing diuretics that promote sodium and water excretion while retaining potassium. These effects occur because these agents bind to receptors at the aldosterone-dependent sodium-potassium exchange site in the distal renal tube.

DRUG ALERT: Spironolactone (Aldactone)
- Monitor potassium levels during treatment.
- Use with caution in patients taking digoxin, since hyperkalemia may reduce the effects of digoxin.
- Instruct patient to avoid foods high in potassium (e.g., bananas, oranges, dried apricots).
- Assess male patients for gynecomastia, a common side effect of long-term use of spironolactone.

β-Adrenergic Blockers. β-Adrenergic blockers directly block the negative effects of the SNS (e.g., increased HR) on the failing

❀ COMPLEMENTARY & ALTERNATIVE THERAPIES

Hawthorn

Scientific Evidence*
- Strong evidence for its use in mild to moderate heart failure
- May inhibit angiotensin-converting enzyme
- May have a diuretic effect
- May reduce incidence of sudden cardiac death in patients with ejection fraction >25%

Nursing Implications
- May add to the effects of cardiac glycosides, antihypertensives, and cholesterol-lowering drugs
- Potentially beneficial treatment for patients who cannot or will not take prescription drugs and may offer additive benefits to established therapies

*Based on a systematic review of scientific literature. Retrieved from *www.naturalstandard.com*.

heart. They can also help in reducing the effect of renin.[19] Because β-blockers can reduce myocardial contractility, care must be taken to start slowly. Dosage is increased every 2 weeks as tolerated by the patient. Major adverse effects include edema, worsening of HF, hypotension, fatigue, and bradycardia. Three β-blockers are approved for use in HF patients: carvedilol (Coreg), bisoprolol (Zebeta), and metoprolol CR/XL (Toprol XL).[1,18]

DRUG ALERT: Carvedilol (Coreg)
- Overdosage can produce profound bradycardia, hypotension, bronchospasm, and cardiogenic shock.
- Obtain standing BP 1 hr after dosing to assess tolerance.
- Abrupt withdrawal may result in sweating, palpitations, and headaches.

Vasodilators

Nitrates. Nitrates cause vasodilation by acting directly on the smooth muscle of the vessel wall. Nitrates can be used in combination with hydralazine (Apresoline) for chronic HF management in patients who cannot tolerate ACE inhibitors or ARBs. Nitrates are of particular benefit in the management of myocardial ischemia related to HF because they promote vasodilation of the coronary arteries.

One specific problem with the use of nitrates in HF is nitrate tolerance. In addition, men with HF may experience erectile dysfunction and as a result take an erectile agent (e.g., sildenafil [Viagra]). Erectile agents are contraindicated in patients taking nitrates, since together they produce symptomatic hypotension.

BiDil. A combination drug containing isosorbide dinitrate and hydralazine (BiDil) is used for the treatment of HF in African Americans who are already being treated with standard therapy. The drug is only approved for use with this ethnic group.[20] How these two drugs work together is not fully known. As an antihypertensive agent, hydralazine relaxes the arteries and decreases the work of the heart. The antianginal agent isosorbide dinitrate relaxes the veins as well as the arteries. Isosorbide seems to work by releasing nitric oxide at the blood vessel wall, but its effect usually wears off after half a day. Hydralazine may prevent this loss of effect. Common side effects of isosorbide/hydralazine are headache and dizziness.

Positive Inotropes. Digitalis preparations (e.g., digoxin [Lanoxin]) increase the force of cardiac contraction (*inotropic action*). They also decrease the HR (*chronotropic action*). These actions allow for more complete emptying of the ventricles,

reducing the volume remaining in the ventricles during diastole. CO increases due to the increased stroke volume from improved contractility.[19]

Patients taking a digitalis preparation are at risk for digitalis toxicity. Hypokalemia, secondary to the use of potassium-depleting diuretics (e.g., thiazides, loop diuretics), is one of the most common causes of digitalis toxicity. Low serum potassium enhances the action of digitalis, causing a therapeutic dose to reach toxic levels. Similarly, hyperkalemia inhibits the action of digitalis, resulting in a subtherapeutic dose. Both hypokalemia and hyperkalemia also cause dysrhythmias. Monitor serum potassium levels of all patients taking digitalis preparations and potassium-depleting and potassium-sparing diuretics. Other electrolyte imbalances, such as hypercalcemia and hypomagnesemia, can also precipitate digitalis toxicity. (Manifestations of electrolyte imbalances are discussed in Chapter 17.)

DRUG ALERT: Digoxin (Lanoxin)
- Monitor for signs of hypokalemia and hyperkalemia, since these can increase or decrease the effects of digoxin, respectively.
- Monitor for early signs of toxicity: anorexia, nausea and vomiting, fatigue, headache, depression, visual changes.
- Monitor for late signs of toxicity: dysrhythmias (e.g., bradycardia, atrioventricular block).

Diseases of the kidney and liver increase the risk of digitalis toxicity because most preparations are metabolized and eliminated by these organs. An older adult is especially prone to digitalis toxicity. This is because digitalis accumulation occurs sooner with decreased liver and kidney function and slowed body metabolism.

The usual treatment of toxicity consists of withholding the drug until the symptoms subside. In the case of life-threatening toxicity, IV digoxin immune Fab (ovine) (Digibind) is an antidote. The treatment of life-threatening dysrhythmias is instituted as needed (see Chapter 36).

Nutritional Therapy

Poor adherence to a low-sodium diet and failure to take prescribed medications as directed are the two most common reasons for readmissions of HF patients to the hospital.[21] Therefore it is critical that you accurately assess a patient's diet.

Diet teaching and weight management are essential to the patient's control of chronic HF. You or a dietitian should obtain a detailed diet history. Determine not only what foods the patient eats but also when, where, and how often the patient dines out. In addition, assess the sociocultural value of food. Use this information to assist the patient in making appropriate dietary choices when developing a diet plan. The National Heart, Lung, and Blood Institute provides helpful dietary guidelines for heart-healthy food preparation for people of various cultures (e.g., Hispanics, Native Americans, Asian Americans, African Americans). These are available online at *www.nhlbi.nih.gov/health/index.htm#recipes*. Diet and weight management recommendations must be individualized and culturally sensitive if the necessary changes are to be made.

The edema associated with chronic HF is often treated by dietary restriction of sodium. Teach the patient what foods are low and high in sodium and ways to enhance food flavors without the use of salt (e.g., substituting lemon juice, various spices). The degree of sodium restriction depends on the severity of the HF and the effectiveness of diuretic therapy. The Dietary Approaches to Stop Hypertension (DASH) diet is effective as a first-line therapy for many individuals with hyperten-

TABLE 35-8   NUTRITIONAL THERAPY

Low-Sodium Diets

General Principles

Do not add salt or seasonings containing sodium when preparing foods.*

Do not use salt at the table.*

Avoid high-sodium foods (e.g., canned soups, processed meats, cheese, frozen meals).

Limit milk products to 2 cups daily.

Sample Menu Plans for 2400-mg Sodium Diet

Breakfast	Sodium (mg)
⅔ cup bran cereal	161
(⅔ cup Shredded Wheat cereal)†	3
1 slice whole-wheat bread	149
1 medium banana	1
6 oz fruit yogurt, fat free	85
1 cup fat-free milk	126
2 tbs jelly	5
Coffee, 8 oz	5

Lunch	
Chicken breast sandwich	
2 slices (3 oz) chicken breast, skinless	65
2 slices whole wheat bread	299
1 slice (¾ oz) American cheese	328
(1 slice [¾ oz] Swiss cheese, natural)†	54
Large-leaf romaine lettuce	1
2 slices tomato	90
1 Tbsp mayonnaise, low fat	90
1 medium peach	7

Dinner	
¾ cup vegetarian spaghetti sauce	459
(6 oz no-salt-added tomato paste)†	260
1 cup spaghetti	1
3 tbs parmesan cheese	349
Spinach salad	
1 cup fresh spinach leaves	24
¼ cup fresh carrots (grated)	10
¼ cup fresh mushrooms (sliced)	1
2 Tbsp vinaigrette dressing	0
½ cup canned pears, juice pack	4
½ cup corn, cooked from frozen	4

Snack	
⅓ cup almonds	4
¼ cup dried apricots	3
6 oz fruit yogurt, fat free	85

*1 tsp of salt equals 2.3 g of sodium.

†Substitutes to reduce to 1500-mg sodium diet.

Chicken Noodle Soup

Nutrition Facts

Serving Size 1/2 cup (120 mL) condensed soup
Servings Per Container about 2.5

Amount Per Serving		
Calories 60	Calories from Fat 15	
		% Daily Value*
Total Fat 1.5 g		2%
Saturated Fat 0.5 g		3%
Trans Fat 0 g		
Cholesterol 15 mg		
Sodium 890 mg		37%
Total Carbohydrate 8 g		3%
Dietary Fiber 1 g		4%
Sugars 1 g		
Protein 3 g		

Vitamin A	4%	**Calcium**	0%
Vitamin C	0%	**Iron**	2%

*Percent Daily Values are based on a 2,000 calorie diet. Your Daily Values may be higher or lower depending on your calorie needs.

		Calories	2000	2500
Total Fat	Less than		65 g	80 g
Sat Fat	Less than		20 g	25 g
Cholesterol	Less than		300 g	300 g
Sodium	Less than		2400 mg	2400 mg
Total Carbohydrate			300 g	375 g
Dietary Fiber			25 g	30 g

FIG. 35-5 Typical nutrition label. Note that a single serving (½ cup) provides more than one third of the daily recommended intake of sodium.

sion (see eTable 33-1: Your Guide to Lowering Your Blood Pressure With DASH). This diet is now also widely used for the patient with HF, with or without hypertension.

The average American adult's daily intake of sodium ranges from 7 to 15 g. A commonly prescribed diet for a patient with HF is a 2-g sodium diet (Table 35-8). All foods high in sodium (over 400 mg/serving) should be avoided. On this diet, processed meats, cheese, bread, cereals, canned soups, and canned vegetables must be limited. Teach the patient and caregiver how to read labels to look for sodium content (Fig. 35-5). The patient and caregiver should also be aware of the high sodium content of most restaurant foods.

Fluid restrictions are not commonly prescribed for the patient with mild to moderate HF. However, in moderate to severe HF and renal insufficiency, fluids are limited to less than 2 L/day.[18] Helping patients deal with thirst as a side effect of the medications is important. Suggest ice chips, gum, hard candy, or ice pops.

To monitor fluid status, instruct patients to weigh themselves at the same time each day, preferably before breakfast and using the same scale, while wearing the same type of clothing. This helps ensure valid comparisons from day to day and helps identify early signs of fluid retention. For patients with visual limitations, suggest scales with larger numbers or an audible response. Instruct patients to call the primary care provider if they see a weight gain of 3 lb (1.4 kg) over 2 days or a 3- to 5-lb (2.3-kg) gain over a week.[18,19]

NURSING MANAGEMENT
HEART FAILURE

NURSING ASSESSMENT

Subjective and objective data that you should obtain from a patient with HF are presented in Table 35-9. Carefully review the patient's current prescription and over-the-counter medications. Assess for use of any nonsteroidal antiinflammatory drugs (NSAIDs), since they can contribute to sodium retention. In addition, review the patient's dietary habits to identify issues related to an exacerbation of HF. The patient's chronic health problems may act as exacerbating factors, affecting the plan of care and the timing and selection of therapies. For example, a patient with sleep apnea may not regularly use his or her continuous positive airway pressure device at night. This can worsen pulmonary or systemic hypertension and lead to an exacerbation of HF.

TABLE 35-9 NURSING ASSESSMENT

Heart Failure

Subjective Data
Important Health Information
Past health history: CAD (including recent MI), hypertension, cardiomyopathy, valvular or congenital heart disease, diabetes mellitus, hyperlipidemia, renal disease, thyroid or lung disease, rapid or irregular heart rate
Medications: Use of and adherence with any heart medications; use of diuretics, estrogens, corticosteroids, nonsteroidal antiinflammatory drugs, over-the-counter drugs, herbal supplements

Functional Health Patterns
Health perception–health management: Fatigue, depression, anxiety
Nutritional-metabolic: Usual sodium intake; nausea, vomiting, anorexia, stomach bloating; weight gain, ankle swelling
Elimination: Nocturia, decreased daytime urine output, constipation
Activity-exercise: Dyspnea, orthopnea, cough (e.g., dry, productive); palpitations; dizziness, fainting
Sleep-rest: Number of pillows used for sleeping; paroxysmal nocturnal dyspnea, insomnia
Cognitive-perceptual: Chest pain or heaviness; RUQ pain, abdominal discomfort; behavioral changes; visual changes

Objective Data
Integumentary
Cool, diaphoretic skin; cyanosis or pallor; peripheral edema (right-sided heart failure)

Respiratory
Tachypnea, crackles, rhonchi, wheezes; frothy, blood-tinged sputum

Cardiovascular
Tachycardia, S_3, S_4, murmurs; pulsus alternans, PMI displaced inferiorly and posteriorly, lifts and heaves, jugular venous distention

Gastrointestinal
Abdominal distention, hepatosplenomegaly, ascites

Neurologic
Restlessness, confusion, decreased attention or memory

Possible Diagnostic Findings
Altered serum electrolytes (especially Na+ and K+), ↑ BUN, creatinine, or liver function tests; ↑ NT-proBNP or BNP; chest x-ray demonstrating cardiomegaly, pulmonary congestion, and interstitial pulmonary edema; echocardiogram showing increased chamber size, decreased wall motion, decreased EF or normal EF with evidence of diastolic failure; atrial and ventricular enlargement on ECG; ↓ O_2 saturation

BNP, b-Type natriuretic peptide; *BUN,* blood urea nitrogen; *EF,* ejection fraction; *NT-proBNP,* N-terminal prohormone of BNP; *PMI,* point of maximal impulse; *RUQ,* right upper quadrant.

NURSING DIAGNOSES

Nursing diagnoses for the patient with HF include, but are not limited to, those presented in Nursing Care Plan 35-1.

PLANNING

The overall goals for the patient with HF include (1) a decrease in symptoms (e.g., shortness of breath, fatigue), (2) a decrease in peripheral edema, (3) an increase in exercise tolerance, (4) adherence with the medical regimen, and (5) no complications related to HF.

NURSING IMPLEMENTATION

HEALTH PROMOTION. Communication and joint decision making among the patient, caregiver, and health care team are integral to selection and delivery of high-quality, patient-centered care. Currently, there is a campaign to aggressively identify and treat risk factors for HF to prevent or slow the progression of the disease.[22] For example, teach a patient with hypertension or hyperlipidemia measures to manage BP or cholesterol with medication, diet, and exercise. Patients with valvular disease should have valve replacement planned before lung congestion develops. Coronary revascularization procedures should be considered in patients with CAD. The use of antidysrhythmic drugs or pacing therapy is indicated for patients with serious dysrhythmias or conduction disturbances. In addition, encourage patients with HF to obtain vaccinations against the flu and pneumonia.

ACUTE INTERVENTION. Many persons with HF experience one or more episodes of ADHF. When they do, they are usually admitted through the ED, initially stabilized, and then managed in an ICU, an intermediate care unit, or a specialized HF unit with continuous ECG monitoring capability.

Successful HF management depends on several important principles: (1) HF is a progressive disease, and treatment plans are established along with quality-of-life goals; (2) symptom management is controlled by the patient with self-management tools (e.g., daily weights, drug regimens, diet and exercise plans); (3) salt and, at times, water must be restricted; (4) energy must be conserved; and (5) support systems are essential to the success of the entire treatment plan.[23] Nursing Care Plan 35-1 applies to the patient with stabilized ADHF or chronic HF.

Reduction of anxiety is an important nursing function, since anxiety may increase the SNS response and further increase myocardial workload. Reducing anxiety may be facilitated by a variety of nursing interventions and the use of sedatives (e.g., benzodiazepines).

The Joint Commission has selected core measures in the management of patients with HF to reflect standards of evidence-based care[24] (available at *www.jointcommission.org/assets/1/6/Heart%20Failure.pdf*). The AHA has developed a program, Get With the Guidelines—Heart Failure, to improve adherence to standards of evidence-based care of patients hospitalized with HF.[25] Together, these approaches work to ensure high-quality care for patients with HF.

AMBULATORY AND HOME CARE. HF is a chronic illness for most persons. When a patient is diagnosed with HF, care should focus on slowing the progression of the disease. Your important nursing responsibilities include (1) teaching the patient about the physiologic changes that have occurred, (2) helping the patient adapt to both physiologic and psychologic changes, and (3) integrating the patient and the caregiver in the overall care plan. Review the signs and symptoms of HF exacerbations with the patient and caregiver and provide them with a clear action plan should symptoms occur.[18] Early detection of worsening HF may help prevent an acute episode requiring hospitalization. A patient and caregiver guide for the patient with HF is presented in Table 35-10 on p. 782.

Patients with HF are at risk for anxiety and depression.[10] Emphasize to the patient that it is possible to live a productive life with this chronic health problem. Patients with HF are usually required to take medication for the rest of their lives. This often becomes difficult because a patient may be asymp-

◎ NURSING CARE PLAN 35-1

Patient With Heart Failure

NURSING DIAGNOSIS*	**Impaired gas exchange** *related to* increased preload and alveolar-capillary membrane changes *as evidenced by* abnormal oxygen saturation, hypoxemia, dyspnea, tachypnea, tachycardia, restlessness, and patient's statement, "I am so short of breath"
PATIENT GOAL	Maintains adequate O_2/CO_2 exchange at the alveolar-capillary membrane to meet O_2 needs of the body

Outcomes (NOC) | **Interventions (NIC) and *Rationales***

Respiratory Status: Gas Exchange
- Cognitive status _____
- Ease of breathing _____
- O_2 saturation _____
- PaO_2 _____

Measurement Scale
1 = Severely compromised
2 = Substantially compromised
3 = Moderately compromised
4 = Mildly compromised
5 = Not compromised

- Dyspnea with exertion _____
- Dyspnea at rest _____
- Restlessness _____

Measurement Scale
1 = Severe
2 = Substantial
3 = Moderate
4 = Mild
5 = None

Respiratory Monitoring
- Monitor pulse oximetry, respiratory rate, rhythm, depth, and effort of respirations *to evaluate changes in respiratory status.*
- Auscultate breath sounds, noting areas of decreased or absent ventilation and presence of adventitious sounds *to detect presence of pulmonary edema.*
- Monitor for increased restlessness, anxiety, and work of breathing *to detect increasing hypoxemia.*

Oxygen Therapy
- Administer supplemental O_2 or other noninvasive ventilator support (e.g., bilevel positive airway pressure [BiPAP]) as needed *to maintain adequate O_2 levels.*
- Monitor the O_2 liter flow rate and placement of O_2 delivery device *to ensure O_2 is adequately delivered.*
- Change O_2 delivery device from mask to nasal prongs during meals as tolerated *to sustain O_2 levels while eating.*
- Monitor the effectiveness of O_2 therapy *to identify hypoxemia and establish range of O_2 saturation.*

Positioning
- Position patient to alleviate dyspnea (e.g., semi-Fowler's position), as appropriate, *to improve ventilation by decreasing venous return to the heart and increasing thoracic capacity.*

NURSING DIAGNOSIS	**Decreased cardiac output** *related to* altered contractility, altered preload, and/or altered stroke volume *as evidenced by* decreased ejection fraction, increased CVP, decreased peripheral pulses, jugular venous distention, orthopnea, chest pain, S_3 and S_4 sounds, and oliguria
PATIENT GOAL	Maintains adequate blood pumped by the heart to meet metabolic demands of the body

Outcomes (NOC) | **Interventions (NIC) and *Rationales***

Cardiac Pump Effectiveness
- Ejection fraction _____
- Systolic BP _____
- Diastolic BP _____
- Apical heart rate _____
- 24-hr I/O balance _____
- CVP _____
- Peripheral pulses _____

Measurement Scale
1 = Severely compromised
2 = Substantially compromised
3 = Moderately compromised
4 = Mildly compromised
5 = Not compromised

- Neck vein distention _____
- Abnormal heart sounds _____
- Dysrhythmia _____
- Dyspnea _____
- Peripheral edema _____
- Pulmonary edema _____

Measurement Scale
1 = Severe
2 = Substantial
3 = Moderate
4 = Mild
5 = None

Cardiac Care
- Perform a comprehensive assessment of peripheral circulation (e.g., check peripheral pulses, edema, capillary refill, color, and temperature of extremity) *to determine circulatory status.*
- Note signs and symptoms of decreased cardiac output (e.g., chest pain, S_3, S_4, jugular venous distention) *to detect changes in status.*
- Monitor fluid balance (e.g., I/O and daily weight) *to evaluate renal perfusion.*
- Continuously monitor cardiac rhythm *to detect dysrhythmias.*
- Monitor for dyspnea, fatigue, tachypnea, and orthopnea *to identify involvement of respiratory system.*
- Instruct patient and caregivers on activity restriction and progression *to allay fears and anxiety.*
- Establish a supportive relationship with the patient and caregiver(s) *to promote adherence to the treatment plan.*
- Inform the patient of the purpose for and benefits of the prescribed activity and exercise.

*Nursing diagnoses are listed in order of priority.

NURSING CARE PLAN 35-1—cont'd
Patient With Heart Failure

NURSING DIAGNOSIS **Excess fluid volume** *related to* increased venous pressure and decreased renal perfusion secondary to heart failure *as evidenced by* rapid weight gain, edema, adventitious breath sounds, oliguria, and patient's statement, "My ankles are so swollen"

PATIENT GOAL Experiences reduction or absence of edema and stable baseline weight

Outcomes (NOC)	Interventions (NIC) and *Rationales*
Fluid Balance	**Hypervolemia Management**

Fluid Balance
- Stable body weight _____
- Peripheral pulses _____
- Serum electrolytes _____
- BP _____
- CVP _____
- 24-hr I/O balance _____

Measurement Scale
1 = Severely compromised
2 = Substantially compromised
3 = Moderately compromised
4 = Mildly compromised
5 = Not compromised

- Ascites _____
- Neck vein distention _____
- Peripheral edema _____
- Adventitious breath sounds _____

Measurement Scale
1 = Severe
2 = Substantial
3 = Moderate
4 = Mild
5 = None

Hypervolemia Management
- Administer prescribed diuretics, as appropriate, *to treat hypervolemia.*
- Monitor for therapeutic effect of diuretic (e.g., increased urine output, decreased CVP, decreased adventitious breath sounds) *to assess response to treatment.*
- Monitor potassium levels after diuresis *to detect excessive electrolyte loss.*
- Weigh patient daily and monitor trends *to evaluate effect of treatment.*
- Monitor intake and output *to assess fluid status.*
- Monitor respiratory pattern for symptoms of respiratory difficulty *to detect pulmonary edema.*
- Monitor hemodynamic status, including CVP, MAP, PAWP, if available, *to evaluate effectiveness of therapy.*
- Monitor changes in peripheral edema *to assess response to treatment.*

NURSING DIAGNOSIS **Activity intolerance** *related to* imbalance between O_2 supply and demand secondary to cardiac insufficiency and pulmonary congestion *as evidenced by* dyspnea, shortness of breath, weakness, increase in heart rate on exertion, and patient's statement, "I am too tired to get out of bed; I have no energy"

PATIENT GOAL Achieves a realistic program of activity that balances physical activity with energy-conserving activities

Outcomes (NOC)	Interventions (NIC) and *Rationales*

Activity Tolerance
- Pulse rate with activity _____
- O_2 saturation with activity _____
- Respiratory rate with activity _____
- Systolic BP with activity _____
- Diastolic BP with activity _____
- Ease of breathing with activity _____
- Ease of performing ADLs _____
- Skin color _____

Measurement Scale
1 = Severely compromised
2 = Substantially compromised
3 = Moderately compromised
4 = Mildly compromised
5 = Not compromised

Energy Management
- Encourage alternate rest and activity periods *to reduce cardiac workload and conserve energy.*
- Provide calming diversionary activities to promote relaxation *to reduce O_2 consumption and to relieve dyspnea and fatigue.*
- Monitor patient's O_2 response (e.g., pulse rate, cardiac rhythm, and respiratory rate) to self-care or nursing activities *to determine level of activity that can be performed.*
- Teach patient and caregiver techniques of self-care *that will minimize O_2 consumption (e.g., self-monitoring and pacing techniques for performance of ADLs).*

Activity Therapy
- Collaborate with occupational and/or physical therapists *to plan and monitor activity or exercise program.*
- Determine patient's commitment to increasing frequency and/or range of activities or exercise *to provide patient with obtainable goals.*

ADLs, Activities of daily living; *CVP,* central venous pressure; *I/O,* intake and output; *HF,* heart failure; *MAP,* mean arterial pressure; *PaO₂,* partial pressure of O_2 in arterial blood; *PAWP,* pulmonary artery wedge pressure.

tomatic when HF is under control. You must stress that the disease is chronic, and that medication must be continued to keep the HF under control.

Teach the patient the expected actions of the prescribed drugs and the signs of drug toxicity. Also teach the patient and caregiver how to take a pulse rate. The pulse rate should always be taken for 1 full minute. A pulse rate less than 50 beats/minute may be a contraindication to taking β-adrenergic blocker or a digitalis preparation unless directed by the health care provider. However, in the absence of symptoms (e.g., heart block, ven-

tricular ectopy, syncope), a pulse rate less than 50 beats/minute may be acceptable. Include clear information about when a drug, especially β-blockers and digitalis, should be held and a health care provider called.

Teach the patient the symptoms of hypokalemia and hyperkalemia if diuretics that deplete or spare potassium are ordered. Frequently the patient who takes thiazide or loop diuretics is given supplemental potassium. It may also be appropriate to instruct patients in home BP monitoring, especially for those HF patients with hypertension.

TABLE 35-10   PATIENT & CAREGIVER TEACHING GUIDE

Heart Failure

Include the following instructions when teaching the patient and caregiver about the management of heart failure.

Dietary Therapy
- Consult the written diet plan and list of permitted and restricted foods.
- Examine labels to determine sodium content. Also examine the labels of over-the-counter drugs such as laxatives, cough medicines, and antacids for sodium content.
- Avoid using salt when preparing foods or adding salt to foods.
- Weigh yourself at the same time each day, preferably in the morning, using the same scale and wearing the same or similar clothes.
- Eat smaller, more frequent meals.

Activity Program
- Increase walking and other activities gradually, provided they do not cause fatigue or dyspnea. Consider a cardiac rehabilitation program.
- Avoid extremes of heat and cold.

Ongoing Monitoring
- Know the signs and symptoms of worsening heart failure (see eTable 35-1: Who Is the Patient With Heart Failure? Think FACES [**F**atigue, limitation of **A**ctivities, chest **C**ongestion/cough, **E**dema, and **S**hortness of breath]).
- Recall the symptoms experienced when illness began. Reappearance of previous symptoms may indicate a recurrence.
- Report immediately to health care provider any of the following:
  - Weight gain of 3 lb (1.4 kg) in 2 days, or 3-5 lb (2.3 kg) in a wk
  - Difficulty breathing, especially with exertion or when lying flat
  - Waking up breathless at night
  - Frequent dry, hacking cough, especially when lying down
  - Fatigue, weakness
  - Swelling of ankles, feet, or abdomen; swelling of face or difficulty breathing (if taking ACE inhibitors)
  - Nausea with abdominal swelling, pain, and tenderness
  - Dizziness or fainting

- Follow up with health care provider on regular basis.
- Consider joining a local support group with your family members and/or caregiver(s).

Health Promotion
- Obtain annual flu vaccination.
- Obtain pneumococcal vaccine (e.g., Pneumovax) and revaccination after 5 yr (for people at high risk of infection or serious disease).
- Develop plan to reduce risk factors (e.g., BP control, smoking cessation, weight reduction).

Rest
- Plan a regular daily rest and activity program.
- After exertion, such as exercise and ADLs, plan a rest period.
- Shorten working hours or schedule rest period during working hours.
- Avoid emotional upsets. Verbalize any concerns, fears, feelings of depression, etc., to health care provider.

Drug Therapy
- Take each drug as prescribed.
- Develop a system (e.g., daily chart, weekly pillbox) to ensure medications have been taken.
- Take pulse rate each day before taking medications (if appropriate). Know the parameters that your health care provider wants for your heart rate.
- Take BP at determined intervals (if appropriate). Know your target BP limits.
- Know signs and symptoms of orthostatic hypotension and how to prevent them (see Table 33-12).
- Know signs and symptoms of internal bleeding (bleeding gums, increased bruises, blood in stool or urine) and what to do if taking anticoagulants.
- Know own INR if taking warfarin (Coumadin) and how often to have blood monitored.

ACE, Angiotensin-converting enzyme; *INR,* international normalized ratio.

The physical therapist, occupational therapist, or you can instruct the patient in energy-conserving and energy-efficient behaviors after an evaluation of daily activities has been done. For example, once you understand the patient's daily routine, make suggestions to simplify work or modify an activity.

Exercise training (e.g., cardiac rehabilitation) improves symptoms of chronic HF but is often underprescribed. Exercise for patients with HF has been found to be safe and to improve the overall sense of well-being. It has also been correlated with mortality reduction.[25,26]

Frequently the patient needs a prescription for rest after an activity. Many hard-driving persons need the "permission" to not feel "lazy." Sometimes the patient may need to stop an activity that he or she enjoys. In such situations, help the patient explore alternative activities that cause less physical stress. Changes may be needed if situations produce an increased cardiac workload (e.g., frequent climbing of stairs). Help a patient identify areas where changes can be made and outside assistance obtained if needed.

Managing HF patients out of the hospital is a priority. Effective home health care can prevent or limit future hospitalizations by providing ongoing assessments (e.g., monitoring vital signs and weight, evaluating response to therapies).[23,27] Many agencies offer specialized programs dedicated to managing HF patients at home. For example, these programs may include the

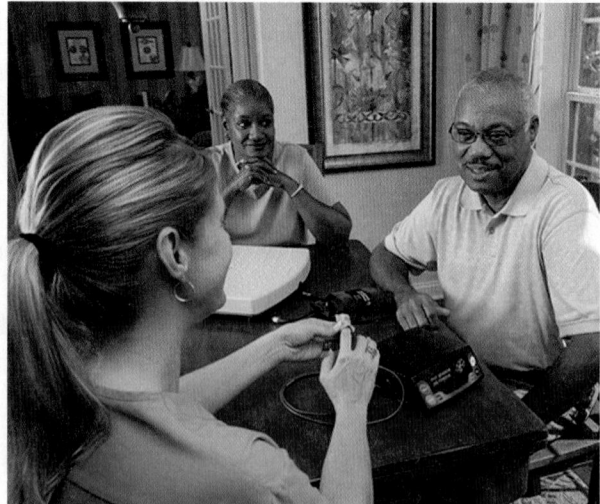

FIG. 35-6 Home-based telehealth monitoring unit.

use of telehealth monitoring technology (e.g., electronic scale, BP cuff, pulse oximeter) to collect physiologic data (Fig. 35-6). The technology may also audibly ask the patient questions such as, "Are you short of breath today?" Results are transmitted telephonically or by computer to the agency. After the data are received and reviewed, the patient may be called to further assess the situation or schedule a visit.

Home health nurses frequently work with protocols set up with the patient's health care team. The protocols enable you and the patient to identify problems, such as an increase in weight or dyspnea, as evidence of worsening HF. To prevent hospitalization, interventions can be started such as changing medications and restricting fluids. Home health nursing care of HF patients is vital in reducing the number of hospitalizations, increasing functional capacity, and improving the quality of life.

PALLIATIVE AND END-OF-LIFE CARE. Health care providers are often reluctant to refer patients with advanced HF for palliative and end-of-life care. One reason is the difficulty in assessing the prognosis of the disease and the unpredictable trajectory of HF during the last few months of life.[28] In addition, patients and caregivers may have a poor understanding of the disease and may fail to recognize HF as a terminal illness.[29]

The ACCF/AHA provides guidelines for patients with end-stage HF (stage D).[1] Health care providers in collaboration with the patient and caregiver can select either extraordinary treatment interventions (e.g., experimental surgery or drugs) or palliative and hospice care. The guidelines recommend (1) ongoing patient and caregiver education regarding prognosis and survival, (2) patient and caregiver education about options for formulating advance directives (e.g., deactivation of ICD), and (3) continuity of medical care (e.g., continuous infusion of inotropes for symptom control).[1]

Patients are eligible for hospice when a physician certifies that they are likely to have a life expectancy of 6 months or less. Unfortunately, many eligible patients are not referred to hospice. There are a number of reasons for this, including a lack of understanding of the role of hospice, lack of an identifiable terminal phase for HF, and concerns about meeting hospice referral criteria.[30] African American and Hispanic patients with HF use hospice less than whites.[31]

The seriousness of the prognosis and the actual knowledge of the expected short life span are misunderstood by many HF patients and caregivers. Many health care providers and HF patients overestimate the life expectancy.[30] When caring for these patients, attempt to identify those who may be eligible for hospice and initiate a discussion among the patient, caregiver, and health care provider.

Because patients with end-stage HF may have multiple symptoms, your care should involve ongoing assessment and evaluation of interventions for effectiveness. Strategies involve patient and caregiver support, drug therapies, and nondrug therapies. Medications are continued unless they are not tolerated. The goals of providing comfort and relieving suffering remain priorities in the care of patients with end-stage HF. (Palliative and end-of-life care are discussed in Chapter 10.)

EVALUATION

The expected outcomes for the patient with HF are presented in Nursing Care Plan 35-1.

CARDIAC TRANSPLANTATION

Cardiac transplantation is the transfer of a healthy donor heart to a patient with a diseased heart. This surgery is used to treat a variety of terminal or end-stage heart conditions (Table 35-11). Retransplantation (i.e., a second or third heart transplant) is also done. In the United States, more than 2000 cardiac

TABLE 35-11	INDICATIONS AND CONTRAINDICATIONS FOR CARDIAC TRANSPLANTATION*

Indications
- End-stage heart failure refractory to medical care
- Severe, decompensated, inoperable, valvular heart disease
- Recurrent life-threatening dysrhythmias not responsive to maximal interventions, including defibrillators
- Any other cardiac abnormalities that severely limit normal function and/or have a mortality risk of more than 50% at 2 yr

Absolute Contraindications
- Chronologic age over 70 yr or physiologic age over 65 yr
- Life-threatening illness (e.g., malignancy) that will limit survival to less than 5 yr despite therapy
- Advanced cerebral or peripheral vascular disease not amenable to correction
- Active infection, including HIV infection
- Severe pulmonary disease that will likely result in the patient being ventilator dependent after transplant

Relative Contraindications
- Uncontrolled diabetes mellitus with vascular and neurologic complications
- Irreversible liver or kidney dysfunction not explained by heart failure
- Morbid obesity
- Active substance abuse (e.g., alcohol, drugs, tobacco)
- Evidence of noncompliance with accepted medical practices
- Psychologic impairment
- Lack of social support network that can make long-term commitment for patient's welfare
- Unrealistic expectations by the patient or caregiver regarding transplant, its risks, and its benefits

*These are representative examples from various heart transplant centers.

transplants are done each year. However, thousands more adults would benefit from a heart transplant if more donated hearts were available. The 1-year transplant survival rate is 88% for males and 86% for females. The 5-year survival rate is 73% for males and 69% for females.[32]

Criteria for Selection

A careful selection process ensures that hearts are distributed fairly and to those who will benefit most from the donor heart. The United Network for Organ Sharing (UNOS) is in charge of a system that gives organs fairly to people. (UNOS is discussed in Chapter 14.)

Indications and contraindications for cardiac transplantation are identified in Table 35-11. Once an individual meets the criteria for cardiac transplantation, a complete physical examination and diagnostic workup are done. In addition, the patient and caregiver undergo a comprehensive psychologic evaluation. This includes assessing coping skills, support systems, and commitment to follow the rigorous regimen that is essential to a successful transplantation. The complexity of the transplant process may be overwhelming to a patient with inadequate support systems and a poor understanding of the lifestyle changes needed after transplant.

Donor and recipient matching is based on body and heart size and an immunologic evaluation. The immunologic assessment includes ABO blood type, antibody screen, panel-reactive antibody (PRA) level, and human leukocyte antigen typing (explained in Chapter 14).

ETHICAL/LEGAL DILEMMAS

Competence

Situation

M.T., a 60-year-old man, has been awaiting heart transplantation for 6 mo. He has been a patient in intensive care for 1 mo, since he has required a ventricular assist device for his failing heart. He recently suffered a stroke, which is a complication of the device. It left him paralyzed on his right side. He is only able to answer yes/no questions by shaking his head. He has required mechanical ventilation since his stroke. For the past 2 wk, hemodialysis has been required because of renal failure. Recently, when you suction him, he has tried to prevent the ventilator tubing from being reconnected by turning his head and biting down on the endotracheal tube. Although he does not have an advance directive, his wife and daughter tell you that, on numerous occasions before these events, he expressed that he would not want to live if he lost his independence. His wife and daughter request to have the mechanical ventilator withdrawn.

Ethical/Legal Points for Consideration

- Decisional capacity for informed consent related to treatment decisions involves four elements: (1) information provided about possible treatment options must be understandable to the patient; (2) possible outcomes of the various treatment options must be explained; (3) the patient must have the capacity to deliberate about the treatment choices and their consequences; and (4) the patient's treatment decision must be freely chosen and made without coercion.
- Legal competence, as determined by the courts, has a fairly low threshold. The ability to respond to questions by signaling a yes or no may be enough to demonstrate understanding of the questions, ability to discriminate between choices, and ability to communicate choices, providing that the answers make sense and are appropriate.
- Next of kin are the legal decision makers in the absence of advance directives if he is unable to make decisions for himself. However, decisional capacity should be tested without assuming it is absent.
- Some courts have accepted past assertions of preferences, past behavior, and assertions of their parties as evidence to support end-of-life preferences in the absence of advance directives.
- You need to be knowledgeable of your hospital or agency's documentation about the local jurisdiction's laws and regulations regarding informed consent and end-of-life decision making.

Discussion Questions

1. What would you do next given M.T.'s behavior and the information you obtained from his wife?
2. What are your feelings and concerns about participating in the care of a patient for whom withdrawal of treatment will result in death?

Once a person is accepted as a transplant candidate (this may happen quickly during an acute illness or after a longer period), he or she is placed on a transplant list. Patients may wait at home and receive ongoing medical care if their condition is stable. If not, they may require hospitalization for more intensive therapy. Unfortunately, the overall waiting period for a new heart is long. Many patients die while waiting for a transplant (see Ethical/Legal Dilemmas box above).

Bridge to Transplantation

Several devices are available as a bridge to transplantation, but only two have received U.S. Food and Drug Administration (FDA) approval for heart recovery after a life-threatening cardiac event. The AB5000 Circulatory Support System and the BVS 5000 Biventricular Support System provide temporary support for one or both sides of the heart in situations where the heart has failed but has the potential to recover (e.g., reversible HF, myocarditis, acute MI). The Thoratec VAD system can also support one or both ventricles, and it is approved as a bridging device for transplantation and for recovery of the heart after cardiac surgery.

Surgical Procedure

The surgical procedure actually involves multiple surgeries. First, the donor heart is retrieved. The donor is usually someone who has suffered irreversible brain injury *(brain death)*. Most donor hearts are obtained at sites distant from the institution performing the transplant. A team of physicians, nurses, and technicians goes to the hospital of the donor to remove donated organs once brain death has been determined. The retrieved organs are transported on ice until they can be implanted. For the heart, this is optimally less than 4 hours. Often the donor heart is flown to the recipient's hospital.

Next, the donated heart is implanted into the recipient. Two different approaches are used in this surgery. In the biatrial approach the recipient's damaged heart is removed at the midatrial level and the donor heart connected at the left atrium, pulmonary artery, aorta, and right atrium. In the bicaval approach the right atrium of the recipient's heart (with the sinoatrial node and maintenance of atrial conduction) is preserved, and then the donor heart is connected. Cardiopulmonary bypass is needed during the surgical procedure to maintain oxygenation and perfusion to vital organs.

Posttransplantation

After the transplant a variety of complications can occur, including a risk for SCD. Acute rejection is an immediate posttransplant complication, and immunosuppressive therapy is the key in posttransplant management. In the first year after transplantation the major causes of death are acute rejection and infection. Later on, malignancy (especially lymphoma) and cardiac vasculopathy (accelerated CAD) are major causes of death.[32]

Most immunosuppressive regimens include corticosteroids, calcineurin inhibitors (cyclosporine [Sandimmune, Neoral], tacrolimus (Prograf), and antiproliferative drugs (mycophenolate mofetil [CellCept]). (The mechanisms of action and side effects of these and other immunosuppressants are discussed in Chapter 14 and Table 14-16.) Because of the use of immunosuppressive therapy, infection is a primary complication after transplant surgery. On a long-term basis, immunosuppressive therapy increases the risk for cancer.[32]

To detect rejection, an EMB is obtained on a weekly basis for the first month, monthly for the following 6 months, and yearly thereafter. In this procedure, a catheter is inserted into the jugular vein and moved into the RV. The catheter uses a bioptome, a device with two small cups that can be closed, to remove small samples of heart muscle.[2,32]

Nursing management throughout the posttransplant period focuses on promoting patient adaptation to the transplant process, monitoring cardiac function, managing lifestyle changes, and providing ongoing teaching of the patient and the caregiver.

CASE STUDY

Heart Failure

iStockphoto/
Thinkstock

Patient Profile

J.E. is a 70-year-old Hispanic woman who was admitted to the intermediate care unit with complaints of increasing shortness of breath, fatigue, and weight gain.

Subjective Data

- History of hypertension for 20 yr
- History of MI at 58 yr of age
- Has experienced increasing shortness of breath, fatigue, and an unexplained 11-lb weight gain during the past 2 wk
- Had a respiratory tract infection 2 wk ago; has persistent cough and edema in legs
- Cannot climb a flight of stairs without getting short of breath
- Sleeps with head elevated on three pillows
- Lives alone, does not always remember to take medication

Objective Data

Physical Examination

- In respiratory distress, use of accessory muscles, respiratory rate 36 breaths/min
- Systolic heart murmur
- Bilateral crackles in all lung fields
- Cyanotic lips and extremities
- Skin cool and diaphoretic

Diagnostic Studies

- Chest x-ray results: cardiomegaly with right and left ventricular hypertrophy; fluid in lower lung fields
- Echocardiogram results: EF 20%

Collaborative Care

- Furosemide (Lasix) 40 mg IV bid
- Potassium 40 mEq PO bid
- Enalapril (Vasotec) 5 mg/day PO
- Nesiritide (Natrecor) 2 mcg/kg IV bolus followed by a continuous infusion of 0.01 mcg/kg/min
- Continuous ECG monitoring
- 2-g sodium diet
- Titrate O_2 to keep O_2 saturation >93%
- Monitor intake and output, and daily weights
- Serum electrolytes; cardiac enzymes q8hr × 3

Discussion Questions

1. Explain the pathophysiology of J.E.'s heart disease and symptomatology.
2. What clinical manifestations of ADHF did J.E. exhibit?
3. What is the significance of the findings of the diagnostic studies?
4. How would a serum NT-proBNP be beneficial in the diagnosis of ADHF?
5. Provide the rationale for each of the medical orders prescribed for J.E.
6. **Priority Decision:** Based on the assessment data presented, what are the priority nursing diagnoses? Identify any collaborative problems.
7. **Priority Decision:** What are your priority nursing interventions for J.E.?
8. **Delegation Decision:** Which of the interventions could be delegated to unlicensed assistive personnel (UAP)?
9. **Priority Decision:** What priority patient teaching measures should be instituted to prevent recurrence of ADHF and prepare J.E. for discharge?
10. **Evidence-Based Practice:** J.E. asks you why it is so important to "watch her salt." She tells you that food tastes better with salt. How would you respond to her?

ⓔvolve Answers and a corresponding concept map available at *http://evolve.elsevier.com/Lewis/medsurg.*

BRIDGE TO NCLEX EXAMINATION

The number of the question corresponds to the same-numbered outcome at the beginning of the chapter.

1. The nurse recognizes that primary manifestations of systolic failure include
   a. ↓ EF and ↑ PAWP.
   b. ↓ PAWP and ↑ EF.
   c. ↓ pulmonary hypertension associated with normal EF.
   d. ↓ afterload and ↓ left ventricular end-diastolic pressure.

2. A compensatory mechanism involved in HF that leads to inappropriate fluid retention and additional workload of the heart is
   a. ventricular dilation.
   b. ventricular hypertrophy.
   c. neurohormonal response.
   d. sympathetic nervous system activation.

3. You are caring for a patient with ADHF who is receiving IV dobutamine (Dobutrex). You know that this drug is ordered because it *(select all that apply)*
   a. increases SVR.
   b. produces diuresis.
   c. improves contractility.
   d. dilates renal blood vessels.
   e. works on the β_1-receptors in the heart.

4. A patient with chronic HF and atrial fibrillation is treated with a digitalis glycoside and a loop diuretic. To prevent possible complications of this combination of drugs, what does the nurse need to do *(select all that apply)*?
   a. Monitor serum potassium levels.
   b. Teach the patient how to take a pulse rate.
   c. Keep an accurate measure of intake and output.
   d. Teach the patient about dietary restriction of potassium.
   e. Withhold digitalis and notify health care provider if heart rate is irregular.

5. Patients with a heart transplantation are at risk for which complications in the first year after transplantation *(select all that apply)*?
   a. Cancer
   b. Infection
   c. Rejection
   d. Vasculopathy
   e. Sudden cardiac death

1. a, 2. c, 3. c, e, 4. a, b, c, 5. b, c, e

ⓔvolve

For rationales to these answers and even more NCLEX review questions, visit *http://evolve.elsevier.com/Lewis/medsurg.*

REFERENCES

*1. Yancy CW, Jessup M, Bozkurt B, et al: 2013 ACCF/AHA guideline for the management of heart failure: executive summary, *Circulation* 128:e1, 2013.

2. Urden LD, Stacy KM, Lough ME: *Critical care nursing: diagnosis and management*, ed 6, St Louis, 2010, Mosby.

3. Go AS, Mozaffarian D, Roger VL, et al: Heart disease and stroke statistics—2013 update: a report from the American Heart Association, *Circulation* 127:e6, 2013.

4. Jorde LB, Carey JC, Bamshad M: *Medical genetics*, ed 4, Philadelphia, 2010, Mosby.

5. Huether S, McCance K: *Understanding pathophysiology*, ed 5, St Louis, 2012, Mosby.

*6. Silver MA, Maisel A, Yancy CW, et al: BNP Consensus Panel 2004: a clinical approach for the diagnostic, prognostic, screening, treatment monitoring, and therapeutic roles of natriuretic peptides in cardiovascular diseases, *Congest Heart Fail* 10(5 Suppl 3):1, 2004. (Classic)

7. Heart Failure Society of America: Who is the patient with heart failure? Think FACES, 2002. Retrieved from *www.hfsa.org/pdf/faces_card.pdf*. (Classic)

*8. Cooper LT, Baughman KL, Feldman AM, et al: The role of endomyocardial biopsy in the management of cardiovascular disease: a scientific statement from the American Heart Association, the American College of Cardiology, and the European Society of Cardiology, *Circulation* 116(19):2216, 2007.

9. Costanzo MR, Guglin ME, Saltzberg MT, et al: Ultrafiltration versus intravenous diuretics for patients hospitalized for acutely decompensated HF, *J Am Coll Cardiol* 49:675, 2007.

10. Diefenbeck CA: Psychosocial risk and protective factors for cardiovascular health and illness, *DNA Reporter* 34:11, 2009.

11. O'Connor C: Depression, not SSRIs linked to increased mortality in heart failure patients, *Arch Intern Med* 168:2232, 2008.

12. Mullens W, Abahams Z, Francis G, et al: Sodium nitroprusside for advanced low-output heart failure, *J Am Coll Cardiol* 52:200, 2008.

13. Dakin CL: New approaches to heart failure in the ED, *Am J Nurs* 108:68, 2008.

14. Peacock WF, Hollander JE, Diercks DB, et al: Morphine and outcomes in acute decompensated heart failure: an ADHERE analysis, *Emerg Med J* 25:205, 2009.

15. Kee JL, Hayes ER, McCuistion LE: *Pharmacology*, ed 7, St Louis, 2012, Mosby.

16. Garg R, Yusuf S: Collaborative Group on ACE Inhibitor Trials: overview of randomized trials of angiotensin-converting enzyme inhibitors on mortality and morbidity in patients with heart failure, *JAMA* 273:1450, 1995. (Classic)

17. Held ML, Sturtz M: Managing acute decompensated heart failure, *Am Nurse Today* 4:18, 2009.

*18. Lindenfeld J, Albert NM, Boehmer JP, et al: Executive summary: HFSA 2010 comprehensive heart failure practice guidelines, *J Card Fail* 16:475, 2010.

19. Ramani GV, Uber PA, Mehra MR: Chronic heart failure, *Mayo Clin Proc* 85:180, 2010.

*20. Mitchell JE, Tam SW, Trivedi K, et al: Atrial fibrillation and mortality in African American patients with heart failure: results from the African American Heart Failure Trial (A-HeFT), *Am Heart J* 162:154, 2011.

*21. Chung M, Lennie T, DeJong M, et al: Patients differ in their ability to self-monitor adherence to a low-sodium diet versus medication, *J Card Fail* 14:114, 2008.

*22. Schocken DD, Benjamin EJ, Fonarow G, et al: Prevention of heart failure: a scientific statement from the American Heart Association councils on epidemiology and prevention, clinical cardiology, cardiovascular nursing, and high blood pressure research, *Circulation* 117:2544, 2008.

*23. Hebert PL, Sisk JE, Wang JJ, et al: Cost-effectiveness of nurse-led disease management for heart failure in an ethnically diverse urban community, *Ann Intern Med* 149:540, 2008.

24. The Joint Commission: Heart failure core measure set. Retrieved from *http://www.jointcommission.org/assets/1/6/Heart%20Failure.pdf*.

25. American Heart Association: Get with the guidelines—heart failure: fact sheet. Retrieved from *www.heart.org/idc/groups/heart-public/@wcm/@hcm/@gwtg/documents/downloadable/ucm_309013.pdf*.

*26. O'Connor CM, Whellan DJ, Lee KL, et al: Efficacy and safety of exercise training in patients with chronic heart failure: HF-ACTION randomized controlled trial, *JAMA* 301:1439, 2009.

*27. Padula CA, Yeaw E, Mistry S: A home-based nurse-coached inspiratory muscle training intervention in heart failure, *Appl Nurs Res* 22:18, 2009.

28. Huynh B, Rovner A, Rich M: Identification of older patients with heart failure who may be candidates for hospice care: development of a simple four-item risk score, *J Am Geriatr Soc* 56:1111, 2008.

*29. Hemani S, Letizia M: Providing palliative care in end-stage heart failure, *J Hosp Palliat Nurs* 10:100, 2008.

30. Adler ED, Goldfinger JZ, Kalman J, et al: Palliative care in the treatment of advanced heart failure, *Circulation* 120:2597, 2009.

31. Givens JL, Tjia J, Zhou C, et al: Racial and ethnic differences in hospice use among patients with heart failure, *Arch Intern Med* 170:427, 2010.

32. Taylor D, Meiser B, Webber S, et al: The International Society of Heart and Lung Transplantation Guidelines for the Care of Heart Transplant Recipients: task force 2: immunosuppression and rejection, 2010. Retrieved from *www.ishlt.org/ContentDocuments/ISHLT_GL_TaskForce2_110810.pdf*.

RESOURCES

American Association of Cardiovascular and Pulmonary Rehabilitation
www.aacvpr.org

American Association of Heart Failure Nurses
www.aahfn.org

American College of Cardiology
www.acc.org

American Heart Association
www.heart.org

Council on Cardiovascular Nursing
www.my.americanheart.org/professional/Councils/CVN/Council-on-Cardiovascular-Nursing_UCM_320474_SubHomePage.jsp

Heart Failure Society of America
www.hfsa.org

International Society for Heart and Lung Transplantation
www.ishlt.org

Mended Hearts
www.mendedhearts.org

National Heart, Lung, and Blood Institute
www.nhlbi.nih.gov

*Evidence-based information for clinical practice.

It is only with the heart that one can see rightly; what is essential is invisible to the eye.
Saint-Exupery

Nursing Management
Dysrhythmias

Linda Bucher

LEARNING OUTCOMES

1. Examine the nursing management of patients requiring continuous electrocardiographic (ECG) monitoring.
2. Differentiate the clinical characteristics and ECG patterns of normal sinus rhythm, common dysrhythmias, and acute coronary syndrome (ACS).
3. Compare the nursing and collaborative management of patients with common dysrhythmias and ECG changes associated with ACS.
4. Differentiate between defibrillation and cardioversion, including indications for use and physiologic effects.
5. Describe the management of patients with pacemakers and implantable cardioverter-defibrillators.
6. Select appropriate interventions for patients undergoing electrophysiologic testing and radiofrequency catheter ablation therapy.

KEY TERMS

asystole, p. 795
atrial fibrillation, p. 796
atrial flutter, p. 795
automatic external defibrillator (AED), p. 802

cardiac pacemaker, p. 803
complete heart block, p. 798
dysrhythmias, p. 787
premature atrial contraction (PAC), p. 794

premature ventricular contraction (PVC), p. 799
telemetry monitoring, p. 790
ventricular fibrillation (VF), p. 800
ventricular tachycardia (VT), p. 799

This chapter describes basic principles of electrocardiographic monitoring and recognition and treatment of common dysrhythmias. In addition, it presents ECG changes that are associated with acute coronary syndrome (ACS).

RHYTHM IDENTIFICATION AND TREATMENT

Your ability to recognize normal and abnormal cardiac rhythms, called dysrhythmias, is an essential nursing skill.[1] Prompt assessment of dysrhythmias and the patient's response to the rhythm is critical.

Conduction System

Four properties of cardiac cells enable the conduction system to start an electrical impulse, send it through the cardiac tissue, and stimulate muscle contraction (Table 36-1). The heart's conduction system consists of specialized neuromuscular tissue located throughout the heart (Fig. 32-4, *A*). A normal cardiac impulse begins in the sinoatrial (SA) node in the upper right atrium. It spreads over the atrial myocardium via interatrial and internodal pathways, causing atrial contraction. The impulse then travels to the atrioventricular (AV) node, through the bundle of His, and down the left and right bundle branches. It ends in the Purkinje fibers, which transmit the impulse to the ventricles.

Nervous Control of the Heart

The autonomic nervous system plays an important role in the rate of impulse formation, the speed of conduction, and the strength of cardiac contraction. The components of the auto-

---

Reviewed by Katrina Allen, RN, MSN, CCRN, Nursing Instructor, Faulkner State Community College: Division of Nursing, Fairhope and Bay Minette, Alabama; Barbara Pope, RN, MSN, PPCN, CCRN, Critical Care Educator, Independent Consultant, Albert Einstein Healthcare Network (retired), Philadelphia, Pennsylvania; and Regina Kukulski, RN, MSN, ACNS, BC, Nurse Educator Consultant, Thomas Edison State College, Capital Health Medical Center, Trenton, New Jersey.

nomic nervous system that affect the heart are the vagus nerve fibers of the parasympathetic nervous system and nerve fibers of the sympathetic nervous system.

Stimulation of the vagus nerve causes a decreased rate of firing of the SA node and slowed impulse conduction of the AV node. Stimulation of the sympathetic nerves increases SA node firing, AV node impulse conduction, and cardiac contractility.[2]

Electrocardiographic Monitoring

The *electrocardiogram* (ECG) is a graphic tracing of the electrical impulses produced in the heart. The waveforms on the ECG represent electrical activity produced by the movement of ions across the membranes of myocardial cells, representing depolarization and repolarization.

The membrane of a cardiac cell is semipermeable. This allows it to maintain a high concentration of potassium and a low concentration of sodium inside the cell. Outside the cell a high concentration of sodium and a low concentration of potassium exist. The inside of the cell, when at rest, or in the polarized state, is negative compared with the outside. When a cell or groups of cells are stimulated, the cell membrane changes its permeability. This allows sodium to move rapidly into the cell, making the inside of the cell positive compared with the outside *(depolarization)*. A slower movement of ions across the membrane restores the cell to the polarized state, called *repolarization*. Fig. 36-1 describes the phases of the cardiac action potential.

The ECG has 12 recording leads. Six of the leads measure electrical forces in the frontal plane. These are bipolar (positive or negative) leads I, II, and III; and unipolar (positive) leads aVR, aVL, and aVF (Fig. 36-2, *A* and *B*). The remaining six unipolar leads (V₁ through V₆) measure the electrical forces in the horizontal plane (precordial leads) (Fig. 36-2, *C*). The 12-lead ECG may show changes suggesting structural changes, conduction disturbances, damage (e.g., ischemia, infarction), electrolyte imbalance, or drug toxicity. Obtaining 12 ECG views of the heart is also helpful in the assessment of dysrhythmias. Fig. 36-3 is an example of a normal 12-lead ECG.

One or more ECG leads can be used to continuously monitor a patient. The most common leads selected are leads II and V₁ (Fig. 36-4). A modified chest lead (MCL₁) is used when only three leads are available for monitoring (eFig. 36-1, showing MCL₁ lead placement, is available on the website for this chapter). MCL₁ is similar to V₁. Accurate interpretation of an ECG depends on the correct placement of the leads on the patient. The monitoring leads used are determined by the patient's clinical status.[3,4]

TABLE 36-1	PROPERTIES OF CARDIAC CELLS
Property	**Definition**
Automaticity	Ability to initiate an impulse spontaneously and continuously
Excitability	Ability to be electrically stimulated
Conductivity	Ability to transmit an impulse along a membrane in an orderly manner
Contractility	Ability to respond mechanically to an impulse

FIG. 36-1 Phases of the cardiac action potential. The electrical potential, measured in millivolts (mV), is indicated along the vertical axis of the graph. Time, measured in seconds (sec), is indicated along the horizontal axis. The action potential has five phases, labeled *0* through *4*. Each phase represents a particular electrical event or combination of electrical events. Phase 0 is the upstroke of rapid depolarization and corresponds with ventricular contraction. Phases 1, 2, and 3 represent repolarization. Phase 4 is known as complete repolarization (or the polarized state) and corresponds to diastole. *RP,* Resting membrane potential; *TP,* threshold membrane potential.

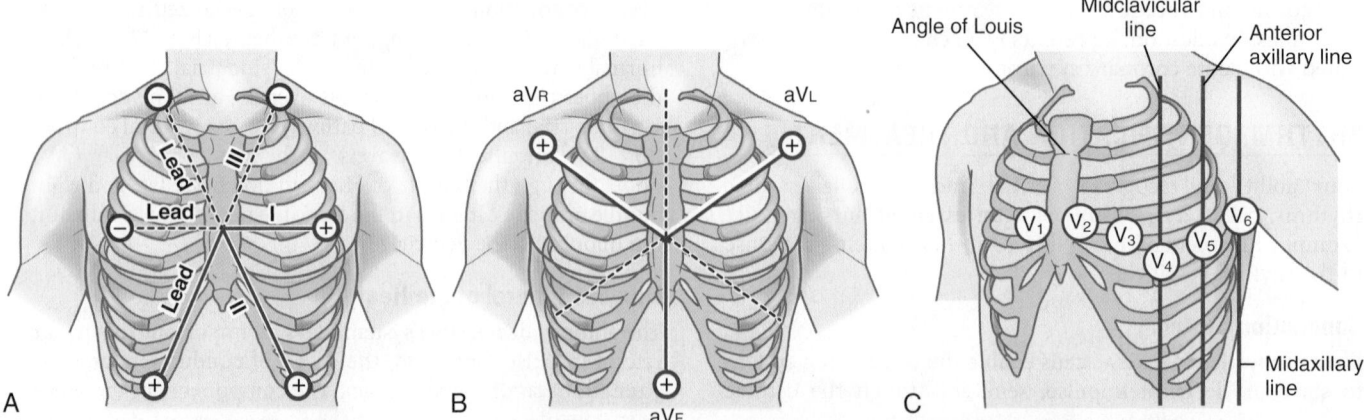

FIG. 36-2 **A,** Limb leads I, II, and III. These bipolar leads are located on the extremities. Illustrated are the angles from which these leads view the heart. **B,** Limb leads aVR, aVL, and aVF. These unipolar leads use the center of the heart as their negative electrode. **C,** Placement for the unipolar chest leads: *V₁,* fourth intercostal space at the right sternal border; *V₂,* fourth intercostal space at the left sternal border; *V₃,* halfway between V₂ and V₄; *V₄,* fifth intercostal space at the left midclavicular line; *V₅,* fifth intercostal space at the left anterior axillary line; *V₆,* fifth intercostal space at the left midaxillary line.

FIG. 36-3 Twelve-lead electrocardiogram showing a normal sinus rhythm.

FIG. 36-4 A, Lead placement for V₁ or V₆ using a five-lead system. **B,** Typical ECG tracing in lead V₁. *C,* Chest; *LA,* left arm; *LL,* left leg; *RA,* right arm; *RL,* right leg.

FIG. 36-5 Time and voltage on the electrocardiogram; 6-sec strip.

The monitor continuously displays the heart rhythm. ECG paper attached to the monitor records the ECG (i.e., rhythm strip). This provides a record of the patient's rhythm. It also allows for measurement of complexes and intervals and for assessment of dysrhythmias.

To correctly interpret an ECG, you measure time and voltage on the ECG paper. ECG paper consists of large (heavy lines)

and small (light lines) squares (Fig. 36-5). Each large square consists of 25 smaller squares (five horizontal and five vertical). Horizontally, each small square (1 mm) represents 0.04 second. This means that one large square equals 0.20 second and that 300 large squares equal 1 minute. Vertically, each small square (1 mm) represents 0.1 millivolt (mV). This means that one large square equals 0.5 mV. Use these squares to calculate the heart rate (HR) and measure time intervals for the different ECG complexes.

You can use a variety of methods to calculate the HR from an ECG. The most accurate way is to count the number of QRS complexes in 1 minute. However, because this method is time consuming, a simpler process is used. Note that every 3 seconds a marker appears on the ECG paper (see Fig. 36-5). Count the number of R-R intervals in 6 seconds and multiply that number by 10. (An R wave is the first upward [or positive] wave of the QRS complex.) This is the estimated number of beats per minute (Fig. 36-6).

Another method is to count the number of small squares between one R-R interval. Divide this number into 1500 to get the HR. Last, you can count the number of large squares between one R-R interval and divide this number into 300 to get the HR (see Fig. 36-6). All these methods are most accurate when the rhythm is regular.[1]

An additional way to measure distances on the ECG strip is to use calipers. Many times a P or an R wave will not fall directly on a light or heavy line. Place the fine points of the calipers exactly on the parts you need to measure and then move to another part of the strip for a more precise time measurement.

ECG leads consist of an electrode pad fixed with electrical conductive gel. Before placing these on the patient, you must properly prepare the skin. Clip excessive hair on the chest wall with scissors. Gently rub the skin with dry gauze until slightly pink. If the skin is oily, wipe with alcohol first. If the patient is diaphoretic, apply a skin protectant before placing the electrode.

You will see artifact on the monitor when leads and electrodes are not secure, or when there is muscle activity (e.g., shivering) or electrical interference. *Artifact* is a distortion of the baseline and waveforms seen on the ECG (Fig. 36-7). Accurate interpretation of heart rhythm is difficult when artifact is present. If artifact occurs, check the connections in the equipment. You may need to replace the electrodes if the conductive gel has dried out.

Telemetry Monitoring. Telemetry monitoring is the observation of a patient's HR and rhythm at a site distant from the

FIG. 36-6 When the rhythm is regular, heart rate can be easily determined. The estimated heart rate is 70 beats/min. NOTE: Recorded from lead II.

FIG. 36-7 Artifact. **A,** Muscle tremor. **B,** Loose electrodes.

---

patient. The use of this technology can help rapidly diagnose dysrhythmias, ischemia, or infarction. Two types of systems are used for telemetry monitoring. The first type, a centralized monitoring system, requires you or a telemetry technician to continuously observe a group of patients' ECGs at a central location. The second system of telemetry monitoring does not require constant surveillance. These systems have the capability of detecting and storing data. Advanced alarm systems provide different levels of detection of dysrhythmias, ischemia, or infarction.

Assessment of Cardiac Rhythm

When assessing the cardiac rhythm, make an accurate interpretation and immediately evaluate the patient's clinical status. Assess the patient's hemodynamic response to any change in rhythm. This information will guide the selection of your interventions. Determination of the cause of dysrhythmias is a priority. For example, tachycardias may be the result of fever and may cause a decrease in cardiac output (CO) and hypotension. Electrolyte disturbances can cause dysrhythmias and, if not treated, can lead to life-threatening dysrhythmias. At all times, the patient, not the "monitor," must be assessed and treated.

Normal sinus rhythm refers to a rhythm that starts in the SA node at a rate of 60 to 100 times per minute and follows the normal conduction pathway (Fig. 36-8). Fig. 36-9 shows the components of a normal ECG tracing. Table 36-2 describes ECG waveforms and intervals, normal durations, and possible sources of disturbances in these features.

Electrophysiologic Mechanisms of Dysrhythmias

Dysrhythmias result from disorders of impulse formation, conduction of impulses, or both. The heart has specialized cells in the SA node, atria, AV node, and bundle of His and Purkinje fibers (His-Purkinje system), which can fire (discharge) spontaneously. This is termed *automaticity*. Normally, the SA node

FIG. 36-8 Normal sinus rhythm. NOTE: Recorded from lead II.

is the pacemaker of the heart. It spontaneously fires 60 to 100 times per minute (Table 36-3). A secondary pacemaker from another site may fire in two ways. If the SA node fires more slowly than a secondary pacemaker, the electrical signals from the secondary pacemaker may "escape." The secondary pacemaker will then fire automatically at its intrinsic rate. These secondary pacemakers may start from the AV node at a rate of 40 to 60 times per minute or the His-Purkinje system at a rate of 20 to 40 times per minute.

Another way that secondary pacemakers can start is when they fire more rapidly than the normal pacemaker of the SA node. *Triggered beats* (early or late) may come from an *ectopic focus* or *accessory pathway* (area outside the normal conduction pathway) in the atria, AV node, or ventricles. This results in a dysrhythmia, which replaces the normal sinus rhythm.

The impulse started by the SA node or an ectopic focus must be conducted to the entire heart. The property of myocardial tissue that allows it to be depolarized by a stimulus is called *excitability.* This is an important part of the transmission of the

FIG. 36-9 The ECG tracing as seen in normal sinus rhythm. *1,* P wave; *2,* PR interval; *3,* QRS complex: Q wave, R wave, S wave; *4,* ST segment; *5,* T wave; *6,* QT interval. Isoelectric (flat) line or baseline represents the absence of electrical activity in the cardiac cells. (See Table 36-2 for timing of intervals.)

TABLE 36-2 ECG WAVEFORMS AND INTERVALS*

Description	Normal Duration (sec)	Source of Possible Variation
P Wave Represents time for the passage of the electrical impulse through the atrium causing atrial depolarization (contraction). Should be upright.	0.06-0.12	Disturbance in conduction within atria
PR Interval Measured from beginning of P wave to beginning of QRS complex. Represents time taken for impulse to spread through the atria, AV node and bundle of His, bundle branches, and Purkinje fibers, to a point immediately preceding ventricular contraction.	0.12-0.20	Disturbance in conduction usually in AV node, bundle of His, or bundle branches but can be in atria as well
QRS Complex *Q wave:* First negative (downward) deflection after the P wave, short and narrow, not present in several leads.	<0.03	MI may result in development of a pathologic Q wave that is wide (≥0.03 sec) and deep (≥25% of the height of the R wave)
R wave: First positive (upward) deflection in the QRS complex.	Not usually measured	
S wave: First negative (downward) deflection after the R wave.	Not usually measured	
QRS Interval Measured from beginning to end of QRS complex. Represents time taken for depolarization (contraction) of both ventricles (systole).	<0.12	Disturbance in conduction in bundle branches or in ventricles
ST Segment Measured from the S wave of the QRS complex to the beginning of the T wave. Represents the time between ventricular depolarization and repolarization (diastole). Should be isoelectric (flat).	0.12	Disturbances (e.g., elevation, depression) usually caused by ischemia, injury, or infarction
T Wave Represents time for ventricular repolarization. Should be upright.	0.16	Disturbances (e.g., tall, peaked; inverted) usually caused by electrolyte imbalances, ischemia, or infarction
QT Interval Measured from beginning of QRS complex to end of T wave. Represents time taken for entire electrical depolarization and repolarization of the ventricles.	0.34-0.43	Disturbances usually affecting repolarization more than depolarization and caused by drugs, electrolyte imbalances, and changes in heart rate

*Heart rate influences the duration of these intervals, especially those of the PR and QT intervals (e.g., QT interval shortens in duration as heart rate increases).
AV, Atrioventricular.

TABLE 36-3	INTRINSIC RATES OF THE CONDUCTION SYSTEM

Part of Conduction System	Rate
SA node	60-100 times/min
AV node	40-60 times/min
Bundle of His, Purkinje fibers	20-40 times/min

AV, Atrioventricular; *SA,* sinoatrial.

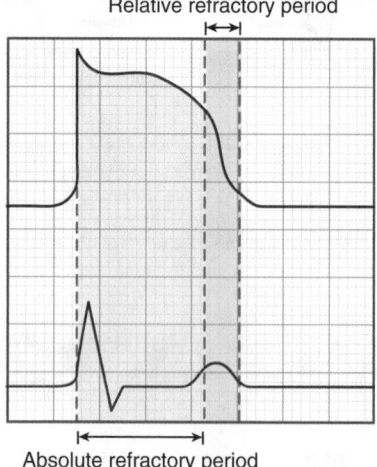

FIG. 36-10 Absolute and relative refractory periods correlated with the cardiac muscle's action potential and with an ECG tracing.

impulse from one cell to another. The level of excitability is determined by the length of time after depolarization that the tissues can be restimulated. The recovery period after stimulation is the *refractory phase* or period. The *absolute refractory phase* or period occurs when excitability is zero and the heart cannot be stimulated. The *relative refractory period* occurs slightly later in the cycle, and excitability is more likely. In states of *full excitability,* the heart is completely recovered. Fig. 36-10 shows the relationship between the refractory period and the ECG.

If conduction is depressed and some areas of the heart are blocked (e.g., by infarction), the unblocked areas are activated earlier than the blocked areas. When the block is unidirectional, this uneven conduction may allow the initial impulse to reenter areas that were previously not excitable but have recovered. The reentering impulse may be able to depolarize the atria and ventricles, causing a premature beat. If the reentrant excitation continues, tachycardia occurs.

Evaluation of Dysrhythmias

Dysrhythmias occur as the result of various abnormalities and disease states. The cause of a dysrhythmia influences the patient's treatment. Table 36-4 presents common causes of dysrhythmias. Table 36-5 presents a systematic approach to assessing a heart rhythm.

Dysrhythmias occurring in nonmonitored settings present management challenges. If the patient becomes symptomatic (e.g., chest pain), determination of the rhythm by cardiac monitoring is a high priority. Activate the emergency medical services (EMS) system. Table 36-6 outlines emergency care of the patient with a dysrhythmia.

In addition to continuous ECG monitoring during hospitalization, several other tests can assess dysrhythmias and the effectiveness of antidysrhythmia drug therapy. An electrophys-

TABLE 36-4	COMMON CAUSES OF DYSRHYTHMIAS*

Cardiac Conditions	Other Conditions
• Accessory pathways	• Acid-base imbalances
• Cardiomyopathy	• Alcohol
• Conduction defects	• Caffeine, tobacco
• Heart failure	• Connective tissue disorders
• Myocardial ischemia, infarction	• Drug effects (e.g., antidysrhythmia drugs, stimulants, β-adrenergic blockers) or toxicity
• Valve disease	• Electric shock
	• Electrolyte imbalances (e.g., hyperkalemia, hypocalcemia)
	• Emotional crisis
	• Herbal supplements (e.g., areca nut, wahoo root bark, yerba maté)
	• Hypoxia
	• Metabolic conditions (e.g., thyroid dysfunction)
	• Near-drowning
	• Sepsis, shock
	• Toxins

*List is not all-inclusive.

TABLE 36-5	APPROACH TO ASSESSING HEART RHYTHM

When assessing a heart rhythm, use a consistent and systematic approach. One such approach includes the following:
1. Look for the P wave. Is it upright or inverted? Is there one for every QRS complex or more than one? Are atrial fibrillatory or flutter waves present?
2. Evaluate the atrial rhythm. Is it regular or irregular?
3. Calculate the atrial rate.
4. Measure the duration of the PR interval. Is it normal duration or prolonged?
5. Evaluate the ventricular rhythm. Is it regular or irregular?
6. Calculate the ventricular rate.
7. Measure the duration of the QRS complex. Is it normal duration or prolonged?
8. Assess the ST segment. Is it isoelectric (flat), elevated, or depressed?
9. Measure the duration of the QT interval. Is it normal duration or prolonged?
10. Note the T wave. Is it upright or inverted?

Additional questions to consider include the following:
1. What is the dominant or underlying rhythm and/or dysrhythmia?
2. What is the clinical significance of your findings?
3. What is the treatment for the particular rhythm?

iologic study, Holter monitoring, event monitoring (or loop recorder), exercise treadmill testing, and signal-averaged ECG can be performed on an inpatient or outpatient basis (see Table 32-6 for nursing care related to these tests).

An *electrophysiologic study* (EPS) can identify the causes of heart blocks, tachydysrhythmias (dysrhythmias with rates greater than 100 beats/minute), bradydysrhythmias (dysrhythmias with rates less than 60 beats/minute), and syncope. An EPS study can also locate accessory pathways and determine the effectiveness of antidysrhythmia drugs.

The Holter monitor continuously records the ECG while the patient is ambulatory and performing daily activities. The patient keeps a diary and records activities and any symptoms.

✚ TABLE 36-6   EMERGENCY MANAGEMENT

Dysrhythmias

Etiology	Assessment Findings	Interventions
See Table 36-4	• Irregular rate and rhythm; tachycardia, bradycardia • Decreased or increased blood pressure • Decreased O₂ saturation • Chest, neck, shoulder, back, jaw, or arm pain • Dizziness, syncope • Dyspnea • Extreme restlessness, anxiety • Decreased level of consciousness, confusion • Feeling of impending doom • Numbness, tingling of arms • Weakness and fatigue • Cold, clammy skin • Diminished peripheral pulses • Diaphoresis • Pallor • Palpitations • Nausea and vomiting	**Initial** • Ensure ABCs. • Administer O₂ via nasal cannula or non-rebreather mask. • Obtain baseline vital signs, including O₂ saturation. • Obtain 12-lead ECG. • Initiate continuous ECG monitoring. • Identify underlying rate and rhythm. • Identify dysrhythmia. • Establish IV access. • Obtain baseline laboratory studies (e.g., CBC, electrolytes). **Ongoing Monitoring** • Monitor vital signs, level of consciousness, O₂ saturation, and cardiac rhythm. • Anticipate need for administration of antidysrhythmia drugs and analgesics. • Anticipate need for intubation if respiratory distress is evident. • Prepare to initiate advanced cardiac life support (e.g., CPR, defibrillation, transcutaneous pacing).

ABCs, Airway, breathing, circulation.

Events in the diary are correlated with any dysrhythmias seen on the ECG. Use of event monitors has improved the evaluation of dysrhythmias in outpatients. Event monitors are recorders that the patient activates only when he or she experiences symptoms. New technology using smart phones can obtain and save ECG recordings and even detect atrial fibrillation.

Exercise treadmill testing evaluates the patient's heart rhythm during exercise. If exercise-induced dysrhythmias or ECG changes occur, they are analyzed and drug therapy evaluated.

The signal-averaged ECG identifies *late potentials* strongly suggesting that the patient may be at risk for developing serious ventricular dysrhythmias. Chapter 32 discusses the diagnostic procedures for assessment of the cardiovascular system and related nursing care.

Types of Dysrhythmias

Figs. 36-11 to 36-19 provide examples of the ECG tracings of common dysrhythmias. Table 36-7 presents the descriptive characteristics.

Sinus Bradycardia. In *sinus bradycardia* the conduction pathway is the same as that in sinus rhythm but the SA node fires at a rate less than 60 beats/minute (Fig. 36-11, *A*). *Symptomatic bradycardia* refers to an HR that is less than 60 beats/minute and is inadequate for the patient's condition, causing the patient to experience symptoms (e.g., chest pain, syncope).

Clinical Associations. Sinus bradycardia may be a normal sinus rhythm in aerobically trained athletes and in some people during sleep. It also occurs in response to carotid sinus massage, Valsalva maneuver, hypothermia, increased intraocular pressure, vagal stimulation, and administration of certain drugs (e.g., β-adrenergic blockers, calcium channel blockers). Common disease states associated with sinus bradycardia are hypothyroidism, increased intracranial pressure, hypoglycemia, and inferior myocardial infarction (MI).

ECG Characteristics. In sinus bradycardia, HR is less than 60 beats/minute and the rhythm is regular. The P wave precedes each QRS complex and has a normal shape and duration. The PR interval is normal, and the QRS complex has a normal shape and duration.

Clinical Significance. The clinical significance of sinus bradycardia depends on how the patient tolerates it. Signs of symp-

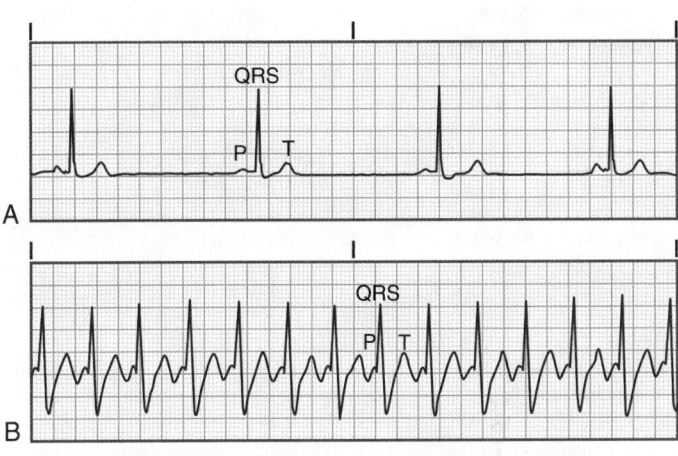

FIG. 36-11 A, Sinus bradycardia. **B,** Sinus tachycardia.

tomatic bradycardia include pale, cool skin; hypotension; weakness; angina; dizziness or syncope; confusion or disorientation; and shortness of breath.

Treatment. For the patient with symptoms, treatment consists of administration of atropine (an anticholinergic drug). If atropine (AtroPen) is ineffective, transcutaneous pacing, or a dopamine (Intropin) or epinephrine (Adrenalin) infusion is considered. Permanent pacemaker therapy may be needed. If bradycardia is due to drugs, these may need to be held, discontinued, or given in reduced dosages.

Sinus Tachycardia. The conduction pathway is the same in *sinus tachycardia* as that in normal sinus rhythm. The discharge rate from the sinus node increases because of vagal inhibition or sympathetic stimulation. The sinus rate is 101 to 200 beats/minute (Fig. 36-11, *B*).

Clinical Associations. Sinus tachycardia is associated with physiologic and psychologic stressors such as exercise, fever, pain, hypotension, hypovolemia, anemia, hypoxia, hypoglycemia, myocardial ischemia, heart failure (HF), hyperthyroidism, anxiety, and fear. It can also be an effect of drugs such as epinephrine, norepinephrine (Levophed), atropine, caffeine, theophylline (Theo-Dur), or hydralazine (Apresoline). In addition, many over-the-counter cold remedies have active ingredients (e.g., pseudoephedrine [Sudafed]) that can cause tachycardia.

TABLE 36-7   CHARACTERISTICS OF COMMON DYSRHYTHMIAS

Pattern	Rate and Rhythm	P Wave	PR Interval	QRS Complex
Normal sinus rhythm	60-100 beats/min and regular	Normal	Normal	Normal
Sinus bradycardia	<60 beats/min and regular	Normal	Normal	Normal
Sinus tachycardia	101-200 beats/min and regular	Normal	Normal	Normal
Premature atrial contraction	Usually 60-100 beats/min and irregular	Abnormal shape	Normal	Normal (usually)
Paroxysmal supraventricular tachycardia	150-220 beats/min and regular	Abnormal shape, may be hidden in the preceding T wave	Normal or shortened	Normal (usually)
Atrial flutter	*Atrial:* 200-350 beats/min and regular *Ventricular:* > or <100 beats/min and may be regular or irregular	Flutter (F) waves (sawtoothed pattern); more flutter waves than QRS complexes; may occur in a 2:1, 3:1, 4:1, etc., pattern	Not measurable	Normal (usually)
Atrial fibrillation	*Atrial:* 350-600 beats/min and irregular *Ventricular:* > or <100 beats/min and irregular	Fibrillatory (f) waves	Not measurable	Normal (usually)
Junctional dysrhythmias	40-180 beats/min and regular	Inverted, may be hidden in QRS complex	Variable	Normal (usually)
First-degree AV block	Normal and regular	Normal	>0.20 sec	Normal
Second-degree AV block				
• Type I (Mobitz I, Wenckebach heart block)	*Atrial:* Normal and regular *Ventricular:* Slower and irregular	Normal	Progressive lengthening	Normal QRS width, with pattern of one nonconducted (blocked) QRS complex
• Type II (Mobitz II heart block)	*Atrial:* Usually normal and regular *Ventricular:* Slower and regular or irregular	More P waves than QRS complexes (e.g., 2:1, 3:1)	Normal or prolonged	Widened QRS, preceded by ≥2 P waves, with nonconducted (blocked) QRS complex
Third-degree AV block (complete heart block)	*Atrial:* Regular but may appear irregular due to P waves hidden in QRS complexes *Ventricular:* 20-60 beats/min and regular	Normal, but no connection with QRS complex	Variable	Normal or widened, no relationship with P waves
Premature ventricular contraction (PVC)	Underlying rhythm can be any rate, regular or irregular rhythm, PVCs occur at variable rates	Not usually visible, hidden in the PVC	Not measurable	Wide and distorted
Ventricular tachycardia	150-250 beats/min and regular or irregular	Not usually visible	Not measurable	Wide and distorted
Accelerated idioventricular rhythm	40-100 beats/min and regular	Not usually visible	Not measurable	Wide and distorted
Ventricular fibrillation	Not measurable and irregular	Absent	Not measurable	Not measurable

AV, Atrioventricular.

ECG Characteristics. In sinus tachycardia, HR is 101 to 200 beats/minute and the rhythm is regular. The P wave is normal, precedes each QRS complex, and has a normal shape and duration. The PR interval is normal, and the QRS complex has a normal shape and duration.

Clinical Significance. The clinical significance of sinus tachycardia depends on the patient's tolerance of the increased HR. The patient may have dizziness, dyspnea, and hypotension because of decreased CO. Increased myocardial oxygen consumption is associated with an increased HR. Angina or an increase in infarction size may accompany sinus tachycardia in patients with coronary artery disease (CAD) or an acute MI.

Treatment. The underlying cause of tachycardia guides the treatment. For example, if the patient is experiencing tachycardia from pain, effective pain management is important to treat the tachycardia. In clinically stable patients, vagal maneuvers can be attempted. In addition, IV β-adrenergic blockers (e.g.,

metoprolol [Lopressor]), adenosine (Adenocard), or calcium channel blockers (e.g., diltiazem [Cardizem]) can be given to reduce HR and decrease myocardial oxygen consumption. In clinically unstable patients, synchronized cardioversion is used. (Cardioversion is discussed on p. 802.)

Premature Atrial Contraction. A **premature atrial contraction (PAC)** is a contraction starting from an ectopic focus in the atrium (i.e., a location other than the SA node) and coming sooner than the next expected sinus beat. The ectopic signal starts in the left or right atrium and travels across the atria by an abnormal pathway. This creates a distorted P wave (Fig. 36-12). At the AV node, it may be stopped (nonconducted PAC), delayed (lengthened PR interval), or conducted normally. If the signal moves through the AV node, in most cases it is conducted normally through the ventricles.

Clinical Associations. In a normal heart a PAC can result from emotional stress or physical fatigue or from the use

FIG. 36-12 Premature atrial contractions (arrows).

of caffeine, tobacco, or alcohol. A PAC can also result from hypoxia; electrolyte imbalances; and disease states such as hyperthyroidism, chronic obstructive pulmonary disease (COPD), and heart disease, including CAD and valvular disease.

ECG Characteristics. HR varies with the underlying rate and frequency of the PAC, and the rhythm is irregular. The P wave has a different shape from that of a P wave originating in the SA node, or it may be hidden in the preceding T wave. The PR interval may be shorter or longer than the PR interval coming from the SA node, but it is within normal limits. The QRS complex is usually normal. If the QRS interval is 0.12 second or more, abnormal conduction through the ventricles occurs.

Clinical Significance. In persons with healthy hearts, isolated PACs are not significant. Patients may report palpitations or a sense that their hearts "skipped a beat." In persons with heart disease, frequent PACs may indicate enhanced automaticity of the atria or a reentry mechanism. Such PACs may warn of or start more serious dysrhythmias (e.g., supraventricular tachycardia).

Treatment. Treatment depends on the patient's symptoms. Withdrawal of sources of stimulation such as caffeine or sympathomimetic drugs may be needed. β-Adrenergic blockers may be used to decrease PACs.

Paroxysmal Supraventricular Tachycardia. *Paroxysmal supraventricular tachycardia* (PSVT) is a dysrhythmia starting in an ectopic focus anywhere above the bifurcation of the bundle of His (Fig. 36-13). Identification of the ectopic focus is often difficult even with a 12-lead ECG, since it requires recording the dysrhythmia as it starts.

PSVT occurs because of a reentrant phenomenon (reexcitation of the atria when there is a one-way block). Usually a PAC triggers a run of repeated premature beats. *Paroxysmal* refers to an abrupt onset and ending. Termination is sometimes followed by a brief period of asystole (absence of all cardiac electrical activity). Some degree of AV block may be present. PSVT can occur in the presence of Wolff-Parkinson-White (WPW) syndrome, or "preexcitation." In this syndrome, there is extra conduction or accessory pathways.

Clinical Associations. In the normal heart, PSVT is associated with overexertion, emotional stress, deep inspiration, and stimulants such as caffeine and tobacco. PSVT is also associated

with rheumatic heart disease, digitalis toxicity, CAD, and cor pulmonale.

ECG Characteristics. In PSVT the HR is 150 to 220 beats/minute, and the rhythm is regular or slightly irregular. The P wave is often hidden in the preceding T wave. If seen, it may have an abnormal shape. The PR interval may be shortened or normal, and the QRS complex is usually normal.

Clinical Significance. The clinical significance of PSVT depends on the associated symptoms. A prolonged episode and HR greater than 180 beats/minute will cause decreased CO because of reduced stroke volume. Symptoms often include hypotension, palpitations, dyspnea, and angina.

Treatment. Treatment for PSVT includes vagal stimulation and drug therapy. Common vagal maneuvers include Valsalva, carotid massage, and coughing. IV adenosine is the drug of choice to convert PSVT to a normal sinus rhythm. This drug has a short half-life (10 seconds) and is well tolerated.[5] IV β-adrenergic blockers, calcium channel blockers, and amiodarone (Cordarone) can also be used. If vagal stimulation and drug therapy are ineffective and the patient becomes hemodynamically unstable, synchronized cardioversion is used.[6] (Cardioversion is discussed on p. 802.)

DRUG ALERT: Adenosine (Adenocard)
- Injection site should be as close to the heart as possible (e.g., antecubital area).
- Give IV dose rapidly (over 1-2 sec) and follow with a rapid 20 mL normal saline flush.
- Monitor patient's ECG continuously. Brief period of asystole is common.
- Observe patient for flushing, dizziness, chest pain, or palpitations.

If PSVT recurs in patients with WPW syndrome, radiofrequency catheter ablation of the accessory pathway is the treatment of choice.[7] (Catheter ablation therapy is discussed on p. 805.)

Atrial Flutter. Atrial flutter is an atrial tachydysrhythmia identified by recurring, regular, sawtooth-shaped flutter waves that originate from a single ectopic focus in the right atrium or, less commonly, the left atrium (Fig. 36-14, *A*).

Clinical Associations. Atrial flutter rarely occurs in a healthy heart. It is associated with CAD, hypertension, mitral valve disorders, pulmonary embolus, chronic lung disease, cor

FIG. 36-13 Paroxysmal supraventricular tachycardia (PSVT). *Arrows* indicate beginning and ending of PSVT.

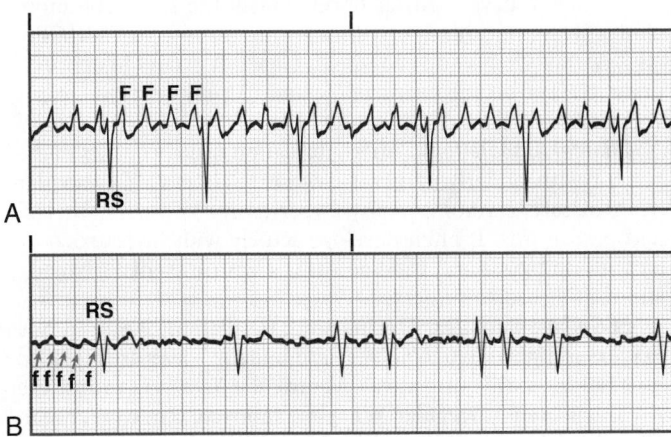

FIG. 36-14 **A,** Atrial flutter with a 4:1 conduction (four flutter *[F]* waves to each QRS complex). **B,** Atrial fibrillation with a controlled ventricular response. Note the chaotic fibrillatory *(f)* waves *(arrows)* between the RS complexes. NOTE: Recorded from lead V₁.

pulmonale, cardiomyopathy, hyperthyroidism, and the use of drugs such as digoxin, quinidine, and epinephrine.

ECG Characteristics. Atrial rate is 200 to 350 beats/minute. The ventricular rate varies based on the conduction ratio. In 2:1 conduction, the ventricular rate is typically found to be approximately 150 beats/minute. Atrial rhythm is regular, and ventricular rhythm is usually regular. The atrial flutter waves represent atrial depolarization followed by repolarization. The PR interval is variable and not measurable. The QRS complex is usually normal. Because the AV node can delay signals from the atria, there is usually some AV block in a fixed ratio of flutter waves to QRS complexes.

Clinical Significance. The high ventricular rates (greater than 100 beats/minute) and loss of the atrial "kick" (atrial contraction reflected by a sinus P wave) that are associated with atrial flutter decrease CO. This can cause serious consequences such as HF, especially in the patient with underlying heart disease. Patients with atrial flutter have an increased risk of stroke because of the risk of thrombus formation in the atria from the stasis of blood. Warfarin (Coumadin) is given to prevent stroke in patients who have atrial flutter.[6,7]

Treatment. The primary goal in treatment of atrial flutter is to slow the ventricular response by increasing AV block. Drugs used to control ventricular rate include calcium channel blockers and β-adrenergic blockers. Electrical cardioversion may be performed to convert the atrial flutter to sinus rhythm in an emergency (i.e., when the patient is clinically unstable) and electively. Antidysrhythmia drugs are used to convert atrial flutter to sinus rhythm (e.g., ibutilide [Corvert]) or to maintain sinus rhythm (e.g., amiodarone, flecainide [Tambocor], dronedarone [Multaq]).[5]

Radiofrequency catheter ablation is the treatment of choice for atrial flutter.[8] The procedure is done in the EPS laboratory and involves placing a catheter in the right atrium. With use of a low-voltage, high-frequency form of electrical energy, the tissue is ablated (or destroyed), the dysrhythmia is ended, and normal sinus rhythm is restored. (Catheter ablation is discussed on p. 802.)

Atrial Fibrillation. Atrial fibrillation is characterized by a total disorganization of atrial electrical activity because of multiple ectopic foci, resulting in loss of effective atrial contraction (Fig. 36-14, *B*). The dysrhythmia may be paroxysmal (i.e., beginning and ending spontaneously) or persistent (lasting more than 7 days).[9] Atrial fibrillation is the most common, clinically significant dysrhythmia with respect to morbidity and mortality rates and economic impact. It occurs in approximately 6% of people over age 65, and its prevalence increases with age.[10]

Clinical Associations. Atrial fibrillation usually occurs in the patient with underlying heart disease, such as CAD, valvular heart disease, cardiomyopathy, hypertensive heart disease, HF, and pericarditis. It often develops acutely with thyrotoxicosis, alcohol intoxication, caffeine use, electrolyte disturbances, stress, and cardiac surgery.

ECG Characteristics. During atrial fibrillation, the atrial rate may be as high as 350 to 600 beats/minute. P waves are replaced by chaotic, fibrillatory waves. Ventricular rate varies, and the rhythm is usually irregular. When the ventricular rate is between 60 and 100 beats/minute, it is atrial fibrillation with a *controlled ventricular response.* Atrial fibrillation with a ventricular rate greater than 100 beats/minute is atrial fibrillation with a *rapid (or uncontrolled) ventricular response.* The PR interval is not

measurable, and the QRS complex usually has a normal shape and duration. At times, atrial flutter and atrial fibrillation may coexist.[1]

Clinical Significance. Atrial fibrillation results in a decrease in CO because of ineffective atrial contractions (loss of atrial kick) and/or a rapid ventricular response. Thrombi (clots) form in the atria because of blood stasis. An embolized clot may develop and move to the brain, causing a stroke. Atrial fibrillation accounts for as many as 17% of all strokes.[10]

Treatment. The goals of treatment include a decrease in ventricular response (to less than 100 beats/minute), prevention of stroke, and conversion to sinus rhythm, if possible. Ventricular rate control is a priority for patients with atrial fibrillation. Drugs used for rate control include calcium channel blockers (e.g., diltiazem), β-adrenergic blockers (e.g., metoprolol), dronedarone, and digoxin (Lanoxin).

For some patients, pharmacologic or electrical conversion of atrial fibrillation to a normal sinus rhythm may be considered

---

EVIDENCE-BASED PRACTICE
Applying the Evidence

G.D. is an 82-year-old woman with a new onset of atrial fibrillation and a history of mitral stenosis (high-risk factor). Her physician has ordered warfarin (Coumadin) to be started. You begin to teach her about the purpose and side effects of warfarin. She stops you and states that she will not take the medicine—she has heard too many stories about people bleeding from this medication. Furthermore, she tells you that she does not want to deal with the blood tests that are needed nor worry about what she eats. She states that she will continue to take her aspirin once a day as usual.

Best Available Evidence	Clinician Expertise	Patient Preferences and Values
Warfarin (Coumadin) is the drug of choice to treat patients with atrial fibrillation who have one or more high-risk factors in order to prevent stroke.	Bleeding is a potential and serious side effect of warfarin and of dual antiplatelet therapy (ASA and clopidogrel).	G.D. does not want to take warfarin or clopidogrel because she is afraid of bleeding.
For patients for whom oral anticoagulation with warfarin is considered unsuitable (e.g., patient preference), the addition of clopidogrel (Plavix) to ASA reduces the risk of major vascular events (especially stroke) but increases the risk of major hemorrhage.	When taking warfarin, INR blood levels need to be checked on a regular basis. Patients should avoid drastic changes in diet, especially foods high in vitamin K (interfere with the action of warfarin).	In addition, she does not want to change her lifestyle to accommodate the changes that would be needed to use warfarin.

Your Decision and Action
You explain the risks of not taking the prescribed medicine (warfarin) or adequate medication (adding clopidogrel to her ASA therapy). She tells you that she understands completely. You support her choice and inform the physician of her decision.

Reference for Evidence
Wann LS, Curtis AB, January CT, et al: 2011 ACCF/AHA/HRS focused update on the management of patients with atrial fibrillation (updating the 2006 guideline): a report of the American College of Cardiology Foundation/American Heart Association Task Force on Practice Guidelines, *J Am Coll Cardiol* 57:223, 2011.

ASA, Acetylsalicylic acid; *INR,* international normalized ratio.

TABLE 36-8 DRUG THERAPY

Anticoagulant Therapy for Atrial Fibrillation

Risk Category	Recommended Therapy
No risk factors	Aspirin, 81-325 mg/day
One moderate-risk factor	Aspirin, 81-325 mg/day, or warfarin*† (target INR 2.0-3.0)
Any high-risk factor or >1 moderate-risk factor	Warfarin* (target INR 2.0-3.0‡)

Level of Risk	Risk Factors
Moderate-risk factors	Age ≥75 yr Heart failure Hypertension LV ejection fraction ≤35% Diabetes mellitus
High-risk factors	Previous stroke, TIA, or embolism Mitral stenosis Prosthetic heart valve‡

Source: Wann LS, Curtis AB, January CT, et al: 2011 ACCF/AHA/HRS focused update on the management of patients with atrial fibrillation (updating the 2006 guideline): a report of the American College of Cardiology Foundation/American Heart Association Task Force on Practice Guidelines, *J Am Coll Cardiol* 57:223, 2011.
*Dabigatran (Pradaxa), a direct thrombin inhibitor, and apixaban (Eliquis) and rivaroxaban (Xarelto), factor Xa inhibitors, are oral anticoagulants approved for use in the treatment of nonvalvular atrial fibrillation only. To date, these drugs have not been incorporated into the guidelines.
†Clopidogrel (Plavix) may be added to aspirin therapy to reduce the risk of major vascular events in patients with atrial fibrillation if warfarin is considered unsuitable (e.g., patient preference, physician determines that patient cannot maintain adequate anticoagulation).
‡If prosthetic heart valve, target INR 2.5-3.5.
INR, International normalized ratio; *LV,* left ventricular; *TIA,* transient ischemic attack.

FIG. 36-15 Junctional escape rhythm. P wave is hidden in the RS complex. NOTE: Recorded from lead V_1.

(e.g., reduced exercise tolerance with rate control drugs, contraindications to warfarin). The most common antidysrhythmia drugs used for conversion to and maintenance of sinus rhythm include amiodarone and ibutilide.[9]

Electrical cardioversion may convert atrial fibrillation to a normal sinus rhythm. If a patient is in atrial fibrillation for longer than 48 hours, anticoagulation therapy with warfarin is needed for 3 to 4 weeks before the cardioversion and for several weeks after successful cardioversion.[5] Anticoagulation therapy is necessary because the procedure can cause the clots to dislodge, placing the patient at risk for stroke. A transesophageal echocardiogram may be performed to rule out clots in the atria. If no clots are present, anticoagulation therapy may not be required before the cardioversion procedure.

If drugs or cardioversion does not convert atrial fibrillation to normal sinus rhythm, long-term anticoagulation therapy is required (Table 36-8). Warfarin is the drug of choice, and patients are monitored for therapeutic levels (e.g., international normalized ratio [INR]). Recently, alternatives to warfarin have been approved for anticoagulation therapy in patients with nonvalvular atrial fibrillation. These drugs do not require routine laboratory testing and include dabigatran (Pradaxa), apixaban (Eliquis), and rivaroxaban (Xarelto). (See Chapter 38 for discussion of anticoagulation therapy.)

For patients with drug-refractory atrial fibrillation or those who do not respond to electrical conversion, radiofrequency catheter ablation (similar to procedure for atrial flutter) and the Maze procedure are further options.[9] The Maze procedure is a surgical intervention that stops atrial fibrillation by interrupting the ectopic electrical signals that are responsible for the dysrhythmia. Incisions are made in both atria, and *cryoablation*

(cold therapy) is used to stop the formation and conduction of these signals and restore normal sinus rhythm.[7]

Junctional Dysrhythmias. *Junctional dysrhythmias* refer to dysrhythmias that start in the area of the AV node. They result because the SA node fails to fire or the signal is blocked. When this occurs, the AV node becomes the pacemaker of the heart. The impulse from the AV node usually moves in a retrograde (backward) fashion. This produces an abnormal P wave that occurs just before or after the QRS complex or that is hidden in the QRS complex. The impulse usually moves normally through the ventricles. Junctional premature beats may occur, and they are treated in a manner similar to that for PACs. Other junctional dysrhythmias include junctional escape rhythm (Fig. 36-15), accelerated junctional rhythm, and junctional tachycardia. These dysrhythmias are treated according to the patient's tolerance of the rhythm and the patient's clinical condition.

Clinical Associations. Junctional dysrhythmias are often associated with CAD, HF, cardiomyopathy, electrolyte imbalances, inferior MI, and rheumatic heart disease. Certain drugs (e.g., digoxin, nicotine, amphetamines, caffeine) can also cause junctional dysrhythmias.

ECG Characteristics. In junctional escape rhythm the HR is 40 to 60 beats/minute. It is 61 to 100 beats/minute in accelerated junctional rhythm and 101 to 180 beats/minute in junctional tachycardia. Rhythm is regular. The P wave is abnormal in shape and inverted, or it may be hidden in the QRS complex (see Fig. 36-15). The PR interval is less than 0.12 second when the P wave precedes the QRS complex. The QRS complex is usually normal.

Clinical Significance. Junctional escape rhythms serve as a safety mechanism when the SA node has not been effective. Escape rhythms such as this should not be suppressed. Accelerated junctional rhythm is due to sympathetic stimulation to improve CO. Junctional tachycardia indicates a more serious problem. This rhythm may reduce CO, causing the patient to become hemodynamically unstable (e.g., hypotensive).

Treatment. Treatment varies according to the type of junctional dysrhythmia. If a patient has symptoms with a junctional escape rhythm, atropine can be used. In accelerated junctional rhythm and junctional tachycardia caused by drug toxicity, the drug is stopped. In the absence of digitalis toxicity, β-adrenergic blockers, calcium channel blockers, and amiodarone are used for rate control. Cardioversion should not be used.

First-Degree AV Block. *First-degree AV block* is a type of AV block in which every impulse is conducted to the ventricles but the time of AV conduction is prolonged (Fig. 36-16, *A*). After the impulse moves through the AV node, the ventricles usually respond normally.

Clinical Associations. First-degree AV block is associated with MI, CAD, rheumatic fever, hyperthyroidism, electrolyte imbalances (e.g., hypokalemia), vagal stimulation, and drugs such as digoxin, β-adrenergic blockers, calcium channel blockers, and flecainide.

A

PR interval

Blocked QRS

B

PR interval   PR interval
0.24 sec   0.32 sec

Blocked QRS   Blocked QRS

C

D

FIG. 36-16 Heart block. **A,** First-degree atrioventricular (AV) block with a PR interval of 0.40 sec. **B,** Second-degree AV block, type I, with progressive lengthening of the PR interval until a QRS complex is blocked. **C,** Second-degree AV block, type II, with constant PR intervals and variable blocked QRS complexes. **D,** Third-degree AV block. Note that there is no relationship between P waves and QRS complexes.

ECG Characteristics. In first-degree AV block, HR is normal and rhythm is regular. The P wave is normal, the PR interval is prolonged (greater than 0.20 second), and the QRS complex usually has a normal shape and duration.

Clinical Significance. First-degree AV block is usually not serious but can be a sign of higher degrees of AV block. Patients with first-degree AV block are asymptomatic.

Treatment. There is no treatment for first-degree AV block. Changes to potentially causative situations may be considered. Monitor patients for any new changes in heart rhythm (e.g., more serious AV block).

Second-Degree AV Block, Type I. *Type I second-degree AV block (Mobitz I or Wenckebach heart block)* includes a gradual lengthening of the PR interval. It occurs because of a prolonged AV conduction time until an atrial impulse is nonconducted and a QRS complex is blocked (missing) (Fig. 36-16, *B*). Type I AV block most commonly occurs in the AV node, but it can also occur in the His-Purkinje system.

Clinical Associations. Type I AV block may result from drugs such as digoxin or β-adrenergic blockers. It may also be associated with CAD and other diseases that can slow AV conduction.

ECG Characteristics. Atrial rate is normal, but ventricular rate may be slower because of nonconducted or blocked QRS

complexes resulting in bradycardia. Once a ventricular beat is blocked, the cycle repeats itself with progressive lengthening of the PR intervals until another QRS complex is blocked. The rhythm appears on the ECG in a pattern of grouped beats. Ventricular rhythm is irregular. The P wave has a normal shape. The QRS complex has a normal shape and duration.

Clinical Significance. Type I AV block is usually a result of myocardial ischemia or inferior MI. It is generally transient and well tolerated. However, in some patients (e.g., acute MI) it may be a warning sign of a more serious AV conduction disturbance (e.g., complete heart block).

Treatment. If the patient is symptomatic, atropine is used to increase HR, or a temporary pacemaker may be needed, especially if the patient has had an MI. If the patient is asymptomatic, the rhythm is closely observed with a transcutaneous pacemaker on standby. Bradycardia is more likely to become symptomatic when hypotension, HF, or shock is present.

Second-Degree AV Block, Type II. In *type II second-degree AV block (Mobitz II heart block)*, a P wave is nonconducted without progressive PR lengthening. This usually occurs when a block in one of the bundle branches is present (Fig. 36-16, *C*). On conducted beats, the PR interval is constant. Type II second-degree AV block is a more serious type of block in which a certain number of impulses from the SA node are not conducted to the ventricles. This occurs in ratios of 2:1, 3:1, and so on (i.e., two P waves to one QRS complex, three P waves to one QRS complex). It may occur with varying ratios.

Clinical Associations. Type II AV block is associated with rheumatic heart disease, CAD, anterior MI, and drug toxicity.

ECG Characteristics. Atrial rate is usually normal. Ventricular rate depends on the intrinsic rate and the degree of AV block. Atrial rhythm is regular, but ventricular rhythm may be irregular. The P wave has a normal shape. The PR interval may be normal or prolonged in duration and remains constant on conducted beats. The QRS complex is usually greater than 0.12 second because of bundle branch block.

Clinical Significance. Type II AV block often progresses to third-degree AV block and is associated with a poor prognosis. The reduced HR frequently results in decreased CO with subsequent hypotension and myocardial ischemia. Type II AV block is an indication for therapy with a permanent pacemaker.

Treatment. Insertion of a temporary pacemaker may be necessary before the insertion of a permanent pacemaker if the patient becomes symptomatic (e.g., hypotension, angina).[6,8] (Temporary pacemakers are discussed on pp. 804-805.)

Third-Degree AV Block. Third-degree AV block, or complete heart block, constitutes one form of AV dissociation in which no impulses from the atria are conducted to the ventricles (Fig. 36-16, *D*). The atria are stimulated and contract independently of the ventricles. The ventricular rhythm is an escape rhythm, and the ectopic pacemaker may be above or below the bifurcation of the bundle of His.

Clinical Associations. Third-degree AV block is associated with severe heart disease, including CAD, MI, myocarditis, cardiomyopathy, and some systemic diseases such as amyloidosis and progressive systemic sclerosis (scleroderma). Some drugs can also cause third-degree AV block, such as digoxin, β-adrenergic blockers, and calcium channel blockers.

ECG Characteristics. The atrial rate is usually a sinus rate of 60 to 100 beats/minute. The ventricular rate depends on the site of the block. If it is in the AV node, the rate is 40 to 60 beats/

FIG. 36-17 Various forms of premature ventricular contractions (PVCs).

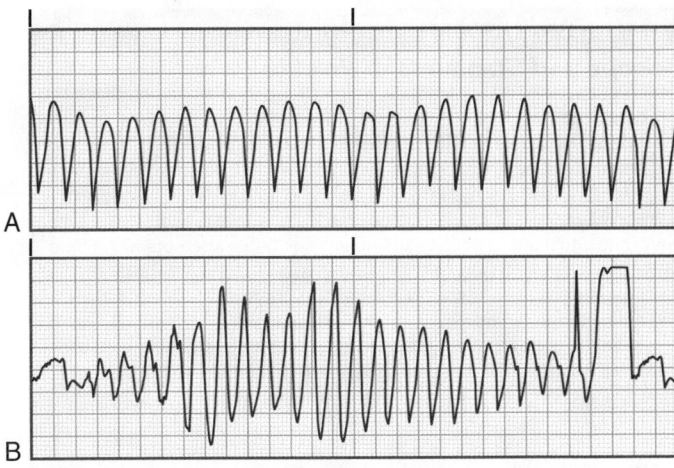

FIG. 36-18 Ventricular tachycardia. **A,** Monomorphic. **B,** Torsades de pointes (polymorphic).

minute, and if it is in the His-Purkinje system, it is 20 to 40 beats/minute. Atrial and ventricular rhythms are regular but unrelated to each other. The P wave has a normal shape. The PR interval is variable, and there is no relationship between the P wave and the QRS complex. The QRS complex is normal if an escape rhythm is initiated at the bundle of His or above. It is widened if an escape rhythm is initiated below the bundle of His.

Clinical Significance. Third-degree AV block usually results in reduced CO with subsequent ischemia, HF, and shock. Syncope from third-degree AV block may result from severe bradycardia or even periods of asystole.

Treatment. For symptomatic patients, a transcutaneous pacemaker is used until a temporary transvenous pacemaker can be inserted.[8] (Types of temporary pacemakers are discussed on pp. 804-805.) The use of drugs such as atropine, dopamine, and epinephrine is a temporary measure to increase HR and support blood pressure (BP) until temporary pacing is started. Patients need a permanent pacemaker as soon as possible.

Premature Ventricular Contractions. A **premature ventricular contraction (PVC)** is a contraction coming from an ectopic focus in the ventricles. It is the premature (early) occurrence of a QRS complex. A PVC is wide and distorted in shape compared with a QRS complex coming down the normal conduction pathway (Fig. 36-17). PVCs that arise from different foci appear different in shape from each other and are called *multifocal* PVCs. PVCs that have the same shape are called *unifocal* PVCs. When every other beat is a PVC, the rhythm is called *ventricular bigeminy.* When every third beat is a PVC, it is called *ventricular trigeminy.* Two consecutive PVCs are called a *couplet.*

Ventricular tachycardia (VT) occurs when there are three or more consecutive PVCs. *R-on-T phenomenon* occurs when a PVC falls on the T wave of a preceding beat. This is especially dangerous because the PVC is firing during the relative refractory phase of ventricular repolarization. Excitability of the cardiac cells increases during this time, and the risk for the PVC to start VT or ventricular fibrillation (VF) is great.

Clinical Associations. PVCs are associated with stimulants such as caffeine, alcohol, nicotine, aminophylline, epinephrine, isoproterenol, and digoxin. They are also associated with electrolyte imbalances, hypoxia, fever, exercise, and emotional stress. Disease states associated with PVCs include MI, mitral valve prolapse, HF, and CAD.

ECG Characteristics. HR varies according to intrinsic rate and number of PVCs. Rhythm is irregular because of premature beats. The P wave is rarely visible and is usually lost in the QRS complex of the PVC. Retrograde conduction may occur, and the P wave may be seen after the ectopic beat. The PR interval is not measurable. The QRS complex is wide and distorted in shape, lasting more than 0.12 second. The T wave is generally large and opposite in direction to the major direction of the QRS complex.

Clinical Significance. PVCs are usually not harmful in the patient with a normal heart. In heart disease, PVCs may reduce the CO and lead to angina and HF depending on frequency. Because PVCs in CAD or acute MI indicate ventricular irritability, assess the patient's physiologic response to PVCs. Obtain the patient's apical-radial pulse rate, since PVCs often do not generate a sufficient ventricular contraction to result in a peripheral pulse. This can lead to a pulse deficit.

Treatment. Treatment relates to the cause of the PVCs (e.g., oxygen therapy for hypoxia, electrolyte replacement). Assessment of the patient's hemodynamic status is important to determine if treatment with drug therapy is needed. Drug therapy includes β-adrenergic blockers, procainamide (Pronestyl), or amiodarone.

Ventricular Tachycardia. A run of three or more PVCs defines **ventricular tachycardia (VT).** It occurs when an ectopic focus or foci fire repeatedly and the ventricle takes control as the pacemaker. Different forms of VT exist, depending on QRS configuration. *Monomorphic* VT (Fig. 36-18, *A*) has QRS complexes that are the same in shape, size, and direction. *Polymorphic* VT occurs when the QRS complexes gradually change back and forth from one shape, size, and direction to another over a series of beats. *Torsades de pointes* (French for "twisting of the points") is polymorphic VT associated with a prolonged QT interval of the underlying rhythm (Fig. 36-18, *B*).

VT may be sustained (longer than 30 seconds) or nonsustained (less than 30 seconds). The development of VT is an ominous sign. It is a life-threatening dysrhythmia because of decreased CO and the possibility of development of VF, which is lethal.

Clinical Associations. VT is associated with MI, CAD, significant electrolyte imbalances, cardiomyopathy, mitral valve prolapse, long QT syndrome, drug toxicity, and central nervous system disorders. This dysrhythmia can be seen in patients who have no evidence of cardiac disease.

ECG Characteristics. Ventricular rate is 150 to 250 beats/minute. Rhythm may be regular or irregular. AV dissociation may be present, with P waves occurring independently of the QRS complex. The atria may be depolarized by the ventricles in a retrograde fashion. The P wave is usually buried in the QRS complex, and the PR interval is not measurable. The QRS complex is distorted in appearance and wide (greater than 0.12 second in duration). The T wave is in the opposite direction of the QRS complex (see Fig. 36-18).

Clinical Significance. VT can be stable (patient has a pulse) or unstable (patient is pulseless). Sustained VT causes a severe decrease in CO because of decreased ventricular diastolic filling times and loss of atrial contraction. This results in hypotension, pulmonary edema, decreased cerebral blood flow, and cardiopulmonary arrest. The dysrhythmia must be treated quickly, even if it occurs only briefly and stops abruptly. Episodes may recur if prophylactic treatment is not started. VF may also develop.

Treatment. Precipitating causes (e.g., electrolyte imbalances, ischemia) must be identified and treated. If the VT is monomorphic and the patient is clinically stable (i.e., pulse is present) and has preserved left ventricular function, IV procainamide, sotalol, or amiodarone is used. These drugs can also be used if the VT is polymorphic with a normal baseline QT interval.

Polymorphic VT with a prolonged baseline QT interval is treated with IV magnesium, isoproterenol, phenytoin (Dilantin), or antitachycardia pacing (discussed later in this chapter). Drugs that prolong the QT interval (e.g., dofetilide [Tikosyn]) should be discontinued. Cardioversion is used if drug therapy is ineffective.

VT without a pulse is a life-threatening situation. It is treated in the same manner as VF. Cardiopulmonary resuscitation (CPR) and rapid defibrillation are the first lines of treatment, followed by the administration of vasopressors (e.g., epinephrine) and antidysrhythmics (e.g., amiodarone) if defibrillation is unsuccessful.[6]

An *accelerated idioventricular rhythm* (AIVR) can develop when the intrinsic pacemaker rate (SA node or AV node) becomes less than that of a ventricular ectopic pacemaker. The rate is between 40 and 100 beats/minute. It is most commonly associated with acute MI and reperfusion of the myocardium after thrombolytic therapy or angioplasty of coronary arteries. It can be seen with digitalis toxicity. In the setting of acute MI, AIVR is usually self-limiting and well tolerated, and it requires no treatment. If the patient becomes symptomatic (e.g., hypotensive, chest pain), atropine can be considered. Temporary pacing may be required. Drugs that suppress ventricular rhythms (e.g., amiodarone) should not be used, since these can terminate the ventricular rhythm and further reduce the HR.

Ventricular Fibrillation. Ventricular fibrillation (VF) is a severe derangement of the heart rhythm characterized on ECG by irregular waveforms of varying shapes and amplitude (Fig. 36-19). This represents the firing of multiple ectopic foci in the ventricle. Mechanically the ventricle is simply "quivering," with no effective contraction, and consequently no CO occurs. VF is a lethal dysrhythmia.

Clinical Associations. VF occurs in acute MI and myocardial ischemia and in chronic diseases such as HF and cardiomyopathy. It may occur during cardiac pacing or cardiac catheterization procedures because of catheter stimulation of the ventricle. It may also occur with coronary reperfusion

FIG. 36-19 Ventricular fibrillation.

after thrombolytic therapy. Other clinical associations are electric shock, hyperkalemia, hypoxemia, acidosis, and drug toxicity.

ECG Characteristics. HR is not measurable. Rhythm is irregular and chaotic. The P wave is not visible, and the PR interval and the QRS interval are not measurable.

Clinical Significance. VF results in an unresponsive, pulseless, and apneic state. If it is not rapidly treated, the patient will not recover.

Treatment. Treatment consists of immediate initiation of CPR and advanced cardiac life support (ACLS) with the use of defibrillation and definitive drug therapy (e.g., epinephrine, vasopressin [Pitressin]). There should be no delay in using a defibrillator once available.

Asystole. Asystole represents the total absence of ventricular electrical activity. Occasionally, P waves are seen. No ventricular contraction occurs because depolarization does not occur. Patients are unresponsive, pulseless, and apneic. Asystole is a lethal dysrhythmia that requires immediate treatment. VF may masquerade as asystole. Always assess the rhythm in more than one lead. The prognosis of a patient with asystole is extremely poor.

Clinical Associations. Asystole is usually a result of advanced cardiac disease, a severe cardiac conduction system disturbance, or end-stage HF.

Clinical Significance. Generally the patient with asystole has end-stage heart disease or has a prolonged arrest and cannot be resuscitated.

Treatment. Treatment consists of CPR with initiation of ACLS measures. These include definitive drug therapy with epinephrine and/or vasopressin, and intubation.

Pulseless Electrical Activity. *Pulseless electrical activity* (PEA) is a situation in which organized electrical activity is seen on the ECG, but there is no mechanical activity of the ventricles and the patient has no pulse. It is the most common dysrhythmia seen after defibrillation. Prognosis is poor unless the underlying cause is quickly identified and treated. The most common causes of PEA include hypovolemia, hypoxia, metabolic acidosis, hyperkalemia, hypokalemia, hypoglycemia, hypothermia, toxins (e.g., drug overdose), cardiac tamponade, thrombosis (e.g., MI, pulmonary embolus), tension pneumothorax, and trauma. Treatment begins with CPR followed by drug therapy (e.g., epinephrine) and intubation. Correcting the underlying cause is critical to prognosis.

Sudden Cardiac Death. The term *sudden cardiac death* (SCD) refers to death from a cardiac cause. Most SCDs result from ventricular dysrhythmias, specifically VT or VF. (SCD is discussed in Chapter 34.)

Prodysrhythmia. Antidysrhythmia drugs can cause life-threatening dysrhythmias similar to those for which they are given. This concept is termed *prodysrhythmia*. The patient who has severe left ventricular dysfunction is the most susceptible to prodysrhythmias. Digoxin and class IA, IC, and III antidysrhythmia drugs can cause a prodysrhythmic response.[5] The first several days of drug therapy are the vulnerable period for developing prodysrhythmias. For this reason, many oral antidysrhythmia drug regimens are started in a monitored hospital setting.

Antidysrhythmia Drugs

Table 36-9 categorizes antidysrhythmia drugs by their primary effects on the cardiac cells and the ECG.

TABLE 36-9 DRUG THERAPY

Antidysrhythmia Drugs

Drug	Actions*	Effects on ECG
Class I: Sodium Channel Blockers	Decrease impulse conduction in the atria, ventricles, and His-Purkinje system	—
Class IA disopyramide (Norpace) procainamide (Pronestyl) quinidine (Quinora)	Delay repolarization	Widened QRS and prolonged QT interval
Class IB mexiletine (Mexitil) phenytoin (Dilantin)	Accelerate repolarization	Little or no effect on ECG
Class IC flecainide (Tambocor) propafenone (Rythmol)	Decrease impulse conduction	Pronounced prodysrhythmic actions, widened QRS, prolonged QT interval
Class II: β-Adrenergic Blockers esmolol (Brevibloc) metoprolol (Lopressor) propranolol (Inderal)	Decrease automaticity of the SA node, slow impulse conduction in AV node, reduce atrial and ventricular contractility	Bradycardia, prolonged PR interval, AV block
Class III: Potassium Channel Blockers amiodarone (Cordarone) bretylium (Bretylol) dofetilide (Tikosyn) ibutilide (Corvert) sotalol† (Betapace)	Delay repolarization, resulting in prolonged duration of action potential and refractory period	Prolonged PR and QT intervals, widened QRS, bradycardia
Class IV: Calcium Channel Blockers diltiazem (Cardizem) verapamil (Calan)	Decrease automaticity of SA node, delay AV node conduction; reduce myocardial contractility	Bradycardia, prolonged PR interval, AV block
Other Antidysrhythmia Drugs adenosine (Adenocard) digoxin (Lanoxin)	Decrease conduction through AV node, reduce automaticity of SA node	Prolonged PR interval, AV block
dronedarone (Multaq)‡	Suppresses atrial dysrhythmias though mechanism is unknown	Prolonged QT interval
Magnesium	Decreases impulse conduction through AV node	AV block

*Antidysrhythmia drugs have a direct effect on the various phases of the action potential (see Fig. 36-1).
†Sotalol has both class II and class III properties.
‡Dronedarone has class I-IV properties.
AV, Atrioventricular; *SA*, sinoatrial.

Defibrillation

Defibrillation is the treatment of choice to end VF and pulseless VT. It is most effective when the myocardial cells are not anoxic or acidotic. Rapid defibrillation (within 2 minutes) is critical to a successful patient outcome. Defibrillation involves the passage of an electric shock through the heart to depolarize the cells of the myocardium. The goal is that the following repolarization

FIG. 36-20 Paddle placement and current flow in monophasic defibrillation **(A)** and biphasic defibrillation **(B)**.

FIG. 36-21 LifePak contains a monitor, defibrillator, and transcutaneous pacemaker.

of myocardial cells will allow the SA node to resume the role of pacemaker.

Defibrillators deliver energy using a monophasic or biphasic waveform. Monophasic defibrillators deliver energy in one direction, and biphasic defibrillators deliver energy in two directions (Fig. 36-20). Biphasic defibrillators deliver successful shocks at lower energies and with fewer postshock ECG abnormalities than monophasic defibrillators.

The output of a defibrillator is measured in *joules*, or watts per second. The recommended energy for initial shocks in defibrillation depends on the type of defibrillator. Biphasic defibrillators deliver the first and any successive shocks using 120 to 200 joules. Recommendations for monophasic defibrillators include an initial shock at 360 joules. After the first shock, start CPR immediately beginning with chest compressions. (CPR is discussed in Appendix A of this book.)

Rapid defibrillation can be performed using a manual or automatic device (Fig. 36-21). Manual defibrillators require you to interpret heart rhythms, determine the need for a shock, and deliver a shock. An **automatic external defibrillator (AED)** can detect heart rhythms and advise the user to deliver a shock using hands-free defibrillator pads. Proficiency in use of the AED is part of the basic life support course for health care providers. You should be familiar with the operation of the type of defibrillator used in your clinical setting.

The following general steps are taken for defibrillation: (1) CPR should be in progress until the defibrillator is available; (2) turn the defibrillator on, and select the proper energy level;

(3) check to see that the synchronizer switch is turned off (discussed below); (4) apply conductive materials (e.g., defibrillator gel pads) to the chest, one to the right of the sternum just below the clavicle, and the other to the left of the apex; (5) charge the defibrillator using the button on the defibrillator or the paddles; (6) position the paddles firmly on the chest wall over the conductive material (see Fig. 36-20); (7) call and look to see that everyone is "all clear" to ensure that personnel are not touching the patient or the bed at the time of discharge; and (8) deliver the charge by depressing buttons on both paddles simultaneously.

Hands-free, multifunction defibrillator pads are available and are placed on the chest as described above. Connect the cables from the pads to the defibrillator. Charge and discharge the defibrillator using buttons on the defibrillator. It is still essential to ensure that all personnel are clear before discharging the defibrillator.

Synchronized Cardioversion. *Synchronized cardioversion* is the therapy of choice for the patient with ventricular tachydysrhythmias (e.g., VT with a pulse) or supraventricular tachydysrhythmias (e.g., atrial fibrillation with a rapid ventricular response). A synchronized circuit in the defibrillator delivers a shock that is programmed to occur on the R wave of the QRS complex of the ECG. The synchronizer switch must be turned on when cardioversion is planned.

The procedure for synchronized cardioversion is the same as for defibrillation with the following exceptions. If synchronized cardioversion is done on a nonemergency basis (i.e., the patient is awake and hemodynamically stable), the patient is sedated (e.g., IV midazolam [Versed]) before the procedure. Strict attention to maintaining the patient's airway is critical. If a patient with supraventricular tachycardia or VT with a pulse becomes hemodynamically unstable, synchronized cardioversion should be performed as quickly as possible. Start the initial energy for synchronized cardioversion at 50 to 100 joules (biphasic defibrillator) and 100 joules (monophasic defibrillator), and increase if needed. If the patient becomes pulseless or the rhythm changes to VF, turn the synchronizer switch off and perform defibrillation.

SAFETY ALERT: Defibrillation and Cardioversion
- Check that the synchronizer switch is OFF when defibrillation is planned.
- Turn the synchronizer switch ON when cardioversion is planned.
- Be certain that personnel are "all clear" before discharging the device.

A   B   Right ventricle

FIG. 36-24 A, A dual-chamber rate-responsive pacemaker from Medtronic, Inc., is designed to treat patients with chronic heart problems in which the heart beats too slowly to adequately support the body's circulation needs. **B,** Pacing leads in both the atrium and the ventricle enable a dual-chamber pacemaker to sense and pace in both heart chambers.

FIG. 36-25 Temporary external, dual-chamber demand pacemaker.

have two distinct features: (1) a sensing device that inhibits the pacemaker when the HR is adequate and (2) a pacing device that triggers the pacemaker when no QRS complexes occur within a preset time.[1,13]

In addition to antibradycardia pacing, devices now include antitachycardia and overdrive pacing. *Antitachycardia pacing* involves the delivery of a stimulus to the ventricle to end tachydysrhythmias (e.g., VT). Overdrive pacing involves pacing the atrium at rates of 200 to 500 impulses per minute in an attempt to terminate atrial tachycardias (e.g., atrial flutter with a rapid ventricular response). You can refer to texts on pacemaker therapy for more detailed information[13] and to eTable 36-1 for the Five Letter Pacemaker Code on the website for this chapter.

Permanent Pacemaker. A *permanent pacemaker* is implanted totally within the body (Fig. 36-24). The power source is placed subcutaneously, usually over the pectoral muscle on the patient's nondominant side. The pacing leads are placed transvenously to the right atrium and/or one or both ventricles and attached to the power source. Common reasons for insertion of a permanent pacemaker are found in Table 36-11.

Cardiac Resynchronization Therapy. *Cardiac resynchronization therapy* (CRT) is a pacing technique that resynchronizes the cardiac cycle by pacing both ventricles *(biventricular pacing).* This promotes improvement in ventricular function (see Fig. 35-4). Most HF patients have intraventricular conduction delays causing abnormal ventricular contraction. This causes dyssynchrony between the right and left ventricles and results in reduced systolic function, pump inefficiency, and worsened HF. For patients with severe left ventricular dysfunction, CRT is

combined with an ICD for maximum therapy.[14] (HF is discussed in Chapter 35.)

Temporary Pacemaker. A *temporary pacemaker* is one that has the power source outside the body (Fig. 36-25). There are three types of temporary pacemakers: transvenous, epicardial, and transcutaneous. Table 36-12 lists common reasons for temporary pacing.

A *transvenous pacemaker* consists of a lead or leads that are threaded transvenously to the right atrium and/or right ventricle and attached to the external power source (Fig. 36-26). Most temporary transvenous pacemakers are inserted in emergency departments and critical care units in emergent situations. They provide a bridge to insertion of a permanent pacemaker or until the underlying cause of the dysrhythmia is resolved.

Epicardial pacing involves attaching an atrial and ventricular pacing lead to the epicardium during heart surgery. The leads are passed through the chest wall and attached to the external power source. Epicardial pacing leads are placed prophylactically should any bradydysrhythmias or tachydysrhythmias occur in the early postoperative period.[8]

A *transcutaneous pacemaker* (TCP) is used to provide adequate HR and rhythm to the patient in an emergency situation. Placement of the TCP is a noninvasive, temporary procedure used until a transvenous pacemaker is inserted or until more definitive therapy is available.[8]

TABLE 36-11	INDICATIONS FOR PERMANENT PACEMAKERS

- Acquired AV block
- Second-degree AV block
- Third-degree AV block
- Atrial fibrillation with a slow ventricular response
- Bundle branch block
- Cardiomyopathy
  - Dilated
  - Hypertrophic
- Heart failure
- SA node dysfunction
- Tachydysrhythmias (e.g., ventricular tachycardia)

AV, Atrioventricular; *SA,* sinoatrial.

TABLE 36-12	INDICATIONS FOR TEMPORARY PACEMAKERS*

- Maintenance of adequate HR and rhythm during special circumstances such as surgery and postoperative recovery, during cardiac catheterization or coronary angioplasty, during drug therapy that may cause bradycardia, and before implantation of a permanent pacemaker
- As prophylaxis after open heart surgery
- Acute anterior MI with second- or third-degree AV block or bundle branch block
- Acute inferior MI with symptomatic bradycardia and AV block
- Electrophysiologic studies to evaluate patient with bradydysrhythmias and tachydysrhythmias

*List is not all-inclusive.
AV, Atrioventricular; *HR,* heart rate; *MI,* myocardial infarction.

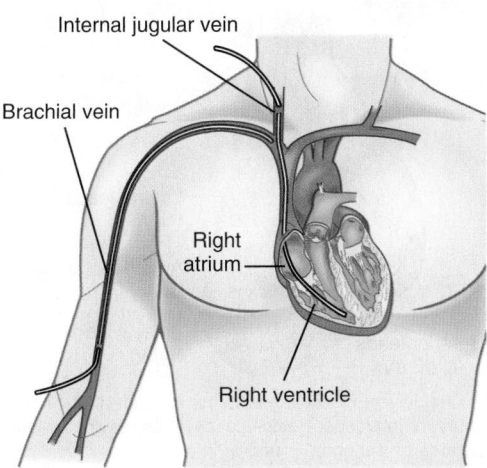

FIG. 36-26 Temporary transvenous pacemaker catheter insertion. A single lead is positioned in the right ventricle through the brachial, subclavian, jugular, or femoral vein.

FIG. 36-27 Transcutaneous pacemaker. Pacing electrodes are placed on the patient's anterior (A) and posterior (B) chest walls and attached to an external pacing unit (C).

The TCP consists of a power source and a rate- and voltage-control device that attaches to two large, multifunction electrode pads. Position one pad on the anterior part of the chest, usually on the V_4 lead position, and the other pad on the back between the spine and the left scapula at the level of the heart (Fig. 36-27). Always use the lowest current that results in a ventricular contraction (capture) to minimize patient discomfort.

Before initiating TCP therapy, it is important to tell the patient what to expect. Explain that the muscle contractions created by the pacemaker when the current passes through the chest wall are uncomfortable. Reassure the patient that the TCP is temporary and that it will be replaced by a transvenous pacemaker as soon as possible. Whenever possible, provide analgesia and/or sedation while the TCP is in use.

Monitoring of Patients With Pacemakers. Patients with temporary or permanent pacemakers are ECG monitored to evaluate the status of the pacemaker. Pacemaker malfunction primarily involves a failure to sense or a failure to capture. *Failure to sense* occurs when the pacemaker fails to recognize spontaneous atrial or ventricular activity, and it fires inappropriately. This can result in the pacemaker firing during the excitable period of the cardiac cycle, resulting in VT. Failure to sense is caused by pacer lead damage, battery failure, sensing set too high, or dislodgment of the electrode. *Failure to capture* occurs when the electrical charge to the myocardium is insufficient to produce atrial or ventricular contraction. This can result in serious bradycardia or asystole. Failure to capture is caused by pacer lead damage, battery failure, dislodgment of the electrode, electrical charge set too low, or fibrosis at the electrode tip.

Complications of invasive temporary (i.e., transvenous) or permanent pacemaker insertion include infection and hematoma formation at the insertion site, pneumothorax, failure to sense or capture, perforation of the atrial or ventricular septum by the pacing lead, and appearance of "end-of-life" battery power on testing the pacemaker. Several measures can prevent or assess for complications. These include prophylactic IV antibiotic therapy before and after insertion, postinsertion chest x-ray to check lead placement and to rule out a pneumothorax, careful observation of insertion site, and continuous ECG monitoring of the patient's rhythm.

After the pacemaker has been inserted, the patient can be out of bed once stable. Have the patient limit arm and shoulder activity on the operative side to prevent dislodging the newly implanted pacing leads. Observe the insertion site for signs of bleeding, and check that the incision is intact. Note any temperature elevation or pain at the insertion site and treat as ordered. Most patients are discharged the next day if stable.

Provide teaching in addition to observing for complications after pacemaker insertion. The patient with a newly implanted pacemaker and the caregiver may have questions about activity restrictions and fears concerning body image after the procedure. The goals of pacemaker therapy include enhancing physiologic functioning and quality of life. Emphasize this to the patient and the caregiver, and provide specific advice on activity restrictions. Table 36-13 outlines patient and caregiver teaching for the patient with a pacemaker.

After discharge, patients need to check pacemaker function on a regular basis. This can include outpatient visits to a pacemaker clinic or home monitoring using telephone transmitter devices. Another method to evaluate pacemaker performance is noninvasive program stimulation. This procedure is done on an outpatient basis in the EPS laboratory.

Radiofrequency Catheter Ablation Therapy

Radiofrequency catheter ablation therapy uses electrical energy to "burn" or ablate areas of the conduction system as definitive treatment of tachydysrhythmias. Ablation therapy is done after EPS has identified the source of the dysrhythmia. An electrode-tipped ablation catheter ablates accessory pathways or ectopic sites in the atria, the AV node, and the ventricles. Catheter ablation is considered the nonpharmacologic treatment of choice for atrial dysrhythmias resulting in rapid ventricular rates and AV nodal reentrant tachycardia refractory to drug therapy.[7,9]

The ablation procedure is successful with a low complication rate. Care of the patient after ablation therapy is similar to that of a patient undergoing cardiac catheterization (see Chapter 32 and Table 32-6).

TABLE 36-13	PATIENT & CAREGIVER TEACHING GUIDE

Pacemaker

Include the following information in the teaching plan for a patient with a pacemaker and the patient's caregiver.

1. Maintain follow-up care with your cardiologist to begin regular pacemaker function checks.
2. Report any signs of infection at incision site (e.g., redness, swelling, drainage) or fever to your cardiologist immediately.
3. Keep incision dry for 4 days after implantation, or as ordered.
4. Avoid lifting arm on pacemaker side above shoulder until approved by your cardiologist.
5. Avoid direct blows to pacemaker site.
6. Avoid close proximity to high-output electric generators, since these can interfere with the function of the pacemaker.
7. You should not have a magnetic resonance imaging (MRI) scan unless the pacemaker is approved as MRI safe or there is a protocol in place for patient safety during the procedure.
8. Microwave ovens are safe to use and do not interfere with pacemaker function.
9. Avoid standing near antitheft devices in doorways of department stores and public libraries. You should walk through them at a normal pace.
10. Air travel is not restricted. Inform airport security of presence of pacemaker because it may set off the metal detector. If hand-held screening wand is used, it should not be placed directly over the pacemaker. Manufacturer information may vary regarding the effect of metal detectors on the function of the pacemaker.
11. Monitor pulse and inform cardiologist if it drops below predetermined rate.
12. Carry pacemaker information card and a current list of your medications at all times.
13. Obtain and wear a Medic Alert ID or bracelet at all times.

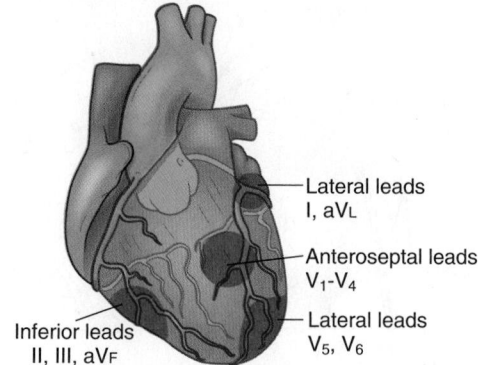

FIG. 36-28 Definitive ECG changes occur in leads that face the area of ischemia, injury, or infarction. Reciprocal changes may occur in leads facing opposite the area of ischemia, injury, or infarction.

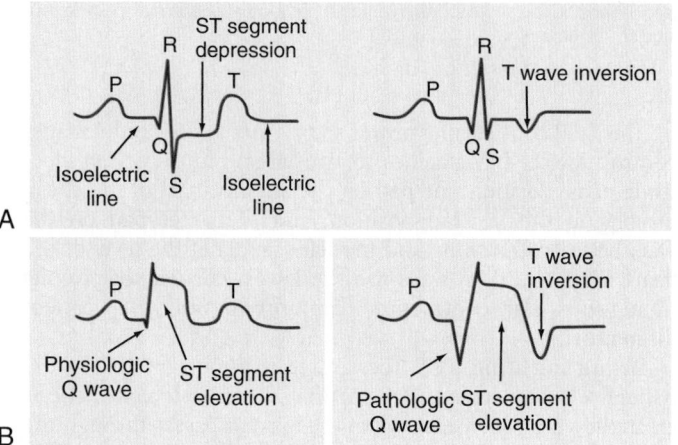

FIG. 36-29 ST segment, T wave, and Q wave changes associated with myocardial ischemia **(A)**, injury **(B)**, and infarction **(C)**.

ECG CHANGES ASSOCIATED WITH ACUTE CORONARY SYNDROME

The 12-lead ECG is a major diagnostic tool used to evaluate patients with ACS. ECG changes that occur with ACS direct many treatment decisions. The ECG changes are in response to ischemia, injury, or infarction (necrosis) of heart cells. The leads facing the area of involvement demonstrate the definitive ECG changes (Fig. 36-28). The leads facing opposite the area involved in ACS often demonstrate reciprocal (opposite) ECG changes. In addition, the pattern of ECG changes among the 12 leads provides information on the coronary artery involved in ACS (Table 36-14).

Ischemia

Typical ECG changes that are seen in myocardial ischemia include ST segment depression and/or T wave inversion (Fig. 36-29, *A*). ST segment depression is significant if it is at least 1 mm (one small box) below the isoelectric line in at least two contiguous (neighboring) leads (see Fig. 36-5). The isoelectric line is flat and represents those normal times in the cardiac cycle when the ECG is not recording any electrical activity in the heart. These times are as follows: (1) from the end of the P wave to the start of the QRS complex, (2) during the entire ST segment, and (3) from the end of the T wave to the start of the next P wave (see Fig. 36-9). Depression in the ST segment and/or T wave inversion occurs in response to an inadequate supply of blood and oxygen, which causes an electrical disturbance in the myocardial cells.[6,7] Once the patient is treated (adequate blood flow is restored), the ECG changes resolve, and the ECG returns to the patient's baseline. (See Chapter 34 for a complete discussion of ACS.)

TABLE 36-14	ECG EVIDENCE IN ACUTE CORONARY SYNDROME		
Left Ventricle Involvement	**ECG Evidence**		**Associated Coronary Artery**
	Leads Facing Area	**Leads Opposite Area (Reciprocal Changes)**	
Septal wall	V_1, V_2	II, III, aV$_F$	Left anterior descending
Anterior wall	V_2-V_4	II, III, aV$_F$	Left anterior descending
Lateral wall, low	V_5, V_6	II, III, aV$_F$	Left anterior descending or circumflex
Lateral wall, high	I, aV$_L$	II, III, aV$_F$	Circumflex
Inferior wall	II, III, aV$_F$	I, aV$_L$, V_5, V_6	Right coronary artery, posterior descending coronary artery

FIG. 36-30 ECG findings with anteroseptal lateral wall myocardial infarction. Normally, leads I, aV$_L$, and V$_1$ to V$_3$ have a positive R wave. Note the pathologic Q waves in these leads and the ST segment elevation in leads V$_2$ to V$_5$ *(arrows)*.

Injury and Infarction

Myocardial injury represents a worsening stage of ischemia that is potentially reversible but may evolve to MI. The typical ECG change seen during injury is ST segment elevation. ST segment elevation is significant if it is 1 mm or more above the isoelectric line in at least two contiguous leads (Fig. 36-29, *B*). If treatment is prompt and effective, it is possible to restore oxygen to the myocardium and avoid or limit infarction. The absence of serum cardiac markers confirms this.

In addition to ST segment elevation, a pathologic Q wave may be seen on the ECG in patients with infarction (Fig. 36-29, *C*). A physiologic Q wave is the first negative deflection (wave) following the P wave. It is normally very short and narrow (see Fig. 36-9 and Table 36-2). A pathologic Q wave that develops during MI is wide (greater than 0.03 second in duration) and deep (greater than or equal to 25% of the height of the R wave).[1,7] This is referred to as a *Q wave MI.* The pathologic Q wave may be present on the ECG indefinitely.

T wave inversion related to MI occurs within hours following the event and may persist for months. The ECG changes seen in injury and MI reflect electrical disturbances in the myocardial cells caused by a prolonged lack of blood and oxygen leading to necrosis (Fig. 36-30).

Patient Monitoring

Monitoring guidelines for patients who are suspected of having ACS include continuous, multilead ECG and ST segment monitoring.[3] The leads selected for monitoring should minimally include the leads that reflect the area of ischemia, injury, or infarction.

SYNCOPE

Syncope, a brief lapse in consciousness accompanied by a loss in postural tone (fainting), is a common diagnosis of patients coming to the emergency department. The causes of syncope can be cardiovascular or noncardiovascular. The most common cause of syncope is cardioneurogenic syncope, or "vasovagal" syncope (e.g., carotid sinus sensitivity). Other cardiovascular causes relate to dysrhythmias (e.g., tachycardias, bradycardias), prosthetic valve malfunction, pulmonary emboli, and HF. Noncardiovascular causes vary and include stress, hypoglycemia, dehydration, stroke, and seizure.[14]

A diagnostic workup for a patient with syncope from a suspected cardiac cause begins with ruling out structural and ischemic heart disease. This is done with echocardiography and stress testing. In the older patient, who is more likely to have structural and ischemic heart disease, EPS is used to diagnose atrial and ventricular tachydysrhythmias and conduction disturbances causing bradydysrhythmias, all of which can cause syncope. These problems can be treated with antidysrhythmia drug therapy, pacemakers, ICDs, and/or catheter ablation therapy.

In patients without structural heart disease or in whom EPS testing is not diagnostic, the *head-up tilt-test* may be performed. Normally, an upright position results in gravity displacing 300 to 800 mL of blood to the lower extremities. Specialized nerve fibers called mechanoreceptors are located throughout the vascular system. These respond to the increased blood volume by starting a reflex increase in sympathetic stimulation and decrease in parasympathetic output. The end results are a slight increase in HR and diastolic BP, and a slight decrease in systolic BP.[15]

In cardioneurogenic syncope, the increase in venous pooling that occurs in the upright position reduces venous return to the heart. This results in a sudden, compensatory increase in ventricular contraction. This is mistaken by the brain as a hypertensive state, and consequently sympathetic stimulation is withdrawn. This produces a paradoxic vasodilation and bradycardia (vasovagal response). The end results are bradycardia, hypotension, cerebral hypoperfusion, and syncope.

In the head-up tilt-test the patient is placed on a table supported by a belt across the torso and feet. Baseline ECG, BP, and HR are obtained in the horizontal position. Next, the table is tilted 60 to 80 degrees and the patient is kept in this upright position for 20 to 60 minutes. ECG and HR are recorded continuously and BP is measured every 3 minutes throughout the test.

If the patient's BP and HR responses are abnormal and clinical symptoms are reproduced (e.g., faintness), the test is considered positive. If after 30 minutes there is no response, the table is returned to the horizontal position and an IV infusion of low-dose isoproterenol may be started in an attempt to provoke a response.

Additional diagnostic tests for syncope can include various recording devices (e.g., Holter monitor or event monitor/loop recorder, which are discussed in Chapter 32 and Table 32-6), blood volume determination, hemodynamic testing, and autonomic reflex testing. About 30% of those who have one episode of syncope experience a recurrence. The underlying cause of syncope and the patient's age and co-morbidities affect the patient's treatment and prognosis.[15]

CASE STUDY

Dysrhythmia

iStockphoto/Thinkstock

Patient Profile
J.M., a 68-year-old retired white postal worker, was admitted to the telemetry unit with a diagnosis of acute decompensated heart failure (HF). He experienced a cardiac arrest (pulseless ventricular tachycardia [VT]) and was successfully defibrillated after one shock. He is transferred to the cardiac care unit. J.M. is awake but lethargic, and responds appropriately to questions.

Subjective Data
- History of hypertension, coronary artery disease, two MIs, and chronic HF
- Reports shortness of breath at rest and even in an upright position

Objective Data
Physical Examination
- Appears weak, anxious
- BP 102/60 mm Hg, pulse 70/min, respirations 26/min
- Lungs: bilateral coarse crackles in the bases
- Heart: S_3 gallop at apex

Diagnostic Studies
- Continuous ECG monitoring

- Echocardiogram: severe left ventricular dysfunction with ejection fraction of 25%
- Serum potassium: 2.9 mEq/L (2.9 mmol/L)
- Serum cardiac markers: negative
- Serum b-type natriuretic peptide (BNP): 1852 pg/mL

Collaborative Care
- Amiodarone (Cordarone) infusion
- Scheduled for electrophysiologic study (EPS)

Discussion Questions
1. Why is J.M. at risk for sudden cardiac death?
2. Explain the rationale for using amiodarone after cardiac arrest.
3. What methods are used to assess the effectiveness of the antidysrhythmia therapy?
4. Interpret the rhythm strip and explain the significance of the other diagnostic studies.
5. Why would J.M. be a candidate for CRT and an ICD?
6. *Priority Decision:* Based on the assessment data provided, what are the priority nursing diagnoses?
7. *Priority Decision:* Based on these nursing diagnoses, what are the priority nursing interventions for J.M.?
8. *Delegation Decision:* Which tasks could be delegated to unlicensed assistive personnel (UAP)?
9. *Evidence-Based Practice*: Once J.M. is stable, he is scheduled for the insertion of a CRT/ICD. On your rounds, he asks you why he needs two devices.

⊜volve Answers available at *http://evolve.elsevier.com/Lewis/medsurg.*

▌ BRIDGE TO NCLEX EXAMINATION

The number of the question corresponds to the same-numbered outcome at the beginning of the chapter.

1. A patient admitted with ACS has continuous ECG monitoring. An examination of the rhythm strip reveals the following characteristics: atrial rate 74 beats/min and regular; ventricular rate 62 beats/min and irregular; P wave normal shape; PR interval lengthens progressively until a P wave is not conducted; QRS normal shape. The priority nursing intervention would be to
   a. perform synchronized cardioversion.
   b. administer epinephrine 1 mg IV push.
   c. observe for symptoms of hypotension or angina.
   d. apply transcutaneous pacemaker pads on the patient.

2. The nurse is monitoring the ECG of a patient admitted with ACS. Which ECG characteristics would be most suggestive of myocardial ischemia?
   a. Sinus rhythm with a pathologic Q wave
   b. Sinus rhythm with an elevated ST segment
   c. Sinus rhythm with a depressed ST segment
   d. Sinus rhythm with premature atrial contractions

3. The ECG monitor of a patient in the cardiac care unit after an MI indicates ventricular bigeminy with a rate of 50 beats/min. The nurse would anticipate
   a. performing defibrillation.
   b. treating with IV amiodarone.
   c. inserting a temporary transvenous pacemaker.
   d. assessing the patient's response to the dysrhythmia.

4. The nurse prepares a patient for synchronized cardioversion knowing that cardioversion differs from defibrillation in that
   a. defibrillation requires a lower dose of electrical energy.
   b. cardioversion is indicated to treat atrial bradydysrhythmias.
   c. defibrillation is synchronized to deliver a shock during the QRS complex.
   d. patients should be sedated if cardioversion is done on a non-emergency basis.

5. Which patient teaching points should the nurse include when providing discharge instructions to a patient with a new permanent pacemaker and the caregiver (select all that apply)?
   a. Avoid or limit air travel.
   b. Take and record a daily pulse rate.
   c. Obtain and wear a Medic Alert ID or bracelet at all times.
   d. Avoid lifting arm on the side of the pacemaker above shoulder.
   e. Avoid microwave ovens because they interfere with pacemaker function.

6. Important teaching for the patient scheduled for a radiofrequency catheter ablation procedure includes explaining that
   a. ventricular bradycardia may be induced and treated during the procedure.
   b. a catheter will be placed in both femoral arteries to allow double-catheter use.
   c. the procedure will destroy areas of the conduction system that are causing rapid heart rhythms.
   d. a general anesthetic will be given to prevent the awareness of any "sudden cardiac death" experiences.

1. c, 2. c, 3. d, 4. d, 5. b, c, d, 6. c

⊜volve

For rationales to these answers and even more NCLEX review questions, visit *http://evolve.elsevier.com/Lewis/medsurg*.

REFERENCES

1. Wesley K: *Huszar's basic dysrhythmias and acute coronary syndrome*, ed 4, St Louis, 2011, Mosby Jems.
2. Patton KT, Thibodeau GA, Douglas MM: *Essentials of anatomy and physiology*, St Louis, 2012, Mosby.
*3. American Association of Critical-Care Nurses: AACN practice alert: ST segment monitoring. Retrieved from *www.aacn.org/wd/practice/content/st-segment-practice-alert.pcms?menu=practice*.
*4. American Association of Critical-Care Nurses: AACN practice alert: dysrhythmia monitoring. Retrieved from *www.aacn.org/wd/practice/content/dysrhythmia-monitoring-practice-alert.pcms?menu=practice*.
5. Lehne RA: *Pharmacology for nursing care*, ed 7, St Louis, 2010, Mosby.
6. Sinz E, Navarro K, Soderberg ES, editors: *Advanced cardiovascular life support: provider manual*, Dallas, 2011, American Heart Association.
7. Carlson KK: *Advanced critical care nursing*, St Louis, 2009, Saunders.
8. American Association of Critical-Care Nurses: *Core curriculum for progressive care nurses*, St Louis, 2010, Saunders.
*9. Wann LS, Curtis AB, January CT, et al: 2011 ACCF/AHA/HRS focused update on the management of patients with atrial fibrillation (updating the 2006 guideline): a report of the American College of Cardiology Foundation/American Heart Association task force on practice guidelines, *J Am Coll Cardiol* 57:223, 2011.

10. Go AS, Mozaffarian D, Roger VL, et al: Heart disease and stroke statistics—2013 update: a report from the American Heart Association, *Circulation* 127:e6, 2013.
*11. Tracy CM, Epstein AE, Darbar D, et al: 2012 ACCF/AHA/HRS focused update of the 2008 guidelines for device-based therapy of cardiac rhythm abnormalities: a report of the American College of Cardiology Foundation/American Heart Association Task Force on Practice Guidelines, *Circulation* 126:1784, 2012.
12. Dunbar SB, Dougherty CM, Sears SF, et al: Educational and psychological interventions to improve outcomes for recipients of implantable cardioverter defibrillators and their families: a scientific statement from the American Heart Association, *Circulation* 126:2146, 2012.
13. Barold SS, Stroobandt RX, Sinnaeve AF: *Cardiac pacemakers and resynchronization step-by-step*, ed 2, Hoboken, NJ, 2010, Wiley-Blackwell.
*14. McAlister FA, Ezekowitz J, Dryden DM, et al: Cardiac resynchronization therapy and implantable cardiac defibrillators in left ventricular systolic dysfunction, AHRQ Pub No 07-E009. Retrieved from *www.ahrq.gov/downloads/pub/evidence/pdf/defib/defib.pdf*. (Classic)
15. Cleveland Clinic: Syncope care and treatment. Retrieved from *http://my.clevelandclinic.org/heart/disorders/electric/syncope.aspx*.

RESOURCES

Additional resources for this chapter are listed after Chapter 34 on p. 765 and Chapter 35 on p. 786.

*Evidence-based information for clinical practice.

*One of the hardest things is having words in
your heart that you can't utter.*
James Earl Jones

Nursing Management
Inflammatory and Structural Heart Disorders

Nancy Kupper and De Ann F. Mitchell

⊖volve WEBSITE

http://evolve.elsevier.com/Lewis/medsurg

- NCLEX Review Questions
- Key Points
- Pre-Test
- Answer Guidelines for Case Study on p. 830
- Rationales for Bridge to NCLEX Examination Questions
- Case Study
  - Patient With Rheumatic Fever and Heart Disease

- Nursing Care Plans (Customizable)
  - eNCP 37-1: Patient With Infective Endocarditis
  - eNCP 37-2: Patient With Valvular Heart Disease
- Concept Map Creator
- Glossary
- Content Updates

- Audio
  - Pericardial Friction Rub

eFigures
- eFig. 37-1: Mitral stenosis and vegetation
- eFig. 37-2: Mitral stenosis with classic "fish mouth" orifice
- eFig. 37-3: Types of cardiomyopathy

LEARNING OUTCOMES

1. Differentiate the etiology, pathophysiology, and clinical manifestations of infective endocarditis and pericarditis.
2. Describe the collaborative care and nursing management of the patient with infective endocarditis and pericarditis.
3. Describe the etiology, pathophysiology, and clinical manifestations of myocarditis.
4. Describe the collaborative care and nursing management of the patient with myocarditis.
5. Differentiate the etiology, pathophysiology, and clinical manifestations of rheumatic fever and rheumatic heart disease.
6. Describe the collaborative care and nursing management of the patient with rheumatic fever and rheumatic heart disease.
7. Relate the pathophysiology to the clinical manifestations and diagnostic studies for the various types of valvular heart disease.
8. Describe the collaborative care and nursing management of the patient with valvular heart disease.
9. Relate the pathophysiology to the clinical manifestations and diagnostic studies for the different types of cardiomyopathy.
10. Compare the nursing and collaborative management of patients with different types of cardiomyopathy.

KEY TERMS

aortic regurgitation (AR), p. 823
aortic stenosis (AS), p. 822
cardiac tamponade, p. 815
cardiomyopathy (CMP), p. 826
chronic constrictive pericarditis, p. 817
dilated cardiomyopathy, p. 827

hypertrophic cardiomyopathy, p. 828
infective endocarditis (IE), p. 811
mitral valve prolapse (MVP), p. 822
myocarditis, p. 817
pericardiocentesis, p. 816

pericarditis, p. 814
regurgitation, p. 821
rheumatic fever (RF), p. 818
rheumatic heart disease, p. 818
stenosis, p. 821

Reviewed by Katrina Allen, RN, MSN, CCRN, Nursing Instructor, Faulkner State Community College: Division of Nursing, Fairhope and Bay Minette, Alabama; Tracy H. Knoll, RN, MSN, Nursing Instructor, Chamberlain College of Nursing, St. Louis, Missouri; and Tammy Ann Ramon, RN, MSN, Nursing Instructor, Delta College, University Center, Michigan.

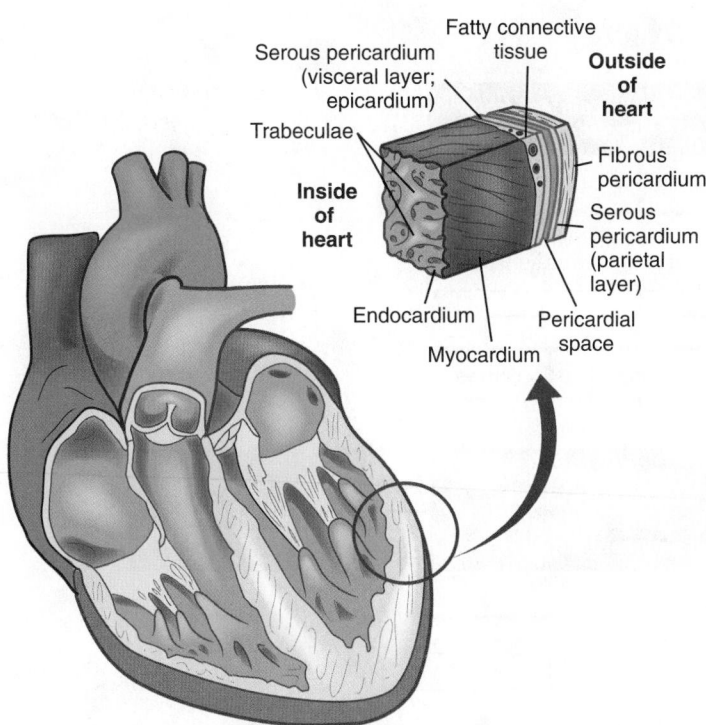

FIG. 37-1 Layers of the heart muscle and pericardium. The section of the heart wall shows the fibrous pericardium, the parietal and visceral layers of the serous pericardium (with the pericardial sac between them), the myocardium, and the endocardium.

FIG. 37-2 Bacterial endocarditis of the mitral valve. The valve is covered with large, irregular vegetations *(arrow)*.

TABLE 37-1	RISK FACTORS FOR ENDOCARDITIS*

Cardiac Conditions
- Prior endocarditis
- Prosthetic heart valves
- Acquired valve disease (e.g., mitral valve prolapse with regurgitation, calcified aortic stenosis)
- Cardiac lesions (e.g., ventricular septal defect, asymmetric septal hypertrophy)
- Rheumatic heart disease (e.g., mitral valve regurgitation)
- Congenital heart disease
- Pacemakers
- Marfan's syndrome
- Cardiomyopathy

Noncardiac Conditions
- Hospital-acquired bacteremia
- IV drug abuse

Procedure-Associated Risks
- Intravascular devices (e.g., pulmonary artery catheters)
- Procedures listed in Table 37-2

*List is not all-inclusive.

This chapter describes the pathophysiology and management of patients experiencing select inflammatory and structural heart disorders. In addition, the nursing care required to manage the needs of these patients is presented.

INFLAMMATORY DISORDERS OF HEART

INFECTIVE ENDOCARDITIS

Infective endocarditis (IE) is an infection of the endocardial layer of the heart. The *endocardium* is the innermost layer of the heart (Fig. 37-1) and heart valves. Therefore IE affects the valves. Treatment of IE with antibiotic therapy has improved the prognosis of this disease. Though relatively uncommon, an estimated 10,000 to 15,000 new cases of IE are diagnosed in the United States each year.[1]

Classification

IE can be classified as subacute or acute. The *subacute form* typically affects those with preexisting valve disease and has a clinical course that may extend over months. In contrast, the *acute form* typically affects those with healthy valves and manifests as a rapidly progressive illness. IE can also be classified based on the cause (e.g., IV drug abuse IE [IVDA IE], fungal endocarditis) or site of involvement (e.g., prosthetic valve endocarditis [PVE]).

Etiology and Pathophysiology

The most common causative organisms of IE, *Staphylococcus aureus* and *Streptococcus viridans*, are bacterial. Other possible pathogens include fungi and viruses.[2] IE occurs when blood turbulence within the heart allows the causative organism to infect previously damaged valves or other endothelial surfaces. This can occur in individuals with a variety of underlying cardiac and noncardiac conditions (Table 37-1).

Vegetations, the primary lesions of IE, consist of fibrin, leukocytes, platelets, and microbes that stick to the valve surface or endocardium (Fig. 37-2). The loss of parts of these fragile vegetations into the circulation results in *emboli.* As many as 50% of patients with IE experience systemic embolization. This occurs from left-sided heart vegetation moving to various organs (e.g., brain, kidneys, spleen) and to the extremities, causing limb infarction. Right-sided heart lesions move to the lungs, resulting in pulmonary emboli.

The infection may spread locally and damage the valves or their supporting structures. This causes dysrhythmias, valve dysfunction, and eventual invasion of the myocardium, leading to heart failure (HF), sepsis, and heart block (Fig. 37-3).

At one time rheumatic heart disease was the most common cause of IE. However, now it accounts for less than 20% of cases. The main contributing factors to IE include (1) aging (more than 50% of older people have aortic stenosis [AS]), (2) IVDA, (3) use of prosthetic valves, (4) use of intravascular devices resulting in health care–associated infections (e.g., methicillin-resistant *S. aureus* [MRSA]), and (5) renal dialysis.[3]

PATHOPHYSIOLOGY MAP

FIG. 37-3 Pathogenesis of infective endocarditis.

Clinical Manifestations

The clinical manifestations of IE are nonspecific and can involve multiple organ systems. Low-grade fever occurs in more than 90% of patients. Other nonspecific manifestations include chills, weakness, malaise, fatigue, and anorexia. Arthralgias, myalgias, back pain, abdominal discomfort, weight loss, headache, and clubbing of fingers may occur in subacute forms of endocarditis.

Vascular manifestations of IE include *splinter hemorrhages* (black longitudinal streaks) that may occur in the nail beds. Petechiae may result from fragmentation and microemboliza- tion of vegetative lesions. They can occur in the conjunctivae, lips, buccal mucosa, and palate and over the ankles, feet, and antecubital and popliteal areas. *Osler's nodes* (painful, tender, red or purple, pea-size lesions) may be found on the fingertips or toes. *Janeway's lesions* (flat, painless, small, red spots) may be seen on the palms and soles. Funduscopic examination may reveal hemorrhagic retinal lesions called *Roth's spots.*

The onset of a new or changing murmur is noted in most patients with IE. The aortic and mitral valves are most often affected. Murmurs are usually absent in tricuspid endocarditis because right-sided heart sounds are too low to be heard. HF occurs in up to 80% of patients with aortic valve endocar- ditis and in approximately 50% of patients with mitral valve endocarditis.[4]

Clinical manifestations secondary to embolization may be present in various body organs. Embolization to the spleen may cause sharp, left upper quadrant pain and splenomegaly, local tenderness, and abdominal rigidity. Embolization to the kidneys may cause flank pain, hematuria, and renal failure. Emboli may lodge in small peripheral blood vessels of the arms and legs and may cause ischemia and gangrene. Embolization to the brain may cause neurologic damage resulting in hemiplegia, ataxia, aphasia, visual changes, and change in the level of conscious- ness. Pulmonary emboli may occur in right-sided endocarditis and cause dyspnea, chest pain, hemoptysis, and respiratory arrest.

Diagnostic Studies

The patient's recent health history is important in assessing IE. Ask patients if they have had any recent (within the past 3 to 6 months) dental, urologic, surgical, or gynecologic procedures, including normal or abnormal obstetric delivery. Document any previous history of IVDA, heart disease, recent cardiac catheterization, cardiac surgery, intravascular device placement, renal dialysis, or infections (e.g., skin, respiratory, urinary tract).

Two blood cultures drawn 30 minutes apart from two differ- ent sites will be positive in more than 90% of patients. Culture- negative endocarditis is often associated with antibiotic usage within the previous 2 weeks, or results from a pathogen not easily detected by standard culture procedures. Negative cul- tures should be kept for 3 weeks if the clinical diagnosis remains endocarditis because of the possibility of slow-growing organ- isms. A mild leukocytosis occurs in acute IE (uncommon in subacute). The erythrocyte sedimentation rate (ESR) and C-reactive protein (CRP) levels may also be elevated.

Major criteria to diagnose IE include at least two of the following: positive blood cultures, new or changed heart murmur, or intracardiac mass or vegetation noted on echocardiography.[5] Echocardiography is valuable in the diagnostic workup for a patient with IE when the blood cultures are negative, or for the patient who is a surgical candidate and has an active infection. Transesophageal echocardiogram and two- or three-dimensional (2-D or 3-D) transthoracic echocardiograms can detect vegetations on the heart valves.[6]

A chest x-ray is done to detect *cardiomegaly* (an enlarged heart). An electrocardiogram (ECG) may show first- or second-degree atrioventricular (AV) block. Heart block occurs because the cardiac valves lie close to conductive tissue, especially the AV node. Cardiac catheterization may be used to evaluate valve functioning and to assess the coronary arteries when surgical intervention is being considered.[7]

Collaborative Care

Prophylactic Treatment. The situations and conditions requiring antibiotic prophylaxis are presented in Table 37-2.

Drug Therapy. Accurate identification of the infecting organism is the key to successful treatment of IE. Long-term treatment is necessary to kill dormant bacteria within the valvular vegetations. Complete elimination of the organism generally takes weeks, and relapses are common.

Initially, patients are hospitalized and IV antibiotic therapy, based on blood cultures, is started. The effectiveness of therapy is assessed with subsequent blood cultures. Cultures that remain positive indicate inadequate or inappropriate selection of antibiotic, aortic root or myocardial abscess, or the wrong diagnosis (e.g., an infection elsewhere).

Fungal endocarditis and PVE respond poorly to antibiotic therapy alone. Early valve replacement followed by prolonged (6 weeks or more) antibiotics is recommended in these situations. Valve replacement (discussed later in this chapter) has become an important adjunct procedure in the management of IE.

Fever may persist for several days after treatment has been started and can be treated with aspirin, acetaminophen (Tylenol), ibuprofen (Motrin), fluids, and rest. Complete bed rest is usually not indicated unless the temperature remains elevated or there are signs of HF. Endocarditis coupled with HF responds poorly to drug therapy and valve replacement and is often life threatening.

NURSING MANAGEMENT INFECTIVE ENDOCARDITIS

NURSING ASSESSMENT

Subjective and objective data that you should obtain from a patient with IE are presented in Table 37-3. Assess vital signs together with heart sounds to detect a murmur, a change in a preexisting murmur, and extra sounds (e.g., S_3).

Arthralgia, which is common in IE, may involve multiple joints and be accompanied by myalgias. Assess the patient for joint tenderness, decreased range of motion (ROM), and muscle tenderness. Examine the patient for petechiae, splinter hemorrhages, and Osler's nodes. Complete a general systems assessment to determine any hemodynamic or embolic complications.

NURSING DIAGNOSES

Nursing diagnoses for the patient with IE may include, but are not limited to, the following:
- Decreased cardiac output *related to* altered heart rhythm, valvular insufficiency, and fluid overload
- Activity intolerance *related to* generalized weakness, arthralgia, and alteration in oxygen transport secondary to valvular dysfunction

Additional information on nursing diagnoses is presented in eNursing Care Plan 37-1 available on the website for this chapter.

PLANNING

The overall goals for the patient with IE include (1) normal or baseline heart function, (2) performance of activities of daily living (ADLs) without fatigue, and (3) knowledge of the therapeutic regimen to prevent recurrence of endocarditis.

NURSING IMPLEMENTATION

HEALTH PROMOTION. The incidence of IE can be decreased by identifying individuals who are at risk for the disease (see Tables 37-1 and 37-2). Assessment of the patient's history and an understanding of the disease process are crucial for planning and implementing appropriate health promotion strategies.

Teaching the patient at high risk for IE helps reduce the incidence and recurrence of the disease. Teaching is crucial for the patient's understanding of and adherence to the treatment

TABLE 37-2   ANTIBIOTIC PROPHYLAXIS TO PREVENT ENDOCARDITIS

Target Groups for Prophylactic Antibiotics
People with the following heart conditions should receive prophylactic antibiotics when they have the conditions or procedures listed below.
- Prosthetic heart valve or prosthetic material used to repair heart valve
- Previous history of infectious endocarditis
- Congenital heart disease (CHD)*
  - Unrepaired cyanotic CHD (including palliative shunts and conduits)
  - Repaired congenital heart defect with prosthetic material or device for 6 mo after the procedure
  - Repaired CHD with residual defects at the site or adjacent to the site of prosthetic patch or prosthetic device
- Cardiac transplantation recipients who develop heart valve disease

Conditions or Procedures Requiring Antibiotic Prophylaxis
When the target groups have the following conditions or procedures, they need prophylactic antibiotics.
- Oral
  - Dental manipulation involving the gums or roots of the teeth
  - Dental manipulation involving puncture of the oral mucosa
  - Dental extractions or implants
  - Prophylactic teeth cleaning with expected bleeding
- Respiratory
  - Respiratory tract incisions (e.g., biopsy)
  - Tonsillectomy and adenoidectomy
- Gastrointestinal and genitourinary
  - Wound infection
  - Urinary tract infection

*Except for the conditions listed above, prophylaxis is no longer recommended for any form of CHD.
Source: Habib G, Hoen B, Tornos P, et al: Guidelines on the prevention, diagnosis and treatment of infective endocarditis (new version 2009): the Task Force on the Prevention, Diagnosis, and Treatment of Infective Endocarditis of the European Society of Cardiology (ESC), *Eur Heart J* 30:2369, 2009.

TABLE 37-3   NURSING ASSESSMENT

Infective Endocarditis

Subjective Data
Important Health Information
Past health history: Valvular, congenital, or syphilitic cardiac disease, including valve repair or replacement; previous endocarditis, childbirth, staphylococcal or streptococcal infections, hospital-acquired bacteremia
Medications: Immunosuppressive therapy
Surgery or other treatments: Recent obstetric or gynecologic procedures; invasive techniques, including catheterization, cystoscopy, intravascular procedures; recent dental or surgical procedures; GI procedures (e.g., endoscopy)

Functional Health Patterns
Health perception–health management: IV drug abuse, alcohol abuse; malaise
Nutritional-metabolic: Weight gain or loss; anorexia; chills, diaphoresis
Elimination: Bloody urine
Activity-exercise: Exercise intolerance, generalized weakness, fatigue; cough, dyspnea on exertion, orthopnea; palpitations
Sleep-rest: Night sweats
Cognitive-perceptual: Chest, back, or abdominal pain; headache; joint tenderness, muscle tenderness

Objective Data
General
Fever

Integumentary
Osler's nodes on extremities; splinter hemorrhages under nail beds; Janeway's lesions on palms and soles; petechiae of skin, mucous membranes, or conjunctivae; purpura; peripheral edema, finger clubbing

Respiratory
Tachypnea, crackles

Cardiovascular
Dysrhythmia, tachycardia, new murmurs, S_3, S_4; retinal hemorrhages

Possible Diagnostic Findings
Leukocytosis, anemia, ↑ ESR, ↑ CRP and cardiac enzymes; positive blood cultures; hematuria; echocardiogram showing chamber enlargement, valvular dysfunction, and vegetations; chest x-ray showing cardiomegaly and pulmonary infiltrates; ECG demonstrating ischemia and conduction defects; signs of systemic embolization or pulmonary embolism

CRP, C-reactive protein; *ESR,* erythrocyte sedimentation rate.

regimen. Tell the patient to avoid people with infection, especially upper respiratory tract infection, and to report cold, flu, and cough symptoms. Stress the importance of avoiding excessive fatigue and the need to plan rest periods before and after activity. Good oral hygiene, including daily care and regular dental visits, is also important. Instruct the patient to inform health care providers performing certain invasive procedures of the history of IE. Be certain the patient understands the importance of prophylactic antibiotic therapy before certain invasive procedures. Refer the patient with a history of IVDA for drug rehabilitation.

AMBULATORY AND HOME CARE. A patient with IE has many problems that require nursing management (see eNursing Care Plan 37-1 on the website for this chapter). IE generally requires treatment with antibiotics for 4 to 6 weeks. After initial treat-

ment in the hospital, the patient may continue treatment at home if hemodynamically stable and adherent. Assess the home setting for adequate support. Patients who receive outpatient IV antibiotics require vigilant home nursing care.

Assessment findings are often nonspecific (see Table 37-3) but can help with the treatment plan. Fever, chronic or intermittent, is a common early sign. Instruct the patient or caregiver about the importance of monitoring body temperature. Persistent temperature elevations may mean that the drug therapy is ineffective. Patients with IE are at risk for life-threatening complications, such as stroke, pulmonary edema, and HF. Teach patients and caregivers to recognize signs and symptoms of these complications (e.g., change in mental status, dyspnea, chest pain, unexplained weight gain).

The patient with IE needs adequate periods of physical and emotional rest. Bed rest may be necessary when the patient has fever or complications (e.g., heart damage). Otherwise the patient may ambulate and perform moderate activity. To prevent problems related to reduced mobility, tell the patient to wear elastic compression stockings, perform ROM exercises, and deep breathe and cough every 2 hours.

The patient may experience anxiety and fear associated with the illness. You must recognize this and implement strategies to help the patient cope with the illness.

Monitor laboratory data to determine the effectiveness of the antibiotic therapy. Ongoing monitoring of the patient's blood cultures is necessary to ensure destruction of the infecting organism. Assess IV lines for patency and signs of complications (e.g., phlebitis). Administer antibiotics as scheduled, and monitor the patient for any adverse drug reactions.

Management also focuses on teaching the patient and caregiver the nature of the disease and on reducing the risk of reinfection. Explain to the patient the relationship of follow-up care, good nutrition, and early treatment of common infections (e.g., colds) to maintain health. Instruct the patient about symptoms that may indicate recurrent infection (e.g., fever, fatigue, chills). Tell the patient to notify the health care provider if any of these symptoms occur. Finally, inform the patient about the importance of prophylactic antibiotic therapy before certain invasive procedures (see Table 37-2).

▌EVALUATION
The expected outcomes are that the patient with IE will
- Maintain adequate tissue and organ perfusion
- Maintain normal body temperature
- Report an increase in physical and emotional comfort

Additional information on expected outcomes for the patient with IE are presented in eNursing Care Plan 37-1 on the website for this chapter.

ACUTE PERICARDITIS

Pericarditis is a condition caused by inflammation of the pericardial sac (the pericardium). The pericardium is composed of the inner serous membrane (visceral pericardium) and the outer fibrous (parietal) layer (see Fig. 37-1). The pericardial space is the cavity between these two layers. Normally it contains 10 to 15 mL of serous fluid. The pericardium serves an anchoring function, provides lubrication to decrease friction during systolic and diastolic heart movements, and assists in preventing excessive dilation of the heart during diastole. It may be congenitally absent or surgically removed.

TABLE 37-4	COMMON CAUSES OF PERICARDITIS

Infectious
- Viral: Coxsackie A and B virus, echovirus, adenovirus, mumps, hepatitis, Epstein-Barr, varicella zoster, human immunodeficiency virus
- Bacterial: Pneumococci, staphylococci, streptococci, *Neisseria gonorrhoeae, Legionella pneumophila, Mycobacterium tuberculosis,* septicemia from gram-negative organisms
- Fungal: *Histoplasma, Candida* species
- Others: Toxoplasmosis, Lyme disease

Noninfectious
- Uremia
- Acute myocardial infarction
- Neoplasms: Lung cancer, breast cancer, leukemia, Hodgkin's lymphoma, non-Hodgkin's lymphoma
- Trauma: Thoracic surgery, pacemaker insertion, cardiac diagnostic procedures
- Radiation
- Dissecting aortic aneurysm
- Myxedema

Hypersensitive or Autoimmune
- Dressler syndrome
- Postpericardiotomy syndrome
- Rheumatic fever
- Drug reactions (e.g., procainamide [Pronestyl], hydralazine [Apresoline])
- Rheumatologic diseases: Rheumatoid arthritis, systemic lupus erythematosus, systemic sclerosis (scleroderma), ankylosing spondylitis

FIG. 37-4 Acute pericarditis. Note shaggy coat of fibers covering surface of heart.

Etiology and Pathophysiology

Common causes of acute pericarditis are listed in Table 37-4. Most often the cause of acute pericarditis is *idiopathic* (unknown), with a variety of suspected viral causes. The coxsackie B virus is the most commonly identified virus.[8]

Pericarditis in the patient with an MI may be described as two distinct syndromes. The first is *acute pericarditis,* which may occur within the initial 48 to 72 hours after an MI. The second is *Dressler syndrome* (late pericarditis), which appears 4 to 6 weeks after an MI (see Chapter 34). An inflammatory response is the characteristic pathologic finding in acute pericarditis. There is an influx of neutrophils, increased pericardial vascularity, and eventually fibrin deposition on the epicardium (Fig. 37-4).

Clinical Manifestations

In acute pericarditis, clinical manifestations include progressive, frequently severe, sharp chest pain. The pain is generally worse with deep inspiration and when lying supine. It is relieved by sitting up and leaning forward. The pain may radiate to the neck, arms, or left shoulder, making it difficult to differentiate from angina. One distinction is that the pain from pericarditis can be referred to the trapezius muscle (shoulder, upper back), since the phrenic nerve innervates this region. The dyspnea that accompanies acute pericarditis is related to the patient's need to breathe in rapid, shallow breaths to avoid chest pain and may be aggravated by fever and anxiety.

The hallmark finding in acute pericarditis is the *pericardial friction rub.* The rub is a scratching, grating, high-pitched sound believed to result from friction between the roughened pericar-dial and epicardial surfaces. It is best heard with the stethoscope placed at the lower left sternal border of the chest with the patient leaning forward. Since it is difficult to distinguish a pericardial friction rub from a pleural friction rub, ask the patient to hold his or her breath. If you still hear the rub, then it is cardiac. It may require frequent attempts to identify because pericardial friction rubs are often intermittent and short lived.

Complications

Two major complications that may result from acute pericarditis are pericardial effusion and cardiac tamponade. *Pericardial effusion* is a build-up of fluid in the pericardium. It can occur rapidly (e.g., chest trauma) or slowly (e.g., tuberculosis pericarditis). Large effusions may compress nearby structures. Pulmonary tissue compression can cause cough, dyspnea, and tachypnea. Phrenic nerve compression can induce hiccups, and compression of the laryngeal nerve may result in hoarseness. Heart sounds are generally distant and muffled, although blood pressure (BP) usually is maintained.

Cardiac tamponade develops as the pericardial effusion increases in volume. This results in compression of the heart. The speed of fluid accumulation affects the severity of clinical manifestations. Cardiac tamponade can occur acutely (e.g., rupture of heart, trauma) or subacutely (e.g., secondary to renal failure, malignancy).

The patient with cardiac tamponade may report chest pain and is often confused, anxious, and restless. As the compression of the heart increases, there is decreased cardiac output (CO), muffled heart sounds, and narrowed pulse pressure. The patient develops tachypnea and tachycardia. Neck veins usually are markedly distended because of increased jugular venous pressure, and pulsus paradoxus is present. *Pulsus paradoxus* is a decrease in systolic BP during inspiration that is exaggerated in cardiac tamponade. (See Table 37-5 for the measurement technique.) In a patient with a slow onset of a cardiac tamponade, dyspnea may be the only clinical manifestation.

Diagnostic Studies

The ECG is useful in the diagnosis of acute pericarditis, with changes noted in approximately 90% of the cases. The most

FIG. 37-5 A, X-ray of a normal chest. **B,** Pericardial effusion is present, and the cardiac silhouette is enlarged with a globular shape *(arrows).*

TABLE 37-5	MEASUREMENT OF PULSUS PARADOXUS

1. Position the patient in a semirecumbent position.
2. Instruct patient to breathe normally.*
2. Using a manually operated blood pressure (BP) cuff, determine systolic BP.
3. Inflate BP cuff at least 20 mm Hg above systolic BP.
4. Deflate cuff slowly until you hear the first Korotkoff sound during expiration, and note the pressure.
5. Continue to slowly deflate cuff until you hear sounds throughout the respiratory cycle (inspiration and expiration), and note the pressure.
6. Determine the difference between the measurements taken in steps 4 and 5. This will equal the amount of paradox:

Sounds heard on expiration at	110 mm Hg
Sounds heard throughout cycle at	– 82 mm Hg
Amount of paradox	28 mm Hg

The difference is normally <10 mm Hg. If the difference is >10 mm Hg, cardiac tamponade may be present.

*Ask the patient to breathe slowly and deeply to reveal this finding when pulsus paradoxus is not severe.

TABLE 37-6	COLLABORATIVE CARE

Acute Pericarditis

Diagnostic
- History and physical examination: pericardial friction rub, pulsus paradoxus
- Laboratory: CRP, ESR, white blood cell count
- Electrocardiogram
- Chest x-ray
- Echocardiogram
- Computed tomography
- Magnetic resonance imaging
- Pericardiocentesis, pericardial window
- Pericardial biopsy

Collaborative Therapy
- Treatment of underlying disease
- Bed rest
- Nonsteroidal antiinflammatory drugs
- Corticosteroids
- Pericardiocentesis (for tamponade)
- Pericardial window (for tamponade or ongoing pericardial effusion)

CRP, C-reactive protein; *ESR,* erythrocyte sedimentation rate.

sensitive ECG changes include diffuse (widespread) ST segment elevations. This reflects the abnormal repolarization that develops secondary to the pericardial inflammation. You need to differentiate these changes from the ST changes seen with MI. (See Chapter 36 for more information on ECG monitoring.)

Echocardiographic findings are most useful in determining the presence of a pericardial effusion or cardiac tamponade. Methods such as Doppler imaging and color M-mode assess diastolic function and diagnose constrictive pericarditis (discussed later in the chapter). Computed tomography (CT) and magnetic resonance imaging (MRI) provide for visualization of the pericardium and pericardial space. Chest x-ray findings are generally normal, but cardiomegaly may be seen in a patient who has a large pericardial effusion (Fig. 37-5).

Common laboratory findings include leukocytosis and elevation of CRP and ESR. Troponin levels may be elevated in patients with ST segment elevation and acute pericarditis, which could indicate concurrent myocardial damage. The fluid obtained during pericardiocentesis or the tissue from a pericardial biopsy may be studied to determine the cause of the pericarditis.

Collaborative Care

Management of acute pericarditis is aimed at identifying and treating the underlying problem and symptoms (Table 37-6). Antibiotics treat bacterial pericarditis, and nonsteroidal antiinflammatory drugs (NSAIDs) (e.g., salicylates [aspirin], ibuprofen) control the pain and inflammation. Corticosteroids are generally reserved for patients with pericarditis secondary to systemic lupus erythematosus, patients already taking corticosteroids for rheumatologic or other autoimmune conditions, or patients who do not respond to NSAIDs. They are used cautiously because of their numerous side effects (see Chapter 50). Colchicine (Colsalide), an antiinflammatory drug used for gout, can be used for patients who have recurrent pericarditis.[9]

Pericardiocentesis is usually performed for pericardial effusion with acute cardiac tamponade, purulent pericarditis, and suspected neoplasm. Hemodynamic support for the patient being prepared for the pericardiocentesis may include administration of volume expanders and inotropic agents (e.g., dopamine [Intropin]) and the discontinuation of any anticoagulants. The procedure is performed rapidly and safely using a percutaneous approach that is guided by echocardiography (Fig. 37-6). A needle is inserted into the pericardial space to remove fluid for analysis and to relieve cardiac pressure. Complications from pericardiocentesis include dysrhythmias, further cardiac tam-

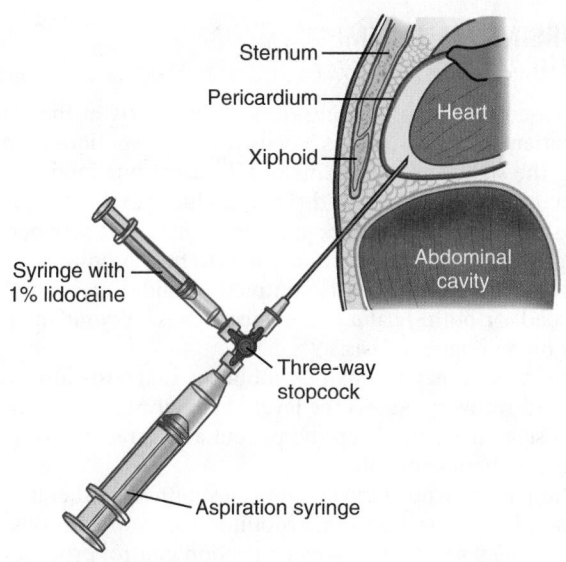

FIG. 37-6 Pericardiocentesis performed under sterile conditions in conjunction with electrocardiogram (ECG) and hemodynamic measurements.

ponade, pneumomediastinum, pneumothorax, myocardial laceration, and coronary artery laceration.

A *pericardial window* can be used for diagnosis or for drainage of excess fluid. It involves cutting a "window" or portion of the pericardium. This allows the fluid to drain continuously into the peritoneum or chest.

NURSING MANAGEMENT
ACUTE PERICARDITIS

The management of the patient's pain and anxiety during acute pericarditis is your primary nursing consideration. Assess the pain to distinguish the pain of myocardial ischemia (angina) from the pain of pericarditis (see Table 34-7). Pericarditic pain is usually located in the precordium or left trapezius region and has a sharp, pleuritic quality that increases with inspiration. Pain is often relieved when the patient sits up or leans forward, and is worse when lying supine. The ECG can aid in distinguishing these types of pain. In acute pericarditis there are diffuse ST segment elevations. In myocardial ischemia there are usually localized ST segment changes. In addition, in acute pericarditis serial ECGs do not show evolving changes like those with MI.

Pain relief measures include keeping the patient on bed rest with the head of the bed elevated to 45 degrees and providing an overbed table for support. Antiinflammatory medications can help control the pain. However, because of the risk of gastrointestinal (GI) bleeding, administer these drugs with food or milk and instruct the patient to avoid alcohol. Other medications, such as a proton pump inhibitor (e.g., pantoprazole [Protonix]), may be ordered to decrease stomach acid.

Anxiety-reducing measures for the patient with acute pericarditis include providing simple, complete explanations of all procedures and possible causes of the pain. These explanations are particularly important for the patient whose diagnosis of acute pericarditis is being established and for the patient who has previously experienced angina or an acute MI.

The patient with acute pericarditis is at risk for cardiac tamponade and decreased CO. Monitor for the signs and symptoms of tamponade and prepare for possible pericardiocentesis.

CHRONIC CONSTRICTIVE PERICARDITIS
Etiology and Pathophysiology

Chronic constrictive pericarditis results from scarring with consequent loss of elasticity of the pericardial sac. It usually begins with an initial episode of acute pericarditis and is characterized by fibrin deposition with a clinically undetected pericardial effusion. Reabsorption of the effusion slowly follows, with progression toward the chronic stage. This involves fibrous scarring, thickening of the pericardium from calcium deposition, and eventual destruction of the pericardial space. The fibrotic, thickened, and adherent pericardium encases the heart, thereby impairing the ability of the atria and ventricles to stretch adequately.

Clinical Manifestations and Diagnostic Studies

Manifestations of chronic constrictive pericarditis occur over time and mimic those of HF and cor pulmonale. Decreased CO accounts for many of the clinical manifestations, including dyspnea on exertion, peripheral edema, ascites, fatigue, anorexia, and weight loss. The most prominent finding on physical examination is jugular venous distention (JVD). Unlike with cardiac tamponade, the presence of pulsus paradoxus (greater than 10 mm Hg) is not common.

ECG changes are often nonspecific in chronic constrictive pericarditis. The heart on the chest x-ray may be normal or enlarged depending on the degree of pericardial thickening and the presence of a pericardial effusion. 2-D echocardiography findings may reveal a thickened pericardium, but without a large pericardial effusion. CT and MRI provide measurement of pericardial thickness and assessment of diastolic filling patterns.

NURSING AND COLLABORATIVE MANAGEMENT
CHRONIC CONSTRICTIVE PERICARDITIS

Unless the patient is free of symptoms or the condition is inoperable, the treatment of choice for chronic constrictive pericarditis is a *pericardiectomy*. This involves complete resection of the pericardium through a median sternotomy with the use of cardiopulmonary bypass (see Chapter 34). Some patients show immediate improvement after surgery, but others may take weeks. The prognosis improves when surgery is performed before the patient becomes clinically unstable.

MYOCARDITIS
Etiology and Pathophysiology

Myocarditis is a focal or diffuse inflammation of the myocardium. Possible causes include viruses, bacteria, fungi, radiation therapy, and pharmacologic and chemical factors. Coxsackie A and B viruses are the most common etiologic agents. Autoimmune disorders (e.g., polymyositis) also have been associated with the development of myocarditis. It may also be idiopathic. Myocarditis is frequently associated with acute pericarditis, particularly when it is caused by coxsackie B virus.[10]

When the myocardium becomes infected, the causative agent invades the myocytes and causes cellular damage and necrosis. The immune response is activated, and cytokines and oxygen free radicals are released. As the infection progresses, an autoimmune response is activated. This causes further destruction of myocytes. Myocarditis results in cardiac dysfunction and has been linked to the development of dilated cardio-myopathy (discussed later in this chapter).

Clinical Manifestations

The clinical features of myocarditis are variable, ranging from a benign course without any overt manifestations to severe heart involvement or sudden cardiac death (SCD). Fever, fatigue, malaise, myalgias, pharyngitis, dyspnea, lymphadenopathy, and nausea and vomiting are early systemic manifestations of the viral illness.

Early cardiac signs appear 7 to 10 days after viral infection. These include pleuritic chest pain with a pericardial friction rub and effusion because pericarditis often accompanies myocarditis. Late cardiac signs relate to the development of HF and may include an S_3 heart sound, crackles, JVD, syncope, peripheral edema, and angina.

Diagnostic Studies and Collaborative Care

The ECG changes for a patient with myocarditis are often non-specific but may reflect associated pericardial involvement (e.g., diffuse ST segment changes). Dysrhythmias and conduction disturbances may be present. Laboratory findings are often inconclusive. They may include mild to moderate leukocytosis and atypical lymphocytes, increased ESR and CRP levels, elevated levels of myocardial markers such as troponin, and elevated viral titers. The virus is generally present in tissue and pericardial fluid samples only during the initial 8 to 10 days of illness.

Histologic confirmation of myocarditis is through an *endomyocardial biopsy.* A biopsy done during the first 6 weeks of acute illness is most diagnostic. This is the period in which lymphocytic infiltration and myocyte damage are present. Nuclear scans, echocardiography, and MRI are used to assess cardiac function.

The treatment for myocarditis consists of managing associated heart symptoms. Angiotensin-converting enzyme (ACE) inhibitors and β-adrenergic blockers are used if the heart is enlarged or to treat HF (see Chapter 35). Diuretics reduce fluid volume and decrease preload. If hypotension is not present, IV medications such as nitroprusside (Nitropress) and milrinone (Primacor) reduce afterload and improve CO by decreasing systemic vascular resistance. Digoxin (Lanoxin) improves myocardial contractility and reduces the heart rate. However, it is used cautiously in patients with myocarditis because of the heart's increased sensitivity to the adverse effects of this drug (e.g., dysrhythmias) and the potential toxicity. Anticoagulation therapy reduces the risk of thrombus formation from blood stasis in patients with a low ejection fraction (EF).

DRUG ALERT: Digoxin (Lanoxin)
- Use cautiously in patients with myocarditis, since the condition predisposes patients to drug-related dysrhythmias and toxicity.

Because myocarditis may have an autoimmune basis, immunosuppressive agents have been used to reduce myocardial inflammation and prevent irreversible myocardial damage. However, the use of these agents for the treatment of myocarditis remains controversial.[11]

General supportive measures for management of myocarditis include oxygen therapy, bed rest, and restricted activity. In cases of severe HF, intraaortic balloon pump therapy and ventricular assist devices may be required (see Chapters 35 and 66).

NURSING MANAGEMENT
MYOCARDITIS

Decreased CO is an ongoing nursing diagnosis in the care of the patient with myocarditis. Focus your interventions on managing the signs and symptoms of HF. Select nursing measures to decrease cardiac workload. These include placing the patient in a semi-Fowler's position, spacing activity and rest periods, and providing a quiet environment. Carefully monitor medications that increase the heart's contractility and decrease preload, afterload, or both. Evaluate the effectiveness of your interventions on an ongoing basis.

The patient may be anxious about the diagnosis of myocarditis and recovery. Assess the level of anxiety, take measures to decrease anxiety, and keep the patient and caregiver informed about the therapeutic plan.

The patient who receives immunosuppressive therapy is at increased risk for infection. Monitor for complications and provide the patient with proper infection control procedures.

Most patients with myocarditis recover spontaneously, although some may develop dilated cardiomyopathy (discussed later in this chapter). If severe HF occurs, the patient may require heart transplantation.

RHEUMATIC FEVER AND RHEUMATIC HEART DISEASE

Rheumatic fever (RF) is an acute inflammatory disease of the heart potentially involving all layers (endocardium, myocardium, and pericardium). Rheumatic heart disease is a chronic condition resulting from RF that is characterized by scarring and deformity of the heart valves.

Etiology and Pathophysiology

RF is a complication that occurs as a delayed result (usually after 2 to 3 weeks) of a group A streptococcal pharyngitis. Symptoms of RF appear to be related to an abnormal immunologic response to group A streptococcal cell membrane antigens.[12] RF affects the heart, skin, joints, and central nervous system (CNS).

RF has declined in developed countries because of the effective use of antibiotics to treat streptococcal infections. However, it remains an important public health problem in developing countries.[12] Rheumatic heart disease, caused by RF, primarily affects young adults.

Cardiac Lesions and Valve Deformities. About 40% of RF episodes are marked by carditis, meaning that all layers of the heart (endocardium, myocardium, and pericardium) are involved (see Fig. 37-1). This gives rise to the term *rheumatic pancarditis.*

Rheumatic endocarditis is found mainly in the valves, with swelling and erosion of the valve leaflets. Vegetation forms from deposits of fibrin and blood cells in areas of erosion (see eFig. 37-1 on the website for this chapter). The lesions initially create thickening of the valve leaflets, fusion of commissures and chordae tendineae, and fibrosis of the papillary muscle. Valve leaflets may become calcified, resulting in stenosis. The less mobile valve leaflets may not close properly, resulting in regurgitation. The mitral and aortic valves are most commonly affected.

Nodules, called *Aschoff's bodies,* are formed by a reaction to inflammation with swelling and destruction of collagen fibers. As the Aschoff's bodies age, they become more fibrous, and scar

TABLE 37-7	MODIFIED JONES CRITERIA FOR DIAGNOSING RHEUMATIC FEVER

Major Criteria
- Carditis
- Monoarthritis or polyarthritis
- Sydenham's chorea
- Erythema marginatum
- Subcutaneous nodules

Minor Criteria
- Clinical findings: Fever, polyarthralgia
- Laboratory findings: ↑ ESR, ↑ WBC count, ↑ CRP
- ECG findings: Prolonged PR interval

Evidence of Group A Streptococcal Infection
- Laboratory findings: ↑ Antistreptolysin-O titer, positive throat culture, positive rapid antigen test for group A streptococci

Source: American Heart Association: Scientific statement: proceedings of the Jones criteria workshop, *Circulation* 106:2521, 2002.
CRP, C-reactive protein; *ESR,* erythrocyte sedimentation rate.

TABLE 37-8	COLLABORATIVE CARE

Rheumatic Fever

Diagnostic
- History and physical examination
- Laboratory findings (see Table 37-7)
- Chest x-ray
- Echocardiogram
- Electrocardiogram

Collaborative Therapy
- Bed rest
- Antibiotics
- Nonsteroidal antiinflammatory drugs
- Salicylates
- Corticosteroids

tissue forms in the myocardium. Rheumatic pericarditis develops and affects both layers of the pericardium. The layers become thickened and covered with a fibrinous exudate. A serosanguineous pericardial effusion may develop. When healing occurs, fibrosis and adhesions develop that partially or completely destroy the pericardial sac. These pathophysiologic changes in the heart can begin during an initial attack of RF. Recurrent infections cause further structural damage.

Extracardiac Lesions. The lesions of RF are systemic and involve the skin, joints, and CNS. Painless subcutaneous nodules, arthralgias or arthritis, and chorea may develop.

Clinical Manifestations

A cluster of signs and symptoms, including laboratory findings, leads to the diagnosis of RF. Established criteria provide a basis for diagnosis.[13] The presence of two major criteria or one major and two minor criteria plus evidence of a preceding group A streptococcal infection indicate a high probability of RF (Table 37-7).

Major Criteria. *Carditis* is the most important manifestation of RF and results in three signs: (1) a heart murmur or murmurs of mitral or aortic regurgitation, or mitral stenosis; (2) cardiac enlargement and HF secondary to myocarditis; and (3) pericarditis resulting in muffled heart sounds, chest pain, pericardial friction rub, or signs of effusion.

Monoarthritis or *polyarthritis* is the most common finding in RF. The inflammatory process affects the synovial membranes of the joints, causing swelling, heat, redness, tenderness, and limitation of motion. The larger joints, particularly the knees, ankles, elbows, and wrists, are most frequently affected.

Sydenham's chorea is the major CNS manifestation of RF. It is often a delayed sign occurring several months after the initial infection. It is characterized by involuntary movements, especially of the face and limbs; muscle weakness; and disturbances of speech and gait.

Erythema marginatum lesions are a less common feature of RF. The bright pink, nonpruritic, maplike macular lesions occur mainly on the trunk and proximal extremities, and may be exacerbated by heat (e.g., warm bath).

Subcutaneous nodules, usually associated with severe carditis, are firm, small, hard, painless swellings located over extensor surfaces of joints, particularly the knees, wrists, and elbows.

Minor Criteria. Minor clinical manifestations (see Table 37-7) are frequently present and are helpful in diagnosing the disease. The minor criteria are used as supplemental data to confirm the presence of RF when only one major criterion is present.

Evidence of Infection. In addition to the major and minor criteria, there must also be evidence of a preceding group A streptococcal infection. Table 37-7 lists the various laboratory tests used to confirm evidence of infection.

Complications

A complication that can result from RF is *chronic rheumatic carditis.* It results from changes in valvular structure that may occur months to years after an episode of RF. Rheumatic endocarditis can result in fibrous tissue growth in valve leaflets and chordae tendineae with scarring and contractures. The mitral valve is most frequently involved. The aortic and tricuspid valves may also be affected.

Diagnostic Studies and Collaborative Care

No single diagnostic test exists for RF. An echocardiogram may show valvular insufficiency and pericardial fluid or thickening.[14] A chest x-ray may show an enlarged heart if HF is present. The most consistent ECG change is delayed AV conduction as evidenced by a prolonged PR interval.

Treatment consists of drug therapy and supportive measures (Table 37-8). Antibiotic therapy does not change the course of the acute disease or the development of carditis. It does eliminate residual group A streptococci remaining in the tonsils and pharynx and prevents the spread of organisms to close contacts. Salicylates, NSAIDs, and corticosteroids are the antiinflammatory agents most widely used in the management of RF. All are effective in controlling the fever and joint manifestations. Salicylates or NSAIDs are used when arthritis is the main manifestation, and corticosteroids are used if severe carditis is present.

NURSING MANAGEMENT
RHEUMATIC FEVER AND RHEUMATIC HEART DISEASE

NURSING ASSESSMENT

Table 37-9 presents the subjective and objective data that you should obtain from a patient with RF and rheumatic heart disease.

Inspect the patient's skin for subcutaneous nodules and erythema marginatum. This involves palpating for subcutaneous nodules over all bony surfaces and along extensor tendons of

TABLE 37-9 NURSING ASSESSMENT
Rheumatic Fever and Rheumatic Heart Disease

Subjective Data
Important Health Information
Past health history: Recent streptococcal infection, previous history of rheumatic fever or rheumatic heart disease

Functional Health Patterns
Health perception–health management: Family history of rheumatic fever; malaise
Nutritional-metabolic: Anorexia, weight loss
Activity-exercise: Palpitations; generalized weakness, fatigue; ataxia
Cognitive-perceptual: Chest pain; widespread joint pain and tenderness (especially large joints)

Objective Data
General
Fever

Integumentary
Subcutaneous nodules and erythema marginatum

Cardiovascular
Tachycardia, pericardial friction rub, muffled heart sounds; murmurs; peripheral edema

Neurologic
Chorea (involuntary, purposeless, rapid motions; facial grimaces)

Musculoskeletal
Signs of monoarthritis or polyarthritis, including swelling, heat, redness, limitation of motion (especially of knees, ankles, elbows, shoulders, wrists)

Possible Diagnostic Findings
Cardiomegaly on chest x-ray; prolonged PR interval on ECG; valve abnormalities, chamber dilation, and pericardial effusion on echocardiogram; ↑ antistreptolysin-O titer, positive throat culture, positive rapid antigen test for group A streptococci; ↑ ESR, ↑ CRP, leukocytosis

CRP, C-reactive protein; *ESR*, erythrocyte sedimentation rate.

the hands and feet. The nodules range in size from 1 to 4 cm and are hard, painless, and freely movable. Erythema marginatum can occur on the trunk and inner aspects of the upper arm and thigh. The erythematous maculae do not itch and are flat. Assess for these bright pink maculae in good light because the rash is difficult to observe, especially in dark-skinned patients.

NURSING DIAGNOSES
Nursing diagnoses for the patient with RF and rheumatic heart disease may include, but are not limited to, the following:
- Decreased CO *related to* valve dysfunction or HF
- Activity intolerance *related to* arthralgia or arthritis secondary to joint pain, pain from pericarditis, and HF
- Ineffective self–health management *related to* lack of knowledge concerning possible disease sequelae and the need for long-term prophylactic antibiotic therapy

PLANNING
The goals for a patient with RF and rheumatic heart disease include (1) normal or baseline heart function, (2) resumption of daily activities without joint pain, and (3) verbalization of the ability to manage the disease sequelae.

NURSING IMPLEMENTATION
HEALTH PROMOTION. RF is a preventable cardiovascular disease. It involves early detection and immediate treatment of group A streptococcal pharyngitis. Adequate treatment of streptococcal pharyngitis prevents initial attacks of RF. Treatment with oral penicillin V (Penicillin VK) or amoxicillin (Moxatag) for 10 days is recommended. If the patient is allergic to penicillin, a narrow-spectrum cephalosporin (e.g., cephalexin [Keflex]), clindamycin (Cleocin), or azithromycin (Zithromax) is used.[15] Therapy requires strict adherence to the full course of treatment. Your role is to teach the community to seek medical attention for symptoms of streptococcal pharyngitis and to emphasize the need for prompt and adequate treatment.

ACUTE INTERVENTION. The primary goals of managing a patient with RF are to (1) control and remove the infecting organism; (2) prevent cardiac complications; and (3) relieve joint pain, fever, and other symptoms. Administer antibiotics as ordered to treat the streptococcal infection. Teach the patient that completing the full course of antibiotics is vital to successful treatment. Administer salicylates, NSAIDs, and corticosteroids as prescribed, and monitor fluid intake as appropriate.

Promoting optimal rest is essential to reduce cardiac workload and the body's metabolic needs. A priority nursing goal is relief of joint pain. Position painful joints for comfort and in proper alignment. Heat may be applied and salicylates or NSAIDs administered for joint pain.

After the acute symptoms have subsided, the patient without carditis can ambulate. If the patient has carditis with HF, strict bed rest restrictions apply (see Chapter 35 for care of a patient with HF). Encourage nonstrenuous activities once recovery has begun.

AMBULATORY AND HOME CARE. Secondary prevention aims at stopping the recurrence of RF. Teach the patient with a history of RF about the disease process, possible sequelae, and the need for continuous antibiotic prophylaxis.

Prior history of RF makes the patient more susceptible to a second attack after a streptococcal infection. The best prevention is treatment with prophylactic antibiotics. Patients with RF without carditis require prophylaxis until age 20 and for a minimum of 5 years. Patients with rheumatic carditis and residual heart disease (e.g., persistent valve disease) need longer-term and even life-long prophylaxis.[13]

Teach the patient about good nutrition, hygienic practices, and adequate rest. Caution the patient about the possible development of heart valve disease. Teach the patient to seek medical attention if symptoms such as excessive fatigue, dizziness, palpitations, unexplained weight gain, or exertional dyspnea develop.[16]

EVALUATION
The expected outcomes for the patient with RF and rheumatic heart disease include
- Ability to perform ADLs with minimal fatigue and pain
- Adherence to treatment regimen
- Expression of confidence in managing disease
- Prevention of complications

VALVULAR HEART DISEASE

The heart contains two AV valves (mitral and tricuspid) and two semilunar valves (aortic and pulmonic), which control unidirectional blood flow (see Fig. 32-1). Valvular heart disease is

FIG. 37-7 Valvular stenosis and regurgitation. **A,** Normal position of the valve leaflets, or cusps, when the valve is open and closed. **B,** Open position of a stenosed valve *(left)* and closed position of regurgitant valve *(right)*. **C,** Hemodynamic effect of mitral stenosis. The stenosed valve is unable to open sufficiently during left atrial systole, inhibiting left ventricular filling. **D,** Hemodynamic effect of mitral regurgitation. The mitral valve does not close completely during left ventricular systole, permitting blood to reenter the left atrium. At the same time, blood is moving forward through the aortic valve.

TABLE 37-10	**MANIFESTATIONS OF VALVULAR HEART DISEASE**
Type	**Manifestations**
Mitral valve stenosis	Dyspnea on exertion, hemoptysis; fatigue; atrial fibrillation on ECG, palpitations, stroke; loud, accentuated S_1; low-pitched, diastolic murmur
Mitral valve regurgitation	*Acute:* Generally poorly tolerated; new systolic murmur with pulmonary edema and cardiogenic shock developing rapidly *Chronic:* Weakness, fatigue, exertional dyspnea, palpitations; an S_3 gallop, holosystolic murmur
Mitral valve prolapse	Palpitations, dyspnea, chest pain, activity intolerance, syncope; or holosystolic murmur
Aortic valve stenosis	Angina, syncope, dyspnea on exertion, heart failure; normal or soft S_1, diminished or absent S_2, systolic murmur, prominent S_4
Aortic valve regurgitation	*Acute:* Abrupt onset of profound dyspnea, chest pain, left ventricular failure and cardiogenic shock *Chronic:* Fatigue, exertional dyspnea, orthopnea, PND; water-hammer pulse; heaving precordial impulse; diminished or absent S_1, S_3, or S_4; soft high-pitched diastolic murmur, Austin Flint murmur
Tricuspid and pulmonic stenosis	*Tricuspid:* Peripheral edema, ascites, hepatomegaly; diastolic low-pitched murmur with increased intensity during inspiration *Pulmonic:* Fatigue, loud midsystolic murmur

PND, Paroxysmal nocturnal dyspnea.

defined according to the valve or valves affected and the type of functional alteration: stenosis or regurgitation (Fig. 37-7).

The pressure on either side of an open valve is normally equal. However, in a stenotic valve, the valve opening is smaller. The forward flow of blood is impaired. This creates a difference in pressure on the two sides of the open valve. The amount of stenosis (constriction or narrowing) is seen in the pressure differences (i.e., the higher the difference, the greater the stenosis). In regurgitation (also called *incompetence* or *insufficiency*), incomplete closure of the valve results in the backward flow of blood.

Valve disorders occur in children and adolescents mainly from congenital conditions. Valvular heart disease remains prevalent because of an increased number of older adults who have some form of cardiovascular disease. AS and mitral regurgitation (MR) are common valve disorders in older adults. Other causes of valve disease in adults include disorders related to acquired immunodeficiency syndrome and the use of some antiparkinsonian drugs.[17]

MITRAL VALVE STENOSIS

Etiology and Pathophysiology

Most cases of adult mitral valve stenosis result from rheumatic heart disease. Rheumatic mitral stenosis is widespread in developing countries. Less common causes are congenital mitral stenosis, rheumatoid arthritis, and systemic lupus erythematosus. Rheumatic endocarditis causes scarring of the valve leaflets and the chordae tendineae. Contractures and adhesions develop between the commissures (the junctional areas). The stenotic mitral valve takes on a "fish mouth" shape because of the thickening and shortening of the mitral valve structures (see eFig. 37-2 on the website for this chapter). These deformities block

the blood flow and create a pressure difference between the left atrium and the left ventricle during diastole. Left atrial pressure and volume increase. This causes higher pulmonary vasculature pressure. The overloaded left atrium places the patient at risk for atrial fibrillation. In chronic mitral stenosis, pressure overload occurs in the left atrium, the pulmonary bed, and the right ventricle.

Clinical Manifestations

The primary symptom of mitral stenosis is exertional dyspnea caused by reduced lung compliance (Table 37-10). Heart sounds include a loud first heart sound and a low-pitched, diastolic murmur (best heard at the apex with the stethoscope). Less frequently, patients may have hoarseness (from atrial enlargement pressing on the laryngeal nerve), hemoptysis (from pulmonary hypertension), chest pain (from decreased CO and coronary perfusion), and seizures or a stroke (from emboli). Fatigue and palpitations from atrial fibrillation may also occur. Emboli can arise from blood stasis in the left atrium secondary to atrial fibrillation.[18]

MITRAL VALVE REGURGITATION

Etiology and Pathophysiology

Mitral valve function depends on intact mitral leaflets, mitral annulus, chordae tendineae, papillary muscles, left atrium, and left ventricle. A defect in any of these structures can result in regurgitation. Most cases of mitral regurgitation (MR) are caused by MI, chronic rheumatic heart disease, mitral valve prolapse, ischemic papillary muscle dysfunction, and IE. MI with left ventricular failure increases the risk for rupture of the chordae tendineae and acute MR.

MR allows blood to flow backward from the left ventricle to the left atrium because of incomplete valve closure during systole. Both the left ventricle and left atrium must work harder to preserve an adequate CO. In acute MR the sudden increase in pressure and volume transmits to the pulmonary bed. This results in pulmonary edema and, if untreated, cardiogenic shock. In chronic MR the additional volume results in left atrial enlargement, left ventricular dilation and hypertrophy, and, finally, a decrease in CO.

Clinical Manifestations

The clinical course of MR is determined by the nature of its onset (see Table 37-10). Patients with acute MR have thready, peripheral pulses and cool, clammy extremities. A low CO may mask a new systolic murmur. Rapid assessment (e.g., cardiac catheterization) and intervention (e.g., valve repair or replacement) are critical.

Patients with chronic MR may remain asymptomatic for many years. Initial symptoms of left ventricular failure may include weakness, fatigue, palpitations, and dyspnea that gradually progress to orthopnea, paroxysmal nocturnal dyspnea, and peripheral edema. Increased left ventricular volume leads to an audible third heart sound (S_3), even with normal left ventricular function. The murmur is a loud holosystolic murmur at the apex radiating to the left axilla. Patients with asymptomatic MR must be monitored carefully. Surgery (valve repair or replacement) should be considered before significant left ventricular failure or pulmonary hypertension develops.[19]

MITRAL VALVE PROLAPSE

Etiology and Pathophysiology

Mitral valve prolapse (MVP) is an abnormality of the mitral valve leaflets and the papillary muscles or chordae that allows the leaflets to prolapse, or buckle, back into the left atrium during systole (Fig. 37-8). It is the most common form of valvular heart disease in the United States. It affects both genders equally.[20]

The use of the term *prolapse* can be misleading because it is used even when the valve is working normally. MVP is usually benign, but serious complications can occur, including MR, IE, SCD, HF, and cerebral ischemia.

FIG. 37-8 Mitral valve prolapse. In this valvular abnormality, the mitral leaflets have prolapsed back into the left atrium. They also demonstrate hooding *(arrow)*. The left ventricle is on the right.

🧬 Genetic Link

Although the etiology of MVP is unknown, some patients have an increased familial incidence. The genetic inheritance is frequently autosomal dominant (see Chapter 13). MVP in this group results from a connective tissue defect affecting only the valve, or as part of Marfan's syndrome or other hereditary conditions that affect the structure of collagen in the body.

Clinical Manifestations

MVP covers a broad range of severity. Most patients are asymptomatic and remain so for their entire lives. About 10% of those with MVP become symptomatic. A characteristic of MVP is a murmur from regurgitation that is louder during systole. MVP does not alter S_1 or S_2 heart sounds. Severe MR is an uncommon but serious complication of MVP.

M-mode and 2-D echocardiography are used to confirm MVP. Dysrhythmias, most commonly premature ventricular contractions, paroxysmal supraventricular tachycardia, and ventricular tachycardia, may cause palpitations, light-headedness, and dizziness. IE may occur in patients with MR associated with MVP.

Patients may or may not have chest pain. The cause of the chest pain is not known. It may be the result of abnormal tension on the papillary muscles. If chest pain occurs, episodes tend to occur in clusters, especially during periods of emotional stress. Dyspnea, palpitations, and syncope may occasionally accompany the chest pain and do not respond to antianginal treatment (e.g., nitrates). β-Adrenergic blockers may be prescribed to control palpitations and chest pain. Encourage the patient to stay hydrated, exercise regularly, and avoid caffeine.

Patients with MVP generally have a benign, manageable course unless problems related to MR develop. No accepted medical therapy appears to delay the need for valve surgery in this group.[20] A teaching plan for patients with MVP is presented in Table 37-11.

AORTIC VALVE STENOSIS

Etiology and Pathophysiology

Congenital aortic stenosis (AS) is generally found in childhood, adolescence, or young adulthood. In older adults, AS is a result of RF or degeneration that may have an etiology similar to that of coronary artery disease. It affects 3% of people over

TABLE 37-11	PATIENT & CAREGIVER TEACHING GUIDE

Mitral Valve Prolapse

Include the following information in the teaching plan for a patient with mitral valve prolapse (MVP) and the patient's caregiver.

- Take medications as prescribed (e.g., β-adrenergic blockers to control palpitations, chest pain).
- Adopt healthy eating habits and avoid caffeine because it is a stimulant and may exacerbate symptoms.
- If you use diet pills or other over-the-counter drugs, check for common ingredients that are stimulants (e.g., caffeine, ephedrine), since these can exacerbate symptoms.
- Begin (or maintain) an exercise program to achieve optimal health.
- Contact the health care provider or emergency medical services (EMS) if symptoms develop or worsen (e.g., palpitations, fatigue, shortness of breath, anxiety).

65 years of age.[21] In rheumatic valve disease, fusion of the commissures and secondary calcification cause the valve leaflets to stiffen and retract, resulting in stenosis. If AS occurs due to rheumatic heart disease, mitral valve disease accompanies it. Isolated AS is usually nonrheumatic in origin. The incidence of rheumatic aortic valve disease has been decreasing, but degenerative stenosis is increasing as the population ages.

AS causes obstruction of flow from the left ventricle to the aorta during systole. The effect is left ventricular hypertrophy and increased myocardial oxygen consumption because of the increased myocardial mass. As the disease progresses and compensatory mechanisms fail, reduced CO leads to decreased tissue perfusion, pulmonary hypertension, and HF.

Clinical Manifestations

Symptoms of AS (see Table 37-10) develop when the valve orifice becomes about one third its normal size. Symptoms include the classic triad of angina, syncope, and exertional dyspnea, reflecting left ventricular failure.[21] The prognosis is poor for patients with symptoms and those whose valve obstruction is not fixed. Nitroglycerin is used cautiously to treat angina, since the drug can significantly reduce BP and worsen chest pain. Auscultation of AS typically reveals a normal or soft S_1, a diminished or absent S_2, a systolic murmur, and a prominent S_4.

> **DRUG ALERT: Nitroglycerin (Nitro-Bid)**
> - Use cautiously in patients with AS, since significant hypotension may occur.
> - Chest pain can worsen due to a decrease in preload and drop in BP.

AORTIC VALVE REGURGITATION

Etiology and Pathophysiology

Aortic regurgitation (AR) may be the result of primary disease of the aortic valve leaflets, the aortic root, or both. Trauma, IE, or aortic dissection can cause acute AR, which constitutes a life-threatening emergency. Chronic AR is generally the result of rheumatic heart disease, a congenital bicuspid aortic valve, syphilis, or chronic rheumatic conditions such as ankylosing spondylitis or reactive arthritis.

AR causes retrograde (backward) blood flow from the ascending aorta into the left ventricle during diastole. This results in volume overload. The left ventricle initially compensates for chronic AR by dilation and hypertrophy. Myocardial contractility eventually declines, and blood volume in the left atrium and pulmonary bed increases. This leads to pulmonary hypertension and right ventricular failure.

Clinical Manifestations

Patients with acute AR have sudden manifestations of cardiovascular collapse (see Table 37-10). The left ventricle is exposed to aortic pressure during diastole. The patient develops severe dyspnea, chest pain, and hypotension indicating left ventricular failure and cardiogenic shock, a life-threatening emergency.

Patients with chronic, severe AR develop a *water-hammer pulse* (a strong, quick beat that collapses immediately). Heart sounds may include a soft or absent S_1, S_3, or S_4; and a soft, high-pitched diastolic murmur.

The patient with chronic AR generally remains asymptomatic for years. Exertional dyspnea, orthopnea, and paroxysmal nocturnal dyspnea develop only after considerable heart dysfunction has occurred (see Table 37-10). Angina occurs less frequently than in AS.

TRICUSPID AND PULMONIC VALVE DISEASE

Etiology and Pathophysiology

Diseases of the tricuspid and pulmonic valves are uncommon, with stenosis occurring more frequently than regurgitation. *Tricuspid stenosis* occurs almost exclusively in patients who have RF or who abuse IV drugs. Tricuspid stenosis results in right atrial enlargement and elevated systemic venous pressures. *Pulmonic stenosis* is almost always congenital and results in right ventricular hypertension and hypertrophy (see Table 37-10).

DIAGNOSTIC STUDIES FOR VALVULAR HEART DISEASE

Diagnosis of valvular heart disease includes data from the patient's history and physical examination and a variety of tests (Table 37-12). A CT scan of the chest with contrast is the gold standard for evaluating aortic disorders.[22] An echocardiogram reveals valve structure, function, and heart chamber size. Transesophageal echocardiography and Doppler color-flow imaging help diagnose and monitor valvular heart disease progression. Real-time 3-D echocardiography can help assess mitral valve and congenital heart disease. Chest x-ray reveals the heart size, altered pulmonary circulation, and valve calcification. An ECG identifies heart rate, rhythm, and any ischemia or ventricular hypertrophy. Cardiac catheterization detects pressure changes in the cardiac chambers, records pressure differences across the valves, and measures the size of valve openings.

TABLE 37-12 COLLABORATIVE CARE
Valvular Heart Disease

Diagnostic
- History and physical examination
- Chest x-ray
- CBC
- Electrocardiogram
- Echocardiography (Doppler and transesophageal)
- Cardiac catheterization

Collaborative Therapy
Nonsurgical
- Prophylactic antibiotic therapy (see Table 37-2)
  - Rheumatic fever
  - Infective endocarditis (see Table 37-2)
- Sodium restriction
- Medications to treat or control HF
  - Vasodilators* (e.g., nitrates, ACE inhibitors)
  - Positive inotropes (e.g., digoxin)
  - Diuretics
  - β-Adrenergic blockers
- Anticoagulation therapy (see Table 38-10)
- Antidysrhythmia drugs
- Percutaneous transluminal balloon valvuloplasty
- Percutaneous valve replacement

Surgical
- Valve repair
  - Commissurotomy (valvulotomy)
  - Valvuloplasty
  - Annuloplasty
- Valve replacement

*Use cautiously in patients with aortic stenosis.
ACE, Angiotensin-converting enzyme; *HF*, heart failure.

COLLABORATIVE CARE OF VALVULAR HEART DISEASE

Conservative Therapy

An important aspect of conservative management of valvular heart disease is prevention of recurrent RF and IE (see Table 37-12). Treatment depends on the valve involved and disease severity. It focuses on preventing exacerbations of HF, acute pulmonary edema, thromboembolism, and recurrent endocarditis. HF is treated with vasodilators, positive inotropes, β-adrenergic blockers, diuretics, and a low-sodium diet (see Chapter 35).

Anticoagulant therapy prevents and treats systemic or pulmonary emboli. It is used prophylactically in patients with atrial fibrillation. Atrial dysrhythmias are common and treated with calcium channel blockers, β-adrenergic blockers, antidysrhythmia drugs, or electrical cardioversion (see Chapter 36).

Percutaneous Transluminal Balloon Valvuloplasty. An alternative treatment for some patients with valvular heart disease is the *percutaneous transluminal balloon valvuloplasty* (PTBV) procedure. During PTBV, the fused commissures are split open. Balloon valvuloplasty is used for mitral, tricuspid, and pulmonic stenosis, and less often for AS. The procedure is done in the cardiac catheterization laboratory. It involves threading a balloon-tipped catheter from the femoral artery or vein to the stenotic valve. The balloon is inflated in an attempt to separate the valve leaflets. A single- or double-balloon technique may be used for the PTBV procedure. Currently, the use of a single Inoue balloon with hourglass shape allows sequential inflation (Fig. 37-9). This technique is the most popular because it is easy and has good results with few complications (e.g., left ventricular perforation). The PTBV procedure is generally indicated for older adults and for those who are poor surgery candidates. The long-term results of PTBV are similar to those of surgical commissurotomy.

Similar to PTBV, the Sapien Transcatheter Heart Valve (THV) is approved for select patients with AS. The THV is inserted through the femoral artery and moved to the heart. It is released and expanded with a balloon in the location of the aortic valve. This procedure is limited to patients who are eligible for surgery, but who are at high risk for surgical complications (e.g., patients with multiple comorbidities).[23]

Surgical Therapy. The decision for surgical intervention depends on the patient's clinical state using the New York Heart Association classification system for functional disability (see Table 35-5). The type of surgery can be valve repair or valve replacement. The procedure that is used depends on the valves involved, the pathology and severity of the disease, and the patient's clinical condition. All types of valve surgery are palliative, not curative, and patients require lifelong health care.

Valve Repair. Valve repair is usually the surgical procedure of choice. It has a lower operative mortality rate than valve replacement and is often used in mitral or tricuspid valvular heart disease.[24,25] Although valve repair avoids the risks of replacement, it may not restore total valve function.

Mitral *commissurotomy (valvulotomy)* is the procedure of choice for patients with pure mitral stenosis. The less precise closed method of commissurotomy has generally been replaced by the open method. In the *closed procedure* the surgeon inserts a transventricular dilator through the apex of the left ventricle into the opening of the mitral valve. The direct vision procedure, or *open procedure,* requires the use of cardiopulmonary bypass. The surgeon removes thrombi from the atrium and

FIG. 37-9 Mitral valvuloplasty performed by the Inoue technique. The catheter is placed in the mitral valve and the distal part of the Inoue balloon inflated **(A)**. The balloon is then pulled back in the mitral valve and inflated for 10 to 15 sec under fluoroscopic control **(B)** until the waist of the balloon is no longer visible **(C)** and the balloon falls back into the left atrium.

INFORMATICS IN PRACTICE

Heart Surgery DVD or CD

- Many patients prefer to watch DVDs or listen to CDs instead of reading pamphlets. For a patient facing heart surgery, using a video can be an effective tool to use when teaching the patient and caregiver what to expect before and after the procedure.
- Remember that the DVD or CD is not the teacher.
- Beforehand discuss what the DVD or CD will cover and encourage the patient and caregiver to write down questions or note what they do not understand.
- After the patient and caregiver view or listen to the material, be available to answer any questions they have. Reinforce important information from the DVD or CD.

makes a commissure incision. Next, the fused chordae are separated by splitting the papillary muscle and debriding the calcified valve.

Open surgical *valvuloplasty* involves repair of the valve by suturing the torn leaflets, chordae tendineae, or papillary muscles. It is primarily used to treat mitral or tricuspid regurgitation.

Minimally invasive valvuloplasty surgery involves a mini-sternotomy or parasternal approach. It may include robotic and thoracoscopic surgical systems. Results compare with those of

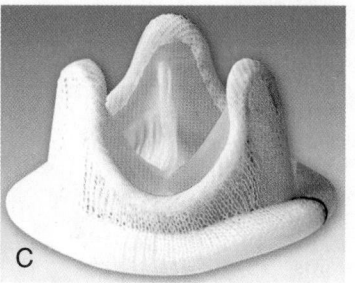

FIG. 37-10 Types of prosthetic heart valves. **A,** Starr-Edwards caged ball valve. **B,** St. Jude bi-leaflet valve. **C,** Carpentier-Edwards porcine valve.

ETHICAL/LEGAL DILEMMAS

Do Not Resuscitate

Situation

J.L., a 68-year-old man, is admitted for a second mitral valve surgery and coronary artery bypass graft surgery. He did not adhere to the treatment plan after his original surgery 7 years ago. You are worried about his future adherence with medications, diet, and exercise. His kidneys are failing and he is on dialysis, making him a high-risk surgical patient. The patient and caregivers want all possible treatment and refuse to discuss Do Not Resuscitate (DNR) orders.

Ethical/Legal Points for Consideration

- Based on their expertise, health care providers have the right to refuse to provide treatment that offers no benefit to the patient.
- Advance directives do not include a DNR order. If the patient is unable to speak for himself or herself, a DNR order can be initiated only by the attending physician or agent and usually depends on evidence of the patient's preferences.
- If there is an advance directive refusing resuscitation, the health care provider is required to act accordingly but is not compelled to enact a DNR without clear direction from the patient or proxy.
- Patient adherence with past treatment plans is not a factor that must be considered in DNR decisions. Many circumstances related to nonadherence are outside the patient's control such as financing, transportation, availability of assistance, and declining physical and medical capabilities.
- If there is disagreement about the patient's treatment plan, a referral can be made to an ethics committee, or the patient can seek treatment from another provider.

Discussion Questions

1. How can a lack of understanding or limited financial resources contribute to nonadherence with the plan of care?
2. What type of information should be provided to a patient and caregiver in discussions about DNR orders? Who should provide this information?
3. Who can initiate a referral to an ethics committee?

Mechanical valves are manufactured from artificial materials and consist of combinations of metal alloys, pyrolytic carbon, and Dacron. *Biologic valves* are constructed from bovine, porcine, and human (cadaver) heart tissue and usually contain some man-made materials. A "decellularizing" process removes the cadaver cells from the valve. This lowers the risk of immune response and tissue rejection. Biologic valves are asymmetric in shape and produce a more natural pattern of blood flow compared with mechanical valves. Asymmetric mechanical valve prototypes are being tested.[27]

Mechanical prosthetic valves are more durable and last longer than biologic valves. However, they have an increased risk of thromboembolism and require long-term anticoagulation therapy. The main complication of mechanical valves is bleeding from the use of anticoagulants. Biologic valves do not require anticoagulation therapy because of their low thrombogenicity. However, they are less durable and tend to cause early calcification, tissue degeneration, and stiffening of the leaflets. Either type of prosthetic valve can leak and cause endocarditis. Minimally invasive aortic valve replacement uses a transcatheter or transapical approach and is the surgical choice for patients at high risk for traditional surgery.[28,29]

Long-term anticoagulation is needed for those patients with biologic valves who have atrial fibrillation. Some patients with biologic valves or annuloplasty with prosthetic rings may need anticoagulation the first few months after surgery until the suture lines are covered by endothelial cells (endothelialized).

The choice of valves depends on many factors. For example, if a patient cannot take an anticoagulant (e.g., women of childbearing age), a biologic valve is considered. A mechanical valve may be best for a younger patient because it is more durable. For patients over age 65, durability is less important than the risks of bleeding from anticoagulants, so most receive a biologic valve.

NURSING MANAGEMENT VALVULAR DISORDERS

NURSING ASSESSMENT

Table 37-13 presents the subjective and objective data to obtain from an individual with valve disease.

NURSING DIAGNOSES

Nursing diagnoses for the patient with valvular heart disease may include, but are not limited to, the following:

- Decreased CO *related to* valvular incompetence
- Excess fluid volume *related to* fluid retention secondary to valvular-induced HF
- Activity intolerance *related to* insufficient oxygenation secondary to decreased CO and pulmonary congestion

the open procedure. In addition, shorter lengths of stay, fewer blood transfusions, less pain, and lower risk of sternal infection and postoperative atrial fibrillation have been reported.[26]

For patients with mitral or tricuspid regurgitation, further valve repair or reconstruction using annuloplasty is an option. *Annuloplasty* involves reconstruction of the annulus, with or without the aid of prosthetic rings (e.g., a Carpentier ring).

Valve Replacement. Valve replacement may be required for mitral, aortic, tricuspid, and occasionally pulmonic valve disease. A wide variety of prosthetic valves are currently available. Desirable valves are nonthrombogenic and durable, and create minimal stenosis. Prosthetic valves are categorized as mechanical or biologic (tissue) valves (Fig. 37-10).

TABLE 37-13   NURSING ASSESSMENT

Valvular Heart Disease

Subjective Data
Important Health Information
Past health history: Rheumatic fever, infective endocarditis; congenital defects, myocardial infarction, chest trauma, cardiomyopathy; syphilis, Marfan's syndrome, streptococcal infections

Functional Health Patterns
Health perception–health management: IV drug abuse; fatigue
Activity-exercise: Palpitations; generalized weakness, activity intolerance; dizziness, fainting; dyspnea on exertion, cough, hemoptysis, orthopnea
Sleep-rest: Paroxysmal nocturnal dyspnea
Cognitive-perceptual: Angina or atypical chest pain

Objective Data
General
Fever

Integumentary
Diaphoresis, flushing, cyanosis, clubbing; peripheral edema

Respiratory
Crackles, wheezes, hoarseness

Cardiovascular
Abnormal heart sounds, including murmurs, S_3, and S_4; dysrhythmias, including atrial fibrillation, premature ventricular contractions; tachycardia; ↑ or ↓ in pulse pressure; hypotension, water-hammer or thready peripheral pulses

Gastrointestinal
Ascites, hepatomegaly, unexplained weight gain

Possible Diagnostic Findings
Cardiomegaly on chest x-ray; ECG abnormalities specific to involved valve; echocardiogram (valve abnormalities and chamber dilation); cardiac catheterization (abnormalities in valves, chamber pressures, cardiac output, and blood flow depending on involved valve)

Additional information on nursing diagnoses is presented in eNursing Care Plan 37-2 available on the website for this chapter.

PLANNING

The overall goals for the patient with valve disease include (1) normal heart function, (2) improved activity tolerance, and (3) an understanding of the disease process and health maintenance measures.

NURSING IMPLEMENTATION

HEALTH PROMOTION. Diagnosing and treating streptococcal infections and providing prophylactic antibiotics for patients with a history of RF are critical to prevent acquired rheumatic valve disease. The patient at risk for endocarditis and any patient with certain cardiac conditions must also receive prophylactic antibiotics (see Table 37-2).

The patient must adhere to prescribed therapies. The individual with a history of RF, endocarditis, and congenital heart disease should know the symptoms of valvular heart disease so early medical treatment may begin.

ACUTE INTERVENTION AND AMBULATORY AND HOME CARE. A patient with progressive valvular heart disease may require outpatient care or hospitalization for management of HF, endocar-

ditis, embolic disease, or dysrhythmias. HF is the most common reason for ongoing medical care.

Your role is to implement therapeutic interventions and evaluate their effects. Design activities considering the patient's limitations. An appropriate exercise plan can increase cardiac tolerance, but activities that cause fatigue and dyspnea should be restricted. Discourage tobacco use. Tell the patient to avoid strenuous physical exercise because damaged valves may not handle the increased CO demand. Your patient's care plan should emphasize conserving energy, setting priorities, and taking planned rest periods. Referral to a vocational counselor may be needed if the patient has a physically or emotionally demanding job.

Perform ongoing cardiac assessments to monitor the effectiveness of medications. Teaching the actions and side effects of drugs is important to increase adherence. The patient must understand the importance of prophylactic antibiotic therapy to prevent IE (see Table 37-2). If the valve disease was caused by RF, ongoing prophylaxis to prevent recurrence is necessary.

When valvular heart disease can no longer be managed medically, surgical intervention is necessary (see Chapter 34 for the care of a patient having heart surgery). The patient who is on anticoagulation therapy (e.g., warfarin [Coumadin]) after surgery for valve replacement must have the international normalized ratio (INR) checked regularly to determine proper dosage and adequacy of therapy. INR values of 2.5 to 3.5 are therapeutic for patients with mechanical valves.

Teaching instructions related to anticoagulation therapy are found in Table 38-14. The patient must know that valve surgery is not a cure, and that regular follow-up with a health care provider is required. Also, teach the patient when to seek medical care. Any manifestations of infection, HF, signs of bleeding, and planned invasive or dental procedures require the patient to notify the health care provider. Finally, encourage patients to obtain and wear a Medic Alert bracelet.

EVALUATION

The expected outcomes for a patient with valvular heart disease are presented in eNursing Care Plan 37-2 available on the website for this chapter.

CARDIOMYOPATHY

Cardiomyopathy (CMP) is a group of diseases that directly affect myocardial structure or function. A diagnosis of CMP is based on the patient's clinical manifestations and noninvasive and invasive diagnostic procedures.

CMP can be classified as primary or secondary. *Primary CMP* refers to those conditions in which the etiology of the disease is idiopathic. The heart muscle in this case is the only part of the heart involved, and other cardiac structures are unaffected. In *secondary CMP* the cause of the myocardial disease is known and is secondary to another disease process. Common causes of secondary CMP are listed in Table 37-14.

Three major types of CMP are dilated, hypertrophic, and restrictive. Each type has its own pathogenesis, clinical presentation, and treatment protocols (Tables 37-15 and 37-16). CMP can lead to cardiomegaly and HF. It is the primary reason that heart transplants are performed.

Takotsubo cardiomyopathy (TCM) is a transient cardiac syndrome that mimics acute coronary syndrome. Patients often are

TABLE 37-14   CAUSES OF CARDIOMYOPATHY

Dilated
- Cardiotoxic agents: alcohol, cocaine, doxorubicin (Adriamycin)
- Coronary artery disease
- Genetic (autosomal dominant)
- Hypertension
- Metabolic disorders
- Muscular dystrophy
- Myocarditis
- Pregnancy
- Valve disease

Hypertrophic
- Aortic stenosis
- Genetic (autosomal dominant)
- Hypertension

Restrictive
- Amyloidosis
- Endomyocardial fibrosis
- Neoplastic tumor
- Post-radiation therapy
- Sarcoidosis
- Ventricular thrombus

TABLE 37-15   COMPARISON OF TYPES OF CARDIOMYOPATHY

	Dilated	Hypertrophic	Restrictive
Major Manifestations	Fatigue, weakness, palpitations, dyspnea	Exertional dyspnea, fatigue, angina, syncope, palpitations	Dyspnea, fatigue
Cardiomegaly	Moderate to severe	Mild to moderate	Mild
Contractility	Decreased	Increased or decreased	Normal or decreased
Valvular Incompetence	Atrioventricular (AV) valves, especially mitral	Mitral valve	AV valves
Dysrhythmias	Sinus tachycardia, atrial and ventricular dysrhythmias	Atrial and ventricular dysrhythmias	Atrial and ventricular dysrhythmias
Cardiac Output	Decreased	Normal or decreased	Normal or decreased
Outflow Tract Obstruction	None	Increased	None

TABLE 37-16   COLLABORATIVE CARE

Cardiomyopathy

Diagnostic
- History and physical examination
- Electrocardiogram
- b-Type natriuretic peptide (BNP)
- Chest x-ray
- Echocardiogram
- Nuclear imaging studies
- Cardiac catheterization
- Endomyocardial biopsy

Collaborative Therapy
- Drug therapy
  - Nitrates (except in hypertrophic CMP)
  - β-Adrenergic blockers
  - Antidysrhythmics
  - ACE inhibitors
  - Diuretics
  - Digitalis (except in hypertrophic CMP unless used to treat atrial fibrillation)
  - Anticoagulants (if indicated)
- Ventricular assist device
- Cardiac resynchronization therapy
- Implantable cardioverter-defibrillator
- Surgical correction
- Heart transplantation

ACE, Angiotensin-converting enzyme; *CMP,* cardiomyopathy.

seen with chest pain, have ST segment elevation on ECG, and have elevated cardiac enzyme levels consistent with an MI. However, when the patient undergoes cardiac angiography, there is no significant coronary artery disease. TCM is an acute, stress-related syndrome that is more common in postmenopausal women. Normal cardiac function returns in days or weeks after supportive therapy.[30]

DILATED CARDIOMYOPATHY

Etiology and Pathophysiology

Dilated cardiomyopathy is the most common type of CMP, with a prevalence of 5 to 8 cases per 100,000 people in the United States. It causes HF in 25% to 40% of cases, occurs more frequently in middle-aged African Americans and men, and has a genetic link in 30% of cases. Dilated CMP often follows an infectious myocarditis. Some evidence links dilated CMP with an autoimmune process.[31] Alcoholic dilated CMP is under-recognized and has unique presentation, treatment, and outcomes.[32] Other common causes of dilated CMP are listed in Table 37-14.

Dilated CMP is characterized by a diffuse inflammation and rapid degeneration of myocardial fibers. This results in ventricular dilation, impaired systolic function, atrial enlargement, and stasis of blood in the left ventricle. SCD from ventricular dysrhythmias is a leading cause of death in idiopathic dilated CMP.[33] *Cardiomegaly* results from ventricular dilation (Fig. 37-11). This causes contractile dysfunction in spite of an enlarged chamber size. In contrast to HF, the walls of the ventricles do not hypertrophy (see eFig. 37-3 on the website for this chapter).

Clinical Manifestations

The signs and symptoms of dilated CMP may develop acutely after a systemic infection or slowly over time. Most people eventually develop HF. Symptoms can include decreased exercise capacity, fatigue, dyspnea at rest, paroxysmal nocturnal dyspnea, and orthopnea. As the disease progresses, the patient may experience dry cough, palpitations, abdominal bloating, nausea, vomiting, and anorexia. Signs can include an abnormal S_3 and/or S_4, dysrhythmias, heart murmurs, pulmonary crackles, edema, weak peripheral pulses, pallor, hepatomegaly, and JVD. Decreased blood flow through an enlarged heart promotes stasis and blood clot formation, and may lead to systemic embolization.

Diagnostic Studies

The diagnosis of dilated CMP is based on the patient's history and exclusion of other causes of HF. Doppler echocardiography is the basis for the diagnosis of dilated CMP in the majority of patients. The chest x-ray may show cardiomegaly with signs of

FIG. 37-11 Dilated cardiomyopathy. The dilated left ventricular wall has thinned *(arrow)*, and the chamber size and volume are increased.

pulmonary venous hypertension and pleural effusion. The ECG may reveal tachycardia, bradycardia, and dysrhythmias with conduction disturbances. Laboratory studies may show elevated serum levels of b-type natriuretic peptide (BNP) in the presence of HF.

Cardiac catheterization confirms or rules out coronary artery disease, and multiple gated acquisition (MUGA) nuclear scan determines EF. EF less than 20% is associated with a 50% mortality rate within 1 year. Endomyocardial biopsy is done at the time of the right-sided heart catheterization to identify any infectious organisms in heart tissue.

NURSING AND COLLABORATIVE MANAGEMENT DILATED CARDIOMYOPATHY

Interventions focus on controlling HF by enhancing myocardial contractility and decreasing preload and afterload. This is similar to the management of chronic HF. Treatment guidelines are based on the specific stage of disease progression (see Table 35-5). Treatment of patients with Class IV (stage D) HF is more palliative than curative.

Several different types of drugs are available to manage HF (see Table 35-7). Nitrates (e.g., nitroglycerin [Nitrol]) and diuretics (e.g., furosemide [Lasix]) decrease preload, and ACE inhibitors (e.g., captopril [Capoten]) reduce afterload. β-Adrenergic blockers (e.g., metoprolol [Lopressor]) and aldosterone antagonists (e.g., spironolactone [Aldactone]) control the neurohormonal stimulation that occurs in HF. Dysrhythmias are treated with antidysrhythmics (e.g., amiodarone) as indicated (see Chapter 36). Anticoagulation therapy reduces the risk of systemic embolization from clots. These may form in the heart chambers secondary to atrial fibrillation.

Drug and nutritional therapy and cardiac rehabilitation may help (1) alleviate symptoms of HF and (2) improve CO and quality of life. A patient with secondary dilated CMP must be treated for the underlying disease process. For example, the patient with alcohol-related dilated CMP must abstain from all alcohol. (See Chapter 11 for a discussion on addictive behaviors and Chapter 35 for a discussion on HF.)

Unfortunately, dilated CMP does not respond well to therapy, and patients experience multiple episodes of HF. Patients are often hospitalized for infusions of dobutamine (Dobutrex) or

milrinone followed by aggressive diuresis. Sometimes these treatments are done on an outpatient basis or in the home under nursing supervision. After treatment, many patients experience an improvement in symptoms that lasts several weeks. The use of statins (e.g., atorvastatin [Lipitor]) in ischemic and idiopathic dilated CMP does increase survival, improve cardiac function, and reduce inflammatory markers[34,35] (see Table 34-5). Additionally, trimetazidine (Vastarel), a metabolic modulator, improves cardiac function and glucose control in diabetic patients with dilated CMP.[36]

Patients also may benefit from nondrug therapies. A ventricular assist device (VAD) allows the heart to rest and recover from acute HF. It may also serve as a bridge to heart transplantation. Additionally, cardiac resynchronization therapy and an implantable cardioverter-defibrillator are used in appropriate patients (see Chapter 35).

The patient with terminal or end-stage CMP may consider heart transplantation. The use of a permanent, implantable VAD, known as destination therapy, is an option for patients with advanced disease who are not candidates for heart transplantation (see Chapter 35). Currently, approximately 50% of heart transplantations are performed for treatment of CMP. Cardiac transplant recipients have a good prognosis. However, donor hearts are difficult to obtain, and many patients with dilated CMP die while awaiting heart transplantation.

Patients with dilated CMP are very ill people with a grave prognosis who need expert nursing care. Observe for signs and symptoms of worsening HF, dysrhythmias, embolic formation, and drug responsiveness. The goals of therapy are to keep the patient at an optimal level of functioning and out of the hospital. Always include caregivers when planning a patient's care. Encourage caregivers to learn cardiopulmonary resuscitation (CPR). Instruct them on when and how to access emergency care.

Home health and hospice nursing can provide the patient and caregiver with palliative care. This includes interventions to maximize and maintain functional status or end-of-life care to prepare for a peaceful death.

HYPERTROPHIC CARDIOMYOPATHY

Etiology and Pathophysiology

Hypertrophic cardiomyopathy is asymmetric left ventricular hypertrophy without ventricular dilation. In one form of the disease the septum between the two ventricles becomes enlarged and obstructs the blood flow from the left ventricle. It is termed *hypertrophic obstructive cardiomyopathy* (HOCMP) or *asymmetric septal hypertrophy* (ASH).

Although hypertrophic CMP can be idiopathic, about half of all cases have a genetic basis characterized by inappropriate myocardial hypertrophy.[37] Early identification is important (see Table 37-14). Hypertrophic CMP occurs less commonly than dilated CMP and is more common in men than in women. It is usually diagnosed in young adults and, most often, in active, athletic individuals. Hypertrophic CMP is the most common cause of SCD in otherwise healthy young people. It accounts for 3% of deaths in young competitive athletes.[38,39]

The four main characteristics of hypertrophic CMP are (1) massive ventricular hypertrophy; (2) rapid, forceful contraction of the left ventricle; (3) impaired relaxation (diastole); and (4) obstruction to aortic outflow (not present in all patients). Ventricular hypertrophy is associated with a thickened intra-

FIG. 37-12 Hypertrophic cardiomyopathy. There is marked left ventricular hypertrophy *(arrow)*, and the chamber size and volume are decreased.

ventricular septum and ventricular wall (Fig. 37-12; also see eFig. 37-3 on the website for this chapter). The end result is impaired ventricular filling as the ventricle becomes noncompliant and unable to relax. The primary defect of hypertrophic CMP is diastolic dysfunction from left ventricular stiffness. Decreased ventricular filling and obstruction to outflow can result in decreased CO, especially during exertion.

Clinical Manifestations

Patients with hypertrophic CMP may be asymptomatic or may have exertional dyspnea, fatigue, angina, and syncope. The most common symptom is dyspnea, which is caused by an elevated left ventricular diastolic pressure. Fatigue occurs because of the resultant decrease in CO and in exercise-induced flow obstruction. Angina can occur and is most often caused by the increased left ventricular muscle mass or compression of the small coronary arteries by the hypertrophic ventricular myocardium. The patient may also have syncope, especially during exertion. Syncope is most often caused by an increase in obstruction to aortic outflow during increased activity. This results in decreased CO and cerebrovascular circulation. Syncope can also be caused by dysrhythmias. Common dysrhythmias include supraventricular tachycardia, atrial fibrillation, ventricular tachycardia, and ventricular fibrillation. Any of these dysrhythmias may lead to syncope or SCD (see Chapters 34 and 36).

Diagnostic Studies

Clinical findings on examination may be unremarkable. However, on palpation of the chest the apical impulse can be exaggerated and displaced to the left. Auscultation may reveal an S_4 and a systolic murmur between the apex and the sternal border at the fourth intercostal space. ECG findings usually indicate ventricular hypertrophy, ST-T wave abnormalities, prominent Q waves in the inferior or precordial leads, left axis deviation, and ventricular and atrial dysrhythmias (see Chapter 36).

The echocardiogram is the primary diagnostic tool to confirm hypertrophic CMP. The echocardiogram may also demonstrate wall motion abnormalities and diastolic dysfunction. Cardiac catheterization and nuclear stress testing may also be helpful in diagnosing and guiding the treatment of hypertrophic CMP.

NURSING AND COLLABORATIVE MANAGEMENT HYPERTROPHIC CARDIOMYOPATHY

Goals of care are to improve ventricular filling by reducing ventricular contractility and relieving left ventricular outflow obstruction. These can be done with the use of β-adrenergic blockers (e.g., metoprolol) or calcium channel blockers (e.g., verapamil [Calan]). Digitalis is considered if needed to treat atrial fibrillation. Amiodarone or sotalol (Betapace) are effective antidysrhythmia medications. However, their use does not prevent SCD. For patients at risk for SCD, a cardioverter-defibrillator is needed (see Chapter 36).

AV pacing is helpful for patients with hypertrophic CMP and outflow obstruction. When the ventricles are paced from the apex of the right ventricle, septal depolarization occurs first. This allows the septum to move away from the left ventricular wall and reduces the degree of obstruction of the outflow tract.

Some patients may be candidates for surgical treatment of their hypertrophied septum. The indications for surgery include severe symptoms unresponsive to therapy with marked obstruction to aortic outflow. The surgery is termed a *ventriculomyotomy and myectomy*. It involves cutting into the thickened septal muscle and removing some of the ventricular muscle. Most patients have an improvement in symptoms and exercise tolerance after surgery.

An alternative nonsurgical procedure to reduce symptoms and the left ventricular outflow obstruction is alcohol-induced, percutaneous transluminal septal myocardial ablation (PTSMA). This procedure consists of injecting alcohol into the first septal artery branching off the left anterior descending artery. This causes ischemia and septal wall infarction. Ablation of the septal wall decreases the obstruction to flow, and the patient's symptoms decrease. The procedure improves HF symptoms and exercise capacity 3 months after ablation.[40] Potential complications of PTSMA include conduction disturbances (e.g., heart block) and MI.

Nursing interventions for hypertrophic CMP focus on relieving symptoms, observing for and preventing complications, and providing emotional support. Focus your teaching on helping patients avoid strenuous activity and dehydration. Any activity that causes an increase in systemic vascular resistance (thus increasing the obstruction to forward flow) is dangerous and should be avoided. Rest and elevation of the feet to improve venous return to the heart can manage chest pain in these patients. Vasodilators such as nitroglycerin may worsen the chest pain by decreasing venous return and further increasing obstruction of blood flow from the heart.

RESTRICTIVE CARDIOMYOPATHY

Etiology and Pathophysiology

Restrictive cardiomyopathy is the least common type of CMP. It is a disease of the myocardium that impairs diastolic filling and stretch (see eFig. 37-3 on the website for this chapter). Systolic function remains unchanged. Although the specific etiology of restrictive CMP is unknown, a number of pathologic processes may be involved in its development. Myocardial fibrosis, hypertrophy, and infiltration produce stiffness of the ventricular wall with loss of ventricular compliance. Secondary causes of restrictive CMP include amyloidosis, endocardial fibrosis, sarcoidosis, fibrosis of different etiology, and radiation to the thorax. With restrictive CMP, the ventricles are resistant to filling and therefore demand high diastolic filling pressures to maintain CO.

Clinical Manifestations and Diagnostic Studies

Classic manifestations of restrictive CMP are fatigue, exercise intolerance, and dyspnea. These occur because the heart cannot increase CO by increasing the heart rate without further compromising ventricular filling. Additional symptoms may include angina, orthopnea, syncope, and palpitations. The patient may have signs of HF, including dyspnea, peripheral edema, weight gain, ascites, hepatomegaly, and JVD.

The chest x-ray may be normal, or it may show cardiomegaly from right and left atrial enlargement. Pleural effusions and pulmonary congestion may be seen in the patient with progression to HF. The ECG may reveal a mild tachycardia at rest. The most common dysrhythmias are supraventricular (atrial fibrillation) or AV block. Echocardiography may reveal a left ventricle that is normal size with a thickened wall, slightly dilated right ventricle, and dilated atria. Endomyocardial biopsy, CT scan, and nuclear imaging may help in the diagnosis.

NURSING AND COLLABORATIVE MANAGEMENT RESTRICTIVE CARDIOMYOPATHY

Currently, there is no specific treatment for restrictive CMP. Interventions are aimed at improving diastolic filling and the underlying disease process. Treatment includes conventional therapy for HF and dysrhythmias. Heart transplant may also be a consideration. Nursing care is similar to the care of a patient with HF. As in the treatment of patients with hypertrophic CMP, teach the patient to avoid situations that impair ventricular filling and increase systemic vascular resistance, such as strenuous activity and dehydration.

Nursing care of a patient with CMP includes individualized teaching based on the patient's clinical manifestations. All patients with CMP are at risk for IE from any procedure that may cause bacteremia. Instruct the patient on the need for prophylactic antibiotics (see Table 37-2). A general patient and caregiver teaching guide is presented in Table 37-17.

TABLE 37-17 PATIENT & CAREGIVER TEACHING GUIDE

Cardiomyopathy

Include the following information in the teaching plan for a patient with cardiomyopathy and the patient's caregiver.

1. Take all medications as prescribed and regularly follow up with health care provider.
2. Follow a low-sodium diet (if ordered) and read all product labels (food and over-the-counter drugs) for sodium content.
3. Drink six to eight glasses of water a day unless fluids are restricted.
4. Achieve and maintain a reasonable weight and avoid large meals.
5. Avoid alcohol, caffeine, diet pills, and over-the-counter cold medicines that may contain stimulants.
6. Balance activity and rest periods.
7. Avoid heavy lifting or vigorous isometric exercises, and check with health care provider for exercise guidelines.
8. Use stress management techniques: relaxation breathing, guided imagery (see Chapter 7).
9. Report any signs of heart failure to health care provider, including weight gain, edema, shortness of breath, and increased fatigue.
10. Encourage caregivers to learn CPR because of the potential for cardiac arrest (see Appendix A).
11. Access emergency medical services according to the health care provider's instructions.

CPR, Cardiopulmonary resuscitation.

CASE STUDY

Valvular Heart Disease

Jupiterimages/
Photos.com/Thinkstock

Patient Profile
R.B., a 50-year-old white man, is admitted to the hospital for valvular heart disease.

Subjective Data
- Reports past history of IV drug abuse
- Reports current regular alcohol intake approximately 1 pint of whiskey per day
- Complains of chest pain with minimal exertion
- Recently unemployed
- States he is short of breath and cannot sleep lying flat
- States he is tired and irritable all the time
- States he cannot afford medications
- Smokes a pack of cigarettes a day

Objective Data
Physical Examination
- Third heart sound (S₃)
- Loud holosystolic murmur of mitral regurgitation
- Edentulous (secondary to periodontal disease)
- Vital signs: temperature 99.0°F (37.2°C); pulse 110, irregular; respirations 24; BP 104/58

Diagnostic Studies
- ECG shows atrial fibrillation with a rapid ventricular response.
- Chest x-ray reveals pulmonary congestion and cardiomegaly.
- Transesophageal echocardiography shows left atrial and ventricular hypertrophy and mitral and aortic regurgitation.

Discussion Questions
1. Identify the cause and course of R.B.'s disease based on his history and current examination.
2. Differentiate between mitral and aortic regurgitation.
3. What medical treatments or surgical procedures will R.B. probably require as his condition worsens?
4. *Priority Decision:* On the basis of the assessment data provided, what are the priority nursing diagnoses?
5. *Priority Decision:* Identify the priority nursing interventions for R.B.
6. *Delegation Decision:* Identify those tasks that you could delegate to unlicensed assistive personnel (UAP).
7. *Evidence-Based Practice:* R.B. asks you why he needs to be on "blood thinners" after his valves are replaced.

BRIDGE TO NCLEX EXAMINATION

The number of the question corresponds to the same-numbered outcome at the beginning of the chapter.

1. Assessment of an IV cocaine user with infective endocarditis should focus on which signs and symptoms (select all that apply)?
   a. Retinal hemorrhages
   b. Splinter hemorrhages
   c. Presence of Osler's nodes
   d. Painless nodules over bony prominences
   e. Painless erythematous macules on the palms and soles

2. The nurse is caring for a patient with chronic constrictive pericarditis. Which assessment finding reflects a more serious complication of this condition?
   a. Fatigue
   b. Peripheral edema
   c. Jugular venous distention
   d. Thickened pericardium on echocardiography

3. A patient is admitted with myocarditis. While performing the initial assessment, the nurse may find which clinical signs and symptoms (select all that apply)?
   a. Angina
   b. Pleuritic chest pain
   c. Splinter hemorrhages
   d. Pericardial friction rub
   e. Presence of Osler's nodes

4. Priority nursing management for a patient with myocarditis includes interventions related to
   a. meticulous skin care.
   b. antibiotic prophylaxis.
   c. tight glycemic control.
   d. oxygenation and ventilation.

5. When teaching a patient about the long-term consequences of rheumatic fever, the nurse should discuss the possibility of
   a. valvular heart disease.
   b. pulmonary hypertension.
   c. superior vena cava syndrome.
   d. hypertrophy of the right ventricle.

6. Which is a priority nursing intervention for a patient during the acute phase of rheumatic fever?
   a. Administration of antibiotics as ordered
   b. Management of pain with opioid analgesics
   c. Encouragement of fluid intake for hydration
   d. Performance of frequent active range-of-motion exercises

7. Which clinical finding would most likely indicate decreased cardiac output in a patient with aortic valve regurgitation?
   a. Reduction in peripheral edema and weight
   b. Carotid venous distention and new-onset atrial fibrillation
   c. Significant pulsus paradoxus and diminished peripheral pulses
   d. Shortness of breath on minimal exertion and a diastolic murmur

8. A patient is diagnosed with mitral stenosis and new-onset atrial fibrillation. Which interventions could the nurse delegate to unlicensed assistive personnel (UAP) (select all that apply)?
   a. Obtain and record daily weight.
   b. Determine apical-radial pulse rate.
   c. Observe for overt signs of bleeding.
   d. Obtain and record vital signs, including pulse oximetry.
   e. Teach the patient how to purchase a Medic Alert bracelet.

9. Which diagnostic study best differentiates the various types of cardiomyopathy?
   a. Echocardiography
   b. Arterial blood gases
   c. Cardiac catheterization
   d. Endomyocardial biopsy

10. The nurse is caring for a patient newly admitted with heart failure secondary to dilated cardiomyopathy. Which intervention would be a priority?
    a. Encourage caregivers to learn CPR.
    b. Consider a consultation with hospice for palliative care.
    c. Monitor the patient's response to prescribed medications.
    d. Arrange for the patient to enter a cardiac rehabilitation program.

1. a, b, c; 2. c; 3. a, b, d; 4. d; 5. a; 6. a; 7. d; 8. a, c; 9. d; 10. c

evolve

For rationales to these answers and even more NCLEX review questions, visit *http://evolve.elsevier.com/Lewis/medsurg*.

REFERENCES

1. Wu K-S, Lee S, Tsai H-C, et al: Non-nosocomial healthcare-associated infective endocarditis in Taiwan: an underrecognized disease with poor outcomes, *BMC Infect Dis* 11(221):1, 2011.

2. Lomas J, Martinez-Marcos F, Plata A, et al: Healthcare-associated infective endocarditis: an undesirable effect of healthcare universalization, *Clin Microbiol Infect* 16(11):1683, 2010.

3. Birchenough E, Moore C, Stevens K, et al: Buttonhole cannulation in adult patients on hemodialysis: an increased risk of infection? *Nephrology Nurs J* 37(5):491, 2010.

4. Cunha B, D'Elia A, Pawar N, et al: Viridans streptococcal (*Streptococcus intermedius*) mitral valve subacute bacterial endocarditis (SBE) in a patient with mitral valve prolapse after a dental procedure: the importance of antibiotic prophylaxis, *Heart Lung* 39(1):65, 2010.

5. Buppert C: NP sued for failure to diagnosis (sic) endocarditis—$1 million settlement, *J Nurs Pract* 7(10):872, 2011.

6. McDermott B, Cunha B, Choi D, et al: Transthoracic echocardiography (TEE): sufficiently sensitive screening test for native valve infective endocarditis (IE), *Heart Lung* 40:358, 2010.

7. Cleveland Clinic: Cardiac catheterization, 2012. Retrieved from *http://my.clevelandclinic.org/heart/services/tests/invasive/ccath.aspx*.

8. Petrov D: Sudden onset of chest pain associated with PR-segment depression in ECG, *Heart Lung* 38(5):440, 2009.

9. Kuo I, Pearson GJ, Koshman SL: Colchicine for the primary and secondary prevention of pericarditis: an update, *Ann Pharmacother* 43(12):2075, 2009.

10. Metzger T, Anderson M: Myocarditis: a defect in central immune tolerance? *J Clin Invest* 121(4):125, 2011.

11. Myocarditis—new treatments, 2011. Retrieved from *www.ccspublishing.com/journals3a/myocarditis.htm.*

12. Parks T: Erratum: underdiagnosis of acute rheumatic fever in primary care settings in a developing country, *Trop Med Int Health* 15(3):384, 2010.

13. Mayo Clinic Staff: Rheumatic fever, 2011. Retrieved from *www.mayoclinic.com/health/rheumatic-fever/DS00250/METHOD+print.*

*14. Simsek Z, Karakelleoglu S, Gündogdu F, et al: Evaluation of left ventricular function with strain/strain rate imaging in patients with rheumatic mitral stenosis, *Anatolian J Cardiol* 10(4):328, 2010.

15. Shulman ST, Bisno AL, Clegg HW, et al: Clinical practice guideline for the diagnosis and management of group A streptococcal pharyngitis: 2012 update by the Infectious Diseases Society of America, *Clin Infect Dis* 55:e86, 2012.

16. Mosby's Nursing Consult, Patient Information: Rheumatic fever, 2012. Retrieved from *www.nursingconsult.com/nursing/patient-education/full-text?handout_id=45551&docId=10087&tab=cond&otherid=48822&english=true&filter_id=47523&filter_by=Rheumatology&sort_by=title&sort_order=asc&page=1&title=&requestUri=filter&story_title=Rheumatic+Fever&parentpage=&secondpage=&searchId=&searchTerm=.*

17. Surapaneni P, Vinales K, Najib M, et al: Valvular heart disease with the use of fenfluramine-phentermine, *Tex Heart Inst J* 38(5):581, 2011.

18. Maganti K, Rigolin V, Sarano M, et al: Valvular heart disease: diagnosis and management, *Mayo Clin Proc* 85(5):483, 2009.

19. Madden S: An alternative treatment approach to mitral regurgitation, *Nurs Stand* 26(13):40, 2011.

20. Gemignani A, Ferri F, Wu W: Mitral valve prolapse. In Ferri F, editor: *Ferri's clinical advisor: 5 books in 1*, Philadelphia, 2012, Mosby.

21. Michelena H, Abel M, Suri R, et al: Intraoperative echocardiography in valvular heart disease: an evidence-based appraisal, *Mayo Clin Proc* 85(7):646, 2010.

22. Bachore T, Hranitzky P, Patel M: Heart disease. In McPhee SJ, Papadakis MA, editors: *Lange 2011 current medical diagnosis and treatment*, ed 50, New York, 2011, McGraw-Hill Medical.

23. U.S. Food and Drug Administration: FDA expands approved use of Sapien artificial heart valve. Retrieved from *www.fda.gov/NewsEvents/Newsroom/PressAnnouncements/ucm323478.htm?source=govdelivery.*

24. Mitral Valve Repair Center at the Mount Sinai Hospital: Mitral valve repair, 2011. Retrieved from *www.mitralvalverepair.org/content/view/64.*

25. Mitral Valve Repair Center at the Mount Sinai Hospital: Mitral valve repair vs. replacement rates, 2011. Retrieved from *www.mitralvalverepair.org/content/view/72.*

26. Mitral Valve Repair Center at the Mount Sinai Hospital: Minimally invasive heart surgery center, 2011. Retrieved from *www.mitralvalverepair.org/content/view/16.*

27. Science Daily: New design for mechanical heart valves, 2011. Retrieved from *www.sciencedaily.com/releases/2011/11/111122113212.htm.*

28. Held ML: Transcatheter aortic valve replacement: new hope for patients with aortic stenosis, *Am Nurse Today* 7(5):11, 2012.

29. Cleveland Clinic: Diseases and conditions—heart valve disease—percutaneous interventions, 2012. Retrieved from *http://my.clevelandclinic.org/heart/percutaneous/percutaneousValve.aspx.*

30. Bradbury B, Cohen F: Early postoperative Takotsubo cardiomyopathy: a case report, *AANA J* 79(3):181, 2011.

31. Xiao H, Wang M, Du Y, et al: Arrhythmogenic autoantibodies against calcium channel lead to sudden death in idiopathic dilated cardiomyopathy, *Eur J Heart Fail* 13:264, 2011.

32. Lamari A, Dattilo G, Morabito G, et al: A dilated alcoholic cardiomyopathy, *Int J Cardiol* 149(3):95, 2009.

33. Samanta S, Vijayverghia R, Vaiphei K: Isolated idiopathic right ventricular dilated cardiomyopathy, *Indian J Pathol Microbiol* 54(1):164, 2011.

*34. Nagueh S, Lombardi R, Tan Y, et al: Atorvastatin and cardiac hypertrophy and function in hypertrophic cardiomyopathy: a pilot study, *Eur J Clin Invest* 40:976, 2010.

35. Kostner K: Statin therapy for hypertrophic cardiomyopathy: too good to be true? *Eur J Clin Invest* 40:965, 2010.

36. Wafa S: Clinical benefits of trimetazidine in diabetic patients with coronary artery disease, *Heart Metab* 48:23, 2010.

37. Wang L, Seidman J, Seidman C: Narrative review: harnessing molecular genetics for the diagnosis and management of hypertrophic cardiomyopathy, *Ann Intern Med* 152(8):513, 2010.

*38. Hypertrophic Cardiomyopathy Association: 2011 ACCF/AHA guidelines for the diagnosis and treatment of hypertrophic cardiomyopathy: a report of the American College of Cardiology Foundation /American Heart Association Task Force on Practice Guidelines. Retrieved from *www.4hcm.org/2011_accf_aha_guidelines.html.*

39. Wilson M, Chandra N, Papadakis M, et al: Hypertrophic cardiomyopathy and ultra-endurance running—two incompatible entities? *J Cardiovasc Magnetic Res* 13(77):1, 2011.

40. Otto A, Aytemir K, Okutucu S, et al: Cyanoacrylate for septal ablation in hypertrophic cardiomyopathy, *J Interv Cardiol* 24(1):77, 2011.

RESOURCES

American Association of Cardiovascular and Pulmonary Rehabilitation
www.aacvpr.org

American College of Cardiology
www.acc.org

American Heart Association
www.heart.org/HEARTORG

Hypertrophic Cardiomyopathy Association
www.4hcm.org

Mayo Clinic
www.mayoclinic.com/health/cardiomyopathy/DS00519

Mended Hearts
www.mendedhearts.org

National Heart, Lung, and Blood Institute
www.nhlbi.nih.gov

Percutaneous Transvenous Mitral Valvuloplasty
www.ptmv.org

YourHeartValve.com
www.yourheartvalve.com

*Evidence-based information for clinical practice.

The best and most beautiful things in the world cannot be seen or even touched. They must be felt within the heart.
Helen Keller

Nursing Management
Vascular Disorders

Deirdre D. Wipke-Tevis and Kathleen A. Rich

evolve WEBSITE

http://evolve.elsevier.com/Lewis/medsurg

- NCLEX Review Questions
- Key Points
- Pre-Test
- Answer Guidelines for Case Study on p. 859
- Rationales for Bridge to NCLEX Examination Questions
- Concept Map Creator
- Glossary
- Content Updates

- Case Studies
  - Patient With Abdominal Aortic Aneurysm
  - Patient With Chronic Peripheral Artery Disease
- Nursing Care Plans (Customizable)
  - eNCP 38-1: Patient With Peripheral Artery Disease of the Lower Extremities
  - eNCP 38-2: Patient After Surgical Repair of the Aorta

eTables
- eTable 38-1: Drugs, Vitamins, Minerals, and Supplements That Interact With Oral Anticoagulants
- eTable 38-2: Sample Venous Thromboembolism Protocol/Order Set

LEARNING OUTCOMES

1. Relate the major risk factors to the etiology and pathophysiology of peripheral artery disease (PAD).
2. Describe the clinical manifestations, collaborative care, and surgical and nursing management of PAD of the lower extremities.
3. Plan appropriate nursing care for the patient with acute arterial ischemic disorders of the lower extremities.
4. Differentiate the pathophysiology, clinical manifestations, collaborative care, and nursing management of thromboangiitis obliterans (Buerger's disease) and Raynaud's phenomenon.
5. Differentiate the pathophysiology, clinical manifestations, and collaborative care of different types of aortic aneurysms.
6. Select appropriate nursing interventions for a patient undergoing an aortic aneurysm repair.

7. Describe the pathophysiology, clinical manifestations, collaborative care, and nursing management of aortic dissection.
8. Evaluate the risk factors predisposing patients to the development of superficial vein thrombosis and venous thromboembolism (VTE).
9. Differentiate between the clinical characteristics of superficial vein thrombosis and VTE.
10. Compare and contrast the collaborative care and nursing management of patients with superficial vein thrombosis and VTE.
11. Prioritize the key aspects of nursing management of the patient receiving anticoagulant therapy.
12. Relate the pathophysiology and clinical manifestations to the collaborative care of patients with varicose veins, chronic venous insufficiency, and venous leg ulcers.

KEY TERMS

acute arterial ischemia, p. 839
aneurysm, p. 841
aortic dissection, p. 845
chronic venous insufficiency (CVI), p. 857
critical limb ischemia, p. 837
deep vein thrombosis (DVT), p. 847

intermittent claudication, p. 834
peripheral artery disease (PAD), p. 833
post-thrombotic syndrome (PTS), p. 849
Raynaud's phenomenon, p. 840
superficial vein thrombosis (SVT), p. 847

thromboangiitis obliterans (Buerger's disease), p. 840
varicose veins, p. 856
venous thromboembolism (VTE), p. 847
venous thrombosis, p. 847
Virchow's triad, p. 847

Problems of the vascular system include disorders of the arteries, veins, and lymphatic vessels. Arterial disorders are classified as atherosclerotic, aneurysmal, and nonatherosclerotic vascular diseases. Atherosclerotic vascular disease is divided into coronary, cerebral, peripheral, mesenteric, and renal artery disease.[1] This chapter discusses peripheral artery disease; aortic aneurysm and dissection; and venous diseases,

specifically venous thromboembolism and chronic venous insufficiency.

PERIPHERAL ARTERY DISEASE

Peripheral artery disease (PAD) involves thickening of artery walls, which results in a progressive narrowing of the arteries

Reviewed by Patricia Hong, RN, MA, Senior Lecturer, University of Washington, School of Nursing, Seattle, Washington; Teri Lynn Kiss, RN, MS, MSSW, CCRN, Director, Medical Unit–2 South and Patient Quality Resources, Fairbanks Memorial Hospital, Fairbanks, Alaska; and Tara McMillan-Queen, RN, MSN, ANP, GNP, Faculty II, Mercy School of Nursing, Charlotte, North Carolina.

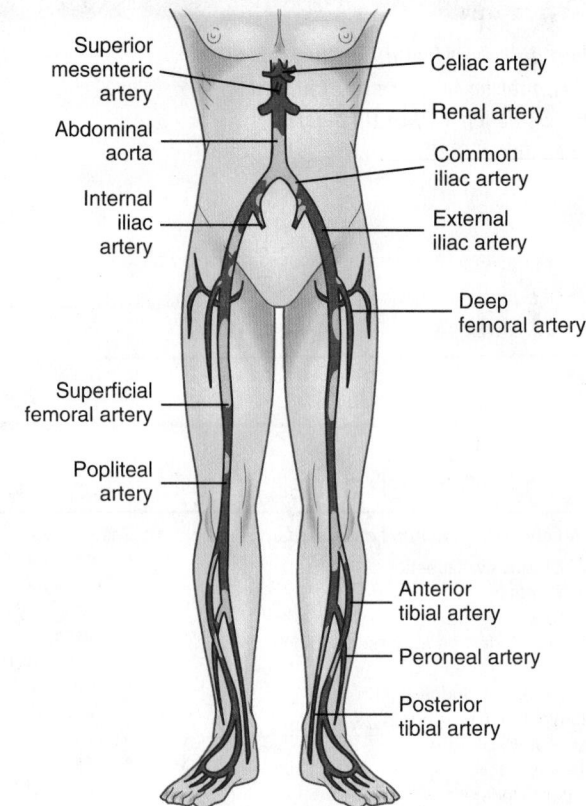

FIG. 38-1 Common anatomic locations of atherosclerotic lesions (shown in *yellow*) of the abdominal aorta and lower extremities.

of the upper and lower extremities. The risk for PAD increases with age; it usually become symptomatic in the sixth to eighth decades of life. In persons with diabetes mellitus, PAD occurs much earlier. About 6% of adults ages 40 years and older and 13% of adults ages 60 years and older have PAD.[2] PAD prevalence is higher in women, and non-Hispanic African Americans.[3,4]

PAD is strongly related to other types of cardiovascular disease (CVD) and their risk factors. Patients with PAD have a significantly higher risk of mortality (in general), CVD mortality, and major coronary events.[5] Thus PAD is a marker of advanced systemic atherosclerosis. Patients with PAD are more likely to have coronary artery disease and/or cerebral artery disease. Unfortunately, most Americans are not familiar with PAD, nor are they aware of PAD risk factors and complications.[6] In general, PAD remains underdiagnosed and undertreated.

Etiology and Pathophysiology

The leading cause of PAD is *atherosclerosis,* a gradual thickening of the *intima* (the innermost layer of the arterial wall) and *media* (middle layer of the arterial wall). This results from the deposit of cholesterol and lipids within the vessel walls and leads to progressive narrowing of the artery. Although the exact cause(s) of atherosclerosis are unknown, inflammation and endothelial injury play a major role (see Chapter 34).

Significant risk factors for PAD include tobacco use, diabetes, hyperlipidemia, elevated C-reactive protein, and uncontrolled hypertension, with the most important being tobacco use. Nicotine is a vasoconstrictor, and tobacco smoke impairs transport and cellular use of oxygen, and increases blood viscosity and homocysteine levels. Other risk factors include family history, hypertriglyceridemia, increasing age, hyperho-

mocysteinemia, hyperuricemia, obesity, sedentary lifestyle, and stress.[4,7] Women with low lifetime recreational activity are at greater risk for PAD than similar men.[8]

Atherosclerosis more commonly affects certain segments of the arterial tree. These include the coronary (see Chapter 34), carotid (see Chapter 58), and lower extremity arteries. Clinical symptoms occur when vessels are 60% to 75% blocked.

PERIPHERAL ARTERY DISEASE OF THE LOWER EXTREMITIES

Lower extremity PAD may affect the iliac, femoral, popliteal, tibial, or peroneal arteries, or any combination of these arteries (Fig. 38-1). The femoral popliteal area is the most common site in nondiabetic patients. Patients with diabetes tend to develop PAD in the arteries below the knee. In advanced PAD, multiple levels of occlusions are found.

Clinical Manifestations

Generally, the severity of the clinical manifestations depends on the site and extent of the blockage and the amount of collateral circulation. The classic symptom of lower extremity PAD is **intermittent claudication,** which is ischemic muscle pain that is caused by exercise, resolves within 10 minutes or less with rest, and is reproducible.[9] The ischemic pain is a result of the buildup of lactic acid from anaerobic metabolism. Once the patient stops exercising, the lactic acid is cleared and the pain subsides. PAD of the iliac arteries produces claudication in the buttocks and thighs. Calf claudication indicates femoral or popliteal artery involvement. Only about 10% of patients with PAD display the classic symptom of intermittent claudication. Older

TABLE 38-1 COMPARISON OF PERIPHERAL ARTERY AND VENOUS DISEASE

Characteristic	Peripheral Artery Disease	Venous Disease
Peripheral pulses	Decreased or absent	Present, may be difficult to palpate with edema
Capillary refill	>3 sec	<3 sec
Ankle-brachial index	≤0.90	>0.90
Edema	Absent unless leg constantly in dependent position	Lower leg edema
Hair	Loss of hair on legs, feet, toes	Hair may be present or absent
Ulcer		
• Location	Tips of toes, foot, or lateral malleolus	Near medial malleolus
• Margin	Rounded, smooth, looks "punched out"	Irregularly shaped
• Drainage	Minimal	Moderate to large amount
• Tissue	Black eschar or pale pink granulation	Yellow slough or dark red, "ruddy" granulation
Pain	Intermittent claudication or rest pain in foot. Ulcer may or may not be painful	Dull ache or heaviness in calf or thigh. Ulcer often painful
Nails	Thickened; brittle	Normal or thickened
Skin color	Dependent rubor, elevation pallor	Bronze-brown pigmentation. Varicose veins may be visible
Skin texture	Thin, shiny, taut	Skin thick, hardened, and indurated
Skin temperature	Cool, temperature gradient down the leg	Warm, no temperature gradient
Dermatitis	Rarely occurs	Frequently occurs
Pruritus	Rarely occurs	Frequently occurs

women experience it less often than men.[10] If PAD involves the internal iliac arteries, erectile dysfunction may result.

Paresthesia, or numbness or tingling, in the toes or feet may result from nerve tissue ischemia. True peripheral neuropathy occurs more often in patients with diabetes (see Chapter 49) and in those with long-standing ischemia. Neuropathy produces severe shooting or burning pain in the extremity. It does not follow particular nerve roots and may be present near ulcerated areas. Gradual, reduced blood flow to neurons produces loss of both pressure and deep pain sensations. Thus patients may not notice lower extremity injuries.

The limb's physical appearance provides important information about blood flow. The skin becomes thin, shiny, and taut, and hair loss occurs on the lower legs. Pedal, popliteal, or femoral pulses are diminished or absent. Pallor (blanching of the foot) develops in response to leg elevation (*elevation pallor*). Conversely, *reactive hyperemia* (redness of the foot) develops when the limb is in a dependent position (*dependent rubor*) (see Table 38-1).

As PAD progresses and involves multiple arterial segments, continuous pain develops at rest. *Rest pain* most often occurs in the foot or toes and is aggravated by limb elevation. Rest pain occurs when blood flow is insufficient to meet basic metabolic requirements of the distal tissues. Rest pain occurs more often at night because cardiac output tends to drop during sleep and the limbs are at the level of the heart. Patients often try to achieve pain relief by dangling the leg over the side of the bed or sleeping in a chair. This allows gravity to maximize blood flow.

The patient with chronic rest pain, ulceration, or gangrene has *critical limb ischemia*. Critical limb ischemia may lead to amputation if untreated. Every attempt is made to save the limb with surgical or endovascular revascularization. If a patient is not a candidate for revascularization and/or if revascularization is not technically possible, medical treatment is required.[11]

Complications

Lower extremity PAD progresses slowly. Prolonged ischemia leads to atrophy of the skin and underlying muscles. Even minor trauma to the feet (e.g., stubbing one's toe, blister from shoes) can result in delayed healing, wound infection, and tissue necrosis, especially in the diabetic patient. Arterial (ischemic) ulcers most often occur over bony prominences on the toes, feet, and lower legs (Table 38-1). Nonhealing arterial ulcers and gangrene are the most serious complications. Amputation may be needed if adequate blood flow is not restored or if severe infection occurs. If PAD is present for an extended period, collateral circulation may prevent gangrene of the extremity. Uncontrolled pain and severe, spreading infection are indicators that an amputation is needed in individuals who are not candidates for revascularization.

Diagnostic Studies

Various tests can assess blood flow and outline the vascular system (Table 38-2). Doppler ultrasound with duplex imaging maps blood flow throughout the entire region of an artery. When palpation of a peripheral pulse is difficult because of severe PAD, the Doppler ultrasound can determine the degree of blood flow. A palpable pulse and a Doppler pulse are not equivalent, and the terms are not interchangeable. *Segmental blood pressures* (BPs) are obtained (using Doppler ultrasound and a sphygmomanometer) at the thigh, below the knee, and at ankle level while the patient is supine. A drop in segmental BP of greater than 30 mm Hg suggests PAD. Angiography and magnetic resonance angiography delineate the location and extent of PAD (see Table 32-6).

The *ankle-brachial index* (ABI) is a PAD screening tool. It is performed using a hand-held Doppler. The ABI is calculated by dividing the ankle systolic BPs by the higher of the left and right brachial systolic BPs. PAD guidelines recommend uniform reporting of ABI results[12] (Table 38-3). In very elderly patients and those with diabetes, the arteries often are calcified and noncompressible. This results in a falsely elevated ABI. ABI measurement is not recommended immediately after revascularization surgery or on distal bypass grafts because of the risk of graft thrombosis.[13]

Collaborative Care

Table 38-2 summarizes the collaborative care for a patient with PAD.

Risk Factor Modification. The first treatment goal in treating PAD is to reduce CVD risk factors in all patients with PAD regardless of the severity of symptoms.[14] Risk factors need to be

TABLE 38-2   COLLABORATIVE CARE

Peripheral Artery Disease

Diagnostic
- Health history and physical examination, including palpation of peripheral pulses
- Doppler ultrasound studies
- Segmental blood pressures
- Ankle-brachial index (see Table 38-3)
- Duplex imaging
- Angiography
- Magnetic resonance angiography

Collaborative Therapy
- Cardiovascular disease risk factor modification
  - Tobacco cessation
  - Regular physical exercise
  - Achieve or maintain ideal body weight
  - Follow Dietary Approaches to Stop Hypertension (DASH) diet (see eTable 33-1)
  - Tight glucose control in diabetics
  - Tight blood pressure control
  - Treatment of hyperlipidemia and hypertriglyceridemia (see Table 34-5)
  - Antiplatelet agent (aspirin or clopidogrel [Plavix])
  - Angiotensin-converting enzyme inhibitors (see Table 33-7)
- Treatment of claudication symptoms
  - Structured walking or exercise program
  - Cilostazol (Pletal)
- Nutrition therapy
- Proper foot care (see Table 49-21)
- Percutaneous transluminal balloon angioplasty with or without stent
- Percutaneous transluminal atherectomy
- Percutaneous transluminal cryoplasty
- Peripheral artery bypass surgery
- Patch graft angioplasty, often in conjunction with bypass surgery
- Endarterectomy (for localized stenosis but rarely done)
- Thrombolytic therapy or mechanical clot extraction therapy (for acute ischemia only)
- Sympathectomy (for pain management only)
- Amputation

TABLE 38-3   INTERPRETATION OF ANKLE-BRACHIAL INDEX RESULTS

Ankle-Brachial Index (ABI)	Clinical Significance
≥1.40	Noncompressible arteries
1.00-1.40	Normal ABI
0.91-0.99	Borderline ABI
≤0.90	Abnormal ABI
Classification of PAD Severity	
0.90-0.71	Mild PAD
0.71-0.41	Moderate PAD
≤40	Severe PAD

PAD, Peripheral artery disease.

modified with both drug therapy and lifestyle changes (see Tables 34-3 to 34-5).

Tobacco cessation is essential to reduce the risk of CVD events, PAD progression, and death. This is a complex and difficult process with a high incidence of smoking relapse. Comprehensive tobacco cessation strategies are recommended (see Tables 11-4 to 11-6).

Diabetes is a major risk factor for PAD and increases the risk of amputation in these patients. It is recommended that diabetic patients maintain a glycosylated hemoglobin (Hb A1C) below 7.0% and, optimally, as near as possible to 6.0%.[15] (Chapter 49 discusses diabetes mellitus.)

Aggressive lipid management is essential for all patients with PAD.[14] Both dietary interventions and drug therapy are needed. Statins (e.g., simvastatin [Zocor]) lower low-density lipoprotein (LDL) and triglyceride levels and reduce CVD morbidity and mortality risks.[16] Unfortunately, as many as 70% of people with PAD do not take a statin and have elevated LDL levels.[2]

Hypertension is a well-known risk factor for PAD progression, as well as other CVD events (e.g., stroke, myocardial infarction [MI], heart failure). Guidelines for the management of hypertension in persons with PAD include BP less than 140/90 mm Hg.[2,14] In PAD patients with diabetes or renal insufficiency, BP less than 130/80 mm Hg is recommended.[15]

Initial antihypertensive therapy includes thiazides and angiotensin-converting enzyme (ACE) inhibitors (e.g., ramipril [Altace]). Lifestyle changes are encouraged and include reducing dietary sodium and following the Dietary Approaches to Stop Hypertension (DASH) diet. (Chapter 33 discusses hypertension.)

Drug Therapy. Antiplatelet agents are considered critical for reducing the risks of CVD events and death in PAD patients. Oral antiplatelet therapy should include 75 to 100 mg/day of aspirin for patients with asymptomatic PAD and 75 to 325 mg/day of aspirin for patients with symptomatic PAD.[11,12] Aspirin-intolerant patients may take clopidogrel (Plavix) daily.

Combination antiplatelet therapy with aspirin and clopidogrel is not typically recommended, but may be used in symptomatic PAD patients at high risk for CVD events.[12] Anticoagulants (e.g., warfarin [Coumadin]) are not recommended for the prevention of CVD events in PAD patients.

> **DRUG ALERT: Clopidogrel (Plavix) and Omeprazole (Prilosec)**
> - Antiplatelet effect of clopidogrel is reduced by about half when given with omeprazole.
> - This increases the risk of MI and stroke.

Two drugs are available to treat intermittent claudication: cilostazol (Pletal) and pentoxifylline (Trental). Cilostazol, a phosphodiesterase inhibitor, inhibits platelet aggregation and increases vasodilation. It is recommended as first-line drug therapy for patients with intermittent claudication who do not respond to exercise therapy or stop using tobacco.[11] Cilostazol does not reduce CVD morbidity and mortality risks, so antiplatelet therapy is also needed.

> **DRUG ALERT: Cilostazol (Pletal)**
> - Contraindicated in patients with heart failure of any severity.

Exercise Therapy. The primary nondrug treatment for intermittent claudication is tobacco cessation in combination with a formal, supervised exercise training program. Exercise improves walking ability. Lack of exercise and impaired walking ability in PAD patients is related to low quality of life.[17] Encouragement of participation in exercise is particularly important for women with PAD, since women experience faster functional decline and greater mobility loss than men with PAD.[17] In addition, women with PAD are more likely to have a history of limited recreational activities.[8]

Walking is the most effective exercise for PAD patients. A supervised PAD rehabilitation program is an effective means of improving exercise performance. Such programs typically include exercise for 30 to 60 minutes/day, 3 to 5 times/week, for 3 to 6 months. Supervised treadmill exercise training improves walking performance and quality of life in PAD patients, whether or not they have claudication.[17]

A home exercise program is an effective alternative to supervised rehabilitation. Encourage slow, progressive physical activity after a warm-up period. Instruct the patient to walk to the point of discomfort, stop and rest, and then resume walking until the discomfort recurs. Walking should be done for 30 to 40 minutes/day, 3 to 5 times/week. An exercise therapy program should also be implemented in PAD patients after surgical interventions (discussed later in this chapter).

Nutritional Therapy. Teach PAD patients to adjust their dietary intake so that their body mass index (BMI) is less than 25 kg/m^2 and their waist circumference is less than 40 inches for men and less than 35 inches for women.[18] Recommend a diet high in fruits, vegetables, and whole grains and low in cholesterol, saturated fat, and salt (see Chapters 34 and 35).

Complementary and Alternative Therapies. Patients taking antiplatelet agents, nonsteroidal antiinflammatory drugs (NSAIDs) (e.g., ibuprofen [Motrin]), and anticoagulants (e.g., warfarin) should consult with their health care provider before taking any dietary or herbal supplements because of potential interactions and bleeding risks[19] (see the Complementary & Alternative Therapies box on p. 851).

Care of the Leg With Critical Limb Ischemia. Critical limb ischemia is a condition characterized by chronic ischemic rest pain lasting more than 2 weeks, arterial leg ulcers, or gangrene of the leg as a result of PAD.[12] Optimal therapy is revascularization via bypass surgery. If this is not feasible, percutaneous transluminal angioplasty (PTA) is recommended in patients with a life expectancy of 2 years or less.[12] Patients with critical limb ischemia who are not candidates for surgery or PTA may be treated with prostanoids (e.g., iloprost [Ventavis]). These drugs may decrease rest pain and improve ulcer healing. Patients with critical limb ischemia should continue CVD risk factor reduction and antiplatelet therapy to reduce the risk of a CVD event.

Conservative management of critical limb ischemia includes protecting the extremity from trauma, decreasing ischemic pain, preventing and controlling infection, and improving perfusion. Carefully inspect, cleanse, and lubricate both feet to prevent cracking of the skin and infection. Avoid soaking the patient's feet to prevent skin *maceration* (or breakdown). If ulceration is present, keep the affected foot clean and dry. Cover any ulcers with a dry, sterile dressing to maintain cleanliness. Deep ulcers can be treated with a variety of wound care products, but healing is unlikely without increased blood flow.

Encourage the patient to select soft, roomy, and protective footwear and avoid extremes of heat and cold. Keep the patient's heels free of pressure. You can do this by placing a pillow under the calves so that the heels are off the mattress. Commercially available devices can also provide heel protection. Administering opioid analgesics and placing the bed in the reverse Trendelenburg position may control pain and increase perfusion to the lower extremities.

Spinal cord stimulation may be helpful in managing pain and preventing amputation in patients with critical limb ischemia. Other promising strategies include gene therapy and endothelial progenitor cell therapy to stimulate blood vessel growth (*angiogenesis*).[20]

Interventional Radiology Catheter-Based Procedures. Interventional radiology catheter-based procedures are alternatives to open surgical approaches for treatment of lower extremity PAD. These procedures take place in a catheterization laboratory rather than in an operating room. Determining which intervention to use depends on blockage location and lesion type and severity.

All these procedures are similar to angiography in that they involve the insertion of a specialized catheter into the femoral artery. The *percutaneous transluminal angioplasty* (PTA) procedure uses a catheter that contains a cylindric balloon at the tip. The end of the catheter is moved to the narrowed (stenotic) area of the artery. The balloon is then inflated, compressing the atherosclerotic intimal lining.[21]

Stents, expandable metallic devices, are positioned within the artery immediately after the balloon angioplasty is done. The stent acts as a scaffold to keep the artery open. The stents may be covered with Dacron or a drug-eluting agent (e.g., paclitaxel) to reduce restenosis by limiting the amount of new tissue growth in the stent.

Atherectomy is the removal of the obstructing plaque. A directional atherectomy device uses a high-speed cutting disk that cuts long strips of the atheroma. Laser atherectomy uses ultraviolet energy to break up the atheroma. Orbital or rotational atherectomy catheters have a diamond-coated tip that rotates at a high speed (similar to a dentist drill). These crush the calcium within the atheroma into particles smaller than a blood cell.

Cryoplasty combines two procedures: PTA and cold therapy. A specialized balloon is filled with liquid nitrous oxide, which changes from liquid to gas as it enters the balloon. Expansion of the gas results in cooling to 14° F (−10° C). The cold limits restenosis by reducing smooth muscle cell activity.[22] Preprocedure and postprocedure nursing care is the same as for a diagnostic angiography. Antiplatelet agents are needed after the procedure to reduce the risk of restenosis. Long-term, low-dose aspirin therapy (75 to 100 mg/day) or clopidogrel (75 mg/day) is recommended. Restenosis rates depend on the procedure performed, lesion type and length, and target vessel characteristics. Immediate postprocedure success rates are high (greater than 95%) for iliac and femoral interventions.[23]

Surgical Therapy. Various surgical approaches can be used to improve blood flow beyond a blocked artery. The most common is peripheral artery bypass surgery with an autogenous (native) vein or synthetic graft to bypass, or carry blood around, the lesion (Fig. 38-2). Synthetic grafts typically are used for long bypasses such as an axillary-femoral bypass. When a person's own vein is not available, human umbilical vein or a composite sequential bypass graft (native vein plus synthetic graft) is an alternative.[14] PTA with stenting may also be used in combination with bypass surgery. Other surgical options include *endarterectomy* (opening the artery and removing the obstructing plaque) and *patch graft angioplasty* (opening the artery, removing plaque, and sewing a patch to the opening to widen the lumen).

Amputation may be required if tissue necrosis is extensive, gangrene or osteomyelitis develops, or all major arteries in the limb are blocked, precluding the possibility of successful surgery.[20] Every effort is made to preserve as much of the limb as possible to improve the potential for rehabilitation. (Amputation is discussed in Chapter 63.)

NURSING MANAGEMENT
LOWER EXTREMITY PERIPHERAL ARTERY DISEASE

NURSING ASSESSMENT

Table 38-4 presents subjective and objective data that you should obtain from a patient with PAD.

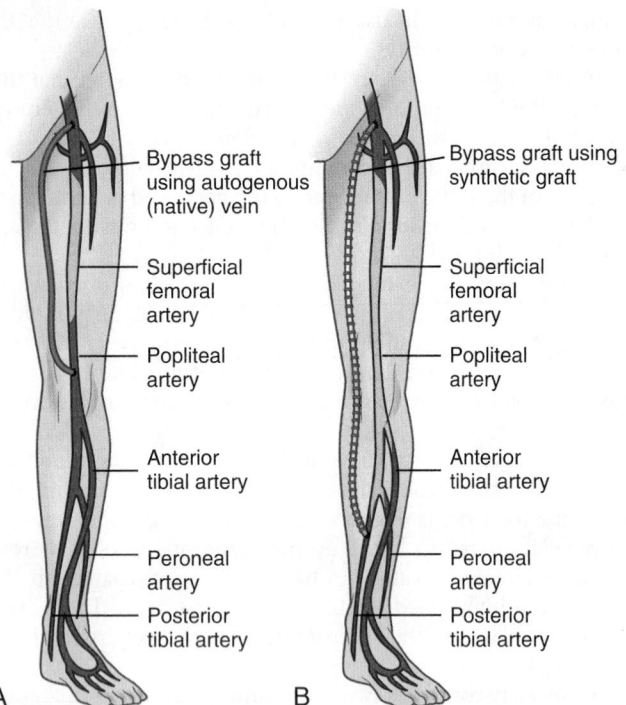

FIG. 38-2 A, Femoral-popliteal bypass graft around an occluded superficial femoral artery. **B,** Femoral–posterior tibial bypass graft around occluded superficial femoral, popliteal, and proximal tibial arteries.

NURSING DIAGNOSES

Nursing diagnoses for the patient with PAD may include, but are not limited to, the following:

- Ineffective peripheral tissue perfusion *related to* deficient knowledge of contributing factors
- Activity intolerance *related to* imbalance between oxygen supply and demand
- Ineffective self-health management *related to* lack of knowledge of disease and self-care measures

Additional information on nursing diagnoses for the patient with PAD of the lower extremities is presented in eNursing Care Plan 38-1 on the website for this chapter.

PLANNING

The overall goals for the patient who has lower extremity PAD include (1) adequate tissue perfusion; (2) relief of pain; (3) increased exercise tolerance; and (4) intact, healthy skin on the extremities.

NURSING IMPLEMENTATION

HEALTH PROMOTION. Assess the patient for CVD risk factors and provide instructions on how to control them (see Tables 34-2 to 34-4). Also teach diet modification to reduce the intake of cholesterol, saturated fat, and refined sugars; proper care of the feet; and avoidance of injury to the extremities. Encourage patients with positive family histories of cardiac, diabetic, or vascular disease to obtain regular follow-up care.

ACUTE INTERVENTION. After surgical or radiologic intervention, the patient is moved to a recovery area for observation. Check the operative extremity every 15 minutes initially and then hourly for color, temperature, capillary refill, presence of peripheral pulses, and sensation and movement. Loss of palpable pulses or a change in the Doppler sound over a pulse requires immediate notification of the physician or radiologist

TABLE 38-4   NURSING ASSESSMENT
Peripheral Artery Disease

Subjective Data
Important Health Information
Past health history: Tobacco use, diabetes mellitus, hypertension, hyperlipidemia, hypertriglyceridemia, hyperuricemia, impaired renal function, obesity; ↑ high-sensitivity C-reactive protein, homocysteine, or lipoprotein (a) [Lp(a)] levels; positive family history, sedentary lifestyle, stress

Functional Health Patterns
Health perception–health management: Family history of cardiovascular disease; tobacco use, including exposure to environmental smoke
Nutritional-metabolic: High sodium, saturated fat, and cholesterol intake; elevated Hb A1C
Activity-exercise: Exercise intolerance
Cognitive-perceptual: Buttock, thigh, or calf pain that is precipitated by exercise and that subsides with rest (intermittent claudication) or progresses to pain at rest; burning pain in forefeet and toes at rest; numbness, tingling, sensation of cold in legs or feet; progressive loss of sensation and deep pain in extremities
Sexuality-reproductive: Erectile dysfunction

Objective Data
Integumentary
Loss of hair on legs and feet; thick toenails; pallor with elevation; dependent rubor; thin, cool, shiny skin with muscle atrophy; skin breakdown and arterial ulcers, especially over bony areas; gangrene

Cardiovascular
Decreased or absent peripheral pulses; feet cool to touch; capillary refill >3 sec; bruits may be present at pulse sites

Neurologic
Mobility or sensation impairment

Possible Diagnostic Findings
Arterial stenosis evident with duplex imaging, ↓ Doppler pressures, ↓ ankle-brachial index, angiography indicative of peripheral atherosclerosis

and prompt intervention. Postoperative ABI measurements are not recommended as they place the patient at risk for graft thrombosis.[13] Compare all assessment findings with the patient's baseline and with findings in the opposite limb.

Many PAD patients have a history of chronic ischemic rest pain and may have developed a tolerance to opioids. Thus aggressive pain management may be needed postoperatively.

After the patient leaves the recovery area, continue to monitor perfusion to the extremities. Assess for potential complications such as bleeding, hematoma, thrombosis, embolization, and compartment syndrome. A dramatic increase in pain, loss of previously palpable pulses, extremity pallor or cyanosis, decreasing ABIs, numbness or tingling, or a cold extremity suggests blockage of the graft or stent. Report these findings to the physician immediately. Women, particularly African American women, experience more graft failure and amputation after lower extremity bypass surgery than men.[6]

Avoid placing the patient in a knee-flexed position except for exercise. Turn the patient and position frequently with pillows to support the incision. On postoperative day 1, assist the patient out of bed several times daily. Discourage prolonged sitting with leg dependency, since it may cause pain and edema, increase the risk of venous thrombosis, and place stress on the suture lines. If edema develops, position the patient supine and elevate the leg above heart level. Occasionally, elastic compression stockings are used to help control leg edema. Walking even short distances is desirable. The use of a walker may be helpful, especially in frail, older patients.

Surgical site infection (SSI) after lower extremity revascularization occurs in about 11% of cases. Women develop SSIs more often than men. Careful postoperative assessment and wound care are important. SSIs are associated with early graft loss, reoperation, and sepsis.[24] If no complications occur, discharge can be anticipated 3 to 5 days after surgery.

AMBULATORY AND HOME CARE. Assess for CVD risk factors and be alert for opportunities to teach health promotion strategies to patients and their caregivers (see Chapters 4 and 34). Continued tobacco use dramatically decreases the long-term patency rates of grafts and stents and increases the risk of an MI or stroke. Long-term therapy with aspirin or clopidogrel is recommended for patients after surgery. Patients having distal peripheral bypass surgery (i.e., below the knee) using synthetic graft materials are given dual antiplatelet therapy (clopidogrel plus aspirin) for 1 year, followed by lifelong single antiplatelet therapy.

Encourage supervised exercise training after a successful revascularization. Explain that exercise improves a number of CVD risk factors, including hypertension, hyperlipidemia, obesity, and glucose levels. Teach foot care to all patients with PAD. Meticulous foot care is especially important in the diabetic patient with PAD (see Table 49-21). Diabetic neuropathy increases the patient's risk for injury and results in delay in seeking treatment. Instruct patients to inspect their legs and feet daily for mottling, changes in skin color or texture, and reduction in hair growth. Show patients how to check skin temperature and capillary refill and to palpate pulses. Emphasize that they must report any changes in these findings or the development of ulceration or inflammation to their health care provider. Thick or overgrown toenails and calluses are potentially serious and require regular attention by a health care provider (e.g., podiatrist). Patients who have poor eyesight, back problems, obesity, or arthritis may need help with foot care. Encourage patients to wear clean, all-cotton or all-wool socks and comfortable shoes with rounded (not pointed) toes and soft insoles. Tell patients to lace shoes loosely and to break in new shoes gradually (Table 38-5).

EVALUATION

The expected outcomes for the patient with PAD of the lower extremities include
- Adequate peripheral tissue perfusion
- Increased activity tolerance
- Knowledge of disease and treatment plan

Additional information on the expected outcomes for the patient with PAD of the lower extremities are presented in eNursing Care Plan 38-1 (available on the website for this chapter).

ACUTE ARTERIAL ISCHEMIC DISORDERS

Etiology and Pathophysiology

Acute arterial ischemia is a sudden interruption in the arterial blood supply to a tissue, an organ, or an extremity that, if left untreated, can result in tissue death. It is caused by embolism, thrombosis of a preexisting atherosclerotic artery, or trauma. *Embolization* of a thrombus from the heart is the most frequent cause of acute arterial occlusion. Heart conditions in which

---

TABLE 38-5 PATIENT & CAREGIVER TEACHING GUIDE

Peripheral Artery Bypass Surgery

Include the following information in the teaching plan for a patient undergoing peripheral artery bypass surgery and the patient's caregiver.

1. Reduce risk factors by stopping the use of all tobacco products, controlling blood glucose levels (if diabetic) and blood pressure, lowering cholesterol and triglyceride levels, achieving or maintaining ideal body weight, and exercising regularly.
2. Provide rationales, basic action, and anticipated duration of medications such as antiplatelets, antihypertensives, lipid-lowering therapy, and pain medication.
3. Eat healthy—it is essential to recovery. Drink plenty of fluids, eat a well-balanced diet (e.g., foods high in protein, vitamins C and A, and zinc; high-fiber foods; fresh fruits and vegetables), eat fewer high-fat foods, and reduce salt intake.
4. Participate in a supervised exercise program or take a daily walk. In the beginning, take several short walks a day and rest between activities. Gradually increase your walking to 30 to 40 min/day, 3 to 5 days/wk.
5. Care for feet and legs. Inspect feet and wash them daily. Wear clean cotton or wool socks and well-fitting shoes. File toenails straight across. Avoid sitting with legs crossed, extreme hot and cold temperatures, and prolonged standing.
6. Follow routine postoperative wound care that includes keeping incision clean and dry; do not disturb Steri-Strips (if present).
7. Monitor for signs and symptoms of impaired healing or infection of the leg incision, and notify health care provider if any of the following occurs:
   - Prolonged drainage or pus from the incision
   - Increased redness, warmth, pain, or hardness along incision
   - Separation of wound edges
   - Temperature >100° F (37.8° C)
8. Keep all follow-up appointments with health care provider.
9. Notify health care provider immediately of increased leg or foot pain or a change in the color or temperature of leg or foot.

---

thrombi can develop include infective endocarditis, mitral valve disease, atrial fibrillation, cardiomyopathies, and prosthetic heart valves. Noncardiac sources of emboli include aneurysms, ulcerated atherosclerotic plaque, recent endovascular procedures, and venous thrombi.

The thrombi become dislodged and may travel anywhere in the systemic circulation if they originate in the left side of the heart. Most emboli block an artery of the lower extremity in areas where vessels branch (e.g., iliofemoral, popliteal, tibial) or there is atherosclerotic narrowing. Sudden local thrombosis may occur at the site of an atherosclerotic plaque. Hypovolemia (e.g., shock), hyperviscosity (e.g., polycythemia), and hypercoagulability (e.g., chemotherapy) predispose an individual to thrombotic arterial occlusion.[25]

Traumatic injury to the extremity itself may cause partial or total blockage. Acute arterial occlusion may also develop as a result of arterial dissection in the carotid artery or aorta or as a result of a procedure-related arterial injury (e.g., after angiography).

Clinical Manifestations

Clinical manifestations of acute arterial ischemia include the *"six Ps": pain, pallor, pulselessness, paresthesia, paralysis,* and *poikilothermia* (adaptation of the limb to the environmental temperature, most often cool). Without immediate intervention, ischemia may progress to tissue necrosis and gangrene within a few hours. If you detect these signs, immediately notify the physician. Paralysis is a late sign of acute arterial ischemia and signals the death of nerves supplying the extremity. Foot drop occurs as a result of nerve damage. Because nerve tissue is extremely sensitive to hypoxia, limb paralysis or ischemic neuropathy may persist even after revascularization.

Collaborative Care

Early treatment is essential to keep the affected limb viable during acute arterial ischemia. Anticoagulant therapy with IV unfractionated heparin (UH) is started to prevent thrombus growth and inhibit further embolization.[11] In patients undergoing embolectomy, UH should be followed by long-term anticoagulation with warfarin (see discussion of other anticoagulant options later in this chapter).

To restore blood flow, the thrombus is removed as soon as possible. Options consist of surgical thrombectomy (recommended procedure), percutaneous catheter-directed thrombolytic therapy, percutaneous mechanical thrombectomy with or without thrombolytic therapy, or surgical bypass.

If surgical thrombectomy is not possible, percutaneous catheter-directed thrombolytic therapy using tissue plasminogen activator (tPA [alteplase]) or urokinase (Kinlytic) is recommended. A catheter is inserted into the femoral artery and moved to the site of the clot, and the thrombolytic drug is infused. Thrombolytic agents work by directly dissolving the clot over a period of 24 to 48 hours. (Chapter 34 discusses thrombolytic therapy.) Another type of catheter may act as a mechanical thrombectomy device, meaning it is also designed to remove or fragment the thrombus.[26] Surgical revascularization may be used in a patient with trauma (e.g., laceration of the artery) or with significant arterial blockage. Amputation is reserved for patients with ischemic rest pain and tissue loss in whom limb salvage is not possible. If the patient remains at risk for further embolization from a persistent source (e.g., chronic atrial fibrillation), long-term oral anticoagulation is recommended to prevent further acute arterial ischemic episodes[27] (see Table 38-10 later in this chapter).

THROMBOANGIITIS OBLITERANS

Thromboangiitis obliterans (Buerger's disease) is a nonatherosclerotic, segmental, recurrent inflammatory disorder of the small- and medium-sized arteries and veins of the upper and lower extremities. Rarely, systemic manifestations of the disease may involve cerebral, coronary, mesenteric, pulmonary, and/or renal arteries. The disease occurs mostly in young men (less than 45 years of age) with a long history of tobacco and/or marijuana use and chronic periodontal infection, but without other CVD risk factors (e.g., hypertension, hyperlipidemia, diabetes).[28]

In the acute phase of Buerger's disease, an inflammatory thrombus forms and blocks the vessel. Over time, the thrombus becomes more organized and the inflammation subsides.[28] During the chronic phase, thrombosis and fibrosis occur in the vessel, causing tissue ischemia. The symptoms of Buerger's disease often are confused with PAD and other autoimmune diseases (e.g., scleroderma). Patients may have intermittent claudication of the feet, hands, or arms. As the disease progresses, rest pain and ischemic ulcerations develop. Other signs and symptoms may include color and temperature changes of the limbs, paresthesia, superficial vein thrombosis, and cold sensitivity.

There are no laboratory or diagnostic tests specific to Buerger's disease. Diagnosis is made based on age of onset; history; clinical symptoms; involvement of distal vessels; presence of ischemic ulcerations; and exclusion of autoimmune disease, diabetes, thrombophilia (inherited tendency to clot), and other source of emboli.[28]

The mainstay of treatment for Buerger's disease is the complete cessation of tobacco and marijuana use in any form. Use of nicotine replacement products is contraindicated. Patients must choose between their tobacco or marijuana and their affected limb, but not both. Conservative management includes avoiding limb exposure to cold temperatures, a supervised walking program, antibiotics to treat any infected ulcers, and analgesics to manage the ischemic pain. Teach patients to avoid trauma to the extremities.

A variety of drugs have been tried to treat Buerger's disease (e.g., calcium channel blockers, cilostazol, sildenafil [Viagra]), but evidence supporting their use is lacking. One promising drug has been IV iloprost. This has been shown to improve rest pain, promote healing of ischemic ulcers, and decrease the need for amputation.[28]

Surgical options include *sympathectomy* (transection of a nerve, ganglion, and/or plexus of the sympathetic nervous system), implantation of a spinal cord stimulator, and bypass surgery. Sympathectomy and implantation of a spinal cord stimulator can improve distal blood flow and reduce pain, but neither alters the inflammatory process. Bypass surgery typically is not an option because of the involvement of smaller, distal vessels but may be used in selected patients with severe ischemia. Painful ulcerations may require finger or toe amputations. Amputation below the knee may occur in severe cases. The rate of amputation in patients who continue tobacco or marijuana use after diagnosis is much higher than in those who stop.[28,29]

RAYNAUD'S PHENOMENON

Raynaud's phenomenon is an episodic vasospastic disorder of small cutaneous arteries, most often involving the fingers and toes. It occurs primarily in young women (typically between 15 and 40 years of age), and it is more common in women than men. The pathogenesis of Raynaud's phenomenon is due to abnormalities in the vascular, intravascular, and neuronal mechanisms that cause an imbalance between vasodilation and vasoconstriction.[30]

Raynaud's phenomenon may occur in isolation or in association with an underlying disease (e.g., rheumatoid arthritis, scleroderma, systemic lupus erythematosus). Other contributing factors include occupation-related conditions, such as use of vibrating machinery or work in cold environments, exposure to heavy metals (e.g., lead), and hyperhomocysteinemia.[30] Diagnosis is based on persistent symptoms for at least 2 years. Patients with Raynaud's phenomenon should have routine follow-up to monitor for development of connective tissue or autoimmune diseases.[31]

Raynaud's phenomenon is characterized by vasospasm-induced color changes of fingers, toes, ears, and nose (white, blue, and red). Decreased perfusion results in pallor (white). The digits then appear cyanotic (bluish purple) (Fig. 38-3). These changes are followed by rubor (red), caused by the hyperemic response that occurs when blood flow is restored. The patient usually describes coldness and numbness in the vasoconstrictive phase. This is followed by throbbing, aching pain,

FIG. 38-3 Raynaud's phenomenon.

FIG. 38-4 Angiography demonstrating fusiform abdominal aortic aneurysm. Note calcification of the aortic wall *(arrows)* and extension of the aneurysm into the common iliac arteries.

tingling, and swelling in the hyperemic phase. An episode usually lasts only minutes but in severe cases may persist for several hours. Exposure to cold, emotional upsets, tobacco use, and caffeine often bring on symptoms.

After frequent, prolonged attacks the skin may become thickened and the nails brittle. Occasionally, complications include *punctate* (small hole) lesions of the fingertips and superficial gangrenous ulcers in advanced stages.

The primary focus of nursing management of Raynaud's phenomenon is patient teaching. Focus your instructions on preventing recurrent episodes. Tell patients to wear loose, warm clothing as protection from the cold, including gloves when handling cold objects. At all times, patients should avoid temperature extremes. Immersing hands in warm water often decreases the vasospasm. The patient should stop using all tobacco products and avoid caffeine and other drugs that have vasoconstrictive effects (e.g., cocaine, amphetamines, ergotamine, pseudoephedrine). Finally, provide patients with stress management strategies as appropriate.

When conservative management is ineffective, drug therapy is considered. Sustained-release calcium channel blockers (e.g., nifedipine [Procardia]) are the first-line drug therapy.[31] Calcium channel blockers relax smooth muscles of the arterioles by blocking the influx of calcium into the cells. This reduces the frequency and severity of vasospastic attacks.

Prompt intervention is needed for patients with digital ulceration and/or critical ischemia. Treatment options include IV prostanoid therapy (e.g., iloprost), antibiotics, analgesics, and possibly an endothelin receptor antagonist (e.g., bosentan [Tracleer]) and surgical debridement of necrotic tissue.[31] Sympathectomy is considered only in advanced cases.

AORTIC ANEURYSMS

The aorta is the largest artery and supplies oxygen, nutrients, and blood to all vital organs. One of the most common problems affecting the aorta is an **aneurysm**, which is a permanent, localized outpouching or dilation of the vessel wall. Aneurysms occur in men more often than in women, and the incidence increases with age. Aneurysms may occur in more than one location. Peripheral artery aneurysms can also develop but are not common.

Etiology and Pathophysiology

Aortic aneurysms may involve the aortic arch and thoracic and/or abdominal aorta. Three fourths of aortic aneurysms occur in

the abdominal aorta (Fig. 38-4) and one fourth in the thoracic aorta. About 1.1 million adults between 55 and 84 years of age have an abdominal aortic aneurysm (AAA).[32] Most AAAs occur below the renal arteries. An abdominal aorta larger than 3 cm in diameter is considered aneurysmal. Growth rates are unpredictable, but the larger the aneurysm, the greater the risk of rupture.

A variety of disorders are associated with aortic aneurysms. The primary causes are classified as degenerative, congenital, mechanical (e.g., penetrating or blunt trauma), inflammatory (e.g., aortitis [Takayasu's arteritis]), or infectious (e.g., aortitis [*Chlamydia pneumoniae,* human immunodeficiency virus]).

Risk factors for aortic aneurysms include age, male gender, hypertension, coronary artery disease, family history, high cholesterol, lower extremity PAD, carotid artery disease, previous stroke, tobacco use, and excess weight or obesity. Male gender, older age, and tobacco use are the most important risk factors. Whites and Native Americans have a higher risk of AAA development than African Americans, Hispanics, and Asian Americans.[32]

Genetic Link

The development of aortic aneurysm and dissection has a strong genetic component. The familial tendency is related to a number of congenital anomalies. Examples include bicuspid aortic valve, coarctation of the aorta, Turner syndrome, autosomal dominant polycystic kidney disease, specific collagen defects (e.g., Ehlers-Danlos syndrome), and premature breakdown of vascular elastic tissue (e.g., Loeys-Dietz syndrome, Marfan's syndrome).[33]

Classification

Aneurysms are classified as true or false aneurysms (Fig. 38-5, *A* to *C*). A *true aneurysm* is one in which the wall of the artery forms the aneurysm, with at least one vessel layer still intact. True aneurysms are further subdivided into fusiform and saccular types. A *fusiform aneurysm* is circumferential and relatively uniform in shape. A *saccular aneurysm* is pouchlike with

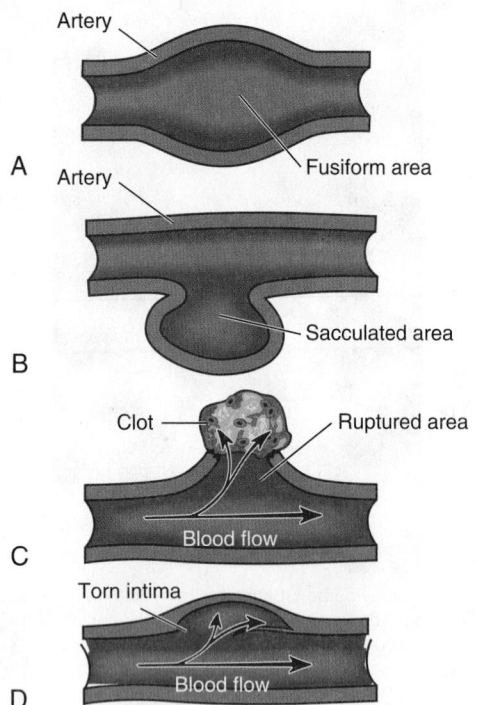

FIG. 38-5 A, True fusiform abdominal aortic aneurysm. **B,** True saccular aortic aneurysm. **C,** False aneurysm, or pseudoaneurysm. **D,** Aortic dissection.

a narrow neck connecting the bulge to one side of the arterial wall.

A *false aneurysm,* or *pseudoaneurysm,* is not an aneurysm but a disruption of all arterial wall layers with bleeding that is contained by surrounding anatomic structures. False aneurysms may result from trauma, infection, peripheral artery bypass graft surgery (at the site of the graft-to-artery anastomosis), or arterial leakage after removal of cannulae (e.g., femoral artery catheters, intraaortic balloon pump devices).[33]

Clinical Manifestations

Thoracic aortic aneurysms (TAAs) are often asymptomatic. When present, symptoms include deep, diffuse chest pain that may extend to the interscapular area. Ascending aorta and aortic arch aneurysms can produce angina from decreased blood flow to the coronary arteries and hoarseness from pressure on the laryngeal nerve. Pressure on the esophagus can cause dysphagia. If the aneurysm presses on the superior vena cava, decreased venous return can result in jugular venous distention (distended neck veins) and edema of the face and the arms.

AAAs also are often asymptomatic and frequently found during routine physical examinations or evaluations for an unrelated problem (e.g., abdominal x-ray, computed tomography [CT] scan). A pulsatile mass in the periumbilical area slightly to the left of the midline may be present. Bruits may be auscultated over the aneurysm. Physical findings may be more difficult to detect in obese individuals.

AAA symptoms may mimic pain associated with abdominal or back disorders. Compression of nearby anatomic structures and nerves may cause symptoms such as back pain, epigastric discomfort, and altered bowel elimination. Occasionally, aneurysms spontaneously embolize plaque, causing *"blue toe syn-*

drome" (patchy mottling of the feet and toes in the presence of palpable pedal pulses).

Complications

Rupture of an aneurysm is the most serious complication. If rupture occurs into the retroperitoneal space, bleeding may be controlled by surrounding anatomic structures, preventing exsanguination and death. In this case the patient often has severe back pain and may or may not have back or flank ecchymosis *(Grey Turner's sign).* If rupture occurs into the thoracic or abdominal cavity, more than 90% of patients will die from massive hemorrhage.[4] The patient who reaches the hospital will be in hypovolemic shock with tachycardia, hypotension, pale clammy skin, decreased urine output, altered level of consciousness, and abdominal tenderness. (Shock is discussed in Chapter 67.) In this situation, simultaneous resuscitation and immediate surgical repair are necessary.

Diagnostic Studies

Chest x-rays are done to reveal abnormal widening of the thoracic aorta. An abdominal x-ray may show calcification within the aortic wall. An electrocardiogram (ECG) may rule out MI, since thoracic aneurysm or dissection symptoms can mimic angina. Echocardiography assesses the function of the aortic valve. Ultrasound is useful for aneurysm screening and to monitor aneurysm size. A CT scan is the most accurate test to determine the length and cross-sectional diameter and the presence of thrombus in the aneurysm. Magnetic resonance imaging (MRI) also may be used to diagnose and assess the location and severity of aneurysms. *Angiography* provides helpful information by using contrast imaging to map the entire aortic system. (Chapter 32 and Table 32-6 discuss angiography.)

Collaborative Care

The goal of both medical and surgical management is to prevent aneurysm rupture. Early detection and prompt treatment are essential. Conservative therapy of small, asymptomatic AAAs (4.0 to 5.5 cm) is the best practice.[34] This consists of risk factor modification (ceasing tobacco use, decreasing BP, optimizing lipid profile) and annual monitoring of aneurysm size using ultrasound, CT, or MRI. Growth rates may be lowered with β-adrenergic blocking agents (e.g. propranolol [Inderal]), statins (e.g., simvastatin), and antibiotics (e.g., doxycycline).[33]

Surgical repair is recommended in patients with asymptomatic aneurysms 5.5 cm in diameter or larger. Surgical intervention may occur sooner if the patient has a genetic disorder (e.g., Marfan's, Ehlers-Danlos syndrome), the aneurysm expands rapidly, it becomes symptomatic, or the risk of rupture is high.[12] A careful review of body systems is necessary to identify any co-morbidities, especially of the lungs, heart, or kidney, because they can influence the patient's surgical risk. Correction of existing carotid or coronary artery blockages may be needed before the aneurysm is repaired.

Surgical Therapy. For elective surgery, the patient is well hydrated, and any electrolyte, coagulation, and hematocrit abnormalities are corrected preoperatively. If the aneurysm has ruptured, emergent surgical intervention is required.

The open aneurysm repair (OAR) involves a large abdominal incision through which the surgeon (1) cuts into the diseased aortic segment, (2) removes any thrombus or plaque, (3) sutures a synthetic graft to the aorta proximal and distal to the aneurysm, and (4) sutures the native aortic wall around the graft to

FIG. 38-6 Surgical repair of an abdominal aortic aneurysm. **A,** Incising the aneurysmal sac. **B,** Insertion of synthetic graft. **C,** Suturing native aortic wall over synthetic graft.

FIG. 38-7 Bifurcated (two-branched) endovascular stent grafting of an aneurysm. **A,** Insertion of a woven polyester tube (graft) covered by a tubular metal web (stent). **B,** The stent graft is inserted through a large blood vessel (e.g., femoral artery) using a delivery catheter. The catheter is positioned below the renal arteries in the area of the aneurysm. **C,** The stent graft is slowly released (deployed) into the blood vessel. When the stent comes in contact with the blood vessel, it expands to a preset size. **D,** A second stent graft can be inserted in the contralateral (opposite) vessel if necessary. **E,** Fully deployed bifurcated stent graft.

act as a protective cover (Fig. 38-6). If the iliac arteries are also aneurysmal, a bifurcated graft replaces the entire diseased segment. With saccular aneurysms, it may be possible to excise only the bulbous lesion, repairing the artery by primary closure (suturing the artery together) or by application of an autogenous or synthetic patch graft.

All OARs require aortic cross-clamping proximal and distal to the aneurysm. Most resections are done in 30 to 45 minutes, after which the clamps are removed and blood flow is restored. If the cross clamp must be applied above the renal arteries, adequate renal blood flow after clamp removal should be determined before closure of the abdominal incision. The risk of postoperative renal complications such as acute kidney injury increases in patients who have OAR of AAAs above the level of the renal arteries.

Endovascular Graft Procedure. Minimally invasive endovascular aneurysm repair (EVAR) is an alternative to conventional OAR. Patients must meet certain eligibility criteria to be candidates for EVAR. These include iliofemoral vessels that will allow for safe graft insertion and vessels of sufficient length and width to support the graft.[33]

EVAR involves the placement of a sutureless aortic graft into the abdominal aorta inside the aneurysm via the femoral artery. The graft, a Dacron cylinder consisting of several sections, is supported with multiple rings of flexible wire (Fig. 38-7). The main section of the graft is bifurcated and delivered through a femoral artery catheter. The second part of the graft is inserted through the opposite femoral artery. When all graft components are in place, they are released (deployed) against the vessel wall by balloon inflation. The blood then flows through the endovascular graft, thus preventing further expansion of the aneurysm. The aneurysmal wall will shrink over time because the blood is now being diverted through the endograft.

Complications. EVAR is less invasive than OAR. However, over time both techniques have similar rates of morbidity and mortality.[12,35]

The most common complication of AAA repair is *endoleak,* the seepage of blood back into the old aneurysm. This may be the result of an inadequate seal at either graft end, a tear through the graft fabric, or leakage between overlapping graft segments. Repair may require coil embolization (insertion of beads) for hemostasis.

Other potential complications include aneurysm growth above or below the graft, aneurysm rupture, aortic dissection, bleeding, renal artery occlusion caused by stent migration, graft thrombosis, incisional site hematoma, and incisional infection. Patients undergoing EVAR must have regular follow-up visits and routine CT or MRI scans for the rest of their lives to monitor for complications. Graft dysfunction may require conversion to an open surgical repair.

A potentially lethal complication in an emergency repair of a ruptured AAA is the development of *intraabdominal hypertension* (IAH) with associated *abdominal compartment syndrome* (ACS).[36] Persistent IAH reduces blood flow to the viscera. ACS refers to the impaired end-organ perfusion caused by IAH and resulting multisystem organ failure.

ACS occurs in about one fourth of cases of ruptured OARs and EVARs. It has a mortality rate up to 70%.[37] IAH is confirmed by measuring the patient's intraabdominal pressure indirectly through a catheter and transducer system, typically by using an indwelling urinary catheter. Treatment goals include control of situations that lead to IAH such as head of bed elevation, hemodynamic instability, and uncontrolled pain and anxiety. A percutaneous catheter decompression may be required in the patient with severe ACS to reduce intraabdominal pressure.[38]

NURSING MANAGEMENT
AORTIC ANEURYSMS

NURSING ASSESSMENT

Begin by performing a thorough history and physical assessment. Because atherosclerosis is a systemic disease, look for signs of coexisting cardiac, pulmonary, cerebral, and lower extremity vascular problems. Monitor the patient for signs of aneurysm rupture, such as diaphoresis; pallor; weakness; tachycardia; hypotension; abdominal, back, groin, or periumbilical pain; changes in level of consciousness; or a pulsating abdominal mass.

Establishing baseline data is critical for comparison with later postoperative assessments. Pay special attention to the character and quality of the patient's peripheral pulses, and renal and neurologic status. Before surgery, mark pedal pulse sites (dorsalis pedis and posterior tibial) with a single-use marker and document any skin lesions on the lower extremities.

PLANNING

The overall goals for a patient undergoing aortic surgery include (1) normal tissue perfusion; (2) intact motor and sensory function; and (3) no complications related to surgical repair, such as thrombosis, infection, or rupture.

NURSING IMPLEMENTATION

HEALTH PROMOTION. To promote overall health, encourage the patient to reduce CVD risk factors (see Table 34-2), including controlling BP, ceasing tobacco use (see Chapter 11), increasing physical activity, and maintaining normal body weight and serum lipid levels. These measures also help ensure continued graft patency after surgical repair.

ACUTE INTERVENTION. During the preoperative period, provide emotional support and teaching to the patient and the caregiver. Preoperative teaching includes a brief explanation of the disease process, the planned surgical procedure(s), preoperative routines, what to expect immediately after surgery (e.g., recovery room, tubes and drains), and usual postoperative timelines. Specific preoperative routines vary by agency and surgeon. In general, aortic surgery patients have a bowel preparation (e.g., laxatives, enemas) and skin cleansing with an antimicrobial agent the day before surgery, have nothing by mouth (NPO) after midnight the day of surgery, and receive IV antibiotics immediately before the incision is made. If appropriate, a preoperative visit to the intensive care unit (ICU) may be helpful to the patient and caregiver. Patients with a history of CVD should receive a β-adrenergic blocker (e.g., metoprolol [Lopressor]) preoperatively to reduce morbidity and mortality.

Postoperatively, aortic surgery patients typically go to an ICU for 24 to 48 hours for close monitoring. When the patient arrives in the ICU, various devices are in place. These include an endotracheal tube for mechanical ventilation, an arterial line, a central venous pressure (CVP) or pulmonary artery (PA) catheter, peripheral IV lines, an indwelling urinary catheter, and a nasogastric (NG) tube. The patient needs continuous ECG and pulse oximetry monitoring. If the thorax is opened during surgery, chest tubes will be in place. Pain medication is given via epidural catheter or patient-controlled analgesia (PCA).

In addition to the usual goals of care for a postoperative patient (e.g., maintaining adequate respiratory function, fluid and electrolyte balance, and pain control [see Chapter 20]), check for graft patency and renal perfusion. Also watch for and intervene to limit or treat cardiac ischemia, dysrhythmias, infections, VTE, and neurologic complications. eNursing Care Plan 38-2 for the patient with an aneurysm repair or other aortic surgery is available on the website for this chapter.

Graft Patency. An adequate BP is important to maintain graft patency. Prolonged low BP may result in graft thrombosis. Administer IV fluids and blood components as ordered to maintain adequate blood flow. Monitor CVP or PA pressures and urine output hourly in the immediate postoperative period to assess the patient's hydration and perfusion status.

Avoid severe hypertension, since it may cause undue stress on the arterial anastomoses, resulting in leakage of blood or rupture at the suture lines. Drug therapy with IV diuretics (e.g., furosemide [Lasix]) or IV antihypertensive agents (e.g., labetalol [Normodyne], metoprolol, hydralazine [Apresoline], sodium nitroprusside [Nipride]) may be indicated.

Cardiovascular Status. Myocardial ischemia or infarction may occur in the perioperative period because of decreased myocardial oxygen supply or increased myocardial oxygen demands. Cardiac dysrhythmias may occur because of electrolyte imbalances, hypoxemia, hypothermia, or myocardial ischemia. Nursing interventions include continuous ECG monitoring; frequent electrolyte and arterial blood gas determinations; administration of oxygen, IV antidysrhythmic and antihypertensive medications, and electrolytes as needed; adequate pain control; and resumption of heart medications.

Infection. A prosthetic vascular graft infection is a relatively rare but potentially life-threatening complication. Nursing interventions to prevent infection include administering a broad-spectrum antibiotic as prescribed. Assess temperature regularly, and promptly report elevations. Monitor laboratory data for an elevated white blood cell (WBC) count, which may be the first indication of an infection. Ensure adequate nutrition, and assess the surgical incision for signs of infection (e.g., redness, swelling, drainage). Keep surgical incisions clean and dry and perform wound care as ordered.

Use strict aseptic technique in the care of all IV, arterial, and CVP or PA catheter insertion sites, since these are ports of entry for bacteria. Meticulous perineal care for the patient with an indwelling urinary catheter and early catheter removal are essential to minimize the risk of urinary tract infection.

Gastrointestinal Status. After OAR, postoperative ileus may develop as a result of anesthesia and the handling of the bowel during surgery. The intestines may become swollen and bruised, and peristalsis ceases for variable intervals. A retroperitoneal surgical approach can be used to decrease the risk of bowel complications.

An NG tube may be placed during surgery and connected to low, intermittent suction to decompress the stomach, prevent aspiration of stomach contents, and decrease pressure on suture lines. Record the amount and character of the NG output. While the patient is NPO, provide oral care frequently. Ice chips or lozenges can help soothe a dry or irritated throat. Assess for bowel sounds every 4 hours. The passing of flatus signals returning bowel function and should be noted. Encourage early ambulation, since this can help the return of bowel function. A postoperative ileus rarely lasts beyond the fourth postoperative day.

If the blood supply to the bowel is disrupted during surgery, temporary ischemia or infarction (death) of intestinal tissue may result. Clinical manifestations of this rare but serious complication include absent bowel sounds, fever, abdominal distention and pain, diarrhea, and bloody stools. If bowel infarction occurs, immediate reoperation is necessary to restore blood flow, with likely resection of the infarcted bowel.

Neurologic Status. Neurologic complications can occur after aortic surgery. When the ascending aorta and aortic arch are involved, assess the patient's level of consciousness, pupil size and response to light, facial symmetry, tongue position, speech, upper extremity movement, and quality of hand grasps (see Chapter 57). When the descending aorta is involved, perform a neurovascular assessment of the lower extremities. Record all assessments and report changes from baseline to the physician immediately.

Peripheral Perfusion Status. The location of the aneurysm determines what type of peripheral perfusion assessment is done. Check and record all peripheral pulses hourly for several hours and then routinely, based on agency policy. When the ascending aorta and aortic arch are involved, assess the carotid, radial, and temporal artery pulses. For surgery of the descending aorta, assess the femoral, popliteal, posterior tibial, and dorsalis pedis pulses (see Fig. 32-6). You may need a Doppler to assess peripheral pulses. Check skin temperature and color, capillary refill time, and sensation and movement of the extremities (see Chapter 32).

Occasionally, lower extremity pulses may be absent for a short time after surgery because of vasospasm and hypothermia. A decreased or absent pulse together with a cool, pale, mottled, or painful extremity may indicate embolization or graft occlusion. Report these findings to the physician immediately. Graft occlusion requires reoperation if identified early. Thrombolytic therapy may also be considered. In some patients, pulses may have been absent before surgery because of coexistent PAD. It is essential to compare your findings with the preoperative status to determine the cause of a decreased or absent pulse and the proper treatment.

Renal Perfusion Status. The patient will have an indwelling urinary catheter after surgery. In the immediate postoperative period, record hourly urine output. Further evaluate renal function by monitoring daily blood urea nitrogen (BUN) and serum creatinine levels. CVP and PA pressures also provide important information about hydration status. Maintain accurate fluid intake and output and record daily weights until the patient resumes a regular diet.

Decreased renal perfusion can occur from embolization of the aortic thrombus or plaque to one or both of the renal arteries. This causes ischemia of one or both kidneys. Hypotension, dehydration, prolonged aortic clamping during surgery, or blood loss also can lead to decreased renal perfusion. Irreversible renal failure may occur after surgery, particularly in high-risk people (e.g., patients with diabetes). (Acute kidney injury is discussed in Chapter 47.)

AMBULATORY AND HOME CARE Instruct the patient and caregiver to gradually increase activities once home. Fatigue, poor appetite, and irregular bowel habits are common. Teach the patient to avoid heavy lifting for 6 weeks after surgery. Any redness, swelling, increased pain, drainage from incisions, or fever greater than 100° F (37.8° C) should be reported to a health care provider.

Teach the patient and caregiver to look for changes in color or warmth of the extremities. Patients and caregivers can learn to palpate peripheral pulses to assess changes in their quality.

Sexual dysfunction in male patients is common after aortic surgery. Preoperatively, document baseline sexual function and recommend counseling as appropriate. A referral to a urologist may be useful if erectile dysfunction occurs.

EVALUATION

Expected outcomes for the patient who undergoes aortic surgery include the following:
- Patent arterial graft with adequate distal perfusion
- Adequate urine output
- No signs of infection

AORTIC DISSECTION

Aortic dissection, often misnamed *"dissecting aneurysm,"* is not a type of aneurysm. Rather, dissection results from the creation of a false lumen between the intima (inner lining) and the media (middle layer) of arterial wall (Figs. 38-5, *D*, and 38-8). Classification of the aortic dissection is based on anatomic location (ascending versus descending aorta) and duration of onset (acute versus chronic). Approximately two thirds of dissections involve the ascending aorta and are acute in onset.[39] Chronic dissections almost always involve the descending aorta.

Etiology and Pathophysiology

Most experts link nontraumatic aortic dissection to degenerated elastic fibers in the arterial wall. Chronic hypertension hastens this process. In aortic dissection a tear develops in the inner layer of the aorta. Blood surges through this tear into the middle layer of the aorta, causing the inner and middle layers to separate (dissect). If the blood-filled channel ruptures through the outside aortic wall, aortic dissection is often fatal.

As the heart contracts, each pulsation increases the pressure on the damaged area, which further increases the dissection. Extension of the dissection may cut off blood supply to critical areas such as the brain, kidneys, spinal cord, and extremities. The false lumen may remain patent, become thrombosed (clotted), rejoin the true lumen by way of a distal tear, or rupture.

Aortic dissection affects men 2 to 5 times more often than women and occurs most frequently in the sixth and seventh decades of life.[39] Predisposing factors include age, aortitis (e.g., syphilis), blunt or iatrogenic trauma, congenital heart disease (e.g., bicuspid aortic valve), connective tissue disorders (e.g., Marfan's syndrome), cocaine or methamphetamine use, history of heart surgery, atherosclerosis, male gender, pregnancy, and hypertension.[33] Younger patients are more likely to have a bicus-

FIG. 38-8 Aortic dissection of the thoracic aorta.

pid aortic valve, Marfan's syndrome, prior aortic valve surgery, or recent trauma. Nearly half of all dissections in women younger than 40 years occur during pregnancy.

Clinical Manifestations

Most patients with an acute ascending aortic dissection report abrupt onset of excruciating chest and/or back pain radiating to the neck or shoulders. Patients with acute descending aortic dissection are more likely to report pain located in their back, abdomen, or legs. The pain is frequently described as "sharp" and "worst ever," or as "tearing," "ripping," or "stabbing."

Dissection pain can be differentiated from MI pain, which is more gradual in onset and has increasing intensity. As the dissection progresses, pain may migrate. Older patients are less likely to have abrupt onset of chest or back pain and more likely to have hypotension and vague symptoms. Some patients have a painless aortic dissection, emphasizing the importance of the physical examination.

If the aortic arch is involved, the patient may exhibit neurologic deficits. These include altered level of consciousness, weakened or absent carotid and temporal pulses, and dizziness or syncope. An ascending aortic dissection usually produces some degree of disruption in blood flow in the coronary arteries and aortic valve insufficiency. The patient may develop angina; MI; and a new high-pitched, heart murmur. In severe cases, these complications can result in left heart failure with the development of dyspnea, orthopnea, and pulmonary edema. When either subclavian artery is involved, radial, ulnar, and brachial pulse quality and BP readings may be different between the left and right arms. As the dissection progresses down the aorta, the abdominal organs and the lower extremities demonstrate evidence of decreased tissue perfusion.

Complications

A severe and life-threatening complication of an acute ascending aortic dissection is *cardiac tamponade*. This occurs when blood from the dissection leaks into the pericardial sac. Clinical manifestations of tamponade include hypotension, narrowed pulse pressure, jugular venous distention, muffled heart sounds, and pulsus paradoxus (see Chapter 37).

The aorta may rupture because it is weakened by the dissection. Hemorrhage may occur into the mediastinal, pleural, or abdominal cavities. Aortic rupture typically results in exsanguination and death. Dissection can lead to occlusion of the blood supply to vital organs. Spinal cord ischemia leads to weakness and decreased sensation to complete lower extremity paralysis. Renal ischemia can lead to renal failure. Abdominal (mesenteric) ischemia can cause abdominal pain, decreased bowel sounds, altered bowel function, and bowel necrosis.

Diagnostic Studies

Diagnostic studies to detect aortic dissection are similar to those for suspected aneurysms (Table 38-6). An ECG can help rule out cardiac ischemia. A chest x-ray may show a widening of the mediastinum and pleural effusion. Three-dimensional (3-D) CT scanning and transesophageal echocardiography (TEE) have become the standard for the diagnosis of acute aortic dissection. A CT scan can provide valuable information on the presence and severity of the dissection. Although an MRI has the highest accuracy for detecting aortic dissection, it is contraindicated in some patients (e.g., those with metal implants, hemodynamically unstable patients).[39]

TABLE 38-6   COLLABORATIVE CARE

Aortic Dissection

Diagnostic	Collaborative Therapy

• Health history and physical examination
• ECG
• Chest x-ray
• CT scan with 3-D reconstruction
• Transesophageal echocardiogram
• Magnetic resonance imaging
	• Bed rest
	• Pain relief with opioids
	• Blood transfusion (if necessary)
	• Drug therapy (see Table 33-7)
	  • IV β-adrenergic blockers (e.g., esmolol [Brevibloc], propranolol [Inderal])
	  • IV calcium channel blockers
	  • Angiotensin-converting enzyme inhibitors
	  • Sodium nitroprusside (Nipride)
	• Surgical aortic resection and repair
	• Endovascular aortic dissection repair

Collaborative Care

Patients with acute aortic dissection are managed in the ICU. The initial goals of therapy for acute aortic dissection without complications are heart rate (HR) and BP control and pain management. HR and BP control reduces aortic wall stress by decreasing systolic BP and myocardial contractility (see Table 38-6). An IV β-adrenergic blocker (e.g., esmolol [Brevibloc]) is titrated to a target HR of 60 beats/minute or less. A calcium channel blocker (e.g., diltiazem [Cardizem], verapamil [Calan]) can be used to lower HR if a β-adrenergic blocker is contraindicated. An IV ACE inhibitor (e.g., enalapril [Vasotec]) may also be used. Reducing the HR, BP, and myocardial contractility limits extension of the dissection. Morphine is the preferred analgesic because it decreases sympathetic nervous system stimulation and relieves pain. Supportive treatment for an acute aortic dissection serves as a bridge to surgery.

Conservative Therapy. The patient with an acute or chronic descending aortic dissection without complications can be treated conservatively. Conservative treatment includes pain relief, HR and BP control, and CVD risk factor modification.

Endovascular Dissection Repair. Endovascular repair of acute descending aortic dissections with complications (e.g., hemodynamic instability) and chronic descending aortic dissection with complications (e.g., peripheral ischemia) is a treatment option. Endovascular dissection repair is similar to EVAR. However, a temporary lumbar drain may be inserted for cerebrospinal fluid removal to reduce spinal cord edema and help prevent paralysis.[40]

Surgical Therapy. An acute ascending aortic dissection is considered a surgical emergency. Otherwise, surgery is indicated when conservative therapy is ineffective or when complications (e.g., heart failure) occur. Open surgical repair is recommended for patients with a chronic dissection who have a connective tissue disorder and a descending thoracic aortic diameter greater than 5.5 cm.[33] The aorta is fragile after dissection. Thus surgery is delayed for as long as possible to allow time for edema to decrease and to permit clotting of the blood in the false lumen. Surgery involves resection of the aortic segment containing the intimal tear and replacement with a synthetic graft. Even with prompt surgical intervention, the in-hospital mortality rate of acute aortic dissection is high.[39] Causes of death include aortic rupture, mesenteric ischemia, MI, sepsis, and multiorgan failure.

NURSING MANAGEMENT
AORTIC DISSECTION

Preoperatively, nursing management includes keeping the patient in bed in a semi-Fowler's position and maintaining a quiet environment. These measures help to keep the HR and the systolic BP at the lowest possible level that maintains vital organ perfusion (typically HR less than 60 beats/minute; systolic BP less than 120 mm Hg). Administer opioids and sedatives as ordered. To prevent extension of the dissection, manage pain and anxiety because they can cause elevations in the HR and systolic BP.

Administration and titration of IV antihypertensive agents require careful supervision, including continuous ECG and intraarterial BP monitoring (see Chapters 36 and 66). Monitor vital signs frequently, sometimes as often as every 2 to 3 minutes, until target HR and BP are reached. Observe for changes in peripheral pulses and signs of increasing pain, restlessness, and anxiety. If the arteries branching off the aortic arch are involved, decreased cerebral blood flow may alter the patient's level of consciousness. Postoperative care is similar to that after OAR (see earlier section on nursing management of aortic aneurysms).

In preparation for discharge, focus on patient and caregiver teaching. All patients with a history of aortic dissection, regardless of location or treatment approach, require long-term medical care to control HR and BP. Patients must understand that they need to take antihypertensive drugs daily for the rest of their lives. β-Adrenergic blockers (e.g., metoprolol) are used to control HR and BP and decrease myocardial contractility. It is important that patients understand the drug regimen and potential side effects (e.g., dizziness, depression, fatigue, erectile dysfunction). Tell the patient to discuss any side effects with the health care provider before discontinuing the drug. Follow-up with regularly scheduled MRIs or CTs is essential. The most common cause of death in long-term survivors is aortic rupture from redissection or aneurysm formation. Instruct patients that if the pain or other symptoms return, they should activate emergency medical services (EMS) for immediate care.

VENOUS DISORDERS

PHLEBITIS

Generally, every hospitalized patient has an IV catheter inserted for giving fluids and/or drugs. *Phlebitis* is inflammation of the walls of small cannulated veins of the hand or arm. Clinical signs and symptoms include pain, tenderness, warmth, erythema, swelling, and a palpable cord.[41] Phlebitis risk factors are mechanical irritation from the catheter, infusion of irritating medications, and catheter location. Phlebitis is rarely infectious and usually resolves quickly after catheter removal. If edema is present, elevate the extremity to promote reabsorption of fluid into the vasculature. Apply warm, moist heat and administer oral NSAIDs (e.g., diclofenac [Voltaren]) or topical NSAIDs (e.g., diclofenac gel [Solaraze]) to relieve pain and inflammation.

VENOUS THROMBOSIS

Venous thrombosis involves the formation of a thrombus in association with inflammation of the vein. It is the most

TABLE 38-7	COMPARISON OF SUPERFICIAL VEIN THROMBOSIS AND VENOUS THROMBOEMBOLISM	
	Superficial Vein Thrombosis	**Venous Thromboembolism (VTE)**
Usual location	Typically, superficial leg veins (e.g., varicosities). Occasionally superficial arm veins.	Deep veins of arms (e.g., axillary, subclavian), legs (e.g., femoral), pelvis (e.g., iliac, inferior or superior vena cava), and pulmonary system.
Clinical findings	Tenderness, itchiness, redness, warmth, pain, inflammation and induration along the course of the superficial vein. Vein appears as a palpable cord. Edema rarely occurs.	Tenderness to pressure over involved vein, induration of overlying muscle, venous distention. Edema. May have mild to moderate pain, deep reddish color to area caused by venous congestion. NOTE: Some patients may have no obvious physical changes in the affected extremity.
Sequelae	If untreated, clot may extend to deeper veins and VTE may occur.	Embolization to lungs (pulmonary embolism) may occur and may result in death.* Pulmonary hypertension and post-thrombotic syndrome with or without venous leg ulceration may develop.

*See Chapter 28 for clinical findings related to pulmonary embolism.

common disorder of the veins and is classified as either superficial vein thrombosis or deep vein thrombosis. Superficial vein thrombosis (SVT) is the formation of a thrombus in a superficial vein, usually the greater or lesser saphenous vein. Deep vein thrombosis (DVT) is a disorder involving a thrombus in a deep vein, most commonly the iliac and femoral veins. Venous thromboembolism (VTE) is the preferred terminology and represents the spectrum of pathology from DVT to pulmonary embolism (PE) (Table 38-7). (Chapter 28 discusses PE.)

SVT has been considered a benign disorder. However, recent data indicate that SVT may be more serious. Nearly 25% of patients with SVT may also have VTE at the time of diagnosis. Further, between 5% and 10% of SVT patients are at risk for developing thromboembolic complications in the future.[42]

Etiology

Three important factors (called Virchow's triad) in the etiology of venous thrombosis are (1) venous stasis, (2) damage of the endothelium (inner lining of the vein), and (3) hypercoagulability of the blood (Fig. 38-9). The patient at risk for the development of VTE usually has predisposing conditions to these three disorders (Table 38-8).

Venous Stasis. Normal venous blood flow depends on the action of muscles in the extremities and the functional adequacy of venous valves, which allow flow in one direction. *Venous stasis* occurs when the valves are dysfunctional or the muscles of the extremities are inactive. Venous stasis occurs more frequently in people who are obese or pregnant, have chronic heart failure or atrial fibrillation, have been traveling on long trips without regular exercise, have a prolonged surgical procedure, or are immobile for long periods (e.g., spinal cord injury, fractured hip, limb paralysis).[43]

FIG. 38-9 Pathophysiology of venous thromboembolism.

TABLE 38-8 RISK FACTORS FOR VENOUS THROMBOEMBOLISM

Venous Stasis	Hypercoagulability of Blood
• Advanced age	• Antiphospholipid antibody syndrome
• Atrial fibrillation	• Antithrombin III deficiency
• Chronic heart failure	• Dehydration or malnutrition
• Obesity	• Elevated (clotting) factor VIII or lipoprotein (a)
• Orthopedic surgery (especially hip or lower extremity)	• Erythropoiesis-stimulating drugs (e.g., epoetin alfa [Procrit])
• Pregnancy and postpartum period	• Factor V Leiden or prothrombin gene mutation
• Prolonged immobility	• High altitudes
• Bed rest	• Hormone therapy
• Fractured leg or hip	• Hyperhomocysteinemia
• Long trips without adequate exercise	• Malignancies (especially breast, brain, hepatic, pancreatic, and gastrointestinal)
• Spinal cord injury or limb paralysis	• Nephrotic syndrome
• Stroke	• Oral contraceptives, especially in women >35 yr who use tobacco
• Varicose veins	• Polycythemia vera
Endothelial Damage	• Pregnancy and postpartum period
• Abdominal and pelvic surgery (e.g., gynecologic or urologic surgery)	• Protein C deficiency
• Caustic or hypertonic IV medications	• Protein S deficiency
• Fractures of the pelvis, hip, or leg	• Sepsis
• History of previous venous thromboembolism	• Severe anemias
• Indwelling, peripherally inserted, central vein catheter	• Tobacco use
• IV drug abuse	
• Trauma	

Endothelial Damage. Damage to the endothelium of the vein may be caused by direct (e.g., surgery, intravascular catheterization, trauma, burns) or indirect (chemotherapy, diabetes, sepsis) injury to the vessel.[43] Damaged endothelium stimulates platelet activation and starts the coagulation cascade. This predisposes the patient to thrombus development.

Hypercoagulability of Blood. Hypercoagulability of blood occurs in many disorders, including severe anemias, polycythemia, malignancies (e.g., cancers of the breast, brain, pancreas, and gastrointestinal tract), nephrotic syndrome, hyperhomocysteinemia, and protein C and S deficiency.[43] A patient with sepsis is predisposed to hypercoagulability because of endotoxins that are released. Some medications (e.g., corticosteroids, estrogens) predispose a patient to thrombus formation.

Women of childbearing age who take estrogen-based oral contraceptives or postmenopausal women on oral hormone therapy (HT) are at increased risk for VTE.[43] Women who use oral contraceptives and tobacco double their risk. Smoking causes hypercoagulability by increasing plasma fibrinogen and homocysteine levels and activating the intrinsic coagulation pathway. Women who use tobacco and oral contraceptives, are over 35 years old, and have a family history of VTE are at an extremely high risk for VTE. In women with a known thrombophilia, the benefits of HT, tamoxifen (Nolvadex), or raloxifene (Evista) must be weighed against the risk for VTE.

Pathophysiology

Localized platelet aggregation and fibrin entrap red blood cells (RBCs), WBCs, and more platelets to form a thrombus. A frequent site of thrombus formation is the valve cusps of veins, where venous stasis occurs. As the thrombus enlarges, increased numbers of blood cells and fibrin collect behind it. This produces a larger clot with a "tail" that eventually blocks the lumen of the vein.

If a thrombus only partially blocks the vein, endothelial cells cover the thrombus and stop the thrombotic process. If the thrombus does not become detached, it undergoes lysis or becomes firmly organized and adherent within 5 to 7 days. The organized thrombus may detach and result in an embolus. Turbulence of blood flow is a major contributing factor to embolization. The thrombus can become an embolus that flows through the venous circulation to the heart and lodges in the pulmonary circulation, becoming a PE (see Fig. 28-11).

Superficial Vein Thrombosis

Clinical Manifestations. The patient with SVT may have a palpable, firm, subcutaneous cordlike vein (see Table 38-7). The area surrounding the vein may be itchy, tender or painful to the touch, reddened, and warm. A mild temperature elevation and leukocytosis may be present. Extremity edema may or may not occur. Lower extremity SVT often involves one or more varicose veins.

Risk factors for SVT include increased age; pregnancy; obesity; malignancy; thrombophilia; estrogen therapy; recent sclerotherapy (e.g., treatment for varicose veins); long-distance travel; and a history of CVI, SVT, or VTE.[42] SVT also can occur in persons with endothelial alterations (e.g., Buerger's disease). SVT also may be unprovoked.

Collaborative Care. Duplex ultrasound is used to confirm the diagnosis (clot 5 cm or larger) and to rule out clot extension to a deep vein.[44,45] For patients with a lower leg SVT, treatment consists of low-molecular-weight heparin (LMWH) for 45 days or a prophylactic dose of fondaparinux (Arixtra).[44] If the SVT affects a very short vein segment (less than 5 cm) and is not near the saphenofemoral junction, anticoagulants may not be necessary and oral NSAIDs can ease symptoms. Additional interventions to relieve SVT symptoms include telling the patient to wear elastic compression stockings, apply topical NSAIDS, and perform mild exercise such as walking.[46]

Venous Thromboembolism

Clinical Manifestations. The patient with lower extremity VTE may or may not have unilateral leg edema, pain, tenderness with palpation, dilated superficial veins, a sense of fullness in the thigh or the calf, paresthesias, warm skin, erythema, or a systemic temperature greater than 100.4° F (38° C) (see Table 38-7). If the inferior vena cava is involved, both legs may be edematous and cyanotic. About 5% to 10% of VTEs involve the upper extremity veins and may extend into the internal jugular vein or superior vena cava.[44] If the superior vena cava is involved, similar symptoms may occur in the arms, neck, back, and face. Diagnosis of an initial VTE is based on clinical assessment combined with D-dimer testing and duplex ultrasound.[47]

Complications. The most serious complications of VTE are PE, post-thrombotic syndrome, and phlegmasia cerulea dolens. (See Chapter 28 for discussion of PE.)

Post-thrombotic syndrome (PTS) occurs in 20% to 50% of patients despite adequate anticoagulant therapy. It results from chronic venous hypertension caused by valvular destruction (from inflammation and scarring), stiff noncompliant vein walls, and persistent venous obstruction. Symptoms include pain, aching, heaviness, swelling, cramps, itching, and tingling.[48,49] Clinical signs include persistent edema, increased pigmentation, eczema, secondary varicosities, and *lipodermatosclerosis* (Fig. 38-10). Venous ulceration can occur with severe PTS. Manifestations of PTS typically begin within 2 years of a

FIG. 38-10 Lipodermatosclerosis. Skin on lower leg becomes scarred, and the leg becomes tapered like an "inverted bottle." Hallmark signs of lipodermatosclerosis are leathery skin, brown discoloration, hyperpigmentation and hypopigmentation, and circumferential or near circumferential scarring and shrinking of the extremity.

VTE.[48,49] Risk factors include persistent leg symptoms 1 month after VTE, VTE located near the iliofemoral junction, extensive VTE, recurrent VTE, obesity, older age, and female gender. Sequential compression devices (SCDs) may be used for patients with severe PTS.[50]

Phlegmasia cerulea dolens (swollen, blue, painful leg), a rare complication, may develop in a patient in the advanced stages of cancer. It results from severe lower extremity VTE(s) that involve the major leg veins, causing near-total occlusion of venous outflow. Patients typically experience sudden, massive swelling; deep pain; and intense cyanosis of the extremity. If untreated, the venous obstruction causes arterial occlusion and gangrene and requires amputation.

Diagnostic Studies. Table 38-9 presents the various diagnostic studies used to determine the site or location and extent of a VTE.

Collaborative Care

Prevention and Prophylaxis. VTE prophylaxis is a core measure of high-quality health care in hospitalized surgical patients. The Joint Commission's core measures for the care of patients with VTE can be found at *www.jointcommission.org/core_measure_sets.aspx*. In addition, it is recommended that hospitals have a thromboprophylaxis policy that addresses VTE prevention on admission of all adult patients. As many as 60% of patients at risk for VTE do not receive appropriate thromboprophylaxis.[51]

In patients at risk for VTE, a variety of interventions are used. These are based on such factors as bleeding and thrombosis risk, past medical history, current medications, medical diagnoses, scheduled procedures, and patient preferences.[52] Early and aggressive mobilization based on the patient's condition is the easiest and most cost-effective method to decrease VTE risk. Patients on bed rest need to change position every 2 hours. Unless contraindicated, teach patients to flex and extend their feet, knees, and hips every 2 to 4 hours while awake. Patients who are able to get out of bed need to be in a chair for meals and ambulate at least four to six times per day as tolerated. Tell the patient and caregiver about the importance of these measures. Early and frequent ambulation is sufficient prophylaxis for very low VTE–risk patients undergoing minor surgical procedures.[53] Anticoagulation and mechanical prophylaxis

TABLE 38-9   DIAGNOSTIC STUDIES

*Venous Thromboembolism**

Study	Description and Abnormal Findings
Blood Laboratory Studies	
ACT, aPTT, INR, bleeding time, Hgb, Hct, platelet count	Alterations if patient has underlying blood dyscrasia (e.g., increased Hgb and Hct in patient with polycythemia).
D-dimer	Fragment of fibrin formed as result of fibrin degradation and clot lysis. Elevated results suggest venous thromboembolism (VTE). *Normal results:* <250 ng/mL (<250 mcg/L)
Fibrin monomer complex	Forms when concentration of thrombin exceeds that of antithrombin. Presence is evidence of thrombus formation and suggests VTE. *Normal results:* <6.1 mg/L
Noninvasive Venous Studies	
Venous compression ultrasound	Evaluation of deep femoral, popliteal, and posterior tibial veins. *Normal finding:* Veins collapse with application of external pressure. *Abnormal finding:* Veins fail to collapse with application of external pressure. Failure to collapse suggests a thrombus.
Duplex ultrasound	Combination of compression ultrasound with spectral and color flow Doppler. Veins examined for respiratory variation, compressibility, and intraluminal filling defects to help determine location and extent of thrombus (most widely used test to diagnose VTE).
Invasive Venous Studies	
Computed tomography venography (CTV)	Uses spiral CT to evaluate veins in the pelvis, thighs, and calves after injection of venous phase contrast material. Uses less contrast material than traditional venography. May be performed simultaneously with CT angiography of pulmonary vessels for patients being evaluated for VTE.
Magnetic resonance venography	Uses magnetic resonance imaging with specialized software to evaluate blood flow through veins. Can be done with or without contrast. Highly accurate for pelvic and proximal veins. Less accurate for calf veins. Can distinguish acute and chronic thrombus.
Contrast venography (phlebogram)	X-ray determination of location and extent of clot using contrast media to outline filling defects. Identifies the presence of collateral circulation. Once the gold standard but currently rarely performed.

*See Table 28-26 for diagnostic studies for pulmonary embolism.
ACT, Activated clotting time; *aPTT,* activated partial thromboplastin time; *INR,* international normalized ratio.

are not recommended for acutely ill medical patients at low risk for VTE.

Elastic compression (antiembolism) stockings (e.g., thromboembolic deterrent [TED] hose) are a part of VTE prevention in hospitalized patients. When fitted correctly (both size and length) and worn properly and consistently from admission until discharge or full mobility, these stockings decrease VTE risk.[54] Proper use means the toe hole is under the toes, the heel patch is over the heel, the thigh gusset is on the inner thigh (thigh length only), and there are no wrinkles. The stockings are not to be rolled down, cut, or otherwise altered. Thigh-length stockings prevent proximal VTE better than knee-length stockings.[55] If the stockings are not fitted and worn correctly, venous return is impeded. This may promote the development of VTE and skin breakdown. VTE prevention is enhanced if elastic compression stockings are used along with anticoagulation.

Sequential compression devices (SCDs) are inflatable garments wrapped around the legs. They apply external pressure to the lower extremities by means of an electric pump. SCDs may or may not be used with elastic compression stockings. Like elastic compression stockings, ensure correct fit by accurately measuring the extremities. SCDs will not be effective if they are not applied correctly; if the fit is incorrect; or if the patient does not wear the device continuously except during bathing, skin assessment, and ambulation. SCDs are not worn when a patient has an active VTE because of the risk of PE. VTE prevention is enhanced if SCDs are used along with anticoagulation.[56]

Drug Therapy. Anticoagulants are used routinely for VTE prevention and treatment. The regimen depends on the patient's VTE risk. The goal of anticoagulant therapy for VTE prophylaxis is to prevent clot formation. The goals for treatment of a confirmed VTE are to prevent new clot development, spread of the clot, and embolization.[57]

Three major classes of anticoagulants are available: (1) vitamin K antagonists (VKA), (2) thrombin inhibitors (both indirect and direct), and (3) factor Xa inhibitors[58] (Table 38-10). Anticoagulant therapy does not dissolve the clot. Clot lysis begins naturally through the body's intrinsic fibrinolytic system (see Chapter 30).

Vitamin K Antagonists. The oral anticoagulant for long-term or extended anticoagulation is warfarin, a VKA. Warfarin inhibits activation of the vitamin K–dependent coagulation factors II, VII, IX, and X, as well as the anticoagulant proteins C and S. (Fig. 30-4 displays the clotting pathways, and clotting factors are listed in Table 30-2.) Warfarin begins to take effect in 48 to 72 hours. It then takes several more days to achieve a maximum effect. Thus an overlap of a parenteral anticoagulant (e.g., UH or LMWH) and warfarin typically is required for 5 days. The level of anticoagulation is monitored daily using the international normalized ratio (INR). The INR is a standardized system of reporting prothrombin time (PT) (Table 38-11, p. 852). The antidote for warfarin-related bleeding is vitamin K or Kcentra (Prothrombin Complex Concentrate [Human]).

Take a careful history before starting warfarin. Do not give antiplatelets or NSAIDs with warfarin, since these drugs

TABLE 38-10 DRUG THERAPY

Anticoagulant Therapy

Drug	Route of Administration	Comments
Vitamin K Antagonists (VKA)		
warfarin (Coumadin)	PO	INR is used for monitoring therapeutic levels. Administer at the same time each day. Variations of certain genes (e.g., *CYP2CP*, *VKORC1*) may influence response to the drug. *Antidote*: Vitamin K. For major VKA-related bleeding, treatment with four-factor prothrombin complex concentrate and IV vitamin K is recommended over fresh frozen plasma.
Thrombin Inhibitors: Indirect		
Unfractionated heparin (UH) heparin sodium (Hep-Lock, Liquaemin, Calciparine)	Continuous IV Intermittent IV Subcutaneous	Therapeutic effects measured at regular intervals by the aPTT or ACT. Monitor complete blood counts at regular intervals and titrate according to parameters. If administering subcutaneously, inject deep into subcutaneous tissue (preferably into the abdominal fatty tissue or above the iliac crest), inserting the entire length of the needle. Hold skinfold during injection but release before removing needle. Do not aspirate. Do not inject intramuscularly. Do not rub site after injection. Rotate sites. *Antidote*: Protamine
Low-molecular-weight heparin (LMWH) enoxaparin (Lovenox) tinzaparin (Innohep) dalteparin (Fragmin) nadroparin (Fraxiparine)	Subcutaneous	Routine coagulation tests typically not required. Monitor complete blood count at regular intervals. Do not expel air bubble before administering subcutaneously. Follow remaining administration guidelines as described above for UH. Reduced dosage needed in patients with renal impairment. Use extreme caution in patients with a history of HIT. *Antidote*: Protamine neutralizes the effects of LMWH.
Thrombin Inhibitors: Direct		
Hirudin derivatives lepirudin (Refludan) bivalirudin (Angiomax) desirudin (Iprivask)	 IV or subcutaneous IV IV or subcutaneous	Therapeutic effect measured by ACT or aPTT. Used in patients with HIT when anticoagulation is still required. *Antidote*: None
Synthetic thrombin inhibitors argatroban (Acova) dabigatran (Pradaxa)	 IV Subcutaneous	Therapeutic effect measured by aPTT. Used in patients at risk for or with HIT. Used for VTE prevention in joint replacement surgery. VTE treatment option and for stroke prevention in nonvalvular atrial fibrillation. *Antidote*: None
Factor Xa inhibitors fondaparinux (Arixtra) rivaroxaban (Xarelto)	 Subcutaneous PO	Routine coagulation tests not required. Monitor complete blood count and creatinine at regular intervals. Do not expel air bubble before administering. Follow remaining administration guidelines as described for UH. Both drugs approved for VTE prophylaxis and treatment. For surgical patients, initial dose should be given no earlier than 6 hr postoperatively. Use with caution in older patients and patients with impaired renal function. May cause thrombocytopenia. If uncontrollable bleeding occurs, treatment with recombinant factor VIIa may be effective. *Antidote*: None

ACT, Activated clotting time; *aPTT,* activated partial thromboplastin time; *HIT,* heparin-induced thrombocytopenia; *INR,* international normalized ratio; *VTE,* venous thromboembolism.

increase bleeding risk.[58] Many other drugs, vitamins, minerals, and dietary and herbal supplements also interact with warfarin (see eTable 38-1, available on the website for this chapter, and the Complementary & Alternative Therapies box on the right). A diet that frequently varies in vitamin K intake (e.g., green leafy vegetables) can make it hard to achieve and maintain a target INR level.

Genetic variants in the genes *VKORC1* and cytochrome P450 2C9 *(CYP2C9)* may influence how some people respond to warfarin (see Table 13-5). Although genetic testing is available, pharmacogenetic-based dosing is not recommended in clinical practice at this time.[59]

Thrombin Inhibitors: Indirect. *Indirect thrombin inhibitors* are divided into two major classes: UH and LMWHs. UH (e.g., heparin [Hep-Lock]) affects both the intrinsic and common pathways of blood coagulation by way of the plasma antithrombin. Antithrombin inhibits thrombin-mediated conversion of fibrinogen to fibrin by affecting factors II (prothrombin), IX, X, XI, and XII (see Fig. 30-4).

🌿 COMPLEMENTARY & ALTERNATIVE THERAPIES

Herbal and Dietary Supplements That May Affect Clotting

Scientific Evidence
There is evidence that the following herbs and dietary supplements may affect blood clotting: bilberry, black cohosh, chamomile, chondroitin sulfate, DHEA, feverfew, garlic, ginger, ginkgo biloba, ginseng, goldenseal, green tea, melatonin, niacin, omega-3 fatty acids, psyllium, red yeast rice extract, saw palmetto, soy, turmeric.

Nursing Implications
- Inform patients that taking these herbs, or dietary supplements may increase their risk of bleeding.
- Caution patients with bleeding disorders about the use of these herbs and dietary supplements. Advise them that they should consult with their health care provider before using these substances.

DHEA, Dehydroepiandrosterone.

TABLE 38-11   TESTS OF BLOOD COAGULATION

Drugs Monitored	Normal Value	Therapeutic Value
International normalized ratio (INR)	0.75-1.25	2-3
Vitamin K antagonists (e.g., warfarin [Coumadin])		
Activated partial thromboplastin time (aPTT)	25-35 sec	46-70 sec
• Unfractionated heparin (e.g., heparin [Hep-Lock])		
• Hirudin derivatives (e.g., bivalirudin [Angiomax])		
• Synthetic thrombin inhibitors (e.g., argatroban [Acova], dabigatran [Pradaxa])		
Activated clotting time (ACT)	70-120 sec*	>300 sec
• Unfractionated heparin		
• Hirudin derivatives		
• Synthetic thrombin inhibitors		
Anti–factor Xa		
• Low-molecular-weight heparin (e.g., enoxaparin [Lovenox])	0 U/mL	0.6-1.0 U/mL
• Factor Xa inhibitors (e.g., fondaparinux [Arixtra], rivaroxaban [Xarelto])	0 U/mL	0.2-1.5 U/mL

*Varies based on type of system and test reagent or activator used.

Heparin can be given subcutaneously for VTE prophylaxis or by continuous IV infusion for VTE treatment. When given IV, heparin requires frequent monitoring of clotting status as measured by activated partial thromboplastin time (aPTT) (see Table 38-11). Protamine sulfate reverses the effect of heparin.

One serious side effect of heparin is *heparin-induced thrombocytopenia* (HIT). HIT is an immune reaction to heparin. It causes a severe, sudden reduction in the platelet count along with a paradoxic increase in venous or arterial thrombosis. HIT is diagnosed by measuring the presence of heparin antibodies in the blood. Treatment requires immediately stopping heparin therapy and, if further anticoagulation is required, using a non-heparin anticoagulant (e.g., fondaparinux).[60] Another side effect of long-term heparin therapy is osteoporosis.

LMWHs (e.g., nadroparin [Fraxiparine]) are derived from UH. They have more bioavailability, more predictable dose response, longer half-life, and fewer bleeding complications than UH. LMWHs are less likely to cause HIT and osteoporosis. LMWHs typically do not require ongoing anticoagulant monitoring and dose adjustment. Protamine neutralizes the effect of LMWH.

Thrombin Inhibitors: Direct. *Direct thrombin inhibitors* are classified as hirudin derivatives or synthetic thrombin inhibitors. Hirudin is manufactured through recombinant deoxyribonucleic acid (DNA) technology. It binds specifically with thrombin and directly inhibits its function without causing plasma protein and platelet interactions. Hirudin derivatives (e.g., lepirudin [Refludan], bivalirudin [Angiomax]) are administered by continuous IV infusion. Lepirudin is approved for prophylaxis or treatment of patients with HIT. Bivalirudin is approved for HIT patients undergoing percutaneous coronary angioplasty. Anticoagulant activity is monitored using aPTT or activated clotting time (ACT) (see Table 38-11). There is no antidote for hirudin derivatives if bleeding occurs.

Argatroban (Acova), a synthetic direct thrombin inhibitor, inhibits thrombin. It is used as an alternative to heparin for the prevention and treatment of HIT and for known HIT patients who require percutaneous coronary interventions. Dabigatran (Pradaxa), an oral direct thrombin inhibitor, is used for VTE prevention after elective joint replacement, for stroke prevention in nonvalvular atrial fibrillation, and as a treatment option in VTE. The effects of argatroban and dabigatran are not reversible. Anticoagulant effect is monitored for both medications using aPTT or ACT.

Factor Xa Inhibitors. *Factor Xa inhibitors* inhibit factor Xa directly or indirectly, producing rapid anticoagulation. Fondaparinux is used for both VTE treatment and prophylaxis. It is given subcutaneously. Coagulation monitoring or dose adjustment is not needed, although the drug's anticoagulant activity can be measured using anti-Xa assays (see Table 38-11). If uncontrollable bleeding occurs, recombinant factor VIIa may be useful. Fondaparinux is contraindicated in patients with renal insufficiency. Rivaroxaban (Xarelto) is an oral factor Xa inhibitor used for VTE prevention.

Anticoagulant Therapy for VTE Prophylaxis. For VTE prophylaxis in the hospitalized medical patient at risk for thrombosis who is not bleeding, low-dose UH, LMWH, or fondaparinux is used. If the patient is at low VTE risk, drug prophylaxis is not needed. Patients with moderate VTE risk (e.g., general, gynecologic, urologic surgery) should receive either UH or LMWH. Patients with high VTE risk (e.g., trauma) should receive UH or LMWH until discharge. Patients having abdominal or pelvic surgery for cancer or major orthopedic surgery (e.g., total knee or hip replacement) should be prescribed VTE prophylaxis for up to 35 days after discharge.[59,61] (See eTable 38-2 for a sample VTE protocol/order set on the website for this chapter.)

Anticoagulant Therapy for VTE Treatment. Patients with confirmed VTE should receive initial treatment with either LMWH, UH, fondaparinux, or rivaroxaban. Oral VKA therapy is also started and continued for 3 months. A therapeutic INR is maintained between 2.0 and 3.0. Daily administration of only LMWH for 3 months is another option. Patients with multiple co-morbidities, complex medical issues, or a very large VTE usually are hospitalized for treatment. Parenteral administration of UH is the typical initial treatment. Depending on the

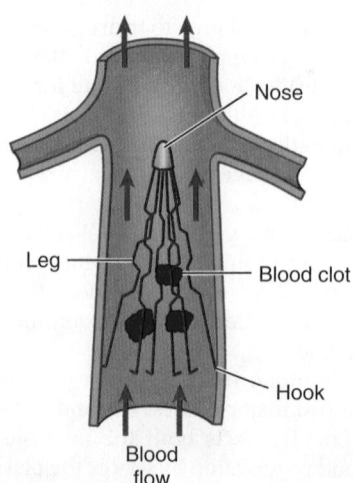

FIG. 38-11 Inferior vena caval interruption technique using Greenfield stainless steel filter to prevent pulmonary embolism. As blood travels up the vena cava, clots are trapped in the filter.

EVIDENCE-BASED PRACTICE

Applying the Evidence

You are caring for H.B., a 78-year-old Native American woman who is being discharged on enoxaparin (Lovenox) following a knee replacement. Her granddaughter will be her primary caregiver. You are preparing to teach her granddaughter how to inject the medication, since H.B. has limited dexterity in her hands because of arthritis. Her granddaughter tells you that H.B. is a modest woman and will not permit her to expose H.B.'s abdomen. She asks if the injection can be given in her arm.

Best Available Evidence	Clinician Expertise	Patient Preferences and Values
Enoxaparin (per the package literature) should be administered by deep subcutaneous injection in the abdomen. Injection sites should be rotated.	Some patients have told you that they used alternate sites for injection of enoxaparin, specifically the thighs and upper arms. You do not have any evidence about the efficacy of the drug when alternate sites are used.	H.B. states she does not want to expose herself to her granddaughter. The granddaughter expresses a desire to support her grandmother's need for modesty.

Your Decision and Action

You discuss the importance of following the drug manufacturer's recommendations regarding site selection with H.B. and her granddaughter. You further explain that there is no evidence on whether alternate sites are equally effective. H.B.'s granddaughter states she is the only one available to do this and she needs to respect her grandmother's wishes. You teach the granddaughter how to inject enoxaparin in H.B.'s upper arms and to alternate the sites and arms. You inform the physician of H.B.'s decision and document your teaching and related conversation.

Reference for Evidence

Lovenox. Retrieved from *www.lovenox.com/consumer/default.aspx*.

TABLE 38-12 NURSING ASSESSMENT
Venous Thromboembolism

Subjective Data
Important Health Information (see Table 38-8)
Past health history: Trauma to vein, intravascular catheter (e.g., peripherally inserted central catheter), varicose veins, pregnancy or recent childbirth, bacteremia, obesity, prolonged bed rest, irregular heartbeat (e.g., atrial fibrillation), COPD, HF, cancer, coagulation disorders and hypercoagulable states, systemic lupus erythematosus, MI, spinal cord injury, stroke, prolonged travel, recent bone fracture, dehydration
Medications: Use of estrogens (including oral contraceptives, hormone therapy), tamoxifen (Nolvadex), raloxifene (Evista), corticosteroids, excessive amounts of vitamin E, erythropoiesis-stimulating drugs
Surgery or other treatments: Any recent surgery, especially orthopedic, gynecologic, gastric, or urologic; previous surgery involving veins; central venous catheter

Functional Health Patterns
Health perception–health management: IV drug abuse, tobacco use, obesity
Activity-exercise: Inactivity
Cognitive-perceptual: Pain in area on palpation or ambulation

Objective Data
General
Fever, anxiety, pain

Integumentary
Increased size of extremity when compared with other side; taut, shiny, warm skin, erythematous, tender to palpation; no physical changes in the affected extremity in some patients

Cardiovascular
Distention and warmth of superficial veins in affected area; edema and cyanosis of extremities, neck, back, and face (if superior vena cava involvement)

Possible Diagnostic Findings
Leukocytosis, abnormal coagulation, anemia or ↑ hematocrit and RBC count, ↑ D-dimer level, positive venous compression on duplex ultrasound study; positive CTV, magnetic resonance venogram, or contrast venogram study

COPD, Chronic obstructive pulmonary disease; *CTV,* computed tomography venogram; *HF,* heart failure; *MI,* myocardial infarction; *RBC,* red blood cell.

---

clinical presentation and home situation, patients may be safely and effectively managed as outpatients.

Thrombolytic Therapy for VTE Treatment. Another treatment option for patients with a thrombus is catheter-directed administration of a thrombolytic drug (e.g., urokinase, tPA). Catheter-directed thrombolysis dissolves the clot(s), reduces the acute symptoms, and decreases the incidence of PTS. Other catheter-based interventions such as angioplasty, stents, or mechanical thrombectomy can be used along with thrombolytic drug therapy. (Chapter 34 discusses thrombolytic therapy.)

Surgical Therapy. Although most patients are managed medically, a small number of patients undergo surgery. Surgical options include open venous thrombectomy and inferior vena cava interruption. *Venous thrombectomy* involves the removal of a thrombus through an incision in the vein. Anticoagulant therapy is recommended after venous thrombectomy.

Vena cava interruption devices (e.g., Greenfield, Vena Tech, TrapEase filters) can be inserted percutaneously through the right femoral or right internal jugular veins. The filter device is opened, and the spokes penetrate the vessel walls (Fig. 38-11). The filters act as a "sieve-type" device, permitting filtration of clots without interruption of blood flow. Complications after the insertion of the device are rare but include air embolism, improper placement, migration of the filter, and perforation of the vena cava with retroperitoneal bleeding. Over time, venous congestion can occur from a buildup of trapped clots. These can clog the filter and completely block the vena cava, requiring filter removal and replacement. A filter device is recommended with proximal VTE of the leg if anticoagulant therapy is contraindicated due to an increased risk of bleeding. Patients with a filter device are at increased risk of developing a VTE. If the bleeding risk resolves, a course of anticoagulant therapy is suggested.[62]

NURSING MANAGEMENT
VENOUS THROMBOEMBOLISM

NURSING ASSESSMENT

Table 38-12 presents the subjective and objective data to obtain from a patient with VTE.

NURSING DIAGNOSES

Nursing diagnoses and collaborative problems for the patient with VTE include, but are not limited to, the following:

- Acute pain *related to* venous congestion, impaired venous return, and inflammation

- Ineffective health maintenance *related to* lack of knowledge about disorder and its treatment
- Risk for impaired skin integrity *related to* altered peripheral tissue perfusion
- Potential complication: bleeding *related to* anticoagulant therapy
- Potential complication: PE *related to* embolization of thrombus, dehydration, and immobility

PLANNING

The overall goals for the patient with VTE include (1) pain relief, (2) decreased edema, (3) no skin ulceration, (4) no bleeding complications, and (5) no evidence of PE.

NURSING IMPLEMENTATION

ACUTE INTERVENTION. Focus your nursing care for the patient with VTE on prevention of emboli formation and reduction of inflammation. Review with the patient any medications, vitamins, minerals, and dietary and herbal supplements being taken that may interfere with anticoagulant therapy (see eTable 38-1 on the website for this chapter and the Complementary & Alternative Therapies box on p. 851). Depending on the anticoagulant ordered, monitor INR, aPTT, ACT, anti–factor Xa levels, complete blood count (CBC), creatinine, factor X levels, hemoglobin, hematocrit, platelet levels, and/or liver enzymes.[63] Monitor platelet counts for patients getting UH or LMWH to assess for HIT. Titrate doses of UH, warfarin, and direct thrombin inhibitors based on results of blood studies and physician-ordered parameters. Direct thrombin inhibitors may need adjustment for patients with renal or liver dysfunction. Always check the results of appropriate tests before starting, giving, or changing anticoagulant therapy.

DRUG ALERT: Anticoagulant Therapy
- Tell patient to avoid taking aspirin, NSAIDs, fish oil supplements, garlic supplements, ginkgo biloba, and certain antibiotics (e.g., sulfamethoxazole and trimethoprim [Bactrim]).
- Instruct patient to report any signs of bleeding (e.g., black or bloody stools, bloody urine, coffee-ground or bloody vomit, nosebleeds).
- Assess for signs of bleeding (e.g., hypotension, tachycardia, hematuria, melena, hematemesis, petechiae, ecchymosis).

Monitor for and reduce the risk of bleeding that may occur with anticoagulant therapy (Table 38-13). Be aware that the risk of bleeding is greater in persons receiving LMWH or UH with an active gastroduodenal ulcer, prior bleeding history, low platelet count, hepatic or renal failure, rheumatic disease, cancer, or age greater than 85 years.[64] Patients receiving warfarin with an INR of 5.0 or more are also at increased risk for bleeding. In the event of anticoagulation above target goals, give reversal agents (e.g., protamine, vitamin K) or make dosage adjustments as ordered. In the event of major VKA-related bleeding, rapid treatment with four-factor prothrombin complex concentrate and IV vitamin K is recommended over fresh frozen plasma.

SAFETY ALERT
- Observe closely for any signs of bleeding:
  - Epistaxis and bleeding gingivae
  - Blood (visible or occult) in emesis, urine, stool, sputum
  - Oozing or visible bleeding from trauma site or surgical incision
  - Excessive menstrual bleeding
- Monitor vital signs for changes: decreased BP, increased HR
- Avoid intramuscular (IM) injections.
- Assess for mental status changes, especially in the older patient, since this may indicate cerebral bleeding.

TABLE 38-13   NURSING INTERVENTIONS FOR PATIENTS TAKING ANTICOAGULANTS

Assessment
- Monitor vital signs as indicated.
- Examine urine and stool for overt and occult signs of blood.
- Inspect skin frequently, especially under any splinting devices.
- Evaluate platelet count for signs of heparin-induced thrombocytopenia.
- Evaluate appropriate laboratory coagulation tests for target therapeutic levels.
- Evaluate lower extremity for ecchymosis or hematoma development if sequential compression device used.
- Perform assessments frequently to observe for signs and symptoms of bleeding (e.g., hypotension, tachycardia) or clotting.
- Notify the health care provider of any abnormalities in assessments, vital signs, or laboratory values.

Injections
- Avoid intramuscular injections.
- Minimize venipunctures.
- Use small-gauge needles for venipunctures unless ordered therapy requires a larger gauge.
- Apply manual pressure for at least 10 min (or longer if needed) on venipuncture sites.

Patient Care
- Avoid restrictive clothing.
- Apply moisturizing lotion to skin.
- Use electric razors, not straight razors.
- Perform physical care in a gentle manner.
- Instruct patient not to forcefully blow nose.
- Avoid removing or disrupting established clots.
- Humidify O_2 source if supplemental O_2 is ordered.
- Use soft toothbrushes or foam swabs for oral care.
- Reposition the patient carefully at regular intervals.
- Limit tape application. Use paper tape as appropriate.
- Administer stool softeners to avoid hard stools and straining.
- Lubricate tubes (e.g., suction catheter) adequately before insertion.
- Avoid restraints if possible. Use only soft, padded restraints if needed.
- Use support pads, mattresses, bed cradles, and therapeutic beds as indicated.
- Apply elastic compression stockings or sequential compression devices as ordered and with attention to proper size, application, and use.
- Perform risk for fall and skin breakdown assessments per agency policy and implement safety measures as needed.

Early ambulation when compared with bed rest does not increase the short-term risk of a PE in patients with VTE. In addition, early ambulation after acute VTE results in a more rapid decrease in edema and limb pain, fewer PTS symptoms, and better quality of life. Teach the patient and caregiver the importance of physical activity and assist the patient to ambulate several times a day. For patients with acute VTE with severe edema and limb pain, bed rest with limb elevation may initially be prescribed.

AMBULATORY AND HOME CARE. Focus discharge teaching on modification of VTE risk factors, use of elastic compression stockings, importance of monitoring laboratory values, medication instructions, and guidelines for follow-up. Once the edema is resolved, measure the patient for custom-fit elastic compression stockings. Stocking use (or sleeves in the case of an upper

DELEGATION DECISIONS

Caring for the Patient With Venous Thromboembolism (VTE)

All members of the health care team have important roles in preventing and managing VTE.

Role of Registered Nurse (RN)
- Assess patients for VTE risk and monitor for VTE in at-risk patients.
- Develop a plan of care to prevent VTE.
- Teach hospitalized patients who are at risk for VTE about preventive measures such as increasing mobility, using elastic compression stockings and sequential compression devices, and taking anticoagulant medications.
- Assess for the use of dietary supplements or herbs that may affect the coagulation status before the initiation of anticoagulant therapy.
- Monitor for adverse effects of anticoagulant use.
- Evaluate the effect of anticoagulant medications by monitoring appropriate laboratory results.
- Assess for complications of VTE, including pulmonary embolism (PE) and chronic venous insufficiency.
- Provide discharge teaching about use of elastic compression stockings and anticoagulant medication instructions (including diet, necessary laboratory testing, and administration of subcutaneous anticoagulants if needed).
- Teach the patient and caregiver the clinical manifestations of PE and the need to contact the EMS if these occur.
- Teach safety precautions to prevent falls or other injuries that might result in bleeding.
- Provide instructions about the use of pressure to stop bleeding and that the EMS should be contacted for persistent bleeding.
- Teach the patient about lifestyle measures to prevent VTE, including leg exercises, ambulation, and avoidance of nicotine and oral contraceptives.

Role of Licensed Practical/Vocational Nurse (LPN/LVN)
- Administer prescribed oral, subcutaneous, and IV anticoagulants (consider state nurse practice act and agency policies regarding administration of high-alert medications and IV medications).
- Measure patients for elastic compression stockings and/or sequential compression devices.

Role of Unlicensed Assistive Personnel (UAP)
- Reposition patients who are on bed rest at least every 2 hr.
- Remind patients about the need to flex and extend the legs and feet every 2 hr while in bed.
- Assist ambulatory patients to ambulate at least 4 to 6 times daily.
- Assist patients with putting on elastic compression stockings.
- Apply sequential compression devices.

TABLE 38-14 PATIENT & CAREGIVER TEACHING GUIDE

Anticoagulant Therapy

Include the following information in the teaching plan for a patient receiving anticoagulant therapy and the patient's caregiver.

1. Give reasons for and action of anticoagulant therapy and how long therapy will last.
2. Take medication at the same time each day (preferably in afternoon or evening).
3. Depending on medication prescribed, obtain blood tests to assess therapeutic effect of the drug and whether change in drug dosage is needed.
4. Contact emergency medical services immediately for any of the following adverse side effects of drug therapy:
   - Blood in urine or stool; or black, tarry stools
   - Vomiting blood, coffee-ground emesis
   - Unusual bleeding from gums, skin, or nose, or heavy menstrual bleeding
   - Severe headaches or stomach pains
   - Chest pain, shortness of breath, palpitations (heart racing)
   - Weakness, dizziness, mental status changes
   - Cold, blue, or painful feet
5. Avoid any trauma or injury that might cause bleeding (e.g., vigorous brushing of teeth, contact sports, rollerblading, use of straight razor).
6. Avoid all aspirin-containing drugs and nonsteroidal antiinflammatory drugs.
7. Limit alcohol intake to small to moderate amounts (12 oz beer, 4 oz wine, 1 oz hard liquor/day).
8. Wear a Medic Alert device indicating what anticoagulant is being taken.
9. Avoid frequent changes in eating habits, such as dramatically increasing foods high in vitamin K (e.g., broccoli, spinach, kale, greens). Do not take supplemental vitamin K.
10. Consult with health care provider before beginning or discontinuing any medication, vitamin, mineral, or dietary or herbal supplement (see Complementary & Alternative Therapies box).
11. Inform all health care providers, including dentist, of anticoagulant therapy.
12. Correct dosing is essential. Provide supervision if patient experiences confusion or cognitive impairment.

---

extremity VTE) is recommended for at least 2 years after a VTE to support the vein walls and valves and decrease swelling and pain.[44,49] Regular use of elastic compression stockings reduces the incidence of mild PTS. Unfortunately, getting the patient to adhere to wearing stockings is a challenge. Address individual risk factors for VTE (e.g., obesity) and barriers to stocking use (e.g., lack of knowledge, depression) to improve patient adherence.[65]

If appropriate, tell the patient to stop smoking and avoid all nicotine products. Instruct the patient to avoid constrictive clothing. If appropriate, tell women with a history of VTE to stop oral contraceptives or HT. Teach patients to limit standing or sitting in a motionless, leg-dependent position. During long train or plane rides, encourage patients to frequently exercise the calf muscles and take short walks around the cabin. For those at high risk for VTE who are planning a long trip, recommend properly fitted, knee-high elastic compression stockings during travel to decrease edema and VTE risk. Aspirin or anticoagulant use is not suggested for long-distance travelers. Teach the patient and caregiver about signs and symptoms of PE such as sudden onset of dyspnea, tachypnea, and pleuritic chest pain. (Chapter 28 discusses PE.) They should contact EMS if these symptoms occur.

Instruct the patient and the caregiver about drug dosage, actions, and side effects; the need for routine blood tests; and what symptoms need immediate medical attention (Table 38-14). Devices are available for home monitoring of INR. Teach patients taking LMWH or fondaparinux and their caregivers how to give the drug subcutaneously. Active or young patients need to avoid contact sports and high-risk (for trauma) activities (e.g., skiing). Teach older patients about safety precautions to prevent falls (e.g., avoid use of throw rugs). Instruct the patient and caregiver to apply pressure for 10 to 15 minutes if bleeding occurs (e.g., nosebleed).

A well-balanced diet is important. Teach patients taking warfarin to follow a consistent diet of foods containing vitamin K and to avoid any supplements containing vitamin K (e.g., vitamins, green tea). Instruct the patient to avoid excessive amounts of vitamin E and alcohol. Encourage proper hydration to prevent additional hypercoagulability of the blood, which may occur with dehydration.

The overweight patient needs to not only limit caloric intake but also increase physical activity to achieve and maintain desired weight. A balanced program of rest and exercise also improves venous return. Help the patient develop an exercise program with an emphasis on walking and swimming. Water exercise is particularly beneficial because of the gentle, even pressure of the water. A 6-month exercise program improves quality of life and reduces PTS.[66]

EVALUATION

The expected outcomes for the patient with VTE include
- Minimal to no pain
- Intact skin
- No signs of hemorrhage or occult bleeding
- No signs of respiratory distress

VARICOSE VEINS

Varicose veins, or *varicosities,* are dilated (3 mm or larger in diameter), tortuous subcutaneous veins commonly found in the saphenous vein system.[67] Varicosities may be small and harmless or large and bulging. *Primary varicose veins* (idiopathic) are due to a congenital weakness of the veins and are more common in women. *Secondary varicose veins* typically result from a previous VTE. Secondary varicose veins also may occur in the esophagus (esophageal varices), vulva, spermatic cords (varicoceles), and anorectal area (hemorrhoids), and as abnormal arteriovenous (AV) connections. *Reticular veins* are smaller varicose veins that appear flat, less tortuous, and blue-green in color. *Telangiectasias* (often referred to as spider veins) are small visible vessels (generally less than 1 mm in diameter) that appear bluish black, purple, or red.

Etiology and Pathophysiology

The etiology of varicose veins is multifactorial. Superficial veins in the lower extremities become dilated and tortuous in response to increased venous pressure. Risk factors include family history of venous disease, weakness of the vein structure, female gender, use of oral contraceptives or HT, tobacco use, increasing age, obesity, pregnancy, history of VTE, venous obstruction resulting from extrinsic pressure by tumors, thrombophilia, or occupations that require prolonged standing or sitting.[67] Although the exact etiology remains unknown, it is thought that the vein valve leaflets are stretched and become incompetent (do not fit together properly). Incompetent vein valves allow backward blood flow, particularly when the patient is standing. This results in increased venous pressure and further venous distention.

Clinical Manifestations and Complications

Discomfort from varicose veins varies among people and tends to be worse after episodes of SVT. Many patients are concerned about cosmetic disfigurement. The most common varicose vein symptoms include a heavy, achy feeling or pain after prolonged standing or sitting, which is relieved by walking or limb elevation. Some patients feel pressure or complain of an itchy, burning, tingling, throbbing, or cramplike leg sensation. Swelling, restless or tired legs, fatigue, and nocturnal leg cramps also may occur.

FIG. 38-12 A, Lateral aspect of varicose veins before treatment. **B,** Lateral aspect of varicose veins 2 years after initial treatment with sclerotherapy.

SVT is the most frequent complication of varicose veins. It may occur spontaneously or after trauma, surgical procedures, or pregnancy. Rare complications include rupture of the varicose veins resulting in external bleeding and skin ulcerations.

Diagnostic Studies and Collaborative Care

Superficial varicose veins can be diagnosed by appearance. A duplex ultrasound can detect obstruction and reflux in the venous system. Treatment usually is not indicated if varicose veins are only a cosmetic problem. If CVI develops, care involves rest with limb elevation; elastic compression stockings; and exercise, such as walking. Two herbal therapies used for varicose vein treatment are horse chestnut seed extract (HCSE) *(Aesculus hippocastanum)* and butcher's broom *(Ruscus aculeatus).*[68] Venoactive drugs (e.g., diosmin, hesperidin, rutosides [Venoruton]) with compression therapy are recommended for patients with varicose veins experiencing pain and swelling.

Sclerotherapy involves the injection of a substance (e.g., hypertonic saline, polidocanol, glycerine) that destroys venous telangiectasias, reticular veins, and superficial varicose veins 5 mm in diameter or smaller (Fig. 38-12). Direct IV injection of a sclerosing agent causes inflammation and results in thrombosis of the vein. This procedure is performed in an office setting and causes minimal discomfort. Potential complications include itching, pain, blistering, edema, inflammation, hyperpigmentation, tissue necrosis, recurrence of varicosities, SVT, and VTE.[69] After injection, a thigh-high elastic compression stocking is worn or an elastic bandage is applied to the leg for several days to maintain pressure over the vein. Long-term compression therapy is advised to help prevent further varicosities.

Other noninvasive options for the treatment of venous telangiectasias include laser therapy and high-intensity pulsed-light therapy. Laser or light therapy is used for isolated small telangiectasias or for patients in whom sclerotherapy is contraindicated or has been ineffective. Laser treatment typically requires more than one session, scheduled at 6- to 12-week intervals. Vascular lasers work by heating the hemoglobin in the vessels, resulting in vessel sclerosis. Potential complications of these therapies include pain, blistering, hyperpigmentation, and superficial erosions.

Surgical intervention is indicated for recurrent SVT or when CVI cannot be controlled with conservative therapy. The traditional surgical intervention involves ligation of the entire vein (usually the greater saphenous vein) and removal of its incompetent branches. An alternative but time-consuming technique is ambulatory phlebectomy. This involves pulling the varicosity through a "stab" incision followed by excision of the vein. Transilluminated powered phlebectomy involves the use of a tissue resector to destroy the varices and removes the pieces via aspiration. Potential complications include bleeding, bruising, and infection. In up to 30% of patients, a new vein forms to replace the one removed.

A less invasive procedure is endovenous ablation of the saphenous vein. Ablation involves the insertion of a catheter that emits energy. This causes collapse and sclerosis of the vein.[70] Potential complications include bruising, tightness along the vein, recanalization (reopening of the vein), and paresthesia. Endovenous ablation also may be done in combination with ligation or phlebectomy.

NURSING MANAGEMENT
VARICOSE VEINS

Prevention is a key factor related to varicose veins. Instruct the patient to avoid sitting or standing for long periods, maintain ideal body weight, take precautions against injury to the extremities, avoid wearing constrictive clothing, and walk daily.

After vein ligation surgery, encourage the patient to deep breathe, which promotes venous return. Check the extremities regularly for color, movement, sensation, temperature, edema, and quality of pedal pulses. Some bruising and discoloration are normal. Postoperatively, elevate the legs 15 degrees to limit edema. Apply elastic compression stockings. Remove them every 8 hours for short periods and then reapply.

Long-term management of varicose veins is directed toward improving circulation and appearance, relieving discomfort, and avoiding complications and ulceration. Varicose veins can recur in other veins after surgery. Teach the patient the proper use and care of custom-fitted elastic compression stockings. The patient should apply stockings in bed before rising in the morning. Emphasize the importance of periodic positioning of the legs above the heart. The overweight patient may need assistance with weight loss. The patient with a job that requires long periods of standing or sitting needs to frequently flex and extend her or his hips, legs, and ankles and change positions.

CHRONIC VENOUS INSUFFICIENCY AND VENOUS LEG ULCERS

Chronic venous insufficiency (CVI), a common problem in women and older adults, is a condition that develops when leg veins and valves fail to keep blood moving forward. This results in *ambulatory venous hypertension*. CVI can lead to *venous leg ulcers* (formerly called *venous stasis ulcers* or *varicose ulcers*). Although CVI and venous leg ulcers are not life-threatening diseases, they are painful, debilitating, and costly conditions that adversely affect the quality of patients' lives.

Etiology and Pathophysiology

Both long-standing primary varicose veins and PTS can progress to CVI. As a result of ambulatory venous hypertension, serous fluid and RBCs leak from the capillaries and venules into the tissue. This produces edema and chronic inflammatory changes. Enzymes in the tissue eventually break down RBCs,

FIG. 38-13 Venous leg ulcer.

causing the release of *hemosiderin,* which causes a brownish skin discoloration. Over time, the skin and subcutaneous tissue around the ankle are replaced by fibrous tissue, resulting in thick, hardened, contracted skin. Although the causes of CVI are known, the exact pathophysiology of venous leg ulcers is unknown.

Clinical Manifestations and Complications

In individuals with CVI the skin of the lower leg is leathery, with a characteristic brownish or "brawny" appearance from the hemosiderin deposition. Edema usually has been persistent for a prolonged period. Eczema, or "stasis dermatitis," is often present, and itching is a common complaint (see Table 38-1).

Venous ulcers classically are located above the medial malleolus (Fig. 38-13). The ulcer is often quite painful, particularly when edema or infection is present. Pain may be worse when the leg is in a dependent position. If the venous ulcer is untreated, the wound becomes wider and deeper, increasing the likelihood of infection. Severe complications can include osteomyelitis and malignant changes.[71] On rare occasions, severe CVI with long-standing nonhealing venous ulcers may result in the need for amputation.

Collaborative Care

Compression is essential for CVI treatment, venous ulcer healing, and prevention of ulcer recurrence. A variety of options are available for compression therapy. These include custom-fitted elastic compression stockings, elastic tubular support bandages, a Velcro wrap (CircAid), SCDs, a paste bandage (Unna boot) with an elastic wrap, and multilayer (three or four) bandage systems (e.g., Profore).[71] There are benefits to each type of compression therapy. Evaluate patients individually when choosing a compression method. Before starting compression therapy, assess the arterial status to make sure that PAD is not also present. An ABI of less than 0.9 suggests PAD, and the patient should not have high levels of compression therapy.

Moist environment dressings are the basis of wound care. A variety of these dressings are available, including transparent film dressings, hydrocolloids, hydrogels, foams, alginates, gauze, and combination dressings.[72] Dressing decisions should be based on wound characteristics, cost, and clinician judgment. (Chapter 12 and Table 12-10 discuss dressings.)

Evaluate the nutritional status of a patient with a venous ulcer. A balanced diet with adequate protein, calories, and nutrients is essential. Foods high in protein (e.g., meat, beans, cheese, tofu), vitamin A (green leafy vegetables), vitamin C (citrus fruits, tomatoes, cantaloupe), and zinc (meat, seafood) are most important for healing. For patients with diabetes, maintaining normal blood glucose levels assists the healing process.

Routine use of antibiotics is not indicated. Clinical signs of infection include change in quantity, color, or odor of the drainage; pus; erythema of the wound edges; change in sensation around the wound; warmth around the wound; increased local pain, edema, or both; dark-colored granulation tissue; induration around the wound; delayed healing; and cellulitis. If signs of infection occur, obtain a wound culture before starting antibiotic therapy. The usual treatment for infection is debridement, wound excision, and systemic antibiotics. A number of antimicrobial dressings (e.g., cadexomer iodine, silver) are available.

If the ulcer does not heal with conservative therapy, pentoxifylline or micronized purified flavonoid fraction (Daflon) is recommended with compression therapy to improve healing.[67] Other treatments may include coverage with a skin replacement or substitute such as split-thickness skin grafts, cultured keratinocyte grafts, or artificial bioengineered skin. When used with compression therapy, a bilayer artificial skin (e.g., Apligraf or Orcel) can increase ulcer healing more than a simple dressing and compression.[73] (Chapter 25 discusses skin grafting.) Although grafts may aid with healing, they do not replace the need for lifelong compression therapy.

An herbal therapy used for CVI treatment is horse chestnut seed extract (HCSE). Escins (the active ingredient) reduce leg pain, itching, and swelling.[68] Minor side effects associated with HCSE include dizziness, gastrointestinal complaints, headache, and pruritus. The value of HCSE in venous ulcer healing and recurrence is not known.

NURSING MANAGEMENT
CHRONIC VENOUS INSUFFICIENCY AND VENOUS LEG ULCERS

Long-term management of venous leg ulcers should focus on teaching the patient self-care measures. Demonstrate the correct application of elastic compression stockings, and have the patient "show back" the skill. Prescription elastic compression stockings should be worn daily to reduce the occurrence of CVI. Stress the importance of regular replacement every 4 to 6 months. Instruct the patient and caregiver to avoid trauma to the limbs, and teach them proper foot and leg care to avoid additional skin trauma. Patients with CVI have dry, flaky, itchy

---

DELEGATION DECISIONS

Caring for the Patient With Chronic Venous Insufficiency

Many patients with chronic venous insufficiency and venous ulcers are cared for in an outpatient setting. In this case the registered nurse (RN) does an initial assessment of the wound, develops the plan of care, and periodically evaluates the patient and venous ulcer. Much of the routine wound care is done by unlicensed assistive personnel (UAP) and licensed practical/vocational nurses (LPN/LVNs).

Role of Registered Nurse (RN)
- Assess patients with venous insufficiency for increases in edema, stasis dermatitis, and venous stasis ulcers.
- Assess patient's diet and nutritional status and make referrals as necessary to a dietitian.
- Choose appropriate options for compression therapy and wound care.
- Evaluate for the effectiveness of therapies and need for alternative approaches.
- Teach patient and family about the pathophysiology, clinical manifestations, complications, and treatment of venous insufficiency.

Role of Licensed Practical/Vocational Nurse (LPN/LVN)
- Administer prescribed analgesics, antibiotics, or other medications.
- Apply compression devices.
- Provide wound care for chronic venous ulcers (consider state nurse practice act and agency policy).

Role of Unlicensed Assistive Personnel (UAP)
- Assist patients in elevating extremities to reduce edema and pain.
- Apply elastic wraps or compression stockings, as directed by the RN.
- Provide wound care for chronic venous ulcers (consider state nurse practice act and agency policy).

---

skin because of stasis dermatitis. Daily moisturizing decreases itching and prevents cracking of the skin. Venous dermatitis may result from contact with sensitizing products such as antibacterial agents (e.g., gentamicin); additives in bandages or dressings (e.g., adhesives); ointments containing lanolin, alcohols, or benzocaine; and over-the-counter creams or lotions with fragrance or preservatives.[71] Assess the wound for signs of infection with each dressing change.

Be certain to discuss activity guidelines and proper limb positioning. Instruct patients with CVI with or without a venous ulcer to avoid standing or sitting for long periods. Standing or sitting with the legs in a dependent position decreases blood flow to the lower extremities. Also instruct patients to frequently elevate their legs above the level of the heart to reduce edema. Encourage patients to begin a daily walking program once an ulcer heals.

CASE STUDY

Peripheral Artery Disease

iStockphoto/Thinkstock

Patient Profile

S.J., a 76-yr-old African American man, is admitted to the hospital with rest pain in both legs and a nonhealing ulcer of the big toe on the right foot.

Subjective Data

- History of a myocardial infarction, stroke, hypertension, heart failure, and type 1 diabetes mellitus
- Underwent a left femoral-popliteal bypass 5 yr ago
- Has a 45 pack-yr history of tobacco use
- Has been using insulin for 30 yr
- Complains of sudden, intense increase in right foot pain for past 2 hr
- Has slept in recliner with right leg in dependent position for several months

Current Medications

- furosemide 40 mg/day PO
- isosorbide dinitrate/hydralazine hydrochloride (BiDil) 1 tablet q8hr
- aspart (NovoLog) insulin with meals
- glargine insulin 50 U/day subcutaneously
- diltiazem sustained release 240 mg/day PO
- aspirin 325 mg/day PO
- Fish oil daily (self-prescribed)

Objective Data

Physical Examination

- BP 148/92 mm Hg; irregular apical HR 90/min, respiratory rate 22/min, temperature 97.9° F (36.6° C)
- Alert and oriented but anxious, no apparent physical or mental deficits from previous stroke
- Has a diminished right femoral pulse, popliteal pulse by Doppler only, posterior tibial pulse by Doppler only, and dorsalis pedis pulse absent (not palpable or present by Doppler); left leg pulses are weakly palpable

- Right leg ABI: 0.20; left leg ABI: 0.68
- Has a 2-cm necrotic ulcer on tip of right big toe
- Has thickened toenails; shiny, thin skin on legs; and hair absent on both lower legs
- Right foot is very cool, pale, and mottled in color with decreased sensation
- No peripheral edema present
- Bedside glucose measurement 298 mg/dL (last meal 4 hr before admission)

Discussion Questions

1. Assess S.J.'s risk factors for peripheral artery disease (PAD).
2. Differentiate S.J.'s signs and symptoms of chronic PAD and acute arterial ischemia.
3. Identify the possible cause(s) for the sudden, intense increase in right foot pain.
4. How would you interpret S.J.'s ABI findings?
5. What additional diagnostic tests can be performed to assess the extent of his PAD?
6. Given the physical examination data, what initial medication(s) would you expect the physician to prescribe?
7. What treatment modalities are possible for S.J.?
8. *Priority Decision:* What are the priority nursing responsibilities in caring for S.J.?
9. *Delegation Decision:* Identify activities that can be delegated to unlicensed assistive personnel.
10. *Priority Decision:* Based on the assessment data presented, what are the priority nursing diagnoses? Are there any collaborative problems?
11. *Evidence-Based Practice:* When teaching S.J., what evidence-based advice would you give him regarding the use of dietary supplements such as fish oil?

⊘volve Answers available at *http://evolve.elsevier.com/Lewis/medsurg.*

BRIDGE TO NCLEX EXAMINATION

The number of the question corresponds to the same-numbered outcome at the beginning of the chapter.

1. A 50-year-old woman weighs 95 kg and has a history of tobacco use, high blood pressure, high sodium intake, and sedentary lifestyle. When developing an individualized care plan for her, the nurse determines that the most important risk factors for peripheral artery disease (PAD) that need to be modified are
   a. weight and diet.
   b. activity level and diet.
   c. tobacco use and high blood pressure.
   d. sedentary lifestyle and high blood pressure.

2. Rest pain is a manifestation of PAD that occurs due to a chronic
   a. vasospasm of small cutaneous arteries in the feet.
   b. increase in retrograde venous blood flow in the legs.
   c. decrease in arterial blood flow to the nerves of the feet.
   d. decrease in arterial blood flow to the leg muscles during exercise.

3. A patient with infective endocarditis develops sudden left leg pain with pallor, paresthesia, and a loss of peripheral pulses. The nurse's initial action should be to
   a. elevate the leg to promote venous return.
   b. start anticoagulant therapy with IV heparin.
   c. notify the physician of the change in peripheral perfusion.
   d. place the bed in reverse Trendelenburg to promote perfusion.

4. Which clinical manifestations are seen in patients with either Buerger's disease or Raynaud's phenomenon *(select all that apply)?*
   a. Intermittent fevers
   b. Sensitivity to cold temperatures
   c. Gangrenous ulcers on fingertips
   d. Color changes of fingers and toes
   e. Episodes of superficial vein thrombosis

5. A patient is admitted to the hospital with a diagnosis of abdominal aortic aneurysm. Which signs and symptoms would suggest that his aneurysm has ruptured?
   a. Sudden shortness of breath and hemoptysis
   b. Sudden, severe low back pain and bruising along his flank
   c. Gradually increasing substernal chest pain and diaphoresis
   d. Sudden, patchy blue mottling on feet and toes and rest pain

6. Priority nursing measures after an abdominal aortic aneurysm repair include
   a. assessment of cranial nerves and mental status.
   b. administration of IV heparin and monitoring of aPTT.
   c. administration of IV fluids and monitoring of kidney function.
   d. elevation of the legs and application of elastic compression stockings.

7. The first priority of collaborative care of a patient with a suspected acute aortic dissection is to
   a. reduce anxiety.
   b. control blood pressure.
   c. monitor for chest pain.
   d. increase myocardial contractility.

8. The patient at highest risk for venous thromboembolism (VTE) is
   a. a 62-year-old man with spider veins who is having arthroscopic knee surgery.
   b. a 32-year-old woman who smokes, takes oral contraceptives, and is planning a trip to Europe.
   c. a 26-year-old woman who is 3 days postpartum and received maintenance IV fluids for 12 hours during her labor.
   d. an active 72-year-old man at home recovering from transurethral resection of the prostate for benign prostatic hyperplasia.

9. Which are probable clinical findings in a person with an acute lower extremity VTE (select all that apply)?
   a. Pallor and coolness of foot and calf
   b. Mild to moderate calf pain and tenderness
   c. Grossly diminished or absent pedal pulses
   d. Unilateral edema and induration of the thigh
   e. Palpable cord along a superficial varicose vein

10. The recommended treatment for an initial VTE in an otherwise healthy person with no significant co-morbidities would include
    a. IV argatroban (Acova) as an inpatient.
    b. IV unfractionated heparin as an inpatient.
    c. subcutaneous unfractionated heparin as an outpatient.
    d. subcutaneous low-molecular-weight heparin as an outpatient.

11. A key aspect of teaching for the patient on anticoagulant therapy includes which instructions?
    a. Monitor for and report any signs of bleeding.
    b. Do not take acetaminophen (Tylenol) for a headache.
    c. Decrease your dietary intake of foods containing vitamin K.
    d. Arrange to have blood drawn routinely to check drug levels.

12. In planning care and patient teaching for the patient with venous leg ulcers, the nurse recognizes that the most important intervention in healing and control of this condition is
    a. sclerotherapy.
    b. using moist environment dressings.
    c. taking horse chestnut seed extract daily.
    d. applying elastic compression stockings.

1. c, 2. c, 3. c, 4. b, c, d, 5. b, 6. c, 7. b, 8. b, 9. b, d, 10. d, 11. a, 12. d

ⓔvolve

For rationales to these answers and even more NCLEX review questions, visit *http://evolve.elsevier.com/Lewis/medsurg.*

REFERENCES

1. Creager MA, Belkin B, Bluth EI, et al: 2012 ACCF/AHA/ACR/SCAI/SIR/STS/SVM/SVN/SVS key data elements and definitions for peripheral atherosclerotic vascular disease: a report of the American College of Cardiology Foundation/American Heart Association Task Force on Clinical Data Standards, *Circulation* 125:395, 2012.

*2. Pande RL, Perlstein TS, Beckman JA, et al: Secondary prevention and mortality in peripheral artery disease National Health and Nutrition Examination Study, 1999 to 2004, *Circulation* 124:17, 2011.

3. Widner JM: Peripheral arterial disease and disability from NHANES 2001-2004 data, *J Vasc Nurs* 29:104, 2011.

4. Go AS, Mozaffarian D, Roger VL, et al: Heart disease and stroke statistics—2013 update: a report from the American Heart Association, *Circulation* 127:e6, 2013.

*5. Arain FA, Ye Z, Bailey KR, et al: Survival in patients with poorly compressible leg arteries, *J Am Coll Cardiol* 59:400, 2012.

*6. Hirsch AT, Allison MA, Gomes AS, et al: A call to action: women and peripheral artery disease: a scientific statement from the American Heart Association, *Circulation* 125:1449, 2012.

*7. Ix JH, Biggs ML, Kizer JR, et al: Association of body mass index with peripheral arterial disease in older adults: the Cardiovascular Health Study, *Am J Epidemiol* 174:1036, 2011.

*8. Wilson AM, Sadrzadeh-Rafie AH, Myers J, et al: Low lifetime recreational activity is a risk factor for peripheral arterial disease, *J Vasc Surg* 54:427, 2011.

9. Huether SE, McCance KL: *Understanding pathophysiology*, ed 5, St Louis, 2012, Mosby.

*10. Egorova NN, Vouyouka AG, Quin J, et al: Analysis of gender-related differences in lower extremity peripheral arterial disease, *J Vasc Surg* 51:372, 2010.

*11. Alonso-Coello P, Bellmunt S, McGorrian C, et al: Antithrombotic therapy in peripheral artery disease: antithrombotic therapy and prevention of thrombosis, ed 9: American College of Chest Physicians evidence-based clinical practice guidelines, *Chest* 141:e669S, 2012. doi: 10.1378/chest.11-2307.

*12. Rooke TW, Hirsch AT, Misra S, et al: 2011 ACCF/AHA focused update of the guideline for the management of patients with peripheral artery disease (updating the 2005 guideline): a report of the American College of Cardiology Foundation/American Heart Association Task Force on Practice Guidelines, *J Am Coll Cardiol* 8:2020, 2012.

13. Aboyans V, Criqui MH, Abraham P, et al: Measurement and interpretation of the ankle-brachial index: a scientific statement from the American Heart Association, *Circulation* 126:2890, 2012.

*14. Hirsch AT, Haskal ZJ, Hertzer NR, et al: ACC/AHA 2005 practice guidelines for the management of patients with peripheral arterial disease (lower extremity, renal, mesenteric, and abdominal aortic): a collaborative report from the American Association for Vascular Surgery/Society for Vascular Surgery, Society for Cardiovascular Angiography and Interventions, Society for Vascular Medicine and Biology,

*Evidence-based information for clinical practice.

Society of Interventional Radiology, and the ACC/AHA Task Force on Practice Guidelines, *Circulation* 113:e463, 2006. (Classic)

15. American Diabetes Association: Standards of medical care in diabetes—2012, *Diabetes Care* 35(Suppl):S11, 2012.

16. Saratzis A, Kitas GD, Saratzis N, et al: Can statins suppress the development of abdominal aortic aneurysms? A review of the current evidence, *Angiology* 61:137, 2010.

17. Hamburg NM, Balady GJ: Exercise rehabilitation in peripheral artery disease: functional impact and mechanisms of benefit, *Circulation* 123:87, 2011.

*18. National Heart, Lung, and Blood Institute: *Clinical guidelines on the identification, evaluation, and treatment of overweight and obesity in adults: the evidence report,* NIH Pub No 98-4083, Bethesda, MD, 1998, National Institutes of Health. (Classic)

19. Tachjian A, Maria V, Jahangir A: Use of herbal products and potential interactions in patients with cardiovascular diseases, *J Am Coll Cardiol* 55:515, 2010.

20. Varu VN, Hogg ME, Kibbe MR: Critical limb ischemia, *J Vasc Surg* 51:230, 2010.

21. Nanjundappa A, Jain A, Cohoon K, et al: Percutaneous management of chronic critical limb ischemia, *Cardiol Clin* 29:395, 2011.

22. Gandhi S, Sakhuja R, Slovut DP: Recent advances in percutaneous management of iliofemoral and superficial femoral artery disease, *Cardiol Clin* 29:381, 2011.

*23. Ahimastos AA, Pappas EP, Bultner PG, et al: A meta-analysis of the outcome of endovascular and noninvasive therapies in the treatment of intermittent claudication, *J Vasc Surg* 64:1511, 2011.

*24. Greenblatt DY, Rajamanickam V, Mell MW: Predictors of surgical site infection after open lower extremity revascularization, *J Vasc Surg* 54:433, 2011.

25. Ouriel K, Kasyap V: Acute limb ischemia. In Jaff M, White C, editors: *Vascular disease: diagnostic and therapeutic approaches,* Minneapolis, 2011, Cardiotext.

26. Lyden SP: Endovascular treatment of acute limb ischemia: review of current plasminogen activators and mechanical thrombectomy devices, *Perspect Vasc Surg* 22:219, 2010.

*27. You JJ, Singer DE, Howard PA, et al: Antithrombotic therapy for atrial fibrillation: antithrombotic therapy and prevention of thrombosis, 9th ed: American College of Chest Physicians evidence-based clinical practice guidelines, *Chest* 141:e531S, 2012.

28. Piazza G, Creager MA: Thromboangiitis obliterans, *Circulation* 121:1858, 2010.

*29. Japanese Circulation Society Joint Working Group: Guideline for management of vasculitis syndrome—JCS 2008, *Circulation* 75:474, 2011.

30. Lazzerini PE, Capecchi PL, Bisogno S, et al: Homocysteine and Raynaud's phenomenon: a review, *Autoimmun Rev* 9:181, 2010.

31. Herrick AL: Contemporary management of Raynaud's phenomenon and digital ischaemic complications, *Curr Opin Rheumatol* 23:555, 2011.

*32. Kent KC, Zwolak RM, Egorova NN, et al: Analysis of risk factors for abdominal aortic aneurysm in a cohort of more than 3 million individuals, *J Vasc Surg* 52:539, 2010.

*33. Hiratzka LF, Bakris GL, Beckman JA, et al: 2010 ACCF/AHA/ AATS/ACR/ASA/SCA/SCAI/SIR/STS/SVM guidelines for the diagnosis and management of patients with thoracic aortic disease: a report of the American College of Cardiology

Foundation/American Heart Association Task Force on Practice Guidelines, American Association for Thoracic Surgery, American College of Radiology, American Stroke Association, Society of Cardiovascular Anesthesiologists, Society for Cardiovascular Angiography and Interventions, Society of Interventional Radiology, Society of Thoracic Surgeons, and Society for Vascular Medicine, *J Am Coll Cardiol* 55:e27, 2010.

*34. Filardo G, Powell JT, Martinez MAM, et al: Surgery for small asymptomatic abdominal aortic aneurysms, *Cochrane Database Syst Rev* 3:CD001835, 2012.

*35. Egorova NN, Vouyouka AG, McKinsey JF, et al: Effect of gender on long-term survival after abdominal aortic aneurysm repair based on results from the Medicare national database, *J Vasc Surg* 54:1, 2011.

36. Ganeshanantham G, Walsh SR, Varty K: Abdominal compartment syndrome in vascular surgery—a review, *Int J Surg* 8:181, 2010.

37. Gidlund KD, Wanhainen A, Björck M: Intra-abdominal hypertension and abdominal compartment syndrome after endovascular repair of ruptured abdominal aortic aneurysm, *Eur J Vasc Endovasc Surg* 41:742e, 2011.

38. Cheatham ML, Safcsak K: Percutaneous catheter decompression in the treatment of elevated intraabdominal pressure, *Chest* 140(6):1428, 2011.

39. Nordon IM, Hinchliffe RJ, Loftus IM, et al: Management of acute aortic syndrome and chronic aortic dissection, *Cardiovasc Intervent Radiol* 34:890, 2011.

*40. Thrumurthy SG, Karthikesalingam A, Patterson BO, et al: A systematic review of mid-term outcomes of thoracic endovascular repair (TEVAR) of chronic type B aortic dissection, *Eur J Vasc Endovasc Surg* 42:632, 2011.

41. Ho KH, Cheung DS: Guidelines on timing in replacing peripheral intravenous catheters, *J Clin Nurs* 21:1499, 2012.

*42. van Langevelde K, Lijfering WM, Rosendaal FR, et al: Increased risk of venous thrombosis in persons with clinically diagnosed superficial vein thrombosis: results from the MEGA study, *Blood* 118:4239, 2011.

43. Reitsma PH, Versteeg HH, Middeldorp S: Mechanistic view of risk factors for venous thromboembolism, *Arterioscler Thromb Vasc Biol* 32:563, 2012.

*44. Kearon C, Akl EA, Comerota AJ, et al: Antithrombotic therapy for VTE disease: antithrombotic therapy and prevention of thrombosis, ed 9: American College of Chest Physicians evidence-based clinical practice guidelines, *Chest* 141:e419S, 2012.

45. Decousus H, Bertoletti L, Frappé P, et al: Recent findings in the epidemiology, diagnosis and treatment of superficial-vein thrombosis, *Thrombosis Res* 127:S81, 2011.

*46. Di Nisio M, Wichers IM, Middeldorp S: Treatment for superficial thrombophlebitis of the leg, *Cochrane Database Syst Rev* 3:CD004982, 2012.

*47. Bates SM, Jaeschke R, Stevens SM, et al: Diagnosis of DVT: antithrombotic therapy and prevention of thrombosis, 9th ed: American College of Chest Physicians evidence-based clinical practice guidelines, *Chest* 141:e351S, 2012.

48. Henke PK, Comerota AJ: An update: etiology, prevention, and therapy of postthrombotic syndrome, *J Vasc Surg* 53:500, 2011.

49. Crumley C: Post-thrombotic syndrome patient education based on the health belief model: self-reported intention to comply with recommendations, *J WOCN* 38:648, 2011.

*50. Cohen J, Akl E, Kahn S: Pharmacologic and compression therapies for postthrombotic syndrome: a systematic review of randomized controlled trials, *Chest* 141(2):308, 2012.

51. Bergmann J-F, Cohen AT, Tapson VF, et al: Venous thromboembolism risk and prophylaxis in hospitalized medically ill patients, *Thromb Haemost* 103:736, 2010.

*52. Kahn SR, Lim W, Dunn AS, et al: Prevention of VTE in nonsurgical patients: antithrombotic therapy and prevention of thrombosis, 9th ed: American College of Chest Physicians evidence-based clinical practice guidelines, *Chest* 141:e195S, 2012.

*53. Gould MK, Garcia DA, Wren SM, et al: Prevention of VTE in nonorthopedic surgical patients: antithrombotic therapy and prevention of thrombosis, 9th ed: American College of Chest Physicians evidence-based clinical practice guidelines, *Chest* 141:e227S, 2012.

*54. Sachdeva A, Dalton M, Amaragiri SV, et al: Elastic compression stockings for prevention of deep vein thrombosis, *Cochrane Database Syst Rev* 7:CD001484, 2010.

*55. CLOTS Trial Collaboration: Thigh-length versus below-knee stockings for deep venous thrombosis prophylaxis after stroke, *Ann Intern Med* 153:553, 2010.

*56. Kakkos SK, Caprini JA, Geroulakos G, et al: Combined intermittent pneumatic leg compression and pharmacological prophylaxis for prevention of venous thromboembolism in high-risk patients, *Cochrane Database Syst Rev* 3:CD005258, 2011.

*57. Garcia DA, Baglin TP, Weitz JI, et al: Parenteral anticoagulants: antithrombotic therapy and prevention of thrombosis, ed 9: American College of Chest Physicians evidence-based clinical practice guidelines, *Chest* 141:e24S, 2012.

*58. Ageno W, Gallus AS, Wittkowsky A, et al: Oral anticoagulant therapy: antithrombotic therapy and prevention of thrombosis, 9th ed: American College of Chest Physicians evidence-based clinical practice guidelines, *Chest* 141:e44S, 2012.

*59. Guyatt GH, Akl EA, Crowther M, et al: Executive summary: antithrombotic therapy and prevention of thrombosis, 9th ed: American College of Chest Physicians evidence-based clinical practice guidelines, *Chest* 141:7S, 2012.

*60. Linkins LA, Dans AL, Moores LK, et al: Treatment and prevention of heparin-induced thrombocytopenia: antithrombotic therapy and prevention of thrombosis, 9th ed: American College of Chest Physicians evidence-based clinical practice guidelines, *Chest* 141:e495S, 2012.

*61. Falck-Ytter Y, Francis CW, Johanson NA, et al: Prevention of VTE in orthopedic surgery patients: antithrombotic therapy and prevention of thrombosis, 9th ed: American College of Chest Physicians evidence-based clinical practice guidelines, *Chest* 141:e278S, 2012.

*62. Young T, Tang H, Hughes R: Vena caval filters for the prevention of pulmonary embolism, *Cochrane Database Syst Rev* 2:CD006212, 2010.

*63. Holbrook A, Schulman S, Witt DM, et al: Evidence-based management of anticoagulant therapy: antithrombotic therapy and prevention of thrombosis, ed 9: American College of Chest Physicians evidence-based clinical practice guidelines, *Chest* 141:e152S, 2012.

*64. Decousus H, Tapson VF, Bergmann JF, et al: Factors at admission associated with bleeding risk in medical patients: findings from the IMPROVE investigators, *Chest* 139:69, 2011.

*65. Finlayson K, Edwards H, Courtney M: The impact of psychosocial factors on adherence to compression therapy to prevent recurrence of venous leg ulcers, *J Clin Nurs* 19:1289, 2010.

*66. Kahn SR, Shrier I, Shapiro S, et al: Six-month exercise training program to treat post-thrombotic syndrome: a randomized controlled two-centre trial, *Can Med Assoc J* 183:37, 2011.

*67. Gloviczki P, Comerota AJ, Dalsing MC, et al: The care of patients with varicose veins and associated chronic venous diseases: clinical practice guidelines of the Society for Vascular Surgery and the American Venous Forum, *J Vasc Surg* 53:2S, 2011.

*68. Pittler MH, Ernst E: Horse chestnut seed extract for chronic venous insufficiency, *Cochrane Database Syst Rev* 9:CD003230, 2010.

*69. Tisi PV, Beverley C, Rees A: Injection sclerotherapy for varicose veins, *Cochrane Database Syst Rev* 5:CD001732, 2011.

*70. Nesbitt C, Eifell RKG, Coyne P, et al: Endovenous ablation (radiofrequency and laser) and foam sclerotherapy versus conventional surgery for great saphenous vein varices, *Cochrane Database Syst Rev* 10:CD005624, 2011.

71. Collins L, Seraj S: Diagnosis and treatment of venous ulcers, *Am Fam Physician* 81:989, 2010.

*72. Palfreyman SSJ, Nelson EA, Lochiel R, et al: Dressings for healing venous leg ulcers, *Cochrane Database Syst Rev* 1:CD001103, 2010.

*73. Jones JE, Nelson EA: Skin grafting for venous leg ulcers, *Cochrane Database Syst Rev* 1:CD001737, 2010.

RESOURCES

American Heart Association
www.heart.org/HEARTORG
American Venous Forum
www.veinforum.org
Cochrane Peripheral Vascular Diseases Group
www.pvd.cochrane.org
Mayo Clinic Heart and Blood Vessels Center: Peripheral Artery Disease
www.mayoclinic.com/health/peripheral-arterial-disease/DS00537/
Society for Clinical Vascular Surgery
http://scvs.org
Society for Vascular Nursing
www.svnnet.org
Society for Vascular Surgery
www.vascularweb.org
Vascular Disease Foundation
www.vdf.org
Venous Disease Coalition
http://venousdiseasecoalition.org

CASE STUDY

Managing Multiple Patients

Introduction
You are working on the cardiovascular stepdown unit and have been assigned to care for the following six patients. You have one LPN and a UAP who are assigned to help you.

Patients

Jupiterimages/Banana-Stock/Thinkstock

L.P. is a 63-year-old Asian American man who was brought to the ED with complaints of chest pain, shortness of breath (SOB), palpitations, and dizziness. L.P.'s CK-MB and troponin levels are within normal limits. His ECG showed atrial fibrillation with a rapid ventricular response. He has been on IV diltiazem (Cardizem) and IV heparin for 24 hours. Although his heart rate has decreased to 102 bpm, the atrial fibrillation persists.

iStockphoto/Thinkstock

J.E. is a 70-year-old Hispanic woman admitted with complaints of increasing shortness of breath, fatigue, and weight gain. She has a systolic murmur and bilateral crackles. Her ejection fraction is 20%. She is currently receiving IV Lasix, oral potassium and enalapril (Vasotec), and a continuous infusion of nesiritide (Natrecor). She is receiving O_2 at 6 L per nasal cannula for an O_2 saturation greater than 93%. Her initial set of cardiac enzymes were normal.

D.M. is a 51-year-old white man who was rushed to the hospital by ambulance after experiencing crushing substernal chest pain that radiated down his left arm. His ECG demonstrated marked ST segment elevation in the inferior leads. Cardiac catheterization within 60 minutes of admission showed a 90% blockage of his LAD. Coronary angioplasty was performed and a stent inserted. He is now 2 days post-PTCA and has no recurrence of his chest pain.

iStockphoto/Thinkstock

R.B. is a 50-year-old white man admitted for valvular heart disease with a history of IV drug use and alcohol abuse. He complains of chest pain with minimal exertion. He has atrial fibrillation with a rapid ventricular response. His rhythm converted to normal sinus rhythm after receiving IV amiodarone. Transesophageal echocardiography shows left atrial and ventricular hypertrophy and mitral and aortic regurgitation.

Jupiterimages/Photos.com/Thinkstock

J.M. is a 68-year-old white man originally admitted 3 days ago with a diagnosis of acute decompensated HF. He had a cardiac arrest (pulseless VT) and was successfully defibrillated after one shock. He underwent electrophysiology studies, culminating in the implantation of an implantable cardiodefibrillator (ICD). He now is being treated for his heart failure.

iStockphoto/Thinkstock

S.J. is a 76-year-old African American man admitted with rest pain in both legs and a nonhealing ulcer of the big toe on the right foot. He has a history of an MI, stroke, hypertension, heart failure, and type 1 diabetes mellitus. He underwent a left femoral-popliteal bypass 5 years ago. His right foot is very cool, pale, and mottled in color with decreased sensation. He has a diminished right femoral pulse, a right popliteal and posterior tibial pulse by Doppler only, and his right dorsalis pedis pulse is absent (not palpable or present by Doppler). His left leg pulses are weakly palpable. His right leg ABI: 0.20; left leg ABI: 0.68.

iStockphoto/Thinkstock

Management Discussion Questions

1. **Priority Decision:** After receiving report, which patient should you see first? Second? Provide a rationale for your decision.
2. **Delegation Decision:** Which tasks could you delegate to the UAP *(select all that apply)*?
   a. Monitor L.P.'s heparin infusion.
   b. Teach D.M. about activity restriction post-PTCA.
   c. Administer prescribed medications to R.B. and J.M.
   d. Report changes in pain or sensation of S.J.'s legs.
   e. Hook up J.M. to 12-lead ECG and monitor for any dysrhythmias.
3. **Priority and Delegation Decision:** As you are assessing L.P., the LPN informs you that S.J. is diaphoretic and complaining of chest pain. Which initial action would be most appropriate?
   a. Ask the LPN to notify S.J.'s health care provider.
   b. Have the LPN administer prescribed nitroglycerin to S.J.
   c. Leave L.P.'s room to perform a focused assessment on S.J.
   d. Finish assessing L.P. while the UAP obtains a 12-lead ECG on S.J.

Case Study Progression
S.J. rates his chest pain as a 9/10. His blood pressure is 110/70, heart rate 110, respiratory rate 26, and O_2 93% on room air. You obtain a 12-lead ECG and administer 0.4 mg SL nitroglycerin with minimal pain relief after 5 minutes. The 12-lead ECG demonstrates new ST elevation in leads II, III, and aVF.

4. Which interventions would you expect the health care provider to order for S.J. *(select all that apply)*?
   a. IV nitroglycerin
   b. IV morphine sulfate
   c. Emergent cardiac catheterization
   d. Furosemide 40 mg IV push STAT
   e. Increase O_2 flow rate to 12 L/minute
5. Which statement would you include in patient teaching regarding ICDs with J.M. and his family?
   a. Avoid air travel.
   b. Avoid driving for 6 weeks.
   c. Avoid any sexual activity in case the ICD discharges.
   d. Avoid standing near antitheft devices in doorways of stores and public buildings.
6. Knowing the mechanism of action for nesiritide, you prioritize monitoring of J.E.'s
   a. blood pressure.
   b. respiratory rate.
   c. b-Natriuretic peptide (BNP) level.
   d. troponin and CK-MB laboratory values.
7. **Management Decision:** You ask the UAP to take D.M.'s vital signs before and after having him walk 300 feet. When reviewing the patient's chart, you note documentation of the patient's walk but not his vital signs. What is your best initial action?
   a. Report the incident to the charge nurse for follow-up.
   b. Talk to the UAP to discuss why the vital signs were not documented.
   c. Walk D.M. yourself again and take his vital signs pre- and post-activity.
   d. Ask the LPN to ambulate D.M. and obtain his vital signs before and after.

Problems of Ingestion, Digestion, Absorption, and Elimination

Peter Bonner

I see my path, but I don't know where it leads. Not knowing where I'm going is what inspires me to travel it.
Rosalia de Castro

It's all right to have butterflies in your stomach. Just get them to fly in formation.
Rob Gilbert

Nursing Assessment
Gastrointestinal System

Paula Cox-North

evolve WEBSITE

http://evolve.elsevier.com/Lewis/medsurg

- NCLEX Review Questions
- Key Points
- Pre-Test
- Answer Guidelines for Case Study in this chapter
- Rationales for Bridge to NCLEX Examination Questions
- Concept Map Creator
- Glossary
- Content Updates
- Animation
  - Rectal Examination

- Videos
  - Auscultation: Abdomen, Bowel Sounds
  - Palpation: Abdomen, Superficial and Deep
  - Percussion: Abdomen
  - Percussion: Liver
  - Percussion: Spleen
  - Physical Examination: Abdomen: Inspection, Auscultation, and Percussion
  - Physical Examination: Abdomen: Palpation

eFigures
- eFig. 39-1: Omentum
- eFig. 39-2: Microscopic structure of liver lobule

LEARNING OUTCOMES

1. Describe the structures and functions of the organs of the gastrointestinal tract.
2. Describe the structures and functions of the liver, gallbladder, biliary tract, and pancreas.
3. Differentiate the processes of ingestion, digestion, absorption, and elimination.
4. Explain the processes of biliary metabolism, bile production, and bile excretion.
5. Link the age-related changes of the gastrointestinal system to the differences in assessment findings.

6. Select significant subjective and objective assessment data related to the gastrointestinal system that should be obtained from a patient.
7. Identify the appropriate techniques used in the physical assessment of the gastrointestinal system.
8. Differentiate normal from abnormal findings of a physical assessment of the gastrointestinal system.
9. Describe the purpose, significance of results, and nursing responsibilities related to diagnostic studies of the gastrointestinal system.

KEY TERMS

bilirubin, p. 870
borborygmi, Table 39-11, p. 878
cheilosis, Table 39-11, p. 878
deglutition, p. 867
endoscopy, p. 882

hematemesis, Table 39-11, p. 878
hepatocytes, p. 869
Kupffer cells, p. 870
melena, Table 39-11, p. 878
pyorrhea, Table 39-11, p. 878

pyrosis, Table 39-11, p. 878
steatorrhea, Table 39-11, p. 878
tenesmus, Table 39-11, p. 878
Valsalva maneuver, p. 869

Reviewed by Phyllis Christianson, MN, APRN-BC, GNP, Senior Lecturer, University of Washington, School of Nursing, Seattle, Washington; and Marian Sawyier, RN, MSN, Staff Nurse, University of New Mexico Hospital, Albuquerque, New Mexico.

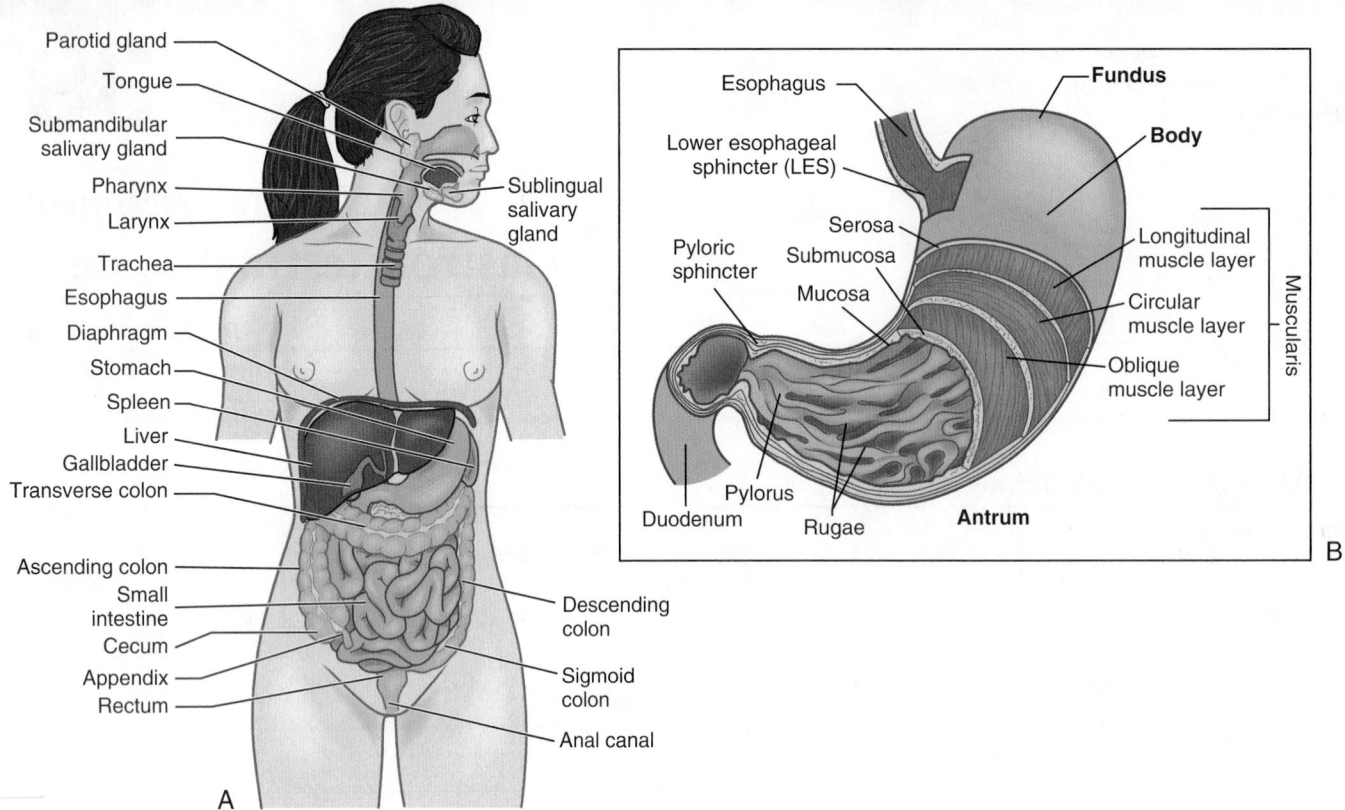

FIG. 39-1 A, Location of organs of the gastrointestinal system. **B,** Parts of the stomach.

The gastrointestinal (GI) system (also called the digestive system) consists of the GI tract and its associated organs and glands. Included in the GI tract are the mouth, esophagus, stomach, small intestine, large intestine, rectum, and anus. The associated organs are the liver, pancreas, and gallbladder (Fig. 39-1).

STRUCTURES AND FUNCTIONS OF GASTROINTESTINAL SYSTEM

The GI tract extends approximately 30 ft (9 m) from the mouth to the anus. It is composed of four common layers. From the inside to the outside, these layers are (1) mucosa, (2) submucosa, (3) muscle, and (4) serosa (see Fig. 39-1). The muscular coat consists of two layers: the circular (inner) layer and the longitudinal (outer) layer.

The GI tract is innervated by the parasympathetic and sympathetic branches of the autonomic nervous system. The parasympathetic (cholinergic) system is mainly excitatory, and the sympathetic (adrenergic) system is mainly inhibitory. For example, peristalsis is increased by parasympathetic stimulation and decreased by sympathetic stimulation. Sensory information is relayed via both sympathetic and parasympathetic afferent fibers.

The GI tract has its own nervous system: the enteric (or intrinsic) nervous system. The enteric nervous system is composed of two nerve layers that lie between the mucosa and the muscle layers. These neurons have receptors for pressure and movement.

The GI tract and accessory organs receive approximately 25% to 30% of the cardiac output at rest and 35% or more after eating. Circulation in the GI system is unique in that venous blood draining the GI tract organs empties into the portal vein, which then perfuses the liver. The vascular supply to the GI tract includes the celiac artery, superior mesenteric artery (SMA), and the inferior mesenteric artery (IMA). The stomach and duodenum receive their blood supply from the celiac axis. The distal small intestine to mid larger intestine receives its blood supply from branches of the hepatic and SMAs. The distal large intestine through the anus receives its blood supply from the IMA. Because such a large percentage of the cardiac output perfuses these organs, the GI tract is a major source from which blood flow can be diverted during exercise, stress, or injury.

The abdominal organs are almost completely covered by the peritoneum. The two layers of the peritoneum are the *parietal layer*, which lines the abdominal cavity wall, and the *visceral layer*, which covers the abdominal organs. The peritoneal cavity is the potential space between the parietal and visceral layers. The two folds of the peritoneum are the mesentery and the omentum. The mesentery attaches the small intestine and part of the large intestine to the posterior abdominal wall and contains blood and lymph vessels. The omentum hangs like an apron from the stomach to the intestines and contains fat and lymph nodes (see eFig. 39-1 on the website for this chapter).

The main function of the GI system is to supply nutrients to body cells. This is accomplished through the processes of (1) *ingestion* (taking in food), (2) *digestion* (breaking down food), and (3) *absorption* (transferring food products into circulation). *Elimination* is the process of excreting the waste products of digestion.

Ingestion

Ingestion is the intake of food. A person's appetite or desire to ingest food influences how much food is eaten. An appetite center is located in the hypothalamus. It is directly or indirectly stimulated by hypoglycemia, an empty stomach, decrease in body temperature, and input from higher brain centers. The hormone *ghrelin* released from the stomach mucosa plays a role in appetite stimulation. Another hormone, *leptin,* is involved in appetite suppression. (Ghrelin and leptin are discussed in Chapter 41.) The sight, smell, and taste of food frequently stimulate appetite. Appetite may be inhibited by stomach distention, illness (especially accompanied by fever), hyperglycemia, nausea and vomiting, and certain drugs (e.g., amphetamines).

Deglutition (swallowing) is the mechanical component of ingestion. The organs involved in the deglutition of food are the mouth, pharynx, and esophagus.

Mouth. The mouth consists of the lips and the oral (buccal) cavity. The lips surround the orifice of the mouth and function in speech. The roof of the oral cavity is formed by the hard and soft palates. The oral cavity contains the teeth, used in mastication (chewing), and the tongue. The tongue is a solid muscle mass and assists in chewing and moving food to the back of the throat for swallowing. Taste receptors (taste buds) are found on the sides and tip of the tongue. The tongue is also important in speech.

Within the oral cavity are three pairs of salivary glands: the parotid, submaxillary, and sublingual glands. These glands produce saliva, which consists of water, protein, mucin, inorganic salts, and salivary amylase.

Pharynx. The pharynx is a musculomembranous tube that is divided into the nasopharynx, the oropharynx, and the laryngeal pharynx. The mucous membrane of the pharynx is continuous with the nasal cavity, mouth, auditory tubes, and larynx. The epiglottis is a lid of fibrocartilage that closes over the larynx during swallowing. During ingestion, the oropharynx provides a route for food from the mouth to the esophagus. When receptors in the oropharynx are stimulated by food or liquid, the swallowing reflex is initiated. The tonsils and the adenoids, composed of lymphoid tissue, assist the body in preventing infection.

Esophagus. The esophagus is a hollow, muscular tube that receives food from the pharynx and moves it to the stomach. It is 7 to 10 in (18 to 25 cm) long and 0.8 in (2 cm) in diameter. The esophagus is located in the thoracic cavity. The upper third of the esophagus is composed of striated skeletal muscle, and the distal two thirds are composed of smooth muscle.

With swallowing, the upper esophageal sphincter (cricopharyngeal muscle) relaxes and a peristaltic wave moves the bolus into the esophagus. Between swallows, the esophagus is collapsed. It is structurally composed of four layers: inner mucosa, submucosa, muscularis propria, and outermost adventitia.

The muscular layers contract *(peristalsis)* and propel the food to the stomach. There are two sphincters: the *upper esophageal sphincter* (UES) at the proximal end of the esophagus and the *lower esophageal sphincter* (LES) at the distal end. The LES remains contracted except during swallowing, belching, or vomiting. The LES is an important barrier that normally prevents reflux of acidic gastric contents into the esophagus.

Digestion and Absorption

Stomach. The stomach's functions are to store food, mix food with gastric secretions, and empty contents in small boluses into the small intestine. The stomach absorbs only small amounts of water, alcohol, electrolytes, and certain drugs.

The stomach is usually J shaped and lies obliquely in the epigastric, umbilical, and left hypochondriac regions of the abdomen (see Fig. 39-5 later in the chapter). It always contains gastric fluid and mucus. The three main parts of the stomach are the fundus (cardia), body, and antrum (see Fig. 39-1). The pylorus is a small portion of the antrum proximal to the pyloric sphincter. Sphincter muscles (the LES and the pyloric sphincter) guard the entrance to and exit from the stomach.

The serous (outer) layer of the stomach is formed by the peritoneum. The muscular layer consists of the longitudinal (outer) layer, circular (middle) layer, and oblique (inner) layer. The mucosal layer forms folds called *rugae* that contain many small glands. In the fundus the glands contain chief cells, which secrete pepsinogen, and parietal cells, which secrete hydrochloric (HCl) acid, water, and intrinsic factor. The secretion of HCl acid makes gastric juice acidic. This acidic pH aids in the protection against ingested organisms. Intrinsic factor promotes cobalamin (vitamin B_{12}) absorption in the small intestine.

Small Intestine. The two primary functions of the small intestine are digestion and *absorption* (uptake of nutrients from the gut lumen to the bloodstream). The small intestine is a coiled tube approximately 23 ft (7 m) in length and 1 to 1.1 in (2.5 to 2.8 cm) in diameter. It extends from the pylorus to the ileocecal valve. The small intestine is composed of the duodenum, jejunum, and ileum. The ileocecal valve prevents reflux of large intestine contents into the small intestine.

The mucosa of the small intestine is thick, vascular, and glandular. The functional units of the small intestine are *villi*, minute, fingerlike projections in the mucous membrane. They contain epithelial cells that produce the intestinal digestive enzymes. The epithelial cells on the villi also have *microvilli*. The circular folds in the mucous and submucous layers, along with the villi and microvilli, increase the surface area for digestion and absorption.

The digestive enzymes on the brush border of the microvilli chemically break down nutrients for absorption. The villi are surrounded by the crypts of Lieberkühn, which contain the multipotent stem cells for the other epithelial cell types. (Stem cells are discussed in Chapter 13.) Brunner's glands in the submucosa of the duodenum secrete an alkaline fluid containing bicarbonate. Intestinal goblet cells secrete mucus that protects the mucosa.

Physiology of Digestion. *Digestion* is the physical and chemical breakdown of food into absorbable substances. Digestion in the GI tract is facilitated by the timely movement of food through the GI tract and the secretion of specific enzymes. These enzymes break down foodstuffs to particles of appropriate size for absorption (Table 39-1).

The process of digestion begins in the mouth, where the food is chewed, mechanically broken down, and mixed with saliva. Approximately 1 L of saliva is produced each day. Saliva facilitates swallowing by lubricating food. Saliva contains amylase (ptyalin), which breaks down starches to maltose. Salivary gland secretion is stimulated by chewing movements and the sight, smell, thought, and taste of food. After swallowing, food is moved through the esophagus to the stomach. No digestion or absorption occurs in the esophagus.

In the stomach the digestion of proteins begins with the release of pepsinogen from chief cells. The stomach's acidic environment results in the conversion of pepsinogen to its active form, pepsin. Pepsin begins the breakdown of proteins. There is minimal digestion of starches and fats. The food is mixed with gastric secretions, which are under neural and hormonal control (Tables 39-2 and 39-3). The stomach also serves as a reservoir for food, which is slowly released into the small intestine. The length of time that food remains in the stomach depends on the composition of the food, but average meals remain from 3 to 4 hours.

In the small intestine, carbohydrates are broken down to monosaccharides, fats to glycerol and fatty acids, and proteins to amino acids. The physical presence and chemical nature of *chyme* (food mixed with gastric secretions) stimulate motility and secretion. Secretions involved in digestion include enzymes from the pancreas, bile from the liver (see Table 39-1), and enzymes from the small intestine. Enzymes on the brush border

of the microvilli complete the digestion process. These enzymes break down disaccharides to monosaccharides and peptides to amino acids for absorption.

Both secretion and motility are under neural and hormonal control. When food enters the stomach and small intestine, hormones are released into the bloodstream (see Table 39-3). These hormones play important roles in the control of HCl acid secretion, production and release of digestive enzymes, and motility.

Absorption is the transfer of the end products of digestion across the intestinal wall to the circulation. Most absorption occurs in the small intestine. The movement of the villi enables the end products of digestion to come in contact with the absorbing membrane. Monosaccharides (from carbohydrates), fatty acids (from fats), amino acids (from proteins), water, electrolytes, vitamins, and minerals are absorbed.

Elimination

Large Intestine. The large intestine is a hollow, muscular tube approximately 5 to 6 ft (1.5 to 1.8 m) long and 2 in (5 cm) in diameter. The four parts of the large intestine are shown in Fig. 39-2.

The most important function of the large intestine is the absorption of water and electrolytes. The large intestine also forms feces and serves as a reservoir for the fecal mass until defecation occurs. Feces are composed of water (75%), bacteria, unabsorbed minerals, undigested foodstuffs, bile pigments, and

TABLE 39-1	GASTROINTESTINAL SECRETIONS	
Daily Amount (mL)	**Secretions, Enzymes**	**Action**
Salivary Glands		
1000-1500	Salivary amylase (ptyalin)	Initiation of starch digestion
Stomach		
2500	Pepsinogen	Protein digestion
	HCl acid	Activation of pepsinogen to pepsin
	Lipase	Fat digestion
	Intrinsic factor	Essential for cobalamin absorption in ileum
Small Intestine		
3000	Enterokinase	Activation of trypsinogen to trypsin
	Amylase	Carbohydrate digestion
	Peptidases	Protein digestion
	Aminopeptidases	Protein digestion
	Maltase	Maltose to two glucose molecules
	Sucrase	Sucrose to glucose and fructose
	Lactase	Lactose to glucose and galactose
	Lipase	Fat digestion
Pancreas		
700	Trypsinogen	Protein digestion
	Chymotrypsin	Protein digestion
	Amylase	Starch to disaccharides
	Lipase	Fat digestion
Liver and Gallbladder		
1000	Bile	Emulsification of fats and aid in absorption of fatty acids and fat-soluble vitamins (A, D, E, K)

TABLE 39-2	PHASES OF GASTRIC SECRETION
Stimulus to Secretion	**Secretion**
Cephalic (nervous)	
Sight, smell, taste of food (before food enters stomach). Initiated in the CNS and mediated by the vagus nerve.	HCl acid, pepsinogen, mucus
Gastric (hormonal and nervous)	
Food in antrum of stomach, vagal stimulation.	Release of gastrin from antrum into circulation to stimulate gastric secretions and motility
Intestinal (hormonal)	
Presence of chyme in small intestine.	*Acidic chyme* (pH <2): Release of secretin, gastric inhibitory polypeptide, cholecystokinin into circulation to decrease HCl acid secretion
	Chyme (pH >3): Release of gastrin from duodenum to increase acid secretion

TABLE 39-3	HORMONES CONTROLLING GI SECRETION AND MOTILITY		
Hormone	**Source**	**Activating Stimuli**	**Function**
Gastrin	Gastric and duodenal mucosa	Stomach distention, partially digested proteins in pylorus	Stimulates gastric acid secretion and motility. Maintains lower esophageal sphincter tone.
Secretin	Duodenal mucosa	Acid entering small intestine	Inhibits gastric motility and acid secretion. Stimulates pancreatic bicarbonate secretion.
Cholecystokinin	Duodenal mucosa	Fatty acids and amino acids in small intestine	Contracts gallbladder and relaxes sphincter of Oddi. Allows increased flow of bile into duodenum; release of pancreatic digestive enzymes.
Gastric inhibitory peptide	Duodenal mucosa	Fatty acids and lipids in small intestine	Inhibits gastric acid secretion and motility.

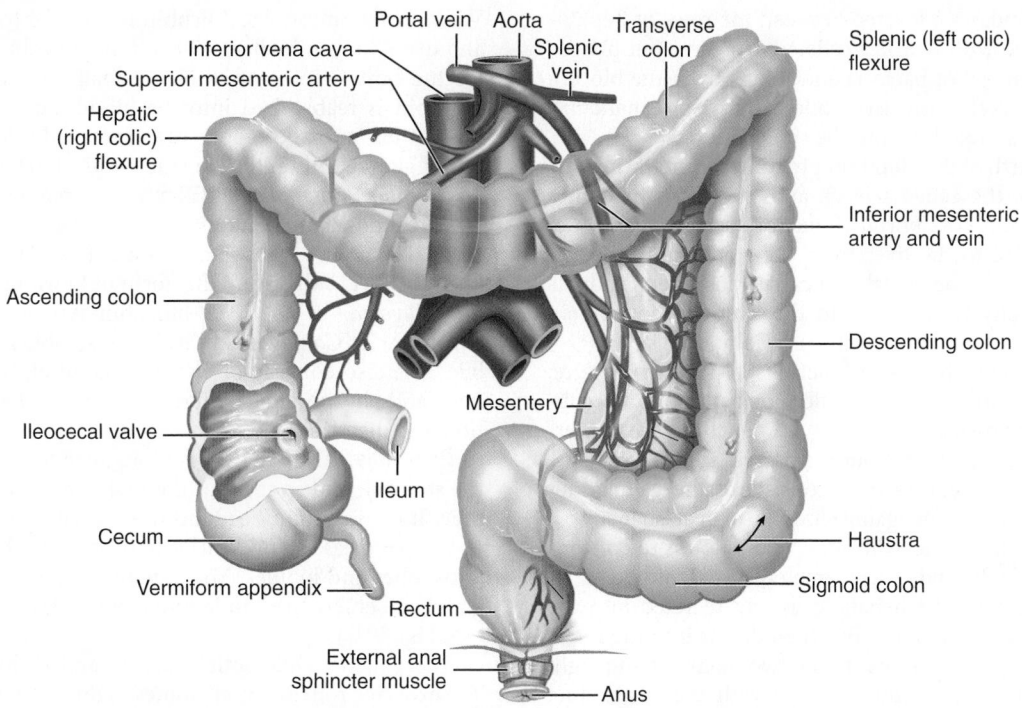

FIG. 39-2 Anatomic locations of the large intestine.

desquamated (shed) epithelial cells. The large intestine secretes mucus, which acts as a lubricant and protects the mucosa.

Microorganisms in the colon are responsible for the breakdown of proteins not digested or absorbed in the small intestine. These amino acids are deaminated by the bacteria, leaving ammonia, which is carried to the liver and converted to urea, which is excreted by the kidneys. Bacteria in the colon also synthesize vitamin K and some of the B vitamins. Bacteria also play a part in the production of flatus.

The movements of the large intestine are usually slow. However, propulsive (mass movements) peristalsis also occurs. When food enters the stomach and duodenum, gastrocolic and duodenocolic reflexes are initiated, resulting in peristalsis in the colon. These reflexes are more active after the first daily meal and frequently result in bowel evacuation.

Defecation is a reflex action involving voluntary and involuntary control. Feces in the rectum stimulate sensory nerve endings that produce the desire to defecate. The reflex center for defecation is in the sacral portion of the spinal cord (parasympathetic nerve fibers). These fibers produce contraction of the rectum and relaxation of the internal anal sphincter. Defecation is controlled voluntarily by relaxing the external anal sphincter when the desire to defecate is felt. An acceptable environment for defecation is usually necessary, or the urge to defecate will be ignored. If defecation is suppressed over long periods, problems can occur, such as constipation or fecal impaction.

Defecation can be facilitated by the **Valsalva maneuver.** This maneuver involves contraction of the chest muscles on a closed glottis with simultaneous contraction of the abdominal muscles. These actions result in increased intraabdominal pressure. The Valsalva maneuver may be contraindicated in the patient with a head injury, eye surgery, cardiac problems, hemorrhoids, abdominal surgery, or liver cirrhosis with portal hypertension.

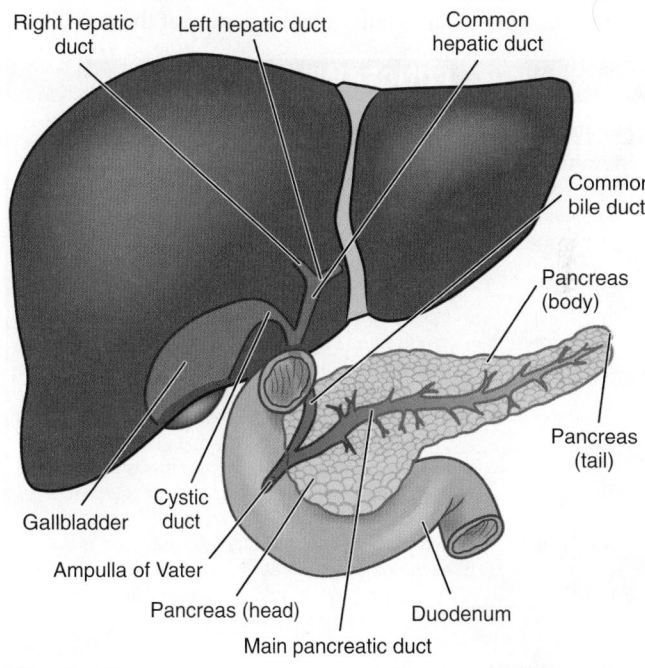

FIG. 39-3 Gross structure of the liver, gallbladder, pancreas, and duct system.

Liver, Biliary Tract, and Pancreas

Liver. The liver is the largest internal organ in the body, weighing approximately 3 lb (1.36 kg). It lies in the right epigastric region (see Fig. 39-5 later in the chapter). Most of the liver is enclosed in peritoneum. It has a fibrous capsule that divides it into right and left lobes (Fig. 39-3).

The functional units of the liver are lobules (see eFig. 39-2 on the website for this chapter). The lobule consists of rows of hepatic cells (**hepatocytes**) arranged around a central vein. The capillaries (sinusoids) are located between the rows of hepatocytes and are lined with Kupffer cells, which carry out phagocytic activity (removal of bacteria and toxins from the blood). Interlobular bile ducts form from bile capillaries (canaliculi). The hepatic cells secrete bile into the canaliculi.

About one fourth of the blood supply comes from the hepatic artery (branch of the celiac artery), and three fourths comes from the portal vein. The portal circulatory system (enterohepatic) brings blood to the liver from the stomach, intestines, spleen, and pancreas. The portal vein carries absorbed products of digestion directly to the liver. In the liver the portal vein branches and comes in contact with each lobule.

The liver is essential for life. It functions in the manufacture, storage, transformation, and excretion of a number of substances involved in metabolism. The liver's functions are numerous and can be classified into four main areas (Table 39-4).

Biliary Tract. The biliary tract consists of the gallbladder and the duct system. The gallbladder is a pear-shaped sac located below the liver. The gallbladder's function is to concentrate and store bile. It holds approximately 45 mL of bile.

Bile is produced by the hepatic cells and secreted into the biliary canaliculi of the lobules. Bile then drains into the interlobular bile ducts, which unite into the two main left and right hepatic ducts. The hepatic ducts merge with the cystic duct from the gallbladder to form the common bile duct (see Fig. 39-3). Most of the bile is stored and concentrated in the gallbladder. It is then released into the cystic duct and moves down the common bile duct to enter the duodenum at the ampulla of Vater. In the intestines, bilirubin is reduced to stercobilinogen and urobilinogen by bacterial action. Stercobilinogen accounts for the brown color of stool. A small amount of conjugated bilirubin is reabsorbed into the blood. Some urobilinogen is reabsorbed into the blood, returned to the liver through the portal circulation (enterohepatic), and excreted in the bile.

Bilirubin Metabolism. Bilirubin, a pigment derived from the breakdown of hemoglobin, is constantly produced (Fig. 39-4). Because it is insoluble in water, it is bound to albumin for transport to the liver. This form of bilirubin is referred to as *unconjugated.* In the liver bilirubin is conjugated with glucuronic acid. *Conjugated* bilirubin is soluble and is excreted in bile. Bile also consists of water, cholesterol, bile salts, electrolytes, and phospholipids. Bile salts are needed for fat emulsification and digestion.

Pancreas. The pancreas is a long, slender gland lying behind the stomach and in front of the first and second lumbar vertebrae. It consists of a head, body, and tail. The anterior surface of the pancreas is covered by peritoneum. The pancreas contains lobes and lobules. The pancreatic duct extends along the gland and enters the duodenum through the common bile duct (see Fig. 39-3).

The pancreas has both exocrine and endocrine functions. The exocrine function contributes to digestion through the production and release of enzymes (see Table 39-1). The endocrine function occurs in the islets of Langerhans, whose β cells secrete insulin and amylin; α cells secrete glucagon; δ cells secrete somatostatin; and F cells secrete pancreatic polypeptide.

TABLE 39-4	FUNCTIONS OF THE LIVER
Function	**Description**
Metabolic Functions	
Carbohydrate metabolism	Glycogenesis (conversion of glucose to glycogen), glycogenolysis (process of breaking down glycogen to glucose), gluconeogenesis (formation of glucose from amino acids and fatty acids).
Protein metabolism	Synthesis of nonessential amino acids, synthesis of plasma proteins (except gamma globulin), synthesis of clotting factors, urea formation from ammonia (NH_3) (NH_3 formed from deamination of amino acids by action of bacteria in colon).
Fat metabolism	Synthesis of lipoproteins, breakdown of triglycerides into fatty acids and glycerol, formation of ketone bodies, synthesis of fatty acids from amino acids and glucose, synthesis and breakdown of cholesterol.
Detoxification	Inactivation of drugs and harmful substances and excretion of their breakdown products.
Steroid metabolism	Conjugation and excretion of gonadal and adrenal corticosteroid hormones.
Bile Synthesis	
Bile production	Formation of bile, containing bile salts, bile pigments (mainly bilirubin), and cholesterol.
Bile excretion	Bile excretion by liver about 1 L/day.
Storage	Glucose in form of glycogen. Vitamins, including fat soluble (A, D, E, K) and water soluble (B_1, B_2, cobalamin, folic acid). Fatty acids. Minerals (iron, copper). Amino acids in form of albumin and beta-globulins.
Mononuclear Phagocyte System	
Kupffer cells	Breakdown of old RBCs, WBCs, bacteria, and other particles. Breakdown of hemoglobin from old RBCs to bilirubin and biliverdin.

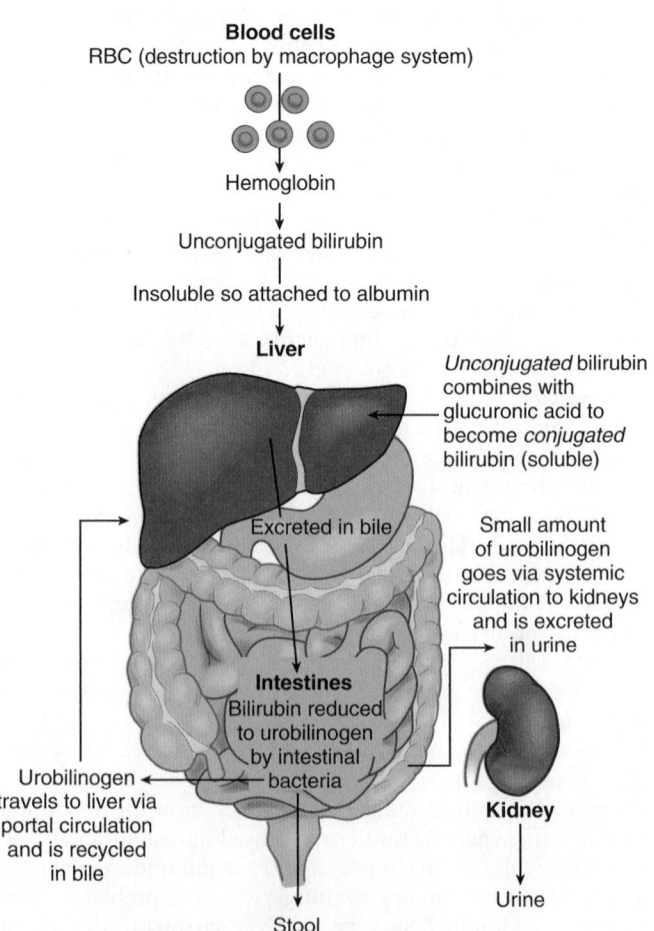

FIG. 39-4 Bilirubin metabolism and conjugation.

GERONTOLOGIC CONSIDERATIONS

EFFECTS OF AGING ON GASTROINTESTINAL SYSTEM

The process of aging changes the functional ability of the GI system (Table 39-5). Diet, alcohol intake, and obesity affect organs of the GI system, making it a challenge to separate the sole effects of aging from lifestyle. *Xerostomia* (decreased saliva production), or dry mouth, affects many older adults and may be associated with difficulty swallowing (dysphagia).[1] Many factors can lead to a decrease in appetite and make eating less

pleasurable. These include a decrease in taste buds and salivary gland secretion, diminished sense of smell, and caries and periodontal disease leading to loss of teeth.

Age-related changes in the esophagus include delayed emptying resulting from smooth muscle weakness and an incompetent LES.[2] Although motility of the GI system decreases with age, secretion and absorption are affected to a lesser extent. The older patient often has a decrease in HCl acid secretion (hypochlorhydria) and a subsequent reduction in the amount of intrinsic factor secreted.

Although constipation is a common complaint of older adults, age-related changes in colonic secretion or motility have not been consistently shown.[3] Factors that may increase the risk for constipation include slower peristalsis, inactivity, decreased dietary fiber, decreased fluid intake, constipating medications, and laxative abuse; neurologic, cognitive, and metabolic disorders may also play a role.[4,5] (Constipation is discussed in Chapter 43.)

The liver size decreases after 50 years of age, but results of liver function tests remain within normal ranges. Age-related enzyme changes in the liver decrease the liver's ability to metabolize drugs and hormones.

The size of the pancreas is unaffected by aging, but it does undergo structural changes such as fibrosis, fatty acid deposits, and atrophy. Both obstructive and nonobstructive gallbladder diseases increase with age.[6]

Older adults, especially those over 85, are at risk for decreased food intake.[7] The economic inability to purchase food supplies affects nutritional intake, especially in the older adult. Economic constraints may also reduce the number of fresh fruits and vegetables consumed and thus the amount of fiber. Immobility limits the ability to obtain and prepare meals. In the United States, approximately one third of people over 60 are obese.[7,8] Age-related changes in the GI system and differences in assessment findings are presented in Table 39-5.

TABLE 39-5   GERONTOLOGIC ASSESSMENT DIFFERENCES

Gastrointestinal System

Expected Aging Changes	Differences in Assessment Findings
Mouth	
Gingival retraction	Loss of teeth, dental implants, dentures, difficulty chewing
Decreased taste buds, decreased sense of smell	Diminished sense of taste (especially salty and sweet)
Decreased volume of saliva	Dry oral mucosa
Atrophy of gingival tissue	Poor-fitting dentures
Esophagus	
Lower esophageal sphincter pressure decreased, motility decreased	Epigastric distress, dysphagia, potential for hiatal hernia and aspiration
Abdominal Wall	
Thinner and less taut	More visible peristalsis, easier palpation of organs
Decreased number and sensitivity of sensory receptors	Less sensitivity to surface pain
Stomach	
Atrophy of gastric mucosa, decreased blood flow	Food intolerances, signs of anemia as result of cobalamin malabsorption, slower gastric emptying
Small Intestines	
Slightly decreased motility and secretion of most digestive enzymes	Complaints of indigestion, slowed intestinal transit, delayed absorption of fat-soluble vitamins
Liver	
Decreased size and lowered position	Easier palpation because of lower border extending past costal margin
Decreased protein synthesis, ability to regenerate decreased	Decreased drug and hormone metabolism
Large Intestine, Anus, Rectum	
Decreased anal sphincter tone and nerve supply to rectal area	Fecal incontinence
Decreased muscular tone, decreased motility	Flatulence, abdominal distention, relaxed perineal musculature
Increased transit time, decreased sensation to defecation	Constipation, fecal impaction
Pancreas	
Pancreatic ducts distended, lipase production decreased, pancreatic reserve impaired	Impaired fat absorption, decreased glucose tolerance

ASSESSMENT OF GASTROINTESTINAL SYSTEM

Subjective Data

Important Health Information

Past Health History. Gather information from the patient about the history or existence of the following problems related to GI functioning: abdominal pain, nausea and vomiting, diarrhea, constipation, abdominal distention, jaundice, anemia, heartburn, dyspepsia, changes in appetite, hematemesis, food intolerance or allergies, indigestion, excessive gas, bloating, lactose intolerance, melena, trouble swallowing, hemorrhoids, or rectal bleeding. In addition, ask the patient about a history or existence of diseases such as reflux, gastritis, hepatitis, colitis, gallstones, peptic ulcer, cancer, diverticuli, or hernias.

Question the patient about weight history. Explore in detail any unexplained or unplanned weight loss or gain within the past 6 to 12 months. Document a history of chronic dieting and repeated weight loss and gain.

Medications. The health history should include an assessment of the patient's past and current use of medications. The names of all drugs, their frequency of use, and their duration of use are important. This is a critical aspect of history taking because many medications may not only have an effect on the GI system but also may be affected by abnormalities of the GI system. The medication assessment should include information about over-the-counter (OTC) medications, prescription

CASE STUDY

Patient Introduction

iStockphoto/Thinkstock

Patient Profile

L.C. is a 58-year-old Native American man from a Pueblo tribe in northern New Mexico. L.C.'s wife and family drove 50 miles to take him to the Indian Health Service hospital. He comes into the emergency department (ED) doubled over in pain. He is grimacing and holding his abdomen with both arms. You are working as the triage nurse that morning.

Critical Thinking

As you read through this chapter, think about L.C.'s symptoms with the following questions in mind:

1. What are the possible causes for L.C.'s acute abdominal pain?
2. What would be your priority assessment?
3. What questions would you ask L.C.?
4. What should be included in the physical assessment? What would you be looking for?
5. What diagnostic studies might you expect to be ordered?

evolve Answers available at *http://evolve.elsevier.com/Lewis/medsurg.*

TABLE 39-6 HEPATOTOXIC CHEMICALS AND DRUGS

- acetaminophen (Tylenol)
- amiodarone (Cordarone)
- arsenic
- azathioprine (Imuran)
- carbamazepine (Tegretol)
- chloroform
- fluconazole (Diflucan)
- gold compounds
- halothane
- isoniazid (INH)
- ketoconazole (Nizoral)
- 6-mercaptopurine (6-MP)
- mercury
- methotrexate
- nevirapine (Viramune)
- niacin
- statins (e.g., simvastatin [Zocor])
- sulfonamides
- thiazide diuretics (e.g., hydrochlorothiazide)
- thiazolidinediones (e.g., pioglitazone [Actos])

TABLE 39-7 SURGERIES OF THE GASTROINTESTINAL SYSTEM

Procedure	Description
Appendectomy	Removal of appendix
Cholecystectomy	Removal of gallbladder
Choledochojejunostomy	Opening between common bile duct and jejunum
Choledocholithotomy	Opening into common bile duct for removal of stones
Colectomy	Removal of colon
Colostomy	Opening into colon
Esophagoenterostomy	Removal of portion of esophagus with segment of colon attached to remaining portion
Esophagogastrostomy	Removal of esophagus and anastomosis of remaining portion to stomach
Gastrectomy	Removal of stomach
Gastrostomy	Opening into stomach
Glossectomy	Removal of tongue
Hemiglossectomy	Removal of half of tongue
Herniorrhaphy	Removal of a hernia
Ileostomy	Opening into ileum
Mandibulectomy	Removal of mandible
Pyloroplasty	Enlargement and repair of pyloric sphincter area
Vagotomy	Resection of branch of vagus nerve

drugs, herbal products, vitamins, and nutritional supplements (see the Complementary & Alternative Therapies box in Chapter 3 on p. 39). Note the use of prescription or OTC appetite suppressants.

Many chemicals and drugs are potentially hepatotoxic (Table 39-6) and result in significant patient harm unless monitored closely. For example, chronic high doses of acetaminophen and nonsteroidal antiinflammatory drugs (NSAIDs) may be hepatotoxic. NSAIDs (including aspirin) may also predispose a patient to upper GI bleeding, with an increasing risk as the person ages. Other medications such as antibiotics may change the normal bacterial composition in the GI tract, resulting in diarrhea. Antacids and laxatives may affect the absorption of certain medications. Ask the patient if laxatives or antacids are taken, including the kind and frequency.

Surgery or Other Treatments. Obtain information about hospitalizations for any problems related to the GI system. Also obtain data related to any abdominal or rectal surgery, including the year, reason for surgery, postoperative course, and possible blood transfusions. Terms related to surgery of the GI system are presented in Table 39-7.

Functional Health Patterns. Key questions to ask a patient with a GI problem are presented in Table 39-8.

Health Perception–Health Management Pattern. Ask about the patient's health practices related to the GI system, such as

maintenance of normal body weight, proper dental care, adequate nutrition, and effective elimination habits.

Query the patient about recent foreign travel with possible exposure to hepatitis or parasitic infestation. Ask about potential risk behaviors for hepatitis C exposure. Document whether the patient has received hepatitis A and B vaccination.

Assess the patient for habits that directly affect GI functioning. The intake of alcohol in large quantities or for long periods has detrimental effects on the stomach mucosa. Chronic alcohol exposure causes fatty infiltration of the liver and can cause damage, leading to cirrhosis and hepatocellular carcinoma. Obtain a history of cigarette smoking. Nicotine is irritating to the GI tract mucosa. Cigarette smoking is related to GI cancers (especially mouth and esophageal cancers), esophagitis, and ulcers. Smoking delays the healing of ulcers.

GENETIC RISK ALERT: Colorectal Cancer

- Colorectal cancer may run in families if first-degree relatives (parents, siblings) or many other family members (grandparents, aunts, uncles) have had colorectal cancer. This is especially true when family members are diagnosed with colorectal cancer before age 50.
- Some genetic conditions associated with an increased risk of colorectal cancer include:
  - Hereditary nonpolyposis colorectal cancer (HNPCC), which is caused by mutations in several different genes.
  - Familial adenomatous polyposis (FAP), which is characterized by multiple polyps that are noncancerous at first, but eventually develop into cancer if not treated. Most cases of FAP are due to mutations of the adenomatous polyposis coli (*APC*) gene.

GENETIC RISK ALERT: Inflammatory Bowel Disease (IBD)

- People with IBD have a genetic predisposition or susceptibility to the disease.
- First-degree relatives have a 5- to 20-fold increased risk of developing IBD.

Family history is an important component of this health pattern. Because of the relationship between colorectal and breast cancer, inquire about a history of either type of cancer in the family. Women with HNPCC also have an increased risk of endometrial and ovarian cancer.

TABLE 39-8   HEALTH HISTORY

Gastrointestinal System

Health Perception–Health Management
- Describe any measures used to treat GI symptoms such as diarrhea or vomiting.
- Do you smoke?* Do you drink alcohol?*
- Are you exposed to any chemicals on a regular basis?* Have you been exposed in the past?*
- Have you recently traveled outside the United States?*

Nutritional-Metabolic
- Describe your usual daily food and fluid intake.
- Do you take any supplemental vitamins or minerals?*
- Have you experienced any changes in appetite or food tolerance?*
- Has there been a weight change in the past 6-12 mo?*
- Are you allergic to any foods?*

Elimination
- Describe the frequency and time of day you have bowel movements. What is the consistency of the bowel movement?
- Do you use laxatives or enemas?* If so, how often?
- Have there been any recent changes in your bowel pattern?*
- Describe any skin problems caused by GI problems.
- Do you need any assistive equipment, such as ostomy equipment, raised toilet seat, commode?

Activity-Exercise
- Do you have limitations in mobility that make it difficult for you to procure and prepare food?*

Sleep-Rest
- Do you experience any difficulty sleeping because of a GI problem?*
- Are you awakened by symptoms such as gas, abdominal pain, diarrhea, or heartburn?*

Cognitive-Perceptual
- Have you experienced any change in taste or smell that has affected your appetite?*
- Do you have any heat or cold sensitivity that affects eating?*
- Does pain interfere with food preparation, appetite, or chewing?*
- Do pain medications cause constipation, diarrhea, or appetite suppression?*

Self-Perception–Self-Concept
- Describe any changes in your weight that have affected how you feel about yourself.
- Have you had any changes in normal elimination that have affected how you feel about yourself?*
- Have any symptoms of GI disease caused physical changes that are a problem for you?*

Role-Relationship
- Describe the impact of any GI problem on your usual roles and relationships.
- Have any changes in elimination affected your relationships?*
- Do you live alone? Describe how your family or others assist you with your GI problems.

Sexuality-Reproductive
- Describe the effect of your GI problem on your sexual activity.

Coping–Stress Tolerance
- Do you experience GI symptoms in response to stressful or emotional situations?
- Describe how you deal with any GI symptoms that result.

Value-Belief
- Describe any culturally specific health beliefs regarding food and food preparation that may influence the treatment of your GI problem.

*If yes, describe.

Nutritional-Metabolic Pattern. A thorough nutritional assessment is essential. Take a diet history and inquire about both content and amount (portion size). Food preferences and preparation may vary by culture. Open-ended questions allow the patient to express beliefs and feelings about the diet. For example, you can say, "Please tell me about your food and beverage intake over the past 24 hours." A 24-hour dietary recall can be used to analyze the adequacy of the diet. Assist the patient in recalling the preceding day's food intake, including early morning and nighttime intake, snacks, liquids, and vitamin supplements. You can then evaluate the diet in relation to recommended servings. The U.S. Department of Agriculture released MyPlate (www.choosemyplate.gov) recommendations for dietary intake. A 1-week recall may provide additional information on usual dietary patterns. Compare weekday and weekend dietary intake patterns in relation to both the quality and quantity of food.

Ask the patient about the use of sugar and salt substitutes, use of caffeine, and amount of fluid and fiber intake. Note any changes in appetite, food tolerance, and weight. Anorexia and weight loss may indicate cancer or inflammation. Decreased food intake can also be the consequence of economic problems and depression.

Ask about food allergies and what GI symptoms occur with the allergic response. Inquire about dietary intolerances, including lactose and gluten.

Elimination Pattern. Elicit a detailed account of the patient's bowel elimination pattern. Note the frequency, time of day, and usual consistency of stool. Document the use of laxatives and enemas, including type, frequency, and results. Investigate any recent change in bowel patterns.

Document the amount and type of fluid and fiber intake because these influence the frequency and consistency of stools. Inadequate intake of fiber can be associated with constipation. Investigate the possible association between a skin problem and a GI problem. Food allergies can cause skin lesions, pruritus, and edema. Diarrhea can result in redness, irritation, and pain in the perianal area. External drainage systems, such as an ileostomy or ileal conduit, may cause local skin irritation.

Activity-Exercise Pattern. Activity and exercise affect GI motility. Immobility is a risk factor for constipation.

Assess ambulatory status to determine if the patient is capable of securing and preparing food. If the patient is unable to do these tasks, determine if a family member or an outside agency is meeting this need.

Note any limitation in patients' ability to feed themselves. Assess for access to a toilet. Identify the use of and access to supplies such as a commode or ostomy supplies.

Sleep-Rest Pattern. GI symptoms can interfere with the quality of sleep. Nausea, vomiting, diarrhea, indigestion, and bloating can produce sleep problems and should be investigated. Ask the patient if GI symptoms affect sleep or rest. For example, a patient with gastroesophageal reflux disease (GERD) may be awakened because of burning, epigastric pain.

A patient may have a bedtime ritual that involves a particular food or beverage. Herbal teas may be sleep inducing. Document individual routines and comply with these whenever possible to avoid sleeplessness. Hunger can prevent sleep and should be relieved by a light, easily digested snack (unless contraindicated).

Cognitive-Perceptual Pattern. Sensory alterations can result in problems related to the acquisition, preparation, and ingestion of food. Changes in taste or smell can affect appetite and eating pleasure. Vertigo can make shopping and standing at a stove difficult and dangerous. Heat or cold sensitivity can make certain foods painful to eat. Problems in expressive communication limit the patient's ability to state personal dietary preferences. If a patient is diagnosed as having a GI disorder, ask questions to determine his or her understanding of the illness and its treatment.

Both acute and chronic pain influence dietary intake. Behaviors associated with pain include avoidance of activity, fatigue, and disruption of eating patterns. Assess patients receiving opioid medications for constipation, nausea, sedation, and appetite suppression.

Self-Perception–Self-Concept Pattern. Many GI and nutritional problems affect the patient's self-perception. Overweight and underweight persons may have problems related to self-esteem and body image. Repeated attempts to achieve a personally acceptable weight can be discouraging and depressing for some people. The way a person recounts a weight history can alert you to potential problems in this area.

The need for external devices to manage elimination, such as a colostomy or an ileostomy, may be challenging for some patients. The patient's willingness to engage in self-care and to discuss this situation provides you with valuable information related to body image and self-esteem.

The altered physical changes often associated with advanced liver disease can be disturbing for the patient. Jaundice and ascites cause significant changes in external appearance. Assess the patient's attitude toward these changes.

Role-Relationship Pattern. Problems related to the GI system such as cirrhosis, hepatitis, ostomies, obesity, and carcinoma may alter the patient's ability to maintain usual roles and relationships. A chronic illness may necessitate leaving a job or reducing work hours. Changes in body image and self-esteem can affect relationships.

Sexuality-Reproductive Pattern. Changes related to sexuality and reproductive status can result from problems of the GI system. For example, obesity, jaundice, anorexia, and ascites could decrease the acceptance of a potential sexual partner. An ostomy could affect the patient's confidence related to sexual activity. Your sensitive questioning can identify potential problems.

Anorexia can affect the reproductive status of a female patient. Obesity leads to reduced fertility and increased miscarriage rates in women.[9]

Coping–Stress Tolerance Pattern. Determine what is stressful for the patient and what coping mechanisms the patient uses. Factors outside the GI tract can influence its functioning. Both psychologic and emotional factors, such as stress and anxiety, influence GI functioning in many people. Stress may be manifested as anorexia, nausea, epigastric and abdominal pain, or diarrhea. Some diseases of the GI system, such as peptic ulcer disease, IBS, and IBD, may be aggravated by stress. However,

GI symptoms should never be attributed solely to psychologic factors.

Value-Belief Pattern. Assess the patient's spiritual and cultural beliefs regarding food and food preparation. Whenever possible, respect these preferences. Determine if any value or belief could interfere with planned interventions. For example, if the patient with anemia is a vegetarian, the prescription of a high-meat diet would be resisted. Thoughtful assessment and consideration of the patient's beliefs and values usually increase adherence and satisfaction.

Objective Data
Physical Examination
Mouth

Inspection. Inspect the mouth for symmetry, color, and size. Observe for abnormalities such as pallor or cyanosis, cracking, ulcers, or fissures. The dorsum (top) of the tongue should have a thin white coating; the undersurface should be smooth. Observe for any lesions. Using a tongue blade, inspect the buccal mucosa and note the color, any areas of pigmentation, and any lesions. Dark-skinned individuals normally have patchy areas of pigmentation. In assessing the teeth and gums, look for caries; loose teeth; abnormal shape and position of teeth; and swelling, bleeding, discoloration, or inflammation of the gingivae. Note any distinctive breath odor.

Inspect the pharynx by tilting the patient's head back and depressing the tongue with a tongue blade. Observe the tonsils, uvula, soft palate, and anterior and posterior pillars. Instruct the patient to say "ah." The uvula and soft palate should rise and remain in the midline.

Palpation. Palpate any suspicious areas in the mouth. Note ulcers, nodules, indurations, and areas of tenderness. The mouth of the older adult requires careful assessment. Give particular attention to dentures (e.g., fit, condition), ability to swallow, the tongue, and lesions. Ask the patient with dentures to remove them during an oral examination to allow for good visualization and palpation of the area.

Abdomen. Two systems are used to anatomically describe the surface of the abdomen. One system divides the abdomen

TABLE 39-9 STRUCTURES LOCATED IN ABDOMINAL REGIONS

Right Upper Quadrant	Left Upper Quadrant	Right Lower Quadrant	Left Lower Quadrant
• Liver and gallbladder	• Left lobe of liver	• Lower pole of right kidney	• Lower pole of left kidney
• Pylorus	• Spleen	• Cecum and appendix	• Sigmoid flexure
• Duodenum	• Stomach	• Portion of ascending colon	• Portion of descending colon
• Head of pancreas	• Body of pancreas	• Bladder (if distended)	• Bladder (if distended)
• Right adrenal gland	• Left adrenal gland	• Right ovary and salpinx	• Left ovary and salpinx
• Portion of right kidney	• Portion of left kidney	• Uterus (if enlarged)	• Uterus (if enlarged)
• Hepatic flexure of colon	• Splenic flexure of colon	• Right spermatic cord	• Left spermatic cord
• Portion of ascending and transverse colon	• Portion of transverse and descending colon	• Right ureter	• Left ureter

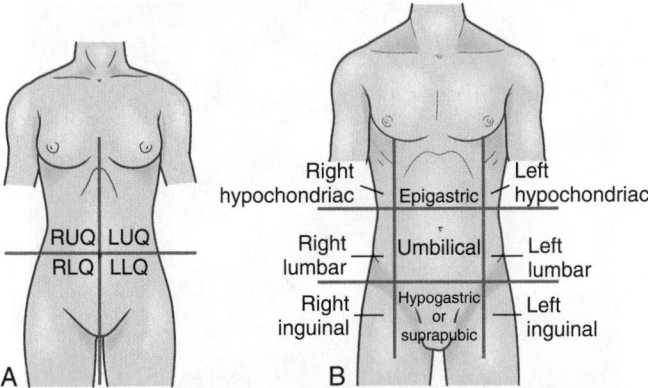

FIG. 39-5 **A,** Abdominal quadrants. **B,** Abdominal regions. *LLQ,* Left lower quadrant; *LUQ,* left upper quadrant; *RLQ,* right lower quadrant; *RUQ,* right upper quadrant.

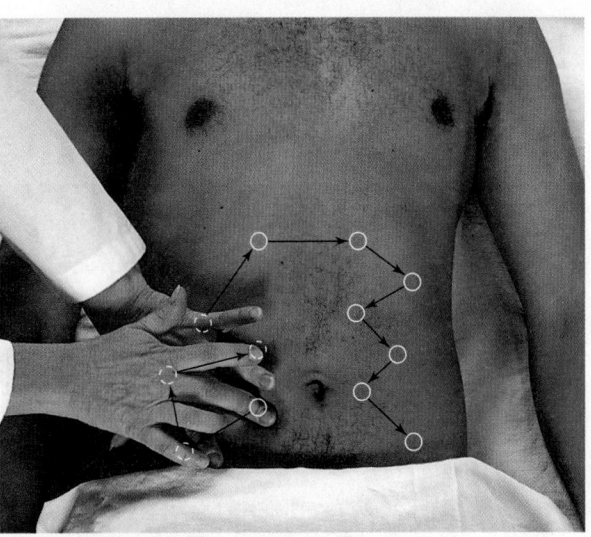

FIG. 39-6 Technique for percussion of the abdomen. Moving clockwise, percuss lightly in all four quadrants. From Jarvis C: *Physical examination and health assessment,* ed 6, St Louis, 2012, Saunders.

into four quadrants by a perpendicular line from the sternum to the pubic bone and a horizontal line across the abdomen at the umbilicus (Fig. 39-5, *A,* and Table 39-9). The other system divides the abdomen into nine regions (Fig. 39-5, *B*), but only the epigastric, umbilical, and suprapubic or hypogastric regions are commonly assessed.

For the abdominal examination, good lighting should shine across the abdomen. The patient should be in the supine position and as relaxed as possible. To help relax the abdominal muscles, have the patient slightly flex the knees and raise the head of the bed slightly. The patient should have an empty bladder. Use warm hands when doing the abdominal examination to avoid eliciting muscle guarding. Ask the patient to breathe slowly through the mouth.

Inspection. Assess the abdomen for skin changes (color, texture, scars, striae, dilated veins, rashes, lesions), umbilicus (location and contour), symmetry, contour (flat, rounded [convex], concave, protuberant, distention), observable masses (hernias or other masses), and movement (pulsations and peristalsis). A normal aortic pulsation may be seen in the epigastric area. Look across the abdomen tangentially (across the abdomen in a line) for peristalsis. Peristalsis is not normally visible in an adult but may be visible in a thin person.

Auscultation. During examination of the abdomen, auscultate before percussion and palpation because these latter procedures may alter the bowel sounds. Use the diaphragm of the stethoscope to auscultate bowel sounds because they are relatively high pitched. Use the bell of the stethoscope to detect lower-pitched sounds. Warm the stethoscope in your hands before auscultating to help prevent abdominal muscle contraction. Listen in the epigastrium and in all four quadrants (start in the lower right quadrant). Listen for bowel sounds for at least

2 minutes. A perfectly "silent abdomen" is uncommon.[10] If you are patient and listen for several minutes, you will frequently find that the sounds are not absent but are hypoactive. If you do not hear bowel sounds, note the amount of time you listened in each quadrant without hearing bowel sounds.

The frequency and intensity of bowel sounds vary depending on the phase of digestion. Normal sounds are relatively high pitched and gurgling. Loud gurgles indicate hyperperistalsis and are termed *borborygmi* (stomach growling). The bowel sounds are more high pitched (rushes and tinkling) when the intestines are under tension, as in intestinal obstruction. Listen for decreased or absent bowel sounds. Terms used to describe bowel sounds include *present, absent, increased, decreased, high pitched, tinkling, gurgling,* and *rushing.*

Also listen for vascular sounds. Normally no aortic bruits should be heard. A *bruit,* best heard with the bell of the stethoscope, is a swishing or buzzing sound and indicates turbulent blood flow.

Percussion. The purpose of percussion of the abdomen is to estimate the size of the liver and determine the presence of fluid, distention, and masses. Sound waves vary according to the density of underlying tissues. Air produces a higher-pitched, hollow sound termed *tympany.* Fluid or masses produce a short, high-pitched sound with little resonance termed *dullness.* Lightly percuss all four quadrants of the abdomen and assess the distribution of tympany and dullness (Fig. 39-6). Tympany is the predominant percussion sound of the abdomen.

FIG. 39-7 **A,** Technique for light palpation of the abdomen. **B,** Technique for deep palpation.

FIG. 39-8 **A,** Technique for liver palpation. **B,** Alternative technique to palpate liver with fingers hooked over the costal region. From Jarvis C: *Physical examination and health assessment,* ed 6, St Louis, 2012, Saunders.

To percuss the liver, start below the umbilicus in the right midclavicular line and percuss lightly upward until dullness is heard, thus determining the lower border of the liver. Next, start at the nipple line in the right midclavicular line and percuss downward between ribs to the area of dullness indicating the upper border of the liver. Measure the height or vertical space between the two borders to determine the size of the liver. The normal range of liver height in the right midclavicular line is 2.4 to 5 in (6 to 12.7 cm).

Palpation. *Light palpation* is used to detect tenderness or cutaneous hypersensitivity, muscular resistance, masses, and swelling. Help the patient relax for deeper palpation. Keep your fingers together and press gently with the pads of the fingertips, depressing the abdominal wall about 0.4 in (1 cm). Use smooth movements and palpate all quadrants (Fig. 39-7, *A*).

Deep palpation is used to delineate abdominal organs and masses (Fig. 39-7, *B*). Use the palmar surfaces of your fingers to press more deeply. Again, palpate all quadrants and note the location, size, and shape of masses, as well as the presence of tenderness. During these maneuvers, observe the patient's facial expression because it will provide nonverbal cues of discomfort or pain.

An alternative method for deep abdominal palpation is the two-hand method. Place one hand on top of the other and apply pressure to the bottom hand with the fingers of the top hand. With the fingers of the bottom hand, feel for organs and masses.

Practice both methods of palpation to determine which one is most effective.

Check a problem area on the abdomen for rebound tenderness by pressing in slowly and firmly over the painful site. Withdraw the palpating fingers quickly. Pain on withdrawal of the fingers indicates peritoneal inflammation. Because assessing for rebound tenderness may produce pain and severe muscle spasm, it should be done at the end of the examination and only by an experienced practitioner.

To palpate the liver, place your left hand behind the patient to support the right eleventh and twelfth ribs (Fig. 39-8). The patient may relax on your hand. Press the left hand forward and place the right hand on the patient's right abdomen lateral to the rectus muscle. The fingertips should be below the lower border of liver dullness and pointed toward the right costal margin. Gently press in and up. The patient should take a deep breath with the abdomen so that the liver drops and is in a better position to be palpated. Try to feel the liver edge as it comes down to the fingertips. During inspiration the liver edge should feel firm, sharp, and smooth. Describe the surface and contour and any tenderness.

To palpate the spleen, move to the patient's left side. Place your right hand under the patient, and support and press the patient's left lower rib cage forward. Place your left hand below the left costal margin, and press it in toward the spleen. Ask the patient to breathe deeply. The tip or edge of an enlarged spleen will be felt by the fingertips. The spleen is normally not palpable. If it is palpable, do not continue because manual compression of an enlarged spleen may cause it to rupture.

TABLE 39-10 NORMAL PHYSICAL ASSESSMENT OF GASTROINTESTINAL SYSTEM

Mouth
- Moist and pink lips
- Pink and moist buccal mucosa and gingivae without plaques or lesions
- Teeth in good repair
- Protrusion of tongue in midline without deviation or fasciculations
- Pink uvula (in midline), soft palate, tonsils, and posterior pharynx
- Swallows smoothly without coughing or gagging

Abdomen
- Flat without masses or scars; no bruises
- Bowel sounds in all quadrants
- No abdominal tenderness; nonpalpable liver and spleen
- Liver 10 cm in right midclavicular line
- Generalized tympany

Anus
- Absence of lesions, fissures, and hemorrhoids
- Good sphincter tone
- Rectal walls smooth and soft
- No masses
- Stool soft, brown, and heme negative

CASE STUDY—cont'd

Objective Data: Physical Examination

iStockphoto/Thinkstock

A focused assessment of L.C. reveals the following: BP 120/74, heart rate 110, respiratory rate 24, temp 100.4°F (38°C). Abdomen firm and slightly distended. High-pitched bowel sounds in upper quadrants. No bowel sounds auscultated in left lower quadrant. Mild abdominal palpation elicits pain.

As you continue to read this chapter, consider diagnostic studies you would anticipate being performed for L.C.

The standard approach for examining the abdomen can be used on the older adult. Palpation is important because it may reveal a tumor. The abdomen may be thinner and more lax unless the patient is obese. If the patient has chronic obstructive pulmonary disease, large lungs, or a low diaphragm, the liver may be palpated 0.4 to 0.8 in (1 to 2 cm) below the right costal margin.

Rectum and Anus. Inspect perianal and anal areas for color, texture, masses, rashes, scars, erythema, fissures, and external hemorrhoids. Palpate any masses or unusual areas with a gloved hand.

For the digital examination of the rectum, place a gloved, lubricated index finger against the anus while the patient gently bears down (Valsalva maneuver). Then, as the sphincter relaxes, insert the finger. Point the finger toward the umbilicus. Try to get the patient to relax. Insert the finger into the rectum as far as possible, and palpate all surfaces. Assess any nodules, tenderness, or irregularities. A sample of stool can be removed with the gloved finger and checked for occult blood. However, a single guaiac-based fecal occult blood test has limited sensitivity in detecting colorectal cancer.

Findings of a normal physical assessment of the GI system are given in Table 39-10. Gerontologic differences in the GI

FOCUSED ASSESSMENT

Gastrointestinal System

Use this checklist to make sure the key assessment steps have been done.

Subjective
Ask the patient about any of the following and note responses.

Loss of appetite	Y	N
Abdominal pain	Y	N
Changes in stools (e.g., color, blood, consistency, frequency)	Y	N
Nausea, vomiting	Y	N
Painful swallowing	Y	N

Objective: Diagnostic
Check the following laboratory results for critical values.

Endoscopy: colonoscopy, sigmoidoscopy, esophagogastroduodenoscopy	✓
CT scan	✓
Radiologic series: upper GI, lower GI	✓
Stool for occult blood or ova and parasites	✓
Liver function tests	✓

Objective: Physical Examination
Inspect

Skin for color, lesions, scars, petechiae, etc.	✓
Abdominal contour for symmetry and distention	✓
Perianal area for intact skin, hemorrhoids	✓

Auscultate*

Bowel sounds	✓

Palpate

Abdominal quadrants using light touch	✓
Abdominal quadrants using a deep technique	✓

*NOTE: Do auscultation before palpation.

system and differences in assessment findings are described in Table 39-5. Assessment abnormalities are presented in Table 39-11. A *focused assessment* is used to evaluate the status of previously identified GI problems and to monitor for signs of new problems (see Table 3-6). A focused assessment of the GI system is presented above.

DIAGNOSTIC STUDIES OF GASTROINTESTINAL SYSTEM

Table 39-12 presents common diagnostic studies of the GI system. Selected diagnostic studies are described in more detail below.

For most diagnostic studies, make sure a signed consent form for the procedure has been completed and is in the medical record. The health care provider doing the procedure is responsible for explaining the procedure and obtaining written consent. However, you play an important role in teaching patients about the procedures. When preparing the patient, it is important to ask about any known allergies to drugs, iodine, shellfish, or contrast media.

Many GI system diagnostic procedures require measures to cleanse the GI tract and the ingestion or injection of a contrast medium or a radiopaque tracer. Often the patient has a series of GI diagnostic tests done. Monitor the patient closely to ensure adequate hydration and nutrition during the testing period.

TABLE 39-11   **ASSESSMENT ABNORMALITIES**

Gastrointestinal System

Finding	Description	Possible Etiology and Significance
Mouth		
Ulcer, plaque on lips or in mouth	Sore or lesion	Carcinoma, viral infections
Cheilosis	Softening, fissuring, and cracking of lips at angles of mouth	Riboflavin deficiency
Cheilitis	Inflammation of lips (usually lower) with fissuring, scaling, crusting	Often unknown
Geographic tongue	Scattered red, smooth (loss of papillae) areas on dorsum of tongue	Unknown
Smooth tongue	Red, slick appearance	Cobalamin deficiency
Leukoplakia	Thickened white patches	Premalignant lesion
Pyorrhea	Recessed gingivae, purulent pockets	Periodontitis
Herpes simplex	Benign vesicular lesion	Herpesvirus
Candidiasis	White, curdlike lesions surrounded by erythematous mucosa	*Candida albicans*
Glossitis	Reddened, ulcerated, swollen tongue	Exposure to streptococci, irritation, injury, vitamin B deficiencies, anemia
Acute marginal gingivitis	Friable, edematous, painful, bleeding gingivae	Irritation from ill-fitting dentures or orthodontic appliances, calcium deposits on teeth, food impaction
Esophagus and Stomach		
Dysphagia	Difficulty swallowing, sensation of food sticking in esophagus	Esophageal problems, cancer of esophagus
Hematemesis	Vomiting of blood	Esophageal varices, bleeding peptic ulcer
Pyrosis	Heartburn, burning in epigastric or substernal area	Hiatal hernia, esophagitis, incompetent lower esophageal sphincter
Dyspepsia	Burning or indigestion	Peptic ulcer disease, gallbladder disease
Odynophagia	Painful swallowing	Cancer of esophagus, esophagitis
Eructation	Belching	Gallbladder disease
Nausea and vomiting	Feeling of impending vomiting, expulsion of gastric contents through mouth	GI infections, common manifestation of many GI diseases; stress, fear, and pathologic conditions
Abdomen		
Distention	Excessive gas accumulation, enlarged abdomen, generalized tympany	Obstruction, paralytic ileus
Ascites	Accumulated fluid within abdominal cavity, eversion of umbilicus (usually)	Peritoneal inflammation, heart failure, metastatic carcinoma, cirrhosis
Bruit	Humming or swishing sound heard through stethoscope over vessel	Partial arterial obstruction (narrowing of vessel), turbulent flow (aneurysm)
Hyperresonance	Loud, tinkling rushes	Intestinal obstruction
Borborygmi	Waves of loud, gurgling sounds	Hyperactive bowel as result of eating
Absent bowel sounds	No bowel sounds on auscultation	Peritonitis, paralytic ileus, obstruction
Absence of liver dullness	Tympany on percussion	Air from viscus (e.g., perforated ulcer)
Masses	Lump on palpation	Tumors, cysts
Rebound tenderness	Sudden pain when fingers withdrawn quickly	Peritoneal inflammation, appendicitis
Nodular liver	Enlarged, hard liver with irregular edge or surface	Cirrhosis, carcinoma
Hepatomegaly	Enlargement of liver, liver edge >1-2 cm below costal margin	Metastatic carcinoma, hepatitis, venous congestion
Splenomegaly	Enlarged spleen	Chronic leukemia, hemolytic states, portal hypertension, some infections
Hernia	Bulge or nodule in abdomen, usually appearing on straining	Inguinal (in inguinal canal), femoral (in femoral canal), umbilical (herniation of umbilicus), or incisional (defect in muscles after surgery)
Rectum and Anus		
Hemorrhoids	Thrombosed veins in rectum and anus (internal or external)	Portal hypertension, chronic constipation, prolonged sitting or standing, pregnancy
Mass	Firm, nodular edge	Tumor, carcinoma
Pilonidal cyst	Opening of sinus tract, cyst in midline just above coccyx	Probably congenital
Fissure	Ulceration in anal canal	Straining, irritation
Melena	Abnormal, black, tarry stool containing digested blood	Cancer, bleeding in upper GI tract from ulcers, varices
Tenesmus	Painful and ineffective straining at stool. Sense of incomplete evacuation	Inflammatory bowel disease, irritable bowel syndrome, diarrhea secondary to GI infection (e.g., food poisoning)
Steatorrhea	Fatty, frothy, foul-smelling stool	Chronic pancreatitis, biliary obstruction, malabsorption problems

Ascending colon Transverse colon Descending colon

Sigmoid colon   Rectum

FIG. 39-9 Barium enema x-ray showing the large intestine.

Some diagnostic studies are especially difficult and uncomfortable for the older adult. Adjustments may be needed during the preparation to avoid dehydration or worsening renal function, and during testing for positioning. Close monitoring is needed to avoid problems such as dehydration from prolonged fluid restriction and diarrhea from bowel-cleansing procedures.

Radiologic Studies

Upper Gastrointestinal Series. An upper GI series with small bowel follow-through provides visualization of the oropharyngeal area, the esophagus, the stomach, and the small intestine via fluoroscopy and x-ray examination. The procedure consists of the patient swallowing contrast medium (a thick barium solution or gastrograffin) and then assuming different positions on the x-ray table. The movement of the contrast medium is observed with fluoroscopy, and several x-rays are taken (see Table 39-12). An upper GI series is used to identify disorders such as esophageal strictures, polyps, tumors, hiatal hernias, foreign bodies, and peptic ulcers.

Lower Gastrointestinal Series. The purpose of a lower GI series (barium enema) examination is to observe by means of fluoroscopy the colon filling with contrast medium and to

---

TABLE 39-12 DIAGNOSTIC STUDIES

Gastrointestinal System

Study	Description and Purpose	Nursing Responsibility
Radiology		
Upper gastrointestinal (GI) or barium swallow	Fluoroscopic x-ray study using contrast medium. Used to diagnose structural abnormalities of esophagus, stomach, and duodenum.	Explain procedure to patient, including the need to drink contrast medium and assume various positions on x-ray table. Keep patient NPO for 8-12 hr before procedure. Tell patient to avoid smoking after midnight before study. After x-ray, take measures to prevent contrast medium impaction (fluids, laxatives). Tell patient that stool may be white up to 72 hr after test.
Small bowel series	Contrast medium is ingested and films taken every 30 min until medium reaches terminal ileum.	Same as for upper GI.
Lower GI or barium enema	Fluoroscopic x-ray examination of colon using contrast medium, which is administered rectally (enema) (see Fig. 39-9). Double-contrast or air-contrast barium enema is test of choice. Air is infused after thick barium flows through transverse colon. Because of the use of endoscopy, not done as frequently.	*Before procedure:* Administer laxatives and enemas until colon is clear of stool evening before procedure. Administer clear liquid diet evening before procedure. Keep patient NPO for 8 hr before test. Instruct patient about being given barium by enema. Explain that cramping and urge to defecate may occur during procedure and that patient may be placed in various positions on tilt table. *After procedure:* Give fluids, laxatives, or suppositories to assist in expelling barium. Observe stool for passage of contrast medium.
Cholangiography		
• Percutaneous transhepatic (PTC)	After local anesthesia and monitored anesthesia care (formerly called conscious sedation), liver is entered with long needle (under fluoroscopy), bile duct is entered, bile withdrawn, and radiopaque contrast medium injected. Fluoroscopy is used to determine filling of hepatic and biliary ducts. IV antibiotics are given prophylactically.	Observe patient for signs of hemorrhage, bile leakage, and infection. Assess patient's medications for possible contraindications, precautions, or complications with use of contrast medium.
• Surgical cholangiogram	Performed during surgery on biliary structures, such as gallbladder. Contrast medium is injected into common bile duct.	Explain to patient that anesthetic will be used. Assess patient's medications for possible contraindications, precautions, or complications with use of contrast medium.
• Magnetic resonance cholangiopancreatography (MRCP)	Uses MRI technology to obtain images of biliary and pancreatic ducts.	Explain procedure to patient. Contraindicated in patient with metal implants (e.g., pacemaker) or one who is pregnant.

Continued

TABLE 39-12   DIAGNOSTIC STUDIES—cont'd

Gastrointestinal System

Study	Description and Purpose	Nursing Responsibility
Radiology—cont'd		
Ultrasound	Used to show the size and configuration of organ. Noninvasive procedure uses high-frequency sound waves (ultrasound waves), which are passed into body structures and recorded as they are reflected (bounded).	
• Abdominal ultrasound	Detects abdominal masses (tumors, cysts), biliary and liver disease, gallstones. A conductive gel (lubricant jelly) is applied to the skin and a transducer is placed on the area.	Instruct patient to be NPO 8-12 hr before ultrasound. Air or gas can reduce quality of images. Food intake can cause gallbladder contraction, resulting in suboptimal study.
• Endoscopic ultrasound (EUS)	Small ultrasound transducer is installed on tip of endoscope. Because EUS transducer gets close to the organ(s) being examined, images obtained are often more accurate and detailed than images provided by traditional ultrasound. Detects and stages esophageal, gastric, rectal, biliary, and pancreatic tumors and abnormalities. Fine-needle aspiration can be used to diagnose dysplasia or cancer.	Same as esophagogastroduodenoscopy (EGD).
• FibroScan or FibroTest	FibroScan (transient elastrography) uses an ultrasound transducer to determine liver stiffness (fibrosis). It is noninvasive and is used in patients with chronic hepatitis C and cirrhosis.	Patient lies in dorsal decubitus position with the right arm in extreme abduction. A probe is positioned in an intercostal space between the ribs.
Nuclear imaging scans (scintigraphy)	Shows size, shape, and position of organ. Functional disorders and structural defects may be identified. Radionuclide (radioactive isotope) is injected IV, and a counter (scanning) device picks up radioactive emission, which is recorded on paper. Only tracer doses of radioactive isotopes are used.	Tell patient that substance to be ingested contains only traces of radioactivity and poses little to no danger. Schedule no more than one radionuclide test on the same day. Explain to patient need to lie flat during scanning.
• Gastric emptying studies	Radionuclide study (scintigraphy) is used to assess ability of stomach to empty solids. Cooked egg containing Tc-99m and toast are eaten with water. Images are obtained at 0, 1, 2, and 4 hr later. Study is used in patients with gastric emptying disorders caused by peptic ulcer, ulcer surgery, diabetes, gastric malignancies, or functional disorders.	Same as above.
• Hepatobiliary scintigraphy (HIDA)	Patient is given IV injection of Tc-99m and positioned under camera to record distribution of tracer in liver, biliary tree, gallbladder, and proximal small intestine. Used to identify obstructions of bile ducts (e.g., gallstones, tumors), diseases of gallbladder, and bile leaks.	Same as above.
• Scintigraphy of GI bleeding	Tc-99m–labeled sulfur colloid or Tc-99m labeling of the patient's own red blood cells (RBCs) to determine the site of active GI blood loss. Sulfur colloid or the patient's RBCs are injected, and images of the abdomen are obtained at intermittent intervals.	Same as above.
Computed tomography (CT)	Noninvasive radiologic examination allows for exposures at different depths. Detects biliary tract, liver, and pancreatic disorders. Use of oral and IV contrast medium accentuates density differences.	Explain procedure to patient. Determine sensitivity to iodine or shellfish if contrast material used.
Magnetic resonance imaging (MRI)	Noninvasive procedure using radiofrequency waves and a magnetic field. Used to detect hepatobiliary disease, hepatic lesions, and sources of GI bleeding and to stage colorectal cancer. IV contrast medium (gadolinium) may be used.	Explain procedure to patient. Contraindicated in patient with metal implants (e.g., pacemaker) or one who is pregnant.
Virtual colonoscopy	Combines CT scanning or MRI with computer virtual reality software to detect intestine and colon diseases, including polyps, colorectal cancer, diverticulosis, and lower GI bleeding. Air is introduced via a tube placed in rectum to enlarge colon to enhance visualization. Images obtained while patient is on back and abdomen. Computer combines images to form 2- and 3-D pictures that are viewed on monitor.	Bowel preparation similar to colonoscopy (see Colonoscopy, below). Unlike conventional colonoscopy, no sedatives are needed and no scope is used. Procedure takes about 15-20 min.

TABLE 39-12 **DIAGNOSTIC STUDIES—cont'd**

Gastrointestinal System

Study	Description and Purpose	Nursing Responsibility
Endoscopy **Esophagogastroduodenoscopy (EGD)**	Directly visualizes mucosal lining of esophagus, stomach, and duodenum with flexible endoscope. Test may use video imaging to visualize stomach motility. Inflammations, ulcerations, tumors, varices, or Mallory-Weiss tears may be detected. Biopsies may be taken and varices can be treated with band ligation or sclerotherapy.	*Before procedure:* Keep patient NPO for 8 hr. Make sure signed consent is on chart. Give preoperative medication if ordered. Explain to patient that local anesthesia may be sprayed on throat before insertion of scope and that patient will be sedated during the procedure. *After procedure:* Keep patient NPO until gag reflex returns. Gently tickle back of throat to determine reflex. Use warm saline gargles for relief of sore throat. Check temperature q15-30min for 1-2 hr (sudden temperature spike is sign of perforation).
Colonoscopy	Directly visualizes entire colon up to ileocecal valve with flexible fiberoptic scope. Patient's position is changed frequently during procedure to assist with advancement of scope to cecum. Used to diagnose or detect inflammatory bowel disease, polyps, tumors, and diverticulosis and dilate strictures. Procedure allows for biopsy and removal of polyps without laparotomy.	*Before procedure:* Bowel preparation is done. This varies depending on physician. For example, patients may be kept on clear liquids 1-2 days before procedure. Cathartic and/or enema given the night before. An alternative is to give 1 gal of polyethylene glycol (GoLYTELY, Colyte) evening before (8-oz glass q10min) or Prepopik, one packet the night before colonoscopy and a second packet morning of colonoscopy. Explain to patient that flexible scope will be inserted while patient in side-lying position. Explain to patient that sedation will be given. *After procedure:* Patient may experience abdominal cramps caused by stimulation of peristalsis because the bowel is constantly inflated with air during procedure. Observe for rectal bleeding and manifestations of perforation (e.g., malaise, abdominal distention, tenesmus). Check vital signs.
Video capsule endoscopy (VCE)	Patient swallows a capsule with camera (approximately the size of a large vitamin), which provides endoscopic visualization of GI tract (see Fig. 39-11). Most commonly used to visualize small intestine and diagnose diseases such as Crohn's disease, small bowel tumors, small bowel injury due to NSAIDs, celiac disease, and malabsorption syndrome and to identify sources of possible GI bleeding in areas not accessible by upper endoscopy or colonoscopy. Camera takes >50,000 images during 8-hr examination. Capsule relays images to monitoring device that patient wears on belt. After examination, images are downloaded to a workstation. Not used in patients with suspected intestinal strictures.	Instruct patient to fast overnight. Patient may have bowel preparation similar to colonoscopy. The video capsule is swallowed, and clear liquids resumed after 2 hr and food and medications after 4 hr. Procedure is comfortable for most patients. Eight hours after swallowing the capsule, the patient returns to have the monitoring device removed. A patency capsule may be used first in patients determined to be high risk for capsule retention due to strictures. Peristalsis causes passage of the disposable capsule with a bowel movement.
Sigmoidoscopy	Directly visualizes rectum and sigmoid colon with lighted flexible endoscope. Sometimes special table is used to tilt patient into knee-chest position. Used to detect tumors, polyps, inflammatory and infectious diseases, fissures, hemorrhoids.	Administer enemas evening before and morning of procedure. Patient may have clear liquids day before, or no dietary restrictions may be necessary. Explain to patient knee-chest position (unless patient is older or very ill), need to take deep breaths during insertion of scope, and possible urge to defecate as scope is passed. Encourage patient to relax and let abdomen go limp. Observe for rectal bleeding after polypectomy or biopsy.
Endoscopic retrograde cholangiopancreatography (ERCP)	Fiberoptic endoscope (using fluoroscopy) is orally inserted into descending duodenum, then common bile and pancreatic ducts are cannulated. Contrast medium is injected into ducts and allows for direct visualization of structures. Technique can also be used to retrieve a gallstone from distal common bile duct, dilate strictures, biopsy, diagnose pseudocysts.	*Before procedure:* Explain procedure to patient, including patient role. Keep patient NPO 8 hr before procedure. Ensure consent form signed. Administer sedation immediately before and during procedure. Administer antibiotics if ordered. *After procedure:* Check vital signs. Check for signs of perforation or infection. Be aware that pancreatitis is most common complication. Check for return of gag reflex.
Endoscopic ultrasound	Combined use of endoscopy and ultrasound using an ultrasound transducer attached to an endoscope. Enables visualization of esophagus, stomach, intestine, liver, pancreas, and gallstones.	Similar to EGD.

Continued

TABLE 39-12   DIAGNOSTIC STUDIES—cont'd

Gastrointestinal System

Study	Description and Purpose	Nursing Responsibility
Endoscopy—cont'd		
Laparoscopy (peritoneoscopy)	Peritoneal cavity and contents are visualized with laparoscope. Biopsy specimen may also be taken. Done with patient in operating room. Double-puncture peritoneoscopy permits better visualization of abdominal cavity, especially liver. Can eliminate need for exploratory laparotomy in many patients.	Make sure signed consent is on chart. Keep patient NPO 8 hr before study. Administer preoperative sedative medication. Ensure that bladder and bowels are emptied. Observe for possible complications of bleeding and bowel perforation after the procedure.
Blood Studies		
Amylase	Measures secretion of amylase by pancreas. Is important in diagnosing acute pancreatitis. Level of amylase peaks in 24 hr and then drops to normal in 48-72 hr. Depending on method, *reference interval* is 30-122 U/L (0.51-2.07 μkat/L).	Obtain blood sample in acute attack of pancreatitis. Explain procedure to patient.
Lipase	Measures secretion of lipase by pancreas. Level stays elevated longer than serum amylase in acute pancreatitis. *Reference interval:* 31-186 U/L (0.5-3.2 μkat/L).	Explain procedure to patient.
Gastrin	Gastrin is a hormone secreted by cells of the antrum of the stomach, the duodenum, and the pancreatic islets of Langerhans. *Reference interval:* 25-100 pg/mL when fasting.	Explain procedure to patient.
Liver Biopsy	Percutaneous procedure uses needle inserted between 6th and 7th or 8th and 9th intercostal spaces on the right side to obtain specimen of hepatic tissue. Often done using ultrasound or CT guidance.	*Before procedure:* Check patient's coagulation status (prothrombin time, clotting or bleeding time). Ensure that patient's blood is typed and crossmatched. Take vital signs as baseline data. Explain holding of breath after expiration when needle is inserted. Ensure that informed consent has been signed. *After procedure:* Check vital signs to detect internal bleeding q15min × 2, q30min × 4, q1hr × 4. Keep patient lying on right side for minimum of 2 hr to splint puncture site. Keep patient in bed in flat position for 12-14 hr. Assess patient for complications such as bile peritonitis, shock, pneumothorax.
Fecal Tests		
Fecal analysis	Form, consistency, and color are noted. Specimen examined for mucus, blood, pus, parasites, and fat content. Tests for occult blood (guaiac test, Hemoccult, Hemoccult II, Hemoccult-SENSA, Hematest) are done. Single DNA test (PreGen-Plus) is a panel of DNA markers used to detect and monitor colorectal cancer.	Observe patient's stools. Collect stool specimens. Check stools for blood. Keep diet free of red meat for 24-48 hr before occult blood test.
Stool culture	Tests for the presence of bacteria, including *Clostridium difficile*.	Collect stool specimen.

observe by x-ray the filled colon. This procedure identifies polyps, tumors, and other lesions in the colon. It consists of administering an enema of contrast medium to the patient. The air-contrast barium enema provides better visualization (Fig. 39-9). Because it requires the patient to retain the barium, it is not tolerated as well in an older or immobile patient.

Virtual Colonoscopy. *Virtual colonoscopy* combines computed tomography (CT) scanning or magnetic resonance imaging (MRI) with computer software to produce images of the colon and the rectum. The test is less invasive than a conventional colonoscopy but does require radiation and prior cleansing of the colon (the technique is described in Table 39-12).

Virtual colonoscopy enables one to better see inside a colon that is narrowed due to inflammation or a growth.[11] However,

if a polyp is discovered using virtual colonoscopy, a conventional colonoscopy will then be needed to obtain a biopsy or remove it. A disadvantage of virtual colonoscopy is that it may be less sensitive in obtaining information on the details and color of the mucosa. In addition, it is less sensitive in detecting small (less than 10 mm) or flat polyps.

Endoscopy

Endoscopy refers to the direct visualization of a body structure through a lighted fiberoptic instrument. The GI structures that can be examined by endoscopy include the esophagus, the stomach, the duodenum, and the colon. The pancreatic, hepatic, and common bile ducts can be visualized with an endoscope. This procedure is called *endoscopic retrograde cholangiopancreatography* (ERCP).

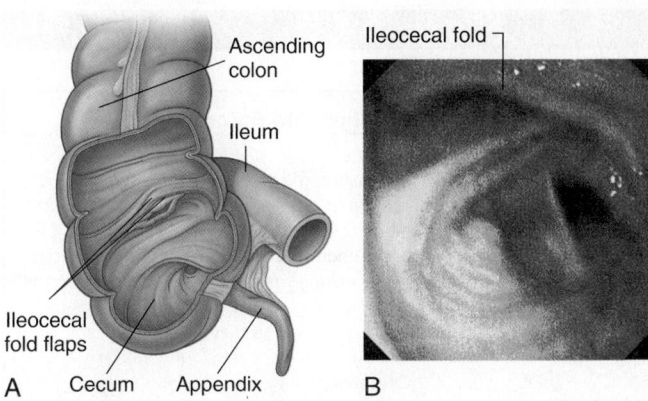

FIG. 39-10 A, Illustration showing the ileocecal junction and the ileocecal fold. **B,** Endoscopic image of the ileocecal fold.

CASE STUDY—cont'd

Objective Data: Diagnostic Studies

iStockphoto/Thinkstock

The ED physician performs a rectal examination and finds a palpable mass. The following diagnostic tests are ordered:
- CBC
- Electrolytes
- Liver function tests
- Urinalysis
- CT scan of the abdomen
- Colonoscopy

The CBC reveals an Hgb of 6.8 g/dL and an Hct of 20%. The white blood cell count is normal. The electrolytes, liver function tests, and urinalysis are within normal limits. The CT scan reveals pockets of gas and fluid in the ascending colon and two medium-sized tumors in the transverse colon.

This case study is continued in Chapter 43 on p. 1003.

The endoscope is an instrument through which biopsy forceps and cytology brushes may be passed. Cameras are attached, and video and still pictures can be taken (Fig. 39-10). Endoscopy is often done in combination with biopsy and cytologic studies.

The major complication of GI endoscopy is perforation through the structure being scoped. All endoscopic procedures require informed, written consent. Specific endoscopy procedures are discussed in Table 39-12. In addition to diagnostic procedures, many invasive and therapeutic procedures may be done with endoscopes. Examples include polypectomy, sclerosis or banding of varices, laser treatment, cauterization of bleeding sites, papillotomy, common bile duct stone removal, and balloon dilation. Many endoscopic procedures require IV short-acting sedation.

Capsule endoscopy is a noninvasive approach to visualize the GI tract (Fig. 39-11). (See Table 39-12 for further discussion of this diagnostic technique.) Its sensitivity in detecting the source of GI bleeding, small lesions, esophageal varices, colonic polyps, and colorectal cancer is under investigation.[12]

FIG. 39-11 Capsule endoscopy. **A,** The video capsule has its own camera and light source. After it is swallowed, it travels through the GI tract and allows visualization of the small intestine. It sends messages to a monitoring device that is worn on a waist belt **(B).** During the 8-hour examination, the patient is free to move about. After the test, the images are viewed on a video monitor.

Liver Biopsy

The purpose of a liver biopsy is to obtain hepatic tissue that can be used in establishing a diagnosis or assessing fibrosis. It may also be useful for following the progress of liver disease, such as chronic hepatitis.

The two types of liver biopsy are open and closed. The *open method* involves making an incision and removing a wedge of tissue. It is done in the operating room with the patient under general anesthesia, often concurrently with another surgical procedure. The *closed,* or *needle, biopsy* is a percutaneous procedure in which the site is infiltrated with a local anesthetic and a needle is inserted between the sixth and seventh or eighth and ninth intercostal spaces on the right side. The patient lies supine with the right arm over the head. Instruct the patient to expire fully and to not breathe while the needle is inserted (see Table 39-12).

Liver Function Studies

Liver function tests (LFTs) are laboratory (blood) studies that reflect hepatic disease. Table 39-13 describes some common LFTs.

TABLE 39-13 **DIAGNOSTIC STUDIES**

Liver Function Tests

Test	Description and Purpose
Bile Formation and Excretion	
Serum bilirubin	Measurement of liver's ability to conjugate and excrete bilirubin, allowing differentiation between unconjugated (indirect) and conjugated (direct) bilirubin in plasma.
• Total	Measurement of direct and indirect total bilirubin. *Reference interval: 0.2-1.2 mg/dL (3-21 μmol/L)*
• Direct	Measurement of conjugated bilirubin. Elevated in obstructive jaundice. *Reference interval: 0.1-0.3 mg/dL (1.7-5.1 μmol/L)*
• Indirect	Measurement of unconjugated bilirubin. Elevated in hepatocellular and hemolytic conditions. *Reference interval: 0.1-1.0 mg/dL (1.7-17 μmol/L)*
Urinary bilirubin	Measurement of urinary excretion of conjugated bilirubin. *Reference interval: 0 or negative*
Protein Metabolism	
Protein (serum)	Measurement of serum proteins manufactured by the liver. • Albumin, *reference interval:* 3.5-5.0 g/dL (35-50 g/L) • Globulin, *reference interval:* 2.0-3.5 g/dL (20-35 g/L) • Total protein, *reference interval:* 6.4-8.3 g/dL (64-83 g/L) • A/G ratio, *reference interval:* 1.5:1-2.5:1
α-Fetoprotein	Indication of hepatocellular cancer. *Reference interval: <10 ng/mL (<10 mcg/L)*
Ammonia	Conversion of ammonia to urea normally occurs in the liver. Increase can result in hepatic encephalopathy secondary to liver cirrhosis. *Reference interval: 15-45 mcg N/dL (11-32 μmol N/L)*

Test	Description and Purpose
Hemostatic Function	
Prothrombin time (PT)	Determination of prothrombin activity. *Reference interval: 11-16 sec*
International normalized ratio (INR)	Standardized system of reporting PT based on a reference calibration model and calculated by comparing the patient's PT with a control value. *Reference interval: In general, 2-3 is the desired therapeutic level with warfarin (Coumadin), depending on laboratory*
Vitamin K	Essential cofactor for many clotting factors. *Reference interval: 0.1-2.2 ng/mL (0.22-4.88 nmol/L)*
Serum Enzymes	
Alkaline phosphatase (ALP)	Originates from bone and liver. Serum levels rise when excretion is impaired as a result of obstruction in the biliary tract. *Reference interval: 38-126 U/L (0.65-2.14 μkat/L), depending on method and age*
Aspartate aminotransferase (AST)	Elevated in liver damage and inflammation. *Reference interval: 10-30 U/L (0.17-0.51 μkat/L)*
Alanine aminotransferase (ALT)	Elevated in liver damage and inflammation. *Reference interval: 10-40 U/L (0.17-0.68 μkat/L)*
γ-Glutamyl transpeptidase (GGT)	Present in biliary tract (not in skeletal or cardiac muscle). Increase in hepatitis and alcoholic liver disease. More sensitive for liver dysfunction than ALP. *Reference interval: 0-30 U/L (0-0.5 μkat/L)*
Lipid Metabolism	
Cholesterol (serum)	Synthesis and excretion by liver. Increase in biliary obstruction. Decrease in cirrhosis and malnutrition. *Reference interval: <200 mg/dL (<5.2 mmol/L), varying with age*

A/G, Albumin/globulin.

BRIDGE TO NCLEX EXAMINATION

The number of the question corresponds to the same-numbered outcome at the beginning of the chapter.

1. A patient is admitted to the hospital with a diagnosis of diarrhea with dehydration. The nurse recognizes that increased peristalsis resulting in diarrhea can be related to
   a. sympathetic inhibition.
   b. mixing and propulsion.
   c. sympathetic stimulation.
   d. parasympathetic stimulation.

2. A patient has an elevated blood level of indirect (unconjugated) bilirubin. One cause of this finding is that
   a. the gallbladder is unable to contract to release stored bile.
   b. bilirubin is not being conjugated and excreted into the bile by the liver.
   c. the Kupffer cells in the liver are unable to remove bilirubin from the blood.
   d. there is an obstruction in the biliary tract preventing flow of bile into the small intestine.

3. As gastric contents move into the small intestine, the bowel is normally protected from the acidity of gastric contents by the
   a. inhibition of secretin release.
   b. release of bicarbonate by the pancreas.
   c. release of pancreatic digestive enzymes.
   d. release of gastrin by the duodenal mucosa.

4. A patient is jaundiced and her stools are clay colored (gray). This is most likely related to
   a. decreased bile flow into the intestine.
   b. increased production of urobilinogen.
   c. increased production of cholecystokinin.
   d. increased bile and bilirubin in the blood.

5. An 80-year-old man states that, although he adds a lot of salt to his food, it still does not have much taste. The nurse's response is based on the knowledge that the older adult
   a. should not experience changes in taste.
   b. has a loss of taste buds, especially for sweet and salt.
   c. has some loss of taste but no difficulty chewing food.
   d. loses the sense of taste because the ability to smell is decreased.

6. When the nurse is assessing the health perception–health maintenance pattern as related to GI function, an appropriate question to ask is
   a. "What is your usual bowel elimination pattern?"
   b. "What percentage of your income is spent on food?"
   c. "Have you traveled to a foreign country in the last year?"
   d. "Do you have diarrhea when you are under a lot of stress?"

7. During an examination of the abdomen the nurse should
   a. position the patient in the supine position with the bed flat and knees straight.
   b. listen in the epigastrium and all four quadrants for 2 minutes for bowel sounds.
   c. use the following order of techniques: inspection, palpation, percussion, auscultation.
   d. describe bowel sounds as absent if no sound is heard in the lower right quadrant after 2 minutes.

8. A normal physical assessment finding of the GI system is/are (select all that apply)
   a. nonpalpable liver and spleen.
   b. borborygmi in upper right quadrant.
   c. tympany on percussion of the abdomen.
   d. liver edge 2 to 4 cm below the costal margin.
   e. finding of a firm, nodular edge on the rectal examination.

9. In preparing a patient for a colonoscopy, the nurse explains that
   a. a signed permit is not necessary.
   b. sedation may be used during the procedure.
   c. only one cleansing enema is necessary for preparation.
   d. a light meal should be eaten the day before the procedure.

1. d, 2. b, 3. b, 4. a, 5. b, 6. c, 7. b, 8. a, c, 9. b

⊖volve

For rationales to these answers and even more NCLEX review questions, visit *http://evolve.elsevier.com/Lewis/medsurg*.

REFERENCES

1. de Mata C, McKenna G, Burke FM: Caries and the older patients, *Dent Update* 38:376, 2011.
2. Gutschow CA, Leers JM, Schroder W, et al: Effect of aging on esophageal motility in patients with and without GERD, *Ger Med Sci* 9:Doc22. doi:10.3205/000145.
3. Rao SS, Go JT: Update on the management of constipation in the elderly: new treatment options, *Clin Interv Aging* 9:163, 2010.
4. Franklin LE, Spain MP, Edlund BJ: Pharmacological management of chronic constipation in older adults, *J Gerontol Nurs* 14:1, 2012.
5. Gallegos-Orozco JR, Foxx-Orenstein AE, Sterler SM, et al: Chronic constipation in the elderly, *Am J Gastroenterol* 107:18, 2012.
6. Holm AN, Gerke H: What should be done with a dilated bile duct? *Curr Gastroenterol Rep* 12:150, 2010.
7. Villareal DT, Chode S, Parimi N, et al: Weight loss, exercise or both and physical function in obese older adults, *N Engl J Med* 364:1218, 2011.
8. Zuchelli T, Myers SE: Gastrointestinal issues in the older female patient, *Gastroenterol Clin North Am* 40:449, 2011.
9. Boots C, Stephenson MD: Does obesity increase the risk of miscarriage in spontaneous conception: a systematic review, *Semin Reprod Med* 29:507, 2011.
10. Jarvis C: *Physical examination and health assessment*, ed 6, St Louis, 2012, Saunders.
11. National Digestive Diseases Information Clearinghouse: Virtual colonoscopy. Retrieved from *http://digestive.niddk.nih.gov/ddiseases/pubs/virtualcolonoscopy/index.aspx#what*.
12. Sieg A: Capsule endoscopy compared with conventional colonoscopy for detection of colorectal neoplasms, *World J Gastrointest Endosc* 3:81, 2011.

RESOURCES

Resources for this chapter are listed in Chapter 40 on p. 905, Chapter 42 on p. 960, Chapter 43 on p. 1004, and Chapter 44 on p. 1043.

40

Nursing Management
Nutritional Problems

Rose DiMaria-Ghalili

> *To eat is a necessity,*
> *but to eat intelligently is an art.*
> **La Rochefoucauld**

LEARNING OUTCOMES

1. Relate the essential components of a well-balanced diet to their impact on health outcomes.
2. Describe the common etiologic factors, clinical manifestations, and management of malnutrition.
3. Describe the components of a nutritional assessment.
4. Explain the indications, complications, and nursing management principles related to the use of enteral nutrition.
5. Explain the indications, complications, and nursing management related to the use of parenteral nutrition.
6. Compare the etiologic factors, clinical manifestations, and nursing management of eating disorders.

KEY TERMS

anorexia nervosa, p. 903
bulimia nervosa, p. 903
enteral nutrition (EN), p. 897

malabsorption syndrome, p. 891
malnutrition, p. 890

parenteral nutrition (PN), p. 901
tube feeding, p. 897

This chapter focuses on problems related to nutrition. A review of normal nutrition provides a basis for evaluating nutritional status. Malnutrition and types of supplemental nutrition, including enteral and parenteral nutrition, are discussed. Obesity is discussed in Chapter 41.

NUTRITIONAL PROBLEMS

Nutrition is the sum of processes by which one takes in and utilizes nutrients.[1] Nutritional status can be viewed as a continuum from undernutrition to normal nutrition to overnutri-

tion. An alteration in the process of nutrient intake or utilization can potentially cause nutritional problems. Nutritional problems occur in all age-groups, cultures, ethnic groups, and socioeconomic classes and across all educational levels.

The nutritional status of a person or a family is influenced by many factors. Attitudes toward the importance of food and eating habits are established early. Cultural or religious preferences and requirements are frequently reflected in dietary intake. The financial status of a family or an individual may influence the type and amount of nutritionally sound food that can be purchased.[2]

Reviewed by Katie Clark, RD, MPH CDE, Assistant Clinical Professor, Nutrition, University of California San Francisco, School of Nursing, San Diego, California; Shellie Simons, RN, PhD, Assistant Professor, University of Massachusetts Lowell, Lowell, Massachusetts; and Patricia Worthington, RN, MSN, CNSC, Nutritional Support Clinical Specialist, Thomas Jefferson University Hospital, Philadelphia, Pennsylvania.

NORMAL NUTRITION

Nutrition is important for energy, growth, and maintenance and repair of body tissues. Optimal nutrition (in the absence of any underlying disease process) results from the ingestion of a balanced diet. The major components of the basic food groups are carbohydrates, fats, proteins, vitamins, minerals, and water. Optimal nutrition and daily physical activity are essential for a healthy lifestyle.

The MyPlate approach to nutritional education (www. choosemyplate.gov) provides a visual guideline for sensible meal planning to help Americans eat healthfully and make good food choices. MyPlate focuses on the proportions of five food groups (grains, protein, fruits, vegetables, and dairy) that you should eat at each meal (Fig. 40-1, Table 40-1). eTables 40-1 and 40-2 (available on the website for this chapter) show the recommended daily amount of food from each food group and sample meal plans.

MyPlate materials have been developed for older adults and are available at *www.nutrition.tufts.edu/research/myplate-older-adults*. Tips on how to be physically active are available at *www. choosemyplate.gov/physical-activity.html*.

A growing number of electronic and print sources are available for determining nutritional information in commonly consumed foods. Nutrition Facts labels are listed on food products (Fig. 40-2). Calories, nutrients, and ingredients of food consumed can be easily tracked for healthy weight management. Consumer and health professional educational materials on the Nutrition Facts labels are available on the U.S. Food and Drug Administration (FDA) website.[3]

A person's daily caloric requirements are influenced by body type, age, gender, medications, physical activity, and the presence or absence of disease. Adjustments in caloric intake are necessary depending on changes in health status and daily activity level. The Mifflin–St. Jeor equation is recommended to estimate daily adult energy (calorie) requirements based on resting metabolic rate for individuals[4,5] (Table 40-2).

A more convenient way to estimate daily calories is based on kilocalories per kilogram (kcal/kg). (Kilocalorie [kcal] is the correct unit to designate caloric intake and expenditure. However, calorie is more commonly used.) An average adult requires an estimated 20 to 35 cal/kg of body weight per day, using an appropriate reference weight.[6] During illness, energy

FIG. 40-1 MyPlate is the primary food group symbol that serves as a reminder to make healthy food choices and to build a healthy plate at mealtimes. It is a visual cue that identifies the five basic food groups from which to select healthy foods. The plate is divided into four slightly different-sized quadrants, with fruits and vegetables taking up half the space and grains and protein making up the other half. The vegetables and grains portions are the largest of the four. Next to the plate is a blue circle for dairy, which could be a glass of milk or a food such as cheese or yogurt. For more information, see *www.choosemyplate.gov*.

TABLE 40-1 **NUTRITIONAL THERAPY**
MyPlate Tips for a Healthy Lifestyle

Making food choices for a healthy lifestyle can be as simple as using these 10 tips. Use the ideas in this list to (1) balance your calories, (2) choose foods to eat more often, and (3) cut back on foods to eat less often.

1.	Balance calories	Find out how many calories you need for a day as a first step in managing your weight. Go to *www.choosemyplate.gov* to find your calorie level. Being physically active also helps you balance calories.
2.	Enjoy your food, but eat less	Take the time to fully enjoy your food as you eat it. Eating too fast or when your attention is elsewhere may lead to eating too many calories. Pay attention to hunger and fullness cues before, during, and after meals. Use them to recognize when to eat and when you have had enough.
3.	Avoid oversized portions	Use a smaller plate, bowl, and glass. Portion out foods before you eat. When eating out, choose a smaller size option, share a dish, or take home part of your meal.
4.	Foods to eat more often	Eat more vegetables, fruits, whole grains, and fat-free or 1% milk and dairy products. These foods have the nutrients you need for health, including potassium, calcium, vitamin D, and fiber. Make them the basis for meals and snacks.
5.	Make half your plate fruits and vegetables	Choose red, orange, and dark-green vegetables like tomatoes, sweet potatoes, and broccoli, along with other vegetables, for your meals. Add fruit to meals as part of main or side dishes or as dessert.
6.	Switch to fat-free or low-fat (1%) milk	They have the same amount of calcium and other essential nutrients as whole milk, but fewer calories and less saturated fat.
7.	Make half your grains whole grains	To eat more whole grains, substitute a whole-grain product for a refined product. For example, eat whole-wheat bread instead of white bread, or brown rice instead of white rice.
8.	Foods to eat less often	Cut back on foods high in solid fats, added sugars, and salt. They include cakes, cookies, ice cream, candies, sweetened drinks, pizza, and fatty meats like ribs, sausages, bacon, and hot dogs. Use these foods as occasional treats, not everyday foods.
9.	Compare sodium in foods	Use the Nutrition Facts label (see Fig. 40-2) to choose lower sodium versions of foods like soup, bread, and frozen meals. Select foods labeled "low sodium," "reduced sodium," or "no salt added."
10.	Drink water instead of sugary drinks	Cut calories by drinking water or unsweetened beverages. Soda, energy drinks, and sports drinks are a major source of added sugar and calories in American diets.

Source: US Department of Agriculture Center for Nutrition Policy and Promotion: Nutrition education series, DG Tips Sheet No 1, June 2011. Retrieved from *www.choosemyplate.gov* and *www.health.gov/dietaryguidelines*.

needs may be greater. Rule-of-thumb estimations are that an individual should consume 20 to 25 cal/kg body weight to lose weight, 25 to 30 cal/kg to maintain body weight, and 30 to 35 cal/kg to gain weight.

Carbohydrates, the body's primary source of energy, yield approximately 4 cal/g. Carbohydrates can be classified as either simple or complex. Simple carbohydrates come in two forms:

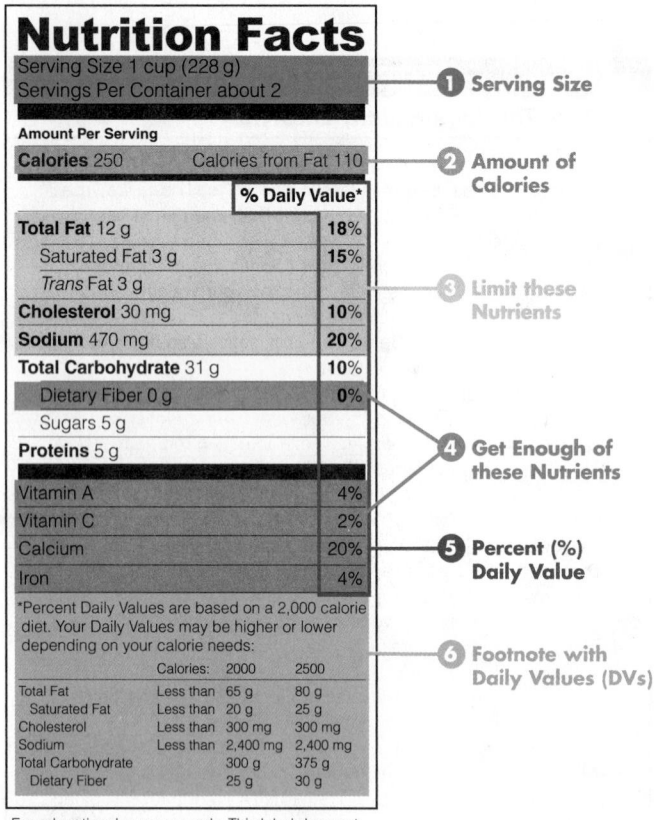

FIG. 40-2 Sample of a Nutrition Facts label.

monosaccharides (e.g., glucose, fructose), which are found in fruits and honey; and disaccharides (e.g., sucrose, maltose, lactose), which are found in foods such as table sugar, malted cereal, and milk, respectively. Complex carbohydrates or polysaccharides include starches, such as cereal grains, potatoes, and legumes.

Carbohydrates are the chief protein-sparing ingredient in a nutritionally sound diet. The Dietary Reference Intake (DRI) recommendations are that 45% to 65% of total calories should come from carbohydrates.[6] Furthermore, individuals should take approximately 14 g of dietary fiber per 1000 calories eaten per day from fruits, vegetables, and whole grains, equating to roughly 28 or 30 g for a typical 2000-calorie diet. Individuals should choose food and beverages with little added sugar or caloric sweeteners.

Fats are a major source of energy for the body. One gram of fat yields 9 calories. Fats are stored in adipose tissue and in the abdominal cavity. Fats also act as carriers of essential fatty acids and fat-soluble vitamins. Fats provide a feeling of satiety after eating. Individuals should limit their fat intake to 20% to 35% of total calories.[7]

Fats in the diet can be divided into (1) potentially harmful (saturated fat and *trans* fat) and (2) healthier dietary fat (monounsaturated and polyunsaturated fat) (see Fig. 34-3). One type of polyunsaturated fat, omega-3 fatty acids, may be especially beneficial to your heart. Omega-3 fatty acids, found in some types of fatty fish, appear to decrease the risk of coronary artery disease.[8]

Diets high in excess calories, usually in the form of fats, contribute to the development of obesity. Individuals should consume less than 10% of calories from saturated fatty acids (approximately 20 g of saturated fat per day in a 2000-calorie diet), limit intake of fat and oils high in *trans*-fatty acids, and limit intake of dietary cholesterol to 300 mg/day.

Proteins, another essential component of a well-balanced diet, are obtained from both animal and plant sources. Ideally, 10% to 35% of daily caloric needs should come from protein.[7] The recommended daily protein intake is 0.8 to 1 g/kg of body weight. One gram of protein yields 4 calories. Amino acids are the fundamental units of protein structure. The 22 amino acids are classified as essential and nonessential. The body is capable of synthesizing nonessential amino acids if an adequate supply of protein is available. However, the nine essential amino acids cannot be synthesized, and their availability depends totally on dietary sources. Protein sources containing all the essential amino acids are called *complete proteins.* Proteins that lack one or more of the essential amino acids are called *incomplete proteins.* Table 40-3 lists good sources of protein. Proteins are essential for tissue growth, repair, and maintenance; body regulatory functions; and energy production.

Vitamins are organic compounds required in small amounts for normal metabolism. Vitamins function primarily in enzyme

TABLE 40-2   ESTIMATING DAILY ENERGY (CALORIE) REQUIREMENTS

Mifflin–St. Jeor Equation

Men: Energy expenditure = 5 + 10 (wt in kg) + 6.25 (ht in cm) − 5 (age)
Women: Energy expenditure = −161 + 10 (wt in kg) + 6.25 (ht in cm) − 5 (age)

To determine total daily calorie needs, the energy expenditure has to be multiplied by the appropriate activity factor, as follows:

1.200 = sedentary (little or no exercise)
1.375 = lightly active (light exercise/sports 1-3 days/wk)
1.550 = moderately active (moderate exercise/sports 3-5 days/wk)
1.725 = very active (hard exercise/sports 6-7 days a wk)
1.900 = extra active (very hard exercise/sports and physical job)

Example

Man: Weight 180 lb, height 5 ft, 10 in, age 50, very active
Energy expenditure = 5 + 10 (82) + 6.25 (178) − 5 (50) × 1.725 = 2911
Woman: Weight 150 lb, height 5 ft,' 6 in", age 60, lightly active
Energy expenditure = −161 + 10 (68) + 6.25 (168) − 5 (60) × 1.375 = 1745

Ht, Height; *wt,* weight.

TABLE 40-3   GOOD SOURCES OF PROTEIN

Complete Proteins	Incomplete Proteins
• Milk and milk products (e.g., cheese)	• Grains (e.g., corn)
• Eggs	• Legumes (e.g., navy beans, soybeans, peas)
• Fish	• Nuts (e.g., peanuts)
• Meats	• Seeds (e.g., sesame seeds, sunflower seeds)
• Poultry	

TABLE 40-4	MAJOR MINERALS AND TRACE ELEMENTS

Major Minerals	Trace Elements
• Calcium	• Chromium
• Chloride	• Copper
• Magnesium	• Fluoride
• Phosphorus	• Iodine
• Potassium	• Iron
• Sodium	• Manganese
• Sulfur	• Molybdenum
	• Selenium
	• Zinc

TABLE 40-5	NUTRITIONAL THERAPY

Foods High in Iron*

Food	Selected Serving Size
Breads, Cereals, and Grain Products	
Farina, regular or quick cooked (enriched)	⅔ cup
Oatmeal, instant, fortified, prepared (enriched)	⅔ cup
Ready-to-eat cereals, fortified (enriched)	1 oz
Meat, Poultry, Fish, and Alternatives	
Beef liver, braised	3 oz
Pork liver, braised	3 oz
Chicken or turkey liver, braised	½ cup diced
Clams: steamed, boiled, or canned (drained)	3 oz
Oysters: baked, broiled, steamed, or canned (undrained)	3 oz
Soybeans, cooked	½ cup

*These foods provide 25%-39% of the Dietary Reference Intake (DRI) of iron.

reactions that facilitate the metabolism of amino acids, fats, and carbohydrates. Vitamins are divided into two categories: *water-soluble* vitamins (vitamin C and the B-complex vitamins) and *fat-soluble* vitamins (vitamins A, D, E, and K). Because the body stores excess fat-soluble vitamins, there is the potential for toxicity when too much is consumed. Upper limits have been established for vitamins A, D, and E.

Mineral salts (e.g., magnesium, iron, calcium) make up approximately 4% of the total body weight. Minerals present in minute amounts are referred to as *trace elements*. Minerals required in amounts greater than 100 mg/day are called *major minerals*. Table 40-4 lists the major minerals and trace elements. Minerals are necessary for the body to build and repair tissues, regulate body fluids, and assist in various functions. Some minerals are stored and can be toxic if taken in excess amounts. The amount of minerals needed in the daily diet varies greatly, from a few micrograms of trace minerals to 1 g or more of the major minerals, such as calcium, phosphorus, and sodium. A well-balanced diet can usually meet the daily requirements of minerals. However, deficiency and excess states can occur.

SPECIAL DIET: VEGETARIAN DIET

The common element among all vegetarians is the exclusion of red meat from the diet. There are many types of vegetarians and no strict definition of the word "vegetarian." Many vegetarians are *vegans,* who are pure or total vegetarians and eat only plants, and *lacto-ovo-vegetarians,* who eat plants and sometimes dairy products and eggs.

Vegetarians can have vitamin or protein deficiencies unless their diets are well planned. Plant protein, although of a lesser quality than that of animal origin, fulfills most of the protein requirements. Combinations of vegetable protein foods (e.g., cornmeal, kidney beans) can increase the nutritional value. Milk made from soybeans or almonds is also an excellent protein source and should be calcium fortified. Other deficiencies that may be present in a vegan diet include calcium, zinc, and vitamins A and D.

The primary deficiency for a strict vegan is lack of cobalamin. This vitamin can be obtained only from animal protein, special supplements, or foods that have been fortified with the vitamin. Vegans not using cobalamin supplements are susceptible to the development of megaloblastic anemia and the neurologic signs of cobalamin deficiency.

Strict vegetarians and lacto-ovo-vegetarians are also at risk for iron deficiency. Table 40-5 lists examples of foods high in iron.

CULTURALLY COMPETENT CARE

NUTRITION

People have unique cultural heritages that may affect eating customs and nutritional status. Each culture has its own beliefs and behaviors related to food and the role that food plays in the etiology and treatment of disease. In addition, culture and religion can influence what food is considered edible, how it is prepared, when it is eaten, and how and who prepares it. For example, some religions, such as Judaism and Islam, have specific laws regarding food. (The websites for Kosher Quest [www.kosherquest.org] and the Islamic Food and Nutrition Council of America [www.ifanca.org] provide detailed information.) Assess the extent to which Jewish or Muslim patients adhere to Kosher or Halal dietary practices to ensure that appropriate meals are served.

Assess the patient's diet history and implement necessary dietary changes. Avoid *cultural stereotyping* by making assumptions or generalizations about diet based on an individual's cultural background. Dietary habits differ considerably within and among ethnic groups. Acculturation, the extent to which immigrants adopt attributes of a new culture, can also affect dietary practices.[9]

It is important to know whether the patient eats "traditional foods" associated with the culture. If traditional foods are eaten, assess their impact on health. For example, "soul foods," which include traditional foods eaten by some African Americans, tend to be high in fat, cholesterol, and sodium.[10] Traditional foods eaten by some Asian Americans may be high in fiber and low in fat and cholesterol, but the diet may also be low in calcium because of limited dairy product intake.[11]

Consideration of cultural beliefs is important when planning and monitoring acceptance of dietary changes. Perception of body weight and size may also be influenced by culture. Ask the patient or family about how culture affects dietary choices and weight maintenance. For example, in some cultures overweight and obesity do not carry the stigma that they do in Western cultures.[12] This may make teaching regarding the necessity of weight reduction more challenging. A Jewish patient who eats only Kosher food may be comforted in knowing that most enteral formulas are manufactured Kosher and are labeled as such. Another example of culturally sensitive planning is adjusting meal service plans for the Muslim patient observing Ramadan (the Islamic month of *fasting*, in which Muslims refrain from eating and drinking during daylight hours).

Teaching related to dietary restrictions and recommended dietary changes should involve the patient's family. Often it is a family member who does the grocery shopping and cooking.

MALNUTRITION

Malnutrition is a deficit, excess, or imbalance of essential nutrients. It may occur with or without inflammation. Malnutrition affects body composition and functional status.[13] Imbalances in macronutrients (carbohydrates, proteins, fat) or micronutrients (electrolytes, minerals, vitamins) occur with malnutrition. Terms such as *undernutrition* and *overnutrition* are also used to describe malnutrition.

Undernutrition describes a state of poor nourishment as a result of inadequate diet or diseases that interfere with normal appetite and assimilation of ingested food. *Overnutrition* refers to the ingestion of more food than is required for body needs, as in obesity.

Malnutrition is a problem in both developing and developed countries across the care continuum (community, hospital, long-term care).[13] Twenty percent to 70% of hospitalized adults are considered malnourished or at nutritional risk.[14] The prevalence of malnutrition in older adults based on the Mini Nutritional Assessment (MNA) ranges from approximately 6% (community-dwelling older adults) to 50% (rehabilitation settings).[15]

Etiology of Malnutrition

Many terms are used to describe the types and etiologies of adult malnutrition.[16,17] Older terms that are still used in some settings include *primary* or *secondary protein-calorie malnutrition* (PCM), *marasmus*, and *kwashiorkor*. Marasmus and kwashiorkor describe forms of malnutrition seen in children in developing countries;[17] these terms should not be used to describe malnutrition in adults.

The following etiology-based terminology is the preferred terminology to use in clinical practice settings, since it indicates the interaction and importance of inflammation on nutritional status.[16,18]

- *Starvation-related malnutrition*, or primary PCM, occurs when nutritional needs are not met (Fig. 40-3). It is a clinical state in which there is chronic starvation without inflammation (e.g., anorexia nervosa).

- *Chronic disease–related malnutrition*, or secondary PCM, is associated with conditions that impose sustained inflammation of a mild to moderate degree.[16] This occurs when tissue needs are not met even though the dietary intake would be satisfactory under normal conditions. Examples of conditions associated with this type of malnutrition include organ failure, cancer, rheumatoid arthritis, obesity, and metabolic syndrome.

- *Acute disease– or injury-related malnutrition* is associated with acute disease or injury states with marked inflammatory response (e.g., major infection, burns, trauma, closed head injury).

Contributing Factors to Malnutrition

Many factors contribute to the development of malnutrition, including socioeconomic factors, physical illnesses, incomplete diets, and food-drug interactions. Table 40-6 lists conditions that increase the risk for malnutrition.

Socioeconomic Factors. *Food security* refers to access by all people, at all times, to sufficient food for an active and healthy lifestyle.[2] Individuals or families with limited financial resources may have *food insecurity* (inadequate access). Food insecurity is problematic because it affects the overall quality of food that is available in both quantity and nutritional value. Families with food insecurity usually choose less expensive "filling" foods, which are more energy dense (high fat) and lack nutritional value. This type of diet increases the risk of nutrient deficiencies.

To help them obtain food, individuals and families may use "safety net programs," including food assistance programs; housing and energy subsidies; and in-kind contributions from relatives, friends, food pantries, or charitable organizations.

Consult with social workers to help patients gain access to government and local programs such as Meals on Wheels that deliver nutritious meals to home-bound individuals. The "heat or eat" phenomenon is problematic, as families with limited economic resources struggle to pay household utility bills or put food on the table. Older adults on a fixed income have an added burden of deciding on whether to pay for medications or food. You and the registered dietitian can assist patients in making food choices that meet nutritional requirements while staying within their limited resources.

Physical Illnesses. Malnutrition is a common consequence of illness, surgery, injury, or hospitalization. The hospitalized patient, especially the older adult, is at risk of becoming malnourished. Prolonged illness, major surgery, sepsis, draining wounds, burns, hemorrhage, fractures, and immobilization can

FIG. 40-3 Patient with malnutrition.

TABLE 40-6	CONDITIONS THAT INCREASE THE RISK FOR MALNUTRITION

- Dementia
- Depression
- Chronic alcoholism
- Excessive dieting to lose weight
- Swallowing disorders (e.g., head and neck cancer)
- Decreased mobility that limits access to food or its preparation
- Nutrient losses from malabsorption, dialysis, fistulas, or wounds
- Drugs with antinutrient or catabolic properties such as corticosteroids and oral antibiotics
- Extreme need for nutrients because of hypermetabolism or stresses such as infection, burns, trauma, or fever
- No oral intake and/or receiving standard IV solutions (5% dextrose) for 10 days (adults) or for 5 days (older adults)

all contribute to malnutrition. Pathologic conditions are frequently aggravated by undernutrition, and an existing deficiency state is likely to become more severe during illness.

Anorexia, nausea, vomiting, diarrhea, abdominal distention, and abdominal cramping may accompany diseases of the GI system. Any combination of these symptoms interferes with normal food consumption and metabolism. In addition, a patient may restrict dietary intake to a few foods or fluids that may not be nutritionally sound out of fear of aggravating an existing GI problem.

Malabsorption syndrome is the impaired absorption of nutrients from the GI tract. Decreases in digestive enzymes or in bowel surface area can quickly lead to a deficiency state. Many drugs have undesirable GI side effects and alter normal digestive and absorptive processes. For example, antibiotics change the normal flora of the intestines, decreasing the body's ability to synthesize biotin.

Fever accompanies many illnesses, injuries, and infections, with a concomitant increase in the body's basal metabolic rate (BMR). Each degree of temperature increase on the Fahrenheit scale raises the BMR by about 7%.[19] Without an increase in caloric intake, body protein stores will be used to supply calories, and protein depletion develops.

Assume responsibility, along with the health care provider and the registered dietitian, for meeting the patient's nutritional needs. Also consider the nutritional requirements of a patient who is not overtly ill but who is undergoing diagnostic studies. This patient may be nutritionally fit on entering the hospital but can develop nutritional problems because of the dietary restrictions imposed by multiple diagnostic studies.

Incomplete Diets. Vitamin deficiencies are rare in most developed countries, except for individuals with eating disorders and chronic abusers of alcohol. Vitamin deficiencies usually involve several vitamins, rather than a single one. The recommended dietary allowances, or DRIs, for essential vitamins and minerals (Table 40-7) can be obtained by eating a diet consisting of foods from the five basic food groups (see Fig. 40-1). DRIs from the Food and Nutrition Board have a safety margin because the levels exceed minimum daily requirements for most people.[20]

When vitamin imbalances do occur, they are usually found among persons with a pattern of alcohol and drug abuse, persons who are chronically ill, and individuals who follow poor dietary practices. Persons who have had surgery on the GI tract may be at risk for vitamin deficiencies. For example, resection of the terminal ileum poses a risk for deficiencies of fat-soluble vitamins. After a gastrectomy, patients require cobalamin supplementation because intrinsic factor (normally made in the stomach) is not available to bind with cobalamin so that this vitamin can be absorbed in the ileum. Followers of fad diets or poorly planned vegetarian diets are also at risk.

Clinical manifestations of vitamin imbalances are most commonly neurologic signs. The recommended DRIs and manifestations of imbalances are presented in eTable 40-3 (available on the website for this chapter).

Food-Drug Interactions. When the patient's health conditions require drug therapy, drug and food interactions may occur. Potential adverse interactions include incompatibilities, altered drug effectiveness, and impaired nutritional status. Food-drug interactions can also occur with the use of over-the-counter drugs and herbs and dietary supplements. Monitor and prevent these potential interactions for patients in the hospital

TABLE 40-7	RECOMMENDED DAILY VITAMIN AND CALCIUM INTAKE*
Vitamin or Mineral	**Dietary Reference Intake**
Fat-Soluble Vitamins	
A	*Men:* 900 mcg/retinol equivalents *Women:* 700 mcg/retinol equivalents
D	*Adults ages 19-70:* 600 IU *Adults age >70:* 800 IU
E	*Adults:* 15 mg
K	*Men:* 120 mcg *Women:* 90 mcg
Water-Soluble Vitamins	
B₁	*Men:* 1.2 mg *Women:* 1.1 mg
B₆	*Men ages 19-50:* 1.3 mg *Men age >51:* 1.7 mg *Women ages 19-50:* 1.3 mg *Women age >51:* 1.5 mg
Cobalamin (B₁₂)	*Adults:* 2-4 mcg
C	*Men:* 90 mg *Women:* 75 mg
Folate (folic acid)	*Adults:* 400 mcg
Minerals	
Calcium	*Men ages 19-70:* 1000 mg *Men age >70:* 1200 mg *Women ages 19-50:* 1000 mg *Women age >51:* 1500 mg

Source: Food and Nutrition Board, Institute of Medicine: *Dietary Reference Intakes (DRIs): recommended dietary allowance and adequate intakes, vitamins,* Washington, DC, 2006, Food and Nutrition Board, National Academies; and Institute of Medicine: *Dietary Reference Intakes for calcium and vitamin D,* Washington, DC, 2010, National Academies Press.
*See eTable 40-3 (on the website for this chapter) for Recommended Dietary Reference Intakes and Manifestations of Imbalance.

and at home. Examples of common food-drug interactions are presented in eTable 40-4 (available on the website for this chapter). Additional information is available at *www.foodmedinteractions.com.*

Pathophysiology of Starvation

Knowing the pathophysiology of the starvation process helps to understand the physiologic changes that occur in malnutrition. Initially, the body selectively uses carbohydrates (glycogen) rather than fat and protein to meet metabolic needs. These carbohydrate stores, found in the liver and the muscles, are minimal and may be totally depleted within 18 hours. During this early phase of starvation, protein is used only in its normal participation in cellular metabolism. However, once carbohydrate stores are depleted, skeletal protein is converted to glucose for energy. Alanine and glutamine are the first amino acids to be used by the liver for the formation of glucose in a process termed *gluconeogenesis.* The resulting available plasma glucose allows the metabolic processes to continue. With these amino acids being used as energy sources, the person may be in negative nitrogen balance (nitrogen excretion exceeds nitrogen intake). Within 5 to 9 days, body fat is fully mobilized to supply much of the needed energy.

In prolonged starvation, up to 97% of calories are provided by fat, and protein is conserved. Depletion of fat stores depends on the amount available, but fat stores are generally used up in

4 to 6 weeks. Once fat stores are used, body or visceral proteins, including those in internal organs and plasma, can no longer be spared and rapidly decrease because they are the only remaining body source of energy available.

If a malnourished patient has surgery, experiences physical trauma, or has an infection, the stress response is superimposed on the starvation response. Protein stores are used for body energy to meet the increased metabolic energy expenditure.

As the protein depletion continues, liver function becomes impaired, and synthesis of proteins decreases. The plasma oncotic pressure is lower because of decreased protein synthesis. A major function of plasma proteins, primarily albumin, is the maintenance of the osmotic pressure of the blood. Because of decreased oncotic pressure, body fluids shift from the vascular space into the interstitial compartment. Eventually albumin leaks into the interstitial space along with the fluid. Edema becomes clinically observable. Often the edema in the patient's face and legs masks the underlying muscle wasting.

As the total blood volume is reduced, the skin appears dry and wrinkled. As fluids shift to the interstitial space, ions also move. Sodium (a predominant extracellular ion) is found in increased amounts within the cell, and potassium (a predominant intracellular ion) and magnesium are shifted to the extracellular space. The sodium-potassium exchange pump has high energy needs, using 20% to 50% of all calories ingested. When the diet is extremely deficient in calories and essential proteins, the pump will fail, leaving sodium inside the cell (along with water), and the cell will expand.

The liver is the body organ that loses the most mass during protein deprivation. It gradually becomes infiltrated with fat secondary to decreased synthesis of lipoproteins. If dietary protein and other necessary constituents are not given, death will rapidly ensue.

Impact of Inflammation. Inflammation affects nutrient metabolism and is an important component of the nutritional status. During the starvation process, there is a decreased BMR, sparing of skeletal muscle, and decreased protein breakdown. However, in inflammatory states, there are alterations in the expression of proinflammatory (e.g., interleukin-6) and antiinflammatory cytokines (e.g., interleukin-10). These cytokine changes result in increased protein and skeletal muscle breakdown, increased BMR, increased glucose turnover, decreased negative acute phase protein (albumin, prealbumin) production, and increased positive acute phase protein (e.g., C-reactive protein [CRP]) production.[16]

Clinical Manifestations

The clinical manifestations of malnutrition range from mild to emaciation (Fig. 40-4) and death. The most obvious clinical signs on physical examination are apparent in the skin (dry and scaly skin, brittle nails, rashes, hair loss), mouth (crusting and ulceration, changes in tongue), muscles (decreased mass and weakness), and CNS (mental changes such as confusion, irritability). The speed at which the malnutrition develops depends on the quantity and quality of the protein intake, caloric value, illness, and the person's age.

Clinical manifestations of malnutrition are the result of numerous interactions at the cellular level. As protein intake is severely reduced, the muscles, which are the largest store of protein in the body, become wasted and flabby, leading to weakness and fatigability. Decreased protein is available for repair, and as a result, wound healing may be delayed. The person is

FIG. 40-4 Severe malnutrition that results in wasting and extensive loss of adipose tissue.

more susceptible to infections. Both humoral and cell-mediated immunity are deficient in malnutrition. There is a decrease in leukocytes in the peripheral blood. Phagocytosis is altered because of the lack of energy necessary to drive the process. Many malnourished individuals are anemic, generally as a result of nutritional deficiencies in iron and folic acid, the necessary building blocks for red blood cells (RBCs). A detailed listing of the clinical manifestations of malnutrition is available in eTable 40-5 (available on the website for this chapter).

Diagnostic Studies

History and Physical Examination. A diet history of foods eaten over the past week reveals a great deal about the patient's dietary habits and knowledge of good nutrition. In addition to the height, weight, and vital signs, assess and document the patient's physical state and each body system. Table 40-8 summarizes the assessment and findings of the patient with malnutrition.

Laboratory Studies. The diagnosis of malnutrition is best determined by body composition, including a thorough history of weight loss, nutrient intake, and measures of functional status and inflammation. Serum albumin has a half-life of approximately 20 to 22 days. In the absence of marked fluid loss, such as from hemorrhage or burns, the serum albumin value lags behind actual protein changes by more than 2 weeks. Therefore albumin is not a good indicator of acute changes in nutritional status.

Prealbumin, a protein synthesized by the liver, has a half-life of 2 days and is a better indicator of recent or current nutritional status. Serum transferrin level is another indicator of protein status. Transferrin, a protein synthesized by the liver and used to transport iron, decreases when protein is deficient.

However, the extent to which visceral proteins, including albumin, prealbumin, and transferrin, are true markers of malnutrition is questionable. Albumin, prealbumin, and transferrin are *negative acute phase proteins,* which mean that during an inflammatory response, the synthesis of these proteins in the liver is decreased. Therefore low or below normal levels of these negative acute phase proteins correspond to an inflammatory state rather than accurately indicating nutritional status.[16,20]

CRP, which is a *positive acute phase protein,* is typically elevated during inflammation and predicts morbidity and mortal-

TABLE 40-8 NURSING ASSESSMENT

Malnutrition

Subjective Data

Important Health Information

Past health history: Severe burns, major trauma, hemorrhage, draining wounds, bone fractures with prolonged immobility, chronic renal or liver disease, cancer, malabsorption syndromes, GI obstruction, infectious diseases (TB, AIDS), acute (e.g., trauma, sepsis) or chronic inflammatory condition (e.g., rheumatoid arthritis)

Medications: Corticosteroids, chemotherapeutic agents, diet pills

Surgery or other treatments: Recent surgery, radiation

Functional Health Patterns

Health perception–health management: Alcohol or drug abuse; malaise, apathy

Nutritional-metabolic: Increase or decrease in weight, weight problems; increase or decrease in appetite, typical dietary intake; food preferences and aversions; food allergies or intolerance; ill-fitting or absent dentures; dry mouth, difficulty in chewing or swallowing; bloating or gas; ↑ sensitivity to cold; delayed wound healing

Elimination: Constipation, diarrhea, nocturia, decreased urine output

Activity-exercise: Increase or decrease in activity patterns; weakness, fatigue, decreased endurance

Cognitive-perceptual: Pain in mouth; paresthesias; loss of position and vibratory sense

Role-relationship: Change in family (e.g., loss of a spouse); financial resources

Sexual-reproductive: Amenorrhea, impotence, decreased libido

Objective Data

General

Listless, cachectic; underweight for height

Integumentary

Dry, brittle, sparse hair with color changes and lack of luster, alopecia; dry, scaly lips, fever blisters, angular crusts and lesions at corners of mouth (cheilosis); brittle, ridged nails; decreased tone and elasticity of skin; cool, rough, dry, scaly skin with brown-gray pigment changes; reddened, scaly dermatitis, scrotal dermatitis; slight cyanosis; peripheral edema

Eyes

Pale or red conjunctivae, gray keratinized epithelium on conjunctiva (Bitot's spots); dryness and dull appearance of conjunctivae and cornea, soft cornea; blood vessel growth in cornea; redness and fissuring of eyelid corners

Respiratory

Decreased respiratory rate, ↓ vital capacity, crackles, weak cough

Cardiovascular

Increased or decreased heart rate, ↓ BP, dysrhythmias

Gastrointestinal

Swollen, smooth, raw, beefy red tongue (glossitis), hypertrophic or atrophic papillae; dental cavities, absent or loose teeth, discolored tooth enamel; spongy, pale, receded gums with a tendency to bleed easily, periodontal disease; ulcerations, white patches or plaques, redness, swelling of oral mucosa; distended, tympanic abdomen; ascites, hepatomegaly, decreased bowel sounds; steatorrhea

Neurologic

Decreased or loss of reflexes, tremor; inattention, irritability, confusion, syncope

Musculoskeletal

Decreased muscle mass with poor tone, "wasted" appearance; bowlegs, knock-knees, beaded ribs, chest deformity, prominent bony structures

Possible Diagnostic Findings

↓ Hemoglobin and hematocrit; ↓ MCV, MCH, or MCHC (iron deficiency); ↓ MCV or MCH (folic acid or cobalamin deficiency); altered serum electrolyte levels, especially hyperkalemia; ↓ BUN and creatinine; ↓ serum albumin, transferrin, and prealbumin; ↓ lymphocytes; ↑ liver enzymes; ↓ serum vitamin levels

MCH, Mean corpuscular hemoglobin; *MCHC,* mean corpuscular hemoglobin concentration; *MCV,* mean corpuscular volume; *TB,* tuberculosis.

---

ity.[21,22] Serum electrolyte levels reflect changes taking place between the intracellular and extracellular spaces. The serum potassium level is often elevated. The RBC count and the hemoglobin level indicate the presence and degree of anemia. The total lymphocyte count decreases with malnutrition. It is calculated by multiplying the percent of lymphocytes times the total white blood cell (WBC) count. Liver enzyme levels, a reflection of liver function, may be elevated during malnutrition. Serum levels of both fat-soluble and water-soluble vitamins are usually decreased. The lowered serum levels of the fat-soluble vitamins correlate with the clinical signs of *steatorrhea* (fatty stools).

Anthropometric Measurements. Anthropometric measurements are gross measures of fat and muscle contents. These measurements tend to be most beneficial when done serially, and by well-trained anthropometrists, to evaluate the long-term effects of malnutrition or responses to nutritional interventions. They consist of measures of skinfold thickness at various sites, which are indicators of subcutaneous fat stores, and midarm muscle circumference, an indicator of protein stores. These measurements are then compared with standards for healthy persons of the same age and gender.

The sites most reflective of body fat are those over the biceps and the triceps, below the scapula, above the iliac crest, and

over the upper thigh. Both skinfold thickness and midarm circumference measurements are decreased in malnutrition. These measurements may also be influenced by shifts in hydration status. The exact relationship of the midarm circumference measure to morbidity and mortality remains to be established.

Waist circumference and hip-to-waist ratio are used more commonly in acute care to reflect nutritional status. These measures are discussed in Chapter 41.

Functional Measurements. Measures of muscle strength are used to assess functional status, an important outcome of nutrition states. Handgrip strength is measured with a hand dynamometer. Functional performance tests such as the Short Physical Performance Battery may be ordered.[23]

NURSING AND COLLABORATIVE MANAGEMENT MALNUTRITION

NURSING ASSESSMENT

As a nurse, you are responsible for nutritional screening across care settings. Nutritional screening identifies individuals who are malnourished or at risk for malnutrition. Nutritional screening is also used to determine if a more detailed nutritional assessment is necessary. The Joint Commission requires nutritional screening for all patients within 24 hours of admission. Many nutritional screening and assessment tools are available.[24,25] Hospital-specific screening tools based on common admission assessment criteria include history of weight loss, prior intake before admission, use of nutritional support, chewing or swallowing issues, and skin breakdown. A standardized approach to nutritional screening is needed to ensure valid and reliable tools are used in the clinical setting.

In older adults the Mini Nutritional Assessment (MNA) is often used[25] (available at *www.mna-elderly.com/forms/mini/mna_mini_english.pdf*). In long-term care the Minimum Data Set (MDS) form is used to obtain information about a person's nutritional status.[26] In home care settings the Outcome and Assessment Information Set (OASIS) prompts you to collect information on diet, oral intake, dental health, swallowing difficulties, and any need for meal assistance.[27]

If the nutritional screening identifies an individual at nutritional risk, a full nutritional assessment is most often needed. A nutritional assessment is a comprehensive approach that includes medical, nutritional, and medication histories; physical examination; anthropometric measurements; and laboratory data (Table 40-9). Nutritional assessment provides the basis for nutritional intervention.

Across all care settings, be aware of the patient's nutritional status. Obtaining an accurate measure of body weight and height and recording this information are critical components of this assessment. When assessing weight, obtain a detailed weight history, noting weight loss. Ask whether the weight loss was intentional or unintentional and the period over which it

took place. A loss of more than 5% of usual body weight over 6 months, whether intentional or unintentional, is a critical indicator for further assessment, especially in the older adult.[28] If an involuntary weight loss exceeds 10% of the usual weight, determine the reason. Unintentional weight loss is also important to consider in the obese individual, since latent malnutrition may be present despite excess body weight. Determine the patient's current weight in relation to ideal body weight.

When possible, measure the patient's actual height rather than using the patient's self-report. Alternatives to standing height (stature) measurements include arm demi-span and knee-height measurements. The *arm demi-span* is the distance from a point on the midline at the suprasternal notch to the web between the middle and ring fingers with the arm horizontally outstretched (*www.mna-elderly.com/forms/mna_guide_english.pdf*). For persons who are confined to bed, the use of a Luft ruler is an alternative to standing height.[29]

Body mass index (BMI) is a measure of weight for height (see Fig. 41-2). A BMI of less than 18.5 kg/m² is considered underweight, normal weight is a BMI between 18.5 and 24.9 kg/m², and overweight is a BMI between 25 and 29.9 kg/m². A BMI of 30 kg/m² or greater is obese. BMIs outside the normal weight range are associated with increased morbidity and mortality.[30]

In addition, obtain a complete diet history from the patient or caregiver. The patient's nutritional state may not be the reason medical care was sought. However, it may be a contributing factor to the disease and have an impact on management and recovery.

TABLE 40-9 COMPONENTS OF NUTRITIONAL ASSESSMENT

Anthropometric Measurements	Diet History
• Height and weight	• Chewing and swallowing ability
• Body mass index (BMI)	• Changes in appetite or taste
• Rate of weight change	• Food and nutrient intake
• Amount of weight loss	• Availability of food
Physical Examination	**Laboratory Data**
• Physical appearance	• Glucose
• Muscle mass and strength	• Electrolytes
• Dental and oral health	• Lipid profile
	• Blood urea nitrogen (BUN)
Health History	**Functional Status**
• Personal and family history	• Ability to perform basic and instrumental activities of daily living
• Acute or chronic illnesses	• Handgrip strength
• Current medications, herbs, supplements	• Performance tests (e.g., timed walk tests)
• Cognitive status, depression	

HEALTHY PEOPLE

Health Impact of a Well-Balanced Diet

- Reduces incidence of anemia
- Maintains normal body weight and prevents obesity
- Maintains good bone health and reduces risk of osteoporosis
- Lowers the risk of developing elevated cholesterol and type 2 diabetes mellitus
- Decreases the risk of heart disease, hypertension, and certain types of cancers

NURSING DIAGNOSES

Nursing diagnoses for the patient with malnutrition include, but are not limited to, the following:

- Imbalanced nutrition: less than body requirements *related to* decreased access, ingestion, digestion, or absorption of food or *related to* anorexia, dysphagia, or increased metabolic needs
- Feeding self-care deficit *related to* decreased strength and endurance, fatigue, and apathy
- Deficient fluid volume *related to* factors affecting access to or absorption of fluids
- Risk for impaired skin integrity *related to* poor nutritional state
- Noncompliance *related to* alteration in perception, lack of motivation, or incompatibility of regimen with lifestyle or resources

PLANNING

The overall goals are that the patient with malnutrition will (1) gain weight, particularly muscle mass; (2) consume a specified number of calories per day (with a diet individualized for the patient); and (3) have no adverse consequences related to malnutrition or nutritional therapies.

NURSING IMPLEMENTATION

HEALTH PROMOTION. You are in a good position to teach and reinforce healthy eating habits with individuals and groups of persons throughout their life span. Use MyPlate, Dietary Guidelines for Americans 2010, and Nutrition Facts food labels to promote healthy nutrition. Free interactive web-based programs are available to track physical activity, calories, and foods eaten (see *www.choosemyplate.gov*).

EVIDENCE-BASED PRACTICE

Translating Research Into Practice

Does Nutritional Education Improve Functional Outcomes in Older Adults?

Clinical Question
In older adults (P) what is the effect of nutritional education (I) on diet, physical and emotional functioning, and quality of life (O)?

Best Available Evidence
- Systematic review of randomized controlled trials (RCTs)

Critical Appraisal and Synthesis of Evidence
- Twenty-three RCTs (n = 12,610) of community-dwelling older adults (65 yr and older) with various diseases. Five trials with nutritional education only; remaining trials with nutritional and lifestyle advice, exercise advice, or screening. Education varied in format and intensity.
- Outcomes included diet, functional outcomes (e.g., strength, balance), hospital readmissions, depression, anxiety, and quality of life.
- Results showed improved body mass index, weight loss, and physical health with decreased depression.
- Brief interventions were as effective as more lengthy ones.

Conclusion
- Nutritional education alone or in combination with other interventions positively influences physical and emotional health.

Implications for Nursing Practice
- Locate nutritional educational resources for older patients residing at home.
- Help patients identify community programs to make positive changes in lifestyle and exercise.

Reference for Evidence
Young K, Bunn F, Trivedi D, et al: Nutritional education for community dwelling older people: a systematic review of randomised controlled trials, *Int J Nurs Stud* 48:751, 2011.

P, Patient population of interest; I, intervention or area of interest; O, outcomes of interest (see p. 12).

ACUTE INTERVENTION. Assess the patient's nutritional state during your assessment of the patient's other physical problems. Identify nutritional risk factors and why they might exist. In states of increased stress, such as surgery, severe trauma, and sepsis, more calories and protein are needed. Wound healing requires increased protein synthesis. For patients undergoing major surgery or those with or at risk for malnutrition, several weeks of increased protein and calorie intake are needed preoperatively to promote healing postoperatively.

When fever is present, the metabolic rate is increased and nitrogen loss is accelerated. Despite the return of body temperature to normal, the rate of protein breakdown and resynthesis may be increased for several weeks. Teach the patient and caregiver the importance of good nutrition and the rationale for recording the daily weight, intake, and output. Daily weights can give an ongoing record of body weight gain or loss. However, rapid gains and losses are usually the result of shifts in fluid balance. The body weight, in conjunction with accurate recording of food and fluid intake, provides a clearer picture of the patient's fluid and nutritional state. To obtain an accurate weight, weigh the patient at the same time each day, on the same scale, with the same type or amount of clothing, and preferably with the bladder recently emptied.

TABLE 40-10 NUTRITIONAL THERAPY*

High-Calorie, High-Protein Diet

Suggestions for high-calorie, high-protein foods include the following.

Breads and Cereals
- Hot cereals (oatmeal, cream of wheat) prepared with milk, added fat (butter or margarine), and sugar
- Potatoes prepared with added fat (butter and whole milk)
- Granola and other cereals with dried fruit
- Croissants, buttermilk biscuits, muffins, banana bread, zucchini bread

Vegetables
- Vegetables prepared with added fat (margarine, butter)
- Fried vegetables

Fruits
- Canned fruit in heavy syrup
- Dried fruit

Meat
- Fried meats
- Meats covered in cream sauces or gravy
- Casseroles

Milk and Milk Products
- Milkshakes
- Whole milk and milk products (yogurt, ice cream, cheese)
- Whipping cream or heavy cream
- Whole milk with added nutritional supplements

*Suggested meal plans for high-calorie, high-protein diet are presented in eTable 40-6 (available on the website for this chapter).

The protein and calorie intake required in the malnourished patient depends on the cause of the malnutrition, the treatment being used, and other stressors affecting the patient. If the patient is able to take food by mouth, obtain a daily calorie count and diet diary to give an accurate record of food intake. You and the registered dietitian can assist the patient and family in selecting high-calorie and high-protein foods (unless medically contraindicated). Preparation of foods preferred by the patient enhances the daily intake. Encourage the family to bring the patient's favorite foods from home while the patient is hospitalized. Table 40-10 gives examples of high-calorie, high-protein foods.

The undernourished patient usually needs to have between-meal supplements. These may consist of items prepared in the dietary department or commercially prepared products. Eating these items between meals provides extra calories, proteins, fluids, and nutrients. If the patient is unable to consume enough nutrition with a high-calorie, high-protein diet, oral liquid nutritional supplements can be added.

Some patients may benefit from appetite stimulants such as megestrol acetate (Megace) or dronabinol (Marinol) to improve nutritional intake. If the patient is still unable to take in enough calories, enteral feedings may be considered. Parenteral nutrition (PN) might need to be initiated if enteral feedings are not feasible.[31] Contraindications for enteral nutrition include GI obstruction, prolonged ileus, severe diarrhea or vomiting, and enterocutaneous fistula.

AMBULATORY AND HOME CARE. With shortened hospital stays, many patients are discharged on a therapeutic diet. Discharge preparation for both the patient and the caregiver is essential. Teach them about the cause of the undernourished state and ways to avoid the problem in the future. Individuals need to be aware that undernourishment, whatever the cause, can recur and that adhering to a diet high in protein and calories for a few weeks cannot fully restore a normal nutritional state. Many months may be needed to reach this goal. Assess the patient's understanding and reinforce the information whenever possible. Assess the patient's and caregiver's ability to comply with the dietary instructions in light of past eating habits, religious and ethnic preferences, age, income, other resources, and state of health. Emphasize the need for continual follow-up care if rehabilitation is to be accomplished and maintained. In the discharge planning, ensure proper follow-up such as visits by the home health nurse and outpatient registered dietitian referrals.

Determine the need for nutritious meals and snacks after discharge from the hospital. The ability of the patient or caregiver to access a registered dietitian may be limited. As a nurse, you may be the primary source of nutritional information. In your assessment, consider the availability and acceptability of community resources that provide meals such as Meals on Wheels, senior congregate feeding sites, and the Supplemental Nutrition Assistance Program (SNAP, formerly known as Food Stamps). Help the patient identify reliable Internet sources that provide evidence-based food and nutrition recommendations.

Keeping a diet diary for 3 days at a time is one way to analyze and reinforce healthful eating patterns. These records are also helpful to the health care team in the follow-up care. Encourage self-assessment of progress by having the patient weigh himself or herself once or twice a week and keep a weight record.

EVALUATION

The expected outcomes are that the patient who is malnourished will
- Achieve and maintain optimal body weight
- Consume a well-balanced diet
- Experience no adverse outcomes related to malnutrition
- Maintain optimal physical functioning

GERONTOLOGIC CONSIDERATIONS

MALNUTRITION

Older adults are particularly vulnerable to malnutrition across care settings.[32] Nutrition affects quality of life, functional status, and health in older adults. Older hospitalized adults with malnutrition are more likely to have poor wound healing, pressure ulcers, infections, decreased muscle strength, postoperative complications, and increased morbidity and mortality risks.[28] You play an important role in assessing the physiologic, functional, environmental, dietary, psychologic, and social factors related to nutritional risk in older adults. Older adults are also less able to regain body weight after periods of undernutrition due to illness or surgery.

Older adults may report little or no appetite, problems with eating or swallowing, inadequate servings of nutrients, and fewer than two meals per day. Limited incomes may cause them to restrict the number of meals or the dietary quality of meals eaten. Social isolation is a problem in older adults. Older adults who live alone may lose their desire to cook and report decreased appetite. Functional limitations may also affect the ability to feed one's self or to purchase food, cook, or prepare meals. Furthermore, older adults may lack transportation to buy food.

Chronic illnesses associated with aging can also affect nutritional status. For example, depression and dysphagia (secondary to stroke) can affect intake. Poor oral health from cavities, gum disease (gingivitis), and missing teeth, as well as *xerostomia* (dry mouth), can impair the older adult's ability to lubricate, masticate, and swallow food. Medications can cause dry mouth, alter the taste of food, or decrease appetite.

Physiologic changes associated with aging include a decrease in lean body mass and redistribution of fat around internal organs, which can lead to a decreased caloric requirement. Furthermore, changes in odor and taste perception (from medications, nutrient deficiencies, or taste-bud atrophy) can alter nutritional status. Sarcopenia is a loss of lean body mass with aging and affects muscle strength and function. Older adults on bed rest or prolonged inactivity lose more lean body mass than younger adults.[30]

Measure weight and height on admission, and routinely assess and document the person's weight. Determine if there is a history of voluntary or involuntary weight loss. Collaborate with the primary care provider and registered dietitian to identify the cause for weight loss and implement appropriate interventions.

Daily requirements for healthy older adults for weight maintenance include 30 cal/kg of body weight, and 0.8 to 1 g/kg of protein per day, with no more than 30% of calories from fat.[28,30] Nutritional requirements may differ depending on the degree of malnutrition and physiologic stress. To prevent loss of muscle mass and maintain function, some experts recommend older adults consume a moderate amount of high-quality protein at each meal.[33] Daily calcium and vitamin D requirements are higher for older adults (see Table 40-7).

Focus your initial care strategies on improving oral intake and providing a stimulating environment for meals. Special strategies, such as adaptive devices (e.g., large-handled eating utensils), often are helpful in increasing dietary intake.

Oral liquid supplements may have a role in improving the nutritional status of older adults.[34] Do not use supplements as meal substitutes, but use them between meals as snacks. In long-term care these beverages may be used instead of water with oral medication administration to increase caloric intake. Some older persons may require nutritional support therapies until their strength and general health improve. Before starting any nutritional support therapy (e.g., enteral or parenteral nutrition) for an older patient unable to give consent, review his or her advance directives regarding the use of artificial nutrition and hydration.

Malnourished or nutritionally at-risk older adults are vulnerable when discharged from the hospital to the home. Older adults may not be able to shop for or prepare foods during the initial recovery period.[35] Consult with the social worker and registered dietitian to ensure that older adults have access to food on discharge. Home-delivered meals or senior congregate feeding programs are an appropriate referral. Many community nutritional programs are available to the older person to make mealtime a pleasant, social event. Improving the social setting of a meal frequently improves dietary intake. The use of SNAP is another alternative that allows low-income households, regardless of age, to buy more food of a greater variety.

Older adults with dementia or a stroke present unique nursing challenges with regard to eating and feeding. (Dementia is discussed in Chapter 60, and strokes are discussed in Chapter 58.)

TYPES OF SPECIALIZED NUTRITIONAL SUPPORT

Oral Feeding

Oral supplements may be used in the patient whose nutritional intake is deficient. This may include milkshakes, puddings, or

FIG. 40-5 Nutritional support algorithm.

commercially available products (e.g., Carnation Instant Breakfast, Ensure, Boost). If patients are unable to maintain or achieve adequate nutritional status, nutritional support may be necessary. For a decision-making plan related to nutritional support, see Fig. 40-5.

Enteral Nutrition

Enteral nutrition (EN), also known as tube feeding, is defined as nutrition (e.g., a nutritionally balanced liquefied food or formula) provided through the GI tract via a tube, catheter, or stoma that delivers nutrients distal to the oral cavity. EN may be ordered for the patient who has a functioning GI tract but is unable to take any or enough oral nourishment, or when it is unsafe to do so.

Indications for EN may include persons with anorexia, oro-facial fractures, head and neck cancer, neurologic or psychiatric conditions that prevent oral intake, extensive burns, or critical illness (especially if mechanical ventilation is required), and those who are receiving chemotherapy or radiation therapy. EN

is considered to be easily administered, safer, more physiologically efficient, and typically less expensive than parenteral nutrition (PN).

Common delivery options are continuous infusion by pump, intermittent infusion by gravity, intermittent bolus by syringe, and cyclic feedings by infusion pump. Continuous infusion is most often used with critically ill patients. Intermittent feeding may be preferred as the patient improves or is receiving EN at home.[36]

Nasally and orally placed tubes (orogastric, nasogastric [NG], nasoduodenal, or nasojejunal) are most commonly used for short-term feeding (less than 4 weeks). Nasoduodenal and nasojejunal tubes are transpyloric tubes. These tubes are used when pathophysiologic conditions such as risk of aspiration warrant feeding the patient below the pyloric sphincter. If the feedings are necessary for an extended time, other tubes are placed in the stomach or small bowel by surgical, endoscopic, or fluoroscopic procedures. (Fig. 40-6 shows the locations of commonly used enteral feeding tubes.)

Orogastric, Nasogastric, and Nasointestinal Tubes. Polyurethane or silicone feeding tubes are long, small in diameter, soft, and flexible, thereby decreasing the risk of mucosal damage from prolonged placement. These tubes are radiopaque, making their position readily identified by x-ray. Placement into the small intestine theoretically decreases the likelihood of regurgitation of contents into the esophagus and subsequent aspiration.[37] With the use of a stylet, these tubes can be placed in a comatose patient because the ability to swallow is not essential during insertion. However, the use of a stylet has been associated with increased risk for perforation.

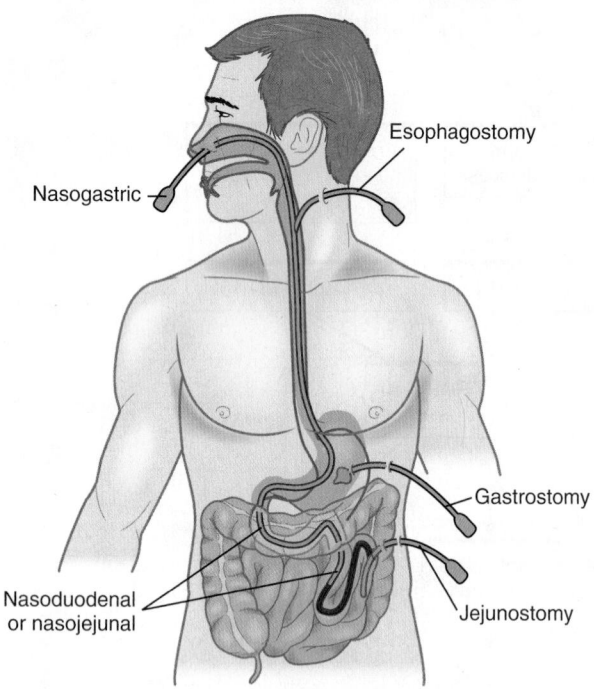

FIG. 40-6 Common enteral feeding tube placement locations.

Although the smaller feeding tubes have many advantages over wider-lumen tubes, such as the standard decompression NG tube, there are some disadvantages. Because of the small diameter, these tubes are more easily clogged when feedings are thick, and the tubes are more difficult to use for checking residual volumes. They are particularly prone to obstruction when oral drugs are not thoroughly crushed and dissolved in water before administration. Failure to flush the tubing before and after both drug administration and residual volume determinations can result in tube clogging. When the tube becomes clogged, it may necessitate removal and insertion of a new tube, adding to cost and patient discomfort. The tubes can become dislodged by vomiting or coughing and can also become knotted or kinked.

Gastrostomy and Jejunostomy Tubes. A gastrostomy tube may be used for a patient who requires EN over an extended time (see Fig. 40-6). Gastrostomy tubes can be placed surgically, radiologically, or endoscopically. The placement of a percutaneous endoscopic gastrostomy (PEG) tube is shown in Fig. 40-7. The patient must have an intact, unobstructed GI tract, and the esophageal lumen must be wide enough to pass the endoscope for PEG tube placement. PEG tube and radiologically placed gastrostomy tube procedures have fewer risks than surgical placement. The procedure requires IV sedation and local anesthesia. IV antibiotics are given before the procedure.

For the patient with chronic reflux, a jejunostomy (J-tube) with continuous feedings may be necessary to reduce the risk of aspiration.[38] Jejunostomy tubes are placed either endoscopically or with open or laparoscopic surgery.

Enteral feedings can be started within 24 to 48 hours after a surgically placed gastrostomy or jejunostomy tube without waiting for flatus or a bowel movement. PEG tube feeding may be started within 2 hours of insertion, although institutionally policies may vary.[39] The feeding tube is either premarked or marked at the skin insertion site. The tube is most often connected to a pump for continuous feeding.

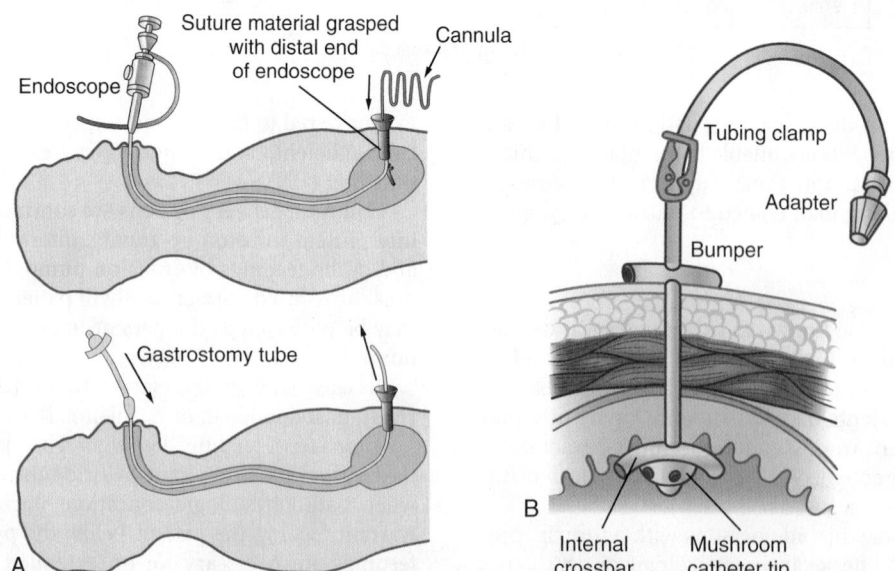

FIG. 40-7 Percutaneous endoscopic gastrostomy. **A,** Gastrostomy tube placement via percutaneous endoscopy. With use of endoscopy, a gastrostomy tube is inserted through the esophagus into the stomach and then pulled through a stab wound made in the abdominal wall. **B,** A retention disk and bumper secure the tube.

TABLE 40-11   PROBLEMS RELATED TO TUBE FEEDINGS

PROBLEMS AND CAUSES	CORRECTIVE MEASURES	PROBLEMS AND CAUSES	CORRECTIVE MEASURES
Vomiting or Aspiration		**Diarrhea**	
Improper placement of tube	• Replace tube in proper position. • Check tube position before beginning feeding and every 8 hr if continuous feedings.	Feeding too fast	• Decrease rate of feeding. • Change to continuous drip feedings.
Delayed gastric emptying, increased residual volume	• If gastric residual volume is ≥250 mL after second gastric residual check, consider a promotility agent. • If gastric residual volume is >500 mL, hold enteral nutrition and reassess patient tolerance.	Medications Low-fiber formula Tube moving distally	• Check for drugs that may cause diarrhea (e.g., sorbitol in liquid medications, antibiotics). • Change to formula with more fiber. • Properly secure tube before beginning feeding. • Check before each feeding or at least every 24 hr if continuous feedings.

Potential for aspiration	• Keep head of bed elevated to 30- to 45-degree angle.
	• Have patient sit up on side of bed or in chair.
	• Encourage ambulation unless contraindicated.
		Contamination of formula	• Refrigerate unused formula and record date opened.
			• Discard outdated formula every 24 hr.
			• Discard formula left standing for longer than manufacturer's guidelines.
			  • 8 hr for ready-to-feed formulas (cans)
			  • 4 hr for reconstituted formula
			  • 24-48 hr for closed-system enteral formulas
			• Use closed system to prevent contamination.
			• Use sterile water for flushes.

Dehydration			
Excessive diarrhea, vomiting	• Decrease rate or change formula. • Check drugs that patient is receiving, especially antibiotics. • Take care to prevent bacterial contamination of formula and equipment.	**Constipation**	
Poor fluid intake	• Increase intake and check amount and number of feedings. • Increase amount of fluid intake if appropriate.	Formula components	• Consult health care provider for change in formula to one with more fiber content. • Obtain laxative order.
High-protein formula	• Change formula.	Poor fluid intake	• Increase fluid intake if not contraindicated. • Give free water as well as formula. • Give total fluid intake of 30 mL/kg body weight.
Hyperosmotic diuresis	• Check blood glucose levels frequently. • Change formula.	Drugs Impaction	• Check for drugs that may be constipating. • Perform rectal examinations to check and manually remove feces if present.

Tube Feedings and Safety. You have a critical role to ensure that tube feedings are administered safely. Nursing management of tube feedings is briefly addressed in eTable 40-7 (available on the website for this chapter). Aspiration and dislodged tubes are two important safety concerns.

Patient Position. Proper patient positioning decreases the risk of aspiration. Elevate the head of bed to a minimum of 30 degrees, but preferably 45 degrees, to prevent aspiration. A reverse Trendelenburg position can be used to elevate the head of the bed, unless contraindicated, when a back rest elevation is not tolerated. If it is necessary to lower the head of the bed for a procedure, return the patient to an elevated position as soon as possible. Check institution policy for suspending feeding while the patient is supine. If intermittent delivery is used, the head should remain elevated for 30 to 60 minutes after feeding.[32]

Aspiration Risk. Evaluate all enterally fed patients for risk of aspiration. Before starting tube feedings, ensure that the tube is in the proper position. Maintain head-of-bed elevation as described above. Checking gastric residual volumes is important when feedings are administered into the stomach. For example, when the infusion rate is 100 mL/hr, the total infused volume of 400 mL may accumulate when gastric emptying is delayed. In addition, gastric secretions can increase the volume beyond 400 mL. With increased residual volume there is increased risk for aspiration of formula into the lungs.[36,37]

Residual Volumes. Check gastric residual volumes every 4 hours during the first 48 hours for gastrically fed patients. After the enteral feeding goal rate is achieved, gastric residual monitoring may be decreased to every 6 to 8 hours in non–critically

ill patients or continued every 4 hours in critically ill patients. (Corrective measures for residual volume are described in Table 40-11.) Feeding tubes may need to be placed below the ligament of Treitz (jejunostomy) when gastric residual volumes consistently measure more than 500 mL. Do not obtain residual volumes for EN delivered through a jejunostomy tube.

Tube Position. Confirm tube position of newly inserted nasal or orogastric tubes before feeding or administering medications. Obtain x-ray confirmation to determine if a blindly placed NG or orogastric tube (small bore or large bore) is properly positioned in the GI tract before administering feedings or medications.

Smaller feeding tubes may be passed directly into the bronchus on insertion without any obvious respiratory manifestations. Do not rely on the auscultation method to differentiate between gastric and respiratory placement, or to differentiate between gastric and small bowel placement. Capnography, a direct monitor of breath-to-breath carbon dioxide level, may be used to detect inadvertent entry of tube into the trachea during insertion. X-ray confirmation is still needed to verify location before feeding. When in doubt, request an x-ray to determine tube location.[37,38]

Maintain proper placement of the tube after feedings are started. A small bowel tube may dislocate upward into the stomach, or the tube's tip can dislocate upward into the esophagus. To determine if a feeding tube has maintained the proper position, mark the exit site of the feeding tube at the time of the initial x-ray and observe for a change in the external tube length during feedings. Recheck the tube insertion length at regular intervals.

Observe for negative pressure when attempting to withdraw fluid from the feeding tube.[39] Negative pressure is more likely felt during attempts to aspirate fluid from a small bowel than from a gastric tube. Observe for unexpected changes in residual volume. An increase in gastric residual volume may indicate displacement of the small intestine tube into the stomach.[39] If a significant increase in the external length is observed, use other bedside tests to help determine whether the tube has become dislocated. These measures include assessment of aspirate color and pH. Because each of these measures has limitations, confirmation is done with more than one single bedside test. Use of technology such as electromagnetic tracking devices along with "tube teams" is associated with reduced tube misplacement.[40]

Complications Related to Tubes and Feedings. The types of problems in patients receiving tube feedings and corrective measures are presented in Table 40-11. When commercial products are used, the concentration, flavor, osmolarity, and amounts of protein, sodium, and fat vary according to the manufacturer. Most commercial formulas are lactose free. The concentrations range from 1 to 2 cal/mL, with most standard formulas providing between 1 and 1.5 cal/mL. Refeeding syndrome, which occasionally occurs with EN, is described below.

Osmolality of the solution is determined by the number and size of particles in solution. In feeding formulas the more hydrolyzed or broken down the nutrients, the greater the osmolality. The more calorically dense the formula, the less water it contains. Protein content greater than 16% can lead to dehydration unless the patient is given supplemental fluids or is sufficiently alert to request additional fluids.

Be aware of this potential problem and provide extra fluids through the feeding tube or, if permitted, by mouth. Tube feedings with high sodium content are contraindicated in the patient with cardiovascular problems, such as heart failure. High fat content is not advocated for a patient with short bowel syndrome or ileocecal resection because of impaired fat absorption.

The registered dietitian is an important health care team member in providing EN. Some institutions have nutritional support teams composed of a physician, nurse, dietitian, and pharmacist. The team's function is to oversee the nutritional support of select inpatients and outpatients. The nutritional support nurse on that team is a key resource for issues regarding patients' nutrition.

In patients receiving gastrostomy or jejunostomy feeding, be alert to two possible problems: (1) skin irritation and (2) dislodgment of the tube. Skin care around the tube site is important because the action of the digestive juices irritates the skin. Assess the skin around the feeding tube daily for signs of redness and maceration. To keep the skin clean and dry, initially rinse it with sterile water and then dry it. Once the site has healed, wash with mild soap and water. A protective ointment (zinc oxide, petroleum gauze) or a skin barrier (karaya, Stomahesive) may be used on the skin around the tube. Other types of drain or tube pouches may be used if the skin is irritated. An enterostomal therapist can provide assistance if these issues arise.

Teach the patient and caregiver how to care for the feeding tube. Accidental tube removal can result in delayed feedings and potential discomfort with tube replacement. Patient teaching includes skin care, care of the tube, and complete information about feeding administration and potential complications.

DELEGATION DECISIONS

Nasogastric and Gastric Tubes and Enteral Feedings

Role of Registered Nurse (RN)
- Insert nasogastric (NG) tube for unstable patient.
- Irrigate NG or gastrostomy tube for unstable patient.
- Insert nasointestinal tube.
- After tube placement is verified, administer bolus or continuous enteral feeding for unstable patient.
- Administer medications through the NG or gastrostomy tube to unstable patient.
- Evaluate nutritional status of patient receiving enteral feedings.
- Monitor for complications related to tubes and enteral feedings.
- Develop plan for gastrostomy or jejunostomy tube care.
- Teach patient and caregiver about home enteral feeding and gastrostomy or jejunostomy tube care.
- Evaluate for therapeutic effect of NG tube connected to suction (e.g., decreased nausea or distention).

Role of Licensed Practical/Vocational Nurse (LPN/LVN)
- Insert NG tube for stable patient.
- Irrigate NG and gastrostomy tubes.
- Administer bolus or continuous enteral feeding for stable patient.
- Remove NG tube.
- Administer medications through NG or gastrostomy tube to stable patient.
- Provide skin care around gastrostomy or jejunostomy tubes.

Role of Unlicensed Assistive Personnel (UAP)
- Provide oral care to patient with NG, gastrostomy, or jejunostomy tube.
- Weigh patient who is receiving enteral feeding.
- Position and maintain patient receiving enteral feeding with the head of bed elevated.
- Notify RN or LPN about patient symptoms (e.g., nausea, diarrhea) that may indicate problems with enteral feedings.
- Alert RN or LPN about enteral feeding infusion pump alarms.
- Empty drainage devices and measure output.

An *enteral feeding misconnection* is an inadvertent connection between an enteral feeding system and a nonenteral system such as an IV line, a peritoneal dialysis catheter, or a tracheostomy tube cuff.[1] With an enteral feeding misconnection, nutritional formula intended for administration into the GI tract is administered via the wrong route, resulting in serious and potentially life-threatening patient complications. Nursing interventions aimed at decreasing the risk of enteral feeding misconnections are found in Table 40-12. eNursing Care Plan 40-1 for patients receiving EN is on the website for this chapter.

GERONTOLOGIC CONSIDERATIONS

ENTERAL NUTRITION
EN strategies, including orogastric, NG, nasointestinal, and gastrostomy feedings, are used in the older patient to improve nutritional status. Because of physiologic changes associated with aging, the older adult is more vulnerable to complications associated with nutritional interventions, especially fluid and electrolyte imbalances. Complications such as diarrhea can leave the patient dehydrated. Decreased thirst perception or impaired cognitive function decreases the patient's ability to seek additional fluids.

With aging, there is an increased risk of glucose intolerance. As a result, the older patient may be more susceptible to hyperglycemia in response to the high carbohydrate load of some

TABLE 40-12	DECREASING RISK OF ENTERAL FEEDING MISCONNECTIONS

1. Teach visitors, LPN/LVNs, and UAP to notify nurse if an enteral feeding line becomes disconnected.
2. Teach visitors, LPN/LVNs, and UAP not to reconnect enteral feeding lines.
3. Do not modify or adapt IV or feeding devices because you may compromise the safety features incorporated into their design.
4. Don't force connections if device parts do not seem to fit properly. Ill-fitting pieces indicate a problem.
5. When making a reconnection, routinely trace lines back to their origins and then ensure that they are secure.
6. When patient arrives on a new unit or setting or during shift handoff, recheck connections and trace all tubes.
7. Route tubes and catheters that have different purposes in unique and standardized directions (e.g., route IV lines toward the patient's head, and route enteral lines toward the feet).
8. Package together all parts needed for enteral feeding and reduce the availability of additional adapters and connectors. This will minimize the availability of dissimilar tubes or catheters that could be improperly connected.
9. Label or color-code feeding tubes and connectors, and teach staff about the labeling or color-coding process in the institution's enteral feeding system.
10. Be sure to identify and confirm the solution's label, since a three-in-one parenteral nutrition solution can appear similar to an enteral nutrition formulation bag. Label the bags with large, bold statements such as "WARNING! For Enteral Use Only—NOT for IV Use."
11. Ensure that all connections are made under proper lighting conditions.
12. Follow your facility's protocol for reporting adverse events and near misses.

Adapted from Millin CJ, Brooks M: Reduce and report enteral feeding tube misconnections, *Nursing* 40:60, 2010; and Guenter P, Hicks RW, Simmons D, et al: Enteral feeding misconnections: a consortium position statement, *Jt Comm J Qual Patient Saf* 34:285, 2008.

enteral feeding formulas. If the older adult has compromised cardiovascular function (e.g., heart failure), he or she will have a decreased ability to handle large volumes of formula. In this situation the use of more concentrated formulas (2.0 cal/mL) may be warranted. The older adult also is at increased risk for aspiration caused by gastroesophageal reflux disease (GERD), delayed gastric emptying, hiatal hernia, or diminished gag reflex. Physical mobility, fine motor movement, and visual system changes associated with aging may contribute to difficulties in managing EN in the home setting.

Parenteral Nutrition

Parenteral nutrition (PN) refers to the administration of nutrients by a route other than the GI tract (e.g., the bloodstream). It is used when the GI tract cannot be used for the ingestion, digestion, and absorption of essential nutrients. PN is a relatively safe and practical method of delivering complete nutritional support.

Regular IV solutions of 5% dextrose (5 g dextrose/dL) in water (D_5W) or 5% dextrose in lactated Ringer's solution (D_5LR) contain no protein and have approximately 170 cal/L. The average adult requires a minimum of 1200 to 1500 cal/day to carry out normal physiologic functions. Patients who sustain severe injury, surgery, or burns and those who are malnourished as a result of medical treatment or disease processes have greatly increased nutritional needs. The volume of regular dextrose

TABLE 40-13	INDICATIONS FOR PARENTERAL NUTRITION*

- Chronic severe diarrhea and vomiting
- Complicated surgery or trauma
- GI obstruction
- Intractable diarrhea
- Severe anorexia nervosa
- Severe malabsorption
- Short bowel syndrome
- GI tract anomalies and fistulae

*This list is not all-inclusive.

solutions needed to meet the caloric requirements exceeds the capacity of the cardiovascular system. Table 40-13 lists common indications for the use of PN.

Composition. Commercially prepared PN base solutions are available. These base solutions contain dextrose and protein in the form of amino acids. The pharmacy adds the prescribed electrolytes (e.g., sodium, potassium, chloride, calcium, magnesium, and phosphate), vitamins, and trace elements (e.g., zinc, copper, chromium, and manganese) to customize and meet the patient's needs. A three-in-one or total nutrient admixture containing an IV fat emulsion, dextrose, and amino acids is widely used.

Calories. Calories in PN are supplied primarily by carbohydrates in the form of dextrose and by fat in the form of fat emulsion. The administration of 100 to 150 g of dextrose daily (1 g provides approximately 3.4 calories, as opposed to oral carbohydrates, which provide 4 calories) has a protein-sparing effect. Adequate nonprotein calories in the form of glucose and fat must be provided to allow use of amino acids for wound healing and not for energy. However, overfeeding can lead to metabolic complications. To minimize these problems, an energy intake of 25 to 35 cal/kg/day in a nonobese patient is often recommended.

The U.S. FDA has approved the use of 10%, 20%, and 30% fat-emulsion solutions. Fat emulsions provide approximately 1 cal/mL (10% solution) or 2 cal/mL (20% solution). The contents of fat emulsion are primarily soybean or safflower triglycerides with egg phospholipids added as an emulsifier.

IV fat emulsions should provide up to 30% of total calories. Most stable patients receive 1 g/kg/day, and the maximum daily lipid dose is 2.5 g/kg/day. Critically ill patients may not tolerate this dose and may receive less than 1 g/kg/day.[31,41] Serum triglyceride levels are determined at the beginning of PN and then monitored closely after that. IV fat emulsions administered separately should be administered over a course of 8 to 10 hours, and the infusion rate should not exceed 0.11 g/kg/hr.[41,42]

It is becoming more common to administer lipid-free PN for the first 3 to 5 days of a critical illness because of the potential for omega-6 fatty acids to produce proinflammatory mediators.[31,41]

Nausea, vomiting, and elevated temperature have been reported, especially when lipids are infused quickly. The administration of fat emulsion is contraindicated in the patient with a disturbance in fat metabolism such as hyperlipidemia. Fat emulsions are used cautiously in the patient at risk for fat embolism (e.g., fractured femur) and the patient with an allergy to eggs or soybeans. Lipid emulsions are also used cautiously in patients with pancreatitis, bleeding disorders, liver failure, and respiratory disease.

Protein. The normal healthy person of average body size needs approximately 45 to 65 g of protein daily. Protein should be provided at the rate of 1 to 1.5 g/kg/day depending on the patient's needs. In a nutritionally depleted patient who is also under the stress of illness or surgery, protein requirements can exceed 150 g/day (1.5 to 2 g/kg/day) to ensure a positive nitrogen balance. Burn patients, who are often on PN, EN, and oral food, may need upward of 2 g/kg protein. Protein needs may be lower than 1 g/kg and restricted in individuals with end-stage renal disease who are not on dialysis.

Electrolytes. Individual requirements should be assessed daily at the beginning of therapy and then several times a week as the treatment progresses. The following are ranges for average daily electrolyte requirements for adult patients without renal or hepatic impairment:[37]

- Sodium: 1 to 2 mEq/kg
- Potassium: 1 to 2 mEq/kg
- Chloride: as needed to maintain acid-base balance
- Magnesium: 8 to 20 mEq
- Calcium: 10 to 15 mEq
- Phosphate: 20 to 40 mmol

The exact amount of electrolytes needed depends on the patient's health problem and on electrolyte levels as determined by blood testing.

Trace Elements and Vitamins. Zinc, copper, chromium, manganese, selenium, molybdenum, and iodine supplements may be added according to the patient's condition and needs. Levels of these elements are monitored in the patient receiving PN, and the health care provider may order additional amounts added to the solutions.

The daily addition of a multivitamin preparation to the PN generally meets the vitamin requirements.

Methods of Administration. PN may be administered as central PN or peripheral parenteral nutrition (PPN). Both central PN and PPN are used in a patient who is not a candidate for EN. The patient receiving PN must be able to tolerate a large volume of fluid.

Central Parenteral Nutrition. *Central PN* is indicated when long-term support is necessary or when the patient has high protein and caloric requirements. Central PN may be given through a central venous catheter that originates at the subclavian or jugular vein and whose tip lies in the superior vena cava (see Fig. 17-18). Central PN can also be given using peripherally inserted central catheters (PICCs) that are placed into the basilic or cephalic vein and then advanced into the distal end of the superior vena cava (see Fig. 17-19).

Peripheral Parenteral Nutrition. *PPN* is administered through a peripherally inserted catheter or vascular access device, which uses a large vein. PPN is used when (1) nutritional support is needed for only a short time, (2) protein and caloric requirements are not high, (3) the risk of a central catheter is too great, or (4) PN is used to supplement inadequate oral intake.

Comparison of Central and Peripheral Parenteral Nutrition. Central PN and PPN differ in tonicity, which is measured in milliosmoles (mOsm; the concentration of particles in a fluid). Blood is isotonic and measures approximately 280 mOsm/L. The standard IV solutions of D₅W and normal saline are essentially isotonic. Central PN solutions are hypertonic, measuring at least 1600 mOsm/L. The high glucose content ranges from 20% to 50%. Central PN must be infused in a large central vein so that rapid dilution can occur. The use of a peripheral vein for hypertonic, central PN solutions would cause irritation and thrombophlebitis. Nutrients can be infused using smaller volumes than PPN. PPN solutions are also hypertonic (as much as 20% glucose), but less so than with central PN, and can be safely administered through a large peripheral vein, although

TABLE 40-14	COMPLICATIONS OF PARENTERAL NUTRITION
Infection	**Catheter-Related Problems**
• Fungus	• Air embolus
• Gram-positive bacteria	• Pneumothorax, hemothorax, and hydrothorax
• Gram-negative bacteria	• Hemorrhage
Metabolic Problems	• Dislodgment
• Hyperglycemia, hypoglycemia	• Thrombosis of vein
• Altered renal function	• Phlebitis
• Essential fatty acid deficiency	
• Electrolyte and vitamin excesses and deficiencies	
• Trace mineral deficiencies	
• Hyperlipidemia	

phlebitis can occur. Another potential complication of PPN is fluid overload.

NURSING MANAGEMENT PARENTERAL NUTRITION

Nursing management of patients receiving PN is presented in eTable 40-8 and eNursing Care Plan 40-2 (available on the website for this chapter).

COMPLICATIONS

Refeeding syndrome is characterized by fluid retention and electrolyte imbalances (hypophosphatemia, hypokalemia, hypomagnesemia) (Table 40-14). Conditions that predispose patients to refeeding syndrome include long-standing malnutrition states such as chronic alcoholism, vomiting and diarrhea, chemotherapy, and major surgery. Refeeding syndrome can occur any time a malnourished patient is started on aggressive nutritional support. Hypophosphatemia is the hallmark of refeeding syndrome and is associated with serious outcomes, including cardiac dysrhythmias, respiratory arrest, and neurologic disturbances (e.g., paresthesias).

HOME NUTRITIONAL SUPPORT

Home PN or EN is an accepted mode of nutritional therapy for the person who does not require hospitalization but who requires continued nutritional support. Some patients have been successfully treated at home for many months and even years. It is important for you to teach the patient and caregiver about catheter or tube care, proper technique in mixing and handling of the solutions and tubing, and side effects and complications.

Home nutritional therapies are expensive. For patients to be reimbursed for expenses, specific criteria must be met. The discharge planning team needs to be involved early in the admission to help plan for such issues. Home nutritional support may also be a burden on the patient and the caregivers and may affect quality of life. Tell the family about support groups such as the Oley Foundation (*www.oley.org*) that provide peer support and advocacy.

EATING DISORDERS

Eating disorders are primarily psychiatric disorders and occur more often in women. Men are also at risk, but are less likely to seek treatment because eating disorders are perceived to be a women's disease.[43] The notion that eating disorders occur more frequently in whites is being challenged. African Americans, Asian Americans, and Mexican Americans are also at risk for eating disorders.[44,45] Patients with eating disorders may be hospitalized for fluid and electrolyte alterations; cardiac dysrhythmias; nutritional, endocrine, and metabolic disorders; and menstrual problems.[46] A number of nutritional problems associated with these disorders require you to implement a nutritional plan of care.

The three most common types of eating disorders are anorexia nervosa, bulimia nervosa, and binge-eating disorder.

Anorexia Nervosa

Anorexia nervosa is characterized by a self-imposed weight loss, endocrine dysfunction, and a distorted psychopathologic attitude toward weight and eating.[47] Anorexia nervosa is a serious mental illness affecting 1.2% to 2.2% of people during their lifetime, and it occurs more frequently in women.[44] Anorexia nervosa clinically manifests as abnormal weight loss, deliberate self-starvation, intense fear of gaining weight, *lanugo* (soft, downy hair covering the body except the palms and soles), refusal to eat, continuous dieting, hair loss, sensitivity to cold, compulsive exercise, absent or irregular menstruation, dry and yellowish skin, and constipation. Signs of malnutrition are noted during the physical examination.

Diagnostic studies often show iron-deficiency anemia and an elevated blood urea nitrogen level that reflects marked intravascular volume depletion and abnormal renal function. Lack of potassium in the diet and loss of potassium in the urine lead to potassium deficiency. Manifestations of potassium deficiency include muscle weakness, cardiac dysrhythmias, and renal failure. Leukopenia, hypoglycemia, hyponatremia, hypomagnesemia, and hypophosphatemia may also be present.

Multidisciplinary treatment must involve a combination of nutritional support and psychiatric care.[48] Nutritional rehabilitation focuses on reaching and maintaining a healthy weight, normal eating patterns, and perception of hunger and satiety. Hospitalization may be necessary if the patient has medical complications that cannot be managed in an outpatient therapy program. Nutritional repletion must be closely supervised to ensure consistent and ongoing weight gains. Refeeding syndrome is a rare but serious complication of refeeding programs. The use of EN or PN may be necessary.

Improved nutrition, however, is not a cure for anorexia nervosa. The underlying psychiatric problem must be addressed by identification of the disturbed patterns of individual and family interactions, followed by individual and family counseling.

Bulimia Nervosa

Bulimia nervosa is a disorder characterized by frequent binge eating and self-induced vomiting associated with loss of control related to eating and a persistent concern with body image.[47] Individuals with bulimia nervosa may have normal weight for height, or their weight may fluctuate with bingeing and purging. They may also abuse laxatives, diuretics, exercise, or diet drugs. They may have signs of frequent vomiting, such as macerated knuckles, swollen salivary glands, broken blood vessels in the eyes, and dental problems. The individual with bulimia nervosa goes to great lengths to conceal abnormal eating habits. Abnormal laboratory parameters, including hypokalemia, metabolic alkalosis, and elevated serum amylase, may occur with frequent vomiting.[47]

The cause of bulimia remains unclear but is thought to be similar to that of anorexia nervosa. Substance abuse, anxiety, affective disorders, and personality disturbances have been reported among persons with bulimia. Over time, problems associated with bulimia become increasingly hard to deal with effectively. A treatment combination of psychologic counseling and diet therapy is essential.[48]

Antidepressants are helpful for some but not all patients with bulimia. Education and emotional support for the patient and family are vital. Support groups such as the National Association of Anorexia Nervosa and Associated Disorders (ANAD) (*www.anad.org*) are helpful to those affected by these disorders.

Binge-eating disorder is less severe than bulimia nervosa and anorexia nervosa. Individuals with binge-eating disorder do not have a distorted body image and are often overweight or obese.[49]

CASE STUDY

Undernutrition

iStockphoto/Thinkstock

Patient Profile
M.S. is a 70-yr-old white woman who is 5 ft, 4 in tall and weighs 100 lb. She was recently admitted to the inpatient medical unit.

Subjective Data
• Reports 30-lb weight loss in past 2 mo
• Recently had a thrombotic stroke with hemiparesis and dysphagia
• Has a history of rheumatoid arthritis
• Has had nothing by mouth for the past 24 hr and just started enteral nutrition via PEG tube
• Lives with her daughter, who is at her bedside

Objective Data
Physical Examination
• Has left-sided weakness
• BP is 150/90 mm Hg
• A PEG tube was recently placed

Laboratory Results
• Serum albumin 2.9 g/dL
• Prealbumin 11.0 mg/dL

Discussion Questions
1. What are M.S.'s risk factors for malnutrition?
2. What is her BMI?
3. What are contributing factors to her developing dysphagia and malnutrition?
4. What should you include in a successful weight gain program for M.S.?
5. Which possible complications of enteral nutrition could M.S. be at risk for developing?
6. *Priority Decision:* What is the priority of the nursing care for M.S.?
7. *Priority Decision:* Based on the assessment data presented, write one or more appropriate nursing diagnoses. Are there any collaborative problems?
8. *Delegation Decision:* How would you use unlicensed assistive personnel (UAP) to care for M.S.?
9. *Evidence-Based Practice:* M.S.'s daughter tells you that her mother's abdomen appears bloated and she wonders if she should massage it.

BRIDGE TO NCLEX EXAMINATION

The number of the question corresponds to the same-numbered outcome at the beginning of the chapter.

1. The percentage of daily calories for a healthy individual consists of
   a. 50% carbohydrates, 25% protein, 25% fat, and <10% of fat from saturated fatty acids.
   b. 65% carbohydrates, 25% protein, 25% fat, and >10% of fat from saturated fatty acids.
   c. 50% carbohydrates, 40% protein, 10% fat, and <10% of fat from saturated fatty acids.
   d. 40% carbohydrates, 30% protein, 30% fat, and >10% of fat from saturated fatty acids.

2. During starvation, the order in which the body obtains substrate for energy is
   a. visceral protein, skeletal protein, fat, glycogen.
   b. glycogen, skeletal protein, fat stores, visceral protein.
   c. visceral protein, fat stores, glycogen, skeletal protein.
   d. fat stores, skeletal protein, visceral protein, glycogen.

3. A complete nutritional assessment including anthropometric measurements is important for the patient who
   a. has a BMI of 25.5 kg/m².
   b. complains of frequent nocturia.
   c. reports a 5-year history of constipation.
   d. reports an unintentional weight loss of 10 lb in 2 months.

4. The nurse confirms initial placement of a blindly inserted small-bore NG feeding tube by
   a. x-ray.
   b. air insufflation.
   c. observing patient for coughing.
   d. pH measurement of gastric aspirate.

5. A patient is receiving peripheral parenteral nutrition. The parenteral nutrition solution is completed before the new solution arrives on the unit. The nurse administers
   a. 20% intralipids.
   b. 5% dextrose solution.
   c. 0.45% normal saline solution.
   d. 5% lactated Ringer's solution.

6. A patient with anorexia nervosa shows signs of malnutrition. During initial refeeding, the nurse carefully assesses the patient for
   a. hyperkalemia.
   b. hypoglycemia.
   c. hypercalcemia.
   d. hypophosphatemia.

1. a, 2. b, 3. d, 4. a, 5. b, 6. d

evolve

For rationales to these answers and even more NCLEX review questions, visit *http://evolve.elsevier.com/Lewis/medsurg.*

REFERENCES

1. ASPEN Board of Directors: Definition of terms, style, and conventions used in ASPEN. Retrieved from *www.nutritioncare.org/Professional_Resources/Guidelines_and_Standards/Guidelines/2010_Definitions_of_Terms,_Style,_and_Conventions_Used_in_A_S_P_E_N__Board_of_Directors.*
2. Holben D: Position of the American Dietetic Association: food insecurity in the United States, *J Am Diet Assoc* 110:1368, 2010.
3. US Food and Drug Administration: Nutrition facts label programs. Retrieved from *www.fda.gov/Food/ResourcesForYou/Consumers/NFLPM/default.htm.*
*4. Academy of Nutrition and Dietetics: Adult weight management evidence-based nutrition practice guideline: executive summary. Retrieved from *www.adaevidencelibrary.com/topic.cfm?cat=3014.*
5. Mifflin MD, St. Jeor ST, Hill LA, et al: A new predictive equation for resting energy expenditure in healthy individuals, *Am J Clin Nutr* 51:242, 1990. (Classic)
6. Wooley JA, Frankenfield D: Energy. In Gotschlich MM, DeLegge MH, Mattox T, et al, editors: *The A.S.P.E.N. nutrition support core curriculum: a case-based approach—the adult patient,* Silver Spring, Md, 2007, ASPEN. (Classic)
7. US Department of Agriculture and US Department of Health and Human Services: *Dietary guidelines for Americans, 2010,* ed 7, Washington, DC, 2010, US Government Printing Office.
8. Mozaffaarian D, Wu JH: Fatty acids and cardiovascular health: are effects of EPA and DHA shared or complementary? *J Nutr* 142:614S, 2012.

9. Satia J: Dietary acculturation and the nutrition transition: an overview, *Appl Physiol Nutr Metab* 35:219, 2010.
10. Spencer A, Jablonski R, Susan SJ: Hypertensive African American women and the DASH diet, *Nurse Pract* 37:41, 2012.
11. Lv N, Brown JL: Impact of a nutrition education program to increase intake of calcium-rich foods by Chinese American women, *J Am Diet Assoc* 111:143, 2011.
*12. Barroso C, Peters RJ, Kelder SH, et al: Beliefs and perceived norms concerning body image among African-American and Latino teenagers, *J Health Psych* 15:858, 2010.
13. Soeters P, Schols A: Advances in understanding and assessing malnutrition, *Curr Opin Clin Nutr Metab Care* 12:487, 2009. (Classic)
14. Heersink J, Brown C, DiMaria-Ghalili R, et al: Undernutrition in hospitalized older adults: patterns and correlates, outcomes, and opportunities for intervention with a focus on processes of care, *J Nutr Elderly* 29:4, 2010.
*15. Kaiser MJ, Bauer JM, Ramsch C, et al: Frequency of malnutrition in older adults: a multinational perspective using the Mini Nutritional Assessment, *J Am Geriatr Soc* 58:1734, 2010.
*16. Jensen GL, Mirtallo J, Compher C, et al: Adult starvation and disease-related malnutrition: a proposal for etiology-based diagnosis in the clinical practice setting from the International Consensus Guideline Committee, *JPEN J Parenter Enteral Nutr* 34:156, 2010.
17. Osorio SN: Reconsidering kwashiorkor, *Top Clin Nutr* 26:10, 2011.
18. Mueller C: Inflammation and malnutrition, *Top Clin Nutr* 26:3, 2011.
19. Wilmore DW: *The metabolic management of the critically ill,* New York, 1977, Plenum. (Classic)

*Evidence-based information for clinical practice.

20. Otten JJ, Hellwig JP, Meyers LD: *Dietary reference intakes: the essential guide to nutrient requirements*, Washington, DC, 2006, National Academies Press. (Classic)

*21. Mueller C, Compher C, Druyan ME, et al: A.S.P.E.N. clinical guidelines: nutrition screening, assessment, and intervention in adults, *JPEN J Parenter Enteral Nutr* 35:16, 2011.

22. Jensen GL: Nutrition assessment and requirements. In Marian M, Russell MK, Shikora SA, editors: *Clinical nutrition for surgical patients*, Boston, 2008, Jones & Bartlett. (Classic)

*23. Skipper A, Ferguson M, Thompson K, et al: Nutrition screening tools: an analysis of the evidence, *JPEN J Parenter Enteral Nutr* 36:292, 2012.

24. DiMaria-Ghalili RA, Guenter PA: The mini-nutritional assessment, *Am J Nurs* 108:50, 2008. (Classic)

25. Dorner B, Posthauer ME, Friedrich EK, et al: Enteral nutrition for older adults in nursing facilities, *Nutr Clin Pract* 26:261, 2011.

26. Guralnik JM, Simonsick EM, Ferrucci L, et al: Short physical performance battery. Retrieved from *www.pt.ntu.edu.tw/mhh/ course/neuro/BS/mmh_geriatric/ShortPhysicalPerformance Battery%5B2%5D.pdf*.

27. Vogelzang JL: Making nutrition sense from OASIS, *Home Healthc Nurse* 21:592, 2003. (Classic)

28. DiMaria-Ghalili RA: Nutrition. In Boltz M, Capezuti E, Fulmer T, et al, editors: *Evidence-based geriatric nursing protocols for best practice*, ed 4, New York, 2012, Springer.

*29. Luft VC, Beghetto M, Castro SMJ, et al: Validation of a new method developed to measure the height of adult patients in bed, *Nutr Clin Pract* 23:424, 2008. (Classic)

*30. Gupta R, Knobel D, Gunabushanam V, et al: The effect of low body mass index on outcome in critically ill surgical patients, *Nutr Clin Pract* 26:593, 2011.

31. Worthington PH, Gilber KA: Parenteral nutrition: risks, complications, and management, *J Infus Nurs* 35:52, 2012.

32. Institute of Medicine: *Retooling for an aging America: building the health care workforce*, Washington, DC, 2008, National Academies Press. (Classic)

33. Locher JL, Wellman NS: "Never the twain shall meet": dual systems exacerbate malnutrition in older adults recently discharged from hospitals, *J Nutr Gerontol Geriatr* 30:24, 2011.

34. English K, Paddon-Jones D: Protecting muscle mass and function in older adults during bed rest, *Curr Opin Clin Nutr Metab Care* 13:34, 2010.

*35. Milne AC, Potter J, Vivanti A, et al: Protein and energy supplementation in elderly people at risk from malnutrition, *Cochrane Database Syst Rev* 2:CD003288, 2009. (Classic)

*36. Enteral Nutrition Practice Recommendations Task Force: Enteral nutrition practice recommendations, *JPEN J Parenter Enteral Nutr* 33:122, 2009. (Classic)

*37. Metheny NA, Stewart BJ, McClave SA: Relationship between feeding tube site and respiratory outcomes, *JPEN J Parenter Enteral Nutr* 35:346, 2011.

38. Bankhead RR, Fang JC: Enteral access devices. In Gotschlich MM, DeLegge MH, Mattox T, et al, editors: *The A.S.P.E.N.*

nutrition support core curriculum: a case-based approach—the adult patient*, Silver Spring, Md, 2007, ASPEN.

39. Boullata J, Carney LN, Guenter P: *A.S.P.E.N. enteral nutrition handbook*, Silver Springs Md, 2010, ASPEN.

40. Koopmann MC, Kudsk KA, Szotkowski MJ, et al: A team-based protocol and electromagnetic technology eliminate feeding tube placement complications, *Ann Surg* 253:287, 2011.

41. Canada T, Crill C, Guenter P: *A.S.P.E.N. parenteral nutrition handbook*, Silver Springs, Md, 2009, ASPEN. (Classic)

*42. ASPEN Board of Directors: Guidelines for the use of parenteral and enteral nutrition in adult and pediatric patients, *JPEN J Parenter Enteral Nutr* 26(Suppl 1):1SA, 2002. (Classic)

43. National Association of Anorexia Nervosa and Associated Disorders: Eating disorders statistics. Retrieved from *www.anad.org/get-information/about-eating-disorders/eating-disorders-statistics*.

44. Talleyrand RM: Eating disorders in African American girls: implications for counselors, *J Counsel Develop* 88:319, 2010.

45. National Eating Disorders Association: Research results on eating disorders in diverse populations. Retrieved from *www.nationaleatingdisorders.org*.

*46. Zhao Y, Encinosa W: *An update on hospitalizations for eating disorders, 1999 to 2009*, HCUP Statistical Brief No 120, Rockville, Md, 2011, Agency for Healthcare Research and Quality.

47. Miller CA, Golder NH: An introduction to eating disorders: clinical presentation, epidemiology, and prognosis, *Nutr Clin Pract* 25:110, 2010.

48. Reiter CS, Graves L: Nutrition therapy for eating disorders, *Nutr Clin Pract* 25:122, 2010.

49. National Institute of Mental Health: Eating disorders. Retrieved from *www.nimh.nih.gov/health/publications/eating-disorders/index.shtml*.

RESOURCES

Academy for Eating Disorders
www.aedweb.org

Academy of Nutrition and Dietetics (formerly American Dietetic Association)
www.eatright.org

American Society for Parenteral and Enteral Nutrition (ASPEN)
www.nutritioncare.org

FDA Food Safety
www.fda.gov/Food/FoodSafety/

Institute of Medicine, Food and Nutrition Board
www.iom.edu/About-IOM/Leadership-Staff/Boards/Food-and-Nutrition-Board.aspx

National Eating Disorder Information Centre
www.nedic.ca

National Eating Disorders Association
www.nationaleatingdisorders.org

U.S. Department of Agriculture, MyPlate
www.choosemyplate.gov

41

Nursing Management
Obesity

Judi Daniels

If you have a dream, don't just sit there.
Gather courage to believe that you can
succeed and leave no stone unturned
to make it a reality.
Rooplean

evolve WEBSITE

http://evolve.elsevier.com/Lewis/medsurg
- NCLEX Review Questions
- Key Points
- Pre-Test
- Answer Guidelines for Case Study on p. 922
- Rationales for Bridge to NCLEX Examination Questions

- Case Study
  - Patient With Obesity and Osteoarthritis
- Concept Map Creator
- Glossary
- Content Updates

eFigure
- eFig. 41-1: Obese women

eTables
- eTable 41-1: Comparison of Fad Diets
- eTable 41-2: Nutritional Therapy: Meal Plans for 1200-Calorie–Restricted Weight-Reduction Diet

LEARNING OUTCOMES

1. Discuss the epidemiology and etiology of obesity.
2. Compare the classification systems for determining a person's body size.
3. Explain the health risks associated with obesity.
4. Discuss nutritional therapy and exercise plans for the obese patient.
5. Describe the different bariatric surgical procedures used to treat obesity.
6. Describe the nursing management related to conservative and surgical therapies for obesity.
7. Describe the etiology, clinical manifestations, and nursing and collaborative management of metabolic syndrome.

KEY TERMS

bariatric surgery, p. 916
body mass index (BMI), p. 906
lipectomy, p. 917

metabolic syndrome, p. 921
obese, p. 906
overweight, p. 906

severely obese, p. 906
waist-to-hip ratio (WHR), p. 907

OBESITY

Obesity is an excessively high amount of body fat or adipose tissue (Fig. 41-1). Obesity is a major health problem because it increases the risk of numerous other diseases such as diabetes and cancer.[1]

Classifications of Body Weight and Obesity

An important part of your patient assessment is to determine and classify a patient's body weight. A number of assessment methods are available, including body mass index (BMI), waist circumference, waist-to-hip ratio (WHR), and body shape. The most widely used and endorsed measures are BMI and waist circumference.[2] These measures are cost-effective with acceptable reliability and are easily used in all practice settings.

Body Mass Index. The most common measure of obesity is the **body mass index (BMI)**. BMI is calculated by dividing a person's weight (in kilograms) by the square of the height in meters (Fig. 41-2). Individuals with a BMI less than 18.5 kg/m² are considered underweight, whereas those with a BMI between 18.5 and 24.9 kg/m² reflect a normal body weight. A BMI of 25 to 29.9 kg/m² is classified as being **overweight,** and those with values at 30 kg/m² or above are considered **obese.** The term **severely** *(morbidly, extremely)* **obese** is used for those with a BMI greater than 40 kg/m² (eFig. 41-1 on the website shows individuals who are severely obese).

Table 41-1 shows the classification of overweight and obesity by BMI. The BMI, which provides an overall assessment of fat mass, must be considered in relation to the patient's age, gender, and body build. For example, a body builder may have a BMI associated with obesity but because of a high

Reviewed by Amanda J. Flagg, PhD, ACNS-BC, CNE, Assistant Clinical Professor, University of Texas Health Science Center at San Antonio School of Nursing, San Antonio, Texas; and Daryle Wane, PhD, ARNP, FNP-BC, Professor of Nursing, Generic Program Track Coordinator, Pasco-Hernando Community College, New Port Richey, Florida.

FIG. 41-1 Obesity is an epidemic in the United States. (iStockphoto/Thinkstock)

$$BMI\ (kg/m^2) = \frac{Weight\ (pounds) \times 703}{Height\ (inches)^2}$$

FIG. 41-2 Body mass index (BMI) chart. Healthy weight: BMI 18 to 24.9 kg/m^2; overweight: BMI 25 to 29.9 kg/m^2; obesity: BMI 30 kg/m^2. BMI = weight (kg)/height (m^2).

muscle mass, the BMI would not be an accurate assessment. In contrast, in individuals who have lost body mass (e.g., older adults), the BMI would underestimate the degree of obesity. For this reason, other measures must be combined with the BMI for an accurate evaluation of a person's weight.

Waist Circumference. *Waist circumference* is another way to assess and classify a person's weight (see Table 41-1). People who have visceral fat with truncal obesity are at an increased risk for cardiovascular disease and metabolic syndrome (discussed later in this chapter). Health risks increase if the waist circumference is greater than 40 inches in men and greater than 35 inches in women.[1]

Waist-to-Hip Ratio. The **waist-to-hip ratio (WHR)** is another tool used to assess obesity. This ratio is a method of describing the distribution of both subcutaneous and visceral adipose tissue. The ratio is calculated by using the waist measurement divided by the hip measurement. A WHR less than 0.8 is optimal, and a WHR greater than 0.8 indicates more truncal fat, which puts the individual at a greater risk for health complications.

Body Shape. *Body shape* is another method of identifying those who are at a higher risk for health problems (Table 41-2). Individuals with fat located primarily in the abdominal area, an *apple-shaped body,* have *android obesity.* Those with fat distribution in the upper legs, a *pear-shaped body,* have *gynoid obesity.* Genetics has an important role in determining a person's body shape. Weight and shape are influenced by genetics.[3]

Epidemiology of Obesity

Currently, more than 35% of adults in the United States are obese. Unless Americans change their ways, 50% of the U.S. population will be obese by 2030.[4] Women having a slightly higher incidence of obesity than men. When those who are

TABLE 41-1	**CLASSIFICATION OF OVERWEIGHT AND OBESITY**			
			Disease Risk Based on Waist Circumference*	
	BMI (kg/m²)	**Obesity Class**	**Men ≤40 in (102 cm)** **Women ≤35 in (89 cm)**	**Men >40 in (102 cm)** **Women >35 in (89 cm)**
Underweight	<18.5	—	—	—
Normal†	18.5-24.9	—	—	—
Overweight	25.0-29.9	—	Increased	High
Obese	30.0-34.9	Class I	High	Very high
	35.0-39.9	Class II	Very high	Very high
Severely obese	≥40.0	Class III	Extremely high	Extremely high

Source: National Heart, Lung, and Blood Institute: Classification of overweight and obesity by BMI, waist circumference, and associated disease risks. Retrieved from *www.nhlbi. nih.gov/health/public/heart/obesity/lose_wt/bmi_dis.htm.*
*Disease risk for type 2 diabetes, hypertension, and cardiovascular disease relative to person of normal weight.
†Increased waist circumference can also be a marker for increased risk in persons of normal weight.
BMI, Body mass index.

TABLE 41-2 RELATIONSHIP BETWEEN BODY SHAPE AND HEALTH RISKS

Body Shape	Characteristics	Health Risks
Gynoid (pear)	• Fat mainly located in the upper legs • Has a better prognosis but difficult to treat	• Osteoporosis • Varicose veins • Cellulite • Subcutaneous fat traps and stores dietary fat • Trapped fatty acids stored as triglycerides

Android (apple)	• Fat primarily located in abdominal area
	• Fat also distributed over upper body (neck, arms, shoulders)
	• Greater risk for obesity-related complications
		• Heart disease
		• Diabetes mellitus
		• Breast cancer
		• Endometrial cancer
		• Visceral fat more active, causing
		  • ↓ Insulin sensitivity
		  • ↑ Triglycerides
		  • ↓ HDL cholesterol
		  • ↑ BP
		  • ↑ Free fatty acid release into blood

HDL, High-density lipoprotein.

🌐 CULTURAL & ETHNIC HEALTH DISPARITIES
Obesity

- African Americans and Hispanics have a higher prevalence of obesity than whites.
- Among women, African Americans have the highest prevalence of being overweight or obese, and 15% are severely obese.
- Among men, Mexican Americans have the highest prevalence of being overweight or obese.
- African American and Hispanic women with low incomes appear to have the greatest likelihood of being overweight when compared with other socioeconomic groups.
- Native Americans have a higher prevalence of being overweight than the general population.
- Among Native Americans ages 45 to 74, more than 30% of women are overweight and more than 40% are obese.
- Asian Americans have the lowest prevalence of being overweight and obese compared with the general population.

overweight are included, the incidence of the adult population with a BMI greater than 25 kg/m² increases to more than 68%.[5]

The highest prevalence of obesity occurs between ages 40 and 59 for women and after 60 years of age for men.[5] African Americans have the highest incidence of obesity followed by Hispanics (see Cultural & Ethnic Health Disparities box above).

Obesity in adulthood is often a problem that begins in childhood or adolescence. Nearly one third of children and teens are currently obese or overweight. It is estimated that almost half of overweight adults were overweight in childhood, and two thirds of obese children remained obese into adulthood.[6] Reversing the childhood obesity crisis is key to addressing the overall obesity epidemic.

HEALTHY PEOPLE
Health Impact of Maintaining a Healthy Weight

- Reduces the risk of developing type 2 diabetes mellitus
- Increases chance of longevity and better quality of life
- Lowers the risk of hypertension and elevated cholesterol
- Reduces the risk of heart disease, stroke, and gallbladder disease
- Reduces the likelihood of breathing problems, including sleep apnea and asthma
- Decreases the risk of developing osteoarthritis, low back pain, and certain types of cancers

Etiology and Pathophysiology

Obesity is an increase in body weight beyond the body's physical requirements. This results in an abnormal increase and accumulation of fat cells. However, the processes leading to and sustaining the obese state are complex and still undergoing investigation.

In obesity, there is an increase in the number of adipocytes *(hyperplasia)* and an increase in their size *(hypertrophy)*. Adipocyte *hypertrophy* is a process by which adipocytes can increase their volume several thousand–fold to accommodate large increases in lipid storage. In addition, preadipocytes are triggered to become adipocytes once storage of existing fat cells is exceeded.[2] This process primarily occurs in the visceral (intraabdominal) and subcutaneous tissues. The process of *hyperplasia* (increase in numbers) of adipocytes is greatest from infancy through adolescence.

The majority of obese persons have *primary obesity,* which is excess calorie intake over energy expenditure for the body's metabolic demands. Others have *secondary obesity,* which can result from various congenital anomalies, chromosomal anomalies, metabolic problems, or central nervous system lesions and disorders.

The cause of obesity involves significant genetic and biologic factors that are highly influenced by environmental and psychosocial factors. Each of these factors can and should be considered individually, but in reality they are interrelated.

🧬 Genetic Link

Studies of twins, adoptees, and families all suggest the existence of genetic factors in obesity.[7,8] The heritability of obesity estimated from twin studies is high, with only slightly lower values in twins raised apart than in those raised together. Similarly, in adoptees the children's BMI correlated with that of their biologic parents rather than their adoptive parents.[9] Estimates of obesity as an inherited problem are more than 50%.[8]

A number of genes have been identified as being linked to obesity. Genes actually may influence how calories are stored and energy released. "Energy-thrifty" genes, once protective against long periods where food was not available, are now maladaptive in societies where food availability is no longer a primary issue.[7] Genes may be responsible for why two individuals living in the same environment can vary considerably in body size.

A strong link exists between a gene known as *FTO* (fat mass and obesity-associated gene) and BMI. Variants of this gene may explain why some people become overweight whereas others do not. People with two copies of a certain allele at the *FTO* gene weigh 7 to 8 lb more and have a greater risk of obesity than those who do not have the risk allele.[10] More research is needed to better understand the role of genes in obesity.

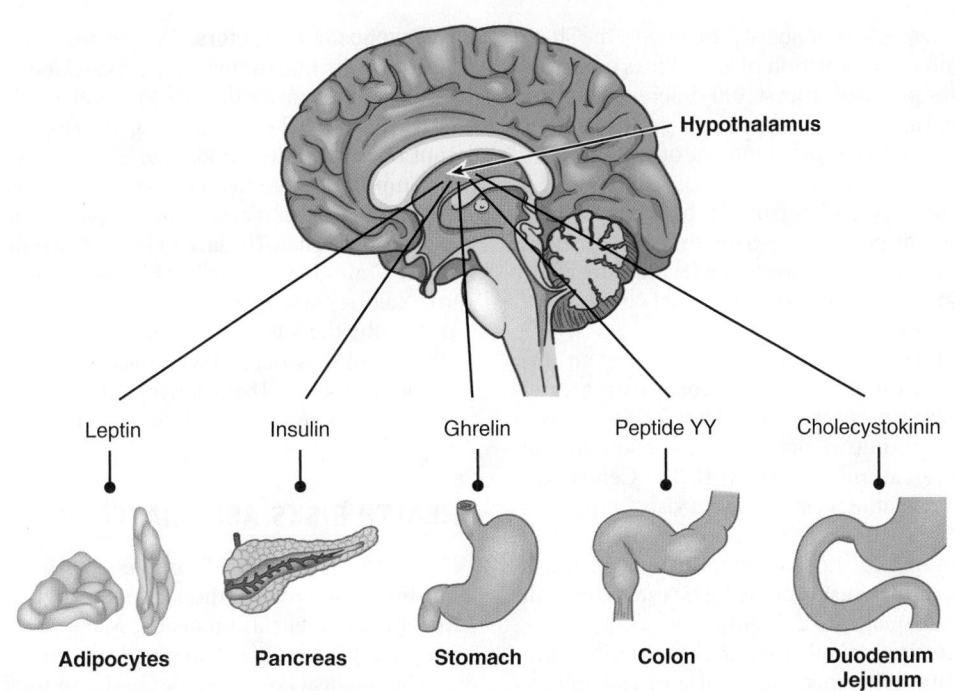

FIG. 41-3 Some of the common hormones and peptides that interact with the hypothalamus to control and influence eating patterns, metabolic activities, and digestion. Obesity disrupts this balance (see Table 41-3).

TABLE 41-3 HORMONES AND PEPTIDES IN OBESITY

Where Produced	Normal Function	Alteration in Obesity	Where Produced	Normal Function	Alteration in Obesity
Neuropeptide Y			**Insulin**		
Hypothalamus	Stimulates appetite	Imbalance causes increased appetite.	Pancreas	Decreases appetite	Increased insulin secretion which stimulates ↑ liver synthesis of triglycerides and ↓ HDL production.
Ghrelin					
Stomach (primarily)	Stimulates appetite ↑ After food deprivation ↓ In response to food in the stomach	Normal postprandial decline does not occur, which can lead to increased appetite and overeating.	**Peptide YY**		
			Colon	Inhibits appetite by slowing GI motility and gastric emptying	Circulating levels are decreased. ↓ Release after eating.
Leptin			**Cholecystokinin**		
Adipocytes	Suppresses appetite and hunger Regulates eating behavior	Obesity is associated with high levels. Leptin resistance develops; thus obese people may lose the effect of appetite suppression.	Duodenum Jejunum	Inhibits gastric emptying and sends satiety signals to hypothalamus	Unknown role

HDL, High-density lipoprotein.

Physiologic Regulatory Mechanisms in Obesity. Research has focused on the physiologic regulatory processes that control eating behavior, energy metabolism, and body fat metabolism. Knowing how appetite is triggered and energy is expended provides important information for understanding obesity and specific targets for the development of drugs.

The hypothalamus, gut, and adipose tissue synthesize hormones and peptides that inhibit or stimulate the appetite (Fig. 41-3). The hypothalamus is a major site for regulating appetite. Neuropeptide Y, produced in the hypothalamus, is a powerful appetite stimulant. When it is imbalanced, it leads to overeating and obesity. Hormones and peptides produced in the gut and adipocyte cells affect the hypothalamus and have a critical role in appetite and energy balance (Table 41-3).

Leptin, secreted from adipocytes when they fill with fat, acts in the hypothalamus to suppress appetite, increase physical activity, and increase fat metabolism. A genetic deficiency of leptin causes extreme obesity. In obesity the level of leptin is actually increased, which has raised the question of whether obese people are insensitive to leptin.[2] Possible causes include failure to produce enough leptin receptors or production of receptors that are faulty.

Ghrelin, a gut hormone, regulates appetite through inhibition of leptin. In a fasting state, ghrelin is increased. Ghrelin acts in the hypothalamus by working on the reward system that triggers overeating. Ghrelin is thought to play a part in compulsive eating. In gastric bypass surgery, ghrelin is decreased significantly, which helps suppress appetite.

The two major consequences of obesity are due to the sheer increase in fat mass and the production of adipokines produced by fat cells. Adipocytes produce at least 100 different proteins. These proteins, secreted as enzymes, adipokines, growth factors, and hormones, contribute to the development of insulin resistance and atherosclerosis.

An increased release of cytokines from fat cells may disrupt immune factors, thus predisposing the person to certain cancers. Because visceral fat accumulation is associated with more alterations of these adipokines, people with abdominal obesity have more complications of obesity.[11]

Environmental Factors. Environmental factors play an important role in obesity. In today's culture, people have greater access to food, particularly prepackaged and fast foods, and soft drinks, which have poor nutritional quality. Portion size of meals has increased dramatically (Table 41-4). The Centers for Disease Control and Prevention has developed visual programs that demonstrate how portions have increased over time.[12] Underestimating portion sizes and therefore caloric intake is common. In addition, eating outside of the home interferes with the ability to control the quality and quantity of food.

Lack of physical exercise is another factor that contributes to weight gain and obesity. With increases in use of technology, labor-saving devices, and cars, Americans are expending less energy in their everyday lives. Elimination of physical education programs in schools, along with increased time spent playing video games and watching TV, has contributed to the increase in sedentary habits.

Socioeconomic status is a known risk factor for obesity in a variety of ways.[13] People with low incomes may attempt to stretch their food dollars by purchasing less expensive foods that often have poor nutritional quality with a greater caloric content. For example, people with low incomes are more likely to purchase pasta, bread, and canned fruit packed with sugar rather than chicken and fresh fruits and vegetables. Low-income residents may also live in environments that do not accommodate outdoor activities (e.g., safe playgrounds, walking tracks, tennis, swimming pools).

Psychosocial Factors. People use food for many reasons besides their nutritional value. Associations with food begin in childhood, such as the use of food for comfort or rewards. Furthermore, when overeating develops at an early age and continues into adulthood, one's ability to sense fullness *(satiety)* is compromised. Whether triggered by specific foods or by the wide variety of choices, some people consume more food than their bodies need. The lack of hunger that drives eating has been termed "mindless eating" and leads to consumption of unnecessary calories and increase in body weight.[13,14]

Finally, the social component of eating begins early in life when food is associated with pleasure and fun at such events as birthday parties, Thanksgiving, and religious holidays. All of these factors must be included when considering the etiology and treatment of obesity.

HEALTH RISKS ASSOCIATED WITH OBESITY

Hippocrates wrote that "corpulence is not only a disease itself, but the harbinger of others," thus recognizing that obesity has major adverse effects on health. Many problems occur in obese people at higher rates than people of normal weight (Fig. 41-4).

The medical cost of adult obesity in the United States is difficult to calculate, but estimates range from $147 billion to nearly $210 billion per year. The bulk of the spending is from treating obesity-related diseases such as diabetes. Obese people spend 42% more on health care costs than healthy-weight people.[4]

Mortality rates rise as obesity increases, especially when obesity is associated with visceral fat. For obese persons, mortality rates from all causes, especially from cardiovascular disease, are increased by 50% to 100% above those of persons with a normal BMI. Being overweight in midlife, once thought to have fewer health consequences than being obese, confers a 20% to 40% increase in mortality rate for both men and women.[11] In addition to these problems, obese patients have a reduced quality of life. Fortunately, most of these conditions can improve if an individual loses weight.

Cardiovascular Problems

Obesity is a significant risk factor for cardiovascular disease in both men and women.[11] Android obesity is the best predictor of these risks and is linked with increased low-density lipoproteins (LDLs), high triglycerides, and decreased high-density lipoproteins (HDLs). Obesity is also associated with hypertension, which can occur because of increased circulating blood volume, abnormal vasoconstriction, increased inflammation (damaging blood vessels), and increased risk of sleep apnea (raises blood pressure [BP]). Altered lipid metabolism and hypertension can increase the long-term risk of heart disease and stroke. Excess body fat can also lead to chronic inflammation throughout the body, especially in blood vessels, thus increasing the risk of heart disease.

Diabetes Mellitus

More than 80% of people with type 2 diabetes are obese or overweight.[4] Hyperinsulinemia and insulin resistance, common features of type 2 diabetes, are also found in obesity, especially when visceral fat is increased. Excess weight decreases the effectiveness of insulin. When insulin does not work effectively, too much glucose stays in the bloodstream. Thus more insulin is made to compensate. Pancreatic β cells (cells that make insulin)

TABLE 41-4	**PORTION SIZES: YESTERDAY VS TODAY**	
	25 Yr Ago	**Today**
Turkey sandwich	320 cal	820 cal
Bagel	3-in diameter, 140 cal	6-in diameter, 350 cal
Cheeseburger	333 cal	590 cal
Soda	6½ oz, 85 cal	20 oz, 250 cal

FIG. 41-4 Health risks associated with obesity.

may get overworked and become worn out. Over time, the pancreas is no longer able to keep blood glucose in normal range. It appears that adiponectin, a peptide that increases insulin sensitivity, is decreased in obese people.

Obesity is a major risk factor for development of type 2 diabetes. Furthermore, obesity complicates the management of type 2 diabetes by increasing insulin resistance and glucose intolerance, which makes drug treatment for diabetes less effective. A weight reduction of 7% can decrease the risk of diabetes by 58%.[15]

Gastrointestinal and Liver Problems

Gastroesophageal reflux disease (GERD) and gallstones are more prevalent in obese people. Gallstones occur due to supersaturation of the bile with cholesterol. Nonalcoholic steatohepatitis (NASH) is a condition in which lipids are deposited in the liver, resulting in a fatty liver. NASH is associated with elevated hepatic glucose production. NASH can eventually progress to cirrhosis and can be fatal. Weight loss can improve NASH.

Respiratory and Sleep Problems

The increased fat mass associated with obesity may lead to sleep apnea and obesity hypoventilation syndrome. The increased distribution of fat around the diaphragm causes a reduced chest

wall compliance, increased work of breathing, and decreased total lung capacity and functional residual capacity. Sleep apnea results from increased fat around the neck, leading to snoring and hypoventilation while sleeping. Weight loss can bring substantial improvement in lung function.

Poor sleep and sleep deprivation may increase appetite. Sleep deprivation has been associated with obesity. Building up a sleep debt over a matter of days can impair metabolism and disrupt hormone levels. The level of leptin falls in people who are sleep deprived, thus promoting appetite.

Musculoskeletal Problems

Obesity is associated with an increased incidence of osteoarthritis because of the stress put on weight-bearing joints, especially the knees and hips. Increased body fat also triggers inflammatory mediators and contributes to deterioration of cartilage. Hyperuricemia and gout are often found in people who are obese and in those who have metabolic syndrome (discussed later in this chapter).

Cancer

Obesity is one of the most important known preventable causes of cancer. About 20% of cancers in women and 15% in men are attributable to obesity.[16] The types of cancer most strongly linked to excess body fat are breast, endometrial, kidney, colorectal, pancreatic, esophageal, and gallbladder cancer.

The underlying mechanisms linking obesity and cancer remain unclear. Breast and endometrial cancer may be due to the increased estrogen levels (estrogen is stored in fat cells) associated with obesity in postmenopausal women. Colorectal cancer has been linked to hyperinsulinemia, and esophageal cancer may be secondary to acid reflux caused by abdominal obesity. Several hormones and factors often present in obese states have been identified as potentiating the risk for cancer. For example insulin, which is a powerful cellular growth factor, is increased in obesity. The resulting hyperinsulinemia may affect cancer cells.

Adipokines (from fat cells) may stimulate or inhibit cell growth. For example, leptin, which is increased in obese people, promotes cell proliferation.

Metabolic Syndrome

Metabolic syndrome is one of the fastest-growing obesity health concerns. It is discussed later in this chapter on p. 921.

Psychosocial Problems

The consequences of obesity extend beyond the physical changes. Stigmatization of obese people, and in some cases discrimination, occurs in three important areas of living: employment, education, and health care. The social stigma associated with obesity has an emotional toll on a person's psychologic well-being. Many obese persons suffer low self-esteem, withdraw from social interaction, and experience major depression.

NURSING AND COLLABORATIVE MANAGEMENT OBESITY

NURSING ASSESSMENT

The first step in the treatment of obesity is to determine whether any physical conditions are present that may be causing or contributing to obesity. This requires a thorough history and physical examination.

Table 41-5 lists information that can assist you in understanding an obese patient and provides a basis for intervention. When assessing an individual who is overweight or obese, be sensitive and nonjudgmental in asking specific and leading questions about weight, diet, and exercise (Table 41-6). In doing so, you can often obtain information that the patient might have withheld out of embarrassment or shyness. Patients need to understand the rationale for questions asked about weight or dietary habits, and you must be ready to respond to their concerns.

When obtaining the history, explore genetic and endocrine factors such as hypothyroidism, hypothalamic tumors, Cushing syndrome, hypogonadism in men, and polycystic ovary syndrome in women. Laboratory tests of liver function and thyroid function, a fasting glucose level, and a lipid panel (triglyceride level, LDL and HDL cholesterol levels) assist in evaluating the cause and effects of obesity. When no organic cause (e.g., hypothyroidism) is associated with obesity, the disorder should be considered a chronic, complex illness.

As part of the initial nursing history and physical examination, examine each body system with particular attention to the organ system in which the patient has expressed a problem or concern. Measurements used with the obese person may include skinfold thickness, waist circumference, height (without

---

TABLE 41-5 NURSING ASSESSMENT
Obese Patient

Subjective Data
Important Health Information
Past health history: Time of obesity onset; diseases related to metabolism and obesity, such as hypertension, cardiovascular problems, stroke, cancer, chronic joint pain, respiratory problems, diabetes mellitus, cholelithiasis, metabolic syndrome
Medications: Thyroid preparations, diet pills, herbal products
Surgery or other treatments: Prior weight-reduction procedures (bariatric surgery)

Functional Health Patterns
Health perception–health management: Family history of obesity; perception of problem; methods of weight loss attempted
Nutritional-metabolic: Amount and frequency of eating; overeating in response to boredom, stress, specific times, or activities; history of weight gain and loss
Elimination: Constipation
Activity-exercise: Typical physical activity; drowsiness, somnolence; dyspnea on exertion, orthopnea, paroxysmal nocturnal dyspnea
Sleep-rest: Sleep apnea, use of continuous positive airway pressure (CPAP)
Cognitive-perceptual: Feelings of rejection, depression, isolation, guilt, or shame; meaning or value of food; adherence to prescribed reducing diets, degree of long-term commitment to a weight loss program
Role-relationship: Change in financial status or family relationships; personal, social, and financial resources to support a reducing diet
Sexuality-reproductive: Menstrual irregularity, heavy menstrual flow in women, birth control practices, infertility; effect of obesity on sexual activity and attractiveness to significant other

Objective Data
General
Body mass index $\geq$30 kg/m^2; waist circumference: woman >35 in (89 cm), man >40 in (102 cm)

Respiratory
Increased work of breathing; wheezing; rapid, shallow breathing

Cardiovascular
Hypertension, tachycardia, dysrhythmias

Musculoskeletal
Decreased joint mobility and flexibility; knee, hip, and low back pain

Reproductive
Gynecomastia and hypogonadism in men

Possible Findings
Elevated serum glucose, cholesterol, triglycerides; chest x-ray demonstrating enlarged heart; electrocardiogram showing dysrhythmia; abnormal liver function tests

---

shoes), weight (obtain in a private location and in a gown if possible), and BMI. Provide specific documentation on these areas. Also assess for any co-morbid diseases associated with obesity (e.g., hypertension, sleep apnea), since these conditions require special treatment.

PLANNING

The overall goals are that the obese patient will (1) modify eating patterns, (2) participate in a regular physical activity program, (3) achieve and maintain weight loss to a specified level, and (4) minimize or prevent health problems related to obesity.

TABLE 41-6 ASSESSING PATIENTS WITH OBESITY

When assessing patients with obesity and before selecting a weight loss strategy, ask the following questions.

- What is your history with weight gain and weight loss?
- What is your motivation for losing weight?
- Would you like to manage your weight differently? If so, how?
- What do you think contributes to your weight?
- What sort of barriers do you think impede your weight loss efforts?
- Are there any major stresses that will make it difficult to focus on weight control?
- What does food mean to you? How do you use food (e.g., to relieve stress, provide comfort)?
- Are other family members overweight?
- How much time can you devote to exercise on a daily or weekly basis?
- How has your health been affected by your body weight?
- What type of support do you have from family and/or friends for losing weight?

TABLE 41-7 COLLABORATIVE CARE

Obesity

Diagnostic
- History and physical examination
- BMI
- Waist-to-hip ratio

Collaborative Therapy
- Nutritional therapy
- Exercise
- Behavior modification
- Support groups
- Drug therapy
  - Appetite-suppressing drugs
  - Nutrient absorption–blocking drugs (orlistat [Xenical])
  - Serotonin agonists (lorcaserin [Belviq])
  - phentermine and topiramate (Qsymia)
- Surgical therapy (see Table 41-9)

BMI, Body mass index.

NURSING IMPLEMENTATION

Obesity is one of the most challenging health crises in the United States. It is a chronic disease, much like hypertension and diabetes. Although obese people can lose weight, they often tend to regain weight. For most patients, lifelong management is indicated.

Together with other members of the health care team, you have a major role in planning for and managing the care of an obese patient. First, examine your own personal beliefs and any potential biases related to obesity. If you associate obesity with a lack of willpower and with overindulgence, the patient can experience shame in a setting that claims to be a caring one. You are in a pivotal position to help overweight and obese individuals. Interventions include helping obese patients explore and deal with their negative experiences and educating other health professionals about stigma and biases experienced by obese patients.

Although health care for obese people has inherently greater demands, health care providers often fail to address these needs, and obese people underutilize health care opportunities available to them. Health care providers are often reluctant to counsel patients about obesity for a variety of reasons, including (1) time constraints during appointments make it difficult, (2) weight management may be viewed as professionally unrewarding, (3) reimbursement for weight management services is difficult to obtain, and (4) many providers do not feel knowledgeable about giving weight loss advice.

Despite the known benefits of weight loss, it is a difficult process for most individuals. Obesity treatment begins with patients understanding their weight history and deciding on a plan that is best for them. In general, the average weight loss program (except for bariatric surgery) results in a 10% reduction of body weight. This average reduction should not be considered a failure, since it is associated with significant health benefits.

Exploring an individual's motivation for weight loss is essential for overall success. Using principles from motivational interviewing (discussed in Chapter 11 on p. 157), you can help patients understand their desire to lose weight and gain confidence in achieving weight loss.[17]

Focusing on the reasons for wanting to lose weight may help patients develop strategies for a weight loss program. Any

supervised plan of care must be directed at two different processes: (1) successful weight loss, which requires a short-term energy deficit; and (2) successful weight control, which requires long-term behavior changes.[18]

A multifaceted approach needs to be used, including nutritional therapy, exercise, behavior modification, and for some, medication or surgical intervention (Table 41-7). Focusing on more than one aspect provides for more effective weight loss and weight control efforts. While doing patient teaching, stress healthy eating habits and adequate physical activity as lifestyle patterns to develop and maintain.

A number of smart phone applications are now available to help patients track eating patterns, calories, and exercise. These tracking systems may provide a patient with immediate access to nutritional information for better dietary decision making.

Even with a comprehensive action plan, there is a high rate of weight regain. This is discouraging when one considers the amount of time, effort, and money expended in attempts to lose weight. For successful management of obesity, it is beneficial to view obesity as a chronic life-long condition that necessitates day-to-day attention.

NUTRITIONAL THERAPY. Restricting dietary intake so that it is below energy requirements is a cornerstone for any weight loss or maintenance program. A good weight loss plan should contain foods from the basic food groups (MyPlate is presented in Fig. 40-1 and Table 40-1). A dietary reduction of at least 500 to 1000 cal/day is recommended for an expected weight loss of 1 to 2 lb/wk.[18] (Table 41-8 presents an example of a 1200-calorie diet.)

A supervised diet plan may be prescribed limiting calories to a total of 800 or less calories per day, but this is not sustainable on a long-term basis. Persons on low-calorie and very-low-calorie diets need frequent professional monitoring because the severe energy restriction places them at risk for multiple nutrient deficiencies.

In general, it is best to recommend a diet that includes adequate amounts of fruits and vegetables, provides enough bulk to prevent constipation, and meets daily vitamin A and vitamin C requirements. Lean meat, fish, and eggs provide sufficient protein and the B-complex vitamins.

It is rare to find an overweight person who has not at some time attempted to lose weight. Some people met with limited

TABLE 41-8   NUTRITIONAL THERAPY

1200-Calorie–Restricted Weight-Reduction Diet*

General Principles
1. Eat regularly. Do not skip meals.
2. Measure foods to determine the correct portion size.
3. Avoid concentrated sweets, such as sugar, candy, honey, pies, cakes, cookies, and regular sodas.
4. Reduce fat intake by baking, broiling, or steaming foods.
5. Maintain a regular exercise program for successful weight loss.

Meal	Exchanges	Menu Plan†
Breakfast	1 meat	1 hard-boiled egg
	2 bread	1 slice toast
		¾ cup dry cereal (unsweetened)
	1 fruit	½ small banana
	1 fat	1 tsp margarine
	1 dairy‡	1 cup low-fat milk
	Beverage	Coffee
Lunch	2 meat	Cheese enchiladas (made with 2 oz
	2 bread	cheese, two corn tortillas, lettuce,
	Vegetable	chili sauce)
	1 fruit	Fresh grapes (12)
	Beverage	Diet soda
Dinner	2 meat	2 oz baked chicken
	1 bread	Corn on the cob with 1 tsp margarine
	Vegetable	Tossed salad and 1 tbs salad dressing
	1 fruit	¾ cup strawberries
	1 milk	1 cup low-fat milk

*For 1000 cal, omit 1 fruit exchange and change low-fat milk to skim milk. For 1500 cal, add 1 meat exchange, 1 fruit exchange, and 2 fat exchanges; change low-fat milk to whole milk. For 1800 cal, add 2 bread exchanges, 3 meat exchanges, 3 fat exchanges, and 1 fruit exchange; change low-fat milk to whole milk.
†Additional sample meal plans are presented in eTable 41-2 available on the website for this chapter.
‡One extra fat exchange allowed for each cup of 2% low-fat milk; 2 extra fat exchanges allowed for each cup of skim milk.

and temporary success, and others have met only with failure. Many individuals attempt weight loss by trying one of the many fad diets that offer the enticement of quick weight loss with little effort (see eTable 41-1 on the website). Often these quick weight-reduction diets (found in the popular media) advocate the elimination of one category of foods (e.g., carbohydrates). Therefore these should be discouraged. Low-carbohydrate diets do produce a rapid weight loss, but reduce the opportunity to get adequate amounts of fiber, vitamins, and minerals. These restrictive diets are difficult to maintain in the long term. It is best to recommend a dietary approach in which calorie restriction includes all food groups. Patients will find it easier to incorporate such a change into their lifestyle and not become as bored with their food options.

The weight loss associated with fad diets is generally short lived. The MyPlate guidelines have longer-lasting results. However, the degree of weight loss strongly depends on the patient's ability to adhere to the diet. The more restrictive the regimen, the greater the demand for intense discipline in the face of an intense desire to eat foods not allowed on the diet.[19]

The degree of success of any reducing diet depends in part on the amount of weight to be lost. A moderately obese person will obviously attain his or her goal more easily than a severely obese person. Because men have a higher percentage of lean body mass, they are often able to lose weight more quickly than women. Women have a higher percentage of body fat, which is metabolically less active than muscle tissue. Postmenopausal women are particularly prone to weight gain, including increased abdominal fat.

Motivation is an essential ingredient for successful weight loss. The obese patient must recognize the advantages of weight loss and weight control. You can assist by helping the patient track eating patterns with a diet diary. Through a frank discussion of eating patterns, the patient often realizes that eating is "mindless" and the result of bad habits picked up over time. These eating behaviors must be changed, or any weight loss will only be temporary.

Setting a realistic and healthy goal, such as losing 1 to 2 lb/wk, should be mutually agreed on at the beginning of counseling. Trying to lose too much too fast usually results in a sense of frustration and failure for the patient. You can help patients understand that losing large amounts of weight in a short period causes skin and underlying tissue to lose elasticity and tone. Slower weight loss offers better cosmetic results.

Inevitably, the patient reaches plateau periods during which no weight is lost. These plateaus may last from several days to several weeks. Remind the patient that plateaus are normal occurrences during weight reduction. A weekly check of body weight is a good method of monitoring progress. Daily weighing is not recommended because of the frequent fluctuations resulting from retained water (including urine) and elimination of feces. Instruct the patient to record the weight at the same time of the day, wearing the same type of clothing.

Experts disagree on the number of meals to be eaten when a person is on a diet. Some nutritionists advocate several small meals per day because the body's metabolic rate is temporarily increased immediately after eating. However, when eating several small meals a day, patients may consume more calories unless they carefully adhere to portion sizes and total daily calorie allotment.

When a person first starts a weight-reduction program, food portion sizes need to be carefully determined to stay within the dietary guidelines. Portion sizes over the past 20 years have increased considerably[12] (see Table 41-4). Food portions can be weighed using a scale, or everyday objects can be used as a visual cue to determine portion sizes. The size of a woman's fist or a baseball is equivalent to a serving of vegetables or fruit. A serving of meat is about the size of a person's palm or a deck of cards. A serving of cheese is about the size of a thumb or six dice. A test on portion sizes is available at *http://hin.nhlbi.nih.gov/portion/index.htm*.

Another aspect of the American diet that needs to be considered is which foods contribute the most calories—animal sources, fruits, grains, or vegetables. Two thirds or more of an individual's diet should be plant-source foods, and the other one third or less should be from animal protein. Being aware of personal consumption habits and striving for the two-thirds to one-third ratio is a simple goal that can be achieved without weighing and measuring foods at every meal. Once this ratio has been adopted into the patient's meal planning, portions can gradually be reduced as activity levels are gradually increased to achieve healthy weight loss. The recommended portion size of animal protein is 3 oz. The standard size for chopped vegetables is ½ cup, according to MyPlate guidelines (see Table 40-1).

A list of healthy or low-calorie foods serves as a good reference and permits an occasional meal to be eaten at a restaurant. Furthermore, the patient who carefully follows the prescribed diet may not need to take vitamin supplements. Encourage the appropriate fluid intake in the form of water. Alcoholic and sugary beverages should be limited or avoided, since they increase caloric intake and are low in nutritional value.

EXERCISE. Exercise is an essential part of a weight control program. Patients should exercise daily, preferably 30 minutes to an hour. There is no evidence that increased activity promotes an increase in appetite or leads to dietary excess. In fact, exercise frequently has the opposite effect. The addition of exercise produces more weight loss than does dieting alone and has a favorable effect on body fat distribution. With regular exercise, WHR is reduced. Finally, exercise is especially important in maintaining weight loss.

When large muscles are involved in the exercise program, a primary benefit is cardiovascular conditioning. Overweight men and women who are active and fit have lower rates of morbidity and mortality than overweight persons who are sedentary and unfit. Therefore exercise is of benefit to overweight persons even if it does not make them lean. Many psychologic benefits can be derived from an increased physical activity program. Exercise decreases tension and stress, promotes better-quality sleep and rest, increases stamina and energy, improves self-concept and self-confidence, improves attitudes, and increases optimism about the future.[18]

Explore with the patient possible ways to incorporate exercise in daily routines. It may be as simple as parking farther from their place of employment or taking the stairs versus an elevator. Encourage individuals to wear a pedometer to track their activity with a goal of 10,000 steps a day. However, success may be walking one third of the recommended steps with incremental increases over time. Although joining a health club can be one way of getting exercise, it is not necessary. Patients can walk, swim, and cycle, all of which have long-term benefits. Stress to patients that engaging in weekend exercise only or in spurts of strenuous activity is not advantageous and can actually be dangerous.

BEHAVIOR MODIFICATION. The assumption behind behavior modification is twofold: (1) obesity is a learned disorder caused by overeating and (2) often the critical difference between an obese person and a person of normal weight is the cues that regulate eating behavior. Therefore most behavior-modification programs deemphasize the diet and focus on how and when to eat.

Teach people to restrict their eating to designated meals and to increase the amount of physical activity in their lives. Persons who participate in a behavioral therapy program are more successful in maintaining their losses over an extended time than those who do not participate in such training.

Various behavioral techniques for patients engaged in a weight loss program include (1) self-monitoring, (2) stimulus control, and (3) rewards. *Self-monitoring* may involve keeping a record of the type and time food was consumed and how the person was feeling when eating. *Stimulus control* is aimed at separating events that trigger eating from the act of eating. *Rewards* may be used as incentives for weight loss. Short- and long-term goals are useful benchmarks for earning rewards. It is important that the reward for a specified weight loss not be associated with food, such as dinner out or a favorite treat. Reward items do not have to have a monetary component. For example, time for a hot bath or an hour of pleasure reading would be an enjoyable reward for many people.

SUPPORT GROUPS. People who are on a weight management plan are often encouraged to join a group where others are also trying to modify their eating habits. Many self-help groups

are available that offer support and information on dieting tips. For example, Take Off Pounds Sensibly (TOPS) (*www.tops. org*) is the oldest nonprofit organization of this type. Behavior modification is an integral part of the program, along with nutrition education. Weight Watchers International, Inc. (*www.weightwatchers.com*) is probably the most successful commercial weight-reduction enterprise. Weight Watchers offers a food plan that is nutritionally balanced and practical to follow. Group leaders, all of whom have successfully lost weight with Weight Watchers, teach members various behavior-modification techniques.

Commercial weight-reduction centers have proliferated across the nation. Many of these programs are staffed by nurses and dietitians. An initial physical examination by a health care provider is required before a candidate is accepted for weight reduction. These weight-reduction centers are cost prohibitive for those with limited financial resources. Many of these programs also offer special prepackaged foods and supplements that must be purchased as part of the weight-reduction plan. Only these prescribed foods and drinks are to be consumed until an agreed-on amount of weight is lost. The patient is encouraged to buy the same type of foods for the maintenance phase of the program, lasting from 6 months to 1 year. Behavior-modification training is incorporated in these programs as well. Individuals must learn how to adjust their diet once they are no longer using the commercial products. This can be challenging for many, and the weight lost may be regained once the restricted food program is completed.

In recent years a number of employers have begun weight loss programs at the workplace. The rationale for such programs is that better health repays the cost of the programs through improved work performance, decreased absenteeism, less hospitalization, and lower insurance costs. Such programs have been well accepted by both employees and employers.

DRUG THERAPY

Drugs should never be used alone. Rather, they should be part of a comprehensive weight-reduction program that includes reduced-calorie diet, exercise, and behavior modification. Drugs should be reserved for adults with a BMI of 30 kg/m^2 or greater (obese), or adults with a BMI of 27 kg/m^2 or greater (overweight) who have at least one weight-related condition such as hypertension, type 2 diabetes, or dyslipidemia.

Appetite-Suppressing Drugs

The sympathomimetic amines suppress appetite by increasing the availability of norepinephrine in the brain, thus stimulating the central nervous system. The sympathomimetics fall into two groups: amphetamines and nonamphetamines. The amphetamines have a much higher abuse potential than the nonamphetamines. Amphetamines are not recommended nor are they approved by the U.S. Food and Drug Administration (FDA) for either short- or long-term weight loss.

Nonamphetamines are not usually recommended for weight loss because of the potential for abuse. If used, these drugs should only be used short term (for 3 months or less). Nonamphetamines include phentermine (Adipex-P, Fastin, Ionamin), diethylpropion (Tenuate), phendimetrazine (Bontril), and benzphetamine (Didrex). Adverse effects of these drugs include palpitations, tachycardia, overstimulation, restlessness, dizziness, insomnia, weakness, and fatigue.

Nutrient Absorption–Blocking Drugs

Orlistat (Xenical) works by blocking fat breakdown and absorption in the intestine. It inhibits the action of intestinal lipases, resulting in undigested fat excreted in the feces. Some fat-soluble vitamin levels may also decrease and may need to be supplemented. Allī, a low-dose form of orlistat, is available for over-the-counter use.

Orlistat is associated with leakage of stool, flatulence, diarrhea, and abdominal bloating, which is accentuated if a high-fat diet is consumed. These side effects limit its acceptance as a weight loss tool. Severe liver injury has been reported in patients using orlistat.[20]

Serotonin Agonist

Lorcaserin (Belviq) is a selective serotonin (5-HT) agonist that suppresses appetite and creates a sense of satiety. Lorcaserin works by activating the serotonin receptor in the brain. Activation of this receptor may help a person eat less and feel full after eating smaller amounts of food. The most common side effects are headache, dizziness, fatigue, nausea, dry mouth, and constipation.

Phentermine and Topiramate (Qsymia)

Qsymia is a combination of two drugs, phentermine and topiramate. Phentermine is a sympathomimetic agent already approved for short-term management of obesity. Topiramate is currently approved for seizure disorders and prophylaxis of migraine. In overweight patients, phentermine suppresses appetite, and topiramate induces a sense of satiety. Qsymia must not be used in patients with glaucoma or hyperthyroidism. Qsymia can increase heart rate, and its effect on the heart rate in patients at high risk for heart attack or stroke is not known.

Nursing Interventions Related to Drug Therapy

Drugs will not cure obesity, and individuals must understand that without substantial changes in food intake and increased physical activity, they will gain weight when drug therapy is stopped. As with any drug treatment, there are side effects. Careful evaluation for other medical conditions can help determine which drugs, if any, would be advisable for a given patient.

Your role related to drug therapy is to teach the patient about proper administration, side effects, and how the drugs fit into the overall weight loss plan. The modification of dosage without consultation with the health care provider can have detrimental effects. Emphasize that diet and exercise regimens are the cornerstones of permanent weight loss. Finally, discourage the purchase of over-the-counter diet aids except for Allī.

SURGICAL THERAPY

Bariatric surgery has become a viable and popular option for treating obesity.[21] Surgery is currently the only treatment that has been found to have a successful and lasting impact for sustained weight loss for severely obese individuals.[22]

The majority of people who undergo bariatric surgery successfully improve their overall quality of life. In addition to losing weight, patients often experience resolution of comorbidities such as diabetes. Although overall mortality is very low, a number of complications can arise from surgery, and the option to have surgery must be carefully considered.

Criteria guidelines for bariatric surgery include having a BMI of 40 kg/m^2 or a BMI of 35 kg/m^2 with one or more severe obesity-related medical complications (e.g., hypertension, type 2 diabetes mellitus, heart failure, sleep apnea). Many insurance carriers do not cover the cost of bariatric surgery. If they do consider reimbursing for the surgery, most of them require documentation of a medically supervised weight loss program for approximately 6 months.[23]

Before being considered candidates for surgery, patients must be screened for psychologic, physical, and behavioral conditions that have been associated with poor surgical outcomes. These include untreated depression, binge eating disorders, and drug and alcohol abuse that may interfere with a commitment to lifelong behavioral changes. Other contraindications to surgery include illnesses that are known to reduce life expectancy and are not likely to be improved with weight reduction. These conditions include advanced cancer; end-stage kidney, liver, and cardiopulmonary disease; severe coagulopathy; or inability to comply with nutritional recommendations.[24]

Bariatric surgeries fall into one of three broad categories: restrictive, malabsorptive, or a combination of malabsorptive and restrictive (Table 41-9 and Fig. 41-5). In *restrictive procedures* the stomach is reduced in size (less food eaten), and in *malabsorptive procedures* the length of the small intestine is decreased (less food absorbed).[21] The majority of procedures are performed laparoscopically, thus decreasing postoperative recuperation as compared to an open procedure. With laparoscopy, patients have fewer wound infections, shorter hospital stays, and a faster recovery period.[23]

Restrictive Surgeries

Restrictive bariatric surgery reduces either the size of the stomach, which causes the patient to feel full more quickly, or the amount allowed to enter the stomach. In these surgeries, digestion is not altered so the risk of anemia or cobalamin deficiency is low. The most common restrictive surgeries include adjustable gastric banding and vertical sleeve gastrectomy.[24]

Adjustable Gastric Banding. Laparoscopic *adjustable gastric banding* (AGB), the most common restrictive procedure done, involves limiting the stomach size with an inflatable band placed around the fundus of the stomach (Fig. 41-5, *A*). This restrictive procedure can be done using a Lap-Band or Realize Band system. The band is connected to a subcutaneous port and can be inflated or deflated (by fluid injection in the health care provider's office) to change the stoma size to meet the patient's needs as weight is lost. The restrictive effect of the band creates a sense of fullness as the upper portion of the stomach now accommodates less than the average stomach. The band then causes a delay in stomach emptying, providing patients with further satiety.

The procedure can be either modified or reversed at a later date if necessary. AGB is the preferred option for patients who are surgical risks because it is a less invasive approach.

Vertical Sleeve Gastrectomy. In the vertical sleeve gastrectomy, about 85% of the stomach is removed, leaving a sleeve-shaped stomach (Fig. 41-5, *B*). Although the stomach is drastically reduced in size, its function is preserved. The procedure is not reversible. The removal of the majority of the stomach also results in the elimination of hormones produced in the stomach that stimulate hunger, such as ghrelin.

Combination of Restrictive and Malabsorptive Surgery

Roux-en-Y Gastric Bypass. The Roux-en-Y gastric bypass (RYGB) procedure is a combination of restrictive and malab-

TABLE 41-9 SURGICAL INTERVENTIONS FOR OBESITY*

Procedure	Anatomic Changes	Advantages	Complications
Restrictive Surgery			
Adjustable gastric banding (AGB) (Lap-Band, Realize Band)	Band encircles the stomach, creating a stoma and a gastric pouch with about 30 mL capacity	• Food digestion occurs through normal process • Band can be adjusted to ↑ or ↓ restriction • Surgery can be reversed • Absence of dumping syndrome • Lack of malabsorption	• Low complication rate • Some nausea and vomiting initially • Problems with adjustment device • Band may slip or erode into stomach wall • Gastric perforation
Vertical sleeve gastrectomy	About 85% of stomach removed, leaving a sleeve-shaped stomach with 60-150 mL capacity	• Function of stomach preserved • No bypass of intestine • Avoids complications of obstruction, anemia, vitamin deficiencies	• Weight loss may be limited • Leakage related to stapling
Vertical banded gastroplasty (VBG)	Band placed around stomach, and staples used above band to create a small gastric pouch	• No surgical anastomosis • More normal anatomy and physiology maintained • Lower risk of infection	• High complication rate • Slow weight loss • Rupture of staple line • Dilated pouch • Dumping syndrome (nausea, vomiting, and/or diarrhea related to ingestion of sweets, high-calorie liquids, or dairy products)
Malabsorptive Surgery			
Biliopancreatic diversion (BPD) with or without duodenal switch	70% of the stomach removed horizontally Anastomosis between the stomach and the intestine Decreases the amount of small intestine available for nutrient absorption Duodenal switch cuts the stomach vertically and is shaped like a tube	• Increased amount of food intake • Less food intolerance • Greater long-term weight loss • Rapid weight loss	• Abdominal bloating, diarrhea, and foul-smelling gas (steatorrhea) • Three or four loose bowel movements a day • Malabsorption of fat-soluble vitamins • Iron deficiency • Protein-calorie malnutrition • Dumping syndrome (with duodenal switch, last two problems are less common)
Combination of Restrictive and Malabsorptive Surgery			
Roux-en-Y gastric bypass (RYGB)	Restrictive surgery on stomach creating pouch Small gastric pouch connected to jejunum Remaining stomach and first segment of small intestine are bypassed	• Better weight loss results than with gastric restrictive procedures • Lower incidence of malnutrition and diarrhea • Rapid improvement of weight-related co-morbidities	• Leak at site of anastomosis • Anemia: iron deficiency, cobalamin deficiency, folic acid deficiency • Calcium deficiency • Dumping syndrome

*See Fig. 41-5.

sorptive surgery. This surgical procedure is the most common bariatric procedure performed in the United States and is considered the gold standard among bariatric procedures.

This procedure, which is irreversible, involves creating a small gastric pouch and attaching it directly to the small intestine using a Y-shaped limb of the small bowel. After the procedure, food bypasses 90% of the stomach, the duodenum, and a small segment of jejunum.

Overall, it has low complication rates, has excellent patient tolerance, and sustains long-term weight loss. Outcomes include improved glucose control with improvement or reversal of diabetes, normalization of BP, decreased total cholesterol and triglycerides, decreased GERD, and decreased sleep apnea.[25]

A complication of the RYGB is *dumping syndrome,* in which gastric contents empty too rapidly into the small intestine, overwhelming its ability to digest nutrients. Symptoms can include vomiting, nausea, weakness, sweating, faintness, and, on occasion, diarrhea. Patients are discouraged from eating sugary foods after surgery to avoid dumping syndrome.[25] Because sections of the small intestine are bypassed, poor absorption of iron can cause iron-deficiency anemia. Patients need to take a multivitamin with iron and calcium supplements. Chronic anemia caused by cobalamin deficiency may also occur. This

problem can usually be managed with parenteral or intranasal cobalamin.

Cosmetic Surgeries to Reduce Fatty Tissue and Skinfolds

Lipectomy. Lipectomy (adipectomy) is performed to remove unsightly flabby folds of adipose tissue (Fig. 41-6). In some patients, up to 15% of the total fat cells can be removed from the breasts, abdomen, and lumbar and femoral areas. There is no evidence that a regeneration of adipose tissue occurs at the surgical sites. However, emphasize to the patient that surgical removal does not prevent obesity from recurring, especially if lifetime eating habits remain the same. Although body image and self-esteem may be enhanced by such procedures, these operations are not without complications. The dangerous effects of anesthesia and the potential for poor wound healing in the obese patient cannot be overemphasized.

Liposuction. Another cosmetic surgical procedure is liposuction, or suction-assisted lipectomy. It is used for cosmetic purposes and not for weight reduction. This surgical intervention helps improve facial appearance or body contours. A good candidate for this type of surgery is a person who has achieved weight reduction but who has excess fat under the chin, along the jaw line, in the nasolabial folds, over the abdomen, or

FIG. 41-5 Bariatric surgical procedures. **A,** Adjustable gastric banding (AGB) uses a band to create a gastric pouch. **B,** Vertical sleeve gastrectomy involves creating a sleeve-shaped stomach by removing about 80% of the stomach. **C,** Vertical banded gastroplasty (VBG) involves creating a small gastric pouch. **D,** Biliopancreatic diversion (BPD) with duodenal switch procedure creates an anastomosis between the stomach and the intestine. **E,** Roux-en-Y gastric bypass procedure involves constructing a gastric pouch whose outlet is a Y-shaped limb of small intestine.

FIG. 41-6 A, Preoperative view of a 37-year-old woman with massive weight loss who had gastric bypass surgery. **B,** Postoperative view 2½ years after abdominoplasty. She also underwent breast surgery, thighlift, backlift with excision of excess skin of the lower back and upper buttocks, and upper arm surgery.

around the waist and upper thighs. A long, hollow, stainless steel cannula is inserted through a small incision over the fatty tissue to be suctioned. This surgical procedure is not usually recommended for the older person because the skin is less elastic and will not accommodate the new underlying shape.

NURSING MANAGEMENT
PERIOPERATIVE CARE OF THE OBESE PATIENT

NURSING IMPLEMENTATION

This section discusses general nursing considerations for the care of the obese patient who is having surgery. Special nursing considerations are described for the patient who is having bariatric surgery. (Care of the surgical patient is discussed in Chapters 18 to 20.)

PREOPERATIVE CARE. Special considerations are necessary for the obese patient, especially the severely obese individual, who is admitted to the hospital for surgery.[26] Before surgery, interview the patient to identify past and current health information and any assistive devices currently in use (e.g., continuous positive airway pressure [CPAP] for sleep apnea). Co-morbidities secondary to obesity increase the risk for complications in the perioperative period. It may be necessary to coordinate care with the patient's cardiologist, pulmonologist, gynecologist, gastroenterologist, or other specialists.

Have a plan in place before the patients arrive so they receive optimal care and do not feel like they are a burden to the nursing staff. Nursing units must have available appropriate size hospital gowns, beds that accommodate an increased body size, and necessary patient transfer equipment. To correctly measure BP in obese people, a larger cuff size is needed to avoid artifactual errors. Ensure that oversized BP cuffs are available and placed in the patient's room.

Consider how the patient will be weighed and transported throughout the hospital. A wheelchair with removable arms that is large enough to safely accommodate the patient and pass easily through doorways should be available.

Preoperative and postoperative assessment of heart, lung, and bowel sounds may require the use of alternative assessment techniques. For example, because of the large chest wall, breath and heart sounds are often distant. Electronic stethoscopes can be used to amplify lung, heart, and bowel sounds. Pulse oximetry may also be used to assess oxygenation status.

Instruct the patient in the proper coughing and deep breathing techniques and methods of turning and positioning to prevent pulmonary complications after surgery. If possible, demonstrate the use of a spirometer before surgery. Use of the spirometer helps prevent and treat postoperative lung congestion. Practicing these strategies preoperatively can help the patient perform them correctly postoperatively. Furthermore, if the patient uses CPAP at home for sleep apnea, make arrangements for the use of a machine while the patient is hospitalized.

Obtaining venous access may be complicated by excess adipose tissue. A longer IV catheter is helpful (longer than 1 in) to go through the overlying tissue to the vein. It is important that the cannula is far enough into the vein to ensure that it is not dislodged or infiltrated.

Special Considerations for Bariatric Surgery. Ensure that the patient scheduled for bariatric surgery understands the surgical procedure. Your teaching depends on the type of procedure and surgical approach.

Prepare the patient before surgery for the possibility of returning with one or more of the following: urinary catheter, IV catheter, compression stockings, and nasogastric tube. Emphasize that vital signs and a general assessment will be conducted frequently to monitor for complications. Further, the patient must understand that he or she will be assisted with ambulation soon after surgery and encouraged to cough and deep breathe to prevent pulmonary complications. Liquids will be started early but only after the patient is fully awake and there is no evidence of any anastomosis leaks.

POSTOPERATIVE CARE. The initial postoperative care focuses on careful assessment and immediate intervention for cardiopulmonary complications, thrombus formation, anastomosis leaks, and electrolyte imbalances. The transfer from surgery may require many trained staff members. During the transfer, the patient's airway should remain stabilized and attention given to managing the patient's pain. Maintain the patient's head at a 35- to 40-degree angle to reduce abdominal pressure and increase lung expansion.

The body stores anesthetics in adipose tissue, thus placing patients with excess adipose tissue at risk for re-sedation. As adipose cells release anesthetics back into the bloodstream, the patient may become sedated after surgery. If this happens, be prepared to perform a head-tilt or jaw-thrust maneuver and keep the patient's oral and nasal airways open.[27]

Diligence in turning and ambulation postoperatively will prevent complications from surgery. Tell the patient that typically he or she will be assisted in walking the evening after surgery and then at least three or four times each day. The patient may be reluctant to move or may not have the stamina to walk even a short distance. In either situation, you will need additional help in facilitating movement in an obese patient.

Obesity can cause a patient's breathing to become shallow and rapid. The extra adipose tissue in the chest and abdomen compresses the diaphragmatic, thoracic, and abdominal structures. This compression restricts the chest's ability to expand, preventing the lungs from working as efficiently as they would otherwise. The patient retains more carbon dioxide with less oxygen delivered to the lungs. This results in hypoxemia, pulmonary hypertension, and polycythemia.

Postoperatively the risk for deep venous thrombosis (DVT) is increased. Venous stasis is common due to the pressure on the veins. Antiembolic stockings or sequential compression stockings may be ordered along with low-dose heparin to minimize the risk of a DVT. Active and passive range-of-motion exercises are a frequent part of daily care.

Wound infection, dehiscence, and delayed healing are potential problems for all obese patients. Assess the patient's skin for any complications related to wound healing. Keep skinfolds clean and dry to prevent dermatitis and secondary bacterial or fungal infections.

Special Considerations for Bariatric Surgery. Patients experience considerable abdominal pain after bariatric surgery. Give pain medications as necessary during the immediate postoperative period (first 24 hours). Be aware that pain could be from an anastomosis leak rather than typical surgical pain.

Abdominal wounds require frequent observation for the amount and type of drainage, condition of the incision, and signs of infection. Protect the incision against undue straining that accompanies turning and coughing. Monitor vital signs to assist in identifying problems such as infection.

If a nasogastric tube is inserted, monitor it for patency and keep it in the correct position. If the patient vomits with a nasogastric tube in place, it may require repositioning; notify the surgeon immediately. The upper gastric pouch is small, and irrigating the tube with too much solution or manipulating the tube position can lead to disruption of the anastomosis or staple line.

During the immediate postoperative period water and sugar-free clear liquids are given (30 mL every 2 hours while awake). Before discharge, instruct patients on a measured amount of a high-protein liquid diet. The patient is taught to eat slowly, stop eating when feeling full, and not consume liquids with solid food. Vomiting is a common complication during this time. A dietitian is usually part of the bariatric team and assists the patient with the transition to the new diet.

AMBULATORY AND HOME CARE

Special Considerations for Bariatric Surgery. The patient who has undergone major surgical treatment for obesity has not been successful in the past in following or maintaining a prescribed diet. Now the patient is forced to reduce oral intake because of the anatomic changes from the surgical procedure. The patient's adherence to a reduced intake is necessary because of the concern for abdominal distention, cramping abdominal pain, and perhaps diarrhea.

Weight loss is considerable during the first 6 to 12 months. During this time the patient must learn to adjust intake sufficiently to maintain a stable weight. Although behavior modification is not necessarily an intended outcome with these surgical procedures, it becomes an unexpected secondary gain. For example, a person who has had bariatric surgery cannot overeat or binge eat without consequences.

The diet generally prescribed should be high in protein and low in carbohydrates, fat, and roughage and consist of six small feedings daily. Fluids should not be ingested with the meal, and in some cases, fluids should be restricted to less than 1000 mL/day. Fluids and foods high in carbohydrate tend to promote diarrhea and symptoms of the dumping syndrome. Generally, calorically dense foods (foods high in fat) should be avoided to permit more nutritionally sound food to be consumed.

The patient must clearly understand the proper diet. Late complications can be anticipated after bariatric surgery, including anemia, vitamin deficiencies, diarrhea, and psychologic problems. Failure to lose weight or loss of too much weight may be caused by the surgical formation of too large a stomach pouch or of an outlet that is much too small, respectively. Peptic ulcer formation, dumping syndrome, and small bowel obstruction may be seen late in the recovery and rehabilitation stage.

Emphasize the importance of long-term follow-up care, in part because of potential complications late in the recovery period. Encourage patients to adhere strictly to the prescribed diet and to inform the health care provider of any changes in their physical or emotional condition. Some patients have been known to overeat when they return home and gain rather than lose weight.

Several potential psychologic problems may arise after surgery. Some patients express guilt feelings that weight loss was achieved by surgical interventions rather than by the "sheer willpower" of reduced dietary intake and exercise. Be ready to provide support and assist the patient in moving away from such negative feelings.

By 6 to 8 months after surgery, considerable weight loss has occurred, and patients are able to see how much their appearance has changed. Discussion of this possible outcome with the patient before surgery and again during the rehabilitation phase facilitates the patient's adjustment to a new body image. Do not hesitate to encourage counseling for unresolved psychologic issues.

Massive weight loss often leaves the patient with large quantities of flabby skin that can result in problems related to altered body image. Reconstructive surgery may alleviate this situation. Reductions of the breasts, upper arms, thighs, and excess abdominal skinfolds are possible solutions.

Often one result of bariatric surgery is the return of fertility in women. Pregnancy complications can result from anemia and nutritional deficiencies. Furthermore, depending on the type of surgery, intestinal obstructions and hernias are commonly experienced in pregnancy.[28] Gallbladder problems may also arise, leading to pancreatitis. Women must carefully consider the risk of pregnancy after bariatric surgery. In general, encourage women to postpone pregnancy for 12 to 18 months after bariatric surgery.[28]

EVALUATION

The expected outcomes are that the obese patient will
- Experience long-term weight loss
- Have improvement in obesity-related co-morbidities

EVIDENCE-BASED PRACTICE

Applying the Evidence

W.G. is a 35-yr-old male patient weighing 367 lb (166.4 kg) with a BMI of 54.3 kg/m^2. He underwent gastric bypass surgery and is now ready for discharge. The bariatric program at your institution recommends the attendance at support groups after surgery. W.G. informs you that he does not feel comfortable in group settings and will not be attending these meetings.

Best Available Evidence	Clinician Expertise	Patient Preferences and Values
Patients attending psychotherapeutic interventions or support groups in combination with bariatric surgery experience greater weight loss results than patients treated with only bariatric surgery.	You have heard from several former bariatric patients who have maintained their weight loss after surgery and attributed this success, in part, to their participation in the support group offered at your facility.	Patient does not feel comfortable in group settings.

Your Decision and Action

You explore W.G.'s feelings about groups and share the reports from former patients with him. He continues to be firm about his unwillingness to attend any support groups. You discuss with him that it is his decision and you will help monitor his progress. Gently remind him that he can change his decision at any time. Inform his physician of his choice.

Reference for Evidence

Beck NN, Johannsen M, Støving RK, et al: Do postoperative psychotherapeutic interventions and support groups influence weight loss following bariatric surgery? A systematic review and meta-analysis of randomized and nonrandomized trials, *Obes Surg* 22(11):1790, 2012.

- Integrate healthy practices into daily routines
- Monitor for adverse side effects of surgical therapy
- Have an improved self-image

GERONTOLOGIC CONSIDERATIONS

OBESITY IN OLDER ADULTS

The prevalence of obesity is increasing in all age-groups, including older people. The number of obese older persons has markedly risen because of increases in both the total number of older persons and the percentage of the older adults who are obese. Obesity is more common in older women than in older men. A decrease in energy expenditure is an important contributor to a gradual increase in body fat with age.

Obesity in older adults can exacerbate age-related declines in physical function and lead to frailty and disability. Obesity is associated with decreased survival. Individuals who are obese live 6 to 7 years less than people of normal weight do.

Many of the changes associated with aging are exacerbated by obesity. Excess body weight places more demands on arthritic joints. The mechanical strain on weight-bearing joints can lead to premature immobility. Excess weight also affects other body systems. Older adults may find that excess intraabdominal weight causes problems with urinary incontinence. In addition, excess weight may contribute to hypoventilation and sleep apnea.

TABLE 41-10	CRITERIA FOR METABOLIC SYNDROME*
Measure	**Criteria**
Waist circumference	≥40 in (102 cm) in men ≥35 in (89 cm) in women
Triglycerides	>150 mg/dL (1.7 mmol/L) OR Drug treatment for elevated triglycerides
High-density lipoprotein (HDL) cholesterol	<40 mg/dL (0.9 mmol/L) in men <50 mg/dL (1.1 mmol/L) in women OR Drug treatment for reduced HDL cholesterol
BP	≥130 mm Hg systolic BP OR ≥85 mm Hg diastolic BP OR Drug treatment for hypertension
Fasting blood glucose	≥110 mg/dL OR Drug treatment for elevated glucose

Source: National Heart, Lung, and Blood Institute: How is metabolic syndrome diagnosed? Retrieved from *www.nhlbi.nih.gov/health/dci/Diseases/ms/ms_diagnosis.html.*
*Any three of the five measures are needed for a diagnosis of metabolic syndrome.

FIG. 41-7 Relationship among insulin resistance, obesity, diabetes mellitus, and cardiovascular disease. *HDL,* High-density lipoprotein.

Obesity affects the quality of life for older adults. Weight loss can improve physical functioning and obesity-related health complications. The same therapeutic approaches for obesity as were discussed earlier also apply to the older adult.

METABOLIC SYNDROME

Metabolic syndrome, also known as *syndrome X, insulin resistance syndrome,* and *dysmetabolic syndrome,* is a collection of risk factors that increase an individual's chance of developing cardiovascular disease, stroke, and diabetes mellitus. It is estimated that around 70 million to 80 million, or about 25%, of Americans have metabolic syndrome.[29] The syndrome is more prevalent in those 60 years of age and older.[30]

Metabolic syndrome is characterized by a cluster of health problems, including obesity, hypertension, abnormal lipid levels, and high blood glucose. Metabolic syndrome is diagnosed if an individual has three or more of the conditions listed in Table 41-10.

Currently health professionals are debating the usefulness of focusing attention on the syndrome itself. The interventions are focused on each risk factor, since there is not one standard treatment for the syndrome itself.[30]

Etiology and Pathophysiology

The main underlying risk factor for metabolic syndrome is insulin resistance related to excessive visceral fat (Fig. 41-7). Insulin resistance is the body's cells diminished ability to respond to the action of insulin. The pancreas compensates by secreting more insulin, resulting in hyperinsulinemia.

Other characteristics of metabolic syndrome include hypertension, increased risk for clotting, and abnormalities in cholesterol levels. The net effect of these conditions is an increased prevalence of coronary artery disease.

Genetics and environment have important roles in the development of metabolic syndrome. African Americans, Hispanics, Native Americans, and Asians are at an increased risk for metabolic syndrome. Environmental factors that influence the chances of having the syndrome are the same involved in the development of obesity. Metabolic syndrome is also associated with aging.

Clinical Manifestations and Diagnostic Studies

The signs of metabolic syndrome are impaired fasting blood glucose, hypertension, abnormal cholesterol levels, and obesity. Medical problems develop over time if the condition remains unaddressed. Patients with this syndrome are at a higher risk of heart disease, stroke, diabetes, renal disease, and polycystic ovary syndrome. Patients who have metabolic syndrome and smoke are at an even higher risk.

NURSING AND COLLABORATIVE MANAGEMENT METABOLIC SYNDROME

Lifestyle modifications are the first-line interventions to reduce the risk factors for metabolic syndrome. Management or reversal of metabolic syndrome can be achieved by reducing the major risk factors of cardiovascular disease: reducing LDL cholesterol, stopping smoking, lowering BP, and reducing glucose levels. For long-term risk reduction, weight should be decreased, physical activity increased, and healthy dietary habits established.

There is no specific management of metabolic syndrome. You can assist patients by providing information on healthy diets, exercise, and positive lifestyle changes. The diet, which should be low in saturated fats, should promote weight loss. Weight reduction and maintenance of a lower weight should be the first priority in those with abdominal obesity and metabolic syndrome.

Because sedentary lifestyles contribute to metabolic syndrome, increasing regular physical activity will lower a patient's risk factors. In addition to assisting in weight reduction, regular

CASE STUDY

Obesity

Hemera/Thinkstock

Patient Profile
S.R. is a 48-yr-old white woman.

Subjective Data
- Reports gradual weight gain of 40 lb during past 40 yr
- Lives in a rural community with no sidewalks
- Spends most of her free time watching television
- Reports health problems related to type 2 diabetes mellitus, shortness of breath, hypertension, and osteoarthritis
- Had knee replacement surgery at age 46 for osteo-arthritis

Objective Data
Physical Examination
- 5 ft, 4 in tall; weighs 210 lb; waist circumference of 39 in
- Has obese, nontender, soft round, abdomen
- BP 160/100 mm Hg

Laboratory Results
- Fasting blood glucose 250 mg/dL (13.9 mmol/L)
- Total cholesterol 205 mg/dL (5.3 mmol/L)
- Triglyceride 298 mg/dL (3.36 mmol/L)
- HDL cholesterol 31 mg/dL (0.8 mmol/L)
- LDL cholesterol 114 mg/dL

Discussion Questions
1. What are S.R.'s risk factors for obesity?
2. What is her estimated BMI?
3. Of the possible complications of obesity, which ones does S.R. have? Why did she develop them?
4. *Priority Decision:* How would you assist S.R. in designing a successful weight loss and weight management program?
5. What are S.R.'s risk factors for metabolic syndrome?
6. Is S.R. a candidate for surgical intervention for obesity? Why or why not?
7. *Evidence-Based Practice:* S.R. tells you that she is motivated to lose weight and thinks that she can "do it on her own." Based on your understanding of the evidence, is this the best approach for her to be successful in losing weight?

Ⓔvolve Answers available at *http://evolve.elsevier.com/Lewis/medsurg.*

---

exercise has been found to decrease the triglyceride level and increase the HDL cholesterol level in patients with metabolic syndrome.

Patients unable to lower risk factors with lifestyle therapies alone or those at high risk for a coronary event or diabetes may be considered for drug therapy. Although there is no specific medication for metabolic syndrome, cholesterol-lowering and antihypertensive drugs can be used. Metformin (Glucophage) has also been used to prevent diabetes by lowering glucose levels and enhancing the cells' sensitivity to insulin.

BRIDGE TO NCLEX EXAMINATION

The number of the question corresponds to the same-numbered outcome at the beginning of the chapter.

1. Which statement best describes the etiology of obesity?
   a. Obesity primarily results from a genetic predisposition.
   b. Psychosocial factors can override the effects of genetics in the etiology of obesity.
   c. Obesity is the result of complex interactions between genetic and environmental factors.
   d. Genetic factors are more important than environmental factors in the etiology of obesity.

2. The obesity classification that is most often associated with cardio-vascular health problems is
   a. primary obesity.
   b. secondary obesity.
   c. gynoid fat distribution.
   d. android fat distribution.

3. Health risks associated with obesity include *(select all that apply)*
   a. colorectal cancer.
   b. rheumatoid arthritis.
   c. polycystic ovary syndrome.
   d. nonalcoholic steatohepatitis.
   e. systemic lupus erythematosus.

4. The best nutritional therapy plan for a person who is obese is
   a. the Zone diet.
   b. the Atkins diet.
   c. Sugar Busters.
   d. foods from the basic food groups.

5. This bariatric surgical procedure involves creating a stoma and gastric pouch that is reversible, and no malabsorption occurs. What surgical procedure is this?
   a. Vertical gastric banding
   b. Biliopancreatic diversion
   c. Roux-en-Y gastric bypass
   d. Adjustable gastric banding

6. A severely obese patient has undergone Roux-en-Y gastric bypass surgery. In planning postoperative care, the nurse anticipates that the patient
   a. may have severe diarrhea early in the postoperative period.
   b. will not be allowed to ambulate for 1 to 2 days postoperatively.
   c. will require nasogastric suction until the incision heals.
   d. may have only liquids orally, and in very limited amounts, during the early postoperative period.

7. Which of the following criteria must be met for a diagnosis of metabolic syndrome *(select all that apply)*?
   a. Hypertension
   b. Elevated triglycerides
   c. Elevated plasma glucose
   d. Increased waist circumference
   e. Decreased low-density lipoproteins

1. c, 2. d, 3. a, c, d, 4. d, 5. d, 6. d, 7. a, b, c, d

Ⓔvolve
For rationales to these answers and even more NCLEX review questions, visit *http://evolve.elsever.com/Lewis/medsurg.*

REFERENCES

1. Achike F, To P, Wang H, et al: Obesity, metabolic syndrome, adipocytes, and vascular function: a holistic viewpoint, *Clin Exper Pharmacol Physiol* 38:1, 2011.

*2. Cornier MA, Depres JP, Davis N, et al: Assessing adiposity: a scientific statement from the American Heart Association, *Circulation* 124(18):1996, 2011.

3. Spanos A: Do weight and shape concerns exhibit genetic effects? Investigating discrepant findings, *Int J Eat Disord* 43(1):29, 2010.

*4. Robert Wood Johnson Foundation: F as in fat: how obesity threatens America's future, Trust for America's Health, 2011. Retrieved from *www.healthyamericans.org/assets/files/TFAH2011FasInFat10.pdf.*

5. Flegal KM, Carroll MD, Ogden C, et al: Prevalence and trends in obesity among US adults, 1999-2008, *JAMA* 303(3):235, 2010.

6. Biro FM, Wien M: Childhood obesity and adult morbidities, *Am J Clin Nutr* 91(5):1499S, 2010.

7. Centers for Disease Control and Prevention: Genomics and health. Retrieved from *www.cdc.gov/genomics/resources/diseases/obesity/obesedit.htm.*

8. Malis C, Rasmussen EL, Foulsen P, et al: Total and regional fat distribution is strongly influenced by genetic factors in young and elderly twins, *Obesity Res* 13:2139, 2005. (Classic)

9. Stunkard A, Sorensen TI, Hanis C, et al: An adoption study of human obesity, *N Engl J Med* 314(4):1483, 1986. (Classic)

10. University of Oxford: Overactive FTO gene does cause overeating and obesity, *Science Daily*, 2010. Retrieved from *www.sciencedaily.com/releases/2010/11/101116220332.htm.*

11. Bray G: Obesity. In Feldman M, Friedman LS, Brandt LJ, editors: *Sleisenger and Fordtran's gastrointestinal and liver disease*, ed 9, Philadelphia, 2010, Saunders.

12. Centers for Disease Control and Prevention: Healthy weight: it's not a diet, it's a lifestyle. Retrieved from *www.cdc.gov/hgov/healthyweight/healthy_eating/portion_size.html.*

13. Davis N, Forges B, Wylie-Rosett J: Role of obesity and lifestyle interventions in the prevention and management of type 2 diabetes, *Minerva Med* 100(3):221, 2009.

14. Popkin BM, Duffey KL: Does hunger and satiety drive eating anymore? Increasing eating occasions and decreasing time between eating occasions in the United States, *Am J Clin Nutr* 91:1342, 2010.

15. Franklin J, Thanavaro J, Ellis P: Body mass index as a guide for diagnosing prediabetes and diabetes, *J Nurse Pract* 7(8):634, 2011.

16. American Institute for Cancer Research: Excess body fat alone causes over 100,000 cancers in US each year. Retrieved from *www.aicr.org/assets/docs/pdf/research/2010pdfs/HarrisonGail_Intro.pdf.*

*17. Appel LJ, Clark JM, Yeh H, et al: Comparative effectiveness of weight-loss interventions in clinical practice, *N Engl J Med* 365(21):1959, 2011.

18. National Heart, Lung, and Blood Institute, North American Association for the Study of Obesity: *The practical guide: identification, evaluation, and treatment of overweight and obesity in adults*, Pub No 00-4084, Washington, DC, 2000, US Department of Health and Human Services.

*19. Sacks F, Bray G, Carey V, et al: Comparison of weight-loss diets with different compositions of fat, protein, and carbohydrates, *N Engl J Med* 360(9):859, 2009.

20. US Food and Drug Administration: Early communication about an ongoing safety review: orlistat (marketed as Alli and Xenical). Retrieved from *www.fda.gov/Drugs/DrugSafety/PostmarketDrugSafetyInformationforPatientsandProviders/DrugSafetyInformationforHealthcareProfessionals/ucm179166.htm.*

21. National Institutes of Health: Bariatric surgery for severe obesity. Retrieved from *http://win.niddk.nih.gov/publications/PDFs/Bariatric_Surgery_508.pdf.*

22. DeMaria EJ: Baseline data from American Society for Metabolic and Bariatric Surgery–designated Bariatric Surgery Centers of Excellence using the Bariatric Outcomes Longitudinal Database, *Surg Obesity Rel Dis* 6(4):347, 2010.

23. Schroeder R, Garrison JM, Johnson MS: Treatment of adult obesity with bariatric surgery, *Am Fam Physician* 84(7):805, 2011.

24. Saver A: Bariatric surgery. Retrieved from *http://emedicine.medscape.com/article/197081-overview#aw2aab6b2b1aa.*

25. Gagnon L, Karwacki Sheff EJ: Outcomes and complications after bariatric surgery, *Am J Nurs* 112:26, 2012.

26. Al-Benna S: Perioperative management of morbid obesity, *J Periop Pract* 21(7):225, 2011.

27. Rowen L, Hunt D, Johnson KL: Managing obese patients in the OR, *OR Nurse* 6:26, 2012.

28. Conrad K, Russell A, Keister K: Bariatric surgery and its impact on childbearing, *Nurs Women's Health* 15(3):228, 2011.

29. Lau DC: Metabolic syndrome: perception or reality? *Curr Atheroscl Rep* 11:264, 2009.

30. Sinclair A, Viljoen A: The metabolic syndrome in older persons, *Clin Geriatr Med* 26(2):261, 2010.

RESOURCES

American Society for Metabolic and Bariatric Surgery
http://asmbs.org
Obesity Society
www.obesity.org
Overeaters Anonymous Headquarters
www.oa.org
Weight Control Information Network
www.win.niddk.nih.gov

---

*Evidence-based information for clinical practice.

CHAPTER
42

When I repress my emotions, my stomach keeps score.
John Powell

Nursing Management
Upper Gastrointestinal Problems

Paula Cox-North

LEARNING OUTCOMES

1. Describe the etiology, complications, collaborative care, and nursing management of nausea and vomiting.
2. Describe the etiology, clinical manifestations, and treatment of common oral inflammations and infections.
3. Describe the etiology, clinical manifestations, complications, collaborative care, and nursing management of oral cancer.
4. Explain the types, pathophysiology, clinical manifestations, complications, and collaborative care (including surgical therapy and nursing management) of gastroesophageal reflux disease (GERD) and hiatal hernia.
5. Describe the pathophysiology, clinical manifestations, complications, and collaborative care of esophageal cancer, diverticula, achalasia, and esophageal strictures.
6. Differentiate between acute and chronic gastritis, including the etiology, pathophysiology, collaborative care, and nursing management.
7. Compare and contrast gastric and duodenal ulcers, including the etiology, pathophysiology, clinical manifestations, complications, collaborative care, and nursing management.
8. Describe the clinical manifestations, collaborative care, and nursing management of stomach cancer.
9. Explain the common etiologies, clinical manifestations, collaborative care, and nursing management of upper gastrointestinal bleeding.
10. Identify common types of foodborne illnesses and nursing responsibilities related to food poisoning.

KEY TERMS

achalasia, p. 940
Barrett's esophagus, p. 932
dysphagia, p. 929
esophageal cancer, p. 937
esophageal diverticula, p. 939
esophagitis, p. 932

gastritis, p. 940
gastroesophageal reflux disease (GERD), p. 931
hiatal hernia, p. 935
Mallory-Weiss tear, p. 925
nausea, p. 924

peptic ulcer disease (PUD), p. 942
stomach cancer, p. 951
stress-related mucosal disease (SRMD), p. 954
vomiting, p. 924

NAUSEA AND VOMITING

Nausea and vomiting are the most common manifestations of gastrointestinal (GI) diseases. Although nausea and vomiting can occur independently, they are usually closely related and treated as one problem. Nausea is a feeling of discomfort in the epigastrium with a conscious desire to vomit. Vomiting is the forceful ejection of partially digested food and secretions (*emesis*) from the upper GI tract.

Vomiting is a complex act that requires the coordinated activities of several structures: closure of the glottis, deep inspiration with contraction of the diaphragm in the inspiratory position, closure of the pylorus, relaxation of the stomach and lower esophageal sphincter (LES), and contraction of the abdominal muscles with increasing intraabdominal pressure. These simultaneous activities force the stomach contents up through the esophagus, into the pharynx, and out the mouth.

Etiology and Pathophysiology

Nausea and vomiting occur in a wide variety of GI disorders and in conditions that are unrelated to GI disease. These include pregnancy; infection; central nervous system (CNS)

Reviewed by Marian Sawyier, RN, MSN, Staff Nurse, University of New Mexico Hospital, Albuquerque, New Mexico.

FIG. 42-1 Stimuli involved in the act of vomiting. *CTZ,* Chemoreceptor trigger zone.

disorders (e.g., meningitis, tumor); cardiovascular problems (e.g., myocardial infarction, heart failure); metabolic disorders (e.g., diabetes mellitus, Addison's disease, renal failure); postoperatively after general anesthesia; side effects of drugs (e.g., chemotherapy, opioids, digitalis); psychologic factors (e.g., stress, fear); and conditions in which the GI tract becomes overly irritated, excited, or distended.

A vomiting center in the brainstem coordinates the multiple components involved in vomiting. This center receives input from various stimuli. Neural impulses reach the vomiting center via afferent pathways through branches of the autonomic nervous system. Receptors for these afferent fibers are located in the GI tract, kidneys, heart, and uterus. When stimulated, these receptors relay information to the vomiting center, which then initiates the vomiting reflex (Fig. 42-1).

The chemoreceptor trigger zone (CTZ) located in the brainstem responds to chemical stimuli of drugs, toxins, and labyrinthine stimulation (e.g., motion sickness). Once stimulated, the CTZ transmits impulses directly to the vomiting center. This action activates the autonomic nervous system, resulting in both parasympathetic and sympathetic stimulation. Sympathetic activation produces tachycardia, tachypnea, and diaphoresis. Parasympathetic stimulation causes relaxation of the LES, an increase in gastric motility, and a pronounced increase in salivation.

Clinical Manifestations

Nausea is a subjective complaint. *Anorexia* (lack of appetite) usually accompanies nausea. When nausea and vomiting occur over a long period, dehydration can develop rapidly. Water and essential electrolytes (e.g., potassium, sodium, chloride, hydrogen) are lost. As vomiting persists, the patient may have severe electrolyte imbalances, loss of extracellular fluid volume, decreased plasma volume, and eventually circulatory failure.

Metabolic alkalosis can result from loss of gastric hydrochloric (HCl) acid. When contents of the small intestine are vomited, metabolic acidosis can occur. However, metabolic acidosis is less common than metabolic alkalosis. Weight loss resulting from fluid loss is evident in a short time when vomiting is severe.

The threat of pulmonary aspiration is a concern when vomiting occurs in older or unconscious patients or in patients with other conditions that impair the gag reflex. To prevent aspiration, put the patient who cannot adequately manage self-care in a semi-Fowler's or side-lying position.

Collaborative Care

The goals of collaborative care are to determine and treat the underlying cause of the nausea and vomiting and to provide symptomatic relief. Assess the patient for precipitating factors, and describe the contents of the emesis. Women are more likely to suffer from nausea and vomiting associated with surgical procedures and motion sickness.[1]

It is important to differentiate among vomiting, regurgitation, and projectile vomiting. *Regurgitation* is an effortless process in which partially digested food slowly comes up from the stomach. Retching or vomiting rarely occurs before it. *Projectile vomiting* is a forceful expulsion of stomach contents without nausea and is characteristic of CNS (brain and spinal cord) tumors.

Emesis containing partially digested food several hours after a meal is indicative of gastric outlet obstruction or delayed gastric emptying. The presence of fecal odor and bile after prolonged vomiting suggests intestinal obstruction below the level of the pylorus. Bile in the emesis may suggest obstruction below the ampulla of Vater. The color of the emesis aids in identifying the presence and source of bleeding. Vomitus with a "coffee ground" appearance is related to gastric bleeding, where blood changes to dark brown as a result of its interaction with HCl acid. Bright red blood indicates active bleeding. This could be due to a **Mallory-Weiss tear** (disruption of the mucosal lining near the esophagogastric junction), esophageal varices, gastric or duodenal ulcer, or neoplasm. A Mallory-Weiss tear is most often related to severe retching and vomiting.

The time of day at which the vomiting occurs is often helpful in determining the cause. Early morning vomiting is common in pregnancy. Emotional stressors with no evident pathologic disorder may elicit vomiting during or immediately after eating.

Drug Therapy. The use of drugs (Table 42-1) in the treatment of nausea and vomiting depends on the cause of the problem. Because the cause cannot always be readily determined, use drugs with caution. Using antiemetics before determining the cause can mask the underlying disease process and delay diagnosis and treatment. Many antiemetic drugs act in the CNS via the CTZ to block the neurochemicals that trigger nausea and vomiting.

DRUG ALERT: Promethazine Injection
- Promethazine should not be administered into an artery or under the skin because of the risk of severe tissue injury, including gangrene.
- When promethazine is administered IV, it can leach out from the vein and cause serious damage to surrounding tissue.
- Deep muscle injection is the preferred route of injection administration.

DRUG ALERT: Metoclopramide (Reglan)
- Chronic use or high doses of metoclopramide carry the risk of tardive dyskinesia.
- Tardive dyskinesia is a neurologic condition characterized by involuntary and repetitive movements of the body (e.g., extremity movements, lip smacking).
- With discontinuation of the drug, the tardive dyskinesia persists.

The serotonin (5-HT$_3$) receptor antagonists are effective in reducing cancer chemotherapy–induced vomiting caused by delayed gastric emptying and also the nausea and vomiting

TABLE 42-1   DRUG THERAPY

Nausea and Vomiting

Drug	Mechanism of Action	Side Effects
Phenothiazines chlorpromazine (Thorazine) perphenazine (Trilafon) prochlorperazine (Compazine) trifluoperazine (Stelazine) promethazine (Phenergan)	Act in the CNS level of the CTZ Block dopamine receptors that trigger nausea and vomiting	Dry mouth, hypotension, sedative effects, rashes, constipation
Antihistamines meclizine (Bonine, Antivert) dimenhydrinate (Dramamine) hydroxyzine (Vistaril) diphenhydramine (Benadryl)	Block the histamine receptors that trigger nausea and vomiting	Dry mouth, hypotension, sedative effects, rashes, constipation
Prokinetic Agents domperidone (Motilium) metoclopramide (Reglan)	Inhibit action of dopamine ↑ Gastric motility and emptying	CNS side effects ranging from anxiety to hallucinations Extrapyramidal side effects, including tremor and dyskinesias (similar to Parkinson's disease)
Serotonin (5-HT$_3$) Antagonists dolasetron (Anzemet) granisetron (Kytril) ondansetron (Zofran) palonosetron (Aloxi)	Block the action of serotonin (substance that causes nausea and vomiting)	Constipation, diarrhea, headache, fatigue, malaise, elevated liver function tests
Anticholinergic (Antimuscarinic) scopolamine transdermal	Blocks the cholinergic pathways to the vomiting center	Xerostomia, somnolence
Butyrophenone droperidol (Inapsine)	Blocks the neurochemicals that trigger nausea and vomiting	Dry mouth, hypotension, sedative effects, rashes, constipation
Others aprepitant (Emend) dexamethasone (Decadron) dronabinol (Marinol) nabilone (Cesamet) thiethylperazine (Torecan) trimethobenzamide (Tigan)		

CTZ, Chemoreceptor trigger zone.

related to migraine headache and anxiety.[2] 5-HT$_3$ antagonists are also used in prevention and treatment of postoperative nausea and vomiting. Dexamethasone (Decadron) is used in the management of both acute and delayed cancer chemotherapy–induced emesis, usually in combination with other antiemetics such as ondansetron (Zofran). Aprepitant (Emend), a substance P/neurokinin-1 receptor antagonist, is used for the prevention of chemotherapy-induced and postoperative nausea and vomiting.

Dronabinol (Marinol) is an orally active cannabinoid that is used alone or in combination with other antiemetics for the prevention of chemotherapy-induced emesis. Because of the potential for abuse, as well as drowsiness and sedation, this drug is used only when other therapies are ineffective.

Nutritional Therapy. The patient with severe vomiting requires IV fluid therapy with electrolyte and glucose replacement until able to tolerate oral intake. In some cases a nasogastric (NG) tube and suction are used to decompress the stomach. Start oral nutrition beginning with clear liquids once symptoms have subsided. Extremely hot or cold liquids are often difficult to tolerate. Carbonated beverages at room temperature and with

the carbonation gone and warm tea are easier to tolerate. The addition of dry toast or crackers may be helpful. Water is the initial fluid of choice for rehydration by mouth. Sipping small amounts of fluid (5 to 15 mL) every 15 to 20 minutes is usually better tolerated than drinking large amounts less frequently. Broth and Gatorade are high in sodium, so administer them with caution.

As the patient's condition improves, provide a diet high in carbohydrates and low in fat. Items such as a baked potato, plain gelatin, cereal, and hard candy are ideal. Coffee, spicy foods, highly acidic foods, and those with strong odors are often poorly tolerated. Tell the patient to eat food slowly and in small amounts to prevent overdistention of the stomach. Liquids taken between meals rather than with meals also reduce overdistention. Consult a dietitian regarding appropriate foods that have nutritional value and are well tolerated by the patient.

Nondrug Therapy. For some patients, acupressure or acupuncture at specific points is effective in reducing postoperative nausea and vomiting.[3] Some patients use herbs such as ginger and peppermint oil. Relaxation breathing exercises, changes in body position, or exercise may be helpful for some patients.

COMPLEMENTARY & ALTERNATIVE THERAPIES
Ginger

Scientific Evidence
- Some evidence that ginger may be effective for nausea and vomiting of pregnancy when used at recommended doses for short periods
- Unclear scientific evidence for the use of ginger for nausea and vomiting related to other conditions

Nursing Implications
- Few adverse effects have been reported with short-term use.
- Ginger may inhibit platelet aggregation and increase risk of bleeding.
- It may lower blood glucose levels.

Source: Based on a systematic review of scientific literature. Retrieved from *www.naturalstandard.com*.

NURSING MANAGEMENT
NAUSEA AND VOMITING

NURSING ASSESSMENT

Each patient with a history of prolonged and persistent nausea or vomiting requires a thorough nursing assessment before you develop a specific plan of care. Although numerous conditions are associated with nausea and vomiting, you should have a basic understanding of the more common conditions and be able to identify the patient who is at high risk. Knowledge of the physiologic mechanisms involved in nausea and vomiting is important in the assessment process. Table 42-2 presents subjective and objective data to be obtained from a patient with nausea and vomiting.

NURSING DIAGNOSES

Nursing diagnoses for the patient with nausea and vomiting may include, but are not limited to, the following:
- Nausea *related to* multiple etiologies
- Deficient fluid volume *related to* prolonged vomiting
- Imbalanced nutrition: less than body requirements *related to* nausea and vomiting

Additional information on nursing diagnoses is presented in eNursing Care Plan 42-1 on the website for this chapter.

PLANNING

The overall goals are that the patient with nausea and vomiting will (1) experience minimal or no nausea and vomiting, (2) have normal electrolyte levels and hydration status, and (3) return to a normal pattern of fluid balance and nutrient intake.

NURSING IMPLEMENTATION

ACUTE INTERVENTION. Most people with nausea and vomiting can be managed at home. When nausea and vomiting persist, hospitalization may be necessary for diagnosis of the underlying problem. Until a diagnosis is confirmed, the patient is on nothing-by-mouth (NPO) status and given IV fluids. An NG tube connected to suction may be needed for the patient with persistent vomiting or when a bowel obstruction or paralytic ileus is suspected. Secure the NG tube to prevent its movement in the nose and back of the throat because this can stimulate nausea and vomiting.

With prolonged vomiting, there is a probability of dehydration and acid-base and electrolyte imbalances. Provide explanations regarding diagnostic tests or procedures performed. Record intake and output, position the patient to prevent

TABLE 42-2 NURSING ASSESSMENT
Nausea and Vomiting

Subjective Data
Important Health Information
Past health history: GI disorders, chronic indigestion, food allergies, pregnancy, infection, CNS disorders, recent travel, bulimia, metabolic disorders, cancer, cardiovascular disease, renal disease
Medications: Antiemetics, digitalis, opioids, ferrous sulfate, aspirin, aminophylline, alcohol, antibiotics; general anesthesia; chemotherapy
Surgery or other treatments: Recent surgery

Functional Health Patterns
Nutritional-metabolic: Amount, frequency, character, and color of vomitus; dry heaves; anorexia; weight loss
Activity-exercise: Weakness, fatigue
Cognitive-perceptual: Abdominal tenderness or pain
Coping–stress tolerance: Stress, fear

Objective Data
General
Lethargy, sunken eyeballs

Integumentary
Pallor, dry mucous membranes, poor skin turgor

Gastrointestinal
Amount, frequency, character (e.g., projectile), content (undigested food, blood, bile, feces), and color of vomitus (red, "coffee ground," green-yellow)

Urinary
Decreased output, concentrated urine

Possible Diagnostic Findings
Altered serum electrolytes (especially hypokalemia), metabolic alkalosis, abnormal upper GI findings on endoscopy or abdominal x-rays

aspiration, and monitor vital signs. Assess for signs of dehydration, and observe for changes in the patient's physical comfort and mentation. Provide physical and emotional support, and maintain a quiet, odor-free environment.

AMBULATORY AND HOME CARE. Teach the patient and the caregiver (1) how to manage the unpleasant sensation of nausea, (2) methods to prevent nausea and vomiting, and (3) strategies to maintain fluid and nutritional intake. You can minimize the occurrence of nausea or vomiting by keeping the immediate environment quiet, free of noxious odors, and well ventilated. Avoiding sudden changes of position and unnecessary activity is also helpful. Use of relaxation techniques, frequent rest periods, effective pain management strategies, and diversional tactics can prevent or reduce nausea and vomiting. Cleansing the face and hands with a cool washcloth and providing mouth care between episodes increase the person's comfort level. When symptoms occur, stop all foods and drugs until the acute phase is over.

If you suspect a medication is the cause, notify the health care provider immediately so that either the dosage can be altered or a new drug prescribed. Advise the patient that stopping the drug without consulting the health care provider may have detrimental effects on the person's health.

When food is the precipitating cause of nausea and vomiting, help the patient identify the specific food. In addition, determine when it was eaten, prior history with that food, and whether anyone else in the family is sick.

A patient may be reluctant to resume fluid intake because of fear of nausea recurring. Suggest that he or she begin with clear liquids or cola beverages, Gatorade, tea or broth, dry crackers or toast, and then plain gelatin. Bland foods, such as pasta, rice, and cooked chicken, are generally well tolerated in small amounts. An antiemetic drug is taken only if prescribed by the health care provider. Taking over-the-counter (OTC) drugs for relief of symptoms may make the problem worse.

EVALUATION

The expected outcomes are that the patient with nausea and vomiting will
- Be comfortable with minimal or no nausea and vomiting
- Have electrolyte levels within normal range
- Be able to maintain adequate intake of fluids and nutrients

GERONTOLOGIC CONSIDERATIONS

NAUSEA AND VOMITING

The older adult experiencing nausea and vomiting requires careful assessment and monitoring, particularly during periods of fluid loss and subsequent rehydration therapy. Older patients are more likely to have cardiac or renal insufficiency that places them at greater risk for life-threatening fluid and electrolyte imbalances. Excessive replacement of fluid and electrolytes may result in adverse consequences for the person who has heart failure or renal disease. The older adult with a decreased level of consciousness may be at high risk for aspiration of vomitus. Close monitoring of the patient's physical status and level of consciousness during episodes of vomiting is important.

Older adults are particularly susceptible to the CNS side effects of antiemetic drugs, since these drugs may produce confusion and increase their risk for falls. Dosages should be reduced and efficacy closely evaluated. Institute safety precautions for these patients (e.g., removing rugs that may cause slipping).

ORAL INFLAMMATION AND INFECTIONS

Oral inflammation and infections may be due to specific mouth diseases or secondary to systemic disorders such as leukemia or vitamin deficiency. Oral inflammation and infections can severely impair oral ingestion. Common inflammations and infections of the oral cavity are presented in Table 42-3. The patient who is immunosuppressed (e.g., receiving chemotherapy for cancer) or using corticosteroid inhalant treatment for asthma is at risk for oral infections (e.g., candidiasis).

TABLE 42-3 INFECTIONS AND INFLAMMATION OF THE MOUTH

Infection or Inflammation	Etiology	Clinical Manifestations	Treatment
Gingivitis	Neglected oral hygiene, malocclusion, missing or irregular teeth, faulty dentistry, eating of soft rather than fibrous foods.	Inflamed gingivae and interdental papillae, bleeding during tooth brushing, development of pus, formation of abscess with loosening of teeth (periodontitis).	Prevention through health teaching, dental care, gingival massage, professional cleaning of teeth, fibrous foods, conscientious brushing habits with flossing.
Vincent's infection (acute necrotizing ulcerative gingivitis, trench mouth)	Fusiform bacteria, Vincent spirochetes; predisposing factors of stress, excessive fatigue, poor oral hygiene, nutritional deficiencies (B and C vitamins).	Painful, bleeding gingivae. Eroding necrotic lesions of interdental papillae, ulcerations that bleed, increased saliva with metallic taste, fetid mouth odor, anorexia, fever, general malaise.	Rest (physical and mental); avoidance of smoking and alcoholic beverages. Soft, nutritious diet. Correct oral hygiene habits. Topical applications of antibiotics. Mouth irrigations with chlorhexidine (Hibiclens) and saline solutions.
Oral candidiasis (moniliasis or thrush)	*Candida albicans* (a yeastlike fungus), debilitation, prolonged high-dose antibiotic or corticosteroid therapy.	Pearly, bluish white "milk-curd" membranous lesions on mucosa of mouth and larynx. Sore mouth, yeasty halitosis.	Miconazole buccal tablets (Oravig), nystatin or amphotericin B as oral suspension or buccal tablets. Good oral hygiene.
Herpes simplex (cold sore, fever blister)*	Herpes simplex virus (type 1 or 2), predisposing factors of upper respiratory tract infections, excessive exposure to sunlight, food allergies, emotional tension, onset of menstruation.	Lip lesions, mouth lesions, vesicle formation (single or clustered). Shallow, painful ulcers.	Spirits of camphor, corticosteroid cream, mild antiseptic mouthwash, viscous lidocaine; removal or control of predisposing factors, antiviral agents (e.g., acyclovir [Zovirax], famciclovir [Famvir], penciclovir [Denavir], valacyclovir [Valtrex]).
Aphthous stomatitis (canker sore)	Recurrent and chronic form of infection secondary to systemic disease, trauma, stress, or unknown causes.	Ulcers of mouth and lips, causing extreme pain. Ulcers surrounded by erythematous base.	Corticosteroids (topical or systemic), tetracycline oral suspension.
Parotitis (inflammation of parotid gland, surgical mumps)	Usually *Staphylococcus* species, *Streptococcus* species occasionally, debilitation and dehydration with poor oral hygiene, NPO status for an extended time.	Pain in area of gland and ear, absence of salivation, purulent exudate from gland, erythema, ulcers.	Antibiotics, mouthwashes, warm compresses; preventive measures such as chewing gum, sucking on hard candy (lemon drops), adequate fluid intake.
Stomatitis (inflammation of mouth)	Trauma, pathogens, irritants (tobacco, alcohol). Renal, liver, and hematologic diseases. Side effect of many cancer chemotherapy drugs and radiation.	Excessive salivation, halitosis, sore mouth.	Removal or treatment of cause, oral hygiene with soothing solutions, topical medications. Soft, bland diet.

*See Table 24-5.

Oral infections may predispose the patient to infections in other body organs. For example, the oral cavity is a potential reservoir for respiratory pathogens. In addition, oral pathogens have been associated with diabetes and heart disease.[4]

Regular and good oral and dental hygiene reduces oral infections and inflammation. Management of these conditions focuses on identification of the cause, elimination of infection, provision of comfort measures, and maintenance of nutritional intake.

ORAL CANCER

There are two types of oral cancer: *oral cavity cancer,* which starts in the mouth, and *oropharyngeal cancer,* which develops in the part of the throat just behind the mouth (called the oropharynx). *Head and neck squamous cell carcinoma* (HNSCC) is a term used for cancers of the oral cavity, pharynx, and larynx, which account for 90% of malignant oral tumors. Annually, oral cancer is diagnosed in 40,250 Americans, and it is estimated that 7850 people die from the disease.[5]

Oral cancer is more prevalent in African American men, and their survival rate is lower than that of white men. Oral cancer is more common after age 35, with 65 years being the average age of diagnosis. It is two times more common in men than in women. The 5-year survival rate is 83% for localized cancer and 61% for all stages of cancer of the oral cavity and pharynx combined.[5]

Most oral malignant lesions occur on the lower lip. Other common sites are the lateral border and undersurface of the tongue, the labial commissure, and the buccal mucosa. Carcinoma of the lip has the most favorable prognosis of any of the oral tumors because lip lesions are usually diagnosed earlier.

Etiology and Pathophysiology

Although the definitive cause of oral cancer is unknown, it has a number of predisposing factors (Table 42-4). The risk of developing oral cancer is related to the duration of tobacco use. A history of frequent alcohol consumption is reported by 75% to 80% of patients who develop oral cancer. More than 30% of patients with cancer of the lip have outdoor occupations, indicating that prolonged exposure to sunlight is a risk factor. Irritation from the pipe stem resting on the lip is a factor in pipe smokers. Human papillomavirus (HPV) contributes to 25% of oral cancer cases.[5] HPV-associated oropharyngeal cancer is associated with multiple sexual partners, especially multiple oral sex partners.[6]

Clinical Manifestations

The common manifestations of oral cancer are shown in Table 42-4. Patients may also report nonspecific symptoms such as chronic sore throat, sore mouth, and voice changes. *Leukoplakia,* called "smoker's patch," is a white patch on the mouth mucosa or tongue. It is often considered a precancerous lesion, although less than 15% of these lesions actually transform into malignant cells. The patch becomes *keratinized* (hard and leathery) and is sometimes described as hyperkeratosis. Leukoplakia is the result of chronic irritation, especially from smoking. *Erythroplasia* (erythroplakia), which is a red velvety patch on the mouth or tongue, is also a precancerous lesion. More than 50% of cases of erythroplakia progress to squamous cell carcinoma.

Cancer of the lip usually appears as an indurated, painless ulcer on the lip. The first sign of carcinoma of the tongue is an ulcer or area of thickening. Soreness or pain of the tongue may occur, especially when eating hot or highly seasoned foods. Cancerous lesions are most likely to develop in the proximal half of the tongue. Some patients experience limitation of movement of the tongue. Later symptoms of cancer of the tongue include increased salivation, slurred speech, **dysphagia** (difficulty swallowing), toothache, and earache. Approximately 30% of patients with oral cancer have an asymptomatic neck mass.

🌐 CULTURAL & ETHNIC HEALTH DISPARITIES
Oral, Pharyngeal, and Esophageal Problems

Nausea and Vomiting
- Asian Americans, Middle Easterners, and African Americans are more likely to experience nausea and vomiting than whites.

Cancers of Oral Cavity and Pharynx
- The incidence and mortality rates are higher in African American men than in whites.
- Death rates as a result of oral cancer are decreasing in whites but increasing in nonwhites.

Esophageal Cancer
- Highest incidence is in non-Hispanic white men.
- Higher incidence occurs in Alaska Natives than in whites.

Stomach Cancer
- Asian Americans and Pacific Islanders, Hispanics, and African Americans have higher rates of stomach cancer than non-Hispanic whites.
- Asian Americans show significantly higher survival rates than other ethnic groups.

TABLE 42-4	**TYPES AND CHARACTERISTICS OF ORAL CANCER**		
Location	**Predisposing Factors**	**Clinical Manifestations**	**Treatment**
Lip	Constant overexposure to sun, ruddy and fair complexion, recurrent herpetic lesions, irritation from pipe stem, syphilis, immunosuppression	Indurated, painless ulcer	Surgical excision, radiation
Tongue	Tobacco, alcohol, chronic irritation, syphilis	Ulcer or area of thickening, soreness or pain. Increased salivation, slurred speech, dysphagia, toothache, earache (later signs)	Surgery (hemiglossectomy or glossectomy), radiation
Oral cavity	Poor oral hygiene, tobacco usage (pipe and cigar smoking, snuff, chewing tobacco), chronic alcohol intake, chronic irritation (jagged tooth, ill-fitting prosthesis, chemical or mechanical irritants), human papillomavirus (HPV)	Leukoplakia, erythroplakia, ulcerations, sore spot, rough area, pain, dysphagia, a lump or thickening in the cheek. A sore throat or a feeling that something is stuck. Difficulty chewing and speaking (later signs)	Surgery (mandibulectomy, radical neck dissection, resection of buccal mucosa), internal and external radiation

TABLE 42-5   COLLABORATIVE CARE

Oral Cancer

Diagnostic	Collaborative Therapy*
• History and physical examination	• Surgery
• Biopsy	• Surgical excision of the tumor
• Oral exfoliative cytology	• Radical neck dissection
• Toluidine blue test	• Radiation (internal or external)
• CT, MRI, PET	• Combined surgical resection with radiation
	• Chemotherapy

*Any of these approaches may be used, depending on the primary lesion and the extent of metastasis.

Diagnostic Studies

Diagnostic tests are performed to identify oral dysplasias, which are precursors to oral cancer. Oral exfoliative cytologic study involves scraping the suspicious lesion and spreading this scraping on a slide for microscopic examination. The toluidine blue test is also used as a screening test for oral cancer. Toluidine blue is applied topically to stain an area, and cancer cells preferentially take up the dye. A negative cytologic smear or negative toluidine blue test does not necessarily rule out a malignant condition. Once cancer is diagnosed, computed tomography (CT), magnetic resonance imaging (MRI), and positron emission tomography (PET) are used in staging the oral cancer.[7]

Collaborative Care

Collaborative care of the patient with oral carcinoma usually consists of surgery, radiation, chemotherapy, or a combination of these (Table 42-5).

Surgical Therapy. Surgery remains the most effective treatment, especially for early-stage disease. Various surgical procedures may be performed, depending on the location and extent of the tumor. Many of the operations are radical procedures involving extensive resections. Some examples are partial *mandibulectomy* (removal of the mandible), *hemiglossectomy* (removal of half of the tongue), *glossectomy* (removal of the tongue), resections of the buccal mucosa and floor of the mouth, and radical neck dissection.

Radical neck dissection includes wide excision of the primary lesion with removal of the regional lymph nodes, the deep cervical lymph nodes, and their lymphatic channels. The following structures may also be removed or transected (depending on the extent of the primary lesion): sternocleidomastoid muscle and other closely associated muscles, internal jugular vein, mandible, submaxillary gland, part of the thyroid and parathyroid glands, and spinal accessory nerve. A tracheostomy is commonly performed along with the radical neck dissection. Drainage tubes are inserted into the surgical area and connected to suction to remove fluid and blood.

Nonsurgical Therapy. Chemotherapy and radiation therapy are used together when there are positive margins, bone erosion, or positive lymph nodes. Chemotherapeutic agents used include 5-fluorouracil (5-FU), methotrexate, cisplatin (Platinol), carboplatin (Paraplatin), paclitaxel (Taxol), docetaxel (Taxotere), cetuximab (Erbitux), and bleomycin (Blenoxane). Combination drug therapies are also used.[8] (Chemotherapy is discussed in Chapter 16.) Brachytherapy with implantations of radioactive seeds may be used to treat early-stage oral cancer.

Palliative treatment is often the best management when the prognosis is poor, the cancer is inoperable, or the patient decides against surgery. Palliation aims to treat the symptoms and make the patient more comfortable. If it becomes difficult for the patient to swallow, a gastrostomy tube may be inserted to allow for adequate nutritional intake. (Enteral nutrition is discussed in Chapter 40.) Analgesic medication should be given freely. Frequent suctioning of the oral cavity is necessary when swallowing becomes difficult. (Other palliative and end-of-life nursing measures are discussed in Chapter 10.)

Nutritional Therapy. Because of depression, alcoholism, or presurgery radiation treatment, patients may be malnourished before surgery. A percutaneous endoscopic gastrostomy (PEG) placement may be considered before radiation treatment or surgery. After radical neck surgery, the patient may be unable to orally ingest nutrients because of mucositis, swelling, location of sutures, or difficulty swallowing. Parenteral fluids are given for the first 24 to 48 hours. After this time, enteral nutrition is given via an NG, gastrostomy, or nasointestinal tube. (PEG and parenteral and enteral feedings are discussed in Chapter 40.) Cervical esophagostomy and pharyngostomy have also been used.

Observe for feeding tolerance and adjust the amount, time, and formula if nausea, vomiting, diarrhea, or distention occurs. Give small amounts of water when the patient can swallow. Observe for choking. Suctioning may be necessary to prevent aspiration.

NURSING MANAGEMENT
ORAL CANCER

NURSING ASSESSMENT

Subjective and objective data to obtain from a patient with oral cancer are presented in Table 42-6.

TABLE 42-6   NURSING ASSESSMENT

Oral Cancer

Subjective Data
Important Health Information
Past health history: Recurrent oral herpetic lesions, human papillomavirus (HPV) infection or vaccination, syphilis, exposure to sunlight
Medications: Immunosuppressants
Surgery or other treatments: Removal of prior tumors or lesions

Functional Health Patterns
Health perception–health management: Use of alcohol and tobacco, pipe smoking; poor oral hygiene
Nutritional-metabolic: Reductions in oral intake, weight loss; difficulty chewing food; increased salivation; intolerance to certain foods or temperatures of food
Cognitive-perceptual: Mouth or tongue soreness or pain, toothache, earache, neck stiffness, dysphagia, difficulty speaking

Objective Data
Integumentary
Indurated, painless ulcer on lip; painless neck mass

Gastrointestinal
Areas of thickening or roughness, ulcers, leukoplakia, or erythroplakia on the tongue or oral mucosa; limited movement of the tongue; increased salivation; drooling; slurred speech; foul breath odor

Possible Diagnostic Findings
Positive exfoliative smear cytology (microscopic examination of cells removed by scraping); positive biopsy

NURSING DIAGNOSES

Nursing diagnoses for the patient with oral cancer may include, but are not limited to, the following:

- Imbalanced nutrition: less than body requirements *related to* oral pain, difficulty chewing and swallowing, surgical resection, and radiation treatment
- Chronic pain *related to* the tumor, surgery, or radiation
- Anxiety *related to* diagnosis of cancer, uncertain future, potential for disfiguring surgery, potential for recurrence, and prognosis
- Ineffective health maintenance *related to* lack of knowledge of disease process and therapeutic regimen and unavailability of a support system

PLANNING

The overall goals are that the patient with carcinoma of the oral cavity will (1) have a patent airway, (2) be able to communicate, (3) have adequate nutritional intake to promote wound healing, and (4) have relief of pain and discomfort.

NURSING IMPLEMENTATION

You have a significant role in early detection and treatment of oral cancer. Identify patients at risk (see Table 42-4) and provide information regarding predisposing factors. Inform the patient who smokes about smoking cessation programs available in the community. Warn adolescents and teenagers about the danger of using snuff or chewing tobacco. (Smoking cessation is discussed in Chapter 11 and Tables 11-4 to 11-6.)

Because early detection of oral cancer is important, teach the patient to report unexplained pain or soreness of the mouth, unusual bleeding, dysphagia, sore throat, voice changes, or swelling or lump in the neck. Refer any individual with an ulcerative lesion that does not heal within 2 to 3 weeks to a health care provider.

Preoperative care for the patient who will have a radical neck dissection involves consideration of the patient's physical and psychosocial needs. Physical preparation is the same as that for any major surgery, with special emphasis on oral hygiene. Explanations and emotional support should include information on postoperative communication and feeding. Explain the surgical procedure, and ensure that the patient understands the information. Radical neck dissection and related nursing management are discussed in Chapter 27 and eNursing Care Plan 27-2.

EVALUATION

The expected outcomes are that the patient with oral cancer will
- Have no respiratory complications
- Be able to communicate
- Maintain an adequate nutritional intake to promote wound healing
- Experience minimal pain and discomfort with eating, drinking, and talking

ESOPHAGEAL DISORDERS

GASTROESOPHAGEAL REFLUX DISEASE

Gastroesophageal reflux disease (GERD) is a chronic symptom of mucosal damage caused by reflux of stomach acid into the lower esophagus. GERD is not a disease but a syndrome. GERD is the most common upper GI problem. Approximately 10% to

HEALTHY PEOPLE
Health Impact of Good Oral Hygiene

- Improves quality of life
- Lowers risk of teeth loss
- Reduces pain and disability
- Decreases cost of care needed from dental professionals
- Assists in early detection of oral and craniofacial cancers
- Decreases risk of developing periodontal disease, gingivitis, and dental caries

FIG. 42-2 Factors involved in the pathogenesis of gastroesophageal reflux disease (GERD). *LES,* Lower esophageal sphincter.

20% of the U.S. population experience GERD symptoms (heartburn or regurgitation) at least once a week.[9]

Etiology and Pathophysiology

GERD has no one single cause (Fig. 42-2). GERD results when the defenses of the esophagus are overwhelmed by the reflux of acidic gastric contents into the esophagus. Gastric HCl acid and pepsin secretions that reflux cause esophageal irritation and inflammation (*esophagitis*). If the refluxate contains intestinal proteolytic enzymes (e.g., trypsin) and bile, this further irritates the esophageal mucosa. The degree of inflammation depends on the amount and composition of the gastric reflux and on the esophagus's mucosal defense mechanisms.

One of the primary etiologic factors in GERD is an incompetent LES. Under normal conditions, the LES acts as an antireflux barrier. An incompetent LES lets gastric contents move from the stomach to the esophagus when the patient is supine or has an increase in intraabdominal pressure.

Decreased LES pressure can be due to certain foods (e.g., caffeine, chocolate, peppermint) and drugs (e.g., anticholinergics). Obesity is a risk factor for GERD, although the specific mechanism remains to be determined.[10] In an obese person the intraabdominal pressure is increased, which can exacerbate GERD. Cigarette and cigar smoking can also contribute to GERD. A common cause of GERD is a hiatal hernia, which is discussed in the next section.

Clinical Manifestations

The symptoms of GERD vary from person to person. The persistence of mild symptoms (i.e., more than twice a week) or moderate to severe symptoms once a week is considered GERD.

TABLE 42-7	FACTORS AFFECTING LOWER ESOPHAGEAL SPHINCTER PRESSURE

Increase Pressure
- bethanechol (Urecholine)
- metoclopramide (Reglan)

Decrease Pressure
- Alcohol
- Anticholinergics
- Chocolate (theobromine)
- Fatty foods
- Nicotine
- Peppermint, spearmint

- Tea, coffee (caffeine)
- Drugs
  - β-Adrenergic blockers
  - Calcium channel blockers
  - diazepam (Valium)
  - morphine sulfate
  - Nitrates
  - progesterone
  - theophylline

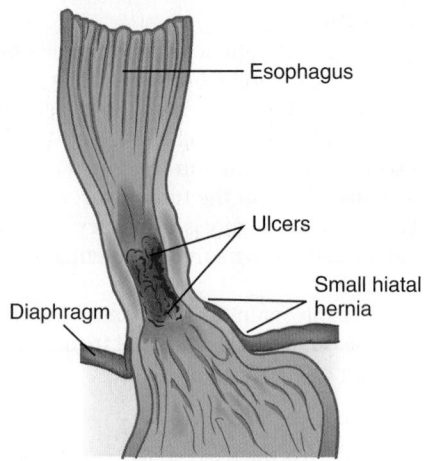

FIG. 42-3 Esophagitis with esophageal ulcerations.

Heartburn *(pyrosis)* is the most common clinical manifestation. Heartburn is a burning, tight sensation felt intermittently beneath the lower sternum and spreading upward to the throat or jaw. Heartburn may occur after ingestion of food or drugs that decrease the LES pressure or directly irritate the esophageal mucosa (Table 42-7). A health care provider should evaluate heartburn that occurs more than twice a week, is rated as severe, occurs at night and wakes a person from sleep, or is associated with dysphagia. Older adults who complain of recent onset of heartburn should receive medical evaluation.

Patients may also complain of dyspepsia. *Dyspepsia* is pain or discomfort centered in the upper abdomen (mainly in or around the midline as opposed to the right or left hypochondrium).

Regurgitation is a fairly common manifestation of GERD. It is often described as hot, bitter, or sour liquid coming into the throat or mouth. Hypersalivation (water brash) may also be reported.

An individual with GERD may also report respiratory symptoms, including wheezing, coughing, and dyspnea. Nocturnal discomfort and coughing can awaken the patient, resulting in disturbed sleep patterns. Otolaryngologic symptoms include hoarseness, sore throat, a *globus sensation* (sense of a lump in the throat), and choking.

GERD-related chest pain can mimic angina and is described as burning; squeezing; or radiating to the back, neck, jaw, or arms. Complaints of chest pain are more common in older adults with GERD. Unlike angina, GERD-related chest pain is relieved with antacids.

Complications

Complications of GERD are due to the direct local effects of gastric acid on the esophageal mucosa. Esophagitis (inflammation of the esophagus) is a common complication of GERD. Esophagitis with esophageal ulcerations is shown in Fig. 42-3. Repeated esophagitis may lead to scar tissue formation, stricture, and ultimately dysphagia.

Another complication of chronic GERD is Barrett's esophagus (esophageal metaplasia). (*Metaplasia* is the reversible change from one type of cell to another type and is generally caused by some sort of abnormal stimulus.) In Barrett's esophagus the flat epithelial cells in the distal esophagus change to columnar epithelial cells. These cell changes are thought to be due primarily to GERD. However, people with no history of reflux symptoms can develop Barrett's esophagus.

Barrett's esophagus is considered a precancerous lesion that increases the patient's risk for esophageal adenocarcinoma.

Approximately 5% to 15% of patients with chronic reflux have Barrett's esophagus.[11] Compared with whites, African Americans and Asians are at lower risk for Barrett's esophagus. Because patients with evidence of metaplasia on an initial endoscopic examination are at risk for esophageal cancer, a surveillance endoscopy every 2 to 3 years is often recommended.[12]

Respiratory complications of GERD include cough, bronchospasm, laryngospasm, and cricopharyngeal spasm. These complications are due to irritation of the upper airway by gastric secretions. Asthma, chronic bronchitis, and pneumonia may develop as a result of aspiration into the respiratory system. Dental erosion, especially in the posterior teeth, may result from acid reflux into the mouth.[12]

Diagnostic Studies

GERD is usually diagnosed on the basis of symptoms and the patient's response to behavioral and drug therapies. Diagnostic tests are done when these therapies are refractory or when complications are suspected. Diagnostic studies performed to determine the cause of the GERD are shown in Table 42-8.

Endoscopy is useful in assessing the LES competence and the degree of inflammation (if present), potential scarring, and strictures. Biopsy and cytologic specimens can differentiate stomach or esophageal carcinoma from Barrett's esophagus. In addition, the degree of dysplasia (low grade versus high grade) is determined. Manometric studies measure pressure in the esophagus and LES and esophageal motility function. Ambulatory esophageal pH monitoring may be done for patients with refractory symptoms and no evidence of mucosal inflammation. Radionuclide tests can also detect reflux of gastric contents and the rate of esophageal clearance.

Collaborative Care

Most patients with GERD can successfully manage this condition through lifestyle modifications and drug therapy. These long-term approaches require patient teaching and adherence to therapies. When these therapies are ineffective, surgery is an option (see Table 42-8).

Lifestyle Modifications. Teach the patient with GERD to avoid factors that trigger symptoms (see Table 42-7). Give particular attention to diet and drugs that may affect the LES, acid secretion, or gastric emptying. Recommend weight reduction if the patient is overweight. A patient and caregiver teaching guide is provided in Table 42-9.

Encourage patients who smoke to stop. If needed, refer the patient to community resources for assistance in stopping smoking. (See Chapter 11 for additional information related to smoking cessation.) If stress seems to cause symptoms, discuss measures to cope with stress. (See Chapter 7 for stress management techniques.)

Nutritional Therapy. Diet does not cause GERD, but food can aggravate symptoms. No specific diet is necessary. Teach patients to avoid foods that decrease LES pressure, such as chocolate, peppermint, tomatoes, fatty foods, coffee, and tea (see Table 42-7), which predispose them to reflux. Also teach patients with GERD to avoid milk, especially at bedtime, since it increases gastric acid secretion. Small, frequent meals help prevent overdistention of the stomach. Saliva production can be increased by chewing gum and oral lozenges, which may help patients with mild symptoms of GERD.

Tell the patient to avoid late evening meals and nocturnal snacking, and to take fluids between rather than with meals to reduce gastric distention. Certain foods (e.g., tomato-based products, orange juice, cola, red wine) may irritate the esophagus.

Drug Therapy. Drug therapy for GERD focuses on decreasing volume and acidity of reflux, improving LES function, increasing esophageal clearance, and protecting the esophageal mucosa[13] (Table 42-10). Proton pump inhibitors (PPIs) and histamine (H_2)-receptor blockers are common and effective treatments for symptomatic GERD. The goal of HCl acid suppression treatment is to reduce the acidity of the gastric refluxate. Patients who are symptomatic with GERD but do not have evidence of esophagitis *(nonerosive GERD)* achieve symptom relief with PPIs and H_2-receptor blockers. The PPIs are more effective in healing esophagitis than H_2-receptor blockers. PPIs are also beneficial in decreasing the incidence of esophageal strictures, a complication of chronic GERD. Omeprazole is available as a prescription as well as an OTC preparation (Prilosec OTC) and in an immediate-release form (Zegerid).

TABLE 42-8 COLLABORATIVE CARE

Gastroesophageal Reflux Disease (GERD) and Hiatal Hernia

Diagnostic
- History and physical examination
- Upper GI endoscopy with biopsy and cytologic analysis
- Esophagram (barium swallow)
- Motility (manometry) studies
- pH monitoring (laboratory or 24 hr ambulatory)
- Radionuclide studies

Collaborative Therapy
Conservative
- Elevation of head of bed on 4- to 6-in blocks
- Avoid reflux-inducing foods (fatty foods, chocolate, peppermint)
- Avoid alcohol
- Reduce or avoid acidic pH beverages (colas, red wine, orange juice)
- Antacids
- Drug therapy (see Table 42-10)
  - Proton pump inhibitors
  - H_2-receptor blockers
  - Prokinetic drug therapy
  - Cholinergic drugs

Surgical
- Nissen fundoplication
- Toupet fundoplication

Endoscopic
- Intraluminal valvuloplasty
- Radiofrequency therapy

LES, Lower esophageal sphincter.

TABLE 42-9 PATIENT & CAREGIVER TEACHING GUIDE

Gastroesophageal Reflux Disease (GERD)

Include the following instructions when teaching the patient and caregiver about management of GERD.
1. Explain the rationale for a low-fat diet.
2. Encourage the patient to eat small, frequent meals to prevent gastric distention.
3. Explain the rationale for avoiding alcohol, smoking (causes an almost immediate, marked decrease in LES pressure), and beverages that contain caffeine.
4. Advise the patient to not lie down for 2-3 hr after eating, wear tight clothing around the waist, or bend over (especially after eating).
5. Have the patient avoid eating within 3 hr of bedtime.
6. Encourage the patient to sleep with head of bed elevated on 4- to 6-in blocks (gravity fosters esophageal emptying).
7. Provide information regarding drugs, including rationale for their use and common side effects.
8. Discuss strategies for weight reduction if appropriate.
9. Encourage patient and caregiver to share concerns about lifestyle changes and living with a chronic problem.

LES, Lower esophageal sphincter.

EVIDENCE-BASED PRACTICE

Translating Research Into Practice

Are Proton Pump Inhibitors Associated With Increased Risk of Diarrhea?

Clinical Question
Among hospitalized patients (P), does the use of proton pump inhibitor drugs (I) increase the risk of *Clostridium difficile*–associated diarrhea (O)?

Best Available Evidence
Meta-analysis of case-control and cohort studies

Critical Appraisal and Synthesis of Evidence
- Twenty-three studies examined hospitalized patient medical records ($n = 300,000$) for proton pump inhibitor (PPI) exposure and confirmation of acute diarrhea due to *C. difficile.*
- Patients taking PPIs have a greater risk (65%) of *C. difficile*–associated diarrhea (CDAD).

Conclusion
- There is a significant positive association between PPIs and the incidence of CDAD.

Implications for Nursing Practice
- Advise patients taking PPIs of the risk for diarrhea and to contact their health care provider if it does not improve.
- Inform patients that CDAD symptoms include watery stool, abdominal pain, and fever.
- Institute infection control procedures in hospitalized patients suspected of having *C. difficile* infection.

Reference for Evidence
Janarthanan S, Ditah I, Adler D, et al: *Clostridium difficile*–associated diarrhea and proton pump inhibitor therapy: a meta-analysis, *Am J Gastroenterol* 107:1001, 2012.

P, Patient population of interest; *I,* intervention or area of interest; *O,* outcomes of interest (see p.12).

TABLE 42-10   DRUG THERAPY

Gastroesophageal Reflux Disease (GERD) and Peptic Ulcer Disease (PUD)

Drug	Mechanism of Action	Side Effects
Proton Pump Inhibitors (PPIs) dexlansoprazole (Dexilant) esomeprazole (Nexium) lansoprazole (Prevacid) omeprazole (Prilosec) pantoprazole (Protonix) rabeprazole (AcipHex)	↓ HCl acid secretion by inhibiting the proton pump ($H^+-K^+-ATPase$) responsible for the secretion of H^+ ↓ Irritation of the esophageal and gastric mucosa	Headache, abdominal pain, nausea, diarrhea, vomiting, flatulence
Histamine (H_2)-Receptor Blockers cimetidine (Tagamet) famotidine (Pepcid) nizatidine (Axid) ranitidine (Zantac)	Blocks the action of histamine on the H_2-receptors to ↓ HCl acid secretion ↓ Conversion of pepsinogen to pepsin ↓ Irritation of the esophageal and gastric mucosa	Headache, abdominal pain, constipation, diarrhea
Prokinetic Agents metoclopramide (Reglan)	Blocks effect of dopamine ↑ Gastric motility and emptying Reduces reflux	CNS side effects ranging from anxiety to hallucinations Extrapyramidal side effects (tremor and dyskinesias similar to Parkinson's disease)
Antiulcer, Protectants sucralfate (Carafate)	Acts to form a protective layer and serves as a barrier against acid, bile salts, and enzymes in the stomach	Constipation
Cholinergic bethanechol (Urecholine)	↑ LES pressure, improves esophageal emptying, increases gastric emptying	Lightheadedness, syncope, flushing diarrhea, stomach cramps, dizziness
Antacids, Acid Neutralizers *Single Substance* aluminum carbonate (Basaljel) aluminum hydroxide (Amphojel) calcium carbonate (Tums, Titralac) magnesium oxide (MagOx) sodium bicarbonate (Alka-Seltzer) sodium citrate (Bicitra) *Aluminum and Magnesium* Gelusil, Maalox, Mylanta, Aludrox aluminum/magnesium trisilicate (Gaviscon)	Neutralizes HCl acid Taken 1-3 hr after meals and at bedtime	*Aluminum hydroxide:* Constipation, phosphorus depletion with chronic use *Calcium carbonate:* Constipation or diarrhea, hypercalcemia, milk-alkali syndrome, renal calculi *Magnesium preparations:* Diarrhea, hypermagnesemia *Sodium preparations:* Milk-alkali syndrome if used with large amounts of calcium; use with caution in patients on sodium restrictions
Prostaglandin (Synthetic) misoprostol (Cytotec)	Protects lining of stomach *Cytoprotective:* Increases production of gastric mucus and mucosal secretion of bicarbonate *Antisecretory:* ↓ HCl acid secretion	Abdominal pain, diarrhea, GI bleeding, uterine rupture if pregnant

LES, Lower esophageal sphincter.

Long-term use of PPIs has been associated with decreased bone density,[14] chronic hypochlorhydria, and increased risk of *Clostridium difficile* in hospitalized patients.[15] Long-term PPI use has also been associated with pneumonia.

DRUG ALERT: Proton Pump Inhibitors (PPIs)
- Long-term use or high doses of PPIs may increase the risk of fractures of hip, wrist, and spine.
- Lower doses or shorter duration of therapy should be considered.
- PPIs are associated with increased risk of *C. difficile* infection in hospitalized patients.

H_2-receptor blockers reduce symptoms and promote esophageal healing in 50% of patients. These drugs are available in OTC and prescription formulations. OTC preparations have lower drug dosages compared with prescription drugs. Some formulations include an H_2-receptor blocker plus antacid combination. For example, Pepcid Complete includes famotidine, calcium carbonate, and magnesium hydroxide. (Antihistamine drugs used to treat allergies are H_1-receptor blockers and have no effect on HCl acid secretion.)

Sucralfate (Carafate), an antiulcer drug, is used in some patients with GERD for its cytoprotective properties. Cholinergic drugs (e.g., bethanechol [Urecholine]) increase LES pressure, improve esophageal emptying in the supine position, and increase gastric emptying. However, cholinergic drugs also increase HCl acid secretion. Prokinetic (motility-enhancing) drugs (metoclopramide [Reglan]) promote gastric emptying and reduce the risk of gastric acid reflux (see Table 42-10) but are not used as primary therapies for GERD.

Antacids produce quick but short-lived relief of heartburn. They should be taken 1 to 3 hours after meals and at bedtime.

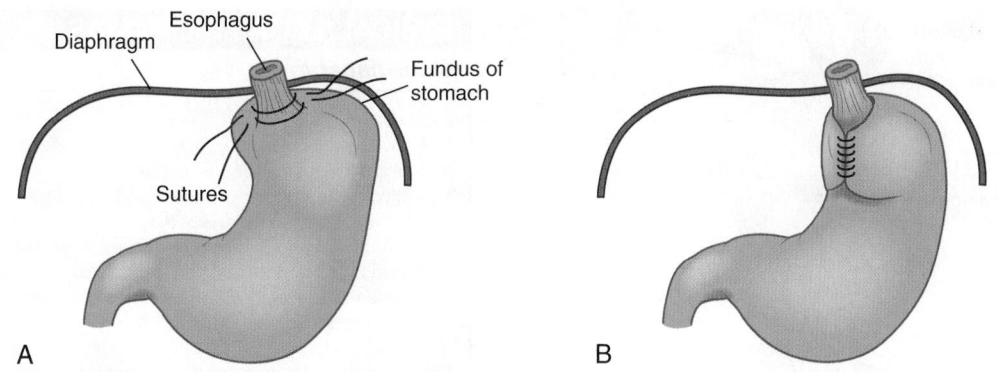

FIG. 42-4 Nissen fundoplication for repair of hiatal hernia. **A,** Fundus of stomach is wrapped around distal esophagus. **B,** The fundus is then sutured to itself.

Antacids with or without alginic acid (e.g., Gaviscon) may be useful in patients with mild, intermittent heartburn. However, in patients with moderate to severe or frequent symptoms or patients with documented esophagitis, antacids are not effective in relieving symptoms or healing lesions.

Surgical Therapy. Surgical therapy (*antireflux* surgery) is reserved for patients with complications of reflux, including esophagitis, intolerance of medications, stricture, Barrett's metaplasia, and persistence of severe symptoms. Most surgical procedures are performed laparoscopically. The goal of surgical interventions is to reduce reflux by enhancing the integrity of the LES. In these procedures the fundus of the stomach is wrapped around the lower portion of the esophagus to reinforce and repair the defective barrier. Laparoscopically performed Nissen and Toupet fundoplications are common antireflux surgeries (Fig. 42-4).

The LINX Reflux Management System is used for patients who continue to have symptoms despite maximum medical management. In this system, titanium beads with a magnetic core are strung together and implanted laparoscopically into the LES. Once implanted, the ring provides strength (augmentation) to a weakened LES. Under resting, nonswallowing conditions the ring tightens due to the magnetic attraction of the beads. When the individual swallows, the force of pressure associated with the movement of the fluids or foods overwhelms the magnetic forces such that the fluid or food passes to the stomach. Adverse events experienced with the system include difficulty swallowing, vomiting, nausea, chest pain, and pain when swallowing food.

Endoscopic Therapy. Alternatives to surgical therapy include endoscopic mucosal resection (EMR), photodynamic therapy, cryotherapy, and radiofrequency ablation (image-guided technique that kills cells through heating). For patients with high-grade dysplasia, EMR can also be used as a diagnostic test to obtain biopsy samples. The results of the biopsy can determine whether adenocarcinoma is present.

NURSING MANAGEMENT
GASTROESOPHAGEAL REFLUX DISEASE

Nursing care for the patient with acute symptoms of GERD consists of encouraging the patient to follow the necessary regimen. The head of the bed is elevated to approximately 30 degrees. This can be done using pillows or with 4- to 6-in blocks under the bed. For 2 to 3 hours after a meal the patient should not be supine. Teach the patient to avoid food and activities that cause reflux (e.g., late-night eating). Instruct patients to contact their health care provider if symptoms persist.

The patient on a PPI needs to take medication before the first meal of the day. Instruct the patient about possible medication side effects (see Table 42-10). Tell the patient on a prescription H_2-receptor agent to take the medication as prescribed and not to stop without checking with his or her health care provider.

Postoperative care focuses on prevention of respiratory complications, maintenance of fluid and electrolyte balance, and prevention of infection. If an open high abdominal incision is used, respiratory complications can occur. Respiratory assessment includes respiratory rate and rhythm, pulse rate and rhythm, and signs of pneumothorax (e.g., dyspnea, chest pain, cyanosis). Deep breathing is essential to fully expand the lungs. Because most procedures are performed laparoscopically, the risk of respiratory complications is reduced. The laparoscopic fundoplication is often performed as an outpatient procedure. However, patients at risk for complications, including those with prior upper abdominal surgeries or co-morbidities (e.g., cardiac disease, obesity), may be hospitalized after the procedure. During the postoperative phase, patients require medications to prevent nausea and vomiting and to control pain. A small percentage of patients experience complications, including gastric or esophageal injury, splenic injury, pneumothorax, perforation, bleeding, infection, and pneumonia.

When peristalsis returns, only fluids are given initially. Measure and record the intake and output. Solids are added gradually with the goal of resuming a normal diet. Teach the patient to avoid foods that are gas forming to prevent gastric distention and to chew food thoroughly.

After surgery, reflux symptoms should decrease. However, the recurrence rate may range from 10% to 30% over a 20-year period. In the first month after surgery the patient may report mild dysphagia caused by edema, but it should resolve. Instruct the patient to report persistent symptoms such as heartburn and regurgitation.

HIATAL HERNIA

Hiatal hernia is herniation of a portion of the stomach into the esophagus through an opening, or hiatus, in the diaphragm. It is also referred to as diaphragmatic hernia and esophageal hernia. It is the most common abnormality found on x-ray examination of the upper GI tract. Hiatal hernias are common in older adults and occur more often in women than in men.

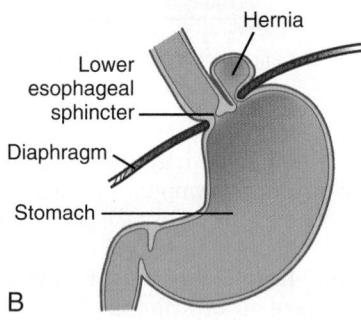

FIG. 42-5 A, Sliding hiatal hernia. **B,** Rolling or paraesophageal hernia.

Hiatal hernias are classified into the following two types (Fig. 42-5):

1. *Sliding:* The junction of the stomach and the esophagus is above the diaphragm, and a part of the stomach slides through the hiatal opening in the diaphragm. This occurs when the patient is supine, and the hernia usually goes back into the abdominal cavity when the patient is standing upright. This is the most common type of hiatal hernia.

2. *Paraesophageal,* or *rolling:* The esophagogastric junction remains in the normal position, but the fundus and the greater curvature of the stomach roll up through the diaphragm, forming a pocket alongside the esophagus. Acute paraesophageal hernia is a medical emergency.

Etiology and Pathophysiology

Many factors contribute to the development of hiatal hernia. Structural changes, such as weakening of the muscles in the diaphragm around the esophagogastric opening, occur with aging. Factors that increase intraabdominal pressure, including obesity, pregnancy, ascites, tumors, intense physical exertion, and heavy lifting on a continual basis, may also predispose patients to development of a hiatal hernia.

Clinical Manifestations and Complications

Some individuals with hiatal hernia are asymptomatic. When present, signs and symptoms of hiatal hernia are similar to those described for GERD on pp. 931-932.

Complications that may occur with hiatal hernia include GERD, esophagitis, hemorrhage from erosion, stenosis (narrowing of the esophagus), ulcerations of the herniated portion of the stomach, strangulation of the hernia, and regurgitation with tracheal aspiration.

Diagnostic Studies

An esophagram (barium swallow) may show the protrusion of gastric mucosa through the esophageal hiatus. Endoscopic visualization of the lower esophagus provides information on the

degree of mucosal inflammation or other abnormalities. Other tests are listed in Table 42-8.

NURSING AND COLLABORATIVE MANAGEMENT HIATAL HERNIA

Conservative therapy of hiatal hernia is similar to that described for GERD (pp. 932-935). Teach the patient to reduce intraabdominal pressure by eliminating constricting garments and avoiding lifting and straining.

Surgical approaches to hiatal hernias can include reduction of the herniated stomach into the abdomen, *herniotomy* (excision of the hernia sac), *herniorrhaphy* (closure of the hiatal defect), an antireflux procedure, and *gastropexy* (attachment of the stomach subdiaphragmatically to prevent rehernation). The goals are to reduce the hernia, provide an acceptable LES pressure, and prevent movement of the gastroesophageal junction. Antireflux surgeries for hiatal hernia are laparoscopically performed Nissen and Toupet techniques (see Fig. 42-4). A thoracic or an open abdominal approach may be done, depending on the patient.

GERONTOLOGIC CONSIDERATIONS

GASTROESOPHAGEAL REFLUX DISEASE AND HIATAL HERNIA

The incidence of hiatal hernia and GERD increases with age. Hiatal hernia is associated with weakening of the diaphragm, obesity, kyphosis, or other factors (e.g., wearing girdles) that increase intraabdominal pressure. Medications commonly taken by older patients decrease LES pressure (e.g., nitrates, calcium channel blockers, antidepressants). Other agents such as nonsteroidal antiinflammatory drugs (NSAIDs) and potassium can irritate the esophageal mucosa (medication-induced esophagitis).

Some older adults with hiatal hernia and GERD are asymptomatic or have less severe symptoms. The first indications may include esophageal bleeding secondary to esophagitis or respiratory complications (e.g., aspiration pneumonia) related to aspiration of gastric contents.

The clinical course and management of GERD and hiatal hernia in the older adult are similar to those for the younger adult. Changes in lifestyle, including eliminating dietary factors (such as caffeine-containing beverages and chocolate) and elevating the head of the bed on blocks, may be challenging for the older adult.

Laparoscopic procedures reduce the risk of surgical repair. An older patient with cardiovascular and pulmonary problems may not be a good candidate for surgical intervention.

ESOPHAGEAL CANCER

Esophageal cancer (malignant neoplasm of the esophagus) is not common. However, the rates are increasing. Annually in the United States approximately 17,460 new cases of esophageal cancer are diagnosed and 15,070 deaths occur from esophageal cancer.[5] The 5-year survival rate is 37% for localized cancer and 18% for regional cancer.

The majority of esophageal cancers are adenocarcinomas, with the remainder being squamous cell tumors. Adenocarcinomas arise from the glands lining the esophagus and resemble cancers of the stomach and small intestine. The incidence of esophageal cancer increases with age, with those between 70 and 84 at greatest risk. There is a higher incidence of esophageal cancer in non-Hispanic white men and Alaska Natives compared with other ethnic groups. The incidence of esophageal cancer is higher in men than in women.

Etiology and Pathophysiology

The cause of esophageal cancer is unknown. Several important risk factors include Barrett's metaplasia, smoking, excessive alcohol intake, and obesity. For example, current smoking or a history of smoking are associated with a 2-fold higher risk of esophageal cancer. Patients with injury to the esophageal mucosa (e.g., from occupational exposure) are at greater risk. Achalasia, a condition in which there is delayed emptying of the lower esophagus, is associated with squamous cell cancer.

Most esophageal tumors are located in the middle and lower portions of the esophagus. The malignant tumor usually appears as an ulcerated lesion and has often advanced by the time the patient experiences symptoms. The tumor may penetrate the muscular layer and even extend outside the wall of the esophagus. Obstruction of the esophagus occurs in the later stages.

Clinical Manifestations and Complications

The onset of symptoms is usually late relative to tumor growth. The majority of patients have advanced disease at diagnosis. Progressive dysphagia is the most common symptom and may be described as a substernal feeling as if food is not passing. Initially the dysphagia occurs only with meat, then with soft foods, and eventually with liquids.

Pain develops late. It is described as occurring in the substernal, epigastric, or back areas and usually increases with swallowing. The pain may radiate to the neck, jaw, ears, and shoulders. If the tumor is in the upper third of the esophagus, symptoms such as sore throat, choking, and hoarseness may occur. Weight loss is fairly common. When esophageal stenosis (narrowing) is severe, regurgitation of blood-flecked esophageal contents is common.

Hemorrhage occurs if the cancer erodes through the esophagus and into the aorta. Esophageal perforation with fistula formation into the lung or trachea sometimes develops. The tumor may enlarge enough to cause esophageal obstruction. The cancer spreads via the lymph system, with the liver and the lung being common sites of metastasis.

Diagnostic Studies

Endoscopic biopsy is necessary to make a definitive diagnosis of carcinoma by identification of malignant cells. Endoscopic ultrasonography (EUS) is an important tool used to stage esophageal cancer. Esophagram (barium swallow) may show narrowing of the esophagus at the tumor site (Table 42-11).

Collaborative Care

The treatment of esophageal cancer depends on the location of the tumor and whether invasion or metastasis has occurred. Esophageal cancer has a poor prognosis, mainly because it is often not diagnosed until the disease is advanced. The best

---

TABLE 42-11 COLLABORATIVE CARE

Esophageal Cancer

Diagnostic
- History and physical examination
- Endoscopy of esophagus with biopsy
- Endoscopic ultrasonography
- Esophagram (barium swallow)
- Bronchoscopy
- CT, MRI

Collaborative Therapy
- Surgery
  - Esophagectomy
  - Esophagogastrostomy
  - Esophagoenterostomy
- Endoscopic procedures
  - Photodynamic therapy
  - Endoscopic mucosal resection
- Radiation therapy
- Chemotherapy
- Palliative treatment
  - Dilation
  - Stent or prosthesis
  - Laser therapy
  - Gastrostomy

results are obtained with a multimodal approach, including surgery, endoscopic ablation, chemotherapy, and radiation therapy. Depending on the location and cancer spread, only chemotherapy and radiation may be used.

Surgery. The types of surgical procedures done are (1) removal of part or all of the esophagus (*esophagectomy*) with use of a Dacron graft to replace the resected part, (2) resection of a portion of the esophagus and anastomosis of the remaining portion to the stomach (*esophagogastrostomy*), and (3) resection of a portion of the esophagus and anastomosis of a segment of colon to the remaining portion (*esophagoenterostomy*). The surgical approaches may be open (thoracic, abdominal incision) or laparoscopic.

Minimally invasive esophagectomy (e.g., laparoscopic vagal nerve–sparing surgery) is being performed more frequently. It has the advantage of using smaller incisions, decreasing intensive care unit (ICU) and hospital stays, and producing fewer pulmonary complications.

Endoscopic Procedures. Endoscopic approaches using photodynamic and/or laser therapy can be performed. In photodynamic therapy, porfimer sodium (Photofrin), which is a photosensitizer, is injected IV. The porfimer is absorbed by most tissues but selectively retained to a greater degree by neoplastic tissue. The light (activator) is transmitted via a fiber passed through the endoscope. Warn patients to avoid direct sunlight for up to 4 weeks after the procedure. Other endoscopic procedures include EMR.

Radiation and Chemotherapy. Most patients with newly diagnosed esophageal cancer have local and advanced disease. Treatment includes chemotherapy with or without radiation therapy. Concurrent radiation and chemotherapy are administered for palliation of symptoms, especially dysphagia, and to increase survival. In some patients, treatment is started before surgery is performed.

Currently, no standard single-agent or combination drug therapy is recommended for esophageal cancer. Single-agent chemotherapeutic agents include bleomycin, mitomycin (Mutamycin), methotrexate, paclitaxel, docetaxel, and irinotecan (Camptosar). Combination regimens include ECF (epirubicin [Ellence], cisplatin, 5-fluorouracil [5-FU]), and taxane- and irinotecan-based combinations. Cisplatin in combination with newer fluoropyrimidine such as tegafur-uracil (Uftoral) (tegafur is a 5-FU prodrug) is also used.

Palliative therapy consists of restoration of the swallowing function and maintenance of nutrition and hydration. Dilation, stent placement, or both can relieve obstruction. Self-expandable metal stents are available with features to prevent stent migration and tumor ingrowth. Dilation is done with various types of dilators. Dilation often relieves dysphagia and allows for improved nutrition. Endoscopic placement of stents or expandable stents may help when dilation is no longer effective.[16] This allows food and liquid to pass through the stenotic segment of the esophagus. Stents may be placed before surgery to improve the patient's nutritional status.

Endoscopic laser therapy of the tumor may be used in combination with dilation. Obstruction recurs as the tumor grows, but laser therapy can be repeated. Sometimes these procedures are combined with radiation therapy. Other measures for palliation include gastrostomy or esophagostomy tube placement for nutritional support and pain management.

Nutritional Therapy. After esophageal surgery, parenteral fluids are given. A jejunostomy feeding tube may be used depending on the type of surgery (e.g., esophagogastrectomy)

performed. A swallowing study is often given before the patient is allowed to have oral fluids. When fluids are permitted, water (30 to 60 mL) is given hourly, with gradual progression to small, frequent, bland meals. The patient should be in an upright position to prevent regurgitation of the fluid. With tube feeding, observe the patient for signs of intolerance to the feeding or leakage of the feeding into the mediastinum. Symptoms that indicate leakage are pain, increased temperature, and dyspnea. A gastrostomy tube may be placed to feed the patient. (Enteral nutrition is discussed in Chapter 40.)

NURSING MANAGEMENT
ESOPHAGEAL CANCER

NURSING ASSESSMENT
Ask the patient about a history of GERD, hiatal hernia, achalasia, Barrett's esophagus, and tobacco and alcohol use. Assess the patient for progressive dysphagia and *odynophagia* (burning, squeezing pain while swallowing). Ask about the type of substances (e.g., meats, soft foods, liquids) that cause dysphagia. Also assess the patient for pain (substernal, epigastric, or back areas), choking, heartburn, hoarseness, cough, anorexia, weight loss, and regurgitation.

NURSING DIAGNOSES
Nursing diagnoses for the patient with esophageal cancer include, but are not limited to, the following:

- Chronic pain *related to* the compression of tumor on surrounding tissues, esophageal stenosis
- Imbalanced nutrition: less than body requirements *related to* dysphagia, odynophagia, weakness, chemotherapy, and radiation therapy
- Ineffective health maintenance *related to* lack of knowledge of disease process and treatment, lack of a support system, and chronic debilitating disease
- Anxiety and grieving *related to* diagnosis of cancer, uncertain future, and poor prognosis

PLANNING
The overall goals are that the patient with esophageal cancer will (1) have relief of symptoms, including pain and dysphagia; (2) achieve optimal nutritional intake; (3) understand the prognosis of the disease; and (4) experience a quality of life appropriate to disease progression.

NURSING IMPLEMENTATION
HEALTH PROMOTION. Counsel the patient with GERD, Barrett's esophagus, or hiatal hernia about the importance of regular follow-up evaluation. Health counseling should focus on elimination of smoking and excessive alcohol intake, as well as other risk factors for GERD (see Table 42-7). Maintenance of good oral hygiene and dietary habits (e.g., intake of fresh fruits and vegetables) is important. Encourage patients to seek medical attention for any esophageal problems, especially dysphagia.

ACUTE INTERVENTION
Preoperative Care. In addition to general preoperative teaching and preparation, pay particular attention to the patient's nutritional needs. Many patients are poorly nourished because of the inability to ingest adequate amounts of food and fluids before surgery. A high-calorie, high-protein diet is recommended. Some patients require a liquid form of this diet. Some patients may need IV fluid replacement or parenteral nutrition. Instruct the patient and caregiver on how to keep an intake and

output record and assess for signs of fluid and electrolyte imbalance. Some treatment protocols necessitate preoperative radiation and chemotherapy.

Meticulous oral care is essential. Cleanse the mouth thoroughly, including the tongue, gingivae, and teeth or dentures. It may be necessary to use swabs or a gauze pad and to scrub the mouth, including the tongue. Milk of magnesia with mineral oil helps remove crust formation.

Teaching should include information about chest tubes (if an open thoracic approach is used), IV lines, NG tubes, pain management, gastrostomy or jejunostomy feeding, turning, coughing, and deep breathing. (General preoperative care is discussed in Chapter 18.)

Postoperative Care. The patient usually has an NG tube in place and may have bloody drainage for 8 to 12 hours. The drainage gradually changes to greenish yellow. Assessment of the drainage, maintenance of the tube, and oral and nasal care are nursing responsibilities. Do not reposition the NG tube or reinsert it without consulting the surgeon.

Because of the location of the surgery and the patient's general condition, emphasize prevention of respiratory complications. Turning and deep breathing should be done every 2 hours. Use of an incentive spirometer helps to prevent respiratory complications.

Cardiac dysrhythmias may result from the proximity of the pericardium to the surgical site. Additional complications that can occur after esophagectomy include esophageal anastomotic leaks, fistula formation, interstitial pulmonary edema, and acute respiratory distress related to the disruption of the mediastinal lymph nodes.

Position the patient in a semi-Fowler's or Fowler's position to prevent reflux and aspiration of gastric secretions. When the patient can drink fluids or eat, maintain the upright position for at least 2 hours after eating to assist with gastric emptying.

AMBULATORY AND HOME CARE. Many patients require long-term follow-up care after surgery for esophageal cancer. The patient may undergo chemotherapy and radiation treatment after surgery. Encourage and assist the patient in maintaining adequate nutrition. A permanent feeding gastrostomy may be required. The patient usually has fears and anxieties about a diagnosis of cancer. Know what the health care provider has told the patient regarding the prognosis and then provide appropriate counseling.

Referral to a palliative care or home health nurse may be needed. (See Chapter 16 for the care of the cancer patient and Chapter 10 for a discussion of palliative and end-of-life care.)

EVALUATION

The expected outcomes are that the patient with esophageal cancer will

- Maintain a patent airway
- Have relief of pain
- Be able to swallow comfortably and consume adequate nutritional intake
- Understand the prognosis of the disease
- Experience a quality of life appropriate to disease progression

OTHER ESOPHAGEAL DISORDERS

Eosinophilic Esophagitis

Eosinophilic esophagitis (EE) is characterized by swelling of the esophagus caused by an infiltration of *eosinophils*. People with EE frequently have a personal or family history of other allergic diseases. The most common food triggers are milk, egg, wheat, rye, and beef. Environmental allergens, such as pollens, molds, cat, dog, and dust mite allergens, may be involved in the development of EE.

Clinical manifestations include severe heartburn, difficulty swallowing, food impaction in the esophagus, nausea, vomiting, and weight loss. The diagnosis is based on the symptoms and biopsy findings of eosinophils infiltrating the esophageal tissue obtained from endoscopy.

Allergy skin testing helps to determine the person's allergens. A trial of avoidance of the foods to which the person has positive allergy tests is the initial form of treatment for EE. A variety of treatment approaches, including acid suppression (see Table 42-10), corticosteroids, and endoscopic dilation, can be used alone or in combination.

Corticosteroids are frequently used to treat EE when avoidance of allergic triggers does not relieve symptoms. Corticosteroids may be used orally (prednisone) or as a topical therapy, such as inhaled corticosteroids (e.g., fluticasone [Flovent]). In asthma, where fluticasone is typically used, it is inhaled. In EE it is swallowed, and this results in the delivery of the drug directly to the esophagus.

Esophageal Diverticula

Esophageal diverticula are saclike outpouchings of one or more layers of the esophagus. They occur in three main areas: (1) above the upper esophageal sphincter (*Zenker's diverticulum*), which is the most common location; (2) near the esophageal midpoint (traction diverticulum); and (3) above the LES (epiphrenic diverticulum) (Fig. 42-6). Pharyngeal pouches (Zenker's diverticula) occur most commonly in individuals over 60 years.

Typical symptoms include dysphagia, regurgitation, chronic cough, aspiration, and weight loss. The patient frequently complains of tasting sour food and smelling a foul odor caused by the stagnant food. Complications include malnutrition, aspiration, and perforation. Endoscopy or barium studies can easily establish a diagnosis.

There is no specific treatment for esophageal diverticula. Some patients find that they can empty the pocket of food that collects by applying pressure at a point on the neck. The diet may need to be limited to foods that pass more readily (e.g., blenderized foods). Treatment via an endoscopic or open approach may be necessary if nutrition is disrupted. Treatment

FIG. 42-6 Possible sites for esophageal diverticula. These hollow outpouchings may occur just above the upper esophageal sphincter (Zenker's, the most common type of pulsion diverticulum), near the midpoint of the esophagus (traction), and just above the lower esophageal sphincter (epiphrenic).

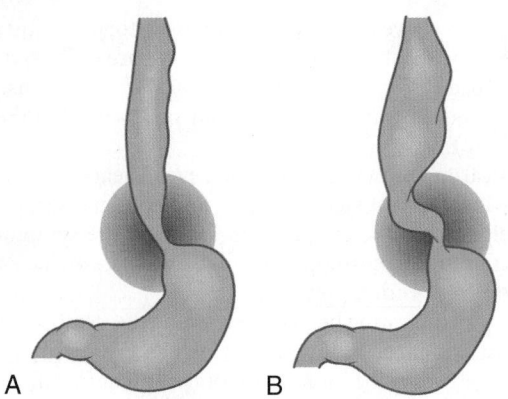

FIG. 42-7 Esophageal achalasia. **A,** Early stage, showing tapering of lower esophagus. **B,** Advanced stage, showing dilated, tortuous esophagus.

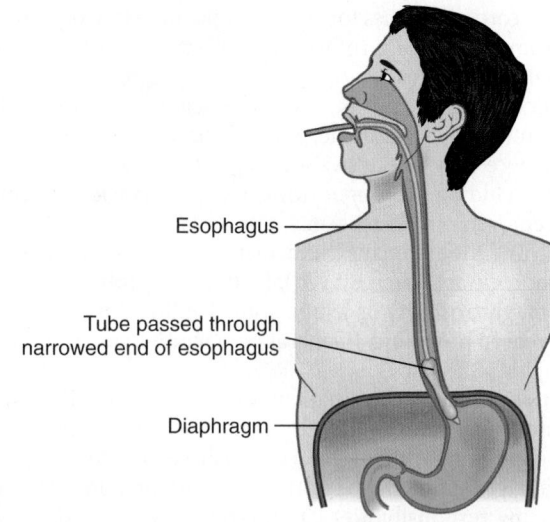

FIG. 42-8 Pneumatic dilation attempts to treat achalasia by maintaining an adequate lumen and decreasing lower esophageal sphincter (LES) tone.

by endoscopic stapling diverticulotomy or diverticulostomy is associated with decreased complications compared with the open approaches. The most serious complication of this treatment is perforation of the esophagus.

Esophageal Strictures

The most common cause of *esophageal strictures* (or narrowing) is chronic GERD. The ingestion of strong acids or alkalis, external beam radiation, and surgical anastomosis can also create strictures. Trauma such as throat lacerations and gunshot wounds may also lead to strictures as a result of scar formation. The strictures can result in dysphagia, regurgitation, and ultimately weight loss.

Strictures can be dilated endoscopically using mechanical *bougies* (dilating instruments) or balloons. The dilation may be performed with or without endoscopy, or with fluoroscopy. Surgical excision with anastomosis is sometimes necessary. The patient may have a temporary or permanent gastrostomy.

Achalasia

In achalasia, peristalsis of the lower two thirds (smooth muscle) of the esophagus is absent. Achalasia is a rare, chronic disorder. With achalasia the pressure in the LES increases along with incomplete relaxation. Obstruction of the esophagus at or near the diaphragm occurs. Food and fluid accumulate in the lower esophagus. The result of this condition is dilation of the lower esophagus proximal to (above) the tapering affected segment of the lower esophagus (Fig. 42-7). There is a selective loss of inhibitory neurons, resulting in unopposed contraction of the LES.

The onset of achalasia is usually insidious. Dysphagia is the most common symptom and occurs with both liquids and solids. Patients may report a globus sensation and/or substernal chest pain (similar to angina pain) that occurs during or immediately after a meal. About a third of the patients experience nocturnal regurgitation. *Halitosis* (foul-smelling breath) and the inability to eructate (belch) are other symptoms. Patients with achalasia also report symptoms of GERD and regurgitation of sour-tasting food and liquids, especially when they are lying down. Weight loss is typical.

Diagnosis is made with esophagram (barium swallow), manometric evaluation (high-resolution manometry), and/or endoscopic evaluation. The exact cause of achalasia is not known, so treatment focuses on symptom management. The goals of treatment are to relieve dysphagia and regurgitation, improve esophageal emptying by disrupting the LES, and

prevent development of megaesophagus (enlargement of the lower esophagus).

Endoscopic pneumatic dilation is done as an outpatient procedure. The LES muscle is disrupted from within using balloons of progressively larger diameter (3.0, 3.5, and 4.0 cm) (Fig. 42-8). If this is ineffective, then a surgical procedure, Heller myotomy, is done laparoscopically. In this procedure the LES is surgically disrupted (myotomy). Because GERD with esophagitis and stricture is a common complication, the patient often has antireflux surgery performed at the same time. The patient can usually return to work 1 to 2 weeks after this procedure.

Medical therapy is less effective than invasive procedures. Smooth muscle relaxants such as nitrates (isosorbide dinitrate [Isordil]) and calcium channel blockers (e.g., nifedipine [Procardia]) taken sublingually 30 to 45 minutes before meals to improve dysphagia may be prescribed. However, side effects (e.g., headache), drug tolerance, and short duration of action limit their use.

The injection of botulinum toxin endoscopically into the LES gives short-term relief of symptoms and improves esophageal emptying. It works by promoting relaxation of the smooth muscle. This treatment is used for older patients for whom surgery and pneumatic dilation may not be appropriate due to other chronic illnesses. Symptomatic treatment consists of eating a semisoft diet, eating slowly and drinking fluid with meals, and sleeping with the head elevated.

Esophageal Varices

Esophageal varices are dilated, tortuous veins occurring in the lower portion of the esophagus as a result of portal hypertension. Esophageal varices are a common complication of liver cirrhosis and are discussed in Chapter 44.

DISORDERS OF THE STOMACH AND UPPER SMALL INTESTINE

GASTRITIS

Gastritis, an inflammation of the gastric mucosa, is one of the most common problems affecting the stomach. Gastritis may be acute or chronic and diffuse or localized.

TABLE 42-12	CAUSES OF GASTRITIS

Drugs
- Aspirin
- Corticosteroids
- Nonsteroidal antiinflammatory drugs (NSAIDs)

Diet
- Alcohol
- Spicy, irritating food

Microorganisms
- *Helicobacter pylori*
- *Salmonella* organisms
- *Staphylococcus* organisms

Environmental Factors
- Radiation
- Smoking

Pathophysiologic Conditions
- Burns
- Large hiatal hernia
- Physiologic stress
- Reflux of bile and pancreatic secretions
- Renal failure (uremia)
- Sepsis
- Shock

Other Factors
- Endoscopic procedures
- Nasogastric tube
- Psychologic stress

Etiology and Pathophysiology

Gastritis occurs as the result of a breakdown in the normal gastric mucosal barrier. This mucosal barrier normally protects the stomach tissue from the corrosive action of HCl acid and pepsin. When the barrier is broken, HCl acid and pepsin can diffuse back into the mucosa. This back diffusion results in tissue edema, disruption of capillary walls with loss of plasma into the gastric lumen, and possible hemorrhage.

Risk Factors. Risk factors and causes of gastritis are listed in Table 42-12. Some of the risk factors are discussed in this section.

Drug-Related Gastritis. Drugs contribute to the development of acute and chronic gastritis. NSAIDs, including aspirin, and corticosteroids inhibit the synthesis of prostaglandins that are protective to the gastric mucosa. Thus the mucosa is more susceptible to injury. NSAID-related gastritis is associated with many drugs, including piroxicam (Feldene), naproxen (Naprosyn), sulindac (Clinoril), indomethacin (Indocin), diclofenac (Voltaren), and ibuprofen (Motrin, Advil).[17]

Risk factors for NSAID-induced gastritis include being female; being over age 60; having a history of ulcer disease; taking anticoagulants, other NSAIDs (including low-dose aspirin), or other ulcerogenic drugs (including corticosteroids); and having a chronic debilitating disorder such as cardiovascular disease. Some drugs such as digitalis (digoxin) and alendronate (Fosamax) have direct irritating effects on the gastric mucosa.

Diet. Dietary indiscretions can also result in acute gastritis. After an alcoholic drinking binge, acute damage to the gastric mucosa can range from localized injury of superficial epithelial cells to destruction of the mucosa with mucosal congestion, edema, and hemorrhage. Prolonged damage induced by repeated alcohol abuse results in chronic gastritis. Eating large quantities of spicy, irritating foods and metabolic conditions such as renal failure can also cause acute gastritis.

Helicobacter pylori. An important cause of chronic gastritis is *Helicobacter pylori* infection. *H. pylori* infection is highest in underdeveloped countries and in people of low socioeconomic status. Infection likely occurs during childhood with transmission from family members to the child, possibly through a fecal-oral or oral-oral route.

In the United States, people born before 1940 are more likely to carry *H. pylori* than people in younger age-groups. *H. pylori* has also been linked to stomach cancer and non-Hodgkin's lymphoma. The role of *H. pylori* in ulcer development is discussed in greater detail in this chapter on p. 943.

Other Risk Factors. Although not as common, other risk factors of chronic gastritis have been identified. Bacterial, viral, and fungal infections, including *Mycobacterium* species, cytomegalovirus (CMV), and syphilis, are associated with chronic gastritis. Gastritis can occur from reflux of bile salts from the duodenum into the stomach as a result of anatomic changes following surgical procedures (e.g., gastroduodenostomy, gastrojejunostomy). Prolonged vomiting may also cause reflux of bile salts. Intense emotional responses and CNS lesions may also produce inflammation of the mucosal lining as a result of hypersecretion of HCl acid.

Autoimmune Gastritis. Autoimmune metaplastic atrophic gastritis (also called autoimmune atrophic gastritis) is an inherited condition in which there is an immune response directed against parietal cells. It most commonly affects women of northern European descent. Patients with autoimmune atrophic gastritis often have other autoimmune disorders. The loss of parietal cells leads to low chloride levels, inadequate production of intrinsic factor, cobalamin (vitamin B_{12}) malabsorption, and pernicious anemia. Atrophic gastritis is associated with an increased risk of stomach cancer.

Clinical Manifestations

In *acute gastritis* the symptoms include anorexia, nausea and vomiting, epigastric tenderness, and a feeling of fullness. Hemorrhage is commonly associated with alcohol abuse and at times is the only symptom. Acute gastritis is self-limiting, lasting from a few hours to a few days, with complete healing of the mucosa expected.

In *chronic gastritis* the manifestations are similar to those described for acute gastritis. Some patients are asymptomatic. However, when the parietal cells are lost as a result of atrophy, the source of intrinsic factor is also lost. The loss of *intrinsic factor*, a substance essential for the absorption of cobalamin in the terminal ileum, ultimately results in cobalamin deficiency. With time, the body's storage of cobalamin in the liver becomes depleted, and a state of deficiency exists. Because it is essential for the growth and maturation of red blood cells (RBCs), the lack of cobalamin results in pernicious anemia and neurologic complications. (Cobalamin deficiency anemia is discussed in Chapter 31.)

Diagnostic Studies

Diagnosis of acute gastritis is most often based on the patient's history of drug and alcohol use. Endoscopic examination with biopsy may be warranted to obtain a definitive diagnosis. Breath, urine, serum, stool, and gastric tissue biopsy tests are available for the determination of *H. pylori* infection. (These diagnostic tests are described in the section on peptic ulcer disease later in this chapter on p. 945.)

Radiologic studies are not helpful because the superficial mucosa is generally involved, and changes will not show clearly on x-ray examination. A complete blood count (CBC) may demonstrate anemia from blood loss or lack of intrinsic factor. Stools are tested for occult blood. Serum tests for antibodies to parietal cells and intrinsic factor may be performed. Tissue biopsy is necessary to rule out gastric carcinoma.

TABLE 42-13   DRUG THERAPY

Helicobacter pylori Infection

Treatment	Duration	Eradication Rate
Triple-Drug Therapy	7-14 days	70%-85%
proton pump inhibitor (PPI)*		
amoxicillin		
clarithromycin (Biaxin)		
Quadruple Therapy	10-14 days	85%
PPI*		
bismuth†		
tetracycline		
metronidazole (Flagyl)		

*See Table 42-10.
†Bismuth is part of a combination capsule (Pylera) containing bismuth, tetracycline, and metronidazole that is used in combination with a PPI (e.g., omeprazole [Prilosec]).

NURSING AND COLLABORATIVE MANAGEMENT GASTRITIS

ACUTE GASTRITIS

Eliminating the cause and preventing or avoiding it in the future are generally all that is needed to treat acute gastritis. The plan of care is supportive and similar to that described for nausea and vomiting. If vomiting accompanies acute gastritis, rest, NPO status, and IV fluids may be prescribed. Dehydration can occur rapidly in acute gastritis with vomiting. Antiemetics are given for nausea and vomiting (see Table 42-1).

In severe cases of acute gastritis, an NG tube may be used (1) to monitor for bleeding, (2) to lavage the precipitating agent from the stomach, or (3) to keep the stomach empty and free of noxious stimuli. Clear liquids are resumed when symptoms have subsided, with gradual reintroduction of solids.

If hemorrhage is considered likely, frequently check vital signs and test the vomitus for blood. All of the management strategies discussed in the section on upper GI bleeding apply to the patient with severe gastritis (see p. 955).

Drug therapy focuses on reducing irritation of the gastric mucosa and providing symptomatic relief. H_2-receptor blockers (e.g., ranitidine, cimetidine) or PPIs (e.g., omeprazole, lansoprazole) reduce gastric HCl acid secretion (see Table 42-10). Teach the patient about the therapeutic effects of PPIs and H_2-receptor blockers.

CHRONIC GASTRITIS

The treatment of chronic gastritis focuses on evaluating and eliminating the specific cause (e.g., cessation of alcohol intake, abstinence from drugs, *H. pylori* eradication). Currently, antibiotic combinations are used to eradicate *H. pylori* (Table 42-13). For the patient with pernicious anemia, cobalamin (administered orally, nasally, or by injections) is needed (see Chapter 31). Discuss the need for lifelong cobalamin therapy with the patient.

The patient undergoing treatment for chronic gastritis may have to adapt to lifestyle changes and strictly adhere to a drug regimen. Some patients find a nonirritating diet consisting of six small feedings a day helpful. Smoking is contraindicated in all forms of gastritis. An interprofessional team approach in which the physician, nurse, dietitian, and pharmacist provide consistent information and support may increase the patient's success in making these alterations.

FIG. 42-9 Peptic ulcers, including an erosion, an acute ulcer, and a chronic ulcer. Both the acute ulcer and the chronic ulcer may penetrate the entire wall of the stomach.

FIG. 42-10 Peptic ulcer of the duodenum.

PEPTIC ULCER DISEASE

Peptic ulcer disease (PUD) is a condition characterized by erosion of the GI mucosa resulting from the digestive action of HCl acid and pepsin. Any portion of the GI tract that comes into contact with gastric secretions is susceptible to ulcer development, including the lower esophagus, stomach, duodenum, and margin of a gastrojejunal anastomosis after surgical procedures. Approximately 350,000 new cases of ulcers are diagnosed each year.

Types

Peptic ulcers can be classified as acute or chronic, depending on the degree and duration of mucosal involvement, and gastric or duodenal, according to the location. The *acute ulcer* (Fig. 42-9) is associated with superficial erosion and minimal inflammation. It is of short duration and resolves quickly when the cause is identified and removed. A chronic ulcer (Fig. 42-10) is one of long duration, eroding through the muscular wall with the formation of fibrous tissue. It is present continuously for many months or intermittently throughout the person's lifetime. Chronic ulcers are more common than acute erosions.

Gastric and duodenal ulcers, although defined as PUD, are different in their etiology and incidence (Table 42-14). Generally, the treatment of all types of ulcers is similar.

Etiology and Pathophysiology

Peptic ulcers develop only in an acid environment. However, an excess of HCl acid may not be necessary for ulcer development. Pepsinogen, the precursor of pepsin, is activated to pepsin in the presence of HCl acid and a pH of 2 to 3. When the stomach acid level is neutralized by food or antacids or acid secretion is

TABLE 42-14	COMPARISON OF GASTRIC AND DUODENAL ULCERS	
Gastric Ulcers	**Duodenal Ulcers**	
Lesion		
Superficial, smooth margins Round, oval, or cone shaped	Penetrating (associated with deformity of duodenal bulb from healing of recurrent ulcers)	
Location of Lesion		
Predominantly antrum, also in body and fundus of stomach	First 1-2 cm of duodenum	
Gastric Secretion		
Normal to decreased	Increased	
Incidence		
Greater in women	Greater in men, but increasing in women (especially postmenopausal)	
Peak age 50-60 yr	Peak age 35-45 yr	
More common in people of lower socioeconomic status	Associated with psychologic stress	
↑ With smoking, drug use (aspirin, NSAID), and alcohol use	↑ With smoking, drug use, and alcohol use	
↑ With incompetent pyloric sphincter and bile reflux	Associated with other diseases (e.g., chronic obstructive pulmonary disease, pancreatic disease, hyperparathyroidism, Zollinger-Ellison syndrome, chronic renal failure)	
Clinical Manifestations		
Burning or gaseous pressure in high left epigastrium and back and upper abdomen	Burning, cramping, pressure-like pain across midepigastrium and upper abdomen. Back pain with posterior ulcers	
Pain 1-2 hr after meals. If penetrating ulcer, aggravation of discomfort with food	Pain 2-4 hr after meals and midmorning, midafternoon, middle of night. Periodic and episodic. Pain relief with antacids and food	
Occasional nausea and vomiting, weight loss	Occasional nausea and vomiting	
Recurrence Rate		
High	High	
Complications		
Hemorrhage, perforation, gastric outlet obstruction, intractability	Hemorrhage, perforation, obstruction	

PATHOPHYSIOLOGY MAP

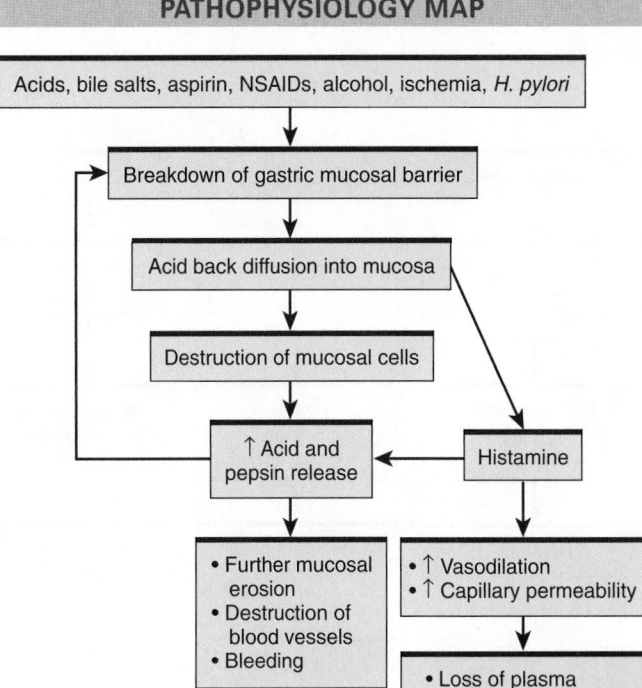

FIG. 42-11 Disruption of gastric mucosa and pathophysiologic consequences of back diffusion of acids.

blocked by drugs, the pH is increased to 3.5 or more. At a pH of 3.5 or more, pepsin has little or no proteolytic activity.

The pathophysiology of ulcer development is outlined in Fig. 42-11. The back diffusion of HCl acid into the gastric mucosa results in cellular destruction and inflammation. Histamine is released from the damaged mucosa, resulting in vasodilation and increased capillary permeability and further secretion of acid and pepsin. Fig. 42-12 depicts the interrelationship between the mucosal blood flow and disruption of the gastric mucosal barrier. As described in the section on gastritis, a variety of agents are known to damage the mucosal barrier.

Helicobacter pylori. In addition to chronic gastritis, *H. pylori* is associated with peptic ulcer development. Approximately two thirds of the world's population is infected with *H. pylori*.[18]

In the stomach the bacteria can survive a long time by colonizing the gastric epithelial cells within the mucosal layer. The bacteria also produce urease, which metabolizes urea-producing ammonium chloride and other damaging chemicals. Urease also activates the immune response with both antibody production and the release of inflammatory cytokines.

The response to *H. pylori* is variable. Not all individuals infected with *H. pylori* go on to develop ulcers. In one scenario, *H. pylori* leads to intestinal metaplasia in the stomach resulting in chronic atrophic gastritis and in some cases stomach cancer. In another scenario, *H. pylori* alters gastric secretion and produces tissue damage, leading to PUD. The response to *H. pylori* is influenced by a variety of factors, including genetics, environment, and diet.

Medication-Induced Injury. Ulcerogenic drugs, such as aspirin and NSAIDs, inhibit synthesis of prostaglandins, increase gastric acid secretion, and reduce the integrity of the mucosal barrier. The use of NSAIDs is responsible for the majority of non–*H. pylori* peptic ulcers. NSAIDs in the presence of *H. pylori* increase the risk of PUD.[17] Patients on corticosteroids, anticoagulants, and selective serotonin reuptake inhibitors (e.g., fluoxetine [Prozac]) are also at increased risk of ulcer development.[19] Corticosteroids affect mucosal cell renewal and decrease its protective effects.

Lifestyle Factors. High alcohol intake is associated with acute mucosal lesions. In addition, alcohol stimulates acid secretion. Coffee (caffeinated and decaffeinated) is a strong stimulant of gastric acid secretion. Psychologic distress, including stress and depression, can negatively influence the healing of ulcers once they have developed. Smoking also delays ulcer healing.

PATHOPHYSIOLOGY MAP

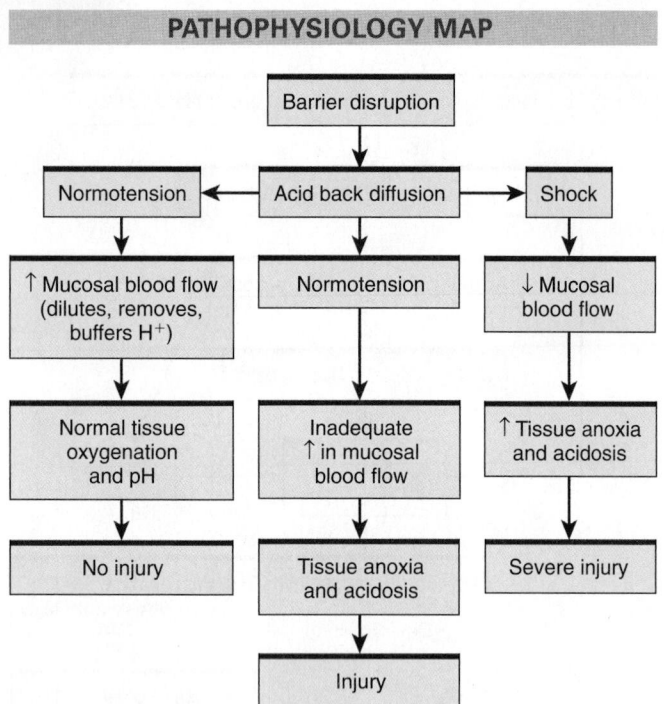

FIG. 42-12 Relationship between mucosal blood flow and disruption of the gastric mucosal barrier.

FIG. 42-13 Duodenal ulcer of the posterior wall penetrating into the head of the pancreas, resulting in walled-off perforation.

Gastric Ulcers. Although gastric ulcers can occur in any portion of the stomach, they are most commonly found in the antrum. Gastric ulcers are less common than duodenal ulcers. Gastric ulcers are more prevalent in women and in older adults. Because the peak incidence of gastric ulcers is in people over 50 years of age, the mortality rate from gastric ulcers is greater than that from duodenal ulcers. Gastric ulcers are more likely than duodenal ulcers to result in obstruction. *H. pylori,* medications, smoking, and bile reflux are risk factors for gastric ulcers.

Duodenal Ulcers. Duodenal ulcers account for about 80% of all peptic ulcers. Duodenal ulcers may occur at any age, but the incidence is especially high between 35 and 45 years of age. Duodenal ulcers can develop in anyone, regardless of occupation or socioeconomic group.

Although many factors are associated with the development of duodenal ulcers, *H. pylori* is most common. *H. pylori* infection is found in approximately 90% to 95% of patients with duodenal ulcers.

The development of duodenal ulcers is often associated with a high HCl acid secretion. Alcohol ingestion and smoking are associated with duodenal ulcer formation because both are known stimulants of acid secretion. Several patient groups are at high risk of duodenal ulcer development, including those with chronic obstructive pulmonary disease, cirrhosis of the liver, chronic pancreatitis, hyperparathyroidism, chronic kidney disease, and *Zollinger-Ellison syndrome* (a rare condition characterized by severe peptic ulceration and HCl acid hypersecretion).

Stress-Related Mucosal Disease (SRMD). SRMD is described later in this chapter in the section on acute upper GI bleeding on p. 954.

Clinical Manifestations

The discomfort generally associated with gastric ulcers is located high in the epigastrium and occurs about 1 to 2 hours after meals. The pain is described as "burning" or "gaseous." If the

ulcer has eroded through the gastric mucosa, food tends to aggravate rather than alleviate the pain. For some patients, the earliest symptoms are due to a serious complication such as perforation.

The symptoms of duodenal ulcers occur when gastric acid comes in contact with the ulcers. With meal ingestion, food is present to help buffer the acid. Symptoms of duodenal ulcers occur generally 2 to 5 hours after a meal. The pain is described as "burning" or "cramplike." It is most often located in the midepigastric region beneath the xiphoid process. Duodenal ulcers can also produce back pain.

Antacids alone or in combination with an H_2-receptor blocker, as well as food, neutralize the acid to provide relief. A characteristic of duodenal ulcer is its tendency to occur continuously for a few weeks or months and then disappear for a time, only to recur some months later.

Not all patients with gastric or duodenal ulcers experience pain or discomfort. *Silent* peptic ulcers are more likely to occur in older adults and those taking NSAIDs. The presence or absence of symptoms is not directly related to the size of the ulcer or the degree of healing.

Complications

The three major complications of chronic PUD are hemorrhage, perforation, and gastric outlet obstruction. All are considered emergency situations and may require surgical intervention.

Hemorrhage. Hemorrhage is the most common complication of PUD. Duodenal ulcers account for a greater percentage of upper GI bleeding episodes than gastric ulcers.

Perforation. Perforation is considered the most lethal complication of PUD. Perforation is commonly seen in large penetrating duodenal ulcers (Fig. 42-13). Even though duodenal ulcers are more prevalent and perforate more often, mortality rates associated with perforation of gastric ulcers are higher. The patient with gastric ulcers is older and often has concurrent medical problems, which accounts for the higher mortality rate.

With perforation, the ulcer penetrates the serosal surface with spillage of either gastric or duodenal contents into the peritoneal cavity. Small perforations seal themselves, resulting in a cessation of symptoms. Larger perforations require immediate surgical closure. Spontaneous sealing occurs as a result of fibrin production in response to the perforation. This can lead to fibrinous fusion of the duodenum or gastric curvature to adjacent tissue (mainly the liver) and strictures that can obstruct the flow of intestinal contents and the passage of stool.

The clinical manifestations of perforation are sudden and dramatic in onset. During the initial phase (0 to 2 hours after perforation) the patient experiences sudden, severe upper abdominal pain that quickly spreads throughout the abdomen. The pain radiates to the back and is not relieved by food or antacids. The abdomen appears rigid and boardlike as the abdominal muscles attempt to protect from further injury. The patient's respirations become shallow and rapid. The heart rate is elevated (tachycardia), and the pulse is weak. Bowel sounds are usually absent. Nausea and vomiting may occur. Many patients report a history of ulcer disease or recent symptoms of indigestion.

The contents entering the peritoneal cavity from the stomach or duodenum may contain air, saliva, food particles, HCl acid, pepsin, bacteria, bile, and pancreatic fluid and enzymes. If the condition is untreated, bacterial peritonitis may occur within 6 to 12 hours. The intensity of the peritonitis is proportional to the amount and duration of the spillage through the perforation. It is difficult to determine from the symptoms alone whether a gastric or duodenal ulcer has perforated because the clinical characteristics of intestinal perforation are the same (see Chapter 43).

Gastric Outlet Obstruction. Both acute and chronic PUD can result in gastric outlet obstruction. Obstruction in the distal stomach and duodenum is the result of edema, inflammation, or pylorospasm and fibrous scar tissue formation. With obstruction the patient reports discomfort or pain that is worse toward the end of the day as the stomach fills and dilates. Relief may be obtained by belching or by self-induced vomiting. Vomiting is common and often projectile. The vomitus contains food particles that were ingested hours or days before the vomiting episode. Constipation occurs because of dehydration and decreased diet intake secondary to anorexia. Over time dilation of the stomach and visible swelling in the upper abdomen may occur.

Diagnostic Studies

The diagnostic tests used to determine the presence and location of an ulcer are similar to those used for acute upper GI bleeding. Endoscopy is the most accurate diagnostic procedure. Endoscopy allows for direct viewing of the gastric and duodenal mucosa (Fig. 42-14). It can be used to determine the degree of ulcer healing after treatment and to confirm the absence of malignancy. During endoscopy, tissue specimens are obtained for identification of *H. pylori* and to rule out stomach cancer.

Several diagnostic tests are available to confirm *H. pylori* infection. These are classified as noninvasive and invasive. Biopsy of the antral mucosa and testing for urease (rapid urease testing) is considered the gold standard for diagnosis of *H. pylori* infection. Noninvasive tests include stool testing or breath testing. Serum or whole blood antibody tests, particularly immunoglobulin G (IgG), do not distinguish between past and current infection. The urea breath test can identify active infection. Urea is a by-product of the metabolism of *H. pylori* bacteria. Although not as accurate as the urea breath test, stool antigen tests can also be performed.

A barium contrast study may be used in the diagnosis of gastric outlet obstruction or for ulcer detection in those patients who cannot undergo endoscopy. The presence of a possible gastrinoma (Zollinger-Ellison syndrome) can be diagnosed by measuring fasting serum gastrin levels. With a gastrinoma, the gastrin levels are elevated. A secretin stimulation test can dif-

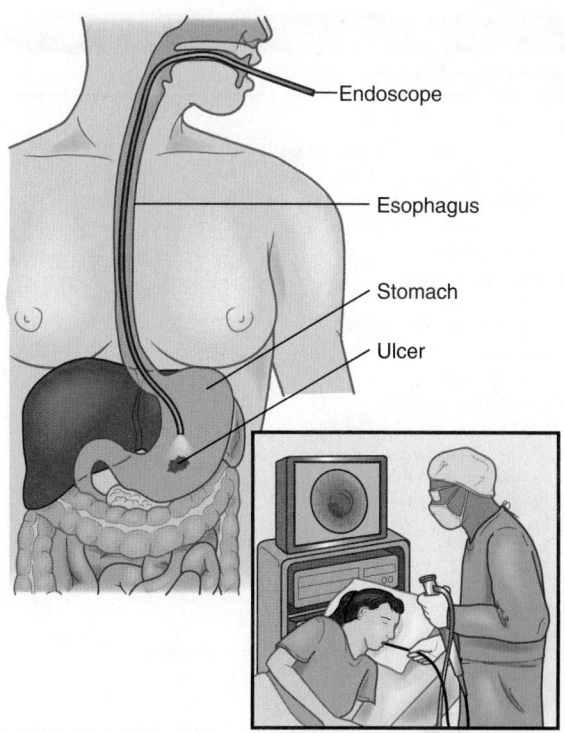

FIG. 42-14 Esophagogastroduodenoscopy (EGD) directly visualizes the mucosal lining of the stomach with a flexible endoscope. Ulcers or tumors can be directly visualized and biopsies taken.

ferentiate patients with gastrinomas from those with other causes of hypergastrinemia.

Laboratory tests, including a CBC, liver enzyme studies, serum amylase determination, and stool examination, should be performed. A CBC may indicate anemia secondary to ulcer bleeding. Liver enzyme studies help detect any liver problems (e.g., cirrhosis) that may complicate ulcer treatment. Stools are routinely tested for blood. A serum amylase determination is done to determine pancreatic function when posterior duodenal ulcer penetration of the pancreas is suspected.

Collaborative Care
Conservative Therapy

When the patient's clinical manifestations and health history suggest the diagnosis of PUD and diagnostic studies confirm it, a treatment regimen is instituted (Table 42-15). The regimen consists of adequate rest, drug therapy, elimination of smoking, dietary modifications (if needed), and long-term follow-up care. The aim of treatment is to decrease gastric acidity and enhance mucosal defense mechanisms.

Patients are generally treated in ambulatory care clinics. Pain disappears after 3 to 6 days, but ulcer healing is much slower. Complete healing may take 3 to 9 weeks, depending on ulcer size, treatment regimen, and patient adherence. Endoscopic examination is the most accurate method to monitor for ulcer healing. The usual follow-up endoscopic evaluation is performed 3 to 6 months after diagnosis and treatment.

Aspirin and nonselective NSAIDs are discontinued for 4 to 6 weeks. When aspirin must be continued, co-administration with a PPI, H_2-receptor blocker, or misoprostol (Cytotec) may be prescribed. Patients with *H. pylori* infection are treated with antibiotics and a PPI. Patients receiving low-dose aspirin for cardiovascular and stroke risk who have a history of ulcer disease or complications may need to receive long-term treatment with a PPI.[20] Enteric-coated aspirin decreases localized

TABLE 42-15   COLLABORATIVE CARE

Peptic Ulcer Disease

Diagnostic
- History and physical examination
- Upper GI endoscopy with biopsy
- *Helicobacter pylori* testing of breath, urine, blood, tissue
- Complete blood cell count
- Liver enzymes
- Serum electrolytes

Collaborative Therapy
Conservative Therapy
- Adequate rest
- Cessation of smoking
- Drug therapy (see Tables 42-9 and 42-13)
  - Proton pump inhibitors
  - H_2-receptor blockers
  - Antibiotics for *H. pylori*
  - Cytoprotective drugs
  - Antacids
  - Anticholinergics (used rarely)
- Stress management (see Chapter 7)

Acute Exacerbation Without Complications
- NPO
- NG suction
- Adequate rest
- IV fluid replacement
- Drug therapy
  - Proton pump inhibitors
  - H_2-receptor blockers
  - Antacids
  - Anticholinergics
  - Sedatives

Acute Exacerbation With Complications (Hemorrhage, Perforation, Obstruction)
- NPO
- NG suction
- IV proton pump inhibitor
- Bed rest
- IV fluid replacement (lactated Ringer's solution)
- Blood transfusions
- Stomach lavage (possible)

Surgical Therapy
- *Perforation:* Simple closure with omentum graft
- *Gastric outlet obstruction:* Pyloroplasty and vagotomy
- *Ulcer removal or reduction*
  - Billroth I and II
  - Vagotomy and pyloroplasty

irritation but has not been proved to reduce the overall risk for GI bleeding.

Smoking has an irritating effect on the mucosa and delays mucosal healing. Smoking should be eliminated completely or severely reduced. (Strategies to enhance patient smoking cessation are discussed in Chapter 11.) Adequate rest, both physical and emotional, is important for ulcer healing and may require some modifications in the patient's daily routine. Avoidance or restriction of alcohol intake will also enhance healing.

Drug Therapy. Drugs are a vital part of therapy (see Table 42-10). Strict adherence to the prescribed regimen of drugs is important. Teach the patient about each drug prescribed, why it is ordered, and the expected benefits.

Because ulcers frequently recur, interruption or discontinuation of therapy can have harmful results. Encourage the patient to adhere to therapy and continue with follow-up care as prescribed. H_2-receptor blockers and PPIs may be stopped after the ulcer has healed or may be prescribed as low-dose maintenance therapy. Teach the patient and the family what to do if pain and discomfort recur or blood is noted in the vomitus or stools.

Histamine (H_2)-Receptor Blockers. H_2-receptor blockers promote ulcer healing. Famotidine, ranitidine, and cimetidine can be given orally or IV, but nizatidine is only available orally. Depending on the specific drug, therapeutic effects last up to 12 hours. The onset of action of H_2-receptor blockers is 1 hour, which is longer than antacids.

Proton Pump Inhibitors. PPIs are more effective than H_2-receptor blockers in reducing gastric acid secretion and promoting ulcer healing. PPIs are also used in combination with antibiotics to treat ulcers caused by *H. pylori*. Omeprazole is available in an OTC formulation at a lower dose and in an immediate-release form.

Antibiotic Therapy. The treatment of *H. pylori* is the most important element of treating PUD in patients positive for *H. pylori*. Antibiotic therapy for *H. pylori* is shown in Table 42-13. Antibiotics are prescribed concurrently with a PPI for 7 to 14 days. Because of the development of antibiotic-resistant organisms, a growing percentage of patients do not have the *H. pylori* eradicated with a single round of therapy.

Antacids. Antacids are used as adjunct therapy for PUD. They increase gastric pH by neutralizing the HCl acid. As a result, the acid content of chyme reaching the duodenum is reduced. In addition, some antacids, such as aluminum hydroxide, can bind to bile salts, thus decreasing the damaging effects of bile on the gastric mucosa. Patients who are at risk for SRMD may be treated prophylactically with antacids along with an antisecretory agent.

The common commercial nonsystemic (poorly absorbed) antacids consist of magnesium hydroxide or aluminum hydroxide as single preparations or in various combinations (see Table 42-10). The neutralizing effects of antacids taken on an empty stomach last only 20 to 30 minutes because they are quickly evacuated. When antacids are taken after meals, the effects may last as long as 3 to 4 hours. Therapy recommending frequent dosing (e.g., hourly) often results in poor adherence.

After the acute phase of bleeding, antacids are generally administered hourly, either orally or through the NG tube. If the tube is in place, the stomach contents should be aspirated and tested periodically for pH level. If pH is less than 5, intermittent suction may be used, or the frequency or dosage of the antacid or antisecretory agent may be increased.

The type and dosage of antacid prescribed depend on side effects and potential drug interactions. Antacids high in sodium (e.g., sodium citrate [Bicitra]) need to be used with caution in older adults and patients with liver cirrhosis, hypertension, heart failure, and renal disease. Magnesium preparations should not be prescribed for patients with renal failure because of the risk of magnesium toxicity. An antacid combination of aluminum and magnesium seems to decrease the side effects of both.

Antacids can interact unfavorably with some drugs. They can enhance the absorption of drugs such as dicumarol and amphetamines. Digitalis preparations can be potentiated when taken in combination with calcium or magnesium antacids. In some instances, antacids decrease the absorption rates of prescribed drugs, such as tetracycline. Before antacid therapy begins, inform the health care provider of any drugs that a patient is taking.

Cytoprotective Drug Therapy. Sucralfate is used for the short-term treatment of ulcers. It provides cytoprotection for the esophagus, stomach, and duodenum. Sucralfate does not have acid-neutralizing capabilities. Its action is most effective at a low pH, and it should be given at least 30 minutes before or after an antacid. Adverse side effects are minimal. However, it does bind with cimetidine, digoxin, warfarin (Coumadin), phenytoin (Dilantin), and tetracycline, causing reduced bioavailability of these drugs.

Misoprostol is a synthetic prostaglandin analog prescribed for the prevention of gastric ulcers caused by NSAIDs and aspirin. It has protective and some antisecretory effects on gastric mucosa. Misoprostol does not interfere with the therapeutic effects of aspirin and NSAIDs. People who require chronic NSAID therapy, such as those with osteoarthritis, may benefit from the use of misoprostol.

Other Drugs. Tricyclic antidepressants (e.g., imipramine [Tofranil], doxepin [Sinequan]) may be prescribed for patients with PUD. Antidepressants may contribute to overall pain relief through their effects on afferent pain fiber transmission. In addition, tricyclic antidepressants have (to varying degrees) some anticholinergic properties, which result in reduced acid secretion. Selective serotonin reuptake inhibitors are associated with a modest risk for upper GI bleeding.[19]

Anticholinergic drugs are used only occasionally for PUD treatment. Anticholinergics are associated with a number of side effects, such as dry mouth, warm skin, flushing, thirst, tachycardia, dilated pupils, blurred vision, and urine retention.

Nutritional Therapy. There is no specific recommended dietary modification for PUD. Patients are taught to eat and drink foods and fluids that do not cause any distressing symptoms. Caffeine-containing beverages and foods can increase symptom distress in some patients. Teach the patient to eliminate alcohol because it can delay healing. Foods that commonly cause gastric irritation include hot, spicy foods; pepper; carbonated beverages; and broth (meat extract).

Therapy Related to Complications of Peptic Ulcer Disease

Acute Exacerbation. An acute exacerbation is frequently accompanied by bleeding, increased pain and discomfort, and nausea and vomiting. Management is similar to that described for upper GI bleeding later in this chapter (see pp. 955-957).

Perforation. The immediate focus of management of a patient with a perforation is to stop the spillage of gastric or duodenal contents into the peritoneal cavity and restore blood volume. An NG tube is inserted into the stomach to provide continuous aspiration and gastric decompression to stop spillage through the perforation. For duodenal aspiration, the tube is placed as near to the perforation site as possible to facilitate decompression.

Circulating blood volume is replaced with lactated Ringer's and albumin solutions. These solutions substitute for the fluids lost from the vascular and interstitial space as the peritonitis develops. Blood replacement in the form of packed RBCs may be necessary. A central venous pressure line and an indwelling urinary catheter may be inserted and monitored hourly. The patient with a history of cardiac disease requires electrocardiographic (ECG) monitoring or placement of a pulmonary artery catheter for accurate assessment of left ventricular function. Broad-spectrum antibiotic therapy is started immediately to treat bacterial peritonitis. Administration of pain medications provides comfort.

Either open or laparoscopic procedures are used for perforation repair depending on the location of the ulcer and the surgeon's preference. The procedure involving the least risk to the patient is simple oversewing of the perforation and reinforcement of the area with a graft of omentum. The excess gastric contents are suctioned from the peritoneal cavity during the surgical procedure.

Gastric Outlet Obstruction. The aim of therapy for obstruction is to decompress the stomach, correct any existing fluid and electrolyte imbalances, and improve the patient's general state of health. An NG tube is used as described previously. With continuous decompression for several days, the ulcer can begin healing, and the inflammation and edema will subside.

After several days of suction, clamp the NG tube and measure gastric residual volume periodically. The frequency and amount of time the tube remains clamped are related to the amount of aspirate obtained and the patient's comfort level. A method commonly followed is to clamp the tube overnight for approximately 8 to 12 hours and then measure the gastric residue in the morning. When the aspirate falls below 200 mL, this is within a normal range and the patient can begin oral intake of clear liquids. Oral fluids begin at 30 mL/hr and then gradually increase in amount. Assess the patient for signs and symptoms of distress or vomiting. As the amount of gastric residue decreases, solid foods are added and the tube removed.

IV fluids and electrolytes are administered according to the degree of dehydration, vomiting, and electrolyte imbalance indicated by laboratory studies. Pain relief results from the decompression. A PPI or H_2-receptor blocker is used if the obstruction is due to an active ulcer as determined by endoscopy. Pyloric obstruction may be treated endoscopically by balloon dilations. Surgical intervention may be necessary to remove scar tissue.

NURSING MANAGEMENT
PEPTIC ULCER DISEASE

NURSING ASSESSMENT
Subjective and objective data to obtain from a patient with PUD are presented in Table 42-16.

NURSING DIAGNOSES
Nursing diagnoses related to PUD may include, but are not limited to, the following:
- Acute pain *related to* increased gastric secretions
- Ineffective self–health management *related to* lack of knowledge of long-term management of PUD
- Nausea *related to* acute exacerbation of disease process

Additional information on nursing diagnoses for the patient with PUD is presented in eNursing Care Plan 42-2 on the website for this chapter.

PLANNING
The overall goals are that the patient with PUD will (1) adhere to the prescribed therapeutic regimen, (2) experience a reduction in or absence of discomfort, (3) exhibit no signs of GI complications, (4) have complete healing of the peptic ulcer, and (5) make appropriate lifestyle changes to prevent recurrence.

NURSING IMPLEMENTATION
HEALTH PROMOTION. You have an important role in identifying patients at risk for PUD. Early detection and effective treat-

TABLE 42-16　NURSING ASSESSMENT

Peptic Ulcer Disease

Subjective Data

Important Health Information

Past health history: Chronic kidney disease, pancreatic disease, chronic obstructive pulmonary disease, serious illness or trauma, hyperparathyroidism, cirrhosis of the liver, Zollinger-Ellison syndrome

Medications: Aspirin, corticosteroids, nonsteroidal antiinflammatory drugs

Surgery or other treatments: Complicated or prolonged surgery

Functional Health Patterns

Health perception–health management: Chronic alcohol abuse, smoking, caffeine use; family history of peptic ulcer disease

Nutritional-metabolic: Weight loss, anorexia, nausea and vomiting, hematemesis, dyspepsia, heartburn, belching

Elimination: Black, tarry stools

Cognitive-perceptual

　Duodenal ulcers: Burning, midepigastric or back pain occurring 2-4 hr after meals and relieved by food; nocturnal pain common

　Gastric ulcers: High epigastric pain occurring 1-2 hr after meals; pain may be precipitated or aggravated by food

Coping-stress tolerance: Acute or chronic stress

Objective Data

General

Anxiety, irritability

Gastrointestinal

Epigastric tenderness

Possible Diagnostic Findings

Anemia; guaiac-positive stools; positive blood, urine, breath, or stool tests for *Helicobacter pylori;* abnormal upper gastrointestinal endoscopic and barium studies

---

ment of ulcers are important aspects of reducing morbidity risks associated with PUD. Patients who are taking ulcerogenic drugs (e.g., aspirin, NSAIDs) are at risk for PUD. Encourage patients to take these drugs with food. Teach patients to report symptoms related to gastric irritation, including epigastric pain, to their health care provider.

ACUTE INTERVENTION. During the acute exacerbation of an ulcer, the patient often complains of increased pain and nausea and vomiting, and some may have evidence of bleeding. Initially many patients attempt to cope with the symptoms at home before seeking medical assistance.

During this acute phase the patient may be NPO for a few days, have an NG tube inserted and connected to intermittent suction, and have IV fluid replacement. Explain to the patient and the caregiver the reasons for these therapies so they understand that the advantages far outweigh any temporary discomfort. Regular mouth care alleviates the dry mouth. Cleansing and lubrication of the nares facilitate breathing and decrease soreness. Analysis of gastric contents may include pH testing and analysis for blood, bile, or other substances. When the stomach is empty of gastric secretions, the ulcer pain diminishes and ulcer healing begins.

The volume of fluid lost, the patient's signs and symptoms, and laboratory test results (hemoglobin, hematocrit, and electrolytes) determine the type and amount of IV fluids administered. Be aware that other health problem (e.g., heart failure) may be adversely affected by the type or amount of fluid used. Take vital signs initially and at least hourly to detect and treat shock.

Physical and emotional rest is conducive to ulcer healing. The patient's immediate environment should be quiet and restful. The use of a mild sedative or tranquilizer has beneficial effects when the patient is anxious and apprehensive. Use good judgment before sedating a person who is becoming increasingly restless because the drug could mask the signs of shock secondary to upper GI bleeding.

If the patient's condition improves without worsening of symptoms (e.g., increased pain, vomiting, hemorrhage), the regimen outlined for conservative therapy is followed. However, complications such as hemorrhage, perforation, and obstruction can occur.

Hemorrhage. Changes in the vital signs and an increase in the amount and redness of the aspirate often signal massive upper GI bleeding. With bleeding, the patient's pain often decreases because the blood helps neutralize the acidic gastric contents. It is important to maintain the patency of the NG tube so that blood clots do not obstruct the tube. If the tube becomes blocked, the patient can develop abdominal distention. Use interventions similar to those described for upper GI bleeding on pp. 955-957.

Perforation. With perforation, the patient complains of sudden, severe abdominal pain. Perforation is manifested by a rigid, boardlike abdomen; severe generalized abdominal and shoulder pain; drawing up of the knees; and shallow, grunting respirations. The bowel sounds that may have been previously normal or hyperactive may diminish and become absent. When the patient with an ulcer demonstrates these changes, suspect perforation and notify the health care provider immediately.

Take vital signs promptly and record them every 15 to 30 minutes. Temporarily stop all oral or NG drugs and feedings until you can notify the health care provider and a definitive diagnosis is made. If perforation does exist, anything taken orally can add to the spillage into the peritoneal cavity and increase discomfort. If you are administering IV fluids at the time of the perforation, maintain the rate or increase it to replace the depleted plasma volume.

When perforation is confirmed, antibiotic therapy begins. When the perforation fails to seal spontaneously, surgical or laparoscopic closure is necessary and is performed as soon as possible. There may not be adequate time to thoroughly prepare the patient and family for the surgical intervention.

Gastric Outlet Obstruction. Gastric outlet obstruction can happen at any time. It is most likely to occur in the patient whose ulcer is located close to the pylorus. The onset of symptoms is usually gradual. Constant NG aspiration of stomach contents can help relieve symptoms. This allows edema and inflammation to subside and permits normal flow of gastric contents through the pylorus.

Regular irrigation of the tube with a normal saline solution per institutional policy may facilitate proper functioning. It may also be helpful to reposition the patient from side to side so that the tube tip is not constantly lying against the mucosal surface.

When the patient has resumed oral feedings and you notice symptoms of obstruction, promptly inform the health care provider. Generally, all that is necessary to treat the problem is to resume gastric aspiration so that the edema and inflammation resulting from the acute episode resolve. IV fluids with electrolyte replacement keep the patient hydrated during this period. To check for ongoing obstruction, clamp the NG tube intermittently and measure the gastric aspirate. It is important to maintain accurate intake and output records, especially of the gastric

TABLE 42-17 PATIENT & CAREGIVER TEACHING GUIDE

Peptic Ulcer Disease (PUD)

Include the following instructions when teaching the patient and caregiver about management of PUD.

1. Follow dietary modifications, including avoidance of foods that may cause epigastric distress. This may include black pepper, spicy foods, and acidic foods.
2. Avoid cigarettes. In addition to promoting ulcer development, smoking delays ulcer healing.
3. Reduce or eliminate alcohol intake.
4. Avoid OTC drugs unless approved by the health care provider. Many preparations contain ingredients, such as aspirin, that should not be taken unless approved by the health care provider. Check with the health care provider regarding the use of nonsteroidal antiinflammatory drugs.
5. Do not interchange brands of antacids, H$_2$-receptor blockers, and proton pump inhibitors that can be purchased OTC without checking with the health care provider. This can lead to harmful side effects.
6. Take all medications as prescribed. This includes both antisecretory and antibiotic drugs. Failure to take medications as prescribed can result in relapse.
7. It is important to report any of the following:
   - Increased nausea or vomiting
   - Increased epigastric pain
   - Bloody emesis or tarry stools
8. Stress can be related to signs and symptoms of PUD. Learn and use stress management strategies (see Chapter 7).
9. Share concerns about lifestyle changes and living with a chronic illness.

aspirate. When conservative treatment is not successful, surgery is performed after the acute phase has passed.

AMBULATORY AND HOME CARE. Patients with PUD have specific needs to prevent recurrence or complications. General instructions should cover aspects of the disease process itself, drugs, possible changes in lifestyle (alcohol intake, smoking), and regular follow-up care. Table 42-17 provides a patient and caregiver teaching guide for PUD.

Knowing the etiology and pathophysiology of PUD may motivate the patient to become involved in care and improve adherence to therapy. Work collaboratively with the dietitian to elicit a dietary history and plan ways to incorporate dietary modifications (if needed) into the patient's home and work setting.

The patient may not be honest about habitual use of alcohol or cigarettes. Provide information about the negative effects of alcohol and cigarettes on PUD and ulcer healing. Teach the patient about prescribed drugs, including their actions, side effects, and dangers if omitted for any reason. Make sure the patient knows why OTC drugs (e.g., aspirin, NSAIDs) should not be taken unless approved by the health care provider.[20] Because you can buy some H$_2$-receptor blockers and PPIs without a prescription, inform the patient that substituting prescription with OTC preparations without checking with the health care provider can lead to harmful side effects.

Try to obtain information about the patient's psychosocial status. Knowledge of lifestyle, occupation, and coping behaviors can be helpful in planning care. The patient may be reluctant to talk about personal subjects, the stress experienced at home or on the job, the usual methods of coping, or dependence on drugs or alcohol.

PUD is often a chronic, recurring disorder. Emphasize the need for long-term follow-up care, and encourage the patient to seek immediate intervention if symptoms return. The patient may be frustrated, especially if the prescribed mode of therapy has been faithfully followed, yet has failed to prevent the recurrence.

Some patients do not adhere to the plan of care, and they experience repeated exacerbations. Patients quickly learn that they often experience no discomfort when they omit prescribed drugs, smoke, or drink alcohol. Consequently, they make no or little alteration in lifestyle. After an acute exacerbation, the patient is likely to be more amenable to following the plan of care and open to suggestions for changes in lifestyle.

Changes, such as smoking cessation and alcohol abstinence, are difficult for many people. The patient may do better in reducing use of these substances rather than totally eliminating them. However, the goal should always be total cessation. Inform the patient with chronic PUD about potential complications, the clinical manifestations indicating their presence, and what to do until the health care provider can be seen.

EVALUATION

Expected outcomes are that the patient with PUD will
- Have pain controlled without the use of analgesics
- Verbalize an understanding of the treatment regimen
- Commit to self-care and management of the disease
- Have no complications (hemorrhage, perforation)

Additional information on expected outcomes for the patient with PUD is presented in eNursing Care Plan 42-2 on the website for this chapter.

Collaborative Care
Surgical Therapy for Peptic Ulcer Disease

With the use of antisecretory and antibiotic agents, surgery for PUD is uncommon. Surgery is performed on patients with complications that are unresponsive to medical management or concerns about stomach cancer.

Surgical procedures include partial gastrectomy, vagotomy, and pyloroplasty. Partial gastrectomy with removal of the distal two thirds of the stomach and anastomosis of the gastric stump to the duodenum is called a *gastroduodenostomy* or *Billroth I* operation (see eFig. 42-1 on the website for this chapter). Partial gastrectomy with removal of the distal two thirds of the stomach and anastomosis of the gastric stump to the jejunum is called a *gastrojejunostomy* or *Billroth II* operation (see eFig. 42-1).

Vagotomy is the severing of the vagus nerve, either totally *(truncal)* or selectively *(highly selective vagotomy)*. These procedures are done to decrease gastric acid secretion. *Pyloroplasty* consists of surgical enlargement of the pyloric sphincter to facilitate the easy passage of contents from the stomach. It is commonly done after vagotomy or to enlarge an opening that has been constricted from scar tissue.

Postoperative Complications. As with all surgeries, acute postoperative bleeding at the surgical site can occur. Monitoring of patients is similar to that described under acute upper GI bleeding. The most common long-term postoperative complications from PUD surgery are (1) dumping syndrome, (2) postprandial hypoglycemia, and (3) bile reflux gastritis.

Dumping Syndrome. *Dumping syndrome* is the direct result of surgical removal of a large portion of the stomach and the pyloric sphincter. Approximately 20% of patients experience dumping syndrome after PUD surgery.

Normally, gastric chyme enters the small intestine in small amounts. However, after surgery the stomach no longer has control over the amount of gastric chyme entering the small intestine. Consequently, a large bolus of hypertonic fluid enters the intestine and results in fluid being drawn into the bowel lumen. This creates a decrease in plasma volume along with distention of the bowel lumen and rapid intestinal transit.

The onset of symptoms occurs within 15 to 30 minutes after eating. The patient usually describes feelings of generalized weakness, sweating, palpitations, and dizziness. These symptoms are due to the sudden decrease in plasma volume. The patient complains of abdominal cramps, *borborygmi* (audible abdominal sounds produced by hyperactive intestinal peristalsis), and the urge to defecate. These manifestations usually last less than 1 hour after eating.

Postprandial Hypoglycemia. *Postprandial hypoglycemia* is considered a variant of dumping syndrome because it is the result of uncontrolled gastric emptying of a bolus of fluid high in carbohydrate into the small intestine. The bolus of concentrated carbohydrate results in hyperglycemia and the release of excessive amounts of insulin into the circulation. This results in reflex hypoglycemia. Symptoms are similar to those of any hypoglycemic reaction and include sweating, weakness, mental confusion, palpitations, tachycardia, and anxiety. Symptoms generally occur 2 hours after eating.

Bile Reflux Gastritis. Gastric surgery that involves the pylorus, with either reconstruction or removal, can result in reflux of bile into the stomach. Prolonged contact with bile causes damage to the gastric mucosa, chronic gastritis, and recurrence of PUD.

The symptoms associated with reflux alkaline gastritis are continuous epigastric distress that increases after meals. Vomiting relieves the distress, but only temporarily. The administration of cholestyramine (Questran), either before or with meals, has been used successfully to treat this problem. Cholestyramine binds with the bile salts that are the source of gastric irritation.

Nutritional Therapy. Start discharge planning and teaching as soon as the immediate postoperative period is successfully passed. The dietitian usually gives dietary instructions, and you need to reinforce them. Because the stomach's reservoir is diminished after gastric resection, patients must reduce their meal size accordingly. Advise the patient to reduce fluids drunk with meals. Dry foods with a low carbohydrate content and moderate protein and fat content are better tolerated initially. Dietary changes, along with a short rest period after each meal, reduce the likelihood of dumping syndrome. Reassure the patient that the unpleasant symptoms are usually of short duration. Following these dietary measures will decrease symptoms within a few months and is essential to long-term adherence.

The immediate ingestion of sugared fluids or candy relieves the hypoglycemic symptoms. To avoid hypoglycemic episodes, instruct the patient to limit the amount of sugar consumed with each meal and to eat small, frequent meals with moderate amounts of protein and fat (Table 42-18). Although only a small percentage of patients experience bile reflux gastritis, caution the patient to notify the health care provider of any continuous epigastric distress after meals.

NURSING MANAGEMENT
SURGICAL THERAPY FOR PEPTIC ULCER DISEASE

PREOPERATIVE CARE

Given the greater use of endoscopic procedures for the treatment of PUD, surgical procedures are used less frequently.

TABLE 42-18 **NUTRITIONAL THERAPY**

Postgastrectomy Dumping Syndrome

Purposes
- To slow the rapid passage of food into the intestine
- To control symptoms of dumping syndrome (dizziness, sense of fullness, diarrhea, tachycardia), which sometimes occurs after a partial or total gastrectomy

Diet Principles
- Divide meals into six small feedings to avoid overloading the stomach and intestine at mealtimes.
- Do not take fluids with meals but at least 30-45 min before or after meals. This helps prevent distention or a feeling of fullness.
- Avoid concentrated sweets (e.g., honey, sugar, jelly, jam, candies, sweet pastries, sweetened fruit) because they sometimes cause dizziness, diarrhea, and a sense of fullness.
- Increase protein and fats to promote rebuilding of body tissues and to meet energy needs. Meat, cheese, and eggs are specific foods to increase in the diet.
- Amount of time these restrictions should be followed varies. The health care provider decides the proper amount of time to remain on this prescribed diet according to the patient's clinical condition and progress.

Surgery can involve either laparoscopic or open surgery techniques. When surgery is planned, the surgeon provides the necessary information about the procedure and the expected outcome so that the patient can make an informed decision. Help the patient and caregiver by clarifying and interpreting their questions. Instruct them on what to expect after surgery, including comfort measures, pain relief, coughing and breathing exercises, use of an NG tube, and IV fluid administration (see Chapter 18).

POSTOPERATIVE CARE

Care of the patient after major abdominal surgery is similar to the postoperative care after abdominal laparotomy (see Chapter 43). An NG tube is used to decompress the remaining portion of the stomach to decrease pressure on the suture line and to allow for resolution of edema and inflammation resulting from surgical trauma.

Observe the gastric aspirate for color, amount, and odor during the immediate postoperative period. The aspirate is usually bright red at first, with a gradual darkening within the first 24 hours after surgery. Normally the color changes to yellow-green within 36 to 48 hours. If the tube becomes clogged during this period, the health care provider may order periodic gentle irrigations with normal saline solution. It is essential that the NG suction is working and that the tube remains patent so that accumulated gastric secretions do not put a strain on the anastomosis. This can lead to distention of the remaining portion of the stomach and result in (1) rupture of the sutures, (2) leakage of gastric contents into the peritoneal cavity, (3) hemorrhage, and (4) possible abscess formation. If the tube must be replaced or repositioned, call the health care provider to perform this task because of the danger of perforating the gastric mucosa or disrupting the suture line.

Observe the patient for signs of decreased peristalsis, including abdominal distention and lower abdominal discomfort, which may indicate intestinal obstruction. Monitor and record accurate intake and output every 4 hours.

Keep the patient comfortable and free of pain by administering prescribed drugs and frequently changing position. In an open surgical approach, the incision is relatively high in the epigastrium and may interfere with deep breathing and coughing. Splinting the area with a pillow while gently and persistently encouraging the patient to deep breathe helps prevent pulmonary complications. Splinting also protects the abdominal suture line from rupturing during coughing. Observe the dressing for signs of bleeding or odor and drainage indicative of an infection. Encourage early ambulation.

While the NG tube is connected to suction, maintain IV therapy. Add potassium and vitamin supplements (as ordered) to the infusion until oral feedings are resumed. Before the NG tube is removed, the patient begins oral feedings of clear liquids to determine the tolerance level. The stomach may be aspirated within 1 or 2 hours to assess the amount remaining and its color and consistency. When fluids are well tolerated, the NG tube is removed and fluids are increased in frequency, with a slow progression to regular foods. The patient begins the regimen of six small meals a day.

Pernicious anemia is a long-term complication of total gastrectomy and may occur after partial gastrectomy. Pernicious anemia is due to the loss of intrinsic factor, which is produced by the parietal cells. The patient may require cobalamin replacement therapy (see Chapter 31). PUD is a chronic problem, and ulcers can recur, especially at the site of the anastomosis.

GERONTOLOGIC CONSIDERATIONS

PEPTIC ULCER DISEASE

The morbidity and mortality rates associated with PUD in the older patient are higher than those for younger adults because of concomitant health problems and a decreased ability to withstand hypovolemia. Monitor older adults who use NSAIDs for osteoarthritis for signs and symptoms of PUD. In older patients, pain may not be the first symptom associated with an ulcer. For some patients the first manifestation is frank gastric bleeding or a decrease in hematocrit.

The treatment and management of PUD in older adults are similar to those in younger adults. An emphasis is placed on prevention of both gastritis and PUD. This includes teaching the patient to take NSAIDs and other gastric-irritating drugs with food, milk, or antacids. Instruct the patient to avoid irritating substances, adhere to the PPI or H$_2$-receptor blocker therapy as prescribed, and report abdominal pain or discomfort to the health care provider.

STOMACH CANCER

Stomach (gastric) cancer is an adenocarcinoma of the stomach wall (Fig. 42-15). The rate of stomach (particularly distal) cancer has been steadily declining in the United States. However, cancer of the cardia and the gastroesophageal junction is increasing. Gastric cancer still accounts for more than 10,540 deaths and 21,320 new cancer cases annually.[5]

Asian Americans and Pacific Islanders, Hispanics, and African Americans have higher rates of stomach cancer than non-Hispanic whites. Stomach cancer is more prevalent in men of the lower socioeconomic class, primarily those living in urban areas. The incidence of stomach cancer increases with age, with the majority being diagnosed between 65 and 80. At the time of diagnosis, only 10% to 20% of patients have disease confined to the stomach, and more than 50% have advanced

FIG. 42-15 Stomach carcinoma. Gross photograph showing an ill-defined, excavated central ulcer surrounded by irregular, heaped-up borders.

metastatic disease. The 5-year survival rate is 80% in patients with early stages (confined to the stomach) and less than 30% in those with advanced disease.[5]

Etiology and Pathophysiology

Many factors have been implicated in the development of stomach cancer, yet no single causative agent has been identified.[21] Stomach cancer probably begins with a nonspecific mucosal injury as a result of infection *(H. pylori)*, autoimmune-related inflammation, repeated exposure to irritants such as bile, antiinflammatory agents, and tobacco use.

Stomach cancer has been associated with diets containing smoked foods, salted fish and meat, and pickled vegetables. Whole grains and fresh fruits and vegetables are associated with reduced rates of stomach cancer. Infection with *H. pylori,* especially at an early age, is a risk factor for stomach cancer. It is possible that *H. pylori* and resulting cell changes can induce a sequence of transitions from dysplasia to cancer. Individuals with lymphoma of the stomach (mucosa-associated lymphoid tissue [MALT]) are at higher risk of stomach cancer.

Other predisposing factors include atrophic gastritis, pernicious anemia, adenomatous polyps, hyperplastic polyps, and achlorhydria. Smoking and obesity both increase the risk of stomach cancer. Although first-degree relatives of patients with stomach cancer are at increased risk, only 8% to 10% of stomach cancers have an inherited familial component.[21]

Stomach cancer spreads by direct extension and typically infiltrates rapidly to the surrounding tissue and liver. Seeding of tumor cells into the peritoneal cavity occurs late in the course of the disease.

Clinical Manifestations

Stomach cancers often spread to adjacent organs before any distressing symptoms occur. The clinical manifestations can include unexplained weight loss, early satiety, indigestion, abdominal discomfort or pain, and signs and symptoms of anemia. The patient may report *early satiety,* or a sense of being full sooner than usual. Anemia, which is common, is caused by chronic blood loss as the lesion erodes through the mucosa or as a result of pernicious anemia (caused by loss of intrinsic factor). The person appears pale and weak and complains of fatigue, weakness, dizziness, and, in extreme cases, shortness of breath. The stool may be positive for occult blood. Supraclavicular lymph nodes that are hard and enlarged suggest metastasis via the thoracic duct. The presence of ascites is a poor prognostic sign.

TABLE 42-19 COLLABORATIVE CARE

Stomach Cancer

Diagnostic	Collaborative Therapy

• History and physical examination
• Endoscopy and biopsy
• CT
• Upper GI barium study (less frequent)
• Exfoliative cytologic study
• Endoscopic ultrasonography
• Complete blood count
• Urinalysis
• Stool examination
• Liver enzymes
• Serum amylase
• Tumor markers
  • Carcinoembryonic antigen (CEA)
  • Carbohydrate antigen (CA)–19-9, CA-125, CA 72-4
  • α-Fetoprotein
	• Surgery
	  • Subtotal gastrectomy—Billroth I or II procedure (see eFig. 42-1)
	  • Total gastrectomy with esophagojejunostomy
	• Adjuvant therapy
	  • Radiation therapy
	  • Chemotherapy
	  • Combination radiation therapy and chemotherapy

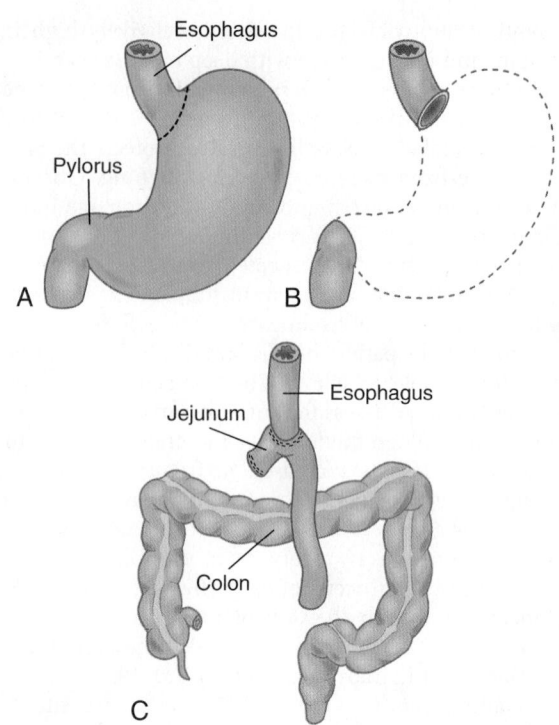

FIG. 42-16 Total gastrectomy for stomach cancer. **A,** Normal anatomic structure of the stomach. **B,** Removal of the stomach (total gastrectomy). **C,** Anastomosis of the esophagus with the jejunum (esophagojejunostomy).

Diagnostic Studies

The diagnostic studies for stomach cancer are presented in Table 42-19. Upper GI endoscopy is the best diagnostic tool. The stomach can be distended with air during the procedure so that the mucosal folds can be stretched. Biopsy of the tissue and subsequent histologic examination are important for the diagnosis of stomach cancer.

Endoscopic ultrasound, CT, and PET scanning can be used to stage the disease. Barium studies do not always detect small lesions of the cardia and the fundus. Laparoscopy is done to determine peritoneal spread.

Blood chemistry studies detect anemia and determine its severity. Elevations in liver enzymes and serum amylase levels may indicate liver and pancreatic involvement. Stool examination provides evidence of occult or gross bleeding.

Collaborative Care

The treatment of choice for stomach cancer is surgical removal of the tumor. Preoperative management of the patient focuses on the correction of nutritional deficits and treatment of anemia. Transfusions of packed RBCs correct the anemia. If a gastric outlet obstruction occurs, gastric decompression may be necessary before surgery. When the tumor has extended into the transverse colon, partial colon resection is required. Preoperative preparation for bowel surgery includes a low-residue diet, enemas to cleanse the bowel, and antibiotics to reduce the intestinal bacteria. Correction of malnutrition is important if surgery is planned.

Surgical Therapy. The surgical intervention used in the treatment of stomach cancer may be the same surgical procedures used for PUD. The location and extent of the lesion, the patient's physical condition, and the surgeon's preference determine the specific surgery used (e.g., open versus laparoscopic). For patients with localized stomach cancer, surgical treatment alone results in a greater than 50% 5-year survival rate. For patients with lymph node–positive cancer, the 5-year survival rate after surgery is 10% to 50% depending on the degree of spread. Survival rates are less when organs adjacent to the stomach show evidence of invasion at the time of surgery.

The surgical aim is to remove as much of the stomach as necessary to remove the tumor and a margin of normal tissue. When the lesion is located in the fundus, a total gastrectomy

with esophagojejunostomy is performed (Fig. 42-16). Lesions located in the antrum or the pyloric region are generally treated by either a Billroth I or II procedure. When metastasis has occurred to adjacent organs, such as the spleen, ovaries, or bowel, the surgical procedure is modified and extended as necessary.

Adjuvant Therapy. The current therapy for localized stomach cancer includes surgical resection and chemotherapy. Agents used in combination include continuous-infusion fluorouracil, epirubicin, cisplatin, etoposide, irinotecan, capecitabine (Xeloda), docetaxel, and oxaliplatin (Eloxatin).

Radiation therapy may be used together with chemotherapy to reduce recurrence and as a palliative measure to decrease tumor mass and provide temporary relief of obstruction. Additional therapies, including intraperitoneal administration of chemotherapeutic agents and immunotherapy, are undergoing evaluation. (These therapies are discussed in Chapter 16.)

NURSING MANAGEMENT
STOMACH CANCER

NURSING ASSESSMENT

The assessment of a person with possible stomach cancer is similar to that for PUD (see Table 42-16). Important data to obtain from the patient and the family include a nutritional assessment, a psychosocial history, the patient's perceptions of the health problem and need for care, and a physical examination of the patient.

The nutritional assessment obtains information regarding appetite and changes in eating patterns over the previous 6 months. Determine the patient's normal weight and any recent changes in it. Unexplained weight loss is common. The patient may report a history of vague abdominal symptoms, including dyspepsia and intestinal gas discomfort or pain. If the patient reports pain, explore where and when it occurs and how it is relieved.

Determine the patient's personal perception of the health problem and method of coping with hospitalization, diagnostic tests, and procedures. The possibility of a diagnosis of cancer and a treatment regimen that may include surgery, chemotherapy, or radiation treatment is stressful.[22] It is important to support the patient and the family. If surgery is probable, assess the patient's expectations regarding surgery (cure or palliation) and how the patient has responded to previous surgical procedures.

Focus your assessment on the patient's current functional abilities, other health problems, and response to therapy. Evaluate the patient's nutritional status. Cachexia may be evident if the nutritional intake has been reduced for an extended period. A malnourished patient does not respond well to chemotherapy or radiation therapy and is a poor surgical risk.

NURSING DIAGNOSES

Nursing diagnoses for the patient with stomach cancer include, but are not limited to, the following:

- Imbalanced nutrition: less than body requirements *related to* inability to ingest, digest, or absorb nutrients
- Anxiety *related to* lack of knowledge of diagnostic tests, unknown diagnostic outcome, disease process, and therapeutic regimen
- Acute pain *related to* underlying disease process and side effects of surgery, chemotherapy, or radiation therapy
- Grieving *related to* perceived unfavorable diagnosis and impending death

PLANNING

The overall goals are that the patient with stomach cancer will (1) experience minimal discomfort, (2) achieve optimal nutritional status, and (3) maintain a degree of spiritual and psychologic well-being appropriate to the disease stage.

NURSING IMPLEMENTATION

HEALTH PROMOTION. Your role in the early detection of stomach cancer is focused on identification of the patient at risk because of specific disorders such as *H. pylori* infection, pernicious anemia, and achlorhydria. Be aware of symptoms associated with stomach cancer, method of spread, and the significant findings on physical examination. Symptoms often occur late and mimic other conditions, such as PUD. Poor appetite, weight loss, fatigue, and persistent stomach distress are symptoms of stomach cancer. Encourage patients who have a positive family history of stomach cancer to undergo diagnostic evaluation if manifestations of anemia, PUD, or vague epigastric distress are present. It is important that you recognize the possible existence of stomach cancer in a patient who is treated for PUD and who fails to have relief after 3 weeks of prescribed therapy.

ACUTE INTERVENTION

Preoperative Care. When the diagnostic tests confirm a malignancy, the patient and the caregiver generally react with shock, disbelief, and depression. Provide emotional and physical support, provide information, clarify test results, and maintain a positive attitude with respect to the patient's immediate recovery and long-term survival.

Because of changes in appetite and early satiety, the patient's current nutritional status may be poor. Surgery may be delayed while the patient becomes more physically able to withstand it.

A positive nutritional state enhances wound healing and the ability to deal with infection and other possible postoperative complications. The patient may be better able to tolerate several small meals a day than three regular meals. The diet may be supplemented by a variety of commercial liquid supplements (see Chapter 40) and vitamins. It may be challenging to persuade the patient to eat when he or she has no appetite and is depressed. Getting the patient's caregiver to assist with meals and encourage intake may be beneficial. If the patient is unable to ingest oral feedings, the health care provider may prescribe enteral (tube feeding) or parenteral nutrition.

If needed, packed RBCs and fluid volume restoration may be given during the preoperative period. Closely observe for reactions to the transfusions. Monitor hemoglobin and hematocrit levels.

The preoperative teaching plan before stomach cancer surgery is similar to that for PUD (see the section on surgical therapy for PUD on pp. 949-951).

Postoperative Care. Postoperative care of the patient with stomach cancer is similar to that following a Billroth I or II procedure (see the section on surgical therapy for PUD earlier in this chapter). When the surgical intervention involves a total gastrectomy, the plan of care is somewhat different. A total gastrectomy requires resection of the lower esophagus, removal of the entire stomach, and anastomosis of the esophagus to the jejunum. If the chest cavity is entered, postoperative drainage is accomplished by the insertion of chest tubes. (Chest surgery and drainage tubes are discussed in Chapter 28.)

After total gastrectomy, the NG tube does not drain a large quantity of secretions because removal of the stomach has eliminated the reservoir capacity. The NG tube is removed when intestinal peristalsis has resumed. Small amounts of clear fluid may then be started. Closely observe the patient for signs of leakage of the fluids at the anastomosis site as evidenced by an elevation in the temperature and increasing dyspnea. When the patient tolerates fluids without distress, fluid intake is increased along with the addition of some solid foods.

As a consequence of a total gastrectomy, a patient experiences the symptoms of dumping syndrome. Weight loss often occurs. Postoperative wound healing may be impaired because of poor nutritional intake. This necessitates IV or oral replacement of vitamins C, D, and K; the B-complex vitamins; and cobalamin. Because these vitamins (with the exception of cobalamin) are normally absorbed in the duodenum, they need to be replaced. For the patient who has had a Billroth I or II procedure (see eFig. 42-1 on the website for this chapter), the postoperative care is similar to that of the patient having this procedure for PUD.

Radiation therapy or chemotherapy is used as an adjuvant to surgery or for palliation. Your role is to provide detailed instructions, reassure the patient, and ensure completion of the designated number of treatments. Start by assessing the patient's knowledge of these therapies. Teach the patient about skin care, the need for nutrition and fluid intake during therapy, and the appropriate use of antiemetic drugs. (Specific care of the patient receiving chemotherapy and radiation therapy is discussed in Chapter 16.)

AMBULATORY AND HOME CARE. Most dietary measures useful after PUD surgery are applicable after surgery for stomach cancer. Make plans for the relief of pain, including comfort measures and the judicious use of analgesics. Teach wound care, if needed, to the primary caregiver in the home setting. Dressings, special equipment, or special services may be required for

TABLE 42-20	TYPES OF UPPER GASTROINTESTINAL BLEEDING

Type	Manifestations
Obvious bleeding	
Hematemesis	Bloody vomitus appearing as fresh, bright red blood or "coffee-ground" appearance (dark, grainy digested blood).
Melena	Black, tarry stools (often foul smelling) caused by digestion of blood in the GI tract. Black appearance is from the presence of iron.
Occult bleeding	Small amounts of blood in gastric secretions, vomitus, or stools not apparent by appearance. Detectable by guaiac test.

TABLE 42-21	COMMON CAUSES OF UPPER GASTROINTESTINAL BLEEDING

Drug Induced
- Corticosteroids
- Nonsteroidal antiinflammatory drugs (NSAIDs)
- Salicylates

Esophagus
- Esophageal varices
- Esophagitis
- Mallory-Weiss tear

Stomach and Duodenum
- Stomach cancer
- Hemorrhagic gastritis
- Peptic ulcer disease
- Polyps
- Stress-related mucosal disease

Systemic Diseases
- Blood dyscrasias (e.g., leukemia, aplastic anemia)
- Renal failure

the patient's care at home. Provide the patient with a list of community agencies (e.g., American Cancer Society) that are available for assistance before the patient goes home.

When chemotherapy or radiation treatment is to be continued after discharge, a referral to the home health nurse may be beneficial. The home health nurse can assist with recovery, determine the degree of patient adherence, and provide consultation to the patient and the caregivers. Encourage the patient to adhere to the prescribed therapies, to keep appointments for chemotherapy administration or radiation treatments, and to keep the health care provider informed of changes in physical condition. (Long-term management of the cancer patient is discussed in Chapter 16.)

EVALUATION

Expected outcomes are that the patient with stomach cancer will

- Experience no or minimal discomfort, pain, or nausea
- Achieve optimal nutritional status
- Maintain a degree of psychologic well-being appropriate to the disease stage

UPPER GASTROINTESTINAL BLEEDING

In the United States approximately 300,000 hospital admissions occur each year for upper GI bleeding.[23] Approximately 60% of these are adults over age 65. Despite advances in drug management of predisposing conditions and identification of risk factors, the mortality rate for upper GI bleeding has remained at approximately 6% to 13% for the past 45 years.[23]

Etiology and Pathophysiology

Although the most serious loss of blood from the upper GI tract is characterized by a sudden onset, insidious occult bleeding can also be a major problem. The severity of bleeding depends on whether the origin is venous, capillary, or arterial. (Types of upper GI bleeding are presented in Table 42-20.) Bleeding from an arterial source is profuse, and the blood is bright red, indicating it has not been in contact with gastric HCl acid secretion. In contrast, "coffee-ground" vomitus indicates that the blood has been in the stomach for some time. A massive upper GI hemorrhage is a loss of more than 1500 mL of blood or 25% of intravascular blood volume. *Melena* (black, tarry stools) indicates slow bleeding from an upper GI source. The longer the passage of blood through the intestines, the darker the stool color because of the breakdown of hemoglobin and the release of iron.

Discovering the cause of the bleeding is not always easy. A variety of areas in the GI tract may be involved. Table 42-21 lists the common causes of upper GI bleeding.

Esophageal Origin. Bleeding from the esophagus is most likely due to chronic esophagitis, Mallory-Weiss tear, or esophageal varices. Chronic esophagitis can be caused by GERD, the ingestion of drugs irritating to the mucosa, alcohol, and cigarette smoking. Esophageal varices most often occur secondary to cirrhosis of the liver. (Esophageal varices are discussed in Chapter 44.)

Stomach and Duodenal Origin. Bleeding peptic ulcers account for 40% of the cases of upper GI bleeding. Drugs (either prescription or OTC) are a major cause of upper GI bleeding. Approximately 25% of people on chronic NSAIDs (e.g., ibuprofen) develop endoscopically determined ulcer disease; of these, 2% to 4% will bleed. Aspirin, NSAIDs, and corticosteroids can cause irritation and disruption of the gastroduodenal mucosa. Even low-dose aspirin is associated with risk for GI bleeding. Many OTC preparations contain aspirin. A careful history of all commonly used drugs is necessary whenever upper GI bleeding is suspected.

Stress-related mucosal disease (SRMD), also called *physiologic stress ulcers,* occurs in patients who have had severe burns or trauma or major surgery. In SRMD, there is either diffuse superficial mucosal injury or discrete deeper ulcers in the fundus and body portions of the stomach (see eFig. 42-2 on the website for this chapter). Patients with coagulopathy and those who experience respiratory failure resulting in mechanical ventilation for more than 48 hours are at highest risk.[24]

Diagnostic Studies

Endoscopy is the primary tool for diagnosing the source (e.g., esophageal or gastric varices, gastritis) of upper GI bleeding (see below). Angiography is used in diagnosing upper GI bleeding when endoscopy cannot be done or when bleeding persists after endoscopic therapy. Angiography is an invasive procedure requiring preparation and setup time and may not be appropriate for a high-risk, unstable patient. In this procedure, a catheter is placed into the left gastric or superior mesenteric artery and advanced until the site of bleeding is discovered.

Laboratory studies include CBC, blood urea nitrogen (BUN), serum electrolytes, prothrombin time, partial thromboplastin time, liver enzymes, arterial blood gases (ABGs), and a type and crossmatch for possible blood transfusions. All vomitus and stools should be tested for gross and occult blood.

Monitor the patient's laboratory studies to estimate the effectiveness of therapy. The hemoglobin and hematocrit values are not of immediate help in estimating the degree of blood loss, but they provide a baseline for guiding further treatment. The initial hematocrit may be normal and may not reflect the loss until 4 to 6 hours after fluid replacement, since initially the loss of plasma and RBCs is equal.

Assess the patient's BUN level. During a significant hemorrhage, blood proteins are broken down by GI tract bacteria, resulting in elevated BUN levels. However, the elevated BUN level may also indicate renal hypoperfusion or renal disease.

Collaborative Care

Although approximately 80% to 85% of patients who have massive hemorrhage spontaneously stop bleeding, the cause must be identified and treatment initiated immediately.

Emergency Assessment and Management. A complete history of events leading to the bleeding episode is deferred until emergency care has been initiated. To facilitate early intervention, the physical examination should focus on early identification of signs and symptoms of shock such as tachycardia, weak pulse, hypotension, cool extremities, prolonged capillary refill, and apprehension. (Shock is discussed in Chapter 67). Monitor vital signs every 15 to 30 minutes.

The patient is at risk for gut perforation and peritonitis, which may be indicated by a tense, rigid, boardlike abdomen. Do a thorough abdominal examination, and note the presence or absence of bowel sounds.

IV lines, preferably two, with a 16- or 18-gauge needle are placed for fluid and blood replacement. The type and amount of fluids infused are dictated by physical and laboratory findings. Generally, an isotonic crystalloid solution (e.g., lactated Ringer's solution) is started. Whole blood, packed RBCs, and fresh frozen plasma may be used for replacement of volume in massive hemorrhage. (The use of blood transfusions and volume expanders is discussed in Chapter 31.)

When upper GI bleeding is less profuse, infusion of isotonic saline solution followed by packed RBCs permits restoration of the hematocrit more quickly and does not create complications related to fluid volume overload. The use of supplemental oxygen delivered by face mask or nasal cannula may help increase blood oxygen saturation.

Urine output is one of the best measures of vital organ perfusion. Therefore an indwelling urinary catheter is inserted so that output can be accurately assessed hourly. A central venous pressure line may be inserted for fluid volume status assessment. If the patient has a history of valvular heart disease, coronary artery disease, or heart failure, a pulmonary artery catheter may be necessary to monitor the patient.

Endoscopic Therapy. The first-line management of upper GI bleeding is endoscopy and endotherapy. Endoscopy performed within the first 24 hours of bleeding is important for diagnosis and the determination of the need for surgical or radiologic intervention.

The goal of endoscopic hemostasis is to coagulate or thrombose the bleeding vessel. Several techniques are used, including (1) thermal (heat) probe, (2) multipolar and bipolar electrocoagulation probe, (3) argon plasma coagulation (APC), and (4) neodymium:yttrium-aluminum-garnet (Nd:YAG) laser. Multipolar electrocoagulation and thermal probe are the two most commonly used procedures. The heat probe coagulates tissue by directly applying a heating element to the bleeding site. The APC is a noncontact coagulation that delivers mono-

TABLE 42-22 DRUG THERAPY

Acute Gastrointestinal Bleeding*

Drug	Source of GI Bleeding	Mechanism of Action
vasopressin (Pitressin)	Esophageal varices	Causes vasoconstriction. ↓ Pressure in the portal circulation and stops bleeding
octreotide (Sandostatin)	Upper GI bleeding, esophageal varices	Somatostatin analog that ↓ blood flow to GI tract ↓ HCl acid secretion by ↓ release of gastrin
epinephrine	Bleeding from ulceration	Injection during endoscopy produces hemostasis Causes tissue edema and pressure on the source of bleeding Injection therapy often combined with other therapies (e.g., laser)

*Other drugs used to treat GI bleeding are antacids, H_2-receptor blockers, and protein pump inhibitors (see Table 42-9).

polar current to tissue. For variceal bleeding, other strategies include variceal ligation, injection sclerotherapy, and balloon tamponade (see Chapter 44).

Surgical Therapy. Surgical intervention is indicated when bleeding continues regardless of the therapy provided and when the site of the bleeding has been identified. Surgical therapy may be necessary when the patient continues to bleed after rapid transfusion of up to 2000 mL of whole blood or remains in shock after 24 hours. The site of the hemorrhage determines the choice of operation. The mortality rates increase considerably in those over 60 years of age.

Drug Therapy. During the acute phase of upper GI bleeding, empiric PPI therapy with high-dose IV bolus and subsequent infusion is often started before endoscopy. This may decrease the amount of bleeding and the need for endoscopic therapy.

During the acute phase, drugs are used to decrease bleeding, decrease HCl acid secretion, and neutralize the HCl acid that is present. Injection therapy with epinephrine (1:10,000 dilution) during endoscopy is effective for acute hemostasis. Epinephrine produces tissue edema and, ultimately, pressure on the source of bleeding (Table 42-22).

Efforts are made to reduce acid secretion because the acidic environment can alter platelet function and interfere with clot stabilization. PPIs or H_2-receptor blockers are administered IV to decrease acid secretion (see Table 42-10). In patients with upper GI bleeding, somatostatin or its long-acting analog octreotide (Sandostatin) may be administered when endoscopy is not available. Both agents reduce blood flow to the GI organs and acid secretion. After an initial bolus, somatostatin is used for 3 to 7 days, whereas octreotide is given for 3 days after the start of bleeding.

NURSING MANAGEMENT
UPPER GASTROINTESTINAL BLEEDING

NURSING ASSESSMENT

A thorough and accurate nursing assessment is an essential first step as you begin care of the patient admitted with upper GI bleeding. The patient may not be able to provide specific information about the cause of the bleeding until immediate physical needs are met. Perform an immediate nursing assessment while you are getting the patient ready for initial treatment. The assessment includes the patient's level of consciousness, vital signs, skin color, and capillary refill. Check the abdomen for distention, guarding, and peristalsis. Immediate determination of vital signs indicates whether the patient is in shock from blood loss and also provides a baseline blood pressure (BP) and pulse for monitoring the progress of treatment. Signs and symptoms of shock include low BP; rapid, weak pulse; increased thirst; cold, clammy skin; and restlessness. Monitor the patient's vital signs every 15 to 30 minutes, and inform the health care provider of any significant changes.

Once the immediate interventions have begun, the patient or caregiver should answer the following questions: Is there a history of previous bleeding episodes? Has the patient received blood transfusions in the past, and were there any transfusion reactions? Are there any other illnesses (e.g., liver disease, cirrhosis) or medications that may contribute to bleeding or interfere with treatment? Does the patient have a religious preference that prohibits the use of blood or blood products?

Subjective and objective data that should be obtained from the patient or caregiver are presented in Table 42-23.

▌NURSING DIAGNOSES

Nursing diagnoses for the patient with upper GI bleeding include, but are not limited to, the following:

- Decreased cardiac output *related to* loss of blood
- Deficient fluid volume *related to* acute loss of blood and gastric secretions
- Ineffective peripheral tissue perfusion *related to* loss of circulatory volume
- Anxiety *related to* upper GI bleeding, hospitalization, uncertain outcome, source of bleeding

▌PLANNING

The overall goals are that the patient with upper GI bleeding will (1) have no further GI bleeding, (2) have the cause of the bleeding identified and treated, (3) experience a return to a normal hemodynamic state, and (4) experience minimal or no symptoms of pain or anxiety.

▌NURSING IMPLEMENTATION

HEALTH PROMOTION. Although not all cases of upper GI bleeding can be anticipated and prevented, you have an important role in identifying patients at high risk. Always consider the patient with a history of chronic gastritis or PUD at high risk. The patient who has had one major bleeding episode is more likely to have another bleed. Patients with cirrhosis and those with previous upper GI bleeding from varices are also at high risk. Instruct the at-risk patient to avoid gastric irritants such as alcohol and smoking, and to take only prescribed medications. OTC drugs can be harmful because they may contain ingredients (e.g., aspirin) that increase the risk of bleeding. Instruct the patient in the methods of testing vomitus or stools for occult blood. Promptly report positive results to the health care provider.

The patient who requires regular doses of drugs that produce gastroduodenal toxicity (peptic ulcer formation, bleeding), such as aspirin, corticosteroids, or NSAIDs, needs to be taught about the potential for GI bleeding. Patients on daily low-dose aspirin to reduce cardiovascular disease risk are at risk for upper GI bleeding, especially patients over 60 with a history of PUD.

TABLE 42-23   NURSING ASSESSMENT

Upper Gastrointestinal Bleeding

Subjective Data
Important Health Information
Past health history: Precipitating events before bleeding episode, previous bleeding episodes and treatment, peptic ulcer disease, esophageal varices, esophagitis, acute and chronic gastritis, stress-related mucosal disease
Medications: Aspirin, nonsteroidal antiinflammatory drugs, corticosteroids, anticoagulants

Functional Health Patterns
Health perception–health management: Family history of bleeding, smoking, alcohol use
Nutritional-metabolic: Nausea, vomiting, weight loss, thirst
Elimination: Diarrhea; black, tarry stools; decreased urine output; sweating
Activity-exercise: Weakness, dizziness, fainting
Cognitive-perceptual: Epigastric pain, abdominal cramps
Coping–stress tolerance: Acute or chronic stress

Objective Data
General
Fever

Integumentary
Clammy, cool, pale skin; pale mucous membranes, nail beds, and conjunctivae; spider angiomas; jaundice; peripheral edema

Respiratory
Rapid, shallow respirations

Cardiovascular
Tachycardia, weak pulse, orthostatic hypotension, slow capillary refill

Gastrointestinal
Red or "coffee-ground" vomitus; tense, rigid abdomen, ascites; hypoactive or hyperactive bowel sounds; black, tarry stools

Urinary
Decreased urine output, concentrated urine

Neurologic
Agitation, restlessness; decreasing level of consciousness

Possible Diagnostic Findings
↓ Hematocrit and hemoglobin; hematuria; guaiac-positive stools, emesis, or gastric aspirate; ↓ levels of clotting factors; ↑ liver enzymes; abnormal endoscopy results

---

Even the lowest dose of aspirin can cause GI bleeding. Taking these drugs with meals or snacks lessens their direct irritation. The co-administration of an NSAID with a PPI or high doses of H_2-receptor blocker can reduce bleeding risk. For the patient at risk for gastric ulcers because of NSAID use, misoprostol may also be prescribed. This prostaglandin analog inhibits acid secretion and reduces upper GI bleeding episodes associated with NSAID use. However, the drug has important side effects, including uterine cramping in women, abdominal cramping, and diarrhea.

When you are working with the patient who has a history of liver cirrhosis with esophageal or gastric varices, provide specific instructions on the importance of avoiding known irritants, such as alcohol and smoking. Emphasize the importance of treating an upper respiratory tract infection promptly. Severe coughing or sneezing can increase pressure on the already fragile varices and may result in massive hemorrhage (see Chapter 44).

Patients with blood dyscrasias (e.g., aplastic anemia) or liver dysfunction or those who are taking cancer chemotherapy drugs are at risk due to a decrease in clotting factors and platelets. Instruct these patients regarding their disease process, drugs, and increased risk of GI bleeding.

ACUTE INTERVENTION. Approach the patient in a calm manner to help decrease the level of anxiety. Use caution when administering sedatives for restlessness because it is one of the warning signs of shock and may be masked by the drugs.

Once an infusion has been started, maintain the IV line for fluid or blood replacement. An accurate intake and output record is essential so that the patient's hydration status can be assessed. Measure the urine output hourly. If the patient has a central venous pressure line or pulmonary artery catheter in place, record these readings every 1 to 2 hours. Hemodynamic monitoring provides an accurate and quick assessment of blood flow and pressure within the cardiovascular system (see Chapter 66).

Observe the older adult or the patient with a history of cardiovascular problems closely for signs of fluid overload. However, volume overload and pulmonary edema are concerns in all patients who are receiving large amounts of IV fluids within a short time. Auscultate breath sounds and closely observe the respiratory effort. Keep the head of the bed elevated to provide comfort and prevent aspiration.

ECG monitoring is also used to evaluate cardiac function. Close monitoring of vital signs, especially in the patient with cardiovascular disease, is important because dysrhythmias may occur.

When an NG tube is inserted, pay special attention to keeping it in proper position and observe the aspirate for blood. Although room-temperature, cool, or iced gastric lavage is used in some institutions, its effectiveness as a treatment for upper GI bleeding is questionable. When lavage is used, approximately 50 to 100 mL of fluid is instilled at a time into the stomach. The lavage fluid may be aspirated from the stomach or drained by gravity. When aspiration is the method used, it is important not to aspirate if resistance is felt. The tip of the NG tube may be up against the gastric mucosal lining. When resistance is a factor, use the gravity method.

Assess the stools for blood (hematochezia, black-tarry, bright red). Black, tarry stools are not usually associated with a brisk hemorrhage but are indicative of prolonged bleeding. Menses and bleeding hemorrhoids should be ruled out as possible sources of blood in the stools. When vomitus contains blood but the stool contains no gross or occult blood, the hemorrhage is considered to have been of short duration.

When oral nourishment is begun, observe the patient for symptoms of nausea and vomiting and a recurrence of bleeding. Feedings initially consist of clear fluids and are given hourly until tolerance is determined. Gradual introduction of foods follows if the patient exhibits no signs of discomfort.

When the hemorrhage is the result of chronic alcohol abuse, closely observe the patient for delirium tremens as withdrawal from alcohol takes place. Symptoms indicating the beginning of delirium tremens are agitation, uncontrolled shaking, sweating, and vivid hallucinations. (Alcohol withdrawal is discussed in Chapter 11.)

AMBULATORY AND HOME CARE. Teach the patient and the caregiver how to avoid future bleeding episodes. Ulcer disease, drug or alcohol abuse, and liver and respiratory diseases can all result in upper GI bleeding. Help the patient and the caregiver be aware of the consequences of not adhering to drug therapy. Emphasize that no drugs (especially aspirin, NSAIDs) other than those prescribed by the health care provider should be taken. Smoking and alcohol should be eliminated because they are sources of irritation and interfere with tissue repair. Long-term follow-up care may be necessary because of possible recurrence. Instruct the patient and family on what to do if an acute hemorrhage occurs in the future.

EVALUATION

The expected outcomes are that the patient with upper GI bleeding will

- Have no upper GI bleeding
- Maintain normal fluid volume
- Experience a return to a normal hemodynamic state
- Understand potential etiologic factors and make appropriate lifestyle modifications

FOODBORNE ILLNESS

Foodborne illness (food poisoning) is a nonspecific term that describes acute GI symptoms such as nausea, vomiting, diarrhea, and cramping abdominal pain caused by the intake of contaminated food or liquids.[25] There are 31 known foodborne pathogens. Each year one out of six Americans, approximately 48 million, experiences a foodborne illness. Of these, 128,000 are hospitalized and approximately 3000 die.[26]

Bacteria account for most of the foodborne illnesses. Raw foods that have become contaminated during growing, harvesting, processing, storing, shipping, or final preparation are the most common source. When food is uncooked and left out for more than 2 hours at room temperature, bacteria can multiply quickly. One example is prepackaged cookie dough. The most common bacterial food poisonings are presented in Table 42-24.

Focus interventions on prevention of infection. Teaching includes correct food preparation and cleanliness, adequate cooking, and refrigeration (Table 42-25). For the hospitalized patient, emphasize correction of fluid and electrolyte imbalance from diarrhea and vomiting. With botulism, additional assessment and care relative to neurologic symptoms are indicated (see Chapter 61).

Escherichia coli O157:H7 Poisoning

Escherichia coli O157:H7 causes hemorrhagic colitis and kidney failure. In the very young and older adults, *E. coli* O157:H7 can be life threatening. *E. coli* O157:H7 is found primarily in undercooked meats, particularly poultry and hamburger.[26] *E. coli* outbreaks have also been observed with contaminated leafy vegetables, fruits, and nuts. Person-to-person contact in families, nursing homes, and child care centers is also an important mode of transmission. Infection can also occur after drinking raw milk, unpasteurized juice, or contaminated fruit juices and after swimming in or drinking sewage-contaminated water.

Most strains of *E. coli* are harmless and live in the intestines of healthy humans and animals. *E. coli* O157:H7 produces a

TABLE 42-24 BACTERIAL FOOD POISONING

Type and Cause	Sources	Clinical Manifestations	Treatment and Prevention
Staphylococcal Toxin from *Staphylococcus aureus*	Meat, bakery products, cream fillings, salad dressings, milk. Skin and respiratory tract of food handlers	*Onset:* 30 min–7 hr Vomiting, nausea, abdominal cramping, diarrhea	*Treat:* Symptomatic, fluid and electrolyte replacement, antiemetics *Prevent:* Immediate refrigeration of foods, monitoring of food handlers
Clostridial *Clostridium perfringens*	Meat or poultry dishes cooked at lower temperature (stew, pot pie), rewarmed meat dishes, gravies, improperly canned vegetables	*Onset:* 8-24 hr Diarrhea, nausea, abdominal cramps, vomiting (rare), midepigastric pain	*Treat:* Symptomatic, fluid replacement *Prevent:* Correct preparation of meat dishes. Serving food immediately after cooking or rapid cooling of food
Salmonella *Salmonella typhimurium* (grows in gut)	Improperly cooked poultry, pork, beef, lamb, and eggs	*Onset:* 8 hr–several days Nausea and vomiting, diarrhea, abdominal cramps, fever and chills	*Treat:* Symptomatic, fluid and electrolyte replacement *Prevent:* Correct preparation of food
Botulism Toxin from *Clostridium botulinum;* ingested toxin absorbed from gut and blocks acetylcholine at neuromuscular junction	Improperly canned or preserved food, home-preserved vegetables (most common), preserved fruits and fish, canned commercial products	*Onset:* 12-36 hr *GI:* Nausea, vomiting, abdominal pain, constipation, distention *Central nervous system:* Headache, dizziness, muscular incoordination, weakness, inability to talk or swallow, diplopia, breathing difficulties, paralysis, delirium, coma	*Treat:* Maintenance of ventilation, polyvalent antitoxin, guanidine hydrochloric acid (enhances acetylcholine release) *Prevent:* Correct processing of canned foods, boiling of suspected canned foods for 15 min before serving
Escherichia coli *E. coli* O157:H7	Contaminated beef, pork, milk, cheese, fish, cookie dough	*Onset:* 8 hr–1 wk (varies by strain) Bloody stools, hemolytic uremic syndrome, abdominal cramping, profuse diarrhea	*Treat:* Symptomatic, fluid and electrolyte replacement *Prevent:* Correct preparation of food

TABLE 42-25 PATIENT & CAREGIVER TEACHING GUIDE

Prevention of Food Poisoning

Include the following instructions when teaching the patient and caregiver how to prevent food poisoning.

1. Cook all ground beef and hamburger thoroughly.
   - Use a digital instant-read meat thermometer to ensure thorough cooking (ground beef can turn brown before disease-causing bacteria are killed).
   - Cook ground beef until a thermometer inserted into several parts of the patty, including the thickest part, reads at least 160° F.
   - People who cook ground beef without using a thermometer can decrease their risk of illness by not eating ground beef patties that are still pink in the middle.
2. If you are served an undercooked hamburger or other ground beef product in a restaurant, send it back for further cooking. Also ask for a new bun and a clean plate.
3. Avoid spreading harmful bacteria. Keep raw meat separate from ready-to-eat foods. Wash hands, counters, and utensils with hot soapy water after they touch raw meat. Never place cooked hamburgers or ground beef on the unwashed plate that held raw patties. Wash meat thermometers in between tests of patties that require further cooking.
4. Drink only pasteurized milk, juice, or cider. Commercial juice with an extended shelf-life that is sold at room temperature (e.g., juice in cardboard boxes, vacuum-sealed juice in glass containers) has been pasteurized. Juice concentrates are also heated sufficiently to kill pathogens.
5. Wash fruits and vegetables thoroughly, especially those that will not be cooked.
6. Do not eat raw food products that are supposed to be cooked. Follow package directions for cooking at proper temperatures.
7. People who are immunocompromised or older adults should avoid eating alfalfa sprouts until the safety of the sprouts can be ensured.

powerful toxin and can cause severe illness. The clinical manifestations of *E. coli* O157:H7 include diarrhea (often bloody) and abdominal cramping pain for 2 to 8 days (average 3 to 4 days) after swallowing the organism. The diarrhea is variable, ranging from mild to bloody. The diarrhea may start out as watery but may progress to bloody. Systemic complications, including hemolytic uremia and thrombocytopenic purpura, and even death can occur.

Infection with *E. coli* O157:H7 is diagnosed by detecting the bacteria in the stool. All people who suddenly have diarrhea with blood should get their stool (stool culture) tested for *E. coli* O157:H7.

Treatment involves supportive care to maintain blood volume. The use of antibiotics remains controversial. Most people recover without antibiotics or other specific treatment. There is no evidence that antibiotics improve the course of disease, and it is thought that treatment with some antibiotics may precipitate kidney complications. Patients should avoid antidiarrheal agents, such as loperamide (Imodium). Other therapies may include dialysis and plasmapheresis.

In approximately 2% to 7% of infections, particularly in young children and older adults, hemolytic uremic syndrome (HUS) occurs, in which the RBCs are destroyed and the kidneys fail. HUS is a life-threatening condition usually treated in an ICU. Blood transfusions and kidney dialysis are often required. Approximately 3% to 5% of patients with HUS die. About one third of people with HUS have abnormal kidney function many years later, and a few require long-term dialysis. Additional long-term complications of HUS include hypertension, seizures, blindness, and paralysis.

CASE STUDY

Peptic Ulcer Disease

iStockphoto/Thinkstock

Patient Profile

F.H., a 40-yr-old male immigrant from Vietnam, has a 1-yr history of epigastric distress. Increasingly, it is not relieved by over-the-counter antacids and cimetidine (Tagamet). He is scheduled for an upper endoscopy this morning.

Subjective Data

- Reports increasing substernal pain, especially 2 to 3 hr after eating
- Currently avoids alcohol and is taking antacids and over-the-counter H_2-receptor blocker
- Smoking history of 1 pack of cigarettes per day for 20 yr
- Complains of increasing fatigue with exercise
- Reports occasional black bowel movement
- Takes Chinese medicine for frequent back pain

Objective Data

Physical Examination

- Height 5 ft, 5 in tall and weight 140 lb

Diagnostic Studies

- Endoscopy reveals a duodenal ulcer
- Hgb 10.2 g/dL; Hct 30%
- Histology of biopsied tissue reveals *Helicobacter pylori* infection

Collaborative Care

- omeprazole 20 mg bid × 10 days
- clarithromycin 500 mg bid × 10 days
- amoxicillin 1 g bid × 10 days

Discussion Questions

1. Explain the pathophysiology of peptic ulcer disease.
2. What are the risk factors for duodenal ulcers? Which of these did F.H. have?
3. What is the pathophysiology of *H. pylori*?
4. What lifestyle changes would you recommend for F.H.?
5. *Priority Decision:* What are the priority nursing interventions for F.H.?
6. *Delegation Decision:* For the interventions that you identified in question 5, which of the following personnel could be responsible for implementing them: registered nurse (RN), licensed practical nurse (LPN), unlicensed assistive personnel (UAP)?
7. *Priority Decision:* Based on the assessment data provided, what are the priority nursing diagnoses? Are there any collaborative problems?
8. *Evidence-Based Decision:* F.H. asks you if the treatment will work and this will be the end of his problems. How will you respond?

ⓔvolve Answers available at *http://evolve.elsevier.com/Lewis/medsurg.*

BRIDGE TO NCLEX EXAMINATION

The number of the question corresponds to the same-numbered outcome at the beginning of the chapter.

1. M.J. calls to tell the nurse that her 85-year-old mother has been nauseated all day and has vomited twice. Before the nurse hangs up and calls the health care provider, she should instruct M.J. to
   a. administer antispasmodic drugs and observe skin turgor.
   b. give her mother sips of water and elevate the head of her bed to prevent aspiration.
   c. offer her mother a high-protein liquid supplement to drink to maintain her nutritional needs.
   d. offer her mother large quantities of Gatorade to drink because older adults are at risk for sodium depletion.

2. The nurse explains to the patient with Vincent's infection that treatment will include
   a. smallpox vaccinations.
   b. viscous lidocaine rinses.
   c. amphotericin B suspension.
   d. topical application of antibiotics.

3. The nurse teaching young adults about behaviors that put them at risk for oral cancer includes
   a. discouraging use of chewing gum.
   b. avoiding use of perfumed lip gloss.
   c. avoiding use of smokeless tobacco.
   d. discouraging drinking of carbonated beverages.

4. The nurse explains to the patient with gastroesophageal reflux disease (GERD) that this disorder
   a. results in acid erosion of the esophagus from frequent vomiting.
   b. will require surgical wrapping or repair of the pyloric sphincter to control the symptoms.
   c. is the protrusion of a portion of the stomach into the esophagus through an opening in the diaphragm.
   d. often involves relaxation of the lower esophageal sphincter, allowing stomach contents to back up into the esophagus.

5. A patient who has undergone an esophagectomy for esophageal cancer develops increasing pain, fever, and dyspnea when a full liquid diet is started postoperatively. The nurse recognizes that these symptoms are most indicative of
   a. an intolerance to the feedings.
   b. extension of the tumor into the aorta.
   c. leakage of fluid or foods into the mediastinum.
   d. esophageal perforation with fistula formation into the lung.

6. The pernicious anemia that may accompany gastritis is due to
   a. chronic autoimmune destruction of cobalamin stores in the body.
   b. progressive gastric atrophy from chronic breakage in the mucosal barrier and blood loss.
   c. a lack of intrinsic factor normally produced by acid-secreting cells of the gastric mucosa.
   d. hyperchlorhydria resulting from an increase in acid-secreting parietal cells and degradation of RBCs.

7. The nurse is teaching the patient and family that peptic ulcers are
   a. caused by a stressful lifestyle and other acid-producing factors such as *H. pylori*.
   b. inherited within families and reinforced by bacterial spread of *Staphylococcus aureus* in childhood.
   c. promoted by factors that tend to cause oversecretion of acid, such as excess dietary fats, smoking, and *H. pylori*.
   d. promoted by a combination of factors that may result in erosion of the gastric mucosa, including certain drugs and alcohol.

8. An optimal teaching plan for an outpatient with stomach cancer receiving radiation therapy should include information about
   a. cancer support groups, alopecia, and stomatitis.
   b. avitaminosis, ostomy care, and community resources.
   c. prosthetic devices, skin conductance, and grief counseling.
   d. wound and skin care, nutrition, drugs, and community resources.

9. The teaching plan for the patient being discharged after an acute episode of upper GI bleeding includes information concerning the importance of *(select all that apply)*
   a. only taking aspirin with milk or bread products.
   b. avoiding taking aspirin and drugs containing aspirin.
   c. only taking drugs prescribed by the health care provider.
   d. taking all drugs 1 hour before mealtime to prevent further bleeding.
   e. reading all OTC drug labels to avoid those containing stearic acid and calcium.

10. Several patients are seen at an urgent care center with symptoms of nausea, vomiting, and diarrhea that began 2 hours ago while attending a large family reunion potluck dinner. You question the patients specifically about foods they ingested containing
    a. beef.
    b. meat and milk.
    c. poultry and eggs.
    d. home-preserved vegetables.

1. b, 2. d, 3. c, 4. d, 5. c, 6. c, 7. d, 8. d, 9. b, c, 10. b

evolve

For rationales to these answers and even more NCLEX review questions, visit *http://evolve.elsevier.com/Lewis/medsurg*.

REFERENCES

1. Buchanan FF, Myles PS, Cicuttini F: Effect of patient sex on general anaesthesia and recovery, *Br J Anaesth* 106:832, 2011.
2. Basch E, Prestrud AA, Hesketh PJ, et al: Antiemetics: American Society of Clinical Oncology clinical practice guideline update, *J Clin Oncol* 29:4189, 2011.
3. Robinson N, Lorenc A, Liao X: The evidence for Shiatsu: a systematic review of Shiatsu and acupressure, *BMC Complement Altern Med* 11:88, 2011.
4. Bensley L, Van Eenwyk J, Ossiander EM: Associations of self-reported periodontal disease with metabolic syndrome and number of self-reported chronic conditions, *Prev Chronic Dis* 8:A50, 2011.
5. American Cancer Society: Cancer facts and figures 2012. Retrieved from *www.cancer.org*.
6. Sanders AE, Slade GD, Patton LL: National prevalence of oral HPV infection and related risk factors in the U.S. adult population, *Oral Dis* 18:430, 2012.
7. Fedele S: Diagnostic aids in the screening of oral cancer, *Head Neck Oncol* 1:5, 2009. (Classic)
8. Bhide SA, Nutting CM: Advances in chemotherapy for head and neck cancer, *Oral Oncol* 46:436, 2010.
9. Sonnenberg A: Effects of environment and lifestyle on gastroesophageal reflux disease, *Dig Dis* 29:229, 2011.
10. Anand G, Katz PO: Gastroesophageal reflux disease and obesity, *Gastroenterol Clin North Am* 39:39, 2010.
11. Robertson L: A new horizon: recommendations and treatment guidelines for Barrett's esophagus, *Gastroenterol Nurs* 32:211, 2009.
12. Ranjitkar S, Kaidonis JA, Smales RJ: Gastroesophageal reflux disease and tooth erosion, *Internat J Dentist* 1:10, 2011.
13. Kahrilas PJ, Shaheen NJ, Vaezi M: American Gastroenterological Association Institute technical review on the management of gastroesophageal reflux disease, *Gastroenterology* 135:1392, 2008. (Classic)
*14. Ngamruengphong S, Leontiadis GI, Radhi S, et al: Proton pump inhibitors and risk of fracture: a systematic review and meta-analysis of observational studies, *Am J Gastroenterol* 106:1209, 2011.
*15. Kwok CS, Arthur AK, Anibueze CI, et al: Risk of *Clostridium difficile* infection with acid suppressing drugs and antibiotics: meta-analysis, *Am J Gastroenterol* 107:1011, 2012.

16. Bower M, Jones W, Vessels B, et al: Role of esophageal stents in the nutrition support of patients with esophageal malignancy, *Nutr Clin Pract* 25:244, 2010.
*17. Lee I, Cryer B: Epidemiology and role of nonsteroidal antiinflammatory drugs in causing gastrointestinal bleeding, *Gastrointest Endosc Clin N Am* 21:597, 2011.
18. Centers for Disease Control and Prevention: *Helicobacter pylori* and peptic ulcer disease: the key to cure. Retrieved from *www.cdc.gov/ulcer/keytocure.htm*.
19. Targownik LE, Bolton JM, Metge CJ, et al: Selective serotonin reuptake inhibitors are associated with a modest increase in the risk of upper gastrointestinal bleeding, *Am J Gastroenterol* 104:1475, 2009.
*20. Thiagarajan P, Jankowski JA: Aspirin and NSAIDs: benefits and harms for the gut, *Best Pract Res Clin Gastroenterol* 26:197, 2012.
21. Blair VR: Familial gastric cancer: genetics, diagnosis, and management, *Surg Oncol Clin N Am* 21:35, 2012.
22. Qian H, Yuan C: Factors associated with self-care self-efficacy among gastric and colorectal cancer patients, *Cancer Nurs* 35:E22, 2012.
23. Holster IL, Kuipers EJ: Management of acute nonvariceal upper gastrointestinal bleeding: current policies and future perspectives, *World J Gastroenterol* 18:1202, 2012.
24. Pilkington KB, Wagstaff MJ, Greenwood JE: Prevention of gastrointestinal bleeding due to stress ulceration: a review of current literature, *Anaesth Intensive Care* 40:253, 2012.
25. National Digestive Diseases Information Clearinghouse: Bacteria and foodborne illness. Retrieved from *http://digestive.niddk.nih.gov/ddiseases/pubs/bacteria*.
26. Centers for Disease Control and Prevention: *Escherichia coli* O157:H7. Retrieved from *www.cdc.gov/ncidod/dbmd/diseaseinfo/escherichiacoli_g.htm*.

RESOURCES

American College of Gastroenterology
   www.acg.gi.org
American Gastroenterological Association
   www.gastro.org
Digestive Disease National Coalition
   www.ddnc.org
National Digestive Diseases Information Clearinghouse
   http://digestive.niddk.nih.gov
Society of Gastroenterology Nurses and Associates (SGNA)
   www.sgna.org

*Evidence-based information for clinical practice.

*Clouds come floating into my life, no longer
to carry rain or usher storm, but to add color
to my sunset.*
Rabindranath Tagore

Nursing Management
Lower Gastrointestinal Problems

Marilee Schmelzer

(e)volve WEBSITE

LEARNING OUTCOMES

1. Explain the common etiologies, collaborative care, and nursing management of diarrhea, fecal incontinence, and constipation.
2. Describe common causes of acute abdominal pain and nursing management of the patient after an exploratory laparotomy.
3. Describe the collaborative care and nursing management of acute appendicitis, peritonitis, and gastroenteritis.
4. Compare and contrast the inflammatory bowel diseases of ulcerative colitis and Crohn's disease, including pathophysiology, clinical manifestations, complications, collaborative care, and nursing management.
5. Differentiate among mechanical and nonmechanical bowel obstructions, including causes, collaborative care, and nursing management.
6. Describe the clinical manifestations and collaborative management of colorectal cancer.
7. Explain the anatomic and physiologic changes and nursing management of the patient with an ileostomy and a colostomy.
8. Differentiate between diverticulosis and diverticulitis, including clinical manifestations, collaborative care, and nursing management.
9. Compare and contrast the types of hernias, including etiology and surgical and nursing management.
10. Describe the types of malabsorption syndromes and collaborative care of celiac disease, lactase deficiency, and short bowel syndrome.
11. Describe the types, clinical manifestations, collaborative care, and nursing management of anorectal conditions.

KEY TERMS

anal fistula, p. 1002
appendicitis, p. 973
celiac disease, p. 997
constipation, p. 966
Crohn's disease, p. 975
diarrhea, p. 962
diverticula, p. 994
fecal incontinence, p. 964

gastroenteritis, p. 975
hemorrhoids, p. 1000
hernia, p. 996
inflammatory bowel disease (IBD), p. 975
intestinal obstruction, p. 982
irritable bowel syndrome (IBS), p. 972
lactase deficiency, p. 999

ostomy, p. 990
paralytic (adynamic) ileus, p. 982
peritonitis, p. 974
short bowel syndrome (SBS), p. 999
steatorrhea, p. 997
stoma, p. 990
ulcerative colitis, p. 975

Reviewed by Carmen Bruni, RN, MSN, Nurse Executive, Assistant Professor of Nursing, Texas A & M International University, Laredo, Texas.

The wide variety of intestinal problems presented in this chapter include the disorders of diarrhea, fecal incontinence, and constipation; inflammatory and infectious bowel disorders; bowel trauma; bowel obstructions; colorectal cancer; abdominal and bowel surgery (including ostomy formation); and malabsorption disorders.

DIARRHEA

Diarrhea is the passage of at least three loose or liquid stools per day. It may be acute, or it is considered chronic if it lasts longer than 4 weeks.[1]

Etiology and Pathophysiology

Ingestion of infectious organisms is the primary cause of acute diarrhea (Table 43-1). Viruses cause most cases of infectious diarrhea in the United States. Although viral infections can be deadly, they are usually short lived (48 hours) and mild. Therefore most patients rarely seek treatment.

Bacterial infections are also common.[2] *Escherichia coli* O157:H7, a type of enterohemorrhagic *E. coli*, is the most common cause of bloody diarrhea in the United States. It is transmitted by inadequately cooked beef or chicken contaminated with the bacteria or in fruits and vegetables exposed to contaminated manure. Other pathologic *E. coli* strains are endemic in developing countries and are common causes of traveler's diarrhea. *Giardia lamblia* is the most common intestinal parasite that causes diarrhea in the United States.

Infectious organisms attack the intestines in different ways.[3] Some organisms (e.g., *Rotavirus A, Norovirus, G. lamblia*) alter secretion and/or absorption of the enterocytes of the small intestine without causing inflammation. Other organisms (e.g., *Clostridium difficile*) impair absorption by destroying cells, cause inflammation in the colon, and produce toxins that also cause damage.

Organisms enter the body in contaminated food (e.g., *Salmonella* organisms in undercooked eggs and chicken) or contaminated drinking water (*G. lamblia* in contaminated lakes or pools). Travelers often get diarrhea, especially if they travel to countries with poorer sanitation than their own. An infection can also be transmitted from one individual to another via the fecal-oral route. For example, adult day care workers can transmit infection from one resident to another if they do not wash their hands thoroughly after changing soiled linen.

An individual's susceptibility to pathogenic organisms is influenced by age, gastric acidity, intestinal microflora, and immunocompetence. Older adults are most likely to suffer life-threatening diarrhea. Since stomach acid kills ingested pathogens, medications designed to decrease stomach acid (e.g., proton pump inhibitors and histamine [H_2]-receptor blockers) increase the likelihood that pathogens will survive.[4]

The healthy human colon contains short-chain fatty acids and bacteria such as *E. coli*. These organisms aid in fermentation and provide a microbial barrier against pathogenic bacteria. Antibiotics kill off the normal flora, making the individual more susceptible to pathogenic organisms. For example, patients receiving broad-spectrum antibiotics (e.g., clindamycin [Cleocin], cephalosporins, fluoroquinolones) are susceptible to pathogenic strains of *C. difficile*. *C. difficile* is the most serious antibiotic-associated diarrhea and is becoming more prevalent. Probiotics, in particular *Saccharomyces boulardii* and *Lactobacillus*, may be helpful in preventing antibiotic-induced diarrhea in some patients.

People who are immunocompromised because of disease (e.g., human immunodeficiency virus [HIV]) or immunosuppressive medications are susceptible to gastrointestinal (GI) tract infection. Patients who are immunocompromised and receiving jejunal enteral nutrition are especially prone to *C. difficile* and other foodborne infections. Jejunostomy and nasointestinal feedings, which bypass the stomach's acid environment, do not contain the poorly digestible fiber that is necessary for the survival of normal colonic bacteria.[5]

Not all diarrhea is due to infection. For example, drugs and specific food intolerances can cause diarrhea. Also, large amounts of undigested carbohydrate in the bowel produce an osmotic diarrhea that promotes rapid transit and prevents absorption of fluid and electrolytes. Lactose intolerance and certain laxatives (e.g., lactulose, sodium phosphate, magnesium

TABLE 43-1	CAUSES OF ACUTE INFECTIOUS DIARRHEA*	
Type of Organism	**Symptoms**
Viral	
Rotavirus (e.g., *Rotavirus A*)	Fever, vomiting, profuse watery diarrhea. Lasts 3-8 days.
Norovirus (also called Norwalk-like virus)	Nausea, vomiting, diarrhea, stomach cramping. Rapid onset. Lasts 1-2 days.
Bacterial	
Enterotoxigenic *Escherichia coli*	Watery or bloody diarrhea. Abdominal cramps. Nausea, vomiting, and fever may be present. Mean duration >60 hr.
Enterohemorrhagic *E. coli* (e.g., *E. coli* O157:H7)	Severe abdominal cramping, bloody diarrhea, vomiting. Low-grade fever. Usually lasts 5-7 days.
Shigella	Diarrhea (sometimes bloody), fever, stomach cramps. Usually lasts 5-7 days. Postinfection arthritis may occur.
Salmonella	Diarrhea, fever, abdominal cramps. Lasts 4-7 days.
Staphylococcus	Nausea, vomiting, abdominal cramps, diarrhea. Usually mild. May cause illness in as little as 30 min. Lasts 1-3 days.
Campylobacter jejuni	Diarrhea, abdominal cramps, fever. Sometimes nausea and vomiting. Lasts about 7 days.
Clostridium perfringens	Diarrhea, abdominal cramps, nausea, vomiting. Occurs 8-24 hr after eating contaminated food and lasts approximately 24 hr.
Clostridium difficile	Watery diarrhea, fever, anorexia, nausea, abdominal pain.
Parasitic	
Giardia lamblia	Abdominal cramps, nausea, diarrhea. May interfere with nutrient absorption.
Entamoeba histolytica	Diarrhea, abdominal cramping. Only 10%-20% are ill, and symptoms are usually mild.
Cryptosporidium	Watery diarrhea. Lasts about 2 wk. May also have abdominal cramps, nausea, vomiting, fever, dehydration, and weight loss. Sometimes no symptoms. Long lasting and may be fatal in those who are immunocompromised (e.g., AIDS).

*An expanded version of this table (eTable 43-1) with source of infection and drug treatment is available on the website for this chapter.

citrate) produce an osmotic diarrhea. Bile salts and undigested fats also lead to excessive fluid secretion in the GI tract. The diarrhea from celiac disease and short bowel syndrome results from malabsorption in the small intestine.

Clinical Manifestations

Infections that attack the upper GI tract (e.g., *Norovirus, G. lamblia*) usually produce large-volume, watery stools; cramping; and periumbilical pain. Patients have either a low-grade or no fever and often experience nausea and vomiting before the diarrhea begins. Infections of the colon and distal small bowel (e.g., *Shigella, Salmonella, C. difficile*) produce fever and frequent bloody diarrhea with a small volume.

Leukocytes, blood, and mucus may be present in the stool, depending on the causative agent (see Table 43-1). Severe diarrhea produces life-threatening dehydration, electrolyte disturbances (e.g., hypokalemia), and acid-base imbalances (metabolic acidosis). *C. difficile* infection can progress to fulminant colitis and intestinal perforation.

Diagnostic Studies

Since most cases of diarrhea resolve quickly, stool cultures are indicated only for patients who are very ill, have a significant fever, or have had diarrhea longer than 3 to 5 days. Stools are examined for blood, mucus, white blood cells (WBCs), and parasites, and cultures are performed to identify infectious organisms. A multiple-pathogen test can simultaneously detect 11 common viral, bacterial, and parasitic causes of infectious gastroenteritis from a single patient sample. Toxins produced by *C. difficile* can usually be detected in a sample of a patient's stool.

Testing for ova and parasites is reserved for people who have had diarrhea more than 2 weeks. The WBC count may be elevated. People with long-standing diarrhea can develop anemia from iron and folate deficiencies. Increased hematocrit, blood urea nitrogen (BUN), and creatinine levels are signs of fluid deficit.

In patients with chronic diarrhea, measurements of stool electrolytes, pH, and osmolality help determine whether the diarrhea is related to decreased fluid absorption or increased fluid secretion. Measurement of stool fat and undigested muscle fibers may indicate fat and protein malabsorption conditions, including pancreatic insufficiency. Some patients with secretory diarrhea have elevated serum levels of GI hormones such as vasoactive intestinal polypeptide and gastrin.

Collaborative Care

Treatment depends on the cause. Foods and drugs that cause diarrhea should be avoided. Acute infectious diarrhea is usually self-limiting. The major concerns are preventing transmission, replacing fluid and electrolytes, and protecting the skin. Patients usually tolerate oral fluids. Solutions containing glucose and electrolytes (e.g., Pedialyte) may be sufficient to replace losses from mild diarrhea. Parenteral administration of fluids, electrolytes, vitamins, and nutrition is necessary if losses are severe.

Antidiarrheal agents are sometimes given to coat and protect mucous membranes, absorb irritating substances, inhibit intestinal transit, decrease intestinal secretions, or decrease central nervous system stimulation of the GI tract (Table 43-2). Antidiarrheal agents are contraindicated in the treatment of some infectious diarrheas because they potentially prolong exposure to the organism. They are used cautiously in inflammatory bowel disease (IBD) because of the danger of *toxic megacolon*

TABLE 43-2 DRUG THERAPY

Antidiarrheal Drugs

Drug	Mechanism of Action
bismuth subsalicylate (Pepto-Bismol)	Decreases secretions and has weak antibacterial activity. Used to prevent traveler's diarrhea.
calcium polycarbophil (Mitrolan)	Bulk-forming agent that absorbs excessive fluid from diarrhea to form a gel. Used when intestinal mucosa cannot absorb fluid.
loperamide (Imodium, Pepto Diarrhea Control)	Inhibits peristalsis, delays transit, increases absorption of fluid from stools.
diphenoxylate with atropine (Lomotil)	Opioid and anticholinergic. Decreases peristalsis and intestinal motility.
paregoric (camphorated tincture of opium)	Opioid. Decreases peristalsis and intestinal motility.
Donnagel-PG (combination of kaolin, pectin, and paregoric)	Decreases peristalsis and intestinal motility.
octreotide acetate (Sandostatin)	Suppresses serotonin secretion, stimulates fluid absorption from GI tract, decreases intestinal motility.

(colonic dilation greater than 5 cm). Regardless of the cause of diarrhea, antidiarrheal drugs should be given only for a short time.

Antibiotics are rarely used to treat acute diarrhea. However, they may be used for certain infections or when the infected individual is severely ill or immunosuppressed. For example, a nonabsorbable antibiotic, rifaximin (Xifaxan), is used to treat traveler's diarrhea that is caused by *E. coli*.

***Clostridium difficile* Infection.** *C. difficile* infection is a particularly hazardous health care–associated infection. Its spores can survive for up to 70 days on objects, including commodes, telephones, thermometers, bedside tables, and floors. *C. difficile* can be transmitted from patient to patient by health care workers who do not adhere to infection control precautions.

The infection is usually treated by stopping antibiotics and starting the patient on either metronidazole (Flagyl) or vancomycin (Vancocin). Metronidazole is the first line of treatment in mild disease because of concerns about vancomycin-resistant enterococcus (VRE). Since recovery rates are substantially better with vancomycin, it is preferred for serious infections. Both drugs are given orally, but metronidazole may also be given IV. Fidaxomicin (Dificid) is generally reserved for patients who are at risk for relapse or have recurrent infections.

Recurrent *C. difficile* infection occurs in about 20% of patients, and the probability of a recurrence rises with each subsequent infection. Feces transplantation is under investigation as a potential therapeutic option for patients with recurrent and resistant *C. difficile* infections.[6] In this procedure healthy person's feces are inserted into the GI tract using an enema or nasogastric tube, or during colonoscopy.

NURSING MANAGEMENT
ACUTE INFECTIOUS DIARRHEA

NURSING ASSESSMENT

Begin the nursing assessment with a thorough history and physical examination (Table 43-3). Ask the patient to describe his or her stool pattern and associated symptoms. Focus on the

TABLE 43-3 NURSING ASSESSMENT
Diarrhea

Subjective Data
Important Health Information
Past health history: Recent travel, infections, stress; diverticulitis or malabsorption; metabolic disorders; inflammatory bowel disease; irritable bowel syndrome
Medications: Laxatives or enemas, magnesium-containing antacids, sorbitol-containing suspensions or elixirs, antibiotics, methyldopa, digitalis, colchicine; OTC antidiarrheal medications
Surgery or other treatments: Stomach or bowel surgery, radiation

Functional Health Patterns
Health perception–health management: Chronic laxative abuse, malaise
Nutritional-metabolic: Ingestion of fatty and spicy foods, food intolerances; anorexia, nausea, vomiting; weight loss; thirst
Elimination: Increased stool frequency, volume, and looseness; change in color and character of stools; steatorrhea, abdominal bloating; decreased urine output
Cognitive-perceptual: Abdominal tenderness, abdominal pain and cramping; tenesmus

Objective Data
General
Lethargy, sunken eyeballs, fever, malnutrition

Integumentary
Pallor, dry mucous membranes, poor skin turgor, perianal irritation

Gastrointestinal
Frequent soft to liquid stools that may alternate with constipation; altered stool color; abdominal distention, hyperactive bowel sounds; pus, blood, mucus, or fat in stools; fecal impaction

Urinary
Decreased output, concentrated urine

Possible Diagnostic Findings
Abnormal serum electrolyte levels; anemia; leukocytosis; eosinophilia; hypoalbuminemia; positive stool cultures; ova, parasites, leukocytes, blood, or fat in stool; abnormal sigmoidoscopy or colonoscopy findings; abnormal lower GI series

duration, frequency, character, and consistency of stool, and the relationship to other symptoms such as pain and vomiting. Inquire about medical conditions that might cause diarrhea and whether the person is taking medications such as antibiotics and laxatives that are known to cause diarrhea, decrease stomach acidity, or cause immunosuppression. Determine whether the patient has traveled to a foreign country or been at a day care facility recently and if family members are also ill. Ask about food preparation practices, food intolerances (e.g., milk), and changes in diet and appetite.

Assess for fever and signs of dehydration (dry skin, low-grade fever, orthostatic changes to pulse and blood pressure, decreased and concentrated urine). Assess the abdomen for distention, pain, and guarding. Inspect the perineal skin for signs of redness and breakdown from the diarrhea.

NURSING DIAGNOSES
Nursing diagnoses for the patient with acute infectious diarrhea may include, but are not limited to, the following:
- Diarrhea *related to* acute infectious process
- Deficient fluid volume *related to* excessive fluid loss and decreased fluid intake

Additional information on nursing diagnoses is presented in eNursing Care Plan 43-1 on the website for this chapter.

PLANNING
The overall goals are that the patient with diarrhea will have (1) no transmission of the microorganism causing the infectious diarrhea; (2) cessation of diarrhea and resumption of normal bowel patterns; (3) normal fluid, electrolyte, and acid-base balance; (4) normal nutritional status; and (5) no perianal skin breakdown.

NURSING IMPLEMENTATION
Consider all cases of acute diarrhea as infectious until the cause is known. Strict infection control precautions are necessary to prevent the illness from spreading to others (see eTable 15-1 on the website for Chapter 15 for CDC Isolation Precautions). Wash your hands before and after contact with each patient and when handling body fluids of any kind. Flush vomitus and stool in the toilet. Teach the patient and caregiver to wash contaminated clothing immediately with soap and water. Also teach them the principles of hygiene, infection control precautions, and the potential dangers of an illness that is infectious to themselves and others. Discuss proper food handling, cooking, and storage with the patient and the caregiver (see Chapter 42, Table 42-24).

Viruses and *C. difficile* spores are extremely difficult to kill. Alcohol-based hand cleaners and ammonia-based disinfectants are ineffective, and even vigorous cleaning with soap and water does not kill everything. Provide private rooms for patients with *C. difficile* infection, and ensure that visitors and health care providers wear gloves and gowns. Infected patients must be given their own disposable stethoscopes and thermometers. Consider all objects in the room contaminated, and ensure they are disinfected with a 10% solution of household bleach.

FECAL INCONTINENCE

Etiology and Pathophysiology
Fecal incontinence is the involuntary passage of stool. It occurs when the normal structures that maintain continence are disrupted. Defecation is a voluntary action when the neuromuscular system is intact (see Chapter 39). Problems with motor function (contraction of sphincters and rectal floor muscles) and/or sensory function (ability to perceive the presence of stool or to experience the urge to defecate) can result in fecal incontinence. Contributing factors to incontinence include weakness or disruption of the internal or external anal sphincter, damage to the pudendal nerve or other nerves that innervate the anorectum, damage to the anal tissue, and trauma to the puborectalis muscle.[7]

For women, obstetric trauma is the most common cause of sphincter disruption. Childbirth, aging, and menopause contribute to the development of fecal incontinence. Other risk factors are listed in Table 43-4. With diarrhea, the likelihood is increased that stool will be accidentally discharged. Chronic constipation can lead to *fecal impaction* (the accumulation of hardened feces in the rectum or sigmoid colon that cannot be expelled). Incontinence occurs as liquid stool seeps around the hardened feces. Fecal impaction is a common problem in older adults with limited mobility. Constipated individuals tend to strain during defecation. Straining contributes to incontinence because it weakens the pelvic floor muscles.

TABLE 43-4 CAUSES OF FECAL INCONTINENCE

Traumatic
- Anorectal surgery for hemorrhoids, fistula, and fissures
- Childbirth injury (episiotomy is a risk factor)
- Perineal trauma or pelvic fracture

Neurologic
- Brain tumor
- Cauda equina nerve injury
- Congenital abnormalities (e.g., spina bifida, myelomeningocele)
- Dementia
- Diabetes mellitus (secondary to neuropathy)
- Multiple sclerosis
- Rectal surgery
- Spinal cord injuries
- Stroke

Inflammatory
- Infection
- Inflammatory bowel disease
- Radiation

Pelvic Floor Dysfunction
- Medications
- Rectal prolapse

Functional
- Physical or mobility impairments affecting toileting ability (e.g., frail older person who cannot get to the bathroom in time)

Other
- Chronic constipation
- Denervation of pelvic muscles from chronic excessive straining
- Fecal impaction
- Loss of rectal elasticity
- Rapid transit of large diarrheal stools

Anorectal surgery such as hemorrhoidectomy and colectomy can damage the sphincters and pudendal nerves. Radiation for prostate cancer decreases rectal compliance. Neurologic conditions, including stroke, spinal cord injury, multiple sclerosis, Parkinson's disease, and diabetic neuropathy, also interfere with defecation. Even people with normally functioning defecation experience incontinence if immobility prevents timely access to a toilet.

Diagnostic Studies and Collaborative Care

The diagnosis and effective management of fecal incontinence require a thorough health history and physical examination. Ask the patient about the number of incontinent episodes per week, stool consistency and volume, and the degree that incontinence interferes with work and social activities. A rectal examination can reveal reduced anal canal muscle tone and contraction strength of the external sphincter, as well as detect internal prolapse, rectocele, hemorrhoids, fecal impaction, and masses. If the impaction is higher in the colon, an abdominal x-ray or a computed tomography (CT) scan may be helpful. Other tests include anorectal manometry, anorectal ultrasonography, and defecography. Sigmoidoscopy or colonoscopy is used to identify inflammation, tumors, fissures, and other pathologic conditions.

Treatment of incontinence depends on the underlying cause. Fecal incontinence from fecal impaction usually resolves after manual disimpaction of the hard feces and cleansing enemas. To prevent recurrence, normal stool consistency is maintained with a bowel management program that includes regular defecation practices, a high-fiber diet, and increased fluid intake. Damage to the anal sphincters may require surgical repair.

Dietary fiber supplements or bulk-forming laxatives such as psyllium in Metamucil increase stool bulk, firm stool consistency, and promote the sensation of rectal filling. Intake of foods that cause diarrhea and rectal irritation may need to be reduced or eliminated. For some patients this may include coffee, dried fruit, onions, mushrooms, green vegetables, fruit with peels, spicy foods, and foods with monosodium glutamate. An antidiarrheal agent (loperamide [Imodium]) is sometimes used to slow intestinal transit.

Kegel exercises (see Table 46-19) are used to strengthen and coordinate the pelvic floor muscles to improve continence. Biofeedback therapy may be recommended to improve awareness of rectal sensation, coordinate internal and external anal sphincters, and increase the strength of external sphincter contraction. Biofeedback training requires intact sensory and motor nerves and motivation to learn. It is a safe, painless, and relatively inexpensive treatment for fecal incontinence.[8]

An injectable treatment, dextranomer/hyaluronic acid gel (Solesta), is reserved for patients who have failed conservative fecal incontinence management. In this treatment, 4 mL of the gel is injected into the deep submucosa of the patient's anal canal. It acts through narrowing of the anal canal. No anesthesia is required. Postinjection pain and bleeding may occur.

Surgery (e.g., sphincter repair procedures) is considered only when nonsurgical conservative treatment fails, the patient has a full-thickness prolapse, and the sphincter needs repair. A colostomy is sometimes necessary.

NURSING MANAGEMENT FECAL INCONTINENCE

NURSING ASSESSMENT

Fecal incontinence is embarrassing, uncomfortable, and irritating to the skin.[9] Its unpredictable nature makes it difficult to maintain school and work activities and hampers social or intimate contact. Be sensitive to the patient's feelings when discussing incontinence. When the underlying cause cannot be corrected, help the patient reestablish a predictable pattern of defecation. Ask about bowel patterns before the incontinence developed; current bowel habits; stool consistency and frequency; and symptoms, including pain during defecation and a feeling of incomplete evacuation (*tenesmus*). Assess whether the patient has defecation urgency and sensation of passing flatus and leaking stool. Check the perineal area for irritation or breakdown. Ask about daily activities (mealtimes and work), diet, and family and social activities. The Bristol Stool Scale is helpful for assessing stool consistency (*www.poopreport.com/Poll/bristol_scale.html*).

Patients who are critically ill and have fecal incontinence are at risk for *incontinence-associated dermatitis* (IAD).[9] IAD is characterized by erythema and skin denudement (erosion) of the perianal or genital areas, buttocks, or upper thighs. It is caused by chemical irritants in feces. Dark-skinned patients may have areas of hypopigmentation. These skin changes place the patient at risk for fungal infection.

NURSING DIAGNOSES

Nursing diagnoses for the patient with fecal incontinence include, but are not limited to, the following:
- Bowel incontinence *related to* inability to control bowel function
- Self-care deficit (toileting) *related to* inability to manage bowel evacuation voluntarily
- Risk for situational low self-esteem *related to* inability to control bowel movements
- Risk for impaired skin integrity *related to* incontinence of stool

PLANNING

The overall goals are that the patient with fecal incontinence will (1) have predictable bowel elimination, (2) maintain perianal skin integrity, (3) participate in work and social activities, and (4) avoid self-esteem problems related to bowel control.

NURSING IMPLEMENTATION

Regardless of the cause of fecal incontinence, bowel training is an effective strategy for many patients. Bowel elimination occurs at regular intervals in most people. Knowing the patient's usual bowel pattern can assist you in planning a bowel program that will achieve optimal stool consistency and predictable bowel elimination patterns. For the hospitalized patient, placement on a bedpan, assistance to a bedside commode, or walks to the bathroom at a regular time daily help to establish regular defecation.[10] For many persons, a good time to schedule elimination is within 30 minutes after breakfast.

If these techniques are ineffective in reestablishing bowel regularity, a bisacodyl (Dulcolax) glycerin suppository or a small phosphate enema may be administered 15 to 30 minutes before the usual evacuation time. These preparations stimulate the anorectal reflex. Since stimulation will not occur unless the suppository or enema touches the rectal wall, first check for stool in the rectum and digitally remove it before inserting the laxative. Once a regular pattern is established, these drugs are discontinued. Digital stimulation is another method for stimulating the anorectal reflex and is commonly included in bowel programs for people with neurogenic bowels (e.g., from spinal cord injury). Irrigation of the rectum and colon (usually with tap water) at regular intervals is another method to achieve continence in patients with neurogenic bowel.[11]

Maintenance of perianal skin integrity is of utmost importance, especially in the bedridden and older adult patient. Incontinence can contaminate wounds, damage the skin, cause bladder infections, and spread infection such as *C. difficile*. Containment of the feces is essential, but it is difficult to maintain a seal with pouching systems and incontinence pads. Avoid the use of rectal tubes and urinary catheters because they can decrease responsiveness of the rectal sphincter and cause ulceration of the rectal mucosa. Fecal management systems such as the Zassi Bowel Management System, Flexi-Seal, and ActiFlo indwelling bowel catheter are designed to contain loose and liquid stools of bedridden patients without damaging the rectum or anal sphincters.[12]

Incontinence briefs may help maintain skin integrity if changed frequently. Implementation of a defined skin care program can reduce IAD. This includes prompt cleansing, moisturizing, and skin protection. The skin is cleaned with a mild soap and rinsed to remove feces, the area is dried, and a protective skin barrier cream is applied. For patients unable to care for themselves at home, teach the caregiver practices to maintain skin integrity.

Teach patients with fecal incontinence to avoid foods such as caffeine that worsen symptoms. In addition, exercising after meals can aggravate symptoms of incontinence.

CONSTIPATION

Normal bowel movements are formed and easy to pass. Frequency varies from three bowel movements daily to one bowel movement every 3 days. Constipation is characterized by absent or infrequent stools and hard, dry stools that are difficult to defecate. Because individuals vary, it is important to compare the current symptoms with the patient's normal pattern of elimination.

Etiology and Pathophysiology

Common causes of constipation include taking in insufficient dietary fiber or fluids, decreasing physical activity, and ignoring the defecation urge. Many drugs, especially opioids, cause constipation.[13] Constipation occurs with diseases that slow GI transit and hamper neurologic function such as diabetes mellitus, Parkinson's disease, and multiple sclerosis. Emotions, including anxiety, depression, and stress, affect the GI tract and can contribute to constipation.[14] Causes of constipation are summarized in eTable 43-2 (available on the website for this chapter).

Some people believe that they are constipated if they do not have a daily bowel movement. This can result in chronic laxative use and subsequent *cathartic colon syndrome*, a condition in which the colon becomes dilated and atonic (lacking muscle tone). Ultimately, the person cannot defecate without a laxative.

Ignoring the urge to defecate for a prolonged period can cause the muscles and mucosa of the rectum to become insensitive to the presence of feces. In addition, the prolonged retention of feces results in drying of stool due to water absorption. The harder and drier the feces, the more difficult it is to expel.

Clinical Manifestations

The clinical presentation of constipation may vary from a chronic discomfort to an acute event mimicking an "acute abdomen." Stools are absent or hard, dry, and difficult to pass. Abdominal distention, bloating, increased flatulence, and increased rectal pressure may also be present.

Hemorrhoids are the most common complication of chronic constipation. They result from venous engorgement caused by repeated *Valsalva maneuvers* (straining) and venous compression from hard impacted stool. Valsalva maneuver may have serious outcomes for patients with heart failure, cerebral edema, hypertension, and coronary artery disease. During straining, the patient inspires deeply and holds the breath while contracting abdominal muscles and bearing down. This increases both intraabdominal and intrathoracic pressures and reduces venous return to the heart. The heart rate decreases (bradycardia) temporarily, the cardiac output decreases, and a transient drop in arterial pressure occurs. When the patient relaxes, thoracic pressure falls, resulting in a sudden flow of blood into the heart, increased heart rate (tachycardia), and an immediate rise in arterial pressure. These changes may be fatal for the patient who cannot compensate for the sudden increased blood flow returning to the heart.

In the presence of *obstipation* (severe constipation when no gas or stool is expelled) or fecal impaction secondary to constipation, colonic perforation may occur. Perforation, which is life threatening, causes abdominal pain, nausea, vomiting, fever, and an elevated WBC count. Rectal mucosal ulcers and fissures may also occur as a result of stool stasis or straining. Diverticulosis is another potential complication of chronic constipation and is described later in this chapter. These complications are most common in older patients.

Diagnostic Studies and Collaborative Care

Perform a thorough history and physical examination so that the underlying cause of constipation can be identified and

TABLE 43-5 DRUG THERAPY
Constipation

Mechanism of Action	Example	Comments
Bulk Forming Absorbs water; increases bulk, thereby stimulating peristalsis *Action:* Usually within 24 hr	methylcellulose (Citrucel) psyllium (Metamucil, Perdiem, Konsyl, Hydrocil, Fiberall)	Contraindicated in patients with abdominal pain, nausea, and vomiting and in patients suspected of having appendicitis, biliary tract obstruction, or acute hepatitis. Must be taken with fluids (≥8 oz); best choice for initial treatment of constipation.
Stool Softeners and Lubricants Lubricate intestinal tract and soften feces, making hard stools easier to pass; do not affect peristalsis *Action:* Softeners in 72 hr, lubricants in 8 hr	*Softeners:* docusate (Colace, Surfak, Peri-Colace) *Lubricants:* mineral oil (Fleet's Oil Retention Enema, Kondremul Plain)	Can block absorption of fat-soluble vitamins such as vitamin K, which may increase risk of bleeding in patients on anticoagulants.
Saline and Osmotic Solutions Cause retention of fluid in intestinal lumen caused by osmotic effect *Action:* Within 15 min–3 hr	Magnesium salts (magnesium citrate, Milk of Magnesia) Sodium phosphates (Fleet Enema, Phospho-soda) lactulose (Constulose) polyethylene glycol (MiraLAX, GoLYTELY, CoLyte)	Magnesium-containing products may cause hypermagnesemia in patients with renal insufficiency.
Stimulants Increase peristalsis by irritating colon wall and stimulating enteric nerves *Action:* Usually within 12 hr	cascara sagrada, senna (Senokot) phenolphthalein: sennosides (Ex-Lax), bisacodyl (Correctol, Feen-a-Mint, Dulcolax), docusate/phenolphthalein (Doxidan)	Cause melanosis coli (brown or black pigmentation of colon). Are most widely abused laxatives. Should not be used in patients with impaction or obstipation.
Selective Chloride Channel Activator Increases intestinal fluid secretion and motility *Action:* Usually within 24 hr	lubiprostone (Amitiza)	Used in the treatment of idiopathic constipation and irritable bowel syndrome with constipation (women only). Contraindicated in patients with history of mechanical GI obstruction.
Intestinal Secretagogue Increases fluid secretion and accelerates intestinal transit. *Action:* Usually within 24 hr	linaclotide (Linzess)	Used in the treatment of idiopathic constipation and irritable bowel syndrome with constipation (men and women).

treatment started. Ask the patient about usual defecation patterns and habits, diet, exercise, use of laxatives, and conditions such as obstetric injuries that could contribute to difficulties with defecation. Abdominal x-rays, barium enema, colonoscopy, sigmoidoscopy, and anorectal manometry may be performed. Many cases of constipation can be prevented by increasing dietary fiber, fluid intake, and exercise. Laxatives (Table 43-5) and enemas may be used to treat acute constipation, but are used cautiously because overuse leads to chronic constipation.[15]

The choice of laxative or enema depends on the severity of the constipation and the patient's health. Daily bulk-forming preparations are used to prevent constipation because they work like dietary fiber and do not cause dependence. Stool softeners are also used to prevent constipation. Bisacodyl tablets and suppositories, milk of magnesia, and lactulose act more rapidly. They are also more likely to cause dependence. Methylnaltrexone (Relistor) is a peripheral μ-opiate receptor antagonist that decreases constipation caused by opioid use. The drug is administered subcutaneously. This agent does not block the analgesic effects.[16]

Enemas are fast acting and beneficial for immediate treatment of constipation, but must be used cautiously. Soapsuds enemas produce inflammation of colon mucosa, tap water enemas can potentially lead to water intoxication, and sodium phosphate (e.g., Fleet) enemas may cause electrolyte imbalances in patients with cardiac and renal problems.

Biofeedback therapy may benefit patients who are constipated as a result of *anismus* (uncoordinated contraction of the anal sphincter during straining). For the patient whose perceived constipation is related to rigid beliefs regarding bowel function, initiate a discussion about these concerns. Give appropriate information on normal bowel function and discuss the adverse consequences of excessive use of laxatives and enemas.

A patient with severe constipation related to bowel motility or mechanical disorders may require more intensive treatment. Diagnostic studies include anorectal manometry, GI tract transit studies, and sigmoidoscopic rectal biopsies. In a patient with unrelenting constipation, a subtotal colectomy with ileorectal anastomosis may be performed.

Nutritional Therapy. Diet is an important factor in the prevention of constipation. Many patients experience improved symptoms when they increase their intake of dietary fiber and fluids. Dietary fiber is found in fruits, vegetables, and grains (Table 43-6). Wheat bran and prunes are especially effective for preventing and treating constipation. Insoluble fiber is found in higher concentrations in whole wheat and bran.[17]

TABLE 43-6 **NUTRITIONAL THERAPY**

High-Fiber Foods

High-fiber foods are especially recommended for patients with diverticulosis, irritable bowel syndrome, constipation, hemorrhoids, atherosclerosis, hyperlipidemia, and diabetes mellitus.

	Fiber/Serving (g)	Serving Size	Calories/Serving
Vegetables			
Asparagus	3.5	½ cup	18
Beans			
• Navy	8.4	½ cup	80
• Kidney	9.7	½ cup	94
• Lima	8.3	½ cup	63
• Pinto	8.9	½ cup	78
• String	2.1	½ cup	18
Broccoli	3.5	½ cup	18
Carrots, raw	1.8	½ cup	15
Corn	2.6	½ medium ear	72
Peas, canned	6.7	½ cup	63
Potatoes			
• Baked	1.9	½ medium	72
• Sweet	2.1	½ medium	79
Squash, acorn	7.0	1 cup	82
Tomato, raw	1.5	1 small	18
Fruits			
Apple	2.0	½ large	42
Blackberries	6.7	¾ cup	40
Orange	1.6	1 small	35
Peach	2.3	1 medium	38
Pear	2.0	½ medium	44
Raspberries	9.2	1 cup	42
Strawberries	3.1	1 cup	45
Grain Products			
Bread, whole wheat	1.3	1 slice	59
Cereal			
• All Bran (100%)	8.4	⅓ cup	70
• Corn Flakes	2.6	¾ cup	70
• Shredded Wheat	2.8	1 biscuit	70
Popcorn	3.0	3 cups	62

Dietary fiber adds to the stool bulk directly and by attracting water. Therefore adequate fluid intake (2 L/day) is essential. Large, bulky stools move through the colon much more quickly than small stools. However, the recommended fluid intake may be contraindicated in the patient with cardiac disease or renal insufficiency or failure. Inform the patient that increasing fiber intake may initially increase gas production because of fermentation in the colon, but this effect decreases with use.

NURSING MANAGEMENT CONSTIPATION

NURSING ASSESSMENT

Subjective and objective data that should be obtained from a patient with constipation are presented in Table 43-7.

NURSING DIAGNOSIS

Nursing diagnoses for the patient with constipation include, but are not limited to, the following:

- Constipation *related to* inadequate intake of dietary fiber and fluid and decreased physical activity

TABLE 43-7 **NURSING ASSESSMENT**

Constipation

Subjective Data
Important Health Information
Past health history: Colorectal disease, neurologic dysfunction, bowel obstruction, environmental changes, cancer, irritable bowel syndrome, diabetes mellitus
Medications: Aluminum and calcium antacids, anticholinergics, antidepressants, antihistamines, antipsychotics, diuretics, opioids, iron, laxatives, enemas

Functional Health Patterns
Health perception–health management: Chronic laxative or enema abuse; rigid beliefs regarding bowel function; malaise
Nutritional-metabolic: Changes in diet or mealtime; inadequate fiber and fluid intake; anorexia, nausea
Elimination: Change in usual elimination patterns; hard, difficult-to-pass stool, decrease in frequency and amount of stools; flatus, abdominal distention; tenesmus, rectal pressure; fecal incontinence (if impacted)
Activity-exercise: Change in daily activity routines; immobility; sedentary lifestyle
Cognitive-perceptual: Dizziness, headache, anorectal pain; abdominal pain on defecation
Coping–stress tolerance: Acute or chronic stress

Objective Data
General
Lethargy

Integumentary
Anorectal fissures, hemorrhoids, abscesses

Gastrointestinal
Abdominal distention; hypoactive or absent bowel sounds; palpable abdominal mass; fecal impaction; small, hard, dry stool; stool with blood

Possible Diagnostic Findings
Guaiac-positive stools; abdominal x-ray demonstrating stool in lower colon

PLANNING

The overall goals are that the patient with constipation will (1) increase dietary intake of fiber and fluids; (2) increase physical activity; (3) pass soft, formed stools; and (4) not have any complications, such as bleeding hemorrhoids.

NURSING IMPLEMENTATION

Nursing management should be based on the patient's symptoms and assessment (see Table 43-7). Teach the patient about the importance of diet in the prevention of constipation. A patient and caregiver teaching guide for constipation is presented in Table 43-8. Emphasize using a high-fiber diet, increasing fluid intake, and exercising regularly. Teach the patient to establish a regular time to defecate and not to suppress the urge to defecate. Discourage the use of laxatives and enemas to achieve fecal elimination.

Defecation is easiest when the person is sitting on a commode with the knees higher than the hips. The sitting position allows gravity to aid defecation, and flexing the hips straightens the angle between the anal canal and the rectum so that stool flows out more easily. Place a footstool in front of the toilet to promote flexion of the thighs. It is challenging to defecate while sitting on a bedpan. For a patient in bed, elevate the head of the bed as high as the patient can tolerate.

TABLE 43-8 PATIENT & CAREGIVER TEACHING GUIDE

Constipation

Include the following instructions when teaching the patient and caregiver about management of constipation.

1. Eat Dietary Fiber

Eat 20-30 g of fiber per day. Gradually increase the amount of fiber eaten over 1-2 wk. Fiber softens hard stool and adds bulk to stool, promoting evacuation.
- Foods high in fiber: raw vegetables and fruits, beans, breakfast cereals (All Bran, oatmeal)
- Fiber supplements: Metamucil, Citrucel, FiberCon

Eat prunes or drink prune juice daily. Prunes stimulate defecation.

2. Drink Fluids

Drink 3 quarts per day. Drink water or fruit juices. Avoid caffeinated coffee, tea, and cola. Fluid softens hard stools. Caffeine stimulates fluid loss through urination.

3. Exercise Regularly

Walk, swim, or bike at least three times per wk. Contract and relax abdominal muscles when standing or by doing sit-ups to strengthen muscles and prevent straining. Exercise stimulates bowel motility and moves stool through the colon.

4. Establish a Regular Time to Defecate

First thing in the morning or after the first meal of the day is a good time because people often have the urge to defecate at this time.

5. Do Not Delay Defecation

Respond to the urge to have a bowel movement as soon as possible. Delaying defecation results in hard stools and a decreased "urge" to defecate. Water is absorbed from stool by the intestine over time. The colon becomes less sensitive to the presence of stool in the rectum.

6. Record Your Bowel Elimination Pattern

Develop a habit of recording when you have a bowel movement on your calendar. Regular monitoring of bowel movement will assist in early identification of a problem.

7. Avoid Laxatives and Enemas

Do not overuse laxatives and enemas because they cause dependence. People who overuse them are unable to have a bowel movement without them.

TABLE 43-9 CAUSES OF ACUTE ABDOMINAL PAIN

- Abdominal compartment syndrome
- Acute pancreatitis
- Appendicitis
- Bowel obstruction
- Cholecystitis
- Diverticulitis
- Gastroenteritis
- Pelvic inflammatory disease
- Perforated gastric or duodenal ulcer
- Peritonitis
- Ruptured abdominal aneurysm
- Ruptured ectopic pregnancy

Most people are embarrassed by the sights and sounds of defecation, so provide as much privacy as possible. Encourage patients to exercise abdominal muscles and to contract abdominal muscles several times a day. Sit-ups and straight-leg raises can also help improve abdominal muscle tone.

Teach patients taking bulking products to follow product recommendations in terms of fluid intake. Patients may initially experience an increase in flatus that will decrease with use.

ACUTE ABDOMINAL PAIN

Etiology and Pathophysiology

Acute abdominal pain is pain of recent onset. It may signal a life-threatening problem and therefore requires immediate attention.[18] Causes include damage to organs in the abdomen and pelvis, which leads to inflammation, infection, obstruction, bleeding, and perforation (Fig. 43-1). The most common causes of acute abdominal pain are listed in Table 43-9. Perforation of the GI tract also results in irritation of the *peritoneum* (serous membrane lining the abdominal cavity) and peritonitis. Hypovolemic shock occurs from bleeding or when obstruction and

peritonitis cause large amounts of fluid to move from the vascular space into the abdomen (third spacing).

Clinical Manifestations

Pain is the most common symptom of an acute abdominal problem. The patient may also complain of nausea, vomiting, diarrhea, constipation, flatulence, fatigue, fever, and bloating.

Diagnostic Studies and Collaborative Care

Diagnosis begins with a complete history and physical examination. Description of the pain (frequency, timing, duration, location), accompanying symptoms, and sequence of symptoms (e.g., pain before or after vomiting) provide vital clues about the origin of the problem. Note the patient's position. The fetal posture is common with peritoneal irritation (e.g., appendicitis), a supine posture with outstretched legs is seen with visceral pain, and restlessness and a seated posture commonly occur with bowel obstructions and obstructions from kidney stones and gallstones.

Physical examination includes examination of the abdomen, rectum, and pelvis. A complete blood count (CBC), urinalysis, abdominal x-ray, and electrocardiogram are done, along with an ultrasound or CT scan. A pregnancy test is performed in women of childbearing age with acute abdominal pain to rule out ectopic pregnancy (see Table 43-9).

Emergency management of the patient with acute abdominal pain is presented in Table 43-10. The goal of management is to identify and treat the cause, and monitor and treat complications, especially shock. Careful use of pain medications (e.g., morphine) provides pain relief without interfering with diagnostic accuracy when patients have nontraumatic acute abdominal pain.

An immediate surgical consult is needed. The surgeon may perform a diagnostic laparoscopy to inspect the surface of abdominal organs, obtain biopsy specimens, perform laparoscopic ultrasounds, and remove organs. A laparotomy is used when laparoscopic techniques are inadequate. If the cause of the acute abdomen can be surgically removed (e.g., inflamed appendix) or surgically repaired (e.g., ruptured abdominal aneurysm), surgery is considered definitive therapy.

NURSING MANAGEMENT ACUTE ABDOMINAL PAIN

NURSING ASSESSMENT

For the patient complaining of acute abdominal pain, take vital signs immediately and again at frequent intervals. Increased pulse and decreasing blood pressure indicate impending shock. An elevated temperature suggests an inflammatory or infectious process. Intake and output measurement provides essential information about the adequacy of vascular volume. Altered

Etiology	Life-Threatening Effect

Inflammation
- Gastroenteritis
- Appendicitis
- Pancreatitis
- Diverticulitis
- Cholecystitis

- Risk of perforation (→ peritonitis)
- Fluid shifts to area of inflammation
- Unable to ingest fluid

Peritonitis
- Perforated peptic ulcers
- Ruptured diverticula
- Ruptured appendix
- Intestinal perforation

- Overwhelming infection
- Fluid shifts to area of inflammation
- Unable to ingest fluid

Septic shock

Obstruction
- Bowel obstruction
- Biliary obstruction
- Mesenteric vascular occlusion

- Strangulation risk
- Fluid trapped in bowel
- Fluid shifts to interstitial space
- Unable to ingest fluid

Hypovolemic shock

Internal Bleeding
- Trauma
- Ruptured abdominal aneurysm
- GI bleed

- Blood lost from vascular space
- Unable to ingest fluid

FIG. 43-1 Etiology of acute abdominal pain and pathophysiologic sequelae.

mental status indicates poor cerebral perfusion. Skin color and temperature and peripheral pulse strength provide information about skin perfusion. Inspect the abdomen for distention, masses, abnormal pulsation, symmetry, hernias, rashes, scars, and pigmentation changes. Auscultate bowel sounds. Bowel sounds that are diminished or absent in a quadrant may indicate a bowel obstruction, acute peritonitis, or paralytic ileus. Palpation should be gentle. Determine pain from peritoneal irritation by asking the person to cough, palpating the abdomen gently, or gently shaking the bed.

Ask the patient about the onset, location, intensity, duration, frequency, and character of pain. Note whether the pain has spread or moved to new sites (quadrants) and what makes the pain worse or better. Is the pain associated with other symptoms, such as nausea, vomiting, changes in bowel and bladder habits, or vaginal discharge in women? Assessment of vomiting includes the amount, color, consistency, and odor of the emesis. Also ask about usual and changes in bowel patterns and habits.

NURSING DIAGNOSES

Nursing diagnoses for the patient with acute abdominal pain include, but are not limited to, the following:
- Acute pain *related to* inflammation of the peritoneum and abdominal distention
- Risk for deficient fluid volume *related to* collection of fluid in peritoneal cavity secondary to inflammation or infection
- Anxiety *related to* pain and uncertainty of cause or outcome of condition

PLANNING

The overall goals are that the patient with acute abdominal pain will have (1) relief of abdominal pain, (2) resolution of inflammation, (3) freedom from complications (especially hypovolemic shock), and (4) normal nutritional status.

NURSING IMPLEMENTATION

General care for the patient with acute abdominal pain involves management of fluid and electrolyte imbalances, pain, and anxiety. Assess the quality and intensity of pain at regular intervals, and provide medication and other comfort measures. Maintain a calm environment and provide information to help allay anxiety. A nasogastric (NG) tube may be used to decrease vomiting and relieve discomfort from gastric distention. Conduct ongoing assessments of vital signs, intake and output, and level of consciousness, which are key indicators of hypovolemic shock.

ACUTE INTERVENTION

Preoperative Care. Preoperative care includes the emergency care of the patient described in Table 43-10 and general care of the preoperative patient (see Chapter 18).

Postoperative Care. Postoperative care depends on the type of surgical procedure performed. In some cases a laparotomy is necessary. When appropriate, a laparoscopic approach is used. Laparoscopic procedures result in lower rates of postoperative complications (poor wound healing and paralytic ileus), earlier diet advancement, and shorter hospital stays compared with open surgical procedures. eNursing Care Plan 20-1, a general plan for the postoperative patient, is presented on the website for Chapter 20.

✚ TABLE 43-10 **EMERGENCY MANAGEMENT**

Acute Abdominal Pain

Etiology	Assessment Findings	Interventions
Inflammation • Appendicitis • Cholecystitis • Crohn's disease • Gastritis • Pancreatitis • Pyelonephritis • Ulcerative colitis	**Abdominal and Gastrointestinal Findings** • Diffuse, localized, dull, burning, or sharp abdominal pain or tenderness • Rebound tenderness • Abdominal distention • Abdominal rigidity • Nausea and vomiting • Diarrhea • Hematemesis • Melena	**Initial** • Ensure patent airway. • Administer O_2 via nasal cannula or non-rebreather mask. • Establish IV access with large-bore catheter and infuse warm normal saline or lactated Ringer's solution. Insert additional large-bore catheter if shock present. • Obtain blood for CBC and electrolyte levels. • Anticipate order for amylase level, pregnancy tests, clotting studies, and type and crossmatch as appropriate. • Insert indwelling urinary catheter. • Obtain urinalysis. • Insert NG tube as needed.
Vascular Problems • Ruptured aortic aneurysm • Mesenteric vascular occlusion	**Hypovolemic Shock** • ↓ Blood pressure • ↓ Pulse pressure • Tachycardia • Cool, clammy skin • ↓ Level of consciousness • ↓ Urine output (<0.5 mL/kg/hr)	**Ongoing Monitoring** • Monitor vital signs, level of consciousness, O_2 saturation, and intake/output. • Assess quality and amount of pain. • Assess amount and character of emesis. • Anticipate surgical intervention. • Keep patient NPO.
Gynecologic Problems • Pelvic inflammatory disease • Ruptured ectopic pregnancy • Ruptured ovarian cyst		
Infectious Disease • *Escherichia coli* O157:H7 • *Giardia* • *Salmonella*		
Other • Obstruction or perforation of abdominal organ • Gastrointestinal bleeding or ischemia • Trauma		

Postoperatively an NG tube with low suction may be used in selected patients to empty the stomach and prevent gastric dilation. If the upper GI tract has been entered, drainage from the NG tube may be dark brown to dark red for the first 12 hours. Later it should be light yellowish brown, or it may have a greenish tinge because of bile. If a dark red color continues or if bright red blood is observed, notify the surgeon because of the possibility of hemorrhage. "Coffee-ground" granules in the drainage indicate blood that has been modified by acidic gastric secretions.

Nausea and vomiting are common after a laparotomy and may be caused by the surgery, decreased peristalsis, or pain medications. Antiemetics such as ondansetron (Zofran), trimethobenzamide (Tigan), and prochlorperazine (Compazine) may be ordered. Management of nausea and vomiting is discussed in Chapter 42. Monitor fluid and electrolyte status along with blood pressure, heart rate, and respirations.

Swallowed air and reduced peristalsis from decreased mobility, manipulation of the abdominal organs during surgery, and anesthesia can result in abdominal distention and gas pains. Early ambulation helps restore peristalsis and eliminate flatus and gas pain. Gradually, as intestinal activity increases, distention and gas pain disappear.

AMBULATORY AND HOME CARE. Preparation for discharge begins soon after surgery. Teach the patient and caregiver about any modifications in activity, care of the incision, diet, and drug therapy. Clear liquids are given initially after surgery and, if tolerated, the patient progresses to a regular diet.

Early ambulation speeds recovery, but normal activities are resumed gradually, with planned rest periods. After surgery the patient is generally instructed not to lift anything heavier than a few pounds. The patient and caregiver should be aware of possible complications after surgery. Teach them to notify the surgeon immediately if fever, vomiting, pain, weight loss, incisional drainage, or changes in bowel function occur.

❚ **EVALUATION**

The expected outcomes are that the patient with acute abdominal pain will have
- Resolution of the cause of the acute abdominal pain
- Relief of abdominal pain and discomfort
- Freedom from complications (especially hypovolemic shock and septicemia)
- Normal fluid, electrolyte, and nutritional status

❚ **CHRONIC ABDOMINAL PAIN**

Chronic abdominal pain may originate from abdominal structures or may be referred from a site with the same or a similar nerve supply. The pain is often described as dull, aching, or diffuse. Common causes of chronic abdominal pain include irritable bowel syndrome (IBS), peptic ulcer disease, chronic pancreatitis, hepatitis, pelvic inflammatory disease, and vascular insufficiency. (Some of these disorders are discussed in this chapter).

Diagnosis of the cause of chronic abdominal pain begins with a thorough history and description of specific pain characteristics, including severity, location, frequency, duration, and onset. The assessment also includes factors that increase or decrease the pain, such as meals, defecation, and activities.

Endoscopy, CT scan, magnetic resonance imaging (MRI), laparoscopy, and barium studies may be done. Treatment for chronic abdominal pain depends on the underlying cause.

IRRITABLE BOWEL SYNDROME

Irritable bowel syndrome (IBS) is a common, chronic functional disorder, meaning that no organic cause is currently known.[19] Symptoms of IBS, including abdominal pain or discomfort and alterations in bowel patterns, are intermittent and may occur for years. Patients often report a history of GI infections and food intolerances. However, the role of food allergies in IBS is unclear. Other dietary factors that may contribute to symptoms include fermentable oligo-, di-, and monosaccharides and polyols (FODMAPs).[20] Examples include fructans (found in wheat), galactans, lactose, fructose, sorbitol, and xylitol.

Psychologic stressors (e.g., depression, anxiety, sexual abuse, posttraumatic stress disorder) are associated with development and exacerbation of IBS.[19] IBS is more frequently diagnosed in women than in men. In addition to abdominal pain and diarrhea or constipation, patients commonly experience abdominal distention, excessive flatulence, bloating, urgency, and sensation of incomplete evacuation. Non-GI symptoms may include fatigue and sleep disturbances.

There are no specific physical findings with IBS. The key to accurate diagnosis is a thorough history and physical examination. Ask patients to describe symptoms, past health history (including psychosocial factors such as stress and anxiety), family history, and drug and diet history. Determine if and how IBS symptoms interfere with school, work, or recreational activities. Diagnostic tests are selectively used to rule out other disorders such as colorectal cancer, IBD, endometriosis, and malabsorption disorders (lactose intolerance, celiac disease). Symptom-based criteria for IBS have been standardized and are referred to as the Rome criteria III (see eTable 43-3 on the website for this chapter).

Treatment is directed at psychologic and dietary factors and drugs to regulate stool output. Patients are more likely to improve with treatment if they have a trusting relationship with their health care provider. Encourage the patient to verbalize concerns. Since treatment is often focused on symptoms, patients may benefit from keeping a diary of symptoms, diet, and episodes of stress to help identify factors that seem to trigger the IBS symptoms. If tolerated, encourage the patient to have a dietary fiber intake of at least 20 g/day (see Table 43-6) or to use a stool bulking agent. Increases in dietary fiber should be started gradually to avoid bloating and abdominal discomfort from gas.

Advise the patient whose primary symptoms are abdominal distention and flatulence to avoid common gas-producing foods such as broccoli and cabbage. Yogurt may be better tolerated than milk products. Probiotics may be used because alterations in intestinal bacteria are believed to exacerbate the condition.[19]

Loperamide, a synthetic opioid that slows intestinal transit, may be used to treat diarrhea when it occurs. Alosetron (Lotronex), a serotonergic antagonist, is used for IBS patients with severe symptoms of pain and diarrhea. Because of serious side effects (e.g., severe constipation, ischemic colitis), alosetron is available only in a restricted access program for women who have not responded to other IBS therapies. Lubiprostone (Amitiza) is approved for the treatment of IBS with constipation in women. Linaclotide (Linzess) is approved for the treatment of IBS with constipation in men and women.

> **DRUG ALERT: Alosetron (Lotronex)**
> - Patients may experience severe constipation and ischemic colitis (reduced blood flow to intestines).
> - If constipation occurs, drug should be discontinued.
> - Symptoms of ischemic colitis include abdominal pain and blood in stool.

Psychologic therapies include cognitive-behavioral therapy, stress management techniques, acupuncture, and hypnosis. Low doses of tricyclic antidepressants seem beneficial, possibly because they decrease peripheral nerve sensitivity. No single therapy has been found to be effective for all patients with IBS.

ABDOMINAL TRAUMA

Etiology and Pathophysiology

Injuries to the abdominal area usually are a result of blunt trauma or penetrating injuries. Common injuries of the abdomen include lacerated liver, ruptured spleen, mesenteric artery tears, diaphragm rupture, urinary bladder rupture, great vessel tears, renal or pancreas injury, and stomach or intestine rupture. *Blunt trauma* commonly occurs with motor vehicle accidents, beatings, and falls and may not be obvious because it does not leave an open wound. Both compression injuries (e.g., direct blow to the abdomen) and shearing injuries (e.g., rapid deceleration in a motor vehicle crash allowing some tissue to move forward while other tissues are held stationary) occur with blunt trauma. *Penetrating injuries* occur when a gunshot or stabbing produces an obvious, open wound into the abdomen.[21]

When solid organs (liver, spleen) are injured, bleeding can be profuse, resulting in hypovolemic shock. When contents from hollow organs (e.g., bladder, stomach, intestines) spill into the peritoneal cavity, the patient is at risk for peritonitis. In addition, abdominal compartment syndrome can develop.

Abdominal compartment syndrome is excessively high pressure in the abdomen (abdominal hypertension). Anything that increases the volume in the abdominal cavity—including edematous organs, bleeding, and third spacing caused by obstruction and inflammation—increases abdominal pressure.[22] High abdominal pressure restricts ventilation, potentially leading to respiratory failure. The high pressure also decreases cardiac output, venous return, and arterial perfusion of organs. Decreased perfusion to the kidneys can lead to renal failure.

Clinical Manifestations

Careful assessment provides important clues to the type and severity of injury. Intraabdominal injuries are often associated with low rib fractures, fractured femur, fractured pelvis, and

---

TABLE 43-11 EMERGENCY MANAGEMENT

Abdominal Trauma

Etiology	Assessment Findings	Interventions
Blunt	**Hypovolemic Shock**	**Initial**
• Falls	• ↓ Level of consciousness	• Ensure patent airway.
• Motor vehicle collisions	• Tachypnea	• Administer O_2 via non-rebreather mask.
• Pedestrian event	• Tachycardia	• Control external bleeding with direct pressure or sterile
• Assault with blunt object	• ↓ Blood pressure	pressure dressing.
• Crush injuries	• ↓ Pulse pressure	• Establish IV access with two large-bore catheters and
• Explosions		infuse warm normal saline or lactated Ringer's solution.
	Surface Findings	• Obtain blood for type and crossmatch and CBC.
Penetrating	• Abrasions or ecchymoses on abdominal wall, flank,	• Remove clothing.
• Knife	or peritoneum	• Stabilize impaled objects with bulky dressing—*do not*
• Gunshot wounds	• Open wounds: lacerations, eviscerations, puncture	*remove.*
• Other missiles	wounds, gunshot wounds	• Cover protruding organs or tissue with sterile saline
	• Impaled object	dressing.
	• Healed incisions or old scars	• Insert indwelling urinary catheter if there is no blood at
		the meatus, pelvic fracture, or boggy prostate.
	Abdominal and Gastrointestinal Findings	• Obtain urine for urinalysis.
	• Nausea and vomiting	• Insert NG tube if no evidence of facial trauma.
	• Hematemesis	• Anticipate diagnostic peritoneal lavage.
	• Absent or decreased bowel sounds	
	• Bloody urine (hematuria)	**Ongoing Monitoring**
	• Abdominal distention	• Monitor vital signs, level of consciousness, O_2
	• Abdominal rigidity	saturation, and urine output.
	• Abdominal pain with palpation	• Maintain patient warmth using blankets, warm IV
	• Rebound tenderness	fluids, or warm humidified O_2.
	• Pain radiation to shoulder and back	

---

thoracic injury. If the patient was in an automobile accident, a contusion or abrasion across the lower abdomen may indicate internal organ trauma due to seat belt use. Seat belts can produce blunt trauma to abdominal organs by pressing the intestine and pancreas into the spinal column.

Clinical manifestations of abdominal trauma are (1) guarding and splinting of the abdominal wall (indicating peritonitis); (2) a hard, distended abdomen (indicating intraabdominal bleeding); (3) decreased or absent bowel sounds; (4) contusions, abrasions, or bruising over the abdomen; (5) abdominal pain; (6) pain over the scapula caused by irritation of the phrenic nerve by free blood in the abdomen; (7) hematemesis or hematuria; and (8) signs of hypovolemic shock (Table 43-11). Ecchymosis around the umbilicus (Cullen's sign) or flanks (Grey Turner's sign) may indicate retroperitoneal hemorrhage. Loss of bowel sounds occurs with peritonitis. If present, bowel sounds are heard in the chest when the diaphragm ruptures. Auscultation of bruits is indicative of arterial damage.

Diagnostic Studies

Laboratory tests include a baseline CBC and urinalysis. Even when bleeding, the patient will have normal hemoglobin and hematocrit because fluids are lost at the same rate as the red blood cells. Deficiencies are evident after fluid resuscitation begins. Blood in the urine may be a sign of damage to the kidney or bladder. Additional laboratory work includes arterial blood gases, prothrombin time, electrolytes, BUN and creatinine, and type and crossmatch (in anticipation of possible blood transfusions). An abdominal CT scan and focused abdominal sonography are the most common diagnostic methods, but the patient must be stable before going for CT. Diagnostic peritoneal lavage can be used to detect blood, bile, intestinal contents, and urine in the peritoneal cavity, but is generally used only for unstable patients to identify blood in the peritoneum.[22]

NURSING AND COLLABORATIVE MANAGEMENT
ABDOMINAL TRAUMA

Emergency management of abdominal trauma focuses on establishing a patent airway and adequate breathing, fluid replacement, and prevention of hypovolemic shock (see Table 43-11). IV lines are inserted, and volume expanders or blood is given if the patient is hypotensive. An NG tube is inserted to decompress the stomach and prevent aspiration. Frequent ongoing assessment is necessary to monitor fluid status, detect deterioration in condition, and determine the necessity for surgery. An impaled object should never be removed until skilled care is available. Removal may cause further injury and bleeding. The decision about whether to do surgery depends on clinical findings, diagnostic test results, and the patient's response to conservative management.

INFLAMMATORY DISORDERS

APPENDICITIS

Appendicitis is inflammation of the appendix, a narrow blind tube that extends from the inferior part of the cecum (Fig. 43-2).

Etiology and Pathophysiology

In the United States, about 1 in 15 people will get appendicitis. It is most common in individuals 10 to 30 years of age. It is the most common cause of acute abdominal pain.[23] A common cause of appendicitis is obstruction of the lumen by a fecalith (accumulated feces) (see Fig. 43-2). Obstruction results in distention; venous engorgement; and the accumulation of mucus and bacteria, which can lead to gangrene, perforation, and peritonitis.

FIG. 43-2 In appendicitis the blood supply of the appendix is impaired by inflammation and bacterial infection in the wall of the appendix, which may result in gangrene.

Clinical Manifestations

Diagnosis can be difficult because many patients do not have classic symptoms. Typically appendicitis begins with periumbilical pain, followed by anorexia, nausea, and vomiting. The pain is persistent and continuous, eventually shifting to the right lower quadrant and localizing at McBurney's point (halfway between the umbilicus and the right iliac crest). Further assessment reveals localized tenderness, rebound tenderness, and muscle guarding. Coughing, sneezing, and deep inhalation magnify the pain. The patient usually prefers to lie still, often with the right leg flexed. Low-grade fever may or may not be present.[23] The older adult may report less severe pain, slight fever, and discomfort in the right iliac fossa.

Diagnostic Studies and Collaborative Care

Examination of the patient includes a complete history, physical examination, and a differential WBC count. The WBC count is mildly to moderately elevated in most cases. A urinalysis is done to rule out genitourinary conditions that mimic the manifestations of appendicitis. CT scan is the preferred diagnostic procedure, but ultrasound is also used.

If diagnosis and treatment are delayed, the appendix can rupture, and the resulting peritonitis can be fatal. The treatment of appendicitis is immediate surgical removal (*appendectomy*) if the inflammation is localized. Surgery, generally performed laparoscopically, is done as soon as the diagnosis is made. Antibiotics and fluid resuscitation are administered before surgery.

If the appendix has ruptured and there is evidence of peritonitis or an abscess, parenteral fluids and antibiotic therapy are given for 6 to 8 hours before the appendectomy to prevent dehydration and sepsis.

▌NURSING MANAGEMENT
▌APPENDICITIS

Encourage the patient with abdominal pain to see a health care provider and to avoid self-treatment. Laxatives and enemas are especially dangerous because the resulting increased peristalsis may cause perforation of the appendix. To ensure that the stomach is empty in case surgery is needed, keep patients on nothing-by-mouth (NPO) status until they can be seen by a health care provider.

TABLE 43-12	CAUSES OF PERITONITIS
Primary	**Secondary**
• Blood-borne organisms	• Appendicitis with rupture
• Genital tract organisms	• Blunt or penetrating trauma to abdominal organs
• Cirrhosis with ascites	• Diverticulitis with rupture
	• Ischemic bowel disorders
	• Pancreatitis
	• Perforated intestine
	• Perforated peptic ulcer
	• Peritoneal dialysis
	• Postoperative (breakage of anastomosis)

Postoperative nursing management for the patient who has an appendectomy is similar to postoperative care of the patient after laparotomy. Ambulation begins the day of surgery or the first postoperative day. The diet is advanced as tolerated. The patient is usually discharged on the first or second postoperative day and resumes normal activities 2 to 3 weeks after surgery.

PERITONITIS

Etiology and Pathophysiology

Peritonitis results from a localized or generalized inflammatory process of the peritoneum. Causes of peritonitis are listed in Table 43-12. Primary peritonitis occurs when blood-borne organisms enter the peritoneal cavity. For example, the ascites that occurs with cirrhosis of the liver provides an excellent liquid environment for bacteria to flourish. Organisms can also enter the peritoneum during peritoneal dialysis. (Peritoneal dialysis is described in Chapter 47.)

Secondary peritonitis is much more common. It occurs when abdominal organs perforate or rupture and release their contents (bile, enzymes, and bacteria) into the peritoneal cavity. Common causes include a ruptured appendix, perforated gastric or duodenal ulcer, severely inflamed gallbladder, and trauma from gunshot or knife wounds.

Intestinal contents and bacteria irritate the normally sterile peritoneum and produce an initial chemical peritonitis, which is followed a few hours later by a bacterial peritonitis. The resulting inflammatory response leads to massive fluid shifts (peritoneal edema) and adhesions as the body attempts to wall off the infection.

Clinical Manifestations

Abdominal pain is the most common symptom of peritonitis. A universal sign of peritonitis is tenderness over the involved area. Rebound tenderness, muscular rigidity, and spasm are other signs of irritation of the peritoneum. Patients may lie still and take only shallow breaths because movement causes pain. Abdominal distention, fever, tachycardia, tachypnea, nausea, vomiting, and altered bowel habits may also be present. These manifestations vary depending on the severity and acuteness of the underlying condition. Complications of peritonitis include hypovolemic shock, sepsis, intraabdominal abscess formation, paralytic ileus, and acute respiratory distress syndrome. If treatment is delayed, peritonitis can be fatal.

Diagnostic Studies and Collaborative Care

A CBC is done to determine elevations in WBC count and hemoconcentration from fluid shifts (Table 43-13). Peritoneal

TABLE 43-13 COLLABORATIVE CARE

Peritonitis

Diagnostic
- History and physical examination
- CBC, including WBC differential
- Serum electrolytes
- Abdominal x-ray
- Abdominal paracentesis and culture of fluid
- CT scan or ultrasound
- Peritoneoscopy

Collaborative Therapy
Preoperative or Nonoperative
- NPO status
- IV fluid replacement
- Antibiotic therapy
- NG suction
- Analgesics (e.g., morphine)
- Oxygen PRN
- Preparation for surgery to include the above and parenteral nutrition

Postoperative
- NPO status
- NG tube to low-intermittent suction
- Semi-Fowler's position
- IV fluids with electrolyte replacement
- Parenteral nutrition as needed
- Antibiotic therapy
- Blood transfusions as needed
- Sedatives and opioids

aspiration may be performed and the fluid analyzed for blood, bile, pus, bacteria, fungus, and amylase content. An x-ray of the abdomen may show dilated loops of bowel consistent with paralytic ileus, free air if perforation has occurred, or air and fluid levels if an obstruction is present. Ultrasound and CT scans may be useful in identifying ascites and abscesses. Peritoneoscopy may be helpful in the patient without ascites. Direct examination of the peritoneum can be obtained along with biopsy specimens for diagnosis.

Patients with milder cases of peritonitis or those who are poor surgical risks may be managed medically. Treatment consists of antibiotics, NG suction, analgesics, and IV fluid administration. Surgery is indicated to locate the cause of the inflammation, drain purulent fluid, and repair any damage (e.g., perforated organs).

NURSING MANAGEMENT
PERITONITIS

NURSING ASSESSMENT

Assessment of the patient's pain, including the location, is important and may help in determining the cause of peritonitis. Assess the patient for the presence and quality of bowel sounds, increasing abdominal distention, abdominal guarding, nausea, fever, and manifestations of hypovolemic shock.

NURSING DIAGNOSES

Nursing diagnoses for the patient with peritonitis include, but are not limited to, the following:
- Acute pain *related to* inflammation of the peritoneum and abdominal distention

- Risk for deficient fluid volume *related to* fluid shifts into the peritoneal cavity secondary to trauma, infection, or ischemia
- Anxiety *related to* uncertainty of cause or outcome of the condition and pain

PLANNING

The overall goals are that the patient with peritonitis will have (1) resolution of inflammation, (2) relief of abdominal pain, (3) freedom from complications (especially sepsis and hypovolemic shock), and (4) normal nutritional status.

NURSING IMPLEMENTATION

The patient with peritonitis is extremely ill and needs skilled supportive care. An IV line is inserted to replace vascular fluids lost to the peritoneal cavity and as an access for antibiotic therapy. Monitor the patient for pain and response to analgesics. The patient may be positioned with knees flexed to increase comfort. Sedatives may be given to allay anxiety.

Accurate monitoring of fluid intake and output and electrolyte status is necessary to determine replacement therapy. Monitor vital signs frequently. Antiemetics may be administered to decrease nausea and vomiting and prevent further fluid and electrolyte losses. The patient is placed on NPO status and may need an NG tube to decrease gastric distention and further leakage of bowel contents into the peritoneum. Low-flow oxygen therapy may be needed.

If the patient has an open surgical procedure, drains are inserted to remove purulent drainage and excess fluid. Postoperative care is similar to that for the patient with an exploratory laparotomy.

GASTROENTERITIS

Gastroenteritis is an inflammation of the mucosa of the stomach and small intestine. Acute gastroenteritis is defined as sudden diarrhea accompanied by nausea, vomiting, and abdominal cramping. Viruses are the most common cause of gastroenteritis. Other causes are presented in Table 43-1.

Norovirus is a leading cause of gastroenteritis from foodborne disease outbreaks in the United States. The Ridascreen Norovirus 3rd Generation EIA is used when a number of people have simultaneously contracted gastroenteritis and there is a clear avenue for virus transmission, such as a shared location or food.

Most cases of gastroenteritis are self-limiting. However, older adults and chronically ill patients may be unable to consume sufficient fluids orally to compensate for fluid loss. If dehydration occurs, IV fluid replacement may be necessary. As soon as tolerated, oral fluids containing glucose and electrolytes (e.g., Pedialyte) should be given. Nursing management of the patient with gastroenteritis is the same as for the patient with acute diarrhea (see pp. 963-964).

INFLAMMATORY BOWEL DISEASE

Inflammatory bowel disease (IBD) is a chronic inflammation of the GI tract. It is characterized by periods of remission interspersed with periods of exacerbation. The exact cause is unknown, and there is no cure. IBD is classified as either **Crohn's disease** or **ulcerative colitis** based on clinical manifestations (Table 43-14). As the name suggests, ulcerative colitis is

TABLE 43-14   COMPARISON OF ULCERATIVE COLITIS AND CROHN'S DISEASE

Characteristic	Ulcerative Colitis	Crohn's Disease
Clinical		
Usual age at onset	Teens to mid-30s*	Teens to mid-30s*
Diarrhea	Common	Common
Abdominal cramping pain	Common	Common
Fever (intermittent)	During acute attacks	Common
Weight loss	Rare	Common, may be severe
Rectal bleeding	Common	Infrequent
Tenesmus	Common	Rare
Malabsorption and nutritional deficiencies	Minimal incidence	Common
Pathologic		
Location	Usually starts in rectum and spreads in a continuous pattern up the colon	Occurs anywhere along GI tract in characteristic skip lesions. Most frequent site is terminal ileum
Distribution	Continuous areas of inflammation	Healthy tissue interspersed with areas of inflammation (skip lesions)
Depth of involvement	Mucosa and submucosa	Entire thickness of bowel wall (transmural)
Granulomas (noted on biopsy)	Occasional	Common
Cobblestoning of mucosa	Rare	Common
Pseudopolyps	Common	Rare
Small bowel involvement	Minimal	Common
Complications		
Fistulas	Rare	Common
Strictures	Occasional	Common
Anal abscesses	Rare	Common
Perforation	Common (because of toxic megacolon)	Common (because inflammation involves entire bowel wall)
Toxic megacolon	Relatively more common	Rare
Carcinoma	Increased incidence of colorectal cancer after 10 yr of disease	Increased incidence of small intestinal cancer. Increased incidence of colorectal cancer but not as much as with ulcerative colitis
Recurrence after surgery	Cure with colectomy	Common at site of anastomosis

*Second peak in incidence after age 60.

usually limited to the colon. Crohn's disease can involve any segment of the GI tract from the mouth to the anus.

Both ulcerative colitis and Crohn's disease commonly occur during the teenage years and early adulthood, and both have a second peak in the sixth decade. IBD is more prevalent in industrialized countries and in Ashkenazi Jews. Many people with IBD have a family member with the disorder.

Etiology and Pathophysiology

IBD is an autoimmune disease involving an immune reaction to a person's own intestinal tract. Some agent or a combination of agents triggers an overactive, inappropriate, sustained immune response. The resulting inflammation causes widespread tissue destruction.

Evidence suggests that IBD is caused by a combination of factors, including environmental factors, genetic predisposition, and alterations in the function of the immune system.[24] Environmental factors such as diet, hygiene, stress, smoking, and nonsteroidal antiinflammatory drugs (NSAIDs) increase susceptibility by influencing the environment of the microbial flora and the immune system. IBD is more prevalent in industrialized regions of the world. Whether diet or other factors unique to Western countries contribute to the development of IBD is not known.[25,26] Specific dietary components have not been identified. However, high dietary intake of total fats, polyunsaturated fatty acid (PUFA), omega-6 fatty acids, and meat is associated with an increased risk of IBD.[26] High fiber and fruit intake is associated with decreased risk of Crohn's disease,

 CULTURAL & ETHNIC HEALTH DISPARITIES

Inflammatory Bowel Disease

- Incidence is about four times higher among whites than in other ethnic groups.
- It has the highest incidence among the Ashkenazi Jewish people and those of middle European origin.

whereas vegetable intake is associated with decreased risk of ulcerative colitis.[27]

Genetic Link

IBD occurs more frequently in whites (particularly those of Jewish descent) and in family members of persons with IBD (especially monozygotic twins). Genetic predisposition has been confirmed by numerous genome-wide association studies.[24] Certain genetic mutations are associated with Crohn's disease, others are associated with ulcerative colitis, and many are associated with both.

Recently, the first gene associated with Crohn's disease, the *NOD2* gene, was identified. Research is ongoing to understand how defects in the *NOD2* gene lead to Crohn's disease and into finding the other genes that cause IBD.

The discovery of numerous gene variations suggests that IBD is a group of diseases that produce similar types of destruction of the mucosa. A genetically susceptible person who is never exposed to the triggering agent will not become ill, and a person

Inflammatory Bowel Disease (IBD)

Crohn's disease   Ulcerative colitis

FIG. 43-3 Comparison of distribution patterns of Crohn's disease and ulcerative colitis.

TABLE 43-15	EXTRAINTESTINAL COMPLICATIONS OF IBD

- Joints
  - Peripheral arthritis (colitic)
  - Ankylosing spondylitis
  - Sacroiliitis
  - Finger clubbing
- Skin
  - Erythema nodosum
  - Pyoderma gangrenosum
- Mouth
  - Aphthous ulcers
- Eye
  - Conjunctivitis
  - Uveitis
  - Episcleritis
- Gallstones
- Kidney stones
- Liver disease: primary sclerosing cholangitis
- Osteoporosis
- Thromboembolism

who is not genetically susceptible will not develop IBD even if exposed to the triggering agent. The pathway from genetic mutation to abnormal immune responses varies depending on which gene or genes are affected. This genetic variation may explain differences in patient responses to various pharmacologic therapies for IBD.

Pattern of Inflammation in Ulcerative Colitis Versus Crohn's Disease. The pattern of inflammation differs between Crohn's disease and ulcerative colitis (Fig. 43-3). In Crohn's disease the inflammation involves all layers of the bowel wall. Crohn's disease can occur anywhere in the GI tract from the mouth to the anus, but occurs most commonly in the terminal ileum and colon. Furthermore, segments of normal bowel can occur between diseased portions, the so-called skip lesions (see Table 43-14). Typically, ulcerations are deep and longitudinal and penetrate between islands of inflamed edematous mucosa, causing the classic cobblestone appearance. Strictures at the areas of inflammation may cause bowel obstruction. Since the inflammation goes through the entire wall, microscopic leaks can allow bowel contents to enter the peritoneal cavity and form abscesses or produce peritonitis.

In Crohn's disease, fistulas can develop between adjacent areas of bowel, between the bowel and the bladder, and between the bowel and the vagina. Fistulas can also form a tract through the skin to the outside of the body. Urinary tract infections are usually the first sign of a bowel or bladder fistula, and feces is sometimes seen in the urine. Fistulas between the bowel and the vagina allow feces to leak out through the vagina, and feces leaks onto the skin if there is a skin fistula.

Ulcerative colitis usually starts in the rectum and moves in a continual fashion toward the cecum. Although sometimes mild inflammation occurs in the terminal ileum, ulcerative colitis is a disease of the colon and rectum (see Fig. 43-3). The inflammation and ulcerations occur in the mucosal layer, the innermost layer of the bowel wall. Since it does not extend through all bowel wall layers, fistulas and abscesses are rare. Water and electrolytes cannot be absorbed through inflamed

mucosa. Diarrhea with large fluid and electrolyte losses is a characteristic feature of damage to the colonic mucosa epithelium. Breakdown of cells results in protein loss through the stool. Areas of inflamed mucosa form *pseudopolyps,* tongue-like projections into the bowel lumen.

Clinical Manifestations

In ulcerative colitis and Crohn's disease, manifestations are often the same (diarrhea, bloody stools, weight loss, abdominal pain, fever, and fatigue). Bloody stools are more common with ulcerative colitis, and weight loss is more common in Crohn's disease because inflammation of the small intestine impairs nutrient absorption. Both forms of IBD are chronic disorders with mild to severe acute exacerbations that occur at unpredictable intervals over many years.

In Crohn's disease, diarrhea and crampy abdominal pain are common symptoms. If the small intestine is involved, weight loss occurs from malabsorption. Rectal bleeding sometimes occurs with Crohn's disease, although not as often as with ulcerative colitis.

In ulcerative colitis, the primary manifestations are bloody diarrhea and abdominal pain. Pain may vary from the mild lower abdominal cramping associated with diarrhea to severe, constant pain associated with acute perforations. With *mild disease,* diarrhea may consist of no more than four semiformed stools daily that contain small amounts of blood. The patient may have no other manifestations. In *moderate disease* the patient has increased stool output (up to 10 stools/day), increased bleeding, and systemic symptoms (fever, malaise, mild anemia, anorexia). In *severe disease,* diarrhea is bloody, contains mucus, and occurs 10 to 20 times a day. In addition, fever, rapid weight loss greater than 10% of total body weight, anemia, tachycardia, and dehydration are present.

Complications

Patients with IBD experience both local (confined to the GI tract) and systemic (extraintestinal) complications (Table 43-15). GI tract complications include hemorrhage, strictures, perforation (with possible peritonitis), fistulas, and colonic dilation (toxic megacolon). Patients with toxic megacolon are at risk of perforation and may need an emergency colectomy. Toxic megacolon is more common with ulcerative colitis. Hemorrhage may lead to anemia and is corrected with blood transfusions and iron supplements. Perineal abscess and fistulas occur in up to a third of patients with Crohn's disease. Some patients develop skin tags around the anus. The incidence and severity of C. difficile infection in patients with IBD are increasing.[27]

Nutritional problems are especially common in Crohn's disease when the terminal ileum is involved. Bile salts and cobalamin are exclusively absorbed in the terminal ileum. Thus disease in the terminal ileum can result in fat malabsorption and anemia.

Patients with a history of IBD are considered at increased or high risk for colorectal cancer. In addition, those with Crohn's disease are at increased risk for small intestinal cancer. Screening for cancer at regular intervals is important in persons with IBD.[28]

Some people with IBD suffer from systemic complications, including joint, eye, mouth, kidney, bone, vascular, and skin problems (see Table 43-15). Circulating factors such as cytokines trigger inflammation in these areas. Routine liver function tests are important because primary sclerosing cholangitis, a complication of IBD, can lead to liver failure.

Diagnostic Studies

The diagnosis of IBD includes ruling out other diseases with similar symptoms and then determining whether the patient has Crohn's disease or ulcerative colitis. In early Crohn's disease the symptoms can be similar to those of IBS. Diagnostic studies also provide information about disease severity and complications. A CBC typically shows iron-deficiency anemia from blood loss. An elevated WBC count may be an indication of toxic megacolon or perforation. Decreased serum sodium, potassium, chloride, bicarbonate, and magnesium levels are due to fluid and electrolyte losses from diarrhea and vomiting. Hypoalbuminemia is present with severe disease as a result of poor nutrition or protein loss. Elevated erythrocyte sedimentation rate, C-reactive protein, and WBCs reflect inflammation. Stool cultures are obtained to determine if infection is present. The stool is examined for blood, pus, and mucus.

Imaging studies such as double-contrast barium enema, small bowel series (small bowel follow through), transabdominal ultrasound, CT, and MRI are useful for the diagnosis of IBD. Colonoscopy allows for examination of the entire large intestine lumen and sometimes the most distal ileum. The extent of inflammation, ulcerations, pseudopolyps, and strictures is determined, and biopsy specimens are taken for a definitive diagnosis. Since a colonoscope can enter only the distal ileum, capsule endoscopy (see Chapter 39) may be used in the diagnosis of Crohn's disease in the small intestine.[29] However, biopsies cannot be obtained with either capsule endoscopy or barium enema.

Collaborative Care

The goals of treatment are to (1) rest the bowel, (2) control the inflammation, (3) combat infection, (4) correct malnutrition, (5) alleviate any stress, (6) provide symptomatic relief, and (7) improve quality of life. Since the cause is unknown, treatment relies on drugs to treat the inflammation and maintain a remission. A variety of drugs are available to treat IBD (Tables 43-16 and 43-17). Hospitalization is indicated if the patient fails to respond to drug therapy, if the disease is severe, and if complications are suspected. Since recurrence rate is high after surgical treatment of Crohn's disease, drugs are the preferred treatment.

Drug Therapy. The goals of drug treatment for IBD are to induce and then maintain a remission. Five major classes of medications used to treat IBD are aminosalicylates, antimicrobials, corticosteroids, immunosuppressants, and biologic and targeted therapy (see Table 43-17). Drugs are chosen based on

TABLE 43-16 COLLABORATIVE CARE
Inflammatory Bowel Disease

Diagnostic
- History and physical examination
- CBC, erythrocyte sedimentation rate
- Serum chemistries
- Testing of stool for occult blood
- Testing of stool for infection
- Capsule endoscopy
- Radiologic studies with barium contrast
- Sigmoidoscopy and colonoscopy with biopsy

Collaborative Therapy
- High-calorie, high-vitamin, high-protein, low-residue, lactose-free (if lactase deficiency) diet
- Drug therapy (see Table 43-17)
  - Aminosalicylates
  - Antimicrobials
  - Corticosteroids
  - Immunosuppressants
  - Biologic and targeted therapy (immunomodulator)
- Elemental diet or parenteral nutrition
- Physical and emotional rest
- Referral for counseling or support group
- Surgery (see Table 43-18)

the location and severity of inflammation. Depending on the severity of the disease, patients are treated with either a "step-down" or "step-up" approach. The step-up approach uses less toxic therapies (e.g., aminosalicylates and antimicrobials) first, and more toxic medications (e.g., biologic and targeted therapy) are started when initial therapies do not work. The step-down approach uses biologic and targeted therapy first.

Sulfasalazine (Azulfidine) contains sulfapyridine and 5-aminosalicylic acid (5-ASA). The 5-ASA accounts for its therapeutic benefits for IBD. Its exact mechanism of action is unknown, but topical application to the intestinal mucosa suppresses proinflammatory cytokines and other inflammatory mediators. When given orally, 5-ASA alone is absorbed before it reaches the lower GI tract where it is needed. When combined with sulfapyridine, 5-ASA reaches the colon. Because many people cannot tolerate sulfapyridine, preparations such as olsalazine (Dipentum), mesalamine (Pentasa), and balsalazide (Colazal) deliver 5-ASA to the terminal ileum and the colon. These drugs are as effective as sulfasalazine and better tolerated when administered orally.

DRUG ALERT: Sulfasalazine (Azulfidine)
- May cause yellowish orange discoloration of skin and urine.
- Avoid exposure to sunlight and ultraviolet light until photosensitivity is determined.

Preparations with 5-ASA can be administered rectally as suppositories, enemas, and foams. Topical treatment offers the advantage of delivering the 5-ASA directly to the tissue where it is needed and minimizes systemic effects. Aminosalicylates are also first-line therapies for mild to moderate Crohn's disease, especially when the colon is involved, but are more effective for ulcerative colitis. These drugs are recommended for both achieving and maintaining a remission.

Although no specific infectious agent has been identified, antimicrobials (e.g., metronidazole, ciprofloxacin [Cipro]) are used to treat IBD. Corticosteroids such as prednisolone and budesonide (Entocort) are used to achieve remission in IBD.

TABLE 43-17 DRUG THERAPY

Inflammatory Bowel Disease

Class	Action	Examples
5-Aminosalicylates (5-ASA)	Decrease GI inflammation through direct contact with bowel mucosa	*Systemic:* sulfasalazine (Azulfidine), mesalamine (Asacol, Pentasa), olsalazine (Dipentum), balsalazide (Colazal) *Topical:* 5-ASA enema (Rowasa), mesalamine suppositories (Canasa)
Antimicrobials	Prevent or treat secondary infection	metronidazole (Flagyl), ciprofloxacin (Cipro), clarithromycin (Biaxin)
Corticosteroids	Decrease inflammation	*Systemic:* corticosteroids (prednisone, budesonide [Entocort] (oral); hydrocortisone or methylprednisolone (IV for severe IBD) *Topical:* hydrocortisone suppository or foam (Cortifoam) or enema (Cortenema)
Immunosuppressants	Suppress immune response	azathioprine (Imuran), 6-mercaptopurine (6-MP), methotrexate, cyclosporine
Biologic and targeted therapy (immunomodulators)	Inhibit the cytokine tumor necrosis factor (TNF) Prevent migration of leukocytes from bloodstream to inflamed tissue	infliximab (Remicade), adalimumab (Humira), certolizumab pegol (Cimzia), golimumab (Simponi) natalizumab (Tysabri)
Antidiarrheals	Decrease GI motility*	diphenoxylate with atropine (Lomotil), loperamide (Imodium)
Hematinics and vitamins	Correct iron-deficiency anemia and promote healing	oral ferrous sulfate or gluconate, iron dextran injection (Imferon), cobalamin, zinc, folate

*Used with caution during severe disease because of potential to produce toxic megacolon.

TABLE 43-18 INDICATIONS FOR SURGICAL THERAPY FOR IBD

- Drainage of abdominal abscess
- Failure to respond to conservative therapy
- Fistulas
- Inability to decrease corticosteroids
- Intestinal obstruction
- Massive hemorrhage
- Perforation
- Severe anorectal disease
- Suspicion of carcinoma

Corticosteroids are given for the shortest possible time because of side effects associated with long-term use. Patients with disease in the left colon, sigmoid, and rectum can be given suppositories, enemas, and foams that deliver the corticosteroid directly to the inflamed tissue with minimal systemic effects. Oral prednisone is given to patients with mild to moderate disease who do not respond to either 5-ASA or topical corticosteroids. IV corticosteroids are reserved for those with severe inflammation. Corticosteroids must be tapered to very low levels when surgery is planned to prevent postoperative complications (e.g., infection, delayed wound healing).

Immunosuppressants (6-mercaptopurine, azathioprine [Imuran]) are given to maintain remission after corticosteroid induction therapy. These drugs require regular CBC monitoring because they can suppress the bone marrow and lead to inflammation of the pancreas or gallbladder. They have a delayed onset of action and are therefore useful for maintenance of remission but not for acute flare-ups.

Methotrexate has also been found to be effective for treatment of Crohn's disease, but patients may suffer flu-like symptoms, bone marrow depression, and liver dysfunction. CBCs and liver enzymes are monitored. Methotrexate should not be used in women who are pregnant because it causes birth defects and fetal death.

Currently there are five major biologic and targeted medications.[30] Four are antitumor necrosis factor (TNF) agents: infliximab (Remicade), adalimumab (Humira), certolizumab pegol (Cimzia) and golimumab (Simponi). The fifth, natalizumab (Tysabri), inhibits leukocyte adhesion by blocking α_4-integrin,

an adhesion molecule. TNF is a proinflammatory cytokine that is released during inflammation. Infliximab is a monoclonal antibody to TNF. It is given IV to induce and maintain remission in patients with Crohn's disease and in patients with draining fistulas who do not respond to conventional drug therapy. Adalimumab and certolizumab pegol have effects similar to those of infliximab. Adalimumab is self-administered subcutaneously every 1 to 2 weeks, and certolizumab pegol must be administered subcutaneously by a health care provider every 4 weeks. Golimumab is administered subcutaneously twice the first month and then every 4 weeks. Natalizumab is administered by IV infusion every 28 days.

The biologic and targeted agents do not work for everyone. They are costly and may produce allergic reactions.[30] The anti-TNF agents are immunogenic, meaning that patients receiving them frequently produce antibodies against them. Immunogenicity leads to an acute infusion reaction and delayed hypersensitivity-type reactions. The drugs are most effective when given at regular intervals and must not be discontinued unless the patient cannot tolerate them. If the drug is stopped and then restarted, infusion reactions are likely. Natalizumab is associated with increased risk of infection, hepatotoxicity, and hypersensitivity reactions. Its use requires a special safety monitoring program.

The anti-TNF agents have similar side effects. The most common adverse effects are upper respiratory and urinary tract infections, headaches, nausea, joint pain, and abdominal pain. More serious effects include reactivation of hepatitis and tuberculosis (TB); opportunistic infections; and malignancies, especially lymphoma. Patients must be tested for TB and hepatitis before treatment begins and cannot receive live virus immunizations. Patients must be informed of these risks before beginning therapy and taught methods to prevent infection and recognize early signs and symptoms (e.g., fever, cough, malaise, dyspnea).

Surgical Therapy
Ulcerative Colitis. Indications for surgery for ulcerative colitis are presented in Table 43-18. Since ulcerative colitis affects only the colon, a total proctocolectomy is curative. Surgical procedures used to treat ulcerative colitis include

(1) total proctocolectomy with ileal pouch/anal anastomosis and (2) total proctocolectomy with permanent ileostomy. Surgical procedures for ulcerative colitis can be performed laparoscopically.

Total Proctocolectomy With Ileal Pouch/Anal Anastomosis (IPAA). The most commonly used surgical procedure for ulcerative colitis is a total proctocolectomy with ileal pouch/anal anastomosis (IPAA). In this procedure a diverting ileostomy is performed, and an ileal pouch is created and anastomosed directly to the anus (Fig. 43-4). The two surgical procedures are performed approximately 8 to 12 weeks apart. The initial procedure includes colectomy, rectal mucosectomy, ileal pouch (reservoir) construction, ileoanal anastomosis, and temporary ileostomy. The second surgery involves closure of the ileostomy to direct stool toward the new pouch. Adaptation of the pouch occurs over the next 3 to 6 months, which usually results in a decreased number of bowel movements. The patient is able to control defecation at the anal sphincter. The major complication of this procedure is acute or chronic pouchitis.

Total Proctocolectomy With Permanent Ileostomy. A proctocolectomy with a permanent ileostomy is a one-stage operation involving the removal of the colon, rectum, and anus with closure of the anal opening. The end of the terminal ileum is brought out through the abdominal wall and forms a stoma, or ostomy. The stoma is usually placed in the right lower quadrant below the belt line. With a permanent ileostomy, continence is not possible.

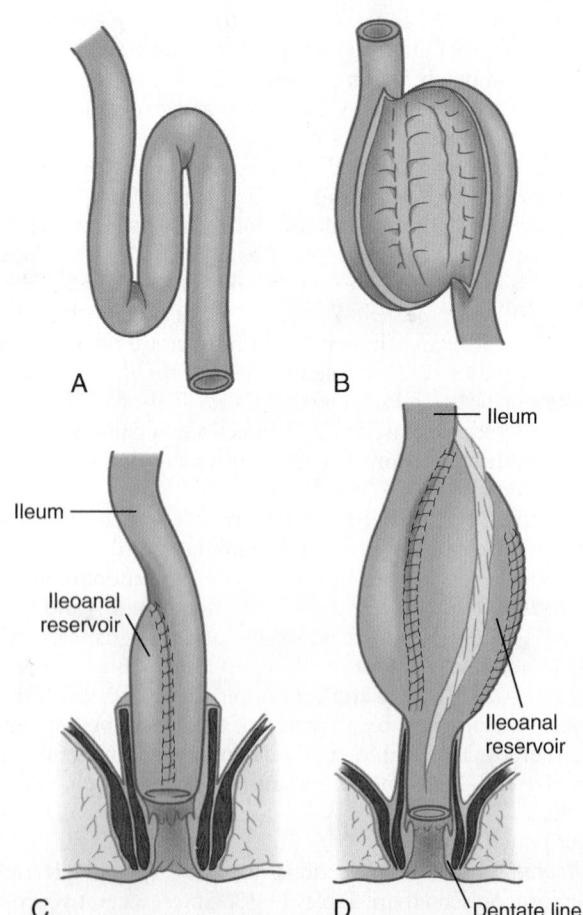

FIG. 43-4 Ileoanal pouch (reservoir). **A,** Formation of a pouch. **B,** Posterior suture lines completed. **C,** J-shaped configuration for ileoanal pouch (J-pouch). **D,** S-shaped configuration for ileoanal pouch (S-pouch).

Crohn's Disease. Surgery for Crohn's disease is usually performed for complications such as strictures, obstructions, bleeding, and fistula (see Table 43-16). Most patients with Crohn's disease eventually require surgery. When segments of the intestine are removed, the remaining intestine is reanastomosed. Unfortunately, the disease often recurs at the anastomosis site.

Repeated removal of sections of small intestine can lead to short bowel syndrome. *Short bowel syndrome* occurs when either surgery or disease leaves too little small intestine surface area to maintain life. Lifetime parenteral nutrition is necessary for survival. (Short bowel syndrome is discussed in this chapter on p. 999.

Conservative surgery is advocated instead of resective surgery in patients with Crohn's disease. Strictures obstructing the bowel can be widened with strictureplasty. If perforation allows bowel contents to drain into the abdominal cavity, the surgeon drains the purulent material, irrigates the abdomen, and makes a temporary ostomy. Abscesses are surgically drained.

Postoperative Care. Postoperative care after surgical procedures for IBD is similar to that described in the general nursing care plan for the postoperative patient (see eNursing Care Plan 20-1 on the website for Chapter 20). If an ileostomy is formed, stoma viability, the mucocutaneous juncture (the area where the mucous membrane of the bowel interfaces with the skin), and peristomal skin integrity must be monitored. (Stoma care is presented later in this chapter on pp. 991-992.)

After surgery, ileostomy output initially may be as high as 1500 to 2000 mL/24 hr. Observe the patient for signs of hemorrhage, abdominal abscess, small bowel obstruction, dehydration, and other related complications. If an NG tube is used, remove it when bowel function returns. Patients, especially those with Crohn's disease, are at risk of early (within 30 days) postoperative bowel obstruction.[31]

Transient incontinence of mucus is a result of intraoperative manipulation of the anal canal. Initial drainage through the ileoanal anastomosis will be liquid. Kegel exercises may help strengthen the pelvic floor and sphincter muscles (see Table 46-19). However, they are not recommended in the immediate postoperative period. Perianal skin care is important to protect the epidermis from mucous drainage and maceration. Instruct the patient to gently clean the skin with a mild cleanser, rinse well, and dry thoroughly. A moisture barrier ointment and a perineal pad may be used.

Nutritional Therapy. Diet is an important component in the treatment of IBD. Consult a dietitian regarding dietary recommendations. The goals of diet management are to (1) provide adequate nutrition without exacerbating symptoms, (2) correct and prevent malnutrition, (3) replace fluid and electrolyte losses, and (4) prevent weight loss.

Nutritional deficiencies are due to decreased oral intake, blood loss, and, depending on the location of the inflammation, malabsorption of nutrients. Patients may reduce food intake in an effort to reduce diarrhea. Inflammatory mediators reduce appetite. Bloody diarrhea leads to iron-deficiency anemia, which is treated with supplemental iron (ferrous sulfate or ferrous gluconate). Parenteral iron may be needed for patients who cannot tolerate oral iron. Iron dextran (Imferon) given intramuscularly by Z-track or IV injection may be necessary if anemia is severe.

Disease of the terminal ileum reduces absorption of cobalamin and bile acids. Reduced cobalamin contributes to anemia, and bile salts are important for fat absorption and contribute to osmotic diarrhea. Cobalamin is available in injection form, given monthly, or as a daily oral or nasal spray. Cholestyramine, an ion-exchange resin that binds unabsorbed bile salts, helps control the diarrhea. Zinc deficiency can result from severe or chronic diarrhea, and supplementation may be necessary.

Medications can contribute to nutritional problems. Patients receiving sulfasalazine should receive folate (folic acid) daily. Those receiving corticosteroids are prone to osteoporosis and need calcium supplements. Potassium supplements may also be necessary with corticosteroids. Corticosteroids lead to sodium retention, loss of potassium (hypokalemia), and potential toxic megacolon. Vitamin D deficiency is more common in persons with IBD. This may be due to malabsorption due to inflammation, surgical resection of intestine, reduced sunlight exposure, and decreased dietary intake.[32]

Overall, it is essential that people with IBD eat a balanced, healthy diet with sufficient calories, protein, and nutrients. Patients can use MyPlate guidelines to ensure that they get adequate portions from all of the food groups (see Fig. 40-1 and Table 40-1). The diet for each patient must be individualized.

During an acute exacerbation, patients with IBD may not be able to tolerate a regular diet. Liquid enteral feedings are preferred over parenteral nutrition because atrophy of the gut and bacterial overgrowth occur when the GI tract is not used. (Enteral and parenteral nutrition are discussed in Chapter 40.) Enteral nutrition is high in calories and nutrients, lactose free, and easily absorbed. Enteral feedings help achieve remission and improve nutritional status. When regular foods are restarted, they are added gradually to help identify food intolerances or sensitivities.

There are no universal food triggers for IBD, but individuals may find that certain foods cause diarrhea. A food diary helps to identify problem foods to avoid. Because many patients with IBD are lactose intolerant, symptoms improve when milk and milk products are avoided. Lactose-intolerant patients can use yogurt as a substitute. High-fat foods also tend to trigger diarrhea. Cold foods and high-fiber foods (cereal with bran, nuts, raw fruits with peels) may promote diarrhea. Smoking stimulates the GI tract (increases motility and secretion) and should be avoided.

NURSING MANAGEMENT
INFLAMMATORY BOWEL DISEASE

NURSING ASSESSMENT

Subjective and objective data that should be obtained from a patient with IBD are presented in Table 43-19.

NURSING DIAGNOSES

Nursing diagnoses for the patient with IBD include, but are not limited to, the following:

- Diarrhea *related to* bowel inflammation and intestinal hyperactivity
- Imbalanced nutrition: less than body requirements *related to* decreased absorption and increased nutrient loss through diarrhea
- Ineffective coping *related to* chronic disease, lifestyle changes, inadequate confidence in ability to cope

Additional information on nursing diagnoses is presented in eNursing Care Plan 43-2 on the website for this chapter.

PLANNING

The overall goals are that the patient with IBD will (1) have fewer and less severe acute exacerbations, (2) maintain normal

---

TABLE 43-19 NURSING ASSESSMENT

Inflammatory Bowel Disease

Subjective Data
Important Health Information
Past health history: Infection, autoimmune disorders
Medications: Antidiarrheal medications

Functional Health Patterns
Health perception–health management: Family history of ulcerative colitis or Crohn's disease; fatigue, malaise
Nutritional-metabolic: Nausea, vomiting; anorexia; weight loss
Elimination: Diarrhea; blood, mucus, or pus in stools
Cognitive-perceptual: Lower abdominal pain (worse before defecation), cramping, tenesmus

Objective Data
General
Intermittent fever, emaciated appearance, fatigue

Integumentary
Pale skin with poor turgor, dry mucous membranes; skin lesions; anorectal irritation, skin tags, cutaneous fistulas

Gastrointestinal
Abdominal distention, hyperactive bowel sounds, abdominal cramps

Cardiovascular
Tachycardia, hypotension

Possible Diagnostic Findings
Anemia; leukocytosis; electrolyte imbalance; hypoalbuminemia; vitamin and trace metal deficiencies; guaiac-positive stool; abnormal sigmoidoscopic, colonoscopic, and/or barium enema findings

---

fluid and electrolyte balance, (3) be free from pain or discomfort, (4) adhere to medical regimens, (5) maintain nutritional balance, and (6) have an improved quality of life.

NURSING IMPLEMENTATION

During the acute phase, focus your attention on hemodynamic stability, pain control, fluid and electrolyte balance, and nutritional support. Maintain accurate intake and output records, and monitor the number and appearance of stools. It is important to establish rapport and encourage the patient to talk about self-care strategies. An explanation of all procedures and treatment helps to build trust and decrease apprehension.

Because of the relationship between emotions and the GI tract, teach the patient strategies for managing stress (see Chapter 7). Remember that patients experiencing a relapse have been managing their disease and need to feel in control. Ask them what you can do to facilitate their self-care. Once you have established a therapeutic relationship, talk with smokers about quitting, since smoking exacerbates the disease.

IBD is a chronic illness. Given the chronicity and uncertainty related to frequency and severity of flares, the patient may experience frustration, depression, and anxiety. Psychotherapy and behavioral therapies may help the patient experiencing psychologic distress in managing his or her symptoms. Assist the patient in accepting the chronicity of IBD and learning strategies to cope with its recurrent, unpredictable nature. Inadequate coping mechanisms are sometimes result of the childhood onset of the disease before the person has the emotional and developmental maturity needed to cope. Patients may suffer severe fatigue, which limits energy for physical activity. Rest is important. Patients may lose sleep because of frequent episodes of diarrhea and abdominal pain. Nutritional deficiencies and anemia leave the patient feeling weak and listless. Schedule activities around rest periods.

Until diarrhea is controlled, help the patient stay clean, dry, and free of odor. Place a deodorizer in the room. Meticulous perianal skin care using plain water (no harsh soap) together with a skin barrier cream prevents skin breakdown. Dibucaine (Nupercainal), witch hazel, or other soothing compresses or prescribed ointment and sitz baths may reduce irritation and discomfort of the anus.

In the majority of patients with IBD the disease is characterized by intermittent exacerbation and remission of symptoms. The patient and caregiver may need help setting realistic short- and long-term goals. Teaching includes (1) the importance of rest and diet management, (2) perianal care, (3) drug action and side effects, (4) symptoms of recurrence of disease, (5) when to seek medical care, and (6) use of diversional activities to reduce stress. Excellent teaching resources written in easily comprehensible language are available from the Crohn's and Colitis Foundation of America (*www.ccfa.org*).

▌ EVALUATION

The expected outcomes are that the patient with IBD will
- Experience a decrease in the number of diarrhea stools
- Maintain body weight within a normal range
- Be free from pain and discomfort
- Demonstrate the use of effective coping strategies

Additional information on expected outcomes is presented in eNursing Care Plan 43-2 on the website for this chapter.

▌ GERONTOLOGIC CONSIDERATIONS

INFLAMMATORY BOWEL DISEASE

Although IBD is considered a disease of teenagers and young adults, a second peak in occurrence is in the sixth decade. The etiology, natural history, and clinical course of IBD are similar to those observed in younger patients. However, in the older patient with ulcerative colitis, the distal colon (proctitis) is usually involved. Diagnosis is sometimes difficult in older adults, since IBD can be confused with *C. difficile* infection and the colitis associated with diverticulosis or NSAID ingestion. Older adults receive the same medical treatment as younger patients and have similar results after ileoanal reservoir surgery.[33] However, they are more prone to complications from corticosteroids than younger adults.

Collaborative care of the older patient with IBD is similar to care of the younger patient. However, because of increased risk of cardiovascular and pulmonary complications, older adults tend to have increased morbidity associated with surgical procedures.

In addition to Crohn's disease and ulcerative colitis, older adults are also vulnerable to inflammation of the colon (colitis) from drug use and systemic vascular disease. Drugs such as NSAIDs, digitalis, sumatriptan (Imitrex), vasopressin, estrogen, and allopurinol (Zyloprim) have been associated with the development of colitis in the older patient. Colitis may also be secondary to ischemic bowel disease related to atherosclerosis and heart failure.

Older adults, particularly those with diminished renal and cardiovascular function, are more vulnerable to the volume depletion consequences of diarrhea. In older adults with IBD,

focus on careful assessment of fluid and electrolyte status and evaluation of the replacement therapies.

INTESTINAL OBSTRUCTION

Intestinal obstruction occurs when intestinal contents cannot pass through the GI tract. The obstruction may occur in the small intestine or colon and can be partial or complete, simple or strangulated.[34] A partial obstruction usually resolves with conservative treatment, whereas a complete obstruction usually requires surgery. A simple obstruction has an intact blood supply, and a strangulated one does not.

TYPES OF INTESTINAL OBSTRUCTION

The causes of intestinal obstruction can be classified as mechanical or nonmechanical.

Mechanical

Mechanical obstruction is a detectable occlusion of the intestinal lumen. Most intestinal obstructions occur in the small intestine.[34] Surgical adhesion is the most common cause of small bowel obstructions and can occur within days of surgery or several years later (Fig. 43-5). Other causes of intestinal obstruction are hernia, strictures from Crohn's disease, and intussusception following bariatric abdominal surgery. The most common cause of colon obstruction is cancer, followed by diverticular disease.

Nonmechanical

Nonmechanical obstruction may result from a neuromuscular or vascular disorder. Paralytic (adynamic) ileus (lack of intestinal peristalsis and bowel sounds) is the most common form of nonmechanical obstruction. It occurs to some degree after any abdominal surgery. It can be difficult to know whether postoperative obstruction is due to paralytic ileus or adhesions. One clue is that bowel sounds usually return before postoperative adhesions develop. Other causes of paralytic ileus include peritonitis, inflammatory responses (e.g., acute pancreatitis, acute appendicitis), electrolyte abnormalities (especially hypokalemia), and thoracic or lumbar spinal fractures.

Pseudo-obstruction is a mechanical obstruction of the intestine without demonstration of obstruction by radiologic methods. Collagen vascular diseases and neurologic and endocrine disorders may cause pseudo-obstruction, but many times the cause is unknown.

Vascular obstructions are rare and are the result of an interference with the blood supply to a portion of the intestines. The most common causes are emboli and atherosclerosis of the mesenteric arteries. Emboli may originate from thrombi in patients who have chronic atrial fibrillation, diseased heart valves, and prosthetic valves. Venous thrombosis may be seen in conditions of low blood flow, such as heart failure and shock.

Etiology and Pathophysiology

About 6 to 8 L of fluid enter the small intestine daily. Most of the fluid is absorbed before it reaches the colon. Approximately 75% of intestinal gas is swallowed air. When an obstruction occurs, fluid, gas, and intestinal contents accumulate proximal to the obstruction, and the distal bowel collapses. The distention reduces the absorption of fluids and stimulates intestinal secretions. The proximal bowel becomes increasingly distended, and

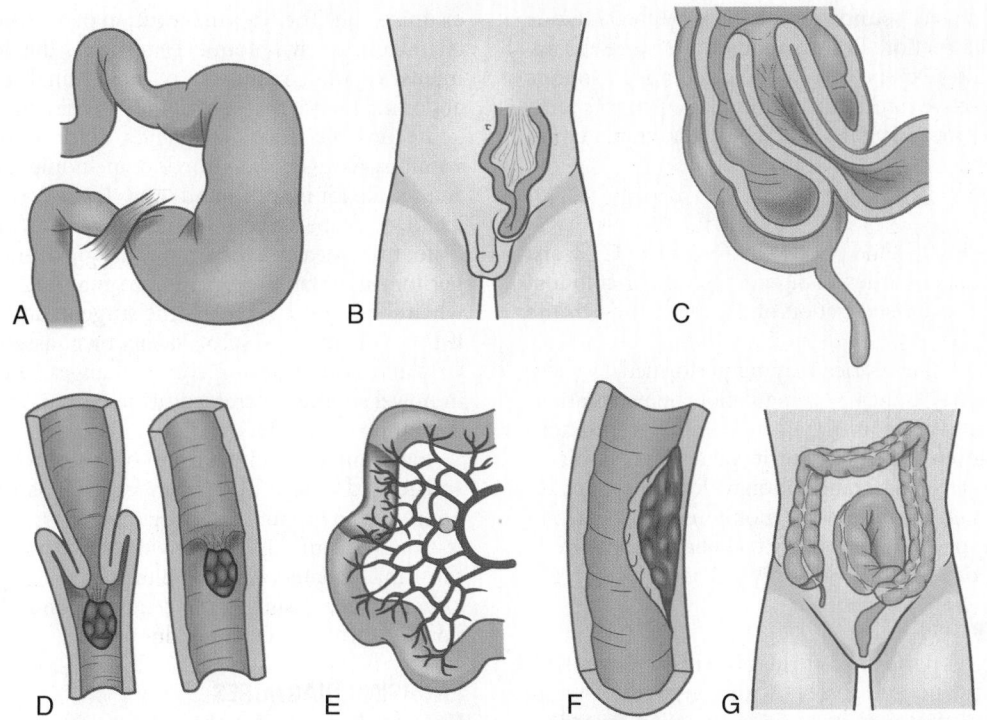

FIG. 43-5 Bowel obstructions. **A,** Adhesions. **B,** Strangulated inguinal hernia. **C,** Ileocecal intussusception. **D,** Intussusception from polyps. **E,** Mesenteric occlusion. **F,** Neoplasm. **G,** Volvulus of the sigmoid colon.

intraluminal bowel pressure rises. The increased pressure leads to an increase in capillary permeability and extravasation of fluids and electrolytes into the peritoneal cavity. Retention of fluids in the intestine and peritoneal cavity (third spacing) leads to a severe reduction in circulating blood volume and results in hypotension and hypovolemic shock.

If blood flow is inadequate, bowel tissue becomes ischemic, then necrotic, and the bowel may perforate. In the most dangerous situation the bowel becomes so distended that the blood flow stops, causing edema, cyanosis, and gangrene of a bowel segment. This is called *intestinal strangulation* or *intestinal infarction.* If it is not corrected quickly, the bowel will become necrotic and rupture, leading to infection, septic shock, and death.

The location of the obstruction determines the extent of fluid, electrolyte, and acid-base imbalances. If the obstruction is high (e.g., upper duodenum), metabolic alkalosis may result from the loss of gastric hydrochloric (HCl) acid through vomiting or NG intubation and suction. When the obstruction is located in the small intestine, dehydration occurs rapidly. Dehydration and electrolyte imbalances do not occur early in large bowel obstruction. If the obstruction is below the proximal colon, solid fecal material accumulates until symptoms of discomfort appear.

Some small intestine obstructions, especially those due to surgical adhesions, may resolve without surgery.[34] Other small intestine obstructions, such as strangulated obstructions, require emergency surgery for survival. *Volvulus* is an intestinal obstruction that occurs by the bowel twisting on itself (see Fig. 43-5). Malignant bowel obstructions are associated with colorectal and ovarian cancer.

Clinical Manifestations

The clinical manifestations of intestinal obstruction vary, depending on its location (Table 43-20). The most important

TABLE 43-20	MANIFESTATIONS OF SMALL AND LARGE INTESTINAL OBSTRUCTIONS	
Manifestation	**Small Intestine**	**Large Intestine**
Onset	Rapid	Gradual
Vomiting	Frequent and copious	Rare
Pain	Colicky, cramplike, intermittent pain	Low-grade, cramping abdominal pain
Bowel movement	Feces for a short time	Absolute constipation
Abdominal distention	Greatly increased	Increased

early manifestations of a small bowel obstruction are colicky abdominal pain, nausea, vomiting, and abdominal distention. Constipation and decreased flatus occur later. Patients with obstructions in the proximal small intestine rapidly develop nausea and vomiting, which is sometimes projectile and contains bile. Vomiting from more distal obstructions of the small intestine is more gradual in onset. Foul-smelling vomitus that looks like stool indicates a long-standing obstruction requiring immediate surgery. Signs of colonic obstruction include abdominal distention, constipation (new onset), and lack of flatus.

Vomiting usually relieves abdominal pain in higher intestinal obstructions. Persistent, colicky abdominal pain is seen in patients with lower intestinal obstruction. With mechanical obstruction, pain generally comes and goes in waves. In contrast, paralytic ileus produces a more constant, generalized abdominal discomfort. Strangulation causes severe, constant pain that is rapid in onset. Abdominal distention is usually absent or minimally noticeable in proximal small intestine obstructions and markedly increased in lower intestinal obstructions. Abdominal tenderness and rigidity are usually absent unless strangulation or peritonitis has occurred.

Auscultation of bowel sounds reveals high-pitched sounds above the area of obstruction. Bowel sounds may also be absent. The patient often notes *borborygmi* (audible abdominal sounds produced by hyperactive intestinal motility). The patient's temperature rarely rises above 100° F (37.8° C) unless strangulation or peritonitis occurs.

Diagnostic Studies

Perform a thorough history and physical examination. CT scans and abdominal x-rays are ordered. Sigmoidoscopy or colonoscopy may provide direct visualization of an obstruction in the colon.

A CBC and blood chemistries may be performed. An elevated WBC count may indicate strangulation or perforation. Elevated hematocrit values may reflect hemoconcentration. Decreased hemoglobin and hematocrit values may indicate bleeding from a neoplasm or strangulation with necrosis. Serum electrolytes, BUN, and creatinine are monitored frequently to assess the degree of dehydration. Metabolic alkalosis can develop as a result of vomiting.

Collaborative Care

Emergency surgery is performed if the bowel is strangulated, but many bowel obstructions resolve with conservative treatment. Initial medical treatment of bowel obstruction caused by adhesions includes placing the patient on NPO status, inserting an NG tube for decompression, providing IV fluid therapy with either normal saline or lactated Ringer's solution (since fluid losses from the GI tract are isotonic), adding potassium to IV fluids after verifying renal function, and administering analgesics for pain control.

The treatment goal for the patient with a malignant bowel obstruction is to regain patency and resolve the obstruction. Stents can be placed via endoscopic or fluoroscopic procedures. They can be used for palliative purposes or until surgery can be performed. Corticosteroids that have antiemetic properties and decrease edema and inflammation may be used in combination with stent placement. A venting gastrostomy tube may be placed endoscopically or percutaneously.[35]

If the obstruction does not improve within 24 hours or if the patient's condition deteriorates, surgery is performed to relieve the obstruction. In some cases, parenteral nutrition may be used to improve the patient's nutritional status before surgery and promote postoperative healing. Surgery may involve simply resecting the obstructed segment of bowel and anastomosing the remaining healthy bowel back together. Partial or total colectomy, colostomy, or ileostomy may be required when extensive obstruction or necrosis is present.

Occasionally obstructions can be removed nonsurgically. A colonoscope can be used to remove polyps, dilate strictures, and remove and destroy tumors with a laser.

NURSING MANAGEMENT INTESTINAL OBSTRUCTION

NURSING ASSESSMENT

Intestinal obstruction is a potentially life-threatening condition. Major concerns are prevention of fluid and electrolyte deficiencies and early recognition of deterioration in the patient's condition (e.g., hypovolemic shock, bowel strangulation). Nursing assessment begins with a detailed patient history and physical

examination. The type and location of obstruction usually cause characteristic symptoms. Determine the location, duration, intensity, and frequency of abdominal pain and whether abdominal tenderness or rigidity is present.

Record the onset, frequency, color, odor, and amount of vomitus. Assess bowel function, including the passage of flatus. Auscultate for bowel sounds and document their character and location. Inspect the abdomen for scars, visible masses, and distention. Measure the abdominal girth, and check for signs of peritoneal irritation (e.g., muscle guarding, rebound pain, pain when the bed is shaken). If the surgeon decides to wait and see if the obstruction resolves on its own, assess the patient regularly and notify the surgeon of changes in vital signs, changes in bowel sounds, decreased urine output, increased abdominal distention, and pain.

Maintain a strict intake and output record, including emesis and tube drainage. A urinary catheter is ordered to monitor hourly urine outputs. Immediately report if the urine output is less than 0.5 mL/kg of body weight per hour because this indicates inadequate vascular volume and the potential for acute kidney injury. Rising serum creatinine and BUN levels are additional indicators of acute kidney injury.

NURSING DIAGNOSES

Nursing diagnoses for the patient with intestinal obstructions include, but are not limited to, the following:
- Acute pain *related to* abdominal distention and increased peristalsis
- Deficient fluid volume *related to* a decrease in intestinal fluid absorption, third space fluid shifts into the bowel lumen and peritoneal cavity, NG suction, and vomiting

PLANNING

The overall goals are that the patient with an intestinal obstruction will have (1) relief of the obstruction and return to normal bowel function, (2) minimal to no discomfort, and (3) normal fluid and electrolyte and acid-base status.

NURSING IMPLEMENTATION

Monitor the patient closely for signs of dehydration and electrolyte imbalances. Administer IV fluids as ordered. Watch for signs and symptoms of fluid overload, since some patients, especially older adults, may not tolerate rapid fluid replacement. Monitor serum electrolyte levels closely. A patient with a high intestinal obstruction is more likely to have metabolic alkalosis. A patient with a low obstruction is at greater risk for metabolic acidosis. The patient is often restless and constantly changes position to relieve the pain. Provide comfort measures and promote a restful environment. Nursing care of the patient after surgery for an intestinal obstruction is similar to care of the patient after a laparotomy (see pp. 970-971).

With an NG tube in place, oral care is extremely important. Vomiting leaves an unpleasant taste in the patient's mouth, and fecal odor may be present. The patient breathes through the mouth, drying the mouth and lips. Encourage and help the patient to brush the teeth frequently. Mouthwash and water for rinsing the mouth and water-soluble lubricant for the lips should be readily available to the patient. Check the nose for signs of irritation from the NG tube. Clean and dry this area daily, apply water-soluble lubricant, and retape the tube. Check the NG tube every 4 hours for patency.

FIG. 43-6 Endoscopic image of pedunculated polyp in descending colon.

POLYPS OF LARGE INTESTINE

Colonic polyps arise from the mucosal surface of the colon and project into the lumen. They may be *sessile* (flat, broad based, and attached directly to the intestinal wall) or *pedunculated* (attached to the intestinal wall by a thin stalk). Polyps tend to be sessile when small and become pedunculated as they enlarge (Fig. 43-6). They may be found anywhere in the large intestine but are most commonly found in the rectosigmoid area. Rectal bleeding and occult blood in the stool are the most common signs. Most patients with polyps are asymptomatic.

Types of Polyps

The most common types of polyps are hyperplastic and adenomatous. *Hyperplastic polyps* are nonneoplastic growths. They rarely grow larger than 5 mm and never cause clinical symptoms. Other benign (nonneoplastic) polyps include inflammatory polyps, lipomas, and juvenile polyps.

    Adenomatous polyps are neoplastic. They are closely linked to colorectal adenocarcinoma. The risk of cancer increases with polyp size. Removing adenomatous polyps decreases the occurrence of colorectal cancer.

Genetic Link

Familial adenomatous polyposis (FAP) is the most common polyposis syndrome (see the Genetics in Clinical Practice box). FAP is a genetic disorder characterized by hundreds or sometimes thousands of polyps in the colon that eventually become cancerous, usually by age 40. Since it is autosomal dominant, 50% of the offspring of a patient with FAP carry the FAP gene. Anyone with a family history of FAP should undergo genetic testing during childhood. If the FAP gene is present, colorectal screening begins at puberty, and annual colonoscopy begins at age 16. Since cancer is inevitable, the colon and rectum are removed, usually by age 25, and proctocolectomy with an IPAA or an ileostomy is performed (see p. 980). Patients with FAP are also at risk for cancers of the thyroid, small bowel, liver, and brain, so lifetime cancer surveillance is essential.[36]

Diagnostic Studies and Collaborative Care

Colonoscopy, sigmoidoscopy, barium enema, and virtual colonoscopy (CT or MRI colonography) are used to discover polyps. All polyps are considered abnormal and should be removed. Colonoscopy is preferred because it allows evaluation of the total colon, and polyps can be removed immediately (*polypectomy*). Polyps can be detected but not removed during barium

GENETICS IN CLINICAL PRACTICE
Familial Adenomatous Polyposis (FAP)

Genetic Basis
- Classic form of disease
  - Autosomal dominant disorder.
  - Mutations in adenomatous polyposis coli *(APC)* gene.
  - Normally this is a tumor suppressor gene involved in DNA repair.
  - Normally this gene produces a special substance (a protein) that keeps polyps from developing in the colon.
- Autosomal recessive FAP
  - Autosomal recessive disorder.
  - Mutations in the *mutY* homolog *(MUTYH)* gene.
  - Normally this gene is involved in DNA repair.

Incidence
- Affects 1 in 6800 to 30,000 people.
- Men and women are affected equally.

Genetic Testing
- DNA testing is available.

Clinical Implications
- Accounts for at least 1% of all colorectal cancers.
- Classic FAP is characterized by colorectal polyps (usually hundreds to thousands).
- Polyps are not present at birth but appear during adolescence and early adulthood.
- Autosomal recessive FAP is characterized by fewer polyps, typically <100.
- If untreated, classic FAP almost always results in the development of colorectal cancer before age 40.
- With classic FAP, other benign and malignant tumors are sometimes found, especially in the duodenum, stomach, bones, skin, and other tissues.
- Many deaths related to FAP could be prevented with early and aggressive monitoring and treatment, including frequent colonoscopies and total colectomy.
- Individuals with a family history of FAP could benefit from genetic counseling.

enema and virtual colonoscopy. If the polyp is not removable during the colonoscopy, a biopsy specimen is taken to stage the cancer in preparation for surgery. After polypectomy, observe the patient for rectal bleeding, fever, severe abdominal pain, and abdominal distention, which may indicate hemorrhage or perforation.

COLORECTAL CANCER

Colorectal cancer (CRC) is the third most common form of cancer and responsible for 9% of cancer deaths. It is estimated that annually about 103,170 Americans are diagnosed with CRC.[28] The incidence of CRC is presented in eFig. 43-1 on the website for this chapter.

    CRC is more common in men than in women. Mortality rates are highest among African American men and women. The risk of CRC increases with age, with about 90% of new CRC cases detected in people older than 50. However, the incidence of CRC in individuals over 50 is decreasing due to increased screening to detect precancerous lesions.

Etiology and Pathophysiology

Risk factors for CRC include a diet high in red or processed meat, obesity, physical inactivity, alcohol, long-term smoking,

TABLE 43-21	RISK FACTORS FOR COLORECTAL CANCER

- Family history of colorectal cancer (first-degree relative)
- Personal history of inflammatory bowel disease
- Personal history of colorectal cancer
- Family or personal history of familial adenomatous polyposis (FAP)
- Family or personal history of hereditary nonpolyposis colorectal cancer (HNPCC) syndrome
- Obesity (body mass index ≥30 kg/m²)
- Red meat (≥7 servings/wk)
- Cigarette smoking
- Alcohol (≥4 drinks/wk)

and low intake of fruits and vegetables.[28] Genetic conditions such as FAP and a personal history of IBD place an individual at risk for CRC. About one third of cases of CRC occur in patients with a family history of CRC.

Hereditary diseases (e.g., FAP) account for about 5% to 10% of CRC cases. Hereditary nonpolyposis colorectal cancer (HNPCC) syndrome (also called Lynch syndrome) is the most common form of hereditary CRC (see the Genetics in Clinical Practice box).

Physical exercise and a diet with large amounts of fruits, vegetables, and grains may decrease the risk of CRC. Long-term use of NSAIDs (e.g., aspirin) is associated with reduced CRC risk. (See Table 43-21 for a list of risk factors.)

Adenocarcinoma is the most common type of CRC. Typically it begins as adenomatous polyps. Approximately 85% of CRCs arise from adenomatous polyps (see Fig. 43-6).

As the tumor grows, the cancer invades and penetrates the muscularis mucosae (see eFig. 43-2 on the website for this chapter). Eventually tumor cells gain access to the regional lymph nodes and vascular system and spread to distant sites. (The stages of tumor growth are shown in Fig. 43-7.) Since

GENETICS IN CLINICAL PRACTICE

Hereditary Nonpolyposis Colorectal Cancer (HNPCC) or Lynch Syndrome

Genetic Basis
- Autosomal dominant disorder.
- Mutations in *MSH2, MLH1, MSH6, PMS2* genes.
- These genes are involved in repair of mistakes when DNA is replicated.

Incidence
- Affects 1 in 500 to 2000 people.

Genetic Testing
- DNA testing is available.

Clinical Implications
- Accounts for 5% of all colorectal cancers.
- Individual with genetic mutation has 80% to 90% lifetime risk of developing colorectal cancer.
- People with HNPCC have an increased risk of cancers of stomach, small intestine, liver, gallbladder, upper urinary tract, brain, skin, and prostate. Occasionally, people with HNPCC also have colon polyps, which occur at an earlier age than do colon polyps in the general population and are more prone to become malignant.
- Individuals with known genetic mutations need to be monitored with colonoscopy every year.
- Women with HNPCC also have a greatly increased risk of endometrial and ovarian cancer.
- Examination by pelvic ultrasound and endometrial biopsy should also be considered to screen for endometrial cancer.

venous blood leaving the colon and rectum flows through the portal vein and the inferior rectal vein, the liver is a common site of metastasis. The cancer spreads from the liver to other sites, including the lungs, bones, and brain. CRC can also spread directly into adjacent structures.

Clinical Manifestations

CRC has an insidious onset, and symptoms do not appear until the disease is advanced. Common clinical manifestations include iron-deficiency anemia, rectal bleeding, abdominal pain, change in bowel habits, and intestinal obstruction or perforation.

Physical findings may include the following:
- *Early disease:* Nonspecific findings (fatigue, weight loss) or none at all
- *More advanced disease:* Abdominal tenderness, palpable abdominal mass, hepatomegaly, ascites

Right-sided lesions are more likely to bleed and cause diarrhea, while left-sided tumors are usually detected later and could present with bowel obstruction (Fig. 43-8).

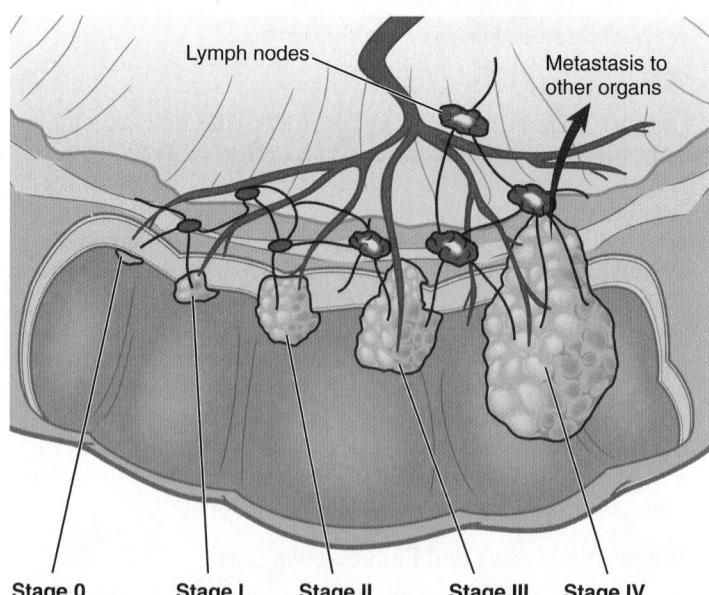

FIG. 43-7 The five stages of colorectal cancer. Stage 0 cancer has not grown beyond the mucosal layer. Stage I cancer has grown beyond the mucosa into the submucosa, but no lymph nodes are involved. Stage II cancer has grown beyond the submucosa into the muscle but there is no lymph node involvement or metastasis. Stage III cancer is any tumor with lymph node involvement but no metastasis. Stage IV cancer is any tumor with lymph node involvement and metastasis.

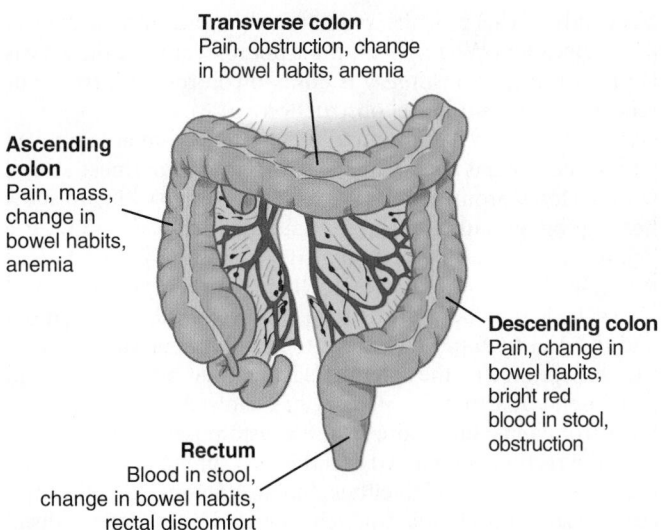

Transverse colon
Pain, obstruction, change
in bowel habits, anemia

Ascending colon
Pain, mass,
change in
bowel habits,
anemia

Descending colon
Pain, change in
bowel habits,
bright red
blood in stool,
obstruction

Rectum
Blood in stool,
change in bowel habits,
rectal discomfort

FIG. 43-8 Signs and symptoms of colorectal cancer by location of primary cancer.

Due to increased emphasis on screening practices, colon cancer is now often detected during screening procedures. Complications of CRC include obstruction, bleeding, perforation, peritonitis, and fistula formation.

Diagnostic Studies

Obtain a thorough history with close attention to family history (Table 43-22). Since symptoms of CRC do not become evident until the disease is advanced, regular screening is advocated to detect and remove polyps before they become cancerous. Beginning at age 50, both men and women at average risk for developing CRC should have screening tests to detect both polyps and cancer based on one of these testing schedules.[28]

Tests that find polyps and cancer include the following:
- Flexible sigmoidoscopy (done every 5 years)
- Colonoscopy (done every 10 years)
- Double-contrast barium enema (done every 5 years)
- CT colonography (virtual colonoscopy) (done every 5 years)

Tests that primarily find cancer include the following:
- Fecal occult blood test (FOBT) (done every year)
- Fecal immunochemical test (FIT) (done every year)

Colonoscopy is the gold standard for CRC screening because the entire colon is examined (only 50% of CRCs are detected by

sigmoidoscopy), biopsies can be obtained, and polyps can be immediately removed and sent to the laboratory for examination. People at average risk of CRC should have a colonoscopy every 10 years beginning at age 50, except for African Americans, who should have the first colonoscopy at age 45.[37]

Less favorable, but acceptable, screening methods include testing the stool for fecal blood. The FOBT and FIT look for blood in the stool. Stool tests must be done frequently, since tumor bleeding occurs at intervals and may easily be missed if a single test is done.

Persons at risk (see Table 43-21) should begin screening earlier and have screening done more often. Those who have a first-degree relative who developed CRC before age 60 or have two first-degree relatives with CRC should have a colonoscopy every 5 years beginning at age 40 or 10 years earlier than the youngest relative developed cancer. However, those who have one first-degree relative who had CRC after age 60 should have the same screening as the average at-risk person.

Once colonoscopy and tissue biopsies confirm the diagnosis of CRC, additional laboratory studies are done, including a CBC to check for anemia, coagulation studies, and liver function tests. A CT scan or MRI of the abdomen may be helpful in detecting liver metastases, retroperitoneal and pelvic disease, and depth of penetration of tumor into the bowel wall. However, liver function tests may be normal even when metastasis has occurred.

Carcinoembryonic antigen (CEA) is a complex glycoprotein sometimes produced by CRC cells. It may be used to monitor for disease recurrence after surgery or chemotherapy, but is not a good screening tool because of the large number of false positives.

Collaborative Care

The prognosis and treatment of CRC correlate with pathologic staging of the disease. The most commonly used staging system is the tumor, node, metastasis (TNM) staging (Table 43-23). As with other cancers, prognosis worsens with greater size and

---

TABLE 43-22 COLLABORATIVE CARE

Colorectal Cancer

Diagnostic	Collaborative Therapy
• History and physical examination	• Surgery
• Digital rectal examination	• Right hemicolectomy
• Testing of stool for occult blood	• Left hemicolectomy
• Barium enema	• Abdominal-perineal resection
• Sigmoidoscopy	• Laparoscopic colectomy
• Colonoscopy	• Chemotherapy
• CBC	• Targeted therapy
• Liver function tests	• Radiation therapy
• CT scan of abdomen	
• MRI	
• Ultrasound	
• Carcinoembryonic antigen (CEA) test	

TABLE 43-23 TNM CLASSIFICATION OF COLORECTAL CANCER

T	Primary Tumor
T_x	Primary tumor cannot be assessed because of incomplete information.
T_{is}	Carcinoma in situ. Cancer is in earliest stage and has not grown beyond mucosa layer.
T_1	Tumor has grown beyond mucosa into the submucosa.
T_2	Tumor has grown through submucosa into muscularis propria.
T_3	Tumor has grown through the muscularis propria into the subserosa but not to neighboring organs or tissues.
T_4	Tumor has spread completely through the colon or rectal wall and into nearby tissues or organs.

N	Lymph Node Involvement
N_x	Lymph nodes cannot be assessed.
N_0	No regional lymph node involvement is found.
N_1	Cancer is found in one to three nearby lymph nodes.
N_2	Cancer is found in four or more nearby lymph nodes.

M	Metastasis
M_x	Presence of distant metastasis cannot be assessed.
M_0	No distant metastasis is seen.
M_1	Distant metastasis is present.

Stage*	TNM†		Duke's	Prognosis‡
0	$T_{is} N_0 M_0$			>96%
I	$T_1 N_0 M_0$	A		>90%
	$T_2 N_0 M_0$	B_1		85%
II	$T_3 N_0 M_0$	B_2		70%-80%
III	Any T, $N_1 M_0$	C		64%
IV	Any T, any N, M_1	D		8%

TABLE 43-24   CLASSIFICATION SYSTEM USED TO STAGE COLORECTAL CANCER

*Staging system is shown in Fig. 43-7. Staging is based on TNM classification.
†See Table 43-23.
‡Estimated 5-yr survival rates.

depth of tumor, lymph node involvement, and metastasis (Table 43-24).

Surgical Therapy. Goals of surgical therapy include (1) complete resection of the tumor together with adequate margins of healthy tissue, (2) a thorough exploration of the abdomen to determine if the cancer has spread, (3) removal of all lymph nodes that drain the area where the cancer is located, (4) restoration of bowel continuity so that normal bowel function will return, and (5) prevention of surgical complications.

Some polyps can be removed during colonoscopy, whereas others require surgery. Polypectomy during colonoscopy can be used to resect CRC in situ and is considered successful when the resected margin of the polyp is free of cancer, the cancer is well differentiated, and there is no apparent lymphatic or blood vessel involvement.

Reduction of colonic bacteria is recommended before surgery to prevent anastomotic leakage of bacteria and to decrease postoperative infection and abscess formation. The bowel is typically cleansed with a polyethylene glycol lavage solution (e.g., MiraLAX, GoLYTELY), and oral antibiotics are given to further decrease the amount of colonic and rectal bacteria.

The site of the CRC dictates the site of the resection (e.g., right hemicolectomy, left hemicolectomy). Surgical removal of stage I cancer includes removal of the tumor and at least 5 cm of intestine on either side of the tumor, plus removal of nearby lymph nodes. The remaining cancer-free ends are sewn back together. Laparoscopic surgery is sometimes used for stage I tumors, especially those in the left colon. Low-risk stage II tumors are treated with wide resection and reanastomosis, but chemotherapy is used in addition to surgery for high-risk stage II tumors.[38] Stage III tumors are treated with surgery and chemotherapy.

Once the cancer has spread to distant sites (stage IV), surgery is palliative and chemotherapy is directed at controlling the spread. Radiation may be used to provide pain relief.

If a patient has a perforation or peritonitis or is hemodynamically unstable, a temporary colostomy may be done. Then later the ends of the colon can be surgically reconnected.

In rectal cancer the surgeon has three major options: (1) local excision, (2) abdominal-perineal resection (APR) with a permanent colostomy, and (3) low anterior resection (LAR) to preserve sphincter function. The surgical decision is based on the location and staging of the cancer and ability to restore normal bowel function and continence. Most patients with rectal cancer require an APR or LAR. The LAR is used more

frequently because of the potential for more normal control over defecation. When the tumor is not resectable or metastasis is present, palliative surgery is done to control hemorrhage or relieve a malignant bowel obstruction.

In APR, both the tumor and the entire rectum are removed and the person has a permanent colostomy. The perineal wound may be closed around a drain or left open with packing to allow healing by granulation. Complications that can occur are delayed wound healing, hemorrhage, persistent perineal sinus tracts, infections, and urinary tract and sexual dysfunctions.

An LAR may be indicated for tumors of the rectosigmoid and the mid to upper rectum. If the tumor is far enough from the anal sphincters, the sphincters may be left intact. The use of end-to-end anastomosis staplers has allowed lower (less than 5 cm from anus) and more secure anastomoses.

If the rectum is removed and the anal sphincters remain, an alternative reservoir with either a colonic J-pouch or coloplasty can be made. The colonic J-pouch is created by folding the distal colon back on itself and suturing it to form a pouch, which replaces the rectum as a reservoir for stool. The patient has a temporary colostomy to allow the J-pouch sutures time to heal before stool enters it. *Coloplasty* is an alternative to the pouch. It is created by slitting the side of a section of colon a short distance proximal to the anus, stretching the colon transversely to make it wider, and then suturing it closed in the new widened position. Patients with sphincter-sparing procedures may experience diarrhea, constipation, and incontinence even years after the procedure. The colonic J-pouch has decreased diarrhea and incontinence problems, but patients may have difficulty evacuating stool.

Chemotherapy and Targeted Therapy. Chemotherapy can be used to shrink the tumor before surgery, as an adjuvant therapy after colon resection, and as palliative treatment for nonresectable cancer. Adjuvant chemotherapy is recommended for patients with stage III tumors and high-risk stage II tumors. Current chemotherapy protocols include 5-fluorouracil (5-FU) and folinic acid (leucovorin) alone or in combination with oxaliplatin (Eloxatin). The preferred protocol includes oxaliplatin, but it may be omitted for patients who have too many side effects. Oral fluoropyrimidines (e.g., capecitabine [Xeloda]) have been found as effective as 5-FU/folinic acid monotherapy and can also be given in combination with oxaliplatin.[38]

DRUG ALERT: Capecitabine (Xeloda)
- Instruct patient not to get immunizations without physician's approval.
- Report temperature >100.4° F (38° C) immediately.

A variety of targeted therapies are used to treat metastatic CRC. Angiogenesis inhibitors, which inhibit the blood supply to tumors, include bevacizumab (Avastin) and ziv-aflibercept (Zaltrap). Regorafenib (Stivarga) is a multi-kinase inhibitor that blocks several enzymes that promote cancer growth. Cetuximab (Erbitux) and panitumumab (Vectibix) block the epidermal growth factor receptor.

Bevacizumab can also be used in combination with chemotherapy (e.g., fluoropyrimidine-oxaliplatin or fluoropyrimidine-irinotecan) to treat metastatic CRC. (Chemotherapy and targeted therapy are discussed in more detail in Chapter 16.)

Radiation Therapy. Radiation therapy may be used postoperatively as an adjuvant to surgery and chemotherapy or as a palliative measure for patients with metastatic cancer. As a palliative measure, its primary objective is to reduce tumor size and provide symptomatic relief. (Radiation therapy is described in Chapter 16.)

TABLE 43-25 NURSING ASSESSMENT
Colorectal Cancer

Subjective Data
Important Health Information
Past health history: Previous breast or ovarian cancer, familial polyposis, villous adenoma, adenomatous polyps, inflammatory bowel disease
Medications: Use of any medications affecting bowel function (e.g., laxatives, antidiarrheal drugs)

Functional Health Patterns
Health perception–health management: Family history of colorectal, breast, or ovarian cancer; weakness, fatigue
Nutritional-metabolic: High-calorie, high-fat, low-fiber diet; anorexia, weight loss; nausea and vomiting
Elimination: Change in bowel habits; alternating diarrhea and constipation, defecation urgency; rectal bleeding; mucoid stools; black, tarry stools; increased flatus, decrease in stool caliber; feelings of incomplete evacuation
Cognitive-perceptual: Abdominal and low back pain, tenesmus

Objective Data
General
Pallor, cachexia, lymphadenopathy (later signs)

Gastrointestinal
Palpable abdominal mass, distention, ascites, and hepatomegaly (liver metastasis)

Possible Diagnostic Findings
Anemia; guaiac-positive stools, palpable mass on digital rectal examination; positive sigmoidoscopy, colonoscopy, barium enema, or CT scan; positive biopsy

NURSING MANAGEMENT
COLORECTAL CANCER

NURSING ASSESSMENT
Subjective and objective data that should be obtained from a patient with CRC are presented in Table 43-25.

NURSING DIAGNOSES
Nursing diagnoses for the patient with CRC include, but are not limited to, the following:
- Diarrhea or constipation *related to* altered bowel elimination patterns
- Fear and anxiety *related to* diagnosis of CRC, surgical or therapeutic interventions, and possible terminal illness
- Ineffective coping *related to* diagnosis of cancer and side effects of treatment

PLANNING
The overall goals are that the patient with CRC will have (1) normal bowel elimination patterns, (2) quality of life appropriate to disease progression, (3) relief of pain, and (4) feelings of comfort and well-being.

NURSING IMPLEMENTATION
HEALTH PROMOTION. Encourage all persons over 50 to have regular CRC screening. Help identify those at high risk who need screening at an earlier age. Participate in early cancer screening to help decrease mortality rates. Realize that barriers exist, including lack of information and fear of diagnosis.

Endoscopic and radiographic procedures can only reveal polyps when the bowel has been adequately prepared to eliminate stool. Provide teaching about bowel cleansing for outpatient diagnostic procedures, and administer cleansing preparations to inpatients. Generally, the patient is placed on a clear liquid diet for 24 to 48 hours before the procedure and is given 4 L of oral polyethylene glycol (PEG) lavage solution the evening before the procedure. Drinking 2 L the evening before and 2 L the morning of the procedure provides better cleansing, especially for endoscopy scheduled for the afternoon. Because many people find the PEG lavage solution difficult to drink and experience nausea and bloating, manufacturers have modified the PEG solutions to improve taste and palatability. Magnesium citrate solution or bisacodyl tablets are sometimes given before the PEG lavage to remove the bulk of stool so only 2 L of PEG are needed. Encourage the patient to drink all of the solution. Stools will be clear or clear yellow liquid when the colon is clean.

ACUTE INTERVENTION. Acute nursing care for the patient with a colon resection is similar to care of the patient having a laparotomy (see pp. 970-971). If the cancer was resected and the ends reanastomosed, bowel function is maintained and routine postoperative care is appropriate. Inform patients about prognosis and future screening. Provide support for dealing with the diagnosis of cancer. Patients who have an APR will have a permanent ostomy and need emotional support to cope with their prognosis and the radical change in body appearance and function.

Patients with more extensive surgery (e.g., APR) may have an open wound and drains (e.g., Jackson-Pratt, Hemovac) and a permanent stoma. Postoperative care includes sterile dressing changes, care of drains, and patient and caregiver teaching about the stoma. Consult with a wound, ostomy, and continence (WOC) nurse before surgery to select the ostomy site on the abdomen, and then provide follow-up care and teaching.

A patient who has open and packed wounds requires meticulous postoperative care. Reinforce dressings and change them frequently during the first several hours postoperatively when drainage is likely to be profuse. Carefully assess all drainage for amount, color, and consistency. The drainage is usually serosanguineous. Examine the wound regularly and record bleeding, excessive drainage, and unusual odor. Use aseptic technique with dressing changes.

If the patient's wound is closed or partially closed, assess the incision for suture integrity and signs and symptoms of wound inflammation and infection. Examine the drainage for amount, color, and characteristics. Observe the skin around the drain for signs of inflammation, and keep the area around the drain clean and dry. Monitor for edema, erythema, and drainage around the suture line, as well as fever and an elevated WBC count.

The patient may experience phantom rectal sensation because the sympathetic nerves responsible for rectal control are not severed during the surgery. Be astute in distinguishing phantom sensations from perineal abscess pain.

Sexual dysfunction is a possible complication of an APR. Although the likelihood of sexual dysfunction depends on the surgical technique used, the surgeon should discuss the possibility with the patient. Members of the health care team should be available to address the patient's questions and concerns. Erection, ejaculation, and orgasm involve different nerve pathways, and a dysfunction of one does not mean complete sexual dysfunction. The WOC nurse is an important source of information concerning sexual dysfunction resulting from an APR.

AMBULATORY AND HOME CARE. Psychologic support for the patient and caregiver is important. The cancer could return. Patients need much emotional support because recurrent cancer is painful, debilitating, and demoralizing. (The special needs of the cancer patient are discussed in Chapter 16.) Issues surrounding palliative care, end-of-life preparation, and hospice need to be addressed (see Chapter 10).

Patients with colostomies need to know how to care for them. Even when patients do not have stomas, they may experience diarrhea, constipation, incontinence, or difficulty passing stool depending on the section of the colon removed and the surgical procedure performed. Patients need to know about diet; incontinence products; and strategies for managing bloating, diarrhea, and bowel evacuation. Often a combination of dietary changes and drugs is used to control diarrhea and constipation.

Patients with sphincter-sparing surgery frequently experience diarrhea and incontinence of feces and gas. They often need antidiarrheal drugs or bulking agents to control the diarrhea, but may overuse them and become constipated. Consultation with a dietitian would help patients and caregivers understand how to choose foods that are less likely to cause diarrhea and odor and could help them discover which foods are problematic for them.

EVALUATION

The expected outcomes for the patient with CRC are that the patient will have
- Minimal alterations in bowel elimination patterns
- Balanced nutritional intake
- Quality of life appropriate to disease progression
- Feelings of comfort and well-being

OSTOMY SURGERY

Types

An **ostomy** is a surgical procedure that allows intestinal contents to pass from the bowel through an opening in the skin on the abdomen. The opening is called a **stoma.** The stoma is created when the intestine is brought through the abdominal wall and sutured to the skin. The intestinal contents then empty through the hole on the surface of the abdomen rather than being eliminated through the anus.

An ostomy is used when the normal elimination route is no longer possible. For example, if the person has CRC, the diseased portion is removed together with a certain margin of healthy tissue. Most stage I to III tumors of the colon can be resected, leaving enough healthy tissue to immediately *anastomose* the two remaining ends of healthy bowel, and no ostomy is necessary. If the tumor involves the rectum and is large enough to necessitate the removal of the anal sphincters, the

TABLE 43-26	COMPARISON OF ILEOSTOMY AND COLOSTOMY			
		Colostomy		
Characteristic	**Ileostomy**	**Ascending**	**Transverse**	**Sigmoid**
Stool consistency	Liquid to semiliquid	Semiliquid	Semiliquid to semiformed	Formed
Fluid requirement	Increased	Increased	Possibly increased	No change
Bowel regulation	No	No	No	Yes (if there is a history of a regular bowel pattern)
Pouch and skin barriers	Yes	Yes	Yes	Dependent on regulation
Irrigation	No	No	No	Possibly every 24-48 hr (if patient meets criteria)
Indications for surgery	Ulcerative colitis, Crohn's disease, diseased or injured colon, familial polyposis, trauma, cancer	Perforating diverticulum in lower colon, trauma, rectovaginal fistula, inoperable tumors of colon, rectum, or pelvis	Same as for ascending	Cancer of the rectum or rectosigmoidal area, perforating diverticulum, trauma

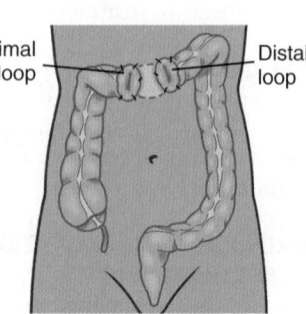

Ileostomy | Ascending colostomy | Descending colostomy | Sigmoid colostomy single-barreled | Transverse colostomy double-barreled

FIG. 43-9 Types of ostomies.

anus is sutured shut and a permanent ostomy is created. Patients at high risk for CRC, such as those with FAP, and patients with ulcerative colitis may have a total colectomy.

Ostomies are described according to location and type (Fig. 43-9). An ostomy in the ileum is called an *ileostomy*. An ostomy in the colon is called a *colostomy*. The ostomy is further characterized by its anatomic site (e.g., sigmoid or transverse colostomy). The more distal the ostomy, the more the intestinal contents resemble feces that are eliminated from an intact colon and rectum. Output from an ileostomy has not entered the colon and thus is liquid. The ileostomy drains continuously, and the patient must constantly wear a bag to collect the drainage. In contrast, output from a sigmoid colostomy resembles normal formed stool, and some patients are able to regulate emptying time so they do not need to wear a collection bag. (See Colostomy Irrigations later in this chapter.) A comparison of colostomies and ileostomies is shown in Table 43-26.

Ostomies may be temporary or permanent. For example, the person with a draining fistula may need a temporary ostomy to prevent stool from reaching the diseased area. Patients who have trauma to the intestines (e.g., gunshot wound, stabbing) may need a temporary ostomy. Cancer involving the rectum requires a permanent ostomy because all bowel distal to the ostomy is removed.

The major types of ostomies are end stoma, double-barreled, and loop ostomy.

End Stoma. An end stoma is surgically constructed by dividing the bowel and bringing out the proximal end as a single stoma. The distal portion of the GI tract is surgically removed, or the distal segment is oversewn and left in the abdominal cavity with its mesentery intact. An end colostomy or ileostomy is then constructed. When the distal bowel is oversewn rather than removed, the procedure is known as a Hartmann's pouch (Fig. 43-10). In this procedure the potential exists for the bowel to be reanastomosed and the stoma to be closed (referred to as a *takedown*). If the distal bowel is removed, the stoma is permanent.

Loop Stoma. A loop stoma is constructed by bringing a loop of bowel to the abdominal surface and then opening the anterior wall of the bowel to provide fecal diversion. This results in one stoma with a proximal opening for feces and a distal opening for mucus drainage (from the distal colon). An intact posterior wall separates the two openings. The loop of bowel is

frequently held in place with a plastic rod for 7 to 10 days after surgery to prevent it from slipping back into the abdominal cavity (Fig. 43-11). A loop stoma is usually temporary.

Double-Barreled Stoma. When the bowel is divided, both the proximal and distal ends are brought through the abdominal wall as two separate stomas (see Fig. 43-9). The proximal one is the functioning stoma. The distal, nonfunctioning stoma is referred to as the mucus fistula. The double-barreled stoma is usually temporary.

NURSING MANAGEMENT OSTOMY SURGERY

Two major aspects of nursing care are (1) emotional support as the patient copes with a radical change in body image and (2) patient and caregiver teaching about stoma care and the ostomy.[39] People with ostomies lose control over flatus and feces and worry about odor and leakage of feces from around the bag.[40] With time people learn to manage the stoma and make adjustments in work, social interactions, and sexual activities. People with new ostomies may be reluctant to return to work and avoid being around other people. Initially, patients may feel unattractive to their partners and unwilling to engage in sexual activities. However, with emotional support and teaching, patients can learn to manage the ostomy and return to their previous lifestyle.

PREOPERATIVE CARE

Major aspects of preoperative care that are unique to ostomy surgery include (1) psychologic preparation for the ostomy, (2) selection of a flat site on the abdomen that allows secure attachment of the collection bag, and (3) selection of a stoma site that will be clearly visible to the patient who will be taking care of it and is appropriate for clothing habits and activities.[41] Psychologic preparation and emotional support are particularly important as the person copes with the change in body image, the loss of control over elimination, and the odors. Provide the patient opportunities for verbalization of concerns and questions. This will enhance the patient's feelings of control and thus ability to cope.

A WOC nurse should select the site where the ostomy will be positioned and mark the abdomen preoperatively.[41-43] The site should be within the rectus muscle on a flat surface that the patient is able to see. Stomas placed outside the rectus muscle increase the chance of developing a hernia. A flat site makes it much easier to create a good seal and avoid leakage from

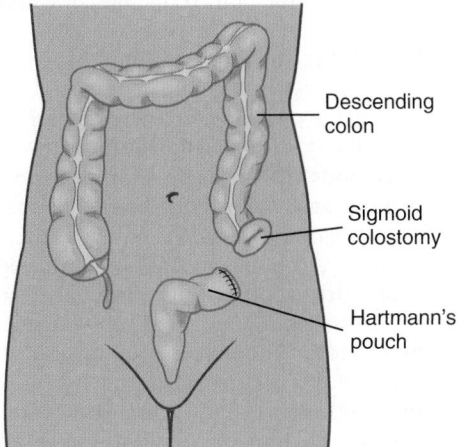
FIG. 43-10 Sigmoid colostomy. Distal bowel is oversewn and left in place to create Hartmann's pouch.

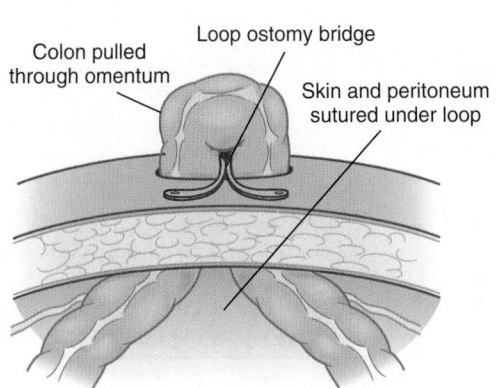
FIG. 43-11 Loop colostomy.

the bag. Patients who cannot see the stoma are unable to care for it.

The patient and caregiver usually have many questions concerning the procedures. If available, a WOC nurse should visit with the patient and the caregiver to determine the patient's ability to perform self-care, identify support systems, and determine any modifications that could facilitate learning during rehabilitation. The patient and the caregiver should understand the extent of surgery, the type of stoma, and related care.

Ask the patient if he or she would like to meet with a person who has adjusted to an ostomy. This gives the patient and caregiver an opportunity to question a person who has adjusted well to an ostomy and who has experienced some of the same feelings and concerns that they have.

POSTOPERATIVE CARE

Postoperative nursing care includes assessment of the stoma and provision of an appropriate pouching system that protects the skin and contains drainage and odor. The stoma should be dark pink to red. A dusky blue stoma indicates ischemia, and a brown-black stoma indicates necrosis. Assess and document stoma color every 4 hours and ensure that there is no excessive bleeding. Teach the patient that the stoma is mildly to moderately swollen the first 2 to 3 weeks after surgery (Table 43-27). A smaller pouch opening will be needed as the swelling goes down to accommodate the stoma's changing size. Determine the size of the stoma with a stoma-measuring card.

The colostomy starts functioning when peristalsis returns. When a temporary colostomy is performed on a colon that was not cleaned out before surgery, stool will drain when peristalsis returns. However, if the bowel was cleansed preoperatively, it will not begin producing stool until days after the surgery when the patient is eating again.

An appropriate pouching system is vital to protect the skin and provide dependable drainage collection. The various pouching systems all have an adhesive skin barrier and a bag or pouch to collect the feces. Flatus is expelled from the bag through a charcoal filter that helps control odor. The skin barrier is a piece of pectin-based or karaya wafer that has a measurable thickness and hydrocolloid adhesive properties. The adhesion occurs in two phases. First, the wafer's backing has adhesive material that forms an immediate bond with the skin. Second, the hydrocolloids interface with the moisture on the skin to form a tighter seal. If the abdominal stoma site has bends or creases, it is difficult to get a good seal and the skin barrier will pull away faster. Also, the weight of drainage from the stoma pulls the wafer away from the skin. For this reason, ostomy bags should be emptied when one-third full.

In the postoperative period an open-ended, transparent, plastic, odor-proof pouch is used to observe the stoma and collect the drainage. Record the volume, color, and consistency of the drainage. Each time the pouch is changed, observe the condition of the skin for irritation. Never place a pouch directly on irritated skin without the use of a skin barrier.

Teach the patient to perform a pouch change, provide appropriate skin care, control odor, care for the stoma, and identify signs and symptoms of complications. Instruct the patient about the importance of fluids and a healthy diet. Provide the names and addresses of United Ostomy Associations of America, and instruct the patient on when to seek health care. Home care and outpatient follow-up by a WOC nurse are highly recommended. Patients should be discharged with written information about their particular ostomy, instructions for pouch changes, a list of supplies and where to purchase them (including names and phone numbers of retailers), outpatient follow-up appointments with the surgeon and WOC nurse, and phone numbers of the surgeon and nurse. Patient and caregiver teaching guidelines are presented in Table 43-28.

Teaching is often complicated by the emotional responses to the stoma. Emotional support, interventions from skillful WOC nurses, and visits from people who have successfully learned to manage their ostomies will help patients learn to cope with and manage the new stoma.

COLOSTOMY CARE

Nursing care for the patient with a colostomy is presented in eNursing Care Plan 43-3 on the website. A colostomy in the ascending and transverse colon has semiliquid stools. Instruct the patient to use a drainable pouch. A colostomy in the sigmoid or descending colon has semiformed or formed stools and can sometimes be regulated by the irrigation method. For these patients, a drainage pouch may or may not be needed. Gas filters are available for both drainable and nondrainable pouches.

A well-balanced diet and adequate fluid intake are important, and most patients with colostomies can eat anything they choose. However, dietary modifications are helpful for decreasing gas production and odor. eTable 43-4 (on the website for this chapter) lists foods and their effects on stoma output.

Colostomy Irrigations. Colostomy irrigations may be used to stimulate emptying of the colon. When the colon is irrigated and emptied on a regular basis, no stool is eliminated between irrigation sessions. Irrigation requires manual dexterity and adequate vision. However, if bowel control is achieved, little or no spillage should occur between irrigations, and the patient may need to wear only a pad or small pouch over the stoma. Regularity is possible only when the stoma is in the distal colon. Irrigation is not used for more proximal ostomies. People who irrigate regularly should still have ostomy bags readily available in case they develop diarrhea from foods or illness. The proce-

TABLE 43-27	CHARACTERISTICS OF STOMA
Characteristic	**Description or Cause**
Color*	
Rose to brick-red	Viable stoma mucosa.
Pale	May indicate anemia.
Blanching, dark red to purple	Indicates inadequate blood supply to the stoma or bowel.
Edema†	
Mild to moderate edema	Normal in the initial postoperative period. Trauma to the stoma.
Moderate to severe edema	Obstruction of the stoma, allergic reaction to food, gastroenteritis.
Bleeding	
Small amount	Oozing from the stoma mucosa when touched is normal because of its high vascularity.
Moderate to large amount	Could indicate lower gastrointestinal bleeding, coagulation factor deficiency, stomal varices secondary to portal hypertension.

*Report sustained color changes to surgeon.
†Closely observe and report to the surgeon and adjust the stoma opening size in the pouch.

TABLE 43-28	**PATIENT & CAREGIVER TEACHING GUIDE**

Ostomy Self-Care

Include the following instructions when teaching the patient and/or caregiver about self-care of an ostomy.
1. Explain what an ostomy is and how it functions.
2. Describe the underlying condition that resulted in the need for an ostomy.
3. Demonstrate and allow the patient and caregiver to practice the following activities:
   - Remove the old skin barrier, cleanse the skin, and correctly apply new skin barriers.
   - Apply, empty, clean, and remove the pouch.
   - Empty the pouch before it is one-third full to prevent leakage.
   - Irrigate the colostomy to regulate bowel elimination (optional).
4. Explain how to contact the wound, ostomy, and continence (WOC) nurse with questions.
5. Describe how to obtain additional ostomy supplies.
6. Explain dietary and fluid management.
   - Identify a well-balanced diet and dietary supplements to prevent nutritional deficiencies.
   - Identify foods to avoid to reduce diarrhea, gas, or obstruction (with ileostomy).
   - Promote fluid intake of least 3000 mL/day to prevent dehydration (unless contraindicated).
   - Increase fluid intake during hot weather, excessive perspiration, and diarrhea to replace losses and prevent dehydration.
   - Describe symptoms of fluid and electrolyte imbalance.
   - Explain how to contact the registered dietitian with questions.
   - Explain how to recognize problems (fluid and electrolyte deficits, fever, diarrhea, skin irritation, stomal problems) and how to contact the appropriate health care provider.
7. Describe community resources to assist with emotional and psychologic adjustment to the ostomy.
8. Explain the importance of follow-up care.
9. Describe the ostomy's potential effects on sexual activity, social life, work, and recreation and strategies to manage these changes.

TABLE 43-29	**PATIENT & CAREGIVER TEACHING GUIDE**

Colostomy Irrigation

Include the following instructions when teaching the patient and caregiver to perform a colostomy irrigation.

Equipment*
Lubricant
Irrigation set (1000- to 2000-mL container, tubing with irrigating stoma cone, clamp)
Irrigating sleeve with adhesive or belt
Toilet tissue to clean around the stoma
Disposal sack for soiled dressing

Procedure
1. Place 500-1000 mL of lukewarm water (not to exceed 105° F [40.5° C]) in container. Titrate the volume for the individual; use enough irrigant to distend the bowel but not enough to cause cramping pain. Most adults use 500-1000 mL of water.
2. Ensure a comfortable position. Patient may sit in chair in front of toilet or on the toilet if the perineal wound is healed.
3. Clear tubing of all air by flushing it with fluid.
4. Hang container on hook or IV pole (18-24 in) above stoma (about shoulder height).
5. Apply irrigating sleeve and place bottom end in toilet bowl.
6. Lubricate stoma cone, insert cone tip gently into the stoma, and hold tip securely in place. The cone is designed to prevent perforation, control the depth of insertion, and prevent water from coming out of the stoma.
7. Allow irrigation solution to flow in steadily for 5-10 min.
8. If cramping occurs, stop the flow of solution for a few seconds, leaving the cone in place.
9. Clamp the tubing and remove irrigating cone when the desired amount of irrigant has been delivered or when the patient senses colonic distention.
10. Allow 30-45 min for the solution and feces to be expelled. Initial evacuation is usually complete in 10-15 min. Close off the irrigating sleeve at the bottom to allow ambulation.
11. Clean, rinse, and dry peristomal skin well.
12. Replace the colostomy drainage pouch or desired stoma covering.
13. Wash and rinse all equipment and hang to dry.

*Commercial sets usually have all the equipment that you will need.

dure for colostomy irrigation is similar to an enema and is presented in Table 43-29.

ILEOSTOMY CARE

An ileostomy stoma protrusion of at least 1 to 1.5 cm makes care easier. When the stoma is flat, seepage occurs, resulting in altered skin integrity. Drainage is frequent and extremely irritating to the skin. Since regularity cannot be established with an ileostomy, a pouch must be worn at all times. An open-ended, drainable pouch is preferable so drainage can be easily emptied. The drainable pouch is usually worn for 4 to 7 days before being changed, unless leakage occurs. In that case, the pouch should be promptly removed, the skin cleansed, and a new pouch applied. A solid skin barrier should always be used.

A transparent pouch should be used in the initial postoperative period to facilitate assessment of stoma viability and pouch application by the patient. Later on patients may prefer opaque pouches. (eNursing Care Plan 43-3 [on the website for this chapter] presents care of the patient with an ileostomy.)

Observe the patient with an ileostomy for signs and symptoms of fluid and electrolyte imbalance, particularly potassium, sodium, and fluid deficits. In the first 24 to 48 hours after surgery the amount of drainage from the stoma may be negligible. Patients with new ileostomies lose the absorptive functions provided by the colon and the delay provided by the ileocecal valve. As a result, they may experience a period of high-volume output of 1000 to 1800 mL/day when peristalsis returns. Later, as the proximal small bowel adapts, the average amount can be 500 mL/day. If the small bowel has been shortened by surgery, drainage from the ileostomy may be greater. Patients need to increase fluid intake to at least 2 to 3 L/day, or more when there are excessive fluid losses from heat and sweating. They may also need to ingest additional sodium. Patients must learn signs and symptoms of fluid and electrolyte imbalance so that they can take appropriate action.

A low-fiber diet is ordered initially, and fiber-containing foods are reintroduced gradually. The ileostomy patient is susceptible to obstruction because the lumen is less than 1 in in diameter and may narrow further at the point where the bowel passes through the fascia/muscle layer of the abdomen. Foods such as popcorn, coconut, mushrooms, olives, stringy vegetables, foods with skins, dried fruits, and meats with casings must be chewed extremely well before swallowing. The goal is for the patient to return to a normal, presurgical diet. If the terminal ileum has been removed, the patient may need cobalamin treatment.

DELEGATION DECISIONS

Ostomy Care

Although licensed practical/vocational nurses (LPN/LVNs) and unlicensed assistive personnel (UAP) provide much of the ostomy care for patients with established ostomies, patients with new ostomies have complex needs and require frequent assessment, planning, intervention, and evaluation by a registered nurse (RN).

Role of Registered Nurse (RN)
- Assess and document stoma appearance.
- For patient with a new ostomy, assess patient's psychologic preparation for ostomy care.
- Choose appropriate ostomy pouching system (skin barrier and bag or pouch) for patient.
- Place ostomy pouching system for a new ostomy.
- Develop plan of care for skin care around the ostomy.
- Teach ostomy care and skin care to patient and caregiver.
- Irrigate new colostomy.
- Teach colostomy irrigation to patient and caregiver.
- Teach patient and caregivers about appropriate dietary choices.
- Consult with wound, ostomy, and continence (WOC) nurse.

Role of Licensed Practical/Vocational Nurse (LPN/LVN)
- Monitor the volume, color, and odor of the ostomy drainage.
- Monitor the skin around the ostomy for breakdown.
- Provide skin care around the ostomy.
- Irrigate colostomy in stable patient.

Role of Unlicensed Assistive Personnel (UAP)
- Empty ostomy bag and measure liquid contents.
- Place the ostomy pouching system for an established ostomy.
- Assist stable patient with colostomy irrigation.

The stoma bleeds easily when it is touched because it has a high vascular supply. Tell the patient that minimal oozing of blood is normal.

ADAPTATION TO AN OSTOMY

Patients experience a grief reaction from the loss of a body part and an alteration in body image. They may feel like they are no longer normal and may experience shame and social isolation. People commonly feel anxiety and fear about stool leaking and the smells and sounds of flatus and stool entering the pouch. They are concerned about how the stoma will affect their lifestyle, including work, eating, sports, sex, and sleeping. They may be angry, depressed, or resentful.

Discuss the psychologic impact of the stoma and how it affects the patient's body image and self-esteem. Assist the patient in identifying ways of coping with depression and anxiety resulting from illness, surgery, or postoperative problems.[44]

Support from the caregiver, family, and friends is vitally important and reassures the patient that he or she is cherished and valued despite having the ostomy. Encourage patients to share their concerns and ask questions, provide information in a manner that is easily understood, recommend support services, and help patients develop confidence and competence in managing the stoma.

The patient can resume activities of daily living within 6 to 8 weeks but should avoid heavy lifting. The patient's physical condition determines when sports may be resumed. Some health care providers recommend avoiding participation in sports where direct trauma to the stoma is likely. Bathing and swimming may be done with or without the pouching system in place because water does not harm the stoma.

Patients want to know how to manage gas and body odors and how to choose clothing that will hide the stoma. Refer patients to the United Ostomy Associations of America (www.ostomy.org) for (1) practical information about living with an ostomy (e.g., ostomy products, irrigation, travel, sex), (2) contact information for local support groups, and (3) opportunities for online communication with other people with ostomies.

SEXUAL FUNCTION AFTER OSTOMY SURGERY

The patient with a stoma may fear rejection by a partner or that others will not find him or her desirable. Incorporate a discussion of sexuality and sexual function in the plan of care. Help the patient understand that sexual function or sexual activity may be affected, but sexuality does not have to be altered. Help the patient realize that it takes time to adjust to the pouch and to body changes before feeling secure in his or her sexual functioning. Also, a woman with an ostomy can still become pregnant.

Pelvic surgery can disrupt nerve and vascular supplies to the genitalia. Radiation therapy, chemotherapy, and medications can also alter sexual function. The patient's overall physical health influences sexual desire. Generalized fatigue caused by illness can also influence desire. Understanding this information can help patients better plan the timing of their sexual activity.

Erection of the penis depends on intact parasympathetic nerves and adequate blood supply to the pelvis and to pudendal nerves that transmit sensory responses from the genital area. Nerve-sparing surgical techniques are used when possible to preserve sexual function. Unfortunately, any pelvic surgery that removes the rectum has the potential of damaging the parasympathetic nerve plexus. Pelvic radiation can reduce blood flow to the pelvis by causing scarring in the small blood vessels. Muscle contraction and genital pleasure that occur during orgasm are not disrupted by pelvic surgery. If the sympathetic nerves in the male's presacral area are damaged, ejaculation may be disrupted. This can occur with the APR procedure.

DIVERTICULOSIS AND DIVERTICULITIS

Diverticula are saccular dilations or outpouchings of the mucosa that develop in the colon (Fig. 43-12). Multiple noninflamed diverticula are present in diverticulosis (see eFig. 43-3 on the website for this chapter). Diverticulitis is inflammation of the diverticula, resulting in perforation into the peritoneum. Clinically, diverticular disease covers a spectrum from asymptomatic, uncomplicated diverticulosis to diverticulitis with complications such as perforation, abscess, fistula, and bleeding.

Etiology and Pathophysiology

Diverticula are common, especially in older adults, but most people never develop diverticulitis.[45] Diverticula may occur anywhere in the GI tract but are most commonly found in the left (descending, sigmoid) colon. The etiology of diverticulosis of the sigmoid colon is thought to be associated with high luminal pressures from a deficiency in dietary fiber intake. The disease is more prevalent in Western, industrialized populations that consume diets low in fiber and high in refined carbohydrates. Diverticula are uncommon in vegetarians. Inadequate dietary fiber slows transit time, and more water is absorbed

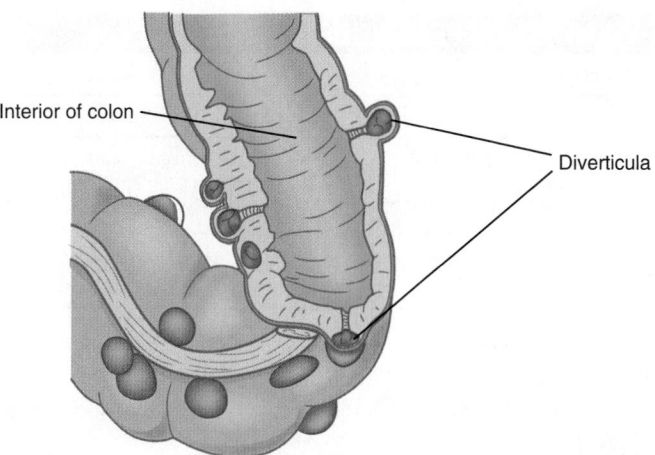

FIG. 43-12 Diverticula are outpouchings of the colon. When they become inflamed, the condition is diverticulitis. The inflammatory process can spread to the surrounding area in the intestine.

from the stool, making it more difficult to pass through the lumen. Decreased stool size raises intraluminal pressure, thus promoting diverticula formation.

Clinical Manifestations and Complications

The majority of patients with diverticulosis have no symptoms. Those with symptoms typically have abdominal pain, bloating, flatulence, or changes in bowel habits. In more serious situations, the diverticula bleed or diverticulitis develops. Diverticulitis is characterized by inflamed diverticula and increased luminal pressures that cause erosion of the bowel wall, and thus perforation into the peritoneum (Fig. 43-13). The most common symptoms of diverticulitis are acute pain in the left lower quadrant (location of sigmoid colon), a palpable abdominal mass, and systemic symptoms of infection (fever, increased C-reactive protein, and leukocytosis with a shift to the left).[45] Older adults with diverticulitis may be afebrile, with a normal WBC count and little, if any, abdominal tenderness. A localized abscess develops when the body is able to wall off the area of perfora-

PATHOPHYSIOLOGY MAP

Diverticulitis

Acute / Chronic

Hemorrhage, Perforation, Pericolic abscess, Stricture

General peritonitis, Local suppuration, Fistula, Intestinal obstruction

FIG. 43-13 Complications of diverticulitis.

TABLE 43-30   COLLABORATIVE CARE
Diverticulosis and Diverticulitis

Diagnostic
- History and physical examination
- Testing of stool for occult blood
- Barium enema
- Sigmoidoscopy
- Colonoscopy
- CBC
- Urinalysis
- Blood culture
- CT scan with oral contrast
- Abdominal x-ray
- Chest x-ray

Collaborative Therapy
Conservative Therapy
- High-fiber diet
- Dietary fiber supplements
- Stool softeners
- Anticholinergics
- Bed rest
- Clear liquid diet
- Oral antibiotics
- Mineral oil
- Bulk laxatives
- Weight reduction (if overweight)

Acute Care: Diverticulitis
- Antibiotic therapy
- NPO status
- IV fluids
- Bed rest
- NG suction
- Surgery
  - Possible resection of involved colon for obstruction or hemorrhage
  - Possible temporary colostomy

tion. Peritonitis develops if it cannot be contained. Bleeding can be extensive, but usually stops spontaneously.

Diagnostic Studies

Diverticular disease can be asymptomatic and is typically discovered during routine sigmoidoscopy or colonoscopy. Diagnosis of diverticulitis is based on the history and physical examination (Table 43-30). Abdominal and chest x-ray rule out other causes of acute abdominal pain, but the preferred diagnostic test is a CT scan with oral contrast.

NURSING AND COLLABORATIVE MANAGEMENT DIVERTICULOSIS AND DIVERTICULITIS

A high-fiber diet, mainly from fruits and vegetables, and decreased intake of fat and red meat are recommended for preventing diverticular disease. High levels of physical activity also seem to decrease the risk. A high-fiber diet (see Table 43-6) is also recommended once diverticular disease is present. Currently there is no evidence to support the theory that diverticulitis can be prevented by avoiding nuts and seeds.

Weight reduction is important for the obese person. A patient with diverticular disease should avoid increased intraabdominal pressure because it may precipitate an attack. Factors that increase intraabdominal pressure are straining at stool, vomiting, bending, lifting, and wearing tight restrictive clothing.

In acute diverticulitis the goal of treatment is to let the colon rest and the inflammation subside. Some patients can be managed at home with oral antibiotics and a clear liquid diet. Hospitalization is necessary if symptoms are severe, the patient is unable to tolerate oral fluids, or the patient has co-morbid diseases.

Patients who are older, are immunosuppressed, or have systemic manifestations of infection (fever, significant leukocytosis) are hospitalized. If hospitalized, the patient is kept on NPO status and bed rest, and fluids and IV antibiotics are given. Observe for signs of abscess, bleeding, and peritonitis, and monitor the WBC count. When the acute attack subsides, give oral fluids first and then progress the diet to semisolids. Ambulation is allowed.

Surgery is reserved for patients with complications such as an abscess or obstruction that cannot be managed medically. The usual surgical procedures involve resection of the involved colon with either a primary anastomosis if adequate bowel cleansing is feasible or a temporary diverting colostomy. The colostomy is reanastomosed after the colon heals.

Provide the patient with diverticular disease with a full explanation of the condition. Patients who understand the disease process well and adhere to the prescribed regimen are less likely to experience an exacerbation of the disease and its complications.

HERNIAS

A **hernia** is a protrusion of the viscus (internal organ such as the intestine) through an abnormal opening or a weakened area in the wall of the cavity in which it is normally contained. A hernia may occur in any part of the body, but it usually occurs within the abdominal cavity (Fig. 43-14). Hernias that easily return to the abdominal cavity are called *reducible*. The hernia can be reduced manually or may reduce spontaneously when the person lies down. If the hernia cannot be placed back into the abdominal cavity, it is known as *irreducible* or *incarcerated*. In this situation the intestinal flow may be obstructed. When the hernia is irreducible and the intestinal flow and blood supply are obstructed, the hernia is strangulated. The result is an acute intestinal obstruction.

Types

The *inguinal hernia* is the most common type of hernia and occurs at the point of weakness in the abdominal wall where

the spermatic cord (in men) or the round ligament (in women) emerges (see Fig. 43-14, *C*). Inguinal hernias are more common in men.

A *femoral hernia* occurs when there is a protrusion through the femoral ring into the femoral canal. It appears as a bulge below the inguinal ligament. It easily becomes strangulated. It occurs more often in women (see Fig. 43-14, *B*). The *umbilical hernia* occurs when the rectus muscle is weak (as with obesity) or the umbilical opening fails to close after birth (see Fig. 43-14, *A*).

Ventral or *incisional hernias* are due to weakness of the abdominal wall at the site of a previous incision. They occur most commonly in patients who are obese, have had multiple surgical procedures in the same area, or have had inadequate wound healing because of poor nutrition or infection.

Clinical Manifestations

A hernia may be readily visible, especially when the person tenses the abdominal muscles. There may be some discomfort as a result of tension. If the hernia becomes strangulated, the patient will have severe pain and symptoms of a bowel obstruction such as vomiting, cramping abdominal pain, and distention. Strangulated hernias or painful, inflamed hernias that cannot be reduced require emergency surgery.[46]

NURSING AND COLLABORATIVE MANAGEMENT
HERNIAS

Diagnosis is based on history and physical examination findings. Laparoscopic surgery is the treatment of choice for hernias. The surgical repair of a hernia, known as a *herniorrhaphy*, is usually an outpatient procedure. Reinforcement of the weakened area with wire, fascia, or mesh is known as a *hernioplasty*.

A   B   C

FIG. 43-14 A, Umbilical hernia. **B,** Femoral hernias (note swelling below the inguinal ligaments). **C,** Right inguinal hernia.

Strangulated hernias are treated immediately with resection of the involved area or a temporary colostomy so that necrosis and gangrene do not occur.

After a hernia repair, the patient may have difficulty voiding. Measure intake and output and observe for a distended bladder. Scrotal edema is a painful complication after an inguinal hernia repair. A scrotal support with application of an ice bag may help relieve pain and edema. Encourage deep breathing, but not coughing. Teach patients to splint the incision and keep their mouths open when coughing or sneezing are unavoidable. The patient may be restricted from heavy lifting for 6 to 8 weeks.

MALABSORPTION SYNDROME

Malabsorption results from impaired absorption of fats, carbohydrates, proteins, minerals, and vitamins. The stomach, small intestine, liver, and pancreas regulate normal digestion and absorption. Digestive enzymes ordinarily break down nutrients so that absorption can take place. If this process is interrupted at any point, malabsorption may occur. Several problems can cause malabsorption (Table 43-31). Lactose intolerance is the most common malabsorption disorder, followed by IBD, celiac disease, tropical sprue, and cystic fibrosis.

The most common signs of malabsorption are weight loss, diarrhea, and steatorrhea (bulky, foul-smelling, yellow-gray, greasy stools with putty-like consistency) (Table 43-32). Steatorrhea does not occur with lactose intolerance.

Tests used to determine the cause of malabsorption include qualitative examination of stool for fat (e.g., Sudan III stain), a 72-hour stool collection for quantitative measurement of fecal fat, serologic testing for celiac disease, and fecal elastase testing to determine if there is pancreatic insufficiency. Near-infrared reflectance analysis (NIRA) for fecal fat is available at some centers in the United States.

Other diagnostic studies include a CT scan and endoscopy to obtain a small bowel biopsy specimen. A small bowel barium enema may be performed to identify abnormal mucosal patterns. Capsule endoscopy can be used to assess the small intestine for alterations in mucosal integrity and inflammation. Tests for carbohydrate malabsorption include the D-xylose test and the lactose tolerance test. Laboratory studies that are frequently ordered include a CBC, measurement of prothrombin time (to see if vitamin K absorption is adequate), serum vitamin A and carotene levels, serum electrolytes, cholesterol, and calcium.

CELIAC DISEASE

Celiac disease is an autoimmune disease characterized by damage to the small intestinal mucosa from the ingestion of wheat, barley, and rye in genetically susceptible individuals.[47] It is a relatively common disease that occurs at all ages and has a wide variety of symptoms. *Celiac sprue* and *gluten-sensitive enteropathy* are other names for celiac disease.

Celiac disease is not the same disease as *tropical sprue*, a chronic disorder acquired in tropical areas that is characterized

TABLE 43-31 CAUSES OF MALABSORPTION

Biochemical or Enzyme Deficiencies
- Lactase deficiency
- Biliary tract obstruction
- Pancreatic insufficiency
- Cystic fibrosis
- Chronic pancreatitis
- Zollinger-Ellison syndrome

Disturbed Lymphatic and Vascular Circulation
- Lymphoma
- Ischemia
- Lymphangiectasia
- Heart failure

Bacterial Proliferation
- Tropical sprue
- Parasitic infection

Small Intestinal Mucosal Disruption
- Celiac disease
- Whipple's disease
- Crohn's disease

Surface Area Loss
- Billroth II gastrectomy
- Short bowel syndrome
- Distal ileal resection, disease, or bypass

TABLE 43-32 MANIFESTATIONS OF MALABSORPTION

Manifestations	Pathophysiology
Gastrointestinal	
Weight loss	Malabsorption of fat, carbohydrates, and protein leading to loss of calories. Marked reduction in caloric intake or increased use of calories.
Diarrhea	Impaired absorption of water, sodium, fatty acids, bile salts, and carbohydrates.
Flatulence	Bacterial fermentation of unabsorbed carbohydrates.
Steatorrhea	Undigested and unabsorbed fat.
Glossitis, cheilosis, stomatitis	Deficiency of iron, riboflavin, cobalamin, folic acid, and other vitamins.
Hematologic	
Anemia	Impaired absorption of iron, cobalamin, and folic acid.
Hemorrhagic tendency	Vitamin C deficiency. Vitamin K deficiency inhibiting production of clotting factors II, VII, IX, and X.
Musculoskeletal	
Bone pain	Osteoporosis from impaired calcium absorption. Osteomalacia secondary to hypocalcemia, hypophosphatemia, inadequate vitamin D.
Tetany	Hypocalcemia, hypomagnesemia.
Weakness, muscle cramps	Anemia, electrolyte depletion (especially potassium).
Muscle wasting	Protein malabsorption.
Neurologic	
Altered mental status	Dehydration.
Paresthesias	Cobalamin deficiency.
Peripheral neuropathy	Cobalamin deficiency.
Night blindness	Thiamine deficiency, vitamin A deficiency.
Integumentary	
Bruising	Vitamin K deficiency.
Dermatitis	Fatty acid deficiency, zinc deficiency, niacin and other vitamin deficiencies.
Brittle nails	Iron deficiency.
Hair thinning and loss	Protein deficiency.
Cardiovascular	
Hypotension	Dehydration.
Tachycardia	Hypovolemia, anemia.
Peripheral edema	Protein malabsorption, protein loss in diarrhea.

by progressive disruption of jejunal and ileal tissue, resulting in nutritional difficulties. Tropical sprue is treated with folic acid and tetracycline.

Celiac disease is most common in people of European ancestry and affects about 1% of the population of the United States. High-risk groups include first- or second-degree relatives of someone with celiac disease and people with disorders associated with the disease such as migraine and myocarditis. It is slightly more common in women, and symptoms often begin in childhood.

Etiology and Pathophysiology

Three factors necessary for developing celiac disease are genetic predisposition, gluten ingestion, and an immune-mediated response.

Genetic Link

About 90% to 95% of patients with celiac disease have human leukocyte antigen (HLA) alleles HLA-DQ2, and the other 5% to 10% have HLA-DQ8. However, not everyone with these genetic markers develops celiac disease, and some people with celiac disease do not have these HLA alleles. (HLAs are discussed in Chapter 14.)

As with other autoimmune diseases, the tissue destruction that occurs with celiac disease is the result of chronic inflammation. Inflammation is activated by the ingestion of gluten found in wheat, rye, and barley. Gluten contains specific peptides called prolamines. In genetically susceptible individuals, partial digestion of gluten releases prolamine peptides, which are absorbed into the intestinal submucosa. The peptides then bind to HLA-DQ2 and/or HLA-DQ8 and activate an inflammatory response. Inflammation damages the microvilli and brush border of the small intestine, ultimately decreasing the amount of surface area available for nutrient absorption. Damage is most severe in the duodenum, probably because it has more exposure to gluten. The inflammation lasts as long as gluten ingestion continues.

Clinical Manifestations

Classic manifestations of celiac disease include foul-smelling diarrhea, steatorrhea, flatulence, abdominal distention, and malnutrition.[48] Some people have no obvious GI symptoms and may instead have atypical signs and symptoms such as decreased bone density and osteoporosis, dental enamel hypoplasia, iron and folate deficiencies, peripheral neuropathy, and reproductive problems. A pruritic, vesicular skin lesion, called *dermatitis herpetiformis,* is sometimes present and occurs as a rash on the buttocks, scalp, face, elbows, and knees.[48] Celiac disease is also associated with other autoimmune diseases, particularly rheumatoid arthritis, type 1 diabetes mellitus, and thyroid disease. The link between celiac disease and reproductive problems is less clear.

Protein, fat, and carbohydrate absorption is affected. Weight loss, muscle wasting, and other signs of malnutrition may be present. Abnormal serum folate, iron, and cobalamin levels can occur. Iron-deficiency anemia is one of the most common manifestations of celiac disease. Patients may exhibit lactose intolerance and need to refrain from lactose-containing products until the disease is under control. Inadequate calcium intake and vitamin D absorption can lead to decreased bone density and osteoporosis.

Diagnostic Studies and Collaborative Care

Early diagnosis and treatment can prevent complications. Screening is recommended for close relatives of patients known to have the disease, young patients with decreased bone density, those with anemia once other causes are ruled out, and certain autoimmune diseases.

Celiac disease is confirmed by (1) histologic evidence of the disease when a biopsy is taken from the small intestine and (2) the symptoms and histologic evidence disappearing when the person eats a gluten-free diet. Diagnostic testing must be done before the person is placed on a gluten-free diet, since the diet will alter the results. Serologic testing for immunoglobulin A (IgA) antitissue transglutaminase and IgA endomysial antibody provides good sensitivity and specificity. Histologic evidence remains the gold standard for confirming the diagnosis. Biopsies show flattened mucosa and noticeable losses of villi. Genotyping involves testing for HLA-DQ2 and/or HLA-DQ8 antigens. Many people spend years seeking treatment for nonspecific complaints before celiac disease is eventually diagnosed.

Treatment with a gluten-free diet (Table 43-33) halts the process. Most patients recover completely within 3 to 6 months of treatment, but they need to maintain a gluten-free diet for the rest of their lives. If the disease is untreated, chronic inflammation and hyperplasia continue. Individuals with celiac disease have an increased risk of non-Hodgkin's lymphoma and GI cancers.

Teach the patient to avoid wheat, barley, oats, and rye products. Although pure oats do not contain gluten, oat products can become contaminated with wheat, rye, and barley during the milling process. Gluten is also found in some medications and in many food additives, preservatives, and stabilizers. A combination of corticosteroids and a gluten-free diet is used to treat individuals with refractory celiac disease who do not respond to a gluten-free diet alone.

Maintenance of a gluten-free diet is difficult, particularly when traveling or eating in restaurants.[49-51] Therefore dietary consultation is imperative. The patient needs to know where to purchase gluten-free products. Gluten-free products are sold in health food stores, in many grocery stores, and through Internet

TABLE 43-33	**NUTRITIONAL THERAPY**

Celiac Disease

Foods to Eat*	Foods to Avoid
• Eggs	• Wheat
• Potatoes	• Barley
• Butter	• Oats
• Cheese, cottage cheese	• Rye
• Meat, fish, poultry (not marinated or breaded)	• Flour (unless it says gluten-free flour, or is made purely from a nongluten source, such as rice flour)
• Yogurt	• Baked goods, including muffins, cookies, cakes, pies
• Fresh fruits	
• Tapioca	
• Corn tortillas	• Bread, including wheat bread, white bread, "potato" bread
• Flax, corn, and rice	
• Soy products	• Pasta, pizza, bagels
• Gluten-free breads, crackers, pasta, and cereals	
• Unflavored milk	
• Peanut butter	
• Coffee, tea, and cocoa	

*Read food labels to look for gluten stabilizers or ingredients that contain gluten.

sites. Check the Internet to get a list of grocery stores that sell gluten-free products. Patients may need referral for financial assistance, since gluten-free products are more expensive than regular foods. The Celiac Sprue Association website (www. csaceliacs.info) and the Celiac Disease Foundation (www. celiac.org) provide suggestions for maintaining a gluten-free diet and living with celiac disease.

Continually encourage and motivate patients to continue the gluten-free diet. Reinforce that nonadherence to the diet will result in chronic inflammation, which can lead to complications such as anemia and osteoporosis.

LACTASE DEFICIENCY

Lactase deficiency is a condition in which the lactase enzyme is deficient or absent. Lactase is the enzyme that breaks down lactose into two simple sugars: glucose and galactose. Primary lactase insufficiency is most commonly a result of genetic factors. Certain ethnic or racial groups, especially those with Asian or African ancestry, develop low lactase levels in childhood. Less common causes include low lactase levels resulting from premature birth and congenital lactase deficiency, a rare genetic disorder. Lactose malabsorption can also occur when conditions leading to bacterial overgrowth promote lactose fermentation in the small bowel, and when intestinal mucosal damage interferes with absorption. The latter occurs with IBD and celiac disease.

The symptoms of lactose intolerance include bloating, flatulence, cramping abdominal pain, and diarrhea. Symptoms generally occur within 30 minutes to several hours after drinking a glass of milk or ingesting a milk product. The diarrhea of lactose intolerance results from fluid secretion into the small intestine, responding to the osmotic action of undigested lactose.

Many lactose-intolerant persons are aware of their milk intolerance and avoid milk and milk products. Lactose intolerance is diagnosed with a lactose tolerance test, a lactose hydrogen breath test, or genetic testing.

Treatment consists of eliminating lactose from the diet by avoiding milk and milk products and/or replacing lactase with commercially available preparations. Milk and ice cream contain more lactose than cheese. Live culture yogurt is an alternative source of calcium, but the patient needs to be sure that milk products have not been added to the yogurt.

A lactose-free diet is given initially and may be gradually advanced to a low-lactose diet as tolerated by the patient. Teach the patient that adherence to the diet is important. Many lactose-intolerant persons may not exhibit symptoms if lactose is taken in small amounts. In some persons, lactose may be tolerated better if taken with meals. Since avoidance of milk and milk products can lead to calcium deficiency, supplements may be necessary to prevent osteoporosis. Lactase enzyme (Lactaid) is available commercially as an over-the-counter (OTC) product. It is mixed with milk and breaks down the lactose before the milk is ingested.

SHORT BOWEL SYNDROME

Short bowel syndrome (SBS) is a condition in which the small intestine does not have adequate surface area to absorb enough nutrients. Thus the person is unable to meet energy, fluid, electrolyte, and nutritional needs on a standard diet. Causes of SBS include diseases that damage the intestinal mucosa, surgical removal of too much small intestine (primarily in patients with Crohn's disease), and congenital defects. Without adequate surface area, lifetime parenteral nutrition is necessary for survival.

Resections of up to 50% of the small intestine cause little disturbance of bowel function, especially if the terminal ileum and ileocecal valve remain intact. The remaining intestine undergoes adaptive changes that are more pronounced in the ileum. The villi and crypts increase in size, and the absorptive capacity of the remaining intestine increases.

Clinical Manifestations

The predominant manifestations of SBS are diarrhea and steatorrhea (unabsorbed fat in the stool). Signs of malnutrition as well as vitamin and mineral deficiencies include weight loss, cobalamin and zinc deficiency, and hypocalcemia. The patient may develop lactase deficiency and bacterial overgrowth. Oxalate kidney stones may form because of increased colonic absorption of oxalate.

Collaborative Care

The overall goals of treatment are that the patient with SBS will have fluid and electrolyte balance, normal nutritional status, and control of diarrhea. In the period immediately following massive bowel resection, patients receive parenteral nutrition to replace fluid, electrolyte, and nutrient losses and to rest the bowel. An antisecretory agent (histamine [H_2]-blocker or proton pump inhibitor) may be given to decrease gastric acid secretion.

A diet high in carbohydrate and low in fat supplemented with soluble fiber, pectin, and the amino acid glutamine is often recommended. The patient with SBS is encouraged to eat at least six meals per day to increase the time of contact between food and the intestine. Oral intake can be supplemented with elemental nutrient formulas and tube feeding during the night. For patients with severe malabsorption, parenteral nutrition (see Chapter 40) may be used.[52] Oral supplements of calcium, zinc, and multivitamins are typically recommended.

Teduglutide (Gattex) is used in SBS in patients who need additional nutrition from parenteral nutrition. It is a subcutaneous injection given once daily that helps to improve intestinal absorption of fluids and nutrients, reducing the frequency and volume of parenteral nutrition.

Opioid antidiarrheal drugs are the most effective in decreasing intestinal motility (see Table 43-2). For patients who have limited ileal resections (less than 39 in [99 cm]), cholestyramine (Questran) reduces diarrhea resulting from unabsorbed bile acids by increasing their excretion in feces. Bile acids stimulate intestinal fluid secretion and reduce colonic fluid absorption.

Intestinal transplantation is a procedure performed at a few specialized transplant centers in the United States. Candidates for this procedure are patients with SBS, dependence on parenteral nutrition, and chronic liver disease. It is often considered a last-resort treatment option for patients with intestinal failure who develop life-threatening complications from parenteral nutrition. Transplantation may include the intestine alone, liver and intestine, or multivisceral combinations (stomach, duodenum, jejunum, ileum, colon, and pancreas).

GASTROINTESTINAL STROMAL TUMORS

Gastrointestinal stromal tumors (GISTs) are a rare form of cancer that originates in cells found in the wall of the GI tract.[53] These cells, known as interstitial cells of Cajal, help control the movement of food and liquid through the stomach and intestines. About 55% of GISTs are found in the stomach; 35% are found in the small intestine; 5% are found in the rectum; and the rest are found in the esophagus, colon, or peritoneum.[53] GISTs are most frequently diagnosed in people between the ages of 50 and 70. Most GISTs are caused by genetic mutations.

The manifestations of GISTs depend on the part of the GI tract affected. Early manifestations are often subtle, including early satiety, bloating, nausea, and vomiting. Because these manifestations are similar to those of many other GI problems, the cancer is difficult to detect early. Later manifestations may include GI bleeding and obstruction caused by growth of the tumor. Often the GIST is found during evaluation (e.g., endoscopy, x-ray) for other problems such as CRC or stomach cancer. The diagnosis of GIST is based on histologic examination of biopsied tissue. Endoscopic ultrasound can be used to determine the extent of the tumor.

Patients initially undergo surgery to remove the tumor, but the GIST has often metastasized by the time of diagnosis or commonly recurs. GISTs are unresponsive to conventional chemotherapy. However, discovery of genetic mutations led to the development of tyrosine kinase inhibitor drugs (e.g., imatinib mesylate [Gleevec]) that are highly effective against GISTs.[43] (Targeted drug therapies are discussed in Chapter 16.)

ANORECTAL PROBLEMS

HEMORRHOIDS

Hemorrhoids are dilated hemorrhoidal veins. They may be internal (occurring above the internal sphincter) or external (occurring outside the external sphincter) (Figs. 43-15 and 43-16). Symptoms include rectal bleeding, pruritus, prolapse, and pain. In affected persons, hemorrhoids appear periodically, depending on the amount of anorectal pressure.

Etiology and Pathophysiology

Hemorrhoids develop as a result of increased anal pressure and weakened connective tissue that normally supports the hemorrhoidal veins. When supporting tissues in the anal canal weaken, usually as a result of straining at defecation, venules become dilated. In addition, blood flow through the veins of the hemorrhoidal plexus is impaired. An intravascular clot in the venule results in a thrombosed external hemorrhoid.

Hemorrhoids are the most common reason for bleeding with defecation. The amount of blood lost at one time may be small, but over time it may lead to iron-deficiency anemia. Hemorrhoids may be precipitated by many factors, including pregnancy, prolonged constipation, straining in an effort to defecate, heavy lifting, prolonged standing and sitting, and portal hypertension (as found in cirrhosis).

Clinical Manifestations

The classic manifestations of hemorrhoidal disease include bleeding, anal pruritus, prolapse, and pain. The patient with internal hemorrhoids may be asymptomatic. However, when internal hemorrhoids become constricted, the patient will

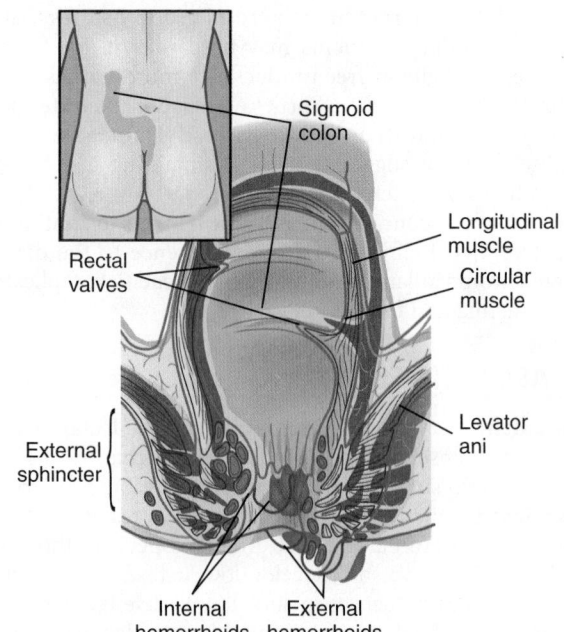

FIG. 43-15 Anatomic structures of the rectum and anus with external and internal hemorrhoids.

report pain. Internal hemorrhoids can bleed, resulting in blood on toilet paper after defecation or blood on the outside of stool. The patient may report a chronic, dull, aching discomfort, particularly when the hemorrhoids have prolapsed.

External hemorrhoids are reddish blue and seldom bleed. Blood clots in external hemorrhoids cause pain and inflammation, and the hemorrhoids are described as thrombosed. External hemorrhoids cause intermittent pain, pain on palpation, itching, and burning. Patients also report bleeding associated with defecation. Constipation or diarrhea can aggravate these symptoms.

Diagnostic Studies and Collaborative Care

Internal hemorrhoids are diagnosed by digital examination, anoscopy, and sigmoidoscopy. External hemorrhoids can be diagnosed by visual inspection and digital examination.

Therapy is directed toward the causes and the patient's symptoms. A high-fiber diet and increased fluid intake prevent constipation and reduce straining, which allows engorgement of the veins to subside. The resulting stool bulk may also decrease stool leakage and therefore itching. Ointments such as dibucaine; creams, suppositories, and impregnated pads that contain

FIG. 43-16 Thrombosed external hemorrhoids.

antiinflammatory agents (e.g., hydrocortisone); or astringents and anesthetics (e.g., witch hazel, benzocaine) may be used to shrink the mucous membranes and relieve discomfort. The use of topical corticosteroids such as hydrocortisone agents should be limited to 1 week or less to prevent side effects such as contact dermatitis and mucosal atrophy. Stool softeners may be ordered to keep the stools soft, and sitz baths help relieve pain.

External hemorrhoids are usually managed by conservative therapy unless they become thrombosed. For internal hemorrhoids, nonsurgical approaches (rubber band ligation, infrared coagulation, cryotherapy, laser treatment) can be used. Rubber band ligation is the most widely used technique. An anoscope is inserted so the hemorrhoid can be identified and then ligated with a rubber band. The rubber band around the hemorrhoid constricts circulation, and the tissue becomes necrotic, separates, and sloughs off. There is some local discomfort with this procedure, but no anesthetic is required. Aspirin or acetaminophen is usually given for discomfort. Infrared coagulation can be used to treat bleeding internal hemorrhoids. In this procedure, either infrared or electric current produces local inflammation. Cryotherapy involves rapid freezing of the hemorrhoid.

A *hemorrhoidectomy* is the surgical excision of hemorrhoids. Surgery is indicated when there is prolapse, excessive pain or bleeding, or large hemorrhoids. In general, hemorrhoidectomy is reserved for patients with severe symptoms related to multiple thrombosed hemorrhoids or marked protrusion. Surgical removal may be done by cautery, clamp, or excision. One surgical approach is to leave the area open so that healing takes place by secondary intention. In another approach, the hemorrhoids are removed, the tissue is sutured, and wound healing takes place by primary intention.

NURSING MANAGEMENT
HEMORRHOIDS

Conservative nursing management for the patient with hemorrhoids includes teaching measures to prevent constipation, avoid prolonged standing or sitting, and properly use OTC drugs for hemorrhoidal symptoms. Teach the patient to seek medical care for severe symptoms of hemorrhoids (e.g., excessive pain and bleeding, prolapsed hemorrhoids). Sitz baths (15 to 20 minutes) two or three times each day for 7 to 10 days may help reduce discomfort and swelling associated with hemorrhoids.

Pain caused by sphincter spasm is a common problem after a hemorrhoidectomy. Be aware that although the procedure is minor, the pain is severe. Opioids are usually given initially. Postoperatively, topical nitroglycerin preparations may be used to decrease pain and subsequent opioid use.

Sitz baths are started 1 or 2 days after surgery. A warm sitz bath provides comfort and keeps the anal area clean. A sponge ring in the sitz bath helps relieve pressure on the area. Initially, the patient should not be left alone because of the possibility of weakness or fainting.

Packing may be inserted into the rectum to absorb drainage, with a T-binder used to hold the dressing in place. If packing is inserted, it usually is removed on the first or second postoperative day. Assess for rectal bleeding. The patient may be embarrassed when the dressing is changed, and privacy should be provided. The patient usually dreads the first bowel movement and often resists the urge to defecate. Pain medication may be given before the bowel movement to reduce discomfort.

A stool softener such as docusate (Colace) is usually ordered for the first few postoperative days. If the patient does not have a bowel movement within 2 or 3 days, an oil-retention enema is given. Teach the patient the importance of diet, care of the anal area, symptoms of complications (especially bleeding), and avoidance of constipation and straining. Sitz baths are recommended for 1 to 2 weeks. The health care provider may order a stool softener to be taken for a time. Hemorrhoids may recur. Occasionally, anal strictures develop and dilation is necessary. Regular checkups are important to prevent any further problems.

ANAL FISSURE

An *anal fissure* is a skin ulcer or a crack in the lining of the anal wall that is caused by trauma, local infection, or inflammation (Fig. 43-17). Fissures are considered either primary or secondary based on their etiology. *Primary fissures* usually occur as a result of local trauma, such as vaginal delivery. High pressure in the internal anal sphincter can result in ischemia, which can lead to fissuring. *Secondary fissures* are due to a variety of conditions, including IBD, prior anal surgery, and infection (syphilis; tuberculosis; gonorrhea; or infection with *Chlamydia*, herpes simplex virus, or HIV).

Anal tissue ulcerates because of ischemia caused by a combination of high resting anal sphincter tone and poor blood supply to the area. The ischemic tissue may ulcerate spontaneously or when traumatized by factors such as hard stools that would not normally cause tissue breakdown. If ischemia is not corrected, the anal fissures will not be able to heal.

The major symptoms are anal pain and bleeding. Pain is especially severe during and after defecation and has been described as "passing broken glass."[54] Bleeding is bright red and usually slight. Constipation results because of fear of pain associated with bowel movements.

Anal fissures are diagnosed through physical examination. Conservative care with fiber supplements, adequate fluid intake, sitz baths, and topical analgesics is successful in some cases, especially if the situation is acute. Topical preparations, including nitrates and calcium channel blockers, are used to decrease rectal anal pressure to allow the fissure to heal without sphincter damage. Local injections of botulinum toxin are also used to decrease rectal anal pressure, and are most effective when

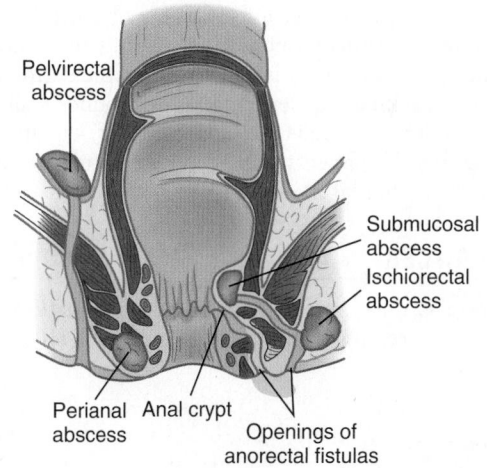

FIG. 43-17 Common sites of anorectal abscesses and fistula formation.

combined with nitrates. Pain may be decreased by softening stools with mineral oil or stool softeners. Warm sitz baths (15 to 20 minutes, three times per day) and anal anesthetic suppositories with hydrocortisone (Anusol-HC) are also ordered.

If topical medications are ineffective, a lateral internal sphincterotomy is the recommended surgical procedure, but it carries the risk of postoperative incontinence. Postoperative nursing care is the same as the care for the patient who has had a hemorrhoidectomy.

ANORECTAL ABSCESS

An *anorectal abscess* is a collection of perianal pus (see Fig. 43-17). The abscess is the result of obstruction of the anal glands, leading to infection and subsequent abscess formation. Abscess formation can occur secondary to anal fissures, trauma, or IBD. The most common causative organisms are *Escherichia coli*, staphylococci, and streptococci. Clinical manifestations include local severe pain and swelling, foul-smelling drainage, tenderness, and elevated temperature. Sepsis can occur as a complication. Anorectal abscesses are diagnosed by rectal examination.

Surgical therapy consists of drainage of abscesses. If packing is used, it should be impregnated with petroleum jelly, and the area should be allowed to heal by granulation. The packing is changed every day, and moist, hot compresses are applied to the area. Care must be taken to avoid soiling the dressing during urination or defecation. A low-fiber diet is given. The patient may leave the hospital with the wound still open. Teach the patient about wound care and the importance of sitz baths, thorough cleaning after bowel movements, and follow-up visits to a health care provider.

ANAL FISTULA

An **anal fistula** is an abnormal tunnel leading from the anus or rectum. It may extend to the outside of the skin, vagina, or buttocks and often precedes an abscess. Anal fistulas are a complication of Crohn's disease and may resolve when drug treatment (i.e., with infliximab) achieves remission of the disease. About 50% of anal fistulas are due to anorectal abscess.

Feces may enter the fistula and cause an infection. There may be persistent, blood-stained, purulent discharge or stool leakage from the fistula. The patient may need to wear a pad to avoid staining clothes.

Surgical therapy involves a fistulotomy or a fistulectomy. In a fistulotomy the fistula is opened, and healthy tissue is allowed to granulate. A fistulectomy is an excision of the entire fistulous tract. Gauze packing is inserted, and the wound is allowed to heal by granulation. Care is the same as that given after a hemorrhoidectomy. In patients with complex fistulas, fibrin glue may be injected to seal the fistula.

ANAL CANCER

Anal cancer is uncommon in the general population, but the incidence is increasing. Human papillomavirus (HPV) is associated with about 80% of the cases of anal cancer. The American Cancer Society estimates that about 7100 people are diagnosed with anal cancer each year in the United States, with more women diagnosed than men.[55] Risk factors include having many sexual partners, genital warts (which are caused by HPV), smoking, receptive anal sex, and HIV infection. The average age at diagnosis is 60. Anal cancer is more common in African Americans than in whites.

Most frequently the initial symptom is rectal bleeding. Other symptoms include rectal pain and sensation of a rectal mass. Some patients have no symptoms, which leads to delayed diagnosis and treatment.

It is especially important to screen high-risk individuals. A swab of the anal mucosa can be obtained during a digital rectal examination. Identification of cell changes (e.g., dysplasia, neoplasia) can be determined. High-resolution anoscopy allows for visualization of the mucosa and biopsy. An endo-anal (*endorectal*) *ultrasound* may also be done.

The use of condoms to reduce the transmission of HPV is recommended. The HPV vaccine Gardasil is used for the prevention of anal cancer and associated precancerous lesions caused by HPV types 6, 11, 16, and 18. Gardasil is also approved for the prevention of cervical, vulvar, and vaginal cancer and the associated precancerous lesions caused by HPV in women. (It is also approved for the prevention of genital warts in men and women.) Another HPV vaccine, Cervarix, may also be useful in the prevention of HPV-associated anal cancer. After vaccination with HPV vaccine, patients at risk need to continue their recommended screening program.

Treatment of anal cancer depends on the size and depth of the lesions. Topical therapy with bichloroacetic or trichloroacetic acid may be used to kill the HPV virus. Imiquimod (Aldara), an immunomodulator, is also used as a topical agent. Therapy also includes surgery, radiation, and chemotherapy. Chemotherapy may include mitomycin, cisplatin (Platinol), and 5-FU.

PILONIDAL SINUS

A *pilonidal sinus* is a small tract under the skin between the buttocks in the sacrococcygeal area. It is thought to be of congenital origin. It may have several openings and is lined with epithelium and hair, hence the name *pilonidal* ("a nest of hair"). The skin is moist, and movement of the buttocks causes the short, wiry hair to penetrate the skin. The irritated skin becomes infected and forms a pilonidal cyst or abscess. There are no symptoms unless there is an infection. If it becomes infected, the patient complains of pain and swelling at the base of the spine.

The formed abscess requires incision and drainage. The wound may be closed or left open to heal by secondary intention. The wound is packed, and sitz baths are ordered. Nursing care includes warm, moist heat applications when an abscess is present. The patient is usually more comfortable lying on the abdomen or side. Teach the patient to avoid contaminating the dressing when urinating or defecating and to avoid straining whenever possible.

CASE STUDY

Colorectal Cancer

iStockphoto/Thinkstock

Patient Profile

L.C., a 58-year-old Native American man, is from a Pueblo tribe in northern New Mexico. L.C.'s wife and family drove 50 miles to take him to the Indian Health Service hospital because of his deteriorating health (see the case study in Chapter 39).

Subjective Data

See the case study in Chapter 39 on p. 874.

Objective Data

Physical Examination

See the case study in Chapter 39 on p. 877.

Laboratory Tests

- CT scan and colonoscopy show two medium-sized tumors in the transverse colon

Collaborative Care

Surgical Procedure

- Transverse hemicolectomy performed and lymph node biopsies taken
- Pathology results indicate that the adenocarcinoma tumor has invaded the muscle wall of colon and 2 out of 5 lymph nodes are positive for cancer

Postoperative

- Feels like his life has ended and does not want to leave hospital.
- States that there is no one to take care of him at his home and he is far away from the hospital.

Follow-Up Treatment

- Scheduled for outpatient chemotherapy

Discussion Questions

1. What are the signs and symptoms of colorectal cancer that L.C. manifested (see the case study in Chapter 39 on p. 874)?
2. What types of diagnostic information are available from a colonoscopy versus a sigmoidoscopy?
3. What stage of CRC does L.C. probably have? What treatment is recommended for this stage of CRC?
4. How could you provide emotional support to L.C. and his family?
5. What is a culturally sensitive way for you to support L.C. and his family in making decisions about his continued health care?
6. *Priority Decision:* Based on the assessment data, what are the priority nursing diagnoses? Are there any collaborative problems?
7. *Priority Decision:* What are the priority nursing interventions for L.C. at this stage of his illness?
8. *Evidence-Based Practice:* L.C. had not had a previous colonoscopy. He is worried that other members of his family may have colon cancer. What can you tell him about the recommendations for colorectal cancer screening?

evolve   Answers available at *http://evolve.elsevier.com/Lewis/medsurg.*

BRIDGE TO NCLEX EXAMINATION

The number of the question corresponds to the same-numbered outcome at the beginning of the chapter.

1. The appropriate collaborative therapy for the patient with acute diarrhea caused by a viral infection is to
   a. increase fluid intake.
   b. administer an antibiotic.
   c. administer antimotility drugs.
   d. quarantine the patient to prevent spread of the virus.

2. When a 35-year-old female patient is admitted to the emergency department with acute abdominal pain, which possible diagnosis should you consider that may be the cause of her pain (*select all that apply*)?
   a. Gastroenteritis
   b. Ectopic pregnancy
   c. Gastrointestinal bleeding
   d. Irritable bowel syndrome
   e. Inflammatory bowel disease

3. Assessment findings suggestive of peritonitis include
   a. rebound abdominal pain.
   b. a soft, distended abdomen.
   c. dull, continuous abdominal pain.
   d. observing that the patient is restless.

4. In planning care for the patient with Crohn's disease, the nurse recognizes that a major difference between ulcerative colitis and Crohn's disease is that Crohn's disease
   a. frequently results in toxic megacolon.
   b. causes fewer nutritional deficiencies than ulcerative colitis.
   c. often recurs after surgery, whereas ulcerative colitis is curable with a colectomy.
   d. is manifested by rectal bleeding and anemia more frequently than is ulcerative colitis.

5. The nurse performs a detailed assessment of the abdomen of a patient with a possible bowel obstruction, knowing that manifestations of an obstruction in the large intestine are (*select all that apply*)
   a. persistent abdominal pain.
   b. marked abdominal distention.
   c. diarrhea that is loose or liquid.
   d. colicky, severe, intermittent pain.
   e. profuse vomiting that relieves abdominal pain.

6. A patient with stage I colorectal cancer is scheduled for surgery. Patient teaching for this patient would include an explanation that
   a. chemotherapy will begin after the patient recovers from the surgery.
   b. both chemotherapy and radiation can be used as palliative treatments.
   c. follow-up colonoscopies will be needed to ensure that the cancer does not recur.
   d. a wound, ostomy, and continence nurse will visit the patient to identify an abdominal site for the ostomy.

7. The nurse explains to the patient undergoing ostomy surgery that the procedure that maintains the most normal functioning of the bowel is
   a. a sigmoid colostomy.
   b. a transverse colostomy.
   c. a descending colostomy.
   d. an ascending colostomy.

8. In contrast to diverticulitis, the patient with diverticulosis
   a. has rectal bleeding.
   b. often has no symptoms.
   c. has localized cramping pain.
   d. frequently develops peritonitis.

9. A nursing intervention that is most appropriate to decrease postoperative edema and pain after an inguinal herniorrhaphy is
   a. applying a truss to the hernia site.
   b. allowing the patient to stand to void.
   c. supporting the incision during coughing.
   d. applying a scrotal support with ice bag.

10. The nurse determines that the goals of dietary teaching have been met when the patient with celiac disease selects from the menu
    a. scrambled eggs and sausage.
    b. buckwheat pancakes with syrup.
    c. oatmeal, skim milk, and orange juice.
    d. yogurt, strawberries, and rye toast with butter.

11. What should a patient be taught after a hemorrhoidectomy?
    a. Take mineral oil before bedtime.
    b. Eat a low-fiber diet to rest the colon.
    c. Administer oil-retention enema to empty the colon.
    d. Use prescribed pain medication before a bowel movement.

1. a, 2. a, b, c, d, e, 3. a, 4. c, 5. a, b, 6. c, 7. a, 8. b, 9. d, 10. a, 11. d

Ⓔvolve

For rationales to these answers and even more NCLEX review questions, visit *http://evolve.elsevier.com/Lewis/medsurg.*

REFERENCES

1. Navaneethan U, Giannella RA: Definition, epidemiology, pathophysiology, clinical classification, and differential diagnosis of diarrhea. In Guandalini S, Vaziri H, editors: *Diarrhea diagnostic and therapeutic advances*, New York, 2011, Humana.

2. McClarren RL, Lynch B, Nyayapati N: Acute infectious diarrhea, *Prim Care Clin Office Pract* 38:539, 2011.

3. Newton JM, Surawicz CM: Infectious gastroenteritis and colitis. In Guandalini S, Vaziri H, editors: *Diarrhea diagnostic and therapeutic advances*, New York, 2011, Humana.

4. Guandalini S: Probiotics for diarrheal disease. In Guandalini S, Vaziri H, editors: *Diarrhea diagnostic and therapeutic advances*, New York, 2011, Humana.

5. O'Keefe SJD: Tube feeding, the microbiota, and *Clostridium difficile* infection, *World J Gatroenterol* 16:139, 2010.

6. Weissman JS, Coyle W: Stool transplants: ready for prime time? *Curr Gastroenterol Rep* 14:313, 2012.

7. Hurnauth C: Management of faecal incontinence in acutely ill patients, *Nurs Stand* 25:48, 2011.

8. Fargo MV, Latimer KM: Evaluation and management of common anorectal conditions, *Am Fam Physician* 15:624, 2012.

*9. Bliss DZ, Savik K, Thorson MAL, et al: Incontinence-associated dermatitis in critically ill adults: time to development, severity, and risk factors, *J Wound Ostomy Continence Nurs* 38:433, 2011.

10. Chipps T: Using behavioural methods to manage faecal incontinence, *Br J Nurs* 20:1172, 2011.

11. Emmanuel A: Review of the efficacy and safety of transanal irrigation for neurogenic bowel dysfunction, *Spinal Cord* 48:664, 2010.

12. Marchetti F, Corallo JP, Ritter J, et al: Retention cuff pressure study of three indwelling stool management systems: randomized study of 10 healthy subjects, *J Wound Ostomy Continence Nurs* 38:569, 2011.

13. Apau D: Assessing the cause of constipation and appropriate interventions, *Gastrointestinal Nurs* 8:24, 2010.

*14. Zhou L, Lin Z, Lin L, et al: Functional constipation: implications for nursing interventions, *J Clin Nurs* 19:1838, 2010.

15. Roerig JL, Steffen KJ, Mitchell JE, et al: Laxative abuse: epidemiology, diagnosis, and management, *Drugs* 70:503, 2010.

*16. Michna E, Blonsky ER, Schulman S, et al: Subcutaneous methylnaltrexone for treatment of opioid-induced constipation in patients with chronic, nonmalignant pain: a randomized controlled study, *J Pain* 12:554, 2011.

17. Suares NC, Ford AC: Systematic review: the effects of fibre in the management of chronic idiopathic constipation, *Aliment Pharmacol Ther* 33:895, 2011.

18. Schein M: The acute abdomen. In Schein M, Rogers P, Assalia A, editors: *Schein's common sense emergency abdominal surgery*, Berlin, 2010, Springer Verlag.

19. Harris LA, Heitkemper MM: Practical considerations for recognizing and managing severe irritable bowel syndrome, *Gastroenterol Nurs* 35:12, 2012.

20. Gibson PR, Shepherd SJ: Evidence-based dietary management of functional gastrointestinal symptoms: the FODMAP approach, *J Gastroenterol Hepatol* 25:252, 2010.

21. Saadia R: Penetrating abdominal trauma. In Schein M, Rogers P, Assalia A, editors: *Schein's common sense emergency abdominal surgery*, Berlin, 2010, Springer Verlag.

22. Schein M: Abdominal compartment syndrome. In Schein M, Rogers P, Assalia A, editors: *Schein's common sense emergency abdominal surgery*, Berlin, 2010, Springer Verlag.

23. National Digestive Diseases Information Clearinghouse: Appendicitis. Retrieved from *http://digestive.niddk.nih.gov/ddiseases/pubs/appendicitis/appendicitis_508.pdf.*

24. Kaser A, Zeissig S, Blumberg RS: Inflammatory bowel disease, *Ann Rev Immunol* 28:573, 2010.

25. Lomer MCE: Symposium 7: nutrition in inflammatory bowel disease: dietary and nutritional considerations for inflammatory bowel disease, *Proc Nutr Soc* 70:329, 2011.

26. Hou JK, Abraham B, El-Serag H: Dietary intake and risk of developing inflammatory bowel disease: a systematic review of the literature, *Am J Gastroenterol* 106:563, 2011.

27. Berg AM, Kelly CP, Farraye FA: *Clostridium difficile* infection in the inflammatory bowel disease patients, *Inflamm Bowel Dis*, 19:194, 2013.

28. American Cancer Society: Colorectal cancer. Retrieved from *www.cancer.org/Cancer/ColonandRectumCancer/DetailedGuide/colorectal-cancer-detection.*

29. Fisher LR, Hasler WL: New vision in video capsule endoscopy: current status and future directions, *Nat Rev Gastroenterol Hepatol* 9:392, 2012.

30. Yanai H, Hanauer SB: Assessing response and loss of response to biological therapies in IBD, *Am J Gastroenterol* 106:685, 2011.

31. Masoomi H, Kang CY, Chaudhry O, et al: Predictive factors of early bowel obstruction in colon and rectal surgery: data from the Nationwide Inpatient Sample, 2006-2008, *J Am Coll Surg* 214:831, 2012.

32. Garq M, Lubel JS, Sparrow MP, et al: Review article: vitamin D and inflammatory bowel disease—established concepts and future directions, *Aliment Pharmacol Ther* 36:324, 2012.

*Evidence-based information for clinical practice.

33. del Val JH: Old-age inflammatory bowel disease onset: a different problem? *World J Gastroenterol* 17:2734, 2011.

34. Schein M: Small bowel obstruction. In Schein M, Rogers P, Assalia A, editors: *Schein's common sense emergency abdominal surgery*, Berlin, 2010, Springer Verlag.

35. Dolan EA: Malignant bowel obstruction: a review of current treatment strategies, *Am J Hospice Palliat Med* 28:576, 2011.

36. Framp A: Working toward understanding the impact of hereditary cancers, *Gastroenterol Nurs* 33:400, 2010.

37. American College of Gastroenterology: Colorectal cancer screening for African Americans. Retrieved from *http:// s3.gi.org/patients/ccrk/ColonCancerFinal.pdf*.

38. Labianca R, Nordlinger B, Beretta GD, et al: Primary colon cancer: ESMO clinical practice guidelines for diagnosis, adjuvant treatment and follow-up, *Ann Oncol* 21(Suppl 5):v70, 2010.

39. Landers M, Savage E, McCarthy G, et al: Self-care strategies for the management of bowel symptoms following sphincter-saving surgery for rectal cancer, *Clin J Oncol Nurs* 15:E105, 2011.

*40. Pittman J: Characteristics of the patient with an ostomy, *J Wound Ostomy Continence Nurs* 38:271, 2011.

41. Deitz D, Gates J: Basic ostomy management, part 1, *Nursing* 40:61, 2010.

42. Ostomy Guidelines Task Force: Management of the patient with a fecal ostomy: best practice guidelines for clinicians, *J Wound Ostomy Continence Nurs* 37:596, 2010.

43. United Ostomy Associations of America: Intimacy after ostomy surgery. Retrieved from *www.ostomy.org/ostomy_info/pubs/ uoaa_sexuality_en.pdf*.

44. Burch J: Resuming a normal life: holistic care of the person with an ostomy, *Br J Community Nurs* 16:366, 2011.

45. Weizman AV, Nguyen GC: Diverticular disease: epidemiology and management, *Can J Gastroenterol* 35:385, 2011.

*46. Mason RJ, Moazzez A, Sohn HJ, et al: Laparoscopic versus open anterior abdominal wall hernia repair: 30-day morbidity and mortality using the ACS-NSQIP data base, *Ann Surg* 254:641, 2011.

47. Ryan M, Grossman S: Celiac disease: implications for patient management, *Gastroenterol Nurs* 34:225, 2011.

48. Gainer CL: Celiac disease: helping patient live gluten-free, *Nurse Pract* 36:14, 2011.

*49. Smith MM, Goodfellow L: The relationship between quality of life and coping strategies of adults with celiac disease adhering to a gluten-free diet, *Gastroenterol Nurs* 34:460, 2011.

50. Armstrong MJ, Hegade V: Advances in coeliac disease, *Curr Opin Gastroenterol* 28:104, 2012.

51. Lee AR, Ng DL, Diamond B, et al: Living with celiac disease: survey from the USA, *J Hum Nutr Diet* 25:233, 2012.

52. Burns DL, Gill BM: Reversal of parenteral nutrition–associated liver disease with a fish oil–based lipid emulsion (Omegaven) in an adult dependent on home parenteral nutrition, *J Parenter Enteral Nutr* 37:274, 2013.

53. Joensuu H, DeMatteo RP: The management of gastrointestinal stromal tumors: a model for targeted and multidisciplinary therapy of malignancy, *Ann Rev Med* 63:247, 2012.

54. Fargo MW, Latimer KM: Evaluation and management of common anorectal conditions, *Am Fam Physician* 15:624, 2012.

55. American Cancer Society: Anal cancer. Retrieved from www.cancer.org/cancer/analcancer/detailedguide/anal-cancer -what-is-key-statistics.

RESOURCES

American Gastroenterological Association
   www.gastro.org
American Society for Gastrointestinal Endoscopy (ASGE)
   www.asge.org
Celiac Sprue Association
   www.csaceliacs.info
Crohn's and Colitis Foundation of America (CCFA)
   www.ccfa.org
International Ostomy Association
   www.ostomyinternational.org
Society of Gastroenterology Nurses and Associates
   www.sgna.org
Wound, Ostomy, and Continence Nurses Society
   www.wocn.org

Life loves the liver of it.
Anne Elizabeth Alice Louise

Nursing Management
Liver, Pancreas, and Biliary Tract Problems

Anne Croghan

℮volve WEBSITE

http://evolve.elsevier.com/Lewis/medsurg

- NCLEX Review Questions
- Key Points
- Pre-Test
- Answer Guidelines for Case Study on p. 1041
- Rationales for Bridge to NCLEX Examination Questions
- Case Studies
  - Patient With Acute Pancreatitis and Septic Shock
  - Patient With Cholelithiasis/ Cholecystitis

- Patient With Cirrhosis
- Patient With Hepatitis
- Nursing Care Plans (Customizable)
  - eNCP 44-1: Patient With Acute Viral Hepatitis
  - eNCP 44-2: Patient With Cirrhosis
  - eNCP 44-3: Patient With Acute Pancreatitis
- Concept Map Creator
- Concept Map for Case Study on p. 1041
- Glossary
- Content Updates

eFigures
- eFig. 44-1: Sengstaken-Blakemore tube
- eFig. 44-2: Total portal diversion after transjugular intrahepatic portosystemic shunt (TIPS)
- eFig. 44-3: X-ray of a gallbladder with gallstones

eTable
- eTable 44-1: Drug Therapy: Side Effects of Interferon, Ribavirin, Telaprevir, and Boceprevir

LEARNING OUTCOMES

1. Differentiate among the types of viral hepatitis, including etiology, pathophysiology, clinical manifestations, complications, and collaborative care.
2. Describe the nursing management of the patient with viral hepatitis.
3. Describe the pathophysiology, clinical manifestations, complications, and collaborative care of the patient with nonalcoholic fatty liver disease.
4. Explain the etiology, pathophysiology, clinical manifestations, complications, collaborative care, and nursing management of the patient with cirrhosis of the liver.
5. Describe the clinical manifestations and management of liver cancer.
6. Differentiate between acute and chronic pancreatitis related to pathophysiology, clinical manifestations, complications, collaborative care, and nursing management.
7. Explain the clinical manifestations, collaborative care, and nursing management of the patient with pancreatic cancer.
8. Describe the pathophysiology, clinical manifestations, complications, and collaborative care of gallbladder disorders.
9. Describe the nursing management of the patient undergoing surgical treatment of cholecystitis and cholelithiasis.

KEY TERMS

acute liver failure, p. 1027
acute pancreatitis, p. 1030
ascites, p. 1019
asterixis, p. 1021
biliary sludge, p. 1030
cholecystitis, p. 1036
cholelithiasis, p. 1036
chronic pancreatitis, p. 1034

cirrhosis, p. 1017
esophageal varices, p. 1019
gastric varices, p. 1019
hepatic encephalopathy, p. 1021
hepatitis, p. 1007
hepatorenal syndrome, p. 1021
jaundice, p. 1009

nonalcoholic fatty liver disease (NAFLD), p. 1016
nonalcoholic steatohepatitis (NASH), p. 1016
paracentesis, p. 1022
portal hypertension, p. 1019
spider angiomas, p. 1018

Reviewed by Paula Cox-North, RN, PhD, NP-C, Harborview Medical Center, Seattle, Washington; Trevah A. Panek, RN, MSN, CCRN, Assistant Professor of Nursing, Saint Francis University, Loretto, Pennsylvania; and Sally P. Scavone, RN, MS, Professor of Nursing, Erie Community College, Buffalo, New York.

Nursing management of patients with liver, pancreatic, and gall-bladder problems is the focus of this chapter. Viral hepatitis, cirrhosis, acute pancreatitis, cholecystitis, and cholelithiasis are described in detail.

DISORDERS OF THE LIVER

HEPATITIS

Hepatitis is a broad term that means inflammation of the liver. Hepatitis is most commonly caused by viruses but can also be caused by drugs (alcohol), chemicals (see Table 39-6), autoimmune diseases, and metabolic abnormalities.

Viral Hepatitis

The types of viral hepatitis are A, B, C, D, and E. They differ in their modes of transmission and clinical manifestations (Table 44-1). The different hepatitis viruses can be responsible for both acute and chronic liver disease.

Other less common viruses can also cause liver disease. These include cytomegalovirus (CMV), Epstein-Barr virus (EBV), herpesvirus, coxsackievirus, and rubella virus.

Hepatitis A Virus. Hepatitis A viral infection can cause a mild flu-like illness or acute hepatitis with jaundice. It can also cause acute liver failure. It does not result in a chronic (long-term) infection. In the United States the incidence of hepatitis A viral infection has declined since vaccination was recommended for at-risk persons and children (at the age of 1 year).[1]

Hepatitis A virus (HAV) is a ribonucleic acid (RNA) virus that is transmitted primarily through the fecal-oral route. It frequently occurs in small outbreaks caused by fecal contamination of food or drinking water. Poor hygiene, improper handling of food, crowded situations, and poor sanitary conditions are contributing factors. Transmission occurs between family members, institutionalized individuals, and children in day care centers. Foodborne hepatitis A outbreaks are usually due to food contaminated by an infected food handler.

The virus is present in feces during the incubation period, so it can be carried and transmitted by persons who have undetectable, subclinical infections. The greatest risk of transmission occurs before clinical symptoms are apparent. HAV is found in feces 2 or more weeks before the onset of symptoms and up to 1 week after the onset of jaundice (Fig. 44-1). It is present only briefly in blood. Anti-HAV (antibody to HAV) immunoglobulin (Ig) M appears in the serum as the stool becomes negative for the virus. Detection of hepatitis A IgM indicates acute hepatitis. Although not commonly tested clinically, hepatitis A IgG indicates past infection. IgG antibody

FIG. 44-1 Jaundiced patient.

TABLE 44-1 CHARACTERISTICS OF HEPATITIS VIRUSES

Incubation Period and Mode of Transmission	Sources of Infection	Infectivity
Hepatitis A Virus (HAV) 15-50 days (average 28) Fecal-oral (primarily fecal contamination and oral ingestion)	Crowded conditions (e.g., day care, nursing home). Poor personal hygiene. Poor sanitation. Contaminated food, milk, water, shellfish. Persons with subclinical infections, infected food handlers; sexual contact, IV drug users.	Most infectious during 2 wk before onset of symptoms. Infectious until 1-2 wk after the start of symptoms.
Hepatitis B Virus (HBV) 45-180 days (average 56-96) Percutaneous (parenteral) or permucosal exposure to blood or blood products Sexual contact Perinatal transmission	Contaminated needles, syringes, and blood products. Sexual activity with infected partners. Asymptomatic carriers. Tattoos or body piercing with contaminated needles.	Before and after symptoms appear. Infectious for 4-6 mo. Carriers continue to be infectious for life.
Hepatitis C Virus (HCV) 14-180 days (average 56) Percutaneous (parenteral) or mucosal exposure to blood or blood products High-risk sexual contact Perinatal contact	Blood and blood products. Needles and syringes. Sexual activity with infected partners.	1-2 wk before symptoms appear. Continues during clinical course. 75%-85% go on to develop chronic hepatitis C and remain infectious.
Hepatitis D Virus (HDV) 2-26 wk HBV must precede HDV Chronic carriers of HBV always at risk	Same as HBV. Can cause infection only when HBV is present. Routes of transmission same as for HBV.	Blood infectious at all stages of HDV infection.
Hepatitis E Virus (HEV) 15-64 days (average 26-42 days) Fecal-oral route Outbreaks associated with contaminated water supply in developing countries	Contaminated water, poor sanitation. Found in Asia, Africa, and Mexico. Not common in United States.	Not known. May be similar to HAV.

provides lifelong immunity (Fig. 44-2). Hepatitis A vaccination and thorough hand washing are the best measures to prevent outbreaks.

Hepatitis B Virus. Hepatitis B virus (HBV) can cause either acute or chronic disease. Transmission occurs when the virus (from infected blood or body fluids) enters the body of an uninfected person who has not received the HBV vaccine. Since the 1990s, the incidence of HBV infection has decreased because of the widespread use of the HBV vaccine.[1]

About 12 million Americans have been infected with HBV. In the majority of adults with acute hepatitis B, the infection completely resolves. Of the more than 1 million Americans who develop chronic infections, liver impairment may range from a normal liver to severe liver disease. Approximately 15% to 25% of chronically infected persons die from chronic liver disease.

HBV is a deoxyribonucleic acid (DNA) virus. It can be transmitted perinatally by mothers infected with HBV; percutaneously (e.g., IV drug use, accidental needle-stick punctures); or

by mucosal exposure to infectious blood, blood products, or other body fluids (e.g., semen, vaginal secretions, saliva). In people with HBV, hepatitis B surface antigen (HBsAg) has been detected in almost every body fluid. Infected semen and saliva contain much lower concentrations of HBV than blood, but the virus can be transmitted via these secretions. If gastrointestinal (GI) bleeding occurs, feces can be contaminated with the virus from the blood. There is no evidence that urine, feces (without GI bleeding), breast milk, tears, and sweat are infective. Organ and tissue transplantation is another potential source of infection. In some patients with acute hepatitis B, there is no readily identifiable risk factor.[1]

Sexual transmission is a common mode of HBV transmission. Men who have sex with men (especially those practicing unprotected anal intercourse) are at risk for HBV infection. Although the risk of transmission is much lower, kissing and sharing food items may spread the virus via saliva. Other at-risk individuals include those who live with chronically infected persons, hemodialysis patients, and health care and public safety workers. HBV can live on a dry surface for at least 7 days; it is much more infectious than human immunodeficiency virus (HIV).

HBV is a complex structure with three distinct antigens: the surface antigen (HBsAg), the core antigen (HBcAg), and the e antigen (HBeAg). HBsAg in the serum for 6 months or longer after infection indicates chronic HBV infection. Each antigen has a corresponding antibody that may develop in response to HBV infection. The presence of hepatitis B surface antibody (anti-HBs) in the blood indicates immunity from the HBV vaccine or from past HBV infection (Fig. 44-3).

Hepatitis C Virus. Infection with the hepatitis C virus (HCV) can result in both acute and chronic illness. Acute hepatitis C, which is usually asymptomatic, can be difficult to detect unless diagnosed with laboratory testing. The most common causes of acute hepatitis C are injection drug use and outbreaks among HIV-positive men who have sex with men.

The majority of patients who acquire hepatitis C usually develop chronic infection.[2] Most are unaware of their infection. Chronic HCV results in a potentially progressive liver disease, with 20% to 30% of these patients developing cirrhosis. Hepa-

FIG. 44-2 Course of infection with hepatitis A virus *(HAV)*. *ALT,* Alanine aminotransferase.

FIG. 44-3 Course of infection with hepatitis B virus *(HBV)*. *ALT,* Alanine aminotransferase; *anti-HBc,* antibody to hepatitis B core antigen; *anti-HBe,* antibody to HBeAg; *anti-HBs,* antibody to HBsAg; *HBeAg,* hepatitis B e antigen; *HBsAg,* hepatitis B surface antigen.

titis C is the most common cause of chronic liver disease and the most common indication for liver transplantation in the United States.[3]

HCV is an RNA virus that is primarily transmitted percutaneously. The most common mode of HCV transmission is the sharing of contaminated needles and equipment among IV drug users.

The proportion of cases attributed to high-risk sexual behavior (e.g., unprotected sex, multiple partners) has increased in recent years. In the United States, 10% of all cases of HCV infection are due to occupational exposure, hemodialysis, and perinatal transmission.[2] Some patients with HCV cannot identify a source. The risk of perinatal HCV transmission is higher in women who are co-infected with both HIV and HCV.

Patients given blood or blood products before 1992 (when blood product testing for HCV began) may be at risk for chronic HCV infection and should be tested. Because of the 15- to 20-year delay between infection and the clinical appearance of liver damage, long-term effects of HCV infection pose important future health care challenges. Chronic HBV and HCV account for 80% of the cases of hepatocellular cancer.

Persons at risk for HCV infection are also at risk for HBV and HIV infections. About 30% to 40% of HIV-infected patients also have HCV. This high rate of co-infection is primarily related to IV drug use. Co-infection with HIV and HCV places the patient at greater risk for progression to cirrhosis.

Hepatitis D Virus. Hepatitis D virus (HDV), also called *delta virus,* is a defective single-stranded RNA virus that cannot survive on its own. It requires hepatitis B to replicate. It can be acquired at the same time as HBV, or a person with HBV can be infected with HDV at a later time. HDV is transmitted percutaneously, similar to HBV. It can cause a spectrum of illness ranging from an asymptomatic chronic carrier state to acute liver failure. There is no vaccine for HDV. However, vaccination against HBV reduces the risk of HDV co-infection.

Hepatitis E Virus. Hepatitis E virus (HEV) is an RNA virus transmitted by the fecal-oral route. The usual mode of transmission is drinking contaminated water. Hepatitis E infection occurs primarily in developing countries, with epidemics reported in India, Asia, Mexico, and Africa. Only a few cases of HEV have been reported in the United States, primarily in persons who recently traveled to an HEV-endemic area.

Pathophysiology

Liver. During an acute viral hepatitis infection, liver damage is mediated by cytotoxic cytokines and natural killer cells that cause lysis of infected hepatocytes. Inflammation can interrupt bile flow (cholestasis). After resolution of an acute infection, liver cells can regenerate and, if no complications occur, resume their normal appearance and function.

A chronic viral hepatitis infection causes chronic inflammation and can cause fibrosis that (over decades) can progress to cirrhosis. (Cirrhosis is discussed later in this chapter.)

Systemic Effects. The antigen-antibody complexes between the virus and its corresponding antibody may form circulating immune complexes in the early phases of hepatitis. The circulating immune complexes activate the complement system (see Chapter 12). The clinical manifestations of this activation are rash, angioedema, arthritis, fever, and malaise. *Cryoglobulinemia* (abnormal proteins found in the blood), glomerulonephritis, and vasculitis have also been found secondary to immune complex activation.

TABLE 44-2	**MANIFESTATIONS OF HEPATITIS**
Acute Hepatitis	**Chronic Hepatitis**
• Anorexia	• Malaise
• Nausea, vomiting	• Easy fatigability
• Right upper quadrant discomfort	• Hepatomegaly
• Constipation or diarrhea	• Myalgias and/or arthralgias
• Decreased sense of taste and smell	• Elevated liver enzymes (aspartate aminotransferase [AST] and alanine aminotransferase [ALT])
• Malaise	
• Headache	
• Fever	
• Arthralgias	
• Urticaria	
• Hepatomegaly	
• Splenomegaly	
• Weight loss	
• Jaundice	
• Pruritus	
• Dark urine	
• Bilirubinuria	
• Light stools	
• Fatigue	
• Continued hepatomegaly with tenderness	
• Weight loss	

Clinical Manifestations

The clinical manifestations of viral hepatitis can be classified into acute and chronic phases (Table 44-2). A large number of patients with acute hepatitis have no symptoms. As a result, infection during the acute phase may not be detected in all patients. However, others may have intermittent or ongoing malaise, fatigue, myalgias, arthralgias, and hepatomegaly.

The acute phase usually lasts from 1 to 4 months. During the incubation period, symptoms may include malaise, anorexia and weight loss, fatigue, nausea, occasional vomiting, and abdominal (right upper quadrant) discomfort. The patient may find food repugnant, and smokers may have distaste for cigarettes. There is also a decreased sense of smell. Other symptoms may include headache, low-grade fever, arthralgias, and skin rashes. Physical examination may reveal hepatomegaly, lymphadenopathy, and sometimes splenomegaly. The acute phase is the period of maximal infectivity.

The acute phase may be *icteric* (jaundice) or anicteric. (Types of jaundice are presented in Table 44-3.) Jaundice, a yellowish discoloration of body tissues, results from an alteration in normal bilirubin metabolism or flow of bile into the hepatic or biliary duct systems. (Normal bilirubin metabolism is presented in Fig. 39-4.) The urine may darken because of excess bilirubin being excreted by the kidneys. If conjugated bilirubin cannot flow out of the liver because of obstruction or inflammation of the bile ducts, the stools will be light or clay colored. *Pruritus* (intense chronic itching) sometimes accompanies jaundice. The pruritus occurs as a result of the accumulation of bile salts beneath the skin.

The convalescent phase following the acute phase begins as jaundice fades and lasts for weeks to months, with an average of 2 to 4 months. During this period, the patient's major complaint is malaise and easy fatigability. Hepatomegaly remains for several weeks, but splenomegaly subsides during this period.

Prior infection with HAV or HBV can provide immunity to that virus *(homologous immunity).* However, the patient can still

TABLE 44-3 CLASSIFICATION OF JAUNDICE

	Hemolytic Jaundice	Hepatocellular Jaundice	Obstructive Jaundice
Causes	• Blood transfusion reactions, sickle cell crisis, hemolytic anemia.	• Hepatitis, cirrhosis, hepatocellular carcinoma.	• Hepatitis, cirrhosis, hepatocellular carcinoma. Common bile duct obstruction from stone(s), biliary strictures, sclerosing cholangitis, and pancreatic cancer.
Description	• Caused by increased breakdown of RBCs, which produces an increased amount of unconjugated bilirubin in blood. • Liver is unable to handle increased load.	• Results from liver's altered ability to take up bilirubin from the blood or to conjugate or excrete it. • In hepatocellular disease, damaged hepatocytes leak bilirubin.	• Results from decreased or obstructed flow of bile through liver or biliary duct system. • Obstruction may occur in intrahepatic or extrahepatic bile ducts. Intrahepatic obstructions are due to swelling or fibrosis of the liver's canaliculi and bile ducts.
Diagnostic Findings ***Serum Bilirubin*** Unconjugated (indirect) Conjugated (direct)	↑ Normal	↑ ↑ or ↓ (severe disease)	Somewhat ↑ Moderately ↑
Urine Bilirubin	Negative	↑	↑
Urobilinogen Stool Urine	↑ ↑	Normal, ↓ Normal, ↑	↓ ↓

be infected with another type of viral hepatitis. An individual with hepatitis C can be reinfected with another strain of HCV.

Complications

Most patients with acute viral hepatitis recover completely. The overall mortality rate for acute hepatitis is less than 1%. The mortality rate is higher in older adults and those with underlying debilitating illnesses (including chronic liver disease). Complications that can occur include acute liver failure, chronic hepatitis, cirrhosis of the liver, and hepatocellular carcinoma.

Almost all cases of acute hepatitis A resolve, although a small number may have a viral relapse in the first 2 to 3 months after the infection. The disappearance of jaundice does not mean the patient has totally recovered. Some HBV infections and the majority of HCV infections result in chronic (lifelong) viral infection.

Chronic HBV is more likely to develop in infants born to infected mothers and in those who acquire the infection before age 5 than in those who acquire the virus after age 5.[1] Alterations in the patient's cellular immune response may be important in the development of the chronic HBsAg carrier state and the progression of acute HBV to chronic HBV. These immune system alterations may explain why the patient with chronic kidney disease who is undergoing dialysis when hepatitis B is acquired is more at risk for developing chronic infection.[4] Persons with chronic kidney disease have a depressed cellular immune response.

HCV infection is more likely than HBV to become chronic.[5] As previously mentioned, many patients with chronic HCV infection develop chronic liver disease, cirrhosis, and hepatocellular cancer.[6] Risk factors for progression to cirrhosis include male gender, alcohol consumption, and excess iron deposition in the liver. Elevated cholesterol or triglycerides, obesity, and diabetes mellitus are also risk factors for the progression of HCV to cirrhosis.

Diagnostic Studies

The only definitive way to distinguish among the various forms of viral hepatitis is by testing the patient's blood for the specific antigen or antibody. In some types of viral hepatitis, the blood can be tested for the viral level (also known as the *viral load*). Tests for the different types of viral hepatitis are presented in Table 44-4. In viral hepatitis, many of the liver function tests show significant abnormalities. The common abnormalities are shown in Table 44-5.

Several tests are available to determine the presence of HCV. Initial testing for HCV infection includes HCV antibody testing. If the antibody test is positive, HCV RNA testing should be obtained to assess for chronic infection; a positive result confirms chronic infection. A small number of patients may have a false-positive HCV antibody test with a negative HCV RNA test. If recent HCV infection is suspected, HCV RNA testing is usually obtained because it may take several weeks or longer for HCV antibodies to develop. This testing may also be helpful in the immunocompromised patient (e.g., patient with HIV). Because of altered or delayed antibody response to HCV, these patients may not have detectable antibody levels even though they are infected with HCV.

Viral genotype testing is done in patients undergoing drug therapy for HBV or HCV infection. HBV has at least eight different genotypes (A to H). In some centers, HBV genotyping is performed before starting treatment. HBV genotype may be useful in predicting disease and treatment outcomes.[6]

HCV has six genotypes and more than 50 subtypes. In the United States, 75% of HCV infections are caused by HCV genotype 1. Genotype is one of the strongest predictors of response to drug therapy.[7] For patients who test positive for HCV, genotyping is obtained before drug therapy is started.

Physical assessment may reveal hepatic tenderness, hepatomegaly, and splenomegaly. The liver is palpable. A liver biopsy is not indicated in acute hepatitis unless the diagnosis is in doubt. In chronic hepatitis a liver biopsy may be done. Biopsy of liver tissue allows for histologic examination of liver cells and characterization of the degree of inflammation, fibrosis, or cirrhosis that may be present. A patient who has a bleeding disorder may not be an appropriate candidate for biopsy because of the risk of bleeding. In these patients a transjugular biopsy may be an option.

TABLE 44-4   TESTS FOR VIRAL HEPATITIS

Virus	Tests	Significance
A	Anti-HAV immunoglobulin M (IgM)	Acute infection.
	Anti-HAV immunoglobulin G (IgG)	Previous infection or immunization. Not routinely done in clinical practice.
B	HBsAg (hepatitis B surface antigen)	Marker of infectivity.
		Present in acute or chronic infection.
		Positive in chronic carriers.
	Anti-HBs (hepatitis B surface antibody)	Indicates previous infection with HBV or immunization.
	HBeAg (hepatitis B e antigen)	Indicates high infectivity.
		Used to determine the clinical management of patients with chronic hepatitis B.
	Anti-HBe (hepatitis B e antibody)	Indicates previous infection.
		In chronic hepatitis B, indicates a low viral load and low degree of infectivity.
	Anti-HBc (antibody to hepatitis B core antigen) IgM	Indicates acute infection.
		Does not appear after vaccination.
	Anti-HBc IgG	Indicates previous infection or ongoing infection with hepatitis B.
		Does not appear after vaccination.
	HBV DNA quantitation	Indicates active ongoing viral replication.
		Best indicator of viral replication and effectiveness of therapy in patient with chronic hepatitis B.
	HBV genotyping	Indicates the genotype of HBV.
C	Anti-HCV (antibody to HCV)	Marker for acute or chronic infection with HCV.
	HCV RNA quantitation	Indicates active ongoing viral replication.
	HCV genotyping	Indicates the genotype of HCV.
D	Anti-HDV	Present in past or current infection with HDV.
	HDV Ag (hepatitis D antigen)	Present within a few days after infection.
E*	Anti-HEV IgM and IgG	Present 1 wk–2 mo after illness onset.
	HEV RNA quantitation	Indicates active ongoing viral replication.

*Currently, no serologic tests to diagnose HEV infection are commercially available in the United States. However, diagnostic tests are available in research laboratories to detect IgM and IgG anti-HEV and HEV RNA levels.
A, Hepatitis A virus (HAV); *B*, hepatitis B virus (HBV); *C*, hepatitis C virus (HCV); *D*, hepatitis D virus (HDV); *E*, hepatitis E virus (HEV).

TABLE 44-5   DIAGNOSTIC FINDINGS IN ACUTE HEPATITIS

Test	Abnormal Finding	Etiology
Transaminases (aminotransferases)		
• Aspartate aminotransferase (AST)	Increased in acute phase	Liver cell injury
	Decreases as jaundice disappears	
• Alanine aminotransferase (ALT)	Increased in acute phase	Liver cell injury
	Decreases as jaundice disappears	
γ-Glutamyl transpeptidase (GGT)	Increased	Liver cell injury
Alkaline phosphatase	Moderately increased	Impaired excretory function of the liver
Serum proteins		
• γ-Globulin	Normal or increased	Impaired clearance from liver
• Albumin	Normal or decreased	Liver cell damage
Serum bilirubin (total)	Increased to about 8-15 mg/dL (137-257 μmol/L)	Liver cell damage
Urinary bilirubin	Increased	Conjugated hyperbilirubinemia
Urinary urobilinogen	Increased 2-5 days before jaundice	Diminished reabsorption of urobilinogen
Prothrombin time	Prolonged	Decreased prothrombin production by liver

Techniques for noninvasive assessment of liver fibrosis may eventually replace the need for liver biopsy. Options include the FibroScan, which uses an ultrasound transducer to determine liver fibrosis. FibroSure (FibroTest) is a biomarker that uses the results of serum tests (e.g., liver enzyme levels) to assess the degree of hepatic fibrosis.[8]

Collaborative Care

There is no specific treatment or therapy for acute viral hepatitis. Most patients can be managed at home. Emphasis is on measures to rest the body and assist the liver in regenerating (Table 44-6). Adequate nutrition and rest seem to be most beneficial for healing and liver cell regeneration. Rest reduces the metabolic demands on the liver and promotes cell regeneration. The degree of rest ordered depends on the severity of symptoms, but usually alternating periods of activity and rest are adequate. Counseling should include the importance of avoiding alcohol and notification of possible contacts for testing and prophylaxis, if indicated.

Drug Therapy. There are no drug therapies for the treatment of acute hepatitis A infection. Treatment of acute hepatitis B is indicated only in patients with severe hepatitis and liver failure. In persons with acute hepatitis C, treatment with pegylated interferon within the first 12 to 24 weeks of infection decreases the development of chronic hepatitis C.[2] Supportive drug therapy may include antiemetics for nausea, such as prochlorperazine (Compazine), promethazine (Phenergan), or ondansetron (Zofran).

Chronic Hepatitis B. Drug therapy for chronic HBV is focused on decreasing the viral load and liver enzymes and slowing the rate of disease progression. Long-term goals are prevention of cirrhosis, liver failure, and hepatocellular cancer.

TABLE 44-6   COLLABORATIVE CARE
Viral Hepatitis

Diagnostic
- History and physical examination
- Liver function studies
- Alanine aminotransferase (ALT)
- Aspartate aminotransferase (AST)
- Serum bilirubin
- Prothrombin time (PT) and INR
- Alkaline phosphatase
- γ-Glutamyl transpeptidase
- Hepatitis testing:
  - *Hepatitis A:* Anti-HAV IgM
  - *Hepatitis B:* HBsAg, anti-HBs, HBeAg, anti-HBe, anti-HBc IgM and IgG, HBV DNA quantitation, HBV genotyping
  - *Hepatitis C:* Anti-HCV, HCV RNA quantitation, HCV genotyping
  - *Hepatitis D:* Anti-HDV, HDV Ag
- FibroScan
- FibroSure (FibroTest)

Collaborative Therapy
Acute and Chronic
- Well-balanced diet
- Vitamin supplements
- Rest (degree of strictness varies)
- Avoidance of alcohol intake and drugs detoxified by the liver

Chronic HBV
- Standard interferon (Intron A)
- Pegylated interferon (PegIntron, Pegasys)
- Nucleoside and nucleotide analogs
  - lamivudine (Epivir)
  - adefovir (Hepsera)
  - entecavir (Baraclude)
  - telbivudine (Tyzeka)
  - tenofovir (Viread)

Chronic HCV
- Pegylated interferon
- ribavirin (Rebetol, Copegus)
- Protease inhibitors
  - telaprevir (Incivek)
  - boceprevir (Victrelis)

HAV, hepatitis A virus; *HB,* hepatitis B; *HBeAg,* hepatitis B e antigen; *HBsAg,* hepatitis B surface antigen; *HBV,* hepatitis B virus; *HCV,* hepatitis C virus; *HDV Ag,* hepatitis D antigen; *HDV,* hepatitis D virus; *INR,* international normalized ratio.

COMPLEMENTARY & ALTERNATIVE THERAPIES
Milk Thistle (Silymarin)

Scientific Evidence
- Previous studies suggested that milk thistle may benefit the liver by protecting and promoting the growth of liver cells and inhibiting inflammation. These studies were small and not well designed.
- Two rigorously designed studies found no real benefit from using milk thistle:
  - Silymarin was no better than placebo for chronic hepatitis C in people who had not responded to standard antiviral treatment.*
  - Hepatitis C patients who used silymarin had fewer and milder symptoms of liver disease and somewhat better quality of life but no change in virus activity or liver inflammation.†

Nursing Implications
- Appears to be well tolerated in recommended doses for up to 6 yr.
- May lower blood glucose.
- May interfere with the liver's cytochrome P450 enzyme system.

*Fried MW, Navarro VJ, Afdhal N, et al: Effect of silymarin (milk thistle) on liver disease in patients with chronic hepatitis C who failed interferon therapy: a randomized, placebo-controlled trial, *JAMA* 308(3):274, 2012.
†Seeff LB, Curto TM, Szabo G, et al: Herbal product use by persons enrolled in the hepatitis C Antiviral Long-Term Treatment Against Cirrhosis (HALT-C) Trial, *Hepatology* 47(2):605, 2008.

Current drug therapies for chronic HBV do not eradicate the virus, but work well to suppress viral replication and prevent complications of hepatitis B.[9] First-line therapies include pegylated interferon and nucleoside and nucleotide analogs (see Table 44-6).

Interferon. Interferon has multiple effects on the viral replication cycle. After binding to receptors on host cell membranes, the drug blocks viral entry into cells, synthesis of viral proteins, and viral assembly and release (see Fig. 14-4). There are two forms of interferon: standard (Intron A) and pegylated. Standard (conventional) interferon has a short half-life, necessitating frequent subcutaneous administrations (three times per week). In contrast, the long-acting preparations (pegylated interferons) are administered subcutaneously less frequently (just once per week), making them more convenient. In addition, with the long-acting preparations, blood levels remain high between doses, and therefore clinical responses are better.

The long-acting preparations are made by conjugating a standard interferon with polyethylene glycol (PEG), in a process known as *pegylation.* Therapeutic effects of the pegylated products (Pegasys and PegIntron) are due solely to its interferon component. The PEG component serves only to delay elimination of the drug. Because of their convenience and superior efficacy, these products are preferred to standard interferon and are used in both hepatitis B and hepatitis C treatment.

In patients with HBV receiving interferon, one third will have a significant reduction of serum HBV DNA levels, normalization of alanine aminotransferase (ALT) levels, and loss of HBeAg. The response to treatment may vary based on viral genotype. Interferon treatment is associated with a number of side effects (see eTable 44-1 on the website for this chapter). These side effects are dose related and tend to decrease in severity with continued treatment. Patients receiving interferon should have blood counts and liver function tests performed every 4 to 6 weeks.

Nucleoside and Nucleotide Analogs. HBV reproduces by making copies of its viral DNA nucleosides and nucleotides. The nucleoside and nucleotide analog drugs fool the virus into thinking they are normal building blocks for DNA. Thus the virus is unable to reproduce.

Nucleoside and nucleotide analogs do not prevent all viral reproduction, but they can substantially lower the amount of virus in the body. These medications include lamivudine (Epivir), adefovir (Hepsera), entecavir (Baraclude), telbivudine (Tyzeka), and tenofovir (Viread). These oral medications are used in the treatment of chronic HBV when there is evidence of active viral replication.

Nucleoside and nucleotide analogs have beneficial effects in terms of reducing viral load, decreasing liver damage, and decreasing liver enzymes. Most patients with HBV require long-term treatment with these medications.[10] When these drugs are stopped, the majority of patients (except those who have seroconverted) have HBV DNA and liver enzyme levels that return to pretreatment levels.

Severe exacerbations of hepatitis B have developed after discontinuation of treatment. If these drugs are discontinued, monitor liver function closely for several months.

Chronic Hepatitis C. Drug therapy is directed at eradicating the virus and preventing HCV-related complications.[11] Treatment for HCV includes pegylated interferon given with ribavirin (Rebetol, Copegus). Patients who have HCV genotype 1 also receive either telaprevir (Incivek) or boceprevir (Victrelis), which are HCV protease inhibitors.[11] Protease is an enzyme that is essential in viral replication.

Treatment of chronic hepatitis C is individualized and based on the genotype, the severity of liver disease, potential side effects, presence of co-morbid conditions, patient's readiness for treatment, and presence of other health problems (e.g., HIV). Pegylated interferon is injected once a week, and ribavirin is taken orally twice daily. Both boceprevir and telaprevir are taken orally every 8 hours. Ribavirin, given in combination with pegylated interferon, has a synergistic effect and reduces the rate of relapse following hepatitis C treatment. Ribavirin has a number of side effects (see eTable 44-1 on the website for this chapter).

> **DRUG ALERT: Ribavirin (Rebetol, Copegus)**
> • During treatment, pregnancy must be avoided both by women taking the drug and by women whose male partners are taking the drug.

Many patients with HIV also have HCV. Patients who have stable HIV and relatively intact immune systems (CD4+ counts greater than 200/μL) are treated for HCV with the goal of eradicating HCV and reducing the risk of progression to cirrhosis. HCV treatment may reduce CD4+ counts, and increase the patient's risk for anemia and leukopenia.

Patients who have advanced fibrosis or cirrhosis can be treated with drug therapy as long as liver decompensation (e.g., ascites, esophageal hemorrhage, jaundice, wasting, encephalopathy) is not present.

Depression or mood changes are common in patients receiving treatment for HCV. Patients need to be screened for depression and other mood disorders before starting interferon-based treatment and monitored frequently while on therapy.[12]

Nutritional Therapy. No special diet is required in the treatment of viral hepatitis. Emphasis is placed on a well-balanced diet that the patient can tolerate. During acute viral hepatitis, adequate calories are important because the patient usually loses weight. If fat content is poorly tolerated because of decreased bile production, it should be reduced. Vitamin supplements, particularly B-complex vitamins and vitamin K, are frequently used. If anorexia, nausea, and vomiting are severe, IV solutions of glucose or supplemental enteral nutrition therapy may be used. Fluid and electrolyte balance must be maintained.

NURSING MANAGEMENT
VIRAL HEPATITIS

NURSING ASSESSMENT
Subjective and objective data that should be obtained from a person with hepatitis are presented in Table 44-7.

NURSING DIAGNOSES
Nursing diagnoses for the patient with viral hepatitis may include, but are not limited to, the following:
• Imbalanced nutrition: less than body requirements *related to* anorexia and nausea
• Activity intolerance *related to* fatigue and weakness
• Risk for impaired liver function *related to* viral infection

---

TABLE 44-7 NURSING ASSESSMENT
*Hepatitis**

Subjective Data
Important Health Information
Past health history: Hemophilia; exposure to infected persons; ingestion of contaminated food or water; exposure to benzene, carbon tetrachloride, or other hepatotoxic agents; crowded, unsanitary living conditions; exposure to contaminated needles; recent travel; organ transplant recipient; exposure to new drug regimens, hemodialysis, transfusion of blood or blood products before 1992; HIV status (if known)
Medications: Use and misuse of acetaminophen, new prescription, over-the-counter, or herbal medications or supplements

Functional Health Patterns
Health perception–health management: IV drug and alcohol abuse; malaise, distaste for cigarettes (in smokers), high-risk sexual behaviors
Nutritional-metabolic: Weight loss, anorexia, nausea, vomiting; feeling of fullness in right upper quadrant
Elimination: Dark urine; light-colored stools, constipation or diarrhea; skin rashes, hives
Activity-exercise: Fatigue, arthralgias, myalgias
Cognitive-perceptual: Right upper quadrant pain and liver tenderness, headache; pruritus
Role-relationship: Exposure as health care worker, long-term care institution resident, incarceration, homeless

Objective Data
General
Low-grade fever, lethargy, lymphadenopathy

Integumentary
Rash or other skin changes, jaundice, icteric sclera, injection sites

Gastrointestinal
Hepatomegaly, splenomegaly

Possible Diagnostic Findings
Elevated liver enzyme levels; ↑ serum total bilirubin, hypoalbuminemia, anemia, bilirubin in urine and increased urobilinogen, prolonged prothrombin time, positive tests for hepatitis, including anti-HAV IgM, HBsAg, anti-HBs, HBeAg, anti-HBe, anti-HBc IgM and IgG, HBV DNA quantitation, anti-HCV, HCV RNA quantitation, anti-HDV; HDV Ag; abnormal liver scan; abnormal results on liver biopsy

*Hepatitis includes both viral and nonviral causes.
HAV, Hepatitis A virus; *HBcAg,* hepatitis B core antigen; *HBeAg,* hepatitis B e antigen; *HBsAg,* hepatitis B surface antigen; *HBV,* hepatitis B virus; *HCV,* hepatitis C virus; *HDV Ag,* hepatitis D antigen; *HDV,* hepatitis D virus.

Additional information is presented on nursing diagnoses for the patient with viral hepatitis in eNursing Care Plan 44-1 (on the website for this chapter).

PLANNING
The overall goals are that the patient with viral hepatitis will (1) have relief of discomfort, (2) be able to resume normal activities, and (3) return to normal liver function without complications.

NURSING IMPLEMENTATION
HEALTH PROMOTION. Viral hepatitis is a public health problem. Your role is important in the prevention and control of this disease. It is helpful to understand the epidemiology of the different types of viral hepatitis before considering appropriate control measures. Preventive and control measures for hepatitis A, B, and C are summarized in Table 44-8.

TABLE 44-8	PREVENTIVE MEASURES FOR VIRAL HEPATITIS*

Hepatitis A	**Hepatitis B and C**
General Measures	**Percutaneous Transmission**
• Hand washing	Screening of donated blood
• Proper personal hygiene	• *HBV:* HBsAg
• Environmental sanitation	• *HCV:* Anti-HCV
• Control and screening (signs, symptoms) of food handlers	Use of disposable needles and syringes
• Serologic screening for those carrying virus	**Sexual Transmission**
• Active immunization: HAV vaccine	• Acute exposure: HBIG administration to sexual partner of HBsAg-positive person
Use of Immune Globulin	• HBV vaccine series administered to uninfected sexual partners
• Early administration (1-2 wk after exposure) to those exposed	• Condoms used for sexual intercourse
• Prophylaxis for travelers to areas where hepatitis A is common if not vaccinated with HAV vaccine	**General Measures**
	• Hand washing
Special Considerations for Health Care Personnel	• Avoid sharing toothbrushes and razors
• Wash hands after contact with a patient or removal of gloves	• HBIG administration for one-time exposure (needle stick, contact of mucous membranes with infectious material)
• Use infection control precautions†	• Active immunization: HBV vaccine
	Special Considerations for Health Care Personnel
	• Use infection control precautions†
	• Reduce contact with blood or blood-containing secretions
	• Handle the blood of patients as potentially infective
	• Dispose of needles properly
	• Use needleless IV access devices when available

*A suggested guideline for general practice to prevent you from contracting viral hepatitis from diagnosed and undiagnosed patients and carriers is for you to wear disposable gloves, goggles, and gowns (sometimes) when fecal or blood contamination is likely in handling (1) soiled bedpans, urinals, and catheters; and (2) when the patient's bed linens are soiled by body excreta or secretions.
†See eTable 15-1 available on the website.
HAV, Hepatitis A virus; *HBIG,* hepatitis B immune globulin; *HBsAg,* hepatitis B surface antigen; *HBV,* hepatitis B virus; *HCV,* hepatitis C virus.

Hepatitis A. Outbreaks of viral hepatitis are usually due to HAV. Preventive measures include personal and environmental hygiene and health education to promote good sanitation. Hand washing is probably the most important precaution. Teach about careful hand washing after bowel movements and before eating.

Vaccination is the best protection against HAV. All children at 1 year of age should receive the vaccine. Adults at risk should also receive the vaccine. These include people who travel to areas with increased rates of hepatitis A, men who have sex with men, injecting and noninjecting drug users, persons with clotting factor disorders (e.g., hemophilia), and persons with chronic liver disease.[1]

There are currently several forms of the HAV vaccine, including Havrix, Vaqta, and Avaxim. HAV vaccine is inactivated HAV. Primary immunization consists of a single dose administered intramuscularly (IM) in the deltoid muscle. A booster is recommended 6 to 12 months after the primary dose to ensure adequate antibody titers and long-term protection. The primary immunization provides immunity within 30 days after a single dose in more than 95% of those vaccinated.

Twinrix, a combined HAV and HBV vaccine, is available for people over 18 years of age. Immunization consists of three doses, given on a 0-, 1-, and 6-month schedule, the same schedule as that used for the single HBV vaccine. Twinrix may be given to high-risk individuals, including patients with chronic liver disease, users of illicit IV drugs, patients on hemodialysis, men who have sex with men, and people with clotting factor disorders who receive therapeutic blood products. The side effects of the vaccine are mild and usually limited to soreness and redness at the injection site.

Isolation is not required for HAV infection. For a patient with HAV infection, use infection control precautions (see eTable 15-1 available on the website for that chapter). A private room is indicated if the patient is incontinent of stool or has poor personal hygiene.

Both hepatitis A vaccine and immune globulin (IG) are used for prevention of HAV infection after exposure to an infected person *(postexposure prophylaxis).* The vaccine is used for preexposure prophylaxis, and IG can be used either before or after exposure. IG provides temporary (1 to 2 months) passive immunity and is effective for preventing hepatitis A if given within 2 weeks after exposure. IG is recommended for persons who do not have anti-HAV antibodies and are exposed as a result of close (household, day care center) contact with persons who have HAV or foodborne exposure. Because patients with HAV are most infectious just before the onset of symptoms (the preicteric phase), those exposed through household contact or foodborne outbreaks should receive IG. Although IG may not prevent infection in all persons, it may modify the illness to a subclinical infection. When hepatitis A occurs in a food handler, IG should be administered to all other food handlers at the establishment. Patrons may also need to be given IG.

Persons who have received a dose of HAV vaccine more than 1 month previously or who have a history of laboratory-confirmed HAV infection do not require IG.

Hepatitis B. The best way to reduce HBV infection is to identify those at risk, screen them for HBV, and vaccinate those who are not infected. Teach individuals at high risk of contracting HBV to reduce risks. Good hygienic practices, including hand washing and using gloves when expecting contact with blood, are important. Patients should not share razors, toothbrushes, and other personal items. Teach patients to use a condom for sexual intercourse, and the partner should be vaccinated.

The HBV vaccine is the best means of prevention. The HBV vaccines (Recombivax HB, Engerix-B) contain HBsAg, which promotes the synthesis of specific antibodies directed against HBV. The vaccine is given in a series of three IM injections in the deltoid muscle. The second dose is administered within 1 month of the first one, and the third within 6 months of the first. The vaccine is more than 95% effective. Only minor adverse reactions have been reported with vaccination, including transient fever and soreness at the injection site. The vaccine is not contraindicated in pregnancy.

The first dose of hepatitis B vaccine should be given at birth, with the vaccine series completed by age 6 to 18 months. Older children and adolescents who did not previously receive the hepatitis B vaccine should also be vaccinated.[13] It is also important to vaccinate adults in the at-risk groups discussed above. Household members of the patient with HBV should be tested and vaccinated if they are HBsAg and antibody negative. Hepatitis vaccination is recommended for patients with chronic kidney disease before they start dialysis. Dialysis patients should routinely have their antibody titer levels checked to determine the need for revaccination.[13]

For postexposure prophylaxis, the HBV vaccine and hepatitis B immune globulin (HBIG) are used. HBIG contains antibodies to HBV and confers temporary passive immunity. HBIG is prepared from plasma of donors with a high titer of anti-HBs. HBIG is recommended for postexposure prophylaxis in cases of needle stick, mucous membrane contact, or sexual exposure and for infants born to mothers who are positive for HBsAg. Ideally HBIG should be given within 24 hours of exposure. The vaccine series should also be started.

According to Centers for Disease Control and Prevention (CDC) guidelines, follow infection control precautions for the patient with HBV. This includes using disposable needles and syringes and disposing of them in puncture-resistant units without recapping, bending, or breaking. (See eTable 15-1 on the website for that chapter for various types of infection control precautions.)

Hepatitis C. No vaccine is currently available for hepatitis C. The primary measures to prevent HCV transmission include screening of blood, organ, and tissue donors; use of infection control precautions; and modification of high-risk behavior. Identify individuals at high risk for contracting HCV and teach methods to reduce risks. Because of the number of people with hepatitis C who have not been diagnosed, the CDC recommends that all persons born between 1945 and 1965 undergo HCV testing regardless of risk factor status.[14] The CDC does not recommend IG or antiviral agents such as interferon for postexposure prophylaxis (e.g., needle-stick exposure from an infected patient) for HCV infection. After an acute exposure (e.g., needle stick), the person should have anti-HCV testing done. For the person exposed to HCV, baseline anti-HCV and ALT levels should be measured, with follow-up testing at 4 to 6 months. Testing for HCV RNA may be performed at 4 to 6 weeks.[15,16]

ACUTE INTERVENTION. In patients with hepatitis, assess for the presence and degree of jaundice. In light-skinned persons, jaundice is usually observed first in the sclera of the eyes and later in the skin. In dark-skinned persons, jaundice is observed in the hard palate of the mouth and inner canthus of the eyes. The urine may have a dark brown or brownish red color because of bilirubin. Comfort measures to relieve pruritus (if present), headache, and arthralgias are helpful (see eNursing Care Plan 44-1 on the website for this chapter).

Ensuring that the patient receives adequate nutrition is not always easy. The anorexia and distaste for food cause nutritional problems. Assess the patient's tolerance of specific foods and eating pattern. Small, frequent meals may be preferable to three large ones and may also help prevent nausea. Often a patient with hepatitis finds that anorexia is not as severe in the morning, so it is easier to eat a good breakfast than a large dinner. Measures to stimulate the appetite, such as mouth care, antiemetics, and attractively served meals in pleasant surroundings, should be included in your nursing care plan. Drinking carbonated beverages and avoiding very hot or very cold foods may help alleviate anorexia. Adequate fluid intake (2500 to 3000 mL/day) is important.

Rest is an important factor in promoting hepatocyte regeneration. Assess the patient's response to the rest and activity plan, and modify it accordingly. Liver function tests and symptoms are used as a guide to activity.

Psychologic and emotional rest is as essential as physical rest. Limited activity may produce anxiety and extreme restlessness in some patients. Diversional activities, such as reading and hobbies, may help.

AMBULATORY AND HOME CARE. Most patients with viral hepatitis are cared for at home, so you need to assess the patient's knowledge of nutrition and provide the necessary dietary teaching. Caution the patient about overexertion and the need to follow the health care provider's advice about when to return to work. Teach the patient and the caregiver how to prevent transmission to other family members. Also teach what symptoms should be reported to the health care provider.

Assess the patient for manifestations of complications. Bleeding tendencies with increasing prothrombin time values, symptoms of encephalopathy, or elevated liver function tests indicate problems.

Instruct the patient to have regular follow-up for at least 1 year after the diagnosis of hepatitis. Because relapses occur with hepatitis B and C, teach the patient the symptoms of recurrence and the need for follow-up evaluations. All patients with chronic HBV or HCV should avoid alcohol, since it can accelerate disease progression.

The patient who is receiving interferon for the treatment of HBV or HCV requires education regarding this drug. Because interferon is administered subcutaneously, the patient or the caregiver needs to be taught how to administer the drug. The numerous side effects with the therapy, including flu-like symptoms (e.g., fever, malaise, fatigue), make adherence to therapy challenging for some patients. Patients who are positive for HBsAg (chronic carrier status) or HCV antibody should not be blood donors.

EVALUATION
Expected outcomes are that the patient with hepatitis will
- Maintain food and fluid intake adequate to meet nutritional needs
- Demonstrate gradual increase in activity tolerance
- Perform daily activities with scheduled rest periods

Additional information on expected outcomes for the patient with hepatitis is provided in eNursing Care Plan 44-1 on the website for this chapter.

DRUG- AND CHEMICAL-INDUCED LIVER DISEASES

Alcohol consumption is a frequent cause of both acute and chronic liver disease. It can cause a spectrum of symptoms, ranging from mild elevation in liver enzymes (aspartate aminotransferase [AST] and ALT); to acute alcoholic hepatitis; to advanced fibrosis and cirrhosis, which usually occurs after decades of excessive alcohol intake. Patients may have serious liver disease caused by another chronic disease (e.g., chronic HCV infection) in combination with alcoholic liver disease.

Acute alcoholic hepatitis is a syndrome of enlarged liver (hepatomegaly), jaundice, elevation in liver enzyme tests (AST, ALT, alkaline phosphate), low-grade fever, and possibly ascites and prolonged prothrombin time. These symptoms may improve with cessation of alcohol intake.

Patients may have undetected liver disease and be seen with complications of cirrhosis. Even at this stage, abstinence can result in significant reversal in some patients. If liver function does not recover after abstaining from alcohol for several months or longer, liver transplantation may be considered.

Chemical hepatotoxicity is due to systemic poisons (e.g., carbon tetrachloride, gold compounds). However, because of their declining use, the incidence of these reactions has declined since the 1980s.

Drug-induced liver injury (DILI) is one of the more common causes of jaundice.[17] Many medications (prescription, over-the-counter [OTC], and herbal supplements) can cause an increase in liver enzymes and, in severe cases, jaundice and acute liver failure. The pattern of injury depends on the drug causing the reaction. The most common cause of DILI is acetaminophen.

> **DRUG ALERT: Acetaminophen (Tylenol)**
> - Drug is safe if taken at recommended levels. However, its prevalence in a variety of pain relievers, fever reducers, and cough medicines may mean that patients do not realize they are taking several drugs that all contain acetaminophen.
> - Many Americans each year experience acute liver failure as a result of taking acetaminophen. About 100 people die annually from overdosing, either intentionally or unintentionally.
> - Combining the drug with alcoholic beverages increases the risk of liver damage.

AUTOIMMUNE, GENETIC, AND METABOLIC DISEASES

Autoimmune Hepatitis

Autoimmune hepatitis is a chronic inflammatory disorder of the liver of unknown cause. It is characterized by the presence of autoantibodies, high levels of serum immunoglobulins, and frequent association with other autoimmune diseases. The majority of patients with autoimmune hepatitis are women. Laboratory tests are used to distinguish it from other forms of hepatitis. Serologic markers are often useful in the diagnosis. These include antinuclear antibodies (ANAs) and anti-DNA antibodies.

The disease process involves an autoimmune reaction against normal hepatocytes. Although it can cause acute liver failure, the course of the disease is variable, with most patients developing chronic hepatitis. Untreated autoimmune hepatitis can progress to cirrhosis. Prednisone with or without azathioprine (Imuran) is the recommended treatment for active autoimmune hepatitis. Cyclosporine (Gengraf), tacrolimus (Prograf, FK506), budesonide (Entocort), methotrexate, and mycophenolate mofetil (CellCept) have also been used in patients who do not respond to prednisone and azathioprine.

Wilson's Disease

Wilson's disease is an autosomal recessive defect in cellular copper transport. A defect in biliary excretion leads to accumulation of copper in the liver, causing progressive liver injury and cirrhosis. Approximately one in 40,000 people have Wilson's disease. It affects both men and women equally. Symptoms appear between ages 5 and 35.[18]

Once cirrhosis occurs, copper leaks into the plasma; accumulates in and damages other tissues; and can cause neurologic, hematologic, and renal disease. The hallmark of Wilson's disease is corneal Kayser-Fleischer rings. These are brownish red rings that can be seen in the cornea near the limbus on eye examination. Low serum ceruloplasmin levels and measurable copper concentrations from liver biopsy samples are also present. Diag-

nosis is based on clinical findings, including the corneal rings and neurologic symptoms. First-degree relatives of patients with Wilson's disease should be screened for the disease.

The recommended initial treatment of symptomatic patients or those with active disease is with chelating agents such as D-penicillamine (Cuprimine) or trientine (Syprine), which promote the excretion of urinary copper. Zinc acetate (Galzin), which has also been used as therapy, interferes with the absorption of copper. Liver transplantation may be required in patients who develop cirrhosis.

Hemochromatosis

Hemochromatosis is an iron overload disorder. Although it is primarily caused by a genetic defect *(hereditary hemochromatosis)*, it may also be caused by liver disease and chronic blood transfusions that are used to treat thalassemia and sickle cell disease. (Hemochromatosis is discussed in Chapter 31.)

Primary Biliary Cirrhosis

Primary biliary cirrhosis (PBC) is a chronic disease of the small bile ducts of the liver. In PBC, there is a T-cell–mediated attack of the small bile duct cells resulting in loss of bile ducts and ultimately *cholestasis* (blockage of bile flow). Over time, this leads to liver fibrosis and cirrhosis.

Most patients diagnosed with PBC are women between ages 30 and 65. The disease is associated with other autoimmune disorders such as rheumatoid arthritis, Sjögren's syndrome, and scleroderma. Elevated serum alkaline phosphatase levels, antimitochondrial antibodies (AMAs), ANAs, and serum lipid levels are seen in patients with PBC.

The goals of treatment are the suppression of ongoing liver damage, prevention of complications, and symptom management. The only approved drug for PBC is ursodeoxycholic acid (ursodiol [Actigall]). Management focuses on malabsorption, skin disorders such as pruritus and xanthomas (cholesterol deposits in the skin), hyperlipidemia, vitamin deficiencies, anemia, and fatigue. Cholestyramine (Questran) is used to treat pruritus. Patients are monitored for progression to cirrhosis. Liver transplantation is a treatment option for end-stage liver disease in patients with PBC.

Primary Sclerosing Cholangitis

Primary sclerosing cholangitis (PSC) is a disease of unknown etiology characterized by chronic inflammation, fibrosis, and strictures (narrowing) of the medium and large bile ducts. The majority of patients with PSC also have ulcerative colitis. Complications of PSC can include cholangitis, cholestasis with jaundice, cholangiocarcinoma (bile duct cancer), and cirrhosis.

Drug therapy has not been beneficial. Treatment is directed at reducing the incidence of biliary complications and screening for bile duct and colorectal cancer, which is related to the high incidence of ulcerative colitis. Patients with advanced liver disease may require liver transplantation.

Nonalcoholic Fatty Liver Disease and Nonalcoholic Steatohepatitis

Nonalcoholic fatty liver disease (NAFLD) refers to a wide spectrum of *liver diseases* ranging from a fatty liver (steatosis) to nonalcoholic steatohepatitis (NASH) to *cirrhosis*. In the spectrum of NAFLD, the common characteristic is the accumulation of fatty infiltration in the hepatocytes. In NASH the fat accumulation is associated with varying degrees of inflammation and fibrosis of the liver. NASH is a serious liver disease that can cause cirrhosis, hepatocellular cancer, and liver failure.

The term *nonalcoholic* is used because NAFLD and NASH occur in individuals who do not consume excessive amounts of alcohol. However, a pathologic analysis of liver cells in NAFLD is similar to that in alcoholic liver disease.

Currently, NAFLD affects about 10% to 20% of the U.S. population. This percentage is increasing because of the growing number of people who are obese. NAFLD should be considered in patients with risk factors such as obesity, diabetes, hyperlipidemia, and hypertension. NASH affects 2% to 5% of the U.S. population.[19] Elevations in liver function tests (ALT, AST) are often the first signs of NAFLD. Definitive diagnosis is by liver biopsy. Ultrasound and computed tomography (CT) scans are also used to diagnose NAFLD.

There is no definitive treatment, and therapy is directed at reduction of risk factors. This includes treatment of diabetes, reduction in body weight, and management of hyperlipidemia.

CIRRHOSIS

Cirrhosis is a chronic progressive disease of the liver characterized by extensive degeneration and destruction of the liver cells (Fig. 44-4). The development of cirrhosis is an insidious, prolonged course, usually after decades of chronic liver disease. Cirrhosis (combined with chronic liver diseases) ranks as the eighth leading cause of death in the United States. Cirrhosis is twice as common in men as in women.

Etiology and Pathophysiology

Any chronic liver disease, including disease from excessive alcohol intake and NAFLD, can cause cirrhosis. The specific cause of cirrhosis may not be determined in all patients. The most common causes of cirrhosis in the United States are chronic hepatitis C infection and alcohol-induced liver disease. In patients with alcohol-induced liver disease, some controversy exists as to whether the cause is the alcohol or the malnutrition that often coexists with alcoholism. A common problem in people who abuse alcohol is protein malnutrition. Some cases of nutrition-related cirrhosis have resulted from extreme dieting, malabsorption, and obesity. Environmental factors and genetic predisposition may also lead to the development of cirrhosis, regardless of dietary or alcohol intake.

Approximately 20% of patients with chronic hepatitis C and 10% to 20% of those with chronic hepatitis B develop cirrhosis.

FIG. 44-4 Cirrhosis that developed secondary to alcoholism. The characteristic diffuse nodularity of the surface is due to the combination of regeneration and scarring of the liver.

Chronic inflammation and cell necrosis result in fibrosis and, ultimately, cirrhosis. Chronic hepatitis combined with alcohol ingestion is synergistic in accelerating liver damage.

Biliary causes of cirrhosis include primary biliary cirrhosis (PBC) and primary sclerosing cholangitis (PSC). Both are described earlier in this chapter on the facing page.

Cardiac cirrhosis includes a spectrum of hepatic derangements that result from long-standing, severe, right-sided heart failure. The treatment is aimed at managing the patient's underlying heart failure.

In cirrhosis the liver cells attempt to regenerate, but the regenerative process is disorganized, resulting in abnormal blood vessel and bile duct architecture. The overgrowth of new and fibrous connective tissue distorts the liver's normal lobular structure, resulting in lobules of irregular size and shape with impeded blood flow. Eventually, irregular and disorganized liver regeneration, poor cellular nutrition, and hypoxia (from inadequate blood flow and scar tissue) result in decreased functioning of the liver.

Clinical Manifestations

Early Manifestations. The onset of cirrhosis is usually insidious. Early symptoms include fatigue. Many patients with normal liver function (compensated cirrhosis) may not be aware of their liver condition. The diagnosis may not be discovered until later, when they manifest symptoms of more advanced liver disease.

Later Manifestations. Later symptoms may be severe and result from liver failure and portal hypertension (Fig. 44-5). Jaundice, peripheral edema, and ascites develop gradually. Other late symptoms include skin lesions, hematologic disorders, endocrine disturbances, and peripheral neuropathies (Fig. 44-6). In the advanced stages, the liver becomes small and nodular.

Jaundice. Jaundice results from the functional derangement of liver cells and compression of bile ducts by connective tissue overgrowth. Jaundice occurs as a result of the decreased ability to conjugate and excrete bilirubin (see Table 44-3). (Normal bilirubin metabolism is presented in Fig. 39-4.) The jaundice

PATHOPHYSIOLOGY MAP

FIG. 44-5 Continuum of liver dysfunction in cirrhosis and resulting manifestations. *ADH,* Antidiuretic hormone; *ALT,* alanine aminotransferase; *AST,* aspartate aminotransferase.

may be minimal or severe, depending on the degree of liver damage.

Skin Lesions. Various skin manifestations are commonly seen in cirrhosis. Spider angiomas (*telangiectasia* or *spider nevi*) are small, dilated blood vessels with a bright red center point and spiderlike branches. They occur on the nose, cheeks, upper trunk, neck, and shoulders. *Palmar erythema* (a red area that blanches with pressure) is located on the palms of the hands. Both of these lesions are attributed to an increase in circulating estrogen as a result of the damaged liver's inability to metabolize steroid hormones.

Hematologic Problems. Hematologic problems include thrombocytopenia, leukopenia, anemia, and coagulation disorders. Thrombocytopenia, leukopenia, and anemia are probably caused by the splenomegaly that results from backup of blood from the portal vein into the spleen (portal hypertension). Overactivity of the enlarged spleen results in increased

removal of blood cells from circulation. Anemia is also due to inadequate red blood cell (RBC) production and survival, poor diet, poor absorption of folic acid, and bleeding from varices.

The coagulation problems result from the liver's inability to produce prothrombin and other factors essential for blood clotting. Coagulation problems are manifested by hemorrhage or bleeding tendencies, such as epistaxis, purpura, petechiae, easy bruising, gingival bleeding, and heavy menstrual bleeding.

Endocrine Problems. Normally the liver is important in the metabolism of adrenocortical hormones, estrogen, and testosterone. In men with cirrhosis, gynecomastia (benign growth of the glandular tissue of the male breast), loss of axillary and pubic hair, testicular atrophy, and impotence with loss of libido may occur because of increased estrogen levels. Younger women with cirrhosis may develop amenorrhea, and older women may have vaginal bleeding. The liver fails to metabolize aldosterone

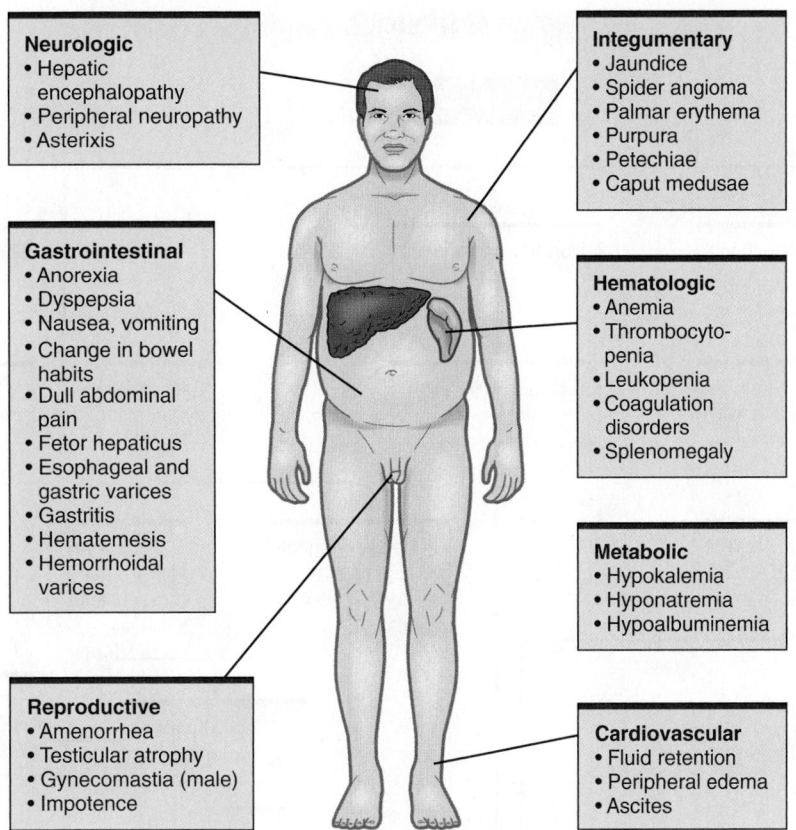

Neurologic
- Hepatic encephalopathy
- Peripheral neuropathy
- Asterixis

Gastrointestinal
- Anorexia
- Dyspepsia
- Nausea, vomiting
- Change in bowel habits
- Dull abdominal pain
- Fetor hepaticus
- Esophageal and gastric varices
- Gastritis
- Hematemesis
- Hemorrhoidal varices

Reproductive
- Amenorrhea
- Testicular atrophy
- Gynecomastia (male)
- Impotence

Integumentary
- Jaundice
- Spider angioma
- Palmar erythema
- Purpura
- Petechiae
- Caput medusae

Hematologic
- Anemia
- Thrombocyto-penia
- Leukopenia
- Coagulation disorders
- Splenomegaly

Metabolic
- Hypokalemia
- Hyponatremia
- Hypoalbuminemia

Cardiovascular
- Fluid retention
- Peripheral edema
- Ascites

FIG. 44-6 Systemic clinical manifestations of liver cirrhosis.

adequately, resulting in hyperaldosteronism with subsequent sodium and water retention and potassium loss.

Peripheral Neuropathy. Peripheral neuropathy is a common finding in alcoholic cirrhosis and is probably due to a dietary deficiency of thiamine, folic acid, and cobalamin. The neuropathy usually results in mixed nervous system symptoms, but sensory symptoms may predominate.

Complications

Major complications of cirrhosis are portal hypertension with resultant esophageal and gastric varices, peripheral edema and ascites, hepatic encephalopathy (mental status changes, including coma), and hepatorenal syndrome. Patients without complications of cirrhosis have *compensated cirrhosis.* Those who have one or more complications of their liver disease have *decompensated cirrhosis.*

Portal Hypertension and Esophageal and Gastric Varices. Structural changes in the liver result in compression and destruction of the portal and hepatic veins and sinusoids. These changes cause obstruction to the normal flow of blood through the portal system, resulting in portal hypertension. Portal hypertension is characterized by increased venous pressure in the portal circulation, splenomegaly, large collateral veins, ascites, and gastric and esophageal varices. Collateral circulation develops in an attempt to reduce high portal pressure and the increased plasma volume and lymphatic flow. The collateral channels commonly form in the lower esophagus (the anastomosis of the left gastric vein and the azygos veins), anterior abdominal wall, parietal peritoneum, and rectum. Varicosities may develop in areas where the collateral and systemic circulations communicate, resulting in esophageal and gastric varices,

caput medusae (ring of varices around the umbilicus), and hemorrhoids.

Esophageal varices are a complex of tortuous veins at the lower end of the esophagus, which are enlarged and swollen as a result of portal hypertension. Gastric varices are located in the upper portion (cardia, fundus) of the stomach. These varices contain little elastic tissue and are fragile. They tolerate high pressure poorly and, as a result, bleed easily. Large varices are more likely to bleed. Esophageal varices are responsible for approximately 80% of variceal hemorrhages. The remaining 20% of variceal hemorrhages are due to gastric varices.

Bleeding esophageal varices are the most life-threatening complication of cirrhosis. The patient may have melena or hematemesis. There may be slow oozing or massive hemorrhage. Massive hemorrhage is a medical emergency.

Peripheral Edema and Ascites. Peripheral edema sometimes precedes ascites, but in some patients its development coincides with or occurs after ascites. Edema results from decreased colloidal oncotic pressure from impaired liver synthesis of albumin and increased portacaval pressure from portal hypertension. Peripheral edema occurs as ankle and presacral edema.

Ascites is the accumulation of serous fluid in the peritoneal or abdominal cavity. It is a common manifestation of cirrhosis. With portal hypertension, proteins shift from the blood vessels via the larger pores of the sinusoids (capillaries) into the lymph space (Fig. 44-7). When the lymphatic system is unable to carry off the excess proteins and water, they leak through the liver capsule into the peritoneal cavity. The osmotic pressure of the proteins pulls additional fluid into the peritoneal cavity (Table 44-9).

PATHOPHYSIOLOGY MAP

FIG. 44-7 Mechanisms for development of ascites.

TABLE 44-9	FACTORS INVOLVED IN ASCITES
Factor	**Mechanism**
Portal hypertension	Increase in resistance of blood flow through liver.
Increased flow of hepatic lymph	Leaking of protein-rich lymph from surface of cirrhotic liver. Intrahepatic blockage of lymph channels.
Decreased serum colloidal oncotic pressure	Impairment of liver synthesis of albumin. Loss of albumin into peritoneal cavity.
Hyperaldosteronism	Increase in aldosterone secretion stimulated by decreased renal blood flow. Decreased liver metabolism of aldosterone.
Impaired water excretion	Reduction in renal blood flow and high serum levels of antidiuretic hormone (ADH).

FIG. 44-8 Gross ascites.

A second mechanism of ascites formation is hypoalbuminemia resulting from the liver's inability to synthesize albumin. The hypoalbuminemia results in decreased colloidal oncotic pressure. A third mechanism is hyperaldosteronism, which occurs when aldosterone is not metabolized by damaged hepatocytes. The increased level of aldosterone causes increased sodium reabsorption by the renal tubules. This retention of sodium, combined with an increase in antidiuretic hormone, causes additional water retention. Because of edema formation, there is decreased intravascular volume and, subsequently, decreased renal blood flow and glomerular filtration.

Ascites is manifested by abdominal distention with weight gain (Fig. 44-8). If the ascites is severe, the umbilicus may be everted. Abdominal striae with distended abdominal wall veins may be present. The patient has signs of dehydration (e.g., dry tongue and skin, sunken eyeballs, muscle weakness) and a decrease in urine output. Hypokalemia is common and is due to an excessive loss of potassium caused by hyperaldosteronism. Low potassium levels can also result from diuretic therapy used to treat the ascites.

Because of alterations in immune function associated with cirrhosis, patients with ascites are at risk for *spontaneous bacterial peritonitis* (SBP). SBP is a bacterial infection of the ascites fluid. This occurs in approximately 15% to 25% of hospitalized patients with cirrhosis and ascites and is particularly common after variceal hemorrhage.[20] The bacteria most frequently found are gram-negative enteric pathogens such as *Escherichia coli*.

Hepatic Encephalopathy. Hepatic encephalopathy is a neuropsychiatric manifestation of liver disease. The pathogenesis is multifactorial and includes the neurotoxic effects of ammonia, abnormal neurotransmission, astrocyte swelling, and inflammatory cytokines. A major source of ammonia is the bacterial and enzymatic deamination of amino acids in the intestines. The ammonia that results from this deamination process normally goes to the liver via the portal circulation and is converted to urea, which is then excreted by the kidneys. When blood is shunted past the liver via the collateral vessels or the liver is unable to convert ammonia to urea, the levels of ammonia in the systemic circulation increase. The ammonia crosses the blood-brain barrier and produces neurologic toxic manifestations. Factors that increase ammonia in the circulation may precipitate hepatic encephalopathy (Table 44-10).

TABLE 44-10 FACTORS PRECIPITATING HEPATIC ENCEPHALOPATHY

Factor	Mechanism
GI hemorrhage	Increase in ammonia in GI tract.
Constipation	Increase in ammonia from bacterial action on feces.
Hypokalemia	Potassium is needed by brain to metabolize ammonia.
Hypovolemia	Increase in blood ammonia because of hepatic hypoxia. Impairment of cerebral, hepatic, and renal function because of decreased blood flow.
Infection	Increase in catabolism and increase in cerebral sensitivity to toxins.
Cerebral depressants (e.g., opioids)	Decrease in metabolism by liver, causing higher drug levels and cerebral depression.
Metabolic alkalosis	Facilitation of transport of ammonia across blood-brain barrier. Increase in renal production of ammonia.
Paracentesis	Loss of sodium and potassium ions. Decrease in blood volume.
Dehydration	Potentiation of ammonia toxicity.
Increased metabolism	Increase in workload of liver.
Uremia (renal failure)	Retention of nitrogenous metabolites.

Hepatic encephalopathy can occur after placement of transjugular intrahepatic portosystemic shunt (TIPS), which is used to treat portal hypertension.[21]

Clinical manifestations of encephalopathy are changes in neurologic and mental responsiveness; impaired consciousness; and inappropriate behavior, ranging from sleep disturbances to lethargy to deep coma.[21] Changes may occur suddenly because of an increase in ammonia in response to bleeding varices or infection or gradually as blood ammonia levels slowly increase. A grading system is often used to classify the stages of hepatic encephalopathy (Table 44-11).

A characteristic manifestation of hepatic encephalopathy is asterixis (flapping tremors). This may take several forms, with the most common involving the arms and hands. When asked to hold the arms and hands stretched out, the patient is unable to hold this position and performs a series of rapid flexion and extension movements of the hands. Impairments in writing involve difficulty in moving the pen or pencil from left to right and *apraxia* (the inability to construct simple figures). Other signs include hyperventilation, hypothermia, and grimacing and grasping reflexes.

Fetor hepaticus (musty, sweet odor of the patient's breath) occurs in some patients with encephalopathy. This odor is from the accumulation of digestive by-products that the liver is unable to degrade.

Hepatorenal Syndrome. Hepatorenal syndrome can occur in patients with decompensated cirrhosis. It is a type of renal failure with advancing azotemia, oliguria, and intractable ascites. In this syndrome the kidneys have no structural abnormality. The etiology is complex, but the final common pathway is likely to be portal hypertension along with liver decompensation resulting in splanchnic and systemic vasodilation and decreased arterial blood volume. As a result, renal vasoconstriction occurs, and renal failure follows. This renal failure can be reversed by liver transplantation. In the patient with cirrhosis, hepatorenal syndrome frequently follows diuretic therapy, GI hemorrhage, or paracentesis.

Diagnostic Studies

Patients with cirrhosis have abnormalities in most of the liver function studies. Enzyme levels, including alkaline phosphatase, AST, ALT, and γ-glutamyl transpeptidase (GGT), are initially elevated because of their release from damaged liver cells. However, in end-stage liver disease AST and ALT levels may be normal. Patients with cirrhosis have decreased total protein, decreased albumin, increased serum bilirubin, and increased globulin levels. Fat metabolism abnormalities are reflected by decreased cholesterol levels. The prothrombin time is prolonged, and bilirubin metabolism is altered (see Table 44-3). A liver ultrasound may be used to assess the severity of cirrhosis. A liver biopsy may be done to identify liver cell changes and

TABLE 44-11 GRADING SCALE FOR HEPATIC ENCEPHALOPATHY

Grade	Level of Consciousness	Intellectual Function	Neurologic Findings
0	Insomnia, sleep disturbances	Subtle change in computational skills	Impaired handwriting, tremor
1	Lack of awareness, personality change	Short attention span, mild confusion, depression	Incoordination, asterixis
2	Lethargy, drowsiness, inappropriate behavior	Disoriented	Asterixis, abnormal reflexes
3	Asleep, rousable	Loss of meaningful conversation, marked confusion, incomprehensible speech	Asterixis, abnormal reflexes
4	Not rousable	Absent	Decerebrate May be responsive to painful stimuli

TABLE 44-12   COLLABORATIVE CARE

Cirrhosis of the Liver

Diagnostic
- History and physical examination
- Liver function studies
- Liver biopsy (percutaneous needle)
- Upper endoscopy (esophagogastroduodenoscopy)
- CT scan, multiphase
- Liver ultrasound (e.g., FibroScan for stiffness)
- Serum electrolytes
- Prothrombin time
- Serum albumin
- Complete blood count

Collaborative Therapy
Conservative Therapy
- Rest
- Administration of B-complex vitamins
- Avoidance of alcohol
- Minimization or avoidance of aspirin, acetaminophen, and NSAIDs

Ascites
- Low-sodium diet
- Diuretics
- Paracentesis (if indicated)

Esophageal and Gastric Varices
- Drug therapy
  - Nonselective β-blocker (e.g., propranolol [Inderal])
  - octreotide (Sandostatin)
  - vasopressin (Pitressin)
- Endoscopic band ligation or sclerotherapy
- Balloon tamponade
- Transjugular intrahepatic portosystemic shunt (TIPS)

Hepatic Encephalopathy
- Antibiotics (rifaximin [Xifaxan])
- lactulose (Cephulac)

alterations in the lobular structure. Differential analysis of ascitic fluid may help confirm the cause of cirrhosis.

Collaborative Care

The goal of treatment is to slow the progress of cirrhosis and prevent and treat any complications. Collaborative care measures are listed in Table 44-12. Management of specific problems associated with cirrhosis is described next.

Ascites. Management of ascites focuses on sodium restriction, diuretics, and fluid removal. The amount of sodium restriction is based on the degree of ascites. Initially the patient may be encouraged to limit sodium intake to 2 g/day.[22] Patients with severe ascites may need to restrict their sodium intake to 250 to 500 mg/day. Very low sodium intake can result in reduced nutritional intake and subsequent problems associated with malnutrition. The patient is usually not on restricted fluids unless severe ascites develops. Accurately assess and monitor fluid and electrolyte balance. Albumin infusion may be used to help maintain intravascular volume and adequate urine output by increasing plasma colloid osmotic pressure.

Diuretic therapy is an important part of management. Often a combination of drugs that work at multiple sites in the nephron is more effective. Spironolactone (Aldactone) is an effective diuretic, even in patients with severe sodium retention. Spironolactone is an antagonist of aldosterone and is potassium

sparing. Other potassium-sparing diuretics include amiloride (Midamor) and triamterene (Dyrenium). A high-potency loop diuretic, such as furosemide (Lasix), is frequently used in combination with a potassium-sparing drug.

Tolvaptan (Samsca), a vasopressin-receptor antagonist, is used to correct hyponatremia in patients with cirrhosis. It causes an increase in water excretion, resulting in an increase in serum sodium concentrations.[23]

A paracentesis (needle puncture of the abdominal cavity) may be performed to remove ascitic fluid or to test the fluid for infection (spontaneous bacterial peritonitis). However, this procedure is reserved for the patient with impaired respiration or abdominal pain caused by severe ascites. It is only a temporary measure because the fluid tends to reaccumulate.

TIPS (discussed later in this section) is used to alleviate ascites that does not respond to diuretics. Peritoneovenous shunt is a surgical procedure that provides continuous reinfusion of ascitic fluid into the venous system. Its use has almost been eliminated because of the high rate of complications.

Esophageal and Gastric Varices. The main therapeutic goal for esophageal and gastric varices is to prevent bleeding and hemorrhage. The patient who has esophageal varices should avoid ingesting alcohol, aspirin, and nonsteroidal antiinflammatory drugs (NSAIDs).

All patients with cirrhosis should have an upper endoscopy (esophagogastroduodenoscopy [EGD]) to screen for varices. The diagnosis of esophageal or gastric variceal bleeding needs to be made by endoscopic examination as soon as possible. Patients with varices at risk of bleeding are started on a nonselective β-blocker (nadolol [Corgard] or propranolol [Inderal]) to reduce the incidence of hemorrhage. β-Blockers decrease high portal pressure.

When variceal bleeding occurs, the first step is to stabilize the patient and manage the airway. IV therapy is initiated and may include administration of blood products. Management that involves a combination of drug therapy and endoscopic therapy is more successful than either approach alone.

Drug therapy for bleeding varices may include the somatostatin analog octreotide (Sandostatin) or vasopressin (VP). The main goal of drug therapy is to stop bleeding so that treatment measures can be initiated. IV administration of VP produces vasoconstriction of the splanchnic arterial bed, decreases portal blood flow, and decreases portal hypertension. However, VP has many side effects, including decreased coronary blood flow, dysrhythmias, and increased BP. Because of this, IV nitroglycerin is often given in combination with VP. The nitroglycerin reduces the adverse effects of the VP while enhancing its beneficial effect. VP should be avoided or used cautiously in the older adult because of the risk of cardiac ischemia.

At the time of endoscopy, band ligation or sclerotherapy may be used to prevent rebleeding. Endoscopic variceal ligation (EVL, or "banding") is performed by placing a small rubber band (elastic O-ring) around the base of the *varix* (enlarged vein). Sclerotherapy involves injection of a sclerosant solution into the varices through an injection needle that is placed through the endoscope.

Balloon tamponade may be used in patients with acute esophageal or gastric variceal hemorrhage that cannot be controlled on initial endoscopy. Balloon tamponade controls the hemorrhage by mechanical compression of the varices. Different types of tubes are available. The Sengstaken-Blakemore tube has two balloons, gastric and esophageal, with three lumens: one for the gastric balloon, one for the esophageal balloon, and one for gastric aspiration (see eFig. 44-1 on the website for this chapter). Two other types of balloons are the Minnesota tube (a modified Sengstaken-Blakemore tube with an esophageal suction port above the esophageal balloon) and the Linton-Nachlas tube.

SAFETY ALERT
- Label each lumen to avoid confusion.
- Deflate balloons for 5 min every 8-12 hr per institutional policy to prevent tissue necrosis.

Supportive measures during an acute variceal bleed include administration of fresh frozen plasma and packed RBCs, vitamin K, and proton pump inhibitors (e.g., pantoprazole [Protonix]). Lactulose (Cephulac) and rifaximin (Xifaxan) may be administered to prevent hepatic encephalopathy from breakdown of blood and the release of ammonia in the intestine. Antibiotics are given to prevent bacterial infection.

Because of the high incidence of recurrent bleeding with each bleeding episode, continued therapy is necessary. Long-term management of patients who have had an episode of bleeding includes nonselective β-blockers, repeated band ligation of the varices, and portosystemic shunts in patients who develop recurrent bleeding.

Shunting Procedures. Nonsurgical and surgical methods of shunting blood away from the varices are available. Shunting procedures tend to be used more after a second major bleeding episode than during an initial bleeding episode. *Transjugular intrahepatic portosystemic shunt (TIPS)* is a nonsurgical procedure in which a tract (shunt) between the systemic and portal venous systems is created to redirect portal blood flow (see eFig. 44-2 on the website for this chapter). A catheter is placed in the jugular vein and then threaded through the superior and inferior vena cava to the hepatic vein. The wall of the hepatic vein is punctured, and the catheter is directed to the portal vein. Stents are positioned along the passageway, overlapping in the liver tissue and extending into both veins.

This procedure reduces portal venous pressure and decompresses the varices, thus controlling bleeding. TIPS does not interfere with a future liver transplantation. Limitations of the procedure include the increased risk of hepatic encephalopathy and stenosis of the stent. TIPS is contraindicated in patients with severe hepatic encephalopathy, hepatocellular carcinoma, severe hepatorenal syndrome, and portal vein thrombosis.

Various surgical shunting procedures may be used to decrease portal hypertension by diverting some of the portal blood flow while allowing adequate liver perfusion. Currently, the surgical shunts most commonly used are the portacaval shunt and the distal splenorenal shunt (Fig. 44-9).

Hepatic Encephalopathy.
The goal of management of hepatic encephalopathy is the reduction of ammonia formation. Ammonia formation in the intestines is reduced with lactulose, a drug that traps ammonia in the gut. It can be given orally, as an enema, or through a nasogastric (NG) tube. The laxative effect of the drug expels the ammonia from the colon. Antibiotics such as rifaximin may also be given, particularly in patients who do not respond to lactulose. Constipation should be prevented.

Control of hepatic encephalopathy also involves treatment of precipitating causes (see Table 44-10). This includes controlling GI bleeding and removing the blood from the GI tract to decrease the protein in the intestine.

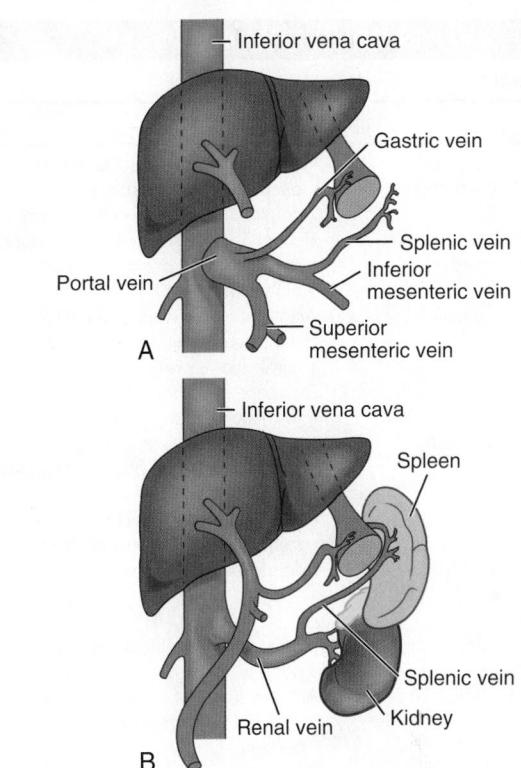

FIG. 44-9 Portosystemic shunts. **A,** Portacaval shunt. The portal vein is anastomosed to the inferior vena cava, diverting blood from the portal vein to the systemic circulation. **B,** Distal splenorenal shunt. The splenic vein is anastomosed to the renal vein. The portal venous flow remains intact while esophageal varices are selectively decompressed. (The short gastric veins are decompressed.) The spleen conducts blood from the high pressure of the esophageal and gastric varices to the low-pressure renal vein.

Drug Therapy.
There is no specific drug therapy for cirrhosis. However, a number of drugs are used to treat symptoms and complications of advanced liver disease (Table 44-13).

Nutritional Therapy.
The diet for the patient who has cirrhosis without complications is high in calories (3000 cal/day) with high carbohydrate content and moderate to low levels of fat. Protein restriction may be appropriate in some patients immediately after a severe flare of symptoms (i.e., episodic hepatic encephalopathy). However, protein restriction is rarely justified in patients with cirrhosis and persistent hepatic encephalopathy. Malnutrition is a more serious clinical problem than hepatic encephalopathy for many of these patients.[24]

A patient with alcoholic cirrhosis frequently has protein-calorie malnutrition. Enteral formula supplements containing protein from branched-chain amino acids that are metabolized by the muscles may be recommended. These supplements provide protein that is more easily metabolized by the liver. Parenteral nutrition or enteral nutrition therapy may be required.

The patient with ascites and edema is on a low-sodium diet. The degree of sodium restriction depends on the patient's condition. The patient needs instruction regarding the degree of restriction. Table salt is a well-known source of sodium, but sodium is also present in baking soda and baking powder. Foods that are high in sodium content include canned soups and vegetables, many frozen foods, salted snacks (e.g., potato chips), nuts, smoked meats and fish, crackers, breads, olives, pickles, ketchup, and beer. Advise the patient to read labels. The patient and the caregiver may need assistance in making the diet

TABLE 44-13   DRUG THERAPY

Cirrhosis

Drug	Mechanism of Action
vasopressin (Pitressin) octreotide (Sandostatin)	Hemostasis and control of bleeding in esophageal and gastric varices, constriction of splanchnic arterial bed
propranolol (Inderal) nadolol (Corgard)	Reduction of portal venous pressure, reduction of esophageal varices bleeding
lactulose (Cephulac)	Acidification of feces in bowel and trapping of ammonia, causing its elimination in feces
rifaximin (Xifaxan) neomycin sulfate	Decrease in bacterial flora, decreased formation of ammonia
magnesium sulfate	Magnesium replacement, hypomagnesemia possible with liver dysfunction
Vitamin K	Correction of clotting abnormalities from decreased levels of this vitamin
Proton pump inhibitors (e.g., pantoprazole [Protonix])	Decrease in gastric acidity
Diuretics	
• spironolactone (Aldactone)	Blocks action of aldosterone, potassium sparing
• furosemide (Lasix)	Acts on distal tubule and loop of Henle to decrease reabsorption of sodium and water

more palatable by using seasonings such as garlic, parsley, onion, lemon juice, and spices.

NURSING MANAGEMENT
CIRRHOSIS

NURSING ASSESSMENT

Subjective and objective data that should be obtained from an individual with cirrhosis are presented in Table 44-14.

NURSING DIAGNOSES

Nursing diagnoses for the patient with cirrhosis include, but are not limited to, the following:

- Imbalanced nutrition: less than body requirements *related to* anorexia, nausea, and impaired utilization and storage of nutrients
- Impaired skin integrity *related to* peripheral edema, ascites, and pruritus
- Excess fluid volume *related to* portal hypertension and hyperaldosteronism
- Ineffective self-health management *related to* ineffective coping and abuse of alcohol

Additional information on nursing diagnoses for the patient with cirrhosis is presented in eNursing Care Plan 44-2 (available on the website for this chapter).

PLANNING

The overall goals are that the patient with cirrhosis will (1) have relief of discomfort, (2) have minimal to no complications (ascites, esophageal varices, hepatic encephalopathy), and (3) return to as normal a lifestyle as possible.

NURSING IMPLEMENTATION

HEALTH PROMOTION. Common risk factors for cirrhosis include alcoholism, malnutrition, viral hepatitis, biliary obstruction, obesity, and right-sided heart failure. Prevention and early

TABLE 44-14   NURSING ASSESSMENT

Cirrhosis

Subjective Data
Important Health Information
Past health history: Previous viral, toxic, or idiopathic hepatitis; NASH, chronic biliary obstruction and infection; severe right-sided heart failure
Medications: Adverse reaction to any medication; use of anticoagulants, aspirin, NSAIDs, acetaminophen

Functional Health Patterns
Health perception–health management: Chronic alcoholism; weakness, fatigue
Nutritional-metabolic: Anorexia, weight loss, dyspepsia, nausea and vomiting; gingival bleeding
Elimination: Dark urine, decreased urine output; light-colored or black stools, flatulence, change in bowel habits; dry, yellow skin, bruising
Cognitive-perceptual: Dull, right upper quadrant or epigastric pain; numbness, tingling of extremities; pruritus
Sexuality-reproductive: Impotence, amenorrhea

Objective Data
General
Fever, cachexia, wasting of extremities

Integumentary
Icteric sclera, jaundice, petechiae, ecchymoses, spider angiomas, palmar erythema, alopecia, loss of axillary and pubic hair, peripheral edema

Respiratory
Shallow, rapid respirations, epistaxis

Gastrointestinal
Abdominal distention, ascites, distended abdominal wall veins, palpable liver and spleen, foul breath; hematemesis; black, tarry stools; hemorrhoids

Neurologic
Altered mentation, asterixis

Reproductive
Gynecomastia and testicular atrophy (men), impotence (men), loss of libido (men and women), amenorrhea or heavy menstrual bleeding (women)

Possible Diagnostic Findings
Anemia, thrombocytopenia; leukopenia; ↓ serum albumin, potassium; abnormal liver function studies; ↑ INR, ↓ platelets, ↑ ammonia, and ↑ bilirubin levels; abnormal abdominal ultrasound or MRI

INR, International normalized ratio; *NASH,* nonalcoholic steatohepatitis.

treatment of cirrhosis focus on reducing or eliminating these risk factors. Alcoholism must be treated. Urge patients to avoid alcohol ingestion, and support their efforts. (The treatment of alcohol dependence is discussed in Chapter 11.)

Adequate nutrition, especially for the alcoholic and other individuals at risk for cirrhosis, is essential to promote liver regeneration. Identify and treat acute hepatitis early so that it does not progress to chronic hepatitis and cirrhosis. Bariatric surgery for morbidly obese individuals has been shown to reduce the incidence of liver disease.[25]

ACUTE INTERVENTION. Nursing care for the patient with cirrhosis focuses on conserving the patient's strength while maintaining muscle strength and tone (see eNursing Care Plan 44-2 on the website for this chapter). When the patient requires complete bed rest, implement measures to prevent pneumonia, thromboembolic problems, and pressure ulcers. Modify the activity and rest schedule according to signs of clinical improvement (e.g., decreasing jaundice, improvement in liver function studies).

Anorexia, nausea and vomiting, pressure from ascites, and poor eating habits all interfere with adequate intake of nutrients. Oral hygiene before meals may improve the patient's taste sensation. Make between-meal snacks available so the patient can eat them at times when he or she can best tolerate them. Provide food preferences whenever possible. Explain the reason for any dietary restrictions to the patient and caregiver.

Nursing assessment and care should include the patient's physiologic response to cirrhosis. Is jaundice present? Where is it observed—sclera, skin, hard palate? What is the progression of jaundice? If the jaundice is accompanied by pruritus, carry out measures to relieve itching. Cholestyramine or hydroxyzine (Atarax) may be ordered to help relieve the pruritus. Other measures to alleviate pruritus include baking soda or Alpha Keri baths, lotions containing calamine, antihistamines, soft or old linens, and control of the temperature (not too hot and not too cold). Keep the patient's nails short and clean. Teach patients to rub with their knuckles rather than scratch with their nails when they cannot resist scratching.

Note the color of urine and stools. When jaundice is present, the urine is often dark brown and foamy when shaken. The stool is gray or tan.

Edema and ascites are frequent manifestations of cirrhosis and require nursing assessments and interventions. Accurate calculation and recording of intake and output, daily weights, and measurements of extremities and abdominal girth help in the ongoing assessment of the location and extent of the edema. Mark the abdomen with a permanent marker so the girth is measured at the same location each time.

Immediately before a paracentesis have the patient void to prevent a puncture of the bladder. When a paracentesis is done, the patient sits on the side of the bed or is placed in high Fowler's position. After the procedure, monitor for hypovolemia and electrolyte imbalances and check the dressing for bleeding and leakage.

Dyspnea is a frequent problem for the patient with severe ascites and can lead to pleural effusions. A semi-Fowler's or Fowler's position allows for maximal respiratory efficiency. Use pillows to support the arms and chest to increase the patient's comfort and ability to breathe.

Meticulous skin care is essential because the edematous tissues are subject to breakdown. Use an alternating-air pressure mattress or other special mattress. A turning schedule (minimum of every 2 hours) must be adhered to rigidly. Support the abdomen with pillows. If the abdomen is taut, cleanse it gently. The patient tends to move little because of abdominal discomfort and dyspnea. Range-of-motion exercises are helpful. Implement measures such as coughing and deep breathing to prevent respiratory problems. The lower extremities may be elevated. If scrotal edema is present, a scrotal support provides some comfort.

When the patient is taking diuretics, monitor the serum levels of sodium, potassium, chloride, and bicarbonate. Monitor renal function (blood urea nitrogen [BUN], serum creatinine) routinely and with any change in the diuretic dosage. Observe for signs of fluid and electrolyte imbalance, especially hypokalemia. Hypokalemia may be manifested by cardiac dysrhythmias, hypotension, tachycardia, and generalized muscle weakness. Water excess is manifested by muscle cramping, weakness, lethargy, and confusion.

Observe for and provide nursing care for any hematologic problems (bleeding tendencies, anemia, increased susceptibility to infection) (see eNursing Care Plan 44-2 on the website for this chapter).

Assess the patient's response to altered body image resulting from jaundice, spider angiomas, palmar erythema, ascites, and gynecomastia. The patient may experience anxiety and embarrassment about these changes. Explain these phenomena and be a supportive listener. Provide nursing care with concern and warmth to help the patient maintain self-esteem.

Bleeding Varices. If the patient has esophageal or gastric varices, observe for any signs of bleeding from the varices, such as hematemesis and melena. If hematemesis occurs, assess the patient for hemorrhage, call the physician, and be ready to assist with treatment used to control the bleeding. The patient will be admitted to the intensive care unit (ICU). The patient's airway must be maintained.

Balloon tamponade may be used in patients who have bleeding that is unresponsive to band ligation or sclerotherapy. When balloon tamponade is used, the initial nursing task is to explain the use of the tube and how it will be inserted. Check the balloons for patency. It is usually the physician's responsibility to insert the tube by either the nose or the mouth (see eFig. 44-1). Then the gastric balloon is inflated with approximately 250 mL of air, and the tube is retracted until resistance (lower esophageal sphincter) is felt. The tube is secured by placement of a piece of sponge or foam rubber at the nostrils (nasal cuff). For continued bleeding, the esophageal balloon is then inflated. A sphygmomanometer is used to measure and maintain the

ETHICAL/LEGAL DILEMMAS
Rationing

Situation

T.H., a 43-yr-old patient with cirrhosis of the liver, is frequently admitted to the hospital. She has been told that her continued drinking will inevitably lead to her death. Now she has been admitted for gastrointestinal bleeding and needs blood transfusions. She has a rare blood type, and it is frequently difficult to get compatible blood. Should you call an ethics consultation?

Ethical/Legal Points for Consideration

* *Rationing,* or the controlled distribution of scarce resources, is a difficult ethical problem. The needs of an individual patient or group of patients are weighed against the needs of many patients, who may have a greater chance of recovery, and the availability of the needed resources.
* Health interests can supercede the interests or rights of an individual. For example, in anticipation of an anthrax attack, the government could confiscate all relevant antibiotics and restrict their use to treatment of the disease.
* Two individual rights that must be considered with regard to rationing are the constitutional right to privacy and the right to consent to or refuse medical procedures and therapy.
* The competent adult is the only person who may consent to or refuse treatment for his or her health care problems.
* In the situation of T.H., if she consents to a blood transfusion, the ability of an intervening party to refuse that treatment would be permitted only given substantial intervening circumstances, and not as a threat to compel compliant behavior in the future.

Discussion Questions

1. What are your feelings about patients with diseases, such as substance abuse, that have a behavioral component? Do these patients deserve aggressive treatment?
2. How would you proceed to make a decision in T.H.'s case? Would you request an ethics committee consultation?

EVIDENCE-BASED PRACTICE

Applying the Evidence

You have been assigned to care for M.K., a 58-yr-old Hispanic man, who is being admitted with alcohol-related cirrhosis. As a part of his admission assessment, you ask about his current use of alcohol. He tells you that he has been "drinking more" since he lost his job. His admission blood alcohol concentration was 295 mg/dL. You ask if he has ever tried to stop drinking. He tells you many times, but "it never lasts." When asked if he has ever been to Alcoholics Anonymous (AA), he states that that "scene" is not for him. M.K. tells you that he knows he will not live very long and he sees no reason to stop drinking at this point.

Best Available Evidence	Clinician Expertise	Patient Preferences and Values
Although treatment strategies for alcohol dependency include inpatient and outpatient treatment programs for the individual, often they are not effective. Another approach is family therapy, which has been shown to decrease the incidence of alcohol-related disease and inpatient hospital stays.	Abstinence from the use of alcohol is critical in the treatment of cirrhosis. You have known many patients who have attended AA and are "recovering alcoholics." You also know that the family is an essential part of the effectiveness of treatment. You ask M.K. if you could meet with him and his family to discuss treatment options.	M.K. is not motivated to consider any treatment approaches for alcohol dependency. M.K. prefers to continue to use alcohol and he tells you that he knows the consequences.

Your Decision and Action

You acknowledge M.K.'s comments about his continued use of alcohol at this time but reassess his decision throughout his hospitalization. You also plan a meeting with key family members to discuss the issue. Based on the results of meeting with the family, you will try to set up a meeting with M.K., the family, and an appropriate therapist.

Reference for Evidence

Meads C, Ting S, Dretzke J, et al: A systematic review of the clinical and cost-effectiveness of psychological therapy involving family and friends in alcohol misuse or dependence, *Database Abstracts Rev Effects* 3, 2012.

desired pressure at 20 to 40 mm Hg. The position of the balloons is verified by x-ray.

Nursing care includes monitoring for complications of rupture or erosion of the esophagus, regurgitation and aspiration of gastric contents, and occlusion of the airway by the balloon. If the gastric balloon breaks or is deflated, the esophageal balloon will slip upward, obstructing the airway and causing asphyxiation. If this happens, cut the tube or deflate the esophageal balloon. Keep scissors at the bedside. Minimize regurgitation by oral and pharyngeal suctioning and by keeping the patient in a semi-Fowler's position.

The patient is unable to swallow saliva because of the inflated esophageal balloon occluding the esophagus. Encourage the patient to expectorate, and provide an emesis basin and tissues. Frequent oral and nasal care provides relief from the taste of blood and irritation from mouth breathing.

Hepatic Encephalopathy. Nursing care of the patient with hepatic encephalopathy focuses on maintaining a safe environment, sustaining life, and assisting with measures to reduce the formation of ammonia. Assess (1) the patient's level of responsiveness (e.g., reflexes, pupillary reactions, orientation), (2) sensory and motor abnormalities (e.g., hyperreflexia, asterixis, motor coordination), (3) fluid and electrolyte imbalances, (4) acid-base imbalances, and (5) the effect of treatment measures.

Assess the neurologic status, including an exact description of the patient's behavior, at least every 2 hours. Plan your care of the patient with neurologic problems based on the severity of the encephalopathy.

Institute measures to prevent constipation to reduce ammonia production. Give drugs, laxatives, and enemas as ordered. Encourage fluids, if not contraindicated. Any GI bleeding may worsen encephalopathy. Assess the patient taking lactulose for diarrhea and excessive fluid and electrolyte losses.

Control factors known to precipitate encephalopathy as much as possible, including anything that may cause constipation (e.g., dehydration, opioid medications).

AMBULATORY AND HOME CARE. The patient with cirrhosis may be faced with a prolonged course and the possibility of life-threatening problems and complications. The patient and caregiver need to understand the importance of continual health care and medical supervision. Supportive measures include proper diet, rest, avoidance of potentially hepatotoxic OTC drugs such as acetaminophen, and abstinence from alcohol.[25] Abstinence from alcohol is important and results in improvement in most patients. However, some patients find abstinence difficult. Explore your own attitude regarding the patient whose cirrhosis is attributed to alcohol abuse. Provide care without rejection or moralizing. Treat the patient with a caring attitude (see Chapter 11).

Cirrhosis is a chronic disease. The patient is affected not only physically but also psychologically, socially, and economically. Major lifestyle changes may be required, especially if alcohol abuse is the primary etiologic factor. Provide information regarding community support programs, such as Alcoholics Anonymous, for help with alcohol abuse.

When you know a patient's diagnosis is cirrhosis, do not assume the cause is excess alcohol intake. Because cirrhosis has many different causes, it is important for you to find out the primary etiology before jumping to conclusions about the patient.

Teach the patient and caregiver about manifestations of complications and when to seek medical attention. Explain both verbally and in writing information about fluid or possible dietary changes (Table 44-15). Include instructions about adequate rest periods, how to detect early signs of complications, skin care, drug therapy precautions, observation for bleeding, and protection from infection. Counseling information regarding sexual problems may be needed. Referral to a community or home health nurse may be helpful to ensure patient adherence to prescribed therapy. Home care for the patient with cirrhosis should emphasize helping the patient maintain the highest level of wellness possible and initiate and maintain necessary lifestyle changes.

EVALUATION

Expected outcomes are that the patient with cirrhosis will

- Maintain food and fluid intake adequate to meet nutritional needs
- Maintain skin integrity with relief of edema and pruritus
- Experience normalization of fluid balance as a result of medical and nursing interventions
- Acknowledge and get treatment for a substance abuse problem

TABLE 44-15	PATIENT & CAREGIVER TEACHING GUIDE

Cirrhosis

When teaching the patient and caregiver about management of cirrhosis, do the following.

1. Explain that cirrhosis is a chronic illness and the importance of continual health care.
2. Teach the symptoms of complications and when to seek medical attention to enable prompt treatment of complications.
3. Teach the patient to avoid potentially hepatotoxic over-the-counter drugs (see Table 39-6) because the diseased liver is unable to metabolize these drugs.
4. Encourage abstinence from alcohol because continued use of alcohol will increase the risk of liver complications.
5. Instruct the patient to avoid aspirin and NSAIDs to prevent hemorrhage when esophageal or gastric varices are present.
6. Teach the patient to avoid activities that increase portal pressure, such as straining at stool, coughing, sneezing, and retching and vomiting. These activities may increase the risk of variceal hemorrhage in patients with portal hypertension and varices.

Additional information on expected outcomes for the patient with cirrhosis is presented in eNursing Care Plan 44-2 (available on the website for this chapter).

ACUTE LIVER FAILURE

Acute liver failure, or *fulminant hepatic failure*, is a clinical syndrome characterized by severe impairment of liver function associated with hepatic encephalopathy. The most common cause is drugs, usually acetaminophen in combination with alcohol.[26] People who abuse alcohol are particularly susceptible to detrimental effects of acetaminophen on the liver. Other drugs that can cause acute liver failure include isoniazid, halothane, sulfa-containing drugs, and NSAIDs. Drugs can cause liver cell failure by disrupting essential intracellular processes or causing an accumulation of toxic metabolic products.

Viral hepatitis, in particular HBV, is the second most common cause of acute liver failure. Hepatitis A is a less common cause.

Acute liver failure is characterized by the rapid onset of severe liver dysfunction in someone with no prior history of liver disease. Although the disease can run its course over 8 weeks, it can last as long as 26 weeks. With improved intensive care, the prognosis is much better now than in the past, with survival rates of approximately 60%.[27]

Clinical Manifestations and Diagnostic Studies

Manifestations include jaundice, coagulation abnormalities, and encephalopathy. In acute liver failure, changes in mentation are the first clinical sign. Patients are susceptible to a wide variety of complications, including cerebral edema, renal failure, hypoglycemia, metabolic acidosis, sepsis, and multiorgan failure.

Serum bilirubin is elevated, and the prothrombin time is prolonged. Liver enzyme levels (AST, ALT) are often markedly elevated. Additional laboratory tests include blood chemistries (especially glucose, since hypoglycemia may be present and require correction), complete blood counts (CBCs), acetaminophen level and screening for other drugs and toxins, viral hepatitis serologies (especially HAV and HBV), serum ceruloplasmin (enzyme synthesized in liver) levels, α_1-antitrypsin levels, iron levels, and autoantibodies (antinuclear and anti–smooth muscle antibodies). Plasma ammonia levels may also be obtained.

CT or magnetic resonance imaging (MRI) is helpful in providing information about the liver size and contour, presence of ascites, tumors, and patency of the blood vessels.

NURSING AND COLLABORATIVE MANAGEMENT ACUTE LIVER FAILURE

Since acute liver failure may progress rapidly, with hour-by-hour changes in consciousness, early transfer to the ICU is preferred once the diagnosis is made. Planning for transfer to a transplant center should begin in patients with grade 1 or 2 encephalopathy because they may worsen rapidly. Early transfer is important because the risks involved with patient transport may increase or even preclude transfer once stage 3 or 4 encephalopathy develops (see Table 44-11).

Renal failure is a frequent complication in patients with liver failure and may be due to dehydration, hepatorenal syndrome, or acute tubular necrosis. The frequency of renal failure may be even greater with acetaminophen overdose or other toxins, where direct renal toxicity occurs. Although few patients die of renal failure alone, it often increases the mortality risk and may worsen the prognosis. Protect renal function by maintaining adequate fluid balance, avoiding nephrotoxic agents (e.g., aminoglycosides, NSAIDs), and promptly identifying and treating infection.

Liver transplantation is the treatment of choice for and increases survival rates in patients with acute liver failure. Cerebral edema, cerebellar herniation, and brainstem compression are the most common causes of death. Treatment of cerebral edema is described in Chapter 57. Monitoring and management of hemodynamic and renal function, as well as glucose, electrolytes, and acid-base status, are critical. Conduct frequent neurologic evaluations for signs of elevated intracranial pressure. Position the patient with the head elevated at 30 degrees. Avoid patient stimulation. Maneuvers that cause straining or Valsalva-like movements may increase intracranial pressure (ICP).

Avoid the use of any sedatives because of their effects on mental status. Only minimal doses of benzodiazepines should be used due to their delayed metabolism by the failing liver. ICP monitoring is discussed in Chapter 57. Additional measures include padding bedrails to avoid injury from possible seizures, closely observing the patient to prevent injuries, monitoring intake and output for renal function, and providing good skin and oral care to avoid breakdown and infection.

Alterations in level of consciousness may compromise nutritional intake. Factors such as coagulation problems may influence whether enteral nutrition is initiated. An NG tube may be irritating to the nasal and esophageal mucosa, thus causing bleeding.[28]

LIVER CANCER (HEPATOCELLULAR CANCER)

Primary liver cancer (hepatocellular carcinoma [HCC] or malignant hepatoma) is the fifth most common cancer and second most common cause of cancer death worldwide.[29] It is the most common cause of death in patients with cirrhosis. The incidence of HCC is rising in the United States because of the large number of patients infected with chronic hepatitis C. Cirrhosis caused by hepatitis C is the most common cause of HCC in the United States, followed by alcoholic cirrhosis.[30] Other

FIG. 44-10 Multiple hepatic metastases from a primary colon cancer. **A,** Gross specimen showing outside of liver. **B,** Liver section showing metastatic lesions.

primary liver tumors are cholangiomas or bile duct cancers (cholangiocarcinoma).

Metastatic carcinoma of the liver is more common than primary carcinoma (Fig. 44-10). The liver is a common site of metastatic growth because of its high rate of blood flow and extensive capillary network. Cancer cells in other parts of the body are commonly carried to the liver via the portal circulation.

In liver cancer, lesions may be singular or numerous and nodular or diffusely spread over the entire liver. Some tumors infiltrate other organs such as the gallbladder or move into the peritoneum or the diaphragm. Primary liver tumors commonly metastasize to the lung.

Clinical Manifestations and Diagnostic Studies

Liver cancer can be difficult to diagnose and differentiate from cirrhosis. They have similar clinical manifestations (e.g., hepatomegaly, splenomegaly, jaundice, weight loss, peripheral edema, ascites, portal hypertension). Other common manifestations of liver cancer include dull abdominal pain in the epigastric or right upper quadrant region, anorexia, nausea and vomiting, and increased abdominal girth. Patients with advanced HCC can have pulmonary emboli and portal vein thrombosis.

Tests used to screen and diagnose liver cancer are ultrasound, CT, and MRI. A percutaneous biopsy is performed when the results of diagnostic imaging studies are inconclusive or tissue is needed to guide treatment. Risks of biopsy include bleeding and potential tumor cell spread. Serum α-fetoprotein (AFP) levels are elevated in approximately 60% of patients with HCC. The level of elevation may not correlate with the clinical features of HCC (e.g., stage or prognosis). (AFP is discussed in Chapter 16.)

NURSING AND COLLABORATIVE MANAGEMENT LIVER CANCER

Prevention of liver cancer focuses on identifying and treating chronic hepatitis B and C viral infections. Treatment of chronic alcohol ingestion may also lower the risk of liver cancer. Screening for at-risk patients usually involves a combination of serum AFP and either CT, MRI, or ultrasound imaging of the liver, usually obtained every 6 to 12 months.

Treatment of liver cancer depends on the size and number of tumors, any spreading beyond the liver, and the patient's age and overall health. In general, the management is similar to that for cirrhosis. Surgical excision (partial hepatectomy) is performed when there is no evidence of invasion of hepatic blood vessels. Surgical resection is possible in only about 15% of patients because the cancer is usually too advanced when the patient is diagnosed. However, surgical interventions offer the best chance for cure of HCC. Liver transplantation is performed when the tumor is localized. Other treatment options are radiofrequency ablation, chemoembolization, and alcohol injection.

In *radiofrequency ablation* (RFA), a thin needle is inserted into the core of the tumor. Then electrical energy is used to create heat in a specific location for a limited time. The end result is destruction of tumor cells. This procedure can be done percutaneously, laparoscopically, or through an open incision. RFA can be used to treat tumors that are less than 5 cm in size and for palliative purposes. Complications are not common but can include infection, bleeding, dysrhythmias, and skin burn.

Chemoembolization (sometimes called transarterial chemoembolization [TACE]) is a minimally invasive procedure frequently performed in the interventional radiology department. A catheter is placed in the arteries to the tumor and an embolic agent is administered, mixed with one or more chemotherapy agents. The embolic agent reduces the blood supply, thus allowing greater exposure of liver cells to the chemotherapy drugs.

With the technique of alcohol injection, surgeons or interventional radiologists identify (with the use of ultrasound) the location of the liver tumor(s). They insert a needle into the tumor and inject a liquid containing a high concentration of alcohol. The concentrated alcohol kills cells, mostly liver cancer cells. This form of treatment is most effective in treating small liver tumors (less than 3 cm).

Systemic chemotherapy is not used for patients with HCC because of the poor response rates. Sorafenib (Nexavar), a targeted therapy, is used to treat metastatic liver cancer. It inhibits new blood vessel growth to tumors (see Table 16-13).

Nursing intervention for the patient with liver cancer focuses on keeping the patient as comfortable as possible. Because this patient manifests the same problems as any patient with advanced liver disease, the nursing interventions discussed for cirrhosis of the liver apply. (See Chapter 16 for care of the patient with cancer.)

The prognosis for patients with liver cancer is poor. The cancer grows rapidly, and death may occur within 6 to 12 months as a result of hepatic encephalopathy or massive blood loss from GI bleeding.

LIVER TRANSPLANTATION

Liver transplantation has become a practical therapeutic option for many people with end-stage liver disease or localized HCC. Liver disease related to chronic viral hepatitis is the leading indication for liver transplantation. Other indications include congenital biliary abnormalities (biliary atresia), inborn errors of metabolism, liver cancer, sclerosing cholangitis, acute liver failure, and chronic end-stage liver disease. Liver transplants are not recommended for the patient with widespread malignant disease. Currently about 17,000 people are waiting for liver transplants. However, only 6000 transplants are performed annually.[31]

Liver transplant candidates must go through a rigorous pre-surgery screening. This is done to confirm the diagnosis of end-stage liver disease and to assess for other co-morbid conditions (e.g., cardiovascular disease, chronic kidney disease) that may affect the patient's surgical outcome. The evaluation includes physical examination, laboratory tests (CBC, liver function tests), cardiac and pulmonary evaluations, endoscopy, CT scan, and psychologic testing. Potential recipients receive counseling regarding cigarette smoking and alcohol abstinence. Contraindications for liver transplant include severe extrahepatic disease, advanced hepatocellular carcinoma or other cancer, ongoing drug or alcohol abuse, and inability to comprehend or comply with the rigorous posttransplant course.

Liver transplantation is performed using both deceased (cadaver) and live donor livers. (See Chapter 14 for a general discussion of organ transplants.) The live donor liver transplant was developed initially for children whose parents wanted to serve as donors. Today, some liver transplant centers are performing live liver transplant procedures for adults. In this procedure, the living person donates a portion of his or her liver to another. However, live liver donation poses potential risks to the donor, including biliary problems, hepatic artery thrombosis, wound infection, postoperative ileus, and pneumothorax.

Because of the scarcity of available livers, a donor liver may be divided into two parts (split liver transplant) and implanted into two recipients. The decision to use a split donor liver is based on the donor's size and health. The recipients of the split liver generally are smaller than the donor. The success rate associated with split liver transplantation is somewhat lower than that associated with whole organ transplantation because of complications.

Postoperative complications of liver transplant include bleeding, infection, and rejection. However, the liver is subject to a less aggressive immunologic attack than other organs such as the kidneys. (Transplants and immunosuppressive therapy are discussed in Chapter 14.)

Immunosuppressive therapy generally involves a combination of corticosteroids (prednisone), a calcineurin inhibitor (cyclosporine or tacrolimus), and an antiproliferative agent (e.g., azathioprine). (Immunosuppressive therapy is presented in Table 14-16.) Tacrolimus appears to be superior to cyclosporine in liver transplantation and is being used in many centers. Standard regimens often change during the course of a liver transplant recipient's life. In addition, corticosteroid withdrawal, which has been shown to be relatively safe in liver transplant recipients, has been done in some centers.

Approximately 78% of patients survive more than 5 years after liver transplant. Long-term survival depends on the cause of liver failure (e.g., localized liver cancer, chronic hepatitis B or C, biliary disease). Patients who have liver disease secondary to viral hepatitis often experience reinfection of the transplanted liver with hepatitis B or C. For patients with HBV, treatment after surgery with IV HBIG and one of the nucleoside or nucleotide analogs (used to treat HBV infection) has reduced the rates of reinfection of the transplanted liver.

Patients with HCV have lower survival rates than other patient groups. Factors that may contribute to recurrent HCV include the donor's advanced age, HCV genotype 1, high HCV RNA levels before the transplant, and co-infection with other viruses (e.g., cytomegalovirus). Although the recurrence of HCV is nearly universal after liver transplantation, avoidance of changes in immunosuppressive regimen helps to prevent clinically aggressive disease. Because of adverse effects associated with its use, antiviral therapy for hepatitis C after transplant is initiated on an individual basis.

The patient who has had a liver transplant requires highly skilled nursing care, either in an ICU or in some other specialized unit. Postoperative nursing care includes assessing neurologic status; monitoring for signs of hemorrhage; preventing pulmonary complications; monitoring drainage, electrolyte levels, and urine output; and monitoring for signs and symptoms of infection and rejection. Common respiratory problems are pneumonia, atelectasis, and pleural effusions. To prevent these complications, encourage the patient to use measures such as coughing, deep breathing, incentive spirometry, and repositioning. Measure the drainage from the Jackson-Pratt drain, NG tube, and T tube, and note the color and consistency of the drainage.

The first 2 months after the surgery are critical for monitoring for infection. Infection can be viral, fungal, or bacterial. Fever may be the only sign of infection. Emotional support and teaching for the patient and caregiver are essential.

GERONTOLOGIC CONSIDERATIONS

LIVER DISEASE IN THE OLDER ADULT

The incidence of liver disease increases with age. With aging, the liver's size and metabolism of drugs decrease, and hepatobiliary function is altered. The liver has a decreased ability to respond to injury, particularly to regenerate after injury.[32] Transplanted livers take longer to regenerate in the older adult compared with the younger adult.

Older adults are particularly vulnerable to drug-induced liver injury. This is due to several factors, including increased use of prescription and OTC drugs, which can lead to drug interactions and potential drug toxicity. Age-related decreases in liver function caused by decreased liver blood flow and enzyme activity result in decreased drug metabolism. In addition, with aging the liver is less able to recover from drug-induced injury.

A growing number of older adults have chronic hepatitis C and subsequent cirrhosis. HCV and elevated liver enzymes may be found during a routine health assessment. Because older adults have more co-morbid conditions, liver transplant following liver failure may not be an option.

Lifetime health behaviors may also influence the development of chronic liver disease in the older adult. Chronic alcohol abuse and obesity can contribute to cirrhosis, fatty liver inflammation (NASH), and subsequent liver failure. Because of co-morbid cardiovascular and pulmonary diseases, the older adult is less able to tolerate variceal bleeding. In the older adult

PATHOPHYSIOLOGY MAP

Etiologic factors		Activation of pancreatic enzymes		Autodigestive effects of pancreatic enzymes

Etiologic factors
- Alcoholism
- Biliary tract disease
- Trauma
- Infection
- Drugs
- Postoperative GI surgery
- Unknown

Activation of pancreatic enzymes

Injury to pancreatic cells

Autodigestive effects of pancreatic enzymes

Trypsin
- Edema
- Necrosis
- Hemorrhage

Elastase
- Hemorrhage

Phospholipase A and lipase
- Fat necrosis

Kallikrein
- Edema
- Vascular permeability
- Smooth muscle contraction
- Shock

FIG. 44-11 Pathogenic process of acute pancreatitis.

with liver disease, hepatic encephalopathy may be misdiagnosed as dementia.

DISORDERS OF THE PANCREAS

ACUTE PANCREATITIS

Acute pancreatitis is an acute inflammation of the pancreas. The degree of inflammation varies from mild edema to severe hemorrhagic necrosis. Acute pancreatitis is most common in middle-aged men and women. On an annual basis, approximately 210,000 persons are admitted to the hospital with acute pancreatitis. It affects women and men equally. The rate of pancreatitis in African Americans is three times higher than in whites.

Etiology and Pathophysiology

Many factors can cause injury to the pancreas. In the United States the most common cause is gallbladder disease (gallstones), which is more common in women. The second most common cause is chronic alcohol intake, which is more common in men.

Smoking is an independent risk factor for acute pancreatitis. **Biliary sludge** or microlithiasis, which is a mixture of cholesterol crystals and calcium salts, is found in 20% to 40% of patients with acute pancreatitis. The formation of biliary sludge is seen in patients with bile stasis. Acute pancreatitis attacks are also associated with hypertriglyceridemia (serum levels over 1000 mg/dL). Other less common causes of acute pancreatitis include trauma (postsurgical, abdominal), viral infections (mumps, coxsackievirus B, HIV), penetrating duodenal ulcer, cysts, abscesses, cystic fibrosis, Kaposi sarcoma, certain drugs (corticosteroids, thiazide diuretics, oral contraceptives, sulfonamides, NSAIDs), metabolic disorders (hyperparathyroidism, renal failure), and vascular diseases.[33]

Pancreatitis may occur after surgical procedures on the pancreas, stomach, duodenum, or biliary tract. Pancreatitis can also develop following endoscopic retrograde cholangiopancreatography (ERCP). In some cases the cause is unknown (idiopathic).

The most common pathogenic mechanism is autodigestion of the pancreas (Fig. 44-11). The etiologic factors injure pancreatic cells or activate the pancreatic enzymes in the pancreas rather than in the intestine. This may be due to reflux of bile

FIG. 44-12 In acute pancreatitis, the pancreas appears edematous and is commonly hemorrhagic *(H)*.

acids into the pancreatic ducts through an open or distended sphincter of Oddi. This reflux may be caused by blockage created by gallstones. Obstruction of pancreatic ducts results in pancreatic ischemia.

Trypsinogen is an inactive proteolytic enzyme produced by the pancreas. It is released into the small intestine via the pancreatic duct. In the intestine it is activated to trypsin by enterokinase. Normally, trypsin inhibitors in the pancreas and plasma bind and inactivate any trypsin that is inadvertently produced. In pancreatitis, activated trypsin in the pancreas can digest the pancreas and produce bleeding.

The exact mechanism by which chronic alcohol intake predisposes a person to pancreatitis is not known. It is thought that alcohol increases the production of the digestive enzymes in the pancreas. Approximately 5% to 10% of alcohol abusers develop pancreatitis. This suggests that environmental (high-fat diet, smoking) and genetic factors may also contribute.

The pathophysiologic involvement of acute pancreatitis is classified as either *mild pancreatitis* (also known as edematous or interstitial pancreatitis) or *severe pancreatitis* (also called *necrotizing pancreatitis*) (Fig. 44-12). In severe pancreatitis, approximately half the patients have permanent decreases in endocrine and exocrine function. Patients with severe pancreatitis are also at high risk of developing pancreatic necrosis, organ failure, and septic complications, resulting in a 25% mortality rate.[33,34]

Clinical Manifestations

Abdominal pain is the predominant manifestation of acute pancreatitis. The pain is due to distention of the pancreas, peritoneal irritation, and obstruction of the biliary tract. The pain is usually located in the left upper quadrant, but it may be in the midepigastrium. It commonly radiates to the back because of the retroperitoneal location of the pancreas. The pain has a sudden onset and is described as severe, deep, piercing, and continuous or steady. The pain is aggravated by eating and frequently has its onset when the patient is recumbent. It is not relieved by vomiting. The pain may be accompanied by flushing, cyanosis, and dyspnea. The patient may assume various positions involving flexion of the spine in an attempt to relieve the severe pain. Other manifestations of acute pancreatitis include nausea and vomiting, low-grade fever, leukocytosis, hypotension, tachycardia, and jaundice.

Abdominal tenderness with muscle guarding is common. Bowel sounds may be decreased or absent. Paralytic ileus may occur and causes marked abdominal distention. The lungs are frequently involved, with crackles present. Intravascular damage from circulating trypsin may cause areas of cyanosis or greenish to yellow-brown discoloration of the abdominal wall. Other areas of ecchymoses are the flanks (*Grey Turner's spots* or *sign*, a bluish flank discoloration) and the periumbilical area (*Cullen's sign*, a bluish periumbilical discoloration). These result from seepage of blood-stained exudate from the pancreas and may occur in severe cases.

Shock may occur because of hemorrhage into the pancreas, toxemia from the activated pancreatic enzymes, or hypovolemia as a result of fluid shift into the retroperitoneal space (massive fluid shifts).

Complications

The severity of the disease varies according to the extent of pancreatic destruction. Some patients recover completely, others have recurring attacks, and others develop chronic pancreatitis. Acute pancreatitis can be life threatening.

Two significant local complications of acute pancreatitis are pseudocyst and abscess. A pancreatic pseudocyst is an accumulation of fluid, pancreatic enzymes, tissue debris, and inflammatory exudates surrounded by a wall. Manifestations of pseudocyst are abdominal pain, palpable epigastric mass, nausea, vomiting, and anorexia. The serum amylase level frequently remains elevated. CT, MRI, and endoscopic ultrasound (EUS) may be used in the detection of a pseudocyst. The cysts usually resolve spontaneously within a few weeks but may perforate, causing peritonitis, or rupture into the stomach or the duodenum. Treatment options include surgical drainage, percutaneous catheter placement and drainage, and endoscopic drainage.

A *pancreatic abscess* is a collection of pus. It results from extensive necrosis in the pancreas. It may become infected or perforate into adjacent organs. Manifestations of an abscess include upper abdominal pain, abdominal mass, high fever, and leukocytosis. Pancreatic abscesses require prompt surgical drainage to prevent sepsis.

The main systemic complications of acute pancreatitis are pulmonary (pleural effusion, atelectasis, pneumonia, and acute respiratory distress syndrome [ARDS]) and cardiovascular (hypotension) complications and tetany caused by hypocalcemia. The pulmonary complications are likely due to the passage of exudate containing pancreatic enzymes from the peritoneal cavity through transdiaphragmatic lymph channels. Enzyme-induced inflammation of the diaphragm occurs with the end result being atelectasis caused by reduced diaphragm movement. Trypsin can activate prothrombin and plasminogen,

increasing the patient's risk for intravascular thrombi, pulmonary emboli, and disseminated intravascular coagulation. When hypocalcemia occurs, it is a sign of severe disease. It is due in part to the combining of calcium and fatty acids during fat necrosis. The exact mechanisms of how or why hypocalcemia occurs are not well understood.

Patients with severe acute pancreatitis are at risk for abdominal compartment syndrome as a result of intraabdominal hypertension and edema. Abdominal compartment syndrome is discussed in Chapter 43.

Diagnostic Studies

The primary diagnostic tests for acute pancreatitis are serum amylase and lipase (Table 44-16). The serum amylase level is usually elevated early and remains elevated for 24 to 72 hours. Serum lipase level, which is also elevated in acute pancreatitis, is an important test because other disorders (e.g., mumps, cerebral trauma, renal transplantation) may increase serum amylase levels. Other findings include an increase in liver enzymes, triglycerides, glucose, and bilirubin and a decrease in calcium.

Diagnostic evaluation of acute pancreatitis is also directed at determining the cause. An abdominal ultrasound, x-ray, or contrast-enhanced CT scan can be used to identify pancreatic problems. CT scan is the best imaging test for pancreatitis and related complications such as pseudocysts and abscesses. ERCP is used (although ERCP can cause acute pancreatitis), along with EUS, magnetic resonance cholangiopancreatography (MRCP), and angiography. Chest x-rays may show pulmonary changes, including atelectasis and pleural effusions.

Collaborative Care

Goals of collaborative care for acute pancreatitis include (1) relief of pain; (2) prevention or alleviation of shock; (3) reduction of pancreatic secretions; (4) correction of fluid and electrolyte imbalances; (5) prevention or treatment of infections; and (6) removal of the precipitating cause, if possible (Table 44-17).

Conservative Therapy. Treatment is primarily focused on supportive care, including aggressive hydration, pain management, management of metabolic complications, and minimization of pancreatic stimulation. Treatment and control of pain are very important. IV morphine may be used. Pain medications may be combined with an antispasmodic agent. However, atropine and other anticholinergic drugs should be avoided when paralytic ileus is present because they can decrease GI mobility, thus contributing to the problem. Other medications that relax smooth muscles (spasmolytics), such as nitroglycerin or papaverine, may be used. Supplemental oxygen is provided to maintain oxygen saturation greater than 95%. In patients with severe pancreatitis, serum glucose levels are closely monitored for hyperglycemia.

TABLE 44-16 DIAGNOSTIC STUDIES

Acute Pancreatitis

Laboratory Test	Abnormal Finding
Serum amylase	↑
Serum lipase	↑
Urinary amylase	↑
Blood glucose	↑
Serum calcium	↓
Serum triglycerides	↑

TABLE 44-17 COLLABORATIVE CARE
Acute Pancreatitis

Diagnostic
- History and physical examination
- Serum amylase
- Serum lipase
- Blood glucose
- Serum calcium
- Serum triglycerides
- Flat plate of the abdomen
- Abdominal ultrasound
- Endoscopic ultrasound (EUS)
- Contrast-enhanced CT of pancreas
- Magnetic resonance cholangiopancreatography (MRCP)
- Endoscopic retrograde cholangiopancreatography (ERCP)
- Chest x-ray

Collaborative Therapy
- Pain medication (e.g., morphine)
- NPO with NG tube to suction
- Albumin (if shock present)
- IV calcium gluconate (10%) (if tetany present)
- Lactated Ringer's solution
- Proton pump inhibitor (e.g., omeprazole [Prilosec])
- Antibiotics (if necrotizing pancreatitis)

TABLE 44-18 DRUG THERAPY
Acute and Chronic Pancreatitis

Drug	Mechanism of Action
Acute Pancreatitis	
morphine	Relief of pain
Antispasmodics (e.g., dicyclomine [Bentyl])	↓ Vagal stimulation, motility, pancreatic outflow (↓ volume and concentration of bicarbonate and enzyme secretion)
	Contraindicated in paralytic ileus
Carbonic anhydrase inhibitor (acetazolamide [Diamox])	↓ Volume and bicarbonate concentration of pancreatic secretion
Antacids	Neutralization of gastric hydrochloric (HCl) acid secretion
	↓ Production and secretion of pancreatic enzymes and bicarbonate
Proton pump inhibitors (omeprazole [Prilosec])	↓ HCl acid secretion (HCl acid stimulates pancreatic activity)
Chronic Pancreatitis	
Pancreatic enzyme products (pancrelipase [Pancrease, Zenpep, Creon, Viokase])	Replacement therapy for pancreatic enzymes
Insulin	Treatment for diabetes mellitus or hyperglycemia, if needed

If shock is present, blood volume replacements are used. Plasma or plasma volume expanders such as dextran or albumin may be given. Fluid and electrolyte imbalances are corrected with lactated Ringer's solution or other electrolyte solutions. Central venous pressure readings may be used to assist in determining fluid replacement requirements. Vasoactive drugs such as dopamine (Intropin) may be used to increase systemic vascular resistance in patients with ongoing hypotension.

It is important to reduce or suppress pancreatic enzymes to decrease stimulation of the pancreas and allow it to rest. This is accomplished in several ways. First, the patient is NPO (taking nothing by mouth). Second, NG suction may be used to reduce vomiting and gastric distention and to prevent gastric acidic contents from entering the duodenum. In addition, certain drugs may be used to suppress gastric acid secretion (Table 44-18). With resolution of the pancreatitis, the patient resumes oral intake. For the patient with severe acute pancreatitis who does not resume oral intake, enteral nutrition support may be initiated.

The inflamed and necrotic pancreatic tissue is a good medium for bacterial growth. In patients with acute necrotizing pancreatitis, infection is the leading cause of morbidity and mortality. Therefore it is important to prevent infections. Because many of the organisms come from the intestine, enteral feeding reduces the risk of necrotizing pancreatitis. Monitor the patient closely so that antibiotic therapy can be instituted early if necrosis and infection occur. Endoscopic- or CT-guided percutaneous aspiration with Gram stain and culture may be performed.

Surgical Therapy. When the acute pancreatitis is related to gallstones, an urgent ERCP plus endoscopic *sphincterotomy* (severing of the muscle layers of the sphincter of Oddi) may be done. This may be followed by laparoscopic cholecystectomy to reduce the potential for recurrence. Surgical intervention may also be indicated when the diagnosis is uncertain and for patients who do not respond to conservative therapy. Those with severe acute pancreatitis may require drainage of necrotic fluid collections. This is done either surgically, under CT guid-

ance, or endoscopically. Percutaneous drainage of a pseudocyst can be performed, and a drainage tube is left in place.

Drug Therapy. Several different drugs are used to prevent and treat problems associated with pancreatitis (see Table 44-18). Currently there are no drugs that cure pancreatitis.

Nutritional Therapy. Initially the patient with acute pancreatitis is on NPO status to reduce pancreatic secretion. Depending on the severity of the pancreatitis, enteral feedings via nasojejunal tube are initiated. Because of infection risk, parenteral nutrition is reserved for patients who cannot tolerate enteral nutrition (see Chapter 40). If IV lipids are ordered, blood triglyceride levels need to be monitored. In cases of moderate to severe pancreatitis, the patient may require enteral feeding via a jejunal feeding tube. When food is allowed, small, frequent feedings are given. The diet is usually high in carbohydrate content because that is the least stimulating to the exocrine portion of the pancreas. Suspect intolerance to oral foods when the patient reports pain, has increasing abdominal girth, or has elevations in serum amylase and lipase levels. The patient needs to abstain from alcohol. Supplemental fat-soluble vitamins may be given.

NURSING MANAGEMENT ACUTE PANCREATITIS

NURSING ASSESSMENT
Subjective and objective data that should be obtained from a person with acute pancreatitis are presented in Table 44-19.

NURSING DIAGNOSES
Nursing diagnoses for the patient with acute pancreatitis may include, but are not limited to, the following:
- Acute pain *related to* distention of pancreas, peritoneal irritation, obstruction of biliary tract, and ineffective pain and comfort measures
- Deficient fluid volume *related to* nausea, vomiting, restricted oral intake, and fluid shift into the retroperitoneal space

TABLE 44-19 NURSING ASSESSMENT

Acute Pancreatitis

Subjective Data
Important Health Information
Past health history: Biliary tract disease, alcohol use, abdominal trauma, duodenal ulcers, infection, metabolic disorders
Medications: Thiazides, nonsteroidal antiinflammatory drugs
Surgery or other treatments: Surgical procedures on the pancreas, stomach, duodenum, or biliary tract; endoscopic retrograde cholangiopancreatography (ERCP)

Functional Health Patterns
Health perception–health management: Alcohol abuse; fatigue
Nutritional-metabolic: Nausea and vomiting; anorexia
Activity-exercise: Dyspnea
Cognitive-perceptual: Severe midepigastric or left upper quadrant pain that may radiate to the back, aggravated by food and alcohol intake and unrelieved by vomiting

Objective Data
General
Restlessness, anxiety, low-grade fever

Integumentary
Flushing, diaphoresis, discoloration of abdomen and flanks, cyanosis, jaundice; decreased skin turgor, dry mucous membranes

Respiratory
Tachypnea, basilar crackles

Cardiovascular
Tachycardia, hypotension

Gastrointestinal
Abdominal distention, tenderness, and muscle guarding; diminished bowel sounds

Possible Diagnostic Findings
↑ Serum amylase and lipase, leukocytosis, hyperglycemia, hypocalcemia, abnormal ultrasound and CT scans of pancreas, abnormal ERCP or MRCP

- Imbalanced nutrition: less than body requirements *related to* anorexia, dietary restrictions, nausea, loss of nutrients from vomiting, and impaired digestion
- Ineffective self-health management *related to* lack of knowledge of preventive measures, diet restrictions, alcohol restriction intake, and follow-up care

Additional information on nursing diagnoses for the patient with acute pancreatitis is presented in eNursing Care Plan 44-3 (available on the website for this chapter).

PLANNING

The overall goals are that the patient with acute pancreatitis will have (1) relief of pain, (2) normal fluid and electrolyte balance, (3) minimal to no complications, and (4) no recurrent attacks.

NURSING IMPLEMENTATION

HEALTH PROMOTION. The major factors involved in health promotion are (1) assessment of the patient for predisposing and etiologic factors and (2) encouragement of early treatment of these factors to prevent acute pancreatitis. Encourage early diagnosis and treatment of biliary tract disease, such as cholelithiasis. Encourage the patient to eliminate alcohol intake, especially if he or she has had any previous episodes of pancre-

atitis. Attacks of pancreatitis become milder or disappear with the discontinuance of alcohol use.

ACUTE INTERVENTION. During the acute phase, it is important to monitor vital signs. Hemodynamic stability may be compromised by hypotension, fever, and tachypnea. Monitor the response to IV fluids. Also closely monitor fluid and electrolyte balance. Frequent vomiting, along with gastric suction, may result in decreased chloride, sodium, and potassium levels.

Respiratory failure may develop in the patient with severe acute pancreatitis. Assess respiratory function (e.g., lung sounds, oxygen saturation levels). If ARDS develops, the patient may require intubation and mechanical ventilatory support.

SAFETY ALERT
- Assess for respiratory distress in the patient with severe acute pancreatitis.
- Listen to lung sounds and monitor O_2 saturation on a regular basis.

Because hypocalcemia can also occur, observe for symptoms of tetany, such as jerking, irritability, and muscular twitching. Numbness or tingling around the lips and in the fingers is an early indicator of hypocalcemia. Assess the patient for a positive Chvostek's sign or Trousseau's sign (see Fig. 17-15). Calcium gluconate (as ordered) should be given to treat symptomatic hypocalcemia. Hypomagnesemia may also develop, necessitating the monitoring of serum magnesium levels.

Because abdominal pain is a prominent symptom of pancreatitis, a major focus of your care is the relief of pain (see eNursing Care Plan 44-3). Pain and restlessness can increase the metabolic rate and subsequent stimulation of pancreatic enzymes. In addition, acute pain can contribute to hemodynamic instability. Morphine may be used for pain relief. Assess and document the duration of pain relief. Measures such as comfortable positioning, frequent changes in position, and relief of nausea and vomiting assist in reducing the restlessness that usually accompanies the pain. Assuming positions that flex the trunk and draw the knees up to the abdomen may decrease pain. A side-lying position with the head elevated 45 degrees decreases tension on the abdomen and may help ease the pain.

For the patient who is on NPO status or has an NG tube, provide frequent oral and nasal care to relieve the dryness of the mouth and nose. Oral care is essential to prevent parotitis. If the patient is taking anticholinergics to decrease GI secretions, the mouth will be especially dry. If the patient is taking antacids to neutralize gastric acid secretion, they should be sipped slowly or inserted in the NG tube.

Observe for fever and other manifestations of infection in the patient with acute pancreatitis. Respiratory tract infections are common because the retroperitoneal fluid raises the diaphragm, which causes the patient to take shallow, guarded abdominal breaths. Measures to prevent respiratory tract infections include turning, coughing, deep breathing, and assuming a semi-Fowler's position.

Other important assessments are observation for signs of paralytic ileus, renal failure, and mental changes. Determine the blood glucose level to assess damage to the β cells of the islets of Langerhans in the pancreas.

After pancreatic surgery, the patient may require special wound care for an anastomotic leak or a fistula. To prevent skin irritation, use skin barriers (e.g., Stomahesive, Karaya Paste, or Colly-Seel), pouching, and drains. In addition to protecting the skin, pouching also permits a more accurate determination of fluid and electrolyte losses and increases patient comfort.

Sterile pouching systems are available. Consult with a clinical specialist or wound, ostomy, and continence (WOC) nurse, if available.

AMBULATORY AND HOME CARE. After acute pancreatitis, the patient may require home care follow-up. Because of loss of physical and muscle strength, physical therapy may be needed. Continued care to prevent infection and detect any complications is important. Counseling regarding abstinence from alcohol is important to prevent the patient from experiencing future attacks of acute pancreatitis and development of chronic pancreatitis. Because cigarettes can stimulate the pancreas, smoking should be avoided.

Dietary teaching should include restriction of fats because they stimulate the secretion of cholecystokinin, which then stimulates the pancreas. Carbohydrates are less stimulating to the pancreas and are encouraged. Instruct the patient to avoid crash dieting and bingeing because they can precipitate attacks.

Instruct the patient and the caregiver to recognize and report symptoms of infection, diabetes mellitus, or steatorrhea (foul-smelling, frothy stools). These changes indicate possible ongoing destruction of pancreatic tissue. Teach the patient and caregiver about the prescribed regimen, including the importance of taking the required medications and following the recommended diet.

EVALUATION

The expected outcomes are that the patient with acute pancreatitis will
- Have adequate pain control
- Maintain adequate fluid balance
- Be knowledgeable about treatment regimen to restore health
- Get help for alcohol dependence (if appropriate)

CHRONIC PANCREATITIS

Chronic pancreatitis is a continuous, prolonged, inflammatory, and fibrosing process of the pancreas. The pancreas is progressively destroyed as it is replaced by fibrotic tissue. Strictures and calcifications may also occur in the pancreas.

Etiology and Pathophysiology

Chronic pancreatitis can be due to alcohol abuse; obstruction caused by cholelithiasis (gallstones), tumor, pseudocysts, or trauma; and systemic diseases (e.g., systemic lupus erythematosus), autoimmune pancreatitis, and cystic fibrosis. Some patients may not have an identifiable risk factor (idiopathic pancreatitis). Chronic pancreatitis may follow acute pancreatitis, but it may also occur in the absence of any history of an acute condition.

The most common cause of obstructive pancreatitis is inflammation of the sphincter of Oddi associated with cholelithiasis. Cancer of the ampulla of Vater, duodenum, or pancreas can also cause this type of chronic pancreatitis.

In nonobstructive pancreatitis there is inflammation and sclerosis, mainly in the head of the pancreas and around the pancreatic duct. This type of chronic pancreatitis is the most common form. In the United States, chronic pancreatitis is found almost exclusively in individuals who abuse alcohol. A genetic factor may predispose a person who drinks to the direct toxic effect of the alcohol on the pancreas.

Clinical Manifestations

As with acute pancreatitis, a major manifestation of chronic pancreatitis is abdominal pain. The patient may have episodes of acute pain, but it usually is chronic (recurrent attacks at intervals of months or years). The attacks may become more and more frequent until they are almost constant, or they may diminish as pancreatic fibrosis develops. The pain is located in the same areas as in acute pancreatitis, but is usually described as a heavy, gnawing feeling or sometimes as burning and cramplike. The pain is not relieved with food or antacids.

Other clinical manifestations include symptoms of pancreatic insufficiency, including malabsorption with weight loss, constipation, mild jaundice with dark urine, steatorrhea, and diabetes mellitus. The steatorrhea may become severe, with voluminous, foul-smelling, fatty stools. Urine and stool may be frothy. Some abdominal tenderness may be present.

Chronic pancreatitis is also associated with a variety of complications, including pseudocyst formation, bile duct or duodenal obstruction, pancreatic ascites or pleural effusion, splenic vein thrombosis, pseudoaneurysms, and pancreatic cancer.

Diagnostic Studies

Confirming the diagnosis of chronic pancreatitis can be challenging. The diagnosis is based on the patient's signs and symptoms, laboratory studies, and imaging. In chronic pancreatitis the levels of serum amylase and lipase may be elevated slightly or not at all, depending on the degree of pancreatic fibrosis. Serum bilirubin and alkaline phosphatase levels may be increased. There is usually mild leukocytosis and an elevated sedimentation rate.

ERCP is used to visualize the pancreatic and common bile ducts. Imaging studies such as CT, MRI, MRCP, abdominal ultrasound, and EUS are useful in patients with chronic pancreatitis. These procedures show a variety of changes, including calcifications, ductal dilation, pseudocysts, and pancreatic enlargement.

Stool samples are examined for fecal fat content. Deficiencies of fat-soluble vitamins and cobalamin, glucose intolerance, and possibly diabetes may also be found in those with chronic pancreatitis. A secretin stimulation test may be used to assess the degree of pancreatic function (see Chapter 39).

Collaborative Care

When the patient with chronic pancreatitis experiences an acute attack, the therapy is identical to that for acute pancreatitis. At other times the focus is on prevention of further attacks, relief of pain, and control of pancreatic exocrine and endocrine insufficiency. It sometimes takes frequent doses of analgesics (morphine or fentanyl patch [Duragesic]) to relieve the pain if dietary measures and enzyme replacement are not effective.

Diet, pancreatic enzyme replacement, and control of diabetes are ways to control the pancreatic insufficiency. Small, bland, frequent meals that are low in fat content are recommended to decrease pancreatic stimulation. Smoking is associated with accelerated progression of chronic pancreatitis. Teach the patient not to consume alcohol and caffeinated beverages.

Pancreatic enzyme products (PEPs) such as pancrelipase (Pancrease, Zenpep, Creon, Viokase) contain amylase, lipase, and trypsin and are used to replace the deficient pancreatic enzymes. They are usually enteric coated to prevent their breakdown or inactivation by gastric acid. Bile salts are sometimes given to facilitate the absorption of the fat-soluble vitamins (A,

D, E, and K) and prevent further fat loss. If diabetes develops, it is controlled with insulin or oral hypoglycemic agents. Acid-neutralizing drugs (e.g., antacids) and acid-inhibiting drugs (e.g., H_2-receptor blockers, proton pump inhibitors) may be given to decrease hydrochloric acid (HCl) secretion but have little overall effect on patient outcomes. Antidepressants, such as nortriptyline (Aventyl), have been shown to reduce the neuropathic pain associated with chronic pancreatitis.

Treatment of chronic pancreatitis sometimes requires endoscopic therapy or surgery. When biliary disease is present or obstruction or pseudocyst develops, surgery may be indicated. Surgical procedures can divert bile flow or relieve ductal obstruction. A choledochojejunostomy diverts bile around the ampulla of Vater, where there may be spasm or hypertrophy of the sphincter. In this procedure the common bile duct is anastomosed into the jejunum. Another type of surgical diverting procedure is the Roux-en-Y pancreatojejunostomy, in which the pancreatic duct is opened and an anastomosis is made with the jejunum. Pancreatic drainage procedures can relieve ductal obstruction and are often done with ERCP. Some patients may undergo ERCP with sphincterotomy and/or stent placement at the site of obstruction. These patients require follow-up procedures such as ERCP to either exchange or remove the stent.

NURSING MANAGEMENT CHRONIC PANCREATITIS

Except during an acute episode, nursing management focuses on chronic care and health promotion. Instruct the patient to take measures to prevent further attacks. Dietary control, along with consistency of other treatment measures, such as taking pancreatic enzymes, is essential. The enzymes are usually taken with meals or a snack. Observe the patient's stools for steatorrhea to help determine the effectiveness of the enzymes. Instruct the patient and the caregiver to observe the stools.

If diabetes has developed, instruct the patient regarding testing of blood glucose levels and drug therapy (see Chapter 49). Ensure that the patient who is taking antisecretory agents or antacids takes them as ordered to control gastric acidity. Antacids should be taken after meals and at bedtime.

The patient must avoid alcohol and may need assistance with this problem. If the patient is dependent on alcohol, referral to other agencies or resources may be necessary (see Chapter 11).

PANCREATIC CANCER

Annually in the United States an estimated 42,500 people are diagnosed with pancreatic cancer, and 35,300 people die from pancreatic cancer.[34] It is the fourth leading cause of death from cancer in the United States. The risk increases with age, with the peak incidence occurring between 65 and 80 years of age.

Most pancreatic tumors are adenocarcinomas originating from the epithelium of the ductal system. More than half of the tumors occur in the head of the pancreas. As the tumor grows, the common bile duct becomes obstructed, and obstructive jaundice develops. Tumors starting in the body or the tail often remain silent until their growth is advanced. The majority of cancers have metastasized at the time of diagnosis. The signs and symptoms of pancreatic cancer are often similar to those of chronic pancreatitis. The prognosis of a patient with cancer of the pancreas is poor. The majority of patients die within 5 to 12

months of the initial diagnosis, and the 5-year survival rate is less than 5%.

Etiology and Pathophysiology

The cause of pancreatic cancer remains unknown. Risk factors for pancreatic cancer include chronic pancreatitis, diabetes mellitus, age, cigarette smoking, family history of pancreatic cancer, high-fat diet, and exposure to chemicals such as benzidine. African Americans have a higher incidence of pancreatic cancer than whites. The most firmly established environmental risk factor is cigarette smoking. Smokers are two to three times more likely to develop pancreatic cancer than nonsmokers. The risk is related to both the duration and amount of cigarettes smoked.

Clinical Manifestations

Common manifestations of pancreatic cancer include abdominal pain (dull, aching), anorexia, rapid and progressive weight loss, nausea, and jaundice. The most common manifestations of cancer of the head of the pancreas are pain, jaundice, and weight loss. Pruritus may accompany obstructive jaundice. In general, pain is common and is related to the location of malignancy. Extreme, unrelenting pain is related to extension of the cancer into the retroperitoneal tissues and nerve plexuses. The pain is frequently located in the upper abdomen or left hypochondrium and often radiates to the back. It is commonly related to eating, and it also occurs at night. Weight loss is due to poor digestion and absorption caused by lack of digestive enzymes from the pancreas.

Diagnostic Studies

Abdominal ultrasound or EUS, spiral CT scan, ERCP, MRI, and MRCP are the most commonly used diagnostic imaging techniques for pancreatic diseases, including cancer. EUS involves imaging the pancreas with the use of an endoscope positioned in the stomach and the duodenum. EUS also allows for fine-needle aspiration of the tumor. CT scan is often the initial study and provides information on metastasis and vascular involvement. ERCP allows visualization of the pancreatic duct and the biliary system. When ERCP is used, pancreatic secretions and tissue can be collected for analysis of different tumor markers. MRI and MRCP may also be used for diagnosing and staging pancreatic cancer. A positron emission tomography (PET) scan or PET/CT scan may also be obtained but usually does not provide additional clinical information.

Tumor markers are used both for establishing the diagnosis of pancreatic adenocarcinoma and for monitoring the response to treatment. Cancer-associated antigen 19-9 (CA 19-9) is elevated in pancreatic cancer and is the most commonly used tumor marker. CA 19-9 can also be elevated in gallbladder cancer or in benign conditions such as acute and chronic pancreatitis, hepatitis, and biliary obstruction.

Collaborative Care

Surgery provides the most effective treatment of cancer of the pancreas. Only 15% to 20% of patients have resectable tumors. The classic surgery is a *radical pancreaticoduodenectomy,* or *Whipple procedure* (Fig. 44-13). This procedure involves resection of the proximal pancreas (proximal pancreatectomy), adjoining duodenum (duodenectomy), distal portion of the stomach (partial gastrectomy), and distal segment of the common bile duct. An anastomosis of the pancreatic duct, common

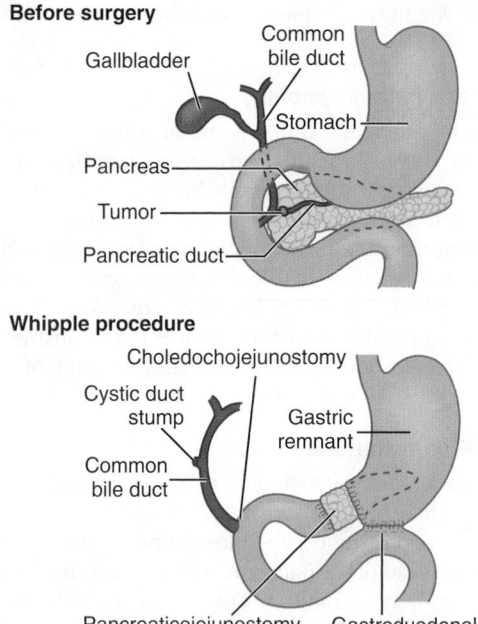

FIG. 44-13 Whipple procedure or radical pancreaticoduodenectomy. This surgical procedure involves resection of the proximal pancreas, adjoining duodenum, distal portion of the stomach, and distal portion of the common bile duct. An anastomosis of the pancreatic duct, common bile duct, and stomach to the jejunum is done.

bile duct, and stomach to the jejunum is done. A total pancreatectomy is performed in some institutions. Sometimes a simple bypass procedure, such as a cholecystojejunostomy to relieve biliary obstruction, may be used as a palliative measure. Some surgeons suggest a more radical resection, such as a total pancreaticoduodenectomy with splenectomy. Endoscopically placed biliary stents can be used as a palliative measure when tumors compress the bile duct.

Radiation therapy alone has little effect on survival, but may be effective for pain relief. External radiation is usually used, but implantation of internal radiation seeds into the tumor has also been used. The current role of chemotherapy in pancreatic cancer is limited. Chemotherapy usually consists of fluorouracil (5-FU) and gemcitabine (Gemzar) either alone or in combination with agents such as capecitabine (Xeloda) or erlotinib (Tarceva). Erlotinib is a targeted therapy (see Table 16-13).

NURSING MANAGEMENT
PANCREATIC CANCER

Because the patient with pancreatic cancer has many of the same problems as the patient with pancreatitis, nursing care includes many of the same measures (see sections on acute and chronic pancreatitis). Provide symptomatic and supportive nursing care. This includes administration of medications and comfort measures to relieve pain. Psychologic support is essential, especially during times of anxiety or depression.

Adequate nutrition is an important part of the nursing care plan. Frequent and supplemental feedings may be necessary. Measures to stimulate the appetite as much as possible and to overcome anorexia, nausea, and vomiting should be included in the nursing care. Because bleeding can result from impaired vitamin K production, assess for bleeding from body orifices

FIG. 44-14 Cholesterol gallstones in a gallbladder that was removed.

and mucous membranes. If the patient is undergoing radiation therapy, observe for adverse reactions, such as anorexia, nausea, vomiting, and skin irritation.

The prognosis for a patient with pancreatic cancer is poor. A significant component of the nursing care is helping the patient and caregiver through the grieving process. Chapter 10 provides information on palliative and end-of-life care.

DISORDERS OF THE BILIARY TRACT

CHOLELITHIASIS AND CHOLECYSTITIS

The most common disorder of the biliary system is **cholelithiasis** (stones in the gallbladder) (Fig. 44-14 and eFig. 44-3 on the website for this chapter). The stones may be lodged in the neck of the gallbladder or in the cystic duct. **Cholecystitis** (inflammation of the gallbladder) is usually associated with cholelithiasis. Cholecystitis may be acute or chronic. Cholelithiasis and cholecystitis usually occur together.

Gallbladder disease is a common health problem in the United States. Approximately 8% to 10% of American adults have cholelithiasis. The actual number is not known because many persons with stones are asymptomatic. *Cholecystectomy* (removal of the gallbladder) ranks among the most common surgical procedures performed in the United States.

The incidence of cholelithiasis is higher in women, especially multiparous women, and persons over 40 years of age. Postmenopausal women on estrogen therapy are at somewhat greater risk of having gallbladder disease than are women who are taking birth control pills. Oral contraceptives affect cholesterol production and increase the likelihood of gallbladder cholesterol saturation. Other factors that increase the occurrence of gallbladder disease are a sedentary lifestyle, a familial tendency, and obesity. Obesity causes increased secretion of cholesterol in bile.

Gallbladder disease is more common in Asian Americans and African Americans than in whites. The incidence is especially high in the Native American population, particularly in the Navajo and Pima tribes.

Etiology and Pathophysiology

Cholelithiasis. The cause of gallstones is unknown. Cholelithiasis develops when the balance that keeps cholesterol, bile salts, and calcium in solution is altered so that these substances precipitate. Conditions that upset this balance include infection

GENDER DIFFERENCES

Cholelithiasis

Men	Women
• Incidence of cholelithiasis is lower in men than in women. • Gender differences in incidence decrease after age 50.	• Pregnancy is the greatest risk factor for increased prevalence in women. • Obesity increases the risk, especially for women.

TABLE 44-20	MANIFESTATIONS OF OBSTRUCTED BILE FLOW

Manifestation	Etiology
Obstructive jaundice	No bile flow into duodenum
Dark amber urine, which foams when shaken	Soluble bilirubin in urine
No urobilinogen in urine	No bilirubin reaching small intestine to be converted to urobilinogen
Clay-colored stools	Same as above
Pruritus	Deposition of bile salts in skin tissues
Intolerance for fatty foods (nausea, sensation of fullness, anorexia)	No bile in small intestine for fat digestion
Bleeding tendencies	Lack of or decreased absorption of vitamin K, resulting in decreased production of prothrombin
Steatorrhea	No bile salts in duodenum, preventing fat emulsion and digestion

and disturbances in the metabolism of cholesterol. In patients with cholelithiasis, the bile secreted by the liver is supersaturated with cholesterol (lithogenic bile). The bile in the gallbladder also becomes supersaturated with cholesterol. When bile is supersaturated with cholesterol, precipitation of cholesterol occurs.

Other components of bile that precipitate into stones are bile salts, bilirubin, calcium, and protein. Mixed cholesterol stones, which are predominantly cholesterol, are the most common gallstones.

Changes in the composition of bile are probably significant in the formation of gallstones. Stasis of bile leads to progression of the supersaturation and changes in the chemical composition of the bile (biliary sludge). Immobility, pregnancy, and inflammatory or obstructive lesions of the biliary system decrease bile flow. Hormonal factors during pregnancy may cause delayed emptying of the gallbladder, resulting in stasis of bile.

The stones may remain in the gallbladder or migrate to the cystic duct or the common bile duct. They cause pain as they pass through the ducts, and they may lodge in the ducts and produce an obstruction. Small stones are more likely to move into a duct and cause obstruction. Table 44-20 depicts the changes and manifestations that occur when the stones obstruct the common bile duct. If the blockage occurs in the cystic duct, the bile can continue to flow into the duodenum directly from the liver. However, when the bile in the gallbladder cannot escape, this stasis of bile may lead to cholecystitis.

Cholecystitis. Cholecystitis is most commonly associated with obstruction caused by gallstones or biliary sludge. Cholecystitis in the absence of obstruction (acalculous cholecystitis) occurs most frequently in older adults and in patients who are critically ill. Acalculous cholecystitis is also associated with pro-

longed immobility and fasting, prolonged parenteral nutrition, and diabetes mellitus. Bacteria reaching the gallbladder via the vascular or lymphatic route, or chemical irritants in the bile, can also produce cholecystitis. E. coli, streptococci, and salmonellae are common causative bacteria. Other etiologic factors include adhesions, neoplasms, anesthesia, and opioids.

Inflammation is the major pathophysiologic condition and may be confined to the mucous lining or involve the entire wall of the gallbladder. During an acute attack of cholecystitis, the gallbladder is edematous and hyperemic, and it may be distended with bile or pus. The cystic duct is also involved and may become occluded. The wall of the gallbladder becomes scarred after an acute attack. Decreased functioning occurs if large amounts of tissue are fibrosed.

Clinical Manifestations

Cholelithiasis may produce severe symptoms or none at all. Many patients have "silent cholelithiasis." The severity of symptoms depends on whether the stones are stationary or mobile and whether obstruction is present. When a stone is lodged in the ducts or when stones are moving through the ducts, spasms may result. The gallbladder spasms occur in response to the stone. This sometimes produces severe pain, which is termed *biliary colic* even though the pain is rarely colicky. The pain is more often steady. The pain can be excruciating and accompanied by tachycardia, diaphoresis, and prostration. The severe pain may last up to an hour, and when it subsides, there is residual tenderness in the right upper quadrant. The attacks of pain frequently occur 3 to 6 hours after a high-fat meal or when the patient lies down. When total obstruction occurs, symptoms related to bile blockage are manifested (see Table 44-20).

Manifestations of cholecystitis vary from indigestion to moderate to severe pain, fever, and jaundice. Initial symptoms of acute cholecystitis include indigestion and pain and tenderness in the right upper quadrant, which may be referred to the right shoulder and scapula. The pain may be acute and be accompanied by nausea and vomiting, restlessness, and diaphoresis. Manifestations of inflammation include leukocytosis and fever. Physical findings include right upper quadrant tenderness and abdominal rigidity. Manifestations of chronic cholecystitis include a history of fat intolerance, dyspepsia, heartburn, and flatulence.

Complications. Complications of cholelithiasis and cholecystitis include gangrenous cholecystitis, subphrenic abscess, pancreatitis, *cholangitis* (inflammation of biliary ducts), biliary cirrhosis, fistulas, and rupture of the gallbladder, which can produce bile peritonitis. In older patients and those with diabetes, gangrenous cholecystitis and bile peritonitis are the most common complications of cholecystitis. *Choledocholithiasis* (stone in the common bile duct) may occur, producing symptoms of obstruction.

Diagnostic Studies

Ultrasonography is commonly used to diagnose gallstones (see Table 39-12). It is especially useful for patients with jaundice (because it does not depend on liver function) and for patients who are allergic to contrast medium. ERCP allows for visualization of the gallbladder, the cystic duct, the common hepatic duct, and the common bile duct. Bile taken during ERCP is sent for culture to identify possible infecting organisms.

Percutaneous transhepatic cholangiography is the insertion of a needle directly into the gallbladder duct followed by injection of contrast materials. It is generally done after ultrasonography indicates a bile duct blockage.

Laboratory tests reveal an increased white blood cell (WBC) count as a result of inflammation. Both direct and indirect bilirubin levels are elevated, as is the urinary bilirubin level if an obstructive process is present (see Table 44-3). If the common bile duct is obstructed, no bilirubin will reach the small intestine to be converted to urobilinogen. Serum enzymes, such as alkaline phosphatase, ALT, and AST, may be elevated. Serum amylase is increased if there is pancreatic involvement.

Collaborative Care

Once gallstones become symptomatic, definitive surgical intervention with cholecystectomy is usually indicated. However, in some cases, conservative therapy may be considered.

Conservative Therapy

Cholelithiasis. The treatment of gallstones depends on the stage of disease. Bile acids (cholesterol solvents) such as ursodeoxycholic acid (ursodiol) and chenodeoxycholic acid (chenodiol) are used to dissolve stones. However, the gallstones may recur. Gallstones are not usually treated with drugs because of the high use and success of laparoscopic cholecystectomy.

ERCP with endoscopic sphincterotomy (papillotomy) may be used for stone removal (Fig. 44-15). ERCP allows for visualization of the biliary system, dilation (balloon sphincteroplasty), and placement of stents and sphincterotomy if warranted. Special catheters with wire baskets or inflatable balloon tip may be used for stone removal.[34] The endoscope is passed to the duodenum. With an electrodiathermy knife attached to the endoscope, the stone is commonly left in the duodenum to pass naturally in the stool. When a stent is placed, it is generally removed or changed after a few months.

Extracorporeal shock-wave lithotripsy (ESWL) is an alternative treatment employed when stones cannot be removed by endoscopic approaches. In ESWL a lithotriptor uses high-energy shock waves to disintegrate gallstones once they have been located by ultrasound. It usually takes 1 to 2 hours to disintegrate the stones. After they are broken up, the fragments pass through the common bile duct and into the small intestine. Usually ESWL and oral dissolution therapy are used together.

Cholecystitis. During an acute episode of cholecystitis, treatment focuses on pain control, control of possible infection with antibiotics, and maintenance of fluid and electrolyte balance (Table 44-21). Treatment is mainly supportive and symptomatic. If nausea and vomiting are severe, NG tube insertion and gastric decompression may be used to prevent further gallbladder stimulation. A cholecystostomy may be used to drain purulent material from the obstructed gallbladder. NSAIDs (e.g., ketorolac [Toradol]) are given for pain management. Anticholinergics may be administered to decrease secretion and counteract smooth muscle spasms.

Surgical Therapy. Laparoscopic cholecystectomy is the treatment of choice for symptomatic cholelithiasis. Approximately 90% of cholecystectomies are done laparoscopically. In this procedure, the gallbladder is removed through one to four small punctures in the abdomen. A laparoscope, which has a camera attached, and grasping forceps are inserted into the abdomen through the punctures. (The incision sites may vary.) Using closed-circuit monitors to view the abdominal cavity, the surgeon retracts and dissects the gallbladder and removes it with grasping forceps. This is a safe procedure with minimal morbidity.

Most patients have minimal postoperative pain and are discharged the day of surgery or the day after. They are usually able to resume normal activities and return to work within 1 week. The main complication is injury to the common bile duct. The

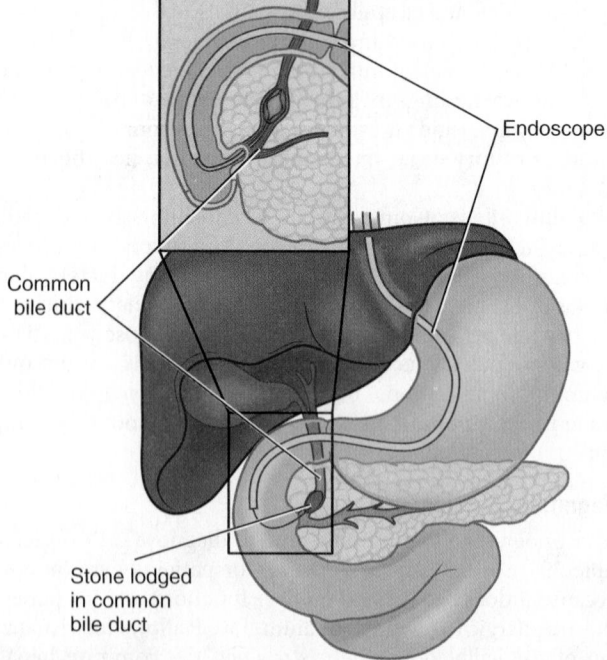

FIG. 44-15 During endoscopic sphincterotomy, an endoscope is advanced through the mouth and stomach until its tip sits in the duodenum opposite the common bile duct. *Inset,* After widening the duct mouth by incising the sphincter muscle, the physician advances a basket attachment into the duct and snags the stone.

TABLE 44-21	**COLLABORATIVE CARE**

Cholelithiasis and Acute Cholecystitis

Diagnostic
- History and physical examination
- Ultrasound
- Endoscopic retrograde cholangiopancreatography (ERCP)
- Percutaneous transhepatic cholangiography
- Liver function studies
- White blood cell count
- Serum bilirubin

Collaborative Therapy
Conservative Therapy
- IV fluid
- NPO with NG tube, later progressing to low-fat diet
- Antiemetics
- Analgesics
- Fat-soluble vitamins (A, D, E, and K)
- Anticholinergics (antispasmodics)
- Antibiotics (for secondary infection)
- Transhepatic biliary catheter
- ERCP with sphincterotomy (papillotomy)
- Extracorporeal shock-wave lithotripsy

Dissolution Therapy
- ursodeoxycholic acid (ursodiol [Actigall])

Surgical Therapy
- Laparoscopic cholecystectomy
- Incisional (open) cholecystectomy

few contraindications to laparoscopic cholecystectomy include peritonitis, cholangitis, gangrene or perforation of the gallbladder, portal hypertension, and serious bleeding disorders.

On selected patients an incisional (open) cholecystectomy may be performed. This involves removal of the gallbladder through a right subcostal incision. A T tube may be inserted into the common bile duct during surgery when a common bile duct exploration is part of the surgical procedure (Fig. 44-16). This ensures patency of the duct until the edema produced by the trauma of exploring and probing the duct has subsided. It also allows the excess bile to drain while the small intestine is adjusting to receiving a continuous flow of bile.

Transhepatic Biliary Catheter. The transhepatic biliary catheter can be used preoperatively in biliary obstruction and in hepatic dysfunction secondary to obstructive jaundice. It can also be inserted for palliative care when inoperable liver, pancreatic, or bile duct carcinoma obstructs bile flow. The catheter is used when endoscopic drainage has been unsuccessful. The catheter is inserted percutaneously and allows for decompression of obstructed extrahepatic bile ducts so that bile can flow freely. After insertion, the catheter is connected to a drainage bag. The skin around the catheter insertion site is cleansed daily with an antiseptic. Observe for bile leakage at the insertion site. The patient may be discharged with it in place.

Drug Therapy. The most common drugs used in the treatment of gallbladder disease are analgesics, anticholinergics (antispasmodics), fat-soluble vitamins, and bile salts. Morphine may be used initially for pain management. NSAIDs (e.g., ketorolac) have also been shown to be helpful in pain management. Anticholinergics such as atropine and other antispasmodics may be used to relax the smooth muscle and decrease ductal tone.

If the patient has chronic gallbladder disease or any biliary tract obstruction, fat-soluble vitamins (A, D, E, and K) may need to be given. Bile salts may be administered to facilitate digestion and vitamin absorption.

Cholestyramine may provide relief from pruritus. Cholestyramine is a resin that binds bile salts in the intestine, increasing their excretion in the feces. It is administered in powder form, mixed with milk or juice. Side effects include nausea, vomiting, diarrhea or constipation, and skin reactions.

Nutritional Therapy. People have fewer problems if they eat smaller, more frequent meals with some fat at each meal to promote gallbladder emptying. If obesity is a problem, a reduced-calorie diet is indicated. The diet should be low in saturated fats (e.g., butter, shortening, lard) and high in fiber and calcium. Rapid weight loss should be avoided because it can promote gallstone formation.

After a laparoscopic cholecystectomy, instruct the patient to have liquids for the rest of the day and eat light meals for a few days. If an incisional cholecystectomy is done, the patient will progress from liquids to a regular diet once bowel sounds have returned. The amount of fat in the postoperative diet depends on the patient's tolerance of fat. A low-fat diet may be helpful if the flow of bile is reduced (usually only in the early postoperative period) or if the patient is overweight. Sometimes the patient is instructed to restrict fats for 4 to 6 weeks. Otherwise, no special dietary instructions are needed other than to eat nutritious meals and avoid excessive fat intake.

NURSING MANAGEMENT
GALLBLADDER DISEASE

NURSING ASSESSMENT

Subjective and objective data that should be obtained from a person with gallbladder disease are presented in Table 44-22.

TABLE 44-22 NURSING ASSESSMENT

Cholecystitis or Cholelithiasis

Subjective Data
Important Health Information
Past health history: Obesity, multiparity, infection, cancer, extensive fasting, pregnancy
Medications: Estrogen or oral contraceptives
Surgery or other treatments: Previous abdominal surgery

Functional Health Patterns
Health perception–health management: Positive family history; sedentary lifestyle
Nutritional-metabolic: Weight loss, anorexia; indigestion, fat intolerance, nausea and vomiting, dyspepsia; chills
Elimination: Clay-colored stools, steatorrhea, flatulence; dark urine
Cognitive-perceptual: Moderate to severe pain in right upper quadrant that may radiate to the back or scapula; pruritus

Objective Data
General
Fever, restlessness

Integumentary
Jaundice, icteric sclera; diaphoresis

Respiratory
Tachypnea, splinting during respirations

Cardiovascular
Tachycardia

Gastrointestinal
Palpable gallbladder, abdominal guarding and distention

Possible Diagnostic Findings
↑ Serum liver enzymes, alkaline phosphatase, and bilirubin; absence of urobilinogen in urine, ↑ urinary bilirubin; leukocytosis, abnormal gallbladder ultrasound

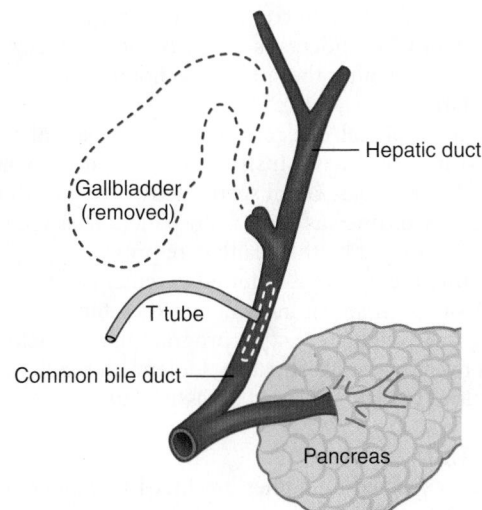

FIG. 44-16 Placement of T tube. *Dotted lines* indicate parts removed.

NURSING DIAGNOSES

Nursing diagnoses for the patient with gallbladder disease treated surgically include, but are not limited to, the following:

- Acute pain *related to* surgical procedure
- Ineffective self-health management *related to* lack of knowledge of diet and postoperative management

PLANNING

The overall goals are that the patient with gallbladder disease will have (1) relief of pain and discomfort, (2) no complications postoperatively, and (3) no recurrent attacks of cholecystitis or cholelithiasis.

NURSING IMPLEMENTATION

HEALTH PROMOTION. Be aware of predisposing factors for gallbladder disease in general health screening. Teach patients from ethnic groups in which the disease is more common, such as Native Americans, the initial manifestations and to see their health care provider if these manifestations occur. Patients with chronic cholecystitis may not have acute symptoms and may not seek help until jaundice and biliary obstruction occur. Earlier detection in these patients is beneficial so that they can be managed with a low-fat diet and monitored more closely.

ACUTE INTERVENTION. Nursing goals for the patient undergoing conservative therapy include treating pain, relieving nausea and vomiting, providing comfort and emotional support, maintaining fluid and electrolyte balance and nutrition, making accurate assessments to ensure effective treatment, and observing for complications.

The patient with acute cholecystitis or cholelithiasis frequently has severe pain. Give the drugs ordered to relieve the pain as required, before it becomes more severe. Assess what drugs relieve the pain and how much medication is required. Observe for side effects of the drugs as part of the continued assessment. Nursing comfort measures, such as a clean bed, comfortable positioning, and oral care, are appropriate.

Some patients have more severe nausea and vomiting than others. For these patients, it may be necessary to insert an NG tube and use gastric decompression. Eliminating intake of food and fluids also prevents further stimulation of the gallbladder. Oral hygiene, care of nares, accurate intake and output measurements, and maintenance of suction should be a part of the nursing care plan for this patient. For patients with less severe nausea and vomiting, antiemetics are usually adequate. When the patient is vomiting, provide comfort measures such as frequent mouth rinses. Remove any vomitus immediately from the patient's view.

If pruritus occurs with jaundice, measures to relieve itching are necessary (see earlier discussion on p. 1025 and eNCP 44-1).

Assess for progression of the symptoms and development of complications. Observe for signs of obstruction of the ducts by stones. These include jaundice; clay-colored stools; dark, foamy urine; steatorrhea; fever; and increased WBC count.

When manifestations of obstruction are present (see Table 44-20), bleeding may result from decreased prothrombin production. Common sites to observe for bleeding are the mucous membranes of the mouth, nose, gingivae, and injection sites. If injections are given, use a small-gauge needle and apply gentle pressure after the injection. Know the patient's prothrombin time and use it as a guide in the assessment process.

Assessment for infections includes monitoring vital signs. A temperature elevation with chills and jaundice may indicate choledocholithiasis.

Your care of the patient after ERCP with papillotomy includes assessment to detect complications such as pancreatitis, perforation, infection, and bleeding. Monitor the patient's vital signs. Abdominal pain and fever may indicate pancreatitis. The patient should be on bed rest for several hours and should be NPO until the gag reflex returns. Teach the patient the need for follow-up if the stent is to be removed or changed.

Postoperative Care. Postoperative nursing care after a laparoscopic cholecystectomy includes monitoring for complications such as bleeding, making the patient comfortable, and preparing the patient for discharge. A common postoperative problem is referred pain to the shoulder because of the carbon dioxide that is used to inflate the abdominal cavity during surgery. It may not be released or absorbed by the body. The carbon dioxide can irritate the phrenic nerve and the diaphragm, causing some difficulty in breathing. Placing the patient in the Sims' position (on left side with right knee flexed) helps move the gas pocket away from the diaphragm. Encourage deep breathing along with movement and ambulation. The pain can usually be relieved by NSAIDs or codeine. The patient is allowed clear liquids and can walk to the bathroom to void. Most patients go home the same day.

Postoperative nursing care for incisional cholecystectomy focuses on adequate ventilation and prevention of respiratory complications. Other nursing care is the same as general postoperative nursing care (see Chapter 20).

If the patient has a T tube (see Fig. 44-16), you need to maintain bile drainage and observe for T-tube functioning and drainage. The T tube is connected to a closed gravity drainage system. If the Penrose or Jackson-Pratt drain or the T tube is draining large amounts, it is helpful to use a sterile pouching system to protect the skin.

AMBULATORY AND HOME CARE. When the patient has conservative therapy, nursing management depends on the patient's symptoms and on whether surgical intervention is planned. Dietary teaching is usually necessary. The diet is usually low in fat, and sometimes a weight-reduction diet is also recommended. The patient may need to take fat-soluble vitamin supplements. Instruct the patient on observations that indicate obstruction (e.g., stool and urine changes, jaundice, pruritus). Explain the importance of continued health care follow-up.

The patient who undergoes a laparoscopic cholecystectomy is discharged soon after the surgery, so home care and teaching are important (Table 44-23).

After an incisional cholecystectomy, the patient is usually discharged in 2 or 3 days. Instruct the patient to avoid heavy lifting for 4 to 6 weeks. Usual sexual activities, including intercourse, can be resumed as soon as the patient feels ready, unless otherwise instructed by the health care provider.

Sometimes the patient is required to remain on a low-fat diet for 4 to 6 weeks. If so, an individualized dietary teaching plan is necessary. A weight-reduction program may be helpful if the patient is overweight. Most patients tolerate a regular diet with no difficulties but should avoid excessive fats.

EVALUATION

The overall expected outcomes are that the patient with gallbladder disease will

Liver, Pancreas, Gallbladder

- Appear comfortable and verbalize pain relief
- Verbalize knowledge of activity level and dietary restrictions

GALLBLADDER CANCER

Primary cancer of the gallbladder is uncommon. The majority of gallbladder carcinomas are adenocarcinomas. Annually an estimated 9810 new cases of gallbladder cancer occur with an estimated 3200 deaths. A relationship exists between cancer of the gallbladder and chronic cholecystitis and cholelithiasis.

The early symptoms of carcinoma of the gallbladder are insidious and are similar to those of chronic cholecystitis and cholelithiasis, which makes the diagnosis difficult. Later symptoms are usually those of biliary obstruction. Gallbladder cancer is twice as common in women as in men.[35]

Diagnosis and staging of gallbladder cancer are done using EUS, abdominal ultrasound, CT, MRI, and/or MRCP. Unfortunately, gallbladder cancer often is not detected until the disease is advanced. When it is found early, surgery can be curative. Several factors influence successful surgical outcomes, including the depth of cancer invasion, extent of liver involvement, venous or lymphatic invasion, and lymph node metastasis. Extended cholecystectomy with lymph node dissection has improved the outcomes for patients with gallbladder cancer.

When surgery is not an option, endoscopic stenting of the biliary tree can be done to reduce obstructive jaundice. Adjuvant therapies, including radiation therapy and chemotherapy, may be used depending on the disease state. Overall, cancer of the gallbladder has a poor prognosis.

Nursing management involves palliative care with special attention to nutrition, hydration, skin care, and pain relief. Nursing care measures used for patients with cholecystitis and cholelithiasis are frequently applied, as well as nursing care measures for the patient with cancer (see Chapter 16).

TABLE 44-23	**PATIENT & CAREGIVER TEACHING GUIDE**

Postoperative Laparoscopic Cholecystectomy

Include the following instructions in the patient's postoperative teaching plan.
1. Remove the bandages on the puncture site the day after surgery and you can shower.
2. Notify your surgeon if any of the following signs and symptoms occurs:
   - Redness, swelling, bile-colored drainage or pus from any incision
   - Severe abdominal pain, nausea, vomiting, fever, chills
3. You can gradually resume normal activities.
4. Return to work within 1 wk of surgery.
5. You can resume your usual diet, but a low-fat diet is usually better tolerated for several weeks after surgery.

CASE STUDY

Cirrhosis of the Liver

Patient Profile
M.B. is a 55-yr-old Native American man admitted with a diagnosis of cirrhosis of the liver. He has been vomiting for 2 days and noticed blood in the toilet when he vomits.

Subjective Data
- Has had cirrhosis for 12 yr
- Acknowledges that he had been drinking heavily for 20 yr but has been sober for the past 2 yr
- Complains of anorexia, nausea, and abdominal discomfort

Objective Data
Physical Examination
- Thin and malnourished
- Has moderate ascites
- Has jaundice of sclera and skin
- Has 4+ pitting edema of the lower extremities
- Liver and spleen are palpable

Laboratory Values
- Total bilirubin: 15 mg/dL (257 mmol/L)
- AST: 190 U/L (3.2 μkat/L)
- ALT: 210 U/L (3.5 μkat/L)
- ECG is at right:

Discussion Questions
1. What are possible causes of cirrhosis? What type of cirrhosis does M.B. probably have?

2. Describe the pathophysiologic changes that occur in the liver as cirrhosis develops.
3. List M.B.'s clinical manifestations of liver failure. For each manifestation, explain the pathophysiologic basis.
4. Explain the significance of the results of his laboratory values and ECG findings.
5. If M.B. begins to manifest signs and symptoms of hepatic encephalopathy, what would you monitor? What measures should be instituted to control or decrease the encephalopathy?
6. What are possible causes of his gastrointestinal bleeding?
7. *Priority Decision:* Based on the assessment data, what are the priority nursing diagnoses? Are there any collaborative problems?
8. *Priority Decision:* What are the priority nursing interventions for the patient at this stage of his illness?
9. *Evidence-Based Practice:* M.B. discusses his prognosis with you. He says, "There is no hope. I might as well keep drinking." How would you respond to his question?

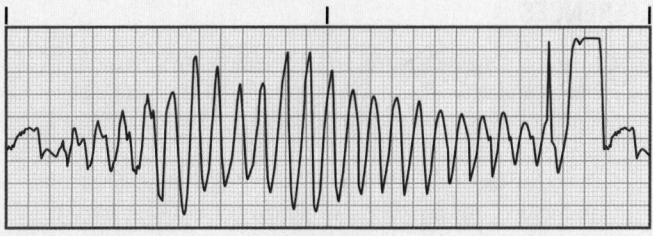

BRIDGE TO NCLEX EXAMINATION

The number of the question corresponds to the same-numbered outcome at the beginning of the chapter.

1. A patient with hepatitis A is in the acute phase. The nurse plans care for the patient based on the knowledge that
   a. pruritus is a common problem with jaundice in this phase.
   b. the patient is most likely to transmit the disease during this phase.
   c. gastrointestinal symptoms are not as severe in hepatitis A as they are in hepatitis B.
   d. extrahepatic manifestations of glomerulonephritis and polyarteritis are common in this phase.

2. A patient with acute hepatitis B is being discharged in 2 days. In the discharge teaching plan the nurse should include instructions to
   a. avoid alcohol for the first 3 weeks.
   b. use a condom during sexual intercourse.
   c. have family members get an injection of immunoglobulin.
   d. follow a low-protein, moderate-carbohydrate, moderate-fat diet.

3. A patient has been told that she has elevated liver enzymes caused by nonalcoholic fatty liver disease (NAFLD). The nursing teaching plan should include
   a. having genetic testing done.
   b. recommending a heart-healthy diet.
   c. the necessity to reduce weight rapidly.
   d. avoiding alcohol until liver enzymes return to normal.

4. The patient with advanced cirrhosis asks why his abdomen is so swollen. The nurse's response is based on the knowledge that
   a. a lack of clotting factors promotes the collection of blood in the abdominal cavity.
   b. portal hypertension and hypoalbuminemia cause a fluid shift into the peritoneal space.
   c. decreased peristalsis in the GI tract contributes to gas formation and distention of the bowel.
   d. bile salts in the blood irritate the peritoneal membranes, causing edema and pocketing of fluid.

5. In planning care for a patient with metastatic liver cancer, the nurse should include interventions that
   a. focus primarily on symptomatic and comfort measures.
   b. reassure the patient that chemotherapy offers a good prognosis.
   c. promote the patient's confidence that surgical excision of the tumor will be successful.
   d. provide information necessary for the patient to make decisions regarding liver transplantation.

6. Nursing management of the patient with acute pancreatitis includes (*select all that apply*)
   a. checking for signs of hypocalcemia.
   b. providing a diet low in carbohydrates.
   c. giving insulin based on a sliding scale.
   d. observing stools for signs of steatorrhea.
   e. monitoring for infection, particularly respiratory tract infection.

7. A patient with pancreatic cancer is admitted to the hospital for evaluation of possible treatment options. The patient asks the nurse to explain the Whipple procedure that the surgeon has described. The explanation includes the information that a Whipple procedure involves
   a. creating a bypass around the obstruction caused by the tumor by joining the gallbladder to the jejunum.
   b. resection of the entire pancreas and the distal portion of the stomach, with anastomosis of the common bile duct and the stomach into the duodenum.
   c. removal of part of the pancreas, part of the stomach, the duodenum, and the gallbladder, with joining of the pancreatic duct, the common bile duct, and the stomach into the jejunum.
   d. radical removal of the pancreas, the duodenum, and the spleen, and attachment of the stomach to the jejunum, which requires oral supplementation of pancreatic digestive enzymes and insulin replacement therapy.

8. The nursing management of the patient with cholecystitis associated with cholelithiasis is based on the knowledge that
   a. shock-wave therapy should be tried initially.
   b. once gallstones are removed, they tend not to recur.
   c. the disorder can be successfully treated with oral bile salts that dissolve gallstones.
   d. laparoscopic cholecystectomy is the treatment of choice in most patients who are symptomatic.

9. Teaching in relation to home management after a laparoscopic cholecystectomy should include
   a. keeping the bandages on the puncture sites for 48 hours.
   b. reporting any bile-colored drainage or pus from any incision.
   c. using over-the-counter antiemetics if nausea and vomiting occur.
   d. emptying and measuring the contents of the bile bag from the T tube every day.

1. a, 2. b, 3. b, 4. b, 5. a, 6. a, e, 7. c, 8. d, 9. b

⊝volve

For rationales to these answers and even more NCLEX review questions, visit *http://evolve.elsevier.com/Lewis/medsurg*.

REFERENCES

1. Centers for Disease Control and Prevention: Viral hepatitis statistics and surveillance—United States, 2010. Retrieved from *www.cdc.gov/hepatitis/Statistics/2010Surveillance/index.htm*.
2. Centers for Disease Control and Prevention: National hepatitis C prevention strategy 2001: a comprehensive strategy for the prevention and control of hepatitis C virus infection and its consequences. Retrieved from *www.cdc.gov/hepatitis/HCV/Strategy/PDFs/NatHepCPrevStrategy.pdf*.
3. Ly KN, Xing J, Klevens RM, et al: The increasing burden of mortality from viral hepatitis in the United States between 1999 and 2007, *Ann Intern Med* 156:271, 2012.
4. Edey M, Barraclough K, Johnson DW: Review article: hepatitis B and dialysis, *Nephrology (Carlton)* 15:137, 2010.
5. Ghany MG, Strader DB, Thomas DL, et al: Diagnosis, management, and treatment of hepatitis C: an update, *Hepatology* 49:1335, 2009.
6. Chevaliez S, Rodriguez C, Pawlotsky JM: New virologic tools for management of chronic hepatitis B and C, *Gastroenterology* 142:1303, 2012.

7. Estrabaud E, Vidaud M, Marcellin P, et al: Genomics and HCV infection: progression of fibrosis and treatment response, *J Hepatol* 57(5):1110, 2012.

8. Stevenson M, Lloyd-Jones M, Morgan MY, et al: Non-invasive diagnostic assessment tools for the detection of liver fibrosis in patients with suspected alcohol-related liver disease: a systematic review and economic evaluation, *Health Technol Assess* 16:1, 2012.

9. Lee H, Park W, Yang JH, et al: Management of hepatitis B virus infection, *Gastroenterol Nurs* 33:120, 2010.

10. Kwon H, Lok AS: Hepatitis B therapy, *Nat Rev Gastroenterol Hepatol* 8:275, 2011.

*11. Poordad F, Dieterich D: Treating hepatitis C: current standard of care and emerging direct-acting antiviral agents, *J Viral Hepat* 19:449, 2012.

12. Rosedale MT, Strauss SM: Depression, interferon therapy, hepatitis C, and substance use: potential treatments and areas for research, *J Am Psychiatr Nurses Assoc* 17:205, 2011.

*13. Centers for Disease Control and Prevention: Advisory Committee for Immunization Practices recommendations. Retrieved from *www.cdc.gov/vaccines/pubs/acip-list.htm.*

14. Centers for Disease Control and Prevention: *CDC announces first ever National Hepatitis Testing Day and proposes that all baby boomers be tested once for hepatitis C (press release),* May 2012. Retrieved from *www.cdc.gov/nchhstp/newsroom/ HepTestingRecsPressRelease2012.html.*

15. Boesecke C, Vogel M: HIV and hepatitis C co-infection: acute HCV therapy, *Curr Opin HIV AIDS* 6:459, 2011.

*16. Ghany MG, Nelson DR, Strader DB, et al: An update on treatment of genotype 1 chronic hepatitis C virus infection: 2011 practice guideline by the American Association for the Study of Liver Diseases, *Hepatology* 54:1433, 2011.

17. Sedky K, Nazir R, Joshi A, et al: Which psychotropic medications induce hepatotoxicity? *Gen Hosp Psychiatry* 34:53, 2012.

18. National Digestive Diseases Information Clearinghouse: Wilson disease, May 2009. Retrieved from *www.digestive.niddk.nih.gov/ ddiseases/pubs/wilson.*

19. National Digestive Diseases Information Clearinghouse: Nonalcoholic steatohepatitis, November 2006. Retrieved from *www.digestive.niddk.nih.gov/ddiseases/pubs/nash.*

20. Bajaj JS, O'Leary JG, Reddy KR, et al: Second infections independently increase mortality in hospitalized cirrhotic patients: the NACSELD experience, *Hepatology* 56:2328, 2012.

21. Riggio O, Nardelli S, Moscucci F, et al: Hepatic encephalopathy after transjugular intrahepatic portosystemic shunt, *Clin Liver Dis* 16:133, 2012.

22. Kashani A, Landaverde C, Medici V, et al: Fluid retention in cirrhosis: pathophysiology and management, *QJM* 101:71, 2008.

23. Habib S, Boyer TD: Vasopressin V2-receptor antagonists in patients with cirrhosis, ascites and hyponatremia, *Therap Adv Gastroenterol* 5:189, 2012.

24. Tsien CD, McCullough AJ, Dasarathy S: Late evening snack: exploiting a period of anabolic opportunity in cirrhosis, *J Gastroenterol Hepatol* 27:430, 2012.

25. Page Acnp-Bc J: Nonalcoholic fatty liver disease: the hepatic metabolic syndrome, *J Am Acad Nurse Pract* 24:345, 2012.

*26. Lee WM, Stravitz TR, Larson AM: Introduction to the Revised American Association for the Study of Liver Diseases position paper on acute liver failure 2011. Retrieved from *www.aasld.org/ practiceguidelines/Documents/AcuteLiverFailureUpdate2011.pdf.*

27. Sood GK: Acute liver failure. Retrieved from *http://emedicine. medscape.com/article/177354-overview#aw2aab6b2b5aa.*

28. Fisher EM, Brown DK: Hepatorenal syndrome: beyond liver failure, *AACN Adv Crit Care* 21:165, 2010.

29. Jemal A, Bray F, Center MM, et al: Global cancer statistics, *CA Cancer J Clin* 61:69, 2011.

30. Forner A, Llovet JM, Bruix J: Hepatocellular carcinoma, *Lancet* 379:1245, 2012.

31. American Liver Foundation: More about organ donation. Retrieved from *www.liverfoundation.org/patients/organdonor/ about.*

32. Carrion AF, Martin P: Viral hepatitis in the elderly, *Am J Gastroenterol* 107:691, 2012.

33. National Digestive Disease Information Clearinghouse: Pancreatitis. Retrieved from *www.digestive.niddk.nih.gov/ ddiseases/pubs/pancreatitis.*

34. Bruesehoff MP: Understanding endoscopic retrograde cholangiopancreatography, *OR Nurse* 6:40, 2012.

35. American Cancer Society: Gallbladder cancer. Retrieved from *www.cancer.org/Cancer/GallbladderCancer/DetailedGuide/ gallbladder-risk-factors.*

RESOURCES

American Association for the Study of Liver Diseases (AASLD)
www.aasld.org
American Gastroenterological Association
www.gastro.org
American Liver Foundation
www.liverfoundation.org
American Pancreatic Association
www.american-pancreatic-association.org
National Pancreas Foundation
www.pancreasfoundation.org
Pancreatic Cancer Action Network
www.pancan.org

*Evidence-based information for clinical practice.

CASE STUDY

Managing Multiple Patients

Introduction

You are working on the medical-surgical unit and have been assigned to care for the following five patients. You have one LPN who is assigned to help you and a UAP who is assigned to assist you and another RN.

Patients

iStockphoto/Thinkstock

L.C. is a 58-year-old Native American man admitted from the emergency department (ED) with acute abdominal pain. A CBC showed a Hgb of 9.0 g/dL and Hct of 26%. The WBC count is normal. A CT scan and colonoscopy indicated two medium-sized tumors in the transverse colon. A hemicolectomy was performed. The adenocarcinoma had spread to the muscle of the colon wall and there were two positive lymph nodes.

iStockphoto/Thinkstock

M.S. is a 70-year-old white woman who was recently admitted to the unit with generalized weakness and malnutrition. She is 5 feet 4 inches tall and weighs 100 lb, with a 30-lb weight loss in past 2 months. Her PMH includes a recent thrombotic stroke with hemiparesis and dysphagia. She has had nothing by mouth for the past 24 hours and just started enteral nutrition via PEG tube.

Hemera/Thinkstock

S.R. is a 48-year-old white woman admitted with complaints of chest pain and shortness of breath. She has a history of type 2 diabetes mellitus, hypertension, and osteoarthritis. She is 5 feet 4 inches tall and weighs 210 lb. Her most recent BP was 160/110 mm Hg. Her morning laboratory results reveal elevations in fasting blood glucose, total cholesterol, LDL cholesterol, and triglycerides. Her HDL cholesterol is low. Her cardiac enzymes and ECG are all within normal limits. She is scheduled to undergo a cardiac stress test at 10 AM.

iStockphoto/Thinkstock

F.H., a 40-year-old male immigrant from Vietnam, has a 1-year history of epigastric distress. He underwent an upper endoscopy a few weeks ago that revealed a duodenal ulcer and *H. pylori*. He was started on omeprazole, clarithromycin, and amoxicillin for 10 days. He came to the ED yesterday with complaints of severe epigastric pain. His Hgb was 8.2 g/dL and Hct was 24%. He was admitted and put on a pantoprazole (Protonix) continuous infusion and is scheduled for a repeat EGD today.

M.B. is a 55-year-old Native American man admitted with a diagnosis of upper GI bleeding. He has been vomiting for 2 days and noticed blood in the toilet when he vomits. He has had cirrhosis for 12 years and admits to drinking heavily for 20 years but has been sober for the past 2 years. He currently complains of anorexia, nausea, and abdominal discomfort. He is thin and malnourished, has moderate ascites, jaundice of sclera and skin, 4+ pitting edema of the lower extremities, and palpable liver and spleen. His bilirubin, serum ammonia level, and liver enzymes are all elevated. His morning laboratory test results demonstrate a Hct of 20% and Hgb of 6.8 g/dL.

Management Discussion Questions

1. ***Priority Decision:*** After receiving report, which patient should you see first? Provide a rationale for your decision.

2. ***Delegation Decision:*** Which tasks could you delegate to the LPN *(select all that apply)*?
   a. Assess L.C.'s pain level and bowel sounds.
   b. Administer oral medications to S.R. with a sip of water.
   c. Provide enteral tube feeding for M.S. if gastric residual <500 mL.
   d. Call M.B.'s health care provider regarding the morning laboratory results.
   e. Because she understands Vietnamese, teach F.H.'s wife about his disease.

3. ***Priority and Delegation Decision:*** As you are assessing M.B., the LPN informs you that F.H. just vomited a large amount of bright red blood. What initial action would be most appropriate?
   a. Have the LPN administer an antiemetic to F.H.
   b. Ask the LPN to notify F.H.'s health care provider.
   c. Leave M.B.'s room to perform a focused assessment on F.H.
   d. Ask the UAP to obtain a unit of packed red blood cells from the blood bank.

Case Study Progression

When you enter F.H.'s room, he tells you that his pain actually feels somewhat relieved since he vomited. However, you note that his skin is cool and clammy, his BP is 90/54 mm Hg, and his heart rate is 116 bpm. You notify his health care provider.

4. Which interventions would you expect the health care provider to order for F.H. *(select all that apply)*?
   a. Stat hemoglobin and hematocrit
   b. Emergent endoscopic and endotherapy
   c. Discontinue the pantoprazole (Protonix) infusion
   d. Start a second IV site and administer 500 mL normal saline over 30 minutes

5. ***Priority Decision:*** After administering a bolus feeding of enteral nutrition to M.S., it would be most important to
   a. assess for gastric residual.
   b. obtain an abdominal x-ray.
   c. keep head of bed elevated 30-45 degrees.
   d. record the total amount of fluid administered.

6. Which intervention to treat ascites might you expect the health care provider to order for M.B. *(select all that apply)*?
   a. Paracentesis
   b. Diuretic therapy
   c. 2 g sodium diet
   d. 1800 mL/day fluid restriction
   e. Shunt insertion from peritoneum to heart

7. ***Management Decision:*** As you enter the nurse's station, you overhear derogatory comments made by the UAP to the LPN about S.R.'s weight. Which response would be most appropriate?
   a. Report the incident to charge nurse for follow-up.
   b. Talk to the UAP to discuss possible HIPAA violation.
   c. Talk to S.R. to assess impact of UAP's bias on her self-image.
   d. Provide education to help staff members recognize obesity as a disease process.

SECTION 9

Problems of Urinary Function

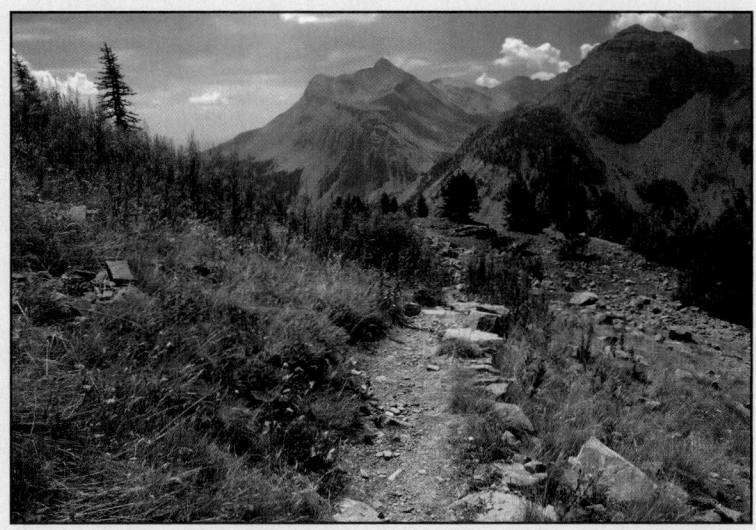

Hemera/Thinkstock

The road to success is always under construction.
Lily Tomlin

Bones can break, muscles can atrophy, glands can loaf,
even the brain can go to sleep without immediate danger to survival.
But should the kidneys fail . . . neither bone, muscle, gland,
nor brain could carry on.
Homer Smith

Nursing Assessment
Urinary System

Betty Jean Reid Czarapata

LEARNING OUTCOMES

1. Differentiate among the anatomic location and functions of the kidneys, ureters, bladder, and urethra.
2. Explain the physiologic events involved in the formation and passage of urine from glomerular filtration to voiding.
3. Select significant subjective and objective data related to the urinary system that should be obtained from a patient.
4. Link the age-related changes of the urinary system to the differences in assessment findings.
5. Select appropriate techniques to use in the physical assessment of the urinary system.
6. Differentiate normal from abnormal findings of a physical assessment of the urinary system.
7. Describe the purpose, significance of results, and nursing responsibilities related to diagnostic studies of the urinary system.
8. Differentiate the normal from the abnormal findings of a urinalysis.

KEY TERMS

costovertebral angle (CVA), p. 1054
creatinine, Table 45-8, p. 1057
cystometrogram, Table 45-8, p. 1060
cystoscopy, Table 45-8, p. 1060

glomerular filtration rate (GFR), p. 1048
glomerulus, p. 1047
intravenous pyelogram (IVP), Table 45-8, p. 1058

nephron, p. 1047
renal biopsy, Table 45-8, p. 1061

Adequate kidney function is essential to the maintenance of a healthy body. If a person has complete kidney failure and treatment is not provided, death is inevitable. This chapter discusses the structures and functions, assessment, and diagnostic studies of the urinary system.

STRUCTURES AND FUNCTIONS OF URINARY SYSTEM

The *upper urinary system* consists of two kidneys and two ureters. The *lower urinary system* consists of a urinary bladder and a urethra (Fig. 45-1). Urine is formed in the kidneys, drains through the ureters to be stored in the bladder, and then passes from the body through the urethra.

Kidneys

The kidneys are the principal organs of the urinary system. The primary functions of the kidneys are to (1) regulate the volume and composition of extracellular fluid (ECF) and (2) excrete waste products from the body. The kidneys also function to control blood pressure, produce erythropoietin, activate vitamin D, and regulate acid-base balance.

Macrostructure. The paired kidneys are bean-shaped organs located retroperitoneally (behind the peritoneum) on either side of the vertebral column at about the level of the twelfth thoracic (T12) vertebra to the third lumbar (L3) vertebra. Each kidney weighs 4 to 6 oz (113 to 170 g) and is about 5 in (12.5 cm) long. The right kidney, positioned at the level of the twelfth rib, is lower than the left. An adrenal gland lies on top of each kidney.

Reviewed by Barbara S. Broome, RN, PhD, FAAN, Associate Dean and Chair, Community/Mental Health, University of South Alabama, College of Nursing, Mobile, Alabama; Marci Langenkamp, RN, MS, Assistant Professor of Nursing, Edison Community College, Piqua, Ohio; and Phyllis A. Matthews, RN, MS, ANCP-BC, CUNP, Urology Nurse Practitioner, Denver VA Medical Center, Denver, Colorado.

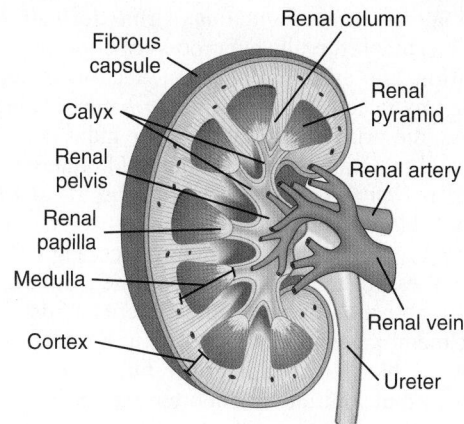

FIG. 45-2 Longitudinal section of the kidney.

FIG. 45-1 Organs of the urinary system. **A,** Upper urinary tract in relation to other anatomic structures. **B,** Male urethra in relation to other pelvic structures. **C,** Female urethra.

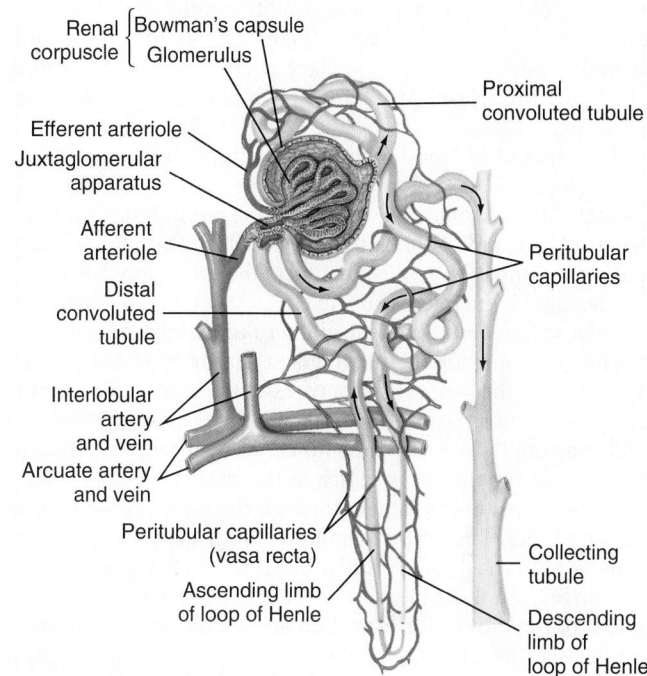

FIG. 45-3 The nephron is the basic functional unit of the kidney. This illustration of a single nephron unit also shows the surrounding blood vessels.

Each kidney is surrounded by a considerable amount of fat and connective tissue that cushions, supports, and maintains its position. A thin, smooth layer of fibrous membrane called the *capsule* covers the surface of each kidney. The capsule protects the kidney and serves as a shock absorber when this area is traumatized from a sudden force or strike. The *hilus* on the medial side of the kidney serves as the entry site for the renal artery and nerves, and as the exit site for the renal vein and ureter.

The parenchyma (actual tissue) of the kidney can be visualized on a longitudinal section of the kidney (Fig. 45-2). The outer layer is the *cortex,* and the inner layer is the *medulla.* The medulla consists of a number of pyramids. The apices (tops) of these pyramids are called *papillae,* through which urine passes to enter the calyces. The minor calyces widen and merge to form major calyces, which form a funnel-shaped sac called the *renal pelvis.* The minor and major calyces transport urine to the renal pelvis, from which it drains through the ureter to the bladder. The renal pelvis can store a small volume of urine (3 to 5 mL).

Microstructure. The **nephron** is the functional unit of the kidney. Each kidney contains approximately 1 million nephrons. Each nephron is composed of the glomerulus, Bowman's capsule, and a tubular system. The tubular system consists of the proximal convoluted tubule, loop of Henle, distal convoluted tubule, and collecting tubules (Fig. 45-3). The glomerulus, Bowman's capsule, proximal tubule, and distal tubule are located

in the cortex of the kidney. The loop of Henle and collecting tubules are located in the medulla. Several collecting tubules join to form a single collecting duct. The collecting ducts eventually merge into a pyramid that empties via the papilla into a minor calyx.

Blood Supply. Blood flow to the kidneys, approximately 1200 mL/min, accounts for 20% to 25% of the cardiac output. Blood reaches the kidneys via the renal artery, which arises from the aorta and enters the kidney through the hilus. The renal artery divides into secondary branches and then into still smaller branches, each of which forms an afferent arteriole. The afferent arteriole divides into a capillary network, the **glomerulus,** which is a tuft of up to 50 capillaries (see Fig. 45-3). The capillaries of the glomerulus unite in the efferent arteriole. This efferent arteriole splits to form a capillary network, the peritubular capillaries, which surround the tubular system. All peritubular capillaries drain into the venous system; the renal vein empties into the inferior vena cava.

Physiology of Urine Formation. Urine formation is the outcome of a complex, multistep process of filtration, reabsorption, secretion, and excretion of water, electrolytes, and metabolic waste products. Although urine formation is the result of this process, the primary functions of the kidneys are to filter the blood and maintain the body's internal homeostasis.

Glomerular Function. Urine formation begins at the glomerulus, where blood is filtered. The glomerulus is a semipermeable membrane that allows filtration (see Fig. 45-3). The hydrostatic pressure of the blood within the glomerular capillaries causes a portion of blood to be filtered across the semipermeable membrane into Bowman's capsule, where the filtered portion of the blood (the glomerular filtrate) begins to pass down to the tubule. Filtration is more rapid in the glomerulus than in ordinary tissue capillaries because the glomerular membrane is porous. The ultrafiltrate is similar in composition to blood except that it lacks blood cells, platelets, and large plasma proteins. Under normal conditions, the capillary pores are too small to allow the loss of these large blood components. In many kidney diseases, capillary permeability is increased, which permits plasma proteins and blood cells to pass into the urine.

The amount of blood filtered each minute by the glomeruli is expressed as the **glomerular filtration rate (GFR)**. The normal GFR is about 125 mL/min. The peritubular capillary network reabsorbs most of the glomerular filtrate before it reaches the end of the collecting duct. Therefore only 1 mL/min (on average) is excreted as urine.

Tubular Function. Since the glomerular membrane is a selective filtration membrane that filters primarily by size, provision is made for the reabsorption of essential materials and the excretion of nonessential ones (Table 45-1). The tubules and collecting ducts carry out these functions by means of reabsorption and secretion. *Reabsorption* is the passage of a substance from the lumen of the tubules through the tubule cells and into the capillaries. This process involves both active and passive transport mechanisms. Tubular *secretion* is the passage of a substance from the capillaries through the tubular cells into the lumen of the tubule. Reabsorption and secretion cause numerous changes in the composition of the glomerular filtrate as it moves through the entire length of the tubule.

In the proximal convoluted tubule, about 80% of the electrolytes are reabsorbed. Normally, all the glucose, amino acids, and small proteins are reabsorbed. Although most reabsorption

occurs by active transport, hydrogen ions (H^+) and creatinine are secreted into the filtrate.

As reabsorption continues in the loop of Henle, water is conserved, which is important for concentrating the filtrate. The descending loop is permeable to water and moderately permeable to sodium, urea, and other solutes. In the ascending limb, chloride ions (Cl^-) are actively reabsorbed, followed by passive reabsorption of sodium ions (Na^+). About 25% of the filtered sodium is reabsorbed in the ascending limb.

Two important functions of the distal convoluted tubules are final regulation of water balance and acid-base balance. Antidiuretic hormone (ADH) is required for water reabsorption in the kidney and is important in water balance. ADH makes the distal convoluted tubules and the collecting ducts permeable to water. This allows water to be reabsorbed into the peritubular capillaries and eventually returned to the circulation.

Decreases in plasma osmolality are detected in the anterior hypothalamus by osmoreceptors. These osmoreceptors send neural input to *superoptic nuclei cells* in the hypothalamus. These superoptic nuclei cells have neuronal axons that terminate in the posterior pituitary gland and act to inhibit secretion of ADH. In the absence of ADH, the tubules are essentially impermeable to water. Thus any water in the tubules leaves the body as urine.

Aldosterone (released from the adrenal cortex) acts on the distal tubule to cause reabsorption of Na^+ and water. In exchange for Na^+, potassium ions (K^+) are excreted. The secretion of aldosterone is influenced by both circulating blood volume and plasma concentrations of Na^+ and K^+.

Acid-base regulation involves reabsorbing and conserving most of the bicarbonate (HCO_3^-) and secreting excess H^+. The distal tubule has different ways to maintain the pH of ECF within a range of 7.35 to 7.45 (see Chapter 17).

Myocyte cells in the right atrium secrete a hormone, atrial natriuretic peptide (ANP), in response to atrial distention, which is a result of an increase in plasma volume. ANP acts on the kidneys to increase sodium excretion. At the same time ANP inhibits renin, ADH, and the action of angiotensin II on the adrenal glands, thereby suppressing aldosterone secretion. These combined effects of ANP result in the production of a large volume of dilute urine. Furthermore, secretion of ANP causes relaxation of the afferent arteriole, thus increasing the GFR.

The renal tubules are also involved in calcium balance. Parathyroid hormone (PTH) is released from the parathyroid gland in response to low serum calcium levels. PTH maintains serum calcium levels by causing increased tubular reabsorption of calcium ions (Ca^{2+}) and decreased tubular reabsorption of phosphate ions (PO_4^{2-}). In kidney disease the effects of PTH may have a major effect on bone metabolism.

Vitamin D is a hormone that can be obtained in the diet or synthesized by the action of ultraviolet radiation on cholesterol in the skin. These forms of vitamin D are inactive and require two more steps to become metabolically active. The first step in activation occurs in the liver; the second step occurs in the kidneys. Active vitamin D is essential for the absorption of calcium from the gastrointestinal (GI) tract. The patient with kidney failure (also called renal failure) has a deficiency of the active metabolite of vitamin D and manifests problems of altered calcium and phosphate balance (see Chapter 47).

In summary, the basic function of nephrons is to cleanse blood plasma of unnecessary substances. After the glomerulus

TABLE 45-1	FUNCTIONS OF NEPHRON SEGMENTS
Component	**Function**
Glomerulus	Selective filtration.
Proximal tubule	Reabsorption of 80% of electrolytes and water, glucose, amino acids, HCO_3^-. Secretion of H^+ and creatinine.
Loop of Henle	Reabsorption of Na^+ and Cl^- in ascending limb and water in descending loop. Concentration of filtrate.
Distal tubule	Secretion of K^+, H^+, ammonia. Reabsorption of water (regulated by ADH) and HCO_3^-. Regulation of Ca^{2+} and PO_4^{2-} by parathyroid hormone. Regulation of Na^+ and K^+ by aldosterone.
Collecting duct	Reabsorption of water (ADH required).

ADH, Antidiuretic hormone.

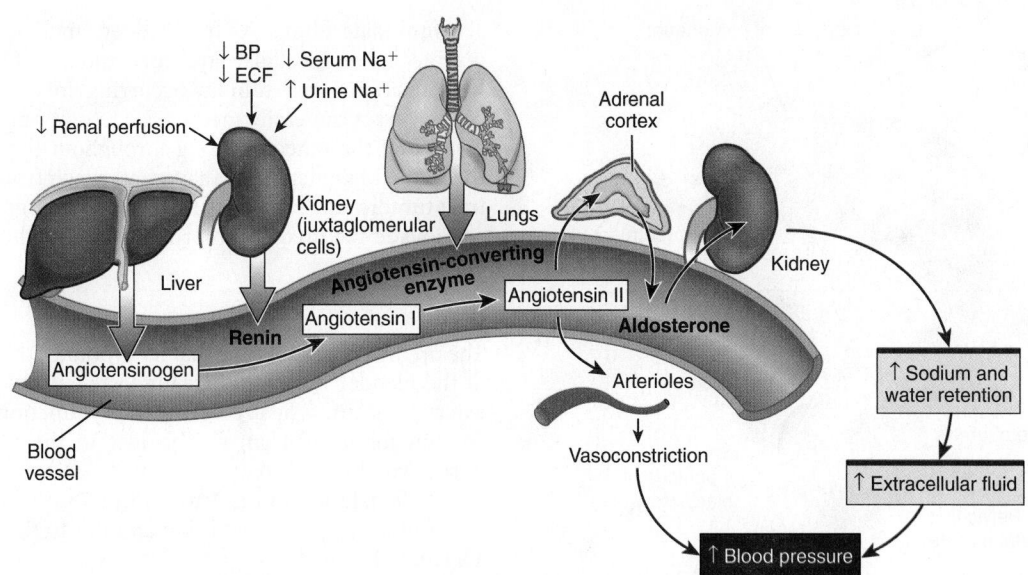

FIG. 45-4 Renin-angiotensin-aldosterone system.

has filtered the blood, the tubules select the unwanted from the wanted portions of tubular fluid. Essential constituents are returned to the blood, and dispensable substances pass into urine.

Other Functions of Kidneys. The kidneys perform vital functions through participation in red blood cell (RBC) production and blood pressure regulation. Erythropoietin is a hormone produced in the kidneys and secreted in response to hypoxia and decreased renal blood flow. Erythropoietin stimulates RBC production in the bone marrow. A deficiency of erythropoietin occurs in kidney failure, leading to anemia.

Renin is important in the regulation of blood pressure. Renin is produced and secreted by the kidney's juxtaglomerular cells (Fig. 45-4). Renin is released into the bloodstream in response to decreased renal perfusion, decreased arterial blood pressure, decreased ECF, decreased serum Na$^+$ concentration, and increased urinary Na$^+$ concentration. The plasma protein angiotensinogen (from the liver) is activated to angiotensin I by renin. Angiotensin I is subsequently converted to angiotensin II by angiotensin-converting enzyme (ACE). ACE is located on the inner surface of all blood vessels, with particularly high levels in the vessels of the lungs. Angiotensin II stimulates the release of aldosterone from the adrenal cortex, which causes Na$^+$ and water retention, leading to increased ECF volume. Angiotensin II also causes increased peripheral vasoconstriction. Release of renin is inhibited by an elevation in blood pressure. Excessive renin production caused by impaired renal perfusion may be a contributing factor in the etiology of hypertension (see Chapters 33 and 47).

Most body tissues synthesize prostaglandins (PGs) from the precursor, arachidonic acid, in response to appropriate stimuli. (See Chapter 12 and Fig. 12-2 for a more detailed discussion of PGs.) In the kidney, PG synthesis (primarily PGE$_2$ and PGI$_2$) occurs primarily in the medulla. These PGs have a vasodilating action, thus increasing renal blood flow, and promote Na$^+$ excretion. They counteract the vasoconstrictor effect of substances such as angiotensin and norepinephrine. Renal PGs may have a systemic effect in lowering blood pressure by decreasing systemic vascular resistance. The significance of renal PGs is related to the kidneys' role in causing hypertension. In renal

failure with a loss of functioning tissue, these renal vasodilator factors are also lost, which may contribute to hypertension (see Chapter 47).

Ureters

The ureters are tubes that carry urine from the renal pelvis to the bladder (see Fig. 45-1). Arranged in a meshlike outer layer, circular and longitudinal smooth muscle fibers contract to promote the peristaltic, one-way flow of urine through the ureters. Distention, neurologic and endocrine influences, and drugs can affect these muscle contractions. Each ureter is approximately 10 to 12 in (25 to 30.5 cm) long and 0.08 to 0.3 in (0.2 to 0.8 cm) in diameter.

The narrow area where each ureter joins the renal pelvis is termed the *ureteropelvic junction* (UPJ). Subsequently, the ureters insert into either side of the bladder base at the *ureterovesical junctions* (UVJs). Ureteral lumens are narrowest at the UVJs. These junctions, the UPJ and UVJ, are often sites of obstruction. The narrow ureteral lumens can be easily obstructed internally (e.g., urinary calculi) or externally (e.g., tumors, adhesions, inflammation). Sympathetic and parasympathetic nerves, along with the vascular supply, surround the mucosal lining of the ureters. Stimulation of these nerves during passage of a stone or clot may cause acute, severe pain, termed *renal colic*.

Because the renal pelvis holds only 3 to 5 mL of urine, kidney damage can result from a backflow of more than that amount of urine. The UVJ relies on the ureter's angle of bladder penetration and muscle fiber attachments with the bladder to prevent the backflow *(reflux)* of urine and ascending infection. The distal ureter enters the bladder laterally at its base, courses along obliquely through the bladder wall for about 1.5 cm, and intermingles with muscle fibers of the bladder base. Circular and longitudinal bladder muscle fibers adjacent to the imbedded ureter help secure it. When bladder pressure rises (e.g., during voiding or coughing), muscle fibers that the ureter shares with the bladder base contract first, promoting ureteral lumen closure. Next, the bladder contracts against its base, ensuring UVJ closure and prevention of urine reflux through the junction.

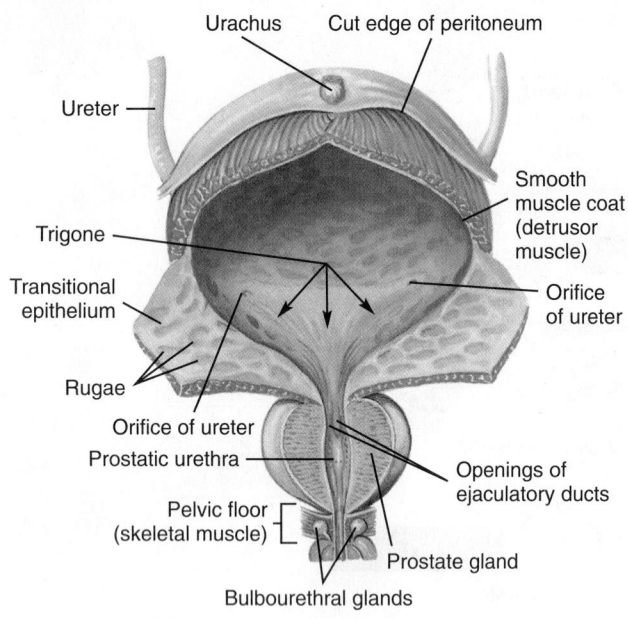

FIG. 45-5 Urinary bladder of a male.

Labels on figure: Urachus · Cut edge of peritoneum · Ureter · Trigone · Transitional epithelium · Rugae · Orifice of ureter · Prostatic urethra · Pelvic floor (skeletal muscle) · Bulbourethral glands · Smooth muscle coat (detrusor muscle) · Orifice of ureter · Openings of ejaculatory ducts · Prostate gland

Bladder

The urinary bladder is a stretchable (able to fill at relatively low pressures) organ positioned behind the symphysis pubis and anterior to the vagina and rectum (Fig. 45-5). Its primary functions are to serve as a reservoir for urine and to eliminate waste products from the body. Normal adult urine output is approximately 1500 mL/day, which varies with food and fluid intake. The volume of urine produced at night is less than half of that formed during the day because of hormonal influences (e.g., ADH). This diurnal pattern of urination is normal. Typically, an individual will urinate five or six times during the day and occasionally at night.

The *trigone* is the triangular area formed by the two ureteral openings and the bladder neck at the base of the bladder. The trigone is affixed to the pelvis by many ligaments and does not change its shape during bladder filling or emptying. The bladder muscle *(detrusor)* is composed of layers of intertwined smooth muscle fibers capable of considerable distention during bladder filling and contraction during emptying. It is attached to the abdominal wall by an umbilical ligament, the *urachus.* As a result of this attachment, as the bladder fills, it rises toward the umbilicus. The dome and the anterior and lateral aspects of the bladder expand and contract.

On average, 200 to 250 mL of urine in the bladder cause moderate distention and the urge to urinate. When the quantity of urine reaches approximately 400 to 600 mL, the person feels uncomfortable. Bladder capacity varies with the individual, but generally ranges from 600 to 1000 mL. Evacuation of urine is termed *urination, micturition,* or *voiding.*

The bladder has the same mucosal lining as that of the renal pelvises, ureters, and bladder neck. The bladder is lined by transitional cell epithelium and is referred to as the *urothelium.* The urothelium is unique to the urinary tract. Transitional cell epithelium is resistant to absorption of urine. Therefore urinary wastes produced by the kidneys do not leak out of the urinary system after they leave the kidneys. Microscopically, transitional cell epithelium is several cells deep. However, as urine enters the bladder, these cells stretch out to only a few cells deep to accommodate filling. As the bladder empties, the urothelium resumes its multicellular layer formation.

Transitional cell tumors occurring in one section of the urinary tract can easily metastasize to other urinary tract areas given that the mucosal lining throughout the urinary tract is the same. Malignant cells may move down from upper urinary tract tumors and embed in the bladder, or large bladder tumors can invade the ureter. Tumor recurrence within the bladder is common.

Urethra

The urethra is a small tube that incorporates the smooth muscle of the bladder neck and extends to the striated muscle of the external meatus. The urethra's primary function is to serve as a conduit for urine from the bladder to the outside the body during voiding and to control voiding.

The female urethra is 1 to 2 in (2.5 to 5 cm) long and lies behind the symphysis pubis but anterior to the vagina (see Fig. 45-1, *C*). The male urethra, which is about 8 to 10 in (20 to 25 cm) long, originates at the bladder neck and extends the length of the penis (see Fig. 45-1, *B*).

Urethrovesical Unit

Together, the bladder, urethra, and pelvic floor muscles form what is called the urethrovesical unit. Voluntary control of this unit is defined as *continence.* Stimulating and inhibiting impulses are sent from the brain through the thoracolumbar (T11 to L2) and sacral (S2 to S4) areas of the spinal cord to control voiding. Distention of the bladder stimulates stretch receptors within the bladder wall. Impulses are transmitted to the sacral spinal cord and then to the brain, causing a desire to urinate. If the time to void is not appropriate, inhibitor impulses in the brain are stimulated and transmitted back through the thoracolumbar and sacral nerves innervating the bladder. In a coordinated fashion, the detrusor muscle accommodates to the pressure (does not contract) while the sphincter and pelvic floor muscles tighten (contract) to resist bladder pressure. If voiding is appropriate, cerebral inhibition is voluntarily suppressed, and impulses are transmitted via the spinal cord for the bladder neck, sphincter, and pelvic floor muscles to relax and for the bladder to contract. The sphincter closes and the detrusor muscle relaxes when the bladder is empty.

Any disease or trauma that affects the function of the brain, spinal cord, or nerves that directly innervate the bladder, bladder neck, external sphincter, or pelvic floor can affect bladder function. These conditions include diabetes mellitus, multiple sclerosis, paraplegia, and tetraplegia (quadriplegia). Drugs affecting nerve transmission also can affect bladder function.

GERONTOLOGIC CONSIDERATIONS

EFFECTS OF AGING ON URINARY SYSTEM

Anatomic changes in the aging kidney include a 20% to 30% decrease in size and weight between ages 30 and 90 years. By the seventh decade of life, 30% to 50% of glomeruli have lost their function. Atherosclerosis accelerates the decrease of renal size with age. Despite these changes, older individuals maintain body fluid homeostasis unless they encounter diseases or other physiologic stressors.[1]

Physiologic changes in the aging kidney include decreased renal blood flow, due in part to atherosclerosis, resulting in a

TABLE 45-2 GERONTOLOGIC ASSESSMENT DIFFERENCES

Urinary System

Gerontologic Changes	Differences in Assessment Findings
Kidney	
• ↓ Amount of renal tissue	• Less palpable
• ↓ Number of nephrons and renal blood vessels; thickened basement membrane of Bowman's capsule and glomeruli	• ↓ Creatinine clearance, ↑ BUN level, ↑ serum creatinine
• ↓ Function of loop of Henle and tubules	• Alterations in drug excretion, nocturia, loss of normal diurnal excretory pattern because of ↓ ability to concentrate urine; less concentrated urine
Ureter, Bladder, and Urethra	
• ↓ Elasticity and muscle tone	• Palpable bladder after urination because of retention
• Weakening of urinary sphincter	• Stress incontinence (especially during Valsalva maneuver), dribbling of urine after urination
• ↓ Bladder capacity and sensory receptors	• Frequency, urgency, nocturia, overflow incontinence
• Estrogen deficiency leading to thin, dry vaginal tissue	• Stress or overactive bladder, dysuria
• ↑ Prevalence of unstable bladder contractions	• Overactive bladder
• Prostatic enlargement	• Hesitancy, frequency, urgency, nocturia, straining to urinate, retention, dribbling

FOCUSED ASSESSMENT
Urinary System

Use this checklist to ensure that the key assessment steps have been done.

Subjective
Ask the patient about any of the following and note responses.

Painful urination	Y	N
Changes in color of urine (blood, cloudy)	Y	N
Change in characteristics of urination (diminished, excessive)	Y	N
Problems with frequent nighttime urination (nocturia)	Y	N

Objective: Diagnostic
Check the following laboratory results for critical values.

Blood urea nitrogen	✓
Serum creatinine	✓
Urinalysis	✓
Urine culture and sensitivity	✓

Objective: Physical Examination
Inspect

Abdomen	✓
Urinary meatus for inflammation or discharge	✓

Palpate

Abdomen for bladder distention, masses, or tenderness	✓

Percuss

Costovertebral angle for tenderness	✓

Auscultate

Renal arteries for bruits	✓

decreased GFR. Alterations in hormone levels, including ADH, aldosterone, and ANP, result in decreased urinary concentrating ability and alterations in the excretion of water, sodium, potassium, and acid. Under normal conditions, the aging kidney is able to maintain homeostasis. However, after abrupt changes in blood volume, acid load, or other insults, the kidney may not be able to function effectively because much of its renal reserve has been lost.

Physiologic changes also occur in the aging urethra and bladder. The female urethra, bladder, vagina, and pelvic floor undergo a loss of elasticity and muscle support. Consequently, older women are more prone to bladder infections and incontinence.

The prostate surrounds the proximal urethra. As men age, the prostate enlarges and may affect urinary patterns, causing hesitancy, retention, slow stream, and bladder infections.[2]

Constipation, a complaint often expressed by older adults, can also affect urination. Partial urethral obstruction may occur because of the rectum's close proximity to the urethra.

Age-related changes in the urinary system and differences in assessment findings are presented in Table 45-2.

ASSESSMENT OF URINARY SYSTEM

Subjective Data

Important Health Information

Past Health History. Question the patient about the presence or history of diseases that are related to renal or other urologic problems. Some of these diseases are hypertension, diabetes

CASE STUDY
Patient Introduction

iStockphoto/Thinkstock

A.K. is a 28-yr-old African American man who comes to the emergency department (ED) in acute distress with complaints of severe abdominal pain. The pain began about 6 hr ago after he finished a 10-mile run as part of his training for a marathon. He says that the pain has steadily increased, he is nauseated, and his urine is a dark, smoky color.

Critical Thinking
As you read through this assessment chapter, think about A.K.'s symptoms with the following questions in mind:

1. What are the possible causes of A.K.'s abdominal pain, nausea, and urine color?
2. What would be your priority assessment of A.K.?
3. What questions would you ask A.K.?
4. What should be included in the physical assessment? What would you be looking for?
5. What diagnostic studies might you expect to be ordered?

evolve Answers available at *http://evolve.elsevier.com/Lewis/medsurg*.

mellitus, gout and other metabolic problems, connective tissue disorders (e.g., systemic lupus erythematosus, systemic sclerosis [scleroderma]), skin or upper respiratory tract infections of streptococcal origin, tuberculosis, viral hepatitis, congenital disorders, neurologic conditions (e.g., stroke, back injury), or trauma. Note specific urinary problems such as cancer, infections, benign prostatic hyperplasia, and calculi.

TABLE 45-3   POTENTIALLY NEPHROTOXIC AGENTS

Antibiotics	Other Drugs	Other Agents
amikacin (Amikin)	captopril (Capoten)	Gold
amphotericin B	cimetidine (Tagamet)	Heavy metals
bacitracin	cisplatin (Platinol)	
cephalosporins	cocaine	
gentamicin	cyclosporine	
kanamycin	ethylene glycol	
neomycin	heroin	
polymyxin B	lithium	
streptomycin	methotrexate	
sulfonamides	nitrosoureas (e.g., carmustine)	
tobramycin (Nebcin)	Nonsteroidal antiinflammatory drugs (e.g., ibuprofen, indomethacin)	
vancomycin	phenacetin	
	quinine	
	rifampin	
	Salicylates (large quantities)	

Medications. An assessment of the patient's current and past use of medications is important. This should include over-the-counter drugs, prescription medications, and herbs. Drugs affect the urinary tract in several ways. Many drugs are known to be nephrotoxic (Table 45-3). Certain drugs may alter the quantity and character of urine output (e.g., diuretics). A number of drugs such as phenazopyridine (Pyridium) and nitrofurantoin (Macrodantin) change the color of urine. Anticoagulants may cause hematuria. Many antidepressants, calcium channel blockers, antihistamines, and drugs used for neurologic and musculoskeletal disorders affect the ability of the bladder or sphincter to contract or relax normally.

Surgery or Other Treatments. Ask the patient about previous hospitalizations related to renal or urologic diseases and all urinary problems during past pregnancies. Inquire about the duration, severity, and patient's perception of any problem and its treatment. Document past surgeries, particularly pelvic surgeries, or urinary tract instrumentation (e.g., catheterization). Ask the patient about any radiation or chemotherapy treatment for cancer.

Functional Health Patterns. Key questions to ask a patient with problems related to the renal system are listed in Table 45-4.

TABLE 45-4   HEALTH HISTORY
Urinary System

Health Perception–Health Management
- How is your energy level compared with 1 yr ago?
- Do you notice any visual changes?*
- Have you ever smoked? If yes, how many packs per day?

Nutritional-Metabolic
- How is your appetite?
- Has your weight changed over the past yr?*
- Do you take vitamins, herbs, or any other supplements?*
- How much and what kinds of fluids do you drink daily?
- How many dairy products and how much meat do you eat?
- Do you drink coffee? Colas? Tea?
- Do you eat chocolate?
- Do you spice your food heavily?*

Elimination
- Are you able to sit through a 2-hr meeting or ride in a car for 2 hr without urinating?
- Do you awaken at night with the desire to urinate? If so, how many times does this occur during an average night?
- Do you ever notice blood in your urine?* If so, at what point in the urination does it occur?
- Do you ever pass urine when you do not intend to? When?
- Do you use special devices or supplies for urine elimination or control?*
- How often do you move your bowels?
- Do you ever experience constipation?
- Do you frequently experience diarrhea? Do you ever have problems controlling your bowels? If so, do you have problems controlling the passage of gas? Watery or liquid stool? Solid stool?

Activity-Exercise
- Have you noticed any changes in your ability to do your usual daily activities?*
- Do certain activities aggravate your urinary problem?*
- Has your urinary problem caused you to alter or stop any activity or exercise?*
- Do you require assistance in moving or getting to the bathroom?*

Sleep-Rest
- Do you awaken at night from an urge to urinate?*
- Do you awaken at night from pain or other problems and urinate as a matter of routine before returning to sleep?*
- Do you experience daytime sleepiness and fatigue as a result of nighttime urination?*

Cognitive-Perceptual
- Do you ever have pain when you urinate?* If so, where is the pain?

Self-Perception–Self-Concept
- How does your urinary problem make you feel about yourself?
- Do you perceive your body differently since you have developed a urinary problem?

Role-Relationship
- Does your urinary problem interfere with your relationships with family or friends?*
- Has your urinary problem caused a change in your job status or affected your ability to carry out job-related responsibilities?*

Sexuality-Reproductive
- Has your urinary problem caused any change in your sexual pleasure or performance?*
- Do you have hygiene problems related to sexual activities that cause you concern?*

Coping–Stress Tolerance
- Do you feel able to manage the problems associated with your urinary problem? If not, explain.
- What strategies are you using to cope with your urinary problem?

Values-Beliefs
- Has your present illness affected your belief system?*
- Are your treatment decisions related to your urinary problem in conflict with your value system?*

*If yes, describe.

Health Perception–Health Management Pattern. Ask about the patient's general health, particularly when a disorder affecting the kidneys is suspected. Abnormal kidney function may be suggested by changes in weight or appetite; excess thirst; fluid retention; and complaints of headache, pruritus, blurred vision, or "feeling tired all the time." Similarly, an older patient may report malaise and nonlocalized abdominal discomfort as the only symptoms of a urinary tract infection (UTI). Family members may report disorientation or increased confusion that may be a sign of UTI in older adults.

Take an occupational history because exposure to certain chemicals can affect the kidneys and urinary system. Phenol and ethylene glycol are examples of nephrotoxic chemicals. Aromatic amines and some organic chemicals may increase the risk of bladder cancers. Textile workers, painters, hairdressers, and industrial workers have a high incidence of bladder tumors.

Get a smoking history. Cigarette smoking is a major risk factor for bladder cancer. Tumors occur more frequently in cigarette smokers than in nonsmokers.

Obtain information about places where a patient has lived. It has been shown that persons living in certain parts of the United States (Great Lakes, Southwest, Southeast) have a higher than normal incidence of urinary calculi, possibly caused by the higher mineral content of the soil and water. A person living in Middle Eastern countries or Africa can acquire certain parasites that can cause cystitis or bladder cancer.

GENETIC RISK ALERT
- Polycystic kidney disease and congenital urinary tract abnormalities (e.g., Alport syndrome [congenital nephritis]) are genetic disorders.
- A family history of certain renal or urologic problems increases the likelihood of similar problems occurring in the patient.
- Ask about family members who have had any of the diseases that the patient mentions in the past health history.

Nutritional-Metabolic Pattern. The usual quantity and types of fluid a patient drinks are important in relation to urinary tract disease. Dehydration may contribute to UTIs, calculi formation, and kidney failure. Large intake of particular foods, such as dairy products or foods high in proteins, may also lead to calculi formation. Asparagus may cause the urine to smell musty, and red urine caused by beet ingestion may be mistaken for bloody urine. Caffeine, alcohol, carbonated beverages, some artificial sweeteners, or spicy foods often aggravate urinary inflammatory diseases. Green tea and some herbal teas also cause diuresis. An unexplained weight gain may be the result of fluid retention secondary to a renal problem. Anorexia, nausea, and vomiting can dramatically affect fluid status and require careful assessment. Obtain information on vitamin and mineral

supplements and herbal therapies. The patient may not think of these supplements and therapies when listing over-the-counter drugs.

Elimination Pattern. Questions about urine elimination patterns are the cornerstone of the health history in the patient with a lower urinary tract disorder. This line of inquiry begins with a question of how the patient manages urine elimination. Most patients eliminate urine by spontaneous voiding. Therefore ask about daytime (diurnal) voiding frequency and the frequency of nocturia. Pelvic organ prolapse, particularly advanced anterior vaginal prolapse, may cause suprapubic pressure, frequency, urgency, and incontinence secondary to urinary retention. Query patients about additional bothersome lower urinary tract symptoms, including urgency, incontinence, or urinary retention. Table 45-5 lists some of the common manifestations of urinary tract disorders.

CASE STUDY—cont'd
Subjective Data

iStockphoto/Thinkstock

A focused subjective assessment of A.K. revealed the following information:
PMH: History of one isolated incidence of possible gout 6 yr ago. He stopped drinking alcohol with no further occurrence. Appendectomy 12 yr ago.
Medications: None.
Health Perception–Health Management: A.K. states that he is usually healthy. He does not smoke or drink alcohol. He has never experienced this type of pain before. Describes the pain as being sharp and colicky (coming in waves). Rates the pain as 9 on a scale of 0-10.
Nutritional-Metabolic: A.K. is currently on a high-protein diet as he trains for the marathon. He eats a lot of chicken, beef, and seafood. He drinks milk-based protein shakes and water after exercising but admits that he does not think he drinks enough to replace fluid loss in perspiration. He drinks coffee for energy but denies eating chocolate or other sweets. He also avoids sodas.
Elimination: Denies any history of difficulty with urination or constipation or diarrhea. This is the first time he has ever noticed a change of color in his urine.
Activity-Exercise: Prides himself in his ability to exercise and run without difficulty.
Sleep-Rest: Does not awaken at night to urinate.
Cognitive-Perceptual: Denies pain on urination.
Self-Perception–Self-Concept: Believes he is able to monitor self and maintain healthy lifestyle.
Coping–Stress Tolerance: Worried that this pain may interfere with his marathon training.

TABLE 45-5 MANIFESTATIONS OF URINARY SYSTEM DISORDERS

General Manifestations	Specific Manifestations Related to Urinary System				
	Edema	Pain	Patterns of Urination	Urine Output	Urine Composition
Fatigue	Facial (periorbital)	Dysuria	Frequency	Anuria	Concentrated
Headaches	Ankle	Flank or	Urgency	Oliguria	Dilute
Blurred vision	Ascites	costovertebral	Hesitancy of stream	Polyuria	Hematuria
Elevated blood pressure	Anasarca	angle	Change in stream		Pyuria
Anorexia	Sacral	Groin	Retention		Color (red, brown,
Nausea and vomiting		Suprapubic	Dysuria		yellowish green)
Chills			Nocturia		
Itching			Incontinence		
Excessive thirst			Stress incontinence		
Change in body weight			Dribbling		
Cognitive changes					

Changes in the color and appearance of urine are often significant and should be evaluated. If blood is visible in the urine, determine if it occurs at the beginning of, throughout, or at the end of urination.

Investigate bowel function. Problems with fecal incontinence may signal neurologic causes for bladder problems because of shared nerve pathways. Constipation and fecal impaction can partially obstruct the urethra, causing inadequate bladder emptying, overflow incontinence, and infection.

Determine the patient's method of handling a urinary problem. A patient may already be using a catheter or collection device. Sometimes a patient has to assume a particular position to urinate or perform maneuvers such as pressing on the lower abdomen (Credé's method) or straining (Valsalva maneuver) to empty the bladder.

Activity-Exercise Pattern. Assess the patient's level of activity. A sedentary person is more likely to have stasis of urine than an active individual and thus can be predisposed to infection and calculi. Demineralization of bones in an individual with limited physical activity can cause increased urine calcium precipitation.

An active person may find that increasing activity aggravates the urinary problem. The patient who has had prostate surgery or who has weakened pelvic floor muscles may leak urine when attempting particular activities such as running. Some men develop chronic inflammatory prostatitis or epididymitis after heavy lifting or long-distance driving.

Sleep-Rest Pattern. Nocturia is a common and a particularly bothersome lower urinary tract symptom that often leads to sleep deprivation, daytime sleepiness, and fatigue. It occurs in multiple disorders affecting the lower urinary tract, including urinary incontinence, urinary retention, and interstitial cystitis. Nocturia also may be related to polyuria secondary to kidney disease, poorly controlled diabetes mellitus, alcoholism, excessive fluid intake, or obstructive sleep apnea.[3]

When assessing nocturia, determine whether the need to urinate causes the person to arise from sleep or whether pain or some other symptom interrupts sleep and the person urinates as a matter of habit before returning to bed. Up to one episode of nocturia is considered normal in younger adults, and up to two episodes are acceptable among adults ages 65 years or older. If the older adult has more than two voidings during the night, assess the amount and timing of fluid intake. This information will help determine whether further investigation is needed.

Cognitive-Perceptual Pattern. Level of mobility, visual acuity, and dexterity are important factors to determine for a patient with urologic problems when managing his or her own care at home, particularly when urine retention or incontinence is a problem. Determine if the patient is alert, is able to understand instructions, and can recall the instructions when necessary.

If urinary incontinence is present, elicit a thorough history of the problem to help determine the type of incontinence. Document what the patient has previously tried to manage the problem. Incontinence is a distressing problem and calls for great sensitivity on your part to obtain accurate information.

A frequent symptom of renal and urologic problems is pain, including dysuria, groin pain, costovertebral pain, and suprapubic pain. Assess pain and document the location, character, and duration. The absence of pain when other urinary symptoms exist is also significant. Many urinary tract tumors are painless in the early stages.

Self-Perception–Self-Concept Pattern. Problems associated with the urinary system, such as incontinence, urinary diversion procedures, and chronic fatigue (may indicate anemia), can result in loss of self-esteem and a negative body image.

Role-Relationship Pattern. Urinary problems can affect many aspects of a person's life, including the ability to work and relationships with others. These factors have important implications for future treatment and management of the patient's condition.

Urinary system problems may be serious enough to cause problems in job-related and social situations. Chronic dialysis therapy often makes regular employment or full-time homemaking difficult. Concurrent poor health and negative body image can seriously alter existing roles.

Sexuality-Reproductive Pattern. Question the patient about the effect of a renal or urologic problem on her or his sexual patterns and satisfaction. Problems related to personal hygiene and fatigue can seriously affect a sexual relationship. Although urinary incontinence is not directly associated with sexual dysfunction, it often has a devastating effect on self-esteem and social and intimate relationships. Counseling of both the patient and partner may be indicated.

Objective Data

Physical Examination

Inspection. Assess for changes in the following:

Skin: Pallor, yellow-gray cast, excoriations, changes in turgor, bruises, texture (e.g., rough, dry skin) (see Table 23-6 for assessment of dark-skinned individuals)

Mouth: Stomatitis, ammonia breath odor

Face and extremities: Generalized edema, peripheral edema, bladder distention, masses, enlarged kidneys

Abdomen: Skin changes described earlier, striae, abdominal contour for midline mass in lower abdomen (may indicate urinary retention) or unilateral mass (occasionally seen in adult, indicating enlargement of one or both kidneys from large tumor or polycystic kidney)

Weight: Weight gain secondary to edema; weight loss and muscle wasting in kidney failure

General state of health: Fatigue, lethargy, and diminished alertness

Palpation. The kidneys are posterior organs protected by the abdominal organs, the ribs, and the heavy back muscles. A landmark useful in locating the kidneys is the **costovertebral angle (CVA)** formed by the rib cage and the vertebral column. The normal-sized left kidney is rarely palpable because the spleen lies directly on top of it. Occasionally the lower pole of the right kidney is palpable.

To palpate the right kidney, place your left (anterior) hand behind and support the patient's right side between the rib cage and the iliac crest (Fig. 45-6). Elevate the right flank with the left hand. Use your right hand to palpate deeply for the right kidney. The lower pole of the right kidney may be felt as a smooth, rounded mass that descends on inspiration. If the kidney is palpable, note its size, contour, and tenderness. Kidney enlargement is suggestive of neoplasm or other serious renal pathologic conditions.

The urinary bladder is normally not palpable unless it is distended with urine. If the bladder is full, it may be felt as a smooth, round, firm organ and is sensitive to palpation.

Percussion. Tenderness in the flank area may be detected by fist percussion (*kidney punch*). This technique is performed by

FIG. 45-6 Palpating the right kidney.

striking the fist of one hand against the dorsal surface of the other hand, which is placed flat along the posterior CVA margin (Fig. 45-7). Normally a firm blow in the flank area should not elicit pain. If CVA tenderness and pain are present, it may indicate a kidney infection or polycystic kidney disease.

A bladder is not normally percussible until it contains 150 mL of urine. If the bladder is full, dullness is heard above the symphysis pubis. A distended bladder may be percussed as high as the umbilicus.

Auscultation. The bell of the stethoscope may be used to auscultate over both CVAs and in the upper abdominal quadrants. With this technique, auscultate the abdominal aorta and renal arteries for a *bruit* (an abnormal murmur), which indicates impaired blood flow to the kidneys. Use the diaphragm of the stethoscope to auscultate the bowels, since they may also affect the urinary system.

Table 45-6 shows how to record the normal physical assessment findings of the urinary system. Table 45-7 presents assessment abnormalities of the urinary system. Assessment

FIG. 45-7 Indirect fist percussion of the costovertebral angle (CVA). To assess the kidney, place one hand over the twelfth rib at the CVA on the back. Thump that hand with the ulnar edge of the other fist. (From Jarvis C: *Physical examination and health assessment,* ed 6, St Louis, 2012, Saunders.)

TABLE 45-6	NORMAL PHYSICAL ASSESSMENT OF URINARY SYSTEM

- No costovertebral angle tenderness
- Nonpalpable kidney and bladder
- No palpable masses

findings may vary in the older adult. Table 45-2 shows the age-related changes in the urinary system and differences in assessment findings. Use a *focused assessment* to evaluate the status of previously identified urinary system problems and to monitor for signs of new problems (see Table 3-6). A focused assessment of the urinary system is presented in the box on p. 1051.

DIAGNOSTIC STUDIES OF URINARY SYSTEM

Numerous diagnostic studies are available to locate and assess problems of the urinary system. Tables 45-8 and 45-9 describe the most common studies, and select studies are described in more detail in the following text.

The accuracy of these diagnostic studies is influenced by (1) adherence to the proper procedures; and (2) the patient's cooperation in terms of fluid restriction, urine specimen collection, study preparations procedures, ability to remain positioned on examination table, or following of other instructions.

Many radiologic studies require the use of a bowel preparation the evening before the study to clear the lower GI tract of feces and flatus. Because the kidneys lie in a retroperitoneal location, the contents of the colon may obstruct visualization of the urinary tract. If the bowel preparation fails to adequately evacuate the lower tract, the study may be unsuccessful and have to be rescheduled. Commonly used bowel preparations include enemas, castor oil, magnesium citrate, and bisacodyl (Dulcolax) tablets or suppositories. Some bowel preparations, such as magnesium citrate and Fleet enema, are contraindicated because magnesium cannot be excreted by the kidneys in patients with kidney failure (see Chapter 47).

When a patient has had diagnostic studies on consecutive days, it is important to prevent dehydration. Often the patient takes nothing by mouth (NPO) after midnight, spends an

Text continued on p. 1061

CASE STUDY—cont'd

Objective Data: Physical Examination

iStockphoto/Thinkstock

A focused assessment of A.K. reveals the following:

A.K. is lying on the ED stretcher with his knees bent and drawn to his abdominal area. He appears restless and keeps moving from back to side in an effort to reduce his discomfort. Vital signs as follows: BP 156/70, apical pulse 108, respiratory rate 24, temperature 37.4° C, O₂ saturation 96% on room air. Awake, alert, and oriented × 3. Lungs clear to auscultation. Apical pulse regular. Abdomen nondistended with + bowel sounds in all 4 quadrants. No rebound tenderness. Positive costovertebral tenderness. Voiding small amounts of dark, smoky urine.

As you continue to read this chapter, consider diagnostic studies you would anticipate being performed for A.K.

TABLE 45-7 ASSESSMENT ABNORMALITIES

Urinary System

Finding	Description	Possible Etiology and Significance
Anuria	Technically no urination (24-hr urine output <100 mL)	Acute kidney injury, end-stage kidney disease, bilateral ureteral obstruction
Burning on urination	Stinging pain in urethral area	Urethral irritation, urinary tract infection
Dysuria	Painful or difficult urination	Sign of urinary tract infection, interstitial cystitis, and wide variety of pathologic conditions
Enuresis	Involuntary nocturnal urination	Symptomatic of lower urinary tract disorder
Frequency	Increased incidence of urination	Acutely inflamed bladder, retention with overflow, excess fluid intake, intake of bladder irritants
	Blood in the urine	Cancer of genitourinary tract, blood dyscrasias, kidney disease, urinary tract infection, stones in kidney or ureter, medications (anticoagulants)
Hesitancy	Delay or difficulty in initiating urination	Partial urethral obstruction, benign prostatic hyperplasia
Incontinence	Inability to voluntarily control discharge of urine	Neurogenic bladder, bladder infection, injury to external sphincter
Nocturia	Frequency of urination at night	Kidney disease with impaired concentrating ability, bladder obstruction, heart failure, diabetes mellitus, finding after renal transplant, excessive evening and nighttime fluid intake
Oliguria	Diminished amount of urine in a given time (24-hr urine output of 100-400 mL)	Severe dehydration, shock, transfusion reaction, kidney disease, end-stage kidney disease
Pain	Suprapubic pain (related to bladder), urethral pain (irritation of bladder neck), flank (CVA) pain	Infection, urinary retention, foreign body in urinary tract, urethritis, pyelonephritis, renal colic or stones
Pneumaturia	Passage of urine containing gas	Fistula connections between bowel and bladder, gas-forming urinary tract infections
Polyuria	Large volume of urine in a given time	Diabetes mellitus, diabetes insipidus, chronic kidney disease, diuretics, excess fluid intake, obstructive sleep apnea
Retention	Inability to urinate even though bladder contains excessive amount of urine	Finding after pelvic surgery, childbirth, catheter removal, anesthesia; urethral stricture or obstruction; neurogenic bladder
Stress incontinence	Involuntary urination with increased pressure (sneezing or coughing)	Weakness of sphincter control, lack of estrogen, urinary retention

CVA, Costovertebral angle.

TABLE 45-8 DIAGNOSTIC STUDIES

Urinary System

Study	Description and Purpose	Nursing Responsibility
Urine Studies		
Urinalysis	General examination of urine to establish baseline information or provide data to establish a tentative diagnosis and determine whether further studies are needed (see Table 45-9).	Try to obtain first urinated morning specimen. Ensure specimen is examined within 1 hr of urinating. Before collecting, wash perineal area (if soiled with menses or fecal material).
Creatinine clearance	Creatinine is a waste product of protein breakdown (primarily body muscle mass). Clearance of creatinine by kidney approximates the GFR. Creatinine clearance is calculated as follows: $$\text{Creatinine clearance} = \frac{\text{Urine creatinine (mg/dL)} \times \text{Urine volume (mL/min)}}{\text{Serum creatinine (mg/dL)}}$$ *Reference interval:* 70-135 mL/min/1.73 m^2 (corrected for body surface area).	Collect 24-hr urine specimen. Discard first urination when test is started. Save urine from all subsequent urinations for 24 hr. Instruct patient to urinate at end of 24 hr and add specimen to collection. Ensure that serum creatinine is determined during 24-hr period.
Composite urine collection	Measures specific components, such as electrolytes, glucose, protein, 17-ketosteroids, catecholamines, creatinine, and minerals. Composite urine specimens are collected over a period ranging from 2 to 24 hr.	Instruct the patient to urinate and discard this first urine specimen. Note this time as the start of the test. Save all urine from subsequent urinations in a container for designated period. At end of period, ask patient to urinate, and this urine is added to container. Remind patient to save all urine during study period. Specimens may have to be refrigerated, or preservatives may have to be added to container used for collecting urine.

GFR, Glomerular filtration rate.

TABLE 45-8   DIAGNOSTIC STUDIES—cont'd

Urinary System

Study	Description and Purpose	Nursing Responsibility
Urine culture ("**clean catch**," "**midstream**")	Confirms suspected urinary tract infection and identifies causative organisms. *Normally,* bladder is sterile, but urethra contains bacteria and a few WBCs. *Reference interval:* If properly collected, stored, and handled: $<10^3$ organisms/mL usually indicates no infection. 10^3-10^5/mL is usually not diagnostic and test may have to be repeated. $>10^5$/mL indicates infection.	Use sterile container for collection of urine. Touch only outside of container. For women, separate labia with one hand and clean meatus with other hand, using at least three sponges (saturated with cleansing solution) in a front-to-back motion. For men, retract foreskin (if present) and cleanse glans with at least three cleansing sponges. After cleaning, instruct patient to start urinating and then continue voiding in sterile container. (The initial voided urine flushes out most contaminants in the urethra and perineal area.) Catheterization may be needed if patient is unable to cooperate with procedure.
Concentration test	Evaluates renal concentration ability. Measured by specific gravity readings. *Reference interval:* 1.003-1.030.	Instruct patient to fast after given time in evening (in usual procedure). Collect three urine specimens at hourly intervals in morning.
Residual urine	Determines amount of urine left in bladder after urinating. Finding may be abnormal in problems with bladder innervation, sphincter impairment, BPH, or urethral strictures. *Reference interval:* ≤50 mL urine (increases with age).	Immediately after patient urinates, catheterize patient or use bladder ultrasound equipment. If a large amount of residual urine is obtained, health care provider may want catheter left in bladder.
Protein determination		
• Dipstick (Albustix, Combistix)	Test detects protein (primarily albumin) in urine. *Reference interval:* 0-trace.	Dip end of stick in urine and read result by comparison with color chart on label as directed. Grading is from 0 to 4+. Interpret with caution. Positive result may not indicate significant proteinuria. Some medications may give false-positive readings.
• Quantitative protein test	A 24-hr collection gives a more accurate indication of amount of protein in urine. Persistent proteinuria usually indicates glomerular kidney disease. *Reference interval:* <150 mg/24 hr (mainly albumin).	Perform 24-hr urine collection as above.
Urine cytologic study	Identifies abnormal cellular structures that occur with bladder cancer. Also used to follow the progress of bladder cancer after treatment.	Obtain specimens by voiding, catheterization, or bladder irrigation. Do not use morning's first voided specimen because epithelial cells may change in appearance in urine held in bladder overnight. As with urinalysis, the specimen should be fresh or brought to laboratory within the hour. An alcohol-based fixative is then added to preserve the cellular structure.
Blood Studies		
Blood urea nitrogen (BUN)	Used to detect renal problems. Concentration of urea in blood is regulated by rate at which kidney excretes urea. *Reference interval:* 6-20 mg/dL (2.1-7.1 mmol/L).	When interpreting BUN, be aware that nonrenal factors may cause increase (e.g., rapid cell destruction from infections, fever, GI bleeding, trauma, athletic activity and excessive muscle breakdown, corticosteroid therapy).
Creatinine	More reliable than BUN as a determinant of renal function. Creatinine is end product of muscle and protein metabolism and is released at a constant rate. *Reference interval:* 0.6-1.3 mg/dL (53-115 μmol/L).	Explain test and watch for postpuncture bleeding.
BUN/creatinine ratio	An increased ratio may be due to conditions that decrease blood flow to kidneys (e.g., heart failure, dehydration), GI bleeding, or increased dietary protein. A decreased ratio may occur with liver disease (due to decreased urea formation) and malnutrition. *Reference interval:* 12:1 to 20:1.	
Uric acid	Used as screening test primarily for disorders of purine metabolism but can also indicate kidney disease. Values depend on renal function, rate of purine metabolism, and dietary intake of food rich in purines. *Female:* 2.3-6.6 mg/dL (137-393 μmol/L). *Male:* 4.4-7.6 mg/dL (262-452 μmol/L).	Explain test and watch for postpuncture bleeding.
Sodium	Main extracellular electrolyte determining blood volume. Usually values stay within normal range until late stages of renal failure. *Reference interval:* 135-145 mEq/L (135-145 mmol/L).	Explain test and watch for postpuncture bleeding.

BPH, Benign prostatic hyperplasia.

Continued

TABLE 45-8   DIAGNOSTIC STUDIES—cont'd

Urinary System

Study	Description and Purpose	Nursing Responsibility
Blood Studies—cont'd		
Potassium	Kidneys are responsible for excreting majority of body's potassium. In kidney disease, K^+ determinations are critical because K^+ is one of the first electrolytes to become abnormal. Elevated K^+ levels >6 mEq/L can lead to muscle weakness and cardiac dysrhythmias. *Reference interval:* 3.5-5.0 mEq/L (3.5-5.0 mmol/L).	Explain test and watch for postpuncture bleeding.
Calcium (total)	Main mineral in bone and aids in muscle contraction, neurotransmission, and clotting. In kidney disease, decreased reabsorption of Ca^{2+} leads to renal osteodystrophy. *Reference interval:* 8.6-10.2 mg/dL (2.15-2.55 mmol/L).	Explain test and watch for postpuncture bleeding.
Phosphorus	Phosphorus balance is inversely related to Ca^{2+} balance. In kidney disease, phosphorus levels are elevated because the kidney is the primary excretory organ. *Reference interval:* 2.4-4.4 mg/dL (0.78-1.42 mmol/L).	Explain test and watch for postpuncture bleeding.
Bicarbonate	Most patients in renal failure have metabolic acidosis and low serum HCO_3^- levels. *Reference interval:* 22-26 mEq/L (22-26 mmol/L).	Explain test and watch for postpuncture bleeding.
Radiologic Procedures		
Kidneys, ureters, bladder (KUB)	X-ray examination of abdomen and pelvis delineates size, shape, and position of kidneys. Radiopaque stones and foreign bodies can be seen.	Perform bowel preparation (if ordered).
Intravenous pyelogram (IVP)	Visualizes urinary tract after IV injection of contrast media. Presence, position, size, and shape of kidneys, ureters, and bladder can be evaluated. Cysts, tumors, lesions, and obstructions cause a distortion in normal appearance of these structures. Patient with significantly decreased renal function should not have IVP because contrast media can be nephrotoxic and worsen renal function.*	Evening before procedure, give cathartic or enema to empty colon of feces and gas. Before procedure, assess patient for iodine sensitivity to avoid anaphylactic reaction. Inform patient that procedure involves lying on table and having serial x-rays taken. Advise patient that during injection of contrast material, warmth, a flushed face, and a salty taste may be experienced. After procedure, force fluids (if permitted) to flush out contrast media.
Renal arteriogram (angiogram)	Visualizes renal blood vessels. Can assist in diagnosing renal artery stenosis (Fig. 45-8), additional or missing renal blood vessels, and renovascular hypertension. Can assist in differentiating between a renal cyst and a renal tumor. Also included in workup of a potential renal transplant donor. A catheter is inserted into the femoral artery and passed up the aorta to the level of the renal arteries (Fig. 45-9). Contrast media is injected to outline the renal blood supply.*	*Before procedure:* Prepare patient the prior evening by giving cathartic or enema. Before injection of contrast material, assess for iodine sensitivity. The patient may experience a transient warm feeling along the course of the blood vessel when contrast media is injected. *After procedure:* Place a pressure dressing over femoral artery injection site. Observe site for bleeding. Have patient maintain bed rest with affected leg straight. Take peripheral pulses in the involved leg every 30-60 min to detect occlusion of blood flow caused by a thrombus. Observe for complications, including thrombus, embolus, local inflammation, hematoma.

*N-acetylcysteine (Mucomyst), a renal vasodilator and antioxidant, is sometimes administered to reduce the incidence of contrast-induced nephropathy; can be given by oral or IV route.

FIG. 45-8 Renal arteriogram showing stenosis of the right renal artery *(arrow).*

FIG. 45-9 Catheter insertion for a renal arteriogram.

TABLE 45-8 DIAGNOSTIC STUDIES—cont'd

Urinary System

Study	Description and Purpose	Nursing Responsibility
Antegrade pyelogram (nephrostogram)	Evaluates upper urinary tract when patient has allergy to contrast media, decreased renal function, or abnormalities that prevent passage of a ureteral catheter. Contrast media may be injected percutaneously into renal pelvis or via a nephrostomy tube that is already in place when determining tube function or ureteral integrity after trauma or surgery.*	Explain procedure and prepare patient as for IVP. Watch for signs of complications (e.g., hematuria, infection, hematoma).
Retrograde pyelogram	X-ray of urinary tract taken after injection of contrast material into kidneys. It may be done if an IVP does not visualize the urinary tract or if patient is allergic to contrast media or has decreased renal function. A cystoscope is inserted and ureteral catheters are inserted through it into renal pelvis. Contrast media is injected through catheters.*	Prepare patient as for IVP. Inform patient that pain may be experienced from distention of pelvis and discomfort from cystoscope. Inform patient that anesthesia may be given for procedure. Complications are similar to those for cystoscopy (see cystoscopy later in table).
Renal ultrasound	Used to detect renal or perirenal masses, differential diagnosis of renal cysts, solid masses, and identification of obstructions. Small external ultrasound probe is placed on patient's skin. Conductive gel is applied to skin. Noninvasive procedure involves passing sound waves into body structures and recording images as they are reflected back. Computer interprets tissue density based on sound waves and displays it in picture form. It can be used safely in patients with renal failure.	Explain procedure to patient. Because radiation exposure is avoided, a number of images can be obtained and repeat studies can be done over a brief period. Images can be obtained from both prone and supine positions. A bowel preparation is not required.
Computed tomography (CT) scan (CT urogram)	Provides excellent visualization of kidneys. Kidney size can be evaluated. Tumors, abscesses, suprarenal masses (e.g., adrenal tumors, pheochromocytomas), and obstructions can be detected. Advantage of CT over ultrasound is its ability to distinguish subtle differences in density. Use of IV-administered contrast media during CT accentuates density of renal tissue and helps differentiate masses.*	Explain procedure to patient. Ask patient about iodine sensitivity. Instruct the patient to lie still during the procedure while the machine takes precise transaxial images. Sedation may be required if patient is unable to cooperate.
Magnetic resonance imaging (MRI)	Useful for visualization of kidneys. Not proven useful for detecting urinary calculi or calcified tumors. Computer-generated films rely on radiofrequency waves and alteration in magnetic field.	Explain procedure to patient. Have patient remove all metal objects. Patients with a history of claustrophobia may need to be sedated. Contraindications: presence of implanted magnetic clips or prosthesis and pacemakers.
Magnetic resonance angiography	Allows visualization of renal vasculature. Gadolinium-enhanced studies allow visualization of the renal artery.	Same as above. Does not require femoral artery puncture.
Cystogram	Visualizes bladder and evaluates vesicoureteral reflux. Also evaluates patients with neurogenic bladder and recurrent urinary tract infections. Can also delineate abnormalities of the bladder (e.g., diverticula, calculi, tumors). Contrast media is instilled into bladder via cystoscope or catheter.	Explain procedure to patient. If done via cystoscope, follow nursing care related to cystoscopy.
Urethrogram	Similar to a cystogram. Contrast media is injected retrograde into the urethra to identify strictures, diverticula, or other urethral pathologic conditions. When urethral trauma is suspected, a urethrogram is done before catheterization.	Explain procedure to patient.
Voiding cystourethrogram (VCUG)	Voiding study of the bladder opening (bladder neck) and urethra. The bladder is filled with contrast media. Fluoroscopic films are taken to visualize the bladder and urethra. After urination, another film is taken to assess for residual urine. Can detect abnormalities of the lower urinary tract, urethral stenosis, bladder neck obstruction, and prostatic enlargement.	Explain procedure to patient.
Loopogram	Detects obstructions, anastomotic leaks, stones, reflux, and other uropathologic features when patient has a urinary pouch or ileal conduit. Because urinary diversions are created with bowel, there is risk of absorption of contrast media.	Explain procedure to patient. Closely monitor patient for reactions to the contrast media.

*N-acetylcysteine (Mucomyst), a renal vasodilator and antioxidant, is sometimes administered to reduce the incidence of contrast-induced nephropathy; can be given by oral or IV route.

Continued

TABLE 45-8 DIAGNOSTIC STUDIES—cont'd

Urinary System

Study	Description and Purpose	Nursing Responsibility
Endoscopy		
Cystoscopy	Inspects interior of bladder with a tubular lighted scope (cystoscope) (Fig. 45-10). Can be used to insert ureteral catheters, remove calculi, obtain biopsy specimens of bladder lesions, and treat bleeding lesions. Lithotomy position is used. Procedure may be done using local or general anesthesia, depending on patient's needs and condition. Complications include urinary retention, urinary tract hemorrhage, bladder infection, and perforation of the bladder.	*Before procedure:* Force fluids or give IV fluids if general anesthesia is to be used. Ensure consent form is signed. Explain procedure to patient. Give preoperative medication. *After procedure:* Explain that burning on urination, pink-tinged urine, and urinary frequency are expected effects. Observe for bright red bleeding, which is not normal. Do not let patient walk alone immediately after procedure because orthostatic hypotension may occur. Offer warm sitz baths, heat, mild analgesics to relieve discomfort.
Urodynamic Studies		
Urine flow study (uroflow)	Measures urine volume in a single voiding expelled in a period of time. Used to (1) assess the degree of outflow obstruction caused by such conditions as BPH or stricture, (2) assess bladder or sphincter dysfunction effects on voiding, and (3) evaluate effects of treatment for lower urinary tract problems. Graphic displays can illustrate straining and intermittent flow patterns or other abnormal voiding disorders. *Normal maximum flow rate:* men: 20-25 mL/sec; women: 25-30 mL/sec. Volume voided and the patient's age can affect the flow rate.	Explain procedure to patient. Ask the patient to start the test with a comfortably full bladder, urinate into a special container, and try to empty completely. Measure residual urine volume immediately after a urinary flow study because this will help identify the degree of chronic urinary retention that is often associated with abnormal flow patterns.
Cystometrogram	Evaluates bladder's capacity to contract and expel urine. Involves insertion of catheter and instillation of water or saline solution into bladder. Measurements of pressure exerted against bladder wall are recorded. If abdominal pressure is measured, a second tube is inserted into the rectum or vagina. This tube is attached to a small fluid-filled balloon to allow pressure recording.	Explain procedure to patient. During the infusion, ask patient about sensations of bladder filling, usually including the first desire (urge) to urinate, a strong desire to urinate, and perception of bladder fullness. Observe patient for manifestations of urinary tract infection after procedure.
Sphincter electromyography (EMG)	Recording of electrical activity created when nervous system stimulates muscle tissue. By placing needles, percutaneous wires, or patches near the urethra, the clinician can assess the pelvic floor muscle activity. During the cystometrogram, sphincter EMG is used to identify voluntary pelvic floor muscle contractions and the response of these muscles to bladder filling, coughing, and other provocative maneuvers.	Explain procedure to patient.
Voiding pressure flow study	Combines a urinary flow rate, cystometric pressures (intravesical, abdominal, and detrusor pressures), and a sphincter EMG for detailed evaluation of micturition. It is completed by assisting the patient to a specialized toilet to urinate while the various pressure tubes and EMG apparatus remain in place.	Explain procedure to patient.
Videourodynamics	Combination of cystometrogram, sphincter EMG, and/or urinary flow study with anatomic imaging of the lower urinary tract, typically via fluoroscopy. Used in selected cases to identify an obstructive lesion and characterize anatomic changes in the bladder and lower urinary tract.	Explain procedure to patient.

A   B

FIG. 45-10 Cystoscopic examination of the bladder in a man. **A,** Flexible cystonephroscope. **B,** Scope inserted into bladder.

TABLE 45-8 DIAGNOSTIC STUDIES—cont'd

Urinary System

Study	Description and Purpose	Nursing Responsibility
Radionuclide cystography (RNC)	Detects and grades vesicoureteral reflux. Similar to VCUG with a small dose of radioisotope tracer instilled into the bladder via urethral catheter. More sensitive than VCUG, and radiation dose is 1/1000 that of the VCUG.	Explain procedure to patient as in VCUG.
Whitaker study	Measures the pressure differential between the renal pelvis and the bladder. Ureteral obstruction can be assessed. Percutaneous access is gained to the renal pelvis by placing a catheter in the renal pelvis. A catheter is also placed in the bladder. Fluid is perfused through the percutaneous tube or needle at a rate of 10 mL/min. Pressure data are then collected. Pressure measurements are combined with fluoroscopic imaging to identify the level of obstruction.	Explain procedure to patient.
Renal Scan	Evaluates anatomic structures, perfusion, and function of kidneys. Radioactive isotopes are injected IV. Radiation detector probes are placed over kidney, and scintillation counter monitors radioactive material in kidney. Radioisotope distribution in kidney is scanned and mapped. Shows location, size, and shape of kidney and, in general, assesses blood flow, glomerular filtration, tubular function, and urinary excretion. Abscesses, cysts, and tumors may appear as cold spots because of nonfunctioning tissue. Also monitors function of a transplanted kidney.	Requires no dietary or activity restriction. Inform patient that no pain or discomfort should be felt during test.
Renal Biopsy	Obtains renal tissue for examination to determine type of kidney disease or to follow progress of kidney disease. Technique is usually done as a skin (percutaneous) biopsy through needle insertion into lower lobe of kidney. Can be performed with CT or ultrasound guidance. Absolute contraindications are bleeding disorders, single kidney, and uncontrolled hypertension. Relative contraindications include suspected renal infection, hydronephrosis, and possible vascular lesions.	Type and crossmatch patient for blood. Ensure consent form is signed. *Before procedure:* Ascertain coagulation status through patient history, medication history, CBC, hematocrit, prothrombin time, and bleeding and clotting time. Patient should not be taking aspirin or warfarin (Coumadin). *After procedure:* Apply pressure dressing and keep patient on affected side for 30-60 min. Bed rest for 24 hr. Vital signs every 5-10 min, first hour. Assess for flank pain, hypotension, decreasing hematocrit, ↑ temperature, chills, urinary frequency, dysuria, and serial urine specimens (gross or microscopic hematuria). Urine dipstick can be used to test for bleeding in urine. Inspect biopsy site for bleeding. Instruct patient to avoid lifting heavy objects for 5-7 days and to not take anticoagulant drugs until allowed by health care provider.

extended time in the x-ray department, is too tired to eat, sleeps the rest of the day, and is NPO after midnight again because of studies scheduled for the next day. Severe dehydration, especially in a diabetic, debilitated, or older patient, may lead to acute kidney injury. When a patient is scheduled for diagnostic studies, ensure that the patient is properly hydrated and given adequate nourishment between studies. Also check with the health care provider regarding insulin dosage for diabetic patients who are placed on NPO status.

Urine Studies

Urinalysis. *Urinalysis* (see Tables 45-8 and 45-9) is one of the first studies done to evaluate disorders of the urinary tract. Results from the urinalysis may indicate possible abnormalities, suggest the need for further studies, or provide evidence of progression in a previously diagnosed disorder.

Although a specimen may be collected at any time of the day for a routine urinalysis, it is best to obtain the first specimen

urinated in the morning. This concentrated specimen is more likely to contain abnormal constituents if they are present in the urine. The specimen should be examined within 1 hour of urinating. Otherwise, bacteria multiply rapidly, RBCs hemolyze, *casts* (molds of renal tubules) disintegrate, and the urine becomes alkaline as a result of urea-splitting bacteria. If it is not possible to send the specimen to the laboratory immediately, refrigerate it. However, to obtain the best results, coordinate specimen collection with routine laboratory hours.

Creatinine Clearance. A common test used to analyze urinary system disorders is creatinine clearance. Creatinine is a waste product produced by muscle breakdown. Urinary excretion of creatinine is a measure of the amount of active muscle tissue in the body, not of body weight. Therefore individuals with larger muscle mass have higher values.[4] Because almost all creatinine in the blood is normally excreted by the kidneys, creatinine clearance is the most accurate indicator of renal function. The result of a creatinine clearance test closely approxi-

TABLE 45-9   **DIAGNOSTIC STUDIES**

Urinalysis

Test	Normal	Abnormal Finding	Possible Etiology and Significance
Color	Amber yellow	Dark, smoky color Yellow-brown to olive green Orange-red or orange-brown Cloudiness of freshly voided urine Colorless urine	Hematuria. Excessive bilirubin. phenazopyridine (Pyridium). Infection. Excessive fluid intake, kidney disease, or diabetes insipidus.
Odor	Aromatic	Ammonia-like odor Unpleasant odor	Urine allowed to stand. Urinary tract infection.
Protein	Random protein (dipstick): 0-trace 24-hr protein (quantitative): <150 mg/day	Persistent proteinuria	Characteristic of acute and chronic kidney disease, especially involving glomeruli. Heart failure. In absence of disease: high-protein diet, strenuous exercise, dehydration, fever, emotional stress, contamination by vaginal secretions.
Glucose	None	Glycosuria	Diabetes mellitus, low renal threshold for glucose reabsorption (if blood glucose level is normal). Pituitary disorders.
Ketones	None	Present	Altered carbohydrate and fat metabolism in diabetes mellitus and starvation; dehydration, vomiting, severe diarrhea.
Bilirubin	None	Present	Liver disorders. May appear before jaundice is visible (see Chapter 44).
Specific gravity	1.003-1.030 Maximum concentrating ability of kidney in morning urine (1.025-1.030)	Low High Fixed at about 1.010	Dilute urine, excessive diuresis, diabetes insipidus. Dehydration, albuminuria, glycosuria. Renal inability to concentrate urine; end-stage kidney disease.
Osmolality	300-1300 mOsm/kg (300-1300 mmol/kg)	<300 mOsm/kg >1300 mOsm/kg	Tubular dysfunction. Kidney lost ability to concentrate or dilute urine (not part of routine urinalysis).
pH	4.0-8.0 (average, 6.0)	>8.0 <4.0	Urinary tract infection. Urine allowed to stand at room temperature (bacteria decompose urea to ammonia). Respiratory or metabolic acidosis.
RBCs	0-4/hpf	>4/hpf	Calculi, cystitis, neoplasm, glomerulonephritis, tuberculosis, kidney biopsy, trauma.
WBCs	0-5/hpf	>5/hpf	Urinary tract infection or inflammation.
Casts	None Occasional hyaline	Present	Molds of the renal tubules that may contain protein, WBCs, RBCs, or bacteria. Noncellular casts (hyaline in appearance) occasionally found in normal urine.
Culture for organisms	No organisms in bladder <10^4 organisms/mL result of normal urethral flora	Bacteria counts >10^5/mL	Urinary tract infection; most common organisms are *Escherichia coli*, enterococci, *Klebsiella*, *Proteus*, and streptococci.

hpf, High-powered field.

mates that of the GFR. A blood specimen for serum creatinine determination should be obtained during the period of urine collection.

Creatinine levels remain remarkably constant for each person because they are not significantly affected by protein ingestion, muscular exercise, water intake, or rate of urine production. Normal creatinine clearance values range from 70 to 135 mL/min (see Table 45-8). After age 40, the creatinine clearance rate decreases at a rate of about 1 mL/min/yr.

Urodynamic Studies

Urodynamic studies measure urinary tract function. Urodynamic tests study the storage of urine within the bladder and the flow of urine through the urinary tract to the outside of the body.[5-7] A combination of techniques may be used for a detailed assessment of urinary function (see Table 45-8).

CASE STUDY—cont'd

Objective Data: Diagnostic Studies

iStockphoto/Thinkstock

The health care provider orders the following initial diagnostic studies for A.K.:
- CBC, basic metabolic panel (electrolytes, BUN, creatinine)
- Urinalysis, culture if indicated
- Renal ultrasound

Although A.K.'s laboratory results are all within normal limits, his renal ultrasound identifies calculi in the left ureter. There is no hydronephrosis at present. The health care provider prescribes parenteral opioids for pain management and admits A.K. to a medical unit for further observation.

BRIDGE TO NCLEX EXAMINATION

The number of the question corresponds to the same-numbered outcome at the beginning of the chapter.

1. A renal stone in the pelvis of the kidney will alter the function of the kidney by interfering with
   a. the structural support of the kidney.
   b. regulation of the concentration of urine.
   c. the entry and exit of blood vessels at the kidney.
   d. collection and drainage of urine from the kidney.

2. A patient with kidney disease has oliguria and a creatinine clearance of 40 mL/min. These findings most directly reflect abnormal function of
   a. tubular secretion.
   b. glomerular filtration.
   c. capillary permeability.
   d. concentration of filtrate.

3. The nurse identifies a risk for urinary calculi in a patient who relates a past health history that includes
   a. hyperaldosteronism.
   b. serotonin deficiency.
   c. adrenal insufficiency.
   d. hyperparathyroidism.

4. Diminished ability to concentrate urine, associated with aging of the urinary system, is attributed to
   a. a decrease in bladder sensory receptors.
   b. a decrease in the number of functioning nephrons.
   c. decreased function of the loop of Henle and tubules.
   d. thickening of the basement membrane of Bowman's capsule.

5. During physical assessment of the urinary system, the nurse
   a. palpates an empty bladder as a small nodule.
   b. auscultates over each CVA to detect impaired renal blood flow.
   c. finds a dull percussion sound when 100 mL of urine is present in the bladder.
   d. palpates above the symphysis pubis to determine the level of urine in the bladder.

6. Normal findings expected by the nurse on physical assessment of the urinary system include (select all that apply)
   a. nonpalpable left kidney.
   b. auscultation of renal artery bruit.
   c. CVA tenderness elicited by a kidney punch.
   d. no CVA tenderness elicited by a kidney punch.
   e. palpable bladder to the level of the pubic symphysis.

7. A diagnostic study that indicates renal blood flow, glomerular filtration, tubular function, and excretion is a(n)
   a. IVP.
   b. VCUG.
   c. renal scan.
   d. loopogram.

8. On reading the urinalysis results of a dehydrated patient, the nurse would expect to find
   a. a pH of 8.4.
   b. RBCs of 4/hpf.
   c. color: yellow, cloudy.
   d. specific gravity of 1.035.

1. d, 2. b, 3. d, 4. c, 5. b, 6. a, d, 7. c, 8. d

ⓔvolve

For rationales to these answers and even more NCLEX review questions, visit *http://evolve.elsevier.com/Lewis/medsurg.*

REFERENCES

1. Nguyen TV, Goldfarb DS: The older adult patient and kidney function, *Consult Pharm* 27(6):431, 2012.
2. van Doorn B, Bosch JL: Nocturia in older men, *Maturitas* 71(1):8, 2012.
3. Cornu JN, Abrams P, Chapple CR, et al: Contemporary assessment of nocturia: definition, epidemiology, pathophysiology, and management—a systematic review and meta-analysis, *Eur Urol* 62(5):877, 2012.
4. Lascano ME, Poggio ED: Kidney function assessment by creatinine-based estimation equations. Retrieved from *www.clevelandclinicmeded.com/medicalpubs/diseasemanagement/nephrology/kidney-function.*
5. Gray M: Traces: making sense of urodynamics testing, part 9: evaluation of sensations detrusor response to bladder filling, *Urol Nurs* 32(1):21, 2012.
6. Farag FF, Heesakkers JP: Non-invasive techniques in the diagnosis of bladder storage disorders, *Neurourol Urodyn* 30(8):1422, 2011.
7. Al Afraa T, Mahfouz W, Campeau L, et al: Normal lower urinary tract assessment in women, part I: uroflowmetry and post-void residual, pad tests, and bladder diaries, *Int Urogynecol J* 23(6):681, 2012.

RESOURCES

Resources for this chapter are listed in Chapter 46 on p. 1100 and Chapter 47 on p. 1131.

46

Tears shed for self are tears of weakness, but tears shed for others are a sign of strength.
Billy Graham

Nursing Management

Renal and Urologic Problems

Betty Jean Reid Czarapata

evolve WEBSITE

http://evolve.elsevier.com/Lewis/medsurg

- NCLEX Review Questions
- Key Points
- Pre-Test
- Answer Guidelines for Case Study on p. 1098
- Rationales for Bridge to NCLEX Examination Questions

- Case Studies
  - Patient With Bladder Cancer and Urinary Diversion
  - Patient With Glomerulonephritis and Kidney Disease
- Nursing Care Plans (Customizable)
  - eNCP 46-1: Patient With a Urinary Tract Infection
  - eNCP 46-2: Patient With Urinary Tract Calculi

- eNCP 46-3: Patient With an Ileal Conduit
- Concept Map Creator
- Glossary
- Content Updates

eTables
- eTable 46-1: Staging of Kidney Cancer
- eTable 46-2: Staging of Bladder Cancer

LEARNING OUTCOMES

1. Differentiate the pathophysiology, clinical manifestations, collaborative care, and drug therapy of cystitis, urethritis, and pyelonephritis.
2. Explain the nursing management of urinary tract infections.
3. Describe the immunologic mechanisms involved in glomerulonephritis.
4. Differentiate the clinical manifestations and nursing and collaborative management of acute poststreptococcal glomerulonephritis, Goodpasture syndrome, and chronic glomerulonephritis.
5. Describe the common causes, clinical manifestations, collaborative care, and nursing management of nephrotic syndrome.

6. Compare and contrast the etiology, clinical manifestations, collaborative care, and nursing management of various types of urinary calculi.
7. Differentiate the common causes and management of renal trauma, renal vascular problems, and hereditary kidney diseases.
8. Describe the clinical manifestations and nursing and collaborative management of kidney cancer and bladder cancer.
9. Describe the common causes and management of urinary incontinence and urinary retention.
10. Differentiate among urethral, ureteral, suprapubic, and nephrostomy catheters with regard to indications for use and nursing responsibilities.
11. Explain the nursing management of the patient undergoing nephrectomy or urinary diversion surgery.

KEY TERMS

calculus, p. 1077
cystitis, p. 1065
glomerulonephritis, p. 1073
Goodpasture syndrome, p. 1074
hydronephrosis, p. 1076

hydroureter, p. 1076
ileal conduit, p. 1095
interstitial cystitis (IC), p. 1071
lithotripsy, p. 1079
nephrolithiasis, p. 1076
nephrosclerosis, p. 1082

nephrotic syndrome, p. 1075
polycystic kidney disease (PKD), p. 1082
pyelonephritis, p. 1065
renal artery stenosis, p. 1082
stricture, p. 1081

urethritis, p. 1065
urinary incontinence (UI), p. 1086
urinary retention, p. 1090
urosepsis, p. 1065

Renal and urologic disorders encompass a wide spectrum of problems. The diverse causes of these disorders may involve infectious, immunologic, obstructive, metabolic, collagen-vascular, traumatic, congenital, neoplastic, and neurologic mechanisms. This chapter discusses specific disorders of the upper urinary tract (kidneys and ureter) and lower urinary tract (bladder and urethra). Acute kidney injury and chronic kidney disease are discussed in Chapter 47.

INFECTIOUS AND INFLAMMATORY DISORDERS OF URINARY SYSTEM

URINARY TRACT INFECTION

Urinary tract infections (UTIs) are the most common bacterial infection in women. During their lifetime, at least 20% of women develop at least one UTI.[1] More than 100,000 people

Reviewed by Barbara S. Broome, RN, PhD, FAAN, Associate Dean and Chair, Community/Mental Health, University of South Alabama, College of Nursing, Mobile, Alabama; Marci Langenkamp, RN, MS, Assistant Professor of Nursing, Edison Community College, Piqua, Ohio; and Phyllis A. Matthews, RN, MS, ANCP-BC, CUNP, Urology Nurse Practitioner, Denver VA Medical Center, Denver, Colorado.

TABLE 46-1   CAUSES OF URINARY TRACT INFECTIONS

- *Escherichia coli**
- *Enterococcus*
- *Klebsiella*
- *Enterobacter*
- *Proteus*
- *Pseudomonas*
- *Staphylococcus*
- *Serratia*
- *Candida albicans*†

*Causative microorganism for urinary tract infection (UTI) in 80% of cases without urinary tract structural abnormalities or calculi.
†Typically identified as the causative microorganism for UTI associated with the use of broad-spectrum antibiotic therapy or in patients with an indwelling catheter.

🌐 CULTURAL & ETHNIC HEALTH DISPARITIES
Urologic Disorders

- Urinary tract calculi are more common among whites than African Americans.
- Uric acid stones are more common in Jewish men.
- Bladder cancer has a higher incidence among white men than African American men.
- In all ethnic groups, bladder cancer affects men about three times more often than women.
- Urinary incontinence is underreported because culturally it is seen as a social hygiene problem causing patient embarrassment.

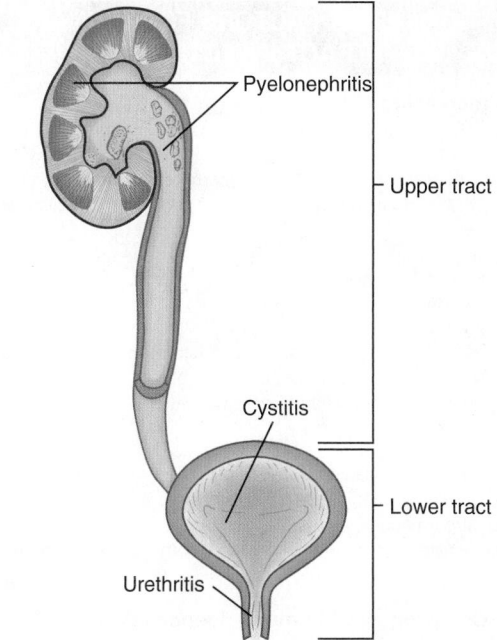

FIG. 46-1 Sites of infectious processes in the upper and lower urinary tracts.

are hospitalized annually for UTIs. More than 15% of patients who develop gram-negative bacteremia die, and one third of these cases are caused by bacterial infections originating in the urinary tract.[2]

Inflammation of the urinary tract may be caused by a variety of disorders, but bacterial infection is by far the most common. The bladder and its contents are free from bacteria in the majority of healthy persons. Nevertheless, a minority of otherwise healthy individuals have some bacteria colonizing the bladder. This condition is called *asymptomatic bacteriuria* and does not justify screening or treatment except in pregnant women.

Escherichia coli is the most common pathogen causing a UTI (Table 46-1) and is primarily seen in women. Bacterial counts of 10^5 colony-forming units per milliliter (CFU/mL) or higher typically indicate a clinically significant UTI. However, counts as low as 10^2 to 10^3 CFU/mL in a person with signs and symptoms are indicative of UTI.

Although fungal and parasitic infections may also cause UTIs, this is uncommon. UTIs from these causes are sometimes found in patients who are immunosuppressed, have diabetes mellitus, or have undergone multiple courses of antibiotic therapy. These types of UTIs may also be found in persons who live in or have traveled to certain developing countries.

Classification of Urinary Tract Infection

A UTI can be broadly classified as an upper or lower UTI according to its location within the urinary system (Fig. 46-1). Infection of the upper urinary tract (involving the renal parenchyma, pelvis, and ureters) typically causes fever, chills, and flank pain, whereas a UTI confined to the lower urinary tract does not usually have systemic manifestations. Specific terms are used to further delineate the location of a UTI. For example, **pyelonephritis** implies inflammation (usually caused by infection) of the renal parenchyma and collecting system, **cystitis** indicates inflammation of the bladder, and **urethritis** means inflammation of the urethra. **Urosepsis** is a UTI that has spread

systemically and is a life-threatening condition requiring emergency treatment.

Classifying a UTI as complicated or uncomplicated is also useful. *Uncomplicated* UTIs occur in an otherwise normal urinary tract and usually involve only the bladder. *Complicated* UTIs include those infections with coexisting obstruction, stones, or catheters; diabetes or neurologic diseases; or pregnancy-induced changes. The term also applies to a recurrent infection. The individual with a complicated infection is at risk for pyelonephritis, urosepsis, and renal damage.

Etiology and Pathophysiology

The urinary tract above the urethra is normally sterile. Several mechanical and physiologic defense mechanisms assist in maintaining sterility and preventing UTIs. These defenses include normal voiding with complete emptying of the bladder, ureterovesical junction competence, and ureteral peristaltic activity that propels urine toward the bladder. Antibacterial characteristics of urine are maintained by an acidic pH (less than 6.0), high urea concentration, and abundant glycoproteins that interfere with the growth of bacteria. An alteration in any of these defense mechanisms increases the risk for a UTI (Table 46-2).

The organisms that usually cause UTIs are introduced via the ascending route from the urethra and originate in the perineum. Most infections are caused by gram-negative bacilli normally found in the gastrointestinal (GI) tract, although gram-positive organisms such as streptococci, enterococci, and *Staphylococcus saprophyticus* can also cause UTIs.

A common factor contributing to ascending infection is urologic instrumentation (e.g., catheterization, cystoscopic examinations).[3] Instrumentation allows bacteria that are normally present at the opening of the urethra to enter into the urethra or bladder. Sexual intercourse promotes "milking" of bacteria from the vagina and perineum and may cause minor urethral trauma that predisposes women to UTIs.

Rarely do UTIs result from a hematogenous route, where blood-borne bacteria secondarily invade the kidneys, ureters,

TABLE 46-2	**RISK FACTORS FOR URINARY TRACT INFECTIONS**

Factors Increasing Urinary Stasis
- Intrinsic obstruction (stone, tumor of urinary tract, urethral stricture, BPH)
- Extrinsic obstruction (tumor, fibrosis compressing urinary tract)
- Urinary retention (including neurogenic bladder and low bladder wall compliance)
- Renal impairment

Foreign Bodies
- Urinary tract calculi
- Catheters (indwelling, external condom catheter, ureteral stent, nephrostomy tube, intermittent catheterization)
- Urinary tract instrumentation (cystoscopy, urodynamics)

Anatomic Factors
- Congenital defects leading to obstruction or urinary stasis
- Fistula (abnormal opening) exposing urinary stream to skin, vagina, or fecal stream
- Shorter female urethra and colonization from normal vaginal flora
- Obesity

Factors Compromising Immune Response
- Aging .
- Human immunodeficiency virus infection
- Diabetes mellitus

Functional Disorders
- Constipation
- Voiding dysfunction with detrusor sphincter dyssynergia

Other Factors
- Pregnancy
- Hypoestrogenic state (menopause)
- Multiple sex partners (women)
- Use of spermicidal agents or contraceptive diaphragm (women)
- Poor personal hygiene
- Habitual delay of urination ("nurse's bladder," "teacher's bladder")

TABLE 46-3	**LOWER URINARY TRACT SYMPTOMS (LUTS)**

Symptoms	Description
Emptying Symptoms	
Hesitancy	• Difficulty starting urine stream • Delay between initiation of urination (because of urethral sphincter relaxation) and beginning of flow of urine • Diminished urinary stream
Intermittency	• Interruption of urinary stream while voiding
Postvoid dribbling	• Urine loss after completion of voiding
Urinary retention or incomplete emptying	• Inability to empty urine from bladder • Caused by atonic bladder or obstruction of urethra • Can be acute or chronic
Dysuria	• Painful or difficult urination
Storage Symptoms	
Urinary frequency	• >8 times in 24-hr period • Often <200 mL each voiding
Urgency	• Sudden, strong, or intense desire to void immediately • Commonly accompanied by frequency
Incontinence	• Involuntary or accidental urine loss or leakage
Nocturia	• Awakened by urge to void 2 or more times during sleep • May be diurnal or nocturnal depending on sleep schedule
Nocturnal enuresis	• Adults: loss of urine during sleep

or bladder from elsewhere in the body. There must be prior injury to the urinary tract, such as obstruction of the ureter, damage caused by stones, or renal scars, for a kidney infection to occur from hematogenous transmission.

An important source of UTIs is health care–associated infections (HAIs), previously called *nosocomial* infections, which account for 31% of all HAIs.[2,4] The cause of HAIs is often *E. coli* and, less frequently, *Pseudomonas* organisms. Catheter-acquired urinary tract infections (CAUTIs) are the most common HAIs and are caused by development of bacterial biofilms that are found on the catheter's inner surface. Most often these infections are underrecognized and undertreated, leading to complications such as renal abscesses, epididymitis, periurethral gland infections, and bacteremia.

Clinical Manifestations

Lower urinary tract symptoms (LUTS) are experienced in patients who have UTIs of the upper urinary tract, as well as those confined to the lower tract. Symptoms are related to either bladder storage or bladder emptying. These symptoms are presented in Table 46-3.

These symptoms include dysuria, frequent urination (more than every 2 hours), urgency, and suprapubic discomfort or pressure. The urine may contain grossly visible blood (hematuria) or sediment, giving it a cloudy appearance. Flank pain, chills, and fever indicate an infection involving the upper urinary tract (pyelonephritis). People with significant bacteriuria may have no symptoms or may have nonspecific symptoms such as fatigue or anorexia.

Remember that these symptoms, considered characteristic of a UTI, are often absent in older adults. Older adults tend to experience nonlocalized abdominal discomfort rather than dysuria and suprapubic pain. In addition, they may have cognitive impairment or generalized clinical deterioration. Because older adults are less likely to experience a fever with a UTI, the value of body temperature as an indicator of a UTI is unreliable.

Multiple factors may produce LUTS similar to the symptoms of a UTI. For example, patients with bladder tumors or those receiving intravesical chemotherapy or pelvic radiation usually experience urinary frequency, urgency, and dysuria. Interstitial cystitis/painful bladder syndrome (discussed on p. 1071) also produces urinary symptoms that are similar to and sometimes confused with a UTI.

Diagnostic Studies

In a patient suspected of having a UTI, initially obtain a dipstick urinalysis to identify the presence of nitrites (indicating bacteriuria), white blood cells (WBCs), and leukocyte esterase (an enzyme present in WBCs indicating pyuria). These findings can be confirmed by microscopic urinalysis. After confirmation of bacteriuria and pyuria, a urine culture may be obtained. A urine culture is indicated in complicated or HAI UTIs, persistent bacteriuria, or frequently recurring UTIs (more than two or three episodes per year). Urine may also be cultured when the infection is unresponsive to empiric therapy or the diagnosis is questionable.[5]

A voided midstream technique (*clean-catch urine sample*) is preferred for obtaining a urine culture in most circumstances. For women, teach them to spread the labia and wipe the periurethral area from front to back using a moistened, clean gauze sponge (no antiseptic is used because it could contaminate the specimen and cause false positives). Then tell them to keep the labia spread, start voiding, and collect the specimen 1 to 2 seconds after voiding starts. For men, instruct them to wipe the glans penis around the urethra and collect the specimen 1 to 2 seconds after voiding begins.

Refrigerate urine immediately on collection. The urine should be cultured within 24 hours of refrigeration. A specimen obtained by catheterization provides more accurate results than a clean-catch specimen. When an adequate clean-catch specimen cannot be readily obtained, a catheterization may be necessary.

A urine culture is accompanied by *sensitivity testing* to determine the bacteria's susceptibility to a variety of antibiotic drugs. The results of this test allow the health care provider to select an antibiotic known to be capable of destroying the bacteria causing a UTI in a specific patient.

Imaging studies of the urinary tract are indicated in selected cases. A computed tomography (CT) urogram or ultrasound may be obtained when obstruction of the urinary system is suspected or UTIs recur.

Collaborative Care

Once a UTI has been diagnosed, appropriate antimicrobial therapy is initiated. An antibiotic may be selected based on the health care provider's best judgment (*empiric therapy*) or the results of sensitivity testing.[6] The collaborative care and drug therapy of UTIs are summarized in Table 46-4. Uncomplicated cystitis can be treated by a short-term course of antibiotics, typically for 1 to 3 days. In contrast, complicated UTIs require longer-term treatment, lasting 7 to 14 days or longer.[7,8]

Many residents of long-term care facilities, especially women, have chronic asymptomatic bacteriuria. However, usually only symptomatic UTIs are treated.

First-choice drugs to empirically treat uncomplicated or initial UTIs are trimethoprim/sulfamethoxazole (TMP/SMX) (Bactrim, Septra), nitrofurantoin (Macrodantin), and fosfomycin (Monurol). TMP/SMX has the advantages of being relatively inexpensive and being taken twice daily. A disadvantage is *E. coli* resistance to TMP/SMX, which is an increasing problem in the United States. Nitrofurantoin is normally given three or four times daily, but a long-acting preparation (Macrobid) is available that is taken twice daily.

Other antibiotics that may be used to treat uncomplicated UTI include ampicillin, amoxicillin, and cephalosporins. The fluoroquinolones are used to treat complicated UTIs. These drugs include ciprofloxacin (Cipro), levofloxacin (Levaquin), norfloxacin (Noroxin), ofloxacin (Floxin), and gatifloxacin (Tequin). In patients with UTIs secondary to fungi, amphotericin or fluconazole (Diflucan) is the preferred therapy.

> **DRUG ALERT: Nitrofurantoin (Furadantin, Macrodantin)**
> - Avoid sunlight. Use sunscreen, and wear protective clothing.
> - Notify health care provider immediately if fever, chills, cough, chest pain, dyspnea, rash, or numbness or tingling of fingers or toes develops.

A urinary analgesic such as oral phenazopyridine (Azo-Standard, Pyridium) may relieve discomfort caused by severe

TABLE 46-4 COLLABORATIVE CARE
Urinary Tract Infection

Diagnostic
- History and physical examination
- Urinalysis (obtain midstream, "clean-catch" voided specimen)
- Urine for culture and sensitivity (if indicated)
- Imaging studies of urinary tract (if indicated)
  - CT urogram
  - Intravenous pyelogram (IVP)
  - CT/IVP
  - Cystoscopy
  - Ultrasound

Collaborative Therapy
Uncomplicated UTI
- Antibiotics
  - trimethoprim/sulfamethoxazole (Bactrim, Septra)
  - trimethoprim alone in patients with sulfa allergy
  - nitrofurantoin (Macrodantin, Macrobid)
  - fosfomycin (Monurol)
- Patient teaching
- Adequate fluid intake (six 8-oz glasses/day)

Recurrent, Uncomplicated UTI
- Repeat urinalysis
- Urine culture and sensitivity testing
- Imaging study of urinary tract (if indicated)
- Antibiotic: trimethoprim/sulfamethoxazole, nitrofurantoin
- Sensitivity-guided antibiotic therapy: ampicillin, amoxicillin, first-generation cephalosporin, fluoroquinolones
- Consider 3- to 6-mo trial of suppressive or prophylactic antibiotic regimen
- Consider postcoital antibiotic prophylaxis: trimethoprim/sulfamethoxazole, nitrofurantoin, cephalexin
- Adequate fluid intake (six 8-oz glasses/day)
- Repeat patient teaching

dysuria. Phenazopyridine is an azo dye excreted in urine, where it exerts a topical analgesic effect on the urinary tract mucosa.

Prophylactic or *suppressive antibiotics* are sometimes given to patients who have repeated UTIs. A low dose of TMP/SMX, nitrofurantoin, or another antibiotic may be taken daily to prevent recurring UTIs, or a single dose may be taken before an event likely to provoke a UTI, such as sexual intercourse. Although suppressive therapy is often effective on a short-term basis, this strategy is limited because of the risk of antibiotic resistance, which ultimately leads to breakthrough infections with increasingly virulent pathogens.

NURSING MANAGEMENT
URINARY TRACT INFECTION

NURSING ASSESSMENT

Subjective and objective data that should be obtained from a patient with a UTI are presented in Table 46-5.

NURSING DIAGNOSES

Nursing diagnoses for the patient with a UTI may include, but are not limited to, the following:
- Impaired urinary elimination *related to* the effects of UTI
- Readiness for enhanced self-health management

Additional information on nursing diagnoses for the patient with a UTI is presented in eNursing Care Plan 46-1 (on the website for this chapter).

TABLE 46-5   NURSING ASSESSMENT
Urinary Tract Infection

Subjective Data
Important Health Information
Past health history: Previous urinary tract infections; urinary calculi, stasis, reflux, strictures, or retention; neurogenic bladder; pregnancy; benign prostatic hyperplasia; sexually transmitted infection; bladder cancer
Medications: Antibiotics, anticholinergics, antispasmodics
Surgery or other treatments: Recent urologic instrumentation (catheterization, cystoscopy, surgery)

Functional Health Patterns
Health perception–health management: Urinary hygiene practices; lassitude, malaise
Nutritional-metabolic: Nausea, vomiting, anorexia; chills
Elimination: Urinary frequency, urgency, hesitancy; dysuria, nocturia
Cognitive-perceptual: Suprapubic or low back pain, costovertebral tenderness; bladder spasms, dysuria, burning on urination
Sexuality-reproductive: Multiple sex partners (women), use of spermicidal agents or contraceptive diaphragm (women)

Objective Data
General
Fever, chills, dysuria
Atypical presentation in older adults: afebrile, absence of dysuria, loss of appetite, altered mental status

Urinary
Hematuria; cloudy, foul-smelling urine; tender, enlarged kidney

Possible Diagnostic Findings
Leukocytosis; UA positive for bacteria, pyuria, RBCs, WBCs, and nitrites; positive urine culture; IVP, CT scan, US, VCUG, and cystoscopy indicating urinary tract abnormalities

IVP, Intravenous pyelogram; *VCUG,* voiding cystourethrogram.

PLANNING

The overall goals are that the patient with a UTI will have (1) relief from bothersome LUTS, (2) prevention of upper urinary tract involvement, and (3) prevention of recurrence.

NURSING IMPLEMENTATION

HEALTH PROMOTION. It is important to recognize individuals who are at risk for a UTI. These people include debilitated persons, older adults, patients who are immunocompromised (e.g., cancer, human immunodeficiency virus [HIV], diabetes mellitus), and patients treated with immunosuppressive drugs or corticosteroids. Health promotion activities, particularly for these individuals, can help decrease the frequency of infections and provide for early detection of infection. Health promotion activities include teaching preventive measures such as (1) emptying the bladder regularly and completely, (2) evacuating the bowel regularly, (3) wiping the perineal area from front to back after urination and defecation, and (4) drinking an adequate amount of liquid each day.

To estimate the amount of fluid intake a person should have in 24 hours, take the person's weight in pounds and divide that number in half. The result is the number of ounces of fluid a person should have per day. Thus a 150-pound person would require 75 oz/day. The person will obtain about 20% of this fluid from food, which leaves 60 oz (1775 mL) obtained by drinking, or just over seven 8-oz glasses of fluid.

Daily intake of cranberry juice or cranberry tablets or capsules may reduce the number of UTIs (see Evidence-Based

EVIDENCE-BASED PRACTICE
Translating Research Into Practice

Do Cranberry Products Prevent Urinary Tract Infections?
Clinical Question
Among adults and children (P), what is the effect of cranberry-containing products (I) vs. placebo vs. nonplacebo control (C) in preventing urinary tract infections (O)?

Best Available Evidence
Systematic review of randomized controlled trials (RCTs)

Critical Appraisal and Synthesis of Evidence
- Thirteen RCTs (*n* = 1616) of patients at high risk for recurrent urinary tract infections (UTIs), including women, older adults, patients with neuropathic bladder, and pregnant women. Children were also studied.
- Cranberry products were juice, capsules, or tablets given for 6 mo in most cases.
- Cranberry-containing products had a positive effect in preventing symptomatic UTIs.
- These products showed greater effect in women (especially those with recurrent UTIs), children, cranberry juice drinkers, and those taking the products more than twice daily.

Conclusion
- Cranberry-containing products can prevent UTIs.
- Cranberry juice was more effective than cranberry capsules. This may be due to increased hydration from the juice.

Implications for Nursing Practice
- Inform patients who are at an increased risk for recurrent UTIs that cranberry products have a protective effect in reducing UTIs.
- Cranberry juice works by preventing the attachment of bacteria to the epithelial cells in the bladder wall.
- Emphasize the importance of adequate fluid intake, including drinking cranberry juice.

Reference for Evidence
Wang C, Fang C, Chen N, et al: Cranberry-containing products for prevention of urinary tract infections in susceptible populations: a systematic review and meta-analysis of randomized controlled trials, *Arch Intern Med* 172:988, 2012.

P, Patient population of interest; *I,* intervention or area of interest; *C,* comparison of interest or comparison group; *O,* outcomes of interest (see p. 12).

Practice box). It is thought that enzymes found in cranberries inhibit attachment of urinary pathogens (especially *E. coli*) to the bladder wall.[9]

All patients undergoing instrumentation of the urinary tract are at risk for developing an HAI UTI. You have a major role in the prevention of these infections.[10-12] Avoidance of unnecessary catheterization and early removal of indwelling catheters are the most effective means for reducing HAI UTIs. Always follow aseptic technique during these procedures. Wash your hands before and after contact with each patient.[13] Wear gloves for care involving the urinary system. When a catheter has been inserted, use special measures, as explained in the section on urethral catheterization later in this chapter on p. 1092.

Routine and thorough perineal hygiene is important for all hospitalized patients, especially when a bedpan is used, after a bowel movement, or if fecal incontinence is present. Answer call lights quickly and offer the bedpan or urinal to bedridden patients at frequent intervals. These measures can prevent incontinence and decrease the number of incontinent episodes.

ACUTE INTERVENTION. Acute intervention for a patient with a UTI includes ensuring adequate fluid intake if it is not contraindicated. Maintaining adequate fluid intake may be difficult because of the patient's perception that fluid intake will worsen the discomfort and urinary frequency associated with a UTI. Tell patients that fluids will increase frequency of urination at first but will also dilute the urine, making the bladder less irritable. Fluids will help flush out bacteria before they have a chance to colonize in the bladder. Caffeine, alcohol, citrus juices, chocolate, and highly spiced foods or beverages should be avoided because they are potential bladder irritants.

Application of local heat to the suprapubic area or lower back may relieve the discomfort associated with a UTI. Advise the patient to apply a heating pad (turned to its lowest setting) against the back or suprapubic area. A warm shower or sitting in a tub of warm water filled above the waist can also provide temporary relief.

Instruct the patient about the prescribed drug therapy, including side effects. Emphasize the importance of taking the full course of antibiotics. Often patients stop antibiotic therapy once symptoms disappear. This can lead to inadequate treatment and recurrence of infection or bacterial resistance to antibiotics.

Sometimes a second drug or a reduced dosage of drug is ordered after the initial course to suppress bacterial growth in patients susceptible to recurrent UTI. Instruct the patient to monitor for signs of improvement (e.g., cloudy urine becomes clear) and a decrease in or cessation of symptoms. Teach patients to promptly report any of the following to their health care provider: (1) persistence of bothersome LUTS beyond the antibiotic treatment course, (2) onset of flank pain, or (3) fever.

AMBULATORY AND HOME CARE. Home care for the patient with a UTI should emphasize the importance of adhering to the drug regimen. Your responsibility is to teach the patient and caregiver about the need for ongoing care (Table 46-6). This includes taking antimicrobial drugs as ordered, maintaining adequate daily fluid intake, voiding regularly (approximately every 3 to 4 hours), urinating before and after intercourse, and temporarily discontinuing the use of a diaphragm.

TABLE 46-6 PATIENT & CAREGIVER TEACHING GUIDE

Urinary Tract Infection

When teaching a patient and caregiver measures to prevent a recurrence of a urinary tract infection (UTI), include the following.

1. Take all antibiotics as prescribed. Symptoms may improve after 1-2 days of therapy, but organisms may still be present.
2. Practice appropriate hygiene, including the following:
   - Carefully clean the perineal region by separating the labia when cleansing.
   - Wipe from front to back after urinating.
   - Cleanse with warm soapy water after each bowel movement.
3. Empty the bladder before and after sexual intercourse.
4. Urinate regularly, approximately every 3-4 hr during the day.
5. Maintain adequate fluid intake.
6. Avoid vaginal douches and harsh soaps, bubble baths, powders, and sprays in the perineal area.
7. Report to the health care provider symptoms or signs of recurrent UTI (e.g., fever, cloudy urine, pain on urination, urgency, frequency).
8. Consider drinking unsweetened cranberry juice (8 oz three times a day) or taking cranberry extract tablets 300-400 mg/day for UTI prevention.

If treatment is complete and the symptoms are still present, instruct the patient to get follow-up care. Recurrent symptoms because of bacterial persistence or inadequate treatment typically occur within 1 to 2 weeks after completion of therapy. If the patient has followed the treatment regimen, a relapse indicates the need for further evaluation.[14]

EVALUATION

The expected outcomes are that the patient with a UTI will
- Experience normal urinary elimination patterns
- Report relief of bothersome urinary tract symptoms
- Verbalize knowledge of treatment regimen

Additional information on the expected outcomes for the patient with a UTI is presented in eNursing Care Plan 46-1 (on the website for this chapter).

ACUTE PYELONEPHRITIS

Etiology and Pathophysiology

Pyelonephritis is an inflammation of the renal parenchyma (Fig. 46-2) and collecting system (including the renal pelvis). The most common cause is bacterial infection, but fungi, protozoa, or viruses can also infect the kidney.

Urosepsis is a systemic infection arising from a urologic source. Its prompt diagnosis and effective treatment are critical because it can lead to septic shock and death in 15% of cases unless promptly eradicated. Septic shock is the outcome of unresolved bacteremia involving a gram-negative organism. (Septic shock is discussed in Chapter 67.)

Pyelonephritis usually begins with colonization and infection of the lower urinary tract via the ascending urethral route. Bacteria normally found in the intestinal tract, such as *E. coli* or *Proteus, Klebsiella,* or *Enterobacter* species, frequently cause pyelonephritis. A preexisting factor is often present such as *vesicoureteral reflux* (retrograde, or backward, movement of urine from lower to upper urinary tract) or dysfunction of the lower urinary tract (e.g., obstruction from benign prostatic hyperplasia [BPH], a stricture, a urinary stone). For residents of long-term care facilities, urinary tract catheterization is a common cause of pyelonephritis and urosepsis.

FIG. 46-2 Acute pyelonephritis. Cortical surface shows grayish white areas of inflammation and abscess formation *(arrows).*

Acute pyelonephritis commonly starts in the renal medulla and spreads to the adjacent cortex. One of the most important risk factors for acute pyelonephritis is pregnancy-induced physiologic changes in the urinary system. Recurring episodes of pyelonephritis, especially in the presence of obstructive abnormalities, can lead to *chronic pyelonephritis* (discussed below).

Clinical Manifestations and Diagnostic Studies

The clinical manifestations of acute pyelonephritis vary from mild fatigue to the sudden onset of chills; fever; vomiting; malaise; flank pain; and the LUTS characteristic of cystitis, including dysuria, urgency, and frequency. *Costovertebral tenderness* to percussion (costovertebral angle [CVA] pain) is typically present on the affected side. Although the clinical manifestations may subside within a few days, even without specific therapy, bacteriuria and pyuria usually persist.

Urinalysis results indicate pyuria, bacteriuria, and varying degrees of hematuria. WBC casts may be found in the urine, indicating involvement of the renal parenchyma. A complete blood count shows leukocytosis and a shift to the left with an increase in bands (immature neutrophils). Urine cultures must be obtained when pyelonephritis is suspected. In patients with more severe illness who are hospitalized, blood cultures are usually obtained as well.

Ultrasonography of the urinary system may be performed to identify anatomic abnormalities, hydronephrosis, renal abscesses, or an obstructing stone. CT urograms are also used to assess for signs of infection in the kidney and complications of pyelonephritis, such as impaired renal function, scarring, chronic pyelonephritis, or abscesses.

Collaborative Care

The diagnostic tests and collaborative therapy of acute pyelonephritis are summarized in Table 46-7. Patients with severe infections or complicating factors such as nausea and vomiting with dehydration require hospitalization.

The patient with mild symptoms may be treated as an outpatient with antibiotics for 14 to 21 days (see Table 46-7). Parenteral antibiotics are often given initially in the hospital to rapidly establish high serum and urinary drug levels. When initial treatment resolves acute symptoms and the patient is able to tolerate oral fluids and drugs, the person may be discharged on a regimen of oral antibiotics for an additional 14 to 21 days. Symptoms and signs typically improve or resolve within 48 to 72 hours after starting therapy.

Relapses may be treated with a 6-week course of antibiotics. Antibiotic prophylaxis may also be used for recurrent infections. The effectiveness of therapy is evaluated based on the presence or absence of bacterial growth on urine culture.

Urosepsis is characterized by bacteriuria and bacteremia (bacteria in blood). Close observation and vital sign monitoring are essential. Prompt recognition and treatment of septic shock may prevent irreversible damage or death.

NURSING MANAGEMENT
ACUTE PYELONEPHRITIS

NURSING ASSESSMENT

Subjective and objective data that should be obtained from a patient with pyelonephritis are similar to those for the patient with a UTI (see Table 46-5).

TABLE 46-7   COLLABORATIVE CARE

Acute Pyelonephritis

Diagnostic
- History and physical examination
- Urinalysis
- Urine for culture and sensitivity
- Imaging studies: ultrasound (initially), CT scan, IVP, CT/IVP, VCUG, radionuclide imaging
- CBC count with WBC differential
- Blood culture (if bacteremia is suspected)
- Percussion for flank (costovertebral angle [CVA]) pain

Collaborative Therapy
Mild Symptoms (Uncomplicated Infection)
- Outpatient management or short hospitalization
  - Empirically selected broad-spectrum antibiotics: ampicillin, vancomycin combined with an aminoglycoside (e.g., tobramycin [Nebcin], gentamicin [Garamycin])
  - Switch to sensitivity-guided therapy: trimethoprim/sulfamethoxazole (Bactrim, Septra) when results of urine and blood culture are available
- Fluoroquinolones: ciprofloxacin (Cipro), ofloxacin (Floxin), norfloxacin (Noroxin), gatifloxacin (Tequin)
- Adequate fluid intake
- Nonsteroidal antiinflammatory drugs (NSAIDs) or antipyretic drugs
- Follow-up urine culture and imaging studies

Severe Symptoms
- Hospitalization
- Parenteral antibiotics
  - Empirically selected broad-spectrum antibiotics: ampicillin, vancomycin combined with an aminoglycoside (e.g., tobramycin, gentamicin)
  - Switch to sensitivity-guided antibiotic therapy when results of urine and blood culture are available
- Oral antibiotics when patient tolerates oral intake
- Adequate fluid intake (parenteral initially; switch to oral fluids as nausea, vomiting, and dehydration subside)
- NSAIDs or antipyretic drugs to reverse fever and relieve discomfort
- Urinary analgesics (as above)
- Follow-up urine culture and imaging studies

IVP, Intravenous pyelogram; *VCUG,* voiding cystourethrogram.

NURSING DIAGNOSES

Nursing diagnoses for the patient with pyelonephritis include, but are not limited to, those for the patient with a UTI (see p. 1067).

PLANNING

The overall goals are that the patient with pyelonephritis will have (1) normal renal function, (2) normal body temperature, (3) no complications, (4) relief of pain, and (5) no recurrence of symptoms.

NURSING IMPLEMENTATION

Health promotion and maintenance measures are similar to those for cystitis (see p. 1072). Early treatment for cystitis can prevent ascending infections. Because patients with structural abnormalities of the urinary tract are at high risk for infection, stress the need for regular medical care.

Nursing interventions vary depending on the severity of symptoms. These interventions include teaching the patient about the disease process with emphasis on (1) continuing medications as prescribed, (2) having a follow-up urine culture, and (3) recognizing manifestations of recurrence or relapse (see

Table 46-6). In addition to antibiotic therapy, encourage the patient to drink at least eight glasses of fluid every day, even after the infection has been treated. Rest will increase patient comfort. The patient who has frequent relapses or reinfections may be treated with long-term, low-dose antibiotics. Making certain the patient understands the rationale for therapy is important to increase adherence.

EVALUATION

The expected outcomes for the patient with pyelonephritis are the same as for UTI (see p. 1069).

CHRONIC PYELONEPHRITIS

In *chronic pyelonephritis* the kidneys become small, atrophic, and shrunken and lose function due to fibrosis (scarring). Chronic pyelonephritis is usually the result of recurring infections involving the upper urinary tract. However, it may also occur in the absence of an existing infection, recent infection, or history of UTIs.

Radiologic imaging and a biopsy, rather than clinical features, are used to confirm the diagnosis of chronic pyelonephritis. Imaging studies reveal a small, fibrotic kidney. The collecting system may be small or hydronephrotic. Biopsy results indicate the loss of functioning nephrons, infiltration of the parenchyma with inflammatory cells, and fibrosis.

The level of renal function in chronic pyelonephritis depends on whether one or both kidneys are affected, the extent of scarring, and the presence of coexisting infection. Chronic pyelonephritis often progresses to end-stage kidney (renal) disease (ESKD) even if the underlying infection is successfully treated. Nursing and collaborative management of the patient with chronic kidney disease is discussed in Chapter 47.

URETHRITIS

Urethritis is an inflammation of the urethra. Causes of urethritis include a bacterial or viral infection, *Trichomonas* and monilial infection (especially in women), chlamydial infection, and gonorrhea (especially in men).

In men the causes of urethritis are usually sexually transmitted. Purulent discharge usually indicates a gonococcal urethritis, whereas a clear discharge typically signifies a nongonococcal urethritis. (Sexually transmitted infections are discussed in Chapter 53.) Urethritis also produces bothersome LUTS, including dysuria, urgency, and frequent urination, similar to those seen with cystitis.

In women, urethritis is difficult to diagnose. It frequently produces bothersome LUTS, but urethral discharge may not be present.

Treatment of urethritis is based on identifying and treating the cause and providing symptomatic relief. Drugs used for bacterial infections include TMP/SMX and nitrofurantoin. Metronidazole (Flagyl) and clotrimazole (Mycelex) may be used for treating *Trichomonas* infection. Drugs such as nystatin (Mycostatin) or fluconazole may be prescribed for monilial infections. In chlamydial infections, doxycycline (Vibramycin) may be used. Women with negative urine cultures and no pyuria usually do not respond to antibiotics.

Warm sitz baths may temporarily relieve bothersome symptoms. Instruct the patient to avoid using vaginal deodorant sprays, properly cleanse the perineal area after bowel move-

ments and urination, and avoid sexual intercourse until symptoms subside. Teach patients with sexually transmitted urethritis to refer their sex partners for evaluation and testing if they had sexual contact in the 60 days preceding the onset of the patient's symptoms or diagnosis.

URETHRAL DIVERTICULA

Urethral diverticula are localized outpouchings of the urethra. Most often they result from enlargement of obstructed periurethral glands. In women, who have a higher incidence than men, the diverticula protrude into the anterior vaginal wall. The rare cases reported in males generally have been associated with lower urinary tract congenital anomalies or surgical trauma.

The periurethral glands are found along the entire length of the urethra, with the majority draining into the distal third of the urethra. Skene's glands are the largest of these glands. Causes of urethral diverticuli include urethral trauma from childbearing, urethral instrumentation, urethral dilation, and infection with gonococcal organisms.

Symptoms include dysuria, postvoid dribbling, frequent urination (more often than every 2 hours), urgency, suprapubic discomfort or pressure, dyspareunia, and a feeling of incomplete bladder emptying. Urinary incontinence is frequently present. However, many women have no symptoms.

The urine may contain gross blood (hematuria) or sediment, which gives it a cloudy appearance. An anterior vaginal wall mass may be felt on physical examination. When palpated, the mass is often quite tender and expresses purulent discharge through the urethra.

Radiographic studies such as voiding cystourethrography (VCUG) can be used to confirm the diagnosis. Additional studies include ultrasound and magnetic resonance imaging (MRI) to determine the size of the diverticulum in relation to the urethral lumen.

Surgical options include transurethral incision of the diverticular neck, marsupialization (creation of a permanent opening) of the diverticular sac into the vagina (often referred to as a Spence procedure), and surgical excision. Stress urinary incontinence is a potential complication of the surgery.

INTERSTITIAL CYSTITIS/
PAINFUL BLADDER SYNDROME

Interstitial cystitis (IC) is a chronic, painful inflammatory disease of the bladder characterized by symptoms of urgency, frequency, and pain in the bladder and/or pelvis. *Painful bladder syndrome* (PBS) is suprapubic pain related to bladder filling. The term *IC/PBS* refers to cases of urinary pain that cannot be attributed to other causes such as infection or urinary calculi.

IC/PBS is more common in women than men. It affects about 3.3 million women and 1.6 million men.[15]

The etiology of IC/PBS remains unknown and is likely multifactorial. Possible causes include neurogenic hypersensitivity of the lower urinary tract, alterations in mast cells in the muscle and/or mucosal layers of the bladder, infection with an unusual organism (e.g., slow-growing virus), or production of a toxic substance in the urine.[16]

The bladder wall may be irritated and inflamed, and can become scarred. *Glomerulations* (superficial ulcerations with pinpoint bleeding) often occur on the bladder wall.

Clinical Manifestations and Diagnostic Studies

The two primary clinical manifestations of IC/PBS are pain and bothersome LUTS (e.g., frequency, urgency). The pain is usually located in the suprapubic area but may involve the vagina, labia, or entire perineal region, including the rectum and anus. The pain varies from moderate to severe and is exacerbated by bladder filling, postponed urination, physical exertion, pressure against the suprapubic area, certain foods, or emotional distress. The pain is transiently relieved by urination. Bothersome LUTS are similar to a UTI, and the condition is often misdiagnosed as a recurring or chronic UTI or, in men, chronic prostatitis.

The patient experiences periods of remission and exacerbation of the pain and bothersome voiding symptoms. Women often report that pain occurs premenstrually and is aggravated by sexual intercourse or emotional stress. Some patients experience symptoms that disappear altogether after a period of weeks to months, whereas others have persistent symptoms over months to years.

IC/PBS is a diagnosis of exclusion.[17] A careful history and physical examination are necessary to rule out other disorders that produce similar symptoms, such as UTI or endometriosis. Urine cultures do not find any bacteria or other organisms in the urine. Furthermore, people with IC/PBS do not respond to antibiotic therapy. Cystoscopic examination may reveal a small bladder capacity and glomerulations, but these findings are frequently not present in patients with IC/PBS.

Collaborative Care

Because the etiology of IC/PBS is unknown, no single treatment consistently reverses or relieves symptoms. Various therapies have been effective, including nutritional and drug therapy.[18,19] Surgical therapy is rarely indicated.

Elimination of foods and beverages that are likely to irritate the bladder may provide some relief from symptoms. Typical bladder irritants include caffeine; alcohol; citrus products; aged cheeses; nuts; foods containing vinegar, curries, or hot peppers; and foods or beverages, including fruits (cranberries), likely to lower urinary pH. Recipes and menus for a well-balanced diet that is specifically designed to avoid bladder-irritating foods and beverages are available at the website for the Interstitial Cystitis Association (*www.ichelp.org*).

Advise patients that an over-the-counter (OTC) dietary supplement called calcium glycerophosphate (Prelief) alkalinizes the urine and can provide relief from the irritating effects of certain foods. This agent may be particularly helpful when dining away from home, where the patient has less control over food preparation.

Because stress can exacerbate or cause flare-ups of IC/PBS symptoms, stress management techniques such as relaxation breathing and imagery (see Chapter 7) may be helpful. Using lubrication or altering positions may decrease pain associated with sexual intercourse.

Two tricyclic antidepressants, amitriptyline (Elavil) and nortriptyline (Aventyl), are used to reduce the burning pain and urinary frequency. Pentosan (Elmiron) is the only oral agent approved for the treatment of patients with symptoms of IC. It enhances the protective effects of the glycosaminoglycan layer of the bladder, and is thought to relieve pain associated with IC/PBS by reducing the irritative effects of urine on the bladder wall. These drugs are used to provide relief over time (weeks to months), but do not provide the immediate relief that may be needed for an acute exacerbation of symptoms. A short course of opioid analgesics may be used for immediate relief.

Dimethyl sulfoxide (DMSO) can be directly instilled into the bladder through a small catheter. This drug desensitizes pain receptors in the bladder wall. Heparin and hyaluronic acid also may be instilled into the bladder to relieve IC/PBS symptoms. Like pentosan, they are thought to enhance the protective properties of the glycosaminoglycan layer of the bladder. Instillations are often administered with lidocaine, which rapidly desensitizes the bladder wall, helping the patient tolerate instillation of additional heparin or hyaluronic acid and providing transient relief from pain.

Several surgical procedures can be used to relieve severe, debilitating pain. Surgical urinary diversion, such as an ileal conduit, is used when other measures fail. Unfortunately, some patients have reported pain within the urinary diversion, possibly indicating that some factor in the urine may contribute to IC/PBS in certain cases.

NURSING MANAGEMENT
INTERSTITIAL CYSTITIS/
PAINFUL BLADDER SYNDROME

Assess the characteristics of the pain associated with IC/PBS. Ask the patient about specific dietary or lifestyle factors that exacerbate or alleviate pain, and assess the intensity of the pain. Instruct the patient to keep a bladder log or voiding diary over a period of at least 3 days to determine voiding frequency and patterns of nocturia. Keeping a pain record at the same time may be useful.

A UTI may occur during the course of IC/PBS management because of diagnostic instrumentation and frequent bladder instillations. A UTI is likely to produce an acute exacerbation of bothersome LUTS and urinary frequency, as well as dysuria (not typically associated with IC/PBS) and odorous urine, possibly with hematuria.

Instruct the patient to maintain good nutrition, particularly in light of the broad dietary restrictions often necessary to control IC-related pain. Advise the patient to take a multivitamin containing no more than the recommended dietary allowance for essential vitamins and to avoid high-potency vitamins because they may irritate the bladder. Advise the patient to avoid clothing that creates suprapubic pressure, including pants with tight belts or restrictive waistlines.

Written educational materials about diet, ways to cope with the need for frequent urination, and strategies for coping with the emotional burden of IC/PBS are available from the Interstitial Cystitis Association (*www.ichelp.com*). Reassurance that IC/PBS is a real condition experienced by others and that it can be treated may relieve the anxiety, anger, guilt, and frustration related to experiences of chronic pain and voiding dysfunction in the absence of a clear-cut diagnosis and treatment strategy.

RENAL TUBERCULOSIS

Renal tuberculosis (TB) is rarely a primary lesion. It is usually secondary to TB of the lung. In a small percentage of patients with pulmonary TB, the tubercle bacilli reach the kidneys via the bloodstream. Onset occurs 5 to 8 years after the primary lung infection.[20] When the kidney is initially infected with bacilli, the patient is often asymptomatic. Sometimes the patient complains of fatigue and develops a low-grade fever. As the lesions ulcerate, infection descends to the bladder and other genitourinary organs. Then the patient experiences cystitis, frequent urination, burning on voiding, and epididymitis (in men).

Symptoms of a UTI are the first manifestations in the majority of patients with renal TB. Renal lesions may calcify as they heal. Infrequently, renal colic, lumbar and iliac pain, and hematuria may be present.

Tuberculin skin test results are positive in most patients, but this finding only indicates that the person has had previous inhalation of mycobacteria rather than active disease. A diagnosis of renal TB is based on finding tubercle bacilli in the urine.

Radiographic tests that may be done include CT urogram, CT/intravenous pyelogram (IVP), and voiding cystourethrogram (VCUG). These studies help determine the extent and severity of the disease.

Long-term complications of renal TB depend on the duration of the disease. Scarring of the renal parenchyma and the development of ureteral strictures occur. The earlier treatment is initiated, the less likely renal failure will develop. The patient may require long-term urologic follow-up. Nursing and col-laborative management for the patient with TB is discussed in Chapter 28.

IMMUNOLOGIC DISORDERS OF KIDNEY

GLOMERULONEPHRITIS

Immunologic processes involving the urinary tract predominantly affect the renal glomerulus. The disease process results in glomerulonephritis (inflammation of the glomeruli), which affects both kidneys equally and is the third leading cause of ESKD in the United States. Although the glomerulus is the primary site of inflammation, tubular, interstitial, and vascular changes also occur.

A variety of conditions can cause glomerulonephritis, ranging from kidney infections to systemic diseases (Table 46-8). Glomerulonephritis can be acute or chronic. With *acute glomerulonephritis*, symptoms come on suddenly and may be temporary or reversible. An example of this is acute poststreptococcal glomerulonephritis (discussed in the next section).

TABLE 46-8 CAUSES OR RISK FACTORS FOR GLOMERULONEPHRITIS

Cause or Risk Factor	Description	Cause or Risk Factor	Description
Infections		IgA nephropathy	• Results from deposits of immunoglobulin A (IgA) in the glomeruli.
Poststreptococcal glomerulonephritis	• GN may develop 1-2 wk after a streptococcal throat infection or, rarely, a skin infection (impetigo).		• Characterized by recurrent episodes of hematuria.
	• Antibodies (Ab) to strep antigen (Ag) develop and the Ag-Ab deposit in the glomeruli, causing inflammation.	**Vasculitis**	
		Polyarteritis	• Autoimmune disease that affects small and medium blood vessels.
Infective endocarditis	• Bacteria can cause an infection of one or more of the heart valves (see Chapter 37).		• Can affect any organ but common in heart, kidneys, and intestines.
	• People at risk include those with a heart defect, such as a damaged or artificial heart valve.	Wegener's granulomatosis	• Form of vasculitis affecting small and medium blood vessels.
	• Bacterial endocarditis is associated with GN, but the exact cause is not known.		• Most commonly affects kidneys, lungs, and upper respiratory tract.
Viral infections	• Viral infections can trigger GN.	**Conditions Causing Scarring of Glomeruli**	
	• Common viruses include human immunodeficiency virus (HIV) and hepatitis B and hepatitis C viruses.	Diabetic nephropathy	• Primary cause of end-stage kidney disease in the United States (see Chapter 47).
			• Microvascular changes of diffuse glomerulosclerosis involving thickening of the glomerular basement membrane.
Immune Diseases		Hypertension	• Nephrosclerosis is a complication of hypertension.
Systemic lupus erythematosus (SLE)	• Autoimmune disorder characterized by the involvement of several tissues and organs, particularly joints, skin, and kidneys (see Chapter 65).		• GN can also cause hypertension.
	• GN frequently occurs in SLE and has a poor prognosis.	Focal segmental glomerulosclerosis	• Characterized by scattered scarring of some of the glomeruli.
			• May result from another disease or occur for unknown reasons.
Scleroderma	• Disease of unknown etiology characterized by widespread alterations of connective tissue and by vascular lesions in many organs (see Chapter 65).	**Other Causes**	
	• In the kidney, vascular lesions are associated with fibrosis. Severity of renal involvement varies.	Amyloidosis	• Caused by infiltration of tissues with amyloid (hyaline substance).
			• Hyaline bodies consist largely of protein.
Goodpasture syndrome	• Autoimmune disorder that causes lung and kidney disease.		• Kidney involvement is common, and proteinuria is often the first clinical manifestation.
	• Causes bleeding into the lungs and GN.	Illegal drug use	• People who use these drugs are at increased risk for GN.

GN, Glomerulonephritis.

Chronic glomerulonephritis is slowly progressive glomerulonephritis generally leading to irreversible renal failure (discussed later in this chapter).

Acute Poststreptococcal Glomerulonephritis

Acute poststreptococcal glomerulonephritis (APSGN) is a common type of acute glomerulonephritis. It is most common in children and young adults, but all age-groups can be affected. APSGN develops 5 to 21 days after an infection of the tonsils, pharynx, or skin (e.g., streptococcal sore throat, impetigo) by nephrotoxic strains of group A β-hemolytic streptococci. The person produces antibodies to the streptococcal antigen. Although the specific mechanism is not known, tissue injury occurs as the antigen-antibody complexes are deposited in the glomeruli, complement is activated (see Chapter 12), and inflammation results.

The clinical manifestations of APSGN include generalized body edema, hypertension, oliguria, hematuria with a smoky or rusty appearance, and proteinuria. Fluid retention occurs as a result of decreased glomerular filtration. Initially edema appears in low-pressure tissues, such as those around the eyes (periorbital edema), but later it progresses to involve the total body as ascites or peripheral edema in the legs. Smoky urine indicates bleeding in the upper urinary tract. The degree of proteinuria varies with the severity of the glomerulonephropathy. Hypertension primarily results from increased extracellular fluid volume. The patient with APSGN may have abdominal or flank pain. At times the patient has no symptoms, with the problem found on routine urinalysis.

More than 95% of patients with APSGN recover completely or improve rapidly with conservative management. Accurate recognition and assessment are critical, since chronic glomerulonephritis develops in 5% to 15% of the affected persons, and irreversible renal failure occurs in 1% of patients.[21]

The diagnosis of APSGN is based on a complete history and physical examination. An immune response to the streptococci is often demonstrated by assessment of antistreptolysin-O (ASO) titers. The finding of decreased complement components (especially C3 and CH50) indicates an immune-mediated response. A renal biopsy may be done to confirm the disease.

Dipstick urinalysis and urine sediment microscopy reveal erythrocytes in significant numbers. Erythrocyte casts are highly suggestive of APSGN. Proteinuria may range from mild to severe. Blood tests include blood urea nitrogen (BUN) and serum creatinine to assess the extent of renal impairment.

NURSING AND COLLABORATIVE MANAGEMENT
ACUTE POSTSTREPTOCOCCAL GLOMERULONEPHRITIS

The management of APSGN focuses on symptomatic relief. Rest is recommended until the signs of glomerular inflammation (proteinuria, hematuria) and hypertension subside. Edema is treated by restricting sodium and fluid intake and by administrating diuretics. Severe hypertension is treated with antihypertensive drugs. Dietary protein intake may be restricted if there is evidence of an increase in nitrogenous wastes (e.g., elevated BUN). The dietary protein restriction varies with the degree of proteinuria. Low-protein, low-sodium, fluid-restricted diets are discussed in Chapter 47.

Antibiotics should be given only if the streptococcal infection is still present. Corticosteroids and cytotoxic drugs have not been shown to be of value in the treatment of APSGN.

One of the most important ways to prevent APSGN is to encourage early diagnosis and treatment of sore throats and skin lesions. If streptococci are found in the culture, treatment with appropriate antibiotic therapy (usually penicillin) is essential. Encourage the patient to take the full course of antibiotics to ensure that the bacteria have been eradicated. Good personal hygiene is an important factor in preventing the spread of cutaneous streptococcal infections.

In most cases, recovery from the acute glomerulonephritis is complete. However, if progressive involvement occurs and chronic glomerulonephritis develops, ESKD results.

Goodpasture Syndrome

Goodpasture syndrome is an autoimmune disease characterized by circulating antibodies against glomerular and alveolar basement membrane. Damage to the kidneys and lungs results when binding of the antibody causes an inflammatory reaction mediated by complement activation (see Chapter 12).

Goodpasture syndrome is a rare disease that is mostly found in young male smokers. The clinical manifestations include flu-like symptoms with pulmonary symptoms such as cough, mild shortness of breath, hemoptysis, crackles, rhonchi, and pulmonary insufficiency. Renal involvement causes hematuria, weakness, pallor, anemia, and renal failure. Pulmonary hemorrhage usually occurs and may precede glomerular abnormalities by weeks or months.

Current management includes corticosteroids, immunosuppressive drugs (e.g., cyclophosphamide [Cytoxan], azathioprine [Imuran]), plasmapheresis (see Chapter 14), and dialysis. Plasmapheresis removes the circulating anti–glomerular basement membrane (GBM) antibodies, and immunosuppressive therapy inhibits further antibody production. Renal transplantation can be attempted after the circulating anti-GBM antibody titer decreases. Although the disease may recur in the transplanted kidney, this is not a contraindication to transplantation.

Nursing management appropriate for a critically ill patient who is experiencing acute kidney injury (see Chapter 47) and respiratory distress (see Chapter 68) is instituted. Death is often secondary to hemorrhage in the lungs and respiratory failure.

Rapidly Progressive Glomerulonephritis

Rapidly progressive glomerulonephritis (RPGN) is a type of glomerular disease characterized by rapid, progressive loss of renal function over days to weeks. In contrast, chronic glomerulonephritis develops insidiously and progresses over many years. The manifestations of RPGN are hypertension, edema, proteinuria, hematuria, and red blood cell (RBC) casts.

RPGN can occur in a variety of situations: (1) as a complication of inflammatory or infectious disease (e.g., APSGN), (2) as a complication of a systemic disease (e.g., systemic lupus erythematosus), (3) as an idiopathic disease, or (4) with the use of certain drugs (e.g., penicillamine).

Treatment is directed toward correction of fluid overload, hypertension, uremia, and inflammatory injury to the kidney. Treatment includes corticosteroids, cytotoxic agents, and plasmapheresis. Dialysis therapy and transplantation are used as maintenance therapy for the patient with RPGN. After kidney transplantation, RPGN may recur.

Chronic Glomerulonephritis

Chronic glomerulonephritis is a syndrome that reflects the end stage of glomerular inflammatory disease. Most types of glomerulonephritis and nephrotic syndrome can eventually lead to chronic glomerulonephritis. Some people who develop chronic glomerulonephritis have no history of kidney disease. Frequently the cause of chronic glomerulonephritis is not found. Infrequently, it is an inherited disorder (e.g., Alport syndrome [see p. 1083]).

With chronic glomerulonephritis, symptoms develop slowly over time. Patients are often unaware that progressive kidney impairment is occurring. They do not realize that they have severe kidney impairment until a diagnostic evaluation is done. Chronic glomerulonephritis is often discovered coincidentally with the finding of an abnormality on a urinalysis or elevated blood pressure (BP).

The syndrome is characterized by proteinuria, hematuria, and the slow development of uremia (see Chapter 47) as a result of decreasing renal function. Chronic glomerulonephritis progresses insidiously toward renal failure in 2 to 30 years.

Clinical manifestations of glomerulonephritis include varying degrees of hematuria (ranging from microscopic to gross) and urinary excretion of various formed elements, including RBCs, WBCs, and casts. Proteinuria and elevated BUN and serum creatinine levels are other findings. Sometimes fatigue may be a presenting symptom.

The patient's history provides important information related to glomerulonephritis. Assess exposure to drugs, immunizations, microbial infections, and viral infections such as hepatitis. Also evaluate the patient for more generalized conditions involving immune disorders, such as systemic lupus erythematosus and scleroderma. Commonly the patient has no recollection or history of any renal problems.

Ultrasound and CT scanning are generally preferred as diagnostic measures. However, a renal biopsy may be performed to determine the exact cause of the glomerulonephritis.

Treatment is supportive and symptomatic. Management of chronic kidney disease is discussed in Chapter 47.

NEPHROTIC SYNDROME

Nephrotic syndrome results when the glomerulus is excessively permeable to plasma protein, causing proteinuria that leads to low plasma albumin and tissue edema.

Etiology and Clinical Manifestations

Some of the common causes of nephrotic syndrome are listed in Table 46-9. About one third of patients with nephrotic syndrome have a systemic disease such as diabetes or systemic lupus erythematosus.

The characteristic manifestations of nephrotic syndrome include peripheral edema, massive proteinuria, hypertension, hyperlipidemia, and hypoalbuminemia. Characteristic laboratory findings include decreased serum albumin, decreased total serum protein, and elevated serum cholesterol. The increased glomerular membrane permeability found in nephrotic syndrome is responsible for the massive excretion of protein in the urine. This results in decreased serum protein and subsequent edema formation. Ascites and *anasarca* (massive generalized edema) develop if there is severe hypoalbuminemia.[22]

The diminished plasma oncotic pressure from the decreased serum proteins stimulates hepatic lipoprotein synthesis, which results in hyperlipidemia. Initially, cholesterol and low-density lipoproteins are elevated. Later the triglyceride level is also

TABLE 46-9	CAUSES OF NEPHROTIC SYNDROME
Primary Glomerular Disease • Membranous proliferative glomerulonephritis • Primary nephrotic syndrome • Focal glomerulonephritis • Inherited nephrotic disease **Extrarenal Causes** **Multisystem Disease** • Systemic lupus erythematosus • Diabetes mellitus • Amyloidosis **Infections** • Bacterial (streptococcal, syphilis) • Viral (hepatitis, human immunodeficiency virus) • Protozoal (malaria)	**Neoplasms** • Hodgkin's lymphoma • Solid tumors of lungs, colon, stomach, breast • Leukemias **Allergens** • Bee sting • Pollen **Drugs** • penicillamine • Nonsteroidal antiinflammatory drugs (NSAIDs) • captopril (Capoten) • heroin

increased. Fat bodies (fatty casts) commonly appear in the urine.

Immune responses, both humoral and cellular, are altered in nephrotic syndrome. As a result, infection is a primary cause of morbidity and mortality. Calcium and skeletal abnormalities may occur, including hypocalcemia, blunted calcium response to parathyroid hormone, hyperparathyroidism, and osteomalacia.

With nephrotic proteinuria, hypercoagulability results from the urinary loss of anticoagulant proteins. Hypercoagulability with thromboembolism is a serious complication of nephrotic syndrome. The renal vein is the most common site for thrombus formation. Pulmonary emboli occur in about 40% of nephrotic patients with thrombosis.

NURSING AND COLLABORATIVE MANAGEMENT NEPHROTIC SYNDROME

Specific treatment of nephrotic syndrome depends on the cause. The goals are to cure or control the primary disease and relieve the symptoms. Corticosteroids and cyclophosphamide may be used for the treatment of nephrotic syndrome. Prednisone has been effective to varying degrees for some causes of nephrotic syndrome (e.g., membranous glomerulonephritis, lupus nephritis). Management of diabetes and treatment of edema are measures used for nephrotic syndrome related to diabetes.

Management of the edema includes the cautious use of angiotensin-converting enzyme inhibitors; nonsteroidal antiinflammatory drugs (NSAIDs); and a low-sodium (2 to 3 g/day), moderate-protein (1 to 2 g/kg/day) diet. If urine protein losses are high (more than 10 g/day), additional protein may be recommended.

Dietary salt restrictions are a key to managing edema. Some individuals may need thiazide or loop diuretics.

The treatment of hyperlipidemia includes lipid-lowering agents, such as colestipol (Colestid) and lovastatin (Mevacor) (see Table 34-5). If thrombosis is detected, anticoagulant therapy may be needed.

A major nursing intervention for a patient with nephrotic syndrome focuses on the management of edema. Assess the edema by weighing the patient daily, accurately recording intake and output, and measuring abdominal girth or extremity size. Compare this information on a daily basis to assess the effectiveness of treatment. Clean the edematous skin carefully. Avoid trauma to the skin. Monitor the effectiveness of diuretic therapy.

Patients with nephrotic syndrome are usually anorexic and have the potential to become malnourished from the excessive loss of protein in the urine. Serve small, frequent meals in a pleasant setting to encourage better dietary intake.

Because the patient with nephrotic syndrome is susceptible to infection, teach the patient to avoid exposure to persons with known infections. Support for the patient, in terms of coping with an altered body image, is essential because of the embarrassment and shame often associated with the edematous appearance.

OBSTRUCTIVE UROPATHIES

Urinary obstruction refers to any anatomic or functional condition that blocks or impedes the flow of urine (Fig. 46-3). It may be congenital or acquired. Damaging effects from urinary tract obstruction affect the system above the level of the obstruction. The severity of these effects depends on the location, duration of obstruction, amount of pressure or dilation, and presence of urinary stasis or infection. Infection increases the risk of irreversible damage.

When obstruction occurs at the level of the bladder neck or prostate, significant bladder changes can occur. Detrusor muscle fibers *hypertrophy* (increase in size) to contract harder to push urine out a narrower pathway. Over a long period, the detrusor loses its ability to compensate for this resistance, eventually leading to large residual urine volume in the bladder.

When *bladder outlet obstruction* is present, pressure increases during bladder filling or storage and can be transmitted to the ureter. This pressure leads to *reflux* (a backflow of urine), **hydroureter** (ureteral dilation and distention), vesicoureteral reflux (backflow, or backward movement, of urine from the lower to upper urinary tract), and **hydronephrosis** (dilation or enlargement of the renal pelvises and calyces) (Fig. 46-4). Chronic pyelonephritis and renal atrophy may develop. If only one kidney is obstructed, the other kidney may try to compensate by hypertrophy.

Partial obstruction may occur in the ureter or at the ureteropelvic junction (UPJ). If the pressure remains low or moderate, the kidney may continue to dilate with no noticeable loss of function. The risk of pyelonephritis is increased because of urinary stasis and reflux. If only one kidney is involved and the other kidney is functioning, the patient may be asymptomatic.

If both kidneys or only one functioning kidney is involved (e.g., if the patient has only one kidney), alterations in renal function (e.g., increased BUN or serum creatinine levels) are found. Progressive obstruction can lead to renal failure. Treatment requires location and relief of the blockage. This can include insertion of a tube (e.g., urethral or ureteral), surgical correction of the primary problem, or diversion of the urinary stream above the level of blockage.

URINARY TRACT CALCULI

Each year an estimated 1 million to 2 million people in the United States have **nephrolithiasis** (kidney stone disease). In the United States the incidence of urinary stone disease is highest in the Southeast and Southwest, followed by the Midwest. Except for struvite (magnesium ammonium phosphate) stones associated with UTI, stone disorders are more common in men than in women. The majority of patients are between 20 and 55 years of age.[4]

Stone formation is more frequent in whites than in African Americans. The incidence is also higher in persons with a family history of stone formation. Stones can recur in up to 50% of patients. Stone formation occurs more often in the summer months, thus supporting the role of dehydration in this process.

Etiology and Pathophysiology

Many factors are involved in the incidence and type of stone formation, including metabolic, dietary, genetic, climatic, life-

Pelvis
• Calculi
• Tumor

Ureter (intrinsic)
• Calculi
• Tumor
• Clot
• Inflammation

Foreign body (calculi)

Ureter (extrinsic)
• Pregnancy
• Tumor (e.g., cervix)

Ureteral stricture

Bladder
• Calculi
• Tumors
• Functional (e.g., neurogenic)

Narrowing of ureterovesical junction

Prostate
• Hyperplasia
• Carcinoma
Urethral stricture

FIG. 46-3 Sites and causes of upper and lower urinary tract obstruction.

FIG. 46-4 Hydronephrosis of the kidney. Note the marked dilation of the pelvis and calyces and thinning of the renal parenchyma.

FIG. 46-5 A, Renal staghorn calculus. The renal pelvis is filled with a large calculus that is shaped to its contours, resembling the horns of a stag *(S)*. **B,** Imbedded staghorn calculus *(arrow)* in hydronephrotic, infected, nonfunctioning kidney.

style, and occupational influences (Table 46-10). Although many theories have been proposed, no single theory can account for stone formation in all cases. Crystals, when in a supersaturated concentration, can precipitate and unite to form a stone. Keeping urine dilute and free flowing reduces the risk of recurrent stone formation in many individuals. A mucoprotein is formed in the kidneys as a matrix for the stone. Urinary pH, solute load, and inhibitors in the urine affect the formation of stones. The higher the pH (alkaline), the less soluble are calcium and phosphate. The lower the pH (acidic), the less soluble are uric acid and cystine. When a substance is not very soluble in fluid, it is more likely to precipitate out of solution.[23]

TABLE 46-10	RISK FACTORS FOR URINARY TRACT CALCULI

Metabolic
- Abnormalities that result in increased urine levels of calcium, oxaluric acid, uric acid, or citric acid

Climate
- Warm climates that cause increased fluid loss, low urine volume, and increased solute concentration in urine

Diet
- Large intake of dietary proteins that increases uric acid excretion
- Excessive amounts of tea or fruit juices that elevate urinary oxalate level
- Large intake of calcium and oxalate
- Low fluid intake that increases urinary concentration

Genetic Factors
- Family history of stone formation, cystinuria, gout, or renal acidosis
- Lifestyle
- Sedentary occupation, immobility

Other important factors in the development of stones include obstruction with urinary stasis and UTI with urea-splitting bacteria (e.g., *Proteus, Klebsiella, Pseudomonas,* and some species of staphylococci). These bacteria cause the urine to become alkaline and contribute to the formation of struvite stones. Infected stones, entrapped in the kidney (Fig. 46-5), may assume a staghorn configuration as the stone branches to occupy a large portion of the collecting system. These stones can lead to a renal infection, hydronephrosis, and loss of kidney function. Genetic factors may also contribute to urine stone formation. Cystinuria, an autosomal recessive disorder, is characterized by a markedly increased excretion of cystine.

Types of Urinary Calculi

The term calculus refers to the stone, and *lithiasis* refers to stone formation. The five major categories of stones are (1) calcium phosphate, (2) calcium oxalate, (3) uric acid, (4) cystine, and (5) struvite (magnesium ammonium phosphate) (Table 46-11). Although calcium stones are the most common, stone composition may be mixed. Calculi can be found in various locations in the urinary tract (see Figs. 46-3 and 46-5).

Clinical Manifestations

The first symptom of a kidney stone is usually severe pain that begins suddenly. Typically, a person feels a sharp pain in the flank area, back, or lower abdomen. People describe the pain as the most excruciating that a person can endure. *Renal colic* is the term used for the sharp, severe pain, which results from the stretching, dilation, and spasm of the ureter in response to the obstructing stone. Nausea and vomiting may occur due to the severe pain.[24]

Urinary stones cause clinical manifestations when they obstruct urinary flow. Common sites of obstruction are at the UPJ (where the renal pelvis narrows into the ureter) and at the ureterovesical junction (UVJ). The type of pain is determined by the location of the stone. If the stone is nonobstructing, pain may be absent. If the obstruction is in a calyx or at the UPJ, the patient may experience dull costovertebral flank pain or renal colic. Pain resulting from the passage of a calculus down the ureter is intense and colicky.

Patients with renal colic have a hard time being still. They go from walking to sitting to lying down, and then they

TABLE 46-11 TYPES OF URINARY TRACT CALCULI

Characteristics	Predisposing Factors	Treatment
Calcium Oxalate* Small, often possible to get trapped in ureter. More frequent in men than in women. *Incidence*: 35%-40%	Idiopathic hypercalciuria, hyperoxaluria, independent of urinary pH, family history	Increase hydration. Reduce dietary oxalate.† Give thiazide diuretics. Give cellulose phosphate to chelate calcium and prevent GI absorption. Give potassium citrate to maintain alkaline urine. Give cholestyramine to bind oxalate. Give calcium lactate to precipitate oxalate in GI tract. Reduce daily sodium intake.
Calcium Phosphate Mixed stones (typically), with struvite or oxalate stones. *Incidence*: 8%-10%	Alkaline urine, primary hyperparathyroidism	Treat underlying causes and other stones.
Struvite (Magnesium Ammonium Phosphate) Three or four times as common in women as men. Always associated with urinary tract infections. Large staghorn type (usually) (see Fig. 46-5). *Incidence*: 10%-15%	Urinary tract infections (usually *Proteus*)	Administer antimicrobial agents, acetohydroxamic acid. Use surgical intervention to remove stone. Take measures to acidify urine.
Uric Acid Predominant in men, high incidence in Jewish men. *Incidence*: 5%-8%	Gout, acidic urine, inherited condition	Reduce urinary concentration of uric acid. Alkalinize urine with potassium citrate. Administer allopurinol. Reduce dietary purines.†
Cystine Genetic autosomal recessive defect. Defective absorption of cystine in GI tract and kidney, excess concentrations causing stone formation. *Incidence*: 1%-2%	Acidic urine	Increase hydration. Give α-penicillamine and tiopronin to prevent cystine crystallization. Give potassium citrate to maintain alkaline urine.

*Calcium stones can exist as calcium oxalate, calcium phosphate, or a mixture of both. Calcium stones account for the majority of all stones.
†See Table 43-12: Causes of Peritonitis.

repeat the process. Some people refer to this as the *kidney stone dance.*

The patient may be in mild shock with cool, moist skin. As a stone nears the UVJ, pain moves around toward the abdomen and down toward the lower quadrant. Men may experience testicular pain, whereas women may complain of labial pain. Both men and women may experience pain in the groin. The patient may also have manifestations of UTI with dysuria, fever, and chills.

Diagnostic Studies

Noncontrast spiral CT, also called a CT/KUB (kidneys, ureters, bladder), is the diagnostic study commonly used in patients with renal colic. It is quick and noninvasive and requires no IV contrast. In some situations, ultrasound and IVP are used. A complete urinalysis helps confirm the diagnosis of a urinary stone by assessing for hematuria, crystalluria, and urinary pH.

Retrieval and analysis of the stones are important in the diagnosis of the underlying problem contributing to stone formation. The patient's serum calcium, phosphorus, sodium, potassium, bicarbonate, uric acid, BUN, and creatinine levels are also measured. A careful history should include any previous episodes of stone formation, prescribed and OTC medications, dietary supplements, and family history of urinary calculi. Measurement of urine pH is useful in the diagnosis of struvite stones and renal tubular acidosis (tendency to alkaline or high pH) and uric acid stones (tendency to acidic or low pH). Patients who are recurrent stone formers should undergo a 24-hour urinary measurement of calcium, phosphorus, magnesium, sodium, oxalate, citrate, sulfate, potassium, uric acid, and total volume.

Collaborative Care

Evaluation and management of a patient with renal calculi consist of two concurrent approaches. The first approach is directed toward management of the acute attack by treating the pain, infection, and/or obstruction. Administer opioids to relieve renal colic pain. Most stones are 4 mm or less in size and will probably pass spontaneously. However, it may take weeks for a stone to pass.

Tamsulosin (Flomax) or terazosin (Hytrin), α-adrenergic blockers that relax the smooth muscle in the ureter, can be used to facilitate stone passage. These drugs are also used to relax the muscle tissue in the prostate in men with BPH.

The second approach is directed toward evaluation of the cause of the stone formation and the prevention of further stone development. Obtain information from the patient, including a family history of stone formation; geographic residence; nutritional assessment, including the intake of vitamins A and D; activity pattern (active or sedentary); history of prolonged illness with immobilization or dehydration; and any history of disease or surgery involving the GI or genitourinary tract.

Therapy for active stone formers requires a comprehensive management approach, with the primary emphasis on teaching. Adequate hydration, dietary sodium restrictions, dietary changes, and drugs are employed to minimize urinary stone formation (see Table 46-11). Various drugs are prescribed, depending on the specific problem underlying the stone formation. These drugs prevent stone formation in various ways, including altering urine pH, preventing excessive urinary excretion of a substance, or correcting a primary disease (e.g., hyperparathyroidism).

Treatment of struvite stones requires control of infection. This may be difficult if the stone remains in place. In addition

FIG. 46-6 **A,** Calcium oxalate stones. **B,** Plain abdominal x-ray showing large bladder calculus.

to antibiotics, acetohydroxamic acid may be used to treat kidney infections that result in the continual formation of struvite stones. Acetohydroxamic acid inhibits the chemical action caused by the persistent bacteria and thus retards struvite stone formation. The stone may have to be removed surgically if the infection cannot be controlled.

Indications for endourologic, lithotripsy, or open surgical stone removal include the following: (1) stones too large for spontaneous passage (usually greater than 7 mm); (2) stones associated with bacteriuria or symptomatic infection; (3) stones causing impaired renal function; (4) stones causing persistent pain, nausea, or paralytic ileus; (5) inability of patient to be treated medically; and (6) patient with only one kidney.

Endourologic Procedures. If the stone is located in the bladder, a cystoscopy is done to remove small stones. For large stones (Fig. 46-6), a *cystolitholapaxy* is done. In this procedure, large stones are broken up with an instrument called a lithotrite (stone crusher). The bladder is then irrigated and the crushed stones washed out. A *cystoscopic lithotripsy* uses an ultrasonic lithotrite to pulverize (break up) stones. Complications associated with these cystoscopic procedures include hemorrhage, retained stone fragments, and infection.

Flexible *ureteroscopes,* inserted via a cystoscope, can be used to remove stones from the renal pelvis and upper urinary tract. Ultrasonic, laser, or electrohydraulic lithotripsy may be used in conjunction with the ureteroscope to pulverize the stone.

In *percutaneous nephrolithotomy,* a nephroscope is inserted into the kidney pelvis through a track (using a sheath) in the skin. The track is created in the patient's back. The kidney stones can be fragmented using ultrasound, electrohydraulic, or laser lithotripsy. The stone fragments are removed, and the pelvis is irrigated. A percutaneous nephrostomy tube is usually left in place to make sure that the ureter is not obstructed. Complications include bleeding, injury to adjacent structures, and infection.

Lithotripsy. Lithotripsy is a procedure used to eliminate calculi from the urinary tract. Lithotripsy techniques include (1) laser lithotripsy, (2) extracorporeal shock-wave lithotripsy (ESWL), (3) percutaneous ultrasonic lithotripsy, and (4) electrohydraulic lithotripsy. *Laser lithotripsy* is used to fragment ureteral and large bladder stones (bladder stones are described above). To access ureteral stones, a ureteroscope is used to get close to the stone. A small fiber is inserted up the endoscope so that the tip (which emits the laser energy) can come in contact

with the stone. A holmium laser in direct contact with the stone is commonly used. The intense energy breaks the stone into small pieces, which can be extracted or flushed out. Because of the type of laser energy, no other tissue is affected. This minimally invasive treatment usually requires general anesthesia.[25]

In *extracorporeal shock-wave lithotripsy (ESWL),* a noninvasive procedure, the patient is anesthetized (spinal or general) to ensure that he or she maintains the same position during the procedure. Fluoroscopy or ultrasound is used to focus the lithotripter on the affected kidney, and a high-voltage spark generator produces high-energy acoustic shock waves that shatter the stone without damaging the surrounding tissues. The stone is broken into fine sand *(steinstrasse)* and excreted in the urine.

In *percutaneous ultrasonic lithotripsy* an ultrasonic probe is placed in the renal pelvis via a percutaneous nephroscope inserted through a small incision in the flank, and is then positioned against the stone. The patient is given general or spinal anesthesia for this procedure. The probe produces ultrasonic waves, which break the stone into sandlike particles.

In *electrohydraulic lithotripsy* the probe is positioned directly on a stone, but it breaks the stone into small fragments that are removed by forceps or by suction. A continuous saline irrigation flushes out the stone particles, and all of the outflow drainage is strained so that the particles can be analyzed. The calculi can also be removed by basket extraction. Complications are rare but they include hemorrhage, sepsis, and abscess formation. Postoperatively, the patient usually complains of moderate to severe colicky pain. The first few times that the patient urinates, the urine is bright red. As the bleeding subsides, the urine becomes dark red or a smoky color. Antibiotics are usually administered after the procedure to reduce the risk of infection.

Hematuria is common after lithotripsy procedures. A self-retaining ureteral stent is often placed after the procedure to facilitate passage of sand (shattered stone) and prevent sand buildup within the ureter, which might lead to obstruction. The stent is typically removed within 2 weeks following lithotripsy. If a stone is large or positioned in the mid or distal ureter, additional treatment, such as surgery, may be necessary.

Surgical Therapy. A small group of patients require open surgical procedures. The primary indications for surgery include pain, infection, and obstruction. The type of open surgery performed depends on the location of the stone. A *nephrolithotomy* is an incision into the kidney to remove a stone. A *pyelolithot-*

TABLE 46-12 NUTRITIONAL THERAPY
Urinary Tract Calculi

Depending on the type of calculi, modify the diet to decrease foods that are high in the substance that is the cause of the calculi. Listed below are foods that are moderate or high in purine, calcium, or oxalate content.

Purine*
High: Sardines, herring, mussels, liver, kidney, goose, venison, meat soups, sweetbreads
Moderate: Chicken, salmon, crab, veal, mutton, bacon, pork, beef, ham

Calcium
High: Milk, cheese, ice cream, yogurt, sauces containing milk; all beans (except green beans), lentils; fish with fine bones (e.g., sardines, kippers, herring, salmon); dried fruits, nuts; Ovaltine, chocolate, cocoa

Oxalate
High: Dark roughage, spinach, rhubarb, asparagus, cabbage, tomatoes, beets, nuts, celery, parsley, runner beans; chocolate, cocoa, instant coffee, Ovaltine, tea; Worcestershire sauce

*Uric acid is a waste product from purine in food.

TABLE 46-13 NURSING ASSESSMENT
Urinary Tract Calculi

Subjective Data
Important Health Information
Past health history: Recent or chronic UTI; bed rest; immobilization; previous urinary tract stones, obstruction, or kidney disease with urinary stasis; gout; benign prostatic hyperplasia (BPH); hyperparathyroidism, chronic diarrhea
Medications: Prior use of medication for prevention of stones or treatment of UTI; allopurinol, analgesics, loop diuretics
Surgery or other treatments: External urinary diversion, long-term indwelling urinary catheter

Functional Health Patterns
Health perception–health management: Family history of renal calculi; sedentary lifestyle
Nutritional-metabolic: Nausea, vomiting; dietary intake of purines, excessive calcium ingestion, salt excess, oxalates, phosphates; low fluid intake; chills
Elimination: Decreased urine output, urinary urgency, frequency, feeling of bladder fullness
Cognitive-perceptual: Acute, severe, colicky pain in flank, back, abdomen, groin, or genitalia; burning on urination, dysuria; anxiety

Objective Data
General
Guarding, back pain, fever, dehydration

Integumentary
Warm, flushed skin or pallor with cool, moist skin (mild shock)

Gastrointestinal
Abdominal distention, absence of bowel sounds

Urinary
Oliguria, hematuria, tenderness on palpation of renal areas, passage of stone or stones

Possible Diagnostic Findings
↑ BUN and serum creatinine levels; RBCs, WBCs, pyuria, crystals, casts, minerals, bacteria on urinalysis; ↑ uric acid, calcium, phosphorus, oxalate, or cystine values on 24-hr urine sample; calculi or anatomic changes on IVP or KUB x-ray; direct visualization of obstruction on cystoureteroscopy

IVP, Intravenous pyelogram; *KUB,* kidneys, ureters, bladder; *UTI,* urinary tract infection.

omy is an incision into the renal pelvis for stone removal. If the stone is located within the ureter, a *ureterolithotomy* is performed. A *cystotomy* may be indicated for bladder calculi. For open surgery on the kidney or ureter, a flank incision directly below the diaphragm and across the side is usually preferred. The most common complications after surgical procedures for stone removal are related to hemorrhage.

Nutritional Therapy. To manage an obstructing stone, have the patient drink adequate fluids to avoid dehydration. Forcing excessive fluids is not advised, since this has not proved effective in facilitating spontaneous passage (excretion) of stones via the urine. Forcing fluids may also increase the pain or precipitate the development of renal colic.

After an episode of urolithiasis, encourage a high fluid intake (approximately 3 L/day) to produce a urine output of at least 2 L/day. High urine output prevents supersaturation of minerals (i.e., dilutes the concentration of urine) and promotes excretion of minerals within the urine, thus preventing stone formation. Increasing the fluid intake is particularly important for patients at risk for dehydration, including those who (1) are active in sports, (2) live in a dry climate, (3) perform physical exercise, (4) have a family history of stone formation, or (5) work outside or in an occupation that requires a great deal of physical activity. Water is the preferred fluid. Limit consumption of colas, coffee, and tea because high intake of these beverages tends to increase the risk of recurring urinary calculi.

A low-sodium diet is recommended, since high-sodium intake increases calcium excretion in the urine. Foods high in calcium, oxalate, and purines are presented in Table 46-12.

NURSING MANAGEMENT
URINARY TRACT CALCULI

NURSING ASSESSMENT

Subjective and objective data that should be obtained from a patient with urinary tract calculi are presented in Table 46-13.

NURSING DIAGNOSES

Nursing diagnoses for the patient with urinary tract calculi include, but are not limited to, the following:

- Impaired urinary elimination *related to* trauma or obstruction of ureters or urethra
- Acute pain *related to* effects of stones and inadequate pain control or comfort measures
- Deficient knowledge *related to* unfamiliarity with information resources and lack of experience with urinary stones

Additional information on nursing diagnoses for the patient with urinary tract calculi is presented in eNursing Care Plan 46-2 (on the website for this chapter).

PLANNING

The overall goals are that the patient with urinary tract calculi will have (1) relief of pain, (2) no urinary tract obstruction, and (3) knowledge of ways to prevent recurrence of stones.

NURSING IMPLEMENTATION

Most people who have had urinary stones can lower their risk of recurrence by changing their lifestyle and dietary habits. Adequate fluid intake is important to produce a urine output of approximately 2 L/day. Consult with the health care provider about recommendations for fluid intake in a given patient. The moderately active, ambulatory person should drink about 3 L/day. Fluid intake needs to be higher in the active patient who works outdoors or who regularly engages in athletic activities. In contrast, fluid intake is less for the sedentary or immobile person. Preventive measures related to the person who is on bed rest or is relatively immobile for a prolonged time include maintaining an adequate fluid intake, turning the patient every 2 hours, and helping the patient sit or stand, if possible, to maximize urinary flow.

Additional preventive measures focus on reducing metabolic or secondary risk factors. For example, dietary restriction of purines may be helpful for the patient at risk for developing uric acid stones. Teach the patient the dosage, scheduling, and potential side effects of drugs used to reduce the risk of stone formation (see Table 46-11). Some patients may be taught to self-monitor urinary pH or urine output.

Pain management and patient comfort are primary nursing responsibilities when managing an obstructing stone and renal colic (see eNursing Care Plan 46-2). To ensure that any spontaneously passed stones are retrieved, strain all urine voided by the patient using a gauze or a urine strainer. Encourage ambulation to promote movement of the stone from the upper to the lower urinary tract. To ensure safety, tell the patient not to walk unattended while experiencing acute renal colic, particularly if opioid analgesics are being given.

EVALUATION

The expected outcomes are that the patient with urinary calculi will

- Maintain free flow of urine with minimal hematuria
- Report satisfactory pain relief
- Verbalize understanding of disease process and measures to prevent recurrence

Additional information on expected outcomes for the patient with urinary calculi is presented in eNursing Care Plan 46-2 (on the website for this chapter).

STRICTURES

A **stricture** is a narrowing of the lumen of the ureter or urethra.

Ureteral Strictures

Ureteral strictures can affect the entire length of the ureter, from the UPJ to the UVJ. These strictures are usually an unintended result of surgical intervention or secondary to adhesions or scar formation, or they may be due to extrinsic factors such as large tumors in the peritoneal cavity. Depending on its severity, ureteral obstruction can threaten the function of the kidney.

Clinical manifestations of a ureteral stricture include mild to moderate colic. This pain may be moderate to severe in intensity if the patient consumes a large volume of fluids (such as alcohol) over a brief period. Infection is unusual unless a calculus or foreign object such as a stent or nephrostomy tube is present.

The discomfort and obstruction of a ureteral stricture may be temporarily bypassed by placing a stent using endoscopy or by diverting urinary flow via a nephrostomy tube inserted into the renal pelvis of the affected kidney. Definitive correction requires dilation with a balloon or catheter. If the stricture is severe or recurs after initial balloon or catheter dilation, it is surgically incised using an endoscopic procedure *(endoureterotomy)*. In selected cases an open surgical approach may be required to excise the stenotic area and reanastomose the ureter to the contralateral ureter *(ureteroureterostomy)* or to the renal pelvis. Alternatively, distal ureteral strictures may be treated by a *ureteroneocystostomy* (reimplantation of the ureter into the bladder wall).

Urethral Strictures

A *urethral stricture* is the result of fibrosis or inflammation of the urethral lumen. Causes of urethral strictures include trauma, urethritis (particularly after gonococcal infection), surgical intervention or repeated catheterizations (iatrogenic), or a congenital defect of the urethra. Once the process of inflammation and fibrosis begins, the lumen of the urethra narrows, and its compliance (ability to close or open in response to bladder filling or micturition) is compromised. Meatal stenosis, a narrowing of the urethral opening, is also common.

Clinical manifestations associated with a urethral stricture include a diminished force of the urinary stream, straining to void, sprayed stream, postvoid dribbling, or a split urine stream. The patient may report feelings of incomplete bladder emptying with urinary frequency and nocturia. Moderate to severe obstruction of the bladder outlet may lead to acute urinary retention. The patient may report a history of urethritis, difficulty with insertion of a urinary catheter, or trauma involving the penis or the perineum. However, many patients are unable to recall any such events, thus leading to a diagnosis of an idiopathic stricture. A history of UTI is common, particularly if the stricture involves the distal urethra. Retrograde urethrography (RUG) and VCUG are used to identify stricture length, location, and caliber.

Initial management of a stricture is focused on dilation. A metal instrument (urethral sound) may be placed, or a series of progressively large stents (filiforms and followers) can be placed into the urethra to expand its lumen in a stepwise fashion. Although this process is initially successful, stenosis frequently recurs. Recurrences may be managed by teaching the patient to repeatedly dilate the urethra by self-catheterization using a soft (coudé-tip, red rubber) catheter every few days. Alternatively, an endoscopic or open surgical procedure *(urethroplasty)* may be a more definitive therapy for an obstructive urethral stricture. Shorter strictures may be treated by resection of the fibrotic area followed by reanastomosis of the urethra. Longer strictures may require the use of a skin flap as a substitute urethral segment.

RENAL TRAUMA

Renal trauma can be blunt or penetrating. *Blunt trauma* is the most common cause. Injury to the kidney should be considered in sports injuries, motor vehicle collisions, and falls. Renal trauma is especially likely when the patient injures the abdomen, flank, or back. *Penetrating injuries* may result from violent encounters (e.g., gunshot or stabbing incidents). The majority of incidents occur in men younger than 30 years of age.

Clinical findings include a history of trauma to the area of the kidneys. Gross or microscopic hematuria may be present.

Diagnostic studies include urinalysis, ultrasound, CT, or MRI evaluation. Renal arteriography may also be used. Both the injured kidney and the uninvolved kidney should be evaluated. The severity of renal trauma depends on the extent of the injury. Treatments range from bed rest, fluids, and analgesia to exploratory surgery and repair or nephrectomy.

Nursing interventions depend on the type of renal trauma and the extent of any associated injuries. Interventions related to renal trauma include the following: (1) assess the cardiovascular status and monitor for shock, especially in a penetrating injury; (2) ensure adequate fluid intake and monitor intake and output; (3) provide for pain relief and comfort measures; and (4) assess for hematuria and myoglobinuria.

RENAL VASCULAR PROBLEMS

Vascular problems involving the kidney include (1) nephrosclerosis, (2) renal artery stenosis, and (3) renal vein thrombosis.

NEPHROSCLEROSIS

Nephrosclerosis is sclerosis of the small arteries and arterioles of the kidney. The decreased blood flow results in ischemia and necrosis of parts of the kidney. *Benign nephrosclerosis,* which usually occurs in adults 30 to 50 years of age, is caused by vascular changes resulting from hypertension and from the atherosclerosis process. Atherosclerotic vascular changes account for most of the loss of renal function associated with aging. The degree of nephrosclerosis is directly related to the severity of hypertension. In the early stages, the patient with benign nephrosclerosis may have normal renal function, with the only detectable abnormality being hypertension.

Accelerated nephrosclerosis (malignant nephrosclerosis) is associated with malignant hypertension, which is characterized by a sharp increase in BP with a diastolic pressure greater than 130 mm Hg. The patient is usually a young adult, with a male-to-female predominance of 2:1. Renal insufficiency progresses rapidly.

Treatment for benign nephrosclerosis is the same as that for essential hypertension (see Chapter 33). Malignant nephrosclerosis is treated with aggressive antihypertensive therapy (see Chapter 33). The availability and use of antihypertensive drugs have improved the prognosis for patients with benign and malignant nephrosclerosis. Kidney disease, and subsequent renal failure, is a major complication of hypertension. The prognosis for a patient with untreated or refractory malignant hypertension is poor, with the major cause of death related to renal failure.

RENAL ARTERY STENOSIS

Renal artery stenosis is a partial occlusion of one or both renal arteries and their major branches. It can be due to atherosclerotic narrowing or fibromuscular hyperplasia. Renal artery stenosis, which accounts for 1% to 2% of all cases of hypertension, is a cause of secondary hypertension.

When hypertension develops rather abruptly, renal artery stenosis should be considered as a possible cause, especially in patients under 30 or over 50 years of age and in patients with no family history of hypertension. This contrasts with the age distribution for primary hypertension, which is 30 to 50 years of age. Diagnostic tests used to assess for renal artery stenosis

include a renal ultrasound, CT scan, MRI scan, and renal arteriogram (the best diagnostic tool).

The goals of therapy are to control the BP and restore perfusion to the kidney. Percutaneous transluminal renal angioplasty is the procedure of choice, especially in older patients who are poor surgical risks. Surgical revascularization of the kidney is indicated when decreased blood flow causes renal ischemia or when renovascular hypertension is present. Revascularization of the kidney may result in the patient becoming normotensive. The surgical procedure usually involves anastomoses between the kidney and another major artery, usually the splenic artery or aorta. In selected cases of unilateral renal involvement, unilateral nephrectomy may be indicated.

RENAL VEIN THROMBOSIS

Renal vein thrombosis may occur unilaterally or bilaterally. Causes include trauma, extrinsic compression (e.g., tumor, aortic aneurysm), renal cell cancer, pregnancy, contraceptive use, and nephrotic syndrome.

The patient has symptoms of flank pain, hematuria, or fever or has nephrotic syndrome. Anticoagulation (e.g., heparin, warfarin [Coumadin]) is important to treat the high incidence of pulmonary emboli. Corticosteroids may be used for the patient with nephrotic syndrome. Surgical thrombectomy may be performed instead of or along with anticoagulation.

HEREDITARY KIDNEY DISEASES

Hereditary kidney (or renal) diseases involve developmental abnormalities of the renal parenchyma. Most inherited structural abnormalities are cystic. However, cysts may also develop as a result of obstructive uropathies, metabolic problems, or neurologic diseases. Cysts may be evaluated to rule out tumors.

POLYCYSTIC KIDNEY DISEASE

Polycystic kidney disease (PKD) is the most common life-threatening genetic disease in the world, affecting 600,000 people in the United States. PKD accounts for 10% to 15% of chronic kidney disease.[26]

 Genetic Link

PKD has two hereditary forms: it may be manifested in childhood or adulthood. The childhood form of PKD is a rare autosomal recessive disorder that is often rapidly progressive (see the Genetics in Clinical Practice box). The adult form of PKD is an autosomal dominant disorder (see Figs. 13-4 and 13-5). If one parent has the disease, there is a 50% chance that the disease will pass to the child.

Adult PKD is latent for many years and is usually manifested between 30 and 40 years of age. It involves both kidneys and occurs in both men and women. The cortex and the medulla are filled with large, thin-walled cysts that are several millimeters to several centimeters in diameter (Fig. 46-7). The cysts enlarge and destroy surrounding tissue by compression. The cysts are filled with fluid and may contain blood or pus. PKD kidneys examined during autopsy appear as if they are filled with golf balls.

Early in the disease patients are generally asymptomatic. Symptoms appear when the cysts begin to enlarge. Often the first manifestations of PKD are hypertension; hematuria (from

Polycystic Kidney Disease (PKD)

	Adult	Child
Genetic basis	• Autosomal dominant	• Autosomal recessive
Incidence	• 1 in 400-1000	• 1 in 10,000-20,000
Gene location	• *PKD1* gene on chromosome 16 and *PKD2* gene on chromosome 4 • Genes code for polycystins (proteins that promote normal kidney development and function) • Mutations in genes lead to formation of thousands of cysts that disrupt the normal function of kidneys and other organs	• Polycystic kidney and hepatic disease *(PKHD1)* gene on chromosome 6 • Gene codes for fibrocystin • Mutations in gene leads to cyst formation
Genetic testing	• DNA testing available	• DNA testing available*
Age of onset	• Ages 30-40	• Infancy or childhood
Clinical implications	• Multisystem involvement • Systemic hypertension occurs in 60%-80% of patients • Increased risk for cerebral aneurysms • Families at risk should be screened	• Up to 30%-50% of affected newborns die shortly after birth • If infant survives the newborn period, chances of survival are good, but about one third need dialysis or transplantation by age 10 yr

*Genetic testing is also available on fertilized embryos before implantation. This allows embryos free of the disorder to be placed into the uterus.

FIG. 46-7 A, Comparison of polycystic kidney with normal kidney. **B,** Cysts in the liver.

rupture of cysts); or a feeling of heaviness in the back, side, or abdomen. However, the first manifestations can also be a UTI or urinary calculi. Chronic pain is one of the most common problems experienced by individuals with PKD. The pain can be constant and severe. Bilateral, enlarged kidneys are often palpable on physical examination. Many people have no symptoms, and the disease is not diagnosed.

PKD can also affect the liver (liver cysts [see Fig. 46-7]), heart (abnormal heart valves), blood vessels (aneurysms), and intestines (diverticulosis). The most serious complication is a cerebral aneurysm, which can rupture.

Diagnosis is based on clinical manifestations, family history, ultrasound (best screening measure), or CT scan. The disease usually progresses from loss of kidney function to ESKD by age 60 in 50% of patients.[27]

NURSING AND COLLABORATIVE MANAGEMENT
POLYCYSTIC KIDNEY DISEASE

There is no specific treatment for PKD. A major aim of treatment is to prevent or treat infections of the urinary tract. Nephrectomy may be necessary if pain, bleeding, or infection becomes a chronic, serious problem. Dialysis and kidney transplant may be needed to treat ESKD (see Chapter 47).

When the patient begins to experience progressive renal failure, the interventions depend on the remaining renal function. Nursing measures are those used for management of ESKD. They include diet modification, fluid restriction, drugs (e.g., antihypertensives), and assistance for the patient and family in coping with the chronic disease process and financial concerns.

The patient who has adult PKD often has children by the time the disease is diagnosed. The patient needs appropriate counseling regarding plans for having more children. In addition, genetic counseling should be provided for the children.

MEDULLARY CYSTIC DISEASE

Medullary cystic disease is a hereditary disorder that occurs in two forms. The *autosomal recessive form* is associated with renal failure before age 20. The *autosomal dominant form* is associated with renal failure after age 20.

Most cysts are located in the medulla. The kidneys are asymmetric in shape and are significantly scarred. Defects in the kidneys' concentrating ability result in polyuria. Other clinical manifestations include hypertension, progressive renal failure, severe anemia, and metabolic acidosis. Genetic counseling may be helpful in family planning. Treatment measures are those related to ESKD (see Chapter 47).

ALPORT SYNDROME

Alport syndrome, also known as *chronic hereditary nephritis,* has two forms: (1) classic Alport syndrome, which is inherited as a sex-linked disorder with hematuria, sensorineural deafness, and deformities of the anterior surface of the lens; and (2) nonclassic Alport syndrome, which is inherited as an autosomal disorder that causes hematuria but not deafness or lens deformities.

Men are affected earlier and more severely than women. The disease is often diagnosed in the first decade of life. The basic defect is a mutation in a gene for collagen that results in altered synthesis of the GBM. Most commonly the patient has hematuria and progressive uremia. Treatment is supportive. Corticosteroids and cytotoxic drugs are not effective. The disease does not recur after kidney transplantation.

URINARY TRACT TUMORS

KIDNEY CANCER

Kidney cancers arise from the cortex or pelvis (and calyces). Tumors from these areas may be benign or malignant. However, malignant tumors are more common. In the United States, about 65,000 new cases of kidney cancer are diagnosed each year and about 13,570 people die from kidney cancer. The incidence of kidney cancer is increasing, but the reason for this is not known.[28]

Renal cell carcinoma (adenocarcinoma) is the most common type of kidney cancer (Fig. 46-8). This type of tumor occurs twice as often in men as in women and is typically discovered when the person is 50 to 70 years of age. Cigarette smoking is the most significant risk factor for the development of renal cell carcinoma. An increased incidence has also been found in first-degree relatives of people who have or had renal cell carcinoma. Other risk factors include obesity; hypertension; and exposure to asbestos, cadmium, and gasoline. Risk for kidney cancer is also increased in individuals who have acquired cystic disease of the kidney associated with ESKD (see Chapter 47).[29]

Clinical Manifestations and Diagnostic Studies

Kidney cancer has no characteristic early symptoms, so many patients go undiagnosed until the disease has significantly progressed. Kidney tumors can cause symptoms by compressing, stretching, or invading structures near or within the kidney. The most common presenting manifestations are hematuria, flank pain, and a palpable mass in the flank or abdomen. Other clinical manifestations include weight loss, fever, hypertension, and anemia.

About 30% of patients have metastasis at the time of diagnosis. Local extension of kidney cancer into the renal vein and vena cava is common (see Fig. 46-8). The most common sites of metastases include lungs, liver, and long bones. Many kidney cancers are diagnosed as incidental findings on imaging studies used to evaluate symptoms for unrelated conditions.

CT scan is commonly used in the diagnosis and can detect small kidney tumors. Ultrasound examinations have improved

FIG. 46-8 Cross section of kidney with renal cell carcinoma. The carcinoma *(black arrow)* is on the pole of the kidney. Note that the renal vein is involved and thrombosed *(white arrow)*.

the ability to differentiate between a solid mass tumor and a cyst. This is significant because the majority of masses detected on imaging are cysts. Angiography, biopsy, and MRI are also used in the diagnosis of renal tumors. Radionuclide isotope scanning is used to detect metastases.

NURSING AND COLLABORATIVE MANAGEMENT KIDNEY CANCER

Preventive measures, such as quitting smoking, maintaining a healthy weight, controlling BP, and reducing or avoiding exposure to toxins, can help reduce the incidence of kidney cancer. Patients in high-risk groups should be aware of their increased risk for kidney cancer. Teach them about early symptoms (e.g., hematuria, hypertension). A cure for kidney cancer is possible when it is detected early and treated.

Collaborative care of the patient with kidney cancer is presented in Table 46-14. Staging of renal carcinoma provides a basis for determining treatment options. A detailed listing of staging is presented in eTable 46-1 (on the website for this chapter). The following is a simple description of staging of kidney cancer:

Stage I: The tumor can be up to 7 cm in diameter but is confined to the kidney.
Stage II: The tumor is larger than a stage I tumor, but is still confined to the kidney.
Stage III: The tumor extends beyond the kidney to the surrounding tissue and may also have spread to a nearby lymph node.
Stage IV: Cancer spreads outside the kidney to multiple lymph nodes or to distant parts of the body, such as bones, brain, liver, or lung.

The treatment of choice for some renal cancers is a partial nephrectomy (for smaller tumors) or a radical nephrectomy (for larger tumors). Radical nephrectomy involves removal of the kidney, adrenal gland, surrounding fascia, part of the ureter, and draining lymph nodes. Nephrectomy can be performed by a conventional (open) approach or laparoscopically (see discussion of nephrectomy on p. 1095). Radiation therapy is used palliatively in inoperable cases and when there is metastasis to bone or lungs.

Other treatment options include cryoablation (freezing technique) and radiofrequency ablation (destroying tumor by using radiofrequency heat). These procedures can be used when surgery is not an option (e.g., patient has co-morbid conditions).

Chemotherapy is used as a treatment in metastatic disease. These drugs include 5-fluorouracil (5-FU), floxuridine (FUDR),

TABLE 46-14 **COLLABORATIVE CARE**
Renal Cell Carcinoma

Diagnostic	Collaborative Therapy
• History and physical examination	• Surgical treatment
• Urinalysis	• Partial nephrectomy
• Ultrasound	• Radical nephrectomy
• CT scan	• Ablation
• MRI	• Cryoablation
• Renal biopsy	• Radiofrequency ablation
• Renal scan	• Radiation therapy
• Angiography	• Chemotherapy
	• Biologic therapy
	• Targeted therapy

and gemcitabine (Gemzar). However, renal cell carcinoma is refractory to most chemotherapy drugs.

Biologic therapy, including α-interferon and interleukin-2 (IL-2), is another treatment in metastatic disease. (The use of α-interferon and IL-2 is discussed in Chapter 16.)

Targeted therapy is the preferred treatment for metastatic kidney cancer. Kinase inhibitors, one class of targeted therapies, block certain proteins (kinases) that play a role in tumor growth and cancer progression. Kinase inhibitors include sunitinib (Sutent), sorafenib (Nexavar), and axitinib (Inlyta). Bevacizumab (Avastin) and pazopanib (Votrient) inhibit the formation of new blood vessel growth to the tumor. Temsirolimus (Torisel) and everolimus (Afinitor) inhibit a specific protein known as the mammalian target of rapamycin (mTOR). These drugs are presented in Table 16-13, and the mechanisms of action are shown in Fig. 16-16.

The diagnosis of cancer is a shock. In kidney cancer the disease can already be metastasized by the time a person is diagnosed. (The nursing care of the patient with cancer is discussed in Chapter 16.)

BLADDER CANCER

About 73,000 new cases of bladder cancer are diagnosed annually, and about 15,000 deaths related to bladder cancer occur every year.[28] Bladder cancer accounts for nearly 1 in every 20 cancers diagnosed in the United States. The most frequent malignant tumor of the urinary tract is transitional cell carcinoma of the bladder. Most bladder tumors are papillomatous growths within the bladder (Fig. 46-9).

Cancer of the bladder is most common between ages 60 and 70 years and is at least three times more common in men than in women. Risk factors for bladder cancer include cigarette smoking, exposure to dyes used in the rubber and other industries, and chronic abuse of phenacetin-containing analgesics. Phenacetin, once a popular analgesic, has been removed from the market. Women treated with radiation for cervical cancer, patients who received cyclophosphamide, and patients who take the diabetes drug pioglitazone (Actos) also have an increased risk for bladder cancer.

FIG. 46-9 A, Papillary transitional cell carcinoma *(T)* seen arising from the dome of the bladder as a cauliflower-like lesion *(arrow).* **B,** Opened bladder showing bladder cancer at an advanced stage. Yellow areas represent ulcerations and necrosis *(arrows).*

Individuals with chronic, recurrent renal calculi (often bladder) and chronic lower UTIs have an increased risk of squamous cell cancer of the bladder. Patients who have indwelling catheters for long periods are also at an increased risk to develop bladder cancer.

Clinical Manifestations and Diagnostic Studies

Microscopic or gross, painless hematuria (chronic or intermittent) is the most common clinical manifestation of bladder cancer. Bladder irritability with dysuria, frequency, and urgency may also occur. When cancer is suspected, obtain urine specimens to identify any neoplastic or atypical cells. Exfoliated cells from the bladder's epithelial surface can be detected in voided specimens. Other urine tests assess for specific factors associated with bladder cancer, such as bladder tumor antigens.

Bladder cancers can be detected using CT, ultrasound, or MRI. The presence of cancer is confirmed by cystoscopy and biopsy. Cystoscopy with biopsy is the most reliable test for detecting bladder tumors.

NURSING AND COLLABORATIVE MANAGEMENT BLADDER CANCER

The majority of bladder cancers are diagnosed at an early stage when the cancer is treatable. Before a treatment regimen is started, bladder cancers are graded based on the cell type and staged based on the extent and invasiveness of the cancer. A grading system is used to classify the malignant potential of tumor cells, using a scale from well differentiated (closely resembling the normal tissue) to undifferentiated (poorly differentiated) (see p. 254 in Chapter 16).

The clinical staging of bladder cancer is determined by the depth of invasion of the bladder wall and surrounding tissue. Staging of bladder cancer is presented in detail in eTable 46-2 (on the website for this chapter). The following is a simple description of staging of bladder cancer:

Stage I: Cancer is in the inner lining of the bladder but has not invaded the bladder muscle wall.

Stage II: Cancer has invaded the bladder wall but is still confined to bladder.

Stage III: Cancer has spread through the bladder wall to surrounding tissue. It may also have spread to the prostate in men or the uterus or vagina in women.

Stage IV: Cancer has spread to the lymph nodes and other organs, such as lungs, bones, or liver.

Eighty percent of bladder tumors are *superficial,* meaning they do not invade the bladder wall. Low-grade, low-stage bladder cancers are the most responsive to treatment, which includes instillation of intravesical chemotherapy. Although patients with superficial tumors are more easily cured, periodic surveillance is important, since two thirds of patients have tumor recurrence within 5 years and nearly 95% have recurrence by 15 years.

Collaborative care of bladder cancer includes surgery, radiation, chemotherapy, and intravesical therapy (Table 46-15).

SURGICAL THERAPY

Surgical therapies include a variety of procedures. *Transurethral resection of the bladder tumor* (TURBT) is used for superficial lesions of the bladder's inner lining. A wire loop inserted through the cystoscope is used to cauterize (with electric current or laser) and kill the cancer cells. This procedure is also used to

TABLE 46-15 COLLABORATIVE CARE
Bladder Cancer

Diagnostic	Collaborative Therapy

• History and physical examination
• Urinalysis
• Urine cytology studies
• Intravenous pyelogram (IVP)
• Cystoscopy with biopsy
• Ultrasound
• CT scan
	• Surgical treatment
	  • Transurethral resection with fulguration
	  • Laser photocoagulation
	  • Open loop resection with fulguration
	  • Cystectomy (segmental, partial, or radical)
	• Radiation therapy
	• Intravesical immunotherapy
	  • Bacille Calmette-Guérin (BCG)
	  • α-interferon (Roferon-A, Intron A)
	• Intravesical chemotherapy
	  • thiotepa (Thioplex)
	  • valrubicin (Valstar)
	• Systemic chemotherapy

control bleeding in the patient who is a poor operative risk or who has advanced tumors. The primary disadvantage of this approach is destruction of the tumor so pathologic evaluation for grading and staging cannot be completed.

A *segmental cystectomy (partial cystectomy)* is used to treat larger tumors or those that only involve one area of the bladder. A portion of the bladder wall containing the tumor is removed along with a margin of normal tissue.

When the tumor is invasive or involves the trigone (the area where the ureters insert into the bladder) and the patient is free from metastasis beyond the pelvic area, a radical cystectomy is the treatment of choice. A *radical cystectomy* involves removal of the bladder, prostate, and seminal vesicles in men and the bladder, uterus, cervix, urethra, and ovaries in women. After a radical cystectomy, a new way needs to be created for urine to leave the body. This surgical technique is called a urinary diversion (discussed on p. 1095 later in this chapter).

Postoperative instructions for any of these surgical procedures include drinking a large volume of fluid for the first week after the procedure. Teach the patient to self-monitor the color and consistency of the urine. The urine is pink for the first several days after the procedure, but it should not be bright red or contain blood clots. Approximately 7 to 10 days after tumor resection, the patient may observe dark red or rust-colored flecks in the urine. These may be from the healing tumor resection site.

Administer opioid analgesics for a brief period after the procedure, along with stool softeners. Also help the patient and family cope with fears about cancer, surgery, and sexuality. Emphasize the importance of regular follow-up care. Follow-up cystoscopies are required on a regular basis after surgery for bladder cancer.

RADIATION THERAPY AND CHEMOTHERAPY
Radiation therapy can be used in combination with cystectomy or as the primary therapy when the cancer is inoperable or the patient refuses surgery. Chemotherapy drugs used in treating invasive bladder cancer include cisplatin (Platinol), vinblastine (Velban), doxorubicin (Adriamycin), and methotrexate.

INTRAVESICAL THERAPY
Chemotherapy with local instillation of chemotherapeutic or immune-stimulating agents can be delivered directly into the

GENDER DIFFERENCES
Urinary Incontinence

Men	Women
• Urinary incontinence is a common manifestation of benign prostatic hyperplasia and prostate cancer in men. • Urinary incontinence in men most often is overflow incontinence caused by urinary retention.	• Prevalence of urinary incontinence is higher in women than men. • Women more frequently experience stress and urge incontinence than men.

bladder by a urethral catheter.[30] *Intravesical therapy* is usually initiated at weekly intervals for 6 to 12 weeks. The chemotherapy drug is instilled directly into the patient's bladder and retained for about 2 hours. The patient's bladder must be empty before instillation. Change the patient's position every 15 minutes for maximum contact in all areas of the bladder. Maintenance therapy after the initial induction regimen may be beneficial.

Bacille Calmette-Guérin (BCG), a weakened strain of *Mycobacterium bovis*, is the treatment of choice for carcinoma in situ. BCG stimulates the immune system rather than acting directly on cancer cells in the bladder. When BCG fails, α-interferon in addition to BCG may be used. Other treatments that can be used when BCG fails include thiotepa (Thioplex), an alkylating agent, and valrubicin (Valstar), a chemotherapy antibiotic.

Most patients have irritative voiding symptoms and hemorrhagic cystitis after intravesical therapy. Thiotepa can significantly reduce WBC and platelet counts in some individuals when absorbed into the circulation from the bladder wall. BCG may cause flu-like symptoms, increased urinary frequency, hematuria, or systemic infection. Other side effects of chemotherapy (e.g., nausea, vomiting, hair loss) are not experienced with intravesical chemotherapy.

Encourage patients to increase their daily fluid intake and to quit smoking. Assess the patient for secondary UTI, and stress the need for routine urologic follow-up. The patient may have fears or concerns about sexual activity or bladder function that need to be addressed. Because of the high rate of disease recurrence and progression in bladder cancer, follow-up studies are very important.

BLADDER DYSFUNCTION

URINARY INCONTINENCE

Urinary incontinence (UI) is an involuntary leakage of urine. Approximately 17 million people in the United States suffer from UI. The prevalence is 30% to 40% among young adult to middle-aged women, and increases to 30% to 50% in older women. In contrast, the incidence of UI in men tends to be considerably lower, ranging from 1% to 5% in young adult men and increasing to 9% to 34% in older men.[31] Although incontinence is more prevalent among older women and older men, it is not a natural consequence of aging. UI has traditionally been viewed as a social or hygienic problem, but it also has a major effect on quality of life and contributes to serious health problems, especially in older adults.

Etiology and Pathophysiology
UI occurs when bladder pressure exceeds urethral closure pressure. Anything that interferes with bladder or urethral sphincter

TABLE 46-16 DRUG THERAPY

Drugs Affecting Lower Urinary Tract Function

Drug	Effect
Alcohol	Polyuria, frequency, urgency, sedation, delirium
α-Adrenergic receptor agonists: pseudoephedrine (Sudafed), ephedrine	Urethral constriction and urinary retention (males)
α-Adrenergic receptor antagonists: prazosin (Minipress), terazosin (Hytrin), doxazosin (Cardura)	Urethral relaxation and stress urinary incontinence in females
ACE inhibitors: captopril (Capoten), lisinopril (Zestril), enalapril (Vasotec)	Cough triggering stress urinary incontinence
Anticholinergics: H$_1$-antihistamines, antiparkinsonian agents	Urinary retention, overflow incontinence, fecal impaction
Tricyclic antidepressants	Anticholinergic effect, α-adrenergic receptor antagonist effect
β-Adrenergic receptor antagonists: propranolol (Inderal), metoprolol (Toprol, Lopressor), atenolol (Tenormin)	Urinary retention
Calcium channel blockers: verapamil (Calan), diltiazem (Cardizem), nifedipine (Procardia)	Urinary retention, fecal impaction
Opioids	Urinary retention, fecal impaction, sedation, delirium
Sedative-hypnotics	Sedation, delirium, muscle relaxation
Diuretics: loop diuretics such as furosemide (Lasix)	Polyuria, frequency, urgency
Methylxanthines (caffeine, theophylline)	Polyuria, bladder irritation
Antiseizure agents: thioridazine (Mellaril), chlorpromazine (Thorazine)	Anticholinergic effect, sedation

ACE, Angiotensin-converting enzyme.

control can result in UI. Using the acronym *DRIP*, the causes can include *D:* delirium, dehydration, depression; *R:* restricted mobility, rectal impaction; *I:* infection, inflammation, impaction; and *P:* polyuria, polypharmacy. (Table 46-16 lists drugs that can affect the lower urinary tract.) Patients may have more than one type of incontinence (Table 46-17).

Diagnostic Studies

The basic evaluation for UI includes a focused history, a physical assessment, and a bladder log or voiding record whenever possible. Obtain information on the onset of UI, factors that provoke urinary leakage, and associated conditions. Pay special attention to factors known to produce transient UI, particularly when the onset of urine loss is relatively sudden. Begin the physical examination with an assessment of general health and functional issues associated with urination, including mobility, dexterity, and cognitive function.

A pelvic examination includes careful inspection of the perineal skin for signs of erosion or rashes related to UI and existence of pelvic organ prolapse. Also evaluate local innervation and pelvic floor muscle strength, including a digital examination of the pelvic floor muscle to determine weakness or tension. Whenever possible, ask the patient to keep a bladder log or

COMPLEMENTARY & ALTERNATIVE THERAPIES

Biofeedback

Scientific Evidence
Biofeedback has been shown to be helpful in treating a variety of medical conditions: urinary incontinence, asthma, Raynaud's disease, irritable bowel syndrome, hot flashes, nausea and vomiting associated with chemotherapy, headaches, hypertension, and seizure disorders.*

Nursing Implications
- Feedback from monitoring equipment can teach patients to control certain involuntary body responses, such as urinary incontinence.
- Although biofeedback is considered safe, patients should consult a qualified professional before using biofeedback.

*Based on a systematic review of scientific literature. Retrieved from *www. naturalstandard.com.*

voiding diary documenting the timing of urinations, episodes of urinary leakage, and frequency of nocturia for a period of 1 to 7 days. This record can be kept by nursing staff if the person is in an inpatient or long-term care facility.

A urinalysis is used to identify possible factors contributing to transient UI (e.g., UTI, diabetes mellitus). Measure postvoid residual (PVR) urine in the patient undergoing evaluation for UI. The PVR volume is obtained by asking the patient to urinate, followed by catheterization or use of a bladder ultrasound within a relatively brief period (preferably 10 to 20 minutes).

Urodynamic testing is indicated in selected cases of UI. Imaging studies of the upper urinary tract (e.g., ultrasound) are obtained when UI is associated with UTIs or evidence of upper urinary tract involvement.

Collaborative Care

An estimated 80% of incontinence can be cured or significantly improved.[32] Transient, reversible factors are corrected initially, followed by management of the type of UI (see Table 46-17). In general, less invasive treatments are attempted before more invasive methods (e.g., surgery). Nevertheless, the choice of the initial treatment is individualized, based on patient preference, the type and severity of UI, and associated anatomic defects.

Several behavioral therapies may be used to improve UI (Table 46-18). Pelvic floor muscle training (Kegel exercises) is used to manage stress, urge, or mixed UI (Table 46-19). Biofeedback is used to help the patient identify, isolate, contract, and relax the pelvic muscles (see the Complementary & Alternative Therapies box on this page).

Drug Therapy. Drug therapy varies according to the UI type (Table 46-20 on p. 1091). In stress UI, drugs have a limited role in the management. α-Adrenergic agonists can be used to increase bladder sphincter tone and urethral resistance, but have limited benefit.

In urge and reflex UI, drugs play a key management role. Anticholinergic drugs and muscarinic receptor antagonists relax the bladder muscle and inhibit overactive detrusor contractions. Several preparations of these drugs are available, including immediate and extended-release tolterodine (Detrol, Detrol LA); immediate, extended-release, and transdermal oxybutynin (Ditropan XL, Oxytrol Transdermal System [also available over-the-counter]); twice-daily trospium chloride (Sanctura); extended-release solifenacin (VESIcare); darifenacin (Enablex); and fesoterodine (Toviaz). Side effects of these drugs include dry mouth, dry eyes, constipation, blurred vision, and somnolence.

TABLE 46-17	**TYPES OF URINARY INCONTINENCE**	
Description	**Causes**	**Treatment**
Stress Incontinence* Sudden increase in intraabdominal pressure causes involuntary passage of urine. Can occur during coughing, laughing, sneezing, or physical activities such as heavy lifting, exercising. Leakage usually is in small amounts and may not be daily.	Found most commonly in women with relaxed pelvic floor musculature (from delivery, use of instrumentation during vaginal delivery, or multiple pregnancies). Structures of the female urethra atrophy when estrogen decreases. Prostate surgery for BPH or prostate cancer.	Pelvic floor muscle exercises (e.g., Kegel exercises), weight loss if patient is obese, cessation of smoking, topical estrogen products, external condom catheters or penile clamp in men, surgery Urethral inserts, patches, or bladder neck support devices (e.g., incontinence pessary) to correct underlying problem
Urge Incontinence* Condition occurs randomly when involuntary urination is preceded by urinary urgency. Seen with overactive bladder symptoms of urgency and frequency. Leakage is periodic but frequent and usually in large amounts. Nocturnal frequency and incontinence are common.	Condition is caused by uncontrolled contraction or overactivity of detrusor muscle. Bladder escapes central inhibition and contracts reflexively. Conditions include: • Central nervous system disorders (e.g., cerebrovascular disease, Alzheimer's disease, brain tumor, Parkinson's disease) • Bladder disorders (e.g., carcinoma in situ, radiation effects, interstitial cystitis) • Interference with spinal inhibitory pathways (e.g., malignant growth in spinal cord, spondylosis) • Bladder outlet obstruction or conditions of unknown etiology	Treatment of underlying cause Biobehavioral interventions, including bladder retraining with urge suppression, decrease in dietary irritants, bowel regularity, and pelvic floor muscle exercises Anticholinergic drugs (e.g., oxybutynin [Ditropan XL, Oxytrol], tolterodine [Detrol, Detrol LA], trospium chloride [Sanctura], solifenacin [VESIcare], and darifenacin [Enablex]); imipramine (Tofranil) at bedtime; calcium channel blockers Containment devices (e.g., external condom catheters) Vaginal estrogen creams Absorbent products
Overflow Incontinence Condition occurs when the pressure of urine in overfull bladder overcomes sphincter control. Leakage of small amounts of urine is frequent throughout the day and night. Urination may also occur frequently in small amounts. Bladder remains distended and is usually palpable.	Disorder is caused by bladder or urethral outlet obstruction (bladder neck obstruction, urethral stricture, pelvic organ prolapse) or by underactive detrusor muscle caused by myogenic or neurogenic factors (e.g., herniated disc, diabetic neuropathy). May also occur after anesthesia and surgery (e.g., hemorrhoidectomy, herniorrhaphy, cystoscopy). Neurogenic bladder (flaccid type).	Urinary catheterization to decompress bladder Implementation of Credé or Valsalva maneuver α-Adrenergic blocker (doxazosin [Cardura], terazosin [Hytrin], tamsulosin [Flomax], alfuzosin [Uroxatral]) 5α-Reductase inhibitors (e.g., finasteride [Proscar]) to decrease outlet resistance bethanechol (Urecholine) to enhance bladder contractions Intravaginal device such as a pessary to support prolapse Intermittent catheterization Surgery to correct underlying problem
Reflex Incontinence Condition occurs when no warning or stress precedes periodic involuntary urination. Urination is frequent, is moderate in volume, and occurs equally during the day and night.	Spinal cord lesion above S2 interferes with central nervous system inhibition. Disorder results in detrusor hyperreflexia and interferes with pathways coordinating detrusor contraction and sphincter relaxation.	Treatment of underlying cause Bladder decompression to prevent ureteral reflux and hydronephrosis Intermittent self-catheterization diazepam (Valium) or baclofen (Lioresal) to relax external sphincter Prophylactic antibiotics Surgical sphincterotomy
Incontinence After Trauma or Surgery In women, vesicovaginal or urethrovaginal fistula may occur. In men, alteration in continence control involves proximal urethral sphincter (bladder neck and prostatic urethra) and distal urethral sphincter (external striated muscle).	Fistulas may occur during pregnancy, after delivery of baby, as a result of hysterectomy or invasive cancer of cervix, or after radiation therapy. Incontinence is a postoperative complication of transurethral, perineal, or retropubic prostatectomy.	Surgery to correct fistula Urinary diversion surgery to bypass urethra and bladder External condom catheter Penile clamp Placement of artificial implantable sphincter
Functional Incontinence Loss of urine resulting from cognitive, functional, or environmental factors.	Older adults often have problems that affect balance and mobility.	Modifications of environment or care plan that facilitates regular, easy access to toilet and promotes patient safety (e.g., better lighting, removal of scatter rugs, ambulatory assistance equipment, clothing alterations, timed voiding, different toileting equipment)

*Patients can have a combination of stress and urge incontinence, referred to as mixed incontinence.

Botox (onabotulinumtoxin A) can be used in the treatment of UI as a result of detrusor overactivity. Botox is injected into the bladder, resulting in relaxation of the bladder, an increase in its storage capacity, and a decrease in UI.

DRUG ALERT: Tolterodine (Detrol)
- Overdosage can result in severe anticholinergic effects.
- These effects include GI cramping, diaphoresis, blurred vision, and urinary urgency.

Surgical Therapy. Surgical techniques also vary depending on the type of UI. Surgical correction of stress UI is aimed at making the urinary structures more receptive to intraabdominal pressure and augmenting the urethral resistance of the internal sphincter. It may involve repositioning the urethra and/or creating a backboard of support to stabilize the urethra and bladder neck and make them more receptive to changes in intraabdominal pressure. Another technique for stress UI augments the urethral resistance of the intrinsic sphincter with a sling or periurethral injectables.

Retropubic colposuspension and pubovaginal sling placement appear to be most effective. Typically, both procedures are performed through low transverse incisions. Complications specific to the retropubic suspensions include postoperative voiding dysfunction, urgency, and vaginal prolapse.

Placement of a suburethral sling, using the person's own fascia, cadaveric fascia, or a synthetic material, is also used to correct stress UI in women. Complications include vascular and bowel injury, urinary retention, mesh or sling erosion, infection, urgency, and bladder perforation. Suburethral slings have success rates comparable to those of colposuspensions or slings and are associated with shorter recovery periods. An artificial urethral sphincter can be used in men with intrinsic sphincter deficiency and severe stress UI.

Alternatively, one of several bulking agents can be injected underneath the mucosa of the urethra to correct stress UI in women or men. Bulking agents include glutaraldehyde cross-linked bovine collagen (GAX collagen), small silicone beads (Durasphere), or polytetrafluoroethylene (Teflon). Because of the risk of migration of Teflon particles, GAX collagen or Durasphere injections are most commonly used today. Although treatment with suburethral compounds avoids the risk associated with open surgery, reinjection is typically required after several years.

Injecting autologous stem cells into the rhabdosphincter and urethral submucosa of women is a recent experimental therapy for stress UI. This technique increases urethral closure pressure and periurethral electromyography activity. However, the injection requires use of transurethral ultrasonography for correct placement of the stem cells.[33]

NURSING MANAGEMENT
URINARY INCONTINENCE

It is important to recognize both the physical and the emotional problems associated with UI. Maintain and enhance the patient's dignity, privacy, and feelings of self-worth. This is a two-step approach: (1) containment devices to manage existing urinary leakage and (2) a definitive plan to reduce or resolve the factors leading to UI.

Management options are reviewed in Tables 46-18 and 46-19. They include lifestyle interventions such as teaching the patient about consumption of an adequate volume of fluids and reduction or elimination of bladder irritants (particularly

TABLE 46-18	INTERVENTIONS FOR URINARY INCONTINENCE
Intervention	**Description**
Lifestyle Modifications	Self-management strategies to reduce or eliminate risk factors, including the following: • Smoking cessation • Weight reduction • Good bowel regimen • Reduction of bladder irritants (e.g., caffeine, aspartame artificial sweetener, citrus juices) • Fluid modifications for those with urge incontinence
Scheduled Voiding Regimens	
Timed voiding	Toileting on a fixed schedule (typically every 2-3 hr during waking hours).
Habit retraining	Scheduled toileting with adjustments of voiding intervals (longer or shorter) based on the individual's voiding pattern.
Prompted voiding	Scheduled toileting that requires prompts to void from a caregiver (typically every 3 hr). Used in conjunction with operant conditioning techniques to reward individuals for maintaining continence and appropriate toileting.
Bladder retraining and urge-suppression strategies	Scheduled toileting with progressive voiding intervals. Includes teaching of urge-control strategies using relaxation and distraction techniques, self-monitoring, reinforcement techniques, and other strategies such as conscious contraction of pelvic floor muscles.
Pelvic Floor Muscle Rehabilitation	
Pelvic floor muscle (Kegel) exercises or training	See Table 46-19.
Vaginal weight training	Active retention of increasing vaginal weights at least twice a day. Typically used in combination with pelvic floor muscle exercises.
Biofeedback	See Complementary & Alternative Therapies box on p. 1087.
Electrical stimulation	Application of low-voltage electric current to sacral and pudendal afferent fibers through vaginal, anal, or surface electrodes. Used to inhibit bladder overactivity and improve awareness, contractility, and efficiency of pelvic muscle contraction.
Anti-Incontinence Devices	
Intravaginal support devices (pessaries and bladder neck support prostheses)	Devices support bladder neck, relieve minor pelvic organ prolapse, and change pressure transmission to the urethra.
Intraurethral occlusive device (urethral plug)	Single-use device that is worn in the urethra to provide mechanical obstruction to prevent urine leakage. Removed for voiding.
Penile compression device	Mechanical fixed compression applied to the penis to prevent any flow or leakage via the urethra. Must be released hourly to void.
Containment Devices	
External collection devices	External catheter (condom) systems (e.g., penile sheaths) direct urine into a drainage bag. Most commonly used by men.
Absorbent products	Variety of reusable and disposable pads and undergarment systems.

TABLE 46-19   PATIENT TEACHING GUIDE

Pelvic Floor Muscle (Kegel) Exercises

Include the following instructions when teaching the patient to perform Kegel exercises.

What Is the Pelvic Floor Muscle?

- Your pelvic floor muscle provides support for your bladder and rectum and, in women, the vagina and the uterus.
- If it weakens or is damaged, it cannot support these organs and their position can change.
- This causes problems with the normal bladder and rectal function.
- If you have a weak pelvic floor muscle, you might want to do special exercises to make the muscle stronger, prevent unwanted urine leakage, and lessen urinary urgency.

Finding the Pelvic Floor Muscle

- Without tensing the muscles of your leg, buttocks, or abdomen, imagine that you are trying to control the passing of gas or pinching off a stool.
- Or imagine you are in an elevator full of people and you feel the urge to pass gas. What do you do?
- You tighten or pull in the ring of muscle around your rectum—your pelvic floor muscle.
- You should feel a lifting sensation in the area around the vagina or a pulling in of your rectum.

How to Do the Exercises

There are two different kinds of exercises—short squeezes and long squeezes.

1. To do the *short squeezes,* tighten your pelvic floor muscle quickly, squeeze hard for 2 sec, and then relax the muscle. Also, when you have strong urinary urges, try to tighten your pelvic floor muscle quickly and hard several times in a row until the urge passes.
2. To do the *long squeezes,* tighten the muscle for 5-10 sec before you relax.

Do both of these exercises 40-50 times each day.

When to Do These Exercises

- You can do these exercises anytime and anywhere.
- You can do these exercises in any position, but sitting or lying down may be the easiest.

How Long Does It Take Before I Notice a Change?

After 4-6 wk of doing these exercises, you should start to see less urine leakage and urinary urgency.

MALE

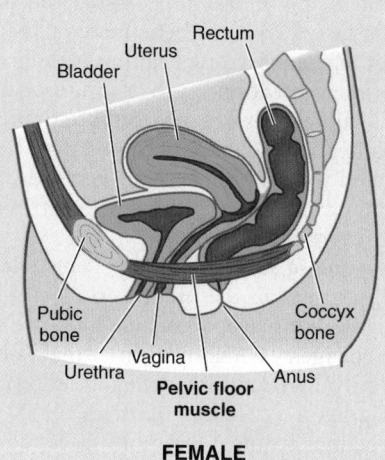

FEMALE

Courtesy Diane Newman.

caffeine and alcohol) from the diet. Advise the patient to maintain a regular, flexible schedule of urination (usually every 2 to 3 hours while awake). Advise patients to quit smoking because this habit increases the risk of stress UI. Counsel patients about the relationship among constipation, UI, and urinary retention. Aggressive management of constipation is recommended, beginning with ensuring adequate fluid intake, increasing dietary fiber, lightly exercising, and judiciously using stool softeners. (The management of constipation is discussed in Chapter 43.)

Behavioral treatments include scheduled voiding regimens (timed voiding, habit training, and prompted voiding), bladder retraining, and pelvic floor muscle training. Assess strategies that the patient uses to contain UI and offer alternative devices when indicated. When attempting to manage UI, many women use feminine hygiene pads, and many men and women use household products such as rags, paper towels, or folded toilet tissue. Unfortunately, none of these products is adequately designed to wick urine away from the skin, prevent soiling of clothing, and reduce or eliminate odor.

Instead, provide information on products specifically designed to contain urine. For example, patients with mild to moderate UI often benefit from incontinent pads containing superabsorbent material, designed to absorb many times its weight in water. Patients with higher-volume urine loss or those with both urinary and fecal incontinence may benefit from disposable or reusable incontinence protective underwear, briefs, or pad/pant systems.

In inpatient or long-term care facilities, nursing management of UI includes maximizing toilet access. This assistance may take the form of offering the urinal or bedpan or assisting the patient to the bathroom every 2 to 3 hours or at scheduled times. Ensure that toilets are accessible to patients and provide privacy to allow effective urine elimination.

URINARY RETENTION

Urinary retention is the inability to empty the bladder when a person voids (micturition) or the accumulation of urine in the bladder because of an inability to urinate. In certain cases, it is

TABLE 46-20 DRUG THERAPY
Voiding Dysfunction*

Class and Mechanism of Action	Drug
Muscarinic Receptor Antagonists and Anticholinergics	
Reduce overactive bladder contractions in urge urinary incontinence and overactive bladder	oxybutynin (Ditropan IR, Ditropan XL, Oxytrol Transdermal System) tolterodine (Detrol, Detrol LA) trospium chloride (Sanctura) solifenacin (VESIcare) darifenacin (Enablex) hyoscyamine (Levsin, Levbid) dicyclomine (Bentyl) flavoxate (Urispas) propantheline (Pro-Banthine) fesoterodine (Toviaz)
α-Adrenergic Antagonists	
Reduce urethral sphincter resistance to urinary outflow	doxazosin (Cardura) terazosin (Hytrin) tamsulosin (Flomax) alfuzosin (Uroxatral)
5α-Reductase Inhibitors	
Androgen suppression that results in epithelial atrophy and a decrease in total prostate size	finasteride (Proscar) dutasteride (Avodart)
α-Adrenergic Agonists	
Increase urethral resistance	phenylpropanolamine pseudoephedrine
β₃-Adrenergic Agonist	
Improves the bladder's storage capacity by relaxing the bladder muscle during filling	mirabegron (Myrbetriq)
Tricyclic Antidepressants	
Reduce sensory urgency and burning pain of interstitial cystitis Reduce overactive bladder contractions	imipramine (Tofranil) amitriptyline (Elavil)
Calcium Channel Blockers	
Reduce smooth muscle contraction strength May reduce burning pain of interstitial cystitis	nifedipine (Adalat) diltiazem (Cardizem) verapamil (Calan, Isoptin)
Hormone Therapy	
Local application reduces urethral irritation and increases host defenses against UTI	estrogen cream (Premarin, Estrace) estrogen vaginal ring (Estring) estrogen vaginal tablets (Vagifem)

*The type of drug therapy depends on the type of incontinence.

DELEGATION DECISIONS
Caring for the Incontinent Patient

All members of the health care team are responsible for decreasing the risk for incontinence and preventing complications such as skin breakdown in patients who are experiencing incontinence.

Role of Registered Nurse (RN)
- Assess for risk factors for incontinence or urinary retention.
- Determine type of incontinence that patient is experiencing.
- Develop plan of care to decrease incontinence.
- Teach patient ways to decrease incontinence such as pelvic floor muscle (Kegel) exercises.
- Assist patient in choosing appropriate products to contain urine.

Role of Licensed Practical/Vocational Nurse (LPN/LVN)
- Use bladder scanner to estimate the postvoid residual volume (PVR).
- Catheterize patient and measure PVR.
- Administer medications to decrease incontinence or urinary retention.

Role of Unlicensed Assistive Personnel (UAP)
- Assist incontinent patient to commode or bedpan at regular intervals.
- Clean patient and provide skin care.
- Notify RN about new-onset incontinence in a previously continent patient.

further evaluation. Even smaller volumes may justify further evaluation when the patient has recurring UTIs or lower urinary tract symptoms suggestive of UTI.

Etiology and Pathophysiology

Urinary retention is caused by two different dysfunctions of the urinary system: bladder outlet obstruction and deficient detrusor (bladder muscle) contraction strength. *Bladder outlet obstruction* leads to urinary retention when the blockage is so severe that the bladder can no longer evacuate its contents despite a detrusor contraction. A common cause of obstruction in men is an enlarged prostate.

Deficient detrusor contraction strength leads to urinary retention when the muscle is no longer able to contract with enough force or for a sufficient time to completely empty the bladder. Common causes of deficient detrusor contraction strength are neurologic diseases affecting sacral segments 2, 3, and 4; long-standing diabetes mellitus; overdistention; chronic alcoholism; and drugs (e.g., anticholinergic drugs).

Diagnostic Studies

The diagnostic studies for urinary retention are the same as the ones for UI (see pp. 1066-1067).

Collaborative Care

Behavioral therapies that were described for UI may also be used in the management of urinary retention. Scheduled toileting and double voiding may be effective in chronic urinary retention with moderate PVR volumes. *Double voiding* is an attempt to maximize bladder evacuation. The patient is asked to urinate, sit on the toilet for 3 to 4 minutes, and urinate again before exiting the bathroom.

For acute or chronic urinary retention, catheterization may be required. Intermittent catheterization allows the patient to remain free of an indwelling catheter with its associated risk of UTI and urethral irritation. In some situations, an indwelling catheter is preferred (e.g., if the patient is unwilling or unable

associated with urinary leakage or postvoid dribbling, called *overflow UI. Acute urinary retention* is the total inability to pass urine via micturition. It is a medical emergency. *Chronic urinary retention* is an incomplete bladder emptying despite urination. The postvoid residual (PVR) volumes in patients with chronic urinary retention vary widely. Normal PVR is between 50 and 75 mL. Findings over 100 mL indicate the need to repeat the measurement. An abnormal PVR in the older patient of more than 200 mL obtained on two separate occasions requires to perform intermittent catheterization). An indwelling catheter is also used when urethral obstruction makes intermittent catheterization uncomfortable or infeasible.

Drug Therapy. Several drugs may be administered to promote bladder evacuation. For the patient with obstruction at the level of the bladder neck, an α-adrenergic blocker may be prescribed. These drugs relax the smooth muscle of the bladder neck, the prostatic urethra, and possibly the rhabdosphincter, diminishing urethral resistance. Examples of α-adrenergic blocking agents are listed in Table 46-20. They are indicated in patients with BPH, bladder neck dyssynergia (muscle incoordination), or detrusor sphincter dyssynergia.

Surgical Therapy. Surgical interventions are used to manage urinary retention caused by obstruction. Transurethral or open surgical techniques are used to treat benign or malignant prostatic enlargement, bladder neck contracture, urethral strictures, or dyssynergia of the bladder neck. Pelvic reconstruction using an abdominal or transvaginal approach can correct bladder outlet obstruction in women with severe pelvic organ prolapse.

Unfortunately, surgery has a minimal role in the management of urinary retention caused by deficient detrusor contraction strength. Attempts to create a bladder stimulator (implanted device capable of stimulating micturition) have proved largely unsuccessful because of the difficulty in achieving a coordinated detrusor contraction associated with pelvic muscle and striated sphincter relaxation.

NURSING MANAGEMENT
URINARY RETENTION

Acute urinary retention is a medical emergency that requires prompt recognition and bladder drainage. Insert a catheter (as ordered) unless otherwise directed. Use a catheter with a retention balloon in anticipation of the need for an indwelling catheter.

Teach the patient with acute urinary retention (and the patient predisposed to these episodes) strategies to minimize risk, including avoiding intake of large volumes of fluid over a brief period. Instead, advise the patient to drink small amounts throughout the day. In addition, instruct the patient (if chilled) to warm up before attempting to urinate and to avoid excessive alcohol intake because it leads to polyuria and a diminished awareness of the need to urinate until the bladder is distended.

Advise the patient who is unable to urinate to drink a cup of coffee or brewed caffeinated tea to create or maximize urinary urgency. Tell patients that sitting in a tub of warm water or taking a warm shower may also help them urinate. If these measures do not lead to successful urination, advise the patient to seek immediate care.

Patients with chronic urinary retention may be managed by behavioral methods, indwelling or intermittent catheterization, surgery, or drugs. Scheduled toileting and double voiding are the primary behavioral interventions used for chronic retention. Scheduled toileting is used to reduce rather than expand bladder capacity. In this case, ask the patient to void every 3 to 4 hours regardless of the desire to urinate. This intervention is particularly useful in the patient with chronic overdistention, diabetes mellitus, or chronic alcoholism characterized by a large bladder capacity and diminished or delayed sensations of bladder filling and urgency.

TABLE 46-21	INDICATIONS FOR URINARY CATHETERIZATION

Indwelling Catheter
- Relief of urinary retention caused by lower urinary tract obstruction, paralysis, or inability to void
- Bladder decompression preoperatively and operatively for lower abdominal or pelvic surgery
- Facilitation of surgical repair of urethra and surrounding structures
- Splinting of ureters or urethra to facilitate healing after surgery or other trauma in area
- Accurate measurement of urine output in critically ill patient
- Contamination of stage III or IV pressure ulcers with urine that has impeded healing, despite appropriate personal care for the incontinence
- Terminal illness or severe impairment, which makes positioning or clothing changes uncomfortable, or which is associated with intractable pain

Intermittent (Straight, In and Out) Catheter
- Study of anatomic structures of urinary system
- Urodynamic testing
- Collection of sterile urine sample in selected situations
- Instillation of medications into bladder
- Measurement of residual urine after urination (postvoid residual [PVR]) if portable ultrasound not available

CATHETERIZATION

INDICATIONS FOR AND COMPLICATIONS OF CATHETERIZATION

Indications for short-term urinary catheterization are listed in Table 46-21. Two unacceptable reasons for catheterization are (1) routine acquisition of a urine specimen for laboratory analysis and (2) convenience of the nursing staff or the patient's family. The risks of HAI are too high to allow catheterization of a patient for the convenience of hospital personnel or family members.

Complications that are seen more frequently with long-term use (more than 30 days) of indwelling catheters include HAIs, bladder spasms, periurethral abscess, pain, urosepsis, UTIs, urethral trauma or erosion, fistula or stricture formation, and stones. Catheterization for sterile urine specimens may occasionally be necessary when patients have a history of complicated UTI. A catheter should be the final resort to provide the patient with a dry environment to prevent skin breakdown and protect dressings or skin lesions.

Urinary catheterization is commonly used in the management of the hospitalized patient. However, it is not without serious complications. The urinary tract is the most common site of HAIs. Urinary catheterization is a major cause of UTIs. Scrupulous aseptic technique is mandatory when a urinary catheter is inserted. After insertion, maintenance and protection of the closed drainage system are major nursing responsibilities. Do not routinely irrigate the catheter; this should be done only if ordered.

While the patient has a catheter in place, maintain patency of the catheter, manage fluid intake, provide for the patient's comfort and safety, and prevent infection. Address the psychologic implications of urinary drainage. Patient concerns can include embarrassment related to exposure of the body, an altered body image, and fear that care of the catheter will result in increased dependency.

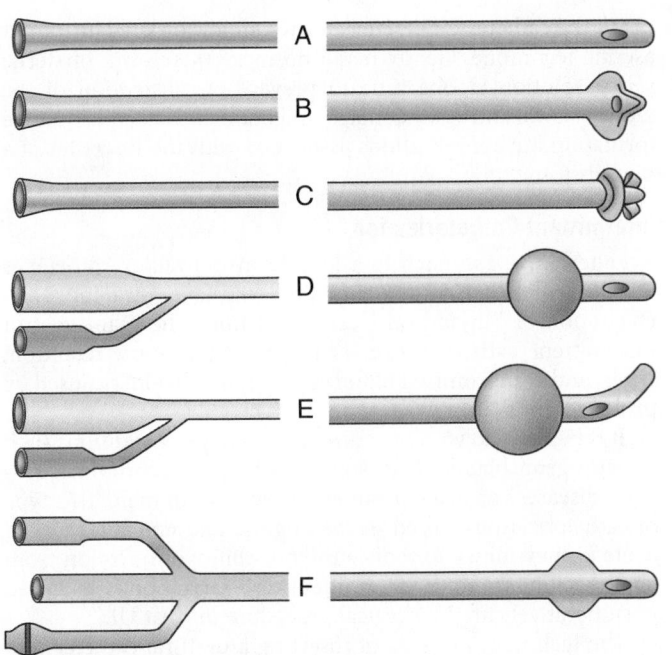

FIG. 46-10 Types of urinary catheters. **A,** Simple urethral catheter. **B,** Mushroom-tip de Pezzer catheter (can be for suprapubic catheterization). **C,** Wing-tip Malecot catheter. **D,** Indwelling urethral catheter with inflated balloon. **E,** Indwelling Tiemann catheter with coudé-tip–inflated balloon. **F,** Three-way indwelling catheter (third lumen can be used for irrigation).

CATHETER CONSTRUCTION

Catheter materials include Teflon-coated latex, silicone elastomer, and hydrogel-coated silicone. Catheters coated with silver or antimicrobial agents may prevent UTIs.

Catheters vary in construction materials, tip shape (Fig. 46-10), and size of the lumen. A coudé-tip catheter is commonly used in men. Catheters are sized according to the French scale. Each French unit (F) equals 0.33 mm of diameter. The diameter listed is the internal diameter of the catheter. The size used varies with the patient's size and the purpose of catheterization. In women, urethral catheter sizes 14F to 16F are the most common. In men, sizes 14F to 18F are used. Balloon sizes are either 5 or 30 mL. The primary problem resulting from too large a catheter is tissue erosion secondary to excessive pressure on the meatus or urethra.

TYPES OF CATHETERS

Four routes are used for urinary tract catheterization: urethral, ureteral, suprapubic, and via a nephrostomy tube.

Urethral Catheters

Urethral catheterization, the most common route of catheterization, involves the insertion of a catheter through the external meatus into the urethra, past the internal sphincter, and into the bladder. Consider the following principles in the management of the patient with an indwelling urethral catheter:

- Teach catheter care to the catheterized patient, particularly one who is ambulatory.
- Use a sterile, closed drainage system in short-term catheterization. Do not disconnect the distal urinary catheter and the proximal drainage tube except for necessary catheter irrigation. Maintain unobstructed downhill flow.

Empty the collecting bag regularly, and keep it below the level of the bladder. Replace a poorly functioning catheter.
- Provide perineal care (once or twice a day and when necessary), including cleaning the meatus-catheter junction with soap and water. Do not use lotion or powder near the catheter.
- Anchor catheters using some type of securement device. It is recommended that the catheter be anchored to the upper thigh in women and to the lower abdomen in men to prevent catheter movement and urethral tension.
- Use sterile technique whenever the collecting system is open. If frequent irrigations are necessary in short-term catheterization to maintain catheter patency, a triple-lumen catheter may be preferable, permitting continuous irrigations within a closed system.
- Aspirate small volumes of urine for culture from the catheter sampling port by means of a sterile syringe and a needle. First prepare the puncture site with a tincture of iodine or alcohol solution.
- When the patient is catheterized for less than 2 weeks, routine catheter change is not necessary. For long-term use of an indwelling catheter, replace the catheter based on patient assessment and not on a routine changing schedule.
- With long-term use of a catheter, a leg bag may be used. If the collection bag is reused, wash it in soap and water and rinse thoroughly. When it is not reused immediately, fill it with ½ cup of vinegar and drain. The vinegar is effective against *Pseudomonas* and other organisms and eliminates odors.
- Remove the catheter as early as possible. Intermittent catheterization and external catheters are alternatives that may be associated with fewer cases of bacteriuria and UTI than chronic indwelling urethral catheters.

Ureteral Catheters

The *ureteral catheter* is placed through the ureters into the renal pelvis. The catheter is inserted either (1) by being threaded up the urethra and bladder to the ureters under cystoscopic observation or (2) by surgical insertion through the abdominal wall into the ureters. The ureteral catheter is used after surgery to splint the ureters and to prevent them from being obstructed by edema. Record the urine volume from the ureteral catheter separately from that of other urinary catheters.

The patient is often kept on bed rest while a ureteral catheter is in place until specific orders indicate that ambulation is permitted. The self-retaining ureteral catheter is often inserted after a lithotripsy procedure or when ureteral obstruction from adjacent tumors or fibrosis threatens renal function. The double-J ureteral catheter is frequently used and allows the patient to ambulate. One end coils up in the kidney pelvis, while the other coils in the bladder.

Check the placement of the ureteral catheter frequently, and avoid tension on the catheter. The catheter drains urine from the renal pelvis, which has a capacity of 3 to 5 mL. If the volume of urine in the renal pelvis increases, tissue damage to the pelvis will result from pressure. Do not clamp the ureteral catheter. If the physician orders irrigation of the ureteral catheter, use strict aseptic technique. If the output is decreased, notify the physician immediately. Check the drainage often (at least every 1 or 2 hours). It is normal for some urine to drain around the ureteral catheter into the bladder. Accurately record the urine output from both the ureters and the urethral catheter. Sometimes a ureteral catheter may be used as a stent and is not expected to drain. It is important to check with the physician as to the type of catheter and what to expect.

Suprapubic Catheters

Suprapubic catheterization is the simplest and oldest method of urinary diversion. The two methods of insertion of a suprapubic catheter into the bladder are (1) through a small incision in the abdominal wall and (2) by the use of a trocar. A suprapubic catheter is placed while the patient is under general anesthesia for another surgical procedure or at the bedside with a local anesthetic. The catheter may be sutured into place. Tape the catheter to prevent dislodgment. The care of the tube and catheter is similar to that of the urethral catheter. A pectin-base skin barrier (e.g., Stomahesive) is effective in protecting the skin around the insertion site from breakdown.

The suprapubic catheter is used in temporary situations such as bladder, prostate, and urethral surgery. The suprapubic catheter is also used on a long-term basis in selected patients.

A suprapubic catheter is prone to poor drainage because of mechanical obstruction of the catheter tip by the bladder wall, sediment, and clots. To ensure patency of the tube (1) prevent tube kinking by coiling the excess tubing and maintaining gravity drainage, (2) have the patient turn from side to side, and (3) milk the tube. If these measures are not effective, obtain a physician order to irrigate the catheter using sterile technique.

If the patient experiences bladder spasms that are difficult to control, urinary leakage may result. Oxybutynin or other oral antispasmodics or belladonna and opium (B&O) suppositories may be prescribed to decrease bladder spasms.

Nephrostomy Tubes

The *nephrostomy tube* (catheter) is inserted on a temporary basis to preserve renal function when a ureter is completely obstructed. The tube is inserted through a small flank incision directly into the pelvis of the kidney and attached to connecting tubing for closed drainage. The principle is the same as with the ureteral catheter—that is, the catheter should never be kinked, compressed, or clamped. If the patient complains of excessive pain in the area or if there is excessive drainage around the tube,

check the catheter for patency. If irrigation is ordered, use strict aseptic technique. Gently instill no more than 5 mL of sterile saline solution at one time to prevent overdistention of the kidney pelvis and renal damage. Infection and secondary stone formation are complications associated with the insertion of a nephrostomy tube.

Intermittent Catheterization

An alternative approach to a long-term indwelling catheter is *intermittent catheterization*, often referred to as "straight" catheterization or "in-and-out" catheterization. The main goal of intermittent catheterization is to prevent urinary retention, stasis, and compromised blood supply to the bladder caused by prolonged pressure.

It is being used with increasing frequency in conditions such as neurogenic bladder (e.g., spinal cord injuries, chronic neurologic diseases) or bladder outlet obstruction in men. This type of catheterization is used in the oliguric and anuric phases of acute kidney injury to reduce the possibility of infection from an indwelling catheter. Intermittent catheterization is also used postoperatively after a surgical procedure to treat UI.

The technique consists of inserting a urethral catheter into the bladder every 3 to 5 hours. Some patients perform intermittent catheterization only once or twice a day to measure residual urine and to ensure an empty bladder.

The techniques and protocols for intermittent catheterization vary. Catheters can be sterile (single use) or clean (multiple use). Catheters can be coated (prelubricated) or uncoated. Available data on intermittent catheterization do not provide convincing evidence that any specific technique (sterile or clean), catheter type (coated or uncoated), method (single-use or multiple-use), person (self or other), or strategy is better than any other for all clinical settings.[34]

The design of single-use, self-lubricating, silicone-coated (closed-sterile) systems is useful for patients who have recurrent UTIs or need to catheterize while at work or during travel. Instruct patients to wash and rinse the catheter and their hands with soap and water before and after catheterization. Lubricant is necessary for men and may make catheterization more comfortable for women. The catheter may be inserted by the patient, caregiver, or health care provider.

Sterile technique is used for catheterization in the hospital or long-term care facility. For home care, a clean technique that includes good hand washing with soap and water is used. Teach the patient to observe for signs of UTI so that treatment can be instituted early. If indicated, some patients are placed on a regimen of prophylactic antibiotics. Urethral damage from intermittent catheterization in men is similar to problems seen with indwelling catheterization. Complications include urethritis, urethral sphincter damage (especially if there is a forceful catheterization against a closed sphincter), urethral stricture, and creation of a false passage.

SURGERY OF THE URINARY TRACT

RENAL AND URETERAL SURGERY

The most common indications for nephrectomy are a renal tumor, polycystic kidneys that are bleeding or severely infected, massive traumatic injury to the kidney, and the elective removal of a kidney from a donor to be transplanted. Surgery involving the ureters and kidneys is most commonly performed to remove calculi that become obstructive, correct congenital anomalies, and divert urine when necessary.

Surgical Procedure

Nephrectomy can be performed by a conventional (open) approach or laparoscopically. In the open approach an incision of about 6 to 10 in is made through several layers of muscle. The incision can be made in the flank or abdominal area.

Laparoscopic Nephrectomy. *Laparoscopic nephrectomy* can be performed in selected situations to remove a diseased kidney. Laparoscopic nephrectomy can also be used to obtain a kidney from a living donor to be transplanted into a person with ESKD. A laparoscopic nephrectomy is performed using five puncture sites. One incision is to view the kidney, and another is to dissect it. The laparoscope contains a miniature camera so that the surgeons can watch what they are doing on a video monitor. Once dissected, the kidney is maneuvered into a nylon impermeable sack and then safely removed from the patient. Compared with conventional nephrectomy, the laparoscopic approach is less painful, involves a shorter hospital stay, and has a much faster recovery.

Preoperative Management

The basic needs of the patient undergoing renal and ureteral surgery are similar to those of any patient who experiences surgery (see Chapters 18 through 20). In addition, it is important preoperatively to ensure adequate fluid intake and a normal electrolyte balance. Tell the patient that, if there is a flank incision, surgery will require a hyperextended, side-lying position. This position frequently causes the patient to experience muscle aches after surgery. If a nephrectomy is planned, it is important that the patient have one working kidney to maintain normal renal function.

Postoperative Management

Specific postoperative needs of a patient are related to urine output, respiratory status, and abdominal distention.

Urine Output. In the immediate postoperative period, measure and record the urine output at least every 1 or 2 hours. Measure drainage from the various catheters and record it separately. Do not clamp or irrigate the catheter or tube without a specific order. The total urine output should be at least 0.5 mL/kg/hr. It is important to assess for urine drainage on the dressing and to estimate this amount. Observe and monitor the color and consistency of urine. Urine with increased amounts of mucus, blood, or sediment may occlude the drainage tubing or catheter.

Weigh the patient daily using the same scale, and have the patient wear similar clothing and dressings each time. A significant change in daily weight can indicate retention of fluids, which places the patient at cardiovascular risk for developing heart failure. Retention of fluids can increase the work required of the remaining kidney to perform its functions.

Respiratory Status. A nephrectomy can be performed through a flank incision just below the diaphragm. Postoperatively, it is important to ensure adequate ventilation. The patient is often reluctant to turn, cough, and deep breathe because of the incisional pain. Give adequate pain medication to ensure the patient's comfort and ability to perform coughing and deep-breathing exercises. Frequently, additional respiratory devices such as an incentive spirometer are used every 2 hours while the patient is awake. In addition, early and frequent ambulation assists in maintaining adequate respiratory function.

Abdominal Distention. Abdominal distention is present to some degree in most patients who have had surgery on their kidneys or ureters. It is most commonly due to paralytic ileus caused by manipulation and compression of the bowel during surgery. Oral intake is restricted until bowel sounds are present (usually 24 to 48 hours after surgery). IV fluids are given until the patient can take oral fluids. Progression to a regular diet follows.

URINARY DIVERSION

Urinary diversion may be performed with or without cystectomy. Urinary diversion procedures are performed to treat cancer of the bladder, neurogenic bladder, congenital anomalies, strictures, trauma to the bladder, and chronic infections with deterioration of renal function. Numerous urinary diversion techniques and bladder substitutes are possible, including an incontinent urinary diversion, a continent urinary diversion catheterized by the patient, or an orthotopic bladder so that the patient voids urethrally.[35] Types of surgical procedures for urinary diversion are presented in Table 46-22 and Fig. 46-11.

Incontinent Urinary Diversion

Incontinent urinary diversion is diversion to the skin, requiring an appliance. The simplest form is the cutaneous ureterostomy, but scarring and strictures of the ureter have led to the use of ileal or colonic conduits. The most commonly performed incontinent urinary diversion procedure is the **ileal conduit** (ileal loop). In this procedure a 6- to 8-in (15- to 20-cm) segment of the ileum is converted into a conduit for urinary drainage. The colon (colon conduit) can be used instead of the ileum. The ureters are anastomosed into one end of the conduit, and the other end of the bowel is brought out through the abdominal wall to form a stoma (Fig. 46-12). Although the segment of bowel remains supported by the mesentery, it is completely isolated from the intestinal tract. The bowel is anastomosed and continues to function normally.

Because there is no valve and no voluntary control over the stoma, drops of urine flow from the stoma every few seconds, requiring a permanent external collecting device. The visible stoma and the need for external collection devices are disadvantages of this procedure. The lifelong need to care for and deal with the stoma and collection devices may be psychologically difficult. These problems have led to the increasing use of continent diversions and orthotopic bladder substitutes.

Continent Urinary Diversions

A *continent urinary diversion* is an intraabdominal urinary reservoir that can be catheterized or that has an outlet controlled by the anal sphincter. Continent diversions are internal pouches created similarly to the ileal conduit. Reservoirs are constructed from the ileum, ileocecal segment, or colon. Large segments of bowel are altered to prevent peristaltic action. A continence mechanism is formed between this large, low-pressure reservoir and the stoma by intussuscepting a portion of bowel. In this way, a patient does not leak involuntarily. The patient with a continent reservoir needs to self-catheterize every 4 to 6 hours but does not need to wear external attachments. Patients may wear a small bandage on the stoma to collect any mucous drainage or excess drainage. Examples of continent diversions are the Kock (Fig. 46-13), Mainz, Indiana, and Florida pouches. The main difference among the various diversions is the segment of

TABLE 46-22   URINARY DIVERSION SURGERY

Description	Advantages	Disadvantages	Special Considerations
Ileal Conduit Ureters are implanted into part of ileum or colon that has been resected from intestinal tract. Abdominal stoma is created.	Relatively good urine flow with few physiologic alterations.	External appliance necessary to continually collect urine.	Surgical procedure is complex. Postoperative complications may be increased. Reabsorption of urea by ileum occurs. Meticulous attention is necessary to care for stoma and collecting device.
Cutaneous Ureterostomy Ureters are excised from bladder and brought through abdominal wall, and stoma is created. Ureteral stomas may be created from both ureters, or ureters may be brought together and one stoma created.	No need for major surgery as required with ileal conduit.	External appliance necessary because of continuous urine drainage. Possibility of stricture or stenosis of small stoma.	Periodic catheterizations may be required to dilate stomas to maintain patency.
Nephrostomy Catheter is inserted into pelvis of kidney. Procedure may be done to one or both kidneys and may be temporary or permanent. It is most frequently done in advanced disease as palliative procedure.	No need for major surgery.	High risk of renal infection. Predisposition to calculus formation from catheter.	Nephrostomy tube may have to be changed every month. Never clamp the catheter.

A   Ileal segment anastomosed to sigmoid colon

Isolated ileal segment with ureters implanted in posterior portion of segment

B   Isolated ileal segment with ureters implanted in posterior portion of segment

Protruding abdominal stoma

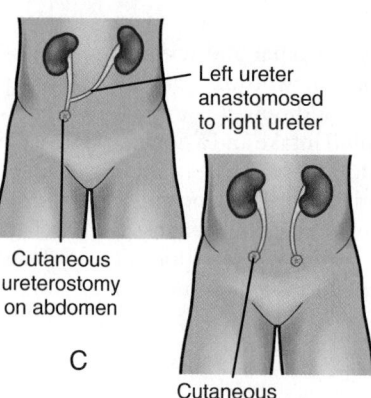

C

Left ureter anastomosed to right ureter

Cutaneous ureterostomy on abdomen

Cutaneous ureterostomy on abdomen

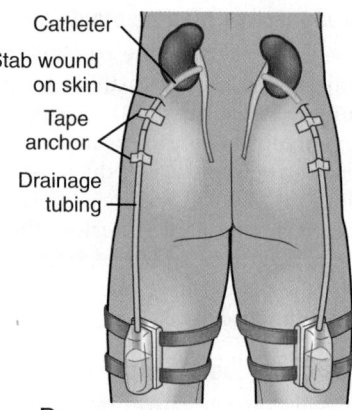

D

Catheter
Stab wound on skin
Tape anchor
Drainage tubing

Bilateral nephrostomy tubes inserted into renal pelvis; catheters exit through an incision on each flank, or there may be just one kidney

FIG. 46-11 Methods of urinary diversion. **A,** Ureteroileosigmoidostomy. **B,** Ileal loop (ileal conduit). **C,** Ureterostomy (transcutaneous ureterostomy and bilateral cutaneous ureterostomies). **D,** Nephrostomy.

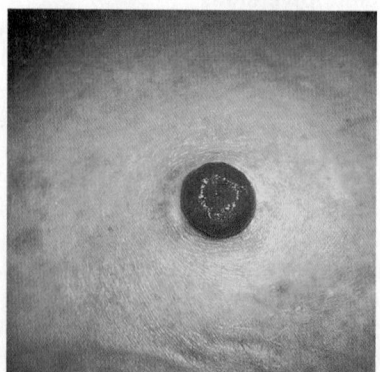

FIG. 46-12 Urinary stoma. Symmetric, no skin breakdown, protrudes about 1.5 cm. Mucosa is healthy red. This configuration is flat when the patient is upright or supine.

Stoma
Pouch
Implantation of ureters

FIG. 46-13 Creation of a Kock pouch with implantation of ureters into one intussuscepted portion of the pouch and creation of a stoma with the other intussuscepted portion.

bowel used. For example, the Indiana pouch uses the right colon as a reservoir and has become a popular form of continent urinary diversion.

Orthotopic Bladder Reconstruction

Orthotopic bladder reconstruction, or orthotopic neobladder, is the construction of a new bladder in the bladder's normal anatomic position, with discharge of urine through the urethra. The reconstruction or neobladder can be derived from various segments of the intestines to create a low-pressure reservoir. An isolated segment of the distal ileum is often preferred. Various procedures include the hemi-Kock pouch, the Studer pouch, and the W-shaped ileoneobladder. In these procedures the bowel is surgically reshaped to become a neobladder. The ureters and urethra are sutured into the neobladder.

Orthotopic bladder reconstruction has become a more viable option for both men and women if cancer does not involve the bladder neck or urethra. Ideal candidates for this procedure have normal renal and liver function, longer than 1- to 2-year life expectancy, adequate motor skills, and no history of inflammatory bowel disease or colon cancer. Obese patients and those with inflammatory bowel disease are not good candidates for this procedure. The advantage of orthotopic bladder substitution is that it allows for natural micturition. Incontinence is a possible problem with this technique, and intermittent catheterization may be required.

NURSING MANAGEMENT
URINARY DIVERSION

PREOPERATIVE MANAGEMENT

Teaching is important for the patient awaiting cystectomy and urinary diversion surgery. Assess the patient's ability and readiness to learn before initiating a teaching program. If the patient is not ready to learn, modify the teaching plan. The patient's anxiety and fear may be decreased by providing more information. However, the anxiety and fear may also interfere with learning. Involve the patient's caregiver and family in the teaching process.

Discuss the psychosocial aspects of living with a stoma (including clothing, changes in body image and sexuality, exercise, and odor). This may allay some fears. Teach the patient with a continent diversion (e.g., Indiana pouch) to catheterize at least every 6 hours and irrigate the pouch daily. The patient with an orthotopic neobladder may have problems with incontinence. Discuss the patient's concerns about sexual activities. A wound, ostomy, and continence (WOC) nurse should be involved in the preoperative phase of the patient's care. A visit from an ostomate or WOC nurse can be helpful. Additional interventions are presented in eNursing Care Plan 46-3 for the patient with an ileal conduit (on the website for this chapter).

POSTOPERATIVE MANAGEMENT

Plan the nursing interventions during the postoperative period (see eNursing Care Plan 46-3 for care after an ileal conduit) to prevent surgical complications such as postoperative atelectasis and shock (see Chapter 20). After pelvic surgery, there is an increased incidence of thrombophlebitis, small bowel obstruction, and UTI. With removal of part of the bowel, the incidence of paralytic ileus and small bowel obstruction is increased, the patient is kept on NPO status, and a nasogastric tube is necessary for a few days.

Prevent injury to the stoma and maintain urine output. Advise the patient that mucus in the urine is a normal occurrence. The mucus is secreted by the mucosa of the intestine (which is used to create the ileal conduit) in response to the irritating effect of urine. Encourage a high fluid intake to "flush" the ileal conduit or continent diversion.

When an ileal conduit is created, provide meticulous care for the skin around the stoma. Alkaline encrustations with dermatitis may occur when alkaline urine comes in contact with exposed skin (Fig. 46-14). The urine is kept acidic to prevent alkaline encrustations. Other common peristomal skin problems include yeast infections, product allergies, and shearing-effect excoriations. Changing appliances (pouches) is described in Table 46-23. A properly fitting appliance is essential to prevent skin problems. The appliance should be about 0.1 in (0.2 cm) larger than the stoma. It is normal for the stoma to shrink within the first few weeks after surgery.

Patients with a neobladder may have postoperative urinary retention and require catheterization. It may take up to 6 months for them to regain bladder control. Patients empty their neo-

TABLE 46-23	PATIENT & CAREGIVER TEACHING GUIDE

Ileal Conduit Appliances

Include the following instructions when teaching a patient or a caregiver how to change an ileal conduit appliance.

Temporary Appliance
1. Cut hole in pouch to fit over stoma (pouch ⅛ in [3.2 mm] larger than stoma).
2. Remove old pouch.
3. Clean area gently and remove old adhesive.
4. Wash area with warm water.
5. Place wick (rolled-up 4 × 4-in pad) over stoma to keep area dry during rest of procedure.
6. Dry skin around stoma.
7. Apply tincture of benzoin or other skin protectant around stoma to area where pouch will be placed.
8. Apply pouch by first smoothing its edges toward side and lower portion of body.
9. Remove wick and complete application of bag.
10. If patient is usually in bed, apply bag so that it lies toward side of body.
11. If patient is ambulatory, apply bag so that it lies vertically.
12. Connect drainage tubing to pouch.
13. Keep drainage pouch on same side of bed as stoma.

Permanent Appliance*
1. Keep appliance in place for 2-14 days.
2. Change appliance when fluid intake has been restricted for several hours.
3. Sit or stand in front of mirror.
4. Moisten edge of faceplate with adhesive solvent and gently remove.
5. Clean skin with adhesive solvent.
6. Wash skin with warm water (may be done while showering).
7. Dry skin and inspect.
8. Place wick (rolled-up 4 × 4-in pad) over stoma to keep skin free of urine.
9. Apply skin cement to faceplate and skin.
10. Place appliance over stoma.
11. Wash removed appliance with soap and lukewarm water; soak in distilled vinegar; rinse with lukewarm water and air dry.

*Many disposable appliances with self-adhesive backing are used as permanent appliances.

FIG. 46-14 Ammonia salt encrustation secondary to alkaline urine.

FIG. 46-15 Retracted urinary stoma with pressure sore from faceplate above stoma *(arrow)*.

bladders by relaxing their outlet sphincter muscles and bearing down with their abdominal muscles. Since there is no longer neurologic feedback between the reservoir and the brain, the patient should not expect a normal desire to void. To avoid bladder overdistention, patients should void at least every 2 to 4 hours, sit during voiding, and practice pelvic floor muscle relaxation to aid voiding. Follow-up x-ray studies include a "pouchogram" 3 to 4 weeks after surgery to assess for healing.

Acceptance of the surgery and of alterations in body image is needed to ensure the patient's best adjustment. Meeting and sharing feelings with similar patients can enhance a patient's adjustment to a urinary diversion. Patient concerns include fear that the stoma will be offensive to others and will interfere with sexual, personal, professional, and recreational activities. Advise the patient that few activities will be restricted as a result of the urinary diversion.

Discharge planning after an ileal conduit includes teaching the patient symptoms of obstruction or infection and care of the ostomy. The patient with an ileal conduit is fitted for a permanent appliance 7 to 10 days after surgery and may need to be refitted at a later time, depending on the degree of stoma healing and shrinkage.

Appliances are made of a variety of products, including natural and synthetic rubbers, plastics, and metals. Most appliances have a faceplate that adheres to the skin, a collecting pouch, and an opening to drain the pouch. The faceplate may be secured to the skin with glues, adhesives, or adherent synthetic wafers. Some appliances do not require adhesives, but their design relies on pressure to keep the pouch in place. If improperly fitted or applied, the faceplate may cause skin problems (Fig. 46-15). Inform the patient and caregiver about where to purchase supplies, emergency telephone numbers, location of ostomy clubs, and follow-up visits with a WOC nurse. Physician follow-up is imperative to monitor the patient's recovery, detect any complications, and assess renal function.

CASE STUDY

Urinary Tract Infection

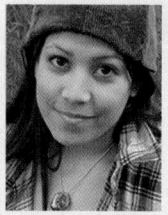

iStockphoto/Thinkstock

Patient Profile
S.U., a 38-yr-old Hispanic woman, was seen in the nurse practitioner's office for a history of painful, frequent urination.

Subjective Data
- Has a history of painful, frequent urination with passage of small volumes of urine for 3 days
- Had intermittent fever, chills, and back pain during these 3 days
- Was frightened when she saw blood in her urine
- Reports this is her third attack of painful urination and back pain in 4 mo
- Is anxious because her father died of kidney cancer
- Remembers having many UTIs as a child
- Has had four pregnancies with difficult vaginal deliveries

Objective Data
Physical Examination
- Complains of bilateral flank pain and abdominal tenderness to palpation
- Temperature is 100.4° F (38° C)

Diagnostic Studies
- Urinalysis: pyuria and hematuria
- Follow-up studies to be done

Discussion Questions
1. What are the most common organisms that cause UTIs?
2. What additional information do you or the nurse practitioner need from S.U.?
3. What factors predispose a patient to a UTI?
4. What is the difference between upper and lower UTIs?
5. *Priority Decision:* What are the priority nursing interventions for S.U.?
6. Why might S.U. be having recurrent bouts of UTIs? What other diagnostic tests may be indicated?
7. *Evidence-Based Practice*: S.U. wants to know what she can do to prevent another UTI. What are you going to tell her?
8. *Priority Decision:* Based on the data presented, write one or more appropriate nursing diagnoses. Are there any collaborative problems?

evolve Answers available at *http://evolve.elsevier.com/Lewis/medsurg.*

BRIDGE TO NCLEX EXAMINATION

The number of the question corresponds to the same-numbered outcome at the beginning of the chapter.

1. In teaching a patient with pyelonephritis about the disorder, the nurse informs the patient that the organisms that cause pyelonephritis most commonly reach the kidneys through
   a. the bloodstream.
   b. the lymphatic system.
   c. a descending infection.
   d. an ascending infection.

2. The nurse teaches the female patient who has frequent UTIs that she should
   a. take tub baths with bubble bath.
   b. urinate before and after sexual intercourse.
   c. take prophylactic sulfonamides for the rest of her life.
   d. restrict fluid intake to prevent the need for frequent voiding.

3. The immunologic mechanisms involved in acute poststreptococcal glomerulonephritis include
   a. tubular blocking by precipitates of bacteria and antibody reactions.
   b. deposition of immune complexes and complement along the GBM.
   c. thickening of the GBM from autoimmune microangiopathic changes.
   d. destruction of glomeruli by proteolytic enzymes contained in the GBM.

4. One of the nurse's most important roles in relation to acute poststreptococcal glomerulonephritis is to
   a. promote early diagnosis and treatment of sore throats and skin lesions.
   b. encourage patients to obtain antibiotic therapy for upper respiratory tract infections.
   c. teach patients with APSGN that long-term prophylactic antibiotic therapy is necessary to prevent recurrence.
   d. monitor patients for respiratory symptoms that indicate the disease is affecting the alveolar basement membrane.

5. The edema that occurs in nephrotic syndrome is due to
   a. increased hydrostatic pressure caused by sodium retention.
   b. decreased aldosterone secretion from adrenal insufficiency.
   c. increased fluid retention caused by decreased glomerular filtration.
   d. decreased colloidal osmotic pressure caused by loss of serum albumin.

6. A patient is admitted to the hospital with severe renal colic. The nurse's first priority in management of the patient is to
   a. administer opioids as prescribed.
   b. obtain supplies for straining all urine.
   c. encourage fluid intake of 3 to 4 L/day.
   d. keep the patient NPO in preparation for surgery.

7. The nurse recommends genetic counseling for the children of a patient with
   a. nephrotic syndrome.
   b. chronic pyelonephritis.
   c. malignant nephrosclerosis.
   d. adult-onset polycystic kidney disease.

8. The nurse identifies a risk factor for kidney and bladder cancer in a patient who relates a history of
   a. aspirin use.
   b. tobacco use.
   c. chronic alcohol abuse.
   d. use of artificial sweeteners.

9. In planning nursing interventions to increase bladder control in the patient with urinary incontinence, the nurse includes
   a. teaching the patient to use Kegel exercises.
   b. clamping and releasing a catheter to increase bladder tone.
   c. teaching the patient biofeedback mechanisms to suppress the urge to void.
   d. counseling the patient concerning choice of incontinence containment device.

10. A patient with a ureterolithotomy returns from surgery with a nephrostomy tube in place. Postoperative nursing care of the patient includes
    a. encouraging the patient to drink fruit juices and milk.
    b. encouraging fluids of at least 2 to 3 L/day after nausea has subsided.
    c. irrigating the nephrostomy tube with 10 mL of normal saline solution as needed.
    d. notifying the physician if nephrostomy tube drainage is more than 30 mL/hr.

11. A patient has had a cystectomy and ileal conduit diversion performed. Four days postoperatively, mucous shreds are seen in the drainage bag. The nurse should
    a. notify the physician.
    b. notify the charge nurse.
    c. irrigate the drainage tube.
    d. chart it as a normal observation.

1. d, 2. b, 3. b, 4. a, 5. d, 6. a, 7. d, 8. b, 9. a, 10. b, 11. d

ⓔvolve

For rationales to these answers and even more NCLEX review questions, visit *http://evolve.elsevier.com/Lewis/medsurg.*

REFERENCES

1. Brusch JL, Bavaro MF, Cunha BA, et al: Cystitis in females. Retrieved from *http://emedicine.medscape.com/article/233101-overview.*

2. Urinary tract infections—adults. Retrieved from *www.ncbi.nlm.nih.gov/pubmedhealth/PMH0001549.*

3. Tambyah PA, Oon J: Catheter-associated urinary tract infection, *Curr Opin Infect Dis* 25(4):365, 2012.

4. National Kidney and Urologic Diseases Information Clearinghouse: Kidney and urologic diseases statistics for the United States. Retrieved from *http://kidney.niddk.nih.gov/kudiseases/pubs/pdf/KUStatistics.pdf.*

*5. Dason S, Dason JT, Kapoor A: Guidelines for the diagnosis and management of recurrent urinary tract infection in women, *Can Urol Assoc J* 5(5):316, 2011.

6. Denes E, Prouzergue J, Ducroix-Roubertou S, et al: Antibiotic prescription by general practitioners for urinary tract infections in outpatients, *Eur J Clin Microbiol Infect Dis* 31(11):3079, 2012.

*Evidence-based information for clinical practice.

7. Hooton TM: Clinical practice: uncomplicated urinary tract infection, *N Engl J Med* 366(11):1028, 2012.

8. Colgan R, Williams M: Diagnosis and treatment of acute uncomplicated cystitis, *Am Fam Physician* 84(7):771, 2011.

*9. Wang C, Fang C, Chen N, et al: Cranberry-containing products for prevention of urinary tract infections in susceptible populations: a systematic review and meta-analysis of randomized controlled trials, *Arch Intern Med* 172:988, 2012.

10. Wenger JE: Reducing rates of catheter-associated urinary tract infection, *Am J Nurs* 110:40, 2010.

11. Dumont C, Wakeman J: Preventing catheter-associated UTIs: survey report, *Nursing* 40(12):24, 2010.

12. Oman KS, Makic MB, Fink R, et al: Nurse-directed interventions to reduce catheter-associated urinary tract infections, *Am J Infect Control* 40(6):548, 2012.

13. Conner BT: Reducing catheter-associated urinary tract infections, *Am Nurse Today* 7:16, 2012.

*14. Nosseir SB, Lind LR, Winkler HA: Recurrent uncomplicated urinary tract infections in women: a review, *J Womens Health* 21(3):347, 2012.

15. National Kidney and Urologic Diseases Information Clearinghouse: Interstitial cystitis/painful bladder syndrome. Retrieved from *http://kidney.niddk.nih.gov/kudiseases/pubs/interstitialcystitis*.

16. Gish BA: Interstitial cystitis/bladder pain syndrome: symptoms, screening, and treatment, *Nurs Womens Health* 15(6):496, 2011.

*17. Hanno P, Burks D, Clemens J, et al: AUA guideline for the diagnosis and treatment of interstitial cystitis/bladder pain syndrome, *J Urol* 185:2162, 2011.

18. Gish BA: Interstitial cystitis/bladder pain syndrome: symptoms, screening and treatment, *Nurs Womens Health* 15(6):496, 2011.

19. Quillin RB, Erickson DR: Management of interstitial cystitis/bladder pain syndrome: a urology perspective, *Urol Clin North Am* 39(3):389, 2012.

20. Soliman MS: Tuberculosis of the genitourinary system. Retrieved from *http://emedicine.medscape.com/article/450651-overview*.

21. Ralph AP, Carapetis JR: Group A streptococcal diseases and their global burden, *Curr Top Microbiol Immunol* 368:1, 2013.

22. Siddall EC, Radhakrishnan J: The pathophysiology of edema formation in the nephrotic syndrome, *Kidney Int* 82(6):635, 2012.

23. Worcester EM, Coe FL: Calcium kidney stones, *N Engl J Med* 363:954, 2010.

24. Stoller ML: Urinary stone disease: symptoms and signs at presentation. Retrieved from *www.urologytoday.net/article/urinary-stone-disease-symptoms-signs-at-presentation*.

*25. Aboumarzouk OM, Kata SG, Keeley FX, et al: Extracorporeal shock wave lithotripsy (ESWL) versus ureteroscopic management for ureteric calculi, *Cochrane Database Syst Rev* 5:CD006029, 2012.

*26. Chandok N: Polycystic liver disease: a clinical review, *Ann Hepatol* 11(6):819, 2012.

*27. Steinman TI: Polycystic kidney disease: a 2011 update, *Curr Opin Nephrol Hypertens* 21(2):189, 2012.

28. American Cancer Society: Cancer facts and figures. Retrieved from *www.cancer.org/research/cancerfactsfigures/index*.

29. Patel C, Ahmed A, Ellsworth P: Renal cell carcinoma: a reappraisal, *Urol Nurs* 32(4):182, 2012.

*30. Houghton BB, Chalasani V, Hayne D, et al: Intravesical chemotherapy plus bacille Calmette-Guérin in non-muscle invasive bladder cancer: a systematic review with meta-analysis, *BJU Int* 111:977, 2013.

31. Schultz JM: Urinary incontinence, *Nursing* 40:33, 2010.

32. Schultz JM: Rethink urinary continence, *Nursing* 42:32, 2012.

33. Stem cell therapy: a future treatment of stress urinary incontinence. Retrieved from *www.medscape.com/viewarticle/735539*.

*34. Newman DK, Willson M: Review of intermittent catheterization and current best practices. Retrieved from *www.medscape.com/viewarticle/745908_7*.

35. Hautmann RE, Abol-Enein H, Davidsson T, et al: ICUD-EAU International Consultation on Bladder Cancer 2012: urinary diversion, *Eur Urol* 63(1):67. 2013.

RESOURCES

American Association of Kidney Patients
www.aakp.org

American Nephrology Nurses' Association
www.annanurse.org

American Urological Association
www.auanet.org

Interstitial Cystitis Association
www.ichelp.org

National Association for Continence (NAFC)
www.nafc.org

National Kidney Foundation
www.kidney.org

National Kidney and Urologic Diseases Information Clearinghouse
www.kidney.niddk.nih.gov

PKD Foundation
www.pkdcure.org

Society of Urologic Nurses and Associates
www.suna.org

United Ostomy Associations of America
www.ostomy.org

Wound, Ostomy, and Continence Nurses Society
www.wocn.org

Also see Resources for Chapter 47 on p. 1131.

Everywhere you go, take a smile with you.
Sasha Azevedo

Nursing Management
Acute Kidney Injury and Chronic Kidney Disease

Carol Headley

Evolve WEBSITE

http://evolve.elsevier.com/Lewis/medsurg

- NCLEX Review Questions
- Key Points
- Pre-Test
- Answer Guidelines for Case Study on p. 1129
- Rationales for Bridge to NCLEX Examination Questions

- Case Studies
  - Patient With Glomerulonephritis and Kidney Disease
  - Patient With Kidney Transplant
- Nursing Care Plan (Customizable)
  - eNCP 47-1: Patient With Chronic Kidney Disease
- Concept Map Creator

- Glossary
- Content Updates

eTables
- eTable 47-1: Manifestations of Acute Kidney Injury
- eTable 47-2: Case Study: Intrarenal Cause of Acute Kidney Injury Following Surgery

LEARNING OUTCOMES

1. Differentiate between acute kidney injury and chronic kidney disease.
2. Identify criteria used in the classification of acute kidney injury using the acronym RIFLE (*R*isk, *I*njury, *F*ailure, *L*oss, *E*nd-stage kidney disease).
3. Describe the clinical course of acute kidney injury.
4. Explain the collaborative care and nursing management of a patient with acute kidney injury.
5. Define *chronic kidney disease* and delineate its five stages based on the glomerular filtration rate.
6. Select risk factors that contribute to the development of chronic kidney disease.
7. Summarize the significance of cardiovascular disease in individuals with chronic kidney disease.
8. Explain the conservative collaborative care for and the related nursing management of the patient with chronic kidney disease.
9. Differentiate among renal replacement therapy options for individuals with end-stage kidney disease.
10. Compare and contrast nursing interventions for individuals on peritoneal dialysis and hemodialysis.
11. Discuss the role of nurses in the management of individuals who receive a kidney transplant.

KEY TERMS

acute kidney injury (AKI), p. 1101
acute tubular necrosis (ATN), p. 1103
arteriovenous fistula (AVF), p. 1120
arteriovenous grafts (AVGs), p. 1120
automated peritoneal dialysis (APD), p. 1119
azotemia, p. 1102

chronic kidney disease (CKD), p. 1107
CKD mineral and bone disorder (CKD-MBD), p. 1110
continuous ambulatory peritoneal dialysis (CAPD), p. 1119
continuous renal replacement therapy (CRRT), p. 1123

dialysis, p. 1117
end-stage kidney (renal) disease (ESKD), p. 1107
hemodialysis (HD), p. 1117
oliguria, p. 1103
peritoneal dialysis (PD), p. 1117
uremia, p. 1108

Kidney failure (also called *renal failure*) is the partial or complete impairment of kidney function. It results in an inability to excrete metabolic waste products and water, and it contributes to disturbances of all body systems. Kidney disease can be classified as acute or chronic (Table 47-1). Acute kidney injury (AKI) has a rapid onset. Chronic kidney disease (CKD) is linked with the development of cardiovascular (CV) disease.

ACUTE KIDNEY INJURY

Acute kidney injury (AKI), previously known as *acute kidney failure*, is the term used to encompass the entire range of the syndrome, ranging from a slight deterioration in kidney function to severe impairment. AKI is characterized by a rapid loss of kidney function. This loss is accompanied by a rise in serum

---

Reviewed by Kay Helzer, RN, MSN, Former Renal/Pancreas Transplant Coordinator, Banner Good Samaritan Medical Center, Phoenix, Arizona; and Marci Langenkamp, RN, MS, Assistant Professor of Nursing, Edison Community College, Piqua, Ohio.

creatinine and/or a reduction in urine output. The severity of dysfunction can range from a small increase in serum creatinine or reduction in urine output to the development of **azotemia** (an accumulation of nitrogenous waste products [urea nitrogen, creatinine] in the blood).

Although AKI is potentially reversible, it has a high mortality rate.[1] AKI usually affects people with other life-threatening conditions[2] (Table 47-2). Most commonly, AKI follows severe, prolonged hypotension or hypovolemia or exposure to a nephrotoxic agent.

AKI can develop over hours or days with progressive elevations of blood urea nitrogen (BUN), creatinine, and potassium with or without a reduction in urine output. Hospitalized patients develop AKI at a high rate (1 in 5) and have a high mortality rate. When AKI develops in patients in intensive care units (ICUs), the mortality rate can be as high as 70% to 80%.[3-5]

Etiology and Pathophysiology

The causes of AKI, which are multiple and complex, are categorized as prerenal, intrarenal (or intrinsic), and postrenal causes (see Table 47-2).

Prerenal. *Prerenal* causes of AKI are factors external to the kidneys. These factors reduce systemic circulation, causing a reduction in renal blood flow. The decrease in blood flow leads to decreased glomerular perfusion and filtration of the kidneys. Although kidney tubular and glomerular function is preserved, glomerular filtration is reduced as a result of decreased perfusion.

It is important to distinguish prerenal oliguria from the oliguria of intrarenal AKI. In prerenal oliguria there is no damage to the kidney tissue (parenchyma). The oliguria is caused by a decrease in circulating blood volume (e.g., severe dehydration, heart failure [HF], decreased cardiac output) and is readily reversible with appropriate treatment. With a decrease in circulating blood volume, autoregulatory mechanisms that increase angiotensin II, aldosterone, norepinephrine, and antidiuretic hormone attempt to preserve blood flow to essential organs. Prerenal azotemia results in a reduction in the excretion of sodium (less than 20 mEq/L), increased sodium and water retention, and decreased urine output.

Prerenal conditions can lead to intrarenal disease if renal ischemia is prolonged. Prerenal conditions account for many cases of intrarenal AKI. If decreased perfusion persists for an extended time, the kidneys lose their ability to compensate and damage to kidney parenchyma occurs (intrarenal damage).

Intrarenal. *Intrarenal* causes of AKI (see Table 47-2) include conditions that cause direct damage to the kidney tissue, resulting in impaired nephron function. The damage from intrarenal causes usually results from prolonged ischemia, nephrotoxins

TABLE 47-1	COMPARISON OF ACUTE KIDNEY INJURY AND CHRONIC KIDNEY DISEASE	
	Acute Kidney Injury	**Chronic Kidney Disease**
Onset	Sudden	Gradual, often over many years
Most common cause	Acute tubular necrosis	Diabetic nephropathy
Diagnostic criteria	Acute reduction in urine output and/or Elevation in serum creatinine	GFR <60 mL/min/1.73m^2 for >3 mo and/or Kidney damage >3 mo
Reversibility	Potentially	Progressive and irreversible
Primary cause of death	Infection	Cardiovascular disease

GFR, Glomerular filtration rate.

TABLE 47-2	COMMON CAUSES OF ACUTE KIDNEY INJURY		
Prerenal	**Intrarenal**	**Postrenal**
Hypovolemia	**Nephrotoxic Injury**	• Benign prostatic hyperplasia
• Dehydration	• Drugs: aminoglycosides (gentamicin, amikacin), amphotericin B	• Bladder cancer
• Hemorrhage	• Contrast media	• Calculi formation
• GI losses (diarrhea, vomiting)	• Hemolytic blood transfusion reaction	• Neuromuscular disorders
• Excessive diuresis	• Severe crush injury	• Prostate cancer
• Hypoalbuminemia	• Chemical exposure: ethylene glycol, lead, arsenic, carbon tetrachloride	• Spinal cord disease
• Burns		• Strictures
	Interstitial Nephritis	• Trauma (back, pelvis, perineum)
Decreased Cardiac Output	• Allergies: antibiotics (sulfonamides, rifampin), nonsteroidal antiinflammatory drugs, ACE inhibitors	
• Cardiac dysrhythmias	• Infections: bacterial (acute pyelonephritis), viral (CMV), fungal (candidiasis)	
• Cardiogenic shock		
• Heart failure		
• Myocardial infarction	**Other Causes**	
	• Prolonged prerenal ischemia	
Decreased Peripheral Vascular Resistance	• Acute glomerulonephritis	
• Anaphylaxis	• Thrombotic disorders	
• Neurologic injury	• Toxemia of pregnancy	
• Septic shock	• Malignant hypertension	
	• Systemic lupus erythematosus	
Decreased Renovascular Blood Flow		
• Bilateral renal vein thrombosis		
• Embolism		
• Hepatorenal syndrome		
• Renal artery thrombosis		

ACE, Angiotensin-converting enzyme; *CMV,* cytomegalovirus.

FIG. 47-1 Acute tubular necrosis. The kidneys are swollen and pale.

	TABLE 47-3	**RIFLE CLASSIFICATION FOR STAGING ACUTE KIDNEY INJURY**	
Stage	**GFR Criteria**	**Urine Output Criteria**
Risk	Serum creatinine increased × 1.5 OR GFR decreased by 25%	Urine output <0.5 mL/kg/hr for 6 hr
Injury	Serum creatinine increased × 2 OR GFR decreased by 50%	Urine output <0.5 mL/kg/hr for 12 hr
Failure	Serum creatinine increased × 3 OR GFR decreased by 75% OR Serum creatinine >4 mg/dL with acute rise ≥0.5 mg/dL	Urine output <0.3 mL/kg/hr for 24 hr (oliguria) OR Anuria for 12 hr
Loss	Persistent acute kidney failure; complete loss of kidney function >4 wk	—
End-stage kidney disease	Complete loss of kidney function >3 mo	—

GFR, Glomerular filtration rate.

(e.g., aminoglycoside antibiotics, contrast media), hemoglobin released from hemolyzed red blood cells (RBCs), or myoglobin released from necrotic muscle cells.

Nephrotoxins can cause obstruction of intrarenal structures by crystallizing or by causing damage to the epithelial cells of the tubules. Hemoglobin and myoglobin can block the tubules and cause renal vasoconstriction. Diseases of the kidney such as acute glomerulonephritis and systemic lupus erythematosus may also cause AKI.

Acute tubular necrosis (ATN) is the most common intrarenal cause of AKI and is primarily the result of ischemia, nephrotoxins, or sepsis (Fig. 47-1). Ischemic and nephrotoxic ATN is responsible for 90% of intrarenal AKI cases.[6,7] Severe kidney ischemia causes a disruption in the basement membrane and patchy destruction of the tubular epithelium. Nephrotoxic agents cause necrosis of tubular epithelial cells, which slough off and plug the tubules. ATN is potentially reversible if the basement membrane is not destroyed and the tubular epithelium regenerates.

ATN is the most common cause of AKI for hospitalized patients. Risks associated with development of ATN while in the hospital include major surgery, shock, sepsis, blood transfusion reaction, muscle injury from trauma, prolonged hypotension, and nephrotoxic agents (see Table 47-2).

Postrenal. *Postrenal* causes of AKI involve mechanical obstruction in the outflow of urine. As the flow of urine is obstructed, urine refluxes into the renal pelvis, impairing kidney function. The most common causes are benign prostatic hyperplasia, prostate cancer, calculi, trauma, and extrarenal tumors. Bilateral ureteral obstruction leads to *hydronephrosis* (kidney dilation), increase in hydrostatic pressure, and tubular blockage, resulting in a progressive decline in kidney function. If bilateral obstruction is relieved within 48 hours of onset, complete recovery is likely. After 12 weeks, recovery is unlikely. Prolonged obstruction can lead to tubular atrophy and irreversible kidney fibrosis. Postrenal causes of AKI account for less than 10% of AKI cases.[7,8]

Clinical Manifestations

Prerenal and postrenal AKI that has not caused intrarenal damage usually resolves quickly with treatment of the cause. However, when parenchymal damage occurs due to either prerenal or postrenal causes, or when parenchymal damage occurs directly as with intrarenal causes, AKI has a prolonged course.

Clinically, AKI may progress through phases: oliguric, diuretic, and recovery. When a patient does not recover from AKI, then CKD may develop.

The RIFLE classification is used to describe the stages of AKI (Table 47-3). *Risk,* the first stage of AKI, is followed by *Injury,* which is the second stage. Then AKI increases in severity to the final or third stage, *Failure.* The two outcome variables are *Loss* and *End-stage kidney disease.* (See eTable 47-2 for a case study showing how RIFLE classification is used.)

Oliguric Phase. Manifestations of AKI are presented in eTable 47-1 (available on the website for this chapter). The most common manifestations are discussed in this section.

Urinary Changes. The most common initial manifestation of AKI is **oliguria,** a reduction in urine output to less than 400 mL/day. Nonoliguria AKI indicates a urine output greater than 400 mL/day. Oliguria usually occurs within 1 to 7 days of the injury to the kidneys. If the cause is ischemia, oliguria often occurs within 24 hours. In contrast, when nephrotoxic drugs are involved, the onset may be delayed for as long as 1 week. The oliguric phase lasts on average about 10 to 14 days but can last months in some cases. The longer the oliguric phase lasts, the poorer the prognosis for complete recovery of kidney function.[1]

About 50% of patients will not be oliguric, making the initial diagnosis more difficult.[5] Changes in urine output generally do not correspond to changes in glomerular filtration rate (GFR). However, changes in urine output are often helpful in differentiating the etiology of AKI. For example, anuria is usually seen with urinary tract obstruction, oliguria is commonly seen with prerenal etiologies, and nonoliguric AKI is seen with acute interstitial nephritis and ATN.[8]

A urinalysis may show casts, RBCs, and white blood cells (WBCs). The casts are formed from mucoprotein impressions of the necrotic renal tubular epithelial cells, which detach or slough into the tubules. In addition, a urinalysis may show a specific gravity fixed at around 1.010 and urine osmolality at about 300 mOsm/kg (300 mmol/kg). This is the same specific gravity and osmolality of plasma, thus reflecting tubular damage with a loss of concentrating ability by the kidney. Proteinuria may be present if kidney failure is related to glomerular membrane dysfunction.

Fluid Volume. Hypovolemia (volume depletion) has the potential to exacerbate all forms of AKI. The reversal of hypovolemia with fluid replacement is often sufficient to treat many forms of AKI, especially prerenal causes.

When urine output decreases, fluid retention occurs. The severity of the symptoms depends on the extent of the fluid overload. In the case of reduced urine output (anuria and oliguria), the neck veins may become distended with a bounding pulse. Edema and hypertension may develop. Fluid overload can eventually lead to HF, pulmonary edema, and pericardial and pleural effusions.

Metabolic Acidosis. In kidney failure the kidneys cannot synthesize ammonia (needed for hydrogen ion excretion) or excrete acid products of metabolism. The serum bicarbonate level decreases because bicarbonate is depleted in buffering hydrogen ions. In addition, defective reabsorption and regeneration of bicarbonate occur. With development of severe acidosis, the patient may develop Kussmaul respirations (rapid, deep respirations) in an effort to compensate by increasing the exhalation of carbon dioxide.

Sodium Balance. Damaged tubules cannot conserve sodium. Consequently, the urinary excretion of sodium may increase, resulting in normal or below-normal levels of serum sodium. Excessive intake of sodium should be avoided because it can lead to volume expansion, hypertension, and HF. Uncontrolled hyponatremia or water excess can lead to cerebral edema.

Potassium Excess. The kidneys normally excrete 80% to 90% of the body's potassium. In AKI the serum potassium level increases because the kidney's normal ability to excrete potassium is impaired. Hyperkalemia is more of a risk if AKI is caused by massive tissue trauma because the damaged cells release additional potassium into the extracellular fluid. Additionally, bleeding and blood transfusions may cause cellular destruction, releasing more potassium into the extracellular fluid. Last, acidosis worsens hyperkalemia as hydrogen ions enter the cells and potassium is driven out of the cells into the extracellular fluid.

Even though patients with hyperkalemia are usually asymptomatic, some patients may complain of weakness with severe hyperkalemia. Acute or rapid development of hyperkalemia may result in clinical signs that are apparent on electrocardiogram (ECG). These changes include peaked T waves, widening of the QRS complex, and ST segment depression. Progressive changes in the ECG that are related to increasing potassium levels are depicted in Fig. 17-14. Because cardiac muscle is intolerant of acute increases in potassium, treatment is essential whenever hyperkalemia develops.[9]

Hematologic Disorders. Several hematologic disorders are seen in patients with AKI. Hospital-acquired AKI often occurs in patients who have multiorgan failure. Leukocytosis is often present with AKI. The most common cause of death in AKI is infection. The most common sites of infection are the urinary and respiratory systems. A complete blood count with evidence of eosinophilia suggests an allergic response and possibly interstitial nephritis, polyarteritis nodosa, or atheroemboli.

Waste Product Accumulation. The kidneys are the primary excretory organs for urea (an end product of protein metabolism) and creatinine (an end product of endogenous muscle metabolism). BUN and serum creatinine levels are elevated in kidney failure. An elevated BUN level must be interpreted with caution because it can also be caused by dehydration; corticosteroids; or catabolism resulting from infections, fever, severe injury, or GI bleeding. The best serum indicator of AKI is creatinine because it is not significantly altered by other factors.

Neurologic Disorders. Neurologic changes can occur as the nitrogenous waste products accumulate in the brain and other nervous tissue. The manifestations can be as mild as fatigue and difficulty concentrating, and then escalate to seizures, stupor, and coma. *Asterixis* (flapping tremor when the wrist is extended) is most common with liver failure, but has been known to occur with advanced and severe kidney dysfunction. The flapping resembles a bird flapping its wings when the hands and wrists are extended outward.

Diuretic Phase. During the diuretic phase of AKI, daily urine output is usually around 1 to 3 L, but may reach 5 L or more. Although urine output is increasing, the nephrons are still not fully functional. The high urine volume is caused by osmotic diuresis from the high urea concentration in the glomerular filtrate and the inability of the tubules to concentrate the urine. In this phase the kidneys have recovered their ability to excrete wastes, but not to concentrate the urine. Hypovolemia and hypotension can occur from massive fluid losses. Patients who develop an oliguric phase will have greater diuresis than patients without oliguria.

Because of the large losses of fluid and electrolytes, the patient must be monitored for hyponatremia, hypokalemia, and dehydration. The diuretic phase may last 1 to 3 weeks. Near the end of this phase, the patient's acid-base, electrolyte, and waste product (BUN, creatinine) values begin to normalize.

Recovery Phase. The recovery phase begins when the GFR increases, allowing the BUN and serum creatinine levels to plateau and then decrease. Although the major improvements occur in the first 1 to 2 weeks of this phase, kidney function may take up to 12 months to stabilize.

The outcome of AKI is influenced by the patient's overall health, the severity of kidney failure, and the number and type of complications. Some individuals do not recover and progress to end-stage kidney disease. The older adult is less likely to have a complete recovery of kidney function. Most patients who recover achieve clinically normal kidney function with no complications (e.g., hypertension). Some scar tissue remains, but loss of function is not clinically significant.

Diagnostic Studies

A thorough history is essential for diagnosing the etiology of AKI. Consider prerenal causes when there is a history of dehydration, blood loss, or severe heart disease. Suspect intrarenal causes if the patient has been exposed to potentially nephrotoxic drugs or has a recent history of a blood transfusion or radiologic study using contrast media. Postrenal causes are suggested by a history of changes in the urinary stream, stones, benign prostatic hyperplasia, or cancer of the bladder or prostate.

Although changes in urine output and serum creatinine occur relatively late in the course of AKI, there are no better criteria for a diagnosis of AKI. An increase in serum creatinine may not be evident until there is a loss of more than 50% of kidney function. The rate of increase in serum creatinine is also important as a diagnostic indicator and in determining the severity of injury.

Urinalysis is an important diagnostic test. Urine sediment containing abundant cells, casts, or proteins suggests intrarenal disorders. The urine osmolality, sodium content, and specific gravity help in differentiating the causes of AKI. Urine sediment may be normal in both prerenal and postrenal AKI. In intrarenal problems, hematuria, pyuria, and crystals may be seen.

To establish a diagnosis of AKI, other testing may be required. A kidney ultrasound is often the first test done, since it provides imaging without exposure to potentially nephrotoxic contrast agents. It is useful for evaluating for possible kidney disease and obstruction of the urinary collection system. A renal scan can assess abnormalities in kidney blood flow, tubular function, and the collecting system. A computed tomography (CT) scan can identify lesions, masses, obstructions, and vascular anomalies. A renal biopsy is considered the best method for confirming intrarenal causes of AKI.

Obtaining a magnetic resonance imaging (MRI) or magnetic resonance angiography (MRA) study with the contrast media gadolinium is not advised in patients with kidney failure unless there is a significant reason to do these tests or unless the ultrasound or CT will not provide the information needed. Administration of gadolinium has been associated with the development of a devastating and potentially lethal disorder, *nephrogenic systemic fibrosis*, in patients with kidney failure. The disease is characterized by skin hyperpigmentation and induration and joint contractures. However, the fibrosis can also develop in other organs.

In patients with normal kidney function, administration of contrast media poses minimal risk. In patients with kidney failure, *contrast-induced nephropathy* (CIN) can occur when contrast media for diagnostic studies causes nephrotoxic injury. The best way to avoid CIN is to avoid exposure to contrast media by using other diagnostic tests such as ultrasound. If contrast media must be administered to a high-risk patient, the patient needs to have optimal hydration and a low dose of the contrast agent. Treatment to prevent CIN remains controversial. Optimal hydration is the goal, but debate continues on whether a bicarbonate or sodium chloride solution with or without the

prophylactic administration of *N*-acetylcysteine (Mucomyst) is beneficial.

Collaborative Care

Because AKI is potentially reversible, the primary goals of treatment are to eliminate the cause, manage the signs and symptoms, and prevent complications while the kidneys recover[2] (Table 47-4). The first step is to determine if there is adequate intravascular volume and cardiac output to ensure adequate perfusion of the kidneys. Diuretic therapy is often administered but not recommended in high doses. Diuretic therapy usually includes loop diuretics (e.g., furosemide [Lasix], bumetanide [Bumex]) or an osmotic diuretic (e.g., mannitol). If AKI is already established, forcing fluids and diuretics will not be effective and may, in fact, be harmful.

Closely monitor fluid intake during the oliguric phase of AKI. The general rule for calculating the fluid restriction is to add all losses for the previous 24 hours (e.g., urine, diarrhea, emesis, blood) plus 600 mL for insensible losses (e.g., respiration, diaphoresis). For example, if a patient excreted 300 mL of urine on Tuesday with no other losses, the fluid allocation on Wednesday would be 900 mL.

Hyperkalemia is one of the most serious complications in AKI because it can cause life-threatening cardiac dysrhythmias. The various therapies used to treat elevated potassium levels are listed in Table 47-5. Both insulin and sodium bicarbonate serve as a temporary measure for treatment of hyperkalemia by promoting a shift of potassium into the cells, but potassium will eventually be released. Calcium gluconate raises the threshold at which dysrhythmias occur, temporarily stabilizing the myocardium. Only sodium polystyrene sulfonate (Kayexalate) and

---

TABLE 47-4 COLLABORATIVE CARE

Acute Kidney Injury

Diagnostic
- History and physical examination
- Identification of precipitating cause
- Serum creatinine and BUN levels
- Serum electrolytes
- Urinalysis
- Renal ultrasound
- Renal scan
- CT scan

Collaborative Therapy
- Treatment of precipitating cause
- Fluid restriction (600 mL plus previous 24-hr fluid loss)
- Nutritional therapy
  - Adequate protein intake (0.6-2 g/kg/day) depending on degree of catabolism
  - Potassium restriction
  - Phosphate restriction
  - Sodium restriction
- Measures to lower potassium (if elevated) (see Table 47-5)
- Calcium supplements or phosphate-binding agents
- Enteral nutrition
- Parenteral nutrition
- Initiation of dialysis (if necessary)
- Continuous renal replacement therapy (if necessary)

TABLE 47-5 THERAPIES FOR ELEVATED POTASSIUM LEVELS

Regular Insulin IV
- Potassium moves into cells when insulin is given.
- IV glucose is given concurrently to prevent hypoglycemia.
- When effects of insulin diminish, potassium shifts back out of cells.

Sodium Bicarbonate
- Therapy can correct acidosis and cause a shift of potassium into cells.

Calcium Gluconate IV
- Generally used in advanced cardiac toxicity (with evidence of hyperkalemic ECG changes).
- Calcium raises the threshold for excitation, resulting in dysrhythmias.

Hemodialysis
- Most effective therapy to remove potassium.
- Works within a short time.

Sodium Polystyrene Sulfonate (Kayexalate)
- Cation-exchange resin is administered by mouth or retention enema.
- When resin is in the bowel, potassium is exchanged for sodium.
- Therapy removes 1 mEq of potassium per gram of drug.
- It is mixed in water with sorbitol to produce osmotic diarrhea, allowing for evacuation of potassium-rich stool from body.

Dietary Restriction
- Potassium intake is limited to 40 mEq/day.
- Primarily used to prevent recurrent elevation; not used for acute elevation.

dialysis actually remove potassium from the body. Never give this drug to a patient with a paralytic ileus because bowel necrosis can occur.

Conservative therapy may be all that is necessary until kidney function improves. Controversy exists about the timing of renal replacement therapy (RRT) in AKI.[10] The most common indications for RRT in AKI are (1) volume overload, resulting in compromised cardiac and/or pulmonary status; (2) elevated serum potassium level; (3) metabolic acidosis (serum bicarbonate level less than 15 mEq/L [15 mmol/L]); (4) BUN level greater than 120 mg/dL (43 mmol/L); (5) significant change in mental status; and (6) pericarditis, pericardial effusion, or cardiac tamponade. Although laboratory values provide rough parameters, the best guide to treatment is good clinical assessment.

If RRT is required, many options are available, but there is no consensus regarding the best approach.[10] Even though peritoneal dialysis (PD) is considered a viable option for RRT, it is not frequently used. Intermittent hemodialysis (HD) (e.g., at intervals of 4 hours either daily, every other day, or 3 or 4 times per week) and *continuous renal replacement therapy* (CRRT) have both been used effectively.

CRRT is provided continuously over approximately 24 hours through cannulation of an artery and vein or cannulation of two veins. CRRT has much slower blood flow rates compared with intermittent HD.

HD is the method of choice when rapid changes are required in a short time. It is technically more complicated because specialized staff and equipment and a vascular access are required. It also requires anticoagulation therapy to prevent the patient's blood from clotting when the blood contacts the foreign material in the extracorporeal dialysis circuit. Rapid fluid shifts during HD may cause hypotension.

RRT and CRRT are discussed later in this chapter on pp. 1123-1124.

Nutritional Therapy. The challenge of nutritional management in AKI is to provide adequate calories to prevent catabolism despite the restrictions required to prevent electrolyte and fluid disorders and azotemia. A primary nutritional goal in AKI is to maintain adequate caloric intake (providing 30 to 35 kcal/kg and 0.8 to 1.0 g of protein per kilogram of desired body weight) to prevent the further breakdown of body protein for energy purposes. Adequate energy should be primarily from carbohydrate and fat sources to prevent ketosis from endogenous fat breakdown and gluconeogenesis from muscle protein breakdown. Supplementation of essential amino acids can be given.

Potassium and sodium are regulated in accordance with plasma levels. Sodium is restricted as needed to prevent edema, hypertension, and HF. Dietary fat intake is increased so that the patient receives at least 30% to 40% of total calories from fat. Fat emulsion IV infusions given as a nutritional supplement provide a good source of nonprotein calories (see Chapter 40).

If a patient cannot maintain adequate oral intake, enteral nutrition is the preferred route for nutritional support (see Chapter 40). When the gastrointestinal (GI) tract is not functional, parenteral nutrition is necessary to provide adequate nutrition. The patient treated with parenteral nutrition may need daily HD or CRRT to remove the excess fluid. Concentrated formulas of parenteral nutrition are available to minimize fluid volume.

NURSING MANAGEMENT
ACUTE KIDNEY INJURY

NURSING ASSESSMENT

Monitor vital signs and fluid intake and output. Daily monitoring of a patient's urine output has prognostic implications and is crucial for determining therapy and daily fluid volume replacement. Examine the urine for color, specific gravity, glucose, protein, blood, and sediment. Assess the patient's general appearance, including skin color, edema, neck vein distention, and bruises.

If a patient is receiving dialysis, observe the access site for inflammation and exudate. Evaluate the patient's mental status and level of consciousness. Examine the oral mucosa for dryness and inflammation. Auscultate the lungs for crackles and rhonchi or diminished breath sounds. Monitor the heart for an S_3 gallop, murmurs, or a pericardial friction rub. Assess ECG readings for dysrhythmias. Review laboratory values and diagnostic test results. All of the previous data are essential for developing a collaborative plan of care.

NURSING DIAGNOSES

Nursing diagnoses and a potential complication for the patient with AKI include, but are not limited to, the following:

- Excess fluid volume *related to* kidney failure and fluid retention
- Risk for infection *related to* invasive lines, uremic toxins, and altered immune responses secondary to kidney failure
- Fatigue *related to* anemia, metabolic acidosis, and uremic toxins
- Anxiety *related to* disease processes, therapeutic interventions, and uncertainty of prognosis
- Potential complication: dysrhythmias *related to* electrolyte imbalances

PLANNING

The overall goals are that the patient with AKI will (1) completely recover without any loss of kidney function, (2) maintain normal fluid and electrolyte balance, (3) have decreased anxiety, and (4) adhere to and understand the need for careful follow-up care.

NURSING IMPLEMENTATION

HEALTH PROMOTION. Prevention and early recognition of AKI are the most important components of care.[11] Prevention is primarily directed toward identifying and monitoring high-risk populations, controlling exposure to nephrotoxic drugs and industrial chemicals, and preventing prolonged episodes of hypotension and hypovolemia. In the hospital the factors that increase the risk for developing AKI are preexisting CKD, older age, massive trauma, major surgical procedures, extensive burns, cardiac failure, sepsis, or obstetric complications.

Careful monitoring of intake and output and fluid and electrolyte balance is essential. Assess and record extrarenal losses of fluid from vomiting, diarrhea, hemorrhage, and increased insensible losses. Prompt replacement of significant fluid losses helps prevent ischemic tubular damage associated with trauma, burns, and extensive surgery. Intake and output records and the patient's weight provide valuable indicators of fluid volume status. Aggressive diuretic therapy for the patient with fluid overload from any cause can lead to a reduction in renal blood flow.[12]

The individual who is taking drugs that are potentially nephrotoxic (see Table 45-3) must have his or her kidney function monitored. Nephrotoxic drugs should be used sparingly in the high-risk patient. When these drugs must be used, they should be given in the smallest effective doses for the shortest possible periods. Caution the patient about abuse of over-the-counter analgesics (especially nonsteroidal antiinflammatory drugs [NSAIDs]) because some of these may worsen kidney function in the patient with mild CKD.

Angiotensin-converting enzyme (ACE) inhibitors can also decrease perfusion pressure and cause hyperkalemia. If other measures such as diet modification, diuretics, and sodium bicarbonate cannot control the hyperkalemia, ACE inhibitors may need to be reduced or eliminated. However, ACE inhibitors are frequently used to prevent proteinuria and progression of kidney disease, especially in diabetic patients.[13]

ACUTE INTERVENTION. The patient with AKI is critically ill and suffers from the effects of not only kidney disease but also co-morbid diseases or conditions (e.g., diabetes, CV disease). Focus on the patient holistically, since he or she will have many physical and emotional needs. Usually the changes caused by AKI arise suddenly. Both the patient and caregiver need assistance in understanding that the whole body's functioning can be disrupted by kidney failure.

You have an important role in managing fluid and electrolyte balance during the oliguric and diuretic phases. Observe and record accurate intake and output. Take daily weights with the same scale at the same time each day to detect excessive gains or losses of body fluid (1 kg is equivalent to 1000 mL of fluid). Assess for the common signs and symptoms of hypervolemia (in the oliguric phase) or hypovolemia (in the diuretic phase), potassium and sodium disturbances, and other electrolyte imbalances that may occur in AKI (see Chapter 17).

Because infection is the leading cause of death in AKI, meticulous aseptic technique is critical. Protect the patient from other individuals with infectious diseases. Be alert for local manifestations of infection (e.g., swelling, redness, pain), as well as systemic manifestations (e.g., fever, malaise, leukocytosis), but realize that the temperature may not always be elevated. Patients with kidney failure have a blunted febrile response to an infection (e.g., pneumonia). If antibiotics are used to treat an infection, the type, frequency, and dosage must be carefully considered because the kidneys are the primary route of excretion for many antibiotics. Dosages need to be considered in light of the patient's level of kidney function if the drug is primarily eliminated by the kidneys. Nephrotoxic drugs (see Table 45-3) should be used judiciously.

Perform skin care and take measures to prevent pressure ulcers because the patient usually develops edema and decreased muscle tone. Mouth care is important to prevent stomatitis, which develops when ammonia (produced by bacterial breakdown of urea) in saliva irritates the mucous membranes.

AMBULATORY AND HOME CARE. Recovery from AKI is highly variable and depends on other organ system failures, the patient's general condition and age, the length of the oliguric phase, and the severity of nephron damage. Protein and potassium intake should be regulated in accordance with kidney function. Follow-up care and regular evaluation of kidney function are necessary. Teach the patient the signs and symptoms of recurrent kidney disease. Emphasize measures to prevent the recurrence of AKI.

The long-term convalescence of 3 to 12 months may cause psychosocial and financial hardships for both the patient and the family. Make appropriate referrals for counseling. If the kidneys do not recover, the patient will need to transition to life on chronic dialysis or possible future transplantation.

EVALUATION

The expected outcomes are that the patient with AKI will
- Regain and maintain normal fluid and electrolyte balance
- Adhere to the treatment regimen
- Experience no complications
- Have a complete recovery

GERONTOLOGIC CONSIDERATIONS

ACUTE KIDNEY INJURY

Older adults are at risk for the same causes of AKI as younger adults. However, they are more susceptible to AKI. Dehydration is a predisposing factor and tends to occur much more frequently in older adults. Dehydration is associated with polypharmacy (diuretics, laxatives, and drugs that suppress appetite or consciousness), acute febrile illnesses, and immobility from being bedridden.

In addition to dehydration, other common causes of AKI in the older adult include hypotension, diuretic therapy, aminoglycoside therapy, obstructive disorders (e.g., prostatic hyperplasia), surgery, infection, and contrast media.

In older adults, impaired function of other organ systems from CV disease or diabetes mellitus can increase the risk of developing AKI. The aging kidney is less able to compensate for changes in fluid volume, solute load, and cardiac output. Mortality rates are similar for older patients and younger patients. However, patients over 65 years of age are less likely to recover from AKI. Despite this, a patient's chronologic age should not be factored into the decision about whether to institute RRT.[9,10]

CHRONIC KIDNEY DISEASE

Chronic kidney disease (CKD) involves progressive, irreversible loss of kidney function. The Kidney Disease Outcomes Quality Initiative (KDOQI) of the National Kidney Foundation defines CKD as either the presence of kidney damage or a decreased GFR less than 60 mL/min/1.73 m² for longer than 3 months. The classification of CKD is presented in Table 47-6. The last stage of kidney failure, end-stage kidney (renal) disease (ESKD), occurs when the GFR is less than 15 mL/min. At this point, RRT (dialysis or transplantation) is required to maintain life.

Although CKD has many different causes, the leading causes are diabetes (about 50%) and hypertension (about 25%). Less common etiologies include glomerulonephritis, cystic diseases, and urologic diseases.[14] (Diseases of the renal system that affect the kidney are discussed in Chapter 46.) CKD is much more

TABLE 47-6	STAGES OF CHRONIC KIDNEY DISEASE	
Description	**GFR (mL/ min/1.73 m²)**	**Clinical Action Plan**
Stage 1 Kidney damage with normal or ↑ GFR	≥90	Diagnosis and treatment CVD risk reduction Slow progression
Stage 2 Kidney damage with mild ↓ GFR	60-89	Estimation of progression
Stage 3 Moderate ↓ GFR	30-59	Evaluation and treatment of complications
Stage 4 Severe ↓ GFR	15-29	Preparation for renal replacement therapy (dialysis, kidney transplant)
Stage 5 Kidney failure	<15 (or dialysis)	Renal replacement therapy (if uremia present and patient desires treatment)

Source: National Kidney Foundation. *www.kidney.org/kidneydisease/aboutckd.cfm.*

🌐 CULTURAL & ETHNIC HEALTH DISPARITIES

Chronic Kidney Disease

- Chronic kidney disease (CKD) has a high incidence in minority populations, especially African Americans and Native Americans.
- Hypertension and diabetes mellitus are also more common in African Americans and Native Americans.

African Americans
- The risk of CKD as a complication of hypertension is significantly increased in African Americans.
- African Americans have the highest rate of CKD, nearly four times that of whites.

Native Americans
- Native Americans have a rate of CKD twice that of whites.
- The rate of CKD is six times higher among Native Americans with diabetes than among other ethnic groups with diabetes.

Hispanics
- The rate of CKD in Hispanics is 1.5 times higher than in non-Hispanic whites.

common than AKI (see Table 47-1). The increasing prevalence of CKD has been partially attributed to the increase in risk factors, including an aging population, rise in rates of obesity, and increased incidence of diabetes and hypertension.[14,15]

More than 26 million American adults have CKD, and a million more are at increased risk. One of every nine Americans has CKD. Over half a million Americans are receiving treatment (dialysis, transplant) for ESKD. Despite all the technologic advances in life-sustaining treatment with dialysis, patients with ESKD have a high mortality rate. As the stage of kidney disease progresses, the mortality rate also increases. Mortality rates are as high as 19% to 24% for individuals with stage 5 CKD on dialysis. About 20% of patients with ESKD receiving dialysis die each year.[14]

Because the kidneys are highly adaptive, kidney disease is often not recognized until there has been considerable loss of nephrons. Because patients with CKD are frequently asymptomatic, CKD is underdiagnosed and undertreated. It has been estimated that about 70% of people with CKD are unaware that they have the disease.[14]

The prognosis and course of CKD are highly variable depending on the etiology, patient's condition and age, and adequacy of health care follow-up. Some individuals live normal, active lives with compensated kidney failure, whereas others may rapidly progress to ESKD (stage 5). Since 1972, the United States has covered the majority of the costs of providing dialysis for those eligible for Medicare benefits. Under Title XVIII of the Social Security Act, ESKD was recognized as a disability. As such, more than 90% of individuals of any age who have ESKD are eligible for financial assistance for treatment through Medicare. Medicare pays for 80% of eligible charges, with the remaining being paid for by state or private insurance or out of pocket.[14]

Clinical Manifestations

As kidney function deteriorates, every body system becomes affected. The clinical manifestations are a result of retained substances, including urea, creatinine, phenols, hormones, electrolytes, and water. Uremia is a syndrome in which kidney function declines to the point that symptoms may develop in multiple body systems (Fig. 47-2). It often occurs when the GFR is 10 mL/min or less.

The manifestations of uremia vary among patients according to the cause of the kidney disease, co-morbid conditions, age, and degree of adherence to the prescribed medical regimen. Many patients are tolerant of the changes because they occur gradually.

Urinary System. In the early stages of CKD, patients usually do not report any change in urine output. Since diabetes is the primary cause of CKD, polyuria may be present, but not necessarily as a consequence of kidney disease. Because most people continue to have sufficient urine output, it is often difficult to convince them that they have kidney disease. As CKD progresses, patients have increasing difficulty with fluid retention and require diuretic therapy. After a period on dialysis, patients may develop anuria.

Metabolic Disturbances

Waste Product Accumulation. As the GFR decreases, the BUN and serum creatinine levels increase. The BUN is increased not only by kidney failure, but also by protein intake, fever, corticosteroids, and catabolism. For this reason, serum creatinine clearance determinations (calculated GFR) are considered more accurate indicators of kidney function than BUN or creatinine. Significant elevations in BUN contribute to development of nausea, vomiting, lethargy, fatigue, impaired thought processes, and headaches.

Altered Carbohydrate Metabolism. Defective carbohydrate metabolism is caused by impaired glucose metabolism, resulting from cellular insensitivity to the normal action of insulin. Mild to moderate hyperglycemia and hyperinsulinemia may occur. Insulin and glucose metabolism may improve (but not to normal values) after the initiation of dialysis.

Patients with diabetes who develop uremia may require less insulin than before the onset of CKD. This is because insulin, which depends on the kidneys for excretion, remains in circulation longer. As a result, a number of patients who required insulin before starting dialysis will be able to discontinue insulin therapy when they start dialysis and their kidney disease pro-

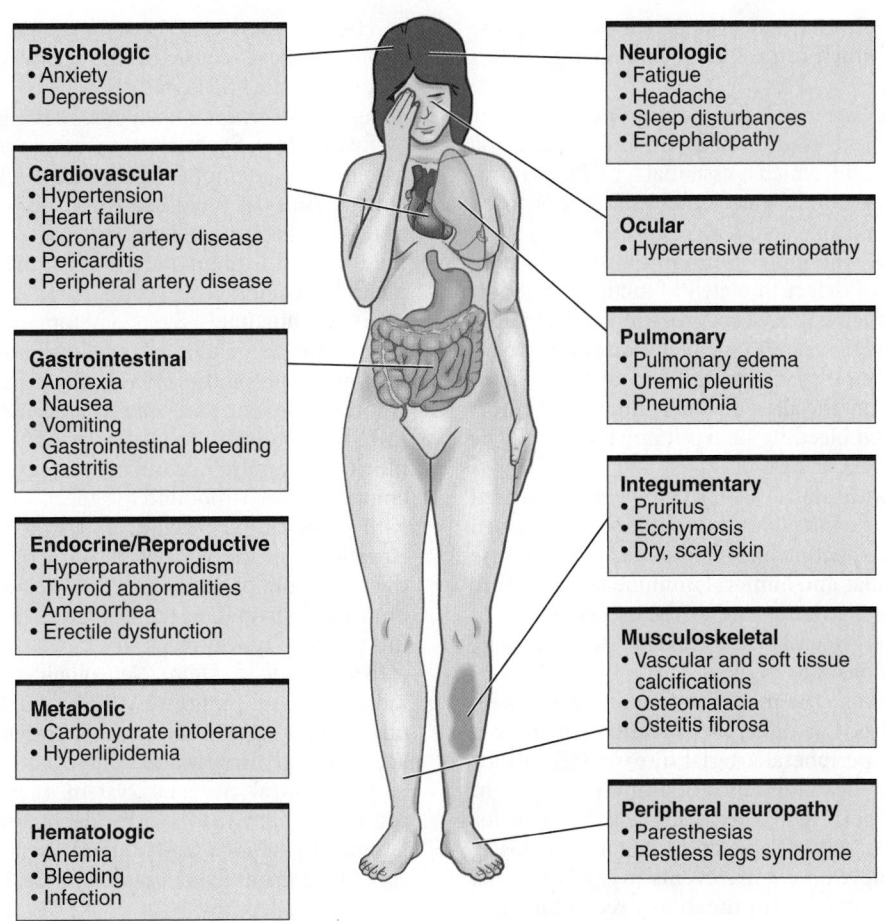

Psychologic
• Anxiety
• Depression

Cardiovascular
• Hypertension
• Heart failure
• Coronary artery disease
• Pericarditis
• Peripheral artery disease

Gastrointestinal
• Anorexia
• Nausea
• Vomiting
• Gastrointestinal bleeding
• Gastritis

Endocrine/Reproductive
• Hyperparathyroidism
• Thyroid abnormalities
• Amenorrhea
• Erectile dysfunction

Metabolic
• Carbohydrate intolerance
• Hyperlipidemia

Hematologic
• Anemia
• Bleeding
• Infection

Neurologic
• Fatigue
• Headache
• Sleep disturbances
• Encephalopathy

Ocular
• Hypertensive retinopathy

Pulmonary
• Pulmonary edema
• Uremic pleuritis
• Pneumonia

Integumentary
• Pruritus
• Ecchymosis
• Dry, scaly skin

Musculoskeletal
• Vascular and soft tissue
  calcifications
• Osteomalacia
• Osteitis fibrosa

Peripheral neuropathy
• Paresthesias
• Restless legs syndrome

FIG. 47-2 Possible clinical manifestations of chronic kidney disease.

gresses. The insulin dosing must be individualized and glucose levels monitored carefully.

Elevated Triglycerides. Hyperinsulinemia stimulates hepatic production of triglycerides. Almost all patients with uremia develop dyslipidemia, with increased very-low-density lipoproteins (VLDLs), increased low-density lipoproteins (LDLs), and decreased high-density lipoproteins (HDLs). The altered lipid metabolism is related to decreased levels of the enzyme lipoprotein lipase, which is important in the breakdown of lipoproteins. Most patients with CKD die from CV disease.[15]

Electrolyte and Acid-Base Imbalances

Potassium. Hyperkalemia is a serious electrolyte disorder associated with kidney disease. Fatal dysrhythmias have been reported when the serum potassium level reaches 7 to 8 mEq/L (7 to 8 mmol/L). Hyperkalemia results from the decreased excretion of potassium by the kidneys, the breakdown of cellular protein, bleeding, and metabolic acidosis. Potassium may also come from the food consumed, dietary supplements, drugs, and IV infusions.

Sodium. Sodium may be elevated, normal, or low in kidney failure. Because of impaired sodium excretion, sodium along with water is retained. If large quantities of water are retained, dilutional hyponatremia occurs. Sodium retention can contribute to edema, hypertension, and HF. Sodium intake must be individually determined but is generally restricted to 2 g/day.

Calcium and Phosphate. Calcium and phosphate alterations are discussed in the section on the musculoskeletal system on p. 1110.

Magnesium. Magnesium is primarily excreted by the kidneys. Hypermagnesemia is generally not a problem unless the

patient is ingesting magnesium (e.g., milk of magnesia, magnesium citrate, antacids containing magnesium). Clinical manifestations of hypermagnesemia can include absence of reflexes, decreased mental status, cardiac dysrhythmias, hypotension, and respiratory failure.

Metabolic Acidosis. Metabolic acidosis results from the kidneys' impaired ability to excrete the acid load (primarily ammonia) and from defective reabsorption and regeneration of bicarbonate. The average adult produces 80 to 90 mEq of acid per day. This acid is normally buffered by bicarbonate. In kidney failure, plasma bicarbonate, which is an indirect measure of acidosis, usually falls to a new steady state at around 16 to 20 mEq/L (16 to 20 mmol/L). The decrease in plasma bicarbonate reflects its use in buffering metabolic acids. The bicarbonate level generally does not progress below this level because hydrogen ion production is usually balanced by buffering from demineralization of the bone (the phosphate buffering system).

Hematologic System

Anemia. A normocytic, normochromic anemia is associated with CKD. The anemia is due to decreased production of the hormone erythropoietin by the kidneys. Erythropoietin normally stimulates precursor cells in the bone marrow to produce RBCs (erythropoiesis). Other factors contributing to anemia are nutritional deficiencies, decreased RBC life span, increased hemolysis of RBCs, frequent blood samplings, and bleeding from the GI tract. For patients receiving maintenance hemodialysis (HD), blood loss in the dialyzer may also contribute to the anemic state. Elevated levels of parathyroid hormone (PTH) (produced to compensate for low serum calcium levels) can inhibit erythropoiesis, shorten survival of RBCs, and cause bone marrow fibrosis, which can result in decreased numbers of hematopoietic cells.

Sufficient iron stores are needed for erythropoiesis. Many patients with kidney failure are iron deficient and require oral iron supplements. Folic acid, which is essential for RBC maturation, is dialyzable because it is water soluble. It needs to be supplemented in the diet (folic acid 1 mg/day).

Bleeding Tendencies. The most common cause of bleeding in uremia is a qualitative defect in platelet function. This dysfunction is caused by impaired platelet aggregation and impaired release of platelet factor III. In addition, alterations in the coagulation system with increased concentrations of both factor VIII and fibrinogen occur. The altered platelet function, hemorrhagic tendencies, and GI bleeding susceptibility can usually be corrected with regular HD or PD.

Infection. Patients with advanced CKD have an increased susceptibility to infection. Infectious complications are caused by changes in leukocyte function and altered immune response and function. Both cellular and humoral immune responses are suppressed. Other factors contributing to the increased risk of infection include hyperglycemia and external trauma (e.g., catheters, needle insertions into vascular access sites).

Cardiovascular System. The most common cause of death in patients with CKD is CV disease. Myocardial infarction, ischemic heart disease, peripheral arterial disease, HF, cardiomyopathy, and stroke are leading causes of death. Even a slight reduction in GFR has been associated with a higher risk for coronary artery disease.[15] CV disease and CKD are so closely linked that if patients develop cardiac events (e.g., myocardial infarction, HF), evaluation of kidney function is recommended.

Traditional CV risk factors such as hypertension and elevated lipids are common in CKD patients. However, CV disease may also be related to nontraditional CV risk factors such as vascular calcification and arterial stiffness, which are major contributors to CV disease in patients with CKD. The calcium deposits in the vascular medial layer are associated with stiffening of the blood vessels. The mechanisms involved are multifactorial. They include (1) vascular smooth muscle cells changing into chondrocytes or osteoblast-like cells, (2) high total body amount of calcium and phosphate resulting from abnormal bone metabolism, (3) impaired renal excretion, and (4) drug therapies to treat the bone disease (e.g., calcium phosphate binders).[16]

Hypertension is highly prevalent in patients with CKD because hypertension is both a cause and a consequence of CKD. Hypertension is aggravated by sodium retention and increased extracellular fluid volume.[17] In some individuals, increased renin production contributes to hypertension (see Fig. 45-4).

Hypertension and diabetes mellitus are contributing risk factors for vascular complications. The vascular changes from long-standing hypertension and the accelerated atherosclerosis contribute to the higher rate of CV disease in CKD. Left ventricular hypertrophy (LVH) is present in about 75% of patients receiving dialysis. Long-standing hypertension, extracellular fluid volume overload, and anemia contribute to development of LVH that may eventually lead to cardiomyopathy and HF.

Patients with CKD are susceptible to cardiac dysrhythmias that result from hyperkalemia and decreased coronary artery perfusion. Uremic pericarditis can develop and occasionally progresses to pericardial effusion and cardiac tamponade. Pericarditis is typically manifested by a friction rub, chest pain, and low-grade fever.

Hypertension can cause retinopathy, encephalopathy, and nephropathy. Because of the many effects of hypertension, blood pressure (BP) control is one of the most important therapeutic goals in the management of CKD.

Respiratory System. With severe acidosis, the respiratory system may attempt to compensate with Kussmaul breathing, which results in increased carbon dioxide removal by exhalation (see Chapter 17). Dyspnea may occur as a manifestation of fluid overload, pulmonary edema, uremic pleuritis (pleurisy), pleural effusions, and respiratory infections (e.g., pneumonia).

Gastrointestinal System. Stomatitis with exudates and ulcerations, a metallic taste in the mouth, and *uremic fetor* (a urinous odor of the breath) are commonly found in CKD. Anorexia, nausea, and vomiting may develop if CKD progresses to ESKD and is not treated with dialysis. Weight loss and malnutrition may also occur. Diabetic *gastroparesis* (delayed gastric emptying) can compound the effects of malnutrition for patients with diabetes. GI bleeding is also a risk because of mucosal irritation and the platelet defect. Constipation may be due to the ingestion of iron salts or calcium-containing phosphate binders. Constipation can be made worse by limitations on fluid intake and physical inactivity.

Neurologic System. Neurologic changes are expected as kidney failure progresses. They are the result of increased nitrogenous waste products, electrolyte imbalances, metabolic acidosis, and atrophy and demyelination of nerve fibers.

The central nervous system (CNS) becomes depressed, resulting in lethargy, apathy, decreased ability to concentrate, fatigue, irritability, and altered mental ability. Seizures and coma may result from a rapidly increasing BUN and hypertensive encephalopathy.

Peripheral neuropathy is initially manifested by a slowing of nerve conduction to the extremities. Individuals with advanced stage 5 CKD may complain of restless legs syndrome (see Chapter 59), described as "bugs crawling inside the leg." Paresthesias are most often experienced in the feet and legs and may be described by the patient as a burning sensation. Eventually, motor involvement may lead to bilateral footdrop, muscular weakness and atrophy, and loss of deep tendon reflexes. Muscle twitching, jerking, *asterixis* (hand-flapping tremor), and nocturnal leg cramps also occur. In patients with diabetes, uremic neuropathy is compounded by the neuropathy associated with diabetes mellitus.

Dialysis should improve general CNS manifestations and may slow or halt the progression of neuropathies. However, motor neuropathy may not be reversible. The treatment for neurologic problems is dialysis or transplantation. Altered mental status, a late manifestation of CKD stage 5, is rarely seen unless the patient has chosen to forgo RRT.

Musculoskeletal System. CKD mineral and bone disorder (CKD-MBD) develops as a systemic disorder of mineral and bone metabolism caused by progressive deterioration in kidney function (Fig. 47-3). As kidney function deteriorates, less vitamin D is converted to its active form, resulting in decreased serum levels. Activated vitamin D is necessary to optimize absorption of calcium from the GI tract; thus low levels of active vitamin D result in decreased serum calcium levels.[18]

Normally serum calcium levels are tightly regulated. PTH is the primary regulator of serum calcium levels. When hypocalcemia occurs, the parathyroid gland secretes PTH, which stimulates bone demineralization, thereby releasing calcium from the bones. Phosphate is released as well, leading to elevated

PATHOPHYSIOLOGY MAP

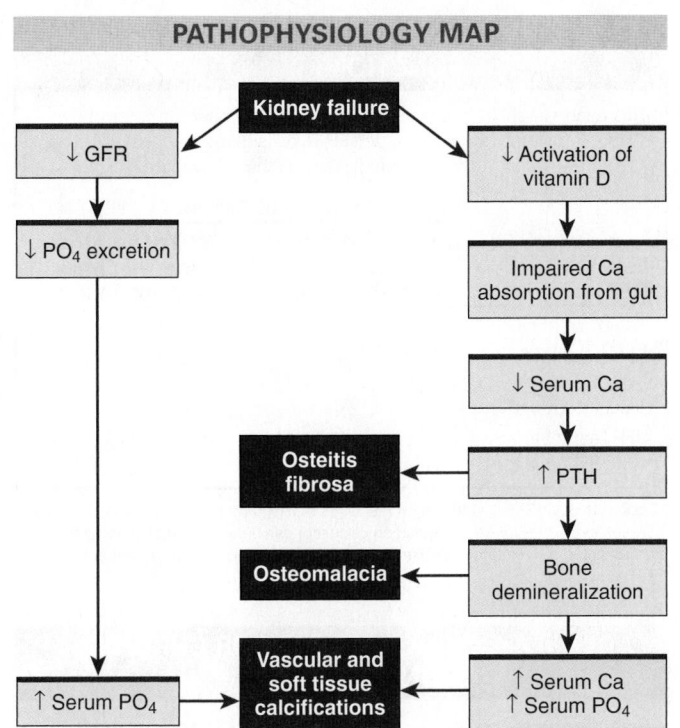

FIG. 47-3 Mechanisms of chronic kidney disease mineral and bone disorder (CKD-MBD). *GFR,* Glomerular filtration rate; *PTH,* parathyroid hormone.

serum phosphate levels. Hyperphosphatemia also results from decreased phosphate excretion by the kidneys. Hyperphosphatemia decreases serum calcium levels and further reduces the kidneys' ability to activate vitamin D.

Low serum calcium, elevated phosphate, and decreased vitamin D contribute to the stimulation of the parathyroid gland and excretion of PTH. The PTH acts on the bone to increase remodeling and increase serum calcium levels. The accelerated rate of bone remodeling causes a weakened bone matrix and places the patient at a higher risk for fractures.

Normally plasma calcium is found ionized or free (physiologically active form) or bound to protein. In kidney failure, it is unusual for hypocalcemia to be symptomatic. The reason for this is that, in the acidotic state associated with renal failure, more calcium is in the ionized form than is bound to protein. However, a low ionized calcium level can lead to tetany (see Chapter 17).

CKD-MBD is a common complication of CKD and results in both skeletal complications and extraskeletal complications (vascular and soft tissue complications). Skeletal complications include *osteomalacia,* which results from demineralization from slow bone turnover and defective mineralization of newly formed bone, and *osteitis fibrosa,* a decalcification of the bone and replacement of bone tissue with fibrous tissue.

Extraskeletal complications result from vascular calcifications. As previously mentioned, vascular calcifications are a significant contributing factor to CV disease. "Uremic red eye" is caused by the irritation from calcium deposits in the eye. Intracardiac calcifications can disrupt the conduction system and cause cardiac arrest. CKD-MBD contributes significantly to a patient's increased morbidity and mortality risks.[18]

Integumentary System. Pruritus is more prevalent in patients receiving dialysis than in the earlier stages of CKD. A small percentage of patients develop refractory pruritus that can have a devastating impact on their well-being and quality of life. Pruritus has multiple causes, including dry skin, calcium-phosphate deposition in the skin, and sensory neuropathy. The itching may be so intense that it can lead to bleeding or infection secondary to scratching. Uremic frost is an extremely rare condition in which urea crystallizes on the skin; this is usually seen only when BUN levels are extremely elevated (e.g., over 200 mg/dL).

Reproductive System. Both men and women can experience infertility and a decreased libido. Women usually have decreased levels of estrogen, progesterone, and luteinizing hormone, causing anovulation and menstrual changes (usually amenorrhea). Menses and ovulation may return after dialysis is started. Men experience loss of testicular consistency, decreased testosterone levels, and low sperm counts.

Sexual dysfunction may also be caused by anemia, which causes fatigue and decreased libido. In addition, peripheral neuropathy can cause impotence in men and anorgasmy in women. Additional factors that may cause changes in sexual function are psychologic problems (e.g., anxiety, depression), physical stress, and side effects of drugs.

Sexual function may improve with maintenance dialysis and may become normal with successful transplantation. Patients that become pregnant while receiving dialysis have been able to carry a fetus to term, but there is significant risk to the mother and infant. Pregnancy in patients with a kidney transplant is more common, but there is still considerable risk to both the mother and fetus.

Psychologic Changes. Personality and behavioral changes, emotional lability, withdrawal, and depression are commonly observed in patients with CKD. Fatigue and lethargy contribute to the feeling of illness. The changes in body image caused by edema, integumentary disturbances, and access devices (e.g., fistulas, catheters) may lead to anxiety and depression. Decreased ability to concentrate and slowed mental activity can give the appearance of dullness and disinterest in the environment. The patient must also deal with significant changes in lifestyle, occupation, family responsibilities, and financial status. Long-term survival depends on medications, dietary restrictions, dialysis, and possibly transplantation. The patient also grieves the loss of kidney function. This can be a prolonged process for some individuals.

Diagnostic Studies

Because persistent proteinuria is usually the first indication of kidney damage, screening for CKD involves a dipstick evaluation of protein in the urine or evaluation for microalbuminuria, which is not detected with routine urinalysis. Patients with diabetes need to have examination of their urine for microalbuminuria if none is detected on routine urinalysis.

A person with persistent proteinuria (1+ protein on standard dipstick testing two or more times over a 3-month period) should have further assessment of risk factors and a diagnostic workup with blood and urine tests to evaluate for CKD. A urine test for albumin-to-creatinine ratio provides an accurate estimate of the protein and albumin excretion rate. A ratio greater than 300 mg albumin per 1 g creatinine signals CKD.

A urinalysis can detect RBCs, WBCs, protein, casts, and glucose. An ultrasound of the kidneys is usually done to detect any obstructions and to determine the size of the kidneys. Other diagnostic studies (Table 47-7) help establish the diagnosis and

TABLE 47-7 COLLABORATIVE CARE
Chronic Kidney Disease

Diagnostic
- History and physical examination
- Identification of reversible kidney disease
- Renal ultrasound
- Renal scan
- CT scan
- Renal biopsy
- BUN, serum creatinine, and creatinine clearance levels
- Serum electrolytes
- Lipid profile
- Protein-to-creatinine ratio in first morning voided specimen
- Urinalysis
- Hematocrit and hemoglobin levels

Collaborative Therapy
- Correction of extracellular fluid volume overload or deficit
- Nutritional therapy*
- Erythropoietin therapy
- Calcium supplementation, phosphate binders, or both
- Antihypertensive therapy
- Angiotensin-converting enzyme (ACE) inhibitors or angiotensin receptor blockers (ARBs)
- Measures to treat hyperlipidemia
- Measures to lower potassium†
- Adjustment of drug dosages to degree of renal function
- Renal replacement therapy (dialysis, kidney transplant)

*See Tables 47-10 and 47-11.
†See Table 47-5.

TABLE 47-8 INDICATORS OF KIDNEY FUNCTION

This example shows why serum creatinine is a poor indicator of kidney function. Calculation of GFR is considered the best index to estimate kidney function as indicated by the following example.

Estimation of GFR	**Type of Patient** 76-Yr-Old African American Woman (Weight 56 kg)	28-Yr-Old African American Man (Weight 74 kg)
Serum creatinine	1.4 mg/dL	1.4 mg/dL
GFR, estimated by the Cockcroft-Gault formula*	30.2 mL/min	82.2 mL/min
GFR, estimated by MDRD equation†	47 mL/min/1.73 m²	64 mL/min/1.73 m²

*Cockcroft-Gault GFR = (140 − Age) × (Weight in kilograms) × (0.85 if female)/(72 × Cr).
†GFR as estimated by MDRD equation calculator can be accessed at www.mdrd.com.
Cr, Creatinine; GFR, glomerular filtration rate; MDRD, modification of diet in renal disease.

TABLE 47-9 RISK FACTORS FOR CHRONIC KIDNEY DISEASE

Risk Factors	Prevention and Management
Diabetes	Achieve optimal glycemic control.
Hypertension	Maintain BP in normal range with angiotensin-converting enzyme (ACE) inhibitors or angiotensin receptor blockers (ARBs).
Age >60 yr	Prevent insult or kidney injury.
Cardiovascular disease	Institute aggressive risk factor reduction.
Family history of CKD	Teach about increased risk and assist with appropriate screening (BP measurement, urinalysis).
Exposure to nephrotoxic drugs	Limit exposure and give sodium bicarbonate as treatment.
Ethnic minority (e.g., African American, Native American)	Teach about increased risk and assist with appropriate screening (BP measurement, urinalysis).

cause of CKD. A kidney biopsy may be necessary to provide a definitive diagnosis.

Many consider serum creatinine the best indicator of kidney function, but in reality serum creatinine alone poorly reflects kidney function. GFR is the preferred measure to determine kidney function. Several GFR calculators are available. The two equations used most frequently to estimate GFR are the Cockcroft-Gault formula and the Modification of Diet in Renal Disease (MDRD) Study equation (Table 47-8). The National Kidney Foundation KDOQI guidelines recommend the MDRD Study equation to estimate GFR.[19]

Collaborative Care

The overall goals of CKD therapy are to preserve existing kidney function, reduce the risks of CV disease, prevent complications, and provide for the patient's comfort (Table 47-9). For many, early recognition, diagnosis, and treatment can deter the progression of kidney disease. It is important that patients with CKD receive appropriate follow-up and referral to a nephrologist early in the course of the disease. Every effort is made to detect and treat potentially reversible causes of kidney failure (e.g., HF, dehydration, infections, nephrotoxins, urinary tract obstruction, glomerulonephritis, renal artery stenosis).

Patients with CKD have a high incidence of CV complications. A higher percentage of patients will die from CV disease than live to need dialysis. When a patient is diagnosed as having CKD, therapy is aimed at treating the CV disease in addition to slowing the progression of kidney disease (see Table 47-7).

A focus on stages 1 through 4 (see Table 47-6) before the need for dialysis (stage 5) includes the control of hypertension, hyperparathyroid disease, anemia, hyperglycemia, and dyslipidemia. The following section focuses primarily on the drug and nutritional aspects of care.

Drug Therapy

Hyperkalemia. Multiple strategies are used to manage hyperkalemia (see Table 47-5). Every effort is made to control hyperkalemia with the restriction of high-potassium foods and drugs. Acute hyperkalemia may require treatment with IV glucose and insulin or IV 10% calcium gluconate. Sodium polystyrene sulfonate, a cation-exchange resin, is commonly used to lower potassium levels in stage 4 and can be administered on an outpatient basis.

Tell the patient to expect some diarrhea because this preparation contains sorbitol, a sugar alcohol that has an osmotic laxative action and ensures evacuation of the potassium from the bowel. Never give sodium polystyrene sulfonate to a patient with a hypoactive bowel (paralytic ileus) because fluid shifts could lead to bowel necrosis. As sodium polystyrene sulfonate exchanges sodium ions for potassium ions, observe the patient for sodium and water retention. If changes appear in the ECG such as peaked T waves and widened QRS complexes, dialysis may be required to remove excess potassium.

Hypertension. For some, the progression of CKD can be delayed by controlling hypertension. (Control and treatment of

Translating Research Into Practice

Can Exercise Improve Physical Fitness in Chronic Kidney Disease?

Clinical Question
For adults with chronic kidney disease (P), what is the effect of exercise (I) on physical fitness and functioning (O)?

Best Available Evidence
Systematic review of randomized controlled trials (RCTs)

Critical Appraisal and Synthesis of Evidence
- Forty-five RCTs ($n = 1863$) of adults with chronic kidney disease (CKD) or kidney transplant. Physical exercise interventions lasted at least 8 wk. Most common intervention was aerobic exercise.
- Fitness and cardiovascular parameters were measured.
- Regular exercise improved muscle strength, walking ability, blood pressure and heart rate, and quality of life.
- Exercise did not significantly affect total cholesterol or triglyceride levels.

Conclusion
- Exercise significantly improved physical fitness (aerobic capacity).

Implications for Nursing Practice
- Encourage regular aerobic exercise to counter muscle strength loss in patients with CKD.
- Maintain contact with patient to promote and encourage adherence to recommended exercise.

Reference for Evidence
Heiwe S, Jacobson SH: Exercise training for adults with chronic kidney disease, *Cochrane Database Syst Rev* 10:CD003236, 2011.

P, Patient population of interest; *I*, intervention or area of interest; *O*, outcomes of interest (see p. 12).

hypertension are discussed in Chapter 33.) It is recommended that the target BP be less than 130/80 mm Hg for patients with CKD and 125/75 mm Hg for patients with significant proteinuria.[17] Treatment of hypertension includes (1) weight loss (if obese), (2) therapeutic lifestyle changes (e.g., exercise, avoidance of alcohol, smoking cessation), (3) diet recommendations (DASH Diet; see eTable 33-1), and (4) administration of antihypertensive drugs. Most patients require two or more drugs to reach target BP.

The antihypertensive drugs most commonly used are diuretics, calcium channel blockers, ACE inhibitors, and angiotensin receptor blocker (ARB) agents. Prescribed medications depend on whether the patient with CKD has diabetes or not. The ACE inhibitors and ARBs are used with diabetics and those with nondiabetic proteinuria because they decrease proteinuria and possibly delay the progression of CKD. However, they must be used cautiously in patients with ESKD because they can further decrease the GFR and increase serum potassium levels.

Periodically measure the BP with the patient in the supine, sitting, and standing positions to monitor the effect of antihypertensive drugs. Teach the patient and caregiver how to monitor the BP at home and what readings require immediate intervention. BP control is essential to slow atherosclerotic changes that could further impair kidney function.

CKD-MBD. Interventions for CKD-MBD include limiting dietary phosphorus, administering phosphate binders, supplementing vitamin D, and controlling hyperparathyroidism.[18] Phosphate intake is not usually restricted until the patient requires RRT. At that time, phosphate is usually limited to about 1 g/day, but dietary control alone is usually inadequate.

Phosphate binders include calcium-based binders: calcium acetate (PhosLo) and calcium carbonate (Caltrate). They bind phosphate in the bowel and are then excreted in the stool. The administration of calcium may increase the calcium load and place the patient at increased risk for vascular calcifications. Therefore, when calcium levels are increased or there is evidence of existing vascular or soft tissue calcifications, consider changing to noncalcium-based phosphate binders, such as lanthanum carbonate (Fosrenol) and sevelamer carbonate (Renvela).

To be most effective, administer phosphate binders with each meal. Constipation is a frequent side effect of phosphate binders and may necessitate the use of stool softeners.

Because bone disease (osteomalacia) is associated with excessive aluminum, aluminum preparations should be used with caution in patients with kidney failure. Do not use magnesium-containing antacids (e.g., Maalox, Mylanta) because magnesium depends on the kidneys for excretion.

Hypocalcemia is a problem in the later stages of CKD because of the inability of the GI tract to absorb calcium in the absence of active vitamin D. If hypocalcemia persists even if the serum phosphate levels are normal, then supplemental calcium and vitamin D should be given. Assess vitamin D levels to determine the need for supplementation. If the levels are low (serum values less than 30 ng/mL), vitamin D supplementation is recommended in the form of cholecalciferol.

Treatment of secondary hyperparathyroidism in ESKD patients requires the activated form of vitamin D because the kidneys no longer possess the ability to activate vitamin D. Active vitamin D is available as oral or IV calcitriol (Rocaltrol, Calcijex), IV paricalcitol (Zemplar), or oral or IV doxercalciferol (Hectorol), and can reduce the elevated levels of PTH.

Hypercalcemia may occur with calcium and vitamin D supplementation. If hypercalcemia occurs, then reduce or discontinue vitamin D and calcium-based phosphate binders. Noncalcium-based phosphate binders can be substituted.

Cinacalcet (Sensipar), a calcimimetic agent, is used to control secondary hyperparathyroidism. Calcimimetics mimic calcium and increase the sensitivity of the calcium receptors in the parathyroid glands. As a result, the parathyroid glands detect calcium at lower serum levels and decrease PTH secretion.

If hyperparathyroid disease becomes severe despite medical management, a subtotal or total parathyroidectomy may be performed to decrease the synthesis and secretion of PTH. In most cases, a total parathyroidectomy is performed, and some parathyroid tissue is transplanted into the forearm. The transplanted cells produce PTH as needed. If production of PTH becomes excessive, some of the cells can be removed from the forearm.

It is difficult to determine what type of bone disease a patient might have by just looking at the serum levels of calcium, phosphorus, PTH, and alkaline phosphatase. The gold standard for diagnosis is a bone biopsy.

Anemia. The most important cause of anemia is a decreased production of erythropoietin. Exogenous erythropoietin (EPO) is used in the treatment. It is available as epoetin alfa (Epogen, Procrit), which can be administered IV or subcutaneously, usually two or three times per week. Darbepoetin alfa (Aranesp) is longer acting and can be administered weekly or biweekly.

A significant increase in hemoglobin and hematocrit levels is usually not seen for 2 to 3 weeks. Higher hemoglobin levels (more than 12 g/dL) and higher doses of EPO are associated with a higher rate of thromboembolic events and increased risk of death from serious CV events (heart attack, HF, stroke). The recommendation is to use the lowest possible dose of EPO to treat anemia. Furthermore, treatment of CKD-related anemia should be individualized with the goal being to reduce the need for blood transfusions. There is no target hemoglobin or widely accepted EPO dosing strategy.[20] Teach people who are prescribed EPO about the risks and benefits and allow them to make an informed decision regarding their individual treatment.

If EPO is used in the management of anemia, recognize that uncontrolled hypertension is a contraindication and that EPO may exacerbate an individual's hypertension. The underlying mechanism is related to the hemodynamic changes (e.g., increased whole blood viscosity) that occur as the anemia is corrected.

Another side effect of EPO therapy is the development of iron deficiency from the increased demand for iron to support erythropoiesis. Iron supplementation is recommended if the plasma ferritin concentrations fall below 100 ng/mL. Some studies have supported the use of parenteral iron with a much higher ferritin value (e.g., 800 ng/mL) in order to optimize treatment. Most CKD patients receive iron supplementation either by mouth or parenterally. Nonadherence may be an issue with oral supplementation because iron has GI side effects such as gastric irritation and constipation. Orally administered iron should not be taken at the same time as phosphate binders because calcium binds the iron, preventing its absorption. Tell the patient that iron may make the stool dark in color.

Most patients receiving HD are prescribed IV iron sucrose injection (Venofer) or sodium ferric gluconate complex in sucrose injection (Ferrlecit). Supplemental folic acid (1 mg/day) is usually given because it is needed for RBC formation and is removed by dialysis.

Blood transfusions should be avoided in treating anemia unless the patient experiences an acute blood loss or has symptomatic anemia (i.e., dyspnea, excess fatigue, tachycardia, palpitations, chest pain). Undesirable effects of transfusions are the increased sensitization and development of antibodies, thus making it more difficult to find a compatible donor for transplantation. Multiple blood transfusions may lead to iron overload because each unit of blood contains about 250 mg of iron.

Dyslipidemia. Dyslipidemia, a known traditional risk factor for CV disease, is a common problem in CKD. Statins (HMG-CoA reductase inhibitors), such as atorvastatin (Lipitor), are used to lower LDL cholesterol levels (see Table 34-5). Evidence supports the use of statins in patients with CKD (especially patients with diabetes) not yet on dialysis. However, simvastatin has been associated with a higher rate of myopathy. It is recommended that patients who develop myopathy on simvastatin be switched to atorvastatin, which has minimal renal clearance and less chance of causing myopathy. The effectiveness of statins in patients on dialysis is still being studied. Fibrates (fibric acid derivatives), such as gemfibrozil (Lopid), are used to lower triglyceride levels (see Table 34-5) and can also increase HDLs. Specific drugs of these classes that are used depend on the individual patient response and physician recommendation.

Complications of Drug Therapy. Many drugs are partially or totally excreted by the kidneys. Delayed and decreased elimination leads to an accumulation of drugs and the potential for drug toxicity. Drug doses and frequency of administration must be adjusted based on the severity of the kidney disease. Increased sensitivity may result as drug levels increase in the blood and tissues. Drugs of particular concern include digoxin, diabetic agents (metformin, glyburide), antibiotics (e.g., vancomycin, gentamicin), and opioid medications.

Nutritional Therapy

Protein Restriction. The current diet is designed to be as normal as possible to maintain good nutrition (Table 47-10). Calorie-protein malnutrition is a potential and serious problem that results from altered metabolism, anemia, proteinuria, anorexia, and nausea. Additional factors leading to malnutrition include depression and complex diets that restrict protein, phosphorus, potassium, and sodium. Frequent monitoring of laboratory parameters, especially serum albumin, prealbumin (may be a better indicator of recent or current nutritional status than albumin), and ferritin, and anthropometric measurements are necessary to evaluate nutritional status. All patients with CKD should be referred to a dietitian for nutritional education and guidance.

For the patient who is undergoing dialysis, protein is not routinely restricted (see Table 47-10). The beneficial role of protein restriction in CKD stages 1 through 4 as a means to reduce the decline in kidney function is being studied.

Historically, dietary counseling often encouraged a restriction of protein for individuals with CKD. Despite some evidence that protein restriction has benefits, many patients find it difficult to adhere to these diets. For CKD stages 1 through 4, many clinicians just encourage a diet with normal protein

TABLE 47-10 NUTRITIONAL THERAPY

*Chronic Kidney Disease**

	Pre–End-Stage Kidney Disease	Hemodialysis	Peritoneal Dialysis
Fluid allowance	As desired or depends on urine output	Urine output plus 600-1000 mL	Unrestricted if weight and blood pressure controlled and residual renal function
Calories	30-35 kcal/kg/day	30-35 kcal/kg/day	25-35 kcal/kg/day (includes calories from dialysate glucose absorption)
Protein	Individualized or 0.6-1.0 g/kg/day (low protein)	1.2 g/kg/day	1.2-1.3 g/kg/day
Sodium	Individualized or 1-3 g/day	Individualized or 2-3 g/day	Individualized or 2-4 g/day
Potassium	Individualized based on laboratory values	Individualized or about 2-4 g/day	Usually not restricted
Phosphorus	Individualized or 1.0-1.8 g/day	Individualized or about 0.6-1.2 g/day	Individualized or about 0.6-1.2 g/day
Calcium	About 1000-1500 mg/day	Individualized	Individualized
Iron	Supplement recommended if receiving erythropoietin	Supplement recommended if receiving erythropoietin	Supplement recommended if receiving erythropoietin

*Diets must be individualized in accordance with needs.

intake. However, teach patients to avoid high-protein diets and supplements because they may overstress the diseased kidneys.

Dietary protein guidelines for PD differ from those for HD because of protein loss in the dialysate. During PD, protein intake must be high enough to compensate for the losses so that the nitrogen balance is maintained. The recommended protein intake is at least 1.2 g/kg of ideal body weight (IBW) per day; this can be increased depending on the patient's individual needs.

For patients with malnutrition or inadequate caloric or protein intake, commercially prepared products that are high in protein but low in sodium and potassium are available (e.g., Nepro, Amin-Aid).[21] As an alternative, liquid or powder breakfast drinks may be purchased at the grocery store.

Water Restriction. Water and any other fluids are not routinely restricted in patients with CKD stages 1 to 5 who are not receiving HD. In an effort to reduce fluid retention, diuretics are often used. Patients on HD have a more restricted fluid intake than patients receiving PD. For those receiving HD, as their urine output diminishes, fluids are restricted. Recommended fluid intake depends on the daily urine output. Generally, 600 mL (from insensible loss) plus an amount equal to the previous day's urine output is allowed for a patient receiving HD.

Foods that are liquid at room temperature (e.g., gelatin, ice cream) should be counted as fluid intake. The fluid allotment should be spaced throughout the day so that the patient does not become thirsty. Patients are advised to limit fluid intake so that weight gains are no more than 1 to 3 kg between dialyses (termed *interdialytic weight gain*).

Sodium and Potassium Restriction. Patients with CKD are advised to restrict sodium. Sodium-restricted diets may vary from 2 to 4 g/day. Do not equate sodium and salt because the sodium content in 1 g of sodium chloride is equivalent to 400 mg of sodium. Instruct the patient to avoid high-sodium foods such as cured meats, pickled foods, canned soups and stews, frankfurters, cold cuts, soy sauce, and salad dressings (see Chapter 35, Table 35-8). Potassium restriction depends on the kidneys' ability to excrete potassium. Most salt substitutes should be avoided if patients have been instructed to restrict potassium because they contain potassium chloride.

Dietary restrictions for potassium range from about 2 to 3 g (39 mg = 1 mEq). Teach patients receiving HD which foods are high in potassium and to avoid them (Table 47-11).

Patients using PD do not usually need potassium restrictions and may even be prescribed oral potassium supplementation because of the loss of potassium with dialysis exchanges.

Phosphate Restriction. As kidney function deteriorates, phosphate elimination by the kidneys is diminished and the patient begins to develop hyperphosphatemia. By the time a patient reaches ESKD, phosphate should be limited to approximately 1 g/day. Foods that are high in phosphate include meat, dairy products (e.g., milk, ice cream, cheese, yogurt), and foods containing dairy products (e.g., pudding). Many foods that are high in phosphate are also high in protein. Since patients on dialysis are encouraged to eat a diet containing protein, phosphate binders are essential to control phosphate.

NURSING MANAGEMENT
CHRONIC KIDNEY DISEASE

NURSING ASSESSMENT

Obtain a complete history of any existing kidney disease or family history of kidney disease. Some kidney disorders,

TABLE 47-11 NUTRITIONAL THERAPY

High-Potassium Foods*

Fruits	Vegetables	Other Foods
• Apricot, raw (medium)	• Baked beans	• Bran or bran products
• Avocado (¼ whole)	• Butternut squash	• Chocolate (1.5-2 oz)
• Banana (¼ whole)	• Refried beans	• Granola
• Cantaloupe	• Black beans	• Milk, all types (1 cup)
• Dried fruits	• Broccoli, cooked	• Nutritional supplements (use only under the direction of physician or dietitian)
• Grapefruit juice	• Carrots, raw	
• Honeydew	• Greens, except kale	
• Orange (medium)	• Mushrooms, canned	• Nuts and seeds (1 oz)
• Orange juice	• Potatoes, white and sweet	• Peanut butter (2 tbs)
• Prunes	• Spinach, cooked	• Salt substitutes, Lite Salt
• Raisins	• Tomatoes or tomato products	• Salt-free broth
	• Vegetable juices	• Yogurt

Source: National Kidney Foundation: Potassium and your CKD diet. *www.kidney.org/atoz/content/potassium.cfm*
*Contain at least 200 mg/portion. Portion = ½ cup unless otherwise noted.

including Alport syndrome and polycystic kidney disease, have a genetic basis. Other disorders that can lead to CKD are diabetes mellitus, hypertension, and systemic lupus erythematosus.

Because many drugs are potentially nephrotoxic, ask the patient about both current and past use of prescription and over-the-counter drugs and herbal preparations. Decongestants and antihistamines that contain pseudoephedrine and phenylephrine cause vasoconstriction and lead to an increase in BP. Also assess the use of antacids. Magnesium and aluminum from antacids can accumulate in the body because they cannot be excreted. Some antacids contain high levels of salt, contributing to hypertension. In addition, antacids may interfere with absorption of other medications.

NSAIDs (aspirin, acetaminophen, ibuprofen, naproxen) can contribute to the development of AKI and progression of CKD, especially when taken in higher doses than recommended. Analgesics in combination and in large quantities have been associated with the development of kidney failure. If taken as prescribed for short periods, these analgesics are usually considered safe.

Assess the patient's dietary habits and discuss any problems regarding intake. Measure the height and weight, and evaluate any recent weight changes.

Recognize that CKD is a lifelong illness. The chronicity of kidney disease and the long-term treatment affect virtually every area of a person's life, including family relationships, social and work activities, self-image, and emotional state. Assess the patient's support systems. The choice of treatment modality may be related to support systems available.

NURSING DIAGNOSES

Nursing diagnoses for CKD may include, but are not limited to, the following:
- Excess fluid volume *related to* impaired kidney function
- Risk for electrolyte imbalance *related to* impaired kidney function resulting in hyperkalemia, hypocalcemia, hyperphosphatemia, and altered vitamin D metabolism
- Imbalanced nutrition: less than body requirements *related to* restricted intake of nutrients (especially protein), nausea, vomiting, anorexia, and stomatitis

Additional information on nursing diagnoses is presented in eNursing Care Plan 47-1 (available on the website for this chapter).

PLANNING

The overall goals are that a patient with CKD will (1) demonstrate knowledge of and ability to comply with the therapeutic regimen, (2) participate in decision making for the plan of care and future treatment modality, (3) demonstrate effective coping strategies, and (4) continue with activities of daily living within physiologic limitations.

NURSING IMPLEMENTATION

HEALTH PROMOTION. Identify individuals at risk for CKD. These include people who have been diagnosed with diabetes or hypertension and people with a history (or a family history) of kidney disease and repeated urinary tract infections. These individuals should have regular checkups along with calculation of the estimated GFR and a routine urinalysis.

People with diabetes need to have their urine checked for microalbuminuria if routine urinalysis is negative for protein. Advise patients with diabetes to report any changes in urine appearance (color, odor), frequency, or volume to the health care provider. If a patient needs a potentially nephrotoxic drug, it is important to monitor kidney function with serum creatinine and BUN.

Individuals identified as at risk need to take measures to prevent or delay the progression of CKD. Most important are measures to reduce the risk or progression of CV disease. These include glycemic control for patients with diabetes (see Chapter 49); BP control; and lifestyle modifications, including smoking cessation.

ACUTE INTERVENTION. Most of the care of the patient with CKD occurs on an outpatient basis. In-hospital care is required for management of complications and for kidney transplantation (if applicable).

AMBULATORY AND HOME CARE. Teach the patient and caregiver about the diet, drugs, and follow-up medical care (Table 47-12). The patient needs to understand the drugs and the common side effects. Because patients with CKD take many medications, a pillbox organizer or a list of the drugs and the times of administration that can be posted in the home may be helpful. Instruct the patient to avoid certain over-the-counter drugs such as NSAIDs and aluminum- and magnesium-based laxatives and antacids. Any over-the-counter medications need to be considered as a risk, since even acetaminophen taken in large doses can be toxic to the kidneys.

Teach the patient to take daily BPs and identify signs and symptoms of fluid overload, hyperkalemia, and other electrolyte imbalances. The dietitian should meet with the patient and caregiver on a regular basis for diet planning. A diet history and consideration of cultural variations facilitate diet planning and adherence.

Motivate patients to the highest level of self-management that is possible for them to achieve. The length of time that a patient can receive conservative medical management for CKD is highly variable. It depends on the rate of progression to kidney failure and the presence of other co-morbid conditions. Specific nursing management of the patient with CKD is presented in eNursing Care Plan 47-1.

Preferably, if the patient is considered a candidate for kidney transplantation, the evaluation can be accomplished before initiation of dialysis. In the best of circumstances, patients can receive a transplant before ever having to start dialysis. Even though transplantation offers the best therapeutic management for patients with kidney failure, the critical shortage of donor organs has limited this treatment option.

Most patients require dialysis, either peritoneal dialysis (PD) or hemodialysis (HD). The majority of patients in the United States choose HD. Clearly explain to the patient and caregiver what is involved in dialysis, transplantation, and even the option for palliative care. Discuss the opportunity for home HD.

Provide information about the treatment options so the patient can be involved in the decision-making process and be given a sense of control over life-altering decisions. Inform the patient that if dialysis is chosen, the option of transplantation still remains. Let the patient know that if a transplanted organ fails, the patient can return to dialysis. Counsel the patient that retransplantation may also be an option.

It is important to respect the patient's choice to not receive treatment.[22] Many times, patients themselves initiate the

---

HEALTHY PEOPLE

Prevention and Detection of Chronic Kidney Disease

- Early detection and treatment are the primary methods for reducing chronic kidney disease.
- Monitor blood pressure to detect elevations so treatment can be started early.
- Treat hypertension appropriately and aggressively, since it is the second leading cause of chronic kidney disease.
- Ensure proper diagnosis and treatment of diabetes mellitus, since it is the leading cause of chronic kidney disease.

TABLE 47-12 PATIENT & CAREGIVER TEACHING GUIDE

Chronic Kidney Disease

Include the following information in the teaching plan for the patient and caregiver.

1. Necessary dietary (protein, sodium, potassium, phosphate) and fluid restrictions.
2. Difficulties in modifying diet and fluid intake.
3. Signs and symptoms of electrolyte imbalance, especially high potassium.
4. Alternative ways of reducing thirst, such as sucking on ice cubes, lemon, or hard candy.
5. Rationales for prescribed drugs and common side effects.
   Examples:
   - Phosphate binders (including calcium supplements used as phosphate barriers) should be taken with meals.
   - Calcium supplements prescribed to treat hypocalcemia directly should be taken on an empty stomach (but not at the same time as iron supplements).
   - Iron supplements should be taken between meals.
6. The importance of reporting any of the following:
   - Weight gain >4 lb (2 kg)
   - Increasing BP
   - Shortness of breath
   - Edema
   - Increasing fatigue or weakness
   - Confusion or lethargy
7. Need for support and encouragement. Share concerns about lifestyle changes, living with a chronic illness, and decisions about type of dialysis or transplantation.

conversation about palliative care. Focus the discussion on moving from the curative approach to promotion of comfort care and consideration of hospice care. Listen to the patient and caregiver, allowing them to do most of the talking, and pay special attention to their hopes and fears. (Palliative and end-of-life care is discussed in Chapter 10.)

EVALUATION

The expected outcomes are that the patient with CKD will maintain

- Fluid and electrolyte levels within normal ranges
- An acceptable weight with no more than a 10% weight loss

Additional information on expected outcomes is presented in eNursing Care Plan 47-1 (available on the website).

DIALYSIS

Dialysis is the movement of fluid and molecules across a semipermeable membrane from one compartment to another. Clinically, dialysis is a technique in which substances move from the blood through a semipermeable membrane and into a dialysis solution *(dialysate)*. It is used to correct fluid and electrolyte imbalances and to remove waste products in kidney failure. It can also be used to treat drug overdoses.

The two methods of dialysis available are peritoneal dialysis (PD) and hemodialysis (HD) (Table 47-13). In PD the peritoneal membrane acts as the semipermeable membrane. In HD an artificial membrane (usually made of cellulose-based or synthetic materials) is used as the semipermeable membrane and is in contact with the patient's blood.

Dialysis is begun when the patient's uremia can no longer be adequately treated with conservative medical management. Generally dialysis is initiated when the GFR is less than 15 mL/min/1.73 m². This criterion can vary widely in different clinical situations, and the physician determines when to start dialysis based on the patient's clinical status. Certain uremic complications, including encephalopathy, neuropathies, uncontrolled hyperkalemia, pericarditis, and accelerated hypertension, indicate a need for immediate dialysis.

Most patients with ESKD are treated with dialysis because (1) there is a lack of donated organs, (2) some patients are physically or mentally unsuitable for transplantation, or (3) some patients do not want transplants. An increasing number of individuals, including older adults and those with complex medical problems, are receiving maintenance dialysis. A patient's chronologic age is not a factor in determining candidacy for dialysis. Factors that are important are the patient's ability to cope and the existing support system.

General Principles of Dialysis

Solutes and water move across the semipermeable membrane from the blood to the dialysate or from the dialysate to the blood in accordance with concentration gradients. The principles of diffusion, osmosis, and ultrafiltration are involved in dialysis (Fig. 47-4). *Diffusion* is the movement of solutes from an area of greater concentration to an area of lesser concentration. In kidney failure, urea, creatinine, uric acid, and electrolytes (potassium, phosphate) move from the blood to the dialysate with the net effect of lowering their concentration in the blood. RBCs, WBCs, and plasma proteins are too large to diffuse through the pores of the membrane. Small-molecular-weight substances can pass from the dialysate into a patient's blood, so the purity of the water used for dialysis is monitored and controlled.

Osmosis is the movement of fluid from an area of lesser concentration to an area of greater concentration of solutes. Glucose is added to the dialysate and creates an osmotic gradient across the membrane, pulling excess fluid from the blood.

TABLE 47-13	COMPARISON OF PERITONEAL DIALYSIS AND HEMODIALYSIS
Advantages	**Disadvantages**
Peritoneal Dialysis (PD)	
• Immediate initiation in almost any hospital	• Bacterial or chemical peritonitis
• Less complicated than hemodialysis	• Protein loss into dialysate
• Portable system with CAPD	• Exit site and tunnel infections
• Fewer dietary restrictions	• Self-image problems with catheter placement
• Relatively short training time	• Hyperglycemia
• Usable in patient with vascular access problems	• Surgery for catheter placement
• Less cardiovascular stress	• Contraindicated in patient with multiple abdominal surgeries, trauma, unrepaired hernia
• Home dialysis possible	• Requires completion of education program
• Preferable for diabetic patient	• Catheter can migrate
	• Best instituted with willing partner
Hemodialysis (HD)	
• Rapid fluid removal	• Vascular access problems
• Rapid removal of urea and creatinine	• Dietary and fluid restrictions
• Effective potassium removal	• Heparinization may be necessary
• Less protein loss	• Extensive equipment necessary
• Lowering of serum triglycerides	• Hypotension during dialysis
• Home dialysis possible	• Added blood loss that contributes to anemia
• Temporary access can be placed at bedside	• Specially trained personnel necessary
	• Surgery for permanent access placement
	• Self-image problems with permanent access

CAPD, Continuous ambulatory peritoneal dialysis.

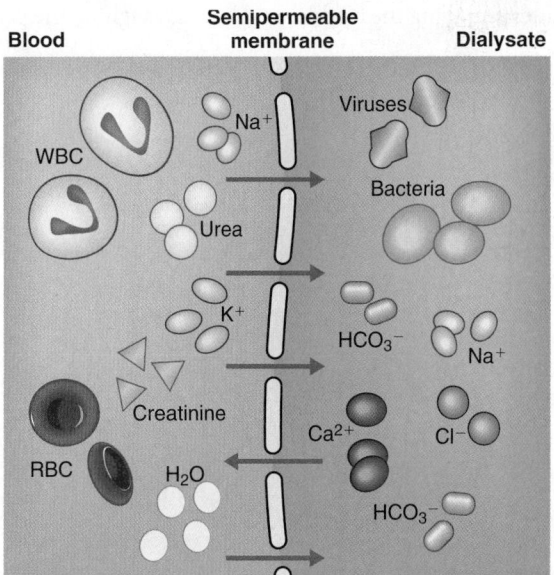

FIG. 47-4 Osmosis and diffusion across a semipermeable membrane.

Excess fluid is removed by creating a pressure differential between the blood and the dialysate solution. *Ultrafiltration* (water and fluid removal) results when there is an osmotic gradient or pressure gradient across the membrane. In PD, excess fluid is removed by increasing the osmolality of the dialysate (osmotic gradient) with the addition of glucose. In HD, the gradient is created by increasing pressure in the blood compartment (positive pressure) or decreasing pressure in the dialysate compartment (negative pressure). Extracellular fluid moves into the dialysate because of the pressure gradient. The excess fluid is removed by creating a pressure differential between the blood and the dialysate solution with a combination of positive pressure in the blood compartment or negative pressure in the dialysate compartment.

PERITONEAL DIALYSIS

Although PD was first used in 1923, it did not come into widespread use for chronic treatment until the 1970s with the development of soft, pliable peritoneal solution bags and the introduction of the concept of continuous PD. In the United States, approximately 12% of patients receiving dialysis treatments are on PD.

Catheter Placement

Peritoneal access is obtained by inserting a catheter through the anterior abdominal wall (Fig. 47-5). The catheter is about 60 cm long and has one or two Dacron cuffs on its subcutaneous and peritoneal portions. The cuffs act as anchors and prevent the migration of microorganisms down the shaft from the skin. Within a few weeks, fibrous tissue grows into the Dacron cuff, holding the catheter in place and preventing bacterial penetration into the peritoneal cavity. The tip of the catheter rests in the peritoneal cavity and has many perforations spaced along the distal end of the tubing to allow fluid to flow in and out of the catheter.

The technique for catheter placement varies. Although it is possible to place a permanent catheter in the peritoneal cavity at the bedside with a trocar, it is usually done via surgery so that its placement can be directly visualized, minimizing potential complications. Preparation of the patient for catheter insertion includes emptying the bladder and bowel, weighing the patient, and obtaining a signed consent form. After placement, PD may be initiated immediately with low volume exchanges, or delayed for 2 weeks pending healing and sealing of the exit site. Once the catheter incision site is healed, the patient may shower and then pat the catheter and exit site dry.

Daily catheter care varies. Some patients just wash with soap and water and go without a dressing (Fig. 47-6), whereas others require daily dressing changes. Teach all patients to examine their catheter site for signs of infection. Showering is preferred to bathing.[23]

Dialysis Solutions and Cycles

PD is accomplished by putting dialysis solution into the peritoneal space. The three phases of the PD cycle are inflow (fill), dwell (equilibration), and drain. The three phases are called an *exchange*. During *inflow*, a prescribed amount of solution, usually 2 L, is infused through an established catheter over about 10 minutes. The flow rate may be decreased if the patient has pain. After the solution has been infused, the inflow clamp is closed before air enters the tubing.

The next part of the cycle is the *dwell* phase, or equilibration, during which diffusion and osmosis occur between the patient's blood and the peritoneal cavity. The duration of the dwell time can last from 20 or 30 minutes to 8 or more hours, depending on the method of PD.

Drain time takes 15 to 30 minutes and may be facilitated by gently massaging the abdomen or changing position. The cycle starts again with the infusion of another 2 L of solution. For manual PD, a period of about 30 to 50 minutes is required to complete an exchange.

Dialysis solutions vary, and the choice of the exchange volume is primarily determined by the size of the peritoneal cavity. A larger person may tolerate a 3-L exchange volume without any difficulty, whereas an average-size person usually tolerates a 2-L exchange. Smaller exchange volumes are used for patients with a smaller body, pulmonary compromise (the added pressure of the large volume may precipitate respiratory difficulty), or inguinal hernias.

Ultrafiltration (fluid removal) during PD depends on osmotic forces, with glucose being the most effective osmotic agent currently available. Dextrose remains the most commonly used osmotic agent in PD solutions. It is relatively safe and inexpensive, but has been associated with high rates of peritoneal glucose absorption leading to problems with hypertriglyceridemia, hyperglycemia, and long-term peritoneal membrane dysfunction.

Alternatives to dextrose PD solution include icodextrin and amino acid solutions. Icodextrin is a commercially available

FIG. 47-5 Peritoneal dialysis showing peritoneal catheter inserted into peritoneal cavity.

FIG. 47-6 Peritoneal catheter exit site.

isoosmolar preparation and induces ultrafiltration by its oncotic effect. Amino acid PD solutions are also available and primarily used for patients requiring nutritional supplementation.

Peritoneal Dialysis Systems

Automated Peritoneal Dialysis. Automated peritoneal dialysis (APD) is the most popular form of PD because it allows patients to do dialysis while they sleep. An automated device called a cycler is used to deliver the dialysate for APD (Fig. 47-7). The automated cycler times and controls the fill, dwell, and drain phases. The machine cycles four or more exchanges per night with 1 to 2 hours per exchange. Alarms and monitors are built into the system to make it safe for the patient to sleep while dialyzing. The patient disconnects from the machine in the morning and usually leaves fluid in the abdomen during the day.

It is difficult to achieve the required solute and fluid clearance solely with nighttime APD. Therefore one or two daytime manual exchanges may also be prescribed to ensure adequate dialysis. Cyclers are about the size of a DVD player and have longer tubing to allow greater mobility.

Continuous Ambulatory Peritoneal Dialysis. Continuous ambulatory peritoneal dialysis (CAPD) is done while the patient is awake during the day. Exchanges are carried out manually by exchanging 1.5 to 3 L of peritoneal dialysate at least four times daily, with dwell times averaging 4 hours. For example, one schedule exchanges at 7 AM, 12 noon, 5 PM, and 10 PM. In this procedure, the person instills 2 to 3 L of dialysate from a collapsible plastic bag into the peritoneal cavity through a disposable plastic tube.

In CAPD the bag and line can be disconnected after the instillation of the fluid. After the equilibration period, the line is reconnected to the catheter, the dialysate (effluent) is drained from the peritoneal cavity, and a new 2- to 3-L bag of dialysate solution is infused. In PD it is critical to maintain aseptic technique to avoid peritonitis. Several tubing connections and devices are commercially available to help in maintaining an aseptic system.

Complications of Peritoneal Dialysis

Exit Site Infection. Infection of the peritoneal catheter exit site is most commonly caused by *Staphylococcus aureus* or *Staphylococcus epidermidis* (from skin flora). Clinical manifestations of an exit site infection include redness at the site, tenderness, and drainage. Superficial exit site infections caused by these organisms are generally resolved with antibiotic therapy. If not treated immediately, subcutaneous tunnel infections usually progress to abscess formation and may cause peritonitis, necessitating catheter removal.

Peritonitis. Peritonitis results from contamination or from progression of an exit site or tunnel infection. Most frequently peritonitis occurs because of improper technique in making or breaking connections for exchanges. Less commonly, peritonitis results from bacteria in the intestine crossing over into the peritoneal cavity. Peritonitis is usually caused by *S. aureus* or *S. epidermidis*.

The primary clinical manifestations of peritonitis are abdominal pain and cloudy peritoneal effluent with a WBC count greater than 100 cells/μL (more than 50% neutrophils) or demonstration of bacteria in the peritoneal effluent by Gram stain or culture. GI manifestations of peritonitis may include diarrhea, vomiting, abdominal distention, and hyperactive bowel sounds. Fever may or may not be present.

Cultures, Gram stain, and a WBC differential of the peritoneal effluent are used to confirm the diagnosis of peritonitis. Antibiotics can be given orally, IV, or intraperitoneally. In most cases, the patient is treated on an outpatient basis. The formation of adhesions in the peritoneum can result from repeated infections and interferes with the peritoneal membrane's ability to act as a dialyzing surface. Repeated infections may require the removal of the peritoneal catheter and termination of PD.

Hernias. Because of increased intraabdominal pressure secondary to the dialysate infusion, hernias can develop in predisposed individuals such as multiparous women and older men. However, in most situations after hernia repair, PD can be resumed after several days using small dialysate volumes and keeping the patient supine.

Lower Back Problems. Increased intraabdominal pressure can cause or aggravate lower back pain. The lumbosacral curvature is increased by intraperitoneal infusion of dialysate. Orthopedic binders and a regular exercise program for strengthening the back muscles have been beneficial for some patients.

Bleeding. After Tenckhoff catheter placement, it is not uncommon for the PD effluent drained after the first few exchanges to be pink or slightly bloody secondary to the trauma associated with catheter insertion. However, bloody effluent over several days or the new appearance of blood in the effluent can indicate active intraperitoneal bleeding. If this occurs, check the BP and hematocrit. Blood may also be present in the effluent of women who are menstruating or ovulating, and this requires no intervention.

Pulmonary Complications. Atelectasis, pneumonia, and bronchitis may occur from repeated upward displacement of the diaphragm, resulting in decreased lung expansion. The longer the dwell time, the greater the likelihood of pulmonary problems. Frequent repositioning and deep-breathing exercises can help. When the patient is lying in bed, elevate the head of the bed to prevent these problems.

Protein Loss. The peritoneal membrane is permeable to plasma proteins, amino acids, and polypeptides. These substances are lost in the dialysate fluid. The amount of loss is usually about 0.5 g/L of dialysate drainage, but it can be as high as 10 to 20 g/day. This loss may increase to as much as 40 g/day during episodes of peritonitis as the peritoneal membrane becomes more permeable. Unresolved peritonitis is associated with exaggerated protein loss that can result in malnutrition and

FIG. 47-7 Automated peritoneal dialysis that can be used while the patient is sleeping.

may indicate the need to terminate PD temporarily or sometimes permanently.

Effectiveness of Chronic Peritoneal Dialysis

Learning the self-management skills required to do PD is usually accomplished in a 3- to 7-day training program. Mortality rates are about equal between in-center HD patients and PD patients for the first few years or possibly even a little lower for patients receiving PD. However, after about 2 years, mortality rates for patients receiving PD are higher, especially for the older person with diabetes and patients with a prior history of CV disease.

The primary advantage of PD is its simplicity and that it is a home-based program, allowing the patient to be in control. There is no need for special water systems, and equipment setup is relatively simple. PD is especially indicated for the individual who has vascular access problems or responds poorly to the hemodynamic stresses of HD.[23]

HEMODIALYSIS

Vascular Access

Obtaining vascular access is one of the most difficult problems associated with HD. To perform HD, a very rapid blood flow is required, and access to a large blood vessel is essential. The types of vascular access include arteriovenous fistulas (AVFs), arteriovenous grafts (AVGs), and temporary vascular access.[24]

Arteriovenous Fistulas and Grafts. A subcutaneous **arteriovenous fistula (AVF)** is usually created in the forearm or upper arm with an anastomosis between an artery and a vein (usually cephalic or basilic) (Figs. 47-8, *A*, and 47-9). The fistula allows arterial blood to flow through the vein. The vein becomes "arterialized" with a larger caliber and thicker walls. The arterial blood flow is essential to provide the rapid blood flow required for HD. As the arterialized vein matures, it is more amenable to repeated venipunctures. Maturation may take 6 weeks to months. AVF should be placed at least 3 months before the need to initiate HD.

Normally, a *thrill* can be felt by palpating the area of anastomosis, and a *bruit* (rushing sound) can be heard with a stethoscope. The bruit and thrill are created by arterial blood moving

at a high velocity through the vein. AVFs are more difficult to create in patients with a history of severe peripheral vascular disease, those with prolonged IV drug use, and obese women. For these individuals, a synthetic graft may be required.

Arteriovenous grafts (AVGs) are made of synthetic materials (polytetrafluoroethylene [PTFE, Teflon]) and form a "bridge" between the arterial and venous blood supplies. Grafts are placed under the skin and are surgically anastomosed between an artery (usually brachial) and a vein (usually antecubital) (Fig. 47-8, *B*). An interval of 2 to 4 weeks is usually necessary to allow the graft to heal, but some centers may use it earlier. Because grafts are made of artificial materials, they are more likely than AVFs to become infected, and they also have a tendency to be thrombogenic. When AVG infections occur, they may require surgical removal, since it is difficult to completely resolve the infection from the synthetic material.

Surgical creation of an arteriovenous access for HD has several risks, including development of distal ischemia *(steal syndrome)* and pain because too much of the arterial blood is being shunted or "stolen" from the distal extremity. Classic manifestations of steal syndrome are pain distal to the access site, numbness or tingling of fingers that may worsen during dialysis, and poor capillary refill. Aneurysms can also develop in the arteriovenous access and can rupture if left untreated.

Never perform BP measurements, insertion of IV lines, and venipuncture in the extremity with the vascular access. These special precautions are taken to prevent infection and clotting of the vascular access.

Temporary Vascular Access. In some situations, when immediate vascular access is required, catheterization of the internal jugular or femoral vein is performed. A flexible Teflon, silicone rubber, or polyurethane catheter is inserted at the bedside into one of these large veins and provides access to the circulation without surgery (Fig. 47-10). The catheters usually have a double external lumen with an internal septum separating the two internal segments. One lumen is used for blood removal and the other for blood return (Fig. 47-11, *A* and *B*). It is now recommended that patients not be discharged from the hospital with a temporary catheter. These catheters have high rates of infection, dislodgment, and malfunction.

Long-term cuffed HD catheters are often used for temporary vascular access. These catheters provide temporary access while the patient is waiting for fistula placement or as long-term access when other forms of access have failed. This type of catheter exits on the upper chest wall and is tunneled subcutaneously to the internal or external jugular vein (Fig. 47-11, *C*). The catheter tip rests in the right atrium. It has one or two

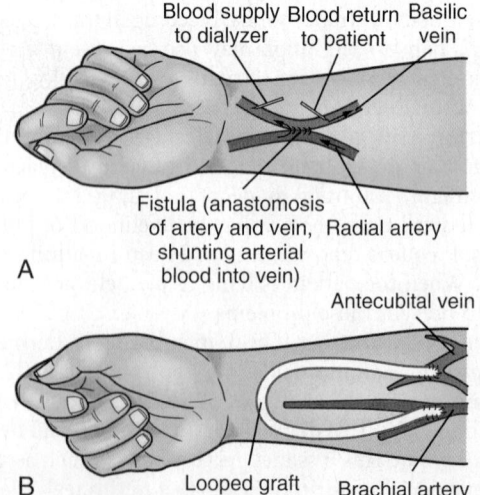

FIG. 47-8 Vascular access for hemodialysis. **A,** Arteriovenous fistula. **B,** Arteriovenous graft.

FIG. 47-9 Arteriovenous fistula created by anastomosing an artery and a vein.

FIG. 47-10 Temporary double-lumen vascular access catheter for acute hemodialysis. **A,** Soft, flexible double-lumen tube is attached to a Y hub. **B,** The distance between the arterial intake lumen and the venous return lumen typically provides recirculation rates of 5% or less.

subcutaneous Dacron cuffs that prevent infection from tracking along the catheter and anchor the catheter, thus eliminating the need for sutures.

Advance planning is essential for management of the patient with kidney failure who is approaching end-stage disease and the need for dialysis. Enough time is needed for evaluation and consideration of the best arteriovenous access for HD and preparation for PD.

Dialyzers. The HD dialyzer is a long plastic cartridge that contains thousands of parallel hollow tubes or fibers. The fibers are semipermeable membranes made of cellulose-based or other synthetic materials. The blood is pumped into the top of the cartridge and is dispersed into all of the fibers. Dialysis fluid *(dialysate)* is pumped into the bottom of the cartridge and bathes the outside of the fibers. Ultrafiltration, diffusion, and osmosis occur across the pores of this semipermeable membrane. When the dialyzed blood reaches the end of the thousands of semipermeable fibers, it converges into a single tube that returns it to the patient. Dialyzers differ in regard to surface area, membrane composition and thickness, clearance of waste products, and removal of fluid.

Procedure for Hemodialysis

The needles used for HD are large bore, usually 14 to 16 gauge, and are inserted into the fistula or graft to obtain vascular access. One needle is placed to pull blood from the circulation to the HD machine, and the other needle is used to return the dialyzed blood to the patient. The needles are attached via tubing to dialysis lines.

If a patient has a catheter, the two blood lines are attached to the two catheter lumens. The needle closer to the fistula (red catheter lumen) is used to pull blood from the patient and send it to the dialyzer with the assistance of a blood pump. Heparin is added to the blood as it flows into the dialyzer because any time blood contacts a foreign substance, it has a tendency to clot. Blood is returned from the dialyzer to the patient through the second needle (blue catheter lumen).

In addition to the dialyzer, a dialysate delivery and monitoring system is used (Fig. 47-12). This system pumps the dialysate through the dialyzer, countercurrent to the blood flow. Dialysis is terminated by flushing the dialyzer with saline solution to

FIG. 47-11 **A,** Right internal jugular placement for a tunneled, cuffed semipermanent catheter. **B,** Temporary hemodialysis catheter in place. **C,** Long-term cuffed hemodialysis catheter.

return the blood in the extracorporeal circuit back to the patient through the vascular access. Then the needles are removed from the patient, and firm pressure is applied to the venipuncture sites until the bleeding stops.

Before beginning treatment, complete an assessment that includes fluid status (weight, BP, peripheral edema, lung and heart sounds), condition of vascular access, temperature, and general skin condition. The difference between the last postdialysis weight and the present predialysis weight determines the ultrafiltration or the amount of weight (from fluid)

FIG. 47-12 Components of a hemodialysis system. Blood is removed via a needle inserted in a fistula or via catheter lumen. It is propelled to the dialyzer by a blood pump. Heparin is infused either as a bolus predialysis or through a heparin pump continuously to prevent clotting. Dialysate is pumped in and flows in the opposite direction of the blood. The dialyzed blood is returned to the patient through a second needle or catheter lumen. Old dialysate and ultrafiltrate are drained and discarded.

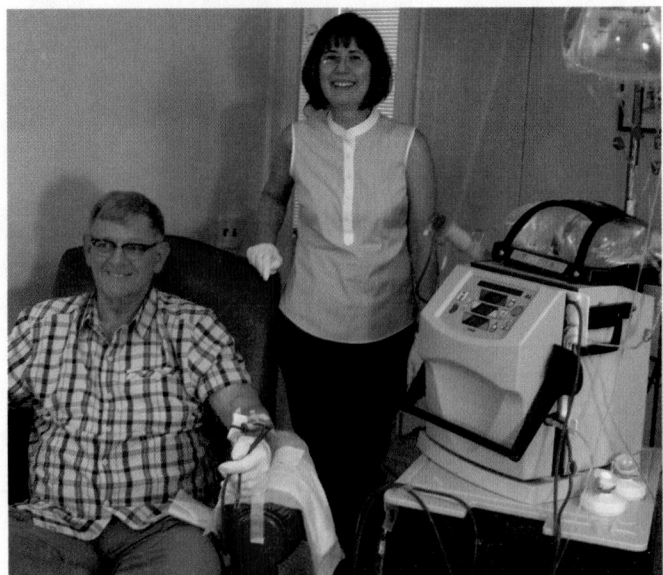

FIG. 47-13 Home hemodialysis is growing in popularity, and machines are more compact.

to be removed. While the patient is on dialysis, take vital signs at least every 30 to 60 minutes because rapid BP changes may occur.

Most maintenance dialysis facilities use reclining chairs that allow for elevation of the feet if hypotension develops. Most people sleep, read, talk, or watch television during dialysis.

Settings and Schedules for Hemodialysis. The majority of HD patients are treated in a community-based center and dialyze for 3 to 4 hours 3 days per week. Other schedule options for HD are short daily HD and long nocturnal HD. In short daily HD, the patient dialyzes for 2½ to 3 hours per session 5 to 6 days per week. Short daily HD is usually done at home.

In-center HD programs have adapted their dialysis schedules so patients can be free during the day. The patient receiving long nocturnal HD has the advantage of sleeping while dialyzing. Each nocturnal treatment lasts 6 to 8 hours, and the patient dialyzes up to six times per week. Patients who choose daily dialysis or nocturnal dialysis tend to feel better, are more in control of their lives, tend to require fewer medications, and have fewer dialysis-related side effects (e.g., hypotension, cramps).

In addition to in-center HD, home HD is available (Fig. 47-13). The option for home HD often depends on a patient's family support. One of the main advantages of home HD is that it allows greater freedom in choosing dialysis times. Daily home HD also offers the potential of significant health benefits. Currently only about 2% of HD patients dialyze at home.

Complications of Hemodialysis

Hypotension. Hypotension that occurs during HD primarily results from rapid removal of vascular volume (hypovolemia), decreased cardiac output, and decreased systemic vascular resistance. The drop in BP during dialysis may precipitate light-

headedness, nausea, vomiting, seizures, vision changes, and chest pain from cardiac ischemia. The usual treatment for hypotension includes decreasing the volume of fluid being removed and infusion of 0.9% saline solution.

Muscle Cramps. The pathogenesis of muscle cramps in HD is poorly understood. Factors associated with the development of muscle cramps include hypotension, hypovolemia, high ultrafiltration rate (large interdialytic weight gain), and low-sodium dialysis solution. Cramps are more frequently seen in the first month after initiation of dialysis than in the subsequent period. Treatment includes reducing the ultrafiltration rate and administering fluids (saline, glucose, mannitol). Hypertonic saline is not recommended, since the sodium load can be problematic. Hypertonic glucose administration is preferred.

Loss of Blood. Blood loss may result from blood not being completely rinsed from the dialyzer, accidental separation of blood tubing, dialysis membrane rupture, or bleeding after the removal of needles at the end of dialysis. If a patient has received too much heparin or has clotting problems, postdialysis bleeding can be significant. It is essential to rinse back all blood, to closely monitor heparinization to avoid excess anticoagulation, and to hold firm but nonocclusive pressure on access sites until the risk of bleeding has passed.

Hepatitis. At one time, hepatitis B had an unusually high prevalence in dialysis patients, but the incidence today is low. Lower transfusion requirements, screening, and recommendations for vaccinations have lowered the incidence. However, outbreaks of hepatitis B still occur, since transmission is attributed to breaks in infection control practices. To prevent transmission, the Centers for Disease Control and Prevention (CDC) has recommended that all patients and personnel in dialysis units receive hepatitis B vaccine.

Currently, hepatitis C virus (HCV) is responsible for the majority of cases of hepatitis in dialysis patients. (Hepatitis is discussed in more detail in Chapter 44.) Approximately 8% to 10% of patients undergoing dialysis in the United States are positive for anti-HCV, which indicates a previous infection. Infection control precautions are mandated in care of the patient with hepatitis C to protect the patient and staff. (Infection control precautions are discussed in Chapter 15.) Currently, no vaccine is available for hepatitis C.[25]

Effectiveness of Hemodialysis

HD is still an imperfect therapy for management of ESKD. It cannot fully replace the normal functions of the kidneys. It can ease many of the symptoms of CKD and, if started early, can prevent certain complications. However, it does not alter the accelerated rate of development of CV disease and the related high mortality rate.

The yearly death rate of patients receiving maintenance dialysis remains high at an estimated 19% to 24%. The majority of deaths are caused by CV disease (stroke or myocardial infarction). Infectious complications are the second leading cause of death.

Individual adaptation to maintenance HD varies considerably. Initially many patients feel positive about the dialysis because it makes them feel better and keeps them alive, but there is often great ambivalence about whether it is worthwhile. Dependence on a machine is a reality. In response to their illness, dialysis patients may be nonadherent or depressed and exhibit suicidal tendencies. The primary nursing goals are to assist the patient in maintaining a healthy self-image and, if possible, rehabilitate with the hopes of returning to work.

CONTINUOUS RENAL REPLACEMENT THERAPY

Continuous renal replacement therapy (CRRT) is an alternative or adjunctive method for treating AKI. It provides a means by which uremic toxins and fluids are removed, while acid-base status and electrolytes are adjusted slowly and continuously in a hemodynamically unstable patient. The patients selected are usually those who do not respond to dietary interventions and drug therapy. The principle of CRRT is to dialyze patients in a more physiologic way over 24 hours, just like the kidneys.

CRRT is contraindicated if a patient has life-threatening manifestations of uremia (hyperkalemia, pericarditis) that require rapid resolution. CRRT can be used in conjunction with HD.

Various types of CRRT are available (Table 47-14). CRRT most commonly uses the venovenous approaches of continuous venovenous hemofiltration (CVVH), continuous venovenous hemodialysis (CVVHD), and continuous venovenous hemodiafiltration (CVVHDF).

Vascular access for CVVH or CVVHD is achieved through the use of a double-lumen catheter (as used in HD [see Fig. 47-10]) placed in the jugular or femoral vein. A blood pump is used to propel the blood through the circuit. A highly permeable, hollow-fiber hemofilter removes plasma water and nonprotein solutes, which are collectively termed *ultrafiltrate*. The ultrafiltration rate (UFR) may range from 0 to 500 mL/hr. Under the influence of hydrostatic pressure and osmotic pressure, water and nonprotein solutes pass out of the filter into the extracapillary space and drain through the ultrafiltrate port into a collection device (drainage bag) (Fig. 47-14). The remaining fluid continues through the filter and returns to the patient via the return port of the double-lumen catheter.

While the ultrafiltrate drains out of the hemofilter, fluid and electrolyte replacements can be infused into the infusion port located after the filter as the blood returns to the patient. This fluid is designed to replace volume and solutes such as sodium, chloride, bicarbonate, and glucose. It also further

TABLE 47-14	CONTINUOUS RENAL REPLACEMENT THERAPIES	
Therapy	**Abbreviation**	**Purpose**
Continuous venovenous hemofiltration	CVVH	Removes both fluid and solutes. Replacement fluid required.
Slow continuous ultrafiltration	SCUF	Simplified version of CVVH. Removes fluid. No fluid replacement required.
Continuous venovenous hemodialysis	CVVHD	Removes both fluids and solutes. Requires both dialysate and replacement fluid.
Continuous venovenous hemodiafiltration	CVVHDF	Removes both fluids and solutes. Requires both dialysate and replacement fluid.

FIG. 47-14 Basic schematic of continuous venovenous therapies. Blood pump is required to pump blood through the circuit. Replacement ports are used for instilling replacement fluids and can be given prefilter or postfilter. Dialysate port is used for infusing dialysis solution. Regardless of modality, ultrafiltrate is drained via the ultrafiltration drain port.

dilutes intravascular fluid, decreasing the concentration of unwanted solutes such as BUN, creatinine, and potassium. The infusion rate of replacement fluid is determined by the degree of fluid and electrolyte imbalance. Replacement fluid may also be infused into the infusion port before the hemofilter. This method allows for greater clearance of urea and can decrease filter clotting.

Anticoagulation is needed to prevent blood clotting during CRRT. Heparin may be infused as a bolus at the initiation of CRRT or through the heparin infusion port before the hemofilter.

Several features of CRRT differ from HD:
- It is continuous rather than intermittent. Large volumes of fluid can be removed over days (24 hours to more than 2 weeks) versus hours (3 to 4 hours).
- Solute removal can occur by *convection* (no dialysate required) in addition to osmosis and diffusion.

- It causes less hemodynamic instability (e.g., hypotension).
- It does not require constant monitoring by a specialized HD nurse but does require a trained ICU nurse.
- It does not require complicated HD equipment, but a blood pump is needed for venovenous therapies.

The type of CRRT can be customized to the patient's needs. Some types involve the introduction of replacement fluids. Large volumes of fluid may be removed hourly (200 to 800 mL), and then a portion of this fluid is replaced. The type of fluid replacement depends on the patient's stability and individual needs. Ultrafiltration and convective losses occur, and solute concentrations in the blood are diluted with the replacement fluid.

The *hemodialysis therapies* (CVVHD and CVVHDF) use dialysate. Dialysis fluid is attached to the distal end of the hemofilter, and the fluid is pumped countercurrent to the blood flow (see Fig. 47-14). As in dialysis, diffusion of solutes and ultrafiltration via hydrostatic pressure and osmosis occur. This is an ideal treatment for a patient who needs both fluid and solute control but cannot tolerate the rapid fluid shifts associated with HD.

CRRT can be continued as long as 30 to 40 days, but the hemofilter should be changed every 24 to 48 hours because of loss of filtration efficiency or potential for clotting. The ultrafiltrate should be clear yellow, and specimens may be obtained for evaluation of serum chemistries. If the ultrafiltrate becomes bloody or blood tinged, a possible rupture in the filter membrane should be suspected, and treatment is suspended immediately to prevent blood loss and infection.

Specific nursing interventions include obtaining weights and monitoring and documenting laboratory values daily to ensure adequate fluid and electrolyte balance. Assessment of hourly intake and output, vital signs, and hemodynamic status is essential. Although reductions in central venous pressure and pulmonary artery pressure are expected, there should be little change in mean arterial pressure or cardiac output. Patency of the CRRT system is assessed and maintained, and the patient's vascular access site is cared for to prevent infection. Treatment is discontinued and the needle(s) removed once the patient's AKI is resolved or there is a decision to withdraw treatment because of patient deterioration.

KIDNEY TRANSPLANTATION

Major progress has been made in kidney transplantation since the first live donor kidney transplant was performed in 1954 in Boston between identical twins. The advances made in organ procurement and preservation, surgical techniques, tissue typing and matching, immunosuppressant therapy, and prevention and treatment of graft rejection have dramatically increased the success of kidney transplantation. (A general discussion of organ transplantation is in Chapter 14, pp. 219-223).

Even though kidney transplantation is by far the best treatment option available to patients with ESKD, fewer than 4% ever receive a transplant. This is because of the high disparity between the supply and demand for kidneys. Every year thousands are waiting for kidney transplantation (more than 93,000 are currently on the list), yet less than one fourth ever receive a kidney. Most die while waiting. Transplantation from a deceased donor usually requires a prolonged waiting period with differences in waiting time depending on age, gender, and race. Average wait times in the United States for a cadaveric kidney to become available usually ranges from 2 to 5 years.[26]

Kidney transplantation is very successful, with 1-year graft survival rates over 90% for deceased donor transplants and 95% for live donor transplants.[26] An advantage of kidney transplantation when compared with dialysis is that it reverses many of the pathophysiologic changes associated with renal failure. It also eliminates the dependence on dialysis and the accompanying dietary and lifestyle restrictions. Transplantation is also less expensive than dialysis after the first year.

Recipient Selection

Appropriate recipient selection is important for a successful outcome. Candidacy is determined by a variety of medical and psychosocial factors that vary among transplant centers. Some transplant programs exclude patients who are morbidly obese or who continue to smoke (despite smoking cessation interventions). A careful evaluation is completed in an attempt to identify and minimize potential complications after transplantation. Certain patients, particularly those with CV disease and diabetes mellitus, are considered high risk and must be carefully evaluated and then monitored closely after the transplantation. For a small number of patients who are approaching ESKD, a *preemptive transplant* (before dialysis is required) is possible if they have a living donor. This approach is most advantageous for patients with diabetes, who have a much higher mortality rate on dialysis than nondiabetics.

Contraindications to transplantation include disseminated malignancies, refractory or untreated cardiac disease, chronic respiratory failure, extensive vascular disease, chronic infection, and unresolved psychosocial disorders (e.g., nonadherence to medical regimens, alcoholism, drug addiction). At one time, patients diagnosed with human immunodeficiency virus (HIV) infection were denied the opportunity for kidney transplantation. However, centers that have included HIV patients demonstrate graft and patient survival rates for patients with HIV that are comparable to those in the HIV-negative population. The presence of hepatitis B or C is not a contraindication to transplantation.[25]

Surgical procedures may be required before transplantation based on the results of the recipient evaluation. Coronary artery bypass or coronary angioplasty may be indicated for advanced coronary artery disease. Cholecystectomy may be necessary for patients with a history of gallstones, biliary obstruction, or cholecystitis. On rare occasions, bilateral nephrectomies are necessary for patients with refractory hypertension, recurrent urinary tract infections, or grossly enlarged kidneys from polycystic kidney disease. In general, the recipient's own kidneys do not need to be removed before he or she receives a kidney transplant.

Histocompatibility Studies

Histocompatibility studies, including human leukocyte antigen (HLA) testing and crossmatching, are discussed in Chapter 14 on pp. 220-221.

Donor Sources

Kidneys for transplantation may be obtained from compatible blood-type deceased donors, blood relatives, emotionally related (close and distant) living donors (e.g., spouses, distant cousins, etc.), and altruistic living donors who are known (friends) or unknown to the recipient.

ETHICAL/LEGAL DILEMMAS

Allocation of Resources

Situation

T.H., a transplant nurse coordinator, is considering her feelings about two patients who are being evaluated for placement on the deceased (cadaveric) kidney transplant waiting list. One patient is a 40-yr-old African American schoolteacher. She is married and has two children. The other patient is a 22-yr-old unemployed white man. He misses three or four dialysis treatments per month and does not take his antihypertensive medications consistently.

Ethical/Legal Points for Consideration

- The foundation of this conflict resides in the Constitution where the founders made education a free public resource and ignored health care as a right. Health care then became a privilege, a resource to be obtained by persons with the funds to pay for it.
- It took almost 200 yr for health entitlement programs to be developed. Medicare is a federally administrated program. Individuals covered by Medicare are protected by Constitutional laws prohibiting discrimination based on race, gender, religion, and ethnic background.
- Medicaid is a federally sponsored program jointly administered by the various states. The states have the right to set coverage eligibility and limits, but may not violate an individual's constitutionally protected rights against discrimination.
- It is highly unlikely that the standard prohibitions against discrimination will change, but it is possible that definitions of unhealthy behavior such as substance abuse, alcoholism, smoking, and obesity might be used to screen out candidates.
- Nurses are concerned about social justice because of their health advocacy role. Today the situation is immensely more complex because of the cost and availability of care.

Discussion Questions

1. What does the 2001 American Nurses Association (ANA) Code of Ethics say about how you as a nurse should view patients?
2. What are your thoughts about which of the patients should receive the next available kidney transplant?

Another option is *paired organ donation* where one donor/recipient pair who are incompatible or poorly matched with each other find another donor/recipient pair with whom they can exchange kidneys. Thus a spouse (person A) who wants to donate a kidney to his wife (person B) but is incompatible is paired with another donor/recipient pair involving a son with ESKD (person C) and his mother (person D). In this example, person A would donate his kidney to person C, and person D would donate her kidney to person B. Paired organ donation is the practice of matching biologically incompatible donor/recipient pairs to permit transplantation of both candidates with a well-matched organ. Expanding the living donor pool is one of the best possibilities for decreasing the size of the waiting list and reducing wait times for people needing a deceased donor.

Live Donors. Live donors undergo an extensive multidisciplinary evaluation to be certain that they are in good health and have no history of disease that would place them at risk for developing kidney failure or operative complications. Psychosocial and financial evaluations are also done. Crossmatches are done at the time of the evaluation and about a week before the transplant to ensure that no antibodies to the donor are present or that the antibody titer is below the allowed level. Advantages of a live donor kidney include better patient and graft survival rates regardless of histocompatibility match, immediate organ availability, immediate function because of minimal *cold time* (kidney out of body and not getting blood supply), and the opportunity to have the recipient in the best possible medical condition because the surgery is elective.

The potential donor sees a nephrologist for a complete history and physical examination and laboratory and diagnostic studies. Laboratory studies include a 24-hour urine study for creatinine clearance and total protein, complete blood count, and chemistry and electrolyte profiles. Hepatitis B and C, HIV, and cytomegalovirus (CMV) testing is done to assess for any transmitted diseases. An ECG and chest x-ray are also done. A renal ultrasound and a renal arteriogram or three-dimensional CT scan is performed to ensure that the blood vessels supplying each kidney are adequate and that there are no anomalies and to determine which kidney will be removed.

A transplant psychologist or social worker determines if the individual is emotionally stable and able to deal with the issues related to organ donation. All donors must be informed about the risks and benefits of donation, the potential short- and long-term complications, and what to expect during the hospitalization and recovery phases. Kidney donation is considered safe without any long-term health consequences. Although the costs of the evaluation and surgery are covered by the recipient's insurance, no compensation is available for lost wages during the posthospitalization recovery period. This period can last 6 weeks or longer.

When there is ABO incompatibility between a donor and recipient, paired donor exchange is a viable alternative. Another option for ABO incompatibility or a positive crossmatch between the donor and recipient is to use plasmapheresis to remove antibodies from the recipient. (Crossmatching is discussed in Chapter 14.) This allows transplant candidates to receive kidneys from live donors with blood types that have traditionally been considered incompatible. After the transplant, the patient undergoes additional plasmapheresis treatments.

Deceased Donors. Deceased (cadaver) kidney donors are relatively healthy individuals who have suffered an irreversible brain injury and are declared brain dead. The most common causes of injury are cerebral trauma from motor vehicle accidents or gunshot wounds, intracerebral or subarachnoid hemorrhage, and anoxic brain damage caused by cardiac arrest. The brain-dead donor must have effective CV function and be supported on a ventilator to preserve the organs. The donor must be free of active IV drug abuse; severe hypertension; longstanding diabetes mellitus; malignancies; sepsis; and communicable diseases, including HIV, hepatitis B and C, syphilis, and tuberculosis.

Even if the donor carried a signed donor card, permission from the donor's legal next of kin is still requested after brain death is determined. That is why it is important for you to talk with your family about your wishes before losing the capacity to convey your desires.

The kidneys are removed and preserved. They can be preserved for up to 72 hours, but most transplant surgeons prefer to transplant kidneys before the cold time (time outside of the body when being transported from the deceased donor to the recipient) reaches 24 hours. Prolonged cold time increases the likelihood that the kidney will not function immediately, and acute tubular necrosis (ATN) may develop.

The United Network for Organ Sharing (UNOS) distributes deceased donor kidneys using an objective computerized point system. The ABO group, HLA typing, age, antibody level, and length of time waiting are entered into the national computer for each candidate. When a donor becomes available, the donor's key information is compared with the data of all patients awaiting transplantation locally and nationwide. Points are given for how close the HLA match is, how long the patient has been waiting, if the antibody level is unusually high, and if the recipient is younger than 19 years old. Extra points are given for high antibody levels because this can severely limit the number of donors with whom the patient will not have a positive crossmatch. The kidney is offered to the recipient with the most points in the local area. If no patients in the local area are suitable, the organ is then offered in the region and then in the nation. When a kidney arrives at the recipient's transplant center, a final crossmatch is done and must be negative for the deceased donor transplantation to proceed. (Crossmatching is discussed in Chapter 14.)

The only exception to the previous plan is if a patient needs an emergency transplant or if a donor and recipient match on all six HLA antigens (zero antigen mismatch). The patient meeting either one of these criteria goes to the top of the list. Emergency transplants are given priority because the patient is facing imminent death if not transplanted (e.g., a patient who had no vascular access sites left and can no longer dialyze). Zero antigen mismatches are given priority because statistically these grafts have better survival rates. If a zero antigen mismatch patient is identified nationally, one of the donor kidneys must be sent to that recipient's transplant center regardless of location.

Surgical Procedure

Live Donor. Living donation accounts for nearly 27% of all kidney transplants in the United States, and most transplant centers regard them as the preferred donation modality. The donor nephrectomy is performed by a urologist or transplant surgeon. The donor's surgery begins 1 to 2 hours before the recipient's surgery. The recipient is surgically prepared for the kidney transplant in a nearby operating room.

Laparoscopic donor nephrectomy is the most common technique for removing a kidney in a living donor. (Laparoscopic nephrectomy is discussed in Chapter 46.) After the kidney has been removed, it is flushed with a chilled, sterile electrolyte solution and prepared for immediate transplant into the recipient. The use of a laparoscopic donor nephrectomy procedure is minimally invasive with fewer risks and shorter recovery time than an open procedure. The laparoscopic approach significantly decreases hospital stay, pain, operative blood loss, debilitation, and length of time off work. For these reasons, the number of people willing to donate a kidney has increased significantly.

For an *open (conventional) nephrectomy,* the donor is placed in the lateral decubitus position on the operating table so that the flank is exposed laterally. An incision is made at the level of the eleventh rib. The rib may have to be removed to provide adequate visualization of the kidney.

Kidney Transplant Recipient. The transplanted kidney is usually placed extraperitoneally in the iliac fossa. The right iliac fossa is preferred to facilitate anastomoses of the blood vessels and ureter and minimize the occurrence of paralytic ileus.

Before any incisions are made, a urinary catheter is placed into the bladder. An antibiotic solution is instilled to distend the bladder and decrease the risk of infection. A crescent-shaped incision is made extending from the iliac crest to the symphysis pubis (Fig. 47-15).

Rapid revascularization is critical to prevent ischemic injury to the kidney. The donor artery is anastomosed to the recipient's internal iliac (hypogastric) or external iliac artery. The donor vein is anastomosed to the recipient's external iliac vein.

When the anastomoses are complete, the clamps are released, and blood flow to the kidney is reestablished. The kidney should become firm and pink. Urine may begin to flow from the ureter immediately.

The donor ureter in most cases is then tunneled through the bladder submucosa before entering the bladder cavity and being sutured in place. This approach is called *ureteroneocystostomy.* This allows the bladder wall to compress the ureter as it contracts for micturition, thereby preventing reflux of urine up the ureter into the transplanted kidney. The transplant surgery takes about 3 to 4 hours.

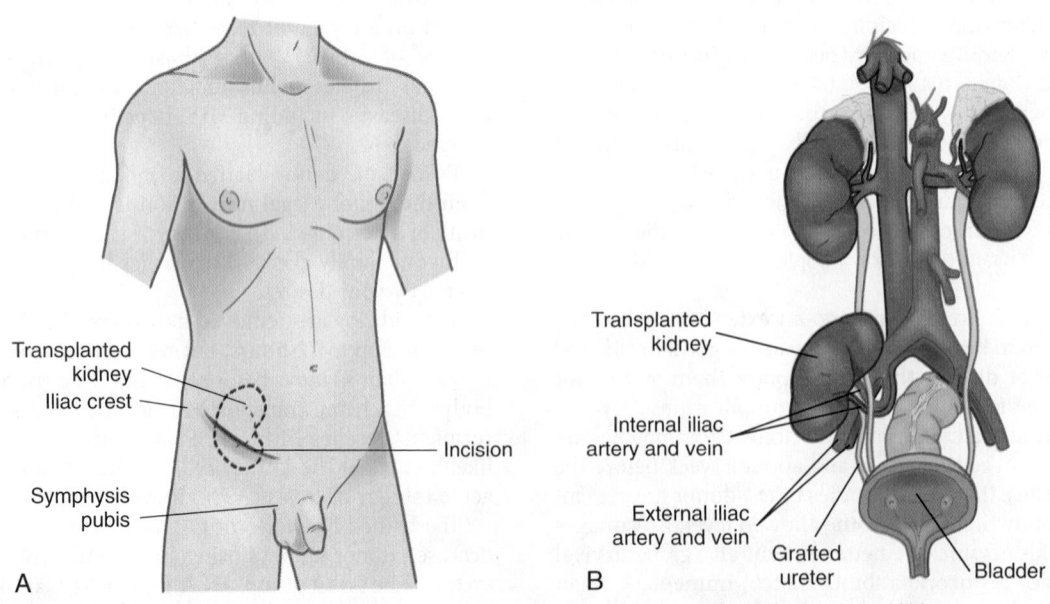

Transplanted kidney
Iliac crest

Symphysis pubis

Incision

A

Transplanted kidney

Internal iliac artery and vein

External iliac artery and vein

Grafted ureter

Bladder

B

FIG. 47-15 A, Surgical incision for a renal transplant. **B,** Surgical placement of transplanted kidney.

NURSING MANAGEMENT
KIDNEY TRANSPLANT RECIPIENT

PREOPERATIVE CARE

Nursing care of the patient in the preoperative phase includes emotional and physical preparation for surgery. Because the patient and caregiver may have been waiting years for the kidney transplant, a review of the operative procedure and what can be expected in the immediate postoperative recovery period is necessary. Stress that there is a chance the kidney may not function immediately, and dialysis may be required for days to weeks. Review the need for immunosuppressive drugs and measures to prevent infection.

To ensure the patient is in optimal physical condition for surgery, an ECG, chest x-ray, and laboratory studies are ordered. Dialysis may be required before surgery for any significant problems such as fluid overload or hyperkalemia. A patient on PD must empty the peritoneal cavity of all dialysate solution before going to surgery. Because dialysis may be required after transplantation, the patency of the vascular access must be maintained. The vascular access extremity should be labeled "dialysis access, no procedures" to prevent use of the affected extremity for BP measurement, blood drawing, or IV infusions.

POSTOPERATIVE CARE

LIVE DONOR. The usual postoperative care for the donor is similar to that following open (conventional) or laparoscopic nephrectomy (see Chapter 46). Closely monitor renal function to assess for impairment, and monitor the hematocrit to assess for bleeding. Donors experience more pain after an open nephrectomy than a laparoscopic procedure. Generally, all donors have more pain than their recipients do. Donors who have had an open surgical approach are ready to be discharged from the hospital in 4 or 5 days and can usually return to work in 6 to 8 weeks. With a laparoscopic approach, donors are discharged from the hospital in 2 to 4 days and can return to work in 4 to 6 weeks. The donor is seen by the surgeon 1 to 2 weeks after discharge.

Nurses caring for the living donor need to acknowledge the precious gift that this person has given. The donor has taken physical, emotional, and financial risks to assist the recipient. It is vital that the donor not be forgotten postoperatively. The donor will need even more support if the donated organ does not work immediately or for some reason fails.

KIDNEY TRANSPLANT RECIPIENT. The first priority during this period is maintenance of fluid and electrolyte balance. Because close monitoring is required, kidney transplant recipients spend the first 12 to 24 hours in the ICU. Very large volumes of urine may be produced soon after the blood supply to the transplanted kidney is reestablished. This diuresis is due to (1) the new kidney's ability to filter BUN, which acts as an osmotic diuretic; (2) the abundance of fluids administered during the operation; and (3) initial renal tubular dysfunction, which inhibits the kidney from concentrating urine normally. Urine output during this phase may be as high as 1 L/hr and gradually decreases as the BUN and serum creatinine levels return toward normal.

Urine output is replaced with fluids milliliter for milliliter hourly for the first 12 to 24 hours. Central venous pressure readings are essential for monitoring postoperative fluid status. Dehydration must be avoided to prevent subsequent renal hypoperfusion and renal tubular damage. Electrolyte monitor-ing to assess for the hyponatremia and hypokalemia often associated with rapid diuresis is critical. Treatment with potassium supplements or infusion of 0.9% normal saline may be indicated. IV sodium bicarbonate may also be required if the patient develops metabolic acidosis from delayed kidney function.

Acute tubular necrosis (ATN) can occur because of prolonged cold times causing ischemic damage and the use of marginal cadaveric donors (those who are medically suboptimal). While the patient is in ATN, dialysis is required to maintain fluid and electrolyte balance. Some patients have high-output ATN with the ability to excrete fluid but not metabolic wastes or electrolytes. Other patients have oliguric or anuric ATN. These patients are at risk for fluid overload in the immediate postoperative period and must be assessed closely for the need for dialysis. The period of ATN can last anywhere from days to weeks, with gradually improving kidney function. Most patients with ATN are discharged from the hospital on dialysis. This is extremely discouraging for the patient, who needs reassurance that renal function usually improves. Dialysis is discontinued when urine output increases and serum creatinine and BUN begin to normalize.

A sudden decrease in urine output in the early postoperative period is a cause for concern. It may be due to dehydration, rejection, a urine leak, or obstruction. A common cause of early obstruction is a blood clot in the urinary catheter. Catheter patency must be maintained, since the catheter remains in the bladder for 3 to 5 days to allow the ureter-bladder anastomosis to heal. If blood clots are suspected, gentle catheter irrigation (if ordered by the health care provider) can reestablish patency.

With a hospital length of stay averaging 4 to 5 days, discharge planning and teaching needs must be identified and addressed early in the hospital course. Postoperative teaching includes how to recognize signs of rejection, infection, and any complications of surgery. Frequent blood tests and clinic visits help detect rejection early. Patient teaching to ensure a smooth transition from the hospital to the home is an integral part of the nursing care.

Immunosuppressive Therapy

The goal of immunosuppression is to adequately suppress the immune response to prevent rejection of the transplanted kidney while maintaining sufficient immunity to prevent overwhelming infection. Immunosuppressive therapy is discussed in Chapter 14 and in Table 14-16.

Complications of Transplantation

Complications of RRTs, including PD, HD, and kidney transplantation, are compared in Table 47-15.

Rejection. Rejection is one of the major problems following kidney transplantation. Rejection can be hyperacute, acute, or chronic. These types of rejection are discussed in Chapter 14 on p. 221. Patients with chronic rejection should be put on the transplant list in the hope that they can be retransplanted before dialysis is required.

Infection. Infection remains a significant cause of morbidity and mortality after transplantation. The transplant recipient is at risk for infection because of suppression of the body's normal defense mechanisms by surgery, immunosuppressive drugs, and the effects of ESKD. Underlying systemic illness such as diabetes mellitus or systemic lupus erythematosus, malnutrition, and older age can further compound the negative effects on the

TABLE 47-15	COMPLICATIONS OF DIALYSIS AND TRANSPLANTATION	
Peritoneal Dialysis (PD)	**Hemodialysis (HD)**	**Transplantation**

• Exit site infection
 • Peritonitis
 • Abdominal pain
 • Catheter outflow
 • Hernias
 • Lower back pain
 • Cardiovascular disease
 • Pulmonary problems
  • Atelectasis
  • Pneumonia
  • Bronchitis
 • Protein loss
 • Carbohydrate abnormalities
 • Lipid abnormalities
 • Encapsulating sclerosing peritonitis
	• Hypotension
	 • Muscle cramps
	 • Exsanguination
	 • Hepatitis
	 • Infection, including sepsis
	 • Disequilibrium syndrome
	 • Cardiovascular disease
		• Rejection of transplant
		  • Hyperacute
		  • Acute
		  • Chronic
		 • Susceptibility to infection
		 • Cardiovascular disease
		 • Malignancies
		 • Recurrence of kidney disease
		 • Corticosteroid-related complications

immune response. At times the signs and symptoms of infection can be subtle. You need to be astute in your observation and assessment of kidney transplant recipients because prompt diagnosis and treatment of infections will improve patient outcomes.

The most common infections observed in the first month after transplantation are similar to those acquired by any postoperative patient, such as pneumonia, wound infections, IV line and drain infections, and urinary tract infections. Fungal and viral infections are not uncommon because of the patient's immunosuppressed state. Fungal infections include *Candida, Cryptococcus,* and *Aspergillus* organisms and *Pneumocystis jiroveci.* Fungal infections are difficult to treat, require prolonged treatment periods, and often involve the administration of nephrotoxic drugs. Transplant recipients usually receive prophylactic antifungal drugs to prevent these infections, such as clotrimazole (Mycelex), fluconazole (Diflucan), and trimethoprim/sulfamethoxazole (Bactrim).

Viral infections, including CMV, Epstein-Barr virus, herpes simplex virus (HSV), varicella-zoster virus, and polyomavirus (e.g., BK virus), can be primary infections or reactivations of existing disease. Primary infections occur as new infections after transplantation from an exogenous source such as the donated organ or a blood transfusion. Reactivation occurs when a virus exists in a patient and becomes reactivated after transplantation because of immunosuppression.

CMV is one of the most common viral infections. If a recipient has never had CMV and receives an organ from a donor with a history of CMV, antiviral prophylaxis will be administered (e.g., ganciclovir [Cytovene], valganciclovir [Valcyte]). If a primary active CMV infection is diagnosed or there is symptomatic reactivation of CMV, IV ganciclovir is given along with an immune globulin that contains CMV antibodies. To prevent HSV infections, oral acyclovir (Zovirax) is given for several months after the transplant.

Cardiovascular Disease. Transplant recipients have an increased incidence of atherosclerotic vascular disease. CV disease is the leading cause of death after renal transplantation. Hypertension, dyslipidemia, diabetes mellitus, smoking, rejection, infections, and increased homocysteine levels can all

contribute to CV disease. Immunosuppressants can worsen hypertension and dyslipidemia. Teach the patient to control risk factors such as elevated cholesterol, triglycerides, and blood glucose and weight gain. Adherence to the prescribed antihypertensive regimen is essential not only to prevent CV events but also to prevent damage to the new kidney. (Hypertension is discussed in Chapter 33.)

Malignancies. The overall incidence of malignancies in kidney transplant recipients is greater than in the general population, primarily because of immunosuppressive therapy. Not only do immunosuppressants suppress the immune system to prevent rejection, but they also suppress the ability to fight infection and the production of abnormal cells such as cancer cells.[27]

The most common types of cancer after transplant are basal and squamous cell carcinoma of the skin, Hodgkin's and non-Hodgkin's lymphoma, and Kaposi sarcoma. Patients are also at risk for cancers of the liver, stomach, oropharynx, anus, vulva, and penis.

Regular screening for cancer is an important part of the transplant recipient's preventive care. Advise the patient to avoid sun exposure by using protective clothing and sunscreens to minimize the incidence of skin cancers.

Recurrence of Original Kidney Disease. Recurrence of the original disease that destroyed the native kidneys occurs in some kidney transplant recipients. It is most common with certain types of glomerulonephritis, immunoglobulin A (IgA) nephropathy, diabetic nephropathy, and focal segmental sclerosis. Disease recurrence can result in the loss of a functioning kidney transplant. Patients must be advised before transplantation if they have a disease known to recur.

Corticosteroid-Related Complications. Aseptic necrosis of the hips, knees, and other joints can result from chronic corticosteroid therapy and renal osteodystrophy. Other significant problems related to corticosteroids include peptic ulcer disease, glucose intolerance and diabetes, cataracts, dyslipidemia, infections, and malignancies. In the first year after transplantation, corticosteroid doses are usually decreased to 5 to 10 mg/day. The use of tacrolimus and cyclosporine has allowed the corticosteroid doses to be much lower than they were in the past.

Many transplant programs have initiated corticosteroid-free drug regimens because of the problems of long-term corticosteroid use. Other centers withdraw patients from corticosteroids over a short period after transplantation. For patients who remain on corticosteroids, vigilant monitoring for side effects and early treatment are essential.

GERONTOLOGIC CONSIDERATIONS

CHRONIC KIDNEY DISEASE

The incidence of CKD in the United States is increasing most rapidly in older patients. The most common diseases leading to renal failure in older people are hypertension and diabetes.

The care of this older population is particularly challenging, not only because of the normal physiologic changes of aging but also because of the disabilities, chronic diseases, and number of co-morbid conditions that develop.[28] Physiologic changes of clinical importance in the older CKD patient include diminished cardiopulmonary function, bone loss, immunodeficiency, altered protein synthesis, impaired cognition, and altered drug metabolism. Malnutrition is common in these patients for a variety of reasons, including lack of mobility, lack of understanding of basic nutritional requirements, social isolation, physical disability, impaired cognitive function, and malabsorption problems.

When conservative therapy for CKD is no longer effective, the older patient needs to consider the best treatment modality based on his or her physical and emotional health, personal preferences, and availability of support. PD allows the patient to be more mobile and to enjoy an increased sense of control over the illness. PD causes less hemodynamic instability than HD but does require self-care or assistance from another person, which may not always be available.

Most individuals 65 years of age or older select treatment with HD, specifically in-center treatment, because of a lack of assistance in the home and reluctance to manage the technology of dialysis. Establishing vascular access for HD may be a concern for an older patient because of atherosclerotic changes. Although transplantation is an option, older patients are less likely to be considered as candidates. Older adults need to be carefully screened to ensure that the benefits of transplantation outweigh the risks.[29] A living donor is preferable so that there is not a prolonged waiting time.

The most common cause of death in older ESKD patients is CV disease (myocardial infarction, stroke), followed by withdrawal from dialysis. If a competent patient decides to withdraw from dialysis, it is essential to support the patient and family. Ethical issues (see the Ethical/Legal Dilemmas box on this page) to consider in this situation include patient competency, benefit versus burden of treatment, and futility of treatment. Withdrawal from treatment is not a failure if the patient is well informed and comfortable with the decision.[30]

The increasing number of older, debilitated ESKD patients receiving dialysis has raised a number of ethical concerns about the use of scarce resources in a population with a limited life expectancy. Dialysis (especially PD) has been successfully used in older adults. Quality of life is good in many older ESKD patients receiving dialysis. There appears to be no justification for excluding the older adult from dialysis programs. Rationing dialysis based on age alone is not supported based on current outcome and quality-of-life data.

ETHICAL/LEGAL DILEMMAS
Withdrawing Treatment

Situation

L.R., a 70-yr-old patient with diabetes mellitus and end-stage kidney disease, has been on dialysis for 10 yr. He tells you that he wants to discontinue his dialysis. His quality of life has diminished during the past 2 yr since his wife died. He is not a transplant candidate.

Ethical/Legal Points for Consideration

- Informed consent includes the legal right to refuse treatment. However, the right to refuse may be more difficult if (1) it is contrary to the wishes of family and friends, (2) the treatment still appears to have some effectiveness, and (3) the treatment has been in place for some time.
- Quality-of-life decisions often outweigh the benefit against the burden of treatment. When a treatment becomes too burdensome, the patient (if competent) may request to withdraw the treatment.
- It must be determined whether some other treatable problem such as depression may be clouding the patient's judgment.
- Some health care professionals become conflicted when they are asked to withdraw treatment, since they may think they are contributing to the patient's untimely death.
- If a decision is made to withdraw treatment, the health care team, patient, and family should develop an appropriate follow-up plan that includes palliative care and hospice support.

Discussion Questions

1. How should you respond to L.R.'s request?
2. What is the American Nurses Association's position on withdrawing or withholding treatment that no longer benefits the patient or causes suffering?

CASE STUDY
Chronic Kidney Disease

iStockphoto/Thinkstock

Patient Profile

M.B. is a 56-yr-old African American college professor. He is seen by his primary care provider for a routine physical examination. He has not been seen by a physician in a little over a year. He complains of generalized malaise, frequent urination, and "increasing thirst." His medical history is significant for borderline hypertension and dyslipidemia. He also smokes at least one pack of cigarettes per day, and his efforts to quit have been unsuccessful.

Subjective Data

- Family history: father died of a heart attack at age 62, brother had coronary artery bypass graft (CABG) at age 50, mother died from complications of diabetes
- Becomes "winded" when walking from his car to his office at the university
- Wakes up at night to urinate and has more frequent urination
- Increasing thirst

Objective Data
Laboratory Data

- Calculated creatinine clearance using the MDRD equation: 42 mL/min/1.73 m²

- Serum creatinine 2.5 mg/dL
- BUN 35 mg/dL
- Serum glucose 264 mg/dL
- Hgb 13 g/dL
- Serum cholesterol 236 mg/dL

Physical Examination

- Weight 220 lb, height 5 ft, 11 in
- Blood pressure 168/104 mm Hg

Discussion Questions

1. What do you think caused M.B.'s kidney failure?
2. What stage of chronic kidney disease does he have?
3. What are the most important treatments for M.B.?
4. Identify the abnormal diagnostic study results and why each would occur.
5. ***Priority Decision:*** What are the priority nursing interventions that would help promote M.B.'s self-management of his disease process?
6. ***Priority Decision:*** Based on the assessment data provided, what are the priority nursing diagnoses? Are there any collaborative problems?
7. ***Evidence-Based Practice:*** M.B. tells you that he has not been taking his blood pressure medications regularly. When he asks you how important they are, what will you tell him?

BRIDGE TO NCLEX EXAMINATION

The number of the question corresponds to the same-numbered outcome at the beginning of the chapter.

1. Which descriptions characterize acute kidney injury (*select all that apply*)?
   a. Primary cause of death is infection.
   b. It almost always affects older people.
   c. Disease course is potentially reversible.
   d. Most common cause is diabetic nephropathy.
   e. Cardiovascular disease is most common cause of death.

2. RIFLE defines three stages of AKI based on changes in
   a. blood pressure and urine osmolality.
   b. fractional excretion of urinary sodium.
   c. estimation of GFR with the MDRD equation.
   d. serum creatinine or urine output from baseline.

3. During the oliguric phase of AKI, the nurse monitors the patient for (*select all that apply*)
   a. hypotension.
   b. ECG changes.
   c. hypernatremia.
   d. pulmonary edema.
   e. urine with high specific gravity.

4. If a patient is in the diuretic phase of AKI, the nurse must monitor for which serum electrolyte imbalances?
   a. Hyperkalemia and hyponatremia
   b. Hyperkalemia and hypernatremia
   c. Hypokalemia and hyponatremia
   d. Hypokalemia and hypernatremia

5. A patient is admitted to the hospital with chronic kidney disease. The nurse understands that this condition is characterized by
   a. progressive irreversible destruction of the kidneys.
   b. a rapid decrease in urine output with an elevated BUN.
   c. an increasing creatinine clearance with a decrease in urine output.
   d. prostration, somnolence, and confusion with coma and imminent death.

6. Nurses need to teach patients at risk for developing chronic kidney disease. Individuals considered to be at increased risk include (*select all that apply*)
   a. older African Americans.
   b. patients more than 60 years old.
   c. those with a history of pancreatitis.
   d. those with a history of hypertension.
   e. those with a history of type 2 diabetes.

7. Patients with chronic kidney disease experience an increased incidence of cardiovascular disease related to (*select all that apply*)
   a. hypertension.
   b. vascular calcifications.
   c. a genetic predisposition.
   d. hyperinsulinemia causing dyslipidemia.
   e. increased high-density lipoprotein levels.

8. Nutritional support and management are essential across the entire continuum of chronic kidney disease. Which statements would be considered true related to nutritional therapy (*select all that apply*)?
   a. Fluid is not usually restricted for patients receiving peritoneal dialysis.
   b. Sodium and potassium may be restricted in someone with advanced CKD.
   c. Decreased fluid intake and a low potassium diet are hallmarks of the diet for a patient receiving hemodialysis.
   d. Decreased fluid intake and a low potassium diet are hallmarks of the diet for a patient receiving peritoneal dialysis.
   e. Increased fluid intake and a diet with potassium-rich foods are hallmarks of a diet for a patient receiving hemodialysis.

9. An ESKD patient receiving hemodialysis is considering asking a relative to donate a kidney for transplantation. In assisting the patient to make a decision about treatment, the nurse informs the patient that
   a. successful transplantation usually provides better quality of life than that offered by dialysis.
   b. if rejection of the transplanted kidney occurs, no further treatment for the renal failure is available.
   c. hemodialysis replaces the normal functions of the kidneys, and patients do not have to live with the continual fear of rejection.
   d. the immunosuppressive therapy following transplantation makes the person ineligible to receive other forms of treatment if the kidney fails.

10. To assess the patency of a newly placed arteriovenous graft for dialysis, the nurse should (*select all that apply*)
   a. monitor the BP in the affected arm.
   b. irrigate the graft daily with low-dose heparin.
   c. palpate the area of the graft to feel a normal thrill.
   d. listen with a stethoscope over the graft to detect a bruit.
   e. frequently monitor the pulses and neurovascular status distal to the graft.

11. A major advantage of peritoneal dialysis is
   a. the diet is less restricted and dialysis can be performed at home.
   b. the dialysate is biocompatible and causes no long-term consequences.
   c. high glucose concentrations of the dialysate cause a reduction in appetite, promoting weight loss.
   d. no medications are required because of the enhanced efficiency of the peritoneal membrane in removing toxins.

12. A kidney transplant recipient complains of having fever, chills, and dysuria over the past 2 days. What is the first action that the nurse should take?
   a. Assess temperature and initiate workup to rule out infection.
   b. Reassure the patient that this is common after transplantation.
   c. Provide warm cover for the patient and give 1 g acetaminophen orally.
   d. Notify the nephrologist that the patient has developed symptoms of acute rejection.

1. a, c, 2. d, 3. b, d, 4. c, 5. a, 6. a, b, d, e, 7. a, b, d, 8. a, b, c, 9. a, 10. c, d, e, 11. a, 12. a

evolve

For rationales to these answers and even more NCLEX review questions, visit *http://evolve.elsevier.com/Lewis/medsurg*.

REFERENCES

1. Workeneh BT: Acute renal failure. Retrieved from *http://emedicine.medscape.com/article/243492-overview.*
2. Kidney Disease: improving Global Outcomes: clinical practice guidelines on acute kidney injury. Retrieved from *www.kdigo.org.*
*3. Murugan R, Kellum JA: Acute kidney injury: what's the prognosis? *Nat Rev Nephrol* 7(4):209, 2011.
*4. Wang HE, Muntner P, Chertow G, et al: Acute kidney injury and mortality in hospitalized patients, *Am J Neph* 35(4):349, 2012.
5. Singbartl K, Kellum J: AKI in the ICU: definition, epidemiology, risk stratification, and outcomes, *Kidney Int* 81(9):819, 2012.
*6. Wu VC, Wang CH, Wang WJ, et al: Sustained low-efficiency dialysis versus continuous veno-venous hemofiltration for postsurgical acute renal failure, *Am J Surg* 199(4):466, 2010.
7. Davies H, Leslie G: Acute kidney injury and the critically ill patient, *Dimens Crit Nurs* 31(3):135, 2012.
8. Yaklin K: Acute kidney injury: an overview of pathophysiology and treatments, *Nephrol Nurs J* 38(1):13, 2011.
9. Dirkes S: Acute kidney injury: not just acute renal failure anymore? *Crit Care Nurse* 31(1):37, 2011.
10. Ostermann M, Dickie H, Barrett N: Renal replacement therapy in critically ill patients with acute kidney injury: when to start, *Nephrol Dial Transplant* 26(13):1027, 2012.
11. Ali B, Gray-Vickrey P: Limiting the damage from acute kidney injury, *Nursing* 41(3):22, 2011.
12. Kellum J, Lameire N: Clinical practice guidelines for acute kidney injury: KDIGO, *Kidney Int* 2(Suppl 1):1, 2012. Retrieved from *www.kdigo.org/clinical_practice_guidelines/pdf/KDIGO%20AKI%20Guideline.pdf.*
13. Thakar CV, Christianson A, Himmelfarb J, et al: Acute kidney injury episodes and chronic kidney disease risk in diabetes mellitus, *Clin J Am Soc Nephrol* 6(11):2567, 2011.
14. US Renal Data System: *USRDS 2012 annual data report: atlas of end-stage renal disease*, Bethesda, Md, 2012, National Institute of Diabetes and Digestive and Kidney Diseases. Retrieved from *www.usrds.org/adr.aspx.*
15. Foody J, Cleary J, Davis L, et al: Chronic kidney disease and cardiovascular risk: a perfect storm, 2011. Retrieved from *www.aapa.org/uploadedFiles/content/CME/PostTest/W175_176%20CKD%20Mono%20JAPPA.pdf.*
16. US Department of Health and Human Services: ESRD: general information, Centers for Medicare and Medicaid Services. Retrieved from *www.cms.hhs.gov/ESRDGeneralInformation.*
17. National Kidney Foundation: High blood pressure and chronic kidney disease. Retrieved from *www.kidney.org/atoz/pdf/hbpandckd.pdf.*
18. Brancaccio D, Cozzolino M: CKD-MBD: an endless story, *J Nephrol* 24(Suppl 18):42, 2011.
19. National Kidney Foundation Kidney Disease Outcomes Quality Initiative (NKF KDOQI). Retrieved from *www.kidney.org/Professionals/kdoqi.*
20. Hasegawa G, Bragg-Gresham J, Pisoni R, et al: Changes in anemia management and hemoglobin levels following revision of a bundling policy to incorporate recombinant human erythropoietin, *Kidney Inter* 79(3):340, 2011.
21. Aparicio M, Bellizzi V, Chauvea P, et al: Protein-restricted diets plus keto/amino acids: a valid therapeutic approach for chronic kidney disease patients, *J Renal Nutr* 22(2 Suppl):S1, 2012.
22. Holley J: Providing optimal care before and after discontinuation, *Semin Dialy* 25(1):33, 2012.
23. National Kidney and Urologic Diseases Information Clearinghouse: Treatment methods for kidney failure: peritoneal dialysis. Retrieved from *http://kidney.niddk.nih.gov/kudiseases/pubs/peritoneal.*
24. National Kidney and Urologic Diseases Information Clearinghouse: Treatment methods for kidney failure: hemodialysis. Retrieved from *http://kidney.niddk.nih.gov/Kudiseases/pubs/hemodialysis.*
25. Abboud O, Becker G, Bellorin-Font E, et al: KDIGO clinical practice guidelines on hepatitis C in chronic kidney disease acknowledged by ISN. Retrieved from *www.kdigo.org/clinical_practice_guidelines/pdf/ISN_HepC_Commentary.pdf.*
26. United Network for Organ Sharing: *2011 annual report: the US scientific registry of transplant recipients and the organ procurement and transplantation network*, Bethesda, Md, 2011, US Department of Health and Human Services.
27. Danovitch GM: *Handbook of kidney transplantation*, ed 5, Philadelphia, 2010, Lippincott Williams & Wilkins.
28. Bleevins C, Toutman M: Successful aging theory and the patient with chronic renal disease: application in the clinical setting, *Nephrol Nurs J* 38(3):255, 2011.
29. Schaeffner E, Rose C, Gill J: Access to kidney transplantation among the elderly in the United States: a glass half full, not half empty, *Clin J Am Soc Nephrol* 5(11):2109, 2010.
*30. Hopkins DJ, Kott MR, Pirozzi J, et al: End-of-life issues and the patient with renal disease: an evidence-based practice project, *Nephrol Nurs J* 38(1):79, 2011.

RESOURCES

American Association of Kidney Patients (AAKP)
www.aakp.org
American Nephrology Nurses' Association
www.annanurse.org
American Organ Transplant Association
www.a-o-t-a.org
International Society of Nephrology (ISN)
www.theisn.org
International Transplant Nurses Society
www.itns.org
Kidney Transplant/Dialysis Association, Inc.
http://ktda.org
National Kidney Disease Education Program
www.nkdep.nih.gov
National Kidney Foundation
www.kidney.org
RenalWEB Patient Education
www.renalweb.com/topics/patiented/patiented.htm
United Network for Organ Sharing
www.unos.org
United States Renal Data System
www.usrds.org/adr.htm

*Evidence-based information for clinical practice.

Urinary System

CASE STUDY

Managing Multiple Patients

Introduction

You are working on the medical-surgical unit and have been assigned to care for the following four patients. You are also assigned to receive a new admission to the clinical unit. You have one UAP on your team to help you.

Patients

iStockphoto/Thinkstock

A.K., a 28-year-old African American man, was admitted for observation after a renal ultrasound identified calculi in the left ureter. A.K. came to the ED with complaints of sharp, colicky left flank pain for which the health care provider prescribed IV opioids. His last pain medication was given 2 hours ago. His current pain level is 4 on a scale of 1-10. He is voiding dark, smoky colored urine. His vital signs are within normal limits. He has positive costovertebral tenderness.

iStockphoto/Thinkstock

S.U., a 38-year-old Hispanic woman, was admitted with acute pyelonephritis following a recent UTI. She complains of bilateral flank pain and has abdominal tenderness to palpation. Her temperature is 100.4° F (38° C). Her urinalysis indicates pyuria and hematuria. Her WBC is elevated at 12,000/µL. Blood culture results are pending. IV antibiotics have been started.

iStockphoto/Thinkstock

M.B., a 56-year-old African American college professor, was admitted with uncontrolled hypertension. He was recently diagnosed with CKD. He smokes at least one pack of cigarettes per day and is experiencing some nicotine withdrawal symptoms. His BP on admission was 224/102 mm Hg. He is receiving IV metoprolol (Lopressor) 5 mg q4hr prn for SBP >180 mm Hg. His most recent BP 3 hr ago was 174/86 mm Hg.

iStockphoto/Thinkstock

D.M., an 82-year-old woman, was admitted to the ED with severe dehydration, heart failure, and acute kidney injury. Her daughter found her unconscious and lying on the floor. She is confused. Her serum potassium level is 5.7 mEq/L. Her urine output for the past 8 hours was 90 mL.

Management Discussion Questions

1. *Priority Decision:* After receiving report, which patient should you see first? Second? Provide a rationale for your decision.
2. *Delegation Decision:* Which tasks could you delegate to the UAP *(select all that apply)?*
   a. Obtain vital signs on M.B.
   b. Strain A.K.'s voided urine.
   c. Report D.M.'s potassium level to health care provider.
   d. Assess S.U. for potential side effects of the IV antibiotics.
   e. Measure D.M.'s urine output and report the results to the RN.

3. *Priority and Delegation Decision:* As you are assessing D.M., the UAP informs you that M.B.'s blood pressure is 190/86. He is asymptomatic. Additionally, the charge nurse informs you that you will be receiving a patient with heart failure from the ED within the next 10 minutes. Which action would be most appropriate?
   a. Ask the charge nurse to assign the new admission to someone else.
   b. Have the UAP admit the new patient while you administer M.B.'s IV metoprolol.
   c. Call the ED and have them hold the new admission until after you have assessed all your patients.
   d. Ask the charge nurse to administer M.B.'s IV metoprolol while you complete your assessment of D.M.

Case Study Progression

As you complete your assessment of D.M., you notice her apical pulse is irregular. She has +1 pitting edema in her lower extremities. Her blood pressure is 160/90 mmHg, heart rate 88 bpm, and respiratory rate 28/min. Her respirations are deep. You notify her health care provider.

4. Which interventions would you expect the health care provider to order for M.B. *(select all that apply)?*
   a. Administer IV Kayexalate.
   b. Obtain arterial blood gas levels.
   c. Place an indwelling urinary catheter.
   d. Perform continuous cardiac monitoring.
   e. Prepare M.B. for hemodialysis and notify her family.
5. *Priority Decision:* Which nursing diagnosis would be of highest priority when planning care for A.K.?
   a. Risk for injury
   b. Impaired comfort
   c. Risk for infection
   d. Ineffective self-health management
6. Which statement would be most appropriate when teaching S.U. about her kidney infection?
   a. "The damage to your kidneys will likely require dialysis."
   b. "Influenza is the most likely cause of your kidney infection."
   c. "You will need to be in the hospital for a 2-week course of IV antibiotics."
   d. "It is very important that you maintain adequate hydration to flush your kidneys."
7. *Management Decision:* As the UAP prepares the room for the patient being admitted from the ED, you overhear her telling a co-worker that she has to do all your work for you. What is your best initial action?
   a. Report the incident to the charge nurse for follow-up.
   b. Ask the UAP to discuss her concerns with you in private.
   c. Tell the UAP how much you appreciate and value her input on your team.
   d. Immediately clarify the situation by telling the UAP all the tasks you are completing.

Problems Related to Regulatory and Reproductive Mechanisms

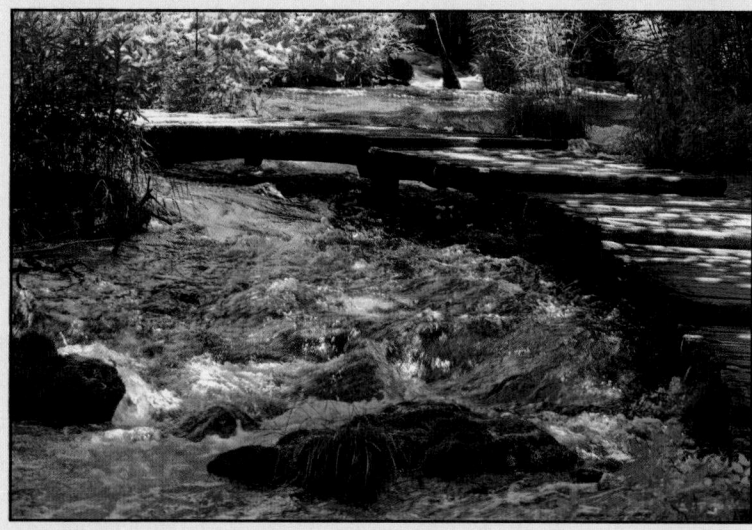

iStockphoto/Thinkstock

We keep moving forward, opening new doors, and doing new things,
because we're curious and curiosity keeps leading us down new paths.
Walt Disney

48

Nursing Assessment
Endocrine System

Susan C. Landis

> *Nobody can go back and start a new
> beginning, but anyone can start today and
> make a new ending.*
> *Maria Robinson*

LEARNING OUTCOMES

1. Describe the common characteristics and functions of hormones.
2. Identify the locations of the endocrine glands.
3. Describe the functions of hormones secreted by the pituitary, thyroid, parathyroid, and adrenal glands and the pancreas.
4. Describe the locations and roles of hormone receptors.
5. Select the significant subjective and objective assessment data related to the endocrine system that should be obtained from a patient.
6. Link age-related changes in the endocrine system to differences in assessment findings.
7. Differentiate normal from common abnormal findings of a physical assessment of the endocrine system.
8. Describe the purpose, significance of results, and nursing responsibilities related to diagnostic studies of the endocrine system.

KEY TERMS

aldosterone, p. 1140
antidiuretic hormone (ADH), p. 1138
catecholamines, p. 1140
circadian rhythm, p. 1137
corticosteroid, p. 1140
cortisol, p. 1140

glucagon, p. 1140
growth hormone (GH), p. 1138
hormones, p. 1134
insulin, p. 1140
islets of Langerhans, p. 1140
melatonin, p. 1139

negative feedback, p. 1137
positive feedback, p. 1137
thyroxine (T$_4$), p. 1139
triiodothyronine (T$_3$), p. 1139
tropic hormones, p. 1138

STRUCTURES AND FUNCTIONS OF ENDOCRINE SYSTEM

Glands

Endocrine glands include the hypothalamus, pituitary, thyroid, parathyroids, adrenals, pancreas, ovaries, testes, and pineal gland (Fig. 48-1). *Exocrine glands* are not part of the endocrine system. They secrete their substances into ducts that then empty into a body cavity or onto a surface. For example, salivary glands produce saliva, which is secreted through salivary ducts into the mouth.

Hormones

Hormones are chemical substances produced in the body that control and regulate the activity of certain target cells or organs. Many are produced in one part of the body and control and regulate the activity of certain cells or organs in another part of the body.

Endocrine glands produce and secrete hormones that travel to affect their specific target tissues. For example, the thyroid gland synthesizes the hormone thyroxine, which affects all body tissues. Some hormones are released directly into the circulation, whereas others may act locally on cells

Reviewed by Saundra J. Hendricks, RN, MS, FNP, BC-ADM, Endocrine Nurses Society, Former President, The Methodist Hospital, Department of Medicine, Houston, Texas; Beth Lucasey, RN, MA, Endocrine Nurses Society Board Member, VP Marketing and Communication, TVAX Biomedical, Kansas City, Missouri; Barbara Lukert, MD, Endocrine Nurses Society Advisor, Endocrinologist, University of Kansas Medical Center, Kansas City, Kansas; and Teresa J. Seright, RN, PhD, CCRN, Assistant Professor of Nursing, Montana State University, Bozeman, Montana.

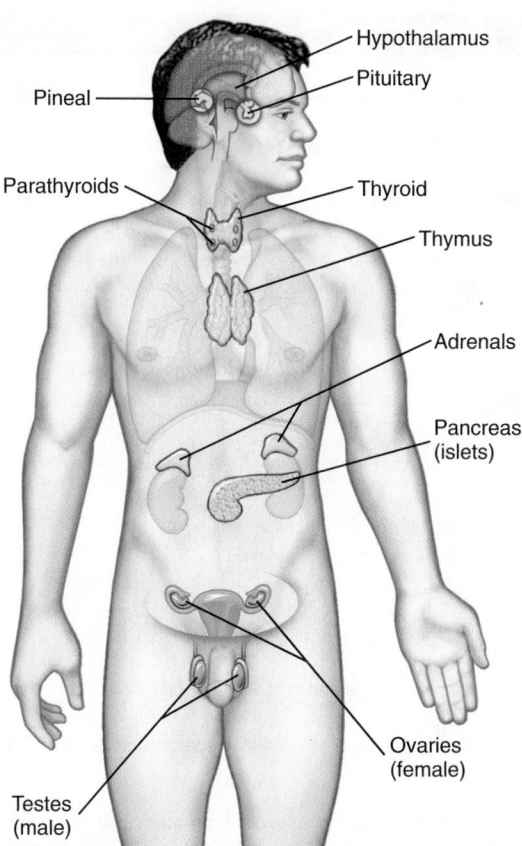

FIG. 48-1 Location of the major endocrine glands. The parathyroid glands lie on the posterior surface of the thyroid gland.

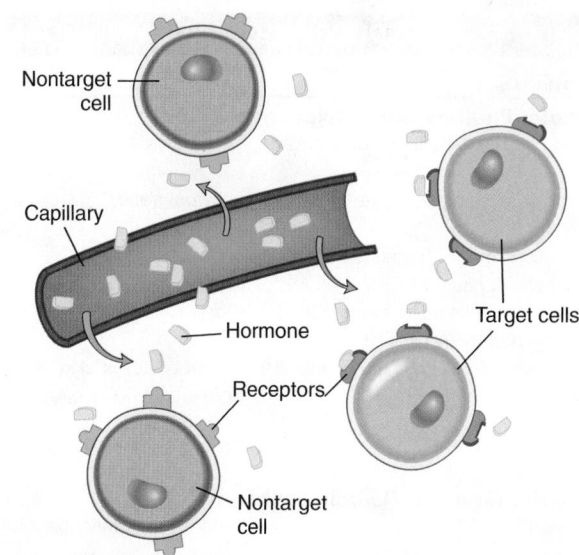

FIG. 48-2 The target cell concept. Hormones act only on cells that have receptors specific to that hormone, since the shape of the receptor determines which hormone can react with it. This is an example of the lock-and-key model of biochemical reactions.

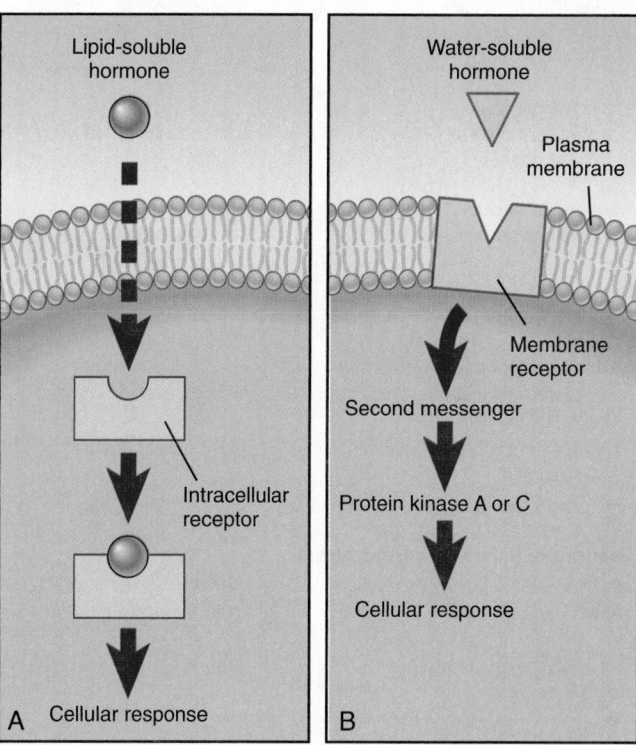

FIG. 48-3 **A,** Lipid-soluble hormones (e.g., steroid hormones) penetrate the cell membrane and interact with intracellular receptors. **B,** Water-soluble hormones (e.g., protein hormones) bind to receptors located in the cell membrane. The hormone-receptor interaction stimulates various cell responses.

where they are released and never enter the bloodstream. This local effect is called *paracrine action.* The action of sex steroids on the ovary is an example of paracrine action.

Most hormones have common characteristics, including (1) secretion in small amounts at variable but predictable rates; (2) regulation by feedback systems; and (3) binding to specific target cell receptors. Table 48-1 summarizes the major hormones, glands or tissues from which they are synthesized, target organs or tissues, and functions.

In addition to important physiologic activities, hormones help regulate the nervous system. For example, catecholamines are hormones when they are secreted by the adrenal medulla, but act as neurotransmitters when secreted by nerve cells in the brain and peripheral nervous system. When epinephrine, a catecholamine, travels through the blood, it is a hormone and affects target tissues. When it travels across synaptic junctions, it acts as a neurotransmitter.[1]

In addition to the endocrine glands, other body organs may secrete hormones. For example, the kidneys secrete erythropoietin, the heart secretes atrial natriuretic peptide, and the gastrointestinal (GI) tract secretes numerous peptide hormones (e.g., gastrin). These hormones are discussed in their respective assessment chapters.

Hormone Receptors. Hormones exert their effects by recognizing their target tissues and attaching to receptor sites in a "lock-and-key" type of mechanism. Therefore a hormone will act only on cells that have a receptor specific for that hormone (Fig. 48-2).

Lipid-Soluble and Water-Soluble Hormones. Hormones are classified by their chemical structure as either lipid soluble or water soluble. The differences in solubility become important in understanding how the hormone interacts with the target cell.

Lipid-soluble hormones are synthesized from cholesterol and are produced by the adrenal cortex, sex glands, and thyroid.[2] Lipid-soluble hormones (steroids, thyroid) are relatively small molecules that cross the target cell membrane by simple diffusion. Steroid and thyroid hormone receptors are located inside the cell (Fig. 48-3). Lipid-soluble hormones are bound to plasma

TABLE 48-1	ENDOCRINE GLANDS AND HORMONES	

Hormones	Target Tissue	Functions
Anterior Pituitary (Adenohypophysis)		
Growth hormone (GH), or somatotropin	All body cells	Promotes protein anabolism (growth, tissue repair) and lipid mobilization and catabolism.
Thyroid-stimulating hormone (TSH), or thyrotropin	Thyroid gland	Stimulates synthesis and release of thyroid hormones, growth and function of thyroid gland.
Adrenocorticotropic hormone (ACTH)	Adrenal cortex	Fosters growth of adrenal cortex. Stimulates secretion of corticosteroids.
Gonadotropic hormones • Follicle-stimulating hormone (FSH) • Luteinizing hormone (LH)*	Reproductive organs	Stimulate sex hormone secretion, reproductive organ growth, reproductive processes.
Melanocyte-stimulating hormone (MSH)	Melanocytes in skin	Increases melanin production in melanocytes to make skin darker.
Prolactin	Ovary and mammary glands in women Testes in men	Stimulates milk production in lactating women. Increases response of follicles to LH and FSH. Stimulates testicular function in men.
Posterior Pituitary (Neurohypophysis)		
Oxytocin	Uterus, mammary glands	Stimulates milk secretion, uterine contractility.
Antidiuretic hormone (ADH), or vasopressin	Renal tubules, vascular smooth muscle	Promotes reabsorption of water, vasoconstriction.
Thyroid		
Thyroxine (T_4)	All body tissues	Precursor to T_3.
Triiodothyronine (T_3)	All body tissues	Regulates metabolic rate of all cells and processes of cell growth and tissue differentiation.
Calcitonin	Bone tissue	Regulates calcium and phosphorus blood levels. Decreases serum Ca^{2+} levels.
Parathyroids		
Parathyroid hormone (PTH), or parathormone	Bone, intestine, kidneys	Regulates calcium and phosphorus blood levels. Promotes bone demineralization and increases intestinal absorption of Ca^{2+}. Increases serum Ca^{2+} levels.
Adrenal Medulla		
Epinephrine (adrenaline)	Sympathetic effectors	Increases in response to stress. Enhances and prolongs effects of sympathetic nervous system.
Norepinephrine (noradrenaline)	Sympathetic effectors	Increases in response to stress. Enhances and prolongs effects of sympathetic nervous system.
Adrenal Cortex		
Corticosteroids (e.g., cortisol, hydrocortisone)	All body tissues	Promote metabolism. Increased in response to stress. Antiinflammatory.
Androgens (e.g., DHEA, androsterone) and estradiol	Reproductive organs	Promote growth spurt in adolescence, secondary sex characteristics, and libido in both sexes.
Mineralocorticoids (e.g., aldosterone)	Kidney	Regulate sodium and potassium balance and thus water balance.
Pancreas (Islets of Langerhans)		
Insulin (from β cells)	General	Promotes movement of glucose out of blood and into cells.
Amylin (from β cells)	Liver, stomach	Decreases gastric motility, glucagon secretion, and endogenous glucose release from liver. Increases satiety.
Glucagon (from α-cells)	General	Stimulates glycogenolysis and gluconeogenesis.
Somatostatin	Pancreas	Inhibits insulin and glucagon secretion.
Pancreatic polypeptide	General	Influences regulation of pancreatic exocrine function and metabolism of absorbed nutrients.
Gonads		
Women: Ovaries		
Estrogen	Reproductive system, breasts	Stimulates development of secondary sex characteristics, preparation of uterus for fertilization and fetal development. Stimulates bone growth.
Progesterone	Reproductive system	Maintains lining of uterus necessary for successful pregnancy.
Men: Testes		
Testosterone	Reproductive system	Stimulates development of secondary sex characteristics, spermatogenesis.

*In men, sometimes referred to as interstitial cell–stimulating hormone (ICSH).
DHEA, Dehydroepiandrosterone.

proteins for transport in the blood. Although lipid-soluble hormones are inactive when bound to plasma proteins, they can be released when appropriate and immediately exert their action at the target tissue.

Water-soluble hormones (insulin, growth hormone [GH], and prolactin) have receptors on or in the cell membrane.[3] Water-soluble hormones circulate freely in the blood to their target tissues, where they act. Water-soluble hormones are not dependent on plasma proteins for transport (see Fig. 48-3).

Regulation of Hormonal Secretion. The regulation of endocrine activity is controlled by specific mechanisms of varying levels of complexity. These mechanisms stimulate or inhibit hormone synthesis and secretion and include feedback, nervous system control, and physiologic rhythms.

Simple Feedback. Negative feedback relies on the blood level of a hormone or other chemical compound regulated by the hormone (e.g., glucose). It is the most common type of endocrine feedback system and results in the gland increasing or decreasing the release of a hormone. Negative feedback is similar to the functioning of a thermostat in which cold air in a room activates the thermostat to release heat, and hot air signals the thermostat to prevent more warm air from entering the room.

The pattern of insulin secretion is a physiologic example of negative feedback between glucose and insulin. Elevated blood glucose levels stimulate the secretion of insulin from the pancreas (see eFig. 48-1 available on the website for this chapter). As blood glucose levels decrease, the stimulus for insulin secretion also decreases. The homeostatic mechanism is considered negative feedback because it reverses the change in blood glucose level. Another example of negative feedback is the relationship between calcium and parathyroid hormone (PTH). Low blood levels of calcium stimulate the parathyroid gland to release PTH, which acts on bone, the intestine, and the kidneys to increase blood calcium levels. The increased blood calcium level then inhibits further PTH release (Fig. 48-4).

Positive feedback is also used to regulate hormone synthesis and release. The female ovarian hormone estradiol operates by this type of feedback. Increased levels of estradiol produced by the follicle during the menstrual cycle result in increased production and release of follicle-stimulating hormone (FSH) by the anterior pituitary. FSH causes further increases in estradiol until the death of the follicle. This results in a drop of FSH serum levels. Thus with this type of feedback, rising hormone levels cause another gland to release a hormone that then stimulates further release of the first hormone. A mechanism for shutting off release of the first hormone (e.g., follicle death) is required or it will continue to be released.

Nervous System Control. In addition to chemical regulation, some endocrine glands are directly affected by the activity of the nervous system. Pain, emotion, sexual excitement, and stress can stimulate the nervous system to modulate hormone secretion. Neural involvement is initiated by the central nervous system (CNS) and implemented by the sympathetic nervous system (SNS). For example, stress is sensed or perceived by the CNS with subsequent stimulation of the SNS. The SNS secretes catecholamines that increase heart rate and blood pressure to deal with stress more effectively. (Effects of stress are discussed in Chapter 7.)

Rhythms. A common physiologic rhythm is the circadian rhythm. This is an endogenous 24-hour rhythm that can be driven and altered by sleep-wake or dark-light 24-hour (diurnal) cycles. Hormone levels fluctuate predictably during these cycles. For example, cortisol rises early in the day, declines toward evening, and rises again toward the end of sleep to peak by morning (Fig. 48-5). GH, thyroid-stimulating hormone (TSH), and prolactin secretions peak during sleep.

The menstrual cycle is an example of a body rhythm that is longer than 24 hours *(ultradian)*. These rhythms must be considered when interpreting laboratory results for hormone levels. (See diagnostic studies section in this chapter and Chapter 51.)

Hypothalamus

Although the pituitary gland has been referred to as the "master gland," most of its functions rely on its interrelationship with the hypothalamus. Two important groups of hormones from the hypothalamus are *releasing* hormones and *inhibiting* hormones. The function of these hormones is to either stimulate the release or inhibit the release of hormones from the anterior pituitary (Table 48-2).

The hypothalamus also contains neurons, which receive input from the CNS, including the brainstem, limbic system, and cerebral cortex. Neurons from the hypothalamus create a circuit to facilitate coordination of the endocrine system and autonomic nervous system (ANS). In addition, the hypothalamus coordinates the expression of complex behavioral responses, such as anger, fear, and pleasure.

Pituitary

The pituitary gland *(hypophysis)* is located in the sella turcica under the hypothalamus at the base of the brain above the sphenoid bone (see Fig. 48-1). The pituitary is connected to the hypothalamus by the infundibular *(hypophyseal)* stalk. This

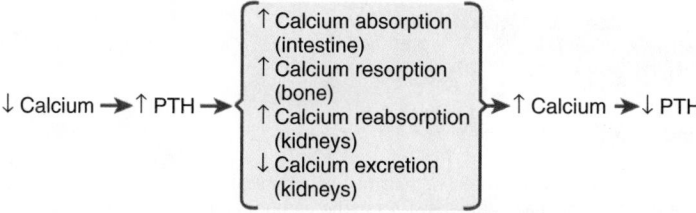

FIG. 48-4 Feedback mechanism between parathyroid hormone *(PTH)* and calcium.

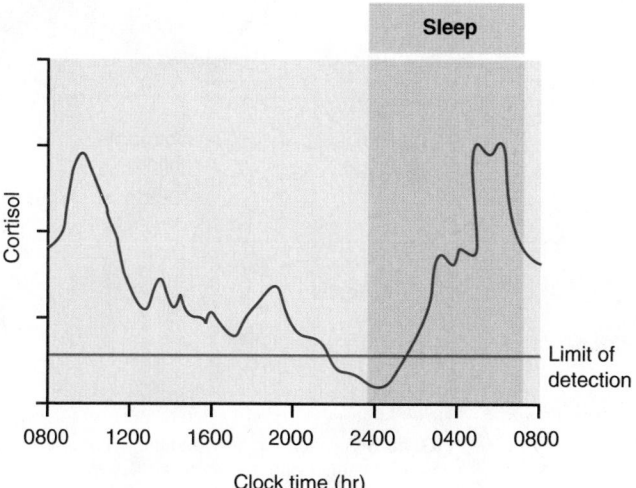

FIG. 48-5 Circadian rhythm of cortisol secretion.

stalk relays information between the hypothalamus and the pituitary. The pituitary consists of two major parts, the anterior lobe *(adenohypophysis)* and the posterior lobe *(neurohypophysis)*. A smaller intermediate lobe produces melanocyte-stimulating hormone.

Anterior Pituitary. The anterior lobe accounts for 80% of the gland by weight and is regulated by the hypothalamus through releasing and inhibiting hormones. These hypothalamic hormones reach the anterior pituitary through a network of capillaries known as the *hypothalamus-hypophyseal portal system.* The releasing and inhibiting hormones in turn affect the secretion of six hormones from the anterior pituitary (Fig. 48-6).

TABLE 48-2	**HORMONES OF THE HYPOTHALAMUS**

The following hormones from the hypothalamus target the anterior pituitary.

Releasing Hormones
- Corticotropin-releasing hormone (CRH)
- Thyrotropin-releasing hormone (TRH)
- Growth hormone–releasing hormone (GHRH), or somatotropin-releasing hormone
- Gonadotropin-releasing hormone (GnRH)
- Prolactin-releasing factor (PRF)

Inhibiting Hormones
- Somatostatin (inhibits growth hormone release)
- Prolactin-inhibiting factor (PIF)

Several hormones secreted by the anterior pituitary are referred to as **tropic hormones.** These are hormones that control the secretion of hormones by other glands. Thyroid-stimulating hormone (TSH) stimulates the thyroid gland to secrete thyroid hormones. Adrenocorticotropic hormone (ACTH) stimulates the adrenal cortex to secrete corticosteroids. Follicle-stimulating hormone (FSH) stimulates secretion of estrogen and the development of ova in women and sperm in men. Luteinizing hormone (LH) stimulates ovulation in women and secretion of sex hormones in both men and women. In men LH is sometimes referred to as interstitial cell–stimulating hormone (ICSH).

Growth hormone (GH) affects the growth and development of all body tissues. It also has numerous biologic actions, including a role in protein, fat, and carbohydrate metabolism. Prolactin stimulates breast development necessary for lactation after childbirth. Prolactin is also referred to as a lactogenic hormone.

Posterior Pituitary. The posterior pituitary is composed of nerve tissue and is essentially an extension of the hypothalamus. Communication between the hypothalamus and posterior pituitary occurs through nerve tracts known as the *median eminence.* The hormones secreted by the posterior pituitary, **antidiuretic hormone (ADH)** and oxytocin, are actually produced in the hypothalamus. These hormones travel down the nerve tracts from the hypothalamus to the posterior pituitary and are stored until their release is triggered by the appropriate stimuli (see Fig. 48-6).

The major physiologic role of ADH (also called arginine vasopressin) is regulation of fluid volume by stimulating

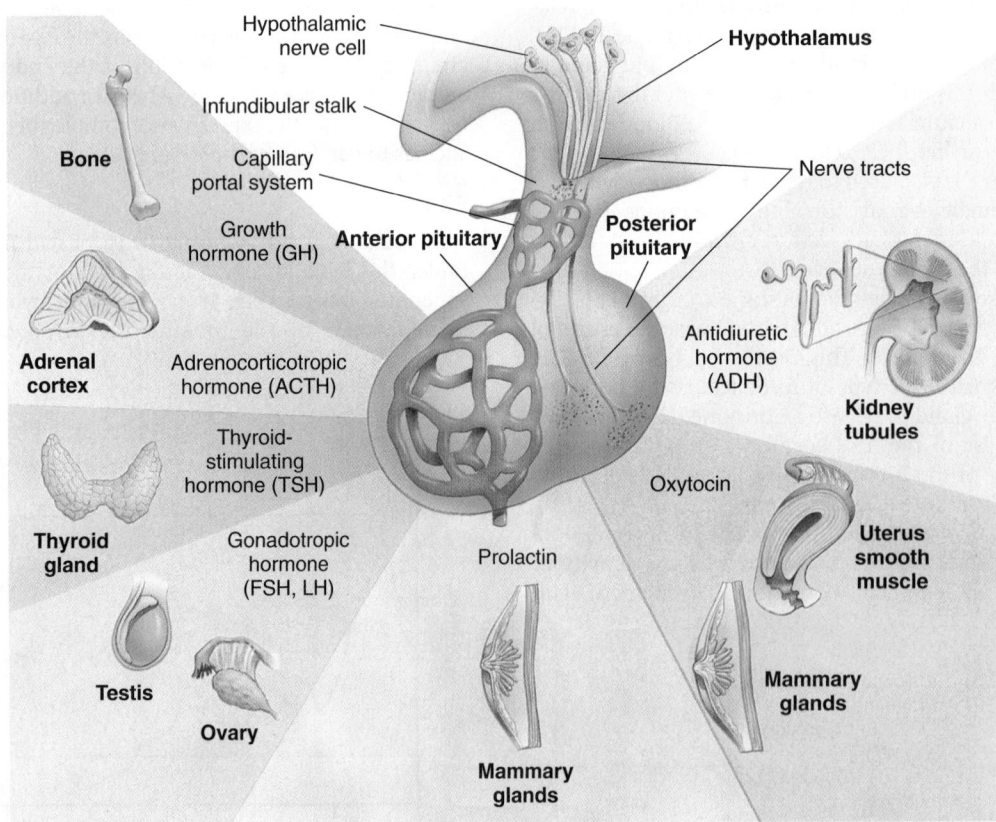

FIG. 48-6 Relationship between the hypothalamus, pituitary, and target organs. The hypothalamus communicates with the anterior pituitary via a capillary system and with the posterior pituitary via nerve tracts. The anterior and posterior pituitary hormones are shown with their target tissues. *FSH,* Follicle-stimulating hormone; *LH,* luteinizing hormone.

FIG. 48-7 Relationship of plasma osmolality to antidiuretic hormone *(ADH)* release and action.

FIG. 48-8 Thyroid and parathyroid glands. Note the surrounding structures.

reabsorption of water in the renal tubules. ADH is also a potent vasoconstrictor. ADH secretion is stimulated by *plasma osmolality* (a measure of solute concentration of circulating blood) and hypovolemia (Fig. 48-7). Plasma osmolality increases when there is a decrease in ECF or an increase in solute concentration. The increased plasma osmolality activates osmoreceptors, which are extremely sensitive, specialized neurons in the hypothalamus. These activated osmoreceptors stimulate ADH release. Volume receptors in large veins, heart atria, and carotid arteries that sense pressure changes also contribute to ADH control. When ADH is released, the renal tubules reabsorb water and the urine becomes more concentrated. When ADH release is inhibited, renal tubules do not reabsorb water, resulting in a more dilute urine excretion.

Oxytocin stimulates ejection of milk into mammary ducts during lactation and contraction of the uterus; it may also affect sperm motility. Oxytocin secretion is increased by stimulation of touch receptors in the nipples of lactating women and vaginal pressure receptors during childbirth.

Pineal Gland

The pineal gland is located in the brain and is composed of photoreceptive cells. The secretion of the hormone melatonin is its primary function. Melatonin secretion is increased in response to exposure to the dark and decreased in response to light. The gland helps to regulate circadian rhythms and the reproductive system at the onset of puberty.

Thyroid Gland

The thyroid gland is located in the anterior portion of the neck in front of the trachea. It consists of two encapsulated lateral lobes connected by a narrow isthmus (Fig. 48-8). The thyroid gland is a highly vascular organ, and its size is regulated by TSH from the anterior pituitary. The three hormones produced and secreted by the thyroid gland are thyroxine (T_4), triiodothyronine (T_3), and calcitonin.

Thyroxine and Triiodothyronine. Thyroxine (T_4) accounts for 90% of thyroid hormone produced by the thyroid gland. However, triiodothyronine (T_3) is much more potent and has greater metabolic effects. About 20% of circulating T_3 is secreted directly by the thyroid gland, and the remainder is obtained by peripheral conversion of T_4. Iodine is necessary for the synthesis of both T_3 and T_4. These two hormones affect metabolic rate, caloric requirements, oxygen consumption, carbohydrate and lipid metabolism, growth and development, brain function, and other nervous system activities. More than 99% of thyroid hormones are bound to plasma proteins, especially thyroxine-binding globulin synthesized by the liver. Only the unbound "free" hormones are biologically active.

Thyroid hormone production and release is stimulated by TSH from the anterior pituitary gland. When circulating levels of thyroid hormone are low, the hypothalamus releases thyrotropin-releasing hormone (TRH), which in turn causes the anterior pituitary to release TSH. High circulating thyroid hormone levels inhibit the secretion of both TRH from the hypothalamus and TSH from the anterior pituitary gland.

Calcitonin. *Calcitonin* is produced by C cells (parafollicular cells) of the thyroid gland in response to high circulating calcium levels. Calcitonin inhibits the transfer of calcium from bone to blood, increases calcium storage in bone, and increases renal excretion of calcium and phosphorus, thereby lowering serum calcium levels. Calcitonin and PTH regulate calcium balance.

Parathyroid Glands

Two pairs of parathyroid glands are usually arranged behind each thyroid lobe (see Fig. 48-8). Although there are usually four glands, their number may range from two to six.

Parathyroid Hormone. The parathyroid glands secrete parathyroid hormone (PTH), also called *parathormone*. Its major role is to regulate the blood level of calcium. PTH acts on bone, the kidneys, and indirectly on the GI tract. PTH stimulates the transfer of calcium from the bone into the blood and inhibits bone formation, resulting in increased serum calcium and phosphate. In the kidney, PTH increases calcium reabsorption and phosphate excretion. In addition, PTH stimulates the renal conversion of vitamin D to its most active form (1,25-dihydroxyvitamin D_3). This active vitamin D promotes absorption of calcium and phosphorus by the GI tract, which ultimately increases bone mineralization. The secretion of PTH is directly regulated by a feedback system. When the serum calcium level is low, PTH secretion increases. When the serum calcium level rises, PTH secretion falls. In addition, high levels of active vitamin D inhibit PTH, and low levels of magnesium stimulate PTH secretion.

FIG. 48-9 The adrenal gland is composed of the adrenal cortex and the adrenal medulla.

Adrenal Glands

The adrenal glands are small, paired, highly vascularized glands located on the upper portion of each kidney. Each gland consists of two parts, the medulla and the cortex (Fig. 48-9). Each part has distinct functions, and the glands act independently from one another.

Adrenal Medulla. The adrenal medulla is the inner part of the gland and consists of sympathetic postganglionic neurons. The medulla secretes the *catecholamines epinephrine* (adrenaline), *norepinephrine* (noradrenaline), and *dopamine*. Catecholamines are synthesized from the amino acid phenylalanine. Catecholamines, usually considered neurotransmitters, are hormones when secreted by the adrenal medulla because they are released into the circulation. They are an essential part of the body's "fight or flight" response to stress (see Chapter 7).

Adrenal Cortex. The adrenal cortex is the outer part of the adrenal gland. It secretes several steroid hormones, including *glucocorticoids, mineralocorticoids,* and *androgens*. Cholesterol is the precursor for steroid hormone synthesis. Glucocorticoids (e.g., cortisol) are named for their effects on glucose metabolism. Mineralocorticoids (e.g., aldosterone) are essential for the maintenance of fluid and electrolyte balance. The term **corticosteroid** refers to hormones synthesized by the adrenal cortex excluding androgens.

Cortisol. Cortisol, the most abundant and potent glucocorticoid, is necessary to maintain life and protect the body from stress. Cortisol is secreted in a diurnal pattern (see Fig. 48-5). The major control of cortisol is through a negative feedback mechanism that involves the secretion of corticotropin-releasing hormone (CRH) from the hypothalamus. CRH stimulates the secretion of ACTH by the anterior pituitary.

One major function of cortisol is the regulation of blood glucose concentration through stimulation of hepatic glucose formation (*gluconeogenesis*). Cortisol decreases peripheral glucose use in the fasting state, inhibits protein synthesis, and stimulates the mobilization of glycerol and free fatty acids. Cortisol also helps maintain vascular integrity and fluid volume through its action on mineralocorticoid receptors. Cortisol levels are increased by stress, burns, infection, fever, acute anxiety, and hypoglycemia.

Glucocorticoids inhibit the inflammatory response and are considered antiinflammatory. Cortisol decreases the inflammatory response by stabilizing the membranes of cellular lysosomes and preventing increased capillary permeability. The lysosomal stabilization reduces the release of proteolytic enzymes and thereby their destructive effects on surrounding tissue. Cortisol can also inhibit production of prostaglandins, thromboxanes, and leukotrienes (see Chapter 12, Fig. 12-2) and alter the cell-mediated immune response.

Aldosterone. Aldosterone is a potent mineralocorticoid that maintains extracellular fluid volume. It acts on the renal tubule to promote renal reabsorption of sodium and excretion of potassium and hydrogen ions. Aldosterone synthesis and secretion are stimulated by angiotensin II, hyponatremia, and hyperkalemia. ANP and hypokalemia inhibit aldosterone synthesis and release.

Adrenal Androgens. The adrenal cortex secretes small amounts of androgens that are converted to sex steroids in peripheral tissues: testosterone in men and estrogen in women. The most common adrenal androgens are dehydroepiandrosterone (DHEA) and androstenedione. In postmenopausal women the major source of estrogen is from the peripheral conversion of adrenal androgen to estrogen. Because they are precursors to other sex steroids, their actions are similar to those of testosterone and estrogen.

Pancreas

The pancreas is a long, tapered, lobular, soft gland located behind the stomach and anterior to the first and second lumbar vertebrae. The pancreas has both exocrine and endocrine functions. The hormone-secreting portion of the pancreas is referred to as the **islets of Langerhans**. The islets account for less than 2% of the gland and consist of four types of hormone-secreting cells: α, β, delta, and F cells. α Cells produce and secrete the hormone glucagon. Insulin and amylin are produced and secreted by β cells. Somatostatin is produced and secreted by the delta cells. Pancreatic polypeptide (PP) is secreted by the F (or PP) cells.

Glucagon. Glucagon is synthesized and released from pancreatic α cells and the gut in response to low levels of blood glucose, protein ingestion, and exercise. Glucagon increases blood glucose by stimulating glycogenolysis, gluconeogenesis, and ketogenesis. Glucagon and insulin function in a reciprocal manner to maintain normal blood glucose levels. In the fasting state, hormones such as catecholamines, cortisol, and glucagon break down stored complex fuels (*catabolism*) to provide glucose as fuel for energy.

Insulin. Insulin is the principal regulator of metabolism and storage of ingested carbohydrates, fats, and proteins. Insulin facilitates glucose transport across cell membranes in most tissues. However, the brain, nerves, lens of the eye, hepatocytes, erythrocytes, and cells in the intestinal mucosa and kidney tubules are not dependent on insulin for glucose uptake. An increased blood glucose level is the major stimulus for insulin synthesis and secretion. Other stimuli to insulin secretion are increased amino acid levels and vagal stimulation. Insulin secretion is usually inhibited by low blood glucose levels, glucagon, somatostatin, hypokalemia, and catecholamines.

A major effect of insulin on glucose metabolism occurs in the liver, where the hormone enhances glucose incorporation into glycogen and triglycerides by altering enzymatic activity and inhibiting gluconeogenesis. After a meal, insulin is responsible for the storage of nutrients (*anabolism*). Another major effect occurs in peripheral tissues, where insulin facilitates glucose transport into cells, transport of amino acids across muscle membranes and their synthesis into protein, and transport of triglycerides into adipose tissue.

GERONTOLOGIC CONSIDERATIONS

EFFECTS OF AGING ON ENDOCRINE SYSTEM

Normal aging has many effects on the endocrine system (Table 48-3). These include (1) decreased hormone production and secretion, (2) altered hormone metabolism and biologic activity, (3) decreased responsiveness of target tissues to hormones, and (4) alterations in circadian rhythms.

Assessment of the effects of aging on the endocrine system may be difficult because the subtle changes of aging may mimic manifestations of endocrine disorders. Endocrine problems may manifest differently in an older adult than in a younger person. Older adults may have multiple co-morbidities and take medications that alter the body's usual response to endocrine

dysfunction. Symptoms of endocrine dysfunction such as fatigue, constipation, or mental impairment are often missed because they are attributed solely to aging. For example, the symptoms of thyroid disease may be attributed to aging, resulting in delayed treatment.

It is important to assess renal function (serum creatinine, blood urea nitrogen [BUN]) in the older adult undergoing diagnostic studies with contrast medium. Older adults with renal dysfunction may be more prone to renal failure with the use of contrast medium.[4]

ASSESSMENT OF ENDOCRINE SYSTEM

Endocrine dysfunction may be the result of hypersecretion or hyposecretion of hormones. The onset of symptoms for specific disorders may be insidious and produce subtle or vague symptoms that are attributed to other physiologic and psychologic causes. Consequently, patients with endocrine dysfunction may be labeled as depressed, malingering, apathetic, or neurotic. In other instances, or in late stages of endocrine dysfunction, the patient may be seen with symptoms that are life threatening and demand immediate intervention.

Subjective Data

Information obtained from the patient can provide important clues as to the functioning of the endocrine system. Obtain a thorough history from the patient or a family member if the patient's mental acuity is compromised (Table 48-4).

Important Health Information

Past Health History. Patients with endocrine disorders often are seen with nonspecific complaints. The chief complaint may relate to not just one but a group of symptoms. The most common presenting problems include fatigue, weakness, menstrual problems, and weight changes. It is important to determine if the onset of symptoms has been gradual or sudden and what the patient has done about them.[5]

Because some of the more general signs of dysfunction are the easiest to overlook, you need to evaluate any reported or observed changes in weight, appetite, skin, libido, mental acuity, emotional stability, or energy levels.

TABLE 48-3 GERONTOLOGIC ASSESSMENT DIFFERENCES

Endocrine System

Changes	Clinical Significance
Thyroid Atrophy of thyroid gland. TSH, T_3, and T_4 secretion are decreased. Increased nodules.	Increased incidence of hypothyroidism with aging. However, most older adults maintain adequate thyroid function. Thyroid hormone replacement dose lower in older adults.
Parathyroid Increased secretion of PTH and increased basal level of PTH.	Increased calcium resorption from bone. Hypercalcemia, hypercalciuria (may reflect defective renal mechanism).
Adrenal Cortex Adrenal cortex becomes more fibrotic and slightly smaller. Decreased metabolism of cortisol. Decreased plasma levels of adrenal androgens and aldosterone.	Decreased metabolic clearance rate for glucocorticoids.
Adrenal Medulla Increased secretion and basal level of norepinephrine. No change in plasma epinephrine levels. Decreased β-adrenergic receptor response to norepinephrine.	Decreased responsiveness to β-adrenergic agonists and receptor blockers. May partly explain increased incidence of hypertension with aging.
Pancreas Increase in fibrosis and fatty deposits in pancreas. Increased glucose intolerance and decreased sensitivity to insulin.	May partly contribute to increased incidence of diabetes mellitus with advanced aging.
Gonads *Women:* Decline in estrogen secretion.	Women experience symptoms associated with menopause and have increased risk for atherosclerosis and osteoporosis.
Men: Decline in testosterone secretion.	Men may or may not experience symptoms.

PTH, Parathyroid hormone; T_3, triiodothyronine; T_4, thyroxine; *TSH,* thyroid-stimulating hormone.

TABLE 48-4   **HEALTH HISTORY**

Endocrine System

Health Perception–Health Management
- What is your usual day like?
- Have you noticed any changes in your ability to perform your usual activities compared with last year? Five yr ago?*

Nutritional-Metabolic
- What is your weight and height?
- How much do you want to weigh?
- Have there been any changes in your appetite or weight?*
- Have you noticed any changes in the distribution of the hair anywhere on your body?*
- Have you noticed any changes in the color of your skin, particularly on your face, neck, hands, or body creases?*
- Has the texture of your skin changed? For example, does it seem thicker and drier than it used to?*
- Have you noticed any difficulty swallowing, throat pain, or hoarseness? Is the top button on your shirt or blouse more difficult to button?*
- Do you feel more nervous than you used to? Do you notice your heart pounding or that you sweat when you do not think you should be sweating?
- Do you have difficulty holding things because of shakiness of your hands?*
- Do you feel that most rooms are too hot or too cold? Do you frequently have to put on a sweater, or feel as though you need to open windows when others in the room seem comfortable?*
- Do you have or have you had any wounds that were slow to heal?*

Elimination
- Do you have to get up at night to urinate? If so, how many times? Do you keep water by your bed at night?
- Have you ever had a kidney stone?*
- Describe your usual bowel pattern. Have you noted any bowel changes?*
- Do you use anything, such as laxatives, to help you move your bowels?*

Activity-Exercise
- What is your usual activity pattern during a typical day?
- Do you have a planned exercise program? If yes, what is it and have you had to make any changes in this routine lately? If so, why and what kinds of changes?
- Do you experience fatigue with or without activity?*
- Have you had any trouble with breathing?*

Sleep-Rest
- How many hours do you sleep at night? Do you feel rested on awakening?
- Are you ever awakened by sweating during the night?*
- Do you have nightmares?*

Cognitive-Perceptual
- How is your memory? Have you noticed any changes?*
- Have you experienced any blurring or double vision?*
- When was your last eye examination?

Self-Perception–Self-Concept
- Have you noticed any changes in your physical appearance or size?*
- Are you concerned about your weight?*
- Do you feel you are able to do what you think you should be capable of doing? If not, why not?
- Does your health problem affect how you feel about yourself?*

Role-Relationship
- Do you have a support system or partner? Are you married? Do you have any children? Do you think you are able to take care of your family and home? If no, why not?
- Where do you work? What kind of work do you do? Are you able to do what is expected of you and what you expect of yourself?
- Are you retired? What type of work did you do before you retired? How do you spend your time now that you've retired?

Sexuality-Reproductive
Women
- When did you start to menstruate? Was this earlier or later than other women in your family?
- When was your last menstrual period? Do you have scant, heavy, or irregular menstrual flows?
- How many children have you had? How much did they weigh at birth? Were you told you had diabetes during any pregnancy?*
- Are you menopausal? If so, for how long?
- Are you attempting to get pregnant but cannot?*
- Are you postmenopausal? If so, do you have any bleeding from your uterus?

Men
- Have you noticed any changes in your ability to have an erection?*
- Are you trying to have children but cannot?*

Coping–Stress Tolerance
- What kind of stressors do you have?
- How do you deal with stress or problems?
- What is your support system? To whom do you turn when you have a problem?

Value-Belief
- Do you think medicine should still be taken even though you feel okay?
- Do any of your prescribed therapies cause any conflict in your value-belief system?*

*If yes, describe.

Medications. Ask about the use of all medications (both prescription and over-the-counter drugs), herbs, and dietary supplements. Ask about the reason for taking the drug, the dosage, and the length of time the drug has been taken. In particular, ask about the use of hormone replacements. Knowing that the patient is currently taking hormone replacements such as insulin, thyroid hormone, or corticosteroids (e.g., prednisone) alerts you to possible problems associated with the use of these agents (e.g., corticosteroids may cause increased blood glucose levels and bone loss with long-term use). The side and adverse effects of many nonhormone medications can contribute to problems affecting endocrine function (e.g., many drugs can affect blood glucose levels) (see eTable 49-1).

Surgery or Other Treatments. Inquire about past medical, surgical, and obstetric history, including number of pregnancies and live births. Ask about traumatic events, birth weight, growth patterns, and stages of physical and emotional development. The depth of information required may vary depending on the presenting condition. For example, data regarding past radiation therapy to the head and neck are especially important when thyroid or pituitary dysfunction is suspected.

Functional Health Patterns. Key questions to ask the patient with an endocrine problem are summarized in Table 48-4.

Health Perception–Health Management Pattern. Ask patients what their usual day is like and how they view their general health. Inquire as to how their perceptions compare to their health a year ago. Ask if their health-related concerns are preventing them from completing things they would like to accomplish.

GENETIC RISK ALERT

Pituitary
- Nephrogenic diabetes insipidus can be inherited as a sex-linked or autosomal disorder.

Thyroid
- Genetics has a role in many cases of hypothyroid and hyperthyroid disorders.
  - Hashimoto's thyroiditis, the most common cause of hypothyroidism, is a chronic autoimmune disorder that has a genetic basis.
  - Graves' disease, a cause of hyperthyroidism, is an autoimmune disease in which genetic factors are involved.

Multiple Endocrine Neoplasia
- Multiple endocrine neoplasia is when two or more different endocrine tumors occur in a person and there is evidence for either a causative mutation or genetic transmission.
- The features of this disorder are relatively consistent within any one family.
- A common endocrine tumor is medullary thyroid carcinoma.
- Some people with this disorder also develop pheochromocytoma.

Diabetes Mellitus
- Genetics has a strong role in the development of type 2 diabetes, and to a lesser extent in type 1 diabetes.

Heredity often plays an important role in the development of endocrine dysfunction. Ask about the occurrence of diabetes mellitus, thyroid disease, and endocrine gland cancers, since these conditions have a familial tendency. A genetic assessment of family members may be appropriate.[5]

Nutritional-Metabolic Pattern. Reported changes in appetite and weight can indicate endocrine dysfunction. Weight loss with increased appetite may indicate hyperthyroidism or diabetes mellitus. Weight gain may indicate hypothyroidism or hypocortisolism. Truncal obesity, purple abdominal striae, and thin extremities occur in patients with hypercortisolism. Obese individuals are more likely to develop type 2 diabetes.

Ask if there have been problems with nausea, vomiting, or diarrhea. Difficulty swallowing or a change in neck size may indicate an enlarged thyroid gland. Increased SNS activity, including nervousness, palpitations, sweating, and tremors, may indicate thyroid dysfunction or a rare tumor of the adrenal medulla *(pheochromocytoma)*. Heat or cold intolerance may indicate hyperthyroidism or hypothyroidism, respectively.

Also ask about changes in the patient's skin, particularly on the face, neck, hands, or body creases. Ask if the patient has noticed any change in the distribution of hair anywhere on the body. Changes in the texture of the skin and whether it seems thicker or drier may indicate endocrine dysfunction. Hair loss can indicate hypopituitarism, hypothyroidism, hyperthyroidism, hypoparathyroidism, or increased testosterone and other androgens. Increased body hair may indicate hypercortisolism. Decreased skin pigmentation can occur in hypopituitarism, hypothyroidism, and hypoparathyroidism, whereas increased skin pigmentation, particularly in sun-exposed areas, can indicate hypocortisolism. A patient with hypothyroidism or excess GH may have skin that feels coarse or leathery. A patient with hyperthyroidism may mention fine, silky hair.

Elimination Pattern. Because maintenance of fluid balance is a major role of the endocrine system, questions related to elimination patterns may uncover endocrine dysfunction. For example, increased thirst and urination can indicate diabetes mellitus (pancreas disorder) or diabetes insipidus (pituitary disorder). Ask about the frequency and consistency of bowel

movements. Frequent defecation may indicate hyperthyroidism or autonomic neuropathy of diabetes mellitus. Constipation is also seen in patients with hypothyroidism, hypoparathyroidism, and hypopituitarism.

Activity-Exercise Pattern. Ask about the usual pattern of activity during a typical day and if the patient has had to make any changes in that activity. Inquire how his or her energy levels compared with past levels. Ask if the patient experiences fatigue with or without activity or if he or she has excessive levels of energy on a daily basis.

Sleep-Rest Pattern. Ask the patient how many hours he or she typically sleeps, and if he or she feels rested on awakening.

Inquire if anything prevents the patient from staying asleep such as nocturia (excessive urination at night), which may indicate diabetes. The patient with type 1 diabetes mellitus on a tight glucose control regimen who complains of sweating or nightmares may be experiencing hypoglycemia. Ask the patient about snoring, which could indicate sleep apnea; this is especially common in men with diabetes mellitus.

Cognitive-Perceptual Pattern. A patient with an endocrine dysfunction may manifest apathy or depression. Question both the patient and family to determine if any cognitive changes are present. Memory deficits and an inability to concentrate are common in endocrine disorders. Visual changes such as blurring or double vision could indicate endocrine problems. Headaches may indicate abnormal pituitary growth.

Self-Perception–Self-Concept Pattern. Endocrine disorders may affect the patient's self-perception because of the associated changes in physical appearance. Determine changes in weight, size of hands and facial features, and level of fatigue. The chronic nature of endocrine disorders and lifelong need for therapy can affect the patient's self-perception. Ask patients to describe how the present illness affects how they feel about themselves.

Role-Relationship Pattern. Ask whether there have been any changes in the patient's ability to maintain roles at home, at work, or in the community. Often the patient with an endocrine disorder is unable to sustain life's roles. However, in most cases the patient can be advised that, with adequate management, previous roles can be resumed. This can be reassuring for the patient and family.

Sexuality-Reproductive Pattern. Document the development of abnormal secondary sex characteristics such as facial hair (*hirsutism*) in women. Ask a detailed history of menstruation and pregnancy. Menstrual dysfunction may be seen in disorders of the ovaries and pituitary, thyroid, and adrenal glands. A history of large-birth-weight babies may indicate gestational diabetes, which may put the patient at a higher risk of developing diabetes mellitus. The inability to lactate may indicate a pituitary disorder.

Male sexual dysfunction may take the form of impotence, decreased libido, infertility, or the lack of development of secondary sexual characteristics. Retrograde ejaculation can occur in diabetes mellitus.

Coping–Stress Tolerance Pattern. Because some endocrine conditions are exacerbated by stress, ask patients about their level of stress and usual coping patterns. Patients' perception of the impact of their condition and treatments on their lifestyle is very important.

Value-Belief Pattern. Determining a patient's ability to make lifestyle changes is an important nursing function. Identify the patient's value-belief patterns so you can help to determine appropriate treatment regimens. This is particularly important in a condition such as diabetes mellitus, which may require major lifestyle changes. Other disorders, such as hypothyroidism or hypocortisolism, may be managed with medications but require lifelong monitoring with the health care provider.

Objective Data

Most endocrine glands (with the exception of the thyroid and testes) are inaccessible to direct examination. Assessment can be accomplished using objective data, including physical examination and diagnostic tests. It is imperative that you understand the actions of hormones so that you can assess the function of a gland by monitoring the target tissue.

Physical Examination. Specific clinical findings for the various endocrine problems are discussed in Chapters 49 and 50. Regardless of the type of endocrine dysfunction, the following general examination should be followed.[6]

Take a full set of vital signs at the beginning of the examination. Variations in temperature, tachycardia, bradycardia, hypotension, or hypertension may be seen with a variety of endocrine-related problems.

Assessment of the endocrine system includes a history of growth and development patterns, weight distribution and changes, and comparisons of these factors with normal findings. Body mass index (BMI) is a height-to-weight ratio used to assess nutritional status (see Chapter 41, Fig. 41-2).

Endocrine disorders may cause changes in mental and emotional status. Throughout the examination, assess the patient's orientation, alertness, memory, affect, personality, and anxiety and the appropriateness of his or her behavior.

Integument. Note the color and texture of the skin, hair, and nails. Note the overall skin color as well as pigmentation and possible ecchymosis (bruise). Hyperpigmentation, or "bronzing" of the skin (particularly on knuckles, elbows, knees, genitalia, and palmar creases), is a classic finding in Addison's disease. Palpate the skin for texture and moisture. Examine hair distribution not only on the head but also on the face, trunk, and extremities. Also assess the appearance and texture of the hair. Dull, brittle hair; excessive hair growth; or hair loss may indicate endocrine dysfunction. Assess any wounds and ask how long they have been present.

Head. Inspect the size and contour of the head. Facial features should be symmetric. Hyperreflexia and facial muscle contraction upon percussion of the facial nerve (*Chvostek's sign*) may occur in hypoparathyroidism. Inspect the eyes for position, symmetry, and shape. Large and protruding eyes (exophthalmos) are associated with hyperthyroidism. Assess visual acuity using a Snellen eye chart. Visual field loss may indicate a pituitary tumor. In the mouth, inspect the buccal mucosa, condition of teeth, and tongue size. Note hair distribution on the scalp and face. Hearing loss is common in acromegaly (from excess GH).[7]

Neck. The thyroid gland is not usually visible during inspection. A feature that distinguishes the thyroid from other masses in the neck is its upward movement on swallowing. Inspect the neck while the patient swallows a sip of water. The neck should appear symmetric without lumps or bulging.

If there is no noticeable enlargement of the thyroid gland, perform palpation using either a posterior or anterior approach. Because palpation may trigger the release of thyroid hormones, it should not be attempted by the inexperienced clinician. This is especially true when examining patients with a diagnosis of goiter or hyperthyroidism. Auscultate the lateral lobes of an enlarged thyroid gland with the stethoscope bell to identify a *bruit,* a soft swishing sound that may indicate a goiter or hyperthyroidism.

The thyroid gland is difficult to palpate and requires practice and validation by a more experienced practitioner. For *anterior palpation,* stand in front of the patient, with the patient's neck flexed. Place your thumb horizontally with the upper edge along the lower border of the cricoid cartilage. Then move your thumb over the isthmus as the patient swallows water. Place your fingers laterally to the anterior border of the sternocleidomastoid muscle, and palpate each lateral lobe before and while the patient swallows water.

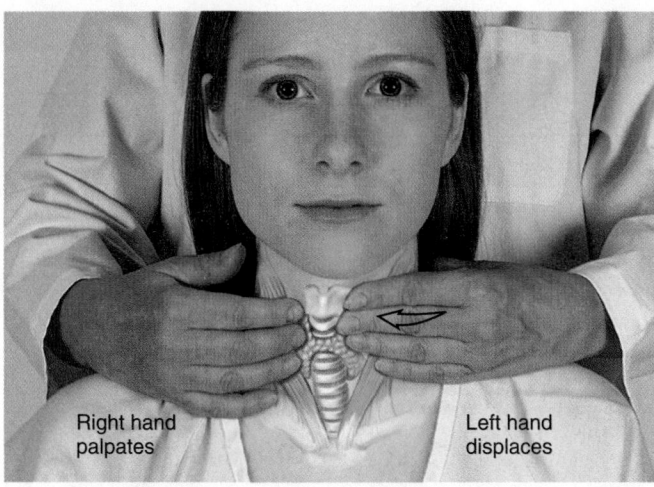

Right hand palpates

Left hand displaces

FIG. 48-10 Posterior palpation of the thyroid gland. (From Jarvis C: *Physical examination and health assessment,* ed 6, St Louis, 2012, Saunders.)

For *posterior palpation,* stand behind the patient (Fig. 48-10). With the thumbs of both hands resting on the nape of the patient's neck, use your index and middle fingers of both hands to feel for the thyroid isthmus and for the anterior surfaces of the lateral lobes. To relax the neck muscles, ask the patient to flex the neck slightly forward and to the right. Displace the thyroid cartilage to the right with your left hand and fingers. Palpate with your right hand after placing the thumb deep and behind the sternocleidomastoid muscle with the index and middle fingers in front of it. Ask the patient to swallow water, and the thyroid will move up.

Repeat this procedure on the left side. Palpate the thyroid for its size, shape, symmetry, and tenderness and for any nodules.

In a normal person, the thyroid is often not palpable. If palpable, it usually feels smooth with a firm consistency, but is not tender with gentle pressure. If nodules, enlargement, asymmetry, or hardness (abnormal findings) are present, refer the patient for further evaluation.

Thorax. Inspect the thorax for shape and characteristics of the skin. Note the presence of breast gynecomastia in men. Auscultate lung sounds and heart sounds, noting any adventitious lung sounds (wheezing, diminished sounds) or extra heart sounds.

FOCUSED ASSESSMENT
Endocrine System

Use this checklist to ensure the key assessment steps have been done.

Subjective
Ask the patient about any of the following and note responses.

Excessive or increased thirst	Y	N
Excessive or decreased urination	Y	N
Excessive hunger	Y	N
Intolerance to heat or cold	Y	N
Excessive sweating	Y	N
Recent weight gain or loss	Y	N

Objective: Diagnostic
Check the following laboratory results for critical values.

Potassium	✓
Glucose	✓
Sodium	✓
Glycosylated hemoglobin (Hb A1C)	✓
Thyroid studies: TSH, T_3, T_4	✓

Objective: Physical Examination
Inspect/Measure

Body temperature	✓
Height and weight	✓
Alertness and emotional state	✓
Skin for changes in color and texture	✓
Hair for changes in color, texture, and distribution	✓

Auscultate

Heart rate, blood pressure	✓

Palpate

Extremities for edema	✓
Skin for texture and temperature	✓
Neck for thyroid size, shape	✓

T_3, Triiodothyronine; T_4, thyroxine; *TSH,* thyroid-stimulating hormone.

Abdomen. Inspect the contour of the abdomen and note the symmetry and color. Cushing syndrome (hypercortisolism) causes the skin to be fragile, resulting in purple-blue striae across the abdomen. Note general obesity or truncal obesity. Auscultate bowel sounds.

Extremities. Assess the size, shape, symmetry, and general proportion of hands and feet. Inspect the skin for changes in pigmentation, lesions, and edema. Evaluate muscle strength and deep tendon reflexes. In the upper extremities, assess for tremors by placing a piece of paper on the outstretched fingers, palm down. Muscular spasms of the hand elicited on application of an occlusive blood pressure cuff for 3 minutes *(Trousseau's sign)* may be noted in hypoparathyroidism.

Genitalia. Inspect the hair distribution pattern, since it may be altered with hormone irregularities. Normally the shape of pubic hair is a diamond in men and an inverted triangle in women.[6] In men, palpate the testes. In women, note any clitoral enlargement.

Assessment abnormalities related to the endocrine system are presented in Table 48-5. A focused assessment of the endocrine system is presented on in the box above.

DIAGNOSTIC STUDIES OF ENDOCRINE SYSTEM

Diagnostic studies of the endocrine system are presented in Table 48-6. The selection of diagnostic studies is guided by

Text continued on p. 1151

CASE STUDY—cont'd
Objective Data: Physical Examination

iStockphoto/Thinkstock

A focused assessment of L.M. reveals the following:

L.M. is sitting on the edge of the examination table. She appears somewhat anxious. Her BP is 190/80, heart rate 84, respiratory rate 20, temp 37° C. Her weight is 182 lb, and she is 5 ft, 3 in tall. L.M.'s face is reddened and puffy, and she appears to have a lump on the back of her neck and shoulders. She has some acne on her face, along with some hair growth on her upper lip and chin area. Her abdomen is protruding but her arms and legs are thin. She has +1 edema in her ankles bilaterally. There are several ecchymotic areas on her upper and lower extremities, as well as purple stretch marks on her abdomen.

As you continue to read this chapter, consider diagnostic studies you would anticipate being performed for L.M.

TABLE 48-5   ASSESSMENT ABNORMALITIES

Endocrine System

Finding	Description	Possible Etiology and Significance
Integument		
Hyperpigmentation	Darkening of the skin, particularly in creases and skinfolds	Addison's disease caused by increased secretion of melanocyte-stimulating hormone; acanthosis nigricans
Depigmentation (vitiligo)	Patchy areas of light skin	May be a marker of autoimmune endocrine disorders
Striae	Purplish red marks below the skin surface. Usually seen on abdomen, breasts, and buttocks	Cushing syndrome
Changes in skin texture	Thick, cold, dry skin	Hypothyroidism
	Thick, leathery, oily skin	Growth hormone excess (acromegaly)
	Warm, smooth, moist skin	Hyperthyroidism
Changes in hair distribution	Hair loss	Hypothyroidism, hyperthyroidism, decreased pituitary secretion
	Diminished axillary and pubic hair	Cortisol deficiency
	Hirsutism (excessive facial hair on women)	Cushing syndrome, prolactinoma (a pituitary tumor)
Skin ulceration	Areas of ulcerated skin, most commonly found on legs and feet	Peripheral neuropathy and peripheral vascular disease, which are contributory factors in the development of diabetic foot ulcers
Edema	Generalized edema	Mucopolysaccharide accumulation in tissue in hypothyroidism
Head and Neck		
Visual changes	Decreased visual acuity and/or decreased peripheral vision	Pituitary gland enlargement or tumor leading to pressure on optic nerve
Exophthalmos	Eyeball protrusion from orbits	Occurs in hyperthyroidism as a result of fluid accumulation in eye and retroorbital tissue
Moon face	Periorbital edema and facial fullness	Cushing syndrome as a result of increased cortisol secretion
Myxedema	Puffiness, periorbital edema, masklike affect	Hydrophilic mucopolysaccharides infiltrating dermis in patients with hypothyroidism
Goiter	Generalized enlargement of thyroid gland	Hyperthyroidism, hypothyroidism, iodine deficiency
Thyroid nodule(s)	Localized enlargement of thyroid gland	May be benign or malignant
Cardiovascular		
Chest pain	Angina caused by increased metabolic demands, effusions	Hyperthyroidism, hypothyroidism
Dysrhythmias	Tachycardia, atrial fibrillation	Hypothyroidism or hyperthyroidism, hypoparathyroidism or hyperparathyroidism, pheochromocytoma
Hypertension	Elevated blood pressure caused by increased metabolic demands and catecholamines	Hyperthyroidism, pheochromocytoma, Cushing syndrome
Musculoskeletal		
Changes in muscular strength or muscle mass	Generalized weakness and/or fatigue	Common symptoms associated with many endocrine problems, including pituitary, thyroid, parathyroid, and adrenal dysfunctions Diabetes mellitus, diabetes insipidus
	Decreased muscle mass	Specifically seen in those with growth hormone deficiency and in Cushing syndrome secondary to protein wasting
Enlargement of bones and cartilage	Coarsening of facial features. Increases in size of hands and feet over a period of several years	Gradual enlargement and thickening of bony tissue occurring with growth hormone excess in adults as seen in acromegaly
Nutrition		
Changes in weight	Weight loss	Hyperthyroidism caused by increases in metabolism, type 1 diabetes mellitus, diabetic ketoacidosis
Altered glucose levels	Weight gain	Hypothyroidism, Cushing syndrome, type 2 diabetes mellitus
	Increased serum glucose	Diabetes mellitus, Cushing syndrome, growth hormone excess
Neurologic		
Lethargy	State of mental sluggishness or somnolence	Hypothyroidism
Tetany	Intermittent involuntary muscle spasms usually involving the extremities	Severe hypocalcemia that can occur with hypoparathyroidism
Seizure	Sudden involuntary contraction of muscles	Consequence of a pituitary tumor
		Fluid and electrolyte imbalance associated with excessive ADH secretion
		Complications of diabetes mellitus, severe hypothyroidism
Increased deep tendon reflexes	Hyperreflexia	Hyperthyroidism, hypoparathyroidism

TABLE 48-5 **ASSESSMENT ABNORMALITIES—cont'd**

Endocrine System

Finding	Description	Possible Etiology and Significance
Gastrointestinal		
Constipation	Passage of infrequent hard stools	Hypothyroidism or calcium imbalances caused by hyperparathyroidism
Reproductive		
Changes in reproductive function	Menstrual irregularities, decreased libido, decreased fertility, impotence	Reproductive function is significantly affected by various endocrine abnormalities, including pituitary hypofunction, growth hormone excess, thyroid dysfunction, and adrenocortical dysfunction
Other		
Polyuria	Excessive urine output	Diabetes mellitus (secondary to hyperglycemia) or diabetes insipidus (associated with decreased ADH)
Polydipsia	Excessive thirst	Extreme water losses in diabetes mellitus (with severe hyperglycemia) and diabetes insipidus, dehydration
Decreased urine output	ADH leading to reabsorption of water from kidney tubules	Syndrome of inappropriate antidiuretic hormone (SIADH)
Thermoregulation	Cold insensitivity	Hypothyroidism caused by a slowing of metabolic processes
	Heat intolerance	Hyperthyroidism caused by excessive metabolism

ADH, Antidiuretic hormone.

TABLE 48-6 **DIAGNOSTIC STUDIES**

Endocrine System

Study	Purpose and Description	Nursing Responsibility
Pituitary Studies *Blood Studies*		
Growth hormone (GH) (somatotropin)	Evaluates GH secretion. Used to identify GH deficiency or GH excess. GH levels are affected by time of day, food intake, and stress. Difficult to interpret significance of isolated GH level. Further evaluation requires stimulation tests (see below). *Men:* <4 ng/mL (<4.0 mcg/L) *Women:* <18 ng/mL (<18 mcg/L) Values >50 ng/mL (>50 mcg/L) suggest acromegaly.	Make sure that patient has been fasting. Emotional and physical stress may alter results. Indicate patient fasting status and recent activity level on the laboratory slip. Send blood sample to laboratory immediately.
Somatomedin C (insulin-like growth factor 1 [IGF-1])	Evaluates GH secretion. Provides a more accurate reflection of mean plasma concentration of GH because it is not subject to circadian rhythm and fluctuations. Low levels indicate GH deficiency. High levels indicate GH excess. *Reference interval:* 135-449 ng/mL	Overnight fasting is preferred but not necessary.
Growth hormone (GH) stimulation	***Insulin tolerance test:*** Regular insulin given IV and blood drawn at −30, 0, 30, 45, 60, and 90 min for measurement of glucose and GH. *Reference interval:* GH >5 mcg/L ***Arginine-GHRH test:*** GHRH bolus followed by 30-min infusion of arginine. *Reference interval:* GH >4.1 mcg/L	Patient must be NPO after midnight. Water is permitted on morning of test. IV access is established for administration of medications and frequent blood sampling. Continually assess for hypoglycemia and hypotension. Keep 50% dextrose and 5% dextrose IV solution at the bedside in case severe hypoglycemia occurs.
Gonadotropins • Follicle-stimulating hormone (FSH) • Luteinizing hormone (LH)	Useful in distinguishing primary gonadal problems from pituitary insufficiency. In women, there are marked differences during menstrual cycle and in postmenopausal period. Levels are low in pituitary insufficiency and high in primary gonadal failure. ***FSH*** *Women:* Follicular phase: 1.37-9.9 mU/mL Ovulatory phase: 6.17-17.2 mU/mL Luteal phase: 1.09-9.2 mU/mL Postmenopause: 19.3-100.6 mU/mL *Men:* 1.42-15.4 mU/mL ***LH*** *Women:* Follicular phase: 1.68-15 IU/L Ovulatory phase: 21.9-56.6 IU/L Postmenopause: 14.2-52.3 IU/L *Men:* 1.24-7.8 IU/L	There is no special preparation of the patient. Only one blood tube is needed for both FSH and LH. Note on the laboratory slip time of menstrual cycle or whether woman is menopausal.

GHRH, Growth hormone–releasing hormone.

Continued

TABLE 48-6   DIAGNOSTIC STUDIES—cont'd

Endocrine System

Study	Purpose and Description	Nursing Responsibility
Pituitary Studies—cont'd **Blood Studies—cont'd**		
Water deprivation (restriction) (ADH stimulation)	Used to differentiate causes of diabetes insipidus (DI), including central DI, nephrogenic DI, and psychogenic polydipsia. ADH (vasopressin) is administered. *Reference interval:* In patients with central DI, urine osmolality increases after ADH. In patients with nephrogenic DI, no or minimal response to ADH.	CAUTION: Patient is NPO for test. Severe dehydration may occur with central or nephrogenic DI during this test. Should be performed only if serum sodium is normal and urine osmolality is <300 mOsm/kg. Obtain baseline weight and urine and plasma osmolality. Assess urine hourly for volume and specific gravity. Send hourly urine samples to laboratory for osmolality determination. Send blood samples for sodium and osmolality every 2 hr. Discontinue test and rehydrate if patient's weight drops >2 kg at any time. Rehydrate with oral fluids. Check orthostatic BP and pulse after rehydration to ensure adequate fluid volume.
Radiologic Studies **Magnetic resonance imaging (MRI)**	Examination of choice for radiologic evaluation of the pituitary gland and hypothalamus. Useful in identifying tumors involving the hypothalamus or pituitary.	Inform patient of the need to lie as still as possible during the test. Explain that tests are painless and noninvasive.
Computed tomography (CT) scan	Used to detect tumor and size of tumor. Oral and/or IV contrast medium may be used.	Inform patient of procedure. Assess renal function before test. Contrast medium may induce renal failure in compromised patients. Patient must lie still during the procedure. If IV contrast is used, check for iodine or shellfish allergy.
Thyroid Studies ***Blood Studies***		
Thyroid-stimulating hormone (TSH) (thyrotropin)	Measures levels of TSH. Considered the most sensitive diagnostic test used for evaluating thyroid dysfunction. *Reference interval:* 0.4-4.2 µU/mL (0.4-4.2 mU/L)	Explain blood draw procedure to the patient. No specific preparations are necessary.
Thyroxine (T_4), total	Measures total serum level of T_4. Useful in evaluating thyroid function and monitoring thyroid therapy. *Reference interval:* 4.6-11.0 mcg/dL (59-142 nmol/L)	See above.
Free thyroxine (FT_4)	Measures active component of total T_4. Because level remains constant, considered better indicator of thyroid function than total T_4. *Reference interval:* 0.8-2.7 ng/dL (10-35 pmol/L)	Instruct patient that FT_4 levels may be measured until symptoms of hyperthyroidism have abated and levels have returned to normal.
Triiodothyronine (T_3), total	Measures serum levels of T_3. Helpful in diagnosing hyperthyroidism if T_4 levels are normal. *Ages 20-50:* 70-204 ng/dL (1.08-3.14 nmol/L) *Ages >50:* 40-181 ng/dL (0.62-2.79 nmol/L)	No specific preparation.
Free triiodothyronine (FT_3)	Measures active component of total T_3. *Reference interval:* 260-480 pg/dL (4.0-7.4 pmol/L)	See above.
T_3 uptake (T_3 resin uptake)	Indirectly measures binding capacity of thyroid-binding globulin. *Reference interval:* 24%-34%	See above.
Thyroid antibodies (Ab) • Thyroid peroxidase (TPO) Ab • Thyroglobulin Ab • Thyroid-stimulating Ab	Measures levels of thyroid antibodies. Assist in the diagnosis of an autoimmune thyroid disease and separate it from other forms of thyroiditis. One or more antibody tests may be ordered depending on symptoms.	See above.
Thyroglobulin	Identifies functioning thyroid tissue or thyroid cancer cells. Primarily used as a tumor marker for patients being treated for thyroid cancer. *Reference interval:* *Men:* 0.5-53 ng/mL *Women:* 0.5-43 ng/mL	See above.
Radiologic Studies **Ultrasound**	Evaluates thyroid nodule(s) to determine if it is a fluid-filled (cystic) or solid tumor and follows change over time.	Explain that gel and a transducer will be used over the neck. The test lasts 15 min. No fasting or sedation required.

ADH, Antidiuretic hormone.

TABLE 48-6 DIAGNOSTIC STUDIES—cont'd

Endocrine System

Study	Purpose and Description	Nursing Responsibility
Thyroid scan and uptake	*Scan:* Used to evaluate nodules of thyroid. Radioactive isotopes are given orally or IV. Scanner passes over thyroid and makes graphic record of radiation emitted. Normal thyroid scan reveals homogeneous pattern with symmetric lobes. Benign nodules appear as warm spots because they take up radionuclide. Malignant tumors appear as cold spots because they tend not to take up radionuclide. *Radioactive iodine uptake (RAIU):* Provides direct measure of thyroid activity. Evaluates function of thyroid nodules. Patient is given radioactive iodine either orally or IV. The uptake by the thyroid gland is measured with a scanner at several time intervals such as 2-4 hr and at 24 hr. The values of RAIU are expressed in percentage of uptake. *Reference interval:* For 2-4 hr, 3%-19% For 24 hr, 11%-30%	Explain procedure to the patient. Reaction to iodine in allergic patients is rare because amount of iodine in preparation is minimal. Instruct patient to drink increased amount of fluids for 24-48 hr unless contraindicated. Radionuclide will be eliminated 6-24 hr.
Parathyroid Studies *Blood Studies* Parathyroid hormone (PTH)	Measures PTH level in serum. Must be interpreted in terms of concomitantly drawn serum calcium level. *Reference interval:* 50-330 pg/mL (50-330 ng/L)	Fasting specimen preferred. Inform patient that blood sample will be drawn. Keep sample on ice.
Calcium (total)	Used to detect bone and parathyroid disorders. Hypercalcemia can indicate primary hyperparathyroidism, and hypocalcemia can indicate hypoparathyroidism. *Reference interval:* 8.6-10.2 mg/dL (2.15-2.55 mmol/L)	See above.
Calcium (ionized)	Free form of calcium unaffected by variable serum albumin levels. *Reference interval:* 4.64-5.28 mg/dL (1.16-1.32 mmol/L)	See above.
Phosphate	Measures inorganic phosphorus. ↑ Levels indicate primary hypoparathyroidism or secondary causes (e.g., renal failure). ↓ Levels indicate hyperparathyroidism. Phosphorus and calcium levels are inversely related. *Reference interval:* 2.4-4.4 mg/dL (0.78-1.42 mmol/L)	See above.
Radiologic Studies Parathyroid scan	Uses radioactive isotopes that are taken up by cells in parathyroid glands to obtain an image of the glands and any abnormally active areas. Assists in identifying the number and location of parathyroid glands.	No food, fluid, or medication restrictions before test.
Adrenal Studies *Blood Studies* Cortisol (total)	Measures amount of total cortisol in serum and evaluates status of adrenal cortex function. *Reference interval:* At 8 AM: 5-23 mcg/dL (138-635 nmol/L) At 4 PM: 3-16 mcg/dL (83-441 nmol/L)	Cortisol has diurnal variation; levels are higher in morning than in evening. Sample should be drawn in morning; evening samples may also be ordered. Note if patient does night shift work. Mark time of blood draw on laboratory slip. Stress and excessive physical activity produce elevated results.
Aldosterone	Used to assess for hyperaldosteronism. *Reference interval:* Upright posture: 7-30 ng/dL (0.19-0.83 nmol/L) Supine position: 3-16 ng/dL (0.08-0.44 nmol/L)	Usually morning blood sample is preferred. Inform patient that the required position, supine or sitting/standing, must be maintained for 2 hr before the specimen is drawn.
Adrenocorticotropic hormone (ACTH) (corticotropin)	Measures plasma level of ACTH. Although ACTH is a pituitary hormone, it controls adrenal cortex secretion, thus helping to determine if underproduction or overproduction of cortisol is caused by dysfunction of the adrenal gland or pituitary gland. *Reference interval:* Morning: <120 pg/mL (<26 pmol/L) Evening: <85 pg/mL (<19 pmol/L)	Patient should be NPO after midnight before morning blood draw between 6-8 AM. Diurnal levels correspond with variation of cortisol levels. Levels are higher in morning, lower in evening. ACTH is unstable; use prechilled blood tube and place on ice and send to laboratory immediately.
ACTH stimulation with cosyntropin	Used to evaluate adrenal function. After baseline cortisol sample is drawn, give cosyntropin (synthetic ACTH) by IV bolus. Cortisol samples are drawn 30 and 60 min after bolus. Plasma cortisol at 60 min should increase by >7 mcg/dL from baseline.	Obtain baseline cortisol level at beginning of cosyntropin infusion. Inject cosyntropin with a plastic syringe and collect blood samples in plastic heparinized tubes. Administer test with continuous-infusion method. Monitor site and rate of IV infusion. Ensure sample collection at appropriate times.

Continued

TABLE 48-6　**DIAGNOSTIC STUDIES—cont'd**

Endocrine System

Study	Purpose and Description	Nursing Responsibility
Adrenal Studies—cont'd		
Blood Studies—cont'd		
ACTH suppression (dexamethasone suppression)	Assesses adrenal function. Especially helpful if hyperactivity (Cushing syndrome) is suspected. *Overnight method:* Dexamethasone (Decadron) 1 mg (low dose) or 4 mg (high dose) is given at 11 PM to suppress secretion of corticotropin-releasing hormone. Plasma cortisol sample is drawn at 8 AM. *Reference interval:* Cortisol level <3 mcg/dL (<0.08 µmol/L) for low dose and <50% of baseline in high dose indicates normal adrenal response.	Ensure that patient has fasted. Inform patient that blood sample will be taken. Observe venipuncture site for bleeding and hematoma formation. Do not test acutely ill patients or those under stress. Stress-stimulated ACTH may override suppression. Screen patient for drugs such as estrogen and corticosteroids that may give false-positive results. Ensure accurate timing of medication and sample collection.
Metanephrine	Screens for pheochromocytoma more accurately than urinary vanillylmandelic acid (VMA) and catecholamine measurements.	Ask about recent history of vigorous exercise, high levels of stress, or starvation (may artificially ↑ levels). Ingestion of caffeine, alcohol, levodopa, lithium, nitroglycerin, acetaminophen, and medications containing epinephrine or norepinephrine can alter test results.
Urine Studies		
17-Ketosteroids	Measures androgen metabolites in urine and evaluates adrenocortical and gonadal function. *Reference interval:* *Men:* 6-20 mg/day (20-70 µmol/day) *Women:* 6-17 mg/day (20-60 µmol/day)	Instruct patient regarding 24-hr urine collection. Tell patient that specimen must be kept refrigerated or iced during entire collection period. Determine whether preservative is required.
Cortisol (free)	Measures free (unbound) cortisol. Preferred test to evaluate hypercortisolism. *Reference interval:* 20-90 mcg/24 hr (55-248 nmol/day)	Instruct patient about 24-hr urine collection and avoidance of stressful situations and excessive physical exercise. Some drugs (e.g., reserpine, diuretics, phenothiazines, insulin, amphetamines) may alter results.
Vanillylmandelic acid (VMA)	Measures urinary excretion of catecholamine metabolite. Levels are increased in pheochromocytoma. *Reference interval:* 1.4-6.5 mg/24 hr (7-33 µmol/day)	Keep 24-hr urine collection at pH <3.0 with HCl acid as preservative. Keep on ice. Consult with laboratory or health care provider about patient discontinuing any drugs 3 days before urine collection.
Radiologic Studies		
Computed tomography (CT)	Abdominal CT is radiologic examination of choice for the adrenal gland. Used to detect tumor and size or metastatic spread. Oral and/or IV contrast medium may be used.	Inform patient of procedure. Patient must lie still during the procedure. Assess renal function if IV contrast is used. Check for iodine or shellfish allergy.
Magnetic resonance imaging (MRI)	Same as MRI above.	Same as MRI above.
Pancreatic Studies		
Blood Studies		
Fasting blood glucose (FBG)	Measures circulating glucose level. *Reference interval:* 70-99 mg/dL (3.9-5.5 mmol/L).	Patient should fast 8-12 hr. Water intake is permitted. Many medications may influence results.
Oral glucose tolerance test (OGTT)	Used to evaluate abnormal FBG levels that do not clearly indicate diabetes. Patient drinks 75 g of glucose; samples for glucose are drawn at baseline and at 30, 60, and 120 min. Test takes 2 hr to complete. *Reference interval:* <100 mg/dL (5.5 mmol/L) at baseline, <200 mg/dL (11.1 mmol/L) at 30 and 60 min, and <140 mg/dL (7.8 mmol/L) at 120 min. Values >200 mg/dL (11.1 mmol/L) at 120 min are considered diagnostic for diabetes mellitus.	Perform test on ambulatory patients after fasting 8-12 hr. Many drugs may influence results, including caffeine and smoking. Ensure that patient's diet 3 days before test includes 150-300 g of carbohydrate with intake of at least 1500 cal/day.
Glycosylated hemoglobin (Hb A1C [A1C])	Indicates the amount of glucose linked to hemoglobin. Assesses long-term glycemic control during previous 3 mo. *Reference interval:* 4.0%-6.0% ADA treatment goal <7%	Inform patient that fasting is not necessary and that blood sample will be drawn. Observe venipuncture site for bleeding or hematoma formation.
Urine Studies		
Glucose	Estimate amount of glucose in urine by using an enzymatic method. Dipstick is dipped into the urine and read for color changes after 1 min. *Reference interval:* Negative	Use freshly voided urine. Many drugs alter glucose readings. Errors are great if directions are not followed exactly.

ADA, American Diabetes Association.

TABLE 48-6 DIAGNOSTIC STUDIES—cont'd

Endocrine System

Study	Purpose and Description	Nursing Responsibility
Ketones	Measures amount of acetone (a type of ketone) excreted in urine as result of incomplete fat metabolism. Tested with a dipstick as described above. Positive result can indicate lack of insulin and diabetic acidosis. *Reference interval:* Negative	Use freshly voided urine specimen. Test is often done with glucose test. Directions must be followed exactly. Certain drugs can produce false-positive or false-negative results.
Radiologic Studies Computed tomography (CT)	Abdominal CT is the radiologic examination of choice for pancreas. Used to identify tumors or cysts. Oral and/or IV contrast medium may be ordered.	Inform patient of procedure. Patient must lie still during the procedure. If IV contrast is used, check for iodine and shellfish allergy. Assess renal function if contrast is used.

ADA, American Diabetes Association; *ADH,* antidiuretic hormone; *GHRH,* growth hormone–releasing hormone.

pertinent findings from the history and physical examination. Laboratory studies may include direct measurement of the hormone level, or they may involve an indirect indication of gland function by evaluating blood or urine components affected by the hormone such as glucose or electrolytes.

Hormones with fairly constant basal levels such as T_4 require a single measurement. Note the time of the sample collection on the laboratory slip. Information about night shift work is important for hormones with circadian or sleep-related secretion (e.g., cortisol). Evaluation of other hormones may require multiple blood samplings such as in suppression tests (e.g., dexamethasone) and stimulation tests (e.g., glucose tolerance). In these situations, it is often necessary to obtain IV access to administer the testing medication and fluids and to draw multiple blood samples.

Disorders associated with the pituitary gland can manifest in a wide variety of ways because of the number of hormones produced. Many diagnostic studies evaluate these hormones either directly or indirectly (see Table 48-6).

A number of tests are available to evaluate thyroid function. The most sensitive and accurate laboratory test is measurement of TSH. Thus it is often recommended as a first diagnostic test for evaluation of thyroid function.[8] Common additional tests ordered in the presence of an abnormal TSH level include total T_4, free T_4, and total T_3. Free T_4 is the unbound thyroxine and is a more accurate reflection of thyroid function than total T_4.

The only hormone secreted by the parathyroid glands is PTH. Because PTH regulates serum calcium and phosphate levels, abnormalities in PTH secretion are reflected in these

CASE STUDY—cont'd

Objective Data: Diagnostic Studies

iStockphoto/Thinkstock

The health care provider orders the following initial diagnostic studies to be drawn in the morning after an 8-hr fast:
- CBC, basic metabolic panel (electrolytes, BUN, creatinine)
- Fasting blood glucose (FBG)
- TSH, free T_4
- Plasma cortisol levels
- Plasma ACTH levels

CBC results reveal a WBC of 12,200/μL and a decreased lymphocyte count at 800 cells/μL. The rest of the CBC is within normal limits (WNL). The FBG is 130 mg/dL. The plasma cortisol and ACTH levels are elevated. Thyroid studies are WNL.

levels. For this reason, diagnostic tests for the parathyroid gland typically include PTH, serum calcium, and serum phosphate levels.

Diagnostic tests associated with the adrenal cortex function focus on the three types of hormones secreted: glucocorticoids, mineralocorticoids, and androgens. These hormone levels can be measured both in blood plasma and in urine. The urine studies often require 24-hour urine collection to eliminate the impact of short-term fluctuations in plasma hormone levels.[9]

The tests found in Table 48-6 are used to evaluate the metabolism of glucose. They are important in the diagnosis and management of diabetes mellitus. (Diagnostic studies for diabetes mellitus are also discussed in Chapter 49.)

BRIDGE TO NCLEX EXAMINATION

The number of the question corresponds to the same-numbered outcome at the beginning of the chapter.

1. A characteristic common to all hormones is that they
   a. circulate in the blood bound to plasma proteins.
   b. influence cellular activity of specific target tissues.
   c. accelerate the metabolic processes of all body cells.
   d. enter a cell to alter the cell's metabolism or gene expression.

2. A patient is receiving radiation therapy for cancer of the kidney. The nurse monitors the patient for signs and symptoms of damage to the
   a. pancreas.
   b. thyroid gland.
   c. adrenal glands.
   d. posterior pituitary gland.

3. A patient has a serum sodium level of 152 mEq/L (152 mmol/L). The normal hormonal response to this situation is
   a. release of ADH.
   b. release of ACTH.
   c. secretion of aldosterone.
   d. secretion of corticotropin-releasing hormone.

4. All cells in the body are believed to have intracellular receptors for
   a. insulin.
   b. glucagon.
   c. growth hormone.
   d. thyroid hormone.

5. When obtaining subjective data from a patient during assessment of the endocrine system, the nurse asks specifically about
   a. energy level.
   b. intake of vitamin C.
   c. employment history.
   d. frequency of sexual intercourse.

6. Endocrine disorders often go unrecognized in the older adult because
   a. symptoms are often attributed to aging.
   b. older adults rarely have identifiable symptoms.
   c. endocrine disorders are relatively rare in the older adult.
   d. older adults usually have subclinical endocrine disorders that minimize symptoms.

7. An abnormal finding by the nurse during an endocrine assessment would be *(select all that apply)*
   a. blood pressure of 100/70 mm Hg.
   b. excessive facial hair on a woman.
   c. soft, formed stool every other day.
   d. 3-lb weight gain over last 6 months.
   e. hyperpigmented coloration in lower legs.

8. A patient has a total serum calcium level of 3 mg/dL (1.5 mEq/L). If this finding reflects hypoparathyroidism, the nurse would expect further diagnostic testing to reveal
   a. decreased serum PTH.
   b. increased serum ACTH.
   c. increased serum glucose.
   d. decreased serum cortisol levels.

1. b, 2. c, 3. a, 4. d, 5. a, 6. a, 7. b, e, 8. a

Ⓔvolve

For rationales to these answers and even more NCLEX review questions, visit *http://evolve.elsevier.com/Lewis/medsurg.*

REFERENCES

1. Huether SE, McCance KL, editors: *Understanding pathophysiology*, ed 5, St Louis, 2013, Mosby.
2. Brashers VL, Heuther SE: Mechanisms of hormonal regulation. In Heuther SE, McCance KL, editors: *Understanding pathophysiology*, ed 5, St Louis, 2013, Mosby.
3. Eliopoulos C: *Gerontological nursing*, ed 7, Philadelphia, 2010, Lippincott Williams & Wilkins.
4. Clark JJ, Wong LL, Lurie F, et al: Proteinuria as a predictor of renal dysfunction in trauma patients receiving intravenous contrast, *Am Surg* 77:1194, 2011.
5. Kirmani S: Molecular genetic testing in endocrinology: a practical guide, *Endocr Pract* 31:1, 2012.
6. Jarvis C: *Physical examination and health assessment*, ed 6, St Louis, 2012, Saunders.
7. Aydin K, Ozturk B, Turkyilmaz MD, et al: Functional and structural evaluation of hearing loss in acromegaly, *Clin Endocrinol* 76:415, 2012.
8. Mitrou P, Raptis SA, Dimitriadis G: Thyroid disease in older people, *Maturitas* 70:5, 2011.
9. Wilson SF, Giddens JF: Health assessment for nursing practice, ed 5, St Louis, 2012, Mosby.

RESOURCES

Resources for this chapter are listed in Chapter 49 on p. 1188 and Chapter 50 on p. 1217.

*What happens is not as important as how
you react to what happens.*
Thaddeus Golas

Nursing Management
Diabetes Mellitus

Janice Lazear

evolve WEBSITE

- NCLEX Review Questions
- Key Points
- Pre-Test
- Answer Guidelines for Case Study on p. 1186
- Rationales for Bridge to NCLEX Examination Questions

- Case Studies
  - Patient With Type 1 Diabetes Mellitus and Diabetic Ketoacidosis
  - Patient With Type 2 Diabetes Mellitus and Hyperosmolar Hyperglycemic Syndrome
- Nursing Care Plans (Customizable)
  - eNCP 49-1: Patient With Diabetes Mellitus
- Concept Map Creator

- Concept Map for Case Study on p. 1186
- Glossary
- Content Updates

eFigure
- eFig. 49-1: Create Your Plate Method

eTable
- eTable 49-1: Effect of Drugs on Blood Glucose Levels

LEARNING OUTCOMES

1. Describe the pathophysiology and clinical manifestations of diabetes mellitus.
2. Differentiate between type 1 and type 2 diabetes mellitus.
3. Describe the collaborative care of the patient with diabetes mellitus.
4. Describe the role of nutrition and exercise in the management of diabetes mellitus.
5. Discuss the nursing management of a patient with newly diagnosed diabetes mellitus.

6. Describe the nursing management of the patient with diabetes mellitus in the ambulatory and home care settings.
7. Relate the pathophysiology of acute and chronic complications of diabetes mellitus to the clinical manifestations.
8. Explain the collaborative care and nursing management of the patient with acute and chronic complications of diabetes mellitus.

KEY TERMS

dawn phenomenon, p. 1163
diabetes mellitus (DM), p. 1153
diabetic ketoacidosis (DKA), p. 1176
diabetic nephropathy, p. 1182
diabetic neuropathy, p. 1182
glycemic index (GI), p. 1166

hyperosmolar hyperglycemic syndrome (HHS), p. 1178
impaired fasting glucose (IFG), p. 1156
impaired glucose tolerance (IGT), p. 1156
insulin resistance, p. 1156

intensive insulin therapy, p. 1158
prediabetes, p. 1156
self-monitoring of blood glucose (SMBG), p. 1167
Somogyi effect, p. 1163

This chapter discusses the pathophysiology, clinical manifestations, complications, and collaborative care of diabetes mellitus. The nurse's role in teaching to promote patient management of diet, activities, and drugs for good control of diabetes is emphasized.

DIABETES MELLITUS

Diabetes mellitus (DM) is a chronic multisystem disease related to abnormal insulin production, impaired insulin uti-lization, or both. Diabetes mellitus is a serious health problem throughout the world, and its prevalence is rapidly increasing. Currently in the United States an estimated 25.8 million people, or 8.3% of the population, have diabetes mellitus, and 79 million more people have prediabetes.[1] Approximately 7 million people with diabetes mellitus have not been diagnosed and are unaware that they have the disease. Diabetes mellitus is the seventh leading cause of death in the United States, but it is likely to be underreported. The annual cost of diabetes exceeds $174 billion, with $116 billion in direct medical costs.[2]

Reviewed by Teressa Sanders Hunter, RN, PhD, Assistant Professor, Langston University, School of Nursing and Health Professions, Langston, Oklahoma; Jane Faith Kapustin, PhD, CRNP, BC-ADM, FAANP, Associate Professor and Assistant Dean for the Master's and DNP Programs and Faculty Practice as Adult NP, Medical Center for Diabetes and Endocrinology, Baltimore, Maryland; Nancy Karnes, RN, MSN, CCRN, CDE, Faculty Nursing Program, Bellevue College, Bellevue, Washington; Lorraine Nowakowski-Grier, MSN, APRN, BC, CDE, Diabetes Nurse Practitioner, Christiana Care Health Services, Newark, Delaware; Susan A. Sandstrom, RN, MSN, BC, CNE, Associate Professor in Nursing (retired), College of Saint Mary, Omaha, Nebraska; and Elaine K. Strouss, RN, MSN, Associate Professor of Nursing, Community College of Beaver County, Monaca, Pennsylvania.

The long-term complications of diabetes make it a devastating disease. Diabetes is the leading cause of adult blindness, end-stage kidney disease, and nontraumatic lower limb amputations. It is also a major contributing factor to heart disease and stroke. Adults with diabetes have heart disease death rates two to four times higher than adults without diabetes. The risk for stroke is also two to four times higher among people with diabetes. In addition, it is estimated that 67% of adults with diabetes have hypertension.[1]

Etiology and Pathophysiology

Current theories link the causes of diabetes, singly or in combination, to genetic, autoimmune, and environmental factors (e.g., virus, obesity). Regardless of its cause, diabetes is primarily a disorder of glucose metabolism related to absent or insufficient insulin supply and/or poor utilization of the insulin that is available.

The American Diabetes Association (ADA) recognizes four different classes of diabetes. The two most common are type 1 and type 2 diabetes mellitus (Table 49-1). The two other classes are gestational diabetes and other specific types of diabetes with various causes.

Normal Insulin Metabolism. Insulin is a hormone produced by the β cells in the islets of Langerhans of the pancreas. Under normal conditions, insulin is continuously released into the bloodstream in small pulsatile increments, with increased release when food is ingested (Fig. 49-1). Insulin lowers blood glucose and facilitates a stable, normal glucose range of approximately 70 to 120 mg/dL (3.9 to 6.66 mmol/L). The average amount of insulin secreted daily by an adult is approximately 40 to 50 U, or 0.6 U/kg of body weight.

Insulin promotes glucose transport from the bloodstream across the cell membrane to the cytoplasm of the cell. The rise in plasma insulin after a meal stimulates storage of glucose as glycogen in liver and muscle, inhibits gluconeogenesis, enhances fat deposition of adipose tissue, and increases protein synthesis. For this reason insulin is an *anabolic*, or storage, hormone. The fall in insulin level during normal overnight fasting facilitates the release of stored glucose from the liver, protein from muscle, and fat from adipose tissue.

Skeletal muscle and adipose tissue have specific receptors for insulin and are considered insulin-dependent tissues. Insulin is required to "unlock" these receptor sites, allowing the transport of glucose into the cells to be used for energy. Other tissues (e.g.,

brain, liver, blood cells) do not directly depend on insulin for glucose transport but require an adequate glucose supply for normal function. Although liver cells are not considered insulin-dependent tissue, insulin receptor sites on the liver facilitate hepatic uptake of glucose and its conversion to glycogen.

Other hormones (glucagon, epinephrine, growth hormone, and cortisol) work to oppose the effects of insulin and are referred to as *counterregulatory hormones*. These hormones increase blood glucose levels by stimulating glucose production and output by the liver and by decreasing the movement of glucose into the cells. The counterregulatory hormones and insulin usually maintain blood glucose levels within the normal range by regulating the release of glucose for energy during food intake and periods of fasting.

TABLE 49-1	COMPARISON OF TYPE 1 AND TYPE 2 DIABETES MELLITUS	
Factor	**Type 1 Diabetes Mellitus**	**Type 2 Diabetes Mellitus**
Age at onset	More common in young people but can occur at any age.	Usually age 35 yr or older but can occur at any age. Incidence is increasing in children.
Type of onset	Signs and symptoms usually abrupt, but disease process may be present for several years.	Insidious, may go undiagnosed for years.
Prevalence	Accounts for 5%-10% of all types of diabetes.	Accounts for 90%-95% of all types of diabetes.
Environmental factors	Virus, toxins.	Obesity, lack of exercise.
Primary defect	Absent or minimal insulin production.	Insulin resistance, decreased insulin production over time, and alterations in production of adipokines.
Islet cell antibodies	Often present at onset.	Absent.
Endogenous insulin	Absent.	Initially increased in response to insulin resistance. Secretion diminishes over time.
Nutritional status	Thin, normal, or obese.	Frequently overweight or obese. May be normal.
Symptoms	Polydipsia, polyuria, polyphagia, fatigue, weight loss.	Frequently none, fatigue, recurrent infections. May also experience polyuria, polydipsia, and polyphagia.
Ketosis	Prone at onset or during insulin deficiency.	Resistant except during infection or stress.
Nutritional therapy	Essential.	Essential.
Insulin	Required for all.	Required for some. Disease is progressive and insulin treatment may need to be added to treatment regimen.
Vascular and neurologic complications	Frequent.	Frequent.

FIG. 49-1 Normal endogenous insulin secretion. In the first hour or two after meals, insulin concentrations rise rapidly in blood and peak at about 1 hour. After meals, insulin concentrations promptly decline toward preprandial values as carbohydrate absorption from the gastrointestinal tract declines. After carbohydrate absorption from the gastrointestinal tract is complete and during the night, insulin concentrations are low and fairly constant, with a slight increase at dawn.

Insulin is synthesized from a precursor, proinsulin. Enzymes split proinsulin to form insulin and C-peptide, and then the two substances are released in equal amounts. Therefore measuring C-peptide in serum and urine is a useful clinical indicator of pancreatic β cell function.

Type 1 Diabetes Mellitus. *Type 1 diabetes mellitus,* formerly known as juvenile-onset diabetes or insulin-dependent diabetes, accounts for approximately 5% of all people with diabetes. Type 1 diabetes generally affects people under 40 years of age, and 40% develop it before 20 years of age. The incidence of type 1 diabetes has increased 3% to 5% over recent decades, and for unknown reasons it is occurring more frequently in younger children.[3]

Etiology and Pathophysiology. Type 1 diabetes is an immune-mediated disease, caused by autoimmune destruction of the pancreatic β cells, the site of insulin production. This eventually results in a total absence of insulin production. Autoantibodies to the islet cells cause a reduction of 80% to 90% of normal function before hyperglycemia and other manifestations occur (Fig. 49-2). A genetic predisposition and exposure to a virus are factors that may contribute to the pathogenesis of immune-related type 1 diabetes.

Genetic Link

Predisposition to type 1 diabetes is related to human leukocyte antigens (HLAs). (See Chapter 14 for a discussion of HLAs and disease associations.) Theoretically, when an individual with certain HLA types is exposed to a viral infection, the β cells of the pancreas are destroyed, either directly or through an auto-immune process. The HLA types associated with an increased risk for type 1 diabetes include HLA-DR3 and HLA-DR4 (see Genetics in Clinical Practice box).

Idiopathic diabetes is a form of type 1 diabetes that is strongly inherited and not related to autoimmunity. It occurs only in a small number of people with type 1 diabetes, most often of Hispanic, African, or Asian ancestry.[3] Latent autoimmune diabetes in adults (LADA), a slowly progressing autoimmune form of type 1 diabetes, usually occurs in people who are over the age of 35 who are not obese.[4]

Type 1 Diabetes Mellitus

Pancreas

- Autoimmune destruction of β cells
- Autoantibodies present for months to years before clinical symptoms
- No production of insulin

Type 2 Diabetes Mellitus

Pancreas

- Defective β cell secretion of insulin
- Insulin resistance stimulates ↑ insulin secretion
- Eventual exhaustion of β cells in many people

Liver

- Excess glucose production
- Inappropriate regulation of glucose production

Adipose tissue

- ↓ Adiponectin and ↑ leptin
- Results in altered glucose and fat metabolism

Muscle

- Defective insulin receptors
- Insulin resistance
- Decreased uptake of glucose by cells resulting in hyperglycemia

FIG. 49-2 Altered mechanisms in type 1 and type 2 diabetes mellitus.

GENETICS IN CLINICAL PRACTICE

Types 1 and 2 Diabetes Mellitus

Type 1 Diabetes Mellitus	Type 2 Diabetes Mellitus	Maturity-Onset Diabetes of the Young (MODY)
Genetic Basis		
• Increased susceptibility (40%-50%) when one has specific human leukocyte antigens (HLA-DR3, HLA-DR4). • Polygenic (>40 genes influence susceptibility).	• Polygenic (>25 genes influence susceptibility).	• Autosomal dominant. • Monogenic (single gene). • Caused by mutations in any of six MODY genes (types 1-6). • Mutations in genes lead to β-cell dysfunction.
Risk to Offspring		
• Risk to offspring of diabetic mothers is 1%-4%. • Risk to offspring of diabetic fathers is 5%-6%. • When one identical twin has type 1 diabetes, the other gets the disease about 30%-40% of the time.	• Risk to offspring is 8%-14%. • When one identical twin gets type 2 diabetes, the other gets it about 60%-75% of the time.	• If one parent has MODY, a child has a 50% chance of developing disease. • If one parent has MODY, a child has a 50% chance of being a carrier.
Clinical Implications		
• Disease is a result of complex interaction of genetic, autoimmune, and environmental factors.	• Disease is a result of complex genetic interactions, which are modified by environmental factors such as body weight and exercise.	• MODY accounts for 1% to 5% of people with diabetes. • Characterized by young age of onset (often before age 25). • Not associated with obesity or hypertension. • Treatment varies depending on the genetic mutation that caused MODY.

Onset of Disease. In type 1 diabetes the islet cell autoantibodies responsible for β-cell destruction are present for months to years before the onset of symptoms. Manifestations of type 1 diabetes develop when the person's pancreas can no longer produce sufficient amounts of insulin to maintain normal glucose. Once this occurs, the onset of symptoms is usually rapid, and patients often are initially seen with impending or actual ketoacidosis. The patient usually has a history of recent and sudden weight loss and the classic symptoms of *polydipsia* (excessive thirst), *polyuria* (frequent urination), and *polyphagia* (excessive hunger).

The individual with type 1 diabetes requires insulin from an outside source *(exogenous insulin)* to sustain life. Without insulin, the patient will develop diabetic ketoacidosis (DKA), a life-threatening condition resulting in metabolic acidosis. Newly diagnosed patients with type 1 diabetes may experience a remission, or "honeymoon period," for 3 to 12 months after treatment is initiated. During this time, the patient requires little injected insulin because β-cell insulin production remains sufficient for glucose control. Eventually, as more β cells are destroyed and blood glucose levels increase, the honeymoon period ends and the patient will require insulin on a permanent basis.

Type 2 Diabetes Mellitus. *Type 2 diabetes mellitus* was formerly known as adult-onset diabetes (AODM) or non–insulin-dependent diabetes (NIDDM). Type 2 diabetes mellitus is, by far, the most prevalent type of diabetes, accounting for approximately 90% to 95% of patients with diabetes.[2] Risk factors for developing type 2 diabetes include being overweight or obese, being older, and having a family history of type 2 diabetes. Although the disease is seen less frequently in children, the incidence is increasing due to the increasing prevalence of childhood obesity. Type 2 diabetes is more prevalent in some ethnic populations. African Americans, Asian Americans, Hispanics, Native Hawaiians or other Pacific Islanders, and Native Americans have a higher rate of type 2 diabetes than whites.[4]

Etiology and Pathophysiology. In type 2 diabetes the pancreas usually continues to produce some *endogenous* (self-made) insulin. However, the insulin that is produced is either insufficient for the needs of the body or is poorly used by the tissues, or both. The presence of endogenous insulin is a major distinction between type 1 and type 2 diabetes. (In type 1 diabetes, there is an absence of endogenous insulin.)

Many factors contribute to the development of type 2 diabetes. The most powerful risk factor is obesity, especially abdominal and visceral adiposity.

🧬 Genetic Link

Although the genetics of type 2 diabetes is not yet fully understood, it is likely multiple genes are involved. Genetic mutations that lead to insulin resistance and a higher risk for obesity have been found in many people with type 2 diabetes. Individuals with a first-degree relative with the disease are 10 times more likely to develop type 2 diabetes.

Four major metabolic abnormalities have a role in the development of type 2 diabetes (see Fig. 49-2). The first factor is **insulin resistance,** a condition in which body tissues do not respond to the action of insulin because insulin receptors are unresponsive, are insufficient in number, or both. Most insulin receptors are located on skeletal muscle, fat, and liver cells. When insulin is not properly used, the entry of glucose into the cell is impeded, resulting in hyperglycemia. In the early stages of insulin resistance, the pancreas responds to high blood glucose by producing greater amounts of insulin (if β-cell function is normal). This creates a temporary state of hyperinsulinemia that coexists with hyperglycemia.

A second factor in the development of type 2 diabetes is a marked decrease in the pancreas's ability to produce insulin, as the β cells become fatigued from the compensatory overproduction of insulin or when β-cell mass is lost. The underlying basis for the failure of β cells to adapt is unknown. It may be linked to the adverse effects of chronic hyperglycemia or high circulating free fatty acids.

A third factor is inappropriate glucose production by the liver. Instead of properly regulating the release of glucose in response to blood levels, the liver does so in a haphazard way that does not correspond to the body's needs at the time.

A fourth factor is altered production of hormones and cytokines by adipose tissue *(adipokines)*. Adipokines secreted by adipose tissue appear to play a role in glucose and fat metabolism and are likely to contribute to the pathophysiology of type 2 diabetes.[5] Adipokines are thought to cause chronic inflammation, a factor involved in insulin resistance, type 2 diabetes, and cardiovascular disease (CVD). The two main adipokines believed to affect insulin sensitivity are adiponectin and leptin.

Individuals with *metabolic syndrome* are at an increased risk for the development of type 2 diabetes. Metabolic syndrome has five components: elevated glucose levels, abdominal obesity, elevated blood pressure (BP), high levels of triglycerides, and decreased levels of high-density lipoproteins (HDLs) (see Table 41-10). An individual with three of the five components is considered to have metabolic syndrome.[6] Overweight individuals with metabolic syndrome can prevent or delay the onset of diabetes through a program of weight loss and regular physical activity. (See Chapter 41 for a discussion of metabolic syndrome.)

Onset of Disease. The disease onset in type 2 diabetes is usually gradual. The person may go for many years with undetected hyperglycemia that might produce few, if any, symptoms. Many people are diagnosed on routine laboratory testing or when they undergo treatment for other conditions, and elevated glucose or glycosylated hemoglobin (A1C or Hb A1C [not commonly used]) levels are found.

Prediabetes. Individuals diagnosed with prediabetes are at increased risk for the development of type 2 diabetes. **Prediabetes** is defined as **impaired glucose tolerance (IGT), impaired fasting glucose (IFG),** or both. It is an intermediate stage between normal glucose homeostasis and diabetes where the blood glucose levels are elevated, but not high enough to meet the diagnostic criteria for diabetes. A diagnosis of IGT is made if the 2-hour oral glucose tolerance test (OGTT) values are 140 to 199 mg/dL (7.8 to 11.0 mmol/L).[3] IFG is diagnosed when fasting blood glucose levels are 100 to 125 mg/dL (5.56 to 6.9 mmol/L).

Persons with prediabetes usually do not have symptoms. However, long-term damage to the body, especially the heart and blood vessels, may already be occurring. It is important for you to encourage patients to undergo screening and to provide instruction about managing risk factors for diabetes. Patients with prediabetes can take action to prevent or delay the development of type 2 diabetes. Those with prediabetes should have their blood glucose and A1C tested regularly and monitor for symptoms of diabetes, such as polyuria, polyphagia, and polydipsia. Maintaining a healthy weight, exercising regularly, and eating a healthy diet have all been found to reduce the risk of developing overt diabetes in people with prediabetes.

Gestational Diabetes. *Gestational diabetes* develops during pregnancy and occurs in about 2% to 10% of pregnancies in the United States.[7] Women with gestational diabetes have a higher risk for cesarean delivery, and their babies have increased risk for perinatal death, birth injury, and neonatal complications. Women who are at high risk for gestational diabetes should be screened at the first prenatal visit.[8] Those at high risk include women who are obese, are of advanced maternal age, or have a family history of diabetes. Women with an average risk for gestational diabetes are screened using an OGTT at 24 to 28 weeks of gestation. Most women with gestational diabetes have normal glucose levels within 6 weeks postpartum. Be aware that women with a history of gestational diabetes have a 35% to 60% chance of developing type 2 diabetes within 10 years.[7] Gestational diabetes and management of the pregnant patient with diabetes are specialized areas not covered in detail in this chapter. Consult an obstetric text for more information.

Other Specific Types of Diabetes. Diabetes occurs in some people because of another medical condition or treatment of a medical condition that causes abnormal blood glucose levels. Conditions that may cause diabetes can result from damage to, injury to, interference with, or destruction of the β-cell function in the pancreas. These include Cushing syndrome, hyperthyroidism, recurrent pancreatitis, cystic fibrosis, hemochromatosis, and parenteral nutrition. Commonly used medications that can induce diabetes in some people include corticosteroids (prednisone), thiazides, phenytoin (Dilantin), and atypical antipsychotics (e.g., clozapine [Clozaril]). Diabetes caused by medical conditions or medications can resolve when the underlying condition is treated or the medication discontinued. (Drugs that can alter blood glucose levels are listed in eTable 49-1 available on the website for this chapter.)

Clinical Manifestations

Type 1 Diabetes Mellitus. Because the onset of type 1 diabetes is rapid, the initial manifestations are usually acute. The classic symptoms are *polyuria, polydipsia,* and *polyphagia.* The osmotic effect of glucose produces the manifestations of polydipsia and polyuria. Polyphagia is a consequence of cellular malnourishment when insulin deficiency prevents utilization of glucose for energy. Weight loss may occur because the body cannot get glucose and turns to other energy sources, such as fat and protein. Weakness and fatigue may result because body cells lack needed energy from glucose. Ketoacidosis, a complication most common in those with untreated type 1 diabetes, is associated with additional clinical manifestations and is discussed later in this chapter.

Type 2 Diabetes Mellitus. The clinical manifestations of type 2 diabetes are often nonspecific, although it is possible that an individual with type 2 diabetes will experience some of the classic symptoms associated with type 1 diabetes, including polyuria, polydipsia, and polyphagia. Some of the more common manifestations associated with type 2 diabetes are fatigue, recurrent infections, recurrent vaginal yeast or candidal infections, prolonged wound healing, and visual changes.

Diagnostic Studies

The diagnosis of diabetes mellitus is made through one of the following four methods.

1. A1C of 6.5% or higher.
2. Fasting plasma glucose (FPG) level greater than or equal to 126 mg/dL (7.0 mmol/L). *Fasting* is defined as no caloric intake for at least 8 hours.
3. Two-hour plasma glucose level greater than or equal to 200 mg/dL (11.1 mmol/L) during an OGTT, using a glucose load of 75 g.
4. In a patient with classic symptoms of hyperglycemia (polyuria, polydipsia, unexplained weight loss) or hyperglycemic crisis, a random plasma glucose greater than or equal to 200 mg/dL (11.1 mmol/L).

If a patient is seen with a hyperglycemic crisis or clear symptoms of hyperglycemia (polyuria, polydipsia, polyphagia) with a random plasma glucose greater than or equal to 200 mg/dL, repeat testing is not warranted.[3] Otherwise, criteria 1 through 3 should be confirmed by repeat testing to rule out laboratory error. It is preferable for the repeat test to be the same test used initially. For example, if a random blood glucose test showed an elevated blood glucose, that same test should be used again when the person is retested.

The accuracy of test results depends on adequate patient preparation and attention to the many factors that may influence the test results. For example, factors that can falsely elevate values include recent severe restrictions of dietary carbohydrate, acute illness, medications (e.g., contraceptives, corticosteroids), and restricted activity such as bed rest. A patient with impaired gastrointestinal absorption or one who has recently taken acetaminophen may have false-negative test results.

A1C measures the amount of glycosylated hemoglobin as a percentage of total hemoglobin (e.g., A1C of 6.5% means that 6.5% of the total hemoglobin has glucose attached to it). The amount of hemoglobin that is glycosylated depends on the blood glucose level. When blood glucose levels are elevated over time, the amount of glucose attached to hemoglobin molecules increases. This glucose remains attached to the red blood cell (RBC) for the life of the cell (approximately 120 days). Therefore the A1C test provides a measurement of glycemic control over the previous 2 to 3 months, with increases in the A1C reflecting elevated blood glucose levels. The A1C has several advantages over the FPG, including greater convenience, since fasting is not required.[3] Diseases affecting RBCs (e.g., iron deficiency anemia or sickle cell anemia) can influence the A1C and should be considered when interpreting test results.

A1C results may be reviewed with patients using the same units (mg/dL or mmol/L) that patients see routinely in blood glucose measurements. An *estimated average glucose* (eAG) can be determined from the A1C. The eAG is $28.7 \times A1C - 46.7$, or the eAG may be obtained by using an online calculator at *http://professional.diabetes.org/glucosecalculator.aspx*. For example, an A1C of 8.0% is equivalent to a glucose level of 183 mg/dL.

All patients with diabetes and prediabetes should have their A1C monitored regularly to determine the success of the current treatment plan and make changes in the plan if glycemic goals are not achieved. The ADA identifies an A1C goal for patients with diabetes of less than 7.0%. The American College of Endocrinology recommends an A1C of less than 6.5%. When the A1C is maintained at near-normal levels, the risk for the development of microvascular and macrovascular complications is greatly reduced. For individuals with prediabetes, monitoring the A1C can detect overt diabetes and provide feedback on efforts to prevent diabetes.

Fructosamine can also be used to assess glucose control. Fructosamine is formed by a chemical reaction of glucose with plasma protein. It reflects glucose control in the previous 1 to 3 weeks. Fructosamine levels may show a change in glucose control before A1C does.

Islet cell autoantibody testing is primarily ordered to help distinguish between autoimmune type 1 diabetes and diabetes from other causes. Autoantibodies can develop to one or several of the autoantigens—GAD65, IA-2, or insulin.

Collaborative Care

The goals of diabetes management are to reduce symptoms, promote well-being, prevent acute complications of hyperglycemia, and prevent or delay the onset and progression of long-term complications. These goals are most likely to be met when the patient is able to maintain blood glucose levels as near to normal as possible. Diabetes is a chronic disease that requires daily decisions about food intake, blood glucose testing, medication, and exercise. Patient teaching, which enables the patient to become the most active participant in his or her own care, is essential to achieve glycemic goals. Nutritional therapy, drug therapy, exercise, and self-monitoring of blood glucose are the tools used in the management of diabetes (Table 49-2).

The three major types of glucose-lowering agents (GLAs) used in the treatment of diabetes are insulin, oral agents (OAs), and noninsulin injectable agents. All individuals with type 1 diabetes require insulin. For some people with type 2 diabetes, a regimen of proper nutrition, regular physical activity, and maintenance of desirable body weight is sufficient to attain optimal blood glucose control. However, eventually most people with type 2 diabetes will require medication management because diabetes is a progressive disease.

TABLE 49-2 COLLABORATIVE CARE

Diabetes Mellitus

Diagnostic
- History and physical examination
- Blood tests, including fasting blood glucose, postprandial blood glucose, A1C, fructosamine, lipid profile, blood urea nitrogen and serum creatinine, electrolytes, islet cell autoantibodies
- Urine for complete urinalysis, microalbuminuria, and acetone (if indicated)
- Blood pressure
- ECG (if indicated)
- Funduscopic examination (dilated eye examination)
- Dental examination
- Neurologic examination, including monofilament test for sensation to lower extremities
- Ankle-brachial index (ABI) (if indicated) (see Table 38-3)
- Foot (podiatric) examination
- Monitoring of weight

Collaborative Therapy
- Patient and caregiver teaching and follow-up programs
- Nutritional therapy (see Table 49-8)
- Exercise therapy (see Tables 49-9 and 49-10)
- Self-monitoring of blood glucose (SMBG) (see Table 49-11)
- Drug therapy
  - Insulin (see Fig. 49-3 and Tables 49-3 and 49-4)
  - Oral and noninsulin injectable agents (see Table 49-7)
  - Enteric-coated aspirin (81-162 mg/day)
  - Angiotensin-converting enzyme (ACE) inhibitors (see Table 33-7)
  - Angiotensin II receptor blockers (ARBs) (see Table 33-7)
  - Antihyperlipidemic drugs (see Table 34-5)

Drug Therapy: Insulin

Exogenous (injected) insulin is needed when a patient has inadequate insulin to meet specific metabolic needs. People with type 1 diabetes require exogenous insulin to survive and may need multiple daily injections of insulin (often four or more) or continuous insulin infusion via an insulin pump to adequately control blood glucose levels. People with type 2 diabetes may require exogenous insulin during periods of severe stress such as illness or surgery. In addition, since type 2 diabetes is a progressive disease, over time the combination of nutritional therapy, exercise, OAs, and noninsulin injectable agents may no longer adequately control blood glucose levels. At that point exogenous insulin would be added as a permanent part of the management plan. People with type 2 diabetes may also need up to four injections per day to adequately control their blood glucose levels. Occasionally insulin pumps are used for patients with type 2 diabetes who have not achieved good glycemic control with other therapies.

Types of Insulin. Today only genetically engineered human insulin made in laboratories is used. The insulin is derived from common bacteria (e.g., *Escherichia coli*) or yeast cells using recombinant deoxyribonucleic acid (DNA) technology (see eFig. 14-1 available on the website for Chapter 14). In the past, insulin was extracted from beef and pork pancreas, but their use was associated with high rates of allergic reactions and complications. These forms of insulin are no longer available.

Insulins differ by their onset, peak action, and duration (Fig. 49-3) and are categorized as rapid-acting, short-acting, intermediate-acting, and long-acting insulin (Table 49-3).

Insulin Regimens. Examples of insulin regimens are presented in Table 49-4. The insulin regimen that most closely mimics endogenous insulin production is the basal-bolus regimen, which uses rapid- or short-acting (bolus) insulin before meals and intermediate- or long-acting (basal) background insulin once or twice a day. The basal-bolus regimen is intensive insulin therapy, consisting of multiple daily insulin injections together with frequent self-monitoring of blood

TABLE 49-3 DRUG THERAPY

Types of Insulin

Classification	Examples	Clarity of Solution
Rapid-acting insulin	lispro (Humalog) aspart (NovoLog) glulisine (Apidra)	Clear
Short-acting insulin	regular (Humulin R, Novolin R)	Clear
Intermediate-acting insulin	NPH (Humulin N, Novolin N)	Cloudy
Long-acting insulin	glargine (Lantus) detemir (Levemir)	Clear
Combination therapy (premixed)	NPH/regular 70/30* (Humulin 70/30, Novolin 70/30) NPH/regular 50/50* (Humulin 50/50) lispro protamine/lispro 75/25* (Humalog Mix 75/25) lispro protamine/lispro 50/50* (Humalog Mix 50/50) aspart protamine/aspart 70/30* (NovoLog Mix 70/30)	Cloudy

*These numbers refer to percentages of each type of insulin.

INSULIN PREPARATION	ONSET, PEAK, DURATION	EXAMPLE
Rapid acting lispro (Humalog) aspart (NovoLog) glulisine (Apidra)	*Onset:* 10–30 min *Peak:* 30 min–3 hr *Duration:* 3–5 hr	6 AM — Noon — 6 PM — Midnight — 6 AM
Short acting Regular (Humulin R, Novolin R)	*Onset:* 30 min–1 hr *Peak:* 2–5 hr *Duration:* 5–8 hr	6 AM — Noon — 6 PM — Midnight — 6 AM
Intermediate acting NPH (Humulin N, Novolin N)	*Onset:* 1.5–4 hr *Peak:* 4–12 hr *Duration:* 12–18 hr	6 AM — Noon — 6 PM — Midnight — 6 AM
Long acting glargine (Lantus) detemir (Levemir)	*Onset:* 0.8–4 hr *Peak:* no pronounced peak *Duration:* 24+ hr	0 — 6 hr — 12 hr — 18 hr — 24 hr

FIG. 49-3 Commercially available insulin preparations showing onset, peak, and duration of action. Individual patient responses to each type of insulin are different and affected by many different factors.

TABLE 49-4 DRUG THERAPY

Insulin Regimens

Regimen	Type of Insulin and Frequency	Action Profile	Comments
Once a day Single dose	Intermediate (NPH) *At bedtime*	7 AM Noon 6 PM Midnight 7 AM	One injection should provide nighttime coverage.
	OR Long-acting (glargine [Lantus], detemir [Levemir]) *In AM or at bedtime*	7 AM Noon 6 PM Midnight 7 AM	One injection will last 24 hr with no peaks and less chance for hypoglycemia. Does not cover postprandial blood glucose levels.
Twice a day Split-mixed dose	NPH and regular or rapid (both regular and rapid are shown on the diagram) *Before breakfast and at dinner*	7 AM Noon 6 PM Midnight 7 AM	Two injections provide coverage for 24 hr. Patient must adhere to a set meal plan.
Three times a day Combination of mixed and single dose	NPH and regular or rapid (both regular and rapid are shown on the diagram) *Before breakfast* + Regular or rapid *Before dinner* + NPH *At bedtime*	7 AM Noon 7 PM 9 PM Midnight 7 AM	Three injections provide coverage for 24 hr, particularly during early AM hours. Decreased potential for 2-3 AM hypoglycemia.
Basal-bolus Multiple dose	Regular or rapid (both regular and rapid are shown on the diagram) *Before breakfast, lunch, and dinner* + Long-acting (glargine or detemir) *Once a day* OR Regular or rapid (both regular and rapid are shown on the diagram) *Before breakfast, lunch, and dinner* + NPH *Twice a day*	7 AM Noon 6 PM Midnight 7 AM 7 AM Noon 6 PM Midnight 7 AM	More flexibility is allowed at mealtimes and for amount of food intake. Good postprandial control. Preprandial blood glucose checks and establishing and following individualized algorithms are necessary. Patients with type 1 diabetes require basal insulin to cover 24 hr. Most physiologic approach, except for pump.

————— Rapid-acting (lispro, aspart, glulisine) insulin.

————— Short-acting (regular) insulin.

- - - - - - Intermediate-acting (NPH) or long-acting (glargine, detemir) insulin.

glucose. The goal is to achieve a near-normal glucose level of 70 to 130 mg/dL before meals.

Other, less intense regimens can also give good glucose control for some people. Ideally, the patient and the health care provider should select a regimen together. The criteria for selection are based on the desired and feasible levels of glycemic control and the patient's lifestyle, diet, and activity patterns. If a less intense regimen is not giving the person optimal control, the health care provider should encourage a more intense approach.

Mealtime Insulin (Bolus). To control postprandial blood glucose levels, the timing of rapid- and short-acting insulin in relation to meals is crucial. Rapid-acting synthetic insulin analogs, which include lispro (Humalog), aspart (NovoLog), and glulisine (Apidra), have an onset of action of approximately 15 minutes and should be injected within 15 minutes of mealtime. The rapid-acting analogs most closely mimic natural insulin secretion in response to a meal.

Short-acting regular insulin has an onset of action of 30 to 60 minutes and should be injected 30 to 45 minutes before a meal to ensure that the onset of action coincides with meal absorption. Because timing an injection 30 to 45 minutes before a meal is difficult for people to incorporate into their lifestyles, the flexibility that rapid-acting insulins offer is preferred by those taking insulin with their meals.[9] Short-acting insulin is also more likely to cause hypoglycemia because of a longer duration of action.

Long- or Intermediate-Acting (Basal) Background Insulin. In addition to mealtime insulin, people with type 1 diabetes must also use a long- or intermediate-acting basal (background) insulin to control blood glucose levels in between meals and overnight. Without 24-hour background insulin, people with type 1 diabetes are more prone to developing DKA.

Many people with type 2 diabetes who use oral medications also require insulin to adequately control blood glucose levels. The long-acting insulins, glargine (Lantus) and detemir (Levemir), are often added to the medication regimen. This type of insulin is released steadily and continuously, and for most people do not have a peak of action (see Fig. 49-3). Although they are typically used for once-daily subcutaneous administration, detemir can be given twice daily. Because they lack peak action time, the risk for hypoglycemia from this type of insulin is greatly reduced. Glargine and detemir must not be diluted or mixed with any other insulin or solution in the same syringe. Mealtime insulin may also be added if oral agents and long-acting insulin are not adequate to achieve glycemic goals.

Intermediate-acting insulin (NPH) is also used as a basal insulin. It has a duration of 12 to 18 hours. The disadvantage of NPH is that it has a peak ranging from 4 to 12 hours, which can result in hypoglycemia. NPH is the only basal insulin that can be mixed with short- and rapid-acting insulins. NPH is a cloudy insulin that must be gently agitated before administration.

Combination Insulin Therapy. For those who want to use only one or two injections per day, a short- or rapid-acting insulin is mixed with intermediate-acting insulin in the same syringe. This allows the patient to have both mealtime and basal coverage without having to administer two separate injections. Although this may be more appealing to the patient, most patients achieve better control with basal-bolus therapy. Patients may mix the two types of insulin themselves or may use a commercially premixed formula or pen (see Table 49-3). Premixed formulas offer convenience to patients, who do not have to draw up and mix insulin from two different vials. This is especially helpful to those who lack the visual, manual, or cognitive skills to mix insulin themselves. However, the convenience of these formulas sacrifices the potential for optimal blood glucose control because there is less opportunity for flexible dosing based on need.

Storage of Insulin. As a protein, insulin requires special storage considerations. Heat and freezing alter the insulin molecule. Insulin vials and insulin pens currently in use may be left at room temperature for up to 4 weeks unless the room temperature is higher than 86° F (30° C) or below freezing (less than 32° F [0° C]). Prolonged exposure to direct sunlight should be avoided. A patient who is traveling in hot climates may store insulin in a thermos or cooler to keep it cool (not frozen). Unopened insulin vials and insulin pens should be stored in the refrigerator.

Patients who are traveling or caregivers of patients who are sight impaired or who lack the manual dexterity to fill their own syringes may prefill insulin syringes. Prefilled syringes containing two different insulins are stable for up to 1 week when stored in the refrigerator, whereas syringes containing only one type of insulin are stable up to 30 days.[10]

Syringes should be stored in a vertical position with the needle pointed up to avoid clumping of suspended insulin in the needle. Before injection, gently roll prefilled syringes between the palms 10 to 20 times to warm the insulin and resuspend the particles. Some insulin combinations are not appropriate for prefilling and storage because the mixture can alter the onset, action, and/or peak times of either of the types. Consult a pharmacy reference as needed when mixing and prefilling different types of insulin.

Administration of Insulin. Routine doses of insulin are usually administered by subcutaneous injection. Regular insulin can be given IV when immediate onset of action is desired. Insulin is not taken orally because it is inactivated by gastric juices.

Insulin Injection. The steps in administering a subcutaneous insulin injection are outlined in Table 49-5. Teach this technique to new insulin users and review periodically with long-term users. Never assume that because the patient already uses insulin, he or she knows and practices the correct insulin injection technique. The patient may not have understood prior instructions, or changes in eyesight may result in inaccurate preparation. The patient may not see air bubbles in the syringe or may improperly read the scale on the syringe. The patient receiving mixed insulins in the same syringe needs to learn the proper technique for combining them if commercially prepared premixed insulins are not used (Fig. 49-4).

The speed with which peak serum concentrations are reached varies with the anatomic site for injection. The fastest subcutaneous absorption is from the abdomen, followed by the arm, thigh, and buttock. Although the abdomen is the preferred injection site, other sites are appropriate as well (Fig. 49-5). Caution the patient about injecting into a site that is to be exercised. For example, the patient should not inject insulin into the thigh and then go jogging. Exercise of the injection site, together with the increased body heat and circulation generated by the exercise, may increase the rate of absorption and speed the onset of insulin action.

Teach patients to rotate the injection within one anatomic site, such as the abdomen, for at least 1 week before using a different site, such as the right thigh. This allows for better

TABLE 49-5 PATIENT & CAREGIVER TEACHING GUIDE

Insulin Therapy

Include the following instructions when teaching the patient and caregiver about insulin therapy.

1. Wash hands thoroughly.
2. Always inspect insulin bottle before using it. Make sure that it is the proper type and concentration, expiration date has not passed, and top of bottle is in perfect condition. The insulin (except for NPH) should look clear and colorless. Discard if it appears discolored or if you see particles in the solution.
3. If insulin solutions are cloudy (see Table 49-3), gently roll the insulin bottle between the palms of hands to mix the insulin.
4. Select proper injection site (see Fig. 49-5).
5. Cleanse the skin with soap and water or alcohol.
6. Pinch up the skin, and push the needle straight into the pinched-up area (90-degree angle). If you are very thin or using a 5/16-in needle, you may need to use a 45-degree angle.
7. Push the plunger all the way down, let go of pinched skin, leave needle in place for 5 sec to ensure that all insulin has been injected, and then remove needle.
8. Destroy and dispose of single-use syringe safely.

1 Wash hands.
2 Gently rotate NPH insulin bottle.
3 Wipe off tops of insulin vials with alcohol sponge.
4 Draw back amount of air into the syringe that equals total dose.

5 Inject air equal to NPH dose into NPH vial. Remove syringe from vial.

36 units

36 U Air NPH insulin (cloudy)

6 Inject air equal to regular dose into regular vial.

12 units

12 U Air Regular insulin (clear)

7 Invert regular insulin bottle and withdraw regular insulin dose.

Regular insulin (clear)

Regular insulin 12 units

8 Without adding more air to NPH vial, carefully withdraw NPH dose and add to regular insulin already in syringe.

NPH insulin (cloudy)

NPH insulin
Regular insulin 36 units
48 units (total dose)

FIG. 49-4 Mixing insulins. This step-order process avoids the problem of contaminating regular insulin with intermediate-acting insulin.

insulin absorption. It may be helpful to think of the abdomen as a checkerboard, with each ½-in square representing an injection site. Injections are rotated systematically across the board, with each injection site at least ½ to 1 in away from the previous injection site.

Most commercial insulin is available as U100, indicating that 1 mL contains 100 U of insulin. U100 insulin must be used with a U100-marked syringe. Disposable plastic insulin syringes are available in a variety of sizes, including 1.0, 0.5, and 0.3 mL. The 0.5-mL size may be used for doses of 50 U or less, and the 0.3-mL syringe can be used for doses of 30 U or less. The 0.5- and 0.3-mL syringes are in 1-U increments. This provides more accurate delivery when the dose is an odd number. The 1.0-mL syringe is necessary for patients who require more than 50 U of insulin. The 1.0-mL syringe is in 2-U increments. When patients change from a 0.3- or a 0.5-mL to a 1.0-mL syringe, make them aware of the dose increment difference.

Insulin syringe needles come in the following lengths: 6 mm (¼ in), 8 mm (5/16 in), and 12.7 mm (½ in).[11] Needle gauges also vary among syringes. The needle gauges available are 28, 29, 30, and 31. The higher the gauge number, the smaller the diameter, thus resulting in a more comfortable injection. Only the person using the syringe should recap the needle; never recap a needle used for a patient. The use of an alcohol swab on the site before self-injection is no longer recommended. Routine hygiene such as washing with soap and rinsing with water is adequate. This applies primarily to patient self-injection technique. When injection occurs in a health care facility, policy may dictate site preparation with alcohol to prevent health care–associated infection (HAI). Perform injections at a 45- to 90-degree angle, depending on the thickness of the patient's fat pad.

An insulin pen is a compact portable device loaded with an insulin cartridge that serves the same function as a needle and syringe (Fig. 49-6). Pen needles are available in lengths of 4 mm (5/32 in), 5 mm (3/16 in), 8 mm (5/16 in), and 12.7 mm (½ in) and in three gauges, 29, 31, and 32. Many patients prefer using insulin pens because of greater convenience and flexibility.[12] They are portable and compact, are more discreet than using a vial and syringe, and provide consistent and accurate dosing.

FIG. 49-5 Injection sites for insulin.

For patients with poor vision, the pen is a better option, since they can hear the clicks of the pen as the dose is selected. Insulin pens come packaged with printed instructions, including pictures of the steps to take when using the pen. These instructions are helpful when teaching new users and reviewing technique with current users of a pen.

Insulin Pump. Continuous subcutaneous insulin infusion can be administered using an *insulin pump*, a small battery-operated device that resembles a standard paging device in size

FIG. 49-6 Parts of insulin pen.

 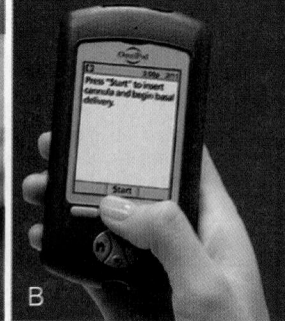

FIG. 49-7 A, OmniPod Insulin Management System. The Pod holds and delivers insulin. **B,** The Personal Diabetes Manager (PDM) wirelessly programs insulin delivery via the Pod. The PDM has a built-in glucose meter. (Courtesy of Insulet Corporation.)

and appearance. Most insulin pumps are worn on the belt or under clothing and loaded with rapid-acting insulin, which is connected via plastic tubing to a catheter inserted into the subcutaneous tissue in the abdominal wall. Insulet Corporation has an insulin pump that is a tubing-free system (Fig. 49-7). All insulin pumps are programmed to deliver a continuous infusion of rapid-acting insulin 24 hours a day, known as the *basal rate.* Basal insulin can be temporarily increased or decreased based on carbohydrate intake, activity changes, or illness. Some individuals require different basal rates at different times of the day.

At mealtime, the user programs the pump to deliver a bolus infusion of insulin appropriate to the amount of carbohydrate ingested and an additional amount, if needed, to bring down high preprandial blood glucose. The insertion site is changed every 2 to 3 days to avoid site infection and to promote good insulin absorption. Insulin pump users must check their blood glucose level at least four times per day. Testing eight times or more per day is common.

A major advantage of the insulin pump is the potential for tight glucose control. This is possible because insulin delivery is similar to the normal physiologic pattern. Pumps offer the benefit of a more normal lifestyle, allowing users more flexibility with meal and activity patterns. Problems and complications of insulin pump therapy are infection at the insertion site, an increased risk for DKA if the insulin infusion is disrupted because of a problem at the infusion site, and the increased cost of the pump and supplies.[13]

Problems With Insulin Therapy. Problems associated with insulin therapy include hypoglycemia, allergic reactions, lipodystrophy, and the Somogyi effect. Hypoglycemia is discussed in detail later in this chapter. (Guidelines for assessing patients treated with insulin and other GLAs are presented in Table 49-6.)

TABLE 49-6	**ASSESSING THE PATIENT TREATED WITH GLUCOSE-LOWERING AGENTS**
Category	**Assessment**
For Patient With Newly Diagnosed Diabetes or for Reevaluation of Drug Regimen	
Cognitive	• Is patient or caregiver able to understand why insulin or OAs are being used as part of diabetes management?
	• Is patient or caregiver able to understand concepts of asepsis, combining insulins, and side effects of medications?
	• Is patient able to remember to take >1 dose/day?
	• Does patient take medications at right times in relation to meals?
Psychomotor	• Is patient or caregiver physically able to prepare and administer accurate doses of the drugs?
Affective	• What emotions and attitudes are patient and caregiver displaying concerning diagnosis of diabetes and insulin or OA treatment?
For Follow-up of GLA-Treated Patient	
Effectiveness of therapy	• Is patient having symptoms of hyperglycemia?
	• Does blood glucose record show good or poor control?
	• Is A1C consistent with glucose records?
Side effects of therapy	• Is atrophy or hypertrophy present at injection sites?
	• Has patient had hypoglycemic episodes? If so, how often? What time of day? What were the symptoms of hypoglycemia?
	• Are there complaints of nightmares, night sweats, or early morning headaches?
	• Has patient had a skin rash or GI upset since taking OAs?
	• Has patient gained or lost weight?
Self-management behaviors	• If patient is having hyperglycemic or hypoglycemic episodes, how are those episodes managed?
	• Has patient analyzed episodes to determine reason for hyperglycemic or hypoglycemic episodes?
	• How much insulin or OA is patient taking and at what time of day? Is patient adjusting insulin dose? Under what circumstances and by how much?
	• Has exercise pattern changed?
	• Is patient adhering to the meal plan? Are meals taken at times corresponding to peak insulin action?

A1C, Glycosylated hemoglobin; *GLA,* glucose-lowering agent; *OA,* oral agent.

Allergic Reactions. Local inflammatory reactions to insulin may occur, such as itching, erythema, and burning around the injection site. Local reactions may be self-limiting within 1 to 3 months or may improve with a low dose of antihistamine. A true insulin allergy is rare. It is manifested by a systemic response with urticaria and possibly anaphylactic shock. Zinc or protamine used as a preservative in the insulin and the latex or rubber stoppers on the vials have been implicated in allergic reactions.

Lipodystrophy. *Lipodystrophy* (atrophy of subcutaneous tissue) may occur if the same injection sites are used frequently. The use of human insulin has significantly reduced the risk for lipodystrophy. *Hypertrophy,* a thickening of the subcutaneous tissue, eventually regresses if the patient does not use the site for at least 6 months. The use of hypertrophied sites may result in erratic insulin absorption.

Somogyi Effect and Dawn Phenomenon. Hyperglycemia in the morning may be due to the Somogyi effect. A high dose of insulin produces a decline in blood glucose levels during the night. As a result, counterregulatory hormones (e.g., glucagon, epinephrine, growth hormone, cortisol) are released, stimulating lipolysis, gluconeogenesis, and glycogenolysis, which in turn produce rebound hyperglycemia. The danger of this effect is that when blood glucose levels are measured in the morning, hyperglycemia is apparent and the patient (or the health care professional) may increase the insulin dose.

If a patient is experiencing morning hyperglycemia, checking blood glucose levels between 2:00 and 4:00 AM for hypoglycemia will help determine if the cause is the Somogyi effect. The patient may report headaches on awakening and recall having night sweats or nightmares. A bedtime snack, a reduction in the dose of insulin, or both can help to prevent the Somogyi effect.

The dawn phenomenon is also characterized by hyperglycemia that is present on awakening. It has been suggested that two counterregulatory hormones, growth hormone and cortisol, excreted in increased amounts in the early morning hours are responsible. The dawn phenomenon affects a majority of people with diabetes and tends to be most severe when growth hormone is at its peak in adolescence and young adulthood.

Careful assessment is required to document the Somogyi effect or dawn phenomenon because the treatment for each differs. The treatment for Somogyi effect is less insulin. The treatment for dawn phenomenon is an increase in insulin or an adjustment in administration time. Your assessment must include insulin dose, injection sites, and variability in the time of meals or insulin administration. Ask the patient to measure and document bedtime, nighttime (between 2:00 and 4:00 AM), and morning fasting blood glucose levels on several occasions. If the predawn levels are less than 60 mg/dL (3.3 mmol/L) and signs and symptoms of hypoglycemia are present, the insulin dosage should be reduced. If the 2:00 to 4:00 AM blood glucose is high, the insulin dosage should be increased. In addition, counsel the patient on appropriate bedtime snacks.

Drug Therapy: Oral and Noninsulin Injectable Agents

OAs and noninsulin injectable agents work to improve the mechanisms by which the body produces and uses insulin and glucose. These drugs work on three defects of type 2 diabetes: (1) insulin resistance, (2) decreased insulin production, and (3) increased hepatic glucose production. These drugs may be used in combination with agents from other classes or with insulin to achieve blood glucose goals. Oral and noninsulin injectable agents are listed in Table 49-7.

Biguanides. The most widely used oral diabetes agent is metformin, the only medication in the biguanide class available in the United States. Forms of metformin include Glucophage (immediate release), Glucophage XR (extended release), Fortamet (extended release), and Riomet (liquid form of metformin). The primary action of metformin is to reduce glucose production by the liver. It also enhances insulin sensitivity at the tissue level and improves glucose transport into the cells. Additionally, it has beneficial effects on plasma lipids.

Metformin is the first-choice drug for most people with type 2 diabetes.[14] Because it may cause moderate weight loss, met-

formin may be useful for people with type 2 diabetes and prediabetes who are overweight or obese. It is also used in the prevention of type 2 diabetes in those with prediabetes who are less than age 60 and have risk factors such as hypertension or a history of gestational diabetes.

Patients who are undergoing surgery or any radiologic procedures that involve the use of a contrast medium are instructed to temporarily discontinue metformin before surgery or the procedure. They should not resume the metformin until 48 hours afterward, once their serum creatinine has been checked and is normal.[10]

DRUG ALERT: Metformin
- Do not use in patients with kidney disease, liver disease, or heart failure. Lactic acidosis is a rare complication of metformin accumulation.
- IV contrast media that contain iodine pose a risk of acute kidney injury, which could exacerbate metformin-induced lactic acidosis.
- To reduce risk of kidney injury, discontinue metformin a day or two before the procedure.
- May be resumed 48 hours after the procedure assuming kidney function is normal.
- Do not use in people who drink excessive amounts of alcohol.

Sulfonylureas. Sulfonylureas include glipizide (Glucotrol, Glucotrol XL), glyburide (Micronase, DiaBeta, Glynase), and glimepiride (Amaryl). The primary action of the sulfonylureas is to increase insulin production by the pancreas. Therefore hypoglycemia is the major side effect with sulfonylureas.

Meglitinides. Like the sulfonylureas, repaglinide (Prandin) and nateglinide (Starlix) increase insulin production by the pancreas. However, because they are more rapidly absorbed and eliminated than sulfonylureas, they are less likely to cause hypoglycemia. When they are taken just before meals, pancreatic insulin production increases during and after the meal, mimicking the normal response to eating. Instruct patients to take meglitinides any time from 30 minutes before each meal right up to the time of the meal. These drugs should not be taken if a meal is skipped.

α-Glucosidase Inhibitors. Also known as "starch blockers," these drugs work by slowing down the absorption of carbohydrate in the small intestine. Acarbose (Precose) and miglitol (Glyset) are the available drugs in this class. Taken with the first bite of each main meal, they are most effective in lowering postprandial blood glucose. Their effectiveness is measured by checking 2-hour postprandial glucose levels.

Thiazolidinediones. Sometimes referred to as "insulin sensitizers," these agents include pioglitazone (Actos) and rosiglitazone (Avandia). They are most effective for people who have insulin resistance. These agents improve insulin sensitivity, transport, and utilization at target tissues. Because they do not increase insulin production, thiazolidinediones do not cause hypoglycemia when used alone. However, these drugs are rarely used today because of their adverse effects. Rosiglitazone is associated with adverse cardiovascular events (e.g., myocardial infarction) and can be obtained only through restricted access programs. Pioglitazone can worsen heart failure and is associated with an increased risk of bladder cancer.

Dipeptidyl Peptidase-4 (DPP-4) Inhibitors. Incretin hormones are released by the intestines throughout the day, but levels increase in response to a meal. When glucose levels are normal or elevated, incretins increase insulin synthesis and release from the pancreas, as well as decrease hepatic glucose production. The incretin hormones are normally inactivated by dipeptidyl peptidase-4 (DPP-4).

TABLE 49-7   DRUG THERAPY

Oral Agents and Noninsulin Injectable Agents

Type	Mechanism of Action	Side Effects
Oral Agents		
Biguanide		
metformin (Glucophage, Glucophage XR, Riomet, Fortamet, Glumetza)	Increases rate of hepatic glucose production; augment glucose uptake by tissues, especially muscles.	Diarrhea, lactic acidosis. Needs to be held 1-2 days before IV contrast media given and for 48 hr after.
Sulfonylureas		
glipizide (Glucotrol, Glucotrol XL)	Stimulate release of insulin from pancreatic islets. Decrease glycogenolysis and gluconeogenesis. Enhance cellular sensitivity to insulin.	Weight gain, hypoglycemia.
glyburide (Micronase, DiaBeta, Glynase PresTab)		
glimepiride (Amaryl)		
Meglitinides		
nateglinide (Starlix)	Stimulate a rapid and short-lived release of insulin from the pancreas.	Weight gain, hypoglycemia.
repaglinide (Prandin)		
α-Glucosidase Inhibitors		
acarbose (Precose)	Delay absorption of glucose from GI tract.	Gas, abdominal pain, diarrhea.
miglitol (Glyset)		
Thiazolidinediones		
pioglitazone (Actos)	Increase glucose uptake in muscle; decrease endogenous glucose production.	Weight gain, edema.
rosiglitazone (Avandia)		*pioglitazone:* increases risk for bladder cancer and exacerbates heart failure.
		rosiglitazone: increases risk for cardiovascular events (e.g., myocardial infarction, stroke).
Dipeptidyl Peptidase-4 (DPP-4) Inhibitors		
linagliptin (Tradjenta)	Enhance activity of incretins, stimulate release of insulin from pancreatic β cells, decrease hepatic glucose production.	Pancreatitis, allergic reactions.
saxagliptin (Onglyza)		
sitagliptin (Januvia)		
alogliptin (Nesina)		
Dopamine Agonist		
bromocriptine (Cycloset)	Activates dopamine receptors in the central nervous system. Unknown how it improves glycemic control.	Orthostatic hypotension.
Combination Therapy		
Glucovance	metformin and glyburide	See side effects for individual drugs.
Metaglip	metformin and glipizide	Same as above.
Avandamet	rosiglitazone and metformin	Same as above.
Duetact	pioglitazone and glimepiride	Same as above.
Actoplus Met, Actoplus Met XR	metformin and pioglitazone	Same as above.
Janumet, Janumet XR	metformin and sitagliptin	Same as above.
Jentadueto	linagliptin and metformin	Same as above.
PrandiMet	metformin and repaglinide	Same as above.
Avandaryl	rosiglitazone and glimepiride	Same as above.
Juvisync	sitagliptin and simvastatin	Same as above.
Kombiglyze	saxagliptin and metformin	Same as above.
Kazano	alogliptin and metformin	Same as above.
Oseni	alogliptin and pioglitazone	Same as above.
Noninsulin Injectable Agents		
Glucagon-Like Peptide-1 (GLP-1) Receptor Agonists*		
exenatide (Byetta)	Stimulate release of insulin, decrease glucagon secretion and gastric emptying; increase satiety.	Nausea, vomiting, hypoglycemia, diarrhea, headache.
exenatide extended-release (Bydureon)		
liraglutide (Victoza)		
Amylin Analog†		
pramlintide (Symlin)	Decreases gastric emptying, glucagon secretion, and endogenous glucose output from liver. Increases satiety.	Hypoglycemia, nausea, vomiting, decreased appetite, headache.

*Administered subcutaneously
†Administered subcutaneously only in abdomen or thigh.

DPP-4 inhibitors (also known as gliptins) include sitagliptin (Januvia), saxagliptin (Onglyza), linagliptin (Tradjenta), and alogliptin (Nesina). DPP-4 inhibitors block the action of the DPP-4 enzyme, which is responsible for inactivating incretin hormones (gastric inhibitory peptide [GIP] and glucagon-like peptide-1 [GLP-1]). The result is an increase in insulin release, decrease in glucagon secretion, and decrease in hepatic glucose production. Since the DPP-4 inhibitors are glucose dependent, they lower the potential for hypoglycemia. The main benefit of these drugs over other medications for diabetes with similar effects is the absence of weight gain as a side effect.

Sodium-Glucose Co-Transporter 2 (SGLT2) Inhibitors. Canagliflozin (Invokana) is the first drug in a new class of drugs known as sodium-glucose co-transporter 2 (SGLT2) inhibitors. It works by blocking the reabsorption of glucose by the kidney, increasing glucose excretion, and lowering blood glucose levels in diabetics.

Dopamine Receptor Agonist. Bromocriptine (Cycloset) is a dopamine receptor agonist that improves glycemic control. The mechanism of action is unknown. Patients with type 2 diabetes are thought to have low levels of dopamine activity in the morning. These low levels of dopamine may interfere with the body's ability to control blood glucose. Bromocriptine increases dopamine receptor activity. It can be used alone or as an add-on to another type 2 diabetes treatment.

Combination Oral Therapy. Many combination drugs are currently available. These drugs combine two different classes of medications to treat diabetes. Examples of these agents are listed in Table 49-7. One advantage of combined therapy is improved patient adherence.

Glucagon-Like Peptide Receptor Agonists. Exenatide (Byetta), exenatide extended-release (Bydureon), and liraglutide (Victoza) simulate GLP-1 (one of the incretin hormones), which is found to be decreased in people with type 2 diabetes. These drugs increase insulin synthesis and release from the pancreas, inhibit glucagon secretion, decrease gastric emptying, and reduce food intake by increasing satiety.

These drugs may be used as monotherapy or adjunct therapy for patients with type 2 diabetes who have not achieved optimal glucose control on OAs. Exenatide and liraglutide are administered using a subcutaneous injection in a prefilled pen. In contrast to exenatide, which is given twice a day, and liraglutide, which is given once daily, Bydureon is given once every 7 days. The delayed gastric emptying that occurs with these medications may affect the absorption of oral medications. Advise patients to take fast-acting oral medications at least 1 hour before injecting exenatide or liraglutide.

DRUG ALERT: Exenatide (Byetta)
• Acute pancreatitis and kidney problems have been associated with its use.

DRUG ALERT: Liraglutide (Victoza)
• Do not use in patients with a personal or family history of medullary thyroid cancer.
• Acute pancreatitis has been associated with its use.

Amylin Analog. Pramlintide (Symlin) is the only available amylin analog. Amylin, a hormone secreted by the β cells of the pancreas in response to food intake, slows gastric emptying, reduces glucagon secretion, and increases satiety.[10] Pramlintide is used in addition to mealtime insulin in patients with type 1 or type 2 diabetes who do not have good glucose control on ideal insulin therapy. It is only used concurrently with insulin and is not a replacement for insulin. Pramlintide is adminis-

tered before major meals subcutaneously into the thigh or abdomen. It cannot be injected into the arm because absorption from this site is too variable. The drug cannot be mixed in the same syringe with insulin.

The concurrent use of pramlintide and insulin increases the risk of severe hypoglycemia during the 3 hours after injection, especially in patients with type 1 diabetes. Instruct patients to eat a meal with at least 250 calories and keep a form of fast-acting glucose on hand in the event that hypoglycemia develops. When pramlintide is used, the bolus dose of insulin should be reduced.

DRUG ALERT: Pramlintide (Symlin)
• Can cause severe hypoglycemia when used with insulin.

Other Drugs Affecting Blood Glucose Levels. Both the patient and the health care provider must be aware of drug interactions that can potentiate hypoglycemic and hyperglycemic effects. For example, β-adrenergic blockers can mask symptoms of hypoglycemia and prolong the hypoglycemic effects of insulin. Thiazide and loop diuretics can potentiate hyperglycemia by inducing potassium loss, although low-dose therapy with a thiazide is usually considered safe. See eTable 49-1 (available on the website) for a list of medications that may influence glycemic control.

Nutritional Therapy

Individualized nutritional therapy, consisting of counseling, education, and ongoing monitoring, is a cornerstone of care for people with diabetes and prediabetes.[15] Adherence to a dietary regimen is challenging for many people. Achieving nutritional goals requires a coordinated team effort that takes into account the person's behavioral, cognitive, socioeconomic, cultural, and religious backgrounds and preferences. Because of these complexities, it is recommended that a dietitian with expertise in diabetes management take the lead. The dietitian should conduct a dietary assessment and develop an individualized food plan. Additional team members may include nurses, certified diabetes educators, clinical nurse specialists, health care providers, and social workers.

Guidelines from the ADA indicate that, within the context of an overall healthy eating plan, a person with diabetes can eat the same foods as a person who does not have diabetes. This means that the same principles of good nutrition that apply to the general population also apply to the person with diabetes. Table 49-8 describes nutritional therapy for patients with diabetes. According to the ADA, the overall goal of nutrition therapy is to assist people with diabetes in making healthy nutritional choices that will lead to improved metabolic control. Additional specific goals include the following:

• Maintain blood glucose levels as near normal as safely possible to prevent or reduce the risk for complications of diabetes.
• Achieve lipid profiles and BP levels that reduce the risk for CVD.
• Prevent or slow the rate of development of chronic complications of diabetes by modifying nutrient intake and lifestyle.
• Address individual nutritional needs while taking into account personal and cultural preferences and respecting the individual's willingness to change eating and dietary habits.
• Maintain the pleasure of eating by allowing as many food choices as appropriate.

TABLE 49-8 NUTRITIONAL THERAPY

Diabetes Mellitus

Component	Recommendations
Total carbohydrate	• Minimum of 130 g/day. • Include carbohydrate from fruits, vegetables, grains, legumes, and low-fat milk. • Monitor by carbohydrate counting, exchange lists, or use of appropriate proportions (eFig. 49-1). • Glycemic index may provide additional benefit. • Sucrose-containing food can be substituted for other carbohydrates in the meal plan. • Fiber intake at 25-30 g/day. • Nonnutritive sweeteners are safe when consumed within FDA daily intake levels.
Protein	• 15%-20% of total calories. • High-protein diets are not recommended for weight loss.
Fat	• Limit saturated fat to <7% of total calories. • *Trans* fat should be minimized. • Dietary cholesterol <200 mg/day. • ≥2 servings of fish per week to provide polyunsaturated fatty acids.
Alcohol	• Limit to moderate amount (maximum 1 drink per day for women and 2 drinks per day for men). • Alcohol should be consumed with food to reduce risk of nocturnal hypoglycemia in those using insulin or insulin secretagogues. • Moderate alcohol consumption has no acute effect on glucose and insulin concentrations, but carbohydrate taken with the alcohol (mixed drink) may raise blood glucose.

Source: American Diabetes Association: Clinical practice recommendations: nutrition recommendations and interventions for diabetes, *Diabetes Care* 31:S61, 2008.

Type 1 Diabetes Mellitus. Meal planning should be based on the individual's usual food intake and preferences and balanced with insulin and exercise patterns. The insulin regimen should be developed with the patient's eating habits and activity pattern in mind. Day-to-day consistency in timing and amount of food eaten is important for those individuals using conventional, fixed insulin regimens. Patients using rapid-acting insulin can adjust the dose before the meal based on the current blood glucose level and the carbohydrate content of the meal. Intensified insulin therapy, such as multiple daily injections or the use of an insulin pump, allows considerable flexibility in food selection and can be adjusted for alterations from usual eating and exercise habits.

Type 2 Diabetes Mellitus. Nutritional therapy in type 2 diabetes should emphasize achieving glucose, lipid, and BP goals. Modest weight loss has been associated with improved insulin resistance. Therefore weight loss is recommended for all individuals with diabetes who are overweight or obese.[15]

No one proven strategy or method can be uniformly recommended. A nutritionally adequate meal plan with appropriate serving sizes, a reduction of saturated and *trans* fats, and low carbohydrates can bring about decreased calorie consumption. Spacing meals is another strategy that spreads nutrient intake throughout the day. A weight loss of 5% to 7% of body weight often improves glycemic control, even if desirable body weight is not achieved. Weight loss is best attempted by a moderate decrease in calories and an increase in caloric expenditure. Regularly exercising and learning new behaviors and attitudes can facilitate long-term lifestyle changes. Monitoring of blood glucose levels, A1C, lipids, and BP provides feedback on how well the goals of nutritional therapy are being met.

Food Composition. The nutrient balance of a diabetic diet is essential to maintain blood glucose levels. Nutritional energy intake should be balanced with the patient's energy output. Each patient's individual meal plan should be constructed with her or his lifestyle and health goals in mind. The following are general recommendations for nutrient balance.

Carbohydrates. Carbohydrates include sugars, starches, and fiber. Carbohydrates provide important sources of energy, fiber, vitamins, and minerals and are therefore important to all people, including those with diabetes. Foods containing carbohydrates from whole grains, fruits, vegetables, and low-fat milk should be included as part of a healthy meal plan. The recommended dietary allowance for carbohydrates is a minimum of 130 g/day.[15]

Glycemic index (GI) is the term used to describe the rise in blood glucose levels after a person has consumed a carbohydrate-containing food. The GI of foods was developed to compare the postprandial responses to carbohydrate-containing foods. Foods with a high GI raise glucose levels faster and higher than foods with a low GI.

GI of 100 refers to the response to 50 g of glucose or white bread in a normal person without diabetes. All other food with an equivalent carbohydrate value is measured against this standard. For example, the GI of an apple is 52, regular milk 27, baked potato 93, cornflake cereal 119, and baked beans 69. An online calculator for GI is available at *www.glycemicindex.com*. The use of GI may provide a modest additional benefit over consideration of total carbohydrates alone.[15]

With all individuals, dietary fiber should be included as part of a healthy meal plan. There is no evidence that a person with diabetes should consume more fiber than an individual who does not have diabetes. The current recommendation for the general population is 25 to 30 g/day.[15]

Nutritive and nonnutritive sweeteners may be included in a healthy meal plan in moderation. Nonnutritive sweeteners include the sugar substitutes saccharine, aspartame, sucralose, neotame, and acesulfame-K.

Fats. Dietary fat provides energy, carries fat-soluble vitamins, and provides essential fatty acids. The ADA recommends limiting saturated fat to less than 7% of total calories. Less than 200 mg/day of cholesterol and limited *trans* fats are also recommended as part of a healthy meal plan. Decreasing fat and cholesterol intake assists in reducing the risk for CVD.

Protein. The amount of daily protein in the diet for people with diabetes and normal renal function is the same as for the general population. The suggested protein intake is 15% to 20% of the total calories consumed. High-protein diets are not recommended as a weight loss method for people with diabetes.

Alcohol. Alcohol inhibits gluconeogenesis (breakdown of glycogen to glucose) by the liver. This can cause severe hypoglycemia in patients on insulin or oral hypoglycemic medications that increase insulin secretion. Encourage patients to honestly discuss their use of alcohol with their health care providers because its use can make blood glucose more difficult to control.

Moderate alcohol consumption can sometimes be safely incorporated into the meal plan if blood glucose levels are well controlled and if the patient is not on medications that will cause adverse effects. Moderate consumption is defined as one drink per day for women and two drinks per day for men. A patient can reduce the risk for alcohol-induced hypoglycemia by eating carbohydrates when drinking alcohol. To decrease the carbohydrate content, recommend using sugar-free mixes and drinking dry, light wines.

Patient Teaching Related to Nutritional Therapy. Most often the dietitian initially teaches the principles of the nutritional therapy regimen. Whenever possible, work with dietitians as part of an interdisciplinary diabetes care team. Some patients who have limited insurance coverage or live in remote areas do not have access to a dietitian. In these cases, you may need to assume responsibility for teaching basic dietary management to patients with diabetes.

Carbohydrate counting is a meal planning technique used to keep track of the amount of carbohydrates eaten with each meal and per day. Often patients are advised to limit carbohydrates to a predetermined number. The amount of total carbohydrates per day depends on previous glycemic control, age, weight, activity level, patient preference, and prescribed medications. A serving size of carbohydrates is 15 g. Patients usually start with 45 to 60 g of carbohydrate per meal. For some patients, insulin regimens are tailored to the number of carbohydrates that a patient will consume at the meal, with a set number of units of insulin given per gram of carbohydrate (e.g., 1 U/15 g carbohydrate, 2 U/25 g carbohydrate). Teach the patient about the foods that contain carbohydrates, how to read food labels, and appropriate serving sizes.

Diabetes exchange lists are another method for meal planning. Instead of counting carbohydrates, the individual is given a meal plan with specific numbers of helpings from a list of exchanges for each meal and snack. The exchanges are starches, fruits, milk, meat, sweets, fats, and free foods. The patient chooses foods from the various exchanges based on the prescribed meal plan. This method may be easier for some patients than carbohydrate counting. Another advantage is that this approach helps the patient limit portion sizes and overall food intake, an important component of weight management.

MyPlate was developed by the U.S. Department of Agriculture (USDA) to represent national nutritional guidelines. This simple method helps the patient visualize the amount of vegetables, starch, and meat that should fill a 9-in plate. For a person with diabetes, each meal needs to have one half of the plate filled with nonstarchy vegetables, one fourth filled with a starch, and one fourth filled with a protein (see eFig. 49-1 available on the website). A glass of nonfat milk and a small piece of fresh fruit complete the meal.[16]

Whenever possible, include family members and caregivers in nutrition education and counseling, particularly the person who cooks for the household. However, the responsibility for maintaining a diabetic diet should not fall to someone other than the person with diabetes. Reliance on another person to make health decisions interferes with the patient's ability to develop self-care skills, which is essential in the management of diabetes. Foster independence, even in patients with visual or cognitive impairment. It is also important to discuss traditional foods with the patient. To improve adherence, the diet needs to be individualized to take into account the patient's preferences and foods that are culturally appropriate.

Exercise

Regular, consistent exercise is an essential part of diabetes and prediabetes management.[17] The ADA recommends that people with diabetes perform at least 150 min/wk (30 minutes, 5 days/

TABLE 49-9	**ACTIVITIES THAT AFFECT CALORIC EXPENDITURE**	
Light Activity (100-200 kcal/hr)	**Moderate Activity (200-350 kcal/hr)**	**Vigorous Activity (400-900 kcal/hr)**
• Driving a car • Fishing • Light housework • Secretarial work • Teaching • Walking casually	• Active housework • Bicycling (light) • Bowling • Dancing • Gardening • Golf • Roller skating • Walking briskly	• Aerobic exercise • Bicycling (vigorous) • Hard labor • Ice skating • Outdoor sports • Running • Soccer • Tennis • Wood chopping

wk) of a moderate-intensity aerobic physical activity (Table 49-9). The ADA also encourages people with type 2 diabetes to perform resistance training three times a week in the absence of contraindications.[18]

Exercise decreases insulin resistance and can have a direct effect on lowering blood glucose levels. It also contributes to weight loss, which further decreases insulin resistance. The therapeutic benefits of regular physical activity may result in a decreased need for diabetes medications to reach target blood glucose goals. Regular exercise may also help reduce triglyceride and low-density lipoprotein (LDL) cholesterol levels, increase high-density lipoprotein (HDL), reduce BP, and improve circulation.[6]

Any new exercise program for diabetic patients should be started only after medical clearance. Patients should start slowly with gradual progression toward the desired goal. Patients who use insulin, sulfonylureas, or meglitinides are at increased risk for hypoglycemia when they increase physical activity, especially if they exercise at the time of peak drug action or eat too little to maintain adequate blood glucose levels. This can also occur if a normally sedentary patient with diabetes has an unusually active day.

The glucose-lowering effects of exercise can last up to 48 hours after the activity, so it is possible for hypoglycemia to occur long after the activity. It is recommended that patients who use medications that can cause hypoglycemia schedule exercise about 1 hour after a meal or that they have a 10- to 15-g carbohydrate snack and check their blood glucose before exercising. They can eat small carbohydrate snacks every 30 minutes during exercise to prevent hypoglycemia. Patients using medications that place them at risk for hypoglycemia should always carry a fast-acting source of carbohydrate, such as glucose tablets or hard candies, when exercising. Table 49-10 describes exercise guidelines for patients with diabetes.

Although exercise is generally beneficial to blood glucose levels, strenuous activity can be perceived by the body as a stress, causing a release of counterregulatory hormones and a temporary elevation of blood glucose. In a person with type 1 diabetes who is hyperglycemic and ketotic, exercise can worsen these conditions. Therefore vigorous activity should be avoided if the blood glucose level is over 250 mg/dL and ketones are present in the urine. If hyperglycemia is present without ketosis, it is not necessary to postpone exercise.[4]

Monitoring Blood Glucose

Self-monitoring of blood glucose (SMBG) is a critical part of diabetes management. By providing a current blood glucose

TABLE 49-10 PATIENT & CAREGIVER TEACHING GUIDE

Exercise for Patients With Diabetes Mellitus

Include the following information in the exercise teaching plan for the patient and caregiver.

1. Exercise does not have to be vigorous to be effective. The blood glucose–reducing effects of exercise can be attained with activity such as brisk walking.
2. The exercises selected should be enjoyable to foster regularity.
3. It is important to have properly fitting footwear.
4. The exercise session should have a warm-up period and a cool-down period. The exercise program should be started gradually and increased slowly.
5. Exercise is best done after meals, when the blood glucose level is rising.
6. Exercise plans should be individualized and monitored by the health care provider.
7. It is important to self-monitor blood glucose levels before, during, and after exercise to determine the effect exercise has on blood glucose level at particular times of the day.
   * *Before exercise, if blood glucose ≤100 mg/dL, eat a 15-g carbohydrate snack. After 15 to 30 min, retest blood glucose levels. Do not exercise if <100 mg/dL.*
   * *Before exercise, if blood glucose ≥250 mg/dL* in a person with type 1 diabetes and ketones are present, avoid vigorous activity.
8. Delayed exercise-induced hypoglycemia may occur several hours after the completion of exercise.
9. Taking a glucose-lowering medication does not mean that planned or spontaneous exercise cannot occur.
10. It is important to compensate for extensive planned and spontaneous activity by monitoring blood glucose levels to make adjustments in the insulin dose (if taken) and food intake.

FIG. 49-8 Blood glucose monitors are used to measure blood glucose levels. Medtronic OneTouch UltraLink glucose meter. (Courtesy of Medtronic Diabetes.)

FIG. 49-9 The MiniMed Paradigm® REAL-Time Revel™ Insulin Pump *(A)* delivers insulin through a thin plastic tubing to an infusion set, which has a cannula *(B)* that sits under the skin. Continuous glucose monitoring occurs through a tiny sensor *(C)* inserted under the skin. Sensor data are sent continuously to the insulin pump through wireless technology giving a more complete picture of glucose levels, which can lead to better treatment decisions and better glucose control. (MiniMed Paradigm® REAL-Time Revel™ Insulin Pump manufactured by the diabetes division of Medtronic, Inc.)

reading, SMBG enables the patient to make decisions regarding food intake, activity patterns, and medication dosages. It also produces accurate records of daily glucose fluctuations and trends, and it alerts the patient to acute episodes of hyperglycemia and hypoglycemia. Furthermore, it provides patients with a tool for achieving and maintaining specific glycemic goals. SMBG is recommended for all insulin-treated patients with diabetes. Other patients with diabetes use SMBG to help achieve and maintain glycemic goals and monitor for acute fluctuations in blood glucose.

The frequency of monitoring depends on several factors, including the patient's glycemic goals, type of diabetes, medication regimen, patient's ability to perform the test independently, and patient's willingness to test. Patients who use multiple insulin injections or insulin pumps should monitor their blood glucose four or more times a day. Patients using less frequent insulin injections, noninsulin therapy, or nutritional therapy will monitor as often as needed to achieve their glycemic goals.[10]

Patients who perform SMBG use portable blood glucose monitors (glucometers). A wide variety of blood glucose monitors are available (Fig. 49-8). Disposable lancets are used to obtain a small drop of capillary blood (usually from a finger stick) that is placed onto a reagent strip. After a specified time, the monitor displays a digital reading of the capillary blood glucose value. The technology of SMBG is rapidly changing, with newer and more convenient systems being introduced on an ongoing basis.

Newer systems allow the user to collect blood from alternative sites such as the forearm or palm. Alternate site testing is

not recommended with rapidly changing blood glucose readings, during pregnancy, or when symptoms of low blood glucose are present. The data from some glucose monitors can be uploaded to a computer and e-mailed to health care providers for review, allowing for more frequent and efficient adjustment of the plan of care if needed.

Continuous glucose monitoring (CGM) systems provide another route for monitoring glucose. The CGM systems available include the (1) Dexcom Seven by Dexcom, (2) MiniMed Paradigm® REAL-Time Revel™ by Medtronic (Fig. 49-9), (3) Guardian REAL-Time by Medtronic, and (4) FreeStyle Navigator by Abbott. Using a sensor inserted subcutaneously, the systems display glucose values that are updated every 1 to 5 minutes. The patient inserts the sensor using an automatic insertion device. Data are sent from the sensor to a transmitter, which displays the glucose value on either an insulin pump (MiniMed Paradigm® REAL-Time Revel™ and Guardian REAL-

Time) or a pager-like receiver (Dexcom Seven and FreeStyle Navigator). The glucose monitor can be used without an insulin pump.

CGMs assist the patient and the health care provider in identifying trends and patterns in glucose levels and are useful for the management of insulin therapy or when continuous blood glucose readings are clinically important. The patient is alerted to episodes of hypoglycemia and hyperglycemia, thus allowing corrective action to be quickly taken. These systems still require finger-stick measurements using a blood glucose monitor to calibrate the sensor and to make treatment decisions.

The blood glucose level reported by a laboratory is sometimes higher than the patient's home glucose monitor or the hospital's portable monitor. This is because some home monitors give capillary blood glucose values from whole blood (via finger stick), whereas tests performed in laboratories provide plasma readings. Plasma samples, or venous samples, are approximately 10% to 12% higher. Most current monitors are automatically calibrated to give a "plasma" test result (even though whole blood was used for the sample) so that the home readings can be more readily compared with laboratory values. It is important to read the literature accompanying a monitor to find out if it is displaying values as whole blood or plasma.

Because errors in monitoring technique can cause errors in management strategies, comprehensive patient teaching is essential. Initial instruction should be followed up with regular reassessment. Review the instructions that accompany each product. Teach patients to use and interpret control solutions. Control solution should be used when first using a glucometer, when a new bottle of strips is used, or when there is a reason to believe that the readings are not correct. Table 49-11 lists the steps to include when teaching the patient how to perform SMBG.

People with type 1 diabetes often test their blood glucose before meals. This is because many patients use insulin pumps or multiple daily injections and base the insulin dose on the carbohydrates in a meal or make adjustments if the preprandial value is above or below target. Testing 2 hours after the first bite of food is taken helps a person see how effectively he or she judged what was eaten or to determine if the bolus insulin dose was adequate for that meal.

Blood glucose testing should be performed whenever hypoglycemia is suspected so that immediate action can be taken. During times of illness, the person should test blood glucose levels at 4-hour intervals to determine the effects of the illness on glucose levels. Teach the patient to test blood glucose before and after exercise to determine the effects of exercise on metabolic control. This is especially important in the patient with type 1 diabetes.

A patient who is visually impaired, cognitively impaired, or limited in manual dexterity needs careful evaluation of the degree to which SMBG can be performed independently. Nurses preparing patients for discharge from the hospital, and nurses working in home health and outpatient settings, may need to identify caregivers who can assume this responsibility. Adaptive devices are available to help patients with certain limitations. These include talking meters and other equipment for the visually impaired.

Bariatric Surgery

Bariatric surgery may be considered for patients with type 2 diabetes who have a body mass index (BMI) greater than 35 kg/m², especially if the diabetes or associated co-morbidities are difficult to control with lifestyle and drug therapy (see Evidence-Based Practice box on p. 1170). Patients with type 2 diabetes who have undergone bariatric surgery need lifelong lifestyle support and monitoring. (Bariatric surgery is discussed in Chapter 41.)

Pancreas Transplantation

Pancreas transplantation can be used as a treatment option for patients with type 1 diabetes. Usually it is done for patients who have end-stage kidney disease and have had or plan to have a kidney transplant. Kidney and pancreas transplants are often performed together, or a pancreas may be transplanted after a kidney transplant. If renal failure is not present, the ADA recommends that pancreas transplantation be considered only for patients who exhibit the following three criteria: (1) a history of frequent, acute, and severe metabolic complications (e.g., hypoglycemia, hyperglycemia, ketoacidosis) requiring medical attention; (2) clinical and emotional problems with the use of exogenous insulin therapy that are so severe as to be incapacitating; and (3) consistent failure of insulin-based management to prevent acute complications.

Successful pancreas transplantation can improve the quality of life for people with diabetes, primarily by eliminating the need for exogenous insulin, frequent blood glucose measurements, and many of the dietary restrictions imposed by the disorder. Transplantation can also eliminate the acute complications commonly experienced by patients with type 1 diabetes (e.g., hypoglycemia, hyperglycemia). However, pancreas transplantation is only partially successful in reversing the long-term renal and neurologic complications of diabetes. The patient will also require lifelong immunosuppression to prevent rejection of the organ. Complications can result from immunosuppressive therapy. (Immunosuppressive therapy is discussed in Chapter 14.)

Pancreatic islet cell transplantation is another potential treatment measure. During this procedure, the islets are harvested

---

TABLE 49-11 PATIENT & CAREGIVER TEACHING GUIDE

Self-Monitoring of Blood Glucose (SMBG)

Include the following instructions when teaching the patient and caregiver about SMBG.

1. Wash hands in warm water. It is not necessary to clean the site with alcohol, and it may interfere with test results. Finger should be dry before puncturing it.
2. If it is difficult to obtain an adequate drop of blood for testing, warm the hands in warm water or let the arms hang dependently for a few minutes before the finger puncture is made.
3. A penlet lancing device is usually used. Place the lancet in the device, following the instructions that come with it. If the puncture is made on the finger, use the side of the finger pad rather than near the center. Fewer nerve endings are along the side of the finger pad. If an alternative site is used (e.g., forearm), special equipment may be needed. Refer to manufacturer's instructions for alternative site use, except during hypoglycemic episodes.
4. Set penlet device to make a puncture just deep enough to obtain a sufficiently large drop of blood. Unnecessarily deep punctures may cause pain and bruising.
5. Follow instructions on monitor for testing the blood.
6. Record results. Compare with personal target blood glucose goals.

EVIDENCE-BASED PRACTICE

Translating Research Into Practice

Bariatric Surgery for Obese Adults With Type 2 Diabetes

Clinical Question

In severely obese adults (P), how do gastric bypass and biliopancreatic diversion (I) compare with medical therapy (C) for remission from type 2 diabetes mellitus (O)?

Best Available Evidence

Systematic review of randomized controlled trials (RCTs)

Critical Appraisal and Synthesis of Evidence

- Sixty adults with type 2 diabetes for ≥5 yr with a BMI ≥35 kg/m² and Hb A1C ≥7.0%.
- Roux-en-Y gastric bypass (n = 20), biliopancreatic diversion (n = 20), or medical therapy (n = 20).
- At 2 yr, more patients in the gastric bypass and biliopancreatic diversion groups achieved diabetes remission than in the medical therapy group.
- Bypass and biliopancreatic diversion each reduced A1C, glucose levels, and BMI more than medical therapy.

Conclusion

- Bariatric surgery (gastric bypass and biliopancreatic diversion) decreases BMI, improves glycemic control, and increases remission from type 2 diabetes more than medical therapy in severely obese adults.

Implications for Nursing Practice

- In addition to behavioral and medical approaches, bariatric surgery often normalizes blood glucose levels, reduces or avoids the need for drugs, and provides a potentially cost-effective approach to treating the disease.
- Bariatric surgery is an appropriate treatment for people with type 2 diabetes and obesity not achieving recommended treatment targets with medical therapies, especially when there are other major co-morbidities.

Reference for Evidence

Mingrone G, Panunzi S, De Gaetano A, et al: Bariatric surgery versus conventional medical therapy for type 2 diabetes, *N Engl J Med* 366: 1577, 2012.

P, Patient population of interest; *I*, intervention or area of interest; *C*, comparison of interest or comparison group; *O*, outcomes of interest (see p. 12).

CULTURAL & ETHNIC HEALTH DISPARITIES

Diabetes Mellitus

- The highest incidence of diabetes is among Native Americans and Alaska Natives (16.5% are being treated for diabetes).
- Pima Indians in Arizona have the highest rate of diabetes in the world (50% of adults have diabetes).
- The rates of diabetes are non-Hispanic whites 7.1%, Asian Americans 8.4%, Hispanics 11.8%, and non-Hispanic blacks 12.6%.
- Diabetes is 1.5 times more likely to cause death in Hispanics and 2.2 times more likely to cause death in African Americans than in non-Hispanic whites.
- Complications from diabetes are a major cause of death among Native Americans. Native Americans have a six times higher rate of end-stage kidney disease and a four times higher rate of amputation than other people with diabetes.
- Treatment for end-stage kidney disease for men with diabetes is 1.6 times higher in Hispanics and 2.7 times higher in African Americans compared with non-Hispanic white men.

Explore the influences of culture on food choices and meal planning with the patient as part of the health history. When giving diet instructions, consider the patient's cultural food preferences. Nutritional resources specifically designed for members of different cultural groups are available from the ADA.

NURSING MANAGEMENT DIABETES MELLITUS

NURSING ASSESSMENT

Table 49-12 provides initial subjective and objective data that should be obtained from a person with diabetes mellitus. After the initial assessment, perform periodic patient assessments on a regular basis.

NURSING DIAGNOSES

Nursing diagnoses related to diabetes mellitus may include, but are not limited to, those found in eNursing Care Plan 49-1.

PLANNING

The overall goals are for the patient with diabetes mellitus to (1) engage in self-care behaviors to actively manage his or her diabetes, (2) experience few or no episodes of acute hyperglycemic or hypoglycemic emergencies, (3) maintain blood glucose levels at normal or near-normal levels, (4) prevent or minimize chronic complications of diabetes, and (5) adjust lifestyle to accommodate the diabetes regimen with a minimum of stress.

NURSING IMPLEMENTATION

HEALTH PROMOTION. Your role in health promotion is to identify, monitor, and teach the patient at risk for diabetes. Obesity is the primary risk factor for type 2 diabetes. The findings from the Diabetes Prevention Program indicated that a modest weight loss of 5% to 7% of body weight and regular exercise of 30 minutes five times a week lowered the risk of developing type 2 diabetes up to 58%.[18]

The ADA recommends routine screening for type 2 diabetes for all adults who are overweight or obese (BMI greater than or equal to 25 kg/m²) or have one or more risk factors. For people who do not have risk factors for diabetes, screening should begin at age 45. Table 49-13 provides criteria to test for prediabetes and diabetes. If results are normal, repeat testing at 3-year

from the pancreas of a deceased organ donor. Most recipients require the use of two or more pancreases. The islets are infused via a catheter through the upper abdomen into the portal vein of the liver. With only the islets transplanted, pain and recovery time are diminished compared with whole pancreas transplants. Currently this procedure is experimental in the United States. Research is continuing to investigate the best ways to implant the islet cells and to prevent their rejection.

CULTURALLY COMPETENT CARE

DIABETES MELLITUS

Because culture can have a strong influence on dietary preferences and meal preparation practices, culturally competent care has special relevance for the patient with diabetes. For example, certain ethnic and cultural groups, such as Hispanics, Native Americans, and African Americans, have a high incidence of diabetes. The increased prevalence can be attributed to genetic predisposition, environmental factors, and dietary choices.

TABLE 49-12 NURSING ASSESSMENT
Diabetes Mellitus

Subjective Data
Important Health Information
Past health history: Mumps, rubella, coxsackievirus or other viral infections; recent trauma, infection, or stress; pregnancy, gave birth to infant >9 lb; chronic pancreatitis; Cushing syndrome; acromegaly; family history of type 1 or type 2 diabetes mellitus
Medications: Use of and adherence to regimen with insulin or OAs; corticosteroids, diuretics, phenytoin (Dilantin)
Surgery or other treatments: Any recent surgery

Functional Health Patterns
Health perception–health management: Positive family history; malaise; date of last eye and dental examination
Nutritional-metabolic: Obesity; weight loss (type 1), weight gain (type 2); thirst, hunger; nausea and vomiting; poor healing (especially involving the feet), adherence to diet in patients with previously diagnosed diabetes
Elimination: Constipation or diarrhea; frequent urination, frequent bladder infections, nocturia, urinary incontinence
Activity-exercise: Muscle weakness, fatigue
Cognitive-perceptual: Abdominal pain; headache; blurred vision; numbness or tingling of extremities; pruritus
Sexuality-reproductive: Erectile dysfunction; frequent vaginal infections; decreased libido
Coping–stress tolerance: Depression, irritability, apathy
Value-belief: Commitment to lifestyle changes involving diet, medication, and activity patterns

Objective Data
Eyes
Soft, sunken eyeballs;* vitreal hemorrhages; cataracts

Integumentary
Dry, warm, inelastic skin; pigmented lesions (on legs); ulcers (especially on feet); loss of hair on toes; acanthosis nigricans

Respiratory
Rapid, deep respirations (Kussmaul respirations)*

Cardiovascular
Hypotension;* weak, rapid pulse*

Gastrointestinal
Dry mouth; vomiting;* fruity breath*

Neurologic
Altered reflexes; restlessness; confusion; stupor; coma

Musculoskeletal
Muscle wasting

Possible Findings
Serum electrolyte abnormalities; fasting blood glucose level ≥126 mg/dL; oral glucose tolerance test >200 mg/dL; random glucose ≥200 mg/dL; leukocytosis; ↑ blood urea nitrogen, creatinine, triglycerides, cholesterol, LDL, VLDL; ↓ HDL; A1C >6.0%; glycosuria; ketonuria; albuminuria; acidosis

*Indicates manifestations of diabetic ketoacidosis.
A1C, Glycosylated hemoglobin; *HDL,* high-density lipoprotein; *LDL,* low-density lipoprotein; *OAs,* oral agents; *VLDL,* very-low-density lipoprotein.

TABLE 49-13 TESTING FOR DIABETES IN ASYMPTOMATIC, UNDIAGNOSED INDIVIDUALS

Who Should Be Tested
1. Testing should be considered in all adults who are overweight (BMI >25 kg/m²) and have additional risk factors:
   - First-degree relative with diabetes
   - Physically inactive
   - Members of a high-risk ethnic population (e.g., African American, Hispanic, Native American, Asian American, Pacific Islander)
   - Women who delivered a baby weighing >9 lb or were diagnosed with gestational diabetes mellitus
   - Hypertensive (≥140/90 mm Hg) or on therapy for hypertension
   - HDL cholesterol level ≤35 mg/dL (0.90 mmol/L) and/or a triglyceride level ≥250 mg/dL (2.82 mmol/L)
   - Women with polycystic ovary syndrome
   - A1C ≥5.7%, IGT, or IFG on previous testing
   - Other clinical conditions associated with insulin resistance (e.g., severe obesity, acanthosis nigricans)
2. In the absence of the above criteria, testing for diabetes should begin at age 45 yr.
3. If results are normal, testing should be repeated at least at 3-yr intervals, with consideration of more frequent testing depending on initial results and risk status.

What Testing Should Be Used
To test for diabetes or to assess risk of future diabetes, A1C, FPG, or 2-hour OGTT is appropriate.

Source: American Diabetes Association: Clinical practice recommendations: standards of medical care, *Diabetes Care* 36 (Suppl):S11, 2013.
A1C, Glycosylated hemoglobin; *BMI,* body mass index; *FPG,* fasting plasma glucose; *HDL,* high-density lipoprotein; *IFG,* impaired fasting glucose; *IGT,* impaired glucose tolerance; *OGTT,* oral glucose tolerance test.

HEALTHY PEOPLE
Prevention and Early Detection of Diabetes Mellitus

- Increase level of exercise because physical activity reduces the risk of type 2 diabetes.
- Maintain a healthy weight because obesity increases the risk of type 2 diabetes.
- If overweight, lose weight and get on a regular exercise program to reduce the risk of diabetes.
- Use a diet that is low in fat content, total calories, and processed foods and high in whole grains, fruits, and vegetables.
- If overweight and over age 45, get a diabetes screening test done.

tes risk test determines if the person is at risk for prediabetes or diabetes based on the number of risk factors present.

ACUTE INTERVENTION. Acute situations involving the patient with diabetes include hypoglycemia, DKA, and hyperosmolar hyperglycemic syndrome (HHS). Nursing management for these situations is discussed in more detail later in this chapter. Other areas of acute intervention relate to management during stress, such as during acute illness and surgery.

Stress of Acute Illness and Surgery. Both emotional and physical stress can increase the blood glucose level and result in hyperglycemia. Because stress is unavoidable, certain situations may require more intense treatment, such as extra insulin, to maintain glycemic goals and avoid hyperglycemia.

Acute illness, injury, and surgery are situations that may evoke a counterregulatory hormone response, resulting in hyperglycemia. Even common illnesses such as a viral upper

intervals.³ Many factors put an individual at an increased risk for diabetes. These include age, ethnicity (being Native American, Hispanic, African American, Asian, Pacific Islander), obesity, having a baby that weighs more than 9 lb, having gestational diabetes, and a family history of diabetes. A diabetes risk test is available at *www.diabetes.org/risk-test.jsp*. The diaberespiratory tract infection or the flu can cause this response. When patients with diabetes are ill, they should check blood glucose at least every 4 hours. An acutely ill patient with type 1 diabetes with a blood glucose greater than 240 mg/dL (13.3 mmol/L) should test his or her urine for ketones every 3 to 4 hours.

Patients should report to the health care provider when glucose levels are over 300 mg/dL for two tests in a row or urine ketone levels are moderate to large. A patient with type 1 diabetes may need an increase in insulin to prevent DKA. Insulin therapy may be required for a patient with type 2 diabetes to prevent or treat hyperglycemic symptoms and avoid an acute hyperglycemic emergency. In critically ill patients, insulin therapy may be started if the blood glucose is persistently greater than 180 mg/dL. These patients have a higher targeted blood glucose goal, which is usually 140 to 180 mg/dL.

Food intake is important during times of stress and illness, when the body requires extra energy. If patients are able to eat normally, they should continue with their regular meal plan while increasing the intake of noncaloric fluids, such as water, diet gelatin, and other decaffeinated beverages, and continue taking OAs, noninsulin injectable agents, and insulin as prescribed. When illness causes patients to eat less than normal, they should continue to take OAs, noninsulin injectable agents, and/or insulin as prescribed while supplementing food intake with carbohydrate-containing fluids. Examples include low-sodium soups, juices, and regular decaffeinated soft drinks. It is important to tell the patient to contact a health care provider if the patient is unable to keep down food or fluid.

During the intraoperative period, adjustments in the diabetes regimen can be planned to ensure glycemic control. The patient is given IV fluids and insulin (if needed) immediately before, during, and after surgery when there is no oral intake. The patient with type 2 diabetes who has been on OAs should understand that this is a temporary measure, not a sign of worsening diabetes.

When caring for an unconscious surgical patient receiving insulin, be alert for hypoglycemic signs such as sweating, tachycardia, and tremors. Frequent monitoring of blood glucose will prevent episodes of severe hypoglycemia.

AMBULATORY AND HOME CARE. Successful management of diabetes requires ongoing interaction among the patient, caregiver, and health care team. It is important that a certified diabetes educator (CDE) be involved in the care of the patient and the family. Because diabetes is a complex chronic condition, a great deal of patient contact takes place in outpatient and home settings. The major goal of patient care in these settings is to enable the patient (with the help of a caregiver) to reach an optimal level of independence in self-care activities. Unfortunately, many patients with diabetes face challenges in reaching these goals. Diabetes increases the risk for other chronic conditions that can affect self-care activities. These include visual impairment, lower extremity problems that affect mobility, and other functional limitations related to a stroke.

An important nursing function is to assess the ability of patients and caregivers in performing activities such as SMBG and insulin injection. Assistive devices for self-administration of insulin include syringe magnifiers, vial stabilizers, and dosing aids for the visually impaired. In some cases, referrals are made to help the patient achieve the self-care goal. These may include an occupational therapist, a social worker, a home care nurse, a home health aide, or a dietitian.

A diagnosis of diabetes affects the patient in many profound ways. Self-management of the disease is demanding. Patients with diabetes continually face lifestyle choices that affect the foods they eat, their activities, and demands on their time and energy. The requirements of scheduled meals, SMBG, medication, and insulin management may interfere with the patient's other responsibilities. Any change in the daily routine is difficult. In addition, they face the challenge of preventing or dealing with the devastating complications of diabetes.

Careful assessment of what it means to the patient to have diabetes should be the starting point of teaching. The goals of teaching should be mutually determined by you and the patient, based on individual needs and therapeutic requirements. Identify the patient's support system, and include them in planning, teaching, and counseling. When family members and other individuals close to the patient are included, they can support the patient's self-care behaviors. Additionally, they can provide care if self-care is not possible. Encourage the family and caregivers to provide emotional support and encouragement as the patient deals with the reality of living with a chronic disease.

Insulin Therapy. Nursing responsibilities for the patient receiving insulin include proper administration, assessment of the patient's response to insulin therapy, and teaching the patient about administration and side effects of insulin (see Table 49-5). Table 49-6 lists guidelines for assessing a patient using glucose-lowering agents, including insulin and OAs.

Assessment of the patient who is a new user of insulin must include an evaluation of his or her ability to safely manage this therapy. This includes the ability to understand the interaction of insulin, diet, and activity and to recognize and treat the symptoms of hypoglycemia appropriately. If the patient does not have the cognitive skills to do these things, identify and teach another responsible person. The patient or caregiver must have the cognitive and manual skills needed to prepare and inject insulin. Otherwise, additional resources will be needed to assist the patient. For patients with cognitive, physical, and other barriers, consider referral to a CDE because he or she has the specialized knowledge and skills to promote self-care behaviors for these patients.

Many patients are fearful when they first begin using insulin.[19] Some find it difficult to self-inject because they are afraid of needles or the pain associated with an injection. Others may think that the insulin is not necessary or that they will experience hypoglycemia after an injection. Explore the patient's underlying fears before beginning the teaching. Assessment of the patient's beliefs and concerns regarding starting insulin will guide the teaching, counseling, and plan of care. Having open discussion with patients, providing educational materials and programs, and working with a diabetes educator are all beneficial for patients starting insulin.

Follow-up assessment of the patient who has been using insulin therapy includes an inspection of injection sites for signs of lipodystrophy and other reactions, review of insulin preparation and injection technique, a history pertaining to the occurrence of hypoglycemic episodes, and assessment of the patient's method for handling hypoglycemic episodes. A review of the patient's recorded blood glucose tests is vital in assessing overall glycemic control and making any needed adjustments.

Oral and Noninsulin Injectable Agents. Your responsibilities for the patient taking oral and noninsulin injectable agents are similar to those for the patient taking insulin. Proper administration of these drugs, assessment of the patient's use of and response to these drugs, and teaching the patient and family are all essential nursing actions.

Your assessment is valuable in determining the most appropriate drug for a patient. Factors such as the patient's mental status, eating habits, home environment, attitude toward diabetes, and medication history all play a significant role in determining the most appropriate drug. For example, frail older adults who live alone are at high risk for severe hypoglycemia because low blood glucose is frequently undetected or untreated in this population. This is especially true if the patient has cognitive impairment. In these cases, an OA that does not cause hypoglycemia, or a shorter-acting OA, would be most appropriate.

Patient teaching is essential. Some patients may assume that their diabetes is not a serious condition if they are only taking a pill for glycemic control. Instruct the patient that these agents will help control blood glucose and help prevent serious long- and short-term complications of diabetes. Teach patients that OAs and noninsulin injectable agents are used in addition to diet and activity as therapy for diabetes and the importance of following their meal and activity plans. Patients should not take extra pills if they have overeaten. If the patient uses sulfonylureas and metformin, instruct the patient about prevention, symptom recognition, and management of hypoglycemia.

Personal Hygiene. The potential for infection requires diligent skin and dental hygiene practices. Because of the susceptibility to periodontal disease, encourage daily brushing and flossing in addition to regular visits to the dentist. When having dental work done, the patient should inform the dentist that he or she has diabetes. Teach patients regarding the importance of sharing their diagnosis with dentists and other health care professionals.

Routine care includes regular bathing, with particular emphasis on foot care. Advise patients to inspect their feet daily, avoid going barefoot, and wear shoes that are supportive and comfortable. If cuts, scrapes, or burns occur, they should be treated promptly and monitored carefully. Wash the area and apply a nonabrasive or nonirritating antiseptic ointment. Cover the area with a dry, sterile pad. Patients should notify the health care provider immediately if the injury does not begin to heal within 24 hours or if signs of infection develop.

Medical Identification and Travel. Instruct the patient to carry medical identification at all times indicating that he or she has diabetes. Police, paramedics, and many private citizens are aware of the need to look for this identification when working with sick or unconscious persons. Every person with diabetes should wear a Medic Alert bracelet or necklace. An identification card (Fig. 49-10) can supply valuable information, such as the name of the health care provider; the type of diabetes; and the type and dosage of insulin, noninsulin injectable agents, or OAs.

Travel for a patient with diabetes requires planning. Being sedentary for long periods may raise the person's glucose level. Encourage the patient to get up and walk at least every 2 hours to lower the risk for deep vein thrombosis and to prevent elevation of glucose levels. The patient should have a full set of diabetes care supplies in the carry-on luggage when traveling by plane, train, or bus. This includes blood glucose monitoring equipment, insulin, noninsulin injectable agents, oral medications, and syringes or insulin pens.

FIG. 49-10 Medical alerts. A patient with diabetes should carry a card and wear a bracelet or necklace that indicates diabetes. If the patient with diabetes is unconscious, these measures will ensure prompt and appropriate attention.

When equipment such as syringes, lancing devices, insulin vials or pens, and insulin pumps are taken onto a commercial airliner, the professional printed pharmaceutical labels should accompany them. A letter from the prescribing health care provider indicating medical necessity may prevent delays at security checkpoints. Notify screeners if an insulin pump is used so they can inspect it while it is on the body, rather than removing it.

For patients who use insulin or OAs that can cause hypoglycemia, snack items and a quick-acting carbohydrate source for treating hypoglycemia should be included in the carry-on luggage. Extra insulin should be available in case a bottle breaks or is lost. For longer trips, the patient should carry a full day's supply of food in the event of canceled flights, delayed meals, or closed restaurants. If the patient is planning a trip out of the country, it is wise to have a letter from the health care provider explaining that the patient has diabetes and requires all the materials, particularly syringes, for ongoing health care.

When travel involves time changes such as traveling coast to coast or across the International Date Line, the patient should contact the health care provider to plan an appropriate insulin schedule. During travel, most patients find it helpful to keep watches set to the time of the city of origin until they reach their destination. The key to travel when taking insulin is to know the type of insulin being taken, its onset of action, the anticipated peak time, and mealtimes.

Patient and Caregiver Teaching. The goals of diabetes self-management education are to match the level of self-management to the patient's individual ability so he or she can become the most active participant possible. Patients who actively manage their diabetes care have better outcomes than those who do not. For this reason, an educational approach that facilitates informed decision making by the patient is advocated. Sometimes this is referred to as the *empowerment approach* to education.

Unfortunately, patients can encounter a variety of physical, psychologic, and emotional barriers when it comes to effectively managing their diabetes. These barriers may include feelings of inadequacy about one's own abilities, unwillingness to make the necessary behavioral changes, ineffective coping strategies, and cognitive deficits. If the patient is not able to manage the disease, a family member may be able to assume part of this role. If the patient or the caregiver cannot make decisions related to diabe-

COMPLEMENTARY & ALTERNATIVE THERAPIES

Herbs and Supplements That May Affect Blood Glucose

Scientific Evidence*
- Herbs and supplements that may lower blood glucose include aloe, α-lipoic acid, cinnamon, chromium, garlic, and ginseng.
- However, many studies have been small and not well designed. Further research is needed.

Nursing Implications
- Teach patients to use herbs and supplements with caution, since they may affect blood glucose.
- Patients with diabetes mellitus should consult their health care provider before using herbs or nutritional supplements.
- Patients who use herbs should monitor their blood glucose levels carefully and regularly.

*Based on a systematic review of scientific literature. Retrieved from *www.naturalstandard.com.*

INFORMATICS IN PRACTICE

Patient Teaching Using Gaming

- Teaching is a critical part of nursing care for patients with diabetes. Put some fun into patient teaching by using gaming applications.
- Try an application with a quiz-show format. The patient answers questions about diabetes and then compares his or her answers in real time to those of other players. The questions (e.g., How does exercise affect insulin?) are written to help the patient learn to manage diabetes on a daily basis.
- Players in online simulations become either a caregiver to or a patient with type 1 diabetes. Players earn rewards by properly managing blood glucose levels.

tes management, consider a referral to a CDE, social worker, or other resources within the community. These resources can assist the patient and the family in outlining a feasible treatment program that meets their capabilities. Patient and health care provider resources are listed at the end of this chapter.

An assessment of the patient's knowledge of diabetes and lifestyle preferences is useful in planning a teaching program. Tables 49-14 and 49-15 present guidelines to use for patient and caregiver teaching. Assess the patient's knowledge base frequently so that gaps in knowledge or incorrect or inaccurate ideas can be corrected.

The ADA offers resources for patients in the form of pamphlets, booklets, books, and a monthly magazine called *Diabetes Forecast.* Affiliates of the ADA are located in all states, and most can be reached by dialing 1-800-DIABETES (800-342-2383). The ADA publishes materials and sponsors conferences for health care professionals concerned with diabetes education, research, and management of patients. The ADA website (*www.diabetes.org*) has extensive information for the public and health care professionals. This organization also recognizes education programs that meet the national standards of diabetes education and can provide a list of these programs. Drug companies manufacturing diabetes-related products also have free educational materials for patients and health care providers.

EVALUATION

The expected outcomes for the patient with diabetes mellitus are addressed in eNursing Care Plan 49-1.

TABLE 49-14 PATIENT & CAREGIVER TEACHING GUIDE

Management of Diabetes Mellitus

Include the following instructions when teaching the patient and caregiver how to manage diabetes mellitus.

Component	What to Teach
Disease Process	• Include an introduction about the pancreas and the islets of Langerhans. • Describe how insulin is made and what affects its production. • Discuss the relationship of insulin and glucose. • Explain the difference between type 1 and type 2 diabetes.
Physical Activity	• Discuss the effect of regular exercise on the management of blood glucose, improvement of cardiovascular function, and general health.
Menu Planning	• Stress the importance of a well-balanced diet as part of a diabetes management plan. • Explain the impact of carbohydrates on the glycemic index and blood glucose levels.
Medication Adherence	• Ensure that the patient understands the proper use of prescribed medication (e.g., insulin [see Table 49-5], OAs, and noninsulin injectables). • Account for a patient's physical limitations or inabilities for self-medication. If necessary, involve the family or the caregiver in proper use of medication. • Discuss all side effects and safety issues regarding medication.
Monitoring Blood glucose	• Teach correct blood glucose monitoring. • Include when blood glucose levels should be checked, how to record them, and how to adjust insulin levels if necessary.
Risk Reduction	• Ensure that the patient understands and appropriately responds to the signs and symptoms of hypoglycemia and hyperglycemia (see Table 49-16). • Stress the importance of proper foot care (see Table 49-21), regular eye examinations, and consistent glucose monitoring. • Inform the patient about the effect that stress can have on blood glucose.
Psychosocial	• Advise the patient of resources that are available to facilitate the adjustment and answer questions about living with a chronic condition such as diabetes (see Resources at end of chapter).

OAs, Oral agents.

ACUTE COMPLICATIONS OF DIABETES MELLITUS

The acute complications of diabetes mellitus arise from events associated with hyperglycemia and hypoglycemia. It is important for the health care provider to distinguish between hyperglycemia and hypoglycemia because hypoglycemia worsens rapidly and constitutes a serious threat if action is not immediately taken. Table 49-16 compares the manifestations, causes, management, and prevention of hyperglycemia and hypoglycemia.

TABLE 49-15 PATIENT & CAREGIVER TEACHING GUIDE

Instructions for Patients With Diabetes Mellitus

Include the following essential instructions for diabetes management.

Do	Do Not
Blood Glucose	
• Monitor your blood glucose at home and record results in a log.	• Skip doses of your insulin, especially when you are sick.
• Take your insulin. OA, and/or noninsulin injectable agent as prescribed.	• Run out of insulin.
• Obtain A1C blood test every 3-6 mo as an indicator of your long-term blood glucose control.	• Ignore the symptoms of hypoglycemia and hyperglycemia.
• Know the symptoms of hypoglycemia and hyperglycemia.	
• Carry some form of rapid-acting glucose at all times so you can treat hypoglycemia quickly.	
• Instruct family members how and when to use glucagon if patient becomes unresponsive because of hypoglycemia.	
Exercise	
• Learn how exercise and food affect your blood glucose levels.	• Forget that exercise will lower your blood glucose level.
• Begin an exercise program after approval from health care provider.	
Diet	
• Have an individualized meal plan created by a dietitian.	• Drink excessive amounts of alcohol because this may lead to unpredictable low blood glucose reactions.
• Follow your diet, eating regular meals at regular times.	
• Choose foods low in saturated and *trans* fat.	• Use a fad diet.
• Limit the amount of alcohol you drink.	• Drink regular soda or lots of fruit juice.
• Know your cholesterol level.	
Other Guidelines	
• Obtain an annual eye examination by an ophthalmologist.	• Smoke cigarettes or use nicotine products.
• Obtain annual urine testing for protein.	
• Examine your feet at home.	• Apply hot or cold directly to your feet.
• Wear comfortable, well-fitting shoes to help prevent foot injury. Break in new shoes gradually.	• Go barefoot.
• Always carry identification that says you have diabetes.	• Put oil or lotion between your toes.
• Have other medical problems treated, especially high blood pressure and high cholesterol.	
• Quit cigarette smoking.	
• Have a yearly influenza vaccination.	

A1C, Glycosylated hemoglobin; *OA,* oral agent.

TABLE 49-16 COMPARISON OF HYPERGLYCEMIA AND HYPOGLYCEMIA

Hyperglycemia	Hypoglycemia
Manifestations*	
Elevated blood glucose†	Blood glucose <70 mg/dL (3.9 mmol/L)
Increase in urination	Cold, clammy skin
Increase in appetite followed by lack of appetite	Numbness of fingers, toes, mouth
	Rapid heartbeat
	Emotional changes
Weakness, fatigue	Headache
Blurred vision	Nervousness, tremors
Headache	Faintness, dizziness
Glycosuria	Unsteady gait, slurred speech
Nausea and vomiting	Hunger
Abdominal cramps	Changes in vision
Progression to DKA or HHS	Seizures, coma
Causes	
Illness, infection	Alcohol intake without food
Corticosteroids	Too little food—delayed, omitted, inadequate intake
Too much food	
Too little or no diabetes medication	Too much diabetic medication
Inactivity	Too much exercise without adequate food intake
Emotional, physical stress	Diabetes medication or food taken at wrong time
Poor absorption of insulin	Loss of weight without change in medication
	Use of β-adrenergic blockers interfering with recognition of symptoms
Treatment	
Get medical care	Follow the Rule of 15 (see p. 1179).
Continue diabetes medication as ordered	See Table 49-19 for treatment of hypoglycemia.
Check blood glucose frequently and check urine for ketones record results	
Drink fluids at least on an hourly basis	
Contact health care provider regarding ketonuria	
Preventive Measures	
Take prescribed dose of medication at proper time	Take prescribed dose of medication at proper time.
Accurately administer insulin, noninsulin injectables, OA	Accurately administer insulin, noninsulin injectables, OA.
Maintain diet	Ingest all recommended foods at proper time.
Adhere to sick-day rules when ill	Provide adequate food intake needed for calories for exercise.
Check blood for glucose as ordered	Be able to recognize and know symptoms and treat them immediately.
Wear diabetic identification	Carry simple carbohydrates.
	Educate family and caregiver about symptoms and treatment.
	Check blood glucose as ordered.
	Wear Medic Alert (diabetic) identification.

*There is usually a gradual onset of symptoms in hyperglycemia and a rapid onset in hypoglycemia.
†Specific clinical manifestations related to elevated levels of blood glucose vary according to the patient.
DKA, Diabetic ketoacidosis; *HHS,* hyperosmolar hyperglycemic syndrome; *OA,* oral agent.

DIABETIC KETOACIDOSIS

Etiology and Pathophysiology

Diabetic ketoacidosis (DKA) is caused by a profound deficiency of insulin and is characterized by hyperglycemia, ketosis, acidosis, and dehydration. It is most likely to occur in people with type 1 diabetes but may be seen in people with type 2 diabetes in conditions of severe illness or stress when the pancreas cannot meet the extra demand for insulin. Precipitating factors include illness and infection, inadequate insulin dosage, undiagnosed type 1 diabetes, poor self-management, and neglect.

When the circulating supply of insulin is insufficient, glucose cannot be properly used for energy. The body compensates by breaking down fat stores as a secondary source of fuel (Fig. 49-11). Ketones are acidic by-products of fat metabolism that can cause serious problems when they become excessive in the blood. Ketosis alters the pH balance, causing metabolic acidosis to develop. Ketonuria is a process that occurs when ketone bodies are excreted in the urine. During this process, electrolytes become depleted as cations are eliminated along with the anionic ketones in an attempt to maintain electrical neutrality.

Insulin deficiency impairs protein synthesis and causes excessive protein degradation. This results in nitrogen losses from the tissues. Insulin deficiency also stimulates the production of glucose from amino acids (from proteins) in the liver and leads to further hyperglycemia. Because of the deficiency of insulin, the additional glucose cannot be used and the blood glucose level rises further, adding to the osmotic diuresis.

If not treated, the patient will develop severe depletion of sodium, potassium, chloride, magnesium, and phosphate. Vomiting caused by the acidosis results in more fluid and electrolyte losses. Eventually, hypovolemia followed by shock will ensue. Renal failure, which may eventually occur from hypovolemic shock, causes the retention of ketones and glucose, and the acidosis progresses. Untreated, the patient becomes comatose as a result of dehydration, electrolyte imbalance, and acidosis. If the condition is not treated, death is inevitable.

Clinical Manifestations

Dehydration occurs in DKA with manifestations of poor skin turgor, dry mucous membranes, tachycardia, and orthostatic hypotension. Early symptoms may include lethargy and weakness. As the patient becomes severely dehydrated, the skin becomes dry and loose, and the eyes become soft and sunken. Abdominal pain may be present and accompanied by anorexia, nausea, and vomiting. *Kussmaul respirations* (rapid, deep breathing associated with dyspnea) are the body's attempt to reverse metabolic acidosis through the exhalation of excess carbon dioxide. Acetone is noted on the breath as a sweet, fruity odor. (See Chapter 17 for a discussion of respiratory compensation of metabolic acidosis.) Laboratory findings include a blood glucose level greater than or equal to 250 mg/dL (13.9 mmol/L), arterial blood pH less than 7.30, serum bicarbonate level less than 16 mEq/L (16 mmol/L), and moderate to large ketones in the urine or serum.[10]

Collaborative Care

Before the advent of SMBG, patients with DKA required hospitalization for treatment. Today, hospitalization may not be required. If fluid and electrolyte imbalances are not severe and blood glucose levels can be safely monitored at home, DKA may be managed on an outpatient basis (Table 49-17). Other factors

---

TABLE 49-17   COLLABORATIVE CARE

Diabetic Ketoacidosis (DKA) and Hyperosmolar Hyperglycemic Syndrome (HHS)

Diagnostic
- History and physical examination
- Blood studies, including immediate blood glucose, complete blood count, pH, ketones, electrolytes, blood urea nitrogen, arterial or venous blood gases
- Urinalysis, including specific gravity, glucose, acetone

Collaborative Therapy
- Administration of IV fluids
- IV administration of short-acting insulin
- Electrolyte replacement
- Assessment of mental status
- Recording of intake and output
- Central venous pressure monitoring (if indicated)
- Assessment of blood glucose levels
- Assessment of blood and urine for ketones
- ECG monitoring
- Assessment of cardiovascular and respiratory status

---

to consider when deciding where the patient is managed include the presence of fever, nausea, vomiting, and diarrhea; altered mental status; the cause of the ketoacidosis; and availability of frequent communication with the health care provider (every few hours). Patients with DKA who have an illness such as pneumonia or a urinary tract infection are usually admitted to the hospital.

DKA is a serious condition that proceeds rapidly and must be treated promptly. Refer to Table 49-18 for the emergency management of a patient with DKA. Because fluid imbalance is potentially life threatening, the initial goal of therapy is to establish IV access and begin fluid and electrolyte replacement. Typically, an infusion of 0.45% or 0.9% NaCl at a rate to restore urine output to 30 to 60 mL/hr and to raise BP constitutes the initial fluid therapy regimen. When blood glucose levels approach 250 mg/dL (13.9 mmol/L), 5% to 10% dextrose is added to the fluid regimen to prevent hypoglycemia and a sudden drop in glucose that can be associated with cerebral edema.[10] Overzealous rehydration, especially with hypotonic IV solutions, can result in cerebral edema.

The aim of fluid and electrolyte therapy is to replace extracellular and intracellular water and to correct deficits of sodium, chloride, bicarbonate, potassium, phosphate, magnesium, and nitrogen. Monitor patients with renal or cardiac compromise for fluid overload. Obtain a serum potassium level before starting insulin. If the patient is hypokalemic, insulin administration will further decrease the potassium levels, making early potassium replacement essential. Although initial serum potassium may be normal or high, levels can rapidly decrease once therapy starts as insulin drives potassium into the cells, leading to life-threatening hypokalemia.

IV insulin administration therapy is directed toward correcting hyperglycemia and hyperketonemia. Insulin is immediately started at 0.1 U/kg/hr by a continuous infusion. It is important to prevent rapid drops in serum glucose to avoid cerebral edema. A blood glucose reduction of 36 to 54 mg/dL/hr (2 to 3 mmol/L/hr) will avoid complications.[10] Insulin allows water and potassium to enter the cell along with glucose and can lead to a depletion of vascular volume and hypokalemia, so monitor the patient's fluid balance and potassium levels.

PATHOPHYSIOLOGY MAP

FIG. 49-11 Metabolic events leading to diabetic ketoacidosis.

✚ TABLE 49-18   EMERGENCY MANAGEMENT

Diabetic Ketoacidosis

Etiology	Assessment Findings	Interventions
• Undiagnosed diabetes mellitus • Inadequate treatment of existing diabetes mellitus • Insulin not taken as prescribed • Infection • Change in diet, insulin, or exercise regimen	• Dry mouth • Thirst • Abdominal pain • Nausea and vomiting • Gradually increasing restlessness, confusion, lethargy • Flushed, dry skin • Eyes appearing sunken • Breath odor of ketones • Rapid, weak pulse • Labored breathing (Kussmaul respirations) • Fever • Urinary frequency • Serum glucose >250 mg/dL (13.9 mmol/L) • Glucosuria and ketonuria	**Initial** • Ensure patent airway. • Administer O₂ via nasal cannula or non-rebreather mask. • Establish IV access with large-bore catheter. • Begin fluid resuscitation with 0.9% NaCl solution 1 L/hr until BP stabilized and urine output 30-60 mL/hr. • Begin continuous regular insulin drip 0.1 U/kg/hr. • Identify history of diabetes, time of last food, and time and amount of last insulin injection. **Ongoing Monitoring** • Monitor vital signs, level of consciousness, cardiac rhythm, O₂ saturation, and urine output. • Assess breath sounds for fluid overload. • Monitor serum glucose and serum potassium. • Administer potassium to correct hypokalemia. • Administer sodium bicarbonate if severe acidosis (pH <7.0).

HYPEROSMOLAR HYPERGLYCEMIC SYNDROME

Hyperosmolar hyperglycemic syndrome (HHS) is a life-threatening syndrome that can occur in the patient with diabetes who is able to produce enough insulin to prevent DKA but not enough to prevent severe hyperglycemia, osmotic diuresis, and extracellular fluid depletion (Fig. 49-12). HHS is less common than DKA. It often occurs in patients over 60 years of age with type 2 diabetes.

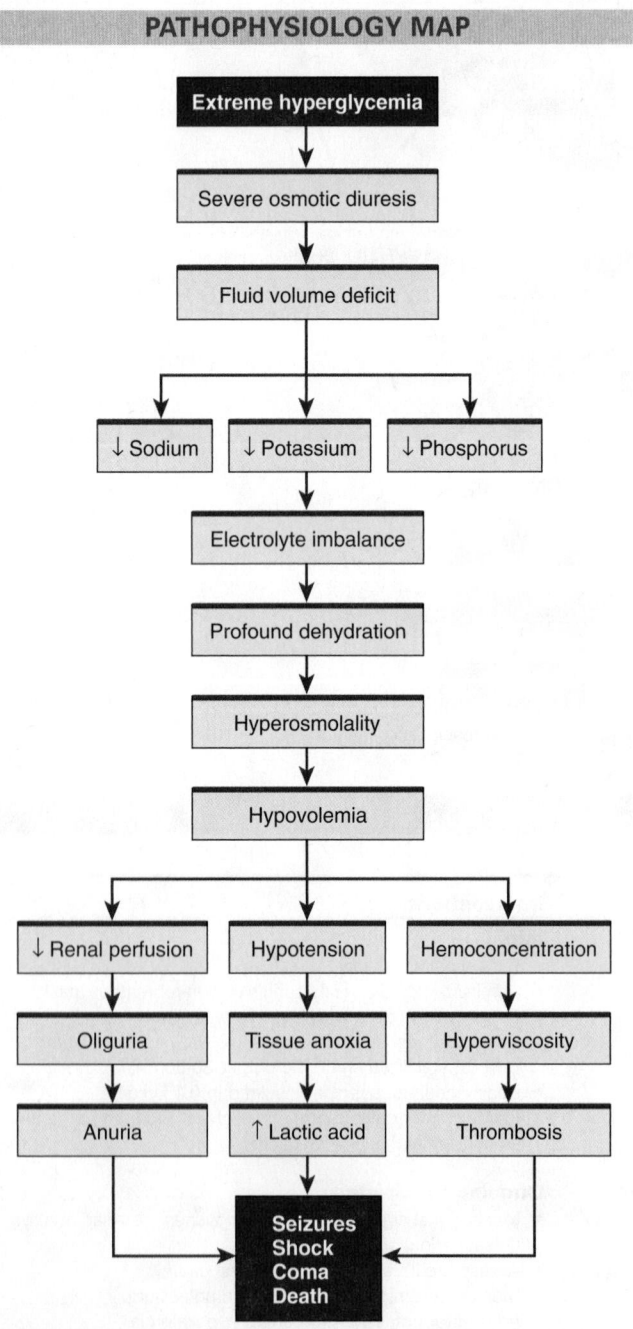

PATHOPHYSIOLOGY MAP

FIG. 49-12 Pathophysiology of hyperosmolar hyperglycemic syndrome.

Common causes of HHS are urinary tract infections, pneumonia, sepsis, any acute illness, and newly diagnosed type 2 diabetes. HHS is often related to impaired thirst sensation and/or a functional inability to replace fluids. There is usually a history of inadequate fluid intake, increasing mental depression, and polyuria.

The main difference between HHS and DKA is that the patient with HHS usually has enough circulating insulin so that ketoacidosis does not occur. Because HHS produces fewer symptoms in the earlier stages, blood glucose levels can climb quite high before the problem is recognized. The higher blood glucose levels increase serum osmolality and produce more severe neurologic manifestations, such as somnolence, coma, seizures, hemiparesis, and aphasia. Since these manifestations resemble a stroke, immediate determination of the glucose level is critical for correct diagnosis and treatment.

Laboratory values in HHS include a blood glucose level greater than 600 mg/dL (33.33 mmol/L) and a marked increase in serum osmolality. Ketone bodies are absent or minimal in both blood and urine.

Collaborative Care

HHS constitutes a medical emergency and has a high mortality rate. The management of DKA and HHS is similar and includes immediate IV administration insulin and either 0.9% or 0.45% NaCl. HHS usually requires greater volumes of fluid replacement (see Table 49-17). This should be accomplished slowly and carefully. Patients with HHS are commonly older and may have cardiac or renal compromise, requiring hemodynamic monitoring to avoid fluid overload during fluid replacement. When blood glucose levels fall to approximately 250 mg/dL (13.9 mmol/L), IV fluids containing glucose are administered to prevent hypoglycemia.

Electrolytes are monitored and replaced as needed. Hypokalemia is not as significant in HHS as it is in DKA, although fluid losses may result in milder potassium deficits that require replacement. Assess vital signs, intake and output, tissue turgor, laboratory values, and cardiac monitoring to check the efficacy of fluid and electrolyte replacement. This includes monitoring serum osmolality and frequently assessing cardiac, renal, and mental status.[10] Once the patient is stabilized, initiate attempts to detect and correct the underlying cause.

NURSING MANAGEMENT
DIABETIC KETOACIDOSIS AND HYPEROSMOLAR HYPERGLYCEMIC SYNDROME

Closely monitor the hospitalized patient with appropriate blood and urine tests. You are responsible for monitoring blood glucose and urine for output and ketones and using laboratory data to determine appropriate patient care.

Monitor the administration of (1) IV fluids to correct dehydration, (2) insulin therapy to reduce blood glucose and serum ketone levels, and (3) electrolytes given to correct electrolyte imbalance. Assess renal status and the cardiopulmonary status related to hydration and electrolyte levels. Monitor the level of consciousness.

Assess for signs of potassium imbalance resulting from hypoinsulinemia and osmotic diuresis (see Chapter 17). When insulin treatment is begun, serum potassium levels may decrease rapidly as potassium moves into the cells once insulin becomes available. This movement of potassium into and out of extracellular fluid influences cardiac functioning. Cardiac monitoring is useful in detecting hyperkalemia and hypokalemia because characteristic changes indicating potassium excess or deficit are observable on electrocardiogram (ECG) tracings (see Fig. 17-14). Assess vital signs often to identify fever, hypovolemic shock, tachycardia, and Kussmaul respirations.

HYPOGLYCEMIA

Hypoglycemia, or low blood glucose, occurs when there is too much insulin in proportion to available glucose in the blood. This causes the blood glucose level to drop to less than 70 mg/dL (3.9 mmol/L). When plasma glucose drops below 70 mg/dL, counterregulatory hormones are released and the autonomic nervous system is activated. Suppression of insulin secretion and production of glucagon and epinephrine provide defense against hypoglycemia. Epinephrine release causes manifestations that include shakiness, palpitations, nervousness, diaphoresis, anxiety, hunger, and pallor. Because the brain requires a constant supply of glucose in sufficient quantities to function properly, hypoglycemia can affect mental functioning. These manifestations are difficulty speaking, visual disturbances, stupor, confusion, and coma. Manifestations of hypoglycemia can mimic alcohol intoxication. Untreated hypoglycemia can progress to loss of consciousness, seizures, coma, and death.

Hypoglycemic unawareness is a condition in which a person does not experience the warning signs and symptoms of hypoglycemia until the glucose levels reach a critical point. Then the person may become incoherent and combative or lose consciousness. This is often related to autonomic neuropathy of diabetes that interferes with the secretion of counterregulatory hormones that produce these symptoms. Patients at risk for hypoglycemic unawareness include those who have had repeated episodes of hypoglycemia, older patients, and patients who use β-adrenergic blockers. Using intensive treatment to get tight blood glucose control in patients who are at risk for hypoglycemic unawareness may not be an appropriate goal because a major drawback is hypoglycemia. These patients are usually managed with blood glucose goals that are somewhat higher than those of patients who are able to detect and manage the onset of hypoglycemia.

Causes of hypoglycemia are often related to a mismatch in the timing of food intake and the peak action of insulin or oral hypoglycemic agents that increase endogenous insulin secretion. The balance between blood glucose and insulin can be disrupted by administering too much insulin or medication, ingesting too little food, delaying the time of eating, and performing unusual amounts of exercise. Hypoglycemia can occur at any time, but most episodes occur when the OA or insulin is at its peak of action or when the patient's daily routine is disrupted without adequate adjustments in diet, medications, and activity. Although hypoglycemia is more common with insulin therapy, it can occur with noninsulin injectable agents and OAs, and it may be severe and persist for an extended time because of the longer duration of action.

Hypoglycemic symptoms may occur when a very high blood glucose level falls too rapidly (e.g., a blood glucose level of 300 mg/dL [16.7 mmol/L] falling quickly to 180 mg/dL [10 mmol/L]). Although the blood glucose level is above normal by definition and measurement, the sudden metabolic shift can evoke hypoglycemic symptoms. Too vigorous management of hyperglycemia with insulin can cause this type of situation.

NURSING AND COLLABORATIVE MANAGEMENT HYPOGLYCEMIA

Hypoglycemia can usually be quickly reversed with effective treatment. At the first sign of hypoglycemia, check the blood glucose if possible. If it is less than 70 mg/dL (3.9 mmol/L), immediately begin treatment for hypoglycemia. If the blood glucose is greater than 70 mg/dL, investigate other possible causes of the signs and symptoms. If the patient has manifestations of hypoglycemia and monitoring equipment is not available or the patient has a history of chronic poor glycemic control, hypoglycemia should be assumed and treatment initiated.

Follow the "Rule of 15" to treat hypoglycemia (Table 49-19). A blood glucose less than 70 mg/dL is treated by ingesting 15 g of a simple (fast-acting) carbohydrate, such as 4 to 6 oz of fruit juice or a regular soft drink. Commercial products such as gels or tablets containing specific amounts of glucose are convenient for carrying in a purse or pocket to be used in such situations. Recheck the blood glucose 15 minutes later. If the value is still less than 70 mg/dL, ingest 15 g more of carbohydrate and recheck the blood glucose in 15 minutes. If no significant improvement occurs after two or three doses of 15 g of simple carbohydrate, contact the health care provider. Because of the potential for rebound hypoglycemia after an acute episode, have the patient ingest a complex carbohydrate after recovery to prevent another hypoglycemic attack.

Avoid treatment with carbohydrates that contain fat, such as candy bars, cookies, whole milk, and ice cream. The fat in those foods will slow the absorption of the glucose and delay the response to treatment. Avoid overtreatment with large quantities of quick-acting carbohydrates so that a rapid fluctuation to hyperglycemia does not occur.

TABLE 49-19 COLLABORATIVE CARE

Hypoglycemia

Diagnostic
- History of hypoglycemic episodes and symptoms.
- Blood glucose—immediately.

Collaborative Therapy
- Determine cause of hypoglycemia (after correction of condition).

Conscious Patient
- Have patient eat or drink 15 g of quick-acting carbohydrate (4-6 oz of regular soda, 8-10 LifeSavers, 1 tbs syrup or honey, 4 tsp jelly, 4-6 oz orange juice, commercial dextrose products [per label instructions]).
- Wait 15 min. Then check blood glucose again.
- If blood glucose is still <70 mg/dL, have patient repeat treatment of 15 g of carbohydrate.
- Once the glucose level is stable and the next meal is more than 1 hr away, give patient additional food of longer-acting combination carbohydrate plus protein or fat (e.g., crackers with peanut butter or cheese) after symptoms subside.
- Immediately notify health care provider or emergency service (if patient outside hospital) if symptoms do not subside after two or three administrations of quick-acting carbohydrate.

Worsening Symptoms or Unconscious Patient
- Subcutaneous or IM injection of 1 mg glucagon. IV administration of 25-50 mL of 50% glucose.

In an acute care setting, patients with hypoglycemia may be treated with 20 to 50 mL of 50% dextrose IV push. Another option, if the patient is not alert enough to swallow and no IV access is available, is to administer 1 mg of glucagon by intramuscular (IM) or subcutaneous injection. An IM injection in a site such as the deltoid muscle will result in a quicker response. Glucagon stimulates a strong hepatic response to convert glycogen to glucose and therefore makes glucose rapidly available. Nausea is a common reaction after glucagon injection. Therefore, to prevent aspiration if vomiting occurs, turn the patient on the side until he or she becomes alert. Patients with minimal glycogen stores will not respond to glucagon. This includes patients with alcohol-related hepatic disease, starvation, and adrenal insufficiency. Teach family members and others likely to be present when a severe hypoglycemic episode occurs when to use and how to inject glucagon.

Once the acute hypoglycemia has been reversed, explore with the patient the reasons why the situation developed. This assessment may indicate the need for additional teaching of the patient and the family to avoid future episodes of hypoglycemia.

CHRONIC COMPLICATIONS OF DIABETES MELLITUS

ANGIOPATHY

Chronic complications of diabetes are primarily those of end-organ disease from damage to blood vessels *(angiopathy)* secondary to chronic hyperglycemia (Fig. 49-13). Angiopathy is one of the leading causes of diabetes-related deaths, with about 68% of deaths caused by CVD and 16% caused by strokes for those ages 65 or older.[2] These chronic blood vessel dysfunctions are divided into two categories: macrovascular complications and microvascular complications.

Several theories exist as to how and why chronic hyperglycemia damages cells and tissues. Possible causes include (1) the accumulation of damaging by-products of glucose metabolism, such as sorbitol, which is associated with damage to nerve cells; (2) the formation of abnormal glucose molecules in the basement membrane of small blood vessels such as those that circulate to the eye and kidney; and (3) a derangement in red blood cell function that leads to a decrease in oxygenation to the tissues.

The Diabetes Control and Complications Trial (DCCT), a landmark study in diabetes management, demonstrated that in patients with type 1 diabetes the risk for microvascular complications could be significantly reduced by keeping blood glucose levels as near to normal as possible for as much of the time as possible *(tight glucose control).*[20] Subjects who maintained tight glucose control reduced their risk of developing retinopathy and nephropathy, some of the most common microvascular complications. Based on these findings, the ADA issued recommendations for the management of diabetes that included treatment goals to maintain blood glucose levels as near to normal as possible. Specific targets for individual patients must take into account the risk for severe or undetected hypoglycemia as a side effect of tight glucose control.

The United Kingdom Prospective Diabetes Study (UKPDS) demonstrated that intensive treatment of type 2 diabetes significantly lowered the risk for developing diabetes-related eye, kidney, and neurologic problems. The findings from this study included a 25% reduction of microvascular disease and a 16%

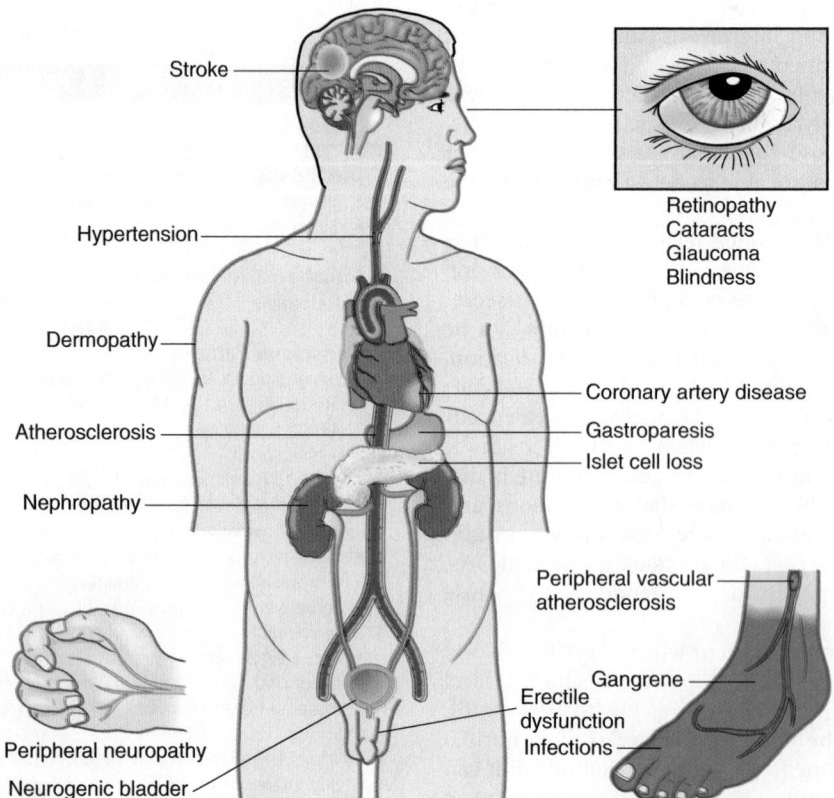

FIG. 49-13 Long-term complications of diabetes mellitus.

reduction in the risk for myocardial infarction in subjects who maintained long-term glycemic control.[21]

Because of the devastating effects of long-term complications, patients with diabetes require scheduled and ongoing monitoring for the detection and prevention of chronic complications. The ADA recommendations for ongoing evaluation are listed in Table 49-20. It is imperative that patients understand the importance of participating in regular follow-up examinations.

Macrovascular Complications

Macrovascular complications are diseases of the large and medium-size blood vessels that occur with greater frequency and with an earlier onset in people with diabetes. Macrovascular diseases include cerebrovascular, cardiovascular, and peripheral vascular disease. Women with diabetes have a four to six times increased risk for CVD, and men with diabetes have a two to three times increased risk for CVD compared with those without diabetes.[4] Patients with diabetes can decrease several risk factors associated with macrovascular complications, such as obesity, smoking, hypertension, high fat intake, and sedentary lifestyle. Smoking, which is detrimental to health in general, is especially injurious to people with diabetes and significantly increases their risk for blood vessel and cardiovascular disease, stroke, and lower extremity amputation. The ADA recommends yearly screening of diabetic patients for CVD risk factors.[10]

Optimizing BP control in patients with diabetes is significant for the prevention of cardiovascular and renal disease. Treating hypertension in diabetic patients results in a decrease in mac-

rovascular and microvascular complications. Hypertension in people with diabetes causes an increase in mortality greater than for those with hypertension without diabetes.[2] A target BP of less than 130/80 mm Hg is recommended for most patients with diabetes.[22]

Patients with diabetes have an increase in lipid abnormalities. This contributes to the increase in CVD seen in this population. The ADA recommends target values of LDL cholesterol less than 100 mg/dL (2.6 mmol/L), triglycerides less than 150 mg/dL (1.7 mmol/L), and HDL cholesterol greater than 40 mg/dL (1.0 mmol/L) in men and greater than 50 mg/dL (1.3 mmol/L) in women.[10] The ADA advocates lifestyle interventions, including nutritional therapy, exercise, weight loss, and smoking cessation to treat hyperlipidemia. Medications (primarily statins) are recommended for those who do not reach lipid goals with lifestyle modifications and for people over 40 years of age with other CVD risk factors regardless of their baseline lipid levels. (Hypertension is discussed in Chapter 33, and coronary artery disease is discussed in Chapter 34.)

Insulin resistance has an important role in the development of CVD and is implicated in the pathogenesis of essential hypertension and dyslipidemia. The role of insulin resistance in the pathogenesis of CVD is not well understood, but it seems to combine with dyslipidemia in contributing to greater risk of CVD in patients with diabetes mellitus. All patients with diabetes should be screened for dyslipidemia at the time diabetes is diagnosed.

Microvascular Complications

Microvascular complications result from thickening of the vessel membranes in the capillaries and arterioles in response to conditions of chronic hyperglycemia. They differ from the macrovascular complications in that they are specific to diabetes. Although microangiopathy can be found throughout the body, the areas most noticeably affected are the eyes (retinopathy), the kidneys (nephropathy), and the skin (dermopathy). Microvascular changes are present in some patients with type 2 diabetes at the time of diagnosis.

DIABETIC RETINOPATHY

Etiology and Pathophysiology

Diabetic retinopathy refers to the process of microvascular damage to the retina as a result of chronic hyperglycemia, nephropathy, and hypertension in patients with diabetes. Diabetic retinopathy is estimated to be the most common cause of new cases of adult blindness.[2]

Retinopathy can be classified as nonproliferative or proliferative. In *nonproliferative retinopathy,* the most common form, partial occlusion of the small blood vessels in the retina causes microaneurysms to develop in the capillary walls. The walls of these microaneurysms are so weak that capillary fluid leaks out, causing retinal edema and eventually hard exudates or intraretinal hemorrhages. Vision may be affected if the macula is involved.

Proliferative retinopathy, the most severe form, involves the retina and the vitreous. When retinal capillaries become occluded, the body compensates by forming new blood vessels to supply the retina with blood, a pathologic process known as *neovascularization.* These new vessels are extremely fragile and hemorrhage easily, producing vitreous contraction. Eventually light is prevented from reaching the retina as the vessels become

TABLE 49-20	MONITORING FOR LONG-TERM COMPLICATIONS OF DIABETES MELLITUS	
Complication	**Type of Examination**	**Frequency**
Retinopathy	• Funduscopic—dilated eye examination • Fundus photography	• Annually
Nephropathy	• Urine for microalbuminuria • Serum creatinine	• Annually
Neuropathy (foot and lower extremities)	• Visual examination of foot	• Daily by patient • Every visit to health care provider

	• Comprehensive foot:
	  • Visual examination
	  • Sensory examination with monofilament and tuning fork
	  • Palpation (pulses, temperature, callus formation)
		• Annually

Cardiovascular disease	• Risk factor assessment: hypertension, dyslipidemia, smoking, family history of premature coronary artery disease, and presence of microalbuminuria or macroalbuminuria	• At least annually
	• Exercise stress testing (may include stress ECG, stress echocardiogram, stress nuclear imaging)	• As needed based on risk factors

Source: Standards of medical care in diabetes, *Diabetes Care* 36 (Suppl):S11, 2013.

torn and bleed into the vitreous cavity. The patient sees black or red spots or lines. If these new blood vessels pull the retina while the vitreous contracts, causing a tear, partial or complete retinal detachment will occur. If the macula is involved, vision is lost. Without treatment, more than half of patients with proliferative diabetic retinopathy will be blind.

Persons with diabetes are also prone to other visual problems. Glaucoma occurs as a result of the occlusion of the outflow channels secondary to neovascularization. This type of glaucoma is difficult to treat and often results in blindness. Cataracts develop at an earlier age and progress more rapidly in people with diabetes.

Collaborative Care

The earliest and most treatable stages of diabetic retinopathy often produce no changes in the vision. Therefore patients with type 2 diabetes should have a dilated eye examination by an ophthalmologist or a specially trained optometrist at the time of diagnosis and annually thereafter for early detection and treatment. A person with type 1 diabetes should have a dilated eye examination within 5 years after the onset of diabetes and then repeated annually.[10]

The best approach to the management of diabetic eye disease is to prevent it by maintaining good glycemic control and managing hypertension. Laser photocoagulation therapy is indicated to reduce the risk of vision loss in patients with proliferative retinopathy or macular edema and in some cases of nonproliferative retinopathy.[23] Laser photocoagulation destroys the ischemic areas of the retina that produce growth factors that encourage neovascularization. A patient who develops vitreous hemorrhage and retinal detachment of the macula may need to undergo vitrectomy. *Vitrectomy* is the aspiration of blood, membrane, and fibers from the inside of the eye through a small incision just behind the cornea. (Photocoagulation and vitrectomy are discussed in Chapter 22.)

Recent research has identified the importance of vascular endothelial growth factor (VEFG) in the development of diabetic retinopathy. Drugs injected into the eye that block the action of VEGF and reduce inflammation are currently being studied for their effectiveness in treating retinopathy.[23]

NEPHROPATHY

Diabetic nephropathy is a microvascular complication associated with damage to the small blood vessels that supply the glomeruli of the kidney. It is the leading cause of end-stage kidney disease in the United States and is seen in 20% to 40% of people with diabetes. Risk factors for diabetic nephropathy include hypertension, genetic predisposition, smoking, and chronic hyperglycemia. Results of the DCCT and UKPDS research have demonstrated that kidney disease can be significantly reduced when near-normal blood glucose control is maintained.[20,21]

Patients with diabetes are screened for nephropathy annually with a random spot urine collection to assess for albuminuria and measure the albumin-to-creatinine ratio. Serum creatinine is also measured to provide an estimation of the glomerular filtration rate and thus the degree of kidney function.

Patients with diabetes who have microalbuminuria or macroalbuminuria should receive either angiotensin-converting enzyme (ACE) inhibitor drugs (e.g., lisinopril [Prinivil, Zestril]) or angiotensin II receptor antagonists (e.g., losartan [Cozaar]).

Both classifications of these drugs are used to treat hypertension and have been found to delay the progression of nephropathy in patients with diabetes.[10] Hypertension significantly accelerates the progression of nephropathy. Therefore aggressive BP management is indicated for all patients with diabetes. Tight blood glucose control is also critical in the prevention and delay of diabetic nephropathy. (See Chapter 33 for a discussion of hypertension and Chapter 47 for a discussion of renal failure.)

NEUROPATHY

Diabetic neuropathy is nerve damage that occurs because of the metabolic derangements associated with diabetes mellitus. About 60% to 70% of patients with diabetes have some degree of neuropathy.[2] The most common type of neuropathy affecting persons with diabetes is sensory neuropathy. This can lead to the loss of protective sensation in the lower extremities, and, coupled with other factors, significantly increases the risk for complications that result in a lower limb amputation. More than 60% of nontraumatic amputations in the United States occur in people with diabetes.[2] Screening for neuropathy should begin at the time of diagnosis in patients with type 2 diabetes and 5 years after diagnosis in patients with type 1 diabetes.[10]

Etiology and Pathophysiology

The pathophysiologic processes of diabetic neuropathy are not well understood. Several theories exist, including metabolic, vascular, and autoimmune factors. The prevailing theory is that persistent hyperglycemia leads to an accumulation of sorbitol and fructose in the nerves that causes damage by an unknown mechanism. The result is reduced nerve conduction and demyelinization. Ischemic damage by chronic hyperglycemia in blood vessels that supply the peripheral nerves is also implicated in the development of diabetic neuropathy. Neuropathy can precede, accompany, or follow the diagnosis of diabetes.

Classification

The two major categories of diabetic neuropathy are *sensory neuropathy*, which affects the peripheral nervous system, and *autonomic neuropathy*. Each of these types can take on several forms.

Sensory Neuropathy. The most common form of sensory neuropathy is distal symmetric polyneuropathy, which affects the hands and/or feet bilaterally. This is sometimes referred to as *stocking-glove neuropathy*. Characteristics of distal symmetric polyneuropathy include loss of sensation, abnormal sensations, pain, and paresthesias. The pain, which is often described as burning, cramping, crushing, or tearing, is usually worse at night and may occur only at that time. The paresthesias may be associated with tingling, burning, and itching sensations. The patient may report a feeling of walking on pillows or numb feet. At times the skin becomes so sensitive (hyperesthesia) that even light pressure from bed sheets cannot be tolerated. Complete or partial loss of sensitivity to touch and temperature is common. Foot injury and ulcerations can occur without the patient ever having pain (Fig. 49-14). Neuropathy can also cause atrophy of the small muscles of the hands and feet, causing deformity and limiting fine movement.

Control of blood glucose is the only treatment for diabetic neuropathy. It is effective in many, but not all, cases. Drug therapy may be used to treat neuropathic symptoms, particu-

FIG. 49-14 Neuropathy: neurotrophic ulceration.

FIG. 49-15 The necrotic toe developed as a complication of diabetes. **A,** Before amputation. **B,** After amputation.

larly pain. Medications commonly used include topical creams (e.g., capsaicin [Zostrix]), tricyclic antidepressants (e.g., amitriptyline [Elavil]), selective serotonin and norepinephrine reuptake inhibitors (e.g., duloxetine [Cymbalta]), and antiseizure medications (e.g., gabapentin [Neurontin], pregabalin [Lyrica]). Capsaicin is a moderately effective topical cream made from chili peppers. It depletes the accumulation of pain-mediating chemicals in the peripheral sensory neurons. The cream is applied three or four times a day. At the start of therapy, symptoms usually increase, followed by relief of pain in 2 to 3 weeks. Tricyclic antidepressants are moderately effective in treating the symptoms of diabetic neuropathy. They work by inhibiting the reuptake of norepinephrine and serotonin, which are neurotransmitters believed to play a role in the transmission of pain through the spinal cord. Duloxetine is thought to relieve pain by increasing the levels of serotonin and norepinephrine, which improves the body's ability to regulate pain. Antiseizure medications decrease the release of neurotransmitters that transmit pain.[24]

Autonomic Neuropathy. Autonomic neuropathy can affect nearly all body systems and lead to hypoglycemic unawareness, bowel incontinence and diarrhea, and urinary retention. *Gastroparesis* (delayed gastric emptying) is a complication of autonomic neuropathy that can produce anorexia, nausea, vomiting, gastroesophageal reflux, and persistent feelings of fullness. Gastroparesis can trigger hypoglycemia by delaying food absorption. Cardiovascular abnormalities associated with autonomic neuropathy are postural hypotension, resting tachycardia, and painless myocardial infarction. Assess patients with diabetes for postural hypotension to determine if they are at risk for falls. Instruct the patient with postural hypotension to change from a lying or sitting position slowly.

Diabetes can affect sexual function in men and women. Erectile dysfunction (ED) in diabetic men is well recognized and common, often being the first manifestation of autonomic neuropathy. ED in diabetes is also associated with other factors, including vascular disease, poor metabolic control, endocrine disorders, psychogenic factors, and medications. Decreased libido is a problem for some women with diabetes. Candidal and nonspecific vaginitis is also common. ED or sexual dysfunction requires sensitive therapeutic counseling for both the patient and the patient's partner. (See Chapter 55 for a further discussion of ED.)

A neurogenic bladder may develop as the sensation in the inner bladder wall decreases, causing urinary retention. A patient with retention has infrequent voiding, difficulty voiding, and a weak stream of urine. Emptying the bladder every 3 hours in a sitting position helps prevent stasis and subsequent infection. Tightening the abdominal muscles during voiding and using the Credé maneuver (mild massage downward over the lower abdomen and bladder) may also help with complete bladder emptying. Cholinergic agonist drugs such as bethanechol (Urecholine) may be used. The patient may also need to learn self-catheterization (see Chapter 46).

COMPLICATIONS OF FEET AND LOWER EXTREMITIES

People with diabetes are at high risk for foot ulcerations and lower extremity amputations.[25] The development of diabetic foot complications can be the result of a combination of microvascular and macrovascular diseases that place the patient at risk for injury and serious infection (Fig. 49-15). Sensory neuropathy and peripheral artery disease (PAD) are risk factors for foot complications. In addition, clotting abnormalities, impaired immune function, and autonomic neuropathy also have a role. Smoking is deleterious to the health of lower extremity blood vessels and increases the risk for amputation.

Sensory neuropathy is a major risk factor for lower extremity amputation in the person with diabetes. *Loss of protective sensation* (LOPS) often prevents the patient from being aware that a foot injury has occurred. Improper footwear and injury from stepping on foreign objects while barefoot are common causes of undetected foot injury in the person with LOPS.[26] Because the primary risk factor for lower extremity amputation is LOPS, annual screening using a *monofilament* is important. This is done by applying a thin, flexible filament to several spots on the plantar surface of the foot and asking the patient to report if it is felt. Insensitivity to a monofilament has been shown to greatly increase the risk for diabetic foot ulcers that can lead to amputation.

PAD increases the risk for amputation by causing a reduction in blood flow to the lower extremities. When blood flow is decreased, oxygen, white blood cells, and vital nutrients are not available to the tissues. Wounds take longer to heal, and the risk for infection increases. Signs of PAD include intermittent claudication, pain at rest, cold feet, loss of hair, delayed capillary filling, and dependent rubor (redness of the skin that occurs when the extremity is in a dependent position). The disease is diagnosed by history, ankle-brachial index (ABI) (see Table 38-3), and angiography. Management includes control or reduction of risk factors, particularly smoking, high cholesterol intake, and hypertension. Bypass or graft surgery is indicated in some patients. (PAD is discussed in Chapter 38.)

If the patient has LOPS or PAD, aggressive measures must be taken to teach the patient how to prevent foot ulcers. These measures include the selection of proper footwear, including prescription shoes. The patient also must carefully avoid injury to the foot, practice diligent skin and nail care, inspect the foot thoroughly each day, and treat small problems promptly.[26] Guidelines for patient teaching are listed in Table 49-21.

Proper care of a diabetic foot ulcer is critical for wound healing. Several forms of treatment can be used. Casting can be done to redistribute the weight on the plantar surface of the foot. Wound control for the ulcer can include debridement, dressings, advanced wound healing products (becaplermin [Regranex]), vacuum-assisted closure, ultrasound, hyperbaric oxygen, and skin grafting.[26]

TABLE 49-21	PATIENT & CAREGIVER TEACHING GUIDE*

Foot Care

Include the following instructions when teaching the patient and caregiver about diabetic foot care.

1. Wash feet daily with a mild soap and warm water. First test water temperature with hands.
2. Pat feet dry gently, especially between toes.
3. Examine feet daily for cuts, blisters, swelling, and red, tender areas. Do not depend on feeling sores. If eyesight is poor, have others inspect feet.
4. Use lanolin on feet to prevent skin from drying and cracking. Do not apply between toes.
5. Use mild foot powder on sweaty feet.
6. Do not use commercial remedies to remove calluses or corns.
7. Cleanse cuts with warm water and mild soap, covering with clean dressing. Do not use iodine, rubbing alcohol, or strong adhesives.
8. Report skin infections or nonhealing sores to health care provider immediately.
9. Cut toenails evenly with rounded contour of toes. Do not cut down corners. The best time to trim nails is after a shower or bath.
10. Separate overlapping toes with cotton or lamb's wool.
11. Avoid open-toe, open-heel, and high-heel shoes. Leather shoes are preferred to plastic ones. Wear slippers with soles. Do not go barefoot. Shake out shoes before putting on.
12. Wear clean, absorbent (cotton or wool) socks or stockings that have not been mended. Colored socks must be colorfast.
13. Do not wear clothing that leaves impressions, hindering circulation.
14. Do not use hot water bottles or heating pads to warm feet. Wear socks for warmth.
15. Guard against frostbite.
16. Exercise feet daily either by walking or by flexing and extending feet in suspended position. Avoid prolonged sitting, standing, and crossing of legs.

*This teaching guide is also appropriate for patients with peripheral vascular problems.

Neuropathic arthropathy, or *Charcot's foot,* results in ankle and foot changes that ultimately lead to joint dysfunction and footdrop. These changes occur gradually and promote an abnormal distribution of weight over the foot, further increasing the chances of developing a foot ulcer as new pressure points emerge. Foot deformity should be recognized early and proper footwear fitted before ulceration occurs.

INTEGUMENTARY COMPLICATIONS

Up to two thirds of persons with diabetes develop skin problems.[10] Diabetic dermopathy, the most common diabetic skin lesion, is characterized by reddish brown, round or oval patches. They initially are scaly, then they flatten out and become indented. The lesions appear most frequently on the shins, but can also be found on the front of the thighs, forearm, side of the foot, scalp, and trunk.

Acanthosis nigricans is a velvety light brown to black skin thickening, predominantly seen on flexures, axillae, and the neck. *Necrobiosis lipoidica diabeticorum* usually appears as red-yellow lesions, with atrophic skin that becomes shiny and transparent revealing tiny blood vessels under the surface (Fig. 49-16). This condition is uncommon and occurs more frequently in young women. It may appear before other clinical signs or symptoms of diabetes. Because the thin skin is prone to injury, special care must be taken to protect affected areas from injury and ulceration.

INFECTION

A person with diabetes is more susceptible to infections because of a defect in the mobilization of white blood cells and an impaired phagocytosis by neutrophils and monocytes. Recurring or persistent infections such as *Candida albicans,* as well as boils and furuncles, in the undiagnosed patient often lead the health care provider to suspect diabetes. Loss of sensation (neuropathy) may delay the detection of an infection.

Persistent glycosuria may predispose patients to bladder infections, especially patients with a neurogenic bladder.

FIG. 49-16 Necrobiosis lipoidica diabeticorum.

Decreased circulation resulting from angiopathy can prevent or delay the immune response. Antibiotic therapy has prevented infection from being a major cause of death in diabetic patients. The treatment of infections must be prompt and vigorous. Teach diabetic patients measures to prevent infection: practicing good hand hygiene, avoiding exposure to individuals who have a communicable illness, and getting an annual influenza vaccine and pneumococcal vaccine (Pneumovax) every 5 years.

PSYCHOLOGIC CONSIDERATIONS

Patients with diabetes have high rates of depression, anxiety, and eating disorders. Depression contributes to poor adherence to diabetes self-care, feelings of helplessness related to chronic illness, and poor outcomes.[10] Assess patients for manifestations of depression.

Persons with type 1 diabetes have an increased risk of developing disordered eating behaviors (DEB).[27] The greatest incidence of eating disorders is seen in females. Adolescent girls

with diabetes are more than twice as likely to develop DEB than those who do not have diabetes.[28] DEBs include anorexia, bulimia, binge eating, excessive restriction of calories, and intense exercise. Patients may intentionally decrease their dose of insulin or omit the dose. This leads to weight loss, hyperglycemia, and glycosuria because the food ingested cannot be used for energy without adequate insulin. Insulin omission and DEBs can have serious consequences, including retinopathy, neuropathy, lipid abnormalities, DKA, and death.[28] Open com-

DELEGATION DECISIONS
Caring for the Patient With Diabetes Mellitus

Oral agents (OAs), noninsulin injectable agents, and insulin can be administered by licensed practical/vocational nurses (LPN/LVNs) (and in some states and settings by unlicensed assistive personnel [UAP]) to stable patients. In patients experiencing acute complications of diabetes mellitus (DM), actions such as insulin administration and infusion of IV fluids should be done or directly supervised by a registered nurse (RN).

Role of Registered Nurse (RN)
- Assess for risk factors for prediabetes and type 1 and type 2 DM.
- Teach the patient and caregiver about self-management of DM, including self-monitoring of blood glucose (SMBG), insulin, noninsulin injectables, OAs, nutrition, physical activity, and recognition and management of hypoglycemia.
- Develop a plan to avoid hypoglycemia or hyperglycemia in the patient with DM who is acutely ill or having surgery.
- Assess for acute complications and implement appropriate actions: hypoglycemia, diabetic ketoacidosis (DKA), and hyperosmolar hyperglycemic syndrome (HHS).
- Assess for chronic complications of diabetes, including cardiovascular disease, retinopathy, nephropathy, neuropathy, and diabetic foot complications.
- Teach patient and caregiver about prevention and management of chronic complications of diabetes.

Role of Licensed Practical/Vocational Nurse (LPN/LVN)
- Administer OAs and routinely scheduled insulin regimens.
- Monitor the diabetic patient for symptoms of hypoglycemia, DKA, and HHS.
- In the ambulatory or home setting, monitor patient self-management of insulin, OAs, nutrition, and physical activity.
- Report concerns with patient self-management in the home setting to the RN.

Role of Unlicensed Assistive Personnel (UAP)
- Check capillary blood glucose (CBG) levels (after being trained and evaluated in this procedure) and report values to the RN.
- Report changes in patient vital signs, urine output, behavior, or level of consciousness to the RN.
- In a community or home care setting, administer OAs and insulin to the stable diabetic patient (consider state nurse practice act and agency policy).

ETHICAL/LEGAL DILEMMAS
Durable Power of Attorney for Health Care

Situation
G.V., a 64-yr-old white woman, is admitted to the intensive care unit with heart failure. She has many complications from a long-term history of type 1 diabetes and hypertension, including a right leg above-the-knee amputation and blindness related to diabetic retinopathy. She severed ties with her family 30 yr ago. She has a life partner of 35 yr whom she designated as her proxy in her signed Durable Power of Attorney. She has stated many times that she would rather die than have renal dialysis. She has been sedated and intubated for 3 days. The physician plans to extubate her and resuscitate her so that dialysis can be initiated. Her brother shows up at the hospital and supports the physician's decision. Her partner disagrees with the decision. The physician refuses to recognize her partner as proxy because she is not a blood relative.

Ethical/Legal Points for Consideration
- The Patient Self-Determination Act (1990) requires all health care facilities receiving Medicare and Medicaid funding to make available advance directives allowing individuals to state their preferences or refusals of health care in the event that they are incapable of consenting for themselves.
- Durable Power of Attorney for health care is one type of advance directive in which people, when they are competent, identify someone else to make decisions for them, should they lose their decision-making ability in the future.
- The Living Will, another type of advance directive, permits individuals to state their own preferences and refusals.
- Many health care providers mistakenly think that proxies must be family members or blood relatives. Lesbian, gay, bisexual, and transgender individuals often have difficulty having their partnership recognized as valid, especially if the patient's family disputes their rights.
- Some families are deeply divided on decisions for their loved ones, and sometimes difficulties occur when money and property are also disputed. The passage of time may be an issue where the original documents were executed and then changes occurred (e.g., divorce, death or disability of the proxy, inability to contact the proxy, inability to find a valid original of the advance directive).
- Within your scope of nursing practice, you need to be informed as to decision-making laws and regulations in your own state and make advance directive documents available to patients. In addition, you need to (1) teach patients and their families about advance directives, (2) make sure that health care providers are aware of the presence of advance directives, (3) assist the patient and family in communicating with the health care providers when a "No Code" order is requested, and (4) assist a conflicted family in obtaining appropriate counseling whenever necessary.

Discussion Questions
1. How would you handle a situation in which the family and surrogate decision maker disagree?
2. How can you assess the patient and family's understanding of durable power of attorney and assist them in understanding their role in decision making?
3. What should you do when a physician orders dialysis to be initiated when you know that this goes against the patient's advance directive?

munication is critical to identify these behaviors early. Patients with eating disorders need to be seen by a mental health professional with expertise in eating disorders and an understanding of diabetes management.

GERONTOLOGIC CONSIDERATIONS

DIABETES MELLITUS

Diabetes is present in more than 25% of persons over 65 years of age, with this age-group being the fastest growing segment of the population developing diabetes.[2] Older people with diabetes have higher rates of premature death, functional disability, and coexisting illnesses such as hypertension and stroke than those without diabetes. The prevalence of diabetes increases with age. A major reason for this is that the process of aging is associated with a reduction in β-cell function, decreased insulin sensitivity, and altered carbohydrate metabolism. Aging is also associated with a number of conditions that are more likely to be treated with medications that impair insulin action (e.g., corticosteroids, antihypertensives, phenothiazines). Undiagnosed and untreated diabetes is more common in older adults, partly because many of the normal physiologic changes of aging resemble those of diabetes, such as low energy levels, falls, dizziness, confusion, and chronic urinary tract infections.

Several factors are taken into account when determining glycemic goals for an older adult. One is that hypoglycemic unawareness is more common in older adults, making these patients more likely to suffer adverse consequences from blood glucose–lowering therapy. They may have delayed psychomotor function that could interfere with the ability to treat hypo-glycemia. Other factors to consider in establishing glycemic goals for the older patient include the patient's own desire for treatment and coexisting medical problems such as cognitive impairment. Compounding the challenge, diabetes has been found to contribute to a greater rate of decline of cognitive function. Although it is generally agreed that treatment is indicated to prevent acute complications and avoid unpleasant symptoms, strict glycemic control may be difficult to achieve.

Diet and exercise are recommended as therapy for older adult patients with diabetes. This should take into account functional limitations that may interfere with physical activity and the ability to prepare meals. Because of the physiologic changes that occur with aging, the therapeutic outcome for the older adult with diabetes who receives OAs may be altered. Assess renal function and creatinine clearance in patients over 80 years of age taking metformin. Monitor those taking sulfonylurea drugs (e.g., glipizide) for hypoglycemia and renal and liver dysfunction. Insulin therapy may be instituted if OAs are not effective. However, it is important to recognize that older adults are more likely to have limitations in the manual dexterity and visual acuity necessary for accurate insulin administration. Insulin pens may be a safer alternative for older adults.

Base patient teaching on the individual's needs, using a slower pace with simple printed or audio materials in patients with cognitive and functional limitations. Include the family or caregivers in the teaching. The patient education issues for the older patient include those related to altered vision, mobility, cognitive status, and functional ability. Consider the patient's financial and social situation and the effect of multiple medications, eating habits, and quality-of-life issues.

CASE STUDY

Diabetic Ketoacidosis

iStockphoto/Thinkstock

Patient Profile
N.B., a 34-yr-old Native American man, was admitted to the emergency department after he was found unconscious by his wife in their home.

Subjective Data (Provided by Wife)
- Was diagnosed with type 1 diabetes mellitus 12 mo ago
- Was taking 50 U/day of insulin: 5 U of lispro insulin with breakfast, 5 U with lunch, and 10 U with dinner plus 30 U of glargine insulin at bedtime
- Has history of gastroenteritis for 1 wk with vomiting and anorexia
- Stopped taking insulin 2 days ago when he was unable to eat

Objective Data
Physical Examination
- Breathing is deep and rapid
- Fruity acetone smell on breath
- Skin flushed and dry

Diagnostic Studies
- Blood glucose level 730 mg/dL (40.5 mmol/L)
- Blood pH 7.26

Discussion Questions
1. Briefly explain the pathophysiology of the development of diabetic ketoacidosis (DKA) in this patient.
2. What clinical manifestations of DKA does this patient exhibit?
3. What factors precipitated this patient's DKA?
4. *Priority Decision:* What is the priority nursing intervention for N.B.?
5. What distinguishes this case history from one of hyperosmolar hyperglycemic syndrome (HHS) or hypoglycemia?
6. *Priority Decision:* What is the priority teaching that should be done with this patient and his family?
7. What role should N.B.'s wife have in the management of his diabetes?
8. *Priority Decision:* Based on the assessment data presented, what are the priority nursing diagnoses? Are there any collaborative problems?
9. *Evidence-Based Practice:* N.B.'s wife asks you if she should have given her husband insulin when he got sick. How would you respond?

ⓔvolve Answers and a corresponding concept map are available at *http://evolve.elsevier.com/Lewis/medsurg.*

BRIDGE TO NCLEX EXAMINATION

The number of the question corresponds to the same-numbered outcome at the beginning of the chapter.

1. Polydipsia and polyuria related to diabetes mellitus are primarily due to
   a. the release of ketones from cells during fat metabolism.
   b. fluid shifts resulting from the osmotic effect of hyperglycemia.
   c. damage to the kidneys from exposure to high levels of glucose.
   d. changes in RBCs resulting from attachment of excessive glucose to hemoglobin.

2. Which statement would be correct for a patient with type 2 diabetes who was admitted to the hospital with pneumonia?
   a. The patient must receive insulin therapy to prevent ketoacidosis.
   b. The patient has islet cell antibodies that have destroyed the pancreas's ability to produce insulin.
   c. The patient has minimal or absent endogenous insulin secretion and requires daily insulin injections.
   d. The patient may have sufficient endogenous insulin to prevent ketosis but is at risk for hyperosmolar hyperglycemic syndrome.

3. Analyze the following diagnostic findings for your patient with type 2 diabetes. Which result will need further assessment?
   a. A1C 9%
   b. BP 126/80 mm Hg
   c. FBG 130 mg/dL (7.2 mmol/L)
   d. LDL cholesterol 100 mg/dL (2.6 mmol/L)

4. Which statement by the patient with type 2 diabetes is accurate?
   a. "I am supposed to have a meal or snack if I drink alcohol."
   b. "I am not allowed to eat any sweets because of my diabetes."
   c. "I do not need to watch what I eat because my diabetes is not the bad kind."
   d. "The amount of fat in my diet is not important. Only carbohydrates raise my blood sugar."

5. You are caring for a patient with newly diagnosed type 1 diabetes. What information is essential to include in your patient teaching before discharge from the hospital (select all that apply)?
   a. Insulin administration
   b. Elimination of sugar from diet
   c. Need to reduce physical activity
   d. Use of a portable blood glucose monitor
   e. Hypoglycemia prevention, symptoms, and treatment

6. What is the priority action for the nurse to take if the patient with type 2 diabetes complains of blurred vision and irritability?
   a. Call the physician.
   b. Administer insulin as ordered.
   c. Check the patient's blood glucose level.
   d. Assess for other neurologic symptoms.

7. A diabetic patient has a serum glucose level of 824 mg/dL (45.7 mmol/L) and is unresponsive. After assessing the patient, the nurse suspects diabetic ketoacidosis rather than hyperosmolar hyperglycemic syndrome based on the finding of
   a. polyuria.
   b. severe dehydration.
   c. rapid, deep respirations.
   d. decreased serum potassium.

8. Which are appropriate therapies for patients with diabetes mellitus (select all that apply)?
   a. Use of statins to treat dyslipidemia
   b. Use of diuretics to treat nephropathy
   c. Use of ACE inhibitors to treat nephropathy
   d. Use of serotonin agonists to decrease appetite
   e. Use of laser photocoagulation to treat retinopathy

1. b, 2. d, 3. a, 4. a, 5. a, d, e, 6. c, 7. c, 8. a, c, e

ⓔvolve

For rationales to these answers and even more NCLEX review questions, visit *http://evolve.elsevier.com/Lewis/medsurg.*

REFERENCES

1. American Diabetes Association: Total prevalence of diabetes and prediabetes. Retrieved from *www.diabetes.org.*
2. Centers for Disease Control and Prevention: National diabetes fact sheet, 2011. Retrieved from *www.cdc.gov/diabetes/pubs/pdf/ndfs_2011.pdf.*
3. American Diabetes Association: Diagnosis and classification of diabetes mellitus, *Diabetes Care* 36 (Suppl):S67, 2013.
4. Centers for Disease Control and Prevention: Diabetes public health resource: groups especially affected, 2012. Retrieved from *www.cdc.gov/diabetes/consumer/groups.htm.*
5. McKenny R, Short D: Tipping the balance: the pathophysiology of obesity and type 2 diabetes mellitus, *Surg Clin North Am* 91:1139, 2011.
*6. Grundy S: Prediabetes, metabolic syndrome, and cardiovascular disease, *J Am Coll Cardiol* 14:635, 2012.

7. National Diabetes Information Clearinghouse: National diabetes statistics, 2011. Retrieved from *http://diabetes.niddk.nih.gov/dm/pubs/statistics.*
*8. HAPO Study Cooperative Research Group: Hyperglycemia and adverse pregnancy outcomes, *N Engl J Med* 358:1991, 2008. (Classic)
*9. Spollett G: Insulin initiation in type 2 diabetes: what are the treatment regimen options and how can we best help patients feel empowered? *JAANP* 24:249, 2012.
10. American Association of Diabetes Educators: *The art and science of self-management education desk reference*, ed 2, Chicago, 2011, The Association.
11. BD Diabetes: Syringe and needle sizes. Retrieved from *www.bd.com/us/diabetes/page.aspx?cat=7001&id=7253.*
12. Magwire M: Addressing barriers to insulin therapy: the role of insulin pens, *Am J Therap* 18:392, 2011.
13. Pickup J: Insulin-pump therapy for type 1 diabetes mellitus, *N Engl J Med* 366:1616, 2012.

*Evidence-based information for clinical practice.

14. Levesque C: Medical management of type 2 diabetes, *J Nurse Pract* 7:492, 2011.

15. American Diabetes Association: Nutrition recommendations and interventions for diabetes, *Diabetes Care* 31:S61, 2008. (Classic)

16. American Diabetes Association: Food and fitness: create your plate. Retrieved from *www.diabetes.org/food-and-fitness/food/planning-meals/create-your-plate*.

17. US Department of Health and Human Services: A report of the surgeon general physical activity and health executive summary. Retrieved from *www.cdc.gov/nccdphp/sgr/index.htm*.

*18. Diabetes Control and Complications Trial Research Group: The effect of intensive treatment of diabetes on the development and progression of long-term complications in insulin-dependent diabetes mellitus, *N Engl J Med* 329:977, 1993. (Classic)

*19. Wang H, Yeh M: Psychological resistance to insulin therapy in adults with type 2 diabetes: mixed-method systematic review, *J Adv Nurs* 68:43, 2012.

20. Boucher J, Hurrell D: Cardiovascular disease and diabetes, *Diabetes Spectrum* 21:154, 2008. (Classic)

*21. UK Prospective Diabetes Study (UKPDS) Group: Intensive blood-glucose control with sulphonylureas or insulin compared with conventional treatment and risk of complications in patients with type 2 diabetes, *Lancet* 352:837, 1998. (Classic)

22. National High Blood Pressure Education Coordinating Committee: The seventh report of the Joint National Committee on Prevention, Detection, Evaluation, and Treatment of High Blood Pressure: the JNC report, *JAMA* 289:2560, 2003. (Classic)

23. Antonetti D, Klein R, Gardner T: Diabetic retinopathy, *N Engl J Med* 366:1227, 2012.

24. Callaghan B, Cheng H, Stables C, et al: Diabetic neuropathy: clinical manifestations and current treatments, *Lancet Neuro* 11:521, 2012.

25. Lipsky B, Berendt A, Cornia P, et al: Infectious Diseases Society of America clinical practice guideline for the diagnosis and treatment of diabetic foot infections, *CID* 54:E132, 2012.

26. Alexiadou K, Doupis J: Management of diabetic foot ulcers, *Diabetes Ther* 3:1, 2012.

27. Young-Hyman D, Davis C: Disordered eating behaviors in individuals with diabetes: importance of context, evaluation and classification, *Diabetes Care* 33:683, 2010.

*28. Jaser S, Yates H, Dumser S, et al: Risk behaviors in adolescents with type 1 diabetes, *Diabetes Educ* 37:756, 2011.

RESOURCES

American Association of Diabetes Educators
www.diabeteseducator.org

American Diabetes Association
www.diabetes.org

Diabetes Monitor
www.diabetesmonitor.com

Diabetes at Work
www.diabetesatwork.org

National Diabetes Education Program
www.ndep.nih.gov

National Diabetes Education Program's Better Diabetes Care
www.betterdiabetescare.nih.gov

National Diabetes Information Clearinghouse
www.diabetes.niddk.nih.gov

The worst thing that can happen to you may be the best thing for you, if you don't let it get the best of you.
Will Rogers

50

Nursing Management
Endocrine Problems

Katherine A. Kelly

⊖volve WEBSITE

http://evolve.elsevier.com/Lewis/medsurg

- NCLEX Review Questions
- Key Points
- Pre-Test
- Answer Guidelines for Case Study on p. 1215
- Rationales for Bridge to NCLEX Examination Questions

- Case Studies
  - Patient With Addison's Disease
  - Patient With Cushing Syndrome
  - Patient With Hyperthyroidism
- Nursing Care Plans (Customizable)
  - eNCP 50-1: Patient With Hyperthyroidism
  - eNCP 50-2: Patient With Hypothyroidism
  - eNCP 50-3: Patient With Cushing Syndrome

- Concept Map Creator
- Glossary
- Content Updates

eFigures
- eFig. 50-1: Hashimoto's thyroiditis
- eFig. 50-2: Thyroid nodule on a scan

LEARNING OUTCOMES

1. Explain the pathophysiology, clinical manifestations, collaborative care, and nursing management of the patient with an imbalance of hormones produced by the anterior pituitary gland.
2. Describe the pathophysiology, clinical manifestations, collaborative care, and nursing management of the patient with an imbalance of hormones produced by the posterior pituitary gland.
3. Explain the pathophysiology, clinical manifestations, collaborative care, and nursing management of the patient with thyroid dysfunction.
4. Describe the pathophysiology, clinical manifestations, collaborative care, and nursing management of the patient with an imbalance of the hormone produced by the parathyroid glands.
5. Identify the pathophysiology, clinical manifestations, collaborative care, and nursing management of the patient with an imbalance of hormones produced by the adrenal cortex.
6. Describe the pathophysiology, clinical manifestations, collaborative care, and nursing management of the patient with an excess of hormones produced by the adrenal medulla.
7. List the side effects of corticosteroid therapy.
8. Describe common nursing assessments, interventions, rationales, and expected outcomes related to patient teaching for management of chronic endocrine problems.

KEY TERMS

acromegaly, p. 1190
Addison's disease, p. 1211
Cushing syndrome, p. 1207
diabetes insipidus (DI), p. 1194
exophthalmos, p. 1197
goiter, p. 1195
Graves' disease, p. 1196

hyperaldosteronism, p. 1214
hyperparathyroidism, p. 1205
hyperthyroidism, p. 1196
hypoparathyroidism, p. 1206
hypopituitarism, p. 1192
hypothyroidism, p. 1201
myxedema, p. 1202

pheochromocytoma, p. 1214
syndrome of inappropriate antidiuretic
 hormone (SIADH), p. 1193
thyroid cancer, p. 1204
thyroiditis, p. 1196
thyrotoxicosis, p. 1197

Reviewed by Dorothy (Dottie) M. Mathers, RN, DNP, CNE, Professor, School of Health Sciences, Pennsylvania College of Technology, Williamsport, Pennsylvania; Teresa J. Seright, RN, PhD, CCRN, Assistant Professor of Nursing, Montana State University, Bozeman, Montana; Daryle Wane, PhD, ARNP, FNP-BC, Professor of Nursing, Generic Program Track Coordinator, Pasco-Hernando Community College, New Port Richey, Florida; Saundra J. Hendricks, RN, MS, FNP, BC-ADM, Department of Medicine, Endocrine Division, The Methodist Hospital, Houston, Texas; Beth Lucasy, RN, MA, VP Marketing and Communications, TVAX Biomedical, Kansas City, Missouri; and Barbara Lukert, MD, Endocrinologist, University of Kansas Medical Center, Kansas City, Kansas.

The endocrine system is made up of a number of organs and glands that are involved in the synthesis and secretion of hormones that affect every body system. Because these hormones have such a wide range of action, endocrine problems are associated with a variety of clinical manifestations. Many aspects of a person's life are affected when an endocrine problem is present.

DISORDERS OF ANTERIOR PITUITARY GLAND

ACROMEGALY

Acromegaly is a rare condition characterized by an overproduction of growth hormone (GH). Approximately six out of every 1 million adults in the United States are diagnosed annually.[1] Both genders are affected equally. The mean age at the time of diagnosis is 40 to 45 years old.

Etiology and Pathophysiology

Acromegaly most often occurs as a result of a benign pituitary tumor (adenoma). The excessive secretion of GH results in an overgrowth of soft tissues and bones in the hands, feet, and face. Because the problem develops after epiphyseal closure, the bones of the arms and legs do not grow longer.

Clinical Manifestations

The changes resulting from excess GH can occur over a number of years and may go unnoticed by family and friends. Patients experience enlargement of hands and feet with joint pain that can range from mild to crippling. Carpal tunnel syndrome may be present. Thickening and enlargement of the bony and soft tissues on the face, feet, and head occur (Fig. 50-1).

Enlargement of the tongue results in speech difficulties, and the voice deepens because of hypertrophy of the vocal cords. Sleep apnea may occur because of upper airway narrowing and obstruction from increased amounts of pharyngeal soft tissues. The skin becomes thick, leathery, and oily. Persons with acromegaly may experience peripheral neuropathy and proximal muscle weakness. Women may develop menstrual disturbances.

Visual changes may occur due to pressure on the optic nerve from a pituitary adenoma. Headaches are common. Since GH antagonizes the action of insulin leading to hyperglycemia,

FIG. 50-1 Progressive development of facial changes associated with acromegaly.

GENDER DIFFERENCES

Endocrine Problems

Men	Women
• Ectopic ACTH production is more common in men.	• Hyperthyroidism and hypothyroidism are more common in women than in men. • Graves' disease affects four to eight times more women than men. • Hyperaldosteronism affects twice as many women as men. • Thyroid nodules and thyroid cancer affect up to four times as many women as men.

ACTH, Adrenocorticotropic hormone.

glucose intolerance and manifestations of diabetes mellitus may occur, including *polydipsia* (increased thirst) and *polyuria* (increased urination).[2] Because GH mobilizes stored fat for energy, it increases free fatty acid levels in the blood and predisposes the patient to atherosclerosis.

The life expectancy of patients with acromegaly is reduced by 5 to 10 years. They are more likely to succumb to cardiac and respiratory diseases, diabetes mellitus, and colorectal cancer.[3] Even when patients are cured or acromegaly is well controlled, manifestations such as joint pain and deformities often remain.

Diagnostic Studies

In addition to the history and physical examination, a diagnosis of acromegaly requires evaluation of plasma insulin-like growth factor 1 (IGF-1) levels and GH response to an oral glucose tolerance test (OGTT). The peripheral actions of GH are mediated by IGF-1. As GH levels rise, so do IGF-1 levels. However, GH is released in a pulsatile fashion, requiring several samples to obtain an accurate measure. Serum IGF-1 levels are more constant, providing a more reliable diagnostic measure of acromegaly.

OGTT is a specific test for acromegaly. Because GH secretion is normally inhibited by glucose, measurement of glucose nonsuppressibility is useful. Two baseline GH levels are obtained before ingestion of 75 or 100 g of oral glucose, and additional GH measurements are made at 30, 60, 90, and 120 minutes. Normally, GH concentration falls during an OGTT. In acromegaly GH levels do not fall, and in some cases GH concentration rises.

Magnetic resonance imaging (MRI) and a high-resolution computed tomography (CT) scan with contrast media are used to detect pituitary tumors. A complete ophthalmologic examination, including visual fields, is done because a tumor may cause pressure on the optic chiasm or optic nerves.

Collaborative Care

The patient's prognosis depends on the age at onset, age when treatment started, and tumor size. The overall goal is to return the patient's GH levels to normal. Treatment consists of surgery, radiation therapy, drug therapy, or a combination of these therapies. With treatment, bone growth can be stopped and tissue hypertrophy reversed. However, sleep apnea and diabetic and cardiac complications may persist.

Surgical Therapy. Surgery (hypophysectomy) is the treatment of choice because it offers the best chance for a cure, especially for smaller pituitary adenomas. Most surgeries are done by an endoscopic *transsphenoidal* approach (Fig. 50-2).

FIG. 50-2 Surgery on the pituitary gland is most commonly performed with the transsphenoidal approach. An incision is made in the inner aspect of the upper lip and gingiva. The sella turcica is entered through the floor of the nose and sphenoid sinuses.

Surgery produces an immediate reduction in GH levels followed by a drop in IGF-1 levels within a few weeks. When the entire pituitary gland is removed, there is permanent loss of all pituitary hormones. Rather than replacing the pituitary (tropic) hormones, which requires parenteral administration, the essential hormones produced by target organs (glucocorticoids, thyroid hormone, and sex hormones) are given. Hormone therapy continues throughout life. Patients with larger tumors or those with GH levels greater than 45 ng/mL may require adjuvant radiation or drug therapy.

Radiation Therapy. Radiation therapy is used when surgery has failed to produce a cure or when patients are poor candidates for surgery. Radiation therapy is usually offered in combination with drugs that reduce GH levels. However, the full effects may not be noted for months to years. Radiation can also be used to reduce the size of a tumor before surgery. Radiation therapy may lead to hypopituitarism, which then requires lifelong hormone replacement therapy.

Stereotactic radiosurgery (gamma knife surgery, proton beam, linear accelerator) may be used for small, surgically inaccessible pituitary tumors or in place of conventional radiation (see Chapter 57). This procedure consists of radiation delivered to one site from multiple angles.

Drug Therapy. Drugs are most commonly used in patients who have had an inadequate response to surgery and/or in combination with radiation therapy. The primary drug used for acromegaly is octreotide (Sandostatin), a somatostatin analog that reduces GH levels to normal in many patients. Octreotide is given by subcutaneous injection three times a week. Two long-acting analogs, octreotide (Sandostatin LAR) and lanreotide SR (Somatuline Depot), are available as intramuscular (IM) injections given every 4 weeks. GH levels are measured every 2 weeks to guide drug dosing, and then every 6 months until the desired response is obtained.

Dopamine agonists (e.g., bromocriptine [Parlodel], pergolide [Permax], cabergoline [Dostinex]) may be given alone or added to somatostatin analogs if complete remission has not been achieved after surgery. These drugs reduce the secretion of GH from the tumor.

GH antagonists (e.g., pegvisomant [Somavert]) reduce the effect of GH in the body by blocking the hepatic production of IGF-1. With the use of drug therapy, most patients achieve normal IGF-1 levels with symptom improvement.[2]

NURSING MANAGEMENT ACROMEGALY

NURSING ASSESSMENT

Assess the patient for signs and symptoms of abnormal tissue growth and evaluate changes in physical size. It is important to question patients about increases in hat, glove, and shoe sizes. Older photographs are helpful to evaluate any changes (see Fig. 50-1). Because physical changes occur slowly and over a long period, the individual may not even be aware of any changes.

NURSING IMPLEMENTATION

Postoperative care after a transsphenoidal hypophysectomy includes elevating the head of the patient's bed at all times to a 30-degree angle. This elevation avoids pressure on the sella turcica and decreases headaches, a frequent postoperative problem. Monitor the pupillary response, speech patterns, and extremity strength to detect neurologic complications. Perform mouth care every 4 hours to keep the surgical area clean and free of debris. Avoid tooth brushing for at least 10 days to protect the suture line. Observe the patient for any signs of bleeding, since hemorrhage may be a complication, particularly when larger tumors are removed by this approach.

Instruct the patient to avoid vigorous coughing, sneezing, and straining at stool (Valsalva maneuver) to prevent cerebrospinal fluid (CSF) leakage. Notify the surgeon, and send any clear nasal drainage to the laboratory to be tested for glucose. A glucose level greater than 30 mg/dL (1.67 mmol/L) indicates CSF leakage from an open connection to the brain. If this happens, the patient is at increased risk for meningitis. Complaints of persistent and severe generalized or supraorbital headache may indicate CSF leakage into the sinuses. A CSF leak usually resolves within 72 hours when treated with head elevation and bed rest. If the leak persists, daily spinal taps may be done to reduce pressure to below-normal levels.

If stereotactic radiosurgery is used, the patient is usually moved from the specialized radiation center to the neurosurgical nursing unit for overnight observation. The patient will be in a stereotactic head frame. Carefully monitor vital signs, neurologic status, and fluid volume status. Possible complications of sterotactic surgery include increased headaches, seizures, nausea, and vomiting. Perform pin-site care according to institutional policy. Instruct family members on pin-site care if the patient is discharged with pins in place.

Observe the patient for transient diabetes insipidus (DI). This may occur because of the loss of antidiuretic hormone (ADH), which is stored in the posterior lobe of the pituitary gland, or cerebral edema related to manipulation of the pituitary during surgery. To assess for DI, closely monitor urine output and serum and urine osmolarity. Clinical manifestations and treatment of DI are discussed in more detail later in this chapter.

If a hypophysectomy is performed or the pituitary gland is damaged, hormone therapy will be necessary. ADH, cortisol, and thyroid hormone replacement will be needed. Surgery may result in permanent loss or deficiencies in follicle-stimulating hormone (FSH) and luteinizing hormone (LH). This can lead to decreased fertility. Assist the patient in working through the grieving process associated with these losses.

If hormones are prescribed, teach the patient about the need for lifelong therapy. Serial photographs to show improvement may be helpful. Patients with acromegaly are at higher risk for colon polyps and colorectal cancer and should have a screening colonoscopy every 3 to 4 years.

EXCESSES OF OTHER TROPIC HORMONES

In addition to GH, the pituitary also secretes prolactin, adrenocorticotropic hormone (ACTH), thyroid-stimulating hormone (TSH), and ADH. An excess of any of these hormones (discussed later in the chapter) can cause significant disturbances in metabolism and general health.

Prolactinomas are among the most common type of pituitary adenomas.[4] Women with prolactinomas frequently experience galactorrhea, anovulation, infertility, oligomenorrhea or amenorrhea, decreased libido, and hirsutism. In men, impotence and decreased sperm density and libido may result. Compression of the optic chiasm can cause visual problems and signs of increased intracranial pressure, including headache, nausea, and vomiting. Because prolactinomas do not typically progress in size, drug therapy is usually the first-line treatment. The dopamine agonists cabergoline and bromocriptine have successfully been used to treat prolactinomas. Surgery may be done depending on the extent and size of the tumor. Radiation therapy may be used to reduce the risk of tumor recurrence for patients with large tumors.

HYPOFUNCTION OF PITUITARY GLAND

Hypopituitarism is a rare disorder that involves a decrease in one or more of the pituitary hormones. The anterior pituitary gland secretes ACTH, TSH, FSH, LH, GH, and prolactin. The posterior pituitary gland secretes ADH and oxytocin. A deficiency of only one pituitary hormone is referred to as *selective hypopituitarism*. Total failure of the pituitary gland results in deficiency of all pituitary hormones—a condition referred to as *panhypopituitarism*. The most common hormone deficiencies associated with hypopituitarism involve GH and gonadotropins (i.e., LH, FSH).

Etiology and Pathophysiology

The usual cause of pituitary hypofunction is a pituitary tumor. Autoimmune disorders, infections, pituitary infarction (Sheehan syndrome), or destruction of the pituitary gland (from trauma, radiation, or surgical procedures) can also cause hypopituitarism. African Americans have a higher incidence of pituitary adenomas than other ethnic groups.[5]

Anterior pituitary hormone deficiencies can lead to end-organ failure. Deficiencies of TSH and ACTH are life threatening. ACTH deficiency can lead to acute adrenal insufficiency and shock. Hypovolemic shock is due to sodium and water depletion. (Acute adrenal insufficiency is discussed later in this chapter on pp. 1211-1212.)

Clinical Manifestations and Diagnostic Studies

The manifestations associated with pituitary hypofunction vary with the type and degree of dysfunction. Early manifestations associated with a space-occupying lesion include headaches, visual changes (decreased visual acuity or decreased peripheral vision), loss of smell, nausea and vomiting, and seizures. Manifestations associated with hyposecretion of the target glands vary widely (Table 50-1).

In addition to a history and physical examination, diagnostic studies such as MRI and CT are used to identify a pituitary

TABLE 50-1	CLINICAL MANIFESTATIONS OF HYPOPITUITARISM
Hormone Deficiency	**Manifestations**
Growth hormone (GH)	Subtle, nonspecific findings. Truncal obesity, decreased muscle mass and strength, weakness, fatigue, depression or flat affect.
Follicle-stimulating hormone (FSH) and luteinizing hormone (LH)	*Women:* Menstrual irregularities, loss of libido, changes in secondary sex characteristics such as decreased breast size. *Men:* Testicular atrophy, diminished spermatogenesis, loss of libido, impotence, decreased facial hair and muscle mass.
Thyroid-stimulating hormone (TSH)	Mild form of primary hypothyroidism: fatigue, cold intolerance, constipation, lethargy, weight gain.
Adrenocorticotropic hormone (ACTH)	Involves a deficiency of cortisol: weakness, fatigue, headache, dry and pale skin, diminished axillary and pubic hair, lowered resistance to infection, fasting hypoglycemia.

tumor. Laboratory tests for diagnosing hypopituitarism vary widely, but generally involve the direct measurement of pituitary hormones (e.g., TSH) or an indirect determination of the target organ hormones (e.g., triiodothyronine [T_3], thyroxine [T_4]). (See Chapter 48 for more information regarding diagnostic studies.)

NURSING AND COLLABORATIVE MANAGEMENT HYPOPITUITARISM

The treatment for hypopituitarism often consists of surgery or radiation therapy followed by lifelong hormone therapy. Surgery and radiation therapy for pituitary tumors are discussed earlier in this chapter on pp. 1190 and 1191. Appropriate hormone therapy is used (e.g., GH, corticosteroids, thyroid hormone, sex hormones). Hormone therapies for thyroid hormone and corticosteroids are discussed later in this chapter on pp. 1202 and 1213.

Somatropin (Omnitrope, Genotropin, Humatrope), which is recombinant human GH, is used for long-term hormone therapy in adults with GH deficiency. These patients respond well to GH replacement and experience increased energy, increased lean body mass, a feeling of well-being, and improved body image. Mild to moderate side effects of GH include fluid retention with swelling in the feet and hands, myalgia, joint pain, and headache. GH is given daily as a subcutaneous injection (preferably in the evening). The dosing is variable because it is adjusted based on symptoms, IGF-1 levels, and the development of adverse effects.

Although gonadal deficiency is not life threatening, hormone therapy is offered to improve sexual function and general well-being. This therapy is contraindicated in individuals with certain medical conditions, such as breast cancer, phlebitis, and pulmonary embolism in women and prostate cancer in men. Estrogen and progesterone replacement therapy may be indicated for hypogonadal women to treat hot flashes, vaginal dryness, and decreased libido. Hormone therapy for women is discussed in Chapter 54. Testosterone is used to treat men with gonadotropin deficiency. The benefits achieved with testoster-

PATHOPHYSIOLOGY MAP

FIG. 50-3 Pathophysiology of syndrome of inappropriate antidiuretic hormone (SIADH).

one therapy include a return of male secondary sex characteristics; improvement in libido; and increased muscle mass, bone mass, and bone density. Hormone therapy for men is discussed in Chapter 55.

DISORDERS OF POSTERIOR PITUITARY GLAND

The hormones secreted by the posterior pituitary, antidiuretic hormone (ADH) and oxytocin, are produced in the hypothalamus and then transported and stored in the posterior pituitary gland. ADH, also referred to as *arginine vasopressin* (AVP) or vasopressin, plays a major role in the regulation of water balance and osmolarity (see Chapter 48).

The two primary problems associated with ADH secretion are a result of either overproduction or underproduction of ADH. Overproduction or oversecretion of ADH results in a condition known as syndrome of inappropriate antidiuretic hormone (SIADH). Underproduction or undersecretion of ADH results in a condition referred to as *diabetes insipidus* (DI).

SYNDROME OF INAPPROPRIATE ANTIDIURETIC HORMONE

Etiology and Pathophysiology

SIADH results from abnormally high production or sustained secretion of ADH. In SIADH, ADH is released despite normal or low plasma osmolarity (Fig. 50-3). This disorder is characterized by fluid retention, serum hypoosmolality, dilutional hyponatremia, hypochloremia, concentrated urine in the presence of normal or increased intravascular volume, and normal renal function.

This syndrome occurs more commonly in older adults. SIADH has various causes (Table 50-2). The most common cause is malignancy, especially small cell lung cancer. Although SIADH tends to be self-limiting when it is caused by head trauma or drugs, it is chronic when associated with tumors or metabolic diseases.

Clinical Manifestations and Diagnostic Studies

ADH increases the permeability of the renal distal tubule and collecting duct, which leads to the reabsorption of water

TABLE 50-2	CAUSES OF SYNDROME OF INAPPROPRIATE ANTIDIURETIC HORMONE
Malignant Tumors • Small cell lung cancer • Pancreatic cancer • Lymphoid cancers (Hodgkin's lymphoma, non-Hodgkin's lymphoma, lymphocytic leukemia) • Thymus cancer • Prostate cancer • Colorectal cancer **Central Nervous System Disorders** • Head injury (skull fracture, subdural hematoma, subarachnoid hemorrhage) • Stroke • Brain tumors • Infection (encephalitis, meningitis) • Cerebral atrophy • Guillain-Barré syndrome • Systemic lupus erythematosus	**Drug Therapy** • carbamazepine (Tegretol) • chlorpropamide (Diabinese) • General anesthesia agents • Opioids • oxytocin • Thiazide diuretics • SSRI antidepressants • Tricyclic antidepressants • Chemotherapy drugs (vincristine [Oncovin], vinblastine [Velban], cyclophosphamide [Cytoxan]) **Miscellaneous Conditions** • Hypothyroidism • Lung infection (pneumonia, tuberculosis, lung abscess) • Chronic obstructive pulmonary disease • Positive pressure mechanical ventilation • HIV • Adrenal insufficiency

SIADH, Syndrome of inappropriate antidiuretic hormone; *SSRI,* selective serotonin reuptake inhibitor.

into the circulation. Consequently, extracellular fluid volume expands, plasma osmolality declines, glomerular filtration rate increases, and sodium levels decline (dilutional hyponatremia).[6] Hyponatremia causes muscle cramping, pain, and weakness. Initially, the patient displays thirst, dyspnea on exertion, and fatigue.

The patient with SIADH experiences low urine output and increased body weight. As the serum sodium level falls (usually below 120 mEq/L [120 mmol/L]), manifestations become more severe and include vomiting, abdominal cramps, muscle twitching, and seizures. As plasma osmolality and serum sodium levels continue to decline, cerebral edema may occur, which leads to lethargy, confusion, headache, seizures, and coma.

The diagnosis of SIADH is made by simultaneous measurements of urine and serum osmolality. Dilutional hyponatremia is indicated by a serum sodium less than 134 mEq/L, serum osmolality less than 280 mOsm/kg (280 mmol/kg), and a urine specific gravity greater than 1.025. A serum osmolality much lower than the urine osmolality indicates the inappropriate excretion of concentrated urine in the presence of dilute serum.

NURSING AND COLLABORATIVE MANAGEMENT SYNDROME OF INAPPROPRIATE ANTIDIURETIC HORMONE

In your assessment of individuals at risk and those who have confirmed SIADH, be alert for low urine output with a high specific gravity, a sudden weight gain without edema, or a decreased serum sodium level. Monitor intake and output, vital signs, and heart and lung sounds. Observe for signs of hyponatremia, including seizures, nausea and vomiting, muscle cramping, and decreased neurologic function.

Once SIADH is diagnosed, treatment is directed at the underlying cause. Medications that stimulate the release of

ADH should be avoided or discontinued (see Table 50-2). If symptoms are mild and serum sodium is greater than 125 mEq/L (125 mmol/L), the only treatment may be a fluid restriction of 800 to 1000 mL/day. This restriction should result in gradual reductions in weight, a progressive rise in serum sodium concentration and osmolality, and symptomatic improvement.

In the acute care setting restrict the patient's total fluid intake to no more than 1000 mL/day (including that taken with medications) and obtain daily weights. Position the head of the bed flat or elevated no more than 10 degrees to enhance venous return to the heart and increase left atrial filling pressure, thereby reducing the release of ADH. Frequent turning, positioning, and range-of-motion exercise (if patient is bedridden) are important to maintain skin integrity and joint mobility. Protect the patient from injury (e.g., assist with ambulation, bed alarm) because of the potential for alterations in mental status. Implement seizure precautions. Provide the patient with frequent oral care and distractions to decrease discomfort related to thirst from the fluid restrictions.

In cases of severe hyponatremia (less than 120 mEq/L), especially in the presence of neurologic manifestations such as seizures, IV hypertonic saline solution (3% to 5%) may be slowly administered. A loop diuretic such as furosemide (Lasix) may be used to promote diuresis, but only if the serum sodium is at least 125 mEq/L (125 mmol/L) because it may promote a further loss of sodium. Because furosemide increases potassium, calcium, and magnesium losses, supplements may be needed. A fluid restriction of 500 mL/day may be indicated for those with severe hyponatremia.

Vasopressin receptor antagonists, tolvaptan (Samsca) and conivaptan (Vaprisol), are used to treat euvolemia-hyponatremia in hospitalized patients. These medications should be initiated in a closely monitored setting to prevent rapid correction of serum sodium.

Assist the patient with chronic SIADH in self-management of the treatment regimen. In chronic SIADH, a fluid restriction of 800 to 1000 mL/day is recommended. Because this degree of restriction may be difficult, demeclocycline (Declomycin) may be administered. This drug blocks the effect of ADH on the renal tubules, resulting in a more dilute urine. The use of ice chips or sugarless chewing gum helps to decrease thirst. Have the patient weigh daily to monitor changes in fluid balance. Teach the patient to supplement the diet with sodium and potassium, especially if loop diuretics are also prescribed. Solutions of these electrolytes must be well diluted to prevent gastrointestinal (GI) irritation or damage. They are best taken at mealtime to allow mixing with and dilution by food. Teach the patient the symptoms of fluid and electrolyte imbalances, especially those involving sodium and potassium (see Chapter 17).

DIABETES INSIPIDUS

Etiology and Pathophysiology

Diabetes insipidus (DI) is caused by a deficiency of production or secretion of ADH or a decreased renal response to ADH. The decrease in ADH results in fluid and electrolyte imbalances caused by increased urine output and increased plasma osmolality (Fig. 50-4). Depending on the cause, DI may be transient or a chronic, lifelong condition.

There are several types of DI (Table 50-3). Central DI is the most common form.

PATHOPHYSIOLOGY MAP

FIG. 50-4 Pathophysiology of diabetes insipidus (DI).

TABLE 50-3	**TYPES OF DIABETES INSIPIDUS**
Type	**Etiology**
Central (neurogenic) DI	Results from an interference with ADH synthesis, transport, or release *Examples:* Brain tumor, head injury, brain surgery, CNS infections
Nephrogenic DI	Results from inadequate renal response to ADH despite presence of adequate ADH *Examples:* Drug therapy (especially lithium), renal damage, hereditary renal disease
Primary DI	Results from excessive water intake *Examples:* Structural lesion in thirst center, psychologic disorder

Clinical Manifestations

DI is characterized by polydipsia and polyuria.[6] The primary characteristic is the excretion of large quantities of urine (2 to 20 L/day) with a very low specific gravity (less than 1.005) and urine osmolality of less than 100 mOsm/kg (100 mmol/kg). Serum osmolality is elevated (usually greater than 295 mOsm/kg [295 mmol/kg]) because of hypernatremia caused by pure water loss in the kidneys. Most patients compensate for fluid loss by drinking large amounts of water so that serum osmolality remains normal or is moderately elevated. The patient may be fatigued from nocturia and experience generalized weakness.

The onset of central DI is usually acute and accompanied by excessive fluid loss. After intracranial surgery, central DI has a triphasic pattern: the acute phase with an abrupt onset of polyuria, an interphase in which urine volume normalizes, and a third phase in which central DI is permanent. The third phase occurs within 10 to 14 days postoperatively. Central DI that results from head trauma is often self-limiting and improves with treatment of the underlying problem. DI following cranial surgery is more likely to be permanent. Although the clinical manifestations of nephrogenic DI are similar to those of central DI, the onset and amount of fluid loss are less dramatic.

If oral fluid intake cannot keep up with urinary losses, severe dehydration results. This is manifested by poor tissue turgor, hypotension, tachycardia, and hypovolemic shock. In addition, the patient may show central nervous system (CNS) manifestations, ranging from irritability and mental dullness to coma, related to increasing serum osmolality and hypernatremia.

Diagnostic Studies

Patients with DI excrete dilute urine at a rate greater than 200 mL/hr with a specific gravity of less than 1.005. Identification of central DI requires a water deprivation test. Before the test, body weight, and urine osmolality, volume, and specific gravity are measured. The patient is deprived of water for 8 to 12 hours, and then given desmopressin acetate (DDAVP) subcutaneously or nasally. Patients with central DI exhibit a dramatic increase in urine osmolality, from 100 to 600 mOsm/kg, and a significant decrease in urine volume. The patient with nephrogenic DI will not be able to increase urine osmolality to greater than 300 mOsm/kg.

Another test to differentiate central DI from nephrogenic DI is to measure the level of ADH after an analog of ADH (e.g., desmopressin) is given. If the cause is central DI, the kidneys will respond to the hormone by concentrating urine. If the kidneys do not respond in this way, then the cause is nephrogenic.

NURSING AND COLLABORATIVE MANAGEMENT DIABETES INSIPIDUS

Nursing management of the patient with DI includes early detection, maintenance of adequate hydration, and patient teaching for long-term management. A therapeutic goal is maintenance of fluid and electrolyte balance.

For central DI, fluid and hormone therapy is the cornerstone of treatment. Fluids are replaced orally or IV, depending on the patient's condition and ability to drink copious amounts of fluids. In acute DI, IV hypotonic saline or dextrose 5% in water (D_5W) is given and titrated to replace urine output. If IV glucose solutions are used, monitor serum glucose levels because hyperglycemia and glycosuria can lead to osmotic diuresis, which increases the fluid volume deficit. Monitoring of blood pressure (BP), heart rate, and urine output and specific gravity is essential and may be required hourly in the patient who is acutely ill. Monitor the level of consciousness and for signs of acute dehydration by assessing alertness, response to stimuli, mucous membranes, tachycardia, and skin turgor. Maintain an accurate record of intake and output and daily weights to determine fluid volume status. Adjustments in fluid replacement should be made accordingly.

DDAVP, an analog of ADH, is the hormone replacement of choice for central DI. Other ADH replacement drugs include aqueous vasopressin (Pitressin) or lysine vasopressin (Diapid). DDAVP can be given orally, IV, subcutaneously, or as a nasal spray. Assess the response to DDAVP (e.g., weight gain, headache, depression, restlessness, hyponatremia). Monitor pulse, BP, level of consciousness, fluid intake and output, and urine specific gravity. Teach the patient about the need for close follow-up. Chlorpropamide (Diabinese) and carbamazepine (Tegretol) are used to help decrease thirst associated with central DI.

Because the kidney is unable to respond to ADH in nephrogenic DI, hormone therapy has little effect. Instead, the treatment includes dietary measures (low-sodium diet) and thiazide diuretics (e.g., hydrochlorothiazide [HydroDIURIL], chlorothiazide [Diuril]), which may reduce flow to the ADH-sensitive distal nephrons. Limiting sodium intake to no more than 3 g/

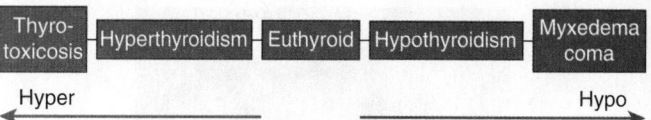

FIG. 50-5 Continuum of thyroid dysfunction.

day often helps decrease urine output. When a low-sodium diet and thiazide drugs are not effective, indomethacin (Indocin) may be prescribed. Indomethacin, a nonsteroidal antiinflammatory drug (NSAID), helps increase renal responsiveness to ADH.

DISORDERS OF THYROID GLAND

Alterations in thyroid function are among the most common endocrine disorders. The thyroid hormones, thyroxine (T_4) and triiodothyronine (T_3), regulate energy metabolism and growth and development. Disorders of the thyroid gland include goiter, benign and malignant nodules, inflammation, hyperthyroidism, and hypothyroidism (Fig. 50-5).

GOITER

A **goiter** is an enlarged thyroid gland. In a person with a goiter the thyroid cells are stimulated to grow, which may result in an overactive thyroid (hyperthyroidism) or an underactive thyroid (hypothyroidism). The most common cause of goiter worldwide is a lack of iodine in the diet. In the United States, where most people use iodized salt, goiter is more often due to the overproduction or underproduction of thyroid hormones or to nodules that develop in the gland itself. *Goitrogens* (foods or drugs that contain thyroid-inhibiting substances) can cause goiter[7] (Table 50-4).

A nontoxic goiter is a diffuse enlargement of the thyroid gland that does not result from a malignancy or inflammatory process. Normal levels of thyroid hormone are associated with this type of goiter. *Nodular goiters* are thyroid hormone–secreting nodules that function independent of TSH stimulation. There may be multiple nodules (multinodular goiter) or a single nodule (solitary autonomous nodule). The nodules are usually benign follicular adenomas. If these nodules are associated with hyperthyroidism, they are termed *toxic nodular goiters*. This type of goiter is commonly found in patients with Graves' disease (Fig. 50-6). Toxic nodular goiters occur equally in men and women. Although they can appear at any age, the frequency is greatest in people over 40 years of age.

TABLE 50-4 GOITROGENS

Thyroid Inhibitors	Foods*
• propylthiouracil (PTU)	• Broccoli
• methimazole (Tapazole)	• Brussels sprouts
• Iodine in large doses	• Cabbage
	• Cauliflower
Other Drugs	• Kale
• Sulfonamides	• Mustard
• Salicylates	• Peanuts
• *p*-Aminosalicylic acid	• Turnips
• lithium	
• amiodarone (Cordarone)	

*List is not all-inclusive.

FIG. 50-6 Exophthalmos and goiter of Graves' disease.

In a person with a goiter, TSH and T_4 levels are measured to determine whether a goiter is associated with normal thyroid function, hyperthyroidism, or hypothyroidism. Thyroid antibodies (e.g., thyroid peroxidase [TPO] antibody) are measured to assess for *thyroiditis* (inflammation of the thyroid). Treatment with thyroid hormone may prevent further thyroid enlargement. Surgery is used to remove large goiters. Goiter as a clinical manifestation of thyroid disorders is further discussed in the following sections.

THYROIDITIS

Thyroiditis, an inflammation of the thyroid gland, is a frequent cause of goiter. *Subacute granulomatous thyroiditis* is thought to be caused by a viral infection. *Acute thyroiditis* is due to bacterial or fungal infection. Subacute and acute forms of thyroiditis have an abrupt onset. The patient complains of pain localized in the thyroid or radiating to the throat, ears, or jaw.[8] Other systemic manifestations include fever, chills, sweats, and fatigue.

Hashimoto's thyroiditis (chronic autoimmune thyroiditis) results in hypothyroidism caused by the destruction of thyroid tissue by antibodies. It is the most common cause of hypothyroid goiters in the United States. Factors placing an individual at higher risk include female gender, a positive family history, older age, and white ethnicity. The goiter, which is the hallmark of Hashimoto's thyroiditis, may develop gradually or rapidly (see eFig. 50-1 available on the website for this chapter). If the thyroid gland enlarges rapidly, structures in the neck (e.g., trachea and laryngeal nerves) may become compressed, thus changing the voice and affecting breathing.

Silent, painless thyroiditis, which may be early Hashimoto's thyroiditis, can occur in postpartum women. This condition, which is usually seen in the first 6 months after delivery, may be due to an autoimmune reaction to fetal cells in the mother's thyroid gland.

T_4 and T_3 levels are initially elevated in subacute, acute, and silent thyroiditis but become depressed with time. In chronic Hashimoto's thyroiditis, thyroid hormone levels are usually low and the TSH level is high. Suppression of radioactive iodine uptake (RAIU) is seen in subacute and silent thyroiditis. Antithyroid antibodies are present in Hashimoto's thyroiditis.

Recovery from acute or subacute thyroiditis may be complete in weeks or months without any treatment. If the thyroiditis is bacterial in origin, treatment may include specific antibiotics or surgical drainage. In the subacute and acute forms, NSAIDs (aspirin or naproxen [Aleve]) are used to relieve symptoms. With more severe pain, corticosteroids (e.g., prednisone up to 40 mg/day) are used to relieve discomfort. This treatment may be required for several months and then should be withdrawn gradually.[9] Propranolol (Inderal) or atenolol (Tenormin) may be used to treat the cardiovascular symptoms related to a hyperthyroid condition. Thyroid hormone therapy is indicated if the patient is hypothyroid.

Nursing care of the patient with thyroiditis includes patient teaching regarding the disease process and course of treatment. Stress the importance of not abruptly discontinuing medications. Instruct the patient to remain under close health care supervision so that progress can be monitored. In addition, teach the patient to report to the health care provider any change in symptoms, such as difficulty breathing or swallowing, swelling to face and extremities, or rapid weight gain or loss.

The patient with Hashimoto's thyroiditis is at risk for other autoimmune diseases such as Addison's disease, pernicious anemia, or Graves' disease. Teach the patient the signs and symptoms of these disorders, particularly Addison's disease. Instruct the patient receiving thyroid hormone about the expected side effects of these drugs and measures to manage them (see p. 1202).

HYPERTHYROIDISM

Hyperthyroidism is hyperactivity of the thyroid gland with sustained increase in synthesis and release of thyroid hormones. Hyperthyroidism occurs in women more than men, with the highest frequency in persons 20 to 40 years old. The most common form of hyperthyroidism is Graves' disease. Other causes include toxic nodular goiter, thyroiditis, excess iodine intake, pituitary tumors, and thyroid cancer.

The term *thyrotoxicosis* refers to the physiologic effects or clinical syndrome of hypermetabolism that results from excess circulating levels of T_4, T_3, or both.[10] Hyperthyroidism and thyrotoxicosis usually occur together, as seen in Graves' disease.

Etiology and Pathophysiology

Graves' Disease. Graves' disease is an autoimmune disease of unknown etiology characterized by diffuse thyroid enlargement and excessive thyroid hormone secretion. Graves' disease accounts for up to 80% of the cases of hyperthyroidism. Women are five times more likely than men to develop Graves' disease. Precipitating factors such as insufficient iodine supply, infection, and stressful life events may interact with genetic factors to cause Graves' disease. Cigarette smoking increases the risk of Graves' disease and the development of eye problems associated with the disease.[11]

In Graves' disease the patient develops antibodies to the TSH receptor. These antibodies attach to the receptors and stimulate the thyroid gland to release T_3, T_4, or both. The excessive release of thyroid hormones leads to the clinical manifestations associated with thyrotoxicosis. The disease is characterized by remissions and exacerbations, with or without treatment. It may progress to destruction of the thyroid tissue, causing hypothyroidism.

TABLE 50-5 CLINICAL MANIFESTATIONS OF THYROID DYSFUNCTION

Hyperfunction	Hypofunction	Hyperfunction	Hypofunction
Cardiovascular System		**Musculoskeletal System**	
• Systolic hypertension	• Increased capillary fragility	• Fatigue	• Fatigue
• Increased rate and force of cardiac contractions	• Decreased rate and force of contractions	• Muscle weakness	• Weakness
• Bounding, rapid pulse	• Varied changes in blood pressure	• Proximal muscle wasting	• Muscular aches and pains
• Increased cardiac output	• Cardiac hypertrophy	• Dependent edema	• Slow movements
• Cardiac hypertrophy	• Distant heart sounds	• Osteoporosis	• Arthralgia
• Systolic murmurs	• Anemia	**Nervous System**	
• Dysrhythmias	• Tendency to develop heart failure, angina, myocardial infarction	• Difficulty focusing eyes	• Apathy
• Palpitations		• Nervousness	• Lethargy
• Atrial fibrillation (more common in the older adult)		• Fine tremor (of fingers and tongue)	• Fatigue
• Angina		• Insomnia	• Forgetfulness
Respiratory System		• Lability of mood, delirium	• Slowed mental processes
• Increased respiratory rate	• Dyspnea	• Restlessness	• Hoarseness
• Dyspnea on mild exertion	• Decreased breathing capacity	• Personality changes of irritability, agitation	• Slow, slurred speech
Gastrointestinal System		• Exhaustion	• Prolonged relaxation of deep tendon muscles
• Increased appetite, thirst	• Decreased appetite	• Hyperactive deep-tendon reflexes	• Stupor, coma
• Weight loss	• Nausea and vomiting	• Depression, fatigue, apathy (in the older adult)	• Paresthesias
• Increased peristalsis	• Weight gain	• Lack of ability to concentrate	• Anxiety, depression
• Diarrhea, frequent defecation	• Constipation	• Stupor, coma	
• Increased bowel sounds	• Distended abdomen	**Reproductive System**	
• Splenomegaly	• Enlarged, scaly tongue	• Menstrual irregularities	• Prolonged menstrual periods or amenorrhea
• Hepatomegaly	• Celiac disease	• Amenorrhea	
Integumentary System		• Decreased libido	• Decreased libido
• Warm, smooth, moist skin	• Dry, thick, inelastic, cold skin	• Impotence in men	• Infertility
• Thin, brittle nails detached from nail bed (onycholysis)	• Thick, brittle nails	• Gynecomastia in men	
• Hair loss (may be patchy)	• Dry, sparse, coarse hair	• Decreased fertility	
• Clubbing of fingers (thyroid acropachy) (see Fig. 50-7)	• Poor turgor of mucosa	**Other**	
• Palmar erythema	• Generalized interstitial edema	• Intolerance to heat	• Increased susceptibility to infection
• Fine silky hair	• Puffy face	• Elevated basal temperature	• Increased sensitivity to opioids, barbiturates, anesthesia
• Premature graying (in men)	• Decreased sweating	• Lid lag, stare	
• Diaphoresis	• Pallor	• Eyelid retraction	• Intolerance to cold
• Vitiligo		• Exophthalmos	• Decreased hearing
• Pretibial myxedema (infiltrative dermopathy)		• Goiter (see Fig. 50-6)	• Sleepiness
		• Rapid speech	• Goiter

Clinical Manifestations

Clinical manifestations of hyperthyroidism are related to the effect of excess circulating thyroid hormone. It directly increases metabolism and tissue sensitivity to stimulation by the sympathetic nervous system.

Palpation of the thyroid gland may reveal a goiter. When the thyroid gland is excessively large, a goiter may be noted on inspection. Auscultation of the thyroid gland may reveal bruits, a reflection of increased blood supply. Another common finding is *ophthalmopathy*, a term used to describe abnormal eye appearance or function. A classic finding in Graves' disease is exophthalmos, a protrusion of the eyeballs from the orbits that is usually bilateral (see Fig. 50-6). Exophthalmos results from increased fat deposits and fluid (edema) in the orbital tissues and ocular muscles. The increased pressure forces the eyeballs outward. The upper lids are usually retracted and elevated, with the sclera visible above the iris. When the eyelids do not close completely, the exposed corneal surfaces become dry and irritated. Serious consequences, such as corneal ulcers and eventual loss of vision, can occur. The changes in the ocular muscles result in muscle weakness, causing diplopia.

Other manifestations of thyroid hyperfunction are summarized in Table 50-5. Abnormal laboratory findings are listed in Table 50-6. A patient in the early stages of hyperthyroidism may exhibit only weight loss and increased nervousness. *Acropachy* (clubbing of the digits) may occur with advanced disease (Fig. 50-7). Manifestations (e.g., palpitations, tremors, weight loss) in older adults with hyperthyroidism do not differ significantly from those of younger adults (Table 50-7). In older patients with reports of confusion and agitation, dementia may be suspected and delay the diagnosis.

Complications

Thyrotoxicosis (also called *thyrotoxic crisis* or *thyroid storm*) is an acute, severe, and rare condition that occurs when excessive amounts of thyroid hormones are released into the circulation. Although it is considered a life-threatening emergency, death is rare when treatment is initiated early. Thyrotoxicosis is thought to result from stressors (e.g., infection, trauma, surgery) in a patient with preexisting hyperthyroidism, either diagnosed or undiagnosed. Patients particularly prone to thyrotoxicosis are those having a thyroidectomy, since manipulation of the

TABLE 50-6 LABORATORY RESULTS FOR HYPERTHYROID AND HYPOTHYROID PATIENTS

Test	Hyperthyroid	Hypothyroid Primary	Hypothyroid Secondary
Thyroid-stimulating hormone (TSH)	↓	↑	↓
T₄ (thyroxine)	↑	↓	↓
Total cholesterol	N	↑	↑
Low-density lipoproteins (LDLs)	↓	↑	↑
Triglycerides	N	↑	↑
Creatine kinase (CK)	N	↑	↑
Basal metabolic rate (BMR)	↑	↓	↓
Thyroid peroxidase (TPO) antibody	N	+ (in autoimmune hypothyroidism)	N

N, Normal; +, positive.

hyperactive thyroid gland results in an increase in hormones released.[11]

In thyrotoxicosis, all the symptoms of hyperthyroidism are prominent and severe. Manifestations include severe tachycardia, heart failure, shock, hyperthermia (up to 105.3° F [40.7° C]), restlessness, irritability, seizures, abdominal pain, vomiting, diarrhea, delirium, and coma. Treatment is aimed at reducing circulating thyroid hormone levels and the clinical manifestations with appropriate drug therapy. Supportive therapy is directed at managing respiratory distress, reducing fever, replacing fluid, and eliminating or managing the initiating stressor(s).

Diagnostic Studies

The two primary laboratory findings used to confirm the diagnosis of hyperthyroidism are decreased TSH levels and elevated free thyroxine (free T₄) levels. Total T₃ and T₄ levels may also

FIG. 50-7 Thyroid acropachy. Digital clubbing and swelling of fingers.

be assessed, but they are not as definitive. Total T₃ and T₄ determine both free and bound (to protein) hormone levels. The free hormone is the only biologically active form of these hormones.

The RAIU test is used to differentiate Graves' disease from other forms of thyroiditis. The patient with Graves' disease shows a diffuse, homogeneous uptake of 35% to 95%, whereas the patient with thyroiditis shows an uptake of less than 2%. The person with a nodular goiter has an uptake in the high normal range.

Collaborative Care

The goal of management of hyperthyroidism is to block the adverse effects of excessive thyroid hormone, suppress oversecretion of thyroid hormone, and prevent complications. There are several treatment options, including antithyroid medications, radioactive iodine therapy, and surgical intervention (Table 50-8). The choice of treatment is influenced by the patient's age and preferences, coexistence of other diseases, and pregnancy status.

Drug Therapy. Drugs used in the treatment of hyperthyroidism include antithyroid drugs, iodine, and β-adrenergic blockers. These drugs are useful in the treatment of thyrotoxic states, but they are not considered curative. Radiation therapy or surgery may ultimately be required.

Antithyroid Drugs. The first-line antithyroid drugs are propylthiouracil (PTU) and methimazole (Tapazole).[12] These drugs

TABLE 50-7 COMPARISON OF HYPERTHYROIDISM IN YOUNGER AND OLDER ADULTS

	Younger Adult	Older Adult
Common causes	Graves' disease in >90% of cases	Graves' disease or toxic nodular goiter
Common symptoms	Nervousness, irritability, weight loss, heat intolerance, warm moist skin	Anorexia, weight loss, apathy, lassitude, depression, confusion
Goiter	Present in >90% of cases	Present in about 50% of cases
Ophthalmopathy	Exophthalmos (see Fig. 50-6) present in 20%-40% of cases	Exophthalmos less common
Cardiac features	Tachycardia and palpitations common, but without heart failure	Angina, dysrhythmia (especially atrial fibrillation), heart failure may occur

TABLE 50-8 COLLABORATIVE CARE

Hyperthyroidism

Diagnostic
- History and physical examination
- Ophthalmologic examination
- ECG
- Laboratory tests
  - TSH levels, serum free T₄
  - Thyroid antibodies (e.g., thyroid peroxidase [TPO] antibody)
  - Total serum T₃ and T₄
- Radioactive iodine uptake (RAIU)

Collaborative Therapy
Drug Therapy
- Antithyroid drugs
  - methimazole (Tapazole)
  - propylthiouracil (PTU)
- Iodine (Lugol's solution, SSKI)
- β-Adrenergic receptor blockers
  - propranolol (Inderal)
  - atenolol (Tenormin) or metoprolol (Toprol)

Radiation Therapy
- Radioactive iodine

Surgical Therapy
- Subtotal thyroidectomy

Nutritional Therapy
- High-calorie, high-protein diet
- Frequent meals

SSKI, Saturated solution of potassium iodine; *TSH,* thyroid-stimulating hormone.

inhibit the synthesis of thyroid hormones. Indications for the use of antithyroid drugs include Graves' disease in the young patient, hyperthyroidism during pregnancy, and the need to achieve a euthyroid state before surgery or radiation therapy. PTU is generally used for patients who are in their first trimester of pregnancy, have an adverse reaction to methimazole, or require a rapid reduction in symptoms. PTU is also considered first line in thyrotoxicosis, since it also blocks the peripheral conversion of T_4 to T_3. The advantage of PTU is that it achieves the therapeutic goal of being euthyroid more quickly, but it must be taken three times per day. In contrast, methimazole is given in a single daily dose.

Individuals vary, but improvement usually begins 1 to 2 weeks after the start of drug therapy. Good results are usually seen within 4 to 8 weeks. Therapy is usually continued for 6 to 15 months to allow for spontaneous remission, which occurs in 20% to 40% of patients. Emphasize to the patient the importance of adherence to the drug regimen. Abrupt discontinuation of drug therapy can result in a return of hyperthyroidism.

Iodine. Iodine is used with other antithyroid drugs to prepare the patient for thyroidectomy or for treatment of thyrotoxicosis. The administration of iodine in large doses rapidly inhibits synthesis of T_3 and T_4 and blocks the release of these hormones into circulation. It also decreases the vascularity of the thyroid gland, making surgery safer and easier. The maximal effect of iodine is usually seen within 1 to 2 weeks. Because of a reduction in the therapeutic effect, long-term iodine therapy is not effective in controlling hyperthyroidism. Iodine is available in the form of saturated solution of potassium iodine (SSKI) and Lugol's solution.

β-Adrenergic Blockers. β-Adrenergic blockers are used for symptomatic relief of thyrotoxicosis. These drugs block the effects of sympathetic nervous stimulation, thereby decreasing tachycardia, nervousness, irritability, and tremors. Propranolol is usually administered with other antithyroid agents. Atenolol is the preferred β-adrenergic blocker for use in the hyperthyroid patient with asthma or heart disease.

Radioactive Iodine Therapy. Radioactive iodine (RAI) therapy is the treatment of choice for most nonpregnant adults. RAI damages or destroys thyroid tissue, thus limiting thyroid hormone secretion. RAI has a delayed response, and the maximum effect may not be seen for up to 3 months. For this reason, the patient is usually treated with antithyroid drugs and propranolol before and for 3 months after the initiation of RAI until the effects of radiation become apparent. Although RAI is usually effective, it has a high incidence of posttreatment hypothyroidism (80% of adequately treated persons), resulting in the need for lifelong thyroid hormone therapy. Teach the patient and the family about the symptoms of hypothyroidism and to seek medical help if these symptoms occur.

RAI therapy is usually administered on an outpatient basis. A pregnancy test is done before initiation of therapy on all women who experience menstrual cycles. Instruct the patient that radiation thyroiditis and parotiditis are possible and may cause dryness and irritation of the mouth and throat. Relief may be obtained with frequent sips of water, ice chips, or a salt and soda gargle three or four times per day. This gargle is made by dissolving 1 tsp of salt and 1 tsp of baking soda in 2 cups of warm water. The discomfort should subside in 3 to 4 days. A mixture of antacid (Mylanta or Maalox), diphenhydramine (Benadryl), and viscous lidocaine can be used to swish and spit, increasing patient comfort when eating. To limit radiation

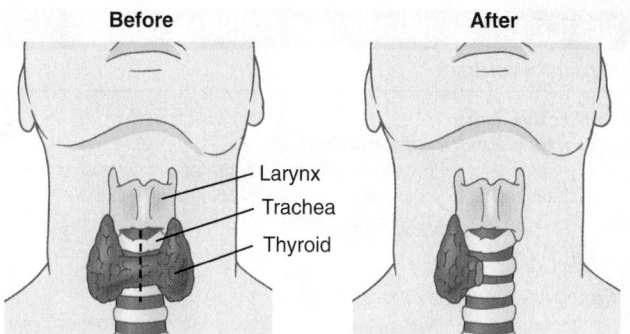

FIG. 50-8 Subtotal thyroidectomy. Part of the thyroid gland is removed.

exposure to others, instruct the patient receiving RAI on the importance of home precautions, including (1) using private toilet facilities if possible and flushing two or three times after each use; (2) separately laundering towels, bed linens, and clothes daily at home; (3) not preparing food for others that requires prolonged handling with bare hands; and (4) avoiding being close to pregnant women or children for 7 days after therapy.

Surgical Therapy. Thyroidectomy is indicated for individuals who have (1) a large goiter causing tracheal compression, (2) been unresponsive to antithyroid therapy, or (3) thyroid cancer (Fig. 50-8). Additionally, surgery may be done when an individual is not a candidate for RAI. One advantage that thyroidectomy has over RAI is a more rapid reduction in T_3 and T_4 levels. A *subtotal thyroidectomy* is often the preferred surgical procedure and involves the removal of a significant portion (90%) of the thyroid gland.

An endoscopic thyroidectomy is a minimally invasive procedure. Several small incisions are made, and a scope is inserted. Instruments are passed through the scope to remove thyroid tissue or nodules. Endoscopic thyroidectomy is an appropriate procedure for patients with small nodules (less than 3 cm) and no evidence of malignancy. Advantages of endoscopic thyroidectomy over open thyroidectomy include less scarring, less pain, and a faster return to normal activity.

Nutritional Therapy. With the increased metabolic rate in hyperthyroid patients, there is a high potential for the patient to have a nutritional deficit. A high-calorie diet (4000 to 5000 cal/day) may be ordered to satisfy hunger, prevent tissue breakdown, and decrease weight loss. This can be accomplished with six full meals a day and snacks high in protein, carbohydrates, minerals, and vitamins. The protein content should be 1 to 2 g/kg of ideal body weight. Increase carbohydrate intake to compensate for increased metabolism. Carbohydrates provide energy and decrease the use of body-stored protein. Teach the patient to avoid highly seasoned and high-fiber foods because these foods can further stimulate the already hyperactive GI tract. Instruct the patient to avoid caffeine-containing liquids such as coffee, tea, and cola to decrease the restlessness and sleep disturbances associated with these fluids. Refer the patient to a dietitian for help in meeting individual nutritional needs.

NURSING MANAGEMENT HYPERTHYROIDISM

NURSING ASSESSMENT

Subjective and objective data that should be obtained from an individual with hyperthyroidism are presented in Table 50-9.

TABLE 50-9 NURSING ASSESSMENT

Hyperthyroidism

Subjective Data
Important Health Information
Past health history: Preexisting goiter; recent infection or trauma, immigration from iodine-deficient area, autoimmune disease
Medications: Thyroid hormones, herbal therapies that may contain thyroid hormone

Functional Health Patterns
Health perception–health management: Positive family history of thyroid or autoimmune disorders
Nutritional-metabolic: Iodine intake; weight loss; increased appetite, thirst; nausea, vomiting
Elimination: Diarrhea; polyuria; sweating
Activity-exercise: Dyspnea on exertion; palpitations; muscle weakness, fatigue
Sleep-rest: Insomnia
Cognitive-perceptual: Chest pain; nervousness; heat intolerance; pruritus
Sexuality-reproductive: Decreased libido; impotence; gynecomastia (in men); amenorrhea (in women)
Coping–stress tolerance: Emotional lability, irritability, restlessness, personality changes, delirium

Objective Data
General Observation
Agitation, rapid speech and body movements; anxiety, restlessness, hyperthermia, enlarged or nodular thyroid gland

Eyes
Exophthalmos, eyelid retraction; infrequent blinking

Integumentary
Warm, diaphoretic, velvety skin; thin, loose nails; fine, silky hair and hair loss; palmar erythema; clubbing; white pigmentation of skin (vitiligo), diffuse edema of legs and feet

Respiratory
Tachypnea, dyspnea on exertion

Cardiovascular
Tachycardia, bounding pulse, systolic murmurs, dysrhythmias, hypertension, bruit over the thyroid gland

Gastrointestinal
Increased bowel sounds; increased appetite, diarrhea, weight loss, hepatosplenomegaly

Neurologic
Hyperreflexia; diplopia; fine tremors of hands, tongue, eyelids

Musculoskeletal
Muscle wasting

Reproductive
Menstrual irregularities, infertility; impotence, gynecomastia in men

Possible Diagnostic Findings
$\uparrow T_3$, $\uparrow T_4$; $\uparrow T_3$ resin uptake; $\downarrow$ or undetectable TSH; chest x-ray showing enlarged heart; ECG findings of tachycardia, atrial fibrillation

TSH, Thyroid-stimulating hormone.

NURSING DIAGNOSES

Nursing diagnoses for the patient with hyperthyroidism include, but are not limited to, the following:

- Activity intolerance *related to* fatigue and heat intolerance
- Imbalanced nutrition: less than body requirements *related to* hypermetabolism and inadequate food intake

Additional information on nursing diagnoses is presented in eNursing Care Plan 50-1 for the patient with hyperthyroidism (available on the website for this chapter).

PLANNING

The overall goals are that the patient with hyperthyroidism will (1) experience relief of symptoms, (2) have no serious complications related to the disease or treatment, (3) maintain nutritional balance, and (4) cooperate with the therapeutic plan.

NURSING IMPLEMENTATION

ACUTE INTERVENTION. Individuals who have hyperthyroidism are usually treated in an outpatient setting. However, patients who develop acute thyrotoxicosis or those who undergo thyroidectomy require hospitalization and acute care.

Acute Thyrotoxicosis. Acute thyrotoxicosis is a systemic syndrome that requires aggressive treatment, often in an intensive care unit. Administer medications (previously discussed) that block thyroid hormone production and the sympathetic nervous system. Provide supportive therapy, including monitoring for cardiac dysrhythmias and decompensation, ensuring adequate oxygenation, and administering IV fluids to replace fluid and electrolyte losses. This is especially important in the patient who experiences fluid losses due to vomiting and diarrhea.

Ensuring adequate rest may be a challenge because of the patient's irritability and restlessness. Provide a calm, quiet room because increased metabolism and sensitivity of the sympathetic nervous system causes sleep disturbances. Other interventions may include (1) placing the patient in a cool room away from very ill patients and noisy, high-traffic areas; (2) using light bed coverings and changing the linen frequently if the patient is diaphoretic; and (3) encouraging and assisting with exercise involving large muscle groups (tremors can interfere with small-muscle coordination) to allow the release of nervous tension and restlessness. It is important to establish a supportive, trusting relationship to facilitate coping by a patient who is irritable, restless, and anxious.

If exophthalmos is present, there is a potential for corneal injury related to irritation and dryness. The patient may have orbital pain. Nursing interventions to relieve eye discomfort and prevent corneal ulceration include applying artificial tears to soothe and moisten conjunctival membranes. Salt restriction may help reduce periorbital edema. Elevate the patient's head to promote fluid drainage from the periorbital area. The patient should sit upright as much as possible.

Dark glasses reduce glare and prevent irritation from smoke, air currents, dust, and dirt. If the eyelids cannot be closed, lightly tape them shut for sleep. To maintain flexibility, teach the patient to exercise the intraocular muscles several times a day by turning the eyes in the complete range of motion. Good grooming can help reduce the loss of self-esteem from an altered body image. If the exophthalmos is severe, treatment options include corticosteroids, radiation of retroorbital tissues, orbital decompression, or corrective lid or muscle surgery.

Thyroid Surgery. When subtotal thyroidectomy is the treatment of choice, the patient must be adequately prepared to avoid postoperative complications. Before surgery, antithyroid drugs, iodine, and β-adrenergic blockers may be administered to achieve a euthyroid state. Iodine reduces vascularization of the thyroid gland, reducing the risk of hemorrhage. Iodine is mixed with water or juice, sipped through a straw, and administered after meals. Assess the patient for signs of iodine toxicity such as swelling of the buccal mucosa and other mucous membranes, excessive salivation, nausea and vomiting, and skin reactions. If toxicity occurs, discontinue iodine administration and notify the health care provider.

Preoperatively, teach the patient about comfort and safety measures. Teach the patient the importance of performing leg exercises. Instruct the patient in how to support the head manually while turning in bed, since this maneuver minimizes stress on the suture line after surgery. The patient should practice range-of-motion exercises of the neck. Explain routine postoperative care such as IV infusions. Tell the patient that talking is likely to be difficult for a short time after surgery.

Postoperative Care. Postoperative complications include hypothyroidism, damage to or inadvertent removal of parathyroid glands causing hypoparathyroidism and hypocalcemia, hemorrhage, injury to the recurrent or superior laryngeal nerve, thyrotoxicosis, and infection.[13] Recurrent laryngeal nerve damage leads to vocal cord paralysis. If both cords are paralyzed, spastic airway obstruction will occur, requiring an immediate tracheostomy.

> **SAFETY ALERT**
> - Although not common, airway obstruction after thyroid surgery is an emergency situation.
> - Oxygen, suction equipment, and a tracheostomy tray should be readily available in the patient's room.

Respiration may also become difficult because of excess swelling of the neck tissues, hemorrhage, and hematoma formation. *Laryngeal stridor* (harsh, vibratory sound) may occur during inspiration and expiration as a result of edema of the laryngeal nerve. Laryngeal stridor may also be related to tetany, which occurs if the parathyroid glands are removed or damaged during surgery, leading to hypocalcemia. To treat tetany, IV calcium salts (e.g., calcium gluconate, calcium gluceptate) should be available.

Important nursing interventions after a thyroidectomy include the following:
- Assess the patient every 2 hours for 24 hours for signs of hemorrhage or tracheal compression such as irregular breathing, neck swelling, frequent swallowing, sensations of fullness at the incision site, choking, and blood on the anterior or posterior dressings.
- Place the patient in a semi-Fowler's position and support the patient's head with pillows. Avoid flexion of the neck and any tension on the suture lines.[13]
- Monitor vital signs and calcium levels. Complete the initial assessment by checking for signs of tetany secondary to hypoparathyroidism (e.g., tingling in toes, fingers, around the mouth; muscular twitching; apprehension) and by evaluating difficulty in speaking and hoarseness. Monitor Trousseau's sign and Chvostek's sign (see Chapter 17, Fig. 17-15). Expect some hoarseness for 3 or 4 days after surgery because of edema.
- Control postoperative pain by giving medication.

If postoperative recovery is uneventful, the patient ambulates within hours after surgery, is permitted to take fluid as soon as tolerated, and eats a soft diet the day after surgery.

The appearance of the incision may be distressing to the patient. Reassure the patient that the scar will fade in color and eventually look like a normal neck wrinkle. A scarf, jewelry, a high collar, or other covering can effectively camouflage the scar.

AMBULATORY AND HOME CARE. The patient, caregiver, and family need to be aware that thyroid hormone balance should be monitored periodically. Most patients experience a period of relative hypothyroidism soon after surgery because of the substantial reduction in the size of the thyroid. However, the remaining tissue usually hypertrophies over time and recovers the capacity to produce hormones. The administration of thyroid hormone is avoided because the exogenous hormone inhibits pituitary production of TSH and delays or prevents the restoration of normal gland function and tissue regeneration.

To prevent weight gain, caloric intake must be reduced substantially below the amount that was required before surgery. Adequate iodine is necessary to promote thyroid function, but excesses can inhibit the thyroid gland. Seafood once or twice a week or normal use of iodized salt should provide sufficient iodine intake. Encourage regular exercise to stimulate the thyroid gland. Teach the patient to avoid high environmental temperatures because they inhibit thyroid regeneration.

Regular follow-up care is necessary. The patient should see the health care provider biweekly for a month and then at least semiannually to assess thyroid function. If a complete thyroidectomy has been performed, instruct the patient about the need for lifelong thyroid hormone replacement. Teach the patient the signs and symptoms of progressive thyroid failure and to seek medical care if these develop. Hypothyroidism is relatively easy to manage with oral administration of thyroid replacement.

EVALUATION

The expected outcomes are that the patient with hyperthyroidism will
- Experience relief of symptoms
- Have no serious complications related to the disease or treatment
- Cooperate with the therapeutic plan

Additional information on expected outcomes is presented in eNursing Care Plan 50-1 for the patient with hyperthyroidism (available on the website for this chapter).

HYPOTHYROIDISM

Hypothyroidism is a deficiency of thyroid hormone that causes a general slowing of the metabolic rate. About 4% of the U.S. population has mild hypothyroidism, with about 0.3% having more severe disease.[14] Hypothyroidism is more common in women than men.

Etiology and Pathophysiology

Hypothyroidism can be classified as primary or secondary. *Primary hypothyroidism* is caused by destruction of thyroid tissue or defective hormone synthesis. *Secondary hypothyroidism* is caused by pituitary disease with decreased TSH secretion or hypothalamic dysfunction with decreased thyrotropin-releasing hormone (TRH) secretion. Hypothyroidism may also be transient and related to thyroiditis or discontinuance of thyroid hormone therapy.

Iodine deficiency is the most common cause of hypothyroidism worldwide. In the United States, the most common cause of primary hypothyroidism is atrophy of the thyroid gland. This atrophy is the end result of Hashimoto's thyroiditis or Graves' disease. These autoimmune diseases destroy the thyroid gland. Hypothyroidism may also develop due to treatment for hyperthyroidism, specifically the surgical removal of the thyroid gland or RAI therapy. Drugs such as amiodarone (Cordarone) (contains iodine) and lithium (blocks hormone production) can cause hypothyroidism.

Hypothyroidism that develops in infancy (*cretinism*) is caused by thyroid hormone deficiencies during fetal or early neonatal life. All infants in the United States are screened for decreased thyroid function at birth.

Clinical Manifestations

Regardless of the cause, hypothyroidism has common features. It has systemic effects characterized by a slowing of body processes. Manifestations vary depending on the severity and the duration of thyroid deficiency, as well as the patient's age at the onset of the deficiency. The onset of symptoms may occur over months to years unless hypothyroidism occurs after a thyroidectomy, after thyroid ablation, or during treatment with antithyroid drugs.

The patient is often fatigued and lethargic and experiences personality and mental changes, including impaired memory, slowed speech, decreased initiative, and somnolence. Many individuals with hypothyroidism appear depressed. Weight gain is most likely a result of a decreased metabolic rate.

Hypothyroidism is associated with decreased cardiac contractility and decreased cardiac output. Thus the patient may experience low exercise tolerance and shortness of breath on exertion. Hypothyroidism may cause significant cardiovascular problems, especially in a person with previous cardiovascular disorders.

Anemia is a common feature of hypothyroidism. Erythropoietin levels may be low or normal. Because the metabolic rate is lower, oxygen demand is reduced. Other hematologic problems are related to cobalamin, iron, and folate deficiencies. The patient may bruise easily. Increased serum cholesterol and triglyceride levels and the accumulation of mucopolysaccharides in the intima of small blood vessels can result in coronary atherosclerosis.

Patients with severe, long-standing hypothyroidism may display myxedema, which alters the physical appearance of the skin and subcutaneous tissues with puffiness, facial and periorbital edema, and a masklike affect. Myxedema occurs due to the accumulation of hydrophilic mucopolysaccharides in the dermis and other tissues (Fig. 50-9). Individuals with hypothyroidism may describe an altered self-image related to their disabilities and altered appearance. Other manifestations of hypothyroidism are summarized in Table 50-5.

In the older adult the typical manifestations of hypothyroidism (including fatigue, cold and dry skin, hoarseness, hair loss,

FIG. 50-9 Common features of myxedema. Dull, puffy skin; coarse, sparse hair; periorbital edema; and prominent tongue.

TABLE 50-10	**COLLABORATIVE CARE**

Hypothyroidism

Diagnostic	**Collaborative Therapy**
• History and physical examination	• Thyroid hormone replacement (e.g., levothyroxine)
• Serum TSH and free T_4	• Monitor thyroid hormone levels and adjust dosage (if needed)
• Total serum T_3 and T_4	• Nutritional therapy to promote weight loss
• Thyroid peroxidase (TPO) antibodies	• Patient and caregiver teaching (see Table 50-11)

TSH, Thyroid-stimulating hormone.

constipation, and cold intolerance) may be attributed to normal aging. For this reason, the patient's symptoms may not raise suspicion of an underlying condition. Older adults who have confusion, lethargy, and depression should be evaluated for thyroid disease.

Complications

The mental sluggishness, drowsiness, and lethargy of hypothyroidism may progress gradually or suddenly to a notable impairment of consciousness or coma. This situation, termed *myxedema coma,* is a medical emergency. Myxedema coma can be precipitated by infection, drugs (especially opioids, tranquilizers, and barbiturates), exposure to cold, and trauma.[14] It is characterized by subnormal temperature, hypotension, and hypoventilation. Cardiovascular collapse can result from hypoventilation, hyponatremia, hypoglycemia, and lactic acidosis. For the patient to survive a myxedema coma, vital functions must be supported and IV thyroid hormone replacement administered.

Diagnostic Studies

The most common and reliable laboratory tests for thyroid function are TSH and free T_4. These values, correlated with symptoms gathered from the history and physical examination, confirm the diagnosis of hypothyroidism. Serum TSH levels help determine the cause of hypothyroidism. Serum TSH is high when the defect is in the thyroid and low when it is in the pituitary or the hypothalamus. The presence of thyroid antibodies suggests an autoimmune origin of the hypothyroidism. Other abnormal laboratory findings are elevated cholesterol and triglycerides, anemia, and increased creatine kinase (see Table 50-6).

Collaborative Care

The treatment goal for a patient with hypothyroidism is restoration of a euthyroid state as safely and rapidly as possible with hormone therapy (Table 50-10). A low-calorie diet is also indicated to promote weight loss or prevent weight gain.

Levothyroxine (Synthroid) is the drug of choice to treat hypothyroidism. In the young and otherwise healthy patient, the maintenance replacement dosage is adjusted according to the patient's response and laboratory findings. When thyroid hormone therapy is initiated, the initial dosages are low to avoid increases in resting heart rate and BP. In the patient with compromised cardiac status, careful monitoring is needed when starting and adjusting the dosage because the usual dose may increase myocardial oxygen demand.[15] The increased oxygen demand may cause angina and cardiac dysrhythmias.

DRUG ALERT: Levothyroxine (Synthroid)
- Carefully monitor patients with cardiovascular disease who take this drug.
- Monitor heart rate and report pulse greater than 100 beats/min or an irregular heartbeat.
- Promptly report chest pain, weight loss, nervousness, tremors, and/or insomnia.

In a patient without side effects, the dose is increased at 4- to 6-week intervals. It may take up to 8 weeks before the full effect of hormone therapy is seen, It is important that the patient regularly take replacement medication. Lifelong thyroid therapy is usually required.

Liotrix is a synthetic mix of levothyroxine (T_4) and liothyronine (T_3) in a 4:1 combination. Levothyroxine has a peak of action of 1 to 3 weeks. In contrast, liotrix has a faster onset of action with a peak of 2 to 3 days. Liotrix can be used in acutely ill individuals with hypothyroidism.

NURSING MANAGEMENT
HYPOTHYROIDISM

NURSING ASSESSMENT
Careful assessment may reveal early and subtle changes in a patient suspected of having hypothyroidism. Note any previous history of hyperthyroidism and treatment with antithyroid medications, radioactive iodine, or surgery. Ask the patient about prescribed iodine-containing medications (see Table 50-4) and any changes in appetite, weight, activity level, speech, memory, and skin such as increased dryness or thickening. Assess for cold intolerance, constipation, and signs of depression. Further assessment should focus on heart rate, tenderness over the thyroid gland, and edema in the extremities and face.

NURSING DIAGNOSES
Nursing diagnoses for the patient with hypothyroidism may include, but are not limited to, the following:
- Imbalanced nutrition: more than body requirements *related to* calorie intake in excess of metabolic rate
- Constipation *related to* GI hypomotility
- Impaired memory *related to* hypometabolism

Additional information on nursing diagnoses is presented in the eNursing Care Plan 50-2 for the patient with hypothyroidism (available on the website for this chapter).

PLANNING
The overall goals are that the patient with hypothyroidism will (1) experience relief of symptoms, (2) maintain a euthyroid state, (3) maintain a positive self-image, and (4) comply with lifelong thyroid therapy.

NURSING IMPLEMENTATION
HEALTH PROMOTION. Currently no consensus exists regarding thyroid function screening. Although hypothyroidism is relatively common, particularly among women over age 50, there does not appear to be strong justification for screening the general population.[16] High-risk populations should be screened for subclinical (asymptomatic) thyroid disease. High-risk individuals include those with a family history of thyroid disease, those with a history of neck radiation, women over 50 years old, and postpartum women.

ACUTE INTERVENTION. Most individuals with hypothyroidism are treated on an outpatient basis. The patient who develops myxedema coma requires acute nursing care, often in an inten-

sive care setting. Mechanical respiratory support and cardiac monitoring are frequently necessary.

Administer thyroid hormone therapy and all other medications IV because paralytic ileus may be present in myxedema coma. Monitor the core temperature because hypothermia often occurs in myxedema coma. Use soap gently and moisturize frequently to prevent skin breakdown. Frequent changes in patient positioning and a low-pressure mattress can also assist in maintaining skin integrity.

Monitor the patient's progress by assessing vital signs, body weight, fluid intake and output, and visible edema. Cardiac assessment is especially important because the cardiovascular response to hormone therapy determines the medication regimen. Note energy level and mental alertness, which should increase within 2 to 14 days and continue to improve steadily to normal levels. The patient's neurologic status and free T_4 levels are used to determine continuing treatment.

AMBULATORY AND HOME CARE. Patient teaching is essential for the patient with hypothyroidism and the caregiver (Table 50-11). Initially the hypothyroid patient may have difficulty processing complex instructions. It is important to provide written instructions, repeat the information often, and assess the patient's comprehension level.

Stress the need for receiving lifelong drug therapy and avoiding abrupt discontinuation of drugs. Instruct the patient in expected and unexpected side effects. In the teaching plan include the signs and symptoms of hypothyroidism or hyperthyroidism that indicate hormone imbalance. Clearly define toxic symptoms. Table 50-5 lists manifestations of hyperthyroidism, which are the same as the toxic manifestations of thyroid hormone replacement.

Teach the patient to immediately contact a health care provider if manifestations of overdose occur, such as orthopnea, dyspnea, rapid pulse, palpitations, chest pain, nervousness, or insomnia. The patient with diabetes mellitus should test his or

TABLE 50-11 PATIENT & CAREGIVER TEACHING GUIDE

Hypothyroidism

Include the following instructions when teaching the patient and caregiver about management of hypothyroidism.
1. Discuss the importance of thyroid hormone therapy.
   - Need for lifelong therapy
   - Taking thyroid hormone in the morning before food
   - Need for regular follow-up care
2. Caution the patient not to switch brands of the hormone unless prescribed, since the bioavailability of thyroid hormones may differ.
3. Emphasize the need for a comfortable, warm environment because of intolerance to cold.
4. Teach measures to prevent skin breakdown. Soap should be used sparingly and lotion applied to skin.
5. Caution the patient, especially if an older adult, to avoid sedatives. If they must be used, suggest that the lowest dose be used. Caregiver should closely monitor mental status, level of consciousness, and respirations.
6. Discuss with the patient and the caregiver measures to minimize constipation, including
   - Gradual increase in activity and exercise
   - Increased fiber in diet
   - Use of stool softeners
   - Regular bowel elimination time
7. Tell patient to avoid using enemas because they produce vagal stimulation, which can be hazardous if cardiac disease is present.

her capillary blood glucose at least daily because the return to the euthyroid state frequently increases insulin requirements. In addition, thyroid drugs potentiate the effects of anticoagulants and decrease the effect of digitalis compounds. Instruct the patient about the toxic signs and symptoms of these medications and the need to remain under close medical observation until stable.

With treatment, striking transformations occur in both appearance and mental function. Most adults return to a normal state. Cardiovascular conditions and (occasionally) psychosis may persist despite corrections of the hormonal imbalance. Relapses occur if treatment is interrupted.

EVALUATION

The expected outcomes are that the patient with hypothyroidism will

- Have relief from symptoms
- Maintain a euthyroid state as evidenced by normal thyroid hormone and TSH levels
- Avoid complications of therapy
- Adhere to lifelong therapy

Additional information on expected outcomes is presented in the eNursing Care Plan 50-2 for the patient with hypothyroidism (available on the website for this chapter).

THYROID NODULES AND CANCER

A *thyroid nodule* (growth in the thyroid gland) may be benign or malignant (thyroid cancer). More than 95% of all thyroid gland nodules are benign. A person's chance of getting a thyroid nodule increases with age. Benign nodules are usually not dangerous, but they can cause tracheal compression if they become too large.

Thyroid cancer is the most common form of an endocrine system cancer. An estimated 56,460 new cases of thyroid cancer are diagnosed annually.[17] The incidence of thyroid cancer has risen significantly in the past 25 years. Thyroid cancer affects more women, and the incidence is higher in Asian Americans.[18]

Radiation exposure significantly increases the risk for thyroid cancer. Adults at higher risk for thyroid cancer include those who were given radiation treatment during childhood for lymphoma, Wilms' tumor, and neuroblastoma. Having a personal or family history of goiter also increases a person's risk.

Types of Thyroid Cancer

The four main types of thyroid cancer are papillary, follicular, medullary, and anaplastic. *Papillary* thyroid cancer is the most common type, accounting for about 70% to 80% of all thyroid cancers. Papillary cancer tends to grow slowly and spreads initially to lymph nodes in the neck.

Follicular thyroid cancer makes up about 15% of all thyroid cancers. It tends to occur in older patients. Follicular cancer first metastasizes into the cervical lymph nodes, then spreads to the neck, lungs, and bones.

Medullary thyroid cancer, which accounts for up to 10% of all thyroid cancers, is more likely to occur in families and to be associated with other endocrine problems. It is diagnosed by genetic testing for a proto-oncogene called *RET*. Medullary thyroid cancer is a type of multiple endocrine neoplasia (see discussion at right). This type of cancer is often poorly differentiated and associated with early metastasis.

Anaplastic thyroid cancer, which is found in less than 2% of patients with thyroid cancer, is the most advanced and aggressive thyroid cancer. It is the least likely to respond to treatment and has a poor prognosis.

Clinical Manifestations and Diagnostic Studies

The primary manifestation of thyroid cancer is a painless, palpable nodule or nodules in an enlarged thyroid gland. Patients or health care providers discover most of these nodules during a routine palpation of the neck. Physical examination may reveal firm, palpable, cervical masses that are suggestive of lymph node metastasis. Hemoptysis and airway obstruction may occur if the trachea is involved.

Nodular enlargement of the thyroid gland or palpation of a mass requires further evaluation. Ultrasound is often the first test used. Follow-up testing may involve CT, MRI, positron emission tomography (PET), and ultrasound-guided fine-needle aspiration (FNA). FNA is indicated when a tissue sample for pathologic examination is necessary. A thyroid scan may also be done to evaluate for possible malignancy. The scan shows whether nodules on the thyroid are "hot" or "cold." Tumors that take up radioactive iodine are called "hot" nodules and are nearly always benign. If the nodule does not take up the radioactive iodine, it appears as "cold" and has a higher risk of being malignant (see eFig. 50-2, available on the website for this chapter).

Elevations in serum calcitonin are associated with medullary thyroid cancer. In papillary and follicular cancers, serum thyroglobulin is elevated. In families with a history of medullary thyroid cancer, encourage family members to get genetic testing done and have thyroid screening on a regular basis.

NURSING AND COLLABORATIVE MANAGEMENT THYROID CANCER

Surgical removal of the tumor is usually indicated for thyroid cancer.[19] Surgical procedures may range from unilateral total lobectomy to near-total thyroidectomy with bilateral lobectomy. Lymph nodes in the neck may be removed with surgery to determine if the cancer has spread. RAI may be given to some patients to destroy any remaining cancer cells after surgery. RAI therapy has been shown to improve survival rates in patients with papillary and follicular thyroid cancer. External beam radiation may be given as palliative treatment for patients with metastatic thyroid cancer.

Many thyroid cancers are TSH dependent, and thyroid hormone therapy in high doses is often prescribed to inhibit pituitary secretion of TSH. Chemotherapy including doxorubicin (Adriamycin), and cyclophosphamide (Cytoxan) may be used for advanced disease. Vandetanib (Caprelsa) and cabozantinib (Cometriq) are targeted therapies used for medullary thyroid cancer that has metastasized. These drugs inhibit tyrosine kinases, which are enzymes that are involved in growth of cancer cells.

Nursing care for the patient with thyroid cancer is similar to that of a patient undergoing thyroidectomy (see p. 1199). Because of the surgical site location and the potential for hypocalcemia, the patient requires frequent postoperative assessment. Assess the patient for airway obstruction, bleeding, and tetany, since the parathyroid gland may have been disturbed or removed during surgery.

MULTIPLE ENDOCRINE NEOPLASIA

Multiple endocrine neoplasia is an inherited condition characterized by hormone-secreting tumors.[20] Multiple endocrine neoplasia is caused by the mutation of one of two genes, *MEN1* or *RET*, that normally control cell growth. Tumors may develop in childhood or later in life.

The two major types of multiple endocrine neoplasia are type 1 and type 2. Both types are commonly inherited as autosomal dominant disorders. Persons with type 1 commonly show signs of parathyroid gland hyperactivity (hyperparathyroidism). Other signs may include hyperactivity of the pituitary gland (prolactinoma) and pancreas (gastrinomas). In most cases the tumors are initially benign, and some tumors later become malignant. Persons with type 2 neoplasia often have clinical manifestations of medullary thyroid carcinoma. They may also develop pheochromocytoma (tumor of the adrenal glands). (Pheochromocytoma is discussed later in this chapter on pp. 1214-1215.)

Treatment of the tumor(s) may include conservative management (watchful waiting), medication to block the effects of excess hormone, and surgical removal of the gland and/or tumor. It is important for patients to have regular screening visits with their health care provider so that new tumors may be detected early and existing tumors carefully monitored.

DISORDERS OF PARATHYROID GLANDS

HYPERPARATHYROIDISM

Etiology and Pathophysiology

Hyperparathyroidism is a condition involving an increased secretion of parathyroid hormone (PTH). PTH helps regulate serum calcium and phosphate levels by stimulating bone resorp-

tion of calcium, renal tubular reabsorption of calcium, and activation of vitamin D. Thus oversecretion of PTH is associated with increased serum calcium levels. Hyperparathyroidism affects approximately 1% of the U.S. population and is more common in women than in men.

Hyperparathyroidism is classified as primary, secondary, or tertiary. *Primary hyperparathyroidism* is due to an increased secretion of PTH leading to disorders of calcium, phosphate, and bone metabolism. The most common cause is a benign tumor (adenoma) in the parathyroid gland. Patients who have previously undergone head and neck radiation may have an increased risk of developing a parathyroid adenoma. Long-term lithium therapy has also been associated with primary hyperparathyroidism. The peak incidence of primary hyperparathyroidism is in the 40s and 50s.

Secondary hyperparathyroidism appears to be a compensatory response to conditions that induce or cause hypocalcemia, the main stimulus of PTH secretion. These conditions include vitamin D deficiencies, malabsorption, chronic kidney disease, and hyperphosphatemia.

Tertiary hyperparathyroidism occurs when there is hyperplasia of the parathyroid glands and a loss of negative feedback from circulating calcium levels. Thus there is autonomous secretion of PTH, even with normal calcium levels. This condition is seen in patients who have had a kidney transplant after a long period of dialysis treatment for chronic kidney disease (see Chapter 47).

Excessive levels of circulating PTH usually lead to hypercalcemia and hypophosphatemia. Multiple body systems are affected (Table 50-12). Decreased bone density can occur

TABLE 50-12 CLINICAL MANIFESTATIONS OF PARATHYROID DYSFUNCTION

Hyperfunction	Hypofunction	Hyperfunction	Hypofunction
Cardiovascular		**Visual**	
• Dysrhythmias	• Decreased contractility of heart muscle	• Corneal calcification on slit-lamp examination	• Eye changes, including lenticular opacities, cataracts, papilledema
• Shortened QT interval on ECG	• Decreased cardiac output		
• Hypertension	• Prolongation of QT and ST intervals on ECG		
	• Dysrhythmias	**Gastrointestinal**	
		• Vague abdominal pain	• Abdominal cramps
Neurologic		• Anorexia	• Fecal incontinence (in older adult)
• Personality disturbances	• Personality changes	• Nausea and vomiting	• Malabsorption
• Emotional irritability	• Psychiatric manifestations of depression, anxiety, psychosis	• Constipation	
• Memory impairment	• Irritability	• Pancreatitis	
• Psychosis, depression	• Memory impairment	• Peptic ulcer disease	
• Delirium, confusion, coma	• Headache, increased intracranial pressure	• Cholelithiasis	
• Poor coordination	• Seizures	• Weight loss	
• Hyperactive deep-tendon reflexes	• Positive Chvostek's sign or Trousseau's phenomenon (see Fig. 17-15)	**Integumentary**	
• Abnormalities of gait	• Tremor	• Skin necrosis	• Dry, scaly skin
• Psychomotor retardation	• Paresthesias of lips, hands, feet	• Moist skin	• Hair loss on scalp and body
• Headache	• Hyperactive deep-tendon reflexes		• Brittle nails, transverse ridging
• Paresthesias	• Disorientation, confusion (in older adult)		• Changes in developing teeth, lack of tooth enamel
		Musculoskeletal	
		• Skeletal pain	• Fatigue
		• Backache	• Weakness
		• Weakness, fatigue	• Painful muscle cramps
		• Pain on weight bearing	• Skeletal x-ray changes, osteosclerosis
		• Osteoporosis	• Soft tissue calcification
Renal		• Pathologic fractures of long bones	• Difficulty walking
• Hypercalciuria	• Urinary frequency	• Compression fractures of spine	
• Kidney stones (nephrolithiasis)	• Urinary incontinence	• Decreased muscle tone, muscle atrophy	
• Urinary tract infections			
• Polyuria			

because of the effect of PTH on osteoclastic (bone resorption) and osteoblastic (bone formation) activity. In the kidneys the excess calcium cannot be reabsorbed, leading to increased levels of calcium in the urine (hypercalciuria). This urinary calcium, along with a large amount of urinary phosphate, can lead to calculi formation.

Clinical Manifestations and Complications

Clinical manifestations range from the asymptomatic individual (diagnosed through testing for unrelated problems) to the patient with overt symptoms.[21] The manifestations are associated with hypercalcemia (see Table 50-12). Muscle weakness, loss of appetite, constipation, fatigue, emotional disorders, and shortened attention span are often noted. Other signs of hyperparathyroidism include osteoporosis, fractures, and kidney stones (nephrolithiasis). Neuromuscular abnormalities are characterized by muscle weakness, particularly in the proximal muscles of the lower extremities. Serious complications of hyperparathyroidism are renal failure; pancreatitis; cardiac changes; and long bone, rib, and vertebral fractures.

Diagnostic Studies

PTH levels are elevated in patients with hyperparathyroidism. Serum calcium levels usually exceed 10 mg/dL (2.50 mmol/L). Because of its inverse relation with calcium, the serum phosphorus level is usually less than 3 mg/dL (0.1 mmol/L). Hypercalcemia in asymptomatic cases is often identified through a routine chemistry panel.

Elevations in other laboratory tests include urine calcium, serum chloride, uric acid, creatinine, amylase (if pancreatitis is present), and alkaline phosphatase (in the presence of bone disease). Bone density measurements may be used to detect bone loss. Conversely, individuals found to have bone loss on a screening dual-energy x-ray absorptiometry (DEXA) scan should be tested for hypercalcemia. MRI, CT, and/or ultrasound may be used for localization of an adenoma.

Collaborative Care

The goal of treatment is to relieve symptoms and prevent complications caused by excess PTH. The choice of therapy depends on the urgency of the clinical situation, the degree of hypercalcemia, and the underlying cause of the disorder.

Surgical Therapy. The most effective treatment of primary and secondary hyperparathyroidism is surgical intervention. Surgery involves partial or complete removal of the parathyroid glands. The most commonly used procedure involves endoscopy and is done on an outpatient basis. Criteria for surgery include elevated serum calcium levels (more than 1 mg/dL above the upper limit of normal), hypercalciuria (greater than 400 mg/day), markedly reduced bone mineral density, overt symptoms (e.g., neuromuscular effects, nephrolithiasis), or those under age 50. Parathyroidectomy leads to a rapid reduction of high calcium levels.

Patients who have multiple parathyroid glands removed may undergo autotransplantation of normal parathyroid tissue in the forearm or near the sternocleidomastoid muscle. This allows PTH secretion to continue with normalization of calcium levels. If autotransplantation is not possible or if it fails, the patient will need to take calcium supplements for life.

Nonsurgical Therapy. A conservative approach is often used in patients who are asymptomatic or have mild symptoms of hyperparathyroidism. Ongoing care includes an annual examination with measurements of serum PTH, calcium, phosphorus, alkaline phosphatase, creatinine and blood urea nitrogen (BUN) (to assess renal function), and urinary calcium excretion. X-rays and DEXA are done to assess for metabolic bone loss. Continued ambulation and the avoidance of immobility are important aspects of management. Dietary measures include high fluid and moderate calcium intake.

Several drugs help lower calcium levels, but they do not treat the underlying problem. Bisphosphonates (e.g., alendronate [Fosamax]) inhibit osteoclastic bone resorption, normalizing serum calcium levels and improving bone mineral density. IV bisphosphonates (e.g., pamidronate [Aredia]) can rapidly lower serum calcium in patients with dangerously elevated levels. Phosphorus is usually supplemented unless contraindicated in a person with an increased risk for urinary calculi formation. Phosphates should be used only if the patient has normal renal function and low serum phosphate levels. Loop diuretics may be given to increase the urinary excretion of calcium.

Calcimimetic agents (e.g., cinacalcet [Sensipar]) increase the sensitivity of the calcium receptor on the parathyroid gland, resulting in decreased PTH secretion and calcium blood levels. Drugs in this class are given for secondary hyperparathyroidism in individuals with chronic kidney disease on dialysis and for patients with parathyroid cancer. Cinacalcet remains under investigation for use in primary hyperparathyroidism.

NURSING MANAGEMENT
HYPERPARATHYROIDISM

Nursing care for the patient after a parathyroidectomy is similar to that for a patient after thyroidectomy. The major postoperative complications are associated with hemorrhage and fluid and electrolyte disturbances. *Tetany,* a condition of neuromuscular hyperexcitability associated with sudden decrease in calcium levels, is another concern. It is usually apparent early in the postoperative period but may develop over several days. Mild tetany, characterized by unpleasant tingling of the hands and around the mouth, may be present but should decrease over time. If tetany becomes more severe (e.g., muscular spasms or laryngospasms), IV calcium may be given. IV calcium gluconate or gluceptate should be readily available for patients after parathyroidectomy in the event that acute tetany occurs.

Monitor intake and output to evaluate fluid status. Assess calcium, potassium, phosphate, and magnesium levels frequently, as well as Chvostek's and Trousseau's signs (see Fig. 17-15). Encourage mobility to promote bone calcification.

If surgery is not performed, treatment to relieve symptoms and prevent complications is initiated. Assist the patient with hyperparathyroidism to adapt the meal plan to his or her lifestyle. A referral to a dietitian may be useful. Because immobility can aggravate the bone loss, emphasize the importance of an exercise program. Encourage the patient to keep the regular follow-up appointments. Instruct the patient regarding the symptoms of hypocalcemia or hypercalcemia, and to report them should they occur. Hypocalcemia and hypercalcemia are discussed in Chapter 17.

HYPOPARATHYROIDISM

Hypoparathyroidism is an uncommon condition associated with inadequate circulating PTH. It is characterized by hypocalcemia resulting from a lack of PTH to maintain serum calcium levels. PTH resistance at the cellular level may also occur *(pseudohypoparathyroidism)*. This is caused by a genetic defect resulting in hypocalcemia in spite of normal or high PTH levels and is often associated with hypothyroidism and hypogonadism.

The most common cause of hypoparathyroidism is iatrogenic. This may include accidental removal of the parathyroid glands or damage to the vascular supply of the glands during neck surgery (e.g., thyroidectomy).[22] Idiopathic hypoparathyroidism resulting from the absence, fatty replacement, or atrophy of the glands is a rare disease that usually occurs early in life and may be associated with other endocrine disorders. Affected patients may have antiparathyroid antibodies. Severe hypomagnesemia (e.g., malnutrition, chronic alcoholism, renal failure) also leads to a suppression of PTH secretion. Other causes of parathyroid deficiency include tumors and heavy metal poisoning.

The clinical features of acute hypoparathyroidism are due to hypocalcemia (see Table 50-12). Sudden decreases in calcium concentration cause tetany, characterized by tingling of the lips and stiffness in the extremities. Painful tonic spasms of smooth and skeletal muscles can cause dysphagia and laryngospasms, which compromise breathing. Lethargy, anxiety, and personality changes may occur. Abnormal laboratory findings include decreased serum calcium and PTH levels and increased serum phosphate levels.

NURSING AND COLLABORATIVE MANAGEMENT HYPOPARATHYROIDISM

Treatment goals for the patient with hypoparathyroidism are to treat acute complications such as tetany, maintain normal serum calcium levels, and prevent long-term complications. Emergency treatment of tetany after surgery requires the administration of IV calcium.

Give IV calcium chloride, calcium gluconate, or calcium gluceptate slowly. Use ECG monitoring during calcium administration because high serum calcium blood levels can cause hypotension, serious cardiac dysrhythmias, or cardiac arrest. The patient who takes digoxin is particularly vulnerable. IV calcium chloride can cause venous irritation and inflammation, and extravasation may cause cellulitis, necrosis, and tissue sloughing. It is important to assess IV patency before administering calcium chloride.

Rebreathing may partially alleviate acute neuromuscular symptoms associated with hypocalcemia such as generalized muscle cramps or mild tetany. Instruct the patient (if cooperative) to breathe in and out of a paper bag or breathing mask. This reduces carbon dioxide excretion from the lungs, increases carbonic acid levels in the blood, and lowers the pH. A lower pH (acidic environment) enhances calcium ionization, which causes more total body calcium to be available in the active form. This will temporarily relieve the manifestations of hypocalcemia.

The patient with hypoparathyroidism needs instruction in the management of long-term drug and nutritional therapy. PTH replacement is not recommended because of the expense and need for parenteral administration. Oral calcium supplements of at least 1.5 to 3 g/day in divided doses are usually prescribed. Hypomagnesemia needs to be corrected in some patients before the hypocalcemia can be treated.

Vitamin D is used in hypocalcemia to enhance intestinal calcium absorption. Vitamin D (e.g., dihydrotachysterol [Hytak-

erol], 1,25-dihydroxycholecalciferol, or calcitriol [Rocaltrol]) raises calcium levels rapidly and is quickly metabolized. Rapid metabolism is desired because vitamin D is a fat-soluble vitamin and toxicity can cause irreversible renal impairment. A high-calcium meal plan includes foods such as dark green vegetables, soybeans, and tofu. Tell the patient to avoid foods containing oxalic acid (e.g., spinach, rhubarb) because they inhibit the absorption of calcium. Instruct the patient about the need for follow-up care, including monitoring of calcium levels three or four times a year.

DISORDERS OF ADRENAL CORTEX

Adrenal cortex steroid hormones have three main classifications: glucocorticoids, mineralocorticoids, and androgens. Glucocorticoids regulate metabolism, increase blood glucose levels, and are critical in the physiologic stress response. The primary glucocorticoid is cortisol. Mineralocorticoids regulate sodium and potassium balance. The primary mineralocorticoid is aldosterone. Androgens contribute to growth and development in both genders and to sexual activity in adult women. The term *corticosteroid* refers to any one of these three types of hormones produced by the adrenal cortex.

CUSHING SYNDROME

Etiology and Pathophysiology

Cushing syndrome is a clinical condition that results from chronic exposure to excess corticosteroids, particularly glucocorticoids.[23] Several conditions can cause Cushing syndrome. The most common cause is iatrogenic administration of exogenous corticosteroids (e.g., prednisone). Approximately 85% of the cases of endogenous Cushing syndrome are due to an ACTH-secreting pituitary adenoma (Cushing disease). Other causes of Cushing syndrome include adrenal tumors and ectopic ACTH production by tumors (usually of the lung or pancreas) outside of the hypothalamic-pituitary-adrenal axis. Cushing disease and primary adrenal tumors are more common in women in the 20- to 40-year-old age-group. Ectopic ACTH production is more common in men.

Clinical Manifestations

Manifestations of Cushing syndrome can be seen in most body systems and are related to excess levels of corticosteroids (Table 50-13). Although signs of glucocorticoid excess usually predominate, symptoms of mineralocorticoid and androgen excess may also be seen.

Corticosteroid excess causes pronounced changes in physical appearance (Fig. 50-10). Weight gain, the most common feature, results from the accumulation of adipose tissue in the trunk, face, and cervical spine area (Fig. 50-11). Hyperglycemia occurs because of glucose intolerance (associated with cortisol-induced insulin resistance) and increased gluconeogenesis by the liver. Muscle wasting causes weakness, especially in the extremities. A loss of bone matrix leads to osteoporosis and back pain. The loss of collagen makes the skin weaker and thinner and more easily bruised. Catabolic processes lead to a delay in wound healing. Irritability, anxiety, euphoria, and occasionally psychosis may also occur.

Mineralocorticoid excess may cause hypertension (secondary to fluid retention), whereas adrenal androgen excess may cause severe acne, virilization in women, and feminization in

TABLE 50-13	CLINICAL MANIFESTATIONS OF ADRENOCORTICAL DYSFUNCTION	
System	**Hyperfunction (Cushing Syndrome)**	**Hypofunction (Addison's Disease)**
Glucocorticoids		
General appearance	Truncal obesity, thin extremities, rounding of face (moon face), fat deposits on back of neck and shoulders (buffalo hump) (see Fig. 50-11).	Weight loss, emaciation.
Integumentary	Thin, fragile skin, purplish red striae (see Fig. 50-12). Petechial hemorrhages, bruises. Florid cheeks (plethora), acne, poor wound healing.	Bronzed or smoky hyperpigmentation of face, neck, hands (especially creases) (see Fig. 50-13), buccal membranes, nipples, genitalia, and scars (if pituitary function normal). Vitiligo, alopecia.
Cardiovascular	Hypervolemia, hypertension, edema of lower extremities.	Hypotension, tendency to develop refractory shock, vasodilation.
Gastrointestinal	Increase in secretion of pepsin and HCl acid, risk of peptic ulcer disease, anorexia.	Anorexia, nausea and vomiting, cramping abdominal pain, diarrhea.
Renal/urinary	Glycosuria, hypercalciuria, risk for kidney stones.	
Musculoskeletal	Muscle wasting in extremities, fatigue, osteoporosis, awkward gait, back pain, weakness, fractures.	Fatigue.
Immune	Inhibition of immune response, suppression of allergic response.	Tendency for coexisting autoimmune diseases.
Metabolic	Hyperglycemia, negative nitrogen balance, dyslipidemia.	Hyponatremia, insulin sensitivity, fever.
Emotional	Euphoria, irritability, depression, insomnia.	Depression, exhaustion or irritability, confusion, delusions.
Mineralocorticoids		
Fluid and electrolytes	Marked sodium and water retention, edema, marked hypokalemia, alkalosis.	Sodium loss, decreased volume of extracellular fluid, hyperkalemia, salt craving.
Cardiovascular	Hypertension, hypervolemia.	Hypovolemia, tendency toward shock, decreased cardiac output.
Androgens		
Integumentary	Hirsutism, acne, hyperpigmentation.	Decreased axillary and pubic hair (in women).
Reproductive	Menstrual irregularities and enlargement of clitoris (in women), gynecomastia and testicular atrophy (in men).	No effect in men, decreased libido in women.
Musculoskeletal	Muscle wasting and weakness.	Decrease in muscle size and tone.

FIG. 50-10 Cushing syndrome. Facies include a rounded face ("moon face") with thin, reddened skin. Hirsutism may also be present.

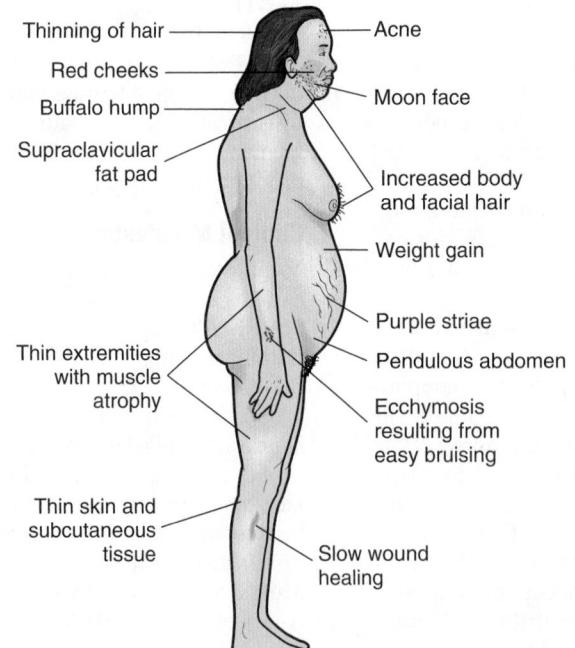

Thinning of hair — Acne
Red cheeks
Buffalo hump — Moon face
Supraclavicular fat pad
Increased body and facial hair
Weight gain
Purple striae
Pendulous abdomen
Thin extremities with muscle atrophy
Ecchymosis resulting from easy bruising
Thin skin and subcutaneous tissue
Slow wound healing

FIG. 50-11 Common characteristics of Cushing syndrome.

FIG. 50-12 Cushing syndrome. Truncal obesity; broad, purple striae; and easy bruising (left antecubital fossa).

men. Menstrual disorders and hirsutism in women and gyne-comastia and impotence in men are seen more commonly in adrenal carcinomas.

The first indication of Cushing syndrome may be the clinical presentation, including (1) centripetal (truncal) obesity or gen-eralized obesity; (2) *"moon face"* (fullness of the face) with facial plethora; (3) purplish red striae (usually depressed below the skin surface) on the abdomen, breast, or buttocks (Fig. 50-12); (4) hirsutism in women; (5) menstrual disorders in women; (6) hypertension; and (7) unexplained hypokalemia.

Diagnostic Studies

Plasma cortisol (the primary glucocorticoid) levels may be elevated, with loss of diurnal variation. When Cushing syn-drome is suspected, a 24-hour urine collection for free cortisol is done. Urine cortisol levels higher than the normal range of 80 to 120 mcg/24 hr indicate Cushing syndrome. If results are borderline, a low-dose dexamethasone suppression test is done. False-positive results can occur in patients with depression and those taking certain medications, including phenytoin (Dilantin) and rifampicin (rifampin [Rifadin]). Urine levels of 17-ketosteroids may be elevated.[24] A CT scan and MRI of the pituitary and adrenal glands may be done.

Plasma ACTH levels may be low, normal, or elevated depend-ing on the underlying cause of Cushing syndrome. High or normal ACTH levels indicate Cushing disease, whereas low or undetectable levels indicate an adrenal or medication etiology. Other findings on diagnostic tests associated with, but not diag-nostic of, Cushing syndrome include leukocytosis, lymphope-nia, eosinopenia, hyperglycemia, glycosuria, hypercalciuria, and osteoporosis. Hypokalemia and alkalosis are seen in ectopic ACTH syndrome and adrenal carcinoma.

Collaborative Care

The primary goal of treatment for Cushing syndrome is to nor-malize hormone secretion. The specific treatment depends on the underlying cause (Table 50-14). If the underlying cause is a pituitary adenoma, the standard treatment is surgical removal of the pituitary tumor using the transsphenoidal approach.[25] (The transsphenoidal approach is discussed earlier in this chapter on pp. 1190-1191.) Radiation therapy may also be used for patients who are not good surgical candidates.

Adrenalectomy is indicated for Cushing syndrome caused by adrenal tumors or hyperplasia. Occasionally, bilateral adrenal-ectomy is necessary. Laparoscopic adrenalectomy is used unless a malignant adrenal tumor is suspected. An open surgical adre-nalectomy is usually performed for adrenal cancer.

Patients with ectopic ACTH-secreting tumors are best managed by locating and removing the tumor (usually lung or pancreas). This is usually possible when the tumor is benign. When a tumor is malignant and it has already metastasized, surgical removal may not be possible or successful.

When the patient is a poor candidate for surgery or prior surgery has failed, then drug therapy may be attempted. The goal of drug therapy is to suppress the synthesis and secretion of cortisol from the adrenal gland (*medical adrenalectomy*). Drugs used include ketoconazole (Nizoral), aminoglutethimide (Cytadren), and mitotane (Lysodren). These are used cautiously because they are often toxic at the dosages needed to reduce cortisol secretion. Hydrocortisone or prednisone may be needed to avoid adrenal insufficiency. Mifepristone (Korlym) may be used to control hyperglycemia in patients with endog-enous Cushing syndrome who have type 2 diabetes.

TABLE 50-14 COLLABORATIVE CARE

Cushing Syndrome

Diagnostic
- History and physical examination
- Mental status examination
- Plasma cortisol levels for diurnal variations
- Plasma ACTH levels
- Complete blood count (CBC) with WBC differential
- Blood chemistries for sodium, potassium, glucose
- Dexamethasone suppression test
- 24-hr urine for free cortisol and 17-ketosteroids
- CT scan, MRI

Collaborative Therapy*
Pituitary Adenoma
- Transsphenoidal resection
- Radiation therapy

Adrenocortical Adenoma, Carcinoma, or Hyperplasia
- Adrenalectomy (open or laparoscopic)
- Drug therapy (e.g., ketoconazole [Nizoral], aminoglutethimide [Cytadren], mitotane [Lysodren], mifepristone [Korlym])

Ectopic ACTH-Secreting Tumor
- Treatment of the tumor (surgical removal or radiation)

Exogenous Corticosteroid Therapy
- Discontinue or alter the dose of exogenous corticosteroids

*Treatment is based on underlying cause.
ACTH, Adrenocorticotropic hormone.

If Cushing syndrome has developed during the course of prolonged administration of corticosteroids (e.g., predni-sone), the following alternatives may be tried: (1) gradual dis-continuance of corticosteroid therapy, (2) reduction of the corticosteroid dose, and (3) conversion to an alternate-day regimen. Gradual tapering of the corticosteroids is necessary to avoid potentially life-threatening adrenal insufficiency. In an alternate-day regimen, twice the daily dosage of a shorter-acting corticosteroid is given every other morning to minimize hypothalamic-pituitary-adrenal suppression, growth suppres-sion, and altered appearance. This regimen is not used when the corticosteroids are given as hormone therapy.

NURSING MANAGEMENT CUSHING SYNDROME

NURSING ASSESSMENT

Subjective and objective data that should be obtained from a patient with Cushing syndrome are presented in Table 50-15.

NURSING DIAGNOSES

Nursing diagnoses for the patient with Cushing syndrome may include, but are not limited to, the following:
- Risk for infection *related to* lowered resistance to stress and suppression of immune system
- Imbalanced nutrition: more than body requirements *related to* increased appetite, high caloric content of foods, and inactivity
- Disturbed body image *related to* change in appearance from disease process
- Impaired skin integrity *related to* excess corticosteroids, immobility, and altered skin fragility

Additional information on nursing diagnoses is presented in eNursing Care Plan 50-3 for the patient with Cushing syndrome (available on the website for this chapter).

TABLE 50-15   NURSING ASSESSMENT

Cushing Syndrome

Subjective Data
Important Health Information
Past health history: Pituitary tumor (Cushing disease); adrenal, pancreatic, or pulmonary neoplasms; GI bleeding; frequent infections
Medications: Corticosteroids

Functional Health Patterns
Health perception–health management: Malaise
Nutritional-metabolic: Weight gain, anorexia; prolonged wound healing, easy bruising
Elimination: Polyuria
Activity-exercise: Weakness, fatigue
Sleep: Insomnia, poor sleep quality
Cognitive-perceptual: Headache; back, joint, bone, and rib pain; poor concentration and memory
Self-perception–self-concept: Negative feelings regarding changes in personal appearance
Sexuality-reproductive: Amenorrhea, impotence, decreased libido
Coping–stress tolerance: Anxiety, mood disturbances, emotional lability, psychosis

Objective Data
General
Truncal obesity, supraclavicular fat pads, buffalo hump, moon face

Integumentary
Plethora; hirsutism of body and face, thinning of head hair; thin, friable skin; acne; petechiae; purpura; hyperpigmentation; purplish red striae on breasts, buttocks, and abdomen; edema of lower extremities

Cardiovascular
Hypertension

Musculoskeletal
Muscle wasting, thin extremities, awkward gait

Reproductive
Gynecomastia, testicular atrophy (in men), enlarged clitoris (in women)

Possible Diagnostic Findings
Hypokalemia, hyperglycemia, dyslipidemia; polycythemia, granulocytosis, lymphocytopenia, eosinopenia; ↑ plasma cortisol; high, low, or normal ACTH levels; abnormal dexamethasone suppression test; ↑ urine free cortisol, 17-ketosteroids; glycosuria, hypercalciuria; osteoporosis on x-ray

ACTH, Adrenocorticotropic hormone.

PLANNING

The overall goals are that the patient with Cushing syndrome will (1) experience relief of symptoms, (2) avoid serious complications, (3) maintain a positive self-image, and (4) actively participate in the therapeutic plan.

NURSING IMPLEMENTATION

HEALTH PROMOTION. Health promotion is focused on identifying patients at risk for Cushing syndrome. Patients receiving long-term, exogenous corticosteroids for a variety of diseases are at risk. Patient teaching related to using medications and monitoring side effects is an important preventive measure.

ACUTE INTERVENTION. The patient with Cushing syndrome is seriously ill. Because the therapy has many side effects, assessment focuses on signs and symptoms of hormone and drug

toxicity and complicating conditions (e.g., cardiovascular disease, diabetes mellitus, infection). Assess and monitor vital signs, daily weight, glucose, and possible infection. Because signs and symptoms of inflammation (e.g., fever, redness) may be minimal or absent, assess for pain, loss of function, and purulent drainage. Monitor for signs and symptoms of abnormal thromboembolic events such as pulmonary emboli (e.g., sudden chest pain, dyspnea, tachypnea).

Another important focus of nursing care is emotional support. Changes in appearance such as centripetal obesity, multiple bruises, hirsutism in women, and gynecomastia in men can be distressing. The patient may feel unattractive, repulsive, or unwanted. You can help by remaining sensitive to the patient's feelings and offering respect and unconditional acceptance. Reassure the patient that the physical changes and much of the emotional lability will resolve when hormone levels return to normal.

If treatment involves surgical removal of a pituitary adenoma, an adrenal tumor, or one or both adrenal glands, nursing care will also focus on preoperative and postoperative care.

Preoperative Care. Before surgery the patient should be brought to optimal physical condition. Hypertension and hyperglycemia must be controlled, and hypokalemia must be corrected with diet and potassium supplements. A high-protein diet helps correct the protein depletion. Preoperative teaching depends on the type of surgical approach planned (hypophysectomy or adrenalectomy) and should include information regarding the anticipated postoperative care. Preoperative management for the patient undergoing a hypophysectomy is discussed earlier in this chapter on pp. 1190-1191.

Postoperative Care. Surgery on the adrenal glands poses greater risks than other operations. Because the adrenal glands are vascular, the risk of hemorrhage is increased. In the postoperative period (for both laparoscopic and open adrenalectomy), patients may have a nasogastric tube, a urinary catheter, IV therapy, central venous pressure monitoring, and leg sequential compression devices to prevent emboli.

Manipulation of glandular tissue during surgery may release large amounts of hormones into the circulation, producing marked fluctuations in the metabolic processes affected by these hormones. Postoperatively, BP, fluid balance, and electrolyte levels may be unstable due to these hormone fluctuations.

High doses of corticosteroids (e.g., hydrocortisone [Solu-Cortef]) are administered IV during surgery and for several days afterward to ensure adequate responses to the stress of the procedure. If large amounts of endogenous hormone have been released into the systemic circulation during surgery, the patient is likely to develop hypertension, increasing the risk of hemorrhage. High levels of corticosteroids increase susceptibility to infection and delay wound healing.

The critical period for circulatory instability ranges from 24 to 48 hours after surgery. During this time you must constantly be alert for signs of corticosteroid imbalance. Report any rapid or significant changes in BP, respirations, or heart rate. Monitor fluid intake and output carefully and assess for potential imbalances. IV corticosteroids are given, and the dosage and flow rate are adjusted to the patient's clinical manifestations and fluid and electrolyte balance. Oral doses are given as tolerated. After IV corticosteroids are withdrawn, keep the IV line open for quick administration of corticosteroids or vasopressors. Obtain morning urine samples (collected at the same time each morning) for cortisol measurement to evaluate the surgery's effectiveness.

If corticosteroid dosage is tapered too rapidly after surgery, acute adrenal insufficiency may develop. Vomiting, increased weakness, dehydration, and hypotension may indicate hypocortisolism. In addition, the patient may complain of painful joints, pruritus, or peeling skin and may experience severe emotional disturbances. Report these signs and symptoms so that drug doses can be adjusted as necessary.

After surgery the patient is usually maintained on bed rest until the BP stabilizes. Be alert for subtle signs of postoperative infection because the usual inflammatory responses are suppressed. To prevent infection, provide meticulous care when changing the dressing and during any other procedures that involve access to body cavities, circulation, or areas under the skin. eNursing Care Plan 50-3 for the patient with Cushing syndrome is available on the website for this chapter.

AMBULATORY AND HOME CARE. Discharge instructions are based on the patient's lack of endogenous corticosteroids and resulting inability to physiologically react to stressors. Consider a home health nurse referral, especially for older adults, because of the need for ongoing evaluation and teaching. Instruct the patient to wear a Medic Alert bracelet at all times and carry medical identification and instructions in a wallet or purse. Teach the patient to avoid exposure to extreme temperatures, infections, and emotional disturbances. Stress may produce or precipitate acute adrenal insufficiency because the remaining adrenal tissue cannot meet an increased hormonal demand. Teach patients to adjust their corticosteroid replacement therapy in accordance with their stress levels. Consult with the patient's health care provider to determine the parameters for dosage changes if this plan is feasible. If the patient cannot adjust his or her own medication or if weakness, fainting, fever, or nausea and vomiting occur, the patient should contact the health care provider for a possible adjustment in corticosteroid dosage. Many patients require lifetime replacement therapy. However, patients should be prepared for it to take several months to adjust the hormone dose satisfactorily.

EVALUATION

The expected outcomes are that the patient with Cushing syndrome will

- Experience no signs or symptoms of infection
- Attain weight appropriate for height
- Verbalize acceptance of appearance and treatment regimen
- Demonstrate healing of skin and maintenance of intact skin

Additional information on expected outcomes is presented in eNursing Care Plan 50-3 for the patient with Cushing syndrome (available on the website for this chapter).

ADRENOCORTICAL INSUFFICIENCY

Etiology and Pathophysiology

Adrenocortical insufficiency (hypofunction of the adrenal cortex) may be from a primary cause (Addison's disease) or a secondary cause (lack of pituitary ACTH secretion). In Addison's disease, all three classes of adrenal corticosteroids (glucocorticoids, mineralocorticoids, and androgens) are reduced. In secondary adrenocortical insufficiency, corticosteroids and androgens are deficient but mineralocorticoids rarely are. ACTH deficiency may be caused by pituitary disease or sup-

pression of the hypothalamic-pituitary axis because of the administration of exogenous corticosteroids.

The most common cause of Addison's disease in the United States is an autoimmune response.[26] Adrenal tissue is destroyed by antibodies against the patient's own adrenal cortex. Often, other endocrine conditions are present and Addison's disease is considered a component of *autoimmune polyglandular syndrome*. This rare syndrome is caused by a mutation in a gene that helps to regulate the immune system. The condition is inherited as an autosomal recessive trait. Addison's disease, if caused by an autoimmune response, is most common in white females.

Although tuberculosis causes Addison's disease worldwide, it is now an uncommon cause in the United States. Other causes include infarction, fungal infections (e.g., histoplasmosis), acquired immunodeficiency syndrome (AIDS), and metastatic cancer. Iatrogenic Addison's disease may be due to adrenal hemorrhage, often related to anticoagulant therapy, chemotherapy, ketoconazole therapy for AIDS, or bilateral adrenalectomy. Adrenal insufficiency most often occurs in adults younger than 60 years of age and affects both genders equally.

Clinical Manifestations

Because manifestations do not tend to become evident until 90% of the adrenal cortex is destroyed, the disease is often advanced before it is diagnosed. The manifestations have a slow (insidious) onset and include progressive weakness, fatigue, weight loss, and anorexia as primary features. Increased ACTH causes the striking feature of a bronze-colored skin hyperpigmentation. It is seen primarily in sun-exposed areas of the body; at pressure points; over joints; and in the creases, especially palmar creases (Fig. 50-13). The changes in the skin are most likely due to increased secretion of β-lipotropin (which contains melanocyte-stimulating hormone [MSH]). This tropic hormone is increased because of decreased negative feedback and subsequent low corticosteroid levels. Other manifestations of adrenal insufficiency are orthostatic hypotension, hyponatremia, salt craving, hyperkalemia, nausea and vomiting, and diarrhea. Irritability and depression may also occur in primary adrenal hypofunction.

Patients with secondary adrenocortical hypofunction may have many signs and symptoms similar to those of patients with Addison's disease. However, they usually do not have hyperpigmented skin because ACTH levels are low.

Complications

Patients with adrenocortical insufficiency are at risk for acute adrenal insufficiency *(addisonian crisis),* a life-threatening

FIG. 50-13 Hyperpigmentation typically seen in Addison's disease.

emergency caused by insufficient adrenocortical hormones or a sudden sharp decrease in these hormones. Addisonian crisis is triggered by (1) stress (e.g., from infection, surgery, psychologic distress), (2) the sudden withdrawal of corticosteroid hormone therapy (which is often done by a patient who lacks knowledge of the importance of this therapy), (3) adrenal surgery, or (4) sudden pituitary gland destruction.

During acute adrenal insufficiency, the patient exhibits severe manifestations of glucocorticoid and mineralocorticoid deficiencies, including hypotension (particularly postural), tachycardia, dehydration, hyponatremia, hyperkalemia, hypoglycemia, fever, weakness, and confusion. Hypotension may lead to shock. Circulatory collapse associated with adrenal insufficiency is often unresponsive to the usual treatment (vasopressors and fluid replacement). GI manifestations include severe vomiting, diarrhea, and pain in the abdomen. Pain may occur in the lower back or the legs.

Diagnostic Studies

Adrenal insufficiency is characterized by depressed serum and urinary cortisol levels. ACTH levels are increased in primary adrenal insufficiency and decreased in secondary disease. Primary adrenal insufficiency is confirmed when cortisol levels fail to rise over basal levels with an ACTH stimulation test. A positive response to ACTH stimulation test indicates a functioning adrenal gland and points to a probable diagnosis of secondary adrenocortical insufficiency related to the pituitary gland. Urine levels of free cortisol are low, as is the urine level of aldosterone.

Other abnormal laboratory findings in some cases include hyperkalemia, hypochloremia, hyponatremia, hypoglycemia, anemia, and increased BUN levels.[25] An ECG may show low voltage and peaked T waves caused by hyperkalemia. CT scans and MRI may be used to identify causes other than autoimmune, including tumors, fungal infections, tuberculosis, or adrenal calcification.

Collaborative Care

Treatment of adrenocortical insufficiency is focused on management of the underlying cause when possible. The mainstay of treatment for the adrenocortical insufficiency is hormone therapy (Table 50-16). Hydrocortisone, the most commonly used form of hormone therapy, has both glucocorticoid and mineralocorticoid properties. During stressful situations the glucocorticoid dosage is increased to prevent addisonian crisis. Mineralocorticoid replacement with fludrocortisone (Florinef) is administered daily. Increased salt needs to be added in the diet.

Addisonian crisis is a life-threatening emergency requiring aggressive management. Treatment must be directed toward shock management and high-dose hydrocortisone replacement. Large volumes of 0.9% saline solution and 5% dextrose are administered to reverse hypotension and electrolyte imbalances until BP returns to normal.

NURSING MANAGEMENT
ADDISON'S DISEASE

NURSING IMPLEMENTATION

ACUTE INTERVENTION. When the patient with Addison's disease is hospitalized, nursing management focuses on monitoring the patient while correcting fluid and electrolyte balance.

TABLE 50-16   **COLLABORATIVE CARE**
Addison's Disease

Diagnostic
- History and physical examination
- Serum cortisol
- Serum ACTH
- Urine cortisol and aldosterone
- Serum electrolytes
- ACTH-stimulation test
- CT scan, MRI

Collaborative Therapy
- Daily glucocorticoid (e.g., hydrocortisone) replacement (two thirds on awakening in morning, one third in late afternoon)*
- Daily mineralocorticoid (fludrocortisone [Florinef]) in morning*
- Salt additives for excess heat or humidity
- Increased doses of cortisol for stress situations (e.g., surgery, hospitalization)

*For conditions of normal daily stress in individuals with usual daytime activity.
ACTH, Adrenocorticotropic hormone.

Assess vital signs and signs of fluid volume deficit and electrolyte imbalance. Monitor trends in serum glucose, sodium, and potassium. Establish baseline data regarding mental status, vital signs, and weight. Obtain a complete medication history to determine drugs that can potentially interact with corticosteroids. These drugs include oral hypoglycemics, cardiac glycosides, oral contraceptives, anticoagulants, and NSAIDs.

Note changes in BP, weight gain, weakness, or other manifestations of Cushing syndrome. In addition, protect against exposure to infection and assist with daily hygiene. Protect the patient from noise, light, and environmental temperature extremes. The patient cannot cope with these stresses because of the inability to produce corticosteroids.

AMBULATORY AND HOME CARE. You have an important role in the long-term management of Addison's disease. The serious nature of the disease and the need for lifelong hormone therapy necessitate a comprehensive teaching plan. Table 50-17 outlines the major areas to include in your teaching plan.

Glucocorticoids are usually given in divided doses, two thirds in the morning and one third in the afternoon. Mineralocorticoids are given once daily, preferably in the morning. This dosage schedule reflects normal circadian rhythm in endogenous hormone secretion and decreases the side effects associated with corticosteroid therapy. Help the patient maintain hormone balance while managing the medication regimen.

The patient with Addison's disease is unable to tolerate physical or emotional stress without additional exogenous corticosteroids. Long-term care revolves around recognizing the need for extra medication and techniques for stress management. Examples of situations requiring corticosteroid adjustment are fever, influenza, extraction of teeth, and rigorous physical activity such as playing tennis on a hot day or running a marathon. If vomiting or diarrhea occurs, as may happen with influenza, notify the health care provider immediately because electrolyte replacement and parenteral administration of cortisol may be necessary. Overall, patients who take their medications consistently can anticipate a normal life expectancy.

Teach the patient about the signs and symptoms of corticosteroid deficiency and excess (Cushing syndrome) and to report these signs to their health care provider so the dose can be adjusted. It is critical that the patient wear an identification

TABLE 50-17 PATIENT & CAREGIVER TEACHING GUIDE

Addison's Disease

Include the following information in the teaching plan for Addison's disease.
1. Names, dosages, and actions of drugs
2. Symptoms of overdosage and underdosage
3. Conditions requiring increased medication (e.g., trauma, infection, surgery, emotional crisis)
4. Course of action to take relative to changes in medication
   - Increase in dose of corticosteroid
   - Administration of large dose of corticosteroid intramuscularly, including demonstration and return demonstration
   - Consultation with health care provider
5. Prevention of infection and need for prompt and vigorous treatment of existing infections
6. Need for lifelong replacement therapy
7. Need for lifelong medical supervision
8. Need for medical identification device
9. Prevention of falls
10. Adverse effects of corticosteroid therapy and prevention techniques
11. Special instruction for patients who are diabetics and management of blood glucose when taking corticosteroids

TABLE 50-18 DRUG THERAPY

Diseases and Disorders Treated With Corticosteroids

Hormone Therapy
Adrenal insufficiency
Congenital adrenal hyperplasia

Therapeutic Effect
Allergic Reactions
- Anaphylaxis
- Bee stings
- Contact dermatitis
- Drug reactions
- Serum sickness
- Urticaria

Collagen Diseases
- Giant cell arteritis
- Mixed connective tissue disorders
- Polymyositis
- Polyarteritis nodosa
- Rheumatoid arthritis
- Systemic lupus erythematosus

Neurologic Diseases
- Prevention of cerebral edema and increased intracranial pressure
- Head trauma

Gastrointestinal Diseases
- Inflammatory bowel disease
- Celiac disease

Endocrine Diseases
- Hypercalcemia
- Hashimoto's thyroiditis
- Thyrotoxicosis

Liver Diseases
- Alcoholic hepatitis
- Autoimmune hepatitis

Pulmonary Diseases
- Aspiration pneumonia
- Asthma
- Chronic obstructive pulmonary disease

Other Diseases or Disorders
- Skin diseases
- Malignancies, leukemia, lymphoma
- Immunosuppression
- Inflammation
- Nephrotic syndrome

bracelet (Medic Alert) and carry a wallet card stating the patient has Addison's disease so that appropriate therapy can be initiated in case of an emergency. Provide verbal instruction and handouts about other medications that can cause a need to increase (e.g., phenytoin, barbiturates, rifampin, antacids) or decrease (e.g., estrogen) glucocorticoid dosage. Instruct patients using mineralocorticoid therapy (fludrocortisone) how to take their BP, increase salt intake, and report any significant changes to their health care provider.

The patient should carry an emergency kit at all times with 100 mg of IM hydrocortisone, syringes, and instructions for use. Instruct the patient and significant others in how to give an IM injection in case the hormone therapy cannot be taken orally. Have the patient verbalize instructions and practice IM injections with saline. Provide written instructions on when the dose should be changed.[27]

CORTICOSTEROID THERAPY

Corticosteroids are used to relieve the signs and symptoms associated with many diseases (Table 50-18). Corticosteroids are effective in treating many diseases and disorders. However, the long-term administration of corticosteroids in therapeutic doses often leads to serious complications and side effects (Table 50-19). For this reason, corticosteroid therapy is not recommended for minor chronic conditions. Therapy should be reserved for diseases that have a risk of death or permanent loss of function, and for conditions in which short-term therapy is likely to produce remission or recovery. The potential benefits of treatment must always be weighed against the risks.

A beneficial effect of corticosteroids in one situation may be a harmful one in another. For example, decreasing inflammation in arthritis is an important therapeutic effect, but increasing the risk for infection is a harmful effect. Suppression of inflammation and the immune response may help save lives in persons with anaphylaxis and in those receiving an organ transplant, but it can reactivate latent tuberculosis and greatly reduces resistance to other infections and cancers. The vasopressive effect of corticosteroids is critical in enabling a person to function in stressful situations, but can produce hypertension when used for drug therapy. Effects and side effects related to corticosteroid therapy are listed in Table 50-19.

DRUG ALERT: Corticosteroids
- Instruct the patient not to abruptly discontinue these drugs.
- Monitor the patient for signs of infection.
- Instruct patients with diabetes to closely monitor blood glucose.

Patients receive corticosteroid therapy for many reasons (see Table 50-18). Detailed instruction is necessary to ensure patient

TABLE 50-19 DRUG THERAPY

Effects and Side Effects of Corticosteroids

- Hypokalemia may develop.
- Patient is predisposed to peptic ulcer disease.
- Skeletal muscle atrophy and weakness occur.
- Mood and behavior changes may be observed.
- Glucose intolerance predisposes patient to diabetes mellitus.
- Fat from extremities is redistributed to trunk and face.
- Hypocalcemia related to anti–vitamin D effect may occur.
- Healing is delayed, with increased risk for wound dehiscence.
- Susceptibility to infection is increased. Infection develops more rapidly and spreads more widely.
- Manifestations of inflammation, including redness, tenderness, heat, swelling, and local edema, are suppressed.
- Pituitary ACTH synthesis is suppressed. Corticosteroid deficiency is likely if hormones are withdrawn abruptly. Taper corticosteroid doses.
- Blood pressure increases because of excess blood volume and potentiation of vasoconstrictor effects. Hypertension predisposes patient to heart failure.
- Protein depletion decreases bone formation, density, and strength, leading to predisposition to pathologic fractures, especially compression fractures of the vertebrae (osteoporosis).

ACTH, Adrenocorticotropic hormone.

adherence. When corticosteroids are used as nonreplacement therapies, they are taken once daily or once every other day. They should be taken early in the morning with food to decrease gastric irritation. Because exogenous corticosteroid administration may suppress endogenous ACTH and therefore endogenous cortisol (suppression is time and dose dependent), emphasize the danger of abrupt cessation of corticosteroid therapy to patients and caregivers. Corticosteroids taken for longer than 1 week will suppress adrenal production, and oral corticosteroids must be tapered. Ensure that increased doses of corticosteroids are prescribed in acute care or home care settings in situations of physical or emotional stress.

Corticosteroid-induced osteoporosis is an important concern for patients who receive corticosteroid treatment for prolonged periods (longer than 3 months).[28] Therapies to reduce the resorption of bone may include increased calcium intake, vitamin D supplementation, bisphosphonates (e.g., alendronate), and a low-impact exercise program. Further instruction and interventions to minimize the side effects and complications of corticosteroid therapy are presented in Table 50-20.

HYPERALDOSTERONISM

Hyperaldosteronism (Conn's syndrome) is characterized by excessive aldosterone secretion. The main effects of aldosterone are (1) sodium retention and (2) potassium and hydrogen ion excretion. Thus the hallmark of this disease is hypertension with hypokalemic alkalosis. *Primary hyperaldosteronism* (PA) is most commonly caused by a small solitary adrenocortical adenoma. Occasionally multiple lesions are involved and are associated with bilateral adrenal hyperplasia. PA affects women more than men and usually occurs between 30 and 60 years of age. A genetic link has been identified in some patients.[29] Up to 2%

TABLE 50-20	**PATIENT & CAREGIVER TEACHING GUIDE**

Corticosteroid Therapy

Include the following instructions when teaching the patient and caregiver to manage corticosteroid therapy.

1. Plan a diet high in protein, calcium (at least 1500 mg/day) and potassium but low in fat and concentrated simple carbohydrates such as sugar, honey, syrups, and candy.
2. Identify measures to ensure adequate rest and sleep, such as daily naps and avoidance of caffeine late in the day.
3. Develop and maintain an exercise program to help maintain bone integrity.
4. Recognize edema and ways to restrict sodium intake to <2000 mg/day if edema occurs.
5. Monitor glucose levels and recognize symptoms of hyperglycemia (e.g., polydipsia, polyuria, blurred vision). Report hyperglycemic symptoms or capillary glucose levels >120 mg/dL (10 mmol/L).
6. Notify health care provider if experiencing heartburn after meals or epigastric pain that is not relieved by antacids.
7. See an eye specialist yearly to assess for cataracts.
8. Use safety measures such as getting up slowly from bed or a chair and use good lighting to avoid accidental injury.
9. Maintain good hygiene practices and avoid contact with persons with colds or other contagious illnesses to prevent infection.
10. Inform all health care providers about long-term corticosteroid use.
11. Recognize need for increased doses of corticosteroids in times of physical and emotional stress.
12. Never abruptly stop the corticosteroids because this could lead to addisonian crisis and possibly death.

of all cases of hypertension are caused by PA. *Secondary hyperaldosteronism* occurs in response to a nonadrenal cause of elevated aldosterone levels such as renal artery stenosis, renin-secreting tumors, and chronic kidney disease.

Elevated levels of aldosterone are associated with sodium retention and excretion of potassium. Sodium retention leads to hypernatremia, hypertension, and headache. Edema does not usually occur because the rate of sodium excretion increases, which prevents more severe sodium retention. The potassium wasting leads to hypokalemia, which causes generalized muscle weakness, fatigue, cardiac dysrhythmias, glucose intolerance, and metabolic alkalosis that may lead to tetany.

Hyperaldosteronism should be suspected in all hypertensive patients with hypokalemia who are not being treated with diuretics. PA is associated with elevated plasma aldosterone levels, elevated sodium levels, decreased serum potassium levels, and decreased plasma renin activity. Adenomas are localized by means of a CT scan or an MRI.[30] If a tumor is not found, plasma 18-hydroxycorticosterone is measured after overnight bed rest. A level greater than 50 ng/dL indicates an adenoma.

NURSING AND COLLABORATIVE MANAGEMENT PRIMARY HYPERALDOSTERONISM

The preferred treatment for PA is surgical removal of the adenoma (adrenalectomy). A laparoscopic approach is most often used. Before surgery, patients should be treated with potassium-sparing diuretics (spironolactone [Aldactone], eplerenone [Inspra]) and antihypertensive agents to normalize serum potassium levels and BP. Spironolactone and eplerenone block the binding of aldosterone to the mineralocorticoid receptor in the terminal distal tubules and collecting ducts of the kidney, thus increasing the excretion of sodium and water and the retention of potassium. Oral potassium supplements and sodium restrictions may also be necessary. However, potassium supplementation and a potassium-sparing diuretic should not be started simultaneously because of the danger of hyperkalemia. Teach patients taking eplerenone to avoid grapefruit juice.

Patients with bilateral adrenal hyperplasia are treated with a potassium-sparing diuretic (e.g., spironolactone, amiloride [Midamor]) or aminoglutethimide, which blocks aldosterone synthesis. Calcium channel blockers may also be used to control BP. Dexamethasone may be used to decrease adrenal hyperplasia.

Nursing care includes careful assessment for signs of fluid and electrolyte balance (especially potassium) and cardiovascular status. Monitor BP frequently before and after surgery because unilateral adrenalectomy is successful in controlling hypertension in only 80% of patients with an adenoma. Instruct patients receiving maintenance therapy with spironolactone or amiloride about the possible side effects of gynecomastia, impotence, and menstrual disorders, as well as the signs and symptoms of hypokalemia and hyperkalemia. Teach patients how to monitor their own BP and the need for frequent monitoring. Stress the need for continued health supervision.

DISORDERS OF ADRENAL MEDULLA

PHEOCHROMOCYTOMA

Pheochromocytoma, which is a rare condition caused by a tumor in the adrenal medulla affecting the chromaffin cells, results in an excess production of catecholamines (epinephrine, norepinephrine). The most dangerous immediate effect of the disease is severe hypertension.[31] If left untreated, it may lead to hypertensive encephalopathy, diabetes mellitus, cardiomyopathy, and death. It is most commonly seen in young to middle-aged adults. Pheochromocytoma may be inherited in persons with multiple endocrine neoplasia.

The most striking clinical features of pheochromocytoma are severe, episodic hypertension accompanied by the classic manifestations of severe, pounding headache; tachycardia with palpitations; profuse sweating; and unexplained abdominal or chest pain. Attacks may be provoked by many medications, including antihypertensives, opioids, radiologic contrast media, and tricyclic antidepressants. The attacks may last from a few minutes to several hours.

Although pheochromocytoma is associated with a number of symptoms, the diagnosis is often missed. Pheochromocytoma is an uncommon cause of hypertension, accounting for only 0.1% of all cases. Consider this condition in patients who do not respond to traditional hypertensive treatments.

The simplest and most reliable diagnostic test for pheochromocytoma is measurement of urinary fractionated metanephrines (catecholamine metabolites) and fractionated catecholamines and creatinine, usually done as a 24-hour urine collection. Values are elevated in at least 95% of persons with pheochromocytoma. Serum catecholamines may be elevated during an "attack." CT scans and MRI are used for diagnosing tumors. Avoid palpating the abdomen of a patient with suspected pheochromocytoma, since it may cause the sudden release of catecholamines and severe hypertension.

NURSING AND COLLABORATIVE MANAGEMENT PHEOCHROMOCYTOMA

The primary treatment of pheochromocytoma is surgical removal of the tumor. Treatment with α- and β-adrenergic receptor blockers is required preoperatively to control BP and prevent an intraoperative hypertensive crisis. The α-adrenergic receptor blocker phenoxybenzamine (Dibenzyline) is given 7 to 10 days preoperatively to reduce BP and alleviate other symptoms of catecholamine excess. After adequate α-adrenergic blockade, β-adrenergic receptor blockers (e.g., propranolol) are used to decrease tachycardia and other dysrhythmias. If β-blockers are started too early, unopposed α-adrenergic stimulation could precipitate a hypertensive crisis. They can also cause orthostatic hypotension. Advise the patient to make postural changes cautiously.

Surgery is most commonly done using a laparoscopic approach. Removal of the adrenal tumor usually cures the hypertension, but hypertension persists in approximately 10% to 30% of patients. If surgery is not an option, metyrosine (Demser) is used to decrease catecholamine production by the tumor.

Case finding is an important nursing role. Any patient with hypertension accompanied by symptoms of sympathoadrenal stimulation should be referred to a health care provider for definitive diagnosis. Assess the patient for the classic triad of symptoms of pheochromocytoma (severe pounding headache, tachycardia, and profuse sweating). Monitor the BP immediately if the patient is experiencing an "attack."

Attempt to make the patient with pheochromocytoma as comfortable as possible. Monitor blood glucose levels to assess for diabetes mellitus. Patients need rest, nourishing food, and emotional support during this period. Preoperative and postoperative care is similar to that for any patient undergoing adrenalectomy except that BP fluctuations from catecholamine excesses tend to be severe and must be carefully monitored. Emphasize the importance of follow-up and routine BP monitoring because hypertension may persist even when the tumor is removed. If metyrosine is being used, instruct the patient to rise slowly and hold onto a secure object, since this drug can cause orthostatic hypotension.

CASE STUDY

Graves' Disease

Jupiterimages/Photos.com/Thinkstock

Patient Profile
R.D., a 47-yr-old white woman, was admitted to the hospital with a high fever. Unable to find a source of infection, the health care provider does an endocrine workup. R.D. is diagnosed with Graves' disease.

Subjective Data
- Reports recent job loss because she is no longer able to tolerate work-related stress
- Reports symptoms including fatigue, unintentional weight loss, insomnia, palpitations, and heat intolerance

Objective Data
Physical Examination
- Fever of 104° F (40° C)
- BP of 150/80 mm Hg, pulse of 116 beats/min, and respiratory rate of 26 breaths/min
- Hot, moist skin
- Fine tremors of the hands
- 4+ deep tendon reflexes and muscle strength of 1 to 2 out of 5

Collaborative Care
- Subtotal thyroidectomy planned for 2 mo later
- Started on propylthiouracil (PTU) and propranolol (Inderal)

Discussion Questions
1. What is the etiology of R.D.'s symptoms?
2. What diagnostic studies would be important in evaluating R.D.'s condition? What results would establish the diagnosis of Graves' disease?
3. Why was surgery delayed?
4. What is the purpose of drug therapy for R.D.?
5. *Priority Decision:* What are the patient's priority teaching needs? What teaching strategies would you use if R.D. could not read?
6. What are the nursing interventions for successful long-term management of R.D. after the subtotal thyroidectomy?
7. *Priority Decision:* Based on the assessment data presented, what are the priority nursing diagnoses pertinent to this patient while hospitalized? Are there any collaborative problems?
8. *Evidence-Based Practice:* Why is R.D. counseled to give up her long-standing cigarette smoking habit?

BRIDGE TO NCLEX EXAMINATION

The number of the question corresponds to the same-numbered outcome at the beginning of the chapter.

1. After a hypophysectomy for acromegaly, postoperative nursing care should focus on
   a. frequent monitoring of serum and urine osmolarity.
   b. parenteral administration of a GH-receptor antagonist.
   c. keeping the patient in a recumbent position at all times.
   d. patient teaching regarding the need for lifelong hormone therapy.

2. A patient with a head injury develops SIADH. Manifestations the nurse would expect to find include
   a. hypernatremia and edema.
   b. muscle spasticity and hypertension.
   c. low urine output and hyponatremia.
   d. weight gain and decreased glomerular filtration rate.

3. The health care provider prescribes levothyroxine (Synthroid) for a patient with hypothyroidism. After teaching regarding this drug, the nurse determines that further instruction is needed when the patient says
   a. "I can expect the medication dose may need to be adjusted."
   b. "I only need to take this drug until my symptoms are improved."
   c. "I can expect to return to normal function with the use of this drug."
   d. "I will report any chest pain or difficulty breathing to the doctor right away."

4. After thyroid surgery, the nurse suspects damage or removal of the parathyroid glands when the patient develops
   a. muscle weakness and weight loss.
   b. hyperthermia and severe tachycardia.
   c. hypertension and difficulty swallowing.
   d. laryngospasms and tingling in the hands and feet.

5. Important nursing intervention(s) when caring for a patient with Cushing syndrome include (select all that apply)
   a. restricting protein intake.
   b. monitoring blood glucose levels.
   c. observing for signs of hypotension.
   d. administering medication in equal doses.
   e. protecting patient from exposure to infection.

6. An important preoperative nursing intervention before an adrenalectomy for hyperaldosteronism is to
   a. monitor blood glucose levels.
   b. restrict fluid and sodium intake.
   c. administer potassium-sparing diuretics.
   d. advise the patient to make postural changes slowly.

7. To control the side effects of corticosteroid therapy, the nurse teaches the patient who is taking corticosteroids to
   a. increase calcium intake to 1500 mg/day.
   b. perform glucose monitoring for hypoglycemia.
   c. obtain immunizations due to high risk of infections.
   d. avoid abrupt position changes because of orthostatic hypotension.

8. The nurse teaches the patient that the best time to take corticosteroids for replacement purposes is
   a. once a day at bedtime.
   b. every other day on awakening.
   c. on arising and in the late afternoon.
   d. at consistent intervals every 6 to 8 hours.

1. a, 2. c, 3. b, 4. d, 5. b, e, 6. c, 7. a, 8. c

ⓔvolve

For rationales to these answers and even more NCLEX review questions, visit *http://evolve.elsevier.com/Lewis/medsurg.*

REFERENCES

1. National Library of Medicine: Acromegaly. Retrieved from *www.ncbi.nlm.nih.gov/pubmedhealth/PMH0001364.*

2. Jones R, Brashers V, Huether S: Alterations of hormonal regulation. In Huether S, McCance K, editors: *Understanding pathophysiology,* ed 5, St Louis, 2012, Mosby.

3. Miller RE, Learned-Miller EG, Trainer P, et al: Early diagnosis of acromegaly: computers versus clinicians, *Clin Endocrinol* 75:226, 2011.

4. Pituitary Network Association. Pituitary disorders: prolactinomas. Retrieved from *www.pituitary.org/disorders/prolactinomas.*

5. McDowell B, Wallace R, Carnahan R, et al: Demographic differences in incidence for pituitary adenoma, *Pituitary* 14:23, 2011.

6. John C, Day MW: Central neurogenic diabetes insipidus, syndrome of inappropriate secretion of antidiuretic hormone, and cerebral salt-wasting syndrome in traumatic brain injury, *Crit Care Nurse* 32:e1, 2012.

7. Medeiros-Neto G, Camargo R, Tomimori E: Approach to and treatment of goiters, *Med Clin North Am* 96:351, 2012.

8. Samuels MH: Subacute, silent, and postpartum thyroiditis, *Med Clin North Am* 96:223, 2012.

9. Li Y, Nishihara E, Kakudo K: Hashimoto's thyroiditis: old concepts and new insights, *Curr Opin Rheumatol* 23:102, 2011.

10. Seigel S, Hodak S: Thyrotoxicosis, *Med Clin North Am* 96:175, 2012.

11. Bahn R, Burch H, Cooper D, et al: Hyperthyroidism and other causes of thyrotoxicosis: management guidelines of the American Thyroid Association and American Association of Clinical Endocrinologists, *Endocr Pract* 17:456 , 2011.

12. Kim M, Ladenson P: Thyroid. In Goldman L, Schafer A, editors: *Goldman: Goldman's Cecil medicine,* ed 24, Philadelphia, 2011, Saunders.

13. Furtado L: Thyroidectomy: postoperative care and common complications, *Nurs Stand* 25:43, 2011.

14. Brent G, Davie T: Hypothyroidism and thyroiditis. In Kronenberg HM, Melmed S, Polonsky KS, et al, editors: *Williams textbook of endocrinology,* ed 12, Philadelphia, 2011, Saunders.

15. Almandoz JP: Hypothyroidism: etiology, diagnosis, and management, *Med Clin North Am* 96:203, 2012.

*16. U.S. Preventive Services Task Force: Screening for thyroid disease: systematic evidence review. Retrieved from *www.ahrq.gov/clinic.*

*Evidence-based information for clinical practice.

17. National Cancer Institute: Thyroid cancer. Retrieved from *www.cancer.gov/cancertopics/types/thyroid*.

18. Popoveniuc G, Jonklaas J: Thyroid nodules, *Med Clin North Am* 96:329, 2012.

19. American Cancer Society: Detailed guide: thyroid cancer. Retrieved from *www.cancer.org*.

20. National Institutes of Health: Genetics home reference: multiple endocrine neoplasia. Retrieved from *ghr.nlm.nih.gov/condition/multiple-endocrine-neoplasia*.

21. Mayo Clinic: Hyperparathyroidism. Retrieved from *www.mayoclinic.com/health/hyperparathyroidism*.

22. Khan MI: Medical management of postsurgical hypoparathyroidism, *Endocr Pract* 17(Suppl 1):18, 2011.

23. Guaraldi F, Salvatori R: Cushing syndrome: maybe not so uncommon of an endocrine disease, *J Am Board Family Med* 25:199, 2012.

24. Pagana KD, Pagana TJ: *Mosby's diagnostic and laboratory test reference*, ed 10, St Louis, 2011, Mosby.

25. Hunt D: Is it Addison's disease or Cushing syndrome? *Am Nurse Today* 7:8, 2012.

26. Bratland E, Husebye E: Cellular immunity and immunopathology in autoimmune Addison's disease, *Molec Cell Endocrinol* 336:180, 2011.

27. National Institute of Diabetes and Digestive and Kidney Diseases: Addison's disease: adrenal insufficiency. Retrieved from *endocrine.niddk.nih.gov/pubs/addison*.

28. Arthritis Foundation: Controlling bone loss when taking steroids. Retrieved from *www.arthritis.org/control-bone-loss-steroids.php*.

29. American Urological Association Foundation: Primary hyperaldosteronism (Conn's syndrome). Retrieved from *www.urologyhealth.org/urology*.

30. Hyperaldosteronism: primary. From F Ferri, editor: *Ferri's clinical advisor*, Mosby, 2013, Mosby.

31. Zuber S: Hypertension in pheochromocytoma: characteristics and treatment, *Endocrinol Metab Clin North Am* 40:295, 2011.

RESOURCES

American Association of Clinical Endocrinologists (AACE)
www.aace.com
American Thyroid Association
www.thyroid.org
Endocrine Nurses Society (ENS)
www.endo-nurses.org
Endocrine Society
www.endo-society.org
Pituitary Network Association
www.pituitary.org
Thyroid Federation International
www.thyroid-fed.org

51

Happiness resides not in possessions and not in gold.
The feeling of happiness dwells in the soul.
Democritus, 420 BC

Nursing Assessment
Reproductive System

Catherine (Kate) Lein

evolve WEBSITE

http://evolve.elsevier.com/Lewis/medsurg

- NCLEX Review Questions
- Key Points
- Pre-Test
- Answer Guidelines for Case Study in this chapter
- Rationales for Bridge to NCLEX Examination Questions
- Concept Map Creator
- Glossary
- Animations
  - Lymphatic Drainage of Breast
  - The Menstrual Cycle

- Videos
  - Inspection and Palpation: Standing Position (Male)—1
  - Inspection and Palpation: Standing Position (Male)—2
  - Inspection: External Genitalia (Female)
  - Inspection: Female Breasts—Sitting Position
  - Inspection: Speculum Examination (Female)
  - Palpation: Bimanual Examination (Female)
  - Palpation: Female Breasts—Supine Position

- Palpation: Inguinal Hernia Evaluation (Male)
- Physical Examination: Abdominal Reflexes, Abdominal Muscles, and Inguinal Area
- Physical Examination: Breasts
- Physical Examination: Breasts and Heart
- Physical Examination: Genitalia and Rectum (Female)
- Physical Examination: Rectum and Prostate Gland (Male)
- Content Updates

LEARNING OUTCOMES

1. Describe the structures and functions of the male and female reproductive systems.
2. Summarize the functions of the major hormones essential for the functioning of the male and female reproductive systems.
3. Explain the physiologic changes during the stages of sexual response for both a man and a woman.
4. Link the age-related changes of the male and female reproductive systems to the differences in assessment findings.
5. Select the significant subjective and objective data related to the male and female reproductive systems and information about sexual function that should be obtained from a patient.

6. Select the appropriate techniques to use in the physical assessment of the male and female reproductive systems.
7. Differentiate normal from common abnormal findings of a physical assessment of the male and female reproductive systems.
8. Describe the purpose, significance of results, and nursing responsibilities related to diagnostic studies of the male and female reproductive systems.

KEY TERMS

amenorrhea, p. 1224
clitoris, p. 1221
ductus deferens, p. 1219
dyspareunia, p. 1228

epididymis, p. 1219
gonads, p. 1218
menarche, p. 1223
menopause, p. 1224

menstrual cycle, p. 1223
mons pubis, p. 1221
nulliparous, p. 1220
spermatogenesis, p. 1219

STRUCTURES AND FUNCTIONS OF MALE AND FEMALE REPRODUCTIVE SYSTEMS

The reproductive system of both males and females consists of primary (or essential) organs and secondary (or accessory) organs. The primary reproductive organs are referred to as **gonads.** The female gonads are the ovaries; the male gonads are the testes. The main responsibility of the gonads is secretion of hormones and production of gametes (ova and sperm).

Secondary (or accessory) organs are responsible for (1) transporting and nourishing the ova and sperm and (2) preserving and protecting the fertilized eggs.

Male Reproductive System

The three primary roles of the male reproductive system are (1) production and transportation of sperm, (2) deposition of sperm in the female reproductive tract, and (3) secretion of hormones. The primary reproductive organs in the male are

Reviewed by Brenda Pavill, RN, PhD, FNP, Associate Professor–Nursing, Misericordia University, Dallas, Pennsylvania.

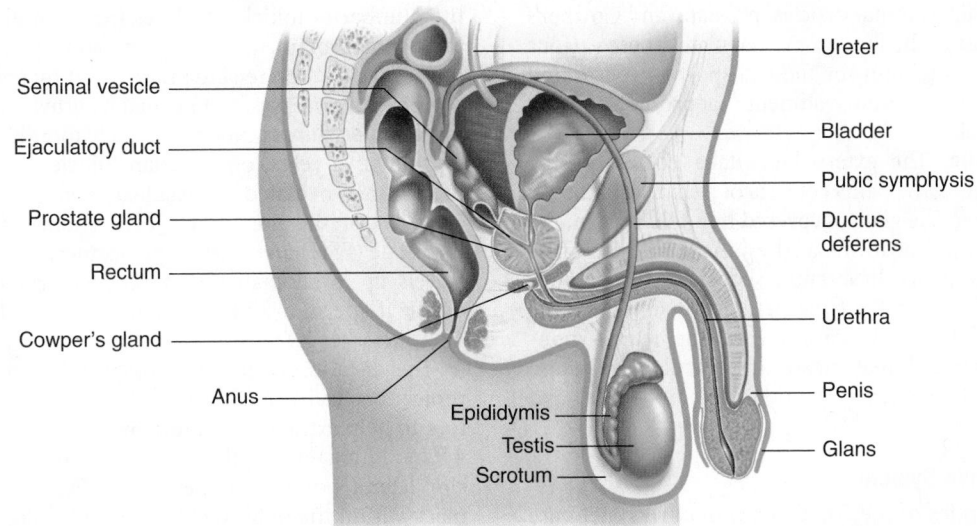

FIG. 51-1 Male reproductive tract.

the testes. Secondary reproductive organs include ducts (epididymis, ductus deferens, ejaculatory duct, and urethra), sex glands (prostate gland, Cowper's glands, and seminal vesicles), and the external genitalia (scrotum and penis)[1] (Fig. 51-1).

Testes. The paired testes are ovoid, smooth, firm organs measuring 1.4 to 2.2 in (3.5 to 5.6 cm) long and 0.8 to 1.2 in (2 to 3 cm) wide. They are within the scrotum, which is a loose protective sac composed of a thin outer layer of skin over a tough connective tissue layer. Within the testes, coiled structures known as seminiferous tubules form *spermatozoa* (immature sperm). The process of sperm production is called **spermatogenesis.** Interstitial cells of the testes lie between the seminiferous tubules and produce the male sex hormone testosterone.

Ducts. Sperm formed in the seminiferous tubules move through a series of ducts. These ducts transport the sperm from the testes to the outside of the body. As sperm exit the testes, they enter and pass through the epididymis, ductus deferens, ejaculatory duct, and urethra.

The **epididymis** is a comma-shaped structure located on the posterosuperior aspect of each testis within the scrotum (see Figs. 51-1 and 51-2). It is a very long, tightly coiled structure that measures about 20 ft in length.[1] The epididymis transports the sperm as they mature. Sperm exit the epididymis through a long, thick tube known as the ductus deferens.

The **ductus deferens** (also known as the *vas deferens*) is continuous with the epididymis within the scrotal sac. It travels upward through the scrotum and continues through the inguinal ring into the abdominal cavity. The spermatic cord is composed of a connective tissue sheath that encloses the ductus deferens, arteries, veins, nerves, and lymph vessels as it ascends up through the inguinal canal (see Fig. 51-2). In the abdominal cavity, the ductus deferens travels up, over, and behind the bladder. Posterior to the bladder the ductus deferens joins the seminal vesicle to form the ejaculatory duct (see Fig. 51-1).

The ejaculatory duct passes downward through the prostate gland, connecting with the urethra. The urethra extends from the bladder, through the prostate, and ends in a slitlike opening (the meatus) on the ventral side of the *glans,* the tip of the penis.

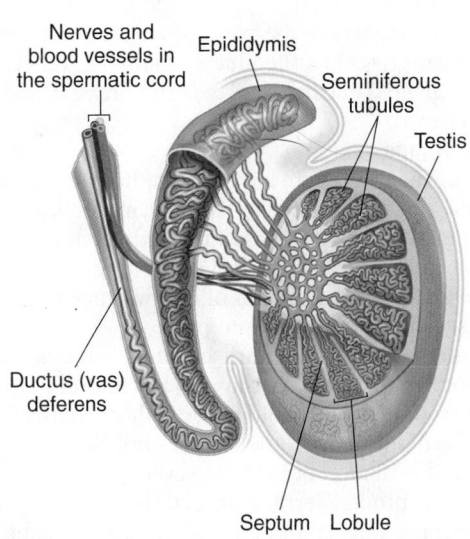

FIG. 51-2 Seminiferous tubules, testis, epididymis, and ductus (vas) deferens in the male.

During the process of ejaculation, sperm travels through the urethra and out of the penis.

Glands. The seminal vesicles, the prostate gland, and Cowper's (bulbourethral) glands are the accessory glands of the male reproductive system. These glands produce and secrete seminal fluid (semen), which surrounds the sperm and forms the *ejaculate.*

The seminal vesicles lie posterior to the bladder and between the rectum and bladder. The ducts of the seminal vesicles fuse with the ductus deferens to form the ejaculatory ducts that enter the prostate gland. The prostate gland lies beneath the bladder. Its posterior surface is in contact with the rectal wall. The prostate normally measures 0.8 in (2 cm) wide and 1.2 in (3 cm) long and is divided into the right and left lateral lobes and an anteroposterior median lobe. Cowper's glands lie on each side of the urethra and slightly posterior to it, just below the prostate. The ducts of these glands enter directly into the urethra.

Secretions from the seminal vesicles, prostate, and Cowper's glands make up most of the fluid in the ejaculate. These various secretions serve as a medium for the transport of sperm and create an alkaline, nutritious environment that promotes sperm motility and survival.

External Genitalia. The external genitalia consist of the penis and the scrotum. The penis consists of a shaft, and the tip is known as the glans. The glans is covered by a fold of skin, the prepuce (or foreskin), that forms at the junction of the glans and the shaft of the penis. In circumcised males the prepuce has been removed. The shaft of the penis consists of erectile tissue composed of the corpus cavernosum, the corpus spongiosum (the fibrous sheath that encases the erectile tissue), and the urethra. The skin covering the penis is thin, loose, and hairless.

Female Reproductive System

The three primary roles of the female reproductive system are (1) production of ova (eggs), (2) secretion of hormones, and (3) protection and facilitation of the development of the fetus in a pregnant female. Like the male, the female has primary and secondary reproductive organs. The primary reproductive organs in the female are the paired ovaries. Secondary reproductive organs include the ducts (fallopian tubes), uterus, vagina, sex glands (Bartholin's glands and breasts), and external genitalia (vulva).

Pelvic Organs

Ovaries. The ovaries are located on either side of the uterus, just behind and below the fallopian (uterine) tubes (Fig. 51-3). The almond-shaped ovaries are firm and solid, approximately 0.6 in (1.5 cm) wide and 1.2 in (3 cm) long. Their functions include ovulation and secretion of the two major reproductive hormones, estrogen and progesterone.

The outer zone of the ovary contains follicles with germ cells, or *oocytes.* Each follicle contains a primordial (immature) oocyte surrounded by granulosa and theca cells. These two layers protect and nourish the oocyte until the follicle reaches maturity and ovulation occurs. However, not all follicles reach maturity. In a process termed *atresia,* most of the primordial follicles become smaller and are reabsorbed by the body. Thus

the number of follicles declines from 2 million to 4 million at birth to approximately 300,000 to 400,000 at menarche. Fewer than 500 oocytes are actually released by ovulation during the reproductive years of the normal healthy woman.

Fallopian Tubes. Normally, each month during a woman's reproductive years, one ovarian follicle reaches maturity, and the ovum is ovulated, or expelled, from the ovary through the stimulus of the gonadotropic hormones, follicle-stimulating hormone (FSH) and luteinizing hormone (LH). The ovum then travels up a fallopian tube where fertilization by sperm may occur, if sperm are present. An ovum can be fertilized up to 72 hours after its release.

The distal ends of the fallopian tubes consist of fingerlike projections called *fimbriae* that "massage" the ovaries at ovulation to help extract the mature ovum. The tubes, which average 4.8 in (12 cm) in length, extend from the fimbriae to the superior lateral borders of the uterus. Fertilization usually takes place within the outer one third of the fallopian tubes.

Uterus. The uterus is a pear-shaped, hollow, muscular organ (see Fig. 51-3). It is located between the bladder and the rectum. In the mature **nulliparous** (never pregnant) woman, the uterus is approximately 2.4 to 3.2 in (6 to 8 cm) long and 1.6 in (4 cm) wide. The uterine walls consist of an outer serosal layer, the *perimetrium;* a middle muscular layer, the *myometrium;* and an inner mucosal layer, the *endometrium.*

The uterus consists of the fundus, body (or corpus), and cervix (see Fig. 51-3). The body makes up about 80% of the uterus and connects with the cervix at the isthmus, or neck. The cervix is the lower portion of the uterus that projects into the anterior wall of the vaginal canal. It makes up about 15% to 20% of the uterus in the nulliparous female. The cervix consists of the *ectocervix,* the outer portion that protrudes into the vagina, and the *endocervix,* the canal in the opening of the cervix. The ectocervix is covered with squamous epithelial cells, which give it a smooth, pinkish appearance. The endocervix contains a lining of columnar epithelial cells, which give it a rough, reddened appearance. The junction at which the two types of epithelial cells meet is termed the *squamocolumnar junction* and contains the optimal types of cells needed for an accurate Papanicolaou (Pap) test to screen for malignancies.

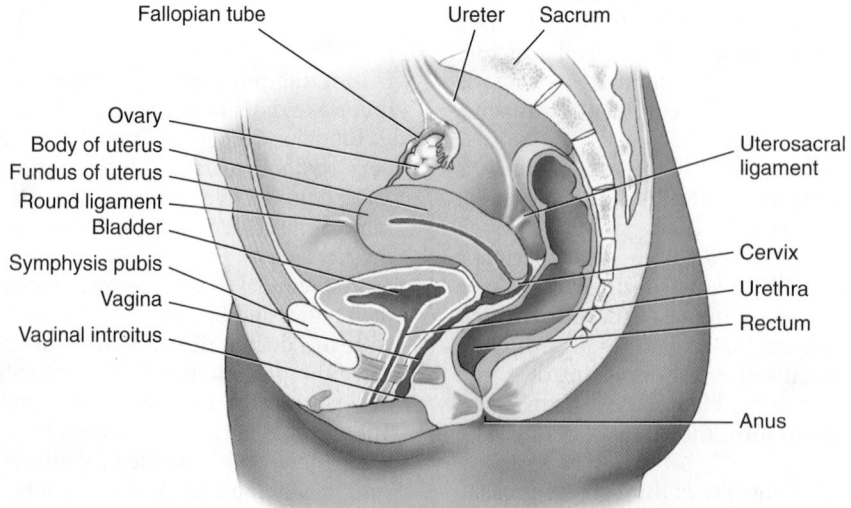

FIG. 51-3 Female reproductive tract.

The cervical canal is 0.8 to 1.6 in (2 to 4 cm) long and is relatively tightly closed. However, the cervix allows sperm to enter the uterus and also allows menses to be expelled. The columnar epithelium, under hormonal influence, provides elasticity during labor for the cervix to stretch to allow passage of a fetus during the birth process. The entrance of sperm into the uterus is facilitated by mucus produced by the cervix under the influence of estrogen. Under normal conditions, the cervical mucus becomes watery, stretchy, and more abundant at ovulation. The postovulatory cervical mucus, under the influence of progesterone, is thick and inhibits sperm passage.

Vagina. The vagina is a tubular structure 3 to 4 in (7.6 to 10 cm) long that is lined with squamous epithelium. The secretions of the vagina consist of cervical mucus, desquamated epithelium, and, during sexual stimulation, a watery secretion. These fluids help protect against vaginal infection. The muscular and erectile tissue of the vaginal walls allows enough dilation and contraction to accommodate the passage of the fetus during labor, as well as penetration of the penis during intercourse. The anterior vaginal wall lies along the urethra and bladder. The posterior vaginal wall is adjacent to the rectum.

Pelvis. The female pelvis consists of four bones (two pelvic bones, sacrum, coccyx) held together by several strong ligaments. The sections of these bones that lie below the iliopectineal line are important during birth and are often a factor determining the ability of a woman to deliver a child vaginally.

External Genitalia. The external portion of the female reproductive system (Fig. 51-4), commonly called the *vulva*, consists of the mons pubis, labia majora, labia minora, clitoris, urethral meatus, Skene's glands, vaginal introitus (opening), and Bartholin's glands.

The mons pubis is a fatty layer lying over the pubic bone. It is covered with coarse hair that lies in a triangular pattern. (The male hair pattern is diamond shaped.) The labia majora are folds of adipose tissue that form the outer borders of the vulva. The hairless labia minora form the borders of the vaginal orifice and extend anteriorly to enclose the clitoris.

The *vestibule* is a boat-shaped fossa between the labia minora, extending from the clitoris at the anterior end to the vaginal opening at the posterior end. The perineum is the area between the vagina and the anus. The vaginal introitus is surrounded by thin membranous tissue called the *hymen*. In the adult woman the hymen usually appears as folds or hymenal tags and separates the external genitalia from the vagina. At the posterior aspect of the vagina, a tense band of mucous membrane connecting the posterior ends of the labia minora is referred to as the *posterior fourchette*.

The clitoris is erectile tissue that becomes engorged during sexual excitation. It lies anterior to the urethral meatus and the vaginal orifice and is usually covered by the prepuce. Clitoral stimulation is an important part of sexual activity for many women.

Ducts of the Skene's glands lie alongside the urinary meatus and are thought to help lubricate the urinary meatus.[2] The Bartholin's glands, located at the posterior and lateral aspects of the vaginal orifice, secrete a thin, mucoid material believed to contribute slightly to lubrication during sexual intercourse. These glands are not usually palpable unless sebaceous-like cysts form or they are swollen in the presence of an infection, such as a sexually transmitted infection (STI).

Breasts. The breasts are a secondary sex characteristic that develops during puberty in response to estrogen and progesterone. Cyclic hormonal changes lead to regular changes in breast tissue to prepare it for lactation when fertilization and pregnancy occur.

The breasts extend from the second to the sixth ribs, with the tail reaching the axilla (Fig. 51-5). The fully mature breast is dome shaped and contains a pigmented center termed the *areola*. The areolar region contains Montgomery's tubercles, which are similar to sebaceous glands and assist in lubricating the nipple. During lactation, the alveoli secrete milk. The milk then flows into a ductal system and is transported to the lactiferous sinuses. The nipple contains 15 to 20 tiny openings through which the milk flows during breastfeeding. The fibrous and fatty tissue that supports and separates the channels of the mammary duct system is primarily responsible for the varying sizes and shapes of the breasts in different individuals.

The breast has a rich lymphatic network that drains into axillary and clavicular channels (see Fig. 52-5). Superficial

FIG. 51-4 External female genitalia.

FIG. 51-5 The lactating female breast. **A,** Glandular structures are anchored to the overlying skin and the pectoralis muscle by suspensory ligaments of Cooper. Each lobule of glandular tissue is drained by a lactiferous duct that eventually opens through the nipple. **B,** Anterior view of a lactating breast. In nonlactating breasts, glandular tissue is less evident with adipose tissue comprising most of the breast.

lymph nodes are located in the axilla and are accessible to examination. This system is often responsible for the metastasis of a malignant tumor from the breast to other parts of the body.

Neuroendocrine Regulation of Reproductive System

The hypothalamus, pituitary gland, and gonads secrete numerous hormones (Fig. 51-6). (Endocrine hormones are discussed in Chapter 48.) These hormones regulate the processes of ovulation, spermatogenesis (formation of sperm), and fertilization and the formation and function of the secondary sex characteristics. The hypothalamus secretes gonadotropin-releasing hormone (GnRH), which stimulates the anterior pituitary gland to secrete its hormones, including FSH and LH. LH in males is sometimes called interstitial cell–stimulating hormone (ICSH). The gonadal hormones are estrogen, progesterone, and testosterone.

In women, FSH production by the anterior pituitary stimulates the growth and maturity of the ovarian follicles necessary for ovulation.[3] The mature follicle produces estrogen, which in turn suppresses the release of FSH. Another hormone, inhibin, is also secreted by the ovarian follicle and inhibits both GnRH and FSH secretion. In men, FSH stimulates the seminiferous tubules to produce sperm.

LH contributes to the ovulatory process because it causes follicles to complete maturation and undergo ovulation. It also affects the development of a ruptured follicle (area where ovum exited during ovulation), which turns into a corpus luteum from which progesterone is secreted. Progesterone maintains the rich vascular state of the uterus (secretory phase) in preparation for fertilization and implantation. In men, LH (or ICSH) triggers testosterone production by the interstitial cells of the testes and thus is essential for the full maturation of sperm.

Prolactin has no known function in men. In women, prolactin stimulates the development and growth of the mammary glands. During lactation, it initiates and maintains milk production.

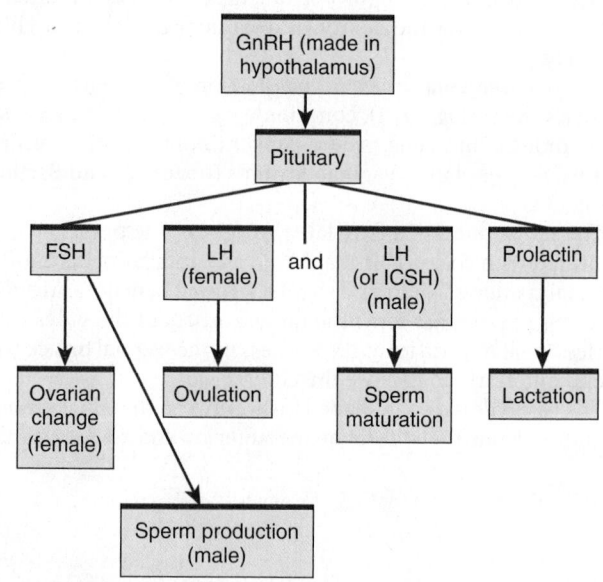

FIG. 51-6 Hypothalamic-pituitary-gonadal axis. Only the major pituitary hormone actions are depicted. *FSH,* Follicle-stimulating hormone; *GnRH,* gonadotropin-releasing hormone; *ICSH,* interstitial cell–stimulating hormone; *LH,* luteinizing hormone.

The gonadal hormones, estrogen and progesterone, are produced by the ovaries in women. Small amounts of an estrogen precursor are also produced in the adrenal cortices. Estrogen is essential to the development and maintenance of the secondary sex characteristics, the proliferative phase of the menstrual cycle immediately after menstruation, and the uterine changes essential to pregnancy. The role and importance of estrogen in men are not well understood. In men, estrogen is produced predominantly in the adrenal cortex.

Progesterone plays a major role in the menstrual cycle but most specifically in the secretory phase. Like estrogen, progesterone is involved in the bodily changes associated with preg-

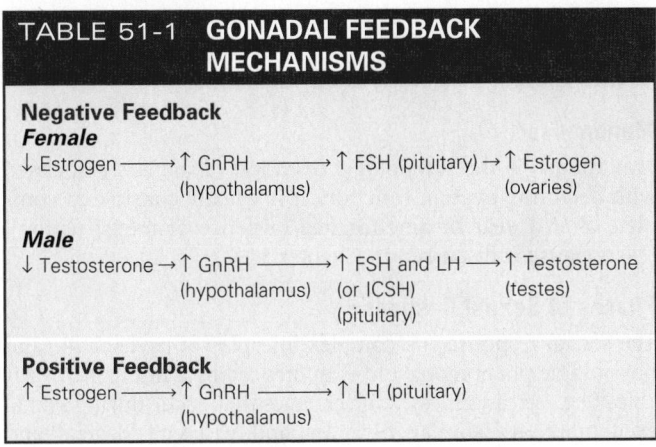

TABLE 51-1	GONADAL FEEDBACK MECHANISMS

Negative Feedback
Female
↓ Estrogen ⟶ ↑ GnRH ⟶ ↑ FSH (pituitary) → ↑ Estrogen
(hypothalamus) (ovaries)

Male
↓ Testosterone → ↑ GnRH ⟶ ↑ FSH and LH ⟶ ↑ Testosterone
(hypothalamus) (or ICSH) (testes)
(pituitary)

Positive Feedback
↑ Estrogen ⟶ ↑ GnRH ⟶ ↑ LH (pituitary)
(hypothalamus)

FSH, Follicle-stimulating hormone; *GnRH,* gonadotropin-releasing hormone; *ICSH,* interstitial cell–stimulating hormone; *LH,* luteinizing hormone.

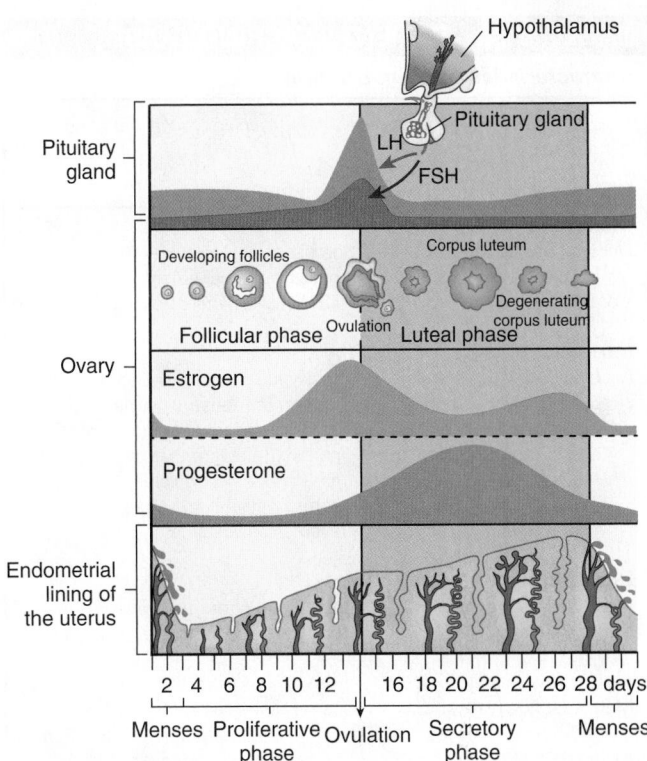

FIG. 51-7 Events of the menstrual cycle. The lines depict the changes in blood hormone levels, the development of the follicles, and the changes in the endometrium during the cycle. *FSH,* Follicle-stimulating hormone; *LH,* luteinizing hormone.

nancy. Adequate progesterone is necessary to maintain an implanted egg.

In men, the major gonadal hormone is testosterone, which is produced by the testes. Testosterone is responsible for the development and maintenance of secondary sex characteristics, as well as for adequate spermatogenesis. In women, androgens are produced in small amounts by the adrenal glands and ovaries.

The circulating levels of gonadal hormones are controlled primarily by a *negative feedback process.* Receptors within the hypothalamus and pituitary are sensitive to the circulating blood levels of the hormones (Table 51-1). Increased levels of hormones stimulate a hypothalamic response to decrease the high circulating levels. Likewise, low circulating levels provoke a hypothalamic response that increases the low circulating levels. For example, if the circulating level of testosterone in men is low, the hypothalamus is stimulated to secrete GnRH. This triggers the anterior pituitary to secrete greater amounts of FSH and LH, which in turn causes an increase in the production of testosterone. The high level of testosterone signals a decrease in the production of GnRH and thus of FSH and LH.

In women, however, there is a slight variation. The circulating levels are controlled through a combination of both a negative and a positive feedback system. A *negative feedback control* mechanism exists similar to that described above. When circulating estrogen levels are low, the hypothalamus is stimulated to increase its production of GnRH. GnRH stimulates the pituitary to secrete greater amounts of FSH and LH, resulting in higher levels of estrogen production by the ovaries. Reciprocally higher levels of circulating estrogen result in a decreasing secretion of GnRH and thus a decrease in the secretion of FSH by the pituitary. Women also have a *positive feedback control* mechanism. Thus with increasing levels of circulating estrogen, a greater level of GnRH is produced, resulting in an increased level of LH from the pituitary. Likewise, lowered levels of estrogen result in a lowered level of LH.

Menarche

Menarche is the first episode of menstrual bleeding, indicating that a girl has reached puberty. Menarche usually occurs at approximately 12 to 13 years of age but can occur as early as 10 years of age in some individuals. Menstrual cycles are often irregular for the first 1 to 2 years after menarche because of *anovulatory cycles* (cycles without ovulation).

Menstrual Cycle

The major functions of the ovaries are ovulation and the secretion of hormones. These functions are accomplished during the normal menstrual cycle, a monthly process mediated by the hormonal activity of the hypothalamus, pituitary gland, and ovaries. Menstruation occurs during each month in which an egg is not fertilized (Fig. 51-7). The endometrial cycle is divided into three phases labeled in relation to uterine and ovarian changes: (1) the *proliferative,* or *follicular, phase;* (2) the *secretory,* or *luteal, phase;* and (3) the *menstrual,* or *ischemic, phase.* The length of the menstrual cycle ranges from 21 to 35 days, with an average of 28 days.[4]

The menstrual cycle begins on the first day of menstruation, which usually lasts 4 to 6 days. Table 51-2 includes characteristics of the menstrual cycle and related teaching. During menstruation, estrogen and progesterone levels are low, but FSH levels begin to increase. During the follicular phase, a single follicle matures fully under the stimulation of FSH. (The mechanism that ensures that usually only one follicle reaches maturity is not known.) The mature follicle stimulates estrogen production, causing a negative feedback with resulting decreased FSH secretion.

Although the initial stage of follicular maturation is stimulated by FSH, complete maturation and ovulation occur only in the presence of LH. When estrogen levels peak on about the twelfth day of the cycle, there is a surge of LH, which triggers ovulation a day or two later. After ovulation (maturation and

TABLE 51-2   PATIENT TEACHING GUIDE

Characteristics of Menstruation

Include the following information when teaching the patient about menstruation.

Characteristic	Teaching
Menarche Occurs between ages 10 and 16 yr. Average age at onset is 12-13 yr.	See health care provider regarding possible endocrine or developmental abnormality when delayed.
Interval Usually is 21-35 days, but regular cycles as short as 17 days or as long as 45 days are considered normal if pattern is consistent for individual.	Keep written record to identify own pattern of menstrual cycle. Expect some irregularity in perimenopausal period. Be aware that drugs (phenothiazines, opioids, contraceptives) and stressful life events can result in missed periods.
Duration Menstrual flow generally lasts 2-8 days.	Realize that pattern is fairly constant but that wide variations do exist.
Amount Menstrual flow varies from 20-80 mL per menses; average is 30 mL. Amount varies among women and in the same woman at different times. It is usually heaviest first 2 days.	Count pads or tampons used per day. The average tampon or pad, when completely saturated, absorbs 20-30 mL. Very heavy flow is indicated by complete soaking of two pads in 1-2 hr. Flow increases and then gradually decreases in perimenopausal period. IUD or drugs such as anticoagulants and thiazides can produce heavy menses.
Composition Menstrual discharge is mixture of endometrium, blood, mucus, and vaginal cells. It is dark red and less viscous than blood and usually does not clot.	Clots indicate heavy flow or vaginal pooling.

IUD, Intrauterine device.

release of an ovum), LH promotes the development of the corpus luteum.

The fully developed corpus luteum continues to secrete estrogen and initiates progesterone secretion. If fertilization occurs, high levels of estrogen and progesterone continue to be secreted because of the continued activity of the corpus luteum from stimulation by human chorionic gonadotropin (hCG). If fertilization does not take place, menstruation occurs because of a decrease in estrogen production and progesterone withdrawal.

During the *follicular phase,* the endometrial lining of the uterus also undergoes change. As more estrogen is produced, the endometrial lining undergoes proliferative changes, including an increase in the length of blood vessels and glandular tissue.

With ovulation and the resulting increased levels of progesterone, the *luteal* (or *secretory*) *phase* begins. If the corpus luteum regresses (when fertilization does not occur) and estrogen and progesterone levels fall, the endometrial lining can no

longer be supported. As a result, the blood vessels contract, and tissue begins to slough (fall away). This sloughing results in the menses and the start of the menstrual phase.[4]

Menopause

Menopause is the physiologic cessation of menses associated with declining ovarian function. It is usually considered complete after 1 year of amenorrhea (absence of menstruation). (Menopause is discussed in Chapter 54.)

Phases of Sexual Response

The sexual response is a complex interplay of psychologic and physiologic phenomena and is influenced by a number of variables (e.g., stress, illness). The changes that occur during sexual excitement are similar for men and women. Masters and Johnson described the sexual response in terms of the excitement, plateau, orgasmic, and resolution phases.[5]

Male Sexual Response. The penis and the urethra are essential to the transport of sperm into the vagina and the cervix during intercourse. This transport is facilitated by penile erection in response to sexual stimulation during the *excitement phase.* Erection results from the filling of the large venous sinuses within the erectile tissue of the penis. In the flaccid state the sinuses hold only a small amount of blood, but during the erection stage they are congested with blood. Because the penis is richly endowed with sympathetic, parasympathetic, and pudendal nerve endings, it is readily stimulated to erection. The loose skin of the penis becomes taut as a result of the venous congestion. This erectile tautness allows for easy insertion into the vagina.

As the man reaches the *plateau phase,* the erection is maintained, and the penis increases in diameter as a result of a slight increase in vasocongestion. Testicle size also increases. Sometimes the glans penis becomes more reddish purple.

The subsequent contraction of the penile and urethral musculature during the *orgasmic phase* propels the sperm outward through the meatus. In this process, termed *ejaculation,* sperm are released into the ductus deferens during contractions. Sperm advance through the urethra, where fluids from the prostate and seminal vesicles are added to the ejaculate. The sperm continue their path through the urethra, receiving a small amount of fluid from the Cowper's glands, and are finally ejaculated through the urinary meatus. *Orgasm* is characterized by the rapid release of the vasocongestion and muscular tension (myotonia) that have developed. The rapid release of muscular tension (through rhythmic contractions) occurs primarily in the penis, prostate gland, and seminal vesicles. After ejaculation, a man enters the *resolution phase.* The penis undergoes involution, gradually returning to its unstimulated, flaccid state.

Female Sexual Response. The changes that occur in a woman during sexual excitation are similar to those in a man. In response to stimulation, the clitoris becomes congested and vaginal lubrication increases from secretions from the cervix, Bartholin's glands, and vaginal walls. This initial response is the excitation phase.

As excitation is maintained in the plateau phase, the vagina expands and the uterus is elevated. In the orgasmic phase, contractions occur in the uterus from the fundus to the lower uterine segment. There is a slight relaxation of the cervical os, which helps the entrance of the sperm, and rhythmic contractions of the vagina. Muscular tension is rapidly released through rhythmic contractions in the clitoris, vagina, and uterus. This phase is followed by a resolution phase in which these organs return to their preexcitation state. However, women do not have to go through the resolution (refractory) recovery state before they can be orgasmic again. They can be multiorgasmic without resolution between orgasms.

GERONTOLOGIC CONSIDERATIONS

EFFECTS OF AGING ON REPRODUCTIVE SYSTEMS

With advancing age, changes occur in the male and female reproductive systems (Table 51-3). In women many of these changes are related to the altered estrogen production that is associated with menopause.[6] A reduction in circulating estrogen along with an increase in androgens in postmenopausal women is associated with breast and genital atrophy, reduction in bone mass, and increased rate of atherosclerosis. Vaginal dryness may occur, which can lead to urogenital atrophy and changes in the composition of vaginal secretions.

A gradual testosterone decline in older men occurs. Manifestations of hormonal decline in men can be physical, psychologic, or sexual. Some of the changes include an increase in prostate size and a decrease in testosterone level, sperm production, muscle tone of the scrotum, and size and firmness of the testicles. Erectile dysfunction and sexual dysfunction occur in some men as a result of these changes.[7]

Gradual changes resulting from advancing age occur in the sexual responses of men and women. The cumulative effects of these changes, as well as the negative social attitude toward sexuality in older adults, can affect the sexual practices of older adults. You have an important role in providing accurate and unbiased information about sexuality and age. Emphasize the normalcy of sexual activity in older adults.

ASSESSMENT OF MALE AND FEMALE REPRODUCTIVE SYSTEMS

Subjective Data

Important Health Information. In addition to general health information, elicit information specifically relating to the reproductive system. Reproduction and sexual issues are often considered extremely personal and private. Develop trust with the patient to elicit such information. A professional demeanor is important when taking a reproductive or sexual history. Be sensitive, use gender-neutral terms when asking about partners, and maintain an awareness of a patient's culture and beliefs. Begin with the least sensitive information (e.g., menstrual history) before asking questions about more sensitive issues such as sexual practices or STIs.

Past Health History. The past health history should include information about major illnesses, hospitalizations, immunizations, and surgeries. Inquire about any infections involving the reproductive system, including STIs. Also take a complete obstetric and gynecologic history from the female patient.

Common pediatric illnesses that affect reproductive function are mumps and rubella. The occurrence of mumps in young men has been associated with an increase in sterility. Bilateral testicular atrophy may occur secondary to mumps-related orchitis. In the health history ask male patients if they have had mumps, been immunized with the mumps vaccine, or have any indications of sterility.

TABLE 51-3 GERONTOLOGIC ASSESSMENT DIFFERENCES

Reproductive Systems

Changes	Differences in Assessment Findings
Male	
Penis	
Decreased subcutaneous fat, decreased skin turgor	Easily retractable foreskin (if uncircumcised). Decrease in size. Fewer sustained erections.
Testes	
Decreased testosterone production	Decrease in size. Change in position (lower).
Prostate	
Benign hyperplasia	Enlargement.
Breasts	
Enlargement	Gynecomastia (abnormal enlargement).
Female	
Breasts	
Decreased subcutaneous fat, increased fibrous tissue, decreased skin turgor	Less resilient, looser, more pendulous tissue. Decreased size. Duct around nipple may feel like stringy strand.
Vulva	
Decreased skin turgor	Atrophy. Decreased amount of pubic hair; decreased size of clitoris and labia.
Vagina	
Atrophy of tissue, decreased muscle tone, alkaline pH	Pale and dry mucosa. Relaxation of outlet, mucosa thins, vagina narrower and shorter, increased potential for infection.
Urethra	
Decreased muscle tone	Cystocele (protrusion of bladder through vaginal wall).
Uterus	
Decreased thickness of myometrium	Decrease in size, uterine prolapse.
Ovaries	
Decreased ovarian function	Nonpalpable ovaries, decreased size.

GENDER DIFFERENCES

Effects of Aging on Sexual Function

Men	Women
• Increased stimulation necessary for erection	• Decreased vaginal lubrication
• Decreased force of ejaculation	• Decreased sensitivity with labia shrinking and more clitoris exposed
• Decreased ability to attain or sustain erection	• Difficulty in maintaining arousal
• Decreased size and rigidity of the penis at full erection	• Difficulty in achieving orgasm after stimulation
• Decreased libido and interest in sex	• Decreased libido and interest in sex

Rubella is of primary concern to women of childbearing age. If rubella occurs during the first 3 months of pregnancy, the possibility of congenital anomalies is increased. For this reason, you should encourage immunization for all women of childbearing age who have not been immunized for rubella or have not already had the disease. (Rubella immunity can be determined by antibody titers.) However, women should not be immunized if they are already pregnant.[8] Advise women not to conceive for at least 3 months after immunization.

Question the patient regarding current health status and any acute or chronic health problems. Problems in other body systems are often related to problems with the reproductive system. Ask questions relating to possible endocrine disorders, particularly diabetes mellitus (DM), hypothyroidism, and hyperthyroidism, because these disorders directly interfere with women's menstrual cycles and with sexual performance. Men who have DM may experience erectile dysfunction and retrograde ejaculation. In women with uncontrolled DM, pregnancy may have significant health risks. Many other chronic illnesses such as cardiovascular disease, respiratory disorders, anemia, cancer, and kidney and urinary tract disorders may affect the reproductive system and sexual functioning.

Determine if the patient has a history of a stroke. In men, strokes may cause physiologic or psychologic erectile dysfunction. Men who have suffered a myocardial infarction (MI) may experience erectile dysfunction because of fear that sexual activity could precipitate another MI. Women share this concern, both as partners of someone who has had an MI and as patients recovering from an MI. Although most patients have concerns about sexual activity after an MI, many are not comfortable expressing these fears to the nurse. Be sensitive to this concern. In women, a history of cardiovascular disease (e.g., hypertension, thrombophlebitis, angina) is associated with a higher incidence of morbidity and mortality with pregnancy or the use of oral contraceptives.

Medications. Document all prescription and over-the-counter medications that the patient is taking, including the reason for the medication, the dosage, and the length of time that the medication has been taken. Ask the patient about the use of herbal products and dietary supplements.

Particularly relevant in the assessment of the reproductive system is the use of diuretics (sometimes prescribed for pre-menstrual edema), psychotropic agents (which may interfere with sexual performance), and antihypertensives (some of which may cause erectile dysfunction). Patients who use drugs such as amlodipine (Norvasc), lisinopril (Prinivil), propranolol (Inderal), and clonidine (Catapres) must be closely assessed for these problems.[9] Also note the use of drugs such as alcohol, marijuana, barbiturates, amphetamines, or phencyclidine hydrochloride (PCP [also called "angel dust"]), which can have serious behavioral or physiologic effects on the reproductive system.

In women, document the use of oral contraceptives or other hormone therapy (HT). The long-term use of both estrogen and progesterone in HT appears to increase the risk of blood clots, cardiovascular disease, stroke, and breast cancer in postmenopausal women.[10] The short-term use of HT appears to be appropriate for women experiencing moderate to severe menopausal symptoms. Women who use tobacco have a much higher risk of clotting disorders. (HT is discussed in Chapter 54.)

A history of cholecystitis and hepatitis is important because these conditions may be contraindications for the use of oral contraceptives. Cholecystitis is often aggravated by oral contraceptives, and chronic active inflammation of the liver generally precludes the use of estrogen products because they are metabolized by the liver. Chronic obstructive pulmonary disease may be a contraindication to oral contraceptive use because progesterone thickens respiratory secretions.

Surgery or Other Treatments.   Note any surgical procedures in the health history. Surgical procedures involving the reproductive system are listed in Table 51-4. Also document any therapeutic or spontaneous abortions.

TABLE 51-4	SURGERIES OF THE REPRODUCTIVE SYSTEMS
Surgery	**Description**
Male	
Herniorrhaphy	Repair of hernia
Orchiectomy	Removal of one or both testes
Prostatectomy	Removal of prostate gland
Repair of testicular torsion	Correction of axial rotation of spermatic cord, which cuts off blood supply to the testicle, the epididymis, and other structures
Varicocelectomy	Repair of varicose vein of scrotum
Vasectomy	Removal of part of ductus (vas) deference. Can be an elective procedure for sterilization or contraception
Female	
Cryosurgery	Use of subfreezing temperature to destroy tissue, especially in treatment of abnormal cells
Dilation and curettage	Dilation of cervix and scraping of endometrium, performed to diagnose disease of uterus, correct heavy or prolonged vaginal bleeding, or empty uterus of products of conception. Also used in the treatment of infertility to correlate state of endometrium and time of cycle
Hysterectomy	Removal of uterus
Mastectomy	Removal of one or both breasts
Oophorectomy	Removal of one or both ovaries
Repair of cystocele	Correction of protrusion of urinary bladder through vaginal wall
Repair of rectocele	Correction of protrusion of rectum into vagina
Salpingectomy	Removal of one or both fallopian tubes
Tubal sterilization	Ligation of fallopian tubes

CASE STUDY

Patient Introduction

iStockphoto/Thinkstock

A.K. is a 68-yr-old Asian American woman who comes to the breast center because she found a large lump in her right breast while showering. She is somewhat anxious, stating "My breasts are typically lumpy, but this feels different!"

Critical Thinking

As you read through this chapter, think about A.K.'s concerns with the following questions in mind:

1. What are the possible causes for a lump in A.K.'s breast?
2. What would be your priority assessment of A.K.?
3. What questions would you ask A.K.?
4. What should be included in the physical assessment? What would you be looking for?
5. What diagnostic studies might you expect to be ordered?

Functional Health Patterns. The key questions to ask a patient with a reproductive problem are presented in Table 51-5.

Health Perception–Health Management Pattern. Two of the primary focuses of this health pattern are the patient's perception of his or her own health and measures that the patient takes to maintain health. Specifically, ask about self-examination practices and screenings. Mammography (based on current guidelines [see Chapter 52]), Pap tests, and breast self-examinations (BSEs) are integral to a woman's health. Testicular self-examination (TSE) should be practiced by all men, starting in adolescence (see Table 55-9). Starting at age 50, men should discuss with their health care provider the risks and benefits of annual prostate cancer screening with specific antigen (PSA) blood testing and a digital rectal examination (DRE)[11] (see Chapter 55). Men at high risk for prostate cancer (i.e., African Americans, men with prostate cancer in first-degree relatives) should begin these discussions earlier with their provider.

 GENETIC RISK ALERT

- Breast, ovarian, uterine, and prostate cancer have known genetic risk factors.
- Having a first-degree relative with any of these cancers significantly increases the risk of cancer for the patient.
- The risk increases if several family members have been affected with these cancers over succeeding generations.
- Individuals with a known hereditary predisposition to breast or ovarian cancer can use this information to make informed decisions about how to minimize their risks.

Family history is also an important component of this health pattern. Inquire about a history of cancer, particularly cancer of the reproductive organs. Determine if the patient has a familial tendency for diabetes mellitus, hypothyroidism, hyperthyroidism, hypertension, stroke, angina, MI, endocrine disorders, or anemia.

Assessment of the reproductive system is incomplete without knowledge of the patient's lifestyle choices. Determine whether a woman uses cigarettes, alcohol, caffeine, or other drugs

---

TABLE 51-5 HEALTH HISTORY

Reproductive System

Health Perception–Health Management
- How would you describe your overall health?
- *Women:* Explain how you examine your breasts. Have you had a Pap test or mammogram recently? If so, what were the results and dates of these tests?
- *Men:* Explain how you examine your testes. Have you had a prostate examination recently? If so, what were the results and date of this examination?
- Describe the health of your family members. Any history of breast, uterine, ovarian, or prostate cancer?
- Do you use tobacco products, alcohol, or drugs?*

Nutritional-Metabolic
- Describe what you usually eat and drink.
- Have you experienced any changes in weight?*
- How do you feel about your current weight?
- Do you take any nutritional supplements such as calcium or vitamins?*
- Do you have any dietary restrictions?*

Elimination
- Do you experience problems with urination (e.g., pain, burning, dribbling, incontinence, frequency)?*
- Have you had bladder infections? If so, when? How often?
- Do you experience problems with bowel movements?* Do you use laxatives?*

Activity-Exercise
- What activities do you typically do each day?
- Do you have enough energy for your desired activities?
- Can you dress yourself? Feed yourself? Walk without help?

Sleep-Rest
- How many hours do you typically sleep each night?
- Do you feel rested after sleep?
- Do you experience any problems associated with sleeping?*

Cognitive-Perceptual
- Are you able to read and write?
- Do you experience problems with dizziness?*
- Do you experience pain? If yes, where?
- Do you experience pain during sexual activity or intercourse?*

Self-Perception–Self-Concept
- How would you describe yourself?
- Have there been any recent changes that have made you feel differently about yourself?*
- Are you experiencing any problems that are affecting your sexuality?*

Role-Relationship
- Describe your living arrangements. Who do you live with?
- Do you have a significant other? If yes, is this relationship satisfying?
- Are you experiencing any role-related problems in your family?* At work?*
- What are the relationships among your family members?

Sexuality-Reproductive
- Are you sexually active? If so, how many partners do you have?
- What kind of sex do you engage in (e.g., oral, vaginal, rectal)?
- How do you protect yourself against sexually transmitted infections and unwanted pregnancy?
- Are you satisfied with your present means of sexual expression? If no, explain.
- Have you experienced any recent changes in your sexual practices?*
- *Women:* Date of last menstruation, description of menstrual flow, problems with menstruation, age of menarche, age of menopause.
- *Women:* Pregnancy history—number of times pregnant, number of living children, number of miscarriages or abortions.

Coping–Stress Tolerance
- Have there been any major changes in your life within the past couple of years?*
- What is stressful in your life right now?
- How do you handle health problems when they occur?

Value-Belief
- What beliefs do you have about your health and illnesses?
- Do you use home remedies?*
- Is religion an important part of your life?*
- Do you think that any of your personal beliefs or values may be compromised because of your treatment?*

*If yes, describe.

because these substances can be detrimental to both mother and fetus. Cigarette smoking may delay conception and can also increase the risk of morbidity in women using oral contraceptives. Smoking in women is also associated with early menopause. These substances may also adversely affect the sperm count in men and cause erectile dysfunction or decreased libido.

Also document if the patient is allergic to sulfonamides, penicillin, rubber, or latex. Sulfonamides and penicillin are used frequently in the treatment of reproductive and genitourinary problems such as vaginitis and gonorrhea. Rubber and latex are commonly used in diaphragms and condoms. An allergy to these substances precludes their use as contraceptive methods.

Nutritional-Metabolic Pattern. Anemia is a common problem in women in their reproductive years, particularly during pregnancy and the postpartum period. Evaluate the adequacy of the diet with this condition in mind.

Take a thorough nutritional and psychologic history to assess for the presence of an eating disorder. Anorexia nervosa can cause amenorrhea and subsequent problems, such as osteoporosis, that are related to menopause. Obesity can be related to polycystic ovarian syndrome and may be a precursor to type 2 diabetes.

From early adolescence, counsel women regarding adequate calcium and vitamin D intake to prevent osteoporosis. Estimate the patient's daily calcium intake to determine whether supplementation is needed. Evaluate folic acid intake for women in their reproductive years because a deficiency can result in spina bifida and other neural tube defects in the fetus.[12]

Elimination Pattern. Many gynecologic problems can result in genitourinary problems. Stress and urge incontinence is common in older women because of relaxation of the pelvic musculature caused by multiple births or advancing age. Vaginal infections predispose patients to chronic or recurrent urinary tract infections. Metastasis of malignant tumors of the reproductive system to the genitourinary system is possible because of their proximity. Benign prostatic hyperplasia is a common problem of older men. It can alter normal urination, causing retention and difficulty in initiating the urinary stream.

Activity-Exercise Pattern. Record the amount, type, and intensity of activity and exercise. Lack of stress on bones secondary to lack of exercise is an important factor in the development of osteoporosis. Weight-bearing exercise decreases the risk of osteoporosis in women. Women who engage in excessive exercise may experience amenorrhea, which may result from decreased estrogen related to a low percentage of body fat (estrogen is stored in fat cells).[13] Anemia can result in fatigue and activity intolerance and can interfere with satisfactory performance of the activities of daily living.

Sleep-Rest Pattern. Sleep patterns may be affected during the postpartum period and also while raising young children. Hot flashes and sweating that are often present during perimenopause can cause serious sleep interruption when the woman awakens in a drenching sweat. The need to change her nightgown and bedding further disrupts her sleep. Insomnia is also a common complaint of perimenopausal women. Daytime fatigue often results from such sleep disruptions. In men, sleep disturbances may be caused by frequent urination at night associated with prostate enlargement or HT for prostate cancer.

Cognitive-Perceptual Pattern. Pelvic pain is associated with various gynecologic disorders such as pelvic inflammatory disease, ovarian cysts, and endometriosis. Dyspareunia (painful intercourse) can be particularly problematic for women. The pain associated with intercourse can create a reluctance to participate in sexual activity and strain relationships with sexual partners. Refer women with dyspareunia to their health care providers.

Self-Perception–Self-Concept Pattern. Changes that occur with aging, such as pendulous breasts and vaginal dryness in women and decreased size of the penis in men, may lead to emotional distress. The subtle changes associated with sexuality and advancing age may alter the self-concept of many persons.

Role-Relationship Pattern. Obtain information regarding the family structure and occupation. Question the patient regarding recent changes in work-related relationships or family conflict. Determine the patient's role in the family as a starting point in determining family dynamics.

Roles and relationships are affected by changes within the family. The addition of a new baby may change family dynamics. Role-relationship patterns change as children begin their careers and move away from home. Another change occurs when people retire.

Sexuality-Reproductive Pattern. The extent and depth of the interview about a patient's sexuality depend primarily on the interviewer's expertise and on the patient's needs and willingness. Before taking a sexual history, assess your comfort with your own sexuality, because any discomfort in questioning becomes obvious to the patient. Carry out interviews in an environment that provides reassurance, confidentiality, and a nonjudgmental attitude. Begin with the least sensitive areas of questioning and then move to more sensitive areas.

For women, obtain a menstrual and an obstetric history. The menstrual history includes the first day of the last menstrual period, description of menstrual flow, age of menarche, and, if applicable, age at menopause. Menstrual history data are used in the detection of pregnancy, infertility, and numerous other gynecologic problems. Have the patient explicitly describe changes in the usual menstrual pattern to determine whether the change is transient and unimportant or connected with a more serious gynecologic problem. *Metrorrhagia* (spotting or bleeding between menstruations), *menorrhagia* (excessive menstrual bleeding), *amenorrhea* (lack of menstruation), and *postcoital bleeding* are examples of such problems.

Identify changes in menstrual patterns associated with the use of contraceptive pills, intrauterine devices (IUDs), birth control patches, vaginal rings, subdermal estrogen-only implants (Jadelle), or medroxyprogesterone (Depo-Provera) injections. Contraceptive pills usually decrease the amount and duration of flow, whereas some IUDs may cause an increase in the amount and duration. Some IUDs also increase the severity of dysmenorrhea. However, newer IUDs contain progestin and may be therapeutic.

The obstetric history includes the number of pregnancies, full-term births, preterm births, and live births. Also include information about any ectopic pregnancies or abortions, either spontaneous or therapeutic. Document any problems that occurred with pregnancy.

A sexual history should include information regarding sexual activity, beliefs, and practices. Explore sexual preference (heterosexual, homosexual, bisexual), the frequency and type of sexual activity (penile-vaginal, penile-rectal, recipient rectal, oral), and the number of partners and protective measures against STIs and pregnancy. Determine the patient's knowledge

TABLE 51-6 SEXUAL HISTORY FORMAT

1. Are you currently in a relationship that involves sexual intercourse? If yes, do you have one or multiple partners?
2. How frequently do you engage in sexual activities? Are you and your partner(s) satisfied with the sexual relationship?
3. How many sexual partners have you had in the past 6 mo?
4. Do you prefer relationships with men, women, or both? (Inquire whether the patient is in a significant relationship.)
5. Has your sex life changed during the past year? If yes, how?
6. Have you ever had a sexually transmitted infection? If yes, what?
7. What are you doing to protect yourself from sexually transmitted infections? If protection is used, what type? Do you use protection every time you have intercourse?
8. Are you currently using any birth control measures? If yes, what type? How long have you been using this product? How effective do you think this has been?
9. Have you ever been in a relationship with anyone who hurt you? Have you ever been forced into sexual acts as a child or an adult?
10. How often have you experienced erectile dysfunction (male) or difficulty with vaginal lubrication (female) or pain with intercourse?

CASE STUDY—cont'd

Subjective Data

iStockphoto/Thinkstock

A focused assessment of A.K. revealed the following information:

PMH: Type 2 diabetes for 5 yr, hypertension, stress incontinence, osteoarthritis. No surgical history.

Medications: metformin (Glucophage) 500 mg PO bid for the past 4 yr, estrogen/medroxyprogesterone (Prempro) 0.3 mg/1.5 mg/day PO for the past 14 yr, lisinopril (Prinivil) 10 mg/day PO for past 3 yr.

Health Perception–Health Management: A.K. has no personal history of breast cancer, but she does have a family history of breast cancer. Her mother was diagnosed at age 60 and her sister at age 40. She is afraid that she may now have cancer. Her last mammogram and clinical breast examination were 2 yr ago. She does not smoke but does enjoy one to two glasses of wine with her dinner every evening.

Nutritional-Metabolic: A.K. is 5 ft, 2 in tall and weighs 166 lb. She reports gaining most of her weight after menopause. She tries to eat a well-balanced meal and watch her carbohydrate intake because of her diabetes.

Elimination: Denies any changes or difficulty with urination or bowel movements except for stress incontinence when she coughs or laughs. States she always wears a panty liner "just in case."

Activity-Exercise: Does not routinely exercise. Occasionally takes a walk around the block with her husband. Otherwise her life is fairly sedentary.

Cognitive-Perceptual: Denies breast pain.

Sexuality-Reproductive: Had onset of menarche at age 11, menopause at age 53. Has two daughters (34 and 32) and a son (30).

of safe sexual practices. A history of multiple sex partners and unprotected sex increases the risk of contracting an STI. For a woman, this can increase the risk of pelvic inflammatory disease, which can compromise her ability to become pregnant.

Table 51-6 outlines specific questions for a sexual history. Only a skilled interviewer should approach some of these questions, and then only with discretion and sensitivity to cultural differences.

Ask both men and women about their general satisfaction with sexuality. The patient's satisfaction with the opportunities for sexual gratification is important information. Question the patient about sexual beliefs and practices and whether orgasm is achieved. Explore any unexplained change in sexual practices or performance. Problems of the reproductive system can cause physiologic or psychologic problems that can lead to painful intercourse, erectile dysfunction, sexual dysfunction, or infertility. Try to determine both the cause and the effect of such problems.

Coping–Stress Tolerance Pattern. The stress related to situations such as pregnancy or menopause increases dependence on support systems. Determine who the support people are in the patient's life. The diagnosis of an STI can cause stress for the patient and the partner. Explore ways to manage this stress.

Value-Belief Pattern. Sexual and reproductive functioning is closely related to cultural, religious, moral, and ethical values. Be aware of your own beliefs in these areas, and recognize and sensitively react to the patient's personal beliefs associated with reproductive and sexuality issues.

Objective Data

Physical Examination: Male. The examination of the male external genitalia includes inspection and palpation. An examination may be performed with the patient lying or standing. The standing position is generally preferred. Sit in front of the standing patient. Use gloves during examination of the male genitalia.

Pubis. Observe the distribution and general characteristics of the pubic hair and the skin. Normally, the hair is in a diamond-shaped pattern and coarser than scalp hair. The absence of hair is not a normal finding unless the man is shaving or waxing the pubic hair. Carefully assess the skin for irritation and inflammation.

Penis. Note the size and skin texture of the penis and any lesions, scars, or swelling. Also note the location of the urethral meatus and the presence or absence of a foreskin. If present, the foreskin should be retracted to note any redness, discharge, irritation, or swelling. Replace the foreskin over the glans after observation. Then compress the glans to note any discharge and its amount, color, and odor if present. Palpate the penile shaft for tenderness or masses and observe the ventral and dorsal aspects.

Scrotum and Testes. This part of the examination is usually not performed by the nurse generalist. The nurse with advanced skills starts by performing a complete skin examination by lifting each testis to inspect all sides of the scrotal sac. Palpate the scrotum to note changes in consistency or any masses. Note if the testes are descended. The left testis usually hangs lower than the right. An undescended testis is a major risk factor for testicular cancer and a potential cause of male infertility.[14]

Inguinal Region and Spermatic Cord. This part of the examination is usually not performed by the nurse generalist. The examiner with advanced skills first inspects the skin overlying the inguinal regions for rashes or lesions. Then ask the patient to bear down or cough. While he is straining, inspect the inguinal area for a bulge. No bulging should be seen.

Examination of the inguinal area continues with palpation. Palpate the right and left inguinal rings using the index or middle finger. Insert the finger into the lower aspect of the scrotum and follow the spermatic cord upward through the triangular, slitlike opening of the inguinal ring. At this point, ask the patient to bear down and cough. Determine whether the strain produces a bulging of the intestines through the ring, indicating a hernia, a condition that requires follow-up. Also palpate the inguinal lymph nodes. Enlargement of the lymph nodes (*lymphadenopathy*) could suggest a pelvic organ infection or malignancy.

Anus and Prostate. Inspect the anal sphincter and perineal regions for lesions, masses, and hemorrhoids. A DRE is required for all men who have symptoms of prostate trouble, such as difficulty initiating urination and the urge to void frequently. This examination should be performed by the health care provider annually for all men 50 years of age and older.

Physical Examination: Female. Physical examination of women often begins with inspection and palpation of the breasts and axillae and then proceeds to the abdomen and genitalia. Examination of the abdomen provides an opportunity to detect pain or any masses that may involve the genitourinary system. Abdominal examination is discussed in Chapter 39.

Breasts. First examine the breasts by visual inspection. With the patient seated, observe the breasts for symmetry, size, shape, skin color, vascular patterns, dimpling, and unusual lesions. Ask the patient to put her arms at her sides, arms overhead, lean forward, and press hands on hips. Observe for any abnormalities during these maneuvers. Palpate the axillae and the clavicular areas for enlarged lymph nodes.

After the patient assumes a supine position, place a pillow under her back on the side to be examined. Ask the patient to put her arm above and behind her head. These maneuvers flatten breast tissue and make palpation easier. Then palpate the breast in a systematic fashion, preferably using a vertical line (see Fig. 52-1). Use the distal finger pads for palpation. Include the axillary tail of Spence in the examination. This area of the breast lies adjacent to the upper outer quadrant, which is where most breast malignancies develop (see Fig. 52-1). Finally, palpate the area around the areolae for masses. Compress the nipple to detect any discharge or masses. Document the color, consistency, and odor of any discharge.

External Genitalia. Use gloves for examination of the external genitalia. Inspect the mons pubis, labia majora, labia minora, posterior fourchette, perineum, and anal region for characteristics of skin, hair distribution, and contour. Note any lesions, inflammation, swelling, and discharge. Separate the labia to fully inspect the clitoris, urethral meatus, and vaginal orifice.

Internal Pelvic Examination. This part of the examination is usually not performed by the nurse generalist. During the speculum examination, the examiner observes the walls of the vagina and the cervix for inflammation, discharge, polyps, and suspicious growths. During this examination, it is possible to obtain a Pap test and collect cells for culture and microscopic examination. After the speculum examination, a bimanual examination is performed to assess the size, shape, and consistency of the uterus and ovaries. The tubes are not normally palpable.

Parts of the pelvic and bimanual examinations are not included in this text, since they are considered advanced skills and are not usually within the scope of the nurse generalist.

Table 51-7 provides an example of a recording format for the physical assessment findings for the male and female reproductive systems. Tables 51-8 through 51-10 summarize assessment abnormalities of the breasts, female reproductive system, and male reproductive system, respectively.

CASE STUDY—cont'd
Objective Data: Physical Examination

Focused assessment of A.K. reveals the following: A palpable, firm, fixed, 1.5-cm mass in upper, outer quadrant of right breast. No dimpling, redness, or swelling noted. No masses palpated in left breast. No lymphadenopathy noted.

As you continue to read this chapter, consider diagnostic studies you would anticipate being performed for A.K.

iStockphoto/Thinkstock

A *focused assessment* is used to evaluate the status of previously identified reproductive problems and to monitor for signs of new problems (see Table 3-6). A focused assessment of the reproductive system is presented in the box above.

DIAGNOSTIC STUDIES OF REPRODUCTIVE SYSTEMS

The most commonly used diagnostic studies in the assessment of the reproductive systems are summarized in Table 51-11 on p. 1233, and select studies are described in more detail below.

Urine Studies

Pregnancy Testing. Pregnancy is generally validated by measuring human chorionic gonadotropin (hCG) in the urine.[15] A solution containing monoclonal antibodies specific for hCG is mixed with a small amount of urine. The presence of hCG causes a change in color of the tested urine.

Home pregnancy test kits use the same assay principle. Positive results are based on the presence of hCG in urine. Some tests can detect pregnancy as early as the first day after a missed menstrual period. These tests are 98% accurate if the test is performed exactly per instructions. A second test is recommended within a week if the first test is negative (assuming menses has not yet occurred).

Hormone Studies. Although estrogen studies are performed on urine, the results are often inaccurate because of variable estrogen levels during the normal cycle and the difficulty in estimating the day of the cycle in women with irregular menses. Adrenal androgens are precursors of estrogens and can be measured in the urine of both men and women. For more information on hormone studies, see Chapter 48.

Blood Studies

Hormone Studies. Serum assays for hCG can detect pregnancy before a woman misses her menstrual period. The prolactin assay is used primarily in the workup of a patient with amenorrhea. High levels of prolactin are normally associated with low levels of estrogen, such as those that occur during lactation. However, the same finding can occur with pituitary adenomas, especially with otherwise unexplained galactorrhea (excessive secretion of breast milk). Serum progesterone and estradiol are sometimes measured to assess ovarian function, particularly for amenorrhea. In addition, hormonal blood studies are essential components of a fertility workup.

Tumor Markers. Biologic tumor markers are used to assess for malignant disease and to monitor therapy (marker levels

TABLE 51-7　NORMAL PHYSICAL ASSESSMENT OF REPRODUCTIVE SYSTEM

Male	Female
Breasts	
Nipples soft. No lumps, nodules, swelling, or enlarged tissue noted.	Symmetric without dimpling. Nipples soft. No drainage, retraction, or lesions noted. No masses or tenderness. No lymphadenopathy.
External Genitalia	
Diamond-shaped hair distribution. No penile lesions or discharge noted. Scrotum symmetric, no masses, descended testes. No inguinal hernia.	Triangular hair distribution. Genitalia dark pink, no lesions, redness, swelling, or inflammation in perineal region. No vaginal discharge noted. No tenderness with palpation of Skene's ducts and Bartholin's glands.
Anus	
No hemorrhoids, fissures, or lesions noted.	No hemorrhoids, fissures, or lesions noted.

TABLE 51-8　ASSESSMENT ABNORMALITIES

Breast

Finding	Description	Possible Etiology and Significance
Nipple inversion or retraction	Recent onset, erythematous, pain, unilateral.	Abscess, inflammation, cancer.
	Recent onset (usually within past year), unilateral presentation, lack of tenderness.	Neoplasm.
Nipple secretions		
• Galactorrhea (female)	Milky, no relationship to lactation, unilateral or bilateral, intermittent or consistent presentation.	Drug therapy, particularly phenothiazines, tricyclic antidepressants, methyldopa. Hypofunction or hyperfunction of thyroid or adrenal glands. Tumors of hypothalamus or pituitary gland. Excessive estrogen. Prolonged suckling or breast foreplay.
• Galactorrhea (male)	Milky, bilateral presentation.	Chorioepithelioma of testes, manifestation of pituitary tumor.
• Purulent	Gray-green or yellow color. Frequent unilateral presentation. Association with pain, erythema, induration, nipple inversion.	Puerperal (after birth) mastitis (inflammatory condition of breast) or abscess.
	Same as above but usually without nipple inversion.	Infected sebaceous cyst.
• Serous discharge	Clear appearance, unilateral or bilateral, intermittent or consistent presentation.	Intraductal papilloma.
• Dark green or multicolored discharge	Thick, sticky, and frequently bilateral.	Ductal ectasia (dilation of mammary ducts).
• Serosanguineous or bloody drainage	Unilateral presentation.	Papillomatosis (widespread development of nipple-like growths), intraductal papilloma, carcinoma (male and female).
Scaling or irritation of nipple	Unilateral or bilateral presentation, crusting, possible ulceration.	Paget's disease, eczema, infection.
Nodules, lumps, or masses	Multiple, bilateral, well-delineated, soft or firm, mobile cysts. Pain. Premenstrual occurrence.	Fibrocystic changes.
	Rubbery consistency, fluid-filled interior, pain.	Ductal ectasia.
	Soft, mobile, well-delineated cyst, absence of pain.	Lipoma, fibroadenoma.
	Erythema, tenderness, induration.	Infected sebaceous cysts, abscesses.
	Usually singular, hard, irregularly shaped, poorly delineated, nonmobile.	Neoplasm.
Dimpling of breast	Unilateral, recent onset, no pain.	Neoplasm.

TABLE 51-9 ASSESSMENT ABNORMALITIES

Female Reproductive System

Finding and Description	Possible Etiology and Significance
Vulvar Discharge	
White, thick, curdy, frequent itching and inflammation, lack of odor or yeast-like smell	Candidiasis (*Candida* or yeast infection), vaginitis
Thin gray or white, copious flow, malodorous or fishy, vulvar irritation	Bacterial vaginosis infection
Frothy green or yellow color; malodorous	*Trichomonas vaginalis*
Bloody discharge	*Chlamydia trachomatis* or *Neisseria gonorrhoeae* infection, menstruation, trauma, cancer
Vulvar Erythema	
Bright or beefy red color, itching	*Candida albicans*, allergy, chemical vaginitis
Reddened base, painful vesicles or ulcerations	Genital herpes
Macules or papules, itching	Chancroid (STI), contact dermatitis, scabies, pediculosis
Vulvar Growths	
Soft, fleshy growth, nontender	Condyloma acuminatum
Flat and warty appearance, nontender	Condyloma latum
Same as either of above, possible pain	Neoplasm
Reddened base, vesicles, and small erosions; pain	Lymphogranuloma venereum, genital herpes, chancroid
Indurated, firm ulcers, no pain	Chancre (syphilis), granuloma inguinale
Abdominal Pain or Tenderness	
Intermittent or consistent tenderness in right or left lower quadrant	Salpingitis (infection of fallopian tube), ectopic pregnancy, ruptured ovarian cyst, PID, tubal or ovarian abscess
Periumbilical location, consistent occurrence	Cystitis, endometritis (inflammation of endometrium), ectopic pregnancy
Abnormal Vaginal Bleeding	
Unusual and inappropriate uterine bleeding	Dysfunctional uterine bleeding, usually anovulatory bleeding, menorrhagia (heavy menstrual bleeding), metrorrhagia (irregular, frequent bleeding), postmenopausal bleeding

PID, Pelvic inflammatory disease.

TABLE 51-10 ASSESSMENT ABNORMALITIES

Male Reproductive System

Finding and Description	Possible Etiology and Significance
Penile Growths or Masses	
Indurated, smooth, disklike appearance; absence of pain; singular presentation	Chancre
Papular to irregularly shaped ulceration with pus, lack of induration	Chancroid
Ulceration with induration and nodularity	Cancer
Flat, wartlike nodule	Condyloma latum
Elevated, fleshy, moist, elongated projections with single or multiple projections	Condyloma acuminatum
Localized swelling with retracted, tight foreskin	Paraphimosis (inability to replace foreskin to its normal position after retraction), trauma
Vesicles, Erosions, or Ulcers	
Painful, erythematous base. Vesicular or small erosions	Genital herpes, balanitis (inflammation of glans penis), chancroid
Painless, singular, small erosion with eventual lymphadenopathy	Lymphogranuloma venereum, cancer
Scrotal Masses	
Localized swelling with tenderness, unilateral or bilateral presentation	Epididymitis (inflammation of epididymis), testicular torsion, orchitis (mumps)
Swelling, tenderness	Incarcerated hernia
Swelling without pain. Unilateral or bilateral presentation. Translucent, cordlike or wormlike appearance	Hydrocele (accumulation of fluid in outer covering of testes), spermatocele (firm, sperm-containing cyst of epididymis), varicocele (dilation of veins that drain testes), hematocele (accumulation of blood within scrotum)
Firm, nodular testes or epididymis. Frequent unilateral presentation	Tuberculosis, cancer
Penile Discharge	
Clear to purulent color, minimal to copious flow	Urethritis or gonorrhea, *Chlamydia trachomatis* infection, trauma
Penile or Scrotal Erythema	
Macules and papules	Scabies, pediculosis
Inguinal Masses	
Bulging unilateral presentation during straining	Inguinal hernia
1- to 3-cm nodules	Lymphadenopathy

rise as disease progresses and fall with disease regression). α-Fetoprotein (AFP), hCG, and CA-125 are sometimes used as tumor markers for reproductive system malignancies. A specific tumor antigen such as PSA is another type of tumor marker, frequently used for prostate cancer.

Serology Tests for Syphilis. The Venereal Disease Research Laboratory (VDRL) test and the rapid plasma reagin (RPR) test detect the presence of antibodies in the serum of patients infected with syphilis. These tests are inexpensive and reliable but have high levels of false-positive results. The fluorescent treponemal antibody absorption (FTA-Abs) test is highly reliable and should be used after a positive VDRL or RPR.

Cultures and Smears

Cultures and smears are most frequently used in the diagnosis of STIs. Specimens for cultures and smears are commonly taken from the vagina, endocervix, and rectum for females and the urethra and rectum for males. For a culture, the specimen is placed on a special culture medium. A smear involves rubbing the specimen on a slide for direct examination. Gram stain smears have been shown to be effective in the diagnosis of *Chlamydia* infection. A nucleic acid amplification test (NAAT)

Text continued on p. 1236

TABLE 51-11 DIAGNOSTIC STUDIES

Male and Female Reproductive Systems

Study	Description and Purpose	Nursing Responsibility
Urine Studies		
Human chorionic gonadotropin (hCG)	Detects pregnancy. Also detects hydatidiform mole and chorioepithelioma (in men and women). *Males and nonpregnant females:* Negative	Obtain menstrual history from patient, including birth control methods. Determine presence or absence of presumptive signs of pregnancy (e.g., breast changes, increased whitish vaginal discharge).
Testosterone	Detects tumors and developmental anomalies of the testes. *Female:* 2-12 mcg/24 hr (6.9-41.6 nmol/24 hr) *Male:* 40-135 mcg/24 hr (139-469 nmol/24 hr)	Instruct patient to collect 24-hr urine specimen and to keep refrigerated.
Follicle-stimulating hormone (FSH)	Indicates gonadal failure because of pituitary dysfunction. *Female:* Follicular phase: 2-15 U/24 hr Midcycle: 8-60 U/24 hr Luteal phase: 2-10 U/24 hr Postmenopause: 35-100 U/24 hr *Male:* 3-11 U/24 hr	Instruct patient to collect 24-hr urine specimen. Indicate phase of menstrual cycle, if menopausal, and if on oral contraceptives or hormones.
Blood Studies		
Prolactin	Detects pituitary dysfunction that can cause amenorrhea. *Female:* 3.8-23.2 ng/mL (3.8-23.2 mg/L) *Male:* 3.0-14.7 ng/mL (3.0-14.7 mg/L)	Observe venipuncture site for bleeding or hematoma formation.
Prostate-specific antigen (PSA)	Detects prostate cancer. Also a sensitive test for monitoring response to therapy. *Reference interval:* <4 ng/mL (<4 mcg/L)	No food or fluid restrictions. Collect 5 mL blood. Observe venipuncture site for bleeding.
hCG	Detects pregnancy. Can also be used as a tumor marker for testicular malignancy. Also used to detect hydatidiform mole. *Males and nonpregnant females:* <5 mIU/mL (<5 IU/L)	Find out where patient is in her menstrual cycle, whether she has missed menses, and if so, how late she is.
Testosterone	Determines whether elevated androgens are due to testicular, adrenal, or ovarian dysfunction or pituitary tumors. Serum testosterone also drawn to assess male infertility and tumors of testicle or ovary. *Male:* 280-1100 ng/dL (10.4-38.17 nmol/L) *Female:* 15-70 ng/dL (0.52-2.43 nmol/L)	Collect health history to eliminate potential sources of interference with accuracy of results (e.g., use of corticosteroids or barbiturates, hypothyroidism or hyperthyroidism).
Progesterone	Determines cause of infertility, monitors success of drugs for infertility or the effect of treatment with progesterone, determines whether ovulation is occurring, and diagnoses problems with the adrenal glands and some types of cancer. *Female:* Follicular phase: 15-70 ng/dL (0.5-2.2 nmol/L) Luteal phase: 200-2500 ng/dL (6.4-79.5 nmol/L) Postmenopause: <40 ng/dL (1.28 nmol/L) *Male:* 13-97 ng/dL (0.4-3.1 nmol/L)	Observe venipuncture site for bleeding or hematoma formation. Include information about last menstrual period and trimester of pregnancy because progesterone levels vary with gestation.
Estradiol	Measures ovarian function. Useful in assessing estrogen-secreting tumors and states of precocious female puberty. May be used to confirm perimenopausal status. Increased serum estradiol levels in men may be indicative of testicular tumors. *Female:* Follicular phase: 20-150 pg/mL (73-1285 pmol/L) Luteal phase: 30-450 pg/mL (110-1652 pmol/L) Postmenopause: ≤20 pg/mL (≤73 pmol/L) *Male:* 10-50 pg/mL (37-184 pmol/L)	Observe venipuncture site for bleeding or hematoma formation.
FSH	Indicates gonadal failure due to pituitary dysfunction. Used to validate menopausal status. *Female:* Follicular phase: 1.37-9.9 mU/mL Ovulatory phase: 6.17-17.2 mU/mL Luteal phase: 1.09-9.2 mU/mL Postmenopause: 19.3-100.6 mU/mL *Male:* 1.42-15.4 mU/mL	No food or fluid restrictions required. State phase of menstrual cycle, if menopausal, or if on oral contraceptive or hormones.
Venereal Disease Research Laboratory (VDRL) (flocculation)	Nonspecific antibody tests used to screen for syphilis. Positive readings can be made within 1-2 wk after appearance of primary lesion (chancre) or 4-15 wk after initial infection. *Reference interval:* Negative or nonreactive	Observe venipuncture site for bleeding or hematoma formation.
Rapid plasma reagin (RPR) (agglutination)	Nonspecific antibody test used to screen for syphilis. *Reference interval:* Negative or nonreactive	Obtain data to identify conditions such as hepatitis, pregnancy, and autoimmune diseases that may interfere with accuracy of results.

Continued

TABLE 51-11 DIAGNOSTIC STUDIES—cont'd

Male and Female Reproductive Systems

Study	Description and Purpose	Nursing Responsibility
Blood Studies—cont'd		
Fluorescent treponemal antibody absorption (FTA-Abs)	Detects syphilis antibodies. Also detects early syphilis with great accuracy. Usually performed if results of VDRL and RPR are questionable. *Reference interval:* Negative or nonreactive	Inform patient that blood sample will be drawn. Observe venipuncture site for bleeding or hematoma formation.
Cultures and Smears		
Dark-field microscopy	Direct examination of specimen obtained from potential syphilitic lesion (chancre) is performed to detect *Treponema pallidum*.	Avoid direct skin contact with open lesion.
Wet mounts	Direct microscopic examination of specimen of vaginal discharge is performed immediately after collection. Determines presence or absence and number of *Trichomonas* organisms, bacteria, white and red blood cells, and candidal buds or hyphae. Other clues or causes of inflammation or infection may be determined.	Explain procedure and purpose to patient. Instruct patient not to douche before examination. Prepare for collection of specimens (glass slide, 10%-20% potassium hydroxide [KOH] solution, sodium chloride [NaCl] solution, and cotton-tipped applicators).
Cultures	Specimens of vaginal, urethral, or cervical discharge are cultured to assess for gonorrhea or *Chlamydia* organisms. Rectal and throat cultures may also be taken, depending on data obtained from sexual history.	Obtain specific contact and sexual history, including oral and rectal intercourse. Instruct against douching before examination. Obtain urethral specimen from men before they void. Instruct sexually active women with multiple partners to have at least a yearly culture for gonorrhea and *Chlamydia*. Instruct sexually active men to have any discharge evaluated immediately to rule out gonorrhea strains that do not cause classic symptoms of dysuria.
Gram stain	Used for rapid detection of gonorrhea. Presence of gram-negative intracellular diplococci generally warrants treatment. Not highly accurate for women. Also a valid alternative for *Chlamydia* testing.	Same as above.
Cytologic Studies		
Papanicolaou (Pap) test	Microscopic study of exfoliated cells via special staining and fixation technique to detect abnormal cells. Most commonly studies cells obtained directly from the endocervix and ectocervix.	Instruct sexually active women to have Pap test according to American Cancer Society guidelines (*www.cancer.org*). Instruct patient not to douche for at least 24 hr before examination. Collect careful menstrual and gynecologic history.
Nipple discharge test	Cytologic study of nipple discharge.	Indicate if patient is taking hormonal preparations or other drugs, is breastfeeding, or has a history of amenorrhea. Instruct patient that nipple discharge should always be evaluated.
Radiologic Studies		
Mammography		
• Screening	X-ray image of breast tissue on radiographic film is used to assess breast tissue. Detects benign and malignant masses.	Instruct patient about the examination and American Cancer Society recommendations for screening (see Chapter 52).
• Diagnostic	Performed when patient has suspicious clinical symptoms or abnormality found on screening mammogram. Additional views of affected breast are taken.	
Ultrasound (abdominal and transvaginal)	Measures and records high-frequency sound waves as they pass through tissues of variable density. In women, useful in detecting masses >3 cm, such as ectopic pregnancy, IUD, ovarian cyst, and hydatidiform mole. In men, used to detect testicular torsion or masses.	Instruct patient that a full bladder may be required depending on reason for the study.
Ultrasound-guided biopsy	Use of ultrasound guidance while performing a biopsy. Ultrasound is used to direct the biopsy needle into the region of interest and obtain a sample of tissue. Removal of small tissue sample to diagnose infection, inflammation, or mass.	Inform patient of purpose for this procedure. It is usually done as an outpatient procedure.
Computed tomography (CT) of pelvis	Detects tumors within the pelvis.	Inform patient of procedure. Patient must lie still during the procedure. If IV contrast medium is used, check for iodine allergy.
Magnetic resonance imaging (MRI)	Radio waves and magnetic field are used to view soft tissue. Useful after an abnormal mammogram or for breast dysplasia. Also used to diagnose abnormalities in the female and male reproductive systems.	Screen patient for metal parts and pacemaker. Inform patient the procedure is painless. Patient must lie still during the procedure.

TABLE 51-11   DIAGNOSTIC STUDIES—cont'd

Male and Female Reproductive Systems

Study	Description and Purpose	Nursing Responsibility
Invasive Procedures		
Breast biopsy	Histologic examination of excised breast tissue, obtained either by needle aspiration or excisional biopsy.	*Before biopsy:* Instruct patient about operative procedures and sedation. *After biopsy:* Perform wound care and instruct patient about breast self-examination.
Hysteroscopy	Allows visualization of uterine lining through insertion of scope through cervix. Used mainly to diagnose and treat abnormal bleeding such as polyps and fibroids. Biopsy may be taken during procedure.	Explain purpose and method of procedure and that it may be done in the physician's office. Inform patient that mild cramping and slight bloody discharge after procedure is normal.
Hysterosalpingogram	Involves instillation of contrast media through cervix into uterine cavity and subsequently through the fallopian tubes. X-ray images taken to detect abnormalities of uterus and its adnexa (ovaries and tubes) as contrast progresses through them. Test may be most useful in diagnostic assessment of fertility (e.g., to detect adhesions near ovary, an abnormal uterine shape, blockage of tubal pathways).	Inform patient about procedure and that it may be fairly uncomfortable. Ask about iodine allergy.
Colposcopy	Direct visualization of cervix with binocular microscope that allows magnification and study of cellular dysplasia and cervix abnormalities. Used as follow-up for abnormal Pap test and for examination of women exposed to DES in utero. Biopsy of cervix may be taken during examination. Valuable in decreasing number of false-negative cervical biopsies.	Instruct patient about this outpatient procedure. Inform patient that this examination is similar to speculum examination.
Conization	Cone-shaped sample of squamocolumnar tissue of cervix is removed for direct study.	Explain purpose and method of procedure and that it requires use of surgical facilities and anesthesia. Instruct patient to avoid sexual intercourse and tampons for about 3-4 wk. Also discuss necessity for 3-wk follow-up.
Loop electrosurgical excision procedure (LEEP)	Excision of cervical tissue via an electrosurgical instrument. Diagnoses and treats cervical dysplasia. Minimizes amount of tissue removed, preserves childbearing ability.	Explain purpose and method of procedure and that it may be done in the physician's office. Patient may feel slight tingling or abdominal cramping during procedure. Discharge, bleeding, and cramping may occur for 1-3 days after procedure.
Culdotomy, culdoscopy, and culdocentesis	*Culdotomy* is an incision made through posterior fornix of cul-de-sac and allows visualization of peritoneal cavity (i.e., uterus, tubes, and ovaries). *Culdoscopy* can then be used to closely study these structures. This technique is valuable in fertility evaluations. Withdrawal of fluid *(culdocentesis)* allows examination of fluid.	Explain purpose and method of procedure. Prepare patient for vaginal operation with preoperative instruction and sedation. Perform assessment of bleeding and discomfort after surgery.
Laparoscopy (peritoneoscopy)	Allows visualization of pelvic structures via fiberoptic scopes inserted through small abdominal incisions. Instillation of CO_2 into cavity improves visualization. Used in diagnostic assessment of uterus, tubes, and ovaries (Fig. 51-8). Can be used in conjunction with tubal sterilization.	Before surgery, instruct patient about procedure, prepare abdomen, and reassure patient about sedation. Inform patient of probability of shoulder pain because of air in the abdomen.
Dilation and curettage (D&C)	Operative procedure dilates cervix and allows curetting of endometrial lining. Used in assessment of abnormal bleeding and cytologic evaluation of lining.	Before surgery, instruct patient about procedure and sedation. Perform postoperative assessment of degree of bleeding (frequent pad check during first 24 hr).
Fertility Studies		
Semen analysis	Semen is assessed for volume (2-5 mL), viscosity, sperm count (>20 million/mL), sperm motility (60% motile), and percent of abnormal sperm (60% with normal structure).	Instruct patient to bring in fresh specimen within 2 hr after ejaculation.
Basal body temperature assessment	Measurement indirectly indicates whether ovulation has occurred. (Temperature rises at ovulation and remains elevated during secretory phase of normal menstrual cycle.)	Instruct woman to take temperature using special basal temperature thermometer (calibrated in tenths of degrees) every morning before getting out of bed. Instruct to record temperature on graph.
Huhner, Sims-Huhner, test	Mucus sample of cervix is examined within 2-8 hr after intercourse. Total number of sperm is assessed in relation to number of live sperm. Used to determine whether cervical mucus is "hostile" to passage of sperm from vagina into uterus.	Instruct couples to have intercourse at estimated time of ovulation and be present for test within 2-8 hr after intercourse.
Endometrial biopsy	Small curette is used to obtain piece of endometrial lining to assess endometrial changes common to progesterone secretion after ovulation. Also used to assess abnormal menstrual or postmenopausal uterine bleeding.	Tell patient test must be performed postovulation. Explain that procedure should cause only short period of uterine cramping and light, bloody vaginal discharge for about 24 hr.
Hysterosalpingogram	Same as operative procedures.	Same as operative procedures.
Serum progesterone	Same as blood studies.	Same as blood studies.

DES, Diethylstilbestrol; *IUD,* intrauterine device.

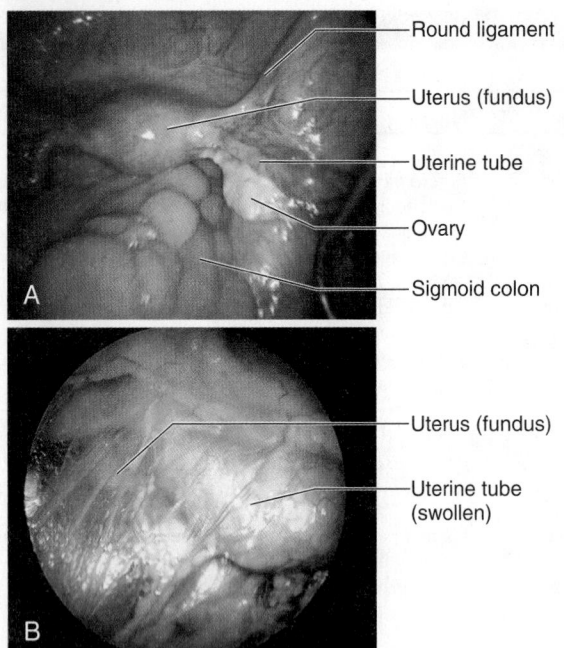

FIG. 51-8 Laparoscopic views of the female pelvis. **A,** Normal image. **B,** Pelvic inflammatory disease. Note reddish inflammatory membrane covering and fixing the ovary and uterus to the surrounding structures.

— Round ligament
— Uterus (fundus)
— Uterine tube
— Ovary
— Sigmoid colon

— Uterus (fundus)
— Uterine tube (swollen)

can screen for both gonorrhea and *Chlamydia* from a wide variety of samples, including vaginal, endocervical, urinary, and urethral specimens. Dark-field microscopy involves the direct examination of a specimen obtained from a chancre for the diagnosis of syphilis.

CASE STUDY—cont'd

Objective Data: Diagnostic Studies

The breast specialist orders the following for A.K.:
• Digital mammography
• Ultrasound of breasts
• MRI of breasts

The mammography reveals an increased density on the right breast. The ultrasound identifies the mass as solid and not fluid filled. The MRI confirms the presence of a suspicious mass in the right breast.

iStockphoto/Thinkstock

The health care provider schedules A.K. for a fine-needle aspiration (FNA) biopsy. The results of the ultrasound-guided FNA biopsy reveal an adenocarcinoma.

Radiologic Studies

Mammography. Mammography, one of the most frequently used diagnostic tools to assess the reproductive system, is used to detect breast masses. Mammography and screening guidelines for mammography are discussed in Chapter 52.

Ultrasound. Ultrasound has many applications for diagnostic studies. Pelvic ultrasound is used to obtain images of the pelvic organs. Transvaginal ultrasound is used to visualize the female genital tract. These types of ultrasound are also used to detect pregnancy in the uterus, ectopic pregnancy, ovarian cysts, and other pelvic masses.

Breast ultrasound is useful in the detection of fluid-filled masses. In men, ultrasound is used to detect testicular masses and testicular torsion. Transrectal ultrasound (TRUS) is useful for diagnosing prostate tumors.

BRIDGE TO NCLEX EXAMINATION

The number of the question corresponds to the same-numbered outcome at the beginning of the chapter.

1. A normal male reproductive function that may be altered in a patient who undergoes a prostatectomy is
   a. sperm production.
   b. production of testosterone.
   c. production of seminal fluid.
   d. release of sperm from the epididymis.

2. Estrogen production by a mature ovarian follicle causes
   a. decreased secretion of FSH and LH.
   b. increased production of GnRH and FSH.
   c. release of GnRH and increased secretion of LH.
   d. decreased release of FSH and decreased progesterone production.

3. Female orgasm is the result of (*select all that apply*)
   a. constriction of the cervical os.
   b. uterine and vaginal contractions.
   c. vaginal enlargement and uterine elevation.
   d. clitoral swelling and increased vaginal lubrication.
   e. rapid release of muscular tension in the reproductive structures.

4. An age-related finding noted by the nurse during the assessment of the older woman's reproductive system is
   a. dyspareunia.
   b. vaginal dryness.
   c. nipple retraction.
   d. increased sensitivity of labia.

5. Significant information about a patient's past health history related to the reproductive system should include
   a. extent of sexual activity.
   b. general satisfaction with sexuality.
   c. previous sexually transmitted infections.
   d. self-image and relationships with others.

6. To evaluate the female patient's breasts, the nurse would use the examination technique of (*select all that apply*)
   a. palpation.
   b. inspection.
   c. percussion.
   d. auscultation.

7. An abnormal finding noted during physical assessment of the male reproductive system is
   a. descended testes.
   b. symmetric scrotum.
   c. slight clear urethral discharge.
   d. the glans covered with prepuce.

8. The nurse is caring for a patient scheduled for an endometrial biopsy who is having difficulty becoming pregnant. The nurse explains to the woman that
   a. the outpatient procedure is usually done preovulation.
   b. bleeding and discharge are common 2 to 4 days after the procedure.
   c. a small sample of tissue is obtained to diagnose and treat cervical dysplasia.
   d. common changes in endometrial cells in relation to progesterone levels will be assessed.

1. c, 2. c, 3. b, c, d, e, 4. b, 5. c, 6. a, b, 7. c, 8. d

⊖volve

For rationales to these answers and even more NCLEX review questions, visit *http://evolve.elsevier.com/Lewis/medsurg*.

REFERENCES

1. Thibodeau G, Patton K: *Structure and function of the body*, ed 14, St Louis, 2012, Mosby.
2. McCance K, Huether S: *Pathophysiology: the biologic basis for disease in adults and children*, ed 6, St Louis, 2010, Mosby.
3. Bulun S: Physiology and pathology of the female reproductive axis. In Melmed S, Polonsky K, Larsen PR, et al, editors: *Williams textbook of endocrinology*, ed 12, St Louis, 2011, Saunders.
4. Rebar R, Erickson G: Reproductive endocrinology and infertility. In Goldman C, Schafer A, editors: *Goldman's Cecil medicine*, ed 24, St Louis, 2011, Saunders.
5. Masters WH, Johnson E: *Human sexual response*, Boston, 1966, Little Brown. (Classic)
6. Mayo Clinic: Menopause. Retrieved from *www.mayoclinic.com/health/menopause*.
7. Laborde E, Brannigan R: Androgen deficiency in the aging male: the tip of the iceberg? *Urol Times* 39:44, 2011.
8. National Institute of Child Health and Human Development: Care before and during pregnancy: prenatal care. Retrieved from *www.nichd.nih.gov/womenshealth*.
9. Saunders 2014 drug reference, St Louis, 2014, Saunders.
10. National Institutes of Health, Women's Health Initiative: Facts about postmenopausal hormonal therapy. Retrieved from *www.nhlbi.nih.gov/health/women*.
11. American Cancer Society: Prostate cancer: early detection. Retrieved from *www.cancer.org*.
*12. Sumar N, McLaren L: Impact on social inequalities of population strategies of prevention for folate intake in women of childbearing age, *Am J Public Health* 101:1218, 2011.
13. Zach K, Smith Machin A, Hoch A: Advances in management of the female athlete triad and eating disorders, *Clin Sports Med* 30:551, 2011.
14. Zoltick B: Shedding light on testicular cancer, *Nurse Pract* 36:32, 2011.
15. US Department of Health and Human Services, Office on Women's Health: Pregnancy tests fact sheet. Retrieved from *www.womenshealth.gov/publications/our-publications/fact-sheet/pregnancy-tests.cfm*.

RESOURCES

Resources for this chapter are listed in Chapter 54 on p. 1306 and Chapter 55 on p. 1332.

*Evidence-based information for clinical practice.

52

What you leave behind is not what is
engraved in stone monuments, but what is
woven into the lives of others.
Pericles

Nursing Management
Breast Disorders

Deborah Hamolsky

evolve WEBSITE

http://evolve.elsevier.com/Lewis/medsurg

- NCLEX Review Questions
- Key Points
- Pre-Test
- Answer Guidelines for Case Study on p. 1258

- Rationales for Bridge to NCLEX Examination Questions
- Case Study
  - Patient With Breast Cancer
- Nursing Care Plan (Customizable)
  - eNCP 52-1: Patient After Mastectomy or Lumpectomy

- Concept Map Creator
- Concept Map for Case Study on p. 1258
- Glossary
- Content Updates

LEARNING OUTCOMES

1. Summarize screening guidelines for the early detection of breast cancer.
2. Describe accurate clinical breast examination techniques, including inspection and palpation.
3. Explain the types, causes, clinical manifestations, and nursing and collaborative management of common benign breast disorders.
4. Assess the risk factors for breast cancer.
5. Describe the pathophysiology and clinical manifestations of breast cancer.

6. Describe the collaborative care and nursing management of breast cancer.
7. Specify the physical and psychologic preoperative and postoperative aspects of nursing management for the patient undergoing a mastectomy.
8. Explain the indications for reconstructive breast surgery, types and complications of reconstructive breast surgery, and nursing management after reconstructive breast surgery.

KEY TERMS

ductal ectasia, p. 1242
fibroadenoma, p. 1242
fibrocystic changes, p. 1241
galactorrhea, p. 1242

gynecomastia, p. 1242
intraductal papilloma, p. 1242
lumpectomy, p. 1247
lymphedema, p. 1249

mammoplasty, p. 1256
mastalgia, p. 1240
mastitis, p. 1240
Paget's disease, p. 1245

Breast disorders are a significant health concern for women. Whether the actual diagnosis is a benign condition or a malignancy, the initial discovery of a lump or change in the breast often triggers intense feelings of anxiety, fear, and denial.

The most frequently encountered breast disorders in women are fibrocystic changes, fibroadenoma, intraductal papilloma, ductal ectasia, and breast cancer. In a woman's lifetime there is a 1 in 8 chance she will be diagnosed with breast cancer.[1] In men, gynecomastia is the most common breast disorder.

ASSESSMENT OF BREAST DISORDERS

Breast Cancer Screening Guidelines

Screening guidelines for the early detection of breast cancer include the following:[2-5]

- Yearly mammograms starting at age 40 and continuing for as long as a woman is in good health. A controversial recommended change is that women at normal risk for breast cancer should begin annual screening at age 50 and stop screening at age 75.[6]

Reviewed by Carole Martz, RN, MS, AOCN, CBCN, Clinical Coordinator, Living in the Future Cancer Survivorship Program, Northshore University Health System, Highland Park Hospital, Highland Park, Illinois; Shannon T. Harrington, RN, PhD, Nursing Lecturer, School of Nursing, Old Dominion University, Norfolk, Virginia; Mary Scheid, RN, MSN, OCN, CBCN, Breast Health Nurse, NCMC Breast Center, North Colorado Medical Center, Greeley, Colorado; and Mary Blessing, RN, MSN, Director, Academic RN Residency Program, University of New Mexico Hospitals, Albuquerque, New Mexico.

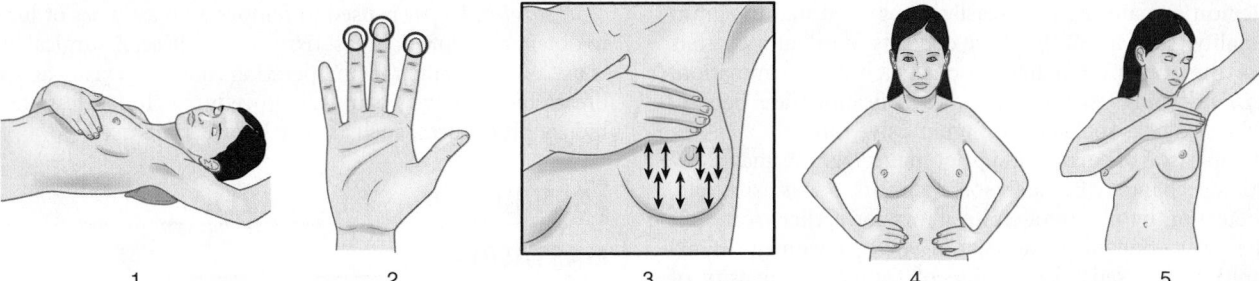

FIG. 52-1 Breast self-examination and patient instruction. *1,* Lie down and place your left arm behind your head. Lying down spreads breast tissue evenly and thinly over the chest wall, making it easier to feel the tissue. *2,* Use finger pads of three middle fingers on your right hand to feel for lumps in left breast. Use overlapping dime-sized circular motions to feel the breast tissue. Use three different levels of pressure to feel the breast tissue. Light pressure to feel tissue closest to the skin; medium pressure to feel a little deeper; and firm pressure to feel tissue closest to the chest and ribs. A firm ridge in the lower curve of each breast is normal. *3,* The up-and-down (vertical) pattern is recommended for examining the entire breast. Move around the breast in an up-and-down pattern starting at an imaginary line straight down your side from the underarm (including the tail of Spence, which is the triangular breast tissue projecting into the axilla), and moving across the breast to the middle of the sternum. Examine the entire breast going down until you feel only ribs and up to the neck or clavicle. Repeat procedure while examining your right breast. *4,* Stand in front of a mirror. Place your hands firmly on your hips, which will tighten the pectoralis muscles. Look at your breasts for size, shape, redness, scaliness, or dimpling of the breast skin or nipple. *5,* Examine each underarm while standing or sitting with arm slightly raised. Check for any lump, hard knot, or thickening of tissue.

- Clinical breast examination (CBE) preferably at least every 3 years for women in their 20s and 30s, and every year for women beginning at age 40.[7]
- Women should report any breast changes promptly to their health care provider. Breast self-examination (BSE) is an option for women starting at age 20.
- Women at increased risk (family history, genetic link, past breast cancer) should talk with their health care provider about the benefits and limitations of starting mammography screening earlier, having additional tests (e.g., breast ultrasound or magnetic resonance imaging [MRI]), or having more frequent examinations.

In recent years there has been some controversy regarding the value of BSE and its role in reducing mortality rates from breast cancer in women. While the benefit of BSE in reducing breast cancer deaths continues to be reviewed, BSE remains a useful technique in helping women develop awareness of how their breasts normally look and feel. Teach women beginning at age 20 the benefits and limitations of BSE and the importance of reporting breast changes (e.g., nipple discharge, a lump) to their health care provider.[8]

When teaching the woman about BSE, include information related to potential benefits, limitations, and harm (chance of a false-positive test result). Allow time for questions about the procedure and a return demonstration. At every periodic health examination, ask the woman who is performing BSE to demonstrate her technique. For women who choose to do BSE, the technique has recently been revised (Fig. 52-1).

BSE is recommended on a monthly schedule. For women who are having regular menstrual periods, this would be right after menstruation when breasts are less lumpy and tender. If menses are irregular or a woman is postmenopausal, advise choosing the same day each month. For women taking oral contraceptives, the first day of a new package may be a helpful reminder.

Diagnostic Studies

Radiologic Studies. Several techniques can be used to screen for breast disease or to help diagnose a suspicious

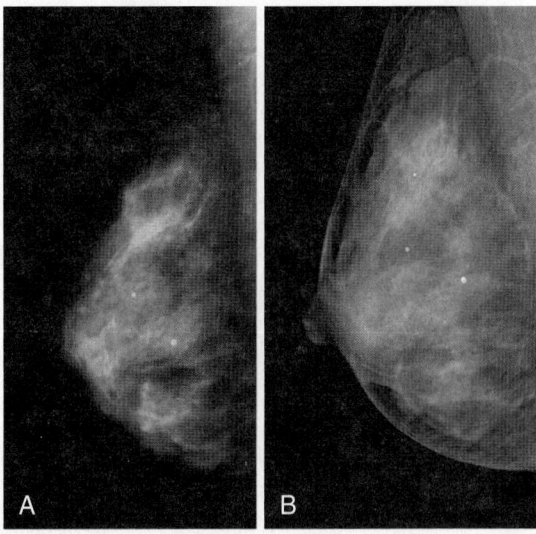

FIG. 52-2 Screening mammogram showing dense breast tissue and benign, scattered microcalcifications of a 57-year-old. **A,** Using conventional x-rays. **B,** Using digital x-rays.

physical finding. *Mammography* is a method used to visualize the breast's internal structure using x-rays (Fig. 52-2). This generally well-tolerated procedure can detect suspicious lumps that cannot be felt. Mammography has significantly improved the early and accurate detection of breast malignancies. Improved imaging technology has also reduced the radiation dose from mammography.

Digital mammography is a technique in which x-ray images are digitally coded into a computer (see Fig. 52-2). It is not clear whether mammogram interpretation has improved with the aid of a computer. The associated costs of using computer-aided detection may also outweigh the benefits.[9]

Three-dimensional (3D) mammography, a new type of mammogram that produces a 3D image of the breast, provides a clearer view of overlapping breast tissue structures. 3-D images help to accurately detect and diagnose breast cancer.

Calcifications are the most easily recognized mammogram abnormality (see Fig. 52-2). These deposits of calcium crystals form in the breast for many reasons, such as inflammation, trauma, and aging. Although most calcifications are benign, they may also be associated with preinvasive cancer.

A comparison of current and prior mammograms may show early tissue changes. Because some tumors metastasize late, early detection by mammography allows for earlier treatment and the prevention of metastasis. In younger women, mammography is less sensitive because of the greater density of breast tissue, resulting in more false-negative results.

About 10% to 15% of all breast cancers cannot be seen on mammography and are detected by palpation or additional diagnostic studies, including ultrasound and MRI. If the clinical findings are suspicious and the mammogram is normal, an ultrasound or MRI may be used. Based on these additional findings, a biopsy may be done.

Ultrasound is used in conjunction with mammography. It may be used to differentiate a solid mass from a cystic mass, to evaluate a mass in a pregnant or lactating woman, or to locate and biopsy a suspicious lesion.

The somo-v ABUS is an ultrasound device for breast cancer screening for use in women with dense breasts. The somo-v ABUS scans a woman's breast, capturing multiple ultrasound images that can be reviewed in 3D. This device is used along with standard mammography in women with a negative mammogram and no breast cancer symptoms.

MRI is recommended as a sensitive screening tool for women who are at high risk for breast cancer, whose mammography or ultrasound is suspicious for malignancy, or who have previously had an occult breast cancer detected by mammogram.

Biopsies. A definitive diagnosis of a suspicious area is made by analyzing biopsied tissue. Biopsy techniques include *fine-needle aspiration* (FNA), core (core needle), vacuum-assisted, and surgical biopsies.

FNA biopsy is performed by inserting a needle into a lesion to sample fluid from a breast cyst, remove cells from intercellular spaces, or sample cells from a solid mass. Before the procedure, the breast area is first locally anesthetized. Then the needle is placed into the breast, and fluid and cells are aspirated into a syringe. Three or four passes are usually made. If the results are negative with a suspicious lesion, an additional biopsy may be necessary. Inform patients that biopsy results are usually available in 1 to 3 days.

A *core (core needle) biopsy* involves removing small samples of breast tissue using a hollow "core" needle. For palpable lesions, this is accomplished by fixing the lesion with one hand and performing a needle biopsy with the other. In the case of nonpalpable lesions, *stereotactic mammography, ultrasound,* or MRI image guidance is used. Stereotactic mammography uses computers to pinpoint the exact location of a breast mass based on mammograms. With ultrasound, the radiologist or surgeon watches the needle on the ultrasound monitor to help guide it to the area of concern. Because a core biopsy removes more tissue than an FNA, it is more accurate.

Vacuum-assisted biopsy is a version of core biopsy that uses a vacuum technique to help collect the tissue sample. In core biopsy, several separate needle insertions are used to acquire multiple samples. During vacuum-assisted biopsy, the needle is inserted only once into the breast, and the needle can be rotated, which allows for multiple samples through a single needle insertion.

A *surgical biopsy* is used to remove a breast mass or lump or to obtain a sample of breast tissue for analysis. A surgical biopsy is usually performed in an operating room. Ten years ago, most breast biopsies were surgical procedures. Today less invasive biopsy procedures, such as core biopsies, are used.

BENIGN BREAST DISORDERS

MASTALGIA

Mastalgia (breast pain) is the most common breast-related complaint in women.[10] The most common form is *cyclic mastalgia,* which coincides with the menstrual cycle. It is described as diffuse breast tenderness or heaviness. Breast pain may last 2 or 3 days or most of the month. The pain is related to hormonal sensitivity. The symptoms often decrease with menopause.

Noncyclic mastalgia has no relationship to the menstrual cycle and can continue into menopause. It may be constant or intermittent throughout the month and last for several years. Symptoms include a burning, aching, or soreness in the breast. The pain may be from trauma, fat necrosis, ductal ectasia, costochrondritis, or arthritic pain in the chest or neck radiating to the breast.

Mammography and targeted ultrasound are frequently done to exclude cancer and provide information on the etiology of mastalgia. Some relief for cyclic pain may occur by reducing intake of caffeine and dietary fat; taking vitamins E, A, and B complex and gamma-linolenic acid (evening primrose oil); and continually wearing a support bra. Compresses, ice, analgesics, and antiinflammatory drugs may also help. Helpful drugs include oral contraceptives and danazol (Danocrine). The androgenic side effects of danazol (acne, edema, hirsutism) may make this therapy unacceptable for many women.

BREAST INFECTIONS

Mastitis

Mastitis is an inflammatory condition of the breast that occurs most frequently in lactating women (Table 52-1). *Lactational mastitis* manifests as a localized area that is erythematous, painful, and tender to palpation. Fever is often present. The infection develops when organisms (usually staphylococci) gain access to the breast through a cracked nipple. In its early stages, mastitis can be cured with antibiotics. Breastfeeding should continue unless an abscess is forming or purulent drainage is noted. The mother may wish to use a nipple shield or to hand-express milk from the involved breast until the pain subsides. The woman should see her health care provider promptly to begin a course of antibiotic therapy. Any breast that remains red, tender, and not responsive to antibiotics requires follow-up care and evaluation for inflammatory breast cancer.[11]

Lactational Breast Abscess

If lactational mastitis persists after several days of antibiotic therapy, a lactational breast abscess may have developed. In this condition, the skin may become red and edematous over the involved breast, often with a corresponding palpable mass, and the patient may have a fever. Antibiotics alone are insufficient treatment for a breast abscess. Ultrasound-guided drainage of the abscess or surgical incision and drainage are necessary. The drainage is cultured, sensitivities are obtained, and therapy with

TABLE 52-1 BENIGN BREAST DISORDERS*

Disorder	Risk Factors	Clinical Manifestations
Lactational mastitis	Occurs in up to 10% of postpartum lactating mothers (both primipara and multipara), usually 2-4 wk after birth.	Warm to touch, indurated, painful, often unilateral, most commonly caused by *Staphylococcus aureus*.
Fibrocystic changes	Most common between ages 35 and 50.	Not usually discrete masses—nodularity instead. Usually accompanied by cyclic pain and tenderness. Mass(es) often cyclic in occurrence (movable, soft).
Cysts	Most common over age 35. Incidence decreases after menopause. Develop in one out of every 14 women.	Palpable fluid-filled mass (movable, soft). Multiple cysts can occur and recur. Rarely associated with breast cancer.
Fibroadenoma	Commonly occurs in 10% of all women ages 15-40.	Palpable mass (firm, movable), usually 2-3 cm in size, rarely associated with breast cancer.
Fat necrosis	Many women report previous history of trauma to breast.	Usually a hard, tender, mobile, indurated mass with irregular borders.
Ductal ectasia	Perimenopausal woman—most common in women in their 50s, previous lactation, inverted nipples.	Fixation of nipple, usually accompanied by nipple discharge of thick gray material. Often associated with breast pain.

*This list is not inclusive; other benign breast disorders are discussed in the text.

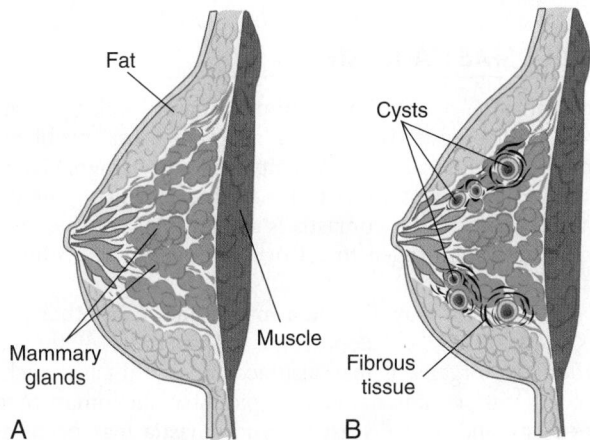

Fat
Cysts
Mammary glands
Muscle
Fibrous tissue
A
B

FIG. 52-3 A, Normal breast tissue. **B,** Fibrocystic breast tissue.

an appropriate antibiotic is begun. Breastfeeding can continue in most cases with ongoing treatment of the abscess.

FIBROCYSTIC CHANGES

Fibrocystic changes in the breast are a benign condition characterized by changes in breast tissue[12] (Fig. 52-3). The changes include the development of excess fibrous tissue, hyperplasia of the epithelial lining of the mammary ducts, proliferation of mammary ducts, and cyst formation. Fibrocystic changes are thought to be due to a heightened responsiveness of breast tissue to circulating estrogen and progesterone. These changes produce pain related to nerve irritation from edema in the connective tissue and to fibrosis that pinches the nerve. Fibrocystic changes are the most common breast disorder.

The use of the term *fibrocystic disease* is incorrect because the cluster of problems is actually an exaggerated response to hormonal influence. The terms *fibrocystic condition* or *fibrocystic complex* are more accurate.

Fibrocystic changes alone are not associated with increased breast cancer risk. Masses or nodularities can appear in both breasts. They are often found in the upper, outer quadrants and usually occur bilaterally.

Fibrocystic changes occur most frequently in women between 35 and 50 years of age but often begin as early as 20 years of age. Pain and nodularity often increase over time but tend to subside after menopause unless high doses of estrogen replacement are used. Fibrocystic changes most commonly occur in women with premenstrual abnormalities, nulliparous women, women with a history of spontaneous abortion, nonusers of oral contraceptives, and women with early menarche and late menopause. Symptoms related to fibrocystic changes often worsen in the premenstrual phase and subside after menstruation.

Manifestations of fibrocystic breast changes include one or more palpable lumps that are often round, well delineated, and freely movable within the breast (see Table 52-1). Discomfort ranging from tenderness to pain may also occur. The lump is usually observed to increase in size and perhaps in tenderness before menstruation. Cysts may enlarge or shrink rapidly. Nipple discharge associated with fibrocystic breasts is often milky, watery-milky, yellow, or green.

Mammography may be helpful in distinguishing fibrocystic changes from breast cancer. However, in some women the breast tissue is so dense that it is difficult to obtain a mammogram. In these situations, ultrasound may be more useful in differentiating a cystic mass from a solid mass.

NURSING AND COLLABORATIVE MANAGEMENT
FIBROCYSTIC CHANGES

With the initial discovery of a discrete mass in the breast by a woman or her health care provider, aspiration or surgical biopsy may be indicated. If the nodularity is recurrent, a wait of 7 to 10 days may be planned in order to note any changes that may be related to the menstrual cycle. With large or frequent cysts, surgical removal may be favored over repeated aspiration. An excisional biopsy may be done if (1) no fluid is found on aspiration, (2) the fluid that is found is hemorrhagic, or (3) a residual mass remains after fluid aspiration. The biopsy is usually performed in an outpatient surgery unit.

Biopsies in women with fibrocystic disease may be indicated if these women have an increased risk for breast cancer. Atypical hyperplasia discovered by breast biopsy increases a woman's risk of developing breast cancer later in life.

Encourage the woman with cystic changes to maintain regular follow-up care. Also teach her BSE to self-monitor changes. Severe fibrocystic changes may make palpation of the breast more difficult. Teach her to report any changes in symptoms or changes found during the BSE so they can be evaluated.

Treatment for a fibrocystic condition is similar to that described earlier for mastalgia. Teach the woman with fibrocystic breasts that she may expect a recurrence of the cysts in one or both breasts until menopause and that the cysts may enlarge or become painful just before menstruation. Additionally, reassure her that the cysts do not "turn into" cancer. Advise her that any new lump that does not respond in a cyclic manner over 1 to 2 weeks should be examined by her health care provider.

FIBROADENOMA

Fibroadenoma is a common cause of discrete benign breast lumps in young women. It generally occurs in women between 15 and 40 years of age. It is the most frequent cause of breast masses in women under 25 years of age.

The possible cause of fibroadenoma may be increased estrogen sensitivity in a localized area of the breast. Fibroadenomas are usually small (but can be large [2 to 3 cm]), painless, round, well delineated, and very mobile. They may be soft but are usually solid, firm, and rubbery in consistency. There is no accompanying retraction or nipple discharge. The lump is often painless. The fibroadenoma may appear as a single unilateral mass, although multiple bilateral fibroadenomas have been reported. Growth is slow and often ceases when the size reaches 2 to 3 cm. Size is not affected by menstruation. However, pregnancy can stimulate dramatic growth.

Fibroadenomas are easily detected by physical examination and may be visible on mammography and ultrasound. However, definitive diagnosis requires FNA, core, or surgical biopsy and tissue examination by a pathologist to exclude other tumors. Treatment of fibroadenomas can include observation with regular monitoring after a malignancy has been ruled out, or surgical excision. In women over 35 years of age, all new lesions should be evaluated by breast ultrasound and possible biopsy.

As an alternative to surgery, tumor removal can be done using *cryoablation*. In this procedure, a cryoprobe is inserted into the tumor using ultrasound guidance. Extremely cold gas is piped into the tumor. The frozen tumor dies and gradually shrinks.

NIPPLE DISCHARGE

Nipple discharge may occur spontaneously or as a result of nipple manipulation. A milky secretion is due to inappropriate lactation (termed **galactorrhea**) and may be a result of problems such as drug therapy, endocrine problems, and neurologic disorders. Nipple discharge may also be idiopathic (no known cause).

Secretions can also be serous, grossly bloody, or brown to green.[13] These secretions may be caused by either benign or malignant disease. A cytology slide may be made of the secretion to determine the specific disease. Diseases associated with nipple discharge include malignancies, cystic disease, intraductal papilloma, and ductal ectasia. Treatment depends on identification of the cause. In most cases, nipple discharge is not related to malignancy.

Intraductal Papilloma

An **intraductal papilloma** is a benign, soft, wartlike growth found in the mammary ducts. It is usually unilateral. Typically, the nipple has a bloody discharge that can be intermittent or spontaneous. Most intraductal papillomas are beneath the areola, and they may be difficult to palpate. They are usually found in women 40 to 60 years of age. A single duct or several ducts may be involved. Treatment includes excision of the pap-

illoma and the involved duct or duct system. Papillomas may be associated with an increased risk of cancer.

Ductal Ectasia

Ductal ectasia (duct dilation) is a benign breast disease of perimenopausal and postmenopausal women involving the ducts in the subareolar area. It usually involves several bilateral ducts. Multicolored, sticky nipple discharge is the primary symptom. Ductal ectasia is initially painless but may progress to burning, itching, and pain around the nipple, as well as swelling in the areolar area. Inflammatory signs are often present, the nipple may retract, and the discharge may become bloody in more advanced disease. Ductal ectasia is not associated with malignancy. If an abscess develops, warm compresses and antibiotics are usually effective treatments. Therapy consists of close follow-up examinations or surgical excision of the involved ducts.

GYNECOMASTIA IN MEN

Gynecomastia, a transient, noninflammatory enlargement of one or both breasts, is the most common breast problem in men. The condition is usually temporary and benign. Gynecomastia in itself is not a risk factor for breast cancer. The most common cause of gynecomastia is a disturbance of the normal ratio of active androgen to estrogen in plasma or within the breast itself.

Gynecomastia may also be a manifestation of other problems. It is seen in developmental abnormalities of the male reproductive organs. It may also accompany diseases such as testicular tumors, adrenal cancer, pituitary adenomas, hyperthyroidism, and liver disease.[14] Gynecomastia may occur as a side effect of drug therapy, particularly with estrogens and androgens, digitalis, isoniazid (INH), ranitidine (Zantac), and spironolactone (Aldactone). The use of heroin and marijuana can also cause gynecomastia.

Senescent Gynecomastia

Senescent gynecomastia occurs in many older men. A probable cause is the elevation in plasma estrogen in older adult men as the result of increased conversion of androgens to estrogens in peripheral circulation. Although initially unilateral, the tender, firm, centrally located enlargement may become bilateral. When gynecomastia is characterized by a discrete, circumscribed mass, it must be biopsied to differentiate it from the rarer breast cancer in males. Senescent hyperplasia requires no treatment and generally regresses within 6 to 12 months.

GERONTOLOGIC CONSIDERATIONS
AGE-RELATED BREAST CHANGES
The loss of subcutaneous fat and structural support and the atrophy of mammary glands often result in pendulous breasts in the postmenopausal woman. Encourage older women to wear a well-fitting bra. Adequate support can improve physical appearance and reduce pain in the back, shoulders, and neck. It can also prevent *intertrigo* (dermatitis caused by friction between opposing surfaces of skin). Sagging breasts can be surgically lifted (mastopexy). This procedure can be done in conjunction with breast reconstruction after a mastectomy is performed.

The decrease in glandular tissue in older women makes a breast mass easier to palpate. This decreased density is likely a result of age-related decreases in estrogen. Rib margins may be palpable in a thin woman and can be confused with a mass. That is why it is so important that women become familiar with their own breasts and what is normal for them. Because the incidence of breast cancer increases with age, encourage older women to continue BSE, to have annual mammograms and CBEs, and to have any breast mass evaluated by their health care provider.

BREAST CANCER

Breast cancer is the most common malignancy in American women except for skin cancer. It is second only to lung cancer as the leading cause of death from cancer in women. In the United States more than 230,480 new cases of invasive breast cancer and more than 57,650 cases of in situ breast cancer are diagnosed annually.[1] About 2140 of those new cases are diagnosed in men. Approximately 39,920 deaths (39,510 women and 410 men) occur each year related to breast cancer.

The incidence of breast cancer is slowly decreasing, with a slight drop in the number of deaths related to breast cancer. This decline may be the result of the decreased use of hormone therapy after menopause.[2] Approximately 2.6 million women are alive in the United States today who are breast cancer survivors.

Patients diagnosed with localized breast cancer with no axillary node involvement have a 5-year survival rate of 98%. Conversely, only 23% of patients diagnosed with advanced-stage breast cancer with metastases to distant sites will survive 5 years or more.[1,2]

Etiology and Risk Factors

Although the etiology is not completely understood, a number of risk factors are related to breast cancer (Table 52-2). Risk factors appear to be cumulative and interacting. Therefore the presence of multiple risk factors may greatly increase the overall risk, especially for people with a positive family history.

Risk Factors for Women. The risk factors most associated with breast cancer include female gender and advancing age. Women are at far greater risk than men, with 99% of breast cancers occurring in women. Increasing age also increases the risk of developing breast cancer. The incidence of breast cancer in women under 25 years of age is very low and increases gradually until age 60. After age 60, the incidence increases dramatically.

Hormonal regulation of the breast is related to the development of breast cancer, but the mechanisms are poorly understood. The hormones estrogen and progesterone may act as tumor promoters to stimulate breast cancer growth if malignant changes in the cells have already occurred. The Women's Health Initiative study showed that the use of combined hormone therapy (estrogen plus progesterone) increases the risk of breast cancer and also the risk of having a larger, more advanced breast cancer at diagnosis.[15] The use of estrogen therapy alone for longer than 10 years (for women with a prior hysterectomy) increases a woman's long-term risk for breast cancer. A link may exist between recent oral contraceptive use and increased risk of breast cancer for younger women.[16]

Modifiable risk factors include excess weight gain during adulthood, sedentary lifestyle, smoking, dietary fat intake, obesity, and alcohol intake.[10] Environmental factors such as radiation exposure may also play a role.

TABLE 52-2	RISK FACTORS FOR BREAST CANCER
Risk Factor	**Comments**
Female	Women account for 99% of breast cancer cases.
Age ≥50 yr	Majority of breast cancers are found in postmenopausal women. After age 60, increase in incidence.
Hormone use	Use of estrogen and/or progesterone as hormone therapy, especially in postmenopausal women.
Family history	Breast cancer in a first-degree relative, particularly when premenopausal or bilateral, increases risk.
Genetic factors	Gene mutations (BRCA1 or BRCA2) play a role in 5%-10% of breast cancer cases.
Personal history of breast cancer, colon cancer, endometrial cancer, ovarian cancer	Personal history significantly increases risk of breast cancer, risk of cancer in other breast, and recurrence.
Early menarche (before age 12), late menopause (after age 55)	A long menstrual history increases the risk of breast cancer.
First full-term pregnancy after age 30, nulliparity	Prolonged exposure to unopposed estrogen increases risk for breast cancer.
Benign breast disease with atypical epithelial hyperplasia, lobular carcinoma in situ	Atypical changes in breast biopsy increase the risk of breast cancer.
Dense breast tissue	Mammograms harder to read and interpret. Dense tissue may be associated with more aggressive tumors.
Weight gain and obesity after menopause	Fat cells store estrogen, which increases the likelihood of developing breast cancer.
Exposure to ionizing radiation	Radiation damages DNA (e.g., prior treatment for Hodgkin's lymphoma).
Alcohol consumption	Women who drink ≥1 alcoholic beverage per day have an increased risk of breast cancer.
Physical inactivity	Breast cancer risk is decreased in physically active women.

🧬 Genetic Link

Family history of breast cancer is an important risk factor, especially if the involved family member also had ovarian cancer, was premenopausal, had bilateral breast cancer, or is a first-degree relative (i.e., mother, sister, daughter). Having any first-degree relative with breast cancer increases a woman's risk of breast cancer 1.5 to 3 times, depending on age. A breast cancer risk assessment tool for health care providers is available through the National Cancer Institute (see Resources at the end of this chapter). About 5% to 10% of all breast cancers are hereditary. This means that specific genetic abnormalities that contribute to the development of breast cancer have been inherited (passed from parent to child). Most inherited cases of breast cancer are associated with mutations in two genes: BRCA1 and BRCA2 (BRCA stands for BReast CAncer). Everyone has BRCA genes. The BRCA1 gene, located on chromosome 17, is a tumor suppressor gene that inhibits tumor development when func-

🧬 GENETICS IN CLINICAL PRACTICE

Breast Cancer

Genetic Basis
- Mutations occur in *BRCA1* and/or *BRCA2* genes.
- Normally these genes are tumor suppressor genes involved in DNA repair.
- Transmission is autosomal dominant.

Incidence
- Approximately 5% to 10% of breast cancers are related to *BRCA1* and *BRCA2* gene mutations.
- Women with *BRCA1* and *BRCA2* gene mutations have a 40% to 80% lifetime risk of developing breast cancer.
- *BRCA1* and *BRCA2* gene mutations are associated with early-onset breast cancer that is more likely to involve both breasts.
- Men with mutations in *BRCA1* and *BRCA2* have an increased risk of breast cancer and prostate cancer.
- Family history of both breast and ovarian cancer increases the risk of having a *BRCA* mutation.

Genetic Testing
- DNA testing is available for *BRCA1* and *BRCA2* gene mutations.

Clinical Implications
- Most breast cancers (about 90%-95%) are not inherited. They are associated with genetic changes that occur after a person is born (somatic mutations). There is no risk of passing on the mutated gene to children.
- Bilateral oophorectomy and/or bilateral mastectomy reduces the risk of breast cancer in women with *BRCA1* and *BRCA2* mutations.
- Mutations in the *BRCA1* and *BRCA2* genes increase the risk of ovarian cancer.
- Genetic counseling and testing for *BRCA* mutations should be considered for women whose personal or family history puts them at high risk for a genetic predisposition to breast cancer.

BRCA, **BR**east **CA**ncer.

tioning normally. Women who have *BRCA1* mutations have a 40% to 80% lifetime chance of developing breast cancer. The *BRCA2* gene, located on chromosome 11, is another tumor suppressor gene. Women with a mutation of this gene have a similar risk of breast cancer.

Mutations in *BRCA* genes may cause as many as 10% to 40% of all inherited breast cancers. As many as 1 in 200 to 400 women in the United States may be carriers for these genetic abnormalities. Women with *BRCA* mutations are also at higher risk for developing ovarian, colon, pancreatic, and uterine cancers.[17]

In addition to *BRCA* gene mutations, many other abnormal genes have been identified that increase a person's risk of developing breast cancer. These include the tumor suppressor gene *p53* (which inhibits tumor development when functioning normally), *ATM* (which helps to repair damaged deoxyribonucleic acid [DNA]), and *CHEK2* (which stops tumor growth).

Most people who develop breast cancer do not inherit an abnormal breast cancer gene, and they do not have a family history of breast cancer. Ongoing research continues to investigate the role of genes in the development of breast cancer.

Risk Factors for Men. Predisposing risk factors for breast cancer in men include hyperestrogenism, a family history of breast cancer, and radiation exposure. A thorough examination of the male breast should be a routine part of a physical examination. Men in *BRCA*-positive families may consider genetic testing. Men with an abnormal *BRCA* gene also have an increased risk of developing prostate cancer.

TABLE 52-3 TYPES OF BREAST CANCER

Type	Frequency of Occurrence
Noninvasive	20%
• Ductal carcinoma in situ	
Invasive/Infiltrating Ductal Carcinoma	70%-75%
• Medullary	
• Tubular	
• Colloid (mucinous)	
• Inflammatory	
• Paget's disease	
Invasive/Infiltrating Lobular Carcinoma	5%-10%

Prophylactic Oophorectomy and Mastectomy. In women with *BRCA1* or *BRCA2* mutations, prophylactic bilateral oophorectomy can decrease the risk of breast cancer and ovarian cancer. Removing the ovaries lowers the risk of breast cancer because the ovaries are the main source of estrogen in a premenopausal woman. Removing the ovaries does not reduce the risk of breast cancer in postmenopausal women because the ovaries are not the main producers of estrogen in these women. A woman who has a high risk of developing breast cancer (i.e., related to factors such as family history and prior tissue biopsies) may choose (in consultation with her physician and genetic counselor) to undergo prophylactic bilateral mastectomy.

Younger women with hereditary (non-*BRCA*) early-stage, estrogen receptor–negative breast cancer may have a higher risk of developing a secondary primary breast cancer in the unaffected (contralateral) breast.[18] These women may also choose to have the unaffected breast removed prophylactically at the time of initial surgery for breast cancer or at a later time.

Pathophysiology

The main components of the breast are lobules (milk-producing glands) and ducts (milk passages that connect the lobules and the nipple). In general, breast cancer arises from the epithelial lining of the ducts *(ductal carcinoma)* or from the epithelium of the lobules *(lobular carcinoma)*. Breast cancers may be *in situ* (within the duct) or invasive (arising from the duct and invading through the wall of the duct).

Metastatic breast cancer is breast cancer that has spread to other organs, with the most common sites being bone, liver, lung, and brain. Cancer growth rates can range from slow to rapid. Factors that affect cancer prognosis are tumor size, axillary node involvement (the more nodes involved, the worse the prognosis), tumor differentiation, estrogen and progesterone receptor status, and *human epidermal growth factor receptor 2* (HER-2) status. HER-2 is a protein that helps regulate cell growth. It is overexpressed in about 25% of patients with breast cancer.[19,20]

Types of Breast Cancer

Breast cancer can be classified as noninvasive or invasive, and ductal or lobular (Table 52-3).

Noninvasive Breast Cancer. An estimated 20% of all diagnosed breast cancers are noninvasive. These intraductal cancers include *ductal carcinoma in situ* (DCIS) and *lobular carcinoma in situ* (LCIS). DCIS tends to be unilateral and may progress to invasive breast cancer if left untreated.

Although the management of DCIS can be controversial, patients should discuss treatment options with their health care provider, including breast-conserving treatment (lumpectomy), mastectomy with breast reconstruction, radiation therapy, and/or hormone therapy (tamoxifen [Nolvadex], anastrozole [Arimidex]).

The term *lobular carcinoma in situ* is somewhat misleading. Although LCIS is a risk factor for developing breast cancer, it is not known to be a premalignant lesion. No surgical or radiation treatment is indicated for LCIS. Hormone therapy may be used as a preventive measure to reduce breast cancer risk for some patients.

Invasive (Infiltrating) Ductal Carcinoma. *Invasive (infiltrating) ductal carcinoma* is the most common type of breast cancer. It starts in the milk duct and then breaks through the wall of the duct, invading the surrounding tissue. From there it may metastasize to other parts of the body.

Types of invasive (infiltrating) ductal carcinoma include *medullary carcinoma,* which accounts for 15% of all breast cancers. It most frequently occurs in women in their late 40s and 50s, manifesting with cells that resemble the medulla of the brain. *Tubular carcinoma* accounts for about 2% of all breast cancers. This type of breast cancer is usually found in women over 50. It has an excellent prognosis. *Colloid (mucinous) carcinoma* accounts for about 1% to 2% of all breast cancer. These tumors, which produce mucus, usually have a favorable prognosis.

Inflammatory Breast Cancer. *Inflammatory breast cancer* is an aggressive and fast-growing breast cancer with a high risk for metastasis. The lymph channels in the skin of the breast become blocked by cancer cells. Because of skin involvement, the breast looks red, feels warm, and has a thickened appearance that is often described as resembling an orange peel *(peau d'orange).*[21] Sometimes the breast develops ridges and small bumps that look like hives. A breast mass may or may not be present.

Paget's Disease. Paget's disease is a rare breast malignancy characterized by a persistent lesion of the nipple and areola with or without a mass. (This is different from Paget's disease of the bone, which is discussed in Chapter 64.) Most women with Paget's disease have underlying ductal carcinoma. Only in rare cases is the cancer confined to the nipple itself.

Itching, burning, bloody nipple discharge with superficial skin erosion and ulceration may be present. Diagnosis of Paget's disease is confirmed by pathologic examination of the lesion. Nipple changes are often diagnosed as an infection or dermatitis, which can lead to treatment delays.

The treatment of Paget's disease is surgical removal of the involved tissue (central lumpectomy or mastectomy). Radiation therapy may also be used after surgery. The prognosis is good when the cancer is confined to the nipple. The nursing care for the patient with Paget's disease is the same as the care for a patient with breast cancer.

Invasive (Infiltrating) Lobular Carcinoma. *Invasive (infiltrating) lobular carcinoma* begins in the lobules (milk-producing glands) of the breast. The cancer cells can break out of the lobule and have the potential to metastasize to other areas of the body. Invasive lobular carcinoma is a type of breast cancer that usually appears as a subtle thickening in the upper outer quadrant of the breast. Often positive for estrogen and progesterone receptors, these tumors respond well to hormone therapy.

Clinical Manifestations

Breast cancer is usually detected as a lump or thickening in the breast or mammographic abnormality. It occurs most often in

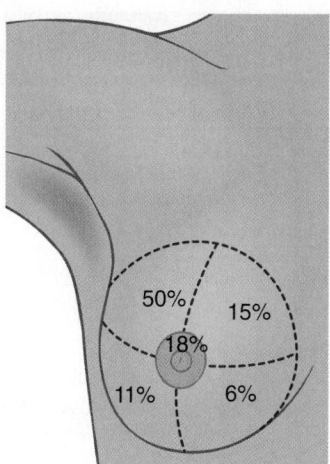

FIG. 52-4 Distribution of where breast cancer occurs.

the upper, outer quadrant of the breast, which is the location of most of the glandular tissue (Fig. 52-4). Breast cancers vary in their growth rate. If palpable, breast cancer is characteristically hard and may be irregularly shaped, poorly delineated, nonmobile, and nontender.

A small percentage of breast cancers cause nipple discharge. The discharge is usually unilateral and may be clear or bloody. Nipple retraction may occur. Peau d'orange may occur due to plugging of the dermal lymphatics. In large cancers, infiltration, induration, and dimpling (pulling in) of the overlying skin may also occur.

Complications

The main complication of breast cancer is recurrence (Table 52-4). Recurrence may be *local* or *regional* (skin or soft tissue near the mastectomy site, axillary or internal mammary lymph nodes) or *distant* (most commonly involving bone, lung, brain, and liver). However, metastatic disease can be found in any site in the body.

Widely disseminated or metastatic disease involves the growth of colonies of cancerous breast cells in parts of the body distant from the breast. Metastases primarily occur through the lymphatics, usually those of the axilla (Fig. 52-5). However, the cancer can spread to other parts of the body without invading the axillary nodes even when the primary breast tumor is small. Even in patients who do not have lymph node involvement (node-negative breast cancer), there is a possibility of distant metastasis.

Diagnostic Studies

In addition to radiologic and biopsy studies used to diagnose breast cancer (see earlier discussion in this chapter on pp. 1239-1240), other tests are used to predict the risk of local or systemic recurrence. These tests include axillary lymph node status, tumor size, estrogen and progesterone receptor status, cell-proliferative indices, and genomic assays.

Axillary lymph node involvement is one of the most important prognostic factors in breast cancer. *Axillary lymph nodes* are often examined to determine if cancer has spread to the axilla on the side of the breast cancer. The more nodes involved, the greater the risk of recurrence.

Lymphatic mapping and *sentinel lymph node dissection* (SLND) help the surgeon identify the lymph node(s) that drain first from the tumor site *(sentinel node).* An SLND is less inva-

TABLE 52-4	SITES OF BREAST CANCER RECURRENCE AND METASTASIS
Site	**Clinical Manifestations**
Local Recurrence	
Skin, chest wall	Firm, discrete nodules. Occasionally pruritic, usually painless, commonly in or near a scar.
Regional Recurrence	
Lymph nodes	Enlarged nodes in axilla or supraclavicular area, usually nontender.
Distant Metastasis	
Skeletal	Localized pain of gradually increasing intensity, percussion tenderness at involved sites, pathologic fracture caused by involvement of bone cortex.
Spinal cord	Progressive back pain, localized and radiating. Change in bladder or bowel function. Loss of sensation in lower extremities.
Brain	Headache described as "different," unilateral sensory loss, focal muscular weakness, hemiparesis, incoordination (ataxia), nausea and vomiting unrelated to medication, cognitive changes.
Pulmonary (including lung nodules and pleural effusions)	Shortness of breath, tachypnea, nonproductive cough (not present in all patients).
Liver	Abdominal distention. Right lower quadrant abdominal pain sometimes with radiation to scapular area. Nausea and vomiting, anorexia, weight loss. Weakness and fatigue. Hepatomegaly, ascites, jaundice. Peripheral edema. Elevated liver enzymes.
Bone marrow	Anemia, infection, increased bleeding, bruising, petechiae. Weakness, fatigue, mild confusion, light-headedness. Dyspnea.

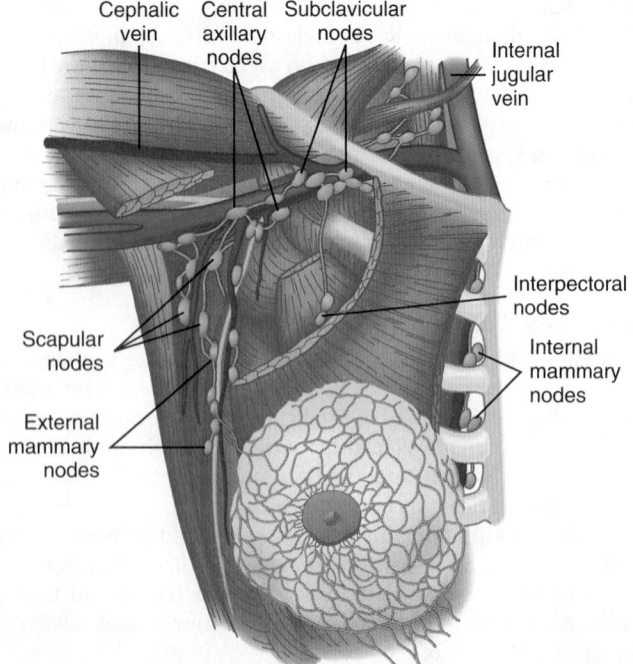

FIG. 52-5 Lymph nodes and drainage in the axilla. The sentinel lymph node is usually found in the external mammary nodes. A complete axillary dissection would remove all nodes.

sive than an axillary lymph node dissection (ALND). In SLND a radioisotope and/or blue dye is injected into the affected breast, and intraoperatively it is determined in which sentinel lymph nodes (SLNs) the radioisotope or dye is located. A local incision is made in the axilla, and the surgeon dissects the blue-stained or radioactive SLNs. Generally, with an SLND, one to four axillary lymph nodes are removed. The nodes may be sent for pathologic analysis. If the SLNs are negative, no further axillary surgery is required. If the SLNs are positive, a complete axillary dissection may be done, depending on the patient's clinical situation. SLND is associated with lower morbidity rates and greater accuracy compared with complete ALND.

Tumor size is a prognostic variable: the larger the tumor, the poorer the prognosis. The wide variety of biologic types of breast cancer explains the variability of disease behavior. In general, the more well differentiated (like the original cell type) the tumor, the less aggressive it is. The cells of poorly differentiated (unlike the original cell type) tumors appear morphologically disorganized, and they are more aggressive.

Estrogen and progesterone receptor status is another diagnostic test useful for decisions about both treatment and prognosis.[12] Receptor-positive tumors (1) commonly show histologic evidence of being well differentiated, (2) frequently have a *diploid* (more normal) DNA content and low proliferative indices, (3) have a lower chance for recurrence, and (4) are frequently hormone dependent and responsive to hormone therapy. Receptor-negative tumors (1) are often poorly differentiated histologically, (2) have a high incidence of *aneuploidy* (abnormally high or low DNA content) and higher proliferative indices, (3) frequently recur, and (4) are usually unresponsive to hormone therapy.

Ploidy status correlates with tumor aggressiveness. Diploid tumors have been shown to have a significantly lower risk of recurrence than aneuploid tumors.

Cell-proliferative indices indirectly measure the rate of tumor cell proliferation. The percentage of tumor cells in the synthesis (S) phase of the cell cycle (see Chapter 16, Fig. 16-1) is another important prognostic indicator. Patients with cells that have high S-phase fractions have a higher risk for recurrence and earlier cancer death.

Another prognostic indicator is the marker HER-2. Overexpression of this receptor has been associated with unusually aggressive tumor growth, a greater risk for recurrence, and a poorer prognosis in breast cancer.[20] About 25% of metastatic breast cancers produce excessive HER-2. The presence of this marker assists in the selection and sequence of drug therapy and predicts the patient's response to treatment.

A patient whose breast cancer tests negative for all three receptors (estrogen, progesterone, and HER-2) has *triple-negative breast cancer*.[22] This subtype of breast cancer accounts for approximately 10% to 20% of cases. The incidence of triple-negative breast cancer is higher in Hispanics, African Americans, younger women, and women with a *BRCA1* mutation. These patients tend to have more aggressive tumors with a poorer prognosis.

A *genomic assay* is a test that uses a sample of the breast cancer tissue to analyze the activity of a group of genes. Knowing whether certain genes are present or absent, or overly active or not active enough, can provide information about the risk of recurrence and the likely benefit of chemotherapy or hormone therapy. Two genomic assays are currently in use for breast cancer: Oncotype DX and MammaPrint. These tests are typically reserved for patients who (1) have early-stage breast cancer with no to few lymph nodes involved; and (2), in the case of Oncotype DX, have estrogen receptor–positive breast cancer that can be treated with hormone therapy.

Cancer markers for breast cancer include CA 15-3 and CA 27-29. These proteins are produced by the *MUC1* gene. Breast cancer cells shed copies of these proteins into the bloodstream. These markers are not specific or sensitive enough to be used as a screening tool to detect early breast cancer. Although not recommended at this time, these markers may be used to monitor a patient's response to treatment of invasive breast cancer and detect recurrence of the disease.

Collaborative Care

A wide range of treatment options is available to the patient and health care providers making critical decisions about how to

TABLE 52-5 COLLABORATIVE CARE

Breast Cancer

Diagnostic
Prediagnosis
- Health history, including risk factors
- Physical examination, including breast and lymph nodes
- Mammography
- Ultrasound
- Breast MRI (if indicated)
- Biopsy

Postdiagnosis
- Lymphatic mapping and sentinel lymph node dissection (SLND)
- Estrogen and progesterone receptor status
- Cell-proliferative indices
- HER-2 marker
- Genetic assays (MammaPrint and Oncotype DX)

Staging
- Complete blood count, platelet count
- Calcium and phosphorus levels
- Liver function tests
- Chest x-ray
- Bone scan (if indicated)
- CT scan of chest, abdomen, pelvis (if indicated)
- MRI (if indicated)
- PET/CT scan (if indicated)

Collaborative Therapy
Surgery
- Breast-conserving surgery (lumpectomy) with SLND and biopsy and/or axillary lymph node dissection
- Modified radical mastectomy (may include immediate or delayed reconstruction)

Radiation Therapy
- Primary radiation therapy
- Brachytherapy
- Palliative radiation therapy

Drug Therapy (see Table 52-8)
- Chemotherapy
- Hormone therapy
- Biologic and targeted therapy
- Chemotherapy
- Hormone therapy
- Biologic and targeted therapy

HER-2, Human epidermal growth factor receptor 2; *PET*, positron emission tomography.

treat breast cancer (Table 52-5). Prognostic factors are considered when treatment decisions are made. The therapeutic regimen is often determined by the clinical stage and biology of the cancer.

Staging of Breast Cancer. The most widely accepted staging method for breast cancer is the TNM system.[23] This system uses tumor size (T), nodal involvement (N), and presence of metastasis (M) to determine the stage of disease. The stage of a breast cancer describes its size and the extent to which it has spread (Table 52-6).

The stages range from 0 to IV, with stage 0 being in situ cancer with no lymph node involvement and no metastasis. Further classification within these stages depends on tumor size and the number of lymph nodes involved. Stage IV indicates metastatic spread, regardless of tumor size or lymph node involvement. The presence or absence of malignant cells in lymph nodes remains a powerful prognostic factor related to local recurrence or metastasis after primary therapy.

Surgical Therapy. Surgery is considered the primary treatment for breast cancer. Table 52-7 describes the most common surgical procedures used to treat breast cancer. The most common surgical options for resectable breast cancer are (1) breast conservation surgery (lumpectomy) and (2) modified radical mastectomy. Most women diagnosed with early-stage breast cancer (tumors smaller than 4 to 5 cm) are candidates for either treatment choice. The overall survival rate with lumpectomy and radiation is about the same as that with modified radical mastectomy.

Breast-Conserving Surgery. Breast-conserving surgery (also called **lumpectomy** or partial mastectomy) usually involves removal of the entire tumor along with a margin of normal surrounding tissue (Fig. 52-6, *A*). After surgery, radiation therapy is delivered to the entire breast, ending with a boost to

TABLE 52-6 STAGING OF BREAST CANCER

Stage	Tumor Size	Lymph Node Involvement	Metastasis
0	TIS*	No	No
I	<2 cm	No	No
II			
A	No evidence of tumor ranging to 5 cm	No, or 1-3 axillary nodes and/or internal mammary nodes	No
B	Ranging from 2 to >5 cm	No, or 1-3 axillary nodes and/or internal mammary nodes	No
III			
A	No evidence of tumor ranging to >5 cm	Yes, 4-9 axillary nodes and/or internal mammary nodes	No
B	Any size with extension to chest wall or skin	Yes, 4-9 axillary nodes and/or internal mammary nodes	No
C	Any size	Yes, ≥10 axillary nodes, internal mammary nodes, or infraclavicular nodes	No
IV	Any size	Any type of nodal involvement	Yes

Modified from American Joint Committee on Cancer: AJCC cancer staging manual, ed 7. Retrieved from *www.cancerstaging.org/staging/changes2010*.
*TIS, Tumor in situ.

TABLE 52-7   SURGICAL PROCEDURES FOR BREAST CANCER

Procedure	Side Effects	Complications	Patient Issues
Breast-Conserving Surgery (Lumpectomy) With Radiation Therapy			
Wide excision of tumor, sentinel lymph node dissection (SLND) and/or axillary lymph node dissection (ALND). Radiation therapy.	Breast soreness Breast edema Skin reactions Arm swelling Sensory changes in breast and arm	*Short-term:* Moist desquamation,* hematoma, seroma, infection *Long-term:* Fibrosis, lymphedema,† myositis, pneumonitis,* rib fractures*	Prolonged treatment* Impaired arm mobility† Change in texture and sensitivity of breast
Modified Radical Mastectomy			
Removal of breast, preservation of pectoralis muscle. SLND and/or ALND.	Chest wall tightness, scar Phantom breast sensations Lymphedema Sensory changes Impaired range of motion	*Short-term:* Skin flap necrosis, seroma, hematoma, infection *Long-term:* Sensory loss, muscle weakness, lymphedema	Loss of breast Incision Body image Need for prosthesis Impaired arm mobility
Tissue Expansion and Breast Implants			
Expander used to slowly stretch tissue. Saline gradually injected into reservoir over weeks to months. Insertion of implant under musculofascial layer of chest wall.	Discomfort Chest wall tightness	*Short-term:* Skin flap necrosis, wound separation, seroma, hematoma, infection *Long-term:* Capsular contractions, displacement of implant	Altered body image Prolonged physician visits to expand implants Potential additional surgeries for nipple construction, symmetry
Breast Reconstruction Tissue Flap Procedures ***Transverse Rectus Abdominis Musculocutaneous (TRAM) Flap***			
Musculocutaneous flap (muscle, skin, fat, blood supply) is transposed from abdomen to the mastectomy site. May be done concurrently with mastectomy.	Pain related to two surgical sites and extensive surgery	*Short-term:* Delayed wound healing, infection, skin flap necrosis, abdominal hernia, hematoma	Prolonged postoperative recovery
Deep Inferior Epigastric Artery Perforator (DIEP) Flap			
Free flap that transfers skin and fat from the abdomen to the chest. Differs from TRAM flap because no muscle is moved.	Requires more time in surgery than TRAM flap Pain related to two surgical sites	If procedure fails, tissue flap may die and have to be completely removed If tissue dies, new reconstruction may not be done for 6-12 mo	Patients may experience less pain and restriction of movement than with a TRAM flap.

*Specific to radiation therapy.
†If ALND (less likely with SLND).

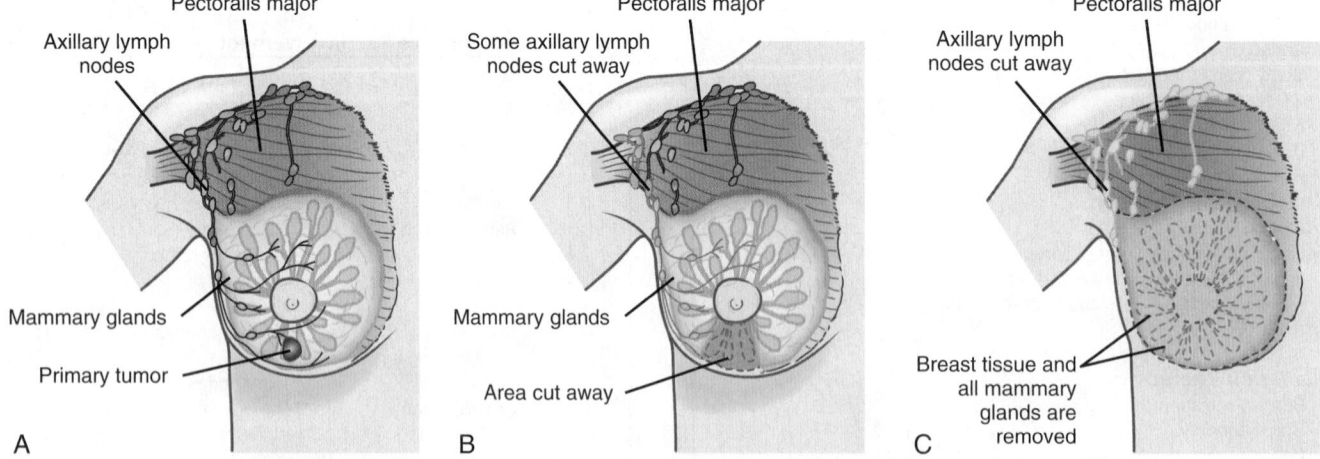

FIG. 52-6 Breast cancer surgery. **A,** Preoperative. **B,** Lumpectomy. **C,** Modified radical mastectomy.

the tumor bed. If evidence exists that the risk for recurrence is high, chemotherapy may be administered before radiation therapy. Contraindications to breast-conserving surgery include the following: breast size is too small in relation to the tumor size to yield an acceptable cosmetic result, masses and calcifications are multifocal (within the same breast quadrant), masses are multicentric (in more than one quadrant), and diffuse cal-

cifications occur in more than one quadrant. Contraindications to radiation therapy (e.g., active lupus or prior radiation therapy in the radiation field) may make mastectomy a better surgical option.

One of the main advantages of breast-conserving surgery and radiation is that it preserves the breast, including the nipple. The goal of the combined surgery and radiation is to maximize

Applying the Evidence

M.S. is a 53-yr-old woman who was diagnosed with breast cancer 2 wk ago. She is recovering from a lumpectomy with negative lymph nodes. Her physician has recommended adjuvant therapy with radiation.

Best Available Evidence	Clinician Expertise	Patient Preferences and Values
The addition of radiation therapy to lumpectomy reduces the risk of local cancer recurrence.	Radiation is recommended even with negative lymph nodes after a lumpectomy. Many patients have minimal or no side effects from radiation therapy. The most common ones are fatigue, malaise, skin reactions, and ulcers or irritation of the skin.	She tells you that she is not sure if she wants to have the radiation treatment because she is afraid of the side effects.

Your Decision and Action
Review the possible side effects and how they can be managed. Then explain the risks of not taking the radiation treatment, which can include recurrence. She tells you that she will discuss it with her husband and possibly reconsider. You understand her concerns and inform the physician of her indecisiveness.

Reference for Evidence
National Cancer Institute: Breast cancer treatment: stage I, II, IIIA, and operable IIIC breast cancer. Retrieved from www.cancer.gov/cancertopics/pdq/treatment/breast/healthprofessional/page6.

FIG. 52-7 Lymphedema. Accumulation of fluid in the tissue after excision of lymph nodes.

the benefits of both cancer treatment and cosmetic outcome while minimizing risks. Disadvantages of this surgery include the increased cost of the surgery plus radiation over surgery alone and the possible side effects of radiation.

Axillary Lymph Node Dissection. Axillary lymph node dissection (ALND) on the same side as the breast cancer is often performed when breast-conserving surgery is done. A typical ALND generally involves the removal of 12 to 20 nodes. Recently, sentinel lymph node dissection (SLND) has become the standard of care, with ALND reserved for patients when clinically indicated (evidence of disease in the axilla) (see Fig. 52-5). Examination of the lymph nodes provides prognostic information and helps determine further treatment (chemotherapy, hormone therapy, or both).

Lymphedema (accumulation of lymph in soft tissue) can occur as a result of the excision or radiation of lymph nodes[24] (Fig. 52-7). When the axillary nodes cannot return lymph fluid to the central circulation, the fluid accumulates in the arm, hand, or breast, causing obstructive pressure on the veins and venous return. The patient may experience heaviness, pain, impaired motor function in the arm, and numbness and paresthesia of the fingers. Fever and a red, painful rash may also be present with infection of the affected arm. These symptoms may indicate the beginning or worsening of lymphedema. Cellulitis and progressive fibrosis of the skin can result from lymphedema. (See further discussion on lymphedema later in this chapter on p. 1254.)

Modified Radical Mastectomy. A *modified radical mastectomy* includes removal of the breast and axillary lymph nodes, but it preserves the pectoralis major muscle (Fig. 52-6, *B*). This surgery would be selected over breast-conserving surgery if the tumor were too large to excise with good margins and attain a

reasonable cosmetic result. Some patients may select this surgical procedure over lumpectomy when presented with a choice.

When a modified radical mastectomy is performed, the patient has the option of breast reconstruction. If the patient chooses to have reconstructive surgery, it can be performed immediately after the mastectomy, or it can be delayed until postoperative recovery is complete.

Postmastectomy Pain Syndrome. *Postmastectomy pain syndrome* can occur in patients after a mastectomy or an axillary node dissection. Common symptoms include chest and upper arm pain, tingling down the arm, numbness, shooting or pricking pain, and unbearable itching that persist beyond the normal 3-month healing time. The most common theory for the onset of this syndrome is injury to intercostobrachial nerves, which are sensory nerves that exit the chest wall muscles and provide sensation to the shoulder and the upper arm.

Treatments include nonsteroidal antiinflammatory drugs, antidepressants, topical lidocaine patches, EMLA (local anesthetics: lidocaine and prilocaine), and antiseizure drugs (e.g., gabapentin [Neurontin]). Other possible treatment modalities include imagery, biofeedback, physical therapy to prevent "frozen shoulder" syndrome as a result of inadequate movement, and psychologic counseling with a therapist trained in the management of chronic pain syndromes.

Radiation Therapy. Radiation therapy is one form of *adjuvant (additional)* therapy that can be used after surgery. Radiation therapy may be used for breast cancer as treatment to (1) prevent local breast cancer recurrences after breast-conserving surgery; (2) prevent local and nodal recurrences after mastectomy; or (3) relieve pain caused by local, regional, or distant recurrence.

Primary Radiation Therapy. When radiation therapy is a primary treatment, it is usually performed after excision of the breast mass. The decision to use radiation therapy after mastectomy is based on the probability that local residual cancer cells are present. The possible presence of residual cells is related to tumor size and biology and number of involved lymph nodes.

In traditional whole breast (and regional lymph nodes in some cases) radiation treatment, the area is radiated 5 days per week over the course of about 5 to 7 weeks. An external beam of radiation is used to deliver an approximate total dose of 45 to 50 Gy (4500 to 5000 cGy or rads). A "boost" is a dose of radiation delivered to the area in which the original tumor was located. It can be given by external beam and adds five to eight more treatments to the total number given.

Studies are examining whether whole breast radiation over 3 weeks and accelerated partial-breast radiation (radiation to area surrounding the tumor site) over 7 days are safe and effective alternatives to traditional radiation. In both these approaches, larger radiation doses are used for each treatment session.[25]

Fatigue, skin changes, and breast edema may be temporary side effects of external beam radiation therapy. Radiation of the axilla and/or supraclavicular nodes may be indicated when lymph nodes are involved to decrease the risk of axillary recurrence. Radiating a localized area will not prevent distant metastasis. Chemotherapy may be used in select cases (e.g., local recurrence after mastectomy). (Nursing management of the patient receiving radiation therapy is discussed in Chapter 16.)

Brachytherapy. *Brachytherapy* (internal radiation) is used for partial-breast radiation as an alternative to traditional external radiation treatment for early-stage breast cancer. Radiation is delivered directly into the cavity left after a tumor is surgically removed by a lumpectomy. This approach is a minimally invasive way to deliver radiation. Because the radiation is concentrated and focused on the area with the highest risk for tumor recurrence, internal radiation only requires 5 days. Traditional external radiation treatments can take 5 to 7 weeks. Internal radiation therapy is primarily delivered using a multicatheter method or balloon-catheter system.

In the *multicatheter method* (e.g., SAVI) many very small catheters are placed in the breast at the site of the tumor. The SAVI is inserted through a small incision, and the catheter bundle expands uniformly. The ends of the catheters stick out through little holes in the skin. Small radioactive seeds are placed in the catheters. The seeds are left in place just long enough to deliver the radiation dose (e.g., 5 to 10 minutes). The tiny radioactive seeds are inserted only during treatment and then removed. The radiation does not remain in the body between treatments or after the final treatment is over.

In the *balloon-catheter system,* the balloon is placed where the tumor is located. The balloon is filled with fluid to keep it in place. Radioactive seeds are inserted (Fig. 52-8). Radiation is emitted by a tiny radioactive seed attached by a wire on the way to an afterloader, a computer-controlled machine. The seed travels through the MammoSite applicator into the inflated balloon. As with the multicatheter system, the radiation does not remain in the body between treatments or after the final treatment is over. Once the final session is completed, the balloon is deflated and the system is removed.

Internal radiation may also be used as a boost therapy in conjunction with external radiation. The long-term effectiveness and safety of brachytherapy is currently under investigation.[25]

Palliative Radiation Therapy. In addition to reducing the primary tumor mass with a resultant decrease in pain, radiation therapy is also used to treat symptomatic metastatic lesions in such sites as bone, soft tissue organs, brain, and chest. Radiation therapy often relieves pain and is successful in controlling recurrent or metastatic disease.

Drug Therapy. Drug therapy, another type of adjuvant therapy, is used to destroy tumor cells that may have spread to

FIG. 52-8 High-dose brachytherapy for breast cancer. The MammoSite system involves the insertion of a single small balloon catheter *(B)* at the time of the lumpectomy or shortly thereafter into the tumor resection cavity (the space that is left after the surgeon removes the tumor). A tiny radioactive seed *(A)* is inserted into the balloon, connected to a machine called an afterloader *(C)*, and delivers the radiation therapy.

distant sites. Drug therapy can decrease the rate of recurrence and increase the length of survival. Because of the risk for recurrent disease, nearly all women with evidence of node involvement, particularly those who are hormone receptor negative, will have some type of drug therapy. Some women, particularly those with a larger or more aggressive tumor, are known to be at higher risk for recurrent or metastatic disease. These women may be recommended for systemic therapy even when there is no evidence of node involvement. Weighing the risks and benefits of drug therapy is a complex process.

Chemotherapy. Chemotherapy refers to the use of cytotoxic drugs to destroy cancer cells. Many breast cancers are responsive to chemotherapy. In some patients, chemotherapy is given preoperatively. Preoperative *(neoadjuvant)* chemotherapy may decrease the size of the primary tumor, with the goal of less extensive surgery.

The use of combinations of drugs is usually superior to the use of a single drug. The benefit of combination treatment results from the use of drugs that have different mechanisms of action and work at different parts of the cell cycle. The more common combination-therapy protocols are (1) CMF—cyclophosphamide (Cytoxan), methotrexate, and 5-fluorouracil (5-FU); (2) AC—doxorubicin (Adriamycin) and cyclophosphamide, with or without the addition of a taxane such as paclitaxel (Taxol) or docetaxel (Taxotere); or (3) CEF or CAF—cyclophosphamide, epirubicin (Ellence) or doxorubicin (Adriamycin), and 5-FU.

DRUG ALERT: Doxorubicin (Adriamycin)
- Monitor for signs of cardiotoxicity and heart failure (e.g., new onset of shortness of breath, pedal edema, decreased activity tolerance, dysrhythmias, ECG changes).
- Instruct patient not to have immunizations without physician's approval.
- Instruct patient to avoid contact with those who recently received live virus vaccine.

Docetaxel, capecitabine (Xeloda), ixabepilone (Ixempra), and an albumin-bound form of paclitaxel (Abraxane) are used in women whose metastatic breast cancer has not responded to standard chemotherapy. Vinorelbine (Navelbine), used to treat metastatic breast cancer, is better tolerated with fewer and milder side effects than other chemotherapy drugs. Eribulin mesylate (Halaven), a microtubule inhibitor, may be used in treating metastatic breast cancer in patients who have received at least two prior chemotherapy regimens.[26]

Because healthy cells are also affected by chemotherapy, a variety of side effects accompany this treatment modality. The incidence and severity of common side effects are influenced by the specific drug combination, drug schedule, and dosage. The most common side effects involve rapidly dividing cells in the gastrointestinal tract (nausea, anorexia, weight loss), bone marrow (anemia), and hair follicles (alopecia [hair loss]).

Cognitive changes during and after treatment, especially with chemotherapy, have been reported in patients with cancer. This phenomenon, called "chemobrain," may affect up to 83% of breast cancer survivors.[27] These changes include difficulties in concentration, memory, focus, and attention. It is not clear if chemobrain is related to specific cancer treatments or is an overall systemic reaction.[28]

Hormone Therapy. Estrogen can promote the growth of breast cancer cells if the cells are estrogen receptor positive. Hormone therapy can block the effect and source of estrogen, thus promoting tumor regression. Hormone therapy may be used as an adjuvant to primary treatment or in patients with recurrent or metastatic cancer.

Both estrogen and progesterone receptor status assays have been developed to identify women whose breast cancers are likely to respond to hormone therapy. These assays reliably predict whether hormone therapy is a treatment option. Chances of tumor regression are significantly greater in women whose tumors contain estrogen and progesterone receptors.

Hormone therapy can (1) block estrogen receptors or (2) suppress estrogen synthesis by inhibiting aromatase, an enzyme needed for estrogen synthesis (Table 52-8). Antiestrogens include tamoxifen, toremifene (Fareston), and fulvestrant (Faslodex).

Estrogen Receptor Blockers. Tamoxifen has been the hormonal agent of choice in estrogen receptor–positive women with all stages of breast cancer over the past 30 years. It is commonly used in early-stage or advanced breast cancer and to treat recurrent disease. Tamoxifen may also be used in high-risk premenopausal and postmenopausal women to prevent breast cancer. Side effects of tamoxifen may include hot flashes, mood swings, vaginal discharge and dryness, and other effects commonly associated with decreased estrogen. It also increases the risk of blood clots, cataracts, stroke, and endometrial cancer in postmenopausal women. Treatment with tamoxifen is generally prescribed for 5 years.

DRUG ALERT: Tamoxifen (Nolvadex)
- Irregular vaginal bleeding or spotting may occur.
- Decreased visual acuity, corneal opacity, and retinopathy can occur in women receiving high doses (240-320 mg/day for >17 mo). These problems may be irreversible.
- Instruct patient to immediately report decreased visual acuity.
- Monitor for signs of deep vein thrombosis, pulmonary embolism, and stroke, including shortness of breath, leg cramps, and weakness.

Toremifene is an antiestrogen agent similar to tamoxifen. It is indicated in the treatment of metastatic breast cancer in postmenopausal women. Fulvestrant may be given to women with advanced breast cancer who no longer respond to tamoxifen. Fulvestrant is given intramuscularly on a monthly basis.

TABLE 52-8   DRUG THERAPY
Breast Cancer

Drug Class	Mechanism of Action	Indications
Hormone Therapy		
Estrogen Receptor Blockers		
tamoxifen (Nolvadex)	Blocks estrogen receptors (ERs)	ER-positive breast cancer in premenopausal and postmenopausal women; Used as a preventive measure in high-risk premenopausal and postmenopausal women
toremifene (Fareston)	Blocks ERs	ER-positive breast cancer in postmenopausal women only
fulvestrant (Faslodex)	Blocks ERs	ER-positive breast cancer in postmenopausal women only
Aromatase Inhibitors		
anastrozole (Arimidex); letrozole (Femara); exemestane (Aromasin)	Prevents production of estrogen by inhibiting aromatase	ER-positive breast cancer in postmenopausal women only
Estrogen Receptor Modulator		
raloxifene (Evista)	In breast blocks the effect of estrogen; In bone promotes effect of estrogen and prevents bone loss	Postmenopausal women
Biologic and Targeted Therapy		
trastuzumab (Herceptin); pertuzumab (Perjeta)	Blocks HER-2 receptor	ER-positive breast cancer in postmenopausal women only
lapatinib (Tykerb)	Inhibits HER-2 tyrosine kinase and EGFR tyrosine kinase	ER-positive breast cancer in postmenopausal women only

EGFR, Epidermal growth factor receptor; *HER-2,* human epidermal growth factor receptor 2.

Common side effects include injection site pain, fatigue, hot flashes, and nausea.

Aromatase Inhibitors. Aromatase inhibitor drugs interfere with the enzyme aromatase, which is needed for the synthesis of estrogen. These drugs, including anastrozole, letrozole (Femara), and exemestane (Aromasin), are used in the treatment of breast cancer in postmenopausal women. Aromatase inhibitors do not block the production of estrogen by the ovaries. Thus they are of little benefit and may be harmful in premenopausal women.

Clinical trials have demonstrated greater disease-free survival when these drugs are given after tamoxifen treatment has ended. They also appear to be more effective than tamoxifen in preventing breast cancer recurrence and possibly more effective in preventing contralateral disease (disease in the other breast).[29]

Aromatase inhibitors have different side effects than tamoxifen. They rarely cause blood clots, and they do not cause endometrial cancer. Because they block the production of estrogen in postmenopausal women, osteoporosis and bone fractures may occur. These drugs have been associated with night sweats, nausea, arthralgias, and myalgias.

Estrogen Receptor Modulator and Others. Raloxifene (Evista) is a selective estrogen receptor modulator that produces both estrogen-agonistic effects on bone and estrogen-antagonistic effects on breast tissue. (Raloxifene is discussed in the section on osteoporosis in Chapter 64.)

Additional drugs that may be used to suppress hormone-dependent breast tumors include megestrol acetate (Megace), diethylstilbestrol (DES), and fluoxymesterone (Halotestin).

Biologic and Targeted Therapy. Trastuzumab (Herceptin) is a monoclonal antibody to HER-2. After the antibody attaches to the antigen, it is taken into the cells and eventually kills them.[20] It can be used alone or in combination with chemotherapy agents such as docetaxel or paclitaxel to treat patients whose tumors overexpress HER-2. Additional genetic testing (e.g., SPoT-Light test) may offer information on which patients are good candidates for treatment with trastuzumab.

> **DRUG ALERT: Trastuzumab (Herceptin)**
> - Use with caution in women with preexisting heart disease.
> - Monitor for signs of ventricular dysfunction and heart failure.

Ado-trastuzumab emtansine (Kadcyla) is trastuzumab connected to a chemotherapy drug called DM1. This antibody-drug combination is a new kind of targeted cancer drug that can attach to certain types of cancer cells and deliver the chemotherapy directly to them.

Pertuzumab (Perjeta) is a new anti-HER-2 therapy that is used for patients who have not received prior treatment for metastatic breast cancer with an anti-HER-2 agent or chemotherapy. Pertuzumab is combined with trastuzumab and docetaxel.

Lapatinib (Tykerb) works inside the cell by blocking the function of the HER-2 protein. It may be used in combination with capecitabine for patients with advanced metastatic disease who are HER-2 positive. The combination treatment is indicated for women who have become resistant to other cancer drugs.

Advanced breast cancer in postmenopausal women who are estrogen and progesterone receptor positive and HER-2 positive may be treated with lapatinib in combination with letrozole. Everolimus (Afinitor) is used in combination with exemestane to treat postmenopausal women with advanced hormone-receptor positive, HER-2-negative breast cancer. The drug combination is intended for use in women with recurrence or progression of their cancer after treatment with letrozole or anastrozole.

Denosumab (Prolia, Xgeva), a monoclonal antibody, may be used to increase bone mass in patients at high risk of fracture from aromatase inhibitor therapy. It is also given to prevent fractures in patients with metastasis to the bone. (The use of biologic and targeted therapies is discussed in Chapter 16.)

Follow-up and Survivorship Care. After treatment for breast cancer, the patient will have ongoing survivorship care. Recommended follow-up examinations generally occur every 3 to 6 months for the first 5 years, and then annually thereafter. Survivorship care plans summarize a patient's care and care plan for ongoing surveillance.[30] In addition, advise women to perform monthly BSE and self–chest wall examination, and report any changes to their health care provider. Local recurrence of breast cancer is usually at the surgical site. The woman should have appropriate breast imaging done at regular inter-

vals (usually 6 months to 1 year) as determined by her risk of recurrence and breast cancer history.

EVIDENCE-BASED PRACTICE
Translating Research Into Practice

What Is the Effect of Physical Activity in Cancer Survivors?

Clinical Question
For cancer survivors (P) does physical activity (I) improve physical and psychologic outcomes (O) after primary treatment completion (T)?

Best Available Evidence
Systematic review of randomized controlled trials (RCTs)

Critical Appraisal and Synthesis of Evidence
- Thirty-four RCTs of cancer survivors; 22 studies were of breast cancer survivors. Intervention was mostly aerobic exercise. Duration of physical activity ranged from 3 to 60 wk (median of 13 wk). Control groups mainly were sedentary or assigned no exercise.
- Breast cancer survivors who did physical activity had an increased ability to bench and leg press, improved quality of life, and decreased fatigue and depression.
- Overall, cancer survivors who exercised showed improved body mass index (BMI), body weight, peak oxygen consumption, distance walked in 6 min, handgrip strength, and quality of life.

Conclusion
- Physical activity has positive effects on physical and psychologic outcomes and quality of life.

Implications for Nursing Practice
- To help patients get interested in physical activity, discuss their favorite forms of exercise, hobbies, and activities.
- Help patients identify physical activity resources (e.g., walking paths, swimming pool, gym).
- Assess the patient's barriers to active participation in exercise.
- When possible, assist patient in adhering to recommended activities.

Reference for Evidence
Fong D, Ho J, Hui B, et al: Physical activity for cancer survivors: meta-analysis of randomized controlled trials, *Br Med J* 344:e70, 2012.

P, Patient population of interest; *I,* intervention or area of interest; *O,* outcomes of interest; *T,* timing (see p. 13).

CULTURALLY COMPETENT CARE

BREAST CANCER

Differences exist in the incidence, mortality rates, and relevant care issues among diverse ethnic groups related to breast cancer (see Cultural & Ethnic Health Disparities box on the facing page). In addition, cultural differences may involve gender roles, health beliefs, religion, and family structure. Other differences may be due to dietary factors and disparities related to access to and use of CBEs and screening mammograms.

Cultural values strongly influence how women respond to and cope with breast cancer and treatment. Health beliefs and behaviors are influenced by diverse cultural norms.[31] Breast cancer screening, diagnosis, and treatment are affected by the cultural values and meanings (body image, sexuality, modesty, motherhood) attached to the breasts. Women may delay screening or treatment for varying reasons, including an acceptance of disease as inevitable fate or "God's will," a mistrust of Western medicine, lack of health care benefits, fear, modesty, or the stigma of a cancer diagnosis.

CULTURAL & ETHNIC HEALTH DISPARITIES
Breast Cancer

- White women have a higher incidence of breast cancer than other ethnic groups.
- African American women have lower survival rates from breast cancer than white women, even when diagnosed at an early stage.
- Triple-negative breast cancer (negative for estrogen, progesterone, and HER-2 receptors) has a higher incidence in Hispanic and African American women.
- Breast cancer incidence and mortality rates are lower among Hispanic and Asian/Pacific Islander women than among white and African American women.
- Breast cancer is the most commonly diagnosed cancer among Hispanic women.
- Hispanic women, especially Mexican Americans, have the lowest rate of cancer screening of any ethnic group.
- Hispanic and African American women are more likely to be diagnosed at a later stage of breast cancer than white women.

HER-2, Human epidermal growth factor receptor 2.

NURSING MANAGEMENT
BREAST CANCER

NURSING ASSESSMENT

Many factors need to be considered when you assess a patient with a breast problem. The history of the breast disorder assists in establishing the diagnosis. Investigate the presence of nipple discharge, pain, rate of growth of the lump, breast asymmetry, and correlation with the menstrual cycle.

Carefully document the size and location of the lump or lumps. Assess the physical characteristics of the lesion, such as consistency, mobility, and shape. If nipple discharge is present, note the color and consistency and whether it occurs from one or both breasts.

Subjective and objective data that should be obtained from an individual suspected of having or diagnosed with breast cancer are presented in Table 52-9.

NURSING DIAGNOSES

Nursing diagnoses related to the care of a patient diagnosed with breast cancer vary. After diagnosis and before a treatment plan has been selected, the following nursing diagnoses would apply:

- Decisional conflict *related to* lack of knowledge about treatment options and their effects
- Fear and/or anxiety *related to* diagnosis of breast cancer
- Disturbed body image *related to* physical and emotional effects of treatment modalities

If a mastectomy or lumpectomy is planned, the nursing diagnoses may include, but are not limited to, those presented in eNursing Care Plan 52-1 (available on the website for this chapter).

PLANNING

The overall goals are that the patient with breast cancer will (1) actively participate in the decision-making process related to treatment, (2) adhere to the therapeutic plan, (3) communicate about and manage the side effects of adjuvant therapy, and (4) access and benefit from the support provided by significant others and health care providers.

TABLE 52-9 NURSING ASSESSMENT
Breast Cancer

Subjective Data
Important Health Information
Past health history: Benign breast disease with atypical changes; previous unilateral breast cancer; menstrual history (early menarche with late menopause); pregnancy history (nulliparity or first full-term pregnancy after age 30); previous endometrial, ovarian, or colon cancer; hyperestrogenism and testicular atrophy (in men)
Medications: Hormones, especially as postmenopausal hormone therapy and in oral contraceptives, infertility treatments
Surgery or other treatments: Exposure to therapeutic radiation (e.g., Hodgkin's lymphoma or thyroid radiation)

Functional Health Patterns
Health perception–health management: Family history of breast cancer (especially mother or sister, young age at diagnosis); history of abnormal mammogram or atypical prior biopsy; palpable change found on BSE; frequent alcohol use
Nutritional-metabolic: Obesity; unexplained severe weight loss (possible indicator of metastasis)
Cognitive-perceptual: Changes in cognition, headache, bone pain (possible indicators of metastasis)
Sexuality-reproductive: Unilateral nipple discharge (clear, milky, or bloody); change in breast contour, size, or symmetry
Coping–stress tolerance: Psychologic stress
Self-perception–self-concept: Anxiety regarding threat to self-esteem
Physical activity: Level of usual activity

Objective Data
General
Axillary and supraclavicular lymphadenopathy

Integumentary
Hard, irregular, nonmobile breast lump most often in upper, outer sector, possibly fixated to fascia or chest wall; thickening of breast; nipple inversion or retraction, erosion; edema ("peau d'orange"), erythema, induration, infiltration, or dimpling (in later stages); firm, discrete nodules at mastectomy site (possible indicator of local recurrence); peripheral edema (possible indicator of metastasis)

Respiratory
Pleural effusions (possible indicator of metastasis)

Gastrointestinal
Hepatomegaly, jaundice; ascites (possible indicators of liver metastasis)

Possible Diagnostic Findings
Finding of mass or change in tissue on breast examination; abnormal mammogram, ultrasound, or breast MRI; positive results of FNA or surgical biopsy or similar results with a needle biopsy

BSE, Breast self-examination; *FNA,* fine-needle aspiration.

NURSING IMPLEMENTATION

HEALTH PROMOTION. Review the risk factors in Table 52-2. A person can reduce her risk factors by maintaining a healthy weight, exercising regularly, limiting alcohol, eating nutritious food, and never smoking (or quitting if she does smoke).

It is important for you to encourage people to adhere to the breast cancer screening guidelines presented on pp. 1238-1239. If a person is at high risk, she needs to develop an individualized plan with the health care provider. Early detection can decrease the morbidity and mortality associated with breast cancer.

Along with these lifestyle choices, there are other risk-reduction options for women at high risk. Genetic testing for *BRCA* gene mutations is available. People with a strong family history of breast cancer should talk with their health care provider about the possibility of genetic testing. Routine screening for genetic abnormalities in women without evidence of a strong family history of breast cancer is not warranted.

In women with an abnormal *BRCA1* or *BRCA2* gene, prophylactic oophorectomy may reduce their risk of developing breast cancer. In deciding whether and when to undergo this surgical procedure, women should receive counseling about the risks and benefits of prophylactic oophorectomy, including fertility issues.

Prophylactic surgery decisions require a great deal of thought, patience, and discussion with the health care provider, genetic counselor, and family. Patients need to consider these options and make decisions with which they feel comfortable. Removing both breasts and ovaries at a young age does not eliminate the risk of breast cancer. A small risk exists that cancer can develop in the areas where the breasts used to be. Close follow-up is necessary, even after prophylactic surgery.

ACUTE INTERVENTION. The times of waiting for the initial biopsy results and waiting for the care provider to make treatment recommendations are difficult for the woman and her family.[32] Even after the health care provider has discussed treatment options, the woman often relies on you to clarify and expand on these options. During this stressful time, the woman may not be coping effectively. Appropriate nursing interventions are to explore the woman's usual decision-making processes, help her evaluate the advantages and disadvantages of the options, provide information relevant to the decision, clarify unresolved issues with the health care provider, and support the patient and family once the decision is made.

Regardless of the surgery planned, provide the patient with sufficient information to ensure informed consent. Some patients seek extensive, detailed information to maintain a sense of control, whereas others avoid information to decrease anxiety and fear. Be sensitive to the individual's need for and preferred type of information. These include (1) preoperative instructions on pain control and what to expect after surgery (e.g., reporting of complications, dressing and drain care, turning, coughing, deep breathing); (2) a review of mobility restrictions and postoperative exercises; and (3) explanation of the recovery period from the time of surgery until the first postoperative visit.

The woman who has breast-conserving surgery usually has an uncomplicated postoperative course with variable pain intensity. Pain primarily depends on the extent of the lymph node dissection performed. If an ALND has been done or if a woman had a mastectomy, drains are generally left in place and patients are discharged home with them. Teach the patient and the family, with a return demonstration, how to manage the drains at home.

Restoring arm function on the affected side after mastectomy and ALND is a key nursing goal. In the hospital, place the woman in a semi-Fowler's position with the arm on the affected side elevated on a pillow. Flexing and extending the fingers should begin in the recovery room with progressive increases in activity encouraged. Postoperative arm and shoulder exercises are instituted gradually (Fig. 52-9). These exercises are designed to prevent contractures and muscle shortening, maintain muscle tone, and improve lymph and blood circulation. The difficulty and pain encountered in performing what used to be simple tasks included in the exercise program may cause frustration and depression. The goal of all exercise is a gradual return to full range of motion within 4 to 6 weeks.

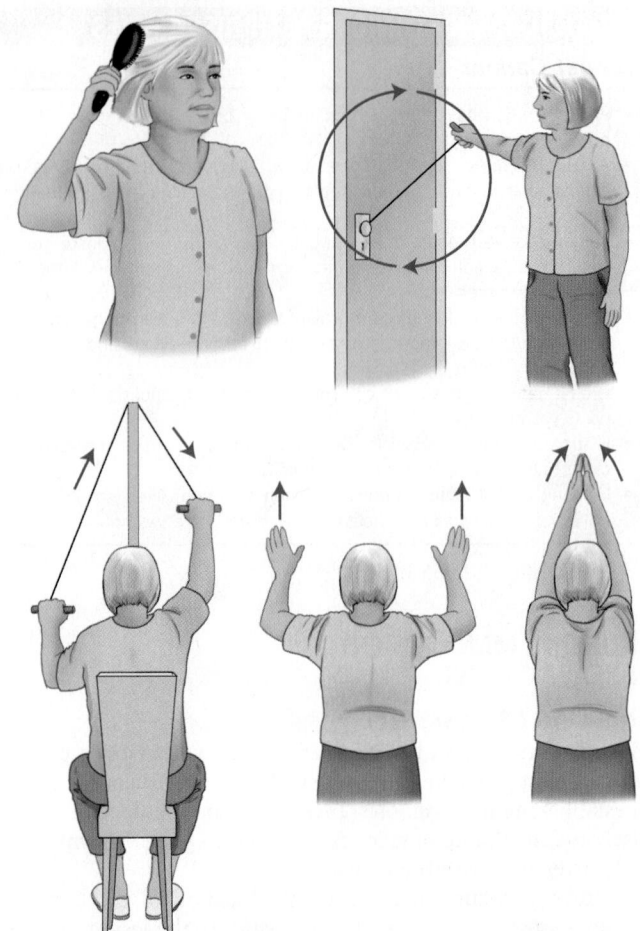

FIG. 52-9 Postoperative exercises for the patient with a mastectomy or lumpectomy with axillary lymph node dissection.

Postoperative discomfort can be minimized by administering analgesics regularly when the patient is in pain and about 30 minutes before initiating exercises. When the patient is able to shower, the warm water on the involved shoulder often relaxes the muscle and reduces joint stiffness. Application of ice, except where contraindicated with plastic surgery procedures, can reduce swelling, inflammation, and pain.

The incidence of arm lymphedema ranges from 2% to 65%, and it can develop 1 to 5 years after surgery.[33] Women who are overweight or obese have a higher risk of developing lymphedema. Teach the woman measures to prevent and reduce lymphedema, including no blood pressure readings, venipunctures, or injections on the affected arm. The affected arm should not be dependent for long periods, and caution should be used to prevent infection, burns, or compromised circulation on the affected side.

If trauma to the arm occurs, the area should be washed thoroughly with soap and water and observed. A topical antibiotic ointment and a bandage or other sterile dressing may be applied.

When the patient's lymphedema is acute (see Fig. 52-7), complete decongestive therapy may be recommended. This therapy consists of a massage-like technique to mobilize the subcutaneous accumulation of fluid. This may then be followed by use of compression bandaging and an intermittent pneumatic compression sleeve. The sleeve applies mechanical massage to the arm and facilitates lymph drainage up toward the heart. Elevation of the arm so that it is level with the heart, diuretics, and isometric exercises may be used to reduce the fluid volume in the arm. To maintain maximum volume reduction, the patient may need to wear a fitted compression sleeve during waking hours and preventively during air travel.

Emotional and Psychologic Care. Throughout history, the female breast has been regarded as a symbol of beauty, femininity, sexuality, and motherhood. The potential loss of a breast, or part of a breast, may be devastating for many women because of the significant psychologic, social, sexual, and body image implications associated with it.

From the time of diagnosis through treatment, survivorship, or metastatic disease, the woman may exhibit signs of distress or tension (e.g., tachycardia, increased muscle tension, sleep disturbances, restlessness, changes in appetite or mood). Assess the woman's body language and affect during periods of high stress and indecision so that appropriate interventions, including referral to a mental health provider, can be initiated.

Remain sensitive to the complex psychologic impact that a diagnosis of cancer and subsequent breast surgery can have on a woman and her family. A relationship in which the woman can express her feelings is therapeutic. With an accepting attitude and the offer of resources, you can help with the feelings of fear, anger, anxiety, and depression. Help to meet the woman's psychologic needs by

- Providing a safe environment for the expression of the full range of feelings.
- Helping her identify sources of support and strength, such as her partner, family, and spiritual or religious practices.
- Encouraging her to identify and learn individual coping strengths.
- Promoting communication between the patient and her family or friends.
- Providing accurate and complete answers to questions about her disease; treatment options; and reproductive, fertility, or lactation issues (if appropriate).
- Making resources available for mental health counseling.
- Offering information about local and national community resources. Referring her to peer support resources, such as Reach to Recovery or local breast cancer organizations, is invaluable. The Reach to Recovery program of the American Cancer Society is a rehabilitation program to help meet the psychologic, physical, and cosmetic needs of women who have had breast surgery. The American Cancer Society and the National Cancer Institute can provide excellent materials to assist you in meeting the special needs of women with breast cancer.

AMBULATORY AND HOME CARE. Explain the specific follow-up plan to the patient and emphasize the importance of ongoing monitoring and self-care. Immediately after surgery, advise the patient to report to the health care provider symptoms such as fever, inflammation at the surgical site, erythema, postoperative constipation, and unusual swelling. Other changes to report are new back pain, weakness, shortness of breath, and change in mental status, including confusion.

For women who have had a mastectomy without breast reconstruction, a variety of products are available. These include garments such as camisoles with soft breast prosthetic inserts or a fitted prosthesis with bra. Should the woman choose a breast prosthesis, a certified fitter can help her select a comfortable, more permanent weighted prosthesis and bra, generally at

COMPLEMENTARY & ALTERNATIVE THERAPIES

Imagery

Imagery is the use of one's mind to generate images that have a calming effect on the body

Scientific Evidence*
- Good evidence for decreasing cancer pain and postoperative pain.
- Good evidence for treatment of migraine or tension headache in conjunction with standard medical care.

Nursing Implications
- Used by nurses to help patients promote relaxation, decrease stress, and manage pain.
- Should be used as a supplemental technique, not a replacement for medical care.

*Based on a systematic review of scientific literature. Retrieved from *www.naturalstandard.com.*

4 to 8 weeks postoperatively. Your role is to present the choices and resources without judgment.

How the loss of part or all of the breast and cancer affect the woman's sexual identity, body image, and relationships can vary. If you are comfortable, initiate a discussion of sexuality by inviting questions about relationships or intimacy concerns. Often the husband, sexual partner, or family members need help dealing with their emotional reactions to the diagnosis and surgery before they can provide effective support for the patient. There are no physical reasons why a mastectomy would prevent sexual satisfaction. The woman taking hormone therapy may have a decreased sexual drive or vaginal dryness. She may need to use lubrication to prevent discomfort during intercourse. Concerns about sexuality are not well addressed by many health care providers.[34] If difficulty in adjustment or other problems develop, counseling may be necessary to deal with the emotional component of a mastectomy and the diagnosis of cancer.

Depression and anxiety may occur with the continued stress and uncertainty of a cancer diagnosis. A woman's self-esteem and identity may also be threatened. The support of family and friends and participation in a cancer support group are important aspects of care that may improve the patient's quality of life.

EVALUATION

The expected outcomes for the patient after a mastectomy or lumpectomy are presented in eNursing Care Plan 52-1 (available on the website for this chapter).

GERONTOLOGIC CONSIDERATIONS

BREAST CANCER

A major risk for breast cancer is increasing age, and more than half of all breast cancers are diagnosed in women who are age 65 or older. Older women are less likely to have mammograms. Screening and treatment decisions for breast cancer should be based on a woman's general health status rather than biologic age, since health status has a greater influence on tolerance to treatment and long-term prognosis. In addition to medical co-morbidities and life expectancy, treatment decisions for the older woman with breast cancer should be based on an assessment of nutritional and functional status; vision, gait, and balance; and the presence of delirium, dementia, or depression.

Breast cancer treatment is similar for older and younger patients, including the use of surgery, radiation therapy, and drug therapy. For healthy older women, breast cancer survival rates are similar to those of younger women when matched by cancer stage.

MAMMOPLASTY

Mammoplasty is the surgical change in the size or shape of the breast. It may be done electively for cosmetic purposes to either enlarge or reduce the size of the breasts. It may also be done to reconstruct the breast after a mastectomy.

A professional, nonjudgmental attitude and clear information about surgical breast options is most useful for women engaged in decision making about mammoplasty. The desire to change the appearance of the breasts has special significance for each woman as she attempts to alter or recreate her body image. Be aware of the cultural value the woman places on the breast. Help the patient set realistic expectations about what mammoplasty can accomplish and about possible complications (e.g., hematoma formation, hemorrhage, infection). If an implant is involved, capsular contracture and loss of the implant are possible.

Breast Reconstruction

Breast reconstructive surgery is done to achieve symmetry and to restore or preserve body image. It may be done simultaneously with a mastectomy or some time afterward. The timing of reconstructive surgery is individualized based on the patient's physical and psychologic needs. Breast reconstruction is also safe and effective for older women.[35]

Indications. The main indication for breast reconstruction is to improve a woman's self-image, regain a sense of normalcy,

and assist in coping with the loss of the breast. Current reconstruction techniques cannot restore lactation, nipple sensation, or erectility. Although the breast will not fully resemble its pre-mastectomy appearance, the reconstructed appearance usually represents an improvement over the mastectomy scar (Fig. 52-10). The contour of the breast is restored without the use of an external prosthesis.

Types of Reconstruction

Breast Implants and Tissue Expansion. A tissue expander can be used to stretch the skin and the muscle at the mastectomy site before inserting permanent implants (Fig. 52-11). The use of tissue expanders and breast implants is the most common breast reconstruction technique currently used. Placement of the expander may be immediate or delayed. The tissue expander is placed in a pocket under the pectoralis muscle, which protects the implant and provides soft tissue coverage. The tissue expander is minimally inflated and then gradually filled by weekly injections of sterile water or saline solution. This procedure stretches the skin and muscle and can be painful. A small magnet is embedded in most expanders to help locate the port where the fluid is injected. Therefore a woman should not have an MRI with a magnet in place. In a second procedure, the expander is surgically removed and a permanent implant is inserted. Some expanders are designed to remain in place and become the implant, eliminating the need for a second surgical procedure. Tissue expansion does not work well in individuals with extensive scar tissue from surgery or radiation therapy.

The body's natural response to the presence of a foreign substance is the formation of a fibrous capsule around the implant. If excessive capsular formation occurs as a result of infection, hematoma, trauma, or reaction to a foreign body, a

FIG. 52-10 A, Appearance of chest after bilateral mastectomy. **B,** Postoperative breast reconstruction before nipple-areolar reconstruction. **C,** Postoperative breast reconstruction after nipple-areolar reconstruction.

FIG. 52-11 A, Tissue expander with gradual expansion. **B,** Tissue expander in place after mastectomy.

contracture can develop, resulting in deformity. Although surgeons differ in their approaches to the prevention of contracture formation, gentle manual massage around the implant is routine. Other adverse outcomes include wrinkling, scarring, asymmetry, pain, and infection at the incision site.[36]

Tissue Flap Procedures. Another choice for breast reconstruction is the use of autologous tissue to recreate a breast mound. If insufficient muscle is left after mastectomy or if the chest wall has been radiated, the person's own tissue may be used to repair the soft tissue defects. Musculocutaneous flaps are most often taken from the back (latissimus dorsi muscle) or the abdomen (transverse rectus abdominis muscle). In the latissimus dorsi musculocutaneous flap, a block of skin and muscle from the patient's back is used to replace tissue removed during mastectomy. A small implant may be needed beneath the flap to gain reasonable breast shape and size. A disadvantage of this technique is an additional scar on the back.

The *transverse rectus abdominis musculocutaneous (TRAM) flap* is a frequently used flap operation. The rectus abdominis muscles are paired flat muscles running from the rib cage down to the pubic bone. Arteries running inside the muscles provide branches at many levels, and these branches supply the fat and skin across a large expanse of the abdomen. With this technique, the surgeon elevates a large block of tissue from the lower abdominal area, but leaves it attached to the rectus muscle (Fig. 52-12). This tissue is then tunneled or placed as "free flaps" under the skin up to the area where the breast will be reconstructed. Then it is molded and fashioned to form a breast. The abdominal incision is closed, giving the patient a result that is similar to having an abdominoplasty ("tummy tuck"). This surgical procedure can last 6 to 8 hours with recovery taking 6 to 8 weeks. Some patients have reported pain and fatigue for up to 3 months. Complications include bleeding, seroma, hernia, infection, and low back pain. An implant may be used in addition to the flap if the flap does not provide the desired cosmetic result alone.

A *deep inferior epigastric artery perforator (DIEP) flap* is a version of the free flap that does not use muscle tissue. With the DIEP flap, only the skin and fat are taken from the same lower abdominal area as the TRAM flap. Patients may experience less pain and restriction of movement with this procedure.

Total skin-sparing mastectomy is the preservation of the skin of the nipple and areola with the removal of underlying breast tissue. It can be done at the same time as immediate breast reconstructive surgery.

Nipple-Areolar Reconstruction. Many patients undergoing breast reconstruction also have nipple-areolar reconstruction. Nipple reconstruction gives the reconstructed breast a much more natural appearance (Fig. 52-10, *C*). Nipple-areolar reconstruction is usually done a few months after breast reconstruction. Tissue to construct a nipple may be taken from the opposite breast or from a small flap of tissue on the reconstructed breast mound. The areola may be grafted from the labia, skin in the area of the groin, or lower abdominal skin, or it may be tattooed with a permanent pigmented dye. In some patients, a small implant may be placed under the completed nipple-areolar reconstruction to add additional projection.

Breast Augmentation

In augmentation mammoplasty (the procedure to enlarge the breasts), an implant is placed in a surgically created pocket between the capsule of the breast and the pectoral fascia, or ideally under the pectoralis muscle. Most implants are silicone envelopes filled with a fluid such as dextran, saline, or silicone. Implants filled with silicone gel most closely resemble the human breast. The U.S. Food and Drug Administration (FDA) has approved the use of silicone gel implants for breast augmentation and reconstruction.[36] Studies continue to collect data on the safety and effectiveness of these implants.

Saline-filled implants are often used in the United States. The silicone shells are filled with normal saline. This implant has an outer shell of silicone that is filled with highly refined soybean oil.

Breast Reduction

For some women, large breasts can be a source of physical and psychologic discomfort. They can interfere with normal daily activities such as walking, using a computer, and driving a car. The weight of large breasts can lead to back, shoulder, and neck problems, including degenerative nerve changes. Overly large breasts can interfere with self-esteem, self-image, and comfort in wearing some clothing. Reduction in the size of the breasts

A   B   C   D

FIG. 52-12 Transverse rectus abdominis musculocutaneous (TRAM) flap. **A,** TRAM flap is planned. **B,** The abdominal tissue, while attached to the rectus muscle, nerve, and blood supply, is tunneled through the abdomen to the chest. **C,** The flap is trimmed to shape the breast. The lower abdominal incision is closed. **D,** Nipple and areola are reconstructed after the breast is healed.

CASE STUDY

Breast Cancer

iStockphoto/Thinkstock

Patient Profile

A.K., a 68-year-old married Asian American woman, has been diagnosed with breast cancer (see Chapter 51 case study on p. 1226). She is scheduled for surgery in the morning for a lumpectomy and sentinel lymph node dissection with possible axillary dissection.

Collaborative Care
Preoperative
- When she is seen in the preoperative clinic 1 week before surgery, she is crying uncontrollably and says, "My husband does not want to look at me anymore. He is afraid of what I am going to look like with a flat chest."
- She says, "I cannot sleep and I just pace the floor at night."
- Expresses concern that her two daughters (34 and 32) and their daughters are going to get "this horrible disease."

Operative Procedure
- A lumpectomy and sentinel lymph node dissection are performed.
- A.K. has cancer cells in her sentinel lymph node.
- Axillary node dissection is then done involving the removal of 12 to 20 nodes.

Postoperative
- Does not want to leave hospital. She wants to stay in bed.
- Fever with swelling and restricted range of motion in right arm.
- Pain not controlled well with pain medication.

Follow-up Findings and Treatment
- Two positive lymph nodes are found.
- Scheduled for outpatient chemotherapy followed by external beam radiation.

Discussion Questions
1. What in A.K.'s breast cancer experience with her family members (see assessment case study in Chapter 51 on p. 1229) might influence her coping response?
2. What information would you provide to A.K. about her surgery?
3. What complication did she develop after her surgery?
4. Which common postoperative exercises will A.K. need to practice after her surgery?
5. *Delegation Decision:* Which of the following personnel should provide this instruction to A.K.: registered nurse, licensed practical/vocational nurse, unlicensed assistive personnel?
6. What community resources are available to help A.K. and her family adjust to the change in her body and to cope with the diagnosis of cancer? How can you access these resources?
7. What information is important for you to provide to A.K. about her radiation treatment and chemotherapy?
8. *Priority Decision:* Based on the assessment data, what are the priority nursing diagnoses? Are there any collaborative problems?
9. What information is important for you to provide to A.K. and her daughters? What early detection measures are important for them to know?
10. *Evidence-Based Practice:* A.K. wants to know what the psychologic benefit may be for her daughters if they decide on a breast cancer genetic risk assessment.

ⓔvolve Answers and a corresponding concept map available at *http://evolve.elsevier.com/Lewis/medsurg.*

---

can have positive effects on the patient's psychologic and physical health.

Reduction mammoplasty is performed by resecting wedges of tissue from the upper and lower quadrants of the breast. The excess skin is removed, and the areola and nipple are relocated on the breast. Lactation can usually be accomplished if massive amounts of tissue are not removed and the nipples are left connected during surgery.

NURSING MANAGEMENT
BREAST AUGMENTATION AND REDUCTION

Breast augmentation and breast reduction may be done in the outpatient surgical area, or they may involve overnight hospitalization. General anesthesia is used. Drains are generally placed in the surgical site to prevent hematoma formation and then removed 2 or 3 days after surgery or when drainage is under 20 to 30 mL/day. The drainage must be examined for color and odor to detect postoperative infection or hemorrhage. Also monitor the woman's temperature. Dressings should be changed as necessary using sterile technique. After surgery, assure the woman that the breast's appearance will improve when healing is completed. Depending on physician preference, the patient may be instructed to wear a bra that provides good support continuously for 2 or 3 days after breast reduction or augmentation. Depending on the extent of the operation, most women resume normal activities within 2 to 3 weeks. Strenuous exercise may not be appropriate until several weeks later.

BRIDGE TO NCLEX EXAMINATION

The number of the question corresponds to the same-numbered outcome at the beginning of the chapter.

1. You are a community health nurse planning a program on breast cancer screening guidelines for women in the neighborhood. To best promote the participants' learning and adherence, you would include *(select all that apply)*
   a. a short audiotape on the BSE procedure.
   b. a packet of articles from the medical literature.
   c. written guidelines for mammography and CBE.
   d. a discussion of the value of early breast cancer detection.
   e. community resources where they can obtain an ultrasound and MRI.

2. In teaching a patient who wants to perform BSE, you inform her that the technique involves both the palpation of the breast tissue and
   a. palpation of cervical lymph nodes.
   b. hard squeezing of the breast tissue.
   c. a mammogram to evaluate breast tissue.
   d. inspection of the breasts for any changes.

3. You are caring for a young woman who has painful fibrocystic breast changes. Management of this patient would include
   a. scheduling a biopsy to rule out malignant changes.
   b. teaching that symptoms will probably subside if she stops using oral contraceptives.
   c. preparing her for surgical removal of the lumps, since they will become larger and more painful.
   d. explaining that restrictions of coffee and chocolate and supplements of vitamin E may relieve some discomfort.

4. When discussing risk factors for breast cancer with a group of women, you emphasize that the greatest known risk factor for breast cancer is
   a. being a woman over age 60.
   b. experiencing menstruation for 30 years or more.
   c. using hormone therapy for 5 years for menopausal symptoms.
   d. having a paternal grandmother with postmenopausal breast cancer.

5. A patient with breast cancer has a lumpectomy with sentinel lymph node dissection that is positive for cancer. You explain that, of the other tests done to determine the risk for cancer recurrence or spread, the results that support the more favorable prognosis are *(select all that apply)*
   a. well-differentiated tumor.
   b. estrogen receptor–positive tumor.
   c. overexpression of HER-2 cell marker.
   d. involvement of two to four axillary nodes.
   e. aneuploidy status from cell proliferation studies.

6. A modified radical mastectomy has been scheduled for your patient with breast cancer. Postoperatively, to restore arm function on the affected side, you would
   a. apply heating pads or blankets to increase circulation.
   b. place daily ice packs to minimize the risk of lymphedema.
   c. teach passive exercises with the affected arm in a dependent position.
   d. emphasize regular exercises for the affected shoulder to increase range of motion.

7. Preoperatively, to meet the psychologic needs of a woman scheduled for a modified radical mastectomy, you would
   a. discuss the limitations of breast reconstruction.
   b. include her significant other in all conversations.
   c. promote an environment for expression of feelings.
   d. explain the importance of regular follow-up screening.

8. To prevent capsular formation after breast reconstruction with implants, teach the patient to
   a. gently massage the area around the implant.
   b. bind the breasts tightly with elastic bandages.
   c. exercise the arm on the affected side to promote drainage.
   d. avoid strenuous exercise until the implant has healed.

1. c, 2. d, 3. d, 4. a, 5. a, b, 6. d, 7. c, 8. a

ⓔvolve

For rationales to these answers and even more NCLEX review questions, visit *http://evolve.elsevier.com/Lewis/medsurg.*

REFERENCES

1. Jemal A, Siegel R, Naishadham D, et al: Cancer statistics 2012, *CA Cancer J Clin* 62:10, 2012.
2. American Cancer Society: Cancer facts and figures 2012. Retrieved from *www.cancer.org.*
3. American Cancer Society: Guidelines for the early detection of cancer. Retrieved from *www.cancer.org.*
*4. National Cancer Institute: Breast cancer screening (PDQ) summary of the evidence. Retrieved from *www.cancer.gov/cancertopics/pdq/screening/breast/healthprofessional.*
5. NCCN Clinical Practice Guidelines in Oncology: Breast cancer. Retrieved from *www.nccn.org.*
6. US Preventive Services Task Force: Screening for breast cancer. Retrieved from *www.uspreventiveservicestaskforce.org/uspstf/uspsbrca.htm.*
7. American Cancer Society: How to examine your breasts. Retrieved from *www.cancer.org/Cancer/BreastCancer/MoreInformation/BreastCancerEarlyDetection/breast-cancer-early-detection-acs-recs-bse.*
8. American Cancer Society: Recommendations for early breast cancer detection in women without breast symptoms. Retrieved from *www.cancer.org.*
*9. Fenton J, Abraham L, Taplin S, et al: Effectiveness of computer-aided detection in community mammography practice, *J Natl Cancer Inst* 103:1152, 2011.
10. Katz V, Dotters D: Breast diseases: diagnosis and treatment of benign and malignant disease. In Lentz G, Lobo R, Gershenson D, et al, editors: *Lentz comprehensive gynecology,* ed 6, St Louis, 2012, Mosby.
11. Robertson F, Bondy M, Yang W, et al: Inflammatory breast cancer, *CA Cancer J Clin* 60:351, 2011.
12. Lewis J, Borgan P: Breast disease. In Bope E, Kellerman R, editors: *Conn's current therapy,* St Louis, 2012, Saunders.
13. Seow J, Metcalf C, Wylie E: Nipple discharge in a screening programme: imaging findings with pathological correlation, *J Med Imaging Radiat Oncol* 55:577, 2011.
14. Ikard RW, Vavra D, Forbes RC, et al: Management of senescent gynecomastia in the Veterans Health Administration, *Breast J* 17:160, 2011.
*15. National Institutes of Health: Women's Health Initiative study. Retrieved from *www.nhlbi.nih.gov/whi.*
16. National Cancer Institute: Oral contraceptives and cancer risk. Retrieved from *www.cancer.gov/cancertopics/factsheet/Risk/oral-contraceptives.*
17. National Cancer Institute: *BRCA1* and *BRCA2:* cancer risk and genetic testing. Retrieved from *www.cancer.gov/cancertopics/factsheet/Risk/BRCA.*
*18. Bedrosian I, Hu C, Chang G: Population-based study of contralateral prophylactic mastectomy and survival outcomes of breast cancer patients, *J Natl Cancer Inst* 102:401, 2010.
*19. Slamon D, Eiermann W, Robert N, et al: Adjuvant trastuzumab in HER-2 positive breast cancer, *N Engl J Med* 365:1273, 2011.
20. Gradishar W: HER-therapy: an abundance of riches, *N Engl J Med* 366:176, 2012.
21. Morris L: Targeting the red-hot danger of inflammatory breast cancer, *Nursing* 40:58, 2010.
22. Lee E, McKean-Cowdin R, Ma H, et al: Characteristics of triple-negative breast cancer in patients with a *BRCA1* mutation: results from a population-based study of young women, *J Clin Oncol* 29:4373, 2011.
23. American Joint Committee on Cancer: *AJCC cancer staging manual,* ed 7. Retrieved from *www.cancerstaging.org/staging/changes2010f.*

*Evidence-based information for clinical practice.

*24. Sherman K, Koelmeyer L: The role of information sources and objective risk status on lymphedema risk-minimization behaviors in women recently diagnosed with breast cancer, *Oncol Nurs Forum* 38:66, 2011.

25. National Cancer Institute: A closer look: studies raise concerns about partial-breast radiation therapy, *NCI Cancer Bull*, January 10, 2012. Retrieved from *www.cancer.gov/ncicancerbulletin/ 01012*.

26. US Food and Drug Administration: FDA approves new treatment option for late-stage breast cancer. Retrieved from *www.fda.gov/NewsEvents/Newsroom/PressAnnouncements/ ucm233863.htm*.

*27. Myers J: Chemotherapy-related cognitive impairment: the breast cancer experience, *Oncol Nurs Forum* 39:69, 2012.

28. National Cancer Institute: Chemotherapy associated with microscopic changes in the brain, *NCI Cancer Bull*, January 10, 2012. Retrieved from *www.cancer.gov/ncicancerbulletin/01012*.

29. National Cancer Institute: Study of raloxifene and tamoxifen (STAR) trial. Retrieved from *www.cancer.gov/clinicaltrials/ noteworthy-trials/star/Page1*.

30. Memorial Sloan-Kettering Cancer Center: Survivorship care plan. Retrieved from *www.mskcc.org/cancer-care/survivorship/ survivorship-care-plan*.

31. Goel M, Gracia G, Baker D: Development and pilot testing of a culturally sensitive multimedia program to improve breast cancer screening in Latina women, *Patient Educ Couns* 84:128, 2011.

*32. Lacovara J, Arzouman J, Kim C, et al: Are patients with breast cancer satisfied with their decision-making? *Clin J Oncol Nurs* 15:320, 2011.

*33. Cemal Y, Pusic A, Mehrara B: Preventative measures for lymphedema: separating fact from fiction, *J Am Coll Surg* 213:543, 2011.

34. Hill E, Sandbo S, Abramsohn E, et al: Assessing gynecologic and breast cancer survivors' sexual health care needs, *Cancer* 117:2643, 2010.

35. Johns Hopkins Medicine: Breast reconstruction improves well-being and quality of life, *HealthAfter50* 24:1, 2012.

36. US Food and Drug Administration: Breast implants. Retrieved from *www.fda.gov/MedicalDevices/ProductsandMedical Procedures/ImplantsandProsthetics/BreastImplants/default.htm*.

RESOURCES

American Cancer Society
    www.cancer.org/cancer/breastcancer/index
CancerCare
    www.cancercare.org
Inflammatory Breast Cancer Research Foundation
    www.ibcresearch.org
Livestrong
    www.livestrong.org
Living Beyond Breast Cancer
    www.lbbc.org
National Breast Cancer Coalition
    www.natlbcc.org
National Cancer Institute
    www.cancer.gov/cancertopics/types/breast
    www.cancer.gov/bcrisktool/about-tool.aspx
National Coalition for Cancer Survivorship (NCCS)
    www.canceradvocacy.org
National Lymphedema Network (NLN)
    www.lymphnet.org
OncoLink (cancer information site)
    www.oncolink.upenn.edu
Oncology Nursing Society
    www.ons.org
Sisters Network (national African American breast cancer survivor group)
    www.sistersnetworkinc.org
Susan G. Komen for the Cure
    www.komen.org
Triple Negative Breast Cancer Foundation
    www.tnbcfoundation.org
Young Survivor Coalition
    www.youngsurvivor.org
Y-ME National Breast Cancer Organization (Y-ME)
    http://en.wikipedia.org/wiki/Y-ME_National_Breast_Cancer _Organization

*The doors we open and close each day decide
the lives we live.*
Flora Whittemore

Nursing Management
Sexually Transmitted Infections

Kay Jarrell

evolve WEBSITE

http://evolve.elsevier.com/Lewis/medsurg

- NCLEX Review Questions
- Key Points
- Pre-Test

- Answer Guidelines for Case Study on p. 1274
- Rationales for Bridge to NCLEX Examination Questions

- Concept Map Creator
- Glossary
- Content Updates

LEARNING OUTCOMES

1. Assess the factors contributing to the high incidence of sexually transmitted infections (STIs).
2. Describe the etiology, clinical manifestations, complications, and diagnostic abnormalities of gonorrhea, syphilis, chlamydial infections, genital herpes, and genital warts.
3. Compare and contrast primary genital herpes with recurrent genital herpes.
4. Explain the collaborative care and drug therapy of gonorrhea, syphilis, chlamydial infections, genital herpes, and genital warts.
5. Integrate the nursing assessment and nursing diagnoses for patients who have an STI.
6. Summarize the nursing role in the prevention and control of STIs.
7. Describe the nursing management of patients with STIs.

KEY TERMS

chancre, Table 53-3, p. 1265
chlamydial infections, p. 1266
genital herpes, p. 1267

genital warts, p. 1269
gonorrhea, p. 1262

sexually transmitted infections (STIs), p. 1261
syphilis, p. 1264

Sexually transmitted infections (STIs) are infectious diseases that are commonly acquired through sexual contact (Table 53-1). They may also be contracted by other routes such as through blood, blood products, perinatal transmission, and autoinoculation. STI is becoming the more common term used for sexually transmitted disease.

Most infections start as lesions on the genitalia and other sexually exposed mucous membranes. Wide dissemination to other areas of the body can then occur. A latent or subclinical phase is present with all STIs. This can lead to a long-term persistent infection and the transmission of disease from an asymptomatic (but infected) person to another person. Having one STI increases the risk of acquiring another. A person can have different STIs at the same time.

In the United States all cases of gonorrhea and syphilis, and in most states chlamydial infection, must be reported to the state or local public health authorities for purposes of surveillance and partner notification. In spite of this requirement, many cases of these infections go unreported. An estimated 65 million Americans are currently infected with one or more STI. Every year an additional 19 million Americans are newly infected with an STI. About 50% of these new cases are in persons 15 to 24 years old.[1]

The most commonly diagnosed STIs are discussed in this chapter. Human immunodeficiency virus (HIV) infection is discussed in Chapter 15. Hepatitis B and C infections are discussed in Chapter 44.

Factors Affecting Incidence of Sexually Transmitted Infections

Many factors contribute to the current STI rates. Earlier reproductive maturity and increased longevity have resulted in a longer sexual life span. The increase in the total population has resulted in an increase in the number of susceptible hosts. Other factors include greater sexual freedom, lack of barrier methods (e.g., condoms) during sexual activity, and the media's increased emphasis on sexuality. Substance abuse contributes to unsafe sexual practices. In addition, increased

Reviewed by Suzanne L. Jed, MSN, FNP-BC, Instructor of Clinical Family Medicine, Keck School of Medicine, University of Southern California, Los Angeles, California; and Danette Y. Wall, ACRN, MSN, MBA/HCM, ISO9001 Lead Auditor, Regional Nurse, Department of Veterans Affairs–Veterans Health Administration, Tampa, Florida.

TABLE 53-1   CAUSES OF SEXUALLY TRANSMITTED INFECTIONS

Sexually Transmitted Infection	Cause
Bacterial	
Gonorrhea	*Neisseria gonorrhoeae*
Syphilis	*Treponema pallidum*
Nongonococcal urethritis (NGU), cervicitis, lymphogranuloma venereum	*Chlamydia trachomatis*
Viral	
Genital herpes	Herpes simplex virus (HSV)
Genital warts. Cervical, vulvar, vaginal, penile, anal, and oropharyngeal cancers	Human papillomavirus (HPV)
Human immunodeficiency virus (HIV) infection, acquired immunodeficiency syndrome (AIDS)	HIV virus (see Chapter 15)
Hepatitis B and C	Hepatitis B and C viruses (see Chapter 44)
Encephalitis, esophagitis, retinitis, pneumonitis in immunocompromised patients	Cytomegalovirus (CMV)

⊕ **CULTURAL & ETHNIC HEALTH DISPARITIES**

Sexually Transmitted Infections

- *Chlamydial infection:* African Americans are 48% of cases.
- *Syphilis:* African Americans are 46% of cases, a rate 60 times higher than that of whites.
- *HSV-2:* More common in African Americans (46%) than whites (18%).
- *Gonorrhea:* African Americans are 77% of reported cases.
- *All STIs:* Hispanics have four times higher rate than whites.

HSV-2, Herpes simplex virus type 2.

Etiology and Pathophysiology

Gonorrhea is caused by *Neisseria gonorrhoeae,* a gram-negative diplococcus. The infection is spread by direct physical contact with an infected host, usually during sexual activity (vaginal, oral, or anal). Mucosal tissues in the genitalia (urethra in men, cervix in women), rectum, and oropharynx are especially sensitive to gonococcal infection. The delicate gonococcus is easily killed by drying, heating, or washing with an antiseptic solution. Consequently, indirect transmission by instruments or linens is rare.

The incubation period is 3 to 8 days. The infection confers no immunity to subsequent reinfection. Gonococcal infection elicits an inflammatory response, which, if left untreated, leads to the formation of fibrous tissue and adhesions. This fibrous scarring is responsible for many complications in women such as strictures and tubal abnormalities, which can lead to tubal pregnancy, chronic pelvic pain, and infertility.

Clinical Manifestations

Men. The initial site of infection in men is usually the urethra. Symptoms of urethritis consist of dysuria and profuse, purulent urethral discharge developing 2 to 5 days after infection (Fig. 53-1). Painful or swollen testicles may also occur. Men generally seek medical evaluation early in the infection because their symptoms are usually obvious and distressing. It is unusual for men with gonorrhea to be asymptomatic.[4]

Women. Many women who contract gonorrhea are asymptomatic or have minor symptoms that are often overlooked, making it possible for them to remain a source of infection. A few women may complain of vaginal discharge, dysuria, or frequency of urination. Changes in menstruation may be a symptom, but the women often disregard these changes. After the incubation period, redness and swelling occur at the site of

leisure time, more national and international travel, and urbanization have brought together people with varying social behaviors and value systems.

Changes in the methods of contraception are also reflected in the incidence of STIs. The condom is considered to be the best form of protection (other than abstinence) against STIs. Although condom use has increased, condoms are still not used frequently in the general population.[2] Commonly used oral contraceptives cause the secretions of the cervix and the vagina to become more alkaline. This change produces a more favorable environment for the growth of organisms that cause STIs at these sites. Women who take oral contraceptives may have a lower risk of pelvic inflammatory disease (PID) as a result of the ability of the cervical mucus to act as a barrier against bacteria. However, the proliferation of *Chlamydia* organisms, the leading cause of nongonococcal PID, may be enhanced by oral contraceptive use.

Whether or not intrauterine device (IUD) users are at increased risk of PID is controversial, but it is clear that IUDs confer no protection against STIs. Long-acting contraceptives such as medroxyprogesterone (Depo-Provera) also offer no protection against STIs. Although these methods do not prevent transmission from partner to partner, they do prevent pregnancy and, therefore, transmission of the infection to the fetus.

▌BACTERIAL INFECTIONS

GONORRHEA

Gonorrhea is the second most frequently reported STI in the United States (chlamydial infections are the most common). In 2009 the gonorrhea rates were the lowest since recording of rates began. Since that time gonorrhea rates have increased slightly. A total of 309,341 cases of gonorrhea have been reported in the United States.[3] Gonorrhea rates are highest in adolescents of all racial and ethnic groups and among African Americans. Most states have enacted laws that permit examination and treatment of minors without parental consent.

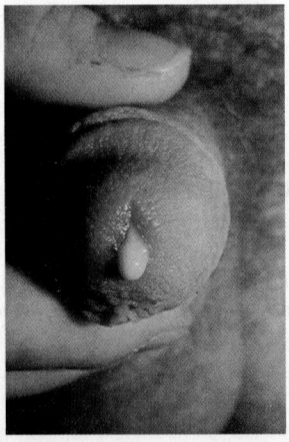

FIG. 53-1 Profuse, purulent drainage in a patient with gonorrhea.

FIG. 53-2 Endocervical gonorrhea. Cervical redness and edema with discharge.

FIG. 53-3 Skin lesions with disseminated gonococcal infection. **A,** On the hand. **B,** On the fifth toe.

contact, which is usually the cervix or urethra (Fig. 53-2). A greenish yellow purulent exudate often develops with a potential for abscess formation. The infection may remain local or can spread by direct tissue extension to the uterus, fallopian tubes, and ovaries. Although the vulva and vagina are uncommon sites for a gonorrheal infection, they may become involved when little or no estrogen is present, as in prepubertal girls and postmenopausal women. Because the vagina acts as a natural reservoir for infectious secretions, transmission is often more efficient from men to women than it is from women to men.

General. Anorectal gonorrhea may be present, usually as a result of anal intercourse. Symptoms may include mucopurulent anal discharge, bleeding, and tenesmus.[5] Most patients with anorectal infections and infections in the throat have few symptoms. A small percentage of individuals develop gonococcal pharyngitis from orogenital sexual contact. When the gonococcus can be demonstrated by a laboratory culture, individuals of either gender are infectious to their sexual partners.

Complications

Because men often seek treatment early in the course of the infection, they are less likely to develop complications. The complications that do occur in men are prostatitis, urethral strictures, and sterility from orchitis or epididymitis. Because women who are asymptomatic seldom seek treatment, complications are more common and usually constitute the reason for seeking medical attention. PID, Bartholin's abscess, ectopic pregnancy, and infertility are the main complications of gonorrhea in women. A small percentage of infected persons, mainly women, may develop a disseminated gonococcal infection (DGI). In DGI the appearance of skin lesions, fever, arthralgia, arthritis, or endocarditis usually causes the patient to seek medical help (Fig. 53-3).

Neonates can develop a gonococcal infection during delivery from an infected mother. Untreated infected infants develop permanent blindness. Almost all states have a health department regulation or law requiring the use of a prophylactic drug such as erythromycin ophthalmic ointment or silver nitrate aqueous solution in the eyes of all newborns. Therefore gonorrheal eye infections in newborns (*ophthalmia neonatorum*) are relatively rare today.

Diagnostic Studies

For men, a presumptive diagnosis of gonorrhea is made if there is a history of sexual contact with a new or infected partner

GENDER DIFFERENCES

Sexually Transmitted Infections

Men	Women
• Syphilis more common, especially in men who have sex with men • More likely to be symptomatic • Easier to diagnose because of less complex anatomy	• Chlamydial infection three times more common • Gonorrhea more common • HSV-2 more common • Have more frequent and serious complications related to STIs (e.g., pelvic inflammatory disease)

HSV-2, Herpes simplex type 2.

followed within a few days by a urethral discharge. Typical clinical manifestations, combined with a positive finding on a Gram-stained smear of the purulent discharge from the penis, give an almost certain diagnosis. A culture of the discharge is indicated for men whose smears are negative in the presence of strong clinical evidence. The nucleic acid amplification test (NAAT) (using ligase or polymerase chain reaction) is a non-culture test with sensitivity similar to culture tests for *N. gonorrhoeae*. It can be done on a wide variety of samples, including vaginal, endocervical, urethral, and urine specimens.[6]

For women, making a diagnosis of gonorrhea on the basis of symptoms is difficult because most women are symptom free or have complaints that may be confused with other conditions. Smears and purulent discharge do not establish a diagnosis of gonorrhea because the female genitourinary tract normally harbors a large number of organisms that resemble *N. gonorrhoeae*. A culture must be performed to confirm the diagnosis. Although the cervix is the most common site of sampling, specimens for culture may also be taken from the urethra, anus, or oropharynx. A urine specimen can reveal gonorrhea if it is present in the cervix or urethra.

Collaborative Care

Drug Therapy. Because of a short incubation period and high infectivity, treatment is generally instituted without awaiting culture results. The treatment of gonorrhea in the early stage is curative with a cephalosporin antibiotic. Treatment for gonorrhea is an intramuscular (IM) dose of ceftriaxone (Rocephin) or cefixime (Suprax) orally (Table 53-2).

Over the years, *N. gonorrhoeae* has developed a resistance to multiple classes of antimicrobial drugs, including fluoroquinolones (ciprofloxacin [Cipro], ofloxacin [Floxin], levofloxacin

TABLE 53-2   COLLABORATIVE CARE

Gonorrhea

Diagnostic

History and physical examination
Gram-stained smears of urethral or endocervical exudate
Culture for *Neisseria gonorrhoeae*
Nucleic acid amplification test (NAAT) to detect *N. gonorrhoeae*
Testing for other STIs (syphilis, HIV, chlamydial infection)

Collaborative Therapy

Uncomplicated gonorrhea: ceftriaxone (Rocephin) IM or cefixime (Suprax) orally
If chlamydial infection is not ruled out: azithromycin (Zithromax) or doxycycline (Vibramycin)
Treatment of sexual contacts
Instruction on abstinence from sexual intercourse and alcohol during treatment
Reexamination if symptoms persist or recur after completion of treatment

Source: Centers for Disease Control and Prevention: Sexually transmitted diseases treatment guidelines, 2010. Retrieved from *www.cdc.gov/STD/treatment.*

[Levaquin]) and tetracyclines (doxycycline [Vibramycin]). Gonococcal resistance to cephalosporin has recently been reported.[7]

The high frequency (up to 20% in men and 40% in women) of coexisting chlamydial and gonococcal infections has led to the addition of azithromycin (Zithromax) or doxycycline to the treatment regimen. Patients with coexisting syphilis are likely to be treated with the same drugs used for gonorrhea.

DRUG ALERT: Doxycycline (Vibramycin)

- Patients on this drug should avoid unnecessary exposure to sunlight.
- Do not take with antacids, iron products, or dairy products.

All sexual contacts of patients with gonorrhea must be evaluated and treated to prevent reinfection after resumption of sexual relations. The "ping-pong" effect of reexposure, treatment, and reinfection can end only when infected partners are treated simultaneously. Additionally, counsel the patient to abstain from sexual intercourse and alcohol during treatment. Sexual intercourse allows the infection to spread and can delay complete healing. Alcohol has an irritant effect on the healing urethral walls. Caution men against squeezing the penis to look for further discharge. Reinfection, rather than treatment failure, is the main cause of infections after treatment has ended.

SYPHILIS

The incidence of syphilis reported in the United States in 2000 was at its lowest rate since reporting started in 1941. During the past decade, syphilis rates increased until 2010 when the rate slightly decreased.[1] Many new cases of syphilis are being seen in men who have sex with men.

Etiology and Pathophysiology

Syphilis is caused by *Treponema pallidum*, a spirochete. This bacterium is thought to enter the body through very small breaks in the skin or mucous membranes. Its entry is facilitated by the minor abrasions that often occur during sexual intercourse. Syphilis is a complex disease in which many organs and tissues of the body can become infected by *T. pallidum*. The infection causes the production of antibodies that also react with normal tissues.

After a short period of protection, antibody levels decrease and a person is susceptible to reinfection. Not all people who are exposed to syphilis acquire the infection, since about one third become infected after intercourse with an infected person. In addition to sexual contact, syphilis may be spread through contact with infectious lesions and sharing of needles among IV drug users.

T. pallidum is extremely fragile and easily destroyed by drying, heating, or washing. The incubation period for syphilis ranges from 10 to 90 days (average 21 days). Congenital syphilis is transmitted from an infected mother to the fetus in utero after the tenth week of pregnancy. An infected pregnant woman has a high risk of a stillbirth or a baby dying shortly after birth.[8] Pregnant women need to be tested for syphilis at their first prenatal visit. Some states require all women to be screened at delivery.

Persons at high risk for acquiring syphilis are also at an increased risk for acquiring HIV infection. Often, both infections are present. Syphilitic lesions (chancres) on the genitalia enhance HIV transmission. Patients with HIV and syphilis appear to be at greatest risk for clinically significant central nervous system (CNS) involvement and may require more intensive treatment than do other patients with syphilis. Therefore the evaluation of all patients with syphilis should also include testing for HIV (with the patient's consent). Conversely, HIV patients should be tested at least annually for syphilis.

Clinical Manifestations

Syphilis has a variety of signs and symptoms that can mimic a number of other diseases. Consequently, compared with other STIs, it is more difficult to recognize syphilis. If it is not treated, specific clinical stages are characteristic of the progression of the disease (Table 53-3).

Complications

Complications of the disease occur mostly in late syphilis. The gummas of benign late syphilis may produce irreparable damage to bone, liver, or skin. In cardiovascular syphilis, the resulting aneurysm may press on structures such as the intercostal nerves, causing pain. The possibility of a rupture exists as the aneurysm increases in size. Scarring of the aortic valve results in aortic valve insufficiency and eventually heart failure.

Neurosyphilis causes degeneration of the brain with mental deterioration. Problems related to sensory nerve involvement are a result of *tabes dorsalis* (progressive locomotor ataxia). There may be sudden attacks of pain anywhere in the body, which can confuse the diagnosis with other conditions. Loss of vision and sense of position in the feet and legs can also occur. Walking may become even more difficult as joint stability is lost. (Late syphilis is also discussed in Chapter 59.)

Diagnostic Studies

The first step in diagnosis is to obtain a detailed and accurate sexual history. Asking if the patient has sex with men, women, or both can be more effective than asking directly about sexual orientation, since some men do not identify themselves as gay or homosexual. In addition, inquire about vaginal, oral, or anal sex. A physical examination should be done to identify any suspicious lesions or other significant signs and symptoms. Since syphilis is "the great imitator" of other conditions, it is easily missed. Oral sex is an important transmission route that is sometimes overlooked.

TABLE 53-3 STAGES OF SYPHILIS

Manifestations	Communicability
Primary Chancre (painless indurated lesion of penis, vulva, lips, mouth, vagina, and rectum) (Fig. 53-4) occurs 10 to 90 days after inoculation. Regional lymphadenopathy (draining of the microorganisms into the lymph nodes). Genital ulcers. *Duration of stage:* 3-8 wk	Exudate from chancre highly infectious; blood is infectious. Most infectious stage, but transmission can occur at any stage if there are moist lesions.
Secondary Occurs a few weeks after chancre appears. Systemic manifestations: flu-like symptoms (e.g., malaise, fever, sore throat, headaches, fatigue, arthralgia, headache, generalized adenopathy). Cutaneous lesions bilateral. Symmetric rash that begins on the trunk and involves the palms and soles. Mucous patches in the mouth (Fig. 53-5), tongue, or cervix. *Condylomata lata* (moist, weeping papules) in the anal and genital area. Weight loss, alopecia. *Duration of stage:* 1-2 yr	Exudate from skin and mucous membrane lesions highly infectious.
Latent Absence of signs or symptoms. Diagnosis based on positive specific treponemal antibody test together with normal CSF and absence of clinical manifestations. *Duration of stage:* Throughout life or progression to late stage	Noninfectious after 4 yr. Possible placental transmission. Almost 25% of persons with latent syphilis develop late syphilis, in some cases many years later.
Late (tertiary)* Appearance 3-20 yr after initial infection. Gummas (chronic, destructive lesions affecting any organ of body, especially skin, bone, liver, mucous membranes) (Fig. 53-6). *Cardiovascular:* Aneurysms, heart valve insufficiency, heart failure, aortitis. *Neurosyphilis:* General paresis (personality changes from minor to psychotic, tremors, physical and mental deterioration), tabes dorsalis (ataxia, areflexia, paresthesias, lightning pains, damaged joints), speech disturbances. *Duration of stage:* Chronic (without treatment), possibly fatal	Noninfectious. Spinal fluid possibly containing organism.

*Several forms such as cardiovascular syphilis and neurosyphilis occur together in approximately 25% of untreated cases.
CSF, Cerebrospinal fluid.

FIG. 53-4 Primary syphilis chancre.

FIG. 53-5 Secondary syphilis. Mucous patch in the mouth.

FIG. 53-6 Destructive skin gummas associated with tertiary syphilis.

Diagnostic studies for syphilis are presented in Table 53-4. The presence of spirochetes on dark-field microscopy and direct fluorescent antibody (DFA) tests of lesion exudate or tissue can confirm a clinical diagnosis of syphilis. However, syphilis is more commonly diagnosed by a serologic test.[4] Tests for syphilis may be classified as those performed for screening and those performed for confirmation of a positive screening test. Nonspecific antitreponemal antibodies can be detected by tests such as the Venereal Disease Research Laboratory (VDRL) test and the rapid plasma reagin (RPR) test. These nontreponemal tests are suitable for screening purposes, and usually become positive 10 to 14 days after the appearance of a chancre. The fluorescent treponemal antibody absorption (FTA-Abs) test and the *T. pallidum* particle agglutination (TP-PA) test detect specific antitreponemal antibodies and are used for confirming the diagnosis.

False-negative and false-positive test results do occur with the nontreponemal tests (VDRL, RPR). A false-negative result may be obtained during primary syphilis if the test is done before the individual has had time to produce antibodies. A false-positive finding may occur if patients have other diseases or conditions such as hepatitis, infectious mononucleosis, collagen diseases (e.g., systemic lupus erythematosus), pregnancy, or aging. Positive nontreponemal test results should be confirmed by more specific treponemal tests to rule out other causes. In the cerebrospinal fluid (CSF), changes such as increased white blood cell count, increased total protein, and a positive treponemal antibody test are diagnostic of neurosyphilis.

TABLE 53-4 COLLABORATIVE CARE

Syphilis

Diagnostic
- History and physical examination
- Dark-field microscopy
- Nontreponemal and/or treponemal serologic testing
- Testing for other STIs (HIV, gonorrhea, chlamydial infection)

Collaborative Therapy
- Antibiotic therapy
  - penicillin G benzathine (Bicillin) or aqueous procaine penicillin G
  - doxycycline (Vibramycin) or tetracycline (when penicillin is contraindicated)
- Confidential counseling and testing for HIV infection
- Surveillance
  - Repeat of nontreponemal tests at 6 and 12 mo
  - Examination of cerebrospinal fluid at 1 yr*

*If treatment involves alternative antibiotics or treatment failure has occurred.

If treatment with antibiotics is initiated early in the course of the disease on the basis of the history and the symptoms, the serologic testing may not indicate syphilis. Once a person has positive serologic findings for syphilis, indicating the presence of antibodies, these findings may remain positive for an indefinite period in spite of successful treatment.

Collaborative Care

Table 53-4 describes collaborative care of syphilis. Specific management is based on the symptoms.

Drug Therapy. Management of syphilis is aimed at eradicating all syphilitic organisms. Penicillin G benzathine (Bicillin) or aqueous procaine penicillin G is the treatment of choice for all stages of syphilis.[9] When penicillin is contraindicated, doxycycline or tetracycline may be used. However, treatment cannot reverse damage that is already present in the late stage of the disease. It is also important that all sexual contacts in the last 90 days be treated.

Patients having persistent or recurring symptoms after drug therapy has ended should be reevaluated. All patients with neurosyphilis must be carefully monitored, with periodic serologic testing, clinical evaluation at 6-month intervals, and repeat CSF examinations for at least 3 years.

CHLAMYDIAL INFECTIONS

Chlamydial infections are the most commonly reported STI in the United States. Infection rates have increased over the past 20 years, with more than 1.3 million cases reported in 2010.[1] This increase may be due in part to better and more intensive screening for the infection. Underreporting is significant because many people are asymptomatic and do not seek testing.

The incidence of chlamydia is higher in women than men, which may be because more women are screened for this infection. Women younger than 25 years old are five times more likely to have a chlamydial infection than women over age 30. Women infected with *Chlamydia* may also be at high risk for acquiring HIV from an infected partner.

Etiology and Pathophysiology

Chlamydial infections are caused by *Chlamydia trachomatis*, a gram-negative bacterium. *Chlamydia* can be transmitted during

TABLE 53-5 RISK FACTORS FOR CHLAMYDIAL INFECTION

- Women and adolescents
- New or multiple sexual partners
- Sexual partners who have had multiple partners
- History of STIs and cervical ectopy
- Coexisting STIs
- Inconsistent or incorrect use of condom

Modified from Centers for Disease Control and Prevention: CDC fact sheet: chlamydia. Retrieved from *www.cdc.gov/std/Chlamydia/STD fact.*

EVIDENCE-BASED PRACTICE

Translating Research Into Practice

What Strategies Improve Screening Rates for Repeat Chlamydial Infections?

Clinical Question
In patients with repeat chlamydial infections (P), what is the effect of reminders and mailed screening kits (I) versus no intervention (C) on rescreening rates (O)?

Best Available Evidence
Systematic review of randomized controlled trials (RCTs) and observational studies

Critical Appraisal and Synthesis of Evidence
- Eight trials (*n* = 25 to 5863/trial) compared patient rescreening rates for repeat chlamydial infections.
- Interventions were mailed screening kits, motivational interviewing, financial incentives, and reminders.
- Rescreening occurred 3 wk to 12 mo after the initial chlamydial infection.
- Mailed screening kits for sample self-collection and phone call, postcard, and e-mail reminders significantly increased rescreening rates.

Conclusion
- Mailed screening kits, reminders, and a combination of both methods increased rescreening rates.

Implications for Nursing Practice
- Repeat chlamydial infections are common and increase the risk of complications.
- Remind patient of importance of rescreening.
- To increase rescreening rates, tailor interventions to meet patient needs and preferences.
- Text message and automated phone calling reminders may also be effective.

Reference for Evidence
Guy R, Hocking J, Low N, et al: Interventions to increase rescreening for repeat chlamydial infection, *Sex Trans Dis* 2:136, 2012.

P, Patient population of interest; I, intervention or area of interest; C, comparison of interest or comparison group; O, outcomes of interest (see p. 12).

vaginal, anal, or oral sex. Numerous different serotypes, or strains, of *C. trachomatis* cause urogenital infections (e.g., non-gonococcal urethritis [NGU] in men and cervicitis in women), ocular trachoma, and lymphogranuloma venereum. Risk factors for chlamydial infection are presented in Table 53-5. As with gonorrhea, chlamydial infections result in a superficial mucosal infection that can become more invasive.

Clinical Manifestations

Chlamydial infection is known as a silent disease because symptoms may be absent or minor in most infected women and in

FIG. 53-7 Chlamydial epididymitis. Red, swollen scrotum.

TABLE 53-6 COLLABORATIVE CARE

Chlamydial Infection

Diagnostic
- History and physical examination
- Nucleic acid amplification test (NAAT)
- Direct fluorescent antibody (DFA) test
- Enzyme immunoassay (EIA)
- Testing for other STIs (gonorrhea, HIV, syphilis)

Collaborative Therapy
- doxycycline (Vibramycin) or azithromycin (Zithromax)
- Alternative regimen: erythromycin, ofloxacin (Floxin), or levofloxacin (Levaquin)
- Instruction on abstinence from sexual intercourse for 7 days after completing treatment
- Treatment of all sexual partners

many men.[10] In men, signs and symptoms include urethritis (dysuria, urethral discharge), proctitis (rectal discharge and pain during defecation), and epididymitis (unilateral scrotal pain, swelling, tenderness, fever) (Fig. 53-7).

In women, signs and symptoms include cervicitis (mucopurulent discharge, hypertrophic ectopy [area that is edematous and bleeds easily]), urethritis (dysuria, frequent urination, pyuria), bartholinitis (purulent exudate), dyspareunia (pain with intercourse), and menstrual abnormalities.

Because chlamydial infections are closely associated with gonococcal infections, clinical differentiation may be difficult. In men, urethritis, epididymitis, and proctitis may occur with both infections. In women, bartholinitis, cervicitis, and salpingitis (inflammation of the fallopian tube) can occur in both chlamydial and gonococcal infections. Therefore both infections are usually treated concurrently even without diagnostic proof. The incubation period of 1 to 3 weeks for chlamydial infection is longer than that for gonorrhea, and the symptoms are often milder.

Complications

Complications often develop from poorly managed, inaccurately diagnosed, or undiagnosed chlamydial infections. The infection is often not diagnosed until complications appear.

In men, epididymitis can lead to rare complications, including abscess, sepsis, infertility, and reactive arthritis (a systemic condition accompanied by skin lesions and inflammation of the eye and urethra).

In women, chlamydial infections can cause fallopian tube damage, a leading cause of ectopic pregnancy and infertility. Complications from chlamydial infections in women may result in PID, which can lead to chronic pelvic pain.[11] PID can also cause nausea, vomiting, fever, malaise, and abnormal vaginal bleeding.

Diagnostic Studies

Chlamydial infections in men and women can be diagnosed by testing urine or collecting swab specimens from the endocervix or vagina (women) or urethra (men). Rectal swab specimens are tested in persons engaging in anal sex. Table 53-6 outlines collaborative care for chlamydial infections.

Cell culture can be used to detect *Chlamydia* organisms. The most common diagnostic tests include the NAAT, DFA test, and enzyme immunoassay (EIA). These tests do not require special handling of specimens and are easier to perform than cell cultures. Amplification tests are the most sensitive diagnostic methods available and require fewer organisms. In addition, these tests can be used with urine samples rather than urethral and cervical swabs.

Collaborative Care

The Centers for Disease Control and Prevention (CDC) recommends that all sexually active women 25 years of age or younger be routinely screened for *Chlamydia*.[9] The CDC further recommends annual screening of all women older than 25 years of age with one or more risk factors for the infection (see Table 53-5).

Drug Therapy. To avoid complications from chlamydial infection, treatment should not be delayed. Doxycycline or azithromycin is used to treat patients and their partners. Treatment of pregnant women usually prevents transmission to the fetus. Patients treated for chlamydial infections should abstain from sexual intercourse for 7 days after treatment and until all sexual partners have completed a full course of treatment. Follow-up care includes advising the patient to return if symptoms persist or recur, treating sexual partners, and encouraging condom use during all sexual contacts.

The high incidence of recurrence may be due to failure to treat the sexual partners of infected people. Because of the high prevalence of asymptomatic infections, screening of high-risk populations is needed to identify those who are infected.

VIRAL INFECTIONS

GENITAL HERPES

Genital herpes is caused by herpes simplex virus (HSV). It is not a reportable infection in most states. Its true incidence is difficult to determine because most people have few to no symptoms. In the United States at least 50 million people are infected with HSV type 2. In people ages 14 to 49 approximately one out of six have genital herpes.[12]

Etiology and Pathophysiology

HSV enters through the mucous membranes or breaks in the skin during contact with an infected person. The virus then reproduces inside the cell and spreads to the surrounding cells. The virus next enters the peripheral or autonomic nerve endings and ascends to the sensory or autonomic nerve ganglion, where it often becomes dormant. Viral reactivation (recurrence) may occur when the virus descends to the initial site of infection, either the mucous membranes or skin. When a person is infected with HSV, the virus usually persists within the individual for life. Transmission of HSV occurs through direct contact with skin or mucous membranes when an infected individual is symptomatic or through asymptomatic viral shedding.

Two different strains of HSV cause infection. In general, HSV type 1 (HSV-1) causes infection above the waist, involving the gingivae, the dermis, the upper respiratory tract, and the CNS. HSV type 2 (HSV-2) most frequently infects the genital tract and the perineum (i.e., locations below the waist). However, either strain can cause infection on the mouth or the genitalia. Although the majority of genital herpes cases are from HSV-2 infection, the incidence of anogenital herpes from HSV-1 is increasing among young women and men who have sex with men.

Clinical Manifestations

Primary Episode. In the *primary (initial) episode* of genital herpes the patient may complain of burning, itching, or tingling at the site of inoculation. Multiple small, vesicular, and sometimes painless lesions may appear on the inner thigh, penis, scrotum, vulva, perineum, perianal region, vagina, or cervix.[13] The vesicles contain large quantities of infectious viral particles (Fig. 53-8). The lesions rupture and form shallow, moist ulcerations. Finally, crusting and epithelialization of the erosions occur. Primary infections tend to be associated with local inflammation and pain, accompanied by systemic manifestations of fever, headache, malaise, myalgia, and regional lymphadenopathy.

Urination may be painful from the urine touching active lesions. Urinary retention may occur as a result of HSV urethri-

tis or cystitis. A purulent vaginal discharge may develop with HSV cervicitis.

Primary lesions are generally present for 17 to 20 days, but new lesions sometimes continue to develop for 6 weeks. The duration of symptoms is longer and the frequency of complications is greater in women. The lesions heal spontaneously unless secondary infection occurs.

Recurrent Episodes. *Recurrent genital herpes* occurs in about 50% to 80% of individuals during the year following the primary episode. Common trigger factors include stress, fatigue, sunburn, general illness, immunosuppression, and menses. Many patients can predict a recurrence by noticing the prodromal symptoms of tingling, burning, and itching at the site where the lesions will eventually appear.[13]

The symptoms of recurrent episodes are less severe, and the lesions usually heal within 8 to 12 days. With time, the recurrent lesions generally occur less frequently. In extreme cases this can indicate immunosuppression and may signal a need to test for HIV.

Complications

Autoinoculation of the virus to extragenital sites such as the fingers and lips ("cold sores") may occur (Fig. 53-9). Although most infections are relatively benign, complications of genital herpes may involve the CNS, causing aseptic meningitis and lower motor neuron damage. Neuron damage may result in atonic bladder, impotence, and constipation. Immunocompromised patients (e.g., HIV-infected patients) should be monitored closely for treatment failure and a slower healing time of HSV lesions.

Women with a primary episode of HSV near the time of delivery have the highest risk of transmitting genital herpes to the neonate. An active genital lesion at the time of delivery is usually an indication for cesarean delivery.[9] Acyclovir (Zovirax) may be given to pregnant women who are at least at 36 weeks of gestation to prevent neonatal transmission.[14]

Diagnostic Studies and Collaborative Care

A diagnosis of genital herpes is usually based on the patient's symptoms and history. Highly accurate serologic tests are available for the diagnosis of HSV-1 and HSV-2. These type-specific immunoassays test for antibodies to HSV. A viral culture of the active lesion can also be used to isolate the virus.

Encourage symptomatic treatment such as using good genital hygiene and wearing loose-fitting cotton undergarments. The lesions should be kept clean and dry. To ensure complete drying of the perineal area, women may use a hair dryer set on a cool setting. Frequent sitz baths may soothe the area and reduce inflammation. Drying agents such as colloidal oatmeal (Aveeno) and aluminum salts (Burow's solution) may

FIG. 53-8 Unruptured vesicles of herpes simplex virus type 2 (HSV-2). **A,** Vulvar area. **B,** Perianal area. **C,** Penile herpes simplex, ulcerative stage.

FIG. 53-9 Autoinoculation of herpes simplex virus (HSV) to the lips.

provide some relief from the burning and itching. Techniques to reduce pain on urination include pouring a pitcher of water onto the perineal area while voiding to dilute the urine, and voiding in a warm tub of water or shower. Pain may require a local anesthetic such as lidocaine (Xylocaine) or systemic analgesics such as codeine and aspirin.

Sexual transmission of HSV can occur during asymptomatic periods, and the use of barrier methods, especially condoms, should be encouraged. When lesions are present, the patient should avoid sexual activity altogether because even barrier protection is not satisfactory in eliminating infection transmission.

Drug Therapy. Treatment of HSV infection should be started before diagnostic results are available because early treatment reduces transmission and duration of the ulcers. Three antiviral agents are available for the treatment of HSV: acyclovir, valacyclovir (Valtrex), and famciclovir (Famvir). These drugs inhibit herpetic viral replication and are prescribed for primary and recurrent infections (Table 53-7). Acyclovir, valacyclovir, and famciclovir are also used to suppress frequent recurrences (six or more episodes per year).

Although not a cure, these drugs shorten the duration of viral shedding and the healing time of genital lesions and reduce outbreaks by 75%.[9] Continued use of oral acyclovir as suppressive therapy for up to 6 years is safe and effective for persons with frequent or severe recurrences. Adverse reactions are mild and include headache, occasional nausea and vomiting, and diarrhea. Acyclovir ointment has no clinical benefit in the treatment of recurrent lesions, either in speed of healing or in resolution of pain, and is not commonly recommended.

IV acyclovir is reserved for severe or life-threatening infections in which hospitalization is required for the treatment of disseminated infections, CNS infections (meningitis), or pneumonitis. Nephrotoxicity has been observed with high-dose IV use. Clinical trials are examining the effectiveness of a vaccine for HSV-2.[15]

TABLE 53-7 COLLABORATIVE CARE

Genital Herpes

Diagnostic
- History and physical examination
- Antibody assay for HSV type
- Viral isolation by tissue culture

Collaborative Therapy
Primary (Initial) Infection
- acyclovir (Zovirax), famciclovir (Famvir), or valacyclovir (Valtrex)

Recurrent Episodic Infection
- acyclovir, famciclovir, or valacyclovir
- Identify triggering factors
- Yearly Pap test
- Abstinence from sexual contact while lesions are present
- Symptomatic care
- Confidential counseling and testing for HIV

Suppressive Therapy
- acyclovir, famciclovir, or valacyclovir

Severe Infection
- acyclovir IV until clinical improvement, followed by oral antiviral therapy

Modified from Centers for Disease Control and Prevention: STD treatment guidelines. Retrieved from *www.cdc.gov/STD/treatment.*

GENITAL WARTS

Genital warts (*Condylomata acuminata*) are caused by the human papillomavirus (HPV). HPV is a highly contagious STI seen frequently in sexually active young adults. There are more than 100 types of papillomaviruses, many of which are sexually transmitted. Ninety percent of genital warts are caused by HPV types 6 and 11. Although genital warts are not malignant, other HPV types (e.g., types 16 and 18) are oncogenic and associated with cervical, vaginal, vulvar, anal, and penile cancers.[16] In most states, genital warts are not a reportable infection.

Minor trauma during intercourse can cause abrasions that allow HPV to enter the body. The epithelial cells infected with HPV undergo transformation and proliferation to form a warty growth. The incubation period of the virus is generally 3 to 4 months, but may be longer.

Clinical Manifestations and Complications

Most individuals who have HPV infection do not know that they are infected because symptoms are often not present. Genital warts are discrete single or multiple papillary growths that are white to gray and pink-flesh colored. They may grow and coalesce to form large, cauliflower-like masses. Most patients have 1 to 10 genital warts.

In men the warts may occur on the penis and scrotum, around the anus, or in the urethra. In women the warts may be located on the inner thighs, vulva, vagina, or cervix and in the perianal area (Fig. 53-10). There are usually no other signs or symptoms. Itching may occur with anogenital warts. Bleeding on defecation may occur with anal warts.

During pregnancy, genital warts tend to grow rapidly and increase in size. An infected mother may transmit the condition to her newborn. Cesarean delivery is not routinely indicated unless the birth canal becomes blocked by massive warts.

Diagnostic Studies and Collaborative Care

Up to two thirds of the early lesions caused by HPV are undetectable by visual examination. A diagnosis of genital warts can be made on the basis of the gross appearance of the lesions. Warts may be confused with condylomata lata of secondary syphilis, carcinoma, or benign neoplasms. Serologic and cytologic testing should be done to rule out these conditions. HPV deoxyribonucleic acid (DNA) tests help determine if women with abnormal Papanicolaou (Pap) test results need further follow-up. Currently, HPV cannot be confirmed by culture.

Prevention of genital warts is hampered by the high proportion of asymptomatic infections and lack of curative treatment. The primary goal when treating visible genital warts is the removal of symptomatic warts.

Treatment consists of chemical or ablative (removal with laser or electrocautery) methods. One common treatment is the use of 80% to 90% trichloroacetic acid (TCA) or bichloroacetic acid (BCA) applied directly to the wart surface. Petroleum jelly is applied to the surrounding normal skin to minimize irritation before a small amount of TCA is applied to the wart with a cotton swab. A sharp stinging pain is often felt with initial acid contact, but this quickly subsides. TCA is not washed off after treatment.

Podophyllin resin (10% to 25%), a cytotoxic agent, is recommended therapy for small external genital warts. When podophyllin is used, it is applied carefully to each wart, avoiding normal tissue, and is then thoroughly washed off in 1 to 4 hours. This substance encourages the sloughing of skin containing

FIG. 53-10 Genital warts. **A,** Severe vulvar warts. **B,** Perineal wart. **C,** Multiple genital warts of the glans penis.

viral particles. Podophyllin has local (e.g., pain, burning) and systemic (e.g., nausea, dizziness, leukopenia, respiratory distress) toxic symptoms. In general, warts located on moist surfaces respond better to topical treatment (e.g., TCA, podophyllin) than do warts on drier surfaces.

Patient-managed treatment is also an option. Podofilox (5%) liquid and gel are available by prescription (Condylox and Condylox Gel). The patient applies the solution or gel for 3 successive days followed by 4 days of no treatment. Treatment can be repeated for up to 4 weeks or until the lesions resolve. Imiquimod (5%) cream (Aldara) is an immune response modifier that is applied once daily at bedtime, three times a week for up to 16 weeks.

The removal of warts may or may not decrease infectivity. Genital warts are difficult to treat and often require multiple office visits.[17] The therapy should be modified if a patient has not improved after three treatments or if the warts have not completely disappeared after six treatments.

If the warts do not regress with any of these therapies, treatments such as cryotherapy with liquid nitrogen, electrocautery, laser therapy, intralesional use of α-interferon, and surgical excision may be indicated. Because treatment does not destroy the virus, merely the infected tissue, recurrences and reinfection are possible, and careful long-term follow-up is advised.

HPV Vaccines. Vaccines are available to protect against HPV types 6, 11, 16, and 18 (Gardasil) and HPV types 16 and 18 (Cervarix). The vaccine is given in three IM doses over a 6-month period and has few side effects.

For females, either Gardasil or Cervarix vaccine is recommended at age 11 or 12 years. It may be given to girls starting at age 9. The vaccine is also recommended for females 13 through 26 years of age who did not get all three doses when they were younger.

For males, Gardasil vaccine is recommended at ages 11 or 12 years. It may be given to boys starting at age 9. This vaccine is recommended for males 13 through 21 years of age who have not completed the three-dose series. This vaccine may be given to men 22 through 26 years of age who have not completed the three-dose series. It is recommended for men through age 26 who have sex with men or whose immune system is weakened because of HIV infection, other illness, or medications.[18]

Because of reported cases of syncope (fainting) during vaccine administration, the patient should remain seated or lying down and be closely observed for 15 minutes after vaccination. These vaccines do not treat active HPV infection. Ideally, individuals should receive the vaccine before the start of sexual activity, but those who are active or even infected still get protection from the HPV types not already acquired. HPV vaccine reduces the risk of anal cancer and may also protect against oropharynx cancer.[19]

NURSING MANAGEMENT
SEXUALLY TRANSMITTED INFECTIONS

NURSING ASSESSMENT
Subjective and objective data that should be obtained from a person with an STI are presented in Table 53-8.

NURSING DIAGNOSES
Nursing diagnoses for the patient with an STI include, but are not limited to, the following:
- Risk for infection *related to* lack of knowledge about mode of transmission, inadequate personal and genital hygiene, and failure to practice precautionary measures
- Anxiety *related to* impact of the condition on relationships, disease outcome, and lack of knowledge of disease
- Ineffective health maintenance *related to* lack of knowledge about disease process, inadequate follow-up measures, and possibility of reinfection

PLANNING
The overall goals are that the patient with an STI will (1) demonstrate understanding of the mode of transmission of STIs and the risk posed by STIs, (2) complete treatment and return for appropriate follow-up, (3) notify or assist in notification of sexual contacts about their need for testing and treatment, (4) abstain from intercourse until infection is resolved, and (5) demonstrate knowledge of safer sex practices.

NURSING IMPLEMENTATION
HEALTH PROMOTION. Many approaches to stopping the spread of STIs have been advocated and have met with varying degrees of success. Be prepared to discuss "safe" sex practices with all patients, not only those who are perceived to be at risk. These practices include abstinence, monogamy, avoidance of certain high-risk sexual practices, and use of condoms and other barriers to limit contact with potentially infectious body fluids or lesions. Sexual abstinence is a certain method of avoiding all

EVIDENCE-BASED PRACTICE

Applying the Evidence

F.C. is a 19-yr-old man who is being seen in the health care center for signs and symptoms of a urinary tract infection. When asked, he shares with you that he is sexually active. After reviewing his health history, you learn that he has not received the human papillomavirus (HPV) vaccine. You discuss the risks and benefits of the vaccine and suggest that he consider getting it.

Best Available Evidence	Clinician Expertise	Patient Preferences and Values
Males ages 9-26 can get vaccinated with Gardasil to reduce the incidence of anogenital HPV infections, which are caused by HPV types 6, 11, 16, or 18. Gardasil protects against the two HPV types (6 and 11) that cause 90% of genital warts.	Approximately 90% of anal cancers have been linked to HPV infection. Males may be unaware of the expanded recommendations for Gardasil, which was originally approved to prevent cervical, vulvar, and vaginal cancer caused by HPV types 6, 11, 16, and 18 in females ages 9 through 26.	F.C. states that he never has unprotected sex and does not like injections.

Your Decision and Action

After listening carefully, F.C. decides to talk to a few of his friends before making a decision about the vaccine. He tells you that he had no idea that he could get HPV infections. If he decides to get the vaccine, he will be back. You document your discussion in his chart.

Reference for Evidence

Advisory Committee on Immunization Practices: Recommendations on the use of quadrivalent human papillomavirus vaccine in males—advisory committee on immunization practices (ACIP) 2011, Centers for Disease Control and Prevention. Retrieved from *www.cdc.gov/mmwr/preview/mmwrhtml/mm6050a3.htm.*

HEALTHY PEOPLE

Health Impact of Responsible Sexual Behavior

- Greatly reduces the risk of contracting sexually transmitted infections, including infection from human immunodeficiency virus, gonorrhea, chlamydial infection, syphilis, and herpes
- Greatly reduces the risk of spreading viruses such as human papillomavirus that could potentially cause cervical, vulvar, vaginal, penile, anal, and oropharyngeal cancers

TABLE 53-8 NURSING ASSESSMENT

Sexually Transmitted Infections

Subjective Data
Important Health Information
Past health history: Contact with individuals with STIs, multiple sexual partners
Medications: Oral contraceptives; allergy to any antibiotics, especially penicillin

Functional Health Patterns
Health perception–health management: Shared needles during IV drug use; malaise
Nutritional-metabolic: Nausea, vomiting, anorexia; pharyngitis, oral lesions, itching at infected site; chills; alopecia
Elimination: Dysuria, urinary frequency, retention; urethral discharge; tenesmus, proctitis
Cognitive-perceptual: Arthralgia; headache; painful, burning lesions
Sexuality-reproductive: Dyspareunia; vaginal discharge, menstrual abnormalities; genital or perianal lesions

Objective Data
General
Fever, lymphadenopathy (generalized or inguinal)

Integumentary
Syphilis: Primary: Painless, indurated genital, oral, or perianal lesions
   Secondary: Bilateral, symmetric rash on palms, soles, or entire body; mucous patches on mouth or tongue; alopecia
Genital herpes: Painful genital or anal vesicular lesions
Genital warts: Single or multiple gray or white genital or anal warts (possibly becoming massive)

Gastrointestinal
Purulent rectal discharge (indicator of gonorrhea), rectal lesions, proctitis

Urinary
Urethral discharge, erythema

Reproductive
Cervical discharge, lesions, inflamed Bartholin's glands

Possible Diagnostic Findings
Gonorrhea: Positive Gram stain, smears, cultures, and DNA amplification for *Neisseria gonorrhoeae*
Syphilis: Positive findings on VDRL and RPR, spirochetes on dark-field microscopy
Chlamydia: Positive culture or DNA amplification for *Chlamydia*
Genital herpes: Positive HSV-1 or HSV-2 antibody titer; positive tissue culture for HSV-1 or HSV-2

DNA, Deoxyribonucleic acid; *HSV-1,* herpes simplex virus type 1; *HSV-2,* herpes simplex virus type 2; *RPR,* rapid plasma reagin; *STIs,* sexually transmitted infections; *VDRL,* Venereal Disease Research Laboratory.

STIs, but few people consider this a feasible alternative to sexual expression. Limiting sexual intimacies outside of a well-established monogamous relationship can reduce the risk of contracting an STI. A teaching guide for the patient with an STI is presented in Table 53-9.

All sexually active women should be screened for cervical cancer using a Pap test. Women with a history of STIs are at greater risk for cervical cancer. Anal Pap tests should also be done for all individuals who are recipients of anal sex. (Pap tests are discussed in Chapter 54.)

Measures to Prevent Infection. An inspection of the sexual partner's genitalia before coitus is recommended. Discharge, sores, blisters, or rash should be viewed with concern. A patient who is aware of specific signs and symptoms of infection can intelligently make the decision to continue the sexual interaction with modifications or elect not to have sexual relations. The patient should remember that, when engaging in sex, he or she is exposed to the infections of everyone with whom the partner has ever had sex.

Tell men that some protection is provided if they void immediately after intercourse and wash their genitalia and the adjacent areas with soap and water. Women may also benefit from postcoital voiding and washing. However, emphasize that these practices do not provide adequate protection against STIs after exposure to infection.

Spermicidal jellies and creams have not been shown to reduce the risk of contracting STIs.[20] These same barriers may serve as supplementary lubrication, thereby decreasing irritation and friction. They also reduce the chance that a minor laceration could serve as the entry point for an infectious organism.

TABLE 53-9 PATIENT TEACHING GUIDE

Sexually Transmitted Infections

When teaching the patient with sexually transmitted infections:

1. Explain precautions to take such as
   - voiding and washing genitalia and surrounding area after coitus to flush out some organisms and reduce the occurrence of infection
   - using condoms
   - being monogamous
   - asking potential partners about sexual history
   - avoiding sex with partners who use IV drugs or who have visible oral, inguinal, genital, perineal, or anal lesions
2. Explain the importance of taking all antibiotics and/or antiviral agents as prescribed. Symptoms will improve after 1-2 days of therapy, but organisms may still be present.
3. Teach patient about the need for treatment of sexual partners to prevent transmission of infection.
4. Instruct patient to abstain from sexual intercourse during treatment and to use condoms when sexual activity is resumed to prevent spread of infection and reinfection.
5. Explain the importance of follow-up examination and reculture at least once after treatment if appropriate to confirm complete cure and prevent relapse.
6. Allow patient and partner to verbalize concerns to clarify areas that need explanation.
7. Instruct patient about symptoms of complications and need to report problems to ensure proper follow-up and early treatment of reinfection.
8. Inform patient regarding state of infectivity to prevent a false sense of security, which might result in careless sexual practices and poor personal hygiene.

Proper use of a condom provides a highly effective mechanical barrier to infection. The condom should be undamaged and correctly in place throughout all phases of sexual activity. A deterrent to barrier usage is alcohol and drug use. Use of barrier contraceptives requires planning and motivation, both of which are impaired with alcohol or drug ingestion. Give specific verbal and written instructions on the proper use of condoms (see eTable 15-4 available at the website for Chapter 15). Partners should discuss any objections to condom usage, such as interference with spontaneity and the presence of a barrier. Information about the mechanics of sexual arousal and incorporating a condom into lovemaking can help in overcoming the individual's or partner's resistance to its use. Female condoms are lubricated polyurethane sheaths designed for vaginal use but are considerably more expensive than male condoms (see eTable 15-5 available at the website for Chapter 15).

Among couples with one infected partner, consistent and scrupulous condom use can reduce transmission to the uninfected partner. Unprotected anal intercourse and other high-risk behaviors should be eliminated, and condoms should be used if sexual contact continues.

Initiate a discussion to assess the risk for contracting an STI. Questions to ask include number of partners, type of birth control used, use of condoms, history of an STI, use of IV drugs, and sexual preference. Instead of asking if a patient is homosexual or asking only about sexual preference, it can be more revealing to ask, "Do you have sex with men or women or both?" Some men who have sex with men do not identify themselves as homosexual or bisexual, which is a major contributor to infection of wives and female or male partners. Although the majority of STIs are transmitted between men having sex with men and heterosexual contact, it is possible to transmit an STI between women.[21]

Plan teaching based on the response to these questions. Interpersonal skills necessary for this interview include respect, compassion, and a nonjudgmental attitude. Tailor your counseling to the individual. Do not assume that older people are not at risk, since an increasing number of older people are becoming infected.

Screening Programs. Screening programs can help prevent certain STIs. For many years, there have been various screening programs to identify cases of syphilis. Many institutions offer voluntary prenatal HIV and syphilis testing and counseling for pregnant women.

Screening programs have been developed and implemented for detection of gonorrhea and chlamydial infection. These programs are targeted to women because women are more likely to have asymptomatic gonorrhea and thereby serve as sources of infection. Routine gonorrheal and chlamydial testing during pelvic examinations and prenatal visits are a major part of these programs. Mass application of screening programs for genital chlamydial infections, genital herpes, and HPV infections (warts) may also be possible with the advent of rapid, cost-effective tests.

Case Finding. Interviewing and case finding are other methods used to control STIs. These activities are directed toward locating and examining all contacts of each known patient with an STI as soon after sexual exposure as possible so that effective treatment can be initiated. Trained interviewers may often find cases even if they are supplied with only limited information. The caseworkers, who are often nurses, are aware of the social implications of these diseases and the need for discretion. Sexual contacts are often not informed about the origin of the information naming them as a contact so that greater cooperation and privacy are ensured.

Partner notification and treatment impose a heavy burden on public health departments and, as a result, the notification often becomes the responsibility of the infected partner. The infected partner may choose not to inform sexual partners, and the partners may choose not to seek treatment. *Expedited partner therapy* (EPT) is a safe, effective tool for treating STIs that allows a health care provider to provide prescriptions or medications to a patient to take to his or her partner, without examining the partner. EPT has been shown to be useful in ensuring partner treatment among men and reducing repeat infections among women.[22] Several states have adopted legislation to allow health care providers to dispense antibiotic therapy for sex partners of individuals with chlamydial infection or gonorrhea. The legality of treating without evaluating the patient is uncertain in some states, and it is illegal in others.

Educational and Research Programs. Actively encourage your community to provide better education about STIs for its citizens. Teenagers, who are known to have a high incidence of infection, should be a prime target for such educational programs. STI rates are also rising in older adults.[23] Older adults are less likely to use condoms and in general have a harder time initiating discussion of sexual health issues.

Knowledge and understanding can decrease the STI epidemic. The HPV vaccine that protects against genital warts and cervical cancer should be encouraged before the start of sexual activity. Accurate and current information may help reduce parental fears related to the vaccine. Consider stressing the prevention of cancer as a reason for the vaccine, which may be more productive and less controversial, thus making the parent and adolescent more receptive. Efforts are being made to develop vaccines for syphilis, gonorrhea, genital herpes, and HIV. Many clinicians view the development of effective vaccines as a prerequisite for the eradication of STIs.

ACUTE INTERVENTION

Psychologic Support. The diagnosis of an STI may be met with a variety of emotions, such as shame, guilt, anger, and a desire for vengeance. Provide counseling and encourage the patient to verbalize feelings. Couples in marital or committed relationships are confronted with an added problem when an STI is diagnosed, and they must face the implication of sexual activity outside the relationship. The acute problem raises other concerns about their relationship and may serve as an incentive for further problem solving. The couple needs support and counseling. A referral for professional counseling to explore the ramifications of an STI in their relationship may be indicated.

A patient who has genital herpes is faced with the fact that repeated infections can occur and that no cure is available. This can be frustrating and disruptive to the patient's physical, emotional, social, and sexual life. Help the patient identify and avoid any factors that may precipitate the condition. Inform the patient that the frequency and severity of recurrences will probably decrease over time.

HPV infections involve a prolonged course of treatment. The patient can become frustrated and distressed because of frequent office visits, associated costs, potential for unpleasant side effects as a result of treatment, and effects of the infection on future health and sexual relationships. Support and a willingness to listen to the patient's concerns are needed. Support groups are also available.

Follow-up. If you work in public health facilities, clinics, or other outpatient settings, you are more likely to care for a patient with an STI than if you work in a hospital setting. Whatever the setting, as a nurse you are in a position to explain and interpret treatment measures such as the purpose and possible side effects of prescribed drugs and the need for follow-up care.

Frequently, single-dose treatment for gonorrhea, chlamydial infection, and syphilis helps prevent the problems associated with nonadherence with drug therapy. Give special instructions to the patient requiring multiple-dose therapy to complete the prescribed regimen. Also inform the patient about problems resulting from nonadherence. All patients should return to the treatment center for a repeat culture from the infected sites or for serologic testing at designated times to determine the effectiveness of the treatment. Explaining to the patient that cures are not always obtained on the first treatment can reinforce the need for a follow-up visit. Also advise the patient to inform sexual partners of the need for testing and treatment, regardless of whether they are free of symptoms or experiencing symptoms.

Hygiene Measures. Emphasize to the patient with an STI the importance of certain hygiene measures. An important component is frequent hand washing and bathing. Bathing and cleaning of the involved areas can provide local comfort and prevent secondary infection. Because douching may spread the infection or undermine local immune responses, it is contraindicated. The synthetic materials used in most undergarments frequently increase or exacerbate local irritations by trapping moisture. Cotton undergarments provide better absorption and are cooler and more comfortable for the patient with an STI.

Sexual Activity. Sexual abstinence is indicated during the communicable phase of the infection. If sexual activity occurs before treatment has been completed, emphasize to the patient

---

ETHICAL/LEGAL DILEMMAS
Confidentiality and HIPAA

Situation

P.H., a 22-yr-old woman, is informed of the positive results of a test for chlamydial infection. You advise her to tell her sexual partners that she has this disease. She refuses to tell her boyfriend because he will know that she has had sex with another partner. You later learn that the nursing student who was in the clinic for the day, who is a friend of the boyfriend, hinted to him that he should have STI testing.

Ethical/Legal Points for Consideration

- Each state has requirements for reporting communicable diseases and other health-related data. Inform the patient of the reporting requirements for communicable diseases.
- Nurses and other health care professionals have both a legal and an ethical obligation to maintain confidentiality of patient information. The Health Insurance Portability and Accountability Act (HIPAA) ensures the privacy of personal health information.
- Your primary obligation is to the patient seeking care. Patient teaching is one way to establish a partnership with this woman. Share information about the effects of the disease if it is not treated, the consequences of reinfection, and the effect of the disease on others who may not know that they are infected. Then encourage the patient to inform her partners of the diagnosis for the good of everyone.

Discussion Questions

1. What are your state's requirements for reportable conditions?
2. In your opinion, what is the best way to balance the needs of an individual patient with those of the general public?
3. What are the risks to the institution for the breach of confidentiality and HIPAA?

---

the importance of using condoms to help prevent the spread of infection and reinfection. Also encourage condom usage after treatment to prevent future exposure to infection. The patient can also choose to relate to a partner in an intimate way that avoids both coitus and oral-genital contact. Note that even single-dose treatments can take up to 1 week to be effective and thus the patient is infectious during this period.

AMBULATORY AND HOME CARE. Because many STIs are cured with a single dose or short course of antibiotic therapy, many persons are casual about the outcome of these infections. The consequences of this attitude can include delays in treatment, nonadherence with instructions, and subsequent development of complications. The complications are serious and costly. They can result in disfigurement and destruction of important tissues and organs.

Surgery and prolonged therapy are indicated for many patients with infection-related complications. Major surgical procedures such as resection of an aneurysm or aortic valve replacement may be necessary to treat cardiovascular problems caused by syphilis. Pelvic surgery and procedures to correct fertility problems secondary to an STI may include lysis of adhesions, dilation of strictures, reconstructive tuboplasty, and in vitro fertilization.

EVALUATION

Expected outcomes for the patient with an STI are that the patient will

- Describe modes of transmission
- Use appropriate hygienic measures
- Experience no reinfection
- Demonstrate compliance with follow-up protocol

CASE STUDY

Gonorrhea and Chlamydial Infection

Eyecandy Images/
Thinkstock

Patient Profile

C.R. is a 24-yr-old Hispanic woman who is seen at the outpatient clinic with complaints of a purulent yellow-white discharge and frequent urination over the past 2 wk. She is sexually active with a new partner after breaking up with a long-term boyfriend. She was treated in the past for *Chlamydia* at age 20.

Subjective Data

- Her sexual partner does not use a condom or spermicide with intercourse
- Her last menstrual period was 3 wk ago
- Her sexual partner was recently treated for epididymitis
- Appears very nervous

Objective Data

- Cervical ectopy noted during Pap test
- Mucopurulent cervical discharge
- Urine pregnancy test is negative
- Nucleic acid amplification test is positive for *Neisseria gonorrhoeae* and *Chlamydia trachomatis*

Collaborative Care

- ceftriaxone 250 mg IM once
- doxycycline 100 mg bid for 7 days

Discussion Questions

1. What were C.R.'s risk factors for acquiring gonorrhea and chlamydial infection?
2. What complications could occur if C.R.'s infections are not treated?
3. *Priority Decision:* What is the priority of care for C.R.?
4. What instructions should C.R. receive to ensure successful treatment? To prevent reinfection? To prevent further transmission of the infection?
5. *Delegation Decision:* Which nursing personnel should be responsible for teaching C.R. what she needs to know about other sexually transmitted infections (STIs): registered nurse, licensed practical/vocational nurse, unlicensed assistive personnel?
6. What impact is her diagnosis likely to have on C.R.'s self-image? On her relationship with her sexual partner?
7. *Priority Decision:* Based on the assessment data presented, what are the priority nursing diagnoses? Are there any collaborative problems?
8. *Evidence-Based Practice:* C.R. mentions she is using the spermicide nonoynol-9 (N-9) to protect herself against STIs. Would you advise her to continue to use it?

ⓔvolve Answers available at *http://evolve.elsevier.com/Lewis/medsurg.*

BRIDGE TO NCLEX EXAMINATION

The number of the question corresponds to the same-numbered outcome at the beginning of the chapter.

1. The individual with the lowest risk for sexually transmitted pelvic inflammatory disease is a woman who uses
   a. oral contraceptives.
   b. barrier methods of contraception.
   c. an intrauterine device for contraception.
   d. a Norplant implant or injectable Depo-Provera for contraception.
2. The nurse is obtaining a subjective data assessment from a woman reported as a sexual contact of a man with chlamydial infection. The nurse understands that symptoms of chlamydial infection in women
   a. are frequently absent.
   b. are similar to those of genital herpes.
   c. include a macular palmar rash in the later stages.
   d. may involve chancres inside the vagina that are not visible.
3. A primary HSV infection differs from recurrent HSV episodes in that *(select all that apply)*
   a. only primary infections are sexually transmitted.
   b. symptoms are less severe during recurrent episodes.
   c. transmission of the virus to a fetus is less likely during primary infection.
   d. systemic manifestations such as fever and myalgia are more common in primary infection.
   e. lesions from recurrent HSV are more likely to transmit the virus than lesions from primary HSV.

4. Explain to the patient with gonorrhea that treatment will include both ceftriaxone and doxycycline because
   a. most patients need both drugs to eradicate the organism.
   b. coverage with more than one antibiotic will prevent reinfection.
   c. no single agent successfully eradicates both primary and recurrent infections.
   d. the high rate of coexisting chlamydial infection and gonorrhea indicates coverage with both drugs.
5. In assessing patients for STIs, the nurse needs to know that many STIs can be asymptomatic. Which STIs can be asymptomatic *(select all that apply)*?
   a. Syphilis
   b. Gonorrhea
   c. Genital warts
   d. Genital herpes
   e. Chlamydial infection
6. To prevent the infection and transmission of STIs, the nurse's teaching plan would include an explanation of
   a. the appropriate use of oral contraceptives.
   b. sexual positions that can be used to avoid infection.
   c. the necessity of annual Pap tests for patients with HPV.
   d. sexual practices that are considered high-risk behaviors.

7. Provide emotional support to a patient with an STI by
   a. offering information on how safer sexual practices can prevent STIs.
   b. showing concern when listening to the patient who expresses negative feelings.
   c. reassuring the patient that the disease is highly curable with appropriate treatment.
   d. helping the patient who received an STI from his or her sexual partner in forgiving the partner.

1. b, 2. a, 3. b, 4. d, 5. a, 6. d, e, c, b, 7. b

Ⓔvolve

For rationales to these answers and even more NCLEX review questions, visit *http://evolve.elsevier.com/Lewis/medsurg*.

REFERENCES

1. Centers for Disease Control and Prevention: STD trends in the United States: 2010 national data for gonorrhea, *Chlamydia*, and syphilis. Retrieved from *www.cdc.gov/std/stats10/trends.htm*.
*2. Reece M, Herbenick D, Schick V, et al: Condom use rates in a national probability sample of males and females ages 14 to 94 in the United States, *J Sex Med* 7(Suppl 5):266, 2010.
3. Centers for Disease Control and Prevention: 2010 Sexually transmitted disease surveillance: gonorrhea. Retrieved from *www.cdc.gov/std/stats10/gonorrhea.htm*.
4. Brill J: Sexually transmitted infections in men, *Prim Care* 37:509, 2010.
5. Knox T, Wanke C: Gastrointestinal manifestations of HIV and AIDS: anorectal diseases. In Goldman L, Schafer A, editors: *Goldman's Cecil medicine*, ed 24, Philadelphia, 2011, Saunders.
6. Borhart J, Birnbaumer D: Emergency department management of sexually transmitted infections, *Emerg Med Clin North Am* 29:587, 2011.
7. Centers for Disease Control and Prevention: Cephalosporin susceptibility among *Neisseria gonorrhoeae* isolates—United States, 2000-2010, *MMWR* 60:873, 2011.
*8. Hawkes S, Matin N, Broutet N, et al: Effectiveness of interventions to improve screening for syphilis in pregnancy: a systematic review and meta-analysis, *Lancet Infect Dis* 11:684, 2011.
9. Centers for Disease Control and Prevention: Sexually transmitted diseases treatment guidelines 2010, *MMWR* 59(#RR-12):1-110, 2010.
10. Champion J, Collins J: Reducing STIs: screening, treatment, and counseling, *Nurse Pract* 37:40, 2012.
11. Haggerty C, Gottlieb S, Taylor B, et al: Risk of sequelae after *Chlamydia trachomatis* genital infection in women, *J Infect Dis* 202(Suppl 2):S134, 2010.
12. Centers for Disease Control and Prevention: Genital herpes: CDC fact sheet. Retrieved from *www.cdc.gov/std/stats10/trends.htm*.
13. Roett M, Mayor M, Uduhiri K: Diagnosis and management of genital ulcers, *Am Fam Physician* 85:254, 2012.

14. Su C, McKay B: Treatment of HSV infection in late pregnancy, *Am Fam Physician* 85:390, 2012.
15. Johnston C, Koelle DM, Wald A: HSV-2: in pursuit of a vaccine, *J Clin Invest* 121:4600, 2011.
16. Hariri S, Unger ER, Sternberg M, et al: Prevalence of genital human papillomavirus among females in the United States: the national health and nutrition examination survey, 2003-2006, *J Infect Dis* 204:566, 2011.
17. American Academy of Dermatology: Genital warts. Retrieved from *www.aad.org/skin-conditions/dermatology-a-to-z/genital-warts*.
18. Centers for Disease Control and Prevention: HPV vaccine (Gardasil): what you need to know. Retrieved from *www.cdc.gov/vaccines/pubs/vis/downloads/vis-hpv-gardasil.pdf*.
19. Palefsky J, Giuliano A, Goldstone S, et al: HPV vaccine against anal HPV infection and anal intraepithelial neoplasia, *N Engl J Med* 365:1576, 2011.
*20. Wilkinson D, Ramjee G, Tholandi M, et al: Nonoxynol-9 for preventing vaginal acquisition of HIV infection by women from men, *Cochrane Database Syst Rev* 4:CD003936, 2002 (republished online 2009, 2012).
21. Ripley V: Promoting sexual health in women who have sex with women, *Nurs Stand* 25:41, 2011.
22. Centers for Disease Control and Prevention: *Expedited partner therapy in the management of sexually transmitted diseases*, Atlanta, 2006, US Department of Health and Human Services. Retrieved from *www.cdc.gov/std/treatment/eptfinalreport2006.pdf*.
23. Jeffers L, DiBartolo M: Raising health care provider awareness of sexually transmitted disease in patients over age 50, *MEDSURG Nurs* 20:285, 2011.

RESOURCES

American Social Health Association
   www.ashastd.org
   (for teens) *www.iwannaknow.org/teens/index.html*
Centers for Disease Control and Prevention, STD/HIV/AIDS
   www.cdc.gov/std
Sexuality Information and Education Council of the United States
   www.siecus.org

*Evidenced-based information for clinical practice.

54

What we have once enjoyed we can never lose.
All that we love deeply becomes a part of us.
Helen Keller

Nursing Management
Female Reproductive Problems

Nancy MacMullen and Laura Dulski

LEARNING OUTCOMES

1. Summarize the etiologies of infertility and the strategies for diagnosis and treatment of the infertile woman.
2. Describe the etiology, clinical manifestations, and nursing and collaborative management of menstrual problems and abnormal vaginal bleeding.
3. Identify the risk factors, clinical manifestations, and collaborative care of ectopic pregnancy.
4. Describe the changes related to menopause and the nursing and collaborative management of the patient with menopausal symptoms.
5. Differentiate among the common problems that affect the vulva, vagina, and cervix and the related nursing and collaborative management.
6. Describe the assessment, collaborative care, and nursing management of women with pelvic inflammatory disease and endometriosis.

7. Explain the clinical manifestations, diagnostic studies, collaborative care, and surgical therapy for cervical, endometrial, ovarian, and vulvar cancers.
8. Summarize the preoperative and postoperative nursing management for the patient requiring surgery of the female reproductive system.
9. Differentiate among the common problems that occur with cystoceles, rectoceles, and fistulas and the related nursing and collaborative management.
10. Summarize the clinical manifestations of sexual assault and the appropriate nursing and collaborative management of the patient who has been sexually assaulted.

KEY TERMS

abortion, p. 1278
amenorrhea, p. 1280
cystocele, p. 1300
dysmenorrhea, p. 1280
ectopic pregnancy, p. 1282

endometriosis, p. 1289
hysterectomy, p. 1282
infertility, p. 1276
leiomyomas, p. 1290
menopause, p. 1283

pelvic inflammatory disease (PID), p. 1287
perimenopause, p. 1283
premenstrual syndrome (PMS), p. 1279

rectocele, p. 1300
sexual assault, p. 1301
uterine prolapse, p. 1300

INFERTILITY

Infertility is the inability to conceive after at least 1 year of regular unprotected intercourse.[1] Approximately 15% of couples in North America are infertile. Understandably, infertility can be both a physical and an emotional crisis.

Etiology and Pathophysiology

Infertility may be caused by either female or male or combined factors. (Conditions that cause male infertility are discussed in Chapter 55.) In some cases, the cause of infertility may not be identified.

The factors usually causing female infertility include problems with ovulation (anovulation or inadequate corpus luteum), tubal obstruction or dysfunction (endometriosis or damage from pelvic infection), and uterine or cervical factors (fibroid tumors or structural anomalies). Risk factors for infertility include tobacco and illicit drug use and being obese or thin. In women the risk for infertility starts about age 30 and increases after age 40.[2]

Reviewed by Brenda Pavill, RN, PhD, FNP, Associate Professor–Nursing, Misericordia University, Dallas, Pennsylvania; and Beth Perry Black, RN, PhD, Professor of Nursing, UNC at Chapel Hill School of Nursing, UNC School of Nursing, Chapel Hill, North Carolina.

TABLE 54-1   COLLABORATIVE CARE

Infertility

Diagnostic
- History and physical examination of both partners, including psychosocial functioning
- Review of menstrual and gynecologic history
- Assessment of possible sexually transmitted infections
- Hormone levels
  - Serum hormone levels (e.g., FSH, LH, prolactin)
  - Urinary LH
- Pap test
- Ovulatory study
- Tubal patency study
  - Hysterosalpingogram
- Postcoital test
  - Cervical mucus
  - Sperm penetration assay
  - Semen analysis
- Pelvic ultrasound
- Genetic screening

Collaborative Therapy
- Hormone therapy
- Drug therapy (see Table 54-2)
- Intrauterine insemination
- Assisted reproductive technologies (ARTs)

FSH, Follicle-stimulating hormone; *LH,* luteinizing hormone.

TABLE 54-2   DRUG THERAPY

Infertility

Drug	Mechanism of Action
Selective Estrogen Receptor Modulator	
clomiphene (Clomid, Serophene)	Stimulates hypothalamus to ↑ production of GnRH, which ↑ release of LH and FSH. End result is stimulation of ovulation.
Menotropins (Human Menopausal Gonadotropin)	
Pergonal Repronex Humegon	Product made of FSH and LH to promote the development and maturation of follicles in the ovaries.
Follicle-Stimulating Hormone Agonists	
urofollitropin (Fertinex, Bravelle) follitropin (Gonal-f, Follistim)	Stimulate follicle growth and maturation by mimicking the body's natural FSH.
GnRH Antagonists	
cetrorelix (Cetrotide) ganirelix (Antagon)	Prevent premature LH surges and premature ovulation in women undergoing ovarian stimulation.
GnRH Agonists	
leuprolide (Lupron) nafarelin (Synarel)	Suppress release of LH and FSH with continuous use. May also be used in the treatment of endometriosis.
Human Chorionic Gonadotropin (hCG)	
Pregnyl Profasi Novarel	Induces ovulation by stimulating the release of eggs from follicles.

FSH, Follicle-stimulating hormone; *GnRH,* gonadotropin-releasing hormone; *LH,* luteinizing hormone.

Diagnostic Studies

A detailed history and a general physical examination of the woman and her partner provide the basis for selecting diagnostic studies (Table 54-1). The possibility of medical, genetic, or gynecologic diseases is explored before tests are performed to determine problems affecting general health and fertility. These tests include hormone levels, ovulatory studies, tubal patency studies, and postcoital studies. Other screening tests for infertility include semen analysis and pelvic ultrasound.

Ovulatory Studies. A basal body temperature record is kept to determine whether there is regular ovulation. The woman is instructed to take and graph her temperature, referred to as basal body temperature, on awakening before any activity. As ovulation approaches, the production of estrogen increases, which may cause a drop in temperature of about 2° F. When ovulation occurs, progesterone is produced, causing a rise in temperature. Thus a temperature graph helps detect ovulation and suggests the timing of intercourse if pregnancy is desired. Ovulation prediction kits are now available for use by women at home. Other tests for ovulation include cervical and vaginal smears, endometrial biopsy, and plasma progesterone levels.

Tubal Patency Studies. Tubal factors (occlusion or deformity) are most commonly assessed using a hysterosalpingogram. This procedure consists of the radiographic visualization of the uterus and fallopian tubes by injecting a radiopaque dye through the cervix. Tubal patency, shape, position, and any distortions of the endometrial cavity can be determined. Laparoscopy may be used when hysterosalpingogram is contraindicated or other pelvic pathologic conditions appear likely.

Postcoital Studies. A postcoital test can determine whether the cervical environment is favorable for the sperm. The couple is asked to have intercourse about the time ovulation is expected and 2 to 12 hours before the office visit. Douching or bathing should be avoided before the test. The cervical and vaginal secretions are aspirated and examined for the number and motility of sperm present.

NURSING AND COLLABORATIVE MANAGEMENT INFERTILITY

The management of infertility problems depends on the cause. If infertility is secondary to an alteration in ovarian function, supplemental hormone therapy to restore and maintain ovulation may be used. Drug therapy to treat infertility is presented in Table 54-2. Chronic cervicitis and inadequate estrogenic stimulation are cervical factors causing infertility. Antibiotic therapy is indicated for cervicitis. Inadequate estrogenic stimulation is treated using estrogen.

When a couple has not succeeded in conceiving while under infertility management, an option is intrauterine insemination with sperm from the partner or a donor. If this technique does not succeed, assisted reproductive technologies (ARTs) may be used. ARTs include in vitro fertilization (IVF), gamete intrafallopian transfer (GIFT), zygote intrafallopian transfer (ZIFT), donor gametes, and embryo cryopreservation. IVF is the removal of mature oocytes from the woman's ovarian follicle via laparoscopy, followed by in vitro fertilization of the ova with the partner's sperm. When fertilization and cleavage have occurred, the resulting embryos are transferred into the woman's uterus. The procedure requires 2 to 3 days to complete and is used in cases of fallopian tube obstruction, diminished sperm count, and unexplained infertility. Frequently, multiple attempts are needed for successful implantation. IVF is financially costly and emotionally stressful.[3]

Assist women experiencing infertility by providing information about the physiology of reproduction and the infertility evaluation, and by addressing the psychologic and social distress that can accompany infertility. Reducing psychologic stress can improve the emotional climate, making it more conducive to achieving a pregnancy.

Teaching and providing emotional support are major responsibilities throughout infertility testing and treatment. Feelings of anger, frustration, grief, and helplessness may heighten as additional diagnostic tests are performed. Infertility can generate great tension in a marriage as the couple exhausts financial and emotional resources. Few insurance carriers cover the high cost of infertility testing and treatment. Encourage couples to participate in a support group for infertile couples, as well as individual therapy.

ABORTION

An **abortion** is the loss or termination of a pregnancy before the fetus has developed to a state of viability (ability to survive outside the uterus). Abortions are classified as *spontaneous* (those occurring naturally) or *induced* (those occurring as a result of mechanical or medical intervention). *Miscarriage* is the common term for the unintended loss of a pregnancy.

Spontaneous Abortion

Spontaneous abortion is the natural loss of pregnancy before 20 weeks of gestation. Fetal chromosomal anomalies may account for many miscarriages before 8 weeks of gestation. Other causes of spontaneous abortions include endocrine abnormalities, maternal infection, acquired anatomic abnormalities (e.g., uterine fibroids, endometriosis), immunologic factors, and environmental factors. About 10% to 15% of all pregnancies end as a result of spontaneous abortion.

Uterine cramping coupled with vaginal bleeding often indicates a spontaneous abortion. Serial measurements of serum β-human chorionic gonadotropin (β-hCG) hormone and vaginal ultrasound examination of the pelvis are the most reliable indicators of viability of the pregnancy.

Treatment to prevent a possible spontaneous abortion is limited. Although bed rest and avoidance of vaginal intercourse are often recommended, there is no evidence that these measures improve the outcome. The woman is advised to report any bleeding to her health care provider. Most women proceed to abortion regardless of treatment. If the products of conception do not pass completely or bleeding becomes excessive, a *dilation and curettage* (D&C) procedure is generally performed.[4] The D&C involves dilating the cervix and scraping the endometrium of the uterus to empty the contents of the uterus.

Women who are experiencing bleeding and cramping during pregnancy may be admitted to the hospital. Vital signs and estimated blood loss are monitored. Women are distressed and experience both physical and emotional pain. Arrange for someone to stay with the patient, since emotional support is important. Be aware of the grieving process that results from the loss of a pregnancy.

Induced Abortion

Induced abortion is an intentional or elective termination of a pregnancy. Induced abortion is done for personal reasons (at the request of the woman) and for medical reasons. Several techniques are used to induce abortion, including menstrual extraction, suction curettage, dilation and evacuation (D&E), and drug therapy (Table 54-3). Deciding on which technique to use to terminate a pregnancy depends on the gestational age (length of the pregnancy) and the woman's condition. Suction curettage may be performed up to 14 weeks of gestation and accounts for more than 90% of abortion procedures.

Drug therapy is another method to induce abortion (medical abortion) early in pregnancy. These agents must be given within the first 49 days of pregnancy (day 1 being the first day of the last menstrual period).

Once the decision is made to have an abortion, the woman and her significant others need support and acceptance.

TABLE 54-3   METHODS FOR INDUCING ABORTION

Method	Length of Pregnancy	Description
Early Abortion		
Menstrual extraction	Usually up to 2 wk after first missed period	Catheter is inserted through cervix into uterus, and suction is applied. Endometrium and contents of uterus are aspirated.
Suction aspiration (curettage)	Up to 14 wk	Cervix is usually dilated, uterine aspirator is introduced, and suction is applied, removing endometrial tissue and implanted pregnancy.
Dilation and evacuation (D&E)	10-16 wk (approximate)	Cervix is dilated, and products of conception are removed by vacuum cannula and use of other instruments as needed.
mifepristone (Mifeprex, RU-486) with misoprostol (Cytotec)	Up to 7 wk	Mifepristone is administered orally. Misoprostol (prostaglandin) is administered orally or intravaginally 2 days later.
methotrexate with misoprostol	Up to 7 wk	Methotrexate is administered intramuscularly. Misoprostol is given intravaginally 5-7 days later.
Late Abortion *Instillation of Drugs*		
Hypertonic saline solution	After 16 wk	About 200 mL of amniotic fluid is withdrawn, with similar amount of 20% normal saline solution injected. Uterus is irritated and begins to contract within 12-36 hr. Contractions may be assisted with IV oxytocin.
Prostaglandins • carboprost (Hemabate) • dinoprostone (Prostin E2, Cervidil)	After 16 wk	Amniocentesis is done, and prostaglandin is inserted into amniotic sac, resulting in stimulation of smooth muscle of uterus. Expulsion of uterine contents occurs within 24 hr.
Hysterotomy	16-20 wk	Miniature cesarean delivery is performed. Incision is made into uterus and contents are removed.

Prepare the patient for what to expect both emotionally and physically. Grief and sadness are normal emotions after an abortion. The patient needs to understand the procedure, including instructions for preprocedure and postprocedure care. Your caring attitude can be a positive factor in the patient's experience.

After the procedure, teach the patient the signs and symptoms of possible complications, such as abnormal vaginal bleeding, severe abdominal cramping, fever, and foul-smelling drainage. Also stress to the patient to avoid intercourse and vaginal insertions until reexamination, which needs to be in 2 weeks. Contraception can be started the day of the procedure or during the patient's return visit in accordance with her needs and desires.

PROBLEMS RELATED TO MENSTRUATION

The normal menstrual cycle is discussed in Chapter 51. The hormonal changes related to the menstrual cycle are shown in Fig. 51-7. Menstruation may be irregular during the first few years after menarche and the years preceding menopause. Once established, a woman's menstrual cycles usually have a predictable pattern. However, considerable normal variation exists among women in cycle length and in duration, amount, and character of the menstrual flow (see Table 51-2).

PREMENSTRUAL SYNDROME

Premenstrual syndrome (PMS) is a symptom complex related to the luteal phase of the menstrual cycle. The symptoms can be severe enough to impair interpersonal relationships or interfere with usual activities. Because many symptoms may be associated with PMS, it is difficult to define. However, PMS symptoms always occur cyclically during the luteal phase before the onset of menstruation and are not present at other times of the month. About 40% of all women have been significantly affected by PMS during their lifetime.[5]

Etiology and Pathophysiology

The etiology and pathophysiology of PMS are not well understood. It may have a biologic trigger with compounding psychosocial factors. Neurotransmitters, such as serotonin, could also be involved. Some women may have a genetic predisposition to PMS. Other proposed causes of PMS include hormone imbalance and nutritional deficiencies. *Premenstrual dysphoric disorder* (PMDD) is the term applied when women with PMS have a severe mood disorder.

Clinical Manifestations

PMS is extremely variable in its clinical manifestations between women and, for an individual woman, from one cycle to another. Common physical symptoms include breast discomfort, peripheral edema, abdominal bloating, sensation of weight gain, episodes of binge eating, and migraine headache. Abdominal bloating and breast swelling are caused by fluid shifts because total body weight does not generally change. Anxiety, depression, irritability, and mood swings are some of the emotional symptoms that women may experience.

Diagnostic Studies and Collaborative Care

PMS can be diagnosed only when other possible causes for the symptoms have been ruled out. A focused health history and

TABLE 54-4 COLLABORATIVE CARE
Premenstrual Syndrome (PMS)
Diagnostic • History and physical examination • Symptom diary

Collaborative Therapy
• Stress management and relaxation therapy
• Nutritional therapy
• Aerobic exercise
• Drug therapy
   • Diuretics
   • Prostaglandin inhibitors (e.g., ibuprofen [Advil, Motrin])
   • Selective serotonin reuptake inhibitors (e.g., sertraline [Zoloft])
   • Combined oral contraceptives

physical examination are done to identify any underlying conditions such as thyroid dysfunction, uterine fibroids, or depression that may account for the symptoms. No definitive diagnostic test is available for PMS. When PMS or PMDD is a possible diagnosis, a woman is given a symptom diary to record her symptoms prospectively for two or three menstrual cycles. Diagnosis is based on an evaluation of the woman's symptoms.

Nondrug and drug strategies can relieve some PMS symptoms (Table 54-4). However, no single treatment is available. The goal of treatment is to reduce the severity of symptoms and enhance the woman's sense of control and quality of life.

Several conservative approaches to managing PMS symptoms are considered helpful, including stress management, diet changes, exercise, education, and counseling. Techniques for stress reduction include yoga, meditation, and biofeedback. To decrease autonomic nervous system arousal, women should avoid caffeine, reduce dietary intake of refined carbohydrates, exercise on a regular basis, and practice relaxation techniques. Eating complex carbohydrates with high fiber, foods rich in vitamin B_6, and sources of tryptophan (dairy and poultry) are thought to promote serotonin production, which improves the symptoms. Vitamin B_6 may be found in such foods as pork, milk, and legumes.

Exercise results in a release of endorphins, leading to mood elevation. Aerobic exercise can also have a relaxing effect. Because fatigue tends to exaggerate the symptoms of PMS, adequate rest in the premenstrual period is a priority.

Explanations about PMS help the woman understand the complexity of the disorder and ways that she can regain a sense of control. Assure the patient that her symptoms are real, PMS exists, and she is not "crazy." Acknowledgment that she has PMS can itself be therapeutic. Teaching the woman's partner about the nature of PMS helps the partner better understand PMS and its effects.

Drug Therapy. Drug therapy is considered when symptoms persist or interfere with daily functioning. Currently no single drug can treat all the symptoms associated with PMS. One therapy may be tried for a time; if no improvement is noted, another approach is tried. Many treatments are symptom specific. For fluid retention, diuretics such as spironolactone (Aldactone) are used. For reducing cramping pain, backache, and migraine headache, prostaglandin inhibitors such as ibuprofen (Motrin, Advil) are used. To improve negative mood, vitamin B_6 supplementation (50 mg/day) may be used. Calcium and magnesium supplementation may also be effective in alleviating psychologic and physiologic symptoms. For anxiety, buspirone

(BuSpar) taken during the luteal phase has helped some women. Women with PMDD may benefit from antidepressants, including fluoxetine (Prozac, Sarafem) and tricyclic antidepressants (e.g., amitriptyline [Elavil]).

Selective serotonin reuptake inhibitors (SSRIs) (e.g., sertraline [Zoloft]) have provided significant relief to women with severe PMS. Other treatments include oral contraceptives containing estrogen and progesterone. Evening primrose oil may help in reducing menstrual cramping for some women.

> **DRUG ALERT: Oral Contraceptives (Both Estrogen and Progesterone)**
> - May increase the risk of cervical, liver, and perhaps breast cancer
> - May elevate blood pressure and cholesterol (related to estrogen)
> - Increase risk of cardiac disease if patient is also smoking
> - May impair effectiveness of concurrent use of antibiotics
> - Are contraindicated in patients with migraine headaches and depression

DYSMENORRHEA

Dysmenorrhea is abdominal cramping pain or discomfort associated with menstrual flow. The degree of pain and discomfort varies with the individual. The two types of dysmenorrhea are *primary* (no pathologic condition exists) and *secondary* (pelvic disease is the underlying cause).[5] Dysmenorrhea is one of the most common gynecologic problems.

Etiology and Pathophysiology

Primary dysmenorrhea is not a disease. It is caused by an excess of prostaglandin $F_{2\alpha}$ ($PGF_{2\alpha}$) and/or an increased sensitivity to it. Stimulation of the endometrium by estrogen, followed by progesterone, results in a dramatic increase in prostaglandin production by the endometrium. With the onset of menses, degeneration of the endometrium releases prostaglandin. Locally, prostaglandins increase myometrial contractions and constriction of small endometrial blood vessels. This causes tissue ischemia and increased sensitization of the pain receptors, resulting in menstrual pain. Primary dysmenorrhea begins in the first few years after menarche, typically with the onset of regular ovulatory cycles.

Secondary dysmenorrhea is usually acquired after adolescence, occurring most commonly at 30 to 40 years of age. Common pelvic conditions that cause secondary dysmenorrhea include endometriosis, chronic pelvic inflammatory disease, and uterine fibroids. Because secondary dysmenorrhea can be caused by many conditions, symptoms vary. However, painful menses is present in all situations.

Clinical Manifestations

Primary dysmenorrhea starts 12 to 24 hours before the onset of menses. The pain is most severe the first day of menses and rarely lasts more than 2 days. Characteristic manifestations include lower abdominal pain that is colicky in nature, frequently radiating to the lower back and upper thighs. The abdominal pain is often accompanied by nausea, diarrhea, fatigue, and headache.

Secondary dysmenorrhea usually occurs after the woman has experienced problem-free periods for some time. The pain, which may be unilateral, is generally more constant and continues longer than in primary dysmenorrhea. Depending on the cause, symptoms such as *dyspareunia* (painful intercourse), painful defecation, or irregular bleeding may occur at times other than menstruation.

NURSING AND COLLABORATIVE MANAGEMENT DYSMENORRHEA

Evaluation begins with distinguishing primary from secondary dysmenorrhea. Obtain a complete health history with special attention to menstrual and gynecologic history. A pelvic examination is performed by the health care provider. The probable diagnosis is primary dysmenorrhea if the history reveals an onset shortly after menarche, symptoms are associated only with menses, and the pelvic examination is normal. If a specific cause of dysmenorrhea is evident, the diagnosis is secondary dysmenorrhea.

Treatment for primary dysmenorrhea includes heat, exercise, and drug therapy. Heat is applied to the lower abdomen or back. Regular exercise is beneficial because it may reduce endometrial hyperplasia and subsequent prostaglandin production. Primary drug therapy is nonsteroidal antiinflammatory drugs (NSAIDs) such as naproxen (Naprosyn), which has antiprostaglandin activity. NSAIDs should be started at the first sign of menses and continued every 4 to 8 hours to maintain a sufficient level of the drug to inhibit prostaglandin synthesis for the usual duration of discomfort.

Oral contraceptives may also be used. They decrease dysmenorrhea by reducing endometrial hyperplasia. Acupuncture and transcutaneous nerve stimulation may be used for women who have inadequate relief from medications or who prefer not to take medications. Patients who are unresponsive to these treatments should be evaluated for chronic pelvic pain (discussed later in this chapter on p. 1289).

Treatment of secondary dysmenorrhea depends on the cause. Some individuals with secondary dysmenorrhea are helped by the approaches used for primary dysmenorrhea.

Instruct women on why dysmenorrhea occurs and how to treat it. This will provide women with a foundation for coping with this common problem and increase feelings of control and self-reliance.

Women often ask what can be done for minor discomforts associated with menstrual cycles. Advise women that during acute pain, relief may be obtained by applying heat to the abdomen or back and taking NSAIDs for analgesia. Also suggest noninvasive pain-relieving practices such as relaxation breathing and guided imagery.

Other health care measures to reduce the discomfort of dysmenorrhea include regular exercise and proper nutritional habits. Avoiding constipation, maintaining good body mechanics, and eliminating stress and fatigue, particularly before menstrual periods, can also decrease discomfort. Staying active and interested in activities may also help.

ABNORMAL VAGINAL BLEEDING

Abnormal vaginal or uterine bleeding is a common gynecologic concern. Abnormalities include *oligomenorrhea* (long intervals between menses, generally greater than 35 days), amenorrhea (absence of menstruation), *menorrhagia* (excessive or prolonged menstrual bleeding), and *metrorrhagia* (irregular bleeding or bleeding between menses). The cause of abnormal bleeding may vary from anovulatory menstrual cycles to more serious conditions such as ectopic pregnancy or endometrial cancer.

The woman's age provides direction for identifying the cause of bleeding. For example, a postmenopausal woman with

CHAPTER 54 Female Reproductive Problems 1281

Reproductive System

abnormal bleeding must always be evaluated for endometrial cancer but does not need to be evaluated for possible pregnancy. For a 20-year-old woman with abnormal bleeding, the possibility of pregnancy must always be considered, and endometrial cancer would be unlikely.

Abnormal bleeding may be caused by dysfunction of the hypothalamic-pituitary-ovarian axis such as a pituitary adenoma. Another possible cause is infection. Changes in lifestyle such as marriage, recent moves, a death in the family, financial stress, and other emotional crises can also cause irregular bleeding. Because psychologic factors can influence endocrine function, they should be considered when the patient is evaluated.

Types of Irregular Bleeding

Oligomenorrhea and Amenorrhea. Anovulation is the most common reason for missing menses once pregnancy has been ruled out. Additional causes of amenorrhea are listed in Table 54-5. *Primary amenorrhea* refers to the failure of menstrual cycles to begin by age 16 years or by age 14 years if secondary sex characteristics are present. *Secondary amenorrhea* refers to the cessation of menstrual cycles once they had been established.

Ovulation is often erratic for several years after menarche and before menopause. Thus oligomenorrhea due to anovulation is common for women at the beginning and end of menstruation. In anovulatory cycles the corpus luteum that produces progesterone does not form. This may result in a situation referred to as *unopposed estrogen*. When unopposed by progesterone, estrogen can cause excessive buildup of the endometrium. Persistent overgrowth of the endometrium increases a woman's risk for endometrial cancer. To reduce this risk, progesterone or oral contraceptives are prescribed to ensure that the patient's endometrial lining is shed at least four to six times per year.

Menorrhagia. The excessive bleeding associated with menorrhagia can be characterized as an increased duration (more than 7 days), increased amount (more than 80 mL), or both. Anovulatory uterine bleeding is the most common cause of menorrhagia. An unopposed estrogen state continues to build up the endometrium until it becomes unstable, resulting in menorrhagia. For young women with excessive bleeding, clotting disorders must be considered. Uterine fibroids (also called *leiomyomas*) and endometrial polyps are common causes of menorrhagia for women in their childbearing years.[6]

Metrorrhagia. Metrorrhagia, also referred to as *spotting* or *breakthrough bleeding*, is bleeding between menstrual periods. For all reproductive-age women, pregnancy complications such as spontaneous abortion or ectopic pregnancy must be considered as a possible cause. Other causes include cervical or endometrial polyps, infection, and cancer. Spotting is common during the first three cycles of oral contraceptives. If spotting continues beyond that, a different pill formulation can be prescribed once other causes of metrorrhagia have been ruled out. Spotting with long-acting progestin therapy (e.g., Mirena intrauterine device [IUD]) or progestin-only pills (medroxyprogesterone [Depo-Provera, Provera]) is also common. For postmenopausal women, endometrial cancer must be considered whenever spotting is experienced. In postmenopausal women, exogenous estrogen administration during hormone therapy is a common cause of metrorrhagia.

Diagnostic Studies and Collaborative Care

Because abnormal vaginal bleeding has multiple causes, the diagnostic and collaborative care varies. A health history and physical examination directed at the most likely causes of vaginal bleeding for the woman's age-group is the first step. These findings provide the basis for selecting laboratory tests and diagnostic procedures. Treatment depends on the etiology of the problem (e.g., menorrhagia, amenorrhea), degree of threat to the patient's health, and whether children are desired in the future.

Combined oral contraceptives may be prescribed for a woman with amenorrhea to ensure regular shedding of the endometrium if she also wants contraception. Tranexamic acid (Lysteda) may be used to treat heavy menstrual bleeding. This drug stabilizes a protein that helps blood to clot. Side effects may include headache, back pain, abdominal pain, muscle and joint pain, anemia, and fatigue. Women using hormonal contraception should take tranexamic acid only if they have a strong medical need, since there is an increased risk of blood clots and stroke. Estradiol valerate/dienogest (Natazia) may be given to women with heavy menstrual bleeding who desire an oral contraceptive to prevent pregnancy.

The treatment goal for women with menorrhagia is to minimize further blood loss. If menorrhagia is the result of anovulatory cycles, the endometrium must be stabilized by a combination of oral estrogen and progesterone.

Balloon thermotherapy is a technique for menorrhagia that involves the introduction of a soft, flexible balloon into the uterus. The balloon is then inflated with sterile fluid (Fig. 54-1). The fluid in the balloon is heated and maintained for 8 minutes, thus causing ablation (removal) of the uterine lining. When the treatment is completed, the fluid is withdrawn from the balloon and the catheter is removed from the uterus. The uterine lining sloughs off in the next 7 to 10 days. Uterine balloon thermotherapy is contraindicated for women who desire to maintain their fertility and for women with any suspected uterine abnormalities such as fibroids, suspected endometrial cancer, prior cesarean delivery, or myomectomy. With severe bleeding, hospitalization is indicated. All patients with menorrhagia should be evaluated for anemia and treated as indicated.

Surgical Therapy. Surgery may be indicated depending on the underlying cause of the abnormal vaginal bleeding. D&C is used only in cases of acute excess bleeding or for older women when endometrial biopsy and ultrasonography have not pro-

---

TABLE 54-5 CAUSES OF AMENORRHEA

Natural Amenorrhea
- Pregnancy
- Breastfeeding
- Menopause

Medications
- Antipsychotics
- Chemotherapy
- Antidepressants

Lifestyle
- Stress
- Excessive exercise
- Low body weight
- Acute and chronic illness

Hormonal Imbalance
- Polycystic ovary syndrome
- Pituitary tumors
- Premature menopause

Structural Problems
- Uterine scarring
- Structural abnormalities of vagina
- Damage to ovaries or uterus from radiation

FIG. 54-1 Balloon thermotherapy for treatment of menorrhagia. **A,** Balloon-tipped catheter is inserted into the uterus through the vagina and the cervix. **B,** The balloon is inflated with a sterile fluid that expands to fit the size and shape of the uterus. The fluid is heated to 188° F (87° C) and maintained for 8 minutes while the uterine lining is treated. **C,** Fluid is withdrawn from the balloon and the catheter is removed. (Courtesy Ethicon, Inc, Cornelia, Ga.)

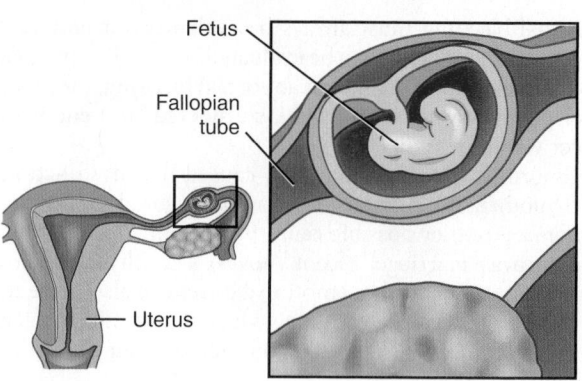

FIG. 54-2 Ectopic pregnancy occurring in the fallopian tube.

vided the necessary diagnostic information. Endometrial ablation for menorrhagia may be done by laser, thermal balloon, cryotherapy, or microwave energy for patients who do not want to have children.

If menorrhagia is caused by uterine fibroids, a **hysterectomy** (surgical removal of the uterus) may be performed. A *myomectomy* (removal of fibroids without removal of the uterus) may be performed if the patient wants to preserve her uterus. The myomectomy is done via laparotomy, laparoscopy, or hysteroscopy. Hormonal regimens and embolization of the blood vessels supplying the fibroid tumor are other treatment options.

NURSING MANAGEMENT
ABNORMAL VAGINAL BLEEDING

Teaching women about the characteristics of the menstrual cycle will enable them to identify normal variations. Table 51-2 includes characteristics of the menstrual cycle and related patient teaching. This knowledge can decrease apprehension and dispel misconceptions about the menstrual cycle. If the patient's menstrual cycle pattern does not fall within the normal range, urge her to discuss this with her health care provider.

The selection of internal or external sanitary protection is a matter of personal preference. Tampons are convenient and make menstrual hygiene easier, whereas pads may provide better protection. Using a combination of tampons and pads and avoiding prolonged use of superabsorbent tampons may decrease the risk of *toxic shock syndrome* (TSS). TSS is an acute life-threatening condition caused by a toxin from *Staphylococcus aureus*. TSS causes high fever, vomiting, diarrhea, weakness, myalgia, and a sunburn-like rash.[7]

Whenever excessive, the amount of the vaginal bleeding should be assessed as accurately as possible. The patient should record and report the number and size of pads or tampons used and the degree of saturation. The patient's fatigue level, along with variations in blood pressure and pulse, should be monitored because anemia and hypovolemia may be present. For the patient requiring a surgical procedure, provide the appropriate preoperative and postoperative care.

ECTOPIC PREGNANCY

An **ectopic pregnancy** is the implantation of the fertilized ovum anywhere outside the uterine cavity. Approximately 3% of all pregnancies are ectopic, and approximately 98% of these occur in the fallopian tube[8] (Fig. 54-2). The remaining 2% to 3% may be ovarian, abdominal, or cervical. Ectopic pregnancy is a life-threatening condition. Earlier identification has contributed to decreased mortality rates.

Etiology and Pathophysiology

Any blockage of the fallopian tube or reduction of tubal peristalsis that impedes or delays the zygote passing to the uterine cavity can result in tubal implantation. After implantation, the growth of the gestational sac expands the tubal wall. Eventually the tube ruptures, causing acute peritoneal symptoms. Less acute symptoms usually begin within 6 to 8 weeks after the last normal menstrual period and weeks before rupture would occur.

Risk factors for ectopic pregnancy include a history of pelvic inflammatory disease, prior ectopic pregnancy, current progestin-releasing IUD, progestin-only birth control failure, and prior pelvic or tubal surgery. Additional risk factors for ectopic pregnancy include procedures used in infertility treatment, including IVF, embryo transfer, and ovulation induction.

Clinical Manifestations

The classic manifestations of ectopic pregnancy are abdominal or pelvic pain, missed menses, and irregular vaginal bleeding. Other manifestations include morning sickness, breast tenderness, gastrointestinal disturbance, malaise, and syncope. Pain is almost always present and is caused by distention of the fallopian tube. It may start unilaterally and then spread to become bilateral. The character of the pain varies among women and can be colicky or vague. If tubal rupture occurs, the pain is intense and may be referred to the shoulder as a result of irritation of the diaphragm by blood released into the abdominal cavity. Symptom severity does not necessarily correlate with the extent of external bleeding present. With rupture, the risk of hemorrhage and hypovolemic shock is present. Suspected rupture is treated as an emergency.

The vaginal bleeding that may accompany ectopic pregnancy is usually described as spotting. However, bleeding may be heavier and can be confused with menses.

Diagnostic Studies

Ectopic pregnancy can be a diagnostic challenge because of its similarity to other pelvic and abdominal disorders, such as salpingitis, spontaneous abortion, ruptured ovarian cyst, appendicitis, and peritonitis. A serum (radioimmunoassay) pregnancy test should be performed. If the test is negative, an ectopic pregnancy is not likely. If ectopic pregnancy cannot be excluded by the pregnancy test, further evaluation is warranted. If the patient is in stable condition, a combination of serial measurements of serum β-hCG and vaginal ultrasonography is used.[9] Absence of a normal intrauterine pregnancy means that the diagnosis is probably a spontaneous abortion or an ectopic pregnancy. With a spontaneous abortion, serial serum β-hCG levels will decrease over time. A complete blood count is obtained when there is any concern regarding the amount of blood loss or if surgery is contemplated.

NURSING AND COLLABORATIVE MANAGEMENT ECTOPIC PREGNANCY

Surgery remains the primary approach for treating ectopic pregnancies and should be performed immediately. However, medical management with methotrexate (Folex) is being used with increasing success in patients who are hemodynamically stable and have a mass less than 3 cm in size.[10] A conservative surgical approach limits damage to the reproductive system as much as possible. Removal of the fetus from the tube is preferred to removing the tube. Laparoscopy is preferable to laparotomy because it decreases blood loss and the length of the hospital stay (Fig. 54-3). If the tube ruptures, conservative surgical approaches may not be possible. The patient may need a blood transfusion and supplemental IV fluid therapy to relieve shock and restore a satisfactory blood volume for safe anesthesia and surgery. The use of laparoscopy has resulted in fewer repeated ectopic pregnancies and a higher rate of future successful pregnancies.

Nursing care depends on the patient's condition. Before the diagnosis has been confirmed, be alert to patient signs of increasing pain and vaginal bleeding, which may indicate that the tube has ruptured. Monitor vital signs closely and observe for signs of shock. Give explanations and prepare the patient for diagnostic procedures when appropriate. Preparation of the patient for abdominal surgery may follow rapidly. Provide reassurance and support for the surgery to the patient and her family. Postoperatively, the patient may express a fear of future ectopic pregnancies and have many questions about the impact of this experience on her fertility.

FIG. 54-3 Laparoscopic treatment of ectopic pregnancy in the right fallopian tube.

PERIMENOPAUSE AND POSTMENOPAUSE

Perimenopause is a normal life transition that begins with the first signs of change in menstrual cycles and ends after cessation of menses.[11] **Menopause** is the physiologic cessation of menses associated with declining ovarian function. It is usually considered complete after 1 year of *amenorrhea* (absence of menstruation). Menopause starts gradually and is usually associated with changes in menstruation, including menstrual flows that are increased, decreased, or irregular. Eventually complete cessation of menses occurs. *Postmenopause* is a term that refers to the time in a woman's life after menopause.

The age at which menopause occurs ranges from 44 to 55 years, with an average age of 51 years. Menopause may occur earlier due to illness, surgical removal of the uterus or both ovaries, side effects of radiation therapy or chemotherapy, or drugs. The age at which menopause occurs is not affected by age at menarche, physical characteristics, number of pregnancies, date of last pregnancy, or oral contraceptive use. However, genetic factors, autoimmune conditions, cigarette smoking, and racial or ethnic factors are related to an earlier age at menopause.

Changes within the ovary start the cascade of events that finally result in menopause. The regression of the follicles within each ovary begins at puberty and accelerates after age 35. With age, fewer follicles remain that are responsive to follicle-stimulating hormone (FSH). FSH normally stimulates the dominant follicle to secrete estrogen. When the follicles can no longer respond to FSH, the production of estrogen and progesterone from the ovary declines. However, perimenopausal women can get pregnant until menopause has occurred, since many women have long anovulatory cycles interspersed with shorter, ovulatory cycles.

With decreased ovarian function, decreased levels of estrogen cause a gradual increase in FSH and luteinizing hormone (LH) as a result of the negative feedback process. By the time menopause occurs, there is a 10- to 20-fold increase in FSH. The elevated FSH level may take several years to return to the premenopausal level. The reduced estrogen level also causes a decrease in the frequency of ovulation and results in changes in the reproductive organs and tissues (e.g., atrophy of vaginal tissue).

Clinical Manifestations

Clinical manifestations of perimenopause and postmenopause are presented in Table 54-6. Perimenopause is a time of erratic hormonal fluctuation. Irregular vaginal bleeding is common.

TABLE 54-6	MANIFESTATIONS OF PERIMENOPAUSE AND POSTMENOPAUSE
Perimenopause	**Postmenopause**
• Irregular menses	• Cessation of menses
• Occasional vasomotor symptoms	• Vasomotor instability (hot flashes and night sweats)
• Atrophy of genitourinary tissue with decreased support	• Atrophy of genitourinary tissue (e.g., vaginal epithelium)
• Stress and urge incontinence	• Stress and urge incontinence
• Osteoporosis	• Breast tenderness
• Mood changes	

TABLE 54-7	MANIFESTATIONS OF ESTROGEN DEFICIENCY	
Vasomotor • Hot flashes • Night sweats		**Musculoskeletal** • Increased fracture rate, especially vertebral bodies but also humerus, distal radius, and upper femur
Genitourinary • Atrophic vaginitis • Dyspareunia secondary to poor lubrication • Incontinence		**Cardiovascular** • Decreased high-density lipoproteins (HDLs) • Increased low-density lipoproteins (LDLs)
Psychologic • Emotional lability • Change in sleep pattern • Decreased REM sleep		**Other** • Diminished collagen content of skin • Breast tissue changes

REM, Rapid eye movement.

With decreasing estrogen, hot flashes and other symptoms begin. The signs and symptoms of diminished estrogen are listed in Table 54-7. The loss of estrogen plays a significant role in the cause of age-related alterations. Changes most critical to a woman's well-being are the increased risks for coronary artery disease (CAD) and osteoporosis (secondary to bone density loss). Other changes include a redistribution of fat, a tendency to gain weight more easily, muscle and joint pain, loss of skin elasticity, changes in hair amount and distribution, and atrophy of external genitalia and breast tissue.

Hallmarks of perimenopause include *vasomotor instability* (hot flashes) and irregular menses. A hot flash (occurs in up to 80% of all women) is described as a sudden sensation of intense heat along with perspiration and flushing.[12] These sensations may last from several seconds to 5 minutes and occur most often at night, thereby disturbing sleep. The cause of hot flashes, or vasomotor instability, is not clearly understood. It has been theorized that temperature regulators in the brain are in proximity to the area where gonadotropin-releasing hormone (GnRH) is released. The lowered estrogen levels are correlated with dilation of cutaneous blood vessels, resulting in hot flashes and increased sweating. The more sudden the withdrawal of estrogen (e.g., surgical removal of the ovaries), the more likely the symptoms will be severe if no hormone replacement is provided. Symptoms usually subside over time and typically last from 5 to 10 years with or without treatment.[13] Hot flashes can be triggered by stress and situations that affect body temperature, such as eating a hot meal, hot weather, or warm clothing. Women who smoke are at higher risk for hot flashes because smoking affects estrogen metabolism. African American women report the highest incidence of hot flashes, whereas Asian American women report the lowest number.[13]

Atrophic vaginal changes secondary to decreased estrogen include thinning of the vaginal mucosa and disappearance of rugae. Vaginal secretions also decrease and become more alkaline. As a result of these changes, the vagina is easily traumatized and more susceptible to infection, including a higher risk for human immunodeficiency virus (HIV) infection if exposed. *Dyspareunia* (painful intercourse) may also occur. This can lead to unnecessary and premature cessation of sexual activity. Dryness is a problem that can be corrected with water-soluble lubricants or, if needed, with hormonal creams or systemic hormone therapy.

Atrophic changes in the lower urinary tract also occur with a decrease in estrogen. Bladder capacity decreases, and the bladder and urethral tissue lose tone. These changes can cause symptoms that mimic a bladder infection (e.g., dysuria, urgency, frequency) when no infection is present.

Whether decreasing estrogen causes the psychologic changes associated with perimenopause is unclear. Depression, irritability, and cognitive problems, which are often attributed to menopause, could result from life stressors or sleep deprivation from hot flashes. Depressive symptoms appear to improve when hormone levels stabilize.

Collaborative Care

The diagnosis of perimenopause should be made only after careful consideration of other possible causes for the woman's symptoms. Depression, thyroid dysfunction, anemia, or anxiety can cause the same symptoms. Review a woman's history of menstrual patterns as part of establishing the diagnosis. Because of the hormonal fluctuations that occur before menopause, routine testing of the serum FSH level to establish a diagnosis is not indicated.

Drug Therapy. Hormone therapy (HT) was once standard therapy in the United States for treating menopausal symptoms. HT includes estrogen for women without a uterus or estrogen and progesterone for women with a uterus. Findings from the Women's Health Initiative (WHI) clinical trials changed this practice.[14] The data showed that women who had taken estrogen plus progestin (Prempro) had an increased risk of breast cancer, stroke, heart disease, and emboli. However, these women had fewer hip fractures and a lower risk of developing colorectal cancer. Women who took only estrogen (Premarin) had an increased risk of stroke and emboli. However, these women had decreased risk for fractures with no increased risk for heart disease or breast or colorectal cancer. A recent systematic review has updated and validated the results of the WHI trials.[15]

If women wish to consider taking HT for the short-term treatment (4 to 5 years) of menopausal symptoms, the risks and benefits of therapy (e.g., minimizes bone loss, hot flashes, vaginal atrophic changes) should be considered carefully. The woman and her health care provider should thoroughly discuss the decision to take HT, and which ones to take. If a woman chooses to use HT, the lowest effective dose should be used. The age that a woman starts HT may determine her risk of heart disease. The risk appears to increase the further a woman moves away from menopause.

The side effects of estrogen include nausea, fluid retention, headache, and breast enlargement. Side effects of progesterone include increased appetite, weight gain, irritability, depression, spotting, and breast tenderness. A commonly used estrogen preparation is 0.625 mg of conjugated estrogen (Premarin) daily. For symptom relief, a higher dose may be needed. To receive the protective benefit of progesterone, 5 to 10 mg of medroxyprogesterone is indicated for 12 days of each month on a cyclic regimen, or 2.5 mg on a continuous regimen. If the estrogen is increased for symptom relief, the progesterone should also be increased. Other forms of progesterone include norethindrone (Aygestin) and micronized progesterone creams, dermal patches, gels, and lotions; rings placed around the cervix; and subcutaneous pellets. Vaginal creams are especially useful for urogenital symptoms (e.g., dryness). Transdermal estrogen (skin patch or spray [EvaMist]) has the advantage of bypassing the liver, but the disadvantage of causing skin irritation.

SSRI antidepressants, including paroxetine (Paxil), fluoxetine, and venlafaxine (Effexor), are an effective alternative to HT in reducing hot flashes. This effect is noted even if the user is not depressed. The mechanism of action is unknown. Clonidine (Catapres), an antihypertensive drug, and gabapentin (Neurontin), an antiseizure drug, have also been shown to relieve hot flashes.

Selective estrogen receptor modulators (SERMs), such as raloxifene (Evista), are also used to treat menopausal problems. These drugs have some of the positive benefits of estrogen, such as preventing bone loss, without the negative effects such as endometrial hyperplasia. Raloxifene competes with estrogen for estrogen receptor sites.[16] It decreases bone loss and serum cholesterol with minimal effects on breast and uterine tissue.

Bisphosphonates, including alendronate (Fosamax) and risedronate (Actonel), are also used to decrease the risk for osteoporosis in postmenopausal women. These drugs enhance bone mineral density by suppressing resorption. SERMs and bisphosphonates are discussed further in Chapter 64 with respect to their role in the management of osteoporosis.

Nonhormonal Therapy. Because of the risks associated with HT, many women try other therapies to relieve menopausal symptoms. Paroxetine (Brisdelle) is a newer nonhormonal treatment that may be used for moderate to severe hot flashes associated with menopause. This drug is a selective serotonin reuptake inhibitor.

Hot flash frequency and severity can be reduced through measures that lead to a decrease in heat production and an increase in heat loss. Keeping a cool environment and limiting caffeine and alcohol intake lower heat production. Relaxation techniques (e.g., relaxation breathing, imagery) may also help. To promote heat loss at night when hot flashes can disrupt sleep, increase air circulation in the room and avoid bedding that traps the heat (e.g., heavy quilts). Loose-fitting clothes do not retain body heat, whereas clothes with tight necks and wrists do. Cool cloths applied to flushed areas also aid in heat loss.

Daily intake of vitamin E in doses up to 800 IU may also help reduce hot flashes in some women. Changing sleep patterns may be helped by avoiding alcohol and controlling hot flashes. Relaxation techniques can promote a better night's sleep by decreasing anxiety. A regular moderate program (three to four times per week) of aerobic and weight-bearing exercises can slow the process of bone loss and a tendency toward weight gain.

Nutritional Therapy. Good nutrition can decrease the risk of cardiovascular disease and osteoporosis in addition to assisting with vasomotor symptoms. A daily intake of about 30 cal/kg of body weight is recommended. A decrease in metabolic rate and careless eating habits can cause the weight gain and fatigue often attributed to menopause. An adequate intake of calcium and vitamin D helps maintain healthy bones and counteracts loss of bone density. Postmenopausal women not receiving supplemental estrogen should have a daily calcium intake of at least 1500 mg, whereas those taking estrogen replacement need at least 1000 mg/day. Calcium supplements are best absorbed when taken with meals. Either dietary calcium or calcium supplements may be used (see Tables 64-14 and 64-15).

COMPLEMENTARY & ALTERNATIVE THERAPIES
Herbs and Supplements for Menopause

Herb	Scientific Evidence	Nursing Implications
Black cohosh	Mixed evidence for use in the treatment of menopausal symptoms*	• Generally well tolerated in recommended doses for up to 6 mo. • Should not be used in people with a liver disorder.
Soy	Mixed evidence for treatment of menopausal symptoms*	• Women with a history of breast, ovarian, or uterine cancer or endometriosis should consult their health care provider before using soy or soy products. • Soy may interact with warfarin. Patients taking warfarin should consult their health care provider before using soy or soy products.

*In general, the evidence for use of these herbs as treatments for menopause symptoms is limited by a lack of well-designed, controlled trials (www.naturalstandard.com).

The diet should be high in complex carbohydrates and vitamin B complex, especially B_6. Phytoestrogens (soy, tofu, chickpeas, sunflower seeds) have been used to reduce menopausal symptoms. Herbal remedies, such as black cohosh, have become popular in treating menopausal symptoms (see Complementary & Alternative Therapies box above). Consultation with an experienced herbal practitioner is recommended before initiating therapy.

NURSING MANAGEMENT
PERIMENOPAUSE AND POSTMENOPAUSE

Foster a positive image of perimenopause as a time of vitality and attractiveness. Perimenopause can provide women with a renewed incentive to enhance self-care and well-being. Provide teaching and reassurance to perimenopausal women who experience difficulty in managing their symptoms. Tell them that symptoms are normal and often are temporary. Discuss nondrug approaches to managing symptoms.

Dry skin can be improved by the use of moisturizing soaps and body lotions. Kegel exercises may help decrease stress incontinence (see Table 46-19). Sexual function can continue with little change in the vast majority of postmenopausal women. Cessation of menstruation and ability to bear children should not be equated with cessation of sexual capability. For some women, menopause may be liberating.

Femininity and libido do not disappear with menopause. A water-soluble lubricant (e.g., Replens, Astroglide, K-Y jelly) is often effective in managing atrophic changes in vaginal epithelium. An active sex life helps increase lubrication and maintains the pliability of vaginal tissues. Provide the patient with an opportunity to candidly discuss concerns related to sexual functioning.

CULTURALLY COMPETENT CARE
MENOPAUSE

Although all women experience menopause, the perception of menopause varies by culture. Ethnic groups have different traditions and beliefs regarding menopause, including the use of complementary and alternative therapies to manage symptoms.[17] Be aware of the attitudes and beliefs regarding menopause among women from various ethnic and cultural backgrounds. In many cultures, menopause is considered a normal part of aging, and little emphasis is placed on the physical and emotional symptoms that accompany the loss of fertility. In cultures where older adults are revered, menopause may be seen as a liberating transition to a state of being a "wise woman."

American culture generally has a negative attitude toward aging and places a high value on youth. Menopause is often considered a disorder that requires treatment. Menopausal symptoms may be viewed as troublesome, with a strong need to treat hot flashes and mood swings. Numerous substances, from HT to herbal preparations, are often used to treat menopausal symptoms.

Menopause is a milestone in a woman's life that is embedded in her own personality and her culture. Approaching the menopausal woman with this understanding is important to provide culturally competent care.

CONDITIONS OF VULVA, VAGINA, AND CERVIX

Etiology and Pathophysiology

Infection and inflammation of the vagina, cervix, and vulva commonly occur when the natural defenses of the acid vaginal secretions (maintained by sufficient estrogen levels) and the presence of *Lactobacillus* are disrupted. The woman's resistance may also be decreased as a result of aging, poor nutrition, and drugs that alter the bacterial flora or mucosa. Organisms gain entrance to the areas through contaminated hands, clothing, douching, and intercourse. Table 54-8 presents the causes, manifestations, diagnostic methods, and collaborative care of common infections and inflammations.

Most lower genital tract infections are related to sexual intercourse. Intercourse can transmit organisms, injure tissues, and alter the acid-base balance of the vagina. Vulvar infections caused by viruses such as herpes and genital warts can be sexually transmitted when no lesions are apparent. Oral contraceptives, antibiotics, and corticosteroids may produce changes in the vaginal pH and trigger an overgrowth of the organisms present. For example, *Candida albicans* may be present in small numbers in the vagina. An overgrowth of this organism causes vulvovaginitis.

Clinical Manifestations

Abnormal vaginal discharge and reddened vulvar lesions are common clinical manifestations. In addition to a thick white curdlike discharge, women with vulvovaginal candidiasis (VVC) often experience intense itching and dysuria, which is the result of urine coming into contact with fissures and irritated areas on the vulva. The hallmark of bacterial vaginosis is the fishy odor of the discharge. Women with cervicitis may notice spotting after intercourse.

Common vulvar lesions include herpes infection and genital warts. Initial or primary herpes infections may be extremely painful. Herpes begins as a small vesicle followed by a superficial red ulcer. Most herpes lesions are painful. Genital warts, caused by the human papillomavirus (HPV), vary in appearance. Irregularly shaped "cauliflower" lesions are common. Genital warts are painless unless traumatized. (Herpes infection and genital warts are discussed in Chapter 53.)

Postmenopausal women may develop gynecologic problems such as *lichen sclerosis*.[18] This chronic inflammatory condition is associated with intense itching in the genital skin area (e.g., labia minora, clitoris). The lesions are white with a "tissue

TABLE 54-8   INFECTIONS OF THE LOWER GENITAL TRACT

Infection and Etiology	Manifestations and Diagnostic Methods	Drug Therapy
Vulvovaginal Candidiasis (VVC) (Monilial Vaginitis)		
Candida albicans (fungus)	Commonly found in mouth, gastrointestinal tract, and vagina. Pruritus, thick white curdlike discharge. KOH microscopic examination: pseudohyphae, pH 4.0-4.7.	Antifungal agents (e.g., miconazole [Monistat], clotrimazole [Gyne-Lotrimin, Mycelex] [available over the counter, in cream or suppository]) Fluconazole (Diflucan).
Trichomonas Vaginitis		
Trichomonas vaginalis (protozoa)	Sexually transmitted. Pruritus, frothy greenish or gray discharge. Hemorrhagic spots on cervix or vaginal walls. Saline microscopic examination: swimming trichomonads, pH >4.5.	Metronidazole (Flagyl) for patient and partner.
Bacterial Vaginosis		
Gardnerella vaginalis *Corynebacterium vaginale*	Mode of transmission unclear. Watery discharge with fishy odor. May or may not have other symptoms. Saline microscopic examination: epithelial cells, pH >4.5.	Oral or vaginal metronidazole (Flagyl) or clindamycin (Clindesse). Examine and treat partner. Lactobacillus acidophilus taken orally by diet (e.g., yogurt, fermented soy products) or supplements can decrease unwanted vaginal bacteria.
Cervicitis		
Chlamydia trachomatis	Sexually transmitted; mucopurulent discharge with postcoital spotting from cervical inflammation. Culture for *Chlamydia* and *Neisseria gonorrhoeae*.	Azithromycin (Zithromax). Treat patient and partner.
Severe Recurrent Vaginitis		
C. albicans (most often)	May be indication of HIV infection. All women who are unresponsive to first-line treatment should be offered HIV testing.	Drug appropriate to opportunistic organism.

KOH, Potassium hydroxide.

paper" appearance initially, although scratching produces changes in the appearance. The cause is unknown. High-potency topical corticosteroid ointment such as clobetasol (Temovate) helps relieve itching.

Collaborative Care

Evaluate genital problems by taking a history, performing a physical examination, and obtaining the appropriate laboratory and diagnostic studies. Because many problems relate to sexual activity, a sexual history is essential. The nature of the problem determines the extent of the evaluation. When ulcerative lesions are present, do a culture for herpes and a blood test for syphilis. Genital warts are usually identified by their clinical appearance. Vulvar dystrophies may be examined via colposcopy with a biopsy taken for diagnosis.

Problems involving vaginal discharge are evaluated by microscopy and cultures. The most common vaginal conditions (i.e., bacterial vaginosis, VVC, and trichomoniasis) are diagnosed by a procedure called a *wet mount*. The findings characteristic of each condition are shown in Table 54-8. To assess for cervicitis, endocervical cultures are obtained for chlamydial infection and gonorrhea. If purulent discharge is observed coming from the cervix, a sample of endocervical cells may be taken to conduct a Gram stain. The Gram-stained slide is examined with a microscope to identify white blood cells and gram-negative diplococci (indicative of gonorrhea). (Sexually transmitted infections [STIs] are discussed in Chapter 53.)

Drug therapy is based on the diagnosis (see Table 54-8). Antibiotics taken as directed will cure bacterial infections. Treatment duration and medications vary with specific STIs. Teach patients how to properly take their medications and to follow up to verify a cure. Partners should be treated so that reinfection does not occur.

Women with vaginal conditions or cervical infection should abstain from intercourse for at least 1 week. Douching should be avoided because it has been adversely linked to pelvic inflammatory disease, STIs, and ectopic pregnancy. Sexual partners must be evaluated and treated if the patient is diagnosed with trichomoniasis, chlamydial infection, gonorrhea, syphilis, or HIV.

Treatment of vulvar dystrophies is symptomatic because no cures are available. Treatment involves controlling the itching and hence the scratching. Interrupting the "itch-scratch cycle" prevents further secondary damage to the skin.

NURSING MANAGEMENT
CONDITIONS OF VULVA, VAGINA, AND CERVIX

Teach women about common genital conditions and how to reduce their risks. Recognize symptoms that indicate a problem, and help women seek care in a timely manner. Discussing problems that concern the patient's genitalia or sexual intercourse is frequently difficult. Use a nonjudgmental attitude to make women feel more comfortable while empowering them to ask questions.

When a woman is diagnosed with a genital condition, ensure that she fully understands the directions for treatment. Taking the full course of medication is especially important to decrease the chance of relapse. Because genitalia are such a private area, the use of graphs and models is especially helpful for patient teaching. When a woman is using a vaginal medication for the first time, show her the applicator and how to fill it. Also

teach where and how the applicator should be inserted using visual aids or models. Vaginal creams should be inserted before going to bed so that the medication will remain in the vagina for a long period. Women using vaginal creams or suppositories may wish to use panty liners during the day when the residual medication may drain out.

PELVIC INFLAMMATORY DISEASE

Pelvic inflammatory disease (PID) is an infectious condition of the pelvic cavity that may involve the fallopian tubes (salpingitis), ovaries (oophoritis), and pelvic peritoneum (peritonitis). A tubo-ovarian abscess may also form (Fig. 54-4). In the United States it is estimated that 1 million women experience an acute episode of PID annually.[19] PID is referred to as "silent" when women do not perceive any symptoms. Other women with PID are in acute distress. PID may also be a cause of chronic pelvic pain (discussed on p. 1289).

Etiology and Pathophysiology

PID is often the result of untreated cervicitis. The organism infecting the cervix ascends higher into the uterus, fallopian tubes, ovaries, and peritoneal cavity. *Chlamydia trachomatis* and *Neisseria gonorrhoeae* are the most common causative organisms of PID. These organisms, as well as anaerobes, mycoplasma, streptococci, and enteric gram-negative rods, gain entrance during sexual intercourse or after pregnancy termination, pelvic surgery, or childbirth. It is important to remember that not all cases of PID are the result of an STI.

Women at increased risk for chlamydial infections (those younger than 24 years of age, who have multiple sex partners, or who have a new sex partner) should be routinely tested for chlamydia. Chlamydial infections can be asymptomatic and unknowingly transmitted during intercourse. Silent PID is a major cause of female infertility.

Clinical Manifestations

Women with PID usually go to a health care provider because they are experiencing lower abdominal pain. The pain typically starts gradually and then becomes constant. The intensity may vary from mild to severe. Movement such as walking can increase the pain. The pain is also frequently associated with intercourse. Spotting after intercourse and purulent cervical or

FIG. 54-4 Pelvic inflammatory disease. Acute infection of the fallopian tubes and the ovaries. The tubes and the ovaries have become an inflamed mass attached to the uterus. A tubo-ovarian abscess is also present.

vaginal discharge may also be noted. Fever and chills may be present. Women with less acute symptoms often notice increased cramping pain with menses, irregular bleeding, and some pain with intercourse. Women who have mild symptoms may go untreated either because they did not seek care or the health care provider misdiagnosed their complaints.

A pelvic examination assists in the diagnosis of PID. Women with PID have lower abdominal tenderness, adnexal tenderness, and positive cervical motion tenderness. Additional criteria useful for diagnosis may include fever and abnormal discharge (vaginal or cervical). Cultures for *N. gonorrhoeae* and *C. trachomatis* are also obtained, and a pregnancy test is done to rule out an ectopic pregnancy. Drug therapy begins when minimal diagnostic criteria are met. Thus treatment is not delayed for culture results. When the patient's pain or obesity compromises the pelvic examination and a tubo-ovarian abscess may be present, a vaginal ultrasound is indicated.

Complications

Immediate complications of PID include septic shock and *Fitz-Hugh-Curtis syndrome*, which occurs when PID spreads to the liver and causes acute perihepatitis. The patient has symptoms of right upper quadrant pain, but liver function tests are normal. Tubo-ovarian abscesses may "leak" or rupture, resulting in pelvic or generalized peritonitis. As the general circulation is flooded with bacterial endotoxins from the infected areas, septic shock may result. Embolisms may occur as the result of thrombophlebitis of the pelvic veins.

PID can cause adhesions and strictures in the fallopian tubes. Ectopic pregnancy may result when a tube is partially obstructed because the sperm can pass through the stricture, but the fertilized ovum cannot reach the uterus. After one episode of PID, the risk of having an ectopic pregnancy increases 10-fold. Further damage can obstruct the fallopian tubes and cause infertility.

Collaborative Care

PID is usually treated on an outpatient basis. The patient is given a combination of antibiotics such as cefoxitin (Mefoxin) and doxycycline (Vibramycin) to provide broad coverage against the causative organisms.[19] With effective antibiotic therapy, the pain should subside. The patient must have no intercourse for 3 weeks. Her partner(s) must be examined and treated. An important part of care is physical rest and oral fluids. Reevaluation in 48 to 72 hours, even if symptoms are improving, is an essential part of outpatient care.

If outpatient treatment is unsuccessful or if the patient is acutely ill or in severe pain, admission to the hospital is indicated. If a tubo-ovarian abscess is present, hospitalization is also indicated. Maximum doses of parenteral antibiotics are given in the hospital. Corticosteroids may be added to the antibiotic regimen to reduce inflammation, allowing for faster recovery and optimizing the chances for subsequent fertility. Application of heat to the lower abdomen or sitz baths may improve circulation and decrease pain. Bed rest in a semi-Fowler's position promotes drainage of the pelvic cavity by gravity and may prevent the development of abscesses high in the abdomen. Analgesics to relieve pain and IV fluids to prevent dehydration are also used.

Surgery is indicated for abscesses that fail to resolve with IV antibiotics. The abscess may be drained by laparoscopy or laparotomy. In extreme cases of infection or severe chronic pelvic pain, a hysterectomy may be performed. When surgery is necessary, the capacity for childbearing is preserved whenever possible.

NURSING MANAGEMENT
PELVIC INFLAMMATORY DISEASE

Subjective and objective data that should be obtained from the woman with PID are presented in Table 54-9. Prevention, early recognition, and prompt treatment of vaginal and cervical infections can help prevent PID and its serious complications. Provide accurate information about factors that place a woman at increased risk for PID. Urge women to seek medical attention for any unusual vaginal discharge or possible infection of their reproductive organs. Inform patients that not all discharge indicates infection, but that early diagnosis and treatment of an infection, if present, can prevent serious complications. Teach patients methods to decrease the risk of getting STIs and to recognize the signs of infection in their partner(s).

The patient may feel guilty about having PID, especially if it is associated with an STI. She may also be concerned about the complications associated with PID, such as adhesions and strictures of the fallopian tubes, infertility, and the increased incidence of ectopic pregnancy. Discuss with the patient her feelings and concerns to help her cope with them more effectively.

For patients requiring hospitalization, you have an important role in implementing drug therapy, monitoring the patient's health status, and providing symptom relief and patient teaching. Record vital signs and the character, amount, color, and odor of the vaginal discharge. Explain the need for limiting

---

TABLE 54-9 NURSING ASSESSMENT
Pelvic Inflammatory Disease

Subjective Data
Important Health Information
Past health history: Use of IUD; previous PID, gonorrhea, or chlamydial infection; multiple sexual partners; exposure to partner with urethritis; infertility
Medications: Use of and allergy to any antibiotics
Surgery or other treatments: Recent abortion or pelvic surgery

Functional Health Patterns
Health perception–health management: Malaise
Nutritional-metabolic: Nausea, vomiting; chills, fever
Elimination: Urinary frequency, urgency
Cognitive-perceptual: Lower abdominal and pelvic pain; low back pain; onset of pain just after a menstrual cycle; dysmenorrhea, dyspareunia, dysuria, vulvar pruritus
Sexuality-reproductive: Abnormal vaginal bleeding and menstrual irregularity; vaginal discharge

Objective Data
Reproductive
Mucopurulent cervicitis, vulvar maceration, vaginal discharge (heavy and purulent to thin and mucoid), tenderness on motion of cervix and uterus; presence of inflammatory masses on palpation

Possible Diagnostic Findings
Leukocytosis; ↑ erythrocyte sedimentation rate; positive culture of secretions or endocervical fluid; pelvic inflammation and positive endometrial biopsy on laparoscopic examination; abscess or inflammation on ultrasonography

IUD, Intrauterine device; *PID,* pelvic inflammatory disease.

activity, being in a semi-Fowler's position, and increasing fluid intake. Assess the degree of abdominal pain to determine the effectiveness of drug therapy.

CHRONIC PELVIC PAIN

Chronic pelvic pain refers to pain in the pelvic region (below the umbilicus and between the hips) that lasts 6 months or longer.[20] It accounts for 10% of all visits to gynecologists and is the reason for 20% to 30% of all laparoscopies. Up to one third of women who have PID have chronic pelvic pain.[21]

The cause of chronic pelvic pain is often hard to find. Many different conditions can cause pelvic pain. Gynecologic etiologies include dysmenorrhea, endometriosis, PID, ovarian cysts, uterine fibroids, pelvic adhesions, and ectopic pregnancies. Abdominal etiologies include irritable bowel syndrome, interstitial cystitis, appendicitis, and colitis. Psychologic factors (e.g., depression, chronic stress, history of sexual or physical abuse) may increase the risk of developing chronic pelvic pain. Emotional distress makes pain worse, and living with chronic pain contributes to emotional distress.

Chronic pelvic pain has many different clinical manifestations, including severe and steady pain, intermittent pain, dull and achy pain, pelvic pressure or heaviness, and sharp pain or cramping. In addition, pain may occur during intercourse or while having a bowel movement.

Determining the cause of chronic pelvic pain often involves a process of elimination. In addition to a detailed history and physical examination (including a pelvic examination), the patient may be asked to keep a journal of the onset of symptoms and any precipitating factors.

Diagnostic tests may include cultures from cervix or vagina (used to detect STIs), ultrasound, computed tomography (CT) scan, or magnetic resonance imaging (MRI) to detect abnormal structures or growths. Laparoscopy may be used to visualize the pelvic organs. This procedure is especially useful in detecting endometriosis and chronic PID.

If the cause of chronic pelvic pain is found, treatment focuses on that cause. If no cause can be found, treatment involves managing the pain. Over-the-counter pain medications (e.g., aspirin, ibuprofen, acetaminophen) may provide some relief. Sometimes stronger pain drugs may be needed. Birth control pills or other hormonal medications may help relieve cyclic pelvic pain related to menstrual cycles. If an infection is the source of the problem, antibiotics are used.

Tricyclic antidepressants (e.g., amitriptyline, nortriptyline [Pamelor]) have pain-relieving and antidepressant effects. These drugs may help improve chronic pelvic pain even in women who do not have depression. The patient may be encouraged to get counseling for any emotional issues.

Laparoscopic surgery may be used to remove pelvic adhesions or endometrial tissue. As a last resort, a hysterectomy may be done.

ENDOMETRIOSIS

Endometriosis is the presence of normal endometrial tissue in sites outside the endometrial cavity.[22] The most frequent sites are in or near the ovaries, uterosacral ligaments, and uterovesical peritoneum (Fig. 54-5). However, endometrial tissues can be in many other locations such as stomach, lungs, intestines, and spleen. The tissue responds to the hormones of the ovarian

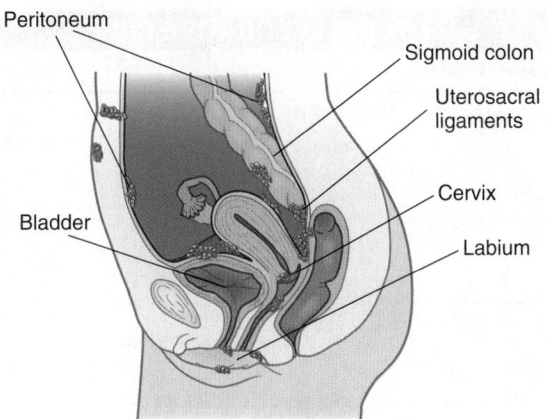

FIG. 54-5 Common sites of endometriosis.

cycle and undergoes a "mini-menstrual cycle" similar to the uterine endometrium.

The typical patient with endometriosis is in her late twenties or early thirties and has never had a full-term pregnancy. Although it is not a life-threatening condition, endometriosis can cause considerable pain. It is also a common cause of infertility and increases the risk of ovarian cancer. Endometriosis is one of the most common gynecologic problems, affecting more than 5.5 million women in North America.[23]

Etiology and Pathophysiology

Although the etiology of endometriosis is poorly understood, many theories have been proposed. A widely held view is that retrograde menstrual flow passes through the fallopian tubes carrying viable endometrial tissues into the pelvis. The tissue attaches to various sites (see Fig. 54-5). Another theory suggests that undifferentiated embryonic peritoneal cavity cells remain dormant in the pelvic tissue until the ovaries produce sufficient hormones to stimulate their growth. Other proposed causes include a genetic predisposition and altered immune function.

Clinical Manifestations

Patients with endometriosis have a wide range of clinical manifestations and severity. The magnitude of a woman's symptoms does not necessarily correlate with the clinical extent of her endometriosis. Dysmenorrhea after years of relatively pain-free menses and infertility may serve as clues to the presence of endometriosis. The most common manifestations are secondary dysmenorrhea, infertility, pelvic pain, dyspareunia, and irregular bleeding. Less common manifestations include backache, painful bowel movements, and dysuria. With menopause, estrogen is no longer produced in the ovaries, and the symptoms may disappear.

When the ectopic endometrial tissues "menstruate," the blood collects in cystlike nodules that have a characteristic bluish black color. When a cyst ruptures, the pain may be acute, and the resulting irritation promotes the formation of adhesions, which attach and fix the affected area to another pelvic structure. Endometrial lesions may become severe enough to cause a bowel obstruction or painful micturition.

Collaborative Care

Endometriosis may be suspected based on a woman's history of the characteristic symptoms and the health care provider's palpation of firm nodular lumps in the adnexa on bimanual

---

TABLE 54-10 COLLABORATIVE CARE

Endometriosis

Diagnostic
- History and physical examination
- Pelvic examination
- Laparoscopy
- Pelvic ultrasound
- MRI

Collaborative Therapy
- Conservative therapy (watch and wait)

Drug Therapy
- Nonsteroidal antiinflammatory drugs (NSAIDs)
- Oral contraceptives
- danazol (Danocrine)
- GnRH agonists (e.g., leuprolide [Lupron])

Surgical Therapy
- Laparotomy to remove implanted tissue and adhesions
- Total abdominal hysterectomy and bilateral salpingo-oophorectomy (TAH-BSO)

GnRH, Gonadotropin-releasing hormone; *MRI,* magnetic resonance imaging.

---

examination. However, laparoscopy is necessary for a definitive diagnosis. The treatment of endometriosis is influenced by the patient's age, desire for pregnancy, symptom severity, and extent and location of the disease. When symptoms are not disruptive, a "watch and wait" approach is used (Table 54-10). When endometriosis is identified as a probable cause of infertility, therapy proceeds more rapidly.

Drug Therapy. Drug therapy is used to reduce symptoms. Pain may be relieved with NSAIDs such as ibuprofen and diclofenac (Voltaren). Drugs to inhibit estrogen production by the ovary are often used to shrink the endometrial tissue. These drugs imitate a state of pregnancy or menopause. Continuous use (for 9 months) of combined oral contraceptives causes regression of endometrial tissue. Ovulation is suppressed by progestin agents such as medroxyprogesterone. Another approach to hormonal treatment is danazol (Danocrine), a synthetic androgen that inhibits the anterior pituitary. This drug causes atrophy of ectopic endometrial tissue. Subjective relief of symptoms is noted within 6 weeks of danazol use. The side effects of weight gain, acne, hot flashes, and hirsutism and the expense of this drug restrict its use.

Another class of drugs used is GnRH agonists (e.g., leuprolide [Lupron], nafarelin [Synarel]). These drugs result in amenorrhea. Side effects are usually the same as those of menopause (hot flashes, vaginal dryness, emotional lability). Loss of bone density has also been reported in women who remain on the therapy longer than 6 months. Endometriosis is controlled but not cured by HT. Persistent lesions give rise to subsequent recurrences once the menstrual cycle is reestablished.

DRUG ALERT: Leuprolide (Lupron)
- Assess patient for pregnancy before initiating therapy.
- Monitor patient for dysrhythmias, palpitations.
- Instruct patient to use nonhormonal contraceptive measures during therapy.

Surgical Therapy. The only cure for endometriosis is surgical removal of all the endometrial implants. Surgical therapy may be conservative or definitive. Conservative surgery is done to confirm the diagnosis or to remove implants. It involves removal or destruction of endometrial implants and lysing or excision of adhesions by means of laparoscopic laser surgery or laparotomy. GnRH agonist therapy (e.g., leuprolide) can be administered for 4 to 6 months to reduce the size of the lesions before surgery. By reducing the extent of the surgery, this preoperative drug treatment helps reduce the development of adhesions that may further threaten fertility. Definitive surgery involves removal of the uterus, fallopian tubes, ovaries, and as many endometrial implants as possible.

For women wishing to get pregnant, conservative surgical therapy is used to remove implants blocking the fallopian tube. Adhesions are removed from the tubes, ovaries, and pelvic structures. Efforts are made to conserve all tissues necessary to maintain fertility.

The individual woman should be actively involved in making the decision about preserving part or all of her ovaries, if surgically possible. Explore her feelings about maintaining her ovarian function. The health care provider should assess the woman's risk for ovarian cancer and provide this information for her consideration.

NURSING MANAGEMENT
ENDOMETRIOSIS

Teach and reassure the patient that endometriosis is not life threatening. This may permit her to accept a conservative and progressive treatment approach. When the symptoms are less severe, teach about nondrug comfort measures that may be helpful. Assist patients in understanding the drugs that have been ordered to treat their condition. Explain the action and possible side effects of the prescribed drug. Psychologic support may be needed for women experiencing severe disabling pain, sexual difficulties secondary to dyspareunia, and infertility.

If conservative surgery is the treatment selected, care is similar to the general preoperative and postoperative care of a patient undergoing laparotomy (see Chapter 43, p. 971). If definitive surgery is planned, the care is similar to that for the patient undergoing an abdominal hysterectomy (see eNursing Care Plan 54-1 on the website for this chapter). Know the extent of the procedure so that appropriate preoperative teaching can be done.

BENIGN TUMORS OF THE FEMALE
REPRODUCTIVE SYSTEM

LEIOMYOMAS

Etiology and Pathophysiology

Leiomyomas (uterine fibroids) are benign smooth-muscle tumors that occur within the uterus. Leiomyomas are common benign tumors of the female genital tract (Fig. 54-6). By 50 years of age, 60% of all women will have had at least one uterine leiomyoma.[24] The cause of leiomyomas is unknown. They appear to depend on ovarian hormones because they grow slowly during the reproductive years and undergo atrophy after menopause.

Clinical Manifestations

The majority of women with leiomyomas do not have any symptoms. When present, the most common symptoms include abnormal uterine bleeding, pain, and symptoms associated with pelvic pressure. Increased bleeding is associated with increased

FIG. 54-6 Leiomyomas. Uterine section showing whorl-like appearance and locations of leiomyomas.

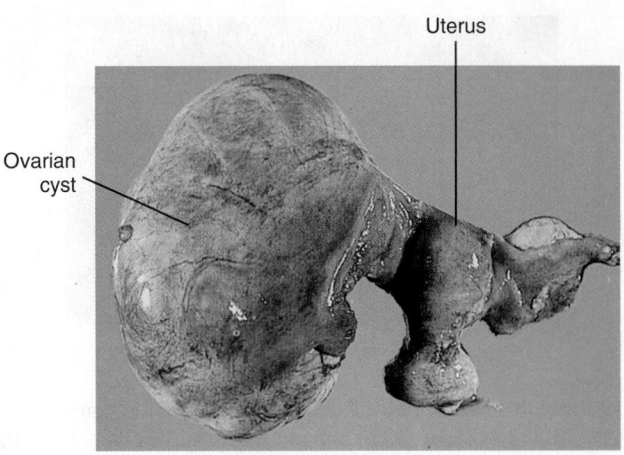

FIG. 54-7 Large ovarian cyst.

endometrial surface area caused by leiomyomas. Pain occurs with infection or twisting of the pedicle from which the tumor is growing. Devascularization and blood vessel compression may also contribute to pain. Pressure on surrounding organs may result in rectal, bladder, and lower abdominal discomfort. Large tumors may cause a general enlargement of the lower abdomen. These tumors are sometimes associated with miscarriage and infertility.

Collaborative Care

Clinical diagnosis is based on the characteristic pelvic findings of an enlarged uterus distorted by nodular masses. Treatment depends on the symptoms, the patient's age, her desire to bear children, and the location and size of the tumors. If the symptoms are minimal, the health care provider may elect to follow the patient closely for a time.

Persistent heavy menstrual bleeding causing anemia and large or rapidly growing tumors are indications for surgery. The leiomyomas are removed by hysterectomy or by myomectomy for women who wish to have children. In this case, only the fibroids are removed to preserve the uterus. Small tumors may be removed using a hysteroscope and laser resection instruments.

Uterine artery embolization is an increasingly used alternative treatment for uterine fibroids.[25] Embolic material (small plastic or gelatin beads) is injected into the uterine artery and carried to the fibroid branches.

Cryosurgery is another option. In cases of large leiomyomas, a GnRH agonist (e.g., leuprolide) may be used preoperatively to shrink the tumor. However, the risks and benefits of this drug should be fully discussed, including the potential for irreversible loss of bone mass. The treatment should not be used on women planning to have children.

Another treatment option uses MRI-guided focused ultrasound to target and destroy uterine fibroids. Treatment requires repeated targeting and heating of the fibroid tissue while the patient lies inside the MRI machine. The procedure can last as long as 3 hours.

CERVICAL POLYPS

Cervical polyps are benign pedunculated lesions that generally arise from the endocervical mucosa and are seen protruding through the cervical os during a speculum examination. Polyps are a characteristic bright cherry-red and are soft and fragile in consistency. They are generally small, measuring less than 3 cm in length, and may be single or multiple. Their cause is unknown.

Symptoms are usually not present, but metrorrhagia and bleeding after straining for a bowel movement and coitus can occur. Polyps are prone to infection. When the polyp is small, it can be excised in an outpatient procedure. If the point of attachment of the polyp cannot be identified and is not accessible to cautery, a polypectomy is performed in an operating room. All tissue removed is sent for pathologic review because polyps occasionally undergo malignant changes.

BENIGN OVARIAN TUMORS

There are many different types of benign tumors. The cause of most of them is unknown. They can be divided into cysts and neoplasms. *Cysts* are usually soft, are surrounded by a thin capsule, and may be detected during the reproductive years. Follicle and corpus luteum cysts are common ovarian cysts (Fig. 54-7). Multiple small ovarian follicles may occur in a condition called *polycystic ovary syndrome* (PCOS) (discussed in the next section). Epithelial ovarian neoplasms may be cystic or solid, and small or extremely large. Cystic teratomas, or dermoid cysts, originate from germ cells and can contain bits of any type of body tissue, such as hair or teeth.

Ovarian masses are often asymptomatic until they are large enough to cause pressure in the pelvis. Constipation, menstrual irregularities, urinary frequency, a full feeling in the abdomen, anorexia, an increase in abdominal girth, and peripheral edema may occur, depending on the tumor's size and location. Pelvic pain may be present if the tumor is growing rapidly. Severe pain results when the cyst twists on its pedicle (ovarian torsion).

In some cases, an ovarian cyst can rupture. A ruptured ovarian cyst is not only extremely painful, but it can lead to serious complications, such as hemorrhage and infection.

Pelvic examination reveals a mass or an enlarged ovary that demands further investigation. If the mass is cystic and smaller than 8 cm, the patient is asked to return for reexamination in 4 to 6 weeks. If the mass is cystic and greater than 8 cm or is solid, laparoscopic surgery or laparotomy is performed. Immediate surgery is necessary if ovarian torsion occurs, causing the ovary to rotate and cutting off circulation. Surgical techniques are used to save as much of the ovary as possible.

Polycystic Ovary Syndrome

Polycystic ovary syndrome (PCOS) is a chronic disorder in which many benign cysts form on the ovaries. It most commonly occurs in women under 30 years old and is a cause of

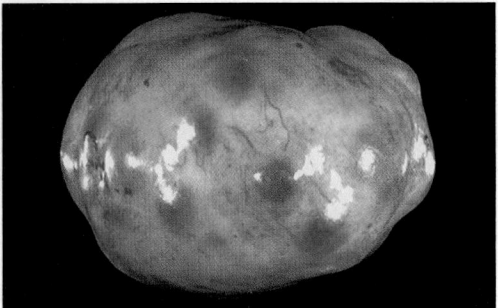

FIG. 54-8 Polycystic ovary syndrome. Multiple fluid-filled cysts in the ovary.

infertility. It affects about 3% to 7% of women of reproductive age.[26] PCOS is due to hormonal abnormalities in which the ovaries produce estrogen and excess testosterone but not progesterone. Fluid-filled cysts develop from mature ovarian follicles that fail to rupture (thereby releasing an egg) each month (Fig. 54-8). This problem affects both ovaries.

Classic manifestations include irregular menstrual periods, amenorrhea, hirsutism, and obesity. Of these manifestations, obesity in particular has been associated with severe symptoms such as excess androgens, oligorrhea, amenorrhea, and infertility. Many women start with normal menstrual periods, which after 1 to 2 years become irregular and then infrequent. If PCOS is left untreated, cardiovascular disease and abnormal insulin resistance with type 2 diabetes mellitus may develop.[27,28]

Pelvic ultrasound reveals enlarged ovaries with multiple small cysts. Successful management includes early diagnosis and treatment to improve quality of life and decrease the risk of complications. Oral contraceptives are useful in regulating menstrual cycles. Hirsutism may be treated with spironolactone. Hyperandrogenism can be treated with flutamide (Eulexin) and a GnRH agonist such as leuprolide. Metformin (Glucophage) reduces hyperinsulinemia and has been shown to improve hyperandrogenism and restore ovulation. For women wishing to become pregnant, fertility drugs (e.g., clomiphene [Clomid]) may be used to induce ovulation. If all other treatments are unsuccessful, a hysterectomy with bilateral salpingectomy and oophorectomy may be performed.

> **DRUG ALERT: Clomiphene (Clomid)**
> Instruct the patient to notify her physician immediately if
> - Lower abdominal pain occurs.
> - Pregnancy is suspected.

Teach the patient the importance of weight management and exercise to decrease insulin resistance. Obesity exacerbates the problems related to PCOS. Monitor lipid profile and fasting glucose levels. Hirsutism is cosmetically distressing for many women. Support the patient as she explores measures to remove unwanted hair (e.g., depilating agents, electrolysis). Stress the importance of regular follow-up care to monitor the effectiveness of therapy and to detect any complications.

CANCERS OF THE FEMALE REPRODUCTIVE SYSTEM

CERVICAL CANCER

Approximately 12,000 women in the United States are diagnosed with cervical cancer and 4200 women die from cervical cancer annually.[29] Noninvasive cervical cancer (in situ) is about

four times more common than invasive cervical cancer. The mortality rate for cervical cancer in the United States is twice as high for African American women as it is for white women. An increased risk of cervical cancer is associated with low socioeconomic status, early sexual activity (before 17 years of age), multiple sexual partners, infection with HPV, immunosuppression, and smoking.

The number of deaths from cervical cancer in the United States has fallen steadily over the past 50 years because of better and earlier diagnosis with the widespread use of the Papanicolaou (Pap) test. In addition to cancer, the Pap test screens for precancerous changes. Treatment of precancerous lesions can prevent progression to cervical cancer.

Etiology and Pathophysiology

The progression from normal cervical cells to dysplasia and then to invasive cervical cancer appears to be related to repeated injuries to the cervix. The progression occurs slowly over years. A strong relationship exists between dysplasia and HPV infections. HPV types 16 and 18 together cause about 70% of cervical cancers. Cancer rates are expected to decline further with vaccines (e.g., Gardasil, Cervarix) now being used for the prevention of HPV.[30]

Clinical Manifestations

Precancerous changes are asymptomatic. This highlights the importance of routine screening. The peak incidence of noninvasive cervical cancer is in women in their early thirties. The average age for women with invasive cervical cancer is 50 (Fig. 54-9). Early cervical cancer is generally asymptomatic, but leukorrhea and intermenstrual bleeding eventually occur. The discharge is usually thin and watery but becomes dark and foul smelling as the disease advances, suggesting an infection. The vaginal bleeding is initially only spotting. As the tumor enlarges, bleeding becomes heavier and more frequent. Pain is a late symptom and is followed by weight loss, anemia, and cachexia.

Diagnostic Studies

The American Cancer Society recommends the following guidelines for annual Pap testing:[31]
- Begin testing at age 21 regardless of when a woman becomes sexually active.

FIG. 54-9 Cervical cancer. View through a speculum inserted into the vagina.

- Women ages 21 to 65 years old should be screened with the Pap test every 3 years.
- Women who have had a total hysterectomy (uterus and cervix removed) for reasons not related to cervical cancer do not need to be tested.
- Women 65 and older should no longer be screened after having two or three consecutive negative Pap tests within the last 2 years.

Women with a history of cervical cancer should continue with screening as recommended by their health care provider for at least 20 years. A woman who has been vaccinated against HPV needs to continue following the screening guidelines for her age-group.

The two types of HPV that have been associated with most cases of cervical cancer (types 16 and 18) can be identified through deoxyribonucleic acid (DNA) testing. HPV DNA tests help determine if women with abnormal Pap test results need further follow-up. Women ages 30 to 65 who have the HPV DNA test and the Pap test (co-testing) can be screened every 5 years rather than every 3 years.

Pap tests are less than 100% accurate in screening for cervical cell abnormalities. Problems occur with both false-positive and false-negative reports. ThinPrep, a liquid-based technique for Pap tests, has reduced the number of inaccurate test results.

The finding of an abnormal Pap test indicates the need for follow-up. Women with minor changes may be followed with a repeated Pap test in 4 to 6 months for 2 years. Up to 80% may revert to normal spontaneously. Women with more prominent changes receive additional procedures, such as colposcopy and biopsy, before a definitive diagnosis can be made. Colposcopy helps identify possible epithelial abnormalities and suggests areas for biopsy. Biopsies are sent for pathologic evaluation. Colposcopy and biopsy have improved diagnosis and allow more focused treatments.

The type and extent of the biopsy vary with the abnormality seen. A punch biopsy may be done on an outpatient basis with a special punch biopsy forceps. The excision of a cone-shaped section of the cervix may be used for both diagnosis and treatment. Conization is accomplished using one of several techniques, depending on the health care provider's experience and the availability of equipment. *Cryotherapy* (freezing) and laser cone vaporization destroy the tissue. Laser cone excision and the *loop electrosurgery excision procedure*

TABLE 54-11   STAGING AND TREATMENT OF CERVICAL CANCER

Stage	Extent	Treatment
0	In situ	Cervical conization, hysterectomy, cryosurgery, laser surgery
I	Confinement to cervix	Radiation, radical hysterectomy
II	Spread beyond cervix to upper two thirds of vagina but not to tissues around uterus	Radiation, cisplatin-based chemotherapy, radical hysterectomy
III	Spread to pelvic wall, involvement of lower third of vagina, and/or has caused kidney problems	Radiation, cisplatin-based chemotherapy
IV	Spread to other parts of the body such as bladder, rectum, liver, lungs, and bones	Radiation, surgery (e.g., pelvic exenteration), cisplatin-based chemotherapy

Modified from National Cancer Institute: Cancer cervical treatment: stages of cervical cancer. Retrieved from *www.cancer.gov/cancertopics/pdq/treatment/cervical/Patient/page2.*

(LEEP) remove the identified tissue and allow for histologic examination to ensure that all microinvasive tissue has been removed. These can be performed as outpatient procedures with mild analgesics or sedation. Complications of these procedures include excessive bleeding and possible cervical stenosis after healing.

Collaborative Care

Vaccines against HPV reduce the incidence of both cervical-related neoplasia and cervical cancer due to infection from HPV types 16 and 18. Vaccination against HPV is recommended for females and males beginning at ages 11 or 12 years. (Vaccines are discussed further in Chapter 53, p. 1270.)

The treatment of cervical cancer is guided by the stage of the tumor and the patient's age and general state of health (Table 54-11). There are four procedures in which fertility can be preserved. Conization may be the only type of therapy needed for noninvasive cervical cancer if analysis of removed tissue demonstrates that a wide area of normal tissue surrounds the excised tissue. Laser treatments can be used in which a directed infrared beam is employed to destroy abnormal tissue. Cautery and cryosurgery may also be used.

Invasive cancer of the cervix is treated with surgery, radiation, and chemotherapy as single treatments or in combination. Surgical procedures include hysterectomy, radical hysterectomy (involving adjacent structures), and, rarely, pelvic exenteration. (Surgical therapy is discussed on p. 1297.) Radiation may be by external (e.g., cobalt) or internal implants (e.g., cesium, radium). Standard radiation treatment is 4 to 6 weeks of external radiation followed by one or two treatments with internal implants (brachytherapy). (Radiation therapy is discussed in Chapter 16.) Cisplatin-based chemotherapy regimens benefit patients with cancer spread beyond the cervix.

ENDOMETRIAL CANCER

Cancer of the endometrium is the most common gynecologic malignancy. Approximately 47,000 newly diagnosed cases of endometrial cancer and 8000 deaths occur annually. Endometrial cancer has a relatively low mortality rate, since most cases are diagnosed early. The survival rate is over 95% if the cancer has not spread at the time of diagnosis.

Etiology and Pathophysiology

The major risk factor for endometrial cancer is estrogen, especially unopposed estrogen.[32] Additional risk factors include increasing age, nulliparity, late menopause, obesity, smoking, diabetes mellitus, and a personal or family history of hereditary nonpolyposis colorectal cancer (HNPCC) (see the Genetics in Clinical Practice box for HNPCC in Chapter 43 on p. 986). Obesity is a risk factor because adipose cells store estrogen, thus increasing endogenous estrogen. Pregnancy and oral contraceptives are protective factors.

Endometrial cancer arises from the lining of the endometrium. Most tumors are adenocarcinomas. The precursor may be a hyperplastic state that progresses to invasive carcinoma. Hyperplasia occurs when estrogen is not counteracted by progesterone. The cancer directly extends into the cervix and through the uterine serosa. As invasion of the myometrium occurs, regional lymph nodes, including the paravaginal and para-aortic, become involved. Hematogenous metastases develop concurrently. The usual sites of metastases are lung, bone, liver, and eventually the brain. Malignant cells can be found in the peritoneal cavity, probably after transport through the fallopian tubes.

Prognostic factors include histologic differentiation, myometrial invasion, peritoneal cytology, lymph node and adnexal metastases, and tumor size. Endometrial cancer grows slowly, metastasizes late, and is curable with therapy if diagnosed early.

Clinical Manifestations

The first sign of endometrial cancer is abnormal uterine bleeding, usually in postmenopausal women. Because perimenopausal women have sporadic periods for a time, it is important that this sign not be ignored or attributed to menopause.

Pain occurs late in the disease process. Other manifestations that may arise are related to metastasis to other organs. Metastatic spread occurs in a characteristic pattern. Spread to the pelvic and para-aortic nodes is common. When distant metastasis occurs, it most commonly involves the lungs, liver, bones, brain, and vagina.

Collaborative Care

Endometrial biopsy is the primary diagnostic test for endometrial cancer. Endometrial biopsy is done on an outpatient basis. Any abnormal or unexpected bleeding in a postmenopausal woman requires obtaining a tissue sample to exclude endometrial cancer. For women who have or are at risk of developing HNPCC, the American Cancer Society recommends annual screening with endometrial biopsy beginning at 35 years of age. The Pap test is not a reliable diagnostic tool for endometrial cancer, but it can rule out cervical cancer.

Most cases of endometrial cancer are diagnosed at an early stage when surgery alone may result in cure. Treatment of endometrial cancer is a total hysterectomy and bilateral salpingo-oophorectomy with lymph node biopsies. The lack of estrogen and progesterone receptors is a poor prognostic indicator. Surgery may be followed by radiation, either to the pelvis or the abdomen externally or intravaginally, to decrease local recurrence.

No tumor markers with high sensitivity and high specificity for endometrial cancer are known at present, although CA-125 is often used in clinical practice. CA-125 has been used in surveillance of advanced endometrial cancer. In patients who have increased CA-125 values pretreatment, this test might prove useful in posttreatment surveillance.

Treatment of advanced or recurrent disease is difficult. Progesterone HT (e.g., megestrol [Megace]) can be used when the progesterone receptor status is positive and the tumor is well differentiated.[32] Tamoxifen (Nolvadex), either alone or in combination with progesterone therapy, is also effective in women with advanced or recurrent endometrial cancer. Chemotherapy is considered when progesterone therapy is unsuccessful. Agents used include doxorubicin (Adriamycin), cisplatin (Platinol), 5-fluorouracil (5-FU), carboplatin (Paraplatin), and paclitaxel (Taxol).

OVARIAN CANCER

Ovarian cancer is a malignant tumor of the ovaries. About 22,280 new cases of ovarian cancer are diagnosed in the United States each year, and about 15,000 women die from the disease annually. It is the fifth leading cause of cancer deaths in women in the United States. Most women with ovarian cancer have advanced disease at diagnosis.[33] It occurs most frequently in women between 55 and 65 years of age. White women are at greater risk for ovarian cancer than African American women.

Etiology and Pathophysiology

Genetic Link

The cause of ovarian cancer is not known. Women who have mutations of the *BRCA* genes have an increased susceptibility

🧬 GENETICS IN CLINICAL PRACTICE
Ovarian Cancer

Genetic Basis
- Mutations in *BRCA1* and/or *BRCA2* genes.
- Normally these genes are tumor suppressor genes involved in DNA repair.
- Autosomal dominant transmission.
- Mutations passed down from either mother or father.

Incidence
- About 10% of cases of ovarian cancer are related to hereditary factors.
- Women with *BRCA1* mutations have a 25%-40% lifetime risk of developing ovarian cancer.
- Women with *BRCA2* mutations have a 10%-20% lifetime risk of developing ovarian cancer.
- Family history of both breast and ovarian cancer increases the risk of having a *BRCA* mutation.
- *BRCA* mutations occur in 10%-20% of patients with ovarian cancer who have no family history of breast or ovarian cancer.

Genetic Testing
- DNA testing is available for *BRCA1* and *BRCA2* genetic mutations.

Clinical Implications
- Bilateral oophorectomy reduces the risk of ovarian cancer in women with *BRCA1* and *BRCA2* mutations.
- Genetic counseling and testing for *BRCA* mutations should be considered for women whose personal or family history puts them at high risk for a genetic predisposition to ovarian cancer.

TABLE 54-12 COLLABORATIVE CARE
Ovarian Cancer

Diagnostic
- History and physical examination
- Pelvic examination
- Abdominal and transvaginal ultrasound
- CA-125 level
- Laparotomy for diagnostic staging

Collaborative Therapy
- Surgery
  - Abdominal hysterectomy and bilateral salpingo-oophorectomy with pelvic lymph node biopsies
  - Debulking for advanced disease
- Chemotherapy
  - Adjuvant and palliative
- Radiation therapy
  - Adjuvant and palliative

---

to ovarian cancer. The *BRCA* genes are tumor suppressor genes that inhibit tumor growth when functioning normally. When they mutate, they lose their tumor suppressor ability. This results in an increased risk for women to develop ovarian or breast cancer (see the Genetics in Clinical Practice box).

The major risk factor for ovarian cancer is family history (one or more first-degree relatives). A family history of breast or colon cancer is also a risk factor. Other risk factors include a personal history of breast or colon cancer and HNPCC (see the Genetics in Clinical Practice box on HNPCC in Chapter 43 on p. 986).

Women who have never been pregnant (nulliparity) are also at higher risk. Other risk factors include increasing age, high-fat diet, increased number of ovulatory cycles (usually associated with early menarche and late menopause), HT, and possibly the use of infertility drugs.

Breastfeeding, multiple pregnancies, oral contraceptive use (more than 5 years), and early age at first birth seem to reduce the risk of ovarian cancer. These factors may have a protective effect because they reduce the number of ovulatory cycles, and thus reduce the exposure to estrogen.

About 90% of ovarian cancers are epithelial carcinomas that arise from malignant transformation of the surface epithelial cells. Germ cell tumors account for another 10%. Histologic grading is an important prognostic determinant. Tumor cells are graded according to the level of differentiation, ranging from well differentiated (grade I) to poorly differentiated (grade III) to undifferentiated (grade IV). Grade IV cells carry a poorer prognosis than the other grades.

Intraperitoneal dissemination is a common characteristic of ovarian cancer. It metastasizes to the uterus, bladder, bowel, and omentum. In advanced disease, it can spread to the stomach, colon, liver, and other parts of the body.

Clinical Manifestations

Symptoms are vague in the early stages. An accumulation of fluid initially causes abdominal enlargement. Nonspecific symptoms that warrant further evaluation include pelvic or abdominal pain, bloating, urinary urgency or frequency, and difficulty eating or feeling full quickly.[33] Women who have one or more of these symptoms, especially if they are new, persistent (occur at least 12 days per month), or worsening, need to see their health care provider. Vaginal bleeding rarely occurs, and pain is not an early symptom. Later signs are increased abdominal girth, unexplained weight loss or gain, and menstrual changes.

Diagnostic Studies

No screening test exists for ovarian cancer. Because early ovarian cancer has vague symptoms, yearly bimanual pelvic examinations should be performed to identify an ovarian mass (Table 54-12). Postmenopausal women should not have palpable ovaries, so a mass of any size should be suspected as possible ovarian cancer. An abdominal or a transvaginal ultrasound can be done to detect ovarian masses. An exploratory laparotomy may be used to establish the diagnosis and stage the disease.

A test called OVA1 can help detect whether a pelvic mass is benign or malignant before it is surgically removed. OVA1 uses a blood sample to test for levels of five biomarkers that change due to ovarian cancer. It is not intended for ovarian cancer screening or for a definitive diagnosis of ovarian cancer.

For women with a high risk for ovarian cancer, screening using a combination of the tumor marker (CA-125) and ultrasound is often recommended in addition to a yearly pelvic examination. CA-125 is positive in 80% of women with epithelial ovarian cancer and is used to monitor the course of the disease. However, levels of CA-125 may be elevated with other malignancies (e.g., pancreatic cancer) or with benign conditions such as fibroids or endometriosis. A large recent clinical trial has reported that screening by CA-125 and ultrasound did not result in fewer deaths from ovarian cancer.[34] Currently only 20% of ovarian cancers are diagnosed at an early stage.

Collaborative Care

Women identified as being at high risk based on family and health history may require counseling regarding options such as prophylactic oophorectomy and oral contraceptives. It is important to note that although oophorectomy significantly reduces the risk of ovarian cancer, it does not completely eliminate the possibility of the disease.

Ovarian cancer staging is critical for guiding treatment decisions. Stage I describes disease limited to the ovaries; stage II, disease limited to the pelvis; stage III, disease limited to the abdominal cavity; and stage IV, distant metastatic disease. The overall survival rate is 90% with early disease, 36% with local spread, and 20% with distant metastases.

Most patients with ovarian cancer have widespread disease at presentation. The initial treatment for all stages of ovarian cancer is surgery, which is usually a total abdominal hysterectomy and bilateral salpingo-oophorectomy with omentectomy and removal of as much of the tumor as possible (i.e., tumor debulking). Surgery facilitates chemotherapy by reducing the number of cells that the chemotherapy has to kill.

Depending on the differentiation of the cells and the stage of cancer, other treatment options include intraperitoneal and systemic chemotherapy, intraperitoneal instillation of radioisotopes, and external abdominal and pelvic radiation therapy. If a patient is clinically free of symptoms after completing treatment, a "second-look" surgical procedure is often performed to determine whether there is any evidence of disease. If no disease is found, the patient is monitored for recurrent disease.

Chemotherapy usually consists of a combination of a platinum compound, such as cisplatin or carboplatin, and a taxane, such as paclitaxel or docetaxel (Taxotere). The typical course of chemotherapy involves three to six cycles. A cycle is a schedule that allows regular doses of a drug, followed by a rest period.

Other chemotherapy drugs used include altretamine (Hexalen), topotecan (Hycamtin), etoposide (VePesid), gemcitabine (Gemzar), and oxaliplatin (Eloxatin). These drugs may be used to treat recurrent disease or as a palliative measure to shrink the tumor to relieve pressure and pain.

VAGINAL CANCER

Primary vaginal cancers are rare, with about 2680 new cases reported annually. The peak incidence is between ages 50 and 70. Vaginal tumors are usually secondary sites or metastases of other cancers such as cervical or endometrial carcinomas. The most common type of vaginal cancer is squamous cell carcinoma. Intrauterine exposure to diethylstilbestrol (DES) places a woman at risk for clear cell adenocarcinoma of the vagina.

Treatment of vaginal cancer depends on the type of cells involved, the stage of the disease, and the size and location of the tumor. Squamous cell carcinomas can be treated with both surgery and radiation.

VULVAR CANCER

Cancer of the vulva is relatively rare, with about 4490 new cases reported annually. Similar to cervical cancer, preinvasive lesions referred to as vulvar intraepithelial neoplasia (VIN) precede invasive vulvar cancer. The invasive form occurs mainly in women over 60 years of age, with the highest incidence being in women in their seventies.

Patients with vulvar neoplasia may have symptoms of vulvar itching or burning, pain, bleeding, or discharge. Women who are immunosuppressed and/or have diabetes mellitus, hypertension, or chronic vulvar dystrophies are at a higher risk for developing vulvar cancers. Several subtypes of HPV have been identified in some but not all vulvar cancers. Vaccines (Gardasil,

Cervarix) are now available to protect against some vaginal and vulvar cancers that are caused by these HPV subtypes. (Vaccines for HPV are discussed in Chapter 53, p. 1270.)

Diagnosis of vulvar cancer is based on physical examination, colposcopy, and biopsy results of the suspicious lesion. VIN can be treated topically with imiquimod cream (Aldara) or surgery.

Laser therapy may be used to kill cancer cells. Surgery is the most common treatment for cancer of the vulva. The goal of surgery is to remove all the cancer without any loss of the woman's sexual function. A local excision with removal of the lesion and surrounding tissue may be done. For more extensive lesions, vulvectomy may be done (various types of vulvectomies are presented in Table 54-13). If the cancer is

TABLE 54-13	SURGICAL PROCEDURES INVOLVING THE FEMALE REPRODUCTIVE SYSTEM
Type of Surgery	**Description**
Abdominal Hysterectomy	
Total hysterectomy	Uterus and cervix removed using large abdominal incision (bikini cut).
Total abdominal hysterectomy and bilateral salpingo-oophorectomy (TAH-BSO)	Uterus, cervix, fallopian tubes, and ovaries removed using large abdominal incision.
Radical hysterectomy	Panhysterectomy, partial vaginectomy, and dissection of lymph nodes in pelvis.
Vaginal Hysterectomy	Uterus and cervix removed through a cut in the top of vagina.
Laparoscopic Hysterectomy	Laparoscope (video camera and small surgical instruments).
Laparoscopic-assisted vaginal hysterectomy (LAVH)	Incision made at top of vagina. Uterus and cervix removed through the vagina. Laparoscope inserted into abdomen to assist in the procedure.
Laparoscopic supracervical hysterectomy	Uterus removed using only laparoscopic instruments. Cervix is left intact.
Robotic-Assisted Surgery	Robot (special machine) used to do surgery through small abdominal incisions. Most often used when a patient has cancer or is very overweight and vaginal surgery is not safe.
Vulvectomy	Surgical procedure to remove part or all of the vulva.
Skinning vulvectomy	Removal of top layer of vulvar skin where the cancer is found. Skin grafts from other parts of the body may be needed to cover the area.
Simple vulvectomy	Entire vulva is removed
Radical vulvectomy	Entire vulva, including clitoris, labia majora and minora, and nearby tissue, is removed. Nearby lymph nodes may also be removed.
Vaginectomy	Removal of vagina.
Pelvic Exenteration	Radical hysterectomy, total vaginectomy, removal of bladder with diversion of urinary system and resection of colon and rectum with colostomy.

extensive, a pelvic exenteration may be done. As adjuvant measures, the patient may have *chemotherapy* or *radiation therapy* after surgery.

SURGICAL PROCEDURES: FEMALE REPRODUCTIVE SYSTEM

A variety of surgical procedures are performed when benign or malignant tumors of the genital tract are found (see Table 54-13). A *hysterectomy* (removal of the uterus) is performed for excision of cancerous tumors of the female reproductive system. A hysterectomy may be done abdominally, vaginally, or laparoscopically. The abdominal route is used when large tumors are present and the pelvic cavity is to be explored or when the tubes and ovaries are to be removed at the same time (Fig. 54-10). The abdominal route can present more postoperative problems because it involves an incision and the opening of the abdominal cavity.

A vaginal route is often used when vaginal repair is done in addition to removal of the uterus. In both vaginal and abdominal hysterectomies, the ligaments that support the uterus are attached to the vaginal cuff to maintain the normal depth of the vagina. Laparoscopic procedures have the advantage of quicker recovery time and fewer complications.[35]

Depending on the findings and reason for the hysterectomy, the cervix may be left in place and not removed. Preserving the cervix may decrease the risk of pelvic floor prolapse and urinary incontinence. The patient needs to continue to get Pap tests if the cervix is left in place or the surgery was done to treat cancer.

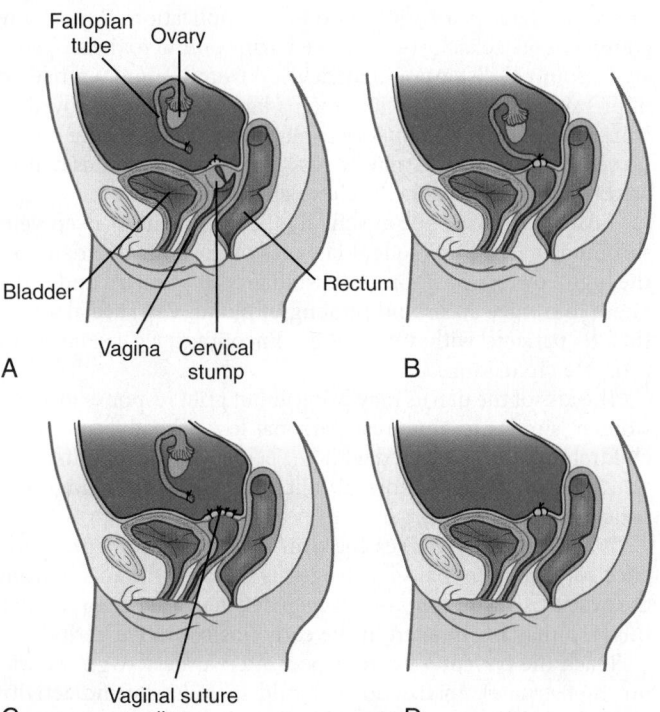

FIG. 54-10 A, Cross section of subtotal hysterectomy. Note that cervical stump, fallopian tubes, and ovaries remain. **B,** Cross section of total hysterectomy. Note that fallopian tubes and ovaries remain. **C,** Cross section of vaginal hysterectomy. Note that fallopian tubes and ovaries remain. **D,** Total hysterectomy, salpingectomy, and oophorectomy. Note that uterus, fallopian tubes, and ovaries are completely removed.

RADIATION THERAPY: CANCERS OF FEMALE REPRODUCTIVE SYSTEM

Radiation is used to cure or control or as a palliative measure for cancers of the female reproductive system, either alone or in combination with other treatments. The goal of radiation therapy is to deliver a specific amount of high-energy (or ionizing) radiation to the cancer with minimal damage to the normal surrounding tissue. Radiation therapy may be external or internal (brachytherapy).

External Radiation Therapy

With external radiation therapy, a source outside of the body delivers electromagnetic radiation in the form of waves. (External radiation therapy and related nursing care are discussed in Chapter 16.)

Brachytherapy

Brachytherapy allows the radiation to be placed internally near or into the tumor. This method can deliver a high dose of radiation directly to the tumor.[36] The dose decreases sharply farther away from the source, causing less damage to the surrounding normal tissue. A variety of forms are used to deliver the therapy, including wires, capsules, needles, tubes, and seeds. Brachytherapy is used in the management of cervical and endometrial cancer because of the accessibility of these body parts and the favorable results obtained. Radium and cesium are two commonly used isotopes.

To prepare the patient for the treatment, give a cleansing enema to prevent straining at stool, which could cause displacement of the isotope. Insert an indwelling catheter to prevent a distended bladder from coming into contact with the radioactive source.

A variety of applicators have been developed for intrauterine treatment. Applicators are inserted into the endometrial cavity and vagina in the operating room. When the applicator contains the radioactive material, this is known as *preloading*. In *afterloading* the applicator is implanted in the operating room but is not loaded with the radioactive material until its correct placement is verified and the patient has returned to her room.

Radiation exposure to the patient is precisely controlled. The radiation exposure to the physician and other personnel involved in the implantation is reduced when the afterload technique is used. The applicator is secured with vaginal packing and is left in place for 24 to 72 hours.

During treatment the patient is placed in a lead-lined private room and is on absolute bed rest. She may be turned from side to side. The presence of an intrauterine applicator produces uterine contractions that may require analgesics. The destruction of cells results in a foul-smelling vaginal discharge, and a deodorizer is helpful. Nausea, vomiting, diarrhea, and malaise may develop as a systemic reaction to the radiation.

At the end of the prescribed period of radiation, the radioactive material and the catheter are removed. The patient is allowed off bed rest and is discharged from the hospital when stable. Late complications that may arise include fistulas (vesicovaginal, ureterovaginal), cystitis, phlebitis, hemorrhage, and fibrosis. If fibrosis occurs, the vaginal wall becomes smaller in diameter and shorter. Dilation of the vagina through intercourse or the use of sequentially sized dilators may be indicated. The patient is urged to report any unusual symptoms or complaints to her physician. (Brachytherapy and related nursing care are discussed in Chapter 16.)

NURSING MANAGEMENT
CANCERS OF FEMALE REPRODUCTIVE SYSTEM

NURSING ASSESSMENT

Malignant tumors of the female reproductive system can be found in the cervix, endometrium, ovaries, vagina, and vulva. A patient with any of these malignant tumors may experience a variety of clinical manifestations, including leukorrhea, irregular vaginal bleeding, vaginal discharge, abdominal pain and pressure, bowel and bladder dysfunction, and vulvar itching and burning. Assessment for these signs and symptoms is an important nursing responsibility.

NURSING DIAGNOSES

Nursing diagnoses for the female patient with cancer of the reproductive system include, but are not limited to, the following:

- Anxiety *related to* threat of a malignancy and lack of knowledge about the disease process and prognosis
- Acute pain *related to* pressure secondary to an enlarging tumor
- Disturbed body image *related to* loss of body part and loss of good health
- Ineffective sexuality pattern *related to* physiologic limitations and fatigue
- Grieving *related to* poor prognosis of advanced disease

PLANNING

The overall goals are that the patient with cancer of the female reproductive system will (1) actively participate in treatment decisions, (2) achieve satisfactory pain and symptom management, (3) recognize and report problems promptly, (4) maintain preferred lifestyle as long as possible, and (5) continue to practice cancer detection strategies.

NURSING IMPLEMENTATION

HEALTH PROMOTION. Through your contact with women in a variety of settings, teach women the importance of routine screening for cancers of the reproductive system. Cancer can be prevented when screening reveals precancerous conditions of the vulva, cervix, endometrium, and, rarely, the ovaries. Also, routine screening increases the chance that a cancer will be found in an early stage. When cancer is identified early, treatment can be more conservative and the woman's prognosis improves. A yearly pelvic examination and Pap test (as indicated) allow the health care provider to detect lesions on the vulva or any uterine or ovarian irregularities and screen for cervical cancer. Encourage women to view routine cancer screening and vaccination against cervical cancer as important self-care activities.

Teaching women about risk factors for cancers of the reproductive system is also important. Limiting sexual activity during adolescence, using condoms, having fewer sexual partners, and not smoking reduce the risk of cervical cancer. When high-risk behaviors are identified, assist women in modifying their lifestyles to decrease risk.

ACUTE INTERVENTION RELATED TO SURGERY. All patients experience a degree of anxiety when contemplating surgery, but the prospect of major gynecologic surgery increases these concerns.

Some women may experience guilt, anger, or embarrassment. Still others may focus on the effect the surgery will have on their reproductive and sexual functions. Some women view the whole process as annoying, whereas others are relieved by the thought of no longer having menstrual periods or becoming pregnant. Try to understand the patient's fears and concerns. Each patient needs to be assessed as an individual. Be willing to listen, since this can provide considerable psychologic support.

Preoperatively, prepare the patient physically for surgery with the standard perineal or abdominal preparation. A vaginal douche and enemas may be given (based on the surgeon's preference). The bladder should be emptied before the patient is sent to the operating room. An indwelling catheter is commonly inserted preoperatively. (See Chapter 18 for discussion of general preoperative patient care.)

Hysterectomy. Postoperatively, the patient who has had an abdominal hysterectomy will have an abdominal dressing. Observe the dressing frequently for any sign of bleeding during the first 8 hours after surgery. (See eNursing Care Plan 54-1 for care of the patient after a total abdominal hysterectomy.)

The patient who has had a vaginal hysterectomy will have a perineal pad. A moderate amount of serosanguineous drainage on the perineal pad is expected. The patient may experience urinary retention postoperatively because of temporary bladder atony resulting from edema or nerve trauma. At times an indwelling catheter is used for 1 to 2 days postoperatively to maintain constant drainage of the bladder and prevent strain on the suture line. If an indwelling catheter is not used, catheterization may be necessary if the patient has not urinated for 8 hours postoperatively. If residual urine is suspected after the removal of an indwelling catheter, catheterization is done to prevent bladder infection caused by pooling of urine. Accidental ligation of a ureter is a serious surgical complication. Report any complaint of backache or decreased urine output to the surgeon.

Abdominal distention may develop from the sudden release of pressure on the intestines when a large tumor is removed or from paralytic ileus secondary to anesthesia and pressure on the bowel. Food and fluids may be restricted if the patient is nauseated. Ambulation will help relieve abdominal flatus.

Take special care to prevent the development of deep vein thrombosis (DVT). Frequent changes of position, avoidance of the high Fowler's position, and avoidance of pressure under the knees minimize stasis and pooling of blood. Pay special attention to patients with varicosities. Encourage leg exercises to promote circulation.

The loss of the uterus may bring about grief response in some women, similar to any great personal loss. The ability to bear children may be associated with her perception of womanhood. Grief from this loss is normal. Elicit the woman's feelings and concerns about her surgery.

When surgery removes the ovaries as well, women experience surgical menopause. Estrogen is no longer available from the ovaries, so symptoms of estrogen deficiency arise. To counter this, HT may be initiated in the early postoperative period.

Teach the patient what to expect after surgery (e.g., she will not menstruate). Instructions should include specific activity restrictions. Intercourse should be avoided until the wound is healed (about 4 to 6 weeks). However, intercourse is not contraindicated once healing is complete. If a vaginal hysterectomy is performed, inform the patient that she may have a temporary loss of vaginal sensation. Reassure her that the sensation will return in several months.

Physical restrictions are limited for a short time. Heavy lifting should be avoided for 2 months. Teach her to avoid activities that may increase pelvic congestion, such as dancing and walking swiftly, for several months. However, activities such as swimming may be both physically and mentally helpful. Assure her that once healing is complete, all previous activity can be resumed.

Many women report a decrease in the quality of their sex lives after cancer treatment.[37] Provide information on what to expect related to their sexual functioning before the treatment and reinforce it afterward.

Salpingectomy and Oophorectomy. Postoperative care of the woman who has undergone removal of a fallopian tube (salpingectomy) or an ovary (oophorectomy) is similar to that for any patient having abdominal surgery. However, if a large ovarian cyst was removed, she may have abdominal distention caused by the sudden release of pressure in the intestines. An abdominal binder may provide relief until the distention subsides.

When both ovaries are removed (bilateral oophorectomy), surgical menopause results. The symptoms are similar to those of regular menopause but may be more severe because of the sudden withdrawal of hormones. Attempts may be made to leave at least a portion of an ovary.

Vulvectomy. Although cancer of the vulva is relatively uncommon, it is important to recognize the extent of the vulvectomy and the significant effect it is likely to have on the patient's life. Having an honest, open attitude with the patient and her partner preoperatively can be most helpful in the postoperative period.

After a vulvectomy (see Table 54-13), the patient has a wound in the perineal area extending to the groin. The wound may be covered or left exposed and frequently has drains attached to portable suction (e.g., Hemovac, Jackson-Pratt). A heavy pressure dressing is often in place for the first 24 to 48 hours. The wound is cleaned with normal saline solution or an antiseptic twice daily. Solutions can be applied with an aseptic bulb syringe or a Waterpik machine. Wound care must be meticulous to prevent infection, which results in delayed healing.

Special attention to bowel and bladder care is needed. A low-residue diet and stool softeners prevent straining and wound contamination. An indwelling catheter is used to provide urinary drainage. Be careful not to dislodge the catheter because extensive edema makes its reinsertion difficult. Heavy, taut sutures are often used to close the wounds, resulting in severe discomfort. In other instances, the wound may be allowed to heal by granulation. Analgesics may be required to control pain. Carefully position the patient using strategically placed pillows to provide comfort. Anticoagulant therapy to prevent DVTs is common.

Because the surgery causes mutilation of the perineal area and the healing process is slow, the patient is likely to become discouraged. Provide opportunities for the patient to express her feelings and concerns about the operation. Teach the patient specific instructions in self-care before discharge. Instruct her to report any unusual odor, fresh bleeding, breakdown of incision, or perineal pain. Home care nursing can benefit the patient during her adjustment period.

Sexual function is often retained. Whether clitoral sensation is retained may be critical to some women, particularly if it was a primary source of orgasmic satisfaction. Discussing alternative methods of achieving sexual satisfaction may be indicated.

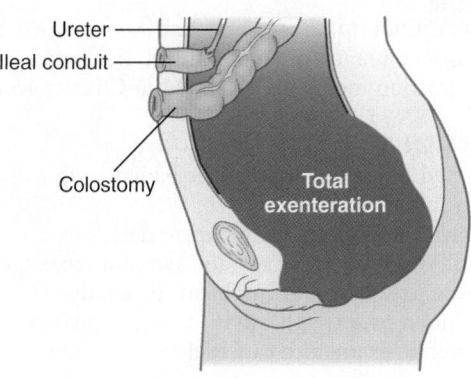

FIG. 54-11 Total exenteration is removal of all pelvic organs with creation of an ileal conduit and a colostomy.

Pelvic Exenteration. When other forms of therapy fail to control the spread of cancer and no metastases have been found outside of the pelvis, pelvic exenteration may be performed. This radical surgery usually involves removal of the uterus, ovaries, fallopian tubes, vagina, bladder, urethra, and pelvic lymph nodes (Fig. 54-11). In some situations, the descending colon, rectum, and anal canal may also be removed. Candidates for this procedure are selected on the basis of their likelihood of surviving the surgery and their ability to adjust to and accept the resulting limitations.

Postoperative care is similar to that of a patient who has had a radical hysterectomy, an abdominal perineal resection, and an ileostomy or a colostomy. The physical, emotional, and social adjustments to life required by the woman and her family are great. There are urinary or fecal diversions in the abdominal wall, a reconstructed vagina, and the onset of menopausal symptoms.

Assess the patient's physical and emotional adjustment to the changes in body image produced by the surgery and her ability to carry out any treatment measures. The patient's rehabilitative process should keep pace with her acceptance of the situation. Much understanding and support are needed from the nursing staff during a long recovery period. Gently encourage the patient to regain her independence. She needs to verbalize her feelings about her altered body structure. Including the family in the plan of care is important. Careful follow-up monitoring is needed so that early recurrence of the cancer can be identified and treated.

ACUTE INTERVENTION WITH RADIATION THERAPY. Instruct the patient who is to receive external radiation to urinate immediately before the treatment to minimize radiation exposure to the bladder. Advise her about radiation side effects, including enteritis and cystitis. These are natural reactions to radiation therapy and do not indicate an overdose. Fully inform the patient of the possible side effects and measures that can be used to reduce their impact.

Nursing management of the patient receiving internal radiation therapy requires special considerations. Do not stay in the immediate area any longer than is necessary to give proper care and attention. No individual nurse should take care of the patient for more than 30 minutes per day. Stay at the foot of the bed or at the entrance to the room to minimize radiation exposure. Instruct visitors to stay 6 ft away from the bed and limit visits to less than 3 hr/day. Efficient organization of nursing care is essential so that you do not stay in the patient's immediate area any longer than is necessary. Fully explain the reasons for these precautions to the patient and her visitors. (A more detailed discussion of nursing care of the patient receiving internal radiation therapy is presented in Chapter 16.)

EVALUATION

The expected outcomes are that the patient with cancer of the female reproductive system will

- Actively participate in treatment decisions
- Achieve satisfactory pain and symptom management
- Recognize and report problems promptly
- Maintain preferred lifestyle as long as possible
- Continue to practice cancer detection strategies

PROBLEMS WITH PELVIC SUPPORT

The most commonly occurring problems with pelvic support are uterine prolapse, cystocele, and rectocele. Although vaginal birth increases the risk for these problems, these conditions can occur in women who have never experienced childbirth. Obesity, chronic coughing, and straining during bowel movements can increase the likelihood of these problems. The decreased estrogen that normally accompanies perimenopause also reduces some connective tissue support.

UTERINE PROLAPSE

Uterine prolapse is the downward displacement of the uterus into the vaginal canal[38] (Fig. 54-12). Prolapse is rated by degrees. In first-degree prolapse the cervix rests in the lower part of the vagina. Second-degree prolapse means the cervix is at the vaginal opening. Third-degree prolapse means the uterus protrudes through the introitus.

Symptoms vary with the degree of prolapse. The patient may describe a feeling of "something coming down." She may have dyspareunia, a dragging or heavy feeling in the pelvis, backache, and bowel or bladder problems if cystocele or rectocele is also present. Stress incontinence is a common and troubling problem. When third-degree uterine prolapse occurs, the

FIG. 54-12 Uterine prolapse. **A,** First-degree prolapse. **B,** Second-degree prolapse. **C,** Third-degree prolapse.

FIG. 54-13 A, Cystocele. **B,** Bladder has prolapsed into the vagina, causing a uterine prolapse.

protruding cervix and vaginal walls are subjected to constant irritation, and tissue changes may occur.

Therapy depends on the degree of prolapse and how much the woman's daily activities have been affected. Pelvic muscle strengthening exercises (Kegel exercises) may be effective for some women (see Table 46-19). If not, a pessary may be used. A *pessary* is a device that is placed in the vagina to help support the uterus. A wide variety of shapes exist, including rings, arches, and balls. Most are made of plastic or wire coated with plastic. When a woman first receives a pessary, she needs instructions for its cleaning and follow-up. Pessaries that are left in place for long periods are associated with erosion, fistulas, and vaginal carcinoma.

If more conservative measures are not successful, surgery is indicated. Surgery generally involves a vaginal hysterectomy with anterior and posterior repair of the vagina and the underlying fascia.

CYSTOCELE AND RECTOCELE

Cystocele occurs when support between the vagina and bladder is weakened (Fig. 54-13). Similarly, a rectocele results from weakening between the vagina and rectum (Fig. 54-14). Cystocele and rectocele are common problems, and in many women they are asymptomatic. With large cystoceles, complete emptying of the bladder can be difficult, predisposing women to bladder infections. A woman with a large rectocele may not be able to completely empty her rectum when defecating unless she helps push the stool out by putting her fingers in her vagina.

As with uterine prolapse, Kegel exercises (see Table 46-19) may be used to strengthen the weakened perineal muscles if the cystocele or rectocele is not too problematic. A pessary may be helpful for cystoceles. Surgery designed to tighten the vaginal

FIG. 54-14 A, Rectocele. **B,** Rectum has prolapsed into the vagina.

wall is generally the method of treatment. A cystocele is corrected with a procedure called an anterior colporrhaphy, whereas a posterior colporrhaphy is done for a rectocele. If further surgery is needed to relieve stress incontinence, procedures to support the urethra and restore the proper angle between the urethra and the posterior bladder wall are used.

NURSING MANAGEMENT
PROBLEMS WITH PELVIC SUPPORT

Assist women in avoiding or decreasing problems with pelvic support by teaching them how to do Kegel exercises. Women of all ages may benefit from these exercises. Instruct the patient to pull in or contract her muscles as if she were trying to stop the flow of urine. She should hold the contraction for several seconds and then relax. Sets of 5 to 10 contractions each should be done several times daily.

If vaginal surgery is necessary, the preoperative preparation usually includes a cleansing douche the morning of surgery. A cathartic and a cleansing enema are usually given when a rectocele repair is scheduled. A perineal shave may be done.

In the postoperative period the goals of care are to prevent wound infection and pressure on the vaginal suture line. This necessitates perineal care at least twice a day and after each urination or defecation. Apply an ice pack locally to help relieve the initial perineal discomfort and swelling. A disposable glove filled with ice and covered with a cloth works well. Later, sitz baths may be used.

After an anterior colporrhaphy, an indwelling catheter is usually left in the bladder for 4 days to allow the local edema to subside. The catheter keeps the bladder empty, preventing strain on the sutures. Twice-daily catheter care with an antiseptic is generally done. After posterior colporrhaphy, straining at stool is avoided by means of a low-residue diet and the prevention of constipation. A stool softener is usually given each night.

Review discharge instructions before the patient leaves the hospital. These include the use of douches or a mild laxative as needed; restrictions on heavy lifting and prolonged standing, walking, or sitting; and avoidance of intercourse until the physician gives permission. There may be a temporary loss of vaginal sensation, which can last for several months.

FISTULA

A *fistula* is an abnormal opening between internal organs or between an organ and the exterior of the body (Fig. 54-15).

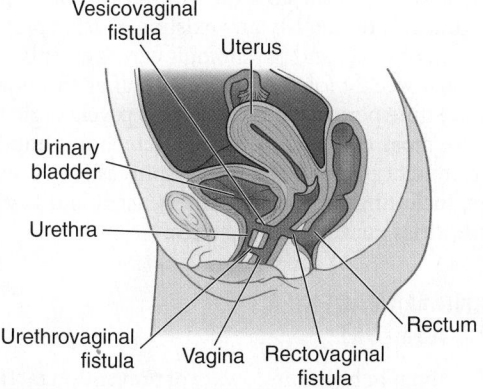

Vesicovaginal fistula
Uterus
Urinary bladder
Urethra
Urethrovaginal fistula
Vagina
Rectovaginal fistula
Rectum

FIG. 54-15 Common fistulas involving the vagina.

Gynecologic procedures cause most urinary tract fistulas. Other causes include injury during childbirth and disease processes, such as cancer. Fistulas may develop between the vagina and the bladder, urethra, ureter, or rectum. When *vesicovaginal* fistulas (between the bladder and the vagina) develop, some urine leaks into the vagina, whereas with *rectovaginal* fistulas (between the rectum and the vagina), flatus and feces escape into the vagina. In both instances, excoriation and irritation of the vaginal and vulvar tissues occur and may lead to severe infections. In addition to wetness, offensive odors may develop, causing embarrassment and severely limiting socialization.

Because small fistulas may heal spontaneously within a matter of months, treatment may not be needed. If the fistula does not heal, surgical excision is required. Inflammation and tissue edema must be eliminated before surgery is attempted, which may involve a wait of up to 6 months. The fistulectomy may result in the patient's having an ileal conduit or temporary colostomy.

NURSING MANAGEMENT
FISTULAS

Perineal hygiene is of great importance both preoperatively and postoperatively. Cleanse the perineum every 4 hours. Warm sitz baths should be taken three times daily if possible. Change perineal pads frequently. Encourage the patient to maintain an adequate fluid intake. Encouragement and reassurance are needed to help the patient cope with her problems.

Postoperatively, emphasize the avoidance of stress on the repaired areas and prevention of infection. Take care so that the indwelling catheter, usually in place for 7 to 10 days, is draining at all times. Urge oral fluids to provide for internal catheter irrigation. Use minimal pressure and strict asepsis if catheter irrigation becomes necessary. The first stool after bowel surgery may be purposely delayed to prevent contamination of the wound. Later, give stool softeners or mild laxatives. (See Chapter 46 for care of a patient with an ileal conduit and Chapter 43 for care of a patient with a colostomy.) Surgical repair of fistulas is not always effective, even in the best conditions. Therefore supportive nursing care for the patient and her significant others is especially important.

SEXUAL ASSAULT

Sexual assault is the forcible perpetration of a sexual act on a person without his or her consent. It can include any of the following actions: sodomy (anal or oral copulation with a person of the same or opposite sex), forced vaginal intercourse, assault with a foreign object, and serial battery.

Sexual assault may be committed by a stranger or by an intimate partner. Intimate partner violence (IPV) is a major health problem in the United States.[39] Survivors can suffer physical trauma and mental health consequences. Pregnancy, STIs, and gynecologic problems can result from IPV. More than half of all female rape victims were raped by an intimate partner. Female victims of IPV frequently report chronic pain, sleep disturbances, poor physical health, and activity limitations.

Clinical Manifestations

Physical. Many women who seek help immediately after the assault will not have any evidence of physical trauma. Evidence of trauma may be limited because women do not resist for fear

✚ TABLE 54-14 EMERGENCY MANAGEMENT

Sexual Assault

Etiology	Assessment Findings	Interventions
• Sexual molestation • Sodomy • Assault involving genitalia (male or female) without consent	• Emotional or physical manifestations of shock • Hysteria • Crying • Anger • Silence • Decreased level of consciousness • Hyperventilation • Oral, vaginal, and rectal injuries • Extragenital injuries • Pain in genital or extragenital area	**Initial** • Treat shock and other urgent medical problems (e.g., head injury, hemorrhage, wounds, fractures). • Assess emotional state. • Contact support person (i.e., social worker, rape advocate, sexual assault nurse examiner). • Do *not* clean the patient until all evidence is collected. Make sure the patient does not wash, douche, urinate, brush teeth, or gargle. • Place sheet on floor. Then have patient stand on sheet to remove clothing. Place sheet with clothing in paper bag. • Obtain forensic evidence per local protocol (e.g., body hair, nail scrapings, tissue, dried semen, vaginal washing, blood samples). • Maintain chain of evidence for all legal specimens. Clearly label evidence and keep in locked cabinet until given to law enforcement agency. • Obtain baseline HIV, syphilis, and other STI screening. • Determine method of contraception, date of last menstrual period, and date of last tetanus immunization. • Consider tetanus prophylaxis if lacerations contain soil or dirt. • Vaccinate against hepatitis B if not already done. **Ongoing Monitoring** • Monitor vital signs and emotional status. • Provide clothing as needed. • Counsel patient regarding confidential HIV and STI testing.

HIV, Human immunodeficiency virus; *STI,* sexually transmitted infection.

of physical danger and injury. When present, physical injuries may include bruising and lacerations to the perineum, hymen, vulva, vagina, cervix, and anus. Fractures, subdural hematomas, cerebral concussions, and intraabdominal injuries may result in the need for hospitalization. Sexual assault also places women at risk for STIs and pregnancy.

Psychologic. Immediately after the assault, women may show shock, numbness, denial, or withdrawal. Some women may seem unnaturally calm; others may cry or express anger. Feelings of humiliation, degradation, embarrassment, anger, self-blame, and fear of another assault are commonly expressed. These symptoms usually decrease after 2 weeks, and victims may appear to have adjusted. Yet any time from 2 to 3 weeks to months or years after the assault, symptoms may return and become more severe. *Rape trauma syndrome* is a classification of posttraumatic stress disorder. Flashbacks, intrusive recall, sleep disturbances, gastrointestinal symptoms, and numbing of feelings are common initial symptoms. Women feel embarrassment, self-blame, and powerlessness. Later symptoms include mood swings, irritability, and anger. Feelings of despair, shame, and hopelessness are often the cause of the anger. These feelings may be internalized and lead to depression. Suicidal ideations may also occur.

Collaborative Care

In the acute care of an assault survivor, ensuring the woman's emotional and physical safety has the highest priority. Table 54-14 outlines the emergency management of the patient who has been sexually assaulted. Most emergency departments (EDs) have identified personnel who have received special training to work with women who have been assaulted.

Many crime-fighting or victim advocate agencies within communities have implemented the position of the sexual assault nurse examiner (SANE).[40] The SANE is a registered

nurse who is certified to provide care to victims of sexual assault, while ensuring evidence is safeguarded. Special procedures are followed in taking the history and conducting the examination to preserve all evidence in case of future prosecution.

When the survivor of an assault is admitted to the ED or clinic, a specific chain of events occurs (Table 54-15). A signed informed consent is obtained from the woman before any data are collected. All materials gathered are well documented, labeled, and given to the appropriate person, such as the pathologist or a police officer. The materials are handled by as few people as possible, and signatures of all responsible for keeping and handling the data are obtained. Many items can be used as evidence if the victim chooses to file a complaint. Consequently, the integrity of the material must be maintained. Your involvement in the medicolegal process depends on the policies of the individual institution and state law.

A gynecologic and sexual history and an account of the assault (who, what, when, and where), as well as a general physical and pelvic examination, add further information about the incident. Laboratory tests are done primarily to look for sperm in the vagina and to identify any existing STIs or pregnancy.

Follow-up physical and psychologic care is essential. Women should return weekly for the first month after the assault. This includes the time period when a woman's psychologic reactions may be the most severe. Provide the telephone numbers and names of contact persons for local resources for sexual assault survivors, including rape crisis centers, legal and law enforcement authorities, and human services.

NURSING MANAGEMENT
SEXUAL ASSAULT

Assist all women in becoming aware of prevention tactics (Table 54-16). Also encourage women to learn some basic techniques

TABLE 54-15 EVALUATION OF ALLEGED SEXUAL ASSAULT

1. Medicolegal
- Valid written consent for examination, photographs, laboratory tests, release of information, and laboratory samples
- Appropriate "chain of evidence" documentation

2. History
- History of assault (who, what, when, where)
- Penetration, ejaculation, extragenital acts
- Activities since assault (e.g., changed clothes, bathed, douched)
- Inquire about safety
- Menstrual and contraceptive history
- Medical history
- Emotional status
- Current symptoms

3. General Physical Examination
- Vital signs and general appearance
- Extragenital trauma—mouth, breasts, neck
- Cuts, bruises, scratches (photographs taken)

4. Pelvic Examination
- Vulvar trauma, erythema; hymen, anal, and rectal status
- Matted hairs or free hairs
- Vaginal examination with unlubricated speculum for discharge, blood, lacerations
- Uterine size
- Adnexa, especially hematomas

5. Laboratory Samples
- Vaginal vault content sampling
- Vaginal smears—microscope evaluation for trichomonads and semen
- Oral or rectal swabs and smears, if indicated
- Blood samples—VDRL serology, pregnancy test; serologic testing for HIV and hepatitis B infection
- Freeze serum sample for later testing
- Cultures—cervix and other areas (if indicated) for gonorrhea and chlamydial infection
- Fingernail scrapings
- Pubic hair scrapings
- Clipping of matted pubic hairs

6. Treatment
- Care of injuries and emotional trauma
- Prophylaxis for STIs, tetanus, and hepatitis B (see appropriate chapters)
- If appropriate, consider levonorgestrel (Plan-B One-Step) emergency contraceptive pill up to 72 hr after assault; follow-up for pregnancy test in 2-3 wk
- Testing for HIV, syphilis, and hepatitis B may be done at 6-8 wk
- Protection of legal rights
- Recommendation of continued follow-up and services of rape crisis center

VDRL, Venereal Disease Research Laboratory.

TABLE 54-16 PATIENT TEACHING GUIDE

Sexual Assault Prevention

Include the following instructions when teaching measures to prevent sexual assault.
1. Be proactive and take a self-defense class.
2. Be aware of date-rape drugs (e.g., GHB, Rohypnol, Ketamine). Never leave your beverage unattended when socializing.
3. Place and maintain lights at all entrances to your home.
4. Keep your doors locked and do not open them to a stranger. Ask for identification if a service person comes to the door.
5. Do not advertise that you live alone. List only your initials with your last name in the telephone directory or on the mailbox. Never reveal to a caller that you are home alone.
6. Avoid walking alone in deserted areas. Walk to the parking lot with a friend; be sure you see each other leave.
7. Have your keys ready as you approach your car or home.
8. Keep all doors locked and the windows up when driving.
9. Never get on an elevator with a suspicious person. Pretend you have forgotten something and get off.
10. Say what you mean in social situations. Be sure your voice and body language reflect your response.
11. Proceed with caution in online correspondence.
12. Carry a loud whistle and use it when you think you are in danger.
13. Yell "Fire!" if you are attacked and run toward a lighted area.

may be inconsistent, confused, and inappropriate. Maintain a nonjudgmental attitude.

The patient usually has many feelings and thoughts about the assault and generally wants to talk about them to an interested listener. Talking may help the patient feel better and gain understanding of her reactions to the incident. When you listen carefully, the patient feels that she is not alone and is better able to gain control over the situation.

Assess the patient's stress level before preparing her for the various procedures that will follow. Let her know what to expect and what is expected of her, as well as why the particular procedure must be done. Because the pelvic examination may trigger a flashback of the attack, answer all related questions before the examination and be a supportive presence during the examination.

After the examination, consider the patient's physical comfort needs. She will need a change of clothing because her original garments may be torn or soiled, or kept as evidence. Most women who have been sexually assaulted feel dirty and need a place to wash and to use a mouthwash, especially if oral sex was involved. Food and drink may also provide comfort to the victim.

Discuss the possibility of pregnancy and offer the patient an emergency contraception pill. Taking a single tablet of levonorgestrel (Plan-B One-Step) within 72 hours after unprotected sexual intercourse reduces the risk of pregnancy. Levonorgestrel is generally effective and safe, and it will not affect an existing pregnancy. Mifepristone (RU-486) is approved for use in early abortions in the United States but not for emergency contraception.

Many sexual assault survivors are unaware of the availability of financial compensation (a law in most states) and appreciate information about the application process. This compensation is to assist them in paying for emergency services and for emotional injuries that may temporarily interfere with their ability to work.

When the patient is discharged, make certain the patient has transportation home. If friends or family members are not

of self-defense. Local high schools and the YWCA usually have self-defense classes for formal instruction. Practicing the various techniques with a friend strengthens a woman's confidence in her ability to fight back. Learning self-defense can make the woman less vulnerable and more self-reliant.

When a sexual assault survivor is brought to the clinic or ED, a quiet, private area should be used for the initial assessment and the examinations that follow. Do not leave the patient alone. Whenever possible, the same nurse should remain with her throughout her stay and provide needed emotional support. The patient's actions and words as she describes the incident

CASE STUDY

Uterine Prolapse and Vaginal Hysterectomy

Jupiterimages/
Photos.com/
Thinkstock

Patient Profile

N.B. is a 65-yr-old white woman who has developed lower pelvic discomfort and stress incontinence. She has type 2 diabetes and hypertension. N.B. is the mother of three children. A second-degree uterine prolapse is diagnosed. N.B. was treated conservatively with a pessary, but her symptoms did not improve. She comes to the hospital for a vaginal hysterectomy and anteroposterior repair.

Subjective Data

- Was initially reluctant about surgery
- Concerned about her dyspareunia and her husband's reaction to the surgery
- Concerned she may have uterine cancer
- States she has stress incontinence and pelvic discomfort

Objective Data

Physical Examination

- Second-degree uterine prolapse on vaginal examination
- BP 150/100 mm Hg, pulse 110 beats/min, respirations 20 breaths/min

Laboratory Studies

- Hemoglobin 10 g/dL (0.10 g/L)
- Hemoglobin A1C 9%

Postoperative Status

- Returned to room with indwelling urinary catheter in place
- Vaginal packing in place
- Sequential compression devices on lower extremities
- Patient-controlled analgesia (PCA) pump for pain management

Discussion Questions

1. What are the common causes of uterine prolapse?
2. N.B. asks you about the effect of the surgery on her sexuality. How would you respond?
3. *Priority Decision:* What are priorities of care for N.B.?
4. What possible complications (including reasons for their development) can occur after a vaginal hysterectomy?
5. *Delegation Decision:* Which nursing personnel should be responsible for teaching N.B. related to her diabetes and hypertension: registered nurse, licensed practical/vocational nurse, unlicensed assistive personnel? What should she be taught?
6. *Priority Decision:* Based on the assessment data presented, what are the priority nursing diagnoses? Are there any collaborative problems?

evolve Answers available at *http://evolve.elsevier.com/Lewis/medsurg.*

available, the hospital or clinic should make arrangements with an appropriate community resource. The patient should not be sent home alone. The victim's partner and family have tremendous potential as both a negative and positive influence. If the partner is the perpetrator of the assault, consultation with the risk management department and law enforcement is necessary to protect the woman.

Many communities today have crisis centers. These public service organizations have trained professional and nonprofessional volunteers who provide an emotional support system on request. Their programs provide advocacy to ensure dignified treatment throughout the medical and police procedures, short-term counseling for the woman and her family, and court assistance and public education on rape-related issues.

BRIDGE TO NCLEX EXAMINATION

The number of the question corresponds to the same-numbered outcome at the beginning of the chapter.

1. In telling a patient with infertility what she and her partner can expect, the nurse explains that
   a. ovulatory studies can help determine tube patency.
   b. a hysterosalpingogram is a common diagnostic study.
   c. the cause will remain unexplained for 40% of couples.
   d. if postcoital studies are normal, infection tests will be done.

2. An appropriate question to ask the patient with painful menstruation to differentiate primary from secondary dysmenorrhea is
   a. "Does your pain become worse with activity or overexertion?"
   b. "Have you had a recent personal crisis or change in your lifestyle?"
   c. "Is your pain relieved by nonsteroidal antiinflammatory medications?"
   d. "When in your menstrual history did the pain with your period begin?"

3. The nurse should advise the woman recovering from surgical treatment of an ectopic pregnancy that
   a. she has an increased risk for salpingitis.
   b. bed rest must be maintained for 12 hours to assist in healing.
   c. having one ectopic pregnancy increases her risk for another.
   d. intrauterine devices and infertility treatments should be avoided.

4. To prevent or decrease age-related changes that occur after menopause in a patient who chooses not to take hormone therapy, the most important self-care measure to teach is
   a. maintaining usual sexual activity.
   b. increasing the intake of dairy products.
   c. performing regular aerobic, weight-bearing exercise.
   d. taking vitamin E and B-complex vitamin supplements.

5. The patient's thick, white, and curdlike vaginal discharge and vulvar pruritus are most consistent with
   a. trichomoniasis.
   b. monilial vaginitis.
   c. bacterial vaginosis.
   d. chlamydial cervicitis.

6. In caring for a patient with pelvic inflammatory disease, the nurse should place her in semi-Fowler's position. The rationale for this measure is to
   a. relieve severe pain.
   b. promote drainage to prevent abscesses.
   c. improve circulation and promote healing.
   d. prevent complication of bowel obstruction.

7. Nursing responsibilities related to the patient receiving brachytherapy for endometrial cancer include
   a. maintaining absolute bed rest.
   b. keeping the patient in high Fowler's position.
   c. allowing visitors if they stay 3 ft (1 m) from the bed.
   d. limiting direct nurse-to-patient contact to 30 minutes per shift.
8. Postoperative goals in caring for the patient who has undergone an abdominal hysterectomy include *(select all that apply)*
   a. monitoring urine output.
   b. changing position frequently.
   c. restricting all food for 24 hours.
   d. observing perineal pad for bleeding.
   e. encouraging leg exercises to promote circulation.
9. Postoperative nursing care for the woman with a gynecologic fistula includes *(select all that apply)*
   a. ambulation.
   b. bladder training.
   c. warm sitz baths.
   d. perineal hygiene.
   e. use of stool softeners.

10. The first nursing intervention for the patient who has been sexually assaulted is to
    a. treat urgent medical problems.
    b. contact support person for the patient.
    c. provide supplies for the patient to cleanse self.
    d. document bruises and lacerations of the perineum and the cervix.

1. b, 2. d, 3. c, 4. c, 5. b, 6. b, 7. a, 8. a, b, e, 9. c, d, 10. a

Ⓔvolve

For rationales to these answers and even more NCLEX review questions, visit *http://evolve.elsevier.com/Lewis/medsurg*.

REFERENCES

1. Sabanegh E, Agarwal A: Definition and demographics of infertility. In Wien A, editor-in-chief: *Campbell-Walsh urology*, ed 10, St Louis, 2011, Saunders.
2. Schmidt L, Sobotka T, Bentzen B, et al: Demographic and medical consequences of the postponement of parenthood, *Hum Reprod Update* 18:29, 2012.
*3. Nachtigall R, MacDougall K, Davis A, et al: Expensive but worth it: older parents' attitudes and opinions about the costs and insurance coverage for in vitro fertilization, *Fertil Steril* 97:82, 2012.
4. Williams D, Pridjian G: Obstetrics. In Rakel R, Rakel D, editors: *Textbook of family medicine*, ed 8, St Louis, 2011, Saunders.
5. Lentz G: Premenstrual syndrome and premenstrual dysphoric disorder. In Lentz G, Lobo R, Gershenson D, et al, editors: *Comprehensive gynecology*, ed 6, St Louis, 2013, Mosby.
6. Mayo Clinic: Menorrhagia (heavy menstrual bleeding). Retrieved from *www.mayoclinic.com/health/menorrhagia*.
7. Centers for Disease Control and Prevention: Toxic shock syndrome. Retrieved from *www.cdc.gov/ncidod/dbmd/diseaseinfo/toxicshock_t.htm*.
8. McQueen A: Ectopic pregnancy: risk factors, diagnostic procedures and treatment, *Nurs Stand* 25:49, 2011.
9. Givens M, Lipscomb G: Diagnosis of ectopic pregnancy, *Clin Obstet Gynecol* 55:387, 2012.
10. Sitka C: Methotrexate: the pharmacology behind medical treatment for ectopic pregnancy, *Clin Obstet Gynecol* 55:433, 2012.
11. Harvard Medical School: Perimenopause: rocky road to menopause, Harvard Health Publications. Retrieved from *www.health.harvard.edu/newsweek/Perimenopause_Rocky_road_to_menopause.htm*.
12. University of California–Berkeley: When a flush is not a winning hand, *Wellness Letter* 27:4, 2011. Retrieved from *www.wellnessletter.com/ucberkeley*.

13. Roush K: Managing menopausal symptoms, *Am J Nurs* 112:28, 2012.
*14. Women's Health Initiative Study: Findings from the WHI post-menopausal hormone therapy trials, Department of Health and Human Services. Retrieved from *www.nhlbi.nih.gov/whi*.
*15. Nelson HD, Walker M, Zakher B, et al: *Menopausal hormone therapy for the primary prevention of chronic conditions: a systematic review to update the U.S. Preventive Services Task Force Recommendations*, AHRQ Pub No 12-05168-EF-1, Washington, DC, 2012, Agency for Healthcare Research and Quality, Department of Health and Human Services.
16. American Cancer Society: Tamoxifen and raloxifene. Retrieved from *www.cancer.org/Cancer/BreastCancer/MoreInformation/MedicinestoReduceBreastCancer*.
17. Im E, Ko Y, Hwang H, et al: "Symptom-specific or holistic": menopausal symptom management, *Health Care Women Int* 33:575, 2012.
18. Stiles M, Redmer J, Paddock E, et al: Gynecologic issues in geriatric women, *J Women's Health* 21:4, 2012.
19. Centers for Disease Control and Prevention: Pelvic inflammatory disease fact sheet. Retrieved from *www.cdc.gov/std/PID/STDFact-PID.htm*.
20. Shin J, Howard F: Management of chronic pelvic pain, *Curr Pain Headache Rep* 15:377, 2011.
21. Apte G, Nelson P, Brisme JM: Chronic female pelvic pain, part 1: clinical pathoanatomy and examination of the pelvic region, *Pain Pract* 12:88, 2012.
22. Donegan C: Caring for women with endometriosis, *Pract Nurse* 42:24, 2012.
23. Cleveland Clinic: Facts about endometriosis. Retrieved from *www.my.clevelandclinic.org/disorders/Endometriosis/hic_Facts_About_Endometriosis*.
24. Munro M: Uterine leiomyomas, current concepts: pathogenesis, impact on reproductive health, and medical, procedural, and surgical management, *Obstet Gynecol Clin North Am* 38:703, 2011.
*25. Gupta J, Sinha A, Lumsden M, et al: Uterine artery embolization for symptomatic uterine fibroids, *Cochrane Database Syst Rev* 5:CD005073, 2012.

*Evidence-based information for clinical practice.

26. Lobo R: Hyperandrogenism. In Lentz G, Lobo R, Gershenson D, et al, editors: *Comprehensive gynecology*, ed 6, St Louis, 2013, Mosby.

*27. Toulis K, Goulis D, Mintziori G, et al: Meta-analysis of cardiovascular disease risk markers in women with polycystic ovary syndrome, *Hum Reprod Update* 17:741, 2011.

28. Androgen Excess and PCOS Society: Polycystic ovary syndrome. Retrieved from *www.ae-society.org/poly_syndrome*.

29. American Cancer Society: *Cancer facts and figures 2012*, Atlanta, 2012, The Society. Retrieved from *www.cancer.org*.

30. National Institutes of Health. National Cancer Institute: Snapshot of cervical cancer. Retrieved from *www.cancer.gov/aboutnci/servingpeople/snapshots/cervical.pdf*.

31. American Cancer Society: American Cancer Society guidelines for the early detection of cancer. Retrieved from *www.cancer.org/Healthy/FindCancerEarly/CancerScreeningGuidelines*.

32. Arora V, Quinn M: Endometrial cancer, *Best Pract Res Clin Obstet Gynaecol* 26:31, 2012.

33. Jelovac D, Armstrong D: Recent progress in the diagnosis and treatment of ovarian cancer, *CA Cancer J Clin* 61:183, 2011.

34. Buys S, Partridge E, Black A, et al: Effect of screening on ovarian cancer mortality: the prostate, lung, colorectal and ovarian (PLCO) cancer screening randomized controlled trial, *JAMA* 305:229, 2011.

35. Koehler C, Gottschalk E, Chiantera V, et al: From laparoscopic assisted radical vaginal hysterectomy to vaginal assisted laparoscopic radical hysterectomy, *BJOG Int J Obstet Gynaecol* 119:254, 2012.

36. Viswanathan A: Advances in the use of radiation for gynecologic cancers, *Hematol Oncol Clin North Am* 26:15, 2012.

*37. Lara L, deAndrade J, Consolo F, et al: Women's poorer satisfaction with their sex lives following gynecological cancer treatment, *Clin J Oncology Nurs* 16:273, 2011.

38. Prasad A, Alvero R: Uterine prolapse. In Ferri F, editor: *Ferri's clinical advisor 2013*, Philadelphia, 2011, Mosby.

39. Cronholm PF, Fogarty CT, Ambuel B, et al: Intimate partner violence, *Am Fam Physician* 83:1165, 2011.

40. Georgia Network to End Sexual Assault: Basic SANE training. Retrieved from *www.gnesa.org*.

RESOURCES

American Congress of Obstetricians and Gynecologists
www.acog.org
American Urological Association
www.auanet.org
Hysterectomy Educational Resources and Services (HERS) Foundation
www.hersfoundation.com
North American Menopause Society
www.menopause.org
Sexuality Information and Education Council of the United States (SIECUS)
www.siecus.org

Only a life lived for others is a life worthwhile.
Albert Einstein

Nursing Management
Male Reproductive Problems

Shannon Ruff Dirksen

LEARNING OUTCOMES

1. Describe the pathophysiology, clinical manifestations, and collaborative care of benign prostatic hyperplasia.
2. Describe the nursing management of benign prostatic hyperplasia.
3. Describe the pathophysiology, clinical manifestations, and collaborative care of prostate cancer.
4. Explain the nursing management of prostate cancer.
5. Specify the pathophysiology, clinical manifestations, and nursing and collaborative management of prostatitis and problems of the penis and scrotum.
6. Explain the clinical manifestations and collaborative care of testicular cancer.
7. Describe the pathophysiology, clinical manifestations, and nursing and collaborative management of problems related to male sexual function.
8. Summarize the psychologic and emotional implications related to male reproductive problems.

KEY TERMS

benign prostatic hyperplasia (BPH), p. 1307
epididymitis, p. 1324
erectile dysfunction (ED), p. 1326
orchitis, p. 1324
paraphimosis, p. 1323

phimosis, p. 1323
prostate cancer, p. 1314
prostatitis, p. 1321
radical prostatectomy, p. 1317
testicular cancer, p. 1325

testicular torsion, p. 1325
transurethral resection of the prostate (TURP), p. 1312
vasectomy, p. 1326

This chapter discusses problems of the male reproductive system. These involve a variety of structures, including the prostate, penis, urethra, ejaculatory duct, scrotum, testes, epididymis, ductus (vas) deferens, and rectum (Fig. 55-1).

PROBLEMS OF THE PROSTATE GLAND

BENIGN PROSTATIC HYPERPLASIA

Benign prostatic hyperplasia (BPH) is a benign enlargement of the prostate gland. It is the most common urologic problem in male adults. About 50% of all men in their lifetime will develop BPH. Of these men, almost half of them will have bothersome lower urinary tract symptoms.[1] Research is not clear about whether having BPH leads to an increased risk of developing prostate cancer.[2,3]

Etiology and Pathophysiology

Although the cause of BPH is not completely understood, it is thought that BPH results from hormonal changes associated with the aging process.[1] One possible cause is excessive accumulation of dihydroxytestosterone (DHT) (the principal intraprostatic androgen) in the prostate cells. This can stimulate cell growth and an overgrowth of prostate tissue. Older

Reviewed by Debra Backus, RN, PhD, CNE, NEA-BC, Associate Professor of Nursing, State University of New York, Canton, New York; and David J. Derrico, RN, MSN, Assistant Clinical Professor, University of Florida, Gainesville, Florida.

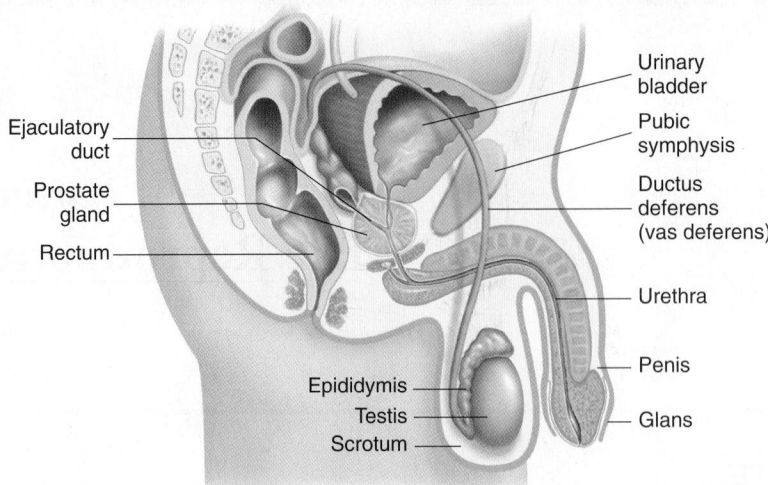

FIG. 55-1 Areas of the male reproductive system in which problems are likely to develop.

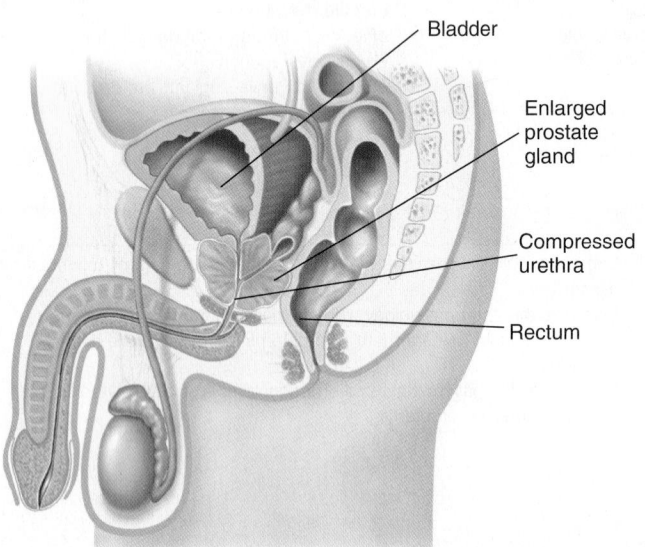

FIG. 55-2 Benign prostatic hyperplasia. The enlarged prostate compresses the urethra.

FIG. 55-3 Views of the prostate by cystoscopy. **A,** Normal appearance. **B,** Moderate benign prostatic hyperplasia with urethral obstruction.

men have a decrease in the blood's testosterone level, but continue to produce and accumulate high levels of DHT in the prostate.

Another possible cause is an increased proportion of estrogen (as compared to testosterone) in the blood. Throughout their lives, men produce both testosterone and small amounts of estrogen. As men age, the amount of active testosterone in the blood decreases, leaving a higher proportion of estrogen. A higher amount of estrogen within the gland increases the activity of substances (e.g., DHT) that promote cell growth.

Typically BPH develops in the inner part of the prostate. (Prostate cancer is most likely to develop in the outer part.) This enlargement gradually compresses the urethra, eventually leading to partial or complete obstruction (Fig. 55-2). The compression of the urethra ultimately leads to the development of clinical symptoms. There is no direct relationship between the size of the prostate and the severity of symptoms or degree of obstruction. The location of the enlargement is most significant in the development of obstructive symptoms (Fig. 55-3). For example, it is possible for mild hyperplasia to cause severe

obstruction, or for extreme hyperplasia to cause few obstructive symptoms.

Risk factors for BPH include aging, obesity (in particular increased waist circumference), lack of physical activity, alcohol consumption, erectile dysfunction, smoking, and diabetes.[4] A positive family history of BPH in first-degree relatives may also be a risk factor.

Clinical Manifestations

Manifestations of BPH are mainly associated with symptoms of the lower urinary tract.[5] The patient's symptoms are usually gradual in onset and may not be noticed until prostatic enlargement has been present for some time. Early symptoms are often minimal because the bladder can compensate for a small amount of resistance to urine flow. The symptoms gradually worsen as the degree of urethral obstruction increases.

Symptoms can be divided into two groups: irritative and obstructive. *Irritative symptoms,* which include nocturia, urinary frequency, urgency, dysuria, bladder pain, and incontinence, are associated with inflammation or infection. Nocturia is often the first symptom that the patient notices.[5]

Obstructive symptoms caused by prostate enlargement include a decrease in the caliber and force of the urinary stream, difficulty in initiating voiding, intermittency (stopping and starting stream several times while voiding), and dribbling at the end of urination. These symptoms are due to urinary retention.

TABLE 55-1 AUA SYMPTOM INDEX TO DETERMINE SEVERITY OF PROSTATIC PROBLEMS

Questions	AUA Symptom Score* (circle one number on each line)					
	Not At All	Less Than 1 Time in 5	Less Than Half the Time	About Half the Time	More Than Half the Time	Almost Always
Over the past month						
1. How often do you have the sensation that your bladder is not completely empty after you finish urinating?	0	1	2	3	4	5
2. How often do you have to urinate again, less than 2 hr after you finish urinating?	0	1	2	3	4	5
3. How often do you stop and start again several times when you urinate?	0	1	2	3	4	5
4. How often do you find it difficult to postpone urination?	0	1	2	3	4	5
5. How often do you have a weak urinary stream?	0	1	2	3	4	5
6. How often do you have to push or strain to begin urination?	0	1	2	3	4	5
7. How many times do you usually get up to urinate from the time you go to bed at night until the time you get up in the morning?	0 (None)	1 (1 time)	2 (2 times)	3 (3 times)	4 (4 times)	5 (5 times or more)
Sum of circled numbers (AUA Symptom Score): _____*						

Source: Barry MJ, Fowler FJ, O'Leary MP, et al: The American Urological Association symptom index for benign prostatic hyperplasia, *J Urol* 148:1549, 1992. Used with permission.
*Score is interpreted as follows: 0-7, mild; 8-19, moderate; 20-35, severe.
AUA, American Urological Association.

The American Urological Association (AUA) symptom index for BPH (Table 55-1) is a widely used tool to assess voiding symptoms associated with obstruction. Although this tool is not diagnostic, it helps determine the extent of symptoms.[6] Higher scores on this tool indicate greater symptom severity.

Complications

Complications of urinary obstruction are relatively uncommon in BPH. Acute urinary retention is a complication that is manifested by the sudden and painful inability to urinate. Treatment involves the insertion of a catheter to drain the bladder. Surgery may also be indicated.

Another complication is urinary tract infection (UTI) and potentially sepsis secondary to UTI. Incomplete bladder emptying (associated with partial obstruction) results in residual urine, which provides a favorable environment for bacterial growth. Calculi may develop in the bladder because of the alkalinization of the residual urine. Bladder stones are more common in men with BPH, although the risk of renal calculi is not significantly increased. Additional complications include renal failure caused by *hydronephrosis* (distention of pelvis and calyces of kidney by urine that cannot flow through the ureter to the bladder), pyelonephritis, and bladder damage if treatment for acute urinary retention is delayed.

Diagnostic Studies

The primary methods used to diagnose BPH include a history and physical examination. (Diagnostic studies are outlined in Table 55-2.) The prostate can be palpated by digital rectal examination (DRE) to estimate its size, symmetry, and consistency. In BPH, the prostate is symmetrically enlarged, firm, and smooth.

Additional diagnostic tests may be indicated, depending on the type and severity of symptoms and clinical findings. A urinalysis with culture is routinely done to identify any infection. Bacteria, white blood cells (WBCs), or microscopic hematuria indicate infection or inflammation.

A prostate-specific antigen (PSA) blood test may be done to rule out prostate cancer. However, PSA levels may be slightly

TABLE 55-2 COLLABORATIVE CARE

Benign Prostatic Hyperplasia

Diagnostic
- History and physical examination
- Digital rectal examination (DRE)
- Urinalysis with culture
- Prostate-specific antigen (PSA)
- Serum creatinine
- Postvoid residual
- Transrectal ultrasound (TRUS)
- Uroflowmetry
- Cystoscopy

Collaborative Therapy
Active Surveillance
Drug Therapy
- 5α-Reductase inhibitors (e.g., finasteride [Proscar], dutasteride [Avodart], dutasteride plus tamsulosin [Jalyn])
- α-Adrenergic receptor blockers (e.g., silodosin [Rapaflo], alfuzosin [Uroxatral], doxazosin [Cardura], prazosin [Minipress], terazosin [Hytrin], tamsulosin [Flomax])
- Erectogenic drugs (e.g., tadalafil [Cialis])

Minimally Invasive Therapy*
- Transurethral microwave thermotherapy (TUMT)
- Transurethral needle ablation (TUNA)
- Laser prostatectomy
- Transurethral electrovaporization of the prostate (TUVP)
- Intraprostatic urethral stents

Invasive (Surgery) Therapy*
- Transurethral resection of the prostate (TURP)
- Transurethral incision of the prostate (TUIP)
- Open prostatectomy

*See Table 55-3.

elevated in patients with BPH. Serum creatinine levels may be ordered to rule out renal insufficiency. Because symptoms of BPH are similar to those of a neurogenic bladder, a neurologic examination may also be performed.

In patients with an abnormal DRE and elevated PSA, a transrectal ultrasound (TRUS) scan is typically indicated. This examination allows for accurate assessment of prostate size and is helpful in differentiating BPH from prostate cancer. Biopsies can be taken during the ultrasound procedure. Uroflowmetry, a study that measures the volume of urine expelled from the bladder per second, is helpful in determining the extent of urethral blockage and thus the type of treatment needed. Postvoid residual urine volume is often measured to determine the degree of urine flow obstruction. Cystoscopy, a procedure allowing internal visualization of the urethra and bladder, is performed if the diagnosis is uncertain and in patients scheduled for prostatectomy.

Collaborative Care

The goals of collaborative care are to (1) restore bladder drainage, (2) relieve the patient's symptoms, and (3) prevent or treat the complications of BPH. Treatment is generally based on the degree to which the symptoms bother the patient or the presence of complications, rather than the size of the prostate. Alternatives to surgical intervention for some patients now include drug therapy and minimally invasive procedures.

The most conservative treatment that may be recommended for some patients with BPH is referred to as *active surveillance,* or watchful waiting.[7] When the patient has no symptoms or only mild ones (AUA symptom scores of 0 to 7), a wait-and-see approach is taken. Because some patients have symptoms that disappear, a conservative approach has value. Making dietary changes (decreasing intake of caffeine, artificial sweeteners, and spicy or acidic foods), avoiding medications such as decongestants and anticholinergics, and restricting evening fluid intake may improve symptoms.

A timed voiding schedule may reduce or eliminate symptoms, thus negating the need for further intervention. If the patient begins to have signs or symptoms that indicate an increase in obstruction, further treatment is indicated.

Drug Therapy. Drugs that have been used to treat BPH with variable degrees of success include 5α-reductase inhibitors and α-adrenergic receptor blockers. Combination therapy using both types of these drugs has been shown to be more effective in reducing symptoms than using one drug alone.

5α-Reductase Inhibitors. These drugs work by reducing the size of the prostate gland. Finasteride (Proscar) blocks the enzyme 5α-reductase, which is necessary for the conversion of testosterone to DHT, the principal intraprostatic androgen. This drug results in regression of hyperplastic tissue through suppression of androgens. Finasteride is an appropriate treatment option for individuals who have a moderate to severe symptom score on the AUA symptom index (see Table 55-1). Although more than 50% of men who are treated with the drug show symptom improvement, it takes about 6 months to be effective. Furthermore, the drug must be taken on a continuous basis to maintain therapeutic results. Serum PSA levels are decreased by almost 50% when taking finasteride. Therefore PSA levels should be doubled when comparing the patient's current levels to premedication levels.

Dutasteride (Avodart) has the same effect on prostatic tissue as finasteride and is a dual inhibitor of 5α-reductase type 1 and 2 isoenzymes. (Finasteride inhibits only the type 2 isoenzyme.) The combination of a 5α-reductase inhibitor (dutasteride) and an α-adrenergic receptor blocker (tamsulosin) is now available in a single oral medication (Jalyn).

In addition to decreasing the symptoms of BPH, finasteride, dutasteride, and Jalyn (finasteride plus tamsulosin) may also

lower the risk of prostate cancer.[8] However, the use of these drugs in prevention of prostate cancer has not been advised because of the increased risk of developing aggressive prostate cancer. Patients with an increased PSA level while taking these medications should be referred to their health care provider. The need for regular prostate cancer screening should also be discussed with the provider.

> **DRUG ALERT: Finasteride (Proscar)**
> • Patient should be aware of the increased risk of orthostatic hypotension with concomitant use of erectile dysfunction drugs.
> • Women who may be or are pregnant should not handle tablets due to potential risk to male fetus (anomaly).

α-Adrenergic Receptor Blockers. α-Adrenergic receptor blockers are another drug treatment option for BPH. These agents selectively block α₁-adrenergic receptors, which are abundant in the prostate and are increased in hyperplastic prostate tissue. Although α-adrenergic blockers are more commonly used for treatment of hypertension, these drugs promote smooth muscle relaxation in the prostate, facilitating urinary flow through the urethra. These agents demonstrate a 50% to 60% efficacy in improvement of symptoms, which occurs within 2 to 3 weeks.

Several α-adrenergic blockers are currently in use, including silodosin (Rapaflo), alfuzosin (Uroxatral), doxazosin (Cardura), prazosin (Minipress), terazosin (Hytrin), and tamsulosin (Flomax). Note that although these drugs offer symptomatic relief of BPH, they do not treat hyperplasia.

Erectogenic Drugs. Tadalafil (Cialis) has been used in men who have symptoms of BPH alone or in combination with erectile dysfunction (ED). The drug has shown to be effective in reducing symptoms for both these conditions (see erectile dysfunction later in this chapter).[9]

Herbal Therapy. Herbal extracts have been used in the management of lower urinary symptoms associated with BPH. In particular, some patients take plant extracts such as saw palmetto *(Serenoa repens)*. However, research indicates that saw palmetto has no benefit over a placebo.[10,11] In a limited number of small trials, herbal preparations such as saxifrage, beta-sitosterol, *Pygeum africanum,* and Cernilton have shown some success in reducing the symptoms of BPH. Advise patients to tell their health care provider about all herbal supplements that they use.

Minimally Invasive Therapy. Minimally invasive therapies are becoming more common as an alternative to watchful waiting and invasive treatment (Table 55-3). They generally do not require hospitalization or catheterization and are associated with few adverse events. Many minimally invasive therapies have outcomes comparable to those of invasive techniques.[12]

Transurethral Microwave Thermotherapy. *Transurethral microwave thermotherapy* (TUMT) is an outpatient procedure that involves the delivery of microwaves directly to the prostate through a transurethral probe to raise the temperature of the prostate tissue to about 113° F (45° C). The heat causes death of tissue, thus relieving the obstruction. A rectal temperature probe is used during the procedure to ensure that the temperature is kept below 110° F (43.5° C) to prevent rectal tissue damage. The procedure takes about 90 minutes.

Postoperative urinary retention is a common complication. Thus the patient is generally sent home with an indwelling catheter for 2 to 7 days to maintain urinary flow and to facilitate the passing of small clots or necrotic tissue. Antibiotics, pain medication, and bladder antispasmodic medications are used to

TABLE 55-3   TREATMENT FOR BENIGN PROSTATIC HYPERPLASIA

Description	Advantages	Disadvantages
Minimally Invasive		
Transurethral Microwave Thermotherapy (TUMT)		
Use of microwave radiating heat to produce coagulative necrosis of the prostate.	Outpatient procedure Erectile dysfunction, urinary incontinence, and retrograde ejaculation are rare	Potential for damage to surrounding tissue Urinary catheter needed after procedure
Transurethral Needle Ablation (TUNA)		
Low-wave radiofrequency used to heat the prostate, causing necrosis.	Outpatient procedure Erectile dysfunction, urinary incontinence, and retrograde ejaculation are rare Precise delivery of heat to desired area Very little pain experienced	Urinary retention common Irritative voiding symptoms Hematuria
Laser Prostatectomy		
Procedure uses a laser beam to cut or destroy part of the prostate. Different techniques are available: • Visual laser ablation of prostate (VLAP) • Contact laser • Photovaporization of prostate (PVP) • Interstitial laser coagulation (ILC)	Short procedure Comparable results to TURP Minimal bleeding Fast recovery time Rapid symptom improvement Very effective	Catheter (up to 7 days) needed after procedure due to edema and urinary retention Delayed sloughing of tissue Takes several weeks to reach optimal effect Retrograde ejaculation
Transurethral Electrovaporization of Prostate (TUVP)		
Electrosurgical vaporization and desiccation are used together to destroy prostatic tissue.	Minimal risks Minimal bleeding and sloughing	Retrograde ejaculation Intermittent hematuria
Intraprostatic Urethral Stents		
Insertion of self-expandable metallic stent into the urethra where enlarged area of prostate occurs.	Safe and effective Low risk	Stent may move Long-term effect is unknown
Invasive (Surgery)		
Transurethral Resection of Prostate (TURP)		
Use of excision and cauterization to remove prostate tissue cystoscopically. Remains the standard for treatment of BPH.	Erectile dysfunction unlikely	Bleeding Retrograde ejaculation
Transurethral Incision of Prostate (TUIP)		
Involves transurethral incisions into prostatic tissue to relieve obstruction. Effective for men with small to moderate prostates.	Outpatient procedure Minimal complications Low occurrence of erectile dysfunction or retrograde ejaculation	Urinary catheter needed after procedure
Open Prostatectomy		
Surgery of choice for men with large prostates, bladder damage, or other complicating factors. Involves external incision with two possible approaches (see Fig. 55-6).	Complete visualization of prostate and surrounding tissue	Erectile dysfunction Bleeding Postoperative pain Risk of infection

treat and prevent postprocedure problems. The procedure is not appropriate for men with rectal problems. Anticoagulant therapy should be stopped 10 days before treatment. Mild side effects include occasional problems of bladder spasm, hematuria, dysuria, and retention.

Transurethral Needle Ablation. Transurethral needle ablation (TUNA) is another procedure that increases the temperature of prostate tissue, thus causing localized necrosis. TUNA differs from TUMT in that low-wave radiofrequency is used to heat the prostate. Only prostate tissue in direct contact with the needle is affected, thus allowing greater precision in removal of the target tissue. The extent of tissue removed by this process is determined by the amount of tissue contact (needle length), amount of energy delivered, and duration of treatment. The majority of the patients undergoing TUNA have an improvement in symptoms.

This procedure is performed in an outpatient unit or physician's office using local anesthesia and IV or oral sedation. The TUNA procedure lasts approximately 30 minutes. The patient typically experiences little pain with an early return to regular activities. Complications include urinary retention, UTI, and irritative voiding symptoms (e.g., frequency, urgency, dysuria). Some patients require a urinary catheter for a short time. Patients often have hematuria for up to a week.

Laser Prostatectomy. The use of laser therapy through visual or ultrasound guidance is an effective alternative to transurethral resection of the prostate (TURP) in treating BPH. The laser beam is delivered transurethrally through a fiber instrument and is used for cutting, coagulation, and vaporization of prostatic tissue. There are a variety of laser procedures using different sources, wavelengths, and delivery systems. Retreatment rates are comparable to those of a TURP.[13]

One common procedure is *visual laser ablation of the prostate* (VLAP), which uses the laser beam to produce deep coagulation necrosis. The affected prostate tissue gradually sloughs in the urinary stream. It takes several weeks before the patient reaches optimal results after this type of laser therapy. At the completion of VLAP, a urinary catheter is inserted to allow for drainage.

Contact laser techniques involve the direct contact of the laser with the prostate tissue, producing an immediate vaporization of the tissue. Blood vessels near the laser tip are immediately cauterized. Thus bleeding during the procedure is rare. A three-way catheter with slow-drip irrigation is placed immediately after the procedure for a short time. Typically the catheter is removed within 6 to 8 hours after the procedure. Advantages of this procedure over TURP include minimal bleeding both during and after the procedure, faster recovery time, and ability to perform the surgery on patients taking anticoagulants.

Photovaporization of the prostate (PVP) uses a high-power green laser light to vaporize prostate tissue. Improvements in urine flow and symptoms are almost immediate after the procedure. Bleeding is minimal, and a catheter is usually inserted for 24 to 48 hours afterward. PVP works well for larger prostate glands.

Another approach to laser prostatectomy is *interstitial laser coagulation* (ILC). The prostate is viewed through a cystoscope. A laser is used to quickly treat precise areas of the enlarged prostate by placement of interstitial light guides directly into the prostate tissue.

Intraprostatic Urethral Stents. Symptoms from obstruction in patients who are poor surgical candidates can be relieved with intraprostatic urethral stents. The stents are placed directly into the prostatic tissue. Complications include chronic pain, infection, and encrustation. The long-term effects are not known.

Invasive Therapy (Surgery). Invasive treatment of symptomatic BPH involves surgery. The choice of the treatment approach depends on the size and location of the prostatic enlargement and patient factors such as age and surgical risk. Invasive treatments are summarized in Table 55-3.

Invasive therapy is indicated when the decrease in urine flow is sufficient to cause discomfort, persistent residual urine, acute urinary retention because of obstruction with no reversible precipitating cause, or hydronephrosis. Intermittent catheterization or insertion of an indwelling catheter can temporarily reduce symptoms and bypass the obstruction. However, avoid long-term catheter use because of the increased risk of infection.

Transurethral Resection of the Prostate. Transurethral resection of the prostate (TURP) is a surgical procedure involving the removal of prostate tissue using a resectoscope inserted through the urethra. TURP has long been considered the gold standard for surgical treatments of obstructing BPH. Although this procedure remains the most common operation performed, the number of TURP procedures done in recent years has declined due to the development of less invasive technologies.[12]

TURP is performed under a spinal or general anesthetic and requires a 1- to 2-day hospital stay. No external surgical incision is made. A resectoscope is inserted through the urethra to excise and cauterize obstructing prostatic tissue (Fig. 55-4). A large three-way indwelling catheter with a 30-mL balloon is inserted into the bladder after the procedure to provide hemostasis and to facilitate urinary drainage. The bladder is irrigated, either

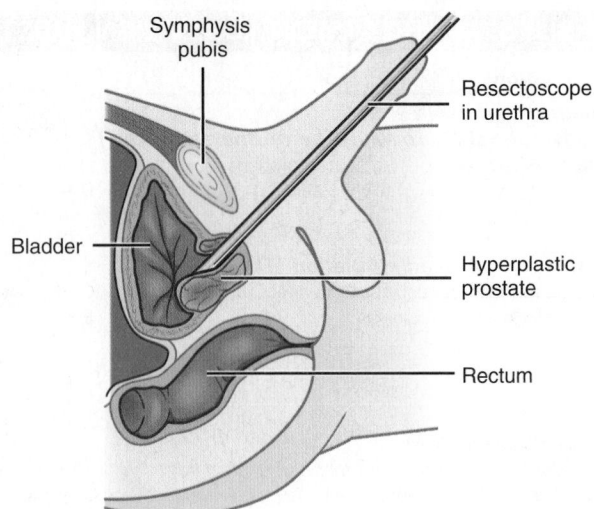

FIG. 55-4 Transurethral resection of the prostate.

continuously or intermittently, usually for the first 24 hours to prevent obstruction from mucus and blood clots.

The outcome for 80% to 90% of patients is excellent, with marked improvements in symptoms and urinary flow rates. Quality of life is also improved. TURP is a surgical procedure with a relatively low risk. Postoperative complications include bleeding, clot retention, and dilutional hyponatremia associated with irrigation. Because bleeding is a common complication, patients taking aspirin, warfarin (Coumadin), or other anticoagulants must discontinue these medications several days before surgery.

Transurethral Incision of the Prostate. Transurethral incision of the prostate (TUIP) is a surgical procedure done under local anesthesia for men with moderate to severe symptoms. Several small incisions are made into the prostate gland to expand the urethra, which relieves pressure on the urethra and improves urine flow. TUIP is an option for patients with a small or moderately enlarged prostate gland. TUIP has similar patient outcomes to TURP in relieving symptoms.

NURSING MANAGEMENT
BENIGN PROSTATIC HYPERPLASIA

Because you will be most directly involved in care of patients with BPH having invasive therapies, the focus of nursing management in this section is on preoperative and postoperative care.

NURSING ASSESSMENT

Subjective and objective data that should be obtained from a patient with BPH are presented in Table 55-4.

NURSING DIAGNOSES

Nursing diagnoses for the patient with BPH preoperatively may include, but are not limited to, the following:

- Acute pain *related to* bladder distention secondary to enlarged prostate
- Risk for infection *related to* an indwelling catheter, urinary stasis, or environmental pathogens

Nursing diagnoses for the patient with BPH who has invasive therapy (surgery) are presented in eNursing Care Plan 55-1 (available on the website for this chapter).

TABLE 55-4 NURSING ASSESSMENT

Benign Prostatic Hyperplasia

Subjective Data
Important Health Information
Medications: Estrogen or testosterone supplementation
Surgery or other treatments: Previous treatment for BPH

Functional Health Patterns
Health perception–health management: Knowledge of the condition
Nutritional-metabolic: Voluntary fluid restriction
Elimination: Urinary urgency, diminution in caliber and force of urinary stream; hesitancy in initiating voiding; postvoid dribbling; urinary retention; incontinence
Sleep: Nocturia
Cognitive-perceptual: Dysuria, sensation of incomplete voiding; bladder discomfort
Sexuality-reproductive: Anxiety about sexual dysfunction

Objective Data
General
Older adult male

Urinary
Distended bladder on palpation; smooth, firm, elastic enlargement of prostate on rectal examination

Possible Diagnostic Findings
Enlarged prostate on ultrasonography; vesicle neck obstruction on cystoscopy; residual urine with postvoiding catheterization; white blood cells, bacteria, or microscopic hematuria with infection; ↑ serum creatinine levels with renal involvement

PLANNING

The overall preoperative goals for the patient having invasive procedures are to have (1) restoration of urinary drainage; (2) treatment of any UTI; and (3) understanding of the upcoming procedure, implications for sexual function, and urinary control. The overall postoperative goals are to have (1) no complications, (2) restoration of urinary control, (3) complete bladder emptying, and (4) satisfying sexual expression.

NURSING IMPLEMENTATION

HEALTH PROMOTION. The cause of BPH is largely attributed to the aging process.[14] Health promotion focuses on early detection and treatment. The American Cancer Society, along with the AUA, recommends a yearly medical history and DRE for men over 50 years of age in an effort to detect prostate problems early. When symptoms of prostatic hyperplasia are present, further diagnostic screening may be necessary (see Table 55-2).

Some men find that the ingestion of alcohol and caffeine tends to increase prostatic symptoms because the diuretic effect increases bladder distention. Compounds found in common cough and cold remedies such as pseudoephedrine (in Sudafed) and phenylephrine (in Allerest PE and Coricidin D) often worsen the symptoms of BPH. These drugs are α-adrenergic agonists that cause smooth muscle contraction. If this happens, the patient should avoid these drugs.

Advise patients with obstructive symptoms to urinate every 2 to 3 hours and when they first feeling the urge. This will minimize urinary stasis and acute urinary retention. Fluid intake should be maintained at a normal level to avoid dehydration or fluid overload. The patient may believe that if he restricts his fluid intake, symptoms will be less severe, but this only increases the chances of an infection. However, if the patient increases his intake too rapidly, bladder distention can develop because of the prostatic obstruction.

ACUTE INTERVENTION. The following discussion focuses on preoperative and postoperative care for the patient undergoing a TURP.

Preoperative Care. Urinary drainage must be restored before surgery. Prostatic obstruction may result in acute retention or inability to void. A urethral catheter such as a coudé (curved-tip) catheter may be needed to restore drainage. In many health care settings, 10 mL of sterile 2% lidocaine gel is injected into the urethra before insertion of the catheter. The lidocaine gel not only acts as a lubricant, but also provides local anesthesia and helps open the urethral lumen. If a sizable obstruction of the urethra exists, the urologist may insert a filiform catheter with sufficient rigidity to pass the obstruction. Aseptic technique is important at all times to avoid introducing bacteria into the bladder. (Urinary catheters are discussed in Chapter 46.)

Antibiotics are usually administered before any invasive procedure. Any infection of the urinary tract must be treated before surgery. Restoring urinary drainage and encouraging a high fluid intake (2 to 3 L/day unless contraindicated) are also helpful in managing the infection.

Patients are often concerned about the impact of the impending surgery on sexual function. Provide an opportunity for the patient and the partner to express their concerns. Inform the patient that surgery may affect sexual function. The ejaculate may be decreased in amount or be totally absent. Most types of prostatic surgery result in some degree of retrograde ejaculation. This may decrease orgasmic sensations felt during ejaculation. Retrograde ejaculation is not harmful because the semen is eliminated during the next urination.

Postoperative Care. The main complications after surgery are hemorrhage, bladder spasms, urinary incontinence, and infection. The plan of care should be adjusted to the type of surgery, the reasons for surgery, and the patient's response to surgery.

After surgery the patient will have a standard catheter or a triple-lumen catheter. Bladder irrigation is typically done to remove clotted blood from the bladder and ensure drainage of urine. The bladder is irrigated either manually on an intermittent basis or more commonly as continuous bladder irrigation (CBI) with sterile normal saline solution or another prescribed solution. If the bladder is manually irrigated (if ordered), instill 50 mL of irrigating solution and then withdraw with a syringe to remove clots that may be in the bladder and catheter. Painful bladder spasms often occur as a result of manual irrigation.

With CBI, irrigating solution is continuously infused and drained from the bladder. The rate of infusion is based on the color of drainage. Ideally the urine drainage should be light pink without clots. Continuously monitor the inflow and outflow of the irrigant. If outflow is less than inflow, assess the catheter patency for kinks or clots. If the outflow is blocked and patency cannot be reestablished by manual irrigation, stop the CBI and notify the physician.

Use careful aseptic technique when irrigating the bladder because bacteria can easily be introduced into the urinary tract. To prevent urethral irritation and minimize the risk of bladder infection, secure the catheter to the leg with tape or a catheter strap. The catheter should be connected to a closed-drainage system. Do not disconnect unless it is being removed, changed, or irrigated. Proper care of the catheter is important. On a daily basis, cleanse the secretions that accumulate around the meatus with soap and water.

Blood clots are expected after prostate surgery for the first 24 to 36 hours. However, large amounts of bright red blood in the urine can indicate hemorrhage. Postoperative hemorrhage may occur from displacement of the catheter, dislodgment of a large clot, or increases in abdominal pressure.

Release or displacement of the catheter dislodges the balloon that provides counterpressure on the operative site. Traction on the catheter may be applied to provide counterpressure (tamponade) on the bleeding site in the prostate, thereby decreasing bleeding. Such traction can result in local necrosis if pressure is applied for too long. Therefore pressure should be relieved on a scheduled basis by qualified personnel. Activities that increase abdominal pressure, such as sitting or walking for prolonged periods and straining to have a bowel movement (Valsalva maneuver), should be avoided in the postoperative recovery period.

Bladder spasms are a distressing complication for the patient after transurethral procedures. They occur as a result of irritation of the bladder mucosa from the insertion of the resectoscope, presence of a catheter, or clots leading to obstruction of the catheter. Instruct the patient not to urinate around the catheter because this increases the likelihood of spasm. If bladder spasms develop, check the catheter for clots. If present, remove the clots by irrigation so that urine can flow freely. Belladonna and opium suppositories or other antispasmodics (e.g., oxybutynin [Ditropan]), along with relaxation techniques, are used to relieve the pain and decrease spasm.

The catheter is often removed 2 to 4 days after surgery. The patient should urinate within 6 hours after catheter removal. If he cannot, reinsert a catheter for a day or two. If the problem continues, instruct the patient to perform clean intermittent self-catheterization (see Chapter 46).

Sphincter tone may be poor immediately after catheter removal, resulting in urinary incontinence or dribbling. This is a common but distressing situation for the patient. Sphincter tone can be strengthened by having the patient practice Kegel exercises (pelvic floor muscle technique) 10 to 20 times per hour while awake. (Kegel exercises are discussed in Table 46-19.) Encourage the patient to practice starting and stopping the stream several times during urination. This facilitates learning the pelvic floor exercises.

It usually takes several weeks to achieve urinary continence. In some instances, control of urine may never be fully regained. Continence can improve for up to 12 months. If continence has not been achieved by that time, refer the patient to a continence clinic. A variety of methods, including biofeedback, have been used to achieve positive results.

You can also instruct the patient to use a penile clamp, a condom catheter, or incontinence pads or briefs to avoid embarrassment from dribbling. In severe cases, an occlusive cuff that serves as an artificial sphincter can be surgically implanted to restore continence. Assist the patient in finding ways to manage the problem that allow him to continue socializing and interacting with others.

Observe the patient for signs of postoperative infection. If an external wound is present (from an open prostatectomy), assess the area for redness, heat, swelling, and purulent drainage. Special care must be taken if a perineal incision is present because of the proximity of the anus. Avoid rectal procedures, such as taking rectal temperatures and administering enemas. The insertion of well-lubricated belladonna and opium suppositories is acceptable.

Dietary intervention and stool softeners are important in the postoperative period to prevent the patient from straining while having bowel movements. Straining increases the intraabdominal pressure, which can lead to bleeding at the operative site. A diet high in fiber facilitates the passage of stool.

AMBULATORY AND HOME CARE. Discharge planning and home care issues are important aspects of care after prostate surgery. Instructions include (1) caring for an indwelling catheter (if one is left in place); (2) managing urinary incontinence; (3) maintaining adequate oral fluid intake; (4) observing for signs and symptoms of urinary tract and wound infection; (5) preventing constipation; (6) avoiding heavy lifting (more than 10 lb [4.5 kg]); and (7) refraining from driving or intercourse after surgery as directed by the physician.

The patient may experience a change in sexual function after surgery. Many men experience *retrograde ejaculation* because of trauma to the internal urethral sphincter. Semen is discharged into the bladder at orgasm and may produce cloudy urine when the patient urinates after orgasm. ED may occur if the nerves are cut or damaged during surgery. The patient may experience anxiety over the change because of a perceived loss of his sex role, self-esteem, or quality of sexual interaction with his partner.

Discuss these changes with the patient and his partner and allow them to ask questions and express their concerns. Sexual counseling and treatment options may be necessary if ED becomes a chronic or permanent problem. (ED is discussed later in this chapter.)

Point out that although some patients experience concerns regarding change in sexual function, this is not a universal concern. Recovery depends on the type of surgery performed and the interval of time between when symptoms first appeared and the date of surgery. It may take up to 1 year for complete sexual function to return.

The bladder may take up to 2 months to return to its normal capacity. Instruct the patient to drink at least 2 to 3 L of fluid per day and urinate every 2 to 3 hours to flush the urinary tract. Teach the patient to avoid or limit the amounts of bladder irritants such as caffeine products, citrus juices, and alcohol. Because the patient may experience incontinence or dribbling, he may incorrectly believe that decreasing fluid intake will relieve this problem.

Urethral strictures may result from instrumentation or catheterization. Treatment may include teaching the patient intermittent clean self-catheterization or having a urethral dilation.

Advise the patient to continue having a yearly DRE if he has had any procedure other than complete removal of the prostate. Hyperplasia or cancer can occur in the remaining prostatic tissue.

EVALUATION

The expected outcomes are that the patient with BPH who has surgery will
- Report satisfactory pain control
- Report improved urinary function with no pain or incontinence

Additional information on expected outcomes for the patient with BPH is presented in eNursing Care Plan 55-1.

PROSTATE CANCER

Prostate cancer is a malignant tumor of the prostate gland. It is estimated that 241,740 new cases of prostate cancer are diagnosed and 28,170 men die annually from the disease in the United States.[15] One of every six men will develop prostate cancer at some point during his life. Prostate cancer is the most common cancer among men, excluding skin cancer. It is the second leading cause of cancer death in men (exceeded only by lung cancer). The majority (more than 60%) of cases occur in men over age 65. However, many cases occur in younger men who sometimes have a more aggressive type of cancer. Almost 2.8 million men in the United States are survivors of prostate cancer.[16]

Etiology and Pathophysiology

Prostate cancer is an androgen-dependent adenocarcinoma that is usually slow growing. It can spread by three routes: direct extension, through the lymph system, or through the bloodstream. Spread by direct extension involves the seminal vesicles, urethral mucosa, bladder wall, and external sphincter. The cancer later spreads through the lymphatic system to the regional lymph nodes. The bloodstream seems to be the mode of spread to pelvic bones, head of the femur, lower lumbar spine, liver, and lungs.

Age, ethnicity, and family history are known risk factors for prostate cancer. (Additional information on ethnicity is presented in the Cultural & Ethnic Health Disparities box on this page.) The incidence of prostate cancer rises markedly after age 50 with a median age at diagnosis of 67 years old.[16] The incidence of prostate cancer worldwide is higher in African Americans than in any other ethnic group (except Jamaican men of African descent).[15] The reasons for the higher rate are unknown. In addition, African American men are likely to have more aggressive tumors at diagnosis and have higher mortality rates from prostate cancer. Differences in survival may be due to body composition, dietary factors, and endogenous hormones.

It is not clear if smoking is a risk factor for prostate cancer. As mentioned earlier, neither is it clear if having BPH increases the risk of developing prostate cancer.[2,3]

Dietary factors and obesity may be associated with prostate cancer. A diet high in red and processed meat and high-fat dairy products along with a low intake of vegetables and fruits may increase the risk of prostate cancer. The role of dietary carotenoids (e.g., lycopene) and antioxidants (e.g., vitamins D and E and selenium) in the risk for prostate cancer is not clear. A large research study found that men who took vitamin E had an increased incidence of prostate cancer, with selenium supplements showing no benefit.[17]

Genetic Link

Currently no known single gene causes prostate cancer. Some genes or gene mutations are more common in men with prostate cancer. From a genetics viewpoint, prostate cancer can be classified into three categories.

Most prostate cancers (about 75%) are considered *sporadic,* which means that damage to the genes occurs by chance after a person is born. Prostate cancer that runs in a family, called *familial prostate cancer,* is less common (about 20%). It occurs because of a combination of shared genes and shared environment or lifestyle factors. Familial prostate cancer is when two or more first-degree relatives (father, brother, son) are diagnosed with prostate cancer.

Hereditary (inherited) prostate cancer is rare (5% to 10%) and occurs when gene mutations are passed down in a family from one generation to the next. In hereditary prostate cancer a family has any of the following characteristics: (1) three or more first-degree relatives with prostate cancer, (2) prostate cancer in three generations on the same side of the family, and (3) two or more close relatives (father, brother, son, grandfather, uncle, nephew) on the same side of the family diagnosed with prostate cancer before age 55.

Only genetic testing can determine whether a man has a genetic mutation. However, no genetic tests are available to determine if a man is predisposed to developing prostate cancer.

Having a family history does not mean that a man will develop prostate cancer; it indicates that he has an increased risk. Men with a family history of prostate cancer should talk with their health care provider about their concerns. It is important for the health care provider to obtain a detailed family history, including a family pedigree (see Figs. 13-4 and 13-5). Depending on the findings of the family history, a referral to a genetic counselor may be appropriate.

Hereditary breast and ovarian cancer (HBOC) syndrome is associated with mutations in the *BRCA1* and/or *BRCA2* genes (BRCA stands for BReast CAncer). HBOC is most commonly associated with an increased risk of breast and ovarian cancer in women. However, men with HBOC also have an increased risk of breast cancer and prostate cancer. Mutations in *BRCA1* and *BRCA2* cause only a small percentage of familial prostate cancers. Genetic testing may be appropriate for families with prostate cancer that also have HBOC.

Clinical Manifestations and Complications

Prostate cancer is usually asymptomatic in the early stages. Eventually the patient may have symptoms similar to those of BPH, including dysuria, hesitancy, dribbling, frequency, urgency, hematuria, nocturia, retention, interruption of urinary stream, and inability to urinate. Pain in the lumbosacral area that radiates down to the hips or the legs, when combined with urinary symptoms, may indicate metastasis.

The tumor can spread to pelvic lymph nodes, bones, bladder, lungs, and liver. Once the tumor has spread to distant sites, the major problem becomes the management of pain. As the cancer spreads to the bones (a common site of metastasis), pain can become severe, especially in the back and the legs because of compression of the spinal cord and destruction of bone (Fig. 55-5).

🌐 CULTURAL & ETHNIC HEALTH DISPARITIES

Cancers of the Male Reproductive System

Prostate Cancer
- African American men have the highest rate of prostate cancer in the world (except Jamaican men of African descent).
- African American men tend to be diagnosed with prostate cancer at an earlier age, have more advanced disease at the time of diagnosis, and have a higher mortality rate than do white men.
- Although the mortality rate for prostate cancer among African American men is higher than that among whites, the mortality rate is declining.
- Asian American men have a lower incidence and lower mortality rates from prostate cancer than white men.

Testicular Cancer
- Testicular cancer occurs more frequently among whites than in other ethnic groups.

FIG. 55-5 Metastasis of prostate cancer to the pelvis and lumbar spine indicated by arrows.

Diagnostic Studies

Most men in the United States with prostate cancer are diagnosed by PSA screening. Health care providers' recommendations for screening vary. Some encourage yearly screening for men over age 50, and some advise men who are at a higher risk for prostate cancer to begin screening at age 40 or 45. Others caution against routine screening.[18] Although specific recommendations regarding PSA screening vary, there is general agreement that men should be informed about the potential risks (e.g., subsequent evaluation and treatment that may be unnecessary) and benefits (early detection of prostate cancer) of PSA screening before being tested.

At the core of the controversy over routine screening is that many men live and die *with* prostate cancer but not *from* it. As screening has become more widespread, smaller cancers are being found in older men. Slow-growing cancers, in most cases, probably do not need to be treated. However, early detection of aggressive cancers by PSA testing has saved lives.

Patients need to discuss the use of PSA screening in their particular situation with their health care provider. This discussion should start earlier for men ages 40 to 45 who are at high risk of developing prostate cancer (e.g., African American, positive family history). After this discussion, men who want to be screened may have an annual DRE and PSA test. On DRE, an abnormal prostate may feel hard, nodular, and asymmetric.

Elevated levels of PSA (normal level, 0 to 4 ng/mL [0 to 4 mcg/L]), a glycoprotein produced by the prostate, does not necessarily indicate prostate cancer. Mild elevations in PSA may occur with aging, BPH, recent ejaculation, or acute or chronic prostatitis or after long bike rides. In addition, cystoscopy, indwelling urethral catheters, and prostate biopsies may also produce elevated PSA levels. Decreases in the PSA level can occur with drugs such as finasteride and dutasteride.

PSA is used not only to detect prostate cancer, but also to monitor the success of treatment. When treatment has been successful in removing prostate cancer, PSA levels should fall to undetectable levels. The regular measurement of PSA levels after treatment is important to evaluate the effectiveness of treatment and possible recurrence of prostate cancer.

An elevated level of prostatic isoenzyme of serum acid phosphatase (prostatic acid phosphatase [PAP]) is another indicator of prostate cancer, especially if there is extracapsular spread. With advanced prostate cancer, serum alkaline phosphatase is increased as a result of bone metastasis. Investigations to locate a serum biomarker for prostate cancer are ongoing.

Neither PSA nor DRE is a definitive diagnostic test for prostate cancer. If PSA levels are continually elevated or if the DRE is abnormal, a biopsy of the prostate tissue is usually indicated. Biopsy of prostate tissue is necessary to confirm the diagnosis of prostate cancer. The biopsy is typically done by a transrectal resection of the prostate (TRUS) because it allows the physician to visualize the prostate and pinpoint abnormalities. When a suspicious area is located, a biopsy needle is inserted into the prostate to obtain a tissue sample. A pathologic examination of the specimen is done to assess for malignant changes. Other tests used to determine the location and extent of the spread of the cancer may include bone scan, computed tomography (CT), and magnetic resonance imaging (MRI) using an endorectal probe.

Collaborative Care

Chemoprevention of prostate cancer is an active area of research. As discussed earlier in this chapter, finasteride and other drugs used to treat BPH may reduce the chance of getting prostate cancer by up to 25%.[8] Which men may benefit from these drugs is unknown given the increased risk of developing aggressive (high-grade) prostate cancer from these drugs. Men who are concerned about prostate cancer should discuss with their health care provider the potential risks and benefits of taking finasteride.

Early recognition and treatment are important to control tumor growth, prevent metastasis, and preserve quality of life. Most patients (90%) with prostate cancer are initially diagnosed when the cancer is in either a local or a regional stage. The 5-year survival rate with an initial diagnosis at this stage is 100%.

The most common classification system for determining the extent of the prostate cancer is the tumor, node, and metastasis (TNM) system (Table 55-5). The tumor is graded on the basis of tumor histology using the Gleason scale.[19] The scale grades the tumor from 1 to 5 based on the degree of glandular differentiation. Grade 1 represents the most well-differentiated or lowest grade (most like the original cells), and grade 5 represents the most poorly differentiated (unlike the original cells) or highest grade. The two most commonly occurring patterns of cells are graded, and then the two scores are added together to create a Gleason score, which ranges from 2 to 10. The PSA level at diagnosis and the patient's Gleason score are used with the TNM system to determine the stage grouping of the tumor.

The collaborative care of the patient with prostate cancer depends on the stage of the cancer and the patient's overall health. At all stages, there is more than one possible treatment option (Table 55-6). The decision of which treatment course to pursue should be made jointly by patients, their partners, and the health care team.[20]

Active Surveillance. Prostate cancer is relatively slow growing. Therefore a conservative approach to management of

TABLE 55-5 STAGE GROUPING OF PROSTATE CANCER

Stage	Tumor Size	Lymph Node Involvement	Metastasis	PSA Level	Gleason Score
I	Not felt on DRE. Not seen by visual imaging.	No	No	<10	≤6
II	Felt on DRE. Seen by imaging. Tumor confined to prostate.	No	No	10-20	6-7
III	Cancer outside prostate. Possible spread to seminal vesicles.	No	No	Any level	Any score
IV	Any size.	Any nodal involvement.	Yes	Any level	Any score

Adapted from American Cancer Society: How is prostate cancer staged? Retrieved from *www.cancer.org/Cancer/ProstateCancer/DetailedGuide/prostate-cancer-staging;* and National Cancer Institute: Stages of prostate cancer. Retrieved from *www.cancer.gov/cancertopics/pdq/treatment/prostate.*
DRE, Digital rectal examination.

TABLE 55-6 COLLABORATIVE CARE
Prostate Cancer

Diagnostic and Staging Workup
- History and physical examination
- Digital rectal examination (DRE)
- Prostate-specific antigen (PSA)
- Prostatic acid phosphatase (PAP)
- Transrectal ultrasound (TRUS)
- Biopsy of prostate and lymph nodes
- Computed tomography (CT)
- Magnetic resonance imaging (MRI)
- Bone scan (to evaluate for metastatic disease)

Collaborative Therapy
Active Surveillance
- Annual PSA and DRE

Surgery
- Radical prostatectomy
- Cryotherapy
- Orchiectomy (for metastatic disease)

Radiation Therapy
- External beam for primary, adjuvant, and recurrent disease
- Brachytherapy

Drug Therapy
- Androgen deprivation therapy (see Table 55-7)
- Chemotherapy for metastatic disease

EVIDENCE-BASED PRACTICE
Applying the Evidence

You are working as an occupational health nurse at a large manufacturing company. G.N. is a 56-yr-old African American who has come to you for his regular blood pressure check. His father and uncle have a history of prostate cancer. He tells you that he has heard that screening for prostate cancer is "all over the news." He has been getting a blood test for prostate-specific antigen (PSA) yearly and asks you if he needs to continue.

Best Available Evidence	Clinician Expertise	Patient Preferences and Values
PSA screening saves lives when performed appropriately in men at high risk of developing prostate cancer.	You know that G.N. is in a high-risk category for prostate cancer. He is African American, is more than 50 yr old, and has first-degree relatives with prostate cancer. Based on these risk factors, you encourage him to continue to get yearly PSA screening.	G.N. wants the best preventive measures to screen for prostate cancer. He was involved in the care of both his father and uncle when they were sick, and does not want that to happen to him.

Your Decision and Action
You encourage G.N. to discuss his concerns about annual PSA testing with his primary health care provider. You also discuss the potential influence of risk factors and diet on developing prostate cancer and teach him about food to avoid or limit (e.g., red meat, high-fat dietary products) and those to increase (e.g., vegetables, fruits).

Reference for Evidence
National Comprehensive Cancer Network: NCCN stresses importance of PSA testing in high-risk men. Retrieved from *www.nccn.org/about/news/newsinfo.asp?NewsID=218.*

prostate cancer is active surveillance, or "watchful waiting." This strategy is appropriate when the patient has (1) a life expectancy of less than 10 years (low risk of dying of the disease); (2) a low-grade, low-stage tumor; and (3) serious coexisting medical conditions. With active surveillance, patients are typically followed with frequent PSA measurements, along with DRE, to monitor the progress of the disease. Significant changes in the PSA level or the DRE, or the development of symptoms, warrant a reevaluation of treatment options.

Surgical Therapy
Radical Prostatectomy. With **radical prostatectomy,** the entire prostate gland, seminal vesicles, and part of the bladder neck (ampulla) are removed. The entire prostate is removed because the cancer tends to be in many different locations within the gland. In addition, a retroperitoneal lymph node dissection is usually done as a separate procedure. Surgery is usually not considered an option for advanced stage disease (except to relieve symptoms associated with obstruction) because metastasis has already occurred.

Traditional surgical approaches for a radical prostatectomy include retropubic and perineal resection (Fig. 55-6). With the *retropubic* approach, a low midline abdominal incision is made to access the prostate gland, and the pelvic lymph nodes can be dissected. With the *perineal* resection, an incision is made between the scrotum and anus.

A *laparoscopic* approach to prostatectomy is being used in some settings. In this method four small incisions are made into the abdomen. It results in less bleeding, less pain, and a faster recovery compared with other approaches.

A *robotic-assisted* (e.g., da Vinci system) prostatectomy is a type of laparoscopy in which the surgeon sits at a computer console while controlling high-resolution cameras and microsurgical instruments. Robotics is being used more, since it allows for increased precision, visualization, and dexterity by the surgeon when removing the prostate gland. Compared with traditional approaches, a robotic-assisted radical prostatectomy

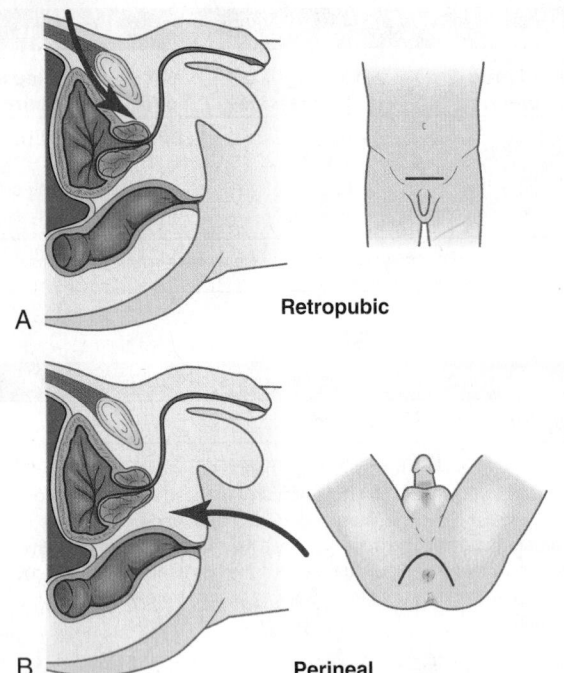

A — Retropubic

B — Perineal

FIG. 55-6 Common approaches used to perform a prostatectomy. **A,** Retropubic approach involves a midline abdominal incision. **B,** Perineal approach involves an incision between the scrotum and the anus.

has resulted in similar surgical outcomes with improved recovery time.[21]

After surgery, the patient has a large indwelling catheter with a 30-mL balloon placed in the bladder via the urethra. A drain is left in the surgical site to aid in the removal of drainage from the area. This drain is typically removed after a couple of days. Because the perineal approach has a higher risk of postoperative infection (because of the location of the incision related to the anus), careful dressing changes and perineal care after each bowel movement are important for comfort and to prevent infection. Depending on the type of surgery, the length of hospital stay postoperatively ranges from 1 to 3 days.

Two major adverse outcomes after a radical prostatectomy are ED and urinary incontinence.[22] The incidence of ED depends on the patient's age, preoperative sexual function, whether nerve-sparing surgery was performed, and the surgeon's expertise. Sexual function after surgery tends to return gradually over at least 24 months or more. Medications such as sildenafil (Viagra) may help improve sexual function.

Problems with urinary control may occur for the first few months after surgery because the bladder must be reattached to the urethra after the prostate is removed. Over time, the bladder adjusts and most men regain control.[23] Kegel exercises strengthen the urinary sphincter and may help improve continence. (Kegel exercises are presented in Table 46-19.) Other complications associated with surgery include hemorrhage, urinary retention, infection, wound dehiscence, deep vein thrombosis, and pulmonary emboli.

Nerve-Sparing Procedure. Near the prostate gland are neurovascular bundles that maintain erectile functioning. The preservation of these bundles during a prostatectomy is possible while still removing all of the cancer. Nerve-sparing prostatectomy is not indicated for patients with cancer outside of the prostate gland. Although the risk of ED is significantly reduced

with this procedure, there is no guarantee that potency will be maintained. However, most men younger than 50 years of age with good preoperative erectile function and low-stage prostate cancer can expect a return of potency after nerve-sparing prostatectomy.

Cryotherapy. *Cryotherapy* (cryoablation) is a surgical technique for prostate cancer that destroys cancer cells by freezing the tissue.[24] It has been used both as an initial treatment and as a second-line treatment after radiation therapy failed. A TRUS probe is inserted to visualize the prostate gland. Probes containing liquid nitrogen are then inserted into the prostate. Liquid nitrogen delivers freezing temperatures, thus destroying the tissue. The treatment takes about 2 hours under general or spinal anesthesia and does not involve an abdominal incision.

Possible complications include damage to the urethra and, in rare cases, a urethrorectal fistula (an opening between the urethra and the rectum) or a urethrocutaneous fistula (an opening between the urethra and the skin). Tissue sloughing, ED, urinary incontinence, prostatitis, and hemorrhage can also occur.

Radiation Therapy. Radiation therapy is another common treatment option for prostate cancer. Radiation therapy may be the only treatment, or it may be used in combination with surgery or with hormone therapy. Salvage radiation therapy given for prostate cancer recurrence after a radical prostatectomy may improve survival in some men.

External Beam Radiation. External beam is the most widely used method of delivering radiation treatments for those with prostate cancer. This therapy can be used to treat patients with prostate cancer confined to the prostate and/or surrounding tissue. Patients are usually treated on an outpatient basis 5 days a week for 4 to 8 weeks. Each treatment lasts only a few minutes.

Side effects from radiation can be acute (occurring during treatment or within 90 days that follow) or delayed (occurring months or years after treatment). The most common side effects involve changes to the skin (dryness, redness, irritation, pain), gastrointestinal tract (diarrhea, abdominal cramping, bleeding), urinary tract (dysuria, frequency, hesitancy, urgency, nocturia), and sexual function (ED).[25] Fatigue may also occur. These problems may lessen 2 to 3 weeks after the completion of radiation therapy. In patients with localized prostate cancer, cure rates with external beam radiation are comparable to those with radical prostatectomy.[15]

Brachytherapy. *Brachytherapy* involves placing radioactive seed implants into the prostate gland, allowing higher radiation doses directly in the tissue while sparing the surrounding tissue (rectum and bladder). The radioactive seeds are placed in the prostate gland with a needle through a grid template guided by TRUS (Fig. 55-7). The grid template and the ultrasound ensure accurate placement of the seeds.

Because brachytherapy is a one-time outpatient procedure, many patients find this more convenient than external beam radiation treatment. Brachytherapy is best suited for patients with early stage disease. The most common side effect is the development of urinary irritative or obstructive problems. Some men may also experience ED. The AUA Symptom Index (see Table 55-1) can be used to measure urinary function for patients undergoing brachytherapy and can be incorporated into postoperative nursing management. For those with more advanced tumors, brachytherapy may be offered in combination with external beam radiation treatment.[26] (Brachytherapy is discussed further in Chapter 16.)

Drug Therapy. The forms of drug therapy available for the treatment of prostate cancer are androgen deprivation (hormone) therapy, chemotherapy, or a combination of both.

Androgen Deprivation Therapy. Prostate cancer growth is largely dependent on the presence of androgens. *Androgen*

FIG. 55-7 A, Prostate brachytherapy. Implantation of radioactive seeds with a needle guided by ultrasound and a template grid. **B,** Radioactive seeds.

deprivation therapy (ADT) reduces the levels of circulating androgens to reduce the tumor growth. Androgen deprivation can be produced by inhibiting androgen production or blocking androgen receptors (Table 55-7).

One of the biggest challenges with ADT is that almost all tumors treated become resistant to this therapy *(hormone refractory)* within a few years. An elevated PSA level is often the first sign that this therapy is no longer effective. Patients taking ADT have an increased risk of cardiovascular side effects, including elevated serum cholesterol and triglyceride levels and coronary artery disease.[27] Research is also examining whether ADT may increase the risk of developing metabolic syndrome.

Osteoporosis and fractures may occur in prostate cancer patients receiving ADT. Drugs recommended to reduce bone mineral loss in these patients include zoledronic acid (Reclast) and raloxifene (Evista).[28] Denosumab (Prolia), a drug that slows the breakdown of bone, may also be used to increase bone mass in men with nonmetastatic prostate cancer.

Androgen Synthesis Inhibitors. The hypothalamus produces luteinizing hormone–releasing hormone (LH-RH), which stimulates the anterior pituitary to produce luteinizing hormone (LH) and follicle-stimulating hormone (FSH). LH stimulates the testicular Leydig cells to produce testosterone. *LH-RH agonists* superstimulate the pituitary. This ultimately results in downregulation of the LH-RH receptors, leading to a refractory condition in which the anterior pituitary is unresponsive to LH-RH. These drugs cause an initial transient increase in LH and testosterone called a *flare*. Symptoms may worsen during this time. However, with continued administration, LH and testosterone levels are decreased.

LH-RH agonists include leuprolide (Lupron, Lupron Depot, Eligard, Viadur,) goserelin (Zoladex), triptorelin (Trelstar), and buserelin (Suprefact) (see Table 55-7). These drugs essentially produce a chemical castration similar to the effects of an orchiectomy. These drugs are given by subcutaneous or intramuscu-

TABLE 55-7 DRUG THERAPY

Androgen Deprivation Therapy for Prostate Cancer

Therapy	Mechanism of Action	Side Effects
Androgen Synthesis Inhibitors **LH-RH Agonists** leuprolide (Lupron, Lupron Depot, Eligard, Viadur) goserelin (Zoladex) triptorelin (Trelstar) buserelin (Suprefact)	Reduce secretion of LH and FSH Decrease testosterone production	Hot flashes, gynecomastia, decreased libido, erectile dysfunction Depression and mood changes
LH-RH Antagonist degarelix	Blocks LH receptors Immediate testosterone suppression	Pain, redness, and swelling at injection site Elevated liver enzymes
CYP17 Enzyme Inhibitor abiraterone (Zytiga)	Inhibits CYP17, an enzyme needed for production of testosterone Inhibits testosterone synthesis from testes, adrenal glands, and prostate cancer cells	Joint swelling, fluid retention, muscle discomfort, hot flashes, diarrhea
Androgen Receptor Blockers bicalutamide (Casodex) flutamide (Eulexin) nilutamide (Nilandron) enzalutamide (Xtandi)	Block action of testosterone by competing with receptor sites	Loss of libido, erectile dysfunction, and hot flashes Breast pain and gynecomastia may also occur

FSH, Follicle-stimulating hormone; *LH,* luteinizing hormone; *LH–RH,* luteinizing hormone–releasing hormone.

lar injections on a regular basis. Viadur is an implant that is placed subcutaneously and delivers leuprolide continuously for 1 year.

Degarelix is an *LH-RH antagonist* that lowers testosterone levels. Unlike the LH-RH agonists, degarelix does not cause a testosterone flare because it acts directly to block LH and FSH receptors. It is given as a subcutaneous injection.

Abiraterone (Zytiga) works by inhibiting an enzyme, CYP17, which is needed for the production of testosterone. This drug is given orally.

Androgen Receptor Blockers. Another classification of anti-androgens is drugs that compete with circulating androgens at the receptor sites. Flutamide (Eulexin), nilutamide (Nilandron), bicalutamide (Casodex), and enzalutamide (Xtandi) are androgen receptor blockers. They are taken daily as an oral medication and can be used in combination with an LH-RH agonist (e.g., goserelin, leuprolide). Combining an androgen receptor blocker with an LH-RH agonist is an often-used treatment, which results in combined androgen blockade.

Chemotherapy. The use of chemotherapy has primarily been limited to treatment for those with hormone-refractory prostate cancer (HRPC) in late-stage disease. In HRPC the cancer is progressing despite treatment. This occurs in patients who have taken an antiandrogen for a certain period. The goal of chemotherapy is mainly palliative.

Some commonly used chemotherapy drugs include docetaxel (Taxotere), cabazitaxel (Jevtana), paclitaxel (Abraxane), mitoxantrone (Novantrone), vinblastine (Velban), cyclophosphamide (Cytoxan), and estramustine (Emcyt).

Men with advanced prostate cancer who have HRPC may receive a vaccine (sipuleucel-T [Provenge]). The vaccine stimulates the patient's system against the cancer and may prolong survival.

Radiotherapy. Radium-223 dichloride (Xofigo) can be used in the treatment of patients with castration-resistant prostate cancer, symptomatic bone metastases, and no known visceral metastatic disease. It is an alpha particle–emitting radiotherapy drug that mimics calcium and forms complexes with hydroxyapatite at areas of increased bone turnover, such as bone metastases.

Orchiectomy. Testosterone, produced by the testes, stimulates growth of the prostate cancer. A bilateral orchiectomy is the surgical removal of the testes that may be done alone or in combination with prostatectomy. For advanced stages of prostate cancer, an orchiectomy is one treatment option for cancer control. Another possible benefit of this procedure is the rapid relief of bone pain associated with advanced tumors. Orchiectomy may also shrink the prostate, thus relieving urinary obstruction in the later stages of disease when surgery is not an option.

After an orchiectomy, the weight gain and loss of muscle mass can alter a man's physical appearance. These physical changes can affect self-esteem, leading to grief and depression. Because this procedure is permanent, many men prefer drug therapy over an orchiectomy.

CULTURALLY COMPETENT CARE

PROSTATE CANCER

You need to be aware of ethnic and cultural considerations when providing information about the risk for prostate cancer and screening recommendations. Consider not only the ethnic

DELEGATION DECISIONS
Caring for the Patient Receiving Bladder Irrigation

Intermittent or continuous bladder irrigation (CBI) is usually required after invasive prostate surgery to prevent bladder obstruction by clots or mucus.

Role of Registered Nurse (RN)
- Assess for bleeding and clots.
- Assess catheter patency by measuring intake and output and presence of bladder spasms.
- Manually irrigate catheter if bladder spasms or decreased outflow occurs.
- Discontinue CBI and notify physician if obstruction occurs.
- Teach patient Kegel exercises after catheter removal.
- Provide care instructions for patient discharged with indwelling catheter.

Role of Licensed Practical/Vocational Nurse (LPN/LVN)
- Monitor catheter drainage for increased blood or clots.
- Increase flow of irrigating solution to maintain light pink color in outflow.
- Administer antispasmodics and analgesics as needed.

Role of Unlicensed Assistive Personnel (UAP)
- Clean around catheter daily.
- Record intake and output.
- Notify RN if large amount of bright red blood in urine.
- Report complaints of pain or bladder spasms to RN.

differences in the incidence of prostate cancer, but also differences in health promotion practices.

African American men have higher mortality rates from prostate cancer than white men. In part this is because their prostate cancer often is more advanced at the time of diagnosis. Despite the availability of early screening measures (PSA and DRE), African American men and those in lower socioeconomic groups frequently do not use them. This is partially related to knowledge levels about prostate cancer. In comparison to white men, African American men with prostate cancer reported more problems with financial access to transportation and health care costs, and they indicated using more religious coping strategies. White men were also perceived as receiving more favorable treatment from their physicians than African Americans.[29]

Although exposure to electronic and print media is successful in informing some men about prostate cancer, the effectiveness differs significantly based on demographic variables such as ethnicity, age, education level, and socioeconomic level. Ideally, all men should be aware of the risks associated with prostate cancer and the screening methods available. Consider the best method to communicate this information to men of all cultures and ethnicities that will result in the greatest degree of understanding and participation in prostate cancer screening.

NURSING MANAGEMENT PROSTATE CANCER

NURSING ASSESSMENT
Subjective and objective data that should be obtained from a patient with prostate cancer are presented in Table 55-8.

NURSING DIAGNOSES
Nursing diagnoses for the patient with prostate cancer depend on the stage of the cancer. General nursing diagnoses may include, but are not limited to, the following.

TABLE 55-8 NURSING ASSESSMENT

Prostate Cancer

Subjective Data
Important Health Information
Medications: Testosterone supplements; use of any medications affecting urinary tract such as morphine, anticholinergics, monoamine oxidase inhibitors, and tricyclic antidepressants

Functional Health Patterns
Health perception–health management: Positive family history; increasing fatigue and malaise
Nutritional-metabolic: High-fat diet; anorexia, weight loss (possible indicators of metastasis)
Elimination: Hesitancy or straining to start stream, urinary urgency, frequency, retention with dribbling, weak stream, hematuria
Sleep: Nocturia
Cognitive-perceptual: Dysuria; low back pain radiating to legs or pelvis, bone pain (possible indicators of metastasis)
Self-perception–self-concept: Anxiety regarding self-concept

Objective Data
General
Older adult male; pelvic lymphadenopathy (late sign)

Urinary
Distended bladder on palpation; unilaterally hard, enlarged, fixed prostate on rectal examination

Musculoskeletal
Pathologic fractures (metastasis)

Possible Diagnostic Findings
Serum PSA; ↑ serum PAP (metastasis); nodular and irregular prostate on ultrasonography, positive biopsy results; anemia

PAP, Prostatic acid phosphatase; *PSA,* prostate-specific antigen.

- Decisional conflict *related to* numerous alternative treatment options
- Acute pain *related to* surgery, prostatic enlargement, bone metastasis, and bladder spasms
- Urinary retention and impaired urinary elimination *related to* obstruction of the urethra by the prostate and loss of bladder tone
- Sexual dysfunction *related to* effects of treatment
- Anxiety *related to* uncertain outcome of disease process on life and lifestyle and effect of treatment on sexual function

PLANNING

The overall goals are that the patient with prostate cancer will (1) be an active participant in the treatment plan, (2) have satisfactory pain control, (3) follow the therapeutic plan, (4) understand the effect of the therapeutic plan on sexual function, and (5) find a satisfactory way to manage the impact on bladder and bowel function.

NURSING IMPLEMENTATION

HEALTH PROMOTION. One of your most important roles in relation to prostate cancer is to encourage patients, in consultation with their health care providers, to have annual prostate screening (PSA and DRE) starting at age 50 (or younger if risk factors are present). Because of their increased risk of prostate cancer, African American men and other men with a family

history of prostate cancer should have an annual PSA and DRE beginning at ages 40 to 45.

ACUTE INTERVENTION. Preoperative and postoperative phases of radical prostatectomy are similar to surgical procedures for BPH (see pp. 1310-1312). Nursing interventions for the patient who undergoes radiation therapy and chemotherapy are discussed in Chapter 16. An additional consideration is the patient's psychologic response to a diagnosis of cancer. Provide sensitive, caring support for the patient and his family to help them cope with the diagnosis. Prostate cancer support groups are available for men and their families to encourage them to be active, informed participants in their own care.

AMBULATORY AND HOME CARE. Teach appropriate catheter care if the patient is discharged with an indwelling catheter in place. Instruct the patient to clean the urethral meatus with soap and water once a day; maintain a high fluid intake; keep the collecting bag lower than the bladder at all times; keep the catheter securely anchored to the inner thigh or abdomen; and report any signs of bladder infection, such as bladder spasms, fever, or hematuria.

If urinary incontinence is a problem, encourage the patient to practice pelvic floor muscle exercises (Kegel exercises) at every urination and throughout the day. Continuous practice during the 4- to 6-week healing process improves the success rate. Products used for incontinence specifically designed for men are available through home care product catalogs and retail stores.

Palliative and end-of-life care is often appropriate and beneficial to the patient with advanced disease and his family (see Chapter 10). Common problems experienced by the patient with advanced prostate cancer include fatigue, bladder outlet obstruction and ureteral obstruction (caused by compression of the urethra and/or ureters from tumor mass or lymph node metastasis), severe bone pain and fractures (caused by bone metastasis), spinal cord compression (from spinal metastasis), and leg edema (caused by lymphedema, deep vein thrombosis, and other medical conditions). Nursing interventions must focus on all of these problems. However, pain management is one of the most important aspects of your care for these patients. Pain control involves ongoing pain assessment, administration of prescribed medications (both opioid and nonopioid agents), and nonpharmacologic methods of pain relief (e.g., relaxation breathing). (Pain management is discussed further in Chapter 9.)

EVALUATION

The outcomes are that the patient with prostate cancer will
- Be an active participant in the treatment plan
- Have satisfactory pain control
- Follow the therapeutic plan
- Understand the effect of the treatment on sexual function
- Find a satisfactory way to manage the impact on bladder or bowel function

PROSTATITIS

Etiology and Pathophysiology

Prostatitis is a broad term that describes a group of inflammatory and noninflammatory conditions affecting the prostate gland. Prostatitis is one of the most common urologic disorders. It is estimated that 12% of all men experience prostatitis in their lifetime.[30] Almost 2 million men are treated for prostatitis every year. The four categories of prostatitis syndromes are (1) acute bacterial prostatitis, (2) chronic bacterial prostatitis, (3) chronic prostatitis/chronic pelvic pain syndrome, and (4) asymptomatic inflammatory prostatitis.

Both acute and chronic bacterial prostatitis generally results from organisms reaching the prostate gland by one of the following routes: ascending from the urethra, descending from the bladder, and invading via the bloodstream or the lymphatic channels. Common causative organisms are *Escherichia coli; Klebsiella, Pseudomonas, Enterobacter,* or *Proteus; Chlamydia trachomatis; Neisseria gonorrhoeae;* and group D streptococci. Chronic bacterial prostatitis differs from acute prostatitis in that it involves recurrent episodes of infection.

Chronic prostatitis/chronic pelvic pain syndrome describes a syndrome of prostate and urinary pain in the absence of an obvious infectious process. The etiology of this syndrome is not known. It may occur after a viral illness, or it may be associated with sexually transmitted infections (STIs), particularly in younger adults. A culture reveals no causative organisms. However, leukocytes may be found in prostatic secretions.

Asymptomatic inflammatory prostatitis is usually diagnosed in individuals who have no symptoms, but are found to have an inflammatory process in the prostate. These patients are usually diagnosed during the evaluation of other genitourinary tract problems. Leukocytes are present in the seminal fluid from the prostate, but the cause of this process is unclear.

Clinical Manifestations and Complications

In acute bacterial prostatitis, common manifestations include fever, chills, back pain, and perineal pain, along with acute urinary symptoms such as dysuria, urinary frequency, urgency, and cloudy urine. The patient may also have acute urinary retention caused by prostatic swelling. With DRE, the prostate is extremely swollen, very tender, and firm. The complications of prostatitis are epididymitis and cystitis. Sexual function may be affected as manifested by postejaculation pain, libido problems, and ED. Prostatic abscess is also a potential, but uncommon, complication.

In chronic bacterial prostatitis and chronic prostatitis/chronic pelvic pain syndrome, manifestations are similar but generally milder than those of acute bacterial prostatitis. These include irritative voiding symptoms (frequency, urgency, dysuria), backache, perineal and pelvic pain, and ejaculatory pain. Obstructive symptoms are uncommon unless there is coexisting BPH. With DRE, the prostate feels enlarged and firm (often described as boggy) and is slightly tender with palpation. Chronic prostatitis can predispose the patient to recurrent UTIs.

The clinical features of prostatitis can mimic those of a UTI. However, it is important to remember that acute cystitis is not common in men.

Diagnostic Studies

Because patients with prostatitis have urinary symptoms, a urinalysis (UA) and urine culture are indicated. Often WBCs and bacteria are present. If the patient has a fever, WBC count and blood cultures are also indicated. The PSA test may be done to rule out prostate cancer. However, PSA levels are often elevated with prostatic inflammation. Thus it is not considered diagnostic in itself.

Microscopic evaluation and culture of expressed prostate secretion are considered useful in the diagnosis of prostatitis.

Expressed prostate secretion is obtained using a premassage and postmassage test.[31] The patient is asked to void into a specimen cup just before and just after a vigorous prostate massage. Prostatic massage (for expressed prostate secretion) should be avoided if acute bacterial prostatitis is suspected, since compression is extremely painful and can increase the risk of bacterial spread. TRUS has not been useful in the diagnosis of prostatitis. However, transabdominal ultrasound or MRI may be done to rule out an abscess on the prostate.

NURSING AND COLLABORATIVE MANAGEMENT
PROSTATITIS

Antibiotics commonly used for acute and chronic bacterial prostatitis include trimethoprim/sulfamethoxazole (Bactrim), ciprofloxacin (Cipro), ofloxacin (Floxin), carbachol (Miostat), carbenicillin (Geocillin), cephalexin (Keflex), and doxycycline (Vibramycin) or tetracycline. These antibiotics may be prescribed for those patients with multiple sex partners. Antibiotics are usually given orally for up to 4 weeks for acute bacterial prostatitis. However, if the patient has high fever or other signs of impending sepsis, hospitalization and IV antibiotics are prescribed. Patients with chronic bacterial prostatitis may be given oral antibiotic therapy for 4 to 12 weeks. Antibiotics may be given for a lifetime if the patient is immunocompromised. A short course of oral antibiotics is usually prescribed for those with chronic prostatitis/chronic pelvic pain syndrome. However, antibiotic therapy often is ineffective for patients whose prostatitis is not due to bacteria.

Although patients with acute and chronic bacterial prostatitis tend to experience a great amount of discomfort, the pain resolves as the infection is treated. Pain management for patients with chronic prostatitis/chronic pelvic pain syndrome is more difficult because the pain persists for weeks to months. No single approach has been shown to provide relief for everyone with this condition. Antiinflammatory agents (e.g., ibuprofen, indomethacin) may be used for pain control in prostatitis, but these drugs provide only moderate pain relief. Warm sitz baths may also help. Relaxation of muscle tissue in the prostate using α-adrenergic blockers (e.g., tamsulosin, alfuzosin) has been shown to be effective in reducing discomfort for some men.

Acute urinary retention can develop in acute prostatitis, requiring insertion of a urinary catheter. However, passage of a catheter through an inflamed urethra is contraindicated in acute prostatitis. The placement of a suprapubic catheter may then be indicated. Repetitive prostatic massage may be recommended as adjunct therapy for prostatitis for men.[31] This measure relieves congestion within the prostate by squeezing out excess prostatic secretions, thus providing pain relief. Prostatic massage is performed using the index finger of a gloved hand and pressing down on the prostate, covering the entire gland's surface in longitudinal strokes. Similar to massage, measures to stimulate ejaculation (masturbation and intercourse) may help to drain the prostate and provide some relief.

Because the prostate can serve as a source of bacteria, fluid intake should be kept at a high level for all patients experiencing prostatitis. Encourage the patient to drink plenty of fluids. This is especially important for those with acute bacterial prostatitis because of the increased fluid needs associated with fever and infection. Management of fever is also an important nursing intervention.

PROBLEMS OF THE PENIS

Health problems of the penis are rare if STIs are excluded (see Chapter 53). Problems of the penis may be classified as congenital, problems of the prepuce, problems with the erectile mechanism, and cancer.

CONGENITAL PROBLEMS

Hypospadias is a urologic abnormality in which the urethral meatus is located on the ventral surface of the penis anywhere from the corona to the perineum. Possible causes are hormonal influences in utero, environmental factors, and genetic factors. Surgical repair of hypospadias may be necessary if it is associated with *chordee* (a painful downward curvature of the penis during erection) or if it prevents intercourse or normal urination. Surgery may also be done for cosmetic reasons or emotional well-being.

PROBLEMS OF PREPUCE

Problems of the prepuce in the United States are not common because circumcision has been a routine procedure for many male infants. Circumcision, the surgical removal of the foreskin of the penis, is a procedure done to male infants for religious or cultural reasons.

Phimosis is a tightness or constriction of the foreskin around the head of the penis, making retraction difficult (Fig. 55-8, *A*). It is caused by edema or inflammation of the foreskin, usually associated with poor hygiene techniques that allow bacterial and yeast organisms to become trapped under the foreskin. The goal of treatment is to return the foreskin to its natural position over the glans penis through manual reduction. One strategy involves pushing the glans back through the prepuce by applying constant thumb pressure while the index fingers pull the prepuce over the glans. Ice and/or hand compression on the foreskin, glans, and penis may be done before this technique to reduce edema. Topical corticosteroid cream applied two or three times daily to the exterior and interior of the tip of the foreskin may also be effective.

Paraphimosis is tightness of the foreskin resulting in the inability to pull it forward from a retracted position and preventing normal return over the glans. An ulcer can develop if the foreskin remains contracted (Fig. 55-8, *B*). Paraphimosis can occur when the foreskin is pulled back during bathing, use of urinary catheters, or intercourse and is not placed back in the forward position. Replacement of the foreskin after careful cleaning helps to prevent this condition. Treatment may include antibiotics; warm soaks; and, in some situations, circumcision or dorsal slit of the prepuce.

PROBLEMS OF ERECTILE MECHANISM

Priapism is a painful erection lasting longer than 6 hours that may constitute a medical emergency. Priapism is caused by complex vascular and neurologic factors that result in an obstruction of venous outflow in the penis. Conditions that may be associated with priapism include sickle cell disease, diabetes mellitus, trauma to the spinal cord, degenerative lesions of the spine, and medications (e.g., cocaine, trazodone). Vasoactive medications (e.g., sildenafil) injected into the corpora cavernosa for ED can also cause priapism.

Complications include penile tissue necrosis caused by lack of blood flow or hydronephrosis from bladder distention. With immediate medical treatment, the risk of permanent ED is low.

Treatment varies depending on the cause. In patients with sickle cell disease, a blood exchange transfusion may be done, whereas other patients may be treated with sedatives, an injection of a smooth muscle relaxant directly into the penis, or aspiration and irrigation of the corpora cavernosa with a large-bore needle.

Peyronie's disease, sometimes referred to as curved or crooked penis, is caused by plaque formation in one of the corpora cavernosa of the penis. The palpable, nontender, hard plaque formation is usually found on the posterior surface. It may occur spontaneously or result from trauma to the penile shaft. The plaque prevents adequate blood flow into the spongy tissue, which results in a curvature during erection. The condition is not dangerous but can result in painful erections, ED, or embarrassment. Patients may improve over time, stabilize, or need surgery.

CANCER OF PENIS

Cancer of the penis is rare, with about 1500 cases diagnosed annually. It occurs more commonly in men who have cancers associated with human papillomavirus (HPV) and in men who were not circumcised as infants.[32] The tumor may appear as a superficial ulceration or a pimple-like nodule. The nontender warty lesion may be mistaken for a venereal wart. The majority of malignancies (95%) are well-differentiated squamous cell carcinomas.

Treatment in the early stages is laser removal of the growth. A radical resection of the penis may be done if the cancer has spread. Surgery, radiation, or chemotherapy may be tried depending on the extent of the disease, lymph node involvement, or metastasis.

PROBLEMS OF SCROTUM AND TESTES

INFLAMMATORY AND INFECTIOUS PROBLEMS

Skin Problems

The skin of the scrotum is susceptible to a number of common skin diseases. The most common are fungal infections, dermatitis (neurodermatitis, contact dermatitis, seborrheic dermatitis), and parasitic infections (scabies, lice). These conditions involve discomfort for the patient but are associated with few severe complications (see Chapter 24).

A   B

FIG. 55-8 **A,** Phimosis: inability to retract the foreskin due to secondary lesions on the prepuce. **B,** Paraphimosis: ulcer with edema from foreskin remaining contracted over the prepuce.

Epididymitis

Epididymitis is an acute, painful inflammatory process of the epididymis (Fig. 55-9), which is often due to an infectious process, trauma, or urinary reflux down the ductus (vas) deferens. It is usually unilateral. Swelling may progress to the point that the epididymis and testis are indistinguishable. In men younger than 40 years of age, the most common cause is gonorrhea or chlamydial infection. UTI and prostatitis are common causes in older men.

The use of antibiotics is important for both partners if the transmission is through sexual contact. Encourage patients to refrain from sexual intercourse during the acute phase. If they do engage in intercourse, a condom should be used. Conservative treatment consists of bed rest with elevation of the scrotum, ice packs, and analgesics. Ambulation places the scrotum in a dependent position and increases pain. Most tenderness subsides within 1 week, although swelling may last for weeks or months.

Orchitis

Orchitis refers to an acute inflammation of the testis. In orchitis, the testis is painful, tender, and swollen. It generally occurs after an episode of bacterial or viral infection such as mumps,

pneumonia, tuberculosis, or syphilis. It can also be a side effect of epididymitis, prostatectomy, trauma, infectious mononucleosis, influenza, catheterization, or complicated UTI. Mumps orchitis is a condition contributing to infertility that could be avoided by childhood vaccination against mumps. Treatment involves the use of antibiotics (if the organism is known), pain medications, or bed rest with the scrotum elevated on an ice pack.

CONGENITAL PROBLEMS

Cryptorchidism (undescended testes) is failure of the testes to descend into the scrotal sac before birth. It is the most common congenital testicular condition. It may occur bilaterally or unilaterally and may be the cause of infertility if corrective surgery is not done by 2 years of age. The incidence of testicular cancer is also higher if the condition is not corrected before puberty. Surgery is performed to locate and suture the testis or testes to the scrotum.

ACQUIRED PROBLEMS

Hydrocele

A *hydrocele* is a nontender, fluid-filled mass that results from interference with lymphatic drainage of the scrotum and swelling of the tunica vaginalis that surrounds the testis (Fig. 55-10; also see Fig. 55-9). Diagnosis is fairly simple because the mass can be seen by shining a flashlight through the scrotum (transillumination). No treatment is indicated unless the swelling becomes large and uncomfortable, in which case aspiration or surgical drainage of the mass is performed.

Spermatocele

A *spermatocele* is a firm, sperm-containing, painless cyst of the epididymis that may be visible with transillumination (see Fig. 55-9). The cause is unknown, and surgical removal is the treatment. It is important for the patient to see his health care provider if he feels any scrotal lumps. He would be unable to distinguish this cyst from cancer when performing self-examination.

Varicocele

A *varicocele* is a dilation of the veins that drain the testes (see Fig. 55-9). The scrotum feels wormlike when palpated. The cause of the problem is unknown. The varicocele is usually located on the left side of the scrotum as a consequence of ret-

FIG. 55-9 Scrotal masses.

FIG. 55-10 Hydrocele.

rograde blood flow from the left renal vein. Surgery is indicated if the patient is infertile, since persistent varicoceles are associated with 40% to 50% of cases of infertility. Sperm is thought to be damaged by varicoceles. Repair of the varicocele may be through injection of a sclerosing agent or by surgical ligation of the spermatic vein.

Testicular Torsion

Testicular torsion involves a twisting of the spermatic cord that supplies blood to the testes and epididymis (see Fig. 55-9). It is most commonly seen in males younger than age 20. It can occur spontaneously, as a result of trauma, or as a result of an anatomic abnormality. The patient experiences severe scrotal pain, tenderness, swelling, nausea, and vomiting. Urinary symptoms, fever, and WBCs or bacteria in the urine are absent. The pain does not usually subside with rest or elevation of the scrotum.

The *cremasteric reflex* is elicited by lightly stroking (with a reflex hammer or tongue blade) the inner aspect of the thigh in a downward direction. The normal response is a contraction of the cremaster muscle that pulls up the scrotum and testis on the side stroked. In testicular torsion, this reflex is absent on the side of the swelling.

Nuclear scan of the testes or Doppler ultrasound is typically performed to assess blood flow within the testicle. Decreased or absent blood flow confirms the diagnosis. Torsion constitutes a surgical emergency because, if the blood supply to the affected testicle is not restored within 4 to 6 hours, ischemia to the testis will occur, leading to necrosis and the possible need for removal. Unless the torsion resolves spontaneously, surgery to untwist the cord and restore the blood supply must be performed immediately.

TESTICULAR CANCER

Etiology and Pathophysiology

Testicular cancer is rare and accounts for less than 1% of all cancers found in males. However, testicular cancer is the most common type of cancer in young men between 15 and 35 years of age.[33] In the United States about 8600 new cases occur annually with a median age at diagnosis of 33 years old.[16] It is one of the most curable types of cancer. Testicular tumors are more common in males who have had undescended testes (cryptorchidism) or a family history of testicular cancer or anomalies. Other predisposing factors include orchitis, human immunodeficiency virus (HIV) infection, maternal exposure to exogenous estrogen, and testicular cancer in the contralateral testis.

Most testicular cancers develop from two types of embryonic germ cells: seminomas and nonseminomas. Although seminoma germ cell cancers are the most common, they are the least aggressive. Nonseminoma testicular germ cell tumors are rare, but very aggressive. Non–germ cell tumors arise from other testicular tissue and include Leydig cell and Sertoli cell tumors. These account for less than 10% of testicular cancers.

Clinical Manifestations and Complications

Testicular cancer may have a slow or rapid onset depending on the type of tumor (see Fig. 55-9). The patient may notice a painless lump in his scrotum, scrotal swelling, and a feeling of heaviness. The scrotal mass usually is nontender and firm. Some patients complain of a dull ache or heavy sensation in the lower abdomen, the perianal area, or the scrotum. Acute pain is the initial symptom in about 10% of patients. Manifestations associated with advanced disease are varied and include lower back or chest pain, cough, and dyspnea.

Diagnostic Studies

Palpation of the scrotal contents is the first step in diagnosing testicular cancer. A cancerous mass is firm and does not transilluminate. Ultrasound of the testes is indicated whenever testicular cancer is suspected (e.g., palpable mass) or when persistent or painful testicular swelling is present. If a testicular neoplasm is suspected, blood is obtained to determine the serum levels of α-fetoprotein (AFP), lactate dehydrogenase (LDH), and human chorionic gonadotropin (hCG).[34] (These tumor markers are discussed in Chapter 16.) A chest x-ray and CT scan of the abdomen and the pelvis are done to detect metastasis. Anemia may be present, and liver function levels may be elevated in metastatic disease.

NURSING AND COLLABORATIVE MANAGEMENT TESTICULAR CANCER

TESTICULAR SELF-EXAMINATION

The scrotum is easily examined, and beginning tumors are usually palpable. Instruct and encourage every male starting at puberty to perform a monthly testicular self-examination for the purpose of detecting testicular tumors or other scrotal abnormalities such as varicoceles. Teach male patients, especially those with a history of an undescended testis or a previous testicular tumor, how to perform self-examination.

The procedure for self-examination is not difficult. The man may indicate some reluctance to examine his own genitalia, but with your encouragement he can learn this simple procedure. Guidelines for self-examination of the scrotum are presented in Table 55-9 and Fig. 55-11 on the following page. Encourage him to perform self-examinations frequently until he is comfortable with the procedure. The scrotum should then be examined once a month. Use teaching aids such as videotapes and illustrations on shower hangers, and introduce students to them during high school or college physical education classes.

COLLABORATIVE CARE

Collaborative care of testicular cancer generally involves a radical orchiectomy (surgical removal of the affected testis, spermatic cord, and regional lymph nodes). Some patients with early stage disease do not need further treatment after an orchiectomy. Retroperitoneal lymph node dissection and removal may also be done in early stage disease. These nodes are the primary route for metastasis.

Postorchiectomy treatment may also involve surveillance, radiation therapy, or chemotherapy, depending on the stage of the cancer. Radiation therapy is mainly used for patients with a seminoma, which is very sensitive to radiation. Radiation does not seem to work well for nonseminomas.

Chemotherapy protocols use a combination of agents, including bleomycin (Blenoxane), etoposide (VePesid), ifosfamide (Ifex), and cisplatin (Platinol). (Testicular germ cell tumors are more sensitive to systemic chemotherapy than any other adult solid tumor.) Retroperitoneal lymph node dissection may be done after chemotherapy as adjunct therapy in patients with advanced testicular cancer.[34]

The prognosis for patients with testicular cancer in recent years has greatly improved, and 95% of the patients obtain

TABLE 55-9   PATIENT TEACHING GUIDE

Testicular Self-Examination

Include the following instructions when teaching a patient testicular self-examination.

1. During a shower or bath is the easiest time to examine the testes. Warm temperatures make the testes hang lower in the scrotum (see Fig. 55-11).
2. Use both hands to feel each testis. Roll the testis between the thumb and first three fingers until the entire surface has been covered. Palpate each one separately.
3. Identify the structures. The testis should feel round and smooth, like a hard-boiled egg. Differentiate the testis from the epididymis. The epididymis is not as smooth as the egg-shaped testis. One testis may be larger than the other. Size is not as important as texture. Check for lumps, irregularities, pain in the testes, or a dragging sensation. Locate the spermatic cord, which is usually firm and smooth and goes up toward the groin.
4. Choose a consistent day of the month (one that is easy to remember, such as a birth date) on which to examine the testes. The examination can be performed more frequently if desired.
5. Notify the health care provider at once if any abnormalities are found.

FIG. 55-11 Testicular self-examination.

FIG. 55-12 Vasectomy procedure. The ductus deferens is ligated or resected for the purpose of sterilization.

complete remission if the disease is detected in the early stages. As a result of treatment successes, a majority of men with testicular cancer are long-term survivors.

However, some of the drugs used to treat testicular cancer can cause serious long-term side effects. These include pulmonary toxicity, kidney damage, nerve damage (which can cause numbness and tingling), and hearing loss (from nerve damage). Secondary malignancies can occur as a result of chemotherapy (see Chapter 16).

All patients with testicular cancer, regardless of pathology or stage, require surveillance and regular physical examinations, chest x-rays, CT scans, and assessment of hCG and AFP. The goal is to detect relapse when the tumor burden is minimal.

Prior infertility or impaired fertility is often present at diagnosis. In treatment of testicular cancer, chemotherapy with cisplatin and/or pelvic irradiation often damages the testicular germ cells.[35] However, spermatogenesis can return in some patients. Because of the high risk for infertility, the cryopreservation of sperm in a sperm bank before treatment begins should be sensitively discussed and recommended for the man with testicular cancer. Ejaculatory dysfunction may result from retroperitoneal lymph node dissection. These issues may be hard to discuss with the newly diagnosed patient. Men may think that the disease is a threat to their maleness and self-worth.

SEXUAL FUNCTION

VASECTOMY

Vasectomy is the bilateral surgical ligation or resection of the ductus deferens performed for the purpose of sterilization (Fig. 55-12). The procedure requires only 15 to 30 minutes and is usually performed with the patient under local anesthesia on an outpatient basis. Although vasectomy is considered a permanent form of sterilization, successful reversals *(vasovasotomy)* have been done.

After vasectomy, the patient should not notice any difference in the look or feel of the ejaculate because its major component is seminal and prostatic fluid. The patient needs to use an alternative form of contraception until semen examination reveals no sperm. This usually requires at least 10 ejaculations or 6 weeks to evacuate sperm distal to the surgical site. Sperm cells continue to be produced by the testes but are absorbed by the body rather than being passed through the ductus deferens. Occasionally postoperative hematoma and swelling of the scrotum occur.

Vasectomy does not affect the production of hormones, ability to ejaculate, or physiologic mechanisms related to erection or orgasm. Psychologic adjustment may be a problem after surgery. It may be difficult for the patient to separate vasectomy from castration at a subconscious level. Some men may develop ED or may feel the need to become more sexually active than they were in the past to prove their masculinity. Careful discussion of the procedure and its outcome before the surgery can help detect patients who may have problems with psychologic adjustment. Surgery should be delayed for these patients.

ERECTILE DYSFUNCTION

Erectile dysfunction (ED) is the inability to attain or maintain an erect penis that allows satisfactory sexual performance. Although sexual function is a topic that many individuals are uncomfortable discussing, health care providers must be able and willing to address ED.[36]

ED is a condition that is significant because of its prevalence, with more than 10 million men in the United States estimated to have ED. It can occur at any age, although the incidence

ETHICAL/LEGAL DILEMMAS
Sterilization

Situation

C.R., a 43-year-old male patient requesting a vasectomy, informs you that he does not wish to discuss this with his wife. The physician's policy is to have the spouse or partner sign a form acknowledging the patient's desire to be sterilized. C.R. explains that although his wife wants to have more children, the one that they already have is all he wants.

Ethical/Legal Points for Consideration

- Legally, for the competent adult, the only person with the right to consent to or refuse health care treatment including sterilization is that competent adult. It is considered a violation of the right to privacy and the Fourteenth Amendment to limit an adult's right to consent or approve by requiring the consent of another.
- Between consenting and competent adults where there is a legally valid marriage contract, there has been some interest in requiring spousal notification of sterilization and abortion.
- Spousal consent or consent of the husband for sterilization of the wife is certainly a common practice in other countries. However, it has never been successfully required in the United States.
- Prior to sterilization procedures, health care providers can require documentation from the other spouse (not having the procedure) that substantiates the informed consent or refusal, including some document showing that the other spouse has been informed of the procedure and the consequences for childbearing.
- The requesting spouse certainly has the right to select another health care provider for the procedure if that spouse wants to avoid creating that documentation.
- In some religions where the ability to terminate a marriage contract by divorce is very limited, the intentional act by one spouse to permanently limit childbearing by sterilization does provide acceptable grounds to break the marriage contract.

Discussion Questions

1. How would you approach this situation?
2. Are there ever circumstances in which deception of a patient or family would be justified?

EVIDENCE-BASED PRACTICE
Translating Research Into Practice

Do Lifestyle Changes and Cardiovascular Medication Improve Erectile Dysfunction?

Clinical Question

For patients with erectile dysfunction (P), what is the effect of lifestyle modifications and drugs for cardiovascular risk factors (I) on severity of dysfunction (O)?

Best Available Evidence

Systematic review and meta-analysis of randomized controlled trials (RCTs)

Critical Appraisal and Synthesis of Evidence

- Six RCTs (n = 740, mean age of 55 yr old) that examined the effect of lifestyle interventions and drugs targeting cardiovascular (CV) risk factors on erectile dysfunction (ED).
- Interventions lasting at least 6 wk included diet, exercise, maintaining an active lifestyle, and drugs to reduce CV risk factors (i.e., statins to lower cholesterol).
- Changes in lifestyle with improved lipid values were related to a decrease in the severity of ED.

Conclusion

- Sexual function was significantly improved in men with ED through lifestyle modification and drugs for CV risk factors.

Implications for Nursing Practice

- Emphasize the importance of a healthy diet and regular physical activity with men experiencing ED.
- Counsel men that declining sexual health should be brought to the attention of the health care provider for early identification of CV risk factors.

Reference for Evidence

Gupta BP, Murad MH, Clifton MM, et al: The effect of lifestyle modification and cardiovascular risk factor reduction on erectile dysfunction: a systematic review and meta-analysis, *Arch Intern Med* 171:1797, 2011.

P, Patient population of interest; *I*, intervention or area of interest; *O*, outcomes of interest (see p. 12).

increases with age. In fact, it is estimated that about 50% of all men between ages 40 and 70 have at least some degree of ED. ED is increasing in all sexually active males regardless of age. In younger men, the increase is attributed to substance abuse (e.g., recreational drugs, alcohol). Middle-aged men are affected by medical conditions (e.g., diabetes, hypertension) or treatment for these conditions (e.g., antihypertensive drugs) that may cause ED.

Etiology and Pathophysiology

ED can result from a large number of etiologic factors (Table 55-10). Common causes include diabetes, vascular disease, side effects from medications, result of surgery (such as prostatectomy), trauma, chronic illness, stress, difficulty in a relationship, or depression. Although studies suggest a link between cardiovascular disease (CVD) and ED, whether ED is a risk factor for CVD is controversial.[37] A reduction in blood flow is a major factor in ED and CVD, and both of these disorders share many of the same risk factors. Physical inactivity may also be linked to ED (see Evidence-Based Practice box).

Normal physiologic age-related changes are associated with changes in erectile function and may be an underlying cause of ED for some men. Table 51-3 lists age-related changes in sexual function. Explain these age-related changes (if necessary) to reassure an anxious older man regarding normal changes in his sexual abilities. (The male sexual response is discussed in Chapter 51.)

Clinical Manifestations and Complications

The typical symptom of ED is a patient's self-report of problems associated with sexual performance. He usually describes an inability to attain or maintain an erection. The symptoms may occur only occasionally, may be continual with a gradual onset, or may occur with a sudden onset. A gradual onset of symptoms is usually associated with physiologic factors, whereas a sudden or rapid onset of symptoms may be associated with psychologic issues.

A man's inability to perform sexually can cause great distress in his interpersonal relationships and may interfere with his concept of himself as a man. It can also affect the relationship between the man and his partner. Problems with ED can lead to a number of personal issues, including anger, anxiety, and depression.

Diagnostic Studies

The first step in diagnosis and management of ED begins with a thorough sexual, health, and psychosocial history. Self-administered assessment and treatment-related questionnaires

TABLE 55-10 RISK FACTORS FOR ERECTILE DYSFUNCTION

Vascular
- Atherosclerosis
- Hypertension
- Peripheral vascular disease

Drug Induced
- Alcohol
- Antiandrogens
- Antilipidemic agents
- Antihypertensives
- Diuretics (chlorothiazide [Diuril], spironolactone [Aldactone])
- Major tranquilizers (diazepam [Valium], alprazolam [Xanax])
- Marijuana, cocaine
- Nicotine
- Tricyclic antidepressants (e.g., amitriptyline [Elavil])

Endocrine
- Diabetes mellitus
- Obesity
- Testosterone deficiency

Genitourinary
- Radical prostatectomy
- Prostatitis
- Renal failure

Neurologic
- Parkinson's disease
- Cerebrovascular disease
- Trauma to the spinal cord
- Tumors or transection of spinal cord

Psychologic
- Stress
- Depression
- Anxiety
- Fear of failure to perform

Other
- Aging

TABLE 55-11 COLLABORATIVE CARE

Erectile Dysfunction

Diagnostic
- History and physical examination
- Sexual history
- Serum glucose and lipid profile
- Testosterone, prolactin, and thyroid hormone levels
- Nocturnal penile tumescence and rigidity testing
- Vascular studies

Collaborative Therapy
- Modify reversible causes
- Drug therapy
  - sildenafil (Viagra)
  - vardenafil (Levitra, Staxyn)
  - tadalafil (Cialis)
  - avanafil (Stendra)
- Vacuum constriction device (VCD)
- Intraurethral medication pellet
- Intracavernosal self-injection
- Penile implants
- Sexual counseling

have been developed and may prove useful as primary screening tools. For example, the International Index of Erectile Function (IIEF) identifies a man's response to five key areas of male sexual function: erectile function, orgasmic function, sexual desire, intercourse satisfaction, and overall satisfaction.[38]

Second, a physical examination should be performed that focuses on secondary sexual characteristics, including size and appearance of the penis and scrotum. A DRE should be done to assess prostate size, consistency, and presence of nodules. Assessment of blood pressure with palpation and auscultation of the femoral arteries and peripheral pulses should also be included.

Further examination or diagnostic testing is typically based on findings from the history and physical examination. A serum glucose and lipid profile is recommended to rule out diabetes mellitus. Hormonal levels for testosterone, prolactin, LH, and thyroid hormones may help identify endocrine-related problems. Blood chemistries (e.g., PSA level) and a complete blood count may help identify systemic diseases.

Other diagnostic tests may be done to diagnose ED. Nocturnal penile tumescence and rigidity testing is a noninvasive method that involves the continuous measurement of penile circumference and axial rigidity during sleep. Such measurements are used to differentiate between physiologic or psychogenic causes of ED and to evaluate the effectiveness of drug therapy. Vascular studies, including penile arteriography, penile blood flow study, and duplex Doppler ultrasound studies, are used to assess penile blood inflow and outflow. Such studies help assess vascular problems interfering with erection.

Collaborative Care

The goal of ED therapy is for the patient and his partner to achieve a satisfactory sexual relationship. The treatment for ED is based on the underlying cause.

A variety of treatment options are available (Table 55-11). Advise patients that none of the options will restore ejaculation

or tactile sensations if they were absent before treatment. The results of these interventions are usually most satisfactory when both partners are involved in the decision-making process and have realistic expectations of the treatment.

It is important to determine if ED is reversible before treatment is started. For example, if ED appears to be a side effect of prescribed drugs, alternative treatments should be explored. With an established diagnosis of testicular failure (hypogonadism), androgen replacement therapy may sometimes be effective. For individuals who have ED that is psychologic in nature, counseling for the patient (and possibly his partner) is recommended. This counseling should be carried out by a qualified therapist.

Erectogenic Drugs. Sildenafil, tadalafil, vardenafil (Levitra, Staxyn), and avanafil (Stendra) are erectogenic drugs.[39] These drugs are phosphodiesterase type 5 (PDE5) inhibitors that cause smooth muscle relaxation and increased blood flow into the corpus cavernosum, thus promoting penile erection. They are taken orally about 30 to 60 minutes before sexual activity, but not more than once a day. These drugs have been found to be generally safe and effective for the treatment of most types of ED.

Side effects include headaches, dyspepsia, flushing, and nasal congestion. Additional rare side effects are blurred or blue-green visual disturbances, sudden hearing loss, and an erection lasting more than 4 hours that will not go away (priapism). Instruct the patient to seek immediate medical attention if any of these rare reactions occur. Because these drugs may potentiate the hypotensive effect of nitrates, they are contraindicated for individuals taking nitrates (e.g., nitroglycerin).

DRUG ALERT: Sildenafil (Viagra)
- Should not be used with nitrates (nitroglycerin) in any form.
- Can potentiate hypotensive effects of nitrates.

Vacuum Constriction Devices. Vacuum constriction devices (VCDs) are suction devices that can be applied to the flaccid penis to produce an erection by pulling blood up into the corporeal bodies. A penile ring or constrictive band is placed around the base of the penis to retain venous blood, thereby preventing the erection from subsiding. (A VCD is shown in eFig. 55-1, available on the website for this chapter.)

Intraurethral Devices. Intraurethral devices include the use of vasoactive drugs administered as a topical gel, an injection into the penis (intracavernosal self-injection), or a medication pellet inserted into the urethra (intraurethral) using a medicated urethral system for erection (MUSE) device. These vasoactive drugs enhance blood flow into the penile arteries. Current vasoactive drugs include papaverine (topical gel or injection), alprostadil (Caverject) (topical gel, transurethral pellet, or injection), and phentolamine (Vasomax). (These devices are shown in eFig. 55-2, available on the website for this chapter.)

Penile Implants. Surgical implants of semirigid or inflatable penile prostheses are shown in eFig. 55-3, available on the website for this chapter. These surgical procedures are highly invasive and associated with potential complications. Thus they are usually indicated for men with severe ED for which other interventions are ineffective.

The devices are implanted into the corporeal bodies to provide an erection firm enough for penetration. The inflatable implant consists of cylinders in the penis, a small pump in the scrotum, and a reservoir in the lower abdomen. The main problems associated with penile prostheses are mechanical failure, infection, and erosions.

Sexual Counseling. Sexual counseling is often recommended before and after treatment. The ability to please both partners enhances satisfaction levels. Counseling should address psychologic or interpersonal factors that may enhance sexual expression, as well as other factors that are of concern. Counseling can be effective for the individual patient, but it is typically best to include his partner, particularly if he is involved in a long-term relationship.[40] Counseling should begin before the start of medical treatment for ED.

NURSING MANAGEMENT
ERECTILE DYSFUNCTION

The man experiencing ED requires a great deal of emotional support for both himself and his partner. Men often do not feel comfortable discussing their problems with others because of society's expectations of a man's sexual abilities. Reassure the patient that confidentiality will be maintained. The majority of men delay seeking medical assistance. They are often highly motivated and expect immediate solutions to their problems. The health care team should provide a support system and accurate information as soon as possible.

Conducting routine health assessments on men seeking any form of medical treatment places you in a unique position. It provides an opportunity to ask the patient questions pertaining to general health, as well as sexual health and function. Given the opportunity, men will be less hesitant to answer these questions when they know that someone cares and can provide them with answers.

ANDROPAUSE

Andropause is a gradual decline in androgen secretion that occurs in most men as they age. The primary male androgen that is reduced is testosterone (Fig. 55-13). Andropause, also called late onset hypogonadism and male menopause, can begin as early as age 40. Factors that determine the rate of decline are not clearly known. Signs and symptoms associated with a lowered level of testosterone include loss of libido, fatigue, ED, depression and mood swings, and sleep disturbances. Symptoms are often attributed to normal aging and frequently are not reported by the patient. The long-term effects, including a loss of muscle mass and strength, may contribute to an increased risk of falls and fractures.[41]

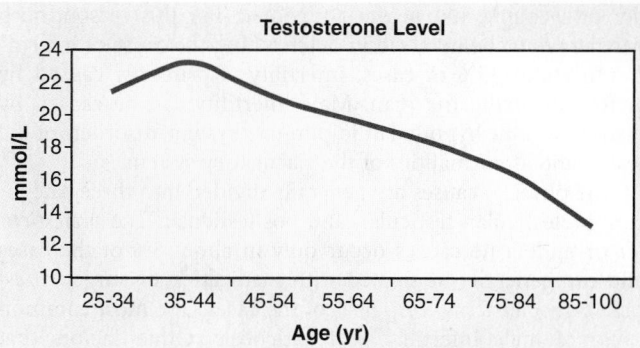

FIG. 55-13 Changes in testosterone plasma level in men as they age.

A diagnosis of andropause is made after a complete physical examination and serum total testosterone levels have been obtained. Normal testosterone levels can range from 280 to 1000 ng/dL. Replacement therapy is generally considered once levels drop below 200 ng/dL.[42] Therapy may be started earlier depending on severity of symptoms. Testosterone replacement therapy (TRT) should not be started until the patient, in consultation with his health care provider, considers the risks and benefits of therapy. Symptoms may improve with TRT, but potential risks include lowered levels of high-density lipoprotein (HDL) cholesterol, increased hematocrit, and worsening sleep apnea. The effect of testosterone on prostatic tissue makes this therapy contraindicated in patients with BPH or prostate cancer. Before treatment is initiated, a DRE and PSA test should be performed. Once TRT begins, patients should be closely monitored by their health care provider.

Replacement therapy is available in different forms. Oral TRT (e.g., methyltestosterone, fluoxymesterone) is not recommended because it is less effective and liver damage can occur with high doses.[43] Intramuscular injections such as cypionate (Depo-Testosterone) and enanthate (Delatestryl) are available in varying doses. These drugs create a cyclic rise and fall in serum testosterone levels with the highest levels 2 or 3 days after the injection. Then the testosterone levels slowly decrease until the next injection. Mood swings can occur with these fluctuations.

Transdermal preparations, including patches and gels (e.g., Androderm, Testim), are more convenient. They are generally applied to the skin daily at various sites, including the back, the arm, and the abdomen. Skin irritation is the most common side effect. Triamcinolone creams (diacetate [Amcort], acetonide [Kenalog]) rubbed into the skin before application of the patch may decrease and prevent irritation. Testosterone may also be given as a buccal tablet (Striant) or as an underarm application (Axiron).

Women of childbearing age and children should avoid direct contact with these products, since they may cause early signs of puberty in young children and changes (virilization) in the external genitalia of a female fetus. Emphasize to the patient the importance of hand washing with soap and water after applying testosterone preparations to the skin. Covering the area with clothing until the preparation has dried is also recommended.

INFERTILITY

Infertility in a couple is defined as the inability to conceive after 1 year of frequent unprotected intercourse. Infertility is a disorder of a couple, not of one individual. For this reason, both partners must be involved in determining the cause of infertility. In about 33% of cases, infertility is primarily caused by factors involving the man. Male infertility can be caused by disorders of the hypothalamic-pituitary system, disorders of the testes, and abnormalities of the ejaculatory system.

The physical causes are generally divided into three categories: pretesticular, testicular, and posttesticular. The *pretesticular* or endocrine causes occur only in about 3% of the cases and can generally be treated with medication or surgery. *Testicular problems* make up 50% of the cases. The most common cause of male infertility is a varicocele. Other factors that influence the testes include infection (e.g., mumps virus, STIs, bacterial infections), congenital anomalies, medications, radiation, substance abuse (alcohol, nicotine, drugs), and environmental hazards. *Posttesticular* causes account for approximately 5% to 7% of the cases, with obstruction, infection, and the result of a surgical procedure being the primary causes. The remaining 40% are classified as *idiopathic,* or of unknown causes.

A careful health history and examination may reveal the cause of a patient's infertility. Thus the history is a starting point for determining cause and treatment. The history should include age; occupation; past injury, surgery, or infections to the genital tract; lifestyle issues such as hot tubs, weight training, or wearing tight undergarments; sexual practices; frequency of intercourse; and emotional factors such as stress levels and the desire for children. Document the use of drugs, such as chemotherapeutic agents, anabolic steroids (testosterone), sulfasalazine (Azulfidine), cimetidine (Tagamet), and recreational drugs, since these drugs can reduce the sperm count. A physical examination can disclose a varicocele, Peyronie's disease, or other physical abnormalities.

The first test in an infertility study is a semen analysis. The test determines the sperm concentration, motility, and morphology. Additional tests that may be helpful in determining the etiology include plasma testosterone and serum LH and FSH measurements. A test for sperm penetration abilities may also be done. The specific cause of infertility is often not determined.

Be concerned and tactful in dealing with the male patient undergoing infertility studies. Many men equate fertility and masculinity.

Treatment options for the man include medications, conservative lifestyle changes (e.g., avoidance of scrotal heat, substance abuse, and high stress), in vitro fertilization techniques, and corrective surgery. Infertility can seriously strain a relationship, and the couple may require counseling and discussion of alternatives if conception is not achieved. (Female infertility is discussed in Chapter 54.)

CASE STUDY

Benign Prostatic Hyperplasia With Acute Urinary Retention

iStockphoto/Thinkstock

Patient Profile

B.G., a 60-yr-old married African American man, comes to the primary health outpatient clinic because of an inability to void for the past 13 hr and pain in the lower abdomen.

Subjective Data

• Complains of the urge to void
• Is restless, anxious, and agitated

Objective Data

• Has prostate enlargement on digital rectal examination
• Has hematuria, bacteria, and WBCs in urine
• Has a tender and palpable bladder above the umbilicus
• PSA test: 8 ng/mL

Collaborative Care

• Indwelling catheter inserted by a urology resident
• Admitted to the hospital

Discussion Questions

1. What risk factors for prostate problems are present in B.G.?
2. Explain the etiology of the objective symptoms B.G. exhibited.
3. Offer possible reasons for B.G.'s elevated PSA level.
4. Discuss the drug and surgical options available to B.G.
5. B.G. asks you about the effect of the various surgical options on his ability to have sex. How would you respond?
6. *Priority Decision:* Based on the assessment data, what are the priority nursing diagnoses? Are there any collaborative problems?
7. *Priority Decision:* What is the priority nursing intervention for B.G.?
8. On further assessment, you note that B.G. has a nursing diagnosis of decisional conflict. How would you help him resolve this conflict related to treatment options?
9. *Evidence-Based Practice:* What information would you offer to B.G. when he asks if he should start taking saw palmetto to prevent future UTIs?

evolve Answers available at *http://evolve.elsevier.com/Lewis/medsurg.*

▌ B R I D G E T O N C L E X E X A M I N A T I O N

The number of the question corresponds to the same-numbered outcome at the beginning of the chapter.

1. An older male patient is experiencing difficulty in initiating voiding and a feeling of incomplete bladder emptying. These symptoms of BPH are primarily caused by
   a. obstruction of the urethra.
   b. untreated chronic prostatitis.
   c. decreased bladder compliance.
   d. excessive secretion of testosterone.

2. Postoperatively, a patient who has had a laser prostatectomy has continuous bladder irrigation with a three-way urinary catheter with a 30-mL balloon. When he complains of bladder spasms with the catheter in place, the nurse should
   a. deflate the catheter balloon to 10 mL to decrease bulk in the bladder.
   b. deflate the catheter balloon and then reinflate to ensure that it is patent.
   c. encourage the patient to try to have a bowel movement to relieve colon pressure.
   d. explain that this feeling is normal and that he should not try to urinate around the catheter.

3. Which factors would place a patient at higher risk for prostate cancer (select all that apply)?
   a. Older than 65 years
   b. Asian or Native American
   c. Long-term use of an indwelling urethral catheter
   d. Father diagnosed and treated for early stage prostate cancer
   e. Previous history of undescended testicle and testicular cancer

4. A patient scheduled for a prostatectomy for prostate cancer expresses the fear that he will have erectile dysfunction. In responding to this patient, the nurse should keep in mind that
   a. erectile dysfunction can occur even with a nerve-sparing procedure.
   b. retrograde ejaculation affects sexual function more frequently than erectile dysfunction.
   c. the most common complication of this surgery is postoperative bowel incontinence.
   d. preoperative sexual function is the most important factor in determining postoperative erectile dysfunction.

5. The nurse explains to the patient with chronic bacterial prostatitis who is undergoing antibiotic therapy that (select all that apply)
   a. all patients require hospitalization.
   b. pain will lessen once treatment has ended.
   c. course of treatment is generally 2 to 4 weeks.
   d. long-term therapy may be indicated in immunocompromised patient.
   e. if the condition is unresolved and untreated, he is at risk for prostate cancer.

6. In assessing a patient for testicular cancer, the nurse understands that the manifestations of this disease often include
   a. acute back spasms and testicular pain.
   b. rapid onset of scrotal swelling and fever.
   c. fertility problems and bilateral scrotal tenderness.
   d. painless mass and heaviness sensation in the scrotal area.

7. The nurse should explain to the patient who has had a vasectomy that
   a. the procedure blocks the production of sperm.
   b. erectile dysfunction is temporary and will return with sexual activity.
   c. the ejaculate will be about half the volume it was before the procedure.
   d. an alternative form of contraception will be necessary for 6 to 8 weeks.

8. To decrease the patient's discomfort over care related to his reproductive organs, the nurse should
   a. relate his sexual concerns to his sexual partner.
   b. arrange to have male nurses care for the patient.
   c. maintain a nonjudgmental attitude toward his sexual practices.
   d. use technical terminology when discussing reproductive function.

1. a, 2. d, 3. a, d, e, 4. a, 5. b, d, 6. d, 7. d, 8. c

ⓔvolve

For rationales to these answers and even more NCLEX review questions, visit *http://evolve.elsevier.com/Lewis/medsurg*.

REFERENCES

1. Roehrborn C: Male lower urinary tract symptoms (LUTS) and benign prostatic hyperplasia (BPH), *Med Clin North Am* 95:8, 2011.

*2. Schenk J, Kristal A, Arnold B, et al: Association of symptomatic benign prostatic hyperplasia and prostate cancer: results from the prostate cancer prevention trial, *Am J Epidemiol* 173:1419, 2011.

*3. Ørsted D, Bojesen S, Nielsen S, et al: Association of clinical benign prostate hyperplasia with prostate cancer incidence and mortality revisited: a nationwide cohort study of 3,009,258 men, *Eur Urol* 60:691, 2011.

4. American Urological Association Foundation: Management of benign prostatic hypertrophy. Retrieved from *www.urology health.org/about*.

5. Gerber G, Brendler C: Evaluation of the urologic patient. In Wien A, editor-in-chief: *Campbell-Walsh urology*, ed 10, St Louis, 2011, Saunders.

6. Barry M, Fowler F, O'Leary M, et al: The American Urologic Association symptom index for benign prostatic hyperplasia, *J Urol* 148:1549, 1992. (Classic)

7. Cleveland Clinic: Benign prostatic hypertrophy. Retrieved from *www.clevelandclinic.org/disorders/benign_prostatic_enlargement_bph*.

8. National Cancer Institute: Prostate cancer prevention trial, National Institutes of Health. Retrieved from *www.cancer.gov*.

9. US Food and Drug Administration: FDA approves Cialis to treat benign prostatic hyperplasia. Retrieved from *www.fda.gov/NewsEvents/Newsroom/PressAnnouncements/2011*.

10. Barry M, Meleth S, Lee J, et al: Effect of increasing doses of saw palmetto extract on lower urinary tract symptoms: a randomized trial, *JAMA* 306:1344, 2011.

*11. MacDonald R, Tacklind J, Rutks I: *Serenoa repens* monotherapy for benign prostatic hyperplasia (BPH): an updated Cochrane systematic review, *BJU Intern* 109:1756, 2012.

*12. Ahyai S, Gilling P, Kaplan S, et al: Meta-analysis of functional outcomes and complications following transurethral procedures for lower urinary tract symptoms resulting from benign prostatic enlargement, *Eur Urol* 58:384, 2010.

*13. Hermann T, Liatsikos E, Nagele U, et al: EAU guidelines on laser technologies, *Eur Urol* 61:783, 2012.

14. National Kidney and Urologic Diseases Information Clearinghouse: Prostate enlargement: benign prostatic hyperplasia, US Department of Health and Human Services. Retrieved from *www.niddk.nih.gov/kudiseases/pubs/prostateenlargemen*.

15. American Cancer Society: Cancer facts and figures 2012. Retrieved from *www.cancer.org*.

16. Siegel R, DeSantis C, Virgo K, et al: Cancer treatment and survivorship statistics, 2012, *CA Cancer J Clin* 62:220, 2012.

*17. Klein E, Thompson I, Tangen C, et al: Vitamin E and the risk of prostate cancer: the selenium and vitamin E cancer prevention trial (SELECT), *JAMA* 306:1549, 2011.

*18. Agency for Healthcare Research and Quality: Screening for prostate cancer: summary of recommendations. Retrieved from *www.uspreventiveservicestaskforce.org/uspstf12/prostate/prostateart.htm*.

19. Cao D: The Gleason score of tumor at the margin in radical prostatectomy is predictive of biochemical recurrence, *Am J Surg Pathol* 34:994, 2010.

*Evidence-based information for clinical practice.

20. National Institutes of Health, National Cancer Institute: Treatment choices for men with early-stage prostate cancer. Retrieved from *www.cancer.gov/cancertopics/treatment/prostate/understanding-prostate-cancer-treatment*.

*21. Quoc-Dien Trinh Q, Sammon J, Sun M, et al: Perioperative outcomes of robot-assisted radical prostatectomy compared with open radical prostatectomy: results from the nationwide inpatient sample, *Eur Urol* 61:679, 2012.

22. Boorjian S, Eastham J, Graefen M, et al: A critical analysis of the long-term impact of radical prostatectomy on cancer control and function outcomes, *Eur Urol* 61:664, 2012.

23. Gandaglia G, Nazareno S, Gallina A, et al: Preoperative erectile function represents a significant predictor of postoperative urinary continence recovery in patients treated with bilateral nerve sparing radical prostatectomy, *J Urol* 187:569, 2012.

24. Dunn M, Kazer M: Prostate cancer overview, *Semin Oncol Nurs* 27:241, 2011.

*25. Cameron S, Springer C, Fox-Wasylyshyn S, et al: A descriptive study of functions, symptoms, and perceived health state after radiotherapy for prostate cancer, *Eur J Oncol Nurs* 16:310, 2012.

*26. Forsythe K, Blacksburg S, Stone N, et al: Intensity-modulated radiotherapy causes fewer side effects than three-dimensional conformal radiotherapy when used in combination with brachytherapy for the treatment of prostate cancer, *Int J Radiat Oncol Biol Phys* 83:630, 2012.

*27. Levine G, D'Amico A, Berger P, et al: Androgen-deprivation therapy in prostate cancer and cardiovascular risk: a science advisory from the American Heart Association, American Cancer Society, and American Urological Association: endorsed by the American Society for Radiation Oncology, *CA Cancer J Clin* 60:194, 2010.

28. VanderWalde A, Hurria A: Aging and osteoporosis, *CA Cancer J Clin* 61:139, 2011.

*29. Dilori C, Steenland K, Goodman M, et al: Differences in treatment-based beliefs and coping between African American and white men with prostate cancer, *J Commun Health* 36:505, 2011.

30. National Institute of Diabetes and Digestive and Kidney Disorders Information Clearinghouse: Prostatitis: disorders of the prostate. Retrieved from *www.niddk.nih.gov/kudiseases/pubs/prostatitis*.

31. Touma N, Nickel J: Prostatitis and chronic pelvic pain syndrome in men, *Med Clin North Am* 95:75, 2011.

32. Lawindy S, Rodriguez A, Horenblas S, et al: Current and future strategies in the diagnosis and management of penile cancer, *Adv Urol* 2011: 593751 (published online 2011 May 30). Retrieved from *www.hindawi.com/journals/au/2011/593751*.

33. National Cancer Institute: Testicular cancer factsheet. Retrieved from *www.nci.nih.gov/cancertopics/factsheet/sites-types/testicular*.

34. Zoltick B: Shedding light on testicular cancer, *Nurse Pract* 36:32, 2011.

35. Bradford B: Chemotherapy-induced infertility in patients with testicular cancer, *Oncol Nurs Forum* 39:27, 2012.

36. Sadovsky R, Brock G, Gerald B, et al: Optimizing treatment outcomes with phosphodiesterase type 5 inhibitors for erectile dysfunction: opening windows to enhanced sexual function and overall health, *J Am Acad Nurse Pract* 23:320, 2011.

*37. Dong J, Zhang Y, Qin L: Erectile dysfunction and risk of cardiovascular disease: meta-analysis of prospective cohort studies, *J Am Coll Cardiol* 58:1378, 2011.

38. Rosen R, Riley A, Wagner G, et al. The International Index of Erectile Function (IIEF): a multidimensional scale for assessment of erectile dysfunction, *Urology* 49:822, 1997. (Classic)

39. Lee M: Focus on phosphodiesterase inhibitors for the treatment of erectile dysfunction in older men, *Clin Therap* 33:1590, 2011.

40. Cleveland Clinic: Erectile dysfunction: sex therapy. Retrieved from *clevelandclinic.org/disorders/erectile_disorder_impotence/hic_sex_therapy.aspx*.

*41. LeBlanc E, Wang P, Lee C, et al: Higher testosterone levels are associated with less loss of lean body mass in older men, *J Clin Endocrinol Metab* 96:3855, 2011.

42. American Association of Clinical Endocrinologists: Medical guidelines for clinical practice for the evaluation and treatment of hypogonadism in adult male patients—2002 update, *Endocrinol Pract* 8:440, 2002. (Classic)

43. Johns Hopkins Medical Letter: Men, should you try testosterone therapy? *HealthAfter50* 22:6, 2011.

RESOURCES

American Cancer Society
www.cancer.org
American Urological Association
www.auanet.org
LiveStrong
www.livestrong.org
National Cancer Institute
www.cancer.gov/cancertopics/types/prostate
National Kidney and Urologic Diseases Information Clearinghouse
www.kidney.niddk.nih.gov
Prostatitis Foundation
www.prostatitis.org
Sexuality Information and Education Council of the United States (SIECUS)
www.siecus.org

CASE STUDY

Managing Multiple Patients

Introduction

You are working on the medical-surgical unit and have been assigned to care for the following six patients. You have one LPN and one UAP on your team to help you.

Patients

iStockphoto/Thinkstock

L.M. is a 35-yr-old Hispanic woman who went to the clinic 3 days ago complaining of "just not feeling well." She was admitted to the hospital for treatment of hypertension caused by newly diagnosed Cushing syndrome. She has been very depressed and crying because of her physical appearance. Her most recent blood pressure was 150/84 mm Hg.

iStockphoto/Thinkstock

N.B. is a 34-yr-old Native American man admitted to the ICU 2 days ago with a diagnosis of diabetic ketoacidosis. He was transferred to the nursing unit yesterday evening. His fasting blood glucose this morning is 296 mg/dL.

iStockphoto/Thinkstock

A.K. is a 68-yr-old Asian American woman recently diagnosed with adenocarcinoma of her right breast. She had a lumpectomy and axillary node dissection yesterday. She has a Jackson-Pratt drain in her right chest. Her last pain medication was administered 1 hour ago, at which time she rated her pain as a 7 on a scale of 0-10.

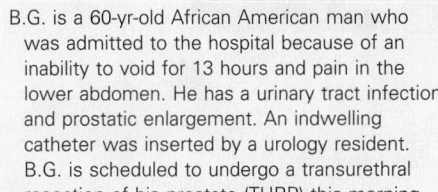

iStockphoto/Thinkstock

B.G. is a 60-yr-old African American man who was admitted to the hospital because of an inability to void for 13 hours and pain in the lower abdomen. He has a urinary tract infection and prostatic enlargement. An indwelling catheter was inserted by a urology resident. B.G. is scheduled to undergo a transurethral resection of his prostate (TURP) this morning.

Jupiterimages/Photos
.com/Thinkstock

R.D. is a 47-yr-old white woman who was diagnosed with Graves' disease 2 months ago. She was treated with antithyroid medication for 2 months and underwent a subtotal thyroidectomy yesterday. She has been complaining of slight numbness and tingling in her fingers.

N.B. is a 65-yr-old white woman who underwent a vaginal hysterectomy and anterior/posterior repair 1 day ago. She has vaginal packing and a urinary catheter in place. Her vital signs are stable and she is not complaining of pain.

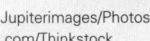

Jupiterimages/Photos
.com/Thinkstock

Management Discussion Questions

1. *Priority Decision:* After receiving report, which patient should you see first? Second? Provide a rationale.
2. *Delegation Decision:* Which tasks could you delegate to UAP *(select all that apply)*?
   a. Assist N.B. to sit out of bed in a chair.
   b. Teach B.G. what to expect postoperatively.
   c. Take R.D.'s vital signs and report the results to you.
   d. Assess A.K.'s mastectomy incision for manifestations of infection.
   e. Listen to L.M. talk about her feelings while helping her with AM care.
3. *Priority and Delegation Decision:* As you are assessing R.D., the LPN informs you that A.K.'s chest dressing is totally saturated with bloody drainage. Which initial action would be most appropriate?
   a. Ask the LPN to call the lab for a stat Hgb and Hct on A.K.
   b. Have the LPN reinforce the dressing with sterile 4 × 4 gauze pads.
   c. Have the LPN stay with R.D. while you assess the patency of A.K.'s Jackson-Pratt drain.
   d. Ask the LPN to stay with A.K. and the UAP to monitor R.D. while you call A.K.'s surgeon.

Case Study Progression

A.K.'s Jackson-Pratt drain was not functioning properly. You get it working and change the chest dressing. The incision is well approximated without signs of infection. When you leave the room, the Jackson-Pratt has a small amount of serosanguineous drainage in it. As you enter R.D.'s room you notice that the patient is having a carpopedal spasm on the same arm that the LPN is taking her blood pressure on. You recognize this as a manifestation of hypocalcemia and notify the health care provider.

4. Which interventions would you expect the health care provider to order for R.D. *(select all that apply)*?
   a. IV calcium gluconate
   b. IV sodium bicarbonate
   c. Have patient hold breath
   d. Rebreathing into paper bag
   e. Parathyroid hormone replacement therapy
5. Which intervention would be most appropriate in caring for L.M.?
   a. Assess her for signs and symptoms of hypoglycemia.
   b. Teach her the need for a high-carbohydrate, low-protein diet.
   c. Administer IV methylprednisolone (Solu-Medrol) over 2 min.
   d. Reassure her that her physical appearance will improve with treatment.
6. B.G. asks you what to expect when he returns from surgery. You explain that he will have a(n)
   a. dressing in his groin as well as a urinary catheter.
   b. 3-way urinary catheter connected to an irrigation system.
   c. patient-controlled analgesia (PCA) pump for pain control.
   d. abdominal and a perineal drain that will be recharged q4h.
7. *Priority and Management Decision:* The LPN is assigned to administer medications to N.B., including his sliding scale Novolog insulin with breakfast. The UAP, who is also a senior nursing student, tells you that the LPN administered N.B.'s insulin at least 30 min after the patient ate his breakfast. What is your best initial action?
   a. Report the incident to the charge nurse for follow-up.
   b. Talk to the LPN about the importance of timely medication administration.
   c. Ask the LPN what time the insulin was given and when the patient ate breakfast.
   d. Ask the UAP to first discuss the concern with the LPN so as to follow proper channels of communication.

SECTION 11

Problems Related to Movement and Coordination

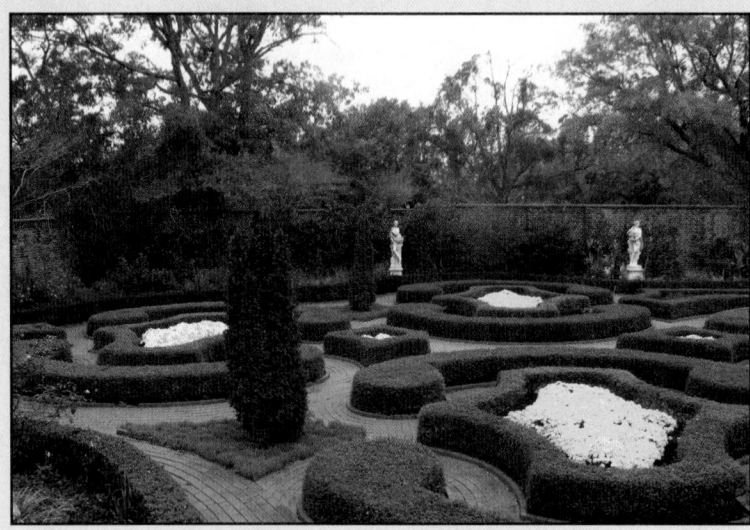

Peter Bonner

If you don't know where you are going, any road will get you there.
Lewis Carroll

The greatest conflicts are not between two people, but between one person and himself.
Garth Brooks

Nursing Assessment
Nervous System

DaiWai Olson

evolve WEBSITE

LEARNING OUTCOMES

1. Differentiate between the functions of neurons and glial cells.
2. Explain the anatomic location and functions of the cerebrum, brainstem, cerebellum, spinal cord, peripheral nerves, and cerebrospinal fluid.
3. Identify the major arteries supplying the brain.
4. Describe the functions of the 12 cranial nerves.
5. Compare the functions of the two divisions of the autonomic nervous system.
6. Link the age-related changes in the neurologic system to the differences in assessment findings.
7. Select significant subjective and objective data related to the nervous system that should be obtained from a patient.
8. Select appropriate techniques to use in the physical assessment of the nervous system.
9. Differentiate normal from abnormal findings of a physical assessment of the nervous system.
10. Describe the purpose, significance of results, and nursing responsibilities related to diagnostic studies of the nervous system.

KEY TERMS

autonomic nervous system (ANS), p. 1340
blood-brain barrier, p. 1342
central nervous system (CNS), p. 1336
cerebrospinal fluid (CSF), p. 1340
cranial nerves (CNs), p. 1340

dermatome, p. 1340
glial cells, p. 1336
lower motor neurons (LMNs), p. 1338
meninges, p. 1342
neurons, p. 1336

neurotransmitters, p. 1337
peripheral nervous system (PNS), p. 1336
reflex, p. 1338
synapse, p. 1337
upper motor neurons (UMNs), p. 1338

Reviewed by Jane A. Madden, RN, MSN, Professor of Nursing, Pikes Peak Community College, Colorado Springs, Colorado.

STRUCTURES AND FUNCTIONS OF NERVOUS SYSTEM

The human nervous system is responsible for the control and integration of the body's many activities. The nervous system can be divided into the central nervous system and the peripheral nervous system. The **central nervous system (CNS)** consists of the brain, spinal cord, and cranial nerves I and II. The **peripheral nervous system (PNS)** consists of cranial nerves III to XII, spinal nerves, and the peripheral components of the autonomic nervous system (ANS).

Cells of Nervous System

The nervous system is made up of two types of cells: neurons and glial cells.

Neurons. Neurons are the primary functional unit of the nervous system, Although neurons come in many shapes and sizes, they share three characteristics: (1) *excitability,* or the ability to generate a nerve impulse; (2) *conductivity,* or the ability to transmit an impulse; and (3) *influence,* or the ability to influence other neurons, muscle cells, or glandular cells by transmitting nerve impulses to them.

A typical *neuron* consists of a cell body, multiple dendrites, and an axon (Fig. 56-1). The cell body containing the nucleus and cytoplasm is the metabolic center of the neuron. *Dendrites* are short processes extending from the cell body that receive impulses from the axons of other neurons and conduct impulses

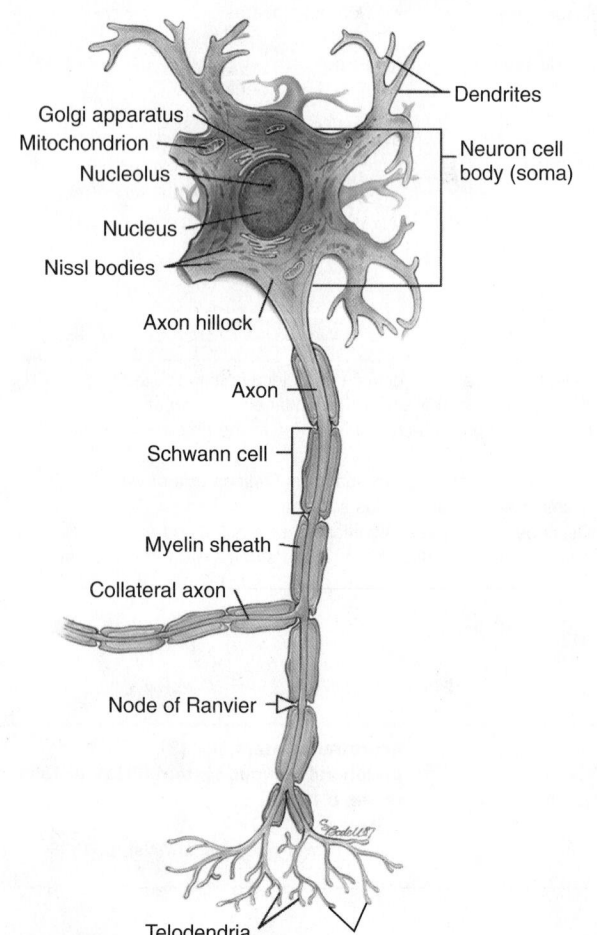

Golgi apparatus
Mitochondrion
Nucleolus
Nucleus
Nissl bodies
Dendrites
Neuron cell body (soma)
Axon hillock
Axon
Schwann cell
Myelin sheath
Collateral axon
Node of Ranvier
Telodendria
Synaptic knobs

FIG. 56-1 Structural features of neurons: dendrites, cell body, and axons.

toward the cell body. The *axon* projects varying distances from the cell body, ranging from several micrometers to more than a meter. The axon carries nerve impulses to other neurons or to end organs. The end organs are smooth and striated muscles and glands.

Many axons in the CNS and PNS are covered by a *myelin sheath,* a white, lipid substance that acts as an insulator for the conduction of impulses. Axons may be myelinated or unmyelinated. Generally, the smaller fibers are unmyelinated.

Neurons have long been thought to be nonmitotic. That is, after being damaged neurons could not be replaced. The discovery of neuronal stem cells now demonstrates that neurogenesis occurs in adult brains after cerebral injury.[1]

Glial Cells. Glial cells (glia or neuroglia) provide support, nourishment, and protection to neurons. Glial cells constitute almost half of the brain and spinal cord mass and are 5 to 10 times more numerous than neurons.

Glial cells are divided into microglia and macroglia. *Microglia,* specialized macrophages capable of phagocytosis, protect the neurons. These cells are mobile within the brain and multiply when the brain is damaged.

Different types of *macroglial cells* include the astrocytes (most abundant), oligodendrocytes, and ependymal cells.[2] *Astrocytes* are found primarily in gray matter and provide structural support to neurons. Their delicate processes form the blood-brain barrier with the endothelium of the blood vessels. They also play a role in synaptic transmission (conduction of impulses between neurons). When the brain is injured, astrocytes act as phagocytes for neuronal debris. They help restore the neurochemical milieu and provide support for repair. Proliferation of astrocytes contributes to the formation of scar tissue *(gliosis)* in the CNS.

Oligodendrocytes are specialized cells that produce the myelin sheath of nerve fibers in the CNS and are primarily found in the white matter of the CNS. (*Schwann cells* myelinate the nerve fibers in the periphery.) *Ependymal cells* line the brain ventricles and aid in the secretion of cerebrospinal fluid (CSF).

Neuroglia are mitotic and can replicate. In general, when neurons are destroyed, the tissue is replaced by the proliferation of neuroglial cells. Most primary CNS tumors involve glial cells. Primary malignancies involving neurons are rare.

Nerve Regeneration

If the axon of the nerve cell is damaged, the cell attempts to repair itself. Damaged nerve cells attempt to grow back to their original destinations by sprouting many branches from the damaged ends of their axons. Axons in the CNS are generally less successful than peripheral axons in regeneration.[3]

Injured nerve fibers in the PNS can regenerate by growing within the protective myelin sheath of the supporting Schwann cells if the cell body is intact. The final result of nerve regeneration depends on the number of axon sprouts that join with the appropriate Schwann cell columns and reinnervate appropriate end organs.

Nerve Impulse

The purpose of a neuron is to initiate, receive, and process messages about events both within and outside the body. The initiation of a neuronal message *(nerve impulse)* involves the generation of an action potential. Once an action potential is initiated, a series of action potentials travels along the axon. When the impulse reaches the end of the nerve fiber, it is transmitted across the junction between nerve cells *(synapse)* by a chemical interaction involving neurotransmitters. This chemical interaction generates another set of action potentials in the next neuron. These events are repeated until the nerve impulse reaches its destination.

Because of its insulating capacity, myelination of nerve axons facilitates the conduction of an action potential. Many peripheral nerve axons have *nodes of Ranvier* (gaps in the myelin sheath) that allow an action potential to travel much faster by jumping from node to node without traversing the insulated membrane segment. This is called *saltatory* (hopping) conduction. In an unmyelinated fiber, the wave of depolarization travels the entire length of the axon, with each portion of the membrane becoming depolarized in turn.

Synapse. A synapse is the structural and functional junction between two neurons. It is the point at which the nerve impulse is transmitted from one neuron to another. The nerve impulse can also be transmitted from neurons to glands or muscles. The essential structures of synaptic transmission are a presynaptic terminal, a synaptic cleft, and a receptor site on the postsynaptic cell.

Neurotransmitters. Neurotransmitters are chemicals that affect the transmission of impulses across the synaptic cleft. (Examples of neurotransmitters are presented in Table 56-1.) Excitatory neurotransmitters activate postsynaptic receptors that increase the likelihood that an action potential will be generated. Inhibitory neurotransmitters activate postsynaptic receptors that inhibit the likelihood that an action potential will be generated.

Each of the hundreds to thousands of synaptic connections of a single neuron has an influence on that neuron. In general, the net effect (excitatory or inhibitory) depends on the number of presynaptic neurons that are releasing neurotransmitters on the postsynaptic cell. A presynaptic cell that releases an excitatory neurotransmitter does not always cause the postsynaptic cell to depolarize enough to generate an action potential.

Neurotransmitters can be affected by drugs and toxins, which can modify their function or block their attachment to receptor sites on the postsynaptic membrane. When many presynaptic cells release excitatory neurotransmitters on a single neuron, the sum of their input is enough to generate an action potential. Neurotransmitters continue to combine with the receptor sites at the postsynaptic membrane until they are inactivated by enzymes, are taken up by the presynaptic endings, or diffuse away from the synaptic region. With the use of cerebral microdialysis (minimally invasive sampling technique), neurotransmitter levels can now be measured in the cerebral cortex.[4]

Central Nervous System

The components of the CNS include the cerebrum (cerebral hemispheres), brainstem, cerebellum, and spinal cord.

Spinal Cord. The spinal cord is continuous with the brainstem and exits from the cranial cavity through the foramen magnum. A cross section of the spinal cord reveals gray matter that is centrally located in an H shape and is surrounded by white matter. The gray matter contains the cell bodies of voluntary motor neurons, preganglionic autonomic motor neurons, and association neurons (interneurons). The white matter contains the axons of the ascending sensory and the descending (suprasegmental) motor fibers. The myelin surrounding these fibers gives them their white appearance. The spinal pathways or tracts are named for the point of origin and the point of

TABLE 56-1 NEUROTRANSMITTERS*

Neurotransmitter	Clinical Relevance
Acetylcholine	A decrease in acetylcholine-secreting neurons is seen in Alzheimer's disease. Myasthenia gravis results from a reduction in acetylcholine receptors.
Amines	
Epinephrine (adrenalin)	Is both a hormone and neurotransmitter. Produced in neurons of CNS and neurosecretory cells of adrenal medulla. Critical component of the fight-or-flight response of SNS.
Norepinephrine	Is both a hormone and neurotransmitter. Has important role as neurotransmitter released from SNS affecting the heart. Along with epinephrine, has important role in fight-or-flight response, increasing heart rate, triggering the release of glucose from energy stores, and increasing blood flow to skeletal muscle.
Serotonin	Primarily found in GI tract, platelets, and CNS. Involved in moods, emotions, and sleep.
Dopamine	Produced in several areas of brain. Involved in emotions and moods and regulating motor control. Parkinson's disease results from destruction of dopamine-secreting neurons.
Amino Acids	
γ-Aminobutyric acid (GABA)	Chief inhibitory neurotransmitter in CNS. Has a role in regulating neuronal excitability throughout the nervous system. Drugs that increase GABA function have been used to treat seizure disorders.
Glutamate and aspartate	Plays key role in learning and memory. Sustained release of glutamate and prolonged excitation is toxic to nerve cells. Glutamate is a destructive factor in amyotrophic lateral sclerosis.
Neuropeptides	
Endorphins and enkephalins	Endogenous opioids that function as neurotransmitters. Produced in pituitary gland and hypothalamus. Produce analgesia and a feeling of well-being. The opioids morphine and heroin bind to endorphin and enkephalin receptors and produce the same effect as the endogenous opioids.
Substance P	Neurotransmitter in pain transmission pathways. Morphine blocks its release.

*These are examples only. Most of the neurotransmitters are also found in other locations and may have additional functions.
CNS, Central nervous system; *SNS,* sympathetic nervous system.

destination (e.g., spinocerebellar tract [ascending], corticospinal tract [descending]).

Ascending Tracts. In general, the ascending tracts carry specific sensory information to higher levels of the CNS. This information comes from special sensory receptors in the skin, muscles and joints, viscera, and blood vessels and enters the spinal cord by way of the dorsal roots of the spinal nerves. The fasciculus gracilis and the fasciculus cuneatus (commonly called the dorsal or posterior columns) carry information and transmit impulses concerned with touch, deep pressure, vibration, position sense, and kinesthesia (appreciation of movement,

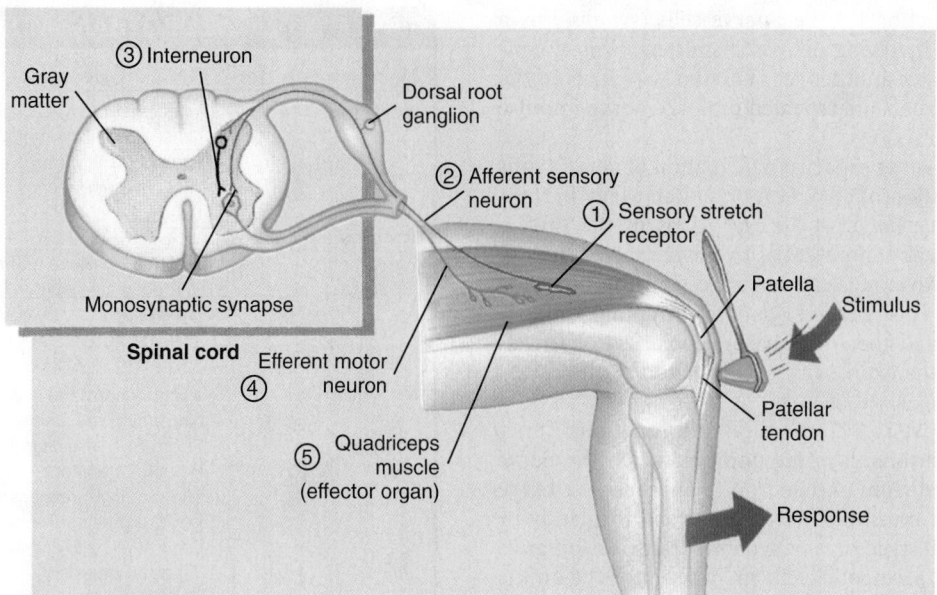

FIG. 56-2 Basic diagram of the patellar "knee jerk" reflex arc, including the *(1)* sensory stretch receptor, *(2)* afferent sensory neuron, *(3)* interneuron, *(4)* efferent motor neuron, and *(5)* quadriceps muscle (effector organ).

weight, and body parts). The *spinocerebellar tracts* carry information about muscle tension and body position to the cerebellum for coordination of movement. The *spinothalamic tracts* carry pain and temperature sensations. Therefore the ascending tracts are organized by sensory modality, as well as by anatomy.

Although the functions of these pathways are generally accepted, other ascending tracts may also carry sensory modalities. The symptoms of various neurologic diseases suggest that additional pathways for touch, position sense, and vibration exist.

Descending Tracts. Descending tracts carry impulses that are responsible for muscle movement. Among the most important descending tracts are the corticobulbar and corticospinal tracts, collectively termed the *pyramidal tract*. These tracts carry volitional (voluntary) impulses from the cerebral cortex to the cranial and peripheral nerves. Another group of descending motor tracts carries impulses from the extrapyramidal system (all motor systems except the pyramidal) concerned with voluntary movement. It includes pathways originating in the brainstem, basal ganglia, and cerebellum. The motor output exits the spinal cord by way of the ventral roots of the spinal nerves.

Lower and Upper Motor Neurons. **Lower motor neurons (LMNs)** are the final common pathway through which descending motor tracts influence skeletal muscle. The cell bodies of LMNs, which send axons to innervate the skeletal muscles of the arms, trunk, and legs, are located in the anterior horn of the corresponding segments of the spinal cord (e.g., cervical segments contain LMNs for the arms). LMNs for skeletal muscles of the eyes, face, mouth, and throat are located in the corresponding segments of the brainstem. These cell bodies and their axons make up the somatic motor components of the cranial nerves. LMN lesions generally cause weakness or paralysis, denervation atrophy, hyporeflexia or areflexia, and decreased muscle tone (flaccidity).

Upper motor neurons (UMNs) originate in the cerebral cortex and project downward. The corticobulbar tract ends in the brainstem, and the corticospinal tract descends into the spinal cord. These neurons influence skeletal muscle movement.

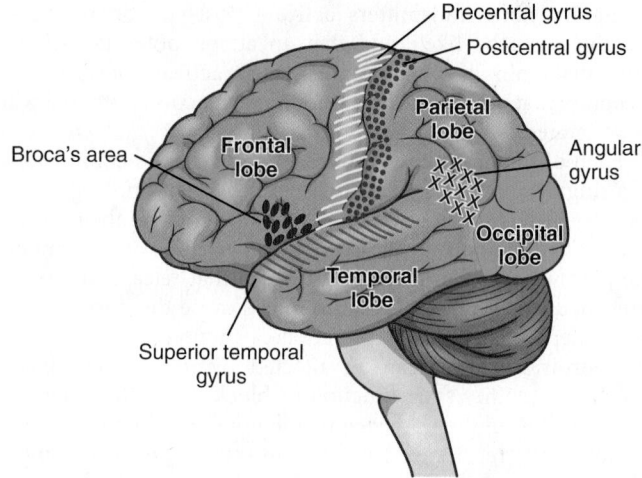

FIG. 56-3 Left hemisphere of cerebrum, lateral surface, showing major lobes and areas of the brain.

UMN lesions generally cause weakness or paralysis, disuse atrophy, hyperreflexia, and increased muscle tone (spasticity).

Reflex Arc. A **reflex** is an involuntary response to stimuli. In the spinal cord, reflex arcs play an important role in maintaining muscle tone, which is essential for body posture. The components of a monosynaptic reflex arc (Fig. 56-2) are a receptor organ, an afferent neuron, an effector neuron, and an effector organ (e.g., skeletal muscle). The afferent neuron synapses with the efferent neuron in the gray matter of the spinal cord. More complex reflex arcs have other neurons (interneurons) in addition to the afferent neuron influencing the effector neuron.

Brain. The term *brain* usually refers to the three major intracranial components: cerebrum, brainstem, and cerebellum.

Cerebrum. The *cerebrum* is composed of the right and left cerebral hemispheres and divided into four lobes: frontal, temporal, parietal, and occipital (Fig. 56-3). The functions of the cerebrum are multiple and complex (Table 56-2). The *frontal lobe* controls higher cognitive function, memory retention, vol-

TABLE 56-2 FUNCTION OF CEREBRUM

Part	Location	Function
Cortical Areas		
Motor		
Primary	Precentral gyrus	Motor control and movement on opposite side of body
Supplemental	Anterior to precentral gyrus	Facilitates proximal muscle activity, including activity for stance and gait, and spontaneous movement and coordination
Sensory		
Somatic	Postcentral gyrus	Sensory response from opposite side of body
Visual	Occipital lobe	Registers visual images
Auditory	Superior temporal gyrus	Registers auditory input
Association areas	Parietal lobe	Integrates somatic and sensory input
	Posterior temporal lobe	Integrates visual and auditory input for language comprehension
	Anterior temporal lobe	Integrates past experiences
	Anterior frontal lobe	Controls higher-order processes (e.g., judgment, reasoning)
Language		
Comprehension	Wernicke's area	Integrates auditory language (understanding of spoken words)
Expression	Broca's area	Regulates verbal expression
Basal Ganglia	Near lateral ventricles of both cerebral hemispheres	Control and facilitate learned and automatic movements
Thalamus	Below basal ganglia	Relays sensory and motor input to and from the cerebrum
Hypothalamus	Below thalamus	Regulates endocrine and autonomic functions
Limbic System	Lateral to hypothalamus	Influences emotional behavior and basic drives such as feeding and sexual behavior

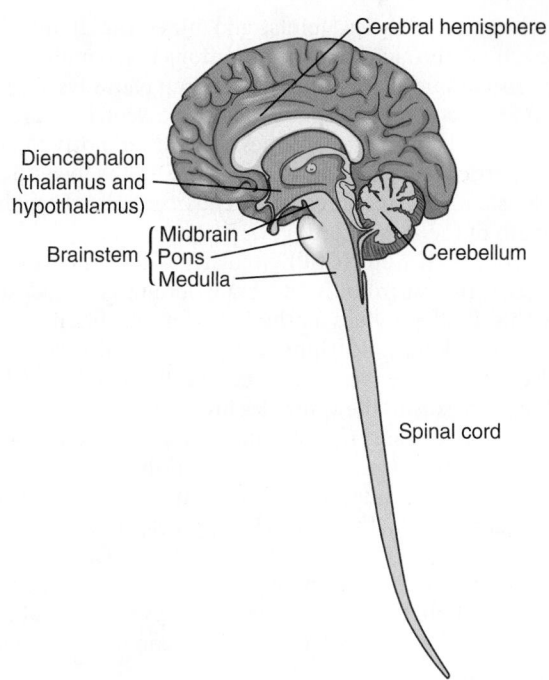

FIG. 56-4 Major divisions of the central nervous system (CNS).

midbrain. Most of them are on both sides of the thalamus. The function of the basal ganglia includes the initiation, execution, and completion of voluntary movements, learning, emotional response, and automatic movements associated with skeletal muscle activity (e.g., swinging the arms while walking, swallowing saliva, and blinking).

The *thalamus* (part of the diencephalon) lies directly above the brainstem (Fig. 56-4) and is the major relay center for afferent inputs to the cerebral cortex. The *hypothalamus* is located just inferior to the thalamus and slightly in front of the midbrain. It regulates the ANS and the endocrine system. The *limbic system* is located near the inner surfaces of the cerebral hemispheres and is concerned with emotion, aggression, feeding behavior, and sexual response.

Brainstem. The *brainstem* includes the midbrain, pons, and medulla (see Fig. 56-4). Ascending and descending fibers to and from the cerebrum and cerebellum pass through the brainstem. The nuclei of cranial nerves III through XII are in the brainstem. The vital centers concerned with respiratory, vasomotor, and cardiac function are located in the medulla.

Also located in the brainstem is the *reticular formation,* a diffusely arranged group of neurons and their axons that extends from the medulla to the thalamus and hypothalamus. The functions of the reticular formation include relaying sensory information, influencing excitatory and inhibitory control of spinal motor neurons, and controlling vasomotor and respiratory activity. The *reticular activating system* (RAS) is a complex system that requires communication among the brainstem, reticular formation, and cerebral cortex. The RAS is responsible for regulating arousal and sleep-wake transitions. The brainstem also contains the centers for sneezing, coughing, hiccupping, vomiting, sucking, and swallowing.

Cerebellum. The *cerebellum* is located in the posterior part of the cranial fossa inferior to the occipital lobe. The cerebellum coordinates voluntary movement and maintains trunk stability and equilibrium. The cerebellum receives information from the

untary eye movements, voluntary motor movement, and speech in Broca's area. The *temporal lobe* integrates somatic, visual, and auditory data and contains Wernicke's speech area. The *parietal lobe* interprets spatial information and contains the sensory cortex. Processing of sight takes place in the *occipital lobe.*

The division of the cerebrum into lobes is useful to delineate portions of the neocortex (gray matter), which makes up the outer layer of the cerebral hemispheres. Neurons in specific parts of the neocortex are essential for various highly complex and sophisticated aspects of mental function, such as language, memory, and appreciation of visual-spatial relationships.

The basal ganglia, thalamus, hypothalamus, and limbic system are also located in the cerebrum. The *basal ganglia* are a group of structures located centrally in the cerebrum and cerebral cortex, muscles, joints, and inner ear. It influences motor activity through axonal connections to the motor cortex, the brainstem nuclei, and their descending pathways.

Ventricles and Cerebrospinal Fluid. The ventricles are four interconnected fluid-filled cavities. The lower portion of the fourth ventricle becomes the central canal in the lower part of the brainstem. The spinal canal extends centrally through the full length of the spinal cord.

Cerebrospinal fluid (CSF) circulates within the subarachnoid space that surrounds the brain, brainstem, and spinal cord. This fluid provides cushioning for the brain and the spinal cord, allows fluid shifts from the cranial cavity to the spinal cavity, and carries nutrients. The formation of CSF in the choroid plexus in the ventricles involves both passive diffusion and active transport of substances. CSF resembles an ultrafiltrate of blood. Although CSF is produced at an average rate of about 500 mL/day, many factors influence CSF production and absorption. The ventricles and central canal are normally filled with an average of 135 mL of CSF. Changes in the rate of production or absorption will result in a change in the volume of CSF that remains in the ventricles and central canal. Excessive buildup of CSF results in a condition known as *hydrocephalus.*

The CSF circulates throughout the ventricles and seeps into the subarachnoid space surrounding the brain and spinal cord. It is absorbed primarily through the *arachnoid villi* (tiny projections into the subarachnoid space), into the intradural venous sinuses, and eventually into the venous system.

The analysis of CSF composition provides useful diagnostic information related to certain nervous system diseases. CSF pressure is often measured in patients with actual or suspected intracranial injury. Increased intracranial pressure, indicated by increased CSF pressure, can force downward (central) herniation of the brain and brainstem. The signs marking this event are part of the herniation syndrome (see Chapter 57).

Peripheral Nervous System

The PNS includes all the neuronal structures that lie outside the CNS. It consists of the spinal and cranial nerves, their associated ganglia (groupings of cell bodies), and portions of the ANS.

Spinal Nerves. The spinal cord can be seen as a series of spinal segments, one on top of another. In addition to the cell bodies, each segment contains a pair of dorsal (afferent) sensory nerve fibers or roots and ventral (efferent) motor fibers or roots, which innervate a specific region of the body. This combined motor-sensory nerve is called a *spinal nerve* (Fig. 56-5). The cell bodies of the voluntary motor system are located in the anterior horn of the spinal cord gray matter. The cell bodies of the autonomic (involuntary) motor system are located in the anterolateral portion of the spinal cord gray matter. The cell bodies of sensory fibers are located in the dorsal root ganglia just outside the spinal cord. On exiting the spinal column, each spinal nerve divides into ventral and dorsal rami, a collection of motor and sensory fibers that eventually goes to peripheral structures (e.g., skin, muscles, viscera).

A **dermatome** is the area of skin innervated by the sensory fibers of a single dorsal root of a spinal nerve (Fig. 56-6). The dermatomes give a general picture of somatic sensory innervation by spinal segments. A *myotome* is a muscle group innervated by the primary motor neurons of a single ventral root. The dermatomes and myotomes of a given spinal segment

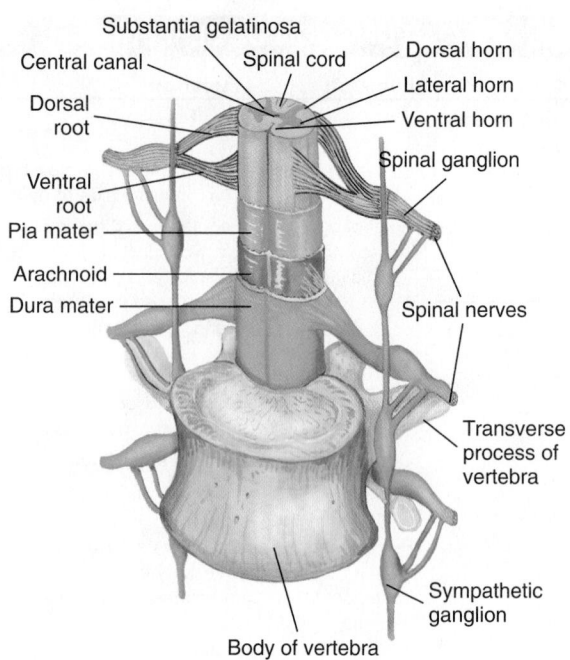

FIG. 56-5 Cross section of spinal cord showing attachments of spinal nerves and coverings of the spinal cord.

overlap with those of adjacent segments because of the development of ascending and descending collateral branches of nerve fibers.

Cranial Nerves. The cranial nerves (CNs) are the 12 paired nerves composed of cell bodies with fibers that exit from the cranial cavity. Unlike the spinal nerves, which always have both afferent sensory and efferent motor fibers, some CNs are only sensory, some only motor, and some both.

Table 56-3 summarizes the motor and sensory components of the CNs. Fig. 56-7 shows the position of the CNs in relation to the brain and spinal cord. Just as the cell bodies of the spinal nerves are located in specific segments of the spinal cord, so are the cell bodies (nuclei) of the CNs located in specific segments of the brain. Exceptions are the nuclei of the olfactory and optic nerves. The primary cell bodies of the olfactory nerve are located in the nasal epithelium, and those of the optic nerve are in the retina.

Autonomic Nervous System. The autonomic nervous system (ANS) is divided into the sympathetic and parasympathetic systems. The ANS governs involuntary functions of cardiac muscle, smooth muscle, and glands through both efferent and afferent pathways. The two systems function together to maintain a relatively balanced internal environment. The preganglionic cell bodies of the *sympathetic nervous system* (SNS) are located in spinal segments T1 through L2. The major neurotransmitter released by the postganglionic fibers of the SNS is norepinephrine, and the neurotransmitter released by the preganglionic fibers is acetylcholine.

The preganglionic cell bodies of the *parasympathetic nervous system* (PSNS) are located in the brainstem and the sacral spinal segments (S2 through S4). Acetylcholine is the neurotransmitter released at both preganglionic and postganglionic nerve endings. (The effects of the SNS and PSNS are compared in eTable 56-1 available on the website for this chapter.)

SNS stimulation activates the mechanisms required for the "fight-or-flight" response that occurs throughout the body. In

TABLE 56-3   CRANIAL NERVES

Nerve	Connection With Brain	Function
I Olfactory	Anterior ventral cerebrum	*Sensory:* from olfactory (smell)
II Optic	Lateral geniculate body of the thalamus	*Sensory:* from retina of eyes (vision)
III Oculomotor	Midbrain	*Motor:* to four eye movement muscles and levator palpebrae muscle *Parasympathetic:* smooth muscle in eyeball
IV Trochlear	Midbrain	*Motor:* to one eye movement muscle, the superior oblique muscle
V Trigeminal		
• Ophthalmic branch	Pons	*Sensory:* from forehead, eye, superior nasal cavity
• Maxillary branch	Pons	*Sensory:* from inferior nasal cavity, face, upper teeth, mucosa of superior mouth
• Mandibular branch	Pons	*Sensory:* from surfaces of jaw, lower teeth, mucosa of lower mouth, and anterior tongue *Motor:* to muscles of mastication
VI Abducens	Pons	*Motor:* to the lateral rectus of the eye
VII Facial	Junction of pons and medulla	*Motor:* to facial muscles of expression and cheek muscle *Sensory:* taste from anterior two thirds of tongue
VIII Vestibulocochlear		
• Vestibular branch	Junction of pons and medulla	*Sensory:* from equilibrium sensory organ, the vestibular apparatus
• Cochlear branch	Junction of pons and medulla	*Sensory:* from auditory sensory organ, the cochlea
IX Glossopharyngeal	Medulla	*Sensory:* from pharynx and posterior tongue, including taste *Motor:* to superior pharyngeal muscles
X Vagus	Medulla	*Sensory:* from much of viscera of thorax and abdomen *Motor:* to larynx and middle and inferior pharyngeal muscles *Parasympathetic:* heart, lungs, most of digestive system
XI Accessory	Medulla and superior spinal segments	*Motor:* to sternocleidomastoid and trapezius muscles
XII Hypoglossal	Medulla	*Motor:* to muscles of tongue

FIG. 56-6 Dermatomes of the body.

FIG. 56-7 The cranial nerves are numbered according to the order in which they leave the brain.

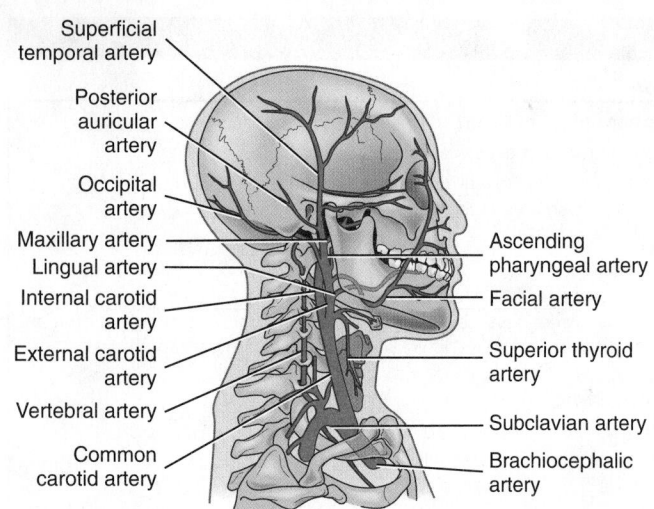

FIG. 56-8 Arteries of the head and neck. Brachiocephalic artery, right common carotid artery, right subclavian artery, and their branches. The major arteries to the head are the common carotid and vertebral arteries.

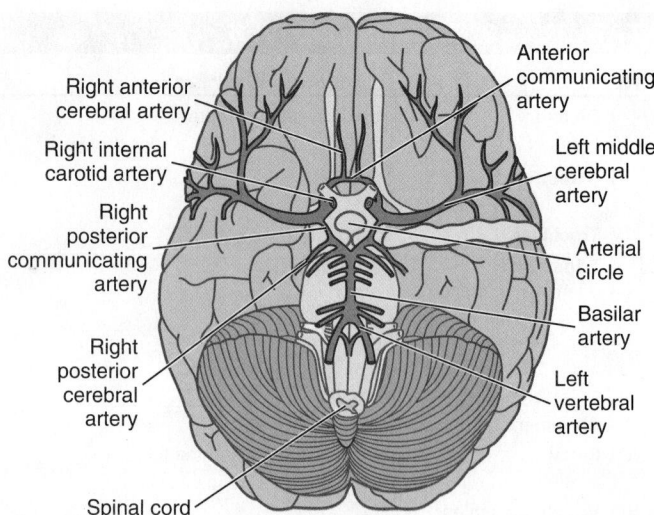

FIG. 56-9 Arteries at the base of the brain. The arteries that compose the circle of Willis are the two anterior cerebral arteries joined to each other by the anterior communicating cerebral artery and to the posterior cerebral arteries by the posterior communicating arteries.

contrast, the PSNS is geared to act in localized and discrete regions. It serves to conserve and restore the body's energy stores. The ANS provides dual and often reciprocal innervation to many structures. For example, the SNS increases the rate and force of heart contraction, and the PSNS decreases the rate and force.

Cerebral Circulation

Knowledge of the distribution of the brain's major arteries is essential for understanding and evaluating the signs and symptoms of cerebrovascular disease and trauma. The brain's blood supply arises from the internal carotid arteries (anterior circulation) and the vertebral arteries (posterior circulation), which are shown in Fig. 56-8.

The internal carotid arteries provide blood flow to the anterior and middle portions of the cerebrum. The vertebral arteries join to form the basilar artery and provide blood flow to the brainstem, cerebellum, and posterior cerebrum. The *circle of Willis* is formed by communicating arteries that join the basilar and internal carotid arteries (Fig. 56-9). The circle of Willis is a safety valve for regulating cerebral blood flow when differential pressures or vascular occlusions are present.

Superior to the circle of Willis, three pairs of arteries supply blood to the left and right hemispheres. The anterior cerebral artery feeds the medial and anterior portions of the frontal lobes. The middle cerebral artery feeds the outer portions of the frontal, parietal, and superior temporal lobes. The posterior cerebral artery feeds the medial portions of the occipital and inferior temporal lobes. Venous blood drains from the brain through the dural sinuses, which form channels that drain into the two jugular veins.

Blood-Brain Barrier. The **blood-brain barrier** is a physiologic barrier between blood capillaries and brain tissue.[5] This barrier protects the brain from harmful agents, while allowing nutrients and gases to enter. The structure of brain capillaries differs from that of other capillaries, so substances that normally pass into most tissues are prevented from entering brain tissue. Lipid-soluble compounds enter the brain easily, whereas water-soluble and ionized drugs enter the brain and the spinal cord slowly. Thus the blood-brain barrier affects the penetration

of drugs. Only certain drugs can enter the CNS from the bloodstream.

Protective Structures

Meninges. The **meninges** consist of three protective membranes that surround the brain and spinal cord: dura mater, arachnoid, and pia mater (see eFig. 56-1 on the website for this chapter). The thick *dura mater* forms the outermost layer. The *falx cerebri* is a fold of the dura that separates the two cerebral hemispheres and slows expansion of brain tissue in conditions such as a rapidly growing tumor or acute hemorrhage. The *tentorium cerebelli* is a fold of dura that separates the cerebral hemispheres from the posterior fossa (which contains the brainstem and cerebellum). Expansion of mass lesions in the cerebrum forces the brain to herniate through the opening created by the brainstem. This is termed *infratentorial herniation* (see Fig. 57-4).

The *arachnoid* layer is a delicate membrane that lies between the dura mater and the *pia mater* (the delicate innermost layer of the meninges). The area between the arachnoid layer and the pia mater is the *subarachnoid space* and is filled with CSF. Structures such as arteries, veins, and cranial nerves passing to and from the brain and the skull must pass through the subarachnoid space. A larger subarachnoid space in the region of the third and fourth lumbar vertebrae is the area used to obtain CSF during a lumbar puncture.

Skull. The skull protects the brain from external trauma. It is composed of eight cranial bones and 14 facial bones. Although the top and sides of the inside of the skull are relatively smooth, the bottom surface is uneven. It has many ridges, prominences, and foramina (holes through which blood vessels and nerves enter the intracranial vault). The largest hole is the *foramen magnum*, through which the brainstem extends to the spinal cord. This foramen offers the only major space for the expansion of brain contents when increased intracranial pressure occurs.

Vertebral Column. The *vertebral column* protects the spinal cord, supports the head, and provides flexibility. The vertebral column is made up of 33 individual vertebrae: 7 cervical, 12 thoracic, 5 lumbar, 5 sacral (fused into one), and 4 coccygeal

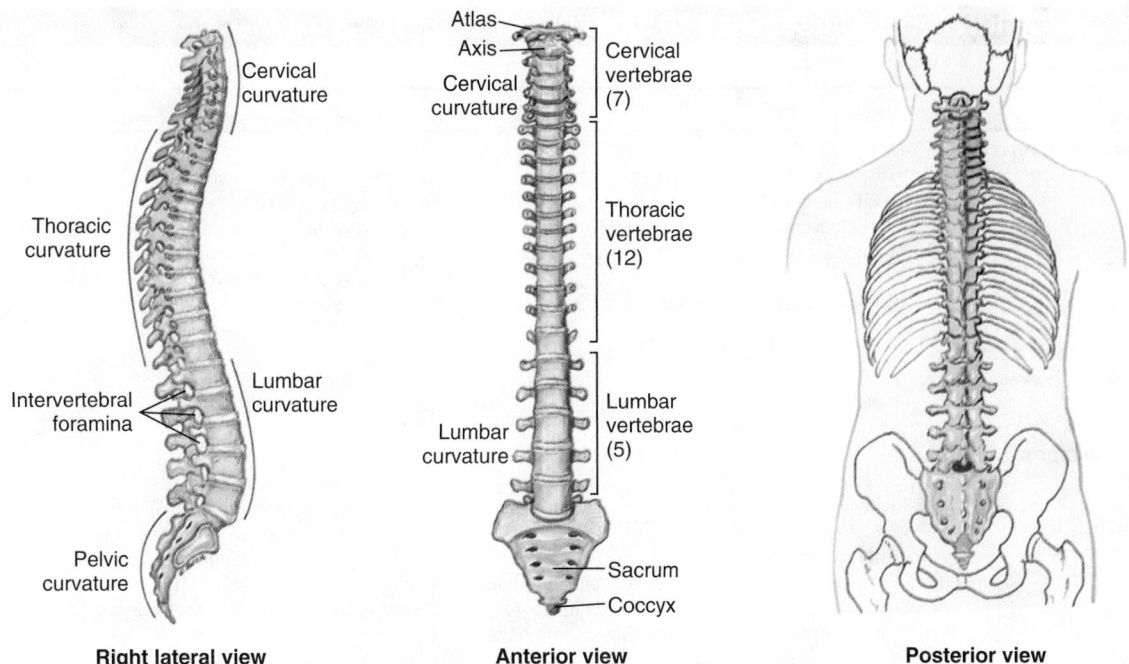

Atlas
Axis
Cervical curvature
Cervical vertebrae (7)

Cervical curvature
Thoracic curvature
Intervertebral foramina
Lumbar curvature
Pelvic curvature

Thoracic vertebrae (12)

Lumbar curvature
Lumbar vertebrae (5)
Sacrum
Coccyx

Right lateral view **Anterior view** **Posterior view**

FIG. 56-10 The vertebral column (three views).

(fused into one). Each vertebra has a central opening through which the spinal cord passes. The vertebrae are held together by a series of ligaments. Intervertebral discs occupy the spaces between vertebrae. Fig. 56-10 shows the vertebral column in relation to the trunk.

GERONTOLOGIC CONSIDERATIONS

EFFECTS OF AGING ON NERVOUS SYSTEM

Several parts of the nervous system are affected by aging. In the CNS the gradual loss of neurons in certain areas of the brainstem, cerebellum, and cerebral cortex begins in early adulthood. With loss of neurons, the ventricles widen or enlarge, brain weight decreases,[6] cerebral blood flow decreases, and CSF production declines.

In the PNS, degenerative changes in myelin cause a decrease in nerve conduction. Coordinated neuromuscular activity, such as the maintenance of blood pressure in response to changing from a lying to a standing position, is altered with aging. As a result, older adults are more likely to experience orthostatic hypotension. Similarly, coordination of neuromuscular activity to maintain body temperature is also less efficient with aging. Older adults are less able to adapt to extremes in environmental temperature and are more vulnerable to both hypothermia and hyperthermia.

Additional relevant changes associated with aging include decreases in memory, vision, hearing, taste, smell, vibration and position sense, muscle strength, and reaction time. Sensory changes, including decreases in taste and smell perception, may result in decreased dietary intake in the older adult. Reduced hearing and vision can result in perceptual confusion. Problems with balance and coordination can put the older adult at risk for falls and subsequent fractures.

Changes in assessment findings result from age-related alterations in the various components of the nervous system (Table 56-4).

ASSESSMENT OF NERVOUS SYSTEM

Subjective Data

Important Health Information

Past Health History. Consider three points when taking a history of a patient with neurologic problems. First, avoid suggesting symptoms or asking leading questions. Second, the mode of onset and the course of the illness are especially important aspects of the history. Often the nature of a neurologic disease process can be described by these facts alone. Obtain all pertinent data in the history of the present illness, especially data related to the characteristics and progression of the symptoms. In some cases the history may include birth injury (e.g., cerebral palsy as a consequence of hypoxia). Third, if the patient is not considered a reliable historian, confirm or obtain the history from someone with firsthand knowledge of the patient.

Medications. Obtain a careful medication history, especially the use of sedatives, opioids, tranquilizers, and mood-elevating drugs. Many other drugs can also cause neurologic side effects.

Surgery or Other Treatments. Inquire about any surgery involving any part of the nervous system, such as head, spine, or sensory organs. If a patient had surgery, determine the date, cause, procedure, recovery, and current status.

Growth and developmental history can be important in ascertaining whether nervous system dysfunction was present at an early age. Specifically inquire about major developmental tasks such as walking and talking.

Functional Health Patterns. Key questions to ask a patient with a neurologic problem are presented in Table 56-5.

Health Perception–Health Management Pattern. Ask about the patient's health practices related to the nervous system, such as substance abuse, smoking, adequate nutrition, blood pressure control, safe participation in physical and recreational activities, and use of seat belts or helmets. Also ask about previous hospitalizations for neurologic problems.

TABLE 56-4 GERONTOLOGIC ASSESSMENT DIFFERENCES

Nervous System

Component	Changes	Differences in Assessment Findings
Central Nervous System **Brain**	↓ Cerebral blood flow and metabolism ↓ Efficiency of temperature-regulating mechanism ↓ Neurotransmitters, loss of neurons ↓ O$_2$ supply Cerebral tissue atrophy and ↑ size of ventricles	Alterations in mental functioning. Impaired ability to adapt to environmental temperature. Conduction of nerve impulses slowed, response time slowed. Changes in gait and ambulation. Diminished kinesthetic sense. Altered balance, vertigo, syncope. ↑ Postural hypotension. Proprioception diminished. ↓ Sensory input.
Peripheral Nervous System **Cranial and spinal nerves**	Loss of myelin and ↓ conduction time Cellular degeneration, death of neurons	↓ Reaction time in specific nerves. ↓ Speed and intensity of neuronal reflexes.
Functional Divisions **Motor** **Sensory***	↓ Muscle bulk ↓ Sensory receptors ↓ Electrical activity Atrophy of taste buds Degeneration and loss of fibers in olfactory bulb Degenerative changes in nerve cells in inner ear, cerebellum, and proprioceptive pathways	Diminished strength and agility. Diminished sense of touch, pain, and temperature. Slowing of or alteration in sensory reception. Signs of malnutrition, weight loss. Diminished sense of smell. Poor ability to maintain balance, widened gait.
Reflexes	↓ Deep tendon reflexes ↓ Sensory conduction velocity	Below-average reflex score. Sluggish reflexes, slowing of reaction time.
Reticular Formation **Reticular activating system**	Modification of hypothalamic function, ↓ stage IV sleep	Disturbances in sleep patterns.
Autonomic Nervous System **Sympathetic nervous system and parasympathetic nervous system**	Morphologic features of ganglia, slowing of autonomic nervous system responses	Orthostatic hypotension, systolic hypertension.

*Specific changes related to the eye are listed in Table 21-1, and specific changes related to the ear are listed in Table 21-7.
ANS, Autonomic nervous system.

CASE STUDY

Patient Introduction

iStockphoto/Thinkstock

A.J. is a 66-yr-old white woman who arrives in the emergency department after falling in the middle of the night when she tried to get up to go to the bathroom. She states that she fell because she could not control her left leg. Her husband brought her to the hospital, but states that he had a really hard time getting her to the car.

Critical Thinking

As you read through this assessment chapter, think about A.J.'s concerns with the following questions in mind:
1. What are the possible causes for her acute leg weakness?
2. What type of assessment would be most appropriate for A.J.: comprehensive, focused, or emergency? What would be your priority assessment?
3. What questions would you ask A.J.?
4. What should be included in the physical assessment? What would you be looking for?
5. What diagnostic studies might you expect to be ordered?

olve Answers available at *http://evolve.elsevier.com/Lewis/medsurg.*

If the patient has an existing neurologic problem, assess how it affects daily living and the ability to carry out self-care. After a careful review of information, ask someone who knows the patient well whether he or she has noticed any mental or physical changes in the patient. The patient with a neurologic problem may not be aware of it or may be a poor historian.

🧬 GENETIC RISK ALERT

- Huntington's disease is a genetically transmitted, autosomal dominant disorder.
- Major neurologic disorders that may have a genetic basis are multiple sclerosis, headaches, Parkinson's disease, and Alzheimer's disease. The presence of these problems in a family history increases the likelihood of similar problems occurring in the patient.
- A careful family history may determine whether a neurologic problem has a genetic basis.

Nutritional-Metabolic Pattern. Neurologic problems can result in poor nutrition. Problems related to chewing, swallowing, facial nerve paralysis, and muscle coordination could make it difficult for the patient to ingest adequate nutrients.[7] Also, certain vitamins such as thiamine (B$_1$), niacin, and pyridoxine (B$_6$) are essential for the maintenance and health of the CNS. Deficiencies in one or more of these vitamins could result in such nonspecific complaints as depression, apathy, neuritis, weakness, mental confusion, and irritability. Cobalamin (vitamin B$_{12}$) deficiency can occur in older adults, who tend to have problems with vitamin absorption from both supplements and natural food sources such as meat, fish, and poultry. Untreated, cobalamin deficiency can cause mental function decline.

Elimination Pattern. Bowel and bladder problems are often associated with neurologic problems such as stroke, head injury, spinal cord injury, multiple sclerosis, and dementia. It is impor-

TABLE 56-5   HEALTH HISTORY

Nervous System

Health Perception–Health Management
- What are your usual daily activities?
- Do you use alcohol, tobacco, or recreational drugs?*
- What safety practices do you perform in a car? On a motorcycle? On a bicycle?
- Do you have hypertension? If so, is it controlled?
- Have you ever been hospitalized for a neurologic problem?*

Nutritional-Metabolic
- Are you able to feed yourself?
- Do you have any problems getting adequate nutrition because of chewing or swallowing difficulties, facial nerve paralysis, or poor muscle coordination?*
- Give a 24-hr dietary recall.

Elimination
- Do you have incontinence of your bowels or bladder?*
- Do you ever experience problems with hesitancy, urgency, retention?*
- Do you postpone defecation?*
- Do you take any medication to manage neurologic problems? If so, what?

Activity-Exercise
- Describe any problems you experience with usual activities and exercise as a result of a neurologic problem.
- Do you have weakness or lack of coordination?*
- Are you able to perform your personal hygiene needs independently?*

Sleep-Rest
- Describe your sleep pattern.
- When you have trouble sleeping, what do you do?

Cognitive-Perceptual
- Have you noticed any changes in your memory?*
- Do you experience dizziness, heat or cold sensitivity, numbness, or tingling?*
- Do you have chronic pain?*
- Do you have any difficulty with verbal or written communication?*
- Have you noticed any changes in vision or hearing?*

Self-Perception–Self-Concept
- How do you feel about yourself, about who you are?
- Describe your general emotional pattern.

Role-Relationship
- Have you experienced changes in roles such as spouse, parent, or breadwinner?*

Sexuality-Reproductive
- Are you dissatisfied with sexual functioning?*
- Are problems related to sexual functioning causing tension in an important relationship?*
- Do you feel the need for professional counseling related to your sexual functioning?*

Coping–Stress Tolerance
- Describe your usual coping pattern.
- Do you think your present coping pattern is adequate to meet the stressors of your life?*
- What needs are unmet by your current support system?

Value-Belief
- Describe any culturally specific beliefs and attitudes that may influence your care.

*If yes, describe.

tant to determine if the bowel or bladder problem was present before or after the neurologic event to plan appropriate interventions. Incontinence of urine and feces and urinary retention are the most common elimination problems associated with a neurologic problem or its treatment.[8] For example, nerve root compression (as occurs in cauda equina conditions) leads to a sudden onset of incontinence. Document key details, such as number of episodes, accompanying sensations or lack of sensations, and measures to control the problem.

Activity-Exercise Pattern. Many neurologic disorders can cause problems in the patient's mobility, strength, and coordination. Neurologic problems can result in changes in the patient's usual activity and exercise patterns. These problems can also result in falls.[9] Assess the person's activities of daily living, since neurologic diseases can affect the ability to perform motor tasks, which increases the possibility of injury.

Sleep-Rest Pattern. Sleep pattern alteration can be both a cause and a response to neurologic problems. Pain and reduced ability to change position because of muscle weakness and paralysis could interfere with sleep quality. Hallucinations resulting from dementia or drugs can also interrupt sleep. Carefully assess and document the patient's sleep pattern and bedtime routines.

Cognitive-Perceptual Pattern. Because the nervous system controls cognition and sensory integration, many neurologic disorders affect these functions. Assess memory, language, calculation ability, problem-solving ability, insight, and judgment.

Ask the patient hypothetical questions such as, "What is a reasonable price for a cup of coffee?" or "What would you do if you saw a car crash outside your house?" Often a structured mental status questionnaire is used to evaluate these functions and provide baseline data.

Delirium is an acute and transient disorder of cognition that can be seen at any time during a patient's illness. As discussed in Chapter 60, delirium is often an early indicator of various illnesses (see Table 60-14). The Confusion Assessment Method tool is used to assess for delirium (see Table 60-16).

Assess a person's ability to use and understand language. Appropriateness of responses is a useful indicator of cognitive and perceptual ability. Determine the patient's understanding and ability to carry out necessary treatments. Neurologic-related cognitive changes can interfere with the patient's understanding of the disease and adherence to related treatment.

Pain is commonly associated with many neurologic problems and is often the reason a patient seeks care. Carefully assess the patient's pain. (Pain and pain assessment are discussed in Chapter 9.)

Self-Perception–Self-Concept Pattern. Neurologic diseases can drastically alter control over one's life and create dependency on others for meeting daily needs. Also, the patient's physical appearance and emotional control can be affected. Sensitively inquire about the patient's evaluation of self-worth, perception of abilities, body image, and general emotional pattern.

Role-Relationship Pattern. Physical impairments such as weakness and paralysis can alter or limit participation in usual roles and activities. Cognitive changes can permanently alter a person's ability to maintain previous roles. These changes can dramatically affect the patient, caregiver, and family. Ask patients if their role (e.g., spouse or breadwinner) has changed as a result of their neurologic problems.

Sexuality-Reproductive Pattern. Assess the person's ability to participate in sexual activity because many neurologic disorders can affect sexual response. Cerebral lesions may inhibit the desire phase or the reflex responses of the excitement phase. The hypothalamus stimulates the pituitary gland to release hormones that influence sexual desire. Brainstem and spinal cord lesions may partially or completely interrupt the desire or ability to have intercourse. Neuropathies and spinal cord lesions may prevent reflex activities of the sexual response or affect sensation and decrease desire. Despite neurologically related changes in sexual function, many persons can achieve satisfying expression of intimacy and affection.

Coping–Stress Tolerance Pattern. The physical sequelae of a neurologic problem can seriously strain a patient's coping patterns. Often the problem is chronic and requires that the patient learn new coping skills. Assess the patient's usual coping pattern to determine if coping skills are adequate to meet the stress of a problem. Also assess the patient's support system.

Value-Belief Pattern. Many neurologic problems have serious, long-term, life-changing effects. Determine what these effects are, since they can strain the patient's belief system. Also determine if any religious or cultural beliefs could interfere with the planned treatment regimen.

Objective Data

Physical Examination. The standard neurologic examination helps determine the presence, location, and nature of disease of the nervous system. The examination assesses six categories of functions: mental status, cranial nerve function, motor function, sensory function, cerebellar function, and reflexes. Develop a consistent pattern of completing the neurologic examination so you remember to include each element every time you examine a patient.

Mental Status. Assessment of mental status (cerebral function) gives a general impression of how the patient is functioning. It involves determining complex and high-level cerebral functions that are governed by many areas of the cerebral cortex. Much of the mental status examination can be assessed as you interact with the patient. For example, assess language and memory when asking the patient for details of the illness and significant past events. Consider the patient's cultural and educational background when evaluating mental status.

The components of the mental status examination include:

- *General appearance and behavior:* This component includes level of consciousness (awake, asleep, comatose), motor activity, body posture, dress and hygiene, facial expression, and speech pattern.
- *Cognition:* Note orientation to time, place, person, and situation, as well as memory, general knowledge, insight, judgment, problem solving, and calculation. Common questions are "Who were the last three presidents?" "Does a rock float on water?" "How much money is a quarter, two dimes, and a nickel?" Consider whether the patient's plans and goals match the physical and mental capabilities. Note the presence of factors affecting intellectual capacity such as cognitive impairment, hallucinations, delusions, and dementia.
- *Mood and affect:* Note any agitation, anger, depression, or euphoria and the appropriateness of these states. Use suitable questions to bring out the patient's feelings.

Cranial Nerves. Testing each CN is an essential part of the neurologic examination (see Table 56-3).

Olfactory Nerve. After determining that both nostrils are patent, test the olfactory nerve (CN I) by asking the patient to close one nostril and identify easily recognized odors (e.g., coffee). Do the same for the other nostril. Chronic rhinitis, sinusitis, and heavy smoking may decrease the sense of smell. Disturbance in ability to smell may be associated with a tumor involving the olfactory bulb, or it may be the result of a basilar skull fracture that has damaged the olfactory fibers as they pass through the delicate cribriform plate of the skull.

Optic Nerve. Assess visual fields and acuity to determine the function of the optic nerve (CN II). Examine each eye independently. Position yourself opposite the patient and ask him or her to look directly at the bridge of your nose and indicate when an object (finger, pencil tip) presented from the periphery of each of the visual fields is seen (Fig. 56-11). Visual field defects may arise from lesions of the optic nerve, optic chiasm, or tracts

Subjective Data

iStockphoto/Thinkstock

A subjective assessment of A.J. revealed the following information:

PMH: Hyperlipidemia, hypertension.
Medications: pravastatin 40 mg/day PO; lisinopril 10 mg/day PO.
Health Perception–Health Management: Smokes one pack of cigarettes per day since she was 28 yr old. Drinks alcohol occasionally. Hypertension controlled when on medication but has not taken her lisinopril for a few weeks because she did not have enough money for the refill and was waiting for her next Social Security check. Has never been hospitalized for a neurologic problem.
Nutritional-Metabolic: A.J. is 5 ft, 3 in tall and weighs 160 lb.
Activity-Exercise: States that up until tonight she was able to walk slowly, but her knees and hips hurt.
Cognitive-Perceptual: States had a brief episode of left-sided weakness and tingling of the face, arm, and hand 3 mo ago. The symptoms totally resolved and she did not seek treatment. Denies dizziness, change in hearing, or memory deficits.
Coping–Stress Tolerance: Is depressed and fearful. Concerned she is having a stroke and she does not know if she has enough money to cover the copay for coming to the emergency department.

FIG. 56-11 A, Nurse checking visual fields. **B,** Nurse checking extraocular movement (EOM).

that extend through the temporal, parietal, or occipital lobes. Visual field changes resulting from brain lesions are usually either a *hemianopsia* (one half of the visual field is affected), a *quadrantanopsia* (one fourth of the visual field is affected), or monocular.

Test visual acuity by asking the patient to read a Snellen chart. Record the number on the lowest line that the patient can read with 50% accuracy. The patient who wears glasses should wear them during testing, unless they are used only for close reading. If a Snellen chart is not available, ask the patient to read newsprint for a gross assessment of acuity. Record the distance from the patient to the newsprint required for accurate reading. Acuity may not be testable by these means if the patient does not read English or is aphasic.

Oculomotor, Trochlear, and Abducens Nerves. Because the oculomotor (CN III), trochlear (CN IV), and abducens (CN VI) nerves all help move the eye, they are tested together. Ask the person to hold the head steady and to follow the movement of your finger, pen, or penlight only with the eyes. Hold the target back about 12 inches so the person can focus on it comfortably. Move the target to each of the six positions (right and up, right, right and down, left and up, left, left and down), hold it momentarily, and then move back to center. Progress clockwise. A normal response is parallel tracking of the object with both eyes.

With weakness or paralysis of one of the eye muscles, the eyes do not move together, and the patient has a *disconjugate gaze*. The presence and direction of *nystagmus* (fine, rapid jerking movements of the eyes) are observed at this time, even though this condition most often indicates vestibulocerebellar problems.

Test other functions of the oculomotor nerve by checking for pupillary constriction and *accommodation* (pupils constricting with near vision). To test pupillary constriction, shine a light into the pupil of one eye and look for ipsilateral constriction of the same pupil and contralateral (consensual) constriction of the opposite eye. Note the size and shape of the pupils. The optic nerve must be intact for this reflex to occur.

Because the oculomotor nerve exits at the top of the brainstem at the tentorial notch, it can be easily compressed by expanding mass lesions. When this occurs, sympathetic input to the pupil is unopposed and the pupil remains dilated. The lack of pupillary constriction is an early sign of central herniation (see Chapter 57).

Two abbreviations commonly used to record the reaction of the pupils are *PERRL* (*P*upils are *E*qual [in size], *R*ound, and *R*eactive to *L*ight) and *PERRLA* (*P*upils are *E*qual, *R*ound, and *R*eactive to *L*ight and *A*ccommodation). The PERRL abbreviation is appropriate when accommodation cannot be assessed such as in an unconscious patient. Convergence and accommodation are tested by having the patient focus on the examiner's finger as it moves toward the patient's nose.

Newly developed tools such as the pupilometer are being explored for their ability to objectively evaluate the pupillary response (Fig. 56-12). The pupilometer measures the pupil's response to a visual stimulus (e.g., light).

Another function of the oculomotor nerve is to keep the eyelid open. Damage to the nerve can cause *ptosis* (drooping eyelid), pupillary abnormalities, and eye muscle weakness.

Trigeminal Nerve. The sensory component of the trigeminal nerve (CN V) is tested with the patient's eyes closed, by having the patient identify light touch and pinprick in each of the three

FIG. 56-12 A pupilometer can be used to measure the pupillary response using a light stimulus.

divisions (ophthalmic, maxillary, and mandibular) of the nerve on both sides of the face. Test the motor component by asking the patient to clench the teeth and palpating the masseter muscles just above the mandibular angle. The corneal reflex test evaluates CN V and CN VII simultaneously. Initially, assess blink-to-threat in the unconscious patient. A drop of saline may be applied to the cornea to assess movement of the eyelid as evidence of corneal reflex. The sensory component of this reflex (corneal sensation) is innervated by the ophthalmic division of CN V. The motor component (eye blink) is innervated by the facial nerve (CN VII).

Facial Nerve. The facial nerve (CN VII) innervates the muscles of facial expression. Test its function by asking the patient to raise the eyebrows, close the eyes tightly, purse the lips, draw back the corners of the mouth in an exaggerated smile, and frown. Note any asymmetry in the facial movements because they can indicate damage to the facial nerve. Although taste discrimination of salt and sugar in the anterior two thirds of the tongue is a function of this nerve, it is not routinely tested unless a peripheral nerve lesion is suspected.

Vestibulocochlear (Acoustic) Nerve. The cochlear portion of the vestibulocochlear nerve (CN VIII) is tested by having the patient close the eyes and indicate when he or she hears the rustling of the examiner's fingertips. For more precise assessment of hearing, perform the Weber and Rinne tests or use an audiometer (see Chapter 21).

The vestibular portion of this nerve is not routinely tested unless the patient complains of dizziness, vertigo, or unsteadiness or has auditory dysfunction. In the unconscious patient the oculocephalic reflex (movement of the eyes when the head is briskly turned to the side) may be assessed.

Glossopharyngeal and Vagus Nerves. The glossopharyngeal and vagus nerves (CN IX and X) are tested together because both innervate the pharynx. Test the gag reflex (bilateral contraction of the palatal muscles) by touching the sides of the posterior pharynx or soft palate with a tongue blade. Assess the sensory component of the glossopharyngeal nerve and the major motor component of the vagus nerve. It is important to assess the gag reflex in patients who have a decreased level of consciousness, a brainstem lesion, or a disease involving the throat musculature. If the reflex is weak or absent, the patient is in danger of aspirating food or secretions. The strength and efficiency of swallowing are important to test in these patients for the same reason.

Another test for the awake, cooperative patient is to have the patient phonate by saying "ah," and note the bilateral symmetry of elevation of the soft palate. If the patient is endotracheally intubated, the cough reflex (elicited when the suction catheter contacts the *carina* of the respiratory tree) is a method of assessing the vagus nerve.

Accessory Nerve. Test the accessory nerve (CN XI) by asking the patient to shrug the shoulders and to turn the head to either side against resistance. There should be smooth contraction of the sternocleidomastoid and trapezius muscles. Also note symmetry, atrophy, or fasciculation of the muscle.

Hypoglossal Nerve. Test the hypoglossal nerve (CN XII) by asking the patient to protrude the tongue. It should protrude in the midline. Next ask the patient to move the tongue up and down and side to side. Finally, the patient should also be able to push the tongue to either side against the resistance of a tongue blade. Again, note any asymmetry, atrophy, or fasciculation.

Motor System. The motor system examination includes assessment of strength, tone, coordination, and symmetry of the major muscle groups. Test muscle strength by asking the patient to push and pull against the resistance of your arm as it opposes flexion and extension of the patient's muscle. Ask the patient to offer resistance at the shoulders, elbows, wrists, hips, knees, and ankles. Mild weakness of the arm is demonstrated by downward drifting of the arm or pronation of the palm (*pronator drift*). Note any weakness or asymmetry of strength between the same muscle groups of the right and left sides.

Test muscle tone by passively moving the limbs through their range of motion. There should be a slight resistance to these movements. Abnormal tone is described as *hypotonia* (flaccidity) or *hypertonia* (spasticity). Note any involuntary movements such as tics, tremor, *myoclonus* (spasm of muscles), *athetosis* (slow, writhing, involuntary movements of extremities), *chorea* (involuntary, purposeless, rapid motions), and *dystonia* (impairment of muscle tone).

Test cerebellar function by assessing balance and coordination. A good screening test for both balance and muscle strength is to observe the patient's stature (posture while standing) and gait. Note the pace and rhythm of the gait and observe for normal symmetric and oppositional arm swing. The patient's ability to ambulate helps to determine the level of nursing care required and the risk of falling.

The finger-to-nose test (having the patient alternately touch the nose, then touch the examiner's finger) and the heel-to-shin test (having the patient stroke the heel of one foot up and down the shin of the opposite leg) test coordination and cerebellar function. Reposition your finger while the patient is touching the nose so that the patient must adjust to a new distance each time your finger is touched. These movements should be performed smoothly and accurately. Other tests include asking the patient to pronate and supinate both hands rapidly and to do a shallow knee bend, first on one leg and then on the other. Note dysarthria or slurred speech because it is a sign of incoordination of the speech muscles.

Sensory System. Several modalities are tested in the somatic sensory examination. Each modality is carried by a specific ascending pathway in the spinal cord before it reaches the sensory cortex. As a rule, perform the examination with the patient's eyes closed and avoid providing the patient with clues. Ask "How does this feel?" rather than "Is this sharp?" In the routine neurologic examination, sensory testing of the anterior torso, posterior torso, and the four extremities is sufficient. However, if a disturbance in sensory function of the skin is identified, the boundaries of that dysfunction should be carefully delineated along the dermatome.

Touch, Pain, and Temperature. Light touch is usually tested first using a cotton wisp or light pin prick. Gently touch each of the four extremities and ask the patient to indicate when he or she feels the stimulus. Test pain by alternately touching the skin with the sharp and dull end of a pin. Tell the patient to respond "sharp" or "dull." Evaluate each limb separately.

Extinction is assessed by simultaneously touching both sides of the body symmetrically. Normally, the simultaneous stimuli are both perceived (sensed). An abnormal response occurs when the patient perceives the stimulus on only one side. The other stimulus is "extinguished."

The sensation of temperature (only to be tested when the response to deep pain is abnormal) can be tested by applying tubes of warm and cold water to the skin and asking the patient to identify the stimuli with the eyes closed. If pain sensation is intact, assessment of temperature sensation may be omitted because both sensations are carried by the same ascending pathways.

Vibration Sense. Assess vibration sense by applying a vibrating tuning fork to the fingernails and the bony prominences of the hands, legs, and feet. Ask the patient if the vibration or "buzz" is felt. Then ask the patient to indicate when the vibration ceases.

Position Sense. Assess position sense (*proprioception*) by placing your thumb and forefinger on either side of the patient's forefinger or great toe and gently moving his or her digit up or down. Ask the patient to indicate the direction in which the digit is moved.

Another test of proprioception is the Romberg test. Ask the patient to stand with feet together and then close his or her eyes. If the patient is able to maintain balance with the eyes open but sways or falls with the eyes closed (i.e., a positive Romberg test), vestibulocochlear dysfunction or disease in the posterior columns of the spinal cord may be indicated. Be aware of patient safety during this test.

Cortical Sensory Functions. Several tests evaluate cortical integration of sensory perceptions (which occurs in the parietal lobes). Assess *two-point discrimination* by placing the two points of a calibrated compass on the tips of the fingers and toes. The minimum recognizable separation is 4 to 5 mm in the fingertips and a greater degree of separation elsewhere. This test is important in diagnosing diseases of the sensory cortex and PNS.

Graphesthesia (ability to feel writing on skin) is tested by having the patient identify numbers traced on the palm of the hands. *Stereognosis* (ability to perceive the form and nature of objects) is tested by having the patient close the eyes and identify the size and shape of easily recognized objects (e.g., coins, keys, safety pin) placed in the hands.

Reflexes. Tendons have receptors that are sensitive to stretch. A reflex contraction of the skeletal muscle occurs when the tendon is stretched. In general, the biceps, triceps, brachioradialis, and patellar and Achilles tendon reflexes are tested. Initiate a simple muscle stretch reflex by briskly tapping the tendon of a stretched muscle, usually with a reflex hammer (Fig. 56-13). The response (muscle contraction of the corresponding muscle) is measured as follows: 0/5 = absent, 1/5 = weak response, 2/5 = normal response, 3/5 = exaggerated response,

FIG. 56-13 The examiner strikes a swift blow over a stretched tendon to elicit a stretch reflex. **A,** Biceps reflex. **B,** Patellar reflex.

and 4/5 = hyperreflexia with clonus. *Clonus,* an abnormal response, is a continued rhythmic contraction of the muscle with continuous application of the stimulus.

Elicit the *biceps reflex,* with the patient's arm partially flexed and palm up, by placing your thumb over the biceps tendon in the antecubital space and striking the thumb with a hammer. The normal response is flexion of the arm at the elbow or contraction of the biceps muscle that can be felt by your thumb.

Elicit the *triceps reflex* by striking the triceps tendon above the elbow while the patient's arm is flexed. The normal response is extension of the arm or visible contraction of the triceps.

Elicit the *brachioradialis reflex* by striking the radius 3 to 5 cm above the wrist while the patient's arm is relaxed. The normal response is flexion and supination at the elbow or visible contraction of the brachioradialis muscle.

Elicit the *patellar reflex* by striking the patellar tendon just below the patella. The patient can be sitting or lying as long as the leg being tested hangs freely. The normal response is extension of the leg with contraction of the quadriceps.

Elicit the *Achilles tendon reflex* by striking the Achilles tendon while the patient's leg is flexed at the knee and the foot is gently dorsiflexed, by the examiner, at the ankle. The normal response is plantar flexion at the ankle.

A *focused assessment* is used to evaluate the status of previously identified neurologic problems and to monitor for signs of new problems (see Table 3-6). A focused assessment of the neurologic system is presented in the box on p. 1351.

Table 56-6 is an example of a normal neurologic physical assessment. Abnormal assessment findings of the neurologic system are presented in Table 56-7.

DIAGNOSTIC STUDIES OF NERVOUS SYSTEM

Numerous diagnostic studies are available to assess the nervous system. Tables 56-8 and 56-9 present the most common studies, and select studies are described in more detail below.

TABLE 56-6	NORMAL PHYSICAL ASSESSMENT OF NERVOUS SYSTEM*	
Parameter	**Findings**
Mental status	• Alert and oriented, orderly thought processes. • Appropriate mood and affect.
Cranial nerves†	• Smell intact to soap or coffee. • Visual fields full to confrontation. • Intact extraocular movements. • No nystagmus. Pupils equal, round, reactive to light and accommodation. • Intact facial sensation to light touch and pinprick. • Facial movements full. • Intact gag and swallow reflexes. Symmetric smile. Midline protrusion of tongue. • Full strength with head turning and shoulder shrugging.
Motor system	• Normal gait and station. Normal tandem walk. Negative Romberg test. • Normal and symmetric muscle bulk, tone, and strength. • Smooth performance of finger-nose, heel-shin movements.
Sensory system	• Intact sensation to light touch, position sense, pinprick, heat and cold.
Reflexes‡	• Biceps, triceps, brachioradialis, patellar, and Achilles tendon reflexes 2/5 bilaterally. • Downgoing toes with plantar stimulation.

*If some portion of the neurologic examination was not done, this should be indicated (e.g., "Smell not tested").
†May also be recorded as "CN I to XII intact."
‡May also be recorded as drawing of stick figure indicating reflex strength at appropriate sites.

CASE STUDY—cont'd

Objective Data: Physical Examination

iStockphoto/Thinkstock

A physical assessment of A.J. reveals the following:
• BP 180/110, HR 94, RR 22, T 37°C
• Alert, oriented, and able to answer questions appropriately but mild slowness in responding
• Left-sided arm weakness (3/5) and leg weakness (4/5)
• NIH Stroke score is 3

As you continue to read this chapter, consider diagnostic studies you would anticipate being performed for A.J.

Cerebrospinal Fluid Analysis

CSF analysis provides information about a variety of CNS diseases. Normal CSF fluid is clear, colorless, odorless, and free of red blood cells and contains little protein. Normal CSF values are listed in Table 56-9. CSF may be obtained through lumbar puncture or ventriculostomy.

Lumbar Puncture. Lumbar puncture is the most common method of sampling CSF. A lumbar puncture is contraindicated in the presence of increased intracranial pressure or infection at the site of puncture.

Before the procedure, have the patient void. Most commonly, the patient is side lying. However, a seated position may also be used. Inform the patient that, as a sterile needle is passed between two lumbar vertebrae, he or she may feel temporary pain radiating down the leg.

TABLE 56-7 **ASSESSMENT ABNORMALITIES**

Nervous System

Finding	Description	Possible Etiology and Significance
Mental Status		
Altered consciousness	Stuporous, mute, diminished response to verbal cues or pain	Intracranial lesions, metabolic disorder, psychiatric disorders
Anosognosia	Inability to recognize bodily defect or disease	Lesions in right parietal cortex
Speech		
Aphasia, dysphasia	Loss of or impaired language faculty (comprehension, expression, or both)	Left cerebral cortex lesion
Dysarthria	Lack of coordination in articulating speech	Cerebellar or cranial nerve lesion Antiseizure drugs, sedatives, hypnotic drug toxicity (including alcohol)
Eyes		
Anisocoria	Inequality of pupil size	Optic nerve injury
Diplopia	Double vision	Lesions affecting nerves of extraocular muscles, cerebellar damage
Homonymous hemianopsia	Loss of vision in one side of visual field	Lesions in the contralateral occipital lobe
Cranial Nerves		
Dysphagia	Difficulty in swallowing	Lesions involving motor pathways of CNs IX, X (including lower brainstem)
Ophthalmoplegia	Paralysis of eye muscles	Lesions in brainstem
Papilledema	"Choked disc," swelling of optic nerve head	Increase in intracranial pressure
Motor System		
Apraxia	Inability to perform learned movements despite having desire and physical ability to perform them	Cerebral cortex lesion
Ataxia	Lack of coordination of movement	Lesions of sensory or motor pathways, cerebellum Antiseizure drugs, sedatives, hypnotic drug toxicity (including alcohol)
Dyskinesia	Impairment of voluntary movement, resulting in fragmentary or incomplete movements	Disorders of basal ganglia, idiosyncratic reaction to psychotropic drugs
Hemiplegia	Paralysis on one side	Stroke and other lesions involving motor cortex
Nystagmus	Jerking or bobbing of eyes as they track moving object	Lesions in cerebellum, brainstem, vestibular system Antiseizure drugs, sedatives, hypnotic toxicity (including alcohol)
Sensory System		
Analgesia	Loss of pain sensation	Lesion in spinothalamic tract or thalamus, specific medications
Anesthesia	Absence of sensation	Lesions in spinal cord, thalamus, sensory cortex, or peripheral sensory nerve Specific medications
Paresthesia	Alteration in sensation	Lesions in the posterior column or sensory cortex
Astereognosis	Inability to recognize form of object by touch	Lesions in parietal cortex
Reflexes		
Extensor plantar response	Upgoing toes with plantar stimulation	Suprasegmental or upper motor neuron lesion
Deep tendon reflexes	Diminished or absent motor response	Lower motor neuron lesions
Spinal Cord		
Bladder dysfunction		
• Atonic (autonomous)	Absence of muscle tone and contractility, enlargement of capacity, no sensation of discomfort, overflow with large residual, inability to voluntarily empty	Early stage of spinal cord injury
• Hypotonic	More ability than atonic bladder but less than normal	Interruption of afferent pathways from bladder
• Hypertonic	Increase in muscle tone, diminished capacity, reflex emptying, dribbling, incontinence	Lesions in pyramidal tracts (efferent pathways)
Paraplegia	Paralysis of lower extremities	Spinal cord transection or mass lesion (thoracolumbar region)
Tetraplegia (quadriplegia)	Paralysis of all extremities	Spinal cord transection or mass lesion (cervical region)

FOCUSED ASSESSMENT

Nervous System

Use this checklist to make sure the key assessment steps have been done.

Subjective
Ask the patient about any of the following and note responses.

Blackouts/loss of memory	Y	N
Weakness, numbness, tingling in arms or legs	Y	N
Headaches, especially new onset	Y	N
Loss of balance/coordination	Y	N
Orientation to person, place, and time	Y	N

Objective: Diagnostic
Check the following laboratory results for critical values.

Lumbar puncture	✓
CT or MRI of brain	✓
EEG	✓

Objective: Physical Examination
Inspect/Observe

General level of consciousness/orientation	✓
Oropharynx for gag reflex and soft palate movement	✓
Peripheral sensation of light touch and pinprick (face, hands, feet)	✓
Smell with an alcohol wipe	✓
Eyes for extraocular movements, PERRLA, peripheral vision, nystagmus	✓
Gait for smoothness and coordination	✓

Palpate

Strength of neck, shoulders, arms, and legs full and symmetric	✓

Percuss

Reflexes	✓

CT, Computed tomography; *EEG,* electroencephalogram; *MRI,* magnetic resonance imaging; *PERRLA,* pupils equal, round, and reactive to light and accommodation.

A manometer is attached to the needle to obtain a CSF pressure. CSF is withdrawn in a series of tubes and sent for analysis. Monitor for headache intensity, meningeal irritation *(nuchal rigidity),* or signs and symptoms of local trauma (e.g., hematoma, pain).

Radiologic Studies

Computed Tomography. Computed tomography (CT) scans provide a rapid means of obtaining radiographic images of the brain (see Fig. 56-15, *A*). When viewed in succession, these images provide a three-dimensional representation of the intracranial contents. Denser material appears white, whereas fluid and air appear dark or black. Brain CT can be completed both with and without contrast media in only a few minutes.

Magnetic Resonance Imaging. Magnetic resonance imaging (MRI) provides greater detail than CT and improved resolution (detail) of the intracranial structures (see Fig. 56-15, *B*). However, MRI requires a longer time to complete and may not be appropriate in life-threatening emergencies. Techniques of functional MRI (fMRI) provide time-related (temporal) images that can be used to evaluate how the brain responds to various stimuli.

Cerebral Angiography. Cerebral angiography is indicated when vascular lesions or tumors are suspected. A catheter is inserted into the femoral (sometimes brachial) artery and

passed through the aortic arch and into the base of a carotid or a vertebral artery for injection of contrast media. Timed-sequence radiographic images are obtained as contrast flows through arteries, smaller vessels, and veins (see Fig. 56-14). This study can help to identify and localize abscesses, aneurysms, hematomas, arteriovenous malformations, arterial spasm, and certain tumors.

Because this is an invasive procedure, adverse reactions may occur. The patient may have an allergic (anaphylactic) reaction to the contrast medium. This reaction usually occurs immediately after injection of the contrast medium and may require emergency resuscitation measures in the procedure room. Once the patient returns to his or her room after the procedure, observe for bleeding at the catheter puncture site (usually the groin).

Electrographic Studies

Electroencephalography. *Electroencephalography* (EEG) involves recording electrical activity of the surface cortical neurons of the brain by electrodes placed on specific areas of the scalp. Specific tests may be done to evaluate the brain's electrical response to lights and loud noises. This test is done to evaluate not only cerebral disease but also the CNS effects of many metabolic and systemic diseases. Among the cerebral diseases assessed by EEG are seizure disorders, sleep disorders, cerebrovascular lesions, and brain injury. Prolonged EEG monitoring is becoming a common test to diagnose and treat seizure disorders.[10] An EEG is noninvasive. Assure patients that there is no risk of electric shock.

Electromyography and Nerve Conduction Studies. *Electromyography* (EMG) is the recording of electrical activity associated with innervation of skeletal muscle. Needle electrodes are inserted into the muscle to record specific motor units because recording from the skin is not sufficient. Normal muscle at rest shows no electrical activity. Electrical activity occurs only when the muscle contracts. This activity may be altered in diseases of muscle itself (e.g., myopathic conditions) or in disorders of muscle innervation (e.g., segmental or LMN lesions, peripheral neuropathic conditions).

Nerve conduction studies involve applying a brief electrical stimulus to a distal portion of a sensory or mixed nerve and recording the resulting wave of depolarization at some point proximal to the stimulation. For example, a stimulus can be applied to the forefinger and a recording electrode placed over the median nerve at the wrist. The time between the stimulus onset and the initial wave of depolarization at the recording electrode is measured. This is termed *nerve conduction velocity.* Damaged nerves have slower conduction velocities.

TABLE 56-8 DIAGNOSTIC STUDIES

Nervous System

Study	Description and Purpose	Nursing Responsibility
Cerebrospinal Fluid Analysis		
Lumbar puncture	CSF is aspirated by needle insertion in L3-4 or L4-5 interspace to assess many CNS diseases (see Table 56-9).	Ensure that patient does not have signs of increased ICP because of the risk of downward herniation from CSF removal. Patient assumes and maintains lateral recumbent position. Use strict aseptic technique. Ensure labeling of CSF specimens in proper sequence. Encourage fluids. Monitor neurologic signs and VS. Administer analgesia as needed.
Radiology		
Skull and spine x-rays	Simple x-ray of skull and spinal column is done to detect fractures, bone erosion, calcifications, abnormal vascularity.	Explain that procedure is noninvasive. Explain positions to be assumed.
Cerebral angiography	Serial x-ray visualization of intracranial and extracranial blood vessels is performed to detect vascular lesions and tumors of brain (Fig. 56-14). Contrast medium is used.	*Preprocedure:* Assess patient for stroke risk before procedure, since thrombi may be dislodged during procedure. Withhold preceding meal. Explain that patient will have hot flush of head and neck when contrast medium is injected. Administer premedication. Explain need to be absolutely still during procedure. *Postprocedure:* Monitor neurologic signs and VS every 15-30 min for first 2 hr, every hour for next 6 hr, then every 2 hr for 24 hr. Maintain bed rest until patient is alert and VS are stable. Report any neurologic status changes.
Computed tomography (CT) scan	Computer-assisted x-ray of multiple cross sections of body parts to detect problems such as hemorrhage, tumor, cyst, edema, infarction, brain atrophy, and other abnormalities (Fig. 56-15, *A*). Contrast media may be used to enhance visualization of brain structures.	Assess for contraindications to contrast media, including allergy to shellfish, iodine, or dye. Explain appearance of scanner. Instruct patient to remain still during procedure.
Magnetic resonance imaging (MRI)	Imaging of brain, spinal cord, and spinal canal by means of magnetic energy (Fig. 56-15, *B*). Used to detect strokes, multiple sclerosis, tumors, trauma, herniation, and seizures. No invasive procedures are required. Contrast media may be used to enhance visualization. Has greater contrast in images of soft tissue structures than CT scan.	Screen patient for metal parts and pacemaker in body. Instruct patient on need to lie very still for up to 1 hr. Sedation may be necessary if patient is claustrophobic.
Magnetic resonance angiography (MRA)	Uses differential signal characteristics of flowing blood to evaluate extracranial and intracranial blood vessels. Provides both anatomic and hemodynamic information. Can be used in conjunction with contrast media.	Similar to MRI (see above).
Positron emission tomography (PET)	Measures metabolic activity of brain to assess cell death or damage. Uses radioactive material that shows up as a bright spot on the image (see Fig. 16-7). Used for patients with stroke, Alzheimer's disease, seizure disorders, Parkinson's disease, and tumors.	Explain procedure to patient. Explain that two IV lines will be inserted. Instruct patient not to take sedatives or tranquilizers. Have patient empty bladder before procedure. Patient may be asked to perform different activities during test.
Single-photon emission computed tomography (SPECT)	A method of scanning similar to PET, but it uses more stable substances and different detectors. Radiolabeled compounds are injected, and their photon emissions can be detected. Images made are accumulation of labeled compound. Used to visualize blood flow or O_2 or glucose metabolism in the brain. Useful in diagnosing strokes, brain tumors, and seizure disorders.	Similar to PET (see above).
Myelogram	X-ray of spinal cord and vertebral column after injection of contrast medium into subarachnoid space. Used to detect spinal lesions (e.g., herniated or ruptured disc, spinal tumor).	*Preprocedure:* Administer sedative as ordered. Instruct patient to empty bladder. Inform patient that test is performed with patient on tilting table that is moved during test. *Postprocedure:* Patient should lie flat for a few hours. Encourage fluids. Monitor neurologic signs and VS. Headache, nausea, and vomiting may occur after procedure.

TABLE 56-8 DIAGNOSTIC STUDIES—cont'd

Nervous System

Study	Description and Purpose	Nursing Responsibility
Electrographic Studies		
Electroencephalography (EEG)	Electrical activity of brain is recorded by scalp electrodes to evaluate seizure disorders, cerebral disease, CNS effects of systemic diseases, brain death.	Inform patient that procedure is noninvasive and without danger of electric shock. Determine whether any medications (e.g., tranquilizers, antiseizure drugs) should be withheld. Resume medications and instruct patient to wash electrode paste out of hair after test.
Magnetoencephalography (MEG)	Uses a biomagnetometer to detect magnetic fields generated by neural activity. It can accurately pinpoint the part of the brain involved in a stroke, seizure, or other disorder or injury. Measures extracranial magnetic fields and scalp electric field (EEG).	MEG, a passive sensor, does not make physical contact with patient. Explain procedure to patient.
Electromyography (EMG) and nerve conduction studies	Electrical activity associated with nerve and skeletal muscle is recorded by insertion of needle electrodes to detect muscle and peripheral nerve disease.	Inform patient that pain and discomfort are associated with insertion of needles.
Evoked potentials	Electrical activity associated with nerve conduction along sensory pathways is recorded by electrodes placed on skin and scalp. Stimulus generates the impulse. Procedure is used to diagnose disease (e.g., multiple sclerosis), locate nerve damage, and monitor function intraoperatively.	Explain procedure to patient.
Ultrasound		
Carotid duplex studies	Combined ultrasound and pulsed Doppler technology. Probe is placed over the carotid artery and slowly moved along the course of the common carotid artery. Frequency of reflected ultrasound signal corresponds to the blood velocity. Increased blood flow velocity can indicate stenosis of a vessel.	Explain procedure to patient. Duplex scanning is a noninvasive study that evaluates the degree of stenosis of the carotid and vertebral arteries.
Transcranial Doppler	Same technology as carotid duplex, but evaluates blood flow velocities of the intracranial blood vessels. Probe is placed on the skin at various "windows" in the skull (areas in the skull that have only a thin bony covering) to register velocities of the blood vessels.	Explain procedure to patient. Noninvasive technique that is useful in assessing vasospasm associated with subarachnoid hemorrhage, altered intracranial blood flow dynamics associated with occlusive vascular disease, presence of emboli, and cerebral autoregulation.

CNS, Central nervous system; *CSF,* cerebrospinal fluid; *ICP,* intracranial pressure.

TABLE 56-9 NORMAL CEREBROSPINAL FLUID VALUES

Parameter	Normal Value
Specific gravity	1.007
pH	7.35
Appearance	Clear, colorless
Red blood cells (RBCs)	None
White blood cells (WBCs)	0-5 cells/μL (0-5 × 10⁶ cells/L)
Protein	
• Lumbar	15-45 mg/dL (0.15-0.45 g/L)
• Cisternal	15-25 mg/dL (0.15-0.25 g/L)
• Ventricular	5-15 mg/dL (0.05-0.15 g/L)
Glucose	40-70 mg/dL (2.2-3.9 mmol/L)
Microorganisms	None
Pressure	60-150 mm H₂O

FIG. 56-14 Cerebral angiogram illustrating an arteriovenous malformation *(arrow).*

FIG. 56-15 Normal images of the brain. **A,** Computed tomography scan. **B,** Magnetic resonance imaging.

Evoked Potentials. *Evoked potentials* are recordings of electrical activity associated with nerve conduction along sensory pathways. The electrical activity is generated by a specific sensory stimulus related to the type of study (e.g., clicking sounds for auditory evoked potentials, mild electrical pulses for somatosensory evoked potentials).[11] Electrodes placed on specific areas of the skin and the scalp record the electrical activity. Increases in the normal time from stimulus onset to a given peak (latency) indicate slowed nerve conduction or nerve damage.

This technique is useful in diagnosing abnormalities of the visual or auditory systems because it reveals whether a sensory impulse is reaching the appropriate part of the brain. Indications for these tests include evaluation of consciousness, multiple sclerosis (optic neuritis), and acoustic neuroma.

BRIDGE TO NCLEX EXAMINATION

The number of the question corresponds to the same-numbered outcome at the beginning of the chapter.

1. In a patient with a disease that affects the myelin sheath of nerves, such as multiple sclerosis, the glial cells affected are the
   a. microglia.
   b. astrocytes.
   c. ependymal cells.
   d. oligodendrocytes.

2. Drugs or diseases that impair the function of the extrapyramidal system may cause loss of
   a. sensations of pain and temperature.
   b. regulation of the autonomic nervous system.
   c. integration of somatic and special sensory inputs.
   d. automatic movements associated with skeletal muscle activity.

3. An obstruction of the anterior cerebral arteries will affect functions of
   a. visual imaging.
   b. balance and coordination.
   c. judgment, insight, and reasoning.
   d. visual and auditory integration for language comprehension.

4. Paralysis of lateral gaze indicates a lesion of cranial nerve
   a. II.
   b. III.
   c. IV.
   d. VI.

5. A result of stimulation of the parasympathetic nervous system is *(select all that apply)*
   a. constriction of the bronchi.
   b. dilation of skin blood vessels.
   c. increased secretion of insulin.
   d. increased blood glucose levels.
   e. relaxation of the urinary sphincters.

6. Assessment of muscle strength of older adults cannot be compared with that of younger adults because
   a. stroke is more common in older adults.
   b. nutritional status is better in young adults.
   c. most young people exercise more than older people.
   d. aging leads to a decrease in muscle bulk and strength.

7. Data regarding mobility, strength, coordination, and activity tolerance are important for the nurse to obtain because
   a. many neurologic diseases affect one or more of these areas.
   b. patients are less able to identify other neurologic impairments.
   c. these are the first functions to be affected by neurologic diseases.
   d. aspects of movement are the most important function of the nervous system.

8. During neurologic testing, the patient is able to perceive pain elicited by pinprick. Based on this finding, the nurse may omit testing for
   a. position sense.
   b. patellar reflexes.
   c. temperature perception.
   d. heel-to-shin movements.
9. A patient's eyes jerk while the patient looks to the left. You will record this finding as
   a. nystagmus.
   b. CN VI palsy.
   c. oculocephalia.
   d. ophthalmic dyskinesia.

10. The nurse is caring for a patient with peripheral neuropathy who is going to have EMG studies tomorrow morning. The nurse should
    a. ensure the patient has an empty bladder.
    b. instruct the patient that there is no risk of electric shock.
    c. ensure the patient has no metallic jewelry or metal fragments.
    d. instruct the patient that she or he may experience pain during the study.

1. d, 2. d, 3. c, 4. d, 5. a, b, c, 6. c, d, 7. a, 8. c, 9. a, 10. b

⊜volve

For rationales to these answers and even more NCLEX review questions, visit *http://evolve.elsevier.com/Lewis/medsurg*.

REFERENCES

1. Gopurappilly R, Pal R, Mamidi MK, et al: Stem cells in stroke repair: current success and future prospects, *CNS Neurol Disorders Drug Targets* 10:741, 2011.
2. Zhang H, Wang FW, Yao LL, et al: Microglia—friend or foe, *Front Biosci (Schol Ed)* 3:869, 2011.
3. Otsuka S, Adamson C, Sankar V, et al: Delayed intrathecal delivery of RhoA siRNA to the contused spinal cord inhibits allodynia, preserves white matter, and increases serotonergic fiber growth, *J Neurotrauma* 28:1063, 2011.
4. Timofeev I, Carpenter KL, Nortje J, et al: Cerebral extracellular chemistry and outcome following traumatic brain injury: a microdialysis study of 223 patients, *Brain* 134:484, 2011.
5. Chen JW, Gombart ZJ, Rogers S, et al: Pupillary reactivity as an early indicator of increased intracranial pressure: the introduction of the neurological pupil index, *Surg Neurol Int* 2:82, 2011.
6. Takahashi R, Ishii K, Kakigi T, et al: Gender and age differences in normal adult human brain: voxel-based morphometric study, *Hum Brain Mapp* 32:1050, 2011.
7. Medin J, Windahl J, von Arbin M, et al: Eating difficulties among stroke patients in the acute state: a descriptive, cross-sectional, comparative study, *J Clin Nurs* 20:2563, 2011.
8. Pinder C, Young C: Adverse cognitive effects of phenytoin in severe brain injury: a case report, *Brain Inj* 25:634, 2011.
9. Hunderfund AN, Sweeney CM, Mandrekar JN, et al: Effect of a multidisciplinary fall risk assessment on falls among neurology inpatients, *Mayo Clinic Proc* 86:19, 2011.
10. Swisher CB, Doreswamy M, Gingrich KJ, et al: Phenytoin, levetiracetam, and pregabalin in the acute management of refractory status epilepticus in patients with brain tumors, *Neurocrit Care* 16(1):109, 2012.
11. Guo L, Gelb AW: The use of motor evoked potential monitoring during cerebral aneurysm surgery to predict pure motor deficits due to subcortical ischemia, *Clin Neurophysiol* 122:648, 2011.

RESOURCES

Resources for this chapter are listed after Chapter 57 on p. 1387, Chapter 58 on p. 1412, Chapter 59 on p. 1442, Chapter 60 on p. 1462, and Chapter 61 on p. 1488.

*Most people do not listen
with the intent to understand;
they listen with the intent to reply.*
Stephen Covey

Nursing Management
Acute Intracranial Problems

Meg Zomorodi

evolve WEBSITE

http://evolve.elsevier.com/Lewis/medsurg

- NCLEX Review Questions
- Key Points
- Pre-Test
- Answer Guidelines for Case Study on p. 1385
- Rationales for Bridge to NCLEX Examination Questions

- Case Studies
  - Patient With Head Injury
  - Patient With Meningitis
- Nursing Care Plans (Customizable)
  - eNCP 57-1: Patient With Increased Intracranial Pressure
  - eNCP 57-2: Patient With Bacterial Meningitis
- Concept Map Creator

- Glossary
- Animation
  - Functional Areas of the Brain
- Content Updates

eFigure
- eFig. 57-1: Systematic approach to nursing assessment of unconscious patient

LEARNING OUTCOMES

1. Explain the physiologic mechanisms that maintain normal intracranial pressure.
2. Describe the common etiologies, clinical manifestations, and collaborative care of the patient with increased intracranial pressure.
3. Describe the collaborative and nursing management of the patient with increased intracranial pressure.
4. Differentiate types of head injury by mechanism of injury and clinical manifestations.

5. Describe the collaborative care and nursing management of the patient with a head injury.
6. Compare the types, clinical manifestations, and collaborative care of patients with brain tumors.
7. Discuss the nursing management of the patient with a brain tumor.
8. Describe the nursing management of the patient undergoing cranial surgery.
9. Differentiate among the primary causes, collaborative care, and nursing management of brain abscess, meningitis, and encephalitis.

KEY TERMS

brain abscess, p. 1381
cerebral edema, p. 1359
coma, p. 1359
concussion, p. 1369
contusion, p. 1370
diffuse axonal injury (DAI), p. 1370

encephalitis, p. 1384
epidural hematoma, p. 1370
Glasgow Coma Scale (GCS), p. 1365
head injury, p. 1368
intracerebral hematoma, p. 1371

intracranial pressure (ICP), p. 1357
meningitis, p. 1381
nuchal rigidity, p. 1382
subdural hematoma, p. 1371
unconsciousness, p. 1359

Acute intracranial problems include diseases and disorders that can increase intracranial pressure (ICP). This chapter discusses the mechanisms that maintain normal ICP and increase ICP. In addition, head injury, brain tumors, and cerebral inflammatory disorders are discussed.

INTRACRANIAL PRESSURE

Understanding the dynamics associated with ICP is important in caring for patients with many different neurologic prob-

lems. The skull is like a closed box with three essential volume components: brain tissue, blood, and cerebrospinal fluid (CSF) (Fig. 57-1). The intracellular and extracellular fluids of brain tissue make up approximately 78% of this volume. Blood in the arterial, venous, and capillary network makes up 12% of the volume, and the remaining 10% is the volume of the CSF.

Primary versus secondary injury is another important concept in understanding ICP. *Primary injury* occurs at the initial time of an injury (e.g., impact of car accident,

---

Reviewed by Sarah Livesay, RN, DNP, ACNP, CNS-A, System Director of Service Line Development, St. Luke's Episcopal Health System, Houston, Texas; Molly M. McNett, RN, PhD, Director, Nursing Research, MetroHealth Medical Center, Cleveland, Ohio; and Susan Yeager, RN, MS, CCRN, ACNP, Neurocritical Care Nurse Practitioner, The Ohio State University Medical Center, Columbus, Ohio.

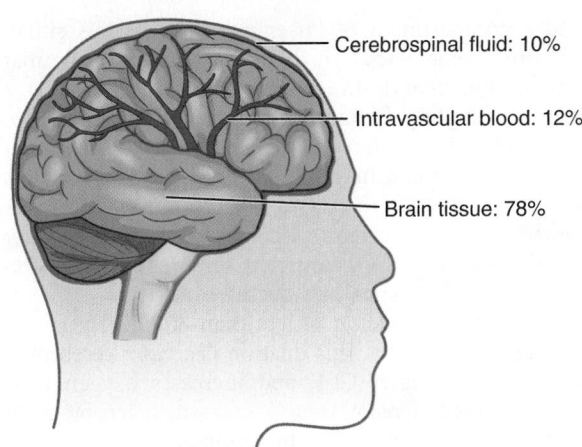

Cerebrospinal fluid: 10%

Intravascular blood: 12%

Brain tissue: 78%

FIG. 57-1 Components of the brain.

TABLE 57-1	CALCULATION OF CEREBRAL PERFUSION PRESSURE

CPP = MAP − ICP

$$MAP = DBP + 1/3\,(SBP - DBP) \text{ or } = \frac{SBP + 2\,(DBP)}{3}$$

Example: Systemic blood pressure = 122/84 mm Hg
MAP = 97 mm Hg
ICP = 12 mm Hg
CPP = 85 mm Hg

CPP, Cerebral perfusion pressure; *DBP,* diastolic blood pressure; *ICP,* intracranial pressure; *MAP,* mean arterial pressure; *SBP,* systolic blood pressure.

blunt-force trauma) that results in displacement, bruising, or damage of the three components. *Secondary injury* is the resulting hypoxia, ischemia, hypotension, edema, or increased ICP that follows the primary injury. Secondary injury, which could occur several hours to days after the initial injury, is a primary concern when managing brain injury. Nursing management of the patient with an acute intracranial problem must include management of secondary injury, and thus increased ICP.

Regulation and Maintenance of Intracranial Pressure

Normal Intracranial Pressure. Intracranial pressure (ICP) is the hydrostatic force measured in the brain CSF compartment. Under normal conditions in which intracranial volume remains relatively constant, the balance among the three components (brain tissue, blood, CSF) maintains the ICP. Factors that influence ICP under normal circumstances are changes in (1) arterial pressure; (2) venous pressure; (3) intraabdominal and intrathoracic pressure; (4) posture; (5) temperature; and (6) blood gases, particularly carbon dioxide levels. The degree to which these factors increase or decrease the ICP depends on the brain's ability to adapt to changes.

The Monro-Kellie doctrine states that the three components must remain at a relatively constant volume within the closed skull structure. If the volume of any one of the three components increases within the cranial vault and the volume from another component is displaced, the total intracranial volume will not change.[1] This hypothesis is only applicable in situations in which the skull is closed. The hypothesis is not valid in persons with displaced skull fractures or hemicraniectomy.

ICP can be measured in the ventricles, subarachnoid space, subdural space, epidural space, or brain tissue using a pressure transducer.[2] Normal ICP ranges from 5 to 15 mm Hg. A sustained pressure greater than 20 mm Hg is considered abnormal and must be treated.

Normal Compensatory Adaptations. In applying the Monro-Kellie doctrine, the body can adapt to volume changes within the skull in three different ways to maintain a normal ICP. First, compensatory mechanisms can include changes in the CSF volume. The CSF volume can be changed by altering CSF absorption or production and by displacing CSF into the spinal subarachnoid space. Second, changes in intracranial blood volume can occur through the collapse of cerebral veins and dural sinuses, regional cerebral vasoconstriction or dilation, and changes in venous outflow. Third, brain tissue volume

compensates through distention of the dura or compression of brain tissue.

Initially an increase in volume produces no increase in ICP as a result of these compensatory mechanisms. However, the ability to compensate for changes in volume is limited. As the volume increase continues, the ICP rises and decompensation ultimately occurs, resulting in compression and ischemia.

Cerebral Blood Flow

Cerebral blood flow (CBF) is the amount of blood in milliliters passing through 100 g of brain tissue in 1 minute. The global CBF is approximately 50 mL/min/100 g of brain tissue.[3] The maintenance of blood flow to the brain is critical because the brain requires a constant supply of oxygen and glucose. The brain uses 20% of the body's oxygen and 25% of its glucose.[4]

Autoregulation of Cerebral Blood Flow. The brain regulates its own blood flow in response to its metabolic needs despite wide fluctuations in systemic arterial pressure. *Autoregulation* is the automatic adjustment in the diameter of the cerebral blood vessels by the brain to maintain a constant blood flow during changes in arterial blood pressure (BP). The purpose of autoregulation is to ensure a consistent CBF to provide for the metabolic needs of brain tissue and to maintain cerebral perfusion pressure within normal limits.

The lower limit of systemic arterial pressure at which autoregulation is effective in a normotensive person is a mean arterial pressure (MAP) of 70 mm Hg. Below this, CBF decreases, and symptoms of cerebral ischemia, such as syncope and blurred vision, occur. The upper limit of systemic arterial pressure at which autoregulation is effective is a MAP of 150 mm Hg.[3] When this pressure is exceeded, the vessels are maximally constricted, and further vasoconstrictor response is lost.

The *cerebral perfusion pressure* (CPP) is the pressure needed to ensure blood flow to the brain. CPP is equal to the MAP minus the ICP (CPP = MAP − ICP) (see example in Table 57-1). This formula is clinically useful, although it does not consider the effect of cerebrovascular resistance. Cerebrovascular resistance, generated by the arterioles within the cranium, links CPP and blood flow as follows: CPP = Flow × Resistance.

When cerebrovascular resistance is high, blood flow to brain tissue is impaired. Transcranial Doppler is a noninvasive technique used in intensive care units (ICUs) to monitor changes in cerebrovascular resistance.

As the CPP decreases, autoregulation fails and CBF decreases. Normal CPP is 60 to 100 mm Hg. A CPP of less than 50 mm Hg is associated with ischemia and neuronal death. A CPP of less than 30 mm Hg results in ischemia and is incompatible with life.

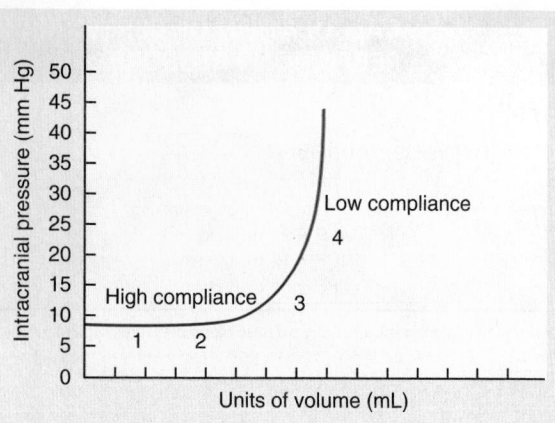

FIG. 57-2 Intracranial pressure-volume curve. (See text for descriptions of *1, 2, 3,* and *4*.)

Normally, autoregulation maintains an adequate CBF and perfusion pressure primarily by adjusting the diameter of cerebral blood vessels and metabolic factors that affect ICP. It is critical to maintain MAP when ICP is elevated.

Remember that CPP may not reflect perfusion pressure in all parts of the brain. There may be local areas of swelling and compression limiting regional perfusion pressure. Thus a higher CPP may be needed for these patients to prevent localized tissue damage. For example, a patient with an acute stroke may require a higher BP, increasing MAP and CPP, in order to increase perfusion to the brain and prevent further tissue damage.

Pressure Changes. The relationship of pressure to volume is depicted in the pressure-volume curve (Fig. 57-2). The curve is affected by the brain's compliance. *Compliance* is the expandability of the brain. It is represented as the volume increase for each unit increase in pressure. With low compliance, small changes in volume result in greater increases in pressure.

$$Compliance = Volume / Pressure$$

The concept of the pressure-volume curve can be used to represent the stages of increased ICP. At stage 1 on the curve, there is high compliance. The brain is in total compensation, with accommodation and autoregulation intact. An increase in volume (in brain tissue, blood, or CSF) does not increase the ICP.

At stage 2, the compliance is beginning to decrease, and an increase in volume places the patient at risk of increased ICP and secondary injury. At stage 3, there is significant reduction in compliance. Any small addition of volume causes a great increase in ICP. Compensatory mechanisms fail, there is a loss of autoregulation, and the patient exhibits manifestations of increased ICP (e.g., headache, changes in level of consciousness or pupil responsiveness).

With a loss of autoregulation, the body attempts to maintain cerebral perfusion by increasing systolic BP. However, decompensation is imminent. The patient's response is characterized by systolic hypertension with a widening pulse pressure, bradycardia with a full and bounding pulse, and altered respirations. This is known as *Cushing's triad* and is a neurologic emergency.

As the patient enters stage 4, the ICP rises to lethal levels with little increase in volume. *Herniation* occurs as the brain tissue is forcibly shifted from the compartment of greater pressure to a compartment of lesser pressure. In this situation, intense pressure is placed on the brainstem, and if herniation continues, brainstem death is imminent.

Factors Affecting Cerebral Blood Flow. Carbon dioxide, oxygen, and hydrogen ion concentration affect cerebral blood vessel tone. An increase in the partial pressure of carbon dioxide in arterial blood ($PaCO_2$) relaxes smooth muscle, dilates cerebral vessels, decreases cerebrovascular resistance, and increases CBF. A decrease in $PaCO_2$ constricts cerebral vessels, increases cerebrovascular resistance, and decreases CBF.

Cerebral oxygen tension of less than 50 mm Hg results in cerebrovascular dilation. This dilation decreases cerebrovascular resistance, increases CBF, and increases oxygen tension. However, if oxygen tension is not increased, anaerobic metabolism begins, resulting in an accumulation of lactic acid. As lactic acid increases and hydrogen ions accumulate, the environment becomes more acidic. Within this acidic environment, further vasodilation occurs in a continued attempt to increase blood flow. The combination of a severely low partial pressure of oxygen in arterial blood (PaO_2) and an elevated hydrogen ion concentration (acidosis), which are both potent cerebral vasodilators, may produce a state where autoregulation is lost and compensatory mechanisms fail to meet tissue metabolic demands.

CBF can be affected by cardiac or respiratory arrest, systemic hemorrhage, and other pathophysiologic states (e.g., diabetic coma, encephalopathies, infections, toxicities). Regional CBF can also be affected by trauma, tumors, cerebral hemorrhage, or stroke. When regional or global autoregulation is lost, CBF is no longer maintained at a constant level but is directly influenced by changes in systemic BP, hypoxia, or catecholamines.

INCREASED INTRACRANIAL PRESSURE

Any patient who becomes unconscious acutely, regardless of the cause, should be suspected of having increased ICP.

Mechanisms of Increased Intracranial Pressure

Increased ICP is a potentially life-threatening situation that results from an increase in any or all of the three components (brain tissue, blood, CSF) within the skull. Elevated ICP is clinically significant because it diminishes CPP, increases risks of brain ischemia and infarction, and is associated with a poor prognosis.[5] Common causes of increased ICP include a mass (e.g., hematoma, contusion, abscess, tumor) and cerebral edema (associated with brain tumors, hydrocephalus, head injury, or brain inflammation).

These cerebral insults, which may result in hypercapnia, cerebral acidosis, impaired autoregulation, and systemic hypertension, increase the formation and spread of cerebral edema. This edema distorts brain tissue, further increasing the ICP, and leads to even more tissue hypoxia and acidosis. Fig. 57-3 illustrates the progression of increased ICP.

It is critical to maintain CBF to preserve tissue and thus minimize secondary injury. Sustained increases in ICP result in brainstem compression and herniation of the brain from one compartment to another.

Displacement and herniation of brain tissue can cause a potentially reversible process to become irreversible. Ischemia and edema are further increased, compounding the preexisting problem. Compression of the brainstem and cranial nerves may be fatal. (Fig. 57-4 illustrates types of herniation.) Herniation

PATHOPHYSIOLOGY MAP

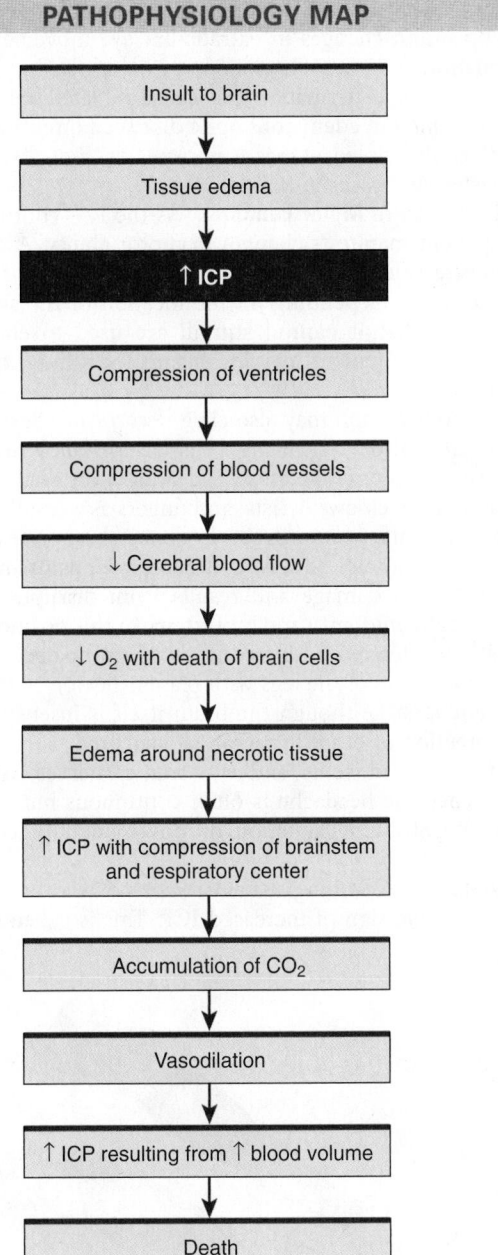

FIG. 57-3 Progression of increased intracranial pressure *(ICP)*.

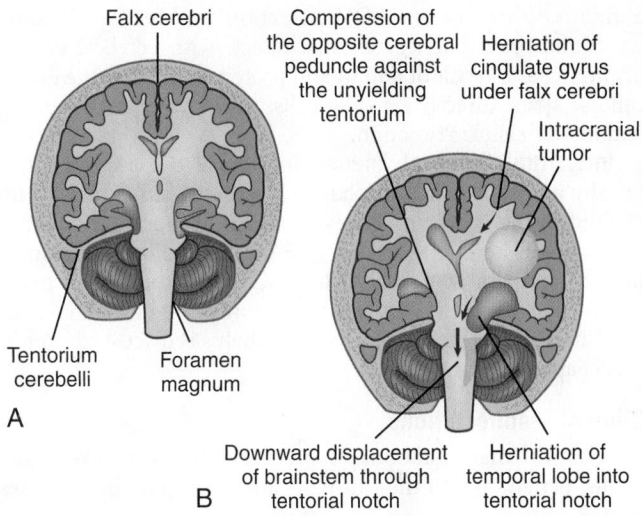

FIG. 57-4 Herniation. **A,** Normal relationship of intracranial structures. **B,** Shift of intracranial structures.

TABLE 57-2	CAUSES OF CEREBRAL EDEMA
Mass Lesions • Brain abscess • Brain tumor (primary or metastatic) • Hematoma (intracerebral, subdural, epidural) • Hemorrhage (intracerebral, cerebellar, brainstem) **Head Injuries and Brain Surgery** • Contusion • Hemorrhage • Posttraumatic brain swelling	**Cerebral Infections** • Meningitis • Encephalitis **Vascular Insult** • Anoxic and ischemic episodes • Cerebral infarction (thrombotic or embolic) • Venous sinus thrombosis **Toxic or Metabolic Encephalopathic Conditions** • Lead or arsenic intoxication • Hepatic encephalopathy • Uremia

forces the cerebellum and the brainstem downward through the foramen magnum. If compression of the brainstem is unrelieved, respiratory arrest will occur due to compression of the respiratory control center in the medulla.

Cerebral Edema

As shown in Table 57-2, there are a variety of causes of **cerebral edema** (increased accumulation of fluid in the extravascular spaces of brain tissue). Regardless of the cause, cerebral edema results in an increase in tissue volume that can increase ICP. The extent and severity of the original insult are factors that determine the degree of cerebral edema.

There are three types of cerebral edema: vasogenic, cytotoxic, and interstitial. The same patient may have more than one type.

Vasogenic Cerebral Edema. *Vasogenic cerebral edema,* the most common type of cerebral edema, occurs mainly in the white matter and is characterized by leakage of macromolecules from the capillaries into the surrounding extracellular space. This results in an osmotic gradient that favors the flow of fluid from the intravascular to the extravascular space. A variety of insults, such as brain tumors, abscesses, and ingested toxins, may cause an increase in the permeability of the blood-brain barrier and produce an increase in the extracellular fluid volume. The speed and extent of the spread of the edema fluid are influenced by the systemic BP, the site of the brain injury, and the extent of the blood-brain barrier defect.

This edema may produce a continuum of symptoms ranging from headache to disturbances in consciousness, including coma (profound state of unconsciousness) and focal neurologic deficits. It is important to recognize that although a headache may seem to be a benign symptom, in cases of cerebral edema it can quickly progress to coma and death. Therefore you must be vigilant in your assessment.

Cytotoxic Cerebral Edema. *Cytotoxic cerebral edema* results from disruption of the integrity of the cell membranes. It develops from destructive lesions or trauma to brain tissue resulting in cerebral hypoxia or anoxia and syndrome of inappropriate antidiuretic hormone (SIADH) secretion. In this type of edema the blood-brain barrier remains intact, with cerebral edema occurring as a result of a fluid and protein shift from the extracellular space directly into the cells, with subsequent swelling and loss of cellular function.

Interstitial Cerebral Edema. *Interstitial cerebral edema* is usually a result of hydrocephalus. *Hydrocephalus* is a build up of fluid in the brain and is manifested by ventricular enlargement. It can be due to excess CSF production, obstruction of flow, or an inability to reabsorb the CSF. Hydrocephalus treatment usually consists of a ventriculostomy or ventriculoperitoneal shunt. (Management of hydrocephalus is discussed later in this chapter.)

Clinical Manifestations

The clinical manifestations of increased ICP can take many forms, depending on the cause, location, and rate of increases in ICP.

Change in Level of Consciousness. The *level of consciousness* (LOC) is the most sensitive and reliable indicator of the patient's neurologic status. Changes in LOC are a result of impaired CBF, which deprives the cells of the cerebral cortex and the reticular activating system (RAS) of oxygen. The RAS is located in the brainstem, with neural connections to many parts of the nervous system. An intact RAS can maintain a state of wakefulness even in the absence of a functioning cerebral cortex. Interruptions of impulses from the RAS or alterations in functioning of the cerebral hemispheres can cause **unconsciousness** (abnormal state of complete or partial unawareness of self or environment).

The patient's state of consciousness is defined by both the behavior and the pattern of brain activity recorded by an electroencephalogram (EEG). A change in consciousness may be dramatic, as in coma, or subtle, such as a flattening of affect, change in orientation, or decrease in level of attention. In the deepest state of unconsciousness (i.e., coma), the patient does not respond to painful stimuli. Corneal and pupillary reflexes are absent. The patient cannot swallow or cough and is incontinent of urine and feces. The EEG pattern demonstrates suppressed or absent neuronal activity.

Changes in Vital Signs. Changes in vital signs are caused by increasing pressure on the thalamus, hypothalamus, pons, and medulla. Manifestations such as *Cushing's triad* (systolic hypertension with a widening pulse pressure, bradycardia with a full and bounding pulse, and irregular respirations) may be present but often do not appear until ICP has been increased for some time or is suddenly and markedly increased (e.g., head trauma). Always recognize Cushing's triad as a medical emergency, since this is a sign of brainstem compression and impending death. A change in body temperature may also occur because increased ICP affects the hypothalamus.

Ocular Signs. Compression of cranial nerve (CN) III, the oculomotor nerve, results in dilation of the pupil on the same side (*ipsilateral*) as the mass lesion, sluggish or no response to light, inability to move the eye upward, and ptosis of the eyelid. These signs can be the result of the brain shifting from midline, compressing the trunk of CN III, and paralyzing the muscles controlling pupillary size and shape. In this situation, a fixed, unilateral, dilated pupil is considered a neurologic emergency that indicates herniation of the brain.

Other cranial nerves may also be affected, such as the optic (CN II), trochlear (CN IV), and abducens (CN VI) nerves. Signs

of dysfunction of these cranial nerves include blurred vision, diplopia, and changes in extraocular eye movements. Central herniation may initially manifest as sluggish but equal pupil response. Uncal herniation may cause a dilated unilateral pupil. *Papilledema* (an edematous optic disc seen on retinal examination) is also noted and is a nonspecific sign associated with persistent increases in ICP.

Decrease in Motor Function. As the ICP continues to rise, the patient manifests changes in motor ability. A *contralateral* (opposite side of the mass lesion) hemiparesis or hemiplegia may develop, depending on the location of the source of the increased ICP. If painful stimuli are used to elicit a motor response, the patient may localize to the stimuli or withdraw from it.

Noxious stimuli may also elicit *decorticate* (flexor) or *decerebrate* (extensor) posturing (Fig. 57-5). Decorticate posture consists of internal rotation and adduction of the arms with flexion of the elbows, wrists, and fingers as a result of interruption of voluntary motor tracts in the cerebral cortex. Extension of the legs may also be seen. A decerebrate posture may indicate more serious damage and results from disruption of motor fibers in the midbrain and brainstem. In this position, the arms are stiffly extended, adducted, and hyperpronated. There is also hyperextension of the legs with plantar flexion of the feet.

Headache. Although the brain itself is insensitive to pain, compression of other intracranial structures, such as the walls of arteries and veins and the cranial nerves, can produce headache. The headache is often continuous but worse in the morning. Straining, agitation, or movement may accentuate the pain.

Vomiting. Vomiting, usually not preceded by nausea, is often a nonspecific sign of increased ICP. This is called unexpected

FIG. 57-5 Decorticate and decerebrate posturing. **A,** Decorticate response. Flexion of arms, wrists, and fingers with adduction in upper extremities. Extension, internal rotation, and plantar flexion in lower extremities. **B,** Decerebrate response. All four extremities in rigid extension, with hyperpronation of forearms and plantar flexion of feet. **C,** Decorticate response on right side of body and decerebrate response on left side of body. **D,** Opisthotonic posturing.

vomiting and is related to pressure changes in the cranium. Projectile vomiting may also occur and is related to increased ICP.

Complications

The major complications of uncontrolled increased ICP are inadequate cerebral perfusion and cerebral herniation (see Fig. 57-4). To better understand cerebral herniation, two important structures in the brain must be described. The *falx cerebri* is a thin wall of dura that folds down between the cortex, separating the two cerebral hemispheres. The *tentorium cerebelli* is a rigid fold of dura that separates the cerebral hemispheres from the cerebellum (see Fig. 57-4). It is called the tentorium (meaning tent) because it forms a tentlike cover over the cerebellum.

Tentorial herniation (central herniation) occurs when a mass lesion in the cerebrum forces the brain to herniate downward through the opening created by the brainstem. *Uncal herniation* occurs when there is lateral and downward herniation. *Cingulate herniation* occurs when there is lateral displacement of brain tissue beneath the falx cerebri.

Diagnostic Studies

Diagnostic studies can identify the cause of increased ICP (Table 57-3). Computed tomography (CT) and magnetic

TABLE 57-3 COLLABORATIVE CARE

Increased Intracranial Pressure

Diagnostic
- History and physical examination
- Vital signs, neurologic assessments, ICP measurements
- Skull, chest, and spinal x-ray studies
- CT scan, MRI, cerebral angiography, EEG, PET
- Transcranial Doppler studies
- Infrascanner
- ECG
- Evoked potential studies
- Laboratory studies, including CBC, coagulation profile, electrolytes, serum creatinine, ABGs, ammonia level, drug and toxicology screen, CSF analysis for protein, cells, glucose*

Collaborative Therapy
- Elevation of head of bed to 30 degrees with head in a neutral position
- Intubation and mechanical ventilation
- ICP monitoring
- Cerebral oxygenation monitoring (PbtO₂, SjvO₂)
- Maintenance of PaO₂ ≥100 mm Hg
- Maintenance of fluid balance and assessment of osmolality
- Maintenance of systolic arterial pressure between 100 and 160 mm Hg
- Maintenance of CPP >60 mm Hg
- Reduction of cerebral metabolism (e.g., high-dose barbiturates)
- Drug therapy
  - Osmotic diuretic (mannitol)
  - Hypertonic saline
  - Antiseizure drugs (e.g., phenytoin [Dilantin])
  - Corticosteroids (dexamethasone [Decadron]) for brain tumors, bacterial meningitis
  - Histamine (H₂)-receptor antagonist (e.g., cimetidine [Tagamet]) or proton pump inhibitor (e.g., pantoprazole [Protonix]) to prevent GI ulcers and bleeding

*A lumbar puncture to obtain CSF for analysis should not be done if there is a possibility of herniation.
CPP, Cerebral perfusion pressure; *ICP,* intracranial pressure; *PaO₂,* partial pressure of oxygen in arterial blood; *PbtO₂,* pressure of oxygen in brain tissue; *SjvO₂,* jugular venous oxygen saturation.

resonance imaging (MRI) have revolutionized the diagnosis of increased ICP. These tests are used to differentiate the many conditions that can cause increased ICP and to assess the effect of treatment.

Additional tests include EEG, cerebral angiography, ICP measurement, brain tissue oxygenation measurement via the LICOX catheter (described later), transcranial Doppler studies, and evoked potential studies. Positron emission tomography (PET) is also used to diagnose the cause of increased ICP. In general, a lumbar puncture is not performed when increased ICP is suspected. The reason for this is that cerebral herniation could occur from the sudden release of the pressure in the skull from the area above the lumbar puncture.

In some institutions a hand-held Infrascanner can be used to detect life-threatening intracranial bleeding. The scanner directs a wavelength of light that can penetrate tissue and bone. Blood from intracranial hematomas absorbs the light differently than other areas of the brain.

Monitoring Intracranial Pressure and Cerebral Oxygenation

Indications for Intracranial Pressure Monitoring. ICP monitoring is used to guide clinical care when the patient is at risk for or has elevations in ICP. It may be used in patients with a variety of neurologic insults, including hemorrhage, stroke, tumor, infection, or traumatic brain injury. ICP should be monitored in patients admitted with a Glasgow Coma Scale (GCS) score of 8 or less and an abnormal CT scan or MRI (hematomas, contusion, edema). (The GCS is presented later in Table 57-5.)

Methods of Measuring Intracranial Pressure. Patients with conditions known to elevate ICP, except those with irreversible problems or advanced neurologic disease, usually undergo ICP monitoring in an ICU. Multiple methods and devices are available to monitor ICP in various sites (Fig. 57-6).

The gold standard for monitoring ICP is the *ventriculostomy,* in which a specialized catheter is inserted into the lateral ventricle and coupled to an external transducer (Figs. 57-7 and 57-8). This technique directly measures the pressure within the ventricles, facilitates removal and/or sampling of CSF, and allows for intraventricular drug administration. In this system the transducer is external, and it is important to ensure that the transducer of the ventriculostomy is level with the foramen of Monro (interventricular foramen). The ventriculostomy system must also be at the ideal height (Fig. 57-9, *A*). A reference point

FIG. 57-6 Coronal section of brain showing potential sites for placement of intracranial pressure monitoring devices.

FIG. 57-7 Intracranial pressure *(ICP)* monitoring can be used to continuously measure ICP. The ICP tracing shows normal, elevated, and plateau waves. At high ICP the P2 peak is higher than the P1 peak, and the peaks become less distinct and plateau.

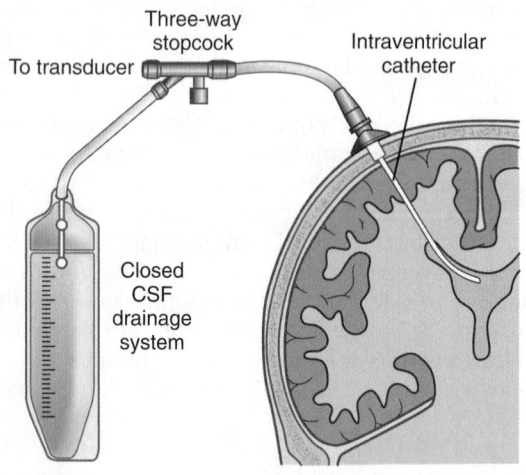

FIG. 57-8 Ventriculostomy in place. Cerebrospinal fluid *(CSF)* can be drained via a ventriculostomy when intracranial pressure (ICP) exceeds the upper pressure parameter set by the physician. Intermittent drainage involves opening the three-way stopcock to allow CSF to flow into the drainage bag for brief periods (30 to 120 seconds) until the pressure is below the upper pressure parameters.

TABLE 57-4	NORMAL INTRACRANIAL PRESSURE WAVEFORMS*	
Waveform	**Meaning**
P1 Percussion wave	Represents arterial pulsations. Normally the highest of the three waveforms.
P2 Rebound wave or tidal wave	Reflects intracranial compliance or relative brain volume. When P2 is higher than P1, intracranial compliance is compromised.
P3 Dicrotic wave	Follows dicrotic notch. Represents venous pulsations. Normally the lowest waveform.

*See Fig. 57-7.

for this foramen is the tragus of the ear. Every time the patient is repositioned, the system needs assessed to ensure it is level.

The *fiberoptic catheter,* an alternative technology, uses a sensor transducer located within the catheter tip. The sensor tip is placed within the ventricle or the brain tissue and provides a direct measurement of brain pressure.

The *subarachnoid bolt* or *screw* is another method of monitoring ICP. It is placed just through the skull between the arach-

noid membrane and the cerebral cortex. It does not allow for CSF drainage but is ideal for patients with mild or moderate head injury. It can easily be converted into a ventriculostomy if the patient decompensates.

Infection is a serious complication with ICP monitoring. Factors that contribute to the development of infection include ICP monitoring more than 5 days, use of a ventriculostomy, a CSF leak, and a concurrent systemic infection. Routinely assessing the insertion site, using aseptic technique, and monitoring the CSF for a change in drainage color or clarity are important nursing interventions.

ICP should be measured as a mean pressure. If a CSF drainage device is in place, the drain must be closed for at least 6 minutes to ensure an accurate reading. Record the waveform strip along with other pressure monitoring waveforms. The normal ICP waveform has three phases (see Fig. 57-7 and Table 57-4). It is important to monitor the ICP waveform, as well as

A   B

FIG. 57-9 **A,** Leveling a ventriculostomy. **B,** Cerebrospinal fluid is drained into a drainage system.

the mean CPP. When ICP is normal, P1, P2, and P3 resemble a staircase.[6] As ICP increases, P2 rises above P1, indicating poor ventricular compliance (see Fig. 57-7). Consider the rate at which changes occur and the patient's clinical condition. Neurologic deterioration might not occur until ICP elevation is pronounced and sustained. Immediately report to the health care provider any ICP elevation, either as a mean increase in pressure or as an abnormal waveform configuration.

Inaccurate ICP readings can be caused by CSF leaks around the monitoring device, obstruction of the intraventricular catheter or bolt (from tissue or blood clot), a difference between the height of the bolt and the transducer, kinks in the tubing, and incorrect height of the drainage system relative to the patient's reference point. Bubbles or air in the tubing can also dampen the waveform.

Cerebrospinal Fluid Drainage. With the ventricular catheter, it is possible to control ICP by removing CSF (see Fig. 57-8). The physician typically orders a specific level at which to initiate drainage (e.g., if ICP is greater than 20 mm Hg) and the frequency of drainage (intermittent or continuous). When the ICP is above the indicated level, the ventriculostomy system is opened by turning a stopcock and allowing the drainage of CSF, thus relieving pressure inside the cranial vault (see Fig. 57-9, *B*).

The two options for CSF drainage are intermittent or continuous. If intermittent drainage is ordered, open the ventriculostomy system at the indicated ICP and allow CSF to drain for 2 to 3 minutes. Then close the stopcock to return the ventriculostomy to a closed system. If continuous ICP drainage is ordered, careful monitoring of the volume of CSF drained is essential, keeping in mind that normal CSF production is about 20 to 30 mL/hr, with a total CSF volume of 90 to 150 mL within the ventricles and subarachnoid space. It is also recommended that a sign be posted above the patient's bed to notify anyone before turning, moving, or suctioning the patient to prevent the removal of too much CSF, which can result in other complications.

Strict aseptic technique during dressing changes or sampling of CSF is imperative to prevent infection. The system must remain intact to ensure that the ICP readings are accurate because treatment is initiated based on the pressures.

Complications of this type of drainage system include ventricular collapse, infection, and herniation or subdural hematoma formation from rapid decompression. Although it is generally recognized that CSF removal decreases ICP and improves CPP, guidelines for CSF removal are not universally accepted, but are typically based on institution or physician preference.[7]

Cerebral Oxygenation Monitoring. Technology is available to measure cerebral oxygenation and assess perfusion. Two such devices used in ICU settings are the *LICOX brain tissue oxygenation catheter* and the *jugular venous bulb catheter*. The LICOX catheter, which measures brain oxygenation and temperature, is placed in viable (healthy) white matter of the brain (Fig. 57-10). The LICOX system provides continuous monitoring of the pressure of oxygen in brain tissue ($PbtO_2$). The normal range for $PbtO_2$ is 20 to 40 mm Hg. A lower than normal $PbtO_2$ level is indicative of ischemia. Another advantage of the LICOX catheter is the ability to measure brain temperature. A cooler brain temperature (96.8° F [36° C]) may produce better outcomes.[8]

The jugular venous bulb catheter is placed in the internal jugular vein and positioned so that the catheter tip is located in the jugular bulb. Placement is verified by an x-ray. This catheter provides a measurement of jugular venous oxygen saturation ($SjvO_2$), which indicates total venous brain tissue extraction of oxygen. This is a measure of cerebral oxygen supply and demand. The normal $SjvO_2$ range is 55% to 75%. Values less than 50% demonstrate impaired cerebral oxygenation.

Collaborative Care

The goals of collaborative care (see Table 57-3) are to identify and treat the underlying cause of increased ICP and to support brain function. The earlier the condition is recognized and treated, the better the patient outcome. A careful history is an important diagnostic aid in the search for the underlying cause. The underlying cause of increased ICP is usually an increase in blood (hemorrhage), brain tissue (tumor or edema), or CSF (hydrocephalus) in the brain.

For any patient with increased ICP, it is important to maintain adequate oxygenation to support brain function. An endo-

A — Catheter

B

FIG. 57-10 **A,** The LICOX brain tissue oxygen system involves a catheter inserted through an intracranial bolt. **B,** The system measures oxygen in the brain (PbtO$_2$), brain tissue temperature, and intracranial pressure. (**B,** Permission granted by Integra LifeSciences Corporation, Plainsboro, NJ.)

tracheal tube or tracheostomy may be necessary to maintain adequate ventilation. Arterial blood gas (ABG) analysis guides the oxygen therapy. The goal is to maintain the PaO$_2$ at greater than or equal to 100 mm Hg and to keep PaCO$_2$ in normal range at 35 to 45 mm Hg. The patient may need to be on a mechanical ventilator to ensure adequate oxygenation.

If increased ICP is caused by a mass lesion (e.g., tumor, hematoma), surgical removal of the mass is the best treatment (see the sections on brain tumors and cranial surgery later in this chapter). Nonsurgical intervention for the reduction of tissue volume related to cerebral tissue swelling and cerebral edema includes the use of diuretics and corticosteroids. In aggressive situations, a craniectomy (removal of part of skull) may be performed to reduce ICP and prevent herniation (see head injury section for further details).

Drug Therapy. Drug therapy plays an important part in the management of increased ICP. Mannitol (Osmitrol) (25%) is an osmotic diuretic given IV. Mannitol acts to decrease the ICP in two ways: plasma expansion and osmotic effect. The immediate plasma-expanding effect reduces the hematocrit and blood viscosity, thereby increasing CBF and cerebral oxygen delivery. A vascular osmotic gradient is created by mannitol. Thus fluid moves from the tissues into the blood vessels, reducing the ICP because of the decrease in the total brain fluid content. Monitor fluid and electrolyte status when osmotic diuretics are used.

Mannitol may be contraindicated if renal disease is present and if serum osmolality is elevated.[5]

Hypertonic saline solution is another drug treatment used to manage increased ICP. It produces massive movement of water out of edematous swollen brain cells and into the blood vessels. This movement of water out of the brain can reduce swelling and improve cerebral blood flow. Hypertonic solution infusion requires frequent monitoring of blood pressure and serum sodium levels because intravascular fluid volume excess can occur. Hypertonic saline infusion has been shown to be just as effective as mannitol when treating increased ICP, and both are often used concurrently when caring for a patient with a severe head injury.[9]

Corticosteroids (e.g., dexamethasone [Decadron]) are used to treat vasogenic edema surrounding tumors and abscesses. However, these drugs are not recommended for head-injured patients. Corticosteroids stabilize the cell membrane and inhibit the synthesis of prostaglandins (see Fig. 12-2), thus preventing the formation of proinflammatory mediators. Corticosteroids also improve neuronal function by improving CBF and restoring autoregulation.

Complications associated with the use of corticosteroids include hyperglycemia, increased incidence of infections, and gastrointestinal (GI) bleeding. Regularly monitor fluid intake and sodium levels, and perform blood glucose monitoring at least every 6 hours until hyperglycemia is ruled out. Patients receiving corticosteroids should concurrently be given antacids or histamine (H$_2$)-receptor blockers (e.g., cimetidine [Tagamet], ranitidine [Zantac]) or proton pump inhibitors (e.g., omeprazole [Prilosec], pantoprazole [Protonix, Protonix IV]) to prevent GI ulcers and bleeding.

Metabolic demands such as fever (greater than 100.4° F [38° C]), agitation or shivering, pain, and seizures can also increase ICP. The health care team should plan to reduce these metabolic demands to lower the ICP in the at-risk patient. Monitor patients for seizure activity. They may need to be placed on prophylactic antiseizure medication. Fever should be well controlled to maintain a temperature of 96.8° to 98.6° F (36° to 37° C) by using antipyretics (e.g., acetaminophen), cool baths, cooling blankets, ice packs, or intravascular cooling devices as necessary. However, avoid letting the patient shiver or shake, since this increases the metabolic workload on the brain. If this occurs, sedatives may be needed or a different cooling method selected.

Manage pain while being careful not to oversedate or overmedicate. Finally, the patient should remain in a quiet, calm environment with minimal noise and interruptions. Observe the patient for signs of agitation, irritation, or frustration. Also teach the caregiver and the family about decreasing stimulation, and coordinate with the health care team to minimize procedures that may produce agitation.

Drug therapy for reducing cerebral metabolism may be an effective strategy to control ICP. Reducing the metabolic rate decreases the CBF and therefore the ICP. High doses of barbiturates (e.g., pentobarbital [Nembutal], thiopental [Pentothal]) are used in patients with increased ICP refractory to other treatments. Barbiturates decrease cerebral metabolism, causing a decrease in ICP and a reduction in cerebral edema.[5] When this treatment is used, monitor the patient's ICP, blood flow, and EEG. Barbiturate dosing is typically based on analysis of the bedside EEG tracing and the ICP. The physician orders the barbiturate infusion at a rate that achieves a desired level of brain wave suppression as a means to control ICP. Total *burst suppression,* recognized by the absence of spikes showing brain activity on the EEG monitor, indicates that maximal therapeutic effect has been achieved.[5]

Nutritional Therapy. Patients must have their nutritional needs met, regardless of their state of consciousness. Because malnutrition promotes continued cerebral edema, maintenance of optimal nutrition is imperative. The patient with increased ICP is in a hypermetabolic and hypercatabolic state that increases the need for glucose as fuel for metabolism of the injured brain. If the patient cannot maintain an adequate oral intake, other means of meeting the nutritional requirements, such as enteral feedings or parenteral nutrition, should be initiated.

Early feeding after brain injury may improve patient outcome.[10] Nutritional replacement should begin within 3 days after injury to reach full nutritional replacement within 7 days after the injury is sustained.[10] (Nutritional therapy is discussed in Chapter 40.) Feedings or supplements should be guided by the patient's fluid and electrolyte status and metabolic needs. The patient should remain in a normovolemic fluid state. Continuously evaluate the patient based on clinical factors such as urine output, insensible fluid loss, serum and urine osmolality, and serum electrolytes.

IV 0.9% sodium chloride is the preferred solution for administration of piggyback medications. If 5% dextrose in water or 0.45% sodium chloride is used, serum osmolarity decreases and an increase in cerebral edema may occur.

NURSING MANAGEMENT
INCREASED INTRACRANIAL PRESSURE

NURSING ASSESSMENT

Subjective data about the patient with increased ICP can be obtained from the patient, caregiver, or family who are familiar with the patient. Learn appropriate neurologic assessment techniques. Describe the LOC by noting the specific behaviors observed. When a deviation from the normal state of consciousness occurs, use a more structured method of observation. This type of systematic approach to nursing assessment is illustrated in eFig. 57-1 (available on the website for this chapter). Assess the LOC using the Glasgow Coma Scale (Table 57-5). Also assess body functions, especially circulation and respiration.

GLASGOW COMA SCALE. The Glasgow Coma Scale (GCS) is a quick, practical, and standardized system for assessing the LOC. The three areas assessed in the GCS are the patient's ability to (1) speak, (2) obey commands, and (3) open the eyes when a verbal or painful stimulus is applied. Specific assessments evaluate the patient's response to varying degrees of stimulus. Three indicators of response are evaluated: (1) opening of the eyes, (2) the best verbal response, and (3) the best motor response (see Table 57-5).

Specific behaviors observed as responses to the testing stimulus are given a numeric value. Your responsibility is to elicit the best response on each of the scales: the higher the scores, the higher the level of brain functioning. The subscale scores are particularly important if a patient is untestable in one area. For example, severe periorbital edema may make eye opening impossible.

TABLE 57-5 GLASGOW COMA SCALE

Appropriate Stimulus	Response	Score
Eyes Open		
• Approach to bedside	Spontaneous response.	4
• Verbal command	Opening of eyes to name or command.	3
• Pain	Lack of opening of eyes to previous stimuli but opening to pain.	2
	Lack of opening of eyes to any stimulus.	1
	Untestable.*	U
Best Verbal Response		
• Verbal questioning with maximum arousal	Appropriate orientation, conversant. Correct identification of self, place, yr, and mo.	5
	Confusion. Conversant, but disorientation in one or more spheres.	4
	Inappropriate or disorganized use of words (e.g., cursing), lack of sustained conversation.	3
	Incomprehensible words, sounds (e.g., moaning).	2
	Lack of sound, even with painful stimuli.	1
	Untestable.*	U
Best Motor Response		
• Verbal command (e.g., "raise your arm, hold up two fingers")	Obedience of command.	6
	Localization of pain, lack of obedience but presence of attempts to remove offending stimulus.	5
• Pain (pressure on proximal nail bed)	Flexion withdrawal,* flexion of arm in response to pain without abnormal flexion posture.	4
	Abnormal flexion, flexing of arm at elbow and pronation, making a fist.	3
	Abnormal extension, extension of arm at elbow usually with adduction and internal rotation of arm at shoulder.	2
	Lack of response.	1
	Untestable.*	U

*Added to the original scale by some centers.

The total GCS score is the sum of the numeric values assigned to each of the three areas evaluated. The highest GCS score is 15 for a fully alert person, and the lowest possible score is 3. A GCS score of 8 or less generally indicates coma. Plot the results of the GCS scores on a graph, which can be used to determine whether the patient is stable, improving, or deteriorating.

The GCS offers several advantages in the assessment of the unconscious patient. It allows different health care professionals to arrive at the same conclusion regarding the patient's status and can be used to discriminate between different or changing states.

Although the GCS is the gold standard assessment tool for LOC, other scales are also used in the clinical setting.[11] In cases of stroke or hemorrhage associated with increased ICP, use the NIH Stroke Scale (see Table 58-9). Other components of the neurologic assessment include cranial nerve assessment and motor and sensory testing.

NEUROLOGIC ASSESSMENT. Compare the pupils with one another for size, shape, movement, and reactivity (Fig. 57-11).

Pupils equal and react normally

Pupil reacts to light (slowly or briskly)

Dilated pupil (compressed cranial nerve III)

Bilateral dilated, fixed pupils (ominous sign)

Pinpoint pupils (pons damage or drugs)

FIG. 57-11 Pupillary check for size and response.

Pattern	Location of Lesion	Description
1. Cheyne-Stokes	Bilateral hemispheric disease or metabolic brain dysfunction	Cycles of hyperventilation and apnea
2. Central neurogenic hyperventilation	Brainstem between lower midbrain and upper pons	Sustained, regular rapid and deep breathing
3. Apneustic breathing	Mid or lower pons	Prolonged inspiratory phase or pauses alternating with expiratory pauses
4. Cluster breathing	Medulla or lower pons	Clusters of breaths follow each other with irregular pauses between
5. Ataxic breathing	Reticular formation of the medulla	Completely irregular with some breaths deep and some shallow. Random, irregular pauses, slow rate

FIG. 57-12 Common abnormal respiratory patterns associated with coma.

If the oculomotor nerve (CN III) is compressed, the pupil on the affected side (ipsilateral) becomes larger until it fully dilates. If ICP continues to increase, both pupils dilate.

Test pupillary reaction with a penlight. The normal reaction is brisk constriction when the light is shone directly into the eye. Also note a consensual response (a slight constriction in the opposite pupil) at the same time. A sluggish reaction can indicate early pressure on CN III. A fixed pupil unresponsive to light stimulus usually indicates increased ICP. However, note that there are other causes of a fixed pupil, including direct injury to CN III, previous eye surgery, administration of atropine, and use of mydriatic eyedrops.

Evaluation of other cranial nerves can be included in the neurologic assessment. Eye movements controlled by CN III, IV, and VI can be examined in the patient who is awake and able to follow commands, and can be used to assess the function of the brainstem. Testing the corneal reflex gives information about the functioning of CN V and VII. If this reflex is absent, initiate routine eye care to prevent corneal abrasion (see Chapters 21 and 22).

Eye movements of the uncooperative or unconscious patient can be elicited by reflex with the use of head movements (oculocephalic) and caloric stimulation (oculovestibular) (see Chapters 21 and 22). To test the oculocephalic reflex (doll's eye reflex), turn the patient's head briskly to the left or right while holding the eyelids open. A normal response is movement of the eyes across the midline in the direction opposite that of the turning. Next, quickly flex and then extend the neck. Eye movement should be opposite to the direction of head movement—up when the neck is flexed and down when it is extended. Abnormal responses can help locate the intracranial lesion. This test should not be attempted if a cervical spine problem is suspected. (The oculovestibular reflex is discussed in Chapter 21.)

Test motor strength by asking the awake and cooperative patient to squeeze your hands to compare strength in the hands. The palmar drift test is an excellent measure of strength in the upper extremities. The patient raises the arms in front of the body with the palms facing upward. If there is any weakness in the upper extremity, the palmar surface turns downward and the arm drifts down. Asking the patient to raise the foot from the bed or to bend the knees up in bed is a good assessment of lower extremity strength. Test all four extremities for strength and for any asymmetry in strength or movement.

Assess the motor response of the unconscious or uncooperative patient by observation of spontaneous movement. If no spontaneous movement is possible, apply a pain stimulus to the patient, and note the response. Resistance to movement during passive range-of-motion exercises is another measure of strength. Do not include hand squeezing as part of the assessment of motor movement in the unconscious or uncooperative patient, since this is a reflex action and can misrepresent the patient's status.

Also record the vital signs, including BP, pulse, respiratory rate, and temperature. Be aware of Cushing's triad, which indicates severely increased ICP. Besides recording respiratory rate, also note the respiratory pattern. Specific respiratory patterns are associated with severely increased ICP (Fig. 57-12).

NURSING DIAGNOSES

Nursing diagnoses for the patient with increased ICP include, but are not limited to, the following:

- Decreased intracranial adaptive capacity *related to* decreased cerebral perfusion or increased ICP
- Risk for ineffective cerebral tissue perfusion *related to* reduction of venous and/or arterial blood flow and cerebral edema
- Risk for disuse syndrome *related to* altered LOC, immobility, and altered nutritional intake

Additional information on nursing diagnoses for patients with increased ICP is presented in eNursing Care Plan 57-1 (available on the website for this chapter).

PLANNING

The overall goals for the patient with increased ICP are to (1) maintain a patent airway; (2) have ICP within normal limits; (3) have normal fluid, electrolyte, and nutritional balance; and (4) prevent complications secondary to immobility and decreased LOC.

NURSING IMPLEMENTATION

ACUTE INTERVENTION

Respiratory Function. Maintaining a patent airway is critical in the patient with increased ICP and is a primary nursing responsibility. As the LOC decreases, the patient is at an increased risk of airway obstruction from the tongue dropping back and occluding the airway or from accumulation of secretions.

SAFETY ALERT
- Be alert to altered breathing patterns.
- Snoring sounds indicate obstruction and require immediate intervention.

Remove accumulated secretions by suctioning as needed. An oral airway facilitates breathing and provides an easier suctioning route in the comatose patient. In general, any patient with a GCS of 8 or less or an altered LOC who is unable to maintain a patent airway or effective ventilation needs intubation and mechanical ventilation.

Prevent hypoxia and hypercapnia to minimize secondary injury. Proper positioning of the head is important. Elevation of the head of the bed to 30 degrees enhances respiratory exchange and aids in decreasing cerebral edema. Suctioning and coughing cause transient decreases in the PaO_2 and increases in the ICP. Keep suctioning to a minimum and less than 10 seconds in duration, with administration of 100% oxygen before and after to prevent decreases in the PaO_2. To avoid cumulative increases in the ICP with suctioning, limit suctioning to two passes per suction procedure, if possible. Patients with elevated ICP are at risk for lower CPP during suctioning. CPP must be maintained above 60 mm Hg to preserve cerebral perfusion.

Try to prevent abdominal distention, since it can interfere with respiratory function. Insertion of a nasogastric tube to aspirate the stomach contents can prevent distention, vomiting, and possible aspiration. However, in patients with facial and skull fractures, a nasogastric tube is contraindicated unless a basilar skull fracture (at base of skull) has been ruled out, and oral insertion of a gastric tube is preferred.

Pain, anxiety, and fear related to the primary injury, therapeutic procedures, or noxious stimuli can increase ICP and BP, thus complicating the management and recovery of the brain-injured patient. The appropriate choice or combination of sedatives, paralytics, and analgesics for symptom management presents a challenge to the ICU team. Administration of these agents may alter the neurologic state, thus masking true neurologic changes. It may be necessary to temporarily suspend drug therapy to appropriately assess neurologic status. The choice, dose, and combination of agents may vary depending on the patient's history, neurologic state, and overall clinical presentation.

Opioids, such as morphine sulfate and fentanyl (Sublimaze), are rapid-onset analgesics with minimal effect on CBF or oxygen metabolism. The IV anesthetic sedative propofol (Diprivan) has gained popularity in the management of anxiety and agitation in the ICU because of its rapid onset and short half-life. An accurate neurologic assessment can be performed soon after turning off the infusion of propofol.[5] A side effect of this drug is hypotension.

Dexmedetomidine (Precedex), an α_2-adrenergic agonist, is used for continuous IV sedation of intubated and mechanically ventilated patients in the ICU setting for up to 24 hours. It is another ideal agent for neurologic patients because of the ease in obtaining a neurologic assessment without altering the dose because of its anxiolytic properties. When using continuous IV sedatives, be aware of the side effects of these drugs, especially hypotension, since this can result in a lower CPP value.

Nondepolarizing neuromuscular blocking agents (e.g., vecuronium [Norcuron], cisatracurium besylate [Nimbex]) are useful for achieving complete ventilatory control in the treatment of refractory intracranial hypertension. Because these agents paralyze muscles without blocking pain or noxious stimuli, they are used in combination with sedatives, analgesics, or benzodiazepines.

Benzodiazepines, although useful for sedation, are usually avoided in the management of the patient with increased ICP because of the hypotensive effect and long half-life, unless they are used as an adjunct to neuromuscular blocking agents.

Frequently monitor and evaluate the ABG values, and take measures to maintain the levels within prescribed or acceptable parameters (see Chapter 26). The appropriate ventilatory support can be ordered on the basis of the PaO_2 and $PaCO_2$ values.

Fluid and Electrolyte Balance. Fluid and electrolyte disturbances can have an adverse effect on ICP. Closely monitor IV fluids with the use of an accurate IV infusion control device or pump. Intake and output, with insensible losses and daily weights taken into account, are important parameters in the assessment of fluid balance.

Make electrolyte determinations daily, and discuss any abnormal values with the physician. It is especially important to monitor serum glucose, sodium, potassium, magnesium, and osmolality.

Monitor urine output to detect problems related to diabetes insipidus and SIADH. Diabetes insipidus is caused by a decrease in antidiuretic hormone (ADH). It results in increased urine output and hypernatremia. The usual treatment of diabetes insipidus is fluid replacement, vasopressin (Pitressin), or desmopressin acetate (DDAVP) (see Chapter 50). If it is not treated, severe dehydration will occur.

SIADH is caused by an excess secretion of ADH. SIADH results in decreased urine output and dilutional hyponatremia. It may result in cerebral edema, changes in LOC, seizures, and coma. (Treatment of SIADH is described in Chapter 50.)

Monitoring Intracranial Pressure. ICP monitoring is used in combination with other physiologic parameters to guide the care of the patient and assess the patient's response to treatment. Valsalva maneuver, coughing, sneezing, suctioning, hypoxemia, and arousal from sleep are factors that can increase ICP. Be alert to these factors and attempt to minimize them.

Body Position. Maintain the patient with increased ICP in the head-up position. Take care to prevent extreme neck flexion, which can cause venous obstruction and contribute to elevated ICP. Adjust the body position to decrease the ICP maximally and to improve the CPP. Elevation of the head of the bed promotes drainage from the head and decreases the vascular congestion that can produce cerebral edema. However, raising the head of the bed above 30 degrees may decrease the CPP by lowering systemic BP. Carefully evaluate the effects of elevation of the head of the bed on both the ICP and the CPP. Position the bed so that it lowers the ICP while optimizing the CPP and other indices of cerebral oxygenation.

Take care to turn the patient with slow, gentle movements because rapid changes in position may increase the ICP. Prevent discomfort in turning and positioning the patient because pain or agitation also increases pressure. Increased intrathoracic pressure contributes to increased ICP by impeding the venous return. Thus coughing, straining, and the Valsalva maneuver should be avoided. Avoid extreme hip flexion to decrease the risk of raising the intraabdominal pressure, which increases ICP. Turn the patient at least every 2 hours.

Decorticate or decerebrate posturing is a reflex response in some patients with increased ICP. Turning, skin care, and even passive range of motion can elicit the posturing reflexes. Provide the physical care to minimize complications of immobility, such as atelectasis and contractures.

Protection From Injury. The patient with increased ICP and decreased LOC needs protection from self-injury. Confusion, agitation, and the possibility of seizures increase the risk for injury. Use restraints judiciously in the agitated patient. If restraints are absolutely necessary to keep the patient from removing tubes or falling out of bed, they should be secure enough to be effective, and the skin area under the restraints should be observed regularly for irritation. Agitation may increase with the use of restraints, which indicates the need for other measures to protect the patient from injury. Light sedation with agents such as midazolam (Versed) or lorazepam (Ativan) may be needed. Having a family member stay with the patient may have a calming effect.

For the patient with seizures or the patient at risk for such activity, institute seizure precautions. Seizures are most likely to occur in the first 7 days after traumatic injury, so prophylactic antiseizure therapy is usually used during this time.[12] Additional seizure precautions include padded side rails, an airway at the bedside, suction readily available, accurate and timely administration of antiseizure drugs, and close observation.

The patient can benefit from a quiet, nonstimulating environment. Always use a calm, reassuring approach. Touch and talk to the patient, even one who is in a coma.

Psychologic Considerations. In addition to carefully planned physical care, also be aware of the psychologic well-being of patients and their families. Anxiety over the diagnosis and the prognosis can be distressing to the patient, caregiver and family, and nursing staff. Your competent and assured manner in performing care is reassuring to everyone involved. Short, simple explanations are appropriate and allow the patient and caregiver to acquire the amount of information they desire. There is a need for support, information, and teaching of both patients and families. Assess the family members' desires to assist in providing care for the patient, and allow for their participation as appropriate. Encourage interdisciplinary management (social work, chaplain, etc.) of the patient and family in decision making as much as possible.

EVALUATION

The expected outcomes are that the patient with increased ICP will

- Maintain ICP and cerebral perfusion within normal parameters
- Experience no serious increases in ICP during or after care activities
- Experience no complications of immobility

Additional expected outcomes for the patient with increased ICP are addressed in eNursing Care Plan 57-1 (available on the website for this chapter).

HEAD INJURY

Head injury includes any injury or trauma to the scalp, skull, or brain. A serious form of head injury is *traumatic brain injury* (TBI). Statistics regarding the occurrence of head injuries are incomplete because many victims die at the injury scene or because the condition is considered minor and health care services are not sought. In U.S. hospital emergency departments, an estimated 1.7 million persons are treated and released with TBI. Fifty thousand people die and 275,000 persons are hospitalized with TBI. Of individuals hospitalized, 20% of the patients die.[13] At least 5.3 million Americans (2% of the U.S. population) currently live with disabilities resulting from TBI (*www.braintrauma.org*).

Motor vehicle collisions and falls are the most common causes of head injury. Other causes of head injury include firearms, assaults, sports-related trauma, recreational injuries, and war-related injuries.[14] Males are twice as likely to sustain a TBI as females.

Head trauma has a high potential for a poor outcome. Deaths from head trauma occur at three points after injury: immediately after the injury, within 2 hours after injury, and approximately 3 weeks after injury.[14] Factors that predict a poor outcome include an intracranial hematoma, older age of the patient, abnormal motor responses, impaired or absent eye movements or pupillary light reflexes, early sustained hypotension, hypoxemia or hypercapnia, and sustained ICP levels greater than 20 mm Hg.[15]

The GCS score on arrival at the hospital is also a strong predictor of survival. A GCS below 8 indicates a 30% to 70% chance of survival, and a score above 8 indicates a greater than 90% survival rate. The majority of deaths after a head injury occur immediately after the injury, either from the direct head trauma or from massive hemorrhage and shock. Deaths occurring within a few hours of the trauma are caused by progressive worsening of the head injury or internal bleeding. Immediate recognition of changes in neurologic status and rapid surgical intervention are critical in the prevention of deaths.[5]

Deaths occurring 3 weeks or more after the injury result from multisystem failure. Expert nursing care in the weeks after the injury is crucial in decreasing the mortality risk and in optimizing patient outcomes.

Types of Head Injuries

Scalp Lacerations. *Scalp lacerations* are an easily recognized type of external head trauma. Because the scalp contains many blood vessels with poor constrictive abilities, most scalp lacerations are associated with profuse bleeding. Even relatively small wounds can bleed significantly. The major complications associated with scalp laceration are blood loss and infection.

Skull Fractures. *Skull fractures* frequently occur with head trauma. Skull fractures can be described in several ways: (1) linear or depressed; (2) simple, comminuted, or compound; and (3) closed or open (Table 57-6). Fractures may be closed or open, depending on the presence of a scalp laceration or extension of the fracture into the air sinuses or dura. The type and severity of a skull fracture depend on the velocity, momentum,

TABLE 57-6 TYPES OF SKULL FRACTURES

Type	Description	Cause
Linear	Break in continuity of bone without alteration of relationship of parts	Low-velocity injuries
Depressed	Inward indentation of skull	Powerful blow
Simple	Linear or depressed skull fracture without fragmentation or communicating lacerations	Low to moderate impact
Comminuted	Multiple linear fractures with fragmentation of bone into many pieces	Direct, high-momentum impact
Compound	Depressed skull fracture and scalp laceration with communicating pathway to intracranial cavity	Severe head injury

TABLE 57-7 MANIFESTATIONS OF SKULL FRACTURES

Location	Manifestations
Frontal fracture	Exposure of brain to contaminants through frontal air sinus, possible association with air in forehead tissue, CSF rhinorrhea, or pneumocranium (air between the cranium and the dura mater)
Orbital fracture	Periorbital ecchymosis (raccoon eyes), optic nerve injury
Temporal fracture	Boggy temporal muscle because of extravasation of blood, oval-shaped bruise behind ear in mastoid region (Battle's sign), CSF otorrhea, middle meningeal artery disruption, epidural hematoma
Parietal fracture	Deafness, CSF or brain otorrhea, bulging of tympanic membrane caused by blood or CSF, facial paralysis, loss of taste, Battle's sign
Posterior fossa fracture	Occipital bruising resulting in cortical blindness, visual field defects, rare appearance of ataxia or other cerebellar signs
Basilar skull fracture	CSF or brain otorrhea, bulging of tympanic membrane caused by blood or CSF, Battle's sign, tinnitus or hearing difficulty, rhinorrhea, facial paralysis, conjugate deviation of gaze, vertigo

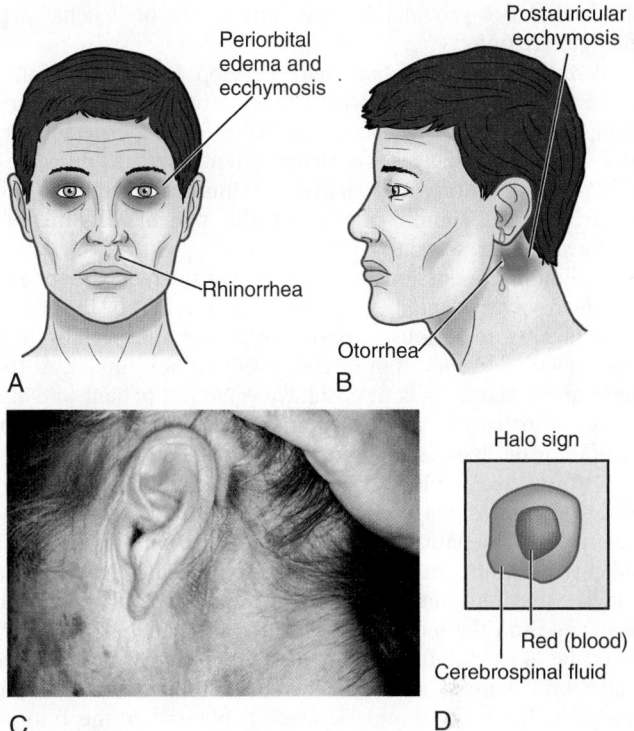

FIG. 57-13 A, Raccoon eyes and rhinorrhea. **B,** Battle's sign (postauricular ecchymosis) with otorrhea. **C,** Battle's sign. **D,** Halo or ring sign (see text).

direction and shape (blunt or sharp) of the injuring agent, and site of impact.

The location of the fracture determines the clinical manifestations (Table 57-7). For example, a basilar skull fracture is a specialized type of linear fracture involving the base of the skull. Manifestations can evolve over the course of several hours; vary with the location and severity of fracture; and may include cranial nerve deficits, Battle's sign (postauricular ecchymosis), and periorbital ecchymosis (raccoon eyes) (Fig. 57-13). This fracture generally is associated with a tear in the dura and subsequent leakage of CSF. *Rhinorrhea* (CSF leakage from the nose) or *otorrhea* (CSF leakage from the ear) generally confirms that the fracture has traversed the dura (see Fig. 57-13). Rhinorrhea may also manifest as postnasal sinus drainage. The significance of rhinorrhea may be overlooked unless the patient is specifically assessed for this finding. The risk of meningitis is high with a CSF leak, and antibiotics should be administered as a preventive measure.

Two methods of testing can be used to determine whether the fluid leaking from the nose or ear is CSF. The first method is to test the leaking fluid with a Dextrostix or Tes-Tape strip to determine whether glucose is present. CSF gives a positive reading for glucose. If blood is present in the fluid, testing for glucose is unreliable because blood also contains glucose. In this event, look for the *halo* or *ring* sign (see Fig. 57-13, *D*). Allow the leaking fluid to drip onto a white gauze pad (4 × 4) or towel, and then observe the drainage. Within a few minutes, the blood coalesces into the center, and a yellowish ring encircles the blood if CSF is present. Note the color, appearance, and amount of leaking fluid because both tests can give false-positive results.

The major potential complications of skull fractures are intracranial infections, hematoma, and meningeal and brain tissue damage. Note that in cases where a basilar skull fracture is suspected, a nasogastric or oral gastric tube should be inserted under fluoroscopy.

Head Trauma. Brain injuries are categorized as diffuse (generalized) or focal (localized). In a *diffuse* injury (e.g., concussion, diffuse axonal injury), damage to the brain cannot be localized to one particular area. In a *focal injury* (e.g., contusion, hematoma), damage can be localized to a specific area of the brain. Brain injury can be classified as *minor* (GCS 13 to 15), *moderate* (GCS 9 to 12), and *severe* (GCS 3 to 8).

Diffuse Injury. Concussion (a sudden transient mechanical head injury with disruption of neural activity and a change in the LOC) is considered a minor diffuse head injury. The patient may or may not lose total consciousness with this injury.

Typical signs of concussion include a brief disruption in LOC, amnesia regarding the event (retrograde amnesia), and headache. The manifestations are generally of short duration. If the patient has not lost consciousness, or if the loss of consciousness lasts less than 5 minutes, the patient is usually discharged from the care facility with instructions to notify the health care provider if symptoms persist or if behavioral changes are noted.

Postconcussion syndrome may develop in some patients, usually anywhere from 2 weeks to 2 months after the injury. Symptoms include persistent headache, lethargy, personality and behavioral changes, shortened attention span, decreased short-term memory, and changes in intellectual ability. This syndrome can significantly affect the patient's abilities to perform activities of daily living.

Although concussion is generally considered benign and usually resolves spontaneously, the symptoms may be the beginning of a more serious, progressive problem, especially in a patient with a history of prior concussion or head injury. At the time of discharge, it is important to give the patient and the caregiver instructions for observation and accurate reporting of symptoms or changes in neurologic status.

Diffuse Axonal Injury. Diffuse axonal injury (DAI) is widespread axonal damage occurring after a mild, moderate, or severe TBI. The damage occurs primarily around axons in the subcortical white matter of the cerebral hemispheres, basal ganglia, thalamus, and brainstem.[16] Initially, DAI was believed to occur from the tensile forces of trauma that sheared axons, resulting in axonal disconnection. There is increasing evidence that axonal damage is not preceded by an immediate tearing of the axon from the traumatic impact, but rather the trauma changes the function of the axon, resulting in axon swelling and disconnection. This process takes approximately 12 to 24 hours to develop and may persist longer.

The clinical signs of DAI are varied, but may include a decreased LOC, increased ICP, decortication or decerebration, and global cerebral edema. Approximately 90% of patients with DAI remain in a persistent vegetative state.[17] Patients with DAI who survive the initial event are rapidly triaged to an ICU, where they will be vigilantly watched for signs of increased ICP and treated accordingly (as previously discussed).

Focal Injury. Focal injury can be minor to severe and can be localized to an area of injury. Focal injury consists of lacerations, contusions, hematomas, and cranial nerve injuries.

Lacerations involve actual tearing of the brain tissue and often occur in association with depressed and open fractures and penetrating injuries. Tissue damage is severe, and surgical repair of the laceration is impossible because of the nature of brain tissue. Medical management consists of antibiotics until meningitis is ruled out, and prevention of secondary injury related to increased ICP. If bleeding is deep into the brain tissue, focal and generalized signs develop.

When major head trauma occurs, many delayed responses are seen, including hemorrhage, hematoma formation, seizures, and cerebral edema. Intracerebral hemorrhage is generally associated with cerebral laceration. This hemorrhage manifests as a space-occupying lesion accompanied by unconsciousness, hemiplegia on the contralateral side, and a dilated pupil on the ipsilateral side. As the hematoma expands, signs of increased ICP become more severe. Prognosis is generally poor for the patient with a large intracerebral hemorrhage. Subarachnoid hemorrhage and intraventricular hemorrhage can also occur secondary to head trauma.

A contusion is bruising of the brain tissue within a focal area. It is usually associated with a closed head injury. A contusion may contain areas of hemorrhage, infarction, necrosis, and edema, and it frequently occurs at a fracture site.

Coup   Contrecoup

Wall   Primary impact   Secondary impact

FIG. 57-14 Coup-contrecoup injury. After the head strikes the wall, a coup injury occurs as the brain strikes the skull (primary impact). The contrecoup injury (the secondary impact) occurs when the brain strikes the skull surface opposite the site of the original impact.

With contusion, the phenomenon of *coup-contrecoup injury* is often noted (Fig. 57-14), and injuries can range from minor to severe. Damage from coup-contrecoup injury occurs when the brain moves inside the skull due to high-energy or high-impact injury mechanisms. Contusions or lacerations occur both at the site of the direct impact of the brain on the skull *(coup)* and at a secondary area of damage on the opposite side away from injury *(contrecoup)*, leading to multiple contused areas. *Contrecoup* injuries tend to be more severe, and overall patient prognosis depends on the amount of bleeding around the contusion site.

Contusions may continue to bleed or rebleed and appear to "blossom" on subsequent CT scans of the brain, which worsens the neurologic outcome. Neurologic assessment may demonstrate focal and generalized manifestation, depending on the contusion's size and location. Seizures are a common complication of brain contusion, especially in the first 7 days after injury.[12] Anticoagulant use and coagulopathy are associated with increased hemorrhage, more severe head injury, and a higher mortality rate.[18] This is especially important when considering older individuals who are taking warfarin (Coumadin) or aspirin at home. If they fall, their contusion is likely to be more severe due to the use of anticoagulants. Thus risk for falls should be assessed (see Table 63-1).

Complications

Epidural Hematoma. An epidural hematoma results from bleeding between the dura and the inner surface of the skull (Figs. 57-15 and 57-16). An epidural hematoma is a neurologic emergency and is usually associated with a linear fracture crossing a major artery in the dura, causing a tear. It can have a venous or an arterial origin. Venous epidural hematomas are associated with a tear of the dural venous sinus and develop slowly. With arterial hematomas, the middle meningeal artery lying under the temporal bone is often torn. Hemorrhage occurs into the epidural space, which lies between the dura and inner surface of the skull (see Fig. 57-15). Because this is an arterial hemorrhage, the hematoma develops rapidly.

Classic signs of an epidural hematoma include an initial period of unconsciousness at the scene, with a brief lucid interval followed by a decrease in LOC. Other manifestations may be a headache, nausea and vomiting, or focal findings. Rapid surgical intervention to evacuate the hematoma and prevent

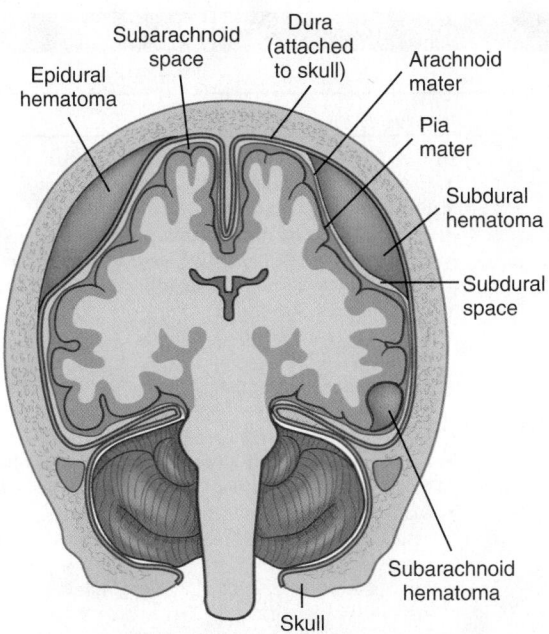

FIG. 57-15 Locations of epidural, subdural, and subarachnoid hematomas.

Epidural hematoma
Subarachnoid space
Dura (attached to skull)
Arachnoid mater
Pia mater
Subdural hematoma
Subdural space
Subarachnoid hematoma
Skull

FIG. 57-16 Epidural hematoma covering a portion of the dura. Multiple small contusions are seen in the temporal lobe.

cerebral herniation, along with medical management for increasing ICP, can dramatically improve outcomes.

Subdural Hematoma. A subdural hematoma occurs from bleeding between the dura mater and the arachnoid layer of the meninges (see Fig. 57-15). A subdural hematoma usually results from injury to the brain tissue and its blood vessels. The veins that drain from the surface of the brain into the sagittal sinus are the source of most subdural hematomas. Because it is usually venous in origin, the subdural hematoma may be slower to develop. However, a subdural hematoma may be caused by an arterial hemorrhage, in which case it develops more rapidly.[19] Subdural hematomas may be acute, subacute, or chronic (Table 57-8).

An *acute subdural hematoma* manifests within 24 to 48 hours of the injury. The signs and symptoms are similar to those associated with brain tissue compression in increased ICP and include decreasing LOC and headache. The size of the hematoma determines the patient's clinical presentation and prognosis. The patient's appearance may range from drowsy and confused to unconscious. The ipsilateral pupil dilates and becomes fixed if ICP is significantly elevated. Blunt force inju-

TABLE 57-8	**TYPES OF SUBDURAL HEMATOMAS**	
Occurrence After Injury	**Progression of Symptoms**	**Treatment**
Acute 24-48 hr after severe trauma.	Immediate deterioration.	Craniotomy, evacuation and decompression.
Subacute 48 hr–2 wk after severe trauma.	Alteration in mental status as hematoma develops. Progression dependent on size and location of hematoma.	Evacuation and decompression.
Chronic Weeks or months, usually >20 days after injury. Often injury seemed trivial or was forgotten by patient.	Nonspecific, nonlocalizing progression. Progressive alteration in LOC.	Evacuation and decompression, membranectomy.

LOC, Level of consciousness.

ries that produce acute subdural hematomas may also cause significant underlying brain injury, resulting in cerebral edema. The resulting increase in ICP from the cerebral edema can cause an increased morbidity and mortality risk despite surgical intervention to evacuate the hematoma.

A *subacute subdural hematoma* usually occurs within 2 to 14 days of the injury. After the initial bleeding, a subdural hematoma may appear to enlarge over time as the breakdown products of the blood draw fluid into the subdural space.

A *chronic subdural hematoma* develops over weeks or months after a seemingly minor head injury. Chronic subdural hematomas are more common in older adults because of a potentially larger subdural space as a result of brain atrophy. With atrophy, the brain remains attached to the supportive structures, but tension is increased, and it is subject to tearing. Because the subdural space is larger, the presenting complaint is focal symptoms, rather than signs of increased ICP.[20] Chronic alcoholics are also prone to cerebral atrophy and subsequent development of subdural hematoma because of an increased incidence of falls.

Diagnosis of a subdural hematoma in the older adult may be delayed because symptoms mimic other health problems in this age-group, such as somnolence, confusion, lethargy, and memory loss. The manifestations of a subdural hematoma are often misinterpreted as vascular disease (stroke, transient ischemic attack [TIA]) and dementia.

Intracerebral Hematoma. Intracerebral hematoma occurs from bleeding within the brain tissue in approximately 16% of head injuries. It usually occurs within the frontal and temporal lobes, possibly from rupture of intracerebral vessels at the time of injury. The size and location of the hematoma are key determinants of the patient's outcome.

Diagnostic Studies and Collaborative Care

CT scan is the best diagnostic test to evaluate for head trauma because it allows rapid diagnosis and intervention in the acute care setting. MRI, PET, and evoked potential studies may also

✚ TABLE 57-9   EMERGENCY MANAGEMENT

Head Injury

Etiology	Assessment Findings	Interventions
Blunt • Motor vehicle collision • Pedestrian event • Fall • Assault • Sports injury **Penetrating** • Gunshot wound • Arrow	**Surface Findings** • Scalp lacerations • Fracture or depressions in skull • Bruises or contusions on face, Battle's sign (bruising behind ears) • Raccoon eyes (dependent bruising around eyes) **Respiratory** • Central neurogenic hyperventilation • Cheyne-Stokes respirations • Decreased O_2 saturation • Pulmonary edema **Central Nervous System** • Unequal or dilated pupils • Asymmetric facial movements • Garbled speech, abusive speech • Confusion • Decreased level of consciousness • Combativeness • Involuntary movements • Seizures • Bowel and bladder incontinence • Flaccidity • Depressed or hyperactive reflexes • Decerebrate or decorticate posturing • GCS score <12 • CSF leaking from ears or nose	**Initial** • Ensure patent airway. • Stabilize cervical spine. • Administer O_2 via non-rebreather mask. • Establish IV access with two large-bore catheters to infuse normal saline or lactated Ringer's solution. • Intubate if GCS score <8. • Control external bleeding with sterile pressure dressing. • Remove patient's clothing. **Ongoing Monitoring** • Maintain patient warmth using blankets, warm IV fluids, overhead warming lights, warm humidified O_2. • Monitor vital signs, level of consciousness, O_2 saturation, cardiac rhythm, GCS score, pupil size and reactivity. • Anticipate need for intubation if gag reflex is impaired or absent. • Assume neck injury with head injury. • Assess for rhinorrhea, otorrhea, scalp wounds. • Administer fluids cautiously to prevent fluid overload and increasing ICP.

GCS, Glasgow Coma Scale, *ICP*, intracranial pressure.

be used in the diagnosis and differentiation of head injuries. An MRI scan is more sensitive than the CT scan in detecting small lesions. Transcranial Doppler studies allow for the measurement of CBF velocity. A cervical spine x-ray series, CT scan, or MRI of the spine may also be indicated, since cervical spine trauma often occurs at the same time as a head injury. In general, the diagnostic studies are similar to those used for a patient with increased ICP (see Table 57-3).

Emergency management of the patient with a head injury is presented in Table 57-9. In addition to measures to prevent secondary injury by treating cerebral edema and managing increased ICP, the principal treatment of head injuries is timely diagnosis and surgery (if necessary). For the patient with concussion and contusion, observation and management of increased ICP are the primary management strategies.

The treatment of skull fractures is usually conservative. For depressed fractures and fractures with loose fragments, a craniotomy is necessary to elevate the depressed bone and remove the free fragments. If large amounts of bone are destroyed, the bone may be removed (craniectomy), and a cranioplasty will be needed later (see the section on cranial surgery later in this chapter).

In cases of large acute subdural and epidural hematomas, or those associated with significant neurologic impairment, the blood must be removed through surgical evacuation. A craniotomy is generally performed to visualize and allow control of the bleeding vessels. Burr-hole openings may be used in an extreme emergency for a more rapid decompression, followed by a craniotomy. A drain may be placed postoperatively for

several days to prevent reaccumulation of blood. In cases where extreme swelling is expected (e.g., DAI, hemorrhage), a craniectomy may be performed, which involves removing a piece of skull to reduce the pressure inside the cranial vault, thus reducing the risk of herniation.

NURSING MANAGEMENT
HEAD INJURY

NURSING ASSESSMENT

A patient with a head injury always has the potential to develop increased ICP. Increased ICP is associated with higher mortality rates and poorer functional outcomes.[6] Objective data are obtained by applying the GCS (see Table 57-5), assessing and monitoring the neurologic status (see eFig. 57-1 on the website for this chapter), and determining whether a CSF leak has occurred. (Nursing assessment related to increased ICP is discussed on pp. 1365-1366.) Nursing assessment of the patient with a head injury is presented in Table 57-10.

NURSING DIAGNOSES

Nursing diagnoses and a potential complication for the patient who has sustained a head injury may include, but are not limited to, the following:

• Risk for ineffective cerebral tissue perfusion *related to* interruption of CBF associated with cerebral hemorrhage, hematoma, and edema
• Hyperthermia *related to* increased metabolism, infection, and hypothalamic injury

TABLE 57-10   NURSING ASSESSMENT

Head Injury

Subjective Data
Important Health Information
Past health history: Mechanism of injury: motor vehicle collision,
   sports injury, industrial incident, assault, falls
Medications: Anticoagulant medications

Functional Health Patterns
Health perception–health management: Alcohol or recreational drugs;
   risk-taking behaviors
Cognitive-perceptual: Headache, mood or behavioral change,
   mentation changes, aphasia, dysphasia, impaired judgment
Coping–stress tolerance: Fear, denial, anger, aggression, depression

Objective Data
General
Altered mental status

Integumentary
Lacerations, contusions, abrasions, hematoma, Battle's sign,
   periorbital edema and ecchymosis, otorrhea, exposed brain matter

Respiratory
Rhinorrhea, impaired gag reflex, inability to maintain a patent airway;
   impending herniation: altered/irregular respiratory rate and pattern

Cardiovascular
Impending herniation: Cushing's triad (systolic hypertension with
   widening pulse pressure, bradycardia with full and bounding pulse,
   irregular respirations)

Gastrointestinal
Vomiting, projectile vomiting, bowel incontinence

Urinary
Bladder incontinence

Reproductive
Uninhibited sexual expression

Neurologic
Altered level of consciousness, seizure activity, pupil dysfunction,
   cranial nerve deficit(s)

Musculoskeletal
Motor deficit/impairment, weakness, palmar drift, paralysis, spasticity,
   decorticate or decerebrate posturing, muscular rigidity or increased
   tone, flaccidity, ataxia

Possible Diagnostic Findings
Location and type of hematoma, edema, skull fracture, and/or foreign
   body on CT scan and/or MRI; abnormal EEG; positive toxicology
   screen or alcohol level, ↓ or ↑ blood glucose level; ↑ ICP

ICP, Intracranial pressure.

- Impaired physical mobility *related to* decreased LOC
- Anxiety *related to* abrupt change in health status, hospital environment, and uncertain future
- Potential complication: increased ICP *related to* cerebral edema and hemorrhage

PLANNING

The overall goals are that the patient with an acute head injury will (1) maintain adequate cerebral oxygenation and perfusion; (2) remain normothermic; (3) achieve control of pain and

ETHICAL/LEGAL DILEMMAS

Brain Death

Situation
The emergency nurse receives a radio call from emergency medical service (EMS) personnel about R.G., a young man involved in a motorcycle crash. He was not wearing a helmet and has a large open skull fracture. Transport from the accident scene was delayed by 45 min as a result of a severe thunderstorm and traffic congestion. On the way to the hospital, R.G. exhibits fixed, dilated pupils and experiences cardiac arrest. Estimated arrival at the hospital is still an additional 45 min as a result of the severe weather. EMS personnel request permission to stop resuscitation efforts.

Ethical/Legal Points for Consideration
- Criteria for brain death include coma or unresponsiveness, absence of brainstem reflexes, and apnea (see Chapter 10).
- The definition of death has changed with the advent of new technology, monitoring devices, and interventions.
- These changes and their effect on the legal diagnosis of death will be accepted by the courts through expert witness testimony.
- Another circumstance that influences the manner in which a state of death is determined is the customary practice or best practice for the specific situation.
- In a situation where the professional responsible for determining a state of death is in remote contact with the patient, but the monitoring devices available provide virtual contact with the patient, a remote diagnosis of death may be legally acceptable.
- Brain death criteria do not address patients in a permanent vegetative state, since the brainstem activity in these patients is adequate to maintain heart and lung function.

Discussion Questions
1. What are your feelings about cessation of brain function vs. cessation of heart and lung function as the criteria for death of a patient?
2. What are your state's laws or practices about stopping cardiopulmonary resuscitation (CPR) efforts by EMS personnel in the field?
3. When brain death has occurred, what is your obligation for education of the family or significant other regarding organ donation?

discomfort; (4) be free from infection; (5) have adequate nutrition; and (6) attain maximal cognitive, motor, and sensory function.

NURSING IMPLEMENTATION

HEALTH PROMOTION. One of the best ways to prevent head injuries is to prevent car and motorcycle collisions. The use of helmets by cyclists has led to fewer TBIs. The use of car seat belts and child car seats is also associated with reduced TBI mortality rates.

Be active in campaigns that promote driving safety, and speak to driver education classes regarding the dangers of unsafe driving and of driving after drinking alcohol and using drugs. Wearing seat belts in cars and helmets for riding on motorcycles is the most effective measure for increasing survival after crashes. Protective helmets should also be worn by lumberjacks, construction workers, miners, horseback riders, bicycle riders, snowboarders, and skydivers. Additionally, individuals who are at risk for falls (e.g., older adults) should be evaluated for safety in the home, since falls are the second leading cause of head injuries.

ACUTE INTERVENTION. Management at the injury scene can have a significant impact on the outcome of the head injury. Emergency management of head injury is presented in Table 57-9. The general goal of nursing management of the head-injured patient is to maintain cerebral oxygenation and perfusion and prevent secondary cerebral ischemia.

Surveillance or monitoring for changes in neurologic status is critically important because the patient's condition may deteriorate rapidly, necessitating emergency surgery. Appropriate preoperative and postoperative nursing interventions are initiated if surgery is anticipated. Because of the close association between hemodynamic status and cerebral perfusion, be aware of any coexisting injuries or conditions.

Explain the need for frequent neurologic assessments to both the patient and the caregiver. Behavioral manifestations associated with head injury can result in a frightened, disoriented patient who is combative and resists help. Your approach should be calm and gentle. A family member may be available to stay with the patient and thus decrease anxiety and fear. One of the most important needs for the caregiver and family members in the acute injury phase is information about the patient's diagnosis, treatment plan, and rationale for the interventions. Other teaching points are presented in Table 57-11.

Perform neurologic assessments at intervals based on the patient's condition. The GCS is useful in assessing the LOC (see Table 57-5). Indications of a deteriorating neurologic state, no matter how subtle, such as a decreasing LOC or decreasing motor strength, should be reported to the health care provider. Monitor the patient's condition closely.[21]

The major focus of nursing care for the brain-injured patient relates to increased ICP (see eNursing Care Plan 57-1). However, some problems may require specific nursing intervention.

Eye problems may include loss of the corneal reflex, periorbital ecchymosis and edema, and diplopia. Loss of the corneal reflex may necessitate administering lubricating eyedrops or taping the eyes shut to prevent abrasion. Periorbital ecchymosis and edema decrease with time, but cold and, later, warm compresses provide comfort and hasten the process. Diplopia can be relieved by use of an eye patch. Consider a consult with an ophthalmologist.

Hyperthermia may occur from injury to or inflammation of the hypothalamus. Elevations in body temperature can result in increased CBF, cerebral blood volume, and ICP. Increased metabolism secondary to hyperthermia increases metabolic waste, which in turn produces further cerebral vasodilation. Avoid hyperthermia with a goal of a temperature of 96.8° to 98.6° F (36° to 37° C) as the standard of care. Use interventions to reduce temperature as previously discussed (see p. 1364) in conjunction with sedation as necessary to prevent shivering.

If CSF rhinorrhea or otorrhea occurs, inform the physician immediately. The head of the bed may be raised to decrease the CSF pressure so that a tear can seal. A loose collection pad may be placed under the nose or over the ear. Do not place a dressing in the nasal or ear cavities. Instruct the patient not to sneeze or blow the nose. Nasogastric tubes should not be used, and nasotracheal suctioning should not be performed on these patients because of the high risk of meningitis.

Nursing measures specific to the care of the immobilized patient, such as those related to bladder and bowel function, skin care, and infection, are also indicated. Nausea and vomiting may be a problem and can be alleviated by antiemetic drugs. Headache can usually be controlled with acetaminophen or small doses of codeine.

If the patient's condition deteriorates, intracranial surgery may be necessary (see the section on cranial surgery later in this chapter). A burr-hole opening or craniotomy may be indicated, depending on the underlying injury that is causing the symptoms. The emergency nature of the surgery may hasten the usual preoperative preparation. Consult with the neurosurgeon to determine specific preoperative nursing measures.

The patient is often unconscious before surgery, making it necessary for a family member to sign the consent form for surgery. This is a difficult and frightening time for the patient's caregiver and family and requires sensitive nursing management. The suddenness of the situation makes it especially difficult for the family to cope.

AMBULATORY AND HOME CARE. Once the condition has stabilized, the patient is usually transferred for acute rehabilitation management. There may be chronic problems related to motor and sensory deficits, communication, memory, and intellectual functioning. Many of the principles of nursing management of the patient with a stroke are appropriate for these patients (see Chapter 58).

Conditions that may require nursing and collaborative management include poor nutritional status, bowel and bladder management, spasticity, dysphagia, deep vein thrombosis, and hydrocephalus. The patient's outward appearance is not a good indicator of how well he or she will ultimately function in the home or work environment. The outward physical appearance does not necessarily reflect what has happened in the brain.

Seizure disorders are seen in approximately 5% of patients with a nonpenetrating head injury. Seizures are most likely to develop during the first week after the head injury,[12] but some patients may not develop a seizure disorder until years later. Antiseizure drugs may be used prophylactically to manage post-traumatic seizure activity.

The mental and emotional sequelae of brain trauma are often the most incapacitating problems. One of the consequences of TBI is that the person may not realize that a brain injury has occurred. Many of the patients with head injuries who have been comatose for more than 6 hours undergo some personality change. They may suffer loss of concentration and

---

TABLE 57-11 PATIENT & CAREGIVER TEACHING GUIDE

Head Injury

Include the following instructions when teaching the patient and caregiver about care during the first 2 or 3 days after a head injury.

1. Notify your health care provider immediately if experiencing signs and symptoms that may indicate complications. These include the following:
   - Increased drowsiness (e.g., difficulty arousing, confusion)
   - Nausea or vomiting
   - Worsening headache or stiff neck
   - Seizures
   - Vision difficulties (e.g., blurring)
   - Behavioral changes (e.g., irritability, anger)
   - Motor problems (e.g., clumsiness, difficulty walking, slurred speech, weakness in arms or legs)
   - Sensory disturbances (e.g., numbness)
   - A heart rate <60 beats/min
2. Have someone stay with you.
3. Abstain from alcohol.
4. Check with your health care provider before taking drugs that may increase drowsiness, including muscle relaxants, tranquilizers, and opioid pain medications.
5. Avoid driving, using heavy machinery, playing contact sports, and taking hot baths.

memory and defective memory processing. Personal drive may decrease. Apathy may increase. Euphoria and mood swings, along with a seeming lack of awareness of the seriousness of the injury, may occur. The patient's behavior may indicate a loss of social restraint, judgment, tact, and emotional control.

Progressive recovery may continue for 6 months or more before a plateau is reached and a prognosis for recovery can be determined. Specific nursing management in the posttraumatic phase depends on specific residual deficits.

In all cases, the family must be given special consideration. They need to understand what is happening and be taught appropriate interaction patterns. Provide guidance and referrals for financial aid, child care, and other personal needs. Assist the family in involving the patient in family activities whenever possible. Help the patient and the family remain hopeful. The family often has unrealistic expectations of the patient as the coma begins to recede. The family expects full return to pretrauma status. In reality, the patient usually experiences a reduced awareness and ability to interpret environmental stimuli. Prepare the family for the patient's emergence from coma and explain that the process of awakening often takes several weeks. Arrange for social work and chaplain consultations for the family in addition to providing open visitation and frequent status updates.

When it is the time for discharge planning, the patient, caregiver, and family may benefit from specific posthospitalization instructions to avoid family-patient friction. Special "no" policies that may be appropriately suggested by the neurosurgeon, neuropsychologist, and nurse include no drinking of alcoholic beverages, no driving, no use of firearms, no working with hazardous implements and machinery, and no unsupervised smoking. Family members, particularly spouses, go through role transition as the role changes from that of spouse to that of caregiver. (The stresses and needs of family caregivers are discussed in Chapter 4.)

▌EVALUATION

The expected outcomes are that the patient with a head injury will

- Maintain normal CPP
- Achieve maximal cognitive, motor, and sensory function
- Experience no infection or hyperthermia

BRAIN TUMORS

The annual rate of newly diagnosed brain tumors in the United States is 22,910, with an estimated 13,700 deaths related to brain tumors. The brain is also a frequent site for metastasis from other sites. The 5-year survival rate for primary site brain tumors is approximately 36%.[22] Males have a slightly higher incidence of brain tumors than females. Brain tumors are more commonly seen in middle-aged persons, but they may occur at any age.

Types

Brain tumors can occur in any part of the brain or spinal cord. Tumors of the brain may be *primary,* arising from tissues within the brain, or *secondary,* resulting from a metastasis from a malignant neoplasm elsewhere in the body.[23] Metastatic brain tumors are the most common brain tumor. The cancers that most commonly metastasize to the brain are lung and breast.

Primary brain tumors are generally classified according to the tissue from which they arise (Table 57-12). Meningiomas represent 34% of all primary brain tumors, making them the most common primary brain tumor. Gliomas (e.g., astrocytoma, glioblastoma multiforme) account for 30% of all brain tumors and 80% of all malignant tumors. Glioblastoma multiforme is the most common form of glioma.

⊕ **CULTURAL & ETHNIC HEALTH DISPARITIES**

Brain Tumors

- Whites have a higher incidence of malignant brain tumors than African Americans.
- White males have the highest incidence of malignant brain tumors.
- African Americans have a higher incidence of benign brain tumors (e.g., meningiomas) than whites.

TABLE 57-12 TYPES OF BRAIN TUMORS

Type	Tissue of Origin	Characteristics
Gliomas		
• Astrocytoma	Supportive tissue, glial cells, and astrocytes	Can range from low-grade to moderate-grade malignancy.
• Glioblastoma multiforme	Primitive stem cell (glioblast)	Highly malignant and invasive. Among the most devastating of primary brain tumors.
• Oligodendroglioma	Oligodendrocytes	Benign (encapsulation and calcification).
• Ependymoma	Ependymal epithelium	Range from benign to highly malignant. Most are benign and encapsulated.
• Medulloblastoma	Primitive neuroectodermal cell	Highly malignant and invasive. Metastatic to spinal cord and remote areas of brain.
Meningioma	Meninges	Can be benign or malignant. Most are benign.
Acoustic neuroma (Schwannoma)	Cells that form myelin sheath around nerves Commonly affects cranial nerve VIII	Many grow on both sides of the brain. Usually benign or low-grade malignancy.
Pituitary adenoma	Pituitary gland	Usually benign.
Hemangioblastoma	Blood vessels of brain	Rare and benign. Surgery is curative.
Primary central nervous system lymphoma	Lymphocytes	Increased incidence in transplant recipients and acquired immunodeficiency syndrome (AIDS) patients.
Metastatic tumors	Lungs, breast	Malignant.

FIG. 57-17 A, A large glioblastoma *(G)* arises from one cerebral hemisphere and has grown to fill the ventricular system. **B,** Meningioma. These two different sections from different levels in the same brain show a meningioma *(M)* compressing the frontal lobe and distorting underlying brain.

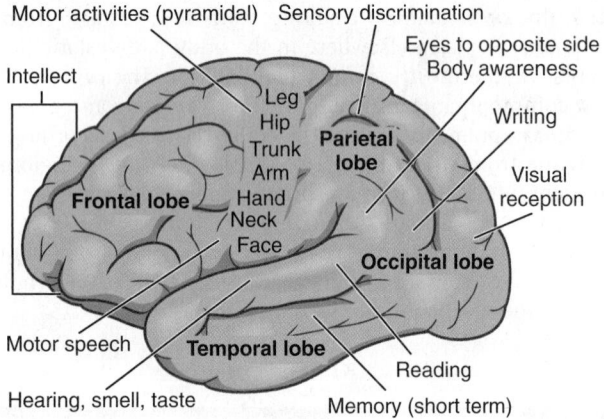

FIG. 57-18 Each area of the brain controls a particular activity.

TABLE 57-13	MANIFESTATIONS OF BRAIN TUMORS
Tumor Location	**Manifestations**
Cerebral hemisphere	
• Frontal lobe (unilateral)	Unilateral hemiplegia, seizures, memory deficit, personality and judgment changes, visual disturbances.
• Frontal lobe (bilateral)	Symptoms associated with unilateral frontal lobe tumors. Ataxic gait.
• Parietal lobe	Speech disturbance (if tumor is in the dominant hemisphere), inability to write, spatial disorders, unilateral neglect.
• Occipital lobe	Vision disturbances and seizures.
• Temporal lobe	Few symptoms. Seizures, dysphagia.
Subcortical	Hemiplegia. Other symptoms may depend on area of infiltration.
Meningeal tumors	Symptoms associated with compression of the brain and depend on tumor location.
Metastatic tumors	Headache, nausea, or vomiting because of ↑ ICP. Other symptoms depend on tumor location.
Thalamus and sellar tumors	Headache, nausea, vision disturbances, papilledema, and nystagmus occur from ↑ ICP. Diabetes insipidus may occur.
Fourth ventricle and cerebellar tumors	Headache, nausea, and papilledema from ↑ ICP. Ataxic gait and changes in coordination.
Cerebellopontine tumors	Tinnitus and vertigo, deafness.
Brainstem tumors	Headache on awakening, drowsiness, vomiting, ataxic gait, facial muscle weakness, hearing loss, dysphagia, dysarthria, "crossed eyes" or other visual changes, hemiparesis.

ICP, Intracranial pressure.

More than half of brain tumors are malignant. They infiltrate the brain tissue and are not amenable to complete surgical removal. Other tumors may be histologically benign but are located such that complete removal is not possible.

Brain tumors rarely metastasize outside the central nervous system (CNS) because they are contained by structural (meninges) and physiologic (blood-brain) barriers. Table 57-12 compares the most common brain tumors. A glioblastoma and meningioma are shown in Fig. 57-17.

Clinical Manifestations and Complications

The clinical manifestations of brain tumors depend mainly on their location and size (Table 57-13). The rate of growth and the appearance of manifestations depend on the location, size, and mitotic rate of the cells of the tissue of origin. Fig. 57-18 illustrates the functional areas of the cerebral cortex and can be used as a guide to correlate the clinical manifestations with the location of the tumor, as indicated by an alteration in the function controlled by the affected area.

Wide ranges of possible clinical manifestations are associated with brain tumors. Headache is a common problem. Tumor-related headaches tend to be worse at night and may awaken the patient. The headaches are usually dull and constant but occasionally throbbing. Seizures are common in gliomas and brain metastases. Brain tumors can cause nausea and vomiting from increased ICP. Cognitive dysfunction, including memory problems and mood or personality changes, is another common manifestation, especially in patients with brain metastases. Muscle weakness, sensory losses, aphasia, and visual-spatial dysfunction are also manifestations of brain tumors.

If the tumor mass obstructs the ventricles or occludes the outlet, ventricular enlargement (hydrocephalus) can occur. As the brain tumor expands, it may also produce manifestations of increased ICP, cerebral edema, or obstruction of the CSF pathways. Unless treated, all brain tumors eventually cause death from increasing tumor volume leading to increased ICP.

Diagnostic Studies

An extensive history and a comprehensive neurologic examination must be done in the workup of a patient with a suspected brain tumor. A careful history and physical examination may provide data with respect to location. New onset of seizures or adult-onset migraines may be indicative of a brain tumor and should be investigated. Diagnostic studies are similar to those used for a patient with increased ICP (see Table 57-3).

The sensitivity of techniques such as MRI and PET scans allows for detection of small tumors and may provide more reliable diagnostic information than a CT scan. CT and brain scanning are used to identify the lesion's location. Other tests include magnetic resonance spectroscopy, functional MRI, and single-photon emission computed tomography (SPECT). The EEG is useful for ruling out seizures, but is of less importance. A lumbar puncture is seldom diagnostic and carries with it the risk of cerebral herniation. Angiography can be used to determine blood flow to the tumor and further localize the tumor. Other studies are done to rule out a primary lesion elsewhere in the body. Endocrine studies are helpful when a pituitary adenoma is suspected (see Chapter 50).

The correct diagnosis of a brain tumor can be made by obtaining tissue for histologic study. In most patients, tissue is obtained at the time of surgery. Computer-guided stereotactic biopsy is also an option. A smear or frozen section can be performed in the operating room for a preliminary interpretation of the histologic type. With this information, the neurosurgeon can make a better decision about the extent of surgery. In some cases, immunohistochemical stains or electron microscopy may be necessary to ascertain the correct diagnosis. Determination of the MIB-1 index, a measure of mitotic rate, is often helpful in assessing the tumor's mitotic activity.

Collaborative Care

Treatment goals are aimed at (1) identifying the tumor type and location, (2) removing or decreasing tumor mass, and (3) preventing or managing increased ICP.

Surgical Therapy. Surgical removal is the preferred treatment for brain tumors (see the section on cranial surgery later in this chapter). Stereotactic surgical techniques are used with greater frequency to perform a biopsy and remove small brain tumors. The outcome of surgical therapy depends on the tumor's type, size, and location. Meningiomas and oligodendrogliomas can usually be completely removed, whereas the more invasive gliomas and medulloblastomas may only be partially removed. Computer-guided stereotactic biopsy, ultrasound, functional MRI, and cortical mapping can be used to localize brain tumors intraoperatively.

Complete surgical removal of brain tumors is not always possible because the tumor is not always accessible or may involve vital parts of the brain. Surgery can reduce tumor mass, which decreases ICP, provides relief of symptoms, and extends survival time.

Ventricular Shunts. Hydrocephalus can be treated with the placement of a ventricular shunt. A catheter with one-way valves is placed in the lateral ventricle and then tunneled through the skin to drain CSF into the jugular vein, peritoneum, or pelvis. Rapid decompression of ICP can cause total body collapse and weakness, including a headache that may be prevented by gradually introducing the patient to the upright position.

Manifestations of shunt malfunction, which are related to increased ICP, include decreasing LOC, restlessness, headache, blurred vision, or vomiting. This may necessitate shunt revision or replacement. Infection may also occur, as exhibited by high fever, persistent headache, and stiff neck. Antibiotics are used to treat the infection. In some situations the shunt must be replaced.

Radiation Therapy and Stereotactic Radiosurgery. Radiation therapy may be used as a follow-up measure after surgery. Radiation seeds can also be implanted into the brain. Cerebral edema and rapidly increasing ICP may be a complication of radiation therapy, but these problems can be managed with high doses of corticosteroids (dexamethasone, prednisone, or methylprednisolone [Solu-Medrol]). (Radiation therapy is discussed in Chapter 16.)

Stereotactic radiosurgery is a method of delivering a highly concentrated dose of radiation to a precise location within the brain. Stereotactic radiosurgery may be used when conventional surgery has failed or is not an option because of the tumor location. (Radiosurgery is discussed on p. 1379.)

Chemotherapy and Targeted Therapy. The effectiveness of chemotherapy has been limited by difficulty getting drugs across the blood-brain barrier, tumor cell heterogeneity, and tumor cell drug resistance. Chemotherapy drugs called nitrosoureas (e.g., carmustine [BCNU], lomustine [CCNU]) are used to treat brain tumors. Normally the blood-brain barrier prohibits the entry of most drugs into the brain. The most malignant tumors cause a breakdown of the blood-brain barrier in the area of the tumor, thus allowing chemotherapy agents to be used to treat the malignancy. Chemotherapy-laden biodegradable wafers (e.g., Gliadel wafer [polifeprosan with carmustine implant]) implanted at the time of surgery can deliver chemotherapy directly to the tumor site. Other drugs being used include methotrexate and procarbazine (Matulane). One method used to deliver chemotherapy drugs directly to the CNS is intrathecal administration via an Ommaya reservoir.

Temozolomide (Temodar) is the first oral chemotherapy agent found to cross the blood-brain barrier. In contrast with many traditional chemotherapy drugs, which require metabolic activation to exert their effects, temozolomide can convert spontaneously to a reactive agent that directly interferes with tumor growth. It does not interact with other drugs commonly taken by patients with brain tumors, such as antiseizure medications, corticosteroids, and antiemetics.

DRUG ALERT: Temozolomide (Temodar)
- Causes myelosuppression. Before using, it is recommended that absolute neutrophil count be ≥1500/µL and platelet count be ≥100,000/µL.
- To reduce nausea and vomiting, take on empty stomach.

Bevacizumab (Avastin) is used to treat patients with glioblastoma multiforme that continues to progress after standard therapy. Bevacizumab is a targeted therapy that inhibits the action of vascular endothelial growth factor, which helps form new blood vessels. These vessels can feed a tumor, helping it to grow, and can also provide a pathway for cancer cells to circulate in the body. (Targeted therapy is discussed in Chapter 16 and Table 16-13.)

Other Therapies. A medical device system, NovoTTF-100A System, is used to treat glioblastoma multiforme that recurs or progresses after receiving chemotherapy and radiation therapy. With this system, electrodes are placed on the surface of the patient's scalp to deliver low-intensity, changing electrical fields called *tumor treatment fields* (TTFs) to the tumor site.

Many techniques to control and treat brain tumors are currently under investigation. Although progress in treatment has increased length and quality of life for patients with brain tumors, outcomes still remain poor for patients with gliomas.[24]

NURSING MANAGEMENT
BRAIN TUMORS

NURSING ASSESSMENT

Structure the initial assessment to provide baseline data of the patient's neurologic status. Use this information to design a realistic, individualized care plan. Assess the patient's LOC, motor abilities, sensory perception, integrated function (including bowel and bladder function), and balance and proprioception, and also assess the coping abilities of the patient, caregiver, and family. Watching a patient perform activities of daily living and listening to the patient's conversation can be part of the neurologic assessment. Having the patient or caregiver explain the problem can be helpful to determine the patient's limitations and obtain information about the patient's insight into the problems. Record all initial data to provide a baseline for comparison to determine whether the patient's condition is improving or deteriorating.

Interview data are as important as the actual physical assessment. Ask questions about the medical history, intellectual abilities and educational level, and history of nervous system infections and trauma. Determine the presence of seizures, syncope, nausea and vomiting, and headaches or other pain to help better plan care for the patient.

NURSING DIAGNOSES

Nursing diagnoses for the patient with a brain tumor may include, but are not limited to, the following:

- Risk for ineffective cerebral tissue perfusion *related to* cerebral edema
- Acute pain (headache) *related to* cerebral edema and increased ICP
- Anxiety *related to* diagnosis and treatment
- Potential complication: seizures *related to* abnormal electrical activity of the brain
- Potential complication: increased ICP *related to* tumor and failure of normal compensatory mechanisms

PLANNING

The overall goals are that the patient with a brain tumor will (1) maintain normal ICP, (2) maximize neurologic functioning, (3) achieve control of pain and discomfort, and (4) be aware of the long-term implications with respect to prognosis and cognitive and physical functioning.

NURSING IMPLEMENTATION

A primary or metastatic tumor of the frontal lobe can cause behavioral and personality changes. Loss of emotional control, confusion, disorientation, memory loss, impulsivity, and depression may be signs of a frontal lobe lesion. These behavioral changes are often not perceived by the patient but can be disturbing and even frightening to the caregiver and family. These changes can also cause a distancing to occur between the family and patient. Assist the caregiver and family in understanding what is happening to the patient, and support the family.

The confused patient with behavioral instability can be a challenge. Protecting the patient from self-harm is an important part of nursing care. Close supervision of activity, use of side rails, judicious use of restraints, appropriate sedative medications, padding of the rails and the area around the bed, and a calm reassuring approach are all essential techniques in the care of these patients.

Perceptual problems associated with frontal and parietal lobe tumors contribute to a patient's disorientation and confusion. Minimize environmental stimuli, create a routine, and use reality orientation for the confused patient.

Seizures, which often occur with brain tumors, are managed with antiseizure drugs. Also use seizure precautions for the patient's protection. Some behavioral changes seen in the patient with a brain tumor are a result of seizure disorders and can improve with adequate seizure control. Patients at risk for seizures may be unable to drive, so be aware of the extra resources needed and collaborate with the social worker and the family. (Seizure disorders are discussed in Chapter 59.)

Motor and sensory dysfunctions interfere with the activities of daily living.[25] Alterations in mobility must be managed. Encourage the patient to provide as much self-care as physically possible. Self-image often depends on the patient's ability to participate in care within the limitations of the physical deficits.

Language deficits can also occur in patients with brain tumors. Motor (expressive) or sensory (receptive) dysphasia may occur. The disturbance in communication can be frustrating for the patient and may interfere with your ability to meet the patient's needs. Make attempts to establish a communication system that can be used by both the patient and the staff.

Nutritional intake may be decreased because of the patient's inability to eat, loss of appetite, or loss of desire to eat. Assess the patient's nutritional status, and ensure adequate nutritional intake. Encourage the patient to eat. Some patients may need enteral or parenteral nutrition (see Chapter 40). The patient with a brain tumor who undergoes cranial surgery requires complex nursing care. This is discussed in the next section.

Although progress is continually being made in helping patients with brain tumors, the prognosis remains grim for those with highly invasive tumors.[24] Provide help and support during the adjustment phase and in long-range planning. Social work and home health nurses may be needed to assist the caregiver with discharge planning and to help the family adjust to role changes and psychosocial and socioeconomic factors. Issues related to palliative and end-of-life care need to be discussed with both the patient and the family (see Chapter 10).

EVALUATION

The expected outcomes are that the patient with a brain tumor will

- Achieve control of pain, vomiting, and other discomforts
- Maintain ICP within normal limits
- Demonstrate maximal neurologic function (cognitive, motor, sensory) given the location and extent of the tumor
- Maintain optimal nutritional status
- Accept the long-term consequences of the tumor and its treatment

TABLE 57-14   INDICATIONS FOR CRANIAL SURGERY

Indication	Cause	Surgical Procedure
Brain abscess	Bacteria that caused intracranial infection	Excision or drainage of abscess
Hydrocephalus	Overproduction of CSF, obstruction to flow, defective reabsorption	Placement of ventriculoatrial or ventriculoperitoneal shunt
Brain tumors	Benign or malignant cell growth	Excision or partial resection of tumor
Intracranial bleeding	Rupture of cerebral vessels because of trauma or stroke	Surgical evacuation through burr holes or craniotomy
Skull fractures	Trauma to skull	Debridement of fragments and necrotic tissue, elevation and realignment of bone fragments
Arteriovenous (AV) malformation	Congenital tangle of arteries and veins (frequently in middle cerebral artery)	Excision of malformation
Aneurysm repair	Dilation of weak area in arterial wall (usually near anterior portion of circle of Willis)	Dissection and clipping or coiling of aneurysm

CSF, Cerebrospinal fluid.

TABLE 57-15   TYPES OF CRANIAL SURGERY

Type	Description
Burr hole	Opening into the cranium with a drill. Used to remove localized fluid and blood beneath the dura.
Craniotomy	Opening into cranium with removal of bone flap and opening the dura to remove a lesion, repair a damaged area, drain blood, or relieve ↑ ICP.
Craniectomy	Excision into the cranium to cut away bone flap.
Cranioplasty	Repair of cranial defect resulting from trauma, malformation, or previous surgical procedure. Artificial material used to replace damaged or lost bone.
Stereotactic procedure	Precise localization of a specific area of the brain using a frame or a frameless system based on three-dimensional coordinates. Procedure is used for biopsy, radiosurgery, or dissection.
Shunt procedures	Alternate pathway to redirect cerebrospinal fluid from one area to another using a tube or implanted device. Examples include ventricular shunt and Ommaya reservoir.

ICP, Intracranial pressure.

CRANIAL SURGERY

The indication for cranial surgery may be related to a brain tumor, CNS infection (e.g., abscess), vascular abnormalities, craniocerebral trauma, seizure disorder, or intractable pain (Table 57-14).

Types

Various types of cranial surgical procedures are presented in Table 57-15.

Craniotomy. Depending on the location of the pathologic condition, a *craniotomy* may be frontal, parietal, occipital, temporal, suboccipital, or a combination of any of these. The surgeon drills a set of burr holes and uses a saw to connect the holes to remove the bone flap. Sometimes operating microscopes are used to magnify the site. After surgery, the bone flap is wired or sutured. Sometimes drains are placed to remove fluid and blood. Patients are usually cared for in an ICU until stable.

Stereotactic Radiosurgery. Stereotactic procedures use precision apparatus (often computer guided) to help the physician precisely target an area of the brain. Stereotactic biopsy can be performed to obtain tissue samples for histologic examination. CT scanning and MRI are used to image the targeted tissue.

With the patient under general or local anesthesia, the surgeon drills a burr hole or creates a bone flap for an entry site and then introduces a probe and biopsy needle. Stereotactic procedures are used for removal of small brain tumors and abscesses, drainage of hematomas, ablative procedures for extrapyramidal diseases (e.g., Parkinson's disease), and repair of arteriovenous malformations. A major advantage of the stereotactic approach is a reduction in damage to surrounding tissue.

Stereotactic radiosurgery is not a form of surgery in the traditional sense. Instead, radiosurgery uses precisely focused radiation to destroy tumor cells and other abnormal growths in the brain. Computers create three-dimensional images of the brain, and these images are used to guide the focused radiation while the patient's head is held still in a stereotactic frame (Fig. 57-19). Radiosurgical techniques can use ionizing radiation generated by a linear accelerator, gamma knife, or CyberKnife. In these procedures, a high dose of cobalt radiation is delivered to precisely targeted tumor tissue. The dose of radiation is delivered in a single treatment lasting a few hours or in multiple sessions. Side effects of stereotactic radiosurgery may include fatigue, headache, and nausea.

In combination with stereotactic procedures to identify and localize tumor sites, surgical lasers can be used to destroy tumors. Three surgical lasers currently used are the carbon dioxide, argon, and neodymium:yttrium-aluminum-garnet (Nd:YAG) lasers. All three work by creating thermal energy, which destroys the tissue on which it is focused. Laser therapy also provides the benefit of reducing damage to surrounding tissue.

NURSING MANAGEMENT
CRANIAL SURGERY

NURSING IMPLEMENTATION

ACUTE INTERVENTION. The general preoperative and postoperative nursing care for the patient undergoing cranial surgery is similar regardless of the cause. Nursing management is similar to that for the patient with increased ICP (presented in eNursing Care Plan 57-1). The patient (if conscious and coherent), caregiver, and family will be concerned about the potential physical and emotional problems that can result from surgery. The uncertainty regarding prognosis and outcome requires compassionate nursing care in the preoperative period.

Preoperative teaching is important in allaying the fears of the patient, caregiver, and family, and also in preparing them for the postoperative period. Provide general information concerning the type of operation that will be performed and what can

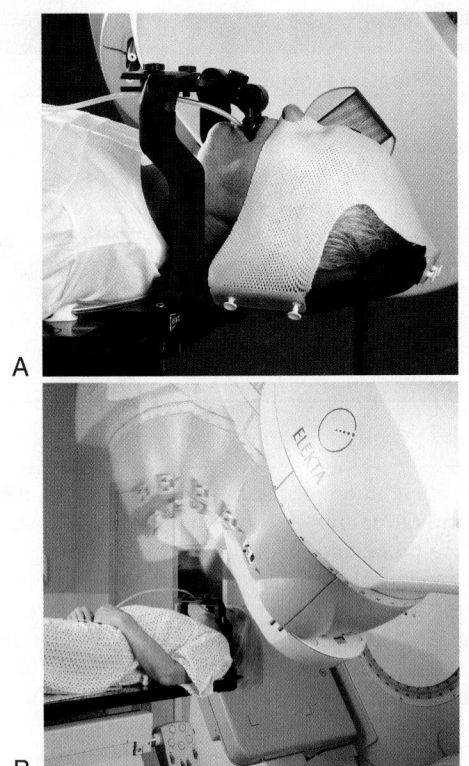

FIG. 57-19 **A,** Patient in a stereotactic frame. **B,** Elekta's Fraxion head frame helps ensure accuracy and precision in stereotactic radiation therapy (SRT) of cancer targets in the brain and cranium. (Courtesy Elekta.)

be expected immediately after the operation. Explain that some hair may be shaved to allow for better exposure and to prevent contamination. The hair is usually removed in the operating room after induction of anesthesia. Also inform the family that the patient will be taken to an ICU or to a special care unit after surgery. The primary goal of care after cranial surgery is prevention of increased ICP. (Nursing management of the patient with increased ICP is presented on pp. 1356-1368.) Frequent assessment of the patient's neurologic status is essential during the first 48 hours. In addition to the neurologic functions, closely monitor fluid and electrolyte levels and serum osmolality to detect changes in sodium regulation, the onset of diabetes insipidus, or severe hypovolemia. Turning and positioning the patient may depend on the site of the operation.

Monitor the patient for pain and nausea. Although the brain itself does not possess pain receptors, patients often report headache caused by edema or pain at the incision site. Control pain with short-acting opioids and monitor neurologic status. Nausea and vomiting are common after surgery and are usually treated with antiemetics. The use of promethazine (Phenergan) is discouraged because it can increase somnolence, thus altering the accuracy of a neurologic assessment.

The surgical dressing is usually in place for a few days. With an incision over the skull in the anterior or middle fossa, the patient will return from the operating room with the head elevated at an angle of 30 to 45 degrees. The head of the bed should remain elevated at least 30 degrees unless the surgical approach is in the posterior fossa or a burr hole has been made. In these cases, the patient is generally kept flat or at a slight elevation (10 to 15 degrees) during the postoperative phase.

If a bone flap has been removed (craniectomy), do not position the patient on the operative side. Observe the dressing for color, odor, and amount of drainage. Notify the surgeon immediately of any excessive bleeding or clear drainage. Checking drains for placement and assessing the area around the dressing are also important. Scalp care should include meticulous care of the incision to prevent wound infection. Cleanse the area and treat it in accordance with hospital protocol or the neurosurgeon's orders. Once the dressing is removed, use an antiseptic soap for washing the scalp. The psychologic impact of hair removal can be alleviated by the use of a wig, turban, scarves, or cap after the incision has completely healed. For the patient who is receiving radiation, instruct the patient to use a sunblock and head covering if any exposure to the sun is anticipated.

AMBULATORY AND HOME CARE. The rehabilitative potential for a patient after cranial surgery depends on the reason for the surgery, the postoperative course, and the patient's general state of health. Base your nursing interventions on a realistic appraisal of these factors. An overall goal is to foster independence for as long as possible and to the highest degree possible.

Specific rehabilitation potential cannot be determined until cerebral edema and increased ICP subside postoperatively. Take care to maintain as much function as possible through measures such as careful positioning, meticulous skin and mouth care, regular range-of-motion exercises, bowel and bladder care, and adequate nutrition.

Referrals may be made to other specialists on the health care team. For example, the speech therapist may be helpful to the patient who has a speech problem, or the physical therapist may

TABLE 57-16 COMPARISON OF CEREBRAL INFLAMMATORY CONDITIONS

	Meningitis	Encephalitis	Brain Abscess
Cause	Bacteria (*Streptococcus pneumoniae, Neisseria meningitidis*, group B streptococci, viruses, fungi)	Bacteria, fungi, parasites, herpes simplex virus (HSV), other viruses (e.g., West Nile virus)	Streptococci, staphylococci through bloodstream
CSF (Reference Interval)			
• Pressure (70-150 mm H$_2$O)	Increased	Normal to slight increase	Increased
• WBC count (0-5 cells/µL)	*Bacterial:* >1000/µL (mainly neutrophils) *Viral:* 25-500/µL (mainly lymphocytes)	500/µL, neutrophils (early), lymphocytes (later)	25-300/µL (neutrophils)
• Protein (15-45 mg/dL [0.15-0.45 g/L])	*Bacterial:* >500 mg/dL *Viral:* 50-500 mg/dL	Slight increase	Normal
• Glucose (40-70 mg/dL [2.2-3.9 mmol/L])	*Bacterial:* Decreased *Viral:* Normal or low	Normal	Low or absent
• Appearance	*Bacterial:* Turbid, cloudy *Viral:* Clear or cloudy	Clear	Clear
Diagnostic Studies	CT scan, Gram stain, smear, culture, PCR*	CT scan, EEG, MRI, PET, PCR, IgM antibodies to virus in serum or CSF	CT scan
Treatment	Antibiotics, dexamethasone, supportive care, prevention of ↑ ICP	Supportive care, prevention of ↑ ICP, acyclovir (Zovirax) for HSV	Antibiotics, incision and drainage Supportive care

*PCR is used to detect viral RNA or DNA.
CSF, Cerebrospinal fluid; *ICP,* intracranial pressure; *PCR,* polymerase chain reaction.

provide an exercise plan to regain functional deficits. Address the needs and problems of each patient individually because many variables affect the plan. The patient's mental and physical deterioration, including seizures, personality disorganization, apathy, and wasting, is difficult for both family and health care professionals to watch. Cognitive and emotional residual deficits are often harder to accept than are motor and sensory losses.

INFLAMMATORY CONDITIONS OF THE BRAIN

Brain abscesses, meningitis, and encephalitis are the most common inflammatory conditions of the brain and spinal cord (Table 57-16). Inflammation can be caused by bacteria, viruses, fungi, and chemicals (e.g., contrast media used in diagnostic tests, blood in the subarachnoid space). CNS infections may occur via the bloodstream, by extension from a primary site, or along cranial and spinal nerves.

The mortality rate for inflammatory conditions of the brain is approximately 2% to 30% in the general population, with higher rates in older patients. Up to 40% of those who recover can have long-term neurologic deficits, including hearing loss.[26]

BRAIN ABSCESS

Brain abscess is an accumulation of pus within the brain tissue that can result from a local or systemic infection. Direct extension from an ear, tooth, mastoid, or sinus infection is the primary cause. Other causes for brain abscess formation include spread from a distant site (e.g., pulmonary infection, bacterial endocarditis), skull fracture, and prior brain trauma or surgery. Streptococci and *Staphylococcus aureus* are the primary infective organisms.

Manifestations of brain abscess, which are similar to those of meningitis and encephalitis, include headache, fever, and nausea and vomiting. Signs of increased ICP may include drowsiness, confusion, and seizures. Focal symptoms may reflect the local area of the abscess. For example, visual field defects or psychomotor seizures are common with a temporal lobe abscess, whereas an occipital abscess may be accompanied by visual impairment and hallucinations. CT and MRI are used to diagnose a brain abscess.

Antimicrobial therapy is the primary treatment for brain abscess. Other manifestations are treated symptomatically. If drug therapy is not effective, the abscess may need to be drained, or removed if it is encapsulated. In untreated cases the mortality rate approaches 100%.

Nursing measures are similar to those for management of meningitis or increased ICP. If surgical drainage or removal is the treatment of choice, nursing care is similar to that described under cranial surgery.

BACTERIAL MENINGITIS

Meningitis is an acute inflammation of the meningeal tissues surrounding the brain and spinal cord. Meningitis usually occurs in fall, winter, or early spring and is often secondary to viral respiratory disease. Older adults and persons who are debilitated are affected more frequently than the general population. College students living in dormitories and individuals living in institutions (e.g., prisoners) are also at a high risk for contracting meningitis.

Bacterial meningitis is considered a medical emergency. Untreated bacterial meningitis has a mortality rate near 100%.

Etiology and Pathophysiology

Streptococcus pneumoniae and *Neisseria meningitidis* are the leading causes of bacterial meningitis. *Haemophilus influenzae* was once the most common cause of bacterial meningitis. However, the use of *H. influenzae* vaccine has resulted in a significant decrease in meningitis related to this organism.

The organisms usually gain entry to the CNS through the upper respiratory tract or the bloodstream. However, they may enter by direct extension from penetrating wounds of the skull or through fractured sinuses in basilar skull fractures.

The inflammatory response to the infection tends to increase CSF production with a moderate increase in ICP. In bacterial meningitis the purulent secretions produced quickly spread to other areas of the brain through the CSF and cover the cranial nerves and other intracranial structures. If this process extends into the brain parenchyma or if concurrent encephalitis is present, cerebral edema and increased ICP become more of a problem. Closely observe all patients with meningitis for manifestations of increased ICP, which is thought to be a result of swelling around the dura and increased CSF volume.

Clinical Manifestations

Fever, severe headache, nausea, vomiting, and nuchal rigidity (neck stiffness) are key signs of meningitis. Photophobia, a decreased LOC, and signs of increased ICP may also be present. Coma is associated with a poor prognosis and occurs in 5% to 10% of patients with bacterial meningitis. Seizures occur in one third of all cases. The headache becomes progressively worse and may be accompanied by vomiting and irritability. If the infecting organism is a meningococcus, a skin rash is common and petechiae may be seen.

Complications

The most common acute complication of bacterial meningitis is increased ICP. Most patients have increased ICP, and it is the major cause of an altered mental status. Another complication of bacterial meningitis is residual neurologic dysfunction.

Dysfunction often occurs involving many cranial nerves. Cranial nerve irritation can have serious sequelae. The optic nerve (CN II) is compressed by increased ICP. Papilledema is often present, and blindness may occur. When the oculomotor (CN III), trochlear (CN IV), and abducens (CN VI) nerves are irritated, ocular movements are affected. Ptosis, unequal pupils, and diplopia are common. Irritation of the trigeminal nerve (CN V) results in sensory losses and loss of the corneal reflex. Irritation of the facial nerve (CN VII) results in facial paresis. Irritation of the vestibulocochlear nerve (CN VIII) causes tinnitus, vertigo, and deafness. The dysfunction usually disappears within a few weeks. However, hearing loss may be permanent after bacterial meningitis.

Hemiparesis, dysphasia, and hemianopsia may also occur. These signs usually resolve over time. If they do not, a cerebral abscess, subdural empyema, subdural effusion, or persistent meningitis is suspected. Acute cerebral edema may cause seizures, CN III palsy, bradycardia, hypertensive coma, and death.

Headaches may occur for months after the diagnosis of meningitis until the irritation and inflammation have completely resolved. It is important to implement pain management for chronic headaches.

A noncommunicating hydrocephalus may occur if the exudate causes adhesions that prevent the normal flow of CSF from the ventricles. CSF reabsorption by the arachnoid villi may also be obstructed by the exudate. In this situation, surgical implantation of a shunt is the only treatment.

Waterhouse-Friderichsen syndrome is a complication of meningococcal meningitis. The syndrome is manifested by petechiae, disseminated intravascular coagulation (DIC), adrenal hemorrhage, and circulatory collapse. DIC and shock, which are some of the most serious complications of meningitis, are associated with meningococcemia. (DIC is discussed in detail in Chapter 31.)

Diagnostic Studies

When a patient has manifestations suggestive of bacterial meningitis, a blood culture and CT scan should be done. Diagnosis is usually verified by doing a lumbar puncture with analysis of the CSF. A lumbar puncture should be completed only after the CT scan has ruled out an obstruction in the foramen magnum in order to prevent a fluid shift resulting in herniation.

Specimens of the CSF, sputum, and nasopharyngeal secretions are taken for culture before the start of antibiotic therapy to identify the causative organism. A Gram stain is done to detect bacteria.

Variations in the CSF depend on the causative organism. Protein levels in the CSF are usually elevated and are higher in bacterial than in viral meningitis. The CSF glucose concentration is commonly decreased in bacterial meningitis but may be normal in viral meningitis. The CSF is purulent and turbid in bacterial meningitis. It may be the same or clear in viral meningitis. The predominant white blood cell type in the CSF during bacterial meningitis is neutrophils (see Table 57-16).

X-rays of the skull may demonstrate infected sinuses. CT scans and MRI may be normal in uncomplicated meningitis. In other cases, CT scans may reveal evidence of increased ICP or hydrocephalus.

Collaborative Care

Bacterial meningitis is a medical emergency. Rapid diagnosis based on history and physical examination is crucial because the patient is usually in a critical state when health care is sought. When meningitis is suspected, antibiotic therapy is instituted after the collection of specimens for cultures, even before the diagnosis is confirmed (Table 57-17).

Ampicillin, penicillin, vancomycin, cefuroxime (Ceftin), cefotaxime (Claforan), ceftriaxone (Rocephin), ceftizoxime (Cefizox), and ceftazidime (Ceptaz) are some commonly prescribed drugs for treating bacterial meningitis. Dexamethasone (a corticosteroid) may also be prescribed before or with the first

---

TABLE 57-17   COLLABORATIVE CARE

Bacterial Meningitis

Diagnostic
- History and physical examination
- Analysis of CSF for protein, glucose, WBC, Gram stain, and culture
- CBC, coagulation profile, electrolyte levels, glucose, platelet count
- Blood culture
- CT scan, MRI, PET scan
- Skull x-ray studies

Collaborative Therapy
- Rest
- IV fluids
- Hypothermia

Drug Therapy
- IV antibiotics
  - ampicillin, penicillin
  - cephalosporin (e.g., cefotaxime [Claforan], ceftriaxone [Rocephin])
- codeine for headache
- dexamethasone (Decadron)
- acetaminophen or aspirin for temperature >100.4° F (38° C)
- phenytoin (Dilantin) IV
- mannitol (Osmitrol) IV for diuresis

CSF, Cerebrospinal fluid; *PET,* positron emission tomography.

dose of antibiotics. Collaborate with the health care provider to manage the headache, fever, and nuchal rigidity often associated with meningitis.

NURSING MANAGEMENT
BACTERIAL MENINGITIS

NURSING ASSESSMENT

Initial assessment should include vital signs, neurologic evaluation, fluid intake and output, and evaluation of the lungs and skin (see eFig. 57-1 available on the website for this chapter).

NURSING DIAGNOSES

Nursing diagnoses for the patient with bacterial meningitis may include, but are not limited to, the following:

- Decreased intracranial adaptive capacity *related to* decreased cerebral perfusion or increased ICP
- Risk for ineffective cerebral tissue perfusion *related to* reduction of blood flow and cerebral edema
- Hyperthermia *related to* infection
- Acute pain *related to* headache and muscle aches

Additional information on nursing diagnoses for the patient with bacterial meningitis is presented in eNursing Care Plan 57-2 (available on the website for this chapter).

PLANNING

The overall goals for the patient with bacterial meningitis are to (1) return to maximal neurologic functioning, (2) resolve the infection, and (3) control pain and discomfort.

NURSING IMPLEMENTATION

HEALTH PROMOTION. Prevention of respiratory tract infections through vaccination programs for pneumococcal pneumonia and influenza is important. Two meningococcal vaccines are available in the United States: meningococcal polysaccharide vaccine (MPSV4) and meningococcal conjugate vaccine (MCV4). MPSV4 has been available since the 1970s. It is the only meningococcal vaccine licensed for people older than 55. MCV4 is the preferred vaccine for people 55 years of age and younger. Two doses of MCV4 are recommended for adolescents 11 through 18 years of age: the first dose at 11 or 12 years of age, with a booster dose at age 16.

Early and vigorous treatment of respiratory tract and ear infections is important. Persons who have close contact with anyone who has bacterial meningitis should be given prophylactic antibiotics.

ACUTE INTERVENTION. The patient with bacterial meningitis is usually acutely ill. The fever is high, and head pain is severe. Irritation of the cerebral cortex may result in seizures. The changes in mental status and LOC depend on the degree of increased ICP. Assess and record vital signs, neurologic status, fluid intake and output, skin, and lung fields at regular intervals based on the patient's condition.

Head and neck pain secondary to movement requires attention. Codeine provides some pain relief without undue sedation for most patients. Assist the patient to a position of comfort, often curled up with the head slightly extended. The head of the bed should be slightly elevated. A darkened room and a cool cloth over the eyes relieve the discomfort of photophobia.

For the delirious patient, additional low lighting may be necessary to decrease hallucinations. All patients suffer some degree of mental distortion and hypersensitivity, and they may be frightened and misinterpret the environment. Make every attempt to minimize environmental stimuli and prevent injury. A familiar person at the bedside may have a calming effect. Be efficient with care but also convey an attitude of caring and of unhurried gentleness. The use of touch and a soothing voice to give simple explanations of activities is helpful. If seizures occur, make appropriate observations and take protective measures. Administer antiseizure drugs such as phenytoin (Dilantin) or levetiracetam (Keppra) as ordered. Problems associated with increased ICP need to be managed (see the section on increased ICP earlier in this chapter).

Fever must be vigorously treated because it increases cerebral edema and the frequency of seizures. In addition, neurologic damage may result from an extremely high temperature over a prolonged time. Acetaminophen or aspirin may be used to reduce fever. However, if the fever is resistant to aspirin or acetaminophen, more vigorous means are necessary, such as a cooling blanket. Take care not to reduce the temperature too rapidly because shivering may result, causing a rebound effect and increasing the temperature. Wrap the extremities in soft towels or a blanket covered with a sheet to reduce shivering (which can raise ICP). If a cooling blanket is not available or desirable, tepid sponge baths with water may be effective in lowering the temperature. Protect the skin from excessive drying and injury and prevent breaks in the skin.

Because high fever greatly increases the metabolic rate and thus insensible fluid loss, assess the patient for dehydration and adequacy of fluid intake. Diaphoresis further increases fluid losses, which should be noted on the output record. Calculate replacement fluids as 800 mL/day for respiratory losses and 100 mL for each degree of temperature above 100.4° F (38° C). Supplemental feeding (e.g., enteral nutrition) to maintain adequate nutritional intake may be necessary. Follow the designated antibiotic schedule to maintain therapeutic blood levels.

Meningitis generally requires respiratory isolation until the cultures are negative. Meningococcal meningitis is highly contagious, whereas other causes of meningitis may pose minimal to no infection risk with patient contact. However, standard precautions are essential to protect the patient and the nurse.

AMBULATORY AND HOME CARE. After the acute period has passed, the patient requires several weeks of convalescence before resuming normal activities. In this period, stress the importance of adequate nutrition, with an emphasis on a high-protein, high-calorie diet in small, frequent feedings.

Muscle rigidity may persist in the neck and the backs of the legs. Progressive range-of-motion exercises and warm baths are useful. Have the patient gradually increase activity as tolerated, but encourage adequate rest and sleep.

Residual effects can result in sequelae such as dementia, seizures, deafness, hemiplegia, and hydrocephalus. Assess vision, hearing, cognitive skills, and motor and sensory abilities after recovery, with appropriate referrals as indicated. Throughout the acute and convalescent periods, be aware of the anxiety and stress experienced by the caregiver and other family members.

EVALUATION

The expected outcomes are that the patient with bacterial meningitis will

- Demonstrate appropriate cognitive function
- Be oriented to person, place, and time
- Maintain body temperature within normal range
- Report satisfaction with pain control

Additional information on expected outcomes for the patient with bacterial meningitis is addressed in eNursing Care Plan 57-2.

VIRAL MENINGITIS

The most common causes of viral meningitis are enteroviruses, arboviruses, human immunodeficiency virus, and herpes simplex virus (HSV). Enteroviruses are most often spread through direct contact with respiratory secretions. Viral meningitis usually manifests as a headache, fever, photophobia, and stiff neck.[26] The fever may be moderate or high.

The Xpert EV test is used to rapidly diagnose viral meningitis. A sample of CSF is used to determine if enterovirus is present, and results are available within hours of symptom onset.[27] An important diagnostic test is examination of the CSF via lumbar puncture. The CSF can be clear or cloudy, and the typical finding is lymphocytosis (see Table 57-16). Organisms are not seen on Gram stain or acid-fast smears. Polymerase chain reaction (PCR) used to detect viral-specific deoxyribonucleic acid (DNA) or ribonucleic acid (RNA) is a highly sensitive method for diagnosing CNS viral infections.

Antibiotics should be administered after the lumbar puncture while awaiting the results of the CSF analysis. Antibiotics are the best defense for bacterial meningitis and can be easily discontinued if the meningitis is found to be viral.[26]

Viral meningitis is managed symptomatically because the disease is self-limiting. Full recovery from viral meningitis is expected. Rare sequelae include persistent headaches, mild mental impairment, and incoordination.

ENCEPHALITIS

Encephalitis, an acute inflammation of the brain, is a serious, and sometimes fatal, disease. In the United States, encephalitis is responsible for about 20,000 cases and 1400 deaths annually.[28]

Encephalitis is usually caused by a virus. Many different viruses have been implicated in encephalitis. Some of the viruses are associated with certain seasons of the year and endemic to certain geographic areas.

Ticks and mosquitoes transmit epidemic encephalitis. Examples include eastern equine encephalitis, La Crosse encephalitis, St. Louis encephalitis, West Nile encephalitis, and western equine encephalitis.[28] Nonepidemic encephalitis may occur as a complication of measles, chickenpox, or mumps. HSV encephalitis is the most common cause of acute nonepidemic viral encephalitis. Cytomegalovirus encephalitis is a common complication in patients with acquired immunodeficiency syndrome (AIDS).

Clinical Manifestations and Diagnostic Studies

The onset of infection is typically nonspecific, with fever, headache, nausea, and vomiting. Encephalitis can be acute or subacute. Signs of encephalitis appear on day 2 or 3 and may vary from minimal alterations in mental status to coma. Virtually any CNS abnormality can occur, including hemiparesis, tremors, seizures, cranial nerve palsies, personality changes, memory impairment, amnesia, and dysphasia.

Early diagnosis and treatment of viral encephalitis are essential for favorable outcomes. Diagnostic findings related to viral encephalitis are shown in Table 57-16. Brain imaging techniques include CT, MRI, and PET. PCR tests allow for early detection of HSV and West Nile encephalitis. West Nile virus should be strongly considered in adults over 50 years old who develop encephalitis or meningitis in summer or early fall. The best diagnostic test for West Nile virus is a blood test that detects viral RNA. This test is also used in screening blood, organs, cells, and tissues that have been donated.

NURSING AND COLLABORATIVE MANAGEMENT ENCEPHALITIS

Prevention of encephalitis requires mosquito control, including cleaning rain gutters, removing old tires, draining bird baths, and removing water where mosquitoes can breed. In addition, insect repellant should be used during mosquito season.

Collaborative and nursing management of encephalitis, including West Nile virus infection, is symptomatic and supportive. In the initial stages of encephalitis, many patients require intensive care.

Acyclovir (Zovirax) and vidarabine (Vira-A) are used to treat encephalitis caused by HSV infection. Acyclovir has fewer side effects than vidarabine and is often the preferred treatment. Use of these antiviral agents has been shown to reduce mortality rates, although neurologic complications may not be reduced. For maximal benefit, antiviral agents should be started before the onset of coma. Treat seizure disorders with antiseizure drugs. Prophylactic treatment with antiseizure drugs may be used in severe cases of encephalitis. Treatment of cytomegalovirus encephalitis in AIDS patients is discussed in Chapter 15.

RABIES

Although 30,000 to 70,000 people die each year from rabies worldwide, only one to three people die annually in the United States. The threat is much greater in developing countries. Rabies vaccine is encouraged for individuals who travel globally, since it remains a serious public health concern.

The etiology of rabies is an RNA virus that causes an acute, progressive viral encephalitis. Although rabies is generally transmitted via saliva from the bite of an infected animal, it can also be spread by scratches, mucous membrane contact with infected secretions, and inhalation of aerosolized virus into the respiratory tract. Any warm-blooded mammal, including livestock, can carry rabies. Throughout the world, rabid dogs are the most common disease vector. However, in developed countries, raccoons, skunks, bats, and foxes are the primary animal carriers.

The rabies virus spreads from the contact site through the CNS via peripheral nerve and possibly muscle fibers. During this time (2 to 14 days after exposure), patients experience flu-like symptoms, pain, paresthesias, or numbness. Then an acute neurologic syndrome occurs 2 to 7 days later and is manifested by agitation, hypersalivation, hydrophobia, dysarthria, vertigo, diplopia, hallucinations, and other neurologic sequelae (e.g., hyperactive reflexes, nuchal rigidity). Coma develops within 7 to 10 days of the neurologic syndrome. Patients experience flaccid paralysis, apnea, hydrophobia, and seizures. Death ensues as a result of respiratory and cardiovascular collapse within a few days after the onset of coma.

Because rabies is nearly always fatal, management efforts are directed at preventing the transmission and onset of the disease. Rabies postexposure prophylaxis is discussed in Chapter 69.

CASE STUDY

Traumatic Brain Injury

Comstock/Thinkstock

Patient Profile

C.G. is a 24-yr-old African American man who has just returned from a 15-mo Army deployment to Afghanistan. He comes to the outpatient clinic with a report of chronic headaches (pain rating of 8/10) and difficulty sleeping. His wife has noticed some personality changes since his return from deployment and is concerned that he has posttraumatic stress disorder (PTSD).

Subjective Data

- Reports that he has been depressed lately but attributes it to headache and difficulty returning home.
- Headache is worse in the morning or when he lies down.
- Uses tobacco and drinks coffee throughout the day.
- Has difficulty sleeping.
- Reports "incidents" of heavy combat and blasts with a loss of consciousness. Cannot remember how many times. Unable to obtain a more through history as he becomes quite agitated.

Objective Data

- During your assessment, you note that C.G. is looking around the room and jumps when the phone rings next door.
- Loss of short-term memory (remembers one of three items).
- Heart rate ranges from 100 to 130 beats/min.
- ECG strip is shown at right:

- Systolic BP ranges from 120 to 160 mm Hg.
- Right pupil, 3 mm sluggishly reactive; left pupil, 3 mm briskly reactive.

Diagnostic Studies

- CT of the head: negative for skull fracture, hematoma, or hemorrhage. Cerebral edema is noted with cingulate herniation on the right side.
- MRI performed following CT; mild diffuse axonal injury noted.

Discussion Questions

1. What could be the cause of C.G.'s hypertension, tachycardia, and ECG rhythm?
2. In addition to PTSD, what do his clinical manifestations suggest?
3. *Priority Decision:* What are the priority nursing interventions that should be implemented?
4. *Priority Decision:* Based on the assessment data presented, what are the priority nursing diagnoses? Are there any collaborative problems?
5. *Evidence-Based Practice:* What interventions and support can help his wife?

⊖volve Answers available at *http://evolve.elsevier.com/Lewis/medsurg.*

BRIDGE TO NCLEX EXAMINATION

The number of the question corresponds to the same-numbered outcome at the beginning of the chapter.

1. Vasogenic cerebral edema increases intracranial pressure by
   a. shifting fluid in the gray matter.
   b. altering the endothelial lining of cerebral capillaries.
   c. leaking molecules from the intracellular fluid to the capillaries.
   d. altering the osmotic gradient flow into the intravascular component.

2. A patient with intracranial pressure monitoring has a pressure of 12 mm Hg. The nurse understands that this pressure reflects
   a. a severe decrease in cerebral perfusion pressure.
   b. an alteration in the production of cerebrospinal fluid.
   c. the loss of autoregulatory control of intracranial pressure.
   d. a normal balance between brain tissue, blood, and cerebrospinal fluid.

3. A nurse plans care for the patient with increased intracranial pressure with the knowledge that the best way to position the patient is to
   a. keep the head of the bed flat.
   b. elevate the head of the bed to 30 degrees.
   c. maintain patient on the left side with the head supported on a pillow.
   d. use a continuous-rotation bed to continuously change patient position.

4. The nurse is alerted to a possible acute subdural hematoma in the patient who
   a. has a linear skull fracture crossing a major artery.
   b. has focal symptoms of brain damage with no recollection of a head injury.
   c. develops decreased level of consciousness and a headache within 48 hours of a head injury.
   d. has an immediate loss of consciousness with a brief lucid interval followed by decreasing level of consciousness.

5. During admission of a patient with a severe head injury to the emergency department, the nurse places the highest priority on assessment for
   a. patency of airway.
   b. presence of a neck injury.
   c. neurologic status with the Glasgow Coma Scale.
   d. cerebrospinal fluid leakage from the ears or nose.

6. A patient is suspected of having a brain tumor. The signs and symptoms include memory deficits, visual disturbances, weakness of right upper and lower extremities, and personality changes. The nurse recognizes that the tumor is most likely located in the
   a. frontal lobe.
   b. parietal lobe.
   c. occipital lobe.
   d. temporal lobe.

7. Nursing management of a patient with a brain tumor includes *(select all that apply)*
   a. discussing with the patient methods to control inappropriate behavior.
   b. using diversion techniques to keep the patient stimulated and motivated.
   c. assisting and supporting the family in understanding any changes in behavior.
   d. limiting self-care activities until the patient has regained maximum physical functioning.
   e. planning for seizure precautions and teaching the patient and the caregiver about antiseizure drugs.

8. The nurse on the clinical unit is assigned to four patients. Which patient should she assess first?
   a. Patient with a skull fracture whose nose is bleeding
   b. Older patient with a stroke who is confused and whose daughter is present
   c. Patient with meningitis who is suddenly agitated and reporting a headache of 10 on a 0-to-10 scale
   d. Patient who had a craniotomy for a brain tumor who is now 3 days postoperative and has had continued vomiting

9. A nursing measure that is indicated to reduce the potential for seizures and increased intracranial pressure in the patient with bacterial meningitis is
   a. administering codeine for relief of head and neck pain.
   b. controlling fever with prescribed drugs and cooling techniques.
   c. keeping the room dark and quiet to minimize environmental stimulation.
   d. maintaining the patient on strict bed rest with the head of the bed slightly elevated.

1. b, 2. d, 3. b, 4. c, 5. a, 6. a, 7. c, e, 8. c, 9. b

⊖volve

For rationales to these answers and even more NCLEX review questions, visit *http://evolve.elsevier.com/Lewis/medsurg.*

REFERENCES

1. Cushing H: *Studies in intracranial physiology and surgery,* London, 1925, Oxford University Press. (Classic)
*2. Vender J, Waller J, Dhandapani K, et al: An evaluation and comparison of intraventricular, intraparenchymal, and fluid-coupled techniques for intracranial pressure monitoring in patients with severe traumatic brain injury, *J Clin Monit Comput* 25:231, 2011.
3. Seidman R: Cerebrovascular disease, Stonybrook University Medical Center. Retrieved from *www.stonybrookmedicalcenter.org/pathology/neuropathology/chapter2.*
4. Oddo M, Villa F, Citerio G: Brain multimodality monitoring: an update, *Curr Opin Crit Care* 18(2):111, 2012.
*5. Haddad S, Arabi Y: Critical care management of severe traumatic brain injury in adults, *Scand J Trauma Resusc Emerg Med* 20:12, 2012.
6. Fan J, Kirkness C, Vicini P, et al: Intracranial pressure waveform morphology and intracranial adaptive capacity, *Am J Crit Care* 17:545, 2008.
*7. Kim G, Amato A, James M, et al: Continuous and intermittent CSF diversion after subarachnoid hemorrhage: a pilot study, *Neurocrit Care* 14:68, 2011.
*8. Choi H, Badjatia N, Mayer S: Hypothermia for acute brain injury: mechanisms and practical aspects, *Nat Rev Neurol* 28:214, 2012.
9. Scalfani M, Dhar R, Zazulia A, et al: Effect of osmotic agents on regional cerebral blood flow in traumatic brain injury, *J Crit Care* 27(5):526.e7, 2012.
10. Justo Meirelles C, de Aguilar-Nascimento J: Enteral or parenteral nutrition in traumatic brain injury: a prospective randomized trial, *Nutricion Hospitalaria* 26:1120, 2011.
11. Kornbluth J, Bhardwaj A: Evaluation of coma: a critical appraisal of popular scoring systems, *Neurocrit Care* 14:134, 2011.

*12. Pieracci F, Moore E, Beauchamp K, et al: A cost-minimization analysis of phenytoin versus levetiracetam for early seizures pharmacoprophylaxis after traumatic brain injury, *J Trauma* 72:276, 2012.
13. Centers for Disease Control and Prevention: Injury prevention and control: traumatic brain injury. Retrieved from *www.cdc.gov/traumaticbraininjury/statistics.html.*
14. Sayer N: Traumatic brain injury and its neuropsychiatric sequelae in war, *Ann Rev Med* 63:405, 2012.
15. American Association of Neurological Surgeons: Traumatic brain injury: fact sheets. Retrieved from *www.aans.org/Patient%20Information/Conditions%20and%20Treatments/Traumatic%20Brain%20Injury.aspx.*
16. Johnson V, Stewart W, Smith D: Axonal pathology in traumatic brain injury, *Exper Neurol* 136(Pt 1):28–42, 2012.
17. Wasserman J, Koenigsberg RA: Diffuse axonal injury. Retrieved from *http://emedicine.medscape.com/article/339912-overview.*
*18. Wong D, Lurie F, Wong L: The effects of clopidogrel on elderly traumatic brain injured patients, *J Trauma* 65:1303, 2008.
19. Phan N, Hemphill J: Management of acute severe traumatic brain injury. Retrieved from *www.uptodate.com/contents/management-of-acute-severe-traumatic-brain-injury.*
20. Chronic subdural hematoma. Retrieved from *www.nlm.nih.gov/medlineplus/ency/article/000781.htm.*
21. Ganz J: Head injury management guidelines for general practitioners, *J Neurosci Rural Pract* 2:198, 2011.
22. National Cancer Institute: Brain tumor, approved by the US National Institutes of Health. Retrieved from *www.cancer.gov/cancertopics/types/brain.*
23. University of Pittsburgh: Types of brain tumors. Retrieved from *www.neurosurgery.pitt.edu/neuro_oncology/brain/types.html.*
24. Wakabayashi T: Clinical trial updates for malignant brain tumors, *Clin Neurol* 51:853, 2011.
25. Davis M, Stoiber A: Glioblastoma multiforme: enhancing survival and quality of life, *Clin J Oncol Nurs* 15:291, 2011.
26. Centers for Disease Control and Prevention: Meningitis questions and answers. Retrieved from *www.cdc.gov/meningitis/about/faq.html.*

*Evidence-based information for clinical practice.

27. Nordqvist C: Rapid test approved by FDA. Retrieved from *www.medicalnewstoday.com/articles/65448.php*.
28. Solomon T, Michael BD, Smith PE, et al: National guideline for the management of suspected viral encephalitis in adults, *J Infect* 64(4):347, 2012.

RESOURCES

American Association of Neuroscience Nurses
www.aann.org
American Brain Tumor Association
www.abta.org
Brain Injury Association of America
www.biausa.org

Brain Trauma Foundation
www.braintrauma.org
Brain Tumor Center
http://btc.mgh.harvard.edu
Centers for Disease Control and Prevention: Traumatic Brain Injury
www.cdc.gov/TraumaticBrainInjury
National Brain Tumor Society
www.braintumor.org
TraumaticBrainInjury.com
www.traumaticbraininjury.com
Tug McGraw Foundation
www.tugmcgraw.org

Motivation is like food for the brain.
You cannot get enough in one sitting.
It needs continual and regular top ups.
Peter Davies

Nursing Management

Stroke

Meg Zomorodi

LEARNING OUTCOMES

1. Describe the incidence of and risk factors for stroke.
2. Explain mechanisms that affect cerebral blood flow.
3. Compare and contrast the etiology and pathophysiology of ischemic and hemorrhagic strokes.
4. Correlate the clinical manifestations of stroke with the underlying pathophysiology.
5. Identify diagnostic studies performed for patients with strokes.
6. Differentiate among the collaborative care, drug therapy, and surgical therapy for patients with ischemic strokes and hemorrhagic strokes.
7. Describe the acute nursing management of a patient with a stroke.
8. Describe the rehabilitative nursing management of a patient with a stroke.
9. Explain the psychosocial impact of a stroke on the patient, caregiver, and family.

KEY TERMS

aneurysm, p. 1392
aphasia, p. 1394
brain attack, p. 1388
cerebrovascular accident (CVA), p. 1388
dysarthria, p. 1394

dysphasia, p. 1394
embolic stroke, p. 1392
hemorrhagic strokes, p. 1392
intracerebral hemorrhage, p. 1392
ischemic stroke, p. 1391

stroke, p. 1388
subarachnoid hemorrhage (SAH), p. 1392
thrombotic stroke, p. 1391
transient ischemic attack (TIA), p. 1391

Stroke occurs when there is (1) *ischemia* (inadequate blood flow) to a part of the brain or (2) hemorrhage into the brain that results in death of brain cells. Functions such as movement, sensation, or emotions that were controlled by the affected area of the brain are lost or impaired. The severity of the loss of function varies according to the location and extent of the brain damage.

The terms **brain attack** and **cerebrovascular accident (CVA)** are also used to describe stroke. The term *brain attack* communicates the urgency of recognizing the clinical manifestations of a stroke and treating this as a medical emergency, as would be done with a heart attack (Table 58-1). After the onset of a stroke, immediate medical attention is crucial to decrease disability and the risk of death.

Stroke is a major public health concern. An estimated 7 million people over the age of 20 in the United States have had a stroke, with 795,000 individuals affected annually.[1] With an aging population, a further increase in the incidence of stroke can be expected. However, stroke can occur at any age. About 28% of strokes occur in people younger than 65 years old.[2]

Stroke is the fourth most common cause of death in the United States, behind cancer, heart disease, and lung disease. More than 275,000 deaths occur annually from stroke. Women are more likely than men to die from a stroke because of the greater number of women over age 65.[1]

Stroke is the leading cause of serious, long-term disability. Of those who survive a stroke, 50% to 70% are functionally independent, and 15% to 30% live with permanent disability.

Reviewed by Carol C. Annesser, RN, MSN, BC, CNE, Assistant Professor, Nursing, Mercy College of Northwest Ohio, Toledo, Ohio; and Molly L. McClelland, RN, PhD, Assistant Professor of Nursing, University of Detroit Mercy, Detroit, Michigan.

Twenty-six percent require long-term care after 3 months.[3] Common long-term disabilities include hemiparesis, inability to walk, complete or partial dependence for activities of daily living (ADLs), aphasia, and depression. In addition to the physical, cognitive, and emotional impact of the stroke on the stroke survivor, the stroke affects the lives of the stroke victim's caregiver and family.[4] A stroke is a lifelong change for both the stroke survivor and the family.

PATHOPHYSIOLOGY OF STROKE

Anatomy of Cerebral Circulation

Blood is supplied to the brain by two major pairs of arteries: the internal carotid arteries (anterior circulation) and the vertebral arteries (posterior circulation). The carotid arteries branch to supply most of the frontal, parietal, and temporal lobes; the basal ganglia; and part of the diencephalon (thalamus and hypothalamus). The major branches of the carotid arteries are the middle cerebral and anterior cerebral arteries. The vertebral arteries join to form the basilar artery, which branches to supply the middle and lower parts of the temporal lobes, occipital lobes, cerebellum, brainstem, and part of the diencephalon. The main branch of the basilar artery is the posterior cerebral artery. The anterior and posterior cerebral circulation is connected at the *circle of Willis* by the anterior and posterior communicating arteries (Fig. 58-1). (Fig. 56-9 illustrates the arteries at the base of the brain.) Genetic variations in this area are common, and all connecting vessels may not be present.

Regulation of Cerebral Blood Flow

The brain requires a continuous supply of blood to provide the oxygen and glucose that neurons need to function. Blood flow must be maintained at 750 to 1000 mL/min (55 mL/100 g of brain tissue), or 20% of the cardiac output, for optimal brain functioning. If blood flow to the brain is totally interrupted (e.g., cardiac arrest), neurologic metabolism is altered in 30 seconds, metabolism stops in 2 minutes, and cellular death occurs in 5 minutes.

The brain is normally well protected from changes in mean systemic arterial blood pressure (BP) over a range from 50 to 150 mm Hg by a mechanism known as *cerebral autoregulation*.

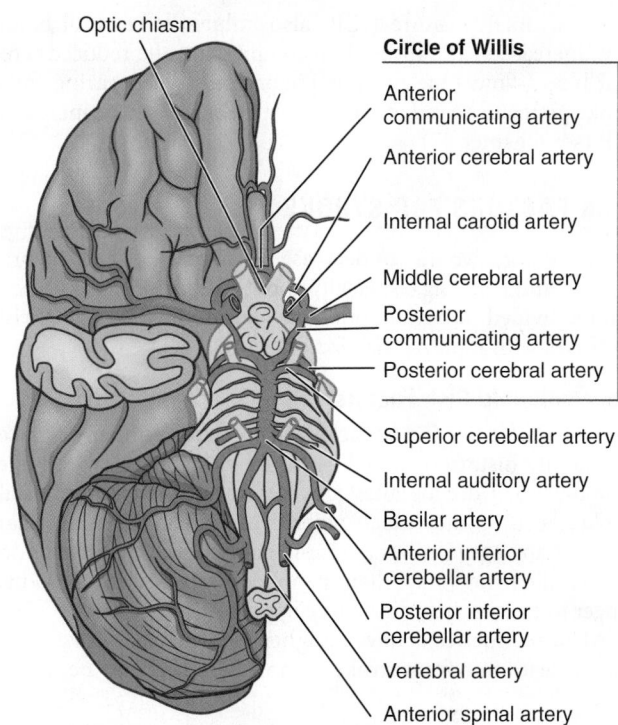

FIG. 58-1 Cerebral arteries and the circle of Willis. The top of the temporal lobe has been removed to show the course of the middle cerebral artery.

Optic chiasm

Circle of Willis
- Anterior communicating artery
- Anterior cerebral artery
- Internal carotid artery
- Middle cerebral artery
- Posterior communicating artery
- Posterior cerebral artery
- Superior cerebellar artery
- Internal auditory artery
- Basilar artery
- Anterior inferior cerebellar artery
- Posterior inferior cerebellar artery
- Vertebral artery
- Anterior spinal artery

This involves changes in the diameter of cerebral blood vessels in response to changes in pressure so that the blood flow to the brain stays constant. When cerebral ischemia occurs, cerebral autoregulation may be impaired, and it is often dependent on changes in BP. Carbon dioxide is a potent cerebral vasodilator, and changes in arterial carbon dioxide levels have a dramatic effect on cerebral blood flow (increased carbon dioxide levels increase cerebral blood flow, and decreased carbon dioxide levels decrease cerebral blood flow). Very low arterial oxygen levels (partial pressure of arterial oxygen less than 50 mm Hg) or increases in hydrogen ion concentration also increase cerebral blood flow.

Factors that affect blood flow to the brain include systemic BP, cardiac output, and blood viscosity. During normal activity, oxygen requirements vary considerably, but changes in cardiac output, vasomotor tone, and distribution of blood flow normally maintain adequate blood flow to the head. Cardiac output has to be reduced by one third before cerebral blood flow is reduced. Changes in blood viscosity affect cerebral blood flow, with decreased viscosity increasing flow.

Collateral circulation may develop over time to compensate for a decrease in cerebral blood flow. An area of the brain can potentially receive blood supply from another blood vessel even if blood supply from the original vessel has been cut off (e.g., because of thrombosis). In other words, the vessels in the brain make an "alternate route" for blood flow to reach damaged areas. Individual differences in collateral circulation partly determine the degree of brain damage and functional loss when a stroke occurs. For example, the bloodstreams of the internal carotid system and the basilar system meet in the posterior communicating arteries. In normal situations the pressure of the arteries is equal and blood will not mix. However, if one of the vessels is blocked, blood will flow from the intact artery to the damaged one, preventing a CVA.

Intracranial pressure (ICP) also influences cerebral blood flow. Increased ICP causes brain compression and reduced cerebral blood flow. One of your major goals when caring for a stroke patient is to reduce secondary injury related to increased ICP (see Chapter 57).

RISK FACTORS FOR STROKE

The most effective way to decrease the burden of stroke is prevention and teaching, especially about risk factors. Risk factors can be divided into nonmodifiable and modifiable. Stroke risk increases with multiple risk factors.

Nonmodifiable Risk Factors

Nonmodifiable risk factors include age, gender, ethnicity or race, and family history or heredity. Stroke risk increases with age, doubling each decade after 55 years of age. Two thirds of all strokes occur in individuals older than 65 years, but stroke can occur at any age. Strokes are more common in men, but more women die from stroke than men. Because women tend to live longer than men, they have more opportunity to suffer a stroke.[1]

African Americans have a higher incidence of stroke and a higher death rate from stroke than whites. This may be related in part to a higher incidence of hypertension, obesity, and diabetes mellitus in African Americans.

Genetic risk factors are important in the development of all vascular diseases, including stroke. A person with a family history of stroke has an increased risk of having a stroke. Genes encoding products involved in lipid metabolism, thrombosis, and inflammation are believed to be potential genetic factors for stroke.

Modifiable Risk Factors

Modifiable risk factors are those that can potentially be altered through lifestyle changes and medical treatment, thus reducing the risk of stroke. Modifiable risk factors include hypertension, heart disease, diabetes mellitus, smoking, excessive alcohol consumption, obesity, sleep apnea, metabolic syndrome, lack of physical exercise, poor diet, and drug abuse.

Hypertension is the single most important modifiable risk factor, but it is still often undetected and inadequately treated. Increases in systolic and diastolic BP independently increase the risk of stroke. Stroke risk can be reduced by up to 50% with appropriate treatment of hypertension.[1-3]

Heart disease, including atrial fibrillation, myocardial infarction, cardiomyopathy, cardiac valve abnormalities, and cardiac congenital defects, is also a risk factor for stroke. Atrial fibrillation is responsible for about 20% of all strokes.[1] The incidence of atrial fibrillation increases with age.

Diabetes mellitus is a significant risk factor for stroke. The risk for stroke in people with diabetes mellitus is five times higher than in the general population.[1]

Increased serum cholesterol and smoking are risk factors for stroke. Smoking nearly doubles the risk of stroke. The risk associated with smoking decreases substantially over time after the smoker quits. After 5 to 10 years of no tobacco use, former smokers have the same risk of stroke as nonsmokers.[5]

The effect of alcohol on stroke risk appears to depend on the amount consumed. Women who drink more than one alcoholic drink per day and men who drink more than two alcoholic drinks per day are at higher risk for hypertension, which increases their chance of stroke. Illicit drug use, especially cocaine use, has been associated with stroke risk.[1]

Abdominal obesity increases ischemic stroke risk in all ethnic groups. In addition, obesity is also associated with hypertension, high blood glucose, and elevated blood lipid levels, all of which increase the risk of stroke.[1] An association of physical inactivity and increased stroke risk is present in both men and women, regardless of ethnicity. Benefits of physical activity can occur with even light to moderate regular activity and may be related to the beneficial impact of exercise on other risk factors. Nutrition teaching is important for the individual at risk for stroke, since a diet high in fat and low in fruits and vegetables may increase stroke risk.

The early forms of birth control pills that contained high levels of progestin and estrogen increased a woman's chance of experiencing a stroke, especially if the woman also smoked heavily. Newer, low-dose oral contraceptives have lower risks for stroke except in those individuals who are hypertensive and smoke.

Other conditions that may increase the risk for strokes include migraine headaches, inflammatory conditions, and hyperhomocysteinemia. Sickle cell disease is another known risk factor for stroke.

GENDER DIFFERENCES

Stroke

Men	Women
• Stroke is more common in men than in women.	• At all ages, more women than men die from strokes.
• In most age-groups, more men than women will have a stroke in a given year.	• Women are more likely to have a hemorrhagic stroke.
• Men are more likely to have a thrombotic stroke.	• Women with atrial fibrillation have an increased risk for stroke.
• Men are more likely to have an embolic stroke.	• Oral contraceptive use and pregnancy contribute to stroke risk.
• Men have a better chance of surviving a stroke than women do.	• tPA is used less frequently to treat women who have strokes.

tPA, Recombinant tissue plasminogen activator.

🌐 CULTURAL & ETHNIC HEALTH DISPARITIES

Stroke

African Americans
• Have a higher incidence of strokes than whites.
• The rate of first strokes is almost twice that of whites.
• Are three times more likely than whites to have an ischemic stroke and four times more likely to have a hemorrhagic stroke.
• High incidence of strokes may be related to their increased rates of hypertension, diabetes mellitus, and sickle cell anemia.
• Have a higher incidence of smoking and obesity than whites, which are two risk factors for stroke.
• Are twice as likely to die from a stroke as whites.

Other Ethnicities
• Hispanics, Native Americans, and Asian Americans have a higher incidence of strokes than whites.
• Diabetes (an important risk factor for strokes) is common among Hispanics.
• Native Americans are more likely than whites to have at least two risk factors for stroke.

Transient Ischemic Attack

Another risk factor associated with stroke is a past history of a **transient ischemic attack (TIA).** A TIA is a transient episode of neurologic dysfunction caused by focal brain, spinal cord, or retinal ischemia, but without acute infarction of the brain. Clinical symptoms typically last less than 1 hour. In the past, TIAs were operationally defined as any focal cerebral ischemic event with symptoms lasting less than 24 hours. However, it is important to teach the patient to seek treatment for any stroke symptoms, since there is no way to predict if a TIA will resolve or if it is in fact the development of a stroke.[6] In general, one third of individuals who experience a TIA do not experience another event, one third have additional TIAs, and one third progress to stroke.[7]

TIAs may be due to microemboli that temporarily block the blood flow. TIAs are a warning sign of progressive cerebrovascular disease. The signs and symptoms of a TIA depend on the blood vessel that is involved and the area of the brain that is ischemic. If the carotid system is involved, patients may have a temporary loss of vision in one eye (*amaurosis fugax*), transient hemiparesis, numbness or loss of sensation, or a sudden inability to speak. Signs of a TIA involving the vertebrobasilar system may include tinnitus, vertigo, darkened or blurred vision, diplopia, ptosis, dysarthria, dysphagia, ataxia, and unilateral or bilateral numbness or weakness.

TIAs should be treated as medical emergencies. Teach people at risk for TIA to seek medical attention immediately with any stroke-like symptom and to identify the time of symptom onset.[8]

TYPES OF STROKE

Unlike a TIA, where ischemia occurs without infarction, a stroke results in infarction and cell death. Strokes are classified as ischemic or hemorrhagic based on the cause and underlying pathophysiologic findings (Fig. 58-2 and Table 58-2).

Ischemic Stroke

An **ischemic stroke** results from inadequate blood flow to the brain from partial or complete occlusion of an artery. Nearly 80% of strokes are ischemic.[1] A TIA attack is usually a precursor to ischemic stroke. Ischemic strokes are further divided into thrombotic and embolic strokes.

Thrombotic Stroke. A **thrombotic stroke** occurs from injury to a blood vessel wall and formation of a blood clot (see Fig. 58-2, *A*). The lumen of the blood vessel becomes narrowed and, if it becomes occluded, infarction occurs. Thrombosis develops readily where atherosclerotic plaques have already narrowed blood vessels. Thrombotic stroke, which is the result of thrombosis or narrowing of the blood vessel, is the most common cause of stroke, accounting for about 60% of strokes.[1] Two thirds of thrombotic strokes are associated with hyperten-

TABLE 58-2 TYPES OF STROKE

Gender and Age	Warning and Onset	Prognosis
Ischemic		
Thrombotic		
Men more than women	*Warning:* TIA (30%-50% of cases)	Stepwise progression, signs and symptoms develop slowly, usually some improvement, recurrence in 20%-25% of survivors.
Oldest median age	*Onset:* Often during or after sleep	
Embolic		
Men more than women	*Warning:* TIA (uncommon)	Single event, signs and symptoms develop quickly, usually some improvement, recurrence common without aggressive treatment of underlying disease.
	Onset: Lack of relationship to activity, sudden onset	
Hemorrhagic		
Intracerebral		
Slightly higher in women	*Warning:* Headache (25% of cases)	Progression over 24 hr. Poor prognosis, fatality more likely with presence of coma.
	Onset: Activity (often)	
Subarachnoid		
Slightly higher in women	*Warning:* Headache (common)	Usually single sudden event, fatality more likely with presence of coma.
Youngest median age	*Onset:* Activity (often), sudden onset, most commonly related to head trauma	

TIA, Transient ischemic attack.

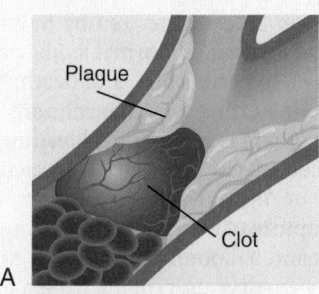

Thrombotic stroke. The process of clot formation (thrombosis) results in a narrowing of the lumen, which blocks the passage of the blood through the artery.

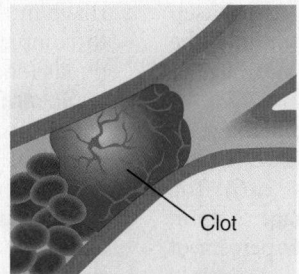

Embolic stroke. An embolus is a blood clot or other debris circulating in the blood. When it reaches an artery in the brain that is too narrow to pass through, it lodges there and blocks the flow of blood.

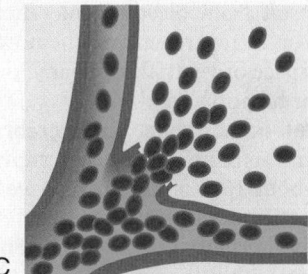

Hemorrhagic stroke. A burst blood vessel may allow blood to seep into and damage brain tissues until clotting shuts off the leak.

FIG. 58-2 Major types of stroke.

sion or diabetes mellitus, both of which accelerate atherosclerosis. In 30% to 50% of individuals, thrombotic strokes are preceded by a TIA.

The extent of the stroke depends on rapidity of onset, the size of the damaged area, and the presence of collateral circulation. Most patients with ischemic stroke do not have a decreased level of consciousness in the first 24 hours, unless it is due to a brainstem stroke or other conditions such as seizures, increased ICP, or hemorrhage. Ischemic stroke symptoms may progress in the first 72 hours as infarction and cerebral edema increase.

Embolic Stroke. Embolic stroke occurs when an embolus lodges in and occludes a cerebral artery, resulting in infarction and edema of the area supplied by the involved vessel (see Fig. 58-2, B). Embolism is the second most common cause of stroke, accounting for about 24% of strokes.[1] Most emboli originate in the endocardial (inside) layer of the heart, with plaque breaking off from the endocardium and entering the circulation. The embolus travels upward to the cerebral circulation and lodges where a vessel narrows or bifurcates (splits). Heart conditions associated with emboli include atrial fibrillation, myocardial infarction, infective endocarditis, rheumatic heart disease, valvular prostheses, and atrial septal defects. Less common causes of emboli include air and fat from long bone (e.g., femur) fractures.

The patient with an embolic stroke commonly has severe clinical symptoms that occur suddenly. Embolic strokes can affect any age-group. Rheumatic heart disease is one cause of embolic stroke in young to middle-aged adults. An embolus arising from an atherosclerotic plaque is more common in older adults.

Warning signs are less common with embolic than with thrombotic stroke. The embolic stroke often occurs rapidly, giving little time to accommodate by developing collateral circulation. The patient usually remains conscious, although he or she may have a headache. Prognosis is related to the amount of brain tissue deprived of its blood supply. The effects of the emboli are initially characterized by severe neurologic deficits, which can be temporary if the clot breaks up and allows blood to flow. Smaller emboli then continue to obstruct smaller vessels, which in turn involve smaller portions of the brain with fewer deficits noted. Recurrence of embolic stroke is common unless the underlying cause is aggressively treated.

Hemorrhagic Stroke

Hemorrhagic strokes account for approximately 15% of all strokes and result from bleeding into the brain tissue itself (intracerebral or intraparenchymal hemorrhage) or into the subarachnoid space or ventricles (subarachnoid hemorrhage or intraventricular hemorrhage).[1]

Intracerebral Hemorrhage. Intracerebral hemorrhage is bleeding within the brain caused by a rupture of a vessel and accounts for about 10% of all strokes (see Fig. 58-2, C). The prognosis of patients with intracerebral hemorrhage is poor, with the 30-day mortality rate at 40% to 80%. Fifty percent of the deaths occur within the first 48 hours.[1]

Hypertension is the most common cause of intracerebral hemorrhage (Fig. 58-3). Other causes include vascular malformations, coagulation disorders, anticoagulant and thrombolytic drugs, trauma, brain tumors, and ruptured aneurysms. Hemorrhage commonly occurs during periods of activity. Most often there is a sudden onset of symptoms, with progression over minutes to hours because of ongoing bleeding.

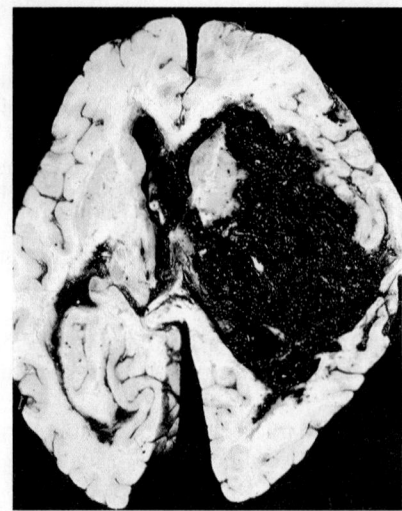

FIG. 58-3 Massive hypertensive hemorrhage rupturing into a lateral ventricle of the brain.

Manifestations include neurologic deficits, headache, nausea, vomiting, decreased level of consciousness (in about 50% of patients), and hypertension. The extent of the symptoms varies depending on the amount, location, and duration of the bleeding. A blood clot within the closed skull can result in a mass that causes pressure on brain tissue, displaces brain tissue, and decreases cerebral blood flow, leading to ischemia and infarction.

Approximately half of intracerebral hemorrhages occur in the putamen and internal capsule, central white matter, thalamus, cerebellar hemispheres, and pons. Initially, patients experience a severe headache with nausea and vomiting. Clinical manifestations of putaminal and internal capsule bleeding include weakness of one side (including the face, arm, and leg), slurred speech, and deviation of the eyes. Progression of symptoms related to a severe hemorrhage includes hemiplegia, fixed and dilated pupils, abnormal body posturing, and coma. Thalamic hemorrhage results in hemiplegia with more sensory than motor loss. Bleeding into the subthalamic areas of the brain leads to problems with vision and eye movement. Cerebellar hemorrhages are characterized by severe headache, vomiting, loss of ability to walk, dysphagia, dysarthria, and eye movement disturbances.

Hemorrhage in the pons is the most serious because basic life functions (e.g., respiration) are rapidly affected. Hemorrhage in the pons can be characterized by hemiplegia leading to complete paralysis, coma, abnormal body posturing, fixed pupils (small in size), hyperthermia, and death.

Subarachnoid Hemorrhage. Subarachnoid hemorrhage (SAH) occurs when there is intracranial bleeding into the cerebrospinal fluid–filled space between the arachnoid and pia mater membranes on the surface of the brain.[9] SAH is commonly caused by rupture of a cerebral aneurysm (congenital or acquired weakness and ballooning of vessels). Aneurysms may be saccular or berry aneurysms, ranging from a few millimeters to 20 to 30 mm in size, or fusiform atherosclerotic aneurysms. The majority of aneurysms are in the circle of Willis. Other causes of SAH include trauma and illicit drug (cocaine) abuse. About 40% of people who have a hemorrhagic stroke due to a ruptured aneurysm die during the first episode. Fifteen percent die from subsequent bleeding.[9] The incidence increases with age and is higher in women than men.

The patient may have warning symptoms if the ballooning artery applies pressure to brain tissue, or minor warning symptoms may result from leaking of an aneurysm before major rupture. In general, cerebral aneurysms are viewed as a "silent killer," since individuals do not have warning signs of an aneurysm until rupture has occurred.

SAFETY ALERT
• Sudden onset of a severe headache that is different from a previous headache and typically the "worst headache of one's life" is a characteristic symptom of a ruptured aneurysm.

Loss of consciousness may or may not occur. The patient's level of consciousness may range from alert to comatose, depending on the severity of the bleed. Other manifestations include focal neurologic deficits (including cranial nerve deficits), nausea, vomiting, seizures, and stiff neck. Despite improvements in surgical techniques and management, many patients with SAH die. Survivors may be left with significant morbidity, including cognitive difficulties.

Complications of aneurysmal SAH include rebleeding before surgery or other therapy is initiated and cerebral vasospasm (narrowing of the blood vessels), which can result in cerebral infarction. Cerebral vasospasm is most likely due to an interaction between the metabolites of blood and the vascular smooth muscle. During the lysis of subarachnoid blood clots, metabolites are released. These metabolites can cause endothelial damage and vasoconstriction. In addition, release of endothelin (a potent vasoconstrictor) may play a major role in the induction of cerebral vasospasm after SAH. Patients with SAH who are at risk for vasospasm are often kept in the intensive care unit for 14 days until the threat of vasospasm is reduced. Peak time for vasospasm occurs 6 to 10 days after the initial bleed.

CLINICAL MANIFESTATIONS OF STROKE

The neurologic manifestations do not significantly differ between ischemic and hemorrhagic stroke. The reason for this is that destruction of neural tissue is the basis for neurologic dysfunction caused by both types of stroke. The clinical manifestations are related to the location of the stroke. Specific manifestations related to the type of stroke are discussed in the previous section. The general clinical manifestations of ischemic and hemorrhagic stroke are discussed together here.

A stroke can affect many body functions, including motor activity, bladder and bowel elimination, intellectual function, spatial-perceptual alterations, personality, affect, sensation, swallowing, and communication. The functions affected are directly related to the artery involved and area of the brain it supplies (Table 58-3). Manifestations related to right- and left-brain damage differ somewhat and are shown in Fig. 58-4.

An additional assessment question that you need to ask is the time of the onset of symptoms. This is important for all types of stroke, especially ischemic strokes, since the time can affect treatment decisions.

Motor Function

Motor deficits are the most obvious effect of stroke. Motor deficits include impairment of (1) mobility, (2) respiratory function, (3) swallowing and speech, (4) gag reflex, and (5) self-care abilities. Symptoms are caused by the destruction of motor neurons in the pyramidal pathway (nerve fibers from the brain that pass through the spinal cord to the motor cells). The characteristic motor deficits include loss of skilled voluntary movement (aki-

TABLE 58-3	STROKE MANIFESTATIONS RELATED TO ARTERY INVOLVEMENT
Artery	**Deficit**
Anterior cerebral	Motor and/or sensory deficit (contralateral), sucking or rooting reflex, rigidity, gait problems, loss of proprioception and fine touch
Middle cerebral	*Dominant side:* Aphasia, motor and sensory deficit, hemianopsia
	Nondominant side: Neglect, motor and sensory deficit, hemianopsia
Posterior cerebral	Hemianopsia, visual hallucination, spontaneous pain, motor deficit
Vertebral	Cranial nerve deficits, diplopia, dizziness, nausea, vomiting, dysarthria, dysphagia, and/or coma

Right-brain damage (stroke on right side of the brain)	**Left-brain damage** (stroke on left side of the brain)
• Paralyzed left side: hemiplegia	• Paralyzed right side: hemiplegia
• Left-sided neglect	• Impaired speech/language aphasias
• Spatial-perceptual deficits	• Impaired right/left discrimination
• Tends to deny or minimize problems	• Slow performance, cautious
• Rapid performance, short attention span	• Aware of deficits: depression, anxiety
• Impulsive, safety problems	• Impaired comprehension related to language, math
• Impaired judgment	
• Impaired time concepts	

FIG. 58-4 Manifestations of right-brain and left-brain stroke.

nesia), impairment of integration of movements, alterations in muscle tone, and alterations in reflexes. The initial *hyporeflexia* (depressed reflexes) progresses to *hyperreflexia* (hyperactive reflexes) for most patients.

Motor deficits after a stroke follow certain specific patterns. Because the pyramidal pathway crosses at the level of the medulla, a lesion on one side of the brain affects motor function on the opposite side of the body (contralateral). The arms and legs of the affected side may be weakened or paralyzed to different degrees depending on which part of and to what extent the cerebral circulation was compromised. A stroke affecting the middle cerebral artery leads to a greater weakness in the upper extremity than the lower extremity. The affected shoulder tends to rotate internally, and the hip rotates externally. The affected foot is plantar flexed and inverted. An initial period of flaccidity may last from days to several weeks and is related to nerve damage. Spasticity of the muscles, which follows the flaccid stage, is related to interruption of upper motor neuron influence.

Communication

The left hemisphere is dominant for language skills in right-handed persons and in most left-handed persons.[10] Language disorders involve expression and comprehension of written and spoken words. The patient may experience aphasia, which may be *receptive aphasia* (loss of comprehension), *expressive aphasia* (inability to produce language), or *global aphasia* (total inability to communicate). Aphasia occurs when a stroke damages the dominant hemisphere of the brain.

Dysphasia refers to impaired ability to communicate. However, in most settings the terms *aphasia* and *dysphasia* are used interchangeably, with aphasia often being the more common term used. (Dysphasia should not be confused with the similarly pronounced *dysphagia,* which is difficulty swallowing.)

Patterns of aphasia may differ, since the stroke affects different portions of the brain. Aphasia may be classified as *nonfluent* (minimal speech activity with slow speech that requires obvious effort) or *fluent* (speech is present but contains little meaningful communication) (Table 58-4). Most types of aphasia are mixed, with impairment in both expression and understanding. A massive stroke may result in global aphasia. Many stroke patients also experience dysarthria, a disturbance in the muscular control of speech. Impairment may involve pronunciation, articulation, and phonation. Dysarthria does not affect the meaning of communication or the comprehension of language, but it does affect the mechanics of speech. Some patients experience a combination of aphasia and dysarthria.

Affect

Patients who have had a stroke may have difficulty controlling their emotions. Emotional responses may be exaggerated or unpredictable. Depression and feelings associated with changes in body image and loss of function can make this worse.[11] Patients may also be frustrated by mobility and communication problems.

An example of unpredictable affect is as follows: a well-respected 63-year-old lawyer has returned home from the hospital after a stroke. During a meal with his family, he becomes frustrated and begins to cry because of the difficulty getting food into his mouth and chewing, something that he was able to do easily before his stroke. His family cannot understand why a previously very competent man is so emotional. As a nurse, it is important for you to help this patient and family understand that frustration and depression are common in the first year after a stroke.

Intellectual Function

Both memory and judgment may be impaired as a result of stroke. These impairments can occur with strokes affecting either side of the brain. A left-brain stroke is more likely to result in memory problems related to language. Patients with a left-brain stroke often are cautious in making judgments. The patient with a right-brain stroke tends to be impulsive and to move quickly.

TABLE 58-4	**TYPES OF APHASIA**
Type	**Characteristics**
Broca's	• A type of nonfluent aphasia. • Damage to frontal lobe of brain. • Frequently speak in short phrases that make sense but are produced with great effort. • Often omit small words such as "is," "and," and "the." • May say, "Walk dog," meaning, "I will take the dog for a walk," or "book book two table," for "There are two books on the table." • Typically understand speech of others fairly well. • Often aware of their difficulties and can become easily frustrated.
Wernicke's	• A type of fluent aphasia. • Damage occurs in left temporal lobe, although it can result from damage to right lobe. • May speak in long sentences that have no meaning, add unnecessary words, and even create made-up words. • May say, "You know that smoodle pinkered and that I want to get him round and take care of him like you want before." • Often difficult to follow what person is trying to say. • Usually have great difficulty understanding speech. • Often unaware of their mistakes.
Global	• A type of nonfluent aphasia. • Results from damage to extensive portions of language areas of brain. • Have severe communication difficulties. • May be extremely limited in ability to speak or comprehend language.
Other	• Results from damage to different language areas in brain. • Some people may have difficulty repeating words and sentences even though they can speak and they understand the meaning of the word or sentence. • Others may have difficulty naming objects even though they know what the object is and what its use is.

An example of behavior in people with right-brain stroke is that they try to rise quickly from a wheelchair without locking the wheels or raising the footrests. On the other hand, people with a left-brain stroke would move slowly and cautiously from the wheelchair. Patients with either type of stroke may have difficulty making generalizations, which interferes with their ability to learn.

Spatial-Perceptual Alterations

Individuals who have had a stroke on the right side of the brain are more likely to have problems with spatial-perceptual orientation. However, this can also occur in people with left-brain stroke.

Spatial-perceptual problems may be divided into four categories. The first is the result of damage of the parietal lobe and causes the patient to have an incorrect perception of self and illness. In this situation, patients may deny their illnesses or their own body parts. The second category occurs when the patient neglects all input from the affected side (erroneous perception of self in space). This may be worsened by *homonymous hemianopsia,* in which blindness occurs in the same half of the visual fields of both eyes. The patient also has difficulty with spatial orientation, such as judging distances. The third spatial-perceptual deficit is *agnosia,* the inability to recognize an object by sight, touch, or hearing. The fourth deficit is *apraxia,* the inability to carry out learned sequential movements on command. Because patients may or may not be aware of their spatial-perceptual alterations, you need to assess for this potential problem, since it will affect rehabilitation and recovery.

Elimination

Most problems with urinary and bowel elimination occur initially and are temporary. When a stroke affects one hemisphere of the brain, the prognosis for normal bladder function is excellent. At least partial sensation for bladder filling remains, and voluntary urination is present. Initially, the patient may experience frequency, urgency, and incontinence. Although motor control of the bowel is usually not a problem, patients are frequently constipated. Constipation is associated with immobility, weak abdominal muscles, dehydration, and diminished response to the defecation reflex. Urinary and bowel elimination problems may also be related to inability to express needs and to manage clothing.

DIAGNOSTIC STUDIES FOR STROKE

When manifestations of a stroke occur, diagnostic studies are done to (1) confirm that it is a stroke and not another brain lesion and (2) identify the likely cause of the stroke (Table 58-5). Tests also guide decisions about therapy.

Important diagnostic tools for patients who have experienced a stroke are a noncontrast computed tomography (CT) scan or magnetic resonance imaging (MRI).[12] These tests can rapidly distinguish between ischemic and hemorrhagic stroke and help determine the size and location of the stroke. Serial CT scans may be used to assess the effectiveness of treatment and to evaluate recovery. Once the individual suspected of TIA or stroke arrives in the emergency department, it is important to rapidly assess and diagnose the patient (usually through a

noncontrast head CT or MRI).[12] Rapid access to these diagnostic tools is important, since the results will determine treatment options for the patient.

CT angiography (CTA) provides visualization of cerebral blood vessels. It can be performed after or at the same time as the noncontrast CT scan. CTA can provide an estimate of perfusion and detect filling defects in the cerebral arteries. Magnetic resonance angiography (MRA) can detect vascular lesions and blockages, similar to CTA. CT/MRI perfusion and diffusion imaging may also be done.

Cardiac imaging is also recommended because many strokes are caused by blood clots from the heart. Angiography can identify cervical and cerebrovascular occlusion, atherosclerotic plaques, and malformation of vessels. Cerebral angiography is a definitive study to identify the source of SAH. Risks of angiography include dislodging an embolus, causing vasospasm, inducing further hemorrhage, and provoking an allergic reaction to contrast media.

Intraarterial digital subtraction angiography (DSA) reduces the dose of contrast material, uses smaller catheters, and shortens the length of the procedure compared with conventional angiography. DSA involves the injection of a contrast agent to visualize blood vessels in the neck and the large vessels of the circle of Willis. It is considered safer than cerebral angiography because less vascular manipulation is required.

Transcranial Doppler (TCD) ultrasonography is a noninvasive study that measures the velocity of blood flow in the major cerebral arteries. TCD is effective in detecting microemboli and vasospasm and is ideal for the patient suspected of having an SAH. Carotid duplex scanning is used not only to detect the cause of the stroke, but also to stratify patients for either medical management or carotid intervention if they have carotid stenoses.

A lumbar puncture may be done to look for evidence of red blood cells in the cerebrospinal fluid if an SAH is suspected but the CT does not show hemorrhage. A lumbar puncture is avoided if the patient is suspected of having an obstruction in the foramen magnum or other signs of increased ICP because of the danger of herniation of the brain downward, leading to pressure on cardiac and respiratory centers in the brainstem and potentially death.

If the suspected cause of the stroke includes emboli from the heart, diagnostic cardiac tests should be done. Blood tests are also done to help identify conditions contributing to stroke and to guide treatment (see Table 58-5).

The LICOX system may be used as a diagnostic tool to evaluate the progression of stroke. LICOX measures brain oxygenation and temperature (see discussion in Chapter 57 on p. 1365 and Fig. 57-10). Secondary brain injury adds significantly to mortality risk and poor functional outcome after a stroke.

COLLABORATIVE CARE FOR STROKE

Preventive Therapy

Primary prevention is a priority for decreasing morbidity and mortality risk from stroke (Table 58-6). The goals of stroke prevention include health promotion for a healthy lifestyle and management of modifiable risk factors to prevent a stroke. Health promotion focuses on (1) healthy diet, (2) weight control, (3) regular exercise, (4) no smoking, (5) limitation on alcohol consumption, and (6) routine health assessments. Patients with known risk factors such as diabetes mellitus, hypertension,

TABLE 58-5 DIAGNOSTIC STUDIES
Stroke

Diagnosis of Stroke (Including Extent of Involvement)
- Computed tomography (CT) scan
- CT angiography (CTA)
- Magnetic resonance imaging (MRI)
- Magnetic resonance angiography (MRA)
- CT/MRI perfusion and diffusion imaging

Cerebral Blood Flow
- Cerebral angiography
- Carotid angiography
- Digital subtraction angiography
- Transcranial Doppler ultrasonography
- Carotid duplex scanning

Cardiac Assessment
- Electrocardiogram
- Chest x-ray
- Cardiac markers (troponin, creatine kinase-MB)
- Echocardiography (transthoracic, transesophageal)

Additional Studies
- Complete blood count, including platelets
- Coagulation studies: prothrombin time, activated partial thromboplastin time
- Electrolytes, blood glucose
- Renal and hepatic studies
- Lipid profile
- Cerebrospinal fluid analysis*

*A lumbar puncture to obtain cerebrospinal fluid is avoided if increased intracranial pressure is suspected.

TABLE 58-6   COLLABORATIVE CARE

Stroke

Diagnostic (see Table 58-5)
- History and physical examination

Collaborative Therapy

Prevention
- Control of hypertension
- Control of diabetes mellitus
- Treatment of underlying cardiac problem
- No smoking
- Limiting alcohol intake

Drug Therapy
- Platelet inhibitors (e.g., aspirin)
- Anticoagulation therapy for patients with atrial fibrillation

Surgical Therapy
- Carotid endarterectomy
- Stenting of carotid artery
- Transluminal angioplasty
- Extracranial-intracranial bypass
- Surgical interventions for aneurysms at risk of bleeding

Acute Care
- Maintenance of airway
- Fluid therapy
- Treatment of cerebral edema
- Prevention of secondary injury

Ischemic Stroke
- Tissue plasminogen activator (tPA) IV or intraarterial
- Stent retrievers
- MERCI retriever

Hemorrhagic Stroke
- Surgical decompression if indicated
- Clipping or coiling of aneurysm

Rehabilitation
- Focus on helping patient achieve independence and functional recovery

MERCI, Mechanical embolus removal in cerebral ischemia.

HEALTHY PEOPLE

Prevention of Stroke

- Reduce salt and sodium intake.
- Maintain a normal body weight.
- Maintain a normal blood pressure.
- Increase level of physical exercise.
- Avoid cigarette smoking or tobacco products.
- Limit consumption of alcohol to moderate levels.
- Follow a diet that is low in saturated fat, total fat, and dietary cholesterol and high in fruits and vegetables.

obesity, high serum lipids, or cardiac dysfunction require close management.

Preventive Drug Therapy. Measures to prevent the development of a thrombus or an embolus are used in patients with TIAs, since they are at high risk for stroke. Antiplatelet drugs are usually the chosen treatment to prevent stroke in patients who have had a TIA. Aspirin is the most frequently used antiplatelet agent, commonly at a dose of 81 to 325 mg/day. Other drugs include ticlopidine (Ticlid), clopidogrel (Plavix), dipyri-

EVIDENCE-BASED PRACTICE

Translating Research Into Practice

Can Mirror Therapy Improve Functioning After Stroke?

Clinical Question

For stroke patients (P), what is the effect of mirror therapy (I) versus control interventions (C) on motor function, activities of daily living (ADLs), and pain (O) at therapy completion and after 6 mo of therapy (T)?

Best Available Evidence

Randomized controlled trials (RCTs) and randomized crossover trials

Critical Appraisal and Synthesis of Evidence

- Fourteen trials (*n* = 567) of patients with stroke comparing mirror therapy to control interventions of no treatment, sham or placebo, or usual care.
- In mirror therapy, which is used to improve motor function after a stroke, a mirror is placed between a person's arms or legs so the image of the unaffected limb gives illusion of normal movement in the affected limb (see Fig. 63-24).
- Mirror therapy has a positive effect on motor function and ADLs in stroke patients, and on relieving pain in patients with complex regional pain syndrome, compared with control interventions.
- The effect of mirror therapy on motor function was stable at a 6-mo follow-up.

Conclusion

- Mirror therapy may improve motor function, ADLs, and pain compared with other interventions with effects lasting after 6 mo.

Implications for Nursing Practice

- Consult with rehabilitation care team if mirror therapy is available as an additional intervention for stroke patients.
- Motivate and encourage patients engaged in mirror therapy to practice as instructed.
- Mirror therapy may be helpful in osteoarthritis and with chronic and phantom limb pain.

Reference for Evidence

Thieme H, Mehrholz J, Pohl M, et al: Mirror therapy for improving motor function after stroke, *Cochrane Database Syst Rev* 3:CD 008449, 2012.

P, Patient population of interest; *I,* intervention or area of interest; *C,* comparison of interest or comparison group; *O,* outcomes of interest; *T,* timing (see p. 12).

damole (Persantine), and combined dipyridamole and aspirin (Aggrenox).[13]

> **DRUG ALERT: Ticlopidine (Ticlid) and Clopidogrel (Plavix)**
> - All health care providers and dentists must be informed that the drug is being taken, especially before scheduling surgery or major dental procedures.
> - Drug may need to be discontinued 10 to 14 days before surgery if antiplatelet effect is not desired.

For patients who have atrial fibrillation, oral anticoagulation can include warfarin (Coumadin), rivaroxaban (Xarelto), and dabigatran etexilate (Pradaxa). The primary advantage of rivaroxaban and dabigatran over warfarin is that these drugs do not need close monitoring or dosage adjustments. Statins (simvastatin [Zocor], lovastatin [Mevacor]) have also been shown to be effective in the prevention of stroke for individuals who have experienced a TIA in the past.[14]

Surgical Therapy for TIA and Stroke Prevention. Surgical interventions for the patient with TIAs due to carotid disease include carotid endarterectomy, transluminal angioplasty, stenting, and extracranial-intracranial (EC-IC) bypass. In a *carotid endarterectomy* (CEA), the atheromatous lesion is removed from the carotid artery to improve blood flow (Fig. 58-5).

Transluminal angioplasty is the insertion of a balloon to open a stenosed artery in the brain and improve blood flow. The balloon is threaded up to the carotid artery via a catheter inserted in the femoral artery.

Stenting involves intravascular placement of a stent in an attempt to maintain patency of the artery (Fig. 58-6). The stent can be inserted during an angioplasty. Once in place, the system can be used with a tiny filter that opens like an umbrella. The filter catches and removes the debris that is stirred up during the stenting procedure before it floats to the brain, where it can trigger a stroke. Stenting is a less invasive strategy for revascularization in patients unable to withstand the CEA because of coexisting medical conditions. Initial research has shown the procedure to be as effective as the CEA.[15]

EC-IC bypass involves anastomosing (surgically connecting) a branch of an extracranial artery to an intracranial artery (most commonly, superficial temporal to middle cerebral artery)

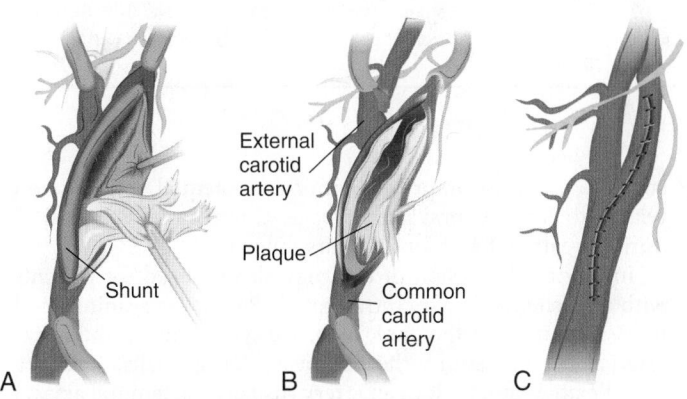

FIG. 58-5 Carotid endarterectomy is performed to prevent impending cerebral infarction. **A,** A tube is inserted above and below the blockage to reroute the blood flow. **B,** Atherosclerotic plaque in the common carotid artery is removed. **C,** Once the artery is stitched closed, the tube can be removed. A surgeon may also perform the technique without rerouting the blood flow.

FIG. 58-6 Brain stent used to treat blockages in cerebral blood flow. **A,** A balloon catheter is used to implant the stent into an artery of the brain. **B,** The balloon catheter is moved to the blocked area of the artery and then inflated. The stent expands due to inflation of the balloon. **C,** The balloon is deflated and withdrawn, leaving the stent permanently in place holding the artery open and improving the flow of blood.

beyond an area of obstruction with the goal of increasing cerebral perfusion. This procedure is generally reserved for patients who do not benefit from other forms of therapy. Postoperatively nursing care for these patients consists of neurovascular assessment, BP management, assessment of stent occlusion or retroperitoneal hemorrhage as complications, and minimization of complications at the insertion site by keeping the patient's leg straight for the prescribed time.

Acute Care for Ischemic Stroke

During initial evaluation, the single most important point in the patient's history is the time of onset of symptoms. The goals for collaborative care during the acute phase are preserving life, preventing further brain damage, and reducing disability.

Table 58-7 outlines the emergency management of the patient with a stroke. Acute care begins with managing circulation, airway, and breathing. Patients may have difficulty keeping an open and clear airway because of a decreased level of consciousness or decreased or absent gag and swallowing reflexes. Maintaining adequate oxygenation is important. Oxygen administration, artificial airway insertion, intubation, and mechanical ventilation may be required. Baseline neurologic assessment is carried out, and patients are monitored closely for signs of increasing neurologic deficit. About 25% of patients worsen in the first 24 to 48 hours.

For emergency care, patients should be transported to the closest certified stroke center or, when such an institution is not available, the closest facility offering emergency stroke care. The American Heart Association recommends that acute care facilities have stroke teams in place. The stroke team generally consists of the registered nurse, neurologist, radiologist, and CT technician.[16]

Elevated BP is common immediately after a stroke and may be a protective response to maintain cerebral perfusion. However, it can also be detrimental. Immediately after an ischemic stroke in those patients who do not receive fibrinolytic therapy (discussed below), the use of drugs to lower BP is recommended only if BP is markedly increased (systolic BP greater than 220 mm Hg or diastolic greater than 120 mm Hg). In a patient who is going to have fibrinolytic therapy, the BP needs to be less than 185/110 mm Hg and then maintained at or below 180/105 mm Hg for at least 24 hours after fibrinolytic therapy. In an acute stroke, IV antihypertensives such as labetalol (Normodyne) and nicardipine (Cardene) are preferred. Although low BP immediately after a stroke is uncommon, hypotension and hypovolemia should be corrected if present.

Fluid and electrolyte balance must be controlled carefully. Generally the goal is to keep the patient adequately hydrated to promote perfusion and decrease further brain injury. Overhydration may compromise perfusion by increasing cerebral edema. Adequate fluid intake during acute care via oral, IV, or tube feedings is a priority. Also monitor urine output to make sure the patient does not become dehydrated.

If secretion of antidiuretic hormone (ADH) increases in response to the stroke, urine output decreases and fluid is retained. Low serum sodium (hyponatremia) may occur. IV solutions with glucose and water are avoided because they are hypotonic and may further increase cerebral edema and ICP. In addition, hyperglycemia may be associated with further brain damage and should be treated. In general, decisions regarding individualized fluid and electrolyte replacement therapy are based on the extent of intracranial edema, symptoms of

TABLE 58-7   EMERGENCY MANAGEMENT

Stroke

Etiology	Assessment Findings	Interventions
• Sudden vascular compromise causing disruption of blood flow to brain • Thrombosis • Trauma • Aneurysm • Embolism • Hemorrhage • Arteriovenous malformation	• Altered level of consciousness • Weakness, numbness, or paralysis of portion of body • Speech or visual disturbances • Severe headache • Heart rate ↑ or ↓ • Respiratory distress • Unequal pupils • Hypertension • Facial drooping on affected side • Difficulty swallowing • Seizures • Bladder or bowel incontinence • Nausea and vomiting • Vertigo	**Initial** • Ensure patent airway. • Call stroke code or stroke team. • Remove dentures. • Perform pulse oximetry. • Maintain adequate oxygenation (SaO_2 >95%) with supplemental O_2, if necessary. • Establish IV access with normal saline. • Maintain BP according to guidelines (e.g., Cardiac Life Support).* • Remove clothing. • Obtain CT scan or MRI immediately. • Perform baseline laboratory tests (including blood glucose) immediately, and treat if hypoglycemic. • Position head in midline. • Elevate head of bed 30 degrees if no symptoms of shock or injury. • Institute seizure precautions. • Anticipate thrombolytic therapy for ischemic stroke. • Keep patient NPO until swallow reflex evaluated. **Ongoing Monitoring** • Monitor vital signs and neurologic status, including level of consciousness (NIH Stroke Scale), motor and sensory function, pupil size and reactivity, SaO_2, and cardiac rhythm. • Reassure patient and family.

*See Appendix A.
NIH, National Institutes of Health; *SaO₂,* arterial oxygen saturation.

increased ICP, central venous pressure levels, laboratory values for electrolytes, and intake and output.

Increased ICP is more likely to occur with hemorrhagic strokes but can occur with ischemic strokes. Increased ICP from cerebral edema usually peaks in 72 hours and may cause brain herniation. Management of increased ICP includes practices that improve venous drainage, such as elevating the head of the bed, maintaining head and neck in alignment, and avoiding hip flexion. Additional measures for reducing ICP include management of hyperthermia (goal temperature of 96.8° to 98.6° F [36° to 37° C]), drug therapy to prevent seizures, pain management, avoidance of hypervolemia, and management of constipation. Cerebrospinal fluid drainage may be used in some patients to reduce ICP. (The specific management of increased ICP is discussed in Chapter 57.)

Drug Therapy for Ischemic Stroke. Fibrinolytic therapy should not be delayed. Recombinant tissue plasminogen activator (tPA) is used to produce localized fibrinolysis by binding to the fibrin in the thrombi. The fibrinolytic action of tPA occurs as the plasminogen is converted to plasmin, whose enzymatic action then digests fibrin and fibrinogen, and thus lyses the clot. Other fibrinolytic agents cannot be substituted for tPA. (Fibrinolytic [thrombolytic] therapy is discussed in Chapter 34.)

tPA is administered IV to reestablish blood flow through a blocked artery to prevent cell death in patients with the acute onset of ischemic stroke. tPA must be administered within 3 to 4½ hours of the onset of clinical signs of ischemic stroke.[16,17] Patients are screened carefully before tPA can be given. Screening includes a noncontrast CT or MRI scan to rule out hemorrhagic stroke; blood tests for glucose level and coagulation disorders; and screening for recent history of gastrointestinal bleeding, stroke, or head trauma within the past 3 months, or major surgery within 14 days.[16,17] If tPA is expected as a treatment option, insert a urinary catheter, nasogastric tube, and multiple IVs before tPA administration. During infusion of the drug, closely monitor the patient's vital signs and neurologic

status to assess for improvement or for potential deterioration related to intracerebral hemorrhage. Control of BP is critical during treatment and for 24 hours following.

Intraarterial infusion of tPA may also be used for patients with an ischemic stroke. Intraarterial tPA can be administered up to 6 hours after the onset of stroke symptoms. In the intraarterial tPA procedure, the neurovascular specialist inserts a thin, flexible catheter into an artery (usually the femoral artery) and guides the catheter to the area of the clot by angiogram. The tPA is administered through the catheter and immediately targets the clot. Less tPA is needed when it is delivered directly to the clot, which can reduce the possibility of intracranial hemorrhage.[17]

The use of anticoagulants (e.g., heparin) in the emergency phase after an ischemic stroke is generally not recommended because of the risk for intracranial hemorrhage. Acetylsalicylic acid (aspirin) at a dose of 325 mg may be initiated within 24 to 48 hours after the onset of an ischemic stroke. Complications of aspirin include gastrointestinal bleeding with higher doses. Aspirin should be administered cautiously if the patient has a history of peptic ulcer disease.[18]

After the patient has stabilized and to prevent further clot formation, patients with strokes caused by thrombi and emboli may be treated with anticoagulants and platelet inhibitors (see discussion on prevention of stroke on pp. 1396-1397). For patients who have atrial fibrillation, oral anticoagulants include warfarin, rivaroxaban, and dabigatran etexilate. Platelet inhibitors include aspirin, ticlopidine, clopidogrel, and dipyridamole. Additionally, the use of statins has been shown to be effective for the patient with an ischemic stroke.[14]

Surgical Therapy for Ischemic Stroke. Stent retrievers (e.g., Solitaire FR, Trevo) are a way of opening blocked arteries in the brain by using a removable stent system. During the procedure, a catheter is used to guide the small stent from the femoral artery in the groin area to the affected artery in the brain. The stent is guided into the part of the artery where a blood clot has

FIG. 58-7 The MERCI retriever removes blood clots in patients who are experiencing ischemic strokes. The retriever is a long, thin wire that is threaded through a catheter into the femoral artery. The wire is pushed through the end of the catheter up to the carotid artery. The wire reshapes itself into tiny loops that latch onto the clot, and the clot can then be pulled out. To prevent the clot from breaking off, a balloon at the end of the catheter inflates to stop blood flow through the artery. *MERCI*, Mechanical embolus removal in cerebral ischemia.

FIG. 58-8 Clipping of aneurysms.

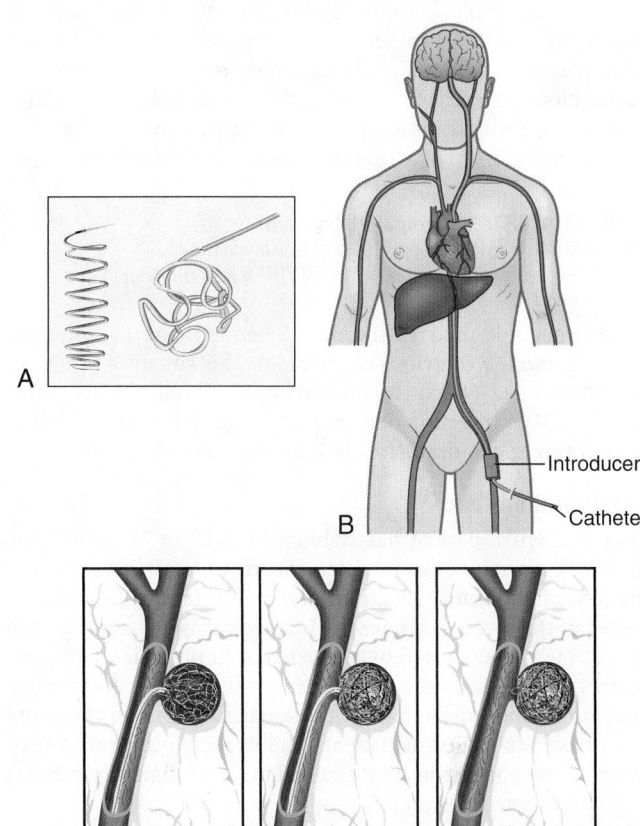

FIG. 58-9 Guglielmi detachable coil (GDC). **A,** A coil is used to occlude an aneurysm. Coils are made of soft, springlike platinum. The softness of the platinum allows the coil to assume the shape of irregularly shaped aneurysms while posing little threat of rupture of the aneurysm. **B,** A catheter is inserted through an introducer (small tube) in an artery in the leg. The catheter is threaded up to the cerebral blood vessels. **C,** Platinum coils attached to a thin wire are inserted into the catheter and then placed in the aneurysm until the aneurysm is filled with coils. Packing the aneurysm with coils prevents the blood from circulating through the aneurysm, reducing the risk of rupture.

formed. The stent expands the interior walls of the artery and allows blood to get to the patient's brain immediately to prevent as much brain damage as possible. The clot seeps into the mesh of the stent. Then, after a few minutes the stent and clot are removed together.

Another surgical approach uses the mechanical embolus removal in cerebral ischemia (MERCI) retriever (Fig. 58-7), which allows the surgeon to go inside the blocked artery of a patient who is experiencing ischemic strokes. The MERCI retriever has a tiny, corkscrew-like device that uses a microcatheter inserted through a femoral artery balloon catheter. Once the corkscrew device reaches the clot in the brain, the device penetrates the clot, allowing it to be removed. A guidewire and the microcatheter are deployed through the balloon catheter and then placed just beyond the clot. The physician then deploys the MERCI retriever device to engage and ensnare the clot. Once the clot is captured, the balloon catheter is inflated to temporarily arrest forward flow while the clot is being withdrawn. The clot is pulled into the balloon catheter and completely out of the body. The balloon is then deflated and blood flow is restored. Research is also being conducted on other mechanical thrombectomy devices for the removal of clots, including acute balloon angioplasty and stenting, snare devices, and ultrasonic aspirators.[19]

Acute Care for Hemorrhagic Stroke

Drug Therapy for Hemorrhagic Stroke. Anticoagulants and platelet inhibitors are contraindicated in patients with hemorrhagic strokes. The main drug therapy for patients with hemorrhagic stroke is the management of hypertension. Oral and IV agents may be used to maintain BP within a normal to high-normal range (systolic BP less than 160 mm Hg). Seizure prophylaxis in the acute period after intracerebral and subarachnoid hemorrhages is situation specific and should be discussed with the collaborative care team.[20]

Surgical Therapy for Hemorrhagic Stroke. Surgical interventions for hemorrhagic stroke include immediate evacuation of aneurysm-induced hematomas or cerebellar hematomas larger than 3 cm. Individuals who have an arteriovenous malformation (AVM) may experience a hemorrhagic stroke if the AVM ruptures. The treatment of AVM is surgical resection and/or radiosurgery (i.e., gamma knife). Both may be preceded by interventional neuroradiology to embolize the blood vessels that supply the AVM.

SAH is usually caused by a ruptured aneurysm. Approximately 20% of patients have multiple aneurysms. Treatment of an aneurysm involves clipping or coiling the aneurysm to prevent rebleeding (Figs. 58-8 and 58-9). In *clipping* the aneurysm, the neurosurgeon places a metallic clip on the neck of the aneurysm to block blood flow and prevent rupture. The clip remains in place for life. In the procedure known as *coiling*, a metal coil is inserted into the lumen of the aneurysm via interventional neuroradiology (see Fig. 58-9). Guglielmi detachable coils (GDCs) provide immediate protection against hemorrhage by reducing the blood pulsations within the aneurysm. Eventually, a thrombus forms within the aneurysm and the aneurysm becomes sealed off from the parent vessel by the formation of an endothelialized layer of connective tissue.

Goals for managing ICP are the same for patients with SAH as they are for patients dealing with acute stroke. After aneurysmal occlusion via clipping or coiling, hyperdynamic therapy (hemodilution-induced hypertension using vasoconstricting agents such as phenylephrine or dopamine [Intropin] and hypervolemia) may be instituted in an effort to increase the mean arterial pressure and increase cerebral perfusion. Volume expansion is achieved via crystalloid or colloid solution.

Interventions to treat cerebral vasospasm either before or after aneurysm clipping or coiling include administration of the calcium channel blocker nimodipine (Nimotop), which is given to patients with SAH to decrease the effects of vasospasm and minimize cerebral damage. Nimodipine restricts the influx of calcium ions into cells by reducing the number of open calcium channels. Although nimodipine is a calcium channel blocker, its exact mechanism of action in reducing vasospasm is not well understood.

DRUG ALERT: Nimodipine (Nimotop)
- Assess BP and apical pulses before administration.
- If pulse is ≤60 beats/min or systolic BP is <90 mm Hg, hold medication and contact physician.

Subarachnoid and intracerebral hemorrhage can involve bleeding into the ventricles of the brain. This situation produces hydrocephalus, which further damages brain tissue from increased ICP. Insertion of a ventriculostomy for cerebrospinal fluid drainage can dramatically improve these situations.[21]

Rehabilitation Care

After the stroke patient has stabilized for 12 to 24 hours, collaborative care shifts from preserving life to lessening disability and attaining optimal function. Many of the interventions discussed in the acute phase are maintained during this phase. The patient may be evaluated by a physiatrist (a physician who specializes in physical medicine and rehabilitation). Remember that some aspects of rehabilitation actually begin in the acute care phase as soon as the patient is stabilized. Specific measures related to rehabilitation are discussed in the section on Ambulatory and Home Care on pp. 1408-1410.

NURSING MANAGEMENT
STROKE

NURSING ASSESSMENT

Subjective and objective data that should be obtained from a person who has had a stroke are presented in Table 58-8. Primary assessment focuses on cardiac and respiratory status and neurologic assessment. If the patient is stable, the nursing history is obtained as follows: (1) description of the current illness with attention to initial symptoms, particularly symptom onset and duration, nature (intermittent or continuous), and changes; (2) history of similar symptoms previously experienced; (3) current medications; (4) history of risk factors and other illnesses such as hypertension; and (5) family history of stroke or cardiovascular diseases. This information is gained through an interview of the patient, family members, significant others, and/or caregiver.

Secondary assessment includes a comprehensive neurologic examination of the patient. This includes (1) level of consciousness, including assessment using the National Institutes of Health (NIH) Stroke Scale (Table 58-9); (2) cognition; (3) motor abilities; (4) cranial nerve function; (5) sensation; (6) proprioception; (7) cerebellar function; and (8) deep tendon reflexes.

TABLE 58-8 NURSING ASSESSMENT
Stroke

Subjective Data
Important Health Information
Past health history: Hypertension; previous stroke, TIA, aneurysm, cardiac disease (including recent myocardial infarction), dysrhythmias, heart failure, valvular disease, infective endocarditis; hyperlipidemia, polycythemia, diabetes, gout; previous head injury, family history of hypertension, diabetes, stroke, or coronary artery disease
Medications: Oral contraceptives; use of and compliance with antihypertensive and anticoagulant therapy; illegal substances and drug use (cocaine)

Functional Health Patterns
Health perception–health management: Positive family history of stroke; alcohol abuse, smoking, drug abuse
Nutritional-metabolic: Anorexia, nausea, vomiting; dysphagia, altered sense of taste and smell
Elimination: Change in bowel and bladder patterns
Activity-exercise: Loss of movement and sensation; syncope; weakness on one side; generalized weakness, easy fatigability
Cognitive-perceptual: Numbness, tingling of one side of the body; loss of memory; alteration in speech, language, problem-solving ability; pain; headache, possibly sudden and severe (hemorrhage); visual disturbances; denial of illness

Objective Data
General
Emotional lability, lethargy, apathy or combativeness, fever

Respiratory
Loss of cough reflex, labored or irregular respirations, tachypnea, rhonchi (aspiration), airway occlusion (tongue), apnea, coughing when eating or delayed coughing

Cardiovascular
Hypertension, tachycardia, carotid bruit

Gastrointestinal
Loss of gag reflex, bowel incontinence, decreased or absent bowel sounds, constipation

Urinary
Frequency, urgency, incontinence

Neurologic
Contralateral motor and sensory deficits, including weakness, paresis, paralysis, anesthesia; unequal pupils, hand grasps; akinesia, aphasia (expressive, receptive, global), dysarthria (slurred speech), agnosias, apraxia, visual deficits, perceptual or spatial disturbances, altered level of consciousness (drowsiness to deep coma) and Babinski's sign, ↓ followed by ↑ deep tendon reflexes, flaccidity followed by spasticity, amnesia, ataxia, personality change, nuchal rigidity, seizures

Possible Diagnostic Findings
Positive CT, CTA, MRI, MRA, or other neuroimaging scans showing size, location, and type of lesion; positive Doppler ultrasonography and angiography indicating stenosis

CTA, Computed tomographic angiography; *MRA,* magnetic resonance angiography; *TIA,* transient ischemic attack.

Clear documentation of initial and ongoing neurologic examinations is essential to note changes in the patient's status.

NURSING DIAGNOSES

Nursing diagnoses for the person with a stroke may include, but are not limited to, those presented in Nursing Care Plan 58-1.

TABLE 58-9   NATIONAL INSTITUTES OF HEALTH STROKE SCALE (NIHSS)

Description

The National Institutes of Health Stroke Scale (NIHSS) is a 15-item neurologic examination used to evaluate the effect of an acute stroke.

Procedure for Use

A trained observer rates the patient's ability to answer questions and perform activities. Ratings for each item are scored and there is an allowance for untestable (UN) items. If an item is left untested, a detailed explanation must be clearly written on the form. Training can be completed free at *www.nihstrokescale.org*.

Item	Scale Definition
Level of consciousness	0 = Alert 1 = Not alert, but arousable by minor stimulation 2 = Not alert, requires repeated stimulation to get attention 3 = Responds only with reflex motor or autonomic effects or totally unresponsive, flaccid, areflexic
Level of consciousness questions	0 = Answers both questions correctly 1 = Answers one question correctly 2 = Answers neither question correctly
Level of consciousness commands	0 = Performs both tasks correctly 1 = Performs one task correctly 2 = Performs neither task correctly
Best gaze	0 = Normal 1 = Partial gaze palsy 2 = Forced deviation, or total gaze paresis
Visual	0 = No visual loss 1 = Partial hemianopsia 2 = Complete hemianopsia 3 = Bilateral hemianopsia or blind
Facial palsy	0 = Normal symmetric movement 1 = Minor paralysis 2 = Partial paralysis 3 = Complete paralysis of one or both sides
Motor and drift (for each extremity)	0 = No drift 1 = Drift 2 = Some effort against gravity 3 = No effort against gravity, limb falls 4 = No movement UN = Amputation
Limb ataxia	0 = Absent 1 = Present in one limb 2 = Present in two limbs
Sensory	0 = Normal 1 = Mild to moderate sensory loss 2 = Severe to total sensory loss
Best language	0 = No aphasia, normal 1 = Mild to moderate aphasia 2 = Severe aphasia 3 = Mute, no usable speech or auditory comprehension
Dysarthria	0 = Normal 1 = Mild to moderate 2 = Severe UN = Intubated or other physical barrier
Extinction or inattention	0 = No abnormality 1 = Inattention or extinction to bilateral stimulation 2 = Does not recognize own hand
Distal motor function	0 = Normal (no flexion after 5 sec) 1 = At least some extension but not fully extended 2 = No voluntary extension after 5 sec

Source: American Stroke Association: NIH stroke scale, 2009. Retrieved from *www.ninds.nih.gov/doctors/NIH_Stroke_Scale.pdf*.

PLANNING

Together with the patient, caregiver, and family, establish the goals of nursing care. Typical goals are that the patient will (1) maintain a stable or improved level of consciousness, (2) attain maximum physical functioning, (3) attain maximum self-care abilities and skills, (4) maintain stable body functions (e.g., bladder control), (5) maximize communication abilities, (6) maintain adequate nutrition, (7) avoid complications of stroke, and (8) maintain effective personal and family coping.

NURSING IMPLEMENTATION

HEALTH PROMOTION. You have a major role in the promotion of a healthy lifestyle. Teaching should focus on stroke prevention, particularly for persons with known risk factors. Nursing measures to reduce risk factors for stroke are similar to those for coronary artery disease (see Chapter 34, Table 34-1) and are discussed earlier in this chapter on pp. 1394-1396.

Uncontrolled or undiagnosed hypertension is the primary cause of stroke. Therefore you need to be involved in BP screening and ensuring that patients adhere to the use of their antihypertensive medications. If a person is a diabetic, it is important that the diabetes is well controlled. If an individual has atrial fibrillation, an anticoagulant (see p. 1398) or aspirin may be used to reduce the risk of stroke. Because smoking is a major risk factor for stroke, you need to be actively involved in helping patients to stop smoking (see Chapter 11, Tables 11-4 to 11-6).

Another important aspect of health promotion is teaching patients and families about early symptoms associated with stroke or TIA. Table 58-1 presents information on when to seek health care for these symptoms.

ACUTE INTERVENTION

Respiratory System. During the acute phase after a stroke, management of the respiratory system is a nursing priority.[22] Stroke patients are particularly vulnerable to respiratory problems. Advancing age and immobility increase the risk for atelectasis and pneumonia.

Risk for aspiration pneumonia is high because of impaired consciousness or dysphagia. Dysphagia after stroke is common.[23] Airway obstruction can occur because of problems with chewing and swallowing, food pocketing (food remaining in the buccal cavity of the mouth), and the tongue falling back. Some stroke patients, especially those with brainstem or hemorrhagic stroke, may require endotracheal intubation and mechanical ventilation initially. Enteral tube feedings also place the patient at risk for aspiration pneumonia. All patients should be screened for their ability to swallow and kept on nothing-by-mouth (NPO) status until dysphagia has been ruled out.

Nursing interventions to support adequate respiratory function are individualized to meet the patient's needs. An oropharyngeal airway may be used in comatose patients to prevent the tongue from falling back and obstructing the airway and to provide access for suctioning. Alternatively, a nasopharyngeal airway may be used to provide airway protection and access. When an artificial airway is required for a prolonged time, a tracheostomy may be performed.

Nursing interventions include frequently assessing airway patency and function, providing oxygenation, suctioning, promoting patient mobility, positioning the patient to prevent aspiration, and encouraging deep breathing. In patients who are on mechanical ventilation, oral care at least every 2 hours reduces the occurrence of ventilator-assisted pneumonia.[24]

⊚ NURSING CARE PLAN 58-1

Patient With Stroke

NURSING DIAGNOSIS* **Decreased intracranial adaptive capacity** *related to* decreased cerebral perfusion pressure of ≤50-60 mm Hg and sustained increase in ICP secondary to thrombus, embolus, or hemorrhage *as evidenced by* baseline ICP ≥15 mm Hg, elevated systolic blood pressure, bradycardia, widened pulse pressure, and increasing NIH Stroke Scale score

PATIENT GOAL Demonstrates signs of stable or improved cerebral perfusion

Outcomes (NOC)	Interventions (NIC) and *Rationales*
Tissue Perfusion: Cerebral	**Cerebral Perfusion Promotion**

Tissue Perfusion: Cerebral
- Intracranial pressure _____
- Systolic blood pressure _____
- Diastolic blood pressure _____

Measurement Scale
1 = Severe deviation from normal range
2 = Substantial deviation from normal range
3 = Moderate deviation from normal range
4 = Mild deviation from normal range
5 = No deviation from normal range

- Restlessness _____
- Decreased level of consciousness _____
- Impaired cognition _____
- Impaired neurologic reflexes _____

Measurement Scale
1 = Severe
2 = Substantial
3 = Moderate
4 = Mild
5 = None

Cerebral Perfusion Promotion
- Consult with physician to determine hemodynamic parameters, and maintain hemodynamic parameters within this range.
- Monitor neurologic status *to detect changes indicative of worsening or improving condition.*
- Calculate and monitor cerebral perfusion pressure (CPP) *to detect change in condition.*
- Monitor respiratory status (e.g., rate, rhythm, and depth of respirations; PaO_2, $PaCO_2$, pH, and bicarbonate levels) *because high $PaCO_2$ and a high hydrogen ion concentration (acidosis) are potent vasodilators that increase cerebral blood flow.*
- Monitor patient's ICP and neurologic responses to care activities, *since changes in positioning and movement can increase ICP.*
- Monitor determinants of tissue oxygen delivery (e.g., $PaCO_2$, SaO_2, hemoglobin levels, and cardiac output) *to ensure adequate cerebral oxygenation.*
- Administer and titrate vasoactive drugs, as ordered, *to maintain hemodynamic parameters.*
- Avoid neck flexion or extreme hip or knee flexion *to avoid obstruction of arterial and venous blood flow.*

NURSING DIAGNOSIS **Risk for aspiration** *related to* decreased level of consciousness and decreased or absent gag and swallowing reflexes

PATIENT GOALS 1. Demonstrates ability to swallow oral foods without aspiration
2. Maintains a clear airway

Outcomes (NOC)	Interventions (NIC) and *Rationales*

Respiratory Status: Airway Patency
- Depth of inspiration _____
- Ability to clear secretions _____

Measurement Scale
1 = Severe deviation from normal range
2 = Substantial deviation from normal range
3 = Moderate deviation from normal range
4 = Mild deviation from normal range
5 = No deviation from normal range

- Adventitious breath sounds _____
- Accumulation of sputum _____

Measurement Scale
1 = Severe
2 = Substantial
3 = Moderate
4 = Mild
5 = None

Aspiration Precautions
- Monitor level of consciousness, cough reflex, gag reflex, and swallowing ability *to determine patient's ability to swallow foods without aspiration.*
- Avoid liquids or use thickening agent *to facilitate swallowing.*
- Feed in small amounts until patient is no longer at risk for aspiration.
- Offer foods or liquids that can be formed into a bolus before swallowing.

Airway Management
- Auscultate breath sounds, noting areas of decreased or absent ventilation and presence of adventitious sounds *to identify airway obstruction and accumulation of secretions.*
- Remove secretions by encouraging coughing or by suctioning *to clear airway.*
- Encourage slow, deep breathing; turning; and coughing *to increase airway clearance without increasing ICP.*
- Assist with incentive spirometer *to open collapsed alveoli, promote deep breathing, and prevent atelectasis.*
- Keep patient NPO until swallow evaluation completed *to prevent aspiration.*

NURSING DIAGNOSIS **Impaired physical mobility** *related to* neuromuscular and cognitive impairment and decreased muscle strength and control *as evidenced by* limited ability to perform gross and fine motor skills, limited range of motion, and difficulty turning

PATIENT GOALS 1. Demonstrates increased muscle strength and ability to move
2. Uses adaptive equipment to increase mobility

Outcomes (NOC)	Interventions (NIC) and *Rationales*

Mobility
- Balance _____
- Muscle movement _____
- Joint movement _____
- Transfer performance _____
- Walking _____

Measurement Scale
1 = Severely compromised
2 = Substantially compromised
3 = Moderately compromised
4 = Mildly compromised
5 = Not compromised

Exercise Therapy: Muscle Control
- Collaborate with physical, occupational, and recreational therapists in developing and executing exercise program *to determine extent of problem and plan appropriate interventions.*
- Determine patient's readiness to engage in activity or exercise protocol *to assess expected level of participation.*
- Apply splints to achieve stability of proximal joints involved with fine motor skills *to prevent contractures.*
- Encourage patient to practice exercises independently *to promote patient's sense of control.*
- Reinforce instructions provided to patient about the proper way to perform exercises *to minimize injury and maximize effectiveness.*
- Provide restful environment for patient after periods of exercise *to facilitate recuperation.*

*Nursing diagnoses listed in order of priority.

⊚ NURSING CARE PLAN 58-1—cont'd

Patient With Stroke

NURSING DIAGNOSIS **Impaired verbal communication** *related to* aphasia *as evidenced by* refusal or inability to speak, difficulty forming words and sentences to express thoughts, and inappropriate verbalization

PATIENT GOALS 1. Uses effective oral and written communication techniques
2. Demonstrates congruency of verbal and nonverbal communication

Outcomes (NOC)	Interventions (NIC) and *Rationales*
Communication	*Communication Enhancement: Speech Deficit*
• Use of spoken language _____	• Listen attentively *to convey the importance of patient's thoughts and to promote a positive environment for learning.*
• Use of written language _____	• Provide positive reinforcement and praise *to build self-esteem and confidence.*
• Use of nonverbal language _____	• Use simple words and short sentences *to avoid overwhelming patient with verbal stimuli.*
• Exchanges messages accurately with others _____	• Perform prescriptive speech-language therapies during informal interactions with patient *to reinforce prescribed therapies.*
Measurement Scale	• Provide verbal prompts and reminders *to help patient to express self.*
1 = Severely compromised	
2 = Substantially compromised	
3 = Moderately compromised	
4 = Mildly compromised	
5 = Not compromised	

NURSING DIAGNOSIS **Unilateral neglect** *related to* visual field cut and loss on one side of body (hemianopsia) and brain injury from cerebrovascular problems *as evidenced by* consistent inattention to stimuli on affected side

PATIENT GOALS 1. Cares for both sides of the body appropriately
2. Uses strategies to minimize unilateral neglect

Outcomes (NOC)	Interventions (NIC) and *Rationales*
Heedfulness of Affected Side	*Unilateral Neglect Management*
• Acknowledges affected side as being integral to self _____	• Monitor for abnormal responses to three types of stimuli: sensory, visual, and auditory *to determine the presence of and degree to which unilateral neglect exists (e.g., inability to see objects on affected side, leaving food on a plate that corresponds to affected side, lack of sensation on affected side).*
• Protects affected side when positioning _____	• Instruct patient to scan from left to right *to visualize the entire environment.*
• Protects affected side when ambulating _____	• Position bed in room so that individuals approach and care for patient on unaffected side.
• Performs activities of daily living to affected side _____	• Rearrange the environment to use the right or left visual field; position personal items, television, or reading materials within view on unaffected side *to compensate for visual field deficits.*
• Arranges environment to compensate for physical or sensory deficits _____	• Touch unaffected shoulder when initiating conversation *to attract patient's attention.*
• Uses visual scanning as a compensatory strategy _____	• Gradually move personal items and activity to affected side as patient demonstrates an ability to compensate for neglect.
Measurement Scale	• Include caregivers in rehabilitation process *to support the patient's efforts and assist with care to promote reintegration with the whole body.*
1 = Never demonstrated	
2 = Rarely demonstrated	
3 = Sometimes demonstrated	
4 = Often demonstrated	
5 = Consistently demonstrated	

NURSING DIAGNOSIS **Impaired urinary elimination** *related to* impaired impulse to void or inability to reach toilet or manage tasks of voiding *as evidenced by* loss of urinary control and involuntary loss of urine at unpredictable times

PATIENT GOALS 1. Perceives impulse to void, removes clothing for toileting, and uses toilet
2. Demonstrates ability to urinate when the urge arises or with a timed schedule

Outcomes (NOC)	Interventions (NIC) and *Rationales*
Urinary Continence	*Urinary Habit Training*
• Recognizes urge to void _____	• Keep a continence specification record for 3 days *to establish voiding pattern and plan appropriate interventions.*
• Maintains predictable pattern of voiding _____	• Establish interval of initial toileting schedule (based on voiding pattern and usual routine) *to initiate process of improving bladder functioning and increased muscle tone.*
• Responds to urge in timely manner _____	• Assist patient to toilet and prompt to void at prescribed intervals *to assist patient in adapting to new toileting schedule.*
• Starts and stops stream _____	• Teach patient to consciously hold urine until the scheduled toileting time *to improve muscle tone.*
Measurement Scale	• Discuss daily record of continence with staff *to provide reinforcement and encourage compliance with toileting schedule.*
1 = Never demonstrated	• Give positive feedback or positive reinforcement to patient when he or she voids at scheduled toileting times, and make no comment when patient is incontinent, *to reinforce desired behavior.*
2 = Rarely demonstrated	
3 = Sometimes demonstrated	
4 = Often demonstrated	
5 = Consistently demonstrated	
• Urine leakage between voidings _____	
• Wets clothing during the day _____	
• Wets clothing or bedding during night _____	
Measurement Scale	
1 = Consistently demonstrated	
2 = Often demonstrated	
3 = Sometimes demonstrated	
4 = Rarely demonstrated	
5 = Never demonstrated	

Continued

NURSING CARE PLAN 58-1—cont'd
Patient With Stroke

NURSING DIAGNOSIS	**Impaired swallowing** *related to* weakness or paralysis of affected muscles *as evidenced by* drooling, difficulty in swallowing, choking
PATIENT GOAL	Demonstrates effective swallowing without choking, coughing, or aspiration

Outcomes (NOC) | **Interventions (NIC) and *Rationales***

Swallowing Status
- Maintains food in mouth _____
- Handles oral secretions _____
- Ability to clear oral cavity _____

Measurement Scale
1 = Severely compromised
2 = Substantially compromised
3 = Moderately compromised
4 = Mildly compromised
5 = Not compromised

- Choking _____
- Coughing _____
- Gagging _____

Measurement Scale
1 = Severe
2 = Substantial
3 = Moderate
4 = Mild
5 = None

Swallowing Therapy
- Collaborate with other members of health care team (e.g., occupational therapist, speech pathologist, dietitian) *to provide continuity in patient's rehabilitative plan.*
- Assist patient to sit in an erect position (as close to 90 degrees as possible) for feeding/exercise *to provide optimal position for chewing and swallowing without aspirating.*
- Assist patient to position head in forward flexion in preparation for swallowing ("chin tuck").
- Assist patient to maintain sitting position for 30 min after completing meal *to prevent regurgitation of food.*
- Instruct patient or caregiver on emergency measures for choking *to prevent complications in the home setting.*
- Check mouth for pocketing of food after eating *to prevent collection and putrefaction of food and/or aspiration.*
- Provide mouth care as needed *to promote comfort and oral health.*
- Monitor body weight *to determine adequacy of nutritional intake.*

NURSING DIAGNOSIS	**Situational low self-esteem** *related to* actual or perceived loss of function and altered body image *as evidenced by* refusal to participate in self-care and expressions of helplessness and uselessness
PATIENT GOALS	1. Expresses positive feelings of self-worth 2. Participates in self-care of affected body parts

Outcomes (NOC) | **Interventions (NIC) and *Rationales***

Self-Esteem
- Verbalizations of self-acceptance _____
- Maintenance of grooming and hygiene _____
- Acceptance of self-limitations _____
- Description of self _____
- Feelings about self-worth _____

Measurement Scale
1 = Never positive
2 = Rarely positive
3 = Sometimes positive
4 = Often positive
5 = Consistently positive

Self-Esteem Enhancement
- Monitor patient's statements of self-worth *to determine effect of stroke on self-esteem.*
- Encourage patient to identify strengths *to facilitate patient's recognition of intrinsic value.*
- Assist in setting realistic goals *to achieve higher self-esteem.*
- Reward or praise patient's progress toward reaching goals.
- Encourage increased responsibility for self *to promote sense of satisfaction, independence, and control, and to reduce frustrations.*
- Monitor levels of self-esteem over time *to determine stressors or situations that trigger low self-esteem and to teach coping mechanisms.*

ICP, Intracranial pressure; *NIH,* National Institutes of Health; *PaCO₂,* partial pressure of carbon dioxide in arterial blood; *PaO₂,* partial pressure of oxygen in arterial blood; *SaO₂,* arterial oxygen saturation.

Patients who have an unclipped or uncoiled aneurysm may experience rebleeding and the possibility of increasing ICP further with coughing or suctioning, so nursing management is aimed at reducing these interventions while maintaining a proper airway.

Interventions related to maintenance of airway function are described in Nursing Care Plan 58-1.

Neurologic System. The primary clinical assessment tool to evaluate and document neurologic status in acute stroke patients is the NIH Stroke Scale (NIHSS),[25] which measures stroke severity (see Table 58-9). The NIHSS is a predictor of both short- and long-term outcomes of stroke patients. Additionally, it serves as a data collection tool for planning patient care and exchanging information among health care providers.

Additional neurologic assessment includes mental status, pupillary responses, and extremity movement and strength. Also closely monitor vital signs. A decreasing level of consciousness may indicate increasing ICP. Monitor ICP and cere-bral perfusion pressure if the patient is in a critical care environment. Record your nursing assessment on flow sheets to communicate the patient's neurologic status to the stroke team.

Cardiovascular System. Nursing goals for the cardiovascular system are aimed at maintaining homeostasis. Many patients with stroke have decreased cardiac reserves secondary to cardiac disease. Cardiac efficiency may be further compromised by fluid retention, overhydration, dehydration, or BP variations. Central venous pressure, pulmonary artery pressure, or hemodynamic monitoring may be used as indicators of fluid balance or cardiac function in the critical care unit.

Nursing interventions include (1) monitoring vital signs frequently; (2) monitoring cardiac rhythms; (3) calculating intake and output, noting imbalances; (4) regulating IV infusions; (5) adjusting fluid intake to individual patient needs; (6) monitoring lung sounds for crackles and rhonchi indicating pulmonary congestion; and (7) monitoring heart sounds for murmurs or for S_3 or S_4 heart sounds. Bedside monitors or telemetry may record cardiac rhythms.

Hypertension is sometimes seen after a stroke as the body attempts to increase cerebral blood flow. It is important to monitor for orthostatic hypotension before ambulating the patient for the first time. Neurologic changes can occur with a sudden decrease in BP.

After a stroke, the patient is at risk for venous thromboembolism (VTE), especially in the weak or paralyzed lower extremity. VTE is related to immobility, loss of venous tone, and decreased muscle pumping activity in the leg. The most effective prevention is to keep the patient moving. Teach the patient active range-of-motion exercises if the patient has voluntary movement in the affected extremity. For the patient with hemiplegia, perform passive range-of-motion exercises several times a day. Additional measures to prevent VTE include positioning to minimize the effects of dependent edema and using elastic compression gradient stockings or support hose. Sequential compression devices may be ordered for bedridden patients. VTE prophylaxis may include low-molecular-weight heparin (e.g., enoxaparin [Lovenox]). The nursing assessment for VTE includes measuring the calf and thigh daily, observing swelling of the lower extremities, noting unusual warmth of the leg, and asking the patient about pain in the calf.

Musculoskeletal System. The nursing goal for the musculoskeletal system is to maintain optimal function by preventing joint contractures and muscular atrophy. In the acute phase, range-of-motion exercises and positioning are important nursing interventions. Passive range-of-motion exercise is begun on the first day of hospitalization. Muscle atrophy secondary to lack of innervation and activity can develop after stroke, so exercise is an important intervention for rehabilitation and recovery.

The paralyzed or weak side needs special attention when the patient is positioned. Position each joint higher than the joint proximal to it to prevent dependent edema. Specific deformities on the weak or paralyzed side that may be present in patients with stroke include internal rotation of the shoulder; flexion contractures of the hand, wrist, and elbow; external rotation of the hip; and plantar flexion of the foot. Subluxation of the shoulder on the affected side is common. Careful positioning and moving of the affected arm may prevent development of a painful shoulder condition. Immobilization of the affected upper extremity may precipitate a painful shoulder-hand syndrome.

Nursing interventions to optimize musculoskeletal function include (1) trochanter roll at the hip to prevent external rotation; (2) hand cones (not rolled washcloths) to prevent hand contractures; (3) arm supports with slings and lap boards to prevent shoulder displacement; (4) avoidance of pulling the patient by the arm to avoid shoulder displacement; (5) posterior leg splints, footboards, or high-top tennis shoes to prevent footdrop; and (6) hand splints to reduce spasticity.

Use of a footboard for the patient with spasticity is controversial. Rather than preventing plantar flexion (footdrop), the sensory stimulation of a footboard against the bottom of the foot increases plantar flexion. Likewise, experts disagree on whether hand splints facilitate or diminish spasticity. The decision regarding the use of footboards or hand splints is made on an individual patient basis.

Integumentary System. The skin of the patient with stroke is particularly susceptible to breakdown related to loss of sensation, decreased circulation, and immobility. This is compounded by advanced age, poor nutrition, dehydration, edema, and incontinence.

DELEGATION DECISIONS

Caring for the Patient With an Acute Stroke

During the first 48 hr after an acute stroke, some nursing activities may be delegated to licensed practical/vocational nurses (LPNs/LVNs) and unlicensed assistive personnel (UAP). The registered nurse (RN) should communicate frequently with these staff members to rapidly intervene based on changes in the patient status.

Role of Registered Nurse (RN)
- Assess clinical manifestations of stroke and determine when clinical manifestations started.
- Screen patient for contraindications for tissue plasminogen activator (tPA) therapy.
- Infuse tPA for patients with ischemic stroke who meet the criteria for tPA administration.
- Assess respiratory status and initiate needed actions such as O_2, oropharyngeal or nasopharyngeal airways, suctioning, and patient positioning to prevent aspiration, obstruction, and atelectasis.
- Assess neurologic status, including intracranial pressure (ICP) if needed.
- Monitor cardiovascular status, including hemodynamic monitoring if needed.
- Assess patient's ability to swallow (in conjunction with the speech therapist).

Role of Licensed Practical/Vocational Nurse (LPN/LVN)
- Administer scheduled anticoagulant and antiplatelet medications.

Role of Unlicensed Assistive Personnel (UAP)
- Obtain vital signs frequently and report these to RN.
- Measure and record urine output.
- Assist with positioning patient and turning patient at least every 2 hr (as directed by RN).
- Perform passive and active range-of-motion exercises (after being trained and evaluated in these procedures).
- Place equipment needed for seizure precautions in patient room.

The nursing plan for prevention of skin breakdown includes (1) pressure relief by position changes, special mattresses, or wheelchair cushions; (2) good skin hygiene; (3) emollients applied to dry skin; and (4) early mobility. An example of a position change schedule is side-backside, with a maximum duration of 2 hours for any position. Position the patient on the weak or paralyzed side for only 30 minutes. If an area of redness develops and does not return to normal color within 15 minutes of pressure relief, the epidermis and dermis are damaged.

Do not massage the damaged area because this may cause additional damage. Control of pressure is the single most important factor in both the prevention and treatment of skin breakdown. Pillows can be used under lower extremities to reduce pressure on the heels. Vigilance and good nursing care are required to prevent pressure sores.

Gastrointestinal System. The most common bowel problem for the stroke patient is constipation. Patients may be prophylactically placed on stool softeners and/or fiber (psyllium [Metamucil]). If a patient has liquid stools, check for stool impaction. Fluid and fiber intake goals should be discussed with the stroke team and are based on the patient's nutritional and fluid status.

Physical activity also promotes bowel function. Laxatives, suppositories, or additional stool softeners may be ordered if the patient does not respond to increased fluid and fiber. Enemas are used only if suppositories and digital stimulation are ineffective because they cause vagal stimulation and increase ICP.

Bowel retraining may be needed and continues into the rehabilitation phase. A bowel management program consists of placing the patient on the bedpan or bedside commode or taking the patient to the bathroom at a regular time daily to reestablish bowel regularity. A good time for the bowel program is 30 minutes after breakfast because eating stimulates the gastrocolic reflex and peristalsis, but timing may need to be adjusted, since individual bowel habits may vary.

Urinary System. In the acute stage of stroke the primary urinary problem is poor bladder control, resulting in incontinence. Take steps to promote normal bladder function and avoid the use of indwelling catheters. If an indwelling catheter must be used initially, remove it as soon as the patient is medically and neurologically stable. Long-term use of an indwelling catheter is associated with urinary tract infections and delayed bladder retraining.

An intermittent catheterization program may be used for patients with urinary retention because of the lower incidence of urinary infections. An alternative to intermittent catheterizations is the external catheter for male patients with urinary incontinence. External catheters do not alleviate the problem of urine retention. Avoid bladder overdistention.

Assist the patient with urinary difficulties or incontinence. Often the patient with stroke has functional incontinence, which is associated with communication difficulties, mobility problems, and dressing or undressing difficulties. A bladder retraining program consists of (1) adequate fluid intake with most of it given between 7:00 AM and 7:00 PM; (2) scheduled toileting every 2 hours using bedpan, commode, or bathroom while encouraging the usual position for urinating (standing for men and sitting for women); (3) observation for signs of restlessness, which may indicate the need for urination; and (4) assessment for bladder distention by palpation.

Assessment of postvoid residual volume is often done using bladder ultrasound. The ultrasound measures how much urine is in the bladder after voiding. If urine remains in the bladder, incomplete emptying is a problem and may cause urinary tract infections. A coordinated program by the entire nursing staff is needed to achieve urinary continence.

Nutrition. The patient's nutritional needs require quick assessment and treatment. The patient may initially receive IV infusions to maintain fluid and electrolyte balance and to administer drugs. Patients with severe impairment may require enteral or parenteral nutrition support. Patients should have their nutritional needs addressed in the first 72 hours of admission to the hospital because nutrition is important for recovery and healing.[26]

SAFETY ALERT
- The first oral feeding should be approached carefully because the gag reflex may be impaired due to dysphagia.

Speech therapists (if available) should perform a swallowing evaluation before patients are started on oral intake. The majority of patients experience dysphagia after a stroke.[23] Before initiating feeding, assess the gag reflex by gently stimulating the back of the throat with a tongue blade. If a gag reflex is present, the patient will gag spontaneously. If it is absent, defer the feeding, and begin exercises to stimulate swallowing. The speech therapist or occupational therapist is usually responsible for designing this program. However, you may be called on to develop the program in some clinical settings.

To assess swallowing ability, elevate the head of the bed to an upright position (unless contraindicated) and give the patient a small amount of crushed ice or ice water to swallow. If the gag reflex is present and the patient is able to swallow safely, you may proceed with feeding.

After careful assessment of swallowing, chewing, gag reflex, and pocketing, oral feedings can be initiated. Mouth care before feeding helps stimulate sensory awareness and salivation and can facilitate swallowing. The patient should remain in a high Fowler's position, preferably in a chair with the head flexed forward, for the feeding and for 30 minutes afterward.

The speech therapist may recommend various dietary items. Foods should be easy to swallow and provide enough texture, temperature (warm or cold), and flavor to stimulate a swallow reflex. Crushed ice can be used as a stimulant. Instruct the patient to swallow and then swallow again. Pureed foods are not usually the best choice because they are often bland and too smooth. Thin liquids are often difficult to swallow and may promote coughing. Thin liquids can be thickened with a commercially available thickening agent (e.g., Thick-It). Avoid milk products because they tend to increase the viscosity of mucus and increase salivation.

Place food on the unaffected side of the mouth. Feedings must be followed by scrupulous oral hygiene because food may collect on the affected side of the mouth. During the acute and rehabilitation phase of the stroke, a dietitian can assist in determining the appropriate daily caloric intake based on the patient's size, weight, and activity level. If the patient is unable to take in an adequate oral diet and dysphagia persists, a percutaneous endoscopic gastrostomy (PEG) tube (see Chapter 40, Fig. 40-7) may be used for nutritional support. Most commercially prepared formulas provide about 1 cal/mL. (Enteral feedings are described in Chapter 40.)

The inability to feed oneself can be frustrating and may result in malnutrition and dehydration. Interventions to promote self-feeding include using the unaffected upper extremity to eat; employing assistive devices such as rocker knives, plate guards, and nonslip pads for dishes (Fig. 58-10); removing unnecessary items from the tray or table, which can reduce spills; and providing a calm environment to decrease sensory overload and distraction. The effectiveness of the dietary program is evaluated in terms of maintenance of weight, adequate hydration, and patient satisfaction. Introduce these interventions in the acute care setting so that maximum rehabilitation can occur once the patient is discharged.

Communication. During the acute stage of stroke, your role in meeting the patient's psychologic needs is primarily supportive. Speech, comprehension, and language deficits are the most difficult problems for the patient and caregiver. Assess the patient for both the ability to speak and the ability to understand. The patient's response to simple questions can guide you in structuring explanations and instructions. If the patient cannot understand words, use gestures to support verbal cues. Collaborate with the speech therapist to assess and formulate a plan of care to enhance communication.

Nursing interventions that support communication include (1) communicating frequently and meaningfully; (2) allowing time for the patient to comprehend and answer; (3) using simple, short sentences; (4) using visual cues; (5) structuring conversation so that it permits simple answers by the patient; and (6) praising the patient honestly for improvements with speech.[27]

An alert patient is usually anxious because of lack of understanding about what has happened and because of difficulty with communication or inability to communicate. The stroke patient with aphasia may easily be overwhelmed by verbal stimuli. Give the patient extra time to comprehend and respond to communication. (Guidelines for communicating with a

FIG. 58-10 Assistive devices for eating. **A,** The curved fork fits over the hand. The rounded plate helps keep food on the plate. Special grips and swivel handles are helpful for some persons. **B,** Knives with rounded blades are rocked back and forth to cut food. The person does not need a fork in one hand and a knife in the other. **C,** Plate guards help keep food on the plate. **D,** Cup with special handle. (Courtesy Sammons Preston, Boling-brook, Ill.)

patient who has aphasia are presented in Table 58-10.) A picture board may be helpful for communicating with the stroke patient. Further evaluation and treatment of language and communication deficits are often done by the speech therapist once the patient has stabilized.

Sensory-Perceptual Alterations. Patients who have had a stroke frequently have perceptual deficits. Patients with a stroke on the right side of the brain usually have difficulty judging position, distance, and rate of movement. These patients are often impulsive and impatient and tend to deny problems related to strokes. They may fail to correlate spatial-perceptual problems with the inability to perform activities, such as guiding a wheelchair through the doorway. The patient with a right-brain stroke (left hemiplegia) is at higher risk for injury because of mobility difficulties. Directions for activities are best given verbally for comprehension. Break the task down into simple steps for ease of understanding. Environmental control, such as removing clutter and obstacles and using good lighting, aids in concentration and safer mobility. Provide nonslip socks at all times. One-sided neglect is common for people with right-brain stroke, so you may assist or remind the patient to dress the weak or paralyzed side or shave the forgotten side of the face.

Patients with a left-brain stroke (right hemiplegia) commonly are slower in organization and performance of tasks. They tend to have impaired spatial discrimination. These patients usually admit to deficits and have a fearful, anxious response to a stroke. Their behaviors are slow and cautious. Nonverbal cues and instructions are helpful for comprehension with patients who have had a left-brain stroke.

Homonymous hemianopsia (blindness in the same half of each visual field) is a common problem after a stroke. Persistent disregard of objects in part of the visual field should alert you to this possibility. Initially, help the patient to compensate by arranging the environment within the patient's perceptual field, such as arranging the food tray so that all foods are on the right side or the left side to accommodate for field of vision (Fig. 58-11). Later, the patient learns to compensate for the visual

FIG. 58-11 Spatial and perceptual deficits in stroke. Perception of a patient with homonymous hemianopsia shows that food on the left side is not seen and thus is ignored.

TABLE 58-10   **COMMUNICATION WITH A PATIENT WITH APHASIA**

1. Decrease environmental stimuli that may be distracting and disrupting to communication efforts.
2. Treat the patient as an adult.
3. Speak with normal volume and tone.
4. Present one thought or idea at a time.
5. Keep questions simple or ask questions that can be answered with "yes" or "no."
6. Let the person speak. Do not interrupt. Allow time for the individual to complete thoughts.
7. Make use of gestures or demonstration as an acceptable alternative form of communication. Encourage this by saying, "Show me . . ." or "Point to what you want."
8. Do not pretend to understand the person if you do not. Calmly say you do not understand and encourage the use of nonverbal communication, or ask the person to write out what he or she wants.
9. Give the patient time to process information and generate a response before repeating a question or statement.
10. Allow body contact (e.g., the clasp of a hand, touching) as much as possible. Realize that touching may be the only way the patient can express feelings.
11. Organize the patient's day by preparing and following a schedule (the more familiar the routine, the easier it will be).
12. Do not push communication if the person is tired or upset. Aphasia worsens with fatigue and anxiety.

defect by consciously attending or by scanning the neglected side. The weak or paralyzed extremities are carefully checked for adequacy of dressing, for hygiene, and for trauma.

In the clinical situation, it is often difficult to distinguish between a visual field cut and a neglect syndrome. Both problems may occur with strokes affecting either the right or the left side of the brain. A person may be unfortunate enough to have both homonymous hemianopsia and a neglect syndrome, which increases the inattention to the weak or paralyzed side. A neglect syndrome results in decreased safety awareness and places the patient at high risk for injury. Immediately after the stroke, anticipate safety hazards and provide protection from injury. Safety measures can include closely observing the patient, elevating side rails, lowering the height of the bed, and using video monitors. Avoid the use of restraints and soft vests because this may agitate the patient.

Other visual problems may include *diplopia* (double vision), loss of the corneal reflex, and *ptosis* (drooping eyelid), especially if the stroke is in the vertebrobasilar distribution. Diplopia is often treated with an eye patch. If the corneal reflex is absent, the patient is at risk for corneal abrasion and should be observed closely and protected against eye injuries. Corneal abrasion can be prevented with artificial tears or gel to keep the eyes moist and an eye shield (especially at night). Ptosis is generally not treated because it usually does not inhibit vision.

Coping. A stroke is usually a sudden, extremely stressful event for the patient, caregiver, family, and significant others. A stroke is often a family disease, affecting the family emotionally, socially, and financially and changing roles and responsibilities within the family.[28] An older couple may perceive the stroke as a threat to life and to accustomed lifestyle. Reactions to this threat vary considerably but may involve fear, apprehension, denial of the severity of stroke, depression, anger, and sorrow. During the acute phase of caring for the stroke patient and the family, nursing interventions designed to facilitate coping involve providing information and emotional support.

Explanations to the patient about what has happened and about diagnostic and therapeutic procedures should be clear and understandable. Decision making and upholding the patient's wishes during this challenging time are of upmost importance. Advance directives should be honored, and family meetings or updates should be held daily about feeding tube placement or tracheostomy.

Give the caregiver and family a careful, detailed explanation of what has happened to the patient. However, if the family is extremely anxious and upset during the acute phase, explanations may need to be repeated at a later time. Because family members usually have not had time to prepare for the illness, they may need assistance in arranging care for family members or pets and for transportation and finances. A social services referral is often helpful.

It is particularly challenging to keep the aphasic patient adequately informed. Tone, demeanor, and touch may also be used to convey support. When communicating with a patient who has a communication deficit, speak in a normal volume and tone, keep questions simple, and present one thought or idea at a time. To decrease frustration, always let the patient speak without interruption and make use of gestures. Do not forget to use writing and communication boards.[27]

AMBULATORY AND HOME CARE. The patient is usually discharged from the acute care setting to home, an intermediate or long-term care facility, or a rehabilitation facility. Ideally, discharge planning with the patient and the caregiver starts early in the hospitalization and promotes a smooth transition from one care setting to another. The stroke team provides guidance for the appropriate care necessary after discharge. If the patient requires a short- or long-term health care facility, the team can make appropriate referrals that allow time to select and arrange for care. A critical factor in discharge planning is the patient's level of independence in performing ADLs. If the patient is returning home, the team can make referrals for needed equipment and services in preparation for discharge.

You have an excellent opportunity to prepare the patient and caregiver for discharge through teaching, demonstration and return demonstration, practice, and evaluation of self-care skills. Total care is considered in discharge planning: medications, nutrition, mobility, exercises, hygiene, and toileting. Follow-up care is carefully planned to permit continuing nursing care; physical, occupational, and speech therapy; and medical care. Identify community resources to provide recreational activities, group support, spiritual assistance, respite care, adult day care, and home assistance based on the patient's needs.

Rehabilitation. *Rehabilitation* is the process of maximizing the patient's capabilities and resources to promote optimal functioning related to physical, mental, and social well-being. The goals of rehabilitation are to prevent deformity and maintain and improve function. Regardless of the care setting, ongoing rehabilitation is essential to maximize the patient's abilities. Most patients see the maximum benefit in the first year of recovery after a stroke.[29]

Rehabilitation requires a team approach so the patient and caregiver can benefit from the combined, expert care of a stroke team. The team must communicate and coordinate care to achieve the patient's goals. As a nurse, you are in a good position to facilitate this process and are often the key to successful rehabilitation efforts. The stroke team is composed of many members, including nurses, physicians, psychiatrist, physical therapist, occupational therapist, speech therapist, registered dietitian, respiratory therapist, vocational therapist, recreational therapist, social worker, psychologist, pharmacist, and chaplain. Physical therapy focuses on mobility, progressive ambulation, transfer techniques, and equipment needed for mobility. Occupational therapy emphasizes retraining for skills of daily living such as eating, dressing, hygiene, and cooking. Occupational therapists are also skilled in cognitive and perceptual evaluation and training. Speech therapy focuses on speech, communication, cognition, and eating abilities.

Many of the nursing interventions outlined in Nursing Care Plan 58-1 for the patient with a stroke are initiated in the acute phase of care and continue throughout rehabilitation. Some of the interventions are independent nursing actions, whereas others involve the entire rehabilitation team.

The rehabilitation nurse assesses the patient, caregiver, and family with attention to (1) the patient's rehabilitation potential, (2) physical status of all body systems, (3) complications caused by the stroke or other chronic conditions, (4) the patient's cognitive status, (5) family resources and support, and (6) expectations of the patient and caregiver related to the rehabilitation program.

Musculoskeletal Function. Initially emphasize the musculoskeletal functions of eating, toileting, and walking for rehabilitation of the patient. Initial assessment consists of determining the stage of recovery of muscle function. If the muscles are still flaccid several weeks after the stroke, the prognosis for regaining function is poor and care focuses on preventing additional loss (Fig. 58-12).

Most patients begin to show signs of spasticity with exaggerated reflexes within 48 hours after the stroke. Spasticity at this phase of stroke denotes progress toward recovery. As improvement continues, small voluntary movements of the hip or shoulder may be accompanied by involuntary movements in the rest of the extremity (*synergy*). The final stage of recovery occurs when the patient has voluntary control of isolated muscle groups.

INFORMATICS IN PRACTICE

Video Games for Stroke Recovery

- Patients dealing with the effects of a stroke often have difficulty performing activities of daily living. Playing active video games, like Nintendo Wii or Xbox Kinect, brings some fun into stroke recovery and may get patients to spend more time in therapy.
- Gaming helps patients regain lost strength, improve motor skills, and improve problem solving and short- and long-term memory.
- Patients can play with their families, including children, making gaming a way to involve others in rehabilitation.

FIG. 58-12 Loss of postural stability is common after stroke. When the nondominant hemisphere is involved, walking apraxia and loss of postural control are usually apparent. The patient is unable to sit upright and tends to fall sideways. Provide appropriate support with pillows or cushions.

Interventions for the musculoskeletal system advance in a manner of progressive activity. Balance training is the initial step and begins with the patient sitting up in bed or dangling the legs over the edge of the bed. Evaluate tolerance by noting dizziness or syncope caused by vasomotor instability.

Also assess whether patients autocorrect their posture when sitting on the edge of the bed. If the patient can straighten his or her posture instead of leaning to the weaker side, the patient may be ready for the next step of transferring from bed to chair. Place the chair beside the bed so that the patient can lead with the stronger arm and leg. The patient sits on the side of the bed, stands, places the strong hand on the far wheelchair arm, and sits down. You may either supervise the transfer or provide minimal assistance by guiding the patient's strong hand to the wheelchair arm, standing in front of the patient while blocking the patient's knees with your knees to prevent knee buckling, and guiding the patient into a sitting position.

In some rehabilitation units the Bobath method is used as an approach to mobility (http://ibita.org). The goal of this approach is to help the patient gain control over patterns of spasticity by inhibiting abnormal reflex patterns. Therapists and nurses use the Bobath approach to encourage normal muscle tone, normal movement, and bilateral function of the body. An example is to have the patient transfer into the wheelchair using the weak or paralyzed side and the stronger side to facilitate more bilateral functioning.

Another approach to stroke rehabilitation is constraint-induced movement therapy (CIMT). CIMT encourages the patient to use the weakened extremity by restricting movement of the normal extremity. Complying with this approach can be challenging for patients and may limit its use. Movement training, skill acquisition, splinting, and exercise are additional therapies offered for rehabilitation of the stroke patient.[29]

Supportive or assistive equipment, such as canes, walkers, and leg braces, may be needed on a short- or long-term basis for mobility. The physical therapist usually selects the most appropriate supportive device(s) to meet individual needs and instructs the patient regarding use. Incorporate physical therapy activities into the patient's daily routine for additional practice and repetition of rehabilitation efforts.

Stroke Survivorship and Coping. Patients who have had strokes often exhibit emotional responses that are not appropriate or typical for the situation. Patients may appear apathetic, depressed, fearful, anxious, weepy, frustrated, and angry. Some patients, especially those with a stroke on the left side of the brain (right hemiplegia), have exaggerated mood swings. The patient may be unable to control emotions and may suddenly burst into tears or laughter. This behavior is out of context and often is unrelated to the patient's underlying emotional state. Nursing interventions for atypical emotional response are to (1) distract the patient who suddenly becomes emotional, (2) explain to the patient and family that emotional outbursts may occur after a stroke, (3) maintain a calm environment, and (4) avoid shaming or scolding the patient during emotional outbursts.

The patient with a stroke may experience many losses, including sensory, intellectual, communicative, functional, role behavior, emotional, social, and vocational losses. The patient, caregiver, and family often go through the process of grief and mourning associated with the losses. Some patients experience long-term depression with symptoms such as anxiety, weight loss, fatigue, poor appetite, and sleep disturbances. In addition, the time and energy required to perform previously simple tasks can result in anger and frustration.

The patient, caregiver, and family need help coping with the losses associated with stroke. Provide assistance by (1) supporting communication between the patient and family; (2) discussing lifestyle changes resulting from stroke deficits; (3) discussing changing roles and responsibilities within the family; (4) being an active listener to allow the expression of fear, frustration, and anxiety; (5) including the family and patient in short- and long-term goal planning and patient care; and (6) supporting family conferences.

Maladjusted dependence with inadequate coping occurs when the patient does not maintain optimal functioning for self-care, family responsibilities, decision making, or socialization. This situation can cause resentment from both the patient and family with a negative cycle of interpersonal dependency and control.[28] Caregivers and family members must cope with three aspects of the patient's behavior: (1) recognition of behavioral changes resulting from neurologic deficits that are not changeable, (2) responses to multiple losses by both the patient and the family, and (3) behaviors that may have been reinforced during the early stages of stroke as continued dependency.

The patient, caregiver, and family may express guilt over not living healthy lifestyles or not seeking professional help sooner. Family therapy is a helpful adjunct to rehabilitation. Open communication, information regarding the total effects of stroke, teaching regarding stroke treatment, and therapy are helpful. Stroke support groups in rehabilitation facilities and in the community are helpful in terms of mutual sharing, education, coping skills, and understanding.

Sexual Function. A patient who has had a stroke may be concerned about the loss of sexual function. Many patients are comfortable talking about their anxieties and fears regarding sexual function if you are comfortable and open to the topic. You may initiate the topic with the patient and spouse or significant other. Common concerns regarding sexual activity are impotence and the occurrence of another stroke during sex. Nursing interventions for sexual activity include teaching about (1) optional positioning of partners, (2) timing for peak energy times, and (3) patient and partner counseling.

Community Integration. Traditionally, successful community integration after stroke has been difficult for the patient because of persistent problems with cognition, coping, physical deficits, and emotional lability that interfere with functioning. Older patients who have had a stroke often have more severe deficits and frequently experience multiple health problems. Failure to continue the rehabilitation regimen at home may result in deterioration and further complications.

Community resources can be an asset to patients and their families. The National Stroke Association provides information, resources, referral services, and quarterly newsletters on stroke. The American Stroke Association, a division of the American Heart Association, has information regarding stroke, hypertension, diet, exercise, and assistive devices. This association sponsors self-help groups in many areas. Easter Seals provides wheelchairs and other assistive devices for stroke patients. Local groups can offer more daily assistance such as meals and transportation. These resources can be identified by nurse case managers, home health nurses, discharge planners, and clinical nurse specialists. (Resources are listed at the end of the chapter.)

GERONTOLOGIC CONSIDERATIONS

STROKE

Stroke is a significant cause of death and disability. The highest incidence of stroke occurs among older adults. Stroke can result in a profound disruption in the life of an older person. The magnitude of disability and changes in total function can leave patients wondering if they can ever return to their "old self," and loss of independence may be a major concern. The ability to perform ADLs may require many adaptive changes because of physical, emotional, perceptual, and cognitive deficits. Home management may be a particular challenge if the patient has an older spouse caregiver who also has health problems. There may be limited family members (including adult children) living in close proximity to provide help.

The rehabilitative phase and helping the older patient deal with the residual deficits of stroke, as well as aging, can provide a challenging nursing experience. Patients may become fearful and depressed because they think they may have another stroke or die. The fear can become immobilizing and interfere with effective rehabilitation.

Changes may occur in the patient-spouse relationship. The dependency resulting from a stroke may threaten the relationship. The spouse may also have chronic medical problems that can affect the ability to take care of the stroke survivor. The patient may not want anyone other than the spouse to provide care, thus putting a significant burden on the spouse.

You have the opportunity to assist the patient and caregiver in the transition through acute hospitalization, rehabilitation, long-term care, and home care. The needs of the patient, the caregiver, and the family require ongoing nursing assessment and adaptation of interventions in response to changing needs to optimize quality of life for all of them.

CASE STUDY

Stroke

iStockphoto/Thinkstock

Patient Profile

A.J., a 66-yr-old white woman, awoke in the middle of the night and fell when she tried to get up and go to the bathroom (see Chapter 56 case study on p. 1344). She fell because she was not able to control her left leg. Her husband took her to the hospital, where she was diagnosed with an acute ischemic stroke. Because she had awakened with symptoms, the actual time of onset was unknown and she was not a candidate for tPA.

Subjective Data

- Left arm and leg are weak and feel numb
- Feeling depressed and fearful
- Requires help with ADLs
- Concerned about having another stroke
- Says she has not taken her medications for high cholesterol and high blood pressure for several weeks
- History of a brief episode of left-sided weakness and tingling of the face, arm, and hand 3 mo earlier, which totally resolved and for which she did not seek treatment

Objective Data

- BP 180/110 mm Hg
- ECG is as follows:

- Left-sided arm weakness (3/5) and leg weakness (4/5)
- Decreased sensation on the left side, particularly the hand
- Left homonymous hemianopsia
- Height 5 ft, 3 in, weight 160 lb
- Alert, oriented, and able to answer questions appropriately but mild slowness in responding

Past Medical History

- Migraines
- Hypertension
- Hyperlipidemia

Discussion Questions

1. How do A.J.'s prior health history and current findings put her at risk for another stroke?
2. How can you address A.J.'s concerns regarding having another stroke?
3. How can A.J. and her family address activity issues such as driving after the stroke?
4. What strategies can you use to help A.J. and her family cope with her depression?
5. *Priority Decision:* What are the priority lifestyle changes that A.J. should make to reduce the likelihood of another stroke?
6. How will homonymous hemianopsia affect A.J.'s hygiene, eating, driving, and community activities?
7. What factors should you assess for related to outpatient rehabilitation for A.J.?
8. *Priority Decision:* What are the priority nursing interventions for A.J.?
9. *Priority Decision:* Based on the assessment data provided, what are the priority nursing diagnoses? Are there any collaborative problems?
10. *Delegation Decision:* What nursing interventions for A.J. can the RN delegate to unlicensed assistive personnel (UAP)?
11. *Evidence-Based Practice:* A.J.'s family wants to know if her atrial flutter caused her stroke and, if so, what she can do to prevent additional problems with her atrial flutter.

BRIDGE TO NCLEX EXAMINATION

The number of the question corresponds to the same-numbered outcome at the beginning of the chapter.

1. Of the following patients, the nurse recognizes that the one with the highest risk for a stroke is a(n)
   a. obese 45-year-old Native American.
   b. 35-year-old Asian American woman who smokes.
   c. 32-year-old white woman taking oral contraceptives.
   d. 65-year-old African American man with hypertension.
2. The factor related to cerebral blood flow that most often determines the extent of cerebral damage from a stroke is the
   a. amount of cardiac output.
   b. oxygen content of the blood.
   c. degree of collateral circulation.
   d. level of carbon dioxide in the blood.
3. Information provided by the patient that would help differentiate a hemorrhagic stroke from a thrombotic stroke includes
   a. sensory disturbance.
   b. a history of hypertension.
   c. presence of motor weakness.
   d. sudden onset of severe headache.
4. A patient with right-sided hemiplegia and aphasia resulting from a stroke most likely has involvement of the
   a. brainstem.
   b. vertebral artery.
   c. left middle cerebral artery.
   d. right middle cerebral artery.
5. The nurse explains to the patient with a stroke who is scheduled for angiography that this test is used to determine the
   a. presence of increased ICP.
   b. site and size of the infarction.
   c. patency of the cerebral blood vessels.
   d. presence of blood in the cerebrospinal fluid.

6. A patient experiencing TIAs is scheduled for a carotid endarterectomy. The nurse explains that this procedure is done to
   a. decrease cerebral edema.
   b. reduce the brain damage that occurs during a stroke in evolution.
   c. prevent a stroke by removing atherosclerotic plaques blocking cerebral blood flow.
   d. provide a circulatory bypass around thrombotic plaques obstructing cranial circulation.
7. For a patient who is suspected of having a stroke, one of the most important pieces of information that the nurse can obtain is
   a. time of the patient's last meal.
   b. time at which stroke symptoms first appeared.
   c. patient's hypertension history and management.
   d. family history of stroke and other cardiovascular diseases.
8. Bladder training in a male patient who has urinary incontinence after a stroke includes
   a. limiting fluid intake.
   b. keeping a urinal in place at all times.
   c. assisting the patient to stand to void.
   d. catheterizing the patient every 4 hours.
9. Common psychosocial reactions of the stroke patient to the stroke include (select all that apply)
   a. depression.
   b. disassociation.
   c. intellectualization.
   d. sleep disturbances.
   e. denial of severity of stroke.

1. d, 2. c, 3. d, 4. c, 5. c, 6. c, 7. b, 8. c, 9. a, d, e

evolve

For rationales to these answers and even more NCLEX review questions, visit *http://evolve.elsevier.com/Lewis/medsurg*.

REFERENCES

1. American Heart Association: AHA statistical update, *Circulation* 125:e2, 2012. Retrieved from *http://circ.ahajournals.org/content/125/1/e2.full#sec-81*.
2. University of Medicine and Dentistry of New Jersey: Stroke statistics. Retrieved from *www.theuniversityhospital.com/stroke/stats.htm*.
3. Centers for Disease Control and Prevention: Faststats: cerebrovascular disease or stroke, 2012. Retrieved from *www.cdc.gov/nchs/fastats/stroke.htm*.
*4. Haley WE, Roth DL, Howard G, et al: Caregiving strain and estimated risk for stroke and coronary heart disease among spouse caregiver: differential effects by race and sex, *Stroke* 41:331, 2010.
5. Centers for Disease Control and Prevention: Health effects of cigarette smoking, 2012. Retrieved from *www.cdc.gov/tobacco/data_statistics/fact_sheets/health_effects/effects_cig_smoking*.
*6. Jakel A, Plested M, Chapman A, et al: Management of patients with transient ischemic attack: insight from real-life clinical practice in Europe and the United States, *Curr Med Res Opin* 28:429, 2012.

7. American Stroke Association: Transient ischemic attack, 2012. Retrieved from *www.strokeassociation.org/STROKEORG/AboutStroke/TIA-Transient-Ischemic-Attack_UCM_310942_Article.jsp*.
8. American Heart Association: The imperative of primary stroke prevention: first things first, 2010. Retrieved from *http://myamericanheart.org/professional/General/The-Imperative-of-Primary-Stroke-Prevention-First-Things-First_UCM_432544_Article.jsp*.
9. Dupont S, Wijdicks E, Lanzino G, et al: Aneurysmal subarachnoid hemorrhage: an overview for the practicing neurologist, *Semin Neurol* 30:545, 2010.
10. McCaffrey P: Neuroanatomy of speech, swallowing and language: the blood supply. Retrieved from *www.csuchico.edu/~pmccaffrey/syllabi/CMSD%20320/362unit11.html*.
*11. Naess H, Lunde L, Brogger J: The triad of pain, fatigue, and depression in ischemic stroke patients: the Bergen Stroke Study, *Cerebrovasc Dis* 33:461, 2012.
*12. Mazzucco S, Turri G, Mirandola R, et al: What is still missing in acute-phase treatment of stroke: a prospective observational study, *Neurol Sci* 34(4):449, 2013.
*13. Kessler C, Thomas K, Kao J: Antiplatelet therapy for secondary prevention of acute coronary syndrome, transient ischemic attack, and noncardioembolic stroke in an era of cost containment, *J Invest Med* 60(5):792, 2012.

*Evidence-based information for clinical practice.

*14. Fisher M, Moonis M: Neuroprotective effects of statins: evidence from preclinical and clinical studies, *Curr Treatment Options Cardiovasc Medicine* 14(3):252, 2012.

*15. Liu Z, Fu W, Guo Z, et al: Updated systematic review and meta-analysis of randomized clinical trial comparing carotid artery stenting and carotid endarterectomy in the treatment of carotid stenosis, *Ann Vasc Surg* 26(4):576, 2012.

*16. Jauch EC, Saver JL, Adams HP, et al: Guidelines for the early management of patients with acute ischemic stroke: a guideline for healthcare professionals from the American Heart Association/American Stroke Association, *Stroke* 44:870, 2013.

*17. Miller J, Hartwell C, Lewandowski C: Stroke treatment using intravenous and intra-arterial tissue plasminogen activator, *Curr Treat Options Cardiovasc Med* 14(3):273, 2012.

*18. Fujita K, Komatsu Y, Sato N, et al: Pilot study of the safety of starting administration of low-dose aspirin and cilostazol in acute ischemic stroke, *Neurol Med Chir* 51:819, 2011.

19. deCarvalho F, deFigueiredo M, Silva G: Acute stroke: post-procedural care and management of complications, *Tech Vasc Interv Radiol* 15:78, 2012.

20. Alberti A: Seizures, *Front Neurol Neurosci* 30:3, 2012.

21. Lazaridis C, Naval N: Risk factors and medical management of vasospasm after subarachnoid hemorrhage, *Neurosurg Clin North Am* 21:353, 2010.

22. Green T, Kelloway L, Davies-Schinkel C, et al: Nurses' accountability for stroke quality of care, part one: review of the literature on nursing-sensitive outcomes, *Can J Neurosci Nurs* 33:13, 2011.

23. Martino R, Martin R, Black S: Dysphagia after stroke and its management, *Can Med Assoc J* 184(10):1127, 2012.

*24. Heck K: Decreasing ventilator-associated pneumonia in the intensive care unit: a sustainable comprehensive quality improvement program, *Am J Infect Control* 40(9):877, 2012.

25. American Stroke Association: NIH stroke scale international, 2011. Retrieved from *www.nihstrokescale.org*.

26. Rowat A: Malnutrition and dehydration after stroke, *Nurs Stand* 26:42, 2011.

27. Borthwick S: Communication impairment in patients following stroke, *Nurs Stand* 26:35, 2011.

28. Smeets S, van Heugten C, Geboers J: Respite care after acquired brain injury: the well-being of caregivers and patients, *Arch Phys Med Rehabil* 93(5):834, 2012.

29. Flansbjer U, Lexell J, Brogardh C: Long term benefits of progressive resistance training in chronic stroke: a 4-year follow up, *J Rehabil Med* 44:218, 2012.

RESOURCES

American Association of Neuroscience Nurses (AANN)
www.aann.org
American Stroke Association
www.strokeassociation.org
Association of Rehabilitation Nurses (ARN)
www.rehabnurse.org
National Institute of Neurological Disorders and Stroke
www.ninds.nih.gov
National Institutes of Health Stroke Scale (NIHSS)
www.nihstrokescale.org
National Stroke Association
www.stroke.org

*If we take care of the moments,
the years will take care of themselves.*
Maria Edgeworth

Nursing Management
Chronic Neurologic Problems

Mariann M. Harding

⊖volve WEBSITE

LEARNING OUTCOMES

1. Compare and contrast the etiology, clinical manifestations, collaborative care, and nursing management of tension-type, migraine, and cluster headaches.
2. Differentiate the etiology, clinical manifestations, diagnostic studies, collaborative care, and nursing management of seizure disorders, multiple sclerosis, Parkinson's disease, and myasthenia gravis.

3. Describe the clinical manifestations and nursing and collaborative management of restless legs syndrome, amyotrophic lateral sclerosis, and Huntington's disease.
4. Explain the potential impact of chronic neurologic disease on physical and psychologic well-being.
5. Outline the major goals of treatment for the patient with a chronic, progressive neurologic disease.

KEY TERMS

This chapter discusses headaches, chronic neurologic disorders, and degenerative neurologic disorders. Chronic neurologic disorders include seizure disorders and restless legs syndrome. Degenerative neurologic disorders include multiple sclerosis, Parkinson's disease, myasthenia gravis, amyotrophic lateral sclerosis, and Huntington's disease.

HEADACHES

Headache is probably the most common type of pain that humans experience. The majority of people have functional headaches, such as migraine or tension-type headaches. The others have organic headaches caused by intracranial or extracranial disease.

Headache pain can arise from both intracranial and extracranial sources. The pain-sensitive structures in the head include venous sinuses, dura, cranial blood vessels, three divisions of the trigeminal nerve (cranial nerve [CN] V), facial nerve (CN VII), glossopharyngeal nerve (CN IX), vagus nerve (CN X), and the first three cervical nerves.

Headaches are classified as primary or secondary headaches. *Primary headaches* are those not caused by a disease or another medical condition. Primary headache classifications include tension-type, migraine, and cluster headaches. The

Reviewed by Margie Francisco, RN, MSN, EdD, Nursing Professor, Illinois Valley Community College, Oglesby, Illinois; and Linda R. Littlejohns, RN, MSN, CNRN, FAAN, Vice President of Clinical Development, Integra Neurosurgery, San Juan Capistrano, California.

TABLE 59-1	COMPARISON OF TYPES OF HEADACHES		
Pattern	**Tension-Type Headache**	**Migraine Headache**	**Cluster Headache**
Site (see Fig. 59-1)	Bilateral, bandlike pressure at base of skull	Unilateral (in 60%), may switch sides, commonly anterior	Unilateral, radiating up or down from one eye
Quality	Constant, squeezing tightness	Throbbing, synchronous with pulse	Severe, bone-crushing
Frequency	Cycles for many years	Periodic, cycles of several months to years	May have months or years between attacks Attacks occur in clusters over a period of 2-12 wk
Duration	30 min–7 days	4-72 hr	5 min–3 hr
Time and mode of onset	Not related to time	May be preceded by prodrome Onset after awakening Gets better with sleep	Nocturnal, commonly awakens patient from sleep
Associated symptoms	Palpable neck and shoulder muscle tension, stiff neck, tenderness	Nausea, vomiting Irritability, sweating Photophobia Phonophobia Prodrome of sensory, motor, or psychic phenomena Family history (in 65%)	Facial flushing or pallor Unilateral lacrimation, ptosis, and rhinitis

type of primary headache is determined using the International Headache Society (IHS) guidelines based on characteristics of the headache (Table 59-1). *Secondary headaches* are caused by another condition or disorder, such as sinus infection, neck injury, and stroke. A patient may have more than one type of headache. The history and neurologic examination are diagnostic keys to determining the type of headache.

TENSION-TYPE HEADACHE

Tension-type headache, also called stress headache, is the most common type of headache. These headaches are characterized by their bilateral location and pressing or tightening quality. Tension-type headaches are usually of mild or moderate intensity and can last from minutes to days. Tension-type headaches are divided by frequency into episodic and chronic types.[1]

Etiology and Pathophysiology

Although the cause of tension-type headaches is not fully understood, the development of this type of headache is believed to be associated with neurovascular factors similar to those involved in migraine headaches. Many patients gradually progress over years from episodic to chronic headaches, with the increasing frequency associated with increasing intensity of the headache.[1]

Clinical Manifestations

Patients usually are initially seen with a bilateral frontal-occipital headache described as a constant, dull pressure, or bandlike headache associated with neck pain and increased tone in the cervical and neck muscles. The headache may involve sensitivity to light (*photophobia*) or sound (*phonophobia*), but does not involve nausea or vomiting. There is no *prodrome* (early manifestation of impending disease), and physical activity does not aggravate symptoms. The headaches may occur intermittently for weeks, months, or even years. Many patients can have a combination of migraine and tension-type headaches, with features of both occurring simultaneously. Patients with migraine headaches may experience tension-type headaches between migraine attacks. Fig. 59-1 shows the location of pain for common headache syndromes.

Diagnostic Studies

Careful history taking is probably the most important tool for diagnosing tension-type headache (Table 59-2). If tension-type headache is present during physical examination, increased

Most frequent site

Less frequent site

Least frequent site

A Tension

B Migraine

C Cluster

FIG. 59-1 Location of pain for common headache syndromes. **A,** Tension headache is often described as feeling of a weight in or on the head or a band squeezing the head. **B,** Migraine headache is described as an intense throbbing or pounding pain that involves one temple. The pain usually is unilateral (on one side of the head), although it can be bilateral. **C,** Cluster headache pain is focused in and around one eye and is often described as sharp, penetrating, or burning.

TABLE 59-2   DIAGNOSTIC STUDIES

Headaches

History and physical examination
- Neurologic examination (often negative)
- Inspection for local infections
- Palpation for tenderness, bony swellings
- Auscultation for bruits over major arteries

Routine laboratory studies
- Complete blood count (CBC)
- Electrolytes
- Urinalysis

Computed tomography (CT) scan of sinuses

Special studies (e.g., CT scan, angiography, EMG, EEG, MRI, MRA, lumbar puncture)

EEG, Electroencephalography; *EMG*, electromyography; *MRA*, magnetic resonance angiography.

GENDER DIFFERENCES

Headaches

Men	Women
• Cluster headaches are more common than in women (6:1). • Exercise-induced headaches are more common than in women.	• Migraine headaches are more common than in men (3:1). • Tension headaches are more common than in men.

resistance to passive movement of the head and tenderness of the head and neck may be present. Electromyography (EMG) may reveal sustained contraction of the neck, scalp, or facial muscles. However, many patients may not show increased muscle tension with this test, even when the test is done during the actual headache.

MIGRAINE HEADACHE

Migraine headache is a recurring headache characterized by unilateral (sometimes bilateral) throbbing pain, a triggering event or factor, and manifestations associated with neurologic and autonomic nervous system dysfunction. The most common age for onset of migraine is between 20 and 30 years. Migraine affects as many as 17% of females and 6% of males in the United States. Migraines are more common in women than men (see Gender Differences box). Risk factors for migraine include family history, low level of education, low socioeconomic status, high workload, and frequent tension-type headaches.[2]

The IHS subdivides migraines into categories. *Migraine without aura* (formerly called common migraine) is the most common type of migraine headache. *Migraine with aura* (formerly called classic migraine) occurs in only 10% of migraine headache episodes.

Etiology and Pathophysiology

Although many theories have addressed the cause of migraine headaches, the exact etiology is not known. The current theory is that a complex series of neurovascular events initiates a migraine headache.[3] People who have migraines have a state of neuronal hyperexcitability in the cerebral cortex, especially in the occipital cortex.

Approximately 70% of those with migraine have a first-degree relative who also had migraine headaches. Migraine is associated with seizure disorders, ischemic stroke, asthma, depression, anxiety, myocardial infarction, Raynaud's syndrome, and irritable bowel syndrome.[3]

In many cases, migraine headaches have no known precipitating events. However, for some patients, specific factors trigger or precipitate a headache. These include foods, menstruation, head trauma, physical exertion, fatigue, stress, missed meals, weather, and drugs. Food triggers include chocolate, cheese, oranges, tomatoes, onions, monosodium glutamate, aspartame, and alcohol (particularly red wine).

Clinical Manifestations

A prodrome and an aura may precede the headache phase by several hours or several days. The *prodrome* may include neurologic (e.g., photophobia), psychologic (e.g., hyperactivity, irritability), and other (e.g., food craving) manifestations. An **aura** is a complex of neurologic symptoms characterized by visual (e.g., bright lights, scotomas [patchy blindness], visual distortions, zigzag lines), sensory (voices or sounds that do not exist, strange smells), and/or motor (e.g., weakness, paralysis, feeling that limbs are moving) phenomena. The aura immediately precedes the headache and may last 10 to 30 minutes before the headache starts.

A migraine headache may last 4 to 72 hours. The headache is described as a steady, throbbing pain that is synchronous with the pulse. Although the headache is usually unilateral, it may switch to the opposite side in another episode. During the headache phase, some patients with migraine may tend to "hibernate." They seek shelter from noise, light, odors, people, and problems.

The presentation of migraine varies in severity. Not all migraine headaches are disabling, and many patients who have migraine headaches do not seek health care treatment for them. In some patients the symptoms of the migraine headaches may become worse over time.

Diagnostic Studies

The diagnosis of migraine headache is usually based on the patient history. The neurologic and other diagnostic examinations are often normal (see Table 59-2).

There is no specific laboratory or radiologic test for migraine headache. Neuroimaging techniques (e.g., head computed tomography [CT], with or without contrast, and magnetic resonance imaging [MRI]) are not recommended for routine evaluation of headache unless the neurologic examination reveals abnormal findings. If atypical features are present, then additional testing is done to rule out a secondary headache.

CLUSTER HEADACHE

Cluster headaches are a rare form of headache, affecting less than 0.1% of the population.[1] Cluster headaches involve repeated headaches that can occur for weeks to months at a time, followed by periods of remission.

Etiology and Pathophysiology

Neither the cause nor the pathophysiologic mechanism of cluster headache is fully known. The trigeminal nerve has a role in the production of pain, but cluster headaches also involve dysfunction of intracranial blood vessels, the sympathetic nervous system, and pain modulation systems. Imaging studies show hypothalamic activation at the onset of cluster headache.[3]

Alcohol is the only dietary trigger. Strong odors, weather changes, and napping are other triggers.[4]

Clinical Manifestations

The cluster headache is one of the most severe forms of headache, with intense pain lasting from a few minutes to 3 hours. The pain of cluster headache is sharp and stabbing, which is in contrast to the pulsing pain of the migraine headache. The pain is generally located around the eye, radiating to the temple, forehead, cheek, nose, or gums. Other manifestations may include swelling around the eye, lacrimation (tearing), facial flushing or pallor, nasal congestion, and constriction of the pupil. During the headache, the patient is often agitated and restless, unable to sit still or relax.

Cluster headaches can occur every other day and as often as eight times a day. The attacks occur in clusters. The clusters occur with regularity, usually at the same time each day, during the same seasons of the year. A cluster typically lasts 2 weeks to 3 months, and then the patient goes into remission for months to years.

Diagnostic Studies

The diagnosis of cluster headache is based on the patient history. Asking patients to keep a headache diary can be useful. CT scan, MRI, or magnetic resonance angiography (MRA) may rule out an aneurysm, a tumor, or an infection. A lumbar puncture may rule out other disorders that may cause similar symptoms.

OTHER TYPES OF HEADACHES

Although tension, migraine, and cluster headaches are by far the most common types of headaches, other types can occur. These headaches may be the first symptom of a more serious illness. Headache can accompany subarachnoid hemorrhage; brain tumors; other intracranial masses; vascular abnormalities; trigeminal neuralgia (tic douloureux); diseases of the eyes, nose, and teeth; and systemic illness (e.g., bacteremia, carbon monoxide poisoning, mountain sickness, polycythemia vera). The symptoms vary greatly. Because of the variety of causes of headache, clinical evaluation must be thorough. It should include an evaluation of personality, life adjustment, environment, and family situation, as well as a comprehensive evaluation of neurologic and physical status.

COLLABORATIVE CARE FOR HEADACHES

If no systemic underlying disease is the cause, the type of headache guides therapy. Table 59-2 outlines the general workup for a patient with headache to rule out any intracranial or extracranial disease. Table 59-3 summarizes the current therapies for prophylaxis and symptom relief of common headaches. These therapies include drugs, meditation, yoga, biofeedback, cognitive-behavioral therapy, and relaxation training.

Cognitive-behavioral therapy and relaxation therapy used alone or in conjunction with drug therapy may be beneficial to some patients. Biofeedback involves the use of physiologic monitoring equipment to give the patient information regarding muscle tension and peripheral blood flow (e.g., skin temperature of the fingers). The patient is trained to relax the muscles and raise the finger temperature, and is given reinforcement (operant conditioning) in accomplishing these changes.

Acupuncture, acupressure, and hypnosis also work well in some patients with headaches. See Chapters 6 and 7 for further description of these therapies.

Drug Therapy

Tension-Type Headache. Drug treatment for tension-type headache usually involves aspirin, acetaminophen (Tylenol), or nonsteroidal antiinflammatory drugs (NSAIDs) used alone or in combination with a sedative, muscle relaxant, or tranquilizer. However, many of these drugs have serious side effects. Caution the patient about the long-term use of aspirin and aspirin-containing drugs because they can cause upper gastrointestinal (GI) bleeding and coagulation abnormalities in susceptible patients. Drugs containing acetaminophen can cause kidney damage with chronic use and liver damage when taking large doses or when combined with alcohol. To decrease the recurrence of tension-type headache, the patient may receive preventive therapy with a tricyclic antidepressant (e.g., amitriptyline [Elavil], nortriptyline) or topiramate (Topamax), divalproex (Depakote), or mirtazapine (Remeron).

Migraine Headache. The aim of drug treatment of an acute migraine attack is terminating or decreasing the symptoms. Many people with mild or moderate migraine can obtain relief with NSAIDs, aspirin, or caffeine-containing combination analgesics. For moderate to severe headaches, the triptans have become the first line of therapy. Triptans (e.g., sumatriptan [Imitrex]) affect selected serotonin receptors, thus reducing neurogenic inflammation of the cerebral blood vessels and producing vasoconstriction (see Table 59-3). They are most effective when taken at the onset of migraine headache or during the aura. Sumatriptan is available in various forms: oral, subcutaneous, nasal spray.

Some patients respond better to one triptan than to others, so health care providers need to be knowledgeable about all of them. Because these drugs cause vasoconstriction, patients with heart disease or stroke should avoid their use. The combination drug sumatriptan/naproxen (Treximet) combines a triptan with an antiinflammatory drug. Risk of serious cardiovascular events such as myocardial infarction, thromboembolic events, and stroke may increase over time with Treximet. When triptans are contraindicated, other drugs can be used (see Table 59-3).

> **DRUG ALERT: Sumatriptan (Imitrex)**
> - Should not be given to patients with the following:
>   - History or manifestations of ischemic cardiac, cerebrovascular, or peripheral vascular problems
>   - Uncontrolled hypertension, since it may increase blood pressure
> - Excess dosage may produce tremor and decrease respirations.

Preventive treatment is important in the management of migraine headaches. The decision to initiate prophylactic treatment is individually determined based on frequency, severity, and any disability related to headaches. Several different classes of medications are used.

Topiramate, an antiseizure drug, taken daily is an effective therapy for migraine prevention. Common side effects include hypoglycemia, paresthesia, weight loss, and cognitive changes. Usually these side effects are mild to moderate and transient. Topiramate must be used for 2 to 3 months to determine its effectiveness. Not all patients will become pain free on this medication. Health care providers must provide adequate teaching regarding topiramate to promote patient adherence.

TABLE 59-3 COLLABORATIVE CARE

Headaches

Tension-Type Headache	Migraine Headache	Cluster Headache
Diagnostic		
History*	History*	History
Collaborative Therapy		
Abortive/Symptomatic Drugs		
Nonopioid analgesics: aspirin, acetaminophen, NSAIDs	Nonopioid analgesics: aspirin, NSAIDs	α-Adrenergic blocker
Analgesic combinations	Serotonin receptor agonists	• ergotamine tartrate
• butalbital/aspirin/caffeine (Fiorinal)	• almotriptan (Axert)	O₂ 100%
• butalbital/acetaminophen/caffeine (Fioricet)	• eletriptan (Relpax)	Serotonin receptor agonists
• dichloralphenazone/acetaminophen/isometheptene (Midrin)	• frovatriptan (Frova)	• almotriptan
Muscle relaxants	• naratriptan (Amerge)	• eletriptan
	• rizatriptan (Maxalt)	• frovatriptan
	• sumatriptan (Imitrex)	• naratriptan
	• zolmitriptan (Zomig)	• rizatriptan
	Combination	• sumatriptan
	• sumatriptan/naproxen (Treximet)	• zolmitriptan
	α-Adrenergic blockers	
	• ergotamine tartrate (Ergomar)	
	• dihydroergotamine (DHE)	
	Analgesic combinations	
	• acetaminophen/caffeine/aspirin	
	• acetaminophen/isometheptene/dichloralphenazone	
	Corticosteroids	
	• dexamethasone (Decadron)	
Preventive/Prophylactic Drugs		
Tricyclic antidepressants	β-Adrenergic blocker	α-Adrenergic blocker
• amitriptyline (Elavil)	• propranolol	• ergotamine tartrate
• nortriptyline (Pamelor)	Antidepressants	Serotonin antagonist
• doxepin (Sinequan)	• amitriptyline	• methysergide
Selective serotonin reuptake inhibitors	• imipramine (Tofranil)	Corticosteroid
• fluoxetine (Prozac)	Antiseizure	• prednisone
• paroxetine (Paxil)	• valproic acid (Depakene)	Calcium channel blocker
β-Adrenergic blocker:	• divalproex	• verapamil
• propranolol (Inderal)	• topiramate (Topamax)	Lithium
Other drugs	• gabapentin (Neurontin)	Biofeedback
• topiramate (Topamax)	Calcium channel blockers	
• divalproex (Depakote)	• verapamil (Calan)	
• mirtazapine (Remeron)	• flunarizine (Sibelium)	
Biofeedback	Serotonin antagonist†	
Psychotherapy	• methysergide (Sansert)	
Muscle relaxation training	Botulinum toxin A (Botox)	
	Biofeedback	
	Relaxation therapy	
	Cognitive-behavioral therapy	

*Diagnostic imaging should be considered in nonacute headache patients with unexplained abnormal neurologic examination, atypical headache, headache features, or an additional risk factor such as immunodeficiency.
†Only for patients suffering from one or more severe headaches per week.

DRUG ALERT: Topiramate (Topamax)
• Instruct patient to do the following:
  • Not abruptly discontinue, since this may cause seizures.
  • Avoid tasks that require alertness until response to drug is established.
  • Take adequate fluids to decrease risk of renal stone development.

Botulinum toxin A (Botox) may be an effective prophylactic treatment for patients who have chronic migraines lasting for 4 hours or more at least 15 days each month, or migraines that do not respond to other medications. Botox is given by multiple injections around the head and neck. Its effects last 2 to 4 months; the injections are repeated every 3 months. The most common adverse reactions are neck pain and headache. There is a slight risk of the toxin migrating from the injection site to other areas of the face and neck, causing swallowing and breath-ing difficulties. Teach the patient to seek immediate medical attention if this occurs.[5]

Additional antiseizure drugs used in migraine prevention are divalproex and gabapentin (Neurontin). Antidepressants used in migraine prophylaxis include tricyclic antidepressants (e.g., amitriptyline) and selective serotonin reuptake inhibitors (e.g., fluoxetine [Prozac]). Other drugs used for migraine headache prevention are listed in Table 59-3.

Cluster Headache. Because cluster headaches occur suddenly, often at night, and do not last long, drug therapy is not as useful as it is for other types of headaches. Acute treatment of cluster headache is inhalation of 100% oxygen delivered at a rate of 6 to 8 L/min for 10 minutes, which may relieve headache by causing vasoconstriction and increasing synthesis of sero-

EVIDENCE-BASED PRACTICE
Translating Research Into Practice

Can Botulinum Toxin A Prevent Headaches?

Clinical Question
For adults with chronic headaches (P), does prophylactic botulinum toxin A (I) vs. placebo vs. medication (C) decrease headache frequency or severity (O)?

Best Available Evidence
Meta-analysis of randomized controlled trials (RCTs) and comparative effectiveness trials

Critical Appraisal and Synthesis of Evidence
- Twenty-seven RCTs (n = 5313) comparing botulinum toxin A (Botox) with placebo, and four trials comparing Botox with medication (amitriptyline [Elavil], topiramate [Topamax], valproic acid [Depakote]).
- Headaches assessed were migraine or tension, episodic (<15 headaches per month) or chronic (>15 headaches per month), and a chronic daily headache.
- Botox resulted in decreased frequency of chronic daily and chronic migraine headaches. It had no effect on episodic migraine or chronic tension-type headaches.
- Botox was not related to fewer migraine headaches when compared with valproic acid, topiramate, or amitriptyline.

Conclusion
- Botox is beneficial for chronic daily headaches and chronic migraine headaches.

Implications for Nursing Practice
- Inform patients that Botox can prevent some types of headaches.
- Advise patients of Botox side effects, including blepharoptosis, paresthesia, neck stiffness and pain, and muscle weakness.

Reference for Evidence
Jackson JL, Kuriyama A, Hayashino Y: Botulinum toxin A for prophylactic treatment of migraine and tension headaches in adults: a meta-analysis, *JAMA* 307:1736, 2012.

P, Patient population of interest; *I*, intervention or area of interest; *C*, comparison of interest or comparison group; *O*, outcomes of interest (see p. 12).

tonin in the central nervous system. This can be repeated after a 5-minute rest. However, a drawback to this treatment is that the patient must have continuous access to the oxygen supply. The triptans (e.g., sumatriptan) are also effective in treating acute cluster headache. Intranasal administration of lidocaine is useful as an adjunctive therapy.[6]

Prophylactic drugs may include verapamil, lithium, ergotamine, divalproex, melatonin, or antiseizure medications. If the cluster headache recurs at a known time, prophylactic methysergide may be used. Options for patients with refractory cluster headaches include invasive nerve blocks, deep brain stimulation, and ablative neurosurgical procedures (e.g., percutaneous radiofrequency).

Other Headaches. Patients with frequent headaches may overuse analgesic drugs. *Medication overuse headache* (MOH) is the term used to describe an analgesic rebound headache. Drugs known to cause this problem are acetaminophen, aspirin, NSAIDs (e.g., ibuprofen), butalbital, sumatriptan, and opioids. Patients with daily headaches may complain of early awakening with decreased appetite, nausea, restlessness, decreased memory, and irritability. Treatment involves abrupt withdrawal of the offending drug (except for opioids, which need to be tapered) and initiation of alternative drugs such as amitriptyline.

TABLE 59-4   NURSING ASSESSMENT
Headaches

Subjective Data
Important Health Information
Past health history: Seizures, cancer, recent fall or trauma, cranial infection, stroke; asthma or allergies; mental illness; relationship of headache to overwork, stress, menstruation, exercise, food, sexual activity, travel, bright lights, or noxious environmental stimuli
Medications: Hydralazine (Apresoline), bromides, nitroglycerin, ergotamine (withdrawal), nonsteroidal antiinflammatory drugs (in high daily doses), estrogen preparations, oral contraceptives, over-the-counter or prescription remedies
Surgery or other treatments: Craniotomy, sinus surgery, facial surgery

Functional Health Patterns
Health perception–health management: Positive family history; malaise
Nutritional-metabolic: Ingestion of alcohol, caffeine, cheese, chocolate, monosodium glutamate, aspartame, lunch meats (nitrites in cured meats), sausage, hot dogs, onions, avocados; anorexia, nausea, vomiting (migraine prodrome); unilateral lacrimation (cluster)
Activity-exercise: Vertigo, fatigue, weakness, paralysis, fainting
Sleep-rest: Insomnia
Cognitive-perceptual
- *Migraine:* Aura; unilateral, severe, throbbing (possible switching of side) headache; visual disturbances; photophobia; phonophobia; dizziness; tingling or burning sensations
- *Cluster:* Unilateral and severe, nocturnal headache; nasal stuffiness
- *Tension-type:* Bilateral, bandlike, dull and persistent, base-of-skull headache, neck tenderness
Self-perception–self-concept: Depression
Coping–stress tolerance: Stress, anxiety, irritability, withdrawal

Objective Data
General
Anxiety, apprehension

Integumentary
Cluster: Forehead diaphoresis, pallor, unilateral facial flushing with cheek edema, conjunctivitis
Migraine: Generalized edema (prodrome), pallor, diaphoresis

Neurologic
Horner's syndrome, restlessness (cluster), hemiparesis (migraine)

Musculoskeletal
Resistance of head and neck movement, nuchal rigidity (meningeal, tension-type), palpable neck and shoulder muscle tension (tension-type)

Possible Diagnostic Findings
Evidence of disease, deformity, or infection on brain imaging (CT, MRI, MRA), cerebral angiogram, lumbar puncture, EEG, EMG; nonspecific brain imaging or laboratory tests

EMG, Electromyography; *MRA,* magnetic resonance angiography.

NURSING MANAGEMENT
HEADACHES

NURSING ASSESSMENT
Table 59-4 outlines subjective and objective data you should obtain from a patient with headache. Because the history provides the key to assessment of headache, it should include specific details of the headache itself, such as the location and type of pain, onset, frequency, duration, relation to events (emotional, psychologic, physical), and time of day of the occurrence. Obtain information about previous illnesses, surgery, trauma, allergies, family history, and response to medication.

Suggest that the patient keep a diary of headache episodes with specific details. This type of record can be of great help in determining the type of headache and the precipitating events. If the patient has a history of migraine, tension-type, or cluster headaches, it is important to determine if the character, intensity, or location of the headache has changed. This may be an important clue as to the cause of the headache.

NURSING DIAGNOSES

Nursing diagnoses for the patient with headache may include, but are not limited to, the following:

- Acute pain *related to* headache
- Ineffective self-health management *related to* drug therapy and lifestyle adjustments

Additional information on nursing diagnoses is presented in eNursing Care Plan 59-1 for the patient with headache (available on the website for this chapter).

PLANNING

The overall goals are that the patient with a headache will (1) have reduced or no pain, (2) demonstrate understanding of triggering events and treatment strategies, (3) use positive coping strategies to deal with pain, and (4) experience increased quality of life and decreased disability.

NURSING IMPLEMENTATION

Patients with chronic headache present a great challenge to health care providers. Since an inability to cope with daily stresses can cause headaches, an effective therapy may be to help patients examine their lifestyle, recognize stressful situations, and learn to cope with them more appropriately. Help the patient identify precipitating factors and develop ways to avoid them. Encourage daily exercise, relaxation periods, and socialization because each can help decrease the recurrence of headache. Suggest alternative ways of handling headache pain through techniques such as relaxation, meditation, and yoga.

In addition to using analgesics and analgesic combinations for symptomatic relief of headache, encourage the migraine sufferer to seek a quiet, dimly lit environment. Massage and moist hot packs to the neck and head can help a patient with tension-type headaches. The patient should learn about the drugs prescribed for preventive/prophylactic and abortive/symptomatic treatment of headache and should be able to describe the purpose, action, dosage, and side effects of the drugs. To prevent accidental overdose, the patient should make a written note of each dose of drug or headache remedy.

For the patient with headaches triggered by food, provide dietary counseling. Encourage the patient to eliminate foods that may provoke headaches, such as chocolate, cheese, oranges, tomatoes, onions, monosodium glutamate, aspartame, alcohol (particularly red wine), excessive caffeine, and fermented or marinated foods. Active challenge and provocative testing with specific foods may be necessary to determine the specific causative agents. However, food triggers may change over time.

Teach patients to avoid smoking and exposure to triggers such as strong perfumes, volatile solvents, and gasoline fumes. Cluster headache attacks may occur at high altitudes with low oxygen levels during air travel. Ergotamine, taken before the plane takes off, may decrease the likelihood of these attacks. See Table 59-5 for a teaching guide for the patient with a headache.

TABLE 59-5 PATIENT & CAREGIVER TEACHING GUIDE

Headaches

Include the following instructions when teaching the patient with a headache and the patient's caregiver.

1. Keep a diary or calendar of headaches and possible precipitating events.
2. Avoid factors that can trigger a headache:
   - Foods containing amines (cheese, chocolate), nitrites (meats such as hot dogs), vinegar, onions, monosodium glutamate
   - Fermented or marinated foods
   - Caffeine
   - Oranges
   - Tomatoes
   - Aspartame
   - Nicotine
   - Ice cream
   - Alcohol (particularly red wine)
   - Emotional stress
   - Fatigue
   - Drugs such as ergot-containing preparations (ergotamine tartrate [Ergomar]) and monoamine oxidase inhibitors (e.g., rasagiline [Azilect])
3. Learn the purpose, action, dosage, and side effects of drugs taken.
4. Self-administer sumatriptan (Imitrex) subcutaneously if prescribed.
5. Use stress management techniques such as relaxation.
6. Participate in regular exercise.
7. Contact health care provider if any of the following occurs:
   - Symptoms become more severe, last longer than usual, or are resistant to medication.
   - Nausea and vomiting (if severe or not typical), change in vision, or fever occurs with the headache.
   - Problems occur with any drugs.

EVALUATION

Expected outcomes are that the patient with headache will

- Report satisfaction with pain relief
- Use drug and nondrug measures appropriately to manage pain

Additional information on expected outcomes for the patient with headache is presented in eNursing Care Plan 59-1 (available on the website for this chapter).

CHRONIC NEUROLOGIC DISORDERS

SEIZURE DISORDERS AND EPILEPSY

Seizure is a paroxysmal, uncontrolled electrical discharge of neurons in the brain that interrupts normal function. Seizures may accompany a variety of disorders, or they may occur spontaneously without any apparent cause. Seizures resulting from systemic and metabolic disturbances are not considered epilepsy if the seizures cease when the underlying problem is corrected. Metabolic disturbances that cause seizures include acidosis, electrolyte imbalances, hypoglycemia, hypoxia, alcohol and barbiturate withdrawal, dehydration, and water intoxication. Extracranial disorders that can cause seizures are heart, lung, liver, or kidney diseases; systemic lupus erythematosus; diabetes mellitus; hypertension; and septicemia.

Epilepsy is a condition in which a person has spontaneous recurring seizures caused by a chronic underlying condition. In the United States, it is estimated that more than 3 million people have active epilepsy, with 200,000 new cases diagnosed each year. National trends show that the incidence of epilepsy is increasing in older adults. New cases of epilepsy are more common in African Americans and in socially disadvantaged populations. Males are slightly more likely to develop epilepsy than females. People at high risk for developing epilepsy include those with Alzheimer's disease or those who have had a stroke. The risk is also increased in the child of a person who has epilepsy.[7]

Etiology and Pathophysiology

Seizure disorders have many possible causes, with the most common causes varying by age. The most common causes of seizure disorder during the first 6 months of life are severe birth injury, congenital defects involving the central nervous system (CNS), infections, and inborn errors of metabolism. In people between 2 and 20 years of age, the primary causes are birth injury, infection, trauma, and genetic factors. In individuals between 20 and 30 years of age, seizure disorder usually occurs as the result of structural lesions, such as trauma, brain tumors, or vascular disease. After 50 years of age, the primary causes of seizure disorders are stroke and metastatic brain tumors. However, nearly 30% of all epilepsy cases are idiopathic, called *idiopathic generalized epilepsy (IGE)*, meaning they are not attributable to a specific cause.

The etiology of recurring seizures (epilepsy) has long been attributed to a group of abnormal neurons *(seizure focus)* that seem to undergo spontaneous firing. This firing spreads by physiologic pathways to involve adjacent or distant areas of the brain. If this activity spreads to involve the whole brain, a generalized seizure occurs. The factor that causes this abnormal firing is not clear. Any stimulus that causes the cell membrane of the neuron to depolarize induces a tendency for spontaneous firing.

Scar tissue (gliosis) is often found in the area of the brain from which the epileptic activity arises. Scarring is believed to interfere with the normal chemical and structural environment of the brain neurons, making them more likely to fire abnormally.

In addition to neuronal alterations, changes in the function of astrocytes may play several key roles in recurring seizures. Activation of astrocytes by hyperactive neurons is one of the crucial factors that predispose neurons nearby to the generation of an epileptic discharge.

⚕ Genetic Link

Genetic abnormalities may be the most important factor contributing to IGE. Some types of epilepsy tend to run in families, suggesting a genetic influence. Other types of IGE are related to abnormalities in specific genes that control the flow of ions in and out of cells and regulate neuron signaling or are involved with protein and carbohydrate metabolism. Some researchers estimate that more than 500 genes could play a role in IGE.[8]

The role of genetics in the etiology of seizure disorders has been difficult to determine because of the problem of separating genetic from environmental or acquired influences. In some forms of epilepsy, families carry a predisposition to seizure disorders in the form of an inherently low threshold to seizure-producing stimuli, such as trauma, disease, and high fever.

Abnormal genes may influence the disorder in subtle ways. For example, a person with epilepsy may have an abnormally active version of a gene that increases resistance to drugs. This may help explain why antiseizure drugs do not work for some people.

TABLE 59-6	CLASSIFICATION OF SEIZURE DISORDERS

Generalized Seizures (Nonfocal Origin)
• Tonic-clonic seizures
• Absence seizures
  • Typical
  • Atypical
  • Absence with special features
• Myoclonic seizures
• Tonic seizures
• Atonic seizures (drop attacks)
• Clonic seizures
	Focal Seizures (Focal Origin)
	• Simple focal seizures (no impairment of consciousness)
	• Complex focal seizures (impairment of consciousness)
	• Focal seizures evolving to secondary generalized seizures
	Unknown

Adapted from Berg AT, Berkovic SF, Brodie MJ, et al: Revised terminology and concepts for organization of seizures and epilepsies: report of the ILAE Commission on Classification and Terminology, 2005-2009, International League Against Epilepsy, *Epilepsia* 5:676, 2010.

Clinical Manifestations

The specific clinical manifestations of a seizure are determined by the site of the electrical disturbance.[9] The preferred method of classifying seizures is presented in Table 59-6. This system, which is based on the clinical and electroencephalographic manifestations of seizures, divides seizures into two major classes: *generalized* and *focal* (Fig. 59-2). Depending on the type, a seizure may progress through several phases: (1) the *prodromal phase,* with signs or activity that precede a seizure; (2) the *aural phase,* with a sensory warning; (3) the *ictal phase,* with full seizure; and (4) the *postictal phase,* the period of recovery after the seizure.

Generalized Seizures. Generalized seizures involve both sides of the brain and are characterized by bilateral synchronous epileptic discharges in the brain from the onset of the seizure. In most cases the patient loses consciousness for a few seconds to several minutes.

Tonic-Clonic Seizures. The most common generalized seizure is the generalized tonic-clonic (formerly known as *grand mal*) seizure. Tonic-clonic seizure is characterized by losing consciousness and falling to the ground if the patient is upright, followed by stiffening of the body (tonic phase) for 10 to 20 seconds and subsequent jerking of the extremities (clonic phase) for another 30 to 40 seconds. Cyanosis, excessive salivation, tongue or cheek biting, and incontinence may accompany the seizure.

In the postictal phase the patient usually has muscle soreness, is tired, and may sleep for several hours. Some patients may not feel normal for several hours or days after a seizure. The patient has no memory of the seizure.

Typical Absence Seizures. The absence seizure (formerly called petit mal) usually occurs only in children and rarely continues beyond adolescence. This type of seizure may cease altogether as the child matures, or it may evolve into another type of seizure. The typical clinical manifestation is a brief staring spell resembling "daydreaming" that lasts only a few seconds, so it often goes unnoticed. When untreated, the seizures may occur up to 100 times a day. The electroencephalogram (EEG) demonstrates a 3-Hz (cycles per second) spike-and-wave pattern that is unique to this type of seizure. Hyperventilation and flashing lights can precipitate absence seizures.

Atypical Absence Seizures. Another type of generalized seizure is *atypical absence seizure,* which is characterized by a

FIG. 59-2 Algorithm for classification of seizures.

staring spell accompanied by other signs and symptoms, including brief warnings, peculiar behavior during the seizure, or confusion after the seizure. It is longer lasting than a typical absence seizure and may be associated with loss of postural tone. The EEG demonstrates atypical spike-and-wave patterns, usually greater or less than 3 Hz.

Other Types of Generalized Seizures. Other generalized seizures are myoclonic, atonic, tonic, and clonic seizures. A *myoclonic seizure* is characterized by a sudden, excessive jerk of the body or extremities. The jerk may be forceful enough to hurl the person to the ground. These seizures are brief and may occur in clusters.

An *atonic* ("drop attack") seizure involves either a tonic episode or a paroxysmal loss of muscle tone and begins suddenly with the person falling to the ground. Consciousness usually returns by the time the person hits the ground, and normal activity can be resumed immediately. Patients with this type of seizure are at a great risk of head injury and often have to wear protective helmets.

A *tonic* seizure involves a sudden onset of maintained increased tone in the extensor muscles. These patients often fall.

Clonic seizures begin with loss of consciousness and sudden loss of muscle tone, followed by limb jerking that may or may not be symmetric.

Focal Seizures. Focal seizures, also called partial or partial focal seizures, are the other major class of seizures (see Table 59-6). Focal seizures begin in one hemisphere of the brain in a specific region of the cortex, as indicated by the EEG. They produce signs and symptoms related to the function of the area of the brain involved. For example, if the discharging focus is located in the medial aspect of the postcentral gyrus, the patient may experience paresthesias and tingling or numbness in the leg on the side opposite the focus. If the discharging focus is located in the part of the brain that governs a particular function, sensory, motor, cognitive, or emotional manifestations may occur.

Focal seizures are divided according to their clinical expression into (1) simple focal seizures (the person remains conscious) and (2) complex focal seizures (the person has a change or loss of consciousness).[8] In a *simple focal seizure,* patients remain conscious but experience unusual feelings or sensations that can take many forms. They may experience sudden and unexplainable feelings of joy, anger, sadness, or nausea. They also may hear, smell, taste, see, or feel things that are not real.

In a *complex focal seizure*, patients have a loss of consciousness or an alteration in their consciousness, producing a dream-like experience. They display strange behavior such as lip smacking and *automatisms* (repetitive movements that may not be appropriate). Patients may continue an activity started before the seizure, such as counting out change or picking items from a grocery shelf, but after the seizure they do not remember the activity performed during the seizure. Other automatisms are less organized, such as picking at clothing, fumbling with objects (real or imaginary), or simply walking away. These seizures usually last just a few seconds.

Focal seizures may be confined to one side of the brain and remain focal (partial) in nature, or they may spread to involve the entire brain, culminating in a generalized tonic-clonic seizure. Any tonic-clonic seizure that is preceded by an aura or warning is a focal seizure that generalizes secondarily. Many tonic-clonic seizures that appear to be generalized from the outset may actually be secondary generalized seizures, but the preceding partial component may be so brief that it is undetected by the patient, by the observer, or even on the EEG. Unlike the primary generalized tonic-clonic seizure, the secondary generalized seizure may result in a transient residual neurologic deficit postictally. This is called *Todd's paralysis* (focal weakness), which resolves after varying lengths of time.

Psychogenic Seizures. Psychogenic seizures, also called pseudoseizures, are seizures that are psychiatric in origin. Since they closely resemble epileptic seizures, psychogenic seizures may be misdiagnosed as epilepsy. Proper diagnosis usually requires video-EEG monitoring to capture a typical episode. Patients with psychogenic seizures frequently have a history of emotional abuse, physical neglect, or a specific traumatic episode.[10]

Complications

Physical. Status epilepticus is a state of continuous seizure activity or a condition in which seizures recur in rapid succession without return to consciousness between seizures. It is the most serious complication of epilepsy and is a neurologic emergency. Status epilepticus can occur with any type of seizure. During repeated seizures the brain uses more energy than can be supplied. Neurons become exhausted and cease to function. Permanent brain damage may result. Tonic-clonic status epilepticus is the most dangerous because it can cause ventilatory insufficiency, hypoxemia, cardiac dysrhythmias, hyperthermia, and systemic acidosis, all of which can be fatal.

Subclinical seizures are a form of status epilepticus in which the sedated patient seizes but without external signs because of sedating medication. For example, a patient under sedation for ventilatory support in the intensive care unit (ICU) could experience a seizure without physical movements. The patient's health care providers could miss the seizure occurrence.

Another complication of seizures is severe injury and even death from trauma suffered during a seizure. Patients who lose consciousness during a seizure are at greatest risk.

Persons with epilepsy have a mortality rate that is two or three times the rate of the general population. Forty percent of these deaths are related to epilepsy because of accidents occurring during seizures, suicide, treatment-related death, death from an underlying disease, and sudden unexplained or unexpected death in epilepsy (SUDEP). SUDEP is higher in males, those on multiple antiseizure medications, and patients with long-standing epilepsy. The direct cause of SUDEP is unknown, but is thought to be related to respiratory dysfunction, cardiac dysrhythmias, or cerebral depression.[11]

Psychosocial. Perhaps the most common complication of seizure disorders is the effect it has on a patient's lifestyle. The patient may develop ineffective coping methods because of the psychosocial problems related to having a seizure disorder. Although attitudes have improved in recent years, epilepsy still carries a social stigma. The patient with epilepsy may experience discrimination in employment and educational opportunities. Transportation may be difficult because of legal sanctions against driving.

Diagnostic Studies

A diagnosis of epilepsy or seizure disorder has many socioeconomic, physical, and psychologic consequences for the patient. Therefore an accurate diagnosis is crucial. The most useful diagnostic tools are an accurate and comprehensive description of the seizures and the patient's health history (Table 59-7). The EEG is a useful diagnostic adjuvant to the history, but only if it shows abnormalities. Abnormal findings help determine the type of seizure and help pinpoint the seizure focus. Ideally, an EEG should be done within 24 hours of a suspected seizure. Unfortunately, only a small percentage of patients with seizure disorders have abnormal findings on the EEG the first time the test is done. Either repeated EEGs or continuous EEG monitoring may be needed to detect abnormalities. An EEG is not a definitive test because some patients who do not have seizure disorders have abnormal patterns on their EEGs, whereas many patients with seizure disorders have normal EEGs between seizures. If abnormal discharges do not occur during the 30 to 40 minutes of sampling during EEG, the test may not indicate an abnormality. Magnetoencephalography may be done in conjunction with the EEG. This test has greater sensitivity in detecting small magnetic fields generated by neuronal activity.

TABLE 59-7 **COLLABORATIVE CARE**
Seizure Disorders and Epilepsy
Diagnostic
History and Physical Examination
• Birth and developmental history
• Significant illnesses and injuries
• Family history
• Febrile seizures
• Comprehensive neurologic assessment
Seizure History
• Precipitating factors
• Antecedent events
• Seizure description (including onset, duration, frequency, postictal state)
Diagnostic Studies
• CBC, urinalysis, electrolytes, creatinine, fasting blood glucose
• Lumbar puncture for CSF analysis
• CT, MRI, MRA, MRS, PET scan
• Electroencephalography (EEG)
Collaborative Therapy
• Antiseizure drugs (see Table 59-9)
• Surgery (see Table 59-10)
• Vagal nerve stimulation
• Psychosocial counseling

MRA, Magnetic resonance angiography; *MRS,* magnetic resonance spectroscopy; *PET,* positron emission tomography.

A complete blood count, serum chemistries, studies of liver and kidney function, and a urinalysis should be done to rule out metabolic disorders. A CT scan or MRI should be done in any new-onset seizure to rule out a structural lesion. Cerebral angiography, single-photon emission computed tomography (SPECT), magnetic resonance spectroscopy (MRS), MRA, and positron emission tomography (PET) may be used in selected clinical situations.

If a patient is diagnosed with a seizure disorder, it is important to classify the seizure type correctly (see Fig. 59-2 and Table 59-6). The choice of treatment depends on the type of seizure.

Collaborative Care

Most seizures do not require professional emergency medical care because they are self-limiting and rarely cause bodily injury. However, if status epilepticus occurs, if significant bodily harm occurs, or if the event is a first-time seizure, medical care should be sought immediately. Table 59-8 summarizes emergency care of the patient with a generalized tonic-clonic seizure, the seizure most likely to warrant professional emergency medical care. Table 59-7 outlines the diagnostic studies and collaborative care of seizure disorders.

Drug Therapy. The primary treatment for seizure disorders is antiseizure drugs (Table 59-9). Because a cure is not possible, the goal of therapy is to prevent seizures with a minimum of toxic side effects from drug therapy. Medications control seizures in about 70% of the patients. Drugs generally act by stabilizing nerve cell membranes and preventing spread of the epileptic discharge. The principle of drug therapy is to begin with a single drug based on the patient's age and weight; type, frequency, and cause of seizure; and then increase the dosage until seizures are controlled or toxic side effects occur.

TABLE 59-8 EMERGENCY MANAGEMENT

Tonic-Clonic Seizures

Etiology	Assessment Findings	Interventions
Head Trauma • Epidural hematoma • Subdural hematoma • Intracranial hematoma • Cerebral contusion • Traumatic birth injury **Drug-Related Processes** • Overdose • Withdrawal of alcohol, opioids, antiseizure drugs • Ingestion, inhalation **Infectious Processes** • Meningitis • Septicemia • Encephalitis **Intracranial Events** • Brain tumor • Subarachnoid hemorrhage • Stroke • Hypertensive crisis • Increased ICP secondary to clogged shunt **Metabolic Imbalances** • Fluid and electrolyte imbalance • Hypoglycemia **Medical Disorders** • Heart, liver, lung, or kidney disease • Systemic lupus erythematosus **Other** • Cardiac arrest • Idiopathic • Psychiatric disorders • High fever	• Aura (peculiar sensations that precede seizure) • Loss of consciousness • Bowel and bladder incontinence • Tachycardia • Diaphoresis • Warm skin • Pallor, flushing, or cyanosis • *Tonic phase:* Continuous muscle contractions • *Hypertonic phase:* Extreme muscular rigidity lasting 5–15 sec • *Clonic phase:* Rigidity and relaxation alternating in rapid succession • *Postictal phase:* Lethargy, altered level of consciousness • Confusion and headache • Repeated tonic-clonic seizures for several min	**Initial** • Ensure patent airway. • Protect patient from injury during seizure. *Do not restrain.* Pad side rails. • Remove or loosen tight clothing. • Establish IV access. • Stay with patient until seizure has passed. • Anticipate administration of phenobarbital, phenytoin (Dilantin), or benzodiazepines (e.g., diazepam [Valium], midazolam [Versed], lorazepam [Ativan]) to control seizures. • Suction as needed. • Assist ventilations if patient does not breathe spontaneously after seizure. Anticipate need for intubation if gag reflex absent. **Ongoing Monitoring** • Monitor vital signs, level of consciousness, O_2 saturation, Glasgow Coma Scale results, pupil size and reactivity. • Reassure and orient the patient after seizure. • Never force an airway between a patient's clenched teeth. • Give IV dextrose for hypoglycemia.

ICP, Intracranial pressure.

If seizure control is not achieved with a single drug, the drug dosage or timing of administration may be changed or a second drug may be added. About one third of patients require a combination regimen for adequate control.

The therapeutic range for each drug indicates the serum level above which most patients experience toxic side effects and below which most continue to have seizures. Therapeutic drug ranges are only guides for therapy. If the patient's seizures are well controlled with a subtherapeutic level, the drug dosage need not be increased. Likewise, if a drug level is above the therapeutic range and the patient has good seizure control without toxic side effects, the drug dosage does not need to be decreased. Serum drug levels are monitored if seizures continue to occur, if seizure frequency increases, or if drug adherence is questioned. Many of the newer drugs do not require drug-level monitoring because the therapeutic range is very large.

The primary drugs to treat generalized tonic-clonic and focal seizures are phenytoin (Dilantin), carbamazepine (Tegretol), phenobarbital, divalproex, and primidone (Mysoline). The drugs used to treat absence and myoclonic seizures include ethosuximide (Zarontin), divalproex, and clonazepam (Klonopin).

TABLE 59-9 DRUG THERAPY

Seizure Disorders and Epilepsy

Generalized Tonic-Clonic and Focal Seizures	Absence and Myoclonic Seizures
• carbamazepine (Tegretol) • divalproex (Depakote) • ezogabine (Potiga) • felbamate (Felbatol) • gabapentin (Neurontin) • lacosamide (Vimpat) • lamotrigine (Lamictal) • levetiracetam (Keppra) • oxcarbazepine (Trileptal) • perampanel (Fycompa) • phenobarbital (Luminal) • phenytoin (Dilantin) • pregabalin (Lyrica) • primidone (Mysoline) • tiagabine (Gabitril) • topiramate (Topamax) • valproic acid (Depakene) • vigabatrin (Sabril) • zonisamide (Zonegran)	• clonazepam (Klonopin) • divalproex (Depakote) • ethosuximide (Zarontin) • zonisamide (Zonegran)

DRUG ALERT: Carbamazepine (Tegretol)
- Do not take with grapefruit juice.
- Instruct patient to report visual abnormalities.
- Abrupt withdrawal after long-term use may precipitate seizures.

Other antiseizure drugs include gabapentin, topiramate, lamotrigine (Lamictal), tiagabine (Gabitril), levetiracetam (Keppra), and zonisamide (Zonegran). Some of these drugs are broad spectrum and appear to be effective for multiple seizure types. Pregabalin (Lyrica) is used as an "add-on" for control of focal seizures that are not successfully managed with a single medication.

Treatment of status epilepticus requires initiation of a rapid-acting IV antiseizure drug. The drugs most commonly used are lorazepam (Ativan) and diazepam (Valium). Because these are short-acting drugs, their administration is followed with long-acting drugs such as phenytoin or phenobarbital.

Because many of the antiseizure drugs (e.g., phenytoin, phenobarbital, ethosuximide, lamotrigine, topiramate) have a long half-life, they can be given in once- or twice-daily doses. This increases the patient's adherence to the drug regimen by simplifying it and avoiding the need to take the drug at work or school.

DRUG ALERT: Antiseizure Drugs
- Abrupt withdrawal after long-term use may precipitate seizures.
- If weaning is to occur, the patient must be seizure free for a prolonged period (e.g., 2 to 5 yr) and have a normal neurologic examination and EEG.

Side effects of antiseizure drugs involve the CNS and include diplopia, drowsiness, ataxia, and mental slowness. Neurologic assessment for dose-related toxicity involves testing the eyes for nystagmus, hand and gait coordination, cognitive functioning, and general alertness.

As a nurse, you need to be knowledgeable about these side effects so that patients can be informed and institute proper treatment. A common side effect of phenytoin is gingival hyperplasia (excessive growth of gingival tissue) and hirsutism, especially in young adults. Good dental hygiene, including regular tooth brushing and flossing, can limit gingival hyperplasia. If gingival hyperplasia is extensive, the hyperplastic tissue may have to be surgically removed (gingivectomy), and phenytoin replaced with another antiseizure drug.

Medication nonadherence can be a problem in persons with a seizure disorder. Take measures to increase patient adherence to the prescribed drug regimens. If made aware of the issue, health care providers can work with the patient to find an acceptable drug regimen. For example, using pregabalin in some cases as an adjunct medication will allow a decreased dose of the primary antiseizure drug, thus decreasing undesirable side effects.

GERONTOLOGIC CONSIDERATIONS

DRUG THERAPY FOR SEIZURE DISORDERS

The incidence of new-onset seizure disorders is high among older adults. Closely consider the relationship between the action of antiseizure drugs and the normal changes that occur with aging. For example, phenytoin is widely used to treat seizure disorders. However, because the liver metabolizes phenytoin, its use can be a problem for older patients with compromised liver function. Age-related changes in liver enzymes decrease the liver's ability to metabolize drugs. Phenobarbital, carbamazepine, and primidone have potential effects on cogni-

TABLE 59-10	SURGERY FOR SEIZURE DISORDERS
Type of Seizure	**Surgical Procedure**
Complex focal seizure of temporal lobe origin	Resectioning of epileptogenic tissue
Focal seizures of frontal lobe origin	Resectioning of epileptogenic tissue (if in resectable area)
Generalized seizures (Lennox-Gastaut syndrome or drop attacks)	Sectioning of corpus callosum
Intractable unilateral multifocal epilepsy associated with infantile hemiplegia	Hemispherectomy or callosotomy

tive function, so their use may be less desirable for the older adult. Carbamazepine, phenytoin, and phenobarbital have many significant drug interactions.[12]

Several of the newer antiseizure medications offer greater treatment benefit to older adults. Compared with older drugs, gabapentin, lamotrigine, oxcarbazepine, and levetiracetam may be safer, have fewer effects on cognitive function, and have fewer interactions with other drugs.[12]

Surgical Therapy. A significant number of patients whose epilepsy is not controlled with drug therapy are candidates for surgical intervention to remove the epileptic focus or prevent spread of epileptic activity in the brain (Table 59-10). The most common surgical intervention is an anterior temporal lobe resection. Approximately 70% of patients are essentially seizure free after this procedure.[8]

The benefits of surgery include cessation or reduction in frequency of the seizures. However, not all types of epilepsy benefit from surgery. An extensive preoperative evaluation is important, including continuous EEG monitoring and other specific tests to ensure precise localization of the focal point. Surgical candidates must meet three requirements: (1) a confirmed diagnosis of epilepsy, (2) an adequate trial with drug therapy without satisfactory results, and (3) a defined electroclinical syndrome (type of seizure disorder).

Other Therapies. Vagal nerve stimulation is used as an adjunct to medications when surgery is not feasible. The exact mechanism of action is unknown, but it is thought to interrupt the synchronization of epileptic brain wave activity and stop excessive discharge of neurons. A surgically implanted electrode in the neck is programmed to deliver the electrical impulse to the vagus nerve. The patient can activate it with a magnet when he or she senses a seizure is imminent. Vagal nerve stimulation can cause adverse effects such as coughing, hoarseness, dyspnea, and tingling in the neck. Battery replacement is required via surgery about every 5 years.

The ketogenic diet is a special high-fat, low-carbohydrate diet that has been used to control seizures in some people with epilepsy. When a person is on this diet, ketones are produced and pass into the brain and replace glucose as an energy source. The diet may be effective for some patients with drug-resistant epilepsy, but the long-term effects of the diet are not clear. Patients on this diet who use anticoagulants need close monitoring for bleeding.[13]

Biofeedback to control seizures is aimed at teaching the patient to maintain a certain brain wave frequency that is refractory to seizure activity. Further trials are needed to assess the effectiveness of biofeedback for seizure control.

NURSING MANAGEMENT
SEIZURE DISORDERS AND EPILEPSY

NURSING ASSESSMENT

Subjective and objective data to obtain from a patient with a seizure disorder are presented in Table 59-11. Obtain data related to a specific seizure episode from a witness.

NURSING DIAGNOSES

Nursing diagnoses for the patient with seizure disorders and epilepsy may include, but are not limited to, the following:
- Ineffective breathing pattern *related to* neuromuscular impairment
- Ineffective self-health management *related to* drug therapy and lifestyle adjustments
- Risk for injury *related to* loss of consciousness during seizure activity and postictal physical weakness

Additional information on nursing diagnoses for the patient with a seizure disorder is presented in eNursing Care Plan 59-2 (available on the website for this chapter).

PLANNING

The overall goals are that the patient with seizures will (1) be free from injury during a seizure, (2) have optimal mental and physical functioning while taking antiseizure drugs, and (3) have satisfactory psychosocial functioning.

NURSING IMPLEMENTATION

HEALTH PROMOTION. Some cases of seizure disorders can be prevented by promoting general safety measures, such as wearing helmets in situations involving risk of head injury. Improved perinatal, labor, and delivery care have reduced fetal trauma and hypoxia and thereby have reduced brain damage leading to seizure disorders.

The patient with a seizure disorder should practice good general health habits (e.g., maintaining a proper diet, getting adequate rest, exercising). Help the patient identify events or situations that precipitate the seizures and provide suggestions for avoiding them or handling them better. Teach the patient to avoid excessive alcohol intake, fatigue, and loss of sleep. Help the patient handle stress constructively.

ACUTE INTERVENTION. Nursing care for a hospitalized patient with a seizure disorder or a patient who has had seizures from metabolic factors involves several responsibilities, including observation and treatment of the seizure, education, and psychosocial intervention.

When a seizure occurs, carefully observe and record details of the event because the diagnosis and subsequent treatment often rest solely on the seizure description. Note all aspects of the seizure. What events preceded the seizure? When did the seizure occur? How long did each phase (aural [if any], ictal, postictal) last? What occurred during each phase?

Both subjective data (usually the only type of data in the aural phase) and objective data are important. Note the exact onset of the seizure (which body part was affected first and how); the course and nature of the seizure activity (loss of consciousness, tongue biting, automatisms, stiffening, jerking, total lack of muscle tone); the body parts involved and their sequence of involvement; and autonomic signs, such as dilated pupils, excessive salivation, altered breathing, cyanosis, flushing, diaphoresis, or incontinence. Assessment of the postictal period should include a detailed description of the level of conscious-

TABLE 59-11   NURSING ASSESSMENT
Seizure Disorders and Epilepsy

Subjective Data
Important Health Information
Past health history: Previous seizures, birth defects or injuries, anoxic episodes; CNS trauma, tumors, or infections; stroke; metabolic disorders, alcoholism; exposure to metals and carbon monoxide; hepatic or renal failure; fever; pregnancy, systemic lupus erythematosus
Medications: Adherence to antiseizure medication regimen; barbiturate or alcohol withdrawal; use and overdose of cocaine, amphetamines, lidocaine, theophylline, penicillin, lithium, phenothiazines, tricyclic antidepressants, benzodiazepines

Functional Health Patterns
Health perception–health management: Positive family history
Cognitive-perceptual: Headaches, aura, mood or behavioral changes before seizure; mentation changes; abdominal pain, muscle pain (postictal)
Self-perception–self-concept: Anxiety, depression; loss of self-esteem, social isolation
Sexuality-reproductive: Decreased sexual drive, erectile dysfunction; increased sexual drive (postictal)

Objective Data
General
Precipitating factors, including severe metabolic acidosis or alkalosis, hyperkalemia, hypoglycemia, dehydration, or water intoxication

Integumentary
Bitten tongue, soft tissue damage, cyanosis, diaphoresis (postictal)

Respiratory
Abnormal respiratory rate, rhythm, or depth; apnea (ictal); absent or abnormal breath sounds, possible airway occlusion

Cardiovascular
Hypertension, tachycardia or bradycardia (ictal)

Gastrointestinal
Bowel incontinence; excessive salivation

Urinary
Incontinence

Neurologic
Generalized
Tonic-clonic: Loss of consciousness, muscle tightening, then jerking; dilated pupils; hyperventilation, then apnea; postictal somnolence
Absence: Altered consciousness (5–30 sec), minor facial motor activity

Focal
Simple: Aura; consciousness; focal sensory, motor, cognitive, or emotional phenomena (focal motor); unilateral "marching" motor seizure (jacksonian)
Complex: Altered consciousness with inappropriate behaviors, automatisms, amnesia of event

Musculoskeletal
Weakness, paralysis, ataxia (postictal)

Possible Diagnostic Findings
Positive toxicology screen or alcohol level; altered serum electrolytes, acidosis or alkalosis, very low blood glucose level, ↑ blood urea nitrogen or serum creatinine, abnormal liver function tests, ammonia; abnormal CT scan or MRI of head, abnormal findings from lumbar puncture; abnormal discharges on EEG

DELEGATION DECISIONS

Caring for the Patient With a Seizure Disorder

Since any nursing staff member may be present when a patient experiences a seizure, all staff members are responsible for maintaining patient safety.

Role of Registered Nurse (RN)
- Teach patient about factors that increase risk for seizures, such as alcohol use, fatigue, inadequate sleep, and stress.
- Teach patient about prescribed antiseizure medications, including drug regimen, side effects, and required monitoring of drug levels.
- Assess and document details of seizure events, including events preceding the seizure; length of each phase of the seizure; course and nature of the seizure activity; and the level of consciousness, vital signs, and activity during the postictal period.
- Assess airway patency and position patient to maintain airway after any seizures.
- Administer IV antiseizure medications to the patient experiencing status epilepticus.
- Make appropriate referrals to the Epilepsy Foundation and community agencies to assist patient with financial problems, work training, employment, and living arrangements.
- Teach family members and caregivers about management of seizures and status epilepticus.
- In the ambulatory and home care setting, evaluate patient self-management of medications and lifestyle.

Role of Licensed Practical/Vocational Nurse (LPN/LVN)
- Administer oral antiseizure medications as scheduled.
- In the ambulatory and home setting, monitor patient adherence with medications and lifestyle changes and report problems to the RN.

Role of Unlicensed Assistive Personnel (UAP)
- Place suction equipment, Ambu bag, and O_2 at the patient bedside.
- Remove potentially harmful objects from the bedside and pad side rails.
- Immediately report any seizure activity to the RN.
- Observe and report events of the seizure to the RN.
- Obtain vital signs during the postictal period.
- Provide oropharyngeal suctioning after a seizure (after being trained and evaluated in this procedure).

TABLE 59-12 PATIENT & CAREGIVER TEACHING GUIDE

Seizure Disorders and Epilepsy

Include the following information in the teaching plan for the patient with a seizure disorder.
1. Take drugs as prescribed. Report any and all side effects of drugs to the health care provider. When necessary, blood is drawn to ensure that therapeutic levels are maintained.
2. Use nondrug techniques, such as relaxation therapy and biofeedback training, to potentially reduce the number of seizures.
3. Be aware of availability of resources in the community.
4. Wear a medical alert bracelet or necklace, and carry an identification card.
5. Avoid excessive alcohol intake, fatigue, and loss of sleep.
6. Eat regular meals and snacks in between if feeling shaky, faint, or hungry.

Caregivers should receive the following information.
1. For first aid treatment of tonic-clonic seizure, it is not necessary to call an ambulance or send the patient to the hospital after a single seizure unless the seizure is prolonged, another seizure immediately follows, or extensive injury has occurred.
2. During an acute seizure, it is important to protect the patient from injury. This may involve supporting and protecting the head, turning the patient to the side, loosening constrictive clothing, and easing the patient to the floor, if seated.

---

ness, vital signs, pupil size and position of the eyes, memory loss, muscle soreness, speech disorders (aphasia, dysarthria), weakness or paralysis, sleep period, and the duration of each sign or symptom.

SAFETY ALERT

During a seizure, you should do the following:
- Maintain a patent airway for the patient.
- Protect the patient's head, turn the patient to the side, loosen constrictive clothing, ease patient to the floor (if seated).
- Do not restrain the patient.
- Do not place any objects in the patient's mouth.

After the seizure the patient may require repositioning to open and maintain the airway, suctioning, and oxygen. A seizure can be frightening for the patient and for others who witnessed it. Assess the level of their understanding and provide information about how and why the event occurred. This is an excellent opportunity for you to dispel many common misconceptions about seizures.

AMBULATORY AND HOME CARE. Prevention of recurring seizures is the major goal in the treatment of epilepsy. For treatment to be effective, drugs must be taken regularly and continuously, often for a lifetime. Ensure that the patient knows this, the specifics of the drug regimen, and what to do if a dose

is missed. Usually the dose is made up if the omission is remembered within 24 hours. Caution the patient not to adjust drug dosages without professional guidance because this can increase seizure frequency and even cause status epilepticus. Encourage the patient to report any medication side effects and to keep regular appointments with the health care provider.

You have an important role in teaching the patient and caregiver. Review the guidelines for teaching shown in Table 59-12. Teach the caregiver, family members, and significant others the emergency management of tonic-clonic seizures (see Table 59-8). Remind them that it is not necessary to call an ambulance or send a person to the hospital after a single seizure unless the seizure is prolonged, another seizure immediately follows, or extensive injury has occurred.

Patients with a seizure disorder may experience concerns or fears related to recurrent seizures, incontinence, or loss of self-control. Support the patient through teaching and by helping him or her use effective coping mechanisms.

Perhaps the greatest challenge for a patient with a seizure disorder is adjusting to the personal and societal limitations imposed by the illness. Discrimination in employment is the most serious problem facing the person with a seizure disorder. For issues relating to job discrimination, refer patients to the state department of vocational rehabilitation or the U.S. Equal Employment Opportunity Commission (EEOC).

Assist the patient who has a specific problem in finding appropriate resources. If you believe that associating with others who have a seizure disorder would be beneficial, refer the patient to the local chapter of the Epilepsy Foundation (EF), a volunteer agency that offers a variety of services to patients with epilepsy. Refer the patient who is an eligible veteran to a Department of Veterans Affairs medical center that provides comprehensive care. If intensive psychologic counseling is needed, refer the patient to a community mental health center.

Social workers and welfare agencies can help with financial problems and living arrangements. State agencies specializing in vocational rehabilitation services can provide vocational assessment, counseling, funding for training, and assistance with job placement for patients whose seizures are not well controlled. They can also offer financial assistance for transportation and medical costs related to vocational rehabilitation or job maintenance.

Driving laws for patients who have had a seizure vary from state to state. For example, some states require a 3-month seizure-free period before issuing or reissuing a driver's license, whereas others require up to 1 year. The EF provides current information on driving laws for each state.

Inform the patient that medical alert bracelets, necklaces, and identification cards are available through the EF, local pharmacies, or companies specializing in identification devices (e.g., Medic Alert). However, the use of these medical identification tags is optional. Some patients have found them beneficial, but others prefer not to be identified as having a seizure disorder.

Encourage the patient to learn more about epilepsy through self-education materials. The EF provides several information pamphlets and may facilitate support groups. Many agencies that offer services to epileptic patients, as well as local chapters of EF, have these available as teaching aids.

EVALUATION

Expected outcomes are that the patient with seizures will
- Experience breathing pattern adequate to meet oxygen needs
- Experience no seizure-related injury
- Express acceptance of seizure disorder by admitting presence of epilepsy and maintaining adherent behavior

Additional expected outcomes are presented in eNursing Care Plan 59-2 available on the website.

RESTLESS LEGS SYNDROME

Etiology and Pathophysiology

Restless legs syndrome (RLS), also called Willis-Ekbom disease, is a relatively common condition characterized by unpleasant sensory (paresthesias) and motor abnormalities of one or both legs. Prevalence rates vary from 5% to 15%. However, the numbers may be higher because the condition is underdiagnosed. RLS is more common in older adults. It is also more common in women than men, and women may have an earlier age of onset.[14]

There are two distinct types of RLS: primary (idiopathic) and secondary. The majority of cases are primary, and many patients with this type of RLS report a positive family history. Secondary RLS can occur with metabolic abnormalities associated with iron deficiency, renal failure, hypertension, diabetes mellitus, or rheumatoid arthritis. Conditions such as anemia, pregnancy, and certain medications can cause or worsen symptoms.

Although the exact pathophysiology of primary RLS is unknown, it is believed that RLS is related to a dysfunction in the brain's basal ganglia circuits that use the neurotransmitter dopamine, which controls movements. In RLS this dysfunction causes the urge to move the legs. Abnormal iron metabolism or brain iron deficiencies may result in abnormalities of the dopamine system, thus leading to RLS.[15]

Clinical Manifestations

The severity of RLS sensory symptoms ranges from infrequent minor discomfort (paresthesias, including numbness, tingling, and "pins and needles" sensation) to severe pain. Sensory symptoms often appear first. Patients describe annoying and uncomfortable (but usually not painful) sensations in the legs. Some describe the sensations like bugs creeping or crawling on the legs. The leg pain is localized within the calf muscles. Patients can also experience pain in the upper extremities and the trunk. The discomfort occurs when the patient is sedentary and is most common in the evening or at night.

The pain at night can disrupt sleep. Physical activity, such as walking, stretching, rocking, or kicking, often relieves the pain. In the most severe cases, patients sleep only a few hours at night, resulting in daytime fatigue and disruption of the daily routine. The motor abnormalities associated with RLS consist of voluntary restlessness and stereotyped, periodic, involuntary movements. The involuntary movements usually occur during sleep. Fatigue further aggravates symptoms. Over time, RLS advances to more frequent and severe episodes.

Diagnostic Studies

RLS is a clinical diagnosis, based in large part on the patient's history or the report of the bed partner related to nighttime activities. The diagnosis of RLS is based on four specific criteria: (1) desire to move the extremities, often associated with paresthesias; (2) motor restlessness; (3) worsening of symptoms at rest with at least temporary relief from activity; and (4) worsening of symptoms in the evening or night.[15]

The patient may undergo polysomnography studies during sleep to distinguish RLS from other clinical conditions that can disturb sleep (e.g., sleep apnea). However, periodic leg movements in sleep are a common feature in RLS patients. Blood tests, such as a complete blood count, serum ferritin levels, and renal function tests (e.g., serum creatinine), may help exclude secondary causes of RLS. A patient's history of diabetes mellitus and its management may provide information to determine whether paresthesias are caused by peripheral neuropathy related to diabetes or RLS.

NURSING AND COLLABORATIVE MANAGEMENT
RESTLESS LEGS SYNDROME

The goal of collaborative management is to reduce patient discomfort and distress and to improve sleep quality. When RLS is secondary to renal failure or iron deficiency, treatment of these conditions will decrease symptoms. Nondrug approaches to RLS management include establishing regular sleep habits; exercising; avoiding activities that cause symptoms; and eliminating aggravating factors such as alcohol, caffeine, and certain drugs (neuroleptics, lithium, antihistamines, antidepressants).

If nondrug measures fail to provide symptom relief, drug therapy is an option. No single medication effectively manages RLS for all patients. The main drugs used in RLS include dopamine precursors (e.g., carbidopa/levodopa [Sinemet]) and dopamine agonists (e.g., ropinirole [Requip], pramipexole [Mirapex]) to increase the amount of dopamine in the brain. The antiseizure drug gabapentin enacarbil (Horizant) is used to decrease the sensory sensations. If the patient has iron deficiency or low serum ferritin levels, iron supplementation is considered.

Other drugs may relieve some symptoms of RLS. These include opioids and benzodiazepines. Low doses of opioids (e.g., oxycodone) are usually reserved for patients with severe symptoms who fail to respond to other drug therapies. The main side effect of opioids is constipation, so the patient may need to take a stool softener or laxative. Clonidine (Catapres) and propranolol (Inderal) are also effective in some patients.

DEGENERATIVE NEUROLOGIC DISORDERS

Degenerative nerve diseases lead to nerve damage that worsens as the disease progresses. These diseases affect many activities, including balance, movement, speech, and respiratory and heart function. There are more than 200 degenerative neurologic disorders. These include the disorders discussed in the remainder of this chapter, as well as disorders such as cerebellar degeneration, Friedreich's ataxia, Creutzfeldt-Jakob disease, and neurofibromatosis. Some have no known cause. However, many of these diseases have a genetic basis. Most degenerative nerve diseases have no cure. Treatment aims to reduce symptoms and help the patient maintain an optimal level of function.

Patients with these diseases have similar concerns and problems. They must deal with not only their disease, but also the impact that the disease has on their quality of life. Many patients have concerns regarding safety, mobility, self-care, and coping. The patient and family often require psychosocial support, especially as the disease progresses and the patient's disability gets worse.

MULTIPLE SCLEROSIS

Multiple sclerosis (MS) is a chronic, progressive, degenerative disorder of the CNS characterized by disseminated demyelination of nerve fibers of the brain and spinal cord. The onset of MS is usually between 20 and 50 years of age, although it can occur in young teens and much older adults. Women are affected two to three times more often than men.

MS is five times more prevalent in temperate climates (between 45 and 65 degrees of latitude), such as those found in the northern United States, Canada, and Europe, as compared with tropical regions. Migration from one geographic area to another may alter a person's risk of developing MS. Immigrants and their descendants tend to take on the risk level (either higher or lower) of the area to which they move. However, the change in risk may not appear immediately. For example, African Americans (in the United States) have a prevalence rate that is 40% that of European Americans, whereas Africans (in Africa) are thought to have a prevalence rate that is approximately 1% that of European Americans. The variations in incidence of MS suggest that geography, ethnicity, and other factors interact in a complex way to cause MS.[16]

Etiology and Pathophysiology

The cause of MS is unknown, although research suggests that it is unlikely MS is related to a single cause. Researchers believe the disease develops in a genetically susceptible person as a result of environmental exposure, like an infection. Multiple genes are believed to be involved in the inherited susceptibility to MS, and first-, second-, and third-degree relatives of patients with MS are at an increased risk.[16]

Possible precipitating factors include infection, smoking, physical injury, emotional stress, excessive fatigue, pregnancy, and a poor state of health. The role of precipitating factors such as exposure to pathogenic agents is controversial. It is possible that their association with MS is random and that there is no cause-and-effect relationship.

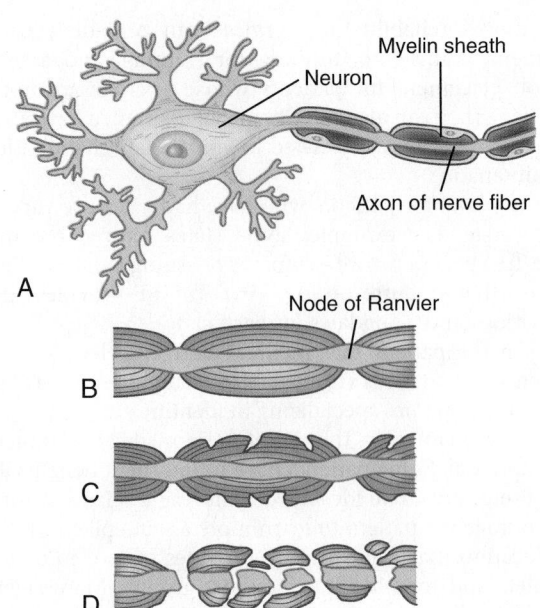

FIG. 59-3 Pathogenesis of multiple sclerosis. **A,** Normal nerve cell with myelin sheath. **B,** Normal axon. **C,** Myelin breakdown. **D,** Myelin totally disrupted; axon not functioning.

Three pathologic processes characterize MS: chronic inflammation, demyelination, and gliosis (scarring) in the CNS. The primary neuropathologic condition is an autoimmune process orchestrated by activated T cells (lymphocytes). An environmental factor or virus in genetically susceptible individuals may initially trigger this process. The activated T cells in the systemic circulation migrate to the CNS, disrupting the blood-brain barrier. This is likely the initial event in the development of MS. Subsequent antigen-antibody reaction within the CNS activates the inflammatory response and leads to the demyelination of axons.

Initially, attacks on the myelin sheaths of the neurons in the brain and spinal cord result in damage to the myelin sheath (Fig. 59-3, *A* to *C*). However, the nerve fiber is not affected. Transmission of nerve impulses still occurs, though transmission is slowed. The patient may complain of a noticeable impairment of function (e.g., weakness). However, the myelin can regenerate, and when it does, symptoms disappear. At that point, the patient experiences a remission.

As ongoing inflammation occurs, the nearby oligodendrocytes are affected, and the myelin loses the ability to regenerate. Eventually damage occurs to the underlying axon. Nerve impulse transmission is disrupted, resulting in the permanent loss of nerve function (Fig. 59-3, *D*). As inflammation subsides, glial scar tissue replaces the damaged tissue, leading to the formation of hard, sclerotic plaques (Fig. 59-4). These plaques are found throughout the white matter of the CNS.

Clinical Manifestations

The onset of MS is often insidious and gradual, with vague symptoms occurring intermittently over months or years that often dissuade the patient from seeking medical attention. Thus the disease may not be diagnosed until long after the onset of the first symptom. The disease is characterized by chronic, progressive deterioration in some patients, and remissions and exacerbations in others. With repeated exacerbations, the overall trend is progressive deterioration in neurologic function.

FIG. 59-4 Chronic multiple sclerosis. Demyelination plaque *(P)* at gray-white junction and adjacent partially remyelinated shadow plaque *(V)*.

TABLE 59-13	PATTERNS OF MULTIPLE SCLEROSIS
Category	**Characteristics**
Relapsing-remitting	• Clearly defined relapses with full recovery or sequelae and residual deficit on recovery. • Approximately 85% of people are initially diagnosed with this type of multiple sclerosis (MS).
Primary-progressive	• Slowly worsening neurologic function from the beginning with no distinct relapses or remissions. • About 10% of people are diagnosed with this type of MS.
Secondary-progressive	• A relapsing-remitting initial course, followed by progression with or without occasional relapses, minor remissions, and plateaus. • New treatments may slow progression. • About 50% of people with relapsing-remitting MS develop this type within 10 yr.
Progressive-relapsing	• Progressive disease from onset, with clear acute relapses, with or without full recovery. Periods between relapses are characterized by continuing progression. • Only 5% of people experience this type of MS.

Since the disease process has a spotty distribution in the CNS, the clinical manifestations vary with each patient according to the areas of the CNS involved. Some patients have severe, long-lasting symptoms early in the course of the disease. Others may experience only occasional and mild symptoms for several years after onset. A classification scheme, with four primary patterns of MS, has been developed based on the clinical course[16,17] (Table 59-13).

Common manifestations of MS include motor, sensory, cerebellar, and emotional problems. Motor symptoms include weakness or paralysis of the limbs, the trunk, or the head; diplopia; scanning speech; and spasticity of the muscles that are chronically affected. Patients with MS experience a variety of sensory abnormalities, including numbness and tingling and other paresthesias, patchy blindness *(scotomas),* blurred vision, vertigo, tinnitus, decreased hearing, and chronic neuropathic pain. Radicular (nerve root) pains may be present, particularly in the low thoracic and abdominal regions. *Lhermitte's sign* is a transient sensory symptom described as an electric shock radiating down the spine or into the limbs with flexion of the neck. Cerebellar signs include nystagmus, ataxia, dysarthria, and dys-

phagia. Many patients have severe fatigue, sometimes with significant disability. The fatigue is aggravated by heat, humidity, deconditioning, and medication side effects.[16]

Bowel and bladder function can be affected if the sclerotic plaque is located in areas of the CNS that control elimination. Problems with defecation usually involve constipation rather than fecal incontinence. Urinary problems are variable. A common problem in MS patients is a *spastic* (uninhibited) bladder. As a result, the bladder has a small capacity for urine, and its contractions are unchecked. This is accompanied by urinary urgency and frequency and results in dribbling or incontinence.

A *flaccid* (hypotonic) bladder indicates a lesion in the reflex arc controlling bladder function. A flaccid bladder has a large capacity for urine because there is no sensation or desire to void, no pressure, and no pain. Generally, the patient has urinary retention, but urgency and frequency may also occur with this type of lesion. Another urinary problem is a combination of the previous two. Urinary problems cannot be adequately diagnosed and treated without urodynamic studies.

Sexual dysfunction occurs in many persons with MS. Physiologic erectile dysfunction may result from spinal cord involvement in men. Women may experience decreased libido, difficulty with orgasmic response, painful intercourse, and decreased vaginal lubrication. Diminished sensation can prevent a normal sexual response in both sexes. The emotional effects of chronic illness and the loss of self-esteem also contribute to loss of sexual response.

Some women with MS who become pregnant experience remission or an improvement in their symptoms during the gestation period. The hormonal changes associated with pregnancy appear to affect the immune system. However, during the postpartum period, women are at greater risk for exacerbation of the disease.

About half of people with MS experience some problems with cognitive function. For most, the problems are difficulties with short-term memory, attention, information processing, planning, visual perception, and word finding. General intellect remains unchanged and intact, including long-term memory, conversational skills, and reading comprehension. In only about 5% to 10% of MS patients, the cognitive changes are so severe that they significantly impair the person's ability to carry out activities of daily living. Most of the time, cognitive difficulties occur later in the course of the disease. However, they can occur much earlier in the disease process, and occasionally they are present at the onset of MS.

Persons with MS may also experience emotional changes such as anger, depression, or euphoria. Physical and emotional trauma, fatigue, and infection may aggravate or trigger signs and symptoms.

The average life expectancy after the onset of symptoms is more than 25 years. Death usually occurs due to infectious complications (e.g., pneumonia) of immobility or because of an unrelated disease.

Diagnostic Studies

Because there is no definitive diagnostic test for MS, factors considered are the history, clinical manifestations, and results of certain diagnostic tests (Table 59-14). An MRI of the brain and spinal cord may show plaques, inflammation, atrophy, and tissue breakdown and destruction. Cerebrospinal fluid (CSF) analysis may show an increase in immunoglobulin G and the

TABLE 59-14 COLLABORATIVE CARE

Multiple Sclerosis

Diagnostic
- History and physical examination
- CSF analysis
- CT scan
- MRI, MRS
- Evoked potential testing
  - Somatosensory evoked potential (SSEP)
  - Auditory evoked potential (AEP)
  - Visual evoked potential (VEP)

Collaborative Therapy
- Drug therapy (see Table 59-15)
- Surgical therapy
  - Thalamotomy (unmanageable tremor)
  - Neurectomy, rhizotomy, cordotomy (unmanageable spasticity)

MRS, Magnetic resonance spectroscopy.

TABLE 59-15 DRUG THERAPY

Multiple Sclerosis

Drug	Patient Teaching
Disease-Modifying Drugs	
Immunomodulators	
β-Interferon (Betaseron, Extavia, Avonex, Rebif)	• Perform self-injection techniques.
glatiramer acetate (Copaxone)	• Report side effects.
teriflunomide (Aubagio)	• Treat flu-like symptoms with an NSAID or acetaminophen.
	• Because it may cause serious liver disease, monitor liver tests.
	• Avoid pregnancy.
Immunosuppressant	
mitoxantrone (Novantrone)	• Report side effects.
dimethyl fumarate (Tecfidera)	• Avoid pregnancy.
	• Avoid contact with large crowds and people who have an infection.
Sphingosine 1-Phosphate Receptor Modulator	
fingolimod (Gilenya)	• Report side effects.
	• Monitor blood pressure regularly.
	• Avoid pregnancy.
Monoclonal Antibody	
natalizumab (Tysabri)	• Report side effects.
	• Avoid pregnancy.
Drugs for Managing Exacerbations	
Corticosteroids	
ACTH	• Restrict salt intake.
prednisone	• Do not abruptly stop therapy.
methylprednisolone	• Know drug interactions.
Drugs for Symptom Management	
Cholinergics	
bethanechol (Urecholine)	• Consult with health care provider before using other drugs, including over-the-counter drugs.
neostigmine (Prostigmin)	
Anticholinergics	
propantheline (Pro-Banthine)	• Consult health care provider before using other drugs, especially sleeping aids, antihistamines (possibly leading to potentiated effect).
oxybutynin (Ditropan)	
Muscle Relaxants	
diazepam (Valium)	• Avoid driving and similar activities because of sedative effects.
baclofen (Lioresal)	
dantrolene (Dantrium)	• Do not abruptly stop therapy.
tizanidine (Zanaflex)	• Avoid use with tranquilizers and alcohol.
Nerve Conduction Enhancer	
dalfampridine (Ampyra)	• Be aware that it may cause seizures, especially at higher doses.
	• Take the tablet whole. Do not take more than 2 in 24 hr.

ACTH, Adrenocorticotropic hormone.

presence of oligoclonal banding.[17] Evoked potential responses are often delayed in persons with MS because of decreased nerve conduction from the eye and the ear to the brain.

To be diagnosed with MS, the patient must have (1) evidence of at least two inflammatory demyelinating lesions in at least two different locations within the CNS, (2) damage or an attack occurring at different times (usually 1 month or more apart), and (3) all other possible diagnoses ruled out.

Collaborative Care

Drug Therapy. Because currently there is no cure for MS, collaborative care is aimed at treating the disease process and providing symptomatic relief (see Table 59-14). Since no two cases of MS are alike, therapy is tailored specifically to the disease pattern and manifestations that the patient is experiencing (Table 59-15).

The initial treatment of MS is the use of immunomodulator drugs to modify the disease progression and prevent relapses. These drugs include interferon β-1b (Betaseron) and glatiramer acetate (Copaxone), which are given subcutaneously every other day, and interferon β-1a (Avonex), which is given intramuscularly (IM). Another formulation of interferon β-1a is Rebif, which is administered subcutaneously three times weekly.

DRUG ALERT: β-Interferon (Avonex, Betaseron, Rebif)
- Rotate injection sites with each dose.
- Assess for depression, suicidal ideation.
- Wear sunscreen and protective clothing while exposed to sun.
- Know that flu-like symptoms are common after initiation of therapy.

Fingolimod (Gilenya) reduces MS disease activity by preventing lymphocytes from reaching the CNS and causing damage. Teriflunomide (Aubagio) is an immunomodulatory agent with antiinflammatory properties. The exact mechanism of action is unknown but may involve a reduction in the number of activated lymphocytes in the CNS. Teriflunomide is specifically indicated for treatment of relapsing forms of MS.

For more active and aggressive forms of MS, IV natalizumab (Tysabri) and mitoxantrone (Novantrone) may be used. Natalizumab, a monoclonal antibody, is given monthly when patients have had an inadequate response to other drugs. Natalizumab increases the risk of progressive multifocal leukoencephalopathy, a potentially fatal viral infection of the brain. Mitoxantrone, an antineoplastic medication, has serious effects, including cardiotoxicity, leukemia, and infertility.[17]

Dimethyl fumarate (Tecfidera) provides a new approach to treating MS by activating the Nrf2 pathway. This pathway provides a way for cells in the body to defend themselves against the inflammation and oxidative stress caused by MS. Dimethyl fumarate is used to treat relapsing-remitting MS.

Corticosteroids (e.g., methylprednisolone, prednisone) are most helpful to treat acute exacerbations of MS. They work by reducing edema and acute inflammation at the site of demyelin-

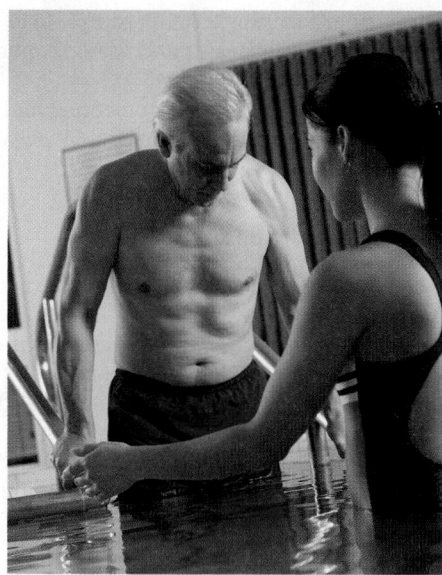

FIG. 59-5 Water therapy provides exercise and recreation for the patient with a chronic neurologic disease. (Photos.com/AbleStock.com/Thinkstock.)

ation. However, these drugs do not affect the ultimate outcome or the degree of residual neurologic impairment from the exacerbation.

Many other drugs are used to treat the various symptoms of MS, which may include fatigue, spasticity, tremor, vertigo or dizziness, depression, pain, bowel problems, bladder problems, sexual dysfunction, and cognitive changes. For example, muscle relaxants are used for spasticity. Amantadine (Symmetrel) and CNS stimulants (pemoline [Cylert], methylphenidate [Ritalin], and modafinil [Provigil]) are used to treat fatigue. Anticholinergics are used to treat bladder symptoms. Tricyclic antidepressants and antiseizure drugs are used for chronic pain syndromes. Dalfampridine (Ampyra) is used to improve walking speed in MS patients. It is a selective potassium channel blocker and improves nerve conduction in damaged nerve segments. It should not be used in patients with a history of seizure disorders or in those with moderate to severe kidney disease.

Other Therapies. Spasticity is primarily treated with muscle relaxants. However, surgery (e.g., neurectomy, rhizotomy, cordotomy), dorsal-column electrical stimulation, or intrathecal baclofen (Lioresal) delivered by pump may be required. Tremors that become unmanageable with drugs are sometimes treated by thalamotomy or deep brain stimulation.

Neurologic dysfunction sometimes improves with physical and speech therapies. Exercise improves the daily functioning for patients with MS not experiencing an exacerbation. Exercise decreases spasticity, increases coordination, and retrains unaffected muscles to substitute for impaired ones. An especially beneficial type of physical therapy is water exercise (Fig. 59-5). Water gives buoyancy to the body and allows the patient to perform activities that would normally be impossible because the patient has more control over the body.

NURSING MANAGEMENT
MULTIPLE SCLEROSIS

NURSING ASSESSMENT

Subjective and objective data that should be obtained from a patient with MS are presented in Table 59-16.

TABLE 59-16   **NURSING ASSESSMENT**
Multiple Sclerosis

Subjective Data
Important Health Information
Past health history: Recent or past viral infections or vaccinations, other recent infections, residence in cold or temperate climates, recent physical or emotional stress, pregnancy, exposure to extremes of heat and cold
Medications: Adherence to regimen of corticosteroids, immunomodulators, immunosuppressants, cholinergics, anticholinergics, antispasmodics

Functional Health Patterns
Health perception–health management: Positive family history; malaise
Nutritional-metabolic: Weight loss; difficulty in chewing, dysphagia
Elimination: Urinary frequency, urgency, dribbling or incontinence, retention; constipation
Activity-exercise: Generalized muscle weakness, muscle fatigue; tingling and numbness, ataxia (clumsiness)
Cognitive-perceptual: Eye, back, leg, joint pain; painful muscle spasms; vertigo; blurred or lost vision; diplopia; tinnitus
Sexuality-reproductive: Impotence, decreased libido
Coping–stress tolerance: Anger, depression, euphoria, social isolation

Objective Data
General
Apathy, inattentiveness

Integumentary
Pressure ulcers

Neurologic
Scanning speech, nystagmus, ataxia, tremor, spasticity, hyperreflexia, decreased hearing

Musculoskeletal
Muscle weakness, paresis, paralysis, spasms, foot dragging, dysarthria

Possible Diagnostic Findings
↓ T suppressor cells, demyelinating lesions on MRI or MRS scans, ↑ IgG or oligoclonal banding in cerebrospinal fluid, delayed evoked potential responses

IgG, Immunoglobulin G; *MRS,* magnetic resonance spectroscopy.

NURSING DIAGNOSES

Nursing diagnoses for the patient with MS may include, but are not limited to, the following:

- Impaired physical mobility *related to* muscle weakness or paralysis and muscle spasticity
- Impaired urinary elimination *related to* sensorimotor deficits
- Ineffective self-health management *related to* knowledge deficit regarding management of MS

Additional information on nursing diagnoses for the patient with MS is presented in the eNursing Care Plan 59-3 (available on the website for this chapter).

PLANNING

The overall goals are that the patient with MS will (1) maximize neuromuscular function, (2) maintain independence in activities of daily living for as long as possible, (3) manage disabling fatigue, (4) optimize psychosocial well-being, (5) adjust to the illness, and (6) reduce factors that precipitate exacerbations.

NURSING IMPLEMENTATION

The patient with MS should be aware of triggers that may cause exacerbations or worsening of the disease. Exacerbations of MS are triggered by infection (especially upper respiratory and urinary tract infections), trauma, immunization, childbirth, stress, and change in climate. Each person responds differently to these triggers. Assist the patient in identifying particular triggers and develop ways to avoid them or minimize their effects.

During the diagnostic phase the patient needs reassurance that, even though there is a tentative diagnosis of MS, certain diagnostic studies must be done to rule out other neurologic disorders. Assist the patient in dealing with the anxiety caused by a diagnosis of a disabling illness. The patient with recently diagnosed MS may need assistance with the grieving process.

During an acute exacerbation, the patient may be immobile and confined to bed. The focus of nursing interventions at this phase is to prevent major complications of immobility, such as respiratory and urinary tract infections and pressure ulcers.

Focus patient teaching on building general resistance to illness, including avoiding fatigue, extremes of heat and cold, and exposure to infection. Encourage vigorous and early treatment of infection when it does occur. Teach the patient to achieve a good balance of exercise and rest; minimize caffeine intake; and eat nutritious, well-balanced meals. A diet high in roughage may help relieve the problem of constipation. Patients should know their treatment regimens, drug side effects, how to watch for and manage side effects, and drug interactions with over-the-counter medications. The patient should consult a health care provider before taking nonprescription drugs.

Bladder control is a major problem for many patients with MS. Although anticholinergics may be beneficial for some patients to decrease spasticity, you may need to teach others self-catheterization (discussed in Chapter 46 on pp. 1092-1094). Bowel problems, particularly constipation, frequently occur in patients with MS. Increasing the dietary fiber intake may help some patients achieve regularity in bowel habits.

The patient with MS and the caregiver need to make many emotional adjustments because of the unpredictability of the disease, the need to change lifestyles, and the challenge of avoiding or decreasing precipitating factors. The National Multiple Sclerosis Society and its local chapters can offer a variety of services to meet the needs of patients with MS.

EVALUATION

The expected outcomes are that the patient with MS will
- Maintain or improve muscle strength and mobility
- Use assistive devices appropriately for ambulation and mobility
- Maintain urinary continence
- Make decisions about health and lifestyle modifications necessary for management of MS

Additional information on expected outcomes for the patient with MS are presented in eNursing Care Plan 59-3 (available on the website for this chapter).

PARKINSON'S DISEASE

Parkinson's disease (PD) is a chronic, progressive neurodegenerative disorder characterized by slowness in the initiation and execution of movement *(bradykinesia)*, increased muscle tone *(rigidity)*, tremor at rest, and gait disturbance. It is the most common form of *parkinsonism* (a syndrome characterized by similar symptoms).

The prevalence of PD is about 160 per 100,000. The diagnosis of PD increases with age, with the condition affecting about 2% of people over 60 years old. However, as many as 15% of those diagnosed with PD are less than 50 years old. PD is more common in men by a ratio of 3:2.[18]

Etiology and Pathophysiology

Although the exact cause of PD is unknown, a complex interplay of environmental and genetic factors is involved. Between 10% and 15% of PD patients have a family history of the disease, indicating a strong genetic basis. In other persons, exposure to toxins or certain viruses may trigger PD.[18]

There are many forms of parkinsonism other than PD. Parkinsonism-like symptoms have occurred after intoxication with a variety of chemicals, including carbon monoxide and manganese (among copper miners) and the product of meperidine analog synthesis, MPTP. Drug-induced parkinsonism can follow therapy with metoclopramide (Reglan), reserpine (Serpasil), methyldopa (Aldomet), lithium, haloperidol (Haldol), and chlorpromazine (Thorazine). Parkinsonism can also be seen after the use of illicit drugs, including amphetamine and methamphetamine. Other causes of parkinsonism include hydrocephalus, MS, encephalitis, infections, stroke, tumor, Huntington's disease, and trauma.[19]

Many changes found in the brains of people with PD may play a role in development of the disease, including a lack of dopamine (DA). The pathologic process of PD involves degeneration of the DA-producing neurons in the substantia nigra of the midbrain (Figs. 59-6 to 59-8), which in turn disrupts the normal balance between DA and acetylcholine (ACh) in the basal ganglia. DA is a neurotransmitter essential for normal functioning of the extrapyramidal motor system, including control of posture, support, and voluntary motion. Manifestations of PD do not occur until 80% of neurons in the substantia nigra are lost.

Lewy bodies, unusual clumps of protein, are found in the brains of patients with PD. It is not known what causes these bodies to form, but their presence indicates abnormal functioning of the brain. Lewy body dementia is discussed in Chapter 60.

Genetic Link

Approximately 20% of PD patients have a family history of PD. Many autosomal dominant and recessive genes have been linked to familial PD. The most common genetic contributor to PD is the *LRRK2* gene. Mutations in this gene also appear to have a role in sporadic, or noninherited, cases of PD. *LRRK2* and mutations in another gene, α-synuclein *(SNCA),* have manifestations similar to those of the common, age-related PD. Other genes involved in familial PD are parkin *(PARK2), DJ-1,* and *PINK1.* Mutations in these genes are often associated with a younger age of onset and have additional manifestations than those typically seen with age-related PD. *PINK1* mutations are related to a rare, early-onset form of PD.[18,20,21]

FIG. 59-6 Nigrostriatal disorders produce parkinsonism. Left-sided view of the human brain showing the substantia nigra and the corpus striatum *(shaded area)* lying deep within the cerebral hemisphere. Nerve fibers extend upward from the substantia nigra, divide into many branches, and carry dopamine to all regions of the corpus striatum.

Clinical Manifestations

The onset of PD is gradual and insidious, with an ongoing progression. It may involve only one side of the body initially. The classic manifestations of PD are a triad of tremor, rigidity, and bradykinesia. In the beginning stages, only a mild tremor, a slight limp, or a decreased arm swing may be evident. Later in the disease the patient may have a shuffling, propulsive gait with arms flexed and loss of postural reflexes. Some patients have a slight change in speech patterns. None of these manifestations alone is sufficient evidence for a diagnosis of the disease.

Tremor. *Tremor,* often the first sign, may be minimal initially, so the patient is the only one who notices it. This tremor can affect handwriting, causing it to trail off, particularly toward the ends of words. Parkinsonian tremor is more prominent at

FIG. 59-8 In Parkinson's disease, positron emission tomography (PET) scan showing reduced fluorodopa uptake in the basal ganglia *(right)* compared with a normal control *(left).*

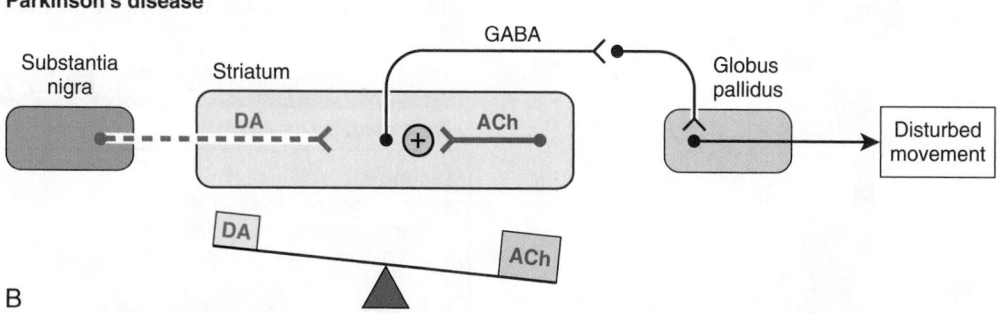

FIG. 59-7 In Parkinson's disease there is a deficit in dopamine. These deficits create an imbalance between dopamine and the excitatory neurotransmitter acetylcholine. **A,** In a healthy person, dopamine *(DA)* released from neurons originating in the substantia nigra inhibits the firing of neurons in the striatum that release γ-aminobutyric acid *(GABA).* Conversely, neurons located within the striatum, which release acetylcholine *(ACh),* excite the GABAergic neurons. Under normal conditions, the inhibitory actions of DA are balanced by the excitatory actions of ACh, and controlled movement results. **B,** In Parkinson's disease, the neurons in the substantia nigra that supply DA to the striatum degenerate. When there is a deficit of DA, the excitatory effects of ACh go unopposed, resulting in disturbed movements (tremor, rigidity).

rest and is aggravated by emotional stress or increased concentration. The hand tremor is described as "pill rolling" because the thumb and forefinger appear to move in a rotary fashion as if rolling a pill, coin, or other small object. Tremor can also involve the diaphragm, tongue, lips, and jaw but rarely causes shaking of the head.

Unfortunately, in many people a benign essential tremor is mistakenly diagnosed as PD. Essential tremor occurs during voluntary movement, has a more rapid frequency than parkinsonian tremor, and is often familial.

Rigidity. *Rigidity,* the second sign of the triad, is the increased resistance to passive motion when the limbs are moved through their range of motion. Parkinsonian rigidity is typified by cogwheel rigidity, or a jerky quality, as if there were intermittent catches in the movement of a cogwheel, when the joint is moved passively. Sustained muscle contraction causes the rigidity and consequently elicits complaints of muscle soreness; feeling tired and achy; or pain in the head, the upper body, the spine, or the legs. Another consequence of rigidity is slowness of movement because it inhibits the alternating of contraction and relaxation in opposing muscle groups (e.g., biceps and triceps).

Bradykinesia. *Bradykinesia* is particularly evident in the loss of automatic movements, which is secondary to the physical and chemical alteration of the basal ganglia and related structures in the extrapyramidal portion of the CNS. In the unaffected patient, automatic movements are involuntary and occur subconsciously. They include blinking of the eyelids, swinging of the arms while walking, swallowing of saliva, self-expression with facial and hand movements, and minor movement of postural adjustment.

The patient with PD does not execute these movements and lacks spontaneous activity. This accounts for the stooped posture, masked face (deadpan expression), drooling of saliva, and shuffling gait *(festination)* that are characteristic of a person with this disease. The posture is that of a slowed "old man" image, with the head and trunk bent forward and the legs constantly flexed (Fig. 59-9).

Postural instability is common. Patients may complain of being unable to stop themselves from going forward (propulsion) or backward (retropulsion). Assessment of postural instability includes the "pull test," in which the examiner stands behind the patient and gives a tug backward on the shoulder, causing the patient to lose his or her balance and fall backward.

In addition to the motor signs of PD, many nonmotor symptoms are common. They include depression, anxiety, apathy, fatigue, pain, constipation, impotence, and short-term memory impairment. Sleep problems are common in patients with PD and include difficulty staying asleep at night, restless sleep, nightmares, and drowsiness or sudden sleep onset during the day.[18]

Complications

As the disease progresses, complications increase. These include motor symptoms (e.g., dyskinesias [spontaneous, involuntary movements], weakness, *akinesia* [total immobility]), neurologic problems (e.g., dementia), and neuropsychiatric problems (e.g., depression, hallucinations, psychosis). As PD progresses, it often results in a severe dementia, which is associated with an increase in mortality.

As swallowing becomes more difficult (dysphagia), malnutrition or aspiration may result. General debilitation may lead to pneumonia, urinary tract infections, and skin breakdown. Orthostatic hypotension may occur in some patients and, along with loss of postural reflexes, may result in falls or other injury.[22]

Diagnostic Studies

Because there is no specific diagnostic test for PD, the diagnosis is based on the history and the clinical features. A firm diagnosis can be made only when at least two of the three signs of the classic triad are present: tremor, rigidity, and bradykinesia. The ultimate confirmation of PD is a positive response to antiparkinsonian drugs. Research is ongoing regarding the role of genetic testing and MRI in diagnosing patients with PD.[23]

Collaborative Care

Because PD has no cure, collaborative care focuses on relieving the symptoms (Table 59-17).

Drug Therapy. Drug therapy for PD is aimed at correcting the imbalance of neurotransmitters within the CNS. Antiparkinsonian drugs either enhance the release or the supply of DA (dopaminergic) or antagonize or block the effects of the overactive cholinergic neurons in the striatum (anticholinergic) (see Fig. 59-7). Levodopa with carbidopa (Sinemet) is often the first drug used. Levodopa is a chemical precursor of DA and can

Blank facial expression

Forward tilt to posture

Slow, monotonous, slurred speech

Tremor

Short, shuffling gait

FIG. 59-9 Characteristic appearance of a patient with Parkinson's disease.

TABLE 59-17   **COLLABORATIVE CARE**
Parkinson's Disease
Diagnostic
• History and physical examination
• Tremor, rigidity, and bradykinesia
• Positive response to antiparkinsonian drugs
• MRI
• Rule out side effects of phenothiazines, reserpine, benzodiazepines, haloperidol
Collaborative Therapy
• Antiparkinsonian drugs (see Table 59-18)
• Deep brain stimulation
• Ablation surgery

cross the blood-brain barrier. It is converted to DA in the basal ganglia. Sinemet is the preferred drug because it also contains carbidopa, an agent that inhibits the enzyme dopa-decarboxylase in the peripheral tissues. Dopa-decarboxylase breaks down levodopa before it reaches the brain. The net result of the combination of levodopa and carbidopa is that more levodopa reaches the brain, and therefore less drug is needed. Levodopa has many side effects and drug interactions. Prolonged use can often result in dyskinesias and "off/on" periods when the medication will unpredictably start or stop working.

DRUG ALERT: Carbidopa/Levodopa (Sinemet)
- Monitor for signs of dyskinesia.
- Effects may be delayed for several weeks to months.
- Instruct patient or caregiver to report any uncontrolled movement of face, eyelids, mouth, tongue, arms, hands, or legs; mental changes; palpitations; severe nausea and vomiting; and difficulty urinating.

Many patients are given Sinemet early in the disease course. It is effective for the management of akinetic symptoms. Tremor and rigidity may also respond to this drug.[21] However, some health care providers believe that, after a few years of therapy, the effectiveness of Sinemet wears off. Therefore they prefer to initiate therapy with a DA receptor agonist. These drugs include bromocriptine (Parlodel), pergolide (Permax), ropinirole (Requip), pramipexole (Mirapex), and rotigotine (Neupro). These drugs directly stimulate DA receptors. Sinemet is then added to the drug regimen when more moderate to severe symptoms are present.

DRUG ALERT: Bromocriptine (Parlodel)
- Patient may become dizzy or faint due to orthostatic hypotension, especially after the first dose.
- Notify physician immediately if a severe headache develops that does not let up or continues to get worse.

Selegiline (Eldepryl) and rasagiline (Azilect), monoamine oxidase type B (MAO-B) inhibitors, are sometimes used in combination with Sinemet. By inhibiting MAO-B, the degradative enzyme for DA, these agents increase the levels of DA and prolong the half-life of levodopa. Rasagiline can also be used alone as therapy in early PD.

Entacapone (Comtan) and tolcapone (Tasmar) block the enzyme catechol O-methyltransferase (COMT), which breaks down levodopa in the peripheral circulation, thus prolonging the effect of Sinemet. These drugs are used only as adjuncts to levodopa.[18]

Anticholinergic drugs such as trihexyphenidyl (Artane) and benztropine (Cogentin) are also used to manage PD. These drugs decrease the activity of ACh, thus providing balance between cholinergic and dopaminergic actions. Antihistamines (e.g., diphenhydramine [Benadryl]) with anticholinergic properties may be used to manage tremors.

The antiviral agent amantadine is also an effective antiparkinsonian drug. Although its exact mechanism of action is not known, amantadine promotes the effect of DA.[18] Rivastigmine (Exelon) or donepezil (Aricept) is used to treat mild to moderate Parkinson's dementia. Amitriptyline may be used to treat depression.

Table 59-18 summarizes the drugs commonly used in PD. The use of only one drug is preferred because fewer side effects occur and the drug dosage is easier to adjust than when several drugs are used. However, as the disease progresses, combination therapy is often required. Excessive amounts of dopaminergic drugs can lead to *paradoxic intoxication* (aggravation rather than relief of symptoms).

TABLE 59-18 DRUG THERAPY

Parkinson's Disease

Drug	Mechanism of Action
Dopaminergics	
Dopamine Precursors	
levodopa (L-dopa)	Converted to dopamine in basal ganglia
levodopa/carbidopa (Sinemet, Parcopa [orally dissolving tablet])	
Dopamine Receptor Agonists	
bromocriptine (Parlodel)	Stimulate dopamine receptors
pergolide (Permax)	
pramipexole (Mirapex)	
ropinirole (Requip, Requip XL)	
rotigotine (Neupro [skin patch])	
Dopamine Agonists	
amantadine (Symmetrel)	Blocks reuptake of dopamine into presynaptic neurons
apomorphine (Apokyn)	Stimulates postsynaptic dopamine receptors
Anticholinergics	
trihexyphenidyl (Artane)	Block cholinergic receptors, thus helping to balance cholinergic and dopaminergic activity
benztropine (Cogentin)	
biperiden (Akineton)	
Antihistamine	
diphenhydramine (Benadryl)	Has anticholinergic effect
Monoamine Oxidase Inhibitors	
selegiline (Eldepryl, Carbex)	Block breakdown of dopamine
rasagiline (Azilect)	
Catechol O-Methyltransferase (COMT) Inhibitors	
entacapone (Comtan)	Block COMT and slow the breakdown of levodopa, thus prolonging the action of levodopa
tolcapone (Tasmar)	

Within 3 to 5 years of standard Parkinson's drug treatments, many patients experience episodes of hypomobility (e.g., inability to rise from chair, to speak, or to walk). The episodes can occur toward the end of a dosing interval with standard medications (so-called end-of-dose wearing off) or at unpredictable times (spontaneous "on/off").

A combination of carbidopa, levodopa, and entacapone (Stalevo) is available for patients with end-of-dose wearing off. Apomorphine (Apokyn) can also be used to treat Parkinson's patients during these episodes of "hypomobility," or "off periods," in which the patient becomes immobile or unable to perform activities of daily living. Apomorphine, which is given by a subcutaneous injection, needs to be taken with an antiemetic drug (e.g., trimethobenzamide [Tigan]) because, when taken alone, it causes severe nausea and vomiting. It must not be taken with the antiemetics in the serotonin (5-HT3) receptor antagonist class (e.g., ondansetron [Zofran]) because the combination of apomorphine and these drugs can lead to very low blood pressure and loss of consciousness.

Surgical Therapy. Surgical procedures are aimed at relieving symptoms of PD and are usually used in patients who are unresponsive to drug therapy or who have developed severe motor complications. Surgical procedures fall into three categories: deep brain stimulation (DBS), ablation (destruction), and transplantation. Today, the most common surgical treatment is

FIG. 59-10 A deep brain stimulator can be used to treat the tremors and uncontrolled movements in Parkinson's disease. Electrodes are surgically placed in the brain and connected to a neurostimulator (pacemaker device) in the chest.

DBS. DBS involves placing an electrode in either the thalamus, globus pallidus, or subthalamic nucleus and connecting it to a generator placed in the upper chest (like a pacemaker) (Fig. 59-10). The device is programmed to deliver a specific current to the targeted brain location. Unlike ablation procedures, DBS can be adjusted to control symptoms better and is reversible (the device can be removed). These ablative and DBS procedures work by reducing the increased neuronal activity produced by DA depletion. DBS has been shown to improve motor function and reduce dyskinesia and medication usage.[18]

Ablation surgery involves stereotactic ablation of areas in the thalamus (*thalamotomy*), globus pallidus (*pallidotomy*), and subthalamic nucleus (*subthalamic nucleotomy*). *Transplantation* of fetal neural tissue into the basal ganglia is designed to provide DA-producing cells in the brains of patients with PD. This form of therapy is still in the experimental stages.

Nutritional Therapy. Diet is of major importance to the patient with PD because malnutrition and constipation can be serious consequences of inadequate nutrition. Patients who have dysphagia and bradykinesia need appetizing foods that are easily chewed and swallowed. The diet should contain adequate roughage and fruit to avoid constipation. Cut food into bite-sized pieces before it is served, and serve it on a warmed plate to preserve its appeal.

Eating six small meals a day may be less exhausting than eating three large meals a day. Plan ample time for eating to avoid frustration. The absorption of levodopa can be impaired by protein ingestion and vitamin B$_6$. Therefore some patients are advised to limit their protein intake to the evening meal to decrease this problem. They also need to consult with their health care provider regarding the possible supplementation of vitamin B$_6$ in their multivitamins and fortified cereals.

NURSING MANAGEMENT
PARKINSON'S DISEASE

NURSING ASSESSMENT

Subjective and objective data that should be obtained from a patient with PD are presented in Table 59-19.

TABLE 59-19	**NURSING ASSESSMENT**

Parkinson's Disease

Subjective Data
Important Health Information
Past health history: Central nervous system trauma, cerebrovascular disorders, exposure to metals and carbon monoxide, encephalitis
Medications: Major tranquilizers, especially haloperidol (Haldol), and phenothiazines, reserpine, methyldopa, amphetamines

Functional Health Patterns
Health perception–health management: Fatigue
Nutritional-metabolic: Excessive salivation, dysphagia; weight loss
Elimination: Constipation, incontinence; excessive sweating
Activity-exercise: Difficulty in initiating movements; frequent falls; loss of dexterity; micrographia (handwriting deterioration)
Sleep-rest: Insomnia, nightmares, daytime sleepiness
Cognitive-perceptual: Diffuse pain in head, shoulders, neck, back, legs, and hips; muscle soreness and cramping
Self-perception–self-concept: Depression; mood swings, hallucinations

Objective Data
General
Blank (masked) faces, slow and monotonous speech, infrequent blinking

Integumentary
Seborrhea, dandruff; ankle edema

Cardiovascular
Postural hypotension

Gastrointestinal
Drooling

Neurologic
Tremor at rest, first in hands (pill rolling), later in legs, arms, face, and tongue; aggravation of tremor with anxiety, absence in sleep; poor coordination; subtle dementia, impaired postural reflexes

Musculoskeletal
Cogwheel rigidity, dysarthria, bradykinesia, contractures, stooped posture, shuffling gait

Possible Diagnostic Findings
No specific tests; diagnosis on basis of history and physical findings and ruling out of other diseases

NURSING DIAGNOSES

Nursing diagnoses for the patient with PD may include, but are not limited to, the following:

- Impaired physical mobility *related to* rigidity, bradykinesia, and akinesia
- Imbalanced nutrition: less than body requirements *related to* inability to ingest food
- Impaired swallowing *related to* neuromuscular impairment (e.g., decreased or absent gag reflex)
- Impaired verbal communication *related to* dysarthria, tremor, and bradykinesia

Additional information on nursing diagnoses for the patient with PD is presented in eNursing Care Plan 59-4 (available on the website for this chapter).

PLANNING

The overall goals are that the patient with PD will (1) maximize neurologic function, (2) maintain independence in activities of daily living for as long as possible, and (3) optimize psychosocial well-being.

NURSING IMPLEMENTATION

Because PD is a chronic degenerative disorder with no acute exacerbations, teaching and nursing care are directed toward maintenance of good health, encouragement of independence, and avoidance of complications such as contractures and falls. Problems secondary to bradykinesia can be alleviated by relatively simple measures.

Promotion of physical exercise and a well-balanced diet are major concerns for nursing care. Exercise can limit the consequences of decreased mobility, such as muscle atrophy, contractures, and constipation. The American Parkinson Disease Association (see Resources at the end of this chapter) publishes a series of booklets and videotapes with helpful exercises that can be used by family members and health care professionals.

A physical therapist may be consulted to design a personal exercise program aimed at strengthening and stretching specific muscles. Overall muscle tone and specific exercises to strengthen the muscles involved with speaking and swallowing should be included. Although exercise will not halt the progress of the disease, it will enhance the patient's functional ability. An occupational therapist can also assist the patient with strategies to increase self-care measures, including eating and dressing.

SAFETY ALERT
- Have patients who are at risk for falling and tend to "freeze" while walking do the following:
  - Consciously think about stepping over imaginary or real lines on the floor.
  - Drop rice kernels and step over them.
  - Rock from side to side.
  - Lift the toes when stepping.
  - Take one step backward and two steps forward.

Work closely with the patient's caregiver and family in exploring creative adaptations that allow maximum independence and self-care. The patient can facilitate getting out of a chair by using an upright chair with arms and placing the back legs of the chair on small (2-in) blocks. Encourage environmental alterations, such as removing rugs and excess furniture to avoid stumbling, using an elevated toilet seat to facilitate getting on and off the toilet, and elevating the legs on an ottoman to decrease dependent ankle edema. Clothing can be simplified by the use of slip-on shoes and Velcro hook-and-loop fasteners or zippers on clothing, instead of buttons and hooks.

Effective management of sleep problems can greatly improve the quality of life for patients with PD. Some PD patients find the use of satin nightwear or satin sheets beneficial. Information on teaching regarding sleep hygiene practices is presented in Chapter 8.

In the early stages of PD, many patients experience depression and anxiety. Patients need to adjust their lifestyle, including work and home responsibilities. As the disease progresses, the impact on the patient's psychologic well-being also increases. Assist the patient by listening, providing teaching, challenging distorted thoughts, and encouraging social interactions. Psychologic therapy and counseling can be helpful.

In the early stage of the disease, the patient has subtle changes in cognitive function, which can progress to dementia. This results in increased caregiver burden and the potential for long-term care placement. Information on care of the patient with dementia is provided in Chapter 60.

Family caregivers (e.g., spouse, children) care for the majority of patients with PD. As the disease progresses, the caregiver burden increases, often while the caregiver's physical and mental health decline. Strategies to reduce caregiver burden are described in Chapter 4. Other interventions for the patient with PD are presented in eNursing Care Plan 59-4 (available on the website for this chapter).

EVALUATION

The expected outcomes are that the patient with PD will
- Perform physical exercise to deter muscle atrophy and joint contractures
- Use assistive devices appropriately for ambulation and mobility
- Maintain nutritional intake adequate for metabolic needs
- Experience safe passage of fluids and/or solids from the mouth to the stomach
- Use methods of communication that meet needs for interaction with others

Additional information on expected outcomes for the patient with PD are presented in eNursing Care Plan 59-4 (available on the website).

MYASTHENIA GRAVIS

Myasthenia gravis (MG) is an autoimmune disease of the neuromuscular junction characterized by the fluctuating weakness of certain skeletal muscle groups. MG occurs in either gender and in persons of any ethnicity. The prevalence rate is 20 per 100,000; currently about 60,000 people have MG in the United States.[24] The peak age at onset in women is during the childbearing years; in men the peak onset of MG is between the ages of 50 and 70 years. However, it does occur in men and women outside of these age ranges.

Etiology and Pathophysiology

MG is caused by an autoimmune process in which antibodies attack acetylcholine (ACh) receptors, resulting in a decreased number of ACh receptor (AChR) sites at the neuromuscular junction. This prevents ACh molecules from attaching and stimulating muscle contraction. Anti-AChR antibodies are detectable in the serum of 90% of patients with generalized MG. In the 10% of patients who lack autoantibodies to AChR, their muscular weakness may be related to autoantibodies to muscle-specific receptor tyrosine kinase, although other autoantibodies may be involved.[25] Thymic tumors are found in about 15% of patients, and abnormal thymus tissue is found in most others.

Clinical Manifestations and Complications

The primary feature of MG is fluctuating weakness of skeletal muscle. The muscles most often involved are those used for moving the eyes and eyelids, chewing, swallowing, speaking, and breathing. These muscles are generally the strongest in the morning and become exhausted with continued activity. A period of rest usually restores strength. Consequently, by the end of the day, muscle weakness is prominent.

In 90% of cases the eyelid muscles or extraocular muscles are involved (Fig. 59-11). Facial mobility and expression can be impaired. The patient may have difficulty chewing and swallowing food. Speech is affected, and the voice often fades after a long conversation. The muscles of the trunk and limbs are less often affected. Of these, the proximal muscles of the neck,

FIG. 59-11 "Peek" sign in myasthenia gravis. During sustained forced eyelid closure he is unable to bury his eyelashes *(left)* and, after 30 sec, he is unable to keep the lids fully closed *(right).*

TABLE 59-20	**COLLABORATIVE CARE**

Myasthenia Gravis

Diagnostic	**Collaborative Therapy**
• History and physical examination	• Drugs
	• Anticholinesterase agents
• Fatigability with prolonged upward gaze (2-3 min)	• Corticosteroids
	• Immunosuppressive
• Muscle weakness	agents
• EMG	• Surgery (thymectomy)
• Tensilon test	• Plasmapheresis
• Acetylcholine receptor antibodies	• IV immunoglobulin G
• Chest x-ray	

EMG, Electromyography.

shoulder, and hip are more often affected than the distal muscles. No other signs of neural disorder accompany MG. There is no sensory loss, reflexes are normal, and muscle atrophy is rare.

The course of this disease is highly variable. Some patients may have short-term remissions, others may stabilize, and others may have severe, progressive involvement.[24] Exacerbations of MG can be precipitated by emotional stress, pregnancy, menses, another illness, trauma, temperature extremes, and hypokalemia. Ingestion of drugs, including aminoglycoside antibiotics, β-adrenergic blockers, procainamide, quinidine, and phenytoin, can aggravate MG. Psychotropic drugs (e.g., lithium carbonate, phenothiazines, benzodiazepines, tricyclic antidepressants) have also been associated with worsening of myasthenia, as have neuromuscular blocking agents (tubocurarine chloride, pancuronium, succinylcholine [Anectine]).

Myasthenic crisis is an acute exacerbation of muscle weakness triggered by infection, surgery, emotional distress, drug overdose, or inadequate drugs. The major complications of MG result from muscle weakness in areas that affect swallowing and breathing. This results in aspiration, respiratory insufficiency, and respiratory tract infection.

Diagnostic Studies

The diagnosis of MG can be made based on history and physical examination. However, other tests may be used if the diagnosis is still in doubt. EMG may show a decreased response to repeated stimulation of the hand muscles, indicative of muscle fatigue. Single-fiber EMG is sensitive in confirming the diagnosis of MG. Use of drugs may also aid in the diagnosis.

The Tensilon test in a patient with MG reveals improved muscle contractility after IV injection of the anticholinesterase agent edrophonium chloride (Tensilon). (Anticholinesterase blocks the enzyme acetylcholinesterase.) This test also aids in the diagnosis of cholinergic crisis (secondary to overdose of anticholinesterase drug), which occurs when there is too much cholinesterase inhibition. Clinical features include muscle fasciculation, sweating, excessive salivation, and constricted pupils. In this condition, Tensilon does not improve muscle weakness but may actually increase it. Atropine, a cholinergic antagonist, should be readily available to counteract the effects of Tensilon when it is used diagnostically. In patients with a confirmed diagnosis of MG, a chest CT scan may be done to evaluate the thymus.

Collaborative Care

Drug Therapy. Drug therapy for MG includes anticholinesterase drugs, alternate-day corticosteroids, and immunosup-

pressants (Table 59-20). Anticholinesterase drugs are aimed at enhancing function of the neuromuscular junction. Acetylcholinesterase is the enzyme that breaks down ACh. Thus inhibition of this enzyme by an anticholinesterase inhibitor will prolong the action of ACh and facilitate transmission of impulses at the neuromuscular junction. Pyridostigmine (Mestinon) is the most successful drug of this group in long-term treatment of MG.

Tailoring the dose to avoid a myasthenic or cholinergic crisis often presents a clinical challenge. Corticosteroids (specifically prednisone) are used to suppress the immune response. Drugs such as azathioprine (Imuran), mycophenolate (CellCept), and cyclosporine (Sandimmune) may also be used for immunosuppression.

Many drugs are contraindicated or must be used with caution in patients with MG. Classes of drugs that should be cautiously evaluated before use include anesthetics, antidysrhythmics, antibiotics, quinine, antipsychotics, barbiturates and sedative-hypnotics, cathartics, diuretics, opioids, muscle relaxants, thyroid preparations, and tranquilizers.

Surgical Therapy. Because the presence of the thymus gland in the patient with MG appears to enhance the production of AChR antibodies, removal of the thymus gland results in improvement in a majority of patients. Thymectomy is indicated for almost all patients with thymoma, for patients with generalized MG between the ages of puberty and about 65 years, and for patients with purely ocular MG.

Other Therapies. Plasmapheresis and IV immunoglobulin G can yield a short-term improvement in symptoms and are indicated for patients in myasthenic crisis or in preparation for surgery when corticosteroids must be avoided. Plasmapheresis directly removes circulating AChR antibodies, leading to a decrease in symptoms. (Plasmapheresis is discussed in Chapter 14.) It is not certain how IV immunoglobulin works, but it is probably related to a decrease in antibody production.[24]

NURSING MANAGEMENT
MYASTHENIA GRAVIS

NURSING ASSESSMENT

Assess the severity of MG by asking the patient about fatigability, what body parts are affected, and how severely they are affected. Assess the patient's coping abilities and strategies and understanding of the disorder. Some patients become so fatigued that they are no longer able to work or even walk.

Objective data should include respiratory rate and depth, oxygen saturation, arterial blood gas analyses, pulmonary function tests, and evidence of respiratory distress in patients with acute myasthenic crisis. Assess muscle strength of all face and limb muscles, swallowing, speech (volume and clarity), and cough and gag reflexes.

NURSING DIAGNOSES

Nursing diagnoses for the patient with MG may include, but are not limited to, the following.

- Ineffective airway clearance *related to* intercostal muscle weakness and impaired cough and gag reflex
- Impaired verbal communication *related to* weakness of the larynx, lips, mouth, pharynx, and jaw
- Activity intolerance *related to* muscle weakness and fatigability
- Disturbed body image *related to* inability to maintain usual lifestyle and role responsibilities

PLANNING

The overall goals are that the patient with MG will (1) have a return of normal muscle endurance, (2) manage fatigue, (3) avoid complications, and (4) maintain a quality of life appropriate to the disease course.

NURSING IMPLEMENTATION

The patient with MG who is admitted to the hospital usually has a respiratory tract infection or is in an acute myasthenic crisis. Nursing care is aimed at maintaining adequate ventilation, continuing drug therapy, and watching for side effects of therapy. Be able to distinguish cholinergic from myasthenic crisis (Table 59-21) because the causes and treatment of the two conditions differ greatly.

As with other chronic illnesses, focus care on the neurologic deficits and their impact on daily living. Teach the patient about a balanced diet that can easily be chewed and swallowed. Semisolid foods may be easier to eat than solids or liquids. Schedul-ing doses of drugs so that peak action is reached at mealtime may make eating less difficult. Arrange diversional activities that require little physical effort and match the patient's interests. Help the patient plan activities of daily living to avoid fatigue. Teaching should focus on the importance of following the medical regimen, complications of the disease, potential adverse reactions to specific drugs, and complications of therapy (crisis conditions) and what to do about them. Explore community resources such as the Myasthenia Gravis Foundation of America and MG support groups.

EVALUATION

The expected outcomes are that the patient with MG will
- Maintain optimal muscle function
- Be free from side effects of drugs
- Not experience complications (myasthenic or cholinergic crises) from the disease
- Maintain a quality of life appropriate to the disease course

AMYOTROPHIC LATERAL SCLEROSIS

Amyotrophic lateral sclerosis (ALS) is a rare progressive neurologic disorder characterized by loss of motor neurons. ALS usually leads to death 2 to 6 years after diagnosis, but a few patients may survive for more than 10 years.[26] This disease became known as Lou Gehrig's disease after the famous baseball player was stricken with it in 1939. The onset is usually between 40 and 70 years of age. ALS is more common in men than women by a ratio of 2:1. Approximately 5000 people in the United States are diagnosed with ALS every year.[26]

For unknown reasons, in ALS motor neurons in the brainstem and the spinal cord gradually degenerate (see eFig. 59-1 available on the website for this chapter). Dead motor neurons cannot produce or transport signals to muscles. Consequently, electrical and chemical messages originating in the brain do not reach the muscles to activate them.

The typical symptoms of ALS are limb weakness, dysarthria, and dysphagia. Muscle wasting and fasciculations result from the denervation of the muscles and lack of stimulation and use. Other symptoms include pain, sleep disorders, spasticity, drooling, emotional lability, depression, constipation, and esophageal reflux.[26] Death usually results from respiratory tract infection secondary to compromised respiratory function.

Unfortunately, there is no cure for ALS. Riluzole (Rilutek) slows the progression of ALS. This drug works to decrease the amount of glutamate (an excitatory neurotransmitter) in the brain.

The illness trajectory for ALS is devastating because the patient remains cognitively intact while wasting away. Guide the patient in the use of moderate-intensity, endurance-type exercises for the trunk and limbs, since this may help reduce ALS spasticity. Nursing interventions include (1) facilitating communication, (2) reducing risk of aspiration, (3) facilitating early identification of respiratory insufficiency, (4) decreasing pain secondary to muscle weakness, (5) decreasing risk of injury related to falls, and (6) providing diversional activities such as reading and companionship,

Support the patient's cognitive and emotional functions. Help the patient and family manage the disease process, including grieving related to the loss of motor function and ultimately death. Discuss with the patient and caregiver issues such as artificial methods of ventilation and advance directives.

TABLE 59-21	COMPARISON OF MYASTHENIC AND CHOLINERGIC CRISES	
Myasthenic Crisis	**Cholinergic Crisis**
Causes	
Exacerbation of myasthenia following precipitating factors or failure to take drug as prescribed or drug dose too low	Overdose of anticholinesterase drugs resulting in increased ACh at the receptor sites, remission (spontaneous or after thymectomy)
Differential Diagnosis	
Improved strength after IV administration of anticholinesterase drugs	Weakness within 1 hr after ingestion of anticholinesterase
Increased weakness of skeletal muscles manifesting as ptosis, bulbar signs (e.g., difficulty swallowing, difficulty articulating words), or dyspnea	Increased weakness of skeletal muscles manifesting as ptosis, bulbar signs, dyspnea
	Effects on smooth muscle include pupillary miosis, salivation, diarrhea, nausea or vomiting, abdominal cramps, increased bronchial secretions, sweating, or lacrimation

ACh, Acetylcholine.

GENETICS IN CLINICAL PRACTICE

Huntington's Disease (HD)

Genetic Basis
- Autosomal dominant disorder.
- Caused by mutation in *HTT* gene located on chromosome 4.

Incidence
- 1 in 10,000.
- Higher incidence in people of European ancestry.
- With each pregnancy a heterozygous affected parent has a 5% chance of having a child with HD.

Genetic Testing
- DNA testing is available.
- DNA testing can be done on fetal cells obtained by amniocentesis or chorionic villus sampling.
- Preimplantation genetic diagnosis can be done on embryos before implantation and pregnancy.
- One copy of altered gene is sufficient to cause HD.
- No test is available to predict when symptoms will develop.

Clinical Implications
- HD is a progressive, degenerative brain disorder.
- Onset of disease usually occurs at 30–50 yr of age. No cure is available.
- Drugs are available to control movements and behavioral problems.
- Genetic counseling may be considered if there is a family history of HD.
- Because HD is an autosomal dominant disorder, individuals who are at risk have a strong motivation to seek genetic testing.
- A positive result is not considered a diagnosis, since it may be obtained decades before the symptoms begin.
- A negative test means that the individual does not carry the mutated gene and will not develop HD.

INFORMATICS IN PRACTICE

Social Networking in Huntington's Disease

- Many patients with Huntington's disease experience social isolation and depression.
- Encourage the patient to participate in an online community where people who have Huntington's disease discuss their condition.
- Social contact and a social network with others who have Huntington's disease will help patients deal better with their illness and improve their quality of life.

the disease progresses. Facial movements involving speech, chewing, and swallowing are affected and may cause aspiration and malnutrition. The gait deteriorates, and ambulation eventually becomes impossible.

Psychiatric symptoms are frequently present in the early stage of the disease, often before the onset of motor symptoms. Depression is common. Other psychiatric symptoms include anxiety, agitation, impulsivity, apathy, social withdrawal, and obsessiveness. Cognitive deterioration is more variable and involves perception, memory, attention, and learning. Eventually all psychomotor processes, including the ability to eat and talk, are impaired.

Death usually occurs 10 to 20 years after the onset of symptoms. The most common cause of death is pneumonia, followed by suicide. Other causes of death include injuries related to a fall and other complications.[27]

Because HD has no cure, collaborative care is palliative. Tetrabenazine (Xenazine) is used to treat the chorea and works to decrease the amount of DA available at synapses in the brain and thus decreases the involuntary movements of chorea.

Other medications used for the movement disorder include neuroleptics such as haloperidol and risperidone (Risperdal), benzodiazepines such as diazepam and clonazepam, and DA-depleting agents such as reserpine and tetrabenazine. Cognitive disorders are treated as needed with nondrug therapies (e.g., counseling, memory books). The psychiatric disorders can be treated with selective serotonin reuptake inhibitors such as sertraline (Zoloft) and paroxetine (Paxil). Antipsychotic medication, such as haloperidol or risperidone, may also be needed.

HD presents a great challenge to health care professionals. The goal of nursing management is to provide the most comfortable environment possible for the patient and caregiver by maintaining physical safety, treating the physical symptoms, and providing emotional and psychologic support.

Because of the choreic movements, caloric requirements are high. Patients may require as many as 4000 to 5000 cal/day to maintain body weight. As the disease progresses, meeting caloric needs becomes a greater challenge when the patient has difficulty swallowing and holding the head still. Depression and mental deterioration can also compromise nutritional intake. Alternative sources of nutrition may be indicated as the disease progresses.

End-of-life issues need to be discussed with the patient and caregiver. These include care in the home or long-term care facility, artificial methods of feeding, advance directives and cardiopulmonary resuscitation (CPR), use of antibiotics to treat infections, and guardianship. These topics should be addressed throughout the course of the disease as the patient and caregiver adapt to increasing disability.

HUNTINGTON'S DISEASE

Huntington's disease (HD) is a genetically transmitted, autosomal dominant disorder that affects both men and women of all races. The offspring of a person with this disease have a 50% risk of inheriting it (see Genetics in Clinical Practice box above). The onset of HD is usually between 30 and 50 years of age. Often the diagnosis is made after the affected individual has had children. About 15,000 Americans are symptomatic, and 150,000 are at risk for HD.[27]

The diagnostic process begins with a review of the family history and clinical symptoms. Genetic testing confirms the disease in a person with symptoms. People who are asymptomatic but who have a positive family history of HD face the dilemma of whether to be genetically tested. If the test is positive, the person will develop HD, but when and to what extent the disease develops cannot be determined.

Like PD, the pathologic process of HD involves the basal ganglia and the extrapyramidal motor system. However, instead of a deficiency of DA, HD involves a deficiency of the neurotransmitters ACh and γ-aminobutyric acid (GABA). The net effect is an excess of DA, which leads to symptoms that are opposite of those of parkinsonism.

The clinical manifestations are a movement disorder and cognitive and psychiatric disorders. The movement disorder is characterized by abnormal and excessive involuntary movements (*chorea*). These are writhing, twisting movements of the face, the limbs, and the body. The movements get worse as

CASE STUDY

Epilepsy With Headache

Purestock/Thinkstock

Patient Profile

J.P. is a 24-yr-old woman who was diagnosed with epilepsy at age 15. At that time, she had a tonic-clonic seizure and was given a prescription for phenytoin (Dilantin). She had a second witnessed seizure 4 mo later, but has since been seizure free. J.P. now has complaints of headaches and says she is afraid that her seizures are going to return. She is single, lives alone, and describes her job as stressful.

Subjective Data

- Describes headache pain on the left side of her forehead as throbbing
- Has vomited with headache
- Describes changes in vision, including flashing lights
- Headache occurs nearly every month on a regular cycle

Objective Data

- Alert and oriented to person
- Neurologic examination negative

- Phenytoin level within normal limits
- EEG normal
- CT of head normal

Discussion Questions

1. What is epilepsy?
2. What is the pathophysiology of epilepsy?
3. What is the significance of the laboratory and diagnostic findings?
4. Is the headache related to seizure activity?
5. **Priority Decision:** What is a priority nursing intervention for J.P.?
6. What should be included in the teaching plan for J.P. regarding the course of the disease?
7. **Priority Decision:** Based on the assessment data, what are the priority nursing diagnoses?
8. **Evidence-Based Practice:** Based on current treatment guidelines, what medication may be effective in managing both J.P.'s epilepsy and her migraine headaches?

⊕volve Answers available at *http://evolve.elsevier.com/Lewis/medsurg.*

▌ BRIDGE TO NCLEX EXAMINATION

The number of the question corresponds to the same-numbered outcome at the beginning of the chapter.

1. A 50-year-old man complains of recurring headaches. He describes these as sharp, stabbing, and located around his left eye. He also reports that his left eye seems to swell and get teary when these headaches occur. Based on this history, you suspect that he has
   a. cluster headaches.
   b. tension headaches.
   c. migraine headaches.
   d. medication overuse headaches.

2. A 65-year-old woman was just diagnosed with Parkinson's disease. The priority nursing intervention is
   a. searching the Internet for educational videos.
   b. evaluating the home for environmental safety.
   c. promoting physical exercise and a well-balanced diet.
   d. designing an exercise program to strengthen and stretch specific muscles.

3. The nurse finds that an 87-year-old woman with Alzheimer's disease is continually rubbing, flexing, and kicking out her legs throughout the day. The night shift reports that this same behavior escalates at night, preventing her from obtaining her required sleep. The next step the nurse should take is to
   a. ask the physician for a daytime sedative for the patient.
   b. request soft restraints to prevent her from falling out of her bed.
   c. ask the physician for a nighttime sleep medication for the patient.
   d. assess the patient more closely, suspecting a disorder such as restless legs syndrome.

4. Social effects of a chronic neurologic disease include *(select all that apply)*
   a. divorce.
   b. job loss.
   c. depression.
   d. role changes.
   e. loss of self-esteem.

5. The nurse is reinforcing teaching with a newly diagnosed patient with amyotrophic lateral sclerosis. Which statement would be appropriate to include in the teaching?
   a. "ALS results from an excess chemical in the brain, and the symptoms can be controlled with medication."
   b. "Even though the symptoms you are experiencing are severe, most people recover with treatment."
   c. "You need to consider advance directives now, since you will lose cognitive function as the disease progresses."
   d. "This is a progressing disease that eventually results in permanent paralysis, though you will not lose any cognitive function."

1. a, 2. c, 3. d, 4. a, b, c, d, e, 5. d

⊕volve

For rationales to these answers and even more NCLEX review questions, visit *http://evolve.elsevier.com/Lewis/medsurg.*

REFERENCES

*1. Mathew PG, Garza I: Headache, *Semin Neurol* 31:5, 2011.
*2. Lipton RB: Chronic migraine, classification, differential diagnosis, and epidemiology, *Headache* 51:77, 2011.

3. Goldman L, Schafer AI: *Goldman's Cecil medicine,* ed 24, St Louis, 2012, Mosby.
*4. Rozen TD, Fishman RS: Cluster headache in the United States of America, *Headache* 52:99, 2012.
*5. Rothrock JF: Onabotulinumtoxin A for the treatment of chronic migraine, *Headache* 51:659, 2011.
*6. Halker R, Vargas B, Dodick DW: Cluster headache: diagnosis and treatment, *Semin Neurol* 30:175, 2010.

*Evidence-based information for clinical practice.

7. Epilepsy Foundation: Epilepsy and seizure statistics. Retrieved from *www.epilepsyfoundation.org/about/statistics.cfm*.

8. National Institute of Neurologic Disorders and Stroke: Seizures and epilepsy. Retrieved from *www.ninds.nih.gov/disorders/epilepsy/detail_epilepsy.htm*.

9. Berg AT, Berkovic SF, Brodie MJ, et al: Revised terminology and concepts for organization of seizures and epilepsies: report of the ILAE Commission on Classification and Terminology, 2005-2009, International League Against Epilepsy, *Epilepsia* 5:676, 2010.

*10. Kranick S, Ekanayake V, Martinez V, et al: Psychopathology and psychogenic movement disorders, *Mov Disord* 26:1844, 2011.

*11. Shorvon S, Tomson T: Sudden unexpected death in epilepsy, *Lancet* 378:2028, 2011.

*12. Stefan H: Epilepsy in the elderly, *Acta Neurol Scand* 124:223, 2011.

*13. Payne NE, Cross JH, Sander JW, et al: The ketogenic and related diets in adolescents and adults, *Epilepsia* 52:1941, 2011.

*14. Cuellar NG: Advances in the science of genomics in restless legs syndrome, *Biol Res Nurs* 12:178, 2010.

15. National Institute of Neurologic Disorders and Stroke: Restless legs syndrome. Retrieved from *www.ninds.nih.gov/disorders/restless_legs/detail_restless_legs.htm*.

16. National Multiple Sclerosis Society: About MS. Retrieved from *www.nationalmssociety.org/about-multiple-sclerosis/index.aspx*.

17. Brodkey MB, Ben-Zacharia AB, Reardon JD: Living well with multiple sclerosis, *Am J Nurs* 111:40, 2011.

18. National Institute of Neurologic Disorders and Stroke: Parkinson's disease. Retrieved from *www.ninds.nih.gov/disorders/parkinsons_disease/detail_parkinsons_disease.htm*.

*19. Vilensky JA, Gilman S, McCall S: A historical analysis of the relationship between encephalitis lethargica and postencephalitic parkinsonism, *Mov Disord* 25:1116, 2010.

*20. Falcone DC, Wood EM, Xie SX, et al: Genetic testing and Parkinson disease: assessment of patient knowledge, attitudes, and interest, *J Genet Counsel* 20:384, 2011.

*21. Bonifati V: Autosomal recessive parkinsonism, *Parkinsonism Relat Disord* 18:S4, 2012.

*22. Gershanik OS: Clinical problems in late-stage Parkinson's disease, *J Neurol* 257:S288, 2010.

*23. Chahine LM, Stern MB: Diagnostic markers for Parkinson's disease, *Curr Opin Neurol* 24:309, 2011.

24. Myasthenia Gravis Foundation of America: What is myasthenia gravis? Retrieved from *www.myasthenia.org/WhatisMG.aspx*.

*25. Vrolix K, Fraussen J, Molenaar PC, et al: The auto-antigen repertoire in myasthenia gravis, *Autoimmunity* 43:380, 2010.

*26. Gordon PH: Amyotrophic lateral sclerosis, *CNS Drugs* 25:1, 2011.

27. National Institute of Neurologic Disorders and Stroke: Huntington's disease. Retrieved from *www.ninds.nih.gov/disorders/huntington/detail_huntington.htm*.

RESOURCES

ALS Association
www.alsa.org

American Association of Neuroscience Nurses (AANN)
www.aann.org

American Headache Society
www.americanheadachesociety.org

American Parkinson Disease Association
www.apdaparkinson.org

Epilepsy Foundation
www.epilepsyfoundation.org

Huntington's Disease Society of America
www.hdsa.org

International Headache Society
www.ihs-headache.org

Myasthenia Gravis Foundation of America
www.myasthenia.org

National Headache Foundation
www.headaches.org

National Institute of Neurological Disorders and Stroke
www.ninds.nih.gov

National Multiple Sclerosis Society
www.nationalmssociety.org

National Parkinson Foundation
www.parkinson.org

Willis-Ekbom Disease Foundation
www.rls.org

*The more you use your brain, the more brain
you have to lose.*
George Dorsey

Nursing Management
Alzheimer's Disease, Dementia, and Delirium

Sharon L. Lewis

ⓔvolve WEBSITE

http://evolve.elsevier.com/Lewis/medsurg

- NCLEX Review Questions
- Key Points
- Pre-Test
- Answer Guidelines for Case Study on p. 1461
- Rationales for Bridge to NCLEX Examination Questions

- Case Study
  - Patient With Alzheimer's Disease
- Nursing Care Plans (Customizable)
  - eNCP 60-1: Patient With Alzheimer's Disease
  - eNCP 60-2: Family Caregivers
- Concept Map Creator

- Glossary
- Content Updates

eTable
- eTable 60-1: Mini-Mental State Examination (MMSE)

LEARNING OUTCOMES

1. Define dementia and describe its impact on society.
2. Compare and contrast different etiologies of dementia.
3. Describe the clinical manifestations, diagnostic studies, and collaborative management of dementia.
4. Describe the clinical manifestations of mild cognitive impairment.
5. Describe the clinical manifestations, diagnostic studies, and collaborative management of Alzheimer's disease.
6. Describe the nursing management of the patient with Alzheimer's disease.
7. Differentiate among other neurodegenerative disorders associated with dementia, including dementia with Lewy bodies, frontotemporal lobar degeneration, Creutzfeldt-Jakob disease, and normal pressure hydrocephalus.
8. Describe the etiology, pathophysiology, clinical manifestations, diagnostic studies, and collaborative management of delirium.

KEY TERMS

Alzheimer's disease (AD), p. 1445
Creutzfeldt-Jakob disease (CJD), p. 1458
delirium, p. 1458
dementia, p. 1443
dementia with Lewy bodies (DLB), p. 1457

familial Alzheimer's disease (FAD), p. 1446
frontotemporal lobar degeneration (FTLD), p. 1458
mild cognitive impairment (MCI), p. 1450
mixed dementia, p. 1458

neurofibrillary tangles, p. 1446
normal pressure hydrocephalus, p. 1458
retrogenesis, p. 1448
sundowning, p. 1454
vascular dementia, p. 1444

This chapter discusses the cognitive disorders of dementia and delirium, with a focus on the nursing management of patients with Alzheimer's disease. The etiology and pathophysiology of dementia and delirium are differentiated, and the collaborative and nursing management of patients with these cognitive disorders are described.

The three most common cognitive problems in adults are dementia, delirium (acute confusion), and depression (Table 60-1). Although this chapter focuses on dementia and delirium, depression is often associated with these conditions.

▌DEMENTIA

Dementia is a syndrome characterized by dysfunction or loss of memory, orientation, attention, language, judgment,

and reasoning. Personality changes and behavioral problems such as agitation, delusions, and hallucinations may occur. Ultimately these problems result in alterations in the individual's ability to work, fulfill social and family responsibilities, and perform activities of daily living. Dementia is often diagnosed when two or more brain functions, such as memory loss or language skills, are significantly impaired.

Fifteen percent of older Americans have dementia. As the average life span increases, the number of those affected with dementia is growing. There are about 100 causes of dementia, with about 60% to 80% of the patients with dementia having a diagnosis of Alzheimer's disease (AD) (Fig. 60-1). In the United States, about half of all patients in long-term care facilities have AD or a related dementia.[1]

Reviewed by Anna M. Bruch, RN, MSN, Professor of Nursing, Illinois Valley Community College, Oglesby, Illinois.

TABLE 60-1   COMPARISON OF DEMENTIA, DELIRIUM, AND DEPRESSION

Feature	Dementia	Delirium	Depression
Onset	Usually insidious.	Rapid, often at night.	Often coincides with life changes. Often abrupt.
Progression	Slow.	Abrupt.	Variable, rapid to slow but may be uneven.
Duration	Years (usually 8-20).	Hours to days to weeks.	Can be several months to years, especially if not treated.
Thinking	Difficulty with abstract thinking, impaired judgment, words difficult to find.	Disorganized, distorted. Slow or accelerated incoherent speech.	Intact but with apathy, fatigue. May be indecisive. Feels sense of hopelessness. May not want to live.
Perception	Misperceptions often present. Delusions and hallucinations.	Distorted. Delusions and hallucinations.	May deny or be unaware of depression. May have feelings of guilt.
Psychomotor behavior	May pace or be hyperactive. As disease progresses, may not be able to perform tasks or movements when asked.	Variable. Can be hyperactive or hypoactive, or mixed.	Often withdrawn and hypoactive.
Sleep-wake cycle	Sleeps during day. Frequent awakenings at night. Fragmented sleep.	Disturbed sleep. Reversed sleep-wake cycle.	Disturbed, often with early morning awakening.

FIG. 60-1 Causes of dementia.

Etiology and Pathophysiology

Dementia is due to both treatable and nontreatable conditions (Table 60-2). The two most common causes of dementia are neurodegenerative conditions (e.g., AD) and vascular disorders. Dementia is sometimes caused by conditions that may initially be reversible (see Table 60-2). However, with prolonged exposure or disease, irreversible changes may occur.

Vascular conditions are the second most common cause of dementia.[1] **Vascular dementia,** also called *multiinfarct dementia,* is loss of cognitive function resulting from ischemic or hemorrhagic brain lesions caused by cardiovascular disease. This type of dementia is the result of decreased blood supply from narrowing and blocking of arteries that supply the brain. Vascular dementia may be caused by a single stroke (infarct) or by multiple strokes.

Risk Factors. The greatest risk factor for dementia is aging, although it is not a normal part of aging. Family history is also an important risk factor, since those with a first-degree relative with dementia are more likely to develop the disease. Those who have more than one first-degree relative with dementia are even at higher risk of developing the disease.[1]

Other risk factors for dementia are diabetes mellitus, obesity, smoking, cardiac dysrhythmias (e.g., atrial fibrillation), hypertension, hypercholesterolemia, and coronary artery disease. Genetic factors (discussed on pp. 1446-1447) also contribute to the risk of dementia.

Diabetes dramatically increases a person's risk of developing AD or other types of dementia. Diabetes can contribute to

TABLE 60-2   CAUSES OF DEMENTIA

Type of Dementia	Cause
Neurodegenerative disorders	• Alzheimer's disease • Dementia with Lewy bodies (DLB) • Frontotemporal lobar degeneration (FTLD) • Down syndrome • Amyotrophic lateral sclerosis (ALS) • Parkinson's disease • Huntington's disease
Vascular diseases	• Vascular (multiinfarct) dementia • Subarachnoid hemorrhage* • Chronic subdural hematoma*
Toxic, metabolic, or nutritional diseases	• Alcoholism • Thiamine (vitamin B_1) deficiency* • Cobalamin (vitamin B_{12}) deficiency* • Folate deficiency* • Hyperthyroidism* • Hypothyroidism*
Immunologic diseases or infections	• Multiple sclerosis • Chronic fatigue syndrome • Infections (e.g., Creutzfeldt-Jakob disease) • Acquired immunodeficiency syndrome (AIDS) • Meningitis* • Encephalitis* • Neurosyphilis* • Systemic lupus erythematosus*
Systemic diseases	• Uremic encephalopathy* • Dialysis dementia* • Hepatic encephalopathy* • Wilson's disease
Trauma	• Head injury*
Tumors	• Brain tumors (primary)* • Metastatic tumors*
Ventricular disorders	• Hydrocephalus*
Drugs†	• Anticholinergics • phenytoin (Dilantin) • Opioids • Hypnotics • Tranquilizers • Antiparkinsonian drugs • Cardiac drugs: digoxin, methyldopa (Aldomet) • Cocaine • Heroin

*Potentially reversible.
†These are examples of drugs that may cause cognitive impairment that is potentially reversible.

dementia in several ways. Insulin resistance, which causes high blood glucose and in some cases leads to type 2 diabetes, may interfere with the body's ability to break down amyloid, a protein that forms brain plaques in AD. High blood glucose also produces oxygen-containing molecules that can damage cells, in a process known as oxidative stress. In addition, high blood glucose along with high cholesterol has a role in atherosclerosis, which contributes to vascular dementia.[2]

Diabetes may contribute to poor memory and diminished mental function in various other ways. The disease causes microangiopathy, which damages small blood vessels throughout the body. Ongoing damage to blood vessels in the brain may be one reason why people with diabetes are at a higher risk of cognitive problems as they grow older. [2]

Head trauma is also a risk factor for dementia. Professional football players and military veterans who had traumatic brain injury or posttraumatic stress disorder have an increased risk for AD and other types of dementia.[3,4]

Clinical Manifestations

Depending on the cause of the dementia, the onset of manifestations may be insidious and gradual or more abrupt. Often dementia associated with neurologic degeneration is gradual and progressive over time. Causes of vascular dementia often result in symptoms that appear suddenly or progress in a stepwise pattern. However, it is difficult to distinguish the etiology of dementia (vascular versus neurodegenerative) based on symptom progression alone. An acute (days to weeks) or subacute (weeks to months) pattern of change may be indicative of an infectious or metabolic cause, including encephalitis, meningitis, hypothyroidism, or drug-related dementia. The manifestations of different types of dementia overlap and can be further complicated by coexisting medical conditions.

Depression is often mistaken for dementia in older adults, and, conversely, dementia for depression. Manifestations of depression (especially in the older adult) include sadness, difficulty thinking and concentrating, fatigue, apathy, feelings of despair, and inactivity. When the depression is severe, poor concentration and attention may result, causing memory and functional impairment. When dementia and depression occur together (as happens in many patients with dementia), the intellectual deterioration can be extreme. Depression, alone or in combination with dementia, is treatable. The challenge is to make an accurate and early assessment and diagnosis (see Table 60-1).

Other clinical manifestations of dementia are discussed in the section on clinical manifestations of AD on pp. 1447-1448.

Diagnostic Studies

The diagnosis of dementia is focused on determining the cause (e.g., reversible versus irreversible factors). An important first step is a thorough medical, neurologic, and psychologic history. A thorough physical examination is performed to rule out other potential medical conditions. Screening for cobalamin (vitamin B_{12}) deficiency and hypothyroidism is often performed. Based on patient history, testing for neurosyphilis (see Chapter 59) may be performed.

Diagnosis of dementia related to vascular causes is based on cognitive loss, vascular brain lesions demonstrated by neuroimaging techniques (computed tomography [CT] or magnetic resonance imaging [MRI]), and the exclusion of other causes of dementia (e.g., AD).

NURSING AND COLLABORATIVE MANAGEMENT DEMENTIA

In many ways, management of the patient with dementia is similar to management of the patient with AD (described later in this chapter). One form of dementia, vascular dementia, can often be prevented. Preventive measures include treatment of risk factors such as hypertension, diabetes, smoking, hypercholesterolemia, and cardiac dysrhythmias. (Stroke is discussed in Chapter 58.) Drugs that are used for patients with AD are also useful in patients with vascular dementia. Drug therapy is discussed on p. 1452 later in this chapter.

ALZHEIMER'S DISEASE

Alzheimer's disease (AD) is a chronic, progressive, degenerative disease of the brain. It is the most common form of dementia, accounting for 60% to 80% of all cases of dementia.[1] AD is named after Alois Alzheimer, a German physician who in 1906 described changes in the brain tissue of a 55-year-old woman who had died of an unusual mental illness.

Approximately 5.2 million Americans suffer from AD. It is estimated that 11% of people age 65 and older, and nearly one third of those over age 85, have AD. Ultimately the disease is fatal, with death typically occurring 4 to 8 years after diagnosis, although some patients live for 20 years. AD is the sixth leading cause of death in the United States.[1] It is the only cause of death among the top 10 in United States that cannot be prevented or cured, or its progression even slowed. The burden of care for the patient with AD on the family, caregivers, and society is staggering. AD has often been referred to as the "long good-bye" or "death in slow motion."

The incidence of AD is slightly higher in African Americans and Hispanic Americans than in whites. AD has been associated with lower socioeconomic status and education level and poor access to health care. Women are more likely than men to develop AD, primarily because they live longer (see the Gender Differences box).

Etiology and Pathophysiology

The exact etiology of AD is unknown, but is likely a combination of genetic and environmental factors. AD is not a normal part of aging, but as with other forms of dementia, age is the most important risk factor for developing AD. Only a small percentage of people younger than 60 years old develop AD. When AD develops in someone younger than 60 years old, it is referred to as *early-onset AD*. AD that becomes evident in individuals more than 60 years old is called *late-onset AD* (see the Genetics in Clinical Practice box).

GENDER DIFFERENCES
Alzheimer's Disease and Dementia

Men	Women
• Men have a higher incidence of vascular dementia than women.	• Nearly two thirds of people with Alzheimer's disease are women. • Women are more likely to develop Alzheimer's disease than men, probably because they live longer. • About twice as many women as men die each year from Alzheimer's disease.

GENETICS IN CLINICAL PRACTICE

Alzheimer's Disease (AD)

Genetic Basis
Early Onset (Familial) (<60 Yr Old at Onset)
- Autosomal dominant disorder.
- Various mutations in the following genes:
  - Amyloid precursor protein *(APP)* gene on chromosome 21
  - Presenilin-1 *(PSEN1)* gene on chromosome 14
  - Presenilin-2 *(PSEN2)* gene on chromosome 1

Late Onset (Sporadic) (>60 Yr Old at Onset)
- Genetically more complex than early-onset form.
- Apolipoprotein E-4 *(ApoE-4)* allele on chromosome 19 increases the likelihood of developing AD.
- Presence of *ApoE-2* allele is associated with a lower risk of AD.

Incidence
Early Onset
- Rare form of AD, accounting for <5% of cases.
- Fifty percent risk of disease for children of affected parents.
- May occur in people as young as 30 yr old.

Late Onset
- *ApoE-4* is present in about 40% of people with late-onset AD. (It is present in 25%–30% of normal population.)
- Many *ApoE-4*-positive people do not develop AD, and many *ApoE-4*-negative people do.

Genetic Testing
Early Onset
- Genetic screening is available for mutations on chromosomes 1, 14, and 21.

Late Onset
- Blood test can identify which *ApoE* allele a person has but cannot predict who will develop disease.*
- *ApoE* testing is mainly used in research to identify people who may have an increased risk of developing AD.

Clinical Implications
- AD is the most common cause of dementia.
- Genetic testing and counseling for family members of patients with early-onset AD may be appropriate.
- If person tests positive for *ApoE-4*, it does not mean that the person will develop AD.

*ApoE testing is useful for studying AD risk in large groups of people, but not for determining an individual's specific risk.

Individuals with a clear pattern of inheritance within a family have **familial Alzheimer's disease (FAD)**. Other cases where no familial connection can be made are termed *sporadic*. FAD is associated with an early onset (before 60 years of age) and a more rapid disease course. In both FAD and sporadic AD, the pathogenesis of AD is similar.

Characteristic findings of AD relate to changes in the brain's structure and function: (1) amyloid plaques, (2) neurofibrillary tangles, (3) loss of connections between neurons, and (4) neuron death. Fig. 60-2 shows the pathologic changes in AD.

As part of aging, people develop some plaques in their brain tissue, but in AD more plaques appear in certain parts of the brain. These plaques consist of clusters of insoluble deposits of a protein called *β-amyloid*, other proteins, remnants of neurons, non-nerve cells such as microglia (cells that surround and digest damaged cells or foreign substances), and other cells such as astrocytes.

FIG. 60-2 Pathologic changes in Alzheimer's disease **A,** Plaque with central amyloid core *(white arrow)* next to a neurofibrillary tangle *(red arrow)* on the histologic specimen from a brain autopsy. **B,** Schematic representation of amyloid plaque and neurofibrillary tangle.

β-Amyloid is cleaved from amyloid precursor protein (APP), which is associated with the cell membrane (Fig. 60-3). The normal function of APP is unknown. In AD, plaques develop first in areas of the brain used for memory and cognitive function, including the hippocampus (a structure that is important in forming and storing short-term memories). Eventually AD attacks the cerebral cortex, especially the areas responsible for language and reasoning.

Neurofibrillary tangles are abnormal collections of twisted protein threads inside nerve cells. The main component of these structures is a protein called *tau*. Tau proteins in the central nervous system (CNS) are involved in providing support for intracellular structure through their support of microtubules. Tau proteins hold the microtubules together like railroad ties hold railroad tracks together. In AD the tau protein is altered, and as a result, the microtubules twist together in a helical fashion (see Fig. 60-3). This ultimately forms the neurofibrillary tangles found in the neurons of persons with AD.

Plaques and neurofibrillary tangles are not unique to patients with AD or dementia. They are also found in the brains of individuals without evidence of cognitive impairment. However, they are more abundant in the brains of individuals with AD.

The other feature of AD is the loss of connections between neurons and neuron death. These processes result in structural damage. Affected parts of the brain begin to shrink in a process called brain atrophy. By the final stage of AD, brain tissue has shrunk significantly (Fig. 60-4).

Genetic Link

Genetic factors may play a critical role in how the brain processes the β-amyloid protein. Overproduction of β-amyloid appears to be an important risk factor for AD. Abnormally high levels of β-amyloid cause cell damage either directly or by eliciting an inflammatory response and ultimately neuron death. Understanding why neurons produce β-amyloid led

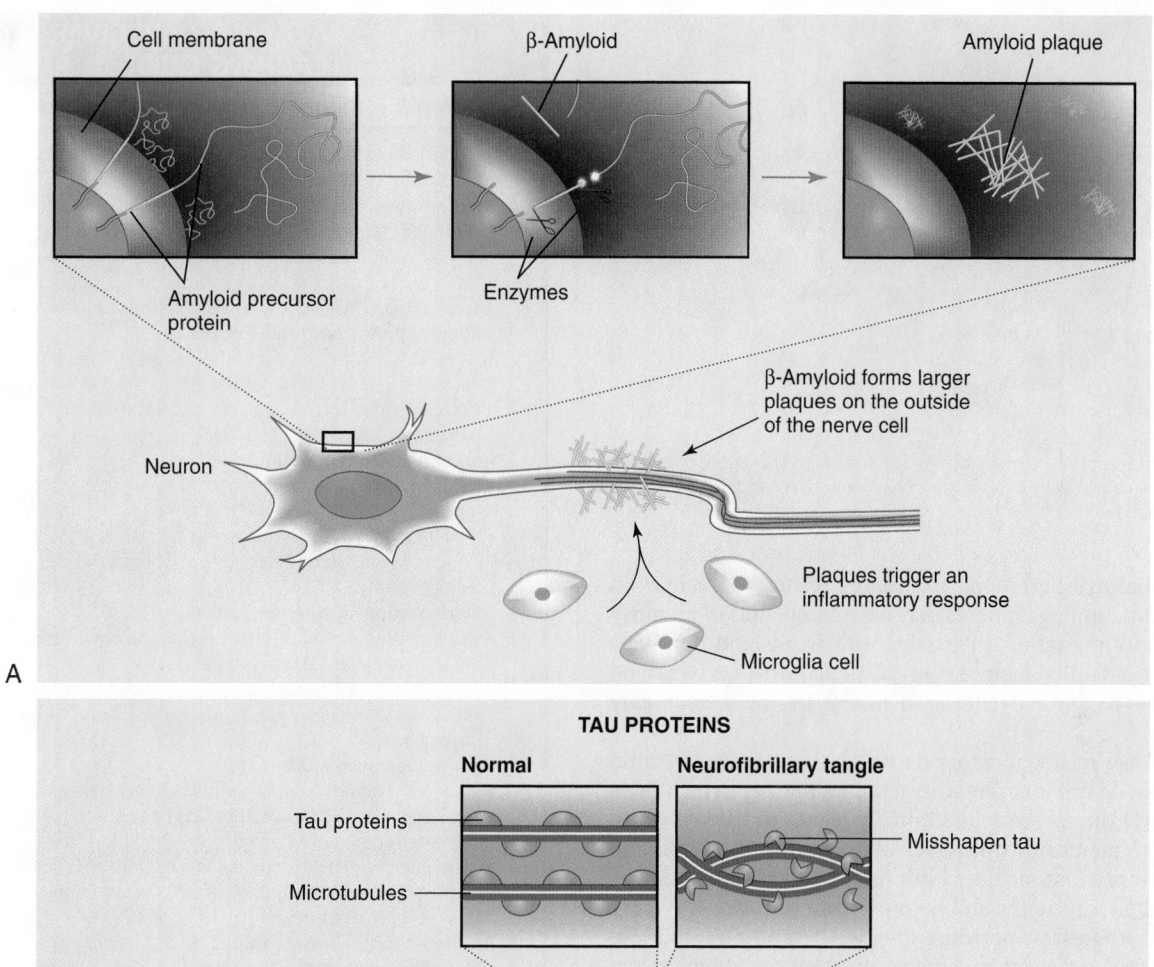

FIG. 60-3 Current etiologic theories for the development of Alzheimer's disease. **A,** Abnormal amounts of β-amyloid are cleaved from the amyloid precursor protein *(APP)* and released into the circulation. The β-amyloid fragments come together in clumps to form plaques that attach to the neuron. Microglia react to the plaque, and an inflammatory response results. **B,** Tau proteins provide structural support for the neuron microtubules. Chemical changes in the neuron produce structural changes in tau proteins. This results in twisting and tangling (neurofibrillary tangles).

researchers to examine the enzymes (and their genes) that are responsible for both the synthesis and processing of APP.

In patients with early-onset AD, three genes have been identified as important in the etiology (see the Genetics in Clinical Practice box on p. 1446). When the *presenilin-1, presenilin-2,* and *APP* genes are mutated, they cause brain cells to overproduce β-amyloid.[5]

The first gene associated with AD was the *epsilon (E)-4* allele of the *apolipoprotein E (ApoE)* gene on chromosome 19. *ApoE* comes in several different alleles or forms, but three alleles occur most commonly. People inherit one allele (i.e., *ApoE-2, ApoE-3, or ApoE-4*) from each parent. *ApoE* contains the instructions to make a protein that helps to carry cholesterol and other types of fat in the bloodstream. *ApoE* may have a role in clearing amyloid plaques. Mutations in this gene result in greater amyloid deposition. The presence of *ApoE-4,* which is a risk-factor gene, increases the risk of a person developing late-onset AD.[5] However, the presence of the gene alone is not adequate to account for AD, since many people with *ApoE-4* do not develop AD.

Environmental Factors. As previously mentioned in the section on risk factors for dementia (pp. 1444-1445), diabetes mellitus, hypertension, current smoking, hypercholesterolemia, obesity, and trauma are associated with an increased risk of dementia, including AD.

Clinical Manifestations

Pathologic changes often precede clinical manifestations of dementia by anywhere from 5 to 20 years.[6] The Alzheimer's Association has developed a list of warning signs that include common manifestations of AD (Table 60-3). The stages of AD can be categorized as mild, moderate, and severe (Table 60-4). The rate of progression from mild to severe is highly variable and ranges from 3 to 20 years.

FIG. 60-4 Effects of Alzheimer's disease on the brain. This figure compares a normal brain *(left)* with a brain that has been affected by Alzheimer's disease *(right)*.

The initial manifestations are usually related to changes in cognitive functioning. Patients may have complaints of memory loss, mild disorientation, or trouble with words and numbers. Often it is a family member, in particular the spouse, who reports the patient's declining memory to the health care provider.

Normal age-related memory decline is characterized by mild changes that do not interfere with activities of daily living (Table 60-5). In AD the memory loss initially relates to recent events, with remote memories still intact. With time and progression of AD, memory loss includes both recent and remote memory and ultimately affects the ability to perform self-care.

As AD progresses, personal hygiene deteriorates, as does the ability to concentrate and maintain attention. Ongoing loss of neurons in AD can cause a person to act in altered or unpredictable ways. Behavioral manifestations of AD (e.g., agitation, aggression) result from changes that take place within the brain. They are neither intentional nor controllable by the individual with the disease. Some patients develop delusions and hallucinations.

With progression of AD, additional cognitive impairments are noted. These include *dysphasia* (difficulty comprehending language and oral communication), *apraxia* (inability to manipulate objects or perform purposeful acts), *visual agnosia* (inability to recognize objects by sight), and *dysgraphia* (difficulty communicating via writing). Eventually long-term memories cannot be recalled, and patients lose the ability to recognize family members and friends. Other problems include aggression and a tendency to wander.

Later in the disease, the ability to communicate and to perform activities of daily living is lost. In the late stages of AD, the patient is unresponsive and incontinent and requires total care.

Retrogenesis. Retrogenesis is the process in AD patients in which degenerative changes occur in the reverse order in which they were acquired.[7] This theory compares the developmental stages in children with the deterioration in AD patients. As seen in Table 60-6, a relationship exists between the developmental stage and deterioration of function. For example, it is appropriate for a person with AD in the moderate stage to feel good about putting together puzzles that belong to his 3-year-old grandson. In fact, they may play well together on the same task or project.

TABLE 60-3 PATIENT & CAREGIVER TEACHING GUIDE

Early Warning Signs of Alzheimer's Disease

Include the following information in the teaching plan for the patient with Alzheimer's disease.

1. **Memory loss that affects job skills**
   - Frequent forgetfulness or unexplainable confusion at home or in the workplace may signal that something is wrong.
   - This type of memory loss goes beyond forgetting an assignment, colleague's name, deadline, or phone number.
2. **Difficulty performing familiar tasks**
   - It is normal for most people to become distracted and to forget something (e.g., leave something on the stove too long).
   - People with AD may cook a meal but then forget not only to serve it but also that they made it.
3. **Problems with language**
   - Most people have trouble finding the "right" word from time to time.
   - Persons with AD may forget simple words or substitute inappropriate words, making their speech difficult to understand.
4. **Disorientation to time and place**
   - Most individuals occasionally forget the day of the week or what they need from the store.
   - People with AD can become lost on their own street, not knowing where they are, how they got there, or how to get back home.
5. **Poor or decreased judgment**
   - Many individuals from time to time may choose not to dress appropriately for the weather (e.g., not bringing a coat or sweater on a cold evening).
   - The person with AD may dress inappropriately in more noticeable ways, such as wearing a bathrobe to the store or a sweater on a hot day.
6. **Problems with abstract thinking**
   - For the person with AD, this goes beyond challenges such as balancing a checkbook.
   - The person with AD may have difficulty recognizing numbers or doing even basic calculations.
7. **Misplacing things**
   - For many individuals, temporarily misplacing keys, purses, or wallets is a normal albeit frustrating event.
   - The person with AD may put items in inappropriate places (e.g., eating utensils in clothing drawers) but have no memory of how they got there.
8. **Changes in mood or behavior**
   - Most individuals experience mood changes.
   - The person with AD tends to exhibit more rapid mood swings for no apparent reason.
9. **Changes in personality**
   - As most individuals age, they may demonstrate some change in personality (e.g., become less tolerant).
   - The person with AD can change dramatically, either suddenly or over time. For example, someone who is generally easygoing may become angry, suspicious, or fearful.
10. **Loss of initiative**
    - The person with AD may become and remain uninterested and uninvolved in many or all of his or her usual pursuits.

Adapted from Alzheimer's Association: *Early warning signs,* Chicago, The Association.

Diagnostic Criteria for Alzheimer's Disease

The original 1984 clinical criteria for AD defined it as having a single stage, dementia, and based the diagnosis solely on clinical symptoms. It assumed that people free of dementia symptoms were disease-free. Since then, research has determined that AD may cause changes in the brain many years before symptoms

TABLE 60-4 STAGES OF ALZHEIMER'S DISEASE

Mild	Moderate	Severe
• Forgetfulness beyond what is seen in a normal person • Short-term memory impairment, especially for new learning • Loss of initiative and interests • May forget recent events or the names of people or things • Small personality changes • May no longer be able to solve simple math problems • Slowly loses the ability to plan and organize	• Memory loss and confusion become more obvious • Has more trouble organizing, planning, and following directions • May need help getting dressed • May start having incontinence • Trouble recognizing family members and friends • Agitation, restlessness • May lack judgment and begin to wander, gets lost • May have trouble sleeping • Delusions, hallucinations, paranoia • Behavioral problems	• Severe impairment of all cognitive functions • Little memory, unable to process new information • Unable to perform self-care activities • Often needs help with daily needs • May not be able to talk • Cannot understand words • May have difficulty eating, swallowing • May not be able to walk or sit up without help • Immobility • Incontinence

TABLE 60-5 COMPARISON OF NORMAL FORGETFULNESS AND MEMORY LOSS

Normal Forgetfulness	Memory Loss in Mild Cognitive Impairment	Memory Loss in Alzheimer's Disease
• Sometimes misplaces keys, eyeglasses, or other items • Momentarily forgets an acquaintance's name • Occasionally has to search for a word • Occasionally forgets to run an errand • May forget an event from the distant past • When driving, may momentarily forget where to turn, but quickly orients self • Jokes about memory loss	• Frequently misplaces items • Frequently forgets people's names and is slow to recall them • Has increasing difficulty finding desired words • Begins to forget important events and appointments • May forget recent events or newly learned information • Becomes temporarily lost more often, may have trouble understanding and following a map • Worries about memory loss, family and friends notice lapses	• Forgets what an item is used for or puts it in an inappropriate place • May not remember knowing a person • Begins to lose language skills and may withdraw from social interaction • Loses sense of time, does not know what day it is • Has seriously impaired recent memory and difficulty learning and remembering new information • Becomes easily disoriented or lost in familiar places, sometimes for hours • May have little or no awareness of cognitive problems

Adapted from Rabins P: Memory. In *The Johns Hopkins white papers,* Baltimore, 2007, Johns Hopkins University.

TABLE 60-6 RETROGENESIS IN ALZHEIMER'S DISEASE

Stage	Alzheimer's Disease	Reisberg Stage*	Developmental Age	Diversion/Distraction Activities
Mild	No difficulty at all.	1	Adult	—
	Some memory trouble begins to affect job and home. Forgets familiar names.	2	—	—
	Much difficulty maintaining job performance. Withdrawal from difficult situations.	3	12+ yr	Can function with understanding. Enjoy things they have always enjoyed—watch TV, play and listen to music, play games.
	Can no longer hold a job, plan and prepare meals, handle personal finances, etc. Driving becomes difficult, although can drive to familiar places.	4	8-12 yr	Can still enjoy simple games, watch TV and videos. Enjoys family photos and memories.
Moderate	Can no longer select proper clothing for occasion or season. Needs help to remain safe in home. Forgets to bathe.	5	5-7 yr	Needs age-appropriate toys and games.
	Requires help with dressing.	6a	5 yr	Needs activities appropriate for preschoolers. Enjoys many of the same activities as preschoolers.
	Requires help with bathing.	6b	4 yr	
	Requires help with toileting.	6c	4 yr	
	Urinary incontinence.	6d	3-4 yr	
	Fecal incontinence.	6e	2-3 yr	
Severe	Speech limited to 5-6 intelligent words/day.	7a	15 mo	Enjoys infant toys, mobiles, dangling ribbons.
	Speech limited to one word/day.	7b	1 yr	
	Can no longer walk without assistance.	7c	1 yr	
	Can no longer sit up without assistance.	7d	6-10 mo	
	Can no longer smile.	7e	2-4 mo	
	Can no longer hold up head.	7f	1-3 mo	

*These stages are based on Functional Assessment Staging. Reisberg B: Functional assessment staging (FAST), *Psychopharmacol Bull* 24:653, 1988.

TABLE 60-7 DIAGNOSTIC CRITERIA FOR ALZHEIMER'S DISEASE*

	Stage and Description	Recommendations for Biomarkers
Preclinical Alzheimer's Disease (AD)	• Brain changes, including amyloid buildup and other early neuron changes, may already be in process. • At this point, significant clinical symptoms are not yet evident. • In some people, amyloid buildup can be detected with positron emission tomography (PET) scans and cerebrospinal fluid (CSF) analysis.	• Use of imaging and biomarker tests at this stage are recommended only for research. • Biomarkers are still being developed and standardized and are not used by clinicians in general practice.
Mild Cognitive Impairment (MCI) due to Alzheimer's Disease	• The MCI stage is marked by symptoms of memory problems, enough to be noticed and measured, but not compromising a person's independence. • People with MCI may or may not progress to Alzheimer's dementia.	• Used primarily by researchers. • May be used in specialized clinical settings to supplement standard clinical tests to help determine possible causes of MCI. • May help confirm that the person's impairment is related to AD.
Dementia due to Alzheimer's Disease	• Characterized by memory, thinking, and behavioral symptoms that impair a person's ability to function in daily life. • Dementia marks the terminal stage of AD. • Encompasses all stages presented in Table 60-4.	• May be used in some cases to increase the level of certainty about a diagnosis of AD. • Also may be used to distinguish AD from other dementias.

Source: Jack CR, Albert MS, Knopman DS, et al: Introduction to the recommendations from the National Institute on Aging–Alzheimer's Association workgroups on diagnostic guidelines for Alzheimer's disease, *Alzheimers Dement* 7:257, 2011.
*Note that these are recommended criteria and guidelines. More research is needed, especially biomarker research, before the new criteria and guidelines can be used in clinical settings.

appear and that symptoms do not always directly relate to abnormal changes in the brain caused by AD.

In 2011 updated criteria and guidelines classified AD as a spectrum, where dementia marks the terminal stage of the disease (Table 60-7). The stages in the new classification spectrum are preclinical AD, mild cognitive impairment, and dementia due to AD.[8] The guidelines address the use of imaging and biomarkers (discussed in section on diagnostic studies below) that may help determine whether changes are due to AD.[9]

Preclinical Stage. A long lag exists between pathologic changes in the brain and manifestations of AD. The future goal would be to modify the disease process of AD before it becomes symptomatic. Once plaques and tangles have formed in sufficient quantity, it may be too late to intervene to prevent the disease or its progression. Although currently all attempts at modifying the disease process have failed, research is ongoing. The model for early intervention is seen in other diseases, such as removing polyps to prevent colon cancer, controlling blood glucose in diabetes before the disease progresses to heart and kidney disease, and treating cardiac risk factors before a person has a myocardial infarction.

Mild Cognitive Impairment. Mild cognitive impairment (MCI), the second stage in the AD spectrum, is a state of cognitive function in which individuals have problems with memory, language, or another essential cognitive function that are severe enough to be noticeable to others and show up on tests, but not severe enough to interfere with activities of daily living. Because the problems do not interfere with daily activities, the person does not meet the criteria for being diagnosed with dementia.[10] To the casual observer, an individual with MCI may seem fairly normal. However, the person with MCI is often aware of a significant change in memory, and family members may observe changes in the individual's abilities (see Table 60-5).

Between 10% and 20% of people 65 years old and older have MCI and are at high risk of developing AD. Some individuals with MCI show no progression and do not go on to develop AD, but an estimated 15% of people with MCI eventually do. Although not in clinical use, biomarkers can be a useful tool to predict who will develop dementia.[10]

No drugs have been approved for the treatment of MCI. Research is being conducted to determine whether patients with MCI would benefit from the medications used in AD (e.g., cholinesterase inhibitors). There is little evidence that cholinesterase inhibitors affect progression to dementia or cognitive test scores in people with MCI.[11]

Currently the primary treatment of MCI consists of ongoing monitoring. Recognize the importance of monitoring the patient with MCI for changes in memory and thinking skills that would indicate a worsening of symptoms or a progression to dementia. It is critical that you understand the 10 early warning signs of AD (see Table 60-3).

Diagnostic Studies

No definitive diagnostic test exists for AD. The diagnosis of AD is primarily a diagnosis of exclusion. In patients with cognitive impairment, there is increased emphasis on early and careful evaluation. As indicated earlier in this chapter, many conditions can cause manifestations of dementia, some of which are treatable or reversible (see Table 60-2).

When all other possible conditions that can cause cognitive impairment have been ruled out, a clinical diagnosis of AD can be made. A comprehensive patient evaluation includes a complete health history, physical examination, neurologic and mental status assessments, and laboratory tests (Table 60-8). Brain imaging tests (e.g., CT or MRI) may show brain atrophy in the later stages of the disease, although this finding occurs in other diseases and can also be seen in persons without cognitive impairment. Positron emission tomography (PET) scanning can be used to differentiate AD from other forms of dementia (Fig. 60-5). Neuroimaging techniques allow for detection of changes early in the disease and monitoring of treatment response. A definitive diagnosis of AD usually requires examination of brain tissue at autopsy and findings of neurofibrillary tangles and neuritic plaques.

The new criteria and guidelines identify two biomarker categories: (1) biomarkers showing the level of β-amyloid accumulation in the brain and (2) biomarkers showing that nerve cells in the brain are injured or actually degenerating. Biomarkers include (1) cerebrospinal fluid (CSF) neurochemical markers:

TABLE 60-8 COLLABORATIVE CARE

Alzheimer's Disease

Diagnostic
- History and physical examination, including psychologic evaluation
- Neuropsychologic testing, including Mini-Cog (Table 60-9), Mini-Mental State Examination (eTable 60-1)
- Brain imaging tests: CT, MRI, MRS, PET
- Complete blood count
- Electrocardiogram
- Serum glucose, creatinine, BUN
- Serum levels of vitamins B_1, B_6, B_{12}
- Thyroid function tests
- Liver function tests
- Screening for depression

Collaborative Therapy
- Drug therapy for cognitive problems (see Table 60-10)
- Behavioral modification
- Moderate exercise
- Assistance with functional independence
- Assistance and support for caregiver

MRS, Magnetic resonance spectroscopy; *PET,* positron emission tomography

FIG. 60-5 Positron emission tomography (PET) scan can be used to assist in the diagnosis of Alzheimer's disease (AD). Radioactive fluorine is applied to glucose (fluorodeoxyglucose), and the yellow areas indicate metabolically active cells. **A,** A normal brain. **B,** Advanced AD is recognized by hypometabolism in many areas of the brain.

β-amyloid and tau proteins and (2) imaging biomarkers: volumetric MRI and PET. The level of tau in the CSF is an indication of neurodegeneration. (Plasma levels of tau or β-amyloid are not of any value in diagnosing AD.) In AD multiple brain structures atrophy and the volume of the brain correlates with neurodegeneration. PET determines brain metabolism using glucose tracers (see Fig. 60-5). PET can also be used to detect amyloid.

Some imaging biomarkers are used in specialized clinical settings. CSF biomarkers are mainly used for research. Biomarkers may be used in some cases to increase the level of certainty about a diagnosis of Alzheimer's dementia and to distinguish Alzheimer's dementia from other dementias. However, more research is needed with biomarkers before they are used routinely in clinical practice.

Neuropsychologic testing with tools such as the Mini-Cog (Table 60-9) and the Mini-Mental State Examination (see eTable 60-1, available on the website for this chapter) can help document the degree of cognitive impairment. The clock drawing

TABLE 60-9 THE MINI-COG

Introduction
The Mini-Cog is used as a brief assessment tool for cognitive impairment. It can be quickly administered and can guide the need for further evaluation.

Administration
1. Instruct the patient to listen carefully to and remember three unrelated words and then to repeat the words. *Example:* apple, table, penny. (This initial step is not scored.)
   The same three words may be repeated to the patient up to three tries to register all three words.
2. Instruct the patient to draw the face of a clock, either on a blank sheet of paper or on a sheet with the clock circle already drawn on the page. After the patient puts the numbers on the clock face, ask him or her to draw the hands of the clock to read a specific time (11:10). The test is considered normal if all numbers are present in the correct sequence and position, and the hands readably display the requested time.
3. Ask the patient to repeat the three previously stated words. Scoring (out of total of 5 points)
   Give 1 point for each recalled word after the clock drawing test.
   - Patients recalling none of the three words are classified as cognitively impaired (score = 0).
   - Patients recalling all three words are classified as not cognitively impaired (score = 3).
   - Patients with intermediate word recall of one or two words are classified on the clock drawing test:
     The clock drawing test is scored 2 if normal and 0 if abnormal.
     Interpretation of results
     0-2: Positive screen for dementia
     3-5: Negative screen for dementia

Source: Borson S, Scanlan J, Brush M, et al: The Mini-Cog: a cognitive "vital signs" measure for dementia screening in multi-lingual elderly, *Intern J Geriatr Psychiatry* 15(11):1021, 2000.

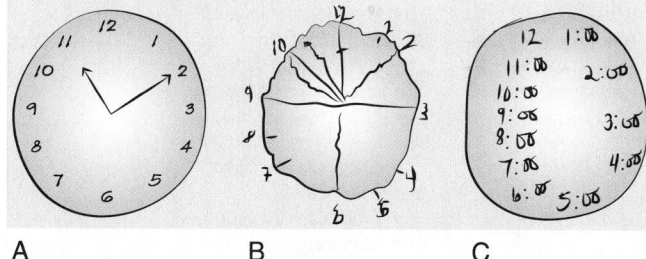

FIG. 60-6 Clock drawing is a simple test that can be used as an assessment technique in dementia. The person undergoing testing is asked to draw a clock, put in all of the numbers, and set the hands at 10 past 11. **A,** Shows a clock drawn by a person with no dementia. **B** and **C** show clocks drawn by people with dementia.

test can be used as part of the Mini-Cog or by itself to assess cognitive function (Fig. 60-6). Neuropsychologic testing is important not only for diagnostic purposes but also to establish a baseline for evaluating changes over time.

Collaborative Care

At this time there is no cure for AD. No treatment is available to stop the deterioration of brain cells in AD. Nothing stops or really slows the progression of the disease.

The collaborative management of AD is aimed at (1) controlling the undesirable behavioral manifestations that the patient may exhibit and (2) providing support for the family caregiver.

Drug Therapy. Although drug therapy for AD is available (Table 60-10), these drugs do not cure or reverse the progression of the disease. Drugs help many people, but not for very long and not very well. The use of drugs may lead to a modest decrease in the rate of decline of cognitive function. However, the drugs have no effect on overall disease progression.[12,13]

Cholinesterase inhibitors block cholinesterase, the enzyme responsible for the breakdown of acetylcholine in the synaptic cleft (Fig. 60-7). Cholinesterase inhibitors include donepezil (Aricept), rivastigmine (Exelon), and galantamine (Razadyne). Rivastigmine is available as a patch.

Memantine (Namenda) protects the brain's nerve cells against excess amounts of glutamate, which is released in large amounts by cells damaged by AD. The attachment of glutamate to N-methyl-D-aspartate (NMDA) receptors permits calcium to flow freely into the cell, which in turn may lead to cell degenera-

tion. Memantine may prevent this destructive sequence by blocking the action of glutamate.

Treating the depression that is often associated with AD may improve cognitive ability. Depression is often treated with selective serotonin reuptake inhibitors, including fluoxetine (Prozac), sertraline (Zoloft), fluvoxamine (Luvox), and citalopram (Celexa). The antidepressant trazodone (Desyrel) may help with problems related to sleep.

Although antipsychotic drugs are approved for treating psychotic conditions (e.g., schizophrenia), they have been used for the management of behavioral problems (e.g., agitation, aggressive behavior) that occur in patients with AD. However, these drugs have been shown to increase the risk of death in older dementia patients.[14] The U.S. Food and Drug Administration (FDA) has warned that antipsychotics are not indicated for the treatment of dementia-related psychosis. However, the warning does not mean that the drugs cannot be used for these patients with dementia.

TABLE 60-10 DRUG THERAPY

Alzheimer's Disease

Problem	Drugs
Decreased memory and cognition	Cholinesterase inhibitors • donepezil (Aricept) • rivastigmine (Exelon) • galantamine (Razadyne) N-methyl-D-aspartate (NMDA) receptor antagonist • memantine (Namenda)
Depression	Selective serotonin reuptake inhibitors (SSRIs) • sertraline (Zoloft) • fluvoxamine (Luvox) • citalopram (Celexa) • fluoxetine (Prozac) Atypical antidepressants • mirtazapine (Remeron) • trazodone (Desyrel)
Behavioral problems (e.g., agitation, physical aggression, disinhibition)	Antipsychotics* • haloperidol (Haldol) • risperidone (Risperdal) • olanzapine (Zyprexa) • quetiapine (Seroquel) • aripiprazole (Abilify) Benzodiazepines • lorazepam (Ativan) • clonazepam (Klonopin)
Sleep disturbances	zolpidem (Ambien)

*The use of these drugs in older patients with dementia is associated with an increased risk of death.

FIG. 60-7 Mechanism of action of cholinesterase inhibitors. **A,** Acetylcholine is released from the nerve synapses and carries a message across the synapse. **B,** Cholinesterase breaks down acetylcholine. **C,** Cholinesterase inhibitors block cholinesterase, thus giving acetylcholine more time to transmit the message.

NURSING MANAGEMENT
ALZHEIMER'S DISEASE

NURSING ASSESSMENT

Subjective and objective data that should be obtained from a person with AD are presented in Table 60-11. Useful questions for the patient and caregiver are, "When did you first notice the memory loss?" and "How has the memory loss progressed since then?"

NURSING DIAGNOSES

Nursing diagnoses for AD may include, but are not limited to, the following:
- Impaired memory *related to* the effects of dementia
- Self-neglect *related to* memory deficit, cognitive impairment, and neuromuscular impairment
- Risk for injury *related to* impaired judgment, gait instability, muscle weakness, and sensory/perceptual alteration
- Wandering *related to* cognitive impairment

Additional information on nursing diagnoses for the patient with AD is presented in eNursing Care Plan 60-1 (available on the website for this chapter).

PLANNING

The overall goals are that the patient with AD will (1) maintain functional ability for as long as possible, (2) be maintained in a safe environment with a minimum of injuries, (3) have personal care needs met, and (4) have dignity maintained. The overall goals for the caregiver of a patient with AD are to (1) reduce caregiver stress; (2) maintain personal, emotional, and physical health; and (3) cope with the long-term effects of caregiving.

NURSING IMPLEMENTATION

HEALTH PROMOTION. Can AD be prevented? Although there is no known definitive way to prevent AD, several steps can help keep your brain healthy:
- *Avoid harmful substances.* Excessive drinking and drug abuse can damage brain cells.
- *Challenge yourself.* Read frequently, do crossword puzzles. Keep mentally active. Learn new skills. This strengthens the brain connections and promotes new ones.
- *Exercise regularly.* Even low to moderate level activity such as walking or gardening three to five times per

TABLE 60-11 NURSING ASSESSMENT

Alzheimer's Disease

Subjective Data
Important Health Information
Past health history: Repeated head trauma, stroke, previous CNS infection, family history of dementia
Medications: Use of any drug to decrease symptoms (e.g., tranquilizers, hypnotics, antidepressants, antipsychotics)

Functional Health Patterns
Health perception–health management: Positive family history; emotional lability
Nutritional-metabolic: Anorexia, malnutrition, weight loss
Elimination: Incontinence
Activity-exercise: Poor personal hygiene; gait instability, weakness; inability to perform activities of daily living
Sleep-rest: Frequent nighttime awakening, daytime napping
Cognitive-perceptual: Forgetfulness, inability to cope with complex situations, difficulty with problem solving (early signs); depression, withdrawal, suicidal ideation (early)

Objective Data
General
Disheveled appearance, agitation

Neurologic
Mild: Loss of recent memory; disorientation to date and time; flat affect; lack of spontaneity; impaired abstraction, cognition, and judgment
Moderate: Agitation; impaired ability to recognize close family and friends; loss of remote memory; confusion, apraxia, agnosia, alexia (inability to understand written language); aphasia; inability to do simple tasks
Severe: Inability to do self-care; incontinence; immobility; limb rigidity; flexor posturing

Possible Diagnostic Findings
Diagnosis by exclusion, cerebral cortical atrophy on CT scan, poor scores on mental status tests, hippocampal atrophy on MRI scan, abnormal changes on PET

week can make you feel better. Daily physical activity, even in older adults, can decrease the risk for cognitive decline.[15]
- *Stay socially active.* Family, friends, church, and a sense of community may all contribute to better brain health.
- *Avoid trauma to the brain.* Because traumatic brain injury may be a risk factor for developing AD, promote safety in physical activities and driving.
- *Treat depression.* Recognize and treat depression early. Depression may cause or worsen memory loss and other cognitive impairment.

Early recognition and treatment of AD are important. You have a responsibility to inform patients and their families regarding the early signs of AD (see Table 60-3).

ACUTE INTERVENTION. The diagnosis of AD is traumatic for both the patient and the family. It is not unusual for the patient to respond with depression, denial, anxiety, fear, withdrawal, and feelings of loss. In the early stages of AD, patients are often aware that their memory is faulty and do things to cover up or mask the problem. See the Resources at the end of this chapter for a link to *What Happens Next?*, a booklet specifically for people dealing with the beginning stages of dementia.

You are in an important position to assess for depression. Antidepressant drugs and counseling may be indicated. Family

caregivers may also be in denial and may not seek medical attention early in the disease. Along with patient assessment, assess family caregivers and their ability to accept and cope with the diagnosis.

Although no current treatment is available for reversing AD, there is a need for ongoing monitoring of both the patient with AD and the patient's caregiver. An important nursing responsibility is to work collaboratively with the caregiver to manage clinical manifestations effectively as they change over time. You are often responsible for teaching the caregiver to perform the many tasks that are required to manage the patient's care. Consider both the patient with AD and the caregiver as patients with overlapping but unique problems.[16]

Patients with AD may be hospitalized for other health problems. Patients with AD are subject to acute and other chronic illnesses and may require surgical interventions. Their inability to communicate symptoms of health problems places the responsibility for assessment and diagnosis on caregivers and health care professionals. Hospitalization of the patient with AD can be a traumatic event for both the patient and caregiver and can precipitate a worsening of the disease or delirium. Patients with AD in the acute care setting need to be observed more closely because of concerns for safety, frequently oriented to place and time, and given reassurance. Anxiety or disruptive behavior may be reduced through the use of consistent nursing staff.

AMBULATORY AND HOME CARE. Currently, family members and friends care for most individuals with AD in their homes. Others with AD reside in various facilities, including long-term care and assisted living facilities. A facility that is good for one person may not be suitable for another. Also, what is helpful for a person at one point in the disease process may be completely different from what is best when the disease progresses.

Patients with AD move through the stages at variable rates. The nursing care required by the patient with AD changes as the disease progresses, emphasizing the need for regular assessment and support. Regardless of the setting, the severity of the problems and the amount of nursing care required intensify over time. The specific manifestations of the disease depend on the area of the brain involved. Nursing care focuses on decreasing clinical manifestations, preventing harm, and supporting the patient and caregiver throughout the disease process.

In the early stages of AD, memory aids (e.g., calendars) may be beneficial. Patients often develop depression during this phase. Depression may be related to the diagnosis of an incurable disorder and the impact of the disease on activities of daily living (e.g., driving, socializing with friends, participating in hobbies or recreational activities).

After the initial diagnosis, patients need to be aware that the progression of the disease is variable. Effective management of the disease may slow the progress of the disease and decrease the burden on the patient, caregiver, and family. However, decisions related to care should be made with the patient, family members, and health care team early in the disease. You have a role in advising the patient and caregiver to initiate health care decisions, including advance directives, while the patient has the capacity to do so. This can ease the burden for the caregiver as the disease progresses.

Adult day care is one of the options available to the person with AD. Although programs vary in size, structure, physical environment, and staff experience, the common goals of all day care programs are to provide respite for the family and a protective environment for the patient. During the early and moderate stages of AD, the person can still benefit from stimulating activities that encourage independence and decision making in a protective environment.[17] The patient returns home tired, content, less frustrated, and ready to be with the family. The respite from the demands of care allows the caregiver to be more responsive to the patient's needs.

As the disease progresses, the demands on the caregiver eventually exceed the resources, and the person with AD may need to be placed in a long-term care facility. Special units to care for persons with AD are becoming increasingly common in long-term care settings. The Alzheimer's unit is designed with an emphasis on safety. For example, many facilities have designated areas that allow the patient to walk freely within the unit, while the unit is secured so that the patient cannot wander outside of it.

As the patient with AD progresses to the late stages (severe impairment) of AD, he or she has increased difficulty with the most basic functions, including walking and talking. Total care is required.

Specific problems relate to the care of the patient with AD in all phases of the disease. These problems are described below.

Behavioral Problems. Behavioral problems occur in about 90% of patients with AD. These problems include repetitiveness (asking the same question repeatedly), delusions (false beliefs), hallucinations, agitation, aggression, altered sleeping patterns, wandering, and resisting care. Many times these behaviors are unpredictable and may challenge caregivers. Caregivers need to be aware that these behaviors are not intentional and are often difficult to control. Behavioral symptoms often lead to the placement of patients in institutional care settings.

These behaviors are often the patient's way of responding to a precipitating factor (e.g., pain, frustration, temperature extremes, anxiety). When these behaviors become problematic, you must plan interventions carefully. Initially assess the patient's physical status. Check the patient for changes in vital signs, urinary and bowel patterns, and pain that could account for behavioral problems. Then assess the environment to identify factors that may trigger behavior disruptions. Extremes in temperature or excessive noise may lead to behavior changes. When the patient is agitated by the environment, either move the patient or remove the stimulus.

When a patient resists or pulls tubes or dressings, cover these items with stretch tube gauze or remove them from the visual field. Reassure the patient that you are present to keep him or her safe. Do not ask the confused or agitated patient challenging "why" questions. If the patient cannot verbalize distress, validate his or her mood. Rephrase the patient's statement to validate its meaning. Closely observe the patient's emotional state.

Nursing strategies that address difficult behavior include redirection, distraction, and reassurance. For the patient who is restless or agitated, redirecting involves changing the patient's focus (e.g., having the patient perform activities such as sweeping, raking, or dusting). Ways to distract the agitated patient may include providing snacks, taking a car ride, sitting on a porch swing or rocker, listening to favorite music, watching videotapes, looking at family photographs, or walking. Reassurance involves communicating to the patient that he or she will be protected from danger, harm, or embarrassment. Use of repetitive activities, songs, poems, music, massage, aromas, or a favorite object can be soothing to patients.[18]

When dealing with the difficult patient, do not threaten to restrain the patient or call the physician. A calming family member can be asked to stay with the patient until the patient becomes calmer. Monitor the patient frequently, and document all interventions. As verbal skills decline, you and the caregiver must rely more on the patient's body language to communicate care needs. The use of positive nurse actions can reduce the use of chemical (drug therapy) restraints.

Disruptive behaviors have been treated with antipsychotic drugs (see Table 60-10). However, as discussed on p. 1452, these drugs have adverse side effects. Before these drugs are used, all other measures of treating behavioral issues should be exhausted.

A specific type of agitation, termed sundowning, is when the patient becomes more confused and agitated in the late afternoon or evening. Behaviors commonly exhibited include agitation, aggressiveness, wandering, resistance to redirection, and increased verbal activity such as yelling. The cause of sundowning is unclear, but several theories propose that it is due to a disruption of circadian rhythms. Other possible causes include fatigue, unfamiliar environment and noise (especially in an acute care setting), medications, reduced lighting, and sleep fragmentation. When a patient experiences sundowning, remain calm and avoid confrontation. Assess the situation for possible causes of the agitation. Nursing interventions that may be helpful include (1) creating a quiet, calm environment; (2) maximizing exposure to daylight (open blinds and turn on lights during the day); (3) evaluating medications to determine if any could cause sleep disturbance; (4) limiting naps and caffeine; and (5) consulting with the health care provider regarding drug therapy. Management of sundowning can be challenging for you, the patient, and the family.

Safety. The person with AD is at risk for problems related to personal safety. Potential hazards include falling, ingesting dangerous substances, wandering, injuring others and self with sharp objects, being burned, and being unable to respond to crisis situations. These concerns require careful attention to the home environment to minimize risk. Supervision is also required. As the patient's cognitive function declines over time, the patient may have difficulty navigating physical spaces and interpreting environmental cues. Assist the caregiver in assessing the home environment for safety risks.

SAFETY ALERT
Teach the caregiver to take the following steps:
- Have stairwells well lit.
- Handrails should be graspable.
- Tack down carpet edges.
- Remove throw rugs and extension cords.
- Use nonskid mats in tub or shower.
- Install handrails in the bath and by the commode.

Wandering is a major concern for caregivers. Wandering may be related to loss of memory or to side effects of drugs, or it may be an expression of a physical or emotional need, restlessness, curiosity, or stimuli that trigger memories of earlier routines. As with other behaviors, observe for factors or events that may precipitate wandering. For example, the patient may be sensitive to stress and tension in the environment. In such cases, wandering may reflect an attempt to leave.[19]

When someone with AD is discovered missing, every second counts. To assist caregivers with locating them, the Alzheimer's Association and the MedicAlert Foundation have created an alliance called MedicAlert + Alzheimer's Association Safe Return.[20] This program includes identification products (e.g.,

DELEGATION DECISIONS

Caring for the Patient With Alzheimer's Disease

All staff members who care for a patient with Alzheimer's disease (AD) are responsible for ensuring the patient's physiologic and psychosocial safety. The registered nurse (RN) is responsible for ongoing assessments of the patient's level of function and for development of the plan of care. Since most patients with AD are cared for at home or in long-term care settings, many routine nursing activities are delegated to licensed practical/vocational nurses (LPN/LVNs), unlicensed assistive personnel (UAP), or family caregivers.

Role of Registered Nurse (RN)
- Assess patient memory and level of function.
- Teach patient and caregivers memory enhancement aids (e.g., calendars, notes).
- Monitor for physiologic problems associated with AD, such as pain, swallowing difficulties, urinary tract infection, pneumonia, skin breakdown, and constipation.
- Assess patient's nutritional and fluid intake and develop a plan to ensure adequate intake.
- Evaluate patient's safety risk factors.
- Determine possible precipitating factors for behavioral changes and develop strategies to address difficult behavior.
- Assess the family caregiver's stress level and coping strategies.
- Make referrals for community services such as adult day care and respite care.

Role of Licensed Practical/Vocational Nurse (LPN/LVN)
- Monitor for behavioral changes that may indicate physiologic problems.
- Check patient environment for potential safety hazards.
- Administer enteral feedings to patients who are unable to swallow (if ordered).
- Administer ordered drug therapy.

Role of Unlicensed Assistive Personnel (UAP)
- Assist patient to use the toilet, commode, or bedpan at frequent intervals.
- Provide personal hygiene, skin care, oral care.
- Help patients with eating.
- Assist patients with daily activities.
- Use bed alarms and surveillance to decrease risk for falls.

bracelet, necklace, wallet cards), a national photo and information database, a 24-hour toll-free emergency crisis line, local chapter support, and wandering behavior education and training for caregivers and families.

Pain Management. Because of difficulties with oral and written language, AD patients may have difficulty expressing physical complaints, including pain. You need to rely on other clues such as the patient's behavior. Pain can result in alterations in the patient's behavior, such as increased vocalization, agitation, withdrawal, and changes in function. Pain should be recognized and treated promptly and the patient's response monitored.

Eating and Swallowing Difficulties. Undernutrition is a problem in the moderate and severe stages of AD, with patients in long-term facilities having the highest incidence of undernutrition. Loss of interest in food and decreased ability to self-feed *(feeding apraxia),* as well as co-morbid conditions, can result in significant nutritional deficiencies in the patient with AD. In long-term care facilities, inadequate assistance with feeding may add to the problem.

Use pureed foods, thickened liquids, and nutritional supplements when chewing and swallowing become problematic for the patient. Patients may need reminders to chew their food

and to swallow. Patients need a quiet and unhurried environment for eating. Avoid distractions at mealtimes, including the television. Low lighting, music, and simulated nature sounds may improve eating behaviors. Easy-grip eating utensils and finger foods may allow the patient to self-feed. Offer liquids frequently.

When oral feeding is not possible, explore alternative routes. Nasogastric (NG) feeding may be used for short periods. However, for the long term the NG tube is uncomfortable and may add to the patient's agitation. A percutaneous endoscopic gastrostomy (PEG) tube provides another option (see Fig. 40-7). However, PEG tubes can be problematic, since patients with AD are particularly vulnerable to aspiration of feeding formula and tube dislodgment. The potential positive outcomes to be gained from nutritional therapies are considered in light of overall outcome goals and potential adverse effects of the specific therapy. Nutritional support therapies are described in Chapter 40.

Oral Care. In the late stages of AD the patient is unable to perform oral self-care. With decreased tooth brushing and flossing, dental problems are likely to occur. Because of swallowing difficulties, patients may retain food in the mouth, adding to the potential for tooth decay. Dental caries and tooth abscess can add to patient discomfort or pain and subsequently may increase agitation. Inspect the mouth regularly and provide mouth care to those patients unable to do self-care.

Infection Prevention. Urinary tract infection and pneumonia are the most common infections in patients with AD. Such infections are ultimately the cause of death in many patients with AD. Because of feeding and swallowing problems, the patient is at risk for aspiration pneumonia. Immobility can also predispose the patient to pneumonia. Reduced fluid intake, prostate hyperplasia in men, poor hygiene, and urinary drainage devices (e.g., catheters) can predispose patients to bladder infection. Any manifestations of infection, such as a change in behavior, fever, cough (pneumonia), or pain on urination (bladder), need prompt evaluation and treatment.

Skin Care. It is important to monitor the patient's skin over time. Note and treat rashes, areas of redness, and skin breakdown. In the late stages, incontinence along with immobility and undernutrition can place the patient at risk for skin breakdown. Keep the skin dry and clean, and change the patient's position regularly to avoid areas of pressure over bony prominences.

Elimination Problems. During the moderate and severe stages of AD, urinary and fecal incontinence lead to increased need for nursing care. When possible, habit or behavioral retraining of bladder and bowel function (e.g., scheduled toileting) may help decrease episodes of incontinence.

Another common elimination problem is constipation. Causes may relate to immobility, dietary intake (e.g., reduced fiber intake), and decreased fluid intake. Increased dietary fiber, fiber supplements, and stool softeners are the first lines of management. The combination of aging, other health problems, and swallowing difficulties may increase the risk of complications associated with the use of mineral oil, stimulants, osmotic agents, and enemas. Management of constipation is discussed in Chapter 43.

Caregiver Support. An estimated 15 million Americans provide unpaid care for people with AD or other dementia.[1] The majority of these are family members providing care in the home (Fig. 60-8). AD is a disease that disrupts all aspects of personal and family life. Caregivers for persons with AD describe it as very

FIG. 60-8 Caregivers of patients with dementia face an incredible challenge that often causes deterioration in their own physical and emotional health. (iStockphoto/Thinkstock.)

TABLE 60-12 FAMILY & CAREGIVER TEACHING GUIDE

Alzheimer's Disease

Include the following instructions when teaching families and caregivers the management of the patient with Alzheimer's disease.

Mild Stage
- Many treatable (and potentially reversible) conditions can mimic dementia (see Table 60-2). Try to get a definitive diagnosis.
- Get the person to stop driving. Confusion and poor judgment can impair driving skills and potentially put others at risk.
- Encourage activities such as visiting with friends and family, listening to music, participating in hobbies, and exercising.
- Provide cues in the home, establish a routine, and determine a specific location where essential items (e.g., glasses) need to be kept.
- Do not correct misstatements or faulty memory.
- Register with MedicAlert + Alzheimer's Association Safe Return, a program established by the MedicAlert Foundation and the Alzheimer's Association to locate individuals who wander from their homes.
- Make plans for the future in terms of advance directives, care options, financial concerns, and personal preference for care.

Moderate Stage
- Install door locks for patient safety.
- Provide protective wear for urinary and fecal incontinence.
- Ensure that the home has good lighting, install handrails in stairways and bathroom, and remove area rugs.
- Label drawers and faucets (hot and cold) to ensure safety.
- Develop strategies such as distraction and diversion to cope with behavioral problems. Identify and reduce potential triggers (e.g., reduce stress, extremes in temperature) for disruptive behavior.
- Provide memory triggers, such as pictures of family and friends.

Severe Stage
- Provide a regular schedule for toileting to reduce incontinence.
- Provide care to meet needs, including oral care and skin care.
- Monitor diet and fluid intake to ensure their adequacy.
- Continue communication through talking and touching.
- Consider placement in a long-term care facility when providing total care becomes too difficult.

stressful (see Table 4-5). These caregivers also exhibit adverse consequences relating to their own emotional and physical health.

The chronic and often severe stress associated with dementia caregiving increases the risk for the development of dementia in spouse caregivers. One mechanism proposed is that the detrimental effects of the chronic stress of caregiving can affect the hippocampus, a region of the brain responsible for memory.[21]

As the disease progresses, the relationship of the caregiver to the patient changes. Family roles may be altered or reversed (e.g., son caring for father). Decisions must be made, including when to tell the patient about the diagnosis, when to have the patient stop driving or doing activities that might be dangerous, when to ask for assistance, and when to place the patient in adult day care or a long-term care facility. With early-onset AD, the patient is affected during his or her most productive years in terms of career and family. The consequences can be devastating for the patient and the family.[22]

Sexual relations for couples are also seriously affected by AD. As the disease progresses, sexual interest may decline for both the patient and partner. A number of reasons account for this, including fatigue, memory impairment, and episodes of incontinence. The patient may also become sexually driven as the disease progresses and the patient becomes more uninhibited.

Work with the caregiver to assess stressors (see Table 4-4) and to identify coping strategies to reduce the burden of caregiving.[23] For example, ask which behaviors are most disruptive to family life at a given time, while remembering that this is likely to change as the disease progresses. Determining what the caregiver views as most disruptive or distressful can help to establish priorities for care. Risk to the safety of the patient and caregiver is given high priority. It is also important to assess what the caregiver's expectations are regarding the patient's behavior. Are the expectations reasonable given the progression of the disease? A family and caregiver teaching guide based on the disease stages is provided in Table 60-12. Other tips for caregivers are listed in Table 60-13. A nursing care plan for the

family caregiver (eNursing Care Plan 60-2) is available on the website for this chapter.

Support groups for caregivers and family members (Fig. 60-9) can provide an atmosphere of understanding and give current information about the disease itself and related topics such as safety, legal, ethical, and financial issues. The needs of family caregivers are discussed in Chapter 4 on pp. 51-52. Strategies related to stress management are discussed in Chapter 7.

The Alzheimer's Association has many educational and support systems available to help family caregivers. The link to a booklet for caregivers, *Caring for a Person With Alzheimer's Disease*, is provided in the Resources section at the end of this chapter.

EVALUATION

Expected outcomes are that the patient with AD will
- Function at the highest level of cognitive ability
- Perform basic personal care activities of daily living, including bathing, dressing, feeding, and toileting by self or with assistance as needed

TABLE 60-13 GUIDELINES FOR DEALING WITH DEMENTIA PATIENTS

Do
- Treat them like adults, with respect and dignity, even when their behavior is childlike.
- Use gentle touch and direct eye contact.
- Remain patient, flexible, calm, and understanding.
- Anticipate challenging behaviors, since the patient's ability to think logically has been affected.
- Give directions using gestures or pictures.
- Simplify tasks. Focus on one thing at a time.
- Avoid questions or topics that require extensive thought, memory, or words.
- Be flexible. If one approach does not work, try another.
- Use distraction, changing the subject, redirecting to another activity.
- Provide reassurance. Praise sincerely for success.

Do Not
- Criticize, correct, or argue.
- Rush or hurry the patient.
- Force participation in activities or events.
- Talk about the patient as if he or she is not there.
- Blame the person with AD. Instead blame the disease.
- Take challenging behaviors personally. These behaviors are due to the patient's disease.
- Use condescending terms, such as "honey" or "sweetie."
- Use threatening gestures.
- Overreact to the person with AD.
- Try to explain "why" or rationalize.

FIG. 60-9 Support groups are an effective way to help caregivers cope. (iStockphoto/Thinkstock.)

- Experience no injury
- Remain in restricted area during ambulation and activity

Additional information on the expected outcomes for the patient with AD is addressed in eNursing Care Plan 60-1 (available on the website for this chapter).

OTHER NEURODEGENERATIVE DISEASES

Parkinson's disease and Huntington's disease are both neurodegenerative diseases (see Chapter 59). Both diseases are chronic, progressive, and incurable. Despite differences in the

etiology and pathophysiology of these diseases, both are associated with the development of dementia in the later stages of disease.

Dementia with Lewy bodies (DLB) is a condition characterized by the presence of Lewy bodies (abnormal deposits of the protein α-synuclein) in the brainstem and cortex. Patients typically have symptoms of parkinsonism, hallucinations, short-term memory loss, unpredictable cognitive shifts, and sleep disturbances. A possible diagnosis of DLB is indicated by dementia plus two of the following symptoms: (1) extrapyramidal signs such as bradykinesia, rigidity, and postural instability, but not always a tremor; (2) fluctuating cognitive ability; and (3) hallucinations. This disease has features of both AD and Parkinson's disease, and it is imperative that a correct diagnosis be reached.

Medications for DLB are determined on an individual basis. Medications may include levodopa/carbidopa and acetylcholinesterase inhibitors. Nursing care for these patients relates to management of the dementia and of problems related to dysphagia and immobility. Swallowing problems can lead to impaired nutrition. These patients are at risk for falls from impaired mobility and balance. Pneumonia is a common complication. The diagnostic criteria for LBD are based on clinical signs and symptoms and confirmed at autopsy by histologic examination of brain tissue.

Frontotemporal lobar degeneration (FTLD) is a clinical syndrome associated with shrinking of the frontal and temporal anterior lobes of the brain. In Pick's disease, one type of FTLD, the brain has abnormal microscopic deposits called Pick bodies (though these are not always present). In FTLD, portions of the frontal and temporal lobes atrophy. FTLD is often misdiagnosed as a psychiatric problem or as AD. However, FTLD tends to occur at a younger age than does AD, typically between ages 40 and 70. The major distinguishing characteristic between these disorders and AD is marked symmetric lobar atrophy of the temporal and/or frontal lobes.

FTLD is characterized by disturbances in behavior, sleep, personality, and eventually memory. The disease progresses relentlessly and may ultimately include language impairment, erratic behavior, and dementia. Because of the strange behavior associated with FTLD, psychiatrists often see these patients first. There is no specific treatment. The diagnosis can be confirmed at autopsy.

Normal pressure hydrocephalus is an uncommon disorder characterized by an obstruction in the flow of CSF, causing a buildup of CSF in the brain. Symptoms of the condition include dementia, urinary incontinence, and difficulty walking. Meningitis, encephalitis, or head injury may cause the condition. If diagnosed early, normal pressure hydrocephalus is treatable by surgery in which a shunt is inserted to divert the fluid away from the brain.

Creutzfeldt-Jakob disease (CJD) is a rare and fatal brain disorder caused by a prion protein. A *prion* is a small infectious pathogen containing protein but lacking nucleic acids. The source of infection of a variant form of CJD (vCJD) is beef obtained from animals contaminated with bovine spongiform encephalopathy, which is also called *mad cow disease*. The risk of contracting vCJD is extremely low.

The earliest symptom of the disease may be memory impairment and behavior changes. The disease progresses rapidly with mental deterioration, involuntary movements (muscle jerks), weakness in the limbs, blindness, and eventually coma. There is no diagnostic test for CJD. Only autopsy and examination of brain tissue can confirm the diagnosis. There is no treatment for CJD.

Mixed dementia occurs when two or more types of dementia are present at the same time. It is characterized by the hallmark abnormalities of Alzheimer's and another type of dementia. Usually the other type of dementia is vascular dementia, but it can be other types, such as DLB.

DELIRIUM

Delirium, a state of temporary but acute mental confusion, is a common, life-threatening, and possibly preventable syndrome. Delirium is the most frequent complication of hospitalization in older patients. In the hospital setting, 15% to 53% of older adults experience delirium postoperatively, and as many as 80% of patients in an intensive care unit (ICU) experience delirium.[24]

TABLE 60-14	FACTORS THAT PRECIPITATE DELIRIUM
Demographic Characteristics • Age 65 yr or older • Male gender **Cognitive Status** • Dementia • Cognitive impairment • History of delirium • Depression **Environmental** • Admission to an intensive care unit • Use of physical restraints • Pain (especially untreated) • Emotional stress • Sleep deprivation **Functional Status** • Functional dependence • Immobility • History of falls **Sensory** • Sensory deprivation • Sensory overload • Visual or hearing impairment	**Decreased Oral Intake** • Dehydration • Malnutrition **Drugs** • Sedative-hypnotics • Opioids • Anticholinergic drugs • Aminoglycosides • Treatment with multiple drugs • Alcohol or drug abuse or withdrawal **Coexisting Medical Conditions** • Severe acute illness • Electrolyte imbalances • Chronic renal or hepatic disease • History of stroke • Neurologic disease • Acute infection, sepsis, fever • Fracture or trauma • Terminal illness **Surgery** • Orthopedic surgery • Cardiac surgery • Prolonged cardiopulmonary bypass • Noncardiac surgery

Etiology and Pathophysiology

The pathophysiologic mechanism of delirium is poorly understood. The main hypothesis is reversible impairment of cerebral oxidative metabolism and multiple neurotransmitter abnormalities. Cholinergic deficiency, excess release of dopamine, and both increased and decreased serotonergic activity may contribute to delirium. Proinflammatory cytokines, including interleukin-1, interleukin-2, interleukin-6, tumor necrosis factor–α (TNF-α), and interferon, appear to play a role. Stress and sleep deprivation have also been linked to the onset of delirium.[25]

Clinically, delirium is rarely caused by a single factor. It is often the result of the interaction of the patient's underlying condition with a precipitating event. Delirium can occur after a relatively minor insult in a vulnerable patient. For example, a patient with underlying health problems such as heart failure, cancer, cognitive impairment, or sensory limitations may develop delirium in response to a relatively minor change (e.g., use of a sleeping medication). In other nonvulnerable patients, it may take a combination of factors (e.g., anesthesia, major surgery, infection, prolonged sleep deprivation) to precipitate delirium. Delirium can also be a symptom of a serious medical illness such as bacterial meningitis.

Understanding factors that can lead to delirium can help in determining effective interventions. Several factors that can precipitate or cause delirium are listed in Tables 60-14 and 60-15. Many of these factors are more common in older patients.[26] In addition, older patients have limited compensatory mechanisms to deal with physiologic insults such as hypoxia, hypoglycemia, and dehydration. Older adults are more susceptible to drug-induced delirium, in part because of their

TABLE 60-15	MNEMONIC FOR CAUSES OF DELIRIUM

Dementia, dehydration
Electrolyte imbalances, emotional stress
Lung, liver, heart, kidney, brain
Infection, intensive care unit
Rx Drugs
Injury, immobility
Untreated pain, unfamiliar environment
Metabolic disorders

TABLE 60-16	CONFUSION ASSESSMENT METHOD (CAM)

Delirium is diagnosed with the presence of features 1 and 2, and either 3 or 4.

Feature 1 *Acute Onset and Fluctuating Course*	Data usually obtained from a family member or nurse. Shown by positive responses to following questions: • Is there evidence of an acute change in mental status from the patient's baseline? • Did the (abnormal) behavior fluctuate during the day (i.e., tend to come and go, or increase and decrease in severity)?
Feature 2 *Inattention*	Shown by positive response to following question: • Did the patient have difficulty focusing attention (e.g., being easily distractible, or having difficulty keeping track of what was being said)?
Feature 3 *Disorganized Thinking*	Shown by a positive response to following question: • Was the patient's thinking disorganized or incoherent, such as rambling or irrelevant conversation, unclear or illogical flow of ideas, or unpredictable switching from subject to subject?
Feature 4 *Altered Level of Consciousness*	Shown by any answer other than "alert" to the following question: • Overall, how would you rate this patient's level of consciousness (alert [normal], vigilant [hyperalert], lethargic [drowsy, easily aroused], stupor [difficult to arouse], or coma [unarousable])?

Adapted from Inouye S, van Dyck C, Alessi C, et al: Clarifying confusion: the Confusion Assessment Method, *Ann Intern Med* 113(12):941, 1990.

increased use of multiple drugs. Many medications, including sedative-hypnotics, opioids (especially meperidine [Demerol]), benzodiazepines, and drugs with anticholinergic properties, can cause or contribute to delirium, especially in older or vulnerable patients. An important risk factor for delirium is pre-existing dementia.[27]

Clinical Manifestations

Patients with delirium can have a variety of manifestations ranging from hypoactivity and lethargy to hyperactivity, agitation, and hallucinations. Patients can also have mixed delirium, manifesting both hypoactive and hyperactive symptoms. Delirium can develop over the course of hours to days. In most patients, delirium usually develops over a 2- to 3-day period. The early manifestations often include inability to concentrate, irritability, insomnia, loss of appetite, restlessness, and confusion. Later manifestations may include agitation, misperception, misinterpretation, and hallucinations.

Acute delirium occurs frequently in hospitalized older adults. This transient condition is characterized by disorganized thinking, difficulty concentrating, and sensory misperceptions that last from 1 to 7 days. However, some delirium manifestations may persist up to and after discharge. Delirium is one of the most frequent consequences of unscheduled surgery on the older adult, especially when the patient has not been stabilized physically or prepared emotionally. Often this patient experiences a decline in ability to perform activities of daily living and an increased risk for falls.

Manifestations of delirium are sometimes confused with those of dementia. A key distinction between delirium and dementia is that the person who exhibits sudden cognitive impairment, disorientation, or clouded sensorium is more likely to have delirium rather than dementia. (A comparison of delirium and dementia is presented in Table 60-1.)

Diagnostic Studies

Diagnosing delirium is complicated because many critically ill patients cannot communicate their needs. A careful medical and psychologic history and physical examination are the first steps in diagnosing delirium. This includes careful attention to medications, both prescription and over-the-counter drugs. The Confusion Assessment Method (CAM) has been extensively studied and is a reliable tool for assessing delirium (Table 60-16). It is important to distinguish whether the delirium is part of an underlying problem of dementia.

Once delirium has been diagnosed, explore potential causes. Carefully review the patient's health history and medication record. Laboratory tests include complete blood count, serum electrolytes, blood urea nitrogen, and creatinine levels; electrocardiogram; urinalysis; liver and thyroid function tests;

and oxygen saturation level. Drug and alcohol levels may be obtained. If unexplained fever or nuchal rigidity is present and meningitis or encephalitis is suspected, a lumbar puncture may be performed. CSF is examined for glucose, protein, and bacteria. If the patient's history includes head injury, appropriate x-rays or scans may be ordered. In general, brain imaging studies such as CT and MRI are used only in situations in which head injury is known or suspected.

NURSING AND COLLABORATIVE MANAGEMENT
DELIRIUM

In caring for the patient with delirium, your roles include prevention, early recognition, and treatment. Prevention of delirium involves recognition of high-risk patients.[28] Patient groups at risk include those with neurologic disorders (e.g., stroke, dementia, CNS infection, Parkinson's disease), sensory impairment, and advanced age. Other risk factors, including hospitalization in an ICU and untreated pain, are listed in Table 60-14.

Care of the patient with delirium focuses on eliminating precipitating factors.[29] If it is drug induced, medications are discontinued. Keep in mind that delirium can also accompany drug and alcohol withdrawal. Depending on patient history, drug screening may be performed. Fluid and electrolyte imbalances and nutritional deficiencies (e.g., thiamine) are corrected

ETHICAL/LEGAL DILEMMAS

Board of Nursing Disciplinary Action

Situation

The State Board of Nursing has received multiple complaints about J.R., a registered nurse (RN) who works in a long-term care facility. J.R. has signed off on three controlled substances count sheets that have been determined to be inaccurate. During an investigation it was discovered that several members of the nursing staff knew about J.R.'s reported behavior, but they did not report their observations to the unit administrator. After the investigation, the board of nursing subpoenas J.R. to a meeting to discuss charges in preparation for a disciplinary hearing.

Ethical/Legal Points for Consideration

- Regulation of professional nursing practice is the right of each of the 50 states, most of which have separate regulatory agencies charged with writing regulations and rules to implement the State Nurse Practice Act. The regulations approved by these agencies carry the weight of law. Failure to behave accordingly places a nurse at risk for disciplinary action.
- The RN who is charged with unprofessional behavior has been charged with an offense and is entitled to the same legal rights as any other individual, including a fair and timely hearing, opportunity to confront the accusers, right to be represented by an attorney, and right to prepare a defense.
- Possible disciplinary actions include temporary suspension of the nursing license, revocation of the nursing license, mandatory rehabilitation for substance abuse, and mandated supervision and evaluation of practice. Sometimes the disciplinary action includes fines and requires re-education. In addition, the State Board of Nursing may report the action to the state attorney general if evidence suggests that a crime has been committed. The RN who has been found guilty of unprofessional practice must report this action on all future applications for nursing positions.
- All RNs should be familiar with their state's nurse practice act and regulations, as well as the composition and actions of the State Board of Nursing. Nurses should pay particular attention to the regulation that lists examples of actionable behavior and disciplinary actions sanctioned by the state.
- RNs have a legal and ethical obligation to report suspected illegal behavior to their administrators and to continue reporting until the situation is resolved. By failing to report, the RN may be charged as an accessory to the act or aiding and abetting the behavior. This RN may be charged with unprofessional behavior and risks losing his or her nursing license. Shifting the obligation to someone else to report or failure to continue reporting each incident does not satisfy this duty.

Discussion Questions

1. How would you handle a situation where retaliation for reporting unprofessional behavior is likely?
2. What would you do if the nurse suspected of illegal behavior is related to someone in the administrative hierarchy?

members to stay at the bedside, providing familiar objects, transferring the patient to a private room or one closer to the nurses' station, and planning for consistent nursing staff if possible. Use reorientation and behavioral interventions in patients with delirium. Provide the patient with reassurance and reorienting information as to place, time, and procedures. Clocks, calendars, and lists of the patient's scheduled activities are also useful in reducing confusion. Reduce environmental stimuli, including noise and light levels.

Personal contact through touch and verbal communication can be an important reorienting strategy. If the patient uses eyeglasses or a hearing aid, they should be readily available because sensory deprivation can precipitate delirium. Avoid the use of restraints. Other interventions, including relaxation techniques, music therapy, and massage, may also be appropriate for some patients with delirium.

Comprehensive, multicomponent interventions to prevent delirium are the most effective and should be implemented through institution-based programs that are interdisciplinary. These interdisciplinary teams may also address issues related to polypharmacy, pain, nutritional status, and potential for incontinence. The patient experiencing delirium is also at risk for the adverse consequences of immobility, including skin breakdown. Give attention to increasing physical activity or providing range-of-motion exercises, when appropriate, and maintaining skin integrity.

Also focus on supporting the family and caregivers during episodes of delirium. Family members need to understand factors that may have precipitated the delirium, as well as the potential outcomes. *Delirium in the ICU: A Guide for Patients and Families* is available in eTable 66-1 (available on the website for Chapter 66).

DRUG THERAPY

Drug therapy is reserved for patients with severe agitation, especially when it interferes with needed medical therapy (e.g., fluid replacement, intubation, dialysis). Agitation can put the patient at risk for falls and injury. Drug therapy is used cautiously because many of the drugs used to manage agitation have psychoactive properties. Drugs should be used only when nonpharmacologic interventions have failed.

Dexmedetomidine (Precedex), an α-adrenergic receptor agonist, has been used in ICU settings for sedation. In addition, low-dose antipsychotics (neuroleptics) may be used such as haloperidol (Haldol), risperidone (Risperdal), olanzapine (Zyprexa), and quetiapine (Seroquel). Haloperidol can be administered IV, intramuscularly, or orally and will produce sedation. In addition to sedation, other side effects of antipsychotics include hypotension; extrapyramidal side effects, including *tardive dyskinesia* (involuntary muscle movements of face, trunk, and arms) and *athetosis* (involuntary writhing movements of the limbs); muscle tone changes; and anticholinergic effects. Carefully monitor older patients receiving antipsychotic agents.

Short-acting benzodiazepines (e.g., lorazepam [Ativan]) can be used to treat delirium associated with sedative and alcohol withdrawal or in conjunction with antipsychotics to reduce extrapyramidal side effects. However, these drugs may worsen delirium caused by other factors and must be used cautiously.

if appropriate. If the problem is related to environmental conditions (e.g., an overstimulating or understimulating environment), changes should be made. If delirium is secondary to infection, appropriate antibiotic therapy is started. Similarly, if delirium is secondary to chronic illness such as chronic kidney disease or heart failure, treatment focuses on these conditions.[30]

Care of the patient experiencing delirium includes protecting the patient from harm. Give priority to creating a calm and safe environment. This may include encouraging family

CASE STUDY

Alzheimer's Disease

iStockphoto/Thinkstock

Patient Profile
M.Y., an 80-yr-old Asian American man, was diagnosed with Alzheimer's disease (AD) 3 yr ago. Today his 78-yr-old wife brings him to the emergency department because he wandered from his home, fell, and injured his left hip.

Subjective Data
- Can state his name
- Confused as to place and time
- Denies memory of wandering or falling
- Agitated, trying to get up
- Denies pain

Objective Data
Physical Examination
- Left leg shorter than right leg
- Tense and anxious

Diagnostic Studies
- X-ray of left hip indicates a fracture
- Mini-Cog testing indicates cognitive impairment

Discussion Questions
1. What is the pathogenesis of AD?
2. What precipitating factors may have resulted in M.Y.'s fall?
3. What precautions need to be taken regarding the inpatient care of M.Y.?
4. *Priority Decision:* What is the priority nursing intervention for M.Y.?
5. What teaching plan should you develop for M.Y. and his wife?
6. Surgery is planned to repair his fractured hip. Why is he at risk for delirium?
7. *Priority Decision:* Based on the assessment data, what are the priority nursing diagnoses? Are there any collaborative problems?
8. *Delegation Decision:* What nursing activities can the RN delegate to unlicensed assistive personnel (UAP)?
9. *Evidence-Based Practice:* M.Y.'s wife asks you if she should give her husband ginkgo to help his memory. How would you respond?

ⓔvolve Answers available at *http://evolve.elsevier.com/Lewis/medsurg.*

▌BRIDGE TO NCLEX EXAMINATION

The number of the question corresponds to the same-numbered outcome at the beginning of the chapter.

1. Dementia is defined as a
   a. syndrome that results only in memory loss.
   b. disease associated with abrupt changes in behavior.
   c. disease that is always due to reduced blood flow to the brain.
   d. syndrome characterized by cognitive dysfunction and loss of memory.

2. Vascular dementia is associated with
   a. transient ischemic attacks.
   b. bacterial or viral infection of neuronal tissue.
   c. cognitive changes secondary to cerebral ischemia.
   d. abrupt changes in cognitive function that are irreversible.

3. The clinical diagnosis of dementia is based on
   a. CT or MRS.
   b. brain biopsy.
   c. electroencephalogram.
   d. patient history and cognitive assessment.

4. Which statement(s) accurately describe(s) mild cognitive impairment *(select all that apply)*?
   a. Always progresses to AD
   b. Caused by variety of factors and may progress to AD
   c. Should be aggressively treated with acetylcholinesterase drugs
   d. Caused by vascular infarcts that, if treated, will delay progression to AD
   e. Patient is usually not aware that there is a problem with his or her memory

5. The early stage of AD is characterized by
   a. no noticeable change in behavior.
   b. memory problems and mild confusion.
   c. increased time spent sleeping or in bed.
   d. incontinence, agitation, and wandering behavior.

6. A major goal of treatment for the patient with AD is to
   a. maintain patient safety.
   b. maintain or increase body weight.
   c. return to a higher level of self-care.
   d. enhance functional ability over time.

7. Creutzfeldt-Jakob disease is characterized by
   a. remissions and exacerbations over many years.
   b. memory impairment, muscle jerks, and blindness.
   c. parkinsonian symptoms, including muscle rigidity and tremors at rest.
   d. increased intracranial pressure secondary to decreased CSF drainage.

8. Which patient is most at risk for developing delirium?
   a. A 50-year-old woman with cholecystitis
   b. A 19-year-old man with a fractured femur
   c. A 42-year-old woman having an elective hysterectomy
   d. A 78-year-old man admitted to the medical unit with complications related to heart failure

1. d, 2. c, 3. d, 4. b, 5. b, 6. a, 7. b, 8. d

ⓔvolve

For rationales to these answers and even more NCLEX review questions, visit *http://evolve.elsevier.com/Lewis/medsurg.*

REFERENCES

1. Alzheimer's Association: 2013 Alzheimer's Association facts and figures report. Retrieved from *www.alz.org/downloads/facts_figures_2013.pdf.*
2. Ohara T, Doi Y, Ninomiya T, et al: Glucose tolerance status and risk of dementia in the community: the Hisayama study, *Neurology* 77:1126, 2011.
3. Lehman EJ, Hein MJ, Baron SL, et al: Neurodegenerative causes of death among retired National Football League players, *Neurology* 79(19):1970, 2012.
4. Yaffe K, Vittinghoff E, Lindquist K, et al: Post-traumatic stress disorder and risk of dementia among U.S. veterans, *Arch Gen Psychiatry* 67(6):608, 2010.
5. Alzheimer's Disease Education and Referral Center: Alzheimer's disease genetics: facts sheet. Retrieved from

www.nia.nih.gov/sites/default/files/alzheimers_disease_genetics_fact_sheet.pdf.

6. Reiman EM, Quiroz YT, Fleisher AS, et al: Brain imaging and fluid biomarker analysis in young adults at genetic risk for autosomal dominant Alzheimer's disease in the presenilin 1 E280A kindred: a case-control study, *Lancet Neurol* 11(12):1048, 2012.

7. Reisberg B, Franssen EH, Souren LE, et al: Evidence and mechanisms of retrogenesis in Alzheimer's and other dementias: management and treatment import, *Am J Alzheimers Dis Other Demen* 17(4):202, 2002. (Classic)

8. Jack CR, Albert MS, Knopmana DS, et al: Introduction to the recommendations from the National Institute on Aging–Alzheimer's Association workgroups on diagnostic guidelines for Alzheimer's disease, *Alzheimers Dement* 7:257, 2011.

9. McKhann GM, Knopman DS, Chertkow H, et al: The diagnosis of dementia due to Alzheimer's disease: recommendations from the National Institute on Aging and the Alzheimer's Association workgroup, *Alzheimers Dement* 7:263, 2011.

*10. Albert MS, DeKoskyb ST, Dickson D, et al: The diagnosis of mild cognitive impairment due to Alzheimer's disease: recommendations from the National Institute on Aging and Alzheimer's Association workgroup, *Alzheimers Dement* 7:270, 2011.

*11. Russ TC, Morling JR: Cholinesterase inhibitors for mild cognitive impairment, *Cochrane Database Syst Rev* 9:CD009132, 2012.

*12. Howard R, McShane R, Lindesay J, et al: Donepezil and memantine for moderate-to-severe Alzheimer's disease, *N Engl J Med* 366(10):893, 2012.

13. Dwolatzky T, Clarfield AM: Cholinesterase inhibitors and memantine in more advanced Alzheimer's disease: the debate continues, *Aging Health* 8(3):233, 2012.

14. Huybrechts KF, Gerhard T, Crystal S, et al: Differential risk of death in older residents in nursing homes prescribed specific antipsychotic drugs: population based cohort study, *BMJ* 344:e977, 2011.

15. Buchman AS, Boyle PA, Yu L, et al: Total daily physical activity and the risk of AD and cognitive decline in older adults, *Neurology* 78:1323, 2012.

16. Levine C: The hospital nurse's assessment of family caregiver needs, *Am J Nurs* 111:47, 2011.

*17. Woods B, Aguirre E, Spector AE, et al: Cognitive stimulation to improve cognitive functioning in people with dementia, *Cochrane Database Syst Rev* 2:CD005562, 2012.

18. Budson AE, Solomon PR: *Memory loss: a practical guide for clinicians*, St Louis, 2011, Saunders.

19. Rowe MA, Greenblum CA, D'Aoust RF: Missing incidents in community-dwelling people with dementia, *Am J Nurs* 112:30, 2012.

20. Alzheimer's Association: MedicAlert + Alzheimer's Association Safe Return. Retrieved from www.alz.org/care/dementia-medic-alert-safe-return.asp.

21. Norton MC, Smith KR, Østbye T: Greater risk for dementia when spouse has dementia? The Cache County study, *J Am Geriatr Society* 58:895, 2010.

22. Lewis SL, Arevalo-Flechas LC, Miner-Williams D: Caregiving. In Giddens J, editor: *Concept-based nursing*, St Louis, 2012, Mosby.

23. Walton MK: Communicating with family caregivers, *Am J Nurs* 111:47, 2011.

24. American Association of Critical-Care Nurses: Delirium assessment and management. Retrieved from www.aacn.org/WD/practice/content/practicealerts/delirium-practice-alert.content.

25. Delirium in the intensive care unit: an under-recognized syndrome of organ dysfunction. Retrieved from www.medscape.com/viewarticle/410883_4.

26. Brooks PB: Postoperative delirium in elderly patients, *Am J Nurs* 112:38, 2012.

27. Fong TG, Jones RN, Marcantonio ER: Adverse outcomes after hospitalization and delirium in persons with Alzheimer's disease, *Ann Intern Med* 156:848, 2012.

*28. Rathier MO, Baker WL: A review of recent clinical trials and guidelines on the prevention and management of delirium in hospitalized older patients, *Hosp Pract* 39(4):96, 2011.

29. Balas MC, Rice M, Chaperon C, et al: Management of delirium in critically ill older adults, *Crit Care Nurse* 32(4):15, 2012.

*30. Neto AS, Nassar AP, Cardoso SO, et al: Delirium screening in critically ill patients: a systematic review and meta-analysis, *Crit Care Med* 40(6):1946, 2012.

RESOURCES

Alzheimer's Association
www.alz.org
Alzheimer's Disease Education and Referral Center
www.alzheimers.org
Caregiver Action Network
http://caregiveraction.org
Lewy Body Dementia Association
www.lewybodydementia.org
National Alliance for Caregiving
www.caregiving.org
National Council on Aging (NCOA)
www.ncoa.org
National Institute of Neurological Disorders and Strokes
www.ninds.nih.gov
National Institute on Aging
www.nia.nih.gov
   Caring for a Person With Alzheimer's Disease
     www.nia.nih.gov/sites/default/files/caring_for_a_person_with_alzheimers_disease_0.pdf
   What Happens Next?
     www.nia.nih.gov/sites/default/files/84206ADEARWhatHappens NextEarlyStageBookletab09OCT01_0.pdf
Stress-Busting Program for Family Caregivers (developed by Sharon Lewis)
www.caregiverstressbusters.org

*Evidence-based information for clinical practice.

So many of our dreams at first seem impossible, then they seem improbable, and then when we summon the will, they soon become inevitable.

Christopher Reeve

Nursing Management
Peripheral Nerve and Spinal Cord Problems

Teresa E. Hills

evolve WEBSITE

http://evolve.elsevier.com/Lewis/medsurg

- NCLEX Review Questions
- Key Points
- Pre-Test
- Answer Guidelines for Case Study on p. 1485
- Rationales for Bridge to NCLEX Examination Questions

- Case Study
  - Patient With Spinal Cord Injury
- Nursing Care Plan (Customizable)
  - eNCP 61-1: Patient With a Spinal Cord Injury
- Concept Map Creator
- Glossary
- Content Updates

eFigures
- eFig. 61-1: Syndromes associated with incomplete cord injuries
- eFig. 61-2: Standard neurologic classification of spinal cord injury

eTable
- eTable 61-1: Comparison of Multiple Sclerosis and Guillain-Barré Syndrome

LEARNING OUTCOMES

1. Explain the etiology, clinical manifestations, collaborative care, and nursing management of trigeminal neuralgia and Bell's palsy.
2. Explain the etiology, clinical manifestations, collaborative care, and nursing management of Guillain-Barré syndrome, botulism, tetanus, and neurosyphilis.
3. Describe the classification of spinal cord injuries and associated clinical manifestations.
4. Describe the clinical manifestations, collaborative care, and nursing management of neurogenic and spinal shock.
5. Relate the clinical manifestations of spinal cord injury to the level of disruption and rehabilitation potential.
6. Describe the nursing management of the major physical and psychologic problems of the patient with a spinal cord injury.
7. Describe the effects of spinal cord injury on the older adult.
8. Explain the types, clinical manifestations, collaborative care, and nursing management of spinal cord tumors.

KEY TERMS

anterior cord syndrome, Table 61-3, p. 1472
autonomic dysreflexia, p. 1479
Bell's palsy, p. 1466
botulism, p. 1468
Brown-Séquard syndrome, Table 61-3, p. 1472
central cord syndrome, Table 61-3, p. 1472
Guillain-Barré syndrome, p. 1467
neurogenic bladder, p. 1480
neurogenic bowel, p. 1481

neurogenic shock, p. 1470
neurosyphilis, p. 1468
paraplegia, p. 1470
posterior cord syndrome, Table 61-3, p. 1472
spinal shock, p. 1470
tetanus, p. 1468
tetraplegia, p. 1470
trigeminal neuralgia, p. 1464

Reviewed by Jean Burt, RN, MSN, Instructor, Wilbur Wright College, Chicago, Illinois; and Fernande E. Deno, RN, MSN, CNE, Instructor, Anoka Ramsey Community College, Coon Rapids, Minnesota.

This chapter discusses peripheral nerve and spinal cord problems, including cranial nerve disorders, polyneuropathies, spinal cord injuries, and spinal cord tumors. A focus of this chapter is the nursing management of the many problems encountered by the patient with a spinal cord injury.

CRANIAL NERVE DISORDERS

Cranial nerve disorders are commonly classified as peripheral neuropathies. The 12 pairs of cranial nerves are considered the peripheral nerves of the brain. The disorders usually involve the motor or sensory (or both) branches of a single nerve (*mononeuropathies*). Causes of cranial nerve problems include tumors, trauma, infections, inflammatory processes, and idiopathic (unknown) causes. Two cranial nerve disorders discussed in this chapter are trigeminal neuralgia and Bell's palsy.

TRIGEMINAL NEURALGIA

Trigeminal neuralgia *(tic douloureux)* is sudden, usually unilateral, severe, brief, stabbing, recurrent episodes of pain in the distribution of the trigeminal nerve. It is diagnosed in approximately 150,000 Americans each year and is the most commonly diagnosed neuralgic condition. It is seen approximately twice as often in women as in men. The majority of cases (more than 90%) are diagnosed in individuals over age 40.[1]

Etiology and Pathophysiology

The trigeminal nerve is the fifth cranial nerve (CN V) and has both motor and sensory branches. In trigeminal neuralgia the sensory or afferent branches, primarily the maxillary and mandibular branches, are involved (Fig. 61-1).

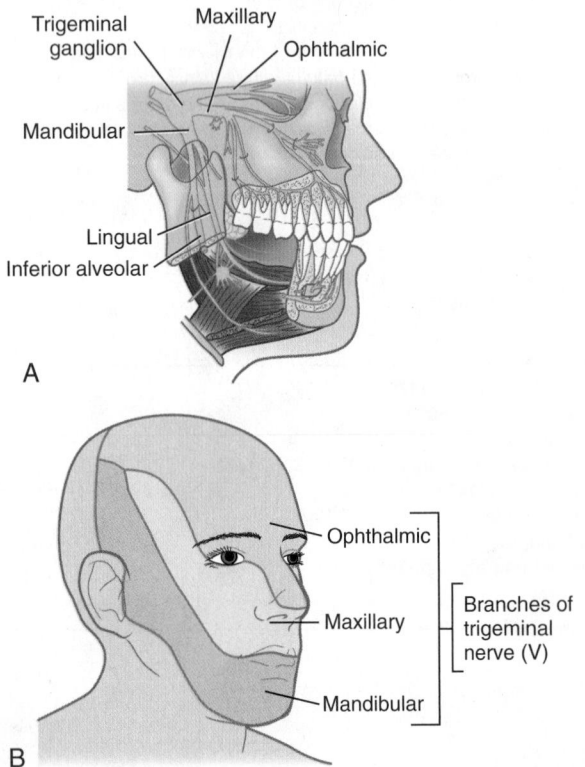

FIG. 61-1 A, Trigeminal (fifth cranial) nerve and its three main divisions: ophthalmic, maxillary, and mandibular nerves. **B,** Cutaneous innervation of the head.

The etiology and pathophysiology of trigeminal neuralgia is not fully understood.[2] One theory is that blood vessels, especially the superior cerebellar artery, become compressed, resulting in chronic irritation of the trigeminal nerve at the root entry zone. This irritation leads to increased firing of the afferent or sensory fibers. Risk factors are multiple sclerosis and hypertension. Other factors that may cause neuralgia include herpesvirus infection, infection of the teeth and jaw, and a brainstem infarct.

Clinical Manifestations

The classic feature of trigeminal neuralgia is an abrupt onset of paroxysms of excruciating pain described as a burning, knifelike, or lightning-like shock in the lips, upper or lower gums, cheek, forehead, or side of the nose. Intense pain, twitching, grimacing, and frequent blinking and tearing of the eye occur during the acute attack (giving rise to the term *tic*). Some patients may also experience facial sensory loss. The attacks are usually brief, lasting only seconds to 2 or 3 minutes, and are generally unilateral.

Recurrences, which are unpredictable, may occur several times a day, or weeks or months apart. After the refractory (pain-free) period, a phenomenon known as clustering can occur. *Clustering* is characterized by a cycle of pain and refractoriness that continues for hours.

The painful episodes are usually initiated by a triggering mechanism of light touch at a specific point *(trigger zone)* along the distribution of the nerve branches. Precipitating stimuli include chewing, tooth brushing, feeling a hot or cold blast of air on the face, washing the face, yawning, or even talking. As a result, the patient may eat improperly, neglect hygienic practices, wear a cloth over the face, and withdraw from interaction with other individuals. The patient may sleep excessively as a means of coping with the pain.

Although this condition is considered benign, the severity of the pain and the disruption of lifestyle can result in almost total physical and psychologic dysfunction or even suicide.

Diagnostic Studies

A computed tomography (CT) scan or magnetic resonance imaging (MRI) of the brain is performed to rule out any lesions (including multiple sclerosis), tumors, or vascular abnormalities. A complete neurologic assessment is done, including audiologic evaluation. The results are usually normal.

Collaborative Care

Once the diagnosis is made, the goal of treatment is relief of pain either medically or surgically (Tables 61-1 and 61-2).

Drug Therapy. Antiseizure drug therapy may reduce pain by stabilizing the neuronal membrane and blocking nerve

TABLE 61-1	COLLABORATIVE CARE
Trigeminal Neuralgia	
Diagnostic	**Collaborative Therapy**

• History and physical examination (including neurologic examination)
 • CT scan
 • MRI
	• Drug therapy
	   • Antiseizure drugs (e.g., carbamazepine [Tegretol], oxcarbazepine [Trileptal])
	   • gabapentin (Neurontin)
	   • Tricyclic antidepressants (e.g., amitriptyline [Elavil])
	 • Local nerve block
	 • Surgical therapy (see Table 61-2)

TABLE 61-2	SURGICAL THERAPY FOR TRIGEMINAL NEURALGIA	
Procedure	**Description**	**Effect**
Peripheral		
Glycerol rhizotomy (injection into one or more branches of the trigeminal nerve)	Chemical ablation	Total pain relief with sparing of touch and corneal reflex.
Intracranial		
Percutaneous radiofrequency rhizotomy	Destruction of sensory fibers by low-voltage current	Total pain relief, sparing of touch and corneal reflex (increased risk for sensory changes).
Microvascular decompression	Lifting of artery pressing on nerve root in posterior fossa with wedge of sponge, leading to removal of pressure at nerve-root entry zone, or removing the involved vessel	Pain relief without loss of sensation.
Gamma knife radiosurgery	Technique that uses high doses of radiation focused on the trigeminal nerve root using stereotactic localization	Pain relief 1 day–4 mo posttreatment. Noninvasive with no loss of sensation.

FIG. 61-2 A, Patient with trigeminal neuralgia having needle placed. **B,** Physician injecting glycerol.

firing.[2] These first-line drugs include carbamazepine (Tegretol), oxcarbazepine (Trileptal), topiramate (Topamax), clonazepam (Klonopin), phenytoin (Dilantin), lamotrigine (Lamictal), and divalproex (Depakote). Gabapentin (Neurontin) or baclofen (Lioresal) can be used in combination with any of the antiseizure drugs if a single agent is not effective. Tricyclic antidepressants such as amitriptyline (Elavil) or nortriptyline (Pamelor, Aventyl) can be used to treat constant burning, or aching pain.[2] Analgesics or opioids are usually not effective in controlling pain.

Conservative Therapy. Nerve blocking with local anesthetics is another treatment option. Relief of pain is temporary, lasting from 6 to 18 months. This treatment is usually tolerated well by older adults.

Some patients use complementary and alternative therapies, usually in combination with drug treatment. These techniques include acupuncture, biofeedback, vitamin therapy, nutritional therapy, and electrical stimulation of the nerves.

Surgical Therapy. If a conservative approach including drug therapy is not effective, surgical therapy is available (see Table 61-2). *Glycerol rhizotomy* is a percutaneous procedure that consists of an injection of glycerol through the foramen ovale into the trigeminal cistern (Fig. 61-2).

Percutaneous radiofrequency rhizotomy is an outpatient procedure consisting of placing a needle into the trigeminal rootlets that are adjacent to the pons and destroying the area by means of a radiofrequency current. This can result in facial numbness (although some degree of sensation may be retained), corneal anesthesia, and trigeminal motor weakness.[3]

Microvascular decompression of the trigeminal nerve is another commonly used procedure for neuralgia. It is done by first performing a small craniotomy behind the ear (suboccipi-

tal craniotomy). The next step involves displacing and repositioning the blood vessels that appear to be compressing the nerve at the root entry zone where it exits the pons. This procedure relieves pain without residual sensory loss, but it is potentially dangerous.[3]

Gamma knife radiosurgery is another surgical treatment that is used to treat trigeminal neuralgia. Radiosurgery (see Chapter 57) using a gamma knife provides precise radiation of the proximal trigeminal nerve identified on high-resolution imaging.

NURSING MANAGEMENT
TRIGEMINAL NEURALGIA

Patients with trigeminal neuralgia are primarily treated on an outpatient basis. Assessment of the attacks, including the triggering factors, characteristics, frequency, and pain management techniques, helps you plan for patient care. The nursing assessment should include the patient's nutritional status, hygiene (especially oral), and behavior (including withdrawal). Evaluate the degree of pain and its effects on the patient's lifestyle, drug use, emotional state, and suicidal tendencies.

Monitor the patient's response to drug therapy and note any side effects. Alternative pain relief measures, such as acupuncture and biofeedback, should be explored for the patient who is not a surgical candidate and whose pain is not controlled by other measures. Environmental management is essential during an acute period to decrease triggering stimuli. The room should be kept at an even, moderate temperature and free of drafts. Many patients prefer to carry out their own care, fearing that someone else will inadvertently injure them.

Teach the patient about the importance of nutrition, hygiene, and oral care and convey understanding if previous oral neglect is apparent. A small, soft-bristled toothbrush or a warm mouthwash assists in promoting oral care. Hygiene activities are best carried out when analgesia is at its peak.

Food should be high in protein and calories and easy to chew. It should be served lukewarm and offered frequently. When oral intake is sharply reduced and the patient's nutritional status is compromised, a nasogastric tube can be inserted on the unaffected side for enteral feedings.

Appropriate teaching related to surgical procedures depends on the type of procedure planned (e.g., percutaneous). Patients need to know that they will be awake during local procedures so that they can cooperate when corneal and ciliary reflexes and facial sensations are checked. After the procedure the patient's pain is compared with the preoperative level. The corneal reflex, extraocular muscles, hearing, sensation, and facial nerve function are evaluated frequently (see Chapter 56). If the corneal reflex is impaired, take special care to protect the eyes. This includes the use of artificial tears or eye shields.

If intracranial surgery is performed, general postoperative nursing care after a craniotomy is appropriate. (Nursing care related to craniotomy is discussed in Chapter 57 on p. 1379.)

After a percutaneous radiofrequency procedure, apply an ice pack to the jaw on the operative side for 3 to 5 hours. To avoid injuring the mouth, the patient should not chew on the operative side until sensation has returned.

Plan for regular follow-up care, and instruct the patient on the dosage and side effects of medications. Although relief of pain may be complete, encourage the patient to keep environmental stimuli to a moderate level and to use stress management techniques. Long-term management after surgical intervention depends on the residual effects of the procedure. If anesthesia is present or the corneal reflex is altered, teach the patient to (1) chew on the unaffected side; (2) avoid hot foods or beverages, which can burn the mucous membranes; (3) check the oral cavity after meals to remove food particles; (4) practice meticulous oral hygiene and continue with semiannual dental visits; (5) protect the face against extremes of temperature; (6) use an electric razor; (7) wear a protective eye shield or avoid rubbing eyes; and (8) examine eye regularly for symptoms of infection or irritation.

BELL'S PALSY

Bell's palsy (peripheral facial paralysis, acute benign cranial polyneuritis) is a disorder characterized by inflammation of the facial nerve (CN VII) on one side of the face in the absence of any other disease such as a stroke. Bell's palsy is an acute, peripheral facial paresis of unknown cause. Each year approximately 40,000 Americans are diagnosed with Bell's palsy. It can affect any age-group. Despite its good prognosis, Bell's palsy leaves more than 8000 people a year in the United States with permanent, potentially disfiguring facial weakness.[4]

Etiology and Pathophysiology

Although the exact etiology is not known, it is believed that a viral infection such as viral meningitis or activation of herpes simplex virus 1 (HSV1) may trigger Bell's palsy. The viral infection causes inflammation, edema, ischemia, and eventual demyelination of the nerve, creating pain and alterations in motor and sensory function. Bell's palsy has also been associated with influenza or a flu-like illness, headaches, chronic middle ear infection, hypertension, diabetes, sarcoidosis, tumors, Lyme disease, and trauma such as skull fracture or facial injury.[4]

Bell's palsy is considered benign, with full recovery in 3 to 6 months, especially if treatment is begun immediately. A small group of patients have long-term facial paralysis.[4]

FIG. 61-3 Facial characteristics of Bell's palsy. **A,** At rest the face may look almost normal, but the patient is not able to wrinkle her forehead on the affected side and the right corner of the mouth droops. **B,** When she is asked to close her eyes and show her teeth, the differences between the affected and unaffected sides become more obvious.

Clinical Manifestations and Diagnostic Studies

The onset of Bell's palsy is often accompanied by an outbreak of herpes vesicles in or around the ear. Patients may complain of pain around and behind the ear. Additional manifestations may include fever, tinnitus, and hearing deficit. Paralysis of the motor branches of the facial nerve typically results in flaccidity of the affected side of the face, with drooping of the mouth accompanied by drooling (Fig. 61-3).

An inability to close the eyelid, with an upward movement of the eyeball when closure is attempted, is also evident. Other manifestations include a widened *palpebral fissure* (the opening between the eyelids); flattening of the nasolabial fold; and inability to smile, frown, or whistle. Unilateral loss of taste is common. Decreased muscle movement may alter chewing ability. Although some patients experience a loss of tearing, many patients complain of excessive tearing. The muscle weakness causes the lower lid to turn out, allowing overflow of normal tear production. Pain may be present behind the ear on the affected side, especially before the onset of paralysis.

Complications include psychologic withdrawal because of changes in appearance, malnutrition, dehydration, mucous membrane trauma, corneal abrasions, muscle stretching, and facial spasms and contractures.

The diagnosis of Bell's palsy is one of exclusion. There is no definitive test. The diagnosis and prognosis are indicated by observing the typical pattern of onset and signs and testing percutaneous nerve excitability by electromyography (EMG).

Collaborative Care

Methods of treatment for Bell's palsy include moist heat, gentle massage, and electrical stimulation of the nerve and prescribed exercises. Stimulation may maintain muscle tone and prevent atrophy. Care is primarily focused on relief of symptoms, prevention of complications, and protection of the eye on the affected side.

Corticosteroids (prednisone) are started immediately, with best results if corticosteroids are initiated before paralysis is complete. When the patient improves to the point that the corticosteroids are no longer necessary, the drug should be tapered over a 2-week period. Because HSV is implicated in approximately 70% of cases of Bell's palsy, treatment with acyclovir (Zovirax), alone or in conjunction with prednisone, may be used. Additional antiviral agents, including valacyclovir

(Valtrex) and famciclovir (Famvir), have also been used in the management of Bell's palsy.

NURSING MANAGEMENT
BELL'S PALSY

The patient with Bell's palsy is treated on an outpatient basis. Mild analgesics can relieve pain. Hot wet packs can reduce the discomfort of herpetic lesions, aid circulation, and relieve pain. Tell the patient to protect the face from cold and drafts because trigeminal *hyperesthesia* (extreme sensitivity to pain or touch) may occur. Maintenance of good nutrition is important. Teach the patient to chew on the unaffected side of the mouth to avoid trapping food and to enjoy the taste of food. Thorough oral hygiene must be carried out after each meal to prevent parotitis, caries, and periodontal disease from accumulated residual food.

The patient may wear dark glasses for protective and cosmetic reasons. Artificial tears (methylcellulose) should be instilled frequently during the day to prevent drying of the cornea. Ointment and an impermeable eye shield can be used at night to retain moisture. In some patients, taping the lids closed at night may be necessary to provide protection. Instruct the patient to report ocular pain, drainage, or discharge.

A facial sling may be helpful to support affected muscles, improve lip alignment, and facilitate eating. The facial sling is usually made and fitted by a physical or occupational therapist. When function begins to return, active facial muscle exercises are performed several times a day.

The change in physical appearance as a result of Bell's palsy can be devastating. Reassure the patient that a stroke did not occur and that chances for a full recovery are good. Enlisting support from family and friends is important. Tell the patient that most patients recover within about 6 weeks of the onset of symptoms.

POLYNEUROPATHIES

GUILLAIN-BARRÉ SYNDROME

Guillain-Barré syndrome (Landry-Guillain-Barré-Strohl syndrome, postinfectious polyneuropathy, ascending polyneuropathic paralysis) is an acute, rapidly progressing, and potentially fatal form of polyneuritis. It is characterized by ascending, symmetric paralysis that usually affects cranial nerves and the peripheral nervous system. The syndrome is rare, affecting an estimated 3000 to 6000 Americans each year. It affects males and females equally.[5,6]

Etiology and Pathophysiology

The etiology of this disorder is unknown. Both cellular and humoral immune mechanisms play a role in the immune reaction directed at the nerves. The result is a loss of myelin (a segmental demyelination) and edema and inflammation of the affected nerves. As demyelination occurs, the transmission of nerve impulses is stopped or slowed down. The muscles innervated by the damaged peripheral nerves undergo denervation and atrophy. In the recovery phase, remyelination occurs slowly, and neurologic function returns in a proximal-to-distal pattern.[6] Guillain-Barré syndrome is similar in presentation to multiple sclerosis (MS), and therefore a full diagnostic workup should be performed to rule out MS (see Chapter 59).

The syndrome is often preceded by immune system stimulation from a viral infection, trauma, surgery, or viral immuniza-

tions. *Campylobacter jejuni* gastroenteritis is thought to precede Guillain-Barré syndrome in approximately 30% of cases.[5-7]

Clinical Manifestations and Complications

Guillain-Barré syndrome is a heterogeneous condition with manifestations ranging from mild to severe. Weakness of the lower extremities (evolving more or less symmetrically) occurs over hours to days to weeks, usually peaking about the fourteenth day. *Paresthesia* (numbness and tingling) is common, with paralysis usually following in the extremities. *Hypotonia* (reduced muscle tone) and *areflexia* (lack of reflexes) are common manifestations.[5-7]

In Guillain-Barré syndrome, autonomic nervous system dysfunction results, with manifestations of orthostatic hypotension, hypertension, and abnormal vagal responses (bradycardia, heart block, asystole). Other autonomic dysfunctions include bowel and bladder dysfunction, facial flushing, and diaphoresis. Patients may also have syndrome of inappropriate antidiuretic hormone (SIADH) secretion.[8] (SIADH is discussed in Chapter 50.) Cranial nerve involvement is manifested as facial weakness, extraocular eye movement difficulties, dysphagia, and paresthesia of the face.

Pain is a common symptom in the patient with Guillain-Barré syndrome. The pain can be paresthesias, muscular aches and cramps, and hyperesthesias. Pain appears to be worse at night. Opioids may be indicated for those experiencing severe pain. Pain may lead to a decrease in appetite and may interfere with sleep.

The most serious complication is respiratory failure, which occurs as the paralysis progresses to the nerves that innervate the thoracic area. Constant monitoring of the respiratory system by checking respiratory rate and depth provides information about the need for immediate intervention, including intubation and mechanical ventilation. Respiratory or urinary tract infections (UTIs) may occur. Immobility from the paralysis can cause problems such as paralytic ileus, muscle atrophy, deep vein thrombosis, pulmonary emboli, skin breakdown, orthostatic hypotension, and nutritional deficiencies.

Diagnostic Studies

Diagnosis is based primarily on the patient's history and clinical signs. Cerebrospinal fluid (CSF) is normal or has a low protein content initially, but after 7 to 10 days it shows an elevated protein level (normal protein is 15 to 45 mg/dL [0.15 to 0.45 g/L]) with a normal cell count. Results of EMG and nerve conduction studies are markedly abnormal (reduced nerve conduction velocity) in the affected extremities. A brain MRI can be done to rule out MS.

NURSING AND COLLABORATIVE MANAGEMENT
GUILLAIN-BARRÉ SYNDROME

Management of Guillain-Barré syndrome is aimed at supportive care, particularly ventilatory support, during the acute phase. Plasmapheresis is used in the first 2 weeks. (Plasmapheresis is discussed in Chapter 14.) IV administration of high-dose immunoglobulin (Sandoglobulin) has been as effective as plasma exchange and is more readily available.

Beyond 3 weeks after disease onset, plasmapheresis and immunoglobulin therapies have little value. Corticosteroids appear to have little effect on the prognosis or duration of the disease.

Assessment of the patient is the most important aspect of nursing care during the acute phase. During the routine assessment, monitor the ascending paralysis; assess respiratory function; monitor arterial blood gases (ABGs); and assess the gag, corneal, and swallowing reflexes. Reflexes are usually decreased or absent.

Monitor blood pressure (BP) and cardiac rate and rhythm during the acute phase because dysrhythmias may occur. Autonomic dysfunction is common and usually takes the form of bradycardia and dysrhythmias. Orthostatic hypotension secondary to muscle atony may occur in severe cases. Vasopressor agents and volume expanders may be needed to treat the low BP. However, the presence of SIADH may require fluid restriction.

The objective of therapy is to support body systems until the patient recovers. Respiratory failure and infection are serious threats. Monitoring the vital capacity and ABGs is essential. If the vital capacity drops to less than 800 mL or the ABGs deteriorate, endotracheal intubation or tracheostomy may be done so that the patient can be mechanically ventilated (see Chapter 68). If fever develops, obtain sputum cultures to identify the pathogen. Appropriate antibiotic therapy is then initiated.

Nutritional needs must be met in spite of possible problems associated with delayed gastric emptying, paralytic ileus, and potential for aspiration if the gag reflex is lost. In addition to testing for the gag reflex, note drooling and other difficulties with secretions that may indicate an inadequate gag reflex. Initially, enteral or parenteral nutrition may be used to ensure adequate caloric intake. Because of delayed gastric emptying, assess residual volumes of the feedings at regular intervals or before feedings (see Chapter 40).

Throughout the course of the illness, provide support and encouragement to the patient, caregiver, and family. Although 85% to 95% of patients almost completely recover, it is generally a slow process that takes months or years. About 30% of those with Guillain-Barré have some residual weakness.[5-7]

BOTULISM

Botulism is rare but the most serious type of food poisoning. It is caused by gastrointestinal (GI) absorption of the neurotoxin produced by *Clostridium botulinum*. This organism is found in the soil, and the spores are difficult to destroy. It can grow in any food contaminated with the spores. Improper home canning of foods is often the cause.[9] It is thought that the neurotoxin destroys or inhibits the neurotransmission of acetylcholine at the myoneural junction, resulting in disturbed muscle innervation.

Neurologic manifestations can develop rapidly or evolve over several days. They include a descending paralysis with muscle incoordination and weakness, difficulty swallowing, seizures, and respiratory muscle weakness that can rapidly deteriorate to respiratory and/or cardiac arrest.

The clinical manifestations, prevention, and treatment are presented in Table 42-24. Patient and caregiving teaching related to food poisoning are presented in Table 42-25. Nursing care during the acute illness is similar to that for Guillain-Barré syndrome. Supportive nursing interventions include rest, activities to maintain respiratory function, adequate nutrition, and prevention of loss of muscle mass.

TETANUS

Tetanus (lockjaw) is a severe infection of the nervous system affecting spinal and cranial nerves. It results from the effects of a potent neurotoxin released by the anaerobic bacillus *Clostridium tetani*. The spores of the bacillus are present in soil, garden mold, and manure. *C. tetani* enters the body through a wound that provides an appropriate low-oxygen environment for the organisms to mature and produce toxin. Examples of possible wounds include IV drug use injection sites, human and animal bites, burns, frostbite, open fractures, and gunshot wounds.[10,11]

Initial manifestations of tetanus include stiffness in the jaw (*trismus*) and neck and signs of infection (e.g., fever). As the disease progresses, the neck muscles, back, abdomen, and extremities become progressively rigid. In severe forms, continuous tonic seizures may occur with *opisthotonos* (extreme arching of the back and retraction of the head). Laryngeal and respiratory spasms cause apnea and anoxia. The slightest noise, jarring motion, or bright light can set off a seizure. These seizures are agonizingly painful. Mortality rate is almost 100% in the severe form.[11]

Tetanus prevention and immunizations, which are the most important factors influencing the incidence of this disease, are summarized in Table 69-6. Adults should receive a tetanus and diphtheria toxoid booster every 10 years. Teach the patient that immediate, thorough cleansing of all wounds with soap and water is important to prevent tetanus. If an open wound occurs and the patient has not been immunized within 5 years, the health care provider should be contacted so that a tetanus booster can be given.

The management of tetanus includes administration of a tetanus toxoid, diphtheria toxoid, and pertussis (Tdap) booster and tetanus immune globulin (TIG) in different sites before the onset of symptoms to neutralize circulating toxins (see Table 69-6). A much larger dose of TIG is administered to patients with clinical manifestations of tetanus.[10-12]

Control of spasms is essential and is managed by sedation and skeletal muscle relaxation, usually with diazepam (Valium), barbiturates, and, in severe cases, neuromuscular blocking agents such as vecuronium (Norcuron) that act to paralyze skeletal muscles. Opioid analgesics such as morphine or fentanyl are also indicated for pain management. A 10- to 14-day course of penicillin, metronidazole, tetracycline, or doxycycline is recommended to inhibit further growth of *C. tetani*.[11]

Because of laryngospasm and the potential need for neuromuscular blocking drugs, a tracheostomy is usually performed early and the patient is maintained on mechanical ventilation. Sedative agents and opioid analgesics are given concomitantly to all patients who are pharmacologically paralyzed. Any recognized wound should be debrided or an abscess drained. Antibiotics may be given to prevent secondary infections.

NEUROSYPHILIS

Neurosyphilis is caused by *Treponema pallidum*, the bacteria that cause syphilis. It usually occurs about 10 to 20 years after a person is first infected with syphilis. Not everyone who has syphilis will develop this complication. It is the result of untreated or inadequately treated syphilis (see Chapter 53). The organism can invade the central nervous system within a few months of the original infection. Untreated neurosyphilis, although not contagious, can be fatal.

Late neurosyphilis results from degenerative changes in the spinal cord (tabes dorsalis) and brainstem (general paresis). *Tabes dorsalis* (progressive locomotor ataxia) is characterized by vague, sharp pains in the legs; ataxia; "slapping" gait; loss of proprioception and deep tendon reflexes; and zones of hyperesthesia. *Charcot's joints,* which are characterized by enlargement, bone destruction, and hypermobility, also occur as a result of joint effusion and edema. Other manifestations of neurosyphilis include seizures, vision and hearing problems, and cognitive impairment.[13]

Management includes treatment with penicillin, symptomatic care, and protection from physical injury.[13] The prognosis after treatment depends on how severe the neurosyphilis is before treatment. The neurologic deficits may remain or progress after treatment.

SPINAL CORD PROBLEMS

SPINAL CORD INJURY

Spinal cord injury (SCI) is caused by trauma or damage to the spinal cord. It can result in either a temporary or permanent alteration in the function of the spinal cord. About 12,000 Americans suffer SCIs each year. About 260,000 persons in the United States are living with SCI.[14,15] With improved treatment strategies, even the very young patient with an SCI can anticipate a long life. The potential for disruption of individual growth and development, altered family dynamics, economic loss in terms of employment, and the high cost of rehabilitation and long-term health care make SCI a major problem.

Young adult men between ages 16 and 30 years have the greatest risk for SCI. Eighty-one percent of people with SCI are male. There has also been an increase in the number of older adults with SCIs. This trend toward older age at time of injury is reflected in the overall increase in mean age of people with SCI from 28 years in the 1970s to 40 years at this time.[15]

Although many people with SCIs can care for themselves independently, those with the highest level of injury may require round-the-clock care at home or in a long-term care facility. Almost 90% of patients with SCI are discharged from the hospital to home or another noninstitutional residence. The remaining 10% are discharged to nursing homes, chronic care facilities, or group homes.

Etiology and Pathophysiology

SCIs are usually a result of trauma. The most common causes are motor vehicle collisions (42%), falls (27%), violence (15%), sports injuries (7%), and other miscellaneous causes (8%).[15]

Types of Injury. The extent of the neurologic damage caused by an SCI results from *primary injury* (actual physical disruption of axons) and *secondary injury* (ischemia, hypoxia, hemorrhage, and edema).

Primary Injury. The spinal cord is wrapped in tough layers of dura and is rarely torn or transected by direct trauma. SCI can be due to cord compression by bone displacement, interruption of blood supply to the cord, or traction resulting from pulling on the cord. Penetrating trauma, such as gunshot and stab wounds, can result in tearing and transection. The initial mechanical disruption of axons as a result of stretch or laceration is referred to as the *primary injury.*

Secondary Injury. *Secondary injury* refers to the ongoing, progressive damage that occurs after the primary injury.[16] Several theories exist on what causes this ongoing damage, including free radical formation, uncontrolled calcium influx, ischemia, and lipid peroxidation. *Apoptosis* (cell death) occurs

---

ETHICAL/LEGAL DILEMMAS
Right to Refuse Treatment

Situation

R.D., a 25-yr-old man, suffered a spinal cord injury (SCI) to C7-8 following a motorcycle accident. He was diagnosed with anterior cord syndrome and has motor paralysis, which may prevent him from riding motorcycles again. He has become extremely depressed and no longer wishes to live. Because of his emotional state, R.D. is now refusing to eat. Can he be forced to receive enteral nutrition (tube feeding)?

Ethical/Legal Points for Consideration
- Withholding treatment in a newly injured but otherwise healthy young adult may present an ethical dilemma for some nurses. They may consider it assisted suicide and believe that it violates an ethical principle.
- A competent adult has the right to consent to or refuse medical treatment under the right to privacy, the Fourteenth Amendment of the Constitution, and case law.*
- Case law has also supported the concept that forced treatment constitutes battery (unlawful use of force on somebody). Furthermore, a mentally competent, physically incapacitated adult can refuse feeding by nasogastric tube and compel the health facility to follow the patient's wishes.†
- To be competent to participate in informed consent or refusal, an adult must be able to understand the information provided about the procedure or treatment, consider choices between alternatives available, and make a choice based on his values and preferences. Depression may not be a determinant in competency to make informed treatment choices.
- If, after adequate treatment for pain, depression, or other medical conditions, the patient persists in his refusal, his wishes must be respected.
- Refusal to eat or drink has never been upheld as illegal, and the alternative—forced eating and drinking—is clearly a violation of patient rights and the criminal act of battery.

Discussion Questions
1. What are your feelings about requests to withhold treatment in a young person with a newly acquired disability?
2. What resources are available to help R.D., his family, and the staff work through this emotionally charged and ethically complex situation?

Cruzan v. Director, Missouri Department of Health, 497 U.S. 261, 1990. Retrieved from *http://supreme.justia.com/cases/federal/us/497/261.*
†*Bouvia v. Superior Court,* 1986. Retrieved from *http://law.justia.com/cases/california/calapp3d/179/1127.html.*

---

and sometimes may continue for weeks or months after the initial injury. Thus the complete cord damage (previously thought to be transection) in severe trauma is related to autodestruction of the cord. Hemorrhagic areas in the center of the spinal cord appear within 1 hour, and by 4 hours there may be infarction in the gray matter.[16] This ongoing destructive process makes it critical that the initial care and management of the patient with an SCI be initiated as soon as possible to limit further destruction of the spinal cord.

Fig. 61-4 illustrates the cascade of events causing secondary injury after traumatic SCI. The resulting hypoxia reduces the oxygen levels below the metabolic needs of the spinal cord. Lactate metabolites and an increase in vasoactive substances, including norepinephrine, serotonin, and dopamine, are noted. At high levels, these vasoactive substances cause vasospasms and hypoxia, leading to subsequent necrosis. Unfortunately, the spinal cord has minimal ability to adapt to vasospasm.

By 24 hours or less, permanent damage may occur because of the development of edema. The edema secondary to the inflammatory response is particularly harmful because of lack

PATHOPHYSIOLOGY MAP

FIG. 61-4 Cascade of metabolic and cellular events that leads to spinal cord ischemia and hypoxia of secondary injury. *RBCs,* Red blood cells; *SCBF,* spinal cord blood flow.

of space for tissue expansion. Therefore compression of the spinal cord occurs. Edema extends above and below the injury, thus increasing the ischemic damage. Because secondary injury progresses over time, the extent of the injury and prognosis for recovery are most accurately determined at least 72 hours or more after injury.

Spinal and Neurogenic Shock. About 50% of people with acute SCI experience a temporary neurologic syndrome known as spinal shock. This type of shock is characterized by decreased reflexes, loss of sensation, and flaccid paralysis below the level of injury.[16] This syndrome lasts days to months and may mask postinjury neurologic function.

Neurogenic shock, in contrast to spinal shock, is due to the loss of vasomotor tone caused by injury and is characterized by hypotension and bradycardia. Loss of sympathetic nervous system innervation causes peripheral vasodilation, venous pooling, and a decreased cardiac output. These effects are generally associated with a cervical or high thoracic injury (T6 or higher).

Classification of Spinal Cord Injury. SCIs are classified by the (1) mechanism of injury, (2) level of injury, and (3) degree of injury.

Mechanisms of Injury. The major mechanisms of injury are flexion, hyperextension, flexion-rotation, extension-rotation, and compression[17] (Fig. 61-5). The flexion-rotation injury is the most unstable of all because the ligamentous structures that stabilize the spine are torn. This injury is most often implicated in severe neurologic deficits.

Level of Injury. *Skeletal level* of injury is the vertebral level where there is the most damage to vertebral bones and ligaments. *Neurologic level* is the lowest segment of the spinal cord

with normal sensory and motor function on both sides of the body. The level of injury may be cervical, thoracic, lumbar, or sacral. Cervical and lumbar injuries are most common because these levels are associated with the greatest flexibility and movement. If the cervical cord is involved, paralysis of all four extremities occurs, resulting in tetraplegia (formerly termed *quadriplegia*). However, when the damage is low in the cervical cord, the arms are rarely completely paralyzed.

If the thoracic, lumbar, or sacral spinal cord is damaged, the result is paraplegia (paralysis and loss of sensation in the legs). Fig. 61-6 shows affected structures and functions at different levels of cord injury.

Degree of Injury. The degree of spinal cord involvement may be either complete or incomplete (partial). *Complete cord involvement* results in total loss of sensory and motor function below the level of injury. *Incomplete cord involvement* results in a mixed loss of voluntary motor activity and sensation and leaves some tracts intact. The degree of sensory and motor loss varies depending on the level of injury and reflects the specific nerve tracts damaged.[16]

Six syndromes are associated with incomplete injuries: central cord syndrome, anterior cord syndrome, Brown-Séquard syndrome, posterior cord syndrome, cauda equina syndrome, and conus medullaris syndrome[16] (Table 61-3).

Clinical Manifestations

The manifestations of SCI are generally the direct result of trauma that causes cord compression, ischemia, edema, and possible cord transection. Manifestations of SCI are related to the level and degree of injury. The patient with an incomplete injury may demonstrate a mixture of manifestations. The higher the injury, the more serious the sequelae because of the proximity of the cervical cord to the medulla and brainstem.[16,17]

American Spinal Injury Association (ASIA) Impairment Scale. The American Spinal Injury Association (ASIA) Impairment Scale is commonly used for classifying the severity of impairment resulting from SCI. It combines assessments of motor and sensory function to determine neurologic level and completeness of injury (Fig. 61-7, and eFig. 61-2, available on the website for this chapter).

The sensory regions are called *dermatomes,* with each segment of the spinal cord innervating a particular area of skin. Each dermatome has a specific point recommended for testing, as shown in eFig. 61-2. A dermatome map is also shown in Fig. 56-6.

The ASIA Impairment Scale is useful for recording changes in neurologic status and identifying appropriate goals for rehabilitation. Movement and rehabilitation potential related to specific locations of the SCI are described in Table 61-4. In general, sensory function closely parallels motor function at all levels.

Respiratory System. Respiratory complications closely correspond to the level of injury. Cervical injuries above the level of C4 present special problems because of the total loss of respiratory muscle function. Mechanical ventilation is required to keep the patient alive. At one time the majority of these patients died at the scene of the injury, but with improved emergency medical services, more of these patients are surviving the initial events of their SCI.

Injury or fracture below the level of C4 results in diaphragmatic breathing if the phrenic nerve is functioning. Even if the injury is below C4, spinal cord edema and hemorrhage can affect the function of the phrenic nerve and cause respiratory insufficiency. Hypoventilation almost always occurs with dia-

FIG. 61-5 Mechanisms of spinal cord injury. Many situations may produce these injuries. This only shows some examples. **A,** Flexion injury of the cervical spine ruptures the posterior ligaments. **B,** Hyperextension injury of the cervical spine ruptures the anterior ligaments. **C,** Compression fractures crush the vertebrae and force bony fragments into the spinal canal. **D,** Flexion-rotation injury of the cervical spine often results in tearing of ligamentous structures that normally stabilize the spine.

phragmatic respirations because of the decrease in vital capacity and tidal volume, a result of impairment of the intercostal muscles.

Cervical and thoracic injuries cause paralysis of abdominal muscles and often the intercostal muscles. Therefore the patient cannot cough effectively enough to remove secretions, leading to atelectasis and pneumonia. An artificial airway provides direct access for pathogens, making bronchial hygiene and chest physiotherapy extremely important measures to reduce infection. Neurogenic pulmonary edema may occur secondary to a dramatic increase in sympathetic nervous system activity at the time of injury, which shunts blood to the lungs. In addition, pulmonary edema may occur in response to fluid overload.

Cardiovascular System. Any cord injury above the level of T6 greatly decreases the affect of the sympathetic nervous system. Bradycardia occurs. Peripheral vasodilation results in hypotension. A relative hypovolemia exists because of the increase in the capacity of the dilated veins. Cardiac monitoring is necessary. In marked bradycardia (heart rate less than 40 beats/minute), appropriate drugs (e.g., atropine) to increase the heart rate and prevent hypoxemia are necessary. The peripheral vasodilation reduces the venous return of blood to the

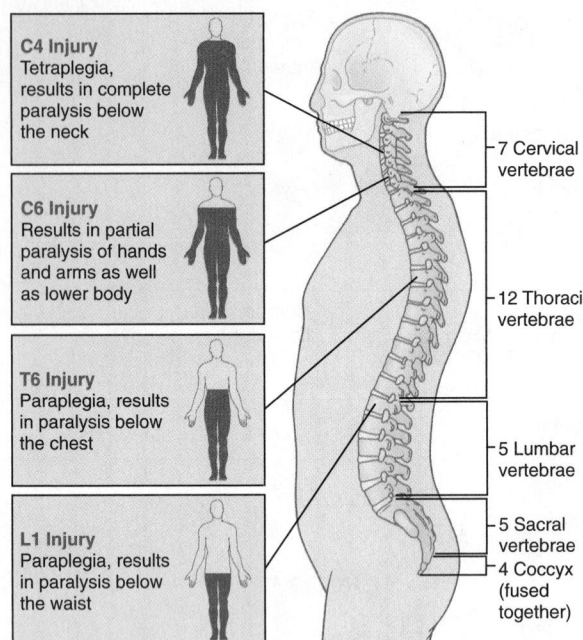

FIG. 61-6 Symptoms, degree of paralysis, and potential for rehabilitation depend on the level of the injury.

American Spinal Injury Association (ASIA) Impairment Scale

☐ **A = Complete:** No motor or sensory function is preserved in the sacral segments S4-5.

☐ **B = Incomplete:** Sensory but not motor function is preserved below the neurologic level and includes the sacral segments S4-5.

☐ **C = Incomplete:** Motor function is preserved below the neurologic level, and more than half of key muscles below the neurologic level have a muscle grade less than 3.

☐ **D = Incomplete:** Motor function is preserved below the neurologic level, and at least half of key muscles below the neurologic level have a muscle grade of 3 or more.

☐ **E = Normal:** Motor and sensory function are normal.

FIG. 61-7 The American Spinal Injury Association Impairment Scale. See eFig. 61-2 on the website for this chapter for standard neurologic classification of spinal cord injury.

TABLE 61-3	INCOMPLETE SPINAL CORD INJURY SYNDROMES
Description	**Manifestations**
Central Cord Syndrome • Caused by damage to the central spinal cord (see eFig. 61-1). • Occurs most commonly in the cervical cord region. • More common in older adults.	• Motor weakness and sensory loss are present in both upper and lower extremities. • Upper extremities are affected more than the lower ones.
Anterior Cord Syndrome • Caused by damage to the anterior spinal artery. • Results in compromised blood flow to the anterior spinal cord. • Typically results from injury causing acute compression of anterior portion of the spinal cord, often a flexion injury (see eFig. 61-1).	• Motor paralysis and loss of pain and temperature sensation below the level of injury. • Because posterior cord tracts are not injured, sensations of touch, position, vibration, and motion remain intact.
Brown-Séquard Syndrome • Results from damage to one half of the spinal cord (see eFig. 61-1). • Typically results from penetrating injury to spinal cord.	• *Ipsilateral* (same side as injury): Loss of motor function and position and vibratory sense, vasomotor paralysis. • *Contralateral* (opposite side of injury): Loss of pain and temperature sensation below the level of injury.
Posterior Cord Syndrome • Results from compression or damage to the posterior spinal artery. • Very rare condition.	• Generally the dorsal columns are damaged, resulting in loss of proprioception. • Pain, temperature sensation, and motor function below the level of injury remain intact.
Conus Medullaris Syndrome and Cauda Equina Syndrome • Result from damage to conus (lowest portion of the spinal cord) and cauda equina (lumbar and sacral nerve roots).	• Flaccid paralysis of the lower limbs and areflexic (flaccid) bladder and bowel.

---

heart and subsequently decreases cardiac output, resulting in hypotension. IV fluids or vasopressor drugs may be required to support the BP.

Urinary System. Urinary retention is a common development in acute SCI and spinal shock. While the patient is in spinal shock, the bladder is atonic and becomes overdistended. An indwelling catheter is inserted to drain the bladder. In the postacute phase the bladder may become hyperirritable, with a loss of inhibition from the brain resulting in reflex emptying. Chronic indwelling catheterization increases the risk of infection.

Gastrointestinal System. If the SCI has occurred above the level of T5, the primary GI problems are related to hypomotility. Decreased GI motor activity contributes to the development of paralytic ileus and gastric distention. A nasogastric tube for intermittent suctioning may relieve the gastric distention. Metoclopramide (Reglan) may be used to treat delayed gastric

emptying. The development of stress ulcers is common because of excessive release of hydrochloric (HCl) acid in the stomach.

Intraabdominal bleeding may occur and is difficult to diagnose because the person with an SCI may experience no pain or tenderness. Continued hypotension in spite of vigorous treatment and decreased hemoglobin and hematocrit may be indications of bleeding. Expanding girth of the abdomen may also be noted.

Loss of voluntary neurologic control over the bowel results in a *neurogenic bowel*. In the early period after injury when spinal shock is present and for patients with an injury level of T12 or below, the bowel is *areflexic* and sphincter tone is decreased. As reflexes return, the bowel becomes *reflexic*, sphincter tone is enhanced, and reflex emptying occurs. Both areflexic and reflexic neurogenic bowel can be managed successfully with a regular bowel program coordinated with the gastrocolic reflex to minimize fecal incontinence.

Integumentary System. A major consequence of lack of movement is the potential for skin breakdown over bony prom-

TABLE 61-4 LEVEL OF SPINAL CORD INJURY AND REHABILITATION POTENTIAL

Movement Remaining	Rehabilitation Potential	Movement Remaining	Rehabilitation Potential
Tetraplegia **C1-3** Often fatal injury. Movement in neck and above, loss of innervation to diaphragm, absence of independent respiratory function.	Ability to drive electric wheelchair equipped with portable ventilator by using chin control or mouth stick, headrest to stabilize head. Computer use with mouth stick, head wand, or noise control. Attendant care 24 hr/day, able to instruct others.	**C7-8** All triceps to elbow extension, finger extensors and flexors, good grasp with some decreased strength, decreased respiratory reserve.	Ability to transfer self to wheelchair. Roll over and sit up in bed. Push self on most surfaces. Perform most self-care. Independent use of wheelchair. Ability to drive car with powered hand controls (in some patients). Attendant care 0-6 hr/day.
C4 Sensation and movement in neck and above. May be able to breathe without a ventilator.	Same as C1-3.	**Paraplegia** **T1-6** Full innervation of upper extremities. Back, essential intrinsic muscles of hand; full strength and dexterity of grasp. Decreased trunk stability, decreased respiratory reserve.	Full independence in self-care and in wheelchair. Ability to drive car with hand controls (in most patients). Independent standing in standing frame.
C5 Full neck, partial shoulder, back, biceps. Gross elbow, inability to roll over or use hands. Decreased respiratory reserve.	Ability to drive electric wheelchair with mobile hand supports. Indoor mobility in manual wheelchair. Able to feed self with setup and adaptive equipment. Attendant care 10 hr/day.	**T6-12** Full, stable thoracic muscles and upper back. Functional intercostals, resulting in increased respiratory reserve.	Full independent use of wheelchair. Ability to stand erect with full leg brace, ambulate on crutches with swing (although gait difficult). Inability to climb stairs.
C6 Shoulder and upper back abduction and rotation at shoulder, full biceps to elbow flexion, wrist extension, weak grasp of thumb, decreased respiratory reserve.	Ability to assist with transfer and perform some self-care. Feed self with hand devices. Push wheelchair on smooth, flat surface. Drive adapted van from wheelchair. Independent computer use with adaptive equipment. Attendant care 6 hr/day.	**L1-2** Varying control of legs and pelvis, instability of lower back.	Good sitting balance. Full use of wheelchair. Ambulation with long leg braces.
		L3-4 Quadriceps and hip flexors, absence of hamstring function, flail ankles.	Completely independent ambulation with short leg braces and canes. Inability to stand for long periods.

inences in areas of decreased or absent sensation. Pressure ulcers can occur quickly and can lead to major infection and sepsis.

Thermoregulation. *Poikilothermism* is the adjustment of the body temperature to the room temperature. This occurs in SCIs because the interruption of the sympathetic nervous system prevents peripheral temperature sensations from reaching the hypothalamus. With spinal cord disruption there is also decreased ability to sweat or shiver below the level of injury, which also affects the ability to regulate body temperature. The degree of poikilothermism depends on the level of injury. Patients with high cervical injuries have a greater loss of ability to regulate temperature than do those with thoracic or lumbar injuries.

Metabolic Needs. Nasogastric suctioning may lead to metabolic alkalosis, and decreased tissue perfusion may lead to acidosis. Electrolyte levels, including sodium and potassium, can be altered by gastric suctioning. Monitor these electrolytes until suctioning is discontinued and a normal diet is resumed. Loss of weight (greater than 10%) is common. The person with an SCI has greater nutritional needs than other patients who are immobilized. A high-protein diet helps prevent skin breakdown and infections and decreases the rate of muscle atrophy.

Peripheral Vascular Problems. Venous thromboembolism (VTE) is a common problem accompanying SCI during the first 3 months.[18] It is more difficult to detect a deep venous thrombosis (DVT) in a person with an SCI because the usual signs and symptoms, such as pain and tenderness, are not present. Pulmonary embolism is one of the leading causes of death in patients with SCI.

Diagnostic Studies

CT scan is the preferred imaging study to diagnose the location and degree of injury and degree of spinal canal compromise. Cervical x-rays are obtained when CT scan is not readily available. However, it is often difficult to visualize C7 and T1 on a cervical x-ray, compromising the ability to fully evaluate cervical spine injury. MRI is used to assess for soft tissue and neurologic changes and for unexplained neurologic deficits or worsening of neurologic status. A comprehensive neurologic examination is performed along with assessment of the head, chest, and abdomen for additional injuries or trauma. Patients with cervical injuries who demonstrate altered mental status may also need a CT angiogram to rule out vertebral artery damage.

Duplex Doppler ultrasound, impedance plethysmography, venous occlusion plethysmography, venography, and the clinical examination are recommended for use as diagnostic tests for DVT.

Collaborative Care

Immediate postinjury goals include maintaining a patent airway, adequate ventilation, and adequate circulating blood volume and preventing extension of cord damage (secondary

✚ TABLE 61-5 EMERGENCY MANAGEMENT

Spinal Cord Injury

Etiology	Assessment Findings	Interventions
Blunt Trauma • Compression, flexion, extension, or rotational injuries to spinal column • Motor vehicle collisions • Pedestrian incidents • Falls • Diving **Penetrating Trauma** • Stretched, torn, crushed, or lacerated spinal cord • Gunshot wounds • Stab wounds	• Pain, tenderness, deformities, or muscle spasms adjacent to vertebral column • Numbness, paresthesias • Alterations in sensation: temperature, light touch, deep pressure, proprioception • Weakness or heaviness in limbs • Weakness, paralysis, or flaccidity of muscles • Spinal shock • Cuts; bruises; open wounds over head, face, neck, or back • Neurogenic shock: hypotension, bradycardia, dry, flushed skin • Bowel and bladder incontinence • Urinary retention • Difficulty breathing • Priapism • Diminished rectal sphincter tone	**Initial** • Ensure patent airway. • Immobilize and stabilize cervical spine.* • Administer O_2 via nasal cannula or non-rebreather mask. • Establish IV access with two large-bore catheters to infuse normal saline or lactated Ringer's solution as appropriate. • Assess for other injuries. • Control external bleeding. • Obtain CT scan or cervical spine x-rays. **Ongoing Monitoring** • Monitor vital signs, level of consciousness, O_2 saturation, cardiac rhythm, urine output. • Keep warm. • Monitor for urinary retention, hypertension. • Anticipate need for intubation if gag reflex absent.

*Spinal immobilization is not recommended in patients who have penetrating trauma.

TABLE 61-6 COLLABORATIVE CARE

Cervical Cord Injury

Diagnostic
- History and physical examination, including complete neurologic examination
- Arterial blood gases
- Serial bedside PFTs
- Electrolytes, glucose level, coagulation profile, hemoglobin and hematocrit levels
- Urinalysis
- CT scan, MRI
- X-rays of spine
- Anteroposterior, lateral, and odontoid spinal x-ray studies
- EMG to measure evoked potentials
- Duplex Doppler ultrasound, impedance plethysmography

Collaborative Therapy
Acute Care
- Immobilization of vertebral column
- Maintenance of heart rate (e.g., atropine) and blood pressure (e.g., dopamine [Intropin])
- Insertion of nasogastric tube and attachment to suction
- Intubation (if indicated by ABGs and PFTs)
- O_2 by high-humidity mask
- Indwelling urinary catheter
- Administration of IV fluids
- Stress ulcer prophylaxis
- Deep vein thrombosis prophylaxis
- Bowel and bladder training

Rehabilitation and Home Care
- Physical therapy
  - Range-of-motion exercises
  - Mobility training
  - Muscle strengthening
- Occupational therapy (splints, activities of daily living training)
- Bowel and bladder training
- Autonomic dysreflexia prevention
- Pressure ulcer prevention
- Recreational therapy
- Patient and caregiver teaching

injury). Table 61-5 outlines the emergency management of the patient with an SCI. Recommended immobilization includes a combination of a rigid cervical collar and supportive blocks on a backboard with straps. Spinal immobilization with sandbags and tape is insufficient and is not recommended. Spinal immobilization in patients with penetrating trauma is not recommended because of increased mortality. The concern during the initial management of patients with potential cervical spinal injuries is that neurologic function may be impaired as a result of movement of the injured vertebrae.[19,20]

Systemic and neurogenic shock must be treated to maintain BP. For injury at the cervical level, all body systems must be maintained until the full extent of the damage can be evaluated.

Collaborative care during the acute phase for a patient with a cervical injury is described in Table 61-6. Compared to cervical injury, patients with SCIs of the thoracic and lumbar vertebrae require less intense support. Respiratory compromise is not as severe, and bradycardia is usually not a problem. Specific problems are treated symptomatically.

After stabilization at the injury scene, the person is transferred to a medical facility. A thorough assessment is done to specifically evaluate the degree of deficit and to establish the level and degree of injury. A history is obtained, with emphasis on how the incident occurred and the extent of injury as perceived by the patient immediately after the event. Assessment involves testing muscle groups rather than individual muscles. Test muscle groups with and against gravity, alone and against resistance, and on both sides of the body. Note spontaneous movement. Ask the patient to move legs and then hands, spread fingers, extend wrists, and shrug shoulders. After assessing motor status, carry out a sensory examination, including touch and pain as tested by pinprick, starting at the toes and working upward toward the head. If time and conditions permit, also assess position sense and vibration.

The types of injury mechanisms that cause spinal cord trauma, especially those involving the cervical cord, may also result in brain injury. Therefore assess for a history of unconsciousness, signs of concussion, and increased intracranial pressure (see Chapter 57). In addition, perform a careful assessment for musculoskeletal injuries and trauma to internal organs.

Because the patient has no muscle, bone, or visceral sensations, the only clue to internal trauma with hemorrhage may be a rapidly increasing BP and pulse. Examine the urine for hematuria, which is also indicative of internal injuries.

Move the patient in alignment as a unit (*logroll*) during transfers and when repositioning to prevent further injury. Monitor respiratory, cardiac, urinary, and GI functions. The patient may go directly to surgery after initial immobilization and stabilization or to the intensive care unit (ICU) for monitoring and management.

Nonoperative Stabilization. Nonoperative treatments involve stabilization of the injured spinal segment and decompression, either through traction or realignment. Stabilization methods eliminate damaging motion at the injury site. These methods are intended to prevent secondary spinal cord damage caused by repeated contusion or compression.

Surgical Therapy. The decision to perform surgery on a patient with an SCI often depends on the particular physician's preference. When cord compression is certain or the neurologic disorder progresses, immediate surgery may be beneficial. Surgery decompresses and stabilizes the spinal column. Early cord decompression may reduce secondary injury to the spinal cord and therefore improve the outcome. Other criteria used in the decision for early surgery include (1) evidence of cord compression, (2) progressive neurologic deficit, (3) compound fracture of the vertebrae, (4) bony fragments (may dislodge and penetrate the cord), and (5) penetrating wounds of the spinal cord or surrounding structures.

Surgery to stabilize the spine can be performed from the back of the spine (*posterior approach*) or from the front of the spine (*anterior approach*). In some cases, both approaches may be needed. A fusion procedure involves attaching metal screws, plates, or other devices to the bones of the spine to help keep them properly aligned. This is usually done when two or more vertebrae have been injured. Small pieces of bone may also be attached to the injured bones to help them fuse into one solid piece. The bone used for this procedure is usually taken from another bone in the body, most often from the hip. (Specific surgical and nursing interventions for these techniques are discussed in Chapter 64 on pp. 1548-1550.)

Drug Therapy. Methylprednisolone (MP), which was used for many years to treat acute SCI, is no longer recommended. It is not approved by the Food and Drug Administration (FDA) for this use and there is no evidence of clinical benefit of MP to treat acute SCI. High-dose MP is associated with harmful side effects including immunosuppression, increased frequency of upper GI bleeding, increased risk of infection, sepsis, longer stays in the ICU, and sometimes death.[21]

Low-molecular-weight heparin (e.g., enoxaparin [Lovenox]) is used to prevent VTE unless contraindicated. Contraindications include internal bleeding and recent surgery. Oral anticoagulation alone is not recommended as a prophylactic treatment strategy.[22]

Vasopressor agents such as dopamine (Intropin) are used in the acute phase as adjuvants to treatment. These agents are used to maintain the mean arterial pressure at a level greater than 90 mm Hg so that perfusion to the spinal cord is improved.

Drug metabolism is altered in patients with an SCI. Therefore drug interactions may occur. The differences in drug metabolism correlate with level and completeness of injury, with greater change apparent in people with cervical cord injury than in those with injury at lower spinal levels.

NURSING MANAGEMENT
SPINAL CORD INJURY

NURSING ASSESSMENT

Subjective and objective data that should be obtained from a patient with a recent SCI are presented in Table 61-7.

NURSING DIAGNOSES

Nursing diagnoses for the patient with an SCI depend on the severity of the injury and the level of dysfunction. The nursing diagnoses for a patient with an SCI may include, but are not limited to, the following:

- Ineffective breathing pattern *related to* respiratory muscle fatigue, neuromuscular paralysis, and/or retained secretions
- Impaired skin integrity *related to* immobility and/or poor tissue perfusion
- Impaired urinary elimination *related to* spinal injury and/or limited fluid intake
- Constipation *related to* neurogenic bowel, inadequate fluid intake, and/or immobility
- Risk for autonomic dysreflexia *related to* reflex stimulation of sympathetic nervous system

Additional information on nursing diagnoses for the patient with an SCI is presented in eNursing Care Plan 61-1 (available on the website for this chapter). The care plan is for a patient with a complete cervical cord injury.

PLANNING

The overall goals are that the patient with an SCI will (1) maintain an optimal level of neurologic functioning; (2) have minimal or no complications of immobility; (3) learn new skills, gain new knowledge, and acquire new behaviors to be able to care for self or successfully direct others to do so; and (4) return to home and the community at an optimal level of functioning.

NURSING IMPLEMENTATION

HEALTH PROMOTION. Nursing interventions for the prevention of an SCI include identification of high-risk populations, counseling, and teaching. Support of legislation related to seat belt use in cars, helmets for motorcyclists and bicyclists, child safety seats, and tougher penalties for drunk-driving offenses is a professional responsibility.

Emphasize the importance of other health promotion and health screening in addition to SCI care. After injury, health-promoting behaviors can have a significant impact on the general health and well-being of the individual with an SCI. Nursing interventions include teaching and counseling; referral to programs such as smoking cessation classes, recreation and exercise programs, and alcohol treatment programs; and performing routine physical examinations for non-neurologic problems. Outpatient health care requires that the facilities for the screening and prevention programs must be accessible to and accommodate people with SCI. Nurses in these clinical settings should advocate for wheelchair-accessible examination rooms, adjustable-height examination tables, and scheduling that allows extra time if needed.

ACUTE INTERVENTION. High cervical cord injury caused by flexion-rotation is the most complex SCI and is discussed in this section. Interventions for this type of injury can be modified for patients with less severe injuries.

TABLE 61-7   NURSING ASSESSMENT
Spinal Cord Injury

Subjective Data
Important Health Information
Health history: Motor vehicle collision, sports injury, industrial incident, gunshot or stabbing injury, falls

Functional Health Patterns
Health perception–health management: Use of alcohol or recreational drugs; risk-taking behaviors
Activity-exercise: Loss of strength, movement, and sensation below level of injury; dyspnea, inability to breathe adequately ("air hunger")
Cognitive-perceptual: Tenderness, pain at or above level of injury; numbness, tingling, burning, twitching of extremities
Coping–stress tolerance: Fear, denial, anger, depression

Objective Data
General
Poikilothermism (unable to regulate body heat)

Integumentary
Warm, dry skin below level of injury (neurogenic shock)

Respiratory
Injury at C1-3: Apnea, inability to cough
Injury at C4: Poor cough, diaphragmatic breathing, hypoventilation
Injury at C5-T6: Decreased respiratory reserve

Cardiovascular
Injury above T5: Bradycardia, hypotension, postural hypotension, absence of vasomotor tone

Gastrointestinal
Decreased or absent bowel sounds (paralytic ileus in injuries above T5), abdominal distention, constipation, fecal incontinence, fecal impaction

Urinary
Retention (for injuries at T1-L2); flaccid bladder (acute stages); spasticity with reflex bladder emptying (later stages)

Reproductive
Priapism, loss of sexual function

Neurologic
Complete: Flaccid paralysis and anesthesia below level of injury resulting in tetraplegia (for injuries above C8) or paraplegia (for injuries below C8), hyperactive deep tendon reflexes, bilaterally positive Babinski test (after resolution of spinal shock)
Incomplete: Mixed loss of voluntary motor activity and sensation

Musculoskeletal
Muscle atony (in flaccid state), contractures (in spastic state)

Possible Diagnostic Findings
Location of level and type of bony involvement on spinal x-ray: injury, edema, compression on CT scan and MRI; positive finding on myelogram

FIG. 61-8 Cervical traction is attached to tongs inserted in the skull.

For cervical injuries, skeletal traction is used less frequently since the development of better surgical stabilization. When skeletal traction is used, the goal is realignment or reduction of the injury. Crutchfield (Fig. 61-8), Vinke, or Gardner-Wells tongs or other types of devices can provide this type of traction, using a rope that extends from the center of the tongs over a pulley and has weights attached at the end. Traction must be maintained at all times. Depending on the type of injury and the goal of treatment, the tongs and traction may be removed 1 to 4 weeks after the injury. One disadvantage of skull tongs is that the skull pins can be displaced. If this occurs, hold the head in a neutral position and get help. Stabilize the head while the physician reinserts the tongs.

Infection at the sites of tong insertion is another potential problem. Preventive care includes cleansing the sites twice a day with normal saline solution and applying an antibiotic ointment, which acts as a mechanical barrier to the entrance of bacteria. The procedures for preventive care of insertion sites may vary depending on individual hospital standards of care.

Special beds are often used in the management of the patient with SCI (Fig. 61-9). Kinetic therapy is the continuous side-to-side rotation of a patient to 40 degrees or more to help prevent pulmonary complications. This lateral rotation also redistributes pressure, helping prevent pressure ulcers.

After cervical fusion or other stabilization surgery, a hard cervical collar or sternal-occipital-mandibular immobilizer brace can be worn (Fig. 61-10). In a stable injury for which surgery is not done, a halo fixation apparatus may be applied. The halo is the most frequently used method of stabilizing cervical injuries. The halo apparatus can be used to apply cervical traction by means of a jacket-like arrangement (Fig. 61-11). Hanging weights, such as those used with tongs, can be incorporated with the halo. In addition, the apparatus can be attached to a body vest, stabilizing the injured area and allowing ambulation if the patient is neurologically intact. Another alternative is to use the halo after the patient has had traction removed. It allows the patient to be more mobile and to begin active rehabilitation.

Patients with thoracic or lumbar spine injuries are immobilized with a custom thoracolumbar orthosis ("body jacket"), which inhibits spinal flexion, extension, and rotation, or with a Jewett brace, which restricts forward flexion.

Immobilization of the neck of the patient with an SCI prevents further injury, but the effects of immobility are profound. Meticulous skin care is critical because decreased sensation and circulation make the patient particularly susceptible to skin breakdown. Remove the patient's backboard as soon as possible

Immobilization. Proper immobilization of the neck involves the maintenance of a neutral position.

SAFETY ALERT
- Use a hard cervical collar, and a backboard to stabilize the neck to prevent lateral rotation of the cervical spine.
- The body should always be correctly aligned.
- Perform turning so that the patient is moved as a unit (i.e., logrolling) to prevent movement of the spine.

FIG. 61-9 The RotoRest Therapy System helps prevent and treat pulmonary complications for immobile patients, including those with unstable cervical, thoracic, and lumbar fractures. Kinetic therapy, the continual side-to-side bilateral rotation of the patient, redistributes pulmonary blood flow and mobilizes secretions to improve ventilation and perfusion matching. The therapy system also helps to prevent pressure ulcers. (Courtesy Arjo Huntleigh, Addison, Ill.)

FIG. 61-10 Sternal-occipital-mandibular immobilizer brace.

Halo ring

Skull pins

Struts

Vest

FIG. 61-11 Halo vest. The halo traction brace immobilizes the cervical spine, which allows the patient to ambulate and participate in self-care.

and replace it with other forms of immobilization to prevent coccygeal and occipital area skin breakdown. Properly fit cervical collars. Inspect the areas under the halo vest or jacket or under braces or orthoses to assess the skin condition.

Respiratory Dysfunction. During the first 48 hours after injury, spinal cord edema may increase the level of dysfunction, and respiratory distress may occur. If the injury is at or above C3, or if the patient is exhausted from labored breathing or ABGs deteriorate (indicating inadequate oxygenation or ventilation), initiate endotracheal intubation or tracheostomy and mechanical ventilation. The possibility of respiratory arrest requires careful monitoring and prompt action should it occur. Pneumonia and atelectasis are potential problems because of reduced vital capacity and the loss of intercostal and abdominal muscle function, resulting in diaphragmatic breathing, pooled secretions, and an ineffective cough.

The older adult has a more difficult time responding to hypoxia and hypercapnia. Therefore aggressive chest physiotherapy, adequate oxygenation, and proper pain management are essential to maximize respiratory function and gas exchange. Other respiratory problems include nasal stuffiness and bronchospasm.

Regularly assess (1) breath sounds, (2) ABGs, (3) tidal volume, (4) vital capacity, (5) skin color, (6) breathing patterns (especially the use of accessory muscles), (7) subjective comments about the ability to breathe, and (8) the amount and color of sputum. A PaO₂ (partial pressure of oxygen in arterial blood) greater than 60 mm Hg and a PaCO₂ (partial pressure of carbon dioxide in arterial blood) less than 45 mm Hg are acceptable values in a patient with uncomplicated tetraplegia. A patient who is unable to count to 10 aloud without taking a breath needs immediate attention.

In addition to monitoring, you can intervene to maintain ventilation. Administer oxygen until ABGs stabilize. Chest physiotherapy and assisted coughing help to clear secretions. Assisted (augmented) coughing simulates the action of the ineffective abdominal muscles during the expiratory phase of a cough. Place the heels of both hands just below the xiphoid process and exert firm upward pressure to the area timed with the patient's efforts to cough (see Fig. 68-7). Perform tracheal suctioning if crackles or rhonchi are present. Incentive spirometry is an additional technique that can be used to improve the patient's respiratory status.

Cardiovascular Instability. Because of unopposed vagal response, the heart rate is slowed, often to less than 60 beats/minute. Any increase in vagal stimulation, such as turning or suctioning, can result in cardiac arrest. Loss of sympathetic nervous system tone in peripheral vessels results in chronic low BP with potential postural hypotension. Lack of muscle tone to aid venous return can result in sluggish blood flow and predispose the patient to DVT.

Frequently assess vital signs. If bradycardia is symptomatic, administer an anticholinergic drug such as atropine. A temporary or permanent pacemaker may be inserted in some patients. Hypotension is managed with a vasopressor agent, such as dopamine or norepinephrine, and fluid replacement.

In the older adult, consider the effects of aging on the cardiovascular system. The older patient is less able to handle the stress of traumatic injury because heart contractions weaken and cardiac output is reduced. Maximum heart rate is also reduced. In addition to the effects of aging, the older person may also have cardiovascular disease.

Sequential compression devices or compression gradient stockings can be used to prevent thromboemboli and to promote venous return. Remove the stockings every 8 hours for skin care. Venous duplex studies may be performed before applying compression devices. Also regularly perform range-of-motion exercises and stretching. Assess the thighs and calves every shift for signs of DVT (e.g., deep reddish color, edema).

If blood loss has occurred from other injuries, monitor hemoglobin and hematocrit levels and administer blood according to protocol. Also monitor the patient for indications of hypovolemic shock secondary to hemorrhage.

Fluid and Nutritional Maintenance. During the first 48 to 72 hours after the injury, the GI tract may stop functioning (paralytic ileus) and a nasogastric tube must be inserted. Because the patient cannot have oral intake, carefully monitor fluid and electrolyte status. Specific solutions and additives are ordered based on individual requirements.

Once bowel sounds are present or flatus is passed, gradually introduce oral food and fluids. Because of severe catabolism, a high-protein, high-calorie diet is necessary for energy and tissue repair. In patients with high cervical cord injuries, evaluate swallowing before starting oral feedings. If the patient is unable to resume eating, enteral nutrition may be used to provide nutritional support (see Chapter 40).

Some patients experience anorexia, which can be due to depression, boredom with institutional food, or discomfort at being fed (often by a hurried nurse). Some patients have a normally small appetite. Occasionally, refusal to eat is a means of maintaining control over the environment because of diminished or absent body control. If the patient is not eating adequately, thoroughly assess the cause.

On the basis of this assessment, make a contract with the patient using mutual goal setting regarding the diet. This gives the patient increased control of the situation and often results in improved nutritional intake. General measures such as providing a pleasant eating environment, allowing adequate time to eat (including any self-feeding the patient can achieve), encouraging the family to bring in special foods, and planning social rewards for eating may be useful. Keep a calorie count, and record the patient's daily weight to evaluate progress. If feasible, the patient should participate in recording calorie intake. Dietary supplements may be necessary to meet nutritional needs. Increased dietary fiber should be included to promote bowel function. Avoid allowing the patient's nutritional intake to become a basis for a power struggle.

Bladder and Bowel Management. Immediately after the injury, urine is retained because of the loss of autonomic and reflex control of the bladder and sphincter. Because there is no sensation of fullness, overdistention of the bladder can result in reflux into the kidney with eventual renal failure. Bladder overdistention may even result in rupture of the bladder. Consequently, an indwelling catheter is usually inserted as soon as possible after injury. Ensure the patency of the catheter by frequent inspection and irrigation if necessary. In some institutions a physician's order is required for this procedure. Strict aseptic technique for catheter care is essential to avoid introducing

EVIDENCE-BASED PRACTICE

Applying the Evidence

You are a nurse working in the rehabilitation unit for patients recovering from spinal cord injuries. K.T., a 26-yr-old man who suffered a spinal cord injury after his 4-wheeler overturned,, has an areflexic bladder. You have discussed the various options for bladder management. He tells you that he would prefer the indwelling catheter. He thinks that this choice would be the least disruptive to his daily schedule of activities.

Best Available Evidence	Clinician Expertise	Patient Preferences and Values
Patients using indwelling catheters, compared with those using intermittent catheters, have similar satisfaction with life and perceived health status. There may be more complications associated with an indwelling catheter (e.g., urinary tract infections) than those associated with intermittent catheterization.	You know that an areflexic bladder is best managed with either an indwelling catheter or intermittent catheterization. You also know that patients may hesitate to select intermittent catheterization for a variety of reasons (e.g., they believe the procedure is painful, they are afraid of performing the procedure incorrectly and possibly hurting themselves, they do not want their lives interrupted by the need to drain their bladder 5-6 times per day).	After reviewing all the information, K.T. indicates that he would prefer an indwelling catheter to intermittent catheterization as the method to self-manage his bladder.

Your Decision and Action

As his nurse, you respect and support his decision. You plan to teach K.T. and his caregiver how to obtain the necessary supplies and care for the catheter once discharged.

References for Evidence

Akkoç Y, Ersöz M, Yıldız N: Effects of different bladder management methods on the quality of life in patients with traumatic spinal cord injury, *Spinal Cord* 51:226, 2013.
Cameron AP, Wallner LP, Forchheimer MB, et al: Medical and psychosocial complications associated with method of bladder management after traumatic spinal cord injury, *Arch Phys Med Rehabil* 92(3):449, 2011.

infection. During the period of indwelling catheterization, a large fluid intake is required. Check the catheter to prevent kinking and ensure free flow of urine.

UTIs are a common problem. The best method for preventing UTIs is regular and complete bladder drainage. After the patient is stabilized, assess the best means of managing long-term urinary function. Usually the patient is started on an intermittent catheterization program. (Intermittent catheterization is discussed on p. 1481 later in this chapter and in Chapter 46.)

Intermittent catheterization should be done every 3 to 4 hours to prevent bacterial overgrowth from urinary stasis. If the appearance or odor of the urine is suspicious or if the patient develops symptoms of a UTI (e.g., chills, fever, malaise), send a specimen for culture.

Consider age-related changes in renal function. The older adult is more likely to develop renal calculi. Older men may have benign prostatic hyperplasia, which may interfere with urinary flow and complicate management of urinary problems.

Constipation is generally a problem during spinal shock because no voluntary or involuntary (reflex) evacuation of the bowels occurs. A bowel program should be started during acute care. This consists of choosing a rectal stimulant (suppository or small-volume enema) to be inserted daily at a regular time, followed by gentle digital stimulation or manual evacuation until evacuation is complete.[23] Initially the program may be done in bed with the patient in the side-lying position, but as soon as the patient has resumed sitting, it should be done in the upright position on a padded bedside commode chair.

Temperature Control. Because there is no vasoconstriction, piloerection, or heat loss through perspiration below the level of injury, temperature control is largely external to the patient. Monitor the environment closely to maintain an appropriate temperature. Also regularly monitor body temperature. Do not overload patients with covers or unduly expose them (such as during bathing). If an infection with high fever develops, more extensive means of temperature control, such as a cooling blanket, may be necessary.

Stress Ulcers. Stress ulcers are a problem for the patient with an SCI because of the physiologic response to severe trauma and psychologic stress. Peak incidence of stress ulcers is 6 to 14 days after injury. Test stool and gastric contents daily for blood, and monitor the hematocrit for a slow drop. Histamine (H_2)-receptor blockers (e.g., ranitidine [Zantac], famotidine [Pepcid]) or proton pump inhibitors (e.g., pantoprazole [Protonix], omeprazole [Prilosec]) may be given prophylactically to decrease the secretion of HCl acid and prevent ulcers during the initial phase.

Sensory Deprivation. You need to compensate for the patient's absent sensations to prevent sensory deprivation. Do this by stimulating the patient above the level of injury. Conversation, music, and interesting foods can be a part of the nursing care plan. Provide prism glasses so that the patient can read and watch television. Make every effort to prevent the patient from withdrawing from the environment.

Patients with SCI often report altered sensorium and vivid dreams during the acute phase of their treatment. Whether this is due to drugs used to manage pain and anxiety is not known. Patients may also experience disrupted sleep patterns as a result of the hospital environment or posttraumatic stress disorder.[24]

Reflexes. Once spinal cord shock is resolved, the return of reflexes may complicate rehabilitation. Lacking control from the higher brain centers, reflexes are often hyperactive and produce exaggerated responses. Penile erections can occur from a variety of stimuli, causing embarrassment and discomfort. Spasms ranging from mild twitches to convulsive movements below the level of injury may also occur. The patient or caregiver may interpret this reflex activity as a return of function. Tactfully explain the reason for the activity. Inform the patient of the positive use of these reflexes in sexual, bowel, and bladder retraining. Spasms may be controlled with the use of antispasmodic drugs such as baclofen, dantrolene (Dantrium), and tizanidine (Zanaflex). Botulism toxin injections may also be given to treat severe spasticity.

Autonomic Dysreflexia. The return of reflexes after the resolution of spinal shock means that patients with an injury level at T6 or higher may develop autonomic dysreflexia. **Autonomic dysreflexia** (also known as *autonomic hyperreflexia*) is a massive uncompensated cardiovascular reaction mediated by the sympathetic nervous system.[25] It involves stimulation of sensory receptors below the level of the SCI. The intact sympathetic nervous system below the level of injury responds to the stimulation with a reflex arteriolar vasoconstriction that increases BP, but the parasympathetic nervous system is unable to directly counteract these responses via the injured spinal cord. Baroreceptors in the carotid sinus and the aorta sense the hypertension and stimulate the parasympathetic system. This results in a decrease in heart rate, but the visceral and peripheral vessels do not dilate because efferent impulses cannot pass through the injured spinal cord.

The most common precipitating cause of autonomic dysreflexia is a distended bladder or rectum. However, autonomic dysreflexia can be caused by any sensory stimulation, including contraction of the bladder or rectum, stimulation of the skin, or stimulation of pain receptors.

Manifestations include hypertension (up to 300 mm Hg systolic), throbbing headache, marked diaphoresis above the level of injury, bradycardia (30 to 40 beats/minute), *piloerection* (erection of body hair) as a result of pilomotor spasm, flushing of the skin above the level of injury, blurred vision or spots in the visual fields, nasal congestion, anxiety, and nausea. It is important to measure BP when a patient with an SCI complains of a headache.

This is a life-threatening condition that requires immediate resolution. If uncorrected, autonomic dysreflexia can lead to status epilepticus, stroke, myocardial infarction, and even death.

Nursing interventions in this serious emergency are elevating the head of the bed 45 degrees or sitting the patient upright, notifying the physician, and determining the cause. The most common cause is bladder irritation. Immediate catheterization to relieve bladder distention may be necessary. Instill lidocaine jelly in the urethra before catheterization. If a catheter is already in place, check it for kinks or folds. If it is plugged, perform small-volume irrigation slowly and gently to open a plugged catheter, or insert a new catheter.

Stool impaction can also result in autonomic dysreflexia. Perform a digital rectal examination only after application of an anesthetic ointment to decrease rectal stimulation and to avoid increasing symptoms. Remove all skin stimuli, such as constrictive clothing and tight shoes. Monitor BP frequently during the episode. If symptoms persist after the source has been relieved, administer an α-adrenergic blocker or an arteriolar vasodilator (e.g., nifedipine [Procardia]). Continue careful monitoring until vital signs stabilize.

Teach the patient and caregiver to recognize the causes and symptoms of autonomic dysreflexia (Table 61-8). They must understand the life-threatening nature of this dysfunction and know how to relieve the cause.

REHABILITATION AND HOME CARE. Rehabilitation of the person with an SCI is complex. With physical and psychologic care and intensive and specialized rehabilitation, the patient with an SCI can learn to function at the highest level of wellness. It is recommended that all patients with a new SCI receive comprehensive inpatient rehabilitation in a rehabilitation unit or center that specializes in spinal cord rehabilitation.

Many of the problems identified in the acute period become chronic and continue throughout life. Rehabilitation focuses on retraining of physiologic processes and extensive patient, caregiver, and family teaching about how to manage the physiologic and life changes resulting from the injury (Fig. 61-12).

Rehabilitation is an interdisciplinary endeavor carried out through a team approach. Team members include rehabilitation nurses, physicians, physical therapists, occupational therapists, speech therapists, vocational counselors, psychologists, therapeutic recreation specialists, prosthetists, orthotists, and dietitians.

Rehabilitation care is organized around the individual patient's goals and needs. Patients are expected to be involved in therapies and learn self-care for several hours each day. Such intensive work at a time when the patient is dealing with the sudden change in health and functional status can be stressful. Progress may be slow. The rehabilitation nurse has a pivotal role in providing encouragement, specialized nursing care, and patient and caregiver teaching, and in helping to coordinate the efforts of the rehabilitation team.

Respiratory Rehabilitation. The patient with a high cervical SCI may have greatly increased mobility with phrenic nerve stimulators or electronic diaphragmatic pacemakers. These devices are not appropriate for all ventilator-dependent patients but may be helpful for those with an intact phrenic nerve. Ventilators are also reasonably portable, and ventilator-dependent tetraplegic patients can be mobile and somewhat independent. Patients and caregivers should be taught all aspects of home ventilator care, with referrals made to appropriate community agencies. Teach patients with cervical-level injuries who are not ventilator dependent assisted coughing, regular use of incentive spirometry, or deep breathing exercises.

Neurogenic Bladder. A **neurogenic bladder** is any type of bladder dysfunction related to abnormal or absent bladder innervation. After spinal cord shock resolves, depending on the completeness of the SCI, patients usually have some degree of neurogenic bladder. Normal voiding requires nervous system coordination of urethral and pelvic floor relaxation with simultaneous contraction of the detrusor muscle. Depending on the injury, a neurogenic bladder may have no reflex detrusor contractions (areflexic, flaccid), may have hyperactive reflex detrusor contractions (hyperreflexic, spastic), or may lack coordination between detrusor contraction and urethral relaxation *(dyssynergia).* Common problems with a neurogenic bladder include urgency, frequency, incontinence, inability to void, and high bladder pressures resulting in reflux of urine into the kidneys.[26]

Types of neurogenic bladder are presented in Table 61-9. Diagnostic and collaborative care of neurogenic bladder is described in Table 61-10. The patient with an SCI and a neurogenic bladder requires a comprehensive program to manage bladder function.

After the patient's overall condition is stable and there is evidence of neurologic reflexes, urodynamic testing (see Table 45-8) and a urine culture are done. Many factors are considered when selecting a bladder management strategy. These include patient preference, upper extremity function, and availability of a caregiver. The type of bladder dysfunction (see Table 61-9) also determines management options.

TABLE 61-8	PATIENT & CAREGIVER TEACHING GUIDE

Autonomic Dysreflexia

For a patient at risk for autonomic dysreflexia, include the following information in the teaching plan for the patient and caregiver.

1. Signs and symptoms
   - Sudden onset of acute headache
   - Elevation in blood pressure and/or reduction in pulse rate
   - Flushed face and upper chest (above the level of injury) and pale extremities (below the level of injury)
   - Sweating above the level of injury
   - Nasal congestion
   - Feeling of apprehension
2. Immediate interventions
   - Raise the person to a sitting position.
   - Remove the noxious stimulus (fecal impaction, kinked urinary catheter, tight clothing).
   - Call the health care provider if above actions do not relieve the signs and symptoms.
3. Measures to decrease the incidence of autonomic dysreflexia
   - Maintain regular bowel function.
   - If manual rectal stimulation is used to promote bowel function, local anesthetics may prevent autonomic dysreflexia.
   - Monitor urine output.
   - Wear a Medic Alert bracelet indicating a history of risk for autonomic dysreflexia.

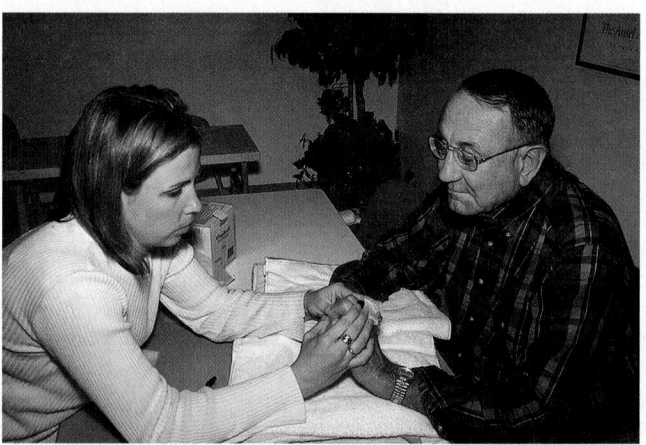

FIG. 61-12 Patient participating in occupational therapy.

TABLE 61-9	TYPES OF NEUROGENIC BLADDER		
	Characteristics	**Causes**	**Manifestations**
Reflexic (spastic, uninhibited)	No inhibitions influence time and place of voiding. Bladder empties in response to stretching of bladder wall.	Results from upper motor neuron injury, corticospinal tract injury. Observed in spinal cord injury, stroke, multiple sclerosis, brain tumor, brain trauma.	Incontinence, frequency, urgency. Voiding is unpredictable and incomplete.
Areflexic (autonomous, flaccid)	Bladder acts as if there were paralysis of all motor functions, fills without emptying.	Results from lower motor neuron injury caused by trauma involving S2-4. Lesions of cauda equina, pelvic nerves.	If sensory function intact, patient feels bladder distention and hesitancy. No control of micturition, resulting in overdistention of bladder and overflow incontinence.
Sensory (lack of sensation of need to urinate)	Damage to sensory limb of bladder spinal reflex arc.	Seen in multiple sclerosis, diabetes mellitus.	Poor bladder sensation, infrequent voiding of large residual volume.

TABLE 61-10	**COLLABORATIVE CARE**

Neurogenic Bladder

Diagnostic
- History and physical examination, including neurologic examination
- Urodynamic testing
- CT urogram
- Intravenous pyelogram
- Urine culture

Collaborative Therapy
- Drug therapy
  - Anticholinergics
  - α-Adrenergic blockers
  - Antispasmodics
- Fluid intake of 1800-2000 mL/day
- Urine drainage
  - Voluntary or reflex voiding
  - Intermittent catheterization
  - Indwelling catheter
- Surgical therapy
  - Sphincterotomy
  - Electrical stimulation
  - Urinary diversion

TABLE 61-11	**PATIENT & CAREGIVER TEACHING GUIDE**

Bowel Management After Spinal Cord Injury

For the patient with a spinal cord injury include the following information about bowel management in the teaching plan for the patient and caregiver.

1. Optimal nutritional intake includes the following:
   - Three well-balanced meals each day
   - Two servings from the milk group
   - Two or more servings from the meat group, including beef, pork, poultry, eggs, fish
   - Four or more servings from the vegetable and fruit groups
   - Four or more servings from the bread and cereal group
2. Fiber intake should be approximately 20-30 g/day. The amount of fiber eaten should be increased gradually over 1-2 wk.
3. Two to three quarts of fluid per day should be consumed unless contraindicated. Water or fruit juices should be used (fluid softens hard stools). Caffeinated beverages such as coffee, tea, and cola should be limited (caffeine stimulates fluid loss through urination).
4. Avoid foods that produce gas (e.g., beans) or upper GI upset (spicy foods).
5. *Timing:* Establish a regular schedule for bowel evacuation. A good time is 30 min after the first meal of the day.
6. *Position:* If possible, an upright position with feet flat on the floor or on a stepstool enhances bowel evacuation. Staying on the toilet, commode, or bedpan for longer than 20-30 min may cause skin breakdown. Based on stability, someone may need to stay with the patient.
7. *Activity:* Exercise is important for bowel function. In addition to improving muscle tone, it also increases GI transit time and increases appetite. Muscles should be exercised. This includes stretching, range-of-motion, position changing, and functional movement.
8. *Drug treatment:* Suppositories may be necessary to stimulate a bowel movement. Manual stimulation of the rectum may also be helpful in initiating defecation. Use stool softeners as needed to regulate stool consistency. Use oral laxatives only if necessary.

Various drugs can be used to treat neurogenic bladders. Anticholinergic drugs (oxybutynin [Ditropan], tolterodine [Detrol]) may be used to suppress bladder contraction. α-Adrenergic blockers (e.g., terazosin [Hytrin], doxazosin [Cardura]) may be used to relax the urethral sphincter, and antispasmodic drugs (e.g., baclofen) may be used to decrease spasticity of pelvic floor muscles.

Numerous drainage methods are possible, including bladder reflex retraining if partial voiding control remains, indwelling catheter, intermittent catheterization, and external catheter (condom catheter). Evaluate the long-term use of an indwelling catheter because of the associated high incidence of UTI, fistula formation, and diverticula. However, for some patients this may be the best option. Patients with indwelling catheters need to have an adequate fluid intake (at least 3 to 4 L/day). Regularly check the patency of the indwelling catheter. The frequency of routine catheter changes ranges widely depending on the type of catheter used and agency policy.

Intermittent catheterization is the most commonly recommended method of bladder management (see Chapter 46). Nursing assessment is important in selecting the time interval between catheterizations. Initially, catheterization is done every 4 hours. Bladder volume can be assessed before catheterization using the portable bladder ultrasound machine. If less than 200 mL of urine is measured, the time interval may be extended. If more than 500 mL of urine is measured, the time interval is shortened. Usually five or six intermittent catheterizations are done per day.

Urinary diversion surgery may be necessary if the patient has repeated UTIs with renal involvement or repeated stones or if therapeutic interventions have been unsuccessful. Surgical treatment of neurogenic bladder includes bladder neck revision (sphincterotomy), bladder augmentation (augmentation cystoplasty), penile prosthesis, artificial sphincter, perineal ureterostomy, cystotomy, vesicotomy, and anterior urethral transplantation. (Urinary diversion procedures are discussed in Chapter 46.)

No matter which bladder management strategy is selected, teach the patient, caregiver, and family how to accomplish successful self-management. Inform them about management techniques, how to obtain necessary supplies, care of supplies and equipment, and when to seek health care. Arrange for resources and referrals for supplies and ongoing care.

Neurogenic Bowel. Careful management of bowel evacuation is necessary in the patient with an SCI because voluntary control of this function may be lost. This condition is called **neurogenic bowel.** The usual measures for preventing constipation include a high-fiber diet and adequate fluid intake (see Table 43-6). Patient and caregiver teaching guidelines related to bowel management are presented in Table 61-11. However, these measures by themselves may not be adequate to stimulate evacuation. In addition, suppositories (bisacodyl [Dulcolax] or glycerin) or small-volume enemas and digital stimulation (performed 20 to 30 minutes after suppository insertion) by the nurse or patient may be necessary. In the patient with an upper motor neuron injury, digital stimulation is necessary to relax the external sphincter to promote defecation. A stool softener such as docusate sodium (Colace) can be used to regulate stool consistency. Oral stimulant laxatives should be used only if absolutely necessary for a day or two and not on a regular basis.

Valsalva maneuver and manual stimulation are useful in patients with lower motor neuron injuries. The Valsalva maneuver requires intact abdominal muscles, so it is used in those patients with injuries below T12. In general, a bowel movement every other day is considered adequate. However, preinjury patterns should be considered. Fecal incontinence can result from too much stool softener or a fecal impaction.

Carefully record bowel movements, including amount, time, and consistency. Timing of defecation may also be an important factor. Planning bowel evacuation for 30 to 60 minutes after the first meal of the day may enhance success by taking advantage of the gastrocolic reflex induced by eating. This reflex may also be stimulated by drinking a warm beverage immediately after the meal. Remember that patient, caregiver, and family teaching is required to promote successful independent bowel management.

Neurogenic Skin. Prevention of pressure ulcers and other types of injury to insensitive skin is essential for every patient with SCI.[27] Nurses in rehabilitation are responsible for teaching these skills and providing information about daily skin care. A comprehensive visual and tactile examination of the skin should be done at least once daily, with special attention given to areas over bony prominences. The areas most vulnerable to breakdown include ischia, trochanters, heels, and sacrum. Initially carefully position and reposition every 2 hours, with gradual increases in the times between turns if no redness over bony prominences is seen at the time of turning. Pressure-relieving cushions must be used in wheelchairs, and special mattresses may also be needed. Movement during turns and transfers should be done carefully to avoid stretching and folding of soft tissues *(shear)*, friction, or abrasion.

Assess nutritional status regularly. Both body weight loss and weight gain can contribute to skin breakdown. Adequate intake of protein is essential for skin health. Measurement of prealbumin, total protein, and albumin can help identify inadequate protein intake. Stress the importance of nutrition to skin health to the patient and caregiver.

Protection of the skin also requires avoidance of thermal injury. Burns can be caused by hot food or liquids, bath or shower water that is too warm, radiators, heating pads, and uninsulated plumbing. Thermal injury also can result from extreme cold (frostbite). Injuries may not be noticed until severe damage is done. Anticipatory guidance about potential risks is essential. Patient and caregiver teaching related to skin care is provided in Tables 61-12 and 61-13.

TABLE 61-12 PATIENT & CAREGIVER TEACHING GUIDE

Skin Care After Spinal Cord Injury

To prevent skin breakdown in a patient with a spinal cord injury, include the following instructions when teaching the patient and caregiver.

Change Position Frequently
- If in a wheelchair, lift self up and shift weight every 15-30 min.
- If in bed, change positions with a regular turning schedule (at least every 2 hr) that includes sides, back, and abdomen.
- Use special mattresses and wheelchair cushions to reduce pressure.
- Use pillows to protect bony prominences when in bed.

Monitor Skin Condition
- Inspect skin frequently for areas of redness, swelling, and breakdown.
- Keep fingernails trimmed to avoid scratches and abrasions.
- If a wound develops, follow standard wound care management procedures.

Sexuality. Sexuality is an important issue regardless of the patient's age or gender. To provide accurate and sensitive counseling and teaching about sexuality, you need to be aware of your own sexuality and understand the human sexual responses. When discussing sexual potential, use scientific terminology rather than slang whenever possible. Knowledge of the level and completeness of injury is needed to understand the male patient's potential for orgasm, erection, and fertility and the patient's capacity for sexual satisfaction.[28]

Men normally have two types of erections: psychogenic and reflex. The process of *psychogenic erections* begins in the brain with sexual thoughts. Signals from the brain are then sent through the nerves of the spinal cord down to the T10-L2 levels. The signals are then relayed to the penis and trigger an erection. A *reflex erection* occurs with direct physical contact to the penis or other erotic areas. A reflex erection is involuntary and can occur without sexually stimulating thoughts. These reflex erections are often short lived and uncontrolled and cannot be maintained or summoned at the time of coitus. The nerves that control a man's ability to have a reflex erection are located in the sacral nerves (S2-4) of the spinal cord.[29]

For men with SCI, the ability to have a psychogenic erection depends on the level and extent of injury. Generally, men with low-level incomplete injuries are more likely to have psychogenic erections than men with higher-level incomplete injuries. Men with complete injuries are less likely to experience psychogenic erections. However, most men with SCI are able to have a reflex erection with physical stimulation regardless of the extent of the injury if the S2-4 nerve pathways are not damaged.

TABLE 61-13 PATIENT & CAREGIVER TEACHING GUIDE

Halo Vest Care

Include the following instructions when teaching the patient and caregiver management of a halo vest.
1. Inspect the pins on the halo traction ring. Report to health care provider if pins are loose or if there are signs of infection, including redness, tenderness, swelling, or drainage at the insertion sites.
2. Clean around pin sites carefully with hydrogen peroxide, water, or alcohol on a cotton swab as directed.
3. Apply antibiotic ointment as prescribed.
4. To provide skin care, the patient should lie down on a bed with his or her head resting on a pillow to reduce pressure on the brace. Loosen one side of the vest. Gently wash the skin under the vest with soap and water, rinse it, and then dry it thoroughly. At the same time, check the skin for pressure points, redness, swelling, bruising, or chafing. Close the open side and repeat the procedure on the opposite side.
5. If the vest becomes wet or damp, carefully dry it with a blow dryer.
6. An assistive device (e.g., cane, walker) may be used to provide greater balance. Flat shoes should be worn.
7. Turn the entire body, not just the head and neck, when trying to view sideways.
8. In case of an emergency, keep a set of wrenches close to the halo vest at all times.
9. Mark the vest strap to maintain consistent buckling and fit.
10. Avoid grabbing bars or vest to assist the patient.
11. Keep sheepskin pad under vest. Change and wash at least weekly.
12. If perspiration or itching is a problem, a cotton T-shirt can be worn under the sheepskin. The T-shirt can be modified with a Velcro seam closure on one side.

Because each SCI is different, the impact of injury on sexual function can also differ.[29]

Treatment for erectile dysfunction includes drugs, vacuum devices, and surgical procedures. Sildenafil (Viagra) has become the treatment of choice in men with SCI. Penile injection of vasoactive substances (papaverine, prostaglandin E) is another medical treatment. Risks include *priapism* (prolonged penile erection) and scarring, so these substances are often considered only after failure of sildenafil. Vacuum suction devices use negative pressure to encourage blood flow into the penis. Erection is maintained by a constriction band placed at the base of the penis. The main surgical option is implantation of a penile prosthesis. (Erectile dysfunction is discussed in Chapter 55.)

Male fertility is affected by SCI, causing poor sperm quality and ejaculatory dysfunction. Recent advances in methods of retrieving sperm (penile vibratory stimulation and electroejaculation) combined with ovulation induction and intrauterine insemination of the female partner have changed the prognosis for men with SCI to father children from unlikely to a reasonable possibility of successful outcomes.

The effect of SCI on female sexual response is less clear. Lubrication is similar to erections in males, with reflex and psychogenic components. Women with upper motor neuron injuries may retain the capacity for reflex lubrication, whereas psychogenic lubrication depends on the completeness of injury. Orgasm is reported by about 50% of women with SCI.[28]

The woman of childbearing age with an SCI usually remains fertile. The injury does not affect the ability to become pregnant or to deliver normally through the birth canal. Menses may cease for as long as 6 months after injury. If sexual activity is resumed, protection against an unplanned pregnancy is necessary. A normal pregnancy may be complicated by UTIs, anemia, and autonomic dysreflexia. Because uterine contractions are not felt, a precipitous delivery is always a danger.

Open discussion with the patient regarding sexual rehabilitation is essential. This important aspect of rehabilitation should be handled by someone specially trained in sexual counseling. A nurse or other rehabilitation professional with such expertise works with the patient and the partner to provide support, with an emphasis on open communication. As a nurse, you should respect every couple's religious and cultural beliefs. Alternative methods of obtaining sexual satisfaction, such as oral-genital sex (cunnilingus and fellatio), may be suggested. Explicit films may also be used, such as a film demonstrating the sexual activities of a patient with paraplegia and a nondisabled partner. Use graphics cautiously because they may be too limiting or focus too much on the mechanics of sex rather than on the relationship.

Care should be taken not to dislodge an indwelling catheter during sexual activity. If an external catheter is used, it should be removed before sexual activity and the patient should refrain from fluids. The bowel program should include evacuation the morning of sexual activity. The partner should be informed that incontinence is always possible. The woman may need a water-soluble lubricant to supplement diminished vaginal secretions and facilitate vaginal penetration.

Grief and Depression. Patients with SCIs may feel an overwhelming sense of loss. They may temporarily lose control over everyday activities and must depend on others for activities of daily living and for life-sustaining measures. Patients may believe that they are useless and burdens to their families. At a stage when independence is often of great importance, they may be totally dependent on others.

The patient's response and recovery differ in some important aspects from those of patients experiencing loss from amputation or terminal illness. First, regression can and does occur at different stages. Working through grief is a difficult, lifelong process with which the patient needs support and encouragement. With recent advances in rehabilitation, patients are often independent physically and discharged from the rehabilitation center before completion of the grief process.

The goal of recovery is related more to adjustment than to acceptance. Adjustment implies the ability to go on with living with certain limitations. Although the patient who is cooperative and accepting is easier to treat, expect a wide fluctuation of emotions from a patient with an SCI. Your role in grief work is to allow mourning as a component of the rehabilitation process. Table 61-14 summarizes the grief response to an SCI and appropriate nursing interventions. Maintaining hope is an important strategy during the grieving process and should not be interpreted as denial. During the shock and denial stage, reassure the patient. During the anger stage, assist the patient in achieving control over the environment, particularly by allowing the patient's input into the plan of care. Do not respond to anger or manipulation or become involved in a power struggle with the patient. As self-care abilities increase, the patient's independence increases.

TABLE 61-14	**GRIEF RESPONSE IN SPINAL CORD INJURY**
Patient Behavior	**Nursing Intervention**
Shock and Denial	
Struggle for survival, complete dependence, excessive sleep, withdrawal, fantasies, unrealistic expectations	• Provide honest information. • Use simple diagrams to explain injury. • Encourage patient to begin road to recovery. • Establish agreement to use and improve all current abilities while not denying the possibility of future improvement.
Anger	
Refusal to discuss paralysis, decreased self-esteem, manipulation, hostile and abusive language	• Coordinate care with patient and encourage self-care. • Support family members. • Use humor appropriately. • Allow patient outbursts. • Do not allow fixation on injury.
Depression	
Sadness, pessimism, anorexia, nightmares, insomnia, agitation, "blues," suicidal preoccupation, refusal to participate in any self-care activities	• Encourage family involvement and the use of community resources. • Plan graded steps in rehabilitation to give success with minimal opportunity for frustration. • Give cheerful and willing assistance with activities of daily living. • Avoid sympathy. • Use firm kindness.
Adjustment and Acceptance	
Planning for future, active participation in therapy, finding personal meaning in experience and continuation of growth, return to premorbid personality.	• Remember that patients have individual personalities. • Balance support systems to encourage independence. • Set goals with patient input. • Emphasize potential.

The patient's caregiver and family also require counseling to avoid promoting dependency in the patient through guilt or misplaced sympathy. The family is also experiencing an intense grieving process. A support group of family members and friends of patients with SCI can help family members increase their participation and knowledge of the grieving process, physical difficulties, rehabilitation plan, and meaning of the disability in society.

During the stage of depression, be patient. Sympathy is not helpful. Treat the patient as an adult and encourage participation in care planning. A primary nurse relationship is helpful. Staff planning and sessions in which staff members can express their feelings help provide consistency of care. To achieve the stage of adjustment, the patient needs continual support throughout the rehabilitation process in the forms of acceptance, affection, and caring. Be attentive when the patient needs to talk and sensitive to needs at the various stages of the grief process.

Although the stage of depression during the grief process usually lasts days to weeks, some individuals may become clinically depressed and require treatment for depression. Evaluation by a psychiatric nurse or psychiatrist is recommended. Treatment may include drugs and therapy.

❚ EVALUATION

Expected outcomes are that the patient with an SCI will
- Maintain adequate ventilation and have no signs of respiratory distress
- Maintain intact skin over bony prominences
- Establish a bowel management program based on neurologic function and personal preference
- Establish a bladder management program based on neurologic function, caregiver status, and lifestyle choices
- Experience no episodes of autonomic dysreflexia

Additional information on expected outcomes for the patient with an SCI is addressed in eNursing Care Plan 61-1 on the website for this chapter.

❚ GERONTOLOGIC CONSIDERATIONS

SPINAL CORD INJURY

Because of increased work and recreational activities of older adults, more older adults are experiencing SCI. Falls are the leading cause of SCI for people 65 and older. Besides having greater mortality rates, older adults with traumatic injuries experience more complications than younger ones, and they are hospitalized longer.

The demographics of patients living with SCI are changing. Given the longer life spans of persons with SCI, an increasing number of older adults are now living with an SCI. Aging is also associated with more chronic illnesses, which can have a serious impact on these older adults. As patients with SCI age, both individual aging changes and length of time since injury can affect functional ability. For example, bowel and bladder dysfunction can increase with the duration and severity of SCI.

Health promotion and screening are important for the older patient with an SCI. Daily skin inspections, UTI prevention measures, and monthly breast examinations for women and regular prostate cancer screening for men are recommended. Cardiovascular disease is the most common cause of morbidity and mortality among older adults with an SCI. The lack of sensation, including chest pain, in those with high-level injuries may mask acute myocardial ischemia. Altered autonomic nervous system function and decreases in physical activity can place the patient at risk for cardiovascular problems, including hypertension.

Health promotion to decrease the risk of injuries includes fall prevention strategies (e.g., using a stepstool or a grab bar to reach high shelves, handrails on stairs). Rehabilitation for the older person who has had an SCI may take longer because of preexisting conditions and poorer health status at the time of the initial injury. An interdisciplinary team approach to rehabilitation is essential in preventing secondary complications associated with SCI, especially in older adults.

SPINAL CORD TUMORS

Spinal cord tumors account for 0.5% to 1% of all neoplasms. These tumors are classified as *primary* (arising from some component of cord, dura, nerves, or vessels) or *secondary* (from primary growths in other places in the body that have metastasized to the spinal cord).

Etiology and Pathophysiology

Spinal cord tumors are further classified as *extradural* (outside the spinal cord), *intradural extramedullary* (within the dura but outside the actual spinal cord), and *intradural intramedullary* (within the spinal cord itself) (Fig. 61-13, Table 61-15).

Extradural tumors are usually metastatic and most often arise in the vertebral bodies.[30] These metastatic lesions can invade intradurally and compress the spinal cord. Tumors that commonly metastasize to the spinal epidural space are those that spread to bone, such as prostate, breast, lung, and kidney cancer.

Because many spinal cord tumors are slow growing, their symptoms are due to the mechanical effects of slow compression and irritation of nerve roots, displacement of the cord, or gradual obstruction of the vascular supply. The slowness of growth does not cause autodestruction (secondary injury) as in traumatic SCIs. Therefore complete functional restoration may be possible when the tumor is removed.

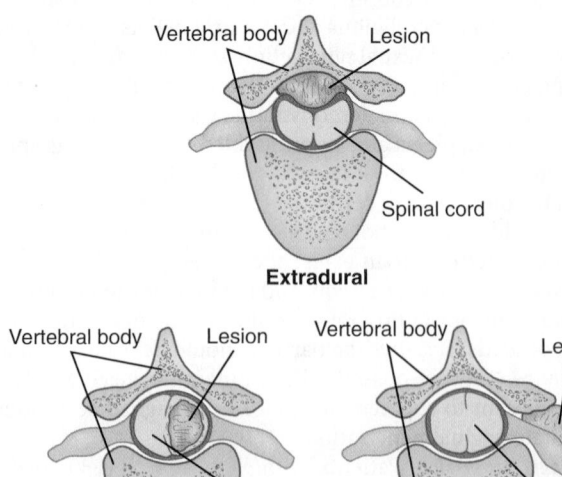

FIG. 61-13 Types of spinal cord tumors.

TABLE 61-15	CLASSIFICATION OF SPINAL CORD TUMORS		
Type	Incidence	Treatment	Prognosis
Extradural			
Outside the spinal cord in extradural space	Ninety percent of all spinal cord tumors. Mostly malignant metastatic lesions.	Relief of cord pressure by surgical laminectomy, radiation, chemotherapy, or combination approach.	Poor. Treatment is usually palliative.
Intradural			
Intradural Extramedullary			
Within dura mater but outside cord	Most frequent of intradural tumors. Mostly benign. Meningiomas, neurofibromas, and schwannomas.	Complete surgical removal of tumor (if possible). Partial removal followed by radiation.	Usually very good if lack of damage to cord from compression.
Intradural Intramedullary			
Within the spinal cord	Least frequent of intradural tumors. Mostly benign. Astrocytomas, ependymomas.	Complete surgical removal of tumor (if possible). Partial removal followed by radiation.	Usually very good if lack of damage to cord from compression. Complete surgical resection of astrocytomas difficult.

Clinical Manifestations

Both sensory and motor problems may result, with the location and extent of the tumor determining the severity and extent of the problem. The most common early symptom of a spinal cord tumor is back pain. The location of the pain depends on the level of compression. The pain worsens with activity, coughing, straining, and lying down. Sensory disruption is later manifested by coldness, numbness, and tingling in an extremity or in several extremities.

Motor weakness accompanies the sensory disturbances and consists of slowly increasing clumsiness, weakness, and spasticity. Paralysis can develop. The sensory and motor disturbances are ipsilateral (on the same side) to the injury. Bladder disturbances are marked by urgency with difficulty in starting the flow and progressing to retention with overflow incontinence.

NURSING AND COLLABORATIVE MANAGEMENT
SPINAL CORD TUMORS

Extradural tumors are seen early on routine spinal x-rays, whereas intradural and intramedullary tumors require MRI or CT scans for detection. CSF analysis may reveal tumor cells.

Compression of the spinal cord is an emergency. Relief of the ischemia related to the compression is the goal of therapy. Corticosteroids are generally prescribed immediately to relieve tumor-related edema. Dexamethasone (Decadron) (often in large doses) is also usually used to treat edema.

Indications for surgery vary depending on the type of tumor. Primary spinal tumors may be removed with the goal of cure. In patients with metastatic tumors, treatment is primarily palliative, with the goal of restoring or preserving neurologic function, stabilizing the spine, and alleviating pain.[30]

Radiation therapy after surgery is fairly effective. Chemotherapy has also been used in conjunction with radiation therapy.

Relief of pain and return of function are the ultimate goals of treatment. Be aware of the patient's neurologic status before and after treatment. Ensuring that the patient receives pain medication as needed is an important nursing responsibility. Depending on the amount of neurologic dysfunction exhibited, the care of the patient may be similar to that of a patient recovering from an SCI. Rehabilitation of patients with spinal cord tumors is similar to rehabilitation for the patient with an SCI.

CASE STUDY

Spinal Cord Injury

iStockphoto/Thinkstock

Patient Profile
Acute Phase

B.V., a 24-yr-old white man, is admitted to the emergency department with the diagnosis of a cervical spinal cord injury (SCI). B.V. was swimming at a neighbor's backyard pool. He dove into the shallow end, striking his head on the bottom of the pool. His friends noticed that he did not resurface. They rescued him and brought him to the side of the pool. They maintained neck immobilization until the rescue crews arrived.

Subjective Data
- Is awake and alert
- Is complaining of neck pain
- Is anxious and asking why he cannot move his legs
- Is asking to see his family

Objective Data
Physical Examination
- Weak biceps movement bilaterally
- No triceps movement bilaterally
- Gross elbow movement present bilaterally
- No movement in bilateral lower extremities
- Decreased sensation from the shoulders down
- No bladder or bowel control
- BP 85/50 mm Hg; pulse 56 beats/min; respirations 32 breaths/min and labored

Diagnostic Studies
- CT C-spine shows C5 subluxation and compression fracture
- MRI C-spine shows a severe spinal cord compression at C5-6

Collaborative Care
- Intubated in the emergency department
- Started on mechanical ventilation
- Placed in tongs and traction on arrival to the ICU

Discussion Questions (Acute Phase)
1. *Priority Decision:* What nursing activities would be a priority on B.V.'s arrival in the ICU?
2. What physiologic problems are causing B.V. to have hypotension and bradycardia?

3. What would be the first line of treatment for B.V.'s hypotension and bradycardia?
4. What signs and symptoms would indicate respiratory distress, and what physiologic problem would cause respiratory distress in B.V.'s injury state?
5. What can you do to decrease B.V.'s anxiety?
6. *Priority Decision:* Based on the assessment data provided, what are the priority nursing diagnoses? Are there any collaborative problems?
7. *Delegation Decision:* Identify activities that can be delegated to unlicensed assistive personnel (UAP).

Patient Profile
Rehabilitation Phase

B.V. is now 1 mo postinjury and is currently at a local inpatient SCI rehabilitation facility. He has since been extubated and uses a wheelchair to mobilize. He eats three meals a day with assistance and is on a strict bowel and bladder program.

Subjective Data
- Awake and alert but anxious
- Complaining of severe headache, blurred vision, and nausea

Objective Data
Physical Examination
- Flushed and diaphoretic above the level of injury
- No bowel movement for 2 days
- BP 235/106 mm Hg, pulse 32 beats/min, respirations 30 breaths/min and labored

Discussion Questions (Rehabilitation Phase)
1. *Priority Decision:* What initial priority nursing interventions would be appropriate?
2. What physiologic problem is causing B.V.'s hypertension and bradycardia?
3. Once the physician has been notified, what other interventions would be appropriate?
4. *Priority Decision:* Based on the assessment data provided, what are the priority nursing diagnoses?
5. Patient and family involvement in the rehabilitation process is vital. What teaching will you provide about bowel management?
6. *Evidence-Based Practice:* B.V. and his family are concerned about the potential risk of autonomic dysreflexia. What information would you provide the patient and family?

evolve Answers available at *http://evolve.elsevier.com/Lewis/medsurg.*

BRIDGE TO NCLEX EXAMINATION

The number of the question corresponds to the same-numbered outcome at the beginning of the chapter.

1. During assessment of the patient with trigeminal neuralgia, the nurse should *(select all that apply)*
   a. inspect all aspects of the mouth and teeth.
   b. assess the gag reflex and respiratory rate and depth.
   c. lightly palpate the affected side of the face for edema.
   d. test for temperature and sensation perception on the face.
   e. ask the patient to describe factors that initiate an episode.

2. During routine assessment of a patient with Guillain-Barré syndrome, the nurse finds the patient is short of breath. The patient's respiratory distress is caused by
   a. elevated protein levels in the CSF.
   b. immobility resulting from ascending paralysis.
   c. degeneration of motor neurons in the brainstem and spinal cord.
   d. paralysis ascending to the nerves that stimulate the thoracic area.

3. A patient is admitted to the ICU with a C7 spinal cord injury and diagnosed with Brown-Séquard syndrome. On physical examination, the nurse would most likely find
   a. upper extremity weakness only.
   b. complete motor and sensory loss below C7.
   c. loss of position sense and vibration in both lower extremities.
   d. ipsilateral motor loss and contralateral sensory loss below C7.

4. A patient is admitted to the hospital with a C4 spinal cord injury after a motorcycle collision. The patient's BP is 84/50 mm Hg, his pulse is 38 beats/minute, and he remains orally intubated. The nurse determines that this pathophysiologic response is caused by
   a. increased vasomotor tone after injury.
   b. a temporary loss of sensation and flaccid paralysis below the level of injury.
   c. loss of parasympathetic nervous system innervation resulting in vasoconstriction.
   d. loss of sympathetic nervous system innervation resulting in peripheral vasodilation.

5. Goals of rehabilitation for the patient with an injury at the C6 level include (select all that apply)
   a. stand erect with leg brace.
   b. feed self with hand devices.
   c. assist with transfer activities.
   d. drive adapted van from wheelchair.
   e. push a wheelchair on a flat surface.

6. A patient with a C7 spinal cord injury undergoing rehabilitation tells the nurse he must have the flu because he has a bad headache and nausea. The nurse's first priority is to
   a. call the physician.
   b. check the patient's temperature.
   c. take the patient's blood pressure.
   d. elevate the head of the bed to 90 degrees.

7. For a 65-year-old woman who has lived with a T1 spinal cord injury for 20 years, which health teaching instructions should the nurse emphasize?
   a. A mammogram is needed every year.
   b. Bladder function tends to improve with age.
   c. Heart disease is not common in persons with spinal cord injury.
   d. As a person ages, the need to change body position is less important.

8. The most common early symptom of a spinal cord tumor is
   a. urinary incontinence.
   b. back pain that worsens with activity.
   c. paralysis below the level of involvement.
   d. impaired sensation of pain, temperature, and light touch.

1. a, d, e, 2. d, 3. d, 4. d, 5. b, c, d, e, 6. c, 7. a, 8. b

ⓔvolve

For rationales to these answers and even more NCLEX review questions, visit *http://evolve.elsevier.com/Lewis/medsurg*.

REFERENCES

1. National Institute of Neurological Disorders and Stroke: Trigeminal neuralgia fact sheet.. Retrieved from *www.ninds.nih.gov/disorders/trigeminal_neuralgia/detail_trigeminal_neuralgia.htm*.
2. Brisman R: Trigeminal neuralgia: diagnosis and treatment, *World Neurosurg* 76(6):533, 2011.
*3. Zakrzewska JM, Akram H: Neurosurgical interventions for the treatment of classical trigeminal neuralgia, *Cochrane Database Syst Rev* 9:CD007312, 2011. DOI:10.1002/14651858.CD007312.pub2.
4. National Institute of Neurological Disorders and Stroke: Bell's palsy fact sheet. Retrieved from *www.ninds.nih.gov/disorders/bells/detail_bells.htm*.
5. National Institute of Neurological Disorders and Stroke: Guillain-Barré syndrome fact sheet. Retrieved from *www.ninds.nih.gov/disorders/gbs/detail_gbs.htm*.
6. Bowyer HR, Glover M: Guillain-Barré syndrome: management and treatment options for patients with moderate to severe progression, *J Neurosci Nurs* 42(5):288, 2010.
7. Lugg J: Recognizing and managing Guillain-Barré syndrome, *Emerg Nurse* 18(3):27, 2010.
8. Saifudheen K, Jose J, Gafoor VA, et al: Guillain-Barré and SIADH, *Neurology* 76(8):1, 2011.
9. Centers for Disease Control and Prevention: Botulism. Retrieved from *http://emergency.cdc.gov/agent/Botulism/clinicians/epidemiology.asp*.
10. Centers for Disease Control and Prevention: Tetanus. Retrieved from *www.cdc.gov/vaccines/pubs/pinkbook/downloads/tetanus.pdf*.

11. Ataro P, Mushatt D, Shagufta A: Tetanus: a review, *South Med J* 104(8):613, 2011.
12. Centers for Disease Control and Prevention. Updated recommendations for use of tetanus toxoid, reduced diphtheria toxoid and acellular pertussis (Tdap) vaccine from the Advisory Committee on Immunization Practices, 2010, *MMWR* 60:13, 2011.
13. National Institute of Neurological Disorders and Stroke: Neurosyphilis information page. Retrieved from *www.ninds.nih.gov/disorders/neurosyphilis/neurosyphilis.htm*.
14. Centers for Disease Control and Prevention, National Center for Injury Prevention and Control: Spinal cord injury (SCI): fact sheet. Retrieved from *www.cdc.gov/ncipc/factsheets/scifacts.htm*.
15. Dawodu ST, Campagnolo DI: Spinal cord injury: definition, epidemiology, pathophysiology. Retrieved from *http://emedicine.medscape.com/article/322480-overview*.
16. Nayduch DA: Back to the basics: identifying and managing acute spinal cord injury, *Nursing* 40(9):24, 2010.
17. Looby S, Flanders A: Spine trauma, *Radiol Clin North Am* 49(1):1, 2011.
*18. Chung SB, Lee SH, Kim ES, et al: Incidence of deep vein thrombosis after spinal cord injury: a prospective study in 37 consecutive patients with traumatic or nontraumatic spinal cord injury treated with mechanical prophylaxis, *J Trauma* 71(4):867, 2011.
*19. Hadley MN, Walters BC: Introduction to the guidelines for the management of acute cervical spine and spinal cord injuries, *Neurosurgery* 72(suppl):1, 2013.
*20. Nicholas T, Hadley MN, Aarabi B, et al: Prehospital cervical spinal immobilization after trauma, *Neurosurgery* 72(suppl):22, 2013.

*Evidence-based information for clinical practice.

*21. Hurlbert RJ, Hadley MN, Walters B, et al: Pharmacological therapy for acute spinal cord injury, *Neurosurgery* 72(suppl):93, 2013.

*22. Dhall SS, Hadley MN, Aarabi B, et al: Deep venous thrombosis and thromboembolism in patients with cervical spinal cord injuries, *Neurosurgery* 72(suppl):244, 2013.

23. Wyndaele JJ: Neurogenic bowel management after spinal cord injury, *Spinal Cord* 48(10):710, 2010.

24. National Spinal Cord Injury Association. Retrieved from *www.spinalcord.org.*

25. Ho CP, Krassioukov AV: Autonomic dysreflexia and myocardial ischemia, *Spinal Cord* 48(9):714, 2010.

26. McGuire EJ: Urodynamics of the neurogenic bladder, *Urol Clin North Am* 37:507, 2010.

*27. Saunders LL, Krause JS, Peters BA, et al: The relationship of pressure ulcers, race, and socioeconomic conditions after spinal cord injury, *J Spinal Cord Med* 33(4):387, 2010.

*28. Consortium for Spinal Cord Medicine: Sexuality and reproductive health in adults with spinal cord injury: a clinical practice guideline for health-care professionals, *J Spinal Cord Med* 33(3):281, 2010.

29. Sexual function for men with SCI. Retrieved from *http://images.main.uab.edu/spinalcord/SCI%20Infosheets%20in%20PDF/Sexual%20Function%20for%20Men%20with%20SCI.pdf.*

30. Spinal Cord Tumor Association. Retrieved from *www.spinalcordtumor.org.*

RESOURCES

American Spinal Injury Association (ASIA)
   www.asia-spinalinjury.org
Christopher and Dana Reeve Foundation
   www.christopherreeve.org
GBS-CIDP Foundation International
   www.gbs-cidp.org
National Institute of Neurological Disorders and Stroke (NINDS)
   www.ninds.nih.gov
National Rehabilitation Information Center (NARIC)
   www.naric.com
National Spinal Cord Injury Association
   www.spinalcord.org
Paralyzed Veterans of America
   www.pva.org
Spinal Cord Society
   www.scsus.org
Spinal Cord Tumor Association, Inc,
   www.spinalcordtumor.org

We must be the change we want to see.
Mahatma Gandhi

Nursing Assessment
Musculoskeletal System

Dottie Roberts

evolve WEBSITE

- NCLEX Review Questions
- Key Points
- Pre-Test
- Answer Guidelines for Case Study in this chapter
- Rationales for Bridge to NCLEX Examination Questions
- Concept Map Creator
- Glossary
- Animations
  - Classification of Joints: Condyloid Joint

- Classification of Joints: Gliding Joint—Hand
- Classification of Joints: Hinge Joint
- Videos
  - Inspection and Palpation: Muscular Development
  - Inspection: Gait in Older Adult
  - Inspection: General Muscular Strength
  - Physical Examination: Abdominal Reflexes, Abdominal Muscles, and Inguinal Area
  - Physical Examination: Anterior Chest, Lungs, and Heart

- Physical Examination: Back and Posterior Chest
- Physical Examination: Feet, Legs, and Hips
- Physical Examination: Musculoskeletal Function
- Physical Examination: Neck
- Physical Examination: Spine
- Physical Examination: Upper Extremities
- Physical Examination: Abdominal Reflexes, Abdominal Muscles, and Inguinal Area
- Content Updates

LEARNING OUTCOMES

1. Describe the gross anatomic and microscopic composition of bone.
2. Explain the classification system for joints and movements at synovial joints.
3. Compare and contrast the types and structure of muscle tissue.
4. Describe the functions of cartilage, muscles, ligaments, tendons, fascia, and bursae.
5. Link age-related changes in the musculoskeletal system to the differences in assessment findings.

6. Select significant subjective and objective data related to the musculoskeletal system that should be obtained from a patient.
7. Select appropriate techniques to use in the physical assessment of the musculoskeletal system.
8. Differentiate normal from abnormal findings of a physical assessment of the musculoskeletal system.
9. Describe the purpose, significance of results, and nursing responsibilities related to diagnostic studies of the musculoskeletal system.

KEY TERMS

ankylosis, Table 62-6, p. 1500
arthrocentesis, p. 1499
arthroscopy, p. 1499
atrophy, Table 62-6, p. 1500
contracture, Table 62-6, p. 1500

crepitation, Table 62-6, p. 1500
isometric contractions, p. 1492
isotonic contractions, p. 1492
kyphosis, Table 62-6, p. 1500
lordosis, Table 62-6, p. 1500

osteons, p. 1490
range of motion, p. 1497
scoliosis, p. 1498
x-ray, p. 1499

This chapter provides a review of the structures and functions of the musculoskeletal system to facilitate nursing assessment and evaluation of the assessment findings of this system. The musculoskeletal system is composed of voluntary muscle and five types of connective tissue: bones, cartilage, ligaments, tendons, and fascia. The purpose of the musculoskeletal system is to protect body organs, provide support and stability for the body, and allow for coordinated movement.

STRUCTURES AND FUNCTIONS OF MUSCULOSKELETAL SYSTEM

Bone

Function. The main functions of bone are support, protection of internal organs, voluntary movement, blood cell production, and mineral storage.[1] Bones provide the supporting framework that keeps the body from collapsing and also

Reviewed by Damien Zsiros, RN, MSN, CNE, CRNP, Nursing Instructor, The Pennsylvania State University School of Nursing, Fayette/The Eberly Campus, Uniontown, Pennsylvania; Jan Foecke, RN, MS, ONC, Director of Programs, National Association of Orthopaedic Nurses, Kansas City, Missouri; and Clemma K. Snider, RN, MSN, Assistant Professor, Associate Degree Nursing, Eastern Kentucky University, Richmond, Kentucky.

allows the body to bear weight. Bones also protect underlying vital organs and tissues. For example, the skull encloses the brain, the vertebrae surround the spinal cord, and the rib cage contains the lungs and heart. Bones serve as a point of attachment for muscles, which are connected to bones by tendons. Bones act as a lever for muscles, and movement occurs as a result of muscle contractions applied to these levers. Bones contain hematopoietic tissue for the production of red and white blood cells. Bones also serve as a site for storage of inorganic minerals such as calcium and phosphorus.

Bone is a dynamic tissue that continuously changes form and composition. It contains both organic material (collagen) and inorganic material (calcium, phosphate). The internal and external growth and remodeling of bone are ongoing processes.

Microscopic Structure. Bone is classified according to structure as *cortical* (compact and dense) or *cancellous* (spongy). In *cortical bone,* cylindric structural units called osteons *(Haversian systems)* fit closely together, creating a dense bone structure (Fig. 62-1, *A*). Within the systems, the Haversian canals run parallel to the bone's long axis and contain the blood vessels that travel to the bone's interior from the periosteum. Surrounding each osteon are concentric rings known as *lamellae,* which characterize mature bone. Smaller canals *(canaliculi)* extend from the Haversian canals to the *lacunae,* where mature bone cells are embedded.

Cancellous bone lacks the organized structure of cortical bone. The lamellae are not arranged in concentric rings but rather along the lines of maximum stress placed on the bone. Cancellous bone tissue is filled with red or yellow marrow, and blood reaches the bone cells by passing through spaces in the marrow.

The three types of bone cells are osteoblasts, osteocytes, and osteoclasts.[2] *Osteoblasts* synthesize organic bone matrix (collagen) and are the basic bone-forming cells. *Osteocytes* are the mature bone cells. *Osteoclasts* participate in bone remodeling by assisting in the breakdown of bone tissue. *Bone remodeling* is the removal of old bone by osteoclasts *(resorption)* and the deposition of new bone by osteoblasts *(ossification).* The inner layer of bone is composed primarily of osteoblasts with a few osteoclasts.

Gross Structure. The anatomic structure of bone is best represented by a typical long bone such as the tibia (see Fig. 62-1, *B*). Each long bone consists of the epiphysis, diaphysis, and metaphysis. The *epiphysis,* the widened area found at each end of a long bone, is composed primarily of cancellous bone. The wide epiphysis allows for greater weight distribution and provides stability for the joint. The epiphysis is also the location of muscle attachment. Articular cartilage covers the ends of the epiphysis to provide a smooth surface for joint movement. The *diaphysis* is the main shaft of the bone. It provides structural support and is composed of compact bone. The tubular structure of the diaphysis allows it to more easily withstand bending and twisting forces. The *metaphysis* is the flared area between the epiphysis and the diaphysis. Like the epiphysis, it is composed of cancellous bone.

The *epiphyseal plate,* or growth zone, is the cartilaginous area between the epiphysis and metaphysis. It actively produces bone to allow longitudinal growth in children. Injury to the epiphyseal plate in a growing child can lead to a shorter extremity that can cause significant functional problems. In the adult, the metaphysis and the epiphysis become joined as this plate hardens to mature bone.

The *periosteum* is composed of fibrous connective tissue that covers the bone. Tiny blood vessels penetrate the periosteum to provide nutrition to underlying bone. Musculotendinous fibers anchor to the outer layer of the periosteum. The inner layer of the periosteum is attached to the bone by bundles of collagen. No periosteum exists on the articular surfaces of long bones. These bone ends are covered by articular cartilage.

The medullary (marrow) cavity is in the center of the diaphysis and contains either red or yellow bone marrow.[3] In the growing child, red bone marrow is actively involved in blood cell production (hematopoiesis). In the adult, the medullary

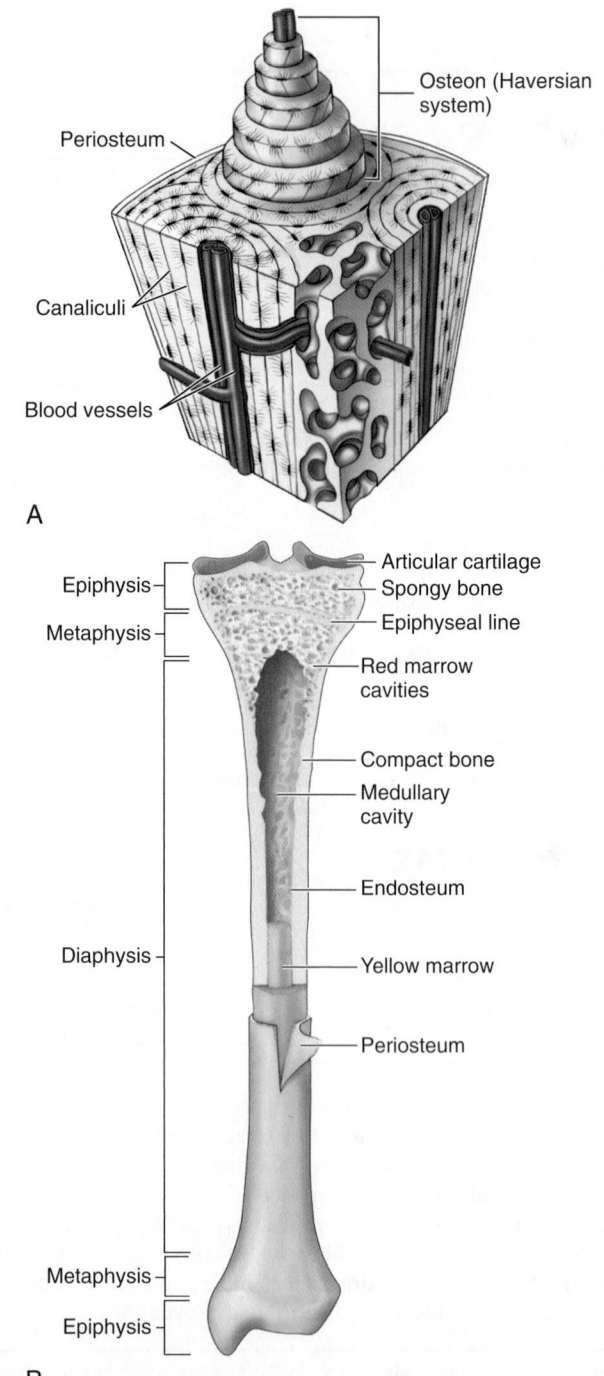

A

B

FIG. 62-1 Bone structure. **A,** Cortical (compact) bone showing numerous structural units called osteons. **B,** Anatomy of a long bone (tibia) showing cancellous and compact bone.

cavity of long bones contains yellow bone marrow, which is mainly adipose tissue. Yellow marrow is involved in hematopoiesis only in times of great blood cell need. In adults, red marrow is found mainly in the *flat bones,* such as the pelvis, skull, sternum, cranium, ribs, vertebrae, and scapulae, and in the *cancellous* ("spongy") material at the epiphyseal ends of long bones such as the femur and the humerus.

Types. The skeleton consists of 206 bones, which are classified according to shape as long, short, flat, or irregular.

Long bones are characterized by a central shaft (diaphysis) and two widened ends (epiphyses) (see Fig. 62-1, *B*). Examples include the femur, humerus, and tibia. *Short bones* are composed of cancellous bone covered by a thin layer of compact bone. Examples include the carpals in the hand and the tarsals in the foot.

Flat bones have two layers of compact bone separated by a layer of cancellous bone. Examples include the ribs, skull, scapula, and sternum. The spaces in the cancellous bone contain bone marrow. *Irregular bones* appear in a variety of shapes and sizes. Examples include the sacrum, mandible, and ear ossicles.

Joints

A *joint* (articulation) is a place where the ends of two bones are in proximity and move in relation to each other. Joints are classified by the degree of movement that they allow (Fig. 62-2).

The most common joint is the freely movable *diarthrodial* (synovial) type. Each joint is enclosed in a capsule of fibrous connective tissue, which joins the two bones together to form a cavity (Fig. 62-3). The capsule is lined by a synovial membrane, which secretes a thick synovial fluid to lubricate the joint, reduce friction, and allow opposing surfaces to slide smoothly over each other. The end of each bone is covered with articular (hyaline) cartilage. Supporting structures (e.g., ligaments, tendons) reinforce the joint capsule and provide limits and stability to joint movement. Types of diarthrodial joints are shown in Fig. 62-4.

Cartilage

The three types of *cartilage* tissue are hyaline, elastic, and fibrous. *Hyaline cartilage,* the most common, contains a moderate amount of collagen fibers. It is found in the trachea, bronchi, nose, epiphyseal plate, and articular surfaces of bones. *Elastic cartilage,* which contains both collagen and elastic fibers, is more flexible than hyaline cartilage. It is found in the ear, epiglottis, and larynx. *Fibrous cartilage* (fibrocartilage) consists mostly of collagen fibers and is a tough tissue that often functions as a shock absorber. It is found between the vertebral discs and also forms a protective cushion between the bones of the pelvic girdle, knee, and shoulder.

Cartilage in synovial joints serves as a support for soft tissue and provides the articular surface for joint movement. It protects underlying tissues. The cartilage in the epiphyseal plate is also involved in the growth of long bones before physical maturity is reached. Because articular cartilage is considered to be avascular, it must receive nourishment by the diffusion of material from the synovial fluid. The lack of a direct blood supply contributes to the slow metabolism of cartilage cells and explains why healing and repair of cartilage tissue occur slowly.

Muscle

Types. The three types of muscle tissue are cardiac (striated, involuntary), smooth (nonstriated, involuntary), and skeletal (striated, voluntary) muscle. *Cardiac muscle* is found in the

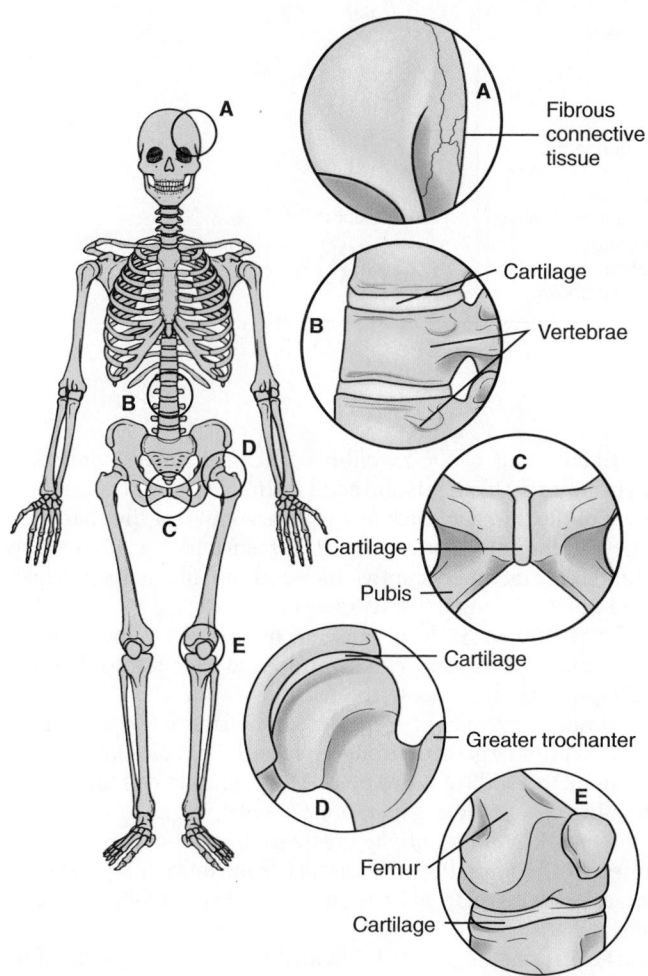

FIG. 62-2 Classification of joints. **A** to **C,** Synarthrotic (immovable) and amphiarthrotic (slightly movable) joints. **D** and **E,** Diarthrodial (freely movable) joints.

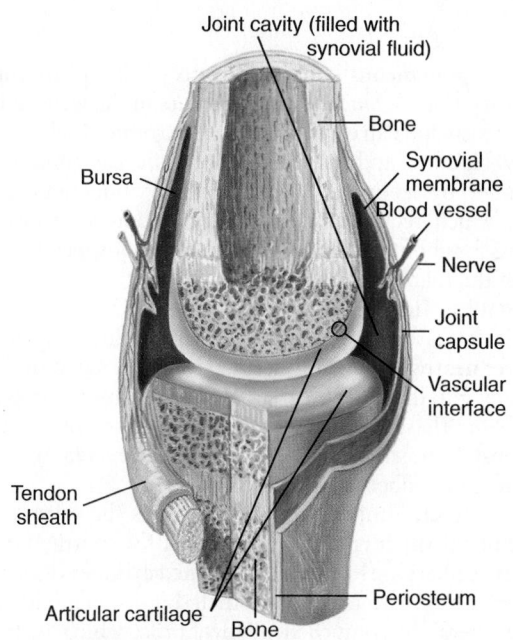

FIG. 62-3 Structure of diarthrodial (synovial) joint.

Joint	Movement	Examples	Illustration
Hinge joint	Flexion, extension	Elbow joint (shown), interphalangeal joints, knee joint	
Ball and socket (spheroidal)	Flexion, extension; adduction, abduction; circumduction	Shoulder (shown), hip	
Pivot (rotary)	Rotation	Atlas-axis, proximal radioulnar joint (shown)	
Condyloid	Flexion, extension; abduction, adduction; circumduction	Wrist joint (between radial and carpals) (shown)	
Saddle	Flexion, extension; abduction, adduction; circumduction, thumb-finger opposition	Carpometacarpal joint of thumb (shown)	
Gliding	One surface moves over another surface	Between tarsal bones, sacroiliac joint, between articular processes of vertebrae, between carpal bones (shown)	

FIG. 62-4 Types of diarthrodial (synovial) joints.

heart. Its spontaneous contractions propel blood through the circulatory system. *Smooth muscle* occurs in the walls of hollow structures such as airways, arteries, gastrointestinal (GI) tract, urinary bladder, and uterus. Smooth muscle contraction is modulated by neuronal and hormonal influences. *Skeletal muscle,* which requires neuronal stimulation for contraction, accounts for about half of a human being's body weight. It is the focus of the following discussion.

Structure. The skeletal muscle is enclosed by the *epimysium,* a continuous layer of deep fascia. The epimysium helps muscles slide over nearby structures. Connective tissue surrounding and extending into the muscle can be subdivided into fiber bundles, or *fasciculi.* These bundles are covered by *perimysium* and an innermost connective tissue layer called the *endomysium* that surrounds each fiber (Fig. 62-5).

The structural unit of skeletal muscle is the muscle cell or muscle fiber, which is highly specialized for contraction. Skeletal muscle fibers are long, multinucleated cylinders that contain many mitochondria to support their high metabolic activity. Muscle fibers are composed of myofibrils, which in turn are made up of contractile filaments (protein). The *sarcomere* is the

contractile unit of the myofibrils. Each sarcomere consists of myosin (thick) filaments and actin (thin) filaments. The arrangement of the thin and thick filaments accounts for the characteristic banding of muscle when it is seen under a microscope. Muscle contraction occurs as thick and thin filaments slide past each other, causing the sarcomeres to shorten.

Contractions. Skeletal muscle contractions allow posture maintenance, body movement, and facial expressions. Isometric contractions increase the tension within a muscle but do not produce movement. Repeated isometric contractions make muscles grow larger and stronger. Isotonic contractions shorten a muscle to produce movement. Most contractions are a combination of tension generation *(isometric)* and shortening *(isotonic).* Muscular *atrophy* (decrease in size) occurs with the absence of contraction that results from immobility, whereas increased muscular activity leads to *hypertrophy* (increase in size).

Skeletal muscle fibers are divided into two groups based on the type of activity they demonstrate. *Slow-twitch muscle fibers* support prolonged muscle activity such as marathon running. Because they also support the body against gravity, they assist

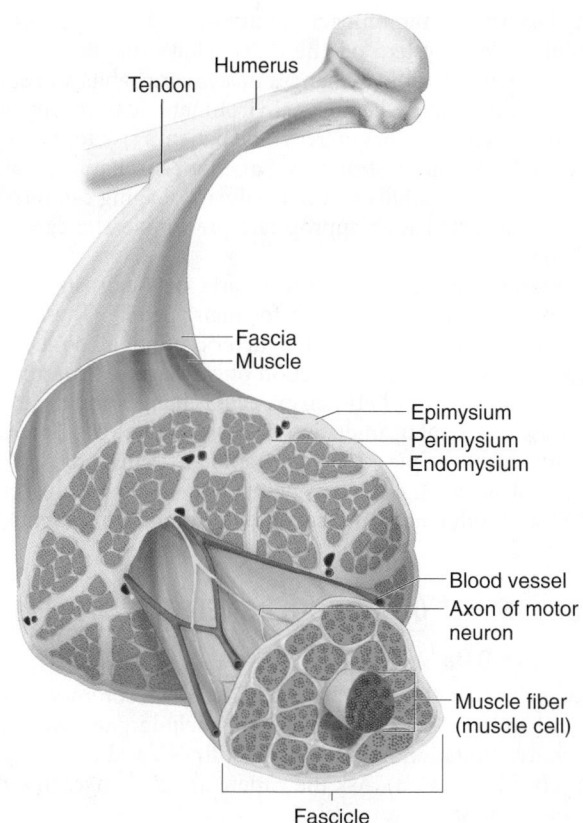

FIG. 62-5 Structure of a muscle.

FIG. 62-6 Neuromuscular junction.

in posture maintenance. *Fast-twitch muscle fibers* are used for rapid muscle contraction required for activities such as blinking the eye, jumping, or sprinting. Fast-twitch fibers tend to tire more quickly than slow-twitch fibers.

Neuromuscular Junction. Skeletal muscle fibers require a nerve impulse to contract. A nerve fiber and the skeletal muscle fibers it stimulates are called a *motor endplate.* The junction between the axon of the nerve cell and the adjacent muscle cell is called the *myoneural* or *neuromuscular junction* (Fig. 62-6).

Acetylcholine is released from the presynaptic neuron and diffuses across the neuromuscular junction to bind with receptors on the motor endplate of the muscle. In response to this stimulation, the sarcoplasmic reticulum releases calcium ions into the cytoplasm. The presence of calcium triggers the contraction in the myofibrils. When calcium is low, *tetany* (involuntary contractions of skeletal muscle) can occur.

Energy Source. The direct energy source for muscle fiber contractions is adenosine triphosphate (ATP). ATP is synthesized by cellular oxidative metabolism in numerous mitochondria located close to the myofibrils. It is rapidly depleted through conversion to adenosine diphosphate (ADP) and must be rephosphorylated. Phosphocreatine provides a rapid source for the resynthesis of ATP, but it is in turn converted to creatine and must be recharged. Glycolysis can serve as a source of ATP when the oxygen supply is inadequate for the metabolic needs of the muscle tissue. Glucose is broken down to pyruvic acid, which can be further converted to lactic acid to make more oxygen available. An accumulation of lactic acid in tissues leads to fatigue and pain.

Ligaments and Tendons

Ligaments and tendons are both composed of dense, fibrous connective tissue that contains bundles of closely packed collagen fibers arranged in the same plane for additional strength. *Tendons* attach muscles to bones as an extension of the muscle sheath that adheres to the periosteum. *Ligaments* connect bones to bones (e.g., tibia to femur at knee joint). They have a higher elastic content than tendons.[4] Ligaments provide stability while permitting controlled movement at the joint.

Ligaments and tendons have a relatively poor blood supply, usually making tissue repair a slow process after injury. For example, the stretching or tearing of ligaments that occurs with a sprain may require a long time to mend.

Fascia

Fascia refers to layers of connective tissue with intermeshed fibers that can withstand limited stretching. Superficial fascia lies immediately under the skin. Deep fascia is a dense, fibrous tissue that surrounds muscle bundles, nerves, and blood vessels. It also encloses individual muscles, allowing them to act independently and to glide over each other during contraction. In addition, fascia provides strength to muscle tissues.

Bursae

Bursae are small sacs of connective tissue lined with synovial membrane and containing viscous synovial fluid. They are typically located at bony prominences or joints to relieve pressure and decrease friction between moving parts.[5] For example, bursae are found between the patella and the skin (prepatellar bursae), between the olecranon process of the elbow and the skin (olecranon bursae), between the head of the humerus and the acromion process of the scapula (subacromial bursae), and between the greater trochanter of the proximal femur and the skin (trochanteric bursae). *Bursitis* is an inflammation of a bursa sac. The inflammation may be acute or chronic.

GERONTOLOGIC CONSIDERATIONS

EFFECTS OF AGING ON MUSCULOSKELETAL SYSTEM

Many of the functional problems experienced by the aging adult are related to changes of the musculoskeletal system. Although some changes begin in early adulthood, obvious signs of musculoskeletal impairment may not appear until later adult years. Alterations may affect the older adult's ability to complete self-care tasks and pursue other customary activities. Effects of musculoskeletal changes may range from mild discomfort and decreased ability to perform activities of daily living to severe, chronic pain and immobility. The risk for falls also increases in the older adult due in part to a loss of strength. Aging can also bring changes in the patient's balance, thus making the person unsteady, and *proprioception* (awareness of self in relation to the environment) may be altered.

The bone remodeling process is altered in the aging adult. Increased bone resorption and decreased bone formation cause a loss of bone density, contributing to the development of osteopenia and osteoporosis (see Chapter 64). Muscle mass and strength also decrease with aging. Almost 30% of muscle mass is lost by age 70. A loss of motor neurons can cause additional problems with skeletal muscle movement. Tendons and ligaments become less flexible, and movement becomes more rigid. Joints in the aging adult are also more likely to be affected by osteoarthritis[6] (see Chapter 65).

Perform a musculoskeletal assessment with a particular emphasis on exercise practices. Obtain information on the type of exercise performed, including frequency and warm-up activ-

ities. Determine the impact of age-related changes of the musculoskeletal system on the older adult's functional status. Specifically inquire about changes in self-care habits and ability to be self-sufficient in the home environment. Identify any musculoskeletal changes that increase the patient's risk for falls, and discuss fall prevention strategies. Functional limitations that are accepted by older adults as a normal part of aging can often be halted or reversed with appropriate preventive strategies (see Table 63-1).

Diseases such as osteoarthritis and osteoporosis are not a normal part of growing older for many people. These metabolic bone diseases involve the deterioration of bone tissue (osteoporosis) and the destruction of cartilage (osteoarthritis). Carefully differentiate between expected changes and the effects of disease in the aging adult. Symptoms of disease can be treated in many cases, helping the older adult to return to a higher functional level. Age-related changes in the musculoskeletal system and differences in assessment findings are presented in Table 62-1.

ASSESSMENT OF MUSCULOSKELETAL SYSTEM

Subjective Data

Important Health Information. The most common symptoms of musculoskeletal impairment include pain, weakness, deformity, limitation of movement, stiffness, and joint crepitation (crackling sound). Ask the patient about changes in sensation or in the size of a muscle.

Past Health History. Because certain illnesses are known to affect the musculoskeletal system either directly or indirectly, question the patient about past medical problems, including tuberculosis, poliomyelitis, diabetes mellitus, parathyroid problems, hemophilia, rickets, soft tissue infection, and neuromuscular disabilities. In addition, past or developing musculoskeletal problems can affect the patient's overall health. Trauma to the musculoskeletal system is a common reason for seeking medical evaluation. Questions should also focus on symptoms of arthritic and connective tissue diseases (e.g., gout, psoriatic arthritis, systemic lupus erythematosus), osteomalacia, osteo-

TABLE 62-1	GERONTOLOGIC ASSESSMENT DIFFERENCES

Musculoskeletal System

Changes	Differences in Assessment Findings
Muscle	
• Decreased number and diameter of muscle cells. Replacement of muscle cells by fibrous connective tissue. • Loss of elasticity in ligaments, tendons, and cartilage. • Reduced ability to store glycogen. Decreased ability to release glycogen as quick energy during stress. • Decreased basal metabolic rate.	• Decreased muscle strength and mass. Abdominal protrusion. Flabby muscles. • Increased rigidity in neck, shoulders, back, hips, and knees. • Decreased fine motor dexterity, decreased agility. • Slowed reaction times and reflexes as a result of slowing of impulse conduction along motor units. Earlier fatigue with activity.
Joints	
• Increased risk for cartilage erosion that contributes to direct contact between bone ends and overgrowth of bone around joint margins. • Loss of water from discs between vertebrae, decreased height of intervertebral spaces.	• Joint stiffness, decreased mobility, limited ROM, possible crepitation on movement. Pain with motion and/or weight bearing. • Loss of height and shortening of trunk from disc compression. Posture change.
Bone	
• Decreased bone density and strength, brittleness. • Slowed remodeling process.	• Loss of height and deformity such as dowager's hump (kyphosis) from vertebral compression and degeneration. • Back pain, stiffness. • Bony prominences more pronounced. • Increased risk of osteopenia and osteoporosis.

CASE STUDY

Patient Introduction

iStockphoto/Thinkstock

T.K. is a 78-yr-old white man brought to the emergency department by ambulance after falling on a patch of ice outside his home. He lay outside in the cold for 2 hr before neighbors found him. He is pale, diaphoretic, and complaining of excruciating pain in his left hip. The paramedics applied O_2 at 2 L via nasal cannula.

Critical Thinking

As you read through this assessment chapter, think about T.K.'s symptoms with the following questions in mind:
1. What is the most likely cause for T.K.'s acute hip pain?
2. What type of assessment would be most appropriate for T.K.: comprehensive, focused, or emergency? What would be your priority assessment(s)?
3. What questions would you ask T.K.?
4. What should be included in the physical assessment? What would you be looking for?
5. What diagnostic studies might you expect to be ordered?

evolve Answers available at *http://evolve.elsevier.com/Lewis/medsurg*.

myelitis, and fungal infection of bones or joints. Ask the patient about possible sources of a secondary bacterial infection, such as ears, tonsils, teeth, sinuses, lungs, or genitourinary tract. These infections can enter the bones, resulting in osteomyelitis or joint destruction. Obtain a detailed account of the course and treatment of any of these problems.

Medications. Question the patient regarding prescription and over-the-counter drugs and herbal products and nutritional supplements (see the Complementary & Alternative Therapies box in Chapter 3 on p. 39). Obtain detailed information about each treatment, including its name, the dose and frequency, length of time it was taken, its effects, and any possible side effects. Inquire about the use of skeletal muscle relaxants, opioids, nonsteroidal antiinflammatory drugs, and systemic and topical corticosteroids. Question the patient who has taken antiinflammatory drugs about GI distress or signs of bleeding.

In addition to drugs taken for treatment of a musculoskeletal problem, ask the patient about drugs that can have detrimental effects on this system. Some of these drugs and their potential side effects include antiseizure drugs (osteomalacia), phenothiazines (gait disturbances), corticosteroids (avascular necrosis, decreased bone and muscle mass), and potassium-depleting diuretics (muscle cramps and weakness). Question women

about their menstrual history. Episodes of premenopausal amenorrhea can contribute to the development of osteoporosis.[7] Ask postmenopausal women about their use of hormone therapy. Inquire about calcium and vitamin D supplements for both women and men.

Surgery or Other Treatments. Obtain information about past hospitalizations related to a musculoskeletal problem. Document the reason for hospitalization; the date and the duration; and the treatment, including ongoing rehabilitation. Also record details of emergency treatment for musculoskeletal injuries. Obtain specific information regarding any surgical procedure, postoperative course, and complications. If the patient experienced a period of prolonged immobilization, consider the possible development of osteoporosis and muscle atrophy.

Functional Health Patterns. The use of functional health patterns assists in organizing the assessment data. Table 62-2 summarizes specific questions to ask in relation to functional health patterns.

Health Perception–Health Management Pattern. Ask about the patient's health practices related to the musculoskeletal system, such as maintenance of a normal body weight, avoidance of excessive stress on muscles and joints, and use of proper body mechanics when lifting objects. Question the patient

---

TABLE 62-2 HEALTH HISTORY

Musculoskeletal System

Health Perception–Health Management Pattern
- Describe your usual daily activities.
- Do you experience any difficulties performing these activities?* Describe what you do if you experience difficulty in dressing, preparing meals and feeding yourself, performing basic hygiene, writing or using the phone, or maintaining your home.
- Do you have to lift heavy objects? Do your work or exercise habits require repetitive motion or joint stress? Describe any specialized equipment you use or wear when you work or exercise that helps protect you from injury.
- Do you take any drugs or herbal products to manage your musculoskeletal problem? If so, what are their names and what are the expected effects?

Nutritional-Metabolic Pattern
- What is your usual daily intake of food and snacks?
- Do you have difficulties preparing your food?
- What dietary supplements do you take? (Ask specifically about calcium, vitamin D supplements, and herbal products.)
- What is your weight? Describe any recent weight loss or gain.

Elimination Pattern
- Does your musculoskeletal problem make it difficult for you to reach the toilet in time?*
- Do you need any assistive devices or equipment to achieve satisfactory toileting?*
- Do you experience constipation related to decreased mobility or to drugs taken for your musculoskeletal problem?*

Activity-Exercise Pattern
- Do you require assistance in completing your usual daily activities because of a musculoskeletal problem?*
- Describe your usual exercise pattern. Do you experience musculoskeletal symptoms before, during, or after exercising?*
- Are you able to move all your joints comfortably through full range of motion?
- Do you use any prosthetic or orthotic devices?*

Sleep-Rest Pattern
- Do you experience any difficulty sleeping because of a musculoskeletal problem?* Do you require frequent position changes at night?*
- Do you wake up at night because of musculoskeletal pain?*
- Do you use complementary and alternative therapies to help you sleep at night?*

Cognitive-Perceptual Pattern
- Describe any musculoskeletal pain you experience. How do you manage your pain? (Ask specifically about adjunctive therapies such as heat and cold or complementary and alternative therapies such as acupuncture.)

Self-Perception–Self-Concept Pattern
- Describe how changes in your musculoskeletal system (posture, walking, muscle strength) and decreased ability to do certain things may affect how you feel about yourself. Have these changes affected your lifestyle?*

Role-Relationship Pattern
- Do you live alone?
- Describe how family, friends, or others assist you with your musculoskeletal problem.
- Describe the effect of your musculoskeletal problem on your work and on your social relationships.

Sexuality-Reproductive Pattern
- Describe any sexual concerns related to your musculoskeletal problem.

Coping–Stress Tolerance Pattern
- Describe how you deal with problems such as pain, weakness, or immobility that have resulted from your musculoskeletal problem.

Value-Belief Pattern
- Describe any cultural practices or religious beliefs that may influence the treatment of your musculoskeletal problem.

*If yes, describe.

specifically about tetanus and polio immunizations. Obtain the most current date and reaction to a tuberculin skin test.

Patients who are good historians can recount numerous minor and major injuries of their musculoskeletal system. Record information chronologically and include the following:

- Mechanism and circumstances of the injury (e.g., twist, crush, stretch)
- Methods and duration of treatment
- Current status related to the injury
- Need for assistive devices
- Interference with activities of daily living

Safety practices can affect the patient's predisposition for certain injuries and illnesses. Therefore ask the patient about safety practices as they relate to the work environment, home life, recreation, and exercise. For example, if the patient is a computer programmer, ask about ergonomic adaptations in the office that decrease the risk of carpal tunnel syndrome or low back pain. Identification of problems in this area will direct your plan for patient teaching.

🧬 GENETIC RISK ALERT
Autoimmune Diseases
- Many autoimmune diseases of the musculoskeletal system have a genetic basis involving human leukocyte antigens (HLAs).
- These diseases include ankylosing spondylitis, rheumatoid arthritis, and systemic lupus erythematosus.

Osteoporosis
- Genetic factors contribute to osteoporosis by influencing not only bone mineral density but also bone size, bone quality, and bone turnover.

Osteoarthritis, Gout, and Scoliosis
- A genetic predisposition is a contributing risk factor in all these diseases.

Muscular Dystrophy
- The most common types of muscular dystrophy are X-linked recessive disorders.

Obtain a family history related to rheumatoid arthritis, systemic lupus erythematosus, ankylosing spondylitis, osteoarthritis, gout, osteoporosis, and scoliosis because a patient may have a genetic predisposition to these or other musculoskeletal disorders.

Nutritional-Metabolic Pattern. The patient's description of a typical day's diet provides clues to areas of nutritional concern that can affect the musculoskeletal system. An adequate intake of vitamins C and D, calcium, and protein is essential for a healthy, intact musculoskeletal system. Abnormal nutritional patterns can predispose individuals to problems such as osteomalacia and osteoporosis. In addition, maintenance of normal weight is an important nutritional goal. Obesity places additional stress on weight-bearing joints such as the knees, hips, and spine, and it predisposes individuals to instability of the ligaments.

Elimination Pattern. Questions about the patient's mobility may reveal difficulty with ambulating to the toilet. Ask the patient if an assistive device such as an elevated toilet seat or a grab bar is necessary to accomplish toileting. Decreased mobility secondary to a musculoskeletal problem can lead to constipation. In addition, musculoskeletal problems can contribute to bowel or bladder incontinence when ambulation is a problem.

Activity-Exercise Pattern. Obtain a detailed account of the type, duration, and frequency of exercise and recreational activities. Compare daily, weekend, and seasonal patterns because occasional or sporadic exercise can be more problematic than regular exercise. Many musculoskeletal problems can affect the patient's activity-exercise pattern. Question the patient about clumsiness or limitations in movement, pain, weakness, crepitus, or any change in the bones or joints that interferes with daily activities.

Extremes of activity related to occupation can also affect the musculoskeletal system. A sedentary occupation can negatively affect muscle flexibility and strength. Jobs that require extreme effort through heavy lifting or pushing can lead to damage of joints and supporting structures. Specifically question the patient about work-related injuries to the musculoskeletal system, including treatment and time lost from work.

Sleep-Rest Pattern. The discomfort caused by musculoskeletal disorders can interfere with the patient's normal sleep pattern. Ask the patient about possible alterations in sleep patterns. If the patient describes sleep interference related to a musculoskeletal problem, inquire further about the type of bedding and pillows used, bedtime routine, sleeping partner, and sleeping positions.

Cognitive-Perceptual Pattern. Fully explore and document any pain experienced by the patient as a result of a musculoskeletal problem. To provide a baseline for later reassessment, ask the patient to describe the intensity of the pain on a numeric scale from 0 to 10 (0 = no pain, 10 = most severe pain imaginable).[8] Reassessments over time assist in determining the effectiveness of any treatment plan. Question the patient about measures used at home for managing pain. Ask about related problems such as joint swelling or muscle weakness and any accommodations that help with the problem. (Pain is discussed in Chapter 9.)

Self-Perception–Self-Concept Pattern. Many chronic musculoskeletal problems lead to deformities and a reduction in activities that can have a serious negative impact on the patient's body image and sense of personal worth. Assess the patient's feelings about these changes and the effect they may have on interactions with family and friends.

Role-Relationship Pattern. Impaired mobility and chronic pain from musculoskeletal problems can negatively affect the patient's ability to perform in roles of spouse, parent, or employee. The ability to pursue and maintain meaningful social and personal relationships can also be affected by musculoskeletal problems. Carefully question the patient about role performance and relationships.

If the patient lives alone, the current musculoskeletal problem and rehabilitation may make it difficult or impossible to continue this arrangement. Determine the degree of assistance available from family, friends, and other caregivers. Find out if additional resources are needed such as physical therapy and home health care.

Sexuality-Reproductive Pattern. The pain of musculoskeletal problems can impede the patient's ability to obtain sexual satisfaction. Explore this area with a sensitive and nonjudgmental attitude. Help the patient feel comfortable discussing any sexual problems related to pain, movement, and positioning. Additional information in obtaining patient data in this area is presented in Chapter 51.

Coping–Stress Tolerance Pattern. Mobility limitations and pain, whether acute or chronic, are serious potential stressors that challenge the patient's coping resources. Recognize the potential for ineffective coping in the patient and family or significant other. Additional questioning will help to determine if a musculoskeletal problem is causing difficulties in coping and adjusting.

CASE STUDY—cont'd

Subjective Data

iStockphoto/Thinkstock

A focused subjective assessment of T.K. revealed the following information:

PMH: Type 2 diabetes for 11 yr. COPD for 15 yr. 40 pack-year smoking history.

Medications: Metformin (Glucophage) 500 mg PO bid; glyburide (DiaBeta) 5 mg/day PO; fluticasone and salmeterol combination (Advair) 250/50 mcg 1 inhalation bid; albuterol 2 puffs q4hr PRN as rescue inhaler.

Health Perception–Health Management: Currently smokes 2 to 3 packs of cigarettes per day. Is trying to quit but finding it difficult. Drinks alcohol at night.

Nutritional-Metabolic: T.K. is 6 ft, 2 in tall and weighs 195 lb. Does not take any nutritional supplements and tends to shy away from milk and other dairy products, since they make him "gassy."

Activity-Exercise: Leads a fairly sedentary lifestyle because of dyspnea on exertion. Until this current fall, has been able to perform ADLs without assistance. Denies any history of musculoskeletal problems.

Cognitive-Perceptual: Rates left hip pain at a 9 on a scale of 0-10. Describes pain as sharp spasms that increase in intensity with any movement.

Coping–Stress Tolerance: Is asking for pain medicine "as strong as you can give me."

Value-Belief Pattern. Ask the patient about cultural or religious beliefs that might influence the patient's acceptance of treatment for the musculoskeletal problem. These may include recommendations for diet, exercise, medication, and lifestyle modifications.

Objective Data

Physical Examination. Examination involves observation, palpation, motion, and muscular assessment. Conduct a general overview, while obtaining data in a careful health history to provide guidance in choosing areas to concentrate on during the local examination. Take specific measurements as indicated by the local examination.

Inspection. A systematic inspection is performed starting at the head and neck and proceeding to the upper extremities, lower extremities, and trunk. The regular use of a systematic approach is important to avoid missing important aspects of the examination. Inspect the skin for general color, scars, or other overt signs of previous injury or surgery. Certain cutaneous lesions require additional investigation because they can indicate underlying disorders. For example, butterfly rash over the cheeks and nose is a characteristic marker of systemic lupus erythematosus.

Note the patient's general body build, muscle configuration, and symmetry of joints. Observe for any swelling, deformity, nodules or masses, and discrepancies in limb length or muscle size. Use the patient's opposite body part for comparison when an abnormality is suspected.

Palpation. Carefully palpate any area that has aroused concern because of a subjective complaint or that appears abnormal on inspection. As with inspection, palpation usually proceeds cephalopedally (head to toe) to examine the neck, shoulders, elbows, wrists, hands, back, hips, knees, ankles, and feet. Both superficial and deep palpation are usually performed consecutively.

Warm your hands to prevent muscle spasm, which can interfere with identification of essential landmarks or soft tissue

FIG. 62-7 A, Goniometer. **B,** Measurement of joint range of motion using a goniometer.

structures. Palpate both muscles and joints to allow for evaluation of skin temperature, local tenderness, swelling, and crepitation. Establish the relationship of adjacent structures, and evaluate the general contour, abnormal prominences, and local landmarks.

Motion. When assessing the patient's joint mobility, carefully evaluate both active and passive **range of motion** (full movement potential of a joint). Measurements should be similar for both active and passive maneuvers. *Active range of motion* means the patient takes his or her own joints through all movements without assistance. *Passive range of motion* occurs when someone else moves the patient's joints without his or her assistance through the full range of motion. Be careful in performing passive range of motion because of the risk of injury to underlying structures. If pain or resistance is encountered, stop manipulation immediately.

If you note deficits in active or passive range of motion, also assess functional range of motion to determine if performance of activities of daily living has been affected by joint changes. This is done by asking the patient if activities such as eating and bathing need to be performed with assistance or cannot be done at all.

Range of motion is most accurately assessed with a goniometer, which measures the angle of the joint (Fig. 62-7). Specific degrees of range of motion of all joints are usually not measured unless a musculoskeletal problem has been identified. A less exact but valuable assessment method is to compare the range of motion of one extremity with that on the opposite side. Common movements that occur at the synovial joints, includ-

TABLE 62-3 SYNOVIAL JOINT MOVEMENTS

Movement	Description
Abduction	Movement of part away from midline of body
Adduction	Movement of part toward midline of body
Circumduction	Combination of flexion, extension, abduction, and adduction resulting in circular motion of a body part
Dorsiflexion	Flexion of the ankle and toes toward the shin
Eversion	Turning of sole outward away from midline of body
Extension	Straightening of joint that increases angle between two bones
External rotation	Movement along longitudinal axis away from midline of body
Flexion	Bending of joint as a result of muscle contraction that results in decreased angle between two bones
Hyperextension	Extension in which angle exceeds 180 degrees
Internal rotation	Movement along longitudinal axis toward midline of body
Inversion	Turning of sole inward toward midline of body
Opposition	Moving the first and fifth metacarpals anteriorly from a flattened palm ("cupping position"); makes it possible to hold objects between the thumb and fingers
Plantar flexion	Flexion of the ankle and toes toward the plantar surface of the foot ("toes pointed")
Pronation	Turning of palm downward
Supination	Turning of palm upward

ing *abduction, adduction, flexion,* and *extension,* are described in Table 62-3.

Muscle-Strength Testing. Grade the strength of individual muscles or groups of muscles during contraction (Table 62-4). Grade normal muscle strength as a 5 bilaterally, with full resistance to opposition. Have the patient apply resistance to the force the examiner is exerting. For example, try to pull the bent arm down while the patient attempts to raise it. Compare muscle strength with the strength of the opposite extremity. Note any subtle variations in muscle strength when comparing the patient's dominant and nondominant sides. Variations in strength also exist when comparing individuals.

Measurement. When length discrepancies or subjective problems are noted, obtain limb length and circumferential muscle mass measurements. For example, measure leg length when gait disorders are observed. Measure the affected limb between the anterosuperior iliac crest and the bottom of the medial malleolus. Then compare it with the similar measure-

ment of the opposite extremity. Measure muscle mass circumferentially at the largest area of the muscle. When recording measurements, document the exact location at which the measurements were obtained (e.g., the quadriceps muscle is measured 15 cm above the patella). This informs the next examiner of the exact area to measure and ensures consistency during reassessment.

Other. Note the patient's use of an assistive device such as a walker or cane. Assess the patient for a proper fit while reviewing the safe and correct technique for using these devices. Regularly review with the patient the use of the assistive device to ensure it remains appropriate and safe.[9] If the patient is able to move independently, assess posture and gait by watching the patient walk, stand, and sit. Musculoskeletal and neurologic problems can result in abnormal gait patterns.

Scoliosis is a lateral S-shaped curvature of the thoracic and lumbar spine. Unequal shoulder and scapula height is usually noted when the patient is observed from the back (Fig. 62-8). Also ask the patient to place the fingertips together as if diving into a swimming pool and slowly bend forward, allowing for assessment of thoracic rib prominence or paravertebral muscle prominence in the lumbar spine. If the deformity is greater than 45 degrees, lung and cardiac function is usually impaired.

The *straight-leg-raising test* is performed on the supine patient with sciatica or leg pain. Passively raise the patient's leg 60 degrees or less. The test is positive if the patient complains of pain along the distribution of the sciatic nerve. A positive test indicates nerve root irritation from intervertebral disc prolapse and herniation, particularly at the level of L4-5 or L5-S1.

Assessment of reflexes is discussed in Chapter 56. Neurovascular assessment is discussed in Chapter 63. Table 62-5 is an example of how to record a normal physical assessment of the musculoskeletal system. Abnormal assessment findings of the musculoskeletal system are presented in Table 62-6.

TABLE 62-4 MUSCLE STRENGTH SCALE

0	No detection of muscular contraction
1	A barely detectable flicker or trace of contraction with observation or palpation
2	Active movement of body part with elimination of gravity
3	Active movement against gravity only and not against resistance
4	Active movement against gravity and some resistance
5	Active movement against full resistance without evident fatigue (normal muscle strength)

FIG. 62-8 Scoliosis in a standing erect posture.

TABLE 62-5	**NORMAL PHYSICAL ASSESSMENT OF THE MUSCULOSKELETAL SYSTEM**

- Normal spinal curvatures
- No muscle atrophy or asymmetry
- No joint swelling, deformity, or crepitation
- No tenderness on palpation of spine, joints, or muscles
- Full range of motion of all joints without pain or laxity
- Muscle strength of 5

FOCUSED ASSESSMENT

Musculoskeletal System

Use this checklist to make sure the key assessment steps have been done.

Subjective
Ask the patient about any of the following and note responses.

Joint pain or stiffness	Y	N
Muscle weakness	Y	N
Bone pain	Y	N

Objective: Diagnostic
Check the results of the following diagnostic studies.

X-ray results	✓
Bone scans	✓
Erythrocyte sedimentation rate	✓

Objective: Physical Examination
Inspect and Palpate

Skeleton and extremities (and compare sides) for alignment, contour, symmetry, size, and gross deformities	✓
Joints for range of motion, tenderness or pain, heat, crepitus, and swelling	✓
Muscles (and compare sides) for size, symmetry, tone, and tenderness or pain	✓
Bones for tenderness or pain	✓

A *focused assessment* is used to evaluate the status of previously identified musculoskeletal problems and to monitor for signs of new problems (see Table 3-6). A focused assessment of the musculoskeletal system is presented in the box above.

DIAGNOSTIC STUDIES OF MUSCULOSKELETAL SYSTEM

Numerous diagnostic studies are available to assess the musculoskeletal system. Table 62-7 presents the most common studies, and select studies are described in more detail below.

The use of studies such as x-rays, magnetic resonance imaging (MRI), and bone scans has greatly improved orthopedic care. The x-ray, or roentgenogram, is the most common diagnostic study used to assess musculoskeletal problems and to monitor the effectiveness of treatment. Because bones are denser than other tissues, x-rays do not penetrate them. Dense areas show as white on the standard x-ray. X-rays provide information about bone deformity, joint congruity, bone density, and calcification in soft tissue. Fracture diagnosis and management are the primary indications for x-rays, but they are also useful in the evaluation of genetic, developmental, infectious, inflammatory, neoplastic, metabolic, and degenerative disorders.

A small fiberoptic tube called an arthroscope is used to directly examine the interior of a joint cavity in a procedure

CASE STUDY—cont'd
Objective Data: Physical Examination

iStockphoto/Thinkstock

A focused assessment of T.K. reveals the following:

BP 166/94, heart rate 98, respiratory rate 36, temp 35.8° C, O_2 saturation 91% on 2 L O_2. Alert and oriented × 3. Left leg shortened and externally rotated. No external bruising noted. +1 Pedal pulses bilaterally. Lungs with bibasilar crackles and expiratory wheezing.

As you continue to read this chapter, consider diagnostic studies you would anticipate being performed for T.K.

FIG. 62-9 Knee arthroscopy in progress. Notice the monitor in the background.

known as **arthroscopy.** After anesthesia has been administered, a large-bore needle is inserted into the joint, and the joint is distended with fluid or air (Fig. 62-9). When the arthroscope is inserted, the surgeon is able to perform extensive, accurate visualization of the joint cavity. Photographs or videotapes can be made through the scope, and a biopsy of the synovium or cartilage can be obtained. Torn tissue can be repaired through arthroscopic surgery, eliminating the need for a larger incision and greatly decreasing the recovery time.

An **arthrocentesis** (joint aspiration) is usually performed for synovial fluid analysis. It may also be done to remove fluid from joints to relieve pain. First, the skin is cleansed and a local anesthetic is given. After an 18-gauge or larger needle is inserted into the joint, the fluid is withdrawn. The appropriate sterile container should be readily available to receive the aspirated fluid, which must be transported immediately to the laboratory. Patients with inflammatory joint conditions (e.g., rheumatoid arthritis, septic arthritis, osteoarthritis) may be treated with an

Text continued on p. 1503

TABLE 62-6 ASSESSMENT ABNORMALITIES

Musculoskeletal System

Finding	Description	Possible Etiology and Significance
Achilles tendonitis	Pain in posterior leg, initially when running or walking. Can progress to pain at rest.	Cumulative stress on Achilles tendon resulting in inflammation.
Ankylosis	Stiffness and fixation of a joint.	Chronic joint inflammation and destruction (e.g., rheumatoid arthritis).
Antalgic gait	Shortened stride with as little weight bearing as possible on the affected side.	Pain or discomfort in the lower extremity on weight bearing. Can be related to trauma or other disorders.
Ataxic gait	Staggering, uncoordinated gait often with sway.	Neurogenic disorders (e.g., spinal cord lesion).
Atrophy	Flabby appearance of muscle leading to decreased function and tone.	Muscle denervation, contracture, prolonged disuse as a result of immobilization.
Boutonnière deformity	Finger abnormality, flexion of proximal interphalangeal (PIP) joint and hyperextension of the distal interphalangeal (DIP) joint of the fingers (see Fig. 65-4, B).	Typical deformity of rheumatoid and psoriatic arthritis caused by rupture of extensor tendons over the fingers.
Contracture	Resistance of movement of muscle or joint as a result of fibrosis of supporting soft tissues.	Shortening of muscle or ligaments, tightness of soft tissue, incorrect positioning of immobilized extremity.
Crepitation (crepitus)	Frequent, audible crackling sound with palpable grating that accompanies movement.	Fracture, dislocation, temporomandibular joint dysfunction, osteoarthritis.
Dislocation	Separation of two bones from their normal position within a joint.	Trauma, disorders of surrounding soft tissues.
Festinating gait	While walking, neck, trunk, and knees flex while the body is rigid. Delayed start with short, quick, shuffling steps. Speed may increase as if patient is unable to stop (festination).	Neurogenic disorders (e.g., Parkinson's disease).
Ganglion cyst	Small fluid-filled bump or mass over a tendon sheath or joint, usually on dorsal surface of wrist or foot.	Inflammation of tissues around a joint, which can increase in size or disappear.
Kyphosis (dowager's hump)	Exaggerated thoracic curvature.	Poor posture, tuberculosis, arthritis, osteoporosis, growth disturbance of vertebral epiphyses.
Lateral epicondylitis (tennis elbow)	Dull ache along outer aspect of elbow, worsens with twisting and grasping motions.	Partial tearing of tendon at its insertion on epicondyle.
Limited range of motion (ROM)	Joint does not achieve the expected degrees of motion.	Injury, inflammation, contracture.
Lordosis (swayback)	Asymmetric scapulae and shoulders, exaggerated lumbar curvature.	Secondary to other spinal deformities, muscular dystrophy, obesity, flexion contracture of hip, congenital dislocation of hip.
Muscle spasticity	Increased muscle tone (rigidity) with sustained muscle contractions (spasms); stiffness or tightness may interfere with gait, movement, speech.	Neuromuscular disorders such as multiple sclerosis (MS) or cerebral palsy.
Myalgia	General muscle tenderness and pain.	Chronic rheumatic syndromes (e.g., fibromyalgia). Overuse, injury, or strain.
Paresthesia	Numbness and tingling, often described as a "pins and needles" sensation.	Compromised sensory nerves, often due to edema in a closed space such as a cast or bulky dressing. May also result from spinal stenosis.
Pes planus (flatfoot)	Abnormal flatness of the sole and arch of the foot.	Hereditary, muscle paralysis, mild cerebral palsy, early muscular dystrophy, injury to posterior tibial tendon.
Plantar fasciitis	Burning, sharp pain on sole of foot; worse in the morning.	Chronic degenerative/reparative cycle resulting in inflammation.
Scoliosis	Asymmetric elevation of shoulders, scapulae, and iliac crests with lateral spine curvature (see Fig. 62-8).	Idiopathic or congenital condition, fracture or dislocation, osteomalacia.
Short-leg gait	A limp, unless corrective footwear used.	Leg length discrepancy of ≥1 in, generally of structural origin (arthritis, fracture).
Spastic gait	Short steps with dragging of foot. Jerky, uncoordinated, cross-knee (scissor) movement.	Neurogenic (e.g., cerebral palsy, hemiplegia).
Steppage gait	Increased hip and knee flexion to clear the foot from the floor. Footdrop is evident, foot slaps down and along walking surface.	Neurogenic disorders (e.g., peroneal nerve injury, paralyzed dorsiflexor muscles).
Subluxation	Partial dislocation of joint.	Instability of joint capsule and supporting ligaments (e.g., trauma, arthritis).
Swan neck deformity	Hyperextension of the PIP joint with flexion of the metacarpophalangeal (MCP) and DIP joints of the fingers (see Fig. 65-4, D).	Typical deformity of rheumatoid and psoriatic arthritis caused by contracture of muscles and tendons.
Swelling	Enlargement, often of a joint due to fluid collection. Generally leads to pain, stiffness.	Trauma or inflammation.
Tenosynovitis	Superficial swelling, pain, and tenderness along a tendon sheath.	Inflammation that often occurs with infection, injury, or overuse.
Torticollis (wryneck)	Neck is twisted in unusual position to one side.	Prolonged contraction of neck muscles, congenital or acquired.
Ulnar deviation (ulnar drift)	Fingers drift to ulnar side of forearm (see Fig. 65-4, A).	Typical deformity of rheumatoid arthritis due to tendon contracture.
Valgum deformity (knock-knees)	When knees are together and there is >1 in (2.5 cm) between the medial malleoli.	Poliomyelitis, congenital deformity, arthritis.
Varum deformity (bowlegs)	When knees are apart and the medial malleoli are together, a space of >1 in (2.5 cm) exists.	Arthritis, congenital deformity.

Musculoskeletal System

TABLE 62-7 DIAGNOSTIC STUDIES

Musculoskeletal System

Study	Description and Purpose	Nursing Responsibility
Radiologic Studies		
Standard x-ray	Determines density of bone. Evaluates structural or functional changes of bones and joints. In anteroposterior view, x-ray beam passes from front to back, allowing one-dimensional view. Lateral position provides two-dimensional view.	Avoid excessive exposure of patient and self. Before procedure, remove any radiopaque objects that can interfere with results. Explain procedure to patient.
Diskogram	X-ray of cervical or lumbar intervertebral disc is done after injection of contrast media into nucleus pulposus. Permits visualization of intervertebral disc abnormalities.	Assess patient for possible allergy to contrast medium. Explain procedure.
Computed tomography (CT) scan	X-ray beam is used with a computer to provide a three-dimensional picture. Used to identify soft tissue abnormalities, bony abnormalities, and various types of musculoskeletal trauma.	Inform patient that procedure is painless. Inform patient of importance of remaining still during procedure. If contrast medium is being used, verify that patient does not have shellfish allergy.
Myelogram with or without CT	Involves injecting a radiographic contrast medium into sac around nerve roots. CT scan may follow to show how the bone is affecting the nerve roots. Sensitive test for nerve impingement and can detect subtle lesions and injuries.	Main risk is the potential for spinal headache. Inform patient that headache should resolve in 1–2 days with rest and fluids, but should be reported to health care provider.
Magnetic resonance imaging (MRI)	Radio waves and magnetic field are used to view soft tissue. Especially useful in the diagnosis of avascular necrosis, disc disease, tumors, osteomyelitis, ligament tears, and cartilage tears. Patient is placed inside scanning chamber. Gadolinium may be injected IV to enhance visualization of structures. Open MRI does not require patient to be placed inside a chamber. Contraindicated in patient with aneurysm clips, metallic implants, pacemakers, electronic devices, hearing aids, and shrapnel.	Inform patient that procedure is painless. Explain that the machine will make loud tapping noises intermittently and there is no cause for alarm. Ear plugs can be requested or music to listen to. Ensure that patient has no metal on clothing (e.g., snaps, zippers, jewelry, credit cards). Inform patient to remain still throughout procedure. Inform patients who are claustrophobic that they may experience symptoms during examination. Administer antianxiety agent if indicated and ordered. Open MRI may be indicated for obese patient or patient with large chest and abdominal girth or severe claustrophobia. ·
Bone Mineral Density (BMD) Measurements		
Dual energy x-ray absorptiometry (DXA)	Measures bone mass of spine, femur, forearm, and total body. Allows assessment of bone density with minimal radiation exposure. Used to diagnose metabolic bone disease and to monitor changes in bone density with treatment.	Inform patient that procedure is painless.
Quantitative ultrasound (QUS)	Evaluates density, elasticity, and strength of bone using ultrasound rather than radiation. Common area assessed is calcaneus (heel).	Same as above.
Radioisotope Studies		
Bone scan	Involves injection of radioisotope (usually technetium [Tc]-99m) that is taken up by bone. A uniform uptake of the isotope is normal. Increased uptake is seen in osteomyelitis, osteoporosis, primary and metastatic malignant lesions of bone, and certain fractures. Decreased uptake is seen in areas of avascular necrosis.	Explain that radioisotope is given 2 hr before procedure. Ensure that bladder is emptied before scan. Inform patient that procedure requires 1 hr while patient lies supine and that no pain or harm will result from isotopes. Increase fluids after the examination.
Endoscopy		
Arthroscopy	Involves insertion of arthroscope into joint (usually knee) for visualization of structure and contents. Can be used for exploratory surgery (removal of loose bodies and biopsy); repair of joint structures; and diagnosis of abnormalities of meniscus, articular cartilage, ligaments, or joint capsule. Other structures that can be visualized through an arthroscope include shoulder, elbow, wrist, jaw, hip, and ankle.	Inform patient that procedure can be performed in outpatient setting and that local or general anesthesia may be used. After procedure, cover wound with sterile dressing. Explain any postprocedure activity restrictions.
Mineral Metabolism		
Alkaline phosphatase	This enzyme, produced by osteoblasts of bone, is needed for mineralization of organic bone matrix. Elevated levels are found in healing fractures, bone cancers, osteoporosis, osteomalacia, and Paget's disease. *Reference interval:* 38-126 U/L (0.65-2.14 μkat/L)	Obtain blood samples by venipuncture. Observe venipuncture site for bleeding or hematoma formation. Inform patient that procedure does not require fasting.
Calcium	Bone is primary organ for calcium storage. Calcium provides bone with rigid structure. Decreased serum level is found in osteomalacia, renal disease, and hypoparathyroidism. Increased level is found in hyperparathyroidism and some bone tumors. *Reference interval:* 8.6-10.2 mg/dL (2.20-2.55 mmol/L)	Same as above.

Continued

TABLE 62-7 DIAGNOSTIC STUDIES—cont'd

Musculoskeletal System

Study	Description and Purpose	Nursing Responsibility
Phosphorus	Amount present is indirectly related to calcium metabolism. Decreased level is found in osteomalacia. Increased level is found in chronic kidney disease, healing fractures, and osteolytic metastatic tumor. *Reference interval:* 2.4-4.4 mg/dL (0.78-1.42 mmol/L)	Same as above.

Serologic Studies

Study	Description and Purpose	Nursing Responsibility
Rheumatoid factor (RF)	Assesses presence of autoantibody (rheumatoid factor) in serum. Factor is not specific for rheumatoid arthritis and is seen in other connective tissue diseases and in a small percentage of normal population. *Reference interval:* Negative or titer <1:17	Same as above.
Erythrocyte sedimentation rate (ESR)	Nonspecific index of inflammation. Measures rapidity with which red blood cells settle from unclotted blood in 1 hr. Results influenced by physiologic factors and diseases. Elevated levels are seen with any inflammatory process (especially rheumatoid arthritis, rheumatic fever, osteomyelitis, and respiratory tract infections). *Reference interval:* <30 mm/hr (some gender variation)	Same as above.
Antinuclear antibody (ANA)	Assesses presence of antibodies capable of destroying nucleus of body's tissue cells. Finding is positive in 95% of patients with systemic lupus erythematosus and may also be positive in individuals with scleroderma or rheumatoid arthritis and in a small percentage of normal population. *Reference interval:* Negative at 1:40 dilution	Same as above.
Anti-DNA antibody	Detects serum antibodies that react with DNA. Most specific test for systemic lupus erythematosus. *Reference interval:* <70 IU/mL	Same as above.
Complement, total hemolytic (CH_{50})	Complement, a normal body protein, is essential to both immune and inflammatory reactions. Complement components used in these reactions are depleted. Complement depletions may be found in patients with rheumatoid arthritis or systemic lupus erythematosus. *Reference interval:* 75-160 U/mL (75-160 kU/L)	Same as above.
Uric acid	End product of purine metabolism is normally excreted in urine. Although not specific, levels are usually elevated in gout. *Male:* 4.4-7.6 mg/dL (262-452 µmol/L) *Female:* 2.3-6.6 mg/dL (137-393 µmol/L)	Same as above.
C-reactive protein (CRP)	Used to diagnose inflammatory diseases, infections, and active widespread malignancy. Synthesized by the liver and is present in large amounts in serum 18-24 hr after onset of tissue damage. *Reference interval:* 6.8-820 mcg/dL (68-8200 mcg/L)	Same as above.
Human leukocyte antigen (HLA)–B27	Antigen often present in autoimmune disorders such as ankylosing spondylitis and rheumatoid arthritis.	Same as above.

Markers of Muscle Injury

Study	Description and Purpose	Nursing Responsibility
Creatine kinase (CK)	Highest concentration found in skeletal muscle. Increased levels found in progressive muscular dystrophy, polymyositis, and traumatic injuries. *Male:* 20-200 U/L *Female:* 20-180 U/L	Same as above.
Potassium	Increased in muscle trauma as cell destruction releases this electrolyte into serum. Cardiac dysrhythmias can be caused by hyperkalemia or hypokalemia. *Reference interval:* 3.5-5.0 mEq/L (3.5-5.0 mmol/L)	Same as above.
Aldolase	Useful in monitoring muscular dystrophy and dermatomyositis. *Reference interval:* 1.5-8.1 U/L	Same as above.

Invasive Procedures

Study	Description and Purpose	Nursing Responsibility
Arthrocentesis	Incision or puncture of joint capsule to obtain samples of synovial fluid from within joint cavity or to remove excess fluid. Local anesthesia and aseptic preparation are used before needle is inserted into joint and fluid aspirated. Useful in diagnosis of joint inflammation, infection, meniscal tears, and subtle fractures.	Inform patient that procedure is usually done at bedside or in examination room. Send samples of synovial fluid to laboratory for examination (if indicated). After procedure apply compression dressing. Observe for leakage of blood or fluid on dressing.

TABLE 62-7 DIAGNOSTIC STUDIES—cont'd

Musculoskeletal System

Study	Description and Purpose	Nursing Responsibility
Electromyogram (EMG)	Evaluates electrical potential associated with skeletal muscle contraction. Small-gauge needles are inserted into certain muscles. Needle probes are attached to leads that feed information to EMG machine. Recordings of electrical activity of muscle are traced on audio transmitter and on oscilloscope and recording paper. Useful in providing information related to lower motor neuron dysfunction and primary muscle disease.	Inform patient that procedure is usually done in EMG laboratory while patient lies supine on special table. Keep patient awake to cooperate with voluntary movement. Inform patient that procedure involves some discomfort from needle insertion. Avoid stimulants, including caffeine, and sedatives 24 hr before procedure.
Miscellaneous		
Duplex venous Doppler	Ultrasound of the veins, usually of the lower extremities, to detect blood flow abnormalities that could indicate deep vein thrombosis.	Inform patient that procedure is painless and noninvasive.
Thermography	Uses infrared detector that measures degree of heat radiating from skin surface. Useful in investigating cause of inflamed joint and in determining patient response to antiinflammatory drug therapy.	Same as above.
Plethysmography	Records variations in volume and pressure of blood passing through tissues. Test is nonspecific.	Same as above.
Somatosensory evoked potential (SSEP)	Evaluates evoked potential of muscle contractions. Electrodes are placed on skin and provide recordings of electrical activity of muscle. Useful in identifying subtle dysfunction of lower motor neuron and primary muscle disease. Measures nerve conduction along pathways not accessible by EMG. Transcutaneous or percutaneous electrodes are applied to the skin and help identify neuropathy and myopathy. Often used during spinal surgery for scoliosis to detect neurologic compromise when patient is under anesthesia.	Inform patient that procedure is similar to EMG but does not involve needles. Electrodes are applied to the skin.

intraarticular injection of corticosteroids after the joint fluid has been aspirated.[10]

The fluid is examined grossly for volume, color, clarity, viscosity, and mucin clot formation. Normal synovial fluid is transparent and colorless or straw colored. It should be scant in amount and of low viscosity. Fluid from an infected joint may be purulent and thick or gray and thin. In gout, the fluid may be whitish yellow. Blood may be aspirated if there is hemarthrosis due to injury or a bleeding disorder. The mucin clot test indicates the character of the protein portion of the synovial fluid. Normally a white, ropelike mucin clot is formed. In the presence of inflammation, the clot fragments easily. The fluid is examined grossly for floating fat globules, which indicate bone injury. In septic arthritis, protein content is elevated and glucose is considerably decreased. Presence of uric acid crystals suggests a diagnosis of gout. A Gram stain and culture may also be done.

CASE STUDY—cont'd

Diagnostic Studies

iStockphoto/Thinkstock

The emergency department physician immediately orders the following diagnostic studies:
• X-ray of left hip
• Chest x-ray
• CBC, electrolytes, aPTT, PT/INR
• Arterial blood gases (ABGs)

The x-ray of the left hip reveals an extracapsular fracture. The chest x-ray findings are consistent with COPD without any evidence of pneumonia at present. Hematocrit is 43%, hemoglobin 15 g/dL, and WBC is 15,100/μL (15.1 × 10⁹/L). The remainder of CBC, electrolytes, aPTT, and PT/INR are WNL. The ABGs demonstrate compensated respiratory acidosis.

This case is continued in Chapter 63 on p. 1536.

BRIDGE TO NCLEX EXAMINATION

The number of the question corresponds to the same-numbered outcome at the beginning of the chapter.

1. The bone cells that function in the resorption of bone tissue are called
   a. osteoids.
   b. osteocytes.
   c. osteoclasts.
   d. osteoblasts.

2. While performing passive range of motion for a patient, the nurse puts the ankle joint through the movements of (select all that apply)
   a. flexion and extension.
   b. inversion and eversion.
   c. pronation and supination
   d. flexion, extension, abduction, and adduction.
   e. pronation, supination, rotation, and circumduction.

3. To prevent muscle atrophy, the nurse teaches the patient with a leg immobilized in traction to perform *(select all that apply)*
   a. flexion contractions.
   b. tetanic contractions.
   c. isotonic contractions.
   d. isometric contractions.
   e. extension contractions.
4. A patient with tendonitis asks what the tendon does. The nurse's response is based on the knowledge that tendons
   a. connect bone to muscle.
   b. provide strength to muscle.
   c. lubricate joints with synovial fluid.
   d. relieve friction between moving parts.
5. The increased risk for falls in the older adult is most likely due to
   a. changes in balance.
   b. decrease in bone mass.
   c. loss of ligament elasticity.
   d. erosion of articular cartilage.
6. While obtaining subjective assessment data related to the musculoskeletal system, it is particularly important to ask a patient about other medical problems such as
   a. hypertension.
   b. thyroid problems.
   c. diabetes mellitus.
   d. chronic bronchitis.

7. When grading muscle strength, the nurse records a score of 3, which indicates
   a. no detection of muscular contraction.
   b. a barely detectable flicker of contraction.
   c. active movement against full resistance without fatigue.
   d. active movement against gravity but not against resistance.
8. A normal assessment finding of the musculoskeletal system is
   a. no deformity or crepitation.
   b. muscle and bone strength of 4.
   c. ulnar deviation and subluxation.
   d. angulation of bone toward midline.
9. A patient is scheduled for an electromyogram (EMG). The nurse explains that this diagnostic test involves
   a. incision or puncture of the joint capsule.
   b. insertion of small needles into certain muscles.
   c. administration of a radioisotope before the procedure.
   d. placement of skin electrodes to record muscle activity.

1. c, 2, a, b, 3. d, 4. a, 5. a, 6. c, 7. d, 8. a, 9. b

⊜volve

For rationales to these answers and even more NCLEX review questions, visit *http://evolve.elsevier.com/Lewis/medsurg.*

REFERENCES

1. Cleveland Clinic: Normal structure and function of the musculoskeletal system. Retrieved from *my.clevelandclinic.org/anatomy/musculoskeletal_system.*
2. Huether S, McCance K: *Understanding pathophysiology,* ed 5, St Louis, 2012, Mosby.
3. Thibodeau GA, Patton KT: *Structure and function of the human body,* ed 14, St Louis, 2012, Mosby.
4. Brinker M, O'Connor D, Almekinders L, et al: Basic science and injury of muscle, tendon, and ligament. In DeLee J, Drez DD, Miller M, editors: *DeLee and Drez's orthopaedic sports medicine,* ed 3, Philadelphia, 2010, Saunders.
5. Jarvis C: *Physical examination and health assessment,* ed 6, St Louis, 2012, Saunders.
6. National Institute of Arthritis and Musculoskeletal and Skin Diseases: Handout on health: osteoarthritis, National Institutes of Health. Retrieved from *www.niams.nih.gov/Health_Info/Osteoarthritis.*

7. Mehler P, Cleary B, Gaudiani J: Osteoporosis in anorexia nervosa, *Eat Disord* 19:194, 2011.
*8. Nworah U: From documentation to the problem: controlling postoperative pain, *Nurs Forum* 47:91, 2012.
9. Thomas S, Halbert J, Mackintosh S, et al: Walking aid use after discharge following hip fracture is rarely reviewed and often inappropriate: an observational study, *J Physiother* 56:267, 2010.
10. Bettencourt RB, Linder M: Arthrocentesis and therapeutic joint injection: an overview for the primary care physician, *Prim Care* 37:691, 2010.

RESOURCES

Resources for this chapter are listed after Chapter 63 on p. 1538, Chapter 64 on p. 1560, and Chapter 65 on p. 1595.

*Evidence-based information for clinical practice.

Dreams are the touchstones of our character.
Henry David Thoreau

Nursing Management
Musculoskeletal Trauma and Orthopedic Surgery

Damien Zsiros and Mary Wollan

evolve WEBSITE

http://evolve.elsevier.com/Lewis/medsurg

- NCLEX Review Questions
- Key Points
- Pre-Test
- Answer Guidelines for Case Study on p. 1536
- Rationales for Bridge to NCLEX Examination Questions

- Case Studies
  - Patient With Musculoskeletal Trauma
  - Patient With Parkinson's Disease and Hip Fracture
- Nursing Care Plans (Customizable)
  - eNCP 63-1: Patient With a Fracture
  - eNCP 63-2: Patient Having Orthopedic Surgery
- Concept Map Creator

- Glossary
- Content Updates

eFigures
- eFig. 63-1: Sagittal section through knee joint
- eFig. 63-2: Stabilization of knee injury with pins in femur and tibia
- eFig. 63-3: Fractures of the humerus

LEARNING OUTCOMES

1. Differentiate among the etiology, pathophysiology, clinical manifestations, and collaborative care of soft tissue injuries, including strains, sprains, dislocations, subluxations, bursitis, repetitive strain injury, carpal tunnel syndrome, and injuries to the rotator cuff, meniscus, and anterior cruciate ligament.
2. Relate the sequential events involved in fracture healing.
3. Compare closed reduction, cast immobilization, open reduction, and traction in terms of purpose, complications, and nursing management.
4. Evaluate the neurovascular assessment of an injured extremity.
5. Explain common complications associated with a fracture and fracture healing.
6. Describe the collaborative care and nursing management of patients with various kinds of fractures.
7. Describe the indications for and the collaborative care and nursing management of the patient with an amputation.
8. Describe the types of joint replacement surgery for arthritis and connective tissue disorders.
9. Prioritize the preoperative and postoperative management of the patient having joint replacement surgery.

KEY TERMS

arthrodesis, p. 1535
arthroplasty, p. 1534
bursitis, p. 1511
carpal tunnel syndrome (CTS), p. 1509
compartment syndrome, p. 1522
dislocation, p. 1508

fat embolism syndrome (FES), p. 1523
fracture, p. 1511
osteotomy, p. 1534
phantom limb sensation, p. 1531
repetitive strain injury (RSI), p. 1508

sprain, p. 1506
strain, p. 1506
subluxation, p. 1508
synovectomy, p. 1534
traction, p. 1514

Musculoskeletal problems resulting from trauma, along with common orthopedic surgical procedures, are discussed in this chapter. The nurse's role in prevention of complications and promotion of function in patients with fractures and orthopedic surgery is emphasized.

The most common cause of musculoskeletal injuries is a traumatic event resulting in fracture, dislocation, and/or soft tissue injuries. Although most of these injuries are not fatal, the cost in terms of pain, disability, medical expense, and lost wages is enormous. For all age-groups, accidents are exceeded

only by heart disease, cancer, chronic lower respiratory tract diseases, and strokes as a cause of death.[1] Accidental injuries (e.g., motor vehicle collisions, drowning, burns) are the leading cause of death in young adults in the United States.

It is important to teach the public about the basic principles of safety and accident prevention. The morbidity associated with accidents can be significantly reduced if people are aware of environmental hazards, use appropriate safety equipment, and apply safety and traffic rules. In the occupational and industrial setting, teach employees and employers about the

Reviewed by Julie Darby, RN, MSN, Assistant Professor, Baptist College of Health Sciences, Memphis, Tennessee.

use of proper safety equipment and avoidance of hazardous working situations.

SAFETY ALERT
- Falls account for many musculoskeletal injuries in the home environment.
- Provide preventive teaching to high-risk individuals (e.g., people with gait instability or visual or cognitive impairment).
- Stress the importance of wearing shoes with functional and stable soles and heels, avoiding wet or slippery surfaces, and removing throw rugs in the home.

TABLE 63-1   PATIENT & CAREGIVER TEACHING GUIDE

Prevention of Musculoskeletal Problems in Older Adults

To prevent musculoskeletal problems, include the following instructions when teaching older adults and their caregivers.

1. Use ramps in buildings and at street corners instead of steps to prevent falls.
2. Eliminate scatter rugs in the home.
3. Treat pain and discomfort from osteoarthritis.
   - Rest in positions that decrease discomfort.
   - Discuss use of medication for pain.
4. Use a walker or cane to help prevent falls.
5. Eat the amount and kind of foods to prevent excess weight gain because obesity adds stress to joints, which may predispose to osteoarthritis.
6. Get regular and frequent exercise.
   - Activities of daily living provide range-of-motion exercises. Tai Chi may also be helpful.
   - Hobbies (e.g., jigsaw puzzles, needlework, model building) exercise finger joints and prevent stiffness.
   - Performing weight-bearing exercise (e.g., walking) is essential and should be done on a daily basis.
7. Use shoes with good support to provide for safety and promote comfort.
8. Gradually initiate activities to promote optimal coordination. Rise slowly to a standing position to prevent dizziness, falls, and fractures.
9. Avoid walking on uneven surfaces and wet floors.

Ways to prevent common musculoskeletal problems in the older adult are listed in Table 63-1.

SOFT TISSUE INJURIES

Soft tissue injuries, which include sprains, strains, dislocations, and subluxations, are usually caused by trauma. The increasing number of people involved in a fitness program or participating in sports has contributed to the increased incidence of soft tissue injuries. Common sports-related injuries are summarized in Table 63-2. The most common sports injuries that result in a visit to the emergency department for younger patients are bruises, sprains and strains, tendinitis, and fractures.[2]

SPRAINS AND STRAINS

Sprains and strains are common injuries from abnormal stretching or twisting forces that may occur during vigorous activities. These injuries tend to occur around joints and in the spinal musculature.

A **sprain** is an injury to the ligamentous structures surrounding a joint, usually caused by a wrenching or twisting motion. Most sprains occur in the ankle, wrist, and knee joints.[3] A sprain is classified according to the degree of ligament damage. A *first-degree (mild) sprain* involves tears in only a few fibers, resulting in mild tenderness and minimal swelling. A *second-degree (moderate) sprain* is partial disruption of the involved tissue with more swelling and tenderness. A *third-degree (severe) sprain* is complete tearing of the ligament in association with moderate to severe swelling. A gap in the muscle may be apparent or palpated through the skin if the muscle is torn. Because areas around joints are rich in nerve endings, the injury can be extremely painful.

A **strain** is an excessive stretching of a muscle, its fascial sheath, or a tendon. Most strains occur in the large muscle groups, including the lower back, calf, and hamstrings. Strains may also be classified as first degree (mild or slightly pulled muscle), second degree (moderate or moderately

---

TABLE 63-2   SPORTS-RELATED INJURIES

Injury	Description	Treatment
Impingement syndrome	Entrapment of soft tissue structures under coracoacromial arch of shoulder.	NSAIDs. Rest until symptoms decrease and then gradual ROM and strengthening exercises.
Rotator cuff tear	Tear within muscle or tendinoligamentous structures around shoulder.	*If minor tear:* Rest, NSAIDs, and gradual mobilization with ROM and strengthening exercises. *If major tear:* Surgical repair.
Shin splints	Inflammation along anterior aspect of calf from periostitis caused by improper shoes, overuse, or running on hard pavement.	Rest, ice, NSAIDs, proper shoes. Gradual increase in activity. If pain persists, x-ray to rule out stress fracture of tibia.
Tendinitis	Inflammation of tendon as a result of overuse or incorrect use.	Rest, ice, NSAIDs. Gradual return to sport activity. Protective brace (orthosis) may be necessary if symptoms recur.
Ligament injury	Tearing or stretching of ligament. Usually occurs as a result of inversion, eversion, shearing, or torque applied to a joint. Characterized by sudden pain, swelling, and instability.	Rest, ice, elevation of extremity if possible, NSAIDs. Protection of affected extremity by use of brace. If symptoms persist, surgical repair may be necessary.
Meniscus injury	Injury to fibrocartilage of knee characterized by popping, clicking, tearing sensation, effusion, and/or swelling.	Rest, ice, elevation of extremity if possible, NSAIDs. Gradual return to regular activities. If symptoms persist, MRI to diagnose meniscus injury and possible arthroscopic surgery.
Anterior cruciate ligament tear	Traumatic tearing of ligament by deceleration forces together with pivoting or odd positions of the knee or leg.	Physical therapy with rehabilitation, knee brace. If knee instability or continued injuries, reconstructive surgery may be done.

torn muscle), and third degree (severely torn or ruptured muscle).

The clinical manifestations of sprains and strains are similar and include pain, edema, decreased function, and contusion. Pain aggravated by continued use is common. Edema develops in the injured area because of the local inflammatory response.

Mild sprains and strains are usually self-limiting, with full function returning within 3 to 6 weeks. X-rays of the affected part may be taken to rule out a fracture. A severe sprain can result in a concomitant *avulsion fracture,* in which the ligament pulls loose a fragment of bone. Alternatively, the joint structure may become unstable and result in subluxation or dislocation. At the time of injury, *hemarthrosis* (bleeding into a joint space or cavity) or disruption of the synovial lining may occur. Severe strains may require surgical repair of the muscle, tendon, or surrounding fascia.

NURSING MANAGEMENT
SPRAINS AND STRAINS

NURSING IMPLEMENTATION

HEALTH PROMOTION. Warming up muscles before exercising and vigorous activity, followed by stretching, may significantly reduce the risk of sprains and strains. Strength, balance, and endurance exercises are also important. Strengthening exercises that involve working against resistance build up muscle strength and bone density. Balance exercises, which may overlap with some strengthening exercises, help to prevent falling. Endurance exercises should start at a low level of effort and progress gradually to a moderate level.[4] Exercise instructions for these types of physical activity are available at *www.weboflife.ksc.nasa.gov/exerciseandaging.*

ACUTE INTERVENTION. If an injury occurs, the immediate care focuses on (1) stopping the activity and limiting movement, (2) applying ice compresses to the injured area, (3) compressing the involved extremity, (4) elevating the extremity, and (5) providing analgesia as necessary (Table 63-3).

RICE (Rest, Ice, Compression, Elevation) may decrease local inflammation and pain for most musculoskeletal injuries. Movement should be restricted and the extremity rested as soon as pain is felt. Unless the injury is severe, prolonged rest is usually not indicated.

Cold (*cryotherapy*) in several forms can be used to produce hypothermia in the involved part. The cold induces physiologic changes in soft tissue, including vasoconstriction and a reduction in the transmission and perception of nerve pain impulses. In addition to pain relief, these changes reduce muscle spasms, inflammation, and edema. Cold is most useful when applied immediately after the injury has occurred. Ice applications should not exceed 20 to 30 minutes per application, and ice should not be applied directly to the skin.

An elastic compression bandage can be wrapped around the injured part. To prevent edema and encourage fluid return, wrap the bandage starting distally (at the point farthest from the midline of the body) and progress proximally (toward the midline of the body). The bandage is too tight if numbness is felt below the area of compression or there is additional pain or swelling beyond the edge of the bandage. The bandage can be left in place for 30 minutes and then removed for 15 minutes. However, some elastic wraps are left on during training, athletic, and occupational activities.

The injured part should be elevated above the heart level to help mobilize excess fluid from the area and prevent further

HEALTHY PEOPLE
Health Impact of Regular Physical Activity

- Assists in weight control.
- Helps maintain bone mass.
- Helps prevent high blood pressure.
- Increases lean muscle and decreases body fat.
- Increases muscle strength, flexibility, and endurance.
- Appears to reduce symptoms of depression and anxiety.
- Reduces the risk of heart disease, diabetes, and colon cancer.
- Enhances psychologic well-being and may reduce risk of depression.

TABLE 63-3 EMERGENCY MANAGEMENT

Acute Soft Tissue Injury

Etiology	Assessment Findings	Interventions
• Falls • Direct blows • Crush injury • Motor vehicle collisions • Sports injuries	• Edema • Ecchymosis, contusion • Pain, tenderness • Decreased sensation with severe edema • Decreased pulse, coolness, and capillary refill >2 sec • Decreased movement • Pallor • Shortening or rotation of extremity • Inability to bear weight when lower extremity involved • Limited or decreased function with upper extremity involvement • Muscle spasms	**Initial** • Ensure airway, breathing, and circulation. • Assess neurovascular status of involved limb. • Elevate involved limb. • Apply compression bandage unless dislocation present. • Apply ice packs to affected area. • Immobilize affected extremity in the position found. Do *not* attempt to realign or reinsert protruding bones. • Anticipate x-rays of injured extremity. • Give analgesia as necessary. • Administer tetanus and diphtheria prophylaxis if there is a break in skin integrity or open fracture. • Administer antibiotic prophylaxis for open fracture, large tissue defects, or mangled extremity injury. **Ongoing Monitoring** • Monitor for changes in neurovascular status. • Eliminate weight bearing when lower extremity involved. • Anticipate compartment pressure monitoring if neurovascular status changes and compartment syndrome suspected.

edema. The injured part should be elevated even during sleep. Mild analgesics and nonsteroidal antiinflammatory drugs (NSAIDs) may be necessary to manage patient discomfort.

After the acute phase (usually 24 to 48 hours), warm, moist heat may be applied to the affected part to reduce swelling and provide comfort. Heat applications should not exceed 20 to 30 minutes, allowing a "cool-down" time between applications. Encourage the patient to use the limb, provided that the joint is protected by means of casting, bracing, taping, or splinting. Movement of the joint maintains nutrition to the cartilage, and muscle contraction improves circulation and resolution of the contusion and swelling.

AMBULATORY AND HOME CARE. Most sprains and strains are treated in the outpatient setting. Instruct the patient to use ice and elevate for 24 to 48 hours after the injury to reduce edema. Encourage the use of mild analgesics to promote comfort. Use of an elastic wrap may provide additional support during activity. Emphasize to the patient the importance of strengthening and conditioning exercises to prevent reinjury.

The physical therapist may help provide pain relief by modalities such as ultrasound. The therapist may also teach the patient exercises to perform for flexibility and strength.

DISLOCATION AND SUBLUXATION

A **dislocation** is a severe injury of the ligamentous structures that surround a joint. Dislocation results in the complete displacement or separation of the articular surfaces of the joint. A **subluxation** is a partial or incomplete displacement of the joint surface. The clinical manifestations of a subluxation are similar to those of a dislocation but are less severe.

Dislocations characteristically result from forces transmitted to the joint that disrupt the soft tissue support structures surrounding it. The joints most frequently dislocated in the upper extremity include the thumb, elbow, and shoulder. In the lower extremity, the hip is vulnerable to dislocation as a result of severe trauma, often associated with motor vehicle collisions (Fig. 63-1). The patella may dislocate because of a sharp blow to the kneecap or after a sudden twisting inward motion while the planted foot is pointed outward.[5]

The most obvious clinical manifestation of a dislocation is deformity. For example, if a hip is dislocated in a posterior (or backward) direction, the limb can be shorter and is often internally rotated on the affected side. Additional manifestations include local pain, tenderness, loss of function of the injured part, and swelling of the soft tissues in the joint region. The major complications of a dislocated joint are open joint injuries, intraarticular fractures, *avascular necrosis* (bone cell death as a result of inadequate blood supply), and damage to adjacent neurovascular tissue.

FIG. 63-1 Soft tissue injury of the hip. **A,** Normal. **B,** Subluxation (partial dislocation). **C,** Dislocation.

X-ray studies are performed to determine the extent of displacement of the involved structures. The joint may also be aspirated to assess for hemarthrosis or fat cells. Fat cells in the aspirate indicate a probable intraarticular (within the joint) fracture.

NURSING AND COLLABORATIVE MANAGEMENT DISLOCATION

A dislocation requires prompt attention and is often considered an orthopedic emergency. It may be associated with significant vascular injury. The longer the joint remains unreduced, the greater the possibility of avascular necrosis. The hip joint is particularly susceptible to avascular necrosis. Compartment syndrome (discussed on p. 1522) may also occur after a dislocation. Neurovascular assessment is critical (see pp. 1517–1518).

The first goal of management is to realign the dislocated portion of the joint in its original anatomic position. This can be accomplished by a closed reduction, which may be performed under local or general anesthesia or IV conscious sedation. Anesthesia is often necessary to relax the muscle so that the bones can be manipulated. In some situations, surgical open reduction may be necessary. After reduction, the extremity is usually immobilized by bracing, splinting, taping, or using a sling to allow the torn ligaments and capsular tissue time to heal.

Nursing management of subluxation or dislocation is directed toward relief of pain and support and protection of the injured joint. After the joint has been reduced and immobilized, motion is usually restricted. A carefully monitored rehabilitation program can prevent fracture instability and joint dysfunction. Gentle range-of-motion (ROM) exercises may be recommended if the joint is stable and well supported. An exercise program slowly restores the joint to its original ROM without causing another dislocation. The patient should gradually return to normal activities.

A patient who has dislocated a joint may be at greater risk for repeated dislocations because of loose ligaments. Activity restrictions may be imposed on the affected joint to decrease the risk of repeated dislocations.

REPETITIVE STRAIN INJURY

Repetitive strain injury (RSI) and *cumulative trauma disorder* are terms used to describe injuries resulting from prolonged force or repetitive movements and awkward postures. RSI is also referred to as repetitive trauma disorder, nontraumatic musculoskeletal injury, overuse syndrome (sports medicine), regional musculoskeletal disorder, and work-related musculoskeletal disorder. Repeated movements strain the tendons, ligaments, and muscles, causing tiny tears that become inflamed. The exact cause of these disorders is unknown. There are no specific diagnostic tests, and diagnosis is often difficult.

Persons at risk for RSI include musicians, dancers, butchers, grocery clerks, vibratory tool workers, and those who frequently use a computer mouse and keyboard. Competitive athletes and poorly trained athletes may also develop RSI. Swimming, overhead throwing (e.g., baseball), weight lifting, gymnastics, tennis, skiing, and kicking sports (e.g., soccer) require repetitive motion, and overtraining compounds the effects of RSI.

In addition to repetitive movements, other factors related to RSI include poor posture and positioning, poor workspace ergonomics, badly designed workplace equipment (e.g., computer keyboard), and repetitive lifting of heavy objects without sufficient muscle rest. The result may be inflammation, swelling, and pain in the muscles, tendons, and nerves of the neck, spine, shoulder, forearm, and hand. Symptoms of RSI include pain, weakness, numbness, or impairment of motor function. RSI can be prevented through education and *ergonomics* (the science that promotes efficiency and safety in the interaction of humans and their work environment). Ergonomic considerations for persons who work at a desk and use a computer include keeping the hips and knees flexed to 90 degrees with the feet flat, keeping the wrist straight to type, having the top of the computer monitor even with the forehead, and taking at least hourly stretch breaks. Once RSI is diagnosed, treatment consists of identification of the precipitating activity; modification of equipment or activity; pain management, including heat or cold application and NSAIDs; rest; physical therapy for strengthening and conditioning exercises; and lifestyle changes.

CARPAL TUNNEL SYNDROME

Carpal tunnel syndrome (CTS) is a condition caused by compression of the median nerve, which enters the hand through the narrow confines of the carpal tunnel (Fig. 63-2). The carpal tunnel is formed by ligaments and bones. CTS is the most common compression neuropathy in the upper extremity. This syndrome is associated with hobbies or occupations that require continuous wrist movement (e.g., musicians, carpenters, computer operators).

This condition is often caused by pressure from trauma or edema caused by inflammation of a tendon (tenosynovitis), neoplasm, rheumatoid arthritis, or soft tissue masses such as ganglia. Hormones may be involved, since initial manifestations of CTS often occur during the premenstrual period, pregnancy, and menopause. Persons with diabetes mellitus, peripheral vascular disease, and rheumatoid arthritis have a higher incidence of CTS because of swelling that changes blood flow to the nerve and narrows the carpal tunnel.[6] Women are more likely than men to develop CTS, possibly because of a smaller carpal tunnel.

The clinical manifestations of CTS are weakness, pain, numbness, or impaired sensation in the distribution of the median nerve (see Fig. 63-2). Numbness and tingling may

awaken the patient at night. Shaking the hands often relieves these symptoms. Clumsiness in performing fine hand movements is also common.

Manifestations of CTS include a positive Tinel's sign and Phalen's sign. *Tinel's sign* can be elicited by tapping over the median nerve as it passes through the carpal tunnel in the wrist. A positive response is a sensation of tingling in the distribution of the median nerve over the hand. *Phalen's sign* can be elicited by allowing the wrists to fall freely into maximum flexion and maintain the position for longer than 60 seconds. A positive response is a sensation of tingling in the distribution of the median nerve over the hand. In late stages there is atrophy of the thenar muscles around the base of the thumb, resulting in recurrent pain and eventual dysfunction of the hand.

NURSING AND COLLABORATIVE MANAGEMENT CARPAL TUNNEL SYNDROME

To prevent CTS, teach employees and employers to identify risk factors. Adaptive devices such as wrist splints may be worn to hold the wrist in a slight extension and relieve pressure on the median nerve. Special keyboard pads and mouses that help prevent repetitive pressure on the median nerve are available for computer users. Other ergonomic changes include workstation modifications, change in body positions, and frequent breaks from work-related activities.

Collaborative care of the patient with CTS is directed toward relieving the underlying cause of the nerve compression. The early symptoms associated with CTS can usually be relieved by stopping the aggravating movement and by resting the hand and wrist by immobilizing them in a hand splint. Splints worn at night help keep the wrist in a neutral position and may reduce night pain and numbness. Physical therapy with hand and wrist exercises may lessen symptom severity. Injection of a corticosteroid drug directly into the carpal tunnel may provide short-term relief. The patient may need to consider a change in occupation because of discomfort and sensory changes.

Carpal tunnel release is generally recommended if symptoms last for more than 6 months. Surgery involves severing the band of tissue around the wrist to reduce pressure on the median nerve (see Fig. 63-2). Surgery is done in the outpatient setting using local anesthesia. The types of carpal tunnel release surgery include open release and endoscopic surgery.[6] In *open release surgery* an incision is made in the wrist and then the carpal ligament is cut to enlarge the carpal tunnel. *Endoscopic carpal tunnel release* is performed through one or more small puncture incisions in the wrist and palm. A camera is attached to a tube, and the carpal ligament is cut. The endoscopic approach may allow for a faster recovery and less postoperative discomfort than traditional open release surgery.

Although symptoms may be relieved immediately after surgery, full recovery may take months. After surgery, assess the hand's neurovascular status. Instruct the patient about wound care and the appropriate assessments to perform at home.

ROTATOR CUFF INJURY

The rotator cuff is a complex of four muscles in the shoulder: the supraspinatus, infraspinatus, teres minor, and subscapularis muscles. These muscles act to stabilize the humeral head in the glenoid fossa while assisting with the ROM of the shoulder joint and rotation of the humerus.

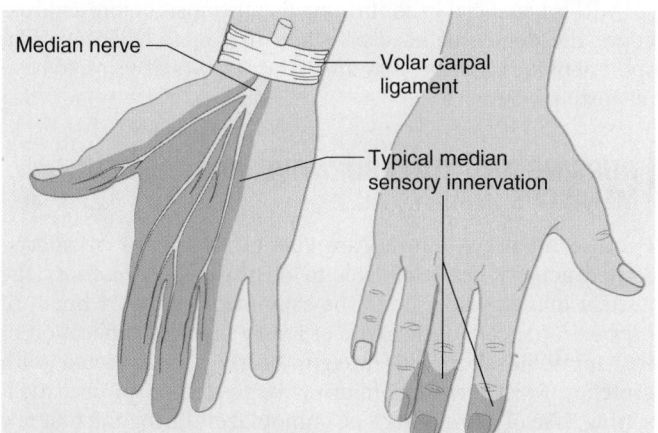

FIG. 63-2 Wrist structures involved in carpal tunnel syndrome. Median nerve distribution. Shaded areas depict the locations of pain in carpal tunnel syndrome.

FIG. 63-3 A torn rotator cuff is repaired using arthroscopic surgery.

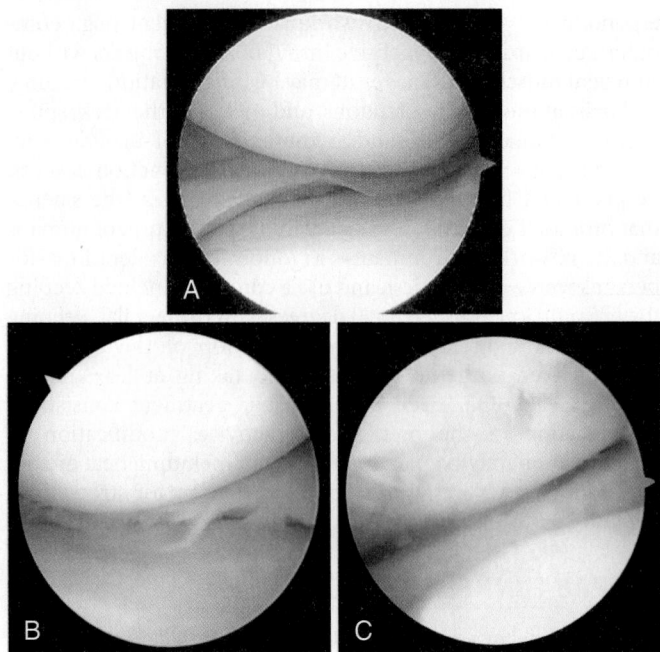

FIG. 63-4 Arthroscopic views of the meniscus. **A,** Normal meniscus. **B,** Torn meniscus. **C,** Surgically repaired meniscus.

A tear in the rotator cuff may occur as a gradual, degenerative process resulting from aging, repetitive stress (especially overhead arm motions), or injury to the shoulder while falling. The rotator cuff can tear as a result of sudden adduction forces applied to the cuff while the arm is held in abduction. In sports, repetitive overhead motions, such as in swimming, weight lifting, and swinging a racquet (tennis, racquetball) often cause injury. Other causes include (1) falling onto an outstretched arm and hand, (2) a blow to the upper arm, (3) heavy lifting, or (4) repetitive work motions.

Manifestations of a rotator cuff injury include shoulder weakness and pain and decreased ROM. The patient usually experiences severe pain when the arm is abducted between 60 and 120 degrees (the painful arc). The *drop arm test,* in which the arm falls suddenly after the patient is asked to slowly lower the arm to the side after it has been abducted 90 degrees, is another sign of rotator cuff injury. An x-ray alone is usually not beneficial in the diagnosis. A tear can usually be confirmed by magnetic resonance imaging (MRI).

The patient with a partial tear or cuff inflammation may be treated conservatively with rest, ice and heat, NSAIDs, corticosteroid injections into the joint, ultrasound, and physical therapy.[7] If the patient does not respond to conservative treatment or if a complete tear is present, surgical repair may be necessary. Most surgical repairs are performed as outpatient procedures through an arthroscope (Fig. 63-3). If the tear is extensive, an *acromioplasty* (surgical removal of part of the acromion to relieve compression of the rotator cuff during movement) may be done. A sling or, more commonly, a shoulder immobilizer may be used immediately after surgery to limit shoulder movement. However, the shoulder should not be immobilized for too long because "frozen" shoulder or arthrofibrosis may occur. Pendulum exercises and physical therapy begin the first postoperative day. Restrictions for lifting weights are usually given, with full recovery taking up to 6 months.

MENISCUS INJURY

The menisci are crescent-shaped pieces of fibrocartilage in the knee. Menisci are also found in other joints. Meniscus injuries are closely associated with ligament sprains common among athletes in sports such as basketball, football, soccer, and hockey.

These activities produce rotational stress when the knee is in varying degrees of flexion and the foot is planted or fixed. A blow to the knee can cause the meniscus to be sheared between the femoral condyles and the tibial plateau, resulting in a torn meniscus. (The knee joint is shown in eFig. 63-1 on the website for this chapter.) People who work in occupations that require squatting or kneeling and older patients may be at risk for degenerative tears.

Meniscus injuries alone do not usually cause significant edema because most of the cartilage is avascular. However, an acutely torn meniscus may be suspected when localized tenderness, pain, and effusion are noted (Fig. 63-4). Pain is elicited by flexion, internal rotation, and then extension of the knee (called *McMurray's test*). The patient may feel that the knee is unstable and often reports that the knee "clicks," "pops," "locks," or "gives way." Quadriceps atrophy is usually evident if the injury has been present for some time. Traumatic arthritis may occur from repeated meniscus injury and chronic inflammation.

MRI is beneficial in confirming the diagnosis before arthroscopy. The degree of knee pain and dysfunction, occupation, sport activities, and age may affect the patient's decision to have or postpone surgery.

NURSING AND COLLABORATIVE MANAGEMENT MENISCUS INJURY

Because meniscus injuries are commonly caused by sports-related activity, teach athletes to do warm-up exercises. The acutely injured knee should be examined within 24 hours of injury. Initial care of this type of injury involves application of ice, immobilization, and weight bearing as tolerated with crutches. Most meniscus injuries are treated in an outpatient setting. Use of a knee brace or immobilizer during the first few days after the injury protects the knee and offers some pain relief. After acute pain has decreased, physical therapy can help the patient regain knee flexion and muscle strength to assist in returning to full function. In older adults with degenerative meniscus tears, progressive exercise therapy may improve neuromuscular function and muscle strength.[8]

Surgical repair or excision of part of the meniscus (meniscectomy) may be necessary (see Fig. 63-4). Meniscal surgery is performed by arthroscopy. Pain relief may include NSAIDs or other analgesics. Rehabilitation starts soon after surgery, including quadriceps and hamstring strengthening exercises and ROM. When the patient's strength is back to its preinjury level, normal activities may be resumed.

ANTERIOR CRUCIATE LIGAMENT INJURY

Knee injuries account for more than 50% of all sport injuries. The most commonly injured knee ligament is the anterior cruciate ligament (ACL). ACL injuries are usually noncontact injuries that occur when the athlete pivots, lands from a jump, or slows down when running. Patients often report coming down on the knee, twisting, and hearing a pop, followed by acute knee pain and swelling. Athletes usually cannot continue playing, and the knee may feel unstable. An injury to the ACL can result in a partial tear, a complete tear, or an *avulsion* (tearing away) from the bone attachments that form the knee (Fig. 63-5).

Examination of the knee with an ACL tear may produce a positive *Lachman's test*.[9] This test is performed by flexing the knee 15 to 30 degrees and pulling the tibia forward while the femur is stabilized. The test is considered positive for an ACL tear if there is forward motion of the tibia with the feeling of a soft or indistinct endpoint. MRI is often used to diagnose coexisting conditions, including a fracture, meniscus tearing, and collateral ligament injuries.

NURSING AND COLLABORATIVE MANAGEMENT ANTERIOR CRUCIATE LIGAMENT INJURY

Prevention programs have been shown to significantly reduce ACL injuries in athletes.[10] Conservative treatment for an intact ACL injury includes rest, ice, NSAIDs, elevation, and ambulation as tolerated with crutches. If there is a tight, painful effu-

sion, it may be aspirated. A knee immobilizer or hinged knee brace may be helpful in supporting the knee. Physical therapy often assists the patient in maintaining knee joint motion and muscle tone.

Reconstructive surgery is usually recommended in physically active patients who have sustained severe injury to the ligament and the meniscus. In reconstruction the torn ACL tissue is removed and replaced with autologous or allograft tissue. ROM is encouraged soon after surgery, and the knee is placed in a brace or immobilizer. Rehabilitation with physical therapy is critical with progressive weight bearing determined by the degree of surgical repair. A safe return to the patient's prior level of physical functioning may take 6 to 8 months.

BURSITIS

Bursae are closed sacs that are lined with synovial membrane and contain a small amount of synovial fluid. They are located at sites of friction, such as between tendons and bones and near the joints. Bursitis (inflammation of the bursa) results from repeated or excessive trauma or friction, gout, rheumatoid arthritis, or infection.

The primary clinical manifestations of bursitis are warmth, pain, swelling, and limited ROM in the affected part. Sites at which bursitis commonly occurs include hands, knees, greater trochanters of the hip, shoulders, and elbows. Improper body mechanics, repetitive kneeling (carpet layers, coal miners, and gardeners), jogging in worn-out shoes, and prolonged sitting with crossed legs are common precipitating activities.

Attempts are made to determine and correct the cause of the bursitis. Rest is often the only treatment needed. The affected part may be immobilized in a compression dressing or splint. Ice and NSAIDs may be used to reduce pain and inflammation.[11] Aspiration of the bursal fluid and intraarticular injection of a corticosteroid may be necessary. If the bursal wall has become thickened and continues to interfere with normal joint function, surgical excision (bursectomy) is often done. Septic bursae usually require surgical incision and drainage.

FRACTURES

Classification

A fracture is a disruption or break in the continuity of the structure of bone. Although traumatic injuries account for the majority of fractures, some fractures are secondary to a disease process (pathologic fractures from cancer or osteoporosis).

Fractures can be classified as *open* (formerly called compound) or *closed* (formerly called simple) depending on communication or noncommunication with the external environment (Fig. 63-6). In an *open fracture* the skin is broken, exposing bone and causing soft tissue injury. In a *closed fracture* the skin has not been ruptured and remains intact.

Fractures can also be classified as complete or incomplete. Fractures are termed *complete* if the break is completely through the bone and *incomplete* if the fracture occurs partly across a bone shaft but the bone is still in one piece. An incomplete fracture is often the result of bending or crushing forces applied to a bone.

Fractures are also described and classified according to the direction of the fracture line. Types include linear, oblique, transverse, longitudinal, and spiral fractures (Fig. 63-7).

FIG. 63-5 Anterior cruciate ligament (ACL) injury. **A,** Partial tear. **B,** Complete tear. **C,** Avulsion.

Open fracture   Closed fracture

FIG. 63-6 Fracture classification according to communication with the external environment.

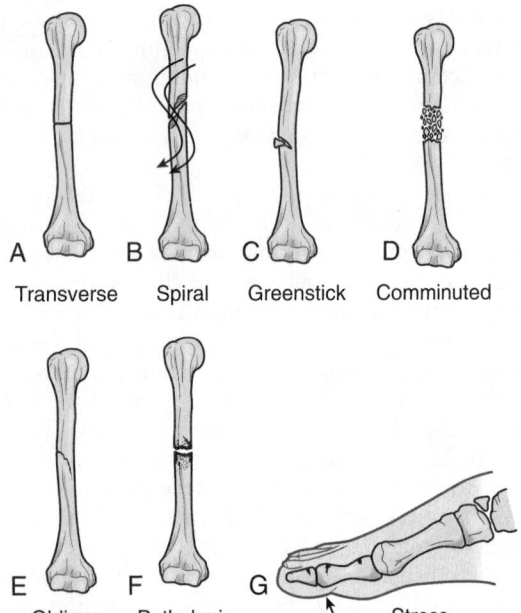

A   B   C   D
Transverse   Spiral   Greenstick   Comminuted

E   F   G
Oblique   Pathologic   Stress

FIG. 63-7 Types of fractures. **A,** Transverse fracture: the line of the fracture extends across the bone shaft at a right angle to the longitudinal axis. **B,** Spiral fracture: the line of the fracture extends in a spiral direction along the bone shaft. **C,** Greenstick fracture: an incomplete fracture with one side splintered and the other side bent. **D,** Comminuted fracture: a fracture with more than two fragments. The smaller fragments appear to be floating. **E,** Oblique fracture: the line of the fracture extends in an oblique direction. **F,** Pathologic fracture: a spontaneous fracture at the site of a bone disease. **G,** Stress fracture: occurs in normal or abnormal bone that is subject to repeated stress, such as from jogging or running.

TABLE 63-4 **MANIFESTATIONS OF FRACTURE**	
Manifestation	**Significance**
Edema and Swelling Disruption and penetration of bone through skin or soft tissues, or bleeding into surrounding tissues.	Unchecked bleeding, swelling, and edema in closed space can occlude circulation and damage nerves (e.g., risk of compartment syndrome).
Pain and Tenderness Muscle spasm as a result of involuntary reflex action of muscle, direct tissue trauma, increased pressure on nerves, movement of fracture parts.	Pain and tenderness encourage splinting of muscle around fracture with reduction in motion of injured area.
Muscle Spasm Irritation of tissues and protective response to injury and fracture.	Muscle spasms may displace nondisplaced fracture or prevent it from reducing spontaneously.
Deformity Abnormal position of extremity or part as result of original forces of injury and action of muscles pulling fragment into abnormal position. Seen as a loss of normal bony contours.	Deformity is cardinal sign of fracture. If uncorrected, it may result in problems with bony union and restoration of function of injured part.
Ecchymosis, Contusion Discoloration of skin as a result of extravasation of blood in subcutaneous tissues.	Ecchymosis may appear immediately after injury and may appear distal to injury. Reassure patient that process is normal and discoloration will eventually resolve.
Loss of Function Disruption of bone or joint, preventing functional use of limb or part.	Fracture must be managed properly to ensure restoration of function to limb or part.
Crepitation Grating or crunching together of bony fragments, producing palpable or audible crunching or popping sensation.	Crepitation may increase chance for nonunion if bone ends are allowed to move excessively. Micromovement of bone-end fragments (postfracture) assists in osteogenesis (new bone growth).

Fractures can also be classified as displaced or nondisplaced. In a *displaced* fracture the two ends of the broken bone are separated from one another and out of their normal positions. Displaced fractures are usually *comminuted* (more than two fragments) or *oblique* (see Fig. 63-7). In a *nondisplaced* fracture the periosteum is intact across the fracture and the bone is still in alignment. Nondisplaced fractures are usually transverse, spiral, or greenstick (see Fig. 63-7).

Clinical Manifestations

The clinical manifestations include immediate localized pain, decreased function, and inability to bear weight on or use the affected part (Table 63-4). The patient guards and protects the extremity against movement. Obvious bone deformity may not be present. If a fracture is suspected, the extremity is immobi-

lized in the position in which it is found. Unnecessary movement increases soft tissue damage and may convert a closed fracture to an open fracture or create further injury to adjacent neurovascular structures.

Fracture Healing

You need to understand the principles of fracture healing (Fig. 63-8) to provide appropriate therapeutic interventions. Bone goes through a complex multistage healing process (termed *union*) that occurs in the following stages:[12]

1. *Fracture hematoma:* When a fracture occurs, bleeding creates a hematoma, which surrounds the ends of the fragments. The hematoma is extravasated blood that changes from a liquid to a semisolid clot. This occurs in the initial 72 hours after injury.

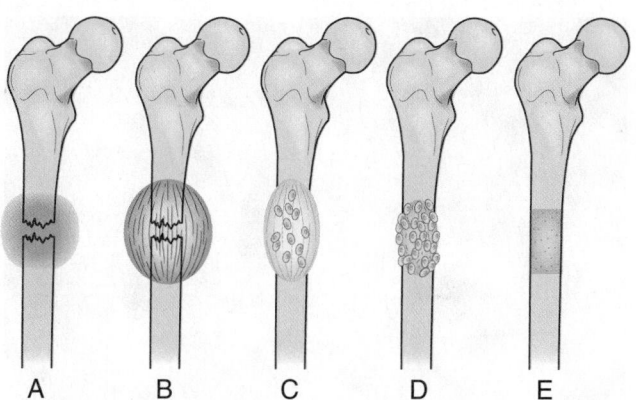

FIG. 63-8 Bone healing (schematic representation). **A,** Bleeding at fractured ends of the bone with subsequent hematoma formation. **B,** Organization of hematoma into fibrous network. **C,** Invasion of osteoblasts, lengthening of collagen strands, and deposition of calcium. **D,** Callus formation: new bone is built up as osteoclasts destroy dead bone. **E,** Remodeling is accomplished as excess callus is resorbed and trabecular bone is laid down.

TABLE 63-5	COMPLICATIONS OF FRACTURE HEALING
Complication	**Description**
Delayed union	Fracture healing progresses more slowly than expected. Healing eventually occurs.
Nonunion	Fracture fails to heal despite treatment. No x-ray evidence of callus formation.
Malunion	Fracture heals in expected time but in unsatisfactory position, possibly resulting in deformity or dysfunction.
Angulation	Fracture heals in abnormal position in relation to midline of structure (type of malunion).
Pseudoarthrosis	Type of nonunion occurring at fracture site in which a false joint is formed with abnormal movement at site.
Refracture	New fracture occurs at original fracture site.
Myositis ossificans	Deposition of calcium in muscle tissue at site of significant blunt muscle trauma or repeated muscle injury.

2. *Granulation tissue:* During this stage, active phagocytosis absorbs the products of local necrosis. The hematoma converts to granulation tissue. Granulation tissue (consisting of new blood vessels, fibroblasts, and osteoblasts) produces the basis for new bone substance called *osteoid* during days 3 to 14 postinjury.

3. *Callus formation:* As minerals (calcium, phosphorus, and magnesium) and new bone matrix are deposited in the osteoid, an unorganized network of bone is formed that is woven about the fracture parts. *Callus* is primarily composed of cartilage, osteoblasts, calcium, and phosphorus. It usually appears by the end of the second week after injury. Evidence of callus formation can be verified by x-ray.

4. *Ossification:* Ossification of the callus occurs from 3 weeks to 6 months after the fracture and continues until the fracture has healed. Callus ossification is sufficient to prevent movement at the fracture site when the bones are gently stressed. However, the fracture is still evident on x-ray. During this stage of *clinical union,* the patient may be allowed limited mobility or the cast may be removed.

5. *Consolidation:* As callus continues to develop, the distance between bone fragments diminishes and eventually closes. During this stage ossification continues. It can be equated with *radiologic union,* which occurs when there is x-ray evidence of complete bony union. This phase can occur up to 1 year after injury.

6. *Remodeling:* Excess bone tissue is resorbed in the final stage of bone healing, and union is complete. Gradual return of the injured bone to its preinjury structural strength and shape occurs. Bone remodels in response to physical loading stress or Wolf's law. Initially, stress is provided through exercise. Weight bearing is gradually introduced. New bone is deposited in sites subjected to stress and resorbed at areas where there is little stress.

Many factors influence the time required for complete fracture healing, including displacement and site of the fracture, blood supply to the area, immobilization, and internal fixation devices (e.g., screws, pins). The ossification process may be arrested by inadequate reduction and immobilization, excessive movement of the fracture fragments, infection, poor nutrition, and systemic disease. Healing time for fractures increases with

TABLE 63-6	COLLABORATIVE CARE

Fractures

Diagnostic
- History and physical examination
- X-ray
- CT scan, MRI

Collaborative Therapy
Fracture Reduction
- Manipulation
- Closed reduction
- Skin traction
- Skeletal traction
- Open reduction

Fracture Immobilization
- Casting or splinting
- Traction
- External fixation
- Internal fixation

Open Fractures
- Surgical debridement and irrigation
- Tetanus and diphtheria immunization
- Prophylactic antibiotic therapy
- Immobilization

age. For example, an uncomplicated midshaft fracture of the femur heals in 3 weeks in a newborn and in 20 weeks in an adult. Smoking also increases fracture healing time. Fracture healing may not occur in the expected time *(delayed union)* or may not occur at all *(nonunion).* Table 63-5 summarizes complications of fracture healing.

Collaborative Care

The overall goals of fracture treatment are (1) anatomic realignment of bone fragments (reduction), (2) immobilization to maintain realignment, and (3) restoration of normal or near-normal function of the injured part. Table 63-6 summarizes the collaborative care of fractures.

Fracture Reduction

Closed Reduction. *Closed reduction* is a nonsurgical, manual realignment of bone fragments to their previous anatomic position. Traction and countertraction are manually applied to the bone fragments to restore position, length, and alignment. Closed reduction is usually performed while the patient is under local or general anesthesia. After reduction, traction, casting, external fixation, splints, or orthoses (braces) immobilize the injured part to maintain alignment until healing occurs.

Open Reduction. *Open reduction* is the correction of bone alignment through a surgical incision. It usually includes internal fixation of the fracture with wires, screws, pins, plates, intramedullary rods, or nails. The type and location of the fracture, patient age, and concurrent disease may influence the decision to use open reduction. The main disadvantages of this form of fracture management are the possibility of infection, complications associated with anesthesia, and effect of preexisting medical conditions (e.g., diabetes).

If open reduction with internal fixation (ORIF) is used for intraarticular fractures, early initiation of ROM of the joint is indicated. Machines that provide continuous passive motion (CPM) to various joints (e.g., knee, shoulder) are used to prevent extraarticular and intraarticular adhesions. The use of CPM results in faster reconstruction of the subchondral (beneath cartilage) bone plate, more rapid healing of the articular cartilage, and decreased incidence of posttraumatic arthritis. ORIF facilitates early ambulation, thus decreasing the risk of complications related to prolonged immobility.

Traction. Traction is the application of a pulling force to an injured or diseased part of the body or an extremity. *Countertraction* pulls in the opposite direction. Traction is used to (1) prevent or reduce pain and muscle spasm associated with low back pain or cervical sprain (e.g., whiplash), (2) immobilize a joint or part of the body, (3) reduce a fracture or dislocation, and (4) treat a pathologic joint condition (e.g., tumor, infection). Traction is also indicated to (1) provide immobilization to prevent soft tissue damage, (2) promote active and passive exercise, (3) expand a joint space during arthroscopic procedures, and (4) expand a joint space before major joint reconstruction.

Traction devices apply a pulling force on a fractured extremity to attain realignment while countertraction pulls in the opposite direction. The two most common types of traction are skin traction and skeletal traction. *Skin traction* is generally used for short-term treatment (48 to 72 hours) until skeletal traction or surgery is possible. Tape, boots, or splints are applied directly to the skin to maintain alignment, assist in reduction, and help diminish muscle spasms in the injured extremity. The traction weights are usually limited to 5 to 10 lb (2.3 to 4.5 kg). A *Buck's traction* boot is a type of skin traction used to immobilize a fracture, prevent hip flexion contractures, and reduce muscle spasms (Fig. 63-9). Pelvic or cervical skin traction may require heavier weights applied intermittently. In skin traction, assessment of the skin is a priority, since pressure points and skin breakdown may develop quickly. Assess key pressure points every 2 to 4 hours.

Skeletal traction, generally in place for longer periods than skin traction, is used to align injured bones and joints or to treat joint contractures and congenital hip dysplasia. It provides a long-term pull that keeps the injured bones and joints aligned. To apply skeletal traction, the physician inserts a pin or wire into the bone, either partially or completely, to align and immobilize the injured body part.[13] Weight for skeletal traction ranges

FIG. 63-9 Buck's traction is most commonly used for fractures of the hip and femur.

from 5 to 45 lb (2.3 to 20.4 kg). The use of too much weight can result in delayed union or nonunion. The major complications of skeletal traction are infection in the area of the bone where the skeletal pin is inserted and the consequences of prolonged immobility.

When traction is used to treat fractures, the forces are usually exerted on the distal fragment to align it with the proximal fragment. Several types of traction are used for this purpose. One of the more common types of skeletal traction is balanced suspension traction (Fig. 63-10). Fracture alignment depends on

DELEGATION DECISIONS

Caring for the Patient With a Cast or Traction

Role of Registered Nurse (RN)
- Perform neurovascular assessments on the affected extremity.
- Assess for clinical manifestations of compartment syndrome.
- Monitor cast during drying for denting or flattening.
- Teach patient and caregiver about cast care and complications of casting.
- Determine correct body alignment to enhance traction.
- Instruct patient and caregiver about traction and correct body positioning.
- Teach patient and caregiver range-of-motion (ROM) exercises.
- Assess for complications associated with immobility or fracture (e.g., wound infection, constipation, deep vein thrombosis, renal calculi, atelectasis).
- Develop plan to minimize complications associated with immobility or fracture.

Role of Licensed Practical/Vocational Nurse (LPN/LVN)
- Check color, temperature, capillary refill, and pulses distal to the cast.
- Mark circumference of any drainage on the cast.
- Monitor skin integrity around cast and at traction connections.
- Pad cast edges and traction connections to prevent skin irritation.
- Monitor pain level and administer prescribed analgesics.
- Notify RN of changes in pain or if pain persists after prescribed analgesics are administered.

Role of Unlicensed Assistive Personnel (UAP)
- Position casted extremity above heart level.
- Apply ice to cast as directed by RN.
- Maintain body position and integrity of traction (after being trained and evaluated in this procedure).
- Assist patient with passive and active ROM exercises.
- Notify RN about patient complaints of pain, tingling, or decreased sensation in the affected extremity.

FIG. 63-10 Balanced suspension skeletal traction. Most commonly used for fractures of the femur, hip, and lower leg. Courtesy Zimmer, Inc.

Short arm cast   Long arm cast

Long leg cast

Short leg cast

FIG. 63-11 Common types of casts.

the correct positioning and alignment of the patient while the traction forces remain constant. For extremity traction to be effective, forces must be pulling in the opposite direction (countertraction). Countertraction is commonly supplied by the patient's body weight or by weights pulling in the opposite direction, and it may be augmented by elevating the end of the bed. It is imperative to maintain traction continuously and to keep the weights off the floor and moving freely through the pulleys.

Fracture Immobilization. Fracture immobilization can be done using casts, braces, splints, immobilizers, and external and internal fixation devices.

Casts. A *cast* is a temporary circumferential immobilization device. Casting is a common treatment following closed reduction. It allows the patient to perform many normal activities of daily living while providing sufficient immobilization to ensure stability. Cast materials are natural (plaster of paris), synthetic acrylic, fiberglass-free, latex-free polymer, or a hybrid of materials. A cast generally incorporates the joints above and below a fracture. Immobilization above and below a joint restricts tendon and ligament movement, thereby assisting with joint stabilization while the fracture heals.

To apply a cast on an extremity, first cover the affected part with a stockinette that is cut longer than the extremity.[14] Then place padding over the stockinette with the bony prominences given extra padding. If plaster of paris casting material is used, it is usually immersed in warm water, then wrapped and molded around the affected part. The number of layers of plaster bandage and the technique of application determine the strength of the cast. The plaster sets within 15 minutes, so the patient may move around without difficulty. However, it is not strong enough for weight bearing until about 24 to 72 hours after application. (The decision about weight bearing is determined by the physician.)

A fresh plaster cast should never be covered because air cannot circulate, heat builds up in the cast that may cause a burn, and drying is delayed. Avoid direct pressure on the cast during the drying period. Handle the cast gently with an open palm to avoid denting the cast. Once the cast is thoroughly dry, the edges may need to be *petaled* to avoid skin irritation from rough edges and to prevent plaster of paris debris from falling into the cast and causing irritation or pressure necrosis. The health care provider places several strips (petals) of tape over the rough areas to ensure a smooth cast edge.

Casts made of synthetic materials are being used more than plaster because they are lightweight, stronger, and relatively waterproof and provide for early weight bearing. The synthetic casting materials (thermolabile plastic, thermoplastic resins, polyurethane, and fiberglass) are activated by submersion in cool or tepid water. Then they are molded to fit the torso or extremity.

Upper Extremity Injuries. Immobilization of an acute fracture or soft tissue injury of the upper extremity is often accomplished by use of a (1) sugar-tong splint, (2) posterior splint, (3) short arm cast, or (4) long arm cast (Fig. 63-11). The *sugar-tong splint* is typically used for acute wrist injuries or injuries that may result in significant swelling. Plaster splints are applied over a well-padded forearm, beginning at the phalangeal joints of the hand, extending up the dorsal aspect of the forearm around the distal humerus, and then extending down the volar aspect of the forearm to the distal palmar crease. The splinting material is wrapped with either elastic bandage or bias stockinette. The sugar-tong posterior splint accommodates postinjury swelling in the fractured extremity.

The *short arm cast* is often used for the treatment of stable wrist or metacarpal fractures. An aluminum finger splint can be incorporated into the short arm cast for concurrent treatment of phalangeal injuries. The short arm cast is a circular cast extending from the distal palmar crease to the proximal forearm. This cast provides wrist immobilization and permits unrestricted elbow motion.

The *long arm cast* is commonly used for stable forearm or elbow fractures and unstable wrist fractures. It is similar to the short arm cast but extends to the proximal humerus, restricting motion at the wrist and elbow. Direct your care in supporting the extremity and reducing the effects of edema by elevating the extremity with a sling. However, when a hanging arm cast is used for a proximal humerus fracture, elevation or a supportive sling is contraindicated because hanging provides traction and maintains fracture alignment.

When a sling is used, ensure that the axillary area is well padded to prevent skin excoriation and maceration associated with direct skin-to-skin contact. Placement of the sling should not put undue pressure on the neck. Encourage movement of the fingers (unless contraindicated) to enhance the pumping action of vascular and soft tissue structures to decrease edema. Also encourage the patient to actively move nonimmobilized joints of the upper extremity to prevent stiffness and contractures.

Vertebral Injuries. The *body jacket brace* is used for immobilization and support for stable spine injuries of the thoracic or lumbar spine. The brace goes around the chest and abdomen and extends from above the nipple line to the pubis. After application of the brace, assess the patient for the development of superior mesenteric artery syndrome *(cast syndrome)*. This condition occurs if the brace is applied too tightly, compressing the superior mesenteric artery against the duodenum. The patient generally complains of abdominal pain, abdominal pressure, nausea, and vomiting. Assess the abdomen for decreased bowel sounds (a window in the brace may be left over the umbilicus). Treatment includes gastric decompression with a nasogastric (NG) tube and suction. Assessment also includes monitoring respiratory status, bowel and bladder function, and areas of pressure over the bony prominences, especially the iliac crest. The brace may need to be adjusted or removed if any complications occur.

Lower Extremity Injuries. Injuries to the lower extremity are often immobilized by a long leg cast, a short leg cast, a cylinder cast, a Robert Jones dressing, or a prefabricated splint or immobilizer. The usual indications for applying a long leg cast are an unstable ankle fracture, soft tissue injuries, a fractured tibia, and knee injuries. The cast usually extends from the base of the toes to the groin and gluteal crease. The short leg cast can be used for a variety of conditions, but primarily for stable ankle and foot injuries. A cylinder cast, which is used for knee injuries or fractures, extends from the groin to the malleoli of the ankle. A Robert Jones dressing is composed of bulky padding materials (absorption dressing and cotton sheet wadding), splints, and an elastic wrap or bias-cut stockinette.

After application of a lower extremity cast or dressing, the extremity should be elevated on pillows above the heart level for the first 24 hours. After the initial phase, a casted extremity should not be placed in a dependent position because of the possibility of excessive edema. After cast application, observe for signs of compartment syndrome (discussed on p. 1522 later in this chapter) and increased pressure, especially in the heel, anterior tibia, head of the fibula, and malleoli. This increased pressure is manifested by pain or a burning feeling in these areas.

Prefabricated knee and ankle splints and immobilizers are used in many settings. This type of immobilization is easy to apply and remove, which permits close observation of the affected joint for swelling and skin breakdown (Fig. 63-12). Depending on the injury, removal of the splint or immobilizer facilitates ROM of the affected joint and a faster return to function.

The *hip spica cast* is now mainly used for femur fractures in children. The purpose of the hip spica cast is to immobilize the affected extremity and the trunk. The hip spica cast extends from above the nipple line to the base of the foot (single spica) and may include the opposite extremity up to an area above the

FIG. 63-12 Knee immobilizer.

knee (spica and a half) or both extremities (double spica). Assess the patient with a hip spica cast for the same problems that are associated with the body jacket brace.

External Fixation. An external fixator is a metallic device composed of metal pins that are inserted into the bone and attached to external rods to stabilize the fracture while it heals. It can be used to apply traction or to compress fracture fragments and to immobilize reduced fragments when the use of a cast or other traction is not appropriate. The external device holds fracture fragments in place similar to a surgically implanted internal device. The external fixator is attached directly to the bones by percutaneous transfixing pins or wires (Fig. 63-13). External fixation is indicated in simple fractures, complex fractures with extensive soft tissue damage, correction of bony defects (congenital), nonunion or malunion, and limb lengthening.

External fixation is often used in an attempt to salvage extremities that otherwise might require amputation. Because the use of an external device is a long-term process, ongoing assessment for pin loosening and infection is critical. Infection signaled by exudate, erythema, tenderness, and pain may require removal of the device. Instruct the patient and caregiver about meticulous pin care. Although each physician has a protocol for pin care cleaning, half-strength hydrogen peroxide with normal saline is often used.

Internal Fixation. Internal fixation devices (pins, plates, intramedullary rods, and metal and bioabsorbable screws) are surgically inserted to realign and maintain bony fragments (Fig. 63-14 and eFig. 63-2 on the website for this chapter). These metal devices are biologically inert and made from stainless steel, vitallium, or titanium. Proper alignment is evaluated by x-ray studies at regular intervals.

Electrical Bone Growth Stimulation. Electrical bone growth stimulation is used to facilitate the healing process for certain types of fractures, especially those with nonunion or delayed healing. The mechanism of action of electrical bone growth stimulation may include (1) increasing the calcium uptake of bone, (2) activating intracellular calcium stores, and (3) increasing the production of bone growth factors (e.g., bone morphogenic protein).

FIG. 63-13 External fixators. **A,** Stabilization of hand injury. **B,** Stabilization of a tibial fracture.

FIG. 63-14 Views of internal fixation devices to stabilize a fractured tibia and fibula.

Noninvasive, semi-invasive, and invasive methods of electrical bone growth stimulation are used. Noninvasive stimulators use direct current or pulsed electromagnetic fields (PEMFs) to generate a weak electrical current. Electrodes are placed over the patient's skin or cast and are used 10 to 12 hours each day, usually while the patient is sleeping. Semi-invasive or percutaneous bone growth stimulators use an external power supply and electrodes that are inserted through the skin and into the bone. Invasive stimulators require surgical implantation of a current generator in an intramuscular or subcutaneous space. An electrode is implanted in the bone fragments.

Drug Therapy. Patients with fractures experience varying degrees of pain associated with muscle spasms. Central and peripheral muscle relaxants, such as carisoprodol (Soma), cyclobenzaprine (Flexeril), or methocarbamol (Robaxin), may be prescribed for relief of pain associated with muscle spasms.[15]

Acute pain management for the patient with a fracture is presented in eNursing Care Plan 63-1 (on the website for this chapter).

In an open fracture the threat of tetanus can be reduced with tetanus and diphtheria toxoid or tetanus immunoglobulin for the patient who has not been previously immunized (see Table 69-6). Bone-penetrating antibiotics, such as a cephalosporin (e.g., cefazolin [Kefzol, Ancef]), are used prophylactically before surgery.

Nutritional Therapy. Proper nutrition is an essential component of the healing process in injured tissue. An adequate energy source is needed to promote muscle strength and tone, build endurance, and provide energy for ambulation and gait-training skills. The patient's dietary requirements must include adequate protein (e.g., 1 g/kg of body weight), vitamins (especially B, C, and D), calcium, phosphorus, and magnesium to ensure optimal soft tissue and bone healing. Low serum protein levels and vitamin C deficiencies interfere with tissue healing. Immobility and bone healing increase calcium needs.

Three well-balanced meals a day usually provide the necessary nutrients. The well-balanced meals should be supplemented by a fluid intake of 2000 to 3000 mL/day to promote optimal bladder and bowel function. Adequate fluid and a high-fiber diet with fruits and vegetables prevent constipation. If immobilized in bed with skeletal traction or in a body jacket brace, the patient should eat six small meals to avoid overeating and thus abdominal pressure and cramping.

NURSING MANAGEMENT FRACTURES

NURSING ASSESSMENT

A brief history of the traumatic episode, the mechanism of injury, and the position in which the victim was found can be obtained from the patient or witnesses. As soon as possible, the patient should be transported to an emergency department where a thorough assessment and treatment can be initiated (Table 63-7). Subjective and objective data that should be obtained from an individual with a fracture are presented in Table 63-8 on p. 1519.

Place special emphasis on the region distal to the site of injury. Document clinical findings before fracture treatment to avoid doubts about whether a problem discovered later was missed during the original examination or was caused by the treatment.

NEUROVASCULAR ASSESSMENT. Musculoskeletal injuries may cause changes in the neurovascular status of an injured extremity. Application of a cast or constrictive dressing, poor positioning, and the physiologic responses to the traumatic injury can cause nerve or vascular damage, usually distal to the injury. The neurovascular assessment should consist of a *peripheral vascular assessment* (color, temperature, capillary refill, peripheral pulses, and edema) and a *peripheral neurologic assessment* (sensation, motor function, and pain). Throughout the neurovascular assessment, compare both extremities to obtain an accurate assessment.

✚ TABLE 63-7 EMERGENCY MANAGEMENT

Fractured Extremity

Etiology	Assessment Findings	Interventions
Blunt Trauma • Motor vehicle collision • Pedestrian event • Falls • Direct blows • Forced flexion or hyperextension • Twisting forces **Penetrating Trauma** • Gunshot • Blast **Other** • Pathologic conditions • Violent muscle contractions (seizures) • Crush injury	• Deformity (loss of normal bony contours) or unnatural position of affected limb • Edema and ecchymosis • Muscle spasm • Tenderness and pain • Warmth at site • Loss of function • Numbness, tingling, loss of distal pulses • Grating (crepitus) • Open wound over injured site, exposure of bone	**Initial** • Treat life-threatening injuries first. • Ensure airway, breathing, and circulation. • Control external bleeding with direct pressure or sterile pressure dressing and elevation of the extremity. • Check neurovascular status distal to injury before and after splinting. • Elevate injured limb if possible. • Do *not* attempt to straighten fractured or dislocated joints. • Do *not* manipulate protruding bone ends. • Apply ice packs to affected area. • Obtain x-rays of affected limb. • Administer tetanus and diphtheria prophylaxis if there is a break in skin integrity. • Mark location of pulses to facilitate repeat assessment. • Splint fracture site, including joints above and below fracture site. **Ongoing Monitoring** • Monitor vital signs, level of consciousness, O_2 saturation, neurovascular status, and pain. • Monitor for compartment syndrome characterized by excessive pain, pain with passive stretch of the affected extremity muscles, pallor, paresthesia, and late signs of paralysis and pulselessness. • Monitor for fat embolism (dyspnea, chest pain, temperature elevation).

Assess an extremity's color (pink, pale, cyanotic) and temperature (hot, warm, cool, cold) in the area of the injury. Pallor or a cool to cold extremity below the injury could indicate arterial insufficiency. A warm, cyanotic extremity could indicate poor venous return. Next assess capillary refill (blanching of the nail bed). The standard for a compressed nail bed to return to its original color is within 3 seconds.

Compare pulses on both the unaffected and injured extremity to identify differences in rate or quality. Pulses are described as strong, diminished, audible by Doppler, or absent. A diminished or absent pulse distal to the injury can indicate vascular dysfunction and insufficiency. Also assess peripheral edema. Pitting edema may be present with severe injury.

Evaluate the ulnar, median, and radial nerves by assessing sensation and motor innervation in the upper extremity. Assess neurovascular status by abduction and adduction of the fingers, opposition of the fingers, and supination and pronation of the hand. In the lower extremity, dorsiflexion and plantar flexion indicate motor function of the peroneal and tibial nerves. Sensory innervation is evaluated for the peroneal nerve on the dorsal part of the foot between the web space of the great and second toes. Tibial nerve assessment is performed by stroking the plantar surface (sole) of the foot. Contralateral evaluation is critical.

Paresthesia (abnormal sensation [e.g., numbness, tingling]) and hypersensation or hyperesthesia may be reported by the patient. Partial or full loss of sensation (paresis or paralysis) may be a late sign of neurovascular damage. Instruct patients to report any changes in their neurovascular status.

▌NURSING DIAGNOSES

Nursing diagnoses for the patient with a fracture may include, but are not limited to, the following:

• Impaired physical mobility *related to* loss of integrity of bone structures, movement of bone fragments, and prescribed movement restrictions

• Risk for peripheral neurovascular dysfunction *related to* vascular insufficiency and nerve compression secondary to edema and/or mechanical compression by traction, splints, or casts
• Acute pain *related to* edema, movement of bone fragments, and muscle spasms
• Readiness for enhanced self–health management

Additional information on nursing diagnoses for the patient with a fracture is presented in eNursing Care Plan 63-1 (on the website for this chapter).

▌PLANNING

The overall goals are that the patient with a fracture will (1) have healing with no associated complications, (2) obtain satisfactory pain relief, and (3) achieve maximal rehabilitation potential.

▌NURSING IMPLEMENTATION

HEALTH PROMOTION. Teach people in the community to take appropriate safety precautions to prevent injuries while at home, at work, when driving, or when participating in sports. Be an advocate for personal actions known to reduce injuries, such as regularly using seat belts; driving within posted speed limits; avoiding distracted driving; warming up muscles before exercise; using protective athletic equipment (helmets and knee, wrist, and elbow pads); using safety equipment at work; and not combining driving and drinking or the use of illicit drugs.

Encourage individuals (especially older adults) to participate in moderate exercise to help maintain muscle strength and balance. To reduce falls, they should wear adequate footwear and assess their living environment for safety (e.g., remove scatter rugs, maintain good lighting, clear paths to the bathroom for nighttime use) (see Table 63-1). Also stress the importance of adequate calcium and vitamin D intake.

ACUTE INTERVENTION. Patients with fractures may be treated in an emergency department or a physician's office and released to home care, or they may require hospitalization for varying

TABLE 63-8 NURSING ASSESSMENT

Fracture

Subjective Data
Important Health Information
Past health history: Traumatic injury; long-term repetitive forces (stress fracture); bone or systemic diseases, prolonged immobility, osteopenia, osteoporosis
Medications: Corticosteroids (osteoporotic fractures); analgesics
Surgery or other treatments: First aid treatment of fracture, previous musculoskeletal surgeries

Functional Health Patterns
Health perception–health management: Estrogen replacement therapy, calcium supplementation
Activity-exercise: Loss of motion or weakness of affected part; muscle spasms
Cognitive-perceptual: Sudden and severe pain in affected area; numbness, tingling, loss of sensation distal to injury; chronic pain that increases with activity (stress fracture)

Objective Data
General
Apprehension, guarding of injured site

Integumentary
Skin lacerations, pallor and cool skin or bluish and warm skin distal to injury; ecchymosis, hematoma, edema at site of fracture

Cardiovascular
Reduced or absent pulse distal to injury, ↓ skin temperature, delayed capillary refill

Neurovascular
Paresthesias, absent or ↓ sensation, hypersensation

Musculoskeletal
Restricted or lost function of affected part; local bony deformities, abnormal angulation; shortening, rotation, or crepitation of affected part; muscle weakness

Possible Diagnostic Findings
Identification and extent of fracture on x-ray, bone scan, CT scan, or MRI

EVIDENCE-BASED PRACTICE

Translating Research Into Practice

Do Vitamin D Supplements Improve Strength in Older Adults?

Clinical Question
In older adults (P) does vitamin D supplementation (I) improve strength, balance, and gait (O)?

Best Available Evidence
Systematic review of randomized controlled trials (RCTs)

Critical Appraisal and Synthesis of Evidence
• Thirteen RCTs (*n* = 2268) of older adults (mainly women) were done to determine the effect of supplemental vitamin D without an exercise intervention on muscle strength, gait, and balance.
• Supplemental vitamin D with daily doses of 800 to 1000 IU consistently demonstrated beneficial effects on strength and balance. An effect on gait was not demonstrated, although further evaluation is recommended.
• Increasing serum vitamin D levels to normal levels resulted in better muscle strength.

Conclusion
• Supplemental vitamin D has beneficial effects on strength and balance in older adults.

Implications for Nursing Practice
• Assess for vitamin D deficiencies and offer strategies to improve nutritional uptake, brief sunlight exposure, and supplementation.
• Discuss the importance of vitamin D in reducing the risk of falls.

Reference for Evidence
Muir SW, Montero-Odasso M: Effect of vitamin D supplementation on muscle strength, gait and balance in older adults: a systematic review and meta-analysis, *J Am Geriatr Soc* 59:2291, 2011.

P, Patient population of interest; *I,* intervention or area of interest; *O,* outcomes of interest (see p. 12).

a significant increase in size of the drainage area. If a wound drainage system is in place, regularly measure the volume of drainage and assess the patency of the system, using aseptic technique to avoid contamination.

Additional nursing responsibilities depend on the type of immobilization used. A blood salvage and reinfusion system that allows for recovery and reinfusion of the patient's own blood may be used. The blood is retrieved from a joint space or cavity, and the patient receives this blood in the form of an autotransfusion. (Autotransfusion is discussed in Chapter 31.) Additional nursing measures for the patient who has had orthopedic surgery are discussed in eNursing Care Plan 63-2 (on the website for this chapter).

Other Measures. Patients often have reduced mobility as a result of the fracture. Plan care to prevent the many complications associated with immobility. Prevent constipation by increased patient activity and maintenance of a high fluid intake (more than 2500 mL/day unless contraindicated by the patient's health status) and a diet high in bulk and roughage (fresh fruits and vegetables). If these measures are not effective in maintaining the patient's normal bowel pattern, warm fluids, stool softeners, laxatives, or suppositories may be necessary. Maintain a regular time for elimination to promote bowel regularity.

Renal calculi can develop as a result of bone demineralization. The hypercalcemia from demineralization causes a rise in

amounts of time. Specific nursing measures depend on the setting and the type of treatment used.

Preoperative Management. If surgical intervention is required to treat a fracture, patients need preoperative preparation. In addition to the usual preoperative nursing measures (see Chapter 18), inform patients of the type of immobilization and assistive devices that will be used and the expected activity limitations after surgery. Assure patients that their needs will be met by the nursing staff until they can resume self-care. Knowing that pain medication will be available if needed is often beneficial.

Postoperative Management. In general, postoperative nursing care and management are directed toward monitoring vital signs and applying the general principles of postoperative nursing care (see Chapter 20). Frequent neurovascular assessments of the affected extremity are necessary to detect early and subtle neurovascular changes. Closely monitor any limitations of movement or activity related to turning, positioning, and extremity support. Pain and discomfort can be minimized through proper alignment and positioning. Carefully observe dressings or casts for any signs of bleeding or drainage. Report urine pH and stone formation from the precipitation of calcium. Unless contraindicated, a fluid intake of 2500 mL/day is recommended. (Renal calculi are discussed in Chapter 46.)

Rapid deconditioning of the cardiopulmonary system can occur as a result of prolonged bed rest, resulting in orthostatic hypotension and decreased lung capacity. Unless contraindicated, these effects can be diminished by having the patient sit on the side of the bed, allowing the patient's lower limbs to dangle over the bedside, and having the patient perform standing transfers. When the patient is allowed to increase activity, assess for orthostatic hypotension. Also assess patients for deep vein thrombosis (DVT) and pulmonary emboli. (DVT is discussed in Chapter 38.)

Traction. When slings are used with traction, inspect exposed skin areas regularly. Pressure over a bony prominence created by the wrinkling of sheets or bedclothes may cause pressure necrosis. Persistent skin pressure may impair blood flow and cause injury to the peripheral neurovascular structures. Observe skeletal traction pin sites for signs of infection. Pin site care varies but usually includes regularly removing exudate with half-strength hydrogen peroxide, rinsing pin sites with sterile saline, and drying the area with sterile gauze.

External rotation of the hip can occur when skin traction is used on the lower extremity. Correct this position by placing a pillow or rolled-up towels along the greater trochanter of the femur. Generally, the patient should be in the center of the bed in a supine position. Incorrect alignment can result in increased pain and nonunion or malunion.

To offset some of the problems associated with prolonged immobility, discuss specific patient activity with the health care provider. If exercise is permitted, encourage patient participation in a simple exercise regimen based on activity restrictions. Activities that the patient should participate in include frequent position changes, ROM exercises of unaffected joints, deep-breathing exercises, isometric exercises, and use of the trapeze bar (if permitted) to raise the body off the bed for linen changes and use of the bedpan. These activities should be performed several times each day. Encourage and help the hospitalized patient to stay connected with friends and family through social media resources (see Informatics in Practice box).

AMBULATORY AND HOME CARE

Cast Care. Because many fractures are treated in an outpatient setting, the patient often requires only a short hospitalization or none at all. Regardless of the type of cast material, a cast can interfere with circulation and nerve function if it is applied too tightly or excessive edema occurs after application. Frequent neurovascular assessments of the immobilized extremity are critical. Teach the patient the signs of cast complications so that they can be reported promptly. Elevation of the extremity above the level of the heart to promote venous return and applications

of ice to control or prevent edema are measures frequently used during the initial phase. (If compartment syndrome is suspected, do not elevate the extremity above the heart.) Instruct the patient to exercise joints above and below the cast. Discourage pulling out cast padding and scratching or placing foreign objects inside the cast because it predisposes the patient to skin breakdown and infection. For itching, instruct the patient that a hair dryer set on a cool setting can be directed under the cast.

Patient and caregiver teaching is important to prevent complications. In addition to specific instructions for cast care and recognition of complications, encourage the patient to contact the health care provider should questions arise. Table 63-9 summarizes patient and caregiver instructions for cast care. Validate the patient's and caregiver's understanding of these instructions before discharge. A follow-up phone call is appropriate, and home care nursing visits are warranted, especially for the patient with a body jacket brace.

The cast is removed in the outpatient setting. Patients often fear being cut by the oscillating blade of the cast saw. Reassure the patient that damage to the skin is unlikely. Teach the patient about possible alterations in the appearance of the extremity (e.g., dry, wrinkled skin, atrophied muscle) that has been beneath the cast. The patient may also have anxiety related to using the injured extremity after the cast is removed.

Psychosocial Problems. Short-term rehabilitative goals are directed toward the transition from dependence to independence in performing simple activities of daily living and preserving or increasing strength and endurance. Long-term rehabilitative goals are aimed at preventing problems associated with musculoskeletal injury (Table 63-10). An important part

---

INFORMATICS IN PRACTICE

Staying Connected While Immobilized

- A patient in traction or other immobilization devices for a long period may feel lonely or isolated.
- There are a number of ways to use a computer or smart phone to ease separation anxiety and help the patient reconnect with family and friends.
- Set up video chat. Encourage personal contact through instant messaging and e-mail. Have the patient catch up on the latest news and blog on social networking sites.

TABLE 63-9   PATIENT & CAREGIVER TEACHING GUIDE

Cast Care

After a cast is applied, include the following instructions when teaching the patient and the caregiver.

Do
1. Apply ice directly over fracture site for first 24 hr (avoid getting cast wet by keeping ice in plastic bag and protecting cast with cloth).
2. Check with health care provider before getting fiberglass cast wet.
3. Dry cast thoroughly after exposure to water.
   - Blot dry with towel.
   - Use hair dryer on low setting until cast is thoroughly dry.
4. Elevate extremity above level of heart for first 48 hr.
5. Move joints above and below cast regularly.
6. Use hair dryer on cool setting for itching.
7. Report signs of possible problems to health care provider.
   - Increasing pain despite elevation, ice, and analgesia.
   - Swelling associated with pain and discoloration of toes or fingers.
   - Pain during movement.
   - Burning or tingling under the cast.
   - Sores or foul odor under the cast.
8. Keep appointment to have fracture and cast checked.

Do Not
1. Get cast wet.
2. Remove any padding.
3. Insert any objects inside cast.
4. Bear weight on new cast for 48 hr (not all casts are made for weight bearing; check with health care provider when unsure).
5. Cover cast with plastic for prolonged periods.

TABLE 63-10   PROBLEMS ASSOCIATED WITH MUSCULOSKELETAL INJURIES

Problem	Description	Nursing Considerations
Muscle atrophy	• Decreased muscle mass normally occurs as a result of disuse after prolonged immobilization. • Loss of nerve innervation can precipitate muscle atrophy.	• Isometric muscle-strengthening exercise regimen within confines of immobilization device assists in reducing amount of atrophy. • Muscle atrophy interferes with and prolongs rehabilitation process.
Contracture	• Abnormal condition of joint characterized by flexion and fixation. • Caused by atrophy and shortening of muscle fibers or by loss of normal elasticity of skin over joint.	• Can be prevented by frequent position change, correct body alignment, and active-passive range-of-motion exercises several times a day. • Intervention requires gradual and progressive stretching of muscles or ligaments in region of joint.
Footdrop	• Plantar-flexed position of the foot (footdrop) occurs when Achilles tendon in ankle shortens because it has been allowed to assume an unsupported position. • Peroneal nerve palsy (a compression neuropathy) can cause footdrop and spinal nerve compression.	• Management of patient with long-term injuries must include preventive measures by supporting foot in neutral position. • Once footdrop has developed, ambulation and gait training may be significantly hindered. • May require splint to keep foot (feet) in neutral position. • High-top athletic shoes may also help.
Pain	• Frequently associated with fractures, edema, and muscle spasm. • Pain varies in intensity from mild to severe and is described as aching, dull, burning, throbbing, sharp, or deep.	• Causes of pain include incorrect positioning and alignment of extremity, incorrect support of extremity, sudden movement of extremity, immobilization device that is applied too tightly or in an incorrect position, constrictive dressings, and motion occurring at fracture site. • Determine causes of pain so that corrective action can be taken.
Muscle spasms	• Caused by involuntary muscle contraction after fracture, muscle strain, or nerve injury and may last several weeks. • Pain associated with muscle spasms is often intense and can last from several seconds to several minutes.	• Measures to reduce the intensity of the muscle spasms are similar to corrective actions for pain control. • Do not massage muscle spasms because it may stimulate muscle tissue contraction that increases spasm and pain. • Thermotherapy, especially heat, may reduce muscle spasm.

of care during the rehabilitative phase is helping the patient adjust to any problems caused by the injury (e.g., separation from family, financial impact of medical care, loss of income from inability to work, potential for lifetime disability). Offer support and encouragement while actively listening to the patient's and the caregiver's concerns.

Ambulation. Know the overall goals of physical therapy in relation to the patient's abilities, needs, and tolerance. Mobility training and instruction in the use of assistive aids (cane, crutches, walker) are major areas of responsibility of the physical therapist. Reinforce these instructions to the patient. The patient with lower extremity dysfunction usually starts mobility training when able to sit in bed and dangle the feet over the side. Collaborate with the physical therapist to coordinate pain management before a physical therapy session.

When the patient begins to ambulate, know the patient's weight-bearing status and the correct technique if the patient is using an assistive device. Weight-bearing ambulation occurs in different degrees: (1) non–weight-bearing (no weight borne) ambulation, (2) touch-down/toe-touch weight-bearing ambulation (contact with floor but no weight borne), (3) partial–weight-bearing ambulation (25% to 50% of patient's weight borne), (4) weight bearing as tolerated (dictated by patient's pain and tolerance), and (5) full–weight-bearing ambulation (no limitations).

Assistive Devices. Devices for ambulation range from a cane (can relieve up to 40% of the weight normally borne by a lower limb) to a walker or crutches (may allow for complete non–weight-bearing ambulation). The health care provider decides which device is appropriate,, balancing the need for maximum stability and safety versus maneuverability (this is required in small spaces such as bathrooms). Discuss with the patient his or her lifestyle requirements and select a device with which each patient feels most secure and independent. The technique for using assistive ambulation devices varies. The involved limb is usually advanced at the same time or immediately after advance

of the device. The uninvolved limb is advanced last. In almost all cases, canes are held in the hand opposite the involved extremity.

Place a transfer belt around the patient's waist to provide stability while he or she is learning to use an assistive device. Discourage the patient from reaching for furniture or relying on another person for support. When there is inadequate upper limb strength or poorly fitted crutches, the patient bears weight at the axilla rather than at the hands, endangering the neurovascular bundle that passes across the axilla. If verbal coaching does not correct the problem, instruct the patient in another form of ambulation (e.g., crutches, walker) until strength is adequate.

Patients who must ambulate without weight bearing require sufficient upper limb strength to lift their own weight at each step. Because the muscles of the shoulder girdle are not accustomed to this work, they require vigorous and diligent training in preparation for this task. Push-ups, pull-ups using the overhead trapeze bar, and weight lifting develop the triceps and biceps. Straight-leg raises and quadriceps-setting exercises strengthen the quadriceps.

Counseling and Referrals. During the rehabilitative process, the patient's caregiver assumes an important role in the provision and follow-through of long-term care plans. Instruct the caregiver in the techniques of strength and endurance exercises, assistance with mobility training, and promotion of activities that enhance the quality of daily living. Also evaluate patients for posttraumatic stress disorder. This is especially important if significant injury to others or fatalities were associated with the patient's injuries.

EVALUATION

The expected outcomes are that the patient with a fracture will
- Report satisfactory relief of pain
- Demonstrate appropriate care of cast or immobilizer
- Experience no peripheral neurovascular dysfunction
- Experience uncomplicated bone healing

COMPLICATIONS OF FRACTURES

The majority of fractures heal without complications. If death occurs after a fracture, it is usually the result of damage to underlying organs and vascular structures or from complications of the fracture or immobility. Complications of fractures may be either direct or indirect. *Direct complications* include problems with bone infection, bone union, and avascular necrosis. *Indirect complications* are associated with blood vessel and nerve damage resulting in conditions such as compartment syndrome, venous thromboembolism, fat embolism, rhabdomyolysis (breakdown of skeletal muscle), and hypovolemic shock. Although most musculoskeletal injuries are not life threatening, open fractures, fractures accompanied by severe blood loss, and fractures that damage vital organs (e.g., lung, heart) are medical emergencies requiring immediate attention.

Infection

Open fractures and soft tissue injuries have a high incidence of infection. An open fracture usually results from the impact of severe external forces. Massive or blunt soft tissue injury often has more serious consequences than the fracture. Devitalized and contaminated tissue is an ideal medium for many common pathogens, including gas-forming (anaerobic) bacilli such as *Clostridium tetani*. Treatment of infection is costly in terms of extended nursing and medical care, time for treatment, and loss of patient income. Osteomyelitis can become chronic[16] (see Chapter 64).

Open fractures require aggressive surgical debridement. The wound is initially cleansed by pulsating saline lavage in the operating room. Gross contaminants are irrigated and mechanically removed. Contused, contaminated, and devitalized tissue such as muscle, subcutaneous fat, skin, and fragments of bone are surgically excised *(debridement)*. The extent of the soft tissue damage determines whether the wound is closed at the time of surgery and whether it requires repeat debridement, closed suction drainage, and skin grafting. Depending on the location and extent of the fracture, reduction may be maintained by external fixation or traction. During surgery the open wound may be irrigated with antibiotic solution. Antibiotic-impregnated beads may also be placed in the surgical site. During the postoperative phase the patient may have antibiotics administered IV for 3 to 7 days. Antibiotics, in conjunction with aggressive surgical management, have greatly reduced the occurrence of infection.

Compartment Syndrome

Compartment syndrome is a condition in which swelling and increased pressure within a limited space (a compartment) press on and compromise the function of blood vessels, nerves, and/or tendons that run through that compartment. Compartment syndrome causes capillary perfusion to be reduced below a level necessary for tissue viability. Compartment syndrome usually involves the leg, but can also occur in the arm, shoulder, and buttock.

Thirty-eight compartments are located in the upper and lower extremities. Two basic causes of compartment syndrome are (1) decreased compartment size resulting from restrictive dressings, splints, casts, excessive traction, or premature closure of fascia; and (2) increased compartment contents related to bleeding, inflammation, edema, or IV infiltration.

Edema can create sufficient pressure to obstruct circulation and cause venous occlusion, which further increases edema. Eventually arterial flow is compromised, resulting in ischemia to the extremity. As ischemia continues, muscle and nerve cells are destroyed over time, and fibrotic tissue replaces healthy tissue. Contracture, disability, and loss of function can occur. Delays in diagnosis and treatment cause irreversible muscle and nerve ischemia, resulting in a functionally useless or severely impaired extremity.

Compartment syndrome is usually associated with trauma, fractures (especially the long bones), extensive soft tissue damage, and crush injury. Fractures of the distal humerus and proximal tibia are the most common fractures associated with compartment syndrome. Compartment injury can also occur after knee or leg surgery. Prolonged pressure on a muscle compartment may result when someone is trapped under a heavy object or a person's limb is trapped beneath the body because of an obtunded state such as drug or alcohol overdose.

Clinical Manifestations. Compartment syndrome may occur initially from the body's physiologic response to the injury, or it may be delayed for several days after the original insult or injury. Ischemia can occur within 4 to 8 hours after the onset of compartment syndrome.

One or more of the following six *P*s are characteristic of compartment syndrome: (1) *pain* distal to the injury that is not relieved by opioid analgesics and *pain* on passive stretch of muscle traveling through the compartment; (2) increasing *pressure* in the compartment; (3) *paresthesia* (numbness and tingling); (4) *pallor*, coolness, and loss of normal color of the extremity; (5) *paralysis* or loss of function; and (6) *pulselessness*, or diminished or absent peripheral pulses.

Collaborative Care. Prompt, accurate diagnosis of compartment syndrome is critical.[17] Perform and document regular neurovascular assessments on all patients with fractures, especially those with an injury of the distal humerus or proximal tibia or soft tissue injuries in these areas. Early recognition and effective treatment of compartment syndrome are essential to avoid permanent damage to muscles and nerves.

Carefully assess the location, quality, and intensity of the pain (see Chapter 9). Evaluate the patient's level of pain on a scale of 0 to 10. Pain unrelieved by drugs and out of proportion to the level of injury is one of the *first* indications of impending compartment syndrome. Pulselessness and paralysis (in particular) are later signs of compartment syndrome. Notify the health care provider immediately of a patient's changing condition.

Because of the possibility of muscle damage, assess urine output. Myoglobin released from damaged muscle cells precipitates and causes obstruction in renal tubules. This condition results in acute tubular necrosis and acute kidney injury. Common signs are dark reddish brown urine and clinical manifestations associated with acute kidney injury (see Chapter 47).

Elevation of the extremity may lower venous pressure and slow arterial perfusion. Therefore the extremity should not be elevated above heart level. Similarly, the application of cold compresses may result in vasoconstriction and exacerbate compartment syndrome. It may also be necessary to remove or loosen the bandage and split the cast in half (bivalving). A reduction in traction weight may also decrease external circumferential pressures.

Surgical decompression (e.g., fasciotomy) of the involved compartment may be necessary (Fig. 63-15). The fasciotomy site is left open for several days to ensure adequate soft tissue

FIG. 63-15 Fasciotomy associated with compartment syndrome. Stabilization of fracture with external fixator.

decompression. Infection resulting from delayed wound closure is a potential problem after a fasciotomy. In severe cases of compartment syndrome, an amputation may be required.

Venous Thromboembolism

The veins of the lower extremities and the pelvis are highly susceptible to thrombus formation after a fracture, especially a hip fracture. Venous thromboembolism (VTE) may also occur after total hip or total knee replacement surgery.[18] In patients with limited mobility, venous stasis is aggravated by inactivity of the muscles that normally assist in the pumping action of venous blood returning to the extremities.

Because of the high risk of VTE in the orthopedic surgical patient, prophylactic anticoagulant drugs such as warfarin (Coumadin), low-molecular-weight heparin (LMWH) such as enoxaparin (Lovenox), fondaparinux (Arixtra), or rivaroxaban (Xarelto) may be ordered. In addition to wearing compression gradient stockings (antiembolism hose) and using sequential compression devices, the patient should move (dorsiflex and plantar flex) the fingers or toes of the affected extremity against resistance and perform ROM exercises on the unaffected lower extremities. (Assessment and management of VTE are discussed in Chapter 38.)

Fat Embolism Syndrome

Fat embolism syndrome (FES) is characterized by systemic fat globules from fractures that are distributed into tissues and organs after a traumatic skeletal injury. FES is a contributory factor in mortality associated with fractures. The fractures that most often cause FES are those of the long bones, ribs, tibia, and pelvis. FES has also been known to occur after total joint replacement, spinal fusion, liposuction, crush injuries, and bone marrow transplantation.

Two theories about fat embolism exist. First, the mechanical theory is that fat emboli may originate from the fat that is released from the marrow of injured bone. The fat then enters the systemic circulation where it embolizes to other organs such as the brain.[19] Microvascular lodging of droplets produces local ischemia and inflammation. Second, the biochemical theory is that hormonal changes caused by trauma or sepsis stimulate the systemic release of free fatty acids such as chylomicrons, which form the fat emboli.

Clinical Manifestations. Early recognition of FES is crucial to prevent a potentially lethal course. Most patients manifest symptoms within 24 to 48 hours after injury. Severe forms have occurred within hours of injury. The fat emboli in the lungs cause a hemorrhagic interstitial pneumonitis that produces signs and symptoms of acute respiratory distress syndrome (ARDS), such as chest pain, tachypnea, cyanosis, dyspnea, apprehension, tachycardia, and decreased partial pressure of arterial oxygen (PaO_2). All of these symptoms are caused by poor oxygen exchange. Because they are frequently the presenting manifestations, changes in mental status (a result of hypoxemia) are important to recognize. Memory loss, restlessness, confusion, elevated temperature, and headache should prompt further investigation so that central nervous system involvement is not mistaken for alcohol withdrawal or acute head injury. The continued change in level of consciousness and petechiae located around the neck, anterior chest wall, axilla, buccal membrane, and conjunctiva of the eye help distinguish fat emboli from other problems. Petechiae may appear due to intravascular thromboses caused by decreased oxygenation.

The clinical course of a fat embolus may be rapid and acute. Frequently the patient expresses a feeling of impending disaster. In a short time, skin color changes from pallor to cyanosis, and the patient may become comatose. No specific laboratory examinations are available to aid in the diagnosis.[19] However, certain diagnostic abnormalities may be present. These include fat cells in blood, urine, or sputum; a decrease of the PaO_2 to less than 60 mm Hg; ST segment changes on ECG; a decrease in the platelet count and hematocrit levels; and a prolonged prothrombin time. A chest x-ray may reveal areas of pulmonary infiltrate or multiple areas of consolidation. This is sometimes referred to as the "white-out effect."

Collaborative Care. Treatment of fat embolism is directed at prevention. Careful immobilization of a long bone fracture is probably the most important factor in prevention of fat embolism. Management of FES is mostly supportive and related to management of symptoms. Treatment includes fluid resuscitation to prevent hypovolemic shock, correction of acidosis, and replacement of blood loss. Encourage coughing and deep breathing. Reposition the patient as little as possible before fracture immobilization or stabilization because of the danger of dislodging more fat droplets into the general circulation.

Use of corticosteroids to prevent or treat fat embolism is controversial. Oxygen is administered to treat hypoxia. Intubation or intermittent positive pressure ventilation may be considered if a satisfactory PaO_2 cannot be obtained with supplemental oxygen alone. Some patients may develop pulmonary edema, ARDS, or both, leading to an increased mortality rate. Most persons survive FES with few sequelae.

TYPES OF FRACTURES

COLLES' FRACTURE

A *Colles' fracture* is a fracture of the distal radius and is one of the most common fractures in adults (Fig. 63-16). The styloid process of the ulna may be involved as well. The injury usually occurs when the patient attempts to break a fall with an outstretched arm and hand. This type of fracture most often occurs in patients over 50 years old whose bones are osteoporotic. A younger person with a Colles' fracture caused by a low-energy force should be referred for an osteoporosis evaluation.

The clinical manifestations of Colles' fracture are pain in the immediate area of injury, pronounced swelling, and dorsal displacement of the distal fragment (silver-fork deformity). This displacement appears as an obvious deformity of the wrist. The major complication associated with a Colles' fracture is vascular insufficiency secondary to edema. Carpal tunnel syndrome can be a later complication.

FIG. 63-16 Colles' fracture. Fracture of the distal radius *(R)* and ulnar *(U)* styloid from patient falling on the outstretched hand.

A Colles' fracture is usually managed by closed manipulation of the fracture and immobilization by either a splint or a cast or, if displaced, by internal or external fixation. Nursing management includes measures to prevent or reduce edema and frequent neurovascular assessments. Provide support and protection of the extremity, and encourage active movement of the thumb and fingers to reduce edema and increase venous return. Instruct the patient to perform active movements of the shoulder to prevent stiffness or contracture.

FRACTURE OF HUMERUS

Fractures involving the shaft of the humerus are common among young and middle-aged adults (see eFig. 63-3 on the website for this chapter). The most common clinical manifestations are an obvious displacement of the humerus shaft, shortened extremity, abnormal mobility, and pain. The major complications associated with fracture of the humerus are radial nerve injury and vascular injury to the brachial artery as a result of laceration, transection, or muscle spasm.

The treatment for a fracture of the humerus depends on the location and displacement of the fracture. Nonoperative treatment may include a hanging arm cast; shoulder immobilizer; or sling and swathe, which is a type of immobilizer that prevents glenohumeral movement. The swathe encircles the trunk and humerus as an additional binder. It is often used after surgical repairs and shoulder dislocation.

When these devices are used, elevate the head of the bed to assist gravity in reducing the fracture. Allow the arm to hang freely when the patient is sitting or standing. Include measures to protect the axilla and prevent skin breakdown. Carefully place absorbable composite dressing pads (i.e., ABD pads) in the axilla and change them twice daily or as needed. Skin or skeletal traction may be used for reduction and immobilization.

During the rehabilitative phase, an exercise program to improve strength and motion of the injured extremity is extremely important. Exercises should include assisted motion of the hand and fingers. The shoulder can also be exercised if the fracture is stable. This helps prevent stiffness secondary to frozen shoulder or fibrosis of the shoulder capsule.

FRACTURE OF PELVIS

Pelvic fractures range from benign to life threatening, depending on the mechanism of injury and associated vascular insult. Although only a small percentage of all fractures are pelvic

fractures, this type of injury is associated with a high mortality rate. Preoccupation with more obvious injuries at the time of a traumatic event may result in an oversight of pelvic injuries.

Pelvic fractures may cause serious intraabdominal injury such as paralytic ileus; hemorrhage; and laceration of the urethra, bladder, or colon. Pelvic fractures can cause acute pelvic compartment syndrome.[20] Patients may survive the initial pelvic injury, only to die from sepsis, FES, or thromboembolism.

Physical examination of the abdomen demonstrates local swelling, tenderness, deformity, unusual pelvic movement, and ecchymosis. Assess the neurovascular status of the lower extremities and manifestations of associated injuries. Pelvic fractures are diagnosed by x-ray and computed tomography (CT) scan.

Treatment of a pelvic fracture depends on the severity of the injury. Stable, nondisplaced fractures require limited intervention, and early mobilization is encouraged. Bed rest for stable pelvic fractures is maintained from a few days to 6 weeks. More complex fractures may be treated with pelvic sling traction, skeletal traction, external fixation, open reduction, or a combination of these methods. ORIF of a pelvic fracture may be necessary if the fracture is displaced. Use extreme care in handling or moving the patient to prevent serious injury from a displaced fracture fragment. Turn the patient only when ordered by the health care provider. Because a pelvic fracture can damage other organs, assess bowel and urinary elimination and distal neurovascular status. Provide back care while the patient is raised from the bed either by independent use of the trapeze or with adequate assistance.

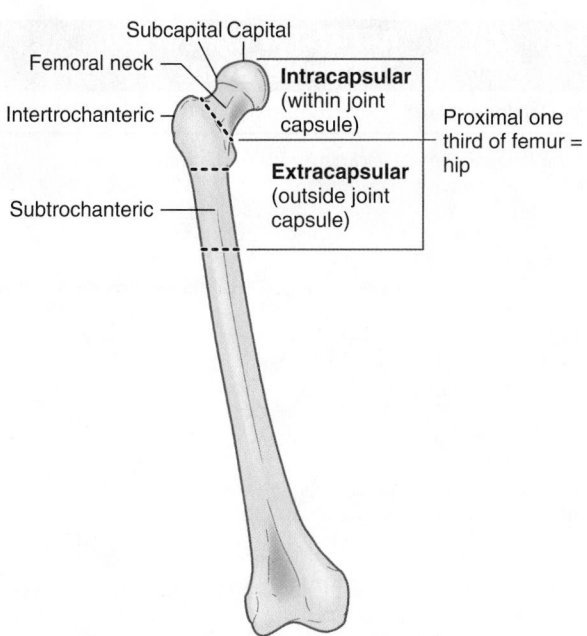

FIG. 63-17 Femur with location of various types of fracture.

FIG. 63-18 Types of surgical repair for a hip fracture.

FIG. 63-19 Total hip replacement (arthroplasty) with a cementless femoral prosthesis of metal alloy with a plastic acetabular socket.

FRACTURE OF HIP

Hip fractures are common in older adults, with 90% of these fractures resulting from a fall.[21] More than 320,000 patients are admitted to hospitals annually because of a hip fracture. By age 90, approximately 33% of all women and 17% of all men will have sustained a hip fracture. In adults more than 65 years old, hip fracture occurs more frequently in women than in men because of osteoporosis.[22] By age 80, one in five women will have a hip fracture. Many older adults with a hip fracture develop disabilities that require long-term care.

A fracture of the hip (Fig. 63-17) refers to a fracture of the proximal (upper) third of the femur, which extends to 5 cm below the lesser trochanter. Fractures that occur within the hip joint capsule are called *intracapsular fractures*. Intracapsular fractures (femoral neck) are further identified by their specific locations: (1) capital (fracture of the head of the femur), (2) subcapital (fracture just below the head of the femur), and (3) transcervical (fracture of the neck of the femur). These fractures are often associated with osteoporosis and minor trauma. *Extracapsular fractures* occur outside the joint capsule. They are termed (1) *intertrochanteric* (in a region between the greater and lesser trochanter) or (2) *subtrochanteric* (below the lesser trochanter). Extracapsular fractures are usually caused by severe direct trauma or a fall.

Clinical Manifestations

The clinical manifestations of hip fractures are external rotation, muscle spasm, shortening of the affected extremity, and severe pain and tenderness around the fracture site. Displaced femoral neck fractures cause serious disruption of blood supply to the femoral head, which can result in avascular necrosis of the femoral head.

Collaborative Care

Initially the affected extremity may be temporarily immobilized by Buck's traction (see Fig. 63-9) until the patient's physical condition is stabilized and surgery can be performed. Buck's traction relieves painful muscle spasms and is used for up to 24 to 48 hours.

Surgical treatment of hip fractures permits early mobilization and decreases the risk of major complications. The type of surgery depends on the location and severity of the fracture and the person's age. Surgical options include (1) repair with internal fixation devices (e.g., hip compression screw, intramedullary devices) (Fig. 63-18), (2) replacement of part of the femur with a prosthesis (partial hip replacement) (see Fig. 63-18), and (3) total hip replacement (involves both the femur and acetabulum) (see Figs. 63-18 and 63-19).

NURSING MANAGEMENT
HIP FRACTURE

NURSING IMPLEMENTATION

PREOPERATIVE MANAGEMENT. The majority of people who have hip fractures are older adults. When planning treatment of the hip fracture, consider the patient's chronic health problems (e.g., diabetes mellitus, cardiac and pulmonary disease). Surgery may be delayed for a brief time until the patient's general health is stabilized.[23]

Before surgery, severe muscle spasms can increase pain. Appropriate analgesics or muscle relaxants, comfortable positioning (unless contraindicated), and properly adjusted traction (if used) can help to manage the spasms.

Teaching is often done in the emergency department because quick surgical intervention is the standard of care today. Many patients do not have an overnight preoperative period in which to receive instructions, or the patient may not have the cognitive abilities to retain this important patient teaching.

When possible, teach the patient the method for exercising the unaffected leg and both arms. Encourage the patient to use the overhead trapeze bar and the opposite side rail to assist in changing positions. A physical therapist can begin to teach out-of-bed and chair transfers. Inform the caregiver about the patient's weight-bearing status after surgery. Plans for discharge begin as soon as the patient enters the hospital because the length of stay postoperatively will only be a few days.

POSTOPERATIVE MANAGEMENT. Similar principles of patient care apply to any of the surgical procedures for hip fractures. The content described in this section is also appropriate for the patient who has a total hip replacement for joint disease.

In the initial postoperative period assess vital signs, intake, and output; monitor respiratory function and deep breathing and coughing; administer pain medication; and observe the dressing and incision for signs of bleeding and infection. eNursing Care Plan 63-2 for the orthopedic surgical patient is presented on the website for this chapter.

In the early postoperative period there is a potential for neurovascular impairment. Assess the patient's extremity for (1) color, (2) temperature, (3) capillary refill, (4) distal pulses, (5) edema, (6) sensation, (7) motor function, and (8) pain. Edema is alleviated by elevating the leg whenever the patient is in a chair. The pain resulting from poor alignment of the affected extremity can be reduced by keeping pillows (or an abductor pillow) between the knees when the patient is turning to either side.

If the hip fracture has been treated by insertion of a prosthesis with a *posterior approach* (accessing the hip joint from the back), measures to prevent dislocation must be used (Table 63-11). Inform the patient and caregiver about positions and activities that predispose the patient to dislocation (more than 90 degrees of flexion, adduction across the midline [crossing of legs and ankles], internal rotation). Many daily activities may reproduce these positions, including putting on shoes and socks; crossing the legs or feet while seated; assuming the side-lying position incorrectly; standing up or sitting down while the body is flexed more than 90 degrees relative to the chair; and sitting on low seats, especially low toilet seats. Until the soft tissue capsule surrounding the hip has healed sufficiently to stabilize the prosthesis, teach the patient to avoid these activities (usually for at least 6 weeks).

Elevated toilet seats and chair alterations (e.g., raising the seat with pillows, maintaining a straight back) are necessary. Towel rolls (i.e., a trochanter roll) or pillows placed on the lateral side of the leg are also used to prevent external rotation. If a foam abduction pillow is used, it should be placed between the legs to prevent dislocation of the new joint (Fig. 63-20). Ensure that the top straps are above the knee to avoid placing pressure on the peroneal nerve at the lateral tibial tubercle.

In addition to teaching the patient and caregiver how to prevent prosthesis dislocation, you should also (1) place an abductor pillow or several pillows between the patient's legs when turning and (2) avoid turning the patient on the affected side until approved by the surgeon. In addition, some health

TABLE 63-11	**PATIENT & CAREGIVER TEACHING GUIDE**

Hip Replacement*

After a hip replacement, include the following instructions when teaching a patient and caregiver.

Do
- Use an elevated toilet seat.
- Place chair inside shower or tub and remain seated while washing.
- Use pillow between legs for first 6 wk after surgery when lying on nonoperative side or when supine.
- Keep hip in neutral, straight position when sitting, walking, or lying.
- Notify surgeon if severe pain, deformity, or loss of function occurs.
- Inform dentist of presence of prosthesis before dental work so that prophylactic antibiotics can be given if indicated.

Do Not
- Force hip into greater than 90 degrees of flexion (e.g., sitting in low chairs or toilet seats).
- Force hip into adduction.
- Force hip into internal rotation.
- Cross legs at knees or ankles.
- Put on own shoes or stockings without adaptive device (e.g., long-handled shoehorn or stocking-helper) until 4-6 wk after surgery.
- Sit on chairs without arms. They are needed to aid rising to a standing position.

*For patients having surgery by a posterior approach.

FIG. 63-20 Maintaining postoperative abduction following total hip replacement.

care providers prefer that the patient keep the leg abductor pillow on except when bathing.

Taking a tub bath and driving a car are not allowed for 4 to 6 weeks. An occupational therapist may teach the patient to use assistive devices, such as reachers or grabbers to avoid bending over to pick something off the floor, long-handled shoehorns, or sock assists. The knees must be kept apart. Instruct the patient to never cross the legs or twist to reach behind.

If the hip fracture has been treated by insertion of a prosthesis with an *anterior approach* (joint reached from front of body), the hip muscles are left intact. This approach generally results in a more stable hip in the postoperative period with a lower rate of complications. Patient precautions related to motion and weight bearing are few and may include instructions to avoid hyperextension.

The physical therapist usually supervises exercises for the affected extremity and ambulation when the surgeon permits it. The patient is usually out of bed on the first postoperative day. In collaboration with the physical therapist, monitor the patient's ambulation status for proper use of crutches or a walker. For the patient to be discharged home, have the patient demonstrate the proper use of crutches or a walker, the ability to transfer into and from a chair and bed, and the ability to ascend and descend stairs.

Weight bearing on the involved extremity varies. Weight bearing of especially fragile fractures may be restricted until x-ray examination indicates adequate healing, usually 6 to 12 weeks.

Complications associated with femoral neck fracture include nonunion, avascular necrosis, dislocation, and degenerative arthritis. As a result of an intertrochanteric fracture, the affected leg may be shortened. A cane or built-up shoe may be required for safe ambulation.

Sudden severe pain, a lump in the buttock, limb shortening, and external rotation indicate prosthesis dislocation. This requires a closed reduction with conscious sedation or open reduction to realign the femoral head in the acetabulum. If this occurs (regardless of the setting), keep the patient on nothing-by-mouth (NPO) status in anticipation of a possible surgical intervention.

Assist both the patient and caregiver in adjusting to the restrictions and dependence imposed by the hip fracture. Anxiety and depression can easily occur, but creative nursing care and awareness of potential problems can help to prevent them. Inform the patient and caregiver about community referral services that can assist in the postdischarge rehabilitation phase.

AMBULATORY AND HOME CARE. Hospitalization averages 3 or 4 days. Patients frequently require care in a subacute unit, at a skilled nursing facility, or in a rehabilitation facility for a few weeks before returning home. Arrange regular follow-up care after discharge, including home health nursing.

Home care considerations include ongoing assessment of pain management, monitoring for infection, and prevention of DVT. The incision may be closed with metal staples, which are removed at the surgeon's office. If warfarin is used to decrease the high risk for thromboembolism, determine prothrombin times weekly and adjust anticoagulation accordingly. Alternatives to warfarin include enoxaparin, fondaparinux, and rivaroxaban. These newer anticoagulants require less monitoring than warfarin. Teach the patient who is receiving an anticoagulant to immediately report signs of bleeding to the health care provider (see Chapter 38).

Exercises designed to restore strength and muscle tone in the quadriceps and muscles about the hip are essential to improve function and ROM. These include quadriceps setting (e.g., tightening the kneecap), gluteal muscle setting (e.g., tightening the buttocks), leg raises in supine and prone positions, and abduction exercises from the supine and standing positions (e.g., swinging the leg out but never crossing midline). The patient continues these exercises for many months after discharge. It is important to teach the exercise program to the caregiver who will be encouraging the patient at home.

A physical therapist assesses ROM, ambulation, and compliance with the exercise regimen. The patient gradually increases the number of repetitions of exercises, adds weights to ankles,

and swims, and may eventually use a stationary bicycle to tone quadriceps and improve cardiovascular fitness. High-impact exercises and sports, such as jogging and tennis, may loosen the implant and should be avoided.

EVALUATION

The expected outcomes are that the patient with a fracture of the hip will
- Report satisfactory pain relief
- Participate in exercise therapy
- Understand prescribed treatment plan

GERONTOLOGIC CONSIDERATIONS

HIP FRACTURE

Factors that increase the risk of a hip fracture in older adults include a tendency to fall, inability to correct a postural imbalance, inadequacy of local tissue shock absorbers (e.g., fat, muscle bulk), and reduced skeletal strength. Factors that increase the older adult's risk of falling include gait and balance problems, decreased vision and hearing, slowed reflexes, orthostatic hypotension, and medication use. Leading hazards of falls are loose rugs and slippery or uneven surfaces.[24]

Many falls are associated with getting in or out of a chair or bed. Falls to the side, the most common type seen in frail older adults, are more likely to result in a hip fracture than a forward fall.[24] External hip protectors may help prevent hip fractures in the frail older patient.[25] Older women often have osteoporosis and accompanying low bone density, which increases their risk of hip and other types of fractures.

Calcium and vitamin D supplementation, estrogen replacement, and bisphosphonate drug therapy decrease bone loss or increase bone density and thus reduce the likelihood of fracture, especially in patients with osteoporosis. (Osteoporosis is discussed in Chapter 64.)

FEMORAL SHAFT FRACTURE

Femoral shaft fracture occurs with a severe direct force because the femur can bend slightly before an actual fracture occurs. Young adults have a higher incidence of this type of fracture. The force exerted to cause the fracture such as from a motor vehicle collision or gunshot wound frequently damages the adjacent soft tissue structures. These injuries may be more serious than the bone injury.

Displacement of the fracture fragments often results in open fracture and increased soft tissue damage. This can lead to considerable blood loss (1 to 1.5 L). The most common types of femoral shaft fracture include transverse, spiral, comminuted, oblique, and open (see Figs. 63-6 and 63-7).

The clinical manifestations of a fracture of the femoral shaft are usually obvious. They include marked deformity and angulation, shortening of the extremity, inability to move either the hip or the knee, and pain. The common complications associated with fracture of the femoral shaft include fat embolism; nerve and vascular injury; and problems associated with bone union, open fracture, and soft tissue damage.

Initial management of a femoral shaft fracture is directed toward stabilization of the patient and immobilization of the fracture. Traction may be used as a temporary measure before surgical treatment or in patients unable to undergo surgery. The method of treatment most often used for a femoral shaft fracture is *intermedullary nailing*.[26] A metal rod is placed into the marrow canal of the femur. The rod passes across the fracture to keep it in position. Internal fixation is preferred because it reduces the hospital stay and the complications associated with prolonged bed rest.

In the postoperative period teach the patient to carefully follow the health care provider's instructions for weight bearing. Promotion and maintenance of strength in the affected extremity usually include gluteal and quadriceps isometric exercises. Ensure that the patient performs ROM and strengthening exercises for all uninvolved extremities in preparation for ambulation. The patient may be allowed to begin non–weight-bearing activities with an ambulatory assistive device (e.g., walker, crutches). Full weight bearing is usually restricted until there is x-ray evidence of union of the fracture fragments.

FRACTURE OF TIBIA

Although the tibia is vulnerable to injury because it lacks a covering of anterior muscle, strong force is required to produce a fractured tibia. As a result, soft tissue damage, devascularization, and open fracture are frequent. The tibia is one of the more common sites of a stress fracture. Complications associated with tibial fractures are compartment syndrome, fat embolism, problems associated with bony union, and possible infection associated with open fracture.

The recommended management for closed tibial fracture is closed reduction followed by immobilization in a long leg cast. ORIF with intramedullary rods, plate fixation, or external fixation is indicated for complex tibial fractures and those with extensive soft tissue damage. Locking plates (screw and plate system) are another type of surgical device. In both types of reduction, the emphasis is on maintaining the strength of the quadriceps.

Assess the neurovascular status of the affected extremity at least every 2 hours during the first 48 hours. Instruct patients to perform active ROM exercises with the uninvolved leg and the upper extremities to build the strength required for crutch walking. When the health care provider has determined that the patient is ready for gait training, instruct the patient in the principles of crutch walking. The patient may be non–weight bearing for 6 to 12 weeks, depending on healing. Home nursing visits can be initiated to augment outpatient appointments and monitor the patient's progress.

STABLE VERTEBRAL FRACTURE

Stable fractures of the vertebral column are usually caused by motor vehicle collisions, falls, diving, or athletic injuries. More than 700,000 vertebral compression fractures occur annually (many of these are stable) in patients with osteoporosis.[27] A stable fracture is one in which the fracture or the fragment is not likely to move or cause spinal cord damage. This type of injury is frequently confined to the anterior element (vertebral body) of the spinal column in the lumbar region, and less frequently involves the cervical and thoracic regions. The vertebral bodies are usually protected from displacement by the intact spinal ligaments.

Most patients with stable spinal fractures experience only brief periods of disability. However, if the ligamentous structures are significantly disrupted, dislocation of the vertebral structures may occur, resulting in instability and injury to the spinal cord (unstable fracture). These injuries generally require

surgery. The most serious complication of vertebral fractures is fracture displacement, which can cause damage to the spinal cord (see Chapter 61). Although stable vertebral fractures are not associated with abnormal spinal cord pathologic conditions, all spinal injuries should be considered unstable and potentially serious until diagnostic tests are performed and the fracture is determined to be stable.

The patient usually complains of pain and tenderness in the affected region of the spine. Sudden loss of function below the level of fracture indicates spinal cord impingement and paraplegia. Stable compression fractures are associated with a kyphotic deformity (flexion angulation of several vertebrae). This deformity may be noted during the physical examination. In patients with a stable vertebral fracture secondary to osteoporosis, several vertebral levels may be involved as evidenced by a *dowager's hump* (abnormal curvature of thoracic spine) (see Fig. 64-9) or *lordosis* (extreme inward curve of lumbar spine). The cervical spine may also be involved. Bowel and bladder dysfunction may indicate an interruption of the autonomic nervous system nerves or injury to the spinal cord.

The overall goal in management of stable vertebral fractures is to keep the spine in good alignment until union has been accomplished. Many nursing interventions are aimed at assessing for the possibility of spinal cord trauma. Regularly evaluate vital signs and bowel and bladder function. Also monitor the motor and sensory status of the peripheral nerves distal to the injured region. Promptly report any deterioration in the patient's neurovascular status.

Treatment includes pain medication followed by early mobilization and bracing. If hospitalized, the patient is usually placed in a standard hospital bed with firm support from the mattress. The aim is to support the spinal column, relax muscles, decrease edema, and prevent potential compression on nerve roots. Teach the patient to keep the spine straight when turning by turning the shoulders and pelvis together. Nursing assistance is necessary for the patient to learn the technique of logrolling. Several days after the initial injury, the health care provider may apply a specially constructed orthotic device (e.g., Milwaukee, Jewett, or Taylor brace), a jacket cast, or a removable corset if there is no evidence of neurologic deficit.

Vertebral compression fractures (which are often due to osteoporosis) may be treated with two outpatient procedures: vertebroplasty or kyphoplasty. *Vertebroplasty* uses radioimaging to guide the injection of bone cement into a fractured vertebral body. The cement (when hardened) serves to stabilize and prevent further vertebral compression. *Kyphoplasty* initially involves inserting a balloon into the vertebral body and then inflating it. This creates a cavity that is filled with bone cement under low pressure. Kyphoplasty results in less leakage of bone cement compared with vertebroplasty and helps restore the height of the vertebral body. Vertebroplasty and kyphoplasty result in improved healing, better pain relief, and decreased complications compared to conservative treatment.[28]

If the fracture is in the cervical spine, the patient may wear a hard cervical collar. Some cervical fractures are immobilized by use of a halo vest (see Fig. 61-11). This consists of a plastic jacket or cast fitted about the chest and attached to a halo that is held in place by skeletal pins inserted into the cranium. These devices immobilize the spine in the fracture area but allow the patient to ambulate.

The patient with a stable vertebral fracture is discharged after (1) regaining ambulation skills, (2) learning care of the cast or orthotic device, and (3) learning how to cope with the safety and security issues imposed by the injury and the treatment. Unstable vertebral fractures and spinal cord injuries are discussed in Chapter 61.

FACIAL FRACTURE

Any bone of the face can be fractured as a result of trauma, such as a motor vehicle collision, assault, or falls.[29] The primary concern after facial injury is to establish and maintain a patent airway and to provide adequate ventilation. Foreign material and blood need to be removed. Suctioning may be necessary. An alternative airway (tracheostomy) may be needed if a patent airway cannot be maintained.

Concurrent facial fractures and cervical spine injuries are common. All patients with facial injuries should be treated as if they have a cervical injury until proven otherwise by examination and imaging studies (e.g., CT scan, x-ray). Table 63-12 describes the clinical manifestations of common facial fractures.

Associated soft tissue injury often makes assessment of a facial injury difficult. Perform oral and facial examinations after the patient has been stabilized and any life-threatening situations have been treated. Careful assessment is made of the ocular muscles and cranial nerve involvement (cranial nerves III, IV, and VI).[30] X-rays are used to determine the extent of the injury. CT scanning helps differentiate between bone and soft tissue.

Suspect injury to the eye when a facial injury occurs, particularly if the injury is near the orbit. If an eye-globe rupture is suspected, stop the examination and place a protective shield over the eye. Signs of globe rupture include the extrusion of vitreous humor, or brown tissue (iris or ciliary body), on the surface of the globe or penetrating through a laceration with an eccentric or teardrop-shaped pupil.

Specific treatment depends on the site and extent of the facial fracture and the associated soft tissue injury. Immobilization or surgical stabilization may be necessary. Maintain a patent airway and adequate nutrition throughout the recovery period.

You need to be sensitive about the alterations in appearance that may occur after a facial fracture. The changes in appearance may be drastic. Edema and discoloration subside with time, but concurrent soft tissue injuries may result in permanent scarring.

Mandibular Fracture

A fracture of the mandible may result from trauma to the face or the jaws. Maxillary fractures may also occur, but they are less common than mandibular fractures. The mandibular fracture may be simple, with no bone displacement, or it may involve loss of tissue and bone. The fracture may require immediate and sometimes long-term treatment to ensure survival and restore satisfactory appearance and function.

Mandibular fracture may also be therapeutically performed to correct an underlying malocclusion problem that cannot be corrected by orthodontic procedures alone. The mandible is resected during surgery and manipulated forward or backward depending on the occlusion problem.

Surgery consists of immobilization, usually by wiring the jaws *(intermaxillary fixation)*. Internal fixation may be done with screws and plates. In a simple fracture with no loss of teeth, the lower jaw is wired to the upper jaw. Wires are placed around the teeth, and then cross-wires or rubber bands are used to hold the lower jaw tight against the upper jaw (Fig. 63-21). Arch bars may be placed on the maxillary and mandibular arches of the teeth. Vertical wires are placed between the arch bars, holding the jaws together. If teeth are missing or bone is displaced, other forms of fixation such as metal arch bars in the mouth or insertion of a pin in the bone may be needed. Bone grafting may also be required. Immobilization is usually necessary for only 4 to 6 weeks because the fractures often heal rapidly.

NURSING MANAGEMENT
MANDIBULAR FRACTURE

Inform the patient preoperatively about the surgical procedure, including what it involves, how the face will look afterward, and alterations caused by the surgery. Reassure the patient about the ability to breathe normally, speak, and swallow liquids. Hospitalization for respiratory monitoring is brief unless there are other injuries or problems.

Postoperative care focuses on a patent airway, oral hygiene, communication, pain management, and adequate nutrition. Two potential problems in the immediate postoperative period are airway obstruction and aspiration of vomitus. Because the patient cannot open the jaws, it is essential that an airway is maintained. Observe for signs of respiratory distress (e.g., dyspnea; alterations in rate, quality, and depth of respirations). Place the patient on the side with the head slightly elevated immediately after surgery.

Tape a wire cutter or scissors (for rubber bands) to the head of the bed and send it with the patient on all appointments and examinations away from the bedside. The wire cutter or scissors may be used to cut the wires or elastic bands in case of an emergency (e.g., cardiac arrest or respiratory distress) requiring

TABLE 63-12	MANIFESTATIONS OF FACIAL FRACTURES
Fracture	**Manifestation**
Frontal bone	Rapid edema that may mask underlying fractures
Periorbital bone	Possible frontal sinus involvement, entrapment of ocular muscles
Nasal bone	Displacement of nasal bones, epistaxis
Zygomatic arch	Depression of zygomatic arch and entrapment of ocular muscles
Maxilla	Segmental motion of maxilla and alveolar fracture of teeth
Mandible	Tooth fractures, bleeding, limited motion of mandible

FIG. 63-21 Intermaxillary fixation.

access to the pharynx or lungs. Information including a picture on the appropriate wires to cut should be included in the care plan. In some cases, cutting the wires may cause the entire facial and upper jaw structure to shift or collapse and worsen the problem. A tracheostomy or endotracheal tray should always be available.

If the patient begins to vomit or choke, try to clear the mouth and airway. Suctioning may be necessary and may be done by the nasopharyngeal or oral route, depending on the extent of injury and the type of repair. An NG tube may be used for decompression to remove fluids and gas from the stomach to help prevent aspiration. An NG tube also helps prevent vomiting. Antiemetics may also be used. The NG tube can later be used as a feeding tube. Teach the patient to clear secretions and vomitus.

Oral hygiene is an extremely important part of nursing care. The mouth should be rinsed frequently, particularly after meals and snacks, to remove food debris. Warm normal saline solution, water, or alkaline mouthwashes may be used. A syringe and soft irrigation catheter or a Water Pik is effective for a thorough oral cleansing. Inspect the mouth several times a day to see that it is clean. Use a tongue depressor to retract the cheeks. Keep the lips, corners of the mouth, and buccal mucosa moist. Dental wax may be used to cover any sharp edges of the wires to prevent irritation of the buccal mucosa.

Communication may be a problem, particularly in the early postoperative period. Establish an effective way of communicating preoperatively (e.g., use of dry erase board, pad and pencil). Usually the patient can speak well enough to be understood, especially after the first few postoperative days.

Ingestion of sufficient nutrients poses a challenge because the diet must be liquid. The patient easily tires of sucking through a straw or laboriously using a spoon. Work with the dietitian and the patient to plan a diet that includes adequate calories, protein, and fluids. Liquid protein supplements may be helpful for improving the nutritional status. The low-bulk, high-carbohydrate diet and the intake of air through the straw create a problem with constipation and flatus. Ambulation, prune juice, and bulk-forming laxatives may help relieve these problems.

The patient is usually discharged with the wires in place. Encourage the patient to verbalize feelings about the altered appearance. Discharge teaching should include oral care, techniques for handling secretions, diet, how and when to use wire cutters or scissors, and when to notify the health care provider about concerns and problems.

AMPUTATION

An *amputation* is the removal of a body extremity by trauma or surgery. An estimated 2 million people in the United States are living with limb loss.[31] The middle and older age-groups have the highest incidence of amputation because of the effects of peripheral vascular disease (PVD), atherosclerosis, and vascular changes related to diabetes mellitus. Amputation in young people is usually secondary to trauma (e.g., motor vehicle crashes, land mines, farm-related injury). In the past decade more than 1600 American military personnel have undergone a service-related amputation.[32]

Clinical Indications

Most amputations are performed due to PVD, especially in older patients with diabetes mellitus. These patients often expe-

TABLE 63-13   **COLLABORATIVE CARE**
Amputation

Diagnostic
- History and physical examination
- Physical appearance of soft tissues
- Skin temperature
- Sensory function
- Presence of peripheral pulses
- Arteriography
- Venography
- Plethysmography
- Transcutaneous ultrasonic Doppler recordings

Collaborative Therapy
Medical
- Appropriate management of underlying disease
- Stabilization of trauma victim

Surgical
- Residual limb management
- Immediate or delayed prosthetic fitting

Rehabilitation
- Coordination of prosthesis-fitting and gait-training activities
- Coordination of muscle-strengthening and physical therapy regimens

rience peripheral neuropathy that progresses to trophic ulcers and subsequent gangrene. Other common reasons for amputation are trauma and thermal injuries, tumors, osteomyelitis, and congenital limb disorders. Although pain is often present, it is not usually the primary reason for an amputation.

Diagnostic Studies

The types of diagnostic studies performed depend on the underlying problem that makes the amputation necessary (Table 63-13). An elevated white blood cell (WBC) count with abnormal differential may indicate infection. Vascular tests such as arteriography, Doppler studies, and venography provide information about the circulatory status of the extremity.

Collaborative Care

If amputation is considered "elective," carefully assess the patient's general health. Chronic illnesses and infection are important considerations before performing an amputation. Help the patient and caregiver understand the need for the amputation and assure them that rehabilitation can result in an active, useful life. If the amputation is performed on an emergency basis as a result of trauma, management of the patient is physically and emotionally more complicated.

The goal of amputation surgery is to preserve extremity length and function while removing all infected, pathologic, or ischemic tissue. (Levels of amputation of upper and lower extremities are illustrated in Fig. 63-22.) The type of amputation depends on the reason for the surgery. A closed amputation is performed to create a weight-bearing *residual limb* (or stump). An anterior skin flap with dissected soft tissue padding covers the bony part of the residual limb. The skin flap is sutured posteriorly so that the suture line will not be positioned in a weight-bearing area. Special care is necessary to prevent accumulation of drainage, which can produce pressure and harbor bacteria that may cause infection.

FIG. 63-22 Location and description of amputation sites of the upper and lower extremities. *AKA,* Above-the-knee amputation.

Disarticulation is an amputation performed through a joint. A *Syme's amputation* is a form of disarticulation at the ankle. An open amputation leaves a surface on the residual limb that is not covered with skin. This type of surgery is generally indicated for control of actual or potential infection. The wound is usually closed later by a second surgical procedure or closed by skin traction surrounding the residual limb. This is often called a *guillotine amputation*.

NURSING MANAGEMENT AMPUTATION

NURSING ASSESSMENT

Assess any preexisting illnesses because most amputations are performed as a result of vascular problems. Assessment of vascular and neurologic status is an important part of the assessment process (see Chapters 32 and 56).

NURSING DIAGNOSES

Nursing diagnoses for the patient with an amputation may include, but are not limited to, the following:
- Disturbed body image *related to* loss of body part and impaired mobility
- Impaired skin integrity *related to* immobility and improperly fitted prosthesis
- Chronic pain *related to* phantom limb sensation or residual limb pain
- Impaired physical mobility *related to* amputation of lower limb

PLANNING

The overall goals are that the patient with an amputation will (1) have adequate relief from the underlying health problem, (2) have satisfactory pain control, (3) reach maximum rehabili-

tation potential with the use of a prosthesis (if indicated), (4) cope with the body image changes, and (5) make satisfying lifestyle adjustments.

NURSING IMPLEMENTATION

HEALTH PROMOTION. Control of causative illnesses such as PVD, diabetes mellitus, chronic osteomyelitis, and pressure ulcers can eliminate or delay the need for amputation. Teach patients with these problems to carefully examine their lower extremities daily for signs of potential problems. If the patient cannot assume this responsibility, the caregiver should help. Instruct patients and their caregivers to report changes in the feet or toes to the health care provider, including changes in skin color or temperature, decrease or absence of sensation, tingling, burning pain, or lesions.

Instruct people in proper safety precautions for recreational activities and potentially hazardous work. This responsibility is especially critical for the occupational health nurse.

ACUTE INTERVENTION. The reasons for an amputation and the rehabilitation potential depend on a person's age, diagnosis, occupation, personality, resources, and support system. It is important for you to recognize the tremendous psychologic and social implications of an amputation. The disruption in body image caused by an amputation often results in a patient going through the grieving process (see Chapter 10). Use therapeutic communication to assist the patient and caregiver through this process to arrive at a realistic attitude about the future.

Preoperative Management. Before surgery, reinforce information that the patient and caregiver have received about the reasons for the amputation, proposed prosthesis, and mobility-training program. To meet the patient's educational needs, know the level of amputation, type of postsurgical dressings to be applied, and type of prosthesis to be used. Instruct the patient in the performance of upper extremity exercises such as push-ups in bed or the wheelchair to promote arm strength. This instruction is essential for crutch walking and gait training. Discuss general postoperative nursing care, including positioning, support, and residual limb care. If a compression bandage is to be used after surgery, instruct the patient about its purpose and how it will be applied. If an immediate prosthesis is planned, discuss general ambulation expectations.

Tell the patient that the amputated limb may feel like it is still present after surgery. This phenomenon, termed **phantom limb sensation,** occurs in many amputees. (Nursing management of phantom limb sensation is discussed in the next section.)

Postoperative Management. General postoperative care for the patient who has had an amputation depends largely on the patient's general state of health, reason for the amputation, and patient's age. Monitor individuals who undergo amputation as a result of a traumatic injury for posttraumatic stress disorder because they have had no time to prepare or perhaps even to participate in the decision to have a limb amputated.

Prevention and detection of complications are important during the postoperative period. Carefully monitor the patient's vital signs and dressings for hemorrhage in the operative area. Careful attention to sterile technique during dressing changes reduces the potential for wound infection.

If an *immediate* postoperative prosthesis has been applied, careful surveillance of the surgical site is required. A surgical tourniquet must always be available for emergency use. If excessive bleeding occurs, notify the surgeon immediately.

FIG. 63-23 A double amputee fitted with prostheses. (Photo courtesy United States Army.)

FIG. 63-24 Mirror therapy, a type of treatment that may reduce phantom limb sensation and pain. (U.S. Navy photo courtesy Mass Communication Specialist Seaman Joseph A. Boomhower.)

The *delayed* prosthetic fitting may be the best choice for patients who have had amputations above the knee or below the elbow, older adults, debilitated individuals, and those with infection (Fig. 63-23). The appropriate timing for use of a prosthesis depends on satisfactory healing of the residual limb and on the patient's general condition. A temporary prosthesis may be used for partial weight bearing once the sutures are removed. Barring any problems, patients can bear full weight on permanent prostheses approximately 3 months after amputation.

Not all patients are candidates for prostheses. The seriously ill or debilitated patient may not have the upper body strength and energy required to use a lower extremity prosthesis. Mobility with a wheelchair may be the most realistic goal for these patients.

Often patients may be extremely anxious about phantom limb sensation because they still perceive pain in the missing portion of the limb. As recovery and ambulation progress, phantom limb sensation and pain usually subside, although the pain may become chronic. The patient may also complain of shooting, burning, or crushing pain and feelings of coldness, heaviness, and cramping,

Mirror therapy reduces phantom limb sensation and pain in some patients[33] (Fig. 63-24). The mirror is thought to provide visual information to the brain, replacing the sensory feedback expected from the missing limb. However, it is unknown why looking in the mirror at the remaining limb would decrease phantom limb sensation and pain. Mirror therapy may also improve patient functioning after a stroke (see Evidence-Based Practice box on p. 1396 in Chapter 58).

Success of the rehabilitation program depends on the patient's physical and emotional health. Chronic illness and deconditioning can complicate rehabilitation efforts. Both physical and occupational therapy must be an integral component of the patient's overall plan of care.

Flexion contractures may delay the rehabilitation process. The most common and debilitating contracture is hip flexion. Hip adduction contracture is rare. To prevent flexion contractures, have patients avoid sitting in a chair for more than 1 hour with hips flexed or having pillows under the surgical extremity. Unless specifically contraindicated, patients should lie on their abdomen for 30 minutes three or four times each day and position the hip in extension while prone.

Proper residual limb bandaging fosters shaping and molding for eventual prosthesis fitting (Fig. 63-25). The physician usually orders a compression bandage to be applied immediately after surgery to support the soft tissues, reduce edema, hasten healing, minimize pain, and promote residual limb shrinkage and maturation. This bandage may be an elastic roll applied to the residual limb or a residual limb shrinker, which is an elastic stocking that fits tightly over the residual limb and lower trunk area.

The compression bandage is initially worn at all times except during physical therapy and bathing. The bandage is taken off and reapplied several times daily, and care is taken to apply it snugly but not so tight as to interfere with circulation. Shrinker bandages should be washed and changed daily. After it is healed, the residual limb is bandaged only when the patient is not wearing the prosthesis. Instruct the patient to avoid dangling the residual limb over the bedside to minimize edema.

As the patient's overall condition improves, an exercise regimen is normally started under the supervision of the health care provider and the physical therapist. Active ROM exercises of all joints should be started as soon after surgery as the patient's pain level and medical status permit. In preparation for mobility, the patient should increase triceps and shoulder strength and lower limb support and learn balance of the altered body. The loss of the weight of an amputated limb requires adaptation of the patient's proprioceptive and coordination mechanisms to prevent falls and injury.

Start of second bandage

FIG. 63-25 Bandaging for the above-the-knee amputation residual limb. Figure-eight style covers progressive areas of the residual limb. Two elastic wraps are required.

Crutch walking is started as soon as the patient is physically able. After an immediate postsurgical fitting, orders related to weight bearing must be carefully followed to avoid injury to the skin flap and delay of tissue healing. Before discharge, instruct the patient and caregiver in residual limb care, ambulation, prevention of contractures, recognition of complications, exercise, and follow-up care (Table 63-14).

AMBULATORY AND HOME CARE. When healing has occurred satisfactorily and the residual limb is well molded, the patient is ready for fitting of the prosthesis. A prosthetist initially makes a mold of the residual limb and measures landmarks for fabrication of the prosthesis. The molded limb socket allows the residual limb to fit snugly into the prosthesis. The limb is covered with a residual limb stocking to ensure good fit and prevent skin breakdown. The residual limb may continue to shrink, causing a loose fit, in which case a new socket has to be fabricated. The patient may need to have the prosthesis adjusted to prevent rubbing and friction between the residual limb and socket. Excessive movement of a loose prosthesis can cause severe skin irritation, breakdown, and gait disturbances.

Artificial limbs become an integral part of the patient's changed body image. Instruct the patient to clean the prosthesis socket daily with a mild soap and rinse thoroughly to remove irritants. Leather and metal parts of the prosthesis should not get wet. Encourage the patient to have regular maintenance of the prosthesis. Consideration of the condition of the shoe is also necessary. A badly worn shoe alters the gait and may damage the prosthesis.

SPECIAL CONSIDERATIONS IN UPPER LIMB AMPUTATION. The emotional implications of an upper limb amputation are often more devastating than those for lower limb amputation. The enforced dependency brought about by one-handedness may be depressing and frustrating to the patient. Because most upper extremity amputations result from trauma, the patient has had little time to adjust psychologically to an amputation or to participate in the decision-making process.

Both immediate and delayed prosthetic fittings are possible for the below-the-elbow amputee. Prosthetic fitting is delayed for the above-the-elbow amputee. The usual functional prosthesis is the arm and hook. A cosmetic hand is available but has limited functional value. As with the lower limb prosthesis, patient motivation and perseverance are major factors contributing to a satisfactory outcome. Technologic advances to improve the functionality of upper limb prostheses are an active area of research.[34]

EVALUATION

The expected outcomes are that the patient with an amputation will

- Accept changed body image and integrate changes into lifestyle
- Have no evidence of skin breakdown
- Have reduction or absence of pain
- Become mobile within limitations imposed by amputation

GERONTOLOGIC CONSIDERATIONS

AMPUTATION

If a lower limb amputation has been performed on an older adult, the patient's previous ability to ambulate may affect the extent of recovery. Use of a prosthesis requires significant strength and energy for ambulation. For example, walking with a below-the-knee prosthesis requires 40% additional energy, and an above-the-knee prosthesis requires 60% more energy than walking on two legs. Older adults whose general health is altered and weakened by disorders such as cardiac or pulmo-

---

TABLE 63-14 PATIENT & CAREGIVER TEACHING GUIDE

Following an Amputation

After an amputation, include the following instructions when teaching the patient and caregiver.

1. Inspect the residual limb daily for signs of skin irritation, especially erythema, excoriation, and odor. Pay particular attention to areas prone to pressure.
2. Discontinue use of the prosthesis if irritation develops. Have the area checked before resuming use of the prosthesis.
3. Wash the residual limb thoroughly each night with warm water and a bacteriostatic soap. Rinse thoroughly and dry gently. Expose the residual limb to air for 20 min.
4. Do not use any substance such as lotions, alcohol, powders, or oil on residual limb unless prescribed by the health care provider.
5. Wear only a residual limb sock that is in good condition and supplied by the prosthetist.
6. Change residual limb sock daily. Launder in a mild soap, squeeze, and lay flat to dry.
7. Use prescribed pain management techniques.
8. Perform ROM to all joints daily. Perform general strengthening exercises, including the upper extremities, daily.
9. Do not elevate the residual limb on a pillow.
10. Lay prone with hip in extension for 30 min three or four times daily.

nary dysfunction may not be candidates for prosthesis use. The patient's ability to ambulate may be limited. If possible, discuss these issues with the patient and caregiver before surgery so that realistic expectations can be set.

COMMON JOINT SURGICAL PROCEDURES

Surgery plays an important role in the treatment and rehabilitation of patients with various types of joint disease. Surgery is aimed at relieving chronic pain, improving joint motion, correcting deformity and malalignment, and removing intraarticular erosion. If decreased functional ability of the joint is not corrected, contraction with permanent limitation of motion often occurs. Limitation of motion at the joint can be demonstrated on physical examination and by joint-space narrowing on x-ray examination.

TYPES OF JOINT SURGERIES

Synovectomy

Synovectomy (removal of synovial membrane) is used as a prophylactic measure and as a palliative treatment of rheumatoid arthritis (RA). Removal of the synovial membrane, thought to be the location of the basic pathologic changes in joint destruction, helps prevent further progression of joint damage. A synovectomy is best performed early in the disease process to prevent serious destruction of joint surfaces. Removal of the thickened synovium prevents extension of the inflammatory process into adjacent cartilage, ligaments, and tendons.

It is impossible to surgically remove all the synovium in a joint. The underlying disease process is still present and will again affect the regenerating synovium. However, the disease appears to be milder after synovectomy, and definite improvements in pain, weight bearing, and ROM can be expected. Common sites for this surgery include the elbow, wrist, and fingers. Synovectomy in the knee is done less frequently because knee joint replacement is usually performed.

Osteotomy

An osteotomy involves removing a wedge or slice of bone to change alignment (joint and vertebral) and to shift weight bearing, thereby correcting deformity and relieving pain. Cervical osteotomy may be used to correct deformity in some patients with ankylosing spondylitis. Halo vests and body jacket braces are worn until fusion occurs (3 to 4 months). Subtrochanteric or femoral osteotomy may provide some relief of pain and improve motion in selected patients with hip osteoarthritis (OA). Osteotomy has proven ineffective in patients with inflammatory joint disease. Osteotomy of the knee (tibia) provides relief of pain in selected patients, but advanced joint destruction is usually corrected by joint replacement surgery.

The postoperative care of the patient with an osteotomy is similar to the treatment of an internal fixation of a fracture at a comparable site (see p. 1519). Internal wires, screws and plates, bone grafts, or an external fixator usually fixes the bone in place.

Debridement

Debridement is the removal of degenerative debris such as loose bodies, osteophytes, joint debris, and degenerated menisci from a joint. This procedure is usually performed on the knee or shoulder using a fiberoptic arthroscope. The procedure is usually done on an outpatient basis. A compression dressing is applied postoperatively. Weight bearing is permitted following knee arthroscopy. Patient teaching includes monitoring for signs of infection, managing pain, and restricting excessive activity for 24 to 48 hours.

Arthroplasty

Arthroplasty is the reconstruction or replacement of a joint to relieve pain, improve or maintain ROM, and correct deformity. The most common uses of arthroplasty are for patients with OA, RA, avascular necrosis, congenital deformities or dislocations, and other systemic problems. There are several types of arthroplasty, including surgical reshaping of the bones of the joints, replacement of part of a joint (hemiarthroplasty), and total joint replacement. Replacement arthroplasty is available for elbows, shoulders, phalangeal joints of the fingers, wrists, hips, knees, ankles, and feet. More than 1 million Americans have knee and hip replacement surgery annually.[35]

Hip Arthroplasty. Total hip arthroplasty (THA) (total hip replacement) provides significant relief of pain and improved function for patients with joint deterioration from OA, RA, and other conditions. Partial and total hip replacements are also used to treat hip fractures.

In THA the prosthesis (implant) replaces the ball and socket joint and upper shaft of the femur (see Fig. 63-19). The socket can be "cemented" in place with polymethyl methacrylate, which bonds to the bone. The socket may also be inserted and not cemented ("cementless"). Cementless THAs may provide longer-term prosthesis stability by facilitating biologic ingrowth of new bone tissue into the porous surface coating of the prosthesis. Although some surgeons use cementless devices for all patients, they are most often recommended for younger, more active patients and patients with good bone quality where bone ingrowth into the components can be readily achieved.

The nursing care for a patient who has a THA is discussed in the section on nursing management of a patient with a hip fracture on pp. 1526–1527.

Hip Resurfacing. An alternative to hip replacement is hip resurfacing, which allows the femoral head to be preserved and reshaped rather than replaced. (In contrast, in a THA the prosthesis replaces the femoral head.) The resurfaced femoral head (ball) is then capped by a metal prosthesis. The metal appears to have a lower rate of wear, and thus the prosthesis may have a longer lifetime. Hip resurfacing is a more favorable option for younger, active patients. After surgery there is generally a 6-month waiting period before strenuous activity until strong muscles are built around the joint. Patients receiving a smaller femoral head (including many women) have a higher failure rate with a resurfaced implant when compared with patients receiving a THA.[36]

Knee Arthroplasty. Unremitting pain and instability as a result of severe destructive deterioration of the knee joint are the main indications for total knee arthroplasty (TKA).[37] Osteoporosis may necessitate bone grafting to augment defects and to correct bone deficiencies. Either part of or the entire knee joint may be replaced with a metal and plastic prosthetic device. A compression dressing may be used to immobilize the knee in extension immediately after the operation. This dressing is removed before discharge and may be replaced with a knee immobilizer or posterior plastic shell, which maintains extension during ambulation and at rest for about 4 weeks. Dislocation is not typical with TKA.

After surgery an emphasis is placed on physical therapy. Isometric quadriceps setting usually begins the first postoperative day. The patient progresses to straight-leg raises and gentle ROM to increase muscle strength and obtain 90-degree knee flexion. Active flexion exercises or passive flexion exercises with a continuous passive motion (CPM) machine may promote joint mobility. Full weight bearing is begun before discharge. An active home exercise program involves progressive ROM with muscle strengthening and flexibility exercises. After TKA, many older patients with advanced OA have shown significant improvement in mobility, motor function tests, and ability to complete daily tasks.

Finger Joint Arthroplasty. A silicone rubber arthroplastic device is used to help restore function in the fingers of the patient with RA. Ulnar deviation is often present, which results in severe functional limitations of the hand. The goal of hand surgery is primarily to restore function related to grasp, pinch, stability, and strength rather than to correct cosmetic deformity. Before surgery the patient is instructed in hand exercises, including flexion, extension, abduction, and adduction of the fingers.

Postoperatively the hand is kept elevated with a bulky dressing in place. After surgery, conduct a neurovascular assessment and look for signs of infection. The success of the surgery depends largely on the postoperative treatment plan, which is usually implemented by an occupational therapist. After the dressing is removed, a guided splinting program is initiated. The patient is discharged with splints to use while sleeping and hand exercises to perform at least three or four times a day for 10 to 12 weeks. Also instruct the patient to avoid lifting heavy objects.

Elbow and Shoulder Arthroplasty. Although available, total replacement of elbow and shoulder joints is not as common as other forms of arthroplasty. Shoulder replacements are performed in patients with severe pain because of RA, OA, avascular necrosis, or previous trauma. The shoulder replacement is usually considered if the patient has adequate surrounding muscle strength and bone stock. If joint replacement is necessary for both elbow and shoulder, the elbow is usually done first because a severely painful elbow interferes with the shoulder rehabilitation program.

Significant pain relief has been achieved after elbow and shoulder arthroplasty, with most patients having no pain at rest or minimal pain with activity. Functional improvements have also resulted in better hygiene and increased ability to perform activities of daily living. However, rehabilitation is longer and more difficult than with other joint surgeries.

Ankle Arthroplasty. Total ankle arthroplasty (TAA) is indicated for RA, OA, trauma, and avascular necrosis. Although the use of TAA is not widespread, it is becoming a viable alternative to fusion for the treatment of severe ankle arthritis in selected patients. Devices available include several fixed-bearing devices and a mobile-bearing cementless prosthesis. This device more closely imitates natural ankle function.

Ankle fusion is often selected over arthroplasty because the result is more durable. However, the patient is left with a stiff foot and the inability to change heel height. TAA is advantageous because it achieves a more normal gait pattern. Postoperatively, the patient may not bear weight for 6 weeks and must elevate the extremity to reduce and prevent edema, be extremely careful to prevent postoperative infection, and maintain immobilization as directed by the physician.

Arthrodesis

Arthrodesis is the surgical fusion of a joint. This procedure is indicated only if articular surfaces are too severely damaged or infected to allow joint replacement or if reconstructive surgery fails. Arthrodesis relieves pain and provides a stable but immobile joint. The fusion is usually accomplished by removal of the articular hyaline cartilage and the addition of bone grafts across the joint surface. The affected joint must be immobilized until bone healing has occurred. Common areas of fusion are wrist, ankle, cervical spine, lumbar spine, and metatarsophalangeal (MTP) joint of the great toe.

Complications of Joint Surgery

Infection is a serious complication of joint surgery, particularly joint replacement surgery.[37] The most common causative organisms are gram-positive aerobic streptococci and staphylococci. Infection may lead to pain and loosening of the prosthesis, generally requiring extensive surgery. Efforts to reduce the incidence of infection include the use of specially designed self-contained operating suites, operating rooms with laminar airflow, and prophylactic antibiotic administration.

Thromboembolism is another potentially serious complication after joint surgeries, particularly those involving the lower extremities. Prophylactic measures such as warfarin, LMWH, and sequential compression devices of the legs are usually instituted. Patients may be followed postoperatively with venous Doppler ultrasound to detect DVT, the source of most pulmonary emboli.

Collaborative Care

Preoperative Management. The primary goal of preoperative assessment is to identify risk factors associated with postoperative complications so that nursing strategies can be implemented to promote optimal positive outcomes. A careful history includes previous medical diagnoses and complications such as diabetes and thromboembolism, pain tolerance and management preferences, current functional status and expectations following surgery, and level of social support and home care needs after discharge. The patient should be free from infection and acute joint inflammation.

If lower extremity surgery is planned, assess upper extremity muscle strength and joint function to determine the type of assistive devices needed postoperatively for ambulation and activities of daily living. Preoperative teaching is important for the patient and caregiver related to the expected hospital course and postoperative management at home. In addition, it prepares them to maximize the usefulness and longevity of the prosthesis. Patients also need to realize that recovery is "not going to happen overnight." Talking with other people who have had a total joint arthroplasty may help the patient better understand the reality of rehabilitation.

Postoperative Management. Postoperatively, perform neurovascular assessment to assess nerve function and circulatory status. Anticoagulation therapy, analgesia, and parenteral antibiotics are administered. In general, the affected joint is exercised and ambulation is encouraged as early as possible to prevent complications of immobility. Specific protocols vary according to the patient, type of prosthesis, and surgeon preference. Pain management techniques may include epidural or intrathecal analgesia, femoral nerve block, patient-controlled IV analgesia, and oral opioids or NSAIDs. Assess patient comfort frequently during the postoperative period.

The hospital stay after arthroplasty is 3 to 5 days depending on the patient's course and need for physical therapy. Physical therapy and ambulation enhance mobility, build muscle strength, and reduce the risk of thromboembolism. If the patient is taking warfarin, therapy starts on the day of surgery, and prothrombin time is measured on a regular basis. For those taking LMWH (e.g., enoxaparin), therapy starts soon after surgery and continues for 2 weeks postoperatively. Daily monitoring of the patient's coagulation status is not necessary when the patient is taking LMWH.

NURSING MANAGEMENT
JOINT SURGERY

The nursing management of the patient undergoing joint surgery begins with preoperative teaching and realistic goal setting. It is important that the patient understands and accepts the limitations of the proposed surgery and realizes that in some cases surgery will not remove or treat the underlying disease. Explain postoperative procedures such as turning, deep breathing, use of bedpan and bedside commode, and use of abductor pillows. Provide opportunities for practice. Reassure the patient that pain relief will be available. Patient-controlled analgesia can be helpful. A preoperative visit from a physical therapist allows practice of postoperative exercises and measurement for crutches or other assistive devices.

Discharge planning begins immediately. Discuss the duration of the hospital stay and the expected postoperative events because the patient and caregiver must prepare. The home environment must be assessed for safety (e.g., scatter rugs, electric cords) and accessibility. Are the bathroom and bedroom on the first floor? Are door frames wide enough to accommodate a walker? Assess the patient's social support. Is a friend or family member available to assist the patient in the home? Will the patient require homemaker or meal services? The older patient may need the rehabilitation services of a subacute or extended care facility for a few weeks postoperatively to progressively develop independent living skills. Nursing interventions for the patient having orthopedic surgery are presented in eNursing Care Plan 63-2 (on the website for this chapter).

Instruct the patient on reporting complications, including infection (e.g., fever, increased pain, drainage) and dislocation of the prosthesis (e.g., pain, loss of function, shortening or malalignment of an extremity). Your role in the home care setting is to act as the liaison between the patient and surgeon, while monitoring for postoperative complications. Also assess the patient's comfort level and ROM at regular intervals to facilitate the goal of improved functional performance.

CASE STUDY

Hip Fracture Surgery

iStockphoto/Thinkstock

Patient Profile
T.K. is a 78-yr-old white man admitted to the hospital through the emergency department. It appears that he may have sustained a fracture to his left hip (see Chapter 62 case study on p. 1494). He is scheduled for a surgical hip repair in the morning.

Subjective Data
See the case study in Chapter 62 on p. 1497.

Collaborative Care
Preoperative
- Pain not relieved by morphine.
- Accompanying T.K. is his wife of 40 yr who is crying and anxious. Her anxiety is also causing T.K. to become anxious.

Operative Procedure
- Left hip repair using hip compression plate and bone screws

Postoperative
- Cefazolin (Ancef) 1 g IV q8hr
- Intake and output for 48 hr
- Morphine via patient-controlled analgesia pump

Discussion Questions
1. How do T.K.'s preexisting medical conditions predispose him to postoperative complications?

2. What actions can you take to help decrease the wife's anxiety?
3. **Priority Decision:** As you plan care for T.K., what are the preoperative and postoperative priority nursing interventions?
4. What are the most likely postoperative complications that T.K. could develop?
5. **Priority Decision:** On assessment of T.K. on the second postoperative day, you note an irregular pulse, which is a new finding. The pulse rate is 66 and the ECG tracing is shown below. You identify this as which dysrhythmia? What is the priority action at this time?

6. **Priority Decision:** What are the priority teaching interventions that should be done before discharge?
7. **Evidence-Based Practice:** Why is satisfactory pain relief an important nursing goal in the postoperative period for T.K?

ⓔvolve   Answers available at *http://evolve.elsevier.com/Lewis/medsurg*.

BRIDGE TO NCLEX EXAMINATION

The number of the question corresponds to the same-numbered outcome at the beginning of the chapter.

1. The nurse suspects an ankle sprain when a patient at the urgent care center relates
   a. being hit by another soccer player during a game.
   b. having ankle pain after sprinting around the track.
   c. dropping a 10-lb weight on his lower leg at the health club.
   d. twisting his ankle while running bases during a baseball game.

2. The nurse explains to a patient with a fracture of the distal shaft of the humerus who is returning for a 4-week checkup that healing is indicated by
   a. formation of callus.
   b. complete bony union.
   c. hematoma at fracture site.
   d. presence of granulation tissue.

3. A patient with a comminuted fracture of the tibia is to have an open reduction with internal fixation (ORIF) of the fracture. The nurse explains that ORIF is indicated when
   a. the patient is unable to tolerate prolonged immobilization.
   b. the patient cannot tolerate the surgery of a closed reduction.
   c. a temporary cast would be too unstable to provide normal mobility.
   d. adequate alignment cannot be obtained by other nonsurgical methods.

4. An indication of a neurovascular problem noted during assessment of the patient with a fracture is
   a. exaggeration of strength with movement.
   b. increased redness and heat below the injury.
   c. decreased sensation distal to the fracture site.
   d. purulent drainage at the site of an open fracture.

5. A patient with a stable, closed fracture of the humerus caused by trauma to the arm has a temporary splint with bulky padding applied with an elastic bandage. The nurse suspects compartment syndrome and notifies the physician when the patient experiences
   a. increasing edema of the limb.
   b. muscle spasms of the lower arm.
   c. rebounding pulse at the fracture site.
   d. pain when passively extending the fingers.

6. A patient with a fracture of the pelvis should be monitored for
   a. changes in urine output.
   b. petechiae on the abdomen.
   c. a palpable lump in the buttock.
   d. sudden increase in blood pressure.

7. During the postoperative period, the nurse instructs the patient with an above-the-knee amputation that the residual limb should not be routinely elevated because this position promotes
   a. hip flexion contractures.
   b. skin irritation and breakdown.
   c. clot formation at the incision site.
   d. increased risk of wound dehiscence.

8. A patient with osteoarthritis is scheduled for a total hip arthroplasty. The nurse explains that the purpose of this procedure is to (select all that apply)
   a. fuse the joint.
   b. replace the joint.
   c. prevent further damage.
   d. improve or maintain ROM.
   e. decrease the amount of destruction in the joint.

9. In teaching a patient scheduled for a total ankle replacement, it is important to tell the patient that after surgery he should avoid
   a. lifting heavy objects.
   b. sleeping on the back.
   c. abduction exercises of the affected ankle.
   d. bearing weight on the affected leg for 6 weeks.

1. d, 2. a, 3. d, 4. c, 5. d, 6. a, 7. a, 8. b, d, 9. d

ⓔvolve

For rationales to these answers and even more NCLEX review questions, visit *http://evolve.elsevier.com/Lewis/medsurg.*

REFERENCES

1. Centers for Disease Control and Prevention: Ten leading causes of death and injury, causes of death by age group. Retrieved from *www.cdc.gov/nchs/fastats/lcod.htm.*

2. National Institute of Arthritis and Musculoskeletal and Skin Diseases: Childhood sports injuries and their prevention: a guide for parents with ideas for kids. Retrieved from *www.niams.nih.gov/health_info/Sports_Injuries/child_sports_injuries.asp.*

3. American Academy of Orthopaedic Surgeons: Sprains, strains, and other soft-tissue injuries. Retrieved from *www.orthoinfo.aaos.org/topic.*

4. National Institute on Aging and the National Aeronautics and Space Administration: Exercise: guide from the National Institute on Aging. Retrieved from *www.weboflife.ksc.nasa.gov/exerciseandaging.*

5. Buttaravoli P, Leffler S: Patellar dislocation. In Buttaravoli P, editor: *Minor emergencies,* ed 3, St Louis, 2012, Saunders.

6. Cleveland Clinic: Get a grip on carpal tunnel syndrome, *Arthritis Advisor* 11:4, 2012.

*7. Agency for Healthcare Research and Quality: Treatment options for rotator cuff tears: a guide for adults and comparative effectiveness of interventions for rotator cuff tears in adults: a guide for clinicians. Retrieved from *http://effectivehealthcare.ahrq.gov/index.cfm/search-for-guides-reviews-and-reports/?productid=544&pageaction=displayproduct.*

*8. Stensrud S, Roos E, Risberg M: A 12-week exercise therapy program in middle-aged patients with degenerative meniscus tears: a case series with 1-year follow-up, *J Orthop Sports Phys Ther* 42:919, 2012.

*9. Meuffels D, Poldervaart M, Diercks R, et al: Guideline on anterior cruciate ligament injury, *Acta Orthop* 83:379, 2012.

*10. Sadoghi P, von Keudell P: Effectiveness of anterior cruciate ligament injury prevention training programs, *J Bone Joint Surg* 94:769, 2012.

11. Aaron D, Patel A, Kayiaros S, et al: Four common types of bursitis: diagnosis and management, *J Am Acad Orthop Surg* 19:359, 2011.

*Evidence-based information for clinical practice.

12. Fazzalari N: Bone fracture and bone fracture repair, *Osteoporosis Int* 22:2003, 2011.

13. Marshall S, Browner B: Emergency care of musculoskeletal injuries. In Townsend C, Beauchamp R, Evers B, et al, editors: *Townsend: Sabiston textbook of surgery*, ed 19, St Louis, 2012, Saunders.

14. Satryb S, Wilson T, Patterson MM: Casting: all wrapped up, *Orthop Nurs* 30:37, 2011.

15. *Saunders nursing drug handbook*, St Louis, 2014, Saunders.

16. Patrice M, Hatch R: General principles of fracture care. In Patrice M, Hatch R, editors: *Eiff: fracture management for primary care*, ed 3, St Louis, 2011, Mosby.

17. Azar F: Traumatic disorders. In Canale S, Beaty J, editors: *Canale and Beaty: Campbell's operative orthopaedics*, ed 12, St Louis, 2012, Mosby.

18. Welle M: Understanding the new emerging oral anticoagulants for venous thromboembolism prophylaxis, *Orthop Nurs* 31:265, 2012.

19. Tzioupis C, Giannoudis P: Fat embolism syndrome: what have we learned over the years? *Trauma* 13:259, 2011.

*20. Ojike N: Pelvic compartment syndrome: a systematic review, *ACTA Orthop Belg* 78:6, 2012.

21. Centers for Disease Control and Prevention: Hip fractures among older adults. Retrieved from *www.cdc.gov/HomeandRecreationalSafety/Falls/adulthipfx.html*.

22. Cummings-Vaughn L: Falls, osteoporosis, and hip fractures, *Med Clin North Am* 95:495, 2011.

*23. Hung W, Egol K, Zuckerman J, et al: Hip fracture management: tailoring care for the older patient, *JAMA* 307:2185, 2012.

24. World Health Organization: WHO global report on falls prevention in older age. Retrieved from *www.who.int/ageing/publications/Falls_prevention7March.pdf*.

*25. Juby A: The challenges of interpreting efficacy of hip protector pads in fracture prevention in high-risk seniors, *Clin Rheumatol* 28:723, 2009. (Classic)

*26. Faucett S, Collinge C, Koval KJ: Is reconstruction nailing of all femoral shaft fractures cost effective? A decision analysis, *J Orthop Trauma* 26:624, 2012.

27. American Academy of Orthopaedic Surgeons: Osteoporosis and spinal fractures. Retrieved from *http://orthoinfo.aaos.org/topic.cfm?topic=A00538*.

28. Asenjo J, Rossel F: Vertebroplasty and kyphoplasty: new evidence adds heat to the debate, *Curr Opin Anesthesiol* 25:577, 2012.

*29. Smith H, Peek-Asa C, Nesheim D, et al: Etiology, diagnosis, and characteristics of facial fracture at a Midwestern level I trauma center, *J Trauma Nurs* 19:57, 2012.

30. Patrice M, Hatch R: Facial and skull fractures. In Patrice M, Hatch R, editors: *Eiff: fracture management for primary care*, ed 3, St Louis, 2011, Mosby.

31. National Limb Loss Information Center: Fact sheet. Retrieved from *www.amputee-coalition.org/fact_sheets/amp_stats_cause*.

32. Fischer H: U.S. Military casualty statistics: Operation New Dawn, Operation Iraqi Freedom, and Operation Enduring Freedom, *Congressional Research Service 5-5700*, September 28, 2010.

*33. Rothgangel A, Brau S, Beurskens A, et al: The clinical aspects of mirror therapy in rehabilitation: a systematic review of the literature, *Int J Rehab Res*, 34:1, 2011.

34. Velez D, Dellefield M: Provide a helping hand to patients with upper extremity prostheses, *Nursing* 41:49, 2011.

35. National Institute of Arthritis and Musculoskeletal and Skin Diseases: Joint replacement surgery: information for multicultural communities. Retrieved from *www.niams.nih.gov/health_info/joint_replacement/default.asp*.

*36. Smith A, Dieppe P, Howard P, et al: Failure rates of metal-on-metal hip resurfacings: analysis of data from the National Joint Registry for England and Wales, *Lancet* 380:1759, 2012.

37. Bartlett D: What you need to know about total knee arthroplasty, *OR Nurse* 6:16, 2012.

RESOURCES

American Academy of Orthopedic Surgeons (AAOS)
www.aaos.org
American Association for Hand Surgery
www.handsurgery.org
American College of Sports Medicine (ACSM)
www.acsm.org
Amputee Coalition
www.amputee-coalition.org
Easter Seals Disability Services
www.easterseals.com
National Amputation Foundation
www.nationalamputation.org
National Association of Orthopaedic Nurses (NAON)
www.orthonurse.org
National Institute of Arthritis and Musculoskeletal and Skin Diseases
www.niams.nih.gov

evolve

For additional Internet resources, see the website for this book at *http://evolve.elsevier.com/Lewis/medsurg*.

Courage is like a muscle.
We strengthen it with use.
Ruth Gordon

Nursing Management
Musculoskeletal Problems

Jerry Harvey

ⓔvolve WEBSITE

http://evolve.elsevier.com/Lewis/medsurg
- NCLEX Review Questions
- Key Points
- Pre-Test
- Answer Guidelines for Case Study on p. 1558
- Rationales for Bridge to NCLEX Examination Questions

- Case Study
  - Patient With Osteoporosis
- Nursing Care Plans (Customizable)
  - eNCP 64-1: Patient With Osteomyelitis
  - eNCP 64-2: Patient With Low Back Pain

- Concept Map Creator
- Glossary
- Content Updates

LEARNING OUTCOMES

1. Describe the pathophysiology, clinical manifestations, collaborative care, and nursing management of osteomyelitis.
2. Differentiate among the types, pathophysiology, clinical manifestations, and collaborative care of bone cancer.
3. Differentiate between the causes and characteristics of acute and chronic low back pain.
4. Explain the conservative and surgical therapy of intervertebral disc damage.
5. Describe the postoperative nursing management of a patient who has undergone vertebral disc surgery.
6. Specify the etiology and nursing management of common foot disorders.
7. Describe the etiology, pathophysiology, clinical manifestations, and collaborative and nursing management of osteomalacia, osteoporosis, and Paget's disease.

KEY TERMS

degenerative disc disease (DDD), p. 1547
herniated disc, p. 1548
low back pain, p. 1544
muscular dystrophy (MD), p. 1544

osteochondroma, p. 1542
osteomalacia, p. 1553
osteomyelitis, p. 1539
osteopenia, p. 1555

osteoporosis, p. 1553
osteosarcoma, p. 1542
Paget's disease, p. 1557
sarcoma, p. 1542

Acute and chronic musculoskeletal problems are a common source of pain and disability. A variety of problems unrelated to trauma that affect the musculoskeletal system are presented in this chapter, including osteomyelitis, bone cancer, muscular dystrophy, foot disorders, and metabolic bone diseases. Management of the patient with both acute and chronic low back pain is addressed, and spinal surgery is discussed as an intervention for a herniated disc. Throughout the discussion of all of these problems, the nurse's role in prevention of injury and maintenance of mobility is emphasized.

OSTEOMYELITIS

Etiology and Pathophysiology

Osteomyelitis is a severe infection of the bone, bone marrow, and surrounding soft tissue. Although *Staphylococcus aureus* is a common cause of infection, a variety of microorganisms may cause osteomyelitis[1] (Table 64-1).

The infecting microorganisms can invade by indirect or direct entry. The *indirect entry* (hematogenous) of microorganisms most frequently affects growing bone in boys younger than 12 years old, and is associated with their higher incidence of blunt trauma. Adults with vascular insufficiency disorders (e.g., diabetes mellitus) and genitourinary and respiratory tract infections are at higher risk for a primary infection to spread via the blood to the bone. The pelvis, tibia, and vertebrae, which are vascular-rich sites of bone, are the most common sites of infection.

Direct entry osteomyelitis can occur at any age when there is an open wound (e.g., penetrating wounds, fractures) and microorganisms gain entry to the body. Osteomyelitis may also occur in the presence of a foreign body such as an implant

Reviewed by Tammy C. Roman, RN, EdD, CNE, Assistant Professor of Nursing, St. John Fisher College, Wegmans School of Nursing, Rochester, New York; and Dianne Travers Gustafson, RN, PhD, Associate Professor, Creighton University School of Nursing, Omaha, Nebraska.

TABLE 64-1	**ORGANISMS CAUSING OSTEOMYELITIS**
Organism	**Predisposing Problem**
Staphylococcus aureus	Pressure ulcer, penetrating wound, open fracture, orthopedic surgery, vascular insufficiency disorders (e.g., diabetes, atherosclerosis)
Staphylococcus epidermidis	Indwelling prosthetic devices (e.g., joint replacements, fracture fixation devices)
Streptococcus viridans	Abscessed tooth, gingival disease
Escherichia coli	Urinary tract infection
Mycobacterium tuberculosis	Tuberculosis
Neisseria gonorrhoeae	Gonorrhea
Pseudomonas	Puncture wounds, IV drug use
Salmonella	Sickle cell disease
Fungi, mycobacteria	Immunocompromised host

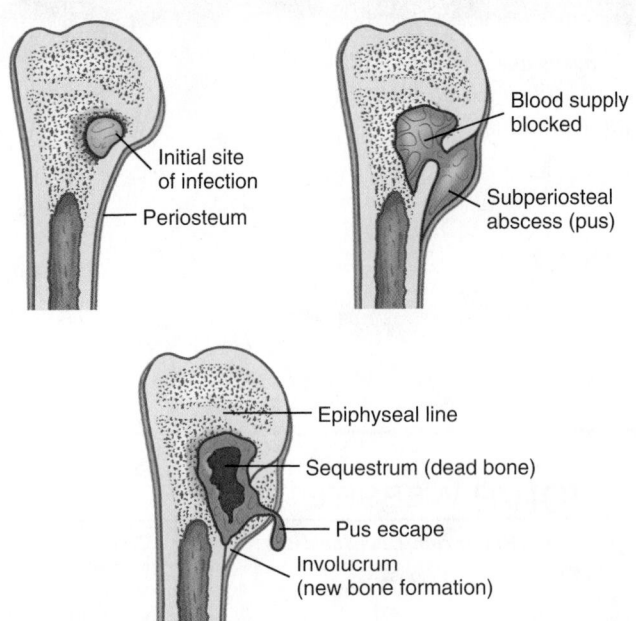

FIG. 64-1 Development of osteomyelitis infection with involucrum and sequestrum.

or an orthopedic prosthetic device (e.g., plate, total joint prosthesis).

After gaining entry into the blood, the microorganisms grow, resulting in an increase in pressure because of the nonexpanding nature of most bone. This increasing pressure eventually leads to ischemia and vascular compromise of the periosteum. The infection spreads through the bone cortex and marrow cavity, ultimately resulting in cortical devascularization and necrosis.

Once ischemia occurs, the bone dies. The area of devitalized bone eventually separates from the surrounding living bone, forming *sequestra*. The part of the periosteum that continues to have a blood supply forms new bone called *involucrum* (Fig. 64-1). It is difficult for blood-borne antibiotics or white blood cells (WBCs) to reach the sequestrum. A sequestrum may become a reservoir for microorganisms that spread to other sites, including the lungs and brain. If the sequestrum does not resolve on its own or is debrided surgically, a sinus tract may develop, resulting in chronic, purulent cutaneous drainage.

Clinical Manifestations and Complications

Acute osteomyelitis refers to the initial infection or an infection of less than 1 month in duration. The clinical manifestations of acute osteomyelitis are both local and systemic. Local manifestations include constant bone pain unrelieved by rest that worsens with activity; swelling, tenderness, and warmth at the infection site; and restricted movement of the affected part. Systemic manifestations include fever, night sweats, chills, restlessness, nausea, and malaise. Later signs include drainage from cutaneous sinus tracts or the fracture site.

Chronic osteomyelitis refers to a bone infection that persists for longer than 1 month or an infection that has failed to respond to the initial course of antibiotic therapy. Chronic osteomyelitis is either a continuous, persistent problem (a result of inadequate acute treatment) or a process of exacerbations and remissions (Fig. 64-2). Systemic signs may be diminished, with local signs of infection more common, including constant bone pain and swelling and warmth at the infection site. Over time, granulation tissue turns to scar tissue. This avascular scar tissue provides an ideal site for continued microorganism growth that cannot be penetrated by antibiotics.

Long-term and mostly rare complications of osteomyelitis include septicemia, septic arthritis, pathologic fractures, and amyloidosis.

Diagnostic Studies

A bone or soft tissue biopsy is the definitive way to determine the causative microorganism. The patient's blood and wound cultures are frequently positive for microorganisms.[2] An elevated WBC count and erythrocyte sedimentation rate (ESR) may also be found. X-ray signs suggestive of osteomyelitis usually do not appear until 10 days to weeks after the initial clinical symptoms, by which time the disease will have progressed. Radionuclide bone scans (gallium and indium) are helpful in diagnosis and are usually positive in the area of infection. Magnetic resonance imaging (MRI) and computed tomography (CT) scans may be used to help identify the extent of the infection.[3]

FIG. 64-2 Resection of femur due to osteomyelitis.

Collaborative Care

Vigorous and prolonged IV antibiotic therapy is the treatment of choice for acute osteomyelitis, as long as bone ischemia has not yet occurred. Cultures or a bone biopsy should be done if possible before initiating drug therapy. If antibiotic therapy is delayed, surgical debridement and decompression are often necessary.

Patients are often discharged to home care or a skilled nursing facility with IV antibiotics delivered via a central venous catheter or peripherally inserted central catheter. IV antibiotic therapy may be started in the hospital and continued at home for 4 to 6 weeks or as long as 3 to 6 months. A variety of antibiotics may be prescribed depending on the microorganism. These drugs include penicillin, nafcillin (Nafcil), neomycin, vancomycin, cephalexin (Keflex), cefazolin (Ancef), cefoxitin (Mefoxin), gentamicin (Garamycin), and tobramycin (Nebcin).

DRUG ALERT: Gentamicin (Garamycin)
- Assess patient for dehydration before starting therapy.
- Ensure renal function testing is done before starting therapy, especially in older patients.
- Monitor peak and trough levels for therapeutic effect and to minimize renal and inner ear toxicity.[4]
- Instruct patient to notify health care provider if any visual, hearing, or urinary problems develop.

In adults with chronic osteomyelitis, oral therapy with a fluoroquinolone (ciprofloxacin [Cipro]) for 6 to 8 weeks may be prescribed instead of IV antibiotics. Oral antibiotic therapy may also be given after acute IV therapy is completed to ensure resolution of the infection. The patient's response to drug therapy is monitored through bone scans and ESR tests.

Treatment of chronic osteomyelitis includes surgical removal of the poorly vascularized tissue and dead bone and the extended use of antibiotics.[5] Antibiotic-impregnated polymethyl methacrylate bead chains may also be implanted at this time to help combat the infection. After debridement of the devitalized and infected tissue, the wound may be closed and a suction irrigation system inserted. Intermittent or constant irrigation of the affected bone with antibiotics may also be initiated. Protection of the limb or the surgical site with casts or braces is often done. Negative-pressure wound therapy (vacuum-assisted wound closure) may be used (see pp. 181-182 in Chapter 12).

Hyperbaric oxygen with 100% oxygen may be given as an adjunct therapy in refractory cases of chronic osteomyelitis. This therapy is thought to stimulate circulation and healing in the infected tissue (see pp. 182-183 in Chapter 12). Orthopedic prosthetic devices, if a source of chronic infection, must be removed. Muscle flaps or skin grafting provides wound coverage over the dead space (cavity) in the bone. Bone grafts may help to restore blood flow. Amputation of the extremity may be indicated when bone destruction is extensive and to save the patient's life or to improve quality of life.

NURSING MANAGEMENT OSTEOMYELITIS

NURSING ASSESSMENT
Subjective and objective data that should be obtained from an individual with osteomyelitis are presented in Table 64-2.

NURSING DIAGNOSES
Nursing diagnoses for the patient with osteomyelitis may include, but are not limited to, the following.
- Acute pain *related to* inflammatory process secondary to infection

TABLE 64-2 NURSING ASSESSMENT
Osteomyelitis

Subjective Data
Important Health Information
Past health history: Bone trauma, open fracture, open or puncture wounds, other infections (e.g., streptococcal sore throat, bacterial pneumonia, sinusitis, skin or tooth infection, chronic urinary tract infection)
Medications: Analgesics or antibiotics
Surgery or other treatments: Bone surgery

Functional Health Patterns
Health perception–health management: IV drug and alcohol abuse; malaise
Nutritional-metabolic: Anorexia, weight loss; chills
Activity-exercise: Weakness, paralysis, muscle spasms around affected bone
Cognitive-perceptual: Local tenderness over affected area, increase in pain with movement of affected bone
Coping–stress tolerance: Irritability, withdrawal, dependency, anger

Objective Data
General
Restlessness; high, spiking temperature; night sweats

Integumentary
Diaphoresis; erythema, warmth, edema at infected bone

Musculoskeletal
Restricted movement; wound drainage; spontaneous fractures

Possible Diagnostic Findings
Leukocytosis, positive blood and/or wound cultures, ↑ erythrocyte sedimentation rate; presence of sequestrum and involucrum on x-rays, radionuclide bone scans, CT, and MRI

- Ineffective self–health management *related to* lack of knowledge regarding long-term management of osteomyelitis
- Impaired physical mobility *related to* pain, immobilization devices, and weight-bearing limitations

Additional information on nursing diagnoses for the patient with osteomyelitis is available in eNursing Care Plan 64-1 (on the website for this chapter).

PLANNING
The overall goals are that the patient with osteomyelitis will (1) have satisfactory pain and fever control, (2) not experience any complications associated with osteomyelitis, (3) cooperate with the treatment plan, and (4) maintain a positive outlook on the outcome of the disease.

NURSING IMPLEMENTATION
HEALTH PROMOTION. The control of infections already in the body (e.g., urinary, respiratory tract, deep pressure ulcers) is important in preventing osteomyelitis. Individuals who are especially at risk for osteomyelitis are those who are immunocompromised, have orthopedic prosthetic devices, or have vascular insufficiencies. Instruct these patients regarding the local and systemic manifestations of osteomyelitis. Also make family members aware of their role in monitoring the patient's health. Instruct patients to immediately report symptoms of bone pain, fever, swelling, and restricted limb movement to the health care provider so treatment can be started.

ACUTE INTERVENTION. Some immobilization of the affected limb (e.g., splint, traction) is usually indicated to decrease pain. Carefully handle the involved limb and avoid excessive manipulation, which increases pain and may cause a pathologic fracture. Assess the patient's pain. Minor to severe pain may be experienced with muscle spasms. Nonsteroidal antiinflammatory drugs (NSAIDs), opioid analgesics, and muscle relaxants may be prescribed to provide patient comfort. Encourage nondrug approaches to pain management (e.g., guided imagery, relaxation breathing) (see Chapters 7 and 9).

Dressings are used to absorb the exudate from draining wounds and to debride devitalized tissue from the wound site. Types of dressings include dry, sterile dressings; dressings saturated in saline or antibiotic solution; and wet-to-dry dressings. Handle soiled dressings carefully to prevent cross-contamination of the wound or spread of the infection to other patients. Sterile technique is essential when changing the dressing.

The patient is frequently on bed rest in the early stages of the acute infection. Good body alignment and frequent position changes prevent complications associated with immobility and promote comfort. Flexion contracture of the lower extremity is a common complication of osteomyelitis because the patient frequently positions the affected extremity in a flexed position to promote comfort. Footdrop can develop quickly if the foot is not correctly supported in a neutral position by a splint or if a splint applies excessive pressure, which can injure the peroneal nerve.

Teach the patient the potential adverse and toxic reactions associated with prolonged and high-dose antibiotic therapy (e.g., tobramycin, neomycin). These reactions include hearing deficit, nephrotoxicity, and neurotoxicity. With cephalosporins (e.g., cefazolin) these reactions include hives, severe or watery diarrhea, blood in stools, and throat or mouth sores.

Tendon rupture (especially the Achilles tendon) can occur with use of the fluoroquinolones (e.g., ciprofloxacin, levofloxacin [Levaquin]). Peak and trough blood levels of most antibiotics should be monitored to avoid adverse effects. Lengthy antibiotic therapy can also result in an overgrowth of *Candida albicans* and *Clostridium difficile* in the genitourinary and gastrointestinal (GI) tract, especially in immunosuppressed and older patients. Instruct the patient to report any changes in the oral cavity such as whitish yellow, curdlike lesions or changes in the genitourinary cavity such as any perianal itching or diarrhea.

The patient, caregiver, and family may be anxious and discouraged because of the serious nature of osteomyelitis, the uncertainty of the outcome, and the cost and lengthy course of treatment. Continued psychologic and emotional support is an integral part of nursing management. A nursing care plan for the patient with osteomyelitis (eNursing Care Plan 64-1) is available on the website for this chapter.

AMBULATORY AND HOME CARE. IV antibiotics can be administered to the patient in a skilled nursing facility or home setting. If at home, instruct the patient and caregiver on the proper care and management of the venous access device. Also teach them how to administer the antibiotic when scheduled and the need for follow-up laboratory testing. Stress the importance of continuing to take antibiotics after the symptoms have subsided. If there is an open wound, dressing changes are often necessary. The patient and caregiver may require supplies and instruction in the technique. If the osteomyelitis becomes chronic, patients need continued physical and psychologic support.

EVALUATION

The expected outcomes are that the patient with osteomyelitis will

- Have satisfactory pain relief
- Follow the recommended treatment regimen
- Verbalize confidence in ability to implement treatment regimen at home
- Demonstrate a consistent increase in mobility and range of motion

BONE TUMORS

Primary bone tumors, both benign and malignant, are relatively rare in adults. They account for only about 3% of all tumors. Metastatic bone cancer in which the cancer has spread from another site is a more common problem.

BENIGN BONE TUMORS

Benign bone tumors are more common than primary malignant tumors. The main types of benign bone tumors are osteochondroma, osteoclastoma, and endochroma (Table 64-3). These types of tumors are often removed by surgery.

Osteochondroma

Osteochondroma is the most common primary benign bone tumor. It is characterized by an overgrowth of cartilage and bone near the end of the bone at the growth plate. It is more commonly found in the long bones of the leg, pelvis, or scapula.

Clinical manifestations include a painless, hard, immobile mass; lower-than-normal height for age; soreness of muscles in close proximity to the tumor; one leg or arm longer than the other; and pressure or irritation with exercise. Patients may also be asymptomatic. Diagnosis is confirmed using x-ray, CT scan, and MRI.

No treatment is necessary for asymptomatic osteochondroma. If the tumor is causing pain or neurologic symptoms because of compression, surgical resection is usually done. Patients should have regular screening examinations for early detection of malignant transformation.

MALIGNANT BONE TUMORS

A sarcoma is a malignant tumor that can develop in bone, muscle, fat, nerve, or cartilage. The most common types of malignant bone tumors are osteosarcoma, chondrosarcoma, and Ewing's sarcoma (see Table 64-3). Annually about 2900 new cases of bone (and joint) cancer occur in the United States, with an estimated 1400 deaths.[6] Primary malignant tumors occur most often during childhood and young adulthood. They are characterized by their rapid metastasis and bone destruction.

Osteosarcoma

Osteosarcoma is a primary malignant bone tumor that is extremely aggressive and rapidly metastasizes to distant sites. It usually occurs in the metaphyseal region of the long bones of extremities, particularly in the regions of the distal femur, proximal tibia, and proximal humerus, as well as the pelvis (Fig. 64-3, *A*). Osteosarcoma is the most common malignant bone tumor affecting children and young adults. It can also occur, but not as commonly, in older adults. It is most often associated with Paget's disease and prior radiation.

Musculoskeletal System

TABLE 64-3	TYPES OF PRIMARY BONE TUMORS
Types	**Description**
Benign	
Osteochondroma	• Most common benign bone tumor • Frequently located in metaphyseal portion of long bones, particularly leg, pelvis, or scapula • Occurs most often in persons ages 10-25 • Malignant transformation may occur (chondrosarcoma)
Osteoclastoma (giant cell tumor)	• Arises in cancellous ends of arm and leg bones • About 10% are locally aggressive and may spread to lungs • High rate of local recurrence after surgery and chemotherapy
Endochroma	• Intramedullary cartilage tumor usually found in cavity of a single hand or foot bone • Rare malignant transformation can occur • If tumor becomes painful, a surgical resection is done • Peak incidence in persons ages 10-20
Malignant	
Osteosarcoma	• Most common primary bone cancer • Occurs mostly in young males between ages 10 and 25 • Most often in bones of arms, legs, or pelvis (see Fig. 64-3, *A*)
Chondrosarcoma	• Occurs in cartilage most commonly in arm, leg, and pelvic bones of older adults ages 50-70 • Can also arise from benign bone tumors (osteochondromas) • Wide surgical resection is mostly done, since tumor rarely responds to radiation and chemotherapy • Survival rate depends on stage, size, and grade of tumor (see Fig. 64-3, *B*)
Ewing's sarcoma	• Develops in medullary cavity of long bones, especially femur, humerus, pelvis, and tibia • Usually occurs in children and teenagers • Use of wide surgical resection, radiation, and chemotherapy has greatly improved the 5-yr survival rate to 60%

FIG. 64-3 A, Osteosarcoma. **B,** Chondrosarcoma.

The use of adjunct chemotherapy after amputation or limb salvage has increased the 5-year survival rate to 70% in people without metastasis. Chemotherapy includes methotrexate, doxorubicin (Adriamycin), cisplatin (Platinol), cyclophosphamide (Cytoxan), etoposide (VePesid), bleomycin (Blenoxane), dactinomycin (Cosmegen), and ifosfamide (Ifex).[7]

Metastatic Bone Cancer

The most common type of malignant bone tumor occurs as a result of metastasis from a primary tumor located at another site. Common sites for the primary tumor include breast, prostate, lungs, kidney, and thyroid. Metastatic cancer cells travel from the primary tumor to the bone via the lymph and blood supply. The metastatic bone lesions are commonly found in vertebrae, pelvis, femur, humerus, or ribs.[8] Pathologic fractures at the site of metastasis are common because of a weakening of the involved bone. High serum calcium levels result as calcium is released from damaged bones.

Once a primary lesion has been identified, radionuclide bone scans are often done to detect the metastatic lesions before they are visible on x-ray. Metastatic bone lesions may occur at any time (even years later) following diagnosis and treatment of the primary tumor. Metastasis to the bone should be suspected in any patient who has local bone pain and a past history of cancer. Treatment may be palliative and consists of radiation and pain management (see Chapter 9). Surgical stabilization of the bone may be indicated if there is a fracture or the patient is at high risk for a fracture. Prognosis depends on the primary type of cancer and any other sites of metastasis.

NURSING MANAGEMENT BONE CANCER

Assess the patient with bone cancer for the location and severity of pain. Also note weakness caused by anemia and decreased mobility. Monitor the site of the tumor for swelling; changes in circulation; and decreased movement, sensation, or joint function.

Clinical manifestations of osteosarcoma are usually associated with the gradual onset of pain and swelling, especially around the knee. A minor injury does not cause the neoplasm but may bring the preexisting condition to medical attention. Metastasis is present in 10% to 20% of individuals when they are diagnosed with osteosarcoma.

Diagnosis is confirmed from tissue biopsy, elevation of serum alkaline phosphatase and calcium levels, x-ray, computed tomography (CT) or positron emission tomography (PET) scans, and magnetic resonance imaging (MRI).

Preoperative (neoadjuvant) chemotherapy may be used in the treatment of osteosarcoma to decrease tumor size before surgery. Limb salvage procedures are usually considered when there is a clear (no cancer present) 6- to 7-cm margin surrounding the lesion. Limb salvage is usually contraindicated if there is major neurovascular involvement, pathologic fracture, infection, or extensive muscle involvement.

Nursing care of the patient with a malignant bone tumor does not differ significantly from the care provided to the patient with a malignant disease of any other body system (see Chapter 16). However, special attention is required to prevent pathologic fractures or to reduce the complications associated with them. It is important to prevent fractures by careful handling and support of the affected extremity and logrolling for those on bed rest.

Treatment for hypercalcemia may need to be initiated if bone decalcification occurs (see Chapter 16, p. 278). The patient is often reluctant to participate in exercise or therapeutic activities because of weakness from the disease and the treatment, fear of falling and fracturing a bone, and fear of pain. Provide regular rest periods between activities.

The pain associated with bone cancer can be severe. The pain is often caused by the tumor pressing against nerves and other organs near the bone. Carefully monitor the patient's pain and ensure that he or she has adequate pain medication. Sometimes radiation therapy is used as a palliative therapy to shrink the tumor and decrease the pain.

Assist the patient and caregiver in accepting the poor prognosis associated with bone malignancies. General principles related to cancer nursing are applicable (see Chapter 16). Special attention is necessary for the problems of pain and disability, side effects of chemotherapy, and postoperative care after surgery such as spinal cord decompression or amputation. As with all types of cancer, stress the importance of follow-up examinations.

MUSCULAR DYSTROPHY

Muscular dystrophy (MD) is a group of genetic diseases characterized by progressive symmetric wasting of skeletal muscles without evidence of neurologic involvement. In all forms of MD an insidious loss of strength occurs with increasing disability and deformity. The types of MD differ in the groups of muscles affected, age of onset, rate of progression, and mode of genetic inheritance (Table 64-4). The most common type of MD is Duchenne.

Genetic Link

Both Duchenne and Becker MD are X-linked recessive disorders usually seen only in males. (X-linked recessive disorders are discussed in Chapter 13.) In Duchenne and Becker MD there is a mutation of the dystrophin gene. Dystrophin in normal muscle cells helps skeletal muscle fibers attach to the basement membrane. Abnormal dystrophin can lead to defects in the plasma membrane of muscle fiber with subsequent muscle fiber degeneration.

A family history can be used to obtain a family pedigree. Family pedigrees for X-linked recessive disorders are shown in Figs. 13-4 and 13-5.

Diagnostic studies for MD include muscle serum enzymes (especially creatine kinase), electromyogram (EMG) testing, muscle fiber biopsy, and electrocardiogram abnormalities reflective of cardiomyopathy. Muscle biopsy confirms the diagnosis with classic findings of fat and connective tissue deposits, degeneration and necrosis of muscle fibers, and a deficiency of the muscle protein dystrophin.

Currently no definitive therapy is available to stop the progressive wasting of MD. The primary goals of treatment are to preserve mobility and independence through exercise, physical

TABLE 64-4	TYPES OF MUSCULAR DYSTROPHY	
Type	**Genetic Basis**	**Manifestations**
Duchenne (pseudohypertrophic)	X-linked Mutation of dystrophin gene	• Onset before age 5 yr • Progressive weakness of pelvic and shoulder muscles • Unable to walk after age 12 yr • Cardiomyopathy • Respiratory failure in teens or 20s • Mental impairment
Becker (benign pseudohypertrophic)	X-linked Mutation of dystrophin gene	• Onset between 5 and 15 yr • Slower course of pelvic and shoulder muscle wasting than Duchenne • Cardiomyopathy • Respiratory failure • May survive into 30s or 40s
Landouzy-Déjérine (facioscapulohumeral)	Autosomal dominant Deletion of chromosome 4q35	• Onset before age 20 • Slowly progressive weakness of face, shoulder muscles, and foot dorsiflexion • Deafness
Erb (limb-girdle)	Autosomal recessive or autosomal dominant	• Onset ranges from early childhood to early adulthood • Slow progressive weakness of shoulder and hip muscles

therapy, and orthopedic appliances. Progressive weakening of muscles around the trunk can lead to spinal collapse. To prevent injuries, the patient may be fitted early with an orthotic jacket to provide stability and prevent further deformity.

Cardiomyopathy often occurs and results in heart failure. Dysrhythmias are a frequent cause of death.[9] Gradual decreases in respiratory function often lead to the use of continuous positive airway pressure (CPAP). Eventually a tracheostomy and mechanical ventilation are necessary to sustain respiratory function. Corticosteroid therapy may significantly halt the disease progression for up to 2 years.[10]

Encourage communication among family members (and parents) to cope with the emotional and physical strains of MD. Teach the patient and caregiver range-of-motion exercises, nutritional therapy, and signs of progression. Genetic testing and counseling may be recommended for individuals with a family history of MD.

Focus your care on keeping the patient active as long as possible. Prolonged bed rest should be avoided because immobility can lead to further muscle wasting. As the disease progresses, the focus shifts to teaching the patient to limit sedentary periods to prevent skin breakdown and respiratory complications. Ongoing medical and nursing care is required throughout the individual's lifetime. The Muscular Dystrophy Association (www.mda.org) is an important resource for health care and support services for MD patients and their caregivers and family.

LOW BACK PAIN

Low back pain is most often due to a musculoskeletal problem. It may be experienced as localized or diffuse. In *localized pain* patients feel soreness or discomfort when they or someone else

GENETICS IN CLINICAL PRACTICE

Duchenne and Becker Muscular Dystrophy (MD)

Genetic Basis
- Caused by different mutations in the same *DMD* gene.
- Gene provides instructions for making dystrophin (protein that keeps muscles intact).
- X-linked recessive disorder.

Incidence
- Between 400 and 600 boys are born with MD each year.
- Together these disorders affect 1 in 3500–5000 newborn males.

Genetic Testing
- DNA testing for mutation in dystrophin gene is available.

Clinical Implications
- Muscular dystrophies are a group of genetic conditions characterized by progressive muscle weakness and atrophy.
- These two conditions differ in their severity, age of onset, and rate of progression (see Table 64-4).
- Few individuals with the disease live to adulthood.
- Genetic testing and counseling should be considered in individuals with a family history of MD.
- Because there are many types of MD with different genetic bases, establishing the type of MD is important to determine treatment and possible genetic counseling recommendations.

palpates or presses on a specific area of the lower back. *Diffuse pain* is spread over a larger area and comes from deep tissue layers.

Low back pain may be radicular or referred. *Radicular pain* is caused by irritation of a nerve root. Sciatica is an example of radicular pain. *Referred pain* is "felt" or perceived in the lower back, but the source of the pain is another location (e.g., kidneys, lower abdomen).

Low back pain is common and has affected about 80% of adults in the United States at least once during their lifetime. Backache is second only to headache as the most common pain complaint. In persons under age 45, low back pain is responsible for more lost working hours than any other medical condition.[11]

Low back pain is a common problem because the lumbar region (1) bears most of the weight of the body, (2) is the most flexible region of the spinal column, (3) contains nerve roots that are vulnerable to injury or disease, and (4) has an inherently poor biomechanical structure. Several risk factors associated with low back pain include lack of muscle tone and excess body weight, stress, poor posture, cigarette smoking, pregnancy, prior compression fractures of the spine, spinal problems since birth, and a family history of back pain. Jobs that require repetitive heavy lifting, vibration (such as a jackhammer operator), and prolonged periods of sitting are also associated with low back pain.

The causes of low back pain of musculoskeletal origin include (1) acute lumbosacral strain, (2) instability of the lumbosacral bony mechanism, (3) osteoarthritis of the lumbosacral vertebrae, (4) degenerative disc disease, and (5) herniation of an intervertebral disc.

Health care personnel who engage in patient care–related tasks are at high risk for the development of low back pain.[12] Lifting and moving patients, excessive time stooping over or leaning forward, and frequent twisting can result in low

back pain that contributes to lost time and productivity and disability.

ACUTE LOW BACK PAIN

Acute low back pain is low back pain that lasts 4 weeks or less. Most acute low back pain is caused by trauma or some type of activity that causes undue stress (often hyperflexion) of the lower back. Examples of trauma or activity that could cause acute back pain are heavy lifting, overuse of the back muscles while working in the yard, a sports injury, or a sudden jolt such as a car accident.

Often symptoms do not appear at the time of injury but develop later (usually within 24 hours) because of a gradual increase in pressure on the nerve by an intervertebral disc. Symptoms may range from muscle ache to shooting or stabbing pain, limited flexibility or range of motion, or an inability to stand straight.

Few definitive diagnostic abnormalities are present with nerve irritation and muscle strain. One test is the straight-leg raise (see Chapter 62, p. 1498). MRI and CT scans are generally not done unless trauma or systemic disease (e.g., cancer, spinal infection) is suspected.

NURSING AND COLLABORATIVE MANAGEMENT
ACUTE LOW BACK PAIN

NURSING ASSESSMENT

Subjective and objective data that should be obtained from the patient with low back pain are summarized in Table 64-5.

NURSING IMPLEMENTATION

HEALTH PROMOTION. As a role model, you need to use proper body mechanics at all times. This includes increasing the patient's bed height, bending at the knees, asking for help in lifting and moving patients, and using lifting devices.

Assess the patient's use of body mechanics and offer advice when the person does activities that could produce back strain (Table 64-6). Some health care providers refer patients with back pain to a program called "Back School." It is a formal program usually taught by health professionals such as physicians, nurses, and physical therapists. It is designed to teach the patient how to minimize back pain and avoid repeat episodes of low back pain. Tips for prevention of back injury are listed in Table 64-6.

Advise patients to maintain appropriate body weight. Excess body weight places additional stress on the lower back and weakens the abdominal muscles that support the lower back. Flat shoes or shoes with low heels and shock-absorbing shoe inserts are recommended for women.

The position assumed while sleeping is also important in preventing low back pain. Tell patients to avoid sleeping in a prone position because it produces excessive lumbar lordosis, placing excessive stress on the lower back. The patient should sleep in either a supine or side-lying position with knees and hips flexed to prevent unnecessary pressure on support muscles, ligaments, and lumbosacral joints. A firm mattress is recommended.

Teach patients the importance of stopping smoking, since it has been associated with low back pain. One reason for this is that nicotine decreases circulation to the intervertebral discs.

TABLE 64-5 NURSING ASSESSMENT

Low Back Pain

Subjective Data
Important Health Information
Past health history: Acute or chronic lumbosacral strain/trauma, osteoarthritis, degenerative disc disease, obesity
Medications: Opioid and nonopioid analgesics, muscle relaxants, nonsteroidal antiinflammatory drugs, corticosteroids; over-the-counter remedies, including herbal products and nutritional supplements
Surgery or other treatments: Previous back surgery, epidural corticosteroid injections

Functional Health Patterns
Health perception–health management: Smoking, lack of exercise
Nutritional-metabolic: Obesity
Activity-exercise: Poor posture, muscle spasms, activity intolerance
Elimination: Constipation
Sleep-rest: Interrupted sleep
Cognitive-perceptual: Pain in back, buttocks, or leg associated with walking, turning, straining, coughing, leg raising; numbness or tingling of legs, feet, toes
Role-relationship: In occupations requiring heavy lifting, vibrations, or extended driving; change in role within family structure due to inability to work and provide income

Objective Data
General
Guarded movement

Neurologic
Depressed or absent Achilles tendon reflex or patellar tendon reflex; positive straight-leg-raising test, positive crossover straight-leg-raising test, positive Trendelenburg test

Musculoskeletal
Tense, tight paravertebral muscles on palpation, ↓ range of motion of spine

Possible Diagnostic Findings
Localization of site of lesion or disorder on myelogram, CT scan, or MRI; determination of nerve root impingement on electromyography

HEALTHY PEOPLE

Prevention of Low Back Pain

- Maintain healthy weight.
- Do not sleep in a prone position.
- Sleep on side with knees flexed and a pillow between the knees.
- Avoid cigarette smoking and tobacco products.
- Obtain regular physical activity, including strength and endurance training.
- Use proper body mechanics to avoid low back strain (e.g., when lifting heavy objects, bend at the knees, not at the waist, and stand up slowly while holding object close to your body).

TABLE 64-6 PATIENT & CAREGIVER TEACHING GUIDE

Low Back Problems

Include the following instructions when teaching the patient and caregiver how to manage low back problems.

Do
- Avoid straining the lower back by placing a foot on a step or stool during prolonged standing.
- Sleep in a side-lying position with knees and hips bent.
- Sleep on back with a lift under knees and legs or on back with 10-in-high pillow under knees to flex hips and knees.
- Regularly exercise 15 min in the morning and evening; begin exercises with 2- or 3-min warm-up period by moving arms and legs, alternately relaxing and tightening muscles; exercise slowly with smooth movements.
- Carry light items close to body.
- Maintain appropriate body weight.
- Use local heat and cold application.
- Use a lumbar roll or pillow for sitting.

Do Not
- Lean forward without bending knees.
- Lift anything above level of elbows.
- Stand in one position for prolonged time.
- Sleep on abdomen or on back or side with legs out straight.
- Exercise without consulting health care provider if having severe pain.
- Exceed prescribed amount and type of exercises without consulting health care provider.

A brief period (1 to 2 days) of rest at home may be necessary for some people, but most patients do better with a continuation of their regular activities. Prolonged bed rest should be avoided.[14] Patients should refrain from activities that aggravate the pain, including lifting, bending, twisting, and prolonged sitting. Most cases of acute low back pain show improvement within 2 weeks and often resolve without treatment.

Teach patients about their health problem and ways to prevent recurrent episodes. Muscle stretching and strengthening exercises may be part of the management plan. (See the Resource section at the end of this chapter for a link to exercises to strengthen the back.) Although the actual exercises are often taught by the physical therapist, it is your responsibility to ensure that the patient understands the type and frequency of exercise prescribed and the rationale for the program.

Other nursing interventions for the patient with low back pain are summarized in eNursing Care Plan 64-2 (on the website for this chapter).

AMBULATORY AND HOME CARE. The goal of management is to make an episode of acute low back pain an isolated incident. If the lumbosacral mechanism is unstable, repeated episodes can be anticipated. The lumbosacral spine may be unable to meet the demands placed on it without strain because of factors such as obesity, poor posture, poor muscle support, older age, or trauma. Intervention is aimed at strengthening the supporting muscles by exercise (see above).

Persistent use of poor body mechanics may also result in repeated episodes of low back pain. If the strain is work related, occupational counseling may be necessary. The frustration, pain, and disability imposed on the patient with low back pain require your emotional support and understanding care.

ACUTE INTERVENTION. If the acute muscle spasms and accompanying pain are not severe and debilitating, the patient may be treated on an outpatient basis with NSAIDs (e.g., acetaminophen) and muscle relaxants (e.g., cyclobenzaprine [Flexeril]). Massage and back manipulation, acupuncture, and the application of cold and hot compresses may help some patients.[13] Severe pain may require a brief course of opioid analgesics.

CHRONIC LOW BACK PAIN

Chronic low back pain is low back pain that lasts more than 3 months or is a repeated incapacitating episode. It is often progressive, and the cause can be difficult to determine. Causes include (1) degenerative conditions such as arthritis or disc disease; (2) osteoporosis or other metabolic bone diseases; (3) prior injury (scar tissue weakens the back); (4) chronic strain on the lower back muscles from obesity, pregnancy, or job-related stooping, bending, or other stressful postures; and (5) congenital abnormalities in the spine.

Spinal Stenosis

Spinal stenosis is a narrowing of the spinal canal (hollow vertical hole that contains the spinal cord). Stenosis in the lumbar area of the spine is a common cause of chronic low back pain. Spinal stenosis can be caused by either acquired or inherited conditions. A common acquired cause is osteoarthritis in the spine. Arthritic changes (bone spurs, calcification of spinal ligaments, degeneration of discs) narrow the space around the spinal canal and nerve roots, eventually leading to compression. Inflammation caused by the compression results in pain, weakness, and numbness.

Other acquired conditions that may lead to spinal stenosis include rheumatoid arthritis, spinal tumors, Paget's disease, and traumatic damage to the vertebral column. Inherited conditions that lead to spinal stenosis include congenital spinal stenosis and scoliosis.

The pain associated with lumbar spinal stenosis often starts in the lower back and then radiates to the buttock and leg. It worsens with walking and, in particular, standing without walking. Numbness, tingling, weakness, and heaviness in the legs and buttocks may also be present. A history of the pain lessening when the patient bends forward or sits down is often a sign of spinal stenosis. In most cases the stenosis slowly progresses and does not cause paralysis.

NURSING AND COLLABORATIVE MANAGEMENT CHRONIC LOW BACK PAIN

Nursing management and treatment of chronic low back pain are similar to those recommended for acute low back pain. Relief of pain and stiffness with mild analgesics, such as NSAIDs, is necessary for the patient's daily comfort. Antidepressants (e.g., duloxetine [Cymbalta]) may help with pain relief and sleep problems. The antiseizure drug gabapentin (Neurontin) may improve walking and relieve leg symptoms.

Weight reduction, sufficient rest periods, local heat or cold application, physical therapy, and exercise and activity throughout the day assist in keeping the muscles and joints mobilized. Cold, damp weather aggravates the back pain, which can be relieved with rest and local heat application. Complementary and alternative therapies such as biofeedback, acupuncture, and yoga may help reduce the pain (see the Evidence-Based Practice box). "Back School" (discussed on p. 1545) can significantly reduce pain and improve body posture for both patients and nurses.[15]

Minimally invasive treatments, such as epidural corticosteroid injections and implanted devices that deliver pain medication, may be used for patients with chronic low back pain that is refractory to the usual therapeutic options. Surgical intervention may be indicated in patients with severe chronic low back

EVIDENCE-BASED PRACTICE
Translating Research Into Practice

Can Yoga Improve Chronic Low Back Pain?
Clinical Question
Among adults with chronic low back pain (P), do interventions of yoga (I) vs. stretching exercises vs. a self-care book (C) improve function and pain (O)?

Best Available Evidence
Randomized controlled trials (RCTs)

Critical Appraisal and Synthesis of Evidence
- One RCT (n = 228) of adults with chronic low back pain comparing 12 weekly classes of yoga (n = 92) or stretching exercises (n = 91) or a self-care book on chronic low back pain (n = 45).
- Outcomes of back-related functional status and pain were assessed at 6, 12, and 26 wk.
- At 12 wk patients doing yoga had better functioning and less pain than patients in the self-care group.
- At 26 wk, functioning for the yoga group remained superior to the self-care group.
- Yoga was not better than stretching exercises at any time point.

Conclusion
- Yoga was more effective than a self-care book in improving function and reducing pain for at least several months. Yoga was no better than stretching classes.

Implications for Nursing Practice
- Assist patients in identifying resources and community classes that focus on stretching exercises and yoga.
- Assess and monitor back pain. Encourage regular participation in complementary and alternative therapies that patients find effective for chronic low back pain.

Reference for Evidence
Sherman KJ, Cherkin DC, Wellman RD, et al: A randomized trial comparing yoga, stretching, and a self-care book for chronic low back pain, *Arch Intern Med* 171:2019, 2011.

P, Patient population of interest; *I*, intervention or area of interest; *C*, comparison of interest or comparison group; *O*, outcomes of interest (see p. 12).

pain who do not respond to conservative care and/or have continued neurologic deficits. (Surgery for low back pain is discussed on pp. 1548-1550.)

INTERVERTEBRAL DISC DISEASE

Intervertebral discs separate the vertebrae of the spinal column and provide shock absorption for the spine. *Intervertebral disc disease* is a condition that involves the deterioration, herniation, or other dysfunction of the intervertebral discs. Disc disorders can involve the cervical, thoracic, and lumbar spine.

Etiology and Pathophysiology

Structural degeneration of discs is often caused by degenerative disc disease (DDD). This progressive degeneration is a normal process of aging and results in the intervertebral discs losing their elasticity, flexibility, and shock-absorbing capabilities.[16] Thinning of the discs occurs as the *nucleus pulposus* (gelatinous center of the disc) starts to dry out and shrink. These changes limit the ability of the discs to distribute pressure loads between the vertebrae. Then these loads are transferred to the *annulus fibrosus* (strong outside portion of the intervertebral disc), causing progressive structural deterioration. With structural damage to the disc, the nucleus pulposus may seep through a torn or stretched annulus. This is called a **herniated disc** *(slipped disc),* a condition in which a spinal disc herniates and bulges outward between the vertebrae (Fig. 64-4).

A herniated disc can be the result of natural degeneration with age or repeated stress and trauma to the spine. The nucleus pulposus may first bulge and then it can herniate, placing pressure on nearby nerves. The most common sites of herniation are the lumbosacral discs, specifically L4-5 and L5-S1. Disc herniation may also occur at C5-6 and C6-7. Disc herniation may be the result of spinal stenosis, in which narrowing of the spinal canal forces the intervertebral disc to bulge.

The spinal nerves emerge from the spinal column through an opening *(intervertebral foramen)* between adjacent vertebrae. Herniated discs can press against these nerves ("pinched nerve") causing *radiculopathy* (radiating pain, numbness, tingling, and diminished strength and/or range of motion).

Osteoarthritis of the spine is associated with DDD and the stresses placed on the vertebrae. The joints, which are not adequately lubricated, rub against each other, leading to damage of the protective cartilage and the formation of painful bone spurs, which are one of the changes found in osteoarthritis.

Clinical Manifestations

In *lumbar disc disease* the most common manifestation is low back pain. Radicular pain that radiates down the buttock and

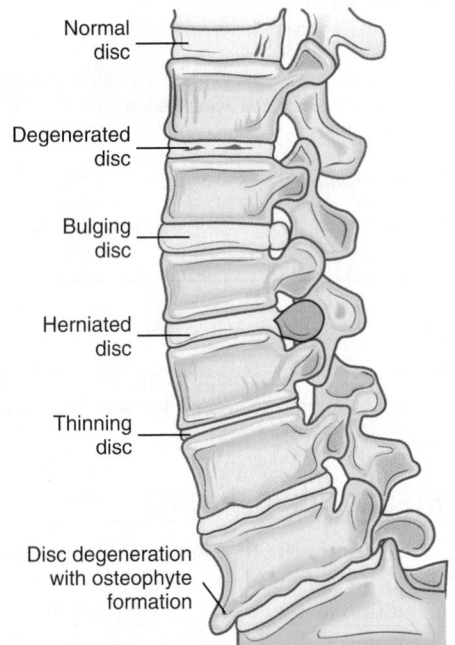

Normal disc

Degenerated disc

Bulging disc

Herniated disc

Thinning disc

Disc degeneration with osteophyte formation

FIG. 64-4 Common causes of degenerative disc damage.

below the knee, along the distribution of the sciatic nerve, generally indicates disc herniation. (Specific manifestations of lumbar disc herniation are summarized in Table 64-7.) The straight-leg-raising test may be positive, indicating nerve root irritation. Back or leg pain may be reproduced by raising the leg and flexing the foot at 90 degrees. Low back pain from other causes may not be accompanied by leg pain. Reflexes may be depressed or absent, depending on the spinal nerve root involved. Paresthesia or muscle weakness in the legs, feet, or toes may occur.

Multiple nerve root *(cauda equina)* compressions from a herniated disc, a tumor, or an epidural abscess may be manifested as bowel and bladder incontinence.[17] This condition is a medical emergency.

In *cervical disc disease* pain radiates into the arms and the hands, following the pattern of the nerve involved. Similar to lumbar disc disease, reflexes may or may not be present, and the handgrip is often weak.

Diagnostic Studies

X-rays are done to detect any structural defects. A myelogram, MRI, or CT scan is helpful in localizing the damaged site. An epidural venogram or diskogram may be necessary if other methods of diagnosis are unsuccessful. An EMG of the extremities can be performed to determine the severity of nerve irritation or to rule out other pathologic conditions such as peripheral neuropathy.

Collaborative Care

The patient with suspected disc damage is usually first managed with conservative therapy (Table 64-8). This includes limitation of extremes of spinal movement (brace, corset, or belt), local heat or ice, ultrasound and massage, traction, and transcutaneous electrical nerve stimulation (TENS). Drug therapy to relieve pain includes NSAIDs, short-term use of opioids, analgesics, muscle relaxants, antiseizure drugs, and antidepressants.[18] Epidural corticosteroid injections may be effective in reducing inflammation and relieving acute pain. If the underlying cause remains, the pain tends to recur.

Once the symptoms subside, back strengthening exercises are begun twice a day and are encouraged for a lifetime. Teach the patient the principles of good body mechanics. Discourage extremes of flexion and torsion. Most patients heal with a conservative treatment plan after 6 months.

Surgical Therapy. If conservative treatment is unsuccessful, radiculopathy becomes progressively worse, or loss of bowel or bladder control (cauda equina) occurs, surgery may then be indicated. Surgery for a damaged disc is generally performed when diagnostic tests indicate that the problem is not responding to conservative treatment and the patient is in constant pain and/or has a persistent neurologic deficit.

TABLE 64-7	**MANIFESTATIONS OF LUMBAR DISC HERNIATION***			
Intervertebral Level	Pain	Affected Reflex	Motor Function	Sensation
L3-4	Back to buttocks to posterior thigh to inner calf	Patellar	Quadriceps, anterior tibialis	Inner aspect of lower leg, anterior part of thigh
L4-5	Back to buttocks to dorsum of foot and big toe	None	Anterior tibialis, extensor hallucis longus, gluteus medius	Dorsum of foot and big toe
L5-S1	Back to buttocks to sole of foot and heel	Achilles	Gastrocnemius, hamstring, gluteus maximus	Heel and lateral foot

*A disc herniation can involve pressure on more than one nerve root.

An *intradiscal electrothermoplasty* (IDET) is a minimally invasive outpatient procedure that may help treat back and sciatica pain. The procedure involves inserting a needle into the affected disc with the guidance of an x-ray. A wire is then threaded down through the needle and into the disc. The wire is heated, which denervates the small nerve fibers that have grown into the cracks and have invaded the degenerating disc. The heat also partially melts the annulus fibrosus, which triggers the body to generate new reinforcing proteins in the fibers of the annulus.

Another outpatient technique is *radiofrequency discal nucleoplasty* (coblation nucleoplasty). A needle is inserted into the disc similar to IDET. Instead of a heating wire, a special radiofrequency probe is used. The probe generates energy that breaks up the molecular bonds of the gel in the nucleus pulposus. The result is that up to 20% of the nucleus is removed, which decompresses the disc and reduces the pressure on both the disc and the surrounding nerve roots. Relief from pain varies among patients.

A third procedure is the use of an *interspinous process decompression system* (X-Stop). This device is made of titanium and fits onto a mount that is placed on vertebrae in the lower back. The X-Stop is used in patients with pain due to lumbar spinal stenosis. The device works by lifting the vertebrae off the pinched nerve.

A common and traditional surgical procedure for lumbar disc disease is a *laminectomy*. It involves the surgical excision of part of the vertebra (referred to as the lamina) to gain access to the protruding disc to remove it. A minimal hospital stay is usually required after the procedure.

A *diskectomy* is another common surgical procedure to decompress the nerve root.[11] Microsurgical diskectomy is a version of the standard diskectomy in which the surgeon uses a microscope to allow better visualization of the disc and disc space during surgery to aid in the removal of the damaged portion. This helps maintain the bony stability of the spine.

A *percutaneous diskectomy* is an outpatient surgical procedure using a tube that is passed through the retroperitoneal soft tissues to the disc with the aid of fluoroscopy. A laser is then used on the damaged portion of the disc. Small stab wounds are used, and minimal blood loss occurs during the procedure. The procedure is effective and safe and decreases rehabilitation time.

The goals of artificial disc replacement surgery are to restore movement and eliminate pain. The *Charité disc* is used in patients with lumbar disc damage associated with DDD. This artificial disc is made up of a high-density core sandwiched between two cobalt-chromium endplates (Fig. 64-5). This device is surgically placed in the spine (usually through a small incision below the umbilicus) after the damaged disc is removed. The disc allows for movement at the level of the implant.

The *ProDisc-L* is another type of artificial lumbar disc that can be used to treat DDD.[19] The *Prestige cervical disc system* may be used in the treatment of DDD of the cervical spine.

A *spinal fusion* may be performed if the spine is unstable. The spine is stabilized by creating an ankylosis (fusion) of contiguous vertebrae with a bone graft from the patient's fibula or iliac crest or from a donated cadaver bone. Metal fixation with rods, plates, or screws may be implanted at the time of spinal surgery to provide more stability and decrease vertebral motion. A posterior lumbar fusion may be performed in patients to provide extra support for bone grafting or a prosthetic device.

Bone morphogenetic protein (BMP), a genetically engineered protein, may be used to stimulate bone growth of the graft in spinal fusions.[20] A dissolvable sponge soaked with BMP is implanted into the spine. The protein on the sponge stimulates the body's own cells to become active and produce bone. BMP begins the process of fusion, which continues even after the protein and sponge dissolve, leaving living bone behind.

TABLE 64-8 COLLABORATIVE CARE

Intervertebral Disc Disease

Diagnostic
- History and physical examination
- X-ray
- CT scan
- MRI
- Myelogram
- Diskogram
- Electromyogram (EMG)

Collaborative Therapy
Conservative
- Restricted activity for several days, limit total bed rest
- Local ice or heat
- Physical therapy
- Drug therapy
  - Analgesics (e.g., tramadol [Ultram, Ryzolt])
  - Nonsteroidal antiinflammatory drugs
  - Muscle relaxants (e.g., cyclobenzaprine [Flexeril])
  - Antiseizure drugs (e.g., gabapentin [Neurontin])
  - Antidepressants (e.g., pregabalin [Lyrica])
  - Epidural corticosteroid injections

Surgical
- Intradiscal electrothermoplasty (IDET)
- Radiofrequency discal nucleoplasty
- Interspinous process decompression system (X-Stop)
- Laminectomy with or without spinal fusion
- Diskectomy
- Percutaneous laser diskectomy
- Artificial disc replacement (e.g., Charité disc)
- Spinal fusion with instrumentation (e.g., plates, screws) or without

FIG. 64-5 The Charité artificial disc, used in degenerative disc disease to replace a damaged intervertebral disc. The Charité artificial disc consists of two cobalt-chromium alloy endplates sandwiched around a movable high-density plastic core. The disc's design helps align the spine and preserve its natural ability to move.

NURSING MANAGEMENT
VERTEBRAL DISC SURGERY

After vertebral disc surgery, postoperative nursing interventions mainly focus on maintaining proper alignment of the spine until it has healed. Depending on the type and extent of surgery and the surgeon's preference, the patient may be able to dangle the legs at the side of the bed, stand, or even ambulate the same day of surgery.

When a patient has had a lumbar fusion, place pillows under the thighs of each leg when supine and between the legs when in the side-lying position to provide comfort and ensure alignment. The patient often fears turning or any movement that increases pain by straining the surgical area. Reassure the patient that the proper technique is being used to maintain body alignment. Sufficient staff should be available to move the patient without undue pain or strain on staff members or the patient.

Postoperatively, most patients require opioids such as morphine IV for 24 to 48 hours. Patient-controlled analgesia (PCA) allows for optimal analgesic levels and is the preferred method of continued pain management during this time. Once fluids are being taken, the patient may be switched to oral drugs such as acetaminophen with codeine, hydrocodone (Vicodin), or oxycodone (Percocet). Diazepam (Valium) may be prescribed for muscle relaxation. Monitor and document pain management and its effectiveness.

Because the spinal canal may be entered during surgery, there is potential for cerebrospinal fluid (CSF) leakage. Immediately report a severe headache or leakage of CSF on the dressing. CSF appears as clear or slightly yellow drainage on the dressing. It has a high glucose concentration and is positive for glucose when tested with a dipstick. Note the amount, color, and characteristics of drainage.

Frequently monitor the patient's peripheral neurologic signs after spinal surgery. Movement of the arms and the legs and assessment of sensation should be unchanged when compared with the preoperative status. These assessments are usually repeated every 2 to 4 hours during the first 48 hours after surgery and compared with the preoperative assessment. Paresthesias, such as numbness and tingling, may not be relieved immediately after surgery. Document any new muscle weakness or paresthesias and report them to the surgeon immediately. Assess extremity circulation using temperature, capillary refill, and pulses.

Paralytic ileus and interference with bowel function may occur for several days and may manifest as nausea, abdominal distention, and constipation. Assess whether the patient is passing flatus; has bowel sounds in all quadrants; and has a flat, soft abdomen. Stool softeners (e.g., docusate [Colace]) may aid in relieving and preventing constipation.

Adequate bladder emptying may be altered because of activity restrictions, opioids, or anesthesia. If allowed by the surgeon, encourage men to dangle the legs over the side of the bed or stand to urinate. Patients should use the commode or ambulate to the bathroom when allowed to promote adequate emptying of the bladder. Ensure that privacy is maintained. Intermittent catheterization or an indwelling catheter may be necessary for patients who have difficulty urinating.

Loss of sphincter tone or bladder tone may indicate nerve damage. Monitor for incontinence or difficulty evacuating the bowel or bladder, and report significant findings to the surgeon immediately.

In addition to the nursing care appropriate for a patient who has had a laminectomy, there are other nursing responsibilities if the patient has also had a spinal fusion. Because a bone graft is usually involved, the postoperative healing time is prolonged compared with that of a laminectomy. Limitations on activity may be necessary over an extended time. A rigid orthosis (thoracic-lumbar-sacral orthosis [TLSO] or chairback brace) is often used during this period. Some surgeons require that the patient be taught to put it on and take it off by logrolling in bed, whereas others allow their patients to apply the brace in a sitting or standing position. Verify the preferred method before initiating this activity.

If surgery is done on the cervical spine, be alert for manifestations of spinal cord edema such as respiratory distress and a worsening neurologic status of the upper extremities. After surgery, the patient's neck may be immobilized in either a soft or hard cervical collar.

In addition to the primary surgical site, regularly assess the donor site for the bone graft. The posterior iliac crest is the most commonly used donor site, although the fibula may also be used. The donor site usually causes greater pain than the spinal fusion area. The donor site is bandaged with a pressure dressing to prevent excessive bleeding. If the donor site is the fibula, neurovascular assessments of the extremity are a postoperative nursing responsibility.

After a spinal fusion the patient may experience some immobility of the spine at the fusion site. Instruct the patient in proper body mechanics and to avoid sitting or standing for prolonged periods. Encourage activities that include walking, lying down, and shifting weight from one foot to the other when standing. Lifting is usually restricted in the postoperative period after spinal surgery. The patient should learn to mentally think through an activity before starting any potentially injurious task such as bending or stooping. Any twisting movement of the spine is contraindicated. Patients should use the thighs and knees, rather than the back, to absorb the shock of activity and movement. A firm mattress or bed board is essential.

▌NECK PAIN

Neck pain occurs almost as frequently as low back pain, affecting up to 50% of adults at some point in their life. Neck pain may be the result of many conditions, both benign (e.g., poor posture) and serious (e.g., herniated cervical disc)[21] (Table 64-9).

Cervical neck sprains and strains occur from hyperflexion and hyperextension injury. Patients have symptoms of stiffness and neck pain and possible pain radiating into the arm and hand. Pain may also radiate into the head, anterior chest, thoracic spine region, and shoulders. Cervical nerve root compression from stenosis, DDD, or herniation may be indicated by weakness or paresthesia of the arm and hand.

The cause of neck pain is diagnosed by history, physical examination, x-ray, MRI, CT scan, and myelogram. An

TABLE 64-9 CAUSES OF NECK PAIN	
• Poor posture	• Spondylosis
• Strain or sprain	• Rheumatoid arthritis
• Degenerative disc disease, including herniation	• Tumor
	• Osteoporosis
• Trauma (e.g., fractures, subluxation)	• Osteomyelitis
	• Meningitis

TABLE 64-10 PATIENT & CAREGIVER TEACHING GUIDE

Neck Exercises

When teaching the patient exercises for neck pain, include the following instructions for the patient and caregiver.

- Bend your head backward until you are looking up at the ceiling. Repeat slowly five times. Stop if experiencing dizziness.
- Bring your head forward so that your chin touches your chest and your face is looking down at the floor. Repeat slowly five times.
- Keep your head facing forward, and bend your ear down toward one shoulder. Alternate this movement with your other ear. Repeat slowly five times on each side.
- Turn your head slowly around to one side as far as it will go. Repeat toward the other side. Repeat exercise five times on each side.

EMG of the upper extremities is done to diagnose cervical radiculopathy.

Conservative treatment for neck pain in patients without an underlying disorder includes head support using a soft cervical collar, heat and ice applications, massage, rest until symptoms subside, ultrasound, and NSAIDs. Therapeutic neck exercises[22] and acupuncture may also be used for pain relief. Most neck pain resolves without surgical intervention.

Preventing neck pain that occurs with everyday activities such as prolonged sitting at a computer or television, sleeping in nonaligned spinal positions, or making jarring movements during exercise is important. Preventive strategies can begin by practicing good posture and maintaining neck flexibility (Table 64-10).

FOOT DISORDERS

The foot is the platform that supports the weight of the body and absorbs considerable shock when the person is ambulating. The foot is a complicated structure composed of bony structures, muscles, tendons, and ligaments. It can be affected by (1) congenital conditions, (2) structural weakness, (3) traumatic and stress injuries, and (4) systemic conditions such as diabetes mellitus and rheumatoid arthritis. Much of the pain, deformity, and disability associated with foot disorders can be directly attributed to or accentuated by improperly fitting shoes, which cause crowding and angulation of the toes and inhibit the normal movement of foot muscles.

The purposes of footwear are to (1) provide support, foot stability, protection, shock absorption, and a foundation for orthoses; (2) increase friction with the walking surface; and (3) treat foot abnormalities. (Table 64-11 summarizes common foot disorders.)

NURSING MANAGEMENT FOOT DISORDERS

NURSING IMPLEMENTATION

HEALTH PROMOTION. Well-constructed and properly fitted shoes are essential for healthy, pain-free feet. The selection of footwear for women is often influenced by fashion styles instead of comfort and support. Stress the importance of having a shoe that conforms to the foot rather than to current fashion trends. The shoe must be long enough and wide enough to avoid crowding the toes and forcing the great toe into a position of

hallux valgus (Fig. 64-6). At the metatarsal head, the shoe should be wide enough to allow foot muscles to move freely and toes to bend. The shank (narrow part of sole under the instep) of the shoe should be rigid enough to give optimal support. The height of the heel should be realistic in relation to the purpose for which the shoe is worn. Ideally, the heel of the shoe should not rise more than 1 in higher than the forefoot support. Wearing higher heeled shoes with a narrow toe box will cause hammertoes and corns over time.[23]

ACUTE INTERVENTION. Many foot problems require a referral to a podiatrist. Depending on the problem, conservative therapies are usually tried first (see Table 64-11). These therapies include NSAIDs, shock-wave therapy, icing, physical therapy, alterations in footwear, stretching, warm soaks, orthotics, ultrasound, and corticosteroid injections. If these methods do not provide relief, then surgery may be recommended.

Depending on the type of surgery performed, pins or wires may extend through the toes, or a protective splint that extends over the end of the foot may be in place. Postoperatively, the foot is usually immobilized by a bulky dressing (Fig. 64-7), short leg cast, slipper (plaster) cast, or a platform "shoe" that fits over the dressing and has a rigid sole (known as a bunion boot).

The foot should be elevated with the heel off the bed to help reduce discomfort and prevent edema. Assess neurovascular status frequently during the immediate postoperative period. The devices inserted may interfere with or preclude assessment for movement. Also be aware that sensation may be hard to evaluate because the patient may have difficulty differentiating pain from surgery and that caused by nerve pressure or circulatory impairment.

A   B

FIG. 64-6 A, Severe hallux valgus with bursa formation. **B,** Postoperative correction.

FIG. 64-7 Postoperative supportive dressing for a moderate forefoot deformity. Dressing must be conforming and binding enough to hold toe in exact position.

TABLE 64-11	COMMON FOOT DISORDERS	
Disorder	**Description**	**Treatment**
Forefoot		
Hallux valgus (bunion)	Painful deformity of great toe consisting of lateral angulation of great toe toward second toe, bony enlargement of medial side of first metatarsal head, swelling of bursa and formation of callus over bony enlargement (see Fig. 64-6).	Conservative treatment includes wearing shoes with wide forefoot or "bunion pocket" and use of bunion pads to relieve pressure on bursal sac. Surgical treatment is removal of bursal sac and bony enlargement and correction of lateral angulation of great toe. May include temporary or permanent internal fixation.
Hallux rigidus	Painful stiffness of first MTP joint caused by osteoarthritis or local trauma.	Conservative treatment includes intraarticular corticosteroids and passive manual stretching of first MTP joint. A shoe with a stiff sole decreases pain in the joint during walking. Surgical treatment is joint fusion or arthroplasty with silicone rubber implant.
Hammer toe	Deformity of the 2nd to 5th toes, including flexion deformity of PIP and DIP joints, hyperextension of MTP joint, flexion deformity of DIP joint alone (mallet toe). Callus formation and flexion of PIP and DIP joint hyperextension (claw toe). Complaints related to hammer toe include burning on bottom of foot and pain and difficulty walking when wearing shoes.	Conservative treatment consists of passive manual stretching of PIP joint and use of metatarsal arch support. Surgical correction consists of resection of base of middle phalanx and head of proximal phalanx and bringing raw bone ends together. Kirschner wire maintains straight position.
Morton's neuroma (Morton's toe or plantar neuroma)	Neuroma in web space between third and fourth metatarsal heads, causing sharp, sudden attacks of pain and burning sensations.	Surgical excision is the usual treatment.
Midfoot		
Pes planus (flatfoot)	Loss of metatarsal arch causing pain in foot or leg.	Symptoms are relieved by use of resilient longitudinal arch supports. Surgical treatment consists of triple arthrodesis or fusion of subtalar joint.
Pes cavus	Elevation of longitudinal arch of foot resulting from contracture of plantar fascia or bony deformity of arch.	Surgical correction is necessary if it interferes with ambulation.
Hindfoot		
Painful heels	Complaint of heel pain with weight bearing. Common causes are plantar bursitis, plantar fasciitis, or bone spur.	Corticosteroids are injected locally into inflamed bursa, and sponge-rubber heel cup is used. Surgical excision of bursa or spur is performed. For plantar fasciitis stretching exercises, ice, shoe heel cup, shock-wave therapy, NSAIDs, and corticosteroids are used.
Calcaneus stress fracture	Complaint of heel pain after moderate walking. Common causes are overtraining, running on hard surfaces, or osteoporosis.	Rest, ice, shoe heel pad, and NSAIDs are used. See health care provider to assess for osteoporosis.
Other Problems		
Corn	Localized thickening of skin caused by continual pressure over bony prominences, especially metatarsal head, frequently causing localized pain.	Corn is softened with warm water or preparations containing salicylic acid and trimmed with razor blade or scalpel. Pressure on bony prominences caused by shoes is relieved.
Soft corn	Painful lesion caused by bony prominence of one toe pressing against adjacent toe. Usual location is web space between toes. Softness caused by secretions keeping web space relatively moist.	Pain is relieved by placing cotton or spacers between toes to separate them. Surgical treatment is excision of projecting bone spur (if present).
Callus	Similar formation to corn but covering wider area and usually located on weight-bearing part of foot.	Same as for corn.
Plantar wart	Painful papillomatous growth caused by virus that may occur on any part of skin on sole of foot. Tend to cluster on pressure points.	Remedies containing salicylic acid (e.g., Compound W), excision with electrocoagulation, or surgical removal. Laser treatments may also be used. May disappear without treatment.

DIP, Distal interphalangeal; *MTP,* metatarsophalangeal; *PIP,* proximal interphalangeal.

The type and extent of surgery determine the degree of ambulation allowed. Crutches, a walker, or a cane may be necessary. The patient may experience pain or a throbbing sensation when starting ambulation. Reinforce instructions given by the physical therapist and the importance of walking with an erect posture and with proper weight distribution. Report dysfunction of gait or continued pain to the physician. Instruct the patient on the importance of frequent rest periods with the foot elevated.

AMBULATORY AND HOME CARE. Foot care should include performing daily hygienic care and wearing clean stockings. Stockings should be long enough to avoid wrinkling and causing pressure areas. Trimming toenails straight across helps prevent ingrown toenails and reduces the possibility of infection. Provide detailed instruction to persons with impaired circulation or diabetes mellitus to prevent serious complications associated with blisters, pressure areas, and infections. (See Table 49-21 for guidelines on foot care.)

GERONTOLOGIC CONSIDERATIONS

FOOT PROBLEMS

The older adult is prone to developing foot problems because of poor circulation, atherosclerosis, and decreased sensation in the lower extremities. This is especially a problem for older patients with diabetes mellitus.[24] A patient may develop an open wound but not feel it because of altered sensation. This may be the result of peripheral vascular disease or diabetic neuropathy. Instruct older adults to inspect their feet daily and report any open wounds or breaks in the skin to their health care provider.[25] If left untreated, wounds may become infected, lead to osteomyelitis, and require surgical debridement. If the infection becomes widespread, lower limb amputation may be necessary. Teach the caregiver of the older adult who needs assistance with hygiene practices the importance of carefully assessing the feet at regular intervals.

METABOLIC BONE DISEASES

Normal bone metabolism is affected by hormones, nutrition, and genetic factors. When dysfunction occurs in any of these factors, a generalized reduction in bone mass and strength may result. Metabolic bone diseases include osteomalacia, osteoporosis, and Paget's disease.

OSTEOMALACIA

Osteomalacia is caused by a vitamin D deficiency, resulting in decalcification and softening of bones. In the United States it is an uncommon disease. This disease is the same as rickets in children except that the epiphyseal growth plates are closed in the adult. Vitamin D is required for the absorption of calcium from the intestine. Insufficient vitamin D intake can interfere with the normal mineralization of bone; with little or no calcification, bone softening results.

Causes of osteomalacia include lack of exposure to ultraviolet rays (which is needed for vitamin D synthesis), GI malabsorption, extensive burns, chronic diarrhea, pregnancy, kidney disease, and drugs such as phenytoin (Dilantin). Morbidly obese persons are at higher risk for developing osteomalacia because of inadequate calcium intake, decreased physical activity, vitamin D deficiency, coexisting chronic diseases (e.g., hyperlipidemia), and the use of medications associated with these diseases (e.g., cholestyramine [Questran]).[26]

Common manifestations of osteomalacia are bone pain, difficulty rising from a chair, and difficulty walking.[27] Other manifestations include muscular weakness, especially in the pelvic girdle; weight loss; and progressive deformities of the spine (*kyphosis*) or extremities. Fractures are common and indicate delayed bone healing.

Laboratory findings commonly include decreased serum calcium or phosphorus levels, decreased serum 25-hydroxyvitamin D, and elevated serum alkaline phosphatase. X-rays may demonstrate the effects of generalized bone demineralization, especially loss of calcium in the bones of the pelvis and associated bone deformity. *Looser's transformation zones* (ribbons of decalcification in bone found on x-ray) are diagnostic of osteomalacia. However, significant osteomalacia may exist without changes noted on x-ray.

Collaborative care of osteomalacia is directed toward correction of the vitamin D deficiency. When vitamin D_3 (cholecalciferol) and vitamin D_2 (ergocalciferol) are used as supplements, the patient often shows a dramatic response. Calcium salts or phosphorus supplements may also be prescribed. Encourage dietary ingestion of eggs, meat, oily fish, and milk and breakfast cereals fortified with calcium and vitamin D. Exposure to sunlight (and ultraviolet rays) is also valuable, along with weight-bearing exercise.

Patients who have bariatric surgery to treat obesity should be assessed for osteomalacia. Any vitamin D deficiencies should be corrected before surgery.[26]

OSTEOPOROSIS

Osteoporosis, or porous bone (fragile bone disease), is a chronic, progressive metabolic bone disease characterized by low bone mass and structural deterioration of bone tissue, leading to increased bone fragility (Fig. 64-8). More than 44 million persons in the United States have decreased bone density or osteoporosis.[28] One in two women and one in four men over age 50 will sustain an osteoporosis-related fracture during their lifetime. Osteoporosis is known as the "silent thief" because it slowly and insidiously over many years robs the skeleton of its banked resources. Bones can eventually become so fragile that they cannot withstand normal mechanical stress.

Osteoporosis is more common in women than in men for several reasons: (1) women tend to have lower calcium intake than men throughout their lives (men between 15 and 50 years of age consume twice as much calcium as women); (2) women have less bone mass because of their generally smaller frames; (3) bone resorption begins at an earlier age in women and is accelerated at menopause; (4) pregnancy and breastfeeding deplete a woman's skeletal reserve unless calcium intake is adequate; and (5) longevity increases the likelihood of osteoporosis.

Current guidelines recommend an initial bone scan in women before the age of 65. If the results are normal and the person is at low risk for osteoporosis, another scan is not needed for 15 years.[29] Testing should start earlier and be done more frequently if a person is at high risk for fractures (e.g., low body weight, smoker, prior fractures). Men should be screened before the age of 70 years old and by age 50 if at high risk for fractures (e.g., low body weight, hypogonadism).[30]

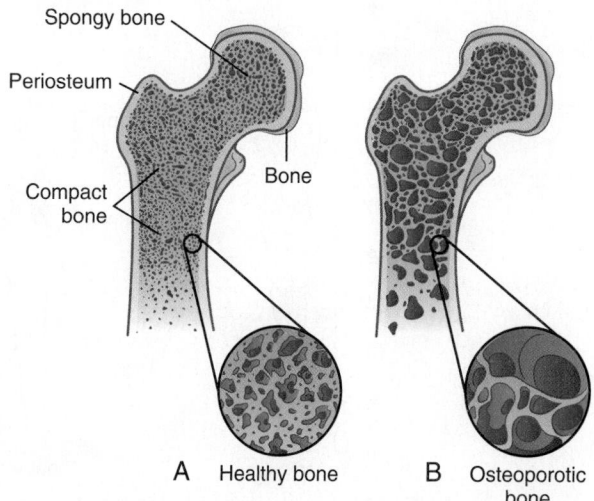

FIG. 64-8 A, Normal bone. **B,** Osteoporotic bone.

Etiology and Pathophysiology

Risk factors for osteoporosis are listed in Table 64-12. Decreased risk is associated with regular weight-bearing exercise and fluoride, calcium, and vitamin D ingestion. Low testosterone levels are a major risk factor in men.

Peak bone mass (maximum bone tissue) is primarily achieved before age 20. It is determined by a combination of four major factors: heredity, nutrition, exercise, and hormone function. Heredity may be responsible for up to 70% of a person's peak bone mass. Bone loss from midlife (ages 35 to 40 years) onward is inevitable, but the rate of loss varies. At menopause, women experience rapid bone loss when the decline in estrogen production is the sharpest. This rate of loss then slows, and eventually matches the rate of bone lost by men 65 to 70 years old.

TABLE 64-12   RISK FACTORS FOR OSTEOPOROSIS

- Advancing age (>65 yr)
- Female gender
- Low body weight
- White or Asian ethnicity
- Current cigarette smoking
- Nontraumatic fracture
- Sedentary lifestyle
- Postmenopausal (estrogen deficiency)
- Family history of osteoporosis
- Diet low in calcium or vitamin D deficiency
- Excessive use of alcohol (>2 drinks/day)
- Low testosterone level in men
- Long-term use of corticosteroids, thyroid replacements, heparin, long-acting sedatives, or antiseizure medications

Genetic factors contribute to osteoporosis by influencing not only bone mineral density but also bone size, bone quality, and bone turnover.

Bone is continuously being deposited by osteoblasts and resorbed by osteoclasts, a process called *remodeling*. Normally the rates of bone deposition and resorption are equal to one another so that the total bone mass remains constant.[31] In osteoporosis, bone resorption exceeds bone deposition.

Specific diseases associated with osteoporosis include inflammatory bowel disease, intestinal malabsorption, kidney disease, rheumatoid arthritis, hyperthyroidism, chronic alcoholism, cirrhosis of the liver, hypogonadism, and diabetes mellitus. Many drugs can interfere with bone metabolism, including corticosteroids, antiseizure drugs (e.g., divalproex sodium [Depakote], phenytoin), aluminum-containing antacids, heparin, certain cancer treatments, and excessive thyroid hormones. At the time one of these drugs is prescribed, inform the patient of this possible side effect. Long-term corticosteroid use is a major contributor to osteoporosis.

Clinical Manifestations

Osteoporosis occurs most commonly in the bones of the spine, hips, and wrists. The usual first manifestations are back pain or spontaneous fractures. The loss of bone substance causes the bone to become mechanically weakened and prone to either spontaneous fractures or fractures from minimal trauma. A person who has one spinal vertebral fracture due to osteoporosis has an increased risk of having a second vertebral fracture within 1 year. Over time, wedging and fractures of the vertebrae produce gradual loss of height and a humped back known as *kyphosis*, or "dowager's hump" (Fig. 64-9).

FIG. 64-9 The effects of osteoporosis. **A,** Comparison of young woman with an older woman. **B,** Severe fixed kyphosis producing a question-mark appearance.

Diagnostic Studies

Osteoporosis often goes unnoticed because it cannot be detected by conventional x-ray until more than 25% to 40% of calcium in the bone is lost. Serum calcium, phosphorus, and alkaline phosphatase levels usually are normal, although alkaline phosphatase may be elevated after a fracture.

Bone mineral density (BMD) measurements are typically expressed as the grams of mineral per unit volume.[32] BMD is determined by peak bone mass and amount of bone loss. (BMD measurements are presented in Table 62-7.) Types of BMD measurement include quantitative ultrasound (QUS) and dual-energy x-ray absorptiometry (DXA). QUS measures bone density with sound waves in the heel, kneecap, or shin. DXA (one of the most common BMD studies) measures bone density in the spine, hips, and forearm (the most common sites of fractures resulting from osteoporosis). DXA studies are also useful to evaluate changes in bone density over time and to assess the effectiveness of treatment.

DXA results are reported as T-scores. The T-score is the number of standard deviations below average for normal bone density. A T-score of −1 or higher indicates normal bone density. Osteoporosis is defined as a BMD of −2.5 or lower (at least 2.5 standard deviations) below the mean BMD of young adults. Osteopenia is defined as bone loss that is more than normal (a T-score between −1 and −2.5), but not yet at the level for a diagnosis of osteoporosis.

Sometimes the health care provider asks for a Z-score instead of a T-score. In this case, a person is compared with someone his or her own age and/or ethnic group instead of an individual in the best of health at 30 years of age. A Z-score that is less than −2.0 indicates a bone density problem.

NURSING AND COLLABORATIVE MANAGEMENT OSTEOPOROSIS

Collaborative care for osteoporosis focuses on proper nutrition, calcium supplementation, exercise, prevention of falls and fractures, and drugs (Table 64-13). The National Osteoporosis Foundation *(www.nof.org)* recommends treatment for osteoporosis for postmenopausal women who have (1) a T-score of less than −2.5, (2) a T-score between −1 and −2.5 with additional risk factors (see Table 64-12), or (3) prior history of a hip or vertebral fracture.

A patient's risk of fracture from osteoporosis can also be calculated with the Fracture Risk Assessment (FRAX) tool *(www.shef.ac.uk/FRAX)*. The FRAX takes into account BMD and additional clinical factors when assessing fracture risk.[33]

Prevention and treatment of osteoporosis focuses on adequate calcium intake (1000 mg/day in premenopausal women and postmenopausal women taking estrogen, and 1500 mg/day in postmenopausal women who are not receiving supplemental estrogen). Foods that are high in calcium content include whole and skim milk, yogurt, turnip greens, cottage cheese, ice cream, sardines, and spinach (Table 64-14). If dietary intake of calcium is inadequate, supplemental calcium may be recommended. Calcium is difficult to absorb in single doses greater than 500 mg.[34] Teach the patient the importance of taking supplemental calcium in divided doses with food. The amount of elemental calcium varies in different calcium preparations (Table 64-15).

Vitamin D is important in calcium absorption and function and may also have a role in bone formation. Most people get

TABLE 64-13 COLLABORATIVE CARE
Osteoporosis

Diagnostic
- History and physical examination
- Serum calcium, phosphorus, alkaline phosphatase, and vitamin D levels
- Bone mineral densitometry
  - Dual-energy x-ray absorptiometry (DXA)
  - Quantitative ultrasound (QUS)

Collaborative Therapy
- Diet high in calcium (see Table 64-14)
- Calcium supplements (see Table 64-15)
- Vitamin D supplements
- Exercise program
- Drug therapy
  - Bisphosphonates
    - alendronate (Fosamax, Binosto)
    - clodronate (Bonefos)
    - etidronate (Didronel)
    - ibandronate (Boniva)
    - pamidronate (Aredia)
    - risedronate (Actonel)
    - tiludronate (Skelid)
    - zoledronic acid (Reclast)
  - salmon calcitonin (Calcimar)
  - Selective estrogen receptor modulator (e.g., raloxifene [Evista])
  - Recombinant form of parathyroid hormone (e.g., teriparatide [Forteo])
  - denosumab (Prolia)
- Minimally invasive procedures
  - Vertebroplasty
  - Kyphoplasty

TABLE 64-14 NUTRITIONAL THERAPY
Sources of Calcium

Food	Calcium (mg)	Food	Calcium (mg)
Good Sources		**Good Sources—cont'd**	
1 cup milk		1 med stalk cooked broccoli	158
• Whole	291	1 cup cooked spinach	200
• Skim	302	1 cup almonds	304
1 oz cheese			
• American	174	**Poor Sources**	
• Cheddar	130	Egg	28
• Cottage	130	3 oz beef, pork, poultry	10
8 oz yogurt	415	Apple, banana	10
1 cup ice cream	176	1 med potato	14
• Soft serve	272	1 med carrot	14
3 oz seafood		¼ head lettuce	27
• Salmon	167		
• Oysters	113		

enough vitamin D from their diet or naturally through synthesis in the skin from exposure to sunlight. Being in the sun for 20 minutes a day is generally enough. However, supplemental vitamin D (800 to 1000 IU) is recommended for postmenopausal women, older men, those who are homebound, and those who get minimal sun exposure.

Regular physical activity is important to build up and maintain bone mass.[35] Exercise also increases muscle strength, coordination, and balance. The best exercises are weight-bearing exercises that force an individual to work against gravity. These

TABLE 64-15 ELEMENTAL CALCIUM CONTENT OF CALCIUM PREPARATIONS

Calcium Preparation	Elemental Calcium Content
Calcium carbonate (Tums 500)	500 mg/tablet
Calcium carbonate + 5 mcg vitamin D_2 (Os-Cal 250)	250 mg/tablet
Calcium gluconate	40 mg/500 mg
Calcium carbonate	400 mg/g
Calcium lactate	80 mg/600 mg
Calcium citrate	40 mg/300 mg

exercises include walking, hiking, weight training, stair climbing, tennis, and dancing. Walking is preferred to high-impact aerobics or running, both of which may put too much stress on the bones, resulting in stress fractures. Walking 30 minutes, three times a week is recommended. Instruct patients to quit smoking and cut down on alcohol intake to decrease the likelihood of losing bone mass.

Although loss of bone cannot be significantly reversed, further loss can be prevented if the patient follows a regimen of calcium and vitamin D supplementation, exercise, and drugs (see Table 64-13) if indicated. Make an effort to keep patients with osteoporosis ambulatory to prevent further loss of bone substance as a result of immobility.

Treatment may also involve the use of a gait aid as needed and to protect areas of potential pathologic fractures. For example, a thoracic-lumbar-sacral orthosis (TLSO) brace may be used to maintain the spine in proper alignment after a fracture or treatment of a vertebral fracture. (Fractures are discussed in Chapter 63.)

Vertebroplasty and *kyphoplasty* are minimally invasive procedures used to treat osteoporotic vertebral fractures[36] (see Chapter 63). In vertebroplasty, bone cement is injected into the collapsed vertebra to stabilize it, but it does not correct the deformity. In kyphoplasty, an air bladder is inserted into the collapsed vertebra and inflated to regain vertebral body height, and then bone cement is injected.

DRUG THERAPY

Estrogen therapy after menopause is no longer given as a primary treatment to prevent osteoporosis because it is associated with an increased risk of heart disease and breast and uterine cancer. If estrogen therapy is being used to treat menopausal symptoms, it also protects the woman against bone loss and fractures of the hip and vertebrae.[37] It is believed that estrogen inhibits osteoclast activity, leading to decreased bone resorption and preventing both cortical and trabecular bone loss.

Bisphosphonates inhibit osteoclast-mediated bone resorption, thereby increasing total bone mass and BMD. These drugs, which are widely used in the treatment of osteoporosis,[38] are listed in Table 64-13. Common side effects are anorexia, weight loss, and gastritis. Instruct patients on the proper administration of a bisphosphonate to aid in its absorption (see Drug Alert). These precautions have been shown to decrease GI side effects (especially esophageal irritation) and increase absorption. A rare and serious side effect of bisphosphonates is jaw osteonecrosis (bone death). The etiology of this side effect is unknown.

EVIDENCE-BASED PRACTICE

Applying the Evidence

R.F. is a 76-yr-old white woman who fell in her home and sustained a hip fracture. Her recent laboratory work shows a vitamin D deficiency. You discuss her options for improving this deficiency. She tells you that she is moving to Arizona to be with her daughter and is planning to spend "many hours in the sun" every day.

Best Available Evidence	Clinician Expertise	Patient Preferences and Values
Postmenopausal women should receive 1500 mg of calcium and 800–1000 IU of vitamin D daily. Dietary sources and supplements should be used to meet these requirements.	You have worked with many patients recovering from fractures related to osteoporosis. You review R.F.'s usual diet and determine that it is deficient in calcium and vitamin D.	Patient prefers sun exposure over changing her diet (she is a vegetarian) or taking supplements.

Your Action and Decision

You discuss the risks associated with daily sun exposure and that sun exposure will not correct a calcium deficiency. R.F. tells you she understands but wants to try before taking "any more pills." You explain the importance of adding foods high in calcium to her diet. You provide her with a list of some choices that meet her vegetarian diet restrictions.

Reference for Evidence

National Institutes of Health: Dietary supplement fact sheet: vitamin D. Retrieved from *www.ods.od.nih.gov/factsheets/VitaminD-Quick Facts.*

DRUG ALERT: Bisphosphonates
- Instruct patient to
  - Take with full glass of water.
  - Take 30 min before food or other medications.
  - Remain upright for at least 30 min after taking.

Alendronate (Fosamax) is available as a once-per-week oral tablet. Ibandronate (Boniva) and risedronate (Actonel) are available as once-per-month oral tablets. Zoledronic acid (Reclast) is approved for a once-yearly IV infusion and can prevent osteoporosis for 2 years after a single infusion. Flu-like symptoms may occur for the first few days after administration of the drug.

Calcitonin is secreted by the thyroid gland and inhibits osteoclastic bone resorption by directly interacting with active osteoclasts. Salmon calcitonin (Calcimar) is available in intramuscular (IM), subcutaneous, and intranasal forms. Administration of the IM or subcutaneous form of the drug at night has been shown to decrease the side effects of nausea and facial flushing associated with this drug. Nausea does not occur with the nasal spray. If patients are using the nasal form, teach them to alternate nostrils daily. Nasal dryness and irritation are the most frequent side effects. When calcitonin is used, calcium supplementation is necessary to prevent secondary hyperparathyroidism.

Another type of drug used in treating osteoporosis is raloxifene (Evista), which is a selective estrogen receptor modulator (SERM). This drug mimics the effect of estrogen on bone by reducing bone resorption without stimulating the tissues of the breast or uterus. Raloxifene in postmenopausal women significantly increases BMD. Side effects included leg cramps, hot flashes, and blood clots. Raloxifene may decrease breast cancer risk. Similar to tamoxifen, it blocks the estrogen receptor sites of cancer cells.

Teriparatide (Forteo), which is a recombinant form of human parathyroid hormone (PTH), increases the action of osteoblasts. This drug is used to treat osteoporosis in men and postmenopausal women at high risk for fractures. Teriparatide is the first drug approved for the treatment of osteoporosis that stimulates new bone formation (most drugs prevent further bone loss). Teriparatide is administered by subcutaneous injection once a day. Side effects include leg cramps and dizziness.

Denosumab (Prolia) may be used for postmenopausal women with osteoporosis who are at high risk for fractures. It is a monoclonal antibody that binds to a protein (RANKL) involved in the formation and function of osteoclasts. Denosumab is given as a subcutaneous injection every 6 months.

Medical management of patients receiving corticosteroids includes prescribing the lowest effective dose and ensuring an adequate intake of calcium and vitamin D, including supplementation when osteoporosis drugs are prescribed. If osteopenia is evident on bone densitometry in people who are taking corticosteroids, treatment with bisphosphonates may be considered.

PAGET'S DISEASE

Paget's disease (osteitis deformans) is a chronic skeletal bone disorder in which excessive bone resorption is followed by replacement of normal marrow by vascular, fibrous connective tissue. The new bone is larger, disorganized, and structurally weaker. The regions of the skeleton commonly affected are pelvis, long bones, spine, ribs, sternum, and cranium. Up to 5% of adults in the United States are affected by Paget's disease.[39] The etiology is unknown, although a viral cause has been proposed. Up to 40% of all patients with Paget's disease have at least one relative with the disorder. Compared with women, men are affected 2:1.

In milder forms of Paget's disease, patients may remain free of symptoms, and the disease may be discovered incidentally on x-ray or serum chemistry findings of a high alkaline phosphatase level.[40] The initial clinical manifestations are usually insidious development of bone pain (which may progress to severe intractable pain), fatigue, and progressive development of a waddling gait. Patients may complain that they are becoming shorter or that their heads are becoming larger. Headaches, dementia, visual deficits, and loss of hearing can result with an enlarged, thickened skull. Increased bone volume in the spine can cause spinal cord or nerve root compression.

Pathologic fracture is the most common complication of Paget's disease and may be the first indication of the disease. Other complications include osteosarcoma, fibrosarcoma, and osteoclastoma (giant cell) tumors.

Serum alkaline phosphatase levels are markedly elevated (indicating high bone turnover) in advanced forms of the disease.[41] X-rays may demonstrate that the normal contour of the affected bone is curved and the bone cortex is thickened and irregular, especially the weight-bearing bones and the cranium. Bone scans using a radiolabeled bisphosphonate demonstrate increased uptake in the affected skeletal areas.

Collaborative care of Paget's disease is usually limited to symptomatic and supportive care and correction of secondary deformities by either surgical intervention or braces. Bisphosphonate drugs (see Table 64-13) are used to retard bone resorption. Zoledronic acid may also be given as a bone-building drug. Calcium and vitamin D are often given to decrease hypocalcemia, a common side effect with these drugs. Drug effectiveness may be monitored by serum alkaline phosphatase levels.

Calcitonin therapy is recommended for patients who cannot tolerate bisphosphonate drugs. Human calcitonin (Cibacalcin) inhibits osteoclastic activity, prevents bone resorption, relieves acute symptoms, and lowers the serum alkaline phosphatase levels. This drug is available as a subcutaneous injection. Salmon calcitonin can also be used as a subcutaneous or IM injection for treating Paget's disease. Salmon calcitonin has a longer half-life and greater milligram potency than human calcitonin. Response to calcitonin therapy is not permanent and often stops when therapy is discontinued.

Pain is usually managed by NSAIDs. Orthopedic surgery for fractures, hip and knee replacements, and knee realignment may be necessary.

A firm mattress should be used to provide back support and relieve pain. The patient may be required to wear a corset or light brace to relieve back pain and provide support when in the upright position. The patient should be proficient in the correct application of such devices and know how to regularly examine areas of the skin for friction damage. Discourage activities such as lifting and twisting. Physical therapy may increase muscle strength. Good body mechanics are essential. A properly balanced nutrition program is important in the management of metabolic disorders of bone, especially pertaining to vitamin D, calcium, and protein, which are necessary to ensure the availability of the components for bone formation. Initiate prevention measures such as patient teaching, use of an assistive device, and environmental changes to prevent falls and subsequent fractures.

SAFETY ALERT
To reduce the risk of patient harm resulting from falls:
- Evaluate patients for fall risk.
- Identify high-risk factors for falls, including medications and uncorrected vision.
- Take action to address any identified risks.

GERONTOLOGIC CONSIDERATIONS

METABOLIC BONE DISEASES
Osteoporosis and Paget's disease are common in older adults. Instruct patients in proper nutritional management to prevent further bone loss. Keep the patient as active as possible to slow demineralization of bone resulting from disuse or extended immobilization.

Because metabolic bone disorders increase the possibility of pathologic fractures, use extreme caution when the patient is turned or moved. Hip fractures in particular can adversely affect quality of life and may lead to admission to a long-term care facility. A supervised exercise program is an essential part of an osteoporosis treatment program. If the patient's condition permits, encourage ambulation without causing fatigue.

CASE STUDY

Osteoporosis

Jupiterimages/
Comstock/Thinkstock

Patient Profile

M.L. is a 58-yr-old white retired nurse who had a total hysterectomy and salpingo-oophorectomy for removal of a benign ovarian cyst 7 yr ago. She also has a history of a seizure disorder since childhood and Addison's disease.

Subjective Data

- Acute, severe lumbar pain and tenderness that radiate to her right hip and lateral thigh after falling and landing on her buttocks last week
- Walking and bending increases pain
- Stress fracture in wrist 5 mo ago
- Reports no noticeable loss of height
- Maternal history of osteoporosis
- Taking corticosteroids and mineralocorticoids for past 6 yr for Addison's disease
- Taking phenytoin (Dilantin) every evening
- Drinks two alcoholic beverages every evening
- Dislikes dairy products

Objective Data

- 5 ft, 7 in tall, 110 lb

Diagnostic Studies

- Tests show decreased bone mineral density at spine and hip
- Lumbar spine radiographs reveal a slightly displaced L4 compression fracture
- Normal serum calcium, phosphorus, and alkaline phosphatase levels

Collaborative Care

- L4 vertebroplasty
- Thoracic-lumbar-sacral orthosis (TLSO) brace postoperatively
- Ibandronate (Boniva) 150 mg/mo PO
- Calcium supplements 1500 mg/day PO
- High-calcium diet
- Reduce alcohol intake
- Regular low-impact weight-bearing exercise program

Discussion Questions

1. What factors increase M.L.'s risk for osteoporosis?
2. Why does walking and bending increase M.L.'s pain?
3. What is the purpose of the TLSO brace prescribed for M.L.?
4. *Priority Decision:* What are the priority teaching needs for M.L.?
5. *Delegation Decision:* Which of the following nursing personnel should be responsible for teaching M.L. related to her osteoporosis and new medication: RN, LPN/LVN, UAP?
6. How might you assist M.L. in increasing her intake of calcium?
7. Why would regular exercise be important for M.L.?
8. *Priority Decision:* Based on the assessment data presented, what are the priority nursing diagnoses? Are there any collaborative problems?
9. *Evidence-Based Practice:* M.L. asks you why taking corticosteroids increases her risk for developing osteoporosis. How would you respond to her?

ⓔvolve Answers available at *http://evolve.elsevier.com/Lewis/medsurg.*

BRIDGE TO NCLEX EXAMINATION

The number of the question corresponds to the same-numbered outcome at the beginning of the chapter.

1. A patient with osteomyelitis is treated with surgical debridement with implantation of antibiotic beads. When the patient asks why the beads are used, the nurse answers *(select all that apply)*
   a. "The beads are used to directly deliver antibiotics to the site of the infection."
   b. "There are no effective oral or IV antibiotics to treat most cases of bone infection."
   c. "This is the safest method of delivering long-term antibiotic therapy for a bone infection."
   d. "The beads are an adjunct to debridement and oral and IV antibiotics for deep infections."
   e. "The ischemia and bone death that occur with osteomyelitis are impenetrable to IV antibiotics."

2. A patient has been diagnosed with osteosarcoma of the humerus. He shows an understanding of his treatment options when he states
   a. "I accept that I have to lose my arm with surgery."
   b. "The chemotherapy before surgery will shrink the tumor."
   c. "This tumor is related to the melanoma I had 3 years ago."
   d. "I'm glad they can take out the cancer with such a small scar."

3. Which individuals would be at high risk for low back pain *(select all that apply)?*
   a. A 63-year-old man who is a long-distance truck driver
   b. A 36-year-old 6 ft, 2 in construction worker who weighs 260 lb
   c. A 28-year-old female yoga instructor who is 5 ft, 6 in and weighs 130 lb
   d. A 30-year-old male nurse who works on an orthopedic unit and smokes
   e. A 44-year-old female chef with prior compression fracture of the spine

4. The nurse's responsibility for a patient with a suspected disc herniation who is experiencing acute pain and muscle spasms is
   a. encouraging total bed rest for several days.
   b. teaching the principles of back strengthening exercises.
   c. stressing the importance of straight-leg raises to decrease pain.
   d. promoting the use of cold and hot compresses and pain medication.

5. In caring for a patient after a spinal fusion, the nurse would immediately report to the physician which patient symptom?
   a. The patient experiences a single episode of emesis.
   b. The patient is unable to move the lower extremities.
   c. The patient is nauseated and has not voided in 4 hours.
   d. The patient complains of pain at the bone graft donor site.

6. Before discharge from the same-day surgery unit, instruct the patient who has had a surgical correction of bilateral hallux valgus to
   a. rest frequently with the feet elevated.
   b. soak the feet in warm water several times a day.
   c. expect the feet to be numb for the next few days.
   d. expect continued pain in the feet, since this is not uncommon.

7. You are teaching a patient with osteopenia. What is important to include in the teaching plan?
   a. Lose weight.
   b. Stop smoking.
   c. Eat a high-protein diet.
   d. Start swimming for exercise.

1. a, 2. b, 3. a, b, d, e, 4. d, 5. b, 6. a, 7. b

evolve

For rationales to these answers and even more NCLEX review questions, visit *http://evolve.elsevier.com/Lewis/medsurg.*

REFERENCES

1. Matteson E, Osmon D: Infections of the bursae, joints, and bones. In Goldman L, Schafer A, editors: *Goldman: Goldman's Cecil medicine,* ed 24, Philadelphia, 2011, Saunders.

2. US National Library of Medicine–PubHealth: Osteomyelitis. Retrieved from *www.ncbi.nlm.nih.gov/pubmedhealth/ PMH0001473.*

3. Merck Manual Home Health Handbook: Osteomyelitis. Retrieved from *www.merckmanuals.com/home/bone _joint_and_muscle_disorders/bone_and_joint_infections/ osteomyelitis.*

4. Lehne R: *Pharmacology for nursing care,* ed 7, Philadelphia, 2012, Saunders.

5. Rao N: Treating osteomyelitis: antibiotics and surgery, *Plast Reconst Surg* 127:117S, 2011.

6. Siegel R, Naishadham D, Jemal A, et al: Cancer statistics 2012, *CA Cancer J Clin* 62:10, 2012.

*7. Anninga J, Gelderblom H, Fiocco M, et al: Chemotherapeutic adjuvant treatment for osteosarcoma: where do we stand? *Eur J Cancer* 47:2431, 2011.

8. American Cancer Society: What is bone metastasis? Retrieved from *www.cancer.org/treatment/understandingyourdiagnosis/ bonemetastasis.*

9. Judge D, Kass D, Thompson W, et al: Pathophysiology and therapy of cardiac dysfunction in Duchenne muscular dystrophy, *Am J Cardiovasc Drugs* 11:287, 2011.

10. Abdel-Hamid H, Clemens P: Pharmacological therapies for muscular dystrophies, *Curr Opin Neurol* 25:604, 2012.

11. National Institute of Neurological Disorders and Stroke: Low back pain, National Institutes of Health. Retrieved from *www.ninds.nih.gov/disorders/backpain.*

*12. Graham P, Dougherty J: Oh, their aching backs! Occupational injuries in nursing assistants, *Orthop Nurs* 31:218, 2012.

13. Cleveland Clinic: Alternative approaches may help ease back pain, *Arthritis Advisor* 11:4, 2012.

14. Casazza B: Diagnosis and treatment of acute low back pain, *Am Fam Physician* 85:343, 2012.

*15. Jaromi M, Nemeth A, Kranicz J, et al: Treatment and ergonomics training of work-related lower back pain and body posture problems for nurses, *J Clin Nurs* 21(11/12):1776, 2012.

16. Johns Hopkins Medicine, Neurology and Neurosurgery: Degenerative disc disease. Retrieved from *www .hopkinsmedicine.org/neurology_neurosurgery/specialty_areas/ spine/conditions/degenerative_disc_disease.html.*

17. Dixit R: Low back pain. In Firestein G, Budd R, Gabriel S, et al, editors: *Kelley's textbook of rheumatology,* ed 9, Philadelphia, 2012, Saunders.

18. Mayo Clinic: Herniated disk. Retrieved from *www.mayoclinic .com/health/herniated-disk.*

*19. Cepoiu-Martin M, Faris P, Lorenzetti D, et al: Artificial cervical disc arthroplasty: a systematic review, *Spine* 36:E1623, 2011.

*20. Deyo R, Ching A, Matsen L, et al: Use of bone morphogenetic proteins in spinal fusion surgery for older adults with lumbar stenosis, *Spine* 37:222, 2012.

21. Cleveland Clinic: Don't let the pain in your neck get you down, *Arthritis Advisor* 10:6, 2011.

*22. Kay T, Gross A, Goldsmith CH, et al: Exercises for mechanical neck disorders, *Cochrane Database Syst Rev* 8:CD004250, 2012.

23. American Academy of Orthopedic Surgeons: Shoes: finding the right fit. Retrieved from *www.orthoinfo.aaos.org.*

24. Turns M: The diabetic foot: an overview for community nurses, *Br J Commun Nurs* 17:422, 2012.

*25. Stolt M, Suhonen R, Puukka P, et al: Foot health and self-care activities of older people in home care, *J Clin Nurs* 21:3082, 2012.

26. Williams S: Metabolic bone disease in the bariatric surgery patient, *J Obesity* 2011:634614, 2011. Retrieved from *www .hindawi.com/journals/jobes/2011/634614.*

27. Bhan A, Rao AD, Rao DS: Osteomalacia as a result of vitamin D deficiency, *Rheum Dis Clin North Am* 38:81, 2012.

28. National Osteoporosis Foundation: Debunking the myths. Retrieved from *www.nof.org/articles.*

*29. Gourlay M, Fine J, Preisser J, et al: Bone-density testing interval and transition to osteoporosis in older women, *N Engl J Med* 366:225, 2012.

*30. Watts N, Adler R, Bilezekian J, et al: Osteoporosis in men: an Endocrine Society clinical practice guideline, *J Clin Endocrinol Metab* 97:1802, 2012.

31. Armas L, Recker R: Pathophysiology of osteoporosis, *Endocrinol Metab Clin North Am* 41:475, 2012.

32. Link T: Osteoporosis imaging: state of the art and advanced imaging, *Radiology* 263:3, 2012.

33. Shuler F, Conjeski J, Kendall D, et al: Understanding the burden of osteoporosis and use of the World Health Organization FRAX, *Orthopedics* 35:798, 2012.

*Evidence-based information for clinical practice.

34. Agency for Healthcare Research and Quality: Diagnosis and treatment of osteoporosis. Retrieved from *www .guideline.gov/content.aspx?id=34270&search=treatment+ of+osteoporosis.*

35. Sutcliffe A: Management and prevention of osteoporosis, *Pract Nurse* 42:32, 2012.

36. Asenjo J, Rossel F: Vertebroplasty and kyphoplasty: new evidence adds heat to the debate, *Curr Opin Anesthesiol* 25:577, 2012.

*37. Schmidt P: The 2012 hormone therapy position statement of the North American Menopause Society, *Menopause* 19:257, 2012.

38. Schuiling K, Robinia K, Nye R: Osteoporosis update, *J Midwifery Womens Health* 56:615, 2011.

39. Chung P, Van Hul W: Paget's disease of bone: evidence for complex pathogenetic interactions, *Semin Arthritis Rheum* 41:619, 2012.

40. Cortis K, Micallef K, Mizzi A: Imaging Paget's disease of bone—from head to toe, *Clin Radiol* 66:662, 2011.

41. Klemm K, Klein M, McPherson R: Biochemical markers of bone metabolism. In Dalton H, Pincus M, editors: *McPherson: Henry's clinical diagnosis and management of laboratory methods*, ed 22, St Louis, 2011, Saunders.

RESOURCES

American Academy of Orthopedic Surgeons (AAOS)
www.aaos.org
Exercises to strengthen the back
http://orthoinfo.aaos.org/topic.cfm?topic=a00302
American College of Foot and Ankle Surgeons (ACFAS)
www.acfas.org
American Podiatric Medical Association
www.apma.org
International Osteoporosis Foundation
www.osteofound.org
Muscular Dystrophy Association (MDA)
www.mda.org
National Association of Orthopaedic Nurses (NAON)
www.orthonurse.org
National Institutes of Health (NIH) Osteoporosis and Related Bone Diseases National Resource Center
www.niams.nih.gov/Health_Info/bone
National Osteoporosis Foundation
www.nof.org
Paget Foundation
www.paget.org

*Most folks are as happy as they make up
their minds to be.*
Abraham Lincoln

Nursing Management
Arthritis and Connective Tissue Diseases

Dottie Roberts

ⓔvolve WEBSITE

http://evolve.elsevier.com/Lewis/medsurg

- NCLEX Review Questions
- Key Points
- Pre-Test
- Answer Guidelines for Case Study on p. 1593
- Rationales for Bridge to NCLEX Examination Questions

- Case Studies
  - Patient With Obesity and Osteoarthritis
  - Patient With Rheumatoid Arthritis
  - Patient With Systemic Lupus Erythematosus
- Nursing Care Plans (Customizable)
  - eNCP 65-1: Patient With Rheumatoid Arthritis
  - eNCP 65-2: Patient With Systemic Lupus Erythematosus

- Concept Map Creator
- Concept Map for Case Study on p. 1593
- Glossary
- Content Updates

eFigure
- eFig. 65-1: Comparison of hands in osteoarthritis and rheumatoid arthritis

LEARNING OUTCOMES

1. Compare and contrast the sequence of events leading to joint destruction in osteoarthritis and rheumatoid arthritis.
2. Detail the clinical manifestations, collaborative care, and nursing management of osteoarthritis and rheumatoid arthritis.
3. Describe the pathophysiology, clinical manifestations, and collaborative care of gout, Lyme disease, and septic arthritis.
4. Summarize the pathophysiology, clinical manifestations, collaborative care, and nursing management of ankylosing spondylitis, psoriatic arthritis, and reactive arthritis.
5. Differentiate the pathophysiology, clinical manifestations, collaborative care, and nursing management of systemic lupus erythematosus, scleroderma, polymyositis, dermatomyositis, and Sjögren's syndrome.
6. Explain the drug therapy and related nursing management associated with arthritis and connective tissue diseases.
7. Compare and contrast the possible etiologies, clinical manifestations, and collaborative and nursing management of fibromyalgia and chronic fatigue syndrome.

KEY TERMS

ankylosing spondylitis (AS), p. 1580
arthritis, p. 1562
chronic fatigue syndrome (CFS), p. 1592
CREST, p. 1587
dermatomyositis (DM), p. 1589
fibromyalgia, p. 1590
gout, p. 1576

Lyme disease, p. 1578
myofascial pain syndrome, p. 1590
osteoarthritis (OA), p. 1562
polymyositis (PM), p. 1589
psoriatic arthritis (PsA), p. 1581
Raynaud's phenomenon, p. 1587
rheumatoid arthritis (RA), p. 1569

septic arthritis, p. 1579
scleroderma, p. 1586
Sjögren's syndrome, p. 1590
spondyloarthropathies, p. 1580
systemic lupus erythematosus (SLE), p. 1582

Reviewed by Cheryl A. Waklatsi, RN, MSN, Assistant Professor Nursing Education, The Christ College of Nursing and Health Sciences, Cincinnati, Ohio; Jerry Harvey, RN, MS, BC, Assistant Professor of Nursing, Liberty University, Lynchburg, Virginia; and Geri B. Neuberger, EdD, APRN-CNS, Professor of Nursing, University of Kansas School of Nursing, Kansas City, Kansas.

This chapter discusses *rheumatic diseases,* which primarily affect body joints, tendons, ligaments, muscles, and bones. These diseases are often characterized by inflammation. Rheumatic diseases result from the loss of function in one or more of the connective or bone structures of the body. There are more than 100 kinds of rheumatic diseases. An estimated 46 million people in the United States have rheumatic conditions.[1]

ARTHRITIS

Arthritis, a type of rheumatic disease, involves inflammation of a joint or joints. Most forms of arthritis affect women more frequently than men.[2] The most common types of arthritis are osteoarthritis, rheumatoid arthritis, and gout.

OSTEOARTHRITIS

Osteoarthritis (OA), the most common form of joint (articular) disease in North America, is a slowly progressive noninflammatory disorder of the diarthrodial (synovial) joints. Currently 27 million Americans are affected by OA, with the numbers expected to greatly increase as the population ages.[1]

Etiology and Pathophysiology

OA involves the formation of new joint tissue in response to cartilage destruction.[3] OA is not considered a normal part of the aging process, but aging is one risk factor for disease development.[4] Cartilage destruction may actually begin between ages 20 and 30, and the majority of adults are affected by age 40. Few patients experience symptoms until after age 50 or 60, but more than half of those over 65 years of age have x-ray evidence of OA in at least one joint. After 55 years of age, women are affected by OA more often than men.[5]

OA is usually caused by a known event or condition that directly damages cartilage or causes joint instability (Table 65-1). The increased incidence of OA in aging women is believed to be due to estrogen reduction at menopause. Modifiable risk factors for OA have been identified, including obesity, which contributes to hip and knee OA. Regular moderate exercise, which also helps with weight control, has been shown to decrease the likelihood of disease development and progression. Anterior cruciate ligament injury, which is associated with quick stops and pivoting as in football and soccer, has been linked to an increased risk of knee OA.[6] Occupations that require frequent kneeling and stooping are also linked to a higher risk of knee OA.

The pathogenesis of OA is complex, with genetic, metabolic, and local factors that interact and cause a process of cartilage deterioration. OA results from cartilage damage at the level of the chondrocytes (Fig. 65-1). Progression of OA causes the normally smooth, white, translucent articular cartilage to become dull, yellow, and granular. Affected cartilage gradually becomes softer, less elastic, and less able to resist wear with heavy use.

The body's attempts at cartilage repair cannot keep up with the destruction that is occurring. Continued changes in the collagen structure of the cartilage lead to fissuring and erosion of the articular surfaces. As the central cartilage becomes thinner, cartilage and bony growth (*osteophytes*) increase at the joint margins. The resulting incongruity in joint surfaces creates an uneven distribution of stress across the joint and contributes to a reduction in motion.

Although inflammation is not characteristic of OA, a secondary synovitis may result when phagocytic cells try to rid the joint of small pieces of cartilage torn from the joint surface. These inflammatory changes contribute to the early pain and stiffness of OA. The pain of later disease results from contact between exposed bony joint surfaces after the articular cartilage has deteriorated completely.

Clinical Manifestations

Systemic. Systemic manifestations, such as fatigue, fever, and organ involvement, are not present in OA. This is an important distinction between OA and inflammatory joint disorders such as rheumatoid arthritis.

Joints. Manifestations of OA range from mild discomfort to significant disability. Joint pain is the predominant symptom and the typical reason that the patient seeks medical attention. Pain generally worsens with joint use. In the early stages of OA, joint pain is relieved by rest. However, in advanced disease the patient may complain of pain at rest or experience sleep disruptions caused by increasing joint discomfort. Pain may also become worse as the barometric pressure falls before inclement weather. As OA progresses, increasing pain can contribute significantly to disability and loss of function. The pain of OA may

TABLE 65-1	CAUSES OF OSTEOARTHRITIS
Cause	**Effects on Joint Cartilage**
Trauma	Dislocations or fractures may lead to avascular necrosis or uneven stress on cartilage.
Mechanical stress	Repetitive physical activities (e.g., sports) cause cartilage deterioration.
Inflammation	Release of enzymes in response to local inflammation can affect cartilage integrity.
Joint instability	Damage to supporting structures causes instability, placing uneven stress on articular cartilage.
Neurologic disorders	Pain and loss of reflexes from neurologic disorders, such as diabetic neuropathy and Charcot's joint, cause abnormal movements that contribute to cartilage deterioration.
Skeletal deformities	Congenital or acquired conditions such as Legg-Calvé-Perthes disease or dislocated hip contribute to cartilage deterioration.
Hematologic or endocrine disorders	Chronic hemarthrosis (e.g., hemophilia) contributes to cartilage deterioration.
Drugs	Drugs such as indomethacin (Indocin), colchicine, and corticosteroids can stimulate collagen-digesting enzymes in joint synovium.

GENDER DIFFERENCES

Osteoarthritis (OA)

Men	Women
• Before age 50, men are affected more often than women.	• After age 50, women are affected twice as often as men.
• After age 55, hip OA is more common in men than in women.	• After age 55, OA in interphalangeal joints and thumb base is more common in women than in men.
• Before age 45, knee OA is more common in men than in women.	• After age 45, knee OA is more common in women than in men.

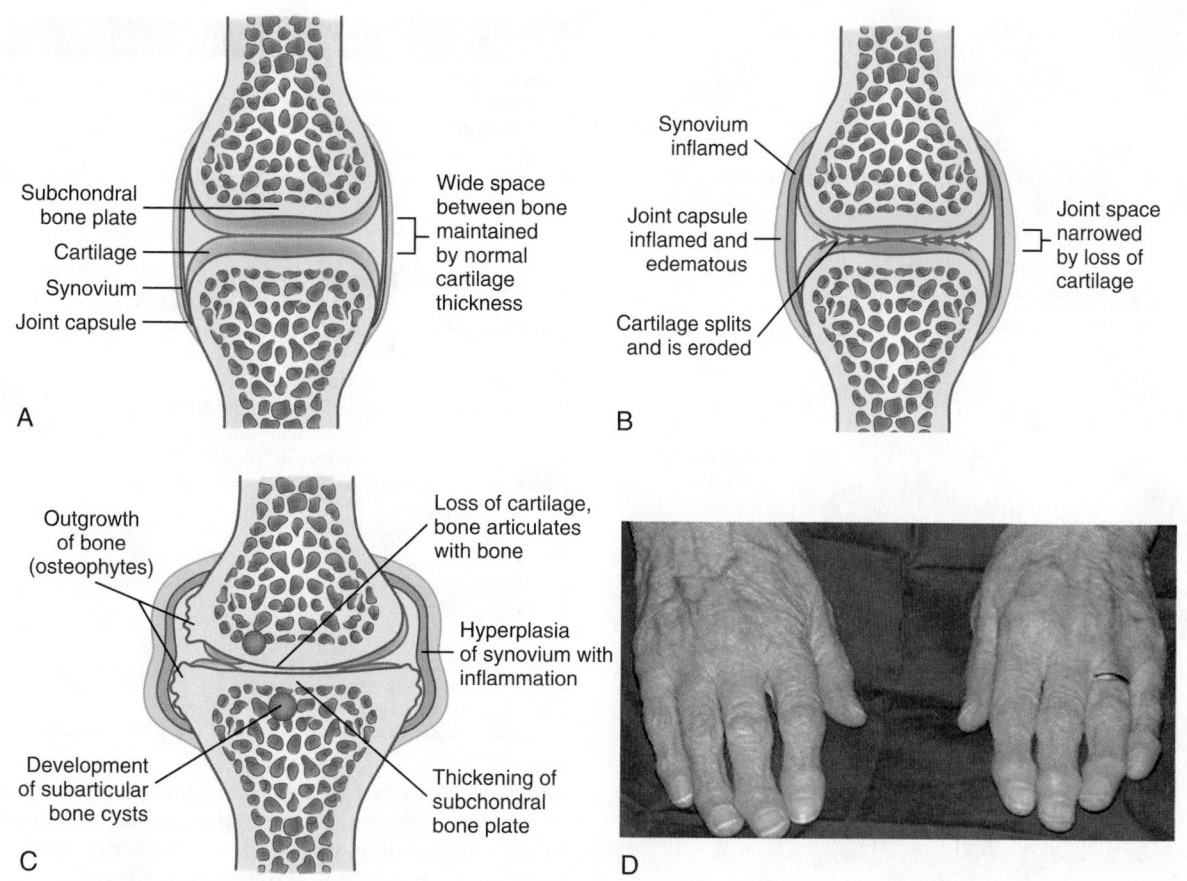

FIG. 65-1 Pathologic changes in osteoarthritis. **A,** Normal synovial joint. **B,** Early change in osteoarthritis is destruction of articular cartilage and narrowing of the joint space. There is inflammation and thickening of the joint capsule and synovium. **C,** With time, thickening of subarticular bone occurs, caused by constant friction of the two bone surfaces. Osteophytes form around the periphery of the joint by irregular overgrowths of bone. **D,** In osteoarthritis of the hands, osteophytes on the distal interphalangeal joints of the fingers, termed *Heberden's nodes,* appear as small nodules.

be referred to the groin, buttock, or medial side of the thigh or knee. Sitting down becomes difficult, as does rising from a chair when the hips are lower than the knees. As OA develops in the intervertebral (apophyseal) joints of the spine, localized pain and stiffness are common.

Unlike pain, which is typically provoked by activity, joint stiffness occurs after periods of rest or static position. Early morning stiffness is common but generally resolves within 30 minutes, a factor distinguishing OA from inflammatory arthritic disorders such as rheumatoid arthritis. Overactivity can cause a mild joint effusion that temporarily increases stiffness. *Crepitation,* a grating sensation caused by loose particles of cartilage in the joint cavity, can also contribute to stiffness. Crepitation is a common sign in patients with knee OA.

OA usually affect joints asymmetrically. The most commonly involved joints are the distal interphalangeal (DIP) and proximal interphalangeal (PIP) joints of the fingers, the metacarpophalangeal (MCP) joint of the thumb, weight-bearing joints (hips, knees), the metatarsophalangeal (MTP) joint of the foot, and the cervical and lower lumbar vertebrae (Fig. 65-2).

Deformity. Deformity or instability associated with OA is specific to the involved joint. For example, *Heberden's nodes* occur on the DIP joints as an indication of osteophyte formation and loss of joint space (see Fig. 65-1, *D*). They can appear as early as age 40 and tend to be seen in family members. *Bouchard's nodes* on the PIP joints indicate similar disease

involvement. Heberden's and Bouchard's nodes are often red, swollen, and tender. Although these bony enlargements usually do not cause significant loss of function, the patient may be distressed by the visible disfigurement.

Knee OA often leads to joint malalignment as a result of cartilage loss in the medial compartment. The patient has a characteristic bowlegged appearance and may develop an altered gait in response to the obvious deformity. In advanced hip OA, one of the patient's legs may become shorter from a loss of joint space.

Diagnostic Studies

A bone scan, computed tomography (CT) scan, or magnetic resonance imaging (MRI) may be useful to diagnose OA because of the sensitivity of these tests in detecting early joint changes. X-rays are helpful in confirming disease and staging the progression of joint damage. As OA progresses, x-rays typically show joint space narrowing, bony sclerosis, and osteophyte formation. However, these changes do not always correlate with the degree of pain that the patient experiences. Despite significant x-ray indications of disease, the patient may be relatively free of symptoms. Conversely, another patient may have severe pain with only minimal x-ray changes.

No laboratory abnormalities or biomarkers have been identified that are specific diagnostic indicators of OA. The erythrocyte sedimentation rate (ESR) is normal except in instances of

FIG. 65-2 Joints most frequently involved in osteoarthritis.

Cervical vertebrae

Lower lumbar vertebrae

Hip

Metacarpophalangeal (MCP)

Proximal interphalangeal (PIP)

Knee

Distal interphalangeal (DIP)

Metatarsophalangeal (MTP)

acute synovitis, when minimal elevations may be noted. Other routine blood tests (e.g., complete blood count [CBC], renal and liver function tests) are useful only in screening for related conditions or for establishing baseline values before the initiation of therapy. Synovial fluid analysis allows differentiation between OA and other forms of inflammatory arthritis. In OA the fluid remains clear yellow with little or no sign of inflammation.

Collaborative Care

Because OA has no cure, collaborative care focuses on managing pain and inflammation, preventing disability, and maintaining and improving joint function (Table 65-2). Nondrug interventions are the foundation for OA management and should be maintained throughout the patient's treatment period. Drug therapy serves as an adjunct to nondrug treatments.

Rest and Joint Protection. The OA patient must understand the importance of a balance of rest and activity. The affected joint should be rested during any periods of acute inflammation and maintained in a functional position with splints or braces if necessary. However, immobilization should not exceed 1 week because of the risk of joint stiffness with inactivity. The patient may need to modify his or her usual activities to decrease stress on affected joints. Teach the patient with knee OA to avoid prolonged periods of standing, kneeling, or squatting. Using an assistive device such as a cane, walker, or crutches can also help decrease stress on arthritic joints.

Heat and Cold Applications. Applications of heat and cold may help reduce complaints of pain and stiffness. Although ice

TABLE 65-2	**COLLABORATIVE CARE**

Osteoarthritis

Diagnostic
- History and physical examination
- Radiologic studies of involved joints (e.g., x-ray, CT scan, MRI, bone scan)
- Synovial fluid analysis

Collaborative Therapy
- Nutritional and weight management counseling
- Rest and joint protection, use of assistive devices
- Therapeutic exercise
- Heat and cold applications
- Complementary and alternative therapies
  - Herbs and nutritional supplements (e.g., glucosamine)
  - Movement therapies (e.g., yoga, Tai Chi)
  - Transcutaneous electrical nerve stimulation (TENS)
  - Acupuncture
- Drug therapy*
  - acetaminophen
  - Nonsteroidal antiinflammatory drugs
  - Antibiotics
  - Intraarticular hyaluronic acid
  - Intraarticular corticosteroids
  - Opioid analgesics
- Reconstructive joint surgery

*See Table 65-3.

is not used as often as heat in the treatment of OA, it can be appropriate if the patient experiences acute inflammation. Heat therapy, including hot packs, whirlpool baths, ultrasound, and paraffin wax baths, is especially helpful for stiffness.

Nutritional Therapy and Exercise. If the patient is overweight, a weight-reduction program is a critical part of the total treatment plan. Help the patient evaluate the current diet to make appropriate changes. (Chapter 41 discusses ways to assist the patient in attaining and maintaining a healthy body weight.) Because the load on the joints and the degree of joint mobilization are essential to the preservation of articular cartilage integrity, exercise is a fundamental part of OA management.[7] Aerobic conditioning, range-of-motion exercises, and specific programs for strengthening the quadriceps have been beneficial for many patients with knee OA.

Complementary and Alternative Therapies. Complementary and alternative therapies for symptom management of arthritis are popular with patients who have failed to find relief through traditional medical care. Acupuncture is effective in decreasing chronic arthritic pain.[8] Other therapies include yoga, massage, guided imagery, and therapeutic touch (see Chapters 6 and 7). Nutritional supplements such as glucosamine and chondroitin may help relieve arthritic pain and improve joint mobility in some patients[9] (see the Complementary & Alternative Therapies boxes on p. 1565).

Drug Therapy. Drug therapy is based on the severity of the patient's symptoms (Table 65-3). The patient with mild to moderate joint pain may get relief from acetaminophen (Tylenol). The patient may receive up to 1000 mg every 6 hours, with the daily dose not to exceed 4 g. A topical agent such as capsaicin cream (Zostrix) may also be beneficial, either alone or in conjunction with acetaminophen. It blocks pain by locally interfering with substance P, which is responsible for the transmission of pain impulses. A concentrated product is available by prescription, but creams of 0.025% to 0.075% capsaicin are available over the counter (OTC). Other OTC products that contain

COMPLEMENTARY & ALTERNATIVE THERAPIES
Acupuncture

Acupuncture is a traditional Chinese medical practice of inserting very fine needles into the skin to stimulate specific anatomic points in the body (called acupoints) for therapeutic purposes.

Scientific Evidence*
Moderately strong for reducing chronic pain from osteoarthritis; chronic headache; and back, neck, and shoulder pain.

Nursing Implications
• Acupuncture is an effective treatment to suggest to patients with chronic pain.
• Refer interested patients to a practitioner who is appropriately trained and licensed (see Chapter 6).

*Source: Vickers A, Cronin A, Maschino A, et al: Acupuncture for chronic pain: individual patient data meta-analysis, *Arch Int Med* 172(19):1444, 2012.

COMPLEMENTARY & ALTERNATIVE THERAPIES
Glucosamine and Chondroitin

Scientific Evidence*
• Both glucosamine and chondroitin provide some relief for moderate to severe arthritic pain but not for mild arthritic pain.
• Pain outcomes over 2 yr were similar to those of patients taking celecoxib (Celebrex) or placebo.

Nursing Implications
• Can be suggested to patients who are unable to take celecoxib or other NSAIDs.
• Discontinue if no effects after consistent use over 90-120 days.
• May decrease effectiveness of insulin or other drugs used to control blood glucose.
• May increase the risk of bleeding.

*Source: National Center for Complementary and Alternative Medicine: Glucosamine/Chondroitin Arthritis Intervention Trial (GAIT): primary and ancillary study results. Retrieved from *www.nccam.nih.gov/research/results/gait*.

TABLE 65-3 DRUG THERAPY
Arthritis and Connective Tissue Disorders*

Drug	Mechanism of Action	Nursing Considerations
Salicylates		
aspirin, salicylate (salsalate [Disalcid]) choline salicylate (Arthropan) choline magnesium trisalicylate (Trilisate)	Antiinflammatory Analgesic Antipyretic Act by inhibiting synthesis of prostaglandins	Administer drug with food, milk, antacids as prescribed, or full glass of water. May use enteric-coated aspirin. Report signs of bleeding (e.g., tarry stools, bruising, petechiae, nosebleeds).
Nonsteroidal Antiinflammatory Drugs (NSAIDs)		
ibuprofen (Motrin, Advil, Novo-Profen) naproxen (Naprosyn, Anaprox, Aleve) ketoprofen (Orudis, Actron) piroxicam (Feldene, Novo-Pirocam) indomethacin (Indocin, Indocid) sulindac (Clinoril, Apo-Sulin, NovoSundac) tolmetin (Tolectin) diclofenac (Voltaren) meclofenamate (Meclomen) nabumetone (Relafen) oxaprozin (Daypro) meloxicam (Mobic) celecoxib (Celebrex)	Antiinflammatory Analgesic Antipyretic Act by inhibiting synthesis of prostaglandins	Administer drug with food, milk, or antacids as prescribed. Report signs of bleeding (e.g., tarry stools, bruising, petechiae, nosebleeds), edema, skin rashes, persistent headaches, visual disturbances. Monitor BP for elevations related to fluid retention. Needs to be used regularly for maximal effect.
Antibiotics		
doxycycline (Vibramycin) minocycline (Minocin)	Decreases action of enzymes on cartilage degradation Antirheumatic effect possibly related to immunomodulatory/antiinflammatory properties	Possible treatment alternative with mild disease.
Topical Analgesics		
capsaicin cream (Zostrix, Capzasin-P) diclofenac sodium (Voltaren Gel)	Depletes substance P from nerve endings, interrupting pain signals to the brain Antiinflammatory Analgesic	Must be used regularly over time for maximal effect. Aloe vera cream may moderate burning sensation. Advise patient not to use cream with external heat source (heating pad) because of risk of burns. Available in OTC and prescriptive strengths. Advise patient to avoid sun and ultraviolet (UV) light exposure. Should not be used in combination with other oral NSAIDs or aspirin due to potential for increased side effects.

*eTable 65-1 presents an enhanced version of this table.
TNF-α, Tumor necrosis factor–alpha.

Continued

TABLE 65-3 DRUG THERAPY—cont'd

Arthritis and Connective Tissue Disorders*

Drug	Mechanism of Action	Nursing Considerations
Corticosteroids *Intraarticular Injections* methylprednisolone acetate (Depo-Medrol) triamcinolone (Aristospan)	Antiinflammatory Analgesic Act by inhibiting synthesis and/or release of inflammatory mediators	Use strict aseptic technique for joint fluid aspiration or corticosteroid injection. Inform patient that joint may feel worse immediately after injection. Inform patient that improvement lasts weeks to months after injection. Advise patient to avoid overusing affected joint immediately after injection.
Systemic hydrocortisone (Solu-Cortef) methylprednisolone (Solu-Medrol) dexamethasone (Decadron) prednisone triamcinolone (Aristocort)	Antiinflammatory Analgesic Act by inhibiting synthesis and/or release of inflammatory mediators	Use only in life-threatening exacerbation or when symptoms persist after treatment with less potent antiinflammatory drugs. Administer for limited time only, tapering dose slowly. Be aware that exacerbation of symptoms occurs with abrupt withdrawal of drug. Monitor BP, weight, CBC, and potassium level. Limit sodium intake. Report signs of infection.
Disease-Modifying Antirheumatic Drugs (DMARDs) methotrexate (Rheumatrex, Trexall)	Antimetabolite Inhibits DNA, RNA, protein synthesis	Monitor CBC and hepatic and renal function. Advise patient to report signs of anemia (fatigue, weakness). Keep patient well hydrated. Teratogenic effects. Inform female patient that contraception should be used during and 3 mo after treatment.
sulfasalazine (Azulfidine, Salazopyrin)	Sulfonamide Antiinflammatory Blocks prostaglandin synthesis	Advise patient that drug may cause orange-yellow discoloration of urine or skin. Space doses evenly around the clock, taking drug after food with 8 oz water. Treatment may be continued even after symptoms are relieved. Monitor CBC.
leflunomide (Arava)	Antiinflammatory Immunomodulatory agent that inhibits proliferation of lymphocytes	Monitor hepatic function. Evaluate for relief of pain, swelling, stiffness, and increase in joint mobility. Advise women of childbearing age to avoid pregnancy.
penicillamine (Cuprimine, Depen)	Antiinflammatory Exact mechanism unknown but may suppress cell-mediated immune response	Monitor WBC count, platelets, urinalysis. Advise patient to take medication 1 hr before or 2 hr after meals or at least 1 hr away from any other drug, food, or milk.
Gold Compounds *Parenteral:* gold sodium thiomalate (Myochrysine), aurothioglucose (Solganal) *Oral:* auranofin (Ridaura)	Alter immune responses, suppressing synovitis of active RA	Rule out pregnancy before beginning treatment. Monitor CBC, urinalysis, and hepatic and renal function. Advise patient that therapeutic response may not occur for 3-6 mo. Advise patient to immediately report pruritus, rash, sore mouth, indigestion, or metallic taste.
Antimalarials hydroxychloroquine (Plaquenil)	Exact mechanism unknown but may suppress formation of antigens	Monitor CBC and hepatic function. Advise patient that therapeutic response may not occur for up to 6 mo. Advise patient to immediately report visual difficulties, muscular weakness, and decreased hearing or tinnitus.
Immunosuppressants azathioprine (Imuran) cyclophosphamide (Cytoxan)	Inhibit DNA, RNA, protein synthesis	Evaluate for relief of pain, swelling, stiffness, and increase in joint mobility. Advise patient to immediately report unusual bleeding or bruising. Advise patient that therapeutic response may take up to 12 wk. Advise women of childbearing age to avoid pregnancy. Encourage increased fluid intake to decrease risk of hemorrhagic cystitis.
mycophenolate mofetil (CellCept)	Inhibits DNA synthesis	Monitor blood count and liver function tests every 2–4 wk for first 3 mo of treatment, thereafter every 1–3 mo. Inform patient of increased infection risk. Instruct patients not to take antacids at same time, since they may interfere with absorption of immunosuppressant.
JAK (Janus Kinase) Inhibitors tofacitinib (Xeljanz)	Inhibits the action of the JAK enzymes, which are signaling pathways inside the cell and have an important role in the inflammation involved in RA	Patients are at increased risk of serious infections, including opportunistic infections. Monitor patient for any sign or symptom of infection so it can be treated early.

TABLE 65-3 DRUG THERAPY—cont'd

Arthritis and Connective Tissue Disorders*

Drug	Mechanism of Action	Nursing Considerations
Biologic and Targeted Therapies		
Tumor Necrosis Factor (TNF) Inhibitors		
etanercept (Enbrel) infliximab (Remicade) adalimumab (Humira) certolizumab (Cimzia) golimumab (Simponi)	Bind to TNF, thus blocking its interaction with TNF cell surface receptors. Decrease inflammatory and immune responses	Evaluate for relief of pain, swelling, stiffness, and increase in joint mobility. Advise patient of increased risk for tuberculosis. Instruct patient to have yearly PPD. Monitor for infection, bleeding, and emergence of malignancies. Advise patient psoriasis may worsen. Advise patient that injection site reaction generally occurs in first month of treatment and decreases with continued therapy. Advise patient to not receive live virus vaccines during treatment.
Interleukin-1 Receptor Antagonist		
anakinra (Kineret)	Blocks the action of interleukin-1, thus decreasing inflammatory response	Evaluate for relief of pain, swelling, stiffness, and increase in joint mobility. Advise patient that injection site reaction generally occurs in first month of treatment and decreases with continued therapy. Evaluate renal function. Monitor for infection. Do not take drug with TNF inhibitors.
Interleukin-6 Receptor Antagonist		
tocilizumab (Actemra)	Blocks action of interleukin-6, thus decreasing inflammatory response	Given to patients with RA who have failed other therapies. Monitor BP and for infection. Advise patient of GI effects (e.g., perforation). Monitor liver enzyme and low-density lipoprotein (LDL) levels.
T Cell Activation Inhibitor		
abatacept (Orencia)	Inhibits T cell activation, thus suppressing immune response	Not recommended for concomitant use with TNF inhibitors. Evaluate for relief of pain, swelling, stiffness, and increase in joint mobility.
B Cell Depleting Agent		
rituximab (Rituxan)	Monoclonal antibody that binds to CD20, an antigen on B cells, destroying B cells and suppressing immune response	Monitor for infection and bleeding. Advise patient to not receive live virus vaccines with treatment. Monitor for low BP if also taking BP medication. Advise patient that fatigue is common with this medication.

camphor, eucalyptus oil, and menthol (e.g., BenGay, Arthricare) may also provide temporary pain relief. Topical salicylates (e.g., Aspercreme) that can be absorbed into the blood are an alternative for patients who are able to take aspirin-containing medication. Because effects of topical agents are not sustained, several applications may be needed daily.

For the patient who fails to obtain adequate pain management with acetaminophen or for a patient with moderate to severe OA pain or signs of joint inflammation, a nonsteroidal antiinflammatory drug (NSAID) may be more effective for pain treatment. NSAID therapy typically is initiated in low-dose OTC strengths (ibuprofen [Motrin, Advil] 200 mg up to four times daily), with the dose increased as symptoms indicate. If the patient is at risk for or experiences gastrointestinal (GI) side effects with a conventional NSAID, supplemental treatment with a protective agent such as misoprostol (Cytotec) may be indicated. Arthrotec, a combination of misoprostol and the NSAID diclofenac, is also available. Diclofenac gel may be applied to the affected joint.

Because traditional NSAIDs block the production of prostaglandins from arachidonic acid by inhibiting the production of cyclooxygenase-1 (COX-1) and cyclooxygenase-2 (COX-2) (see Fig. 12-2), the risk for GI erosion and bleeding is increased. Traditional NSAIDs affect platelet aggregation, leading to a prolonged bleeding time. Patients taking both warfarin (Couma-

din) and an NSAID are at high risk for bleeding. Concerns have also been raised regarding the possible negative effects of long-term NSAID treatment on cartilage metabolism, particularly in older patients who may already have diminished cartilage integrity. As an alternative to traditional NSAIDs, treatment with the COX-2 inhibitor celecoxib (Celebrex) may be considered in selected patients.

When given in equivalent antiinflammatory dosages, all NSAIDs are considered comparable in efficacy but vary widely in cost. Individual responses to the NSAIDs are also variable. Some patients still prefer aspirin, but it is no longer a common treatment and should not be used in combination with NSAIDs because both inhibit platelet function and prolong bleeding time. Intraarticular injections of corticosteroids may be appropriate for the patient with local inflammation and effusion. Four or more injections without relief suggest the need for additional intervention. Systemic use of corticosteroids is not indicated and may actually accelerate the disease process.

Another treatment for mild to moderate knee OA is hyaluronic acid (HA), a type of viscosupplementation. HA is found in normal joint fluid and articular cartilage. It contributes to both the viscosity and elasticity of synovial fluid, and its degradation can result in joint damage. Synthetic and naturally occurring HA derivatives (Orthovisc, Synvisc, Supartz, Nuflexxa, Hyalgan) are administered in three weekly injections directly into the joint space. Synvisc-1, a newer single-injection HA drug, may offer pain relief for up to 6 months. HA may also be added to oral supplements of glucosamine, chondroitin, and methylsulfonylmethane (MSM). Few side effects have been reported with HA.

Medications thought to slow the progression of OA or support joint healing are known as disease-modifying osteoarthritis drugs (DMOADs). To date, no drugs have been approved to modify OA progression despite numerous clinical trials. A variety of molecular targets are under investigation, including the use of anticatabolic agents to stimulate new cartilage growth and slow OA progression.[10]

Surgical Therapy. Symptoms of disease are often managed conservatively for many years, but the patient's loss of joint function, unrelieved pain, and diminished ability to independently perform self-care may prompt a recommendation for surgery. In patients less than 55 years of age, arthroscopic surgery for knee OA may delay the need for more serious surgery, such as a knee replacement. The main indication for arthroscopic surgery for OA is to remove debris (e.g., bits of cartilage known as loose bodies) that may be causing problems with joint motion. Reconstructive surgical procedures (e.g., hip and knee replacements) are discussed in Chapter 63.

NURSING MANAGEMENT
OSTEOARTHRITIS

NURSING ASSESSMENT

Carefully assess and document the type, location, severity, frequency, and duration of the patient's joint pain and stiffness. Also question the patient about the extent to which these symptoms affect the ability to perform activities of daily living. Note pain management practices and question the patient about the duration and success of each treatment. Physical examination of the affected joint or joints includes assessment of tenderness, swelling, limitation of movement, and crepitation. Compare an involved joint with the contralateral joint if it is not affected.

NURSING DIAGNOSES

Nursing diagnoses for the patient with OA may include, but are not limited to, the following:

- Acute and chronic pain *related to* physical activity and lack of knowledge of pain self-management techniques
- Impaired physical mobility *related to* weakness, stiffness, or pain on ambulation
- Imbalanced nutrition: more than body requirements *related to* intake in excess of energy output
- Depression *related to* chronic pain, changing physical appearance, and impaired social and work roles

PLANNING

The overall goals are that the patient with OA will (1) maintain or improve joint function through a balance of rest and activity, (2) use joint protection measures (Table 65-4) to improve activity tolerance, (3) achieve independence in self-care and maintain optimal role function, and (4) use drug and nondrug strategies to manage pain satisfactorily.

NURSING IMPLEMENTATION

HEALTH PROMOTION. Prevention of OA is possible in many cases. Community education should focus on altering modifiable risk factors by losing weight and reducing occupational and

---

TABLE 65-4 PATIENT & CAREGIVER TEACHING GUIDE

Joint Protection and Energy Conservation

Include the following instructions when teaching patients with arthritis to protect joints and conserve energy.

- Maintain appropriate weight.
- Use assistive devices, if indicated.
- Avoid forceful repetitive movements.
- Avoid positions of joint deviation and stress.
- Use good posture and proper body mechanics.
- Seek assistance with necessary tasks that may cause pain.
- Develop organizing and pacing techniques for routine tasks.
- Modify home and work environment to create less stressful ways to perform tasks.

HEALTHY PEOPLE

Prevention of Osteoarthritis

- Avoid trauma to joints.
- Avoid cigarette smoking.
- Maintain healthy weight.
- Use safety measures to protect and decrease risk of injury to joints.
- Exercise regularly, including strength and endurance training.

---

recreational hazards. Athletic instruction and physical fitness programs should include safety measures that protect and reduce trauma to the joints. Traumatic joint injuries should be treated promptly to prevent the development of OA.

ACUTE INTERVENTION. The person with OA most often complains of pain, stiffness, limitation of function, and the frustration of coping with these physical difficulties on a daily basis. The older adult may believe that OA is an inevitable part of aging and that nothing can be done to ease the discomfort and related disability.

The patient with OA is usually treated on an outpatient basis, often by an interdisciplinary team of health care providers that may include an internal medicine physician or family health care provider, a rheumatologist, a nurse, an occupational therapist, and a physical therapist. Health assessment questionnaires are often used to pinpoint areas of decreased function. Complete questionnaires at regular intervals to document disease and treatment progression. Treatment goals can be developed based on data from the questionnaires and the physical examination, with specific interventions to target identified problems. The patient is usually hospitalized only if joint surgery is planned (see Chapter 63).

Drugs are administered for the treatment of pain and inflammation. Nondrug strategies to decrease pain and disability may include gentle exercise, the application of heat (thermal packs) or cold (ice packs), relaxation, and yoga.[11] Splints may be prescribed to rest and stabilize painful or inflamed joints.

Once an acute flare has subsided, a physical therapist can provide valuable assistance in planning an exercise program. Therapists may recommend Tai Chi as a low-impact form of exercise. Tai Chi can be performed by patients of all ages and may be done in a wheelchair. Emphasize the importance of warming up before any exercise to prevent stretch injuries.

Patient and caregiver teaching related to OA is an important nursing responsibility. Provide information about the nature and treatment of the disease, pain management, body mechanics, correct use of assistive devices (e.g., cane, walker), principles of joint protection and energy conservation (see Table 65-4), nutritional choices, weight and stress management, and an exercise program.

Assure the patient that OA is a localized disease and that severe deforming arthritis is not the usual course. The patient can also gain support and understanding of the disease process through community resources such as the Arthritis Foundation's Self-Help Course (*www.arthritis.org*).

AMBULATORY AND HOME CARE. Individualize home management goals to meet the patient's needs. Include the caregiver, family members, and significant others in goal setting and teaching. Home and work environment modification is essential for patient safety, accessibility, and self-care. Measures include removing scatter rugs, providing rails at the stairs and bathtub, using night-lights, and wearing well-fitting supportive shoes. Assistive devices such as canes, walkers, elevated toilet seats, and grab bars also reduce the load on an affected joint and promote safety. Urge the patient to continue all prescribed therapies at home and also be open to new approaches to symptom management.

Sexual counseling may help the patient and significant other to enjoy physical closeness by introducing the idea of alternate positions and timing for sexual activity. Discussion also increases awareness of each partner's needs. Encourage the patient to take analgesics or a warm bath to decrease joint stiffness before sexual activity.

EVALUATION

The expected outcomes are that the patient with OA will
- Experience adequate rest and activity
- Achieve satisfactory pain management
- Maintain joint flexibility and muscle strength through joint protection and therapeutic exercise
- Verbalize acceptance of OA as a chronic disease, collaborating with health care providers in disease management

RHEUMATOID ARTHRITIS

Rheumatoid arthritis (RA) is a chronic, systemic autoimmune disease characterized by inflammation of connective tissue in the diarthrodial (synovial) joints. RA is typically characterized by periods of remission and exacerbation. RA is frequently accompanied by extraarticular manifestations.

RA occurs globally, affecting all ethnic groups. It can occur at any time of life, but the incidence increases with age, peaking between 30 and 50 years old. An estimated 1.3 million adult Americans are affected by RA. Women are more likely than men to have the disease.[12]

Etiology and Pathophysiology

Although the exact cause of RA is unknown, it probably results from a combination of genetics and environmental triggers. An autoimmune etiology, which is currently the most widely accepted theory, suggests that changes associated with RA begin when a genetically susceptible person has an initial immune response to an antigen. Although a bacterium or virus has been proposed as a possible antigen, to date no infection or organism has been identified as the cause.

The antigen, which is probably not the same in all patients, triggers the formation of an abnormal immunoglobulin G (IgG). RA is characterized by autoantibodies against this abnormal

IgG. The autoantibodies are known as rheumatoid factor (RF), and they combine with IgG to form immune complexes that initially deposit on synovial membranes or superficial articular cartilage in the joints. Immune complex formation leads to the activation of complement, and an inflammatory response results. (Complement activation is discussed in Chapter 12, and immune complex formation is discussed in Chapter 14.)

Neutrophils are attracted to the site of inflammation, where they release proteolytic enzymes that can damage articular cartilage and cause the synovial lining to thicken (Fig. 65-3). Other inflammatory cells include T helper (CD4) cells, which are the primary orchestrators of cell-mediated immune responses. Activated CD4 cells stimulate monocytes, macrophages, and synovial fibroblasts to secrete the proinflammatory cytokines interleukin-1 (IL-1), interleukin-6 (IL-6), and tumor necrosis factor (TNF). These cytokines are the primary factors that drive the inflammatory response in RA. If unarrested, the disease progresses through four stages, which are identified in Table 65-5.

TABLE 65-5 ANATOMIC STAGES OF RHEUMATOID ARTHRITIS

Stage	Characteristics
I: Early	No destructive changes on x-ray, possible x-ray evidence of osteoporosis.
II: Moderate	X-ray evidence of osteoporosis, with or without slight bone or cartilage destruction. No joint deformities (although possibly limited joint mobility). Adjacent muscle atrophy. Possible presence of extraarticular soft tissue lesions (e.g., nodules, tenosynovitis).
III: Severe	X-ray evidence of cartilage and bone destruction in addition to osteoporosis. Joint deformity, such as subluxation, ulnar deviation, or hyperextension, without fibrous or bony ankylosis. Extensive muscle atrophy. Possible presence of extraarticular soft tissue lesions (e.g., nodules, tenosynovitis).
IV: Terminal	Fibrous or bony ankylosis with stage III criteria.

Data from American College of Rheumatology: Classification criteria for determining progression of rheumatoid arthritis. Retrieved from *www.hopkins-arthritis.org/physician-corner/education/acr/acr.html#class_rheum*.
NOTE: These findings describe spontaneous remission or drug-induced disease suppression.

FIG. 65-3 Rheumatoid arthritis. **A,** Early pathologic change in rheumatoid arthritis is rheumatoid synovitis. The synovium is inflamed. Lymphocytes and plasma cells increase greatly. **B,** With time, articular cartilage destruction occurs, vascular granulation tissue grows across the surface of the cartilage (pannus) from the edges of the joint, and the articular surface shows loss of cartilage beneath the extending pannus, most marked at joint margins. **C,** Inflammatory pannus causes focal destruction of bone. At edges of the joint there is osteolytic destruction of bone, responsible for erosions seen on x-rays. This phase is associated with joint deformity. **D,** Multiple deformities of the foot associated with rheumatoid arthritis.

Genetic Link

Genetic predisposition is important in the development of RA. For example, a higher concurrence of RA has been noted in identical twins compared with fraternal twins.[13] The strongest evidence for a genetic influence is the role of human leukocyte antigens (HLA), especially the HLA-DR4 and HLA-DR1 antigens. (HLA is discussed in Chapter 14.)

Smoking increases the risk of RA for persons who are genetically predisposed to the disease, and makes successful treatment more difficult.

Clinical Manifestations

Joints. The onset of RA is typically insidious. Nonspecific manifestations such as fatigue, anorexia, weight loss, and generalized stiffness may precede the onset of arthritic complaints. The stiffness becomes more localized in the following weeks to months. Some patients report a history of a precipitating stressful event such as infection, work stress, physical exertion, childbirth, surgery, or emotional upset. However, research has been unable to directly correlate such events with the onset of RA.

Specific articular involvement is manifested by pain, stiffness, limitation of motion, and signs of inflammation (e.g., heat, swelling, tenderness). Joint symptoms occur symmetrically and frequently affect the small joints of the hands (PIP and MCP)

and feet (MTP). Larger peripheral joints such as wrists, elbows, shoulders, knees, hips, ankles, and jaw may also be involved. The cervical spine may be affected, but the axial skeleton (the spine and bones connected to it) is generally spared. Table 65-6 compares RA and OA.

The patient characteristically experiences joint stiffness after periods of inactivity. Morning stiffness may last from 60 minutes to several hours or more, depending on disease activity. MCP and PIP joints are typically swollen. In early disease the fingers may become spindle shaped from synovial hypertrophy and thickening of the joint capsule. Joints become tender, painful, and warm to the touch. Joint pain increases with motion, varies in intensity, and may not be proportional to the degree of inflammation. Tenosynovitis frequently affects the extensor and flexor tendons around the wrists, producing manifestations of carpal tunnel syndrome and making it difficult for the patient to grasp objects.

As disease activity progresses, inflammation and fibrosis of the joint capsule and supporting structures may lead to deformity and disability. Atrophy of muscles and destruction of tendons around the joint cause one articular surface to slip past the other *(subluxation).* Metatarsal head dislocation and subluxation in the feet may cause pain and walking disability (Fig. 65-3, *D*). Typical distortions of the hand include ulnar drift

TABLE 65-6 COMPARISON OF RHEUMATOID ARTHRITIS AND OSTEOARTHRITIS

Parameter	Rheumatoid Arthritis	Osteoarthritis
Age at onset	Young to middle age.	Usually >40 yr.
Gender	Female/male ratio is 2:1 or 3:1. Less marked sex difference after age 60.	Before age 50, more men than women. After age 50, more women than men.
Weight	Lost or maintained weight.	Often overweight.
Disease	Systemic disease with exacerbations and remissions.	Localized disease with variable, progressive course.
Affected joints	Small joints typically first (PIPs, MCPs, MTPs), wrists, elbows, shoulders, knees. Usually bilateral, symmetric joint involvement.	Weight-bearing joints of knees and hips, small joints (MCPs, DIPs, PIPs), cervical and lumbar spine. Often asymmetric.
Pain characteristics	Stiffness lasts 1 hr to all day and may decrease with use. Pain is variable, may disrupt sleep.	Stiffness occurs on arising but usually subsides after 30 min. Pain gradually worsens with joint use and disease progression, relieved with rest.
Effusions	Common.	Uncommon.
Nodules	Present, especially on extensor surfaces.	Heberden's (DIPs) and Bouchard's (PIPs) nodes.
Synovial fluid	WBC count >20,000/μL with mostly neutrophils.	WBC count <2000/μL (mild leukocytosis).
X-rays	Joint space narrowing and erosion with bony overgrowths, subluxation with advanced disease. Osteoporosis related to corticosteroid use.	Joint space narrowing, osteophytes, subchondral cysts, sclerosis.
Laboratory findings	RF positive in 80% of patients. Elevated ESR, CRP indicative of active inflammation.	RF negative. Transient elevation in ESR related to synovitis.

CRP, C-reactive protein; *DIPs,* distal interphalangeal; *ESR,* erythrocyte sedimentation rate; *MCPs,* metacarpophalangeals; *MTPs,* metatarsophalangeals; *PIPs,* proximal interphalangeal; *RF,* rheumatoid factor.

("zig-zag deformity"), swan neck, and boutonnière deformities (Fig. 65-4).

Extraarticular Manifestations. RA can affect nearly every system in the body (Fig. 65-5). Extraarticular manifestations are more likely to occur in the person with high levels of biomarkers such as RF.

Rheumatoid nodules develop in 20% to 30% of all patients with RA.[14] Rheumatoid nodules appear subcutaneously as firm, nontender, granuloma-type masses and are usually located over the extensor surfaces of joints such as fingers and elbows. Nodules at the base of the spine and back of the head are common in older adults. On the skin, these nodules can ulcerate, similar to pressure ulcers. In later disease, cardiopulmonary effects may occur. These may include pleurisy, pleural effusion, pericarditis, pericardial effusion, and cardiomyopathy.

Sjögren's syndrome is seen in 10% to 15% of patients with RA.[14] Sjögren's syndrome can occur by itself or in conjunction with other arthritic disorders such as RA and systemic lupus erythematosus (SLE). Affected patients have diminished lacrimal and salivary gland secretion, leading to a dry mouth; burning, itchy eyes with decreased tearing; and photosensitivity. (Sjögren's syndrome is discussed later in this chapter on p. 1590.)

Felty syndrome occurs most commonly in patients with severe, nodule-forming RA. It is characterized by splenomegaly and leukopenia.

Flexion contractures and hand deformities cause diminished grasp strength and affect the patient's ability to perform self-care tasks. Nodular myositis and muscle fiber degeneration can lead to pain similar to that of vascular insufficiency. Cataract development and loss of vision can result from scleral nodules. Depression may occur, which is often related to the chronic pain associated with RA.[15]

Diagnostic Studies

An accurate diagnosis is essential to the initiation of appropriate treatment and the prevention of unnecessary disability. A diagnosis is often made based on history and physical findings, but some laboratory tests are useful for confirmation and to monitor disease progression (see Tables 65-7 and 65-8). Positive RF

FIG. 65-4 Typical deformities of rheumatoid arthritis. **A,** Ulnar drift. **B,** Boutonnière deformity. **C,** Hallux valgus. **D,** Swan neck deformity.

occurs in approximately 80% of adult RA patients, and titers rise during active disease. ESR and C-reactive protein (CRP) are general indicators of active inflammation. An increase in antinuclear antibody (ANA) titers is also seen in some RA patients. Testing for the anti-citrullinated protein antibody (ACPA) is another important diagnostic test for RA. Levels of ACPA are more specific than those of RF for RA and in some cases may allow for an earlier and more accurate diagnosis.[16]

Synovial fluid analysis in early disease often shows a straw-colored fluid with many fibrin flecks. The enzyme MMP-3 is increased in the synovial fluid of the patient with RA, and it may be a marker of progressive joint damage. The white blood cell (WBC) count of synovial fluid is elevated (up to 25,000/μL). Inflammatory changes in the synovium can be confirmed by tissue biopsy.

X-rays are not specifically diagnostic of RA. They may be inconclusive during early stages of the disease, revealing only soft tissue swelling and possible bone demineralization. In later disease, narrowing of the joint space, destruction of articular

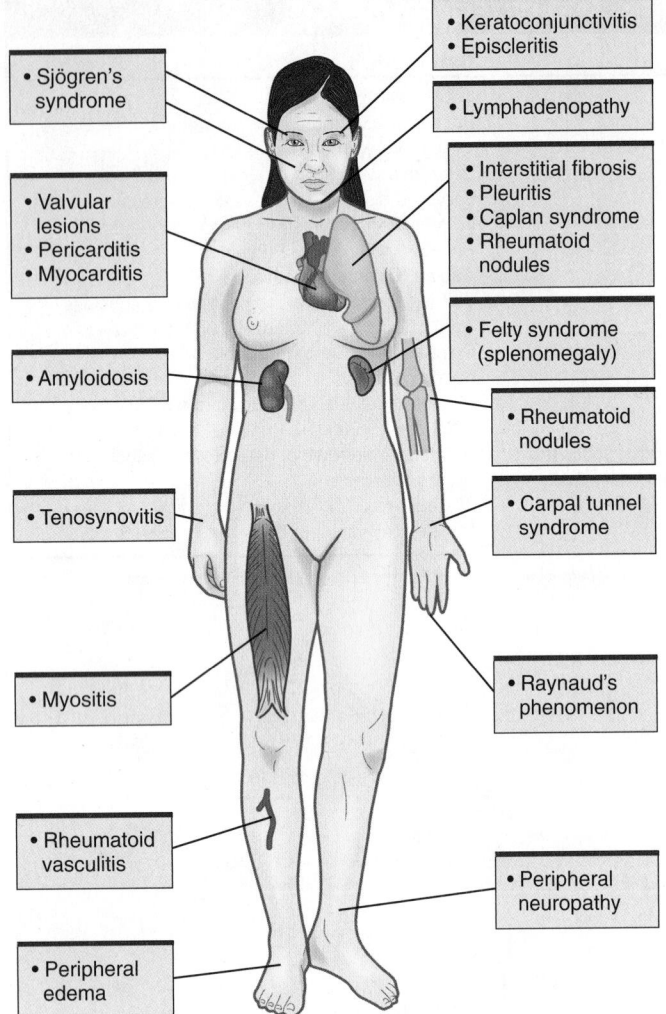

FIG. 65-5 Extraarticular manifestations of rheumatoid arthritis.

Labels on figure:
- Sjögren's syndrome
- Valvular lesions
- Pericarditis
- Myocarditis
- Amyloidosis
- Tenosynovitis
- Myositis
- Rheumatoid vasculitis
- Peripheral edema
- Keratoconjunctivitis
- Episcleritis
- Lymphadenopathy
- Interstitial fibrosis
- Pleuritis
- Caplan syndrome
- Rheumatoid nodules
- Felty syndrome (splenomegaly)
- Rheumatoid nodules
- Carpal tunnel syndrome
- Raynaud's phenomenon
- Peripheral neuropathy

cartilage, erosion, subluxation, and deformity are seen. Malalignment and ankylosis are often evident in advanced disease. Baseline films may be useful in monitoring disease progression and treatment effectiveness. Bone scans are more useful in detecting early joint changes and confirming a diagnosis so that RA treatment can be initiated.

Criteria for the diagnosis of RA in a newly presenting patient are described in Table 65-7.

Collaborative Care

Care of the patient with RA begins with a comprehensive program of education and drug therapy. Teaching regarding drug therapy includes correct administration, reporting of side effects, and frequent medical and laboratory follow-up visits. Teach the patient and the caregiver about the disease process and home management strategies. NSAIDs are prescribed to promote physical comfort. Physical therapy helps the patient maintain joint motion and muscle strength. Occupational therapy develops upper extremity function and encourages joint protection through the use of splints or other assistive devices and strategies for activity pacing.

An individualized treatment plan considers the nature of the disease activity, joint function, age, gender, family and social roles, and response to previous treatment (see Table 65-8). A

TABLE 65-7 DIAGNOSTIC CRITERIA FOR RHEUMATOID ARTHRITIS*

Patients should be tested for RA who initially are seen with:
- At least 1 joint with definite clinical synovitis
- Synovitis not better explained by another disease

	Score
A. Joint Involvement	
• 1 large joint	0
• 2-10 large joints	1
• 1-3 small joints (with or without large joint involvement)	2
• 4-10 small joints (with or without large joint involvement)	3
• >10 joints (at least 1 small joint)	5
B. Serology (at least 1 test result needed for classification)	
• Negative RF *and* negative ACPA	0
• Low-positive RF *or* low-positive ACPA	2
• High-positive RF *or* high-positive ACPA	3
C. Acute Phase Reactants (at least 1 test needed)	
• Normal CRP *and* normal ESR	0
• Abnormal CRP *or* abnormal ESR	1
D. Duration of Symptoms	
• <6 wk	0
• ≥6 wk	1

From Aletaha D, Neogi T, Silman AJ, et al: 2010 Rheumatoid arthritis classification criteria: an American College of Rheumatology/European League Against Rheumatism Collaborative Initiative, *Arthritis Rheum* 62:2569, 2010. Retrieved from *www.rheumatology.org/practice/clinical/classification/ra/2010_revised_criteria_classification_ra.*

SCORING: Add score of categories A-D. Possible scores range from 0-10. A score of ≥6 indicates the definitive presence of RA.

*Used for newly diagnosed patients.

ACPA, Anti-citrullinated protein antibody; *CRP,* C-reactive protein; *ESR,* erythrocyte sedimentation rate; *RF,* rheumatoid factor.

TABLE 65-8 COLLABORATIVE CARE

Rheumatoid Arthritis

Diagnostic
- History and physical examination
- Laboratory studies
  - Complete blood cell (CBC) count
  - Erythrocyte sedimentation rate (ESR)
  - Rheumatoid factor (RF)
  - Anti-citrullinated protein antibody (ACPA)
  - Antinuclear antibody (ANA)
  - C-reactive protein (CRP)
- X-ray studies of involved joints
- Synovial fluid analysis

Collaborative Therapy
- Nutritional and weight management counseling
- Therapeutic exercise
- Psychologic support
- Rest and joint protection, use of assistive devices
- Heat and cold applications
- Complementary and alternative therapies
  - Herbal products
  - Acupuncture
- Drug therapy (See Table 65-3)
  - Disease-modifying antirheumatic drugs (DMARDs)
  - Intraarticular or systemic corticosteroids
  - Nonsteroidal antiinflammatory drugs (NSAIDs)
  - Biologic and targeted therapy
- Reconstructive surgery (e.g., arthroplasty)

caring, long-term relationship with an arthritis health care team can promote the patient's self-esteem and positive coping.

Drug Therapy

Disease-Modifying Antirheumatic Drugs. Drugs remain the cornerstone of RA treatment (see Table 65-3). Because irreversible joint changes can occur as early as the first year of RA, health care providers aggressively prescribe disease-modifying antirheumatic drugs (DMARDs). These drugs have the potential to lessen the permanent effects of RA, such as joint erosion and deformity. The choice of drug is based on disease activity; the patient's level of function; and lifestyle considerations, such as the desire to bear children.

Treatment of early RA often involves DMARD therapy with methotrexate (Rheumatrex).[17] The rapid antiinflammatory effect of methotrexate reduces clinical symptoms in days to weeks. It has a lower toxicity than other drugs. Side effects include bone marrow suppression and hepatotoxicity. Methotrexate therapy requires frequent laboratory monitoring, including CBC and chemistry panel.

Sulfasalazine (Azulfidine) and the antimalarial drug hydroxychloroquine (Plaquenil) may be effective DMARDs for mild to moderate disease. They are rapidly absorbed, relatively safe, and well-tolerated medications. The synthetic DMARD leflunomide (Arava) blocks immune cell overproduction. Its efficacy and side effects are similar to those of methotrexate and sulfasalazine. Because the drug is teratogenic, the possibility of pregnancy in women of childbearing age must be excluded before therapy is initiated.

Tofacitinib (Xeljanz) is a new drug used to treat moderate to severe active RA. This drug is from a new class of medications called JAK (Janus kinase) inhibitors. The drug interferes with the JAK enzymes that contribute to the joint inflammation in RA.

Biologic and Targeted Therapies. Biologic and targeted therapies are also used to slow disease progression in RA. These drugs can be categorized based on their mechanism of action (see Table 65-3). They can be used to treat patients with moderate to severe disease who have not responded to DMARDs, or in combination therapy with an established DMARD such as methotrexate.

Tumor necrosis factor inhibitors include etanercept (Enbrel), infliximab (Remicade), adalimumab (Humira), certolizumab (Cimzia), and golimumab (Simponi). Etanercept is a biologically engineered copy (using recombinant deoxyribonucleic acid [DNA] technology) of the TNF cell receptor. This soluble TNF receptor binds to TNF in circulation before TNF can bind to the cell surface receptor. By inhibiting binding of TNF, etanercept inhibits the inflammatory response. This drug is given as a subcutaneous injection.

DRUG ALERT: Etanercept (Enbrel)
- Increased risk of serious infection and heart failure is a concern.
- Report persistent fever, bruising, bleeding, or other signs of infection.

Infliximab and adalimumab are monoclonal antibodies that bind to TNF, thus preventing the TNF from binding to TNF receptors on cells. Infliximab is given IV, in combination with methotrexate. Adalimumab is given subcutaneously.

Certolizumab and golimumab are TNF inhibitors that improve symptoms in patients with moderate to severe RA. Both drugs are given in combination with methotrexate. When compared to other biologic and targeted therapy, certolizumab stays in the system longer and may also show a more rapid (1

to 2 weeks) and significant reduction in RA symptoms. Certolizumab is also used in treating Crohn's disease.

DRUG ALERT: Tumor Necrosis Factor Inhibitors
- Administer tuberculin test and chest x-ray before initiation of therapy.
- Monitor for signs of infection and stop drug if acute infection develops.
- Instruct patients to avoid live vaccination while taking drug.

Anakinra (Kineret) is a recombinant version of IL-1 receptor antagonist (IL-1Ra). It blocks the biologic activity of IL-1 by competitively inhibiting IL-1 binding to the IL-1 receptor. It is given as a subcutaneous injection. Anakinra is used to reduce the pain and swelling associated with moderate to severe RA. It can be used in combination with DMARDs but not with TNF inhibitors. Concurrent use of these agents can cause serious infection and neutropenia.

Tocilizumab (Actemra) blocks the action of IL-6, a proinflammatory cytokine. It is used to treat patients with moderate to severe RA who have not adequately responded to or cannot tolerate other drugs for RA.

Abatacept (Orencia) blocks T cell activation. It is recommended for patients who have an inadequate response to DMARDs or TNF inhibitors. It is given IV. Like anakinra, it should not be used concomitantly with TNF inhibitors.

Rituximab (Rituxan) is a monoclonal antibody that targets B cells (see Fig. 16-16). It may be used in combination with methotrexate for patients with moderate to severe RA not responding to TNF inhibitors (e.g., etanercept, infliximab). It is given IV.

Other Drug Therapy. Additional medications used infrequently for treating RA include antibiotics (minocycline [Minocin]), immunosuppressants (azathioprine [Imuran]), penicillamine (Cuprimine), and gold preparations (auranofin [Ridaura], gold sodium thiomalate [Myochrysine]).

Corticosteroid therapy can be used for symptom control. Intraarticular injections may temporarily reduce the pain and inflammation associated with disease flare-ups. Long-term use of oral corticosteroids should not be a mainstay of RA treatment because of the risk of complications, including osteoporosis and avascular necrosis. However, low-dose prednisone may be used for a limited time in select patients to decrease disease activity until DMARD therapy is effective.

Various NSAIDs and salicylates continue to be included in the drug regimen to treat arthritic pain and inflammation. Enteric-coated aspirin may be used in high dosages of 3.2 to 5.4 g/day (10 to 18 tablets).[18] NSAIDs have antiinflammatory, analgesic, and antipyretic properties. Some relief may be noted within days of the start of treatment with NSAIDs, but full effectiveness may take 2 to 3 weeks. NSAIDs may be used when the patient cannot tolerate high doses of aspirin. Antiinflammatory drugs that are taken only once or twice a day may improve the patient's ability to follow the treatment regimen (see Table 65-3). The newer-generation NSAIDs, the COX-2 inhibitors, are effective in RA as well as OA. Celecoxib is currently the only available COX-2 inhibitor.

Nutritional Therapy.
Although there is no special diet for RA, balanced nutrition is important. Fatigue, pain, depression, limited endurance, and mobility deficits often accompany RA and may cause a loss of appetite or interfere with the patient's ability to shop for and prepare food. Weight loss may result. The occupational therapist may help the patient modify the home environment and use assistive devices to make food preparation easier.

Corticosteroid therapy or immobility secondary to pain may result in unwanted weight gain. A sensible weight loss program consisting of balanced nutrition and exercise reduces stress on affected joints. Corticosteroids also increase the appetite, resulting in a higher caloric intake. In addition, the patient may become distressed as signs and symptoms of Cushing syndrome, including moon face and the redistribution of fatty tissue to the trunk, change the physical appearance. Encourage the patient to continue to eat a balanced diet and not to alter the corticosteroid dose or stop therapy abruptly. Weight slowly adjusts to normal several months after cessation of therapy.

Surgical Therapy.   Occasionally, surgery is needed to relieve severe pain and improve the function of severely deformed joints. Removal of the joint lining (synovectomy) is one type of surgical therapy. Total joint replacement (arthroplasty) can be done for many different joints in the body. Joint surgery is discussed in Chapter 63.

NURSING MANAGEMENT
RHEUMATOID ARTHRITIS

NURSING ASSESSMENT

Subjective and objective data that should be obtained from the patient with RA are presented in Table 65-9.

NURSING DIAGNOSES

Nursing diagnoses for the patient with RA may include, but are not limited to, the following:
- Impaired physical mobility *related to* joint pain, stiffness, and deformity
- Chronic pain *related to* joint inflammation, misuse of joints, and ineffective pain and/or comfort measures
- Disturbed body image *related to* chronic disease activity, long-term treatment, deformities, stiffness, and inability to perform usual activities

Additional information on nursing diagnoses for the patient with RA is provided in eNursing Care Plan 65-1 (on the website for this chapter).

PLANNING

The overall goals are that the patient with RA will (1) have satisfactory pain management, (2) have minimal loss of functional ability of the affected joints, (3) participate in planning and carrying out the therapeutic regimen, (4) maintain a positive self-image, and (5) perform self-care to the maximum amount possible.

NURSING IMPLEMENTATION

HEALTH PROMOTION.   Prevention of RA is not possible based on the current state of knowledge. However, early treatment can help prevent further joint damage. Community education programs should focus on symptom recognition to promote early diagnosis and treatment of RA. The Arthritis Foundation offers many publications, classes, and support activities to assist affected persons (see Resources at the end of this chapter).

ACUTE INTERVENTION.   The primary goals in the management of RA are the reduction of inflammation, management of pain, maintenance of joint function, and prevention or minimization of joint deformity. Goals may be met through a comprehensive program of drug therapy, balance of rest and activity with joint protection, heat and cold applications, exercise, and patient and caregiver teaching. Work closely with the health care provider,

---

TABLE 65-9   NURSING ASSESSMENT
Rheumatoid Arthritis

Subjective Data
Important Health Information
Past health history: Recent infections; precipitating factors such as emotional upset, infections, overwork, childbirth, surgery; pattern of remissions and exacerbations
Medications: Aspirin, NSAIDs, corticosteroids, DMARDs
Surgery or other treatments: Any joint surgery

Functional Health Patterns
Health perception–health management: Positive family history for rheumatoid arthritis or other autoimmune disorders; malaise, ability to participate in therapeutic regimen; impact of disease on functional ability
Nutritional-metabolic: Anorexia, weight loss; dry mucous membranes of mouth and pharynx
Activity-exercise: Stiffness and joint swelling, muscle weakness, difficulty walking, fatigue
Cognitive-perceptual: Paresthesias of hands and feet, loss of sensation; symmetric joint pain and aching that increases with motion or stress on joint

Objective Data
General
Lymphadenopathy, fever

Integumentary
Keratoconjunctivitis; subcutaneous rheumatoid nodules on forearms, elbows; skin ulcers; shiny, taut skin over involved joints; peripheral edema

Cardiovascular
Symmetric pallor and cyanosis of fingers (Raynaud's phenomenon); distant heart sounds, murmurs, dysrhythmias

Respiratory
Chronic bronchitis, tuberculosis, histoplasmosis, fibrosing alveolitis

Gastrointestinal
Splenomegaly (Felty syndrome)

Musculoskeletal
Symmetric joint involvement with swelling, erythema, heat, tenderness, and deformities; enlargement of proximal phalangeal and metacarpophalangeal joints; limitation of joint movement; muscle contractures, muscle atrophy

Possible Diagnostic Findings
Positive rheumatoid factor, ↑ ESR, anemia; ↑ WBCs in synovial fluid; evidence of joint space narrowing, and bony erosion and deformity on x-ray (osteoporosis with advanced disease)

DMARDs, Disease-modifying antirheumatic drugs; *ESR,* erythrocyte sedimentation rate; *NSAIDs,* nonsteroidal antiinflammatory drugs.

---

physical and occupational therapists, and social worker to help the patient restore function and make appropriate lifestyle adjustments to chronic illness.

The newly diagnosed RA patient is usually treated on an outpatient basis. Hospitalization may be necessary for patients with extraarticular complications or advancing disease requiring reconstructive surgery for disabling deformities.

Intervention begins with a careful physical assessment (e.g., joint pain, swelling, range of motion [ROM], and general health status). Also evaluate psychosocial needs (e.g., family support, sexual satisfaction, emotional stress, financial constraints, vocational and career limitations) and environmental concerns (e.g., transportation, home or work modifications). After identifying the patient's problems, coordinate a carefully planned program for rehabilitation and education with the interdisciplinary health care team.

Suppression of inflammation may be effectively achieved through the administration of NSAIDs, DMARDs, and biologic and targeted therapies. Careful attention to timing of drug administration is critical to sustain a therapeutic drug level and reduce early morning stiffness. Discuss the action and side effects of each prescribed drug and the importance of laboratory monitoring. Because many patients with RA take several different drugs, make the drug regimen as understandable as possible. Encourage patients to develop a method for remembering to take their medications (e.g., pill containers).

Nondrug management may include the use of therapeutic heat and cold, rest, relaxation techniques, joint protection (see Tables 65-4 and 65-10), biofeedback (see Chapter 6), transcutaneous electrical nerve stimulation (see Chapter 9), and hypnosis. Allow the patient and the caregiver to choose therapies that promote optimal comfort within the parameters of their lifestyle.

Lightweight splints may be prescribed to rest an inflamed joint and prevent deformity from muscle spasms and contractures. Remove the splints at regular intervals to give skin care and perform ROM exercises. After assessment has been completed and supportive care has been given, reapply the splints as prescribed. The occupational therapist may help identify additional self-help devices for activities of daily living.

Plan your care and procedures around the patient's morning stiffness. Sitting or standing in a warm shower, sitting in a tub with warm towels around the shoulders, or simply soaking the hands in a basin of warm water may help relieve joint stiffness and allow the patient to perform activities of daily living more comfortably.

AMBULATORY AND HOME CARE

Rest. Alternating scheduled rest periods with activity throughout the day helps relieve fatigue and pain. The amount of rest needed varies according to the severity of the disease and the patient's limitations. The patient should rest before becoming exhausted. Total bed rest rarely is necessary and should be avoided to prevent stiffness and other effects of immobility. However, even a patient with mild disease may require daytime rest in addition to 8 to 10 hours of sleep at night. Help the patient identify ways to modify daily activities to avoid overexertion that can lead to fatigue and exacerbate disease activity. For example, the patient may tolerate meal preparation more easily while sitting on a high stool in front of the sink.

Good body alignment while resting can be maintained through use of a firm mattress or bed board. Encourage positions of extension, and teach the patient to avoid positions of flexion. To decrease the risk of joint contracture, never place pillows under the knees. A small, flat pillow may be used under the head and shoulders.

Joint Protection. Protecting joints from stress is important. Help the patient identify ways to modify tasks to put less stress on joints during routine activities (Table 65-10). Energy conservation requires careful planning. The emphasis is on work simplification techniques. Work should be done in short periods with scheduled rest breaks to avoid fatigue (pacing). Activities should be organized to avoid going up and down stairs repeatedly. Carts should be used to carry supplies, or materials that

TABLE 65-10 PATIENT & CAREGIVER TEACHING GUIDE

Protection of Small Joints

Include the following instructions when teaching the patient with arthritis how to protect small joints.
1. Maintain joint in neutral position to minimize deformity.
   - Press water from a sponge instead of wringing.
2. Use strongest joint available for any task.
   - When rising from chair, push with palms rather than fingers.
   - Carry laundry basket in both arms rather than with fingers.
3. Distribute weight over many joints instead of stressing a few.
   - Slide objects instead of lifting them.
   - Hold packages close to body for support.
4. Change positions frequently.
   - Do not hold book or grip steering wheel for long periods without resting.
   - Avoid grasping pencil or cutting vegetables with knife for extended periods.
5. Avoid repetitive movements.
   - Do not knit for long periods.
   - Rest between rooms when vacuuming.
   - Modify home environment to include faucets and doorknobs that are pushed rather than turned.
6. Modify chores to avoid stress on joints.
   - Avoid heavy lifting.
   - Sit on stool instead of standing during meal preparation.

are used often can be stored in a convenient, easily reached area. Timesaving joint protective devices (e.g., electric can opener) should be used whenever possible. Tasks can also be delegated to other family members.

Patient independence may be increased by occupational therapy training with assistive devices that simplify tasks, such as built-up utensils, buttonhooks, modified drawer handles, lightweight plastic dishes, and raised toilet seats. Wearing shoes with Velcro fasteners and clothing with buttons or a zipper down the front instead of the back makes dressing easier. A cane or a walker offers support and relief of pain when walking.

Heat and Cold Therapy and Exercise. Heat and cold applications can help relieve stiffness, pain, and muscle spasm. Application of ice is especially beneficial during periods of disease exacerbation, whereas moist heat appears to offer better relief of chronic stiffness. Superficial heat sources such as heating pads, moist hot packs, paraffin baths, and warm baths or showers can relieve stiffness to allow participation in therapeutic exercises. Plastic bags of small frozen vegetables (peas or kernel corn), which can easily mold around the shoulder, wrists, or knees, are an effective home treatment. The patient can also use ice cubes or small paper cups of frozen water to massage areas proximal or distal to a painful joint. Heat and cold can be used as often as desired. However, the heat application should not exceed 20 minutes at one time, and the cold application should not exceed 10 to 15 minutes at one time. Alert the patient to the possibility of a burn and the need to avoid the use of a heat-producing cream (e.g., capsaicin) with another external heat device.

Individualized exercise is an integral part of the treatment plan. A physical therapist usually develops a therapeutic exercise program to improve the flexibility and strength of the affected joints and the patient's overall endurance. Reinforce program participation and ensure correct performance of the exercises. Inadequate joint movement can result in progressive joint immobility and muscle weakness, and overaggressive exercise can result in increased pain, inflammation, and joint damage. Emphasize that participating in a recreational exercise program (e.g., walking, swimming) or performing usual daily activities does not eliminate the patient's need for therapeutic exercise to maintain adequate joint motion.

Gentle ROM exercises are usually done daily to keep the joints functional. The patient should have the opportunity to practice the exercises with supervision. Aquatic exercises in warm water (78° to 86° F [25° to 30° C]) allow easier joint movement because of the buoyancy and warmth of the water. At the same time, although movement seems easier, water provides two-way resistance that makes muscles work harder than they would on land. During acute inflammation, exercise should be limited to one or two repetitions.

Psychologic Support. Self-management and adherence to an individualized home treatment program can be accomplished only if the patient has a thorough understanding of RA, the nature and course of the disease, and the goals of therapy. In addition, consider the patient's value system and perception of the disease.

The patient is challenged constantly by problems of limited function and fatigue, loss of self-esteem, altered body image, and fear of disability and deformity. Discuss alterations in sexuality. Chronic pain or loss of function may make the patient vulnerable to believing the claims of false advertising and attempting unproven or even dangerous remedies. Help the patient recognize fears and concerns that are faced by all people who live with chronic illness.

Evaluation of the family support system is important. Financial planning may be necessary. Community resources such as a home care nurse, homemaker services, and vocational rehabilitation may be considered. Self-help groups are beneficial for some patients.

The presence of chronic pain may lead to depression. Strategies that may help to decrease depressive symptoms include listening to music, reading, exercising, and counseling. Hypnosis and biofeedback may also be of value.

GERONTOLOGIC CONSIDERATIONS

ARTHRITIS

The prevalence of arthritis in older adults is high, and the disease is accompanied by problems unique to this age-group. The most problematic areas in older adults include the following:

- The high incidence of OA in older adults often keeps the health care provider from considering other types of arthritis.
- Age alone causes changes in serologic profiles, making interpretation of laboratory values such as RF and ESR more difficult. Drugs taken for co-morbid conditions can also affect laboratory values.
- Polypharmacy in the older adult can result in iatrogenic arthritis.
- Nonorganic musculoskeletal pain syndromes and weakness may be related to depression and physical inactivity.
- Diseases such as SLE, which commonly occurs in younger adults, can develop in a milder form in older adults.

Aging brings many physical and metabolic changes that may increase the older patient's sensitivity to both the therapeutic and toxic effects of some drugs. The older adult who takes NSAIDs has an increased risk for side effects, particularly GI

bleeding and renal toxicity. The use of NSAIDs with a shorter half-life may require more frequent dosing but may also produce fewer side effects in the older patient with altered drug metabolism.

The common occurrence of polypharmacy in the older adult makes the use of additional drugs in RA treatment particularly problematic because of the increased likelihood of untoward drug interactions. The drug regimen should be simplified as much as possible to increase adherence (e.g., limited number of drugs with decreased frequency of administration), particularly for the patient without regular assistance.

A major concern in the older patient relates to the use of corticosteroid therapy. Corticosteroid-induced osteopenia can add to the problem of decreased bone density related to age and inactivity. It also increases the risk of pathologic fractures, especially compression fractures of vertebrae. Corticosteroid-induced myopathy can be minimized or prevented by an age-appropriate exercise program. Although important for all age-groups, an adequate support system for the older adult is a critical factor in the ability to follow a treatment regimen that includes nutritional planning, exercise, general health maintenance, and appropriate therapy.

GOUT

Gout is a type of recurring acute arthritis characterized by the accumulation of uric acid crystals in one or more joints. Characteristic deposits of sodium urate crystals occur in articular, periarticular, and subcutaneous tissues. More than 3 million Americans are affected by gout. The incidence among African American men is nearly twice that of white men.[19]

Gout may be classified as primary or secondary. In *primary gout* a hereditary error of purine metabolism leads to the overproduction or retention of uric acid. Primary gout, which accounts for 90% of cases, occurs predominantly in middle-aged men.

Secondary gout may be related to another acquired disorder (Table 65-11) or may be the result of drugs known to inhibit uric acid excretion. Secondary gout may also be caused by drugs that increase the rate of cell death, such as the chemotherapy agents used in treating leukemia. Hyperuricemia may also develop in patients taking thiazide diuretics, postmenopausal women, and organ transplant recipients who are receiving immunosuppressive agents.

Obesity in men increases the risk of gout. Hypertension, diuretic use, and excessive alcohol consumption are additional risk factors. A diet high in purine-rich foods (e.g., shellfish such as crab and shrimp; vegetables such as lentils, asparagus, and spinach; meats such as beef, chicken, and pork) will not cause gout, but can trigger an acute attack if a person is susceptible to gout.

TABLE 65-11	CAUSES OF HYPERURICEMIA
• Acidosis or ketosis	• Malignant disease
• Alcohol use	• Myeloproliferative disorders
• Atherosclerosis	• Obesity or starvation
• Chemotherapy drugs	• Renal insufficiency
• Diabetes mellitus	• Sickle cell anemia
• Drug-induced renal impairment	• Exposure to lead
• Hyperlipidemia	• Use of certain common drugs (low-dose aspirin, thiazide, diuretics, niacin)
• Hypertension	

Etiology and Pathophysiology

Uric acid is the major end product of purine catabolism and is primarily excreted by the kidneys. Gout is caused by (1) an increase in uric acid production; (2) underexcretion of uric acid by the kidneys; or (3) increased intake of foods containing purines, which are metabolized to uric acid by the body. Underexcretion of uric acid is believed to be the major cause of hyperuricemia in 80% to 90% of affected persons. High dietary intake of purine alone has relatively little effect on uric acid levels. Hyperuricemia may result from prolonged fasting or excessive alcohol drinking because of the increased production of keto acids, which then inhibit uric acid excretion.

Clinical Manifestations and Complications

In the acute phase, gouty arthritis may occur in one or more joints but usually less than four. Affected joints may appear dusky or cyanotic and are extremely tender. Inflammation of the great toe (podagra) is the most common initial problem. Other affected joints may include wrists, knees, ankles, and midtarsal area of the foot. Olecranon bursae may also be involved. Acute gouty arthritis is usually precipitated by trigger events such as trauma, surgery, alcohol ingestion, or systemic infection. The onset of symptoms typically occurs at night with sudden swelling and excruciating pain peaking within several hours, often accompanied by low-grade fever. Individual attacks usually subside, treated or untreated, in 2 to 10 days. The affected joint returns to normal and patients are often free of symptoms between attacks.

Chronic gout is characterized by multiple joint involvement and visible deposits of sodium urate crystals (tophi). These are typically noted in the synovium, subchondral bone, olecranon bursae, and vertebrae; along tendons; and in the skin and cartilage (Fig. 65-6). Tophi are rarely present at the initial attack and are generally noted only many years after the onset of disease.

The severity of gouty arthritis varies. The clinical course may consist of infrequent mild attacks or multiple severe episodes (up to 12 per year) associated with a slowly progressive disability. In general, the higher the serum uric acid level, the earlier the appearance of tophi and the greater the tendency toward more frequent, severe episodes of acute gout. Chronic inflammation may result in joint deformity, and cartilage destruction may predispose the joint to secondary OA. Large and unsightly tophaceous deposits may perforate overlying skin, producing draining sinuses that often become infected.

Excessive uric acid excretion may lead to kidney or urinary tract stone formation. Pyelonephritis associated with intrarenal sodium urate deposits and obstruction may contribute to kidney disease.

Diagnostic Studies

In gout, serum uric acid levels are usually elevated above 6 mg/dL. However, hyperuricemia is not specifically diagnostic of gout because increased levels may be related to a variety of drugs or may exist as an asymptomatic abnormality in the general population. Specimens for 24-hour urine uric acid values may be obtained to determine if the disease is caused by decreased renal excretion or overproduction of uric acid.

Synovial fluid aspiration is a controversial part of patient evaluation because an accurate diagnosis of gout is possible in 80% of patients based on clinical symptoms alone. However, aspiration may have therapeutic value by decompressing a swollen joint capsule. Joint aspiration is also the only reliable method of distinguishing gout from septic arthritis and *pseudogout* (calcium phosphate crystals are formed). Affected fluid characteristically contains needle-like monosodium urate crystals.[20] X-rays appear normal in the early stages of gout. In chronic disease, tophi may appear as eroded areas in the bone.

Collaborative Care

Goals for the care of the patient with gout (Table 65-12) include termination of an acute attack using an antiinflammatory agent such as colchicine. Drug therapy is the primary therapy used in treating acute and chronic gout. In addition, weight reduction

FIG. 65-6 Tophi associated with chronic gout. Nodules are painless and filled with uric acid crystals.

TABLE 65-12 COLLABORATIVE CARE

Gout

Diagnostic
- History and physical examination
- Family history of gout
- Sodium urate crystals in synovial fluid
- Elevated serum uric acid levels
- Elevated 24-hr urine for uric acid levels
- X-ray of affected joints

Collaborative Therapy
- Joint immobilization
- Local application of heat or cold
- Joint aspiration and intraarticular corticosteroids
- Dietary avoidance of food and fluids with high purine content (e.g., anchovies, liver, wine, beer)
- Drug therapy
  - colchicine
  - Nonsteroidal antiinflammatory drugs (e.g., naproxen [Naprosyn])
  - allopurinol (Zyloprim)
  - probenecid (Benemid)
  - febuxostat (Uloric)
  - Corticosteroids (prednisone)
  - Intraarticular corticosteroids (methylprednisolone)
  - Adrenocorticotropic hormone (ACTH)

(as needed) and possible avoidance of alcohol and foods high in purine (red and organ meats) are recommended.

Drug Therapy. Acute gout is treated with colchicine and NSAIDs. Because colchicine has antiinflammatory effects but no analgesic properties, an NSAID is added to the treatment regimen for pain management. Oral administration of colchicine generally produces dramatic pain relief when given within 12 to 24 hours of an attack.[20] Colchicine also has diagnostic merit in that a good response to this drug offers further evidence for the diagnosis of gout.

Future attacks of gout are prevented in part by a maintenance dose of urate-lowering drugs such as a xanthine oxidase inhibitor (allopurinol [Zyloprim, Aloprim]) or a uricosuric drug (probenecid [Benemid, Probalan]). Febuxostat (Uloric), a selective inhibitor of xanthine oxidase, is given for long-term management of hyperuricemia in people with chronic gout.

Patients who cannot take or do not respond to drugs that lower uric acid in the blood may be given pegloticase (Krystexxa). This drug is an enzyme that metabolizes uric acid into a harmless chemical that is excreted in the urine. The drug is given IV. Corticosteroids given either orally or by intraarticular injection can be helpful in treating acute attacks of gout. Systemic corticosteroids may be used only if routine therapies are contraindicated or ineffective. Adrenocorticotropic hormone (ACTH) may also be used for treating acute gout.

For many years, the standard therapy for hyperuricemia caused by urate underexcretion has been uricosuric drugs such as probenecid, which inhibit renal tubular reabsorption of urates. However, these drugs are ineffective when creatinine clearance is reduced, as can occur in patients over 60 years old and those with renal impairment. Aspirin inactivates the effect of uricosuric drugs, resulting in urate retention, and should be avoided while taking uricosuric drugs. Acetaminophen can be used safely if analgesia is required.

Adequate urine volume with normal renal function (2 to 3 L/day) must be maintained to prevent precipitation of uric acid in the renal tubules. Allopurinol, which blocks the production of uric acid, is particularly useful in patients with uric acid stones or renal impairment, in whom uricosuric drugs may be ineffective or dangerous. For patients who cannot tolerate allopurinol because of side effects, oxypurinol can be prescribed. Oxypurinol is the active metabolite of allopurinol. The angiotensin II receptor antagonist losartan (Cozaar) may be especially useful for treatment of older patients with both gout and hypertension. Losartan promotes urate diuresis and may normalize serum urate levels. Combination therapy with losartan and allopurinol may also be given. Regardless of which drugs are prescribed, serum uric acid levels must be checked regularly to monitor treatment effectiveness.

Nutritional Therapy. Dietary restrictions that limit alcohol and foods high in purine help minimize uric acid production (see Table 46-12). Instruct obese patients in a carefully planned weight-reduction program.

NURSING MANAGEMENT
GOUT

Nursing interventions for the patient with an acute episode of gout include supportive care of the inflamed joints. Avoid causing pain by careless handling of an inflamed joint. Bed rest may be appropriate with affected joints properly immobilized. Involvement of a lower extremity may require use of a cradle or footboard to protect the painful area from the weight of bedclothes. Assess the limitation of motion and degree of pain and document treatment effectiveness.

Help the patient and family understand that hyperuricemia and gout are chronic problems that can be controlled with careful adherence to a treatment program.[21] Explain the importance of drug therapy and the need for periodic determination of serum uric acid levels. Teach the patient about precipitating factors that may cause an attack, including excessive caloric intake or overindulgence in purine-containing foods and alcohol, starvation (fasting), drug use (e.g., niacin, aspirin, diuretics), and major medical events (e.g., surgery, myocardial infarction).

LYME DISEASE

Lyme disease is a spirochetal infection caused by *Borrelia burgdorferi* and transmitted by the bite of an infected deer tick. It was first identified in 1975 in Lyme, Connecticut, after an unusual clustering of arthritis in children. It is now the most common vector-borne disease in the United States. The tick typically feeds on mice, dogs, cats, cows, horses, deer, and humans. Wild animals do not exhibit the illness, but clinical Lyme disease does occur in domestic animals. Person-to-person transmission does not occur.

The peak season for human infection is during the summer months. Most U.S. cases occur in three endemic areas: along the northeastern coast from Maryland to Massachusetts, in the Midwestern states of Wisconsin and Minnesota, and along the northwestern coast of California and Oregon. More than 20,000 cases are reported annually in the United States. Reinfection is not uncommon.

Lyme disease symptoms can mimic those of other diseases such as multiple sclerosis, mononucleosis, and meningitis. The most characteristic clinical symptom of early localized disease is *erythema migrans* (EM), a skin lesion ("bull's eye rash") that occurs in 70% to 80% of infected persons at the site of the tick bite within 3 to 30 days after exposure (Fig. 65-7). The lesion begins as a red macule or papule that slowly expands to form a large round lesion of up to 12 in with a bright red border and central clearing. The EM lesion is often accompanied by acute flu-like symptoms, such as low-grade fever, chills, headache, stiff neck, fatigue, swollen lymph nodes, and migratory joint and muscle pain. Of note, loss of tone in facial muscles can manifest as Bell's palsy. Symptoms usually occur in a week, but may be delayed for up to 30 days. The flu-like symptoms generally resolve over a period of weeks or months, even if untreated.

FIG. 65-7 Erythema migrans. Characteristic skin lesion of Lyme disease that occurs at the site of tick bite.

Musculoskeletal System

TABLE 65-13 PATIENT & CAREGIVER TEACHING GUIDE

Prevention and Early Treatment of Lyme Disease

Include the following instructions when teaching patients how to prevent Lyme disease.

- Avoid walking through tall grasses and low brush, and sitting on logs.
- Mow grass. Remove brush around paths, buildings, and campsites to create "tick-safe zones."
- Move woodpiles and bird feeders away from house. Discourage deer (main source of food for adult ticks) from being in the area.
- Wear long pants or nylon tights of tightly woven, light-colored fabric so ticks can be easily seen.
- Tuck pants into boots or long socks, wear long-sleeved shirts tucked into pants, and wear closed shoes when hiking.
- Check often for ticks crawling from pant legs to open skin.
- Thoroughly inspect and wash clothes. Placing clothing in dryer on high heat effectively kills ticks.
- Spray insect repellent containing DEET sparingly on skin or apply permethrin to boots, clothes (especially on lower extremities), and camping gear.
- Have pets wear tick collars, inspect them often, and do not allow pets on furniture or beds.

Include the following instructions when teaching patients and caregivers living in endemic areas.

- Remove attached ticks with tweezers (not fingers). Grasp tick's mouth parts as close to skin as possible and gently pull straight out. Do not twist or jerk. Avoid folk solutions such as painting the tick with nail polish or petroleum jelly.
- Save the tick in a bottle of alcohol (if you need it later for identification).
- Wash bitten area with soap and water and apply antiseptic. Wash hands.
- See a health care provider immediately if flu-like symptoms or a bull's-eye rash appears within 2-30 days after removal of tick.

Adapted from Centers for Disease Control and Prevention: It's spring: time to prevent Lyme disease. Retrieved from *www.cdc.gov/features/lymedisease;* and Centers for Disease Control and Prevention: Tick removal. Retrieved from *www.cdc.gov/lyme/removal/index.html.*
DEET, N,N-diethyl-m-toluamide.

If not treated, the spirochete can disseminate within several weeks or months to the heart, joints, and central nervous system (CNS). Carditis may occur.[22] About 60% of persons with untreated infection develop chronic arthritic pain and swelling in the large joints. Nervous system problems may include severe headaches or poor motor coordination. The accompanying neurologic condition known as tertiary neuroborreliosis results in confusion and forgetfulness.

A diagnosis of Lyme disease is often based on clinical manifestations, in particular the EM lesion, and a history of exposure in an endemic area. CBC and ESR are usually normal. A two-step laboratory testing process is recommended by the Centers for Disease Control and Prevention to confirm the diagnosis.[23] The first step is the enzyme immunoassay (EIA), which will have positive results for most people with Lyme disease. If the EIA is positive or inconclusive, a Western blot test is done to confirm the infection. In individuals with neurologic involvement, cerebrospinal fluid should also be examined.

Active lesions can be treated with oral antibiotics. Doxycycline (Vibramycin), cefuroxime (Ceftin), and amoxicillin are often effective in treating early-stage infection and preventing later stages of the disease. Doxycycline prevents Lyme disease when given within 3 days after the bite of a deer tick. Short-term therapy of 2 to 3 weeks is usually effective for solitary EM, but patients with neurologic or cardiac complications may require IV therapy with ceftriaxone (Rocephin) or penicillin. In most cases, persons with Lyme disease are treated successfully with antibiotics. Approximately 10% to 20% of persons treated with antibiotics for Lyme disease may experience lingering fatigue or joint and muscle pain. This condition, known as post–Lyme disease syndrome, may result from residual damage to tissues and the immune system.[22]

Reducing exposure to ticks is the best way to prevent Lyme disease. Patient and caregiver teaching for people living in endemic areas is outlined in Table 65-13. No vaccine is available for Lyme disease.

SEPTIC ARTHRITIS

Septic arthritis (infectious or bacterial arthritis) is caused by microorganisms invading the joint cavity. Bacteria can travel through the bloodstream from another site of active infection, resulting in hematogenous seeding of the joint. Organisms can also be introduced directly through trauma or surgical incision.

Any bacteria can cause the infection—even nonpathogenic bacteria in the immunocompromised patient. *Staphylococcus aureus* and *Streptococcus hemolyticus* are the most common causative organisms.[24] *Neisseria gonorrhoeae* is the most common cause in sexually active young adults. Factors that increase the risk of infection include (1) diseases in which there is decreased host resistance (e.g., leukemia, diabetes mellitus), (2) treatment with corticosteroids or immunosuppressive drugs, and (3) debilitating chronic illness.

In septic arthritis, large joints such as the knee and hip are most frequently involved. Inflammation of the joint cavity causes severe pain, erythema, and swelling. Because infection has often spread from a primary site elsewhere in the body, fever or shaking chills often accompany articular manifestations. A diagnosis may be made by aspiration of the joint (arthrocentesis) and culture of the synovial fluid. However, WBC counts may be low early in the infectious process, and diagnosis is not possible solely based on WBC counts. Blood cultures for aerobic and anaerobic organisms should also be obtained.

Septic arthritis requires prompt treatment to prevent joint destruction and bone loss.[25] Broad-spectrum antibiotics against gram-negative organisms, pneumococci, and staphylococci are often started before the causative organism is identified. Once the organism is identified, specific treatment can be determined. Infections may respond to treatment within 2 weeks or may take as long as 4 to 8 weeks, depending on the causative organism. Local aspiration and surgical drainage may be required. If diagnosis and treatment are delayed, destruction of articular cartilage can occur, followed by loss of joint function. Chronic infection can also develop. Septic arthritis of the hip can contribute to development of avascular necrosis.

Assess and monitor joint inflammation, pain, and fever. To control pain, use resting splints or traction to immobilize affected joints. Local hot compresses can also help relieve pain. Initiate gentle ROM exercises as soon as tolerated to prevent muscle atrophy and joint contractures. Explain the need for antibiotics and the importance of their continued use until the infection is resolved. Offer support to the patient who requires arthrocentesis or operative drainage. Use strict aseptic technique when assisting with joint aspiration procedures.

SPONDYLOARTHROPATHIES

The **spondyloarthropathies** are a group of interrelated multisystem inflammatory disorders that affect the spine, peripheral joints, and periarticular structures. These disorders are all negative for rheumatoid factor (RF) and thus are often referred to as seronegative arthropathies.

Inheritance of HLA-B27 is strongly associated with these diseases. Both genetic and environmental factors play a role in the development of this group of diseases, which includes ankylosing spondylitis, psoriatic arthritis, and reactive arthritis. (HLAs and their relationship to autoimmune diseases are discussed in Chapter 14.)

The spondyloarthropathies share clinical and laboratory characteristics that may make it difficult to distinguish among them in early disease. These characteristics include absence of antibodies in the serum, inflammatory arthritis of the spine, peripheral joint involvement predominantly of the lower extremities, sacroiliitis, uveitis, enteric mucosal lesions, and skin lesions.[26]

ANKYLOSING SPONDYLITIS

Ankylosing spondylitis (AS) is a chronic inflammatory disease that primarily affects the axial skeleton, including the sacroiliac joints, intervertebral disc spaces, and costovertebral articulations. HLA-B27 antigen is found in approximately 90% of people with AS. Individuals with the antigen have a significantly greater risk of developing a spondyloarthropathy than those who do not.[19] The usual age of onset of AS is before 40 years old. Men are three to five times more likely to develop AS than women. The disease may go undetected in women because of a milder course.

Etiology and Pathophysiology

Genetic predisposition appears to play an important role in the pathogenesis of AS, but the precise mechanisms of the disease are unknown. Aseptic synovial inflammation in the joints and adjacent tissue causes the formation of granulation tissue *(pannus)* and dense fibrous scars that lead to fusion of articular tissues. Extraarticular inflammation can affect the eyes, lungs, heart, kidneys, and peripheral nervous system.

Clinical Manifestations and Complications

AS is characterized by symmetric sacroiliitis and progressive inflammatory arthritis of the axial skeleton. Symptoms of inflammatory spine pain are the first clues to a diagnosis of AS. The patient typically complains of low back pain, stiffness, and limitation of motion that is worse during the night and in the morning but improves with mild activity. In women, early symptoms of disease may manifest as pain and stiffness in the neck rather than the lower back. General symptoms such as fever, fatigue, anorexia, and weight loss are rarely present. *Uveitis* (intraocular inflammation) is the most common nonskeletal symptom. It can appear as an initial presentation of the disease years before arthritic symptoms develop. AS patients may also experience chest pain and sternal/costal cartilage tenderness that can be distressing.

Severe postural abnormalities and deformity can lead to significant disability for the patient with AS (Fig. 65-8). Impaired spinal ROM and fixed kyphosis contribute to altered visual function, raising concerns about safe ambulation. Aortic insuf-

FIG. 65-8 Advanced ankylosing spondylitis. Kyphotic posture causes many patients to have a protuberant abdomen secondary to pulmonary restriction.

🧬 GENETICS IN CLINICAL PRACTICE

Ankylosing Spondylitis

Genetic Basis
- Inheritance of human leukocyte antigen (HLA) B27 increases susceptibility to development of ankylosing spondylitis (AS).

Incidence
- About 80%-90% of white people with AS have HLA-B27 antigen.
- Inheriting HLA-B27 does not mean that a person will develop the disease. Of children who inherit HLA-B27 from a parent with AS, 80% do not develop the disease.
- AS is three to five times more common in men than in women.
- It occurs more often in whites than in other ethnic groups.
- It affects 7 in 100,000 people.

Genetic Testing
- Testing for HLA-B27 antigen available.

Clinical Implications
- Diagnosis of AS usually occurs between ages 18 and 40.
- Multiple genetic and environmental factors play a role in pathogenesis of disease.
- It is not known how HLA-B27 increases the risk of AS.
- AS is present in about 3%-10% of patients with inflammatory bowel disease (IBD).
- About 50%-70% of patients with both AS and IBD are HLA-B27 positive.

ficiency and pulmonary fibrosis are frequent complications. Cauda equina syndrome (compression of the nerves at the end of the spinal cord) can also result, contributing to lower extremity weakness and bladder dysfunction. In addition, the patient is at risk for spinal fracture because of associated osteoporosis.

Diagnostic Studies

X-rays are the most important radiographic technique for the diagnosis and follow-up of AS. However, x-rays are limited in detecting early sacroiliitis or subtle changes in posterior vertebrae. MRI can be useful in assessing early cartilage abnormalities, while CT scan is appropriate in specific situations (e.g., cases with subtle x-ray changes). Changes on later spinal films include the appearance of "bamboo spine," which is the result of calcifications (syndesmophytes) that bridge from one vertebra to another.

Laboratory testing is not specific, but an elevated ESR and mild anemia may be seen. When the suspicion of AS is high, the presence of the HLA-B27 antigen improves the likelihood of this diagnosis.

Collaborative Care

Prevention of AS is not possible. However, families with other diagnosed HLA-B27-positive rheumatic diseases (e.g., acute anterior uveitis, juvenile spondyloarthritis) should be alert to signs of low back pain for early identification and treatment of AS.

Care of the AS patient is aimed at maintaining maximal skeletal mobility while decreasing pain and inflammation. Heat applications can help relieve local symptoms. NSAIDs and salicylates are commonly prescribed. DMARDs such as sulfasalazine or methotrexate have little effect on spinal disease but may help with peripheral joint disease. Local corticosteroid injections may be beneficial in relieving symptoms.

TNF, which promotes inflammation, is found in elevated levels in the blood and certain tissues of patients with AS. Etanercept, a biologic and targeted therapy drug, binds TNF and inhibits its action. Etanercept reduces active inflammation and improves spinal mobility. Additional anti-TNF inhibitors (infliximab, adalimumab, golimumab) may also be effective.

Once pain and stiffness are managed, exercise is essential. Postural control is important to minimize spinal deformity. The exercise regimen should include back, neck, and chest stretches. Hydrotherapy has also been shown to decrease pain and facilitate spinal extension. Surgery may be indicated for severe deformity and mobility impairment. Spinal osteotomy and total joint replacement are the most commonly performed procedures (see Chapter 63).

NURSING MANAGEMENT ANKYLOSING SPONDYLITIS

A key nursing responsibility is to teach the patient with AS about the disease and principles of therapy. The home management program should include regular exercise and attention to posture, local moist heat applications, and knowledgeable use of drugs.

Baseline ROM assessment includes chest expansion (using breathing exercises). Encourage smoking cessation to decrease the risk for lung complications in those with reduced chest expansion. Ongoing physical therapy includes gentle, graded stretching and strengthening exercises to preserve ROM and improve thoracolumbar flexion and extension.

Discourage excessive physical exertion during periods of active flare-up of the disease. Proper positioning at rest is essential. The mattress should be firm, and the patient should sleep on the back with a flat pillow, avoiding positions that encourage flexion deformity. Postural training emphasizes avoiding spinal flexion (e.g., leaning over a desk); heavy lifting; and prolonged walking, standing, or sitting. Encourage sports that facilitate natural stretching, such as swimming and racquet games. Family counseling and vocational rehabilitation are important.

PSORIATIC ARTHRITIS

Psoriatic arthritis (PsA) is a progressive inflammatory disease that affects about 10% of the 3 million people with psoriasis.[27] Psoriasis is a common, benign, inflammatory skin disorder characterized by red, irritated, and scaly patches. Both PsA and psoriasis appear to have a genetic link with the HLA antigens in many patients. Although the exact cause of PsA is unknown, a combination of immune, genetic, and environmental factors is suspected.

PsA can occur in different forms. These include (1) arthritis involving primarily the small joints of the hands and feet (DIP), (2) asymmetric arthritis involving joints of the extremities, (3) symmetric polyarthritis resembling RA, and (4) arthritis of the sacroiliac joints and spine (psoriatic spondylitis).[28]

On x-ray, the cartilage loss and erosion resemble those of RA. Advanced cases of PsA often reveal widened joint spaces. A "pencil in cup" deformity is common in the DIP joints as a result of osteolysis. In this deformity the narrowed end(s) of the metacarpals or phalanges insert into the expanded end of the other (adjacent) bone sharing the joint. Elevated ESR, mild anemia, and elevated blood uric acid levels can be seen in some patients. Therefore the diagnosis of gout must be excluded.

Treatment includes splinting, joint protection, and physical therapy. NSAIDs given early in the course of the disease may help with inflammation. Drug therapy also includes the DMARDs such as methotrexate, which is effective for both articular and cutaneous manifestations. Sulfasalazine and cyclosporine may be used for treating PsA. In addition, biologic and targeted therapy, such as etanercept, golimumab, adalimumab, and infliximab, may also be used.

REACTIVE ARTHRITIS

Reactive arthritis (Reiter's syndrome) occurs more commonly in young men than in young women. It is associated with a symptom complex that includes urethritis, conjunctivitis, and mucocutaneous lesions. Although the exact etiology is unknown, reactive arthritis appears to be a reaction triggered in the body after exposure to specific genitourinary or GI tract infections. Chlamydia trachomatis is most often implicated in sexually transmitted reactive arthritis.[19] Reactive arthritis is also associated with GI infections with Shigella, Salmonella, Campylobacter, or Yersinia species and other microorganisms.

Individuals who are positive for HLA-B27 are at increased risk of developing reactive arthritis after sexual contact or exposure to certain enteric pathogens. This finding supports the likelihood of a genetic predisposition.

Urethritis develops within 1 to 2 weeks after sexual contact or GI infection. In women, symptoms include cervicitis. Low-grade fever, conjunctivitis, and arthritis may occur over the next several weeks. This type of arthritis tends to be asymmetric, frequently involving the large joints of the lower extremities and the toes. Lower back pain may occur with severe disease. Mucocutaneous lesions commonly occur as small, painless, superficial ulcerations on the tongue, oral mucosa, and glans penis. Soft tissue manifestations commonly include Achilles tendinitis or plantar fasciitis. Few laboratory abnormalities occur, although the ESR may be elevated.

Prognosis is favorable, with most patients recovering after 2 to 16 weeks. Because reactive arthritis is often associated with

C. trachomatis infection, treatment of patients and their sexual partners with doxycycline is widely recommended. Conjunctivitis and lesions require no treatment, but topical ophthalmic corticosteroids are typically prescribed for treatment of uveitis. Drug therapy may also include NSAIDs, methotrexate, and sulfasalazine. Physical therapy may be helpful during disease recovery.

Most patients have complete remission with restoration of full joint function. Up to 30% may develop chronic or recurring disease, which can result in major disability.[29] X-ray changes in chronic reactive arthritis closely resemble those of AS. Treatment of chronic reactive arthritis is symptomatic.

SYSTEMIC LUPUS ERYTHEMATOSUS

Systemic lupus erythematosus (SLE) is a multisystem inflammatory autoimmune disease. It is a complex disorder of multifactorial origin resulting from interactions among genetic, hormonal, environmental, and immunologic factors. SLE typically affects the skin, joints, and serous membranes (pleura, pericardium), along with the renal, hematologic, and neurologic systems. SLE is characterized by a chronic unpredictable course marked by alternating periods of exacerbation and remission.

The overall incidence of SLE in the United States is approximately 2 to 8 per 100,000.[30] Most cases of SLE occur in women in their childbearing years. Women are 10 times more likely than men to develop SLE. African Americans (especially), Asian Americans, Hispanics, and Native Americans are more likely than whites to develop the disease.

Etiology and Pathophysiology

The etiology of the abnormal immune response in SLE is unknown.[31] Based on the high prevalence of SLE among family members, a genetic influence is suspected. Multiple susceptibility genes from the HLA complex, including *HLA-DR3*, show associations with SLE.

Hormones are also known to play a role in the etiology of SLE. Onset or exacerbation of disease symptoms sometimes occurs after the onset of menarche, with the use of oral contraceptives, and during and after pregnancy. The disease tends to worsen in the immediate postpartum period.

Environmental factors are believed to contribute to the occurrence of SLE, with sun exposure and sunburns as the most common environmental triggers. Infectious agents may serve as a stimulus for immune hyperactivity. SLE may also be precipitated or aggravated by certain drugs such as procainamide (Pronestyl), hydralazine (Apresoline), and a number of antiseizure drugs.

SLE is characterized by the production of a large variety of autoantibodies against nucleic acids (e.g., single- and double-stranded DNA), erythrocytes, coagulation proteins, lymphocytes, platelets, and many other self-proteins. Autoimmune reactions characteristically are directed against constituents of the cell nucleus (antinuclear antibodies [ANAs]), particularly DNA.

Circulating immune complexes containing antibody against DNA are deposited in the basement membranes of capillaries in the kidneys, heart, skin, brain, and joints. Complement is activated, and inflammation occurs.[32] The overaggressive autoimmune response is also related to activation of B and T cells. The specific manifestations of SLE depend on which cell types

or organs are involved. (SLE is a type III hypersensitivity response [see Chapter 14].)

Clinical Manifestations and Complications

SLE is extremely variable in its severity, ranging from a relatively mild disorder to a rapidly progressive one affecting many body systems (Fig. 65-9). No characteristic pattern occurs in the progressive involvement of SLE. Any organ can be affected by an accumulation of circulating immune complexes. The most commonly affected tissues are the skin and muscle, the lining of the lungs, the heart, nervous tissue, and the kidneys. Generalized complaints such as fever, weight loss, arthralgia, and excessive fatigue may precede an exacerbation of disease activity.

Dermatologic Problems. Cutaneous vascular lesions can appear in any location but are most likely to develop in sun-exposed areas. Severe skin reactions can occur in people who are photosensitive. The classic butterfly rash over the cheeks and bridge of the nose occurs in 50% of patients with SLE (Fig. 65-10). About 20% of patients have *discoid* (round, coin-shaped) lesions. A small number of patients have persistent lesions, photosensitivity, and mild systemic disease in a syndrome referred to as *subacute cutaneous lupus.*

Ulcers of the oral or nasopharyngeal membranes occur in up to one third of patients with SLE. Alopecia is also common, with or without underlying scalp lesions. The hair may grow back during remission, but hair loss may be permanent over lesions. The scalp becomes dry, scaly, and atrophied.

Musculoskeletal Problems. Arthritis occurs in more than 90% of patients with SLE. Polyarthralgia with morning stiffness is often the patient's first complaint and may precede the onset of multisystem disease by many years. Diffuse swelling is accompanied by joint and muscle pain and some stiffness. Lupus-related arthritis is generally nonerosive, but it may cause deformities such as swan neck deformity of the fingers (see Fig. 65-4, *D*), ulnar deviation, and subluxation with hyperlaxity of the joints. Patients with SLE have an increased risk of bone loss and fracture.

Cardiopulmonary Problems. Tachypnea and cough in patients with SLE are suggestive of lung disease. Pleurisy is also possible. Cardiac involvement may include dysrhythmias resulting from fibrosis of the sinoatrial and atrioventricular nodes. This is an ominous sign of advanced disease, contributing significantly to the morbidity and mortality seen in SLE. Pericarditis can also occur. Clinical factors such as hypertension and hypercholesterolemia require aggressive therapy and careful monitoring. In addition, people with SLE are at risk for secondary *antiphospholipid syndrome,* a disorder of coagulation that leads to clots in the arteries and veins with associated risk of stroke, gangrene, and heart attack.

Renal Problems. Lupus nephritis (LN) occurs in approximately 40% of patients with SLE. Renal involvement is usually evident within 5 years after symptoms of SLE appear. Manifestations of renal involvement vary from mild proteinuria to rapidly progressive glomerulonephritis. Scarring and permanent damage can lead to end-stage kidney disease.

The primary goal in treating LN is to slow the progression of nephropathy and preserve renal function by managing the underlying disease. The importance of obtaining a renal biopsy is controversial, but findings can help guide treatment. Although LN may be one of the more serious complications of SLE, effective treatments are available. These typically include corticosteroids, cytotoxic agents (cyclophosphamide [Cytoxan]),

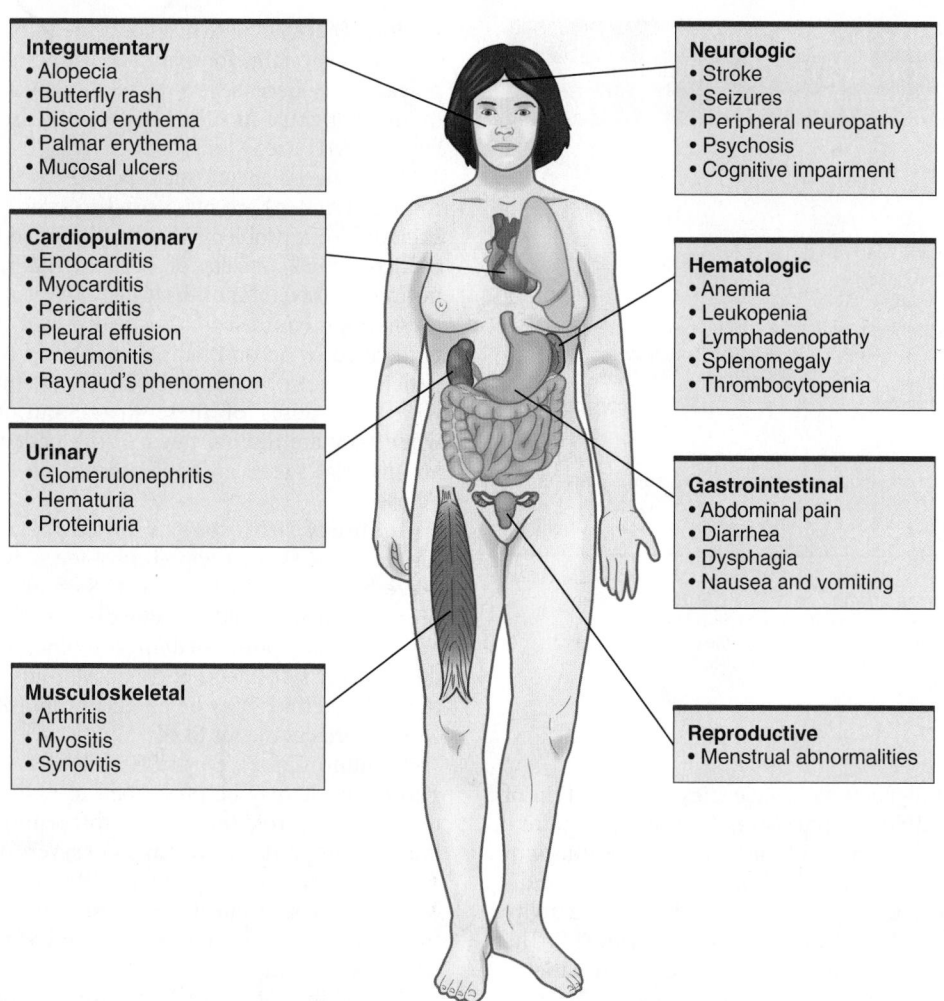

FIG. 65-9 Multisystem involvement in systemic lupus erythematosus.

The figure shows the following system involvements:

Integumentary
- Alopecia
- Butterfly rash
- Discoid erythema
- Palmar erythema
- Mucosal ulcers

Cardiopulmonary
- Endocarditis
- Myocarditis
- Pericarditis
- Pleural effusion
- Pneumonitis
- Raynaud's phenomenon

Urinary
- Glomerulonephritis
- Hematuria
- Proteinuria

Musculoskeletal
- Arthritis
- Myositis
- Synovitis

Neurologic
- Stroke
- Seizures
- Peripheral neuropathy
- Psychosis
- Cognitive impairment

Hematologic
- Anemia
- Leukopenia
- Lymphadenopathy
- Splenomegaly
- Thrombocytopenia

Gastrointestinal
- Abdominal pain
- Diarrhea
- Dysphagia
- Nausea and vomiting

Reproductive
- Menstrual abnormalities

FIG. 65-10 Butterfly rash of systemic lupus erythematosus.

and immunosuppressive agents (azathioprine, cyclosporine, mycophenolate mofetil [CellCept]). Rituximab and eculizumab (Soliris) are being studied as possible treatments. Oral prednisone or pulsed IV methylprednisolone may also be used as an intervention for LN, especially in the initial treatment period when cytotoxic agents have not had time to take effect.

Nervous System Problems. Along with renal involvement, neuropsychiatric manifestations are prevalent in SLE. Generalized or focal seizures are the most common manifestation involving the CNS and occur in as many as 15% of patients with

SLE by the time of diagnosis. Seizures are generally controlled by corticosteroids or antiseizure drugs. Peripheral neuropathy can also occur, leading to sensory and motor deficits.

Cognitive dysfunction, recognized as a CNS manifestation of SLE, may result from the deposition of immune complexes within the brain tissue. It is characterized by disordered thought processes, disorientation, memory deficits, and psychiatric symptoms such as severe depression and psychosis. Various psychiatric disorders are reported in SLE, including mood disorders, anxiety, and psychosis, although they may be related to the stress of having a major illness or to associated drug therapies. Occasionally a stroke or aseptic meningitis may be attributable to SLE. Headaches are also common and can become severe during a flare (exacerbation of disease).

Hematologic Problems. The formation of antibodies against blood cells, such as erythrocytes, leukocytes, thrombocytes, and coagulation factors, is also a common feature of SLE.[32] Anemia, mild leukopenia, and thrombocytopenia are often present. Some patients develop a tendency toward coagulopathy involving either excessive bleeding or blood clot development. A manifestation of antiphospholipid antibody syndrome is a common cause of hypercoagulability in SLE patients, many of whom benefit from high-intensity treatment with warfarin.

Infection. Patients with SLE appear to have increased susceptibility to infections, possibly because of defects in the ability

TABLE 65-14 DIAGNOSTIC CRITERIA FOR SYSTEMIC LUPUS ERYTHEMATOSUS*

- Malar rash
- Discoid rash
- Photosensitivity
- Oral ulcers
- Arthritis: nonerosive, involvement of two or more joints characterized by tenderness, swelling, and effusion
- Serositis: pleuritis or pericarditis
- Renal disorder: persistent proteinuria or cellular casts in urine
- Neurologic disorder: seizures or psychosis (in the absence of causative drugs or known metabolic disorders)
- Hematologic disorder: hemolytic anemia, leukopenia, lymphopenia, or thrombocytopenia
- Immunologic disorder: positive LE preparation, anti-DNA antibody or antibody to Sm nuclear antigen, or false-positive serologic tests for syphilis
- Antinuclear antibody

Source: Tan EM, Cohen AS, Fries JF, et al: The 1982 revised criteria for classification of systemic lupus erythematosus, *Arthritis Rheum* 25:11, 1982. Retrieved from *www.rheumatology.org/practice/clinical/classification/SLE/sle.asp.*
*A person is classified as having SLE if four or more of the criteria are present, serially or simultaneously, during any interval of observation.
LE, Lupus erythematosus; *Sm,* Smith.

to phagocytize invading bacteria, deficiencies in production of antibodies, and the immunosuppressive effect of many antiinflammatory drugs. Infection is a major cause of death, with pneumonia being the most common infection. Fever may indicate an underlying infectious process rather than lupus activity alone. Vaccinations are generally safe for patients with SLE. The exception is the need to avoid live virus vaccines in patients being treated with corticosteroids or cytotoxic agents.

Diagnostic Studies

The diagnosis of SLE is based on distinct criteria revealed through patient history, physical examination, and laboratory findings (Table 65-14). No specific test is diagnostic for SLE, but a variety of abnormalities may be present in the blood. SLE is marked by the presence of ANA in 97% of persons with the disease.

Other antibodies include anti-DNA, antineuronal, anticoagulant, anti-WBC, anti–red blood cell (RBC), antiplatelet, antiphospholipid, and anti–basement membrane. Anti–double-stranded DNA antibodies are found in half the persons with SLE. The anti-Smith (Sm) antibodies are found in 30% to 40% of persons with lupus and are almost always considered diagnostic. The lupus erythematosus (LE) cell prep test is a nonspecific test for SLE and is positive in other rheumatic diseases. ESR and CRP levels are not diagnostic of SLE, but may be used to monitor disease activity and effectiveness of therapy.

Collaborative Care

A major challenge in the treatment of SLE is managing the active phase of the disease while preventing complications of treatments. Survival is influenced by several factors, including age, race, gender, socioeconomic status, accompanying morbid conditions, and severity of disease. The prognosis of SLE can be improved with early diagnosis, prompt recognition of serious organ involvement, and effective therapeutic regimens.

Drug Therapy. NSAIDs continue to be an important intervention, especially for patients with mild polyarthralgias or polyarthritis. Because prolonged therapy is likely, careful patient monitoring must include the potential for GI and renal effects from NSAID use.

Antimalarial agents such as hydroxychloroquine and chloroquine (Aralen) are often used to treat fatigue and moderate skin and joint problems. Unlike the rapid response noted with corticosteroids, effects of antimalarial therapy may not be noticed for several months.[33] Flares may also be prevented with these drugs. Funduscopic and visual field examinations must be performed by an ophthalmologist every 6 to 12 months when patients are on hydroxychloroquine. Retinopathy can develop with high doses of these drugs, but it generally reverses when they are discontinued. If the patient cannot tolerate an antimalarial agent, an antileprosy drug such as dapsone may be used.

The use of corticosteroids should be limited. However, tapering doses of IV methylprednisolone may help control severe exacerbations of polyarthritis. Steroid-sparing immunosuppressants such as methotrexate can serve as an alternative treatment and are prescribed in combination with folic acid to decrease the side effects of corticosteroids. However, high doses of corticosteroids may be especially appropriate for the patient with severe cutaneous SLE.

Immunosuppressive drugs such as azathioprine and cyclophosphamide may be prescribed to reduce the need for long-term corticosteroid therapy. Azathioprine or cyclophosphamide is also appropriate for treatment of severe organ-system disease, especially LN. Close monitoring is necessary to minimize drug toxicity and side effects. Because blood clots can be a life-threatening complication of SLE, anticoagulants such as warfarin or heparin may be prescribed.[33]

Topical immunomodulators are an alternative to corticosteroids for treating serious skin conditions. Tacrolimus (Protopic, Prograf) and pimecrolimus (Elidel) suppress immune activity in the skin, including the butterfly rash and possibly discoid lesions.

Clinical trials are currently investigating the effect of various medications on SLE management. These include biologic and targeted therapy agents that interfere with the immune response such as abatacept, and hormones (prasterone [Prestara]) to combat lupus-induced osteoporosis. Thalidomide as a second-line therapy has been shown to improve cutaneous lupus even in persons who have not responded to other therapies.

When teaching patients about their prescribed drugs, include their indications for use, proper administration, and possible side effects. Help the patient understand that abrupt cessation may exacerbate disease activity.

Disease management is most appropriately monitored by serial anti-DNA titers and serum complement levels (Table 65-15). Simpler and less costly tests such as ESR or CRP may also help in monitoring treatment effectiveness.

NURSING MANAGEMENT
SYSTEMIC LUPUS ERYTHEMATOSUS

NURSING ASSESSMENT

Subjective and objective data that should be obtained from the patient with SLE are presented in Table 65-16. In particular, evaluate the extent to which pain and fatigue influence activities of daily living.

TABLE 65-15 COLLABORATIVE CARE
Systemic Lupus Erythematosus

Diagnostic
- History and physical examination
- Antibodies (e.g., anti-DNA, anti-Sm, ANA)
- Complete blood cell count
- LE cell prep
- Serum complement levels
- Urinalysis
- X-ray of affected joints
- Chest x-ray
- ECG to determine extraarticular involvement

Collaborative Therapy
- NSAIDs for mild disease
- Steroid-sparing drugs (e.g., methotrexate)
- Antimalarials (e.g., hydroxychloroquine [Plaquenil])
- Corticosteroids for exacerbations and severe disease
- Immunosuppressive drugs (e.g., cyclophosphamide [Cytoxan], mycophenolate mofetil [CellCept])

ANA, Antinuclear antibody; *LE,* lupus erythematosus; *Sm,* Smith.

NURSING DIAGNOSES

Nursing diagnoses for the patient with SLE may include, but are not limited to, the following:
- Fatigue *related to* chronic inflammation and altered immunity
- Impaired skin integrity *related to* photosensitivity, skin rash, and alopecia
- Impaired comfort *related to* illness-related symptoms, treatment-related side effects, and the potential for variable and unpredictable progression of the disease

Additional information on nursing diagnoses for the patient with SLE is presented in eNursing Care Plan 65-2 (on the website for this chapter).

PLANNING

The overall goals are that the patient with SLE will (1) have satisfactory pain management, (2) adhere to the therapeutic regimen to achieve maximum symptom management, (3) demonstrate awareness of and avoid activities that exacerbate the disease, and (4) maintain optimal role function and a positive self-image.

NURSING IMPLEMENTATION

HEALTH PROMOTION. Prevention of SLE is not possible at this time. However, education of health professionals and the community should promote a clear understanding of the disease and the need for early diagnosis and treatment.

ACUTE INTERVENTION. As in the majority of rheumatic diseases, the unpredictable nature of SLE presents many challenges to the patient and caregiver. The physical, psychologic, and sociocultural problems associated with the long-term management of SLE require the varied approaches and skills of the multidisciplinary health care team.

During an exacerbation of SLE, the patient may become abruptly and dramatically ill. Nursing interventions include accurately recording the severity of symptoms and documenting the response to therapy. Specifically assess fever pattern, joint inflammation, limitation of motion, location and degree of discomfort, and fatigue. Monitor the patient's weight and fluid intake and output if corticosteroids are prescribed because

TABLE 65-16 NURSING ASSESSMENT
Systemic Lupus Erythematosus

Subjective Data
Important Health Information
Past health history: Exposure to ultraviolet radiation, drugs, chemicals, viral infections; physical or psychologic stress; states of increased estrogen activity, including early onset of menarche, pregnancy, and postpartum period; pattern of remissions and exacerbations
Medications: Oral contraceptives, procainamide (Pronestyl), hydralazine (Apresoline), isoniazid (INH), antiseizure drugs, antibiotics (possibly precipitating symptoms of SLE); corticosteroids, NSAIDs

Functional Health Patterns
Health perception–health management: Family history of autoimmune disorders; frequent infections; malaise; impact of disease on functional ability
Nutritional-metabolic: Weight loss, oral and nasal ulcers; nausea and vomiting; xerostomia (salivary gland dryness), dysphagia; photosensitivity with rash; frequent infections
Elimination: Decreased urine output; diarrhea or constipation
Activity-exercise: Morning stiffness; joint swelling and deformity; shortness of breath, dyspnea; excessive fatigue
Sleep-rest: Insomnia
Cognitive-perceptual: Visual disturbances; vertigo; headache; polyarthralgia; chest pain (pericardial, pleuritic); abdominal pain; joint pain; painful, throbbing, cold fingers with numbness and tingling
Sexuality-reproductive: Amenorrhea, irregular menstrual periods
Coping–stress tolerance: Depression, withdrawal

Objective Data
General
Fever, lymphadenopathy, periorbital edema

Integumentary
Alopecia; dry, scaly scalp; keratoconjunctivitis, malar "butterfly" rash, palmar or discoid erythema, urticaria, periungual erythema, purpura, or petechiae; leg ulcers

Respiratory
Pleural friction rub, decreased breath sounds

Cardiovascular
Vasculitis; pericardial friction rub; hypertension, edema, dysrhythmias, murmurs; bilateral, symmetric pallor and cyanosis of fingers (Raynaud's phenomenon)

Gastrointestinal
Oral and pharyngeal ulcers; splenomegaly

Neurologic
Facial weakness, peripheral neuropathies, papilledema, dysarthria, confusion, hallucination, disorientation, psychosis, seizures, aphasia, hemiparesis

Musculoskeletal
Myopathy, myositis, arthritis

Urinary
Proteinuria

Possible Diagnostic Findings
Presence of anti-DNA, anti-Sm, and antinuclear antibodies; anemia, leukopenia, thrombocytopenia; ↑ erythrocyte sedimentation rate (ESR); positive LE cell prep; ↑ serum creatinine; microscopic hematuria, cellular casts in urine; pericarditis or pleural effusion evident on chest x-ray

Sm, Smith.

of their fluid-retention effect and the possibility of renal failure. Collection of 24-hour urine samples for protein and creatinine clearance may be ordered. Observe for signs of bleeding that result from drug therapy, such as pallor, skin bruising, petechiae, or tarry stools.

Carefully assess the neurologic status. Observe for visual disturbances, headaches, personality changes, seizures, and forgetfulness. Psychosis may indicate CNS disease or may be an effect of corticosteroid therapy. Irritation of the nerves of the extremities (peripheral neuropathy) may produce numbness, tingling, and weakness of the hands and feet.

Explain the nature of the disease, modes of therapy, and all diagnostic procedures. Emotional support for the patient and family is also essential, especially during an exacerbation.

AMBULATORY AND HOME CARE. Emphasize the importance of patient cooperation for successful home management. Help the patient understand that even strong adherence to the treatment plan is no guarantee against exacerbations because the course of the disease is unpredictable. A variety of factors may increase disease activity, such as fatigue, sun exposure, emotional stress, infection, drugs, and surgery. Help the patient and caregiver eliminate or minimize exposure to precipitating factors (Table 65-17).

Lupus and Pregnancy. Because SLE is most common in women of childbearing age, treatment during pregnancy must be considered. The woman's primary health care provider (or rheumatologist) and obstetrician should thoroughly discuss with the woman her desire to become pregnant. Infertility may have resulted from renal involvement and the previous use of high-dose corticosteroid and chemotherapy drugs. The SLE patient should understand that spontaneous abortion, stillbirth, and intrauterine growth retardation are common problems with pregnancy. They occur because of deposits of immune complexes in the placenta and because of inflammatory responses in the placental blood vessels.

Renal, cardiovascular, pulmonary, and central nervous systems (in particular) may be affected during pregnancy. Women who already demonstrate serious SLE involvement in these systems should be counseled against pregnancy. For the best outcome, pregnancy should be planned at a point when the disease activity is minimal. Exacerbation is common during the postpartum period. Therapeutic abortion offers the same risk of postdelivery exacerbation as carrying the fetus to term.

Psychosocial Issues. The patient with SLE confronts many psychosocial issues. Disease onset and symptoms may be vague, and SLE may be undiagnosed for a long time. Supportive therapies may become as important as medical treatment in helping the patient cope with the disease. Counsel the patient and caregiver that SLE has a good prognosis for the majority of people.

Families worry about hereditary aspects and want to know whether their children will also have SLE. Many couples require pregnancy and sexual counseling. Individuals making decisions about marriage and careers worry about how SLE will interfere with their plans. You may have to educate teachers, employers, and co-workers.

The obvious physical effects of skin lesions and alopecia may cause social isolation for the patient with SLE, affecting his or her self-esteem and body image.[34] Consultation with a dermatologist may be recommended for appropriate treatment and cosmetic products to conceal the rash.

Pain and fatigue may interfere with quality of life. Pacing techniques and relaxation therapy can help the patient remain involved in day-to-day activities. Stress the importance of planning both recreational and occupational activities. Young adults may find sun restrictions and physical limitations particularly difficult to follow. Help the patient develop and accomplish reasonable goals for improving or maintaining mobility, energy levels, and self-esteem.

▌EVALUATION

The expected outcomes are that the patient with SLE will
- Use energy conservation techniques
- Adapt lifestyle to energy level
- Maintain skin integrity with the use of topical treatments
- Prevent exacerbations with the use of sunscreens and limited sun exposure

Additional information on expected outcomes for the patient with SLE is presented in eNursing Care Plan 65-2 (on the website for this chapter).

SCLERODERMA

Scleroderma *(systemic sclerosis)* is a disorder of connective tissue characterized by fibrotic, degenerative, and occasionally inflammatory changes in the skin, blood vessels, synovium, skeletal muscle, and internal organs.

Scleroderma occurs in all ethnic groups but is more common in African Americans than whites. Hispanics and Native Americans may also be at higher risk than whites. Although symptoms may begin at any time, the usual age at onset is between 30 and 50 years. Scleroderma is relatively rare, with approximately 75,000 to 100,000 people in the United States affected. Seventy-five percent of cases are women.[35]

Two types of disease exist: *limited cutaneous scleroderma,* which is the more common (80%), and *diffuse scleroderma.* Both forms are systemic with distinct degrees and types of organ involvement and disease progression. The prognosis of patients with limited disease is generally better than for those with diffuse disease.

Etiology and Pathophysiology

The exact cause of scleroderma is unknown. Immunologic dysfunction and vascular abnormalities are believed to play a role

---

TABLE 65-17	PATIENT & CAREGIVER TEACHING GUIDE

Systemic Lupus Erythematosus

Include the following information in the teaching plan for a patient with systemic lupus erythematosus and the caregiver.
- Disease process
- Names of drugs, actions, side effects, dosage, administration
- Pain management strategies
- Energy conservation and pacing techniques
- Therapeutic exercise, use of heat therapy (for arthralgia)
- Avoidance of physical and emotional stress
- Avoidance of exposure to individuals with infection
- Avoidance of drying soaps, powders, household chemicals
- Use of sunscreen protection (at least SPF 15) and protective clothing, with minimal sun exposure from 11:00 AM to 3:00 PM
- Regular medical and laboratory follow-up
- Marital and pregnancy counseling as needed
- Community resources and health care agencies

SPF, Sun protection factor.

Normal skin   **Scleroderma**

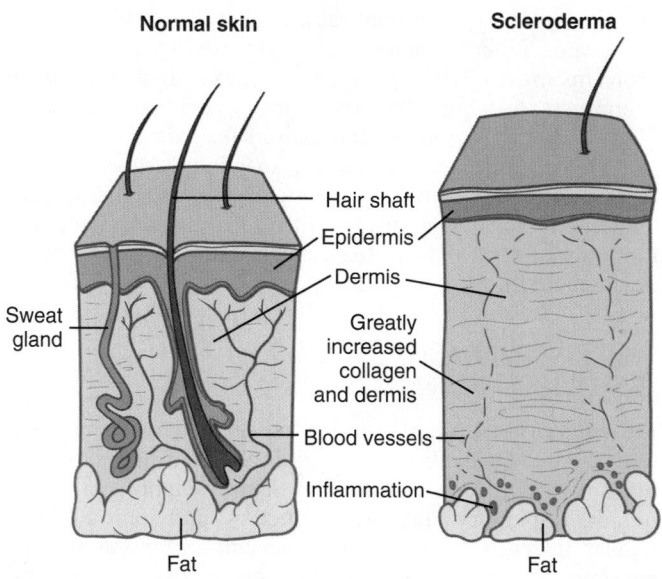

- Hair shaft
- Epidermis
- Dermis
- Greatly increased collagen and dermis
- Blood vessels
- Inflammation

Sweat gland

Fat   Fat

FIG. 65-11 Skin changes in scleroderma.

FIG. 65-12 Hand of a patient with scleroderma showing sclerodactyly.

in the development of widespread systemic disease. Other risk factors associated with skin thickening include environmental or occupational exposure to coal, plastics, and silica dust.

In scleroderma, collagen (protein that gives normal skin its strength and elasticity) is overproduced (Fig. 65-11). Excessive production of collagen leads to progressive tissue fibrosis and occlusion of blood vessels. Proliferation of collagen disrupts the normal functioning of internal organs, such as lungs, kidney, heart, and GI tract.

The vascular alterations, which primarily involve the small arteries and arterioles, are almost always present in scleroderma. These changes are some of the earliest alterations in scleroderma.

Clinical Manifestations

Manifestations of scleroderma range from a diffuse cutaneous thickening with rapidly progressive and widespread organ involvement to the more benign limited cutaneous form. The signs of limited disease appear on the face and hands, whereas diffuse disease initially involves the trunk and extremities. Clinical manifestations of scleroderma can be described by the acronym CREST:

Calcinosis: painful deposits of calcium in the skin

Raynaud's phenomenon: abnormal blood flow in response to cold or stress

Esophageal dysfunction: difficulty with swallowing caused by internal scarring

Sclerodactyly: tightening of the skin on the fingers and the toes

Telangiectasia: red spots on hands, forearms, palms, face, and lips

Raynaud's Phenomenon. Raynaud's phenomenon (paroxysmal vasospasm of the digits) is the most common initial complaint in limited scleroderma. Patients have diminished blood flow to the fingers and toes on exposure to cold (blanching or white phase), followed by cyanosis as hemoglobin releases oxygen to the tissues (blue phase), and then erythema during rewarming (red phase). The color changes are often accompanied by numbness and tingling. Raynaud's phenomenon may precede the onset of systemic disease by months, years, or even

decades. (Raynaud's phenomenon is described in more detail in Chapter 38.)

Skin and Joint Changes. Symmetric painless swelling or thickening of the skin of the fingers and hands may progress to diffuse scleroderma of the trunk. In limited disease, skin thickening generally does not extend above the elbow or above the knee, although the face may be affected. In more diffuse disease, the skin loses elasticity and becomes taut and shiny, producing the typical expressionless facies with tightly pursed lips. Skin changes in the face may also contribute to reduced ROM in the temporomandibular joint. The hands may be affected by sclerodactyly in which the fingers are in a semiflexed position, with tightened skin to the wrist (Fig. 65-12). Reduced peripheral joint function may occur as an early symptom of polyarthritis.

Internal Organ Involvement. About 20% of people with scleroderma develop secondary Sjögren's syndrome, a condition associated with dry eyes and dry mouth. Dysphagia, gum disease, and dental caries can result. Frequent reflux of gastric acid can also occur as a result of esophageal fibrosis. If swallowing becomes difficult, the patient is likely to decrease food intake and loses weight. Additional GI effects include constipation resulting from colonic hypomotility and diarrhea caused by malabsorption from bacterial overgrowth.

Lung involvement includes pleural thickening, pulmonary fibrosis, and pulmonary function abnormalities. The patient develops a cough and dyspnea. Pulmonary arterial hypertension and interstitial lung disease may occur. Pulmonary arterial hypertension is treated with medications such as extended-release nifedipine (Afeditab CR), bosentan (Tracleer), and ambrisentan (Letairis). (Pulmonary artery hypertension is discussed in Chapter 28.) Lung disease is the main cause of death in scleroderma.

Primary heart disease consists of pericarditis, pericardial effusion, and cardiac dysrhythmias. Myocardial fibrosis resulting in heart failure occurs most frequently in patients with diffuse disease.

Renal disease was previously a major cause of death in diffuse scleroderma. Because malignant hypertension associated with rapidly progressive and irreversible renal insufficiency can occur, early recognition of renal involvement and initiation of therapy are critical. Recent improvements in dialysis, bilateral nephrectomy in patients with uncontrollable hypertension, and kidney transplantation have offered some hope to patients with renal failure. In particular, use of angiotensin-converting enzyme (ACE) inhibitors (e.g., lisinopril [Prinivil]) has had a marked impact on the ability to treat renal disease.

Diagnostic Studies

Laboratory findings in scleroderma are relatively normal. Blood studies may reveal a mild hemolytic anemia as a result of RBC damage in diseased small vessels. ANAs are found in most patients.[36] The scleroderma antibody SCL-70 is found in about 30% of patients with diffuse disease, and serum RF is found in 30% of affected patients. An anticentromere antibody is seen in many patients with CREST. If renal involvement is present, urinalysis may show proteinuria, microscopic hematuria, and casts. Serum levels of creatinine may be elevated. X-ray evidence of subcutaneous calcification, distal esophageal hypomotility, or bilateral pulmonary fibrosis is diagnostic of scleroderma. Pulmonary function studies reveal decreased vital capacity and lung compliance.

Collaborative Care

The collaborative care of scleroderma (Table 65-18) offers no specific treatment. Supportive care is directed toward preventing or treating secondary complications of involved organs. Physical therapy helps to maintain joint mobility and preserve muscle strength. Occupational therapy assists the patient in maintaining functional abilities.

Drug Therapy. No specific drug or combination of drugs has been proven effective for the treatment of scleroderma. Vasoactive agents are often prescribed in early disease, and calcium channel blockers (nifedipine [Adalat, Procardia], diltiazem [Cardizem]) are now a common treatment choice for Raynaud's phenomenon. Reserpine (Serpasil), an α-adrenergic blocking agent, increases blood flow to the fingers. Bosentan, an endothelin-receptor antagonist, and epoprostenol (Flolan), a vasodilator, may help prevent and treat digital ulcers while improving exercise capacity and heart and lung dynamics. Losartan, an angiotensin II blocker, may be used to treat Raynaud's phenomenon.

Corticosteroids may have little effect on scleroderma. Topical agents may provide some relief from joint pain. Capsaicin cream may be useful, not only as a local analgesic, but also as a vasodilator. Other therapies prescribed to treat specific systemic problems include tetracycline for diarrhea caused by bacterial overgrowth, histamine (H_2)-receptor blockers (e.g., cimetidine [Tagamet]) and proton pump inhibitors (e.g., omeprazole [Prilosec]) for esophageal symptoms, an antihypertensive agent (e.g., captopril [Capoten], propranolol [Inderal], methyldopa [Aldomet]) for hypertension with renal involvement, and immunosuppressive drugs (e.g., cyclophosphamide, mycophenolate mofetil).

NURSING MANAGEMENT
SCLERODERMA

Prevention of scleroderma is not possible. Nursing interventions for these patients often begin during a hospitalization for diagnostic purposes. Assess vital signs, weight, intake and output, respiratory and bowel function, and joint ROM at regular intervals as indicated by specific symptoms to plan appropriate care. Emotional stress and cold ambient temperatures may aggravate Raynaud's phenomenon. Instruct patients with scleroderma not to have finger-stick blood testing done because of compromised circulation and poor healing of the fingers.

Teaching is an important nursing intervention as the patient and family begin to live with this disease. Obvious changes in the face and hands often lead to poor self-image and the loss of mobility and function. The patient must actively complete therapeutic exercises at home to prevent skin retraction and promote vascularization. Mouth excursion (yawning with an open mouth) is a good exercise to help with temporomandibular joint function. Isometric exercises are most appropriate if the patient has arthropathy because no joint movement occurs. Encourage the use of moist heat applications or paraffin baths to promote skin flexibility in the hands and feet. Teach the patient to use assistive devices as appropriate and organize activities to preserve strength and reduce disability.

Teach the patient to protect the hands and feet from cold exposure and possible burns or cuts that might heal slowly. Smoking should be avoided because of its vasoconstricting effect. Signs of infection should be reported promptly. Lotions may help alleviate skin dryness and cracking, but they must be rubbed in for an unusually long time because of the thick skin.

Dysphagia may be reduced by eating small, frequent meals; chewing carefully and slowly; and drinking fluids. Heartburn may be minimized by using antacids 45 to 60 minutes after each meal and by sitting upright for at least 2 hours after eating. Using additional pillows or raising the head of the bed on blocks may help reduce nocturnal gastroesophageal reflux.

Job modifications are often necessary because of problems with climbing stairs, using a computer, writing, and being exposed to cold. The patient may become socially withdrawn as skin tightening alters the appearance of the face and hands. Dining out may become socially embarrassing because of the patient's small mouth, difficulty swallowing, and reflux. Some individuals with scleroderma wear gloves to protect fingertip ulcers and to provide extra warmth. Emphasize daily oral hygiene because neglect may lead to increased tooth and gingival problems. The patient needs a dentist who is familiar with scleroderma and can deal with a small mouth.

Psychologic support, biofeedback training, and relaxation can reduce stress and improve sleeping habits. Sexual dys-

---

TABLE 65-18 COLLABORATIVE CARE

Scleroderma

Diagnostic
- History and physical examination
- Antinuclear antibody titers
- Anticentromere antibody
- Nail bed capillary microscopy
- X-ray of chest
- Skin or visceral biopsy
- Urinalysis (proteinuria, hematuria, casts)
- Pulmonary function tests
- ECG

Collaborative Therapy
- Physical therapy
- Occupational therapy
- Drug therapy
  - *Vasoactive agents:* reserpine (Serpasil), bosentan (Tracleer), epoprostenol (Flolan)
  - *Calcium channel blockers:* diltiazem (Cardizem), nifedipine (Adalat, Procardia)
  - *Angiotensin-converting enzyme inhibitors:* lisinopril (Prinivil)
  - *Immunosuppressive drugs:* cyclophosphamide (Cytoxan), mycophenolate mofetil (CellCept)

function resulting from body changes, pain, muscular weakness, limited mobility, decreased self-esteem, erectile dysfunction, and decreased vaginal secretions may require sensitive counseling.

POLYMYOSITIS AND DERMATOMYOSITIS

Polymyositis (PM) is diffuse, idiopathic, inflammatory myopathy of striated muscle that produces bilateral weakness, usually most severe in the proximal or limb girdle muscles. When muscle changes associated with PM are accompanied by characteristic skin changes, the disorder is called dermatomyositis (DM).[37]

Although these relatively rare disorders can be similar in signs, symptoms, and treatment, they are two distinct diseases. They typically affect adults ages 45 to 65 years. Both PM and DM occur twice as often in women as in men. Patients with PM generally have more severe disease than those with DM.

Etiology and Pathophysiology

The exact cause of PM and DM is unknown. Theories include an infectious agent, neoplasms, drugs or vaccinations, and stress. Because T cytotoxic cells and macrophages have been found near the damaged muscle fibers of PM, this disease is believed to be caused by cell-mediated injury. In contrast, DM has been associated with B cells (humoral immunity) and destruction of the muscle microvasculature. An autoimmune response to nuclear and cytoplasm self-antigens has also been noted in many persons with these disorders.[38]

Clinical Manifestations and Complications

Muscular. Patients with PM and DM experience weight loss and increasing fatigue, with a gradually developing weakness of the muscles that leads to difficulty performing routine activities. The most commonly affected muscles are those of the shoulders, legs, arms, and pelvic girdle. The patient may have difficulty rising from a chair or bathtub, climbing stairs, combing hair, or reaching into a high cupboard. Neck muscles may become so weak that the patient is unable to raise the head from the pillow. Muscle discomfort or tenderness is uncommon. Muscle examination reveals an inability to move against resistance or even gravity. Weak pharyngeal muscles may produce dysphagia and dysphonia (nasal or hoarse voice).

Dermal. Skin changes of DM include a classic violet-colored, cyanotic, or erythematous symmetric rash *(heliotrope)* with edema around the eyelids. Violet or erythematous papules and small plaques can develop over the DIP or MCP areas, and at elbow or knee joints in about 70% of patients with DM (Gottron's papules) (Fig. 65-13). These early skin changes usually prompt earlier recognition of DM compared with PM, in which a rash does not appear. Reddened, smooth, or scaly patches appear with the same symmetric distribution but sparing the interphalangeal spaces (Gottron's sign). They can be confused with psoriasis or seborrheic dermatitis. An erythematous scaling rash (poikiloderma) may develop as a late finding on the back, buttocks, and a V-shaped area of the anterior neck and chest. Hyperemia and telangiectasias are often present at the nail beds. Calcium nodules (calcinosis cutis), which can develop throughout the skin, are especially common in long-standing DM.

Other Manifestations. Joint redness, pain, and inflammation often occur and contribute to limitations in joint ROM in

FIG. 65-13 Dermatomyositis skin changes. Gottron's papules.

PM and DM. Contractures and muscle atrophy may occur with advanced disease. Weakened pharyngeal muscles can lead to a poor cough effort, difficulty swallowing, and increased risk for aspiration pneumonia in both disorders. Interstitial lung disease occurs in up to 65% of all patients. People with DM also have an increased risk of cancer, which may be present at the time of diagnosis. Both PM and DM may be associated with other connective tissue disorders (e.g., scleroderma).

Diagnostic Studies

A diagnosis of PM or DM is confirmed by MRI, electromyogram (EMG), muscle biopsy, and serum muscle enzyme levels. An EMG suggestive of PM shows bizarre high-frequency discharges and spontaneous fibrillation, with positive spikes at rest. Muscle biopsy reveals necrosis, degeneration, regeneration, and fibrosis with pathologic findings distinct for DM or PM. Markers such as creatinine kinase and myoglobin are elevated. Elevation of the ESR or CRP is also expected with active disease. In addition, more than 50% of persons with PM have positive RF. The typical skin rash seen with DM is not commonly found with other disorders.

NURSING AND COLLABORATIVE MANAGEMENT POLYMYOSITIS AND DERMATOMYOSITIS

PM and DM are treated initially with high-dose corticosteroids. Improvement generally occurs if corticosteroid therapy is instituted promptly. Dosage can be reduced as the patient improves. Long-term corticosteroid therapy may be required because relapses are common when the drug is withdrawn. If corticosteroids are ineffective after 4 weeks of treatment and/or organ involvement is occurring, immunosuppressive drugs (methotrexate, azathioprine, tacrolimus, cyclophosphamide) may also be administered.

DM has been shown to improve with high doses of IV immunoglobulin. Topical corticosteroids and hydroxychloroquine may be prescribed to treat the skin rash.

The role of newer medications such as TNF inhibitors remains unclear, although their use in refractory cases has shown some success. Ongoing clinical trials continue to explore the use of the monoclonal antibody rituximab and interferon α-2a in the treatment of PM and DM.

Physical therapy can be helpful and should be tailored to disease activity. Massage and passive movement are appropriate during active disease. More aggressive exercises should be reserved for periods when disease activity is minimal, as evidenced by low serum enzyme levels.

Teach the patient about the disease, prescribed therapies, diagnostic tests, and the importance of regular medical care. It is important for the patient to understand that the benefits of therapy are often delayed. For example, weakness may increase during the first few weeks of corticosteroid therapy. Pay special attention to patient safety. Encourage the use of assistive devices as a fall prevention strategy. To prevent aspiration, encourage the patient to rest before meals, maintain an upright position when eating, and choose a diet of easily swallowed foods.

Assist the patient in organizing activities and using pacing techniques to conserve energy. Encourage daily ROM exercises to prevent contractures. When active inflammation is not evident, start muscle-strengthening (repetitive) exercises. Home care and bed rest may become necessary during the acute phase of PM because profound muscle weakness results in the patient's inability to complete activities of daily living.

MIXED (OVERLAPPING) CONNECTIVE TISSUE DISEASE

Patients having a combination of clinical features of several rheumatic diseases are described as having *mixed* or *overlapping connective tissue disease.*[38] The term is used to describe a disorder with features of SLE, Sjögren's syndrome, and PM. About 80% of people with this disease are women.

SJÖGREN'S SYNDROME

Sjögren's syndrome is a relatively common autoimmune disease that targets the moisture-producing exocrine glands, which leads to *xerostomia* (dry mouth) and *keratoconjunctivitis sicca* (dry eyes).[39] The nose, throat, airways, and skin can also become dry. The disease may affect other glands as well, including those in the stomach, pancreas, and intestines (extraglandular involvement). The disease is usually diagnosed in people over age 40, with 90% of them women.

In primary Sjögren's syndrome, symptoms can be traced to problems with lacrimal and salivary glands. The patient with primary disease is likely to have antibodies against the cytoplasmic antigens SSA (or Ro) and SSB (or La), as well as ANA. The patient with secondary Sjögren's syndrome typically had another autoimmune disease (e.g., RA, SLE) before Sjögren's developed.

Sjögren's syndrome appears to be caused by genetic and environmental factors. Several genes seem to be involved. One gene predisposes whites to the disease, whereas other genes are linked to the disease in people of Japanese, Chinese, and African American heritage. The trigger may be a viral or bacterial infection that adversely stimulates the immune system. In Sjögren's syndrome, lymphocytes attack and damage the lacrimal and salivary glands.

Dry eyes cause decreased tearing, which leads to a "gritty" sensation in the eyes, burning, blurred vision, and photosensitivity. Dry mouth produces buccal membrane fissures, altered sense of taste, dysphagia, and increased frequency of mouth infections or dental caries. Dry skin and rashes, joint and muscle pain, and thyroid problems may also be present. Other exocrine glands can be affected. For example, vaginal dryness may lead to dyspareunia (painful intercourse).

Autoimmune thyroid disorders, including Graves' disease and Hashimoto's thyroiditis, are common with Sjögren's syndrome. Histologic study reveals lymphocyte infiltration of salivary and lacrimal glands. The disease may become more generalized and involve the lymph nodes, bone marrow, and visceral organs (pseudolymphoma). Persons with severe Sjögren's syndrome have a 5% risk of developing non-Hodgkin's lymphoma.[40]

Ophthalmologic examination (Schirmer's test for tear production), measures of salivary gland function, and lower lip biopsy of minor salivary glands aid in diagnosis. The treatment of Sjögren's syndrome is symptomatic, including (1) instillation of preservative-free artificial tears or ophthalmic antiinflammatory drops (e.g., cyclosporine [Restasis]) as necessary to maintain adequate hydration and lubrication, (2) surgical punctual occlusion, and (3) increased fluids with meals. Dental hygiene is important.

Pilocarpine (Salagen) and cevimeline (Evoxac) can be used to treat symptoms of dry mouth. Increased humidity at home may reduce respiratory tract infections. Vaginal lubrication with a water-soluble product such as K-Y jelly may increase comfort during intercourse.

MYOFASCIAL PAIN SYNDROME

Myofascial pain syndrome is a chronic form of muscle pain. It is characterized as musculoskeletal pain and tenderness, typically in the chest, neck, shoulders, hips, and lower back. Referred pain from these muscle groups can also travel to the buttock, hand, and head, causing severe headaches.

Temporomandibular joint pain may also originate in myofascial pain. Regions of pain are often within the taut bands and fascia of skeletal muscles. When activated by pressure, trigger points are thought to activate a characteristic pattern of pain that can worsen with activity or stress.

Myofascial pain syndrome occurs more often in middle-aged adults, and in women rather than men. Patients complain of the pain as deep and aching and accompanied by a sensation of burning, stinging, and stiffness. Examples of this syndrome include fibromyalgia, myalgia, and myositis.[41]

Physical therapy is one treatment used for myofascial pain syndrome. A typical treatment is the "spray and stretch" method, in which the painful area is iced or sprayed with a coolant such as ethyl chloride and then stretched. Positive results have been seen with topical patches and injection of the trigger points with a local anesthetic (e.g., 1% lidocaine). Massage, acupuncture, biofeedback, and ultrasound therapy have also benefitted some patients.

FIBROMYALGIA

Fibromyalgia is a chronic disorder characterized by widespread, nonarticular musculoskeletal pain and fatigue with multiple tender points. People with fibromyalgia may also experience nonrestorative sleep, morning stiffness, irritable bowel syndrome, and anxiety. Fibromyalgia is a commonly diagnosed musculoskeletal disorder and a major cause of disability. It affects an estimated 5 million Americans, with 75% to 90% of these persons being women.[42] Fibromyalgia and chronic fatigue syndrome share many commonalities (Table 65-19).

Etiology and Pathophysiology

Identifying the underlying causes and pathophysiologic mechanisms of fibromyalgia is an active area of research. There is general agreement that fibromyalgia is a disorder involving neuroendocrine/neurotransmitter dysregulation. The pain amplification experienced by the affected patient is due to abnormal sensory processing in the CNS.

Multiple physiologic abnormalities have been found. They include increased levels of substance P in the spinal fluid, low levels of blood flow to the thalamus, dysfunction of the hypothalamic-pituitary-adrenal (HPA) axis, low levels of serotonin and tryptophan, and abnormalities in cytokine function. Serotonin and substance P play a role in mood regulation, sleep,

and pain perception. Changes in the HPA axis can also negatively affect a person's physical and mental health, leading to an increased incidence of depression and a decreased response to stress. Genetic factors also contribute to the etiology of fibromyalgia, as a familial tendency exists. A recent illness or trauma may serve as a trigger in susceptible people.

Clinical Manifestations and Complications

The patient complains of a widespread burning pain that worsens and improves through the course of a day. It is often difficult for the patient to discriminate whether pain occurs in the muscles, joints, or soft tissues. Head or facial pain often results from stiff or painful neck and shoulder muscles. The pain can accompany temporomandibular joint dysfunction, which affects an estimated one third of patients with fibromyalgia.

Physical examination characteristically reveals point tenderness at 11 or more of 18 identified sites (Fig. 65-14). Patients with fibromyalgia are sensitive to painful stimuli throughout the body, not merely at the identified tender sites. In addition, point tenderness can vary from day to day. On some occasions, the patient may respond to fewer than 11 tender points. At other times, palpation of all sites may elicit pain.

Cognitive effects range from difficulty concentrating to memory lapses and a feeling of being overwhelmed when dealing with multiple tasks. Many individuals report migraine headaches. Depression and anxiety often occur and may require drug therapy. Stiffness, nonrefreshing sleep, fatigue, and numbness or tingling in the hands or feet (paresthesia) often accompany fibromyalgia. Restless legs syndrome is also typical, with the patient describing an irresistible urge to move the legs when at rest or lying down.[43]

Irritable bowel syndrome with manifestations of constipation and/or diarrhea, abdominal pain, and bloating is common. Fibromyalgia patients may also experience difficulty swallowing, perhaps because of abnormalities in esophageal smooth

TABLE 65-19	COMMONALITIES BETWEEN FIBROMYALGIA AND CHRONIC FATIGUE SYNDROME
Commonality	**Description**
Occurrence	Previously healthy, young, and middle-aged women.
Etiology (theories)	Infectious trigger, dysfunction in HPA axis, alteration in CNS.
Clinical manifestations	Generalized musculoskeletal pain, malaise and fatigue, cognitive dysfunction, headaches, sleep disturbances, depression, anxiety, fever.
Course of disease	Variable intensity of symptoms, fluctuates over time.
Diagnosis	No definitive laboratory tests or joint and muscle examinations, mainly a diagnosis of exclusion.
Collaborative therapy	Treatment is symptomatic and may include antidepressant drugs such as amitriptyline (Elavil) and fluoxetine (Prozac). Other measures are heat, massage, regular stretching, biofeedback, stress management, and relaxation training. Patient and caregiver teaching is essential.

HPA, Hypothalamic-pituitary-adrenal.

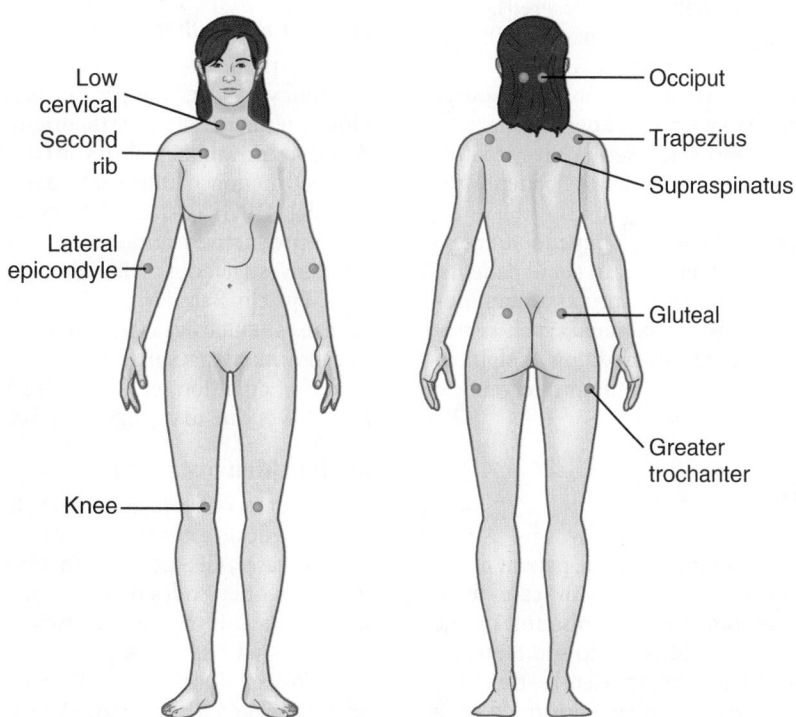

FIG. 65-14 Tender points in fibromyalgia.

Low cervical
Second rib
Lateral epicondyle
Knee

Occiput
Trapezius
Supraspinatus
Gluteal
Greater trochanter

muscle function. Increased frequency of urination and urinary urgency, in the absence of a bladder infection, are typical complaints. Women with fibromyalgia may experience more difficult menstruation, with a worsening of disease symptoms during this time.

Diagnostic Studies

A definitive diagnosis of fibromyalgia is often difficult to establish. Lack of knowledge about the disease and its manifestations among health care providers may also cause delays in diagnosis and treatment.

Laboratory results in most cases serve to rule out other suspected disorders. Occasionally a low ANA titer is seen, but it is not considered diagnostic. Muscle biopsy may reveal a nonspecific moth-eaten appearance or fiber atrophy. The American College of Rheumatology classifies an individual as having fibromyalgia if two criteria are met: (1) pain is experienced in 11 of the 18 tender points on palpation (see Fig. 65-14) and (2) a history of widespread pain is noted for at least 3 months.[44] Widespread pain is defined as pain that occurs on both sides of the body and above and below the waist. In addition, fatigue, cognitive symptoms, and extensive somatic symptoms are considered in establishing a diagnosis.

Collaborative Care

The treatment of fibromyalgia is symptomatic and requires a high level of patient motivation. You have a key role in teaching the patient to be an active participant in the therapeutic regimen. Rest can help the pain, aching, and tenderness.

Drug therapy for the chronic widespread pain associated with fibromyalgia includes pregabalin (Lyrica), duloxetine (Cymbalta), and milnacipran (Savella). Low-dose tricyclic antidepressants, selective serotonin reuptake inhibitors (SSRIs), or benzodiazepines (e.g., diazepam [Valium]) may also be prescribed. If the tricyclic antidepressant amitriptyline (Elavil) is not well tolerated, similar drugs can be substituted (e.g., doxepin [Sinequan], imipramine [Tofranil], trazodone [Desyrel]). SSRI antidepressants (e.g., sertraline [Zoloft] or paroxetine [Paxil]) tend to be reserved for fibromyalgia patients who also have depression. SSRIs may need to be prescribed at higher doses than when used to treat depression. Both antidepressants and muscle relaxants (e.g., cyclobenzaprine [Flexeril]) have sedative effects that can help improve nighttime rest for the patient with fibromyalgia.

Long-acting opioids generally are not recommended unless fibromyalgia is refractory to other therapies. In some patients, pain may be managed with OTC analgesics such as acetaminophen, ibuprofen, or naproxen (Aleve). Nonopioids such as tramadol (Ultram) may also be used. In addition, zolpidem (Ambien) is sometimes prescribed for short-term intervention in the patient with severe sleep problems.

NURSING MANAGEMENT
FIBROMYALGIA

Because of the chronic nature of fibromyalgia, the patient needs consistent support from you and other health care team members. Massage is often combined with ultrasound or the application of alternating heat and cold packs to soothe tense, sore muscles and increase blood circulation. Gentle stretching to relieve muscle tension and spasm can be performed by a physical therapist or practiced by the fibromyalgia patient at

home. Yoga and Tai Chi are often appropriate choices. Low-impact aerobic exercise, such as walking, can help prevent muscle atrophy.

Dietitians often urge fibromyalgia patients to limit their consumption of sugar, caffeine, and alcohol because these substances have been shown to be muscle irritants. Vitamin and mineral supplements may help combat stress, correct deficiencies, and support the immune system. However, unproven "miracle diets" or supplements should be carefully investigated by the patient and discussed with the health care provider before using them. Inform the patient that some foods and supplements can cause serious or even dangerous side effects when mixed with certain drugs.

Pain and the related symptoms of fibromyalgia can cause significant stress. Patients with fibromyalgia may not deal effectively with stress. Effective relaxation strategies include biofeedback, mindfulness meditation, and cognitive behavioral therapy. Patients need to receive initial training for these interventions, but they can then continue to practice in their own homes. (Stress management is discussed in Chapter 7.) Psychologic counseling (individual or group) may also be beneficial for the patient with fibromyalgia.

CHRONIC FATIGUE SYNDROME

Chronic fatigue syndrome (CFS), also called *chronic fatigue and immune dysfunction syndrome* or *myalgic encephalomyelitis,* is a disorder characterized by debilitating fatigue and a variety of associated complaints. CFS is a poorly understood condition that can have a devastating impact on the lives of patients and their families.

An estimated 1 million people in the United States have CFS, but less than 20% of them have been diagnosed. Women are affected more often than men. CFS occurs in all ethnic and socioeconomic groups. The prevalence of CFS is difficult to establish because of the lack of validated diagnostic tests.

Etiology and Pathophysiology

Despite numerous attempts to determine the etiology and pathology of CFS, the precise mechanisms remain unknown. However, there are many theories about the cause of CFS. Neuroendocrine abnormalities have been implicated involving a hypofunction of the HPA axis and hypothalamic-pituitary-gonadal (HPG) axis, which together regulate the stress response and reproductive hormone levels. Several microorganisms have been investigated as etiologic agents, including herpesviruses (e.g., Epstein-Barr virus [EBV], cytomegalovirus [CMV]), retroviruses, enteroviruses, *Candida albicans,* and mycoplasma. Because many patients have cognitive deficits (e.g., decreased memory, attention, concentration), it has also been proposed that CFS is due to changes in the CNS.

Clinical Manifestations

CFS is often difficult to distinguish from fibromyalgia because many clinical features are similar (see Table 65-19). In about half the cases, CFS develops insidiously, or the patient may have intermittent episodes that gradually become chronic. Incapacitating fatigue is the most common symptom of CFS and is the problem that causes the patient to seek health care.

In other situations, CFS arises suddenly in a previously active, healthy individual. An unremarkable flu-like illness or other acute stress is often identified as a triggering event.

Associated symptoms (Table 65-20) may fluctuate in intensity over time.

The patient may become angry and frustrated with the inability of health care providers to diagnose a problem. The disorder may have a major impact on work and family responsibilities. Some individuals may even need help with activities of daily living.

Diagnostic Studies

Physical examination and diagnostic studies can be used to rule out other possible causes of the patient's symptoms. No laboratory test can diagnose CFS or measure its severity. The Centers for Disease Control and Prevention has developed a diagnostic algorithm based on the patient's symptoms[45] (see Table 65-20). In general, CFS remains a diagnosis of exclusion.

TABLE 65-20	DIAGNOSTIC CRITERIA FOR CHRONIC FATIGUE SYNDROME*

Major Criterion
- Unexplained, persistent, or relapsing chronic fatigue of new and definite onset (not lifelong). Not due to ongoing exertion. Not substantially alleviated by rest. Results in substantial reduction in occupational, educational, social, or personal activities.

Minor Criteria
- Impaired memory or concentration
- Frequent or recurring sore throat
- Tender cervical or axillary lymph nodes
- Muscle pain
- Multijoint pain without joint swelling or redness
- Headaches of a new type, pattern, or severity
- Unrefreshing sleep
- Postexertional malaise

Adapted from Centers for Disease Control and Prevention: Chronic fatigue syndrome: revised case definition. Retrieved from *www.cdc.gov/cfs/cfsdefinitionHCP.htm*.
*For a diagnosis to be made, the patient must demonstrate the major criterion, plus four or more of the minor criteria for ≥6 mo. These criteria were prepared by the Centers for Disease Control and Prevention, National Institutes of Health, and International Chronic Fatigue Syndrome Study Group.

NURSING AND COLLABORATIVE MANAGEMENT CHRONIC FATIGUE SYNDROME

Because no definitive treatment exists for CFS, supportive management is essential. Tell the patient what is known about the disease. All complaints should be taken seriously.

NSAIDs can be used to treat headaches, muscle and joint aches, and fever. Because many patients with CFS also have allergies and sinusitis, antihistamines and decongestants can be used to treat allergic symptoms. Tricyclic antidepressants (e.g., doxepin, amitriptyline) and SSRIs (e.g., fluoxetine [Prozac], paroxetine) can improve mood and sleep problems. Clonazepam (Klonopin) can also be used to treat sleep disturbances and panic disorders. The use of low-dose hydrocortisone to decrease fatigue and disability is being studied.

Total rest is not advised because it can potentiate the self-image of being an invalid, while strenuous exertion can exacerbate the exhaustion. Therefore it is important to plan a carefully graduated exercise program. A well-balanced diet, including fiber and fresh dark-colored fruits and vegetables for antioxidant action, is essential in treatment. Behavioral therapy may be used to promote a positive outlook and improve overall disability, fatigue, and other symptoms.

One of the major problems facing many CFS patients is financial instability.[46] When the illness strikes, they cannot work or must decrease the amount of time working. Loss of a job often leads to loss of medical insurance. Obtaining disability benefits can be frustrating because of the difficulty of establishing a definitive diagnosis of CFS. Patients with CFS may experience substantial occupational and psychosocial impairments and loss, including the social pressure and isolation from being characterized as lazy or "crazy."

CFS does not appear to progress. Although most patients recover or at least gradually improve over time, some do not show substantial improvement. Recovery is more common in individuals with a sudden onset of CFS.

CASE STUDY

Rheumatoid Arthritis

iStockphoto/Thinkstock

Patient Profile
K.R., a 42-yr-old married white woman, is seen at the rheumatology clinic with complaints of tenderness and pain in the small joints of her hands.

Subjective Data
- Complains of tenderness, joint pain, and stiffness in her hands for the last 3 mo
- Experiencing fatigue, anorexia, and morning stiffness
- Mother diagnosed with ankylosing spondylitis 8 yr ago
- Expresses doubt about her ability to manage disease

Objective Data
Physical Examination
- Swelling, warmth, and tenderness of third and fourth metacarpophalangeal joints of both hands
- Mild pain with neck motion
- Tenosynovitis

Diagnostic Studies
- Positive ESR, RF, and ACPA
- Moderate bone demineralization evident bilaterally in hand x-rays

Collaborative Care
- Diagnosed with RA
- Started on methotrexate (Rheumatrex) 7.5 mg PO once per week, etanercept (Enbrel) 50 mg subcutaneously once per week, prednisone 10 mg/day

Discussion Questions
1. How will you explain the pathophysiology of RA to K.R.?
2. K.R. asks you if genetic factors are related to a diagnosis of RA. How will you respond?
3. What are some home and work modifications that you can suggest to K.R. to reduce her symptoms?
4. What suggestions can you make to K.R. about coping with fatigue?
5. *Priority Decision:* Based on the assessment data presented, what are the priority nursing diagnoses? Are there any collaborative problems?
6. *Evidence-Based Practice:* Why is an exercise program important in the treatment plan for K.R.?

ᴇvolve Answers and a corresponding concept map available at *http://evolve.elsevier.com/Lewis/medsurg*.

BRIDGE TO NCLEX EXAMINATION

The number of the question corresponds to the same-numbered outcome at the beginning of the chapter.

1. In assessing the joints of a patient with osteoarthritis, the nurse understands that Heberden's nodes
   a. are often red, swollen, and tender.
   b. indicate osteophyte formation at the DIP joints.
   c. are the result of pannus formation at the PIP joints.
   d. occur from deterioration of cartilage by proteolytic enzymes.

2. A patient with rheumatoid arthritis is experiencing articular involvement of the joints. The nurse recognizes that these characteristic changes include (select all that apply)
   a. bamboo-shaped fingers.
   b. metatarsal head dislocation in feet.
   c. noninflammatory pain in large joints.
   d. asymmetric involvement of small joints.
   e. morning stiffness lasting 60 minutes or more.

3. When administering medications to the patient with gout, the nurse would recognize that which drug is used as a treatment for this disease?
   a. Colchicine
   b. Febuxostat
   c. Sulfasalazine
   d. Cyclosporine

4. The nurse should teach the patient with ankylosing spondylitis the importance of
   a. regularly exercising and maintaining proper posture.
   b. avoiding extremes in environmental temperatures.
   c. maintaining usual physical activity during flare-ups.
   d. applying hot and cool compresses for relief of local symptoms.

5. In teaching a patient with SLE about the disorder, the nurse knows that the pathophysiology of SLE includes
   a. circulating immune complexes formed from IgG autoantibodies reacting with IgG.
   b. an autoimmune T-cell reaction that results in destruction of the deep dermal skin layer.
   c. immunologic dysfunction leading to chronic inflammation in the cartilage and muscles.
   d. the production of a variety of autoantibodies directed against components of the cell nucleus.

6. In teaching a patient with Sjögren's syndrome about drug therapy for this disorder, the nurse includes instruction on use of which drug?
   a. Pregabalin (Lyrica)
   b. Etanercept (Enbrel)
   c. Cyclosporine (Restasis)
   d. Cyclobenzaprine (Flexeril)

7. Teach the patient with fibromyalgia the importance of limiting intake of which foods (select all that apply)?
   a. Sugar
   b. Alcohol
   c. Caffeine
   d. Red meat
   e. Root vegetables

1. b, 2. b, e, 3. b, 4. a, 5. d, 6. c, 7. a, b, c

ⓔvolve

For rationales to these answers and even more NCLEX review questions, visit *http://evolve.elsevier.com/Lewis/medsurg.*

REFERENCES

1. National Institute of Arthritis and Musculoskeletal and Skin Disease: Questions and answers about arthritis and rheumatic diseases. Retrieved from *www.niams.nih.gov/health_info/arthritis/arthritis_rheumatic_qa.asp.*

2. Centers for Disease Control and Prevention: Arthritis: meeting the challenge. Retrieved from *www.cdc.gov/nccdphp/publications/aag/arthritis.htm.*

3. Roberts D: Arthritis and connective tissue disorders. In National Association of Orthopaedic Nurses: *NAON core curriculum for orthopaedic nursing,* ed 7, Boston, 2012, Pearson Custom Publishing.

4. Centers for Disease Control and Prevention: Arthritis risk factors. Retrieved from *www.cdc.gov/arthritis/basics/risk_factors.htm.*

5. Arthritis Foundation: Who gets osteoarthritis? Retrieved from *www.arthritis.org/who-gets-osteoarthritis.php.*

6. Antonelli M, Starz T: Assessing for risk and progression of osteoarthritis: the nurse's role, *Am J Nurs* 112:S26, 2012.

7. American College of Rheumatology Subcommittee on Osteoarthritis Guidelines: Recommendations for the medical management of osteoarthritis of the hip and knee. Retrieved from *www.rheumatology.org/practice/clinical/guidelines/oa-mgmt.asp.*

*8. Vickers A, Cronin A, Maschino A, et al: Acupuncture for chronic pain: individual patient data meta-analysis, *Arch Inter Med* 172(19):1444, 2012.

*9. National Center for Complementary and Alternative Medicine: Glucosamine/Chondroitin Arthritis Intervention Trial (GAIT): primary and ancillary study results. Retrieved from *http://nccam.nih.gov/research/results/gait.*

10. LeGraverand-Gastineau MP: Disease-modifying osteoarthritis drugs: facing development challenges and choosing molecular targets, *Curr Drug Targets* 11:528, 2010.

11. Robbins L, Kulsea M: The state of the science in the prevention and management of osteoarthritis, *Am J Nurs* 112:S3, 2012.

12. Centers for Disease Control and Prevention: Rheumatoid arthritis. Retrieved from *www.cdc.gov/arthritis/basics/rheumatoid.htm#6.*

13. Firestein G: Etiology and pathogenesis of rheumatoid arthritis. In G Firestein, R Budd, S Gabriel, et al, editors: *Kelley's textbook of rheumatology,* ed 9, Philadelphia, 2012, Saunders.

14. Johns Hopkins Arthritis Center: Rheumatoid arthritis clinical presentation. Retrieved from *www.hopkins-arthritis.org/arthritis-info/rheumatoid-arthritis/rheum_clin_pres.*

15. Cleveland Clinic: RA doldrums: how to cope with joint pain and depression, *Arthritis Advisor* 11:3, 2012.

16. Besada E, Nikolaissen C, Nossent H: Should rheumatoid factor in rheumatoid arthritis be sent to Davy Jones's locker? *Scand J Rheumatol* 41:85, 2012.

17. Simmons S: Recognizing and managing rheumatoid arthritis, *Nursing* 41:34, 2011.

18. Arthritis Foundation: Arthritis drug chart: NSAIDs. Retrieved from *www.arthritistoday.org/DrugGuide/drug-chart.php?drug_type=NSAIDs.*

*Evidence-based information for clinical practice.

19. *Arthritis Keeping Your Joints Healthy,* Boston, 2011, Harvard Health Publications.

20. Hardy E: Gout diagnosis and management: what NPs need to know, *Nurse Pract* 36:15, 2011.

21. Doghramji PP: Managing your patient with gout: a review of treatment options, *Postgrad Med* 123:56, 2011.

22. Bockenstedt L: Lyme disease. In G Firestein, R Budd, S Gabriel, et al, editors: *Kelley's textbook of rheumatology,* ed 9, Philadelphia, 2012, Saunders.

23. Centers for Disease Control and Prevention: Lyme disease. Retrieved from *www.cdc.gov/lyme/.*

24. Xu B, Katz B: Atypical presentation of *Staphylococcus aureus* septic arthritis in an elderly woman, *Clin Geriatr* 20:43, 2012.

25. Horowitz DL, Katzap E, Horowitz S, et al: Approach to septic arthritis, *Am Fam Physician* 84:653, 2011.

26. Akgul O, Ozgocmen S: Classification criteria for spondyloarthropathies, *World J Orthop* 2:107, 2011.

27. Cleveland Clinic: Psoriatic arthritis: when you feel pain above and below your skin, *Arthritis Advisor* 11:1, 2012.

28. National Psoriasis Foundation: The five types of psoriatic arthritis. Retrieved from *www.psoriasis.org/netcommunity/ learn_psatypes.*

29. Hill Gaston JS: Reactive arthritis and undifferentiated spondyloarthritis. In G Firestein, R Budd, S Gabriel, et al, editors: *Kelley's textbook of rheumatology,* ed 9, Philadelphia, 2012, Saunders.

30. Bernknop A, Rowley K, Bailey T: A review of systemic lupus erythematosus and current treatment options, *Formulary* 46:178, 2011.

31. Ferenkeh-Koroma A: Systemic lupus erythematosus: nurse and patient education, *Nurs Stand* 26:49, 2012.

32. Tsokos GC: Systemic lupus erythematosus, *New Engl J Med* 365:2110, 2011.

33. Lupus Foundation of America: Medications to treat lupus symptoms. Retrieved from *www.lupus.org/webmodules/ webarticlesnet/templates/new_learntreating.aspx?articleid=2246& zoneid=525.*

34. Jolly M, Pickard, A, Mikolaitis R, et al: Body image in patients with systemic lupus erythematosus, *Int J Behav Med* 19:157, 2012.

35. American College of Rheumatology: Scleroderma. Retrieved from *www.rheumatology.org/practice/clinical/patients/diseases_ and_conditions/scleroderma.pdf.*

36. Varga J: Systemic sclerosis (scleroderma). In L Goldman, A Schafer, editors: *Goldman: Goldman's Cecil medicine,* ed 24, Philadelphia, 2011, Saunders.

37. Cedars-Sinai Health System: Polymyositis and dermatomyositis. Retrieved from *www.cedars-sinai.edu/Patients/Health- Conditions/Polymyositis-and-Dermatomyositis.aspx.*

38. von Mühlen C, Nakamura R: Clinical and laboratory evaluation of systemic rheumatic diseases. In R McPherson, M Pincus, editors: *McPherson: Henry's clinical diagnosis and management by laboratory methods,* ed 22, Philadelphia, 2011, Saunders.

39. Jonsson R, Vogelsang P, Volchenkov R, et al: The complexity of Sjögren's syndrome: novel aspects on pathogenesis, *Immunol Lett* 141:1, 2011.

*40. Covelli ME, Lanciano P, Tartaglia M, et al: Rituximab treatment for Sjögren syndrome–associated non-Hodgkin's lymphoma: case series, *Rheum Int* 32:3281, 2012.

41. Belden J, DeFriez C, Huether S: Pain, temperature, sleep, and sensory function. In S Huether, K McCance, editors: *Understanding pathophysiology,* ed 5, St Louis, 2012, Mosby.

42. Cleveland Clinic: Chronic pain: is it fibromyalgia—or something else? *Arthritis Advisor* 10:4, 2011.

*43. Shillam C, Jones K, Miller L: Fibromyalgia symptoms, physical function, and comorbidity in middle-aged and older adults, *Nurs Res* 60:309, 2011.

44. Wolfe F, Clauw DJ, Fitzcharles M, et al: The American College of Rheumatology preliminary diagnostic criteria for fibromyalgia and measurement of symptom severity, *Arthritis Care Res* 62:600, 2010.

45. Centers for Disease Control and Prevention: Chronic fatigue syndrome: revised case definition. Retrieved from *www.cdc.gov/ cfs/cfsdefinitionHCP.htm.*

46. Burns D, Bennett C, McGough A: Chronic fatigue syndrome or myalgic encephalomyelitis, *Nurs Stand* 26:48, 2012.

RESOURCES

American College of Rheumatology
www.rheumatology.org
Arthritis Foundation
www.arthritis.org
International Association for CFS/ME
www.iacfsme.org
Lupus Foundation of America
www.lupus.org
National Fibromyalgia Association
www.fmaware.org
National Institute of Arthritis and Musculoskeletal and Skin Diseases Information Clearinghouse, National Institutes of Health
www.niams.nih.gov
National Psoriasis Foundation
www.psoriasis.org
Scleroderma Foundation
www.scleroderma.org
Sjögren's Syndrome Foundation
www.sjogrens.org
Spondylitis Association of America
www.spondylitis.org

Managing Multiple Patients

You are working on the medical-surgical unit and have been assigned to care for the following five patients. You have one LPN and one UAP on your team to help you.

Patients

iStockphoto/Thinkstock

A.J. is a 66-yr-old white woman who had an ischemic stroke 2 days ago. She has a history of migraines, hypertension, and atrial fibrillation. She is alert, oriented, and able to answer questions appropriately but has mild slowness in responding. She has left-sided arm weakness (3/5) and left leg weakness (4/5). Her vital signs are BP 160/84, HR 88, RR 20, T 37° C. She is receiving ASA 325 mg po daily, Lovenox 80 mg subcutaneously q12hr, lisinopril 10 mg po daily, Cardizem CD 180 mg po daily, and Coumadin 5 mg po daily. Her most recent INR was 1.7. She is scheduled to receive physical therapy today.

Purestock/Thinkstock

J.P. is a 24-yr-old woman who fell and hit her head after experiencing a tonic-clonic seizure. Her boyfriend found her lying semiconscious on the floor in her apartment. She had an emergency evacuation of a subdural hematoma and was initially admitted to the ICU. She was transferred to the medical-surgical unit yesterday and is scheduled for rehabilitation evaluation. She is oriented to person only and is somewhat restless. A safety sitter is with her at all times.

iStockphoto/Thinkstock

M.Y., an 80-yr-old Asian American man, had an ORIF 2 days ago for a fractured left hip. He has a 3-yr history of Alzheimer's disease and is confused to place and time. Although he has a history of agitation, he has been pleasant and cooperative. He has a personal alarm and bed alarm on for safety. His hip dressing is dry and intact and the drainage in the hemovac is minimal.

iStockphoto/Thinkstock

B.V., a 24-yr-old white man, was admitted to the ICU 3 weeks ago after suffering a C5-6 cervical spinal cord injury. B.V. dove into the shallow end of a neighbor's backyard pool and struck his head on the bottom. He was initially placed in cervical traction, intubated, and mechanically ventilated. He has since undergone surgical stabilization and the traction was removed. He was weaned from the ventilator 2 days ago. He was transferred to the medical-surgical unit yesterday. He is currently requesting medication for a "severe headache."

Jupiterimages/Comstock/
Thinkstock

M.L. is a 58-yr-old white retired nurse who suffered an L4 compression fracture after falling 1 week ago. She underwent vertebroplasty yesterday and was kept in the hospital overnight for observation after experiencing some postoperative hypotension. She has a 6-yr history of Addison's disease. She is planning to be discharged home today.

Management Discussion Questions

1. *Priority Decision:* After receiving report, which patient should you see first? Provide a rationale.
2. *Delegation Decision:* Which tasks could you delegate to UAP *(select all that apply)?*
   a. Explain discharge instructions to M.L.
   b. Change the dressing on M.Y.'s left hip.
   c. Obtain vital signs on M.L. before discharge.
   d. Sit with J.P. while the safety sitter takes a break.
   e. Assess A.J.'s ability to swallow before feeding her breakfast.
3. *Priority and Delegation Decision:* When you enter the room to assess B.V., you find him diaphoretic with a flushed face and pale extremities. His BP is 200/102 mm Hg. Which two initial actions would be most appropriate?
   a. Ask the UAP to obtain a stat bladder scan.
   b. Have the LPN administer his oral antihypertensive meds stat.
   c. Elevate the head of the bed while assessing for any noxious stimuli.
   d. Ask the LPN to stay with B.V. while you call B.V.'s health care provider.
   e. Insert rectal suppository after applying lidocaine to the area around the rectum.

Case Study Progression

B.V.'s bladder scan revealed 700 mL of urine. After you have the LPN catheterize him using a local anesthetic gel, his symptoms subside. You take this time to further teach B.V. about the clinical manifestations of autonomic dysreflexia and the need to report any symptom as soon as it appears. You also take the time to discuss bladder training strategies and how to avoid bladder distention in the future. B.V. is grateful for the information and your caring attitude. Just as you are finishing, the UAP informs you that M.Y. has pulled out his hemovac drain.

4. What should be your initial intervention for M.Y.?
   a. Reinsert the hemovac drain.
   b. Assess the incision site for a hematoma.
   c. Notify M.Y.'s surgeon that the drain was removed.
   d. Apply pressure to the incisional site where the drain had been placed.
5. Which intervention would be most appropriate in caring for A.J.?
   a. Place her left arm in a sling for support.
   b. Arrange the food tray so that all foods are on the right side.
   c. Call the health care provider to decrease her Coumadin dosage.
   d. Position her left leg so that the ankle is lower than the knee to prevent contractures.
6. When teaching J.P.'s boyfriend about what to expect during recovery from a head injury, which statement is most accurate?
   a. "You can tell by how great she looks physically that she will ultimately function well at the home."
   b. "One good thing that will come out of this injury is that her seizures should occur less frequently."
   c. "Most patients are usually transferred for acute rehabilitation management to prepare them for going home."
   d. "She can expect a full recovery without any chronic problems, but it may take a few months to achieve that goal."
7. *Priority and Management Decision:* As you enter M.L.'s room to discuss her discharge plans, you find her all packed up and walking out the door. She tells you the UAP already told her what she needed to do. What is your best initial action?
   a. Ask M.L. if she has any further questions.
   b. Call the UAP to M.L.'s room to find out what she told her.
   c. Review discharge instructions with M.L. to ascertain correct understanding.
   d. Give M.L. a telephone number to call in case she has any concerns when she gets home.

Nursing Care in Critical Care Settings

iStockphoto/Thinkstock

If you don't like the road you're walking, start paving another one.
Dolly Parton

*You must have long-range goals to keep you
from being frustrated by short-range failures.*
Charles C. Noble

Nursing Management
Critical Care

Linda Bucher and Maureen A. Seckel

Evolve WEBSITE

LEARNING OUTCOMES

1. Differentiate the various certification opportunities for critical care nurses.
2. Select appropriate nursing interventions to manage common problems and needs of critically ill patients.
3. Develop strategies to manage issues related to caregivers of critically ill patients.
4. Apply the principles of hemodynamic monitoring to the collaborative care and nursing management of patients receiving this intervention.
5. Differentiate the purpose of, indications for, and function of circulatory assist devices and related collaborative care and nursing management.
6. Differentiate the indications for and modes of mechanical ventilation.
7. Select appropriate nursing interventions related to the care of an intubated patient.
8. Relate the principles of mechanical ventilation to the collaborative care and nursing management of patients receiving this intervention.

KEY TERMS

arterial pressure–based cardiac output (APCO), p. 1606
assist-control ventilation (ACV), p. 1619
circulatory assist devices (CADs), p. 1610
continuous positive airway pressure (CPAP), p. 1621
endotracheal (ET) intubation, p. 1613

hemodynamic monitoring, p. 1602
high-frequency oscillatory ventilation (HFOV), p. 1622
intraaortic balloon pump (IABP), p. 1610
mechanical ventilation, p. 1618
negative pressure ventilation, p. 1618

positive end-expiratory pressure (PEEP), p. 1621
positive pressure ventilation (PPV), p. 1618
pressure support ventilation (PSV), p. 1621
ventricular assist device (VAD), p. 1612
volume ventilation, p. 1618
weaning, p. 1625

This chapter focuses on the role of the critical care nurse in the management of the critically ill patient in an intensive care setting. The chapter reviews the concepts related to cardiovascular and respiratory dynamics. It emphasizes nursing management of patients requiring aspects of critical care not addressed in other chapters, such as invasive hemodynamic monitoring, circulatory assist devices, artificial airways, and mechanical ventilation.

CRITICAL CARE NURSING

The American Association of Critical-Care Nurses (AACN) defines *critical care nursing* as that specialty dealing with human responses to life-threatening problems.[1] Critical care nurses care for patients with acute and unstable physiologic problems, and their caregivers. This involves assessing life-threatening conditions, initiating appropriate interventions,

Reviewed by Steven J. Palazzo, RN, PhD, Sauvage Fellow, The Hope Heart Institute, and Nurse Faculty Leadership Academy Fellow, STTI, Seattle University, College of Nursing, Seattle, Washington; and Trevah A. Panek, RN, MSN, CCRN, Assistant Professor of Nursing, Saint Francis University, Loretto, Pennsylvania.

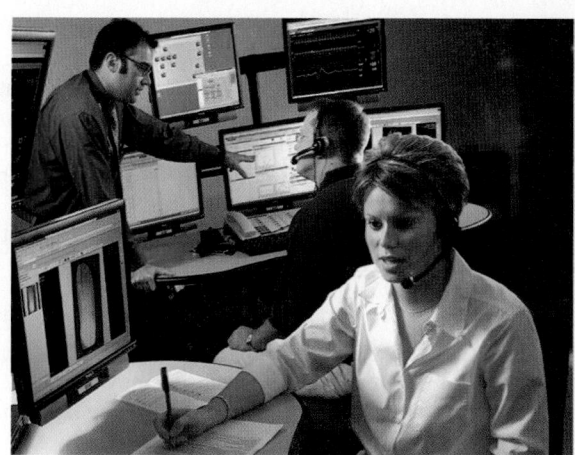

FIG. 66-1 Tele-intensive care unit control room. (From Avera Health, Sioux Falls, S Dak.)

FIG. 66-2 Typical intensive care unit. (Courtesy Spacelabs Medical, Redmond, Wash.)

evaluating the outcomes of the interventions, and providing education and emotional support to caregivers.

Critical Care Units

Critical care units (CCUs) or *intensive care units* (ICUs) are designed to meet the special needs of acutely and critically ill patients. In many hospitals the concept of ICU care has expanded from delivering care in a standard unit to bringing ICU care to patients wherever they might be. For example, the *electronic* or *teleICU* assists the bedside ICU team by monitoring the patient from a remote location (Fig. 66-1).

Similarly, the development of *rapid response teams* (RRTs) provides for the delivery of advanced care by specialized teams usually composed of a critical care nurse, a respiratory therapist, and a critical care physician or an advanced practice registered nurse (APRN). The team brings rapid and immediate care to unstable patients in noncritical care units. Patients often exhibit early and subtle signs of deterioration (e.g., mild confusion, tachypnea) 6 to 8 hours before cardiac or respiratory arrest. Early critical care intervention has made significant contributions to reducing mortality rates in these patients.[2]

The technology available in the ICU is extensive and always evolving. It is possible to continuously monitor the electrocardiogram (ECG), blood pressure (BP), oxygen (O_2) saturation, cardiac output (CO), intracranial pressure, and temperature. More advanced monitoring devices measure cardiac index (CI), stroke volume (SV), stroke volume variation (SVV), ejection fraction (EF), end-tidal carbon dioxide (CO_2), and tissue O_2 consumption. Patients may receive ongoing support from mechanical ventilators, intraaortic balloon pumps (IABPs), circulatory assist devices (CADs), or dialysis machines. Fig. 66-2 shows a typical ICU.

Progressive care units (PCUs), also called intermediate care or step-down units, provide a transition between the ICU and the general care unit or discharge. Generally, PCU patients are at risk for serious complications, but their risk is lower than that of ICU patients. Examples of patients found in PCUs include those scheduled for interventional cardiac procedures (e.g., stent placement), awaiting heart transplant, receiving stable doses of vasoactive IV drugs (e.g., diltiazem [Cardizem]), or being weaned from prolonged mechanical ventilation. Monitoring capabilities in these units include continuous ECG, arterial BP, O_2 saturation, and end-tidal CO_2. The use of PCUs provides

critical care nursing for an at-risk patient population in a more cost-effective environment.

Critical Care Nurse

A critical care nurse has in-depth knowledge of anatomy, physiology, pathophysiology, pharmacology, and advanced assessment skills, as well as the ability to use advanced technology. As a critical care nurse, you perform frequent assessments to monitor trends (patterns) in the patient's physiologic parameters (e.g., BP, ECG). This allows you to rapidly recognize and manage complications while aiding healing and recovery. You must also provide psychologic support to the patient and caregiver. To be effective, you must be able to communicate and collaborate with all members of the interdisciplinary health team (e.g., physician, dietitian, social worker, respiratory therapist, occupational therapist).

As a critical care nurse, you will face ethical dilemmas related to the care of your patients. Moral distress over perceived issues of delivering futile or nonbeneficial care can lead to emotional exhaustion or burnout. Consequently, it is important that all members of the health care team coexist in a healthy work environment.

Specialization in critical care nursing requires formal education combined with a preceptored clinical orientation, often over several months. The AACN Certification Corporation offers critical care certification (CCRN) in adult, pediatric, and neonatal critical care nursing; progressive care certification (PCCN); and teleICU certification (CCRN-E). Subspecialty certifications are available in cardiac medicine (CMC) and cardiac surgery (CSC). The designation requires registered nurse (RN) licensure, practice experience in the related specialty area, and successful completion of a written test. Certification validates basic knowledge of critical or progressive care nursing. It is not the same as advanced practice.

Advanced practice critical care nurses currently have a graduate (master's or doctorate) degree with a proposed transition to a doctor of nursing practice (DNP) by 2015.[3] These nurses function in a variety of roles: patient and staff educators, consultants, administrators, researchers, or expert practitioners. The advanced practice critical care nurse who is a clinical nurse specialist (CNS) typically functions in one or more of these roles. Certification for the CNS in acute and critical care is available through the AACN. Another advanced practice role is the acute care nurse practitioner (ACNP). This APRN provides comprehensive care to select critically ill patients and their caregivers. The ACNP conducts comprehensive assessments, orders and interprets diagnostic tests, manages health problems and disease-related symptoms, prescribes treatments, and coordinates care during transitions in settings. Certification as an ACNP is available through the AACN. Prescriptive authority and licensure regulations for APRNs vary by state.

Critical Care Patient

AACN defines a *critically ill patient* as one who is at high risk for actual or potential life-threatening health problems and who requires intense and vigilant nursing care.[1] A patient is generally admitted to the ICU for one of three reasons. First, the patient may be physiologically unstable, requiring advanced clinical judgments by you and a physician. Second, the patient may be at risk for serious complications and require frequent assessments and often invasive interventions. Third, the patient may require intensive and complicated nursing support related to the use of IV polypharmacy (e.g., sedation, thrombolytics, drugs requiring titration [e.g., vasopressors]) and advanced technology (e.g., mechanical ventilation, intracranial pressure monitoring, continuous renal replacement therapy, hemodynamic monitoring).

ICU patients can be clustered by disease condition (e.g., neurology, pulmonary) or age-group (e.g., neonatal, pediatrics). ICU patients are sometimes clustered by acuity (e.g., acute and unstable versus technology dependent but stable). Patients commonly treated in the ICU include those with respiratory distress, myocardial infarction, or acute neurologic impairment or those receiving care after cardiac surgery or other major surgical procedures (e.g., organ transplantation). Trauma and burn ICUs care for critically injured patients. Patients with medical emergencies (e.g., sepsis, diabetic ketoacidosis, drug overdoses, thyroid crisis) are treated in a medical ICU. The patient who is not expected to recover from an illness is usually not admitted to an ICU. For example, the ICU is not used to manage the patient in a persistent coma or to prolong the natural process of death.

Despite the emphasis on caring for patients who are expected to survive, the incidence of death is higher in ICU patients than in non-ICU patients. In general, nonsurvivors are older, have co-morbidities (e.g., liver disease, obesity), and experience longer ICU stays.[4] Consequently, it is important that you are skilled in palliative and end-of-life care (see Chapter 10).

Common Problems of Critical Care Patients. The patient admitted to the ICU is at risk for numerous complications and special problems. Critically ill patients are usually immobile and at high risk for skin problems (see Chapter 24) and venous thromboembolism (see Chapter 38). The use of multiple, invasive devices predisposes the patient to health care–associated infections (HAIs). Sepsis and multiple organ dysfunction syndrome (MODS) may follow (see Chapter 67). Adequate nutrition for the critically ill patient is essential. Other special problems relate to anxiety, pain, impaired communication, sensory-perceptual problems, and sleep disorders.

Nutrition. Patients often arrive at ICUs with conditions that result in either hypermetabolic states (e.g., burns, sepsis) or catabolic states (e.g., acute kidney injury). Other times, patients are in severely malnourished states (e.g., chronic heart, pulmonary, or liver disease). In general, inadequate nutrition is linked to increased mortality and morbidity rates. One contributing

factor to underfeeding patients is the frequent interruptions in enteral feedings because of medication administration and multiple tests and procedures. Determining who to feed, what to feed, when to feed, and how to feed (e.g., route of administration) is crucial when caring for critically ill patients.[5] Collaborate with the physician and the dietitian to determine how best to meet the nutritional needs of ICU patients.

The primary goal of nutritional support is to prevent or correct nutritional deficiencies. This is usually done by the early provision of enteral nutrition (i.e., delivery of calories via the gastrointestinal [GI] tract) or parenteral nutrition (i.e., IV delivery of calories).[5] Enteral nutrition preserves the structure and function of the gut mucosa and stops the movement of gut bacteria across the intestinal wall and into the bloodstream. In addition, early enteral nutrition is associated with fewer complications and shorter hospital stays and is less expensive than parenteral nutrition.[5] (Enteral and parenteral nutrition are discussed in Chapter 40.)

Parenteral nutrition is used when the enteral route cannot provide adequate nutrition or is contraindicated. Examples of these conditions are paralytic ileus, diffuse peritonitis, intestinal obstruction, pancreatitis, GI ischemia, abdominal trauma or surgery, and severe diarrhea.

Anxiety. Anxiety is a common problem for ICU patients. The primary sources of anxiety include the perceived or anticipated threat to health or life, loss of control of body functions, and an environment that is foreign. Many patients and caregivers feel uncomfortable in the ICU with its complex equipment, high noise and light levels, and intense pace of activity. Pain, impaired communication, sleeplessness, immobilization, and loss of control all enhance anxiety.

To help reduce anxiety, encourage patients and caregivers to express concerns, ask questions, and state their needs. Include the patient and caregiver in all conversations and explain the purpose of equipment and procedures. Be sure to structure the patient's environment in a way that decreases anxiety. For example, encourage caregivers to bring in photographs and personal items. Appropriate use of antianxiety drugs (e.g., lorazepam [Ativan]) and relaxation techniques (e.g., music therapy) may reduce the stress response that can be triggered by anxiety.[6]

Pain. The control of pain in the ICU patient is vital. As many as 70% of ICU patients have moderate to severe unrelieved pain. Inadequate pain control is often linked with agitation and anxiety and is known to add to the stress response. ICU patients at high risk for pain include those who (1) have medical conditions that include ischemic, infectious, or inflammatory processes; (2) are immobilized; (3) have invasive monitoring

---

INFORMATICS IN PRACTICE

Smart Infusion Pumps

- Smart infusion pumps, with preprogrammed drug libraries and wireless technology, calculate medication dose and delivery rates to help prevent IV medication errors and reduce the risk of patient harm.
- Smart pumps provide information used in driving safe practices, such as the total number of infusions programmed using the drug library, how many times pumps were manually overridden, or how often an alert resulted in reprogramming an infusion.
- Remember, if you make a mistake and enter incorrect data, you will get incorrect results. Some drugs (e.g., heparin [Hep-Lock]) require that a second nurse confirm the pump settings. Always use your best nursing judgment when using smart infusion pumps or any other technology and follow agency policy.

devices, including endotracheal tubes; and (4) require invasive or noninvasive procedures.[7]

For some critically ill patients (e.g., those needing mechanical ventilation), continuous IV sedation (e.g., propofol [Diprivan]) and an analgesic agent (e.g., fentanyl [Sublimaze]) are effective strategies for sedation and pain control. However, patients getting deep sedation are unresponsive. This prevents you and other health care providers from fully assessing the patient's neurologic status. To address this problem, guidelines should include a daily, scheduled interruption of sedation, or "sedation holiday." These daily interruptions allow you to awaken the patient to conduct a neurologic examination.[8] (Pain management is discussed in Chapter 9.)

Impaired Communication. Inability to communicate is distressing for patients who cannot speak because of the use of sedative and paralyzing drugs or an endotracheal tube. As part of every procedure, explain what will happen or is happening to the patient. When the patient cannot speak, explore alternative methods of communication, such as picture boards, notepads, magic slates, or computer keyboards. When speaking with the patient, look directly at the patient and use hand gestures when appropriate. For patients and caregivers who do not speak English, an approved translator or translator phone service must be provided (see Chapter 4).

Nonverbal communication is important. High levels of procedure-related touch and lower levels of comfort-related touch often characterize the ICU environment. Patients have different levels of tolerance for being touched, usually related to culture and personal history. If appropriate, use comforting touch with ongoing evaluation of the patient's response. Similarly, encourage caregivers to touch and talk with the patient even if the patient is unresponsive.

Sensory-Perceptual Problems. Acute and reversible sensory-perceptual changes are common in ICU patients. The combination of alterations in mentation (e.g., delusions, short attention span, loss of recent memory), psychomotor behavior (e.g., restlessness, lethargy), and sleep-wake cycle (e.g., daytime sleepiness, nighttime agitation) has been inappropriately called *ICU psychosis*. The patient experiencing these changes is not psychotic but is suffering from *delirium*. It is estimated that the prevalence of delirium in ICU patients is as high as 80%.[9] Significant risk factors for delirium include preexisting dementia, history of baseline hypertension or alcohol abuse, and severe illness on admission. Environmental factors that can contribute to delirium include sleep deprivation, anxiety, sensory overload, and immobilization. Physical conditions such as hemodynamic instability, hypoxemia, hypercarbia, electrolyte disturbances, and severe infections can lead to delirium. Last, certain drugs (e.g., sedatives [benzodiazepines], analgesics [opioids], and antimicrobials [aminoglycosides]) have been linked with the development of delirium.[9] (Chapter 60 discusses delirium.)

Monitor all ICU patients for delirium. Assessment tools include the Confusion Assessment Method for the ICU and the Intensive Care Delirium Screening Checklist[9] (both available at *www.icudelirium.org*). It is critical to address physiologic factors (e.g., correction of oxygenation, perfusion, and electrolyte problems). The use of clocks and calendars can help orient the patient. If the patient demonstrates hyperactivity, insomnia, or delusions, management with sedative drugs with anxiolytic effects (e.g., dexmedetomidine [Precedex]) can be considered.[9] In addition, the presence of a caregiver may help orient the patient and reduce agitation. (See eTable 66-1 on the website for this chapter.)

Sensory overload can also result in patient distress and anxiety. Environmental noise levels are particularly high in the ICU.[10] You can limit noise and assist the patient in understanding noises that cannot be prevented. Conversation is a particularly stressful noise, especially when the discussion concerns the patient and is held in the presence of, but without participation from, the patient.[10] Reduce this source of stress by finding suitable places for patient-related discussions. Whenever possible, include the patient or the caregiver in the discussion.

You can also limit noise levels by muting phones, setting alarms based on the patient's condition, and reducing unnecessary alarms. For example, silence the BP alarm when handling invasive lines and then reset the alarm when done. Similarly, silence ventilator alarms when suctioning. Last, limit overhead paging and all unnecessary noise in patient care areas.

Sleep Problems. Nearly all ICU patients have sleep disturbances. Patients may have difficulty falling asleep or have disrupted sleep because of noise, anxiety, pain, frequent monitoring, or treatment procedures. Sleep disturbance has been associated with delirium and delayed recovery.[8,10] Arrange the environment to promote the patient's sleep-wake cycle. Strategies include scheduling rest periods, dimming lights at nighttime, opening curtains during the daytime, getting physiologic measurements without disturbing the patient, limiting noise, and providing comfort measures (e.g., massage).[11] If necessary, use benzodiazepines (e.g., temazepam [Restoril]) and benzodiazepine-like drugs (e.g., zolpidem [Ambien]) to induce and maintain sleep. (Sleep and sleep disorders are discussed in Chapter 8.)

Issues Related to Caregivers

When someone becomes critically ill, care extends beyond the patient to the patient's caregivers. Caregivers play a valuable role in the patient's recovery and are members of the health care team. They contribute to the patient's well-being by

- Providing a link to the patient's personal life (e.g., news of family, job)
- Advising the patient in health care decisions or functioning as the decision maker when the patient cannot
- Helping with activities of daily living (e.g., bathing, oral suctioning)
- Providing positive, loving, and caring support

To be effective in caring for their loved one, caregivers need your guidance and support. The experience of having a friend or relative in the ICU is physically and emotionally difficult, often to the point of exhaustion. Anxiety and concerns regarding the patient's condition, prognosis, and pain are some of the issues caregivers confront. In addition, caregivers commonly experience anxiety over the financial issues related to the provision of care during a critical illness. Consulting with the case manager or social worker is helpful in these instances.

Caregivers often disrupt their daily routines to support the patient. They may be far from their own home, friends, and relatives. Ultimately, caregivers of the critically ill are in crisis, and family-centered care is essential.[12] To provide family-centered care effectively, you must be skilled in crisis intervention. Conduct a family assessment and intervene as necessary. Strategies include active listening, reduction of anxiety, and support of those who become upset or angry. Acknowledge the caregivers' feelings and accept and support their decisions. Consult other health care team members (e.g., chaplains, psychologists, patient representatives) as necessary to help caregivers cope. The extent to which family-centered care is provided can affect the patient's clinical course in the ICU.

The major needs of caregivers of critically ill patients include information, reassurance, and convenience.[13] Lack of information is a major source of anxiety for the caregivers. Assess the caregiver's understanding of the patient's status, treatment plan, and prognosis and provide information as appropriate. Identify a spokesperson for the family to help coordinate information exchange between the health care team and family.

The caregiver needs reassurance regarding the way in which the patient's care is managed and decisions are made. Invite the caregiver to meet the health care team members. Evaluate the appropriateness of including caregivers in interdisciplinary rounds and patient care conferences. It helps caregivers accept and cope with problems when they see that the health care team is caring and competent, decisions are deliberate, and their input is valued. If the patient has an advance directive, the caregiver needs to see that the patient's wishes are followed. If the patient has designated a durable power of attorney for health care, this person must be involved in the patient's plan of care.

Caregivers of critically ill patients need access to the patient. Limiting visitation does not protect the patient from adverse physiologic consequences.[14] AACN strongly recommends less restrictive, individualized visiting policies. This is accomplished by assessing the patient's and caregiver's needs and preferences and incorporating these into the plan of care.[14]

ETHICAL/LEGAL DILEMMAS

Family Presence and Visitation in the Adult ICU

Situation

B.W., a new nurse, is undergoing orientation in the surgical intensive care unit (ICU). He asks his preceptor why the patients' families are permitted on the unit throughout the day and even the night. B.W. states that, in his last position, visiting hours in the ICU were 10 AM to noon and 4 to 6 PM. He adds that families make him nervous when they watch what he is doing and ask him multiple questions. B.W. states that he intends to tell the visitors to leave the patient's room when he is providing care.

Ethical/Legal Points for Consideration

- The majority of nurses in adult ICUs prefer unrestricted visiting policies, but research indicates that most ICU policies limit visitation.
- Family visitation was thought to cause the patient physiologic stress and interfere with care. Additionally, it was believed that family visitation was mentally exhausting to patients and families, and even contributed to increased infection rates. Evidence does not support any of these beliefs.
- Evidence suggests several positive patient benefits to flexible family visitation: decreases in anxiety, confusion, and agitation; reductions in cardiovascular complications; decreases in length of ICU stay; and reports that patients feel more secure and satisfied with care.
- Similar evidence exists for the benefits of flexible visitation for family members: increases in satisfaction, decreases in anxiety, promotion of better communication, and increases in opportunities for patient and family teaching as the family becomes more involved in care.
- Some conditions may require restricting visitation: a legal reason is documented in the chart; visitor behavior presents a risk to the patient, family, staff, or others; visitor behavior disrupts the functioning of the unit; visitor has a contagious illness or has been exposed to a contagious disease that could endanger the patient's health; or the patient requests fewer or no visitors.

Discussion Questions

1. How should the preceptor respond to B.W.'s statement of his intentions?
2. Does B.W. have an ethical or legal obligation to permit family visitation regardless of his personal concerns? Defend your position.

The first time that caregivers visit it is important for you to prepare them for the experience. Briefly describe the patient's appearance and the physical environment (e.g., equipment, noise).[15] Join caregivers as they enter the room, and observe the responses of both the patient and caregivers. Invite the caregivers to participate in the patient's care if they desire. In some ICUs, visitation includes animal-assisted therapy or pet visitation. The positive benefits of these interventions (e.g., decreases in BP and anxiety) far outweigh the risks (e.g., transmission of infection from animal to patient). They should be a part of the visitation policy.

In addition to traditional visiting, caregivers of patients undergoing invasive procedures (e.g., central line insertion) and cardiopulmonary resuscitation (CPR) want the option of being present at the bedside during these events. Even when the outcomes are not favorable, being present helps caregivers overcome doubts about the patient's condition, reduces their anxiety and fear, meets their need to be together and to support their loved one, and aids the grief process if death occurs. AACN encourages critical care nurses to develop policies and procedures that provide for the option of family presence during invasive procedures and CPR.[16]

CULTURALLY COMPETENT CARE

CRITICAL CARE PATIENTS

Providing culturally competent care to critically ill patients and caregivers is challenging. Often, meeting the patient's physiologic needs is a priority and overshadows the influence of the patient's culture on the illness experience. It remains important to consider the cultural aspects of the meaning of sickness and health, pain, dying and death, and grief when caring for critically ill patients and their caregivers (see Chapter 2).

Cultural perspectives on dying and death are complex. Telling some patients that they are dying as a way of letting them prepare for death may infringe on the family's role. Others view a discussion about advance directives as a legal device to deny care.

Customs surrounding dying and death vary widely. Caregiver requests may range from asking you to leave a window open so the spirit of the dead person can leave, to providing the final bath for the deceased. Ask the caregivers about the family's cultural traditions when caring for the dying patient. Several variables influence the expressions of grief that follow the loss of a loved one. These include the relationship between the grieving person and the deceased, whether the loss is sudden or anticipated, the support systems available to the grieving person, past experiences with loss, and the person's religious and cultural beliefs. Proceed cautiously when approaching patients facing death and their caregivers. Asking patients, "What do you want to know?" and "Who do you want with you when discussing options?" are good starting points.[17] (Chapter 10 provides additional information about end-of-life care.)

HEMODYNAMIC MONITORING

Hemodynamic monitoring is the measurement of pressure, flow, and oxygenation within the cardiovascular system. The purpose of hemodynamic monitoring is to assess heart function, fluid balance, and the effects of fluids and drugs on CO. Both invasive (internally placed devices) and noninvasive (external devices) hemodynamic parameters (values) are obtained. These include systemic and pulmonary arterial pressures, central venous pressure (CVP), pulmonary artery wedge pressure (PAWP) (also known as pulmonary artery occlusive pressure [PAOP]), CO/CI, SV/SV index [SVI], SVV, O_2 saturation of the hemoglobin of arterial blood (SaO_2), and mixed venous oxygen saturation (SvO_2). From these measurements you can calculate several values, including the resistance of the systemic and pulmonary arterial vasculature and O_2 content, delivery, and consumption. When you integrate these data, you get a picture of the patient's hemodynamic status and the effect of therapy over time (trends). Make all measurements with attention to technical accuracy. Inaccurate data can result in unnecessary or inappropriate treatment.

Hemodynamic Terminology

Cardiac Output and Cardiac Index. *Cardiac output* (CO) is the volume of blood in liters pumped by the heart in 1 minute.

Cardiac index (CI) is the measurement of the CO adjusted for body surface area (BSA). It is a more precise measurement of the efficiency of the heart's pumping action. Although minor beat-to-beat variations may occur, generally the left and right ventricles pump the same volume. The volume ejected with each heartbeat is the *stroke volume* (SV). Like CI, *stroke volume index* (SVI) is the measurement of SV adjusted for BSA. CO and the forces opposing blood flow determine BP. *Systemic vascular resistance* (SVR) (opposition encountered by the left ventricle) or *pulmonary vascular resistance* (PVR) (opposition encountered by the right ventricle) is the resistance to blood flow by the vessels. Preload, afterload, and contractility (see Chapter 32) determine SV (and thus CO and BP). It is essential that you understand these concepts and relationships. In addition, you must understand the effects of manipulating each of these variables. Table 66-1 presents the formulas and values for common hemodynamic parameters.

TABLE 66-1 RESTING HEMODYNAMIC PARAMETERS

Indicators	Normal Range
Preload	
Right atrial pressure (RAP) or central venous pressure (CVP)	2-8 mm Hg
Pulmonary artery wedge pressure (PAWP) or left atrial pressure (LAP)	6-12 mm Hg
Pulmonary artery diastolic pressure (PADP)	4-12 mm Hg
Right ventricular end-diastolic volume (RVEDV) $= \dfrac{\text{Stroke volume (SV)}}{\text{Right ventricular ejection fraction (RVEF)}}$	100-160 mL
Afterload	
Pulmonary vascular resistance (PVR) $= \dfrac{(\text{Pulmonary artery mean pressure [PAMP]} - \text{PAWP}) \times 80}{\text{Cardiac output (CO)}}$	<250 dynes/sec/cm^{-5}
Pulmonary vascular resistance index (PVRI) $= \dfrac{(\text{PAMP} - \text{PAWP}) \times 80}{\text{Cardiac index (CI)}}$	160-380 dynes/sec/cm^{-5}/m^2
Systemic vascular resistance (SVR) $= \dfrac{(\text{Mean arterial pressure [MAP]} - \text{CVP}) \times 80}{\text{CO}}$	800-1200 dynes/sec/cm^{-5}
Systemic vascular resistance index (SVRI) $= \dfrac{(\text{MAP} - \text{CVP}) \times 80}{\text{CI}}$	1970-2390 dynes/sec/cm^{-5}/m^2
MAP $= \dfrac{\text{Systolic blood pressure} + 2(\text{Diastolic blood pressure})}{3^*}$	70-105 mm Hg
PAMP $= \dfrac{\text{Pulmonary artery systolic pressure (PASP)} + 2\,\text{PADP}}{3^*}$	10-20 mm Hg
Other	
Stroke volume $= \dfrac{\text{CO}}{\text{Heart rate}}$	60-150 mL/beat
Stroke volume index (SVI) $= \dfrac{\text{CI}}{\text{Heart rate}}$	30-65 mL/beat/m^2
Stroke volume variation (SVV) $= \dfrac{\text{SV}_{max} - \text{SV}_{min}}{\text{SV}_{mean}}$	<13%
Heart rate (HR)	60-100 beats/min
CO $= $ SV $\times$ HR	4-8 L/min
CI $= \dfrac{\text{CO}}{\text{Body surface area (BSA)}}$	2.2-4 L/min/m^2
RVEF $= \dfrac{\text{SV}}{\text{RVEDV} \times 100}$	40%-60%
Arterial hemoglobin O_2 saturation	95%-100%
Mixed venous hemoglobin O_2 saturation	60%-80%
Venous hemoglobin O_2 saturation	70%

*This formula is an approximation because it does not take into consideration the heart rate. The monitor looks at the area under the pressure curve, as well as the heart rate, to calculate MAP and PAMP.

Preload. *Preload* is the volume within the ventricle at the end of diastole. Unfortunately, chamber volume measurements are difficult to obtain. Instead, various pressures are used to estimate the volume. Left ventricular preload is called *left ventricular end-diastolic pressure.* PAWP, a measurement of pulmonary capillary pressure, reflects left ventricular end-diastolic pressure under normal conditions (i.e., when there is no mitral valve dysfunction, intracardiac defect, or dysrhythmia). CVP, measured in the right atrium or in the vena cava close to the heart, is the right ventricular preload or right ventricular end-diastolic pressure when there is no tricuspid valve dysfunction, intracardiac defect, or dysrhythmia.

Frank-Starling's law explains the effects of preload and states that the more a myocardial fiber is stretched during filling, the more it shortens during systole and the greater the force of the contraction. As preload increases, force generated in the subsequent contraction increases, and thus SV and CO increase. The greater the preload, the greater the myocardial stretch and the greater the O_2 requirement of the myocardium. Hence, increases in CO via increased preload require increased delivery of O_2 to the myocardium. Remember that the change in SV with preload comes about because of stretching and recoil of the heart muscle. However, the clinical measurement made is not a direct measurement of the muscle length. The measurement is of the pressure at the time of the peak stretch (end diastole) (see Table 66-1). This pressure indirectly indicates the amount of stretch and the volume. This pressure is also important because it indicates pressure in the blood vessels of the lung or in the blood returning to the heart. Diuresis and vasodilation decrease preload, and fluid administration increases preload.

Afterload. *Afterload* refers to the forces opposing ventricular ejection. These forces include systemic arterial pressure, the resistance offered by the aortic valve, and the mass and density of the blood to be moved. Clinically, although the measures fail to include all the components of afterload, SVR and arterial pressure are indices of left ventricular afterload. Similarly, PVR and pulmonary arterial pressure are indices of right ventricular afterload. Increased afterload often results in a decreased CO. CO can be restored and myocardial O_2 needs reduced by decreasing afterload (i.e., decreasing forces opposing contraction). Vasodilator drug therapy (e.g., milrinone [Primacor]) can reduce afterload.

Vascular Resistance. *Systemic vascular resistance* (SVR) is the resistance of the systemic vascular bed. *Pulmonary vascular resistance* (PVR) is the resistance of the pulmonary vascular bed. Both these measures reflect afterload as described earlier and can be adjusted for body size (see Table 66-1).

Contractility. *Contractility* describes the strength of contraction. Contractility is said to increase when preload is unchanged yet the heart contracts more forcefully. Epinephrine, norepinephrine (Levophed), isoproterenol (Isuprel), dopamine (Intropin), dobutamine (Dobutrex), digitalis-like drugs, calcium, and milrinone increase or improve contractility. These drugs are termed *positive inotropes.* Contractility is reduced by *negative inotropes.* Examples include certain drugs (e.g., alcohol, calcium channel blockers, β-adrenergic blockers) and clinical conditions (e.g., acidosis). Increased contractility results in increased SV and increased myocardial O_2 requirements. There are no direct clinical measures of cardiac contractility. Measuring the patient's preload (PAWP) and CO and graphing the results indirectly indicates contractility. If preload, heart rate, and afterload remain constant yet CO changes, con-

FIG. 66-3 Components of a pressure monitoring system. The cannula, shown entering the radial artery, is connected via pressure (nondistensible) tubing to the transducer. The transducer converts the pressure wave into an electronic signal. The transducer is wired to the electronic monitoring system, which amplifies, conditions, displays, and records the signal. Stopcocks are inserted into the line for specimen withdrawal and for referencing and zero-balancing procedures. A flush system, consisting of a pressurized bag of IV fluid, tubing, and a flush device, is connected to the system. The flush system provides continuous slow (approximately 3 mL/hr) flushing and provides a mechanism for fast flushing of lines.

tractility is changed. Contractility is reduced in the failing heart.

Principles of Invasive Pressure Monitoring

Invasive lines are used in the ICU to measure systemic and pulmonary BPs. Fig. 66-3 shows the components of a typical invasive arterial BP monitoring system. The catheter, pressure tubing, flush system, and transducer are disposable.

Pressure monitoring equipment is referenced and zero balanced to the environment and dynamic response characteristics optimized for accuracy. *Referencing* means positioning the transducer so that the zero reference point is at the level of the atria of the heart. The stopcock nearest the transducer is usually the zero reference for the transducer. To place this level with the atria, use an external landmark, the phlebostatic axis. To identify the *phlebostatic axis,* draw two imaginary lines with the patient supine (Fig. 66-4, *A*). Draw a horizontal line down from the axilla, midway between the anterior and posterior chest walls. Draw a vertical line laterally through the fourth intercos-

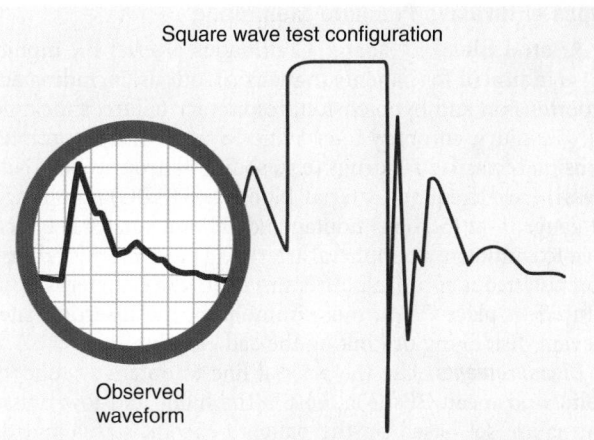

Square wave test configuration

Observed
waveform

When the fast flush of the continuous flush system is activated and quickly released, a sharp upstroke terminates in a flat line at the maximal indicator on the monitor and hard copy. This is then followed by an immediate rapid downstroke extending below baseline with just 1 or 2 oscillations within 0.12 second (minimal ringing) and a quick return to a baseline. The patient's pressure waveform is also clearly defined with all components of the waveform, such as the dicrotic notch on an arterial waveform, clearly visible.

FIG. 66-5 Optimally damped system. Dynamic response test (square wave test) using the fast flush system: normal response. No adjustment in the monitoring system is required.

Phlebostatic
axis   4th intercostal space
Outermost
anterior
chest
Midchest
Outermost
posterior
chest
A

Air-fluid
interface
(zeroing
stopcock)
Transducer   Carpenter level
Phlebostatic axis
B

FIG. 66-4 Identification of the phlebostatic axis. **A,** Phlebostatic axis is an external landmark used to identify the level of the atria in the supine patient. It is defined as the intersection of two imaginary lines: one drawn horizontally from the axilla, midway between the anterior and posterior chest walls, and the other drawn vertically through the fourth intercostal space along the lateral chest wall. **B,** Air-fluid interface (zeroing the stopcock) is level with the phlebostatic axis using a carpenter's or laser level.

tal space along the chest wall. The phlebostatic axis is the intersection of the two imaginary lines. Mark this location on the patient's chest with a permanent marker. Position the port of the stopcock nearest the transducer level with the phlebostatic axis. Tape the transducer to the patient's chest at the phlebostatic axis or mount it on a bedside pole (Fig. 66-4, *B*).

Zeroing confirms that when pressure within the system is zero, the monitor reads zero. To do this, open the reference stopcock to room air (off to the patient) and observe the monitor for a reading of zero. This allows the monitor to use the atmospheric pressure as a reference for zero. Zero the transducer during the initial setup, immediately after insertion of the arterial line, when the transducer has been disconnected from the pressure cable or the pressure cable has been disconnected from the monitor, and when the accuracy of the measurements is questioned. Always follow the manufacturer's guidelines.

Optimizing dynamic response characteristics involves checking that the equipment reproduces, without distortion, a signal that changes rapidly. Perform a *dynamic response test (square wave test)* every 8 to 12 hours and when the system is opened to air or the accuracy of the measurements is questioned. It involves activating the fast flush and checking that the equipment reproduces a distortion-free signal (Fig. 66-5).

Table 66-2 outlines the steps in obtaining BP measurements with an invasive line. Obtain measurements from both digital and printed analog outputs. Readings from a printed pressure tracing at the end of expiration (to limit the effect of the respiratory cycle on arterial BP) are most accurate.[18] Position the patient supine for initial readings. Unless the patient's BP is extremely sensitive to orthostatic changes, values with head-of-bed (HOB) elevation (up to 45 degrees) are generally equal to measurements with the patient supine. Additionally, readings in the prone position are generally accurate. However, there is little support for the accuracy of readings in the lateral posi-

TABLE 66-2	INVASIVE ARTERIAL BLOOD PRESSURE MEASUREMENT

1. Explain the procedure to the patient.
2. Position the patient supine and flat or, if appropriate, with the head of the bed at less than 45 degrees or prone.
3. Confirm that the zero reference (port of the stopcock nearest the transducer) is placed at the level of the phlebostatic axis (see Fig. 66-4). If the reference stopcock is not taped to the patient's chest, use a leveling device to position the stopcock on a bedside pole at the point level with the phlebostatic axis.
4. Observe the monitor tracing and assess the quality of the tracing. Perform a dynamic response test (see Fig. 66-5).
5. Obtain an analog printout, if available, and measure the systolic and diastolic pressures at end expiration (see Fig. 66-6). If no printout is available, freeze the tracing on the oscilloscope screen and use the cursor to measure the pressures at end expiration.
6. Record the pressure measurements promptly, including (if available) the printout marked to identify the points read.

tions.[18] It is not necessary to reposition the patient for each pressure reading. However, it is important to keep the zero reference stopcock level with the phlebostatic axis.

SAFETY ALERT: Positioning the Zero Reference Stopcock
- Mark the location of the phlebostatic axis on the patient's chest with a permanent marker.
- Recheck the leveling of the zero reference stopcock to the phlebostatic axis with any change in the patient's position before obtaining a reading.
- Transducers placed higher than the phlebostatic axis will produce falsely low readings. Transducers placed lower than the phlebostatic axis will produce falsely high readings.

Types of Invasive Pressure Monitoring

Arterial Blood Pressure. Continuous arterial BP monitoring is indicated for patients in many situations, including acute hypertension and hypotension, respiratory failure, shock, neurologic injury, coronary interventional procedures, continuous infusion of vasoactive drugs (e.g., sodium nitroprusside [Nitropress]), and frequent arterial blood gas (ABG) sampling. A 20-gauge, 2-in (5.1-cm) nontapered Teflon catheter is typically used to cannulate a peripheral artery (e.g., radial, femoral) using a percutaneous approach. After insertion, the catheter is usually sutured in place.[18] You must immobilize the insertion site to prevent dislodging or kinking the catheter line.

Measurements. Use the arterial line to obtain systolic, diastolic, and mean BPs (Fig. 66-6). The high- and low-pressure alarms are set based on the patient's current status and then activated. Various patient conditions will change the pressure tracings. In heart failure, the systolic upstroke may be slower. In volume depletion, systolic pressure varies greatly with mechanical ventilation, decreasing during inspiration. Observe simultaneous ECG and pressure tracings with dysrhythmias. Dysrhythmias that significantly diminish arterial BP are more urgent than those that cause only a slight decrease in systolic amplitude.

Complications. Arterial lines carry the risk of hemorrhage, infection, thrombus formation, neurovascular impairment, and loss of limb. Hemorrhage is most likely to occur when the catheter dislodges or the line disconnects. To avoid this serious complication, use Luer-Lok connections, always check the arterial waveform, and activate alarms. If the pressure in the line falls (e.g., when the line is disconnected), the low-pressure alarm sounds immediately, allowing you to promptly correct the problem.

Infection is a risk with any invasive line. To limit the risk of catheter-related infection, inspect the insertion site for local signs of inflammation and monitor the patient for signs of systemic infection. Change the pressure tubing, flush bag, and transducer every 96 hours or according to agency policy. If infection is suspected, remove the catheter and replace the equipment.

Circulatory impairment can result from formation of a thrombus around the catheter, release of an embolus, spasm, or occlusion of the circulation by the catheter. Before inserting a line into the radial artery, perform an *Allen test* to confirm that ulnar circulation to the hand is adequate. In this test, apply pressure to the radial and ulnar arteries simultaneously. Ask the patient to open and close the hand repeatedly. The hand should blanch. Release the pressure on the ulnar artery while maintaining pressure on the radial artery. If pinkness fails to return within 6 seconds, the ulnar artery is inadequate and you should not use the radial artery for line insertion.

To maintain line patency and limit thrombus formation, assess the continuous flush system every 1 to 4 hours to determine that the (1) pressure bag is inflated to 300 mm Hg, (2) flush bag contains fluid, and (3) system is delivering 3 to 6 mL/hr. Because of the risk of heparin-induced thrombocytopenia (HIT), heparinized saline should not be routinely used for the flush solution.[18] (HIT is discussed in Chapter 31.)

Once the catheter is inserted, evaluate the neurovascular status distal to the arterial insertion site hourly. The limb with compromised arterial flow will be cool and pale, with capillary refill time longer than 3 seconds. The patient may have symptoms of neurologic impairment (e.g., paresthesia, pain, paralysis). Neurovascular impairment, which can result in the loss of a limb, is an emergency.

Arterial Pressure–Based Cardiac Output. Arterial pressure–based cardiac output (APCO) monitoring is a minimally invasive technique to determine *continuous CO* (CCO)/*continuous CI* (CCI). In addition to measuring CCO, APCO is used to assess a patient's ability to respond to fluids by increasing SV (*preload responsiveness*). This is determined by using *stroke volume variation* (SVV) or by measuring the percent increase in SV after a fluid bolus[19] (see Table 66-1). This technology uses a specialized sensor that attaches to a standard arterial pressure line and a monitor (Fig. 66-7).

SVV is the variation of the arterial pulsation caused by the heart-lung interaction. It is a sensitive indicator of preload responsiveness when used on select patients. SVV is used only for patients on controlled mechanical ventilation with a fixed

FIG. 66-6 A, Simultaneously recorded electrocardiogram (ECG) tracing and **B,** systemic arterial pressure tracing. Systolic pressure is the peak pressure. The *dicrotic notch* indicates aortic valve closure. Diastolic pressure is the lowest value before contraction. Mean pressure is the average pressure over time calculated by the monitoring equipment.

FIG. 66-7 FloTrac sensor and Vigileo monitor. (Courtesy Edwards Lifesciences, Irvine, Calif.)

respiratory rate and a fixed tidal volume of 8 mL/kg. Also, the APCO monitor may not be able to filter certain dysrhythmias—specifically atrial fibrillation—limiting the use of SVV in these patients. These limitations only apply to SVV, not to the use of APCO for CO monitoring.

Measurements. Arterial pressure is the force generated by the ejection of blood from the left ventricle into the arterial circulation. Pulsatile pressure waves are produced by the heart's contractions (systole). The specialized sensor measures the arterial pulse pressure, which is proportional to SV. APCO monitoring uses the arterial waveform characteristics along with patient demographic data (i.e., gender, age, height, and weight) to calculate SV and pulse rate (PR) to calculate CCO/CCI and SV/SVI every 20 seconds. CO is calculated by multiplying the PR and calculated SV and is displayed on a continuous basis.[20] APCO monitoring is frequently used in conjunction with a central venous oximetry catheter. Together, these allow for continuous monitoring of central venous oxygen saturation ($ScvO_2$) and SVR that is derived from the CVP.

APCO is only indicated in adult patients and cannot be used in patients who are on IABP therapy.[20]

Pulmonary Artery Flow-Directed Catheter. Pulmonary artery (PA) pressure monitoring guides the acute-phase management of patients with select complicated heart and lung problems (Table 66-3). PA diastolic (PAD) pressure and PAWP are sensitive indicators of cardiac function and fluid volume status. PAD pressure and PAWP increase in heart failure and fluid volume overload. They decrease with volume depletion. Fluid therapy based on PA pressures can restore fluid balance while avoiding overcorrection or undercorrection of the problem. Monitoring PA pressures permits precise therapeutic manipulation of preload. This allows CO to be maintained without placing the patient at risk for pulmonary edema.

A PA flow-directed catheter (e.g., Swan-Ganz) is used to measure PA pressures, including PAWP. The standard PA cath-

eter is number 7.5F, 43 in (110 cm) long, with multiple lumens (Fig. 66-8). When properly positioned, the distal lumen port (catheter tip) is within the PA. This port is used to monitor PA pressures and sample mixed venous blood (e.g., to evaluate O_2 saturation).

A balloon connected to an external valve surrounds the distal lumen port. Balloon inflation has two purposes: (1) to allow moving blood to float the catheter forward and (2) to allow PAWP measurement. The catheter has one or two proximal lumens, with exit ports in the right atrium or right atrium and right ventricle (if two). The right atrium port is used for

TABLE 66-3	INDICATIONS AND CONTRAINDICATIONS FOR PULMONARY ARTERY CATHETERIZATION*

Indications
- Assessment of response to therapy in patients with precapillary and mixed types of pulmonary hypertension
- Cardiogenic shock
- Differential diagnosis of pulmonary hypertension
- Myocardial infarction with complications (e.g., heart failure, cardiogenic shock)
- Potentially reversible systolic heart failure (e.g., fulminant myocarditis)
- Severe chronic heart failure requiring inotropic, vasopressor, and vasodilator therapy
- Transplantation work-up

Contraindications
- Coagulopathy
- Endocardial pacemaker
- Endocarditis
- Mechanical tricuspid or pulmonic valve

*List is not all-inclusive.

FIG. 66-8 Pulmonary artery (PA) catheter. **A,** Illustrated catheter has five lumens. When properly positioned, the distal lumen exit port is in the PA and the proximal lumen ports are in the right atrium and right ventricle. The distal and one of the proximal ports are used to measure PA and central venous pressures, respectively. A balloon surrounds the catheter near the distal end. The balloon inflation valve is used to inflate the balloon with air to allow reading of the pulmonary artery wedge pressure. A thermistor located near the distal tip senses PA temperature and is used to measure thermodilution cardiac output when solution cooler than body temperature is injected into a proximal port. **B,** Photo of an actual catheter. (**B,** Courtesy Edwards Critical Care Division, Baxter Healthcare Corporation, Santa Ana, Calif.)

measurement of CVP, injection of fluid for CO determination, and withdrawal of blood specimens. The second proximal port (if available) is used for infusion of fluids and drugs or blood sampling. A thermistor (temperature sensor) is located near the distal tip and is wired to an external connector. This is used to monitor blood or core temperature and for the thermodilution method of measuring CO.[21]

In addition to providing most of the same functions as the standard PA catheter, the advanced technology PA catheter can continuously monitor the patient's SvO_2. This provides a global indicator of the balance between oxygen delivery and oxygen consumption. CCO and right ventricular EF (RVEF) also can be measured using advanced thermodilution technology. RVEF provides information regarding RV function and helps to assess right heart contractility. RV end-diastolic volume is continuously measured by dividing SV by RVEF (see Table 66-1). This serves as a key indicator of preload.

The PA catheter sheath (introducer) usually has a side port that serves as a large-bore IV line. Most catheters have a plastic "sleeve" connected to the sheath. This allows the catheter to be advanced or pulled back while maintaining sterility. The physician or other qualified health care provider (e.g., ACNP) usually manipulates the PA catheter, but this practice varies by agency.

Pulmonary Artery Catheter Insertion. Before PA catheter insertion, note the patient's electrolyte, acid-base, oxygenation, and coagulation status. Imbalances such as hypokalemia, hypomagnesemia, hypoxemia, or acidosis can make the heart more irritable and increase the risk of ventricular dysrhythmia during catheter insertion. Coagulopathy increases the risk of hemorrhage. Preparation for the procedure includes arranging the monitor, cables, and infusion and pressurized flush solutions. The system is zero referenced to the phlebostatic axis. The physician or other health care provider explains the procedure to the patient and obtains informed consent. The patient is positioned supine and flat. The PA catheter is inserted through

a sheath percutaneously into the internal jugular, subclavian, antecubital, or femoral vein using surgical asepsis. Venous cutdown is rarely required. The catheter is advanced through the venous system to the right side of the heart.

Continuously observe the characteristic waveforms on the monitor as the catheter is moved through the heart to the PA (Fig. 66-9). When the tip reaches the right atrium, the balloon is inflated. Inflation of the balloon should not exceed the balloon's capacity (1.5 mL of air). The catheter is then "floated" through the tricuspid valve into the right ventricle and then through the pulmonic valve to the PA. Monitor the ECG continuously during insertion because of the risk for dysrhythmias, particularly when the catheter reaches the right ventricle. Once a typical PAWP tracing is observed, the balloon is deflated, and the PA waveform should return on the monitor. After insertion and before using the PA catheter, a chest x-ray must confirm the catheter's position. To maintain the catheter in its proper position, secure it at the point of entry into the skin. Note and record the measurement at the exit point. Finally, apply an occlusive dressing, and then change it according to agency policy.

Recently, the use of PA pressure monitoring has decreased dramatically. This is due, in part, to risks associated with the technology (e.g., infection) and the development of less invasive techniques (e.g., APCO monitoring). More detailed information about PA pressure monitoring is available as an eSupplement on the website for this chapter.

Central Venous or Right Atrial Pressure Measurement. CVP is a measurement of right ventricular preload and reflects fluid volume problems. It is most often measured with a central venous catheter placed in the internal jugular or subclavian vein. It can be measured with a PA catheter using the proximal lumen located in the right atrium. CVP waveforms (Fig. 66-10) are similar to PAWP waveforms. CVP is measured as a mean pressure at the end of expiration. An elevated CVP indicates

FIG. 66-9 Position of the pulmonary artery flow-directed catheter during progressive stages of insertion with corresponding pressure waveforms.

right ventricular failure or volume overload. A low CVP indicates hypovolemia.

Venous Oxygen Saturation Monitoring. Both CVP and PA catheters can include sensors to measure O_2 saturation of hemoglobin in venous blood. The O_2 saturation of venous blood from the CVP catheter is termed *central venous oxygen saturation* ($ScvO_2$). Similarly, the O_2 saturation of blood from the PA catheter is termed *mixed venous oxygen saturation* (SvO_2). Either measurement is useful in determining the adequacy of tissue oxygenation. $ScvO_2/SvO_2$ reflects the balance between oxygenation of the arterial blood, tissue perfusion, and tissue O_2 consumption. $ScvO_2/SvO_2$ is useful in assessing hemodynamic status and response to treatments or activities when considered in conjunction with arterial O_2 saturation (Table 66-4). Normal $ScvO_2/SvO_2$ at rest is 60% to 80%.

Carefully review sustained decreases and increases in $ScvO_2/SvO_2$. Decreased $ScvO_2/SvO_2$ may indicate decreased arterial oxygenation, low CO, low hemoglobin level, or increased O_2 consumption or extraction. If the $ScvO_2/SvO_2$ falls below 60%, determine which of these factors has changed. Observe for changes in arterial oxygenation (e.g., monitor pulse oximetry or ABGs) and indirectly assess CO and tissue perfusion. This is done by noting any changes in mental status, strength and quality of peripheral pulses, capillary refill, urine output, and skin color and temperature. If arterial oxygenation, CO, and hemoglobin level are unchanged, a fall in $ScvO_2/SvO_2$ indicates increased O_2 consumption or extraction. This could represent an increased metabolic rate, pain, movement, or fever. If O_2 consumption increases without a comparable increase in O_2 delivery, more O_2 is extracted from the blood, and $ScvO_2/SvO_2$ will continue to fall.[22]

Increased $ScvO_2/SvO_2$ is also clinically significant and may indicate a clinical improvement (e.g., increased arterial O_2 saturation, improved perfusion, decreased metabolic rate) or problem (e.g., sepsis). In sepsis, O_2 is not extracted properly at the tissue level, resulting in increased $ScvO_2/SvO_2$.

Your interventions are guided by changes in $ScvO_2/SvO_2$. For example, you might note that the patient's heart rate increased moderately during repositioning but that the $ScvO_2/SvO_2$ remained stable. In this case, you would conclude that the patient tolerated the position change. If the $ScvO_2/SvO_2$ had dropped, this would be an indication to stop the activity until the $ScvO_2/SvO_2$ returns to baseline.

In many cases, as activity or metabolism increases, heart rate and CO increase, and $ScvO_2/SvO_2$ remains constant or varies slightly. However, critically ill patients often have conditions (e.g., heart failure, shock) that prevent substantial increases in CO. In these cases, $ScvO_2/SvO_2$ can be a useful indicator of the balance between O_2 delivery and consumption.

Noninvasive Arterial Oxygenation Monitoring

Pulse oximetry is a noninvasive and continuous method of determining the oxygen saturation of hemoglobin (SpO_2). Monitoring SpO_2 may reduce the frequency of ABG sampling (see Chapter 26). SpO_2 is normally 95% to 100%. Accurate SpO_2 measurements may be difficult to obtain on patients who are hypothermic, receiving IV vasopressor therapy (e.g., norepinephrine), or experiencing hypoperfusion and vasoconstriction (e.g., shock). Consider alternative locations for placement of the pulse oximetry probe (e.g., forehead, earlobe).

FIG. 66-10 Cardiac events that produce the central venous pressure (CVP) waveform with *a*, *c*, and *v* waves. The *a* wave represents atrial contraction. The *x* descent represents atrial relaxation. The *c* wave represents the bulging of the closed tricuspid valve into the right atrium during ventricular systole. The *v* wave represents atrial filling. The *y* descent represents opening of the tricuspid valve and filling of the ventricle.

TABLE 66-4	INTERPRETATION OF $ScvO_2/SvO_2$* MEASUREMENTS	
$ScvO_2/SvO_2$ Measurement	**Physiologic Basis for Change in $ScvO_2/SvO_2$**	**Clinical Diagnosis and Rationale**
High $ScvO_2/SvO_2$ (80%-95%)	Increased O_2 supply Decreased O_2 demand	• Patient receiving more O_2 than required by clinical condition • Anesthesia, which causes sedation and decreased muscle movement • Hypothermia, which lowers metabolic demand (e.g., with cardiopulmonary bypass) • Sepsis caused by decreased ability of tissues to use O_2 at the cellular level • False high positive because pulmonary artery catheter is wedged in a pulmonary capillary (SvO_2 only)
Normal $ScvO_2/SvO_2$ (60%-80%)	Normal O_2 supply and metabolic demand	• Balanced O_2 supply and demand
Low $ScvO_2/SvO_2$ (<60%)	Decreased O_2 supply caused by • Low hemoglobin • Low arterial saturation (SaO_2) • Low cardiac output • Increased O_2 demand	• Anemia or bleeding with compromised cardiopulmonary system • Hypoxemia resulting from decreased O_2 supply or lung disease • Cardiogenic shock caused by left ventricular pump failure • Metabolic demand exceeds O_2 supply in conditions that increase muscle movement and metabolic rate, including physiologic states such as shivering, seizures, and hyperthermia and nursing interventions such as being weighed on a bedside scale and turning

Source: Urden LD, Lough ME, Stacy KM: *Critical care nursing: diagnosis and management,* ed 6, St Louis, 2010, Mosby.
*$ScvO_2$ values are generally slightly higher than SvO_2 values.

A common use for pulse oximetry is to evaluate the effectiveness of O_2 therapy. Decreased SpO_2 indicates inadequate oxygenation of the blood in the pulmonary capillaries. You can correct this by increasing the fraction of inspired oxygen (FIO_2) and evaluating the patient's response. Similarly, use SpO_2 to monitor how the patient tolerates decreases in FIO_2 and responds to interventions. For example, if SpO_2 falls when you position the patient in a left lateral recumbent position, plan position changes that pose less risk for the patient.

Noninvasive Hemodynamic Monitoring: Impedance Cardiography

Impedance cardiography (ICG) is a continuous or intermittent, noninvasive method of obtaining CO and assessing thoracic fluid status. Based on the concepts of *impedance* (the resistance to the flow of electric current [Ω]), ICG uses four sets of external electrodes to deliver a high-frequency, low-amplitude current that is similar to that used in apnea monitors. Blood is an excellent conductor of electricity (lower impedance), and pulsatile blood flow generates electrical impedance changes. ICG measures the change in impedance ($d\Omega$) in the ascending aorta and left ventricle over time (dt) and is represented as $d\Omega/dt$. Ωo is the measurement of the average impedance of the fluid in the thorax. Impedance-based hemodynamic parameters (CO, SV, and SVR) are calculated from Ωo, $d\Omega/dt$, mean arterial pressure (MAP), CVP, and the ECG.

Major indications for ICG include early signs and symptoms of pulmonary or cardiac dysfunction, differentiation of cardiac or pulmonary cause of shortness of breath, evaluation of etiology and management of hypotension, monitoring after discontinuing a PA catheter or justification for insertion of a PA catheter, evaluation of drug therapy, and diagnosis of rejection after cardiac transplantation. ICG is not recommended in patients who have generalized edema or third spacing because the excess volume interferes with accurate signals.

NURSING MANAGEMENT
HEMODYNAMIC MONITORING

Assessment of hemodynamic status requires integrating data from many sources and trending these data over time. Thorough, basic nursing observations provide important clues about the patient's hemodynamic status. Begin by obtaining baseline data regarding the patient's general appearance, level of consciousness, skin color and temperature, vital signs, peripheral pulses, capillary refill, and urine output. Does the patient appear tired, weak, exhausted? There may be too little cardiac reserve to sustain even minimum activity. Pallor, cool skin, and diminished pulses may indicate decreased CO. Changes in mental status may reflect problems with cerebral perfusion or oxygenation. Monitor urine output to determine the adequacy of perfusion to the kidneys. The patient with diminished perfusion to the GI tract may develop hypoactive or absent bowel sounds. If the patient is bleeding and developing shock, BP might initially be relatively stable, yet the patient may become increasingly pale and cool from peripheral vasoconstriction. Conversely, the patient experiencing septic shock may remain warm and pink yet develop tachycardia and BP instability. Elevated heart rates are common in stressed, compromised, critically ill patients. However, sustained tachycardia increases myocardial O_2 demand and can result in decreased CO.

Always correlate observational data with data obtained from biotechnology (e.g., ECG, arterial and PA pressures, $ScvO_2/SvO_2$). Single hemodynamic values are rarely helpful. You must monitor trends in these values and evaluate the whole clinical picture with the goals of recognizing early clues and intervening before problems escalate.

CIRCULATORY ASSIST DEVICES

Mechanical circulatory assist devices (CADs), such as the intraaortic balloon pump (IABP) and left or right ventricular assist device (VAD), are used to decrease cardiac work and improve organ perfusion in patients with heart failure when conventional drug therapy is no longer adequate. The type of device used depends on the extent and nature of the heart problem. CADs provide interim support in three types of situations: (1) the left, right, or both ventricles require support while recovering from acute injury (e.g., postcardiotomy); (2) the patient must be stabilized before surgical repair of the heart (e.g., a ruptured septum); and (3) the heart has failed, and the patient is awaiting cardiac transplantation. All CADs decrease cardiac workload, increase myocardial perfusion, and augment circulation. The most commonly used CAD is the IABP.

Intraaortic Balloon Pump

The intraaortic balloon pump (IABP) provides temporary circulatory assistance to the sick heart by reducing afterload (via reduction in systolic pressure) and augmenting the aortic diastolic pressure, resulting in improved coronary blood flow. Table 66-5 lists the indications for an IABP.

The IABP consists of a sausage-shaped balloon, a pump that inflates and deflates the balloon, a control panel for synchronizing the balloon inflation to the cardiac cycle, and fail-safe fea-

TABLE 66-5	INDICATIONS AND CONTRAINDICATIONS FOR IABP THERAPY*

Indications
- Refractory unstable angina (when drugs have failed)
- Short-term bridge to heart transplantation
- Acute myocardial infarction with any of the following:†
  - Ventricular aneurysm accompanied by ventricular dysrhythmias
  - Acute ventricular septal defect
  - Acute mitral valve dysfunction
  - Cardiogenic shock
  - Refractory chest pain with or without ventricular dysrhythmias
- Preoperative, intraoperative, and postoperative cardiac surgery (e.g., prophylaxis before surgery, failure to wean from cardiopulmonary bypass, left ventricular failure after cardiopulmonary bypass)
- High-risk interventional cardiology procedures

Contraindications
- Irreversible brain damage
- Major coagulopathy (e.g., disseminated intravascular coagulation [DIC])
- Terminal or untreatable diseases of any major organ system
- Abdominal aortic and thoracic aneurysms
- Moderate to severe aortic insufficiency
- Generalized peripheral vascular disease (e.g., aortoiliac disease)‡

*List is not all-inclusive.
†Allows time for emergent angiography and corrective cardiac surgery to be performed.
‡May inhibit placement of balloon and is considered a relative contraindication; sheathless insertion may be used.

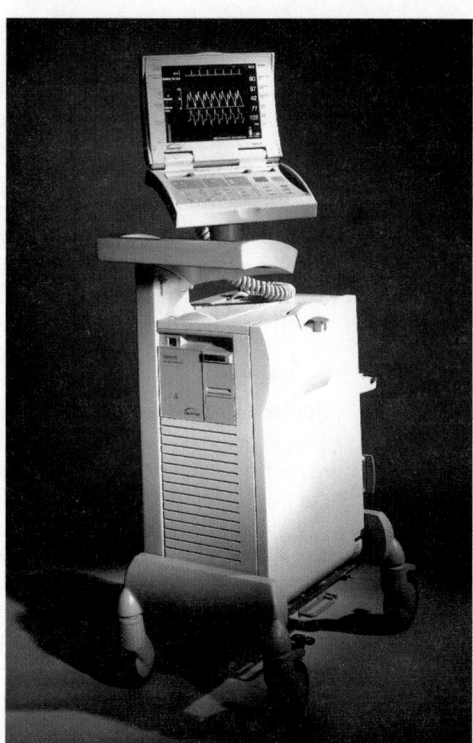

FIG. 66-11 Intraaortic balloon pump machine. (Courtesy Datascope Corp, Fairfield, NJ.)

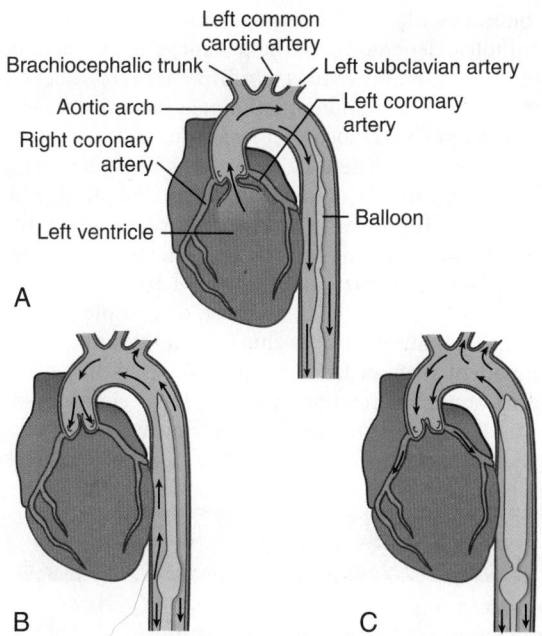

FIG. 66-12 Intraaortic balloon pump. **A,** During systole the balloon is deflated, which facilitates ejection of blood into the periphery. **B,** In early diastole, the balloon begins to inflate. **C,** In late diastole, the balloon is totally inflated, which augments aortic pressure and increases the coronary perfusion pressure with the end result of increased coronary and cerebral blood flow.

tures (Fig. 66-11). The balloon is inserted percutaneously or surgically into the femoral artery. It is moved toward the heart and placed in the descending thoracic aorta just below the left subclavian artery and above the renal arteries (Fig. 66-12). After placement, an x-ray confirms the position. A pneumatic device fills the balloon with helium at the start of diastole (immediately after aortic valve closure) and deflates it just before the next systole. The ECG is the trigger used to start the deflation on the upstroke of the R wave (of the QRS) and inflation on the T wave. The dicrotic notch of the arterial pressure tracing is used to refine timing (see eFig. 66-4 on the website for this chapter). IABP therapy is known as *counterpulsation* because the timing of balloon inflation is opposite to ventricular contraction. The IABP assist ratio is 1:1 in the acute phase of treatment, meaning that one IABP cycle of inflation and deflation occurs for every heartbeat.

Effects of Counterpulsation. In late diastole when the balloon is totally inflated, blood is forcibly displaced distal to the extremities and proximal to the coronary arteries and main branches of the aortic arch. Diastolic arterial pressure rises (diastolic augmentation), increasing coronary artery perfusion pressure and perfusion of vital organs. The rise in coronary artery perfusion pressure causes an increase in blood flow to the myocardium. The balloon is rapidly deflated just before systole. This creates a vacuum that causes aortic pressure to drop. When aortic resistance to left ventricular ejection is reduced (reduced afterload), the left ventricle empties more easily and completely. As with other types of afterload reduction, the SV increases, yet the myocardial O_2 consumption decreases. Table 66-6 summarizes the hemodynamic effects of IABP therapy.

Complications With IABP Therapy. Vascular injuries such as dislodgment of plaque, aortic dissection, and compromised distal circulation are common with IABP therapy. Thrombus

TABLE 66-6	HEMODYNAMIC EFFECTS OF COUNTERPULSATION

Effects of Inflation During Diastole
- Increased diastolic pressure (may exceed systolic pressure)
- Increased pressure in the aortic root during diastole
- Increased coronary artery perfusion pressure
- Improved O_2 delivery to the myocardium
  - Decreased angina
  - Decreased electrocardiographic evidence of ischemia
  - Decreased ventricular ectopy

Effects of Deflation During Systole
- Decreased afterload
- Decreased peak systolic pressure
- Decreased myocardial O_2 consumption
- Increased stroke volume, possibly associated with
  - Improved mentation
  - Warm skin
  - Increased urine output
  - Decreased heart rate
- Increased forward flow of blood, decreasing preload
  - Decreased PA pressures, including PAWP
  - Decreased crackles

PA, Pulmonary artery; *PAWP,* PA wedge pressure.

and embolus formation add to the risk of circulatory compromise to the extremity. The action of the IABP can also destroy platelets and cause thrombocytopenia. Peripheral nerve damage can occur, particularly when a cutdown is performed for insertion. Movement of the balloon can block the left subclavian, renal, or mesenteric arteries. This can result in a weak or absent radial pulse, decreased urine output, and reduced or absent bowel sounds. Patients receiving IABP therapy are prone to infection. Local or systemic signs of infection require catheter removal.[23] To reduce these complications, perform cardiovascular, neurovascular, and hemodynamic assessments every 15 to 60 minutes, depending on the patient's status (Table 66-7).

Mechanical complications from IABP are rare but can occur. Improper timing of balloon inflation may cause increased afterload, decreased CO, myocardial ischemia, and increased myocardial O_2 demand. These complications must be recognized immediately. If the balloon develops a leak, the pump will automatically stop. The catheter is promptly removed to avoid an embolus. Signs of a leak include less effective augmentation, repeated alarms for gas loss, and blood backing up into the catheter. A malfunction of the balloon or console triggers failsafe alarms and automatically shuts down the unit.

The patient with an IABP is relatively immobile, limited to side-lying or supine positions with the HOB elevated less than 45 degrees. The patient may be receiving ventilatory support and will likely have multiple invasive lines that increase the challenge of comfortable positioning. The patient may experience sleeplessness and anxiety. Adequate sedation, pain relief, skin care, and comfort measures are essential.

As the patient improves, circulatory support provided by the IABP is gradually reduced. Weaning involves reducing the IABP assist ratio from 1:1 to 1:2 and assessing the patient's response (see eFig. 66-4 on the website for this chapter). If hemodynamic parameters remain stable, the ratio can be changed from 1:2 to 1:3 until the IABP catheter is removed. Pumping is continued until the line is removed even if the patient is stable. This reduces the risk of thrombus formation around the catheter.

Ventricular Assist Devices

The **ventricular assist device (VAD)** provides short- and long-term support for the failing heart and allows more mobility than the IABP. VADs are inserted into the path of flowing blood to augment or replace the action of the ventricle. Some VADs are implanted internally (e.g., peritoneum), and others are positioned externally. A typical VAD shunts blood from the left atrium or ventricle to the device and then to the aorta. Some VADs provide right or biventricular support (Fig. 66-13).

Failure to wean from cardiopulmonary bypass (CPB) after surgery is a primary indicator for VAD support. VADs are also used to support patients with ventricular failure caused by myocardial infarction and patients awaiting heart transplantation. A VAD is a temporary device that can partially or totally support circulation until the heart recovers or a donor heart is obtained. Cannula sites depend on the type of device used. For support of the right side of the heart, the right atrium and PA are cannulated. The left ventricular apex can be cannulated for left VADs. Direct cannulation of the atria and great vessels occurs in the operating room through a sternotomy.

Appropriate patient selection for VAD therapy is critical. Indications include (1) failure to wean from CPB or postcardiotomy cardiogenic shock, (2) a bridge to recovery or heart transplantation, and (3) patients with New York Heart Association Class IV heart disease (see Table 35-5) who have failed

TABLE 66-7	MANAGING COMPLICATIONS OF IABP THERAPY
Potential Complications	**Nursing Interventions**
Site infection from invasive lines	• Use strict aseptic technique for insertion and dressing changes for all lines. • Cover all insertion sites with occlusive dressings. • Administer prescribed prophylactic antibiotic for entire course of therapy.
Pneumonia associated with immobilization	• Reposition patient q2hr, being careful not to displace balloon. • If patient requires chest physiotherapy, avoid introducing ECG artifact.
Arterial trauma caused by insertion or displacement of balloon	• Evaluate and mark peripheral pulses before insertion of balloon to use as baseline for assessing pulses after insertion. • After insertion of balloon, evaluate perfusion to both upper and lower extremities at least every hour. • Measure urine output at least every hour (occlusion of renal arteries causes severe decrease in urine output). • Observe arterial waveforms for sudden changes. • Keep head of bed no higher than 45 degrees. • Do not flex cannulated leg at the hip. • Immobilize cannulated leg to prevent flexion using a draw sheet tucked under the mattress, soft ankle restraint, or knee immobilizer.
Thromboembolism caused by trauma, balloon obstruction of blood flow distal to catheter	• Administer prophylactic heparin if ordered. • Evaluate pulses, urine output, and level of consciousness at least every hour. • Check circulation, sensation, and movement in both legs at least every hour.
Hematologic complications caused by platelet aggregation along the balloon (e.g., thrombocytopenia)	• Monitor coagulation profiles, hematocrit, and platelet count.
Hemorrhage from insertion site	• Check site for bleeding at least every hour. • Monitor vital signs for signs of hypovolemia with each check.
Balloon leak or rupture	• Prepare for emergent removal and possible reinsertion.

FIG. 66-13 Schematic diagram of a biventricular assist device (BVAD).

medical therapy. Relative contraindications for VAD therapy include (1) BSA less than manufacturer's limit (e.g., 1.3 m^2), (2) renal or liver failure unrelated to a cardiac event, and (3) co-morbidities that would limit life expectancy to less than 3 years.[24]

Implantable Artificial Heart

Every year about 2200 patients receive cardiac transplants, yet the demand for heart transplants far exceeds the supply. Research on mechanical CADs has led to the development of a fully implantable artificial heart that can sustain the body's circulatory system. This device is used to replace the hearts of patients who are not eligible for a transplant and have no other treatment alternative. One major advantage of the artificial heart compared with heart transplantation is decreased costs for implantation and drug therapies. Patients do not require immunosuppression therapy and thus do not experience its inevitable, long-term effects. However, patients do require lifelong anticoagulation.[25]

NURSING MANAGEMENT
CIRCULATORY ASSIST DEVICES

The patient with an IABP requires highly skilled nursing care. Perform frequent and thorough cardiovascular assessments. These include measurement of hemodynamic parameters (e.g., arterial BP, CO/CI, SVR), auscultation of the heart and lungs, and evaluation of the ECG (e.g., rate, rhythm). Assess for adequate tissue perfusion (e.g., skin color and temperature, mental status, capillary refill, peripheral pulses, urine output, bowel sounds) at regular intervals. It is expected that IABP therapy will improve these findings.

Nursing care of the patient with a VAD is similar to that of the patient with an IABP. Observe the patient for bleeding, cardiac tamponade, ventricular failure, infection, dysrhythmias, renal failure, hemolysis, and thromboembolism. Unlike the patient with an IABP, who must remain in bed with limited position change, the patient with VAD may be mobile and require an activity plan. In some cases, patients with VADs may go home. Preparation for discharge is complex and requires in-depth teaching about the device and support equipment

(e.g., battery chargers). A competent caregiver must be present at all times.

Ideally, patients with CADs will recover through ventricular improvement, heart transplantation, or artificial heart implantation. However, many patients die, or the decision to terminate the device is made and death follows. Both the patient and caregiver require emotional support. Consult other members of the health care team, such as social workers or clergy, as appropriate.

ARTIFICIAL AIRWAYS

Patients in the ICU often need mechanical assistance to maintain airway patency. Inserting a tube into the trachea, bypassing upper airway and laryngeal structures, creates an artificial airway. The tube is placed into the trachea via the mouth or nose past the larynx (endotracheal [ET] intubation) or through a stoma in the neck (tracheostomy). ET intubation is more common in ICU patients than a tracheostomy. It is performed quickly and safely at the bedside. Indications for ET intubation include (1) upper airway obstruction (e.g., secondary to burns, tumor, bleeding), (2) apnea, (3) high risk of aspiration, (4) ineffective clearance of secretions, and (5) respiratory distress. Fig. 66-14 shows the parts of an ET tube.

A *tracheotomy* is a surgical procedure that is performed when the need for an artificial airway is expected to be long term. There is ongoing debate regarding the timing of a tracheotomy in the patient requiring an ET tube. Research suggests that early tracheotomy (2 to 10 days) may have advantages over delayed tracheotomy, particularly when mechanical ventilation is predicted to be needed for longer than 10 to 14 days.[26] The situation varies with the patient, physician, and institution. Chapter 27 discusses tracheostomy tubes and related nursing management.

Endotracheal Tubes

In *oral intubation* the ET tube is passed through the mouth and vocal cords and into the trachea with the aid of a laryngoscope or a bronchoscope. In *nasal ET intubation* the ET is placed blindly (i.e., without seeing the larynx) through the nose, nasopharynx, and vocal cords. Oral ET intubation is preferred for

FIG. 66-14 Endotracheal tube. **A,** Parts of an endotracheal tube. **B,** Tube in place with cuff deflated. **C,** Tube in place with the cuff inflated. **D,** Photo of tube before placement.

Translating Research Into Practice

Does Timing of Tracheotomy Affect Critically Ill Patient Outcomes?

Clinical Question
In critically ill patients (P) what is the effect of an early tracheotomy (I) vs. late tracheotomy (C) on short-term mortality and incidence of ventilator-assisted pneumonia (O)?

Best Available Evidence
Systematic review of randomized controlled trials (RCTs)

Critical Appraisal and Synthesis of Evidence
- Seven RCTs (*n* = 1044) of critically ill adult patients requiring prolonged mechanical ventilation. Early tracheotomy was compared with either late tracheotomy or prolonged endotracheal intubation.
- Primary outcomes were short-term mortality and ventilator-assisted pneumonia (VAP).
- Secondary outcomes were long-term mortality, duration of ventilation and sedation, length of ICU and hospital stay, and complications.
- Early tracheotomy did not significantly reduce short–term or long-term mortality or rate of VAP. Tracheotomy timing was not related to reductions in duration of mechanical ventilation or sedation, shorter stays in ICU or hospital, or more complications.

Conclusion
- Clinically significant outcomes are not affected by timing of a tracheotomy.

Implications for Nursing Practice
- The optimal tracheotomy timing (early vs. late) for patients on prolonged mechanical ventilation is not really known.
- Continue to consider benefits of tracheotomy (e.g., increased patient comfort, improved oral hygiene) compared to the risks and complications (e.g., bleeding, wound infection, tracheal stenosis). The risk/benefit of tracheotomy needs to be weighed against the risk/benefit of prolonged endotracheal intubation.

Reference for Evidence
Wang F, Wu Y, Bo L, et al: The timing of tracheotomy in critically ill patients undergoing mechanical ventilation: a systematic review and meta-analysis of randomized controlled trials, *Chest* 140:1456, 2011.

P, Patient population of interest; *I*, intervention or area of interest; *C*, comparison of interest or comparison group; *O*, outcomes of interest (see p. 12).

most emergencies because the airway can be secured rapidly and a larger-diameter tube is used. A larger-bore ET tube reduces the *work of breathing* (WOB) because of less airway resistance. It is easier to remove secretions and perform fiberoptic bronchoscopy if needed. Nasal ET intubation is rarely used but may be needed when head and neck movement is risky.

There are risks associated with oral ET intubation. It is difficult to place an oral tube if head and neck mobility is limited (e.g., suspected spinal cord injury). Teeth can be chipped or accidentally removed during the procedure. Salivation is increased and swallowing is difficult. Patients can obstruct the ET tube by biting down on it. Sedation along with a bite block or oropharyngeal airway may be used to avoid this. The ET tube and bite block (if used) should be secured (separately) to the face. Mouth care is a challenge because of limited space in the oral cavity. Manage this by using smaller or pediatric-sized oral products for tooth brushing, cleaning, and suctioning.

Nasal intubation is contraindicated in patients with facial fractures or suspected fractures at the base of the skull and postoperatively after cranial surgeries. The WOB is greater because the longer, narrower tube offers more airflow resistance

and may kink. Suctioning and secretion removal are more difficult. Finally, nasal tubes have been linked to an increased incidence of sinus infection and ventilator-associated pneumonia (VAP).[27]

Endotracheal Intubation Procedure

Unless ET intubation is emergent, consent for the procedure is obtained. Tell the patient and caregiver the reason for ET intubation, the steps in the procedure, and the patient's role in the procedure (if indicated). Also explain that, while intubated, the patient will not be able to speak, but that you will provide other means of communication. Tell them that the patient's hands may be briefly restrained for safety purposes.

Have a self-inflating *bag-valve-mask* (BVM) (e.g., *Ambu bag*) available and attached to O_2, suctioning equipment ready at the bedside, and IV access. The BVM contains a reservoir that is filled with O_2 so that concentrations of 90% to 95% are delivered. The slower the bag is deflated and inflated, the higher the O_2 concentration that is delivered. Assemble and check the equipment to be used, remove the patient's dentures or partial plates (for oral intubation), and administer medications as ordered. Premedication varies depending on the patient's level of consciousness (e.g., awake, obtunded) and the nature of the procedure (e.g., emergent, nonemergent).

Rapid-sequence intubation (RSI) is the rapid, concurrent administration of both a sedative and a paralytic agent during emergency airway management to decrease the risks of aspiration and injury to the patient. RSI is not indicated in patients who are in cardiac arrest or have a known difficult airway.[28] A sedative-hypnotic-amnesic (e.g., midazolam [Versed], etomidate [Amidate]) is used to induce unconsciousness, along with a rapid-onset opioid (e.g., fentanyl) to blunt the pain of the procedure. A paralytic drug (e.g., succinylcholine [Anectine]) is then given to produce skeletal muscle paralysis. Monitor the patient's oxygenation status during the procedure with pulse oximetry.

For oral intubation, place the patient supine with the head extended and the neck flexed ("sniffing position"). This position permits visualization of the vocal cords. For nasal intubation, the nasal passages may be sprayed with a local anesthetic and vasoconstrictor (e.g., lidocaine [Xylocaine] with epinephrine) to reduce trauma and bleeding. Before intubation is started, preoxygenate the patient using the BVM and 100% O_2 for 3 to 5 minutes. Each intubation attempt is limited to less than 30 seconds. Ventilate the patient between successive attempts using the BVM and 100% O_2.

After intubation, inflate the cuff and confirm the placement of the ET tube while the patient is manually ventilated using the BVM with 100% O_2. Use an end-tidal CO_2 detector to confirm proper placement by noting the presence of exhaled CO_2 from the lungs. Place the detector between the BVM and the ET tube and either observe for a color change (indicating the presence of CO_2) or a number. If no CO_2 is detected, the tube is in the esophagus and needs to be reinserted.[29] Auscultate the lungs for bilateral breath sounds and the epigastrium for the absence of air sounds. Observe the chest for symmetric chest wall movement. In addition, SpO_2 should be stable or improved.

If the findings support proper ET tube placement, connect the tube to an O_2 source and secure per agency policy (Fig. 66-15). Suction the ET tube and pharynx, and insert a bite block as needed. Obtain a chest x-ray immediately to confirm tube location (2 to 6 cm above the carina in the adult). This position

Modified T piece for
ventilator circuit

Irrigation part for
saline lavage

Removable
plug

Thumb control
for suction

Catheter

Catheter
sheath

Ventilator
circuit

To vacuum source

FIG. 66-15 Closed tracheal suction system.

allows the patient to move the neck without moving the tube or causing it to enter the right mainstem bronchus. Once proper positioning is confirmed with x-ray, record and mark the position of the tube at the lip or teeth (usually 21 cm for women and 23 cm for men) or nose. Cut excess tubing to reduce dead air space.

The ET tube is connected to either humidified air, O_2, or a mechanical ventilator. Obtain ABGs immediately after intubation to determine baseline oxygenation and ventilation status. ABG values are reviewed and used to guide oxygenation and ventilation changes. Continuous pulse oximetry and end-tidal CO_2 monitoring provide valuable data related to arterial oxygenation and ventilation.

NURSING MANAGEMENT
ARTIFICIAL AIRWAY

Management of a patient with an artificial airway is often a shared responsibility between you and the respiratory therapist, with specific management tasks determined by agency policy. Nursing responsibilities for the patient with an artificial airway may include some or all of the following: (1) maintaining correct tube placement, (2) maintaining proper cuff inflation, (3) monitoring oxygenation and ventilation, (4) maintaining tube patency, (5) assessing for complications, (6) providing oral care and maintaining skin integrity, and (7) fostering comfort and communication. eNursing Care Plan 66-1 for the patient on a mechanical ventilator is available on the website for this chapter.

MAINTAINING CORRECT TUBE PLACEMENT

Continuously monitor the patient with an ET tube for proper placement. If the tube is dislodged, it could end up in the pharynx or enter the esophagus or the right mainstem bronchus (thus ventilating only the right lung).

SAFETY ALERT: Endotracheal Tube Placement
- Maintain proper ET tube position by placing an "exit mark" on the tube.
- Confirm that the mark remains constant while at rest and during patient care, repositioning, and transport.

Observe for symmetric chest wall movement and auscultate to confirm bilateral breath sounds. If the ET tube is not positioned properly, it is an emergency. Stay with the patient, maintain the airway, support ventilation, and call for the appropriate help to immediately reposition the tube. It may be necessary to ventilate the patient with a BVM and 100% O_2. If a dislodged tube is not repositioned, minimal or no O_2 is delivered to the lungs or the entire tidal volume is delivered to one lung. This places the patient at risk for pneumothorax.

MAINTAINING PROPER CUFF INFLATION

The cuff is an inflatable, pliable sleeve encircling the outer wall of the ET tube (see Fig. 66-14). The high-volume, low-pressure cuff stabilizes and "seals" the ET tube within the trachea and prevents escape of ventilating gases. However, excess volume in the cuff can damage the tracheal mucosa. To avoid this, inflate the cuff with air, and measure and monitor the cuff pressure. To ensure adequate tracheal perfusion, maintain cuff pressure at 20 to 25 cm H_2O.[30] Measure and record cuff pressure after intubation and on a routine basis (e.g., every 8 hours) using the *minimal occluding volume* (MOV) *technique* or *the minimal leak technique* (MLT).

The steps in the MOV technique for cuff inflation are as follows: (1) for the mechanically ventilated patient, place a stethoscope over the trachea and inflate the cuff to MOV by adding air until no air leak is heard at peak inspiratory pressure (end of ventilator inspiration); (2) for the spontaneously breathing patient, inflate until no sound is heard after a deep breath or after inhalation with a BVM; (3) use a manometer to verify that cuff pressure is between 20 and 25 cm H_2O; and (4) record cuff pressure in the chart. If adequate cuff pressure cannot be maintained or larger volumes of air are needed to keep the cuff inflated, there could be a leak in the cuff or tracheal dilation at the cuff site. In these situations, notify the physician to reposition or change the ET tube.

The procedure for MLT is similar with one exception. Remove a small amount of air from the cuff until a slight air leak is auscultated at peak inflation. Both techniques aim to prevent the risks of tracheal damage from high cuff pressures. The use of continuous cuff measurement is being studied.[31]

MONITORING OXYGENATION AND VENTILATION

Vigilantly monitor the patient with an ET tube for adequate oxygenation by assessing clinical findings, ABGs, SpO_2, and, if available, $ScvO_2/SvO_2$. Assess for signs of hypoxemia such as a change in mental status (e.g., confusion), anxiety, dusky skin, and dysrhythmias. Periodic ABGs (specifically PaO_2) and continuous SpO_2 provide objective data regarding oxygenation. Lower values are expected in patients with some disease states, such as chronic obstructive pulmonary disease (COPD). CVP or PA catheters with $ScvO_2$ or SvO_2 capability provide an indirect indication of the patient's tissue oxygenation status (see Table 66-4).

Indicators of ventilation include clinical findings, $PaCO_2$, and continuous partial pressure of end-tidal CO_2 ($PETCO_2$). Assess the patient's respirations for rate, rhythm, and use of accessory muscles. The patient who is hyperventilating will be breathing rapidly and deeply and may experience circumoral and peripheral numbness and tingling. The patient who is hypoventilating will be breathing shallowly or slowly and may appear dusky. $PaCO_2$ is the best indicator of alveolar hyperventilation (e.g., decreased $PaCO_2$, increased pH indicate respira-

Adapted from Chulay M, Seckel M: Suctioning: endotracheal or tracheostomy tube. In Wiegand DL-M, editor: *AACN procedure manual for critical care*, ed 6, St Louis, 2011, Saunders.
*Attach a PEEP valve to the BVM for patients on >5 cm H₂O PEEP.
BVM, Bag-valve-mask; *ECG*, electrocardiogram; *ET*, endotracheal; *FIO₂*, fraction of inspired oxygen; *PEEP*, positive end-expiratory pressure.

TABLE 66-8 SUCTIONING PROCEDURES FOR PATIENT ON MECHANICAL VENTILATOR

General Measures for Open and Closed Suction Techniques

1. Gather all equipment.
2. Wash hands and don personal protective equipment.
3. Explain procedure and patient's role in assisting with secretion removal by coughing.
4. Monitor patient's cardiopulmonary status (e.g., vital signs, SpO₂, SvO₂/ScvO₂, ECG, level of consciousness) before, during, and after the procedure.
5. Turn on suction and set vacuum to 100-120 mm Hg.
6. Pause ventilator alarms.

Open-Suction Technique

7. Open sterile catheter package using the inside of the package as a sterile field. NOTE: Suction catheter should be no wider than half the diameter of the ET tube (e.g., for a 7-mm ET tube, select a 10F suction catheter).
8. Fill the sterile solution container with sterile normal saline or water.
9. Don sterile gloves.
10. Pick up sterile suction catheter with dominant hand. Using nondominant hand, secure the connecting tube (to suction) to the suction catheter.
11. Check equipment for proper functioning by suctioning a small volume of sterile saline solution from the container. **(Go to step 13.)**

Closed-Suction Technique

12. Connect the suction tubing to the closed suction port.
13. Hyperoxygenate the patient for 30 sec using one of the following methods:
    - Activate the suction hyperoxygenation setting on the ventilator using nondominant hand.
    - Increase FIO₂ to 100%. NOTE: Remember to return FIO₂ to baseline level at the completion of the procedure if not done automatically after preset time by ventilator.
    - Disconnect the ventilator tubing from the ET tube and manually ventilate the patient with 100% O₂ using a BVM device.* Administer five or six breaths over 30 sec. NOTE: Use of a second person to deliver the manual breaths significantly increases the tidal volume delivered.
14. With suction off, gently and quickly insert the catheter using the dominant hand. When you meet resistance, pull back ½ in.
15. Apply continuous or intermittent suction using the nondominant thumb. Withdraw the catheter over 10 sec or less.
16. Hyperoxygenate for 30 sec as described in step 13.
17. If secretions remain and the patient has tolerated the procedure, perform two or three suction passes as described in steps 14 and 15. NOTE: Rinse the suction catheter with sterile saline solution between suctioning passes as needed.
18. Reconnect patient to ventilator (open-suction technique).
19. At the completion of ET tube suctioning, rinse the catheter and connecting tubing with the sterile saline solution.
20. Suction oral pharynx. NOTE: Use a separate catheter for this step when using the closed-suction technique.
21. Discard the suction catheter and rinse the connecting tubing with the sterile saline solution (open-suction technique).
22. Reset FIO₂ (if necessary) and ventilator alarms.
23. Reassess patient for signs of effective suctioning.

tory alkalosis) or hypoventilation (e.g., increased PaCO₂, decreased pH indicate respiratory acidosis).

PETCO₂ monitoring (*capnography*) is done by analyzing exhaled gas directly at the patient-ventilator circuit (*mainstream sampling*) or by transporting a sample of gas via a small-bore tubing to a bedside monitor (*sidestream sampling*). Continuous PETCO₂ monitoring can assess the patency of the airway and the presence of breathing. In addition, gradual changes in PETCO₂ values may accompany an increase in CO₂ production (e.g., sepsis, hypoventilation, neuromuscular blockade) or a decrease in CO₂ production (e.g., hypothermia, decreased CO, metabolic acidosis). In patients with normal ventilation-to-perfusion ratios (see Chapter 68), PETCO₂ can be used as an estimate of PaCO₂, with PETCO₂ generally 1 to 5 mm Hg lower than PaCO₂. However, in patients with unusually large dead air space or serious mismatch between ventilation and perfusion, PETCO₂ is not a reliable estimate of PaCO₂.[29]

MAINTAINING TUBE PATENCY

Do not routinely suction a patient. Regularly assess the patient to determine if suctioning is needed. Indications for suctioning include (1) visible secretions in the ET tube, (2) sudden onset of respiratory distress, (3) suspected aspiration of secretions, (4) increase in peak airway pressures, (5) auscultation of adventitious breath sounds over the trachea or bronchi, (6) increase in respiratory rate or sustained coughing, and (7) sudden or gradual decrease in PaO₂ or SpO₂.

Table 66-8 describes two recommended suctioning methods, the *closed-suction technique* (CST) and the *open-suction technique* (OST). The CST uses a suction catheter that is enclosed in a plastic sleeve connected directly to the patient-ventilator circuit (see Fig. 66-15). With the CST, oxygenation and ventilation are maintained during suctioning, and exposure to the patient's secretions is reduced. The CST should be used for patients who (1) require high levels of positive end-expiratory pressure (PEEP) (greater than 10 cm H₂O), (2) have high levels of FIO₂, (3) have bloody or infected pulmonary secretions, (4) require frequent suctioning, and (5) experience clinical instability with the OST.[32]

Potential complications associated with suctioning include hypoxemia, bronchospasm, increased intracranial pressure, dysrhythmias, hypertension, hypotension, mucosal damage, pulmonary bleeding, pain, and infection.[32] Closely assess the patient before, during, and after the suctioning procedure. If the patient does not tolerate suctioning (e.g., decreased SpO₂, increased or decreased BP, sustained coughing, development of dysrhythmias), stop the procedure and hyperoxygenate until equilibration occurs and before attempting another suction pass. Prevent hypoxemia by hyperoxygenating the patient before and after each suctioning pass and limiting each pass to 10 seconds or less (see Table 66-8). Assess both the ECG and SpO₂ before, during, and after the suctioning procedure.

Causes of dysrhythmias during suctioning include (1) hypoxemia resulting in myocardial ischemia; (2) vagal stimulation caused by tracheal irritation; and (3) sympathetic nervous system stimulation caused by anxiety, discomfort, or pain. Dysrhythmias include tachydysrhythmias and bradydysrhythmias, premature beats, and asystole. Stop suctioning if any new dysrhythmias develop. Avoid excessive suctioning in patients with severe hypoxemia or bradycardia.

Tracheal mucosal damage may occur because of excessive suction pressures (greater than 120 mm Hg), overly vigorous catheter insertion, and the characteristics of the suction catheter itself. Blood streaks or tissue shreds in aspirated secretions may indicate that mucosal damage has occurred. Mucosal damage increases the risk of infection and bleeding, particularly if the patient is receiving anticoagulants.[32] Trauma to the mucosa can be prevented by following the steps described in Table 66-8.

Secretions may be thick and difficult to suction because of inadequate hydration, inadequate humidification, infection, or inaccessibility of the left mainstem bronchus or lower airways. Adequately hydrating the patient (e.g., oral or IV fluids) and providing supplemental humidification of inspired gases may assist in thinning secretions. Instillation of normal saline into the ET tube is discouraged and may be harmful. If infection is the cause of thick secretions, give the patient appropriate antibiotics. Mobilization, postural drainage, percussion, and turning the patient every 2 hours may help move secretions into larger airways.

PROVIDING ORAL CARE AND MAINTAINING SKIN INTEGRITY

When an oral ET tube is in place, the patient's mouth is always open. Moisten the lips, tongue, and gums with saline or water swabs to prevent mucosal drying. Proper oral care provides comfort and prevents injury to the gums and plaque formation (Table 66-9). Meticulous care is required to prevent skin breakdown on the face, lips, tongue, and nares because of pressure from the ET tube or bite block or the method used to secure the ET tube to the patient's face. Reposition and retape the ET tube every 24 hours and as needed. This practice may be shared between nursing and respiratory therapy or limited to respiratory therapy.

For the nasally intubated patient, remove the old tape or ties and clean the skin around the ET tube with saline-soaked gauze or cotton swabs. For the orally intubated patient, remove the bite block (if present) and the old tape or ties. Provide oral hygiene and then reposition the ET tube to the opposite side of the mouth. Replace the bite block (if appropriate) and reconfirm

---

TABLE 66-9	ORAL CARE PROCEDURES FOR PATIENT ON MECHANICAL VENTILATOR

General Measures
1. Gather all equipment.
2. Wash hands and don personal protective equipment.
3. Explain procedure to the patient and caregiver, if present.
4. Perform oral care using pediatric or adult soft toothbrushes at least twice a day by gently brushing to clean and remove plaque.
5. Use oral swabs with a 1.5% hydrogen peroxide solution every 2-4 hr.
6. Use 0.12% chlorhexidine oral rinse twice daily.
7. Apply a mouth moisturizer to oral mucosa and lips with each cleaning.
8. Suction oral cavity and pharynx frequently. See Fig. 66-16 for example of an endotracheal tube that can provide continuous or intermittent subglottic suctioning.

NOTE:
• Change all oral suction equipment and suction tubing every 24 hr.
• Rinse nondisposable oral suction apparatus with sterile normal saline after each use and place on a dry paper towel.

Adapted from Vollman KM, Sole ML: Endotracheal tube and oral care. In Wiegand DL-M, editor: *AACN procedure manual for critical care,* ed 6, St Louis, 2011, Saunders; and Institute for Healthcare Improvement: How-to guide: prevent ventilator-associated pneumonia. Retrieved from *http://www.ihi.org.*

---

proper cuff inflation and tube placement. Secure the ET tube again per agency policy (see eFig. 66-5 on the website for this chapter). If a manufactured tube holder is used, loosen the straps, massage the area under the straps, and then reapply the straps. Two staff members should perform the repositioning procedure to prevent accidental dislodgment. Monitor the patient for any signs of respiratory distress throughout the procedure.

FOSTERING COMFORT AND COMMUNICATION

Intubation is a major stressor for the patient.[33,34] The intubated patient may experience anxiety from not being able to talk or knowing what to expect. Communicating with the intubated patient can be frustrating for the patient, caregiver, and you. To communicate more effectively, use a variety of methods[35] (see Common Problems of Critical Care Patients earlier in this chapter on p. 1600).

The physical discomfort associated with ET intubation and mechanical ventilation often requires sedating the patient and giving an analgesic until the ET tube is no longer required. The patient may need morphine, lorazepam, propofol, or other sedatives to blunt the anxiety and discomfort related to intubation. Evaluate the drugs' effectiveness in achieving an acceptable level of patient comfort. In addition, consider using relaxation techniques (e.g., music therapy) to complement drug therapy.

COMPLICATIONS OF ENDOTRACHEAL INTUBATION

Two major complications of ET intubation are unplanned extubation and aspiration. Unplanned *extubation* (i.e., removal of the ET tube from the trachea) can be a catastrophic event and usually complicates the patient's recovery. Unplanned extubations can be due to patient removal of the ET tube or accidental removal during movement or a procedure. Usually the unplanned extubation is obvious (the patient is holding the ET tube). Other times, the tip of the ET tube is in the hypopharynx or esophagus and the extubation is not so obvious.

> **SAFETY ALERT: Unplanned Extubation**
> Observe for signs of unplanned extubation, which can be a life-threatening event:
> • Patient talking
> • Activation of the low-pressure ventilator alarm
> • Diminished or absent breath sounds
> • Respiratory distress
> • Gastric distention

You are responsible for preventing unplanned extubation by ensuring that the ET tube is secured and observing and supporting the ET tube during repositioning, procedures, and patient transfers. Additionally, giving adequate sedation and analgesia and using standardized weaning protocols decrease the incidence of self-extubation.[36] The use of soft wrist restraints or mitts to immobilize the patient's hands has not shown to be an absolute deterrent to self-extubation.[37] Be sure to explain to the patient and caregiver when you use restraints for patient safety. Reassess for the continued need of restraints per agency policy.

Should an unplanned extubation occur, stay with the patient and call for help. Interventions are aimed at maintaining the patient's airway, supporting ventilation (e.g., manually ventilating the patient with a BVM and 100% O_2), securing the appropriate assistance to immediately reintubate the patient (if necessary), and providing psychologic support to the patient.

FIG. 66-16 Continuous subglottal suctioning can be provided by the Hi Lo Evac Tube. A dorsal lumen above the cuff allows for suctioning of secretions from the subglottic area. (Reprinted by permission of Nellcor Puritan Bennett Inc, Pleasanton, Calif.)

FIG. 66-17 Negative pressure ventilator. (Courtesy Lifecare, Westminster, Colo.)

Aspiration is another potential hazard for the patient with an ET tube. The ET tube passes through the epiglottis, splinting it in an open position. Thus the intubated patient cannot protect the airway from aspiration. The high-volume, low-pressure ET or tracheal cuff cannot totally prevent the trickle of oral or gastric secretions into the trachea. Further, secretions collect above the cuff. When the cuff is deflated, those secretions can move into the lungs. Some ET tubes provide continuous suctioning of secretions above the cuff (Fig. 66-16).

Oral intubation increases salivation, yet swallowing is difficult, so suction the patient's mouth frequently. Use a Yankauer (tonsil-tip) suction catheter or a sterile single-use catheter. Other factors contributing to aspiration include improper cuff inflation, patient positioning, and tracheoesophageal fistula. The patient with an ET tube is at risk for aspiration of gastric contents. Even when the cuff is properly inflated, take precautions to prevent vomiting, which can lead to aspiration.[38] Often, a nasogastric (NG) or an orogastric (OG) tube is inserted and connected to low, intermittent suction when a patient is first intubated. An OG tube is preferred over an NG tube to reduce the risk of sinusitis. All patients who are intubated or receiving enteral feedings must have the HOB elevated a minimum of 30 to 45 degrees unless medically contraindicated.

MECHANICAL VENTILATION

Mechanical ventilation is the process by which the FIO$_2$ (21% [room air] or more) is moved in and out of the lungs by a mechanical ventilator. Mechanical ventilation is not curative. It is a means of supporting patients until they recover the ability to breathe independently. It can also serve as a bridge to long-term mechanical ventilation, or until a decision is made to withdraw ventilatory support.

Indications for mechanical ventilation include (1) apnea or impending inability to breathe or protect the airway, (2) acute respiratory failure (see Chapter 68), (3) severe hypoxia, and (4) respiratory muscle fatigue.[39] Patients with chronic pulmonary disease and their caregivers should be given the opportunity to discuss mechanical ventilation before end-stage respiratory disease develops. Encourage all patients, particu-

larly those with chronic illnesses, to discuss the subject with their families and health care providers. They should record and place the results of these discussions in an advance directive. The decision to use, withhold, or withdraw mechanical ventilation must be made carefully, respecting the wishes of the patient and caregiver. When the health care team, patient, and/or caregiver disagree over the plan of care, you need to consult the agency's ethics committee for assistance.

Types of Mechanical Ventilation

The two major types of mechanical ventilation are negative pressure and positive pressure ventilation.

Negative Pressure Ventilation. Negative pressure ventilation involves the use of chambers that encase the chest or body and surround it with intermittent subatmospheric (or negative) pressure. The "iron lung" was the first form of negative pressure ventilation, developed during the polio epidemic. Intermittent negative pressure around the chest wall causes the chest to be pulled outward, reducing intrathoracic pressure. Air rushes in via the upper airway, which is outside the sealed chamber. Expiration is passive. The machine cycles off, allowing chest retraction. This type of ventilation is similar to normal ventilation in that decreased intrathoracic pressures produce inspiration, and expiration is passive. Negative pressure ventilation is delivered by noninvasive ventilation and does not require an artificial airway.

Several portable negative pressure ventilators are available for home use for patients with neuromuscular diseases, central nervous system disorders, diseases and injuries of the spinal cord, and severe COPD (Fig. 66-17). Negative pressure ventilators are not routinely used for acutely ill patients.

Positive Pressure Ventilation. Positive pressure ventilation (PPV) is the primary method used with acutely ill patients (Fig. 66-18). During inspiration the ventilator pushes air into the lungs under positive pressure. Unlike spontaneous ventilation, intrathoracic pressure is raised during lung inflation rather than lowered. Expiration occurs passively as in normal expiration. Modes of PPV are categorized into two groups: volume and pressure ventilation.[39]

Volume Ventilation. With **volume ventilation** a predetermined tidal volume (V$_T$) is delivered with each inspiration, and the amount of pressure needed to deliver the breath varies based on compliance and resistance factors of the patient-ventilator

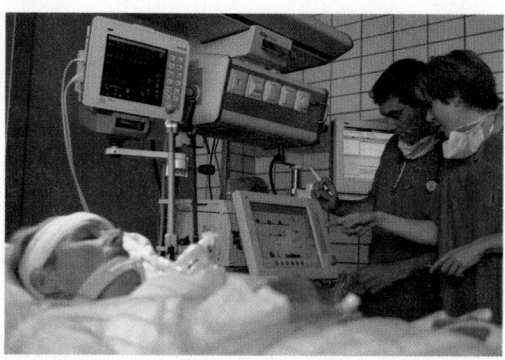

FIG. 66-18 Patient receiving mechanical ventilation. (Courtesy Draeger Medical.)

system. Consequently, the V_T is consistent from breath to breath, but airway pressures vary.

Pressure Ventilation. With *pressure ventilation* the peak inspiratory pressure is predetermined, and the V_T delivered to the patient varies based on the selected pressure and compliance and resistance factors of the patient-ventilator system. With this understanding, careful attention must be given to the V_T to prevent unplanned hyperventilation or hypoventilation. For example, when the patient breathes out of synchrony with the ventilator, the pressure limit may be reached quickly, and the volume of gas delivered may be small. Initially, pressure ventilation was used only in stable patients being weaned from the ventilator. Today, pressure ventilation is frequently used to treat critically ill patients.

Settings of Mechanical Ventilators

Mechanical ventilator settings regulate rate, depth, and other characteristics of ventilation (Table 66-10). Settings are based on the patient's status (e.g., ABGs, ideal body weight, level of consciousness, muscle strength). The ventilator is tuned as finely as possible to match the patient's ventilatory pattern. Settings are evaluated and adjusted frequently until the patient achieves optimal ventilation. Some settings serve as a fail-safe mechanism, alerting staff to problems with ventilation. It is important that you check that all ventilator alarms are always on. Alarms alert the staff to potentially dangerous situations such as mechanical malfunction, apnea, unplanned extubation, or patient asynchrony with the ventilator (Table 66-11). On many ventilators the alarms can be temporarily suspended or silenced for up to 2 minutes for suctioning or testing while a staff member is in the room. After that time, the alarm system automatically becomes functional again.

Modes of Volume Ventilation

The variable methods by which the patient and ventilator interact to deliver effective ventilation are called *ventilator modes*. The selected ventilator mode is based on how much WOB the patient should or can perform. WOB refers to inspiratory effort needed to overcome the elasticity and viscosity of the lungs along with the airway resistance. The mode is determined by the patient's ventilatory status, respiratory drive, and ABGs. Generally, ventilator modes are controlled or assisted.

With controlled ventilatory support, the ventilator does all of the WOB. With assisted ventilatory support, the ventilator and patient share the WOB. Historically, volume modes such as controlled mandatory ventilation (CMV), assist-control ventilation (ACV), and synchronized intermittent mandatory venti-

TABLE 66-10	SETTINGS OF MECHANICAL VENTILATION
Parameter	**Description**
Respiratory rate (f)	Number of breaths the ventilator delivers per minute. *Usual setting:* 6-20 breaths/min
Tidal volume (V_T)	Volume of gas delivered to patient during each ventilator breath. *Usual volume:* 6-10 mL/kg
O_2 concentration (FIO_2)	Fraction of inspired O_2 (FIO_2) delivered to patient. May be set between 21% (essentially room air) and 100%. *Usually adjusted* to maintain PaO_2 level >60 mm Hg or SpO_2 level >90%
Positive end-expiratory pressure (PEEP)	Positive pressure applied at the end of expiration of ventilator breaths. *Usual setting:* 5 cm H_2O
Pressure support	Positive pressure used to augment patient's inspiratory pressure. *Usual setting:* 6-18 cm H_2O
I:E ratio	Duration of inspiration (I) to duration of expiration (E). *Usual setting:* 1:2 to 1:1.5 unless IRV is desired
Inspiratory flow rate and time	Speed with which the V_T is delivered. *Usual setting:* 40-80 L/min and time is 0.8-1.2 sec
Sensitivity	Determines the amount of effort the patient must generate to initiate a ventilator breath. It may be set for pressure triggering or flow triggering. *Usual setting:* A pressure trigger is set 0.5-1.5 cm H_2O below baseline pressure and a flow trigger is set 1-3 L/min below baseline flow
High-pressure limit	Regulates the maximal pressure the ventilator can generate to deliver the V_T. When the pressure limit is reached, the ventilator terminates the breath and spills the undelivered volume into the atmosphere. *Usual setting:* 10-20 cm H_2O above peak inspiratory pressure

Adapted from Urden LD, Lough ME, Stacy KM: *Critical care nursing: diagnosis and management,* ed 6, St Louis, 2010, Mosby.
IRV, Inverse ratio ventilation.

lation (SIMV) have been used to treat critically ill patients. More recently, pressure modes such as pressure support ventilation (PSV) and pressure-control inverse ratio ventilation (PC-IRV) have become more widespread.[39] Table 66-12 describes these ventilator modes.

Assist-Control Mechanical Ventilation. With assist-control ventilation (ACV), the ventilator delivers a preset V_T at a preset frequency. When the patient initiates a spontaneous breath, the ventilator senses a decrease in intrathoracic pressure and then delivers the preset V_T. The patient can breathe faster than the preset rate but not slower. This mode has the advantage of allowing the patient some control over ventilation while providing some assistance. ACV is used in patients with a variety of conditions, including neuromuscular disorders (e.g., Guillain-Barré syndrome), pulmonary edema, and acute respiratory failure.

In the ACV mode, the patient has the potential for hypoventilation and hyperventilation. The spontaneously breathing

TABLE 66-11 INTERPRETING MECHANICAL VENTILATION ALARMS

Alarm	Possible Causes
High-pressure limit	• Secretions, coughing, or gagging • Patient fighting ventilator (ventilator asynchrony) • Condensate (water) in tubing • Kinked or compressed tubing (e.g., patient biting on endotracheal tube [ET] tube) • Increased resistance (e.g., bronchospasm) • Decreased compliance (e.g., pulmonary edema, pneumothorax)
Low-pressure limit	• Total or partial ventilator disconnect • Loss of airway (e.g., total or partial extubation) • ET tube or tracheotomy cuff leak (e.g., patient speaking, grunting)
Apnea	• Respiratory arrest • Oversedation • Change in patient condition • Loss of airway (e.g., total or partial extubation)
High tidal volume, minute ventilation, or respiratory rate	• Pain, anxiety • Change in patient condition • Excess condensate in tubing (i.e., false reading)
Low tidal volume or minute ventilation	• Change in patient's breathing efforts (e.g., rate and volume) • Patient disconnection, loose connection, or leak in circuit • ET tube or tracheotomy cuff leak (e.g., patient speaking, grunting) • Insufficient gas flow
Ventilator inoperative or low battery	• Machine malfunction • Unplugged, power failure, or internal battery not charged

Adapted from Pierce LN: *Management of the mechanically ventilated patient*, ed 2, St Louis, 2007, Saunders.
ET, Endotracheal.

patient can easily be overventilated, resulting in hyperventilation. If the volume or minimum rate is set low and the patient is apneic or weak, the patient will be hypoventilated. Thus these patients require vigilant assessment and monitoring of ventilatory status, including respiratory rate, ABGs, SpO_2, and $ScvO_2$/SvO_2. It is also important that the sensitivity or amount of negative pressure required to initiate a breath is appropriate to the patient's condition. For example, if it is too difficult for the patient to initiate a breath, the WOB is increased and the patient may tire or develop ventilator asynchrony (i.e., the patient "fights" the ventilator).

Synchronized Intermittent Mandatory Ventilation. With *synchronized intermittent mandatory ventilation* (SIMV), the ventilator delivers a preset V_T at a preset frequency in synchrony with the patient's spontaneous breathing. Between ventilator-delivered breaths, the patient is able to breathe spontaneously through the ventilator circuit. Thus the patient receives the preset FIO_2 during the spontaneous breaths but self-regulates the rate and volume of those breaths. This mode of ventilation differs from ACV, in which all breaths are of the same preset volume. It is used during continuous ventilation and during weaning from the ventilator. SIMV may also be combined with PSV (described below). Potential benefits of SIMV include improved patient-ventilator synchrony, lower mean airway pressure, and prevention of muscle atrophy as the patient takes on more of the WOB.

TABLE 66-12 MODES OF MECHANICAL VENTILATION

Volume Modes
Assist-Control (AC) or Assisted Mandatory Ventilation (AMV)
• Requires that rate, V_T, inspiratory time, and PEEP be set for the patient.
• The ventilator sensitivity is also set, and when the patient initiates a spontaneous breath, a full-volume breath is delivered.

Intermittent Mandatory Ventilation (IMV) and Synchronized Intermittent Mandatory Ventilation (SIMV)
• Requires that rate, V_T, inspiratory time, sensitivity, and PEEP are set for the patient.
• In between "mandatory breaths," patients spontaneously breathe at their own rates and V_T. With SIMV, the ventilator synchronizes the mandatory breaths with the patient's own inspirations.

Pressure Modes
Pressure Support Ventilation (PSV)
• Provides an augmented inspiration to a spontaneously breathing patient.
• The clinician selects an inspiratory pressure level, PEEP, and sensitivity.
• When the patient initiates a breath, a high flow of gas is delivered to the preselected pressure level, and pressure is maintained throughout inspiration.
• The patient determines the parameters of V_T, rate, and inspiratory time.

Pressure-Control Inverse Ratio Ventilation (PC-IRV)
• Combines pressure-limited ventilation with an inverse ratio of inspiration to expiration.
• The clinician selects the pressure level, rate, inspiratory time (1:1, 2:1, 3:1, 4:1), and the PEEP level.
• With the prolonged inspiratory times, auto-PEEP may result.
• The auto-PEEP may be a desirable outcome of the inverse ratios.
• Some clinicians use PC without IRV.
• Conventional inspiratory times are used and rate, pressure level, and PEEP are selected.

Airway Pressure Release Ventilation (APRV)
• Provides two levels of continuous positive airway pressure (CPAP) with timed releases, and permits spontaneous breathing throughout the respiratory cycle.
• The clinician selects both pressure high and pressure low along with time high and time low. Tidal volume is not a set variable and depends on the CPAP level, the patient's compliance and resistance, and spontaneous breathing effort.

Positive End-Expiratory Pressure (PEEP) and Continuous Positive Airway Pressure (CPAP)
PEEP
• Creates positive pressure at end exhalation and restores functional residual capacity (FRC).
• The term *PEEP* is used when end-expiratory pressure is provided during ventilator positive pressure breaths.

CPAP
• Similar to PEEP, CPAP restores FRC.
• This pressure is continuous during spontaneous breathing; no positive pressure breaths are present.

Modified from Burns SM: Invasive mechanical ventilation (through an artificial airway) volume and pressure modes. In Wiegand DL-M, editor: *AACN procedure manual for critical care*, ed 6, St Louis, 2011, Saunders.

SIMV also has disadvantages. If spontaneous breathing decreases when the preset rate is low, ventilation might not be adequately supported. Only patients with regular, spontaneous breathing should use low-rate SIMV. Weaning with SIMV demands close monitoring and may take longer because the rate of breathing is gradually reduced. Patients being weaned with SIMV may also have increased muscle fatigue associated with spontaneous breathing efforts.

Modes of Pressure Ventilation

Pressure Support Ventilation. With pressure support ventilation (PSV), positive pressure is applied to the airway only during inspiration and is used in conjunction with the patient's spontaneous respirations. The patient must be able to initiate a breath in this modality. The level of positive airway pressure is preset so that the gas flow rate is greater than the patient's inspiratory flow rate. As the patient initiates a breath, the machine senses the spontaneous effort and supplies a rapid flow of gas at the initiation of the breath and variable flow throughout the breath. With PSV the patient determines inspiratory length, V_T, and respiratory rate. V_T depends on the pressure level and airway compliance.

PSV is used with continuous ventilation and during weaning. PSV may also be used with SIMV during weaning. PSV is not used as a sole ventilatory support during acute respiratory failure because of the risk of hypoventilation. Advantages of PSV include increased patient comfort, decreased WOB (because inspiratory efforts are augmented), decreased O_2 consumption (because inspiratory work is reduced), and increased endurance conditioning (because the patient is exercising respiratory muscles).

Pressure-Control Inverse Ratio Ventilation. *Pressure-control inverse ratio ventilation* (PC-IRV) combines pressure-limited ventilation with an inverse ratio of inspiration (I) to expiration (E). Some clinicians use PC without IRV. The I/E ratio is the ratio of duration of inspiration to the duration of expiration. This value is normally a ratio of 1:2. With IRV, the I/E ratio begins at 1:1 and may progress to 4:1. Prolonged positive pressure is applied, increasing inspiratory time. IRV progressively expands collapsed alveoli. The short expiratory time has a PEEP-like effect, preventing alveolar collapse. Because IRV imposes a nonphysiologic breathing pattern, the patient requires sedation with or without paralysis. PC-IRV is indicated for patients with acute respiratory distress syndrome (ARDS) who continue to have refractory hypoxemia despite high levels of PEEP. Not all patients with poor oxygenation respond to PC-IRV.

Airway Pressure Release Ventilation. *Airway pressure release ventilation* (APRV) permits spontaneous breathing at any point during the respiratory cycle with a preset continuous positive airway pressure (CPAP) with short timed pressure releases. The CPAP level (pressure high, pressure low) is adjusted to maintain oxygenation goals while the timed releases (time high, time low) are increased or decreased to meet ventilation goals. V_T is not a set variable and depends on the CPAP level, the patient's compliance and resistance, and spontaneous breathing effort. The mode is designed for patients with ARDS who need high pressure levels for alveolar recruitment (open collapsed alveoli). One advantage of this mode is the ability to permit spontaneous respirations. This may reduce the need for deep sedation or paralytics.

Other Modes. Increases in ventilator technology have led to the development of additional pressure modes. However, because of the nonstandardization of these options, the names and features are manufacturer specific. The superiority of these modes has not been established. Some examples include *volume-assured pressure ventilation* and *adaptive support ventilation*.

Other Ventilatory Maneuvers

Positive End-Expiratory Pressure. Positive end-expiratory pressure (PEEP) is a ventilatory maneuver in which positive pressure is applied to the airway during exhalation. Normally during exhalation, airway pressure drops to zero, and exhalation occurs passively. With PEEP, exhalation remains passive, but pressure falls to a preset level, often 3 to 20 cm H_2O. Lung volume during expiration and between breaths is greater than normal with PEEP. This increases functional residual capacity (FRC) and often improves oxygenation with restoration of lung volume that normally remains at the end of passive exhalation. The mechanisms by which PEEP increases FRC and oxygenation include increased aeration of patent alveoli, aeration of previously collapsed alveoli, and prevention of alveolar collapse throughout the respiratory cycle.

PEEP is titrated to the point that oxygenation improves without compromising hemodynamics. This is termed *best* or *optimal PEEP*. Often 5 cm H_2O PEEP (referred to as *physiologic PEEP*) is used prophylactically to replace the glottic mechanism, help maintain a normal FRC, and prevent alveolar collapse. PEEP of 5 cm H_2O is also used for patients with a history of alveolar collapse during weaning. PEEP improves gas exchange, vital capacity, and inspiratory force when used during weaning.

In contrast, *auto-PEEP* is not purposely set on the ventilator but is a result of inadequate exhalation time. Auto-PEEP is additional PEEP over what is set by the health care provider. This additional PEEP may result in increased WOB, barotrauma, and hemodynamic instability. However, during some ventilator modes (PC-IRV), auto-PEEP may be desirable. Interventions to limit auto-PEEP include sedation and analgesia, large-diameter ET tube, bronchodilators, short inspiratory times, and decreased respiratory rates. Reducing water accumulation in the ventilator circuit by frequent emptying or use of heated circuits also limits auto-PEEP. In patients with short exhalation times and early airway closure (e.g., asthma), setting PEEP can offset auto-PEEP by splinting the airway open during exhalation and preventing "air trapping."

In general, the major purpose of PEEP is to maintain or improve oxygenation while limiting risk of O_2 toxicity. FIO_2 can often be reduced when PEEP is used. PEEP is indicated in lungs with diffuse disease, severe hypoxemia unresponsive to FIO_2 greater than 50%, and loss of compliance or stiffness. It is used in pulmonary edema to provide a counterpressure opposing fluid extravasation. The classic indication for PEEP therapy is ARDS (see Chapter 68). PEEP is contraindicated or used with extreme caution in patients with highly compliant lungs (e.g., COPD), unilateral or nonuniform disease, hypovolemia, and low CO. In these cases the adverse effects of PEEP may outweigh any benefits.

Continuous Positive Airway Pressure. Continuous positive airway pressure (CPAP) restores FRC and is similar to PEEP. However, the pressure in CPAP is delivered continuously during spontaneous breathing, thus preventing the patient's airway pressure from falling to zero. For example, if CPAP is 5 cm H_2O, airway pressure during expiration is 5 cm H_2O. During inspiration, 1 to 2 cm H_2O of negative pressure is generated, thus reducing airway pressure to 3 or 4 cm H_2O. The patient receiving SIMV with PEEP receives CPAP when breathing spontaneously. CPAP is commonly used in the treatment of obstructive sleep apnea.[40] CPAP can be administered noninvasively by a tight-fitting mask or an ET or tracheal tube. CPAP increases WOB because the patient must forcibly exhale against the CPAP. Therefore it must be used with caution in patients with myocardial compromise.

Automatic Tube Compensation. *Automatic tube compensation* (ATC) is an adjunct designed to overcome WOB through an artificial airway. It is currently available on many ventilators. ATC is increased during inspiration and decreased during expiration. It is set by entering the internal diameter of the patient's airway along with the desired percentage of compensation. ATC may increase auto-PEEP in patients with obstructive disease and should be used cautiously in this population.[41]

Bilevel Positive Airway Pressure. In addition to O_2, *bilevel positive airway pressure* (BiPAP) provides two levels of positive pressure support: higher inspiratory positive airway pressure and lower expiratory positive airway pressure. It is a noninvasive modality and is delivered through a tight-fitting face mask, nasal mask, or nasal pillows. As with PSV delivered through an artificial airway, the patient must be able to spontaneously breathe and cooperate with this treatment.[40] BiPAP is used for COPD patients with heart failure and acute respiratory failure and for patients with sleep apnea. BiPAP may also be used after extubation to prevent reintubation. Patients with shock, altered mental status, or increased airway secretions are not candidates for BiPAP because of the risk of aspiration and the inability to remove the mask.

High-Frequency Oscillatory Ventilation. High-frequency oscillatory ventilation (HFOV) involves delivery of a small V_T (usually 1 to 5 mL/kg of body weight) at rapid respiratory rates (100 to 300 breaths/minute) in an effort to recruit and maintain lung volume and reduce intrapulmonary shunting. One benefit of HFOV is the ability to support gas exchange at a fixed mean airway pressure while limiting the risk of ventilator-induced lung injury. HFOV has been widely accepted in neonatal and pediatric ICUs. It is used in adults for the treatment of refractory hypoxemia and ARDS.[42] Patients receiving HFOV must be sedated and may be paralyzed to suppress spontaneous respiration. All patients must receive concurrent sedation and analgesia if using a paralytic drug (see Chapter 68).

Nitric Oxide. *Nitric oxide* (NO) is a gaseous molecule that is made intravascularly and participates in the regulation of pulmonary vascular tone. Inhibition of NO production results in pulmonary vasoconstriction, and administration of continuous inhaled NO results in pulmonary vasodilation. NO may be administered via an ET tube, a tracheostomy, or a face mask. Currently, NO is used in ARDS, as a diagnostic screening tool for pulmonary hypertension during a cardiac catheterization, and during or after cardiac surgery.

Prone Positioning. *Prone positioning* is the repositioning of a patient from a supine or lateral position to a prone (on the stomach, face down) position. This repositioning improves lung recruitment (reexpansion) through various mechanisms. Gravity reverses the effects of fluid in the dependent parts of the lungs as the patient is moved from supine to prone. The heart rests on the sternum, away from the lungs, contributing to an overall uniformity of pleural pressures. The prone position is a relatively safe (although nurse-intensive), supportive therapy used in critically ill patients with acute lung injury or ARDS to improve oxygenation.[43]

Extracorporeal Membrane Oxygenation. *Extracorporeal membrane oxygenation* (ECMO) is an alternative form of pulmonary support for the patient with severe respiratory failure. It is used more frequently in the pediatric and neonatal populations but is increasingly being used in adults. ECMO is a modification of cardiac bypass and involves partially removing blood from a patient with large-bore catheters, infusing O_2, removing CO_2, and returning the blood to the patient. This intensive therapy requires systemic anticoagulation and is a time-limited intervention. A skilled team of specialists, including a perfusionist, is required continuously at the bedside.[44]

Complications of Positive Pressure Ventilation

Although PPV may be essential to maintain ventilation and oxygenation, it can cause adverse effects. It is often difficult to distinguish complications of mechanical ventilation from the underlying disease.

Cardiovascular System. PPV can affect circulation because of the transmission of increased mean airway pressure to the thoracic cavity. With increased intrathoracic pressure, thoracic vessels are compressed. This results in decreased venous return to the heart, decreased left ventricular end-diastolic volume (preload), decreased CO, and hypotension. Mean airway pressure is further increased if titrating PEEP (greater than 5 cm H_2O) to improve oxygenation.

If the lungs are noncompliant (e.g., ARDS), airway pressures are not as easily transmitted to the heart and blood vessels. Thus effects of PPV on CO are reduced. Conversely, with compliant lungs (e.g., emphysema), there is increased danger of transmission of high airway pressures and negative effects on hemodynamics.

Compromised venous return by PPV is worsened by hypovolemia (e.g., hemorrhage) and decreased venous tone (e.g., sepsis, spinal shock). Restoration and maintenance of the circulating blood volume are important in minimizing cardiovascular complications.

Pulmonary System

Barotrauma. As lung inflation pressures increase, risk of *barotrauma* increases. Patients with compliant lungs (e.g., COPD) are at greater risk for barotrauma. This results when the increased airway pressure distends the lungs and possibly ruptures fragile alveoli or emphysematous blebs. Patients with stiff lungs (e.g., ARDS) who are given high inspiratory pressures and high levels of PEEP (greater than 5 cm H_2O) and patients with lung abscesses resulting from necrotizing organisms (e.g., staphylococci) are also susceptible to barotrauma.

Air can escape into the pleural space from alveoli or interstitium and become trapped. Pleural pressure increases and collapses the lung, causing pneumothorax. (Chapter 28 discusses the clinical manifestations of pneumothorax.) The lungs receive air during inspiration but cannot expel it during expiration. Respiratory bronchioles are larger on inspiration than expiration. They may close on expiration, and air becomes trapped. With PPV, a simple pneumothorax can become a life-threatening tension pneumothorax. The mediastinum and contralateral lung are compressed, reducing CO. Immediate treatment of the pneumothorax is required. For some patients, chest tubes are placed prophylactically.

Pneumomediastinum usually begins with rupture of alveoli into the lung interstitium. Progressive air movement occurs into the mediastinum and subcutaneous neck tissue, and a pneumothorax often follows. New, unexplained subcutaneous emphysema is an indication for immediate chest x-ray. Pneumomediastinum and subcutaneous emphysema may be too small to detect on x-ray or clinically before the development of a pneumothorax.

Volutrauma. The concept of *volutrauma* in PPV relates to the lung injury that occurs when a large V_T is used to ventilate noncompliant lungs. Volutrauma results in alveolar fractures and movement of fluids and proteins into the alveolar spaces. Low-volume ventilation rather than pressure ventilation should be used in ARDS patients to protect the lungs.

Alveolar Hypoventilation. *Alveolar hypoventilation* can be caused by inappropriate ventilator settings, leakage of air from the ventilator tubing or around the ET tube or tracheostomy cuff, lung secretions or obstruction, and low ventilation/perfusion ratio. A low V_T or respiratory rate decreases minute ventilation. This results in hypoventilation and leads to respiratory acidosis. A leaking cuff or tubing that is not secured may cause air leakage, lowering the delivered V_T. Excess lung secretions can cause hypoventilation. Mobilizing the patient, turning the patient every 1 to 2 hours, providing chest physiotherapy to lung areas with increased secretions, encouraging deep breathing and coughing, and suctioning (as needed) may limit this. Atelectasis may develop. Increasing the V_T, adding small increments of PEEP, and adding a preset number of sighs to the ventilator settings reduce the risk of atelectasis.

Alveolar Hyperventilation. Respiratory alkalosis can occur if the respiratory rate or V_T is set too high *(mechanical overventilation)* or if the patient receiving assisted ventilation is *hyperventilating*. It is easy to overventilate a patient on PPV. Particularly at risk are patients with chronic alveolar hypoventilation and CO_2 retention. For example, the patient with COPD may have a chronic $PaCO_2$ elevation (acidosis) and compensatory bicarbonate retention by the kidneys. When the patient is ventilated, the patient's "normal baseline" rather than the standard normal values is the therapeutic goal. If the COPD patient is returned to a standard normal $PaCO_2$, the patient will develop alkalosis because of the retained bicarbonate. Such a patient could move from compensated respiratory acidosis to serious metabolic alkalosis. The presence of alkalosis makes weaning from the ventilator difficult. Alkalosis, especially if the onset is abrupt, can have additional serious consequences, including hypokalemia, hypocalcemia, and dysrhythmias. Neuromuscular irritability, seizures, coma, and death can occur. Usually the patient with COPD who is supported on the ventilator does better with a short inspiratory and longer expiratory time.

If hyperventilation is spontaneous, it is important to determine the cause and treat it. Possible causes include hypoxemia, pain, fear, anxiety, or compensation for metabolic acidosis. Patients who fight the ventilator or breathe out of synchrony may be anxious or in pain. If the patient is anxious and fearful, sitting with the patient and verbally coaching the patient to breathe with the ventilator may help. If these measures fail, manually ventilating the patient slowly with a BVM and 100% O_2 may slow breathing enough to bring it in synchrony with the ventilator.

Ventilator-Associated Pneumonia. The risk for hospital-acquired pneumonia is highest in patients requiring mechanical ventilation because the ET or tracheostomy tube bypasses normal upper airway defenses. In addition, a poor nutritional state, immobility, and the underlying disease process (e.g., immunosuppression, organ failure) make the patient more prone to infection. *Ventilator-associated pneumonia* (VAP) is

pneumonia that occurs 48 hours or more after ET intubation.[45] It occurs in 9% to 27% of all intubated patients, with half of the cases developing within the first 4 days of mechanical ventilation. In addition, patients who develop VAP have significantly longer hospital stays and higher mortality rates than those who do not.

In patients with early VAP (within 96 hours of mechanical ventilation), sputum cultures often grow gram-negative bacteria (e.g., *Escherichia coli, Klebsiella, Streptococcus pneumoniae, Haemophilus influenzae*). Organisms associated with late VAP include antibiotic-resistant organisms such as *Pseudomonas aeruginosa* and oxacillin-resistant *Staphylococcus aureus*. These organisms are abundant in the hospital environment and the patient's GI tract. They can spread in a number of ways, including contaminated respiratory equipment, inadequate hand washing, adverse environmental factors such as poor room ventilation and high traffic flow, and decreased patient ability to cough and clear secretions. Colonization of the oropharynx tract by gram-negative organisms predisposes the patient to gram-negative pneumonia.

Clinical evidence suggesting VAP includes fever, elevated white blood cell count, purulent or odorous sputum, crackles or rhonchi on auscultation, and pulmonary infiltrates noted on chest x-ray. The patient is treated with antibiotics after appropriate cultures are taken by tracheal suctioning or bronchoscopy and when infection is evident.

Guidelines on VAP prevention include (1) HOB elevation at a minimum of 30 to 45 degrees unless medically contraindicated, (2) no routine changes of the patient's ventilator circuit tubing, and (3) the use of an ET tube with a dorsal lumen above the cuff to allow continuous suctioning of secretions in the subglottic area[46] (see Fig. 66-16). Prevention also includes strict hand washing before and after suctioning, whenever ventilator equipment is touched, and after contact with any respiratory secretions (see Nursing Management: Artificial Airway earlier in this chapter). Always wear gloves when in contact with the patient and change gloves between activities (e.g., emptying urinary catheter drainage, hanging an IV drug). Finally, always drain the water that collects in the ventilator tubing away from the patient as it collects.

Sodium and Water Imbalance. Progressive fluid retention often occurs after 48 to 72 hours of PPV, especially PPV with PEEP. Fluid retention is associated with decreased urine output and increased sodium retention. Fluid balance changes may be due to decreased CO, which in turn results in diminished renal perfusion. Consequently, renin release is stimulated with subsequent production of angiotensin and aldosterone (see Chapter 45, Fig. 45-4). This results in sodium and water retention. It is also possible that pressure changes within the thorax are associated with decreased release of atrial natriuretic peptide, which also causes sodium retention. Mild water retention is also associated with PPV. Less insensible water loss occurs via the airway because ventilated delivered gases are humidified with body-temperature water. In addition, as a part of the stress response, release of antidiuretic hormone and cortisol contributes to sodium and water retention.

Neurologic System. In patients with head injury, PPV (especially with PEEP) can impair cerebral blood flow. The increased intrathoracic positive pressure impedes venous drainage from the head, resulting in jugular venous distention. The patient may exhibit increases in intracranial pressure because of the impaired venous return and increase in cerebral volume. Elevating the

HOB and keeping the patient's head in alignment may decrease the harmful effects of PPV on intracranial pressure.

Gastrointestinal System. Patients receiving PPV are stressed because of the serious illness, immobility, or discomforts associated with the ventilator. This places the ventilated patient at risk for developing stress ulcers and GI bleeding. Patients with a preexisting ulcer or those receiving corticosteroids are at an increased risk. Any kind of circulatory compromise, including reduction of CO caused by PPV, may contribute to ischemia of the gastric and intestinal mucosa and possibly increase the risk of translocation of GI bacteria.

To decrease the risk of VAP, guidelines support the use of routine peptic ulcer prophylaxis in mechanically ventilated patients.[46] Peptic ulcer prophylaxis includes the administration of histamine (H_2)-receptor blockers (e.g., ranitidine [Zantac]), proton pump inhibitors (PPIs) (e.g., esomeprazole [Nexium]), and enteral nutrition to decrease gastric acidity and diminish the risk of stress ulcer and hemorrhage. Some evidence suggests that the use of PPIs may be linked to an increase in the development of *Clostridium difficile*–associated diarrhea.[47] (This is discussed in Chapter 42 on p. 933.)

Gastric and bowel dilation may occur because of gas accumulation in the GI tract from swallowed air. The irritation of an artificial airway may cause excessive air swallowing and subsequent gastric dilation. Gastric or bowel dilation may put pressure on the vena cava, decrease CO, and prohibit adequate diaphragmatic excursion during spontaneous breathing. Elevation of the diaphragm as a result of paralytic ileus or bowel dilation leads to compression of the lower lobes of the lungs. This may cause atelectasis and compromise respiratory function. Decompression of the stomach is done by inserting an OG or NG tube.[48]

Immobility, sedation, circulatory impairment, decreased oral intake, use of opioid pain medications, and stress contribute to decreased peristalsis. The patient's inability to exhale against a closed glottis may make defecation difficult. As a result, the ventilated patient is at risk for constipation, and a bowel regimen should be initiated.

Musculoskeletal System. Maintenance of muscle strength and prevention of the problems associated with immobility are important. Adequate analgesia and nutrition can enhance exercise tolerance. Plan for early and progressive mobility of appropriate patients receiving PPV.[49] (See eFig. 66-6 on the website for this chapter.) In collaboration with physical and occupational therapy, perform passive and active exercises to maintain muscle tone in the upper and lower extremities. Simple maneuvers such as leg lifts, knee bends, quadriceps setting, or arm circles are appropriate. Prevent contractures, pressure ulcers, footdrop, and external rotation of the hip and legs by proper positioning and the use of specialized mattresses or beds. Use a portable ventilator or manually ventilate the patient with a BVM and 100% O_2 while ambulating.

Psychosocial Needs. The patient receiving mechanical ventilation often experiences physical and emotional stress. In addition to the problems related to critical care patients discussed at the beginning of this chapter, the patient supported by a mechanical ventilator is unable to speak, eat, move, or breathe normally. Tubes and machines cause pain, fear, and anxiety. Usual activities of daily living such as eating, elimination, and coughing are extremely complicated.

Feeling safe is an overpowering need of patients on mechanical ventilation. In addition, four related needs include the need

to know (information), the need to regain control, the need to hope, and the need to trust. When patients' needs are met, they feel safe. Work to strengthen the various factors that affect feeling safe. Encourage hope, as appropriate, and build trusting relationships with both the patient and caregiver. Involve patients and caregivers in decision making as much as possible.[14,16]

Patients receiving PPV usually require sedation (e.g., propofol) and/or analgesia (e.g., fentanyl) to facilitate optimal ventilation. Before initiating sedation or analgesia in the mechanically ventilated patient who is agitated or anxious, identify the cause of distress. Common problems that can result in patient agitation or anxiety include PPV, nutritional deficits, pain, hypoxemia, hypercapnia, drugs, and environmental stressors (e.g., sleep deprivation). Delirium is an acute change in mental status. It is a marker of cerebral insufficiency and associated with longer hospital stays and higher mortality rates. ICU patients are particularly vulnerable to delirium, and you must make every effort to assess and treat it.[8]

At times, the decision is made to paralyze the patient with a neuromuscular blocking agent (e.g., cisatracurium [Nimbex]) to provide more effective synchrony with the ventilator and improve oxygenation. Remember that the paralyzed patient can hear, see, think, and feel. It is important to administer IV sedation and analgesia concurrently when the patient is paralyzed. Monitoring patients receiving these medications is challenging. Assessment of the patient should include train-of-four (TOF) peripheral nerve stimulation, physiologic signs of pain or anxiety (changes in heart rate and BP), and ventilator synchrony. The TOF assessment involves using a peripheral nerve stimulator to deliver four successive stimulating currents to elicit muscle twitches (Fig. 66-19). The number of twitches varies with the percentage of neuromuscular blockade. The usual goal is one or two twitches out of four. Noninvasive electroencephalogram-based technology can also help guide sedative and analgesic therapy in these patients. Excessive administration of neuromuscular blocking agents may predispose the patient to prolonged paralysis and muscle weakness even after these agents are stopped.

Many patients have few memories of their time in the ICU, whereas others remember vivid details. Although appearing to be asleep, sedated, or paralyzed, patients may be aware of their surroundings, and you should always address them as if they were awake and alert.[50]

FIG. 66-19 Placement of electrodes along ulnar nerve.

Machine Disconnection or Malfunction. Mechanical ventilators may become disconnected or malfunction. When turned on and operative, alarms alert you to problems (see Table 66-11). Most deaths from accidental ventilator disconnection occur while the alarm is off, and most accidental disconnections in critical care settings are discovered by low-pressure alarms. The most frequent site for disconnection is between the tracheal tube and the adapter. Push connections together and then twist to secure more tightly. Be certain that alarms are set at all times, and chart that this is the case. You can pause alarms (not inactivate) during suctioning or removal from the ventilator, but you must reactivate them before leaving the patient's bedside.

Ventilator malfunction may also occur due to several factors. Although most institutions have emergency generators in the event of a power failure and newer ventilators may have battery backup, power failure is always a possibility. Have a plan for manually ventilating all patients who depend on a ventilator. If, at any time, you determine that the ventilator is malfunctioning (e.g., failure of O_2 supply), disconnect the patient from the machine and manually ventilate with a BVM and 100% O_2 until the ventilator is fixed or replaced.

Nutritional Therapy: Patient Receiving Positive Pressure Ventilation

PPV and the hypermetabolism associated with critical illness can contribute to inadequate nutrition. The presence of an ET tube eliminates the normal route for eating. Patients with a tracheostomy may be able to eat normally once the stoma heals. Swallowing studies and a consultation with a speech therapist are done to assess the patient's readiness. When eating with a tracheostomy tube in place, the patient should tilt the head slightly forward to facilitate swallowing and to prevent aspiration. Diet may be restricted to soft foods (e.g., puddings, ice cream) and thickened liquids.

Patients unlikely to be able to eat for 3 to 5 days should have a nutritional assessment and enteral feeding started within 24 to 48 hours of admission.[5] Inadequate nutrition makes the patient receiving prolonged mechanical ventilation prone to poor O_2 transport secondary to anemia and to poor tolerance of minimal exercise. Critically ill patients have frequent interruptions of enteral feedings because of problems with residuals, transportation to and during procedures, and routine nursing care. Poor nutrition and the disuse of respiratory muscles contribute to decreased respiratory muscle strength. In addition, critical illness, trauma, and surgery are associated with hypermetabolism, anxiety, pain, and increased WOB, which greatly increase caloric expenditure. Serum protein levels (e.g., albumin, prealbumin, transferrin, total protein) are usually decreased. Inadequate nutrition can delay weaning, decrease resistance to infection, and slow down recovery. Enteral gastric or small bowel feeding is the preferred method to meet caloric needs of ventilated patients (see Chapter 40 for discussion of enteral feeding).

Verification of feeding tube placement includes (1) x-ray confirmation before initial use, (2) marking and ongoing assessment of the tube's exit site, and (3) ongoing review of routine x-rays and aspirate.[48] The auscultatory method of assessment (i.e., listening for air after injection) is not a reliable method for verifying the placement of feeding tubes.

A concern regarding the nutritional support of patients receiving PPV is the carbohydrate content of the diet. Metabolism of carbohydrates may increase the serum CO_2 levels. This

can result in a higher required minute ventilation and increased WOB. Limiting carbohydrate content in the diet may lower CO_2 production. Consult the dietitian to determine the caloric and nutrient needs of these patients.

Weaning From Positive Pressure Ventilation and Extubation

Weaning is the process of reducing ventilator support and resuming spontaneous ventilation. The weaning process differs for patients requiring short-term ventilation (up to 3 days) versus long-term ventilation (longer than 3 days). Patients requiring short-term ventilation (e.g., after cardiac surgery) experience a linear weaning process. Patients likely to require prolonged PPV (e.g., patients with COPD who develop respiratory failure) often experience a weaning process that consists of peaks and valleys. Preparation for weaning begins when PPV is initiated and involves a team approach (e.g., nurse, physician, patient, caregiver, dietitian, respiratory therapist, physical therapist).

Weaning generally consists of three phases: the *preweaning phase*, the *weaning process*, and the *outcome phase*. The preweaning or assessment phase determines the patient's ability to breathe spontaneously. Assessment in this phase depends on a combination of respiratory (Table 66-13) and nonrespiratory factors. Weaning assessment parameters should include criteria to assess muscle strength (negative inspiratory force) and endurance (spontaneous V_T, vital capacity, minute ventilation, and rapid shallow breathing index). In addition, the patient's lungs should be reasonably clear on auscultation and chest x-ray. Nonrespiratory factors include the patient's neurologic status; hemodynamics; fluid, electrolytes, and acid-base balance; nutrition; and hemoglobin. It is important to have an alert, well-rested, and well-informed patient relatively free from pain and anxiety who can cooperate with the weaning plan. This does not mean complete withdrawal from sedatives or analgesics. Instead,

drugs should be titrated to achieve comfort without causing excessive drowsiness.

A *spontaneous breathing trial* (SBT) is recommended in patients who demonstrate weaning readiness.[51] An SBT should be at least 30 minutes but no more than 120 minutes. It may be done with low levels of CPAP, low levels of PSV, or a T piece. Tolerance of the trial may lead to extubation. Failure to tolerate an SBT should prompt a search for reversible or complicating factors and a return to a nonfatiguing ventilator modality for the patient. The SBT should be reattempted the next day.

The use of a weaning protocol decreases ventilator days (see eFig. 66-7, available on the website for this chapter). The parts of a protocol are not as important as the use of a protocol to prevent delays in weaning. The patient receiving SIMV can have the ventilator breaths gradually reduced as his or her ventilatory status permits. CPAP or PSV can be added to SIMV. PSV is thought to

---

TABLE 66-13 INDICATORS FOR WEANING

Weaning Readiness

Patients receiving mechanical ventilation for respiratory failure should undergo a formal assessment of weaning potential if the following are satisfied:*

1. Reversal of the underlying cause of respiratory failure
2. Adequate oxygenation
   - PaO_2/FIO_2 >150-200
   - SpO_2 ≥90%
   - PEEP ≤5-8 cm H_2O
   - FIO_2 ≤40%-50%
   - pH ≥7.25

3. Hemodynamic stability
   - Absence of myocardial ischemia
   - Absence of clinically significant hypotension (no vasopressor therapy or low dose)
4. Patient ability to initiate an inspiratory effort
5. Optional criteria
   - Hemoglobin ≥7-10 mg/dL
   - Core temperature ≤38° (100.4° F) to 38.5° C (101.3° F)
   - Mental status awake and alert or easily arousable

Weaning Assessment

Measurement	Significance	Normal Values	Indices for Weaning
Spontaneous respiratory rate (f)	Respiratory rate/frequency over 1 min.	12-20 min	<35 min
Spontaneous tidal volume (V_T)	Amount of air exchanged during normal breathing at rest. Measure of muscle endurance.	7-9 mL/kg	≥5 mL/kg
Minute ventilation (V_E)	Tidal volume multiplied by respiratory rate over 1 min. *For example:* 0.350 (V_T) × 28 (f) = 9.8 L/min	5-10 L/min	≤10 L/min
Negative inspiratory force or pressure (NIF, NIP)	Amount of negative pressure that a patient is able to generate to initiate spontaneous respirations. Measured by clinician: After complete occlusion of inspiratory valve, a pressure manometer is attached to airway or mouth for 10-20 sec while negative inspiratory efforts are noted.	–75 to –100 cm H_2O	>–20 cm H_2O The more negative the number, the better indication for weaning.
Positive expiratory pressure (PEP)	Measure of expiratory muscle strength and ability to cough. Measured by clinician: After complete occlusion of expiratory valve, a pressure manometer is attached to the airway or mouth for 10-20 sec while positive expiratory efforts are noted.	60-85 cm H_2O	≥30 cm H_2O
Compliance, rate, oxygenation, and pressure (CROP) index	Combined index that is complex to calculate. $C_{Dyn} \times NIF \times (PaO_2/PAO_2)/f$ C_{Dyn} = Compliance PaO_2/PAO_2 = Oxygenation ratio of arterial O_2/alveolar O_2	Not applicable	>13
Rapid shallow breathing index (f/V_T)	Spontaneous respiratory rate over 1 min divided by tidal volume (in liters). *For example:* 30 (f)/0.400 (V_T) = 75/L	60-105/L	<105/L
Vital capacity (VC)	Maximum inspiration and then measurement of air during maximal forced expiration. Measure of respiratory muscle endurance or reserve or both. Requires patient cooperation.	65-75 mL/kg	≥10-15 mL/kg
Spontaneous breathing trial (SBT)	If patient passes daily weaning screen, assess patient during spontaneous breathing with little or no ventilator assistance. Trial should be at least 30 min to a maximum of 120 min.		Successful completion of trial is based on an integrated patient assessment.

Adapted from A Collective Task Force Facilitated by the American College of Chest Physicians, the American Association for Respiratory Care, and the American College of Critical Care Medicine. Evidence-based guidelines for weaning and discontinuing ventilatory support. Respiratory Care 47:69, 2002; and Burns SM: Weaning process. In Wiegand DL-M, editor: *AACN procedure manual for critical care*, ed 6, St Louis 2011, Saunders.

*The decision to use these criteria must be individualized to the patient.

provide gentle, slow respiratory muscle conditioning. It may be especially beneficial for patients who are deconditioned or have heart problems. Some patients may be weaned by simply providing humidified oxygen (T-piece or flow-by method).

Weaning may be tried at any time of day, although it is usually done during the day, with the patient ventilated at night in a rest mode. The rest mode should be a stable, nonfatiguing, and comfortable form of support for the patient. Regardless of the weaning mode selected, all health care team members should be familiar with the weaning plan. Additionally, it is important to permit the patient's respiratory muscles to rest between weaning trials. Once the respiratory muscles become fatigued, they may require 12 to 24 hours to recover.

The patient being weaned and the caregiver need ongoing emotional support. Explain the weaning process to them and keep them informed of progress. Place the patient in a comfortable sitting or semirecumbent position. Obtain baseline vital signs and respiratory parameters. During the weaning trial, closely monitor the patient for signs and symptoms that may signal intolerance and a need to end the trial (e.g., tachypnea, dyspnea, tachycardia, dysrhythmias, sustained desaturation [SpO_2 less than 91%], hypertension or hypotension, agitation, diaphoresis, anxiety, sustained V_T less than 5 mL/kg, changes in mentation). Document the patient's tolerance throughout the weaning process and include statements regarding the patient's and the caregiver's perceptions.

The weaning outcome phase is the period when the patient is extubated or weaning is stopped because no further progress is being made. The patient who is ready for extubation should receive hyperoxygenation and suctioning (e.g., oropharynx, ET tube). Instruct the patient to take a deep breath, and at the peak of inspiration, deflate the cuff and remove the tube in one motion. After removal, encourage the patient to deep breathe and cough, and suction the oropharynx as needed. Administer supplemental O_2 and provide naso-oral care. Carefully monitor the patient's vital signs, respiratory status, and oxygenation immediately after extubation, within 1 hour, and per institution policy. If the patient does not tolerate extubation, immediate reintubation or a trial of noninvasive ventilation may be necessary.

Chronic Mechanical Ventilation

Mechanical ventilators are no longer limited to the ICU but are now a part of long-term and home care. In some instances, terminally ill, ventilated patients may be discharged to hospice. The emphasis on controlling hospital costs has increased the early discharge of patients and the need to provide highly technical care such as mechanical ventilation in home settings.[52] The success of home mechanical ventilation depends, in part, on careful predischarge assessment and planning for both the patient and caregivers.

Both negative pressure and positive pressure ventilators are used in the home. Negative pressure ventilators do not require an artificial airway and are less complicated to use. Several types of small, portable (battery-powered) positive pressure ventilators are available and can be attached to a wheelchair or placed on a bedside table. Settings and alarms on these ventilators are simpler to use than on the standard ICU ventilators.

Home mechanical ventilation has advantages and disadvantages. Having the patient in the home eliminates the strain that the hospital setting imposes on family dynamics. Caregivers' feelings of helplessness when they first hear about the necessity for long-term mechanical ventilation is frequently balanced by the opportunity to participate in the patient's care in the home

setting. At home the patient may be able to take part in more activities of daily living around an individualized schedule and, because of the smaller size of the home ventilator, be more mobile. Another advantage of home mechanical ventilation is the reduced risk of HAIs.

Disadvantages of home mechanical ventilation include problems related to equipment, reimbursement, caregiver stress and fatigue, and the patient's complex needs. Ventilated patients are usually dependent, requiring extensive nursing care, at least initially. Disposable products may not be reimbursable. Financial resources must be carefully assessed when arranging home mechanical ventilation. Schedule a meeting with the discharge team before initiating a teaching plan for discharge.

Another disadvantage of home mechanical ventilation is its potential impact on the family. Caregivers may seem enthusiastic about caring for their loved one in the home but may be motivated by numerous, complex factors. They may not understand the sacrifices they may have to make financially and in personal time and commitment. Encourage caregivers to consider respite care to periodically relieve their stress and fatigue.

NURSING MANAGEMENT MECHANICAL VENTILATION

eNursing Care Plan 66-1 for the patient receiving mechanical ventilation is available on the website for this chapter.

OTHER CRITICAL CARE CONTENT

Table 66-14 lists additional critical care content presented in other chapters of this book.

TABLE 66-14	CROSS-REFERENCES TO CRITICAL CARE CONTENT
Topic	**Discussed in Chapter**
Acute coronary syndrome	34
Acute heart failure	35
Acute respiratory distress syndrome (ARDS)	68
Acute respiratory failure	68
Basic life support and CPR	Appendix A
Burns	25
Cardiac dysrhythmias	36
Cardiac pacemakers	36
Cardiac surgery	34
Central venous access device (CVAD)	17
Continuous renal replacement therapy (CRRT)	47
Delirium	60
Emergencies	69
End-of-life (EOL) care	10
Enteral nutrition (EN)	40
Head injury, including ICP monitoring	57
Multiple organ dysfunction syndrome (MODS)	67
Myocardial infarction (MI)	34
Oxygen delivery	29
Pain management	9
Parenteral nutrition (PN)	40
Pulmonary edema	35
Renal dialysis	47
Shock	67
Stroke	58
Systemic inflammatory response syndrome (SIRS)	67
Tracheostomy	27
Trauma	69

CPR, Cardiopulmonary resuscitation; *ICP,* intracranial pressure.

CASE STUDY

Critical Care and Mechanical Ventilation

iStockphoto/Thinkstock

Patient Profile

R.K. is a 72-yr-old white man who collapsed on the street. He was unresponsive on admission and remains unresponsive. He has an oral ET tube in place and is receiving mechanical ventilation. He weighs 198 lb (90 kg). A subclavian central line was placed to monitor CVP and administer fluids.

Subjective Data

None. Patient is unresponsive to painful stimuli.

Objective Data

Physical Examination

- Noninvasive BP 100/75 mm Hg; heart rate 128 (atrial fibrillation with a rapid ventricular response); temperature 102° F (38.8° C); SpO$_2$ is 98%
- Purulent secretions from ET tube
- Breath sounds: rhonchi bilaterally, decreased breath sounds on the right

Diagnostic Studies

- Chest x-ray reveals right lower lung consolidation
- ABGs: pH 7.48; PaO$_2$ 94 mm Hg; PaCO$_2$ 30 mm Hg; HCO$_3$ 34 mEq/L
- CT scan is positive for massive hemorrhagic stroke

Collaborative Care

- Positive pressure ventilation settings: assist-control mode
- Settings: FIO$_2$ 70%, V$_T$ 700 mL, respiratory rate 16 breaths/min, PEEP 5 cm H$_2$O
- Enteral feeding at 25 mL/hr via small-bore nasogastric feeding tube
- External condom catheter for urinary drainage
- HOB elevated at 40 degrees
- Reposition every 2 hr
- Azithromycin (Zithromax) 500 mg IV q24hr
- Cefotaxime (Claforan) 2 g IV q6hr
- D$_5$NS with KCl 20 mEq/L at 100 mL/hr

Discussion Questions

1. Identify two reasons for intubating and providing mechanical ventilation for R.K.
2. What do R.K.'s ABGs indicate, and which ventilator setting(s) should be changed?
3. What is his PaO$_2$/FIO$_2$ ratio, and what does it indicate?
4. R.K.'s BP drops to 80 mm Hg. Despite increasing doses of vasopressors and fluid challenges, his BP remains low. A central venous catheter and an arterial line are inserted. APCO monitoring is started. What would be the purpose of hemodynamic monitoring in this patient?
5. **Priority Decision:** What are two priority nursing considerations for a patient with invasive monitoring?
6. R.K.'s pulmonary condition deteriorates. PaO$_2$ drops to 70 mm Hg, and SpO$_2$ is 89%. PEEP is increased to 7.5 cm H$_2$O. What implications does this have for R.K. given his hemodynamic status?
7. **Priority Decision:** Based on the data presented, what are the priority nursing diagnoses? Are there any collaborative problems?
8. **Delegation Decision:** What patient care activities can you delegate to unlicensed assistive personnel?
9. **Evidence-Based Practice:** R.K.'s family wants to know why he is getting tube feedings. What would you tell the family? What is the evidence to support the use of tube feedings?
10. After 4 days, R.K. remains unresponsive and has developed renal failure. The physician believes the patient will not recover from his neurologic injury and wishes to discuss goals of care with the patient's caregiver. What would be your role in this meeting?

ⓔvolve Answers available at *http://evolve.elsevier.com/Lewis/medsurg.*

▌BRIDGE TO NCLEX EXAMINATION

The number of the question corresponds to the same-numbered outcome at the beginning of the chapter.

1. Certification in critical care nursing (CCRN) by the American Association of Critical-Care Nurses indicates that the nurse
   a. is an advanced practice nurse who cares for acutely and critically ill patients.
   b. may practice independently to provide symptom management for the critically ill.
   c. has earned a master's degree in the field of advanced acute and critical care nursing.
   d. has practiced in critical care and successfully completed a test of critical care knowledge.

2. What are the appropriate nursing interventions for the patient with delirium in the ICU (*select all that apply*)?
   a. Use clocks and calendars to maintain orientation.
   b. Encourage round-the-clock presence of caregivers at the bedside.
   c. Sedate the patient with appropriate drugs to protect the patient from harmful behaviors.
   d. Silence all alarms, reduce overhead paging, and avoid conversations around the patient.
   e. Identify physiologic factors that may be contributing to the patient's confusion and irritability.

3. The critical care nurse recognizes that an ideal plan for caregiver involvement includes
   a. a caregiver at the bedside at all times.
   b. allowing caregivers at the bedside at preset, brief intervals.
   c. an individually devised plan to involve caregivers with care and comfort measures.
   d. restriction of visiting in the ICU because the environment is overwhelming to caregivers.

4. To establish hemodynamic monitoring for a patient, the nurse zeros the
   a. cardiac output monitoring system to the level of the left ventricle.
   b. pressure monitoring system to the level of the catheter tip located in the patient.
   c. pressure monitoring system to the level of the atrium, identified as the phlebostatic axis.
   d. pressure monitoring system to the level of the atrium, identified as the midclavicular line.

5. The hemodynamic changes the nurse expects to find after successful initiation of intraaortic balloon pump therapy in a patient with cardiogenic shock include *(select all that apply)*
   a. decreased SV.
   b. decreased SVR.
   c. decreased PAWP.
   d. increased diastolic BP.
   e. decreased myocardial oxygen consumption.
6. The purpose of adding PEEP to positive pressure ventilation is to
   a. increase functional residual capacity and improve oxygenation.
   b. increase FIO_2 in an attempt to wean the patient and avoid O_2 toxicity.
   c. determine if the patient is in synchrony with the ventilator or needs to be paralyzed.
   d. determine if the patient is able to be weaned and avoid the risk of pneumomediastinum.
7. The nursing management of a patient with an artificial airway includes
   a. maintaining ET tube cuff pressure at 30 cm H_2O.
   b. routine suctioning of the tube at least every 2 hours.
   c. observing for cardiac dysrhythmias during suctioning.
   d. preventing tube dislodgment by limiting mouth care to lubrication of the lips.

8. The nurse monitors the patient with positive pressure mechanical ventilation for
   a. paralytic ileus because pressure on the abdominal contents affects bowel motility.
   b. diuresis and sodium depletion because of increased release of atrial natriuretic peptide.
   c. signs of cardiovascular insufficiency because pressure in the chest impedes venous return.
   d. respiratory acidosis in a patient with COPD because of alveolar hyperventilation and increased PaO_2 levels.

1. d, 2. a, c, 3. c, 4. c, 5. b, c, d, e, 6. a, 7. c, 8. c

⊜volve

For rationales to these answers and even more NCLEX review questions, visit *http://evolve.elsevier.com/Lewis/medsurg.*

REFERENCES

1. American Association of Critical-Care Nurses: About critical care nursing. Retrieved from *www.aacn.org/WD/publishing/content/pressroom/aboutcriticalcarenursing.content.*
2. Jones DA, DeVita MA, Bellomo R: Rapid-response teams, *N Engl J Med* 365:139, 2011.
3. American Association of Critical-Care Nurses: Frequently asked questions about APRN Consensus Model implementation for NP programs. Retrieved from *www.aacn.org/WD/Certifications/Content/APRN-NP-FAQs.content.*
4. Wiegand DL-M, Williams LD: End-of-life care. In KK Carlson, editor: *Advanced critical care nursing*, St Louis, 2009, Saunders.
*5. McClave SA, Martindale RG, Vanek VW, et al: Guidelines for the provision and assessment of nutrition support therapy in the adult critically ill patient: Society of Critical Care Medicine and American Society for Parenteral and Enteral Nutrition, *J Parenter Enteral Nutr* 33:277, 2009.
*6. Woods S: Spiritual and complementary therapies to promote healing and reduce stress. In NC Molter, editor: *Protocols for practice: creating healing environments*, ed 2, Sudbury, Mass, 2007, Jones & Bartlett. (Classic)
*7. Arbour RB: Pain management. In NC Molter, editor: *Protocols for practice: creating healing environments*, ed 2, Sudbury, Mass, 2007, Jones & Bartlett. (Classic)
*8. Barr J, Fraser GL, Puntillo K, et al: Clinical practice guidelines for the management of pain, agitation, and delirium in adult patients in the intensive care unit, *Crit Care Med* 41:263, 2013.
*9. American Association of Critical-Care Nurses: Delirium assessment and management. Retrieved from *www.aacn.org/WD/practice/content/practicealerts/delirium-practice-alert.content.*
*10. Lawson N, Thompson K, Saunders G, et al: Sound intensity and noise evaluation in a critical care unit, *Am J Crit Care* 19:e88, 2010.

*11. Hellstrom A, Willman A: Promoting sleep by nursing interventions in health care settings: a systematic review, *Worldviews Evid Based Nurs* 8:128, 2011.
12. Institute for Patient and Family Centered Care: Advancing the practice of patient and family centered care in hospitals: how to get started. Retrieved from *www.ipfcc.org/pdf/getting_started.pdf.*
*13. Leske JS, Pasquale MA: Family needs, interventions and presence. In NC Molter, editor: *Protocols for practice: creating healing environments*, ed 2, Sudbury, Mass, 2007, Jones & Bartlett. (Classic)
*14. American Association of Critical-Care Nurses: AACN practice alert: family presence: visitation in the adult ICU. Retrieved from *www.aacn.org/WD/practice/docs/practicealerts/family-visitation-adult-icu-practicealert.pdf.*
15. Society of Critical Care Medicine: Patient and family resources: ICU issues and answers brochures. Retrieved from *www.myicucare.org/Support_Brochures/Pages/default.aspx.*
*16. American Association of Critical-Care Nurses: AACN practice alert: family presence during CPR and invasive procedures. Retrieved from *www.aacn.org/WD/Practice/Docs/PracticeAlerts/Family%20Presence%2004-2010%20final.pdf.*
*17. Medina J, Puntillo K, editors: *AACN protocols for practice: palliative care and end-of-life issues in critical care*, Sudbury, Mass, 2006, Jones & Bartlett. (Classic)
*18. Shaffer RB: Arterial catheter insertion (assist). In Wiegand DL-M, editor: *AACN procedure manual for critical care*, ed 6, St Louis, 2011, Saunders.
*19. Edwards Lifesciences: Understanding stroke volume variation and its clinical application. Retrieved from *http://ht.edwards.com/presentationvideos/powerpointslides/strokevolumevar/strokevolumevariation.pdf.*
*20. Kern ME: Arterial pressure-based cardiac output monitoring. In DL-M Wiegand, editor: *AACN procedure manual for critical care*, ed 6, St Louis, 2011, Saunders.
*21. Klein DG: Cardiac output measurement techniques (invasive). In DL-M Wiegand, editor: *AACN procedure manual for critical care*, ed 6, St Louis, 2011, Saunders.

*Evidence-based information for clinical practice.

*22. Headley JM, Giuliano KK: Continuous venous oxygenation monitoring. In DL-M Wiegand, editor: *AACN procedure manual for critical care*, ed 6, St Louis, 2011, Saunders.

*23. Castelluci D: Intraaortic balloon pump management. In Wiegand DL-M, editor: *AACN procedure manual for critical care*, ed 6, St Louis, 2011, Saunders.

*24. Puhlman M, Hargraves J: Ventricular assist devices. In Wiegand DL-M, editor: *AACN procedure manual for critical care*, ed 6, St Louis, 2011, Saunders.

25. Abiomed: The AbioCor system. Retrieved from *www.abiomed. com/products/heart-replacement*.

26. Mallick A, Bodenham AR: Tracheostomy in critically ill patients, *Eur J Anaesthesiol* 27:676, 2010.

27. Greene LR, Sposato K: APIC elimination guide: guide to the elimination of ventilator-associated pneumonia. Retrieved from *www.apic.org/Resource_/EliminationGuideForm/18e326ad-b484-471c-9c35-6822a53ee4a2/File/VAP_09.pdf*.

28. Light S: Rapid sequence intubation: stay up to date on this important procedure, *J Am Acad Physician Assistants* 23:37, 2010.

29. Walsh BK, Crotwell DN, Restrepo RD: Capnography/capnometry during mechanical ventilation, *Respir Care* 56:503, 2011.

*30. American Association of Respiratory Care: AARC clinical practice guidelines: endotracheal suctioning of mechanically ventilated patients with artificial airways, *Respir Care* 55:758, 2010.

*31. Sole ML, Su Z, Talbert S, et al: Evaluation of an intervention to maintain endotracheal tube cuff pressure within therapeutic range, *Am J Crit Care* 20:109, 2011.

*32. Chulay M, Seckel MA: Suctioning: endotracheal or tracheostomy tube. In DL-M Wiegand, editor: *AACN procedure manual for critical care*, ed 6, St Louis, 2011, Saunders.

*33. Lusk B, Lash AA: The stress response: psychoneuroimmunology and stress among ICU patients, *Dimens Crit Care Nurs* 24:25, 2005. (Classic)

*34. Thomas LA: Clinical management of stressors perceived by patients on mechanical ventilation, *AACN Clin Issues* 14:73, 2003. (Classic)

35. Jarachovic M, Mason M, Kerber K, et al: The role of standardized protocols in unplanned extubations in a medical intensive care unit, *Am J Crit Care* 20:304, 2011.

*36. Chang L, Wang KK, Yann-Fen C: Influence of physical restraint of unplanned extubation of adult intensive care patient: a case control study, *Am J Crit Care* 17:408, 2008.

*37. Happ MB: Communicating with mechanically ventilated patients: state of the science, *AACN Clin Issues* 12:247, 2001. (Classic)

*38. American Association of Critical-Care Nurses: AACN practice alert: prevention of aspiration. Retrieved from *www.aacn.org/WD/practice/docs/practicealerts/aacn-aspiration-practice-alert.pdf*.

*39. Burns SM: Invasive mechanical ventilation (through an artificial airway): volume and pressure modes. In Wiegand DL-M, editor: *AACN procedure manual for critical care*, ed 6, St Louis, 2011, Saunders.

*40. Burns SM: Noninvasive positive pressure ventilation: continuous positive airway pressure (CPAP) and bilevel positive airway pressure (BiPAP). In DL-M Wiegand, editor: *AACN procedure manual for critical care*, ed 6, St Louis, 2011, Saunders.

*41. Unoki T, Serita A, Grap MJ: Automatic tube compensation during weaning from mechanical ventilation: evidence and clinical implications, *Crit Care Nurs* 28:34, 2008.

42. Ali S, Ferguson ND: High-frequency oscillatory ventilation in ALI/ARDS, *Crit Care Clin* 27:487, 2011.

43. Dickinson S, Park PK, Napolitano LM: Prone-positioning therapy in ARDS, *Crit Care Clin* 27:511, 2011.

44. Park PK, Napolitano LM, Bartlett RH: Extracorporeal membrane oxygenation in adult acute respiratory distress syndrome, *Crit Care Clin* 27:627, 2011.

*45. American Association of Critical-Care Nurses: AACN practice alert: ventilator-associated pneumonia. Retrieved from *ww.aacn.org/WD/Practice/Docs/Ventilator_Associated_Pneumonia_1-2008.pdf*.

46. Institute for Healthcare Improvement: How-to guide: prevent ventilator-associated pneumonia. Retrieved from *www.ihi.org*.

47. FDA Drug Safety Communication: *Clostridium difficile*–associated diarrhea can be associated with stomach acid drugs known as proton pump inhibitors. Retrieved from *www.fda.gov/drugs/drugsafety/ucm290510.htm*.

*48. American Association of Critical-Care Nurses: AACN practice alert: verification of feeding tube placement. Retrieved from *www.aacn.org/wd/practice/content/feeding-tube-practice-alert.pcms?menu=practice*.

49. Vollman KM: Introduction to progressive mobility, *Crit Care Nurse* 30:S3, 2010.

50. Desai SV, Law TJ, Needham DM: Long-term complications of critical care, *Crit Care Med* 39:371, 2011.

*51. Burns SM: Weaning process. In DL-M Wiegand, editor: *AACN procedure manual for critical care*, ed 6, St Louis, 2011, Saunders.

52. American College of Chest Physicians: Home mechanical ventilation resource center. Retrieved from *www.chestnet.org/accp/article/home-mechanical-ventilation-resource-center*.

RESOURCES

American Association of Critical-Care Nurses
www.aacn.org
American Association for Respiratory Care
http://connect.aarc.org/Home
Society of Critical Care Medicine
www.sccm.org

Once you choose hope, anything's possible.
Christopher Reeve

Nursing Management
Shock, Systemic Inflammatory Response Syndrome, and Multiple Organ Dysfunction Syndrome

Maureen A. Seckel

evolve WEBSITE

http://evolve.elsevier.com/Lewis/medsurg

- NCLEX Review Questions
- Key Points
- Pre-Test
- Answer Guidelines for Case Study on p. 1652
- Rationales for Bridge to NCLEX Examination Questions

- Case Studies
  - Patient With Acute Pancreatitis and Septic Shock
  - Patient With Cardiogenic Shock
  - Patient With Sepsis
- Nursing Care Plan (Customizable)
  - eNCP 67-1: Patient in Shock
- Concept Map Creator
- Glossary
- Content Updates

eFigures
- eFig. 67-1: Compensatory stage of shock
- eFig. 67-2: Progressive stage of shock
- eFig. 67-3: Irreversible stage of shock
- eFig. 67-4: Sepsis alert treatment protocol
- eFig. 67-5: Anaphylaxis algorithm

LEARNING OUTCOMES

1. Relate the pathophysiology to the clinical manifestations of the different types of shock: cardiogenic, hypovolemic, distributive, and obstructive.
2. Compare the effects of shock, systemic inflammatory response syndrome, and multiple organ dysfunction syndrome on the major body systems.

3. Compare the collaborative care, drug therapy, and nursing management of patients experiencing different types of shock.
4. Describe the nursing management of a patient experiencing multiple organ dysfunction syndrome.

KEY TERMS

anaphylactic shock, p. 1636
cardiogenic shock, p. 1633
hypovolemic shock, p. 1633
multiple organ dysfunction syndrome (MODS), p. 1649

neurogenic shock, p. 1634
obstructive shock, p. 1637
sepsis, p. 1636
septic shock, p. 1636

shock, p. 1631
systemic inflammatory response syndrome (SIRS), p. 1649

Shock, systemic inflammatory response syndrome (SIRS), and multiple organ dysfunction syndrome (MODS) are serious and interrelated problems (Fig. 67-1). This chapter provides an overview of the different types of shock, SIRS, and MODS, and the related management of each.

SHOCK

Shock is a syndrome characterized by decreased tissue perfusion and impaired cellular metabolism. This results in an imbalance between the supply of and demand for oxygen and nutrients. The exchange of oxygen and nutrients at the cellular level is essential to life. When cells experience hypoperfusion, the demand for oxygen and nutrients exceeds the supply at the microcirculatory level.

Classification of Shock

The four main categories of shock are cardiogenic, hypovolemic, distributive, and obstructive[1,2] (Table 67-1). Although the cause, initial presentation, and management strategies vary

Reviewed by Lori Godaire, RN-BC, MS, CCRN, CNL, Clinical Nurse Leader, Critical Care Services, William W. Backus Hospital, Norwich, Connecticut; Janet E. Jackson, RN, MS, Assistant Professor, Department of Nursing, Bradley University, Peoria, Illinois; and Anna Moore, RN, MS, Associate Professor, J. Sargeant Reynolds Community College, Richmond, Virginia.

FIG. 67-1 Relationship of shock, systemic inflammatory response syndrome, and multiple organ dysfunction syndrome. *CNS*, Central nervous system. (See Table 67-1 for causes of shock states.)

TABLE 67-1 CLASSIFICATION OF SHOCK STATES

Types and Causes	Examples	Types and Causes	Examples
Cardiogenic Shock		**Distributive Shock**	
• Systolic dysfunction: inability of the heart to pump blood forward	Myocardial infarction, cardiomyopathy, blunt cardiac injury, severe systemic or pulmonary hypertension, myocardial depression from metabolic problems	**Neurogenic Shock**	
		• Hemodynamic consequence of spinal cord injury and/or disease at or above T5	Severe pain, drugs, hypoglycemia, injury
• Diastolic dysfunction: inability of the heart to fill	Cardiac tamponade, ventricular hypertrophy, cardiomyopathy	• Spinal anesthesia	
• Dysrhythmias	Bradydysrhythmias, tachydysrhythmias	• Vasomotor center depression	
• Structural factors	Valvular stenosis or regurgitation, ventricular septal rupture, tension pneumothorax	**Anaphylactic Shock**	
		• Hypersensitivity (allergic) reaction to a sensitizing substance	Contrast media, blood or blood products, drugs, insect bites, anesthetic agents, food or food additives, vaccines, environmental agents, latex
Hypovolemic Shock			
Absolute Hypovolemia			
• External loss of whole blood	Hemorrhage from trauma, surgery, GI bleeding	**Septic Shock**	
• Loss of other body fluids	Vomiting, diarrhea, excessive diuresis, diabetes insipidus, diabetes mellitus	• Infection	Pneumonia, peritonitis, urinary tract, invasive procedures, indwelling lines and catheters
Relative Hypovolemia		• At-risk patients	Older adults, patients with chronic diseases (e.g., diabetes mellitus, chronic kidney disease, heart failure), patients receiving immunosuppressive therapy or who are malnourished or debilitated
• Pooling of blood or fluids	Bowel obstruction		
• Fluid shifts	Burn injuries, ascites		
• Internal bleeding	Fracture of long bones, ruptured spleen, hemothorax, severe pancreatitis		
• Massive vasodilation	Sepsis	**Obstructive Shock**	
		• Physical obstruction impeding the filling or outflow of blood resulting in reduced cardiac output	Cardiac tamponade, tension pneumothorax, superior vena cava syndrome, abdominal compartment syndrome, pulmonary embolism

for each type of shock, the physiologic responses of the cells to hypoperfusion are similar.

Cardiogenic Shock. Cardiogenic shock occurs when either systolic or diastolic dysfunction of the heart's pumping action results in reduced cardiac output (CO). Causes of cardiogenic shock are listed in Table 67-1. Mortality rates for patients with cardiogenic shock approach 60%.[3] Decreased filling of the heart results in decreased stroke volume.

The heart's inability to pump the blood forward is called *systolic dysfunction.* Systolic dysfunction primarily affects the left ventricle, since systolic pressure is greater on the left side of the heart. When systolic dysfunction affects the right side of the heart, blood flow through the pulmonary circulation is reduced. The most common cause of systolic dysfunction is acute myocardial infarction (MI). Cardiogenic shock is the leading cause of death from acute MI.[4] Causes of diastolic dysfunction are listed in Table 67-1.

Fig. 67-2 describes the pathophysiology of cardiogenic shock. Whether the initiating event is myocardial ischemia, a structural problem (e.g., valvular disorder, ventricular septal rupture), or dysrhythmias, the physiologic responses are similar: the patient experiences impaired tissue perfusion and cellular metabolism.

The early clinical presentation of a patient with cardiogenic shock is similar to that of a patient with acute decompensated heart failure (see Chapter 35). The patient may have tachycardia and hypotension. Pulse pressure may be narrowed due to the heart's inability to pump blood forward during systole and increased volume during diastole. An increase in systemic vascular resistance (SVR) increases the workload of the heart, thus increasing the myocardial oxygen consumption. The heart's inability to pump blood forward also results in a low CO (less than 4 L/minute) and *cardiac index* (less than 2.5 L/min/m²).

On assessment, the patient is tachypneic and has crackles on auscultation of breath sounds because of pulmonary congestion. The hemodynamic profile demonstrates an increase in the pulmonary artery wedge pressure (PAWP), stroke volume variation (SVV), and pulmonary vascular resistance.

Signs of peripheral hypoperfusion (e.g., cyanosis, pallor, diaphoresis, weak peripheral pulses, cool and clammy skin, delayed capillary refill) are seen. Decreased renal blood flow results in sodium and water retention and decreased urine output. Anxiety, confusion, and agitation may develop as cerebral perfusion is impaired. Tables 67-2 and 67-3 describe the laboratory findings and clinical presentation of a patient with cardiogenic shock.

Hypovolemic Shock. Hypovolemic shock occurs after a loss of intravascular fluid volume (see Table 67-1). The volume is inadequate to fill the vascular space. The volume loss may be either an absolute or a relative volume loss. *Absolute hypovolemia* results when fluid is lost through hemorrhage, gastrointestinal (GI) loss (e.g., vomiting, diarrhea), fistula drainage, diabetes insipidus, or diuresis. In *relative hypovolemia,* fluid volume moves out of the vascular space into the extravascular space (e.g., intracavitary space). This type of fluid shift is called *third spacing.* One example of relative volume loss is leakage of fluid from the vascular space to the interstitial space from increased capillary permeability, as seen in burns (see Chapter 25).

In hypovolemic shock the size of the vascular compartment remains unchanged while the volume of blood or plasma decreases. Whether the loss of intravascular volume is absolute or relative, the physiologic consequences are similar. A reduction in intravascular volume results in a decreased venous return to the heart, decreased preload, decreased stroke volume, and decreased CO. A cascade of events results in decreased tissue perfusion and impaired cellular metabolism, the hallmarks of shock (Fig. 67-3).

The patient's response to acute volume loss depends on a number of factors, including extent of injury, age, and general state of health. However, the clinical presentation of hypovolemic shock is consistent (see Table 67-3). An overall assessment of physiologic reserves may indicate the patient's ability to compensate. A patient may compensate for a loss of up to 15% of the total blood volume (approximately 750 mL). Further loss of volume (15% to 30%) results in a sympathetic nervous system (SNS)–mediated response. This response results in an increase in heart rate, CO, and respiratory rate and depth. The stroke volume, central venous pressure (CVP), and PAWP are decreased because of the decreased circulating blood volume.

The patient may appear anxious, and urine output begins to decrease. If hypovolemia is corrected by crystalloid fluid replacement at this time, tissue dysfunction is generally reversible. If volume loss is greater than 30%, compensatory mechanisms may begin to fail and immediate replacement with blood products should be started. Loss of autoregulation in the microcirculation and irreversible tissue destruction occur with loss of more than 40% of the total blood volume.[5,6] Common laboratory studies and assessments that are done include serial measurements of hemoglobin and hematocrit levels, electrolytes, lactate, blood gases, mixed central venous oxygen saturation (SvO₂), and hourly urine outputs (see Table 67-2).

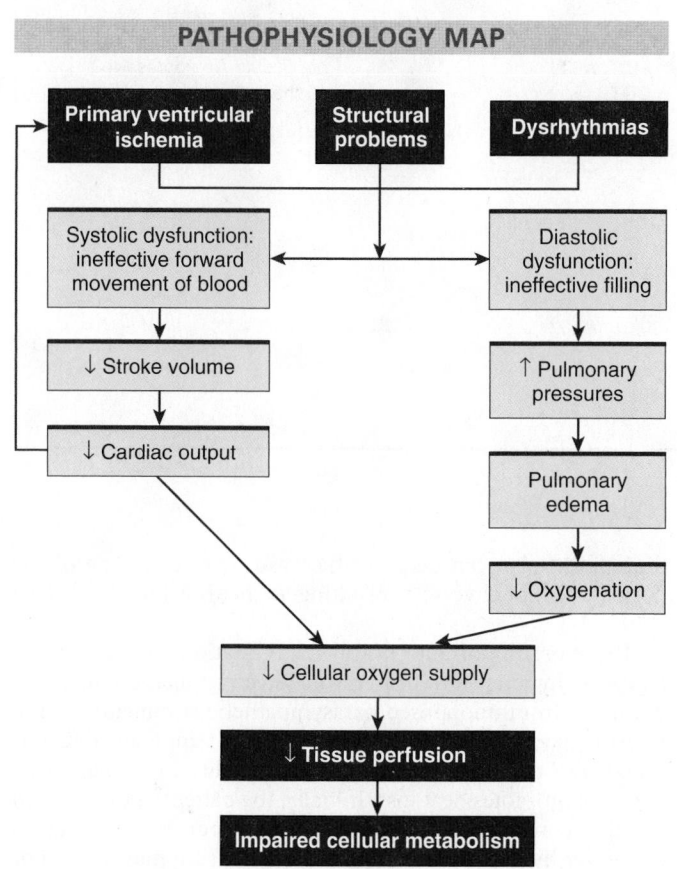

PATHOPHYSIOLOGY MAP

FIG. 67-2 The pathophysiology of cardiogenic shock.

TABLE 67-2   DIAGNOSTIC STUDIES

Laboratory Changes in Shock

Laboratory Study	Finding	Significance of Finding
Red blood cells		
RBC count, hematocrit, hemoglobin	Normal	Remains within normal limits in shock because of relative hypovolemia and pump failure and in hemorrhagic shock before fluid resuscitation.
	↓	Hemorrhagic shock after fluid resuscitation when fluids other than blood are used.
	↑	Nonhemorrhagic shock caused by actual hypovolemia and hemoconcentration.
White blood cells		
WBC count, bands	↑	Infection, septic shock.
DIC screen		Acute DIC can develop within hours to days after an initial assault on the body (e.g., shock).
• Fibrin split products (FSP)	↑	
• Fibrinogen level	↓	
• Platelet count	↓	
• PTT and PT	↑	
• INR	↑	
• Thrombin time	↑	
• D-dimer	↑	
Creatine kinase	↑	Trauma, myocardial infarction in response to cellular damage and/or hypoxia.
Troponin	↑	Increases in myocardial infarction.
BUN	↑	Indicates impaired kidney function caused by hypoperfusion as a result of severe vasoconstriction, or occurs secondary to catabolism of cells (e.g., trauma, infection).
Creatinine	↑	Indicates impaired kidney function caused by hypoperfusion as a result of severe vasoconstriction. Is more sensitive indicator of renal function than BUN.
Glucose	↑	Found in early shock because of release of liver glycogen stores in response to sympathetic nervous system stimulation and cortisol. Insulin insensitivity develops.
	↓	Occurs because of depleted glycogen stores with hepatocellular dysfunction possible as shock progresses.

Laboratory Study	Finding	Significance of Finding
Serum electrolytes		
• Sodium	↑	Found in early shock because of increased secretion of aldosterone, causing renal retention of sodium.
	↓	May occur iatrogenically when excess hypotonic fluid is administered after fluid loss.
• Potassium	↑	Results when cellular death liberates intracellular potassium. Also occurs in acute kidney injury and acidosis.
	↓	Found in early shock because of increased secretion of aldosterone, causing renal excretion of potassium.
Arterial blood gases	Respiratory alkalosis	Found in early shock secondary to hyperventilation.
	Metabolic acidosis	Occurs later in shock when lactate accumulates in blood from anaerobic metabolism.
Base deficit	>−6	Indicates acid production secondary to hypoxia.
Blood cultures	Growth of organisms	May grow organisms in patients who are in septic shock.
Lactate level	↑	Usually increases once significant hypoperfusion and impaired oxygen utilization at the cellular level have occurred. By-product of anaerobic metabolism.
Liver enzymes (ALT, AST, GGT)	↑	Elevations indicate liver cell destruction in progressive stage of shock.

ALT, Alanine aminotransferase; *AST*, aspartate aminotransferase; *BUN*, blood urea nitrogen; *DIC*, disseminated intravascular coagulation; *GGT*, γ-glutamyl transferase; *INR*, international normalized ratio; *PT*, prothrombin time; *PTT*, partial thromboplastin time.

Distributive Shock

Neurogenic Shock. Neurogenic shock is a hemodynamic phenomenon that can occur within 30 minutes of a spinal cord injury at the fifth thoracic (T5) vertebra or above; it can last up to 6 weeks. The injury results in a massive vasodilation without compensation because of the loss of SNS vasoconstrictor tone. This massive vasodilation leads to a pooling of blood in the blood vessels, tissue hypoperfusion, and ultimately impaired cellular metabolism (Fig. 67-4).

In addition to spinal cord injury, spinal anesthesia can block transmission of impulses from the SNS. Depression of the vasomotor center of the medulla from drugs (e.g., opioids, benzo-diazepines) also can decrease the vasoconstrictor tone of the peripheral blood vessels, resulting in neurogenic shock (see Table 67-1).

The most important clinical manifestations in neurogenic shock are hypotension (from the massive vasodilation) and bradycardia (from unopposed parasympathetic stimulation).[7] The patient may not be able to regulate body temperature. Combined with massive vasodilation, the inability to regulate temperature promotes heat loss. Initially, the patient's skin is warm due to the massive dilation. As the heat disperses, the patient is at risk for hypothermia. Later, the patient's skin may be cool or warm depending on the ambient temperature (*poikilothermia—*

TABLE 67-3 CLINICAL PRESENTATION OF TYPES OF SHOCK

		Distributive Shock			
Cardiogenic Shock	**Hypovolemic Shock**	**Neurogenic Shock**	**Anaphylactic Shock**	**Septic Shock**	**Obstructive Shock**
Cardiovascular System					
Tachycardia ↓ BP ↓ Capillary refill Chest pain may or may not be present	↓ Preload ↓ Stroke volume ↓ Capillary refill	↓ BP ↓/↑ Temperature Bradycardia	Chest pain Third spacing of fluid	↓/↑ Temperature Myocardial dysfunction Biventricular dilation ↓ Ejection fraction	↓ BP ↓ Preload
Pulmonary System					
Tachypnea Crackles Cyanosis Rhonchi	Tachypnea → bradypnea (late)	Dysfunction related to level of injury	Shortness of breath Edema of larynx and epiglottis Wheezing Stridor Rhinitis	Hyperventilation Crackles Respiratory alkalosis → respiratory acidosis Hypoxemia Respiratory failure ARDS Pulmonary hypertension	Tachypnea → bradypnea (late) Shortness of breath
Renal System					
↑ Na⁺ and H₂O retention ↓ Renal blood flow ↓ Urine output	↓ Urine output	Bladder dysfunction	Incontinence	↓ Urine output	↓ Urine output
Skin					
Pallor Cool, clammy	Pallor Cool, clammy	↓ Skin perfusion Cool or warm Dry	Flushing Pruritus Urticaria Angioedema	Warm and flushed → cool and mottled (late)	Pallor Cool, clammy
Neurologic System					
↓ Cerebral perfusion: • Anxiety • Confusion • Agitation	↓ Cerebral perfusion: • Anxiety • Confusion • Agitation	Flaccid paralysis below the level of the lesion Loss of reflex activity	Anxiety Feeling of impending doom Confusion ↓ LOC Metallic taste	Alteration in mental status (e.g., confusion) Agitation Coma (late)	↓ Cerebral perfusion: • Anxiety • Confusion • Agitation
Gastrointestinal System					
↓ Bowel sounds Nausea, vomiting	Absent bowel sounds	Bowel dysfunction	Cramping Abdominal pain Nausea Vomiting Diarrhea	GI bleeding Paralytic ileus	↓ to absent bowel sounds
Diagnostic Findings*					
↑ Cardiac markers ↑ b-Type natriuretic peptide (BNP) ↑ Blood glucose ↑ BUN ECG (e.g., dysrhythmias) Echocardiogram (e.g., left ventricular dysfunction) Chest x-ray (e.g., pulmonary infiltrates)	↓ Hematocrit ↓ Hemoglobin ↑ Lactate ↑ Urine specific gravity Changes in electrolytes		Sudden onset History of allergies Exposure to contrast media	↑/↓ WBC ↓ Platelets ↑ Lactate ↑ Blood glucose ↑ Urine specific gravity ↓ Urine Na⁺ Positive blood cultures	Specific to cause of obstruction

*Also see Table 67-2.
ARDS, Acute respiratory distress syndrome; *BUN*, blood urea nitrogen; *LOC*, level of consciousness;

PATHOPHYSIOLOGY MAP

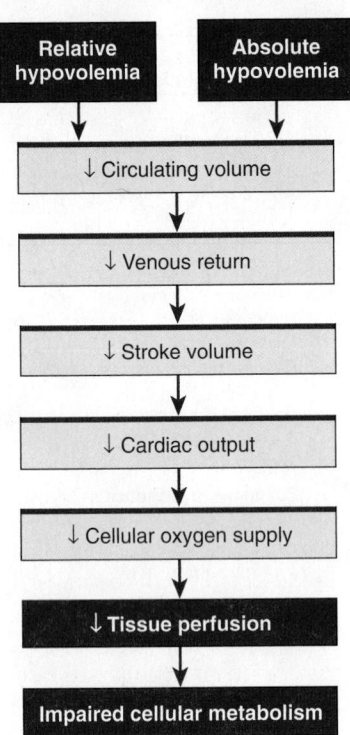

FIG. 67-3 The pathophysiology of hypovolemic shock.

PATHOPHYSIOLOGY MAP

FIG. 67-4 The pathophysiology of neurogenic shock.

taking on the temperature of the environment). In either case, the skin is usually dry. Tables 67-2 and 67-3 further describe the laboratory findings and clinical presentation of a patient with neurogenic shock.

Although spinal shock and neurogenic shock often occur in the same patient, they are not the same disorder. *Spinal shock* is a transient condition that is present after an acute spinal cord injury (see Chapter 61). The patient with spinal shock experiences the absence of all voluntary and reflex neurologic activity below the level of the injury.

Anaphylactic Shock. Anaphylactic shock is an acute, life-threatening hypersensitivity (allergic) reaction to a sensitizing substance (e.g., drug, chemical, vaccine, food, insect venom). The reaction quickly causes massive vasodilation, release of vasoactive mediators, and an increase in capillary permeability. As capillary permeability increases, fluid leaks from the vascular space into the interstitial space. Anaphylactic shock can lead to respiratory distress due to laryngeal edema or severe bronchospasm, and circulatory failure from the massive vasodilation.[8] The patient has a sudden onset of symptoms, including dizziness, chest pain, incontinence, swelling of the lips and tongue, wheezing, and stridor. Skin changes include flushing, pruritus, urticaria, and angioedema. In addition, the patient may be anxious and confused and have a sense of impending doom.

A patient can have a severe allergic reaction, possibly leading to anaphylactic shock, after contact, inhalation, ingestion, or injection with an antigen (allergen) to which the individual has previously been sensitized (see Table 67-1). Parenteral administration of the antigen (allergen) is the route most likely to cause anaphylaxis. However, oral, topical, and inhalation routes can also cause anaphylactic reactions. Tables 67-2 and 67-3

describe the laboratory findings and clinical presentation of a patient in anaphylactic shock. Quick and decisive action is critical to prevent the progression of an allergic reaction to anaphylactic shock. (Anaphylaxis is discussed in Chapter 14.)

Septic Shock. Sepsis is a systemic inflammatory response to a documented or suspected infection (Table 67-4). In as many as 10% to 30% of patients with sepsis, the causative organism is not identified. *Severe sepsis,* defined as sepsis complicated by organ dysfunction, is diagnosed in more than 750,000 patients per year and has mortality rates as high as 28% to 50%.[9-11]

Septic shock is the presence of sepsis with hypotension despite adequate fluid resuscitation, along with inadequate tissue perfusion resulting in tissue hypoxia. The main organisms that cause sepsis are gram-negative and gram-positive bacteria. Parasites, fungi, and viruses can also cause sepsis and septic shock.[12] Fig. 67-5 presents the pathogenesis of septic shock.

When a microorganism enters the body, the normal immune or inflammatory responses are started. However, in severe sepsis and septic shock the body's response to the microorganism is exaggerated. Inflammation and coagulation increase, and fibrinolysis decreases. Endotoxins from the microorganism cell wall stimulate the release of cytokines, including tumor necrosis factor (TNF), interleukin-1 (IL-1), and other proinflammatory mediators that act through secondary mediators such as platelet-activating factor, IL-6, and IL-8.[12] (See Chapter 12 for discussion of the inflammatory response.) The release of platelet-activating factor results in the formation of microthrombi and obstruction of the microvasculature. The combined effects of the mediators

TABLE 67-4   DIAGNOSTIC CRITERIA FOR SEPSIS

Infection, documented or suspected, and some of the following.

General Variables
- Fever (temperature >100.9° F [38.3° C])
- Hypothermia (core temperature <97.0° F [36° C])
- Heart rate >90 beats/min
- Tachypnea
- Altered mental status
- Significant edema or positive fluid balance (>20 mL/kg over 24 hr)
- Hyperglycemia (blood glucose >140 mg/dL) in the absence of diabetes

Inflammatory Variables
- Leukocytosis (WBC count >12,000/µL)
- Leukopenia (WBC count <4000/µL)
- Normal WBC count with >10% immature forms
- Elevated C-reactive protein
- Elevated procalcitonin

Hemodynamic Variables
- Arterial hypotension (SBP <90 mm Hg, MAP <70 mm Hg, or a decrease in SBP >40 mm Hg)

Organ Dysfunction Variables
- Arterial hypoxemia (PaO_2/FIO_2 <300)
- Acute oliguria (urine output <0.5 mL/kg/hr for at least 2 hr despite adequate fluid resuscitation)
- Serum creatinine increase >0.5 mg/dL
- Coagulation abnormalities (INR >1.5 or PTT >60 sec)
- Ileus (absent bowel sounds)
- Thrombocytopenia (platelet count <100,000/µL)
- Hyperbilirubinemia (total bilirubin >4 mg/dL)

Tissue Perfusion Variables
- Hyperlactatemia (>1 mmol/L)
- Decreased capillary refill or mottling

Source: Dellinger RP, Levy MM, Rhodes A, et al: Surviving sepsis campaign: international guidelines for management of severe sepsis and septic shock: 2012, *Crit Care Med* 41:580, 2013.
FIO_2, Fraction of inspired oxygen; *INR*, international normalized ratio; *MAP*, mean arterial pressure; PaO_2, partial pressure of arterial oxygen; *PTT*, partial thromboplastin time; *SBP*, systolic blood pressure.

result in damage to the endothelium, vasodilation, increased capillary permeability, and neutrophil and platelet aggregation and adhesion to the endothelium.

Septic shock has three major pathophysiologic effects: vasodilation, maldistribution of blood flow, and myocardial depression. Patients may be euvolemic, but because of acute vasodilation, relative hypovolemia and hypotension occur. In addition, blood flow in the microcirculation is decreased, causing poor oxygen delivery and tissue hypoxia. The combination of TNF and IL-1 is thought to have a role in sepsis-induced myocardial dysfunction. The ejection fraction is decreased for the first few days after the initial insult. Because of a decreased ejection fraction, the ventricles dilate to maintain the stroke volume. The ejection fraction typically improves, and ventricular dilation resolves over 7 to 10 days. Persistence of a high CO and a low SVR beyond 24 hours is an ominous finding and is often associated with an increased development of hypotension and MODS. Coronary artery perfusion and myocardial oxygen metabolism are not primarily altered in septic shock.

In addition to the cardiovascular dysfunction that accompanies sepsis, respiratory failure is common. The patient initially

hyperventilates as a compensatory mechanism, resulting in respiratory alkalosis. Once the patient can no longer compensate, respiratory acidosis develops. Respiratory failure develops in 85% of patients with sepsis, and 40% develop acute respiratory distress syndrome (ARDS) (see Chapter 68). These patients need to be intubated and mechanically ventilated. Other clinical signs of septic shock include alteration in neurologic status; decreased urine output; and GI dysfunction, such as GI bleeding and paralytic ileus. Table 67-3 gives the clinical presentation of a patient with septic shock.

Obstructive Shock. Obstructive shock develops when a physical obstruction to blood flow occurs with a decreased CO (Fig. 67-6). This can be caused by restricted diastolic filling of the right ventricle from compression (e.g., cardiac tamponade, tension pneumothorax, superior vena cava syndrome). Other causes include *abdominal compartment syndrome* in which increased abdominal pressures compress the inferior vena cava, thus decreasing venous return to the heart (see Chapter 43). Pulmonary embolism and right ventricular thrombi cause an outflow obstruction as blood leaves the right ventricle through the pulmonary artery. This leads to decreased blood flow to the lungs and decreased blood return to the left atrium.

Patients experience a decreased CO, increased afterload, and variable left ventricular filling pressures depending on the obstruction. Other clinical signs include jugular venous distention and pulsus paradoxus (see Table 37-5). Rapid assessment and treatment are important to prevent further hemodynamic compromise and possibly cardiac arrest (see Fig. 67-6).

Stages of Shock

In addition to an understanding of the underlying pathogenesis of the type of shock that the patient is experiencing, monitoring and management are guided by knowing where the patient is on the shock "continuum." This continuum begins with the initial stage of shock that occurs at a cellular level and is usually not clinically apparent. Metabolism changes at the cellular level from aerobic to anaerobic, causing lactic acid buildup. Lactic acid is a waste product that is removed by the liver. However, this process requires oxygen, which is unavailable because of the decrease in tissue perfusion. Shock is categorized into three clinically apparent but overlapping stages: compensatory stage, progressive stage, and irreversible stage.[5]

Compensatory Stage. In the *compensatory stage* the body activates neural, hormonal, and biochemical compensatory mechanisms in an attempt to overcome the increasing consequences of anaerobic metabolism and to maintain homeostasis. (See eFig. 67-1 on the website for this chapter.) The patient's clinical presentation begins to reflect the body's responses to the imbalance in oxygen supply and demand (Table 67-5).

One of the classic signs of shock is a drop in blood pressure (BP), which occurs because of a decrease in CO and a narrowing of the pulse pressure. The baroreceptors in the carotid and aortic bodies immediately respond by activating the SNS. The SNS stimulates vasoconstriction and the release of the potent vasoconstrictors epinephrine and norepinephrine. Blood flow to the most essential (vital) organs, the heart and brain, is maintained, while blood flow to the nonvital organs, such as kidneys, GI tract, skin, and lungs, is diverted or shunted.

The myocardium responds to the SNS stimulation and the increase in oxygen demand by increasing the heart rate and contractility. However, increased contractility increases myocardial oxygen consumption. The coronary arteries dilate in

PATHOPHYSIOLOGY MAP

FIG. 67-5 The pathophysiology of septic shock. *CNS,* Central nervous system.

PATHOPHYSIOLOGY MAP

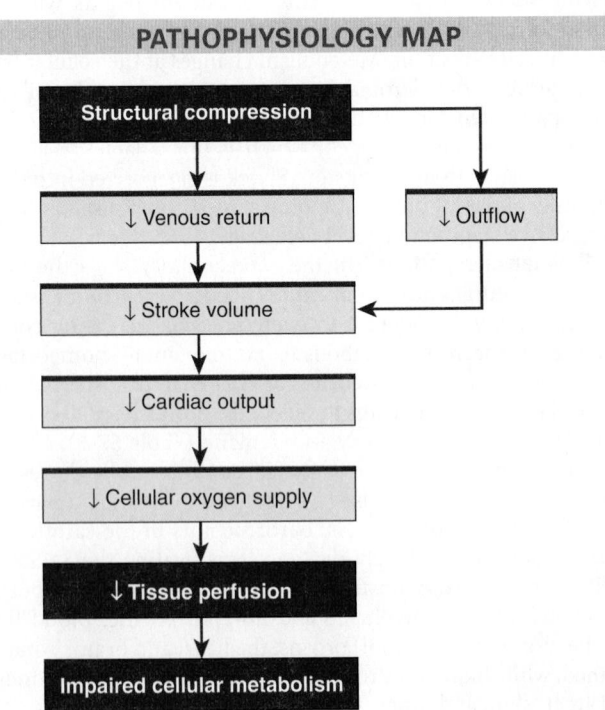

FIG. 67-6 The pathophysiology of obstructive shock.

an attempt to meet the increased oxygen demands of the myocardium.

Shunting blood away from the lungs has an important clinical effect in the patient in shock. Decreased blood flow to the lungs increases the patient's physiologic dead space. *Physiologic dead space* is the anatomic dead space (the amount of air that will not reach gas-exchanging units) and any inspired air that cannot participate in gas exchange. The clinical result of an increase in dead space ventilation is a *ventilation-perfusion mismatch.* Some areas of the lungs that are participating in ventilation will not be perfused because of the decreased blood flow to the lungs. Arterial oxygen levels will decrease, and the patient will have a compensatory increase in the rate and depth of respirations (see Chapter 68).

The shunting of blood from other organ systems also results in clinically important changes. The decrease in blood flow to the GI tract results in impaired motility and a slowing of peristalsis. This increases the risk for the development of a paralytic ileus.

Decreased blood flow to the skin results in the patient feeling cool and clammy. The exception is the patient in early septic shock who may feel warm and flushed because of a hyperdynamic state. Decreased blood flow to the kidneys activates the renin-angiotensin system. Renin stimulates angiotensinogen to produce angiotensin I, which is then converted to angiotensin II (see Fig. 45-4). Angiotensin II is a potent vasoconstrictor that causes both arterial and venous vasoconstriction. The net result is an increase in venous return to the heart and an increase in

TABLE 67-5 MANIFESTATIONS OF STAGES OF SHOCK*

Compensatory Stage	Progressive Stage	Irreversible Stage
Neurologic System		
Oriented to person, place, time	↓ Cerebral perfusion pressure	Unresponsive
Restless, apprehensive, confused	↓ Cerebral blood flow	Areflexia (loss of reflexes)
Change in level of consciousness	↓ Responsiveness to stimuli	Pupils nonreactive and dilated
	Delirium	
Cardiovascular System		
Sympathetic nervous system response:	↑ Capillary permeability → systemic interstitial edema	Profound hypotension
• Release of epinephrine/	↓ Cardiac output → ↓ BP and ↑ HR	↓ Cardiac output
norepinephrine (vasoconstriction)	MAP <60 mm Hg (or 40 mm Hg drop in BP from baseline)	Bradycardia, irregular rhythm
• ↑ MVO$_2$	↓ Coronary perfusion → dysrhythmias, myocardial ischemia,	↓ BP inadequate to perfuse vital organs
• ↑ Contractility	myocardial infarction	
• ↑ HR	↓ Peripheral perfusion → ischemia of distal extremities,	
Coronary artery dilation	diminished pulses, ↓ capillary refill	
Narrowed pulse pressure		
↓ BP		
Respiratory System		
↓ Blood flow to the lungs:	Acute respiratory distress syndrome (ARDS):	Severe refractory hypoxemia
• ↑ Physiologic dead space	• ↑ Capillary permeability	Respiratory failure
• ↑ Ventilation-perfusion mismatch	• Pulmonary vasoconstriction	
• Hyperventilation	• Pulmonary interstitial edema	
• ↑ Minute ventilation (V$_E$)	• Alveolar edema	
• Tachypnea	• Diffuse infiltrates	
	• Tachypnea	
	• ↓ Compliance	
	• Moist crackles	
Gastrointestinal System		
↓ Blood supply	Vasoconstriction and ↓ perfusion → ischemic gut (e.g.,	Ischemic gut
↓ GI motility	stomach, small and large intestines, gallbladder, pancreas)	
Hypoactive bowel sounds	• Erosive ulcers	
↑ Risk for paralytic ileus	• GI bleeding	
	• Translocation of GI bacteria	
	• Impaired absorption of nutrients	
Renal System		
↓ Renal blood flow	Renal tubules become ischemic → acute tubular necrosis	Anuria
↑ Renin resulting in release of	↓ Urine output	
angiotensin (vasoconstrictor)	↑ BUN/creatinine ratio	
↑ Aldosterone resulting in Na$^+$ and H$_2$O	↑ Urine sodium	
reabsorption	↓ Urine osmolality and specific gravity	
↑ Antidiuretic hormone resulting in H$_2$O	↓ Urine potassium	
reabsorption	Metabolic acidosis	
Hepatic System		
	Failure to metabolize drugs and waste products	Metabolic changes from accumulation of
	Cell death (↑ liver enzymes)	waste products (e.g., NH$_3$, lactate, CO$_2$)
	Jaundice (decreased clearance of bilirubin)	
	↑ NH$_3$ and lactate	
Hematologic System		
	DIC	DIC progresses
	• Thrombin clots in microcirculation	
	• Consumption of platelets and clotting factors	
Temperature		
Normal or abnormal	Hypothermia or hyperthermia	Hypothermia
Skin		
Pale and cool	Cold and clammy	Mottled, cyanotic
Warm and flushed		

*Also see Table 67-2 and Table 67-3.
DIC, Disseminated intravascular coagulation; *MAP*, mean arterial pressure; *MVO$_2$*, myocardial oxygen consumption; *NH$_3$*, ammonia.

BP. Angiotensin II also stimulates the adrenal cortex to release aldosterone. This results in sodium and water reabsorption and potassium excretion by the kidneys. The increase in sodium reabsorption raises the serum osmolality and stimulates the release of antidiuretic hormone (ADH) from the posterior pituitary gland. ADH increases water reabsorption by the kidneys, thus further increasing blood volume. The increase in total circulating volume results in an increase in CO and BP.

A multisystem response to decreasing tissue perfusion is initiated in the compensatory stage of shock. At this stage the body is able to compensate for the changes in tissue perfusion. If the cause of the shock is corrected, the patient will recover with little or no residual effects. If the cause of the shock is not corrected and the body is unable to compensate, the patient enters the progressive stage of shock.

Progressive Stage. The *progressive stage* of shock begins as compensatory mechanisms fail. (See eFig. 67-2 on the website for this chapter.) Changes in the patient's mental status are important findings in this stage.

The cardiovascular system is profoundly affected in the progressive stage of shock. CO begins to fall, resulting in a decrease in BP and coronary artery, cerebral, and peripheral perfusion. Continued decreased cellular perfusion and resulting altered capillary permeability are the distinguishing features of this stage. Altered capillary permeability allows leakage of fluid and protein out of the vascular space into the surrounding interstitial space. In addition to the decrease in circulating volume, there is an increase in systemic interstitial edema. The patient may have *anasarca* (diffuse profound edema). Fluid leakage from the vascular space also affects the solid organs (e.g., liver, spleen, GI tract, lungs) and peripheral tissues by further decreasing perfusion.

Sustained hypoperfusion results in weak peripheral pulses, and ischemia of the distal extremities eventually occurs. Myocardial dysfunction from decreased perfusion results in dysrhythmias, myocardial ischemia, and possibly MI. The end result is a complete deterioration of the cardiovascular system.

The pulmonary system is often the first system to display signs of critical dysfunction. During the compensatory stage, blood flow to the lungs is already reduced. In response to the decreased blood flow and the SNS stimulation, the pulmonary arterioles constrict, resulting in increased pulmonary artery (PA) pressure. As the pressure within the pulmonary vasculature increases, blood flow to the pulmonary capillaries decreases and ventilation-perfusion mismatch worsens.

Another key response in the lungs is the movement of fluid from the pulmonary vasculature into the interstitial space. As capillary permeability increases, the movement of fluid to the interstitial spaces results in interstitial edema, bronchoconstriction, and a decrease in functional residual capacity. With further increases in capillary permeability, the fluid moves to the alveoli, with resultant alveolar edema and a decrease in surfactant production. The combined effects of pulmonary vasoconstriction and bronchoconstriction are impaired gas exchange, decreased compliance, and worsening ventilation-perfusion mismatch. Clinically, the patient has tachypnea, crackles, and an overall increased work of breathing.

The GI system is also affected by prolonged decreased tissue perfusion. As the blood supply to the GI tract is decreased, the normally protective mucosal barrier becomes ischemic. This ischemia predisposes the patient to ulcers and GI bleeding (see Chapter 42). It also increases the risk of bacterial migration

from the GI tract to the blood. The decreased perfusion to the GI tract also leads to a decreased ability to absorb nutrients.

The effect of prolonged hypoperfusion on the kidneys is renal tubular ischemia. The resulting acute tubular necrosis may lead to acute kidney injury. This can be worsened by nephrotoxic drugs (e.g., certain antibiotics, anesthetics, diuretics) (see Chapter 47). The patient has decreased urine output and elevated blood urea nitrogen (BUN) and serum creatinine. Metabolic acidosis occurs from the kidneys' inability to excrete acids (especially lactic acid) and reabsorb bicarbonate.

Other organ systems are also affected by the sustained hypoperfusion in the progressive stage of shock. The loss of the functional ability of the liver leads to a failure of the liver to metabolize drugs and waste products (e.g., lactate, ammonia). Jaundice results from an accumulation of bilirubin. As the liver cells die, enzymes become elevated (e.g., alanine aminotransferase, aspartate aminotransferase, γ-glutamyl transferase). The liver also loses its ability to function as an immune organ. Bacteria that may move from the GI tract are no longer destroyed by the Kupffer cells. Instead, they are released into the bloodstream, thus increasing the possibility of bacteremia.[12]

Dysfunction of the hematologic system adds to the complexity of the clinical picture. The patient is at risk for disseminated intravascular coagulation (DIC), in which consumption of the platelets and clotting factors with secondary fibrinolysis results in clinically significant bleeding from many orifices. These include, but are not limited to, the GI tract, lungs, and puncture sites (see Chapter 31). Altered laboratory values in DIC are presented in Table 67-3.

In this stage, aggressive interventions are necessary to prevent the development of MODS.

Irreversible Stage. In the final stage of shock, the *irreversible stage,* decreased perfusion from peripheral vasoconstriction and decreased CO exacerbate anaerobic metabolism. (See eFig. 67-3 on the website for this chapter.) The accumulation of lactic acid contributes to increased capillary permeability and dilation. Increased capillary permeability allows fluid and plasma proteins to leave the vascular space and move to the interstitial space. Blood pools in the capillary beds secondary to the constricted venules and dilated arterioles. The loss of intravascular volume worsens hypotension and tachycardia and decreases coronary blood flow. Decreased coronary blood flow leads to worsening myocardial depression and a further decline in CO. Cerebral blood flow cannot be maintained, and cerebral ischemia results.

The patient in this stage of shock demonstrates profound hypotension and hypoxemia. The failure of the liver, lungs, and kidneys results in an accumulation of waste products, such as lactate, urea, ammonia, and carbon dioxide. The failure of one organ system affects several other organ systems. In this final stage, recovery is unlikely. The organs are in failure and the body's compensatory mechanisms are overwhelmed (see Table 67-5).

Diagnostic Studies

There is no single diagnostic study to determine whether a patient is in shock. Establishing a diagnosis begins with a history and physical examination. Obtaining a thorough medical and surgical history, and a history of recent events (e.g., surgery, chest pain, trauma), provides valuable data.

Decreased tissue perfusion in shock leads to an elevation of lactate and a base deficit (the amount needed to bring the pH back to normal). These laboratory changes may reflect an increase in anaerobic metabolism. Table 67-2 summarizes other laboratory findings seen in shock.

Additional diagnostic studies include a 12-lead electrocardiogram (ECG), continuous ECG monitoring, chest x-ray, continuous pulse oximetry, and hemodynamic monitoring (e.g., arterial pressure, central venous or PA pressure, $ScvO_2/SvO_2$). (Chapter 66 discusses hemodynamic monitoring.)

Collaborative Care: General Measures

Critical factors in the successful management of a patient experiencing shock relate to the early recognition and treatment of the shock state. Prompt intervention in the early stages of shock may prevent the decline to the progressive or irreversible stage. Successful management of the patient in shock includes the following:

1. Identification of patients at risk for developing shock
2. Integration of the patient's history, physical examination, and clinical findings to establish a diagnosis
3. Interventions to control or eliminate the cause of the decreased perfusion
4. Protection of target and distal organs from dysfunction
5. Provision of multisystem supportive care

Table 67-6 provides an overview of the initial assessment findings and interventions for the emergency care of patients in shock.[13,14] General management strategies begin with ensuring that the patient has a patent airway. Once the airway is established, either naturally or with an endotracheal tube, oxygen delivery must be optimized. Supplemental oxygen and mechanical ventilation may be necessary to maintain an arterial oxygen saturation of 90% or more (PaO_2 greater than 60 mm Hg) to avoid hypoxemia (see Chapter 66). The mean arterial pressure (MAP) and circulating blood volume are optimized with fluid replacement and drug therapy.

Oxygen and Ventilation. Oxygen delivery depends on CO, available hemoglobin, and arterial oxygen saturation (SaO_2). Methods to optimize oxygen delivery are directed at increasing supply and decreasing demand. Supply is increased by (1) optimizing the CO with fluid replacement or drug therapy, (2) increasing the hemoglobin through transfusion of whole blood or packed red blood cells (RBCs), and/or (3) increasing the arterial oxygen saturation with supplemental oxygen and mechanical ventilation.

Plan care to avoid disrupting the balance of oxygen supply and demand. Space activities that increase oxygen consumption (e.g., endotracheal suctioning, position changes) appropriately for oxygen conservation. Continuous monitoring of $ScvO_2$ by a central venous catheter or mixed venous oxygen saturation (SvO_2) by a PA catheter is helpful. Both reflect the dynamic balance between oxygen supply and demand. Assess these values along with related hemodynamic measures (e.g., arterial pressure–based cardiac output [APCO], oxygen consumption, hemoglobin) to evaluate the patient's response to treatments or activities (see Chapter 66).

Fluid Resuscitation. The cornerstone of therapy for septic, hypovolemic, and anaphylactic shock is volume expansion with administration of the appropriate fluid. Fluid resuscitation should start using one or two large-bore (e.g., 14- to 16-gauge) IV catheters, preferably in the antecubital veins, or a central venous catheter. Both crystalloids (e.g., normal saline or hypertonic solutions) and colloids (e.g., albumin) have a role in fluid resuscitation (Table 67-7; also see Table 17-17). The choice of fluid for resuscitation remains controversial. Currently, isotonic crystalloids, such as normal saline, are used in the initial resus-

---

⊕ TABLE 67-6 EMERGENCY MANAGEMENT

Shock

Etiology*	Assessment Findings	Interventions
Surgical • Postoperative bleeding • Ruptured organ or vessel • Gastrointestinal bleeding • Aortic dissection • Vaginal bleeding • Ruptured ectopic pregnancy or ovarian cyst **Medical** • Myocardial infarction • Dehydration • Addisonian crisis • Diabetes insipidus • Sepsis • Diabetes mellitus • Pulmonary embolus **Trauma** • Ruptured or lacerated vessel or organ (e.g., spleen) • Fractures, spinal injury • Multiorgan injury	• Restlessness • Confusion • Anxiety • Feeling of impending doom • Decreased level of consciousness • Weakness • Rapid, weak, thready pulses • Dysrhythmias • Hypotension • Narrowed pulse pressure • Cool, clammy skin (warm skin in early onset of septic and neurogenic shock) • Tachypnea, dyspnea, or shallow, irregular respirations • Decreased O_2 saturation • Extreme thirst • Nausea and vomiting • Chills • Pallor • Cyanosis • Obvious hemorrhage or injury • Temperature dysregulation	**Initial** • Assess ABCs. • Stabilize cervical spine as appropriate. • Administer high-flow O_2 (100%) by non-rebreather mask or bag-valve-mask. • Anticipate need for intubation and mechanical ventilation. • Establish IV access with two large-bore catheters (14-16 gauge) or assist with insertion of central line and begin fluid resuscitation with crystalloids (e.g., 30 mL/kg repeated until hemodynamic improvement is noted). • Draw blood for laboratory studies (e.g., blood cultures, lactate, WBC). • Control any external bleeding with direct pressure or pressure dressing. • Assess for life-threatening injuries (e.g., cardiac tamponade, liver laceration, tension pneumothorax). • Consider vasopressor therapy if hypotension persists after fluid resuscitation. • Insert an indwelling bladder catheter and nasogastric tube. • Administer antibiotic therapy after blood cultures if sepsis is suspected. • Obtain 12-lead ECG and treat dysrhythmias. **Ongoing Monitoring** • Level of consciousness • Vital signs, including pulse oximetry; peripheral pulses, capillary refill, skin color and temperature • Respiratory status • Heart rate and rhythm • Urine output

*See Table 67-1 for additional etiologies of shock.
ABCs, Airway, breathing, circulation.

TABLE 67-7   FLUID THERAPY IN SHOCK

Fluid Type	Mechanism of Action	Type of Shock	Nursing Implications
Crystalloids *Isotonic* • 0.9% NaCl (NSS) • Lactated Ringer's (LR)	Fluid primarily remains in the intravascular space, increasing intravascular volume.	Used for initial volume replacement in most types of shock.	Monitor patient closely for circulatory overload. Do not use LR in patients with liver failure. LR may be used if hyperchloremic acidosis develops from use of NSS in fluid resuscitation.
Hypertonic • 1.8%, 3%, 5% NaCl	Fluid remains in the intravascular space, increases serum osmolarity, shifts fluid volume from intracellular space to extracellular space to intravascular space.	May be used for initial volume expansion in hypovolemic shock.	Monitor patient closely for signs of hypernatremia (e.g., disorientation, convulsions). Central line preferred for infusing saline solutions ≥3%, since these may damage veins.
Blood or Blood Products Packed red blood cells	Replaces blood loss, increases O$_2$-carrying capability.	All types of shock.	Same precautions as any blood administration (see Chapter 31).
Fresh frozen plasma	Replaces coagulation factors.		
Platelets	Helps control bleeding caused by thrombocytopenia.		
Colloids Human serum albumin (5% or 25%)	Can increase plasma colloid osmotic pressure. Rapid volume expansion.	All types of shock except cardiogenic and neurogenic shock.	Use 5% solution in hypovolemic patients. Use 25% solution in patients with fluid and sodium restrictions. Monitor for circulatory overload. Mild side effects of chills, fever, and urticaria may develop. More expensive than crystalloids.
dextran (dextran 40)	Hyperosmotic glucose polymer.	Limited use because of side effects, including reducing platelet adhesion, diluting clotting factors.	Increases risk of bleeding. Important to monitor patient for allergic reactions and acute renal failure. Has maximum volume recommendations per manufacturer.

NSS, Normal saline solution.

citation of shock. Lactated Ringer's solution is used cautiously in all shock situations because the failing liver cannot convert lactate to bicarbonate, so serum lactate levels increase. In some cases, hypertonic saline may be considered to expand plasma volume. Colloids are effective volume expanders because the size of their molecules keeps them in the vascular space for a longer time. However, they are costly and no definitive studies have shown that using colloids for resuscitation improves patient outcomes.[15]

The choice of fluid for resuscitation is also based on the type and volume of fluid lost and the patient's clinical status. If the patient does not respond to 2 to 3 L of crystalloids, blood administration and CVP, APCO, or PA pressure monitoring may be started.[16,17] Monitor trends in BP with an automatic BP cuff or an arterial catheter to assess the patient's response. An indwelling bladder catheter monitors urine output and aids in assessing the patient's fluid status during resuscitation.

When large amounts of fluids are required, you must protect the patient against two major complications: hypothermia and coagulopathy. If the patient has persistent hypotension after fluid resuscitation and normalized CVP (8 to 12 mm Hg), a vasopressor (e.g., norepinephrine [Levophed], dopamine [Intropin]) and/or an inotrope (e.g., dobutamine [Dobutrex]) may be added. The goal for fluid resuscitation is restoration of tissue perfusion. Thus decisions on which agent to use should be based on the physiologic goal. Although BP helps determine whether the patient's CO is adequate, an assessment of end-organ perfusion (e.g., urine output, neurologic function, peripheral pulses) provides more relevant information.

SAFETY ALERT
• Warm crystalloid and colloid solutions during massive fluid resuscitation.
• When administering large volumes of packed RBCs, remember that they do not contain clotting factors. Replace these factors based on the clinical situation and laboratory studies.

Drug Therapy. The primary goal of drug therapy for shock is the correction of decreased tissue perfusion. Medications used to improve perfusion in shock are given IV via an infusion pump and central venous line, since many of them have vasoconstrictor properties that would be harmful if the drug extravasated while being infused peripherally (Table 67-8).

Sympathomimetic Drugs. Many of the drugs used in the treatment of shock have an effect on the SNS. Drugs that mimic the action of the SNS are termed *sympathomimetic.* The effects of these drugs are mediated through their binding to α- or β-adrenergic receptors. The various drugs differ in their relative α- and β-adrenergic effects. (See Chapter 33 and Table 33-1.)

Many of the sympathomimetic drugs cause peripheral vasoconstriction and are called vasopressor drugs (e.g., norepinephrine, dopamine, phenylephrine [Neo-Synephrine]). These drugs can cause severe peripheral vasoconstriction and an increase in SVR, further risking tissue perfusion. The increased SVR increases the workload of the heart and can harm a patient in cardiogenic shock by causing further myocardial damage. Use of vasopressor drugs is limited to patients who do not respond to fluid resuscitation. Adequate fluid resuscitation must be achieved before starting vasopressors because the vasoconstric-

TABLE 67-8 DRUG THERAPY

Shock

Drug*	Mechanism of Action	Type of Shock	Nursing Implications
dobutamine (Dobutrex)	↑ Myocardial contractility ↓ Ventricular filling pressures ↓ SVR, PAWP ↑ CO, stroke volume, CVP ↑/↓ HR	Used in cardiogenic shock with severe systolic dysfunction Used in septic shock to increase O₂ delivery and raise ScvO₂/SvO₂ to 70% if Hgb >7 g/dL or Hct ≥30%	Administration via central line is recommended (infiltration leads to tissue sloughing). Do not administer in same line with NaHCO₃. Monitor HR, BP (hypotension may worsen, requiring addition of a vasopressor). Stop infusion if tachydysrhythmias develop.

dopamine (Intropin)	Positive inotropic effects:
	  ↑ Myocardial contractility
	  ↑ Automaticity
	  ↑ Atrioventricular conduction
	↑ HR, CO
	↑ BP, ↑ MAP
	↑ MVO₂
	Can cause progressive vasoconstriction at high doses
		Cardiogenic shock	Administration via central line is recommended (infiltration leads to tissue sloughing).
			Do not administer in same line with NaHCO₃.
			Monitor for tachydysrhythmias.
			Monitor for peripheral vasoconstriction (e.g., paresthesias, coldness in extremities) at moderate to high doses.

epinephrine (Adrenalin)	*Low doses:* β-Adrenergic agonist (cardiac stimulation, bronchodilation, peripheral vasodilation) ↑ HR, contractility, CO ↓ SVR *High doses:* α-Adrenergic agonist (peripheral vasoconstriction) ↑ Stroke volume, SVR ↑ Systolic/↓ diastolic BP, widened pulse pressure ↑ CVP, PAWP	Cardiogenic shock Anaphylactic shock Septic shock requiring additional agent after norepinephrine Cardiac arrest, pulseless ventricular tachycardia, ventricular fibrillation, asystole	Monitor for HR >110 beats/min. Monitor for dyspnea, pulmonary edema. Monitor for chest pain, dysrhythmias secondary to ↑ MVO₂. Monitor for renal failure secondary to ischemia.
hydrocortisone (Solu-Cortef)	Decreases inflammation, reverses increased capillary permeability ↑ BP, HR	Septic shock requiring vasopressor therapy (despite fluid resuscitation) to maintain adequate BP Anaphylactic shock if hypotension persists after initial therapy	Monitor for hypokalemia, hyperglycemia. Consider use as continuous infusion.
norepinephrine (Levophed)	β₁-Adrenergic agonist (cardiac stimulation) α-Adrenergic agonist (peripheral vasoconstriction) Renal and splanchnic vasoconstriction ↑ BP, MAP, CVP, PAWP, SVR ↑/↓ CO	Cardiogenic shock after myocardial infarction Septic shock—first drug of choice for BP unresponsive to adequate fluid resuscitation	Administration via central line is recommended (infiltration leads to tissue sloughing). Monitor for dysrhythmias secondary to ↑ MVO₂ requirements.
phenylephrine (Neo-Synephrine)	α-Adrenergic agonist (peripheral vasoconstriction) Renal, mesenteric, splanchnic, cutaneous, and pulmonary blood vessel constriction ↑ HR, BP, SVR ↑/↓ CO	Neurogenic shock	Monitor for reflex bradycardia, headache, restlessness. Monitor for renal failure secondary to ↓ renal blood flow. Administration via central line is recommended (infiltration leads to tissue sloughing).
nitroglycerin (Tridil)	Venodilation Dilates coronary arteries ↓ Preload, MVO₂, SVR, BP	Cardiogenic shock	Continuously monitor BP and HR, since reflex tachycardia may occur. Glass bottle recommended for infusion.
sodium nitroprusside (Nipride)	Arterial and venous vasodilation ↓ Preload, afterload ↓ CVP, PAWP ↑/↓ CO ↓ BP	Cardiogenic shock with ↑ SVR	Continuously monitor BP. Protect solution from light. Wrap infusion bottle with opaque covering. Administer with D₅W only. Monitor serum cyanide levels and for signs of cyanide toxicity (e.g., metabolic acidosis, tachycardia, altered level of consciousness, seizures, coma, almond smell on breath).
vasopressin (Pitressin, Pressyn)	Antidiuretic hormone Nonadrenergic vasoconstrictor ↑ MAP ↑ Urine output	Shock states (most commonly septic shock) refractory to other vasopressors	Usually administer low dose. Infusions are not titrated. Monitor hemodynamic pressures and urine output.

*Consult individual facility's guidelines, pharmacist, pharmacology references, and drug manufacturer's administration materials for additional information and dosing recommendations.
CO, Cardiac output; *CVP,* central venous pressure; *MAP,* mean arterial pressure; *MVO₂,* myocardial oxygen consumption; *PAWP,* pulmonary artery wedge pressure; *PT,* prothrombin time; *PTT,* partial thromboplastin time; *SVR,* systemic vascular resistance.

tor effects in patients with low blood volume will cause further reduction in tissue perfusion.

The goal of vasopressor therapy is to achieve and maintain a MAP of greater than 65 mm Hg.[9,13] Continuously monitor end-organ perfusion (e.g., urine output, level of consciousness) and serum lactate levels (e.g., every 2 hours for the first 6 hours) to ensure that tissue perfusion is adequate.

Vasodilator Drugs. Patients in cardiogenic shock have decreased myocardial contractility, and vasodilators may be needed to decrease afterload. This reduces myocardial workload and oxygen requirements. Although generalized sympathetic vasoconstriction is a useful compensatory mechanism for maintaining BP, excessive constriction can reduce tissue blood flow and increase the workload of the heart. The rationale for using vasodilator therapy for a patient in shock is to break the harmful cycle of widespread vasoconstriction causing a decrease in CO and BP, resulting in further sympathetic-induced vasoconstriction.

The goal of vasodilator therapy, as in vasopressor therapy, is to maintain the MAP greater than 65 mm Hg. Also monitor hemodynamic parameters (e.g., CVP, APCO, CO, ScvO$_2$/SvO$_2$, PA pressures) so that fluids can be increased or vasodilator therapy decreased if a serious fall in CO or BP occurs. The vasodilator agent most often used for the patient in cardiogenic shock is nitroglycerin (Tridil). Vasodilation may be enhanced with nitroprusside (Nipride) or nitroglycerin in noncardiogenic shock.

Nutritional Therapy. Protein-calorie malnutrition is one of the main manifestations of hypermetabolism in shock. Nutrition is vital to reducing mortality. Enteral nutrition should be started within the first 24 hours.[18] Generally, parenteral nutrition is used if enteral feedings are contraindicated or fail to meet at least 80% of the patient's caloric requirements.[19] (Chapter 40 discusses parenteral and enteral nutrition.) Start the patient on a slow continuous drip of small amounts of enteral feedings (e.g., 10 mL/hr). Early enteral feedings enhance the perfusion of the GI tract and help maintain the integrity of the gut mucosa.

Weigh the patient daily on the same scale at the same time of day. If the patient experiences a significant weight loss, rule out dehydration before adding more calories. Large weight gains are common because of third spacing of fluids. Therefore daily weights serve as a better indicator of fluid status than caloric needs. Serum protein, total albumin, prealbumin, BUN, serum glucose, and serum electrolytes are all used to assess nutritional status.

Collaborative Care: Specific Measures

Cardiogenic Shock. For a patient in cardiogenic shock, the overall goal is to restore blood flow to the myocardium by restoring the balance between oxygen supply and demand. Cardiac catheterization is performed as soon as possible after the initial insult. Specific measures to restore blood flow include angioplasty with stenting, emergency revascularization, and valve replacement (see Chapter 34). Until these interventions are done, the heart must be supported to optimize stroke volume and CO to achieve optimal perfusion (see Tables 67-8 and 67-9).

Hemodynamic management of a patient in cardiogenic shock aims to reduce the workload of the heart through drug therapy and/or mechanical interventions. Drug selection is based on the clinical goal and a thorough understanding of each drug's mechanism of action. Drugs can be used to decrease the workload of the heart by dilating coronary arteries (e.g.,

nitrates), reducing preload (e.g., diuretics), reducing afterload (e.g., vasodilators), and reducing heart rate and contractility (e.g., β-adrenergic blockers).

The patient may also benefit from a circulatory assist device (e.g., intraaortic balloon pump, ventricular assist device [VAD])[20] (see Chapter 66). The goals of this intervention are to decrease the SVR and the left ventricular workload so the heart can heal. A VAD may be used as a temporary measure for the patient in cardiogenic shock who is awaiting heart transplantation. Heart transplantation is an option for a small, select group of patients with cardiogenic shock.

Hypovolemic Shock. The underlying principles of managing patients with hypovolemic shock focus on stopping the loss of fluid and restoring the circulating volume. Fluid resuscitation in hypovolemic shock initially is calculated using a 3:1 rule (3 mL of isotonic crystalloid for every 1 mL of estimated blood loss). Table 67-7 delineates the different types of fluid used for volume resuscitation, the mechanisms of action, and specific nursing implications for each fluid type.

Septic Shock. Patients in septic shock require large amounts of fluid replacement. Volume resuscitation of 30 to 50 mL/kg is usually done with isotonic crytalloids to achieve a target CVP of 8 to 12 mm Hg. Albumin 0.5 to 1 g/kg/dose may be added when patients require substantial volumes. Use of a fluid challenge technique (e.g., to achieve a minimum of 30 mL/kg of crystalloids) is repeated until hemodynamic improvement (e.g., increase in MAP and/or CVP, change in SVV) is noted.[9] (An example of a sepsis alert treatment protocol [eFig. 67-4] is available on the website for this chapter.) Table 67-9 presents predetermined end points of fluid resuscitation. To optimize and evaluate large-volume fluid resuscitation, hemodynamic monitoring with a minimum of a central venous catheter is necessary. The overall goals of fluid resuscitation are to restore the intravascular volume and organ perfusion.

Once the CVP is 8 mm Hg or more, vasopressors may be added. The first drug of choice is norepinephrine. Vasodilation and low CO, or vasodilation alone, can cause low BP in spite of adequate fluid resuscitation. Vasopressin (Pitressin) may be added for patients refractory to vasopressor therapy.[9,10,13] Exogenous vasopressin is used to replace the stores of physiologic vasopressin that are often depleted in septic shock.

> **DRUG ALERT: Vasopressin (Pitressin)**
> - Infuse at low doses (e.g., 0.03 U/min).
> - Do not titrate infusion.
> - Use cautiously in patients with coronary artery disease.

Vasopressor drugs may increase BP but may also decrease stroke volume. An inotropic agent (e.g., dobutamine) is often added to offset the decrease in stroke volume and increase tissue perfusion (see Table 67-8). IV corticosteroids may be considered for patients in septic shock who cannot maintain an adequate BP with vasopressor therapy despite fluid resuscitation.[9] In an attempt to meet the increasing tissue demands coupled with a low SVR, the patient initially demonstrates a normal or high CO. If the patient is unable to achieve and maintain an adequate CO and has unmet tissue oxygen demands, the CO may need to be increased using drug therapy (e.g., dopamine).[9] ScvO$_2$/SvO$_2$ monitoring is used to assess the balance between oxygen delivery and consumption, and the adequacy of the CO[17] (see Chapter 66). If balance is maintained, the tissue demands will be met.

Antibiotics are an important and early component of therapy. They should be started within the first hour of septic shock.

TABLE 67-9   COLLABORATIVE CARE

Shock

Oxygenation	Circulation	Drug Therapies	Supportive Therapies
Cardiogenic Shock • Provide supplemental O₂ (e.g., nasal cannula, non-rebreather mask) • Intubation and mechanical ventilation, if necessary • Monitor ScvO₂/SvO₂	• Restore blood flow with thrombolytics, angioplasty with stenting, emergent coronary revascularization • Reduce workload of the heart with circulatory assist devices: IABP, VAD	• Nitrates (e.g., nitroglycerin) • Inotropes (e.g., dobutamine) • Diuretics (e.g., furosemide) • β-Adrenergic blockers (contraindicated with ↓ ejection fraction)	• Treat dysrhythmias

Hypovolemic Shock
• Provide supplemental O₂
• Monitor ScvO₂/ScvO₂
	• Restore fluid volume (e.g., blood or blood products, crystalloids)
	• Rapid fluid replacement using two large-bore (14-16 gauge) peripheral IV lines or central venous catheter
	• End points of fluid resuscitation:
	  • CVP 15 mm Hg
	  • PAWP 10-12 mm Hg
		• No specific drug therapy	• Correct the cause (e.g., stop bleeding, GI losses)
			• Use warmed IV fluids, including blood products (if appropriate)

Septic Shock
• Provide supplemental O₂
• Intubation and mechanical ventilation, if necessary
• Monitor ScvO₂/SvO₂
	• Aggressive fluid resuscitation (e.g., 30 mL/kg of crystalloids repeated as long as hemodynamic improvement is noted)
	• End points of fluid resuscitation:
	  • CVP 8-12 mm Hg
	  • MAP ≥65 mm Hg
	  • Urine output ≥0.5 mL/kg/hr
	  • Normalized lactate levels
		• Antibiotics as ordered
		• Vasopressors (e.g., norepinephrine)
		• Inotropes (e.g., dobutamine)
		• Anticoagulants (e.g., low-molecular-weight heparin)
			• Obtain cultures (e.g., blood, wound) before beginning antibiotics
			• Monitor temperature
			• Control blood glucose
			• Stress ulcer prophylaxis

Neurogenic Shock • Maintain patent airway • Provide supplemental O₂ • Intubation and mechanical ventilation (if necessary)	• Cautious administration of fluids	• Vasopressors (e.g., phenylephrine) • Atropine (for bradycardia)	• Minimize spinal cord trauma with stabilization • Monitor temperature
Anaphylactic Shock • Maintain patent airway • Optimize oxygenation with supplemental O₂ • Intubation and mechanical ventilation, if necessary	• Aggressive fluid resuscitation with colloids	• Epinephrine (IM or IV) • Antihistamines (e.g., diphenhydramine) • Histamine (H₂)-receptor blockers (e.g., famotidine [Pepcid]) • Bronchodilators: nebulized (e.g., albuterol) • Corticosteroids (if hypotension persists)	• Identify and remove offending cause • Prevent via avoidance of known allergens • Premedicate with history of prior sensitivity (e.g., contrast media)
Obstructive Shock • Maintain patent airway • Provide supplemental O₂ • Intubation and mechanical ventilation, if necessary	• Restore circulation by treating cause of obstruction • Fluid resuscitation may provide temporary improvement in CO and BP	• No specific drug therapy	• Treat cause of obstruction (e.g., pericardiocentesis for cardiac tamponade, needle decompression or chest tube insertion for tension pneumothorax, embolectomy for pulmonary embolism)

CO, Cardiac output; *CVP,* central venous pressure; *IABP,* intraaortic balloon pump; *MAP,* mean arterial pressure; *PAWP,* pulmonary artery wedge pressure; *VAD,* ventricular assist device.

Obtain cultures (e.g., blood, wound exudate, urine, stool, sputum) before antibiotics are started. However, this should not delay the start of antibiotics within the first hour. Broad-spectrum antibiotics are given first, followed by antibiotics that are more specific once the organism has been identified.[9]

Glucose levels should be maintained below 180 mg/dL (10.0 mmol/L) for patients in shock. Intensive glucose control (81 to 108 mg/dL) actually increases mortality.[21] Frequently monitor glucose levels in all patients in septic shock.

Stress ulcer prophylaxis with proton pump inhibitors (e.g., pantoprazole [Protonix]) for patients with bleeding risk factors and venous thromboembolism prophylaxis (e.g., heparin, enoxaparin [Lovenox]) are also recommended for these patients.[9]

Neurogenic Shock. The specific treatment of neurogenic shock is based on the cause. If the cause is spinal cord injury, general measures to promote spinal stability (e.g., spinal precautions, cervical stabilization with a collar) are initially used. Once the spine is stabilized, definitive treatment of the hypotension and bradycardia is essential to prevent further spinal cord damage. Hypotension, which occurs as a result of a loss of sympathetic tone, is associated with peripheral vasodilation and decreased venous return. Treatment involves the use of vasopressors (e.g., phenylephrine) to maintain BP and organ perfusion (see Table 67-8). Bradycardia may be treated with atropine (AtroPen). Infuse fluids cautiously as the cause of the hypotension is not related to fluid loss.[7]

The patient with a spinal cord injury also needs to be monitored for hypothermia caused by hypothalamic dysfunction (see Table 67-9). Although corticosteroids do not have an effect in neurogenic shock, methylprednisolone (Solu-Medrol) is used for patients with a spinal cord injury to prevent secondary spinal cord damage caused by the release of chemical mediators (see Chapter 61).

Anaphylactic Shock. The first strategy in managing patients at risk for anaphylactic shock is prevention. A thorough history is key to avoid the risk factors for anaphylaxis (see Table 67-1). The clinical presentation of anaphylactic shock is dramatic, and immediate intervention is required. (An example of an anaphylaxis algorithm [eFig. 67-5] is available on the website for this chapter.) Epinephrine is the drug of choice to treat anaphylactic shock.[8] It causes peripheral vasoconstriction and bronchodilation and opposes the effect of histamine. IV diphenhydramine (Benadryl) is given to block the massive release of histamine from the allergic reaction.

Maintaining a patent airway is important because the patient can quickly develop airway compromise from laryngeal edema or bronchoconstriction. Nebulized bronchodilators are highly effective. Aerosolized epinephrine can also be used to treat laryngeal edema. Endotracheal intubation or cricothyroidotomy may be necessary to secure and maintain a patent airway.

Hypotension results from leakage of fluid out of the intravascular space into the interstitial space as a result of increased vascular permeability and vasodilation. Aggressive fluid resuscitation, predominantly with colloids, is necessary. IV corticosteroids may be helpful in anaphylactic shock if significant hypotension persists after 1 to 2 hours of aggressive therapy (see Tables 67-8 and 67-9).

Obstructive Shock. The primary strategy in treating obstructive shock is early recognition and treatment to relieve or manage the obstruction (see Table 67-1). Mechanical decompression for pericardial tamponade, tension pneumothorax,

and hemopneumothorax may be done by needle or tube insertion. Obstructive shock from a pulmonary embolism may require thrombolytic therapy. Superior vena cava syndrome, a compression or obstruction of the outflow tract of the mediastinum, may be treated by radiation, debulking, or removal of the mass or cause. A decompressive laparotomy may be indicated for abdominal compartment syndrome for patients with high intraabdominal pressures and hemodynamic instability.

NURSING MANAGEMENT
SHOCK

NURSING ASSESSMENT

Your role is vital in caring for patients who are at risk for developing shock or are in a state of shock. Focus your initial assessment on the ABCs: airway, breathing, and circulation. Next, assess for tissue perfusion. This includes evaluating vital signs, level of consciousness, peripheral pulses, capillary refill, skin (e.g., temperature, color, moisture), and urine output. As shock progresses, the patient's skin becomes cooler and mottled, urine output decreases, peripheral pulses diminish, and neurologic status declines.

To understand the complexity of the patient's clinical status, integrate all of the assessment data. It is essential to obtain a brief history from the patient or caregiver, including a description of the events leading to the shock condition, time of onset and duration of symptoms, and a health history (e.g., medications, allergies, date of last tetanus vaccination, recent travel). In addition, obtain details regarding any care that the patient received before hospitalization.

NURSING DIAGNOSES

Nursing diagnoses for the patient in shock may include, but are not limited to, the following:

- Ineffective peripheral tissue perfusion with risk for decreased cardiac tissue perfusion, ineffective cerebral tissue perfusion, ineffective renal perfusion, impaired liver function, and ineffective GI perfusion *related to* low blood flow or maldistribution of blood
- Anxiety *related to* severity of condition and hypoxemia

Additional information on nursing diagnoses for the patient with shock is presented in eNursing Care Plan 67-1 (available on the website for this chapter).

PLANNING

The overall goals for a patient in shock include (1) evidence of adequate tissue perfusion, (2) restoration of normal or baseline BP, (3) recovery of organ function, (4) avoidance of complications from prolonged states of hypoperfusion, and (5) prevention of health care–acquired complications of disease management and care.

NURSING IMPLEMENTATION

HEALTH PROMOTION. You have an important role in the prevention of shock, beginning with the identification of patients at risk. In general, patients who are older, are immunocompromised, or have chronic illnesses are at an increased risk. Any person who has surgery or trauma is at risk for shock resulting from hemorrhage, spinal cord injury, sepsis, and other conditions (see Table 67-1).

Planning is essential to help prevent shock after you identify an at-risk person. For example, a person with an acute anterior wall MI is at high risk for cardiogenic shock.[22] The primary goal for this patient is to limit the infarct size. This is done by restoring coronary blood flow through percutaneous coronary intervention, thrombolytic therapy, or surgical revascularization. Rest, analgesics, and sedation can reduce the myocardial demand for oxygen. Modify the patient's environment to provide care at intervals that will not increase the patient's oxygen demand. For example, if the patient becomes tired with bathing, perform this care at a time that does not interfere with tests or other activities that may also increase oxygen demand.

A person with a severe allergy to such substances as drugs, shellfish, insect bites, and latex is at increased risk for anaphylactic shock. This risk can be decreased if the patient is carefully questioned about allergies.

SAFETY ALERT
- Always confirm the patient's allergies before administering medications or beginning diagnostic procedures (e.g., computed tomography [CT] scan with contrast media).
- Premedicate (e.g., diphenhydramine, methylprednisolone) patients who need a drug to which they are at high risk for an allergic reaction (e.g., contrast media).
- Encourage patients with allergies to obtain and wear a medical alert tag and report their allergies to their health care providers.
- Instruct patients about the availability of kits that contain equipment and medication (e.g., epinephrine [EpiPen]) for the treatment of acute allergic reactions.

Careful monitoring of fluid balance can help prevent hypovolemic shock. Ongoing monitoring of intake and output and daily weights is important. In addition, monitoring the patient's clinical status is essential because trends in clinical findings are more meaningful than any one piece of clinical information.

Carefully monitor all patients for the development of infection. Progression from an infection to sepsis and septic shock depends on the patient's defense mechanisms. Patients who are immunocompromised are at high risk for opportunistic infections. Strategies to decrease the risk of health care–associated infections (HAIs) include decreasing the number of invasive catheters (e.g., central lines, bladder catheters), using aseptic technique during invasive procedures, and paying strict attention to hand washing. In addition, all equipment must be changed per agency policy and thoroughly cleaned or discarded (if disposable) between patient use.

Evidence-based guidelines are available to reduce the risk of HAIs (e.g., ventilator-associated pneumonia, central line infections, catheter-associated urinary tract infections). These guidelines, called *care bundles,* outline key interventions aimed at reducing infections (see *www.ihi.org/explore/Bundles/Pages/default.aspx*).

ACUTE INTERVENTION. Your role in shock involves (1) monitoring the patient's ongoing physical and emotional status, (2) identifying trends to detect changes in the patient's condition, (3) planning and implementing nursing interventions and therapy, (4) evaluating the patient's response to therapy, (5) providing emotional support to the patient and caregiver, and (6) collaborating with other members of the health team to coordinate care (see Chapter 66).

Neurologic Status. Assess the patient's neurologic status, including orientation and level of consciousness, at least every 1 to 2 hours. The patient's neurologic status is the best indicator of cerebral blood flow. Be aware of the clinical manifestations of neurologic involvement (e.g., changes in behavior, restlessness, hyperalertness, blurred vision, confusion, paresthesias).

Note and report any subtle changes in the patient's mental status (e.g., mild agitation).

Orient the patient to person, place, time, and events on a regular basis. Orientation to the intensive care unit (ICU) environment is particularly important. Minimize noise and light levels to control sensory input. Maintain a day-night cycle of activity and rest as much as possible. Sensory overload and disruption of the patient's diurnal cycle may contribute to delirium (see Chapter 66).

Cardiovascular Status. Most of the therapy for shock is based on information about the patient's cardiovascular status. If the patient is unstable, continuously assess heart rate and rhythm, BP, CVP, and PA pressures, including CO, SVR, and SVV (if available). (Chapter 66 discusses hemodynamic monitoring.) Monitoring trends in hemodynamic parameters provides more important information than single values. Integration of hemodynamic data with physical assessment data is essential in planning strategies to manage the patient with shock.

Patients in shock often have hypotension. There is no definitive research that supports placing patients in the Trendelenburg (head-down) position during hypotensive crisis. Patients in this position may experience compromised pulmonary function and increased intracranial pressure. The Trendelenburg position should not be used to treat hypotension.[23]

Continuously monitor the patient's ECG to detect dysrhythmias that may result from the cardiovascular and metabolic abnormalities associated with shock. Assess heart sounds for an S_3 or S_4 sound or new murmurs. An S_3 sound usually indicates heart failure.

In addition to monitoring the patient's cardiovascular status, give the prescribed therapy to correct the dysfunctions of the cardiovascular system. Assess the patient's response to fluid and medication administration as often as every 10 to 15 minutes. Make appropriate adjustments (e.g., medication titration) as needed. Once tissue perfusion is restored and the patient is stabilized, you can decrease the frequency of monitoring and slowly wean the patient off medications to support BP and tissue perfusion.

Respiratory Status. Frequently assess the respiratory status of the patient in shock to ensure adequate oxygenation, detect complications early, and provide data regarding the patient's acid-base status. Initially monitor the rate, depth, and rhythm of respirations as frequently as every 15 to 30 minutes. Increased rate and depth provide information regarding the patient's attempts to correct metabolic acidosis. Assess breath sounds every 1 to 2 hours and as needed for any changes that may indicate fluid overload or accumulation of secretions.

Use pulse oximetry to continuously monitor oxygen saturation. Pulse oximetry using a patient's finger may not be accurate in a shock state because of poor peripheral circulation. Instead, attach the probe to the ear, nose, or forehead (according to the manufacturer's guidelines). Arterial blood gases (ABGs) provide definitive information on ventilation and oxygenation status and acid-base balance. Initial interpretation of ABGs is often your responsibility. A PaO_2 below 60 mm Hg (in the absence of chronic lung disease) indicates hypoxemia and the need for higher oxygen concentrations or for a different mode of oxygen administration. Low $PaCO_2$ with a low pH and low bicarbonate level may indicate that the patient is attempting to compensate for metabolic acidosis from increasing lactate levels.

A rising $PaCO_2$ with a persistently low pH and PaO_2 indicates the need for advanced pulmonary management. Most patients in shock are intubated and on mechanical ventilation. Maintaining a patent airway and monitoring for ventilator-related complications are critical. (Chapter 66 discusses artificial airways and mechanical ventilation.)

Renal Status. Initially, measure urine output every 1 to 2 hours to assess the adequacy of renal perfusion. Inserting an indwelling bladder catheter facilitates measurements. Urine output below 0.5 mL/kg/hr may indicate inadequate perfusion of the kidneys. Also use trends in serum creatinine values to assess renal function. Serum creatinine is a better indicator of renal function than BUN levels, since BUN is affected by the patient's catabolic state.

Body Temperature and Skin Changes. Monitor temperature every 4 hours if normal. In the presence of an elevated or subnormal temperature, obtain hourly core temperatures (e.g., urinary or PA catheter). Use light covers and control the room temperature to keep the patient comfortably warm. If the patient's temperature rises above 101.5° F (38.6° C) and the patient becomes uncomfortable or experiences cardiovascular compromise, manage the fever with antipyretic drugs (e.g., ibuprofen [Motrin], acetaminophen [Tylenol]) or remove some of the patient's covers.

Monitor the patient's skin (e.g., upper and lower extremities) for signs of adequate perfusion. Changes in temperature, pallor, flushing, cyanosis, diaphoresis, and piloerection may indicate hypoperfusion.

Gastrointestinal Status. Auscultate bowel sounds at least every 4 hours, and monitor for abdominal distention. If a nasogastric tube is present, measure drainage and check for occult blood. Similarly, check all stools for occult blood.

Personal Hygiene. Hygiene is especially important to the patient in shock because impaired tissue perfusion predisposes the patient to skin breakdown and infection. Perform bathing and other nursing measures carefully because a patient in shock is experiencing problems with oxygen delivery to tissues. The increased oxygen demand that occurs during bathing and repositioning of patients with limited oxygen reserves makes the prevention of health care–associated pressure ulcers challenging. Turn the patient at least every 1 to 2 hours and maintain good body alignment to help prevent pressure ulcers. Use a pressure-relieving or pressure-reducing mattress or a specialty bed as needed. Use good clinical judgment in determining priorities of care to limit the demands for increased oxygen. Perform passive range of motion three or four times a day to maintain joint mobility. Monitor trends in oxygen consumption (e.g., SpO_2, $ScvO_2$/SvO_2) during all nursing interventions to assess the patient's tolerance of activity.

Oral care for the patient in shock is essential because mucous membranes may become dry and fragile in the volume-depleted patient. In addition, the intubated patient usually has difficulty swallowing, resulting in pooled secretions in the mouth. Apply a water-soluble lubricant to the lips to prevent drying and cracking. Brush the patient's teeth or gums with a soft toothbrush every 12 hours, and swab the lips and oral mucosa with a moisturizing solution every 2 to 4 hours.[24]

Emotional Support and Comfort. Do not underestimate the effects of fear and anxiety when the patient and caregiver are faced with a critical, life-threatening situation (see Chapter 66). Fear, anxiety, and pain may aggravate respiratory distress and increase the release of catecholamines. When implementing care, monitor the patient's mental state and level of pain. Provide medications to decrease anxiety and pain as appropriate. Continuous infusions of a benzodiazepine (e.g., lorazepam [Ativan]) and an opioid or anesthetic (e.g., morphine, propofol [Diprivan]) are extremely helpful in decreasing anxiety and pain.

Talk to the patient and encourage the caregiver to talk to the patient, even if the patient is intubated, is sedated, or appears comatose. Hearing is often the last sense to decrease, and even if the patient cannot respond, he or she may still be able to hear. If the intubated patient is capable of writing, provide a "magic slate" or a pencil and paper. Alphabet boards or signboards with common requests (e.g., turn, fan, lights) are also useful.

Provide the patient with simple explanations of all procedures before you carry them out, as well as information regarding the current plan of care. If the patient or caregiver asks questions about progress and prognosis, provide simple and honest answers.

Do not overlook the patient's spiritual needs. Patients may desire a visit from a chaplain, priest, rabbi, or minister. One way to provide support is to offer to call a member of the clergy rather than wait for the patient or caregiver to express a wish for spiritual counseling.

Caregivers can have a therapeutic effect on the patient by providing support and comfort. Caregivers (1) link the patient to the outside world; (2) facilitate decision making and advise the patient; (3) assist with activities of daily living; (4) act as liaisons to advise the health care team of the patient's wishes for care; and (5) provide safe, caring, familiar relationships for the patient.[25-27] Most important, caregivers wish to be kept informed of the patient's condition. If possible, the same nurses should continually care for the patient to decrease anxiety, limit conflicting information, and increase trust. If the prognosis becomes grave, support the patient's caregiver when making difficult decisions such as withdrawing life support. The health care team must promote realistic expectations and outcomes. Remember, compassion is as essential as scientific and technical expertise in the total care of the patient and caregiver.

You should ensure that the caregiver is able to spend time with the patient, provided the patient perceives this time as comforting. Explain in simple terms the purpose of any tubes and equipment attached to or surrounding the patient. Inform the caregivers of what they may and may not touch. If possible, place the patient's hands and arms outside the sheets to encourage therapeutic touch. Encourage caregivers to perform simple comfort measures if desired. Provide privacy as much as possible, but assure the patient and caregiver that assistance is readily available should it be needed. Position the call bell in reach of the patient or caregiver at all times.

AMBULATORY AND HOME CARE. Rehabilitation of the patient who has experienced critical illness requires correction of the precipitating cause, prevention or early treatment of complications, and education focused on disease management or prevention of recurrence based on the initial cause of shock. Continue to monitor the patient for indications of complications throughout the recovery period. These may include decreased range of motion, muscle weakness, decreased physical endurance, renal failure following acute tubular necrosis (see Chapter 47), and fibrotic lung disease caused by ARDS (see Chapter 68). Thus patients recovering from shock often require diverse services after discharge. These can include admission to transitional care units (e.g., for mechanical ventilation weaning), rehabilitation centers (inpatient or outpatient), or home health care agencies. Start planning for a safe transition from hospital to home as soon as the patient is admitted to the hospital.

EVALUATION

The expected outcomes for the patient in shock include

- Adequate tissue perfusion with restoration of normal or baseline BP
- Normal organ function with no complications from hypoperfusion
- Decreased fear and anxiety and increased psychologic comfort

Additional information on expected outcomes for the patient with shock is presented in eNursing Care Plan 67-1 (available on the website for this chapter).

SYSTEMIC INFLAMMATORY RESPONSE SYNDROME AND MULTIPLE ORGAN DYSFUNCTION SYNDROME

Etiology and Pathophysiology

Systemic inflammatory response syndrome (SIRS) is a systemic inflammatory response to a variety of insults, including infection (referred to as sepsis), ischemia, infarction, and injury (see Table 67-4). Generalized inflammation in organs remote from the initial insult characterizes SIRS.[12] A systemic inflammatory response can be triggered by many different mechanisms, including the following:

- *Mechanical tissue trauma:* Burns, crush injuries, surgical procedures
- *Abscess formation:* Intraabdominal, extremities
- *Ischemic or necrotic tissue:* Pancreatitis, vascular disease, MI
- *Microbial invasion:* Bacteria, viruses, fungi, parasites
- *Endotoxin release:* Gram-negative and gram-positive bacteria
- *Global perfusion deficits:* Postcardiac resuscitation, shock states
- *Regional perfusion deficits:* Distal perfusion deficits

Multiple organ dysfunction syndrome (MODS) is the failure of two or more organ systems in an acutely ill patient such that homeostasis cannot be maintained without intervention. MODS results from SIRS. These two syndromes represent the ends of a continuum. Transition from SIRS to MODS does not occur in a clear-cut manner[12] (see Fig. 67-1).

Organ and Metabolic Dysfunction. When the inflammatory response is activated, consequences include the release of mediators, direct damage to the endothelium, and hypermetabolism. In addition, vascular permeability increases. This allows mediators and protein to leak out of the endothelium and into the interstitial space. White blood cells begin to digest the foreign debris, and the coagulation cascade is activated (see Chapter 30). Hypotension, decreased perfusion, microemboli, and redistributed or shunted blood flow eventually compromise organ perfusion.

The respiratory system is often the first system to show signs of dysfunction in SIRS and MODS.[9,10,12] Inflammatory mediators have a direct effect on the pulmonary vasculature. The endothelial damage from the release of inflammatory mediators causes increased capillary permeability. This causes movement of fluid from the pulmonary vasculature into the pulmonary interstitial spaces. The fluid then moves to the alveoli, causing alveolar edema. Type I pneumocytes (alveolar cells) are destroyed. Type II pneumocytes are damaged, and surfactant production is decreased. The alveoli collapse. This creates an increase in *shunt* (blood flow to the lungs that does not partici-

pate in gas exchange) and worsening ventilation-perfusion mismatch. The end result is ARDS. Patients with ARDS need aggressive pulmonary management with mechanical ventilation. (See Chapter 68 for a complete discussion of ARDS.)

Cardiovascular changes include myocardial depression and massive vasodilation in response to increasing tissue demands. Vasodilation results in decreased SVR and BP. The baroreceptor reflex causes release of *inotropic* (increasing force of contraction) and *chronotropic* (increasing heart rate) factors that enhance CO. To compensate for hypotension, CO increases by an increase in heart rate and stroke volume. Increases in capillary permeability cause a shift of albumin and fluid out of the vascular space, further reducing venous return and thus preload. The patient becomes warm and tachycardic with a high CO and a low SVR. Other signs include decreased capillary refill, skin mottling, increased CVP and PAWP, and dysrhythmias. $ScvO_2$/SvO_2 may be abnormally high because the patient is perfusing areas not consuming much oxygen (e.g., skin, nonworking muscle) while other areas may have blood shunted away from them. Eventually, either perfusion of vital organs becomes insufficient or the cells are unable to use oxygen and their function is further compromised.

Neurologic dysfunction commonly presents as mental status changes with SIRS and MODS. These acute changes can be an early sign of SIRS or MODS. The patient may become confused and agitated, combative, disoriented, lethargic, or comatose. These mental status changes may be due to hypoxemia, the effects of inflammatory mediators, or impaired perfusion.

Acute kidney injury (AKI) is frequently seen in SIRS and MODS. Hypoperfusion and the effects of the mediators can cause AKI. Decreased perfusion to the kidneys activates the SNS and the renin-angiotensin system. The stimulation of the renin-angiotensin system results in systemic vasoconstriction and aldosterone-mediated sodium and water reabsorption. Another risk factor for the development of AKI is the use of nephrotoxic drugs. Antibiotics commonly used to treat gram-negative bacteria (e.g., aminoglycosides) can be nephrotoxic. Careful monitoring of drug levels is essential to avoid the nephrotoxic effects.

The GI tract also plays a key role in the development of MODS. GI motility is often decreased in critical illness, causing abdominal distention and paralytic ileus. In the early stages of SIRS and MODS, blood is also shunted away from the GI mucosa, making it highly vulnerable to ischemic injury. Decreased perfusion leads to a breakdown of this normally protective mucosal barrier, thus increasing the risk for ulceration, GI bleeding, and bacterial movement from the GI tract into circulation.[12]

Metabolic changes are pronounced in SIRS and MODS. Both syndromes trigger a hypermetabolic response. Glycogen stores are rapidly converted to glucose (glycogenolysis). Once glycogen is depleted, amino acids are converted to glucose (gluconeogenesis), reducing protein stores. Fatty acids are mobilized for fuel. Catecholamines and glucocorticoids are released and result in hyperglycemia and insulin resistance. The net result is a catabolic state, and lean body mass (muscle) is lost.

The hypermetabolism associated with SIRS and MODS may last for several days and results in liver dysfunction. Liver dysfunction in MODS may begin long before clinical evidence of it is present. Protein synthesis is impaired. The liver cannot make albumin, one of the key proteins in maintaining plasma oncotic pressure. Consequently, plasma oncotic pressure is altered, and fluid and protein leak from the vascular spaces to the interstitial space. Administration of albumin does not normalize oncotic pressure in these patients at this point.

As the state of hypermetabolism persists, the patient cannot convert lactate to glucose, and lactate accumulates (lactic acidosis). Despite increases in glycogenolysis and gluconeogenesis, eventually the liver is unable to maintain an adequate glucose level and the patient becomes hypoglycemic. Hypoglycemia can also develop due to acute adrenal insufficiency.

DIC may result from dysfunction of the coagulation system. DIC causes simultaneous microvascular clotting and bleeding because of the depletion of clotting factors and platelets in addition to excessive fibrinolysis. (Chapter 31 discusses DIC.)

Electrolyte imbalances are common and result from the hormonal and metabolic changes and fluid shifts. These changes worsen mental status changes, neuromuscular dysfunction, and dysrhythmias. The release of ADH and aldosterone results in sodium and water retention. Aldosterone increases urinary potassium loss, and catecholamines cause potassium to move into the cell, resulting in hypokalemia. Hypokalemia is associated with dysrhythmias and muscle weakness. Metabolic acidosis results from impaired tissue perfusion, hypoxia, and a shift to anaerobic metabolism with a resultant increase in lactate levels. Progressive renal dysfunction also contributes to metabolic acidosis. Hypocalcemia, hypomagnesemia, and hypophosphatemia are common.

Clinical Manifestations of SIRS and MODS

The clinical manifestations of SIRS and MODS are presented in Table 67-10.

NURSING AND COLLABORATIVE MANAGEMENT SIRS AND MODS

The prognosis for the patient with MODS is poor, with mortality rates of 70% to 80% when three or more organ systems fail.[12] The most common cause of death continues to be sepsis. Survival improves with *early, goal-directed therapy*.[9] (An example of a sepsis alert treatment protocol [eFig. 67-4] is available on the website for this chapter.) Therefore the most important goal is to prevent the progression of SIRS to MODS.

A critical part of your role is vigilant assessment and ongoing monitoring to detect early signs of deterioration or organ dysfunction. Collaborative care for patients with SIRS and MODS focuses on (1) prevention and treatment of infection, (2) maintenance of tissue oxygenation, (3) nutritional and metabolic support, and (4) appropriate support of individual failing organs. Table 67-10 summarizes the management for patients with SIRS and MODS.

PREVENTION AND TREATMENT OF INFECTION
Aggressive infection control strategies are essential to decrease the risk for HAIs. Early, aggressive surgery is recommended to remove necrotic tissue (e.g., early debridement of burn tissue) that can provide a culture medium for microorganisms. Aggressive pulmonary management, including early ambulation, can

reduce the risk of infection. Strict asepsis can decrease infections related to intraarterial lines, endotracheal tubes, indwelling bladder catheters, IV lines, and other invasive devices or procedures. Daily assessment of the ongoing need for invasive lines and other devices is an important strategy to prevent or limit HAIs.

Despite aggressive strategies, infection may develop. Once an infection is suspected, begin interventions to treat the cause. Send appropriate cultures and initiate broad-spectrum antibiotic therapy, as ordered. Therapy is adjusted based on the causative organism, if necessary.

MAINTENANCE OF TISSUE OXYGENATION
Hypoxemia frequently occurs in patients with SIRS and MODS. These patients have greater oxygen needs and decreased oxygen supply to the tissues. Interventions that decrease oxygen demand and increase oxygen delivery are essential. Sedation, mechanical ventilation, analgesia, and rest may decrease oxygen demand and should be considered. Oxygen delivery may be optimized by maintaining normal levels of hemoglobin (e.g., transfusion of packed RBCs) and PaO_2 (80 to 100 mm Hg), using individualized tidal volumes with positive end-expiratory pressure, increasing preload (e.g., fluids) or myocardial contractility to enhance CO, or reducing afterload to increase CO.

NUTRITIONAL AND METABOLIC NEEDS
Hypermetabolism in SIRS or MODS can result in profound weight loss, cachexia, and further organ failure. Protein-calorie malnutrition is one of the primary signs of hypermetabolism in SIRS and MODS. Total energy expenditure is often increased 1.5 to 2.0 times the normal metabolic rate. Because of their relatively short half-life, monitor plasma transferrin and prealbumin levels to assess hepatic protein synthesis.

The goal of nutritional support is to preserve organ function. Providing early and optimal nutrition decreases morbidity and mortality rates in patients with SIRS and MODS. The enteral route is preferred, but if it cannot be used or cannot meet caloric needs, parenteral nutrition should be initiated or added.[18,19] (Chapter 40 discusses enteral and parenteral nutrition.) Attention to glycemic control with a goal of 140 to 180 mg/dL using insulin infusions is important in these patients.[21]

SUPPORT OF FAILING ORGANS
Support of any failing organ is a primary goal of therapy. For example, the patient with ARDS requires aggressive oxygen therapy and mechanical ventilation (see Chapter 68). DIC should be treated appropriately (e.g., blood products) (see Chapter 31). Renal failure may require dialysis. Continuous renal replacement therapy is better tolerated than hemodialysis, especially in a patient with hemodynamic instability (see Chapter 47).

A final consideration may be that further interventions are futile. It is important to maintain communication between the health care team and, in most cases, the patient's caregiver regarding realistic goals and likely outcomes for the patient with MODS. Withdrawal of life support may be the best option for the patient.

TABLE 67-10   MANIFESTATIONS AND MANAGEMENT OF SIRS AND MODS

Manifestations	Management	Manifestations	Management
Respiratory System		**Renal System**	
Development of ARDS (see Chapter 68):	Prevention	*Prenal:* Renal hypoperfusion	Diuretics
• Severe dyspnea	Optimize O_2 delivery and minimize O_2 consumption	• BUN/creatinine ratio >20:1	• Loop diuretics (e.g., furosemide [Lasix])
• Tachypnea	Mechanical ventilation (see Chapter 66)	• ↓ Urine Na^+ <20 mEq/L	• May need to increase dosage due to ↓ glomerular filtration rate
• PaO_2/FIO_2 ratio <200	• Positive end-expiratory pressure	• ↑ Urine specific gravity >1.020	Continuous renal replacement therapy (see Chapter 47)
• Bilateral fluffy infiltrates on chest x-ray	• Lung protective modes (e.g., pressure-control inverse ratio ventilation, low tidal volumes)	• ↑ Urine osmolality	
• PAWP <18 mm Hg	• Permissive hypercapnia	*Intrarenal:* Acute tubular necrosis	
• Ventilation-perfusion (V/Q) mismatch	• Positioning (e.g., continuous lateral rotation therapy, prone positioning)	• BUN/creatinine ratio <10:1-15:1	
• Pulmonary hypertension		• ↑ Urine Na^+ >20 mEq/L	
• Increased minute ventilation		• ↓ Urine osmolality	
• Decreased compliance		• Urine specific gravity ~1.010	
• Refractory hypoxemia			
Cardiovascular System		**Gastrointestinal System**	
Myocardial depression	Volume management	Mucosal ischemia	Stress ulcer prophylaxis
Massive vasodilation	• Central venous or PA catheter for hemodynamic monitoring	• ↓ Intramucosal pH	• Antacids (e.g., Maalox)
↓ SVR, BP	• APCO for minimally invasive hemodynamic monitoring	• Potential translocation of gut bacteria	• Proton pump inhibitors (e.g., omeprazole [Prilosec])
↓ MAP	• ↑ Preload via volume replacement	• Potential abdominal compartment syndrome	• sucralfate (Carafate)
↑ HR, stroke volume	• Arterial pressure monitoring	Hypoperfusion → ↓ peristalsis, paralytic ileus	Monitor abdominal distention, intraabdominal pressures
↑ CO	• Maintain MAP >65 mm Hg	Mucosal ulceration on endoscopy	Dietary consultation
Systolic, diastolic dysfunction	Vasopressors	GI bleeding	Enteral feedings
Biventricular failure	Intermittent or continuous $ScvO_2$/SvO_2 monitoring		• Stimulate mucosal activity
	Balance O_2 supply and demand		• Provide essential nutrients and optimal calories
	Continuous ECG monitoring		
	Circulatory assist devices	**Hepatic System**	
	Venous thromboembolism prophylaxis	Bilirubin >2 mg/dL (34 µmol/L)	Maintain adequate tissue perfusion
		↑ Liver enzymes (ALT, AST, GGT)	Provide nutritional support (e.g., enteral feedings)
		↑ Serum NH_3	Careful use of drugs metabolized by liver
		↓ Serum albumin, prealbumin, transferrin	
Central Nervous System		Jaundice	
Acute change in neurologic status	Evaluate for hepatic or metabolic encephalopathy	Hepatic encephalopathy	
Fever	Optimize cerebral blood flow		
Hepatic encephalopathy	↓ Cerebral O_2 requirements	**Hematologic System**	
Seizures	Prevent secondary tissue ischemia	↑ Bleeding times, ↑ PT, ↑ PTT	Observe for bleeding from obvious and/or occult sites
Confusion, disorientation, delirium	Calcium channel blockers (reduce cerebral vasospasm)	↓ Platelet count (thrombocytopenia)	Replace factors being lost (e.g., platelets)
Failure to wean, prolonged rehabilitation		↑ Fibrin split products	Minimize traumatic interventions (e.g., IM injections, multiple venipunctures)
		↑ D-dimer	
Endocrine System			
Hyperglycemia → hypoglycemia	Provide continuous infusion of insulin and glucose to maintain blood glucose 140-180 mg/dL (7.77-10.0 mmol/L)		

ALT, Alanine aminotransferase; *APCO,* arterial pressure–based cardiac output; *ARDS,* acute respiratory distress syndrome; *AST,* aspartate aminotransferase; *BUN,* blood urea nitrogen; *CO,* cardiac output; *GGT,* γ-glutamyl transferase; *MAP,* mean arterial pressure; *NH₃,* ammonia; *PA,* pulmonary artery; *PAWP,* pulmonary artery wedge pressure; *PT,* prothrombin time; *PTT,* partial thromboplastin time; *ScvO₂,* oxygen saturation in venous blood; *SvO₂,* oxygen saturation in mixed venous blood; *SVR,* systemic vascular resistance.

CASE STUDY

Shock

iStockphoto/Thinkstock

Patient Profile

K.L., a 25-yr-old Korean American, was not wearing his seat belt when he was the driver involved in a motor vehicle crash. The windshield was broken, and K.L. was found 15 ft from his car. He was face down, conscious, and moaning. His wife and daughter were found in the car with their seat belts on. They sustained no serious injuries, but were upset. All passengers were taken to the emergency department (ED). The following information pertains to K.L.

Subjective Data

- States, "I can't breathe"
- Cries out when abdomen is palpated

Objective Data

Physical Examination

- Cardiovascular: BP 80/56 mm Hg; apical pulse 138 but no palpable radial or pedal pulses; carotid pulse present but weak
- ECG as follows:

- Lungs: respiratory rate 38 breaths/min; labored breathing with shallow respirations; asymmetric chest wall movement; absence of breath sounds on left side
- Trachea deviated slightly to the right
- Abdomen: slightly distended and left upper quadrant painful on palpation
- Musculoskeletal: open compound fracture of the lower left leg

Diagnostic Studies

- Chest x-ray: Hemothorax and six rib fractures on left side
- Hematocrit: 28%

Collaborative Care *(in the ED)*

- Left chest tube placed, draining bright red blood
- IV access obtained via one peripheral line and right subclavian central line
- Fluid resuscitation started with crystalloids
- High-flow O_2 via non-rebreather mask

Surgical Procedure

- Splenectomy
- Repair of torn intercostal artery
- Repair of compound fracture

Discussion Questions

1. What types of shock is K.L. experiencing? What clinical manifestations did he display that support your answer?
2. What were the causes of K.L.'s shock states? What are other causes of these types of shock?
3. *Priority Decision:* What are the priority nursing responsibilities for K.L.?
4. *Priority Decision:* What ongoing nursing assessment parameters are essential for this patient?
5. What are his potential complications?
6. *Priority Decision:* Based on the assessment data presented, what are the priority nursing diagnoses?
7. *Delegation Decision:* Identify the tasks that could be delegated to unlicensed assistive personnel (UAP).
8. *Evidence-Based Practice:* You are orienting a new graduate RN. He asks you why crystalloids are used instead of colloids for fluid resuscitation. What is your response?

ⓔvolve Answers available at *http://evolve.elsevier.com/Lewis/medsurg.*

■ BRIDGE TO NCLEX EXAMINATION

The number of the question corresponds to the same-numbered outcome at the beginning of the chapter.

1. A patient has a spinal cord injury at T4. Vital signs include falling blood pressure with bradycardia. The nurse recognizes that the patient is experiencing
   a. a relative hypervolemia.
   b. an absolute hypovolemia.
   c. neurogenic shock from low blood flow.
   d. neurogenic shock from massive vasodilation.

2. A 78-year-old man has confusion and temperature of 104° F (40° C). He is a diabetic with purulent drainage from his right heel. After an infusion of 3 L of normal saline solution, his assessment findings are BP 84/40 mm Hg; heart rate 110; respiratory rate 42 and shallow; CO 8 L/minute; and PAWP 4 mm Hg. This patient's symptoms are most likely indicative of
   a. sepsis.
   b. septic shock.
   c. multiple organ dysfunction syndrome.
   d. systemic inflammatory response syndrome.

3. Appropriate treatment modalities for the management of cardiogenic shock include *(select all that apply)*
   a. dobutamine to increase myocardial contractility.
   b. vasopressors to increase systemic vascular resistance.
   c. circulatory assist devices such as an intraaortic balloon pump.
   d. corticosteroids to stabilize the cell wall in the infarcted myocardium.
   e. Trendelenburg positioning to facilitate venous return and increase preload.

4. The most accurate assessment parameters for the nurse to use to determine adequate tissue perfusion in the patient with MODS are
   a. blood pressure, pulse, and respirations.
   b. breath sounds, blood pressure, and body temperature.
   c. pulse pressure, level of consciousness, and pupillary response.
   d. level of consciousness, urine output, and skin color and temperature.

1. d, 2. b, 3. a, c, 4. d

ⓔvolve

For rationales to these answers and even more NCLEX review questions, visit *http://evolve.elsevier.com/Lewis/medsurg.*

REFERENCES

1. McLean B, Zimmerman JL. Diagnosis and management of shock. In B McLean, JL Zimmerman, editors: *Guide for fundamental critical care support*, ed 4, Mount Pleasant, Ill, 2007, Society of Critical Care Medicine. (Classic)

2. Gallagher JJ: Shock and end points of resuscitation. In KK Carlson, editor: *AACN advanced critical care nursing*, St Louis, 2009, Saunders. (Classic)

3. Patel AK, Hollenberg SM: Cardiovascular failure and cardiogenic shock, *Semin Respir Crit Care Med* 22:598, 2011.

4. McAtee ME: Cardiogenic shock, *Crit Care Nurs Clin North Am* 23:607, 2011.

5. Tuggle D: Optimizing hemodynamics: strategies for fluid and medication titration in shock. In KK Carlson, editor: *AACN advanced critical care nursing*, St Louis, 2009, Saunders. (Classic)

6. Mandel J, Palevsky PM: Treatment of severe hypovolemia or hypovolemic shock in adults, 2012. Retrieved from *www.uptodate.com/contents/treatment-of-severe-hypovolemia-or-hypovolemic-shock-in-adults*.

*7. Casha S, Christie S: A systematic review of intensive cardiopulmonary management after spinal cord injury, *J Neurotrauma* 28:1479, 2011.

*8. Lieberman P, Nicklas RA, Oppenheimer J, et al: The diagnosis and management of anaphylaxis practice parameter: 2010 update, *J Allergy Clin Immunol* 126:477, 2010.

*9. Dellinger RP, Levy MM, Rhodes A, et al: Surviving sepsis campaign: international guidelines for management of severe sepsis and septic shock: 2012, *Crit Care Med* 41:580, 2013.

10. Aitken LM, Williams G, Harvey M, et al: Nursing considerations to complement the surviving sepsis campaign guidelines, *Crit Care Med* 39:1800, 2011.

11. Chalupka AN, Talmor D: The economics of sepsis, *Crit Care Clin* 28:57, 2012.

12. Cheek DJ, Rodgers SC, Schulman CS: Systemic inflammatory response syndrome and multiple organ dysfunction syndrome. In KK Carlson, editor: *AACN advanced critical care nursing*, St Louis, 2009, Saunders. (Classic)

*13. American Association of Critical-Care Nurses: AACN practice alert: severe sepsis. Retrieved from *www.aacn.org/WD/Practice/Docs/Severe_Sepsis_04-2010.pdf*.

14. Strickler J: Halt the downward spiral of traumatic hypovolemic shock, *Nurs 2012 Crit Care* 7:42, 2012.

*15. Perel P, Roberts I, Ker K: Colloids versus crystalloids for fluid resuscitation in critically ill patients, *Cochrane Database Syst Rev* 2:CD000567, 2013.

16. Hata J, Stotts C, Shelsky C: Reduced mortality with noninvasive hemodynamic monitoring of shock, *J Crit Care* 26:e1, 2011.

17. Walley KR: Use of central venous oxygen saturation to guide therapy, *Am J Respir Crit Care Med* 184:514, 2011.

*18. McClave SA, Martindale RG, Vanek VW, et al: Guidelines for the provision and assessment of nutrition support therapy in the adult critically ill patient: Society of Critical Care Medicine and American Society for Parenteral and Enteral Nutrition, *J Parenter Enteral Nutr* 33:277, 2009.

19. Luehrs Hayes G, McKinzie BP, Moore Bullington W, et al: Nutritional supplements in critical illness, *AACN Adv Crit Care* 22:301, 2011.

20. Myers TJ: Temporary ventricular assist devices in the intensive care unit as a bridge to decision, *AACN Adv Crit Care* 23:55, 2012.

21. NICE-SUGAR Study Investigators. Intensive versus conventional glucose control in critically ill patients, *N Engl J Med* 360:1283, 2009.

*22. Wright RS, Anderson JL, Adams CD, et al: 2011 ACCF/AHA focused update of the guidelines for the management of patients with unstable angina/non-ST-elevation myocardial infarction (updating the 2007 guideline), *J Am Coll Cardiol* 57:1920, 2011.

23. Flynn Makic MB, VonRueden KT, Rauen CA, et al: Evidence-based practice habits: putting more sacred cows out to pasture, *Crit Care Nurse* 31:31, 2011.

*24. American Association of Critical-Care Nurses: AACN practice alert: oral care for patients at risk for ventilator-associated pneumonia, 2010. Retrieved from *www.aacn.org/WD/Practice/Docs/Oral_Care_in_the_Critically_Ill.pdf*.

*25. American Association of Critical-Care Nurses: AACN practice alert: family presence during resuscitation and invasive procedures, 2010. Retrieved from *www.aacn.org/WD/Practice/Docs/PracticeAlerts/Family%20Presence%2004-2010%20final.pdf*.

*26. American Association of Critical-Care Nurses: AACN practice alert: family presence: visitation in the adult ICU, 2011. Retrieved from *www.aacn.org/WD/practice/docs/practicealerts/family-visitation-adult-icu-practicealert.pdf*.

*27. Redekopp MA, Leske JS: Family visitation and partnership. In NC Molter, editor: *Protocols for practice: creating healing environments*, ed 2, Sudbury, Mass, 2007, Jones & Bartlett. (Classic)

RESOURCES

Additional resources for this chapter are listed after Chapter 66 on p. 1630 and Chapter 69 on p. 1694.

---

*Evidence-based information for clinical practice.

*What oxygen is to the lungs, such is hope to
the meaning of life.*
Emil Brunner

Nursing Management
Respiratory Failure and
Acute Respiratory Distress Syndrome

Richard Arbour

⊖volve WEBSITE

LEARNING OUTCOMES

1. Compare the pathophysiologic mechanisms and clinical manifestations that result in hypoxemic and hypercapnic respiratory failure.
2. Differentiate between the nursing and collaborative management of the patient with hypoxemic or hypercapnic respiratory failure.
3. Relate the pathophysiologic mechanisms and the clinical manifestations associated with acute lung injury and acute respiratory distress syndrome (ARDS).
4. Select appropriate nursing and collaborative management strategies for the patient with ARDS.
5. Prioritize measures to prevent or reverse complications that may result from acute respiratory failure or ARDS.

KEY TERMS

acute lung injury (ALI), p. 1665
acute respiratory distress syndrome
   (ARDS), p. 1665
alveolar hypoventilation, p. 1657

hypercapnia, p. 1654
hypercapnic respiratory failure, p. 1655
hypoxemia, p. 1654
hypoxemic respiratory failure, p. 1655

hypoxia, p. 1658
refractory hypoxemia, p. 1666
shunt, p. 1656
work of breathing (WOB), p. 1659

This chapter discusses the etiology, pathophysiology, and clinical manifestations of acute respiratory failure and acute respiratory distress syndrome (ARDS). Nursing and collaborative management of patients with respiratory failure and ARDS focuses on interventions to promote adequate oxygenation and ventilation while addressing the underlying causes.

ACUTE RESPIRATORY FAILURE

The major function of the respiratory system is gas exchange. This involves the transfer of oxygen (O_2) and carbon dioxide (CO_2) between atmospheric air and circulating blood within the pulmonary capillary bed (Fig. 68-1). *Respiratory failure* results when one or both of these gas-exchanging functions are inadequate (e.g., insufficient O_2 is transferred to the blood or inadequate CO_2 is removed from the lungs). Diseases that interfere with adequate O_2 transfer result in hypoxemia. This causes a decrease in arterial O_2 (PaO_2) and saturation (SaO_2). Insufficient CO_2 removal results in hypercapnia. This causes an increase in arterial CO_2 ($PaCO_2$).[1-4]

Arterial blood gases (ABGs) are used to assess changes in pH, PaO_2, $PaCO_2$, bicarbonate, and SaO_2. Pulse oximetry is used intermittently or continuously to assess arterial O_2 saturation (SpO_2).

Reviewed by Susan J. Eisel, RN, MSEd, Associate Professor of Nursing, Mercy College of Ohio, Toledo, Ohio; Eleanor Fitzpatrick, RN, MSN, CCRN, Clinical Nurse Specialist, Thomas Jefferson University Hospital, Philadelphia, Pennsylvania; and Amanda Jones Moose, RN, BSN, Nursing Faculty, Caldwell Community College and Technical Institute, Taylorsville, North Carolina.

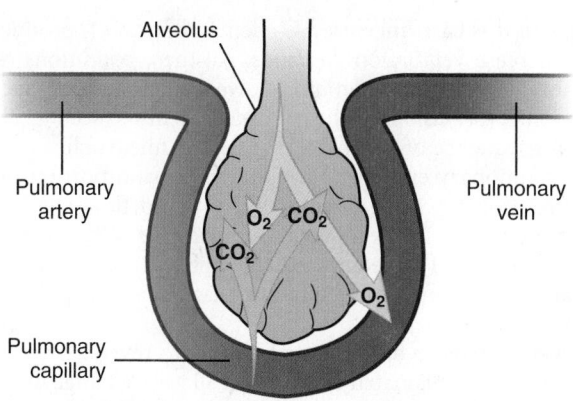

FIG. 68-1 Normal gas exchange unit in the lung.

FIG. 68-2 Classification of respiratory failure.

Respiratory failure is not a disease but a symptom of an underlying pathologic condition affecting lung function, O_2 delivery, cardiac output (CO), or the baseline metabolic state. It is a condition that occurs because of one or more diseases involving the lungs or other body systems (Table 68-1 and eTable 68-1 [available on the website for this text]). Respiratory failure is classified as hypoxemic or hypercapnic (Fig. 68-2). Hypoxemic respiratory failure is also referred to as *oxygenation failure* because the primary problem is inadequate O_2 transfer between the alveoli and the pulmonary capillaries. Although no universal definition exists, **hypoxemic respiratory failure** is commonly defined as a PaO_2 less than 60 mm Hg when the patient is receiving an inspired O_2 concentration of 60% or more. This definition incorporates two important concepts: (1) the PaO_2 level indicates inadequate O_2 saturation of hemoglobin, and (2) this PaO_2 level exists despite administration of supplemental O_2 at a percentage (60%) that is about three times that in room air (21%).[5-7]

Hypercapnic respiratory failure is also referred to as *ventilatory failure* because the primary problem is insufficient CO_2 removal. **Hypercapnic respiratory failure** is commonly defined as a $PaCO_2$ greater than 45 mm Hg in combination with acidemia (arterial pH less than 7.35). This definition incorporates three important concepts: (1) the $PaCO_2$ is higher than normal, (2) there is evidence of the body's inability to compensate for this increase (acidemia), and (3) the pH is at a level where a further decrease may lead to severe acid-base imbalance. (See Chapter 17 for a discussion of acid-base balance.) Numerous disorders can compromise lung ventilation and subsequent carbon dioxide removal (see Table 68-1 and eTable 68-1).

Many patients experience both hypoxemic and hypercapnic respiratory failure.[6-9] Always interpret data within the context of your assessment findings and the patient's baseline. For example, a person with chronic lung disease may have a baseline $PaCO_2$ higher than "normal."

Etiology and Pathophysiology

Hypoxemic Respiratory Failure. Four physiologic mechanisms may cause hypoxemia and subsequent hypoxemic respiratory failure: (1) mismatch between ventilation (V) and perfusion (Q), commonly referred to as V/Q mismatch; (2) shunt; (3) diffusion limitation; and (4) alveolar hypoventilation. The most common causes are V/Q mismatch and shunt.

Ventilation-Perfusion Mismatch. In normal lungs the volume of blood perfusing the lungs each minute (4 to 5 L) is approximately equal to the amount of gas that reaches the alveoli each

TABLE 68-1	CAUSES OF HYPOXEMIC AND HYPERCAPNIC RESPIRATORY FAILURE*
Hypoxemic Respiratory Failure	**Hypercapnic Respiratory Failure**
Respiratory System	**Respiratory System**
• Acute respiratory distress syndrome	• Asthma
• Pneumonia	• COPD
• Toxic inhalation (e.g., smoke inhalation)	• Cystic fibrosis
• Hepatopulmonary syndrome (e.g., low-resistance flow state; V/Q mismatch)	**Central Nervous System**
	• Brainstem injury or infarction
• Massive pulmonary embolism (e.g., thrombus emboli, fat emboli)	• Sedative and opioid overdose
	• Spinal cord injury
• Pulmonary artery laceration and hemorrhage	• Severe head injury
	Chest Wall
• Inflammatory state and related alveolar injury	• Thoracic trauma (e.g., flail chest)
	• Kyphoscoliosis
	• Pain
Cardiac System	• Severe obesity
• Anatomic shunt (e.g., ventricular septal defect)	**Neuromuscular System**
• Cardiogenic pulmonary edema	• Myasthenia gravis
	• Critical illness polyneuropathy
• Shock (decreasing blood flow through pulmonary vasculature)	• Acute myopathy
	• Toxin exposure or ingestion (e.g., tree tobacco, acetylcholinesterase inhibitors, carbamate or organophosphate poisoning)
• High cardiac output states: diffusion limitation	• Amyotrophic lateral sclerosis
	• Phrenic nerve injury
	• Guillain-Barré syndrome
	• Poliomyelitis
	• Muscular dystrophy
	• Multiple sclerosis

*List is not all-inclusive.

minute (4 to 5 L). In a perfectly matched system, each portion of the lung would receive 1 mL of air (ventilation) for each 1 mL of blood flow (perfusion). This match of ventilation and perfusion would result in a V/Q ratio of 1:1, which is expressed as V/Q = 1. When the match is not 1:1, a *V/Q mismatch* occurs.

Although this example implies that ventilation and perfusion are ideally matched in all areas of the lung, this situation does not normally exist. In reality, some regional mismatch occurs. At the lung apex, V/Q ratios are greater than 1 (more ventilation than perfusion). At the lung base, V/Q ratios are less than 1 (less ventilation than perfusion). Because changes at the lung apex balance changes at the base, the net effect is a close overall match (Fig. 68-3).

Many diseases and conditions cause V/Q mismatch (Fig. 68-4). The most common are those in which increased secretions are present in the airways (e.g., chronic obstructive pulmonary disease [COPD]) or alveoli (e.g., pneumonia), and in which bronchospasm is present (e.g., asthma).[5-8] V/Q mismatch may also result from alveolar collapse *(atelectasis)* or as a result of pain. Pain interferes with chest and abdominal wall movement and compromises ventilation. Additionally, it increases muscle tension, producing generalized muscle rigidity. Pain also causes systemic vasoconstriction and activates the stress response. Finally, it increases O_2 consumption and CO_2 produc-

tion.[10] In this case, increased O_2 demand and CO_2 production may increase ventilation demands. All these conditions result in limited airflow *(ventilation)* to alveoli but have no effect on blood flow *(perfusion)* to the gas exchange units (see Fig. 68-1). The consequence of the imbalance is V/Q mismatch.

A pulmonary embolus affects the perfusion portion of the V/Q relationship. The embolus limits blood flow but has no effect on airflow to the alveoli, again causing V/Q mismatch[11] (see Fig. 68-4). If large enough, the embolus can cause hemodynamic compromise due to the blockage of a large pulmonary artery.

O_2 therapy is an appropriate first step to reverse hypoxemia caused by V/Q mismatch because not all gas exchange units are affected. O_2 therapy increases the PaO_2 in blood leaving normal gas exchange units, thus causing a higher than normal PaO_2. The well-oxygenated blood mixes with poorly oxygenated blood, raising the overall PaO_2 of blood leaving the lungs. The optimal approach to treating hypoxemia caused by a V/Q mismatch is directed at the cause.

Shunt. A **shunt** occurs when blood exits the heart without having participated in gas exchange. A shunt can be viewed as an extreme V/Q mismatch (see Fig. 68-4). There are two types of shunt: anatomic and intrapulmonary. An *anatomic shunt* occurs when blood passes through an anatomic channel in the heart (e.g., a ventricular septal defect) and bypasses the lungs. An *intrapulmonary shunt* occurs when blood flows through the pulmonary capillaries without participating in gas exchange. Intrapulmonary shunt is seen in conditions in which the alveoli fill with fluid (e.g., acute respiratory distress syndrome [ARDS], pneumonia).

O_2 therapy alone is often ineffective in increasing the PaO_2 if hypoxemia is due to shunt. Patients with shunt are usually more hypoxemic than patients with V/Q mismatch. They often require mechanical ventilation and a high fraction of inspired O_2 (FIO_2) to improve gas exchange.

Diffusion Limitation. *Diffusion limitation* occurs when gas exchange across the alveolar-capillary interface is compromised by a process that thickens, damages, or destroys the alveolar membrane or affects blood flow through the pulmonary capillaries (Fig. 68-5). Diffusion limitation is worsened by disease states affecting the pulmonary vascular bed such as severe COPD or recurrent pulmonary emboli. Some disease states cause the alveolar-capillary interface to become thicker (fibrotic), which slows gas transport. These include pulmonary fibrosis, interstitial lung disease, and ARDS.[12,13]

V/Q	PaO$_2$	PaCO$_2$	
3.3	132	28	Apex of lung
1.0	108	39	Midpoint of lung
0.63	89	42	Base of lung

FIG. 68-3 Regional V/Q differences in the normal lung. At the lung apex, the V/Q ratio is 3.3, at the midpoint 1.0, and at the base 0.63. This difference causes the PaO$_2$ to be higher at the apex of the lung and lower at the base. Values for PaCO$_2$ are the opposite (i.e., lower at the apex and higher at the base). Blood that exits the lung is a mixture of these values.

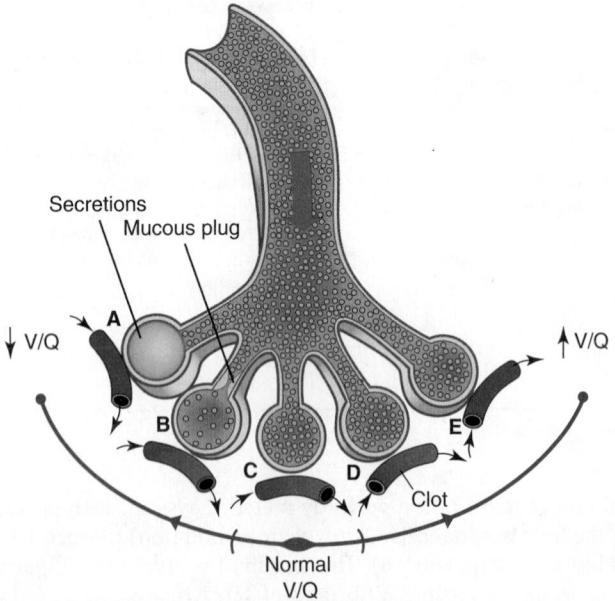

FIG. 68-4 Range of ventilation-to-perfusion (V/Q) relationships. **A,** Absolute shunt, no ventilation because of fluid filling the alveoli. **B,** V/Q mismatch, ventilation partially compromised by secretions in the airway. **C,** Normal lung unit. **D,** V/Q mismatch, perfusion partially compromised by emboli obstructing blood flow. **E,** Dead space, no perfusion because of obstruction of the pulmonary capillary.

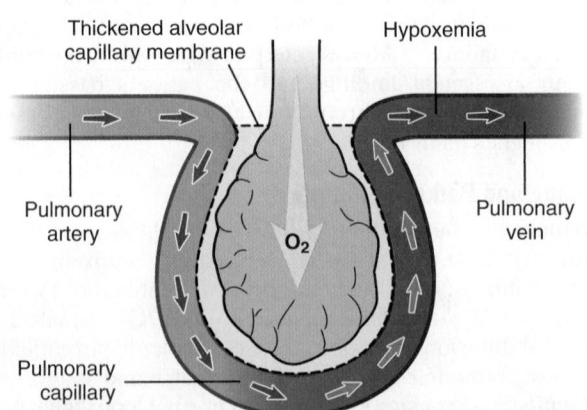

FIG. 68-5 Diffusion limitation. Exchange of CO_2 and O_2 cannot occur because of the thickened alveolar-capillary membrane.

The classic sign of diffusion limitation is hypoxemia that is present during exercise but not at rest. During exercise, blood moves more rapidly through the lungs, decreasing the time for diffusion of O_2 across the alveolar-capillary interface. Diffusion limitation may also occur in a high CO state (e.g., hepatopulmonary syndrome) or other disease states (e.g., inflammatory response seen with pancreatitis or severe brain trauma) unrelated to lung tissue damage. In this situation, CO is markedly elevated and vascular resistance is low. Blood circulates through the pulmonary capillary bed rapidly, allowing less time for gas exchange to occur.[14]

Alveolar Hypoventilation. Alveolar hypoventilation is a generalized decrease in ventilation that results in an increase in the $PaCO_2$ and a consequent decrease in PaO_2. Alveolar hypoventilation may be the result of restrictive lung diseases, central nervous system (CNS) diseases, chest wall dysfunction, acute asthma, or neuromuscular diseases. Although alveolar hypoventilation is primarily a mechanism of hypercapnic respiratory failure, it is mentioned here because it can also cause hypoxemia.[15]

Interrelationship of Mechanisms. Frequently, hypoxemic respiratory failure is caused by a combination of two or more of the following: V/Q mismatch, shunt, diffusion limitation, and alveolar hypoventilation. For example, the patient with acute respiratory failure secondary to pneumonia may have a combination of V/Q mismatch and shunt. In this case, inflammation, edema, and hypersecretion of exudate within the bronchioles and gas exchange units obstruct the airways (V/Q mismatch) and fill the alveoli with exudate (shunt). Additional contributing factors to hypoxemic respiratory failure include increases in O_2 demand such as with severe anxiety or agitation and unrelieved pain.

Hypercapnic Respiratory Failure. Hypercapnic respiratory failure results from an imbalance between ventilatory supply and ventilatory demand. *Ventilatory supply* is the maximum ventilation (gas flow in and out of the lungs) that the patient can sustain without developing respiratory muscle fatigue. *Ventilatory demand* is the amount of ventilation needed to keep the $PaCO_2$ within normal limits. Normally, ventilatory supply far exceeds ventilatory demand. Therefore people with normal lung function can engage in strenuous exercise, which greatly increases CO_2 production without an increase in $PaCO_2$. Patients with lung disease such as severe COPD do not have this advantage and cannot effectively increase lung ventilation in response to exercise or metabolic demands.

Hypercapnia occurs when ventilatory demand exceeds ventilatory supply and $PaCO_2$ cannot be sustained within normal limits. Hypercapnia reflects substantial lung dysfunction. Hypercapnic respiratory failure is sometimes called *ventilatory failure* because the primary problem is the respiratory system's inability to remove sufficient CO_2 to maintain a normal $PaCO_2$. Hypercapnic respiratory failure is also described as acute or chronic respiratory failure. For example, an episode of respiratory failure may represent an acute decompensation in a patient whose underlying lung function has deteriorated to the point that some degree of decompensation is always present (chronic respiratory insufficiency).

Many different diseases can cause a limitation in ventilatory supply (see Table 68-1 and eTable 68-1). These diseases can be grouped into four categories: (1) abnormalities of the airways and alveoli, (2) abnormalities of the CNS, (3) abnormalities of the chest wall, and (4) neuromuscular conditions.[16,17]

Airway and Alveoli Abnormalities. Patients with asthma, COPD, and cystic fibrosis are at high risk for hypercapnic respiratory failure because the underlying pathophysiology of these conditions results in airflow obstruction and air trapping. Ultimately respiratory muscle fatigue and ventilatory failure occur due to the additional work needed to inspire adequate tidal volumes against increased airway resistance and air trapped within the alveoli.[18-21]

Central Nervous System Abnormalities. A variety of CNS problems may suppress the drive to breathe. A common example is an overdose of a respiratory depressant drug (e.g., opioids, benzodiazepines). In a dose-related manner, CNS depressants decrease CO_2 reactivity in the brainstem. This allows arterial CO_2 levels to rise. A brainstem infarction or severe head injury may also interfere with normal function of the respiratory center in the medulla. Patients with these conditions are at risk for respiratory failure because the medulla does not alter the respiratory rate in response to a change in $PaCO_2$. CNS dysfunction may also include high-level spinal cord injuries that limit nerve supply to the respiratory muscles of the chest wall and diaphragm. Apart from direct brainstem dysfunction, metabolic or structural brain injury resulting in decreased or loss of consciousness may interfere with the patient's ability to manage secretions or adequately protect his or her airway.

Chest Wall Abnormalities. Several conditions prevent normal movement of the chest wall and limit lung expansion. In patients with flail chest, fractures prevent the rib cage from expanding normally because of pain, mechanical restriction, and muscle spasm. In patients with kyphoscoliosis, the change in spinal configuration compresses the lungs and prevents normal expansion of the chest wall. In patients with severe obesity, the weight of the chest and abdominal contents may limit lung expansion. These conditions place patients at risk for respiratory failure because they limit lung expansion or diaphragmatic movement and consequently gas exchange.

Neuromuscular Conditions. Various types of neuromuscular diseases may result in respiratory muscle weakness or paralysis (see Table 68-1). For example, patients with Guillain-Barré syndrome, muscular dystrophy, myasthenia gravis (acute exacerbation), or multiple sclerosis are at risk for respiratory failure because the respiratory muscles are weakened or paralyzed as a result of the underlying neuromuscular condition. Therefore they are unable to maintain normal $PaCO_2$ levels.[15-17]

Neuromuscular disorders may be acquired as a consequence of exposure to toxins (e.g., carbamate/organophosphate pesticides, chemical nerve agents) that interfere with the nerve supply to muscles and lung ventilation. Respiratory muscle weakness may also result from muscle wasting during a critical illness, peripheral nerve damage, and/or prolonged effects of neuromuscular blocking agents.

In summary, respiratory failure may occur in three of these categories (CNS, chest wall, neuromuscular conditions) despite the presence of normal lungs. Respiratory failure occurs because the medulla, chest wall, peripheral nerves, or respiratory muscles are not functioning normally. The patient may have no damage to lung tissue but may be unable to inspire a tidal volume sufficient to remove CO_2 from the lungs.

Tissue Oxygen Needs. Remember that even though PaO_2 and $PaCO_2$ determine the definition of respiratory failure, the major cause of respiratory failure is the lung's inability to meet the O_2 needs of the tissues. This failure may occur because of inadequate O_2 delivery to the tissues or because the tissues cannot use the O_2 delivered to them. It may also occur as a result of the stress response and dramatic increases in tissue O_2 consumption.

Tissue O_2 delivery is determined by cardiac output and the amount of O_2 carried in the hemoglobin. Therefore respiratory failure places the patient at greater risk if there are coexisting heart problems or anemia. Failure of O_2 use most commonly occurs in septic shock. Adequate O_2 may be delivered to the tissues, but impaired O_2 extraction or diffusion limitation exists at the cellular level. This results in an abnormally high amount of O_2 returning in the venous blood because it is not used at the tissue level. (Chapter 67 discusses shock.) Acid-base alterations (e.g., alkalosis, acidosis) may also interfere with O_2 delivery to peripheral tissues (see Chapter 17).

Clinical Manifestations

Respiratory failure may develop suddenly (minutes or hours) or gradually (several days or longer). A sudden decrease in PaO_2 or a rapid rise in $PaCO_2$ implies a serious condition, which can rapidly become a life-threatening emergency. An example is the patient with asthma who develops severe bronchospasm and a marked decrease in airflow, resulting in rapid respiratory muscle fatigue, acidemia, and respiratory failure.

A more gradual change in PaO_2 and $PaCO_2$ is better tolerated because compensation can occur. An example is the patient with COPD who develops a progressive increase in $PaCO_2$ over several days after a respiratory tract infection. Because the change occurred over several days, there is time for renal compensation (e.g., retention of bicarbonate), which minimizes the change in arterial pH. The patient will have compensated respiratory acidosis.[3,4] (See Chapter 17 for a discussion of renal compensation for acid-base disorders.)

Manifestations of respiratory failure are related to the extent of change in PaO_2 or $PaCO_2$, the rapidity of change (acute versus chronic), and the patient's ability to compensate for this change. When the patient's compensatory mechanisms fail, respiratory failure occurs. Because clinical manifestations vary, it is important to watch trends in ABGs, pulse oximetry, and assessment findings to fully evaluate the extent of change. Frequently, the first indication of respiratory failure is a change in the patient's mental status. Mental status changes often occur early, before ABG results are obtained. This is because the brain is very sensitive to variations in O_2 and CO_2 levels and acid-base balance. Restlessness, confusion, agitation, and combative behavior suggest inadequate O_2 delivery to the brain and should be fully investigated.

You may detect manifestations of respiratory failure that are specific (primary) (arising from the respiratory system) or nonspecific (secondary) (arising from other body systems) (Table 68-2). Understanding the significance of these manifestations is critical to your ability to detect the onset of respiratory failure and evaluate the effectiveness of treatment.

Tachycardia, tachypnea, and mild hypertension can be early signs of respiratory failure consequent to physiologic stress and elevated catecholamine levels. Such changes can indicate an attempt by the heart and lungs to compensate for decreased O_2 delivery. A severe morning headache may suggest that hypercapnia occurred during the night. Hypercapnia causes cerebral vasodilation, increased cerebral blood flow, and a mild increase in intracranial pressure (ICP) that produces a headache. At night the respiratory rate is slower and the lungs of patients at risk for respiratory failure may remove less $PaCO_2$.[22] Rapid,

TABLE 68-2	MANIFESTATIONS OF HYPOXEMIA AND HYPERCAPNIA*
Specific	**Nonspecific**
Hypoxemia	
Respiratory	**Cerebral**
Dyspnea	Agitation
Tachypnea	Disorientation
Prolonged expiration (I:E = 1:3, 1:4)	Restless, combative behavior
Nasal flaring	Delirium
Intercostal muscle retraction	Confusion
Use of accessory muscles in respiration	↓ Level of consciousness
	Coma (late)
↓ SpO_2 (<80%)	
Paradoxic chest or abdominal wall movement with respiratory cycle (late)	**Cardiac**
	Tachycardia
	Hypertension
	Skin cool, clammy, and diaphoretic
	Dysrhythmias (late)
	Hypotension (late)
Cyanosis (late)	
	Other
	Fatigue
	Inability to speak in complete sentences without pausing to breathe
Hypercapnia	
Respiratory	**Cerebral**
Dyspnea	Morning headache
Use of tripod position	Disorientation
Pursed-lip breathing	Progressive somnolence
↓ Respiratory rate or rapid rate with shallow respirations	Elevated intracranial pressure (if monitored)
	Coma (late)
↓ Tidal volume	
↓ Minute ventilation	**Cardiac**
	Dysrhythmias
	Hypertension
	Tachycardia
	Bounding pulse
	Neuromuscular
	Muscle weakness
	↓ Deep tendon reflexes
	Tremors, seizures (late)

*List is not all-inclusive.
I:E, Inspiratory:expiratory ratio.

shallow breaths suggest that tidal volume may be inadequate to remove CO_2 from the lungs. Cyanosis is an unreliable indicator of hypoxemia and is a late sign of respiratory failure because it does not occur until hypoxemia is severe (PaO_2 of 45 mm Hg or less).

Consequences of Hypoxemia and Hypoxia. *Hypoxemia* occurs when the amount of O_2 in arterial blood is less than the normal value (normal PaO_2 is 80 to 100 mm Hg). Hypoxia occurs when the PaO_2 falls sufficiently to cause signs and symptoms of inadequate oxygenation (see Table 68-2). Hypoxemia can lead to hypoxia if not corrected. If hypoxia or hypoxemia is severe, the cells shift from aerobic to anaerobic metabolism. Anaerobic metabolism uses more fuel, produces less energy, and is less efficient than aerobic metabolism. The waste product of anaerobic metabolism is lactic acid. This is more difficult to remove from the body than CO_2 because it has to be buffered with sodium bicarbonate. When the body does not have enough sodium bicarbonate to buffer the lactic acid produced by anaerobic metabolism, metabolic acidosis, tissue and cellular dysfunction, and cell death may occur. Blood pressure (BP) and cardiac output can fall, and vasoactive or inotropic agents are often less effective in an acidotic environment.

Hypoxia and metabolic acidosis have adverse effects on the vital organs, especially the heart and CNS. The heart tries to compensate for the decreased O_2 level in the blood by increasing the heart rate and cardiac output. A cardiovascular hyperdynamic state may also occur due to catecholamine release that is associated with the physiologic stress response. As the PaO_2 decreases and acidosis increases, the myocardium becomes dysfunctional and cardiac output may decrease. In addition, angina and dysrhythmias may occur. All of these result in a further decrease in O_2 delivery.

Permanent brain damage may occur if the hypoxia is severe and prolonged. Renal function may also be impaired. Sodium retention, edema, acute tubular necrosis, and uremia may occur. Gastrointestinal (GI) system alterations include tissue ischemia, increased permeability of the intestinal wall, and possible migration of bacteria from the GI tract into circulation.

Specific Clinical Manifestations. The patient in respiratory failure may have a rapid, shallow breathing pattern or a respiratory rate that is slower than normal. Both changes predispose the patient to insufficient CO_2 removal. The patient may increase the respiratory rate in an effort to blow off accumulated CO_2. This breathing pattern requires a substantial amount of work and can lead to respiratory muscle fatigue. A change from a rapid rate to a slower rate in a patient in acute respiratory distress such as that seen with acute asthma suggests extreme progression of respiratory muscle fatigue and increased probability of respiratory arrest.[5-7,9]

The patient's position is an indication of the effort associated with **work of breathing (WOB)**, or the effort used for muscle contraction during inhalation to accomplish lung ventilation. The patient may be able to lie down (mild distress), be able to lie down but prefer to sit (moderate distress), or be unable to breathe unless sitting upright (severe distress). A common position used by patients with moderate to severe COPD is to sit with the arms propped on the overbed table or on the knees. This so-called *tripod position* helps decrease the WOB, since propping the arms increases the anteroposterior diameter of the chest and changes pressure in the thorax (Fig. 68-6).

FIG. 68-6 Tripod positioning is used to increase chest and lung expansion and decrease work of breathing for patients with COPD or asthma.

Patients may use pursed-lip breathing (see Table 29-13). This increases SaO_2 because it slows respirations, allows more time for expiration, and prevents the small bronchioles from collapsing, thus helping air exchange. Another assessment parameter is the number of pillows the patient needs to breathe comfortably when lying flat. This is termed *orthopnea* and is documented as one-, two-, three-, or four-pillow orthopnea.

The person who is experiencing dyspnea is working hard to breathe and may be able to speak only a few words at a time between breaths. The patient's ability to speak indicates the severity of dyspnea. The patient may speak in sentences (mild or no distress), short phrases (moderate distress), or only words (severe distress). The number of words is also a clue. The patient may have "two-word" or "three-word" dyspnea, signifying that only two or three words can be spoken before pausing to breathe. There may also be a change in the onset of fatigue with walking. An additional assessment parameter is how far the patient is able to walk without stopping to rest.

The *inspiratory (I) to expiratory (E) (I:E) ratio* may change in patients in respiratory distress. Normally, the I:E ratio is 1:2, which means that expiration is twice as long as inspiration. The ratio may increase to 1:3 or 1:4, which signifies airflow obstruction and that more time is required to empty the lungs.

You may observe *retraction* (inward movement) of the intercostal spaces or the supraclavicular area and use of the accessory muscles (e.g., sternocleidomastoid) during inspiration or expiration. Use of the accessory muscles signifies moderate distress. Paradoxic breathing indicates severe distress. Normally, the thorax and abdomen move outward on inspiration and inward on exhalation. During *paradoxic breathing,* the abdomen and chest move in the opposite manner—outward during exhalation and inward during inspiration. Paradoxic breathing results from maximal use of the accessory muscles of respiration. The patient may also be diaphoretic from the WOB.

Perform auscultation to assess the patient's baseline breath sounds and any changes from baseline. Note and document the presence and location of any abnormal breath sounds. Crackles (generally heard on inspiration) may indicate pulmonary edema. Rhonchi (generally heard on expiration) indicate additional lung secretions and may be symptomatic of pneumonia or COPD. Absent or diminished breath sounds may indicate atelectasis, pleural effusion, or impaired inspiratory effort and hypoventilation. Bronchial breath sounds over the lung periphery often indicate lung consolidation from pneumonia. A pleural friction rub may also be heard in the presence of pneumonia that involves the pleura.

A thorough nursing assessment may result in early detection of respiratory insufficiency, allowing interventions to be started sooner and preventing respiratory failure. Patients with end-stage (severe) chronic lung disease may have low PaO_2 values or elevated $PaCO_2$ levels and crackles as their "normal" baseline. It is especially important to monitor specific and nonspecific signs of respiratory failure in patients with COPD because a small change can cause significant decompensation (see Table 68-2). Immediately report any change in mental status (e.g., agitation, confusion, decreased level of consciousness). This may indicate the onset of rapid deterioration in clinical status and the need for mechanical ventilation.

Diagnostic Studies

After physical assessment, the most common diagnostic studies used to evaluate respiratory failure are chest x-ray and ABG analysis. A chest x-ray helps to identify possible causes of respiratory failure (e.g., atelectasis, pneumonia). ABGs determine the levels of $PaCO_2$, PaO_2, bicarbonate, and pH. In respiratory failure, ABGs are used to evaluate oxygenation (PaO_2) and ventilation ($PaCO_2$) status and acid-base balance. Pulse oximetry monitors oxygenation status, but reveals little about lung ventilation. A catheter may be inserted into an artery to obtain blood for ABGs and monitor BP.

Other diagnostic studies that may be done include a complete blood cell count, serum electrolytes, urinalysis, and electrocardiogram (ECG). Blood and sputum cultures are obtained as necessary to determine sources of possible infection. If pulmonary embolus is suspected, a CT scan or V/Q lung scan may be done. For the patient in severe respiratory failure requiring endotracheal intubation, end-tidal CO_2 ($ETCO_2$) may be used to assess tube placement within the trachea immediately after intubation. (Chapter 66 discusses intubation.) $ETCO_2$ monitoring (capnography) and transcutaneous CO_2 monitoring may also be used during ventilator management to assess trends in lung ventilation.[23] Although not commonly done in acute situations, pulmonary function tests may be performed.

In severe respiratory failure, central venous or PA pressure monitoring or arterial pressure–based CO monitoring is used to measure hemodynamic parameters (e.g., central venous pressure, PA pressures, CO, stroke volume variation, central/mixed venous O_2 saturation [$ScvO_2$/SvO_2]). These data help to determine the adequacy of tissue perfusion and the patient's response to treatment measures. Hemodynamic monitoring can also determine whether the accumulation of fluid in the lungs is the result of heart or lung problems. It can also provide feedback on the physiologic effects of mechanical ventilation on hemodynamic status.[24] (Chapter 66 discusses hemodynamic monitoring in detail.)

NURSING AND COLLABORATIVE MANAGEMENT ACUTE RESPIRATORY FAILURE

Because many different problems cause respiratory failure, specific care of these patients varies. This section discusses general assessment and collaborative care measures that apply to patients with acute respiratory failure. In acute care settings, collaboration between nursing and other health care team members (e.g., respiratory therapists) is essential.

NURSING ASSESSMENT

Table 68-3 presents subjective and objective data that should be obtained from the patient with acute respiratory failure.

NURSING DIAGNOSES

Nursing diagnoses for the patient with acute respiratory failure may include, but are not limited to, the following:

- Impaired gas exchange *related to* alveolar hypoventilation, intrapulmonary shunting, V/Q mismatch, and diffusion impairment
- Ineffective airway clearance *related to* excessive secretions, decreased level of consciousness, presence of an artificial airway, neuromuscular dysfunction, and pain
- Ineffective breathing pattern *related to* neuromuscular impairment of respirations, pain, anxiety, decreased level of consciousness, respiratory muscle fatigue, and bronchospasm

---

TABLE 68-3 NURSING ASSESSMENT

Acute Respiratory Failure

Subjective Data
Important Health Information
Past health history: Chronic lung disease; potential occupational exposures to lung toxins; tobacco use (pack-years); alcohol or drug use; previous hospitalizations related to lung disease; thoracic or spinal cord trauma; severe obesity; altered consciousness; age (physiologic and chronologic)
Medications: Use of home O_2, inhalers (bronchodilators), home nebulization, over-the-counter medications; immunosuppressant (e.g., corticosteroid) therapy, CNS depressants
Surgery or other treatments: Previous intubation and mechanical ventilation; recent thoracic or abdominal surgery

Functional Health Patterns
Health perception–health management: Exercise, self-care activities; immunizations (flu, pneumonia, hepatitis)
Nutritional-metabolic: Eating habits; bloating, indigestion; weight gain or loss; change in appetite; use of vitamins or herbal supplements
Activity-exercise: Fatigue, dizziness; dyspnea at rest or with activity, wheezing, cough (productive or nonproductive); sputum (volume, color, viscosity); palpitations, swollen feet; change in exercise tolerance
Sleep-rest: Changes in sleep pattern; use of CPAP
Cognitive-perceptual: Headache, chest pain or tightness; chronic pain
Coping–stress tolerance: Anxiety, depression, hopelessness; risk of drug, alcohol, or nicotine withdrawal

Objective Data
General
Restlessness, agitation

Integumentary
Pale, cool, clammy skin or warm, flushed skin; peripheral and central cyanosis; peripheral dependent edema

Respiratory
Shallow, increased respiratory rate progressing to decreased rate; use of accessory muscles with evidence of retractions, altered I:E ratio; increased diaphragmatic excursion or asymmetric chest expansion; paradoxic chest and abdominal wall movement; tactile fremitus, crepitus, or deviated trachea on palpation; absent, diminished, or adventitious breath sounds; pleural friction rub; bronchial or bronchovesicular sounds heard in other than normal location; inspiratory stridor

Cardiovascular
Vital signs: Tachycardia progressing to bradycardia, dysrhythmias, extra heart sounds (S_3, S_4); bounding pulse; hypertension progressing to hypotension; pulsus paradoxus; jugular venous distention; pedal edema

Gastrointestinal
Abdominal distention, ascites, epigastric tenderness, hepatojugular reflex

Neurologic
Somnolence, confusion, slurred speech, restlessness, delirium, agitation, tremors, seizures, coma; asterixis, decreased deep tendon reflexes; papilledema

Possible Diagnostic Findings
$\downarrow/\uparrow$ pH, $\uparrow/\downarrow$ $PaCO_2$, $\uparrow/\downarrow$ bicarbonate, $\downarrow$ PaO_2, $\downarrow$ SaO_2, $\downarrow$ PEFR, $\downarrow$ tidal volume, $\downarrow$ forced vital capacity, $\downarrow$ minute ventilation, $\downarrow$ negative inspiratory force; abnormal serum electrolytes, hemoglobin, hematocrit, and white blood cell count; abnormal findings on chest x-ray; abnormal central venous or pulmonary artery pressures, cardiac output

CPAP, Continuous positive airway pressure; *I:E,* inspiratory:expiratory; *PEFR,* peak expiratory flow rate.

Additional information on nursing diagnoses for the patient with acute respiratory failure is presented in eNursing Care Plan 68-1 (available on the website for this chapter).

PLANNING

The overall goals for the patient with acute respiratory failure include (1) normal ABG values or values within the patient's baseline, (2) normal breath sounds or breath sounds within the patient's baseline, (3) no dyspnea or breathing patterns within the patient's baseline, (4) independent maintenance of the airway, and (5) effective cough and ability to clear secretions.

PREVENTION

As part of the plan of care for any patient who may be at risk for respiratory failure, prevention and early recognition of respiratory distress are important. Prevention involves a thorough history and physical assessment to identify the patient at risk for respiratory failure and then the initiation of appropriate nursing interventions. These include teaching the patient about deep breathing and coughing, use of incentive spirometry, and ambulation. Prevention of atelectasis, pneumonia, and complications of immobility, as well as optimization of hydration and nutrition, can potentially decrease the risk of respiratory failure in the acutely or critically ill patient.

RESPIRATORY THERAPY

The major goals of care for acute respiratory failure include maintaining adequate oxygenation and ventilation. Interventions include O_2 therapy, mobilization of secretions, and positive pressure ventilation (PPV) (Table 68-4).

OXYGEN THERAPY. The primary goal of O_2 therapy is to correct hypoxemia. If hypoxemia is secondary to V/Q mismatch, supplemental O_2 administered at 1 to 3 L/minute by nasal cannula, or 24% to 32% by face mask or Venturi mask, should improve the PaO_2 and SaO_2. Hypoxemia secondary to an intrapulmonary shunt is usually not responsive to high O_2 concentrations. In this case, the patient usually requires PPV. PPV provides O_2 therapy and humidification, decreases WOB, and reduces respiratory muscle fatigue. In addition, PPV assists in opening collapsed airways and decreasing shunt. PPV is provided via an endotracheal tube (most frequently) or noninvasively by means of a tight-fitting mask.[25,26] (Chapter 66 discusses mechanical ventilation in detail.)

The patient with acute respiratory failure must be able to tolerate the type of O_2 delivery system chosen. For example, a face mask may cause anxiety from feelings of claustrophobia. The anxiety can cause dyspnea, increase O_2 consumption and CO_2 production, and cause the patient to remove the O_2 device. The selected O_2 delivery system must also maintain PaO_2 at 55 to 60 mm Hg or higher and SaO_2 at 90% or higher at the lowest O_2 concentration possible.

High O_2 concentrations replace the nitrogen gas normally present in the alveoli, thus causing instability and atelectasis. In intubated patients, exposure to 60% or higher FIO_2 for longer than 48 hours poses a significant risk for O_2 toxicity. In nonintubated patients the risk is less clear. The effects of prolonged exposure to high levels of O_2 include increased pulmonary capillary permeability, decreased surfactant production and surfactant inactivation, and fibrotic changes in the alveoli. (Chapter 29 and Table 29-20 discuss O_2 delivery devices.)

Another possible risk of O_2 therapy is specific to patients with chronic hypercapnia (e.g., patients with COPD). Chronic hypercapnia blunts the response of chemoreceptors in the medulla to elevated CO_2 levels as a respiratory stimulant. In this situation, hypoxia stimulates respirations. Provide O_2 to patients with chronic hypercapnia through a low-flow device such as a nasal cannula at 1 to 2 L/minute or a Venturi mask at 24% to 28%. Closely monitor patients for changes in mental status, respiratory rate, and ABG results until their PaO_2 level has reached their baseline normal value.

MOBILIZATION OF SECRETIONS. Retained pulmonary secretions may cause or exacerbate acute respiratory failure. This occurs because the movement of O_2 into the alveoli and removal of CO_2 are blocked. Secretions can be mobilized through effective coughing, adequate hydration and humidification, chest physiotherapy (physical therapy), airway suctioning, and ambulation when possible.

Effective Coughing and Positioning. If secretions are obstructing the airway, encourage the patient to cough. The patient with a

---

TABLE 68-4   COLLABORATIVE CARE

Acute Respiratory Failure

Diagnostic
- Vital signs
- History and physical examination
- Arterial blood gases
- Pulse oximetry
- Chest x-ray
- CBC
- Serum electrolytes and urinalysis
- ECG
- Blood and sputum cultures (if indicated)
- Hemodynamic parameters: CVP, SVV, PAWP

Collaborative Therapy
Respiratory Therapy
- O_2 therapy
- Mobilization of secretions
  - Effective coughing
  - Incentive spirometry
  - Hydration and humidification
  - Chest physiotherapy
  - Airway suctioning
  - Ambulation
  - Positioning: head of bed elevated to assist lung ventilation; tripod positioning for optimal comfort and efficiency during breathing
- Positive pressure ventilation
  - Noninvasive positive pressure ventilation
  - Intubation with positive pressure ventilation

Drug Therapy
- Relief of bronchospasm (e.g., albuterol [Proventil])
- Reduction of airway inflammation (corticosteroids)
- Reduction of pulmonary congestion (e.g., furosemide [Lasix], morphine)
- Treatment of pulmonary infections (e.g., antibiotics)
- Reduction of severe anxiety, pain, and agitation (e.g., lorazepam [Ativan], fentanyl [Sublimaze], morphine)

Medical Supportive Therapy
- Management of the underlying cause of respiratory failure
- Maintenance of adequate cardiac output
- Maintenance of adequate hemoglobin concentration

Nutritional Therapy
- Enteral nutrition support
- Parenteral nutrition support

CVP, Central venous pressure; *PAWP,* pulmonary artery wedge pressure; *SVV,* stroke volume variation.

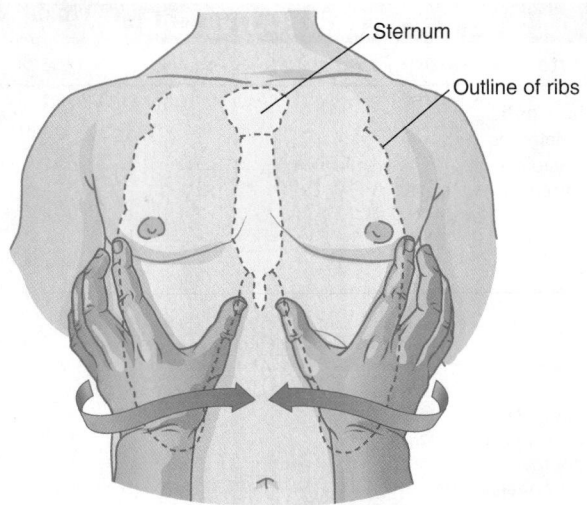

FIG. 68-7 Augmented coughing is performed by placing one or both hands on the anterolateral base of the lungs. After the patient takes a deep inspiration and at the beginning of expiration, move the hand(s) forcefully upward. This increases abdominal pressure and aids in producing a forceful cough.

neuromuscular weakness from a disease or exhaustion may not be able to generate sufficient airway pressures to produce an effective cough. *Augmented coughing (quad coughing)* may be of benefit to these patients. Perform augmented coughing by placing one or both hands on the anterolateral base of the lungs (Fig. 68-7). As the patient ends a deep inspiration and begins the expiration, move your hands forcefully upward, increasing abdominal pressure and facilitating the cough. This measure helps increase expiratory flow and thereby facilitates secretion clearance.

Some patients may benefit from therapeutic cough techniques. *Huff coughing* is a series of coughs performed while saying the word "huff" (see Table 29-23). This technique prevents the glottis from closing during the cough. Patients with COPD generate higher flow rates with a huff cough than is possible with a normal cough. The huff cough is effective in clearing only the central airways, but it may assist in moving secretions upward.

The staged cough also assists in mobilizing secretions. To perform the *staged cough,* the patient assumes a sitting position, breathes three or four times in and out through the mouth, and coughs while bending forward and pressing a pillow inward against the diaphragm.

Positioning the patient upright, either by elevating the head of the bed at least 45 degrees or by using a reclining chair or chair bed, helps maximize thoracic expansion, thereby decreasing dyspnea and improving secretion mobilization. A sitting position improves pulmonary function and assists in venous pooling in dependent body areas such as the lower extremities. When lungs are upright, ventilation and perfusion are best in the lung bases.

Lateral or side-lying positioning may be used in patients with disease involving only one lung. This position, termed *good lung down,* allows for improved V/Q matching in the affected lung. Pulmonary blood flow and ventilation are optimal in dependent lung areas. This position also allows secretions to drain out of the affected lung to the point where they may be removed by suctioning. For example, in patients with significant right-sided pneumonia, optimal positioning would be to place them on their left side to maximize ventilation and perfusion in the "good" lung and facilitate secretion removal from the affected lung (postural drainage). All patients should be side-

lying if there is any possibility that the tongue will obstruct the airway or that aspiration may occur. Keep an oral or nasal airway at the bedside for use if necessary. Airway control with endotracheal intubation and PPV is indicated when patients cannot maintain their airway and lung ventilation.

Hydration and Humidification. Thick and viscous secretions are difficult to expel. Adequate fluid intake (2 to 3 L/day) keeps secretions thin and easier to remove. If the patient is unable to take sufficient fluids orally, IV hydration is used. Thoroughly assess the patient's cardiac and renal status to determine whether he or she can tolerate the IV fluid volume and avoid heart failure and pulmonary edema. Regularly assess for signs of fluid overload by clinical evaluation (e.g., crackles, dyspnea) and invasive monitoring (e.g., increased central venous pressure). These considerations would also apply to the patient with renal dysfunction.

An appropriate humidification device is an adjunct in secretion management. Aerosols of sterile normal saline, administered by a nebulizer, may be used to liquefy secretions. O_2 may also be given by aerosol mask to thin secretions and facilitate their removal. Aerosol therapy may induce bronchospasm and severe coughing, causing a decreased PaO_2. Frequent assessment of patient tolerance to therapy is critical. Mucolytic agents such as nebulized acetylcysteine (Mucomyst) mixed with a bronchodilator may be used to thin secretions. A side effect of these drugs is bronchospasm so they are used only in special situations (e.g., during bronchoscopy to remove thick, copious secretions).

Chest Physiotherapy. Chest physiotherapy is indicated in patients who produce more than 30 mL of sputum per day or have evidence of severe atelectasis or pulmonary infiltrates. Postural drainage, percussion, and vibration to the affected lung segments assist in moving secretions to the larger airways where they are removed by coughing or suctioning. Positioning affects oxygenation. Patients may not tolerate head-down or lateral positioning because of extreme dyspnea or hypoxemia caused by V/Q mismatch. (Chest physiotherapy is discussed in Chapter 29 on p. 594.)

Airway Suctioning. Nasopharyngeal, oropharyngeal, or nasotracheal suctioning (blind suctioning without a tracheal tube in place) is done if the patient is unable to expectorate secretions. Suctioning through an artificial airway (e.g., endotracheal tube) is also performed as needed (see Chapters 27 and 66). A mini-tracheostomy (or mini-trach) is used to suction patients who have difficulty mobilizing secretions and when blind suctioning is difficult or ineffective. The *mini-trach* is a 4-mm indwelling plastic cuffless cannula inserted through the cricothyroid membrane. It is used to instill sterile normal saline solution to elicit a cough and to perform suctioning. Contraindications for a mini-trach include an absent gag reflex, history of aspiration, and the need for long-term mechanical ventilation. At all times, suction cautiously and closely monitor the patient for complications (e.g., hypoxia, increased ICP, dysrhythmias).

POSITIVE PRESSURE VENTILATION. If intensive measures fail to improve ventilation and oxygenation and the patient continues to show signs of acute respiratory failure, ventilatory assistance is needed. PPV may be provided invasively through orotracheal or nasotracheal intubation or noninvasively through a nasal or face mask.[22,26]

Noninvasive positive pressure ventilation (NIPPV) is used for patients with acute or chronic respiratory failure. During NIPPV, a mask is placed tightly over the patient's nose or nose and mouth and the patient breathes spontaneously while PPV

FIG. 68-8 Noninvasive bilevel positive pressure ventilation. A mask is placed over the nose or nose and mouth. Positive pressure from a mechanical ventilator assists the patient's breathing efforts, decreasing the work of breathing.

is delivered. With NIPPV, it is possible to decrease the WOB without the need for endotracheal intubation. Bilevel positive airway pressure (BiPAP) is a form of NIPPV in which different positive pressure levels are set for inspiration and expiration (Fig. 68-8). Continuous positive airway pressure (CPAP) is another form of NIPPV in which a constant positive pressure is delivered to the airway during inspiration and expiration.[27-30]

NIPPV is most useful in managing chronic respiratory failure in patients with chest wall and neuromuscular disease (see Table 68-1). NIPPV has been used in patients with hypoxemic respiratory failure (e.g., ARDS, cardiogenic pulmonary edema), but with less success. NIPPV may also be used for patients who refuse endotracheal intubation but still want some palliative ventilatory support (e.g., patients with end-stage COPD).[31,32] NIPPV is not appropriate for patients who have excessive secretions, decreased level of consciousness, high O_2 requirements, facial trauma, or hemodynamic instability. NIPPV is also used postextubation to avoid reintubation. (Chapter 66 discusses artificial airways, PPV, CPAP, and BiPAP in detail.)

DRUG THERAPY

Goals of drug therapy for patients in acute respiratory failure include (1) relief of bronchospasm; (2) reduction of airway inflammation and pulmonary congestion; (3) treatment of pulmonary infection; and (4) reduction of severe pain, anxiety, and restlessness.

RELIEF OF BRONCHOSPASM. Relief of bronchospasm increases alveolar ventilation. Short-acting bronchodilators, such as metaproterenol (Alupent) and albuterol (Ventolin), reverse bronchospasm. Side effects of these β-adrenergic agonist drugs include tachycardia and hypertension. Prolonged use can increase the risk of dysrhythmias and cardiac ischemia. Monitor ECG and vital signs for any changes with administration of these drugs. Give these drugs using a hand-held nebulizer or a metered-dose inhaler with a spacer. In acute bronchospasm these drugs may be given at 15- to 30-minute intervals until a response occurs. The bronchodilator effects of these medications can sometimes worsen hypoxemia by redistributing the inspired gas to areas of decreased perfusion. Administering the bronchodilator with an oxygen-enriched gas mixture usually reduces this effect.[6,7] (Chapter 29 discusses nursing management related to bronchodilators.)

REDUCTION OF AIRWAY INFLAMMATION. Corticosteroids (e.g., methylprednisolone [Solu-Medrol]) may be used in conjunction with bronchodilating agents for bronchospasm and inflammation. When given IV in acute asthma, corticosteroids speed resolution of airway inflammation and edema. Inhaled corticosteroids require 4 to 5 days for optimum therapeutic effects and are not used for acute respiratory failure.

DRUG ALERT: IV Corticosteroids
- Monitor potassium levels, since corticosteroids exacerbate hypokalemia caused by diuretics.
- Prolonged use causes adrenal insufficiency.

REDUCTION OF PULMONARY CONGESTION. Pulmonary interstitial fluid can accumulate because of direct or indirect injury to the alveolar capillary membrane (e.g., ARDS) or from heart failure. The result is decreased alveolar ventilation and hypoxemia. IV diuretics (e.g., furosemide [Lasix]), morphine, and nitroglycerin (Tridil) are used to decrease the pulmonary congestion caused by heart failure. If atrial fibrillation is also present, calcium channel blockers (e.g., diltiazem [Cardizem]) and β-adrenergic blockers (e.g., metoprolol [Lopressor]) are used to decrease heart rate and improve CO. (Chapter 35 discusses heart failure.)

TREATMENT OF PULMONARY INFECTIONS. Pulmonary infections (e.g., pneumonia, acute bronchitis) result in excessive mucus production; fever; increased O_2 consumption; and inflamed, fluid-filled, or collapsed alveoli. Alveoli that are fluid filled or collapsed cannot participate in gas exchange. Pulmonary infections can either cause or exacerbate acute respiratory failure. IV antibiotics, such as azithromycin (Zithromax) or ceftriaxone (Rocephin), are often given to treat infections. Chest x-rays help identify the location and extent of a suspected infectious process. Sputum cultures help determine the type of organisms causing the infection and their sensitivity to antimicrobial medications.[33]

REDUCTION OF SEVERE ANXIETY, PAIN, AND AGITATION. Anxiety, restlessness, and agitation result from hypoxia. In addition, fear caused by the inability to breathe and a sense of loss of control may increase anxiety. Anxiety, pain, and agitation increase O_2 consumption, which may worsen the hypoxemia. Anxiety, pain, and agitation also increase CO_2 production, affect ventilator management, and increase morbidity. Several strategies can assist the patient in reducing anxiety and pain.

Sedation and analgesia with drug therapy such as propofol (Diprivan) (used for mechanically ventilated patients), benzodiazepines (e.g., lorazepam [Ativan], midazolam [Versed]), and opioids (e.g., morphine, fentanyl [Sublimaze]) are used to decrease anxiety, agitation, and pain. Continued agitation increases the patient's WOB, O_2 consumption, CO_2 production, and risk of injury (e.g., unplanned extubation). Patients receiving these agents are best managed by following an evidence-based protocol that includes a regular "sedation holiday" for ongoing assessment.[34,35] (Sedation holiday is discussed in Chapter 66 on p. 1601.)

SAFETY ALERT
- Monitor patients closely for cardiopulmonary depression when giving any sedative or analgesic agents.
- Agitation is often caused by pain, hypoxemia, electrolyte imbalance, evolution of brain injury, and adverse drug reactions.
- Assess and aggressively treat all potentially reversible causes of agitation.
- Sedative and analgesic agents may have a prolonged effect in critically ill patients, delay weaning from mechanical ventilation, and contribute to increased length of stay.

Address treatable causes of agitation (e.g., hypoxemia, pain, hypercapnia). Patients who breathe asynchronously with mechanical ventilation may also benefit from adjustment of ventilator flow rates and other settings. Patients who remain asynchronous with mechanical ventilation despite aggressive sedative and analgesic dosing may require neuromuscular blockade (paralysis) with agents such as vecuronium (Norcuron) or cisatracurium (Nimbex). These drugs relax skeletal muscles by interfering with neuromuscular transmission and, ultimately, provide synchrony with mechanical ventilation. Neuromuscular blockade may also decrease the patient's risk of lung injury related to excessive inspiratory/intrathoracic pressures. In this way, the ventilator can provide optimal respiratory support. Remember that a patient receiving neuromuscular blockade can appear to be asleep but still possibly be awake and in pain. For this reason, both aggressive sedation and analgesia are essential.

SAFETY ALERT
- Provide concurrent sedation and analgesia to the point of unconsciousness for patients receiving neuromuscular blockade. This eliminates patient awareness, assures patient comfort, and avoids the terrifying experience of being awake and in pain while paralyzed.
- Use neuromuscular blockade for the shortest duration and in the lowest dose possible to avoid complications (e.g., myopathy).

Monitoring levels of sedation in patients receiving neuromuscular blockade is challenging. Noninvasive electroencephalogram-based technology may help guide sedative and analgesic therapy in these patients.[36] Levels of drug paralysis are monitored primarily by clinical assessment of ventilation and whether goals of care are being met. A frequent adjunct to monitoring paralysis is use of a peripheral nerve stimulator (see Fig. 66-19). Clinical assessment is essential to determine the adequacy of sedation, analgesia, and neuromuscular blockade in critically ill patients.

MEDICAL SUPPORTIVE THERAPY

Goals and related interventions to maximize O_2 delivery are essential to improving the patient's oxygenation and ventilation status. The primary goal is to treat the underlying cause of the respiratory failure. Other supportive goals include maintaining an adequate CO and hemoglobin concentration.

TREATING THE UNDERLYING CAUSE. Interventions are directed toward reversing the disease process that caused the acute respiratory failure. Patients with hypoventilation need to be diagnosed and treated rapidly. Patients with V/Q mismatch, shunting, or diffusion limitation are managed differently depending on the underlying cause. In all patient situations, monitoring treatment effects, including trends in ABGs and changes in respiratory status, is an ongoing process.

MAINTAINING ADEQUATE CARDIAC OUTPUT. CO reflects the blood flow reaching the tissues. BP and mean arterial pressure (MAP) are important indicators of the adequacy of CO. Always interpret BP and MAP readings within the context of the physical assessment to determine adequacy of CO and tissue perfusion. Usually a systolic BP of 90 mm Hg or more or a MAP greater than 60 mm Hg is adequate to maintain perfusion to the vital organs. At these levels, changes in mental status may be attributed to the level of O_2 and CO_2 rather than decreased cerebral perfusion. In a patient with chronic, uncontrolled hypertension, a systolic BP of 90 to 100 mm Hg is often inadequate to maintain systemic and cerebral perfusion. Cerebral perfusion may not only tolerate but may require a higher BP

and MAP to prevent episodes of brain ischemia or hypoperfusion to other organs.

Decreased CO is treated by administration of IV fluids, medications, or both. (Chapter 67 discusses drugs used to treat decreased CO and shock.) CO can also be decreased by changes in intrathoracic or intrapulmonary pressures from PPV. Patients experiencing exacerbation of COPD or asthma and those receiving PPV are at risk of alveolar hyperinflation, increased right ventricular afterload, and excessive intrathoracic pressures. These changes can result in limited blood flow from the right side of the heart through the pulmonary vasculature to the left side of the heart and can cause hemodynamic compromise. In addition, blood return from the systemic circulation to the right side of the heart may be impaired, further decreasing preload. Each of these physiologic effects can lead to severe hemodynamic compromise. Consequently, closely monitor BP and clinical indicators of adequate CO and tissue perfusion with initiation of or changes in mechanical ventilation.

MAINTAINING ADEQUATE HEMOGLOBIN CONCENTRATION. Hemoglobin is the primary carrier of O_2 to the tissues. Delivery of O_2 to the tissues is compromised in anemic patients. A hemoglobin of 9 g/dL (90 g/L) or higher typically ensures adequate O_2 saturation of the hemoglobin for tissue oxygenation. Monitor the patient for signs of blood loss (e.g., hypotension, melena). Transfusion with packed red blood cells may be used if an adequate hemoglobin level is not maintained and the patient is symptomatic.

NUTRITIONAL THERAPY

Maintenance of protein and energy stores is especially important in patients with acute respiratory failure. The hypermetabolic state in critical illness increases the caloric requirements needed to maintain body weight and muscle mass. Thus nutritional depletion causes a loss of muscle mass, including the respiratory muscles, and may prolong recovery. The dietitian, in collaboration with the health care team, determines the optimal method of feeding and optimal caloric and fluid requirements. During the acute manifestations of respiratory failure, the risk of aspiration typically prevents oral intake. Ideally, enteral or parenteral nutrition is started within 24 hours in malnourished patients and within 3 days in well-nourished patients. When acute manifestations subside, the patient may resume oral intake as able.

EVALUATION

The expected outcomes are that the patient with respiratory failure will
- Maintain a patent airway with effective removal of secretions
- Achieve normal or baseline respiratory rate and rhythm, and breath sounds
- Maintain adequate oxygenation as indicated by normal or baseline ABGs
- Experience normal hemodynamic status

Additional outcomes are presented in eNursing Care Plan 68-1 (available on the website for this chapter).

GERONTOLOGIC CONSIDERATIONS

RESPIRATORY FAILURE

Older adults are the fastest-growing age-group in the United States, a trend that is increasingly reflected within the patient populations in acute and critical care settings. Multiple factors contribute to an increased risk of respiratory failure in older adults. The reduction in ventilatory capacity that accompanies aging places the older adult at risk for respiratory failure. Physiologic aging of the lung includes alveolar dilation, larger air spaces, and loss of surface area for gas exchange. Diminished elastic recoil within the airways, decreased chest wall compliance, and decreased respiratory muscle strength also occur. In older adults the PaO_2 falls further and the $PaCO_2$ rises to a higher level before the respiratory system is stimulated to alter the rate and depth of breathing. This delayed response can contribute to the development of respiratory failure. In addition, a history of tobacco use is a risk factor that can accelerate age-related respiratory changes. Poor nutritional status and less available physiologic reserve in the cardiopulmonary and autonomic nervous systems increase the risk of additional disease states such as pneumonia and heart disease. These may further compromise respiratory function and lead to respiratory failure. Poor nutrition can also result in a decrease in muscle mass and related respiratory drive.[31,37]

Older adults are more vulnerable to delirium, health care–associated infections, and the adverse effects of polypharmacy. Delirium is an independent risk factor for increased mortality and morbidity rates in critically ill patients. It can complicate ventilator management and weaning by interfering with patient cooperation. Delirium associated with agitation increases CO_2 elimination and O_2 consumption, increases the risk for unplanned extubation and device removal, and extends length of hospital stay and ventilator days.[38,39] (Delirium is discussed in Chapters 60 and 66.)

Adjust assessment parameters for age-related changes. For example, heart rate and BP generally increase with age and the related changes in the cardiovascular system. Therefore you need to know the patient's baseline vital signs. Compare these with the ongoing physical assessment findings to appropriately evaluate changes in cardiopulmonary function in the older adult.

ACUTE RESPIRATORY DISTRESS SYNDROME

Acute respiratory distress syndrome (ARDS) is a sudden and progressive form of acute respiratory failure in which the alveolar-capillary interface becomes damaged and more permeable to intravascular fluid (Fig. 68-9). ARDS exists on a continuum. One way to assess the degree of impairment in gas exchange is to measure the PaO_2/FIO_2 (P/F) ratio. Under normal circumstances (e.g., PaO_2 85 to 100 mm Hg; FIO_2 0.21 [room air]), the P/F ratio would be greater than 400 (e.g., 95/0.21 = 452). With the onset and progression of lung injury and impairment in O_2 delivery through the alveolar-capillary interface, the PaO_2 may remain lower than expected despite increased FIO_2.

The term acute lung injury (ALI) is used when the P/F ratio is 200 to 300 (e.g., 86/0.4 = 215). The term *ARDS* is used when the P/F ratio is less than 200 (e.g., 80/0.8 = 100). In both cases, the alveoli fill with fluid, resulting in severe dyspnea, hypoxemia refractory to supplemental O_2, reduced lung compliance, and diffuse pulmonary infiltrates.[40]

The incidence of ARDS in the United States is estimated at more than 150,000 cases annually. Despite supportive therapy, the mortality rate from ARDS is approximately 50%. Patients who have both gram-negative septic shock and ARDS have a mortality rate of 70% to 90%.

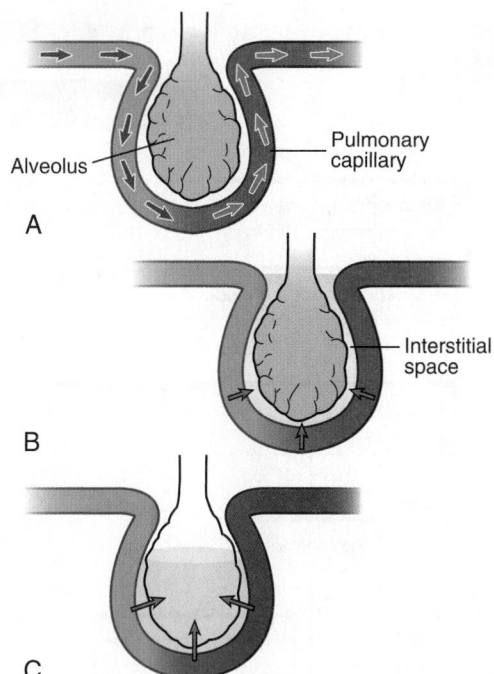

FIG. 68-9 Stages of edema formation in acute respiratory distress syndrome. **A,** Normal alveolus and pulmonary capillary. **B,** Interstitial edema occurs with increased flow of fluid into the interstitial space. **C,** Alveolar edema occurs when the fluid crosses the blood-gas barrier.

TABLE 68-5	PREDISPOSING CONDITIONS TO ARDS	
Direct Lung Injury	**Indirect Lung Injury**
Common Causes	
Aspiration of gastric contents or other substances	Sepsis (especially gram-negative infection)
Viral or bacterial pneumonia	Severe massive trauma
Sepsis	
Less Common Causes	
Chest trauma	Acute pancreatitis
Embolism: fat, air, amniotic fluid, thrombus	Anaphylaxis
Inhalation of toxic substances	Cardiopulmonary bypass
Near-drowning	Disseminated intravascular coagulation
O_2 toxicity	Nonpulmonary systemic diseases
Radiation pneumonitis	Opioid drug overdose (e.g., heroin)
	Severe head injury
	Shock states
	Transfusion-related acute lung injury (e.g., multiple blood transfusions)

Etiology and Pathophysiology

Table 68-5 lists conditions that predispose patients to the development of ARDS. Patients with multiple risk factors are three or four times more likely to develop ARDS.

The most common cause of ARDS is sepsis. Direct lung injury may cause ARDS (Fig. 68-10), or ARDS may develop because of the systemic inflammatory response syndrome (SIRS) (see Fig. 67-1). SIRS may have an infectious or a noninfectious etiology. It is characterized by widespread inflammation or clinical responses to inflammation after a variety of physiologic insults, including severe trauma, gut ischemia, and lung injury.[41,42] ARDS may also develop as a consequence of

PATHOPHYSIOLOGY MAP

FIG. 68-10 Pathophysiology of acute lung injury *(ALI)* and acute respiratory distress syndrome *(ARDS)*.

multiple organ dysfunction syndrome (MODS). MODS results from organ system dysfunction that progressively increases in severity and ultimately results in multisystem organ failure. (Chapter 67 discusses SIRS and MODS.)

An exact cause for the damage to the alveolar-capillary interface is not known, but it is thought to be caused by stimulation of the inflammatory and immune systems, which causes an attraction of neutrophils to the pulmonary interstitium. The neutrophils release biochemical, humoral, and cellular mediators that produce changes in the lung. These include increased pulmonary capillary membrane permeability, destruction of elastin and collagen, formation of pulmonary microemboli, and pulmonary artery vasoconstriction[41,42] (see Fig. 68-10). (Chapters 12 and 14 discuss these mediators.)

The pathophysiologic changes in ARDS are divided into three phases: (1) injury or exudative phase, (2) reparative or proliferative phase, and (3) fibrotic phase.

Injury or Exudative Phase. The *injury or exudative phase* occurs approximately 1 to 7 days (usually 24 to 48 hours) after the initial direct lung injury or host insult. Initially, engorgement of the peribronchial and perivascular interstitial space produces interstitial edema. Next, fluid from the interstitial space crosses the alveolar membrane and enters the alveolar space. Intrapulmonary shunt develops because the alveoli fill with fluid, and blood passing through them cannot be oxygenated (see Figs. 68-4 and 68-9).

Alveolar type I and II cells (which produce surfactant) are damaged by the changes caused by ARDS. This damage, in addition to further fluid and protein accumulation, results in sur-

factant dysfunction. The function of *surfactant* is to maintain alveolar stability by decreasing alveolar surface tension and preventing alveolar collapse. Decreased synthesis of surfactant and inactivation of existing surfactant cause the alveoli to become unstable and collapse *(atelectasis)*. Widespread atelectasis further decreases lung compliance, compromises gas exchange, and contributes to hypoxemia.

Also during this stage, necrotic cells, protein, and fibrin form hyaline membranes that line the alveoli. Hyaline membranes contribute to the development of fibrosis and atelectasis, leading to a decrease in gas exchange capability and lung compliance.

The primary pathophysiologic changes that describe the *injury or exudative phase* of ARDS are interstitial and alveolar edema (noncardiogenic pulmonary edema) and atelectasis. Severe V/Q mismatch and shunting of pulmonary capillary blood result in hypoxemia unresponsive to increasing concentrations of O_2 (termed **refractory hypoxemia**). Diffusion limitation, caused by hyaline membrane formation, worsens the hypoxemia. As the lungs become less compliant because of decreased surfactant, pulmonary edema, and atelectasis, the patient must generate higher airway pressures to inflate "stiff" lungs. Reduced lung compliance greatly increases the patient's WOB. During ventilator management at this stage, increasing inspiratory and plateau pressures may be needed to deliver a controlled ventilation because of worsening lung compliance.[41-43]

Hypoxemia and the stimulation of juxtacapillary receptors in the stiff lung parenchyma *(J reflex)* initially cause an increase in respiratory rate and a decrease in tidal volume. This breathing pattern increases CO_2 removal, producing respiratory alkalosis. CO increases in response to hypoxemia, a compensatory effort to increase pulmonary blood flow. However, as atelectasis, pulmonary edema, and pulmonary shunt increase, compensation fails, and hypoventilation, decreased CO, and decreased tissue O_2 perfusion eventually occur.

Reparative or Proliferative Phase. The *reparative or proliferative phase* of ARDS begins 1 to 2 weeks after the initial lung injury. During this phase, there is an influx of neutrophils, monocytes, and lymphocytes and fibroblast proliferation as part of the inflammatory response. The proliferative phase is complete when the diseased lung is characterized by dense, fibrous tissue. Increased pulmonary vascular resistance and pulmonary hypertension may occur in this stage because fibroblasts and inflammatory cells destroy the pulmonary vasculature. Lung compliance continues to decrease as a result of interstitial fibrosis. Hypoxemia worsens because of the thickened alveolar membrane, causing diffusion limitation and shunting. If the reparative phase persists, widespread fibrosis results. If the reparative phase is stopped, the lesions will resolve.

Fibrotic Phase. The *fibrotic phase* of ARDS occurs approximately 2 to 3 weeks after the initial lung injury. This phase is also called the *chronic* or *late phase* of ARDS. By this time, the lung is completely remodeled by collagenous and fibrous tissues. The diffuse scarring and fibrosis result in decreased lung compliance. In addition, the surface area for gas exchange is significantly reduced because the interstitium is fibrotic, and therefore hypoxemia continues. Pulmonary hypertension results from pulmonary vascular destruction and fibrosis.

Clinical Progression

Progression of ARDS varies among patients. Some survive the acute phase of lung injury. Pulmonary edema resolves, and complete recovery occurs in a few days. The chance for survival is poor in those who enter the fibrotic (chronic or late) stage, which requires long-term mechanical ventilation. It is not known why injured lungs repair and recover in some patients, and in others ARDS progresses. Several factors seem to be important in determining the course of ARDS, including the nature of the initial injury, extent and severity of coexisting diseases, and pulmonary complications (e.g., pneumothorax, O_2 toxicity).

Clinical Manifestations and Diagnostic Studies

The initial presentation of ARDS is often subtle. At the time of the initial injury, and for several hours to 1 or 2 days afterward, the patient may not experience respiratory symptoms or may exhibit only dyspnea, tachypnea, cough, and restlessness. Chest auscultation may be normal or reveal fine, scattered crackles. ABGs usually indicate mild hypoxemia and respiratory alkalosis caused by hyperventilation. (Table 68-6 presents the findings that support a diagnosis of ALI and ARDS.) Respiratory alkalosis results from hypoxemia and the stimulation of juxtacapillary receptors. The chest x-ray may be normal or reveal minimal scattered interstitial infiltrates. Edema may not show on the x-ray until there is a 30% increase in fluid content in the lung.

As ARDS progresses, symptoms worsen because of increased fluid accumulation and decreased lung compliance. Respiratory distress becomes evident as WOB increases. Tachypnea and intercostal and suprasternal retractions may be present. Pulmonary function tests in ARDS reveal decreases in compliance,

TABLE 68-6	DIAGNOSTIC FINDINGS IN ALI AND ARDS

Refractory Hypoxemia
Acute lung injury: PaO_2/FIO_2 ratio between 200-300
Acute respiratory distress syndrome: PaO_2/FIO_2 ratio <200

Chest X-Ray
New bilateral interstitial and alveolar infiltrates

Pulmonary Artery Wedge Pressure
≤18 mm Hg or no clinical evidence of heart failure

FIG. 68-11 Chest x-ray of a patient with acute respiratory distress syndrome (ARDS). The x-ray shows new, bilateral, diffuse, homogeneous pulmonary infiltrates without cardiac failure, fluid overload, chest infection, or chronic lung disease.

lung volumes, and *functional residual capacity* (FRC, the amount of air remaining in the lungs at the end of normal expiration). Tachycardia, diaphoresis, changes in mental status, cyanosis, and pallor may be present. Chest auscultation usually reveals scattered to diffuse crackles and rhonchi. The chest x-ray shows diffuse and extensive bilateral interstitial and alveolar infiltrates. A central venous or PA catheter may be inserted. PA wedge pressure does not increase in ARDS because the cause is noncardiogenic (not related to the heart).

Hypoxemia despite increased FIO_2 by mask, cannula, or endotracheal tube is a hallmark of ARDS. ABGs may initially demonstrate a normal or decreased $PaCO_2$ despite severe dyspnea and hypoxemia. Hypercapnia signifies that respiratory muscle fatigue and hypoventilation are occurring, interfering with optimum gas exchange.

As ARDS progresses, it is associated with profound respiratory distress requiring endotracheal intubation and PPV. The chest x-ray is often termed *whiteout* or *white lung* because consolidation and infiltrates are widespread throughout the lungs, leaving few recognizable air spaces (Fig. 68-11). Pleural effusions may also be present. Severe hypoxemia, hypercapnia, metabolic acidosis, and manifestations of target organ dysfunction may develop if therapy is not promptly started.

Complications

Complications may develop as a result of ARDS itself or its treatment. (Table 68-7 lists the common complications of

ARDS.) The major cause of death in ARDS is MODS, often accompanied by sepsis. The vital organs most commonly involved are the kidneys, liver, and heart. The organ systems most often involved are the CNS, hematologic system, and GI system.

Ventilator-Associated Pneumonia. A frequent complication of ARDS is ventilator-associated pneumonia (VAP), occurring in as many as 68% of patients with ARDS. Risk factors include impaired host defenses, contaminated equipment, invasive monitoring devices, aspiration of GI contents (especially in patients receiving enteral feedings), and prolonged mechanical ventilation. Strategies to prevent VAP include strict infection control measures (e.g., strict hand washing, sterile technique during endotracheal suctioning, frequent mouth care and oral hygiene) and a ventilator bundle protocol[44-48] (Table 68-8). (Chapter 28 discusses pneumonia, and Chapter 66 discusses VAP.)

Barotrauma. *Barotrauma* may result from rupture of overdistended alveoli during mechanical ventilation. The high peak airway pressures required may predispose patients with ARDS to this complication. Barotrauma results in alveolar air reaching locations where it is not usually found. This can lead to pulmonary interstitial emphysema, pneumothorax, subcutaneous emphysema, pneumoperitoneum, pneumomediastinum, pneumopericardium, and tension pneumothorax.[49] (Chapter 28 discusses pneumothorax.)

To avoid barotrauma and minimize the risk associated with elevated plateau and peak inspiratory pressures, the patient with ARDS is often ventilated with smaller tidal volumes (e.g., 6 mL/kg) and varying amounts of positive end-expiratory pressure (PEEP) to minimize O_2 requirements and intrathoracic pressures. This approach, called the Acute Respiratory Distress Syndrome Clinical Network (ARDSNet) protocol, reduces mortality rate and the number of ventilator days for these patients. One result of this protocol is an elevation in $PaCO_2$. This is termed *permissive hypercapnia* because the $PaCO_2$ is allowed to rise above normal limits. It is generally well tolerated as long as the rise in $PaCO_2$ is gradual to allow systemic and brain circulation to compensate, the pH is 7.2 or higher, and the patient does not have preexisting ICP elevation.[49-51]

TABLE 68-7 **COMPLICATIONS ASSOCIATED WITH ARDS**

Infection
- Catheter-related infection (e.g., central and peripheral IV catheters, urinary catheters)
- Sepsis

Respiratory Complications
- O_2 toxicity
- Pulmonary barotrauma (e.g., pneumothorax, pneumomediastinum, subcutaneous emphysema)
- Pulmonary emboli
- Pulmonary fibrosis
- Ventilator-associated pneumonia

Gastrointestinal Complications
- Paralytic ileus
- Pneumoperitoneum
- Stress ulceration and hemorrhage
- Hypermetabolic state, dramatically increased nutrition requirements

Renal Complications
- Acute kidney injury

Cardiac Complications
- Dysrhythmias
- Decreased cardiac output

Hematologic Complications
- Anemia
- Disseminated intravascular coagulation
- Thrombocytopenia
- Venous thromboembolism

Endotracheal Tube Complications
- Laryngeal ulceration
- Tracheal malacia
- Tracheal stenosis
- Tracheal ulceration

Central Nervous System and Psychologic Complications
- Delirium
- Sleep deprivation
- Posttraumatic stress disorder

TABLE 68-8 **COMPONENTS OF A VENTILATOR BUNDLE**

- Elevation of head of the bed 30 to 45 degrees
- Daily "sedation holidays" and assessment of readiness for extubation (see Chapter 66)
- Peptic ulcer disease prophylaxis (see Chapter 42)
- Venous thromboembolism prophylaxis (see Chapter 38)
- Daily oral care with chlorhexidine (0.12%) solution (see Table 66-9)

Source: Institute for Healthcare Improvement: Implement the IHI ventilator bundle. Retrieved from *www.ihi.org/knowledge/Pages/Changes/ImplementtheVentilator Bundle.aspx*.

EVIDENCE-BASED PRACTICE

Translating Research Into Practice

How Effective Is Subglottic Secretion Drainage on Ventilator-Associated Pneumonia?

Clinical Question
In critically ill patients on mechanical ventilation (P), how effective is subglottic secretion drainage (I) on the incidence of ventilator-associated pneumonia (VAP) and length of stay (O)?

Best Available Evidence
- Systematic review and meta-analysis of randomized controlled trials (RCTs)

Critical Appraisal and Synthesis of Evidence
- Sixteen RCTs ($n = 1709$) of critically ill intubated patients receiving intermittent or continuous subglottic secretion drainage. Outcomes were VAP rate, intubation duration, length of ICU and hospital stay, and mortality.
- Subglottic secretions pool immediately above the endotracheal tube cuff.
- Subglottic drainage decreased VAP incidence by 52% and shortened duration on mechanical ventilation by 2 days. Earlier extubation may be related to the 3-day decrease in patient length of ICU stay.
- Subglottic drainage did not affect length of hospital stay or mortality rate.

Conclusion
- Draining subglottic secretions has many positive patient outcomes, including decreased VAP incidence.

Implications for Nursing Practice
- Consult with health care team members regarding the importance of subglottic drainage for patients on mechanical ventilation.

Reference for Evidence
Leasure R, Stirlen J, Lu S: Prevention of ventilator-associated pneumonia through aspiration of subglottic secretions: a systematic review and meta-analysis, *Dimens Crit Care Nurs* 31:102, 2012.

P, Patient population of interest; *I*, intervention or area of interest; *O*, outcomes of interest (see p. 12).

Volutrauma. *Volutrauma* occurs in patients with ARDS or other clinical states requiring mechanical ventilation and large tidal volumes (e.g., 10 to 15 mL/kg) to ventilate noncompliant lungs. Volutrauma results in *alveolar fractures* (damage or tears in the alveoli) and movement of fluids and proteins into the alveolar spaces. To limit this complication, smaller tidal volumes or pressure-control ventilation is recommended in patients with ARDS (see Chapter 66).

Stress Ulcers. Critically ill patients with acute respiratory failure are at high risk for stress ulcers. Bleeding from stress ulcers occurs in 30% of patients with ARDS who require PPV, a higher incidence than other causes of acute respiratory failure. Management strategies include correction of predisposing conditions such as hypotension, shock, and acidosis. Prophylactic management includes antiulcer agents such as proton pump inhibitors (e.g., pantoprazole [Protonix]), and mucosal-protecting agents (e.g., sucralfate [Carafate]). Early initiation of enteral nutrition also helps prevent mucosal damage (see Chapters 40 and 66).

Renal Failure. Renal failure can occur from decreased renal tissue oxygenation because of hypotension, hypoxemia, or hypercapnia. Renal failure may also result from the administration of nephrotoxic drugs (e.g., vancomycin [Vancocin]) used to treat ARDS-related infections.

NURSING AND COLLABORATIVE MANAGEMENT ACUTE RESPIRATORY DISTRESS SYNDROME

The collaborative care for acute respiratory failure (see Table 68-4) and the nursing care plan for acute respiratory failure (eNursing Care Plan 68-1, available on the website for this chapter) apply to patients with ARDS. The following section discusses additional collaborative care measures for the patient with ARDS (Table 68-9).

TABLE 68-9 COLLABORATIVE CARE

Acute Respiratory Distress Syndrome

Diagnostic
See Table 68-6

Collaborative Therapy
Respiratory Therapy
- O₂ administration
- Lateral rotation therapy
- Positive pressure ventilation with PEEP
- Prone positioning
- Permissive hypercapnia
- Alternative modes of mechanical ventilation: pressure-control inverse ratio ventilation, airway pressure release ventilation, high-frequency ventilation (see Chapter 66)

Supportive Therapy
- Identification and treatment of underlying cause
- Hemodynamic monitoring
- Inotropic and vasopressor medications
  - dopamine (Intropin)
  - dobutamine (Dobutrex)
  - norepinephrine (Levophed)
- Diuretics
- IV fluid administration
- Sedation/analgesia
- Neuromuscular blockade

PEEP, Positive end-expiratory pressure.

NURSING ASSESSMENT

Because ARDS causes acute respiratory failure, the subjective and objective data that you should obtain from someone with ARDS are the same as those for acute respiratory failure (see Table 68-3).

NURSING DIAGNOSES

Nursing diagnoses for the patient with ARDS may include, but are not limited to, those described for acute respiratory failure (see p. 1660).

PLANNING

Patients with ARDS are cared for in critical care units. With appropriate therapy, the overall goals include a PaO₂ of 60 mm Hg or higher and adequate lung ventilation to maintain normal pH. The goals for a patient recovering from ARDS include (1) PaO₂ within normal limits for age or baseline values on room air, (2) SaO₂ greater than 90%, (3) patent airway, and (4) clear lungs on auscultation.

OXYGEN ADMINISTRATION. The primary goal of O₂ therapy is to correct hypoxemia. O₂ administered via a face mask or nasal cannula is inadequate to treat refractory hypoxemia that is associated with ARDS. Initially use masks with high-flow systems that deliver higher O₂ concentrations to maximize O₂ delivery. Continuously monitor SpO₂ to assess the effectiveness of O₂ therapy. The general standard for O₂ administration is to give the patient the lowest concentration that results in a PaO₂ greater than 60 mm Hg. The patient's risk for O₂ toxicity increases when the FIO₂ exceeds 60% for more than 48 hours. Patients with ARDS need intubation with mechanical ventilation to maintain the PaO₂ at acceptable levels.

POSITIVE PRESSURE VENTILATION. Endotracheal intubation and PPV provide additional respiratory support. However, even with these interventions it may be necessary to maintain the FIO₂ at 60% or higher to maintain a PaO₂ of at least 60 mm Hg. During PPV, it is common to apply PEEP at 5 cm H₂O to compensate for loss of glottic function caused by the endotracheal tube. In patients with ARDS, higher levels of PEEP (e.g., 10 to 20 cm H₂O) may be used. PEEP increases FRC and opens up collapsed alveoli. PEEP is typically applied in 3 to 5 cm H₂O increments until oxygenation is adequate with FIO₂ less than or equal to 60%. PEEP may improve V/Q in respiratory units that collapse at low airway pressures, thus allowing the FIO₂ to be lowered.

However, PEEP is not a benign therapy. The additional intrathoracic and intrapulmonic pressures can compromise venous return to the right side of the heart, thereby decreasing preload, CO, and BP. High levels of PEEP cause hyperinflation of the alveoli, compression of the pulmonary capillary bed, reduction in blood return to the left side of the heart, and a dramatic reduction in BP. In addition, high levels of PEEP or excessive inspiratory pressures can result in barotrauma and volutrauma.

If hypoxemic respiratory failure persists in spite of high levels of PEEP, alternative modes and therapies may be used. These include airway pressure release ventilation, pressure-control inverse ratio ventilation, high-frequency ventilation, and permissive hypercapnia (low tidal volumes that allow PaCO₂ to increase slowly).[49-51] (Chapter 66 provides additional information on mechanical ventilation and PEEP.)

Extracorporeal membrane oxygenation (ECMO) and extracorporeal CO₂ removal (ECCO₂R) pass blood across a gas-exchanging membrane outside the body and then return oxygenated blood back to the body. $ECCO_2R$ with PPV allows the lungs to heal while the lungs are not functional.[52,53]

Positioning Strategies. Some patients with ARDS have a marked improvement in PaO_2 when turned from the supine to the prone position (e.g., PaO_2 70 mm Hg supine, PaO_2 90 mm Hg prone) with no change in FIO_2[54] (Fig. 68-12). The response may be sufficient to allow a reduction in FIO_2 or PEEP.

In the early phases of ARDS, fluid moves freely throughout the lung. Because of gravity, this fluid pools in dependent regions of the lung. As a result, some alveoli are fluid filled (dependent areas), whereas others are air filled (nondependent areas). In addition, when the patient is supine, the heart and mediastinal contents place more pressure on the lungs than in the prone position. Thus the supine position changes pleural pressure and predisposes the patient to atelectasis. If you turn the patient from supine to prone, air-filled, nonatelectatic alveoli in the ventral (anterior) portion of the lung become dependent. Perfusion may be better matched to ventilation. Not all patients respond to prone positioning with an increase in PaO_2, and there is no reliable way of predicting who will respond. Prone positioning may be considered for patients with refractory hypoxemia who do not respond to other strategies to increase PaO_2.[54]

Other positioning strategies to consider for patients with ARDS include continuous lateral rotation therapy (CLRT) and kinetic therapy. CLRT provides continuous, slow, side-to-side turning of the patient by rotating the actual bed frame less than 40 degrees. The bed's lateral movement is maintained for 18 of

every 24 hours to simulate postural drainage and to help mobilize pulmonary secretions. In addition, the bed may also contain a vibrator pack that provides chest physiotherapy. This feature assists with secretion mobilization and removal (Fig. 68-13). Kinetic therapy is similar to CLRT in that patients are rotated side-to-side 40 degrees or more. It is important to obtain baseline assessments of the patient's pulmonary status (e.g., respiratory rate and rhythm, breath sounds, ABGs, SpO_2) and continue to monitor the patient throughout the therapy.

MEDICAL SUPPORTIVE THERAPY

MAINTENANCE OF CARDIAC OUTPUT AND TISSUE PERFUSION. Patients on PPV and PEEP frequently experience decreased CO. One cause is decreased venous return from the PEEP-induced increase in intrathoracic pressure. Impaired contractility and decreased preload can also decrease CO. Hemodynamic monitoring (e.g., CVP, CO, $ScvO_2$, SvO_2) via central venous or pulmonary artery pressure, or arterial pressure-based CO monitoring, is essential. This allows you to see trends, detect changes, and adjust therapy as needed. An arterial catheter also provides continuous monitoring of BP and sampling of blood for ABGs. If the CO falls, it may be necessary to administer crystalloid fluids or colloid solutions or to lower PEEP. Use of inotropic drugs such as dobutamine (Dobutrex) or dopamine (Intropin) may also be necessary. (Chapter 66 discusses hemodynamic monitoring in detail.)

Packed red blood cells are used to increase hemoglobin and thus the O_2-carrying capacity of the blood. The hemoglobin level is usually kept around 9 to 10 g/dL (90 to 100 g/L) with an SpO_2 of 90% or more (when PaO_2 is greater than 60 mm Hg).

MAINTENANCE OF NUTRITION AND FLUID BALANCE. Maintenance of nutrition and fluid balance is challenging in the patient with ARDS. Consult with a dietitian to determine optimal caloric needs. Enteral or parenteral feedings are started to meet the high energy requirements of these patients. Enteral formulas enriched with omega-3 fatty acids may improve the clinical outcomes of patients with ARDS.[5]

Increasing pulmonary capillary permeability results in fluid in the lungs and causes pulmonary edema. At the same time, the patient may be volume depleted and thus at risk for hypo-

FIG. 68-12 **A,** Turning patient prone on Vollman Prone Positioner. **B,** Patient lying prone on Vollman Prone Positioner. (©2006 Hill-Rom Services, Inc. Reprinted with permission. All rights reserved.)

FIG. 68-13 TotalCare SpO2RT Bed System offers continuous lateral rotation therapy and percussion and vibration therapies. Patients can easily and quickly be repositioned. (©2006 Hill-Rom Services, Inc. Reprinted with permission. All rights reserved.)

tension and decreased CO from mechanical ventilation and PEEP. Monitor hemodynamic parameters (e.g., CVP, stroke volume variation), daily weights, and intake and output to assess the patient's fluid status. Controversy exists as to the benefits of fluid replacement with crystalloids versus colloids. Critics of colloid replacement believe that proteins in colloids may leak into the pulmonary interstitium, increasing the movement of fluid into the alveoli. Advocates of colloid replacement believe that colloids help keep fluid from leaking into the alveoli. The patient is often placed on fluid restriction, and diuretics are used as necessary.

EVALUATION

The expected outcomes for the patient with ARDS are similar to those for a patient with acute respiratory failure (see p. 1664).

CASE STUDY

Acute Respiratory Distress Syndrome

Patient Profile

J.N. is a 55-yr-old white man who was admitted 12 hr ago to a surgical ICU after emergent surgery for an acutely ischemic bowel.

Past Medical History
- Lumbar spine surgery 5 yr ago
- Chronic back pain controlled with oxycodone (Oxy-Contin) 15 mg PO tid

iStockphoto/Thinkstock

The surgical procedure involved extensive abdominal surgery to repair a perforated colon, irrigate the abdominal cavity, and provide hemostasis. During surgery his systolic BP dropped to 70 mm Hg. Seven units of packed red blood cells and 4 L of 0.9% saline were infused. He is receiving 60% O_2 via an aerosol face mask.

Postoperative Orders
- Continuous ECG and pulse oximetry monitoring
- Infuse 0.9% saline at 125 mL/hr via a central venous IV catheter
- Monitor hourly urine output via indwelling bladder catheter
- Pain management via a continuous IV infusion of morphine

J.N.'s pulmonary status worsens. He needs progressively higher FIO_2. Emergent endotracheal intubation and mechanical ventilation are needed. Sedation, analgesia, and neuromuscular blockade are started to achieve anxiolysis, pain control, and ventilator synchrony. Postintubation chest x-ray reveals a pneumothorax, requiring the emergent placement of a chest tube. Immediately after chest tube placement, his O_2 saturation decreased significantly below baseline to 80%-82%. No significant changes were evident in ventilation or lung compliance, and he remained synchronous with mechanical ventilation. ABGs showed $PaCO_2$ increased to 52 mm Hg and PaO_2 decreased to 44 mm Hg. J.N. was tachycardic during and immediately after chest tube insertion. A 10-mg bolus of morphine is given followed by an increase in the continuous infusion. After 30 min, his O_2 saturation improved to 90%-91% and ABGs showed improved oxygenation (PaO_2 63 mm Hg) and ventilation ($PaCO_2$ 45 mm Hg).

Postoperative Day 1

J.N.'s lung function continues to worsen and his hypoxemia is refractory to 100% FIO_2 and high levels of PEEP. He experiences kidney and liver failure. There is little hope of weaning him from mechanical ventilation. He has an advance directive that indicates he does not want to be kept alive by artificial means.

Subjective Data
- Patient is sedated and paralyzed. Unable to communicate.
- His wife and two adult children are at the bedside and voicing concerns and questions regarding his progress.

Objective Data
Physical Assessment
- *General:* Sedated, paralyzed, well-nourished man; head of bed elevated 45 degrees; skin cool with moderate diaphoresis

- *Respiratory:* No accessory muscle use, retractions, or paradoxic breathing; respiratory rate 18 breaths/min and in phase with ventilator; SpO_2 85%; fine crackles at lung bases
- *Cardiovascular:* BP 100/60 mm Hg
- ECG as follows:

- Equal apical-radial pulse; weak peripheral pulses; temperature 101° F (38.3° C) rectally
- *Gastrointestinal:* Surgical dressing dry and intact; colostomy draining serosanguineous drainage
- *Urologic:* Indwelling bladder catheter draining concentrated urine less than 30 mL/hr

Diagnostic Findings
- ABGs: pH 7.15, PaO_2 59 mm Hg, $PaCO_2$ 57 mm Hg, HCO_3 16 mEq/L, O_2 saturation 86%
- PaO_2/FIO_2 ratio <200
- Chest x-ray: new bilateral, scattered interstitial infiltrates compatible with an ARDS pattern as interpreted by the radiologist

Discussion Questions
1. How does the pathophysiology of ARDS predispose the patient to refractory hypoxemia?
2. What clinical manifestations does J.N. exhibit that support a diagnosis of ARDS?
3. What are the possible causes of ARDS in J.N.?
4. What are the possible complications that J.N. is at risk for developing secondary to ARDS?
5. What are possible reasons for J.N.'s sudden decline in pulmonary status during and immediately after chest tube insertion?
6. *Evidence-Based Practice:* You are orienting a new nurse who asks you why you offered J.N.'s family the opportunity to stay at the bedside while the chest tube was placed. How would you respond?
7. What are possible reasons for improved oxygenation and CO_2 levels after administration of additional opioid analgesia?
8. *Priority Decision:* What priority interventions should be implemented to improve J.N.'s respiratory status and hypoxemia?
9. *Priority Decision:* Based on the assessment data presented, what are the priority nursing diagnoses?
10. *Delegation Decision:* When developing the plan of care for J.N., what tasks can you delegate to unlicensed assistive personnel (UAP)?
11. What information should you provide to J.N.'s caregiver(s) given his decline in cardiopulmonary function?
12. Given the guidelines in the patient's advance directive, what ethical/legal issues might you encounter in this patient scenario?

BRIDGE TO NCLEX EXAMINATION

The number of the question corresponds to the same-numbered outcome at the beginning of the chapter.

1. Which signs and symptoms differentiate hypoxemic respiratory failure from hypercapnic respiratory failure *(select all that apply)*?
   a. Cyanosis
   b. Tachypnea
   c. Morning headache
   d. Paradoxic breathing
   e. Use of pursed-lip breathing

2. The O_2 delivery system chosen for the patient in acute respiratory failure should
   a. always be a low-flow device, such as a nasal cannula or face mask.
   b. administer continuous positive airway pressure ventilation to prevent CO_2 narcosis.
   c. correct the PaO_2 to a normal level as quickly as possible using mechanical ventilation.
   d. maintain the PaO_2 at greater than or equal to 60 mm Hg at the lowest O_2 concentration possible.

3. The most common early clinical manifestations of ARDS that the nurse may observe are
   a. dyspnea and tachypnea.
   b. cyanosis and apprehension.
   c. hypotension and tachycardia.
   d. respiratory distress and frothy sputum.

4. Maintenance of fluid balance in the patient with ARDS involves
   a. hydration using colloids.
   b. administration of surfactant.
   c. fluid restriction and diuretics as necessary.
   d. keeping the hemoglobin at levels above 9 g/dL (90 g/L).

5. Which intervention is most likely to prevent or limit barotrauma in the patient with ARDS who is mechanically ventilated?
   a. Decreasing PEEP
   b. Increasing the tidal volume
   c. Use of permissive hypercapnia
   d. Use of positive pressure ventilation

1. a, b, c; 2. d; 3. a, 4. c; 5. c

ⓔvolve

For rationales to these answers and even more NCLEX review questions, visit *http://evolve.elsevier.com/Lewis/medsurg*.

REFERENCES

1. Kaynar AM: Respiratory failure. Retrieved from *http:// emedicine.medscape.com/article/167981-overview*.
2. Myers TR, Tomasio L: Asthma: 2015 and beyond, *Respir Care* 56:1389, 2011.
3. Nee PA, Al-Jubouri MA, Gray AJ, et al: Critical care in the emergency department: acute respiratory failure, *Emerg Med J* 28:94, 2011.
4. Byrd RP: Respiratory acidosis. Retrieved from *http:// emedicine.medscape.com/article/301574-overview*.
5. Harman EH: Acute respiratory distress syndrome. Retrieved from *http://emedicine.medscape.com/article/165139-overview*.
6. Morris MJ: Asthma. Retrieved from *http://emedicine.medscape .com/article/296301-overview*.
7. Jackson DJ, Sykes A, Mallia P, et al: Asthma exacerbations: origin, effect and prevention, *J Allergy Clin Immunol* 128:1165, 2011.
8. Evensen AE: Management of COPD exacerbations, *Am Fam Physician* 81:607, 2010.
9. Abbatecola AM, Fumagalli A, Bonardi D, et al: Practical management problems of chronic obstructive pulmonary disease in the elderly: acute exacerbations, *Curr Opin Pulm Med* 17(Suppl 1):S49, 2011.
10. Patel SB, Kress JP: Sedation and analgesia in the mechanically ventilated patient, *Am J Respir Crit Care Med* 185:486, 2012.
11. Ouellette DR: Pulmonary embolism. Retrieved from *http:// emedicine.medscape.com/article/300901-overview*.
12. Cortes I, Penuelas O, Esteban A: Acute respiratory distress syndrome: evaluation and management, *Minerva Anesthesiol* 78:343, 2012.
13. Demirijian BJ: Emphysema. Retrieved from *http://emedicine. medscape.com/article/298283-overview*.
14. Hemprich U, Papadakos PJ, Lachmann B: Respiratory failure and hypoxemia in the cirrhotic patient including hepatopulmonary syndrome, *Curr Opin Anaesthesiol* 23:133, 2010.
15. Racca F, Del Sorbo L, Mongini T, et al: Respiratory management of acute respiratory failure in neuromuscular diseases, *Minerva Anesthesiol* 76:51, 2010.
16. Mokhlesi B: Obesity hypoventilation syndrome: a state-of-the -art review, *Respir Care* 55:1347, 2010.
17. Fayyaz J: Hypoventilation syndromes. Retrieved from *http:// emedicine.medscape.com/article/304381-overview*.
18. Tzani P, Aiello M, Elia D, et al: Dynamic hyperinflation is associated with a poor cardiovascular response to exercise in COPD patients, *Respir Res* 12:150, 2011.
19. Ortiz JR, Neuzil KM, Victor JC, et al: Influenza-associated cystic fibrosis pulmonary exacerbations, *Chest* 137:852, 2010.
20. Zemanick ET, Harris JK, Conway S, et al: Measuring and improving respiratory outcomes in cystic fibrosis lung disease: opportunities and challenges to therapy, *J Cystic Fibrosis* 9:1, 2010.
21. Brulotte CA, Lang ES: Acute exacerbations of chronic obstructive pulmonary disease in the emergency department, *Emerg Med Clin North Am* 30:223, 2012.
22. Boldrini R, Fasano L, Nava S: Noninvasive mechanical ventilation, *Curr Opin Crit Care* 18:48, 2012.
23. Restrepo RD, Hirst KR, Wittnebel L, et al: AARC clinical practice guideline: transcutaneous monitoring of carbon dioxide, *Respir Care* 57:1955, 2012.
24. Boerrigter B, Trip P, Bogaard HJ, et al: Right atrial pressure affects the interaction between lung mechanics and right ventricular function in spontaneously breathing COPD patients. Retrieved from *http://www.ncbi.nlm.nih.gov/pmc/ articles/PMC3260236/pdf/pone.0030208.pdf*.
25. Russell R, Anzueto A, Weisman I: Optimizing management of chronic obstructive pulmonary disease in the upcoming decade, *Int J COPD* 6:47, 2011.
26. Donahoe M: Acute respiratory distress syndrome: a clinical review, *Pulm Circ* 1:192, 2011.

*27. Keenan SP, Sinuff T, Burns KEA, et al: Clinical practice guidelines for the use of noninvasive positive-pressure ventilation and noninvasive positive airway pressure in the acute care setting, *Can Med Assoc J* 183:E195, 2011.

28. Gursel G, Aydogdu M, Tasyurek G, et al: Factors associated with noninvasive ventilation response in the first day of therapy in patients with hypercapnic respiratory failure, *Ann Thorac Med* 7:92, 2012.

29. Brown LK: Hypoventilation syndromes, *Clin Chest Med* 31:249, 2010.

30. Antonelli M, Azoulay E, Bonten M, et al: Year in review in intensive care medicine 2010, Part III: ARDS and ALI, mechanical ventilation, noninvasive ventilation, weaning, endotracheal intubation, lung ultrasound and paediatrics, *Intens Care Med* 37:394, 2011.

31. Schortgen F, Follin A, Piccari L, et al: Results of noninvasive ventilation in very old patients, *Ann Intens Med* 2:5, 2012.

32. Muir JF, Lamia B, Molano C, et al: Respiratory failure in the elderly patient, *Semin Respir Crit Care Med* 31:634, 2010.

33. Pomares X, Monton C, Espasa M, et al: Long-term azithromycin therapy in patients with severe COPD and repeated exacerbations, *Int J COPD* 6:449, 2011.

*34. DeGrado JR, Anger KE, Szumita PM, et al: Evaluation of a local ICU sedation guideline on goal-directed administration of sedatives and analgesics, *J Pain Res* 4:127, 2011.

*35. Devabhakthuni S: Analgosedation: a paradigm shift in intensive care unit sedation practice, *Ann Pharmacol* 46:530, 2012.

*36. Arbour R, Waterhouse J, Seckel MA, et al: Correlation between the sedation-agitation scale and the bispectral index in ventilated patients in the intensive care unit, *Heart Lung* 38:336, 2009.

37. Permpogkosol S: Iatrogenic disease in the elderly: risk factors, consequences and prevention, *Clin Interven Aging* 6:77, 2011.

*38. Cerejeira J, Mukaetova-Ladinski EB: A clinical update on delirium: from early recognition to effective management. Retrieved from *www.ncbi.nlm.nih.gov/pmc/articles/PMC3169311/pdf/NRP2011-875196.pdf.*

*39. Schreier AM: Nursing care, delirium and pain management for the hospitalized older adult, *Pain Manag Nurs* 11:177, 2010.

40. Villar J: What is the acute respiratory distress syndrome? *Respir Care* 56:1539, 2011.

41. Horlander KT: Imaging in acute respiratory distress syndrome. Retrieved from *http://emedicine.medscape.com/article/362571-overview.*

42. Raghavendran K, Napolitano LM: Definition of ALI/ARDS, *Crit Care Clin* 27:429, 2011.

43. Collins SR, Blank RS: Approaches to refractory hypoxemia in acute respiratory distress syndrome: current understanding, evidence and debate, *Respir Care* 56:1573, 2011.

*44. Crimlisk JT, Gustavson KA, Silva J: Translating guidelines into practice: ventilator-associated pneumonia prevention strategies in an acute rehabilitation unit, *Dimens Crit Care Nurs* 31:118, 2012.

*45. Morris AC, Hay AW, Swann DG, et al: Reducing ventilator-associated pneumonia in intensive care: impact of implementing a care bundle, *Crit Care Med* 39:2218, 2011.

*46. Sole ML, Penoyer DA, Bennett M, et al: Oropharyngeal secretion volume in intubated patients: the importance of oral suctioning, *Am J Crit Care* 20:e141, 2011.

47. Maselli DJ, Restrepo MI: Strategies in the prevention of ventilator-associated pneumonia, *Ther Adv Respir Dis* 5:131, 2011.

*48. Ames NJ: Evidence to support tooth brushing in critically ill patients, *Am J Crit Care* 20:242, 2011.

49. Soo Hoo GW: Barotrauma and mechanical ventilation. Retrieved from *http://emedicine.medscape.com/article/296625-overview.*

50. Hess DR: Approaches to conventional mechanical ventilation of the patient with acute respiratory distress syndrome, *Respir Care* 56:1555, 2011.

51. Pierrakos C, Karanikolas M, Scoletta S, et al: Acute respiratory distress syndrome: pathophysiology and therapeutic options, *J Clin Med Res* 4:7, 2012.

52. Raoof S, Goulet K, Esan A, et al: Severe hypoxemic respiratory failure, part 2: Nonventilatory strategies, *Chest* 137:1437, 2010.

53. Combes A, Bacchetta M, Brodie D, et al: Extracorporeal membrane oxygenation for respiratory failure in adults, *Curr Opin Crit Care* 18:99, 2012.

54. Dickinson S, Park PK, Napolitano LM: Prone-positioning therapy in ARDS, *Crit Care Clin* 27:511, 2011.

RESOURCES

Resources for this chapter are listed after Chapter 66 on p. 1630.

*Evidence-based information for clinical practice.

One of the tests of leadership is the ability to recognize a problem before it becomes an emergency.
Arnold H. Glasow

Nursing Management

Emergency, Terrorism, and Disaster Nursing

Linda Bucher

evolve WEBSITE

http://evolve.elsevier.com/Lewis/medsurg

- NCLEX Review Questions
- Key Points
- Pre-Test
- Answer Guidelines for Case Study on p. 1692

- Rationales for Bridge to NCLEX Examination Questions
- Case Study
  - Patient With Musculoskeletal Trauma
- Concept Map Creator
- Glossary
- Content Updates

eTables
- eTable 69-1: Trauma Verification Levels
- eTable 69-2: Biologic Agents of Terrorism
- eTable 69-3: Chemical Agents of Terrorism by Target Organ or Effect

LEARNING OUTCOMES

1. Apply the steps in triage, the primary survey, and the secondary survey to a patient experiencing a medical, surgical, or traumatic emergency.
2. Relate the pathophysiology to the assessment and collaborative care of select environmental emergencies (e.g., hyperthermia, hypothermia, submersion injury, bites).
3. Relate the pathophysiology to the assessment and collaborative care of select toxicologic emergencies.
4. Select appropriate nursing interventions for victims of violence.
5. Differentiate among the responsibilities of health care providers, the community, and select federal agencies in emergency and mass casualty incident preparedness.

KEY TERMS

emergency, p. 1691
family presence (FP), p. 1678
frostbite, p. 1684
heat cramps, p. 1682
heat exhaustion, p. 1682

heatstroke, p. 1683
hypothermia, p. 1684
jaw-thrust maneuver, p. 1677
mass casualty incident (MCI), p. 1691
primary survey, p. 1676

secondary survey, p. 1678
submersion injury, p. 1686
terrorism, p. 1690
triage, p. 1675

This chapter presents an overview of triage and care of emergency patients not addressed elsewhere in this book. Common emergency situations discussed include heat- and cold-related emergencies, submersion injuries, bites and stings, and various types of poisonings. The chapter concludes with a discussion of terrorism, followed by a description of a mass casualty incident, and the methods of responding to the incident.

The emergency management of various medical, surgical, and traumatic emergencies is discussed throughout the textbook. Tables summarize emergency management of specific problems. Table 69-1 lists each emergency management table by title, chapter number, and page.

Most patients with life-threatening or potentially life-threatening problems arrive at the hospital through the emergency department (ED). More patients report to the ED for less urgent conditions. Every year more than 136 million people visit EDs. This number is increasing for a variety of reasons, including (1) the inability to see a primary care provider, (2) an aging population, (3) shorter hospital stays resulting in frequent readmissions, (4) acute mental health crises, and (5) lack of health insurance (or a primary care provider). These factors, plus the increase in ED closures, result in chronic overcrowding and long wait times.[1,2]

Emergency nurses care for patients of all ages and with a variety of problems. However, some EDs specialize in certain

Reviewed by Janet E. Jackson, RN, MS, Assistant Professor, Department of Nursing, Bradley University, Peoria, Illinois; Lisa A. Webb, RN, MSN, CEN, Instructor of Nursing, Charleston Southern University, Charleston, South Carolina; and Amber Young, RN, MSN, Instructor of Nursing, Bellin College, School of Nursing, Green Bay, Wisconsin.

patient populations or conditions, such as pediatric ED or trauma ED. (See eTable 69-1 for the resources at various levels of trauma designated facilities.) The Emergency Nurses Association (ENA) is the specialty organization aimed at advancing emergency nursing practice. The ENA provides standards of

care for nurses working in the ED, and a certification process that allows nurses to become certified emergency nurses (CENs).[3]

CARE OF EMERGENCY PATIENT

Recognition of life-threatening illness or injury is one of the most important goals of emergency nursing. Initiation of interventions to reverse or prevent a crisis is often a priority before a medical diagnosis is made. This process begins with your first contact with a patient. Prompt identification of patients requiring immediate treatment and determination of appropriate interventions are essential nurse competencies.

Triage

Triage, a French word meaning "to sort," refers to the process of rapidly determining patient acuity. It is one of the most important assessment skills needed by emergency nurses.[4,5] Most often, you will confront multiple patients who have a variety of problems. The triage process works on the premise that patients who have a threat to life must be treated before other patients.

A *triage system* identifies and categorizes patients so that the most critical are treated first. The ENA and American College of Emergency Physicians support the use of a five-level triage system.[6] The *Emergency Severity Index* (ESI) is a five-level triage system that incorporates concepts of illness severity and resource utilization (e.g., electrocardiogram [ECG], laboratory work, radiology studies, IV fluids) to determine who should be treated first[5] (Table 69-2). The ESI includes a triage algorithm that directs you to assign an ESI level to patients coming into the ED. (The triage algorithm can be found in the ESI Implementation Handbook available at *www.ahrq.gov/research/esi*.) Initially, assess the patient for any threats to life (ESI-1) (e.g., Is the patient dying?) or presence of a high-risk situation (ESI-2)

TABLE 69-1 EMERGENCY MANAGEMENT

Emergency Management Tables

Title	Chapter	Page
Abdominal Trauma	43	973
Acute Abdominal Pain	43	971
Acute Soft Tissue Injury	63	1507
Anaphylactic Shock	14	214
Chemical Burns	25	457
Chest Pain	34	750
Chest Trauma	28	541
Cocaine and Amphetamine Toxicity	11	164
Depressant Drug Overdose	11	164
Diabetic Ketoacidosis	49	1177
Dysrhythmias	36	793
Electrical Burns	25	456
Eye Injury	22	390
Fractured Extremity	63	1518
Head Injury	57	1372
Hyperthermia	69	1683
Hypothermia	69	1685
Inhalation Injury	25	456
Sexual Assault	54	1302
Shock	67	1641
Spinal Cord Injury	61	1474
Stroke	58	1398
Submersion Injuries	69	1687
Thermal Burns	25	455
Thoracic Injuries	28	542
Tonic-Clonic Seizures	59	1423

TABLE 69-2   FIVE-LEVEL EMERGENCY SEVERITY INDEX (ESI)

	Level				
Definition	**ESI-1**	**ESI-2**	**ESI-3**	**ESI-4**	**ESI-5**
Stability of vital functions (ABCs)	Unstable	Threatened	Stable	Stable	Stable
Life threat or organ threat	Obvious	Likely but not always obvious	Unlikely but possible	No	No
How soon patient should be seen by physician	Immediately	Within 10 min	Up to 1 hr	Could be delayed	Could be delayed
Expected resource intensity	High resource intensity Staff at bedside continuously Often mobilization of team response	High resource intensity Multiple, often complex diagnostic studies Frequent consultation Continuous monitoring	Medium to high resource intensity Multiple diagnostic studies (e.g., multiple laboratory studies, x-rays) or brief observation Complex procedure (e.g., IV fluids, medications)	Low resource intensity One simple diagnostic study (e.g., x-ray) or simple procedure (e.g., sutures)	Low resource intensity Examination only
Examples	Cardiac arrest, intubated trauma patient, overdose with bradypnea, severe respiratory distress	Chest pain probably resulting from ischemia, multiple trauma unless responsive	Abdominal pain or gynecologic disorders unless in severe distress, hip fracture in older patient	Closed extremity trauma, simple laceration, cystitis	Cold symptoms, minor burn, recheck (e.g., wound), prescription refill

Modified and reprinted with permission. Copyright 1999, Richard C. Wuerz, MD, and David R. Eitel, MD.
ABCs, Airway, breathing, circulation.

TABLE 69-3   EMERGENCY ASSESSMENT: PRIMARY SURVEY

Assessment	Interventions
Airway With Simultaneous Cervical Spine Stabilization and/or Immobilization	
• Assess for respiratory distress. • Assess airway for patency. • Check for loose teeth or foreign bodies. • Assess for bleeding, vomitus, or edema.	• Open airway. • Use jaw-thrust maneuver. • Remove or suction any foreign bodies. • Insert oropharyngeal or nasopharyngeal airway, endotracheal tube, cricothyroidotomy. • Immobilize cervical spine using rigid cervical collar and cervical immobilization device. Secure forehead to backboard.
Breathing	
• Assess ventilation. • Scan chest for signs of breathing. • Look for paradoxic movement of the chest wall during inspiration and expiration. • Note use of accessory muscles or abdominal muscles. • Observe and count respiratory rate. • Note color of nail beds, mucous membranes, skin. • Auscultate lungs. • Assess for jugular venous distention and position of trachea.	• Give supplemental O_2 via appropriate delivery system (e.g., non-rebreather mask). • Ventilate with bag-valve-mask with 100% O_2 if respirations are inadequate or absent. • Prepare to intubate if severe respiratory distress (e.g., agonal breaths) or arrest. • Have suction available. • If absent breath sounds, prepare for needle thoracostomy and chest tube insertion.
Circulation	
• Check carotid or femoral pulse. • Palpate pulse for quality and rate. • Assess skin color, temperature, and moisture. • Check capillary refill. • Assess for external bleeding. • Measure blood pressure.	• If absent pulse, initiate cardiopulmonary resuscitation and advanced life-support measures. • If shock symptoms or hypotensive, start two large-bore (14- to 16-gauge) IVs and initiate infusions of normal saline or lactated Ringer's solution. • Control bleeding with direct pressure and pressure dressings, if appropriate. • Administer blood products if ordered. • Consider autotransfusion if isolated chest trauma. • Consider use of a pneumatic antishock garment or pelvic splint in the presence of pelvic fracture with hypotension. • Obtain blood samples for type and crossmatch.
Disability *Brief Neurologic Assessment*	
• Assess level of consciousness by determining response to verbal and/or painful stimuli (e.g., AVPU, Glasgow Coma Scale). • Assess pupils for size, shape, equality, and reactivity.	• Periodically reassess level of consciousness, mental status, pupil size and reactivity.
Identify Deformities	
• Inspect extremities for any obvious deformities. • Determine range of movement and strength in extremities.	• Immobilize (e.g., splint) any obvious deformities.
Brief Pain Assessment	
• Assess pain (e.g., PQRST [see Table 34-7]).	• Periodically reassess pain using standardized pain scale.
Exposure and Environmental Control	
• Assess full body for additional or related injuries	• Remove clothing for adequate examination. • Keep patient warm with blankets, warmed IV fluids, overhead lights to prevent heat loss, if appropriate. • Maintain privacy.

AVPU, A = alert, *V* = responsive to voice, *P* = responsive to pain, and *U* = unresponsive.

(e.g., Is this a high-risk patient who should not wait to be seen?). Next, evaluate patients who do not meet the criteria for ESI-1 or ESI-2 for the number of anticipated resources they may need. Assign patients to ESI level 3, 4, or 5 based on this determination. Normal vital signs are required for patients assigned to ESI level 3. Patients with abnormal vital signs may be reassigned to ESI level 2.[5] (For practice using the ESI triage system, see the ESI Implementation Handbook available at *www.ahrq.gov/research/esi*.)

After you complete the initial focused assessment to determine the presence of actual or potential threats to life, proceed with a more detailed assessment. A systematic approach to this assessment decreases the time needed to identify potential threats to life and limits the risk of overlooking a life-threatening condition. A primary and secondary survey is the approach used for all trauma patients. For nontrauma patients, the primary survey is followed by a focused assessment. (Focused assessments are discussed in Chapter 3.)

Primary Survey

The **primary survey** (Table 69-3) focuses on airway, breathing, circulation (ABC), disability, and exposure or environmental control. It aims to identify life-threatening conditions so that appropriate interventions can be started. You may identify life-

TABLE 69-4	POTENTIAL LIFE-THREATENING CONDITIONS FOUND DURING PRIMARY SURVEY*

Airway
- Inhalation injury (e.g., fire victim)
- Obstruction (partial or complete) from foreign bodies, debris (e.g., vomitus), or tongue
- Penetrating wounds and/or blunt trauma to upper airway structures

Breathing
- Anaphylaxis
- Flail chest with pulmonary contusion
- Hemothorax
- Pneumothorax (e.g., open, tension)

Circulation
- Direct cardiac injury (e.g., myocardial infarction, trauma)
- Pericardial tamponade
- Shock (e.g., massive burns, hypovolemia)
- Uncontrolled external hemorrhage
- Hypothermia

Disability
- Head injury
- Stroke

*List is not all-inclusive.

FIG. 69-1 Jaw-thrust maneuver is the recommended procedure for opening the airway of an unconscious patient with a possible neck or spinal injury. With the patient lying supine, kneel at the top of the head. Place one hand on each side of the patient's head, resting your elbows on the surface. Grasp the angles of the patient's lower jaw and lift the jaw forward with both hands without tilting the head.

threatening conditions related to ABCs (Table 69-4) at any point during the primary survey. When this occurs, start interventions immediately, before moving to the next step of the survey.

A = Airway With Cervical Spine Stabilization and/or Immobilization. Nearly all immediate trauma deaths occur because of airway obstruction. Saliva, bloody secretions, vomitus, laryngeal trauma, dentures, facial trauma, fractures, and the tongue can obstruct the airway. Patients at risk for airway compromise include those who have seizures, near-drowning, anaphylaxis, foreign body obstruction, or cardiopulmonary arrest. If an airway is not maintained, obstruction of airflow, hypoxia, and death will result.

Primary signs and symptoms in a patient with a compromised airway include dyspnea, inability to speak, gasping (agonal) breaths, foreign body in the airway, and trauma to the face or neck. Airway maintenance should progress rapidly from the least to the most invasive method. Treatment includes opening the airway using the **jaw-thrust maneuver** (avoiding hyperextension of the neck) (Fig. 69-1), suctioning and/or removal of foreign body, insertion of a nasopharyngeal or an oropharyngeal airway (in unconscious patients only), and endotracheal intubation. If intubation is impossible because of airway obstruction, an emergency cricothyroidotomy or tracheotomy is performed (see Chapter 27). Ventilate patients with 100% O₂ using a bag-valve-mask (BVM) device before intubation or cricothyroidotomy.[7]

Rapid-sequence intubation is the preferred procedure for securing an unprotected airway in the ED. It involves the use of sedation (e.g., midazolam [Versed]) or anesthesia (e.g., etomidate [Amidate]) and paralysis (e.g., succinylcholine [Anectine]). These drugs aid intubation and reduce the risk of aspiration and airway trauma.[7] (See Chapter 66 for more information on intubation.)

Suspect cervical spine trauma in any patient with face, head, or neck trauma and/or significant upper chest injuries. Stabilize the cervical spine (head maintained in a neutral position) and/or immobilize during assessment of the airway. At the scene of

the injury, the cervical spine is immobilized with a rigid *cervical collar* (C-collar) and a *cervical immobilization device* (CID) (also known as "head blocks"). Finally, secure the patient's forehead to the backboard. Do not use sandbags because the weight of the bags could move the head if the patient is logrolled.

B = Breathing. Adequate airflow through the upper airway does not ensure adequate ventilation. Many conditions cause breathing changes, including fractured ribs, pneumothorax, penetrating injury, allergic reactions, pulmonary emboli, and asthma attacks. Patients with these conditions may have a variety of signs and symptoms, including dyspnea (e.g., pulmonary emboli), paradoxic or asymmetric chest wall movement (e.g., flail chest), decreased or absent breath sounds on the affected side (e.g., pneumothorax), visible wound to chest wall (e.g., penetrating injury), cyanosis (e.g., asthma), tachycardia, and hypotension.

Every critically injured or ill patient has an increased metabolic and oxygen demand and should have supplemental O₂. Administer high-flow O₂ (100%) via a non-rebreather mask and monitor the patient's response. Life-threatening conditions (e.g., flail chest, tension pneumothorax) can severely and quickly compromise ventilation. Interventions may include BVM ventilation with 100% O₂, needle decompression, intubation, and treatment of the underlying cause.

C = Circulation. An effective circulatory system includes the heart, intact blood vessels, and adequate blood volume. Uncontrolled internal or external bleeding places an individual at risk for hemorrhagic shock (see Chapter 67). Check a central pulse (e.g., carotid) because peripheral pulses may be absent due to direct injury or vasoconstriction. If you feel a pulse, assess the quality and rate. Assess the skin for color, temperature, and moisture. Altered mental status and delayed capillary refill (longer than 3 seconds) are common signs of shock. Take care when evaluating capillary refill in cold environments because cold delays refill.

Insert IV lines into veins in the upper extremities unless contraindicated, such as in a massive fracture or an injury that affects limb circulation. Insert two large-bore (14- to 16-gauge) IV catheters and start aggressive fluid resuscitation using normal saline or lactated Ringer's solution (see Chapter 67 for more information on hypovolemic shock and fluid resuscitation).

Apply direct pressure with a sterile dressing followed by a pressure dressing to any obvious bleeding sites. Obtain blood samples for typing to determine ABO and Rh group. Give type-specific packed red blood cells if needed. In an emergency (life-threatening) situation, give uncrossmatched blood if immediate transfusion is warranted. Pelvic splints or belts for pelvic fracture may be used for bleeding with hypotension.[8]

D = Disability. Conduct a brief neurologic examination as part of the primary survey. The patient's level of consciousness is a measure of the degree of disability. Determine the patient's response to verbal and/or painful stimuli to assess level of consciousness. A simple mnemonic to remember is *AVPU*: *A* = alert, *V* = responsive to voice, *P* = responsive to pain, and *U* = unresponsive. In addition, use the Glasgow Coma Scale (GCS) to determine the level of consciousness (see Table 57-5). Finally, assess the pupils for size, shape, equality, and reactivity.

E = Exposure or Environmental Control. Remove all trauma patients' clothing to perform a thorough physical assessment. This often requires cutting off the patient's clothing. Be careful not to cut through any area that may provide forensic evidence (e.g., bullet hole). Once the patient is exposed, use warming blankets, overhead warmers, and warmed IV fluids to limit heat loss, prevent hypothermia, and maintain privacy.

Secondary Survey

The secondary survey begins after addressing each step of the primary survey and starting any lifesaving interventions. The secondary survey is a brief, systematic process that aims to identify *all* injuries[9] (Table 69-5).

F = Full Set of Vital Signs, Focused Adjuncts, Facilitate Family Presence. Obtain a full set of vital signs, including blood pressure (BP), heart rate, respiratory rate, O_2 saturation, and temperature after the patient is exposed. If the patient has sustained or is suspected of having sustained chest trauma, or if the BP is abnormally high or low, obtain the BP in both arms.

At this point, determine whether to proceed with the secondary survey or to perform additional interventions. The input of other health care team members often influences this decision. The following focused adjuncts are considered for patients who sustain significant trauma or require lifesaving interventions during the primary survey:

- Continuously monitor ECG for heart rate and rhythm.
- Continuously monitor O_2 saturation and end-tidal carbon dioxide (if appropriate) (see Chapter 66).
- Obtain portable chest x-ray to confirm exact placement of tubes (e.g., endotracheal, gastric).
- Insert an indwelling catheter to decompress the bladder, monitor urine output, and check for hematuria. Do not insert an indwelling catheter if blood is present at the urinary meatus (e.g., urethral tear) or if scrotal hematoma or perineal ecchymosis is present. Men with a high-riding prostate gland on rectal examination are at risk for a urethral injury. The physician may order a retrograde urethrogram before inserting a catheter.
- Insert orogastric or nasogastric tube to decompress and empty the stomach, reduce the risk of aspiration, and test the contents for blood. Place an orogastric tube in a patient with significant head or facial trauma, since a nasogastric tube could enter the brain.
- Facilitate laboratory and diagnostic studies (e.g., type and crossmatch, complete blood count and metabolic panel, blood alcohol, toxicology screening, arterial blood

gases [ABGs], coagulation profile, cardiac markers, pregnancy [urine], x-rays, computed tomography [CT] scans, ultrasound).
- Determine the need for tetanus prophylaxis.

Facilitating **family presence (FP)** completes this step of the secondary survey. Research supports the benefits for patients, caregivers, and staff of allowing FP during resuscitation and invasive procedures.[10,11] Patients report that caregivers provide comfort, serve as advocates for them, and help remind the health care team of their "personhood." Caregivers who wish to be present during invasive procedures and resuscitation view themselves as active participants in the care process. They also believe that they comfort the patient and that it is their right to be with the patient. Nurses report that family members serve as "patient helpers" (e.g., provide support) and "staff helpers" (e.g., act as a translator).[10] It is essential to assign a member of the health care team to explain care delivered and answer questions should a caregiver request FP during resuscitation or invasive procedures.

G = Give Comfort Measures. Provision of comfort measures is of paramount importance when caring for patients in the ED. Pain is the primary complaint of most patients who come to the ED.[12] Many EDs have developed pain management guidelines to treat pain early, beginning at triage. Pain management strategies should include a combination of pharmacologic (e.g., nonsteroidal antiinflammatory drugs, IV opioids) and nonpharmacologic (e.g., imagery, distraction, positioning) measures. You play a pivotal role in ongoing pain management because of your frequent contact with patients. General comfort measures such as providing verbal reassurance, listening, reducing stimuli (e.g., dimming lights), and developing a trusting relationship with the patient and caregiver should be provided to all patients in the ED. Additional measures include splinting, elevating, and icing injured extremities as appropriate.

H = History and Head-to-Toe Assessment. The history of the incident, injury, or illness provides clues to the cause of the crisis (e.g., Were the injuries self-inflicted?) and suggests specific assessment and interventions. The patient may not be able to give a history. However, caregivers, friends, witnesses, and prehospital personnel can often provide necessary information. Prehospital information focuses on the mechanism and pattern of injury, injuries suspected, vital signs, treatments initiated, and patient responses.

Details of the incident are extremely important because the mechanism of injury and injury patterns can predict specific injuries. For example, a restrained front-seat passenger may have a head injury or knee, femur, or hip fractures from hitting the dashboard and an abdominal injury from the seat belt. If there were deaths at the scene, the patient is at high risk for significant injury.

Patients who jump from buildings or bridges may have bilateral calcaneal (heel) fractures, bilateral wrist fractures, and lumbar spine compression fractures. They are also at risk for aortic tears. Older patients who have climbed ladders and fallen may have had a stroke or myocardial infarction that led to the fall.

Prehospital personnel provide a detailed description of the patient's general condition, level of consciousness, and apparent injuries. An experienced ED team can complete a history within 5 minutes of the patient's arrival. If the patient is emergently ill, obtain a thorough history from caregivers or friends after the

TABLE 69-5 EMERGENCY ASSESSMENT: SECONDARY SURVEY

Assessment	Interventions
Full Set of Vital Signs	
Establish baseline vital signs	• Obtain vital signs: temperature, heart rate, respiratory rate, oxygen saturation, BP bilaterally.
Focused Adjuncts	
Determine need for additional procedures	• Initiate continuous ECG, O_2 saturation, and end-tidal carbon dioxide monitoring. • Insert urinary catheter (if not contraindicated). • Insert gastric tube. • Obtain blood for laboratory studies. • Arrange for diagnostic studies (e.g., chest x-ray). • Provide tetanus prophylaxis, if appropriate.
Facilitate Family Presence	
Determine caregiver's desire to be present during invasive procedures and/or cardiopulmonary resuscitation	• Assign team member to support caregivers.
Give Comfort Measures	
Assess, treat, and reassess for pain, anxiety	• Provide emotional support to patient and caregiver. • Provide additional comfort measures as appropriate (e.g., distraction, ice, position of comfort, warm blanket, analgesia).
History and Head-to-Toe Assessment	
History	• Obtain details of the incident/illness, mechanism and pattern of injury, length of time since incident occurred, injuries suspected, treatment provided and patient's response, level of consciousness. • Use the mnemonic **AMPLE** to determine **A**llergies, **M**edication history, **P**ast health history (e.g., preexisting medical/psychiatric conditions, last menstrual period), **L**ast meal, and **E**vents/Environment preceding illness or injury.
Head, Neck, and Face	• Note general appearance, including skin color. • Examine face and scalp for lacerations, bone or soft tissue deformity, tenderness, bleeding, and foreign bodies. • Inspect eyes, ears, nose, and mouth for bleeding, foreign bodies, drainage, pain, deformity, ecchymosis, lacerations. • Palpate head for depressions of cranial or facial bones, contusions, hematomas, areas of softness, bony crepitus. • Examine neck for stiffness, pain in cervical vertebrae, tracheal deviation, distended neck veins, bleeding, edema, difficulty swallowing, bruising, subcutaneous emphysema, bony crepitus.
Chest	• Observe rate, depth, and effort of breathing, including chest wall movement and use of accessory muscles. • Palpate for bony crepitus, subcutaneous emphysema. • Auscultate breath sounds. • Obtain 12-lead ECG and chest x-ray. • Inspect for external signs of injury: petechiae, bleeding, cyanosis, bruises, abrasions, lacerations, old scars.
Abdomen and Flanks	• Look for symmetry of abdominal wall and bony structures. • Inspect for external signs of injury: bruises, abrasions, lacerations, punctures, old scars. • Auscultate for bowel sounds. • Palpate for masses, guarding, femoral pulses. • Note type and location of pain, rigidity, or distention of abdomen.
Pelvis and Perineum	• Gently palpate pelvis. • Assess genitalia for blood at the meatus, priapism, ecchymosis, rectal bleeding, anal sphincter tone. • Determine ability to void.
Extremities	• Inspect for signs of external injury: deformity, ecchymosis, abrasions, lacerations, swelling. • Observe skin color and palpate skin for pain, tenderness, temperature, and crepitus. • Evaluate movement, strength, and sensation in arms and legs. • Assess quality and symmetry of peripheral pulses.
Inspect Posterior Surfaces	• Logroll and inspect and palpate back for deformity, bleeding, lacerations, bruises.

patient is taken to the treatment area. The history should include the following questions:

- What is the chief complaint? What caused the patient to seek attention?
- What are the patient's subjective complaints?
- What is the patient's description of pain (e.g., location, duration, quality, character)?
- What are the witnesses' (if any) descriptions of the patient's behavior since the onset?
- What is the patient's health history? The mnemonic *AMPLE* is a memory aid that prompts you to ask about the following:
  - *A:* Allergies to drugs, food, latex, environment
  - *M:* Medication history
  - *P:* Past health history (e.g., preexisting medical or psychiatric conditions, previous hospitalizations or surgeries, smoking history, recent use of drugs or alcohol, tetanus immunization, last menstrual period, baseline mental status)
  - *L:* Last meal
  - *E:* Events or environmental factors leading to the illness or injury

Head, Neck, and Face. Assess the patient for general appearance, skin color, and temperature. Check the eyes for extraocular movements. A disconjugate gaze is an indication of neurologic damage. Battle's sign, or bruising directly behind the ear(s), may indicate a fracture of the base of the posterior portion of the skull. "Raccoon eyes," or periorbital ecchymosis, is usually an indication of a fracture of the base of the frontal portion of the skull. Check the ears for blood and cerebrospinal fluid (see Chapter 57 and Fig. 57-13). Do not block clear drainage from the ear or nose.

Assess the airway for foreign bodies, bleeding, edema, and loose or missing teeth. Check for the ability to open the mouth and swallow. Inspect the neck for bruising, edema, bleeding, or distended neck veins. Palpate the trachea to determine whether it is midline. A deviated trachea may signal a life-threatening tension pneumothorax. Subcutaneous emphysema may indicate laryngotracheal disruption. A stiff or painful neck may signify a fracture of one or more cervical vertebrae. Protect the cervical spine using a C-collar and supine positioning if indicated.

Chest. Inspect the chest for paradoxic chest movements and large sucking chest wounds. Palpate the sternum, clavicles, and ribs for deformity, point tenderness, and crepitus. Auscultate breath sounds and heart sounds. In addition to tension pneumothorax and open pneumothorax, evaluate the patient for rib fractures, pulmonary contusion, blunt cardiac injury, and hemothorax. Obtain a chest x-ray and 12-lead ECG, particularly on a patient with known or suspected heart disease. The ECG is done to detect dysrhythmias and signs of myocardial ischemia or infarction.

Abdomen and Flanks. The abdomen and flanks are more difficult to assess. Frequent evaluation for subtle changes in the abdomen is essential. Motor vehicle collisions and assaults can cause blunt trauma. Penetrating trauma tends to injure specific, solid organs (e.g., spleen) based on their trajectory. Stabilize impaled objects (e.g., knife), since they need to be removed in a controlled environment such as an operating room. Decreased bowel sounds may indicate a temporary paralytic ileus. Bowel sounds in the chest may indicate a diaphragmatic rupture. Percuss the abdomen for distention (e.g., tympany [excessive air], dullness [excessive fluid]) and palpate for tenderness.

If you suspect intraabdominal hemorrhage, a *focused abdominal sonography for trauma* (FAST) to identify blood in the peritoneal space (hemoperitoneum) is preferred. This procedure is noninvasive and performed quickly at the bedside.[13] However, a FAST cannot rule out a retroperitoneal bleed. If one is suspected, a CT scan is usually ordered.

Pelvis and Perineum. Gently palpate the pelvis to determine stability. Do not rock the pelvis. Pain may indicate a pelvic fracture and the need for an x-ray. Inspect the genitalia for bleeding, priapism, and obvious injuries. Assess for bladder distention, hematuria, dysuria, or inability to void. The physician may perform a rectal examination to check for blood, a high-riding prostate gland (e.g., urethral injury), and loss of sphincter tone (e.g., spinal cord injury).

Extremities. Assess the upper and lower extremities for point tenderness, crepitus, and deformities. Splint injured extremities above and below the injury to decrease further soft tissue injury and pain. Grossly deformed, pulseless extremities should be realigned by the physician and then splinted. Check pulses before and after movement or splinting of an extremity. A pulseless extremity is a time-critical vascular or orthopedic emergency. Immobilize and elevate injured extremities, and apply ice packs. Prophylactic antibiotics are ordered for open fractures.

Also, assess extremities for *compartment syndrome.* This occurs as pressure and swelling increase inside a section of an extremity (e.g., anterior compartment of lower leg) over several hours. This compromises the viability of the extremity muscles, nerves, and arteries. Potential causes of compartment syndrome include crush injuries, fractures, edema (e.g., burns), and hemorrhage.

I = Inspect Posterior Surfaces. The trauma patient should always be logrolled (while maintaining cervical spine immobilization) to inspect the patient's posterior surfaces and whenever movement is needed. This often requires three to four or more people with one person supporting the head. Inspect the back for ecchymosis, abrasions, puncture wounds, cuts, and obvious deformities. Palpate the entire spine for misalignment, deformity, and pain.

Intervention and Evaluation

Once the secondary survey is complete, record all findings. Provide tetanus prophylaxis based on vaccination history and the condition of any wounds[14] (Table 69-6).

Regardless of the patient's chief complaint, ongoing monitoring and evaluation of interventions are critical. You are responsible for providing appropriate interventions and assessing the patient's response. The evaluation of airway patency and the effectiveness of breathing will always be the highest priority. Monitor respiratory rate and rhythm, O_2 saturation, and ABGs (if ordered) to evaluate the patient's respiratory status. Also, closely monitor the level of consciousness; vital signs; quality of peripheral pulses; urine output; and skin temperature, color, and moisture for key information about circulation and perfusion.

Depending on the patient's injuries or illness, the patient may be (1) transported for diagnostic tests (e.g., CT scan) or to the operating room for immediate surgery; (2) admitted to an intensive care, telemetry, or general unit; or (3) transferred to another facility. You may go with critically ill patients on transports. You are responsible for monitoring the patient during

TABLE 69-6	**TETANUS VACCINES AND TIG FOR WOUND MANAGEMENT**	
	Type of Wound	
Vaccination History	**Clean, Minor Wounds**	**All Other Wounds**
Age 11–64 Yr*		
Unknown or <3 doses of tetanus toxoid–containing vaccine	Tdap and recommend catch-up vaccination	Tdap and recommend catch-up vaccination TIG
≥3 doses of tetanus toxoid–containing vaccine *and* <5 yr since last dose	No indication	No indication
≥3 doses of tetanus toxoid–containing vaccine *and* 5–10 yr since last dose	No indication	Tdap preferred (if not yet received) or Td
≥3 doses of tetanus toxoid–containing vaccine *and* >10 yr since last dose	Tdap preferred (if not yet received) or Td	Tdap preferred (if not yet received) or Td
Age ≥65 Yr		
Unknown or <3 doses of tetanus toxoid–containing vaccine	Td or Tdap and recommend catch-up vaccination. Tdap preferred if patient has close contact with children <12 mo of age	Td or Tdap and recommend catch-up vaccination. Tdap preferred if patient has close contact with children <12 mo of age TIG
≥3 doses of tetanus toxoid–containing vaccine *and* <5 yr since last dose	No indication	No indication
≥3 doses of tetanus toxoid–containing vaccine *and* 5–10 yr since last dose	No indication	Td or Tdap. Tdap preferred if patient has close contact with children <12 mo of age
≥3 doses of tetanus toxoid–containing vaccine *and* >10 yr since last dose	Tdap preferred (if not yet received) or Td	Td or Tdap. Tdap preferred if patient has close contact with children <12 mo of age

Source: Centers for Disease Control and Prevention: Disaster information: tetanus prevention after a disaster. Retrieved from *www.bt.cdc.gov/disasters/disease/tetanus.asp.*
*Pregnant women: As part of standard wound management care to prevent tetanus, a tetanus toxoid–containing vaccine might be recommended for wound management in a pregnant woman if ≥5 yr have elapsed since last receiving Td. If a tetanus booster is indicated for a pregnant woman who previously has not received Tdap, Tdap should be administered (at any gestational age).
Td, Tetanus-diphtheria toxoid absorbed; *Tdap,* tetanus toxoid, reduced diphtheria toxoid, and acellular pertussis vaccine; *TIG,* tetanus immune globulin (human).

transport, notifying the health care team should the patient's condition become unstable, and initiating basic and advanced life-support measures as needed.

Post–Cardiac Arrest Hypothermia

Many patients arrive at the ED in cardiac arrest. Patients with nontraumatic, out-of-hospital cardiac arrest benefit from a combination of good chest compressions and rapid defibrillation (see Appendix A), therapeutic hypothermia, and supportive care. Therapeutic hypothermia for 24 hours after the return of spontaneous circulation (ROSC) decreases mortality rates

EVIDENCE-BASED PRACTICE
Applying the Evidence

F.P. is a 76-yr-old woman admitted to the emergency department with new-onset atrial fibrillation with a rapid ventricular response (heart rate of 148 beats/min). She has mild shortness of breath and palpitations. As you administer a bolus dose of diltiazem (Cardizem) and prepare the continuous drip, she shares with you that she is concerned about her pets. F.P. lives alone and states that she "must go home" but will "return in the morning" to continue her treatment. She asks you to stop her medication and help her prepare to leave.

Best Available Evidence	**Clinician Expertise**	**Patient Preferences and Values**
Atrial fibrillation results in a decrease in cardiac output because of ineffective atrial contractions and/or a rapid ventricular response. Thrombi (clots) can form in the atria and may pass to the brain, causing cerebral embolic events.	You know that the goals of treatment for this patient include rate control, prevention of stroke, and conversion to sinus rhythm, if possible.	Patient's concerns for her pets are greater than her concerns for her current health situation.
Ventricular rate control (heart rate <100 beats/min) is a priority for patients with atrial fibrillation. If drugs or cardioversion do not convert atrial fibrillation to normal sinus rhythm, long-term anticoagulation therapy is needed.	F.P. is at risk for complications the longer her heart rate remains elevated and she delays treatment of her dysrhythmia.	

Your Decision and Action
You and F.P. fully explore options for the care of her pets. None are acceptable to F.P. You then explain the risk she is taking should she leave the emergency department. F.P. states she understands and will sign the papers needed to be able to leave. You inform the physician and prepare the leaving "Against Medical Advice" papers.

Reference for Evidence
Wann LS, Curtis AB, January CT, et al: 2011 ACCF/AHA/HRS focused update on the management of patients with atrial fibrillation (updating the 2006 guideline): a report of the American College of Cardiology Foundation/American Heart Association task force on practice guidelines, *J Am Coll Cardiol* 57:223, 2011.

and improves neurologic outcomes in many patients.[15] It is recommended for all patients who are comatose or who do not follow commands after ROSC.[16]

Therapeutic hypothermia involves three phases: induction, maintenance, and rewarming. The induction phase begins in the ED. The goal core temperature is 89.6° to 93.2°F (32° to 34°C). A variety of methods are used to cool patients. These include cold saline infusions and cooling devices (e.g., Arctic Sun). Patients require intubation and mechanical ventilation, invasive monitoring (e.g., arterial and central pressures), and continuous assessment during this therapy.[15] Protocols are used to direct the care of these patients. (Sample protocols and procedures are available at *www.med.upenn.edu/resuscitation/hypothermia/protocols.shtml.*)

Death in the Emergency Department

Unfortunately, a number of patients will not benefit from the skill, expertise, and technology available in the ED. It is important for you to deal with your feelings about sudden death so that you can help caregivers begin the grieving process (see Chapter 10).

Recognize the importance of certain hospital rituals to help caregivers grieve. These can include collecting the belongings, arranging for an autopsy (e.g., coroner's case), viewing the body, and making mortuary arrangements. The death must seem real so that the caregivers can begin to accept the death. You play a significant role in providing comfort to the surviving loved ones after a death in the ED. Whenever possible, provide an area for privacy and, if appropriate, arrange for a visit from a chaplain.[17]

Many patients who die in the ED could potentially be candidates for *non-heart-beating donation*. Certain tissues and organs (e.g., corneas, heart valves, skin, bone, kidneys) can be harvested from patients after death. Approaching caregivers about donation after an unexpected death is distressing to both the staff and caregivers. For many, however, the act of donation may be the first positive step in the grieving process. *Organ procurement organizations* (OPOs) assist in the process of screening potential donors, counseling donor families, obtaining informed consent, and harvesting organs from patients who are on life support or who die in the ED.[18]

GERONTOLOGIC CONSIDERATIONS

EMERGENCY CARE

The proportion of the population over age 65 is growing, with most leading active lives. Overall, people older than 65 account for 24% of all ED visits.[19] Regardless of a patient's age, aggressive interventions are warranted for all injuries or illnesses unless the patient has a preexisting terminal illness, an extremely low chance of survival, or an advance directive indicating a different course of action.

The older population is at high risk for injury because of many of the anatomic and physiologic changes that occur with aging (e.g., reduced visual acuity, limited neck rotation, slower gait, reduced reaction time). Of the injury-related admissions for people over 65 years old, most are for fractures, with many of these resulting from falls.[19] The most common causes of falls in older adults are generalized weakness, environmental hazards (e.g., loose mats, furniture), cardiovascular syncope (e.g., dysrhythmias), and orthostatic hypotension (e.g., side effect of medications, dehydration). When assessing a patient who has fallen, determine whether the physical findings may have caused the fall or may be due to the fall itself. For example, a patient may come to the ED with acute confusion. The confusion may be due to a myocardial infarction or stroke that caused the patient to fall, or the patient may have suffered a head injury as a result of a fall from tripping on a rug.

Understanding the physiologic and psychosocial aspects of aging will improve the care delivered to older adults in the ED (see Chapter 5). Unfortunately, many older adults dismiss symptoms as simply "normal for their age." It is important to fully investigate any complaint by an older adult.

ENVIRONMENTAL EMERGENCIES

Increased interest in outdoor activities such as running, cycling, skiing, and swimming has increased the number of environmental emergencies seen in the ED. Illness or injury may be caused by the activity, exposure to weather, or attack from various animals or humans. Specific environmental emer-

TABLE 69-7 RISK FACTORS FOR HEAT-RELATED EMERGENCIES

Age	Prescription Drugs
• Infants	• Anticholinergics
• Older adults	• Antihistamines
	• Antiparkinsonian drugs
Environmental Conditions	• Antispasmodics
• High environmental temperatures	• β-Adrenergic blockers
• High relative humidity	• Butyrophenones
	• Diuretics
	• Phenothiazines
Preexisting Illness	• Tricyclic antidepressants
• Cardiovascular disease	
• Cystic fibrosis	**Alcohol**
• Dehydration	
• Diabetes mellitus	**Street Drugs**
• Obesity	• Amphetamines
• Previous stroke or other central nervous system lesion	• Jimson weed
	• Lysergic acid diethylamide (LSD)
• Skin disorders (e.g., large burn scars)	• Phencyclidine (PCP)
	• 3,4-Methylenedioxymethamphetamine (MDMA, Ecstasy)

Adapted from Howard PK, Steinmann RA, editors: *Sheehy's emergency nursing,* ed 6, St Louis, 2010, Mosby.

gencies discussed in this section include heat-related emergencies, cold-related emergencies, submersion injuries, bites, and stings.

HEAT-RELATED EMERGENCIES

Brief exposure to intense heat or prolonged exposure to less intense heat leads to heat stress. This occurs when thermoregulatory mechanisms such as sweating, vasodilation, and increased respirations cannot compensate for exposure to increased ambient temperatures. Ambient temperature is a product of environmental temperature and humidity. Strenuous activities in hot or humid environments, clothing that interferes with perspiration, high fevers, and preexisting illnesses predispose individuals to heat stress (Table 69-7). Table 69-8 presents the management of heat-related emergencies.

Heat Cramps

Heat cramps are severe cramps in large muscle groups fatigued by heavy work. Cramps are brief and intense and tend to occur during rest after exercise or heavy labor. Nausea, tachycardia, pallor, weakness, and profuse diaphoresis are often present. The condition is seen most often in healthy, acclimated athletes with inadequate fluid intake. Cramps resolve rapidly with rest and oral or parenteral replacement of sodium and water. Elevation, gentle massage, and analgesia minimize pain associated with heat cramps. Instruct the patient to avoid strenuous activity for at least 12 hours. Discharge teaching should emphasize salt replacement during strenuous exercise in hot, humid environments. You can also recommend the use of commercially prepared electrolyte solutions (e.g., sports drinks).

Heat Exhaustion

Prolonged exposure to heat over hours or days leads to heat exhaustion. This is a clinical syndrome characterized by fatigue, nausea, vomiting, extreme thirst, and feelings of anxiety (see

TABLE 69-8 EMERGENCY MANAGEMENT

Hyperthermia

Etiology	Assessment Findings	Interventions
Environmental	**Heat Cramps**	**Initial**
• Lack of acclimatization	• Severe muscle contractions in exerted muscles	• Manage and maintain ABCs.
• Physical exertion, especially during hot weather	• Thirst	• Provide high-flow O₂ via non-rebreather mask or BVM.
• Prolonged exposure to extreme temperatures		• Establish IV access and begin fluid replacement for significant heat injury.
	Heat Exhaustion	• Place patient in a cool environment.
Trauma	• Pale, ashen skin	• For patient with heatstroke, initiate rapid cooling
• Head injury	• Fatigue, weakness	measures: remove patient's clothing, place wet
• Spinal cord injury	• Profuse sweating	sheets over patient, and place in front of fan;
	• Extreme thirst	immerse in a cool water bath; administer cool IV
Metabolic	• Altered mental status (e.g., anxiety)	fluids or lavage with cool fluids.
• Dehydration	• Hypotension	• Obtain 12-lead ECG.
• Diabetes	• Tachycardia	• Obtain blood for electrolytes and CBC.
• Thyrotoxicosis	• Weak, thready pulse	• Insert urinary catheter.
	• Temperature 99.6°-104° F (37.5°-40° C)	
Drugs		**Ongoing Monitoring**
• Amphetamines	**Heatstroke**	• Monitor ABCs, temperature and vital signs, level
• Antihistamines	• Hot, dry skin	of consciousness.
• β-Adrenergic blockers	• Altered mental status (e.g., ranging	• Monitor heart rhythm, O₂ saturation, and urine
• Diuretics	from confusion to coma)	output.
• Phenothiazines	• Hypotension	• Replace electrolytes as needed.
• Tricyclic antidepressants	• Tachycardia	• Monitor urine for development of myoglobinuria.
	• Weakness	• Monitor clotting studies for development of
Other	• Temperature >104° F (40° C)	disseminated intravascular coagulation.
• Alcohol		
• Cardiovascular disease		
• CNS disorders		

ABCs, Airway, breathing, circulation; *BVM,* bag-valve-mask.

Table 69-8). Hypotension, tachycardia, elevated body temperature, dilated pupils, mild confusion, ashen color, and profuse diaphoresis are also present. Hypotension and mild to severe temperature elevation (99.6° to 104° F [37.5° to 40° C]) are caused by dehydration.[20] Heat exhaustion usually occurs in individuals engaged in strenuous activity in hot, humid weather, but it also occurs in sedentary individuals.

Begin treatment by placing the patient in a cool area and removing constrictive clothing. Monitor the patient for ABCs, including cardiac dysrhythmias (caused by electrolyte imbalances). Initiate oral fluid and electrolyte replacement unless the patient is nauseated. Do not use salt tablets because of potential gastric irritation and hypernatremia. Initiate a 0.9% normal saline IV solution if oral solutions are not tolerated. An initial fluid bolus may be needed to correct hypotension. However, correlate fluid replacement to clinical and laboratory findings. Place a moist sheet over the patient to decrease core temperature through evaporative heat loss. Consider hospital admission for the older adult, the chronically ill, or those who do not improve within 3 to 4 hours.

Heatstroke

Heatstroke, the most serious form of heat stress, results from failure of the hypothalamic thermoregulatory processes. It is a medical emergency. Increased sweating, vasodilation, and increased respiratory rate (the body's attempt to lower temperature) deplete fluids and electrolytes, specifically sodium. Eventually, sweat glands stop functioning, and core temperature increases rapidly, within 10 to 15 minutes. The patient has a core temperature greater than 104° F (40° C), altered mentation, absence of perspiration, and circulatory collapse. The skin is hot, dry, and ashen. A range of neurologic symptoms occur

(e.g., hallucinations, loss of muscle coordination, combativeness) because the brain is extremely sensitive to thermal injuries. Cerebral edema and hemorrhage may occur as a result of direct thermal injury to the brain and decreased cerebral blood flow.

Death from heatstroke is directly related to the amount of time that the patient's body temperature remains elevated.[20] Prognosis is related to age, baseline health status, and length of exposure. Older adults and individuals with diabetes mellitus, chronic kidney disease, cardiovascular disease, pulmonary disease, or other physiologic compromise are particularly vulnerable.

Collaborative Care. Treatment of heatstroke focuses on stabilizing the patient's ABCs and rapidly reducing the core temperature. Administration of 100% O₂ compensates for the patient's hypermetabolic state. Ventilation with a BVM or intubation and mechanical ventilation may be required. Correct fluid and electrolyte imbalances and initiate continuous ECG monitoring for dysrhythmias.

Various cooling methods are available, such as removing clothing, covering with wet sheets, and placing the patient in front of a large fan (evaporative cooling), immersing the patient in a cool water bath (conductive cooling), and administering cool fluids or lavaging with cool fluids.[20] Whatever method is selected, closely monitor the patient's temperature and control shivering. Shivering increases core temperature (because of the associated heat generated by muscle activity) and complicates cooling efforts. Chlorpromazine (Thorazine) IV is the drug of choice to control shivering. Aggressive temperature reduction should continue until core temperature reaches 102° F (38.9° C).[20] Antipyretics are not effective in this situation because the elevated temperature is not related to infection.

Monitor the patient for signs of *rhabdomyolysis* (a serious syndrome caused by the breakdown of skeletal muscle). The muscle breakdown leads to myoglobinuria, which places the kidneys at risk for acute kidney injury. Carefully monitor the urine for color (e.g., tea colored), amount, pH, and myoglobin. Finally, obtain clotting studies to monitor the patient for signs of disseminated intravascular coagulation (see Chapter 31).

Patient and caregiver teaching focuses on how to avoid future problems. Provide essential information regarding proper hydration during hot weather and physical exercise. Instruct patients on the early signs of and interventions for heat-related stress.

COLD-RELATED EMERGENCIES

Cold injuries may be localized (frostbite) or systemic (hypothermia). Contributing factors include age, duration of exposure, environmental temperature, homelessness, preexisting conditions (e.g., diabetes mellitus, peripheral vascular disease), medications that suppress shivering (e.g., opioids, psychotropic agents, antiemetics), and alcohol intoxication. Alcohol causes peripheral vasodilation, increases sensation of warmth, and depresses shivering. Smokers have an increased risk of cold-related injury because of the vasoconstrictive effects of nicotine.

Frostbite

Frostbite is true tissue freezing that results in the formation of ice crystals in the tissues and cells. Peripheral vasoconstriction is the initial response to cold stress and results in a decrease in blood flow and vascular stasis. As cellular temperature decreases and ice crystals form in intracellular spaces, the organelles are damaged and the cell membrane destroyed. This results in edema. Depth of frostbite depends on ambient temperature, length of exposure, type and condition (wet or dry) of clothing, and contact with metal surfaces. Other factors that affect severity include skin color (dark-skinned people are more prone to frostbite), lack of acclimatization, previous episodes, exhaustion, and poor peripheral vascular status.

Superficial frostbite involves skin and subcutaneous tissue, usually the ears, nose, fingers, and toes. The skin appearance ranges from waxy pale yellow to blue to mottled, and the skin feels crunchy and frozen. The patient may complain of tingling, numbness, or a burning sensation. Handle the area carefully and never squeeze, massage, or scrub the injured tissue because it is easily damaged. Remove clothing and jewelry because they may constrict the extremity and decrease circulation. Immerse the affected area in a water bath (98.6° to 104° F) [37° to 40° C]).[20] Use warm soaks for the face. The patient often experiences a warm, stinging sensation as tissue thaws. Blisters form within a few hours (Fig. 69-2). The blisters should be debrided and a sterile dressing applied. Avoid heavy blankets and clothing because friction and weight can lead to sloughing of damaged tissue. Rewarming is extremely painful. Residual pain may last weeks or even years. Administer analgesia and tetanus prophylaxis as appropriate (see Table 69-6). Evaluate the patient with superficial frostbite for systemic hypothermia.

Deep frostbite involves muscle, bone, and tendon. The skin is white, hard, and insensitive to touch. The area has the appearance of deep thermal injury with mottling gradually progressing to gangrene (Fig. 69-3). The affected extremity is immersed in

FIG. 69-2 Edema and blister formation 24 hours after frostbite injury occurring in an area covered by a tightly fitted boot.

FIG. 69-3 Gangrenous necrosis 6 weeks after the frostbite injury shown in Fig. 69-2.

a circulating water bath (98.6° to 104° F) [37° to 40° C]) until flushing occurs distal to the injured area.[20] After rewarming, the extremity should be elevated to reduce edema. Significant edema may begin within 3 hours, with blistering in 6 hours to days. IV analgesia is required in severe frostbite because of the pain associated with tissue thawing. Provide tetanus prophylaxis and evaluate the patient for systemic hypothermia. Amputation may be required if the injured area is untreated or treatment is unsuccessful. The patient may be admitted to the hospital for observation with bed rest, elevation of the injured part, and prophylactic antibiotics if the wound is at risk for infection.

Hypothermia

Hypothermia, defined as a core temperature below 95° F (35° C), occurs when heat produced by the body cannot compensate for heat lost to the environment.[20] Most body heat is lost as radiant energy, with the greatest loss from the head, thorax, and lungs (with each breath). Wet clothing increases evaporative heat loss to five times greater than normal; immersion in cold water (e.g., near drowning) increases evaporative heat loss to 25 times greater than normal. Environmental exposure to freezing temperatures, cold winds, and wet terrain plus physical exhaustion, inadequate clothing, and inexperience predisposes individuals to hypothermia. Older adults are more prone to hypothermia because of decreased body fat, dimin-

✚ TABLE 69-9 EMERGENCY MANAGEMENT

Hypothermia

Etiology	Assessment Findings	Interventions

Environmental
• Inadequate clothing for environmental temperature
• Prolonged exposure to cold
• Prolonged immersion or near-drowning
 	
Metabolic
• Hypoglycemia
• Hypothyroidism
 	
Health Care Associated
• Administration of neuromuscular blocking agents
• Blood administration
• Cold IV fluids
• Inadequate warming or rewarming in the ED or operating room
 	
Other
• Alcohol
• Barbiturates
• Phenothiazines
• Shock
• Trauma
	• Core body temperature:
	  • *Mild hypothermia:* 93.2°–96.8°F (34°–36°C)
	  • *Moderate hypothermia:* 86°–93.2°F (30°–34°C)
	  • *Severe hypothermia:* ≤86°F (≤30°C)
	• Shivering, diminished or absent at core body temperatures ≤86°F (30°C)
	• Hypoventilation
	• Hypotension
	• Altered mental status (ranging from confusion to coma)
	• Areflexia (absence of reflexes)
	• Pale, cyanotic skin
	• Blue, white, or frozen extremities
	• Dysrhythmias: bradycardia, atrial fibrillation, ventricular fibrillation, asystole
	• Fixed, dilated pupils
		Initial
		• Remove patient from cold environment.
		• Manage and maintain ABCs.
		• Provide high-flow O₂ via non-rebreather mask or BVM.
		• Anticipate intubation for diminished or absent gag reflex.*
		• Establish IV access with two large-bore catheters for fluid resuscitation
		• Rewarm patient:
		  • *Passive:* Remove wet clothing, apply dry clothing and warm blankets, use radiant lights.
		  • *Active external:* Apply heating devices (e.g., air or fluid-filled warming blankets), use warm water immersion.
		  • *Active internal:* Provide warmed IV fluids; heated, humidified O₂. Peritoneal lavage with warmed fluids. Extracorporeal circulation (e.g., cardiopulmonary bypass, rapid fluid infuser, hemodialysis).
		• Obtain 12-lead ECG.
		• Anticipate need for defibrillation.*
		• Warm central trunk first in patients with severe hypothermia to limit rewarming shock.
		• Assess for other injuries.
		• Keep patient's head covered with warm, dry towels or stocking cap to limit loss of heat.
		• Treat patient gently to avoid increased cardiac irritability.
		
		Ongoing Monitoring
		• Monitor ABCs, temperature, level of consciousness, vital signs.
		• Monitor O₂ saturation, heart rate and rhythm.
		• Monitor electrolytes, glucose.

*NOTE: Medications and defibrillation may not be effective with core temperatures <86°F (30°C).
ABCs, Airway, breathing, circulation; *BVM,* bag-valve-mask.

ished energy reserves, decreased basal metabolic rate, decreased shivering response, decreased sensory perception, chronic medical conditions, and medications that alter body defenses.

Hypothermia mimics cerebral or metabolic disturbances causing ataxia, confusion, and withdrawal, so the patient may be misdiagnosed. Peripheral vasoconstriction is the body's first attempt to conserve heat. As cold temperatures persist, shivering and movement are the body's only mechanisms for producing heat.

Assessment findings in hypothermia are variable and depend on core temperature (Table 69-9). Patients with *mild hypothermia* (93.2° to 96.8°F [34° to 36°C]) have shivering, lethargy, confusion, rational to irrational behavior, and minor heart rate changes. *Moderate hypothermia* (86° to 93.2°F [30° to 34°C]) causes rigidity, bradycardia, slowed respiratory rate, BP obtainable only by Doppler, metabolic and respiratory acidosis, and hypovolemia. Shivering diminishes or disappears at core temperatures of 86°F (30°C).[19]

As core temperature drops, basal metabolic rate decreases two or three times. The cold myocardium is extremely irritable, making it vulnerable to dysrhythmias (e.g., atrial and ventricular fibrillation). Decreased renal blood flow decreases glomerular filtration rate, which impairs water reabsorption and leads to dehydration. The hematocrit increases as intravascular volume decreases. Cold blood becomes thick and acts as a thrombus, placing the patient at risk for stroke, myocardial infarction, pulmonary emboli, and renal failure. Decreased blood flow leads to hypoxia, anaerobic metabolism, lactic acid accumulation, and metabolic acidosis.

Severe hypothermia (at or below 86°F [30°C]) makes the person appear dead and is a potentially life-threatening situation. Metabolic rate, heart rate, and respirations are so slow that they may be difficult to detect. Reflexes are absent, and the pupils fixed and dilated. Profound bradycardia, ventricular fibrillation, or asystole may be present. Every effort is made to warm the patient to at least 86°F (30°C) before the person is pronounced dead.[20] The cause of death is usually refractory ventricular fibrillation.

Collaborative Care. Treatment of hypothermia focuses on managing and maintaining ABCs, rewarming the patient, correcting dehydration and acidosis, and treating cardiac dysrhythmias (see Table 69-9). Use passive or active external rewarming for mild hypothermia. *Passive* or *spontaneous rewarming* involves moving the patient to a warm, dry place; removing damp clothing; using radiant lights; and placing warm blankets on the patient. *Active external* or *surface rewarming* involves fluid- or air-filled warming blankets, or warm (98.6° to 104°F [37° to 40°C]) water immersion.[20] Closely monitor the patient for marked vasodilation and hypotension during rewarming.

Use *active internal* or *core rewarming* for moderate to severe hypothermia. This refers to the application of heat directly to the core. Techniques include (1) heated (up to 111.2°F [44°C]), humidified O₂; (2) warmed IV fluids (up to 98.6°F [37°C]); (3) peritoneal lavage with warmed fluids (up to 113°F [45°C]); and (4) extracorporeal circulation with cardiopulmonary bypass, rapid fluid infuser, or hemodialysis.[20]

Gentle handling is essential to prevent stimulation of the cold myocardium. Carefully monitor core temperature during rewarming procedures. Rewarming places the patient at risk for *afterdrop,* a further drop in core temperature. This occurs when cold peripheral blood returns to the central circulation. Rewarming shock can produce hypotension and dysrhythmias. Thus patients with moderate to severe hypothermia should have the core warmed before the extremities. Discontinue active rewarming once the core temperature reaches 89.6° to 93.2° F (32° to 34° C).[19]

Patient teaching focuses on how to avoid future cold-related problems. Essential information includes dressing in layers for cold weather, covering the head, carrying high-carbohydrate foods for extra calories, and developing a plan for survival should an injury occur.

SUBMERSION INJURIES

Submersion injury results when an individual becomes hypoxic as the result of submersion in a substance, usually water. More than 50,000 submersion events and approximately 4000 deaths from drowning occur each year in the United States. Most of the victims are children younger than 5 years of age or boys and men between ages 15 and 25. The primary risk factors for submersion injury include inability to swim, use of alcohol or drugs, trauma, seizures, hypothermia, stroke, and child neglect.

Drowning is death from suffocation after submersion in water or other fluid. *Near-drowning* is survival from a potential drowning. *Immersion syndrome* occurs with immersion in cold water. This leads to stimulation of the vagus nerve and potentially fatal dysrhythmias (e.g., bradycardia, cardiac arrest).

Some near-drowning victims do not aspirate water (i.e., *dry drowning*) but do develop potentially life-threatening bronchospasm and airway obstruction. Near-drowning victims who do aspirate water develop pulmonary edema. Regardless of what type of fluid is aspirated, the end result is acute respiratory distress syndrome[20] (see Chapter 68). The osmotic gradient caused by aspirated fluid leads to fluid imbalances in the body. Hypotonic freshwater is rapidly absorbed into the circulatory system through the alveoli. Freshwater is often contaminated with chlorine, mud, or algae. This causes the breakdown of lung surfactant, fluid seepage, and pulmonary edema. Hypertonic saltwater draws fluid from the vascular space into the alveoli, impairing alveolar ventilation and resulting in hypoxia. Fig. 69-4 shows the pulmonary effects of saltwater and freshwater aspiration. The body attempts to compensate for hypoxia by shunting blood to the lungs. This results in increased pulmonary pressures and deteriorating respiratory status. More and more blood is shunted through the alveoli. However, the blood is not adequately oxygenated, and hypoxemia worsens. This can result in cerebral injury, edema, and brain death.

Table 69-10 lists the assessment findings of a patient with a submersion injury. Aggressive resuscitation efforts (e.g., airway and ventilation management), especially in the prehospital phase, improve survival of near-drowning victims.[20]

Collaborative Care

Treatment of submersion injuries focuses on correcting hypoxia and fluid imbalances, supporting basic physiologic functions, and rewarming when hypothermia is present. Initial evaluation involves assessment of airway, cervical spine, breathing, and circulation. Table 69-10 lists other interventions.

FIG. 69-4 Pathophysiology of submersion injury.

Mechanical ventilation with positive end-expiratory pressure or continuous positive airway pressure is used to improve gas exchange across the alveolar-capillary membrane when significant pulmonary edema is present. Ventilation and oxygenation are the primary techniques for treating respiratory failure (see Chapters 66 and 68). Mannitol (Osmitrol) or furosemide (Lasix) is used to treat cerebral edema or decrease free water.

Deterioration in neurologic status suggests cerebral edema, worsening hypoxia, or profound acidosis. Near-drowning victims may also have head and neck injuries that cause prolonged alterations in the level of consciousness. Complications can develop in patients who are essentially free of symptoms immediately after the near-drowning episode. This *secondary drowning* refers to delayed death from drowning due to pulmonary complications. Consequently, observe all victims of near-drowning in a hospital for a minimum of 23 hours.[20] Additional observation is needed for patients who have co-morbidities (e.g., heart disease).

Patient teaching focuses on water safety and how to minimize the risks for drowning. Remind patients and caregivers to lock all swimming pool gates; use life jackets on all watercrafts, including inner tubes and rafts; and learn water survival skills (e.g., swimming lessons). Emphasize the dangers of combining alcohol and drugs with swimming and other water sports.

STINGS AND BITES

Animals, spiders, snakes, and insects cause injury and even death by biting or stinging. Morbidity is a result of either direct tissue damage or lethal toxins. Direct tissue damage is a product of animal size, characteristics of the animal's teeth, and strength of the jaw. Tissue is lacerated, crushed, or chewed, while teeth, fangs, stingers, spines, or tentacles release toxins that have local

✚ TABLE 69-10 EMERGENCY MANAGEMENT
Submersion Injuries

Etiology	Assessment Findings	Interventions
• Inability to swim or exhaustion while swimming • Entrapment or entanglement with objects in water • Loss of ability to move secondary to trauma, stroke, hypothermia, myocardial infarction (MI) • Poor judgment due to alcohol or drugs • Seizure while in water	**Pulmonary** • Ineffective breathing • Dyspnea • Respiratory distress • Respiratory arrest • Crackles, rhonchi • Cough with pink-frothy sputum • Cyanosis **Cardiac** • Tachycardia • Bradycardia • Dysrhythmia • Hypotension • Cardiac arrest **Other** • Panic • Exhaustion • Coma • Coexisting illness (e.g., MI) or injury (e.g., cervical spine injury) • Core temperature slightly elevated or below normal depending on water temperature and length of submersion	**Initial** • Manage and maintain ABCs. • Assume cervical spine injury in all near-drowning victims and stabilize or immobilize cervical spine. • Provide 100% O_2 via non-rebreather mask or BVM. • Anticipate need for intubation and mechanical ventilation if airway is compromised (e.g., absent gag reflex). • Establish IV access with two large-bore catheters for fluid resuscitation and infuse warmed fluids if appropriate. • Obtain 12-lead ECG. • Assess for other injuries. • Remove wet clothing and cover with warm blankets. • Obtain temperature and begin rewarming if needed. • Obtain cervical spine and chest x-rays. • Insert gastric tube and urinary catheter. **Ongoing Monitoring** • Monitor ABCs, vital signs, level of consciousness. • Monitor O_2 saturation, heart rate and rhythm. • Monitor temperature and maintain normothermia. • Monitor for signs of acute respiratory failure. • Monitor for signs of secondary drowning.

ABCs, Airway, breathing, circulation; *BVM*, bag-valve-mask.

or systemic effects. Death associated with animal bites is due to blood loss, allergic reactions, or lethal toxins. Injuries caused by select insects, ticks, animals (e.g., dogs, cats), and humans are described here.

Hymenopteran Stings

The *Hymenoptera* family includes bees, yellow jackets, hornets, wasps, and fire ants. Stings can cause mild discomfort or life-threatening anaphylaxis (see Chapter 67). Venom may be cytotoxic, hemolytic, allergenic, or vasoactive. Symptoms may begin immediately or be delayed up to 48 hours. Reactions are more severe with multiple stings.[20] Most hymenopterans sting repeatedly. However, the domestic honey bee stings only once, usually leaving a barbed stinger with an attached venom sac in the skin so that release of venom continues. African honey bees (killer bees), which look like domestic bees, have migrated into North America. If threatened, these bees aggressively swarm and can repeatedly sting their victims (e.g., humans, animals). These attacks can be fatal.

> **SAFETY ALERT: Hymenopteran Stings**
> • Remove the stinger using a scraping motion with a fingernail, knife, or needle.
> • Avoid using tweezers because they may squeeze the stinger and release more venom.
> • Remove rings, watches, or any restrictive clothing around the sting site.

Symptoms vary from stinging, burning, swelling, and itching to edema, headache, fever, syncope, malaise, nausea, vomiting, wheezing, bronchospasm, laryngeal edema, and hypotension. Treatment depends on the severity of the reaction. Treat mild reactions with elevation, cool compresses, antipruritic lotions, and oral antihistamines. More severe reactions require intramuscular or IV antihistamines (e.g., diphenhydramine [Bena-

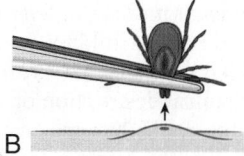

FIG. 69-5 Tick removal. **A,** Use tweezers to grasp the tick close to the skin. **B,** With a steady motion, pull the tick's body up and away from the skin. Do not be alarmed if the tick's mouthparts remain in the skin. Once the mouthparts are removed from the rest of the tick, it can no longer transmit disease.

dryl]), subcutaneous epinephrine, and corticosteroids (e.g., dexamethasone [Decadron]). Chapter 14 discusses allergic reactions and related patient teaching.

Tick Bites

Ticks live throughout the United States, but are most common in the northwestern, Rocky Mountain, and northeastern regions. Emergencies associated with tick bites include Lyme disease, Rocky Mountain spotted fever, and tick paralysis. The infected tick or the release of neurotoxin causes the disease. Ticks release neurotoxic venom as long as the tick head attaches to the body. Therefore safe removal of the tick is essential for effective treatment. Use forceps or tweezers to grasp the tick close to the point of attachment and pull upward in a steady motion (Fig. 69-5). After you remove the tick, clean the skin with soap and water. Do not use a hot match, petroleum jelly, nail polish, or other products to remove the tick, since these measures may cause a tick to salivate, thus increasing the risk for infection.[21]

Lyme disease is the most common tick-borne disease in the United States. Symptoms appear within days of a bite from the *Ixodid* (hard) tick and result from exposure to the spirochete *Borrelia burgdorferi* that lives on the tick. The initial stage of this disease is characterized by flu-like symptoms (e.g., headache, stiff neck, fatigue) and, in some patients, a characteristic bull's eye rash (i.e., an expanding circular area of redness 5 cm or more in diameter). Treatment at this stage includes doxycycline (Vibramycin). The rash will disappear even if the patient is not treated.

Monoarticular arthritis, meningitis, and neuropathies occur days or weeks after the initial symptoms. Recommended treatment includes ceftriaxone (Rocephin).[20] Chronic arthritis, peripheral radiculoneuropathy, and heart disease characterize the later stage of the disease. These illnesses can last several months to years after the initial skin lesion. (Chapter 65 discusses Lyme disease.)

Rocky Mountain spotted fever is caused by *Rickettsia rickettsii*, a bacterium that is spread to humans by the *Ixodid* tick. It has an incubation period of 2 to 14 days. A pink, macular rash appears on the palms, wrists, soles, feet, and ankles within 10 days of exposure. Other symptoms include fever, chills, malaise, myalgias, and headache. Diagnosis is often difficult in the early stages, and without treatment the disease can be fatal.[20] Antibiotic therapy with doxycycline is the treatment of choice.

Tick paralysis occurs 5 to 7 days after exposure to a neurotoxin introduced by a wood tick or dog tick. Classic symptoms are flaccid ascending paralysis, which develops over 1 to 2 days. Without tick removal, the patient dies as respiratory muscles become paralyzed. Tick removal leads to return of muscle movement, usually within 48 to 72 hours.[20]

Animal and Human Bites

Every year more than 5 million animal bites are reported in the United States. Children are at greatest risk. The most significant problems associated with animal bites are infection and mechanical destruction of skin, muscle, tendons, blood vessels, and bone. The bite may cause a simple laceration or be associated with crush injury, puncture wound, or tearing of multiple layers of tissue. The severity of injury depends on animal size, victim size, and anatomic location of the bite. Animal bites from dogs and cats are most common, with wild or domestic rodents (e.g., squirrels, hamsters) following as the third most frequently reported offenders.

Dog bites usually occur on the extremities. However, facial bites are common in small children. Most victims own the dogs that bite them. Dog bites may involve significant tissue damage with deaths reported, usually in children. A plastic surgeon should evaluate all disfiguring wounds of the face.

Cat bites cause deep puncture wounds that can involve tendons and joint capsules and result in a greater incidence of infection than with dog bites. Septic arthritis, osteomyelitis, and tenosynovitis can occur as a result of cat bites. The most common causative organisms of infections from dog and cat bites are from the *Pasteurella* species (e.g., *P. multocida*). Most healthy cats and dogs carry this organism in their mouths.

Human bites also cause puncture wounds or lacerations (Fig. 69-6). These carry a high risk of infection from oral bacterial flora, most commonly *Staphylococcus aureus*, *Streptococcus* organisms, and hepatitis virus. Hands, fingers, ears, nose, vagina, and penis are the most common sites of human bites and are frequently a result of violence or sexual activity. Patients with Boxer's fracture (fracture of the fourth or fifth metacarpal) often have concurrent open wounds on the knuckles from striking teeth. The human jaw has great crushing ability, causing laceration, puncture, crush injury, soft tissue tearing, and even

FIG. 69-6 Probable human bite injury, though denied by patient. Human bites cause extensor tendon injuries, fractures, and joint capsule injuries and can harbor foreign bodies.

amputation. Infection rates are as high as 50% when victims do not seek medical care within 24 hours of injury.

Collaborative Care. Initial treatment for animal and human bites includes cleaning with copious irrigation, debridement, tetanus prophylaxis, and analgesics as needed. Prophylactic antibiotics are used for animal and human bites at risk for infection, such as wounds over joints, those greater than 6 to 12 hours old, puncture wounds, and bites of the hand or foot. Individuals at greatest risk of infection are infants, older adults, immunosuppressed patients, alcoholics, diabetics, and people taking corticosteroids.

Leave puncture wounds open. Splint wounds over joints. Lacerations are loosely sutured. However, initial closure is used for facial wounds. The patient is admitted for IV antibiotic therapy when an infection is present. These patients have an increased incidence of cellulitis, osteomyelitis, and septic arthritis. Report animal and human bites to the police as required.

Consideration of rabies postexposure prophylaxis is an essential component in management of animal bites. A neurotoxic virus found in the saliva of some mammals causes rabies. If untreated, the condition is fatal in humans. Consider rabies exposure if an animal attack was not provoked, involves a wild animal, or involves a domestic animal not immunized against rabies. Always provide rabies postexposure prophylaxis when the animal is not found or a carnivorous wild animal causes the bite. Start the regimen with an initial, weight-based dosage of rabies immune globulin (RIG [HyperRab S/D]) to provide passive immunity. Follow this with a series of five injections of human diploid cell vaccine (HDCV [Imovax Rabies]) on days 0, 3, 7, 14, and 28 to provide active immunity.[22] (Rabies is discussed in Chapter 57.)

DRUG ALERT: Rabies Postexposure Prophylaxis
- Administer the calculated dose of RIG via infiltration around the wound edges.
- Administer any remaining volume of RIG intramuscularly at a site distant from the vaccine site (e.g., gluteal site for bite wounds on the arm).
- Administer the HDCV intramuscularly in the deltoid.

POISONINGS

A poison is any chemical that harms the body. More than 5 million cases of human poisonings occur each year in the United States.[23] Poisonings can be accidental, occupational, recreational, or intentional. Natural or manufactured toxins can be ingested, inhaled, injected, splashed in the eye, or absorbed through the skin. Table 69-11 presents common poisons.

TABLE 69-11   COMMON POISONS

Poison	Manifestations	Treatment
Acetaminophen (Tylenol)	*Phase 1* (within 24 hr of ingestion): Malaise, diaphoresis, nausea and vomiting *Phase 2* (24-28 hr after ingestion): Right upper quadrant pain, decreased urine output, diminished nausea, increase in LFTs *Phase 3* (72-96 hr after ingestion): Nausea and vomiting, malaise, jaundice, hypoglycemia, enlarged liver, possible coagulopathies, including DIC *Phase 4* (7-8 days after ingestion): Recovery, resolution of symptoms, LFTs return to normal	Activated charcoal, *N*-acetylcysteine (oral form may cause vomiting, IV form can be used)
Acids and alkalis • *Acids:* Toilet bowl cleaners, antirust compounds • *Alkalis:* Drain cleaners, dishwashing detergents, ammonia	Excess salivation, dysphagia, epigastric pain, pneumonitis; burns of mouth, esophagus, and stomach	Immediate dilution (water, milk), corticosteroids (for alkali burns), induced vomiting is contraindicated
• Aspirin and aspirin-containing medications	Tachypnea, tachycardia, hyperthermia, seizures, pulmonary edema, occult bleeding or hemorrhage, metabolic acidosis	Activated charcoal, gastric lavage, urine alkalinization, hemodialysis for severe acute ingestion, intubation and mechanical ventilation, supportive care
Bleaches	Irritation of lips, mouth, and eyes, superficial injury to esophagus; chemical pneumonia and pulmonary edema	Washing of exposed skin and eyes, dilution with water and milk, gastric lavage, prevention of vomiting and aspiration
Carbon monoxide	Dyspnea, headache, tachypnea, confusion, impaired judgment, cyanosis, respiratory depression	Removal from source, administration of 100% O_2 via non-rebreather mask, BVM, or intubation and mechanical ventilation; consider hyperbaric O_2 therapy
Cyanide	Almond odor to breath, headache, dizziness, nausea, confusion, hypertension, bradycardia followed by hypotension and tachycardia, tachypnea followed by bradypnea and respiratory arrest	Amyl nitrate (nasally), IV sodium nitrate, IV sodium thiosulfate, supportive care
Ethylene glycol	Sweet aromatic odor to breath, nausea and vomiting, slurred speech, ataxia, lethargy, respiratory depression	Activated charcoal, gastric lavage, supportive care
Iron	Vomiting (often bloody), diarrhea (often bloody), fever, hyperglycemia, lethargy, hypotension, seizures, coma	Gastric lavage, chelation therapy (deferoxamine [Desferal])
Nonsteroidal antiinflammatory drugs	Gastroenteritis, abdominal pain, drowsiness, nystagmus, hepatic and renal damage	Activated charcoal, gastric lavage, supportive care
Tricyclic antidepressants (e.g., amitriptyline [Elavil])	*In low doses:* Anticholinergic effects, agitation, hypertension, tachycardia *In high doses:* Central nervous system depression, dysrhythmias, hypotension, respiratory depression	Multidose activated charcoal, gastric lavage, serum alkalinization with sodium bicarbonate, intubation and mechanical ventilation, supportive care; never induce vomiting
Alcohol, barbiturates, benzodiazepines, cocaine, hallucinogens, stimulants	See Chapter 11	See Chapter 11

BVM, Bag-valve-mask; *DIC,* disseminated intravascular coagulation; *LFTs,* liver function tests.

Chapter 11 discusses other poisonings related to the use of illegal drugs such as amphetamines, opioids, and hallucinogens. Poisoning may also be due to toxic plants or contaminated foods. (Chapter 42 discusses food poisoning.)

Severity of the poisoning depends on type, concentration, and route of exposure. Toxins can affect every tissue of the body, so symptoms can be seen in any body system. Specific management of toxins involves decreasing absorption, enhancing elimination, and implementing toxin-specific interventions. Consult the local poison control center 24 hours a day for the most current treatment protocols for specific poisons.[24]

Options for decreasing absorption of poisons include activated charcoal, dermal cleansing, eye irrigation, and, less frequently, gastric lavage. Gastric lavage involves oral insertion of a large-diameter (36F to 42F) gastric tube for irrigation of copious amounts of saline. Elevate the head of the bed or place the patient on the side to prevent aspiration. Patients with an altered level of consciousness or diminished gag reflex are intubated before lavage. Patients who ingest caustic agents, co-ingest sharp objects, or ingest nontoxic substances should not receive lavage. Perform gastric lavage within 1 hour of ingestion of most poisons to be effective.[23] Problems associated with lavage include esophageal perforation and aspiration.

The most common and effective intervention for management of poisonings is administration of activated charcoal orally or via a gastric tube within 1 hour of poison ingestion.[23] Many toxins adhere to charcoal and pass through the gastrointestinal (GI) tract rather than being absorbed into the circulation. Activated charcoal does not absorb ethanol, hydrocarbons, alkali, iron, boric acid, lithium, methanol, or cyanide. Adults receive 50 to 100 g of charcoal. For some toxins (e.g., phenobarbital, digoxin) multiple-dose charcoal may be required.[25] Contraindications to charcoal administration include diminished bowel sounds, ileus, and ingestion of a substance poorly absorbed by charcoal. Charcoal can absorb and neutralize antidotes (e.g., *N*-acetylcysteine [Mucomyst] for acetaminophen toxicity). Do not give these immediately before, with, or shortly after charcoal.[25]

Skin and ocular decontamination involves removal of toxins from skin and eyes using copious amounts of water or saline.[26] Most toxins, with the exception of mustard gas, can be safely removed with water or saline. Water mixes with mustard gas and releases chlorine gas. As a rule, brush dry substances from the skin and clothing before using water. Do not remove powdered lime with water. It should just be brushed off. Wear personal protective equipment (e.g., gloves, gowns, goggles, respirators) for decontamination to prevent secondary exposure. Decontamination procedures are usually done by those specially trained in hazardous material decontamination before the patient arrives at the hospital and again at the hospital, if necessary. Decontamination takes priority over all interventions except those needed for basic life support.

The administration of cathartics, whole-bowel irrigation, hemodialysis, urine alkalinization, chelating agents, and antidotes increases the elimination of poisons. Cathartics, such as sorbitol, are given together with the first dose of activated charcoal to stimulate intestinal motility and increase elimination.[23] Avoid multiple doses of cathartics because of potentially fatal electrolyte abnormalities. Whole-bowel irrigation is controversial and involves administration of a nonabsorbable bowel evacuant solution (e.g., GoLYTELY). Administer the solution every 4 to 6 hours until stools are clear. This process can be effective for swallowed objects, such as cocaine-filled balloons or condoms, and heavy metals such as lead and mercury.[25] There is a high risk of electrolyte imbalance caused by fluid and electrolyte losses with this approach.

Hemodialysis is reserved for patients who develop severe acidosis from ingestion of toxic substances (e.g., aspirin). Other interventions include alkalinization and chelation therapy. Sodium bicarbonate administration raises the pH (greater than 7.5), which is particularly effective for phenobarbital and salicylate poisoning. Vitamin C is added to IV fluids to enhance excretion of amphetamines and quinidine. Chelation therapy is considered for heavy metal poisoning (e.g., edetate calcium disodium [calcium EDTA] for lead poisoning). A limited number of true antidotes are available, and many of these agents are themselves toxic.[25]

Focus patient teaching for toxic emergencies on how the poisoning occurred. Arrange for an evaluation and follow-up by a mental health professional for all patients who experience poisoning because of a suicide attempt or substance abuse. The Occupational Safety and Health Administration should evaluate all poisoning related to an occupational hazard.[27]

VIOLENCE

Violence is the acting out of the emotions of fear and/or anger to cause harm to someone or something. It may be the result of organic disease (e.g., temporal lobe epilepsy), psychosis (e.g., schizophrenia), or antisocial behavior (e.g., assault, murder). The patient cared for in the ED may be the victim or the perpetrator of violence. Violence can take place in a variety of settings, including the home, community, and workplace. EDs have been identified as high-risk areas for *workplace violence*.[28] Measures to protect staff include the use of on-site security personnel and police officers, metal detectors, surveillance cameras, and locked access doors. The ENA supports comprehensive workplace violence prevention plans and recommends that they be implemented and evaluated in every ED.[28]

Family and intimate partner violence (IPV) is a pattern of coercive behavior in a relationship that involves fear; humiliation; intimidation; neglect; or intentional physical, emotional, financial, or sexual injury (see Chapter 54 for information on sexual assault). The ENA encourages ED nurses to become certified *sexual assault nurse examiners* (SANEs). The SANE nurse provides expert emergency care, collects and documents evidence, participates in staff and community education, and advocates for sexual assault and rape victims.[29]

IPV is found in all professions, cultures, socioeconomic groups, age-groups, and genders. Although men can be victims of family violence and IPV, most victims are women, children, and older adults. Each year, more than 5 million women and 3 million men are treated in EDs for *battery* (assault) by spouses, caregivers, or individuals known to them. As many as 20% of battered women are pregnant at the time of the assault.[29]

In the ED, you need to screen for family violence and IPV (e.g., Do you feel safe at home? Is anyone hurting you?). Routine screening for this risk factor is required.[29] Barriers to conducting effective screening include limited privacy in the ED, lack of time, and lack of knowledge about how to ask about family violence and IPV. The development and implementation of policies, procedures, and staff education programs do improve screening practices.[28]

Initiate appropriate interventions for patients who you suspect or find are victims of abuse. These include making referrals, providing emotional support, and informing victims about their options (e.g., safe house, legal rights).[30] See Resources at the end of this chapter for additional information on family violence and IPV.

AGENTS OF TERRORISM

The threat of terrorism is an ongoing concern. Terrorism involves overt actions such as the dispensing of nuclear, biologic, or chemical (NBC) agents as weapons for the express purpose of causing harm. Prompt recognition and identification of potential health hazards are essential in the preparedness of health care professionals.

Biologic agents most commonly used in terrorist attacks include anthrax, smallpox, botulism, plague, tularemia, and hemorrhagic fever. eTable 69-2 (available on the website for this chapter) summarizes general information regarding select biologic agents of terrorism. Anthrax, plague, and tularemia are treated effectively with antibiotics if sufficient supplies are available and the organisms are not resistant. Smallpox can be prevented or the incidence reduced by vaccination, even when first given after exposure. Botulism is treated with antitoxin though several vaccines are being studied. There is no established treatment for most viruses that cause hemorrhagic fever.[31]

Chemicals are also used as agents of terrorism and are categorized according to their target organ or effect.[32] (See eTable 69-3 on the website for this chapter.) For example, sarin is a highly toxic nerve gas that can cause death within minutes of exposure. It enters the body through the eyes and skin and acts by paralyzing the respiratory muscles. Antidotes for nerve agent poisoning include atropine (AtroPen) and pralidoxime chloride (2-PAM chloride). Multiple doses may be needed to reverse the effects of the nerve agents.

Phosgene is a colorless gas normally used in chemical manufacturing. If inhaled at high concentrations for a long enough period, it causes severe respiratory distress, pulmonary edema, and death. Mustard gas is yellow to brown and has a garlic-like odor. The gas irritates the eyes and causes skin burns and blisters. Protocols to treat victims of chemical exposure vary and relate to the specific agent.[32]

Radiologic or nuclear agents represent another category of agents of terrorism. *Radiologic dispersal devices* (RDDs), also known as "dirty bombs," consist of a mix of explosives and radioactive material (e.g., pellets). When the device is detonated, the blast scatters radioactive dust, smoke, and other material into the surrounding environment, resulting in radioactive contamination.[33]

The main danger from an RRD results from the explosion, which can cause serious injuries to the victims. The radioactive materials used in an RRD (e.g., uranium, iodine-131) do not usually generate enough radiation to cause immediate serious illness, except to those victims who are in close proximity to the explosion. However, the radioactive dust and smoke can spread and cause illness if inhaled. Since radiation cannot be seen, smelled, felt, or tasted, you should initiate measures to limit contamination (e.g., covering the patient's nose and mouth) and provide for decontamination (e.g., shower).[33,34]

Ionizing radiation, such as that from a nuclear bomb or damage to a nuclear reactor, represents a serious threat to the safety of victims and the environment. Exposure to ionizing radiation may or may not include skin contamination with radioactive material. Initiate decontamination procedures immediately if external radioactive contaminants are present. *Acute radiation syndrome* (ARS) develops after a substantial exposure to ionizing radiation and follows a predictable pattern.[32,35] (For additional information on ARS, see *www.bt.cdc.gov/radiation/arsphysicianfactsheet.asp.*)

Explosive devices (e.g., TNT, dynamite) that are used as agents of terrorism result in one or more of the following types of injuries: blast, crush, or penetrating. Blast injuries result from the supersonic overpressurization shock wave caused by the explosion. This shock wave primarily damages the lungs, GI tract, and middle ear. Crush injuries (i.e., blunt trauma) often result from explosions in confined spaces causing structural collapse (e.g., falling debris). Some explosive devices contain materials that are projected during the explosion (e.g., shrapnel), leading to penetrating injuries.

EMERGENCY AND MASS CASUALTY INCIDENT PREPAREDNESS

The term **emergency** usually refers to any extraordinary event (e.g., multi-vehicle crash) that requires a rapid and skilled response and that the community's existing resources can manage. An emergency is differentiated from a **mass casualty incident (MCI)** in that an MCI is a man-made (e.g., involving NBC agents) or natural (e.g., hurricane) event or disaster that overwhelms a community's ability to respond with existing resources. MCIs usually involve large numbers of victims, physical and emotional suffering, and permanent changes within a community. In addition, MCIs always require assistance from resources outside the affected community (e.g., American Red Cross, Federal Emergency Management Agency [FEMA]) (Fig. 69-7).

When an emergency or an MCI occurs, first responders (e.g., police, emergency medical personnel) are sent to the scene. Triage of victims of an emergency or an MCI differs from the usual triage described earlier. Several systems exist, and many

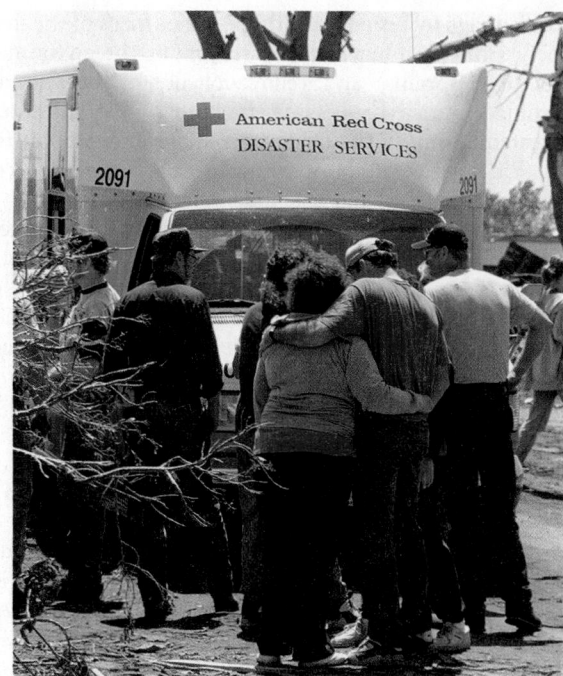

FIG. 69-7 American Red Cross.

ETHICAL/LEGAL DILEMMAS
Good Samaritan

Situation
You are a registered nurse, employed as a charge nurse at a subacute rehabilitation facility. It is midnight and you are driving home from work when you see a motor vehicle collision with a person at the side of the road waving and yelling for help. You stop and call 911 to report the incident. What do you do next?

Ethical/Legal Points for Consideration
- As a licensed health care provider, you are under no legal obligation to stop and render aid.
- If you do stop, you assume an obligation not to leave the scene until sufficiently trained first responders arrive and assume control.
- Between 50 and 75 yr ago, many states moved to encourage trained health care providers to stop and render aid by passing "Good Samaritan" statutes. These statutes, which vary somewhat from state to state, offer immunity from lawsuit for bystanders who offer aid in emergencies except in the case of gross negligence.
- A Good Samaritan must not be in the place of employment or under employment conditions.
- An example of gross negligence might be refusing to assist someone who obviously had a serious hemorrhage in favor of a person with a minor injury because the bleeding person looked old and disheveled.
- Immunity covers only the scene of the accident and not subsequent care under the supervision of health care providers.
- If there is a national disaster, an act of terrorism, or a major emergent need for health care personnel, you may be required to go to an assigned site to offer aid. You would not be covered by the Good Samaritan Act under these circumstances.

Discussion Questions
1. What factors do you think contribute to a health care provider's decision whether to stop to provide aid?
2. What basic aid would you feel comfortable providing if you do not have an emergency or trauma background?
3. Would your professional liability (malpractice) insurance cover you if someone claimed that you acted negligently while providing assistance?

use colored tags to designate both the seriousness of the injury and the likelihood of survival. One system uses green for minor injuries (e.g., sprains) and yellow for urgent, but not life-threatening injuries (e.g., open fractures). Red indicates a life-threatening injury requiring immediate intervention (e.g., shock). Blue indicates those who are expected to die (e.g., massive head trauma), and black identifies the dead.[36]

Triage of victims of an emergency or an MCI must be conducted in less than 15 seconds. In general, two thirds of victims are tagged green or yellow, and the remaining are tagged red, blue, or black. Victims need to be treated and stabilized and, if there is known or suspected contamination, decontaminated at the scene. After this, they are transported to hospitals. Many other victims arrive at hospitals on their own (i.e., walking wounded). The total number of victims a hospital can expect is estimated by doubling the number of victims who arrive in the first hour. Generally, 30% of victims require admission to the hospital, and half of these need surgery within 8 hours.

In addition to the services provided by first responders, many communities have developed *community emergency response teams* (CERTs). CERTs are recognized by FEMA as important partners in emergency preparedness. The CERT training helps citizens understand their personal responsibility in preparing for a natural or man-made disaster. In addition, participants are taught what to expect after a disaster and how to safely help themselves, their family, and their neighbors. Training includes lifesaving skills with emphasis on decision making and rescuer safety. CERTs are an extension of the first responder services. They can offer immediate help to victims and organize untrained volunteers to assist until professional services arrive.[37]

All health care providers have a role in emergency and MCI preparedness. Knowledge of the hospital's *emergency response plan* is essential. This includes individual roles and responsibilities of the members of the response team plus participation in emergency/MCI preparedness drills on a regular basis. Several types of drills can assess a hospital's level of emergency pre-paredness. These include hospital disaster drills, computer simulations, and tabletop exercises. Drills allow health care providers to become familiar with the emergency response procedures.[38]

Response to MCIs often requires the aid of a federal agency. The National Incident Management System (NIMS) is a section within the U.S. Department of Homeland Security. NIMS is responsible for coordinating federal, state, and local government efforts to respond to and manage domestic MCIs.[39] One important aspect of NIMS is the development of the *Incident Command System* (ICS). This standardized organizational structure provides for the management of all incidents. NIMS requires that all emergency services–related disciplines (e.g., hospitals, health care providers, emergency response services) wishing to participate in the emergency management of disasters must be NIMS and ICS trained. You can take courses online and at no cost (*http://training.fema.gov/is/nims.asp*).

The National Disaster Medical System (NDMS) is a part of the U.S. Department of Health and Human Services, Office of Preparedness and Response. The NDMS expands the nation's medical response capability by organizing and training volunteer disaster medical assistance teams (DMATs). Each DMAT consists of members with a variety of health or medical skills and those with specialized support skills (e.g., communications, logistics, security). DMATs are sent to disaster sites with enough supplies and equipment to remain self-sufficient for 72 hours while providing medical care. DMAT personnel are deployed for a period of 2 weeks.[40]

All disasters result in psychologic stress to the individuals involved immediately after the event. This stress can persist for an extended period and is influenced, in part, by the nature of the event, the individual's age, preexisting coping mechanisms, role in the event, and medical and psychologic history. Many hospitals and DMATs have a *critical incident stress management unit*. This unit arranges group discussions to allow participants to share and validate their feelings and emotions about the experience. This is important for emotional recovery.

CASE STUDY

Trauma

iStockphoto/Thinkstock

Patient Profile
D.F., a 20-yr-old Hispanic female trauma patient, is brought to the ED in an ambulance. She was the driver in a motor vehicle collision and was not wearing a seat belt. Two children in the car were pronounced dead at the scene. The paramedics stated that there was significant damage to the car on the driver's side.

Subjective Data
• Patient asks, "What happened? Where am I?"
• Complains of shortness of breath and leg pain

Objective Data
Physical Examination
• Vital signs: blood pressure 85/40 mm Hg, heart rate 140 beats/min, respiratory rate 36 breaths/min; O₂ saturation 85% with 100% non-rebreather mask
• Decreased breath sounds on left side of chest
• Asymmetric chest wall movement

• Glasgow Coma Score = 14; pupils slightly unequal
• Badly deformed left lower leg with significant swelling and a pedal pulse by Doppler only
• 4-cm head laceration, bleeding controlled

Discussion Questions
1. What are D.F.'s most likely life-threatening injuries?
2. *Priority Decision:* What is the priority of care for D.F.?
3. *Priority Decision:* What interventions does this patient need immediately?
4. What other interventions should you consider?
5. *Delegation Decision:* What activities could you delegate to unlicensed assistive personnel (UAP)?
6. Several family members have arrived in the ED, including the mother of one of the children who died. The second child who died was the patient's child. How should you approach the family?
7. *Priority Decision:* Based on assessment data presented, what are the priority nursing diagnoses? Are there any collaborative problems?
8. *Evidence-Based Practice:* What are the best practice guidelines for fluid resuscitation in patients who are experiencing hypovolemic shock?

BRIDGE TO NCLEX EXAMINATION

The number of the question corresponds to the same-numbered outcome at the beginning of the chapter.

1. An older man arrives in triage disoriented and tachypneic. His skin is hot and dry. His wife states that he was fine earlier today. The nurse's next priority would be to
   a. obtain a detailed medical history from his wife.
   b. assess his vital signs, including a rectal temperature.
   c. determine the kind of insurance he has before treating him.
   d. start supplemental oxygen and have the ED physician see him.

2. A patient has a core temperature of 90° F (32.2° C). The most appropriate rewarming technique would be
   a. passive rewarming with warm blankets.
   b. active internal rewarming using warmed IV fluids.
   c. passive rewarming using air-filled warming blankets.
   d. active external rewarming by submersing in a warm bath.

3. Effective interventions to decrease absorption or increase elimination of an ingested poison include which of the following (select all that apply)?
   a. Hemodialysis
   b. Milk dilution
   c. Eye irrigation
   d. Gastric lavage
   e. Activated charcoal

4. An older woman arrives in the ED complaining of severe pain in her right shoulder. The nurse notes that her clothes are soiled with urine and feces. She tells the nurse that she lives with her son and that she "fell." She is tearful and asks you if she can be admitted. What possibility should the nurse consider?
   a. Paranoia
   b. Possible cancer
   c. Family violence
   d. Orthostatic hypotension

5. A chemical explosion occurs at a nearby industrial site. The first responders report that victims are being decontaminated at the scene and approximately 125 workers will need medical evaluation and care. The nurse receiving this report should know that this will first require activation of
   a. a code blue alert.
   b. a disaster medical assistance team.
   c. the local police and fire departments.
   d. the hospital's emergency response plan.

1. b, 2. b, 3. a, d, e, 4. c, 5. d

ⓔvolve

For rationales to these answers and even more NCLEX review questions, visit *http://evolve.elsevier.com/Lewis/medsurg.*

REFERENCES

1. Gilboy N: Triage. In PK Howard, RA Steinmann, editors: *Sheehy's emergency nursing,* ed 6, St Louis, 2010, Mosby.

2. American College of Emergency Physicians: Emergency department wait times, crowding and access fact sheet, 2012. Retrieved from *www.acep.org/uploadedFiles/ACEP/News_Room/ NewsMediaResources/Media_Fact_Sheets/FINAL%20Wait%20 Times%20Crowding%20and%20Access.pdf.*

3. Emergency Nurses Association: Welcome to BCEN. Retrieved from *www.bcencertifications.org/Pages/default.aspx.aspx.*

4. Rund DA, Rausch TS: *Triage,* St Louis, 1981, Mosby. (Classic)

5. Gilboy N, Tanabe P, Travers DA, et al: *Emergency Severity Index (ESI): a triage tool for emergency department, version 4: Implementation handbook 2012 edition,* AHRQ Pub No. 12-0014, Rockville, Md, 2011, Agency for Healthcare Research and Quality. Retrieved from *www.ahrq.gov/research/esi.*

6. Emergency Nurses Association, American College of Emergency Physicians: Standardized ED triage scale and acuity categorization. Retrieved from *www.ena.org/SiteCollection Documents/Position%20Statements/STANDARDIZEDED TRIAGESCALEANDACUITYCATEGORIZATION.pdf.*

7. O'Neal JV: Airway management. In BB Hammond, PG Zimmermann, editors: *Sheehy's manual of emergency care,* ed 7, St Louis, 2013, Mosby.

8. Cerepani MJ: Orthopedic and neurovascular trauma. In PK Howard, RA Steinmann, editors: *Sheehy's emergency nursing,* ed 6, St Louis, 2010, Mosby.

9. Solheim J: Assessment and stabilization of the trauma patient. In BB Hammond, PG Zimmermann, editors: *Sheehy's manual of emergency care,* ed 7, St Louis, 2013, Mosby.

*10. American Association of Critical-Care Nurses: AACN practice alert: family presence during CPR and invasive procedures.

Retrieved from *www.aacn.org/WD/Practice/Docs/PracticeAlerts/ Family%20Presence%2004-2010%20final.pdf.*

11. Emergency Nurses Association: Family presence at the bedside during invasive procedures and resuscitation. Retrieved from *www.ena.org/SiteCollectionDocuments/Position%20Statements/ FamilyPresence.pdf.*

12. American Society for Pain Management Nursing, Emergency Nurses Association, American College of Emergency Physicians, American Pain Society: Optimizing the treatment of pain in patients with acute presentations. Retrieved from *www.ena.org/SiteCollectionDocuments/Position%20Statements/ Pain_Mgmt_pol.pdf.*

13. Harris C: Abdominal trauma. In BB Hammond, PG Zimmermann, editors: *Sheehy's manual of emergency care,* ed 7, St Louis, 2013, Mosby.

14. Centers for Disease Control and Prevention: Disaster information: tetanus prevention after a disaster. Retrieved from *www.bt.cdc.gov/disasters/disease/tetanus.asp.*

15. Bucher L, Buruschkin R, Kenyon D, et al: Improving outcomes with therapeutic hypothermia, *Nurs Crit Care* 7:22, 2012.

*16. O'Gara P, Kushner FG, Ascheim DD, et al: 2013 ACCF/AHA guideline for the management of ST-elevation myocardial infarction, *J Am Coll Cardiol* 61:e78, 2013.

17. Emergency Nurses Association: End-of-life care in the emergency department. Retrieved from *www.ena.org/ SiteCollectionDocuments/Position%20Statements/EndofLife CareintheEmergencyDepartment.pdf.*

18. United Network for Organ Sharing: Professional education. Retrieved from *www.unos.org/resources/UNOSprofessional Resources.asp.*

19. Samaras N, Chevalley T, Samaras D, et al: Older patients in the emergency department: a review, *Ann Emerg Med* 56:261, 2010.

20. Hammond BB, Zimmermann PG, editors: *Sheehy's manual of emergency care,* ed 7, St Louis, 2013, Mosby.

*Evidence-based information for clinical practice.

21. Centers for Disease Control and Prevention: Tick removal. Retrieved from *www.cdc.gov/lyme/removal/index.html*.

22. Denke NJ: Wound management. In PK Howard, RA Steinmann, editors: *Sheehy's emergency nursing*, ed 6, St Louis, 2010, Mosby.

23. Sturt P: Toxicologic emergencies. In PK Howard, RA Steinmann, editors: *Sheehy's emergency nursing*, ed 6, St Louis, 2010, Mosby.

24. National Capital Poison Control Center: Act fast. Retrieved from *www.poison.org/actFast/1800.asp*.

25. Lehne RA: *Pharmacology for nursing care*, ed 7, St Louis, 2010, Mosby.

26. Egging D: Ocular emergencies. In PK Howard, RA Steinmann, editors: *Sheehy's emergency nursing*, ed 6, St Louis, 2010, Mosby.

27. Occupational Health and Safety Administration: Occupational injury and illness recording and reporting requirements. Retrieved from *www.osha.gov/pls/oshaweb/owadisp.show _document?p_table=FEDERAL_REGISTER&p_id=16312*.

28. Emergency Nurses Association: Violence in the emergency setting. Retrieved from *www.ena.org/SiteCollectionDocuments/ Position%20Statements/Violence_in_the_Emergency_Care _Setting_-_ENA_PS.pdf*.

29. Emergency Nurses Association: Intimate partner and family violence, maltreatment, and neglect. Retrieved from *www .ena.org/SiteCollectionDocuments/Position%20Statements/ Violence_-_Intimate_Partner_and_Family_-_ENA_PS.pdf*.

*30. Nelson HD, Bougatsos C, Blazina I: Screening women for intimate partner violence: a systematic review to update the U.S. Preventive Services Task Force recommendation, *Ann Intern Med* 156:796, 2012.

31. Centers for Disease Control and Prevention: Viral hemorrhagic fevers. Retrieved from *www.cdc.gov/ncidod/dvrd/spb/mnpages/ dispages/vhf.htm*.

32. Andress K: Nuclear, biologic, and chemical agents of mass destruction. In PK Howard, RA Steinmann, editors: *Sheehy's emergency nursing*, ed 6, St Louis, 2010, Mosby.

33. Centers for Disease Control and Prevention: Frequently asked questions about dirty bombs. Retrieved from *www.bt.cdc.gov/ radiation/dirtybombs.asp*.

34. Emergency Nurses Association: Hazardous material exposure. Retrieved from *www.ena.org/SiteCollectionDocuments/Position% 20Statements/Hazardous_Material_Exposure_-_ENA_PS.pdf*.

35. Military Medical Operations Armed Forces Radiobiology Research Institute: Medical management of radiological casualties. Retrieved from *www.usuhs.mil/afrri/outreach/ pdf/3edmmrchandbook.pdf*.

*36. Lerner EB, Schwartz RB, Coule PL, et al: Mass casualty triage: an evaluation of the data and development of a proposed national guideline, *Disaster Med Public Health Preparedness* 2:S25, 2008. (Classic)

37. Community Emergency Response Team: About CERT. Retrieved from *www.citizencorps.gov/cert/about.shtm*.

*38. Agency for Healthcare Research and Quality: Evidence report/ technology assessment number 95: training of hospital staff to respond to a mass casualty incident. Retrieved from *archive. ahrq.gov/downloads/pub/evidence/pdf/hospmci/hospmci.pdf*.

39. Robinson KS: Emergency preparedness. In PK Howard, RA Steinmann, editors: *Sheehy's emergency nursing*, ed 6, St Louis, 2010, Mosby.

40. US Department of Health and Human Services: Disaster medical assistance teams. Retrieved from *www.phe.gov/ Preparedness/responders/ndms/teams/Pages/dmat.aspx*.

RESOURCES

American College of Emergency Physicians
www.acep.org
American Nurses Association, Disaster Preparedness and Response
www.nursingworld.org/MainMenuCategories/WorkplaceSafety/DPR
American Red Cross
www.redcross.org
American Trauma Society
www.amtrauma.org
Association of Emergency Physicians (AEP)
www.aep.org
Centers for Disease Control and Prevention, Emergency Preparedness and Response
www.bt.cdc.gov
Emergency Nurses Association (ENA)
www.ena.org
Federal Emergency Management Agency (FEMA)
www.fema.gov
National Capital Poison Center
www.poison.org
National Coalition Against Domestic Violence
www.ncadv.org
National Domestic Violence Hotline
www.ndvh.org
National Response Center
www.nrc.uscg.mil/index.htm
US Department of Health and Human Services, Public Health Emergency
www.ndms.dhhs.gov/index.html
US Department of Justice, Office on Violence Against Women
www.ovw.usdoj.gov

CASE STUDY

Managing Multiple Patients

You are working in a 12-bed intensive care unit and have been assigned to care for the following two patients. There is one UAP available to help as needed.

Patients

iStockphoto/Thinkstock

R.K. is a 72-year-old white man who was admitted with a massive stroke after collapsing on the street. He is unresponsive, even to painful stimuli. He has an oral endotracheal (ET) tube in place and is receiving mechanical ventilation (assist-control mode, FIO$_2$ 70%, VT 700 mL, respiratory rate 16 breaths/min, PEEP 5 cm H$_2$O). His chest x-ray revealed right lower lung consolidation. A subclavian central line was placed to monitor CVP and administer fluids. IV antibiotics have been started. His cardiac rhythm on admission was atrial fibrillation with a rapid ventricular response. He is receiving IV diltiazem (Cardizem) and his ventricular response has slowed to 84 bpm. His temperature is elevated despite receiving acetaminophen q 4 hr. He is also receiving enteral feeding at 25 mL/hr via small-bore nasogastric feeding tube and has an external condom catheter for urinary drainage.

iStockphoto/Thinkstock

J.N. is a 55-year-old white man who was admitted 24 hours ago after emergent surgery for an acutely ischemic bowel. The surgical procedure involved extensive abdominal surgery to repair a perforated colon, irrigate the abdominal cavity, and provide hemostasis. During surgery his systolic BP dropped to 70 mm Hg. Seven units of packed red blood cells and 4 L of 0.9% saline were infused. His pulmonary status worsened within 12 hours of admission to the ICU, requiring an emergent ET intubation. He developed a pneumothorax after intubation and a left-side chest tube was placed at that time. His hypoxemia has rapidly progressed and is currently refractory to 100% FIO$_2$ and high levels of PEEP. His laboratory test results indicate kidney and liver failure. He has an advance directive that indicates he does not want to be kept alive by artificial means, but he has a full code status. He is currently sedated, paralyzed, and unable to communicate. His urinary catheter is draining concentrated urine <30 mL/hr. He has a central line in place and is receiving 0.9% saline at 125 mL/hr. His most recent ABGs are as follows: pH 7.12, PaO$_2$ 50 mm Hg, PaCO$_2$ 62 mm Hg, HCO$_3$ 17 mEq/L, and O$_2$ saturation 84%. His PaO$_2$/FIO$_2$ ratio is <200 and his chest x-ray shows worsening bilateral interstitial infiltrates compatible with an ARDS pattern.

Management Discussion Questions

1. **Priority Decision:** After receiving report, which patient should you see first? Provide rationale.
2. **Delegation Decision:** Which tasks could you delegate to the UAP (*select all that apply*)?
   a. Record vital signs on R.K. and J.N.
   b. Suction R.K. and J.N.'s ET tubes as needed.
   c. Titrate the diltiazem IV drip downward based on R.K.'s heart rate.
   d. Talk to J.N.'s family regarding his advance directive and current code status.
3. **Priority and Delegation Decision:** As you are assessing J.N., the UAP informs you that R.K. just vomited all over his bed. Which initial action would be most appropriate?
   a. Ask the UAP to give R.K. a bath while you finish assessing J.N.
   b. Turn off the enteral tube feeding on R.K. and auscultate his lungs.
   c. Ask the UAP to inform the health care provider about J.N.'s ABG results while you assess R.K.
   d. Finish assessing R.K. and then suction R.K.'s endotracheal tube to remove any aspirated emesis.

Case Study Progression

R.K.'s lungs are clear to auscultation. Evaluation of his gastrointestinal status reveals minimal bowel sounds and a gastric residual of 200 mL even after his emesis. You elevate the head of his bed to 60 degrees, hold the tube feeding, and notify his health care provider.

4. Which intervention would you expect the health care provider to order for R.K.?
   a. Morphine sulfate 2 mg IV stat
   b. Metoclopramide (Reglan) 10 mg IV q6hr
   c. Restart enteral tube feeding while maintaining HOB elevation at 90 degrees
   d. Hold enteral tube feeding for 1 hour and restart with half-strength fluids at same rate
5. J.N.'s ABG results reflect a worsening of his ARDS. You correctly identify that these results demonstrate
   a. uncompensated respiratory acidosis.
   b. uncompensated respiratory alkalosis.
   c. partially compensated respiratory acidosis.
   d. partially compensated respiratory alkalosis.
6. **Management Decision:** You walk into J.N.'s room and find his wife whispering in his ear with her hand on the ventilator tubing, appearing to be ready to disconnect him from life support. What is your best initial action?
   a. Ask J.N.'s wife to leave the room immediately.
   b. Report the incident to the charge nurse and security immediately.
   c. Ask J.N.'s wife if you could talk to her about her husband's condition.
   d. Report the incident to J.N.'s health care provider to address J.N.'s code status.

A

Basic Life Support for Health Care Providers

Linda Bucher

Basic life support (BLS) consists of a series of actions and skills performed by the rescuer(s) based on assessment findings. The first actions the rescuer performs on finding an adult victim are to assess for responsiveness and to look for signs of breathing. This is done by tapping or shaking the victim's shoulder and asking, "Are you all right?" and scanning the victim's chest for signs of breathing. If the victim does not respond, there is no breathing or abnormal breathing (e.g., agonal gasps), and the rescuer is alone, the rescuer shouts for help. If someone responds, the rescuer sends him or her to activate the *emergency response system* (ERS) and get an *automatic external defibrillator* (AED) (if available). If no one responds, the rescuer activates the ERS, gets an AED (if available), returns to the victim, and begins *cardiopulmonary resuscitation* (CPR) and defibrillation if necessary.[1]

CARDIOPULMONARY RESUSCITATION

Cardiac arrest is characterized by the absence of a pulse and breathing in an unconscious victim. The current approach for CPR is the chest *compressions–airway-breathing* (CAB) sequence.[1]

The first step in CPR is to perform a pulse check by palpating the carotid pulse for at least 5 but no more than 10 seconds.

While maintaining a head-tilt position with one hand on the forehead, locate the victim's trachea using two or three fingers of the other hand. Slide these fingers into the groove between the trachea and the neck muscles where the carotid pulse can be felt. The technique is more easily performed on the side nearest you.

If a pulse is felt, give one rescue breath every 5 to 6 seconds (10 to 12 breaths/minute) and recheck the pulse every 2 minutes (see Fig. A-1 and Airway and Breathing below). If no pulse is felt, initiate CAB.[1]

Chest Compressions

The proper technique for providing chest compressions is shown in Fig. A-2. Chest compression technique consists of fast and deep applications of pressure on the sternum. The victim must be in the supine position when the compressions are performed. The victim must be lying on a flat, hard surface, such as a CPR board (specially designed for use in CPR), a headboard from a unit bed, or, if necessary, the floor. Position yourself close to the side of the victim's chest.

Chest compressions are combined with rescue breathing for an effective resuscitation effort of the adult victim of cardiac arrest. The compression-ventilation ratio for one- or two-rescuer CPR is 30 compressions to 2 breaths (Table A-1).

FIG. A-1 The head tilt–chin lift maneuver is used to open the victim's airway to give rescue breaths. **A,** Rescuer places one hand on the victim's forehead and applies firm, backward pressure with the palm to tilt the head back. The chin is lifted and brought forward with the fingers of the other hand. **B,** Mouth-to-barrier device: Rescuer places the device tightly over the victim's mouth and nose and delivers a regular breath. **C,** Mouth-to-mouth technique: Rescuer pinches the victim's nostrils, tightly seals mouth over victim's mouth, and delivers a regular breath. NOTE: Rescuer should observe for a rise in the victim's chest *(blue arrows)*.

Reviewed by Amber Young, RN, MSN, Instructor of Nursing, Bellin College, School of Nursing, Green Bay, Wisconsin.

TABLE A-1   ADULT ONE- AND TWO-RESCUER BASIC LIFE SUPPORT WITH AUTOMATIC EXTERNAL DEFIBRILLATOR (AED)

Assess
- Determine unresponsiveness: tap or shake victim's shoulder; shout, "Are you all right?"
- Check for no breathing or abnormal breathing (e.g., gasping).

Activate Emergency Response System (ERS)
- Activate ERS (e.g., call 911) and get the AED (if available) (outside of hospital).
- Call a code and ask for the AED or crash cart (in hospital).

Check for Pulse
- Feel for carotid pulse (5-10 sec).
- If victim has a pulse but is not breathing or not breathing adequately, begin rescue breathing at a rate of 1 breath every 5-6 sec (see Fig. A-1) and recheck circulation every 2 minutes.

Begin High-Quality CPR
- If there is no pulse, expose the victim's chest and immediately begin chest compressions (see Fig. A-2).
- Deliver compressions at a rate of at least 100/minute.
- Compress the chest at least 2 inches.
- Allow for complete chest recoil after each compression.
- Deliver a compression-ventilation ratio of 30 compressions to 2 breaths.
- Minimize interruptions in compressions by delivering the 2 breaths in <10 sec.

Deliver Effective Breaths
- Open airway adequately (see Fig. A-1, *A*).
- Deliver breath to produce a visible chest rise (see Fig. A-1, *B, C*).
- Avoid excessive ventilation.

Integrate Prompt Use of the AED
- Use AED as soon as possible.
- If rhythm is shockable, deliver one shock and then resume chest compressions immediately after delivery of shock.
- If the rhythm is not shockable, resume CPR and recheck rhythm every five cycles.

Continue CPR
- Continue CPR between rhythm checks and shocks, and until ACLS providers arrive or the victim shows signs of movement.

Source: American Heart Association: *BLS for healthcare providers—student manual,* Dallas, 2011, The Association.
ACLS, Advanced cardiovascular life support; *CPR,* cardiopulmonary resuscitation.

FIG. A-2 Cardiopulmonary resuscitation. **A,** Position of the hands during chest compressions. **B,** When pressure is applied, the sternum is displaced posteriorly with the heel of the hand. **C,** Arms are kept straight and the rescuer pushes deep (at least 2 in) and fast (a rate of at least 100 compressions per minute).

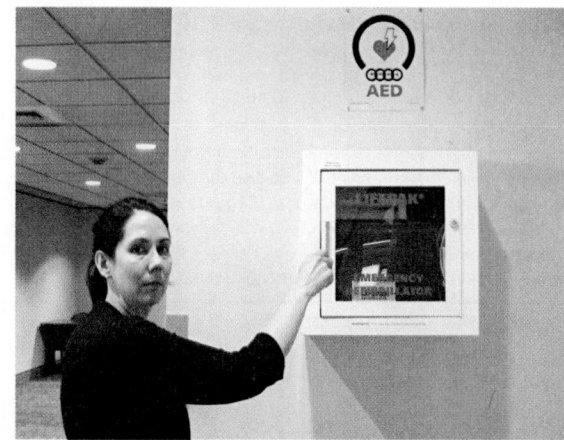

FIG. A-3 Automatic external defibrillator (AED) located in a shopping center.

If the patient has an advanced airway (e.g., endotracheal tube, laryngeal mask airway), do not pause between compressions for breaths.[1]

It is preferable to have two persons performing CPR. One rescuer, positioned at the victim's side, performs chest compressions while the second rescuer, positioned at the victim's head, maintains an open airway and performs ventilations. To maintain the quality and rate of compressions, rescuers should change roles every 2 minutes.[1] Interruptions in CPR should be limited.

Defibrillation

When the AED or advanced cardiovascular life support (ACLS) team arrives, assess the victim's rhythm. If the victim has a shockable rhythm (e.g., ventricular tachycardia, ventricular fibrillation), deliver one shock followed by five cycles of CPR before checking the rhythm again. If the rhythm is not a shockable rhythm, resume CPR and recheck the rhythm every five cycles. CPR should continue between rhythm checks and shocks, and until the ACLS team arrives or the victim shows signs of movement.[1]

The American Heart Association includes training in the use of AEDs with instruction of health care personnel and laypersons in BLS. Survival from cardiac arrest is the highest when immediate CPR is provided and defibrillation occurs within 3 to 5 minutes.[1] AEDs are found in many out-of-hospital, public settings (Fig. A-3).

Airway and Breathing

If a victim has a pulse but is gasping (e.g., agonal breathing) or not breathing, establish an open airway and begin rescue breath-

TABLE A-2 MANAGEMENT OF THE ADULT CHOKING VICTIM

Conscious Adult Choking Victim
Assess Victim for Severe Airway Obstruction
Look for any of the following signs:
- Poor or no air exchange
- Clutching the neck with the hands, making the universal choking sign
- Weak, ineffective cough or no cough at all
- High-pitched noise while inhaling or no noise at all
- Increased respiratory difficulty
- Possible cyanosis

Ask the victim if he or she is choking. If the victim nods yes and cannot talk or has any of the symptoms noted above, severe airway obstruction is present and you must take immediate action.

Abdominal Thrusts (Heimlich Maneuver) With Standing or Sitting Victim (see Fig. A-4)
1. Stand or kneel behind victim and wrap arms around the victim's waist.
2. Make fist with one hand.
3. Place thumb side of fist against victim's abdomen. Position fist midline, slightly above navel and well below breastbone.
4. Grasp fist with other hand and press fist into victim's abdomen with a quick, forceful upward thrust.
5. Give each new thrust with a separate, distinct movement to relieve the obstruction. CAUTION: If victim is pregnant or obese, give chest thrusts instead of abdominal thrusts. Position hands (as described) over lower portion of the breastbone and apply quick backward thrusts.
6. Repeat thrusts until object is expelled or victim becomes unresponsive.

Unconscious Adult Choking Victim
If you see a choking victim collapse and become unresponsive:
1. Activate the emergency response system.
2. Lower the victim to the ground and begin CPR, starting with compressions (do not check for a pulse).
3. Open the victim's mouth wide each time you prepare to give breaths. Look for the object. If you see the object and can easily remove it, do so with your fingers. If you do not see the object, continue with CPR using the chest compression–airway–breathing sequence (see Table A-1).
4. If efforts to ventilate are unsuccessful, continue with CPR.

Source: American Heart Association: *BLS for healthcare providers—student manual,* Dallas, 2011, The Association.

FIG. A-4 Abdominal thrusts (Heimlich maneuver) administered to a conscious (standing) choking victim.

and watch for a rise in the victim's chest. Continue rescue breaths at a rate of 10 to 12 per minute. When the victim has a tracheostomy, give ventilations through the stoma.

If the victim cannot be ventilated, proceed with CPR. When providing the next rescue breaths, look for any objects in the victim's mouth and remove them if visible (Table A-2).

HANDS-ONLY CPR

Hands-only CPR can be used to help adult victims who suddenly collapse from cardiac arrest outside of a health care setting. If you witness this event (as a bystander), you can choose to provide chest compressions only (push fast and deep in the center of the chest) or conventional CPR (described previously). Both methods are effective when done in the first few minutes of an out-of-hospital cardiac arrest.[2]

REFERENCES

1. American Heart Association: *BLS for healthcare providers—student manual,* Dallas, 2011, The Association.
2. American Heart Association: Two steps to staying alive with hands-only CPR. Retrieved from *www.heart.org/HEARTORG/CPRAndECC/HandsOnlyCPR/Hands-Only-CPR_UCM_440559_SubHomePage.jsp.*

RESOURCES

American Heart Association, CPR and Emergency Cardiovascular Care
www.heart.org/cpr
American Heart Association, Hands-Only CPR
http://handsonlycpr.org

ing. Open an adult's airway by hyperextending the head (see Fig. A-1). Use the *head tilt–chin lift maneuver.* This involves tilting the head back with one hand and lifting the chin forward with the fingers of the other hand. Use the *jaw-thrust maneuver* if you suspect a cervical spine injury (see Fig. 69-1). Attempt to ventilate the victim using a mouth-to-barrier (recommended) device (e.g., face mask or bag-valve-mask) or mouth-to-mouth resuscitation[1] (see Fig. A-1, *B, C*).

For mouth-to-mouth resuscitation give ventilations with the victim's nostrils pinched. Take a regular (not deep) breath and tightly seal your lips around the victim's mouth. Give one breath

Nursing Diagnoses

Activity Intolerance
Activity Intolerance, Risk for
Activity Planning, Ineffective
Activity Planning, Risk for Ineffective
Adverse Reaction to Iodinated Contrast Media, Risk for
Airway Clearance, Ineffective
Allergy Response, Risk for
Anxiety
Aspiration, Risk for
Attachment, Risk for Impaired
Autonomic Dysreflexia
Autonomic Dysreflexia, Risk for
Behavior, Disorganized Infant
Behavior, Readiness for Enhanced Organized Infant
Behavior, Risk for Disorganized Infant
Bleeding, Risk for
Blood Glucose Level, Risk for Unstable
Body Image, Disturbed
Body Temperature, Risk for Imbalanced
Breast Milk, Insufficient
Breastfeeding, Ineffective
Breastfeeding, Interrupted
Breastfeeding, Readiness for Enhanced
Breathing Pattern, Ineffective
Cardiac Output, Decreased
Caregiver Role Strain
Caregiver Role Strain, Risk for
Childbearing Process, Ineffective
Childbearing Process, Readiness for Enhanced
Childbearing Process, Risk for Ineffective
Comfort, Impaired
Comfort, Readiness for Enhanced
Communication, Readiness for Enhanced
Confusion, Acute
Confusion, Chronic
Confusion, Risk for Acute
Constipation
Constipation, Perceived
Constipation, Risk for
Contamination
Contamination, Risk for
Coping, Defensive
Coping, Ineffective
Coping, Readiness for Enhanced
Coping, Ineffective Community
Coping, Readiness for Enhanced Community

Coping, Compromised Family
Coping, Disabled Family
Coping, Readiness for Enhanced Family
Death Anxiety
Decision-Making, Readiness for Enhanced
Decisional Conflict
Denial, Ineffective
Dentition, Impaired
Development, Risk for Delayed
Diarrhea
Disuse Syndrome, Risk for
Diversional Activity, Deficient
Dry Eye, Risk for
Electrolyte Imbalance, Risk for
Energy Field, Disturbed
Environmental Interpretation Syndrome, Impaired
Failure to Thrive, Adult
Falls, Risk for
Family Processes, Dysfunctional
Family Processes, Interrupted
Family Processes, Readiness for Enhanced
Fatigue
Fear
Feeding Pattern, Ineffective Infant
Fluid Balance, Readiness for Enhanced
Fluid Volume, Risk for Imbalanced
Fluid Volume, Deficient
Fluid Volume, Excess
Fluid Volume, Risk for Deficient
Gas Exchange, Impaired
Gastrointestinal Motility, Risk For Dysfunctional
Gastrointestinal Motility, Dysfunctional
Gastrointestinal Perfusion, Risk for Ineffective
Grieving
Grieving, Complicated
Grieving, Risk for Complicated
Growth, Risk for Disproportionate
Growth and Development, Delayed
Health, Deficient Community
Health Behavior, Risk-Prone
Health Maintenance, Ineffective
Home Maintenance, Impaired
Hope, Readiness for Enhanced
Hopelessness
Human Dignity, Risk for Compromised
Hyperthermia

Hypothermia
Immunization Status, Readiness for Enhanced
Impulse Control, Ineffective
Incontinence, Functional Urinary
Incontinence, Overflow Urinary
Incontinence, Reflex Urinary
Incontinence, Stress Urinary
Incontinence, Urge Urinary
Incontinence, Risk for Urge Urinary
Incontinence, Bowel
Infection, Risk for
Injury, Risk for
Insomnia
Intracranial Adaptive Capacity, Decreased
Jaundice, Neonatal
Jaundice, Risk for Neonatal
Knowledge, Deficient
Knowledge, Readiness for Enhanced
Latex Allergy Response
Latex Allergy Response, Risk for
Lifestyle, Sedentary
Liver Function, Risk for Impaired
Loneliness, Risk for
Maternal–Fetal Dyad, Risk for Disturbed
Memory, Impaired
Mobility, Impaired Bed
Mobility, Impaired Physical
Mobility, Impaired Wheelchair
Moral Distress
Nausea
Noncompliance
Nutrition, Readiness for Enhanced
Nutrition, Imbalanced: Less Than Body Requirements
Nutrition, Risk for Imbalanced: More Than Body Requirements
Nutrition, Imbalanced: More Than Body Requirements
Oral Mucous Membrane, Impaired
Other-Directed Violence, Risk for
Pain, Acute
Pain, Chronic
Parenting, Impaired
Parenting, Readiness for Enhanced
Parenting, Risk for Impaired
Perioperative Positioning Injury, Risk for
Peripheral Neurovascular Dysfunction, Risk for
Personal Identity, Disturbed
Personal Identity, Risk for Disturbed
Poisoning, Risk for
Post-Trauma Syndrome
Post-Trauma Syndrome, Risk for
Power, Readiness for Enhanced
Powerlessness
Powerlessness, Risk for
Protection, Ineffective
Rape-Trauma Syndrome
Relationship, Ineffective
Relationship, Readiness for Enhanced
Relationship, Risk for Ineffective
Religiosity, Impaired
Religiosity, Readiness for Enhanced
Religiosity, Risk for Impaired
Relocation Stress Syndrome
Relocation Stress Syndrome, Risk for

Renal Perfusion, Risk for Ineffective
Resilience, Impaired Individual
Resilience, Readiness for Enhanced
Resilience, Risk for Compromised
Role Conflict, Parental
Role Performance, Ineffective
Self-Care, Readiness for Enhanced
Self-Care Deficit, Bathing
Self-Care Deficit, Dressing
Self-Care Deficit, Feeding
Self-Care Deficit, Toileting
Self-Concept, Readiness for Enhanced
Self-Directed Violence, Risk for
Self-Esteem, Chronic Low
Self-Esteem, Situational Low
Self-Esteem, Risk for Chronic Low
Self-Esteem, Risk for Situational Low
Self-Health Management, Ineffective
Self-Health Management, Readiness for Enhanced
Self-Mutilation
Self-Mutilation, Risk for
Self-Neglect
Sexual Dysfunction
Sexuality Pattern, Ineffective
Shock, Risk for
Skin Integrity, Impaired
Skin Integrity, Risk for Impaired
Sleep Deprivation
Sleep, Readiness for Enhanced
Sleep Pattern, Disturbed
Social Interaction, Impaired
Social Isolation
Sorrow, Chronic
Spiritual Distress
Spiritual Distress, Risk for
Spiritual Well-Being, Readiness for Enhanced
Spontaneous Ventilation, Impaired
Stress Overload
Sudden Infant Death Syndrome, Risk for
Suffocation, Risk for
Suicide, Risk for
Surgical Recovery, Delayed
Swallowing, Impaired
Therapeutic Regimen Management, Ineffective Family
Thermal Injury, Risk for
Thermoregulation, Ineffective
Tissue Integrity, Impaired
Tissue Perfusion, Ineffective Peripheral
Tissue Perfusion, Risk for Decreased Cardiac
Tissue Perfusion, Risk for Ineffective Cerebral
Tissue Perfusion, Risk for Ineffective Peripheral
Transfer Ability, Impaired
Trauma, Risk for
Unilateral Neglect
Urinary Elimination, Impaired
Urinary Elimination, Readiness for Enhanced
Urinary Retention
Vascular Trauma, Risk for
Ventilatory Weaning Response, Dysfunctional
Verbal Communication, Impaired
Walking, Impaired
Wandering

C

Laboratory Reference Intervals

The tables in this appendix list some of the most common tests, their reference intervals (formally referred to as normal values), and possible etiologies of abnormal results. Laboratory results may vary depending on different techniques or different laboratories. Possible etiologies are presented in alphabetic order. Abbreviations appearing in the tables are defined as follows:

mEq = milliequivalent
mm Hg = millimeter of mercury
mm = millimeter
mOsm = milliosmole

L = liter
dL = deciliter (10^{-1} liter)
mL = milliliter (10^{-3} liter)
μL = microliter (10^{-6} liter, 10^{-3} milliliter)
fL = femtoliter (10^{-15} liter, 10^{-12} milliliter)

g = gram
mg = milligram (10^{-3} gram)
mcg = microgram (10^{-6} gram)
ng = nanogram (10^{-9} gram)
pg = picogram (10^{-12} gram)

U = unit
μU = microunit
IU = international unit

mmol = millimole (10^{-3} mole)
μmol = micromole (10^{-6} mole)
nmol = nanomole (10^{-9} mole)
pmol = picomole (10^{-12} mole)
kPa = kilopascal
μkat = microkatal

Source: Burtis CA, Ashwood ER, Bruns DE: *Tietz textbook of clinical chemistry and molecular diagnostics*, ed 5, St Louis, 2013, Elsevier.

TABLE C-1 SERUM, PLASMA, AND WHOLE BLOOD CHEMISTRIES

| Test | Reference Intervals | | Possible Etiology | |
	Conventional Units	SI Units	Higher	Lower
Acetone			Diabetic ketoacidosis, high-fat diet, low-carbohydrate diet, starvation	
• Quantitative	<2.0 mg/dL	<344 μmol/L		
• Qualitative	Negative	Negative		
Albumin	3.5-5.0 g/dL	35-50 g/L	Dehydration	Chronic liver disease, malabsorption, malnutrition, nephrotic syndrome
Aldolase	1.5-8.1 U/L	1.5-8.1 U/L	Skeletal muscle disease	Renal disease
α₁-Antitrypsin	78-200 mg/dL	0.78-2.0 g/L	Acute and chronic inflammation, arthritis	Chronic lung disease (early onset), malnutrition, nephrotic syndrome
α₁-Fetoprotein	<10 ng/mL	<10 mcg/L	Cancer of testes, ovaries, and liver	
Ammonia	15-45 mcg N/dL	11-32 μmol N/L	Severe liver disease	
Amylase	30-122 U/L (method dependent)	0.51-2.07 μkat/L	Acute and chronic pancreatitis, mumps (salivary gland disease), perforated ulcers	Acute alcoholism, cirrhosis of liver, extensive destruction of pancreas
Bicarbonate	22-26 mEq/L	22-26 mmol/L	Compensated respiratory acidosis, metabolic alkalosis	Compensated respiratory alkalosis, metabolic acidosis
b-Type natriuretic peptide (BNP)	<100 pg/mL	<100 pmol/L	Heart failure	
Bilirubin			Biliary obstruction, impaired liver function, hemolytic anemia, pernicious anemia	
• Total	0.2-1.2 mg/dL	3-21 μmol/L		
• Indirect	0.1-1.0 mg/dL	1.7-17.0 μmol/L		
• Direct	0.1-0.3 mg/dL	1.7-5.1 μmol/L		

Continued

Reviewed by Julie Dittmer, RN, MSN, Eastern Iowa Community College, Bettendorf, Iowa.

TABLE C-1   SERUM, PLASMA, AND WHOLE BLOOD CHEMISTRIES—cont'd

Test	Reference Intervals		Possible Etiology	
	Conventional Units	**SI Units**	**Higher**	**Lower**
Blood gases*				
• Arterial pH	7.35-7.45	7.35-7.45	Alkalosis	Acidosis
• Venous pH	7.32-7.43	7.32-7.43		
• $PaCO_2$	35-45 mm Hg	4.66-5.98 kPa	Compensated metabolic alkalosis	Compensated metabolic acidosis
• $PvCO_2$	38-55 mm Hg	5.06-7.32 kPa	Respiratory acidosis	Respiratory alkalosis
• PaO_2	80-100 mm Hg	10.6-13.33 kPa	Administration of high	Chronic lung disease, decreased
• PvO_2	38-42 mm Hg	5.04-5.57 kPa	concentration of oxygen	cardiac output
Calcium (total)	8.6-10.2 mg/dL	2.15-2.55 mmol/L	Acute osteoporosis, hyperparathyroidism, vitamin D intoxication, multiple myeloma	Acute pancreatitis, hypoparathyroidism, liver disease, malabsorption syndrome, renal failure, vitamin D deficiency
Calcium (ionized)	4.64-5.28 mg/dL	1.16-1.32 mmol/L		
Carbon dioxide (CO_2)	23-29 mEq/L	23-29 mmol/L	Same as bicarbonate	
Carotene	10-85 mcg/dL	0.19-1.58 µmol/L	Cystic fibrosis, hypothyroidism, pancreatic insufficiency	Dietary deficiency, malabsorption disorders
Chloride	96-106 mEq/L	96-106 mmol/L	Metabolic acidosis, respiratory alkalosis, corticosteroid therapy, uremia	Addison's disease, diarrhea, metabolic alkalosis, respiratory acidosis, vomiting
Cholesterol	<200 mg/dL	<5.2 mmol/L	Biliary obstruction, hypothyroidism, idiopathic hypercholesterolemia, renal disease, uncontrolled diabetes	Extensive liver disease, hyperthyroidism, malnutrition, corticosteroid therapy
• High-density lipoproteins (HDLs)	Male: >40 mg/dL Female: >50 mg/dL	>1.04 mmol/L >1.3 mmol/L		

• Low-density lipoproteins (LDLs)	*Recommended:*
	  <100 mg/dL
	Near optimal:
	  100-129 mg/dL
	  (2.6-3.34 mmol/L)
	Moderate risk for CAD:
	  130-159 mg/dL
	  (3.37-4.12 mmol/L)
	High risk for CAD:
	  >160 mg/dL
	  (>4.14 mmol/L)
		Recommended:
		  <2.6 mmol/L
		Near optimal:
		  2.6-3.34 mmol/L
		
		Moderate risk for CAD:
		  3.37-4.12 mmol/L
		
		High risk for CAD:
		  >4.14 mmol/L		

Copper	80-155 mcg/dL	12.6-24.3 µmol/L	Cirrhosis	Wilson's disease
Cortisol	8 AM: 5-23 mcg/dL 8 PM: <10 mcg/dL	0.14-0.63 µmol/L <0.28 µmol/L	Cushing syndrome, pancreatitis	Adrenal insufficiency, panhypopituitary states
Creatine	0.2-1.0 mg/dL	15.3-76.3 µmol/L	Active rheumatoid arthritis, biliary obstruction, hyperthyroidism, renal disorders, severe muscle disease	Diabetes mellitus
Creatine kinase (CK)	*Male:* 20-200 U/L *Female:* 20-180 U/L	Male: 20-200 U/L Female: 20-180 U/L	Musculoskeletal injury or disease, myocardial infarction, severe myocarditis, exercise, numerous IM injections	
• CK-MB	<4%-6% of total CK	<0.4-0.6	Acute myocardial infarction	
Creatinine	0.6-1.3 mg/dL	53-115 µmol/L	Severe renal disease	
Ferritin	10-250 ng/mL	10-250 mcg/L	Sideroblastic anemia, anemia of chronic disease (infection, inflammation, liver disease)	Iron-deficiency anemia
Folate (folic acid)	5-16 ng/mL	11-36 nmol/L	Hypothyroidism	Alcoholism, hemolytic anemia, inadequate diet, malabsorption syndrome, megaloblastic anemia
Gamma-glutamyl transferase (GGT)	0-30 U/L	0-0.5 µkat/L	Liver disease, infectious mononucleosis, pancreatitis, hyperthyroidism	Hypothyroidism
Glucose (fasting)	70-99 mg/dL	3.9-5.5 mmol/L	Acute stress, Cushing disease, diabetes mellitus, hyperthyroidism, pancreatic insufficiency	Addison's disease, hepatic disease, hypothyroidism, insulin overdosage, pancreatic tumor, pituitary hypofunction
Haptoglobin	26-185 mg/dL	260-1850 mg/L	Infectious and inflammatory processes, malignant neoplasms	Hemolytic anemia, mononucleosis, toxoplasmosis, chronic liver disease

TABLE C-1   SERUM, PLASMA, AND WHOLE BLOOD CHEMISTRIES—cont'd

	Reference Intervals		Possible Etiology	
Test	Conventional Units	SI Units	Higher	Lower
Insulin (fasting)	4-24 µU/mL	29-172 pmol/L	Acromegaly, adenoma of pancreatic islet cells, untreated mild case of type 2 diabetes	Inadequately treated type 1 diabetes mellitus
Iron, total	50-175 mcg/dL	9.0-31.3 µmol/L	Excessive RBC destruction	Iron-deficiency anemia, anemia of chronic disease
Iron-binding capacity	250-425 mcg/dL	44.8-76.1 µmol/L	Iron-deficient state, polycythemia	Cancer, chronic infections, pernicious anemia
Lactic acid (L-Lactate)	6.3-22.5 mcg/dL	0.7-2.5 mmol/L	Acidosis, heart failure, shock	
Lactic dehydrogenase (LDH)	140-280 U/L	0.83-2.5 µkat/L	Heart failure, hemolytic disorders, hepatitis, metastatic cancer of liver, myocardial infarction, pernicious anemia, pulmonary embolus, skeletal muscle damage	
Lactic dehydrogenase isoenzymes				
• LDH₁	18%-33%	0.18-0.33	Myocardial infarction, pernicious anemia	
• LDH₂	28%-40%	0.28-0.40	Pulmonary embolus, sickle cell crisis	
• LDH₃	18%-30%	0.18-0.30	Malignant lymphoma, pulmonary embolus	
• LDH₄	6%-16%	0.06-0.16	Systemic lupus erythematosus, pulmonary infarction	
• LDH₅	2%-13%	0.02-0.13	Heart failure, hepatitis, pulmonary embolus and infarction, skeletal muscle damage	
Lipase	31-186 U/L	0.5-3.2 µkat/L	Acute pancreatitis, hepatic disorders, perforated peptic ulcer	
Magnesium	1.5-2.5 mEq/L	0.75-1.25 mmol/L	Addison's disease, hypothyroidism, renal failure	Chronic alcoholism, severe malabsorption
Osmolality	275-295 mOsm/kg	275-295 mmol/kg	Chronic renal disease, diabetes mellitus	Addison's disease, diuretic therapy
Oxygen saturation (arterial) (SaO₂)	>95%	>0.95	Polycythemia	Anemia, cardiac decompensation, respiratory disorders
pH	See Blood gases			
Phenylalanine	0.8-1.8 mg/dL	48-109 µmol/L	Phenylketonuria	
Phosphatase, acid	0-0.6 U/L	0-90 µkat/L	Advanced Paget's disease, cancer of prostate, hyperparathyroidism	
Phosphatase, alkaline	38-126 U/L	0.65-2.14 µkat/L	Bone diseases, marked hyperparathyroidism, obstruction of biliary system, rickets	Excessive vitamin D ingestion, hypothyroidism
Phosphorus (phosphate)	2.4-4.4 mg/dL	0.78-1.42 mmol/L	Healing fractures, hypoparathyroidism, renal disease, vitamin D intoxication	Diabetes mellitus, hyperparathyroidism, vitamin D deficiency
Potassium	3.5-5.0 mEq/L	3.5-5.0 mmol/L	Addison's disease, diabetic ketosis, massive tissue destruction, renal failure	Cushing syndrome, diarrhea (severe), diuretic therapy, gastrointestinal fistula, pyloric obstruction, starvation, vomiting
Progesterone (Female)				
• Follicular phase	15-70 ng/dL	0.5-2.2 nmol/L	Adrenal hyperplasia, choriocarcinoma of ovary, pregnancy, cysts of ovary	Threatened abortion, hypogonadism, amenorrhea, ovarian tumor
• Luteal phase	200-2500 ng/dL	6.4-79.5 nmol/L		
• Postmenopause	<40 ng/dL	1.28 nmol/L		
Prostate-specific antigen (PSA)	<4 ng/mL	<4 mcg/L	Prostate cancer	

Continued

TABLE C-1   SERUM, PLASMA, AND WHOLE BLOOD CHEMISTRIES—cont'd

Test	Reference Intervals Conventional Units	Reference Intervals SI Units	Possible Etiology Higher	Possible Etiology Lower
Proteins			Burns, cirrhosis (globulin fraction), dehydration	Liver disease, malabsorption
• Total	6.4-8.3 g/dL	64-83 g/L		
• Albumin	3.5-5.0 g/dL	35-50 g/L		
• Globulin	2.0-3.5 g/dL	20-35 g/L		
• Albumin/globulin ratio	1.5:1-2.5:1	1.5:1-2.5:1	Multiple myeloma (globulin fraction), shock, vomiting	Malnutrition, nephrotic syndrome, proteinuria, renal disease, severe burns
Sodium	135-145 mEq/L	135-145 mmol/L	Dehydration, impaired renal function, primary aldosteronism, corticosteroid therapy	Addison's disease, diabetic ketoacidosis, diuretic therapy, excessive loss from GI tract, excessive perspiration, water intoxication
Testosterone	Male: 280-1100 ng/dL	Male: 10.4-38.17 nmol/L		Hypofunction of testes, hypogonadism
	Female: 15-70 ng/dL	Female: 0.52-2.43 nmol/L	Polycystic ovary, virilizing tumors	
T_4 (thyroxine), total	4.6-11.0 mcg/dL	59-142 nmol/L	Hyperthyroidism, thyroiditis	Cretinism, hypothyroidism, myxedema
T_4 (thyroxine), free	0.8-2.7 ng/dL	10-35 pmol/L		
T_3 uptake	24%-34%	0.24-0.34	Hyperthyroidism	Hypothyroidism
T_3 (triiodothyronine), total	Ages 20-50: 70-204 ng/dL	1.08-3.14 nmol/L	Hyperthyroidism	Hypothyroidism
	Ages >50: 40-181 ng/dL	0.62-2.79 nmol/L		
Thyroid-stimulating hormone (TSH)	0.4-4.2 µU/mL	0.4-4.2 mU/L	Myxedema, primary hypothyroidism, Graves' disease	Secondary hypothyroidism
Transaminases				
• Aspartate aminotransferase (AST)	10-30 U/L	0.17-0.51 µkat/L	Liver disease, myocardial infarction, pulmonary infarction, acute hepatitis	
• Alanine aminotransferase (ALT)	10-40 U/L	0.17-0.68 µkat/L	Liver disease, shock	
Transferrin	190-380 mg/dL	1.9-3.8 g/L		
Transferrin saturation (%)	15%-50%	15%-50%		
Triglycerides	<150 mg/dL	<1.7 mmol/L	Diabetes mellitus, hyperlipidemia, hypothyroidism, liver disease	Malnutrition
Troponins (cardiac)			Myocardial infarction	
• Troponin T (cTnT)	<0.5 ng/mL (<0.5 mcg/L)			
• Troponin I (cTnI)	<0.1 ng/mL (<0.1 mcg/L)			
Urea nitrogen (BUN)	6-20 mg/dL	2.1-7.1 mmol/L	Increase in protein catabolism (fever, stress), renal disease, urinary tract infection	Malnutrition, severe liver damage
Uric acid	Male: 4.4-7.6 mg/dL	Male: 262-452 µmol/L	Gout, gross tissue destruction, high-protein weight reduction diet, leukemia, renal failure	Administration of uricosuric drugs
	Female: 2.3-6.6 mg/dL	Female: 137-393 µmol/L		
Vitamin A (retinol)	30-80 mcg/dL	1.05-2.80 µmol/L	Excess ingestion of vitamin A	Vitamin A deficiency
Vitamin B_{12} (cobalamin)	200-835 pg/mL	148-616 pmol/L	Chronic myeloid leukemia	Strict vegetarianism, malabsorption syndrome, pernicious anemia, total or partial gastrectomy
Vitamin C (ascorbic acid)	0.4-2.0 mg/dL	23-114 µmol/L	Excessive ingestion of vitamin C	Connective tissue disorders, hepatic disease, renal disease, rheumatic fever, vitamin C deficiency
Zinc	70-120 mcg/dL	10.7-120 µmol/L		Alcoholic cirrhosis

*Because arterial blood gases are influenced by altitude, the value for PaO_2 decreases as altitude increases. The lower value is normal for an altitude of 1 mile.

$PaCO_2$, Partial pressure of CO_2 in arterial blood; $PvCO_2$, partial pressure of CO_2 in venous blood; PaO_2, partial pressure of oxygen in arterial blood; PvO_2, partial pressure of oxygen in venous blood; RBC, red blood cell; SaO_2, arterial oxygen saturation.

TABLE C-2 HEMATOLOGY

Test	Reference Intervals		Possible Etiology	
	Conventional Units	**SI Units**	**Higher**	**Lower**
Bleeding time	2-7 min	120-420 sec	Defective platelet function, thrombocytopenia, von Willebrand disease, aspirin ingestion, vascular disease	
Activated partial thromboplastin time (aPTT)	25-35 sec*	25-35 sec*	Deficiency factors I, II, V, VIII, IX, X, XI, XII; hemophilia, liver disease; heparin therapy	
Prothrombin time (Protime, PT)	11-16 sec*	11-16 sec*	Warfarin therapy; deficiency of factors I, II, V, VII, and X; vitamin K deficiency; liver disease	
Fibrinogen	200-400 mg/dL	2-4 g/L	Burns (after first 36 hr), inflammatory disease	Burns (during first 36 hr), DIC, severe liver disease
Fibrin split (degradation) products	<10 mcg/mL	<10 mg/L	Acute DIC, massive hemorrhage, primary fibrinolysis	
D-Dimer	<250 ng/mL	<250 mcg/L	DIC, myocardial infarction, deep vein thrombosis, unstable angina	
Erythrocyte count† (altitude dependent)	*Male:* 4.3-5.7 × 10⁶/μL *Female:* 3.8-5.1 × 10⁶/μL	*Male:* 4.3-5.7 × 10¹²/L *Female:* 3.8-5.1 × 10¹²/L	Dehydration, high altitudes, polycythemia vera	Anemia, leukemia, posthemorrhage
Red blood indices				
• Mean corpuscular volume (MCV)	80-100 fL	80-100 fL	Macrocytic anemia	Microcytic anemia
• Mean corpuscular hemoglobin (MCH)	27-34 pg	27-34 pg	Macrocytic anemia	Microcytic anemia
• Mean corpuscular hemoglobin concentration (MCHC)	32%-37%	0.32-0.37	Spherocytosis	Hypochromic anemia
Erythrocyte sedimentation rate (ESR)	<30 mm/hr (some gender variation)	<30 mm/hr (some gender variation)	*Moderate increase:* acute hepatitis, myocardial infarction; rheumatoid arthritis *Marked increase:* acute and severe bacterial infections, malignancies, pelvic inflammatory disease	Malaria, severe liver disease, sickle cell anemia
Hematocrit† (altitude dependent)	*Male:* 39%-50% *Female:* 35%-47%	*Male:* 0.39-0.50 *Female:* 0.35-0.47	Dehydration, high altitudes, polycythemia	Anemia, hemorrhage, overhydration
Hemoglobin† (altitude dependent)	*Male:* 13.2-17.3 g/dL *Female:* 11.7-15.5 g/dL	*Male:* 132-173 g/L *Female:* 117-155 g/L	COPD, high altitudes, polycythemia	Anemia, hemorrhage
Hemoglobin, glycosylated (A1C)	4.0%-6.0%	4.0%-6.0%	Poorly controlled diabetes mellitus	Sickle cell anemia, chronic renal failure, pregnancy
Platelets (thrombocytes)	150-400 × 10³/μL	150-400 × 10⁹/L	Acute infections, chronic granulocytic leukemia, chronic pancreatitis, cirrhosis, collagen disorders, polycythemia, postsplenectomy	Acute leukemia, DIC, thrombocytopenic purpura
Reticulocyte count	0.5%-1.5% of RBC	0.5%-1.5% of RBC	Hemolytic anemia, polycythemia vera	Hypoproliferative anemia, macrocytic anemia, microcytic anemia
White blood cell count†	4.0-11.0 × 10³/μL	4.0-11.0 × 10⁹/L	Inflammatory and infectious processes, leukemia	Aplastic anemia, side effects of chemotherapy and irradiation
WBC differential				
• Segmented neutrophils	50%-70%	0.50-0.70	Bacterial infections, collagen diseases, Hodgkin's lymphoma	Aplastic anemia, viral infections
• Band neutrophils	0%-8%	0-0.08	Acute infections	
• Lymphocytes	20%-40%	0.20-0.40	Chronic infections, lymphocytic leukemia, mononucleosis, viral infections	Corticosteroid therapy, whole body irradiation
• Monocytes	4%-8%	0.04-0.08	Chronic inflammatory disorders, malaria, monocytic leukemia, acute infections, Hodgkin's lymphoma	
• Eosinophils	0%-4%	0-0.04	Allergic reactions, eosinophilic and chronic granulocytic leukemia, parasitic disorders, Hodgkin's lymphoma	Corticosteroid therapy
• Basophils	0%-2%	0-0.02	Hypothyroidism, ulcerative colitis, myeloproliferative diseases	Hyperthyroidism, stress

*Values depend on reagent and instrumentation used.
†Components of complete blood count (CBC).
COPD, Chronic obstructive pulmonary disease; *DIC,* disseminated intravascular coagulation; *RBC,* red blood cell; *WBC,* white blood cell.

TABLE C-3   SEROLOGY-IMMUNOLOGY

Test	Reference Intervals		Possible Etiology	
	Conventional Units	**SI Units**	**Higher**	**Lower**
Antinuclear antibody (ANA)	Negative at 1:40 dilution	Negative at 1:40 dilution	Chronic hepatitis, rheumatoid arthritis, scleroderma, systemic lupus erythematosus	
Anti-DNA antibody	<70 IU/mL	<70 IU/mL	Systemic lupus erythematosus	
Anti-Sm (Smith)	Negative	Negative	Systemic lupus erythematosus	
C-reactive protein (CRP)	6.8-820 mcg/dL	68-8200 mcg/L	Acute infections, any inflammatory condition, widespread malignancy	
Carcinoembryonic antigen (CEA)	*Nonsmoker:* <3 ng/mL *Smoker:* <5 ng/mL	*Nonsmoker:* <3 mcg/L *Smoker:* <5 mcg/L	Carcinoma of colon, liver, pancreas; chronic cigarette smoking; inflammatory bowel disease; other cancers	
Complement, total hemolytic (CH$_{50}$)	75-160 U/mL	75-160 kU/L		Acute glomerulonephritis, systemic lupus erythematosus, rheumatoid arthritis, subacute bacterial endocarditis
Direct Coombs or direct antihuman globulin test (DAT)	Negative	Negative	Acquired hemolytic anemia, drug reactions, transfusion reactions	
Fluorescent treponemal antibody absorption (FTA-Abs)	Negative or nonreactive	Negative or nonreactive	Syphilis	
Hepatitis A antibody	Negative	Negative	Hepatitis A	
Hepatitis B surface antigen (HB$_s$Ag)	Negative	Negative	Hepatitis B	
Hepatitis C antibody	Negative	Negative	Hepatitis C	
Monospot or monotest	Negative	Negative	Infectious mononucleosis	
Rheumatoid factor (RF)	Negative or titer <1:17	Negative or titer <1:17	Rheumatoid arthritis, Sjögren's syndrome, systemic lupus erythematosus	
RPR	Negative or nonreactive	Negative or nonreactive	Syphilis, systemic lupus erythematosus, rheumatoid arthritis, leprosy, malaria, febrile diseases, IV drug abuse	
VDRL	Negative or nonreactive	Negative or nonreactive	Syphilis	

RPR, Rapid plasma regain test; *VDRL,* Veneral Disease Research Laboratory test.

TABLE C-4 URINE CHEMISTRY

Test	Specimen	Reference Intervals Units	Reference Intervals SI Units	Possible Etiology Higher	Possible Etiology Lower
Acetone	Random	Negative	Negative	Diabetes mellitus, high-fat and low-carbohydrate diets, starvation	
Aldosterone	24 hr	3-30 mcg/day (low sodium diet increases threefold to fivefold)	0.08-0.83 nmol/day	*Primary aldosteronism:* adrenocortical tumors *Secondary aldosteronism:* cardiac failure, cirrhosis, large dose of ACTH, salt depletion	ACTH deficiency, Addison's disease, corticosteroid therapy
Amylase	24 hr	1-17 U/hr	1-17 U/hr	Acute pancreatitis	
Bence Jones protein	Random	Negative	Negative	Multiple myeloma	
Bilirubin	Random	Negative	Negative	Liver disorders	
Calcium	24 hr	100-250 mg/day	2.5-6.3 mmol/day	Bone tumor, hyperparathyroidism	Hypoparathyroidism, malabsorption of calcium and vitamin D
Catecholamines	24 hr			Pheochromocytoma, progressive muscular dystrophy, heart failure	
• Epinephrine		<20 mcg/day	<109 nmol/day		
• Norepinephrine		15-80 mcg/day	89-473 nmol/day		
Creatine	24 hr	<100 mg/day	<763 µmol/day	Liver cancer, hyperthyroidism, diabetes, Addison's disease, infections, burns, muscular dystrophy, skeletal muscle atrophy	Hypothyroidism
Creatinine	24 hr	0.6-2.0 g/day	5.3-17.7 mmol/day	Anemia, leukemia, muscular atrophy	Renal disease
Creatinine clearance	24 hr	59-137 mL/min/1.73 m²	0.59-1.37 mL/sec/m²		Renal disease
Estrogens	24 hr				
• Female				Gonadal or adrenal tumor	Endocrine disturbance, ovarian dysfunction, menopause
• Premenopause		15-80 mcg/day	15-80 mcg/day		
• Postmenopause		<20 mcg/day	<20 mcg/day		
• Male		15-40 mcg/day	15-40 mcg/day		
Glucose	Random	Negative	Negative	Diabetes mellitus, pituitary disorders	
Hemoglobin	Random	Negative	Negative	Extensive burns, glomerulonephritis, hemolytic anemias, hemolytic transfusion reaction	
5-Hydroxyindole acetic acid (5-HIAA)	24 hr	2-7 mg/day	10.5-36.6 µmol/day	Malignant carcinoid syndrome	
Ketone bodies	24 hr	20-50 mg/day	0.34-0.86 mmol/day	Diabetes mellitus, starvation, dehydration	
Metanephrine	24 hr	92-934 mcg/day	500-5100 nmol/day	Pheochromocytoma	
Myoglobin	Random	Negative	Negative	Crushing injuries, electric injuries, extreme physical exertion	
Osmolality	Random	300-1300 mOsm/kg	300-1300 mmol/kg	Dehydration, tubular dysfunction (kidney lost ability to dilute urine)	Tubular dysfunction (kidney lost ability to concentrate urine)
pH	Random	4.0-8.0	4.0-8.0	Urinary tract infection, urine allowed to stand at room temperature	Respiratory or metabolic acidosis
Protein (dipstick)	Random	0-trace	0-trace	Acute and chronic renal disease, especially involving glomeruli; heart failure	
Protein (quantitative)	24 hr	<150 mg/day	<0.15 g/day	Cardiac failure, inflammatory processes of urinary tract, nephritis, nephrosis, strenuous exercise	
Sodium	24 hr	40-220 mEq/day	40-220 mmol/day	Acute tubular necrosis	Hyponatremia
Specific gravity	Random	1.003-1.030	Same as conventional units	Albuminuria, dehydration, glycosuria	Diabetes insipidus
Uric acid	24 hr	250-750 mg/day	1.5-4.5 mmol/day	Gout, leukemia	Nephritis
Urobilinogen	24 hr	0.5-4.0 mg/day	0.8-6.8 µmol/day	Hemolytic disease, hepatic parenchymal cell damage, liver disease	Complete obstruction of bile duct
Vanillylmandelic acid	24 hr	1.4-6.5 mg/day	7-33 µmol/day	Pheochromocytoma	

ACTH, Adrenocorticotropic hormone.

TABLE C-5   FECAL ANALYSIS

| Test | Reference Intervals | | Possible Etiology |
	Conventional Units	SI Units	Higher
Fecal fat	<6 g/24 hr	Same as conventional units	Chronic pancreatic disease, obstruction of common bile duct, malabsorption syndrome
Mucus	Negative	Negative	Mucous colitis, spastic constipation
Pus	Negative	Negative	Chronic bacillary dysentery, chronic ulcerative colitis, localized abscesses
Blood*	Negative	Negative	Anal fissures, hemorrhoids, malignant tumor, peptic ulcer, inflammatory bowel disease
Color			
• Brown			Various color depending on diet
• Clay			Biliary obstruction or presence of barium sulfate
• Tarry			More than 100 mL of blood in gastrointestinal tract
• Red			Blood in large intestine
• Black			Blood in upper gastrointestinal tract or iron medication

*Ingestion of meat may produce false-positive results. Patient may be placed on a meat-free diet for 3 days before the test.

TABLE C-6   CEREBROSPINAL FLUID ANALYSIS

| Test | Reference Intervals | | Possible Etiology | |
	Conventional Units	SI Units	Higher	Lower
Pressure	60-150 mm H_2O	60-150 mm H_2O	Hemorrhage, intracranial tumor, meningitis	Head injury, spinal tumor, subdural hematoma
Blood	Negative	Negative	Intracranial hemorrhage	
Cell count (age dependent)			Inflammation or infections of CNS	
• WBC	0-5 cells/μL	$0\text{-}5 \times 10^6$ cells/L		
• RBC	Negative	Negative		
Chloride	118-132 mEq/L	118-132 mmol/L	Uremia	Bacterial infections of CNS (meningitis, encephalitis)
Glucose	40-70 mg/dL	2.2-3.9 mmol/L	Diabetes mellitus, viral infections of CNS	Bacterial infections and tuberculosis of CNS
Protein				
• Lumbar	15-45 mg/dL	0.15-0.45 g/L	Guillain-Barré syndrome, poliomyelitis, trauma	
• Cisternal	15-25 mg/dL	0.15-0.25 g/L	Syphilis of CNS	
• Ventricular	5-15 mg/dL	0.05-0.15 g/L	Acute meningitis, brain tumor, chronic CNS infections, multiple sclerosis	

CNS, Central nervous system.

A

absence (petit mal) seizure seizure characterized by a brief staring spell and a very brief loss of consciousness that usually occurs only in children and rarely continues beyond adolescence.

acromegaly a condition caused by excessive secretion of growth hormone characterized by an overgrowth of the bones and soft tissues.

actinic keratosis a slowly developing, localized thickening and scaling of the outer layers of the skin consisting of hyperkeratotic papules and plaques as a result of chronic, prolonged exposure to the sun; also known as solar keratosis.

acute bronchitis an inflammation of the lower respiratory tract that is usually due to infection.

acute hepatic failure a clinical syndrome characterized by severe impairment of liver function associated with hepatic encephalopathy; also referred to as acute liver failure.

acute kidney injury (AKI) clinical syndrome characterized by a rise in serum creatinine and/or a reduction in urine output.

acute lung injury (ALI) a condition that occurs when the patient's PaO_2/FIO_2 ratio is 200–300 (e.g., 86/0.4 = 215).

acute pancreatitis an acute inflammatory process of the pancreas caused by autodigestion and marked by symptoms of an acute condition of the abdomen and escape of pancreatic enzymes into the pancreatic tissues.

acute respiratory distress syndrome (ARDS) a sudden and progressive form of acute respiratory failure in which the alveolar-capillary membrane becomes damaged and more permeable to intravascular fluid.

acute tubular necrosis (ATN) a type of intrarenal acute injury of the kidney that affects the renal tubules, caused by renal ischemia and nephrotoxic injury.

adhesion a band of scar tissue between or around organs.

adventitious sounds extra breath sounds that are not normally heard, such as crackles, rhonchi, wheezes, and pleural friction rubs.

afterload the peripheral resistance against which the left ventricle must pump.

allergic rhinitis the reaction of the nasal mucosa to a specific allergen.

alopecia partial or complete lack of hair resulting from normal aging, endocrine disorder, drug reaction, anticancer medication, or skin disease.

Alzheimer's disease (AD) a chronic, progressive, degenerative disease of the brain.

amyotrophic lateral sclerosis (ALS) a rare progressive neurologic disorder characterized by loss of motor neurons and by weakness and atrophy of the muscles of the hands, forearms, and legs, spreading to involve most of the body and face.

anaphylactic shock an acute and life-threatening hypersensitivity (allergic) reaction to a sensitizing substance, such as a drug, chemical, vaccine, food, or insect venom.

aneurysm congenital or acquired weakness of the arterial wall resulting in dilation and ballooning of the vessel.

angina chest pain that is a clinical manifestation of reversible myocardial ischemia.

ankylosing spondylitis a chronic inflammatory disease that primarily affects the axial skeleton, including the sacroiliac joints, intervertebral disc spaces, and costovertebral articulations.

ankylosis stiffness or fixation of a joint usually resulting from destruction of articular cartilage and subchondral bone.

aortic dissection the result of a tear in the intimal (innermost) lining of the arterial wall that allows blood to enter between the intima and media, thus creating a false lumen.

aphasia an abnormal neurologic condition in which language function is disordered or absent because of an injury to certain areas of the cerebral cortex.

aplastic anemia a disease with a deficiency of all of the formed elements of blood (specifically red blood cells, white blood cells, and platelets), representing a failure of the cell-generating capacity of bone marrow.

appendicitis an inflammation of the appendix that, if undiagnosed, leads rapidly to perforation and peritonitis.

arterial blood pressure a measure of the pressure exerted by blood against the walls of the arterial system.

arteriovenous fistula (AVF) type of vascular access created most commonly in the forearm with an anastomosis between an artery (usually radial or ulnar) and a vein (usually cephalic).

arteriovenous grafts (AVGs) fistula made of synthetic materials that forms a "bridge" between the arterial and venous blood supplies.

arthritis inflammation of a joint; most prevalent types are osteoarthritis, rheumatoid arthritis, and gout.

arthrocentesis incision or puncture of joint capsule to obtain samples of synovial fluid from within joint cavity or to remove excess fluid.

arthrodesis the surgical fusion of a joint.

arthroplasty surgical reconstruction or replacement of a joint.

arthroscopy insertion of an arthroscope into a joint for visualization or surgery.

ascites an abnormal intraperitoneal accumulation of a fluid containing large amounts of protein and electrolytes as a result of portal hypertension.

asterixis flapping tremor (liver flap) commonly affecting the arms and hands that is a manifestation of hepatic encephalopathy.

asthma a chronic inflammatory lung disease that results in airflow obstruction; characterized by recurring episodes of paroxysmal dyspnea, wheezing on expiration, and/or inspiration caused by constriction of the bronchi, coughing, and viscous mucoid bronchial secretions.

asystole represents the total absence of ventricular electrical activity.

atelectasis an abnormal condition characterized by the collapse of alveoli, preventing the respiratory exchange of carbon dioxide and oxygen in a part of the lungs.

atherosclerosis formation of focal deposits of cholesterol and lipids known as atheromas or plaque, primarily within the intimal wall of arteries, that obstruct circulation.

atrial fibrillation a cardiac dysrhythmia characterized by a total disorganization of atrial electrical activity without effective atrial contraction.

atrial flutter an atrial tachydysrhythmia identified by recurring, regular, sawtooth-shaped flutter waves.

atrophy wasting of muscle, characterized by decreased circumference and flabby appearance leading to decreased function and tone.

aura a sensation of light or warmth or other perception that may be a warning of an attack of a migraine or an epileptic seizure.

auscultation the act of listening for sounds within the body to evaluate the condition of the heart, blood vessels, lungs, pleura, intestines, or other organs.

autoimmunity an inappropriate immune reaction to self-proteins.

azotemia an accumulation of nitrogenous waste products such as blood urea nitrogen (BUN) and creatinine.

B

bariatric surgery a surgical procedure used to treat severe obesity.

Barrett's esophagus a precancerous esophageal disorder characterized by metaplastic cell changes.

basal cell carcinoma a malignant epithelial cell tumor arising from epidermal basal cells that begins as a papule and enlarges peripherally, developing a central crater that erodes, crusts, and bleeds.

Bell's palsy a disorder characterized by a disruption of the motor branches of the facial nerve (cranial nerve [CN] VII) on one side of the face in the absence of any other disease such as a stroke.

benign prostatic hyperplasia (BPH) a nonmalignant, noninflammatory enlargement of the prostate gland caused by an increase in the number of epithelial cells and stromal tissue.

biologic therapy treatment using biologic agents such as interferons, interleukins, monoclonal antibodies, and growth factors to modify the relationship between the host and tumor.

borborygmi audible abdominal sounds produced by hyperactive intestinal peristalsis.

botulism a serious food poisoning caused by GI absorption of the neurotoxin produced by *Clostridium botulinum* that results in disturbed muscle innervation.

brachytherapy radiation delivery system that means "closed" treatment and consists of the implantation or insertion of radioactive materials directly into the tumor or in close proximity to the tumor.

brain abscess   an accumulation of pus within the brain tissue that can result from a local or a systemic infection from another source, such as the skull, sinuses, or other structures in the head.

brain attack   term used to describe a stroke.

brain death   a clinical diagnosis of an irreversible loss of all brain functions, including those of the brainstem.

bursitis   inflammation of the bursa.

C

calculus   an abnormal stone formed in body tissues by an accumulation of mineral salts.

carboxyhemoglobinemia   the presence of carboxyhemoglobin in the blood; occurs with carbon monoxide poisoning.

carcinogens   agents capable of producing cellular alterations leading to the development or increasing the incidence of neoplastic growth.

carcinoma in situ   a lesion with all the histologic features of cancer except invasion.

cardiac index (CI)   a measure of the cardiac output of a patient per square meter of body surface area.

cardiac output (CO)   the amount of blood pumped by each ventricle in 1 minute.

cardiac pacemaker   an electronic device used to increase the heart rate in severe bradycardia by electrically stimulating the heart muscle.

cardiac reserve   the ability to respond to demands (exercise, stress, hypovolemia) by altering cardiac output threefold or fourfold.

cardiac tamponade   compression of the heart produced by fluid accumulation in the pericardial sac.

cardiogenic shock   shock occurring when either systolic or diastolic dysfunction of the myocardium results in compromised cardiac output.

cardiomyopathy   a group of diseases that directly affect the structural or functional ability of the myocardium.

carpal tunnel syndrome   a condition caused by compression of the median nerve beneath the transverse carpal ligament within the narrow confines of the carpal tunnel located in the wrist.

cataract   an abnormal progressive condition of the lens of the eye characterized by an opacity within the lens.

celiac disease   an inborn error of metabolism characterized by the inability to hydrolyze peptides contained in gluten.

cell-mediated immunity   immunity that is initiated through specific antigen recognition by T lymphocytes, monocytes/macrophages, and natural killer cells.

cellulitis   a diffuse, acute bacterial infection of the skin and subcutaneous tissue characterized most commonly by local heat, redness, pain, and swelling.

central cord syndrome   damage to the central spinal cord characterized by microscopic hemorrhage, edema of the central spinal cord, and compression on anterior horn cells.

cerebral edema   increased accumulation of fluid in the extravascular spaces of brain tissue that can lead to increased intracranial pressure.

chancre   painless indurated lesions found on the penis, vulva, lips, mouth, vagina, and rectum characteristic of syphilis.

cheilosis   a disorder of the lips and mouth characterized by bilateral scales and fissures, resulting from a deficiency of riboflavin in the diet.

chemotherapy   the treatment of disease with chemical agents.

Cheyne-Stokes respiration   an abnormal breathing pattern characterized by alternating periods of apnea and deep, rapid breathing; usually seen as a person nears death.

cholecystitis   inflammation of the gallbladder.

cholelithiasis   stones in the gallbladder.

chronic bronchitis   obstructive pulmonary disease characterized by excessive production of mucus and chronic inflammatory changes in the bronchi.

chronic fatigue syndrome (CFS)   a disorder characterized by debilitating fatigue and a variety of associated complaints.

chronic kidney disease (CKD)   the presence of kidney damage or decreased glomerular filtration rate for at least 3 months with functional or structural abnormalities, with or without decreased glomerular filtration rate.

chronic kidney disease (CKD) mineral and bone disorder   a systemic disorder of mineral and bone metabolism due to progressive deterioration in kidney function.

chronic pancreatitis   progressive destruction of the pancreas with fibrotic replacement of pancreatic tissue.

chronic stable angina   chest pain that occurs intermittently over a long period with the same pattern of onset, duration, and intensity of symptoms.

cirrhosis   chronic progressive disease of the liver characterized by extensive degeneration and destruction of the liver parenchymal cells.

cluster headaches   repeated headaches that can occur for weeks to months at a time, followed by periods of remission.

collateral circulation   development of arterial branching that occurs within the coronary circulation when occlusion of the coronary arteries occurs slowly over a long period.

coma   a profound state of unconsciousness.

community-acquired pneumonia (CAP)   a lower respiratory tract infection of the lung parenchyma with onset in the community or during the first 2 days of hospitalization.

compartment syndrome   a condition in which elevated intracompartmental pressure within a confined myofascial compartment compromises the neurovascular function of tissues within that space.

complete heart block   third-degree atrioventricular heart block in which no impulses from the atria are conducted to the ventricles.

concussion   a sudden transient mechanical head injury, such as a blow or explosion, with disruption of neural activity and a change in the level of consciousness.

continuous renal replacement therapy (CRRT) provides a means by which solutes and fluids can be removed slowly and continuously in the hemodynamically unstable patient.

contracture   an abnormal, usually permanent condition of a joint, characterized by flexion and fixation.

contusion   the bruising of the brain tissue within a focal area without altering the integrity of the pia mater and arachnoid layers.

coronary artery disease (CAD)   an abnormal condition that may affect the heart's arteries and produce various pathologic effects, especially the reduced flow of oxygen and nutrients to the myocardium.

cor pulmonale   hypertrophy of the right side of the heart, with or without heart failure, resulting from pulmonary hypertension.

crackle   short, low-pitched sound consisting of discontinuous bubbling caused by air passing through the airway intermittently occluded by mucus, an unstable bronchial wall, or a fold of mucosa.

crepitation   crackling sound or grating sensation as a result of friction between bones.

cretinism   hypothyroidism that develops in infancy.

cryosurgery   the use of subfreezing temperatures to perform surgery.

curettage   scraping of material from the wall of a cavity or other surface; performed to remove tumors or other abnormal tissue or to obtain tissue.

Cushing syndrome   a metabolic disorder resulting from the chronic and excessive production of cortisol by the adrenal cortex or by the administration of glucocorticoids in large doses for several weeks or longer.

cystic fibrosis (CF)   an autosomal recessive, multisystem disease characterized by altered function of the exocrine glands involving primarily the lungs, pancreas, and sweat glands.

cystitis   an inflammatory condition of the urinary bladder characterized by pain, urgency, frequency of urination, and hematuria.

cystocele   herniation or protrusion of the urinary bladder through the wall of the vagina, resulting from weakened connective tissue support between the vagina and bladder.

D

death rattle   a sound produced by air moving through mucus that has accumulated in the throat of a dying person who has lost the cough reflex.

debridement   removal of dirt, foreign objects, damaged tissue, and cellular debris from a wound or a burn to prevent infection and promote healing.

deep vein thrombosis (DVT)   a disorder involving a thrombus in a deep vein; most commonly the iliac and femoral veins.

degenerative disc disease (DDD)   progressive degeneration that is a normal process of aging; results in the intervertebral discs losing their elasticity, flexibility, and shock-absorbing capabilities.

dehiscence   the separation and disruption of previously joined wound edges, typically an abdominal incision.

delirium   a state of temporary but acute mental confusion.

dementia a syndrome caused by brain disease, evidenced by chronic personality disintegration, confusion, memory impairment, and deterioration of intellectual capacity and function.

dermatomyositis a disease of the connective tissues characterized by pruritic or eczematous inflammation of the skin and tenderness of the muscles.

diabetes insipidus (DI) a group of conditions associated with deficient production or secretion of antidiuretic hormone (ADH), or a decreased renal response to ADH caused by injury of the neurohypophyseal system.

diabetes mellitus (DM) a multisystem disease related to abnormal insulin production, impaired insulin utilization, or both.

diabetic ketoacidosis (DKA) an acute metabolic complication of diabetes occurring when fats are metabolized in the absence of insulin resulting in formation of acid by-products, such as ketones.

dialysis technique in which substances move from the blood through a semipermeable membrane and into a dialysis solution.

diabetic nephropathy a microvascular complication of diabetes mellitus associated with damage to the small blood vessels that supply the glomeruli of the kidney.

diabetic neuropathy nerve damage caused by the metabolic derangements associated with diabetes mellitus.

dislocation a severe injury of the ligamentous structures that surround a joint resulting in the complete displacement or separation of the articular surfaces of the joint.

disseminated intravascular coagulation (DIC) a grave coagulopathy resulting from the overstimulation of clotting and anticlotting processes in response to disease or injury.

diverticulum a saccular dilation or outpouching of the mucosa through the circular smooth muscle of the intestinal wall.

dysarthria a disturbance in the muscular control of speech resulting from interference in the control and execution over the muscles of speech.

dysmenorrhea abdominal cramping pain or discomfort associated with menstrual flow.

dyspareunia abnormal pain during sexual intercourse.

dysphagia difficulty swallowing.

dysphasia difficulty related to the comprehension or use of language.

dysplastic nevi nevi that are larger than usual with irregular borders and various shades of color; also known as atypical moles.

dyspnea shortness of breath; difficulty breathing that may be caused by certain heart or lung conditions, strenuous exercise, or anxiety.

E

ecchymoses bruising.

ectopic pregnancy the implantation of a fertilized ovum anywhere outside the uterine cavity.

embolic stroke a stroke that occurs when an embolus lodges in and occludes a cerebral artery, resulting in infarction and edema of the area supplied by the involved vessel.

emergence delirium a neurologic alteration in recovery from anesthesia that can include behaviors such as restlessness, agitation, disorientation, thrashing, and shouting.

emphysema an abnormal condition of the pulmonary system characterized by overinflation and destructive changes in alveolar walls.

empyema an accumulation of purulent exudates in a body cavity, especially the pleural space, that results from bacterial infection, such as pleurisy or tuberculosis.

encephalitis an acute inflammation of the brain usually caused by a virus.

endometriosis the presence of normal endometrial tissue in sites outside the endometrial cavity.

endoscopy the direct visualization of a body structure through a lighted instrument (scope).

endotracheal intubation artificial airway created by inserting a tube into the trachea through the mouth or nose, past the larynx, and bypassing the upper airway and laryngeal structures.

enteral nutrition (EN) the administration of a nutritionally balanced, liquefied food or formula through a tube inserted into the stomach, duodenum, or jejunum.

epididymitis acute or chronic inflammation of the epididymis, usually secondary to an infectious process, trauma, or urinary reflux down the vas deferens.

epidural block injection of a local anesthetic into the epidural (extradural) space by either a thoracic or lumbar approach.

epidural hematoma collection of blood between the dura and inner surface of the skull, producing compression of the dura mater and thus of the brain.

epilepsy a condition in which a person has spontaneously recurring seizures caused by a chronic underlying condition.

epistaxis nosebleed.

erectile dysfunction (ED) the inability to attain or maintain an erect penis that allows satisfactory sexual performance.

erythema redness or inflammation of the skin or mucous membranes that result from dilation and congestion of superficial capillaries.

escharotomy incisions into necrotic tissue from a severe burn performed when eschar formation compromises circulation.

esophageal diverticulum saclike outpouching of one or more layers of the esophagus.

esophageal speech a method of swallowing air, trapping it in the esophagus, and releasing it to create sound.

esophageal varices distended, tortuous, fragile veins at the lower end of the esophagus that result from portal hypertension.

esophagitis inflammation of the mucosal lining of the esophagus caused by infection, irritation from a nasogastric tube, or, most commonly, backflow of gastric juice from the stomach.

evisceration the separation and disruption of previously joined wound edges to the extent that an internal organ, typically intestinal contents, protrudes through the wound.

excision and grafting procedure during which eschar is removed down to the subcutaneous

tissue or fascia, depending on the degree of injury; a graft is then placed on clean, viable tissue to achieve good adherence.

exophthalmos protrusion of the eyeballs from the orbits caused by increased fat deposits and fluid in the retroorbital tissues.

external otitis inflammation or infection of the epithelium of the auricle and ear canal.

F

fat embolism syndrome (FES) embolization of fat globules that occurs in a small percentage of patients with fractures.

fibrinolysis a continual process resulting in the dissolution of fibrin to maintain blood in its fluid form.

fibroadenoma a small, painless, round, well-delineated, mobile benign breast tumor commonly found in young women.

fibrocystic changes a benign condition of the breasts characterized by development of excess fibrous tissue, hyperplasia of the epithelial lining of the mammary ducts, proliferation of mammary ducts, and cyst formation.

fibromyalgia a chronic disorder characterized by widespread, nonarticular musculoskeletal pain and fatigue with multiple tender points.

flail chest instability of the chest wall resulting from multiple rib fractures.

focal seizures seizures that begin in a specific region of the cortex and may be confined to one side of the brain and remain partial or focal in nature, or they may spread to involve the entire brain.

fracture a disruption or break in the continuity of the structure of bone.

fremitus vibration of the chest wall produced by vocalization.

frontotemporal lobar degeneration (FTLD) a rare disorder caused by shrinking frontal and temporal lobes of the brain; characterized by disturbances in behavior, sleep, personality, and eventually memory.

frostbite freezing that results in the formation of ice crystals in the tissues and cells.

full-thickness burn destruction of all skin elements and subcutaneous tissues with possible involvement of muscles, tendons, and bones.

G

galactorrhea a milky secretion from the nipple caused by inappropriate lactation.

gastritis inflammation of the gastric mucosa.

gastroenteritis an inflammation of the mucosa of the stomach and small intestine.

gastroesophageal reflux disease (GERD) any clinically significant symptomatic condition or histopathologic alteration presumed to be secondary to reflux of gastric contents into the lower esophagus.

generalized seizures seizures characterized by bilateral synchronous epileptic discharge in the brain with loss of consciousness for a few seconds to several minutes.

genital herpes a sexually transmitted infection caused by the herpes simplex virus type 2 (HSV-2), resulting in painful genital or anal vesicular lesions.

Glasgow Coma Scale assessment tool for altered states of consciousness that evaluates motor responses, verbal responses, and eye opening.

glaucoma a group of disorders characterized by (1) increased intraocular pressure and the consequences of elevated pressure, (2) optic nerve atrophy, and (3) peripheral visual field loss.

glial cells cells in the central nervous system that provide support, nourishment, and protection to neurons.

glomerular filtration rate (GFR) the amount of blood filtered by the glomeruli in a given time.

glomerulonephritis an immune-related inflammation of the glomeruli characterized by proteinuria, hematuria, decreased urine production, and edema.

glycemic index term used to describe the rise in blood glucose levels after a person has consumed a carbohydrate-containing food.

goiter enlargement of the thyroid gland that may be associated with hyperthyroidism, hypothyroidism, or normal thyroid function.

gonorrhea infection of the genitalia, the rectum, and/or the oropharynx by *Neisseria gonorrhoeae*, which, if left untreated, leads to the formation of fibrous tissue and adhesions.

Goodpasture syndrome an example of cytotoxic autoimmune disease characterized by the presence of circulating antibodies against the glomerular basement membrane and alveolar basement membrane.

gout recurrent attacks of acute arthritis associated with increased levels of serum uric acid.

Guillain-Barré syndrome an acute, rapidly progressing, and potentially fatal form of polyneuritis possibly caused by a cell-mediated immunologic reaction directed at the peripheral nerves.

gynecomastia a transient enlargement of one or both breasts in men.

H

heat cramps severe cramps in large muscle groups caused by depletion of both water and salt; usually follow vigorous exertion in an extremely hot environment.

heat exhaustion a clinical syndrome characterized by fatigue, light-headedness, nausea, vomiting, diarrhea, and feelings of impending doom precipitated by prolonged exposure to heat over hours or days.

heatstroke the most serious form of heat stress; results from failure of the central thermoregulatory mechanisms and is considered a medical emergency.

heaves sustained lifts of the chest wall in the precordial area that can be seen or palpated.

hematemesis vomiting of blood that indicates bleeding in the upper GI tract.

hemochromatosis an autosomal recessive disease characterized by increased intestinal iron absorption and, as a result, increased tissue iron deposition.

hemodialysis (HD) dialysis that uses an artificial membrane as the semipermeable membrane through which the patient's blood circulates.

hemolytic anemia an anemia caused by destruction of RBCs at a rate that exceeds production.

hemophilia hereditary bleeding disorders caused by defective or deficient clotting factors.

hemorrhagic stroke a stroke that results from bleeding into the brain tissue itself or into the subarachnoid space or ventricles.

hemorrhoids varicosities in the lower rectum or anus caused by congestion in the veins of the hemorrhoidal plexus.

hemothorax accumulation of blood in the pleural space.

hepatic encephalopathy changes in neurologic and mental function resulting from high levels of ammonia in the blood that a damaged liver cannot detoxify.

hepatitis inflammation of the liver.

hepatorenal syndrome a serious complication of cirrhosis characterized by functional renal failure with advancing azotemia, oliguria, and intractable ascites.

hernia a protrusion of a viscus through an abnormal opening or a weakened area in the wall of the cavity in which it is normally contained.

herniated disc herniation of nuclear material from the intervertebral disc that may compress or place tension on a cervical, lumbar, or sacral spinal nerve root.

hiatal hernia herniation of a portion of the stomach into the esophagus through an opening, or hiatus, in the diaphragm.

histologic grading a categorization of tumors in which the appearance of cells and the degree of differentiation are evaluated pathologically.

Hodgkin's lymphoma a malignant condition characterized by proliferation of abnormal giant, multinucleated cells, called *Reed-Sternberg cells,* which are located in lymph nodes.

hordeolum an infection of the sebaceous glands in the eyelid margin; commonly known as a sty.

hospice a concept of care that provides compassion, concern, and support for the dying person.

human immunodeficiency virus (HIV) a retrovirus that causes HIV infection and acquired immunodeficiency syndrome.

human leukocyte antigens (HLAs) a system consisting of a series of linked genes that occur together on the sixth chromosome in humans and that is used to assess tissue compatibility.

humoral immunity antibody-mediated immunity.

Huntington's disease a genetically transmitted, autosomal dominant disorder that affects both men and women of all races and is characterized by chronic, devastating loss of all neurologic function, resulting in dementia.

hydronephrosis dilation or enlargement of the renal pelvis and calyces resulting from obstruction in the lower urinary tract with backflow of urine to the kidney.

hydrostatic pressure the force that fluid exerts within a compartment.

hydroureter dilation of the renal pelvis due to backflow of urine.

hyperaldosteronism excessive aldosterone secretion caused by an adenoma of the adrenal zona glomerulosa or bilateral adrenal hyperplasia.

hypercapnia greater than normal amounts of carbon dioxide in the blood; also called hypercarbia.

hypercapnic respiratory failure a condition in which the $PaCO_2$ is above normal in combination with acidemia.

hyperopia farsightedness or the inability of the eye to focus on nearby objects.

hyperosmolar hyperglycemic syndrome (HHS) a life-threatening syndrome that can occur in the patient with diabetes who is able to produce enough insulin to prevent diabetic ketoacidosis but not enough to prevent severe hyperglycemia, osmotic diuresis, and extracellular fluid depletion.

hyperparathyroidism a condition involving increased secretion of parathyroid hormone resulting in increased serum calcium levels.

hypertension a common disorder characterized by sustained elevation of blood pressure.

hypertensive crisis a severe and abrupt elevation in blood pressure.

hyperthyroidism a clinical syndrome in which there is a sustained increase in the synthesis and release of thyroid hormones by the thyroid gland.

hypertonic a solution that increases the degree of osmotic pressure on a semipermeable membrane.

hypertrophic scar an inappropriately large, red, raised, and hard scar that occurs when the body produces excess collagen tissue.

hypoparathyroidism a condition of insufficient secretion of the parathyroid glands.

hypopituitarism a rare disorder that involves a decrease in one or more of the pituitary hormones and marked by excessive deposits of fat and persistence or acquisition of adolescent characteristics.

hypothermia a core temperature <95° F (35° C) that occurs when heat produced by the body cannot compensate for heat lost to the environment.

hypothyroidism insufficient circulation of thyroid hormones resulting in a hypometabolic state.

hypotonic a solution that has a lower concentration of solute than another solution, thus exerting less osmotic pressure on a semipermeable membrane.

hypoxemia low oxygen tension in the blood characterized by a variety of nonspecific clinical signs and symptoms.

hypoxemic respiratory failure a condition in which the PaO_2 is 60 mm Hg or less when the patient is receiving an inspired oxygen concentration of 60% or greater.

hypoxia the state in which the PaO_2 has fallen sufficiently to cause signs and symptoms of inadequate oxygenation.

hysterectomy surgical removal of the uterus.

I

ileal conduit urinary diversion procedure in which ureters are implanted into a part of the ileum or colon that has been resected from the intestinal tract and an abdominal stoma is created.

impaired fasting glucose (IFG) an intermediate stage between normal glucose homeostasis and diabetes.

impaired glucose tolerance (IGT) an intermediate stage between normal glucose homeostasis and diabetes where the blood glucose level is 140 mg/dL (7.8 mmol/L) to 199 mg/dL (11 mmol/L) 2 hours after a meal.

infective endocarditis an infection of the endocardial surface of the heart.

infertility the inability to achieve a pregnancy after at least 1 year of regular intercourse without contraception.

inflammatory bowel disease (IBD) chronic, recurrent inflammatory diseases of the intestinal tract that include ulcerative colitis and Crohn's disease.

insulin resistance a condition in which body tissues do not respond to the action of insulin.

intensive insulin therapy multiple daily insulin injections together with frequent self-monitoring of blood glucose.

intermittent claudication ischemic muscle ache or pain precipitated by a consistent level of exercise, resolves within 10 minutes or less with rest, and is reproducible.

interstitial cystitis chronic, painful inflammatory disease of the bladder probably associated with an autoimmune or allergic response.

intraaortic balloon pump (IABP) a temporary circulatory assist device used to enhance the function of a compromised heart by reducing afterload and augmenting the aortic diastolic pressure.

intracerebral hematoma collection of blood within the parenchyma of the brain, possibly from the rupture of an intracerebral vessel at the time of a head injury.

intracerebral hemorrhage a type of hemorrhagic stroke in which bleeding within the brain is caused by a rupture of a blood vessel.

intracranial pressure the hydrostatic force measured in the brain cerebrospinal fluid compartment.

intravenous pyelogram (IVP) a diagnostic study using an IV contrast medium excreted through the urinary system; used to examine the structure and function of the urinary system.

iron-deficiency anemia a microcytic hypochromic anemia caused by inadequate supplies of iron needed to synthesize hemoglobin; characterized by pallor, fatigue, and weakness.

irritable bowel syndrome (IBS) a symptom complex characterized by intermittent and recurrent abdominal pain associated with an alteration in bowel function (diarrhea or constipation).

ischemic stroke a stroke that results from inadequate blood flow to the brain due to partial or complete occlusion of an artery.

isometric contractions muscular contraction that increases tension but does not produce movement.

isotonic contractions muscular contraction with shortening that produces movement.

J

jaundice a symptom of yellowish discoloration of body tissues that results from an increased concentration of bilirubin in the blood.

jaw-thrust maneuver a technique used to maintain an open airway that should be used in emergency situations.

K

keloid an overgrowth of collagenous scar tissue at the site of a skin injury, particularly a wound or a surgical incision; the new tissue is elevated, rounded, and firm.

keratinocytes cells synthesized from epidermal cells in the basal layer; the cells produce a specialized protein, keratin, that is vital to the protective barrier function of the skin.

keratitis an inflammation or infection of the cornea; may be caused by a variety of microorganisms or by other factors.

Korotkoff sounds sounds heard during the taking of a blood pressure reading using a sphygmomanometer and stethoscope.

Korsakoff's psychosis a form of amnesia often seen in people with chronic alcoholism; characterized by loss of short-term memory and an inability to learn.

Kupffer cells a type of macrophage found in the liver that removes bacteria and toxins from the blood.

kyphosis anterior-posterior or forward bending of spine with convexity of curve in posterior direction.

L

lactase deficiency an inherited abnormality in which the amount of the digestive enzyme lactase is inadequate for the normal digestion of milk products, resulting in the inability to digest lactose.

lacunar stroke a stroke resulting from occlusion of a small penetrating artery with development of a cavity in the place of the infarcted brain tissue.

leiomyoma a benign smooth muscle tumor that occurs most commonly within the uterus, stomach, esophagus, or small intestine; uterine fibroid.

leukemia a broad term given to a group of malignant diseases characterized by diffuse replacement of bone marrow with proliferating leukocyte precursors.

leukopenia an abnormal decrease in the number of total white blood cells to <4000/μL.

lichenification the thickening of the skin as a result of proliferation of keratinocytes with accentuation of the normal markings of the skin often caused by repeated scratching of a pruritic lesion.

lithotripsy the use of sound waves to break renal stones into small particles that can be eliminated from the urinary tract.

lordosis lumbar spinal deformity resulting in anterior-posterior curvature with concavity in posterior direction.

lumpectomy breast conserving surgery that involves the removal of the entire tumor along with a margin of normal tissue.

lung abscess a pus-containing lesion of the lung parenchyma that results in a cavity formed by necrosis of lung tissue.

Lyme disease a spirochetal infection caused by *Borrelia burgdorferi* and transmitted by the bite of an infected deer tick; characterized by fever, chills, headache, stiff neck, and migratory joint and muscle pain.

lymphedema accumulation of lymph in soft tissue with swelling resulting from inflammation, obstruction, or removal of lymph channels and nodes.

lymphomas malignant neoplasms originating in the bone marrow and lymphatic structures resulting in the proliferation of lymphocytes.

M

malabsorption syndrome a complex of symptoms resulting from disorders in the intestinal absorption of nutrients, characterized by anorexia, weight loss, abdominal bloating, muscle cramps, bone pain, and steatorrhea.

malignant hyperthermia a rare genetic metabolic disease characterized by hyperthermia with rigidity of skeletal muscles that can result in death.

malignant melanoma a tumor arising in cells producing melanin, usually the melanocytes of the skin.

malignant neoplasm a tumor that tends to grow, invade, and metastasize; usually has an irregular shape and is composed of poorly differentiated cells.

Mallory-Weiss tear a tear that occurs in the esophageal mucosa at the junction of the esophagus and stomach, caused by severe retching and vomiting and results in severe bleeding.

mammoplasty a change in the size or shape of the breast due to surgery.

mass casualty incident a human-caused (e.g., biologic warfare) or natural (e.g., hurricane) event or disaster that overwhelms a community's ability to respond with existing resources.

mastalgia breast pain; can be caused by congestion or "caking" during lactation, an infection, or fibrocystic disease, especially during or before menstruation, or in advanced cancer.

mastectomy surgical removal of the breast.

mastitis an inflammatory condition of the breast that occurs most frequently in lactating women, caused by streptococcal or staphylococcal infection.

mean arterial pressure (MAP) a calculated average of systolic and diastolic blood pressures; calculated by adding the diastolic pressure to one third of the pulse pressure.

medical care–associated pneumonia (MCAP) pneumonia occurring 48 hours or longer after hospital admission and not incubating at the time of hospitalization.

megaloblastic anemias a group of disorders caused by impaired DNA synthesis and characterized by the presence of large red blood cells.

melena black, tarry stools that indicate slow bleeding from an upper GI source.

menarche the first episode of menstrual bleeding; indicates female has reached puberty.

Ménière's disease a disease characterized by symptoms caused by inner ear disease including episodic vertigo, tinnitus, fluctuating sensorineural hearing loss, and aural fullness.

meningitis an acute inflammation of the pia mater and the arachnoid membrane surrounding the brain and the spinal cord.

menopause the physiologic cessation of menses associated with declining ovarian function.

metabolic equivalent (MET) a unit of measurement of heat production by the body; used to determine the energy costs of various exercises.

metabolic syndrome a collection of risk factors that increase an individual's chance of developing cardiovascular disease and diabetes mellitus.

metastasis the spread of the cancer from the initial or primary site to a distant site.

migraine headache a recurring headache characterized by unilateral or bilateral throbbing pain and a triggering event or factor; can occur with and without an aura.

mild cognitive impairment (MCI) a state of cognition and functional ability between normal aging and early Alzheimer's disease.

mixed dementia presentation of two or more types of dementia simultaneously.

mitral valve prolapse (MVP) a structural abnormality of the mitral valve leaflets and the papillary muscles or chordae that allows the leaflets to prolapse, or buckle, back into the left atrium during ventricular systole.

multiple myeloma a condition in which malignant neoplastic plasma cells infiltrate the bone marrow and destroy bone.

multiple organ dysfunction syndrome (MODS) the failure of more than one organ system in an acutely ill patient such that homeostasis cannot be maintained without intervention.

multiple sclerosis (MS) a chronic, progressive, degenerative disorder of the central nervous system characterized by disseminated demyelination of nerve fibers of the brain and spinal cord.

murmur a gentle blowing, fluttering, or humming sound heard on auscultation and produced by turbulent blood flow through the heart or the walls of large arteries.

muscular dystrophy (MD) a group of genetically transmitted diseases characterized by progressive symmetric wasting of skeletal muscle without evidence of neurologic involvement.

myasthenia gravis (MG) an autoimmune disease of the neuromuscular junction characterized by the fluctuating weakness of certain skeletal muscle groups.

myasthenic crisis an acute exacerbation of myasthenia gravis triggered by infection, surgery, emotional distress, or overdose or inadequate medication.

myelodysplastic syndrome (MDS) a group of related hematologic disorders characterized by a change in the quantity and quality of bone marrow elements.

myocardial infarction (MI) an irreversible cardiac cellular death caused by sustained myocardial ischemia.

myocarditis a focal or diffuse inflammation of the myocardium.

myopia nearsightedness or the inability of the eye to focus on objects far away.

myxedema the progression of the mental sluggishness, drowsiness, and lethargy of hypothy-roidism to a notable impairment of consciousness or coma that is a medical emergency.

N

nadir the lowest point, such as the blood cell count after it has been depressed by chemotherapy.

narcolepsy a chronic neurologic disorder caused by the brain's inability to regulate sleep-wake cycles normally; results in fleeting urges to sleep throughout the day.

nasal polyps benign mucous membrane masses that form slowly in response to repeated inflammation of the sinus or nasal mucosa and project into the nasal cavity.

nephrolithiasis the formation of stones in the urinary tract.

nephrosclerosis a vascular disease of the kidney characterized by sclerosis of the small arteries and arterioles of the kidney resulting in renal tissue necrosis.

nephrotic syndrome an abnormal condition of the kidney characterized by peripheral edema, massive proteinuria, hyperlipidemia, and hypoalbuminemia.

neurofibrillary tangles tangled bundles of fibers seen in the cytoplasm of abnormal neurons in those areas of the brain most affected by Alzheimer's disease.

neurogenic bladder any type of bladder dysfunction related to abnormal or absent bladder innervation caused by a lesion of the nervous system.

neurogenic bowel loss of voluntary neurologic control over the bowel.

neurogenic shock neurologic syndrome caused by the loss of vasomotor tone caused by spinal cord injury at the fifth thoracic (T5) vertebra or above and characterized by hypotension, bradycardia, and warm, dry extremities.

neuropathic pain pain caused by damage to nerve cells or changes in spinal cord processing of nervous system input.

neurosyphilis an infection of any part of the nervous system by the organism *Treponema pallidum.*

neutropenia an abnormal reduction of the neutrophil count to <1000/μL.

nociception activation of the primary afferent nerves with peripheral terminals that respond to noxious stimuli.

nociceptive pain pain caused by damage to somatic or visceral tissue; occurs abruptly after an injury or disease, persists until healing occurs, and often is intensified by anxiety or fear.

nonalcoholic fatty liver disease (NAFLD) a group of disorders characterized by hepatic *steatosis* (accumulation of fat in the liver) and is not associated with other causes such as hepatitis, autoimmune disease, or consumption of alcohol.

normal pressure hydrocephalus an uncommon disorder characterized by an obstruction in the flow of cerebrospinal fluid; causes a buildup of this fluid in the brain.

nuchal rigidity resistance to flexion of the neck.

nulliparous never having given birth.

nystagmus an abnormal, involuntary, repetitive movement of the eyes.

O

O₂ toxicity a condition of oxygen overdosage caused by prolonged exposure to a high level of oxygen.

obese the classification used to describe individuals with body mass index values ≥30 kg/m².

obstructive shock develops when a physical obstruction of blood flow occurs with decreased cardiac output.

obstructive sleep apnea (OSA) a condition characterized by partial or complete upper airway obstruction during sleep.

oliguria producing <400 mL of urine in 24 hour.

oncogenes potentially cancer-inducing genes.

oncotic pressure the osmotic pressure of a colloid in solution.

orchitis an acute inflammation of the testis.

orthostatic hypotension abnormally low blood pressure occurring when an individual suddenly assumes a standing position.

osteoarthritis a slowly progressive, noninflammatory disorder of the diarthrodial (synovial) joints.

osteochondroma primary benign bone tumor characterized by an overgrowth of cartilage and bone near the end of the bone at the growth plate.

osteomalacia a rare condition of adult bones associated with vitamin D deficiency, resulting in decalcification and softening of bone.

osteomyelitis a severe infection of the bone, bone marrow, and surrounding soft tissue.

osteon cylindrical-shaped structural units that fit closely together in compact bone, creating a dense bone structure.

osteopenia bone loss that is more than normal (a T-score between −1 and −2.5), but not yet at the level for a diagnosis of osteoporosis.

osteoporosis a metabolic bone disease characterized by low bone mass and structural deterioration of bone tissue, leading to increased bone fragility and pathologic fractures.

osteosarcoma a primary bone tumor that is extremely aggressive and rapidly metastasizes to distant sites; usually occurs in the metaphyseal region of the long bones of the extremities.

osteotomy removing or adding a wedge or slice of bone to change its alignment and shift weight bearing, thereby correcting deformity and relieving pain.

ostomy a surgical procedure in which an opening is made to allow the passage of urine from the bladder or intestinal contents from the bowel through an incision or stoma surgically created in the wall of the abdomen.

otosclerosis a hereditary condition in which irregular ossification occurring on the footplate of the stapes in the oval window results in decreased hearing acuity.

P

Paget's disease of the bone a skeletal bone disorder in which there is excessive bone resorption followed by replacement of normal marrow by vascular, fibrous connective tissue and new bone that is larger, disorganized, and weaker.

Paget's disease of the breast a breast malignancy characterized by a persistent lesion of the nipple and areola with or without a palpable mass.

palliative care an approach that improves the quality of life of patients and their families who face problems associated with life-threatening illness.

palpation a physical examination technique in which the examiner feels the texture, size, consistency, and location of certain body parts with the hands.

pancytopenia a marked decrease in the number of red blood cells, white blood cells, and platelets.

paracentesis a procedure in which fluid is withdrawn from a cavity of the body.

paralytic ileus the lack of intestinal peristalsis.

paraplegia paralysis characterized by motor and/or sensory loss in the lower limbs and trunk.

parasomnias unusual and often undesirable behaviors that occur with sleep or during arousal from sleep, such as enuresis (bed-wetting), hallucinations, and eating.

parenteral nutrition (PN) the administration of nutrients by a route (e.g., bloodstream) other than the GI tract.

Parkinson's disease (PD) a disease of the basal ganglia characterized by a slowing down in the initiation and execution of movement, increased muscle tone tremor at rest, and impaired postural reflexes.

paroxysmal nocturnal dyspnea (PND) sudden attacks of respiratory distress that awaken the sleeper, usually after several hours of sleep in a reclining position.

partial-thickness burn varying degrees of epidermal and dermal skin injury in which some skin elements remain viable for regeneration.

pelvic inflammatory disease (PID) an infectious condition of the pelvic cavity that may involve infection of the fallopian tubes, ovaries, and pelvic peritoneum.

peptic ulcer disease (PUD) erosion of the GI mucosa that results from the digestive action of HCl acid and pepsin.

percussion a physical examination technique in which the examiner taps the body with the fingertips or fist.

percutaneous coronary intervention (PCI) a common intervention for coronary artery disease in which a catheter equipped with an inflatable balloon tip is inserted into a narrowed coronary artery and the balloon is inflated.

pericardiocentesis a procedure in which a 16- to 18-gauge needle is inserted into the pericardial space to remove fluid for analysis and to relieve cardiac pressure.

pericarditis a condition caused by inflammation of the pericardial sac.

perimenopause a normal life transition that begins with the first signs of change in menstrual cycles and ends after cessation of menses.

peripheral artery disease (PAD) the progressive narrowing and degeneration of the arteries of the neck, abdomen, and extremities.

peripheral stem cell transplantation the transplantation of stem cells obtained from the peripheral blood in an outpatient procedure; often takes more than one procedure to obtain enough stem cells.

peritoneal dialysis (PD) dialysis using the peritoneal membrane as the semipermeable membrane.

peritonitis the inflammation of the peritoneum.

pernicious anemia a progressive megaloblastic macrocytic anemia resulting from inadequate gastric secretion of intrinsic factor necessary for absorption of cobalamin.

pertussis a highly contagious infection of the lower respiratory tract with a gram-negative bacillus, *Bordetella pertussis.*

petechiae small purplish lesions.

phantom limb sensation the perception of sensations or pain in an amputated limb.

pharmacogenetics the study of variability of responses to drugs due to variations in single genes.

pharmacogenomics the study of variability of responses to drugs due to variations in and interactions of multiple genes.

pheochromocytoma a rare condition characterized by a tumor of the adrenal medulla that produces excessive catecholamines causing persistent or intermittent hypertension.

phimosis a constriction of the uncircumcised foreskin around the head of the penis making retraction difficult.

pleural effusion an abnormal accumulation of fluid in the intrapleural spaces of the lungs.

pleural friction rub a creaking or grating sound from roughened, inflamed surfaces of the pleura rubbing together, evident during inspiration, expiration, or both and no change with coughing.

pleurisy (pleuritis) inflammation of the pleura.

pneumoconiosis a general term for lung diseases caused by inhalation and retention of dust particles.

pneumonia an acute inflammation of the lungs, often caused by inhaled pneumococci of the species *Streptococcus pneumoniae.*

pneumothorax a collection of air or gas in the pleural space causing the lung to collapse.

point of maximal impulse (PMI) the site on the chest wall where the thrust or pulsation of the left ventricle is most prominent.

polycystic kidney disease (PKD) a genetic kidney disorder in which the cortex and the medulla are filled with thin-walled cysts that enlarge and destroy surrounding tissue.

polycythemia an abnormal condition with excessive levels of red blood cells.

polymyositis diffuse, idiopathic, inflammatory myopathies of striated muscle, producing bilateral weakness usually most severe in the proximal or limb-girdle muscles; some forms of polymyositis are associated with malignancy.

portal hypertension increased venous pressure in the portal circulation caused by compression and destruction of the portal and hepatic veins and sinusoids.

positive end-expiratory pressure (PEEP) a ventilatory maneuver in which positive pressure is applied to the airway during exhalation.

postural drainage the use of various positions to promote gravity drainage of bronchial secretions.

prediabetes impaired glucose tolerance; occurs when a 2-hour plasma glucose level is higher than normal but lower than that considered diagnostic for diabetes.

prehypertension a disorder characterized by a systolic blood pressure of 120 to 139 mm Hg and a diastolic blood pressure of 80 to 89 mm Hg.

preload the volume of blood in the ventricles at the end of diastole before the next contraction.

premature atrial contraction (PAC) contraction originating from an ectopic focus in the atrium in a location other than the sinus node.

premature ventricular contraction (PVC) a contraction originating in an ectopic focus in the ventricles.

premenstrual syndrome (PMS) a common disorder in women in which a group of physical and psychologic symptoms occur during the last few days of the menstrual cycle and before the onset of menstruation.

presbycusis hearing loss associated with aging.

presbyopia a hyperopic shift to farsightedness resulting from a loss of elasticity of the lens of the eye.

pressure ulcer a localized area of tissue necrosis caused by unrelieved pressure that occludes blood flow to the tissues.

primary hypertension an elevated systemic arterial pressure for which no cause can be found and which is often the only significant clinical finding.

Prinzmetal's angina a variant angina; occurs at rest, usually in response to reversible, severe spasm of a major coronary artery.

prostatitis an acute or chronic inflammation of the prostate gland, usually as a result of infection.

pruritus itching.

psoriasis a chronic skin disorder characterized by circumscribed red patches covered by thick, dry, silvery, adherent scales.

pulmonary edema an acute, life-threatening situation in which the lung alveoli become filled with serous or serosanguineous fluid, caused most commonly by heart failure.

pulmonary embolism a thromboembolic occlusion of the pulmonary vasculature resulting from thrombi in the venous circulation or right side of the heart that travel as emboli until lodging in the pulmonary vessels.

pulmonary hypertension elevated pulmonary pressure resulting from an increase in pulmonary vascular resistance to blood flow through small arteries and arterioles.

pulse pressure the difference between the systolic and diastolic pressures.

pursed-lip breathing a technique of exhaling against pursed lips to prolong exhalation, preventing bronchiolar collapse and air trapping.

pyelonephritis a diffuse pyogenic infection of the renal parenchyma and collecting system.

pyrosis a burning sensation in the epigastric or substernal area; heartburn.

R

radical prostatectomy the surgical removal of the entire prostate gland, seminal vesicles, and part of the bladder neck (ampulla).

Raynaud's phenomenon an episodic vasospastic disorder of small cutaneous arteries, most frequently involving the fingers and toes.

rectocele the herniation or protrusion of the rectum through the wall of the vagina resulting from weakened connective tissue support between the vagina and rectum.

refractive error a defect in the ability of the lens of the eye to focus an image accurately on the retina, as occurs in nearsightedness and farsightedness.

renal artery stenosis a partial occlusion of one or both renal arteries and their major branches; is a major cause of abrupt-onset hypertension.

repetitive strain injury (RSI) a cumulative trauma disorder resulting from prolonged, forceful, or awkward movements resulting in strain of tendons, ligaments, and muscles, causing tiny tears that become inflamed.

restless legs syndrome (RLS) the unpleasant sensory and motor abnormalities of one or both legs; characterized by an irritating sensation of uneasiness, tiredness, and itching deep within the muscles of the leg.

retinal detachment a separation of the retina from the retinal pigment epithelium in the back of the eye, allowing the vitreous humor to leak between the two layers.

retinopathy the process of microvascular damage of the retina; may develop slowly or rapidly.

rheumatic fever an inflammatory disease of the heart that potentially involves all layers.

rheumatic heart disease (RHD) the resulting damage to the heart muscle and heart valves from rheumatic fever, a chronic condition characterized by scarring and deformity of the heart valves.

rheumatoid arthritis (RA) a chronic, systemic autoimmune disease characterized by inflammation of connective tissue in the diarthrodial (synovial) joints, typically with periods of remission and exacerbation.

rhinoplasty the surgical reconstruction of the nose.

rhonchi the continuous rumbling, snoring, or rattling sounds from obstruction of large airways with secretions.

S

sarcoma a malignant tumor that originates from embryonal mesoderm that becomes connective tissue, muscle, bone, and fat.

scleroderma a disorder of connective tissue characterized by fibrotic, degenerative, and occasionally inflammatory changes in the skin, blood vessels, synovium, skeletal muscle, and internal organs.

scoliosis a lateral S-shaped curvature of the thoracic and lumbar spine.

secondary hypertension elevated blood pressure associated with any of several primary diseases, such as renal, pulmonary, endocrine, and vascular diseases.

seizure a paroxysmal, uncontrolled electrical discharge of neurons in the brain that interrupts normal function leading to a sudden, violent involuntary series of contractions of a group of muscles.

sepsis a systemic inflammatory response to infection.

septic arthritis infectious or bacterial arthritis caused by invasion of the joint cavity with microorganisms; bacterial inflammation of a joint may be caused by the spread of bacteria through the bloodstream from an infection elsewhere in the body or by contamination of a joint during trauma or surgery.

septic shock the presence of sepsis with hypotension despite adequate fluid resuscitation along with the presence of tissue perfusion abnormalities.

severely obese the classification used to describe individuals with body mass index values >40 kg/m^2.

sexually transmitted infections (STIs) infectious diseases transmitted most commonly through sexual intercourse or genital contact.

shock a syndrome characterized by decreased tissue perfusion and impaired cellular metabolism resulting in an imbalance between the supply of and demand for oxygen and nutrients.

sickle cell disease (SCD) a group of inherited, autosomal recessive disorders characterized by the presence of an abnormal form of hemoglobin in the erythrocyte.

silent ischemia an asymptomatic ischemia that may damage the heart.

Sjögren's syndrome an autoimmune disease that targets moisture-producing glands, leading to the common symptoms of xerostomia (dry mouth) and keratoconjunctivitis sicca (dry eyes).

Somogyi effect a condition in which an excessive dose of insulin causes blood glucose levels to decline during sleep, triggering the release of counterregulatory hormones that increase the blood glucose levels, resulting in high blood glucose levels at morning testing; indicates a need for reduced dose of insulin.

spermatogenesis the formation of sperm.

spider angiomas small, dilated blood vessels with a bright red center point the size of a pinhead from which small blood vessels radiate.

spinal shock the immediate failure of all spinal cord function at the time of injury below the level of cord damage resulting in flaccid paralysis, loss of reflexes, and loss of sympathetic innervation.

spondyloarthropathies a group of interrelated multisystem inflammatory disorders that affect the spine, peripheral joints, and periarticular structures.

status epilepticus a state of continuous seizure activity or a condition in which seizures recur in rapid succession without return to consciousness between seizures.

steatorrhea a greater than normal amount of fat in the feces.

stenosis a constriction or narrowing.

stent an expandable meshlike structure designed to maintain vessel patency by compressing the arterial walls and resisting vasoconstriction.

strabismus a condition in which the individual cannot consistently focus both eyes simultaneously on the same object.

stricture an abnormal temporary or permanent narrowing of the lumen of a hollow organ.

stroke the death of brain cells that occurs when there is ischemia to a part of the brain or hemorrhage into the brain.

subarachnoid hemorrhage a stroke resulting from intracranial bleeding into the cerebrospinal fluid–filled space between the arachnoid and pia mater membranes on the surface of the brain.

subdural hematoma a collection of blood between the dura mater and the arachnoid layer of the meninges of the brain that is generally of venous origin, usually caused by injury.

submersion injury hypoxia resulting from submersion in a substance, usually water.

sudden cardiac death (SCD) unexpected death from cardiac causes.

sundowning a condition in which the individual becomes more confused and agitated in the late afternoon or evening.

surfactant a lipoprotein that lowers the surface tension in the alveoli, reduces the amount of pressure needed to inflate the alveoli, and decreases the tendency of the alveoli to collapse.

syndrome of inappropriate antidiuretic hormone (SIADH) a condition associated with overproduction or oversecretion of ADH.

synovectomy the surgical removal of synovial membrane.

syphilis the infection of organs and tissues of the body by *Treponema pallidum*.

systemic inflammatory response syndrome (SIRS) a systemic inflammatory response to a variety of insults, including infection, ischemia, infarct, and injury.

systemic lupus erythematosus (SLE) a chronic multisystem inflammatory disorder associated with abnormalities of the immune system.

systolic failure a type of ventricular failure caused by impaired contractile function, increased afterload, or mechanical abnormalities.

T

teletherapy radiation therapy administered by a machine positioned at some distance from the patient; the most common form of radiation therapy treatment.

tenesmus the painful spasmodic contraction of the anal sphincter and a persistent desire to empty the bowel.

tension pneumothorax a rapid accumulation of air in the pleural space causing severely high intrapleural pressures with resultant tension on the heart and great vessels.

tension-type headache a headache characterized by a bilateral feeling of pressure around the head.

tetanus lockjaw; an extremely severe polyradiculitis and polyneuritis affecting spinal and cranial nerves that results from the effects of a potent neurotoxin released by the anaerobic bacillus *Clostridium tetani*.

tetraplegia the paralysis of the arms, legs, and trunk occurring with spinal cord damage at C8 or above.

thalassemia an autosomal recessive genetic disorder of inadequate production of normal hemoglobin.

thoracentesis a surgical procedure done to remove fluid from the pleural space.

thoracotomy a surgical opening into the thoracic cavity.

thrombocytopenia a reduction of the platelet count.

thrombocytosis a condition marked by excessive platelets; a disorder that occurs with inflammation and some malignant disorders.

thrombotic stroke a stroke resulting from thrombosis or narrowing of the blood vessel.

thyroiditis an inflammatory process in the thyroid gland.

thyrotoxicosis (also called thyrotoxic crisis) a hypermetabolic state caused by excessive circulating levels of T_4, T_3, or both.

tinnitus a subjective noise sensation, often described as ringing, heard in one or both ears.

tonic-clonic seizure a seizure characterized by loss of consciousness and falling to the ground, followed by stiffening of the body for 10 to 20 seconds and subsequent jerking of the extremities for another 30 to 40 seconds.

tracheostomy a surgical opening into the trachea through which an indwelling tube may be inserted.

tracheotomy a surgical incision into the trachea for the purpose of establishing an airway; performed below a blockage by a foreign body, tumor, or edema of the glottis.

traction the application of a pulling force to an injured or diseased part of the body or an extremity while countertraction pulls in the opposite direction.

transurethral resection of the prostate (TURP) a surgical procedure involving the removal of prostate tissue with the use of a resectoscope inserted through the urethra.

triage a system that identifies and categorizes patients so the most critical are treated first.

trigeminal neuralgia a neurologic condition of the trigeminal facial nerve characterized by paroxysms of flashing, stablike pain radiating along the course of a branch of the nerve from the angle of the jaw.

trigger point a circumscribed hypersensitive area within a tight band of muscle that is caused by acute or chronic muscle strain.

tuberculosis (TB) an infectious disease caused by *Mycobacterium tuberculosis;* usually involves the lungs, but also occurs in the larynx, kidneys, bones, adrenal glands, lymph nodes, and meninges and can be disseminated throughout the body.

tumor angiogenesis the process of the formation of blood vessels within the tumor itself.

tumor-associated antigens the altered cell surface antigens found on cancer cells.

U

ulcerative colitis a chronic inflammatory bowel disease that causes ulceration of the colon and rectum.

unstable angina (UA) an angina that is new in onset, occurs at rest, or has a worsening pattern.

uremia the presence of excessive amounts of urea and other nitrogenous waste products in the blood; renal function declines to the point that symptoms develop in multiple body systems.

urethritis inflammation of the urethra.

urinary incontinence (UI) an uncontrolled leakage of urine; can be caused by anything that interferes with bladder or urethral sphincter control, including confusion or depression, infection, atrophic vaginitis, urinary retention, restricted mobility, fecal impaction, or drugs.

urinary retention the inability to empty the bladder despite micturition, or the accumulation of urine in the bladder because of an inability to urinate.

urosepsis a urinary tract infection that has spread into the systemic circulation; life-threatening condition requiring emergency treatment.

urticaria a pruritic skin eruption characterized by transient wheals of varying shapes and sizes with well-defined erythematous margins and pale centers; usually an allergic phenomenon.

uterine prolapse the downward displacement of the uterus into the vaginal canal as a result of impaired pelvic support.

V

Valsalva maneuver a maneuver that involves contraction of the chest muscles on a closed glottis with simultaneous contraction of the abdominal muscles.

varicose veins the dilated, tortuous subcutaneous veins most frequently found in the saphenous system.

vascular dementia the loss of cognitive function resulting from ischemic, ischemic-hypoxic, or hemorrhagic brain lesions caused by cardiovascular disease.

vasectomy the bilateral surgical ligation or resection of the vas deferens performed for the purpose of sterilization.

ventricular assist device (VAD) a device that is applied externally or internally into the path of flowing blood to augment or replace the action of the ventricle of the heart.

ventricular fibrillation a severe derangement of the heart rhythm characterized on electrocardiogram (ECG) by irregular undulations of varying contour and amplitude.

ventricular tachycardia (VT) a condition that occurs when an ectopic focus or foci fire repetitively and the ventricle takes control as the pacemaker.

vertigo a sensation that a person or objects around the person are moving or spinning; usually stimulated by movement of the head.

vesicants agents that when accidentally infiltrated into the skin cause severe local tissue breakdown and necrosis.

viral load the quantity of viral particles in a biologic sample.

Virchow's triad three important factors in the etiology of venous thrombosis: (1) venous stasis, (2) damage of the endothelium (inner lining of the vein), and (3) hypercoagulability of the blood.

viremia large amounts of virus in the blood, resulting from initial infection with a virus.

W

Wernicke's encephalopathy an inflammatory, hemorrhagic, degenerative condition of the brain resulting from a deficiency of thiamine; is seen in association with chronic alcoholism.

wheezes a form of rhonchus characterized by a continuous high-pitched squeaking sound caused by rapid vibration of bronchial walls.

window period a time period of 2 months after HIV infection during which an infected individual will not test positive for HIV-antibody.

ILLUSTRATION CREDITS

CHAPTER 1

Fig. 1-4, Courtesy Elizabeth Burkhart, RN, MPH, PhD, Chicago, Ill. **Fig. 1-6,** Courtesy Kathryn Bowles. From Moser DK, Riegel B: *Cardiac nursing: a companion to Braunwald's heart disease,* St Louis, 2008, Saunders. **Fig. 1-7,** Adapted from Courtlandt CD, Noonan L, Leonard GF: Model for improvement—part 1: A framework for health care quality, *Pediatric Clinics of North America* 56:757, 2009.

CHAPTER 2

Fig. 2-1, From McGinnis JM, Williams-Russo P, Knickman JR: The case for more active policy attention to health promotion, *Health Affairs* 21:78, 2002. **Fig. 2-2,** From *www.cdc.gov/vitalsigns.* **Fig. 2-9,** From Giger JN: *Transcultural nursing,* ed 6, St Louis, 2013, Mosby.

CHAPTER 3

Figs. 3-1, 3-4, Courtesy Linda Bucher, RN, PhD, CEN, CNE, Staff Nurse, Virtua Memorial Hospital, Mt. Holly, N.J. **Fig. 3-3,** From Seidel HM, Ball JW, Dains JE, Flynn JA: *Mosby's guide to physical examination,* ed 7, St Louis, 2011, Saunders.

CHAPTER 4

Figs. 4-2, 4-3, 4-4, Courtesy Linda Bucher, RN, PhD, CEN, CNE, Staff Nurse, Virtua Memorial Hospital, Mt. Holly, N.J.

CHAPTER 5

Fig. 5-1, From Woog P: *The chronic illness trajectory framework: the Corbin and Strauss nursing model,* New York, 1992, Springer. **Fig. 5-7,** Adapted from Fulmer T: The geriatric nurse specialist role: a new model, *Nursing Management* 22:91, 1991. © Copyright Lippincott Williams & Wilkins, *http://lww.com.* **Fig. 5-10,** Redrawn from Benzon J: Approaching drug regimens with a therapeutic dose of suspicion, *Geriatric Nursing* 12(4):1813, 1991.

CHAPTER 8

Fig. 8-4, Modified from LaFleur Brooks M: *Exploring medical language: a student-directed approach,* ed 8, St Louis, 2012, Mosby. **Fig. 8-5,** From Goldman L, Schafer AI: *Goldman's Cecil medicine,* ed 24, Philadelphia, 2012, Saunders.

CHAPTER 9

Fig. 9-1, Developed by McCaffery M, Pasero C, Paice JA. Modified from M McCaffery, C Pasero: *Pain: clinical manual,* ed 2, St Louis, 1999, Mosby. **Fig. 9-7,** From DeLee JC, Drez D, Miller MD: *DeLee and Drez's orthopaedic sports medicine: principles and practices,* ed 3, Philadelphia, 2009, Saunders.

CHAPTER 10

Fig. 10-1, Courtesy Kathleen A. Pollard, RN, MSN, CHPN, Phoenix, Ariz. **Fig. 10-4,** From Rick Brady, Riva, Md.

CHAPTER 12

Fig. 12-5, From Bale S, Jones V: *Wound care nursing: a patient-centered approach,* ed 2, St Louis, 2006, Mosby. **Fig. 12-6,** From Hayden RJ, Jebson PJL: Wrist arthrodesis, *Hand Clinics,* 21(4): 631-640, 2005. **Figs. 12-7, 12-8,** Reproduced with kind permission from Dr. C. Lawrence, Wound Healing Research Unit, Cardiff. In S Bale, V Jones, editors: *Wound care nursing: a patient-centered approach,* ed 2, St Louis, 2006, Mosby. **Fig. 12-9,** Courtesy Robert B. Babiak, RN, BSN, CWOCN, San Antonio, Tex. **Fig. 12-10,** From Perry AG, Potter PA, Elkin MK: *Nursing interventions and clinical skills,* ed 5, St Louis, 2012, Mosby.

CHAPTER 12 (cont.)

Fig. 12-11, From Abai B, Zickler RW, Pappas PJ, et al: Lymphorrhea responds to negative pressure wound therapy, *Journal of Vascular Surgery* 45(3):610-613, 2007.

CHAPTER 13

Figs. 13-1, 13-2, Adapted from *The New Genetics.* National Institute of General Medical Science. National Institutes of Health. US Department of Health and Human Services.

CHAPTER 14

Figs. 14-8, 14-9, From Morison MJ: *Nursing management of chronic wounds,* Edinburgh, 2001, Mosby. **Fig. 14-13,** From McKenry L, Tessier E, Hogan M: *Mosby's pharmacology in nursing,* St Louis, 2006, Mosby.

CHAPTER 15

Fig. 15-5, From Emond R, Welsby P, Rowland H: *Colour atlas of infectious diseases,* ed 4, Edinburgh, 2003, Mosby. **Fig. 15-6,** From Friedman-Kien AE: *Color atlas of AIDS,* Philadelphia, 1989, Saunders. **Fig. 15-7,** Set of slides published in 1992 by Jon Fuller, MD and Howard Libman, MD at Boston University School of Medicine, Boston, Mass. **Fig. 15-8,** From the Centers for Disease Control and Prevention. Courtesy Jonathan W.M. Gold, MD, New York. **Fig. 15-9,** From James WD, Berger T, Elston D: *Andrews' diseases of the skin: clinical dermatology,* ed 11, St Louis, 2011, Saunders.

CHAPTER 16

Fig. 16-1, Adapted from Kumar V, Abbas AK, Fausto N, et al: *Robbins and Cotran pathologic basis of disease,* ed 8, Philadelphia, 2010, Saunders. **Fig. 16-3,** Adapted from Stevens A, Lowe J: *Pathology: an illustrated review in colour,* ed 2, London, 2000, Mosby. **Fig. 16-4,** Adapted from Fidler IT: The pathogenesis of cancer metastasis: the "seed and soil" hypothesis revisited, *Nature Reviews. Cancer* 3:453-458, 2003. **Fig. 16-7,** From Shimizu N, Masuda H, Yamanaka H, et al: Fluorodeoxyglucose positron emission tomography scan of prostate cancer bone metastases with flare reaction after endocrine therapy, *Journal of Urology* 161(2): 609, 1999. **Fig. 16-11,** From Weinzweig N, Weinzweig J: *The mutilated hand,* Philadelphia, 2005, Mosby. **Figs. 16-12, 16-13,** Courtesy Jormain Cady, Virginia Mason Medical Center, Seattle, Wash. **Fig. 16-18,** From Forbes CD, Jackson WF: *Colour atlas and text of clinical medicine,* ed 3, London, 2003, Mosby.

CHAPTER 17

Fig. 17-1, Modified from Copstead-Kirkhorn LC, Banasik JL: *Pathophysiology,* ed 4, St Louis, 2010, Mosby. **Figs. 17-4, 17-6, 17-7,** From Patton KT, Thibodeau GA: *Anatomy and physiology,* ed 8, St Louis, 2013, Mosby. **Fig. 17-14,** From McCance KL, Huether SE: *Pathophysiology: the biologic basis for disease in adults and children,* ed 6, St Louis, 2010, Mosby.

CHAPTER 18

Fig. 18-1, Courtesy Susan R. Volk, RN, MSN, CCRN, CPAN, Staff Development Specialist, Christiana Care Health System, Newark, Del.

CHAPTER 19

Fig. 19-1, Courtesy Greg McVicar. **Fig. 19-2,** Courtesy Swedish Edmonds Hospital, Edmonds, Wash. Photograph by Amy Wesley. **Fig. 19-4,** Courtesy The Methodist Hospital, Houston, Tex. Photograph by Donna Dahms, RN, CNOR. **Fig. 19-5,** Courtesy Covidien, Mansfield, Mass.

CHAPTER 20

Fig. 20-5, Courtesy Christine R. Hoch, RN, MSN, Nursing Instructor, Delaware Technical Community College, Newark, Del.

CHAPTER 21

Figs. 21-1, 21-3, 21-6, Modified from Patton KT, Thibodeau GA: *Anatomy and physiology,* ed 8, St Louis, 2013, Mosby. **Fig. 21-4,** From Kanski JJ: *Clinical ophthalmology: a synopsis,* ed 2, New York, 2009, Butterworth-Heinemann. **Fig. 21-5,** From Newell FW: *Ophthalmology: principles and concepts,* ed 7, St Louis, 1992, Mosby. **Fig. 21-7, B, C,** from Swartz MH: *Textbook of physical diagnosis: history and examination,* ed 6, Philadelphia, 2010, Saunders.

CHAPTER 22

Figs. 22-1, 22-2, 22-3, 22-4, 22-5, 22-8, Courtesy Cory J. Bosanko, OD, FAAO, Eye Centers of Tennessee, Crossville, Tenn. **Fig. 22-9,** From Flint P, Haughey B, Lund V, Niparko JK, editors: *Cummings otolaryngology: head and neck surgery,* ed 5, St Louis, 2010, Mosby.

CHAPTER 23

Fig. 23-2, From Patton KT, Thibodeau GA, Douglas M: *Essentials of anatomy and physiology,* St. Louis, 2012, Mosby. **Figs. 23-3, 23-6,** From Habif TP: *Clinical dermatology: a color guide to diagnosis and therapy,* ed 5, St Louis, 2009, Mosby. **Figs. 23-4, 23-8,** From Gawkrodger D, Ardern-Jones MR: *Dermatology,* ed 5, Edinburgh, 2012, Churchill Livingstone. **Figs. 23-5, 23-7, 23-10,** From Graham-Brown R, Bourke J, Cunliffe T: *Dermatology: fundamentals of practice,* Edinburgh, 2008, Mosby Ltd. **Fig. 23-9,** From Hurwitz S: *Clinical pediatric dermatology: a textbook of skin disorders of childhood and adolescence,* ed 2, Philadelphia, 1993, Saunders.

CHAPTER 24

Figs. 24-1, 24-11, From Habif TP: *Clinical dermatology: a color guide to diagnosis and therapy,* ed 5, St Louis, 2010, Mosby. **Fig. 24-2,** From The Skin Cancer Foundation, New York, N.Y. **Figs. 24-3, 24-12,** From Graham-Brown R, Bourke J, Cunliffe T: *Dermatology: fundamentals of practice,* Edinburgh, 2008, Mosby Ltd. **Figs. 24-4, 24-8,** From Swartz MH: *Textbook of physical diagnosis: history and examination,* ed 6, Philadelphia, 2010, Saunders. **Figs. 24-5, 24-9,** From Gawkrodger D, Ardern-Jones MR: *Dermatology,* ed 5, Edinburgh, 2012, Churchill Livingstone. **Fig. 24-6,** From Habif TP: *Clinical dermatology: a color guide to diagnosis and therapy,* ed 4, St Louis, 2004, Mosby. **Figs. 24-7, 24-10,** From James WD, Berger T, Elston DMD: *Andrews' diseases of the skin,* ed 11, Philadelphia, 2011, Saunders. **Fig. 24-13,** Courtesy Peter Bonner, Placitas, N. Mex. **Fig. 24-14,** From Pastorek N, Bustillo A: Deep plane facelift, *Facial Plastic Surgery Clinics of North America* 13:433-449, 2005.

CHAPTER 25

Figs. 25-1, 25-2, 25-8, 25-9, 25-11, 25-12, Courtesy Judy A. Knighton, Toronto, Canada. **Fig. 25-6,** From American Association of Critical-Care Nurses: *AACN advanced critical care nursing,* St Louis, 2009, Mosby. **Fig. 25-14,** Courtesy Linda Bucher, RN, PhD, CEN, CNE, Staff Nurse, Virtua Memorial Hospital, Mt. Holly, N.J.

CHAPTER 26

Fig. 26-1, Redrawn from Price SA, Wilson LM: *Pathophysiology: clinical concepts of disease processes,* ed 6, St Louis, 2003, Mosby. **Figs. 26-2, 26-3, 26-8, 26-9,** Redrawn from Thompson JM, McFarland GK, Hirsch JE, Tucker SM: *Mosby's clinical nursing,* ed 5, St Louis, 2002, Mosby. **Fig. 26-4, A,** From Dantzker DR, Bone RC, George RB, editors: *Pulmonary and critical care medicine,* vol 1, St Louis, 1993, Mosby. **Fig. 26-4, B,** From Albertine KH, Williams MC, Hyde DM: Anatomy of the lungs. In RJ Mason, VC Broaddus, JF Murray, et al, editors: *Murray and Nadel's textbook of respiratory medicine,* ed 4, Philadelphia, 2005, Saunders. **Fig. 26-10,** Redrawn from Beare PG, Myers JL: *Adult health nursing,* ed 3, St Louis, 1998,

Mosby. **Fig. 26-11, A,** Courtesy Olympus America Inc, Melville, N.Y. **Fig. 26-12,** Redrawn from Du Bois RM, Clarke SW: *Fiberoptic bronchoscopy in diagnosis and management,* Orlando, 1987, Grune & Stratton.

CHAPTER 27

Fig. 27-1, A, Courtesy Boston Medical, Westborough, Mass. **Fig. 27-1, B,** From Roberts JR, Hedges JR: *Clinical procedures in emergency medicine,* ed 5, Philadelphia, 2009, Saunders. **Fig. 27-4,** From Potter PA, Perry AG: *Basic nursing: essentials for practice,* ed 7, St Louis, 2011, Mosby. **Fig. 27-5, D,** Courtesy Dale Medical Products, Inc, Plainville, Mass. **Fig. 27-8,** Courtesy Passy-Muir, Inc, Irvine, Calif. **Fig. 27-11,** From Eggers G, Flechtenmacher C, Kurzen J, Hassfeld S: Infiltrating basal cell carcinoma of the neck 34 years after irradiation of an haemangioma in early childhood. A case-report, *Journal of Cranio-maxillofacial Surgery* 33:199, 2005. **Fig. 27-12, A,** Courtesy Wade Hampton.

CHAPTER 28

Fig. 28-2, From Damjanov I, Linder J: *Anderson's pathology,* ed 10, St Louis, 1996, Mosby. **Fig. 28-3,** From Kumar V, Abbas AK, Aster JC, Fausto N: *Robbins and Cotran pathologic basis of disease,* ed 8, Philadelphia, 2010, Saunders. **Fig. 28-8,** From Atrium Medical Corporation, Hudson, N.H. **Fig. 28-9, A,** Courtesy and © Copyright Becton, Dickinson and Company. **Fig. 28-11,** From the teaching collection of the Department of Pathology, University of Texas Southwestern Medical School, Dallas, Tex. In V Kumar, AK Abbas, JC Aster, N Fausto, editors: *Robbins and Cotran pathologic basis of disease,* ed 8, Philadelphia, 2010, Saunders.

CHAPTER 29

Fig. 29-1, Adapted from McCance KL, Huether SE, editors: *Pathophysiology: the biologic basis for disease in adults and children,* ed 6, St Louis, 2010, Mosby. **Fig. 29-3,** Redrawn from Price SA, Wilson LM: *Pathophysiology: clinical concepts of disease processes,* ed 6, St Louis, 2003, Mosby. **Fig. 29-4,** Modified from National Heart, Lung, and Blood Institute: *Expert Panel Report 3: Guidelines for the diagnosis and management of asthma.* National Asthma Education and Prevention Program, The Institute, 2007. **Figs. 29-5, 29-7,** From Potter PA, Perry AG, Stockert P, Hall A: *Basic nursing: essentials for practice,* ed 7, St. Louis, 2011, Mosby. **Figs. 29-12, 29-13,** Courtesy Nellcor Puritan Bennett, Inc, Pleasanton, Calif. **Fig. 29-15,** Courtesy Smiths Medical North America. **Fig. 29-17, C,** From Kumar V, Abbas AK, Aster JC, Fausto N: *Robbins and Cotran pathologic basis of disease,* ed 8, Philadelphia, 2010, Saunders.

CHAPTER 30

Figs. 30-1, 30-2, Modified from Patton KT, Thibodeau GA: *Anatomy and physiology,* ed 8, St Louis, 2013, Mosby. **Fig. 30-7,** Modified from Herlihy B, Maebius N: *The human body in health and illness,* ed 4, Philadelphia, 2011, Saunders.

CHAPTER 31

Fig. 31-4, Modified from McCance KL, Huether SE: *Pathophysiology: the biologic basis for disease in adults and children,* ed 6, St Louis, 2010, Mosby. **Figs. 31-6, 31-8, 31-10,** From Forbes CD, Jackson WF: *Colour atlas and text of clinical medicine,* ed 3, London, 2003, Mosby. **Fig. 31-12,** Modified from McKinney ES, James SR, Murray SS, Nelson K: *Maternal-child nursing,* Philadelphia, 2000, Saunders. **Fig. 31-13,** From Hoffman AV, Pettit JE: *Color atlas of clinical hematology,* ed 4, Philadelphia, 2009, Mosby. **Fig. 31-15,** From Cotran RS, Kumar V, Abbas AK: *Robbins pathologic basis of disease,* ed 6, Philadelphia, 1999, Saunders.

CHAPTER 32

Figs. 32-9, 32-12, From Drake RL, Vogl AW, Mitchell AWM: *Gray's anatomy for students,* ed 2, Philadelphia, 2010, Churchill Livingstone. **Fig. 32-10,** From Otto C: *Textbook of clinical echocardiography,* ed 3, St Louis, 2004, Saunders. **Fig. 32-11,** From Libby P et al: *Braunwald's heart disease: a textbook of cardiovascular medicine,* ed 8, St Louis, 2008, Saunders.

CHAPTER 33

Fig. 33-2, From Kumar V, Cotran RS, Robbins SL: *Robbins basic pathology,* ed 8, Philadelphia, 2007, Saunders. **Fig. 33-3,** From US Department of Health and Human Services: *Seventh report of the Joint National Committee on Prevention, Detection, Evaluation, and Treatment of High Blood Pressure (JNC 7),* Washington, DC, 2003, National Institutes of Health. **Fig. 33-4,** From Kliegman RM, Behrman RE, Jenson HB, Stanton B: *Nelson textbook of pediatrics,* ed 18, Philadelphia, 2011, Saunders.

CHAPTER 34

Fig. 34-7, From Zipes DB, Libby P, Bonow RO, Braunwald E: *Braunwald's heart disease: a textbook of cardiovascular medicine,* ed 7, St Louis, 2005, Saunders. **Fig. 34-10,** From Kumar V, Abbas AK, Aster JC, Fausto N: *Robbins and Cotran pathologic basis of disease,* ed 8, Philadelphia, 2010, Saunders.

CHAPTER 35

Fig. 35-2, Modified from Huether SE, McCance KL: *Understanding pathophysiology,* ed 3, St Louis, 2004, Mosby. **Fig. 35-3,** Modified from Urden LD, Stacy KM, Lough ME: *Critical care nursing: diagnosis and management,* ed 6, St Louis, 2010, Mosby. **Fig. 35-6,** Used with permission from Honeywell HomMed.

CHAPTER 36

Fig. 36-5, Modified from Wesley K: *Basic dysrhythmias and acute coronary syndromes,* ed 4, St Louis, 2011, Mosby JEMS. **Fig. 36-10,** Modified from Urden LD, Stacy KM, Lough ME: *Critical care nursing: diagnosis and management,* ed 6, St Louis, 2010, Mosby. **Fig. 36-21,** Courtesy Medtronic Physio-Control, Redmond, Wash. **Figs. 36-22, A, 36-24, A, 36-25,** Courtesy Medtronic, Inc., Minneapolis, Minn. **Fig. 36-29,** From Bucher L, Melander S: *Critical care nursing,* Philadelphia, 1999, Saunders.

CHAPTER 37

Fig. 37-1, Modified from Patton KT, Thibodeau GA: *The human body in health and disease,* ed 5, St Louis, 2010, Mosby. **Figs. 37-2, 37-4,** From Damjanov I, Linder J: *Pathology: a color atlas,* St Louis, 2000, Mosby. **Fig. 37-5,** From Guzzetta CE, Dossey BM: *Cardiovascular nursing: holistic practice,* St Louis, 1992, Mosby. **Fig. 37-7,** From McCance KL, Huether SE: *Pathophysiology: the biologic basis for disease in adults and children,* ed 6, St Louis, 2010, Mosby. **Figs. 37-8, 37-11, 37-12,** From Kumar V, Abbas AK, Aster JC, Fausto N: *Robbins and Cotran pathologic basis of disease,* ed 8, Philadelphia, 2010, Saunders. **Fig. 37-9,** From Crawford MH, DiMarco JP, Paulus WJ: *Cardiology,* ed 3, Edinburgh, 2010, Mosby Ltd. **Fig. 37-10,** From Bonow RO, Mann DL, Zipes DP, Libby P: *Braunwald's heart disease: a textbook of cardiovascular medicine,* ed 9, Philadelphia, 2012, Saunders.

CHAPTER 38

Figs. 38-3, 38-13, From Kamal A, Brockelhurst JC: *Colour atlas of geriatric medicine,* ed 2, 1991, Mosby-Year Book-Europe. **Fig. 38-4,** Courtesy Jo Menzoian, Boston, Mass. **Fig. 38-8,** From Damjanov I, Linder J, editors: *Anderson's pathology,* ed 10, St Louis, 1996, Mosby. **Fig. 38-10,** From Etufugh CN, Phillips TJ: Venous ulcers, *Clinics in Dermatology,* 25(1):125, 2007. **Fig. 38-12,** From Goldman MP, Guex JJ, Weiss RA: *Sclerotherapy: treatment of varicose and telangiectatic leg veins,* ed 5, Philadelphia, 2011, Mosby.

CHAPTER 39

Fig. 39-2, From Patton KT, Thibodeau GA: *Anatomy and physiology,* ed 8, St Louis, 2013, Mosby. **Figs. 39-9, 39-10,** From Drake RL, Vogl

W, Mitchell AWM: *Gray's anatomy for students,* ed 2, Edinburgh, 2010, Churchill Livingstone. **Fig. 39-11,** From Given Imaging, Inc, Norcross, Ga.

CHAPTER 40

Fig. 40-1, US Department of Agriculture, Center for Nutrition Policy and Promotion: Guidance on Use of USDA's MyPlate and Statements about Amounts of Food Groups Contributed by Foods on Food Product Labels, Washington, DC. **Fig. 40-2,** US Department of Health and Human Services, Nutrition Facts Label, Silver Spring, Md. **Fig. 40-3,** From Morgan SL, Weinsier RL: *Fundamentals of clinical nutrition,* ed 2, St Louis, 1998, Mosby. **Fig. 40-4,** From Kamal A, Brockelhurst JC: *Color atlas of geriatric medicine,* ed 2, St Louis, 1991, Mosby. **Fig. 40-5,** Adapted from Ukleja A, Freeman KL, Gilbert K, and the ASPEN Board of Directors: Standards for nutrition support: adult hospitalized patients, *Nutrition in Clinical Practice* 25:403, 2010. **Fig. 40-7,** Redrawn from Mahan LK, Arlin M: *Krause's food, nutrition, and diet therapy,* ed 8, Philadelphia, 1992, Saunders.

CHAPTER 41

Fig. 41-6, From Shermak MA: Contouring the epigastrium, *Aesthetic Surgery Journal* 25:506, 2005.

CHAPTER 42

Fig. 42-1, Modified from McKenry L, Tessier E, Hogan M: *Mosby's pharmacology in nursing,* ed 22, St Louis, 2006, Mosby. **Fig. 42-4,** Modified from Doughty DB, Jackson DB: *Mosby's clinical nursing series: gastrointestinal disorders,* St Louis, 1993, Mosby. **Figs. 42-6, 42-8, 42-9,** Modified from Price SA, Wilson LM: *Pathophysiology: clinical concepts of disease processes,* ed 6, St Louis, 2003, Mosby. **Figs. 42-10, 42-15,** From Kumar V, Abbas AK, Aster JC, Fausto N: *Robbins and Cotran pathologic basis of disease,* ed 8, Philadelphia, 2010, Saunders.

CHAPTER 43

Fig. 43-6, Courtesy David Bjorkman, MD, University of Utah School of Medicine, Department of Gastroenterology. In McCance KL, Huether SE: *Pathophysiology: the biologic basis for disease in adults and children,* ed 6, St Louis, 2010, Mosby. **Fig. 43-8,** Modified from McCance KL, Huether SE: *Pathophysiology: the biologic basis for disease in adults and children,* ed 6, St Louis, 2010, Mosby. **Fig. 43-14, A and B,** From Zitelli BJ, McIntire SC, Nowalk AJ: *Zitelli and Davis' atlas of pediatric physical diagnosis,* ed 6, Philadelphia, 2012, Saunders. **Fig. 43-14, C,** From Swartz MH: *Textbook of physical diagnosis: history and examination,* ed 6, Philadelphia, 2010, Saunders. **Fig. 43-16,** From Townsend CM, Beauchamp RD, Evers BM, et al: *Sabiston textbook of surgery: the biological basis of modern surgical practice,* ed 19, Philadelphia, 2012, Saunders.

CHAPTER 44

Figs. 44-1, 44-8, 44-13, From Butcher GP: *Gastroenterology: an illustrated colour text,* London, 2004, Churchill Livingstone. **Figs. 44-2, 44-3,** From McCance KL, Huether SE: *Pathophysiology: the biologic basis for disease in adults and children,* ed 6, St Louis, 2010, Mosby. **Figs. 44-4, 44-10, B, 44-14,** From Kumar V, Abbas AK, Aster JC, Fausto N: *Robbins and Cotran pathologic basis of disease,* ed 8, Philadelphia, 2010, Saunders. **Figs. 44-5, 44-7,** Adapted from Huether SE, McCance KL: *Understanding pathophysiology,* ed 5, St Louis, 2012, Mosby. **Fig. 44-10, A,** From Kumar V, Abbas AK, Fausto N: *Robbins and Cotran pathologic basis of disease,* ed 7, Philadelphia, 2005, Saunders. **Fig. 44-12,** From Stevens A, Lowe J: *Pathology: illustrated review in colour,* ed 2, London, 2000, Mosby.

CHAPTER 45

Fig. 45-3, Modified from Thibodeau GA, Patton KT: *The human body in health and disease,* ed 4, St Louis, 2005, Mosby. **Fig. 45-4,** Modified from Herlihy B, Maebius N: *The human body in health and disease,* ed 4, Philadelphia, 2011, Saunders. **Fig. 45-5,** Modified from Thibodeau GA, Patton KT: *Anatomy and physiology,* ed 6, St Louis, 2007, Mosby. **Figs. 45-6, 45-8,** From Brundage DJ: *Renal disorders,* St Louis, 1992, Mosby. **Fig. 45-10, A,** Courtesy Circon Corporation, Santa Barbara, Calif.

CHAPTER 46

Figs. 46-2, 46-4, From Kumar V, Abbas AK, Aster JC, Fausto N, et al: *Robbins and Cotran pathologic basis of disease,* ed 8, Philadelphia, 2010, Saunders. **Fig. 46-5, A,** From Stevens A, Lowe JS, Scott I: *Core pathology: illustrated review in color,* ed 3, London, 2009, Mosby Ltd. **Figs. 46-5, B,** and **46-6,** From Bullock N, Doble A, Turner W, Cuckow P: *Urology: an illustrated colour text.* London, 2008, Churchill Livingstone. **Fig. 46-7, A,** From Brundage DJ: *Renal disorders,* St Louis, 1992, Mosby. **Figs. 46-7, B, and 46-8, 46-9, B,** From Kumar V, Abbas AK, Fausto N: *Robbins and Cotran pathologic basis of disease,* ed 7, Philadelphia, 2005, Saunders. **Fig. 46-9, A,** From Stevens A, Lowe J: *Pathology: illustrated review in colour,* ed 2, London, 2000, Mosby. **Figs. 46-12, 46-14, 46-15,** Courtesy Lynda Brubacher, Virginia Mason Hospital, Seattle, Wash.

CHAPTER 47

Fig. 47-1, From Stevens A, Lowe J: *Pathology: illustrated review in colour,* ed 2, London, 2000, Mosby. **Fig. 47-6,** Courtesy Mary Jo Holechek, Baltimore, Md. **Fig. 47-7,** Courtesy Baxter Healthcare Corporation, McGaw Park, Ill. **Figs. 47-9, 47-11, B, C,** Courtesy Dr. Stephen Van Voorst, MD. **Fig. 47-10, A,** Courtesy Quinton Instrument Co., Seattle, Wash. **Fig. 47-13,** From NxStage Medical, Inc, Lawrence, Mass.

CHAPTER 48

Figs. 48-1, 48-6, Modified from Patton KT, Thibodeau GA: *Anatomy and physiology,* ed 8, St Louis, 2013, Mosby. **Fig. 48-3,** Modified from McCance KL, Huether SE: *Pathophysiology: the biologic basis for disease in adults and children,* ed 6, St Louis, 2010, Mosby. **Fig. 48-8,** From Thibodeau GA, Patton KT: *The human body in health and disease,* ed 4, St Louis, 2005, Mosby.

CHAPTER 49

Figs. 49-11, 49-13, From Kumar V, Abbas AK, Aster JC, Fausto N: *Robbins and Cotran pathologic basis of disease,* ed 8, Philadelphia, 2010, Saunders. **Fig. 49-12,** Modified from Urden LD, Stacy KM, Lough ME: *Critical care nursing: diagnosis and management,* ed 6, St Louis, 2010, Mosby. **Figs. 49-15, 49-16,** From Chew SL, Leslie D: *Clinical endocrinology and diabetes: an illustrated colour text,* Edinburgh, 2006, Churchill Livingstone.

CHAPTER 50

Fig. 50-1, Courtesy Linda Haas, Seattle, Wash. **Fig. 50-3,** Modified from Urden LD, Stacy KM, Lough ME: *Critical care nursing: diagnosis and management,* ed 6, St Louis, 2010, Mosby. **Fig. 50-6,** From Forbes CD, Jackson WF: *Colour atlas and text of clinical medicine,* ed 3, London, 2003, Mosby. **Figs. 50-7, 50-12, 50-13,** From Chew SL, Leslie D: *Clinical endocrinology and diabetes: an illustrated colour text,* Edinburgh, 2006, Churchill Livingstone. **Fig. 50-9,** Courtesy Paul W. Ladenson, MD, The Johns Hopkins University and Hospital, Baltimore, Md. From HM Seidel, JW Ball, JE Dains, GW Benedict, editors: *Mosby's guide to physical examination,* ed 6, St Louis, 2006, Mosby. **Fig. 50-10,** From Seidel HM, Ball JW, Dains JE, Benedict GW: *Mosby's guide to physical examination,* ed 6, St Louis, 2006, Mosby.

CHAPTER 51

Figs. 51-1, 51-2, 51-4, 51-5, 51-7, Modified from Patton KT, Thibodeau GA: *Anatomy and physiology,* ed 8, St Louis, 2013, Mosby. **Fig. 51-3,** Modified from McKenry L, Tessier E, Hogan M: *Mosby's pharmacology in nursing,* St Louis, 2006, Mosby. **Fig. 51-8, A,** From Abrahams

P, Marks S, Hutching R: *McMinn's color atlas of human anatomy,* ed 5, Philadelphia, 2003, Saunders. **Fig. 51-8, B,** From Symonds EM, MacPherson MB: *Color atlas of obstetrics and gynecology,* London, 1994, Mosby Wolfe.

CHAPTER 52

Fig. 52-1, Data from American Cancer Society: How to perform a breast self-exam, revised October 2011. *www.cancer.org/Cancer/BreastCancer/MoreInformation/BreastCancerEarlyDetection/breast-cancer-early-detection-acsrecsbse.* **Fig. 52-2,** From Adam A, Dixon AK, Grainger RG, et al: *Grainger and Allison's diagnostic radiology,* ed 5, St Louis, 2008, Churchill Livingstone. **Fig. 52-5,** From Donegan WL, Spratt JS: *Cancer of the breast,* ed 3, Philadelphia, 1988, Saunders. **Fig. 52-7,** From Swartz MH: *Textbook of physical diagnosis: history and examination,* ed 6, Philadelphia, 2010, Saunders. **Fig. 52-10,** Courtesy Brian Davies, MD. From Fortunato N, McCullough S: *Plastic and reconstructive surgery,* St Louis, 1998, Mosby. **Fig. 52-11, A,** Modified from Cameron J: *Current surgical therapy,* ed 5, St Louis, 1995, Mosby. **Fig. 52-11, B,** Courtesy Brian Davies, MD. From Fortunato N, McCullough S: *Plastic and reconstructive surgery,* St Louis, 1998, Mosby.

CHAPTER 53

Fig. 53-1, From Marx J, Walls R, Hockberger R: *Rosen's emergency medicine: concepts and clinical practice,* ed 7, St Louis, 2010, Mosby. **Figs. 53-2, 53-7, 53-8, B,** From Morse S, Moreland A, Holmes K, editors: *Atlas of sexually transmitted diseases and AIDS,* London, 1996, Mosby-Wolfe. **Figs. 53-3, A,** and **53-6,** From Cohen J, Powderly WG: *Infectious diseases,* ed 2, St Louis, 2004, Mosby. **Figs. 53-3, B,** and **53-5,** From Mandell GL, Bennett JE, Dolin R: *Mandell, Douglas, and Bennett's principles and practice of infectious diseases,* ed 7, Philadelphia, 2010, Churchill Livingstone. **Fig. 53-4,** From Forbes CD, Jackson WF. *Color atlas and text of clinical medicine,* ed 3, London, 2003, Mosby. **Figs. 53-8, A, C,** and **53-10, C,** From Centers for Disease Control and Prevention. Courtesy Susan Lindsley. **Fig. 53-9,** From Centers for Disease Control and Prevention. Courtesy Dr. Hermann. **Fig. 53-10, A,** From Centers for Disease Control and Prevention. Courtesy Joe Millar. **Fig. 53-10, B,** From Centers for Disease Control and Prevention. Courtesy Dr. Wiesner.

CHAPTER 54

Fig. 54-3, From Katz V: *Comprehensive gynecology,* ed 5, St Louis, 2007, Mosby. **Fig. 54-4,** From Kumar V, Abbas AK, Aster JC, Fausto N: *Robbins and Cotran pathologic basis of disease,* ed 8, Philadelphia, 2010, Saunders. **Fig. 54-5,** Modified from Stenchever MA, Droegemueller W, Herbst AL, Mishell D Jr: *Comprehensive gynecology,* ed 4, St Louis, 2001, Mosby. **Fig. 54-6,** From McCance KL, Huether SE: *Pathophysiology: the biologic basis for disease in adults and children,* ed 6, St Louis, 2010, Mosby. **Fig. 54-7,** From Symonds EM, McPherson MBA: *Colour atlas of obstetrics and gynecology,* London, 1994, Mosby. **Fig. 54-8,** From Kumar V, Abbas A, Fausto N: *Robbins and Cotran pathologic basis of disease,* ed 7, Philadelphia, 2005, Saunders. **Fig. 54-9,** From Drake RL, Vogl W, Mitchell AWM: *Gray's anatomy for students,* ed 2, Edinburgh, 2010, Churchill Livingstone. **Fig. 54-10,** Modified from Phipps WJ, Sands JK, Marek JF: *Medical-surgical nursing: concepts and clinical practice,* ed 6, St Louis, 1999, Mosby. **Fig. 54-12,** Modified from Seidel HM, Ball JW, Dains JE, Flynn JA: *Mosby's guide to physical examination,* ed 7, St Louis, 2011, Mosby. **Fig. 54-13, B,** From Huffman JW: *Gynecology and obstetrics,* Philadelphia, 1962, Saunders. **Fig. 54-14, B,** From Townsend CM: *Sabiston textbook of surgery,* ed 18, St Louis, 2009, Mosby.

CHAPTER 55

Fig. 55-3, From Townsend CM, Beauchamp RD, Evers BM, Mattox KL: *Sabiston textbook of surgery,* ed 19, Philadelphia, 2012, Saunders. **Fig. 55-5,** From Mettler F: *Essentials of radiology,* ed 2, Philadelphia, 2004, Saunders. **Fig. 55-7, B,** From Abeloff MD, Armitage JO, Niederhuber JE, Kastan MB, editors: *Abeloff's clinical oncology,* ed 4, 2008, Churchill Livingstone. **Fig. 55-10,** From Swartz MH: *Textbook of physical diagnosis,* ed 6, Philadelphia, 2010, Saunders. **Fig. 55-11,** From Seidel HM, Ball JW, Dains JE, Flynn JA: *Mosby's guide to physical examination,* ed 7, St Louis, 2011, Mosby.

CHAPTER 56

Figs. 56-1, 56-8, 56-9, 56-10, Modified from Thibodeau GA, Patton KT: *Anatomy and physiology,* ed 8, St Louis, 2013, Mosby. **Fig. 56-2,** Modified from Thibodeau GA, Patton KT: *Anatomy and physiology,* ed 6, St Louis, 2007, Mosby. **Fig. 56-6,** From Herlihy B: *The human body in health and illness,* ed 4, St Louis, 2011, Saunders. **Fig. 56-7,** Redrawn from McCance KL, Huether SE: *Pathophysiology: the biologic basis for disease in adults and children,* ed 6, St Louis, 2010, Mosby. **Figs. 56-11, 56-12,** Courtesy DaiWai Olson, RN PhD, CCRN, Dallas, Tex. **Fig. 56-14,** From Chipps E, Clanin N, Campbell V: *Neurologic disorders,* St Louis, 1992, Mosby. **Fig. 56-15,** From Fuller G, Manford M: *Neurology: an illustrated colour text,* ed 3, New York, 2010, Churchill Livingstone.

CHAPTER 57

Fig. 57-4, Modified from McCance KL, Huether SE: *Pathophysiology: the biologic basis for disease in adults and children,* ed 6, St Louis, 2010, Mosby. **Fig. 57-7,** Modified from Copstead-Kirkhorn LC, Banasik JL: *Pathophysiology,* ed 5, St Louis, 2013, Mosby. **Fig. 57-9,** Courtesy Meg Zomorodi, RN, PhD, CNL, Raleigh, N.C. **Fig. 57-13, C,** From Bingham BJG, Hawke M, Kwok P: *Clinical atlas of otolaryngology,* St Louis, 1992, Mosby. **Fig. 57-15,** From Copstead-Kirkhorn LC, Banasik JL: *Pathophysiology,* ed 4, St Louis, 2010, Mosby. **Fig. 57-16,** From Kumar V, Abbas AK, Aster JC, Fausto N: *Robbins and Cotran pathologic basis of disease,* ed 8, Philadelphia, 2010, Saunders. **Fig. 57-17,** From Stevens A, Lowe J: *Pathology: illustrated review in colour,* ed 2, London, 2000, Mosby.

CHAPTER 58

Fig. 58-3, From Kumar V, Abbas AK, Aster JC, Fausto N: *Robbins and Cotran pathologic basis of disease,* ed 8, Philadelphia, 2010, Saunders. **Fig. 58-11,** Modified from Hoeman SP: *Rehabilitation nursing,* ed 2, St Louis, 1995, Mosby. **Fig. 58-12,** From Forbes CD, Jackson WF: *Colour atlas and text of clinical medicine,* ed 3, London, 2003, Mosby.

CHAPTER 59

Fig. 59-4, From Stevens A, Lowe J: *Pathology: illustrated review in colour,* ed 2, London, 2000, Mosby. **Fig. 59-7,** From Lehne RA: *Pharmacology for nursing care,* ed 8, St Louis, 2013, Saunders. **Fig. 59-8,** From Aminoff MJ, Daroff RB: *Encyclopedia of the neurological sciences,* Waltham, Mass., 2003, Academic Press. **Fig. 59-11,** From Sanders DB, Massey JM: Clinical features of myasthenia gravis. In AG Engel, editor: *Neuromuscular junction disorders: handbook of clinical neurology,* New York, 2008, Elsevier.

CHAPTER 60

Fig. 60-5, From Roberts GS: *Neuropsychiatric disorders,* London, 1993, Mosby-Wolfe. **Fig. 60-6,** Modified from Stern TA: *Massachusetts General Hospital comprehensive clinical psychiatry,* Philadelphia, 2008, Mosby.

CHAPTER 61

Fig. 61-1, Modified from Patton KT, Thibodeau GA: *Anatomy and physiology,* ed 8, St Louis, 2013, Mosby. **Fig. 61-2,** Courtesy Joe Rothrock, Media, Pa. **Fig. 61-3,** From Forbes CD, Jackson WF: *Color atlas and text of clinical medicine,* ed 3, London, 2003, Mosby. **Fig. 61-4,** Modified from Marciano FF, Greene KA, Apostolides PJ, et al: Pharmacologic management of spinal cord injury: review of the literature, *BNI Quarterly* 11(2):11, 1995. In KL McCance, SE Huether, editors: *Pathophysiology: the biologic basis for disease in*

adults and children, ed 5, St Louis, 2006, Mosby. **Fig. 61-5, A, B, C,** From Copstead-Kirkhorn LC, Banasik JL: *Pathophysiology,* ed 5, St Louis, 2014, Mosby. **Fig. 61-7,** From American Spinal Injury Association/International Medical Society of Paraplegic (ASIA/IMOSP): *International standards for neurological functional classification of spinal cord injury patients* (revised), Chicago, 2002, The Association. **Figs. 61-8, 61-12,** Courtesy Michael S. Clement, MD, Mesa, Ariz. **Fig. 61-11,** Modified from Urden LD, Stacy KM, Lough ME: *Priorities in critical care nursing,* ed 6, St Louis, 2012, Mosby.

CHAPTER 62

Fig. 62-1, A, From Herlihy B, Maebius N: *The human body in health and illness,* ed 4, Philadelphia, 2011, Saunders. **Figs. 62-1, B, 62-6,** From Patton KT, Thibodeau GA: *Anatomy and physiology,* ed 8, St Louis, 2013, Mosby. **Fig. 62-5,** From Patton KT, Thibodeau GA, Douglas M: *Essentials of anatomy and physiology,* St Louis, 2012, Mosby. **Fig. 62-7, A,** From Wilson SF, Giddens JF: *Health assessment for nursing practice,* ed 5, St Louis, 2013, Mosby. **Fig. 62-7, B,** From Barkauskas V, Baumann L, Stoltenberg-Allen K, et al: *Health and physical assessment,* ed 2, St Louis, 1998, Mosby. **Fig. 62-8,** From Zitelli BJ, McIntire SC, Nowalk AJ: *Zitelli and Davis' atlas of pediatric physical diagnosis,* ed 6, St Louis, 2012, Mosby. **Fig. 62-9,** From Miller MD, Howard RF, Plancher KD: *Surgical atlas of sports medicine,* Philadelphia, 2003, Saunders.

CHAPTER 63

Fig. 63-2, From Buttaravoli P: *Minor emergencies,* ed 3, Philadelphia, Saunders, 2012. **Fig. 63-4, A,** From David Lintner, MD, Houston, Tex., www.drlintner.com. **Fig. 63-4, B, C,** Courtesy Peter Bonner, Placitas, N. Mex. **Figs. 63-9, 63-20,** Courtesy Mary Wollan, RN, BAN, ONC, Spring Park, Minn. **Fig. 63-12,** From Maher AB, Salmond SW, Pellino T, editors: *Orthopaedic nursing,* ed 3, Philadelphia, 2002, Saunders. **Fig. 63-13, A,** Courtesy Howmedica, Inc, Allendale, Pa. **Fig. 63-13, B,** From Canale ST, Beaty JH: *Campbell's operative orthopaedics,* ed 12, Philadelphia, 2013, Mosby. **Fig. 63-14,** From Jeremy Lewis, MD. Dallas, Tex. **Fig. 63-15,** From Browner BD, Jupiter JB, Levine AM, Trafton P: *Skeletal trauma: fractures, dislocations, ligamentous injuries,* ed 4, Philadelphia, 2009, Saunders. **Fig. 63-16,** Mettler FA: *Essentials of radiology,* ed 2, Philadelphia, 2005, Saunders. **Fig. 63-21,** Courtesy R.A. Weinstein, Denver, Colo.

CHAPTER 64

Fig. 64-2, From Thibodeau GA, Patton KT: *The human body in health and disease,* ed 5, St Louis, 2010, Mosby. **Fig. 64-3,** From Damjanov I, Linder J: *Anderson's pathology,* ed 10, St Louis, 1996, Mosby. **Figs. 64-6, 64-7,** From Canale ST, Beaty JH: *Campbell's operative orthopaedics,* ed 12, Philadelphia, 2013, Mosby. **Fig. 64-9, A,** From Phillips N: *Berry & Kohn's operating room technique,* ed 12, St Louis, 2013, Mosby. **Fig. 64-9, B,** Courtesy MA Mir. In Kanski JJ: *Clinical diagnosis in ophthalmology,* St Louis, 2006, Mosby.

CHAPTER 65

Fig. 65-1, D, From Forbes CD, Jackson WF: *Color atlas and text of clinical medicine,* ed 3, London, 2003, Mosby. **Fig. 65-3, D,** From Canale ST, Beaty JH: *Campbell's operative orthopaedics,* ed 12, Philadelphia, 2013, Mosby. **Fig. 65-6,** Courtesy John Cook, MD. From Goldstein, BG, Goldstein AE: *Practical dermatology,* ed 2, St Louis, 1997, Mosby. **Fig. 65-7,** From Marx J, Hockberger R, Walls R: *Rosen's emergency medicine,* ed 7, Philadelphia, 2009, Mosby. **Fig. 65-8,** From Kim DH, Henn J, Vaccaro AR, Dickman C: *Surgical anatomy and techniques to the spine,* Philadelphia, 2006, Saunders. **Figs. 65-10, 65-13,** From Firestein GS, Budd RC, Gabriel SE, McInnes IB: *Kelley's textbook of rheumatology,* ed 9, Philadelphia, 2012, Saunders. **Fig. 65-12,** From Zitelli BJ, Davis HW: *Atlas of pediatric physical diagnosis,* ed 4, St Louis, 2002, Mosby.

Glycosuria, 1062t
Glycosylated hemoglobin (A1C), in diabetes
     mellitus, 1147t-1151t, 1156-1158
Glynase (glyburide), for diabetes mellitus, 1163,
     1164t
Glyset (miglitol), for diabetes mellitus, 1163, 1164t
Goiter, 1146t-1147t, 1195-1196, 1195f, 1196f
Gold compounds, for rheumatoid arthritis,
     1565t-1567t, 1573
Golimumab (Simponi), for rheumatoid arthritis,
     1573
Gonad, 1218
Gonadal hormones, 1222f, 1230
Gonadotropin-releasing hormone, 1222, 1222f
Gonadotropin-releasing hormone agonists
     for endometriosis, 1290, 1290b
     for infertility, 1277t
Gonadotropin-releasing hormone antagonists, for
     infertility, 1277t
Gonadotropins, measurement of, 1147t-1151t
Goniometer, 1497-1498, 1497f
Gonorrhea, 1262-1264. See also Sexually
     transmitted infections.
     case study of, 1274b
     septic arthritis in, 1579
     vs. chlamydial infection, 1267
Good lung down, 1662
Good Samaritan laws, 1691b
Goodpasture syndrome, 212, 1073t, 1074
Goserelin (Zoladex), for prostate cancer,
     1319-1320, 1319t
Gout, 1576-1578, 1576t
Gowning, preoperative, 338
Graft(s)
     arteriovenous, for hemodialysis, 1120, 1120f
     coronary artery bypass, 752-753, 752f, 757-758
     endovascular, for aortic aneurysms, 843, 843f
     skin. See Skin grafts.
Graft rejection, 221, 221f
     in renal transplantation, 1127
Graft-versus-host disease, 223-224, 276
Granulation tissue, 178, 178t, 180t
     excessive, 180t
Granulocyte, 614f, 615-616
Granulocyte colony-stimulating factor, for
     neutropenia, 662
Granulocyte-macrophage colony-stimulating
     factor, for neutropenia, 662
Granulocytopenia, 660
Granulocytosis, 615-616
Granulomas, in tuberculosis, 528-529
Graphesthesia, 1348
Graves' disease, 1195-1196, 1196f. See also
     Hyperthyroidism.
     case study of, 1215b
Great toe, gout in, 1577
Greenstick fractures, 1512, 1512f
Grey Turner's sign, 842, 1031
Grief, 143-144, 143t, 144f
     in spinal cord injury, 1483-1484, 1483t
Grief Wheel, 144, 144f
Grotton's papules, in dermatomyositis, 1589, 1589f
Growth factors
     hematopoietic, for cancer, 273-274, 274t
     in hematopoietic stem cell transplant, 275
Growth hormone, 1136t, 1138
     deficiency of, in hypopituitarism, 1192
     excess of, in acromegaly, 1190-1191
     measurement of, 1147t-1151t
Growth hormone stimulation, 1147t-1151t
Guardianship, 936b
Guglielmi detachable coil, 1399, 1399f
Guided imagery, 94-95, 94t-95t
Guided meditation, 94
Guillain-Barré syndrome, 1467

Gynecomastia, 1242
Gynoid obesity, 907, 907f

H

H₂-receptor blockers
     for GERD, 934, 934t
     for nausea and vomiting, 925-926, 926t
     for peptic ulcers, 946
Haemophilus influenzae meningitis, 1381, 1381t
Hair, 415
     age-related changes in, 417, 417t
     assessment of, 417-423. See also Integumentary
          system, assessment of.
Hair loss. See Alopecia.
Hairy leukoplakia, HIV-related, 234, 235f
Halal foods, 889-890
Halitosis, in achalasia, 940
Hallucinogens, overdose of, 1689t
Hallux rigidus, 1552t
Hallux valgus, 1551f, 1552t
     in rheumatoid arthritis, 1570-1571, 1571f
Halo sign, 1369, 1369f
Halo vest, 1476, 1477f, 1528
     patient teaching for, 1482t
Haloperidol (Haldol), for delirium, 1460
Halothane (Fluothane), 343t
Hamartomas, pulmonary, 541
Hammer toe, 1552t
Hand
     burns of, 462
     deformities of, in rheumatoid arthritis,
          1570-1571, 1571f
Hand massage, 84, 84f
Hand washing, preoperative, 338
Hand-foot syndrome, in cancer, 269-270
Handoff procedures, 5, 15t, 328, 335, 362t
Hardiness, 89
Hartmann's pouch, 991, 991f
Hartmann's solution, 308t
Hashimoto's thyroiditis, 1196
Haversian systems, 1490, 1490f
Hawthorn, 82t, 777b
Hay fever, 210
Head and neck cancer, 512-514, 929-930
     case study of, 519b
     chemotherapy for, 930
     clinical manifestations of, 512-513, 929
     collaborative care in, 513-514, 930, 930t
     cultural aspects of, 929b
     diagnosis of, 513, 930
     etiology of, 929
     nursing management of, 514-518, 930-931
          assessment in, 515t, 930, 930t
          evaluation in, 518, 931
          implementation in, 515-518, 931
          nursing diagnoses in, 515, 931
          planning in, 515, 515t, 931
     nutritional therapy for, 514, 930
     pathophysiology of, 929
     prevention of, 515
     radiation therapy for, 515-516, 930
     staging of, 513
     surgery for, 930
     swallowing problems in, 266t-267t, 268, 514
     treatment of, 513-514, 513f
     types of, 929t
Head injuries, 1368-1372
     ambulatory and home care for, 1374-1375
     brain injuries in, 1369-1370
     collaborative care in, 1371-1372
     complications of, 1370-1371
          long-term, 1374-1375
     concussions in, 1369-1370
     dementia and, 1445
     diagnosis of, 1371-1372

Head injuries (Continued)
     emergency management of, 1372-1374, 1372t
     epidural hematoma in, 1370-1371
     family concerns in, 1375
     health promotion for, 1373-1375
     nursing management of, 1372-1378, 1373t
     patient teaching for, 1374t
     scalp lacerations in, 1368
     seizures after, 1370, 1374
     skull fractures in, 1368-1369, 1369f, 1369t
     types of, 1368-1370
Head lice, 437, 437t
Head tilt-chin lift, in CPR, 1696f, 1697-1698
Headache, 1413-1418
     biofeedback for, 1416
     cluster, 1414f, 1414t
     collaborative care for, 1416-1418
     diagnosis of, 1415t
     drug therapy for, 1416-1418, 1417t
     gender differences in, 1415b
     in increased ICP, 1360
     medication overuse, 1418
     migraine, 1414f, 1414t
     nursing management of, 1418-1419, 1418t
     patient teaching for, 1419t
     primary vs. secondary, 1413-1414
     in subarachnoid hemorrhage, 1393b
     in systemic disease, 1416
     tension-type, 1414-1415, 1414f, 1414t
Head-up tilt-test, 807-808
Healing. See Wound healing.
Healing touch, 85
Health care
     access to, 20-23, 20b. See also Health disparities.
     conventional model of, 79, 80t, 85
     integrative model of, 79, 80t
     rationing of, 1025b
Health care financing, 4-5
Health care providers. See also Nurse(s).
     HIV infection in, 230, 230t, 232, 241
Health care workplace, cultural diversity in, 25-26
Health care–associated infections, 230, 230t
     urinary tract, 1066, 1068
Health care–associated pneumonia, 523. See also
     Pneumonia.
Health, determinants of, 19-20, 20f
Health disparities, 20-23, 20b
     age and, 22
     bias and discrimination and, 23
     case study of, 33b
     education and, 22
     ethnicity and race and, 21
     factors and conditions leading to, 20-23, 21b,
          21t
     gender and, 22
     income and, 22, 22f
     legal/ethical issues in, 20b
     occupation and, 22
     place and, 21-22
     provider attitudes and, 23
     reduction of, 31-33, 31t
     in rural populations, 66-67
     sexual orientation and, 22-23
Health equity, 20
Health history. See History.
Health Insurance Portability and Accountability
     Act (HIPAA), 10
     social networking and, 4b
Health literacy, 22, 53
Health maintenance organizations (HMOs), 4-5
Health perception–health management pattern, 39
Health promotion
     models of, 48-49, 49t
     for older adults, 72
     prevention and, 63

Health status, 19
Health-related beliefs and practices, 24, **26-30**, 26t
Healthy People 2020, 5, 5t, 20
Hearing aids, 409-410, 409t, 411b
Hearing loss, 406-408
 assessment of, **379-382**
 assistive devices/techniques for, 409-410, 409t, 411b
 causes of, 407f
 central, 377, 407
 in chronic otitis media, **404**
 classification of, 407, 407t
 clinical manifestations of, 407-408
 communication in, 409-410, 410t
 conductive, 406-407
 cultural aspects of, 388b
 diagnosis of, **382-384**, 383t
 drug-related, 380-381, 408-409
 in Ménière's disease, **405**, 406t
 mixed, 407
 noise levels and, 408, 408f
 nursing management of, 408-410
 in older adults, 410-411
 prevention of, 408, 408b
 sensorineural, 377, 407
 tinnitus and, 407-408
 viral infections and, 408-409
Hearing tests, **382-384**, 383t
Heart. *See also under* Cardiac.
 blood flow through, 687, 687f
 implantable artificial, 1613
 layers of, 811f
 neural control of, 787-788
 in older adults, 691, 691t
 structures and functions of, 687-689, 687f-688f, 811f
Heart attack. *See* Myocardial infarction.
Heart disease. *See also* Cardiovascular disorders.
 atherosclerotic. *See* Coronary artery disease.
 in cancer, 266t-267t, 270
 chest pain in, **740-747.** *See also* Angina.
 in chronic kidney disease, 1110
 electrical injury and, 452
 hypertensive, 713-714, 714f, 714t
 inflammatory, **811-813**
 obesity and, 910, 911f
 postoperative, **355-356**
 rheumatic. *See* Rheumatic heart disease.
 stroke and, 1390
 sudden cardiac death in, 762
 syncope in, **807-808**
 valvular, **820-825.** *See also* Valvular heart disease.
Heart failure, 766-786
 acute decompensated, 769-770, 772-775
 acute interventions for, 779
 ambulatory and home care for, 779-783
 case study of, 785b
 chronic, 770-771
 circulatory assist devices for, 773, 1610-1613
 classification of, 772, 772t
 clinical manifestations of
  in acute decompensated failure, 769-770, 770t, 771f
  in chronic failure, 770-771
  in right- vs. left-sided failure, 770t
 collaborative care for
  in acute decompensated failure, 772-775
  in chronic failure, 775-777
 compensated, 768, 780
 complications of, 771-772

Heart failure *(Continued)*
 counterregulatory mechanisms in, 768-769
 cultural aspects of, 767b
 diagnosis of, 772, 773t
 diastolic, 767
 in dilated cardiomyopathy, **827-828**
 drug therapy for
  in acute decompensated failure, 773-775, 774t
  in chronic failure, 774t, 776-777
 etiology of, 767, 767t
 gender differences in, 768b
 genetic factors in, 767-769
 left-sided, 769, 771t
 mixed systolic-diastolic, 767-768
 after myocardial infarction, 748
 nursing care plan for, 9b, 780b-781b
 nursing management of, 778-783
  assessment in, 778, 779t
  implementation in, 780
  nursing diagnoses in, 779
  planning in, 780
 nutritional therapy for, 777-778, 778t
 palliative and end-of-life care in, 783
 pathophysiology of, 767
 patient teaching for, 779-783, 782t
 right-sided, 769, 771t
 systolic, 767
 transplantation for, **783-784**, 783t
Heart murmurs. *See* Murmurs.
Heart rate
 calculation of, 789-790
 monitoring of. *See also* Electrocardiography (ECG).
  telemetric, 790
 regulation of, 690
Heart sounds, 697-698, 697f
Heart transplantation, **783-784**, 783t
Heart valves
 disorders of. *See* Valvular heart disease.
 prosthetic, 825, 825f
Heartburn, in GERD, 932
Heart-lung transplantation, 556
Heat cramps, 1682
Heat exhaustion, 1682-1683
Heat therapy, 132-133, 133t
 for osteoarthritis, 1564
 for rheumatoid arthritis, 1575-1576
 in RICE therapy, 177
 for soft tissue injuries, 1508
Heatstroke, 1683-1684
Heaves, 695-697
Heberden's nodes, 1563
Heel pain, 1552t
Height, measurement of, in nutritional assessment, 894
Heimlich maneuver, 1698f, 1698t
Heimlich valve, 545, 545f
***Helicobacter pylori* infection**
 diagnosis of, 945
 drug therapy for, 942t, 946
 gastric cancer and, 951
 gastritis and, 941-942
 peptic ulcers and, 943-944
Heliotrope rash, in dermatomyositis, 1589
Hemangioblastoma, 1375
Hemarthrosis, 1507
 in hemophilia, 655, 656f, 657
Hematemesis, 483, 620, 878t, 954t
Hematocrit, 625
 normal values for, 626t
 in respiratory assessment, 491t-493t
Hematologic disorders, 623t-624t, 632-683

Hematologic system, 613-631
 assessment of, **619-625**
  bone marrow biopsy in, 628-630, 629t, 630f
  case study of, 613, 620b, 622b, 625b
  diagnostic studies in, **625-630**, 626t-627t
  focused, 625, 625b
  functional health patterns in, 620-622
  health history in, 619, 621t
  molecular cytogenetics and gene analysis in, 629t, 630
  physical examination in, 622-625
  radiologic studies in, 628, 629t
 blood in, 614-616
 bone marrow in, 613-614
 clotting in, 616-618
 iron metabolism in, 616
 liver in, 619
 lymph system in, 618-619
 in older adults, 619, 619t
 spleen in, 618
 structures and functions of, **613-619**, 614f
Hematology, reference intervals for, 1705t
Hematomas, 422t
 epidural, 1370-1372, 1371f
 fracture, 1512, 1513f
 intracerebral, 1370-1371
 subdural, 1371-1372, 1371t-1372t
Hematopoiesis, 613-614, 614f
 in bone marrow, 1490-1491
 in spleen, 618
Hematopoietic growth factors, for cancer, **273-274**, 274t
Hematopoietic stem cells, **200**, 613-614, 614f
 transfusion of, for leukemia, 667-668
 transplantation of, **200**, **274-276**, 274t, 275f
  for sickle cell disease, 647
  for urinary incontinence, 1089
Hematuria, 1056t
Hemianopsia, 1346-1347
 homonymous, 1350t, 1407, 1407f
Hemiplegia, 1350t, 1407-1408
Hemochromatosis, 647-648, 648b, 1016
Hemodiafiltration, continuous venovenous, 1123
Hemodialysis. *See also* Dialysis.
 for acute kidney injury, 1106
 complications of, 1122-1123, 1128t
 continuous, 1106
  venovenous, 1123-1124, 1123f, 1123t
 effectiveness of, 1123
 in-center, 1122
 in-home, 1122, 1122f
 intermittent, 1106
 for poisoning, 1690
 procedure for, 1121-1122
 settings and schedules for, 1122
 system components for, 1121, 1122f
 vascular access for, 1120-1121
  arteriovenous fistulas/grafts for, 1120, 1120f
  dialyzers for, 1121
  temporary, 1120-1121, 1121f
 vs. peritoneal dialysis, 1117t
Hemodynamic monitoring, 699t-703t, **1602-1610**
 afterload in, 1604
 of arterial blood pressure, 1606
 cardiac index in, 1603, 1606
 of cardiac output, 1603, 1606
  arterial pressure–based, 1606-1607, 1606f
 of central venous pressure, 1608-1609
 complications of, 1606
 contractility in, 1604
 dynamic response test in, 1605, 1605f
 equipment for, 1604-1605, 1604f
 impedance cardiography in, 1610

X-Stop (interspinous process decompression
system), 1549
Xtandi (enzalutamide), for prostate cancer, 1319t,
1320

Y

Yoga, 83b, 83f
  for back pain, 1547b
Young-old adults, 64

Z

Zafirlukast (Accolate), for asthma, 570t-571t,
  571-572
Zaleplon (Sonata), 104
Zanaflex (tizanidine), for pain, 127, 128t
Zanamivir (Relenza), for influenza, 504

Zelboraf (vemurafenib), pharmacogenetics of, 198,
  199f
Zenapax (daclizumab), for transplant
  immunosuppression, 222t, 223
Zenker's diverticula, 939-940, 939f
Zetia (Ezetimibe), 739t, 740
Ziagen (abacavir), pharmacogenetics of, 198,
  199f
Zileuton (Zyflo), for asthma, 570t-571t
Zinc, 82t
  for colds, 505b
Zocor (simvastatin), 739b, 739t
Zoladex (goserelin), for prostate cancer,
  1319-1320, 1319t
Zoledronic acid (Zometa), for multiple myeloma,
  674, 674b

Zoledronic acid (Reclast), for osteoporosis, 1556
Zollinger-Ellison syndrome, 944-945
Zolpidem (Ambien), for insomnia, 104
Zonule, 369
Zoonosis, 228
Zortess (everolimus), for transplant
  immunosuppression, 222t, 223
Zoster, 436t
Zostrix. See Capsaicin (Zostrix).
Z-scores, 1555
Zyban (buproprion), 158, 158t
Zydonel (hydrocodone), 124, 125t
Zygote intrafallopian transfer, 1277-1278
Zyloprim (allopurinol), for gout, 1578
Zytiga (abiraterone), for prostate cancer, 1319t,
  1320

ABBREVIATIONS

ABG	arterial blood gas
ACE	angiotensin-converting enzyme
ACLS	advanced cardiac life support
ACS	acute coronary syndrome
ACTH	adrenocorticotropic hormone
ADH	antidiuretic hormone
AED	automatic external defibrillator
AIDS	acquired immunodeficiency syndrome
AKA	above-knee amputation
AKI	acute kidney injury
ALI	acute lung injury
ALL	acute lymphocytic leukemia
ALS	amyotrophic lateral sclerosis
AMI	acute myocardial infarction
ANA	antinuclear antibody
ANS	autonomic nervous system
AORN	Association of periOperative Room Nurses
APD	automated peritoneal dialysis
aPTT	activated partial thromboplastin time
ARDS	acute respiratory distress syndrome
ATN	acute tubular necrosis
BCLS	basic cardiac life support
BKA	below-knee amputation
BMI	body mass index
BMR	basal metabolic rate
BMT	bone marrow transplantation
BPH	benign prostatic hyperplasia
BSE	breast self-examination
BUN	blood urea nitrogen
CABG	coronary artery bypass graft
CAD	coronary artery disease; circulatory assist device
CAPD	continuous ambulatory peritoneal dialysis
CAVH	continuous arteriovenous hemofiltration
CBC	complete blood count
CCU	coronary care unit; critical care unit
CDC	Centers for Disease Control and Prevention
CIS	carcinoma in situ
CKD	chronic kidney disease
CLL	chronic lymphocytic leukemia
CML	chronic myelocytic leukemia
CMP	cardiomyopathy
CN	cranial nerve
CNS	central nervous system
CO	cardiac output
COPD	chronic obstructive pulmonary disease
CPAP	continuous positive airway pressure
CPR	cardiopulmonary resuscitation
CRRT	continuous renal replacement therapy
CRNA	certified registered nurse anesthetist
CSF	cerebrospinal fluid
CT	computed tomography
CVA	cerebrovascular accident; costovertebral angle
CVAD	central venous access device
CVI	chronic venous insufficiency
CVP	central venous pressure
D&C	dilation and curettage
DDD	degenerative disk disease
DI	diabetes insipidus
DIC	disseminated intravascular coagulation
DJD	degenerative joint disease
DKA	diabetic ketoacidosis
DM	diabetes mellitus; diastolic murmur
DRE	digital rectal examination
DVT	deep vein thrombosis
ECF	extracellular fluid
ECG	electrocardiogram
ED	emergency department; erectile dysfunction
EEG	electroencephalogram
EMG	electromyogram
EMS	emergency medical services
ENT	ear, nose, and throat
ERCP	endoscopic retrograde cholangiopancreatography
ERT	estrogen replacement therapy
ESKD	end-stage kidney disease
ESR	erythrocyte sedimentation rate
ET	endotracheal
FEV	forced expiratory volume
FRC	functional residual capacity
FUO	fever of unknown origin
GCS	Glasgow Coma Scale
GERD	gastroesophageal reflux disease
GFR	glomerular filtration rate
GH	growth hormone
GI	glycemic index
GTT	glucose tolerance test
GU	genitourinary
GYN, Gyn	gynecologic
HAI	health care–associated infection
HAV	hepatitis A virus
Hb, Hgb	hemoglobin
HBV	hepatitis B virus
Hct	hematocrit
HCV	hepatitis C virus
HD	hemodialysis, Huntington's disease
HDL	high-density lipoprotein
HF	heart failure
HIV	human immunodeficiency virus
H&P	history and physical examination
HPV	human papillomavirus
HSCT	hematopoietic stem cell transplantation
IABP	intraaortic balloon pump
IBS	irritable bowel syndrome
ICP	intracranial pressure
I&D	incision and drainage
IE	infective endocarditis
IFG	impaired fasting glucose
IGT	impaired glucose tolerance
INR	international normalized ratio
IOP	intraocular pressure
IPPB	intermittent positive-pressure breathing
ITP	idiopathic thrombocytopenic purpura
IUD	intrauterine device
IV	intravenous
IVP	intravenous push; intravenous pyelogram
JVD	jugular venous distention
KS	Kaposi sarcoma
KUB	kidney, ureters, and bladder (x-ray)
KVO	keep vein open
LAD	left anterior descending
LDL	low-density lipoprotein